BRIEF CONTENTS OF VOLUME 2

W9-ATF-873

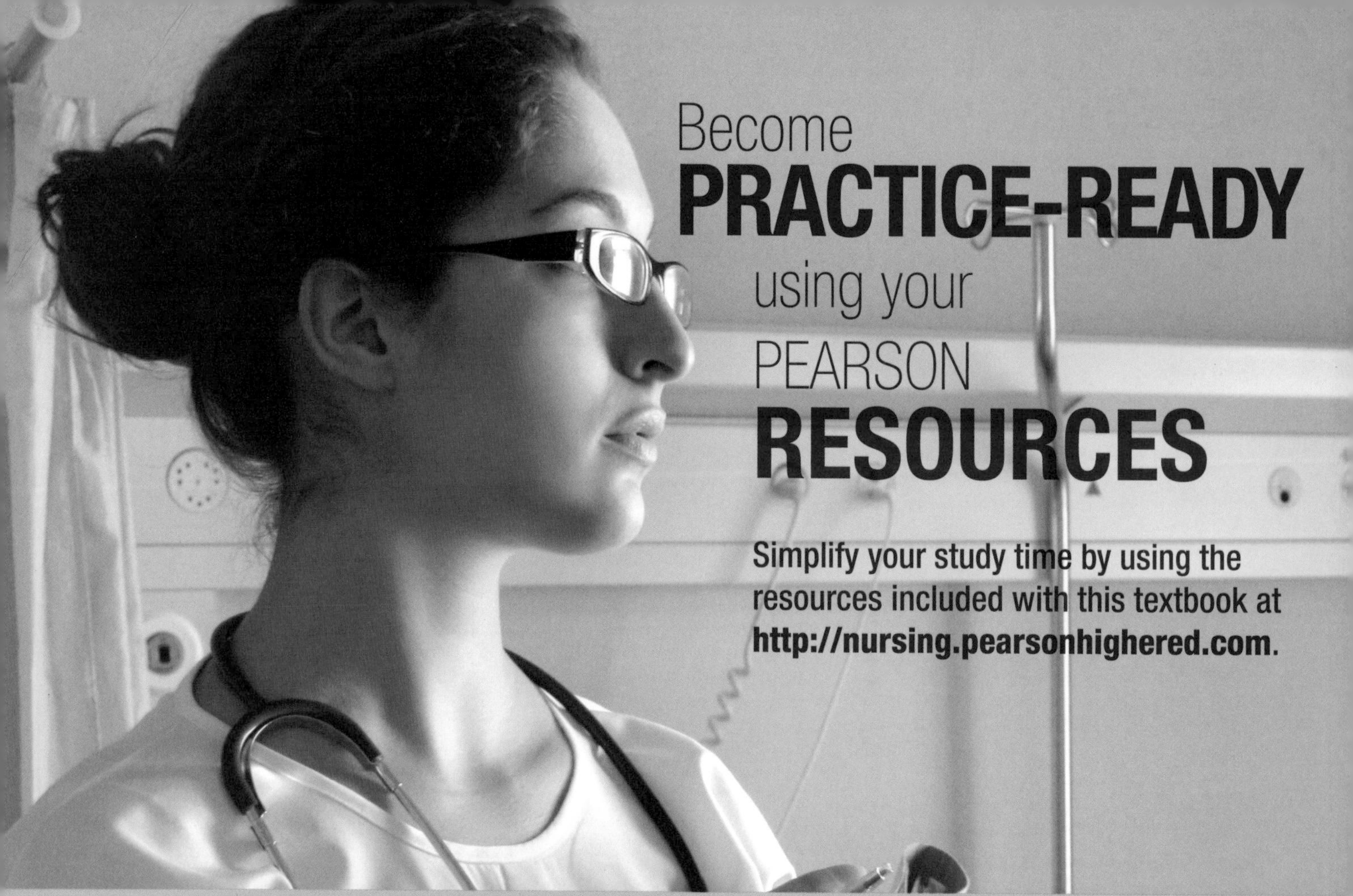

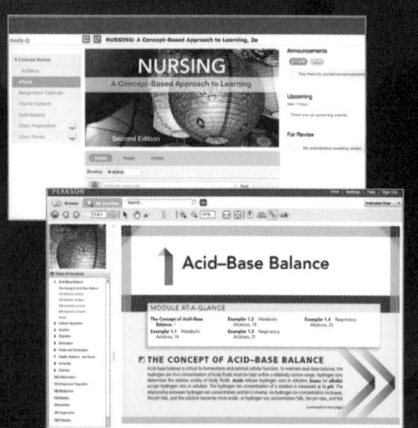
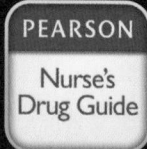
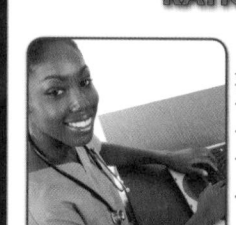

VOLUME 1

NURSING

A Concept-Based Approach to Learning

SECOND EDITION

PEARSON

Boston   Columbus   Indianapolis   New York   San Francisco   Upper Saddle River
Amsterdam   Cape Town   Dubai   London   Madrid   Milan   Munich   Paris   Montreal   Toronto
Delhi   Mexico City   Sao Paulo   Sydney   Hong Kong   Seoul   Singapore   Taipei   Tokyo

Publisher: Julie Alexander
Executive Editor: Kelly Trakalo
Development Editors: Laura S. Horowitz and Adelaide R. McCulloch
Program Manager: Melissa Bashe
Editorial Assistants: Erin Rafferty and Kevin Wilson
Director of Marketing: David Gesell
Senior Marketing Manager: Phoenix Harvey
Marketing Specialist: Michael Sirinides
Director, Product Management Services: Etain O'Dea
Project Management Team Lead: Patrick Walsh
Project Manager: Maria Reyes
Manufacturing Manager: Maura Zaldivar-Garcia
Art Director/Cover and Interior Design: Mary Siener
Cover Art: Aaron Craven/Vetta/Getty Images
Lead Digital Project Manager: Karen Bretz
Digital Project Manager: Tanika Henderson
Full-Service Project Management: Kelly Ricci
Composition: Aptara®, Inc.
Manufactured in the United States by RR Donnelley
Cover Printer: RR Donnelley

Library of Congress Cataloging-in-Publication Data
Nursing (Pearson : 2015)
    Nursing : a concept-based approach to learning.—Second edition.
        p. ; cm.
    Includes bibliographical references and index.
    ISBN-13: 978-0-13-293426-8 (v. 1)
    ISBN-10: 0-13-293426-4 (v. 1)
    I. Title.
    [DNLM: 1. Nursing.   2. Nursing Care. WY 100.1]
    RT40
    610.73—dc23
                                        2013045274

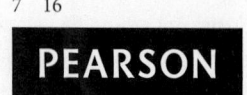

ISBN 13: 978-0-13-293426-8

ISBN 10:   0-13-293426-4

ACKNOWLEDGMENTS

We would like to extend our heartfelt thanks to more than 80 of our colleagues from schools of nursing across the country who have given their time generously during the past few years to help us create this concept-based learning package. The talented faculty on our Concepts Advisory Panel, and all of the Contributors and Reviewers helped us to develop this second version through contributions and answering a myriad of questions right up to the time of publication. *Nursing: A Concept-Based Approach to Learning*, Second Edition, has benefited immeasurably from their efforts, insights, suggestions, objections, encouragement, and inspiration, as well as from their vast experience as faculty and practicing nurses.

We would like to thank the editorial team, especially Julie Alexander, Publisher, for her continual support throughout this process; Kim Norbuta, the editor that started us off and Kelly Trakalo, the Executive Editor who came in at the end. Kevin Wilson and Erin Rafferty, editorial assistants, for helping to keep all the balls in the air; Melissa Bashe for keeping us organized and most of all Laura Horowitz and Addy McCulloch, development editors, for their dedication and attention to detail that promoted an excellent outcome once again. Many thanks to the Pearson production team of Maria Reyes and Patrick Walsh, and to Kelly Ricci and the Aptara team for producing this book with precision. Finally, a special thanks to the design team, led by Mary Siener, for the thoughtful and integrated design of our concepts solution.

CONCEPTS ADVISORY PANEL

Janet B. Arthurs, EdD, MSN, RNC
Gaston College
Dallas, NC

Colleen Coletta Burgess, EdD, PMHCNS-BC, MSN, RN
Cabarrus College
Concord, NC

Michelle Byrne, PhD, RN, CNOR, CNE
University of West Georgia
Carrollton, GA

Barbara Callahan, MEd, RN, NCC, CHSE
Lenoir Community College
Kinston, NC

Karen Carlson, PhD, RN
University of New Mexico
Albuquerque, NM

Linda K. Daley, PhD, RN, ANEF
The Ohio State University
Columbus, OH

Kathy Magorian, EdD, RN
University of South Dakota
Vermillion, SD

Pamela Phillips, PhD, RN
Blue Ridge Community College
Flat Rock, NC

T. Kim Rodehorst, PhD, RN, AE-C
University of Nebraska Medical Center–Scottsbluff Campus
Scottsbluff, NE

Susan Wilhelm, PhD, RNC
University of Nebraska Medical Center
Omaha, NE

CONTRIBUTORS

Barbara Hope Arnoldussen, MBA, BSN, RN, CPHQ
International Technological University
San Jose, CA

Cynthia D. Booher, MSN, CNRN, RN
Guilford Technical Community College
Jamestown, NC

Colleen Coletta Burgess, EdD, PMHCNS-BC, MSN, RN
Cabarrus College
Concord, NC

Michelle Byrne, PhD, CNOR, CNE, RN
University of West Georgia
Carrollton, GA

Barbara Callahan, MEd, RN, NCC, CHSE
Lenoir Community College
Kinston, NC

Patricia Caudle, DNSc, CNM, FNP-BC
Frontier Nursing University
Hyden, KY

Amy Mitchell Corbitt, MSN, RN
ECPI University
Newport News, VA

Deborah Duchesneau, FNP-BC, MSN, BSN, BACS
Carolina East Internal Medicine
Pollocksville, NC

Brigette Dupuch-Knudsen, MS, RN, CNOR
University of North Georgia
Northside Hospital
Atlanta, GA

Carolyn Gersch, MSN, CNE, RN
Kettering College
Kettering, OH

Camella G. Marcom, MSN, RN
Vance-Granville Community College
Henderson, NC

Jeanne Marie Papa, MBE, MSN, ACNP-BC, CCRN
Neumann University
Aston, PA

Cynthia A. Parkman, PhD, RN
National University
San Diego, CA

Carole Rae-Reed, PhD, RN, APN, PMHCNS
The Richard Stockton College of New Jersey
Galloway, NJ

Amanda C. Reichert, MS(NEd), MS, RN
Georgia Gwinnett College
Lawrenceville, GA

Barbara Sittner, PhD, RN, APRN-CNS
Bryan College of Health Sciences
Lincoln, NE

Margaret M. Slusser, PhD, RN
The Richard Stockton College of New Jersey
Galloway, NJ

Sharon Souter, PhD, CNE, RN
University of Mary Hardin-Baylor
Belton, TX

Sharon L. Stewart, RN, CPHQ
Baltimore, MD

Susan Wilhelm, PhD, RNC
University of Nebraska Medical Center
Omaha, NE

REVIEWERS

The following reviewers gave valuable feedback on drafts of the modules:

Linda Alfieri, MSN, CNE
Cayuga Community College
Auburn, NY

Jacqueline Bencker, BSN, RN, CNOR
St. Mary Medical Center
Langhorne, PA

Lorraine Buchanan, MSN, RN
University of Kansas School of Nursing
Kansas City, KS

Cara Busenhart, MSN, APRN, CNM
University of Kansas School of Nursing
Kansas City, KS

Michelle Byrne, PhD, RN, CNE, CNOR
University of North Georgia
Dahlonega, GA

Karen Carlson, PhD, RN
University of New Mexico
Albuquerque, NM

Rachel Choudhury, MSN, RN, CNE
Chamberlain College of Nursing
Columbus, Ohio

Marilyn Cox, MSN, RN, CDE, BC-ADM
Children's Medical Center Dallas
Dallas, TX

Ann Crawford, PhD, MSN, BSN
University of Mary Hardin-Baylor
Belton, TX

Judy Flowers, MSN, MEd, RN
Catawba Valley Community College
Hickory, NC

J. Kaye Fuson, BSN, RN
Davidson County Community College
Mocksville, NC

Lance Hadley, DNP, MSN, BSN
West Texas A&M University
Canyon, TX

Robin Harris, MSN, MSEd, BSN, RN
College of The Albemarle
Elizabeth City, NC

Fairuz Lutz, MSN, BSN, RN
Wesley College
Dover, DE

Kathy Magorian, EdD, MSN, RN
University of South Dakota
Vermillion, SD

Steven A. Marinos, MSN, RN
Johnston Community College
Smithfield, NC

Sue Ellen Miller, MSN, RN, CNE
Forsyth Technical Community College
Winston-Salem, NC

Geri Neuberger, EdD, APRN-CNS
University of Kansas School of Nursing
Kansas City, KS

Martha Olson, MSN, RN
University of Nebraska Medical Center
Omaha, NE

Karen Panunto, EdD, MSN, RN, APN
Wesley College
Dover, DE

Pamela Phillips, PhD, MSN, BSN, AB
Blue Ridge Community College
Weyers Cave, VA

Theresa Pietsch, PhD, RN, CRRN, CNE
Neumann University
Aston, PA

Sharon Rappold, MSN, RN, BC
Wharton County Junior College
Wharton, TX

Jean Robley, MSN, PHN, BSN
Alexandria Technical and Community College
Alexandria, MN

Judith Rolph, MSN, RN
MassBay Community College
Framingham, MA

T. Kim Rodehorst-Weber, PhD, RN
University of Nebraska Medical Center
College of Nursing
Omaha, NE

Dana K. Samson, MSN, RN
University of Nebraska Medical Center
Omaha, NE

Patricia Sharpnack, DNP, RN, CNE, NEA-BC
Ursuline College
Pepper Pike, OH

Debbie Stevenson, MSN, BSN, RN
Lincoln Technical Institute
Fern Park, FL

Ferquita Stokes, MSN-Ed, BSN, RN
Herzing University
Orlando, FL

Karen Tarnow, PhD, RN
University of Kansas School of Nursing
Kansas City, KS

Gerry Walker, DHEd, MSN, BSN, RN
Park University
Parkville, MO

Arthur West, MPA, MSN, BSN, CCRN, ADN
Southeastern Community College
Whiteville, NC

Jackie Williams, PhD, MEd, MSN, BSN
Georgia Perimeter College
Clarkston, GA

FIRST EDITION ADVISORS AND CONTRIBUTORS

Charlotte Blackwell, MSEd, BSN, RN
Wake Technical Community College

Carol Hardin Boles, MSN, RN
Surry Community College

Catherine Borysewicz, MSN, RN, BC, CNE
Carolinas College of Health Sciences

Colleen Burgess, EdD, MSN, RN, APRN, BC
Catawba Valley Community College

Barbara Callahan, MEd, BSN, RN, NCC
Lenoir Community College

Sheryl Cornelius, MSN, RN
Mitchell Community College

Rachelle Denney, MSNC, RN, BSN
Fayetteville Technical Community College

Cathy L. H. Franklin-Griffin, PhD, RN
Surry Community College

Delia Frederick, MSNEd, RN
Southwestern Community College

Martha Freeze, MSN, ACNSBC
Rowan Cabarrus Community College

Robin Harris, MSED, BSN, RN
College of the Albemarle

Barbara Knopp, MSN, RN
North Carolina Board of Nursing

June Martin, MSN, RN
Forsyth Technical Community College

Debra S. McKinney, MSN, MBA/HCM, RN
University of Phoenix Online

Katherine K. Phillips, MSN, RN
Guilford Technical Community College

Camille Reese, EdD, MSN, RNC
Mitchell Community College

Linda Smith, MSN, RN
Johnston Community College

Marilyn Springle, MSN, RN, FNPBC
Carteret Community College

Renee Taylor, BSN, RN
Robeson Community College

Kathy Williford, MSN, RN
NEWH Nursing Consortium

Linda Wright, MSN, RN
Western Piedmont Community College

PREFACE

Nursing: A Concept-Based Approach to Learning, Second Edition, represents the cutting edge in nursing education. This uniquely integrated solution provides students with a consistent design of content and assessment that specifically supports a concept-based curriculum. Available as a fully integrated digital experience or in print format, this solution meets the needs of today's nursing student.

The goal of this program is to help students learn the essential knowledge they will need for client care.

▶ CONTENT ORGANIZATION

Fifty-one concepts have been chosen in three domains. Some nursing programs will use this program in its entirety, others will choose some concepts and supplement with additional materials. To learn more about how to develop a concept-based program, see the *Faculty Guide to Concept-Based Learning* and *Student Guide to Concept-Based Learning* at nursing.pearsonhighered.com.

The content is organized as shown in the following chart:

DOMAIN	COMPETENCIES
Individual Parts I, II, and III of text	Developmentally appropriate client-centered care, collaboration, cultural competence, evidence-based practice, assessment, and communication
Nursing Part IV of text	Professional behavior, assessment, communication, clinical decision making, and other National League for Nursing Accreditation Committee (NLNAC) competencies for graduates of associate degree programs
Healthcare Part V of text	Quality improvement, evidence-based practice, informatics, and other elements essential to nursing within the healthcare system

Within each domain, the curriculum presents information that is critical to the practice of nursing. Each domain is divided into modules that include a concept and its essential exemplars. Within the individual domain, the concept model delineates human systems of functioning, first describing the normal process of each system and then presenting common alterations from normal that are related to the system. These alterations are referred to as *exemplars.* For example, in the module on Oxygenation, the normal process of ventilation and gas exchange is presented in The Concept of Oxygenation, followed by five frequently seen alterations, or exemplars: Acute Respiratory Distress Syndrome, Asthma, Chronic Obstructive Pulmonary Disease, Respiratory Syncytial Virus/Bronchiolitis, and Sudden Infant Death Syndrome. The information is provided in such a way that students will be able to apply informa-

tion learned to other alterations in oxygenation in addition to those presented in the curriculum.

Further, the individual domain presents each concept with the underlying premise that no one concept functions without input from various other concepts. As such, this model provides opportunities for students to link concepts and their interactions together. For example, how does the concept of oxygenation link to the concept of perfusion? To the concept of cognition?

The curriculum addresses traditional therapies and treatments as well as newer complementary and alternative therapies. It provides information about diagnostic testing, assessment interviews, case studies and discussion questions, as well as critical thinking questions to promote linking of concepts, which helps students understand that all of the concepts are integrated.

▶ NEW TO THE SECOND EDITION

The Second Edition reflects feedback from users of the First Edition and extensive discussion and work by the Concepts Advisory Panel. It has been significantly updated and rewritten and reflects a consistent approach to learning.

Three New Concepts!
- *Digestion*
- *Nutrition*
- *Perioperative Care*

13 New Exemplars!
- Gastroesophageal Reflux Disease, Hepatitis, Malabsorption Disorders, Pancreatitis, and Pyloric Stenosis (within the Digestion Module)
- Diabetes in Children (within the Metabolism Module)
- Adjustment Disorder with Depressed Mood (within the Mood and Affect Module)
- Nursing Plan of Care and Prioritizing Care (supporting the Clinical Decision Making Module)
- Groups and Group Communication (within the Communication Module)
- Just Culture (within the Legal Module)
- Safety Considerations Across the Life Span and Workplace Safety (within the Safety Module)

- *New! Concepts Related To . . .* tables appear in each module to clearly show how concepts can be integrated.
- *New! Case Studies.* Each module contains one to four multipart longitudinal case studies.

■ *New! Community-Based Care feature.* These special boxes show how nurses can help clients manage their care in the community.

▶ ADDITIONAL RESOURCES

eText. For a fully integrated experience, the eText version of the content contains interactive self-assessments and links to additional content and multimedia. The highlighting, notes, search tools, and more provide a completely interactive experience. Look for these icons:

 MiniModules and Charts. These online features provide additional content on enrichment topics such as anatomy and physiology, additional Nursing Care Plans, and extra case studies to supplement student learning.

 Videos, animations and narrated lectures are placed throughout the content to help students understand key topics and concepts.

 NCLEX® Review. Learners can access the practice NCLEX® style questions that are an extension of their textbook experience.

 Relate and Reflect. Critical thinking questions link together concepts and exemplars. Case Studies provide practical nursing situations with critical thinking questions.

MyNursingLab. Specifically created to support a concept-based approach, this assessment tool provides a guided learning path proven to help students synthesize vast amounts of information. Each concept is broken into a series of short lessons and each lesson contains a pretest, personalized study tools, and a post-test. Robust reporting tools help students and instructors gauge progress.

Nursing: A Concept-Based Approach to Skills Manual. This companion skills book has been specifically designed to meet the needs of a concept-based curriculum.

The Neighborhood 2.0. Created by Dr. Jean Giddens in response to a need within a concept-based curriculum, The Neighborhood 2.0 is a virtual community of characters that engages students and provides a rich foundation of information that supports concepts and exemplars.

Instructor Resources

Annotated Instructor's eText. The instructors version of the eText contains detailed outlines and suggestions for classroom and clinical activities. Use the whiteboard feature to bring content into your classroom! Icons visible only to the instructor include:

 Learning Outcomes. This icon provides a link to where in the concept the learning outcome is met.

 Lecture Outlines. This icon provides a link to an outline that educators can use to frame their lectures.

 Activities. Individual, group and clinical activity suggestions are provided to enhance learning.

 The Neighborhood 2.0. The Neighborhood is an online virtual community that helps students bridge the gap between lecture and clinical experience for a deeper understanding of the entire context of patient care. Students get to know the unfolding nature of health and illness of all these characters with text, photos, video clips and medical records. Cases from The Neighborhood are presented in various concepts and exemplars.

Class Preparation Resources. This resource provides instructors with a searchable database of activities, lecture PowerPoints, Clicker Questions, Images, and more!

ClassMaster. This online wizard maps course topics, concepts, and exemplars, to corresponding activities, resources, and reading assignments.

Test Bank. The test bank consists of NCLEX®-style questions with complete rationales for correct and incorrect answers. Available in a variety of formats.

FEATURES

▶ CONSISTENT STRUCTURE!

Each module is consistently formatted and color-coded to promote learning.

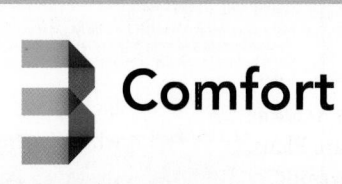

3 Comfort

MODULE AT-A-GLANCE

The Concept of Comfort, 141
Exemplar 3.1
   Acute and Chronic Pain, 152

Exemplar 3.2
   End-of-Life Care, 174
Exemplar 3.3
   Fatigue, 185

Exemplar 3.4
   Fibromyalgia, 190
Exemplar 3.5
   Sleep–Rest Disorders, 194

> Each concept begins with **The Concept of** providing a general description of the "concept" portion of the module.

⬚ THE CONCEPT OF COMFORT

Comfort in health care is defined by Katharine Kolcaba's Comfort Theory as "the immediate state of being strengthened by having the needs for relief, ease, and transcendence addressed in the four contexts of holistic human experience: physical, psychospiritual, sociocultural, and environmental." In this definition, clients achieve *relief* when their needs are met, *ease* is a state of contentment, and *transcendence* allows clients to rise above their problems. In addition, *physical* comfort is related to bodily sensations and homeostatic mechanisms, *psychospiritual* comfort is related to the individual awareness of oneself and one's relationship to a higher being, *sociocultural* comfort is related to family and societal relationships, and *environmental* comfort is related to the external surroundings (Kolcaba, Tilton, & Drouin, 2006).

Increased comfort, reduced stress, and a healing environment are linked to increased client satisfaction and shorter hospital stays (Geimer-Flanders, 2009; HermanMiller, 2010; Seifert & Hickman, 2005). Stressors can include anything from pain to lack of natural lighting to fear of the unknown. Providing a healing environment in which stressors are reduced through adequate comfort measures allows clients to maintain normal vital signs, receive adequate sleep–rest and nutrition, and feel a sense of control over their healing process. «

> **Concept Learning Outcomes** provide a structured outline for learning.

Concept Learning Outcomes

After reading about this concept, you will be able to:

1. Summarize the physiology of comfort.
2. Examine the relationship between comfort and other concepts/systems.
3. Identify commonly occurring alterations in comfort and their related therapies.
4. Differentiate common assessment procedures used to examine comfort across the life span.
5. Describe diagnostic and laboratory tests to determine the individual's comfort status.
6. Explain management of comfort and prevention of discomfort.
7. Demonstrate the nursing process in providing culturally competent and caring interventions across the life span for individuals with common alterations in comfort.
8. Compare and contrast common independent and collaborative interventions for clients with alterations in comfort.

Concept Key Terms

Acute fatigue, 145
Acute pain, 143
Breathing exercises, 150
Chronic fatigue, 145
Chronic fatigue
  syndrome, 145
Chronic pain, 143
Comfort, 141
End-of-life care, 145
Fatigue, 145
Fibromyalgia, 145
Imagery, 150

Insomnia, 145
Movement techniques, 151
Muscle relaxation, 150
Narcolepsy, 145
Pain, 143
Parasomnia, 145
Polysomnography (PSG), 148
Restless leg syndrome, 145
Sleep apnea, 145
Sleep hygiene, 149
Sleep loss, 145
Tender points, 145

141

> **Concept Key Terms** list provides a study tool for learning new vocabulary specific to the concept. Page numbers are included for easy reference.

Normal Presentation and Alterations to the Concept: Across the Lifespan!

▶ NORMAL PRESENTATION OF COMFORT

Comfort is a relative feeling based on expectations and past experiences. Therefore, a "normal" level of comfort may be different for every client. However, there are some elements of comfort that are common to all individuals.

Physiology Review

An individual experiences comfort when each level of Maslow's hierarchy of needs is fulfilled (**Figure 3–1** ●). The most basic physiological needs of oxygen, shelter, food, water, and sleep are met, and the individual feels safe and free from anxiety, fear, and pain. The individual who experiences true comfort senses love and belonging from family and friends. For individuals seeking health care, comfort also includes participating in a healthy nurse–client relationship. In addition, individuals experience comfort in the areas of self-esteem and self-actualization by giving and receiving respect, feeling confident, and accepting reality.

Because comfort is subjective, the nurse should aim to understand what is "comfortable" or "normal" for the client. Some clients have difficulty articulating this or have such a high tolerance for discomfort that it is difficult to determine an appropriate baseline. For example, a woman who has worked for the Peace Corps in Africa for several years may be unperturbed by an extra day's stay in the hospital, but an Olympic athlete might find the extra day of confinement and rest intolerable.

Signs of comfort can sometimes be determined from client assessment for sympathetic nervous system responses such as heart and respiratory rate, blood pressure, and body and skin temperature. However, "normal" vital signs are not always reli-

Each concept begins with an overview of the **Normal Presentation** including a review of physiology and genetic and lifespan considerations.

▶ ALTERATIONS TO COMFORT

Very few people meet the criteria for comfort stated by Kolcaba. What aspects of discomfort are most commonly encountered by nurses? This chapter focuses on five common sources of discomfort: pain, end-of-life care, fatigue, fibromyalgia, and sleep–rest disorders. Read Concepts Related to Comfort to see how Comfort is interrelated with other concepts.

Alterations and Manifestations

Pain, fatigue, and sleep–rest disorders are basic alterations in comfort caused by disease, illness, or injury; fibromyalgia is a classic example of a disease characterized by these three types of discomfort. Discomfort is also a reality at the end of life, and nurses must provide comfort for clients and families during end-of-life care. These alterations in comfort will be summarized here and explored in depth in the exemplar sections (also see the Alterations and Therapies feature).

Alterations to the concept include prevalence, genetic considerations, and nonmodifiable risk factors.

Alterations and Therapies summarize commonly seen alterations and possible treatments.

Lifespan Considerations Comfort

Infants/Toddlers

- Infants verbalize discomfort by crying. Ask the parents for descriptions of the infant's manifestations of pain, including suspected location and how the pain influences eating, sleeping, and behavior.
- Discomfort in otherwise healthy infants may be related to milk components. Bottle-fed infants may need a specialized formula. For breastfed infants, the mother's diet may need to be modified.
- Infants and toddlers should be comforted by being held, rocking, murmuring soothing words, and rubbing or patting the torso or extremities.
- Many pain medications have no dosing instructions for children under 2 years old. Warn parents to follow physician's orders for all medications given to infants and toddlers.

Children

- Involve the child in describing any discomfort, but also ask the parent(s) or guardian about the child's behaviors related to discomfort.
- Before performing any procedures or tests, explain the procedure to the child to help decrease anxiety. When possible, it may also help to demonstrate the procedure on the parent before performing the procedure on the child.
- Depending on age and personality, children may be comforted by being held, hugging, holding hands, or receiving a treat like a sucker, sticker, or small toy.
- If you must perform a painful procedure such as an injection, engage the parent in the child's care by asking the parent to offer comfort or distraction.

Adolescents

- Adolescents may respond to treatment and comfort better if you interact with them as adults rather than as children.
- Some adolescents may reject any offer of comfort.

Adults

- If diagnosed with a chronic or fatal disease, adults may find comfort in knowledge. Take the time to describe the disease and what to expect for tests, medications, and other interventions, and to answer any questions they have.
- Comfort is a subjective experience, so listen carefully when the client is describing any feelings of discomfort, and care for the client accordingly.

Pregnant Women

- Pregnant women, especially first-time mothers, may be very anxious about their health and the health of their baby. Take time to explain the expected growth and development of the fetus and expected maternal changes. Answer any questions.
- Provide tips about self-care, physical activity, and sleeping positions that will help ease discomfort. Encourage adequate nutrition, hydration, and sleep–rest.

Older Adults

- Older adults are more likely to suffer from chronic conditions such as diabetes, chronic pain, heart disease, cancer, and arthritis. Provide a safe and comfortable environment for regular appointments, and foster a healthy nurse–client relationship to promote comfort.
- Explain procedures and medications at each visit; some older adult clients have memory deficits. Provide written instructions and explanations. Provide assistance with movement as needed, especially for clients with chronic pain or arthritis.

End of Life

- Provide adequate pain relief with pharmacologic agents as ordered.
- Promote psychosocial comfort by offering to arrange a visit from a spiritual leader and/or loved ones.
- Facilitate referrals for grief counseling for the family and other loved ones.
- Honor the client's and family's decisions about end-of-life care.

Lifespan Considerations highlight concept considerations specific to infants, children, adolescents, pregnancy, and older adults.

Alterations and Therapies Comfort

ALTERATION	DESCRIPTION/ DEFINITION	MANIFESTATIONS	INTERVENTIONS AND THERAPIES
Acute pain	Pain of varying severity, location, and etiology that lasts fewer than 6 months.	■ Elevated blood pressure ■ Increased heart rate ■ Nausea and vomiting ■ Sweating ■ Rapid/shallow respirations ■ Anxiety ■ Decreased function in activities of daily living	Pharmacologic pain management: ■ Opioid analgesics ■ Nonsteroidal anti-inflammatory drugs (NSAIDs) ■ Nonopioid analgesics Nonpharmacologic therapy: ■ Massage ■ Diversionary therapies (music, involvement in hobbies, aroma therapy) ■ Application of heat and cold
Chronic pain	Pain of varying severity, location, and etiology that lasts 6 months or more (even if intermittent).	■ Depression ■ Irritability ■ Impaired mobility and/or activity ■ Sleep disturbance	Pharmacologic pain management: ■ Nonopioid analgesics ■ Antidepressants ■ NSAIDs ■ Muscle relaxants ■ Opioid analgesics Nonpharmacologic therapy: ■ Guided imagery ■ Massage ■ Nerve stimulation units ■ Chiropractic interventions ■ Physical therapy ■ Relaxation techniques ■ Positioning
End-of-life care	Care that takes place when death is imminent	■ Loss of muscle tone ■ Slowing of circulation ■ Change in respirations ■ Sensory impairments ■ Impaired metabolic processes	■ Palliative or aggressive care as chosen by client and family ■ Maintenance of comfort ■ Maintenance of hygiene ■ Psychosocial support for client and family
Fatigue	Lack of energy or motivation with or without drowsiness	■ Tiredness ■ Depression ■ Anxiety ■ Irritability ■ Decreased cognition	Pharmacologic therapy: ■ Sleeping aids ■ Stimulants ■ Antidepressants ■ Pain management Nonpharmacologic therapy: ■ Improved sleep hygiene

Concepts Related to **Comfort**

Promotion of comfort is an integral part of nursing care. The exemplars included in this module explore several common manifestations of discomfort, including pain, fatigue, and sleep–rest disorders. However, alterations in comfort are not limited to these specific manifestations. The concept of comfort is interrelated to numerous other physiological and psychosocial concepts. For example, one of the classic symptoms of inflammation is pain. Therefore, nurses can offer comfort to clients with inflammation by administering pain medications as ordered and providing nonpharmacologic comfort measures such as cold therapy. Clients with pain, especially joint pain, lower back pain, or trauma pain, often experience decreased mobility. Nursing interventions for these clients may include ambulation assistance and hygiene care. Impaired tissue integrity is a common cause of discomfort and can also lead to more serious complications, such as infection. Comfort measures may include assessing the client for infection, providing hygiene care for the wound, and assisting with repositioning for immobile clients.

Promotion of comfort includes both physical and psychosocial wellness. Individuals suffering grief over a lost loved one or lost personal health may need emotional comfort in the form of therapeutic communication or referrals to support groups. Comfort care is also closely tied to ethical issues for many clients, such as individuals with drug addiction who need opioid treatment for severe pain or the family deciding about withdrawing or withholding of life-sustaining treatments for a client at the end of life. The relationship between comfort and the concepts of inflammation, mobility, tissue integrity, grief and loss, and ethics are summarized in the following table.

CONCEPT	RELATIONSHIP TO COMFORT	NURSING IMPLICATIONS
Inflammation		
■ Assessment interview: Inflammation ■ Independent interventions and therapies	Inflammation → pain.	■ Assess pain in clients with inflammation; provide pharmacologic treatments as ordered. ■ Offer comfort measures such as ice or heat; promote adequate sleep and rest.
Mobility		
■ Mobility assessment ■ Assessment interview: Mobility	↓ mobility is often caused by pain, injury, or disease.	■ Assist with ambulation and activities of daily living; encourage adequate sleep and rest. ■ Offer pharmacologic treatments as ordered.
Tissue Integrity		
■ Integumentary assessment ■ Pressure ulcers	↓ tissue integrity = ↑ risk for pain, inflammation, and infection.	■ Assess for skin breakdown; promote mobility. ■ Assist with repositioning as needed; monitor for signs and symptoms of infection.
Grief and Loss		
■ Assessment interview: Grief and loss	Loss or expected loss of a loved one is emotionally distressing.	■ Use therapeutic communication techniques; encourage expression of emotions; facilitate referrals to counselors and support groups.
Ethics		
	Physicians may be reluctant to prescribe opioids based on race, ethnicity, or history of addiction.	■ Advocate for the provision of adequate pain relief to all clients; provide culturally sensitive care; offer nonpharmacologic comfort measures to all clients.

▶ INTERVENTIONS AND THERAPIES

For the client experiencing alterations in comfort, initial interventions are directed at identifying the source of the discomfort. For clients with physical pain, while pain relief is a priority, masking the pain through analgesic administration can make identifying the underlying cause much more difficult. For this reason, especially until the cause of the client's discomfort is identified, interventions to promote comfort may focus on nonpharmacologic measures. These include simple interventions such as applying heat or cold as

Independent

Promotion of comfort includes teaching clients about lifestyle changes that can help decrease their symptoms of pain, depression, or fatigue. Three basic independent categories of teaching include sleep hygiene, psychosocial well-being, and relaxation therapy.

Collaborative

For the client experiencing discomfort, collaborative therapies include both pharmacologic and nonpharmacologic interventions. Pharmacologic interventions involve the administration of medications, examples of which are listed in the Medications feature. Nonpharmacologic therapies may be either alternative therapies, which are used instead of pharmacologic therapies, or complementary therapies, which are used in addition to pharmacologic therapies. Common nonpharmacologic therapies, such as acupuncture and herbal supplements, are discussed in the specific exemplars.

Medications **Sleep**

CLASSIFICATION AND DRUG EXAMPLES	MECHANISM OF ACTION	NURSING CONSIDERATIONS
Hypnotics/Sedatives ■ Benzodiazepines ■ Nonbenzodiazepines *Drug examples:* Temazepam, zolpidem, eszopiclone	Produces CNS depression by acting on the limbic, thalamic, and hypothalamic regions of the CNS (benzodiazepines). Interacts with GABA receptor (nonbenzodiazepines).	Monitor older adults for paradoxical reaction. Do not use in depressed, suicidal, or pregnant clients. Tolerance and addiction may result from benzodiazepine use; slowly taper dosage when discontinuing therapy; drugs should not be used for more than 4–6 months.

Complementary and Alternative Therapy Herbal Supplements for Sleep Disorders

Herbal supplements may be an alternative for individuals who do not tolerate pharmacologic therapy because of side effects. Two herbs that are traditionally used to aid sleep are valerian (*Valeriana officinalis*) and chamomile (*Matricaria recutita*). Valerian usually has to be taken for 2 or 3 weeks before it produces an effect, and clinical trials have not proven its effectiveness. Possible side effects of valerian include indigestion, headache, palpitations, and dizziness. Chamomile, often taken as a tea, has a soothing effect that may induce sleep and decrease restlessness, although this effect has not been proven in clinical studies. It is safe for both adults and children except individuals who are allergic to ragweed or daisies.

Melatonin is a sleep hormone produced by the pineal gland. Synthetic melatonin is sold in many pharmacies and health food stores and may be taken to regulate sleep patterns. It is often helpful for sleep disturbances related to shift work or jet lag. It has been proven effective in treating sleep disorders in children with autism (Rossignol & Frye, 2011) and children with ADHD (Hoebert et al., 2009). It may also be helpful for older adults with insomnia when combined with magnesium and zinc supplements (Rondanelli et al., 2011).

New! Concepts Related to feature helps you understand how concepts are integrated, how a client with an alteration in one concept will likely have alterations in other concepts as well.

Interventions and Therapies sections divide therapies into *Independent* (those nurses can perform on their own) and *Collaborative* (those done with primary care providers or other members of the healthcare team)

Medication boxes provide specific drug information and nursing considerations.

Complementary and Alternative Therapy boxes provide additional information on herbal and other nonpharmacologic therapies.

Clinical Reasoning, Client-Focused Nursing Care, and Evidence-Based Practice

New! Longitudinal Case Studies consisting of three parts appear in the individual domain section. These case studies follow a single client through varies levels of acuity of a particular alteration. Case studies end with two sets of questions. Level I questions can be answered using the material covered in the Concept. Level II questions require additional information from elsewhere in the Concepts program, from the student's own experience, or from research.

CASE STUDY \\ PART 1

April Daves is a 34-year-old Black female who was in a severe motor vehicle accident 6 months ago. All of her injuries have healed, but when she continues to have chronic pain in several of her joints and muscles, her primary care physician refers her to an orthopedic specialist. As the nurse at the orthopedic clinic, you are responsible for obtaining Ms. Daves's medical history and making the initial assessment. You learn that Ms. Daves broke her left fibula near the knee, dislocated her left shoulder, and suffered whiplash. She reports almost constant burning pain and stiffness in her left knee, shoulder, and neck, but sometimes she also feels pain in her right knee and in her hips. She figures it is just "sympathy pain," but the combined pain makes movement difficult. She rates her current pain at a 5 on a scale of 0–10, but if she has to move around a lot, it increases to a 7. Her vital signs are temperature 97.2°F oral; pulse 86 bpm; respirations 20/min; and BP 146/82 mmHg. Ms. Daves reports she has been trying to manage her pain with acetaminophen and ibuprofen. However, they aren't always effective, and she often has trouble sleeping at night because of the pain. Her boss is starting to notice a drop in productivity at work because she has trouble staying awake when sitting at her desk.

After the physician reviews Ms. Daves's health history and performs a physical assessment, he sends her for x-rays on her left knee and shoulder. Although the x-rays do not show any obvious abnormalities, he suspects Ms. Daves may have developed osteoarthritis. The physician asks you to schedule Ms. Daves for a CT scan of her left knee and left shoulder. He prescribes meloxicam (Mobic) as an analgesic and recommends that the client return for a follow up visit after her CT scans are completed.

Clinical Reasoning Questions Level I

1. During her client history, what alterations in comfort does Ms. Daves reveal?
2. Based on Ms. Daves's vital signs, what assumptions can you make about her level of discomfort?
3. Why might Ms. Daves's other joints be feeling "sympathy pain," as she describes it?

Clinical Reasoning Questions Level II

4. What nonpharmacologic therapies could you suggest for pain management? Fatigue?

CASE STUDY \\ PART 2

Two days before April Daves is scheduled to return to her orthopedic physician, she is awakened by severe pain. Because she is unable to get out of bed, Ms. Daves calls 911. She is transferred to the hospital by ambulance. As her emergency department (ED) nurse, you assess Ms. Daves. Her only complaint is pain, which she rates as a 9 on a scale of 0 to 10. Ms. Daves reports she has been taking her NSAIDs as prescribed. Her heart rate, respiratory rate, and blood pressure are all slightly elevated. Ms. Daves further reports that the pain has prevented her from sleeping more than 3–4 hours each night. Aside from her motor vehicle crash, Ms. Daves has no history of illness or trauma. You report your findings to the ED physician.

After reviewing Ms. Daves's medical history and performing a physical assessment, the physician orders a complete blood count (CBC) and a urinalysis, the results of which are normal. He also obtains the results of Ms. Daves's CT scans, which are normal. The ED physician suspects that Ms. Daves may have fibromyalgia. Using the 2010 fibromyalgia criteria, the ED physician determines that Ms. Daves's widespread pain index is 8 and her symptom severity scale score is 9. The physician diagnoses Ms. Daves with fibromyalgia and prescribes milnacipran (Savella). He instructs her to visit her primary care physician for follow up as soon as possible.

Clinical Reasoning Questions Level I

1. What causes fibromyalgia?
2. What nursing interventions can you implement immediately to help relieve Ms. Daves's pain?
3. For the client with fibromyalgia, what findings would you expect to be revealed by the CBC and urinalysis?

Clinical Reasoning Questions Level II

4. Refer to the exemplar on Fibromyalgia in this module. Based on your knowledge of Ms. Daves's clinical signs and symptoms, what somatic symptoms is she likely to be experiencing?
5. Why did the physician choose milnacipran instead of duloxetine or pregabalin for Ms. Daves's fibromyalgia?
6. What client teaching topics should you review with Ms. Daves before her discharge?

REFLECT Case Study \\ Part 3

Ms. Daves has been visiting her primary care provider as recommended for follow up care. Six months after beginning treatment with milnacipran (Savella), Ms. Daves returns for a regular checkup. As you review her chart, you note that Ms. Daves's physician confirmed the ED physician's diagnoses of fibromyalgia. Upon assessment, Ms. Daves's vital signs are normal, and her pain intensity is a 3 on a scale of 0–10. She also reports that she is sleeping better at night, although she occasionally has insomnia even though the pain is manageable. When you ask how Savella is working for her, she says that it has helped her pain and stiffness but her mouth has been really dry since she started taking it and she sometimes has slight nausea.

Clinical Reasoning Questions Level I

1. What suggestions can you give Ms. Daves to help decrease her dry mouth and nausea?
2. What further assessment should be included to help determine the cause of Ms. Daves's insomnia?
3. Can you suggest other therapies to help decrease Ms. Daves's pain even further?

Clinical Reasoning Questions Level II

4. What nursing interventions can you implement to help prevent future flare-ups of Ms. Daves's fibromyalgia?
5. What information should you give Ms. Daves about milnacipran (Savella) and drug–drug interactions?
6. What coping techniques would be useful for Ms. Daves as she deals with fibromyalgia?

▶ PREVENTION

Prevention of discomfort begins with the client. Personal preferences, lifestyle habits, and culture are all factors in the development of chronic diseases and other contributors to discomfort, and only the client can change behaviors that increase the risk of discomfort. However, nurses provide essential client education that can encourage clients to change their behaviors to decrease the risk of developing a chronic disease or experiencing an acute illness or injury.

Lifestyle habits that predispose individuals to chronic health alterations, such as poor nutrition, smoking, excessive alcohol consumption, and poor sleep hygiene, all increase an individual's risk for experiencing discomfort. Poor nutrition can include both overeating and undernutrition. Eating a healthy diet in combination with good sleep hygiene can help prevent the development of many chronic diseases that lead to symptoms of discomfort.

Smoking, alcohol consumption, and illicit drug use can also lead to alterations in comfort. Because nicotine, alcohol, and illicit drugs are addictive, quitting drug use is associated with withdrawal symptoms. Emotional withdrawal symptoms include anxiety, irritability, insomnia, and depression. Physical withdrawal symptoms include sweating, palpitations, nausea, and difficulty breathing.

Other lifestyle habits that may lead to discomfort are working at a job that requires heavy lifting, long hours, or repetitive movement, which increases the risk of injury and fatigue. Participation in physical activities such as team sports or extreme sports also increases susceptibility to injury and consequent discomfort.

Sections on **Prevention** and **Assessment** cover modifiable risk factors, screenings, nursing assessments, and diagnostic tests.

▶ ASSESSMENT

The nursing assessment should explore not only the client's level of discomfort but also the degree to which discomfort is affecting the client's daily life. Some clients may not even realize the extent to which discomfort is impacting their lifestyle and overall well-being.

Comfort Assessment

ASSESSMENT/METHOD	NORMAL FINDINGS	ABNORMAL FINDINGS	LIFESPAN OR DEVELOPMENTAL CONSIDERATIONS
Interview Client History			
Client description of symptoms. Pain scale. Depression assessment.	The client should report no signs or symptoms of discomfort.	▪ Client reports mild to severe pain. ▪ Client reports disrupted sleep patterns. ▪ Client reports or displays signs of nausea or vomiting. ▪ Client reports lack of appetite or ravenous appetite. ▪ Client reports lack of motivation, feelings of despair, or feelings of anxiety.	▪ Look for nonverbal signs of discomfort such as crying, shielding an injured area, lack of affect, or withdrawal in nonverbal children and mentally impaired clients. ▪ Signs of depression and anxiety in children may indicate abuse, and assessment of the child in the absence of the parent(s) may be warranted. ▪ Gastrointestinal discomfort can be a physiological response to disease or it can be a side effect of medication. Check client history for current medications and known drug allergies. ▪ Depression and anxiety can be primary or secondary conditions. Be sure to assess the depressed or anxious client for symptoms of chronic conditions.
Physical Assessment			
Vital signs. Visual inspection. Polysomnography (PSG) for identification of suspected sleep disorders. Blood and urine analysis.	Client should have normal vital signs, and no obvious external injuries or infections. Results of all clinical tests should be within normal limits.	▪ Severe pain may be accompanied by sympathetic nervous system findings such as increased heart rate, sweating, and nausea. ▪ PSG indicates abnormal REM/NREM cycles or severe apnea (Mayo Clinic, 2011a). ▪ Client appears depressed, nervous, or confused. ▪ Abnormal blood and urine analysis may indicate illness or malnutrition.	▪ Children may be fearful of physical assessment. To promote comfort during ical adu asse

Assessment and ***Assessment Interview*** features summarize normal and abnormal findings and questions to ask the client.

Assessment Interview Discomfort (Pain, Depression, Anxiety, Appetite, Sleep Disorder)

Current Problem

▪ When did your discomfort start?

▪ How would you describe your discomfort?

▪ On a scale of 0 to 10, with 0 meaning no pain and 10 meaning the worst pain you can imagine, how would you rate your current pain intensity?

▪ Which activities make the discomfort better or worse?

▪ How long have you had this discomfort?

▪ How does this discomfort affect your activities of daily living?

▪ What do you do to alleviate your discomfort?

▪ Are you currently taking any medications to alleviate your discomfort?

▪ Does your discomfort affect your sleep pattern or your mood?

▪ Does your discomfort affect your appetite?

▪ Does eating or drinking make your discomfort better or worse?

▪ Do you feel that your discomfort is related to another disease or condition?

▪ Do you feel sad frequently?

▪ Do you have trouble motivating yourself to participate in daily activities?

▪ Have you had thoughts of suicide?

▪ Have you had any changes in daily habits that increased your symptoms of discomfort?

Client History

▪ Have you had this discomfort in the past?

▪ How often does this symptom of discomfort occur?

▪ Have you taken medications for this problem in the past?

▪ Have you had past experiences that affect the way you view this discomfort?

Lifestyle

▪ Do you drink alcohol? If so, how much? Do you feel this contributes to your symptoms?

▪ Do you smoke? If so, how much? Do you feel this contributes to your symptoms?

▪ Do you exercise? Is your condition related to your participation in physical activity?

▪ Describe your average daily food and drink intake. Do you feel that your diet contributes to your symptoms?

Evidence-Based Practice Overcoming Barriers to Adequate Pain Management

Problem

Pain is a major reason that clients seek health care and take medications, and it accounts for a substantial portion of lost work productivity and disability. However, clients in pain are often underdiagnosed and undertreated, especially racial and ethnic minorities, people of lower socioeconomic status, women, children, older adults, military veterans, surgery and cancer clients, and people at the end of life (IOM, 2011).

Evidence

Pain management remains ineffective due to attitudes and educational deficits of healthcare providers and clients and limitations of pharmacologic agents. Attitudes of healthcare providers can be influenced by both medical evidence and clients' psychosocial influences. In particular, providers are more likely to suggest clients are feigning pain in the absence of medical evidence, and they are less likely to take clients' report of pain into account, if psychosocial influences are present (De Ruddere et al., 2013). Methods of pain management also need to be improved. Using multiple pain medications with different mechanisms of action and side effects will improve efficacy in relieving pain and decrease the incidence of adverse reactions compared to single drug therapies (Sinatra, 2010). In addition, compared to no intervention, physical and psychosocial nonpharmacologic interventions for pain can significantly improve clients' pain level (Park & Hughes, 2012).

Implications

Healthcare professionals need to have a better understanding of pain and pain management. The perception of pain involves both physiological and psychosocial aspects, and pain management should include adequate pharmacologic interventions as well as complementary nonpharmacologic methods to reduce physiological pain and increase psycho-

social well-being. Education for healthcare providers should include training programs that offer standardized information about pain, guidelines related to caring for clients in pain, and experience in caring for clients in pain (IOM, 2011). Education should also include information about the proper use of opioids. Opioids, which are the most effective pain medications, are often underprescribed because of prejudices, misconceptions, and fears about their use (Notcutt & Gibbs, 2010). All healthcare providers should be encouraged to keep their knowledge current by participating in continuing education courses, and certification examinations should assess providers' knowledge about pain (IOM, 2011).

Critical Thinking Application

1. Do you have any biases that may hinder your ability to provide adequate pain management for clients? Think about a variety of situations that may present opportunities for bias, including caring for clients of different cultures, clients with drug addiction, young children and older adults, and clients at the end of life.

2. You are caring for a 72-year-old woman with osteoarthritis who is receiving inadequate pain control. How will you act as an advocate to provide better pain management for your client?

3. You are caring for a 19-year-old male who is a known gang member. During a recent altercation, he sustained a stab wound. He is sleeping restlessly and moaning. It is time for his next dose of opioids, but your nurse manager tells you to give him only half the prescribed dose because he is probably a drug addict and you don't want to feed his addiction. What should you do?

4. What are three ways in which you can stay up-to-date on current pain management nursing standards?

Evidence-Based Practice features demonstrate how research informs practice.

Pathophysiology and Etiology sections occur in most exemplars and include risk factors and prevention.

▶ PATHOPHYSIOLOGY AND ETIOLOGY

Pain is triggered by the peripheral nervous system, which lies outside the brain and spinal cord. There are two types of neurons in the peripheral nervous system: sensory and motor neurons. **Nociceptors**, or sensory receptors that respond to pain, send a signal along the sensory neurons to the spinal cord, where the signal is transmitted to the brain for interpretation. The brain then sends a signal back to the site of pain via motor neurons, causing the body to respond to the painful stimuli. This process happens so rapidly that the individual may reflexively withdraw from the painful stimuli even before becoming aware of the pain.

Nociceptors (**Figure 3–3 ●**) are specialized pain receptors that are present on all body tissues, with the exception of the brain. Skin and muscles contain many nociceptors, whereas internal organs have relatively few nociceptors. Categories of pain stimuli include biological, chemical, electrical, mechanical, and thermal (**Table 3–1 ●**). The duration of exposure and magnitude of the stimuli determine the intensity of the pain response.

In addition to being stimulated by external factors, cellular injury can trigger the local release of biochemicals that stimulate nociceptors, including prostaglandins, serotonin, bradykinin, and hydrogen ions. These mediators act on ion channels and G protein–coupled receptors to directly or indirectly initiate a pain impulse (Fein, 2012).

A clients' culture influences their response to and beliefs about pain. Some common cultural differences related to pain are listed here.

Arabs/Muslims

- May not request pain medicine but instead thank Allah for pain if it is the result of a healing medical procedure.
- Pain is considered a test of faith. Therefore Muslim clients must endure pain as a sign of faith in return for forgiveness and mercy. However, Muslims must seek pain relief when necessary because needless pain and suffering are frowned upon.
- Arabs and Muslims prefer to be with family when in pain and may express pain more freely around family.

Asians

- Chinese clients may not ask for medication because they do not want to take the nurse away from a more important task.
- Clients from Asian cultures often value stoicism as a response to pain. A client who complains openly about pain is thought to have poor social skills.
- Filipino clients may not take pain medication because they view pain as being the will of God.
- Indians who follow Hindu practices believe that pain must be endured in preparation for a better life in the next cycle.

Blacks

- Blacks often report higher pain intensity than other cultures.
- They believe suffering and pain are inevitable.

- They believe in prayer and laying on of hands to heal pain and believe that relief is proportional to faith.

Jews

- Jews may be vocal and demanding of assistance.
- They believe that pain must be shared and validated by others.

Hispanics

- Hispanics may believe that pain is a form of punishment and that suffering must be endured if they are to enter heaven.
- They vary widely in their expression of pain: Some are stoic and some are expressive.
- Catholic Hispanics may turn to religious practices to help them endure the pain.

Native Americans

- Native Americans may prefer to receive medications that have been blessed by a tribal shaman They believe such a blessing allows the client to be more at peace with the creator and makes the medicine stronger.
- They tend to be less expressive both verbally and nonverbally.
- They usually tolerate a high level of pain without requesting pain medication.
- They may pick a sacred number when asked to rate pain on a numerical pain scale.

Sources: Based on Munoz, C., & Luckmann, J. (2005). *Transcultural communication in nursing* (2nd ed.). Clifton Park, NY: Delmar Learning; Andrews, M. M., & Boyle, J. S. (2003). *Transcultural concepts in nursing care* (4th ed.). Philadelphia, PA: Lippincott Williams & Wilkins; Al-Atiyyat, N. M. H. (2009). Cultural diversity and cancer pain. *Journal of Hospice and Palliative Nursing*, 11(3), 154–164; Davidhizar, R., & Giger, J. N. (2004). A review of the literature on care of clients in pain who are culturally diverse. *International Nursing Review*, 51(1), 47–55.

Focus on Diversity and Culture features provide additional information to extend the foundational content.

Stay Current: Visit **www.childpain.org**, the Web site of the *Special Interest Group on Pain in Childhood*, to learn more on this topic.

Stay Current: The Hartford Institute of Geriatric Nursing offers *Try This, a site with assessment tools for use on older adults.* **http://hartfordign.org/resources/try_this_series/**

New! Stay Current alerts direct you to current research, guidelines, or organizations that relate to the concept.

▶ CLINICAL MANIFESTATIONS

Often, the body responds to severe, acute pain by activating the sympathetic nervous system's fight-or-flight response. The sympathetic response causes an increase in blood pressure, pulse, and respiratory rate, diaphoresis, pallor, and dilated pupils. Nurses may also recognize visible symptoms of pain such as crying, grimacing, shielding the site of injury, compensatory posturing, and slow movements. In addition, the client may express anxiety about the condition that is causing acute pain. Some clients may not manifest physiological or behavioral signs of pain even while experiencing moderate to severe pain, and not all clients have the same physiological response to the same intensity of pain.

As the body adapts to pain, visible and physiological symptoms of pain may be harder to detect. The sympathetic response returns to baseline levels unless the client experiences breakthrough pain, and some visible signs of pain, such as crying, cease. Pain fibers may become sensitized, so that the intensity and perception of pain increase over time. Therefore clinical manifestations of chronic pain may include compensatory posturing, muscle spasms or tense muscles, limited mobility, groaning during movements, and clenched teeth. Chronic pain is also often accompanied by psychosocial manifestations, such as depression, withdrawal from previously enjoyable activities, fatigue, and resignation to dealing with constant pain.

Uncontrolled pain has multiple detrimental effects on the body. Compensatory posturing can lead to muscle atrophy, neuropathies, and contractures. To make up for this weakened area, the body overuses another area, occasionally causing pain in that area as well (Tennant, 2008). Possible alterations in insulin and lipid metabolism contribute to the development of atherosclerosis. Changes in the endocrine system may cause immune suppression, increasing the risk of infection and slowing wound healing (Tennant, 2004). Other effects of uncontrolled pain include changes in appetite, sleep disruption, decreased circulating oxygen levels, and increased risk of thrombosis. If allowed to

Clinical Manifestations sections cover the signs and symptoms seen in alterations of the concept.

Clinical Manifestations and Therapies Acute and Chronic Pain

ETIOLOGY	CLINICAL MANIFESTATIONS	CLINICAL THERAPIES
Acute pain	■ Client report of acute pain ■ Elevated vital signs ■ Nausea and vomiting ■ Restlessness and anxiety ■ Behavioral indications (crying, grimacing, shielding)	■ Pharmacologic therapy ■ Heat/ice ■ Movement restriction ■ Distraction ■ Family support
Chronic pain	■ Client report of chronic pain ■ Normal vital signs ■ Depression ■ Irritability ■ Impaired mobility and/or activity ■ Sleep disturbances	■ Pharmacologic therapy ■ Injections ■ Surgery ■ Massage ■ Chiropractic interventions ■ Cognitive-behavioral therapy ■ Positive attitude ■ Religious rituals ■ Support (family, friends, groups)

Clinical Manifestations and Therapies features summarize content in an easy-to-read table.

Multisystem Effects of Leukemia

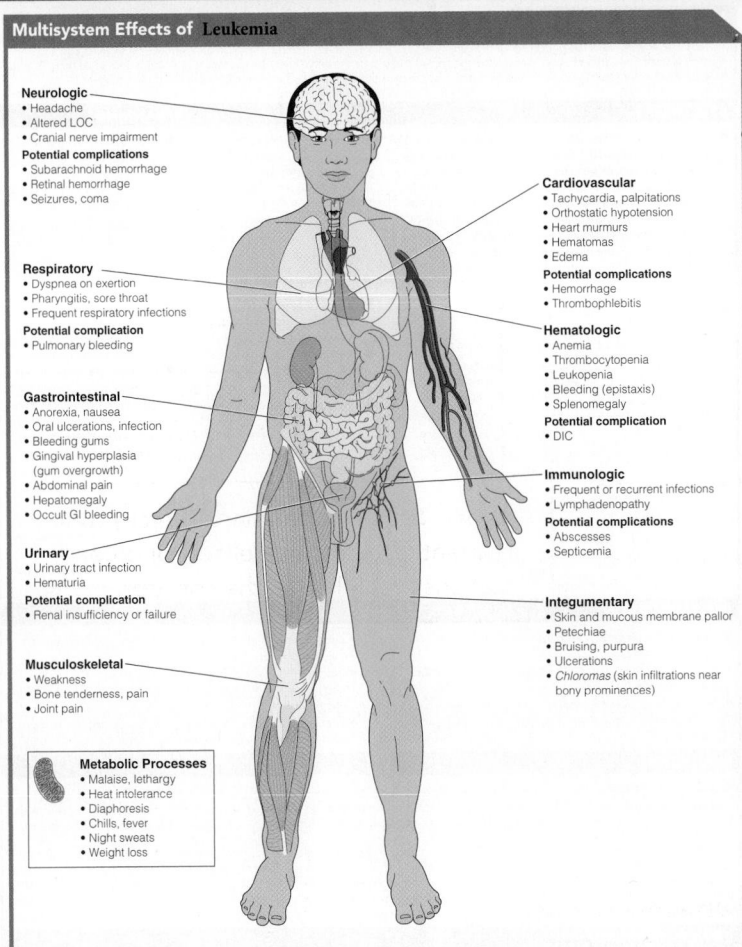

Neurologic
• Headache
• Altered LOC
• Cranial nerve impairment
Potential complications
• Subarachnoid hemorrhage
• Retinal hemorrhage
• Seizures, coma

Respiratory
• Dyspnea on exertion
• Pharyngitis, sore throat
• Frequent respiratory infections
Potential complication
• Pulmonary bleeding

Gastrointestinal
• Anorexia, nausea
• Oral ulcerations, infection
• Bleeding gums
• Gingival hyperplasia (gum overgrowth)
• Abdominal pain
• Hepatomegaly
• Occult GI bleeding

Urinary
• Urinary tract infection
• Hematuria
Potential complication
• Renal insufficiency or failure

Musculoskeletal
• Weakness
• Bone tenderness, pain
• Joint pain

Metabolic Processes
• Malaise, lethargy
• Heat intolerance
• Diaphoresis
• Chills, fever
• Night sweats
• Weight loss

Cardiovascular
• Tachycardia, palpitations
• Orthostatic hypotension
• Heart murmurs
• Hematomas
• Edema
Potential complications
• Hemorrhage
• Thrombophlebitis

Hematologic
• Anemia
• Thrombocytopenia
• Leukopenia
• Bleeding (epistaxis)
• Splenomegaly
Potential complication
• DIC

Immunologic
• Frequent or recurrent infections
• Lymphadenopathy
Potential complications
• Abscesses
• Septicemia

Integumentary
• Skin and mucous membrane pallor
• Petechiae
• Bruising, purpura
• Ulcerations
• *Chloromas* (skin infiltrations near bony prominences)

Multisystem Effects features show how certain alterations affect many body systems.

► COLLABORATION

In order to treat pain effectively, nurses collaborate with other healthcare providers. Pharmacologic therapies are nonopioids, NSAIDs, opioids, and coanalgesics. Nonpharmacologic therapies include nerve blocks, spinal cord stimulation, physical therapy, and nutritional supplements, among others. For clients with severe chronic pain, pain clinics offer the expertise needed to discover the right combination of treatments to provide consistent pain relief.

Diagnostic Tests

While laboratory and diagnostic tests may be performed to determine the cause of pain, no laboratory tests are available to directly measure a client's pain level. Instead, pain scales such as a faces pain scale or a numeric pain scale are available to help gauge a client's pain level. Changes in vital signs can also be an indication of pain, although these changes are also seen with other conditions. In addition, the body releases stress hormones in response to pain, which may be detected by blood tests. The most prevalent stress hormones are cortisol and catecholamines.

Surgery

Depending upon the pain's etiology, surgery may be a viable treatment option. For example, surgical repair of a bone fracture may be the first major step toward alleviating severe pain. Recovery from surgery often brings about its own pain, but that pain is usually short-lived compared to the pain that would result from not performing the surgery. In addition, clients may

Collaboration sections cover diagnostic tests, pharmacologic, and nonpharmacologic therapies used to address the alteration.

Client Teaching Sleep Hygiene

Fatigue is often the result of inadequate sleep. Nurses should promote and teach good sleep hygiene to all clients with fatigue, sleep–rest disorders, and acute and chronic illnesses that could cause fatigue. Good sleep hygiene includes

■ Practicing bedtime rituals that are calming, such as reading, taking a bath, praying, and listening to music.
■ Maintaining a restful environment that is free of distractions (e.g., lights and noise), is a comfortable temperature, and has appropriate ventilation.
■ Wearing loose-fitting sleepwear.
■ Using clean and dry linens.
■ Sleeping in a position that aids in muscle relaxation and supports injured areas.

■ Scheduling medications to promote sleep (i.e., taking medications that cause alertness in the morning and medications that cause drowsiness at night).
■ Avoiding naps during the day.
■ Avoiding stimulants such as caffeine and alcohol, especially in the evening; also avoiding heavy meals late in the evening.
■ Using the bed for sleep, not other activities such as watching TV.
■ Setting consistent times for sleeping and waking, and allowing adequate hours for sleep.
■ Exercising in the morning or afternoon rather than the evening.

Client Teaching, Community-Based Care, and **Safety Alerts** broaden the scope of content and provide necessary nursing information.

Community-Based Care Managing Chronic Pain at Home

Clients with chronic pain have to live at home and care for themselves in spite of their pain. Teaching clients and their family how to administer drugs, watch for side effects, and perform nonpharmacologic interventions will help enhance both the clients' and the caregivers' lives. See **Table 3–6 ●** for an overview of medications used for the management of chronic pain. Discussions should include the following topics:

■ Describe the drugs to be taken, including dose, frequency, route of administration, side effects, and potential drug, food, or herbal interactions.
■ Discuss the importance of taking drugs around the clock rather than prn.

■ Dispel any myths or misconceptions about opioid analgesics, including teaching clients that the risk of addiction is very low when pain medications are taken as prescribed.
■ Help clients and their family choose appropriate nonpharmacologic interventions to decrease pain, and teach them how to perform the interventions correctly.
■ Teach clients and their family the importance of adequate sleep and rest and not overusing the area in pain.
■ Provide information about community resources, including support groups, pain clinics, and the American Pain Society.

SAFETY ALERT
Studies have shown that taking short breaks can reduce fatigue and improve performance. Nurses should be vigilant about taking adequate breaks (i.e., 10 minutes every 2 hours, 30 minutes for meals, free of client care responsibilities) to prevent fatigue and errors that may occur because of fatigue (Rogers, 2008).

SAFETY ALERT
All clients on opioids should be monitored for sedation and respiratory depression during the first 24 hours (especially after surgery), during the peak effect, after increasing or decreasing a dose, before additional doses of opioids are given, or when changing opioids or routes of administration. If the respiratory rate falls below 8–10/min, the client should be aroused and naloxone therapy should be considered (Jarzyna et al., 2011).

■ NURSING PROCESS

Current studies estimate that 43% of American adults—or approximately 100 million Americans—suffer from chronic pain. This presents an economic burden of $560–$635 billion per year in both healthcare costs and lost work productivity. Because of the overwhelming prevalence of pain, nurses are constantly caring for clients in pain.

Uncontrolled pain can lead to comorbidities such as depression, sleep disturbances, and obesity; changes in the nervous system's response to painful stimuli; accelerated disease progression; and increased length of hospital stay. Proper application of the nursing process provides information needed for appropriate care, attainable and measurable client goals for pain management, effective nursing interventions for pain relief, and evaluation of the client's pain level for potential revision of the nursing care plan.

Assessment

Unless a client's physiological needs require priority attention (e.g., severe burns, complex fracture, gunshot wound), all clients should be asked whether they are experiencing pain. Many clients do not voluntarily complain about pain even when pain is present, and persistent pain can contribute to a poor prognosis.

Client Interview

The client interview should begin with eliciting a description of the client's pain. Ask questions about

- **Location.** "Where does it hurt?"
- **Intensity.** "On a scale of 0 to 10, with 0 representing no pain and 10 representing the worst possible pain, how would you rate the intensity of your pain now?"

Nursing Process sections within each exemplar cover assessment, diagnosis, planning, implementation, and evaluation of clients with a particular alteration.

Nursing Care Plans focusing on one client with an alteration are provided with many exemplars.

NURSING CARE PLAN   A Client With Chronic Pain

James Grier, age 28, visits the pain clinic with chronic low back pain. He states that he worked in a warehouse three years ago and injured his back while lifting heavy boxes. Although he was treated for the initial injury, he has had chronic back pain since then. During severe flare-ups, he can barely move, and he misses work approximately five days per month because of his back pain.

ASSESSMENT

■ In an interview with Kenneth Hill, RN, regarding his pain, Mr. Grier rates his pain as a 7 on a scale of 0–10. Flare-ups usually last about a week before his pain is controlled to a 5. Mr. Grier describes his constant pain as a dull ache, but it throbs during flare-ups with sharp piercing sensations during movement. Nothing seems to relieve the pain except lying completely still, although the pain keeps him from falling asleep. He is currently taking ibuprofen as needed, which is usually 400 mg q4h. In the past, he has taken Vicodin, 5–10 mg q4–6h, with moderate success, although it gives him slight nausea and drowsiness.

■ Upon observation, Mr. Hill notes that Mr. Grier has no obvious external sources of pain, but he does have beads of sweat on his forehead. Mr. Hill also notices that Mr. Grier grimaces and holds his breath during movement, and his movements are very slow. A physical assessment indicates a pulse of 92bpm, respiratory rate of 20/min with shallow breaths, blood pressure of 130/84 mmHg, and temperature of 100.8°F.

DIAGNOSIS

- *Chronic Pain* related to lower back pain as evidenced by behavioral and sympathetic reactions and the client's report.
- *Impaired Physical Mobility* related to severe lower back pain as evidenced by slow movements and grimacing during movement.
- *Disturbed Sleep Pattern* related to lower back pain as evidenced by client's report.
- *Readiness for Enhanced Knowledge* about pain management.
- *Fear* about potential job loss.

(NANDA-I © 2012)

PLANNING

- After 3 days on the pain medication, the client will report a decrease in pain intensity from a 7 to a 3 or 4 on the numerical scale.
- The client will report increased physical mobility with no increase in pain intensity over baseline during movement.
- The client will demonstrate an understanding of good sleep hygiene and will report receiving adequate sleep.
- The client will demonstrate knowledge about nonpharmacologic methods of pain relief.
- The client will choose three methods of nonpharmacologic pain relief to implement.
- The client will report decreased pain as a result of nonpharmacologic therapies.
- The client will report a decrease in lost workdays as a result of lower back pain.

IMPLEMENTATION

- Consult with a physician about opioid and nonopioid analgesic therapies for Mr. Grier.
- Teach Mr. Grier the importance of taking pain medications around the clock.
- Teach Mr. Grier about nonpharmacologic interventions, including heat, distractions, acupuncture, massage, and mild exercise.

- Encourage Mr. Grier to talk about his pain, and validate his pain experience.
- Provide Mr. Grier with contact information for the pain clinic and encourage him to call the clinic if his prescribed therapies are ineffective.
- Encourage Mr. Grier to set regular follow up appointments to help manage his pain effectively over time.

EVALUATION

Four days after Mr. Grier's appointment, Mr. Hill calls Mr. Grier to assess his pain. Mr. Grier reports that he has been taking his pain medications as prescribed. He is applying heat to his back for 30 minutes three times a day, and he is performing strengthening exercises for his back. When the pain is most severe, he listens to music to help distract him from the pain. Mr. Grier reports that with this new therapy, his pain is now a 4 on a scale of 0–10.

One month after his appointment, Mr. Grier returns to the pain clinic for a follow up appointment. He reports that his pain has been a 2 or 3 for the past week, and he has missed only one day of work in the past month. He continues to take the nonopioid analgesics as instructed and performs strengthening exercises three times a week. His boss has noticed an increase in his work productivity. To maintain pain control without opioids, Mr. Hill recommends alternating acetaminophen and ibuprofen and adding a monthly back massage to Mr. Grier's therapeutic regimen.

CRITICAL THINKING

1. Mr. Grier asks you why he needs to continue the strengthening exercises and include back massages in his therapy. What do you tell him?
2. If Mr. Grier reports excessive nausea in response to his opioid medication, what suggestions will you give him to decrease his nausea and provide comfort?
3. How would you adapt this care plan to a client with knee pain instead of back pain?

Relating Concepts and Exemplars: Practical Applications

▌REVIEW The Concept of Comfort

RELATE Link the Concepts

Linking the concept of comfort with the concept of elimination:

1. How can you help clients with "embarrassing" symptoms such as bowel incontinence feel more comfortable talking about their condition?
2. Describe comfort measures for a client who requires catheterization for treatment of urinary retention.

Linking the concept of comfort with the concept of violence:

3. Explain the psychosocial considerations related to promoting comfort during the care and assessment of a rape victim.
4. When assessing a child who is believed to have been abused, what comfort measures can be used to reduce the child's anxiety and promote trust?

READY Go to Companion Skills Manual

REFER Go to Pearson Student Nursing Resources
nursing.pearsonhighered.com

- Additional review materials

REFLECT Case Study \\ Part 3

Ms. Daves has been visiting her primary care provider as recommended for follow up care. Six months after beginning treatment with milnacipran (Savella), Ms. Daves returns for a

regular checkup. As you review her chart, you note that Ms. Daves's physician confirmed the ED physician's diagnoses of fibromyalgia. Upon assessment, Ms. Daves's vital signs are normal, and her pain intensity is a 3 on a scale of 0–10. She also reports that she is sleeping better at night, although she occasionally experiences chronic pain even though the pain is manageable. When you ask how Savella is working for her, she says that it has helped her pain and stiffness but her mouth has been really dry since she started taking it and she sometimes has slight nausea.

Clinical Reasoning Questions Level I

1. What suggestions can you giv[e] her dry mouth and nausea?
2. What further assessment shou[ld] mine the cause of Ms. Daves's
3. Can you suggest other therapie[s] pain even further?

Clinical Reasoning Questions Lev[el II]

4. What nursing interventions ca[n] vent future flare-ups of Ms. Da[ves]
5. What information should you giv[e] (Savella) and drug–drug interact[ion]
6. What coping techniques wou[ld] she deals with fibromyalgia?

New! Each ***Concept*** section ends with a Review section that includes critical thinking questions that link concepts together, a list of additional resources, and Part 3 of the longitudinal case study.

▌REVIEW Acute and Chronic Pain

RELATE Link the Concepts and Exemplars

Linking the exemplar of acute and chronic pain with the concept of culture and diversity:

1. When you are caring for a client who appears to be in pain but denies it, how might understanding of the client's culture help you interpret the dichotomy between body language and reported pain?
2. How might interpretations and interventions for pain differ among cultures?

Linking the exemplar of acute and chronic pain with the concept of stress and coping:

3. What alterations in stress and coping would you anticipate when a client experiences chronic pain?
4. When caring for a mother with acute pain over the past few weeks, the client relates she has just not had the energy to deal with her children. How is pain impacting this mother's ability to cope with her children's needs?

READY Go to Companion Skills Manual

REFER Go to Pearson Student Nursing Resources
nursing.pearsonhighered.com

- Additional review material
- Chart: Printable pain management flow sheet
- Minimodule: Neonates and Pain

REFLECT Case Study

Mr. Backwater is a 48-year-old Cherokee Indian. His history includes nicotine abuse, lung cancer, arthritis in both knees, and headaches. Mr. Backwater has trouble breathing, especially after exertion. During a routine checkup, the nurse's assessment reveals that Mr. Backwater is experiencing severe pain in his right side when inhaling, and he has painful mouth sores as a result of his chemotherapy treatment. Between the chemotherapy and the mouth sores, Mr. Backwater is losing weight because of inadequate food intake.

1. What cultural influences do you need to consider when assessing Mr. Backwater's pain?
2. Should Mr. Backwater's history of nicotine abuse influence which pharmacologic agents are prescribed for his pain? Why or why not? How can you advocate for Mr. Backwater if inadequate pain medications are prescribed?
3. What cultural practices can you recommend as nonpharmacologic therapy for Mr. Backwater's pain?

Each ***Exemplar*** section ends with a similar Review section. Critical thinking questions link together concepts and exemplars. Case Studies provide practical nursing situations with critical thinking questions. Additional resources are also listed.

TO THE INSTRUCTOR

▶ INTRODUCTION

Nursing education is evolving. As the nursing profession has developed to encompass a variety of roles at all levels of society, including direct client care, advocacy, and leadership at the local, state, and national levels, nursing education is changing to help nursing students prepare to enter a more robust, demanding, and rewarding profession. Societal forces that have created the climate for transforming nursing education include, but are not limited to, the global economy, technological advances, and changes in healthcare delivery systems. Tried and true teaching methods now seem antiquated as faculty compete for students' attention with a variety of new and engaging sources of information and entertainment. In addition, the overwhelming discovery of new knowledge in the "information age" has resulted in nursing students feeling overwhelmed by the quantity of knowledge and skills they must gain in order to become practicing nurses.

University and college nursing programs across the United States have begun evaluating how their programs can meet the needs of today's nursing students. Many are moving to the model of concept-based learning in an effort to meet the challenges facing nursing students and nurses today. This model provides the impetus for educators to transition away from traditional methods of faculty-centered teaching and passive learning toward active, focused, participative, and collaborative teaching and learning. *Nursing: A Concept-Based Approach to Learning,* Second Edition, is designed to assist nursing faculty to provide students with a broader perspective while promoting a deeper understanding of content in a focused, participative, and collaborative learning environment.

▶ WHAT IS CONCEPT-BASED LEARNING?

Concept-based learning is a paradigm for learning that classifies essential content into categories that have common relevant features, reinforces those concepts by teaching exemplars, and then encourages learners to determine whether each concept does or does not apply to a given situation. The goal is to teach the concepts well enough that students can recognize them in any context. Concept-based learning is more student centered and student directed than traditional education models. Students are expected to delve into the content and learn how to access information independently. In concept-based learning, the instructor is more of a facilitator of learning than an expert imparting knowledge to students.

Using this approach involves drawing attention to conceptual lenses, that is, to concepts that force students to think at the integration level and relate topics to broader contexts. *Nursing: A Concept-Based Approach to Learning,* Second Edition, uses the individual client as a conceptual lens, focusing on human systems functioning and providing examples of common deviations from health across the life span, and then making links to how concepts are related and interrelated. Professional behavior and healthcare system concepts are interwoven with the human system concepts to guide care decisions and delivery systems for individuals, families, and communities.

With the conceptual lens of the individual client across the life span identified, essential concepts have been selected that reflect critical areas of nursing practice. These concepts are the "big ideas" that reflect different aspects of the conceptual lens. Generalizations, or central ideas of enduring understanding, are derived from the concepts and assist the learner to apply the concept. Generalizations coupled with learning outcomes clarify what students should be able to do when they complete the unit of instruction and help guide all other activities. Exemplars have been selected based on incidence, prevalence, or broad applicability to other concepts (see below). Topics, processes, and skills reflect content that is needed to complete the performance outcome. As a result, faculty and learners keep reflecting back on the "big ideas" and performance outcomes to increase understanding of the whole, and then the part, and then back to the whole again.

The benefit of concept-based learning is that organized and sequenced conceptual structures create stable and usable bodies of knowledge that promote independent and critical thinking. This in turn promotes the higher-order thinking necessary to meet the demands of our constantly changing world. As students become more actively engaged in learning rather than simply memorizing facts, they begin to see patterns and to use those patterns to think about the facts they learn. For example, when a student is involved in a clinical simulation centered around a child who has respiratory distress, the student has the opportunity to auscultate abnormal breath sounds, inspect the chest to see retractions and rapid breathing, observe the child with cyanosis, and see an oxygen saturation level that is below normal, while also thinking about developmental issues, the effects of stress, and the safety of the child. Through multiple ways of learning (e.g., clinical experience, discussion of case studies with peers), these patterns become a part of the student's learning repertoire, which is based on a full experience rather than memorization of facts. An added benefit of connecting essential facts to a broader context is that it helps learners retain information. The facts become more meaningful when students can relate them to their own lives and experiences. A concept-process approach also helps students make connections between other related subject areas. *A goal in this type of learning is to build a conceptual understanding of nursing that will be transferable to future knowledge and developments in a variety of related client-care situations.*

A concept-based approach also helps students develop critical thinking skills and integrate new knowledge with what they have already learned to attain a level of constructed knowledge. As learners progress to higher levels of knowing, then the higher level critical thinking/clinical reasoning skills can be added, including (1) assumptions about a healthcare situation that must be questioned, and (2) evidence utilization to determine the outcome including empirical data, expert opinions, professional standards, and personal experiences. Implications, the highest level of critical thinking/clinical reasoning skills, are best applied with real-world situations or simulations. This skill is related to the constructed, conceptual knowing level in which the learner integrates all aspects of the healthcare situation.

In summary, a conceptual approach to teaching provides nursing students with a deeper understanding of their field that is transferable to a broader spectrum of both current and future practice.

▶ BASIS FOR SELECTION OF CONCEPTS AND EXEMPLARS

Nursing: A Concept-Based Approach to Learning examines the professional requirements of nursing care through the lens of the human life span, and categorizes content into three domains: the individual domain, the nursing domain, and the healthcare domain. Within each of these domains, content is organized into modules, which include the concept and specific exemplars that contain relevant critical or essential content that illustrates the concept.

For the First Edition, faculty advisors from the state of North Carolina identified concepts and exemplars based on a number of national initiatives, feedback from clinical partners, and other considerations. Prior to developing the Second Edition, a Concepts Advisory Panel consisting of nursing faculty from throughout the country, representing both two- and four-year programs, was selected to guide the revision. They reviewed the First Edition text, studied feedback from faculty using the text as well as those representing programs not using the text, and identified workplace trends and national priorities to develop a new template and modify and select the concepts and exemplars for *Nursing: A Concept-Based Approach to Learning,* Second Edition.

Like its predecessor, this Second Edition takes into consideration the need for nurses to practice safe, effective care within today's healthcare environments, and the need for nursing students to be "floor ready" when they graduate. To that extent, concepts and exemplars included in this text have their basis in a number of national initiatives and identified priorities, including:

- Reports from the Institute of Medicine, including *Crossing the Quality Chasm: A New Health System for the 21st Century* (2001)

- *Healthy People 2020*
- Prevalence rates determined by the Centers for Disease Control and Prevention, the National Institutes of Health, the American Psychiatric Association, and other government and professional organizations
- Priorities, standards of practice, and codes of behavior established by the American Nurses Association, the National Council of State Boards of Nursing, the American Association of Colleges of Nursing, the National League for Nursing, and other professional nursing organizations
- Federal legislation that impacts healthcare providers and agencies, such as the Health Insurance Portability and Accountability Act, and federal agencies that administer federal regulations, such as the Centers for Medicare and Medicaid Services and the Occupational Safety and Health Administration
- QSEN and KSA competencies
- NCLEX-RN examination priorities
- Workplace expectations and requirements.

▶ ORGANIZATION OF MATERIAL

Nursing: A Concept-Based Approach to Learning, Second Edition, offers 51 concepts and their exemplars organized into modules.

Parts I, II, and III: The Individual Domain

All of the concepts related to the holistic individual, family, and community are presented in the modules in Parts I, II, and III, which encompass the Individual Domain. These modules address the biological, physical, cognitive, and psychosocial processes and their alterations that most frequently bring the individual into contact with the nursing and healthcare domains. Each concept within the individual domain addresses the impact of that concept on individuals across the life span, inclusive of cultural, gender, and developmental considerations. Part I includes the biological and physical concepts (e.g., Acid–Base Balance and Elimination). Part II includes the primarily psychosocial concepts (e.g., Family and Mood and Affect). Part III is devoted to the concept of Reproduction.

Part IV: The Nursing Domain

Part IV, the Nursing Domain, contains concepts related to competencies for graduates of nursing programs such as Assessment, Clinical Decision Making, Collaboration, and Professional Behaviors.

Part V: The Healthcare Domain

Part V, the Healthcare Domain, contains such IOM and QSEN competencies as Evidence-Based Practice, Informatics, and Safety, as well as additional elements essential to nursing, including Advocacy, Ethics, and Legal Issues.

▶ CONCLUSION

Written by nurses, and based on a strong foundation of adult learning, this concept-based curriculum provides a focal point to direct learning through concepts, examples of alterations via exemplars, faculty and student activities, and collaborative group exercises. In addition to input from the Concepts Advisory Panel and content written by nurses, academicians from across the United States provided peer reviews of the concepts and exemplars.

This curriculum provides many opportunities for student nurses to learn collaboratively through skill development, case studies and discussions, group examination of resources and technology, and student–faculty interactions. By working together, faculty and students will become partners in learning, promoting greater acquisition of knowledge and understanding, and greater skill development—all of which will produce the most successful, empathetic, informed, and skilled graduates of nursing programs.

TO THE STUDENT

▶ CONCEPT-BASED LEARNING

The practice of nursing occurs in complex environments. Nurses must be able to take the knowledge they have learned in school and in practice and transfer it to new situations. Nurses must become lifelong learners to stay current with new disorders, new treatments, and evidence-based practice. To help you achieve these goals, your school or instructor has chosen a new way to help you learn to be a nurse. You will be taking a concept-based approach to learning. Concept-based learning is a student-centered approach to learning. Students participate actively in the learning environment, assuming responsibility for their own knowledge as they learn to integrate concepts, apply information, and use clinical reasoning to provide client-centered care. So instead of memorizing 3,000 alterations to the body systems in a lecture-driven platform as is done in traditional programs, you are going to learn more in-depth knowledge of selected alterations, using critical thinking skills so that you will be able to transfer your knowledge to new situations and client presentations.

You will learn:

- 51 concepts that affect all ages (such as Oxygenation, Mobility, Communication, and Safety)
- 235 exemplars (that is, disorders or examples) of those concepts that cover the life span
- How to integrate your knowledge of the 51 concepts in order to provide care for clients of all ages
- How to learn on your own to evaluate and use evidence and to stay current with new standards so you can take excellent care of your clients.

▶ THE MODULES

Each of the 51 concepts is combined with its exemplars in a module. As examples, consider the modules on Oxygenation and Communication. See the section on Features starting on page vii for samples of these sections and features.

The Concept of Oxygenation

The beginning section of the module on Oxygenation is *The Concept of Oxygenation*, and in this section you will learn about

- *Normal Oxygenation*. What does normal oxygenation look like and sound like in a client? What are the genetic and lifespan considerations for normal oxygenation?

- *Alterations to Oxygenation* and how they manifest in clients such as a decreased level of oxygen in the blood (hypoxemia), breathing too fast (tachypnea), and shortness of breath (dyspnea).
- The relationship of oxygenation to other concepts in a feature called *Concepts Related to Oxygenation.* For example, if a client has altered oxygenation, she may also have altered Acid–Base Balance, altered Cognition, and altered Perfusion.
- *Prevention* of poor oxygenation in your clients.
- *Assessment* of oxygenation in a client including taking a history and performing a physical assessment.
- *Interventions and Therapies* used to help the client with altered oxygenation. These are divided into *Independent* therapies (those you can do on your own such as elevating the head of the client's bed to allow him to breathe more easily) and *Collaborative* (those that need orders from a physician, such as medication, or are performed by other members of the healthcare team, such as a respiratory therapist).

In addition, a three-part *Case Study* of a client with altered oxygenation helps you see how nursing care is provided.

The Oxygenation Exemplars

After you have learned about The Concept of Oxygenation, you'll move on to study the oxygenation *Exemplars.* There are five exemplars for Oxygenation: Acute Respiratory Distress Syndrome (ARDS), Asthma, Chronic Obstructive Pulmonary Disease (COPD), Respiratory Syncytial Virus (RSV)/Bronchiolitis, and Sudden Infant Death Syndrome (SIDS). These five exemplars were chosen for a variety of reasons:

- Some are very common (asthma, COPD) and you will likely see them often in practice.
- Some (ARDS, asthma, COPD) have been identified by national standards or organizations (e.g., the Institute of Medicine, *Healthy People 2020,* The Joint Commission) as priorities to be addressed.
- They cover the life span: Asthma is seen at all ages, SIDS occurs in infants, COPD is a disorder primarily seen in older adults, and RSV is seen in both infants/toddlers and older adults.
- Some are treated mostly in the doctor's office or at home (asthma), and others are treated almost exclusively in hospitals (ARDS).

Once you learn about these exemplars in detail, you will be able to apply that knowledge to care for clients with other disorders that include alterations in oxygenation.

The Concept of Communication

The Concept of Communication starts with a description of the communication process and then covers modes of communication (verbal, nonverbal, electronic, and written). The next topic is factors that influence the communication process such as development, gender, and sociocultural characteristics, including features to help you communicate with children, teens, and older adults. The next main topic is barriers to communication (such as being defensive), and the final section is on types of communicators (aggressive, passive, and assertive) with special emphasis on how to be an assertive communicator. Other features include the following.

- The *Concepts Related to Communication* feature shows how Communication is integrated with Oxygenation, Grief and Loss, Safety, and Advocacy.
- A *Nursing Process* section shows you how communication is an integral part of the nursing process.
- Two *Case Studies* help you see communication in action and prompt you to think about how you would communicate in those situations.

The Communication Exemplars

The module on Communication has four exemplars:

- *Groups and Group Communications* covers different types of groups, their functions, and how groups communicate with an emphasis on healthcare groups such as teams, task forces, and therapy groups.
- *Therapeutic Communication* covers therapeutic communication techniques (such as empathizing, attentive listening, and confronting), barriers to communication, the phases of and development of therapeutic relationships, and communicating with children and families.
- *Documentation* covers the purposes of documentation, various documentation methods and systems, the legal and ethical considerations in documentation, how to document nursing activities, facility-specific documentation, and general guidelines for recording.
- *Reporting* covers the topic of communicating specific information to a person or group of people including handoff communication, telephone reports, care plan conferences, and nursing rounds.

▶ INTEGRATING THE CONCEPTS

As mentioned above, the body works as a unified whole. A disturbance in one part of the body impacts the entire individual. That is, a client who has altered Oxygenation will most likely have additional alterations that impact care. For example, a client with chronic obstructive pulmonary disease (COPD) may have altered Cognition, because his brain is not getting enough oxygen. He may have issues with Safety because he is using supplemental oxygen (which is flammable) at home, and he still wants to smoke. He may have altered Fluids and Electrolytes because he is not drinking enough because his Mobility is limited

and he has trouble getting to the kitchen and does not want to have to get up too often to urinate. And his nurse may have difficulty with Communication because his Cognition is altered.

To help you integrate the concepts, the *Concepts Related to …* feature gives examples of other concepts that are often altered when the concept being studied is altered. The end of each concept and each exemplar has a *Review* section that contains sets of questions designed to help you think through the links that exist with other concepts and exemplars. These questions promote deep thinking, which you need for nursing practice. For example, in the review section for *The Concept of Oxygenation,* the linking questions are:

Linking the concept of oxygenation with the concept of infection:

1. Why would alterations in oxygenation lead to an increased risk of certain infections?
2. What are some ways to decrease the risk of infections that are caused by alterations in oxygenation?

Linking the concept of oxygenation with the concept of mobility:

3. How might alterations in oxygenation affect mobility?
4. What are some nursing interventions that can decrease the risk of altered mobility for clients with alterations in oxygenation?

Linking the concept of oxygenation with the concept of perfusion:

5. How are the concepts of oxygenation and perfusion related?
6. What disease processes related to oxygenation can affect the body's ability to perfuse adequately?

Linking the concept of oxygenation with the concept of cognition:

7. How might an alteration in oxygenation impact an individual's orientation?
8. How might lack of oxygenation to the brain be detected?

And in the *Review* section for the exemplar on *Therapeutic Communication* in the module on Communication, the linking questions are:

Linking the exemplar of therapeutic communication with the concept of advocacy:

1. How do strong therapeutic communication skills contribute to the nurse's role as a client advocate?
2. How do strong therapeutic communication skills contribute to the nurse's ability to work within groups to advocate for clients?

Linking the exemplar of therapeutic communication with the concept of teaching and learning:

3. The nurse is preparing to teach a client who is newly diagnosed with diabetes about self-care. Describe the three phases of the therapeutic relationship as it applies to the client teaching plan.
4. While teaching the client with diabetes, the nurse accidentally creates a barrier to the therapeutic relationship by misspeaking. What should the nurse do next?

And most important of all, your instructors will coach you in learning to integrate the concepts, and eventually, you will learn to do so on your own.

Even though the concepts in this book are integrated, you will learn them one at a time. The order in which you learn them may depend on the region where you live, your school's curriculum, and the clients you serve. If your instructor chooses to teach Oxygenation as your first concept, you would need to know a little bit about Acid–Base Balance, Cellular Regulation, Cognition, Comfort, Infection, Mobility, and Perfusion just to understand the Concepts Related to Oxygenation feature and to answer the linking questions in the Review section. You can do this in several ways:

■ Use the knowledge you already have. Think about the anatomy and physiology of the cardiovascular system to remember how Perfusion might affect Oxygenation. Think about the older adults in your life to consider how Mobility might affect Oxygenation.

■ You can read ahead: If you have a linking question about a concept you have not yet studied in class, read that module, or at least skim the Normal Presentation section to help you remember what you already know about the concept in question.

■ You should research the topics on your own and revisit the content often. The more exposure you have to the content, the deeper your learning will be.

We hope you enjoy *Nursing: A Concept-Based Approach to Learning,* Second Edition.

CONTENTS

Available online at nursing.pearsonhighered.com and within the interactive e-text:

Appendix B: Diagnostic Values and Laboratory Tests

Part I

Biophysical Modules

Part I consists of the biophysical modules within the individual domain. Each module presents a biophysical concept—such as oxygenation or perfusion—and selected alterations of that concept presented as exemplars. In the concept of oxygenation, for example, exemplars include asthma and chronic obstructive pulmonary disease. Each module addresses the impact of that concept and selected alterations on individuals across the life span, inclusive of cultural, gender, and developmental considerations.

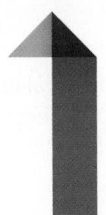

Acid–Base Balance

◨ THE CONCEPT OF ACID–BASE BALANCE

Acid–base balance is critical to homeostasis and optimal cellular function. To maintain acid–base balance, the hydrogen ion (H+) concentration of body fluids must be kept within a relatively narrow range. Hydrogen ions determine the relative acidity of body fluids. **Acids** release hydrogen ions in solution; **bases** (or **alkalis**) accept hydrogen ions in solution. The hydrogen ion concentration of a solution is measured as its **pH**. The relationship between hydrogen ion concentration and pH is inverse: As hydrogen ion concentration increases, the pH falls, and the solution becomes more acidic; as hydrogen ion concentration falls, the pH rises, and the

(continued on next page)

Concept Learning Outcomes

After reading about this concept, you will be able to:

1. Summarize the physiology of acid–base balance.
2. Examine the relationship between acid–base balance and other concepts/systems.
3. Identify commonly occurring alterations in acid–base balance and their related therapies.
4. Differentiate common assessment procedures used to examine acid–base balance across the life span.
5. Describe diagnostic and laboratory tests to determine the individual's acid–base balance status.
6. Explain management of acid–base balance and prevention of acid–base imbalance.
7. Demonstrate the nursing process in providing culturally competent and caring interventions across the life span for individuals with common alterations in acid–base balance.
8. Compare and contrast common independent and collaborative interventions for clients with alterations in acid–base balance.

Concept Key Terms

Acidosis, 4
Acids, 3
Alkalis, 3
Alkalosis, 4
Allen test, 10
Arterial blood gases (ABGs), 6
Base excess (BE), 6
Bases, 3

Buffers, 4
Hypercapnia, 6
Hypocapnia, 6
Hypoxemia, 6
$PaCO_2$, 6
PaO_2, 6
pH, 3
Serum bicarbonate, 6
Volatile acid, 4

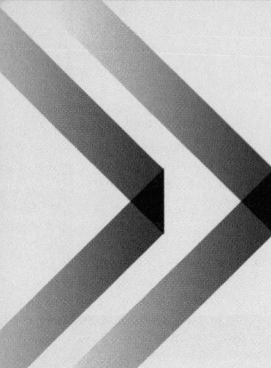

solution becomes more alkaline or basic. The normal pH of body fluids is slightly basic, ranging from 7.35 to 7.45. (A pH of 7 is neutral.) Normal pH indicates acid–base balance.

Acid–base imbalance results from any one of several underlying causes and can be an important clue in diagnosing illness or disease. Failure to restore acid–base balance can lead to impairment of organs and critical bodily functions. The body's tolerance for alterations in acid–base levels is very narrow; a pH below 7.00 or above 7.6 for even a short time can result in quick death. **<<**

▶ NORMAL ACID–BASE BALANCE

Metabolic processes in the body continuously produce acids, which fall into two categories: volatile acids and nonvolatile acids. A **volatile acid** can be eliminated from the body as a gas. Carbonic acid (H_2CO_3) is the only volatile acid produced in the body. It dissociates (separates) into carbon dioxide (CO_2) and water (H_2O); the lungs eliminate the carbon dioxide. All other acids produced in the body are *nonvolatile acids* that must be metabolized or excreted in fluid. Examples are lactic acid (resulting from cellular destruction), hydrochloric acid (found in stomach secretions), phosphoric acid (from the oxidation of phospholipids and phosphoproteins), and sulfuric acid (formed by oxidation of sulfur containing amino acids). Most acids and bases in the body are weak; that is, they neither release nor accept a significant number of hydrogen ions.

Despite the body's continuous acid production, three systems work together to maintain pH within a normal range: buffer systems, the respiratory system, and the renal system.

Physiology Review

BUFFER SYSTEMS   **Buffers** are substances that prevent major changes in pH by releasing hydrogen ions. When excess acid is present in body fluid, buffers bind with hydrogen ions to minimize the change in pH. If body fluids become too basic or alkaline, buffers release hydrogen ions, restoring the pH. Although buffers act within a fraction of a second, their capacity to maintain pH is limited. The body's major buffer systems are the bicarbonate–carbonic acid buffer system, the phosphate buffer system, and protein buffers.

The normal serum bicarbonate level is 24–28 mEq/L; that of carbonic acid is 1.2 mEq/L. Thus the ratio of bicarbonate (HCO_3) to carbonic acid (H_2CO_3) is 20:1. Although the amounts of bicarbonate and carbonic acid in the body vary somewhat, as long as this ratio is maintained, the pH remains within the 7.35–7.45 range (**Figure 1–1 ●**).

Bicarbonate (HCO_3) is a weak base; when an acid is added to the system, the hydrogen ion in the acid combines with bicarbonate and the pH changes only slightly. Carbonic acid (H_2CO_3) is a weak acid produced when carbon dioxide dissolves in water. When a base is added to the system, it combines with carbonic acid and the pH remains within the normal range.

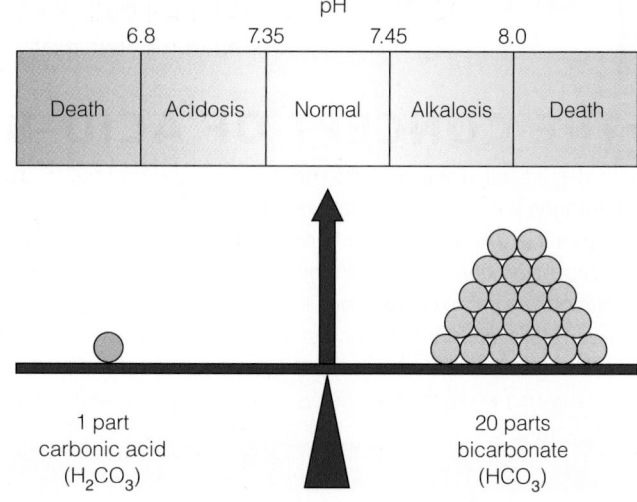

Figure 1–1 ● The normal ratio of bicarbonate to carbonic acid is 20:1. As long as this ratio is maintained, the pH remains within the normal range of 7.35–7.45.

Adding a strong acid to extracellular fluid (ECF) depletes bicarbonate, changing the 20:1 ratio and causing the pH to drop below 7.35. This is known as **acidosis**. Adding a strong base depletes carbonic acid as it combines with the base, again disrupting the 20:1 ratio. The pH rises above 7.45, a condition known as **alkalosis**.

RESPIRATORY SYSTEM   The respiratory system (and the brain's respiratory center) regulates carbonic acid by eliminating or retaining carbon dioxide. Carbon dioxide is a potential acid; when combined with water, it forms carbonic acid, a volatile acid. Acute increases in carbon dioxide or hydrogen ions in the blood stimulate the brain's respiratory center, increasing both the rate and depth of respiration. As a result, carbon dioxide is eliminated and carbonic acid levels fall, bringing the pH to a more normal range. Although this compensation for increased hydrogen ion concentration occurs within minutes, it becomes less effective over time. For example, clients with chronic lung disease (such as chronic obstructive pulmonary disease, COPD) may have consistently high carbon dioxide levels in their blood.

Alkalosis, by contrast, depresses the respiratory center, decreasing both the rate and depth of respiration and causing

Concepts Related to **Acid–Base Balance**

While the human body is made up of numerous systems that can be studied individually, no system is truly isolated. Instead, the function of one body system can greatly affect the function of one or more other body systems. For example, changes in acid–base balance can result in decreased tissue perfusion, leading to cardiac arrest. Acidosis or alkalosis may result in a decreasing level of consciousness, and clients with acute respiratory acidosis may also experience irritability and altered mental status. Chronic respiratory acidosis can manifest in impaired memory and/or personality changes. Metabolic acidosis resulting from fluid or electrolyte imbalance can be particularly dangerous, especially in the case of diabetic ketoacidosis (DKA). Some of the concepts related to acid–base balance are outlined below.

CONCEPT	RELATIONSHIP TO ACID–BASE BALANCE	NURSING IMPLICATIONS
Communication		
	Acid–base imbalances may impair communication.	■ Speak in terms clients can understand. ■ Let client know what is occurring. ■ Watch for nonverbal communication. ■ Demonstrate compassion.
Cognition		
	↓ O_2 can cause changes in cognition.	■ Maintain adequate oxygenation. ■ Monitor closely for change in level of consciousness (LOC). ■ LOC changes can lead to stupor and coma.
Fluids and Electrolytes		
■ Fluid and electrolyte imbalance	Metabolic results from another primary disorder	■ Focus treatment on primary disorder, reduce the effects of acidosis on cardiac function, and restore fluid levels in the body. ■ Administer intravenous (IV) bicarbonate as ordered. ■ Administer IV fluids with insulin to correct acidosis in clients with DKA. ■ Rapid administration of sodium bicarbonate leads to metabolic alkalosis and hypokalemia. ■ Monitor ABG values.
Perfusion		
	↓ tissue perfusion from shock, cardiac arrest	■ Administer oxygen therapy as ordered. ■ Correct underlying problem and improve tissue perfusion and restore life.
Oxygenation		
	Hypoventilation: ↓ respirations r/t reduced alveolar ventilation so the carbon dioxide pressures increase above normal.	■ Monitor respiration in all clients. ■ Monitor vital signs, pulse oximetry. ■ Give special attention when respirations are 12 breaths per minute or less. ■ Underlying cause will determine course of treatment. ■ Severe hypoventilation will require opioid antagonist (e.g., Naloxone). Monitor respiration in all clients.
	Hyperventilation: ↑ respirations r/t increased alveolar ventilation so the carbon dioxide pressures decrease above normal.	■ Monitor vital signs, pulse oximetry. ■ Underlying cause will determine course of treatment. ■ Calm client if cause is panic. ■ Speak in a slow, calm voice.

carbon dioxide retention. The retained carbon dioxide then combines with water to restore carbonic acid levels and bring the pH back within the normal range.

RENAL SYSTEM The renal system is responsible for the long-term regulation of acid–base balance. The kidneys normally eliminate the excess nonvolatile acids produced during metabolism. The kidneys also regulate bicarbonate levels in ECF by regenerating or reabsorbing bicarbonate ions in the renal tubules. Although the kidneys respond more slowly to changes in pH (over hours to days), they can generate bicarbonate and selectively excrete or retain hydrogen ions as needed. In acidosis, when excess hydrogen ions are present and the pH falls, the kidneys excrete hydrogen ions and retain bicarbonate. In alkalosis, the kidneys retain hydrogen ions and excrete bicarbonate to restore acid–base balance.

The **$PaCO_2$** measures the pressure exerted by dissolved carbon dioxide in the blood and reflects the respiratory component of acid–base regulation and balance because it is regulated by the lungs. The normal value is 35–45 mmHg. A $PaCO_2$ of less than 35 mmHg is known as **hypocapnia**; a $PaCO_2$ greater than 45 mmHg is known as **hypercapnia.**

The abbreviations $PaCO_2$ and PaO_2 are used interchangeably with pCO_2 and pO_2. The *P* stands for partial pressure: the pressure exerted by the gas dissolved in the blood. The *a* indicates that the sample is arterial blood. Because these measurements are rarely done on venous or capillary blood, the *a* is often deleted from the abbreviation.

The **PaO_2** is a measure of the pressure exerted by oxygen that is dissolved in the plasma. Only about 3% of oxygen in the blood is transported in solution; most is combined with hemoglobin. However, it is the dissolved oxygen that is available to the cells for metabolism. As dissolved oxygen diffuses out of plasma into the tissues, more is released from hemoglobin. The normal value for PaO_2 is 75–100 mmHg. A PaO_2 of less than 80 mmHg indicates **hypoxemia**. The PaO_2 is valuable for evaluating respiratory function, but it is not used as a primary measurement in determining acid–base status. The **serum bicarbonate** (HCO_3) reflects the renal regulation of acid–base balance. The normal HCO_3 value is 24–28 mEq/L.

The **base excess (BE)** is a calculated value also known as *buffer base capacity*. The BE measures substances that can accept or combine with hydrogen ions. It reflects the degree of acid–base imbalance by indicating the status of the body's total buffering capacity. It represents the amount of acid or base that must be added to a blood sample to achieve a pH of 7.4 and is essentially a measure of increased or decreased bicarbonate. The normal value for BE for arterial blood is +2 to −2 mEq/L.

Acid–base balance is assessed primarily by measuring **arterial blood gases (ABGs)**. Arterial blood is most often used because it reflects acid–base balance throughout the entire body better than venous or capillary blood that has dispersed oxygen into the tissues and has collected carbon dioxide. However, venous blood gases are occasionally ordered when frequent ABGs have resulted in damage to normal arterial gas sampling sites. Arterial blood also provides information about the effectiveness of the lungs in oxygenating blood.

✳ Go to **nursing.pearsonhighered.com** to see Appendix B for information on normal and abnormal values and on how to evaluate ABG measurements.

▶ ALTERATIONS TO ACID–BASE BALANCE

Acid–base imbalances fall into two major categories: acidosis and alkalosis. As noted previously, acidosis occurs when the hydrogen ion concentration increases above normal (pH below 7.35). Alkalosis occurs when the hydrogen ion concentration falls below normal (pH above 7.45). It is important to remember that alterations in acid–base balance affect other concepts/body systems. See "Concepts Related to Acid–Base Balance" for examples.

Alterations and Manifestations

Acid–base imbalances are further classified as *metabolic* or *respiratory* disorders. In metabolic disorders, the primary change is in the concentration of bicarbonate. In *metabolic acidosis*, the amount of bicarbonate decreases in relation to the amount of acid in the body (**Figure 1–2A ●**). This condition can develop from abnormal bicarbonate losses or from excess nonvolatile acids in the body. The pH falls below 7.35, and the bicarbonate concentration is less than 24 mEq/L. *Metabolic alkalosis*, by contrast, occurs when there is an excess of bicarbonate in relation to the amount of hydrogen ion (Figure 1–2B). The pH is above 7.45, and the bicarbonate concentration is greater than 28 mEq/L.

In respiratory disorders, the primary change is in the concentration of carbonic acid. *Respiratory acidosis* occurs when carbon dioxide is retained, increasing the amount of carbonic acid in the body (**Figure 1–3A ●**). As a result, the pH falls to less than 7.35, and the $PaCO_2$ is greater than 45 mmHg. When too much carbon dioxide is lost, carbonic acid levels fall and *respiratory alkalosis* develops (Figure 1–3B). The pH rises to above 7.45, and the $PaCO_2$ is less than 35 mmHg. It is important to remember that any condition that causes hypoventilation may result in respiratory acidosis and hypoxemia, while any condition that causes hyperventilation often results in respiratory alkalosis.

Acid–base disorders are further defined as *primary* (simple) and *mixed*. Primary disorders usually have one cause. For example, respiratory failure often causes respiratory acidosis due to retained carbon dioxide; renal failure usually causes metabolic acidosis due to retained hydrogen ion and impaired bicarbonate production. **Table 1–1 ●** summarizes primary acid–base imbalances with the common causes of each. Mixed disorders occur from combinations of respiratory and metabolic disturbances. For example, a client in cardiac arrest develops a mixed respiratory and metabolic acidosis due to lack of ventilation (and retained CO_2) and hypoxia of body tissues that leads to anaerobic metabolism and acid by-products (excess nonvolatile acids).

Compensation

With primary acid–base disorders, compensatory changes in other parts of the regulatory system occur to restore a normal

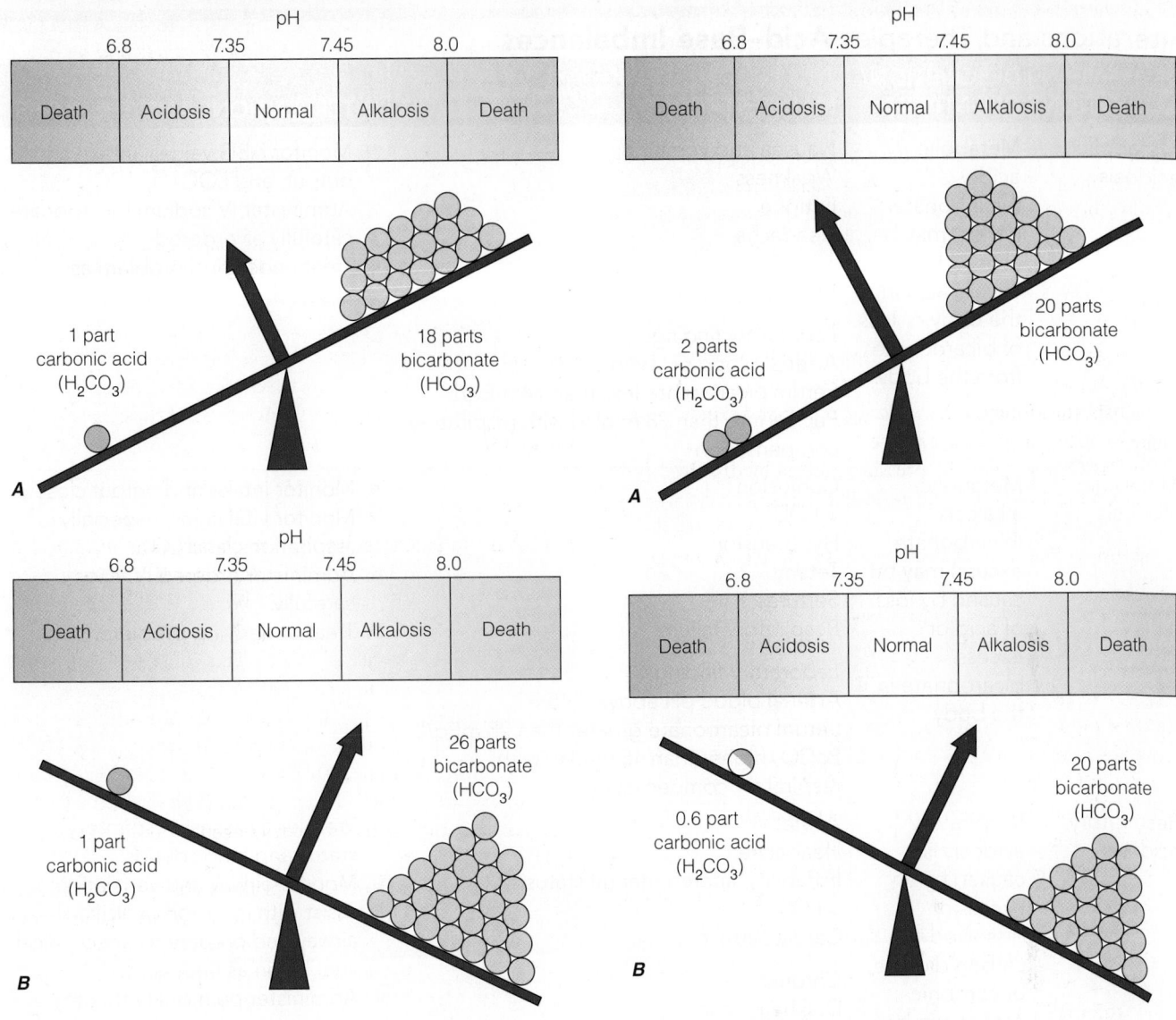

Figure 1–2 ● Metabolic acid–base imbalances. *A*, Metabolic acidosis. *B*, Metabolic alkalosis.

Figure 1–3 ● Respiratory acid–base imbalances. *A*, Respiratory acidosis. *B*, Respiratory alkalosis.

pH and homeostasis. In metabolic acid–base disorders, the change in pH affects the rate and depth of respirations, which, in turn, affect carbon dioxide elimination and the $PaCO_2$ and helps restore the ratio of carbonic acid to bicarbonate. The kidneys compensate for simple respiratory imbalances. The change in pH affects both bicarbonate conservation and hydrogen ion elimination (**Table 1–2** ●).

Compensatory changes in respirations occur within minutes of a change in pH. These changes, however, become less effective over time. The renal response takes longer to restore the pH, but it is a more effective long-term mechanism. If the pH is restored to within normal limits, the disorder is said to be *fully compensated*. When these changes are reflected in ABG values but the pH remains outside normal limits, the disorder is said to be *partially compensated*.

Risk Factors

Acid–base imbalances occur in critically ill clients. There are many underlying causes of these disturbances. Each acid–base

disorder is treated separately, with the underlying cause considered in the critically ill clients. Particular issues of which nurses should be aware include the following:

- Metabolic acidosis occurs in clients with insulin-dependent diabetes mellitus and chronic renal failure. Metabolic acidosis from severe diarrhea can occur at any age, but children and older adults are at greatest risk.

- Metabolic alkalosis occurs in clients in acute care. Older adults are at risk because of their fragile fluid and electrolyte status.

- Clients of all ages are at risk for respiratory acidosis when alveolar hypoventilation occurs. Clients with COPD are at the highest risk for chronic respiratory acidosis.

- Older adults and young children are at risk for respiratory alkalosis with large-dose salicylate ingestion. Respiratory alkalosis is often misidentified in the older adult because its early symptoms, hyperventilation and altered mental status, are attributed to other disease processes.

Alterations and Therapies **Acid–Base Imbalances**

ALTERATION	DESCRIPTION/ DEFINITION	MANIFESTATIONS	INTERVENTIONS AND THERAPIES
Metabolic acidosis	Metabolic acidosis (bicarbonate deficit) may be caused by excess acid in the body or loss of bicarbonate from the body.	Nausea and vomiting Weakness Fatigue Headache ↓ LOC Hyperventilation *Laboratory findings:* Arterial blood pH below 7.35 Serum bicarbonate less than 24 mEq/L $PaCO_2$ less than 38 mmHg with respiratory compensation	▪ Monitor ABG values, intake and output, and LOC. ▪ Administer IV sodium bicarbonate carefully as ordered. ▪ Treat underlying problem as ordered.
Metabolic alkalosis	Metabolic alkalosis (bicarbonate excess) may be caused by loss of acid or excess bicarbonate in the body.	Confusion ↓ LOC Hypotension Tetany Seizures Respiratory failure *Laboratory findings:* Arterial blood pH above 7.45 Serum bicarbonate greater than 28 mEq/L $PaCO_2$ higher than 45 mmHg with respiratory compensation	▪ Monitor intake and output closely. ▪ Monitor vital signs, especially respirations, and LOC. ▪ Administer ordered IV fluids carefully. ▪ Treat underlying problem.
Respiratory acidosis	Respiratory acidosis is caused by an excess of dissolved carbon dioxide, or carbonic acid; it can be acute or chronic.	*Acute:* Headache Irritability, altered mental status ↓ LOC Cardiac arrest *Chronic:* Dull headache Impaired memory Personality changes Weakness *Laboratory findings:* Arterial blood pH less than 7.35 $PaCO_2$ above 45 mmHg HCO_3 normal or slightly elevated in acute; above 28 mEq/L in chronic	▪ Frequently assess respiratory status and lung sounds. ▪ Monitor airway and ventilation; assist with insertion of artificial airway and prepare for mechanical ventilation as necessary. ▪ Administer pulmonary therapy measures such as inhalation therapy, percussion and postural drainage, bronchodilators, and antibiotics as ordered. ▪ Monitor fluid intake and output, vital signs, and ABGs. ▪ Administer narcotic antagonists as indicated. ▪ Maintain adequate hydration (2–3 L of fluid per day unless contraindicated by other health conditions).
Respiratory alkalosis	Respiratory alkalosis is caused by hyper-ventilation, leading to a carbon dioxide deficit.	Hyperventilation Dizziness Palpitations Anxiety–panic Tetany ↓ LOC *Laboratory findings (in uncompensated respiratory alkalosis):* Arterial blood pH above 7.45 $PaCO_2$ less than 35 mmHg	▪ Monitor vital signs and ABGs. ▪ Teach client to breathe more slowly. ▪ Reduce stimuli in environment and speak in calm, quiet voice.

TABLE 1–1 Common Causes of Primary Acid–Base Imbalances

IMBALANCE	COMMON CAUSES
Metabolic acidosis pH < 7.35 HCO_3 < 24 mEq/L Critical values pH < 7.20 HCO_3 < 10 mEq/L	↑ Acid production ■ Lactic acidosis ■ Ketoacidosis related to diabetes, starvation, or alcoholism ■ Salicylate toxicity ↓ Acid excretion ■ Renal failure ↑ Bicarbonate loss ■ Diarrhea, ileostomy drainage, intestinal fistula ■ Biliary or pancreatic fistulas ↑ Chloride ■ Sodium chloride IV solutions ■ Renal tubular acidosis ■ Carbonic anhydrase inhibitors
Metabolic alkalosis pH > 7.45 HCO_3 > 28 mEq/L Critical values pH > 7.60 HCO_3 > 40 mEq/L	↑ Acid loss or excretion ■ Vomiting, gastric suction ■ Hypokalemia ↑ Bicarbonate ■ Alkali ingestion (bicarbonate of soda) ■ Excess bicarbonate administration
Respiratory acidosis pH < 7.35 $PaCO_2$ > 45 mmHg Critical values pH < 7.20 $PaCO_2$ > 77 mmHg	Acute respiratory acidosis ■ Acute respiratory conditions (pulmonary edema, pneumonia, acute asthma) ■ Opiate overdose ■ Foreign body aspiration ■ Chest trauma Chronic respiratory acidosis ■ Chronic respiratory conditions (COPD, cystic fibrosis) ■ Multiple sclerosis, other neuromuscular diseases ■ Stroke
Respiratory alkalosis pH > 7.45 $PaCO_2$ < 35 mmHg Critical values pH > 7.60 $PaCO_2$ < 20 mmHg	■ Anxiety-induced hyperventilation (e.g., anxiety) ■ Fever ■ Early salicylate intoxication ■ Hyperventilation with mechanical ventilator

CASE STUDY \\ A

Jay James is a 24-year-old male who was rock climbing with his friends at a national park 25 miles from the nearest hospital when he suddenly lost his footing and slid 20 feet to the ground. Mr. James was alert and oriented when his friends reached him, and he could move all extremities quite easily. He had multiple scrapes over his anterior chest and a large gash over his left thigh (near the groin), which was bleeding profusely. His friends made a makeshift tourniquet, which slowed the bleeding. They immediately contacted the park ranger, who secured a helicopter to evacuate Mr. James to the nearest hospital.

Two large-bore IVs were placed in each arm in-flight, and normal saline was administered. The flight medic placed a 100% nonrebreathing mask on Mr. James. Mr. James became disoriented and confused during the flight. Mr. James arrived in the emergency department (ED) in 45 minutes after the fall.

On arrival in the ED, Mr. James is lethargic but responsive to painful stimuli. He has multiple abrasions over his chin and neck. His pulse oximetry is 99% on the nonrebreather mask, so the ED team replaces the mask with a nasal cannula at 4 L/m. A repeat pulse oximeter reads 95% saturation.

Vital signs are as follows: HR 130 bpm, BP 100/60 mmHg, R 30/min, and T_O 99.1°F. Skin is cool and clammy, nail beds are pale, and mucous

TABLE 1–2 Compensation for Simple Acid–Base Imbalances

PRIMARY DISORDER	CAUSE	COMPENSATION	EFFECT ON ABGs
Metabolic acidosis	Excess nonvolatile acids; bicarbonate deficiency	Rate and depth of respirations increase, eliminating additional CO_2.	↓ pH ↓ HCO_3 ↓ $PaCO_2$
Metabolic alkalosis	Bicarbonate excess	Rate and depth of respirations decrease; CO_2 is retained.	↑ pH ↑ HCO_3 ↑ $PaCO_2$
Respiratory acidosis	Retained CO_2 and excess carbonic acid	Kidneys conserve bicarbonate to restore carbonic acid:bicarbonate ratio of 1:20.	↓ pH ↑ $PaCO_2$ ↑ HCO_3
Respiratory alkalosis	Loss of CO_2 and deficient carbonic acid	Kidneys excrete bicarbonate and conserve H^+ to restore carbonic acid:bicarbonate ratio.	↑ pH ↓ $PaCO_2$ ↓ HCO_3

membranes are dry. All pulses are palpable but weak and thready. Lungs are clear, heart sounds regular. Output via urinary catheter for the last hour is 20 mL.

Clinical Reasoning Questions Level I

1. What is the most likely cause of Mr. James's high heart rate and low blood pressure?
2. If you were the nurse assigned to Mr. James, what would be your primary concerns at this time?

Clinical Reasoning Questions Level II

3. What is the priority nursing diagnosis for Mr. James at this time?
4. Why is Mr. James exhibiting confusion and disorientation?
5. What diagnostic tests would you expect to be ordered for Mr. James?

▶ ASSESSMENT

Nursing Assessment

Focused assessment data related to acid–base imbalances include the following:

- **Health history.** Acid–base balance is a function of the chemical and physiological components of the body. A complete health history is necessary to determine the underlying acid–base imbalance. Each specific disorder has different symptoms. It is important to identify the prescribed and over-the-counter medications that the client is currently

taking, as well as any complementary therapies, such as vitamins and herbal supplements.

- **Physical assessment.** Vital signs are taken, including pulse oximetry. It is important to correlate the results of the pulse oximeter with ABG results.

Lifespan and Cultural Considerations

Infants, children, and older adults are at risk for acid–base disorders related to fluid and electrolyte imbalances. See the Lifespan Considerations box below. Considerations particular to pregnant women are discussed in the module on Reproduction.

Diagnostic Tests

Arterial blood gases evaluate the client's acid–base balance and oxygenation. The examiner must perform an **Allen test** before drawing arterial blood gases. An Allen test is a measurement of radial or ulnar patency; the examiner digitally compresses either the radial or the ulnar artery after the client has forced the blood out of the hand by clenching it into a fist. Failure of the blood to diffuse into the hand when it is opened indicates occlusion of whichever artery was not compressed (Stedman, 2011). In such a case, the circulation is inadequate and no ABG is drawn. Blood gases may be drawn by respiratory therapists, healthcare providers, or nurses with specialized skills (intensive-care-trained). Because blood is drawn from a high-pressure artery, it is important to apply pressure to the puncture site for 10 minutes (more than 10–15

Lifespan Considerations Acid–Base Imbalance

Infants and Children
- Infants and children are at high risk for fluid and electrolyte imbalance because of their immature kidneys, which cannot concentrate urine.
- Infants have rapid respiratory rates, which can lead to insensible losses, and they cannot actively seek fluid.

Older Adults
- Older adults are at high risk for fluid and electrolyte imbalance because of the decreased ability of their kidneys to concentrate urine, their decreased thirst sensation, and decreased levels of intracellular fluid.
- Older adults have more comorbidities, such as hypertension, heart disease, renal impairment, and dementia. All of these conditions contribute to electrolyte imbalance.

Box 1–1   Interpreting ABGs

1. Look at the pH.
   - pH < 7.35 = acidosis
   - pH > 7.45 = alkalosis
2. Look at the $PaCO_2$.
   - $PaCO_2$ < 35 mmHg = hypocapnia; more carbon dioxide is being exhaled than normal.
   - $PaCO_2$ > 45 mmHg = hypercapnia; carbon dioxide is being retained.
3. Evaluate the pH–$PaCO_2$ relationship for a possible respiratory problem.
   - If the pH is < 7.35 (acidosis) and the $PaCO_2$ is > 45 mmHg (hypercapnia), retained carbon dioxide is causing increased H^+ concentration and respiratory acidosis.
   - If the pH is > 7.45 (alkalosis) and the $PaCO_2$ is < 35 mmHg (hypocapnia), low carbon dioxide levels and decreased H^+ concentration are causing respiratory alkalosis.
4. Look at the bicarbonate.
   - If the HCO_3 is < 24 mEq/L, bicarbonate levels are lower than normal.
   - If the HCO_3 is > 28 mEq/L, bicarbonate levels are higher than normal.
5. Evaluate the pH, HCO_3 and BE for a possible metabolic problem.
   - If the pH is < 7.35, the HCO_3 is < 24 mEq/L, and the BE is < −2 mEq/L, then low bicarbonate levels and high H^+ concentrations are causing metabolic acidosis.
   - If the pH is > 7.45, the HCO_3 is > 28 mEq/L, and the BE is > +2 mEq/L, then high bicarbonate levels are causing metabolic alkalosis.
6. Look for compensation.
   - Renal compensation
     a. In respiratory acidosis (pH < 7.35, $PaCO_2$ > 45 mmHg), the kidneys retain HCO_3 to buffer the excess acid, so the HCO_3 is > 28 mEq/L.
     b. In respiratory alkalosis (pH > 7.45, $PaCO_2$ < 35 mmHg), the kidneys excrete HCO_3 to minimize the alkalosis, so the HCO_3 is < 24 mEq/L.
   - Respiratory compensation
     a. In metabolic acidosis (pH < 7.35, HCO_3 < 24 mEq/L), the rate and depth of respirations increase, increasing carbon dioxide elimination, so the $PaCO_2$ is < 35 mmHg.
     b. In metabolic alkalosis (pH > 7.45, HCO_3 > 28 mEq/L), respirations slow and carbon dioxide is retained, so the $PaCO_2$ is > 45 mmHg.
7. Evaluate oxygenation.
   - PaO_2 < 75 mmHg = hypoxemia; possible hypoventilation.
   - PaO_2 > 100 mmHg = hyperventilation.

minutes if the client is receiving anticoagulant therapy) after the procedure to reduce the risk of bleeding or bruising. A systematic approach is important in the analysis of ABG results. First, evaluate each individual measurement; then analyze the interrelationships to determine the client's acid–base status (**Box 1–1 ●**).

CASE STUDY \\ B

Anna Zemakis is a 49-year-old female admitted to the hospital with severe vomiting and muscle weakness. She fell two weeks ago and reports not feeling well since. Four days ago, she developed abdominal discomfort with vomiting. The vomiting has been severe, and she has not been able to eat or drink very much. She says she has lost a significant amount of weight. She has felt very weak, anorexic, and lethargic. She has not had diarrhea or urinary symptoms. There is no significant past medical history, and she reports she is not on any prescribed medications or taking anything "over-the-counter."

Ms. Zemakis's vital signs are as follows: HR 84 bpm, BP 90/58 mmHg (sitting), BP 110/60 mmHg (lying), R 18/min, T_O 98.9°F, and pulse oximetry 98% on room air. Her lungs are clear, and her heart sounds normal. You observe she has dry mucous membranes. Initial examination reveals slight abdominal tenderness.

Clinical Reasoning Questions Level I

1. What is Ms. Zemakis's primary health problem?
2. As the nurse assigned to Ms. Zemakis, what are your concerns at this time?

Clinical Reasoning Questions Level II

3. What nursing diagnoses are appropriate for Ms. Zemakis at this time? Which takes priority?

4. What therapies would assist Ms. Zemakis in returning to homeostasis?
5. Referring to the module on Perfusion, what is the significance of the different blood pressure readings in different positions?

▶ INTERVENTIONS AND THERAPIES

The goal of treatment is to restore or maintain normal body balance. Treatment of acid–base imbalance depends on identification and treatment of the underlying cause; collaborative care for an acid–base imbalance also depends on identification of the underlying cause. When taking the client's health history, consider conditions potentially related to culture and developmental stages.

Independent

Interventions related to acid–base management may include the following:

- Daily weight
- Monitoring of intake and output
- Assessing respiratory and renal function
- Maintaining a patent airway
- Monitoring oxygen saturation
- Taking vital signs
- Assessing level of consciousness and neurological function
- Prompt reporting of changes in client condition

Collaborative

The nurse approaches acid–base imbalances by taking vital signs and taking a thorough client history, which includes risk factors, cardiac, renal, pulmonary, current medications, medical conditions, and symptoms. For clients in severe distress, family members may need to be consulted for critical information, including recent eating habits and history of vomiting. There is ongoing collaboration with the healthcare team for all clients.

PHARMACOLOGIC THERAPIES Specific pharmacologic therapies are available to treat acidosis and alkalosis. Careful monitoring of ABG levels prevents overtreatment that causes pH to alter in the opposite direction, changing alkalosis to acidosis or acidosis to alkalosis.

In clients with acidosis, the therapeutic goal is to reverse the effects of excess acids in the blood and return the client to normal pH levels as quickly as possible. The pharmacologic treatment of choice for acute acidosis is sodium bicarbonate infusions, provided that the bicarbonate level is low. The bicarbonate ion acts quickly as a base to neutralize acids in the blood and other body fluids. Carefully monitor the client's ABGs during infusions and watch for signs of alkalosis; this drug can "overcorrect" the acidosis, causing blood pH to turn alkaline. Symptoms of alkalosis include irritability, confusion, cyanosis, slow respirations, irregular pulse, and muscle weakness. If these symptoms occur, withhold the medication and notify the healthcare provider.

The nurse's role in sodium bicarbonate therapy involves carefully monitoring a client's condition and educating the client and family about the prescribed treatment. Sodium bicarbonate is given to neutralize acidotic states; so first analyze the ABG reports of pH, carbon dioxide levels ($PaCO_2$), bicarbonate levels (HCO_3), and oxygenation status (PaO_2 and O_2 saturation). Assess the client for symptoms associated with acidosis, such as sleepiness, coma, disorientation, dizziness, headache, seizures, and hypoventilation. Also assess the client for causative factors that could produce acidosis, such as diabetes mellitus, shock, and diarrhea. Successful management of the underlying disease condition frequently corrects acidosis.

Several contraindications and precautions are related to the administration of sodium bicarbonate. Because of the sodium content of this drug, use it judiciously in clients with cardiac disease and renal impairment.

Sodium bicarbonate is also used to alkalinize the urine and speed the excretion of acidic substances. This process is useful in treating overdoses of certain acidic medications such as aspirin and phenobarbital and is useful as adjunctive therapy for certain chemotherapeutic drugs such as methotrexate. Sodium bicarbonate is also used in chronic renal failure to neutralize the metabolic acidosis that occurs when the kidneys cannot excrete hydrogen ion. Intravenous (IV) sodium bicarbonate causes the urine to become more alkaline. Less acid is reabsorbed in the renal tubules, so more acid and acidic medicine is excreted. This process is known as *ion trapping*. Monitor the client's acid–base status closely and report symptoms of imbalance. Provide care directed toward supporting critical body functions such as cardiovascular, respiratory, and neurological status, which may be impaired secondary to the drug overdose.

Sodium bicarbonate (baking soda) is used as a home remedy to neutralize gastric acid, relieving heartburn and sour stomach. Although occasional use is acceptable, nurses should be aware that clients may misinterpret cardiac symptoms as

Client Teaching Sodium Bicarbonate

Include the following points when teaching clients and their families about sodium bicarbonate:

- Immediately contact the primary healthcare provider if gastric discomfort continues or is accompanied by chest pain, dyspnea, or diaphoresis.
- Use nonsodium antacids to prevent the absorption of excess sodium or bicarbonate into the systemic circulation.
- Do not use any antacid, including sodium bicarbonate, for longer than 2 weeks without consulting your healthcare provider.

heartburn, and overuse of sodium bicarbonate may lead to systemic alkalosis.

Client education as it relates to sodium bicarbonate should include the goals of therapy, the reasons for obtaining baseline data such as vital signs and electrolyte levels, and possible drug side effects.

AIRWAY MANAGEMENT Clients experiencing respiratory distress may require intubation. Although there is no specific rule for when to intubate, generally intubation is indicated if the client has a $PaCO_2$ greater than 77 mmHg, PaO_2 less than 60 mmHg, and a pH less than 7.20. Clients with chronic hypercarbia require care to correct their status slowly, as correcting $PaCO_2$ too quickly may result in metabolic alkalosis due to excessive retention of bicarbonate. Clients who are hypoxemic may also require supplemental oxygen, which has been shown to improve outcomes and reduce mortality rates (Feller-Kopman & Schwartzstein, 2012). Mechanical ventilation and oxygen administration are discussed in detail in the concept of Oxygenation.

CASE STUDY \\ C

John Quinland is a 60-year-old male with a 45-year history of smoking two packs of cigarettes a day. Over the past year, he has become increasingly short of breath. At first, he noticed this only when exercising, but now he is short of breath even at rest. Over the past year, he has had several infections of the lower respiratory tract that were treated successfully with antibiotics at the local emergency department. His shortness of breath has not subsided, and he uses his accessory muscles of respiration to assist him in breathing. Mr. Quinland does not have a primary care provider and does not get physical examinations. He had his last physical over 20 years ago to meet a work requirement. Mr. Quinland goes to the nearest hospital when he has a respiratory infection. The ED physician advises Mr. Quinland to find a healthcare provider because he needs routine checkups. But Mr. Quinland does not take the advice.

Clinical Reasoning Questions Level I

1. If you were the nurse taking Mr. Quinland's health history during his latest trip to the emergency department, what would be your primary concerns?

2. What nursing diagnoses are appropriate for Mr. Quinland at this time?

3. Is Mr. Quinland's smoking the priority consideration at this time? Why or why not?

Clinical Reasoning Questions Level II

4. Refer to the exemplar on COPD in the module on Oxygenation. What signs/symptoms of COPD does Mr. Quinland exhibit? What risk factors does he have?

5. Refer to the exemplar on Nicotine Use in the module on Addiction. Why/how does smoking result in alterations such as chronic hypercapnia and COPD?

6. What client teaching would you attempt to provide Mr. Quinland prior to discharge?

REVIEW The Concept of Acid–Base Balance

RELATE Link the Concepts

Linking the concept of acid–base balance with the concept of oxygenation:

1. What oxygenation changes are seen in clients with acidosis and alkalosis?

2. Why does hypoventilation decrease oxygenation? Why does hyperventilation increase oxygenation?

Linking the concept of acid–base balance with the concept of communication:

3. How might an acid–base imbalance impair a client's ability to communicate?

4. Give some examples of therapeutic communication techniques to use when addressing concerns of clients whose communication is limited due to severity of illness?

Linking the concept of acid–base balance with the concept of safety:

5. It is always important to guard against medication errors. In particular, why would this be important in caring for a client with acid–base imbalance?

6. In what situations or for what clients might it be necessary to arrange for a home safety assessment prior to discharge?

READY Go to Companion Skills Manual

REFER Go to Pearson Nursing Student Resources

nursing.pearsonhighered.com

- Additional review materials

REFLECT Case Study \\ D

Maria Hernandez is an 80-year-old female (weight 40 kg) who is admitted to the intensive care unit following a motor vehi-cle collision. She was driving and wearing her seat belt when she ran her car off the road and hit a tree. She remembers the collision and did not lose consciousness. Her injuries include a left anterior flail segment of the lung, a fractured left shoulder, and facial bruising. She is hemodynamically stable but has respiratory distress with paradoxical movement of her left anterior chest wall. She has no head or neck injury. Recently she has had several unexplained blackouts. She takes a beta blocker daily for hypertension.

She was intubated and ventilated in the ED because of respiratory distress. Initial ventilation was tidal volume 700 mLs at a rate of 12 breaths with 100% oxygen. Peripheral perfusion was good. An intravenous infusion of lactated Ringer solution was started at 100 ml per hour. Arterial blood gases were obtained half an hour later.

At this time, Ms. Hernandez's vital signs are T_O 98.8°F, HR 110 bpm, BP 120/60 mmHg, R 16/min, and pulse oximeter 99% on 100% oxygen. Her ABG values are pH 7.55, pCO_2 25 mmHg, pO_2 50 mmHg, HCO_3 21 mEq/L.

Clinical Reasoning Questions Level I

1. What is Ms. Hernandez's primary problem?

2. What is the cause of her respiratory distress?

3. What do her ABG results indicate?

Clinical Reasoning Questions Level II

4. Refer to the concept of Oxygenation. What will you need to monitor Ms. Hernandez for while she is intubated?

5. Refer to the concept of Oxygenation. How will you help Ms. Hernandez communicate while she is intubated?

6. Refer to the concept of Legal Issues. Ms. Hernandez's nephew calls to inquire about her condition? What regulations or policies apply when another individual calls seeking information about a client. How do you respond to the nephew?

EXEMPLAR 1.1 Metabolic Acidosis

EXEMPLAR KEY TERMS

Kussmaul respirations, 15
Metabolic acidosis, 14

EXEMPLAR LEARNING OUTCOMES

After reading about this exemplar, you will be able to:

1. Describe the pathophysiology, etiology, clinical manifestations, and direct and indirect causes of metabolic acidosis.

2. Identify risk factors and prevention methods associated with metabolic acidosis.

3. Illustrate the nursing process in providing culturally sensitive care across the life span for individuals with metabolic acidosis.

4. Formulate priority nursing diagnoses appropriate for an individual with metabolic acidosis.

5. Summarize therapies used by interdisciplinary teams in the collaborative care of an individual with metabolic acidosis.

6. Plan evidence-based care for an individual with metabolic acidosis and his or her family in collaboration with other members of the healthcare team.

7. Evaluate expected outcomes for an individual with metabolic acidosis.

▶ OVERVIEW

Metabolic acidosis (bicarbonate deficit) is characterized by a low pH (<7.35) and a low bicarbonate (<24 mEq/L). It may be caused by excess acid in the body or loss of bicarbonate from the body. When metabolic acidosis develops, the respiratory system attempts to return the pH to normal by increasing the rate and depth of respirations. Carbon dioxide elimination increases, and the $PaCO_2$ falls (<35 mmHg).

▶ PATHOPHYSIOLOGY AND ETIOLOGY

Three basic mechanisms can cause metabolic acidosis:

1. Accumulation of metabolic acids
2. Excess loss of bicarbonate
3. An increase in chloride levels.

An accumulation of metabolic acids can result from excess acid production or impaired renal elimination of metabolic acids. Lactic acidosis develops due to tissue hypoxia and a shift to anaerobic metabolism by the cells. Lactate and hydrogen ions are produced, forming lactic acid. Both oxygen and glucose are necessary for normal cell metabolism. When intracellular glucose is inadequate due to starvation or a lack of insulin to move it into cells, the body breaks down fatty tissue to meet its metabolic needs. In this process, fatty acids are released and converted to ketones; ketoacidosis results. Aspirin (acetylsalicylic acid) breaks down into salicylic acid in the body. Substances such as aspirin, methanol (wood alcohol), and ethylene (contained in antifreeze and solvents) cause a toxic increase in body acids by either breaking down into acid products (salicylic acid) or stimulating metabolic acid production (Porth & Matfin, 2009). Renal failure impairs the body's ability to excrete excess hydrogen ions and form bicarbonate.

Excess metabolic acids increase the hydrogen ion concentration of body fluids. The buffering of excess acid by bicarbonate, leads to what is known as a *high anion gap acidosis*.

The pancreas secretes bicarbonate-rich fluid into the small intestine. Intestinal suction, severe diarrhea, ileostomy drainage, or fistulas can lead to excess losses of bicarbonate. Hyperchloremic acidosis can develop when excess of a chloride solution (such as NaCl) is infused, causing a rise in chloride concentrations. It also may be related to renal disease or administration of carbonic anhydrate inhibitor diuretics. The anion gap remains normal in metabolic acidosis due to bicarbonate loss or excess chloride.

Acidosis depresses cell membrane excitability, affecting neuromuscular function. It also increases the amount of free calcium in ECF by interfering with protein binding. Severe acidosis (pH of 7.0 or less) depresses myocardial contractility, leading to decreased cardiac output. If kidney function is normal, acid excretion and ammonia production increase to eliminate excess hydrogen ions.

Acid–base imbalances also affect electrolyte balance. In acidosis, potassium is retained as the kidney excretes excess hydrogen ions. Excess hydrogen ions also enter the cells, displacing potassium from the intracellular space to maintain the balance of cations and anions within the cells. The effect of both processes is to increase serum potassium levels. Also in acidosis, calcium is released from its bonds with plasma proteins, increasing the amount of ionized (free) calcium in the blood. Magnesium levels may fall in acidosis.

Risk Factors

Metabolic acidosis is rarely a primary disorder; it usually develops during the course of another disease, as follows:

- Acute lactic acidosis usually results from tissue hypoxia due to shock or cardiac arrest.
- Clients with type 1 diabetes mellitus are at risk for developing diabetic ketoacidosis.

Clinical Manifestations and Therapies **Metabolic Acidosis**

ETIOLOGY	CLINICAL MANIFESTATIONS	CLINICAL THERAPIES
Conditions that increase nonvolatile acids in the blood (e.g., renal impairment, diabetes mellitus, starvation)	▪ Diminished appetite	▪ Monitor ABG values, intake and output, and LOC.
Conditions that decrease bicarbonate (e.g., prolonged diarrhea)	▪ Nausea and vomiting	▪ Position client to facilitate chest expansion.
Excessive infusion of chloride-containing IV fluids (e.g., NaCl)	▪ Abdominal pain	▪ Provide oral care for dry mouth.
Excessive ingestion of acids (e.g., salicylates)	▪ Weakness	▪ Administer IV sodium bicarbonate carefully if ordered.
Cardiac arrest	▪ Fatigue	▪ Treat underlying problem as ordered.
	▪ Headache	
	▪ General malaise	
	▪ Decreasing LOCs	
	▪ Dysrhythmias	
	▪ Bradycardia	
	▪ Warm, flushed skin	
	▪ Skeletal problems	
	▪ Hyperventilation (Kussmaul's respirations)	
	▪ Dyspnea	

- Acute or chronic renal failure impairs the excretion of metabolic acids.
- Diarrhea, intestinal suction, or abdominal fistulas increase the risk for excess bicarbonate loss.

Other common causes of metabolic acidosis are listed in Table 1–1 on page 9.

▶ CLINICAL MANIFESTATIONS

Metabolic acidosis affects the function of many body systems. Its general manifestations include weakness and fatigue, headache, and general malaise. The effects on gastrointestinal function cause diminished appetite, nausea, vomiting, and abdominal pain. The level of consciousness may decline into stupor and coma. Cardiac dysrhythmias develop, and cardiac arrest may occur. The skin is often warm and flushed. Skeletal problems may develop in chronic acidosis, as calcium and phosphate are released from the bones. Manifestations of compensatory mechanisms are seen. The deep and rapid respirations that are seen are known as **Kussmaul respirations**. The client may complain of shortness of breath, or dyspnea.

▶ COLLABORATION

Metabolic acidosis normally results from another primary disorder. Therefore the focus is on treating the primary disorder, reducing the effects of acidosis on cardiac function, and ensuring adequate oxygenation. Diagnostic tests include ABGs, serum electrolytes, and tests as indicated by the underlying primary disorder.

Pharmacologic Therapy

To reduce the effects of acidosis on cardiac function, an alkalinizing solution such as bicarbonate may be given if the pH is less than 7.2. Sodium bicarbonate is the most commonly used alkalinizing solution; others include lactate, citrate, and acetate solutions (which are metabolized to bicarbonate). Alkalinizing solutions are given intravenously for severe acute metabolic acidosis. In chronic metabolic acidosis, the oral route is used.

Carefully monitor the client treated with bicarbonate. Rapid correction of the acidosis may lead to metabolic alkalosis and hypokalemia. Hypernatremia and hyperosmolality may develop as well, leading to water retention and fluid overload.

> **SAFETY ALERT**
> As metabolic acidosis is corrected, potassium shifts back into the intracellular space. This shift can lead to hypokalemia and cardiac dysrhythmias. Carefully monitor serum potassium levels during treatment.

Treatment for diabetic ketoacidosis includes intravenous insulin and fluid replacement. Alcoholic ketoacidosis is treated with saline solutions and glucose. Treatment for lactic acidosis from decreased tissue perfusion (e.g., shock, cardiac arrest) focuses on correcting the underlying problem and improving tissue perfusion. Clients with chronic renal failure and mild or moderate metabolic acidosis may or may not require treatment, depending on their pH and bicarbonate levels. When metabolic acidosis is due to diarrhea, treatment includes correcting the underlying cause and providing fluid and electrolyte replacement.

■ NURSING PROCESS

Nurses frequently provide care for clients with metabolic acidosis, although the focus of care is usually the underlying disorder (e.g., diabetes mellitus, renal failure) rather than the acidosis itself. For this reason, it is vital for the nurse to be aware of the effects of acidosis and its implications for nursing care.

To promote health in clients at risk for metabolic acidosis, discuss management of the underlying disease process (e.g., type 1 diabetes, renal failure) to help them prevent complications such as diabetic ketoacidosis and metabolic acidosis. Because early manifestations of metabolic acidosis (e.g., fatigue, general malaise, diminished appetite, nausea, abdominal pain) resemble those of common viral disorders such as influenza, stress the importance of promptly seeking treatment if these symptoms develop.

Assessment

- *Health history.* Current manifestations, including diminished appetite, nausea, vomiting, abdominal discomfort, fatigue, lethargy, and other symptoms; duration of symptoms and any precipitating factors such as diarrhea and ingestion of a toxin such as aspirin, methanol, or ethylene; chronic diseases such as diabetes or renal failure, cirrhosis of the liver, or endocrine disorders; current medications.
- *Physical assessment.* Mental status and LOC; vital signs including respiratory rate and depth; apical and peripheral pulses; skin color and temperature; abdominal contour and distention; bowel sounds; urine output.

Diagnosis

Although the focus of nursing management is on the primary disorder, the acidosis itself has effects that require care. Possible nursing diagnoses for the client with metabolic acidosis are the following:

- *Decreased Cardiac Output*
- *Risk for Excess Fluid Volume*
- *Risk for Injury*

(NANDA-I © 2012)

Planning

Planning for the client with metabolic acidosis involves identification and treatment of the underlying cause and restoration and maintenance of acid–base balance. (Refer to other concepts for a discussion of interventions specific to the underlying disorder.) Potential goals for the client with metabolic acidosis may be the following:

- Client will describe and demonstrate preventive measures related to chronic disease process.
- pH will remain within normal range.
- Disease process causing acid–base imbalance will be controlled to reduce acid production or alkaline loss.
- Client will maintain vital signs within normal range for age and condition.

- Client will maintain baseline cardiac rhythm.
- Client will maintain or regain normal serum electrolyte levels.

Implementation

Metabolic acidosis affects cardiac output by decreasing myocardial contractility, slowing the heart rate, and increasing the risk for dysrhythmias. The accompanying hyperkalemia increases the risk for decreased cardiac output as well. (See the module on Fluids and Electrolytes for discussion about hyperkalemia.)

Monitor Cardiac Status

- Monitor vital signs, including peripheral pulses and capillary refill. Hypotension, diminished pulse strength, and slowed capillary refill may indicate decreased cardiac output and impaired tissue perfusion. Poor tissue perfusion can increase the risk for lactic acidosis.
- Monitor the ECG pattern for dysrhythmias and changes characteristic of hyperkalemia. Notify the physician of changes. Progressive ECG changes such as widening of the QRS complex indicate an increasing risk of dysrhythmias and cardiac arrest. Dysrhythmias further decrease cardiac output, possibly intensifying the degree of acidosis.
- Monitor laboratory values, including ABGs, serum electrolytes, and renal function studies (serum creatinine and BUN). Frequent monitoring of laboratory values allows evaluation of the effectiveness of treatment as well as early identification of potential problems.

SAFETY ALERT
Administering bicarbonate to correct acidosis increases the risk for hypernatremia, hyperosmolality, and fluid volume excess.

Monitor Potential for Excess Fluid Volume

- Monitor and maintain fluid replacement as ordered. Monitor serum sodium levels and osmolality.
- Monitor heart and lung sounds, central venous pressure (CVP), and respiratory status. Increasing dyspnea, adventitious lung sounds, a third heart sound (S_3) due to the volume of blood flow through the heart, and high CVP readings indicate hypervolemia and should be reported to the care provider.
- Assess for edema, particularly in the back, sacral, and periorbital areas. Initially, edema affects dependent tissues—the back and sacrum in clients who are bedridden. Periorbital edema indicates more generalized edema.
- Assess urine output hourly. Maintain accurate intake and output records. Note urine output less than 30 mL/hour or a positive fluid balance on 24-hour total intake and output calculations. Heart failure and inadequate renal perfusion may lead to decreased urine output.
- Obtain daily weights using consistent conditions (same time of day, clothing, and scale). Daily weights are an accurate indicator of fluid balance.
- Administer prescribed diuretics as ordered, monitoring the client's response to therapy. Loop or high-ceiling

diuretics such as furosemide can lead to further electrolyte imbalances, especially hypokalemia. This is a significant risk like that seen during correction of metabolic acidosis.

Reduce Risk for Injury

Mental status and brain function are affected by acidosis, increasing the risk for injury. The nurse working with clients who exhibit altered mental status related to acidosis should

- Monitor neurological function, including mental status, LOC, and muscle strength. As the pH falls, the resulting decline in mental functioning leads to confusion, stupor, and a decreasing LOC.
- Institute safety precautions as necessary: Keep the bed in its lowest position with side rails raised. These measures help protect the client from injury resulting from confusion or disorientation.
- Keep clocks, calendars, and familiar objects at bedside. Orient to time, place, and circumstances as needed. Allow significant others to remain with the client as much as possible. An unfamiliar environment and altered thought processes can further increase the risk for injury. Significant others provide a sense of security and reduce anxiety.

Care in the Community

When preparing the client with metabolic acidosis for discharge, consider the cause of the acidosis and any underlying factors. Discharge planning and teaching focus on the underlying cause of the imbalance. The client who has developed ketoacidosis as a result of diabetes mellitus, starvation, or alcoholism needs interventions and teaching to prevent future episodes of acidosis. Diet, medication management, and alcohol dependency treatment are vital teaching areas. When metabolic acidosis is related to renal failure, the client should be referred for management of the renal failure itself. Clients who have experienced diarrhea or excess ileostomy drainage leading to bicarbonate loss need information about appropriate diarrhea treatment strategies and need to know when to call their primary care provider. Provide teaching to the client and family about the following:

- Using appropriate resources to get medical assistance.
- Contacting their primary care provider immediately if they experience, dizziness, nausea, vomiting, and fatigue.

Evaluation

Expected outcomes of nursing care relate to prevention of acidosis and restoration of normal body balance during disease processes. During the recovery period, frequently monitor pH levels and vital signs, and reassess the client's condition to revise care plans as necessary. Expected outcomes include the following:

- Client maintains pH within normal range.
- Client's vital signs remain within normal range based on age and condition.
- Client maintains adequate oxygenation of tissues.
- Client is able to describe or demonstrate measures to control the disease process to prevent future complications of pH imbalance.

REVIEW **Metabolic Acidosis**

RELATE Link the Concepts and Exemplars

The ambulance arrives with a client who presents with Kussmaul respirations and a history of diabetes mellitus.

Linking the exemplar of metabolic acidosis with the concept of metabolism:

1. Based on the client's history, what impact does the nurse expect to find on acid–base balance?
2. When the nurse is assessing this client, what symptoms of diabetic ketoacidosis would be directly related to alterations in pH?

Linking the exemplar of metabolic acidosis with the concept of fluids and electrolytes:

3. When assessing the client, what electrolyte imbalances should the nurse monitor in acidosis?
4. What signs of dehydration related to diabetes mellitus will the nurse observe in a client in acute metabolic acidosis?

Linking the exemplar of metabolic acidosis with the concept of safety:

5. What precautions would the nurse implement for the client with metabolic acidosis to prevent potential injury?
6. The client with metabolic acidosis becomes confused and disoriented. What nursing care will the nurse provide to this client to maintain safety?

READY Go to Companion Skills Manual

REFER Go to Pearson Nursing Student Resources

nursing.pearsonhighered.com
- Additional review materials

REFLECT Case Study

Reread Case Study A on page 9. Mr. James's arterial blood gas values were pH 7.28, $PaCO_2$ 31 mmHg, PaO_2 95 mmHg, and HCO_3 15 mEq/L. Central venous pressure or right atrial pressure (RAP) ranged from 1 to 3 cm H_2O pressure. ECG revealed sinus tachycardia with ST depression in most leads. Two units of packed red blood cells were ordered and rapidly transfused into the client. His hemoglobin was 10 gm/dl and his hematocrit was 40% before the transfusion.

1. What is the priority nursing diagnosis for Mr. James at this time? Why?
2. What is the interpretation of the arterial blood gas results?
3. How is the client compensating for the acidosis?
4. Refer to the module on Perfusion. Why was the CVP catheter placed in this client? What are normal CVP values?
5. Why is the hematocrit falsely elevated?
6. What safety precautions should be implemented for Mr. James at this time?

EXEMPLAR 1.2 **Metabolic Alkalosis**

EXEMPLAR KEY TERM
Metabolic alkalosis, 17

EXEMPLAR LEARNING OUTCOMES
After reading about this exemplar, you will be able to:

1. Describe the pathophysiology, etiology, clinical manifestations, and direct and indirect causes of metabolic alkalosis.
2. Identify risk factors and prevention methods associated with metabolic alkalosis.
3. Illustrate the nursing process in providing culturally sensitive care across the life span for individuals with metabolic alkalosis.
4. Formulate priority nursing diagnoses appropriate for an individual with metabolic alkalosis.
5. Summarize therapies used by interdisciplinary teams in the collaborative care of an individual with metabolic alkalosis.
6. Plan evidence-based care for an individual with metabolic alkalosis and his or her family in collaboration with other members of the healthcare team.
7. Evaluate expected outcomes for an individual with metabolic alkalosis.

▶ OVERVIEW

Metabolic alkalosis (bicarbonate excess) is characterized by a high pH (>7.45) and a high bicarbonate (>28 mEq/L). It may be caused by loss of acid or excess bicarbonate in the body. When metabolic alkalosis develops, the respiratory system attempts to return the pH to normal by slowing the respiratory rate. Carbon dioxide is retained, and the $PaCO_2$ increases (>45 mmHg).

▶ PATHOPHYSIOLOGY AND ETIOLOGY

Hydrogen ions may be lost through the kidneys or via gastric secretions or because of a shift of H+ into the cells. Metabolic alkalosis due to loss of hydrogen ions usually occurs because of vomiting or gastric suction. Gastric secretions are highly acidic (pH 1–3). When these are lost through vomiting or gastric suction, the alkalinity of body fluids increases. This increased alkalinity results from the loss of acid and from selective retention of bicarbonate by the kidneys as chloride is depleted. (Chloride is the major anion in ECF; when it is lost, bicarbonate is retained as a replacement anion.)

Increased renal excretion of hydrogen ions can be prompted by hypokalemia as the kidneys try to conserve potassium, excreting hydrogen ions instead. Hypokalemia contributes to metabolic alkalosis in another way as well. When potassium shifts out of cells to maintain extracellular potassium levels, hydrogen ions shift into the cells to maintain the balance between cations and anions within the cells.

Clinical Manifestations and Therapies Metabolic Alkalosis

ETIOLOGY	CLINICAL MANIFESTATIONS	CLINICAL THERAPIES
Excessive acid losses due to vomiting or gastric suction Excessive use of potassium-losing diuretics Excessive adrenal corticoid hormones due to ■ Cushing's syndrome ■ Hyperaldosteronism ■ Excessive bicarbonate intake from antacids ■ Parenteral sodium bicarbonate infusion	■ Confusion ■ Decreasing level of consciousness ■ Hyperreflexia ■ Tetany ■ Dysrhythmias ■ Hypotension ■ Seizures ■ Respiratory failure	■ Monitor intake and output closely. ■ Monitor vital signs, especially respirations and LOC. ■ Administer ordered IV fluids carefully. ■ Administer oxygen as ordered. ■ Treat underlying problem.

Excess bicarbonate usually occurs as a result of ingesting antacids that contain bicarbonate (such as soda bicarbonate or Alka-Seltzer) or overzealous administration of bicarbonate to treat metabolic acidosis. Common causes of metabolic alkalosis are summarized in Table 1–1.

In alkalosis, more calcium combines with serum proteins, reducing the amount of ionized (physiologically active) calcium in the blood. This reduction in ionized calcium accounts for many of the common manifestations of metabolic alkalosis. Alkalosis also affects potassium balance: Hypokalemia not only can cause metabolic alkalosis (see above), but also can result from metabolic alkalosis. Hydrogen ions shift out of the intracellular space to help restore the pH, prompting more potassium to enter the cells and depleting ECF potassium. The high pH depresses the respiratory system as the body retains carbon dioxide to restore the ratio of carbonic acid to bicarbonate.

Risk Factors

Like other acid–base imbalances, metabolic alkalosis rarely occurs as a primary disorder. Risk factors include hospitalization, hypokalemia, and treatment with alkalinizing solutions (e.g., bicarbonate).

▶ CLINICAL MANIFESTATIONS

Manifestations of metabolic alkalosis result from decreased calcium ionization and are similar to those of hypocalcemia. They include numbness and tingling around the mouth, fingers, and toes; dizziness; Trousseau's sign; and muscle spasm. As the respiratory system compensates for metabolic alkalosis, respirations are depressed and respiratory failure with hypoxemia and respiratory acidosis may develop.

▶ COLLABORATION

Metabolic alkalosis typically arises as a consequence of an underlying primary disorder. The plan of care and therapeutic regimen are aimed at controlling alkalosis while treating the underlying cause.

Pharmacologic Therapy

Treatment of metabolic alkalosis includes restoring normal fluid volume and administering potassium chloride and sodium chloride solution. The potassium restores serum and intracellular potassium levels, allowing the kidneys to conserve hydrogen ions more effectively. Chloride promotes renal excretion of bicarbonate. Sodium chloride solutions restore fluid volume deficits that can contribute to metabolic alkalosis. In severe alkalosis, an acidifying solution such as dilute hydrochloric acid or ammonium chloride may be administered. In addition, drugs may be used to treat the underlying cause of the alkalosis.

Laboratory and Diagnostic Tests

The following laboratory and diagnostic tests may be ordered:

- ***ABGs*** show a pH greater than 7.45 and bicarbonate level greater than 28 mEq/L. With compensatory hypoventilation, carbon dioxide is retained and the $PaCO_2$ is greater than 45 mmHg.

- ***Serum electrolytes*** often demonstrate decreased serum potassium (<3.5 mEq/L) and decreased chloride (<95 mEq/L) levels. The serum bicarbonate level is high. Although the total serum calcium may be normal, the ionized fraction of calcium is low.

- ***Urine pH*** may be low (pH 1–3) if metabolic alkalosis is caused by hypokalemia. The kidneys selectively retain potassium and excrete hydrogen ion to restore ECF potassium levels. Urinary chloride levels may be normal or greater than 250 mEq/24 hours.

- ***The ECG pattern*** shows changes similar to those seen with hypokalemia. (See the concept of Fluids and Electrolytes for more information related to symptoms of hypokalemia.) These changes may be due to hypokalemia or to the alkalosis.

◼ NURSING PROCESS

Health promotion activities focus on teaching clients the risks of using sodium bicarbonate as an antacid to relieve heartburn or gastric distress. Stress the availability of other effective antacid preparations and the need to seek medical evaluation for persistent gastric symptoms.

In the hospital setting, carefully monitor laboratory values for clients at risk for developing metabolic alkalosis, particularly clients undergoing continuous gastric suction.

Assessment

Focused assessment data related to metabolic alkalosis include the following:

- **Health history.** Current manifestations such as numbness and tingling, muscle spasms, dizziness, or other symptoms; duration of symptoms and any precipitating factors such as bicarbonate ingestion, vomiting, diuretic therapy, or endocrine disorders; current medications
- **Physical assessment.** Vital signs, including apical pulse and rate and depth of respirations; muscle strength; deep tendon reflexes
- **Diagnostic tests.** ABGs, serum electrolytes

Diagnosis

As with metabolic acidosis, nursing care of the client with metabolic alkalosis often focuses on intervening for client responses to the primary problem rather than the alkalosis itself. However, the risk for impaired gas exchange is a priority problem, especially with severe metabolic alkalosis. Possible nursing diagnoses for the client with metabolic alkalosis include the following:

- *Risk for Impaired Gas Exchange*
- *Deficient Fluid Volume*
- *Risk for Injury*

(NANDA-I © 2012)

Planning

Planning for the client with metabolic alkalosis depends on identification and treatment of the underlying cause. Restoring and maintaining normal acid–base balance is the desired outcome. Nursing care will also include measures to treat the underlying disorder, such as hypokalemia. (Refer to other modules for a discussion of interventions specific to the underlying disorder.) Appropriate outcomes will include resolution of the underlying cause and the client's return to

- Oxygen saturation level of 93% or greater.
- Normal or near normal fluid and electrolyte volumes.

Implementation

Nursing care of the client with metabolic alkalosis is focused on controlling pH while treating the underlying causative disorder and preventing complications.

Monitor for Impaired Gas Exchange

Respiratory compensation for metabolic alkalosis depresses the respiratory rate and reduces the depth of breathing to promote carbon dioxide retention. As a result, the client is at risk for impaired gas exchange, especially in the presence of underlying lung disease.

- Monitor respiratory rate, depth, and effort. Monitor oxygen saturation continuously, reporting an oxygen saturation level of less than 93% (or as ordered). The depressed respiratory drive associated with metabolic alkalosis can lead to hypoxemia and impaired oxygenation of tissues. Oxygen saturation levels of less than 90% indicate significant oxygenation problems.
- Assess skin color; note and report cyanosis around the mouth. Central cyanosis, seen around the mouth and oral mucous membranes, indicates significant hypoxia and is a late sign.
- Monitor mental status and LOC. Report decreasing LOC or behavior changes such as restlessness, agitation, or confusion. Changes in mental status or behavior may be early signs of hypoxia.
- Place in semi-Fowler or Fowler position as tolerated. Elevating the head of the bed facilitates alveolar ventilation and gas exchange.
- Administer oxygen as ordered or as necessary to maintain oxygen saturation levels. Supplemental oxygen can help maintain blood and tissue oxygenation despite depressed respirations.
- Schedule nursing care activities to allow rest periods. The client who is hypoxemic has limited energy reserves, necessitating frequent rest and limited activities.

Monitor for Fluid Volume Deficit

Clients with metabolic alkalosis often have an accompanying fluid volume deficit.

- Assess intake and output accurately, monitoring fluid balance. In acute situations, hourly intake and output assessment may be indicated. Urine output of less than 30 mL/hour indicates inadequate tissue perfusion, inadequate renal perfusion, and an increased risk for acute renal failure.
- Assess vital signs, CVP, and peripheral pulse volume at least every 4 hours. Hypotension, tachycardia, low CVP, and weak, easily obliterated peripheral pulses indicate hypovolemia.
- Weigh daily under standard conditions (time of day, clothing, and scale). Rapid weight changes accurately reflect fluid balance.
- Administer intravenous fluids as prescribed using an electronic infusion pump. If rapid fluid replacement is ordered, monitor for the following indicators of fluid overload: dyspnea, tachypnea, tachycardia, increased CVP, jugular vein distension, and edema. Rapid fluid replacement may lead to hypervolemia, resulting in pulmonary edema and cardiac failure, particularly in clients with compromised cardiac and renal function.
- Monitor serum electrolytes, osmolality, and ABG values. Rehydration and administration of potassium chloride affect both acid–base and fluid and electrolyte balance. Careful monitoring is important to identify changes.

Care in the Community

When preparing the client with metabolic alkalosis for discharge, consider the cause of the alkalosis and any underlying factors. For example, provide teaching to the client and family about the following:

- Using appropriate antacids for heartburn and gastric distress
- Using potassium supplements as ordered or eating high-potassium foods to prevent hypokalemia if taking a potassium-wasting diuretic or if aldosterone production is impaired
- Contacting the primary care provider if uncontrolled or extended vomiting develops.

Evaluation

Expected outcomes of nursing care relate to restoration of normal body balance. Revisions in the care plan may need to be made if the client does not respond to some aspect of the plan. Nurses may need to follow up with clients released from hospital care to determine whether they are continuing to follow instructions for self-monitoring and self-care. Possible outcomes for the client with metabolic alkalosis include the following:

- Client reports use of antacids that are acceptable for use and that reduce risk of recurrence of metabolic alkalosis.
- Client describes proper self-administration procedure for oral potassium supplements.
- Client describes when to notify provider related to changes in daily weight.
- Client's arterial pH returns to normal range.
- Client's serum electrolyte values are within normal range.

REVIEW Metabolic Alkalosis

RELATE Link the Concepts and Exemplars

Linking the exemplar of metabolic alkalosis with the concept of fluids and electrolytes:

1. What pathophysiological process is involved with metabolic alkalosis that leads to a decrease in mental function?
2. What changes in serum electrolyte levels could indicate a risk for metabolic alkalosis?

Linking the exemplar of metabolic alkalosis with the concept of tissue integrity:

3. What impact might the client with full thickness burns over 50% of the body experience in regard to acid–base balance?
4. What caring interventions might be implemented (independently by the nurse or collaboratively by the healthcare team) to prevent metabolic alkalosis?

Linking the exemplar of metabolic alkalosis with the concept of communication:

5. What information about the client with metabolic alkalosis should the nurse include in the end-of-shift report?
6. The client with metabolic alkalosis becomes confused and disoriented. What strategies will help promote communication with this client?

READY Go to Companion Skills Manual

REFER Go to Pearson Nursing Student Resources
nursing.pearsonhighered.com

- Additional review questions

REFLECT Case Study

Reread Case Study B on page 11. Ms. Zemakis's initial labs reveal Na 130, K 2.0, Cl 103, Mg 1.4, BUN 10, and creatinine 1.2 mmol/l. ABG values are pH 7.47, $PaCO_2$ 26 mmHg, PaO_2 88 mmHg, HCO_3 29 mEq/L.

Ms. Zemakis is transferred to the intensive care step-down unit for fluid and electrolyte replacement with ECG monitoring.

1. What are the priority nursing interventions for Ms. Zemakis at this time?
2. What is the interpretation of the ABG results?
3. What is the cause of her muscle weakness?
4. Why is ECG monitoring necessary?
5. Why does this client need closer monitoring in the intensive care step-down unit?

EXEMPLAR 1.3   Respiratory Acidosis

EXEMPLAR KEY TERMS
Hypercapnia, *21*
Hypoxemia, *21*
Respiratory acidosis, *21*
Ventilation, *21*

EXEMPLAR LEARNING OUTCOMES
After reading about this exemplar, you will be able to:

1. Describe the pathophysiology, etiology, clinical manifestations, and direct and indirect causes of respiratory acidosis.
2. Identify risk factors and prevention methods associated with respiratory acidosis.
3. Illustrate the nursing process in providing culturally sensitive care across the life span for individuals with respiratory acidosis.
4. Formulate priority nursing diagnoses appropriate for an individual with respiratory acidosis.
5. Summarize therapies used by interdisciplinary teams in the collaborative care of an individual with respiratory acidosis.
6. Plan evidence-based care for an individual with respiratory acidosis and his or her family in collaboration with other members of the healthcare team.
7. Evaluate expected outcomes for an individual with respiratory acidosis.

▶ OVERVIEW

Respiratory acidosis is caused by an excess of dissolved carbon dioxide, or carbonic acid. It is characterized by a pH less than 7.35 and a $PaCO_2$ greater than 45 mmHg. Respiratory acidosis may be acute or chronic. In chronic respiratory acidosis, the bicarbonate is higher than 26 mEq/L as the kidneys compensate by retaining bicarbonate.

▶ PATHOPHYSIOLOGY AND ETIOLOGY

Both acute and chronic respiratory acidosis result from carbon dioxide retention caused by alveolar hypoventilation. **Hypoxemia** (decreased oxygen) frequently accompanies respiratory acidosis.

Acute Respiratory Acidosis

Acute respiratory acidosis results from a sudden failure of **ventilation** (the exchange of oxygen and carbon dioxide). Chest trauma, aspiration of a foreign body, acute pneumonia, and overdoses of narcotic or sedative medications can lead to this condition. Because acute respiratory acidosis occurs with the sudden onset of hypoventilation—for example, with cardiac arrest—the $PaCO_2$ rises rapidly and the pH falls markedly. A pH of 7 or lower can occur within minutes, resulting in death if not corrected (Metheny, 2009). Initially, the serum bicarbonate level is unchanged because the compensatory response of the kidneys continues over hours to days.

Hypercapnia (increased carbon dioxide levels) affects neurological function and the cardiovascular system. Carbon dioxide rapidly crosses the blood–brain barrier. Cerebral blood vessels dilate, and if the condition continues, intracranial pressure increases and *papilledema* (swelling and inflammation of the optic nerve where it enters the retina) develops (Porth & Matfin, 2009). Peripheral vasodilation also occurs, and the pulse rate increases to maintain cardiac output.

Chronic Respiratory Acidosis

Chronic respiratory acidosis is associated with chronic respiratory or neuromuscular conditions such as COPD, asthma, cystic fibrosis, and multiple sclerosis. These conditions affect alveolar ventilation because of airway obstruction, structural changes in the lung, and limited chest wall expansion. Most clients with chronic respiratory acidosis have COPD with chronic bronchitis and emphysema. In chronic respiratory acidosis, the $PaCO_2$ increases over time and remains elevated. The kidneys retain bicarbonate, increasing bicarbonate levels, and the pH often remains close to the normal range because of adequate metabolic compensation.

The acute effects of hypercapnia may not develop when carbon dioxide levels rise gradually, allowing compensatory changes to occur. When carbon dioxide levels are chronically elevated, the respiratory center becomes less sensitive to the gas as a stimulant of the respiratory drive. The PaO_2 provides the primary stimulus for respirations. Clients with chronic respiratory acidosis are at risk for developing *carbon dioxide narcosis* (with manifestations of acute respiratory acidosis) if the respiratory center is suppressed by the administration of excess supplemental oxygen. Manifestations include confusion, tremors, and convulsions; coma can occur if blood levels of CO_2 reach 70 mmHg or higher. Clients with chronic respiratory acidosis can tolerate CO_2 levels that are much higher than normal.

> **SAFETY ALERT**
> Carefully monitor neurological and respiratory status in clients with chronic respiratory acidosis who are receiving oxygen therapy. Immediately report a decreasing LOC or depressed respirations.

Risk Factors

Acute or chronic lung disease (e.g., pneumonia, COPD) or trauma is the primary risk factor for respiratory acidosis. Other conditions that depress or interfere with ventilation, such as excess narcotic analgesics, airway obstruction, and neuromuscular disease, also are risk factors for respiratory acidosis. Selected causes of respiratory acidosis are listed in Table 1–1 on page 9.

▶ CLINICAL MANIFESTATIONS

The manifestations of acute and chronic respiratory acidosis differ. In acute respiratory acidosis, the rapid rise in $PaCO_2$ levels causes manifestations of hypercapnia. Cerebral vasodilation causes manifestations such as headache, blurred vision, irritability, and mental cloudiness. If the condition continues, the LOC progressively decreases. Rapid and dramatic changes in ABGs can lead to unconsciousness and ventricular fibrillation, a potentially lethal cardiac dysrhythmia. The skin of the client with acute respiratory acidosis may be warm and flushed, and the pulse rate is elevated.

The manifestations of chronic respiratory acidosis include weakness and a dull headache. Sleep disturbances, daytime sleepiness, impaired memory, and personality changes also may be manifestations of chronic respiratory acidosis. Clients with acute respiratory failure require treatment in the emergency department or intensive care unit. The focus is on restoring adequate ventilation and gas exchange.

Acute respiratory acidosis is often the result of inadequate breathing patterns resulting in retained carbon dioxide and inadequate intake of oxygen. As a result, hypoxemia often accompanies hypercapnia, requiring administration of supplemental oxygen. The administration of oxygen to the client with chronic hypercapnia, such as the client with COPD, must be delivered with caution to prevent removing the respiratory drive in those who breathe as a result of minor hypoxia. See the exemplar on COPD in the concept of Oxygenation, for more information about the administration of oxygen to those with chronic hypercapnia.

▶ COLLABORATION

Care of the client experiencing respiratory acidosis involves the efforts of the entire healthcare team. A respiratory therapist may provide breathing treatments and related therapies as ordered. Consultation with the pharmacist and the client's pri-

Clinical Manifestations and Therapies Respiratory Acidosis

ETIOLOGY	CLINICAL MANIFESTATIONS	CLINICAL THERAPIES
Acute lung conditions that impair alveolar gas exchange (e.g., pneumonia, acute pulmonary edema, aspiration of foreign body, near-drowning) Chronic lung disease (e.g., asthma, cystic fibrosis, emphysema) Overdose of narcotics or sedatives that depress respiratory rate and depth Brain injury that affects the respiratory center Airway obstruction Mechanical injury	*Acute respiratory acidosis:* ■ Headache ■ Warm, flushed skin ■ Elevated pulse ■ Blurred vision ■ Irritability, altered mental status ■ Decreasing LOC ■ Cardiac arrest *Chronic respiratory acidosis:* ■ Weakness ■ Dull headache ■ Sleep disturbances with daytime sleepiness ■ Impaired memory ■ Personality changes	■ Frequently assess respiratory status and lung sounds. ■ Evaluate mental status; document and report changes in alertness. ■ Place in semi-Fowler's to Fowler's position as tolerated. ■ Encourage the client with chronic respiratory acidosis to use pursed-lip breathing. ■ Monitor airway and ventilation; insert artificial airway and prepare for mechanical ventilation as necessary. ■ Administer pulmonary therapy measures such as inhalation therapy, percussion and postural drainage, bronchodilators, and antibiotics as ordered. ■ Monitor fluid intake and output, vital signs, and ABGs. ■ Administer narcotic antagonists as indicated.

mary care provider prevents administration of medications that may be contraindicated. Clients who are using accessory muscles to breathe may require increased caloric intake and the participation of a dietician.

Diagnostic Tests

The following diagnostic tests may be ordered:

■ **ABGs** show a pH of less than 7.35 and a $PaCO_2$ of more than 45 mmHg. In acute respiratory acidosis, the bicarbonate level is initially within normal range but increases to greater than 28 mEq/L if the condition persists. In chronic respiratory acidosis, both the $PaCO_2$ and the HCO_3 may be significantly elevated.

■ **Serum electrolytes** may show hypochloremia (chloride level <95–105 mEq/L) in chronic respiratory acidosis.

■ **Pulmonary function tests** may be done to determine whether chronic lung disease is the cause of the respiratory acidosis. However, these studies are not done during the acute period.

Additional diagnostic tests may be done to identify the underlying cause of the respiratory acidosis. Chest X-ray and sputum studies (cytology and culture) may be ordered to identify an acute or chronic lung disorder. If drug overdose is suspected, serum levels of the drug may be obtained.

Pharmacologic Therapy

Bronchodilator drugs may be administered to open the airways and antibiotics prescribed to treat respiratory infections. If excess narcotics or anesthetic has caused acute respiratory aci-

dosis, narcotic antagonists such as naloxone may be given to reverse the effects.

Respiratory Support

Treatment of respiratory acidosis, either acute or chronic, focuses on improving alveolar ventilation and gas exchange. Clients with severe respiratory acidosis and hypoxemia may require intubation and mechanical ventilation. The $PaCO_2$ level is lowered slowly to prevent complications such as cardiac dysrhythmias and decreased cerebral perfusion. In clients with chronic respiratory acidosis, oxygen is administered cautiously to prevent carbon dioxide narcosis.

Pulmonary hygiene measures may be instituted, such as deep breathing and coughing exercises, breathing treatments, and percussion and drainage. Adequate hydration is important to promote removal of respiratory secretions.

◼ NURSING PROCESS

Nursing care of clients with respiratory acidosis is focused on improving breathing patterns and maintaining a patent airway. Because of the link between smoking and chronic pulmonary diseases, nursing care may include teaching clients how to make healthier lifestyle choices.

Assessment

■ *Health history.* Current manifestations (including headache, irritability, and lethargy), difficulty thinking, blurred vision, and other symptoms; duration of symptoms and any precipitating factors such as drug use or respiratory infection;

chronic diseases such as cystic fibrosis or COPD; current medications
- **Physical examination.** Mental status and LOC; vital signs; skin color and temperature; rate and depth of respirations, pulmonary excursion, and lung sounds

Diagnosis

Restoring effective alveolar ventilation and gas exchange is the priority of interdisciplinary and nursing care for clients with respiratory acidosis. Possible nursing diagnoses for the client with respiratory acidosis include the following:

- *Impaired Gas Exchange*
- *Ineffective Airway Clearance*
- *Anxiety*
- *Risk for Injury*

(NANDA-I © 2012)

Planning

Planning for the client with respiratory acidosis involves both restoration of acid–base balance and appropriate treatment for any underlying disease or cause. Expected outcomes include resolution of the underlying illness and the client's maintaining

- Adequate fluid intake.
- Oxygenation saturation greater than 90%.
- Normal $PaCO_2$ levels
- pH balance.

Implementation

Frequently assess respiratory status, including rate, depth, effort, and oxygen saturation levels. Decreasing respiratory rate and effort along with decreasing oxygen saturation levels may signal worsening respiratory failure and respiratory acidosis.

SAFETY ALERT Frequently assess LOC. A decline in LOC may indicate increasing hypercapnia and the need for increasing ventilatory support (such as intubation and mechanical ventilation).

Promote Gas Exchange

- Promptly evaluate and report ABG results to the physician and respiratory therapist. Rapid changes in carbon dioxide or oxygen levels may necessitate modification of the treatment plan to prevent complications of overcorrection of respiratory acidosis.
- Place in semi-Fowler's to Fowler's position as tolerated. Elevating the head of the bed promotes lung expansion and gas exchange.
- Administer oxygen as ordered. Carefully monitor response. Reduce the oxygen flow rate or percentage and immediately report increasing somnolence. Supplemental oxygen can suppress the respiratory drive in clients with chronic respiratory acidosis.

Promote Effective Airway Clearance

- Frequently auscultate breath sounds (whether the client is on or off a mechanical ventilator). Increasing adventitious sounds or decreasing breath sounds (faint or absent) may indicate worsening airway clearance due to obstruction or fatigue.
- Encourage the client with chronic respiratory acidosis to use pursed-lip breathing. Pursed-lip breathing helps maintain open airways throughout exhalation, promoting carbon dioxide elimination. See the Client Teaching feature on Effective Coughing in the module on Oxygenation for detailed instructions on purse-lipped breathing.
- Frequently reposition and encourage ambulation as tolerated. Repositioning, sitting at the bedside, and ambulation promote airway clearance and lung expansion.
- Encourage fluid intake. Fluids help liquefy secretions and hydrate respiratory mucous membranes, promoting airway clearance.
- Administer medications such as inhaled bronchodilators as ordered. Inhaled bronchodilators help relieve bronchial spasm, dilating airways.
- Provide percussion, vibration, and postural drainage as ordered. Pulmonary hygiene measures such as these help loosen respiratory secretions.

Reduce Anxiety Levels

Anxiety is a common result of both hypoxia and hypercapnia triggered by the neurons' insufficient oxygen supply. Clients with respiratory disorders commonly experience anxiety that is eliminated by improved ventilation and oxygenation. The nurse can help the client reduce anxiety levels through the following interventions:

- Remain with the client and monitor for changes in condition.
- Explain procedures and treatments using short, simple sentences. Providing clearly understood information reduces fear of the unknown.
- Reduce environmental stimuli, and use a calm, reassuring manner. These measures help reduce anxiety.
- Allow supportive family members to remain with the client as much as possible to provide further reassurance.

Reduce Risk for Injury

Clients with respiratory acidosis may experience blurred vision and an altered level of consciousness, putting them at risk for injuries. Nurses working with these clients should:

- Assess LOC, mental status, orientation frequently.
- Place call alarm controls within reach.
- Manage rest and activity patterns to improve gas exchange and reduce oxygen demands.
- Administer supplemental oxygen as needed to prevent cellular hypoxia and tissue damage.

Care in the Community

Planning and teaching for home care focus on the problem that caused the respiratory acidosis.

- Teach the client and family about preventive measures and equipment that may be used in the home. The client who developed acute respiratory acidosis as a result of acute pneumonia or chest trauma may require only teaching to prevent future problems.
- If acute respiratory acidosis occurred secondarily to a narcotic overdose, determine whether the drug was prescribed for pain or whether it was an illicit street drug. Provide teaching to the client who requires continuous narcotic medication. Refer the client using illicit drugs to a substance abuse counselor, treatment center, or Narcotics Anonymous, as appropriate; refer the family to support groups as well.
- For clients with chronic lung disease and their families, discuss ways to avoid future episodes of acute respiratory failure. Encourage the client to receive immunization against pneumococcal pneumonia and influenza. Discuss with the client and family ways to avoid acute respiratory infections, such as good hand washing, crowd avoidance, and cough etiquette.
- Provide instructions regarding measures to take when respiratory status is further compromised. The client and family should be alerted that symptoms such as headache accompanied by blurred vision or weakness, irritability and confusion, or sleep disturbances and memory impairments warrant immediate medical attention. Shortness of breath or activity intolerance are often the earliest symptoms of worsening respiratory status. Wheezing, grunting, use of accessory muscles, and cyanosis are often late signs.

Evaluation

The evaluation of nursing care is based on the client's progress in meeting goals, and the nurse revises the plan of care as indicated by outcomes. Expected outcomes of nursing care for a client with respiratory acidosis include the following:

- Client maintains patent airway.
- Client maintains appropriate breathing patterns to meet oxygen demands.
- Client remains conscious and does not display anxiety indicating potential hypoxia.
- ABG reflects pH and $PaCO_2$ within an acceptable range for the client.

REVIEW Respiratory Acidosis

RELATE Link the Concepts and Exemplars

Linking the exemplar of respiratory acidosis with the concept of perfusion:

1. Describe the pathophysiological process that leads from cardiac arrest to respiratory acidosis.
2. Describe how pulmonary embolism might impact the client's pH.

Linking the exemplar of respiratory acidosis with the concept of mobility:

3. Regarding the care of an older adult with a hip fracture that was repaired in surgery earlier today, how might the client's reduced mobility increase the risk of respiratory acidosis?
4. What independent and collaborative nursing interventions might be initiated to prevent respiratory acidosis in this client?

Linking the exemplar of respiratory acidosis with the concept of safety:

5. What precautions would the nurse implement for the client with respiratory acidosis to prevent potential injury?
6. The client with respiratory acidosis becomes confused and disoriented. What is the first intervention needed?

READY Go to Companion Skills Manual

REFER Go to Pearson Nursing Student Resources
nursing.pearsonhighered.com

- Additional review materials

REFLECT Case Study

Reread Case Study C on page 12. Mr. Quinland's vitals were as follows: HR 125 bpm, BP 150/90 mmHg, R 32/min, and T_O 101.1°F. Arterial blood gases were immediately drawn by the respiratory therapist. ABG values were pH 7.32, $PaCO_2$ 50 mmHg, PaO_2 78 mmHg, HCO_3 45 mEq/L. The nurse auscultated decreased breath sounds with scattered rhonchi in the right upper and middle lobes. The client was placed on a 2L nasal cannula, and pulse oximetry was 90%. The respiratory therapist administered a nebulizer treatment, and a chest x-ray was performed.

The hospital admitted Mr. Quinland overnight. The chest x-ray revealed hyperinflation with flattened diaphragm and right lobular bacterial pneumonia. He was started on antibiotics and remained on low-flow oxygen. A pulmonologist consult was ordered, and Mr. Quinland was discharged after seeing the pulmonary physician. He was scheduled for pulmonary function studies after the pneumonia cleared. The discharge medications were antibiotics, respiratory inhalers, and oxygen. Discharge teaching included information on smoking cessation. Unfortunately Mr. Quinland was not able to wean to room air, and he was discharged on a 2L nasal cannula with oximetry of 91%. Home care services have been arranged for Mr. Quinland.

1. What is the interpretation of the ABG results?
2. How is the client compensating for the acidosis?
3. How can you determine if this is a chronic problem?
4. Mr. Quinland's pO_2 is clearly below the normal range. An instinct might be to give 100% oxygen. Why would this be dangerous for him?
5. Why is it important for the client to follow up with the pulmonologist?

EXEMPLAR 1.4 Respiratory Alkalosis

EXEMPLAR KEY TERMS

Hyperventilation, 25
Respiratory alkalosis, 25

EXEMPLAR LEARNING OUTCOMES

After reading about this exemplar, you will be able to:

1. Describe the pathophysiology, etiology, clinical manifestations, and direct and indirect causes of respiratory alkalosis.
2. Identify risk factors and prevention methods associated with respiratory alkalosis.
3. Illustrate the nursing process in providing culturally sensitive care across the life span for individuals with respiratory alkalosis.
4. Formulate priority nursing diagnoses appropriate for an individual with respiratory alkalosis.
5. Summarize therapies used by interdisciplinary teams in the collaborative care of an individual with respiratory alkalosis.
6. Plan evidence-based care for an individual with respiratory alkalosis and his or her family in collaboration with other members of the healthcare team.
7. Evaluate expected outcomes for an individual with respiratory alkalosis.

▶ OVERVIEW

Respiratory alkalosis is characterized by a pH greater than 7.45 and a $PaCO_2$ of less than 35 mmHg. It is always caused by **hyperventilation** (unusually fast respirations, or overbreathing), leading to a carbon dioxide deficit.

▶ PATHOPHYSIOLOGY AND ETIOLOGY

In acute respiratory alkalosis, the pH rises rapidly as the $PaCO_2$ falls. Because the kidneys are unable to adapt rapidly to the change in pH, the bicarbonate level remains within normal limits. Anxiety-based hyperventilation is the most common cause of acute respiratory alkalosis. Other physiological causes of hyperventilation include high fever, hypoxia, gram-negative bacteremia, and thyrotoxicosis (excessive amounts of thyroid hormones). Early salicylate intoxication (aspirin overdose), encephalitis, and high progesterone levels in pregnancy directly stimulate the respiratory center, potentially leading to hyperventilation and respiratory alkalosis. Hyperventilation also can occur during anesthesia and mechanical ventilation if the rate and tidal volume (depth) of ventilation are excessive.

If hyperventilation continues, the kidneys compensate by eliminating bicarbonate to restore the ratio of bicarbonate to carbonic acid. The bicarbonate level is lower than normal in chronic respiratory alkalosis, and the pH may be close to the normal range.

Alkalosis increases binding of extracellular calcium to albumin, reducing ionized calcium levels. As a result, neuromuscular excitability increases, and manifestations similar to hypocalcemia develop. Low carbon dioxide levels in the blood cause vasoconstriction of cerebral vessels, increasing the neurological manifestations of the disorder.

Risk Factors

Anxiety with hyperventilation is the most common cause of respiratory alkalosis; therefore anxiety disorders increase the risk for this acid–base imbalance. In the client who is critically ill, mechanical ventilation is a risk factor for respiratory alkalosis if breaths per minute or peak pressures are set too high for the client's needs.

▶ CLINICAL MANIFESTATIONS

The manifestations of respiratory alkalosis include light-headedness, a feeling of panic and difficulty concentrating, circumoral and distal extremity paresthesias (numbness or tingling), tremors, and positive Chvostek sign (a type of facial spasm, usually indicative of hypocalcemia) and Trousseau sign (a spasm of the hand and forearm). The client also may experience tinnitus, a sensation of chest tightness, and palpitations (cardiac dysrhythmias). Seizures and loss of consciousness may occur.

ABGs generally show a pH greater than 7.45 and a $PaCO_2$ of less than 35 mmHg. In chronic hyperventilation, there is a compensatory decrease in serum bicarbonate to less than 24 mEq/L, and the pH may be near normal.

▶ COLLABORATION

Management of respiratory alkalosis focuses on correcting the imbalance and treating the underlying cause. It is important to create a calm, quiet, low-stimulation environment to reduce the client's anxiety or panic. ABGs must be ordered prior to administration of medications or oxygen therapy.

Pharmacologic Therapy

A sedative or antianxiety agent may be necessary to relieve anxiety and restore a normal breathing pattern. Additional drugs may be ordered to correct underlying problems other than anxiety-induced hyperventilation.

Respiratory Therapy

Historically, use of paper bags has been a recommended treatment for hyperventilation. While use of paper bags helps to raise carbon dioxide levels in clients with true hyperventilation syndrome, it can also cause hypoxia. Other diseases can mimic hyperventilation (such as myocardial infarction), and hypoxia induced by the use of a paper bag will cause further cellular damage (Cho, 2013). Elevated carbon dioxide levels have been found to trigger panic attacks, which can further exacerbate hyperventilation. The best treatment for suspected hyperventilation is to teach breathing exercises, encouraging the client to take slow, regular breaths.

Clinical Manifestations and Therapies **Respiratory Alkalosis**

ETIOLOGY	CLINICAL MANIFESTATIONS	CLINICAL THERAPIES
Hyperventilation due to	Dizziness	▪ Monitor vital signs, LOC, and ABGs.
▪ Extreme anxiety	Numbness and tingling around mouth, hands, and feet	▪ Encourage client to breathe more slowly; teach breathing and stress reduction techniques.
▪ Elevated body temperature	Palpitations	▪ Administer sedative or antianxiety agent as ordered.
▪ Overventilation with a mechanical ventilator	Dyspnea	▪ Monitor ventilator settings.
▪ Hypoxia	Chest tightness	▪ Administer oxygen as ordered.
▪ Salicylate overdose	Anxiety/panic	▪ Maintain fluid status.
▪ Brain stem injury	Tremors	
▪ Fever	Tetany	
▪ Increased basal metabolic rate	Seizures, loss of consciousness	

◼ NURSING PROCESS

Nursing care is focused on reducing anxiety through manipulation of the environment to reduce stimuli and to create a sense of peace. This restful environment will help the client breathe more slowly and effectively.

Assessment

▪ *Health history.* Anxiety disorders; the triggering event for the onset of hyperventilation; mental health disorders; coping mechanisms; support systems available to the client.

▪ *Physical examination.* Breath sounds; neurological function; respiratory and cardiac status; any changes in LOC

Diagnosis

Possible nursing diagnoses for the client with respiratory alkalosis include the following:

▪ *Ineffective Breathing Pattern*
▪ *Anxiety*
▪ *Risk for Injury*

(NANDA-I © 2012)

Planning

Planning for the client with respiratory alkalosis involves identification and treatment of its underlying cause and the restoration of acid–base balance. Appropriate outcomes include resolution of the underlying cause and that the client will

▪ Manifest normal respiratory rate and rhythm.
▪ Maintain safety.
▪ Maintain appropriate fluid status.

Implementation

The usual cause of hyperventilation and respiratory alkalosis is psychological, although physiological disorders also can lead to hyperventilation. It is important not only to address the hyperventilation but also to identify the underlying cause.

▪ Assess respiratory rate, depth, and ease. Monitor vital signs (including temperature) and skin color. Assessment data can help identify the underlying cause, such as a fever or hypoxia.

▪ Obtain subjective assessment data such as the circumstances leading up to the current situation, current health and recent illnesses or medication use, and current manifestations. Subjective data provide clues to the cause and circumstances of the hyperventilation response.

▪ Reassure the client that the symptoms do not indicate a heart attack and that will resolve when breathing returns to normal. Manifestations of hyperventilation and respiratory alkalosis such as dyspnea, chest tightness or pain, and palpitations can mimic those of a heart attack.

▪ Instruct the client to maintain eye contact and breathe with you to slow the respiratory rate. These measures help make the client aware of respirations and provide a sense of support and control (Ackley & Ladwig, 2011). Be aware that some clients are uncomfortable making eye contact for cultural reasons.

▪ Protect the client from injury. If hyperventilation continues to the point where the client loses consciousness, respirations will return to normal, as will acid–base balance.

▪ Refer for counseling a client who has experienced repeated episodes of hyperventilation or who has a chronic anxiety disorder. Counseling can help the client develop alternative strategies for dealing with anxiety.

Planning and teaching for home care are directed toward the underlying cause of hyperventilation. If anxiety precipitated the episode, discuss anxiety and stress management strategies with the client. Teach the client how to identify a hyperventilation reaction and provide self-care, and when to seek medical intervention.

Evaluation

The evaluation of care is based on the client's ability to meet goals set during the planning stage and the outcomes achieved. Nursing care is reformulated as needed if outcomes are not met.

Expected outcomes for the client with respiratory alkalosis include the following:

- Client experiences no subsequent episodes of hyperventilation.
- Client describes strategies for coping with anxiety in the future.

- Family displays ability to contribute to calming client during times of anxiety.
- Client and/or family participate in support groups that will help the client cope with an anxiety disorder.

REVIEW Respiratory Alkalosis

RELATE Link the Concepts and Exemplars

Linking the exemplar of respiratory alkalosis with the concept of oxygenation:

1. Why is oxygenation often a concern when dealing with a client with respiratory alkalosis?
2. For the mechanically ventilated client, what ventilator settings need to be adjusted if the ABGs returned demonstrate respiratory alkalosis?

Linking the exemplar of respiratory alkalosis with the concept of anxiety:

3. What would be an expected outcome for a client with hyperventilation syndrome?
4. What occurs if the client loses consciousness from hyperventilation related to anxiety?

Linking the exemplar of respiratory alkalosis with the concept of safety:

5. What would be the nurse's specific concerns regarding safety for a client with respiratory alkalosis?

6. What safety precautions might the nurse employ to prevent injury to the client with respiratory alkalosis related to hyperventilation caused by anxiety?

READY Go to Companion Skills Manual

REFER Go to Pearson Nursing Student Resources
nursing.pearsonhighered.com

- Additional review questions

REFLECT Case Study

Reread Case Study D on page 13. The respiratory therapist made changes to Ms. Hernandez's ventilator. A half hour after the ventilator changes were made, the ABG values were pH 7.42, $PaCO_2$ 35 mmHg, PaO_2 100 mmHg, and HCO_3 24 mEq/L.

1. What is the interpretation of the arterial blood gas results?
2. Why is it important to wait 20–30 minutes after making ventilator changes to draw ABGs?
3. Refer to the concept of Oxygenation. What are some signs that Ms. Hernandez is ready to be weaned from the ventilator?

■ REFERENCES

Ackley, B. J., & Ladwig, G. B. (2011). *Nursing diagnosis handbook: A guide to planning care* (10th ed.). St. Louis, MO: Mosby.Berman, A., & Kozier, B. (Eds.). (2011). *Kozier & Erb's fundamentals of nursing: Concepts, process, and practice* (9th ed.). Upper Saddle River, NJ: Pearson Prentice Hall.

Cho, K. C. (2013). Electrolyte and acid–base disorders. In M. A. Papadakis, S. J. McPhee, M. W. Rabow (Eds.), *Current medical diagnosis and treatment 2013*. Retrieved

January 20, 2013 from http://www.accessmedicine.com/content.aspx?aID=10909.

Feller-Kopman, D. J., & Schwartzstein, R. M. (2012). Use of oxygen in patients with hypercapnia. *UpToDate*. Retrieved from http://www.uptodate.com/contents/use-of-oxygen-in-patients-with-hypercapnia.

Metheny, N. M. (2009). *Fluid and electrolyte balance: Nursing considerations* (5th ed.). Philadelphia, PA: Lippincott Williams & Wilkins.

Porth, C. M., & Matfin, G. (2009). *Pathophysiology: Concepts of altered health states* (8th ed.). Philadelphia, PA: Lippincott Williams & Wilkins.

Stedman, T. L. (2011). *Stedman's medical dictionary for the health professions and nursing* (7th ed.). Philadelphia, PA: Lippincott Williams & Wilkins.

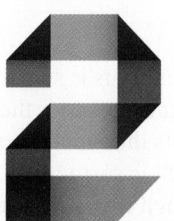 # Cellular Regulation

MODULE AT-A-GLANCE

THE CONCEPT OF CELLULAR REGULATION

The cell is the basic unit of life and the working unit of all living systems. Although life begins with just a single cell, by adulthood, nearly 75 trillion cells combine to form the human body (Roberts, 2010). The body's many types of specialized cells function differently depending on their location. For example, pancreatic cells have a very different function than nerve cells. All cells share common features, such as a nucleus containing 46 chromosomes and organelles such as mitochondria.

Cell reproduction, proliferation, and growth are regulated by the body. Alterations in cellular regulation can have devastating consequences for body tissues and functions. This concept and its exemplars provide essential information about the nature of the alterations, risk factors, clinical manifestations, and interventions and treatment options. The exemplars that follow discuss selected alterations in greater detail. **<<**

Concept Learning Outcomes

After reading about this concept, you will be able to:

1. Summarize the physiology of the hematological system related to cellular regulation.

2. Examine the relationship between cellular regulation and other concepts/systems.

3. Identify commonly occurring alterations in cellular regulation and their related therapies.

4. Differentiate common assessment procedures used to examine cellular regulation across the life span.

5. Describe diagnostic and laboratory tests to determine the individual's cellular regulation status.

6. Explain management of cellular regulation and prevention of alterations in cellular regulation.

7. Demonstrate the nursing process in providing culturally competent and caring interventions across the life span for individuals with common alterations in cellular regulation.

8. Compare and contrast common independent and collaborative interventions for clients with alterations in cellular regulation.

Concept Key Terms

Anaplasia, *32*

Autosomes, *31*

Cell cycle, *32*

Chromosomes, *31*

Deoxyribonucleic acid (DNA), *30*

Differentiation, *32*

Dysplasia, *32*

Genome, *31*

Homologous chromosomes, *31*

Hyperplasia, *32*

Meiosis, *32*

Metaplasia, *32*

Mitosis, *32*

Ribonucleic acid (RNA), *30*

Sex chromosomes, *31*

Somatic cells, *32*

▶ NORMAL CELLULAR REGULATION

Practically all of the cells in the human body are microscopic. Although often called building blocks, cells are not brick-shaped objects. They can be flat, round, threadlike, or irregularly shaped. Cells vary greatly in size, shape, and function, but they all share certain common features. Any change in or disturbance to one or more of these common features can result in abnormal cell development or replication. To understand alterations in cellular function, nurses must first understand the common characteristics of cells.

Physiology Review

Exploration of cellular regulation begins with a discussion of the cell, which is the site of numerous metabolic and regulatory processes.

CELL MEMBRANE   Every cell, regardless of its shape or function, must have a cell membrane in order to maintain its integrity and survive. The membrane is a defined boundary that possesses a definite shape and holds the cell contents together. The cell membrane acts as a protective covering and is responsible for allowing materials in and out of the cell.

The cell membrane, however, allows only certain things to move in or out of the cell. Because the membrane determines what may pass through, it is a selectively permeable (or semipermeable) membrane. Substances are transported across cell membrane in various ways (**Table 2–1 ●**).

The cell membrane also has identification markers to show that it comes from a specific individual. If a foreign cell shows up (e.g., in a transplanted organ), the body signals an attack on that cell or group of cells.

CYTOPLASM   Inside the cell is a watery soup of proteins, nucleic acids, gases, salts, and other substances that are essential for life. This internal environment of the cell, known as the cytoplasm, must be maintained in balance in order for the cell to survive.

NUCLEUS AND NUCLEOLUS   The nucleus is sometimes described as the brain of the cell. Within the nucleus is the biological "software" that regulates and directs the activities of the organelles in the cell. The nucleus of a cell is surrounded by a double-walled nuclear membrane. Although this membrane is composed of two layers, it has large pores that allow certain materials to pass in and out.

Chromatin is tightly wound into bundles called chromosomes and is the material found in the nucleus that contains **deoxyribonucleic acid (DNA)**. Coded into DNA are instructions that determine the individual's inherited characteristics, such as hair and eye color, as well as the production of every protein needed by the body. These instructions are called *genes*.

The nucleolus, a spherical body made up of dense fibers, is found within the cell nucleus. Its major function is to synthesize the **ribonucleic acid (RNA)** that forms ribosomes.

Centrosomes are tubular structures usually found in pairs in the nucleus. They contain centrioles, which are involved in cell division.

RIBOSOMES   Ribosomes are organelles found on the endoplasmic reticulum or floating around in the cytoplasm. Ribosomes are made of RNA and assist in the production of enzymes and other proteins needed for cell repair and reproduction.

ENDOPLASMIC RETICULUM   The endoplasmic reticulum is a series of channels set up in the cytoplasm; these channels are formed from folded membranes. The endoplasmic reticulum has two distinct forms. The rough endoplasmic reticulum, which has a sandpaper-like appearance due to the ribosomes on its surface, is responsible for the synthesis of protein. Once the protein is synthesized, it is sent to the Golgi apparatus for processing. The

TABLE 2–1	Methods of Cellular Transportation
CELLULAR TRANSPORTATION METHODS	DESCRIPTION
Passive Transportation (no energy required)	
Diffusion	Movement of a substance from an area of high concentration to an area of low concentration
Facilitated diffusion	Movement of a substance that is assisted via a "revolving door" in the direction it was already traveling, from an area of high concentration to an area of low concentration
Osmosis	Movement of water across a membrane from an area that has a low concentration of a solute to an area that has a higher concentration until the concentration is the same on both sides of the membrane
Filtration	Application of pressure to force water and dissolved materials across a membrane
Active Transport (energy required)	
Active transport pumps	A method that requires additional energy (in the form of adenosine triphosphate) to move substances against the concentration gradient (from low concentration to high concentration)
Endocytosis	Ingestion of substances that are too large to diffuse across the cell membrane
Phagocytosis	Form of endocytosis in which solid particles are brought into the cell via vesicles
Pinocytosis	Form of endocytosis in which liquid is brought into the cell via vesicles
Exocytosis	Transportation of material outside of the cell

smooth endoplasmic reticulum has no ribosomes on its surface, making it appear smooth. This endoplasmic reticulum synthesizes lipids (fats) and steroids.

MITOCHONDRIA   Mitochondria are tiny, bean-shaped organelles that act as the cell's power plant, providing up to 95% of the body's energy needs for cellular repair, movement, and reproduction. Special enzymes in the mitochondria help to take in oxygen and turn it into energy.

GOLGI APPARATUS   The Golgi apparatus looks like a bunch of flattened, membranous sacs. Once a protein is received from the endoplasmic reticulum, a portion of the Golgi apparatus envelops the protein, which is pinched off and moved to the cell membrane to be released or secreted. The cells of organs with a high level of secretion or storage, such as the digestive system, contain a larger Golgi apparatus. Salivary glands and pancreatic glands, for example, are made of cells containing a large Golgi apparatus.

LYSOSOMES   Lysosomes are vesicles containing powerful enzymes that clean up intercellular debris and other waste. They also aid in maintaining health by destroying unwanted bacteria through the process of phagocytosis (process by which microorganisms and cellular debris are engulfed and destroyed).

Genetic and Lifespan Considerations

As with many disorders and diseases, certain factors predispose an individual for the development of alterations in cellular regulation. Even before birth, certain genetic processes are already at work in determining whether any number of alterations will be present.

DNA AND GENES   New developments in research seek to provide treatment to the individual client based on genetic components specific to the client's cellular makeup and disease characteristics. While knowledge of the cell, DNA, cell division, chromosomes, and genes has always been important for nurses, it is becoming more essential as the nursing profession begins to deliver a genetic standard of care to the adult client (**Figure 2–1 ●**).

All human cells except mature red blood cells contain a complete set of DNA molecules. DNA molecules consist of long sequences of nucleotides, or bases, represented by the letters A, G, T, and C. The order of these bases dictates the exact instructions for the functioning of that particular cell. Writing the correct order of the bases using A, G, T, and C represents the sequence of the bases in DNA. All of the DNA in a human cell is referred to as the human **genome**, or the complete set of inheritance for an individual. The human genome includes the DNA in the cell nucleus as well as the DNA in the mitochondria. Each individual's genome is unique.

The cell nucleus contains about 6 feet of DNA that is tightly wound and packaged into 23 pairs of **chromosomes** (threadlike strands of DNA in the cell that carry the genes), making a complete set of 46 chromosomes. The structure and number of chromosomes can be shown by a karyotype, or picture, of an individual's chromosomes. There are two copies of each chromosome. One copy, or half of the complete set of these

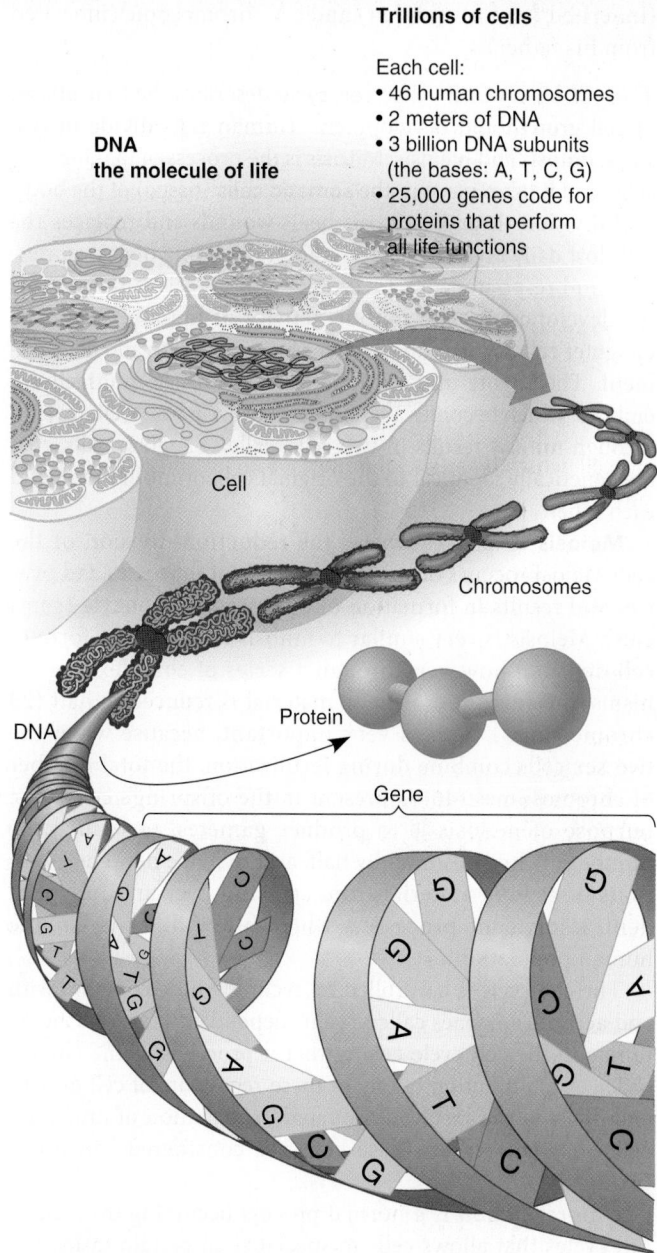

Trillions of cells

Each cell:
• 46 human chromosomes
• 2 meters of DNA
• 3 billion DNA subunits (the bases: A, T, C, G)
• 25,000 genes code for proteins that perform all life functions

DNA the molecule of life

Cell

Chromosomes

DNA

Protein

Gene

Figure 2–1 ● Each cell nucleus throughout the body contains the genes, DNA, and chromosomes that make up the majority of an individual's genome. The remaining portion of the human genome is in the mitochondria.

46 chromosomes, is inherited from the mother, and the other copy, or the other half of the 46 chromosomes, is inherited from the father. For example, an individual will have two of chromosome 1 (one inherited from the mother and one inherited from the father). These two copies or pairs of inherited chromosomes are called **homologous chromosomes**.

Chromosomes are numbered according to size, with chromosome 1 being the largest and chromosome 22 being the smallest. The first 22 pairs of chromosomes, known as **autosomes**, are alike in males and females. The 23rd pair, the **sex chromosomes**, determines an individual's gender. A female has two copies of the X chromosomes (one copy inherited from each parent), and a male has one X chromosome (inherited from his mother) and a Y chromosome (inherited from his father).

THE CELL CYCLE   The **cell cycle** describes the four phases of cell growth and development. Human cells divide in two ways, mitosis and meiosis. **Mitosis** is the process of making new cells, and it takes place in the **somatic cells** (tissue) of the body. Cell division through mitosis heals wounds and replaces the cells lost daily on skin surfaces and in the lining of gastrointestinal and respiratory tracts. In addition, mitosis is responsible for development. The mitotic activity of the zygote and its daughter cells is the foundation for human growth and development. The zygote undergoes mitosis to form a multicellular embryo, which becomes a fetus and then an infant. Cell division through mitosis results in two cells, called daughter cells, that are genetically identical to the original cell, or mother cell, and each other.

Meiosis is also known as the reduction division of the cell. Meiosis occurs only in the sex cells of the testes and ovaries and results in formation of the sperm and oocyte (gametes). Meiosis is very similar to mitosis in that it is a form of cell division; however, through a series of complex mechanisms, the amount of genetic material is reduced in half (23 chromosomes). This is very important, because when the two sex cells combine during fertilization, the total number of chromosomes (46) is present in the offspring's cells. The purpose of meiosis is to produce gametes, to reduce the number of chromosomes by half, and to make new combinations of genetic material from crossing-over and independent assortment processes, which allow diversity in the human population.

The cell cycle is controlled by cyclins, which combine with and activate enzymes called cyclin-dependent kinases. Checkpoints in the cell cycle ensure that it proceeds in the correct order. A malfunction of any of these regulators of cell growth and division can result in the rapid proliferation of immature cells. In some cases, these cells are considered cancerous (malignant).

Differentiation is a normal process occurring over many cell cycles that allows cells to specialize in certain tasks. For example, some epithelial cells lining the lungs develop into tall columnar cells with cilia. These columnar cells sweep potentially dangerous debris out of the lungs. When adverse conditions occur in body tissues during differentiation, protective adaptations can produce alterations in cells. Some of these alterations are helpful, but in other cases, the cells mutate beyond usefulness and become liabilities (Porth & Matfin, 2010).

▶ ALTERATIONS TO CELLULAR REGULATION

A number of potentially undesirable cellular alterations can occur during cell differentiation. These include the following:

- **Hyperplasia** is an increase in the number or density of normal cells. Hyperplasia occurs in response to stress, increased metabolic demands, or elevated levels of hormones. Exam-

ples include the hyperplasia of myocardial cells in response to a prolonged increase in the body's demand for oxygen, and hyperplasia of uterine cells in response to rising levels of estrogen during pregnancy. Hyperplastic cells are under normal DNA control.

- **Metaplasia** is a change in the normal pattern of differentiation such that dividing cells differentiate into cell types not normally found at that location in the body. The metaplastic cell is normal for its particular type, but it is not in its normal location. Some metaplastic cells are less functional than the cells they replace. Metaplasia is a protective response to adverse conditions, often the result of inflammation. Metaplastic cells are under normal DNA control and are reversible when the stressor or other disruptive condition ceases. An example of metaplasia often occurs in the lungs of smokers where normal columnar ciliated epithelium may be replaced by a squamous stratified epithelium known as squamous metaplasia (Wang et al., 2010).

- **Dysplasia** represents a loss of DNA control over differentiation occurring in response to adverse conditions. Dysplastic cells show abnormal variations in size, shape, and appearance and a disturbance in their usual arrangement. Examples of dysplasia include changes in the cervix in response to continued irritation, such as from the human papillomavirus, or leukoplakia on oral mucous membranes in response to chronic irritation from smoking.

- **Anaplasia** is the regression of a cell to an immature or undifferentiated cell type. Anaplastic cell division is no longer under DNA control. Anaplasia usually occurs when a damaging or transforming event takes place inside the dividing, still undifferentiated cell, leading to loss of useful function. Anaplasia may occur in response to overwhelmingly destructive conditions inside the cell or in surrounding tissue (Porth & Matfin, 2010). It is often associated with malignancies and is one of the criteria used to grade the aggressiveness of cancer cells.

Although hyperplasia, metaplasia, and dysplasia often reverse after the irritating factor is eliminated, they can lead to malignancy under certain conditions. This is especially true of dysplasia, which represents a loss of DNA control. Anaplasia is not reversible, and the degree of anaplasia determines the potential risk for cancer.

Any one of these alterations in cellular regulation has the potential to become cancerous or cause any one of many disorders that can compromise client health. The most common of these are cancer, anemia, sickle cell disease, leukemia, and polycythemia (see the Alterations and Therapies table and the exemplars that follow). Others you may see, such as endometriosis and HIV, are discussed in other modules.

Although the human body's numerous systems can be studied individually, no system is truly isolated. Instead, the function of one body system can greatly affect the function of one or more other body systems. Likewise, psychosocial factors can impact a number of body systems and physiological processes. For more information on how the concepts are integrated, see Concepts Related to Cellular Regulation.

Alterations and Therapies **Cellular Regulation**

ALTERATION	DESCRIPTION	MANIFESTATIONS	INTERVENTIONS AND THERAPIES
Cancer (e.g., breast, colon, lung, ovarian, prostate, and testicular)	Abnormal and rapid growth of body cells that may invade surrounding body tissues and spread (metastasize) to other sites	Variable, depending on the location and size of the growth, as well as on whether other tissues and organs are affected. Surrounding blood vessels and organs may also be affected, producing varying effects. General signs and symptoms may include lethargy, fever, and weight loss (American Cancer Society [ACS], 2012e).	■ Identify and treat the affected organ(s) and/or tissue(s). Conventional treatments may include chemotherapy, radiation, and surgical removal of the affected organ/tissue. Alternative treatments may include relaxation therapy, guided imagery, and certain homeopathic supplements.
Anemia (e.g., aplastic, hemolytic, and iron deficiency)	Deficiency of hemoglobin or reduction of number of red blood cells (RBCs) that leads to inadequate delivery of oxygenation to cells, tissues, and organs. May also be caused by blood loss, impaired RBC production, or excessive RBC destruction.	Variable, depending on the underlying cause. General signs and symptoms may include lethargy, pallor, dyspnea, dizziness, and confusion.	■ Identify and treat the underlying cause. Medical interventions may include blood transfusions and surgical measures to stop internal bleeding. Nutritional supplements may include iron (for treatment of iron deficiency anemia) and folate or vitamin B_{12} (for treatment of anemia due to vitamin deficiency). ■ When possible, aplastic anemia is treated through elimination of the known cause. Pharmacologic treatments may include medications that induce RBC production, such as erythropoietin and colony-stimulating factors. Other treatments include blood and marrow stem cell transplants (National Heart, Lung, and Blood Institute [NHLBI], 2012a).
Leukemia	Form of cancer in which abnormal and rapid formation of white blood cells (WBCs) leads to circulation of increased numbers of abnormal, immature WBCs	Fatigue, pallor, weight loss, bruising, unusual bleeding, recurrent infections, joint or bone pain, weakness	■ Varies depending on type of leukemia, client age, and other factors. Conventional treatments may include chemotherapy, radiation, biological therapy, bone marrow transplantation (BMT), and surgical removal of the spleen (splenectomy) (Mayo Clinic, 2012c). Alternative treatments may include relaxation therapy, guided imagery, and certain homeopathic supplements.

(continued on next page)

Alterations and Therapies **Cellular Regulation** (continued)

ALTERATION	DESCRIPTION	MANIFESTATIONS	INTERVENTIONS AND THERAPIES
Sickle cell disease	Inherited alteration of hemoglobin (Hgb S) that results in deformed (sickle-shaped) RBCs	Trapping of deformed RBCs in blood vessels may cause vascular occlusion, leading to reduced or blocked blood flow to organs and tissues. Symptoms may include anemia, pain, recurrent infections, growth retardation. In infants, hand-foot syndrome (swollen hands and feet due to blockage of blood flow) may be the first sign of this disorder (Mayo Clinic, 2012d).	■ Supplemental oxygen, IV fluids (for hydration), and analgesics may be administered during an acute crisis. Long-term management may include RBC transfusion therapy. General pharmacologic management may include antibiotics and immunizations for infection prevention (Pack-Mabien, 2009). Hydroxyurea may be administered to stimulate production of fetal hemoglobin (which appears to help prevent the formation of sickle cells) (Mayo Clinic, 2012d).
Polycythemia	Abnormal increase in the production of erythrocytes (RBCs) leading to increased blood viscosity	Increased coagulability of blood, leading to increased risks for injury, including myocardial infarction (MI), cerebrovascular accident, and heart failure (Mayo Clinic, 2012b)	■ Phlebotomy (to reduce RBC count) ■ Hydration with IV fluids. Hydroxyurea may be administered to decrease RBC and platelet production. Aspirin may be administered for analgesia and to reduce blood coagulability (Mayo Clinic, 2012b).

Prevalence

Although disorders of cellular regulation affect millions throughout the world, certain populations tend to be more susceptible to certain disorders.

CANCER According to the National Cancer Institute, on January 1, 2009, the United States was home to more than 12.5 million survivors of some form of cancer. This population was comprised of more women (6,742,240) than men (5,811,097). Although the age of onset varies for different forms of cancer, of the men and woman born today, an estimated 41.24% will be diagnosed with cancer at some point in their lives (Howlader et al., 2012).

Stay Current: *For current statistics related to the prevalence of cancer, visit the National Cancer Institute's Web site at* **http://seer.cancer.gov/faststats**.

ANEMIA As opposed to being a primary disease, anemia is the result of an underlying pathological process. For this reason, the prevalence of anemia depends on its cause. Most often, this condition is linked to blood loss, impaired production of RBCs, or increased destruction of RBCs (Osborn et al., 2013), all of which will be discussed in greater detail in the exemplar on Anemia.

SICKLE CELL DISEASE An estimated 70,000 to 100,000 people in the United States are affected by sickle cell disease (NHLBI, 2012b). Although its prevalence is greater among Blacks/African Americans, development of this disorder is not limited to these populations. Throughout the world, sickle cell disease affects millions of people from a variety of cultural backgrounds. However, this condition is more prevalent among those whose ancestral origins include Africa, South or Central America, the Caribbean, Saudi Arabia, India, and certain Mediterranean regions (NHLBI, 2012b).

Genetic Considerations and Nonmodifiable Risk Factors

CANCER According to the National Cancer Institute (NCI) (2013c), certain forms of cancer may have a genetic component. For example, skin cancer (melanoma), ovarian cancer, breast cancer, and cancers of the prostate and colon tend to occur more commonly in some families. Regardless of genetics, for all forms of cancer, socioeconomic factors have a major impact. In general, a low socioeconomic status and lack of healthcare coverage are associated with an increased risk for developing cancer (U.S. Department of Health and Human Services, 2011).

ANEMIA Genetic considerations and nonmodifiable risk factors for anemia depend on the underlying cause of the disorder. For example, because of menstruation, women are at greater risk for development of anemia that results from blood loss. Considerations related to some of the more common forms of anemia are discussed in the exemplar on Anemia.

SICKLE CELL DISEASE The development of sickle cell disease depends entirely on genetics. People with this disease are born with two sickle hemoglobin genes, one gene coming from each parent. If only one sickle hemoglobin gene is inherited, the individual has a condition called sickle cell trait. Although people with sickle cell trait do not have sickle cell disease, they may pass the sickle hemoglobin gene to their offspring (NHLBI, 2012b).

Concepts Related to **Cellular Regulation**

To illustrate this concept, consider the impact of the body's inflammatory response on the activity of white blood cells (WBCs). In a healthy individual, any type of trauma can trigger the inflammatory process, causing a number of responses at the cellular level. (For a detailed discussion of the inflammatory process, see the module on Inflammation.) One response to trauma involves the recruitment of WBCs to the site of the injury. At the injury site, WBCs fight infection, increase blood flow to the injured area, and even summon additional WBCs to the site.

Infection, which can result from the introduction of bacteria, viruses, fungi, or other foreign substances into the body, activates the body's immune response. As with inflammation, infection also causes an increase in WBC production.

To further explore the relationships between concepts, consider the effects of oxidative stress (OS), which is the body's physiological response to both external and internal stress factors. OS occurs when the body is unable to adequately manage or neutralize molecules called *free radicals* (Osborn et al., 2013). A number of factors can lead to the production of free radicals. For example, free radicals may be end products of food breakdown. They also may be produced when the body is exposed to certain environmental toxins, such as radiation and tobacco smoke (MedlinePlus, 2013a). Psychosocial factors, such as anxiety disorders and depression, may also cause OS (Bouayed, Rammal, & Soulimani, 2009). In turn, research suggests the cellular damage caused by OS is linked to a number of disorders and diseases, including cancer, diabetes, and Alzheimer disease (Roberts & Sindhu, 2009). The relationship between OS and disease development reflects the relationship between the concepts of Stress and Coping and Cellular Regulation.

CONCEPT	RELATIONSHIP TO CELLULAR REGULATION	NURSING IMPLICATIONS
Inflammation		
■ The inflammatory process ■ Stages of inflammation ■ Mediators of inflammation	Trauma → activation of inflammatory response → recruitment of WBCs to site of injury and increased WBC production	■ Assess for signs and symptoms of inflammation, including redness and swelling. Be aware that fever may accompany inflammatory processes, even in the absence of infection. ■ Anticipate administration of anti-inflammatory medications, possible application of ice to inflamed area, and, if possible, elevation of injured site. ■ Be aware that an increased WBC count may indicate an inflammatory process, infection, or a combination of both.
Infection		
■ Types of infections ■ Chain of infection ■ Stages of infectious process ■ Prevention	Introduction of bacteria, viruses, fungi, or foreign substances → activation of immune response → increased production of WBCs	■ Assess for signs and symptoms of infection, including redness, swelling, and draining from the injured site. Be aware that fever often accompanies infectious processes. ■ Anticipate potential need for blood and/or wound cultures and administration of antibiotics. ■ Antipyretics may also be indicated. ■ Be aware that increased WBC count may indicate an inflammatory process, infection, or a combination of both.
Stress and Coping		
■ Stressors and the coping process ■ Manifestations of stress ■ Alterations from normal coping responses	Physical and/or emotional stress → oxidative stress (OS) → production of free radicals → increased risk for development of diseases and disorders	■ Assess psychosocial factors that impact the client. ■ Recognize the potential health effects of physical and emotional stressors. ■ Anticipate the need for client teaching related to coping and relaxation. When indicated, referral to other healthcare professionals may be appropriate for both disease prevention and health promotion.

CASE STUDY \\ PART 1

Andrew, an 8-year-old Native American male, is brought to the emergency department (ED) by his mother. On arrival, Andrew is pressing a bloody towel against his nose. As the triage nurse, you direct the boy and his mother to the assessment station. Andrew's mother explains that Andrew's nose began bleeding "about an hour ago" during a baseball tournament. Andrew denies any traumatic injury and his mother reports that her son's game had not yet begun when the bleeding began. Andrew appears to be in no acute distress. His respiratory rate is 28 breaths per minute, and his respirations are regular and not labored. Andrew's pulse rate is 136, which is elevated. As you apply a blood pressure cuff to Andrew's arm, you notice light, scattered bruising along his forearm. His blood pressure is 118/71, which is slightly elevated. Although Andrew denies any additional complaints, during further exploration of his health status, his mother reports that her son has seemed "really tired lately" and that he "seems like he's been bruising very easily."

Clinical Reasoning Questions Level I

1. Considering your assessment of Andrew, which findings might suggest an alteration in cellular regulation?
2. Why might Andrew's blood pressure and pulse rate be elevated?
3. What is the relationship between bleeding and bruising?

Clinical Reasoning Questions Level II

4. At this time, presuming Andrew has lost a significant amount of blood, what is the priority nursing diagnosis for this client?
5. *Refer to the exemplar on Leukemia within this module.* Which blood test do you expect to be ordered for further assessment of Andrew's condition?

▶ PREVENTION

Although genetic factors play a part in the development of some illnesses caused by impaired cellular regulation, an individual's health is also affected by the many personal choices he or she makes. Wellness promotion and simple health practices can significantly affect the risk for developing disorders of cellular regulation.

Modifiable Risk Factors

Several important areas of client teaching address basic health practices that may help clients reduce their risk for certain cancers. Examples include the following:

1. *Have clients, especially children, increase intake of fruits and vegetables.* Most people do not eat enough of these foods, and increased intake is associated with lower rates of many cancers. Aim for a minimum of five servings daily.
2. *Encourage sunscreen use.* Early excessive exposure to sun and one or more severe sunburns during childhood increase chances of skin cancers developing in adulthood. Clients who work outdoors, athletes, coaches, and others who spend time outside regularly should use sunscreen daily, regardless of the climate in which they live.
3. *Discourage smoking* and emphasize the importance of protecting children from exposure to tobacco smoke.
4. *Have homes tested for radon.* Be alert for exposure to any potential hazardous substances in the home or on clients' clothes if they work in industries with chemicals or other harmful substances.

Screenings

When there is a familial history of cancer, encourage the family to learn more about the cancer and teach children to receive regular surveillance as they enter young adulthood. Inform adolescent and adult clients in all families about screenings, such as the Papanicolaou test, breast self-examination, and testicular examination, that can lead to early detection.

▶ ASSESSMENT

The assessment of the client with alterations in cellular regulation is highly dependent on the specific alteration and the organ systems involved. For example, when the alteration involves cells directly related to the transport of oxygen, an important assessment includes oxygenation and breathing patterns.

Ongoing assessment of all clients with alterations in cellular regulation includes assessment of stress and coping abilities and psychosocial supports. This includes assessing spouse, parent, and caregiver stress levels and coping abilities and how they are accessing support groups, financial resources, and spiritual and other supports.

Assessment of the client with cancer also includes assessment of the client's nutrition and hydration status. Please refer to the exemplar on Cancer, for a discussion of nutrition and hydration assessment.

Nursing Assessment

Because early intervention and treatment of cancer improve client outcomes, nurses should assess all clients for early warning signs of cancer and teach clients those signs to watch for and report. The early warning signs include change in bowel or bladder habits, a sore that does not heal, unusual bleeding or discharge, thickening or lump in the breast or elsewhere, indigestion or difficulty swallowing, obvious change in wart or mole, or a nagging cough or hoarseness (ACS, 2012e).

Clients with alterations in cellular function may commonly display activity intolerance, which can result in reduced activity, risk for injury, and alterations in skin integrity. Assessing activity tolerance, promoting safety, and helping the client remain as active as possible all play a role in the client's eventual outcome.

Developmental Assessment of Children

Assessment of the child's physical and neurological development helps in determining the progress made during treatment and provides a baseline for evaluating the long-term effects of treatment. Developmental assessment of children should be performed regularly during treatment for cancer, at times when the child feels well so that the results are accurate. Children under 6 years of age who have cancer should receive regular developmental assessment with a standardized tool such as the Denver II Developmental Screening Test (see the module on Development). Recommend referral to a neuropsychologist for testing early in treatment and if changes in developmental performance are noted. Observe developmental milestones at each contact with the child and refer for further assessment if regression is observed. Performance in school and social activities with friends provides important information about expected developmental milestones in older children.

Diagnostic Tests

Clients with disorders of cellular regulation may need diagnostic tests or procedures to assist in decision making and treatment. Useful tests may include the following:

- Biopsy
- Bone marrow aspiration
- Computed tomography or computed axial tomography
- Magnetic resonance imaging
- Positron-emission tomography
- Radiograph (x-ray)
- Scans
- Ultrasound
- Complete blood count (CBC)
- Red blood indices
- Serum chemistry panel
- Tumor markers
- Urinalysis
- Lumbar puncture.

CASE STUDY \\ PART 2

Andrew is admitted to the ED. During the ED physician's assessment, Andrew tells the physician he feels "a little short of breath," especially when he runs. Andrew's mother reports he has been treated for strep throat three times and has had several ear infections within the past 6 months. The physician orders a CBC with differential for Andrew. After the phlebotomist draws Andrew's blood, she has to apply pressure to the puncture site for nearly 2 minutes before the site stops bleeding. You return to check on Andrew's status. The physician tells you he suspects Andrew may have developed leukemia.

Clinical Reasoning Questions Level I

1. Which two components of the CBC will be most useful for evaluation of Andrew's shortness of breath with physical activity?
2. Based on Andrew's recurrent nosebleeds and his delayed clotting response after venipuncture, which particular blood component would you expect to be impaired?

3. Describe methods by which you could explain venipuncture to Andrew. How could you involve his mother when explaining the procedure?

Clinical Reasoning Questions Level II
Refer to the exemplar on Leukemia within this module.

4. If Andrew has developed leukemia, what results would you expect the CBC to reveal?
5. To further evaluate Andrew for leukemia, for which invasive diagnostic test might he be scheduled?
6. Explain the relationship between frequent/recurrent infections and leukemia.

▶ INTERVENTIONS AND THERAPIES

For the client with alterations in cellular regulation, nursing interventions focus on reducing complications and maintaining optimal homeostasis. Interventions common to clients with cellular alterations include those directed at nutrition, activity, breathing, fatigue, and comfort. Nurses also provide interventions and client teaching to help clients manage side effects and provide clients and their families with psychosocial support. These interventions are critical to the client's successful recovery.

Independent

For the client with impaired cellular regulation, independent nursing interventions include providing education about the disease and offering emotional support to the client and family members. In many cases, clients can greatly improve their health status by recognizing and avoiding situations that exacerbate their condition. In addition to teaching about the client's condition and treatments, the nurse should also focus on helping the client and family understand how to prevent complications.

PROVIDING PSYCHOSOCIAL SUPPORT   A diagnosis of cancer or sickle cell disease can create a whirlwind of emotions. Initially, family members may experience shock and anger. They need basic information about the disease and the purpose of the tests that will be performed. Instructions often need to be repeated because clients and family members may not process information the first time it is presented due to their increased stress levels. For pediatric clients, assist the parents to plan how and when to tell the child the diagnosis. What the child needs to know is based on his or her developmental level and understanding.

After progressing from the initial state of shock about the diagnosis, the family needs to learn more about the disease, including the pathophysiology, treatment, and expected outcome or the prognosis. Clarify the family's understanding of these areas and be ready to answer questions. Provide both verbal explanations and written material. Clients and family members may talk with friends, purchase books, or search the Internet for information. Find out where they are getting information and provide additional resources when appropriate. Correct misconceptions and misinformation. Knowing what to expect can help decrease anxiety.

As the client experiences remissions and exacerbations or complications, the family feels alternately hopeful and discouraged. Help the family to identify support systems, and intervene as needed to enhance these systems. Facilitate contact with extended family members who might be of help, faith-based or spiritual connections, social service agencies, and other resources such as the Internet and parent and caregiver support groups. Assist clients and caregivers who are concerned about job obligations and financial concerns.

Provide opportunities for clients to express thoughts and feelings. During this process, clients can disclose their fears. During these times, the nurse may simply listen, educate, or dispel fears that stem from lack of understanding. Suggest clients make use of area support groups and provide referrals as appropriate. Although sometimes clients are not ready to talk with others, sharing with others who have had similar experiences can reduce anxiety and provide much needed support.

Promoting Healthy Grieving   Clients with cancer and their families may experience anticipatory grieving. Clients who lose a body part or function experience great loss and will go through a grieving process. Nurses listen attentively to expressions of grief and watch for nonverbal cues (e.g., failure to make eye contact, crying, and silence). Not all clients will express grief clearly; sometimes unspoken grief is the most painful. Grief is relieved only when expressed in a nonthreatening environment.

Nurses can be helpful to clients and their families by explaining that it is normal to have periods of depression, anger, and denial after breast surgery. All these feelings are appropriate expressions of grief.

If the client wishes to do so, involve the partner in helping the client cope with her or his loss. Remember that the partner may also be grieving. Not all clients want to share their grief, and not all partners are interested and supportive.

Considerations for the Pediatric Client and Family
Support for the child with cancer and his or her family includes considering the impact on siblings. They may alternately resent and feel guilty about the sibling's illness. They may not understand the treatments or disease. School progress may be slowed and teachers may not be aware of the sibling's stress.

The child undergoing treatment for cancer needs support appropriate to his or her developmental stage and cognitive level (**Figure 2–2 ●**). (See the module on Development for developmental levels and effective support strategies for children of different ages.) Younger children primarily need support during painful procedures and separation from parents. Older children need intervention strategies to assist in working through feelings related to treatments (**Figure 2–3 ●**). A major developmental task of adolescence is to attain independence and control, but cancer often interferes with adolescents' ability to achieve this task. Therefore, plan nursing strategies that empower adolescents as much as possible. This might include

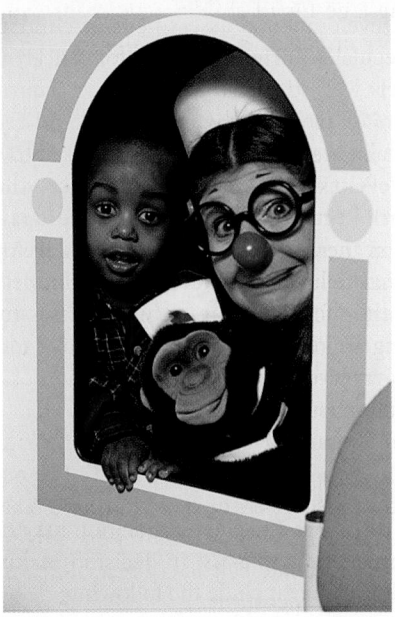

Figure 2–2 ● Clowns from the Big Apple Clown Care Unit can help to ease the stress of hospitalization for seriously ill children and their families. Here, a clown doctor and her puppet distract a toddler who is waiting for his clinic appointment.

asking them whether they prefer morning or afternoon appointments, being placed on a teen unit where they can receive treatments with other teens, and encouraging parents to allow them choices about issues at home.

Talk with the child's teachers before the return to school after treatment to explain the child's condition and assist with plans to prepare the other children. Role-play with the child how to tell friends about any changes in appearance. A nurse or child-life specialist could attend the class of a young child to explain what the child is experiencing. Arrange for tutors if necessary to assist the child with schoolwork during hospitalization and home care. Explore the option of summer camp for children with cancer. The Make-a-Wish Foundation strives to make

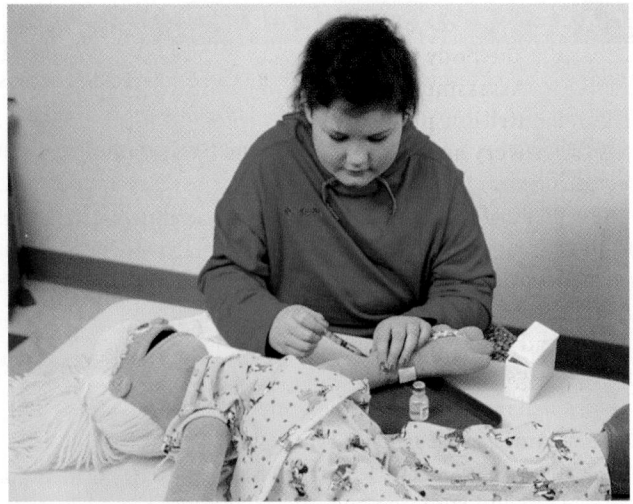

Figure 2–3 ● A child in a pediatric oncology clinic gives injections to a doll. This type of play therapy helps children deal with fear, thus lowering their stress level.

dreams come true for ill children by sponsoring them for a desired activity or outing. Refer the child to this foundation if appropriate.

PROMOTING BALANCED NUTRITION, ACTIVITY, AND REST   The high metabolic rate of cancer growth depletes the client's nutritional stores so that many clients are cachectic at the time of diagnosis. In addition, the catabolic effect of chemotherapy and radiation on normal cells necessitates additional cellular replacement. Nurses working with clients being treated for cancer promote healthy nutritional status by performing ongoing assessments, providing client teaching, and initiating interventions to improve nutrition and hydration. Client teaching about a well-rounded diet, including all of the macro- and micronutrients, is an important caring intervention (see the module on Nutrition). Along with balanced nutrition, the client should also be encouraged to seek a balance between activity and rest. Clients frequently report fatigue, and nurses can promote an adequate balance of rest, sleep, and activity in order to maintain homeostasis.

Stay Current: *For more information on nutrition in cancer care, go to the National Cancer Institute at* **www.cancer.gov/ cancertopics/pdq/supportivecare/nutrition/Patient/page1**.

Collaborative

Nurses will provide appropriate pain management interventions, both pharmacologic and nonpharmacologic, to clients experiencing discomfort as the result of rapid cellular reproduction (cancer) placing pressure on healthy cells or alterations in cellular function that may result in inadequate oxygenation of tissues (anemias). Clients with cancer who require surgery or radiation will require careful management related to these interventions. These requirements are discussed in the respective cancer exemplars and in the module on Perioperative Care. Clients with alterations in cellular regulation will require some assistance from members of the healthcare team in managing nutrition and hydration and managing treatment side effects.

NUTRITION AND HYDRATION   Cells cannot function properly if the body is not provided with all of the essential nutrients. Assessment of nutritional status and promotion of good nutrition play important roles in supporting the client's recovery as well as reducing the likelihood of cellular alterations.

The goals of nutrition therapy during treatment for cancer are to prevent or reverse any nutritional deficiencies, preserve the client's lean body mass, minimize any side effects that influence nutritional state, allow for the growth needs of pediatric clients, and improve overall quality of life. Administer antiemetic drugs to lessen nausea from chemotherapy. Offer frequent, small meals. It may be helpful to offer the client's favorite foods at times when nausea and vomiting are decreased. Ask family members what treatments they use to decrease the client's nausea and vomiting and inform them of techniques that may enhance intake. Perform 24-hour dietary recalls to assess the client's intake, and evaluate height and weight regularly. Special nutritional products may be given orally, nasogastric or

nasoduodenal tube feedings may be given, or total parenteral nutrition may be necessary. When the client's nutritional status is deteriorating or parenteral nutrition is used, perform weekly studies of serum electrolytes, liver chemistry, glucose, and triglycerides. Partner with both the oncologist and the dietitian to plan interventions appropriate for meeting the needs of individual clients.

Hydration management can be challenging, because the client may not be thirsty but is excreting large numbers of cell fragments and other substances as a result of treatment. Children in particular are at risk for dehydration due to a higher concentration of fluid within the body, Offer frequent, small amounts of fluid. Include frozen ice pops or other fluid-containing foods such as Jell-O, fruit, or soups. Caution should be taken to avoid citrus fruits because acidic foods can exacerbate complications of chemotherapy such as stomatitis. Measure intake and output. To ensure adequate excretion, a number of chemotherapy drugs are given with intravenous fluids. It is important to administer fluids as ordered and to ensure that the recommended urinary output excretion rate is maintained after drug administration.

MANAGE TREATMENT SIDE EFFECTS   All cancer treatments affect some normal body cells as well as cancer cells, causing a wide variety of side effects. Clients and their caregivers should be taught that some side effects may not develop until after therapy is completed. Emphasize the importance of all follow-up visits for monitoring of late effects.

A frequent occurrence is *myelosuppression* or suppression of blood cell production in the bone marrow. Suppression of the immune response may lead to increased susceptibility to infection. *Neutropenia* is present when the absolute neutrophil count (ANC) is less than 500 cells/mm^3 or if between 500 and 1,000 cells/mm^3 when chemotherapy is being given and falling levels are anticipated. At these levels, clients will be given a broad-spectrum antibiotic; granulocyte colony-stimulating factor (G-CSF) may be given. Take the client's temperature, isolate the client from others with infections, and perform serum laboratory studies as ordered.

Protect the client from bruises and be alert for hemorrhage or signs of bleeding such as petechiae, nosebleeds, dark-colored or bloody stools, and the presence of blood in vomit and urine, which may occur due to thrombocytopenia. The client may need to receive infusions of platelets if thrombocytopenia is severe. If thrombocytopenia develops, minimize needlesticks and other intrusive procedures. Report any bleeding episodes to the oncologist. Be sure parents and caregivers know that the client should avoid contact sports or other rough activities and that any healthcare provider, such as a dentist, should be informed of the client's treatment and condition.

PHARMACOLOGIC THERAPY   Pharmacologic therapies play an important role in treating alterations in cellular regulation. Because of the toxicity of antineoplastic medications, administration of chemotherapy often requires the nurse to obtain advanced training. Special gloves are worn to provide greater protection should the medication spill or splash during administration.

Medications Cellular Regulation

CLASSIFICATION AND DRUG EXAMPLES	MECHANISMS OF ACTION	NURSING CONSIDERATIONS
Antineoplastics: Alkylating Agents *Drug examples:* busulfan, carboplatin, carmustine, cisplatin, chlorambucil, cyclophosphamide, ifosfamide, lomustine, melphalan	Interfere with DNA production, causing cellular death. Not cell specific, so both cancerous and noncancerous cells are destroyed.	■ Monitor CBC with differential, platelet count, uric acid levels, and kidney and liver function studies. ■ Monitor temperature; avoid rectal temperature assessment. ■ Assess mentation and neurological status. ■ Concurrent administration with drugs that are toxic to kidneys or liver is contraindicated. ■ Contraindicated in clients with liver, kidney, or gastrointestinal disorders.
Antineoplastics: Antitumor Antibiotics *Drug examples:* bleomycin, dactinomycin, daunorubicin, doxorubicin epirubicin, idarubicin mitomycin	Interfere with production and action of nucleic acids to inhibit DNA and RNA replication.	■ Monitor CBC with differential and electrolytes. ■ Monitor neurological status. ■ Monitor for bleeding and protect client from traumatic injury. ■ Monitor for signs of infection. ■ Contraindicated in clients with liver, kidney, cardiac, pulmonary, gastrointestinal, or lung disease.
Antineoplastics: Antimetabolites *Drug examples:* capecitabine, cytarabine, fluorouracil, methotrexate, pemetrexed, pralatrexate	Interfere with pyrimidine and purine synthesis, which are essential for DNA production.	■ Monitor CBC with differential, electrolytes, and kidney and liver function studies. ■ Monitor for bleeding and protect client from traumatic injury. ■ Monitor for signs of infection. ■ Monitor for dyspnea and cough.
Hormones and Hormone Agonists *Drug examples:* *Hormones:* dexamethasone, diethylstilbestrol, estradiol, ethinyl, medroxyprogesterone, prednisone *Hormone antagonists:* abiraterone, anastrozole, bicalutamide, exemestane	Help block cancerous cells from utilizing the hormones that promote their growth and inhibit the body's natural production of hormones that promote growth of the cancerous cells.	■ Monitor CBC with differential. ■ Monitor blood pressure. ■ Monitor for signs of bleeding and protect client from traumatic injury. ■ Monitor for signs of infection. ■ Advise client to discontinue this medication only when advised to do so by the healthcare provider.
Biological Response Modifiers *Drug examples:* interferon alfa-2b, interferon alfacon-1, peginterferon alfa-2a	Stimulate immune function or block tumor growth; block cellular replication.	■ Monitor electrolytes and assess for signs of dehydration. ■ Monitor for signs of infection. ■ Monitor for capillary leak syndrome (hypotension, generalized edema, decreased urine output).
Natural Products: Vinca Alkaloids *Drug examples:* vinblastine, vincristine, vinorelbine	Cause immediate cellular death by inhibition of mitosis.	■ Monitor CBC with differential and liver function studies. ■ Monitor for bleeding and protect client from traumatic injury. ■ Monitor for signs of infection. ■ Monitor neurological status.
Antianemic Agents: Iron Supplements *Drug examples:* ferrous fumarate, ferrous gluconate, ferrous sulfate	Provide additional iron intake for the purpose of correcting RBC abnormalities caused by iron deficiency. Do not stimulate RBC production (erythropoiesis).	■ Monitor hemoglobin and reticulocyte counts. ■ To avoid staining teeth, thoroughly dilute liquid preparations and administer by using a straw or a dropper to apply medication to the back of the tongue. ■ Advise client of potential side effects, including black or dark green stools and constipation.
Antianemic Agents *Drug examples:* folic acid (vitamin B_9 or folate) and vitamin B_{12} (cyanocobalamin)	Folic acid stimulates production of RBCs, WBCs, and platelets in clients with megaloblastic anemia. Vitamin B_{12} (cyanocobalamin) is necessary for the production of RBCs and is used to treat vitamin B_{12} deficiency and pernicious anemia.	■ Monitor CBC with reticulocyte count, vitamin B_{12}, and serum folate levels. ■ Monitor serum potassium for 48 hours following initiation of cyanocobalamin treatment. ■ Especially in clients with cardiovascular disease, monitor for signs and symptoms of pulmonary edema.

Sources: Data from Osborn, K. S., Wraa, C. E., Watson, A., & Holleran, R. S. (2013). *Medical-surgical nursing: Preparation for practice* (2nd ed.). Upper Saddle River, NJ: Pearson; Wilson, B. A., Shannon, M. T., & Shields, K. M. (2013). *Pearson nurse's drug guide.* Upper Saddle River, NJ: Pearson; American Cancer Society (ACS). (2013c). *Chemotherapy principles: An in-depth discussion of the techniques and its role in cancer treatment.* Retrieved from http://www.cancer.org/acs/groups/cid/documents/webcontent/002995-pdf.pdf.

▨ REVIEW The Concept of Cellular Regulation

RELATE Link the Concepts

Linking the concept of cellular regulation with the concept of infection:

1. How does impaired cellular regulation influence a client's susceptibility to infection?

2. What can the nurse do to help reduce the likelihood of infection in clients with disorders related to impaired cellular regulation?

Linking the concept of cellular regulation with the concept of stress and coping:

3. What is the relationship between poor coping abilities and disorders of cellular regulation?

4. Which personality types are most often correlated with a risk for ineffective coping?

5. Is there a relationship between personality and impaired cellular regulation? Explain your answer.

Linking the concept of cellular regulation with the concept of safety:

6. Identify three safety concerns specific to the client with a disorder related to impaired cellular regulation.

7. Based on QSEN competencies, how can the nurse promote safety for the client with a disorder of cellular regulation?

READY Go to Companion Skills Manual

REFER Go to Pearson Student Nursing Resources
nursing.pearsonhighered.com

- Additional review materials
- Additional case study

REFLECT Case Study \\ Part 3

Andrew's laboratory results are available. His CBC results include the following:

WBC: 37.8 (normal = 4.5–10 K/μL)
RBC: 3.2 (normal = 4.6–6 M/μL)
PLT (platelets): 90 (normal = 150–400 K/μL)
Lymphocytes: 70 (normal = 25%–35%)

Per the ED physician's request, the pediatric oncologist arrives to examine Andrew and review his laboratory test results. Afterward, she suspects Andrew's signs and symptoms may be caused by acute lymphoblastic leukemia (ALL). Andrew is admitted to the hospital for further evaluation and treatment.

Clinical Reasoning Questions Level I

1. What diagnostic test will likely be included in Andrew's plan of care in order to confirm the suspected diagnosis of ALL?

2. Which component of Andrew's CBC suggests thrombocytopenia?

3. In reacting to the potential diagnosis of cancer, what response(s) might you anticipate from Andrew and his family members?

Clinical Reasoning Questions Level II

Refer to the exemplar on Leukemia within this module.

4. What does Andrew's lymphocyte measurement suggest about his body's ability to fight infection?

5. As you prepare to transfer Andrew to the pediatric oncology unit, he asks you why he has to stay in the hospital. How should you respond?

6. Formulate three nursing diagnoses that are appropriate for inclusion in the nursing plan of care for Andrew and his family.

EXEMPLAR 2.1 **Cancer**

EXEMPLAR KEY TERMS
Benign, *42*
Cachexia, *48*
Cancer, *41*
Carcinogenesis, *45*
Carcinogens, *45*
Chemotaxis, *43*
Chemotherapy, *56*
Grading, *53*
Invasion, *43*
Malignant, *42*
Metastasis, *42*
Neoplasm, *42*
Oncogenes, *45*
Oncology, *42*
Palliation, *57*
Staging, *53*
Tumor lysis syndrome (TLS), *49*
Tumor marker, *54*
Xerostomia, *61*

EXEMPLAR LEARNING OUTCOMES
After reading about this exemplar, you will be able to:

1. Describe the pathophysiology, etiology, clinical manifestations, and direct and indirect causes of cancer.

2. Identify risk factors and prevention methods associated with cancer.

3. Illustrate the nursing process in providing culturally competent care across the life span for individuals with cancer.

4. Formulate priority nursing diagnoses appropriate for an individual with cancer.

5. Summarize therapies used by interdisciplinary teams in the collaborative care of an individual with cancer.

6. Plan evidence-based care for an individual with cancer and his or her family in collaboration with other members of the healthcare team.

7. Evaluate expected outcomes for an individual with cancer.

▶ OVERVIEW

Cancer refers to a group of complex diseases whose manifestations depend on the affected body system and the type of cells involved. It is marked by uncontrolled growth and the spread of abnormal cells. Cancer can affect people of any age, gender, ethnicity, or geographic region. Although the incidence and mortality rates of cancer have continued to decline since 1990, it remains one of the most feared diseases. Even the suggestion of a cancer diagnosis often evokes feelings of hopelessness and helplessness.

Cancer results when normal cells mutate into abnormal, deviant cells that then perpetuate within the body. Cancer can affect any body tissue. Nursing care of the client with cancer is holistic and comprehensive, focusing on cancer not as one disease but as a constellation of many diseases. The nurse recognizes that cancer is a disruptive and life-threatening process that affects the whole individual and any significant others. Nursing interventions are based on the understanding that cancer is a chronic disease with acute episodes, that the client is often treated in the home, and that the client is usually treated with a combination of therapeutic modalities. Equally important, the nurse recognizes that caring for the client with cancer involves prevention, early detection, treatment, supportive care, long-term follow-up, and, for some clients, end-of-life care (Oncology Nursing Society, 2012).

Oncology is the study of cancer. The term is derived from the Greek word *oncoma* ("bulk"). Oncologists specialize in caring for clients with cancer; they may be medical doctors, surgeons, radiologists, immunologists, or researchers. The oncology nurse has received specialized training in cancer care and treatment and is an important and significant member of the oncology team. Oncology nurses have special skills in assisting the client and family with the psychosocial issues associated with cancer and terminal illness. Collaboration among healthcare professionals (e.g., surgeons, oncologists, nurses, social workers) ensures the most effective care and treatment for the client with cancer.

▶ PATHOPHYSIOLOGY AND ETIOLOGY

A **neoplasm** is a mass of new tissue (a collection of cells) that grows independently of its surrounding structures and has no physiological purpose. The term *neoplasm* is often used interchangeably with *tumor* (from the Latin word meaning "swelling"). Neoplasms are said to be autonomous for these reasons:

- They grow at a rate uncoordinated with the needs of the body.
- They share some of the properties of the parent cells but with altered size and shape.

- They do not benefit the host and, in some cases, are actively harmful.

Neoplasms are not completely autonomous, however, because they require a blood supply with nutrients and oxygen to sustain their growth. Neoplasms typically are classified as benign or malignant based on their potential to damage the body and their growth characteristics.

A neoplasm may be classified as benign or malignant. **Benign** means that a growth does not endanger life or health; it tends to not recur after treatment. **Malignant** means that if not treated, a growth will recur, continue to grow, and spread to other sites in the body, ending in death.

Benign Neoplasms

Benign neoplasms are localized growths. They form a solid mass, have well-defined borders, and are frequently encapsulated. Benign neoplasms tend to respond to the body's homeostatic controls. Thus, they often stop growing when they reach the boundaries of another tissue (a process called contact inhibition). They grow slowly and often remain stable in size. Because they are usually encapsulated, benign neoplasms often are easily removed and tend not to recur.

Although typically harmless, benign neoplasms can be destructive if they crowd surrounding tissue and obstruct the function of organs. For example, a benign meningioma (from the meninges of the brain and spinal cord) can cause severely increased intracranial pressure, which progressively impairs the individual's cerebral function. Unless the meningioma can be successfully removed, the steadily rising intracranial pressure will eventually lead to coma and death.

Malignant Neoplasms

In contrast to benign neoplasms, malignant neoplasms grow aggressively and do not respond to the body's homeostatic controls. Malignant neoplasms are not cohesive, and they present with an irregular shape. Instead of slowly crowding other tissues aside, malignant neoplasms cut through surrounding tissues, causing bleeding, inflammation, and necrosis (tissue death) as they grow. This invasive quality of malignant neoplasms is reflected in the origin of the word *cancer* (from the Greek *karkinos*, meaning "crab"). Healthcare professionals are referring to a malignant neoplasm when they use the term *cancer*.

Malignant cells from the primary tumor may travel through the blood or lymph to invade other tissues and organs of the body and form a secondary tumor. The spreading of malignant neoplasms to other areas of the body—perhaps their most destructive trait—is called **metastasis**. Malignant neoplasms can recur after surgical removal of the primary and secondary tumors and after other treatments. **Table 2–2** ● compares benign and malignant neoplasms.

Malignant neoplasms vary in their degree of differentiation from the parent tissue. Highly differentiated cancer cells try to mimic the specialized function of the parent tissue, but undifferentiated cancers, consisting of immature cells, have almost no resemblance to the parent tissue and so perform no useful function. To make matters worse, undifferentiated cancers rob the body of its energy and nutrition as they grow. Undifferentiated anaplastic cells have little structural or functional relation-

TABLE 2–2 Comparison of Benign and Malignant Neoplasms

BENIGN	MALIGNANT
Local	Invasive
Cohesive	Noncohesive
Well-defined borders	Does not stop at tissue border
Pushes other tissues out of the way	Invades and destroys surrounding tissues
Slow growth	Rapid growth
Encapsulated	Metastasizes to distant sites
Easily removed	Not always easy to remove
Does not recur	Can recur

Box 2–1 Characteristics of Malignant Cells

- Loss of regulation of mitotic rate
- Loss of cell specialization
- Loss of contact inhibition
- Progressive acquisition of the cancerous phenotype and immortality
- Irreversibility of cancerous phenotype to greater aggressiveness
- Altered cell structure: differences in cell nucleus and cytoplasm
- Simplified metabolic activity
- Transplantability (metastasis)
- Ability to promote own survival

ship to the parent cells and are the basis of many malignant neoplasms. The degree of differentiation of anaplastic cells is a consideration in the classification and staging of neoplasms.

CHARACTERISTICS OF MALIGNANT CELLS Malignant neoplasms may be identified by the following predictable cellular characteristics:

- **Loss of regulation of the rate of mitosis.** This results in rapid cell division and growth of the neoplasm.

- **Loss of specialization and differentiation.** Malignant cells do not perform typical cellular functions. Many produce hormones and enzymes similar to those of the parent tissue, but usually in excessive amounts, possibly revealing their presence.

- **Loss of contact inhibition.** Malignant cells do not respect other cellular boundaries. They easily invade and destroy other tissues.

- **Progressive acquisition of a cancerous phenotype.** Cellular mutation seems to be a sequential process involving successive generations of cells, with each generation becoming more deviant than the previous one. Additionally, malignant cells seem to be "immortal"—that is, they do not stop growing and die, as do normal cells, which have a genetically determined life span.

- **Irreversibility.** The transformation into a malignant cell is irreversible. Rarely does a malignant neoplasm revert to a benign state.

- **Altered cell structure.** Cytological examination of malignant cells reveals distinct differences in the cell nucleus and cytoplasm as well as an overall cell shape that differs from that of normal cells of the particular tissue type.

- **Simplified metabolic activities.** The work of malignant cells is simpler than that of normal cells; they show an increased synthesis of substances needed for cell division, and they have no need to create proteins for the specialized functions of the tissues they invade.

- **Transplantability.** Malignant cells often break away from the primary tissue site and travel to other locations in the body, where they establish new growths.

- **Ability to promote their own survival.** Malignant cells may create ectopic sites to produce the hormones they need for their growth. By their very presence and their ability to

initiate vascular permeability, malignant cells promote the development of nonneoplastic stroma, a connective tissue framework consisting of collagen and other components, which then supports the neoplasm. They may also create their own blood supply. Through a process called angiogenesis, tumor cells secrete a polypeptide angiogenic growth factor that stimulates blood vessels from surrounding normal tissue to grow into the tumor. Finally, malignant cells divert nutrition from the host to meet their own needs, by diffusion when the tumor is less than 1 mm and by means of the newly formed blood vessels thereafter. If unchecked, malignant cells eventually destroy their host (**Box 2–1 ●**).

TUMOR INVASION AND METASTASIS Cancer cells may overtake adjacent tissues (**invasion**) and spread from their primary site to distant organs (metastasis).

Invasion Aggressive tumors possess several qualities that facilitate invasion:

- **Ability to cause pressure atrophy.** The pressure of a growing tumor can cause atrophy and necrosis of adjacent tissues. The malignancy then moves into the vacated space.

- **Ability to disrupt the basement membrane of normal cells.** Many cancer cells can bind to elements of the basement membrane and secrete enzymes that degrade that physical barrier, thus facilitating their movement into normal tissues, lymph, and blood circulation.

- **Motility.** Because malignant cells are less tightly bound to each other than normal cells (reduced adhesiveness), they easily separate from the neoplasm and move into surrounding body fluids and tissues.

- **Response to chemical signals from adjacent tissues. Chemotaxis** (the movement of cells in response to a chemical stimulus) draws the tumor cells into the normal tissues, possibly as a result of the degrading of the basement membranes of the normal cells. This breakdown of normal cellular membranes releases the chemical stimulus physiologically designed to draw normal phagocytic cells to clean up the debris. Malignant cells are also known to respond chemotactically to the end product of cellular metabolism. Some cancer cells even produce a substance called autocrine motility factor, which calls other malignant cells to a normal tissue. The first invading cells produce this substance, which then actively draws other malignant cells from the primary tumor into the invaded normal tissue.

Metastasis   The factors that favor invasion also contribute to the process of metastasis. Metastasis can occur by means of one or more mechanisms, including embolism in the blood or lymph or spread by way of body cavities.

A blood- or lymph-borne metastasis allows a new tumor to be established in a distant organ. **Figure 2–4 ●** shows metastasis through the bloodstream. A tumor's ability to metastasize in this manner requires the following steps:

1. Intravasation of malignant cells through blood or lymphatic vessel walls and into the circulation
2. Survival of the malignant cells in the blood (to survive, the cells must escape the notice of the body's immune surveillance; only about 1 in 1,000 cells does so)
3. Extravasation from the circulation and implantation in a new tissue.

The tumor cells tend to clump together, forming an embolus, and continue growing until their size prevents further travel in the vessel or lymph channel. The growing neoplastic mass then uses its invasive abilities (secreting enzymes and motility factor) to move into the nearest organ.

Approximately 60% of metastatic lesions tend to occur in a schema reflecting the pattern of blood or lymph circulation. Some malignant cells, however, defy a bloodborne pattern and actually target specific organs to which they prefer to metastasize. For example, lung cancer frequently metastasizes to the adrenal glands, and breast cancer frequently metastasizes to bone.

Malignant cells that gain access to the lymph channels may travel to a preferred organ and then move into it the same way

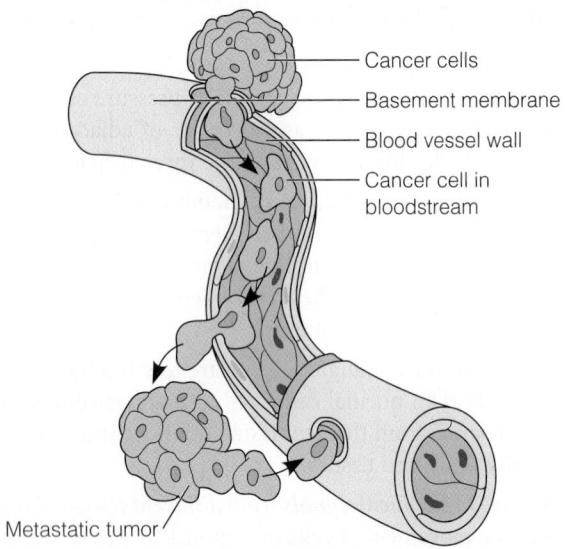

- Cancer cells
- Basement membrane
- Blood vessel wall
- Cancer cell in bloodstream

Metastatic tumor

Figure 2–4 ● Metastasis through the bloodstream. Cancer cells secrete enzymes and a motility factor that disrupt the basement membrane in the blood vessel. In this way, the cancer cells gain access to the circulation. Once in the blood, only about 1 cell in 1,000 escapes immune detection, but that can be enough. Undetected cells move out of the blood, again secreting enzymes and cutting through the vessel wall into new tissue. The tissue selected for establishing a new tumor may be downstream from the original tumor, or a chemical attraction may cause the malignant cells to target a specific site. Once in the new site, the malignant cells multiply and establish a metastatic tumor.

they emigrate through blood vessels. Alternatively, the malignant cells may become trapped in the lymph node and continue to grow. Eventually, the malignant cells replace the node's tissues. At this point, emboli from the cancerous node disseminate to other nodes, creating a cascade reaction. The malignant cascade causes widespread transfer of the tumor to uncharacteristic sites.

A malignant tumor may break through the walls of the organ in which it is primarily housed, in the process shedding cells into the nearby body cavity. Those cells are then free to establish new tumors in a distant area of that cavity. For example, malignant cells from a colon cancer may be seeded into the peritoneal cavity, establishing a new tumor in the mesenteric epithelium.

Metastatic lesions are differentiated from primary neoplasms by cell morphology: Metastatic cells do not resemble the tissue in which they reside. The most common sites of metastasis are the lymph nodes, liver, lungs, bones, and brain.

For metastasis to occur, the cancerous cells must avoid detection by the immune system. Thus, impairment of the immune system is a major factor in the establishment of metastatic lesions. Cells may escape detection in several different ways:

- Aggressive cancer cells may compile a large mass (>1 cm) so rapidly that the immune system is unable to overcome the tumor before it takes hold in a new tissue.

- For tumor cells to be recognized as foreign by the immune system, they must display on their surface a special antigen called *tumor-associated antigen* (TAA). TAA marks tumor cells for destruction by the lymphocytes. Some oncogenic viruses depress the expression of TAA on infected cells. Also, some tumors in advanced stages of growth no longer display TAA. Thus, such tumor cells escape detection as they travel through the blood or lymph.

- If the individual's immune response is weakened or altered, then a metastatic tumor may take hold with little opposition.

An estimated 50%–60% of all cancers have already metastasized by the time the primary tumor is identified. This may account for the current ACS (2013b) estimated 28% mortality rate due to cancer, and it certainly supports the need for client education to facilitate early diagnosis. The time it takes for metastasis to occur is extremely variable and often difficult to predict. Some cancers, such as basal cell carcinomas, do not metastasize. The aggressiveness and location of the tumor, and the state of the individual's immune system, determine whether and how rapidly metastasis takes place.

Immune System Response

When the immune system discovers a neoplasm, it tries to destroy it using the resources of the body. The body mounts an all-out assault on the foreign invader, calling on many resources:

- Chemical mediators
- Hormones and enzymes
- Blood cells
- Antibodies
- Proteins
- Inflammatory and immune responses.

These protective responses also mobilize the fluid, electrolyte, and nutritional systems. This massive effort requires tremendous energy. (See the module on Fluids and Electrolytes for specific information on these systems.) If the neoplasm is small enough (i.e., microscopic), the immune system can destroy it, and a tumor will never manifest. A neoplasm of 1 cm is large enough to overwhelm most immune systems; however, the body will continue trying to fight until it reaches the stage of exhaustion and is no longer capable (Selye, 1984). Thus, many clients with cancer present with fatigue, weight loss, anemia, dehydration, and electrolyte imbalances.

Etiology

Theories of **carcinogenesis** (the production or origin of cancer) include the involvement of cellular mutation, oncogenes, and tumor suppressor genes. Central to these theories are two important concepts about the etiology of cancer. First, damaged DNA, whether inherited or from external sources, sets up the necessary initial step for cancer to occur. Second, impairment of the human immune system, from whatever cause, lessens its ability to destroy abnormal cells.

CELLULAR MUTATION   The theory of cellular mutation suggests that **carcinogens** (cancer-causing substances) cause mutations in cellular DNA. It is believed that the carcinogenic process has three stages: (1) initiation, (2) promotion, and (3) progression. The initiation stage involves permanent damage in the cellular DNA as a result of exposure to a carcinogen (e.g., radiation or chemicals) that was not repaired or that had a defective repair. Promotion may last for years and includes conditions, such as smoking or alcohol use, that act repeatedly on the already affected cells. In the progression stage, further inherited changes acquired during cell replication develop into a cancer.

ONCOGENES   **Oncogenes** are genes that promote cell proliferation and are capable of triggering cancerous characteristics. Oncogenes can be classified according to their overall function. Several oncogenes and their relationship to human cancers have been identified. For example, *BRCA1* and *BRCA2* are associated with breast cancer (NCI, 2013a).

A decrease in the body's immune surveillance may allow the expression of oncogenes; this can occur during times of stress or in response to certain carcinogens. For example, cytomegaloviruses (CMVs), which frequently occur in clients who are HIV positive, are associated with a higher incidence of Kaposi sarcoma (Osborn et al., 2013).

TUMOR SUPPRESSOR GENES   Tumor suppressor genes normally suppress oncogenes. They can become inactive by deletion or mutation. Inherited cancers have been associated with tumor suppressor genes. An example is p53, a suppressor gene that has been associated with sarcoma and cancer of the breast and brain.

Causative Agents

A number of agents are known to cause cancer, or at least are strongly linked to certain kinds of cancers. These carcinogens are both external (e.g., chemicals, radiation, and viruses) and internal (e.g., hormones, immune conditions, and inherited

mutations). Causal factors may act together or in sequence to initiate or promote carcinogenesis. Ten or more years often pass between exposures or mutations and detectable cancer.

Carcinogens can be categorized in two groups: genotoxic carcinogens, which directly alter DNA and cause mutations, and promoter substances, which cause other adverse biological effects, such as cytotoxicity, hormonal imbalances, altered immunity, or chronic tissue damage. Promoter substances do not cause cancer in the absence of previous cell damage (initiation), and they often require high-level and long-term contact with the altered cells.

Although everyone comes into contact with a vast number of substances that are considered carcinogenic, not everyone develops cancer. Other factors, such as genetic predisposition, impairment of the immune response, and repeated exposure to the carcinogen, are necessary for a cancer to develop.

Several viruses have been associated with the development of cancer. These viruses damage cells and induce hyperplastic cell growth. Viral infection may play a role in cell mutation that can progress to malignant cells. Normal aging and immune system dysfunction increase an individual's susceptibility to viral carcinogens (Osborn et al., 2013). **Box 2–2** ● identifies these viruses and the cancers with which they are associated.

In addition, viruses play a significant role in weakening immunological defenses against neoplasms. For example, human immunodeficiency virus, which infects helper T lymphocytes and monocytes, impairs an individual's protection against certain cancers, such as lymphoma and Kaposi sarcoma.

Risk Factors

Risk factors make an individual or a population vulnerable to a specific disease or other unhealthy outcome. Risk factors can be divided into those that are controllable and those that are not

---

Box 2–2   Cancers Associated With Viral Etiology

HERPES SIMPLEX VIRUS TYPES 1 AND 2 (HSV-1 AND HSV-2)
- Carcinoma of the lip
- Cervical carcinoma
- Kaposi sarcoma

HUMAN CYTOMEGALOVIRUS (HCMV)
- Kaposi sarcoma
- Prostate cancer

EPSTEIN-BARR VIRUS (EBV)
- Burkitt lymphoma

HUMAN HERPESVIRUS 6 (HHV-6)
- Lymphoma

HEPATITIS B VIRUS (HBV)
- Primary hepatocellular cancer

PAPILLOMAVIRUS
- Malignant melanoma
- Cervical, penile, and laryngeal cancers

HUMAN T-LYMPHOTROPIC VIRUSES (HTLV)
- Adult T-cell leukemia and lymphoma
- T-cell variant of hairy-cell leukemia
- Kaposi sarcoma

controllable. Knowledge and assessment of risk factors are especially important in counseling clients and families about measures to prevent cancer.

HEREDITY It is estimated that 5%–10% of cancers may have a hereditary component (ACS, 2011). The familial pattern of some breast and colon cancers has been well documented. Lung, ovarian, and prostate cancers have also shown some familial relationships. For most cancers, however, research has yet to distinguish true genetic transfer from environmental causes. So although further research is needed to identify cancers that are caused by the inheritance of defective genes, familial predisposition to malignancies should be counted among risk factors. This allows people at risk to reduce behaviors that promote cancer. For example, a client with a family history of lung cancer should be counseled to avoid smoking, to avoid areas where smoking is allowed, and to avoid working in an occupation that may expose the client to inhaled carcinogens.

AGE Cancer is a disease associated with aging; approximately 77% of cancer diagnoses occur after age 55 (ACS, 2013b). A number of factors are associated with this increased risk in older adults. One possible factor is that at least five cycles of genetic mutations seem necessary to cause permanent damage to the afflicted cells. In addition, long-term exposure to high doses of promotional agents is usually necessary to allow the cancer to take hold. Another factor may be the immune system's decline with aging (Osborn et al., 2013). Another problem is that free radicals (molecules resulting from the body's metabolic and oxidative processes) tend to accumulate in the cells over time, causing damage and mutation.

Hormonal changes that occur with aging can be associated with cancer. Postmenopausal women receiving exogenous estrogen have an increased risk for breast and uterine cancers. Older men are at risk for prostate cancer, possibly as a result of the breakdown of testosterone into carcinogenic forms.

GENDER Gender is a risk factor for certain types of cancer. Breast cancer is the most frequently diagnosed cancer in women; prostate cancer is the most frequently diagnosed cancer in men. The incidence of bladder cancer is approximately three times higher in men than in women, whereas thyroid cancer occurs more commonly among women (ACS, 2013b).

POVERTY Individuals living in poverty are at higher risk for cancer than the population in general. Inadequate access to health care, especially preventive screening and counseling, may be a major factor. Although other factors that may be involved, such as diet and stress, usually come under the category of controllable risks, these risks are frequently uncontrollable in this population.

STRESS Although some studies suggest a direct link between stress and cancer development, other studies are unable to establish such a link. Perhaps more easily supported is a link between cancer risks and unhealthy coping mechanisms that may emerge under stressful conditions. Unhealthy coping behaviors such as overeating, smoking, and alcohol abuse may lead to physical conditions that are associated with higher risks for developing cancer (NCI, 2013d).

DIET Some foods are considered genotoxic, such as the nitrosamines and nitrous indoles found in preserved meats and pickled, salted foods. Other foods, such as high-fat, low-fiber foods—the mainstay of many American diets—promote colon, breast, and sex hormone–dependent tumors. When fish and meat are excessively fried or broiled, potent carcinogenic compounds can form that may cause tumors in the mammary glands, colon, liver, pancreas, and bladder. Also, repeatedly using fat to fry foods at high temperatures produces high levels of polycyclic hydrocarbons, which increase the risk for cancer considerably. Other food-related substances believed to increase cancer risk include sodium saccharine, red food dyes, and both regular and decaffeinated coffee.

OCCUPATION Occupational risk might be considered either controllable or uncontrollable. For many people, both education and ability limit their choice of occupation; moreover, during times of high unemployment, changing occupation because it poses risk factors may not be a viable option. Federal standards are designed to protect workers from hazardous substances, but many believe that these standards are not strict enough, and that inspections are not frequent enough, to prevent violations.

Specific risks vary according to the occupation. For example, those who work outdoors, such as farmers and construction workers, are exposed to solar radiation. Healthcare workers, such as x-ray technicians and biomedical researchers, are exposed to ionizing radiation and carcinogenic substances.

INFECTION Because a number of viruses have been linked to some cancers, avoiding those specific infections will decrease risk. Although some infections may be unavoidable—Epstein-Barr, for example—others, such as genital herpes and papillomavirus-induced genital warts, can often be avoided by following safer sex practices (e.g., the use of condoms).

TOBACCO USE Lung cancer is considered highly preventable because of its relationship to smoking. The genotoxic carcinogenic substances in tobacco are considered weak; therefore, stopping smoking can reverse the damage it causes. However, many other substances in tobacco are highly promotional, so the larger the dose and the longer the use, the higher the risk for developing cancer. Research has shown a significantly lower risk for death from lung cancer among former smokers compared to current smokers. For smokers who quit before 40 years of age, the risk of death due to conditions associated with continued smoking is reduced by approximately 90% (Jha et al., 2013).

Smokers also face an increased risk for oropharyngeal, esophageal, laryngeal, gastric, pancreatic, and bladder cancers. Pipe and cigar smokers are especially susceptible to oropharyngeal and laryngeal cancers. Oral and esophageal cancers are more common among those who chew tobacco or use snuff. Smokers who have a genetic decrease in α_1-antitrypsin (an enzyme that protects lung tissue) that results in emphysema face an even higher risk for cancer than smokers without this defect.

Secondhand tobacco smoke has also been identified as a cause of cancer. According to some researchers, among adults, secondhand smoke may increase the risk of developing breast cancer, as well as nasal sinus cavity and nasopharyngeal cancer. In children, secondhand smoke is believed to increase the risk of developing brain tumors, lymphoma, and leukemia (NCI, 2013e).

ALCOHOL USE   Alcohol promotes cancer by enhancing the contact between carcinogens, such as those in tobacco, and the stem cells that line the oral cavity, larynx, and esophagus (Porth & Matfin, 2010). People who both smoke and drink a considerable amount of alcohol daily have an increased risk for oral, esophageal, and laryngeal cancers.

RECREATIONAL DRUG USE   Recreational drug use often promotes an unhealthy lifestyle that increases an individual's general risk for cancer; for example, habitual drug users often do not maintain adequate nutrition. Furthermore, recreational drugs are implicated as promoters because of their suppressive effect on the immune system. Recent research findings suggest marijuana use is linked to the development of testicular cancer (Trabert et al., 2011). Although some studies suggest smoking marijuana may increase the risk for developing lung cancer, the results of these studies are often confounded by the subjects' concurrent cigarette smoking. What is known is that marijuana smoke and tobacco smoke contain many of the same carcinogens, some of which are found in higher concentrations in marijuana smoke (Hall & Degenhardt, 2009).

OBESITY   Excessive body fat has been linked to an increased risk for hormone-dependent cancers. Because sex hormones are synthesized from fat, people who are obese often have excessive amounts of the hormones that feed hormone-dependent malignancies of the breast, bowel, ovary, endometrium, and prostate.

SUN EXPOSURE   As the protective ozone layer thins, more of the sun's damaging ultraviolet radiation reaches the earth. As a consequence, the rate of skin cancers has increased. Sun-related skin cancers are now considered a problem for all people, regardless of skin color, but people of northern European extraction with very fair skin, blue or green eyes, and light-colored hair are most vulnerable. Older adults with decreased pigment, even those with darker skin, are also more at risk.

Prevention

Cancer prevention centers around making healthy lifestyle choices, such as avoiding smoking and limiting alcohol consumption, as well as eating a balanced diet. A healthy diet combined with regular exercise is an effective means of avoiding obesity, which is a risk factor for several types of cancer. Good physical health also allows for optimal immune function, reducing the risk of infection and thereby reducing the risk for developing certain types of cancer. Wearing sunscreen and avoiding prolonged sun exposure are simple but effective preventive steps for avoiding skin cancer. In the occupational setting, it is especially important to follow safety protocols, including those designed to prevent exposure to carcinogens.

▶ CLINICAL MANIFESTATIONS

Much of the nursing care for clients with cancer is related to the generalized effects of cancer on the body and to the side effects of the treatments used to remove or destroy the cancer. Although the pathophysiological effects of a cancer vary with the type and location of the cancer, the effects detailed in this section are common among many types of cancer.

Disruption of Function

Physiological functioning can be upset by obstruction or pressure. For example, a large tumor in the bowel can stop intestinal motility, resulting in a bowel obstruction. Prostatic tumors can obstruct the bladder neck or urethra, resulting in urine retention. Intracranial pressure can be dangerously increased by a glioma.

Obstruction or pressure can cause anoxia and necrosis of surrounding tissues, which in turn cause a loss of function of the involved organ or tissue. For example, a kidney tumor may progress to renal failure. Pressure against the superior vena cava from an adjacent lung tumor or tumor-infiltrated lymph nodes can interrupt the blood flow to the heart.

In the liver, either a primary hepatocellular cancer or metastatic lesion can have several significant effects:

■ In liver parenchymal tissue, it can impair the multiple life-sustaining functions of the liver, such as carbohydrate metabolism, synthesis of plasma proteins, detoxification, and immunological functions. These functional impairments result in severe nutritional, hormonal, hematological, and immunological problems.

■ Because more than 1 L of blood per minute passes through the liver via the portal vein, obstruction to this flow by a tumor can cause portal hypertension. This results in backup of fluid and increased pressure in the splanchnic circulation. The end result is ascites (third-spaced fluid in the peritoneal cavity) and varices (friable, overdistended blood vessels) of the esophageal, gastric, mesenteric, and hemorrhoidal vessels.

Hematological Alterations

Hematological alterations can impair the normal function of blood cells. For example, in leukemia, a malignant proliferative disease of the hematopoietic (blood cell–producing) system, the immature leukocytes cannot perform the normal protective phagocytic functions, and immunity is compromised. Additionally, the excessive numbers of immature leukocytes in the bone marrow impair erythrocyte (RBC) and thrombocyte (platelet) production, resulting in secondary anemia and clotting disorders (American Society of Hematology, 2011).

Other examples of hematological alteration include the following:

■ Gastrointestinal tumors disrupt the absorption of vitamin B_{12} and iron.

■ Growing tumors need purines and folate and have a unique ability to accumulate and store these substances. Thus, the tumor deprives the bone marrow of these substances, which are needed for erythropoiesis (RBC production).

■ Renal cell carcinoma produces its own erythropoietin hormone, which causes an excessively large number of RBCs to be produced and dumped into the bloodstream. The resulting polycythemia causes viscous blood, which impairs circulation, plugs small capillaries, and promotes thrombus formation.

Infection

If the tumor invades and connects two incompatible organs, such as the bowel and the bladder, and thus creates a fistula, infection becomes a serious problem. As they destroy viable tissue and thus their own source of nutrition, tumors may become necrotic; septicemia may result. Some tumors are less efficient in creating capillaries; as a consequence, the center of the tumor may become necrotic and infected. When a tumor grows near the surface of the body, it may erode through to the surface, thus breaking down the natural defenses of intact skin and mucous membranes and providing a site for the entry of microorganisms. Any malignant involvement of the organs or tissues of immunity—such as the liver, bone marrow, Peyer patches in the small intestine, spleen, or lymph nodes—can seriously impair the immune response, allowing infections to develop in vulnerable tissues.

Hemorrhage

Tumor erosion through blood vessels can cause extensive bleeding, giving rise to severe anemia. Hemorrhage can be serious enough to cause life-threatening hypovolemic shock.

Anorexia-Cachexia Syndrome

A characteristic feature of cancer is the wasted appearance of its victims, called **cachexia**. In many cases, unexplained rapid weight loss is the first symptom that brings the client to a healthcare provider. This can result from a variety of problems associated with cancer, such as pain, infection, depression, or the side effects of chemotherapy and radiation. Usually, however, the emaciation, malnutrition, and loss of energy are attributed to the anorexia-cachexia syndrome.

This syndrome is specific to cancer because of the effect of cancer cells on the host's metabolism. The neoplastic cells divert nutrition to their own use while causing changes that reduce the client's appetite. Early in the disease, glucose metabolism is altered, causing an increase in serum glucose levels. Through the process of negative feedback, anorexia (loss of appetite) results. In addition, the tumor secretes substances that decrease appetite by altering taste and smell and by producing early satiety. Pain, infection, and depression also contribute to anorexia. Some types of cancers cause specific food aversions, such as to red meat, coffee, or chocolate.

Avaricious cancer cells support their growth through widespread catabolism of the body's tissue and muscle proteins. This catabolism, coupled with inadequate nutrient intake, results in the typical cachexia. Normally, a starvation state reduces the body's basal metabolic rate. However, in many people with cancer, the metabolic rate is increased, probably because of the hyperactive metabolic and reproductive activities of the malignant cells. One theory suggests that cytokinins the body produces in response to the tumor are responsible for both early satiety and cachexia. One specific cytokine, called tumor necrosis factor alpha or cachectin, is believed to enhance the increased metabolic consumption of nutrients. Cancers of the gastrointestinal system further promote anorexia-cachexia by decreasing absorption and use of nutrients; the side effects of some treatment modalities enhance this effect. **Figure 2–5** ● shows the characteristic appearance of a cachectic individual.

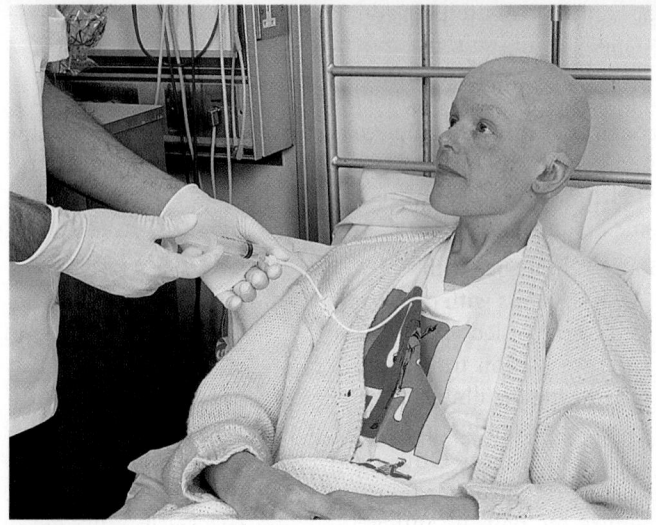

Figure 2–5 ● Cachectic individual. Cancer robs its host of nutrients and increases body catabolism of fat and muscle to meet its metabolic needs.
Source: Simon Fraser/SPL/Science Source.

Paraneoplastic Syndromes

Paraneoplastic syndromes are disorders resulting from the production of biologically active chemicals (such as hormones) by physiological sites that are separate from the primary cancer site and to which cancer has not metastasized (Pelosof & Gerber, 2010). These syndromes may be early warning signs of cancer, indicate complications, or suggest the return of a malignancy. Examples of paraneoplastic syndromes include the following:

- Breast, ovarian, and renal cancers may set up ectopic parathyroid hormone sites, causing severe hypercalcemia.
- Oat cell and other lung cancers may produce ectopic secretions of insulin (causing hypoglycemia), parathyroid hormone, antidiuretic hormone (causing excessive fluid retention, hypertension, and peripheral edema), and adrenocorticotropic hormone.

Paraneoplastic syndromes can affect practically any body system.

Pain

Pain is ranked as one of the most serious concerns of clients, families, and oncology healthcare professionals. Because pain management for people with cancer has a reputation as being ineffective, the anticipation of pain may engender fear in even the most stoic people. Most individuals fear pain and suffering even more than possible death, although pain management strategies have improved tremendously. Despite international acceptance of World Health Organization guidelines that outline the management of cancer-related pain, inadequate pain management is still a significant issue for this population (Fairchild, 2010).

TYPES OF CANCER PAIN   Cancer pain can be divided into two main categories, acute and chronic, with subgroupings. These classifications serve to indicate appropriate therapeutic approaches. Acute pain has a well-defined pattern of onset, exhibits common signs and symptoms, and is often identified with hyperactivity of the autonomic system. Chronic pain, which lasts more than 6 months, frequently lacks the objective manifestations of acute pain, primarily because the autonomic nervous system adapts to this chronic stress. Unfortunately, chronic pain often results in personality changes, alterations in functional abilities, and lifestyle disruptions that can seriously affect compliance with treatment and the quality of life.

Most clients with cancer who cite acute pain as the primary symptom that led to the diagnosis tend to associate pain with the introduction to their disease. If these clients experience pain during the illness or after therapy, they often perceive the pain as the introduction to another cancer or as a recurrence of the original cancer. Other clients report experiencing pain as a component of cancer therapy. These clients often are able to endure the pain in anticipation of a successful outcome of treatment.

Chronic pain may be related to treatment or may indicate progression of the disease. Identifying the pain as treatment related rather than tumor related is extremely important, because it has a definite effect on the client's psychological outlook. For the client whose pain is caused by advancement of the disease, psychological factors play an even more important role. Hopelessness and fear of impending death intensify physiological pain and contribute to overall suffering (which goes well beyond just physical pain).

Three other categories used to classify clients with cancer pain are worth mentioning: clients with preexisting pain, those with a history of drug abuse, and dying clients with cancer-related pain. The first two groups may have altered perceptions of pain and may not have the anticipated response to pain medication. For the dying client, pain is strongly associated with both the client's and family's confrontation of issues of hopelessness and death. Confronting these issues can intensify the perception of pain.

CAUSES OF CANCER PAIN

Direct tumor involvement is the primary cause of the pain experienced by people with cancer. This includes metastatic bone disease, nerve compression, and involvement of visceral organs. The pain from tumor involvement is believed to be mechanical, resulting from stretching of tissues and compression. Chemicals from ischemia or tumor metabolites and toxins that activate and sensitize nociceptors and mechanoreceptors are also responsible for tumor pain.

Side effects or toxic effects of cancer therapies (e.g., surgery, radiation, and chemotherapy) may also cause cancer pain. These are usually the result of traumatized tissue; one example is the oropharyngeal ulcerations that occur with some types of chemotherapy. However, these therapies may also be used to manage pain, such as radiation to decrease pain associated with bone metastasis.

Psychological Stress

People confronted with a cancer diagnosis exhibit a variety of psychological and emotional responses. Some people see cancer as a death sentence and experience overwhelming grief, often giving up. Others may feel guilt, considering the cancer a punishment for past behaviors, such as smoking, unhealthy eating habits, or delaying diagnosis or treatment. The client may experience anger, especially if the individual believes that he or she had been practicing a healthful lifestyle; beneath that anger may reside feelings of powerlessness. Fear is common: fear of the outcome of the illness, fear of the effects of treatment, fear of pain, and fear of death. Some people feel isolated because of the stigma of cancer and old beliefs about contagion. Body image concerns and sexual dysfunction may be present but often unexpressed, especially if the cancer is of the breast or sexual organs or causes visible body changes.

Oncological Emergencies

Clients may experience oncological emergencies resulting from the cancer itself or as a side effect of treatment. Oncological emergencies can be organized into three groups: metabolic, hematological, and those involving space-occupying lesions. Overall, the most common oncological emergencies are tumor lysis syndrome, septic shock, brain herniation, spinal cord compression, and superior vena cava compression from a superior mediastinal mass.

METABOLIC EMERGENCIES

Metabolic emergencies result from the lysis (dissolving or decomposing) of tumor cells, a process called **tumor lysis syndrome (TLS)**. In TLS, cellular lysis leads to the release of intracellular contents into the circulation, causing hyperkalemia, hyperuricemia, and hyperphosphatemia. Consequences of this syndrome may include cardiac arrhythmias, renal failure, and death. Although usually associated with rapid cell lysis due to chemotherapy, TLS may also occur spontaneously, without any apparent cause. TLS is most often seen in cancers with high growth rates, acute leukemias, and lymphomas (Bercovitz, Greffe, & Hunger, 2010; Osborn et al., 2013).

A second type of metabolic emergency is septic shock. During periods of immune suppression, the client is vulnerable to overwhelming infection. Systemic infection that progresses to septic shock may lead to circulatory failure and death. For these clients, prompt, aggressive treatment is critical to survival. (See the exemplar on Sepsis in the module on Infection for a full description of septicemia and septic shock.)

A third type of metabolic emergency involves the development of cancer-related hypercalcemia (elevated calcium in the serum). When bone breaks down due to cancer, the calcium released from the bone into the circulation may lead to hypercalcemia. However, there are also other potential causes. For example, certain types of tumors release proteins that mimic parathyroid hormone, causing bones to release calcium. Treatment depends on the cause of the hypercalcemia and may include administration of medications such as bisphosphonates, which stop bone breakdown (American Society of Clinical Oncology [ASCO], 2012b).

HEMATOLOGICAL EMERGENCIES

Hematological emergencies result from bone marrow suppression or infiltration of brain and respiratory tissue with high numbers of leukemic blast cells (hyperleukocytosis). Bone marrow suppression results in anemia and *thrombocytopenia* (decreased platelets) with resultant coagulation disturbance. Idiopathic bleeding, which is bleeding due to unknown causes, may be a sign of thrombocytopenia. Examples of external idiopathic bleeding include epistaxis (bleeding from the nose) that is not due to trauma and bleeding from the gums after brushing the teeth. Thrombocytopenia may also lead to bruising easily or bruising that is not related to injury. Disseminated intravascular coagulation (DIC), which occurs when the body's intricate clotting mechanisms are impaired, occurs in some cases. DIC may lead to rapid, profuse blood loss and is a life-threatening complication. Gastrointestinal and central nervous system bleeding (strokes) are common. Disruption of normal WBC production and resulting hyperleukocytosis can lead to obstruction of small blood vessels throughout the body.

Treatment of DIC may include infusion of packed red blood cells for anemia, platelet transfusion, and administration of vitamin K and fresh frozen plasma for thrombocytopenia and hemorrhage. Management of hyperleukocytosis may include transfusion of platelets, hemodialysis, administration of hydroxyurea and urate oxidase, and leukapheresis if needed (Sung et al., 2012).

SPACE-OCCUPYING LESIONS   Extensive tumor growth may result in spinal cord compression, increased intracranial pressure, brain herniation, seizures, massive hepatomegaly, gastrointestinal obstruction, cardiac and respiratory complications, and superior vena cava syndrome (obstruction of the superior vena cava by tumor). These emergencies are often caused by neuroblastoma, medulloblastoma, astrocytoma, Hodgkin disease, or lymphoma. After biopsy of the mass, treatment involves radiation therapy, antineoplastic agents (chemotherapy), and corticosteroids.

Lifespan and Cultural Considerations

A diagnosis of cancer can be devastating to a child and his family or to a woman who is pregnant. Each of these clients faces specific challenges related to psychosocial needs and treatment considerations.

CHILDREN AND ADOLESCENTS   Nurses caring for the child or adolescent with cancer provide family-centered care—that is, they provide care for the entire family. Care ranges from assessing the child's physiological and psychological status at the bedside or during an office visit to assessing the parent's need for respite or additional resources and the sibling's need for a more predictable schedule. In particular, nurses need to be knowledgeable about the client and family's psychosocial needs and issues related to survival and treatment of children with cancer.

Psychosocial Needs   The diagnosis of cancer is devastating for families. While attempting to cope with the diagnosis, parents must simultaneously gather resources to support the child, make treatment decisions, and adjust family life to integrate the needs of the child with cancer. Some families need to travel a great distance for the child's treatments, and others may have financial constraints that make healthcare costs a major concern. For nearly everyone, parental work schedules and arrangements for other children must be adjusted. Both father and mother should be included in plans of care; extended family members may also be important sources of help. Most cancer treatments last for a minimum of several months and may last several years, necessitating nearly constant adaptation by the child and family. A child's developmental stage significantly impacts his reaction to the illness:

- Infants and toddlers are unaware of the severity of the disease and deal with issues such as pain and separation from parents.
- Preschoolers are beginning to understand illness. However, they may think they caused their illness, and may be confused about why the parent cannot make the illness go away.
- School-age children can understand a diagnosis of cancer and benefit from opportunities to talk about the experience.
- Adolescents find contact with others who have gone through their experience reassuring and supportive.

Nearly all children are hospitalized after diagnosis. Care should include being in proximity to parents, involvement in self-care appropriate for age, positive relationships with staff, and emotional care (Tomlinson & Kline, 2010). Programs such as group therapy sessions, computer programs about cancer and treatment, and school reintegration can assist youth who are adjusting to cancer.

Understandably, a diagnosis of cancer followed by hospitalization can be traumatic for a child, and may evoke a variety of emotional responses, including anxiety and depression. Some medications used in the treatment of cancer can cause depression as well (Tomlinson & Kline, 2010). Careful assessment and monitoring of the child's psychosocial status before and throughout treatment are essential.

Cancer Survival   Children with cancer, as well as their families, are dealing with a complex illness that will influence their lives for years. During the past 30 years, treatment for childhood cancers has been increasingly successful. From 1969 to 2008, mortality rates for children with cancer declined by 66% (ACS, 2012a). The success of new modalities and treatment combinations has, however, created special healthcare needs for many survivors.

Treatment of Cancer in Children   The short- and long-term effects of surgery are numerous and depend on the nature of the procedure. If surgical intervention is necessary, in addition to her illness, the child must cope with fears related to surgery and anesthesia, as well as with challenges associated with postoperative recovery. Whenever possible and appropriate, the nurse should encourage the child to take part in decision-making processes and to actively participate in her plan of care. Allowing the pediatric client to play an active role in her care gives her a sense of control and promotes effective coping (Salmela et al., 2010).

Likewise, radiation has both immediate and long-term effects. According to the American Cancer Society, radiation can impair the growth of bones and teeth, leading to conditions such as leg length discrepancy, osteoporosis, or poor dental health. Chronic pain can result from skeletal toxicity. Hypothyroidism can be observed in those who have had head and neck radiation. Cardiotoxicity and pulmonary toxicity can result from mediastinal radiation, and delayed puberty and sterility can result from radiation effects to the cranium and spinal regions. Impaired neurocognitive performance may occur as long-term effects of treatment, especially with higher doses of radiation (ACS,

2012c). Some studies have found lower behavioral and social competence in treated children, and higher rates of posttraumatic stress syndrome (Tomlinson & Kline, 2010).

Chemotherapy can cause a wide variety of effects, both during its administration and for years afterward. Cardiomyopathy can occur with some drugs, especially the anthracyclines. Temporary or permanent pulmonary toxicity and renal complications can develop. Certain chemotherapy drugs and antibiotics, as well as radiation to the ear or brain, can lead to hearing loss. Radiation to the eye and certain chemotherapy medications can cause cataracts and other eye problems. Learning disabilities and change in intelligence quotient (IQ) occur in some children. Infertility may also result (ACS, 2012c).

Secondary cancers, most commonly solid tumors, occur in some survivors. Secondary cancers are also called second malignant neoplasms (SMNs), and are those that occur subsequent to the primary cancer and treatment but are of a different histological type. Cancer treatment during childhood may predispose the client to developing SMNs. For example, survivors of childhood cancer tend to have a higher risk for developing cancer in areas that were previously treated with radiation. Although radiation is responsible for most secondary tumors, some chemotherapy drugs have also been implicated.

Survivors of childhood cancer are also at higher risk for developing cancers commonly seen in adults, such as colon, breast, or prostate cancer (ACS, 2012c). Reproductive health can pose problems as the survivor reaches young adulthood and wishes to have children.

The diagnosis and stress of treatment, along with the risk of recurrence, are significant stressors for the child with cancer. Families may find it difficult to obtain full insurance coverage for the child who has had a prior cancer. Employment can be a potential problem for cancer survivors if employers have concerns about the earlier cancer diagnosis. Most people with cancer report fear of recurrence of the disease, which is a stressor. Research suggests survivors of childhood cancer may demonstrate higher rates of depression and suicidal ideation (Recklitis et al., 2010). Conversely, hopefulness and the sense of having an added purpose in life can be positive outcomes for many cancer survivors. Some meet with others who have a recent diagnosis, and both children and their families sometimes work on fundraising events that financially support cancer research. The highest risk for long-term psychological distress in adult survivors of childhood cancer occurs in those with poor health status, low income, low education, and unemployment (Recklitis et al., 2010). A group of physician researchers identified the following barriers to optimal care for cancer survivors:

■ Lack of knowledge about survivorship by healthcare professionals

■ Lack of knowledge about risks and care recommendations by the cancer survivor

■ Limitations to follow-up care due to issues related to healthcare coverage and insurability

■ Inadequate access to psychological services geared toward promoting the transition to independence in adulthood.

Therefore, additional education of healthcare professionals and the public, as well as research into survivor issues, is recommended (Henderson, Friedman, & Meadows, 2010).

Focus on Diversity and Culture
The Client With Cancer

A client's cultural background may impact care in a variety of ways. Cultural preferences, values, and beliefs may determine who makes the decisions regarding the client's care, the extent to which the client wants to explore complementary and alternative therapies, and the client's dietary preferences (see the module on Culture and Diversity). Whenever possible, the healthcare team considers clients' cultural and religious practices (e.g., not scheduling procedures or treatments on religious holy days). Although some research supports the use of complementary therapies such as acupuncture, yoga, and meditation to manage treatment side effects, research in this area remains limited. More importantly, some herbal and over-the-counter vitamins and supplements (e.g., St. John's wort and high doses of vitamins) may adversely impact treatment (National Center for Complementary and Alternative Medicine [NCCAM], 2012b).

PREGNANT WOMEN Approximately 1 out of 1,000 pregnant women will simultaneously battle cancer. While some cancers are capable of spreading to the placenta, most cancers are unable to spread to the fetus. Naturally, recognition and treatment of cancer remains a critical concern for both mother and baby (ASCO, 2013).

Because cancer-related symptoms may be similar to those that normally accompany pregnancy, delayed diagnosis may be an issue. For example, frequent headaches and abdominal bloating, which are commonly associated with pregnancy, may be overlooked or accepted as being normal pregnancy-related manifestations. Likewise, because most pregnant women do not undergo mammogram screenings, breast cancer may develop undetected. However, the converse is also true: Pregnancy can lead to detection of cancerous conditions that otherwise may not have been recognized; for example, a prenatal ultrasound may reveal ovarian cancer (ASCO, 2013).

Although surgery is considered to be the safest treatment option for pregnant women with cancer, certain types of chemotherapy may be administered during the second and third trimester. Generally, treatment with radiation is avoided, due to potentially harmful fetal effects (ASCO, 2013). When a pregnancy is involved, the approach to treating cancer becomes even more complex. Nursing considerations include acknowledging the immense physical and psychosocial stress these clients face, as well as being aware of the latest treatment approaches for the specific form of cancer involved.

🌐 *Stay Current: To learn more about the management of breast cancer in pregnant women, visit the National Cancer Institute's Web site at* **www.cancer.gov/cancertopics/pdq/ treatment/breast-cancer-and-pregnancy/HealthProfessional/ page1/AllPages**.

For an overview of the treatment of other forms of cancer in pregnant women, visit the National Institutes of Health Web site at **www.nlm.nih.gov/medlineplus/cancerandpregnancy.html**.

Clinical Manifestations and Therapies **Cancer**

ETIOLOGY	CLINICAL MANIFESTATION	CLINICAL THERAPIES
Direct tumor involvement with the tissues often results in pain.	■ Pain, often severe in nature and described as any type, depending on the tissue involved	■ Pain management usually requires narcotic analgesics with escalating dosages as tolerance develops.
Anorexia-cachexia syndrome often results from rapid growth and reproduction of cancer cells and their need for increased nutrients.	■ Muscle wasting, weight loss, emaciated appearance, with resulting weakness and fatigue	■ Nutritional counseling ■ Increase caloric intake ■ Reduction in activity level ■ Vitamin and mineral supplementation ■ Dietary supplements, such as liquid formulas, may help provide extra calories between meals.
Risk for infection may increase as a result of bone marrow suppression secondary to both the tumor growth and treatments.	■ Fever, malaise, fatigue with minor infections ranging to septicemia with systemic infection	■ Teach infection prevention techniques, including hand hygiene, cough etiquette, and crowd avoidance. ■ Antimicrobial medications to treat existing infections ■ Monitor and maintain hydration.
Paraneoplastic syndrome often results from tumor growth that usually involves the endocrine system but may also involve the kidney, skin, neurological, or other systems.	■ Manifestations depend on the system involved. Increased hormone production from ectopic tumor sites will produce symptoms similar to those seen in hypersecretion of hormone.	■ Surgery to remove tumor ■ Palliative treatment of symptoms until tumor reduction therapies diminish impact of tumor ■ Supportive treatment

▶ COLLABORATION

A team approach is essential to the care of clients diagnosed with cancer. Education is a key factor in the prevention and treatment of cancer. For some forms of cancer, including breast and colorectal, early diagnosis is associated with treatment that is both more successful and less extensive in nature (ACS, 2012a). For the client with cancer, diagnosis, treatment, and aftercare are complex processes that require all members of the healthcare team to combine knowledge with compassion throughout each phase of care.

Diagnostic Tests

Several procedures are used to diagnose cancer. X-ray imaging, computed tomography (CT), ultrasonography, and magnetic resonance imaging (MRI) can locate abnormal tissues or tumors. However, only microscopic histological examination of the tissue reveals the type of cell and its structural difference from the parent tissue. Tissue samples are acquired through biopsy, shed cells (e.g., Papanicolaou smear), or collections of secretions (e.g., sputum). Lymph nodes are also biopsied to determine whether metastasis has begun. Simple screening procedures can be used to pick up substances secreted by the tumor, such as the prostate-specific antigen (PSA) blood test now being used to identify early prostate cancers. Increases in enzymes or hormones released by normal tissues when they are damaged can also contribute to the diagnosis. Increased alkaline phosphatase noted in bone metastases and osteosarcoma is one example of an enzyme increase associated with cancer. Recent research also has identified tumor markers, which are used for early diagnosis, tracking responses to therapy, and devising immunological treatments.

Some investigators studying chemical mediators of the immune system have noted that communication seems to occur between the chemical mediators and the emotional centers of the brain. Healthcare providers should listen carefully to the client who states "I feel I have cancer" and investigate thoroughly.

To help standardize diagnosis and treatment protocols, an elaborate identification system has been developed. This consists of naming the tumor (classification) and describing its aggressiveness (grading) and spread within or beyond the tissue of origin (staging).

Tumors are classified and named by the tissue or cell of origin. Tumor nomenclature often incorporates the Latin stem identifying the tissue from which the tumor arises. For example, a carcinoma arises from epithelial tissue; adjectives are added to further specify the location. A glandular malignancy arising from epithelial tissue is classified as an adenocarcinoma. A tumor arising from supportive tissues is called a sarcoma; the specific type of tissue is added as a prefix. For example, a cancer of fibrous connective tissue is called a fibrosarcoma, and a smooth muscle cancer is a leiomyosarcoma. A tumor from seminal or germ tissue is called a seminoma. **Table 2–3** ● compares the nomenclature of benign and malignant neoplasms.

Other names for tumors incorporate the name of the discoverer of that particular cancer, such as Burkitt lymphoma or Hodgkin disease. Hematopoietic malignancies (also known as liquid tumors) are usually named by the type of immature blood cell that dominates. For example, myelocytic leukemia is

TABLE 2–3   Nomenclature for Benign and Malignant Neoplasms

	TISSUE OF ORIGIN	BENIGN	MALIGNANT
Ectoderm/endoderm	Epithelium	Papilloma	Carcinoma
	Gland	Adenoma	Adenocarcinoma
	Liver cells	Hepatocellular adenoma	Hepatocellular carcinoma
	Neuroglia	Glioma	Glioma
	Melanocytes	Melanoma	Malignant melanoma
	Basal cells		Basal cell carcinoma
	Germ cells	Tetroma	Seminoma
Mesoderm	Connective tissue		
	Adipose tissue	Lipoma	Liposarcoma
	Fibrous tissue	Fibroma	Fibrosarcoma
	Bone tissue	Osteoma	Osteosarcoma
	Cartilage	Chondroma	Chondrosarcoma
	Muscle		
	Smooth muscle	Leiomyoma	Leiomyosarcoma
	Striated muscle	Rhabdomyoma	Rhabdomyosarcoma
	Neural tissue		
	Nerve cells	Ganglioneuroma	Neuroblastoma
	Endothelial tissues		
	Blood vessels	Hemangioma	Angiosarcoma
			Kaposi sarcoma
	Meninges	Meningioma	Malignant meningioma
Hematopoietic tissues	Granulocytes	Granulocytosis	Leukemia
	Plasma cells		Multiple myeloma
	Lymphocytes		Lymphomas

named for the immature form of the granulocyte that is predominant in this malignancy.

GRADING AND STAGING   **Grading** evaluates the amount of differentiation (level of functional maturity) of the cell and estimates the rate of growth based on the mitotic rate. Cells that are the most differentiated—that is, cells that are most like the parent tissue and therefore the least malignant—are classified as grade 1 and are associated with a better prognosis. Grade 4 is reserved for the least differentiated and most aggressively malignant cells. Because of the differences inherent in tumor appearance and biological behavior, grading criteria may vary with different locations and types of tumors.

Staging is used to classify solid tumors and refers to the relative size of the tumor and extent of the disease. The TNM staging system is internationally recognized: The T stands for the relative tumor size, depth of invasion, and surface spread; N indicates the presence and extent of lymph node involvement; and M denotes the presence or absence of distant metastases. **Table 2–4** ● shows the basic outline of the TNM system; however, other systems are also used to differentiate types and locations of tumors (e.g., melanomas, cervical cancer, and Hodgkin disease).

CYTOLOGICAL EXAMINATION   For the malignant tissues to be identified by name, grade, and stage, they must first be subjected to histological and cytological examination by light or electron microscopy. Specimens are collected by three basic methods:

1. **Exfoliation from an epithelial surface.** Examples include scraping cells from the cervix (Pap smear) or bronchial washings.
2. **Aspiration of fluid from body cavities or blood.** Examples include WBCs for evaluation of hematopoietic cancers, pleural fluid, and cerebrospinal fluid.
3. **Needle aspiration of solid tumors.** This could include the breast, lung, or prostate.

TABLE 2–4   The TNM Staging System

	STAGE	MANIFESTATIONS
Tumor	T0	No evidence of primary tumor
	Tis	Tumor in situ
	T1, T2, T3, T4	Ascending degrees of tumor size and involvement
Nodes	N0	No abnormal regional nodes
	N1a, N2a	Regional nodes—no metastasis
	N1b, N2b, N3b	Regional lymph nodes—metastasis suspected
	Nx	Regional nodes cannot be assessed clinically
Metastasis	M0	No evidence of distant metastasis
	M1, M2, M3	Ascending degrees of metastatic involvement of the host, including distant nodes

Cytological examination is also carried out on specimens from biopsied tissues or tumors and on collected body secretions, such as sputum or urine.

After collection, specimens are spread on a glass slide, fixed, and stained if necessary. The morphological features of the cells are examined, with special attention to the nucleus and cytoplasm. Other special pathological procedures can be carried out on the specimen, but they must be ordered ahead of time if special preparations of the specimen are necessary.

TUMOR MARKERS A **tumor marker** is a protein molecule detectable in serum or other body fluids. This marker is used as a biochemical indicator for the presence of a malignancy. Small amounts of tumor marker proteins are found in normal body tissues or benign tumors and are not specific for malignancy. However, high levels are suspicious and mandate follow-up diagnostic studies.

Tumor marker tests are currently in the developmental and investigational phase and are most useful for monitoring the client's response to therapy and for detecting residual disease. However, one marker, PSA, has received a great deal of media attention as a detector of prostate cancer. As a result, many healthcare practitioners recommend screening for it in men over age 40, much as Pap smears and mammograms are recommended for women.

Tumor markers fall into two general categories: those derived from the tumor itself and those associated with host (immune) response to the tumor. Examples of tumor markers include the following:

- **Antigens.** These are present in fetal tissue but normally are suppressed after birth. Thus, their presence in large amounts may reflect an anaplastic process in tumor cells. Alpha-fetoprotein and carcinoembryonic antigen (CEA) are oncofetal antigens.

- **Hormones.** Hormones are, of course, present in human blood and tissues in considerable amounts, but very high levels not related to other conditions may signify the presence of a hormone-secreting malignancy. Some common hormones seen as tumor markers include human chorionic gonadotropin, antidiuretic hormone, parathyroid hormone, calcitonin, and catecholamines.

- **Proteins.** These narrow down the type of tissue that may be malignant, although they can also be increased in hyperplastic disorders. Examples of tissue-specific proteins include serum immunoglobin and beta$_2$-microglobulin.

- **Enzymes.** Rapid, excessive growth of a tissue may cause some of the enzymes and isoenzymes normally present in that particular tissue to spill into the bloodstream. Elevated levels can point to either hyperplasia of the tissue or cancer. Prostatic acid phosphatase and neuron-specific enolase are examples. Table 2–5 ● compares selected tumor-derived markers with their presence in neoplasms and other conditions.

TABLE 2–5 Selected Tumor-Derived Markers Associated With Specific Neoplasms

	TUMOR MARKER	ASSOCIATED NEOPLASM
Oncofetal antigens	Carcinoembryonic antigen (CEA)	Adenocarcinomas of colon, lung, breast, ovary, stomach, pancreas
	Alpha-fetoprotein (AFP)	Primary liver cell cancer, ovarian cancer, gonadal germ cell tumors
Hormones	Human chorionic gonadotropin (HCG)	Gonadal germ cell tumors
	Calcitonin	Medullary cancer of thyroid
	Catecholamines/metabolites	Pheochromocytoma
Enzymes	Lactate dehydrogenase	Leukemia, lymphoma, gonadal germ cell tumors, melanoma, neuroblastoma
Isoenzymes	Prostatic acid phosphatase (PAP)	Adenocarcinoma of prostate
	Neuron-specific enolase (NSE)	Small-cell lung carcinoma, neuroblastoma
Specific proteins	Prostate-specific antigen (PSA)	Adenocarcinoma of prostate
	Immunoglobin	Multiple myeloma
	CA 125	Epithelial ovarian cancer
	CA 19-9	Adenocarcinoma of pancreas, colon
	CA 15-3	Breast cancer
	CA 27-29	Breast cancer
	Bladder tumor antigen (BTA)	Bladder cancer
	Epidermal growth factor receptor (EGFR), also known as	Non-small-cell, lung, head and neck, colon, pancreas, breast cancers
	HER1	Breast cancer
	HER2	Breast cancer

Source: Based on American Society of Clinical Oncology. (2013). What to know: ASCO's guideline on tumor markers for testicular cancer and extragonadal germ cell tumors in teenage boys and men. Retrieved from http://www.cancer.net/publications-and-resources/what-know-ascos-guidelines/what-know-ascos-guideline-tumor-markers-testicular-cancer-and-extragonadal-germ-cell-tumors-teenage; MedLine Plus. (2013). Lactate dehydrogenase test. Retrieved from http://www.nlm.nih.gov/medlineplus/ency/article/003471.htm; American Cancer Society. (2012). Tumor specific markers. Retrieved from http://www.cancer.org/treatment/understandingyour-diagnosis/examsandtestdescriptions/tumormarkers/tumor-markers-specific-markers.

ONCOLOGICAL IMAGING Because physical assessment usually cannot detect cancer until the tumor has reached a size that poses a major risk for metastasis, radiological examination is extremely important in early diagnosis. This diagnostic process may involve routine x-ray imaging (usually for screening only), CT, MRI, ultrasonography, nuclear imaging, angiography, and positron-emission tomography.

X-Ray Imaging Considered the least expensive and least invasive diagnostic procedure, film screen imaging (standard x-ray imaging) is the method of choice for screening such body areas as the breast (mammography), lung, and bone to identify changes in tissue density that may indicate malignancies. X-ray studies are limited in that they do not easily distinguish among calcifications, benign cystic growths, and true malignancies. However, as a screening tool, x-ray imaging can usually reassure the client if findings are negative or encourage follow-up studies if findings are suspicious. X-ray imaging is still the method of choice for lung cancer. Unfortunately, it does not usually reveal tumors until they have reached about 1 cm in size, which is late in their development.

Computed Tomography By applying computers and mathematics to diagnostic imaging, CT allows for visualization of cross sections of the anatomy. Because CT scans reveal subtle differences in tissue densities, they provide much greater accuracy in tumor diagnosis than traditional x-rays. CT is useful in screening for some cancers such as renal cell and most gastrointestinal tumors and in evaluating possible lymph node involvement.

Magnetic Resonance Imaging Like CT, MRI involves computerized mathematical technology. The client is placed within a strong magnetic field, pulsed radio waves are directed at the client, and transmitted signals based on tissue characteristics are analyzed by a computer. Related diagnostic imaging procedures—positron-emission tomography and single-photon-emission computed tomography—create visible images by measuring electrical impulses from different body structures. Despite its expense, MRI is the diagnostic tool of choice for both screening and follow-up of cranial as well as head and neck tumors.

Ultrasonography Ultrasonography is relatively safe and noninvasive. It measures sound waves as they bounce off various body structures, giving an image of normal anatomy as well as revealing abnormalities that indicate tumors. Ultrasonography has been adapted for diagnosing some specific tumors. For example, transrectal ultrasonography has provided excellent imaging of early prostate cancers and is used to guide needle biopsy. Ultrasound imaging is also more useful for detecting masses in the denser breast tissue of young women.

Nuclear Imaging Nuclear imaging involves the use of a special scintillation scanner in conjunction with the ingestion or injection of specific radioactive isotopes. This is an invasive, but usually safe, diagnostic method for identifying tumors in various body tissues. For the client with a newly diagnosed cancer, the procedure is often used to check for possible bone or other organ metastases. This evaluation helps the healthcare provider determine appropriate treatment.

The principle underlying the technology is that certain isotopes have an affinity for specific tissues; for example, radioactive iodine (I-131) has an affinity for the thyroid gland. Malignancies in these tissues sequester an abnormally large amount of the isotope, which then can be traced and measured by the scintillation scanner. This procedure is considered safe, because the amount of isotope used is small enough not to damage normal cells.

Usually, the procedure is only minimally distressing for clients. Drinking the isotope solution is not pleasant but is tolerable; some anxious clients may have difficulty lying still during the scan. Antianxiety medication may help. Some clients may experience nausea from drinking the isotope and require antiemetic drugs to complete the procedure. Client preparation may include complete restriction of fluids and food by mouth or allowing only clear fluids after midnight.

Angiography An expensive and invasive procedure, angiography is used infrequently for tumor diagnosis. Angiography is performed when the precise location of the tumor cannot be identified or the tumor's extent needs to be visualized before surgery.

The procedure involves injecting a radiopaque dye into a major blood vessel proximal to the organ or tissue to be examined. The movement of the dye through the vasculature of the organ or tissue is then traced by means of fluoroscopy or serial x-ray films. In some cases, small catheters are threaded through the vein under fluoroscopy to ensure the specific placement of the dye. Blockage to the flow of the dye indicates the tumor's location. Dye may also be used to identify blood vessels supplying a tumor, allowing the surgeon to know where to safely ligate vessels.

Angiography requires preparation similar to that for minor surgery. This includes ensuring that the client takes in only fluids on the day of the examination, performing skin preparation at the insertion site, and administering sedative drugs before the procedure. Clients should be informed that injection of the dye used to enhance imaging may cause a hot, flushing sensation or nausea and vomiting. Although angiography is usually done on an outpatient basis, the client will be kept in a short-stay unit for several hours and monitored for such complications as bleeding at the catheter insertion site.

DIRECT VISUALIZATION Procedures for direct visualization are invasive but do not require the use of radiography. Examples include the following:

- Sigmoidoscopy (viewing the sigmoid colon with a fiberoptic flexible sigmoidoscope)
- Cystoscopy (viewing the urethra and bladder)
- Endoscopy (viewing the upper gastrointestinal tract)
- Bronchoscopy (inspecting the tracheobronchial tree).

These methods allow visual identification of the organs within the limits of the scope and usually permit biopsy of suspicious lesions or masses. Flexible fiberoptic scopes may be more useful, because they allow deeper penetration than traditional scopes. These procedures all require some client preparation, cause moderate to considerable discomfort, and may require sedation or even anesthesia, as in the case of bronchoscopy. Some procedures, such as sigmoidoscopy and cystoscopy, may be performed in the physician's office rather than a hospital and therefore cost less, making them more accessible screening procedures.

Client preparation includes a thorough bowel cleansing before the sigmoidoscopy and cystoscopy; the client may ingest only liquids the morning of the procedure. Because anesthesia may be required, clients undergoing bronchoscopy and endoscopy may be instructed to have nothing by mouth from midnight until the procedure.

A more radical method of direct visualization for suspected malignancies is exploratory surgery with biopsy. In this method, the client undergoes the usual preoperative preparation for the type of surgery anticipated. When the tumor is exposed, a sample of tissue (biopsy) is sent to the pathology laboratory for a "frozen-section" histological examination. This can be done rapidly, while the client remains on the operating table under anesthesia. If the initial report is negative, the benign mass is usually removed to prevent further symptoms. If the report is positive for cancer, the tumor and, often, the adjacent lymph nodes are resected, along with any other suspicious tissue. The tumor, nodes, and any other specimens are sent to the pathology laboratory for more in-depth analysis. The client then receives the usual postoperative care.

LABORATORY TESTS   Most laboratory tests of blood, urine, and other body fluids are used to rule out nutritional disorders and other noncancerous conditions that may be causing the client's symptoms. For example, a CBC helps screen for such problems as anemia, infection, and impaired immunity. Blood chemistries can point out nutritional disturbances and electrolyte imbalances. When combined with other diagnostic tests, routine laboratory tests can be used to form a differential diagnosis and, in certain forms of cancer, can also give clues about disease progression. These tests include evaluating levels of enzymes such as alanine aminotransferase, aspartate aminotransferase, and lactic dehydrogenase for liver metastases. Special protein tumor markers, such as PSA for prostate cancer and CEA for colon cancer, are also used.

✳ Go to **nursing.pearsonhighered.com** to see a table listing common laboratory tests, their normal values, and their possible indications.

Surgery

In many cases, the primary treatment is surgical removal of the cancerous lesion along with a portion of the normal surrounding tissue. The nature of the surgery depends on the location of the cancer, as well as on whether or not the cancer has metastasized. Surgery may also be used for diagnostic confirmation (e.g., a biopsy) and to relieve secondary effects of the cancer, including pain and obstruction of other organs or impairment of physiological processes.

Pharmacologic Therapy

Pharmacologic treatment of cancer, commonly referred to as **chemotherapy**, is the administration of chemicals that destroy cancer cells. Chemotherapeutic medications attack growing cells. Compared to normal cells, cancer cells usually replicate at a faster rate; as a result, cancerous cells are particularly suscep-

tible to these medications. However, the attack on cancer cells is accompanied by unavoidable damage to normal, healthy cells, as manifested by side effects associated with these drugs (ASCO, 2012c). Chemotherapy medications may be administered via numerous routes, including oral, intravenous, subcutaneous, intramuscular, topical, arterial, and intrathecal. Certain chemotherapeutic agents may be administered intraperitoneally (directly into the abdominal cavity) (ASCO, 2012c).

Total pharmacologic eradication of cancer cells is nearly impossible. Rather, the goal of chemotherapy is to kill the greatest possible number of cancer cells, and then to allow the client's immune system to complete the process (Osborn et al., 2013). In addition to being used as a primary treatment in certain cases, chemotherapy may be administered prior to surgery or radiation therapy to cause tumor shrinkage. Following surgery or radiation therapy, chemotherapeutic agents may be administered to help kill remaining cancer cells (ASCO, 2012c).

A simple method of classifying this complex group of drugs includes the following six categories:

- Alkylating agents
- Antitumor antibiotics
- Antimetabolites
- Hormones and hormone agonists
- Biological response modifiers
- Natural products.

For an overview of select chemotherapeutic medications, including their mechanism of action and important nursing considerations for each drug category, see the Medications feature in The Concept of Cellular Regulation section earlier in this module.

SAFETY ALERT
Workplace exposure to antineoplastic agents is believed to be linked to the development of cancer, as well as potentially causing adverse reproductive effects, including infertility, spontaneous abortion, and birth defects. Pharmacists who prepare chemotherapy agents and the nurses who administer the drugs are included among the individuals at greatest risk for exposure to antineoplastic agents (CDC, 2012b). Adherence to safety regulations regarding the preparation and handling of antineoplastic agents remains voluntary; however, nurses and other individuals who are exposed to antineoplastic agents are urged to follow all established safety guidelines and standards (Nelson, 2010).

Radiation Therapy

More than half of all clients diagnosed with cancer will be treated with radiation therapy (Osborn et al., 2013). Radiation therapy is the application of high-energy x-rays or particles for the purpose of damaging or killing cancer cells. Rather than being systemic in nature, as is the case with many forms of chemotherapy, radiation therapy is a localized treatment intended to affect only one body region. Goals of therapy include tumor shrinkage prior to surgery, prevention of postoperative tumor recurrence, and eradication of cancer cells in other parts of the body (ACSO, 2012c). Radiation therapy may also be used for **palliation**, which aims not to cure the disease, but to relieve disease-related symptoms and enhance the client's quality of life (Osborn et al., 2013).

Most commonly, external-beam radiation therapy, during which radiation is administered from a source outside the body, is administered. In addition to using x-rays, external-beam radiation therapy may incorporate the use of high-energy protons, which can kill cancer cells. Internal radiation therapy delivered by way of implants is called brachytherapy (ASCO, 2012c).

■ NURSING PROCESS

Nursing care is vitally important to the client's recovery. The client, family, and loved ones are often very frightened by the diagnosis of cancer and require emotional as well as physical support. It is not unusual for clients to become very sick during treatment as a result of complications or if the neoplasm does not respond to treatment. Nursing care focuses on teaching clients about self-care to avoid complications and minimize side effects of treatment as well as on providing emotional, spiritual, and psychological support.

Assessment

Assessment of the client suspected of having cancer begins with a focused assessment of the organ system involved but then broadens to include a full assessment to determine sites of possible metastasis. For example, the client presenting with a lump in the breast will have a focused assessment looking for changes in the breast that may indicate the cause of the lump. However, once the client is diagnosed with cancer, a more thorough assessment will be required that looks for any abnormality that could indicate metastasis, side effects of treatment, or complications of therapy.

The client interview generally progresses from exploration of the client's current complaint to a broader health history and physical status. In addition, for clients who are diagnosed with cancer, functional limitations, psychosocial considerations, and the client's understanding of the treatment plan should be discussed. (See the Assessment Interview feature.)

Assessment Interview Cancer

The following are appropriate questions to ask the client during the initial interview and at subsequent assessments:

- *"What brought you in to see the doctor?"* Asking open-ended, introductory questions may elicit more information than asking specific questions. The answer should elicit not only data about the signs and symptoms but also fears or concerns. For clients who offer insufficient information in response to this open-ended question, more specific questions may be necessary, such as "Did you have pain or any specific physical problems that caused you to seek health care?"

- *"Do you have any history of other medical conditions or health problems?"* Thorough knowledge of the client's health history is essential to the client's overall care and can also help you anticipate problems and formulate potential nursing diagnoses related to other diseases that may interact with the cancer.

- *"What kinds of physical problems are you having at this time? Do you have pain? Are you nauseated? Have you lost a great deal of weight? Are you so tired you have difficulty carrying on your daily activities? Are you feeling blue or discouraged because of your illness?"* For each positive response, ask follow-up questions to narrow down or define the exact nature of the problem.

- *"What options has your physician suggested for treating your cancer?"* The answer will indicate clients' knowledge about their treatment and, possibly, their communication with the physician. Often, under the stress of a cancer diagnosis, clients do not hear or understand what the physician is saying and are afraid to ask questions. Lack of knowledge indicates a need to collaborate with the physician to explain the information to the client so that the client can absorb and understand it. If the client has a good understanding of the treatment plan, discussing how he feels about it can be useful in exposing fears, concerns, and emotional responses.

- *"What do you expect to happen as a result of this treatment?"* The client's answer may be used to gauge his expectations, as well as to determine education needs regarding the goals and effects of the treatment.

- *"What effect is the disease and/or treatment having on your ability to carry on with your usual daily activities?"* Additional questions may also be needed to pinpoint the types of limitations. The response to this question should provide information regarding the client's functional status.

- *"Who is available to help you at home and run errands for you? Who can provide transportation for you to get to your appointments or treatments? Who can you rely on to be a good listener when you're sad or just to be a comfortable companion? Is there someone you would like to make healthcare decisions for you if there is a time when you are unable to make them for yourself?"* It often seems that the client with cancer is the one who takes care of everyone else; asking for help may be difficult. This information can identify how much support and help the client has or needs. The last question introduces the concept of advanced directives and durable power of attorney regarding health care (see the module on Legal Issues).

- *"How do you manage your stress or your feelings of discomfort? What helps you feel better? Do you think these measures work well for you?"* The responses to these questions provide information about the client's coping strategies and may identify maladaptive strategies, such as alcohol or drug use. Lack of appropriate coping methods can interfere with the client's response to treatment and decrease overall quality of life.

Other assessment questions may be useful at different stages of the client's illness. For example, if the client is not expected to survive the cancer, it is important to ask whether the client has made decisions about last wishes (e.g., for a funeral and burial), whether these have been discussed with significant others, and whether the client has made out a will.

Nurses face a major challenge in educating clients about preventive measures and lifestyle changes to reduce the risk of cancer. At the same time, all clients with cancer must be treated with full respect and dignity, regardless of past lifestyle choices or health behaviors.

Once a cancer diagnosis is established, nurses help clients recover and support them during the rehabilitation phase. In cases of terminal cancer, nurses provide comfort and facilitate positive growth for the client and significant others.

Physical Assessment

When screening for cancer, nurses should keep in mind the American Cancer Society's guidelines for early detection (Box 2–3 ●).

As soon as the client is admitted to the healthcare service or agency, conduct a complete physical assessment to establish a baseline against which to evaluate changes. It is especially important to document the nutritional status of the client using anthropomorphic measurements (i.e., frame size, height, weight, body fat, and muscle mass), and to evaluate laboratory results and note any specific signs and symptoms. For discussion of assessment of nutritional status, refer to the module on Nutrition.

It is also important to assess the client's hydration status, especially if the client is not taking oral food and fluids well or is having bouts of vomiting. (See the module on Fluids and Electrolytes for information on assessment of fluid status.)

Diagnosis

Relevant nursing diagnoses vary depending on the individual client, as well as the client's stage of care. Examples of nursing diagnoses that may be appropriate for inclusion in the plan of care for the client with cancer may include the following:

- *Risk for Infection*
- *Risk for Injury*
- *Imbalanced Nutrition: Less Than Body Requirements*
- *Impaired Tissue Integrity*
- *Acute Pain*
- *Anxiety*
- *Disturbed Body Image*
- *Anticipatory Grieving.*

(NANDA-I © 2012)

Planning

Nursing goals focus on supporting the whole individual and managing specific problems, such as pain, poor nutrition, dehydration, fatigue, adverse emotional responses, altered individual and family coping, and the side effects of medical treatment. Nursing goals may include the following:

- The client will demonstrate no signs or symptoms of infection.
- The client will sustain no injuries.
- Using a predetermined pain rating scale in which 0 represents "no pain" and 10 represents "the worst possible pain," the client will consistently rate her pain at a level of 3 or less.
- The client will maintain weight within normal range based on height and body type.
- The client will remain hydrated, as evidenced by assessment of skin turgor and mucous membranes.

Box 2–3   Selected Cancer Screening Guidelines for Asymptomatic Individuals of Average Risk

COLORECTAL CANCER (MALES AND FEMALES)

- Fecal occult blood test (FOBT) or immunochemical FOBT annually beginning at age 50 or stool DNA test (interval of testing uncertain).
- As alternatives to fecal testing, beginning at age 50, either a flexible sigmoidoscopy every 5 years, double contrast barium enema every 5 years, colonoscopy every 10 years, or CT colonography every 5 years.

BREAST CANCER (FEMALES)

- The client may or may not opt to perform monthly breast self-examination (BSE) beginning at age 20. Either choice is acceptable. Regardless, education should emphasize benefits and limitations of BSE, as well as the importance of immediately reporting any changes or symptoms to a healthcare provider.
- Clinical breast examination (CBE) preferably every 1–3 years from age 20 to 39 and then annually beginning at age 40.
- Mammogram annually beginning at age 40.

CERVICAL AND UTERINE CANCER (FEMALES)

- Papanicolaou (Pap) smear and HPV test every 3 years for women ages 21–29.

- For women ages 30 to 65, screening with both HPV testing and Pap smear (preferred) every 3–5 years.
- Screening may be discontinued in women ages 65 or older who demonstrate three or more consecutive negative Pap tests and no positive Pap test in the last 10 years.
- Cervical cancer screening may be discontinued following total hysterectomy.

PROSTATE CANCER (MALES)

- Men ages 50 years or older should be educated as to the benefits and limitations of prostate-specific antigen (PSA) testing and digital rectal examination. Screening should be completed only in conjunction with an informed decision-making process.

HEALTH COUNSELING AND CANCER CHECKUP (MALES AND FEMALES)

- Upon periodic examination, cancer-related screening should include assessment for cancers of the thyroid, testicles, ovaries, lymph nodes, oral region, and skin. Education and counseling should be provided regarding sun exposure, nutrition and diet, tobacco, sexual behaviors, and occupational and environmental exposures, as well as any other risk factors.

Source: Based on National Cancer Institute. (2013). *PDQ cancer information summaries: Screening/detection (testing for cancer).* Retrieved from http://www.cancer.gov/cancertopics/pdq/screening; MD Anderson Center. (2013). *Cancer screening guidelines.* Retrieved from http://www.mdanderson.org/patient-and-cancer-information/cancer-information/cancer-topics/prevention-and-screening/cancer-screening-guidelines/index.html; American Cancer Society. (2013). *Cancer facts and figures 2013.* Atlanta, GA: Author.

- The client and family will vocalize feelings related to cancer diagnosis and seek support from others to improve coping.
- The client will relate potential side effects of chosen therapies and list strategies for minimizing or coping with symptoms.

Implementation

Nursing interventions are evidence-based strategies geared toward helping the client meet the measurable goals associated with each nursing diagnosis. As with all elements of the care plan, the selection and implementation of nursing interventions must be tailored to reflect the individual client's needs. For the client diagnosed with cancer, nursing interventions also vary significantly depending on the type and location of the cancer cells.

In addition to physical care, clients diagnosed with cancer have critical comfort-related and psychosocial needs that must be addressed in order to promote recovery. While management of life-threatening physiological conditions always takes priority over pain management, in the stable client, treatment of pain remains a priority concern. Analgesics should be administered as ordered; collaboration with the prescribing provider may be needed to achieve a pain management regimen that affords the client consistently acceptable pain relief. (For a detailed discussion of the nurse's role in pain management, see the Comfort module.) In addition to effectively managing pain, nursing interventions relevant to the physiological and psychosocial care of the client with cancer are discussed next.

Prevent Infection

Clients with cancer face multiple risks for infection including malnutrition, tumor necrosis, suppression of WBCs from chemotherapy or radiation, anorexia resulting from nausea and other treatment side effects. Bone marrow depression resulting from certain types of cancer and chemotherapy undermines the body's ability to respond to infection. The client may exhibit the classic signs of infection: lassitude, fever, anorexia, pain in the affected area, and physical evidence of infection, such as a purulent, draining lesion or wound. If the bone marrow is compromised, the usual signs and symptoms of infection may be absent or reduced.

- Monitor vital signs. Fever and sympathetic nervous system responses, such as increased pulse and respiration, are the usual early signs of infection. However, clients with severe immunosuppression may be unable to mount a fever; therefore, the absence of fever cannot rule out infection.
- Monitor WBC counts frequently, especially if the client is receiving chemotherapy known to cause bone marrow suppression. This allows the nurse to notify the physician at the first sign of diminishing WBC counts so that corrective action can be taken.
- Teach the client to avoid crowds, small children, and people with infections when his WBC count is at nadir (lowest point during chemotherapy) and to practice scrupulous personal hygiene. During periods of leukopenia, clients may lose immunity to their own natural flora. Careful attention to hygiene reduces the risk of infection. Small children should be avoided, because they often have microbes to which most people are usually immune but that the client may not be able to resist.
- Protect skin and mucous membranes from injury. Teach appropriate skin care measures, such as good hygiene, use of a moisturizing lotion to prevent dryness and cracking, frequent changes of position for individuals who are bed bound, and immediate attention to skin breaks or lesions. Ensuring intact skin strengthens the first line of defense against infection.
- Encourage the client to consume a diet high in protein, minerals, and vitamins, especially vitamin C. Improving nutrition decreases the risk of infection. Vitamin C has been shown to help prevent certain types of infection, such as colds.

Prevent Injury

In addition to infection, cancer can pose a risk for injury from, for example, obstruction by a large tumor or one located in a limited body space (e.g., in the brain, bowel, or bronchial airways). If the cancer is one that creates ectopic sites of hormones, elevated levels of hormones that are not under the control of the pituitary gland can injure the client in a variety of ways. Signs of obstruction depend on the organ involved: Bowel obstruction presents with pain, distention, and cessation of bowel activities; obstruction in the brain gives signs of increased intracranial pressure or personality/behavioral change; bronchial obstruction manifests as respiratory distress, cyanosis, and altered arterial blood gases. Ectopic production of parathyroid hormone manifests as high serum calcium levels as well as signs of hypercalcemia; ectopic production of antidiuretic hormone causes fluid retention and manifests as hypertension and peripheral and pulmonary edema.

- Assess frequently for signs and symptoms indicating problems with organ obstruction. Early detection of major problems allows the nurse to seek medical help before the problem evolves into a physiological crisis.
- Teach the client to differentiate minor problems from those of a serious nature. Encourage the client to consult with the nurse or physician if in doubt or to call 911 if she becomes very ill. The Community-Based Care feature provides guidelines to help clients identify serious problems. Having guidelines for when to call the physician provides an anxiety-reducing safety net for the client and family and promotes early detection of complications.
- Monitor laboratory values that may indicate the presence of ectopic functioning and report abnormal findings to physician immediately. **Table 2-6** ● provides laboratory indicators of ectopic functioning. Refer to the respective modules for specific signs and symptoms of alterations in acid-base,

TABLE 2-6 Laboratory Indicators of Ectopic Functioning

HORMONE	SPECIFIC LABORATORY TEST
Antidiuretic hormone (ADH)	Serum and urine osmolality
Adrenocorticotropic hormone (ACTH)	Plasma ACTH, ACTH suppression test, ACTH stimulation test, urine catecholamines
Calcitonin	Serum calcitonin
Insulin	Serum glucose, glucose tolerance test
Parathyroid hormone (PTH)	Serum PTH serum calcium
Thyroxine (T_4)	Serum thyroid-stimulating hormone (TSH), triiodothyronine, T_4

Community-Based Care When Clients With Cancer Should Call for Help

Instruct the client or family member to call the nurse or physician if any of the following signs or symptoms occurs:

- Oral temperature greater than 38.6°C (101.5°F)
- Severe headache
- Significant increase in pain at the usual site, especially if the pain is not relieved by the medication regimen; or severe pain at a new site
- Difficulty breathing
- New bleeding from any site, such as rectal or vaginal bleeding
- Confusion, irritability, or restlessness
- Withdrawal, greatly decreased activity level, or frequent crying
- Verbalizations of deep sadness or a desire to end life

- Changes in body functioning, such as the inability to void or severe diarrhea or constipation
- Changes in eating patterns, such as refusal to eat, extreme hunger, or a significant increase in nausea and vomiting
- Appearance of edema in the extremities or significant increase in edema already present.

Instruct the client or family member to call 911 if the client:

- Is having much difficulty breathing or if the lips or face has a bluish tinge
- Becomes unconscious or has a convulsion
- Exhibits unmanageable behavior, such as being physically abusive, hurting self, or engaging in uncontrollable activity.

---

electrolytes, and endocrine function. Early detection promotes early medical intervention and prevents serious consequences from the ectopic secretion.

Promote Balanced Nutrition

The anorexia-cachexia syndrome (described earlier in this exemplar) is a common cause of malnutrition in clients with cancer. Metabolism increases in response to increased cancer cell production, while the cancer's parasitic activity reduces the nutrients available to the body. Loss of appetite, food aversion, nausea and vomiting, and painful oral lesions from chemotherapy or radiation may contribute to impaired nutrition. Tumors of the gastrointestinal tract that affect absorption also contribute to the problem. Manifestations include wasted appearance, considerable weight loss over a relatively short period of time, anthropometric measurements below 85% of standard for fat and muscle tissue, decreases in serum proteins, and negative responses to antigen testing.

- Assess current eating patterns, including usual likes and dislikes, and identify factors that impair food intake. This allows for a more individualized plan based on needs and preferences.
- Evaluate degree of malnutrition:
  a. Check laboratory values for total serum protein, serum albumin and globins, total lymphocyte count, serum transferrin, hemoglobin, and hematocrit. These values represent the laboratory values that are most likely to decrease with malnutrition.
  b. Calculate nitrogen balance and creatinine-height index. Calculate skeletal muscle mass, and compare findings to normal ranges. Urinary creatinine is an index of lean body mass and decreases in malnutrition. Lean muscle mass is catabolized for energy in clients with cancer.
  c. Take anthropometric measurements, and compare them to standards: height, weight, elbow breadth, arm circumference, triceps skinfold thickness, and arm muscle mass. This estimates the degree of wasting; findings below 85% of standard are considered malnutrition.
- Teach the principles of maintaining good nutrition by using the federal government's MyPlate recommendations and

adapting the diet to medical restrictions and current preferences. This tailors the food plan to the client's needs and thereby promotes compliance.

- Manage problems that interfere with eating:
  a. Encourage eating whatever is appealing, and consider adding nutritional supplements, such as Ensure Plus or Isocal, to the diet. It is better to eat something, even if it is not nutritionally balanced.
  b. Eat small, frequent meals. These are more easily digested and absorbed and usually better tolerated by the client with anorexia.
  c. Encourage the client to try icy-cold foods (e.g., ice cream) or those that are more highly seasoned if food has no taste. Chemotherapy and radiation therapy may harm taste buds and prevent distinguishing the taste of foods. Strong seasonings and coldness make food more enjoyable to the client with diminished taste. However, spicy foods are not recommended for clients with stomatitis.
  d. Encourage cold and bland, semisoft and liquid foods for clients with painful oropharyngeal ulcers; use an anesthetic, alcohol-free mouthwash before eating. These foods are less irritating to sensitive mucous membranes; deadening the pain can make chewing and swallowing easier.
  e. Manage nausea and vomiting by administering antiemetic drugs (around-the-clock medication may be an effective preventive measure). Encourage the client to eat small, frequent, low-fat meals with dry foods (e.g., crackers and toast), to avoid liquids with meals, and to sit upright for an hour after meals. Remove emesis basins, and encourage oral hygiene before eating. Dry, low-fat foods are more readily tolerated when nauseated. Removing vomiting cues, such as odor and supplies associated with vomiting, can reduce nausea.

Client teaching related to nutrition focuses on the following:

- Supplement meals with products such as Ensure Plus or Isocal and take multivitamin and mineral tablets with meals.
- Increase calorie intake by adding ice cream or frozen yogurt to liquid supplements and commercial protein powders to milk or juice.

Box 2–4 Manifestations of Alterations in Tissue Integrity

- Small ulcers occur on the tongue and mucous membranes in the mouth and throat.
- Herpes simplex type 1 lesions or vesicles evolve into ulcerations.
- Fungal infections, such as thrush (resulting from *Candida* infections), are manifested by a white, yellow, or tan coating with dry, red, fissured tissue underneath.
- Red, swollen, friable gums bleed with minimal or no trauma.
- **Xerostomia** is excessive dryness of the mucous membranes (caused by chemotherapy or radiation).

- Keep a food diary to document food intake. By seeing how little is being consumed, the client may eat more.
- Administer parenteral nutrition via central line or other venous access device (VAD). For these clients, teach safety measures, care of the VAD, and explain how the pump delivering solution works. Provide an emergency phone number for help with administration problems.

Protect Tissue Integrity

The most common impairment of tissue integrity occurs in the oral-pharyngeal-esophageal mucous membranes. It is secondary to the effects of some chemotherapeutic drugs and radiation treatment to the head and neck. The oral-pharyngeal-esophageal tissues are lined with cells that have a high mitotic turnover rate and are therefore vulnerable to many chemotherapeutic drugs. Leukemias, bone marrow transplants, and herpes viral infections are other etiological factors in the disruption of oral-pharyngeal-esophageal tissue. **Box 2–4** ● lists manifestations of this problem.

- Carefully assess and evaluate the type of tissue impairment present. Identify possible sources, such as chemotherapy or radiation therapy to head and neck. This allows the nurse to implement corrective measures appropriate to the type of problem.
- Implement and teach measures for preventing oropharyngeal infection:
  a. Encourage cleaning teeth gently and using a nonalcohol mouthwash several times a day. Reducing the oral flora by performing frequent hygiene decreases the risk of infection.
  b. Culture any oral lesions and report the problem to the physician. Herpes lesions may not follow a typical pattern in clients who are immunosuppressed. Identifying the cause of the infection, whether viral, fungal, or bacterial, allows the physician to prescribe the appropriate treatment.
- Implement and teach measures for reducing trauma to delicate tissues:
  a. Counteract dry mouth with lubricating and moisturizing agents, such as Gatorade, sugarless gum, and Blistex. This protects mucous membranes from infection and trauma.
  b. Avoid putting sharp instruments in the mouth. Use smooth plastic spoons and forks for eating, especially with a bleeding disorder. Dental work should be done by dental oncologists.
  c. Brush teeth with a very soft toothbrush, and obtain a new toothbrush monthly. If gums are friable and bleeding, clean teeth with a soft cloth placed over a finger or with

toothpaste on the finger. Chlorhexidine mouthwash (Peridex) may be used. This protects gums from trauma and decreases the risk of hemorrhage.

- Administer specific medications as ordered to control infection and/or pain:
  a. Acyclovir is often used to treat viral infections.
  b. Systemic antibiotics are used to treat bacterial infections.
  c. Nystatin or clotrimazole solution for "swish and swallow" or lozenges that dissolve slowly in the mouth are used for fungal infections.
  d. Use viscous Xylocaine or various combination mouthwashes before meals and as needed. These agents reduce pain and inflammation. Review the contents of each mouthwash and assist in client teaching to prevent hypersensitivity reactions to ingredients (e.g., to lidocaine).

Promote Healthy Coping

Early in the disease continuum—for example, during diagnosis and treatment—threats to or changes in health status, physical comfort, role functioning, or even socioeconomic status can cause anxiety. Later, anxiety may result from the anticipation of pain, disfigurement, or the threat of death. In particular, clients whose coping skills have been poor in the past (e.g., in managing anger) may find themselves at a loss to manage this current crisis. The client may manifest overt signs of anxiety: trembling, restlessness, irritability, hyperactivity, stimulation of the sympathetic nervous system (e.g., increased blood pressure, pulse, respiration, excessive perspiration, and pallor), withdrawal, worried facial expressions, and poor eye contact. The client may report insomnia and feelings of tension and apprehension or express concerns regarding perceived changes brought about by the disease and fear of future events.

- Carefully assess the client's level of anxiety (moderate anxiety, severe anxiety, or panic) and the reality of the threats represented in the client's current situation. The level of anxiety and the reality of the perceived threat influence the type of intervention that is appropriate for the client. A client in panic may need medical intervention with appropriate medications, whereas those with moderate or severe anxiety are often managed by the nurse through counseling and teaching new coping skills.
- Establish a therapeutic relationship by conveying warmth and empathy and by listening nonjudgmentally. A client who feels safe in the relationship with the nurse more easily expresses feelings and thoughts. The client will be able to trust the nurse and perhaps be willing to try new behaviors as suggested.
- Encourage the client to acknowledge and express feelings, no matter how inappropriate they may seem to the client. Just by expressing their feelings, clients often can significantly diminish anxiety. Expressing feelings also allows the client to direct energy toward healing and thus has a positive therapeutic effect. Moreover, by acknowledging feelings, especially those the client considers unacceptable, the client can lay the groundwork for new coping behaviors.
- Review the coping strategies the client has used in the past, and build on past successful behaviors, introducing new strategies as appropriate. Explain why inappropriate strategies, such as repressing anger or turning to alcohol, are not helpful. The client will be more willing to make changes that

Client Teaching Parents of Children With Cancer

It is a gross understatement to say that the diagnosis and treatment of a child with cancer causes great anxiety for the parents. Client teaching can help alleviate some of the anxiety parents experience by providing information about key aspects of treatment. Depending on the stage and type of treatment, the following suggestions may be helpful for parents:

- Children in radiation and chemotherapy experience fatigue. Provide extra rest periods with shorter activity periods between them.
- Have an overnight bag ready in case the child develops a complication and needs to be taken to stay in the hospital for a few days. Several hospital stays of a few days are normal during treatment.

- When concerned about a symptom in the child, ask the care provider. Parents are often key in identifying problems early.
- Because poor appetite can interfere with nutrition intake, children with cancer need to eat when they express hunger.
- Remember that children are still at the normal developmental age. Treat them as a reflection of their ages, not as if they are older or younger.
- Try to maintain contact with the child's peer group and family members.
- Seek information from other parents and resources on cancer care.
- Parents need time for relaxation so that their own energy remains high and they are better able to deal with the child's therapy.

build on what has already worked in the past. The client will also be more willing to reject inappropriate strategies if he is given a persuasive reason why they have not had the desired effect in managing previous crises.

- Provide a safe, calm, and quiet environment for the client in panic. Remain with the client, and administer antianxiety medications as ordered. Staying with the client and displaying calmness and confidence can protect the client from injury and prevent further panic. If the panic does not subside with the nurse's presence and support, referral to the physician for medication management may be necessary.

Promote Healthy Body Image

Cancer and cancer treatments frequently result in major physiological and psychological changes in body image. Loss of a body part (e.g., amputation, prostatectomy, or mastectomy), skin changes and hair loss from chemotherapy or radiation therapy, disfigurement (e.g., lymphedema in the affected upper and lower extremities), or creation of unnatural openings on the body for elimination (e.g., colostomy or ileostomy) may have a major effect on the individual's self-image. The gaunt, wasted appearance of the client with cachexia or of the draining, malodorous lesions that result when cancer breaks through the skin also have a significant impact on a client's body image. Visible changes or disfigurement may also give rise to fear of rejection, which plays a major role in sexual dysfunction. Typical client responses including verbalizing negative feelings about the body and/or fear of rejection by others, refusing to look at the affected site, and depersonalizing the body change or lost part (e.g., by calling the colostomy "that thing").

- Discuss the meaning of the loss or change with the client. Doing so helps the nurse discover the best approach for this particular client and involves the client more actively in interventions. A small, seemingly trivial loss may have a big impact, especially when viewed in light of the other changes that are occurring in the client's life. Likewise, a major loss may not be as important as the nurse might imagine. To ensure more appropriate and individualized care, evaluate each situation in terms of the reactions of the specific client.

- Observe and evaluate the client's interaction with significant others. People who are important to the client may unintentionally reinforce negative feelings about body image; on the other hand, the client may perceive rejection where none exists.
- Allow denial, but do not participate in the denial; for example, if a client does not want to look at the wound, the nurse may say, "I am going to change the dressing on your breast incision now." During the initial stage of shock at the loss of a body part, denial is a protective mechanism and should not be challenged, nor should it be promoted. A matter-of-fact approach and an empathetic attitude will go far to facilitate the eventual acceptance of the change.
- Assist the client and significant others to cope with the changes in appearance:
  a. Provide a supportive environment.
  b. Encourage the client and significant others to express feelings about the situation.

Lifespan Considerations
Children With Cancer and Hair Loss

For many parents, the loss of the child's hair during treatment can be devastating. Ask the parents and the child what this issue is like for them. Prepare them for the fact that hair loss can be rapid or slow. Find out how they plan to cope. Some children want their hair cut very short so its loss will not be as traumatic. Offer resources for wigs, hats, or other ideas. Put them in touch with children who have lost hair and with those who have regrown theirs.

Talk with the child's teachers before the return to school after treatment. Explain the child's condition and assist with plans to prepare the other children. Role-play with the child how to tell friends about any changes in appearance. A nurse or child-life specialist could attend the class of a young child to explain what the client is experiencing.

Provide client teaching about the need for the child with hair loss to cover the head, wear sunscreen when outside, and avoid the sun as much as possible to minimize chance of burn to the head, which is prone to burning due to lack of prior sun exposure.

c. Give matter-of-fact responses to questions and concerns.

d. Identify new coping strategies to resolve feelings.

e. Enlist family and friends in reaffirming the client's worth.

A supportive, safe environment in which feelings are respected and new coping strategies can be tried promotes acceptance, as does reaffirming that the client's worth is not diminished by any physical changes.

■ Teach the client or significant others to participate in the care of the afflicted body area. Support and validate their efforts. Active involvement in providing care, such as changing a dressing or emptying a colostomy bag, empowers the client and/or significant others. This intimate involvement also desensitizes feelings about disfigurement and promotes acceptance. Provide positive reinforcement to promote continued participation.

■ Teach strategies for minimizing physical changes, such as providing skin care during radiation therapy and dressing to enhance appearance and minimize the change in the body part. Early intervention can limit the negative side effects of treatment and actually promote recovery. Involving the client provides an additional way for the client to be in control of a difficult situation.

■ Teach ways to reduce the alopecia that results from chemotherapy and to enhance appearance until the hair grows back:

a. Discuss the pattern and timing of hair loss. This allows the client to cope with changes and incorporate them into daily activities.

b. Encourage wearing cheerful, brightly colored head coverings; assist in color coordinating them with usual clothing. Attractive head coverings protect the bald head while allowing the client to feel stylish and well dressed.

c. Refer to a good wig shop before hair loss is experienced. Hair color and texture can be matched to minimize obvious changes in appearance.

d. Refer to support programs such as "Look Good . . . Feel Better," which is sponsored by the ACS and the Cosmetic, Toilet, and Fragrance Association Foundation. A support group can diminish feelings of isolation and provide practical tips for managing problems.

e. Reassure that hair will grow back after chemotherapy is discontinued, but also inform that the color and texture of the new hair may be different. Hair loss can be devastating for clients. Interventions to reduce that loss can have a significant impact on body image concerns. Moreover, knowing what to expect may decrease anxiety and distress.

Promote Healthy Grief Responses

Overall, only 50% of people with cancer fully recover, and certain types of cancer have a much higher death rate. Thus, the client with cancer is often confronted with facing death and making preparations for it. This can be a healthy response that allows the client and family to work through the dying process and achieve growth in the final stage of life. Perceived changes in body image and lifestyle also can prompt anticipatory grieving. The client or significant others may show sorrow, anger, depression, or withdrawal, expressing distress at the potential loss or verbalizing concern about unfinished life business.

■ Use the therapeutic communication skills of active listening, silence, and nonverbal support to provide an open environment for the client and significant others to discuss their feelings realistically and to express anger or other negative feelings appropriately.

■ Answer questions about illness and prognosis honestly, but always encourage hope. This allows for realistic appraisal of the situation and planning, and it also helps combat feelings of hopelessness and depression.

■ Encourage the client who is dying to make funeral and burial plans ahead of time and to be sure her will is in order. Make sure the necessary phone numbers can be easily located. This gives a sense of control and relieves family members of these concerns.

■ Encourage the client to continue taking part in activities she enjoys, including maintaining employment as long as possible. This gives a sense of continuity of life even in the face of severe losses.

Evaluation

When evaluating the client's response to therapy, it is important to remember that while hopeful outcomes would always include client recovery and absence of complications, this is not realistic for every individual diagnosed with cancer. In some cases, outcomes may include the client's acceptance of and preparedness for death. Other expected outcomes may include the following:

■ The client demonstrates no evidence of infection.

■ Using a predetermined pain rating scale, the client reports pain level of 3 or less, allowing for adequate rest and performance of ADLs.

■ The client reports reduction in side effects of treatment regimen.

■ The client demonstrates appropriate dietary choices to increase caloric intake.

REVIEW Cancer

RELATE Link the Concepts and Exemplars

Linking the exemplar of cancer with the concept of evidence-based practice:

1. How does evidence-based practice impact cancer screening guidelines?

2. In what ways can the nurse ensure that he is adhering to current principles of evidenced-based practice?

Linking the exemplar of cancer with the concept of healthcare systems:

3. Suggest rationales for why reducing cancer-causing lifestyle choices as suggested by the federal government's *Healthy People 2020* program is so important to reducing costs within the healthcare system.

4. How do cancer diagnoses impact the healthcare system?

READY Go to Companion Skills Manual

REFER Go to Pearson Nursing Student Resources
nursing.pearsonhighered.com

- Additional review materials
- Laboratory Tests Used for Cancer Diagnosis
- Nursing Care Plan: A Client With Cancer

REFLECT Case Study

Mandy Leno, 63 years old, has lived with bipolar disorder since young adulthood. She has recently been diagnosed with pancreatic cancer. Following her diagnosis of cancer, Ms. Leno experiences an acute manic episode and is admitted to an inpatient psychiatric unit for evaluation and treatment. She is currently pacing up and down the hall, stating that she will conquer her cancer without drugs or surgery. She is refusing all medications. She has been sleeping little and has deep circles under her eyes. She has eaten very little in the past few days. Her urine output is low, she is disheveled, and her clothes are dirty. Mandy is divorced and has no other family nearby. She has a daughter who lives across the country and has three small children.

1. What are the priorities of care for Ms. Leno?
2. Is Ms. Leno capable of giving consent for surgery? Is surgical consent needed? Why or why not?
3. Should Ms. Leno's daughter be contacted? Explain your answer.

EXEMPLAR 2.2   Anemia

EXEMPLAR KEY TERMS

Anemia, 64
Aplastic anemia, 69
Hemolytic anemia, 68
Iron deficiency anemia, 66
Neonatal anemia, 69
Pernicious anemia, 66
Physiological anemia of infancy, 69
Thalassemia, 68

EXEMPLAR LEARNING OUTCOMES

After reading about this exemplar, you will be able to:

1. Describe the pathophysiology, etiology, clinical manifestations, and direct and indirect causes of anemia.

2. Identify risk factors and prevention methods associated with anemia.
3. Illustrate the nursing process in providing culturally competent care across the life span for individuals with anemia.
4. Formulate priority nursing diagnoses appropriate for an individual with anemia.
5. Summarize therapies used by interdisciplinary teams in the collaborative care of an individual with anemia.
6. Plan evidence-based care for an individual with anemia and his or her family in collaboration with other members of the healthcare team.
7. Evaluate expected outcomes for an individual with anemia.

▶ OVERVIEW

The red blood cell (RBC or erythrocyte) carries oxygen throughout the body. Oxygen binds to hemoglobin, which is the main component of the RBC. **Anemia** occurs when oxygen delivery is inadequate due to a deficient volume of healthy RBCs or a decreased amount of normal hemoglobin. In some cases, even though the number of RBCs is adequate, a defect in the structure and function of the RBC prevents adequate oxygen transport, which causes anemia. Symptoms of anemia can be very vague; in many cases, fatigue is the first symptom of this disorder.

Anemia that occurs due to a decreased volume of RBCs (hematocrit) may be caused by blood loss, inadequate RBC production, or increased RBC destruction. Insufficient or defective hemoglobin may occur due to nutritional deficiencies and physiological disorders.

▶ PATHOPHYSIOLOGY AND ETIOLOGY

Because RBCs are needed to carry oxygen throughout the body, all types of anemia, regardless of their cause, reduce the oxygen-carrying capacity of the blood. Therefore, anemia results in less oxygen reaching cells and tissues, which can lead to tissue hypoxia.

When the onset of anemia is slow, compensatory mechanisms may prevent or mask the appearance of symptoms. However, when oxygen demands increase, such as during exercise or with infection, the symptoms of anemia may become more apparent.

During these times, as blood is redistributed to the vital organs, the skin, mucous membranes, conjunctiva, and nail beds may develop pallor (**Figure 2–6 ●**). Tissue hypoxia triggers a compensatory increase in heart rate and respiratory rate. Increased heart rate promotes an increase in cardiac output, while increased respiratory rate allows for greater delivery of oxygen to the lungs

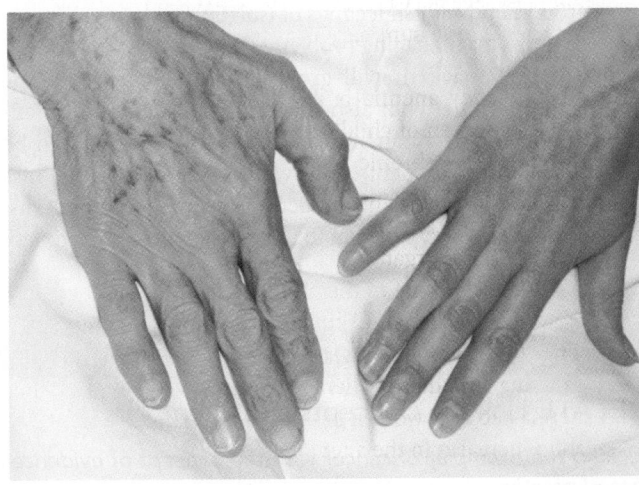

Figure 2–6 ● The skin of the client with anemia appears pale beside that of an individual with a normal hemoglobin and hematocrit.
Source: Westminster Hospital/Science Source.

Box 2–5 Pathophysiological Mechanisms of Anemia

DECREASED RED BLOOD CELL PRODUCTION	INCREASED RED BLOOD CELL LOSS OR DESTRUCTION

■ Altered hemoglobin synthesis:
  a. Iron deficiency
  b. Thalassemia
  c. Chronic inflammation
■ Altered DNA synthesis:
  a. Vitamin B_{12} malabsorption or deficiency
  b. Folic acid malabsorption or deficiency
■ Bone marrow failure:
  a. Aplastic anemia (stem cell dysfunction)
  b. Red cell aplasia
  c. Myeloproliferative leukemias
  d. Cancer metastasis, lymphoma
  e. Chronic infection or inflammation, physical and emotional fatigue
	■ Acute or chronic blood loss:
	  a. Hemorrhage or trauma
	  b. Chronic gastrointestinal bleeding, menorrhagia
	■ Increased hemolysis:
	  a. Hereditary cell membrane disorders
	  b. Defective hemoglobin—sickle cell anemia or trait
	  c. Pyruvate kinase or glucose-6-phosphate dehydrogenase deficiency affecting glycolysis or cell oxidation
	  d. Immune mechanisms and disorders (e.g., blood reaction, hypersensitivity responses, and autoimmune disorders)
	  e. Splenomegaly and hypersplenism
	  f. Infection
	  g. Erythrocyte trauma (e.g., caused by cardiopulmonary bypass, hemolytic uremic syndrome)

and, subsequently, to the blood. Tissue hypoxia may cause angina, fatigue, dyspnea on exertion, and night cramps. It also stimulates erythropoietin release; in turn, increased erythropoietin activity stimulates RBC production in the bone marrow and may lead to bone pain. Cerebral hypoxia can lead to headache, dizziness, and visual disturbances. Severe anemia may cause heart failure.

Etiology

Although a number of different pathological mechanisms can lead to anemia, iron deficiency is the most common cause (**Box 2–5 ●**). Except in infants, inadequate dietary iron intake is rarely a causative factor of iron deficiency anemia. A healthy diet usually provides more than the recommended daily amount of iron, which is 1 mg/day in adults and 2 mg/day in menstruating women (University of Maryland Medical Center [UMMC], 2009a). Excessive iron loss as a result of chronic bleeding is the usual cause of iron deficiency anemia in adults. In menstruating women, excessive blood loss due to heavy menstrual periods (menorrhagia) is the most common cause. See the Clinical Manifestations and Therapies feature on page 72 for a summary of common causes of iron deficiency anemia.

Iron deficiency anemia is particularly common in older adults and in women of childbearing age. Iron deficiency anemia can result from chronic, occult (hidden) blood loss caused by slowly bleeding peptic ulcers, gastrointestinal inflammation, hemorrhoids, and cancer. Depending on its severity, anemia may affect all major organ systems.

Iron deficiency is one of the most common nutritional deficiencies seen in children (Suskind, 2009). Pica (consumption of or cravings for nonfood items) also is associated with iron deficiency anemia in pediatric clients. Lead poisoning is associated with anemia and may worsen in those with anemia because lead absorption increases in the anemic state.

Risk Factors

Clients who do not eat a well-balanced diet rich in fresh fruits and vegetables are at increased risk for those anemias caused by nutrient deficiency, including iron deficiency anemia. During childbearing years, women lose blood during menstruation. Inadequate intake of iron can result in reduced production of RBCs, increasing the risk of anemia due to iron deficiency.

Prevention

Several forms of anemia are genetic in origin and cannot be prevented. However, for those cases of anemia that are caused by iron deficiency, adequate nutrition is a major factor. General guidelines include a balanced diet that combines iron-rich foods with vegetables, fruits, whole grains, low-fat milk products, eggs, lean meat, and fish. Legumes, which include lentils and certain types of peas and beans, are also recommended as sources of nonheme (not from a meat source) iron. Ideally, meals should combine nonheme iron sources with foods that are rich in vitamin C, which promotes the absorption of nonheme iron (Centers for Disease Control and Prevention [CDC], 2011a). Likewise, anemia that is due primarily to insufficient intake of vitamin B_{12} can be treated (and in some cases, reversed) through dietary modifications. Foods rich in vitamin B_{12} include eggs, cheese, milk, meat, and fortified cereals.

▶ CLINICAL MANIFESTATIONS

Anemia is categorized by cause: blood loss, nutritional, hemolytic, and bone marrow suppression (aplastic). A neonatal anemia also is recognized. Each type has its own specific pathophysiology and manifestations.

Blood Loss Anemia

All bleeding involves the loss of RBCs and other blood components. However, the effects and manifestations related to this process depend on the volume and rate of blood loss, as well as on whether the bleeding is acute or chronic.

Acute loss of a significant volume of blood triggers compensatory mechanisms (including an increase in heart rate and constriction of peripheral blood vessels) that help maintain cardiac output. Vessels in the liver, a blood storage organ, also constrict, increasing circulating volume. Fluid shifts from the interstitial spaces into the vascular compartment to maintain blood volume, diluting the cellular components of the blood and reducing its viscosity. If hemorrhage continues, compensatory mechanisms become less effective, increasing the risk for hypovolemic shock and circulatory failure. Initial manifestations of hypovolemic shock include tachycardia and tachypnea; the skin may be pale, cool, and clammy as peripheral vessels constrict to maintain blood flow to the heart and brain. With continued blood loss, hypotension, increased tachycardia, decreased level of consciousness, and oliguria develop.

With chronic bleeding that does not involve the acute loss of significant blood volume, fluid shifts from the interstitial spaces into the vessels. This compensatory shift prevents the development of hypovolemia. However, blood viscosity is reduced, which may result in a systolic heart murmur.

In acute blood loss, circulating RBCs are of normal size and shape (normocytic). Early in the hemorrhage, the red blood cell count, hemoglobin, and hematocrit may be normal; as fluid shifts from the interstitial space into the vascular space to maintain circulating volume, however, the RBC count, hemoglobin, and hematocrit fall. If sufficient iron is available, the number of circulating RBCs and hemoglobin levels return to normal within 3–4 weeks after the bleeding episode. Chronic blood loss, on the other hand, depletes iron stores as RBC production attempts to maintain the RBC supply. The resulting RBCs are small (microcytic) and pale (hypochromic).

Nutritional Anemias

A number of different nutrients are required for normal RBC development (erythropoiesis). Iron is a key nutrient necessary for hemoglobin synthesis. In addition, adequate supplies of protein (and its building blocks, amino acids), vitamins, and other minerals are required. The B vitamins, particularly B_{12} (cobalamin) and folate, play a key role in RBC development. Vitamins C and E also are necessary.

Nutritional anemias result from nutrient deficits that affect RBC formation or hemoglobin synthesis. The nutrient deficit may be caused by inadequate diet, malabsorption of the nutrient, or increased need for the nutrient. The most common types of nutritional anemias are iron deficiency anemia, vitamin B_{12} deficiency anemia, and folic acid deficiency anemia. Vitamin B_{12} and folic acid anemias are sometimes called megaloblastic anemias, because enlarged, nucleated RBCs (megaloblasts) are seen in these anemias.

IRON DEFICIENCY ANEMIA   **Iron deficiency anemia** develops when the body's supply of iron is inadequate for optimal RBC formation. The body cannot synthesize hemoglobin without iron. Normally, the body efficiently recycles and stores iron, reusing much of the iron contained in RBCs that are removed from circulation because of age or damage. However, small amounts of iron are continually lost in the feces; therefore, adequate iron intake is necessary for normal hemoglobin synthesis and RBC production.

Iron deficiency anemia results in fewer numbers of RBCs and in microcytic, hypochromic, and malformed RBCs (poikilocytosis) (**Figure 2–7 ●**). Chronic iron deficiency may lead

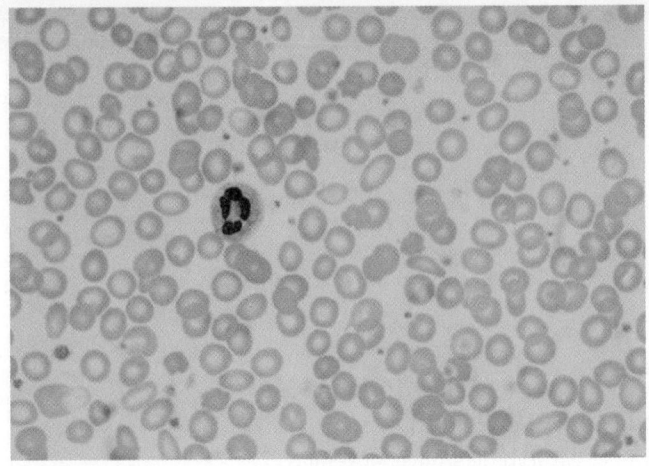

to brittle, spoon-shaped nails; cheilosis (cracks at the corners of the mouth); a smooth, sore tongue; and pica.

VITAMIN B_{12} DEFICIENCY ANEMIA   Vitamin B_{12} is necessary for DNA synthesis and is found almost exclusively in foods derived from animals. Vitamin B_{12} deficiency occurs when inadequate vitamin B_{12} is consumed or, more commonly, when it is poorly absorbed from the gastrointestinal tract. Deficiency of this vitamin impairs cell division and maturation of the cell nucleus, especially in rapidly proliferating RBCs. As a result, macrocytic (large), misshapen (oval rather than concave) RBCs with thin membranes are produced. Great numbers of these large, immature RBCs enter the circulation. These cells are fragile, incapable of carrying adequate amounts of oxygen, and have a shortened life span.

Failure to absorb dietary vitamin B_{12} produces **pernicious anemia**. It develops from lack of gastric intrinsic factor (IF), which is a substance secreted by the gastric mucosa. Intrinsic factor binds with vitamin B_{12} and travels with it to the ileum, where the vitamin is absorbed. In the absence of IF, the body cannot absorb vitamin B_{12}.

Vitamin B_{12} deficiency may also result from other malabsorption disorders and dietary factors. Resection of the stomach or ileum, loss of pancreatic secretions, and chronic gastritis can affect vitamin B_{12} absorption. Dietary deficiencies of vitamin B_{12} are rare, usually occurring only among strict vegetarians.

Manifestations of vitamin B_{12} deficiency anemia develop gradually as body stores of the vitamin are depleted. Pallor or slight jaundice and weakness develop. In pernicious anemia, a smooth, sore, beefy red tongue and diarrhea may occur. Because vitamin B_{12} is important for neurological function, paresthesias (altered sensations, such as numbness or tingling) in the extremities and problems with proprioception (the sense of one's position in space) develop. These manifestations may progress to difficulty maintaining balance as a result of spinal cord damage. The degree to which neurological abnormalities can be reversed depends on both the severity and duration of the abnormalities. Earlier treatment generally produces better outcomes (Stabler, 2013).

Multisystem Effects of Anemia

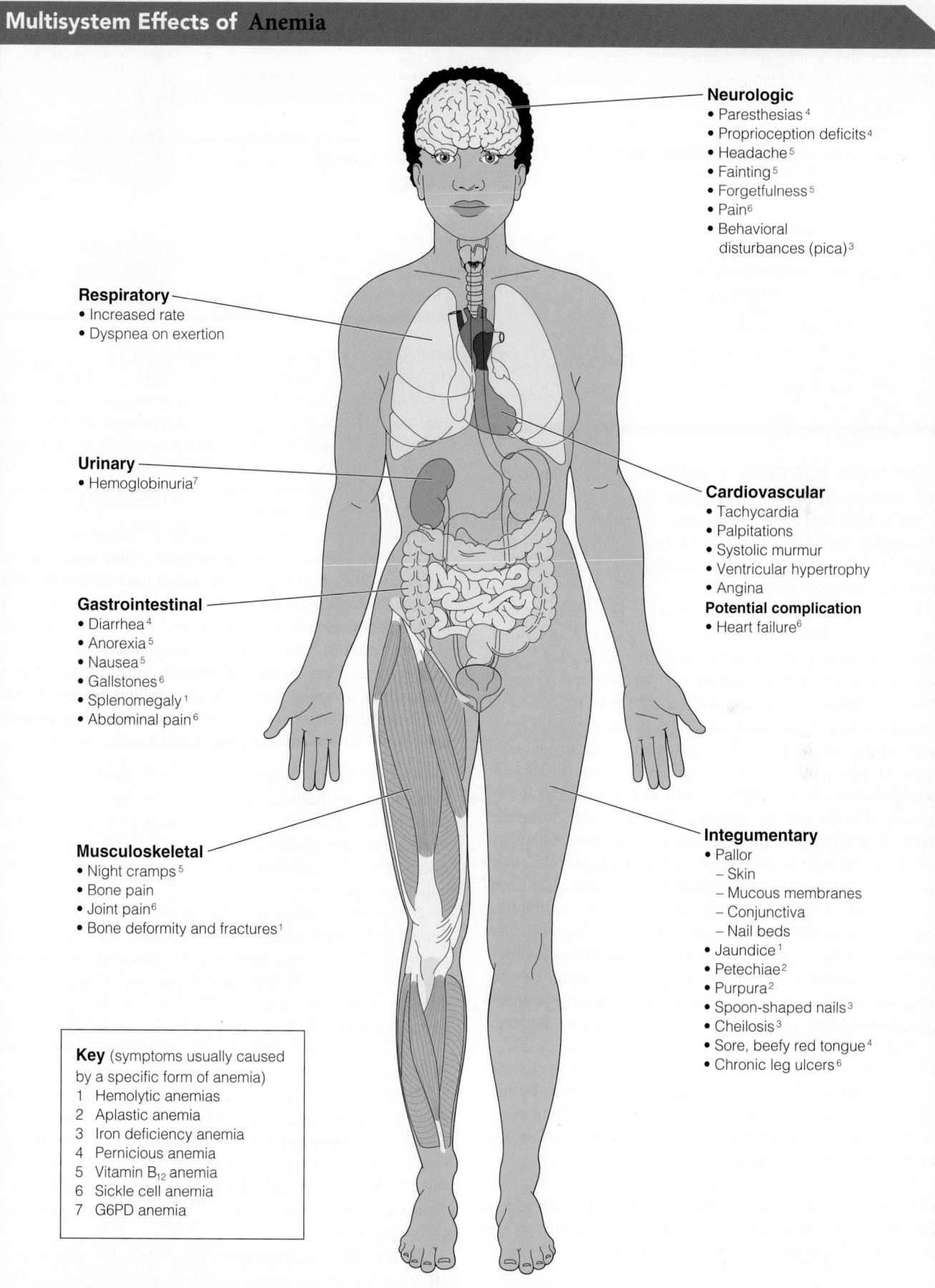

Neurologic
- Paresthesias [4]
- Proprioception deficits [4]
- Headache [5]
- Fainting [5]
- Forgetfulness [5]
- Pain [6]
- Behavioral disturbances (pica) [3]

Respiratory
- Increased rate
- Dyspnea on exertion

Urinary
- Hemoglobinuria [7]

Cardiovascular
- Tachycardia
- Palpitations
- Systolic murmur
- Ventricular hypertrophy
- Angina
Potential complication
- Heart failure [6]

Gastrointestinal
- Diarrhea [4]
- Anorexia [5]
- Nausea [5]
- Gallstones [6]
- Splenomegaly [1]
- Abdominal pain [6]

Musculoskeletal
- Night cramps [5]
- Bone pain
- Joint pain [6]
- Bone deformity and fractures [1]

Integumentary
- Pallor
  - Skin
  - Mucous membranes
  - Conjunctiva
  - Nail beds
- Jaundice [1]
- Petechiae [2]
- Purpura [2]
- Spoon-shaped nails [3]
- Cheilosis [3]
- Sore, beefy red tongue [4]
- Chronic leg ulcers [6]

Key (symptoms usually caused by a specific form of anemia)
1 Hemolytic anemias
2 Aplastic anemia
3 Iron deficiency anemia
4 Pernicious anemia
5 Vitamin B_{12} anemia
6 Sickle cell anemia
7 G6PD anemia

Box 2–6   Causes of Folic Acid Deficiency Anemia

- Inadequate dietary intake
At risk:
  a. Older adults
  b. Clients with alcoholism
  c. Clients receiving total parenteral nutrition

- Increased metabolic requirements
At risk:
  a. Pregnant women
  b. Infants and teenagers
  c. Clients undergoing hemodialysis
  d. Clients with forms of hemolytic anemia

- Folic acid malabsorption and impaired metabolism
  a. Celiac sprue
  b. Chemotherapeutic agents, folate antagonists (methotrexate, pentamidine), or anticonvulsants
  c. Alcoholism

Box 2–7   Causes of Hemolytic Anemia

INTRINSIC
- Red blood cell membrane defects
- Hemoglobin structure defects (e.g., sickle cell disease, thalassemia)
- Inherited enzyme defects (e.g., glucose-6-phosphate dehydrogenase deficiency)

EXTRINSIC
- Drugs, chemicals
- Toxins and venoms
- Bacterial and other infections
- Trauma, burns
- Mechanical damage (prosthetic heart valves)

FOLIC ACID DEFICIENCY ANEMIA   Like vitamin B_{12}, folic acid is required for DNA synthesis and normal maturation of RBCs. Folic acid deficiency anemia is characterized by fragile, megaloblastic (large and immature) cells. Folic acid is found in green leafy vegetables, fruits, cereals, and meats, and it is absorbed from the intestines.

Folic acid deficiency anemia as a result of inadequate intake is more common among people who are chronically undernourished. This includes older adults and those with alcohol or drug addictions. Those with alcoholism are especially at risk because alcohol suppresses folate metabolism, which forms folic acid. Because increased folic acid levels also may lead to anemia, pregnant women are at greater risk for anemia due to increased intake of folic acid to promote fetal development. Infants and teenagers can develop temporary folic acid deficiencies during periods of rapid growth. Impaired folic acid absorption and metabolism can cause folic acid deficiency anemia. Malabsorption disorders, such as celiac sprue (a hereditary gastrointestinal disorder characterized by the inability to metabolize amino acids found in gluten), and certain medications, such as methotrexate and some chemotherapeutic agents, may be implicated. Causes of folic acid deficiency anemia are summarized in **Box 2–6** ●.

The manifestations of folic acid deficiency anemia develop gradually, as folic acid stores are depleted. Signs and symptoms may include pallor, progressive weakness and fatigue, shortness of breath, and heart palpitations. Manifestations similar to those associated with vitamin B_{12} anemia, such as glossitis, cheilosis, and diarrhea, are common. No neurological symptoms occur with folic acid deficiency anemia, helping to differentiate it from vitamin B_{12} deficiency anemia. These two nutritional anemias do, however, sometimes coexist.

Maternal folic acid deficiency is strongly associated with neural tube defects, such as meningomyelocele. The neural tube develops early in the process of fetal development, often before pregnancy is recognized.

Hemolytic Anemias

Hemolytic anemias are characterized by premature destruction (lysis) of RBCs. When RBCs break down, iron and other by-products of their destruction remain in the plasma. RBC lysis (hemolysis) may occur within the circulatory system or as a result of phagocytosis by WBCs, such as circulating monocytes and macrophages in the spleen. In response to hemolysis, the hematopoietic activity of bone marrow increases, leading to increased reticulocytes (immature RBCs) in circulating blood. Most types of hemolytic anemia are characterized by normocytic and normochromic RBCs.

There are many different causes of hemolytic anemias (**Box 2–7** ●). The cause may be intrinsic, arising from disorders within the RBC itself, or extrinsic, originating outside the RBC. Intrinsic disorders include cell membrane defects, defects in hemoglobin structure and function, and inherited enzyme deficiencies. Extrinsic causes of hemolytic anemia include drugs, bacterial and other toxins, and trauma. This section discusses thalassemia, acquired hemolytic anemia, and glucose-6-phosphate dehydrogenase anemia. (For details regarding sickle cell anemia, see the exemplar on Sickle Cell Disease.)

THALASSEMIA   **Thalassemia** refers to inherited disorders of hemoglobin synthesis in which either the alpha or beta chains of the hemoglobin molecule are missing or defective. This leads to deficient hemoglobin production and fragile hypochromic, microcytic RBCs called target cells because of their distinctive bull's-eye appearance.

Thalassemia is more prevalent among certain populations. People of Mediterranean descent (southern Italy and Greece) are more likely to have beta-defect thalassemia (often called Cooley anemia or Mediterranean anemia). People of Asian ancestry, especially those from Thailand, the Philippines, and China, more often have alpha-defect thalassemia. Africans and African Americans may have both alpha- and beta-defect thalassemia.

Children with thalassemia major require blood transfusions throughout their lives. However, lifelong blood transfusions create additional health risks, including the potential for iron overload. As a result of iron-related cardiac problems, these individuals usually die by 30 years of age (Muncie & Campbell, 2009). Individuals with thalassemia minor often are asymptomatic.

Manifestations of thalassemia major include mild to moderate anemia, mild splenomegaly, bronze skin coloring, and bone marrow hyperplasia. The major form of the disease causes severe anemia, heart failure, and liver and spleen enlargement from increased red cell destruction. Fractures of the long bones, ribs, and vertebrae may result from bone marrow expansion and thinning as a result of increased hematopoiesis. Jaundice, hepatomegaly, and splenomegaly may develop because of hemolysis. Accumulation of iron in the heart, liver, and pancreas following repeated transfusions for treatment may eventually cause failure of these organs.

ACQUIRED HEMOLYTIC ANEMIA Acquired hemolytic anemia is caused by hemolysis resulting from factors outside of the RBCs. Causes of acquired hemolytic anemias include the following:

- Mechanical trauma to RBCs produced by prosthetic heart valves, severe burns, hemodialysis, or radiation
- Autoimmune disorders
- Bacterial or protozoal infection
- Immune system–mediated responses, such as transfusion reactions
- Drugs, toxins, chemical agents, or venoms.

The manifestations of acquired hemolytic anemia depend on the extent of hemolysis and the body's ability to replace destroyed red blood cells. The anemia itself often is mild to moderate as erythropoiesis increases to replace the destroyed RBCs. The spleen enlarges as it removes damaged or destroyed RBCs. If the breakdown of heme units exceeds the liver's ability to conjugate and excrete bilirubin, jaundice develops. When the condition is severe, bone marrow expands, and bones may be deformed or may develop pathological fractures. The severity of generalized manifestations of anemia (e.g., tachycardia and pallor) depends on the degree of anemia and deficiency of tissue oxygenation.

GLUCOSE-6-PHOSPHATE DEHYDROGENASE ANEMIA Glucose-6-phosphate dehydrogenase (G6PD) anemia is caused by a hereditary defect in RBC metabolism. It is relatively common in people of African and Mediterranean descent. The defective gene is located on the X chromosome and therefore affects more males than females. There are many variations of this genetic defect.

Glucose-6-phosphate dehydrogenase is an enzyme that catalyzes glycolysis, the process in which an RBC derives cellular energy. A defect in G6PD action causes direct oxidation of hemoglobin, damaging the RBC. Hemolysis usually occurs only when the affected individual is exposed to stressors (e.g., drugs such as aspirin, sulfonamides, or vitamin K derivatives) that increase the metabolic demands on RBCs. The G6PD deficiency impairs the necessary compensatory increase in glucose metabolism and causes cellular damage. Damaged RBCs are destroyed over a period of 7–12 days.

When the client is exposed to a stressor that triggers G6PD anemia, symptoms develop within several days. These may include pallor, jaundice, hemoglobinuria (hemoglobin in the urine), and an elevated reticulocyte count. As new RBCs develop, counts return to normal.

Aplastic Anemia

In **aplastic anemia**, the bone marrow fails to produce all three types of blood cells, leading to pancytopenia, a deficiency in both red and white blood cells. Normal bone marrow is replaced by fat. Fortunately, aplastic anemia is rare.

A rare form of aplastic anemia, Fanconi anemia, is caused by defects of DNA repair. For approximately 50% of acquired aplastic anemias, however, the underlying cause is unknown (idiopathic aplastic anemia). Other cases of aplastic anemia follow stem cell damage caused by exposure to radiation or certain chemical substances, such as benzene, arsenic, pesticides, certain antibiotics (especially chloramphenicol), and chemotherapeutic drugs (NHLBI, 2012d). Aplastic anemia also may occur with viral infections, such as mononucleosis, hepatitis C, and HIV disease (Porth & Matfin, 2010).

In aplastic anemia, the number of stem cells in the bone marrow is significantly reduced. The stem cell pool may be less than 1% of normal when the disease is recognized. Anemia develops as the bone marrow fails to replace RBCs that have reached the end of their life span. Remaining RBCs may be normochromic and normocytic, or they may be large, with increased mean corpuscular volume.

Manifestations of aplastic anemia vary with the severity of the pancytopenia. Its onset usually is insidious, but it may be sudden. Manifestations include fatigue, pallor, progressive weakness, exertional dyspnea, headache, and ultimately, tachycardia and heart failure. Platelet deficiency leads to bleeding problems; bleeding gums, excessive bruising, and nosebleeds may be the initial symptoms. A deficiency of WBCs increases the risk of infection, causing manifestations such as sore throat and fever.

Lifespan and Cultural Considerations

Neonatal anemia may be caused by blood loss, hemolysis/erythrocyte destruction, and impaired RBC production (Janus & Moerschel, 2010). Blood loss (hypovolemia) occurs in utero from placental bleeding (placenta previa or abruptio placentae). Intrapartum blood loss may be fetomaternal, fetofetal, or the result of umbilical cord bleeding. Birth trauma to abdominal organs (adrenal hemorrhage) or the cranium (subgaleal bleed) may produce significant blood loss, and cerebral bleeding may occur because of hypoxia.

Excessive hemolysis of RBCs is usually a result of blood group incompatibilities, but it may be caused by infections. The most common cause of impaired RBC production is a genetically transmitted deficiency in G6PD.

Physiological anemia of infancy occurs as a result of the normal, gradual drop in hemoglobin for the first 6–12 weeks of life. When the amount of hemoglobin decreases in term infants, the bone marrow begins production of RBCs again, and the anemia disappears.

▶ COLLABORATION

Ensuring adequate tissue oxygenation is the priority of care in treating anemia. Specific therapy is determined by the underlying cause of the disorder. Anemia that results from nutritional deficiencies is addressed through dietary counseling. Some cases of anemia may be treated with drugs. In severe cases, the client with anemia may need a blood transfusion. (For an overview of treatments used in the management of various types of anemia, see the Clinical Manifestations and Therapies feature on page 72.) Members of the interdisciplinary healthcare team may include pharmacists and nutritionists or dietitians in addition to nurses, physicians, and other healthcare professionals.

Diagnostic Tests

The diagnosis of anemia is established on the basis of laboratory studies. The complete blood count (CBC), which is a routine diagnostic test, measures both RBCs and hemoglobin and is useful in identification of anemia related to inadequate RBC count or hemoglobin. However, additional analysis is needed to confirm adequate RBC structure and function. A diet history and analysis can provide information related to food intake. Tests that may be ordered include the following:

- CBC
- Hemoglobin and hematocrit
- Hemoglobin electrophoresis
- Serum iron
- Serum ferritin
- Iron-binding capacity
- Microscopic analysis
- Schilling test
- Bone marrow examination
- Quantitative assay of G6PD.

Surgery

For the client diagnosed with anemia that is due to blood loss, treatment focuses on identifying the source of the bleeding and, if possible, surgically repairing the damaged organ or tissues. Treatment of aplastic anemia resulting from damaged bone marrow may include a stem cell transplant (also referred to as a bone marrow transplant). The client with pernicious anemia may require surgical exploration to assess for disorders such as celiac disease, Crohn disease, and diverticuli, which are conditions known to decrease the production of gastric intrinsic factor (Osborn et al., 2013). Splenectomy may be indicated in treatment of the client with thalassemia major.

Pharmacologic Therapy

Medications used to treat anemia depend on the underlying cause. Pharmacologic agents used to treat and manage anemia include vitamin B_{12}, ferrous sulfate (or other iron sources), and folic acid.

For treatment of symptomatic iron deficiency anemia that does not respond to dietary modifications alone, supplemental iron may be administered orally or parenterally. Intravenous (IV) and intramuscular (IM) administration of iron are becoming more common, particularly in clients with an acute deficiency or an anemia associated with chronic gastrointestinal blood loss, chronic renal failure, and other chronic conditions that increase the need for blood cell production (e.g., cancers). Critical side effects associated with parenterally administered iron preparations range from hypersensitivity reactions to anaphylaxis (Wysowski et al., 2010). For this reason, clients who receive IV iron supplementation must be closely observed for signs and symptoms of an adverse reaction. For oral preparations, common side effects include constipation, nausea, and heartburn.

Parenteral vitamin B_{12} is given when malabsorption or lack of intrinsic factor leads to vitamin B_{12} deficiency anemia.

Folic acid is ordered for women of childbearing age, pregnant women, and clients with folic acid deficiency or sickle cell disease to meet the increased demands of the bone marrow. Hydroxyurea, a drug that promotes fetal hemoglobin production, may be prescribed for clients with sickle cell disease, particularly those with frequent crises or severe disease. Resulting increased levels of fetal hemoglobin interfere with the sickling process and reduce the incidence of painful crises (UMMC, 2009c).

Erythropoietin may be ordered for clients with low erythropoietin levels (e.g., clients with chronic renal failure) and for people who have anemia associated with other chronic diseases. Erythropoietin is given subcutaneously, and it may be given as often as three times a week in chronic renal failure. Because erythropoietin stimulates RBC production, adequate iron must be present. Clients receiving erythropoietin may require regular IV iron therapy as well.

Immunosuppressive therapy with antithymocyte globulin, corticosteroids, and cyclosporine may be used to treat aplastic anemia. Androgens may stimulate blood cell production in some clients with aplastic anemia.

SAFETY ALERT
In rare cases, parenteral iron administration may cause anaphylaxis. Should signs and symptoms of anaphylaxis develop, discontinue the infusion, remain with the client, closely monitor for signs and symptoms of airway compromise and other complications, and notify the primary care provider immediately.

Nonpharmacologic Therapy

Good nutrition and awareness of the signs and symptoms related to exacerbations of anemia are essential to health promotion for clients diagnosed with this disorder. Because of the inherent relationship between anemia and impaired oxygenation, activity tolerance is a primary consideration for these clients, and a healthy balance between rest and activity is also essential.

NUTRITION   Dietary modifications are recommended for nutritional deficiency anemias, such as iron deficiency anemia, vitamin B_{12} deficiency anemia, or folic acid deficiency anemia. **Box 2–8 ●** identifies good sources of dietary iron, folic acid, and vitamin B_{12}. For individuals whose condition cannot be managed or reversed strictly through diet, good nutrition is still extremely important for optimizing energy levels and promoting general wellness.

BLOOD TRANSFUSION   Blood transfusions may be indicated to treat anemias resulting from major blood loss, such as from trauma or major surgery, and severe anemia regardless of cause. In acute hemorrhage, whole blood may be given to replace both blood cells and volume. A unit of packed RBCs may be given when anemia is severe and the client demonstrates cardiovascular instability or compromise. Treatment of aplastic anemia may also incorporate blood transfusions. For individuals diagnosed with thalassemia, blood transfusions will be required throughout their life span.

Box 2–8   Dietary Sources of Iron, Folic Acid, and Vitamin B$_{12}$

IRON

Iron in the diet comes from two sources. The first, heme iron, makes up about one half of the iron from animal sources. The second, nonheme iron, includes the remaining iron from animal sources and all the iron from plants, legumes, and nuts. Heme iron promotes absorption of nonheme iron from other foods when both forms are consumed at the same time. Absorption of nonheme iron is enhanced by vitamin C and is inhibited by tea and coffee.

SOURCES OF HEME IRON

- Beef
- Chicken
- Egg yolk
- Clams, oysters
- Pork loin
- Turkey
- Veal

SOURCES OF NONHEME IRON

- Bran flakes
- Brown rice
- Whole-grain breads
- Dried beans
- Dried fruits
- Greens
- Oatmeal

SOURCES OF FOLIC ACID

- Green leafy vegetables
- Broccoli
- Organ meats
- Eggs
- Wheat germ
- Asparagus
- Milk
- Yeast
- Kidney beans

SOURCES OF VITAMIN B$_{12}$

- Liver
- Fresh shrimp and oysters
- Eggs
- Milk
- Kidney
- Meats (muscle)
- Cheese

■ NURSING PROCESS

Nursing care includes screening clients at risk for anemia in order to promote early intervention and to prevent complications. Acute exacerbations and crises related to anemia warrant emergent care, such as oxygen administration and administration of IV fluid, as described earlier in this exemplar. Long-term care for the client with anemia centers around prevention of complications and optimization of health and wellness. Client teaching is directed toward self-care and will often include dietary counseling.

Assessment

Assessment data to collect for clients with suspected anemia include the following:

- **Health history.** Complaints of shortness of breath with activity, fatigue, weakness, dizziness or fainting, palpitations; history of previous anemia, bleeding episodes; menstrual history (if appropriate); medications; chronic diseases; usual diet and patterns of alcohol intake or cigarette smoking.

Complementary and Alternative Therapy
Plant Enzymes for Nutritional Anemias

Complementary healthcare practitioners may recommend specific plant enzymes to treat nutritional anemias. Plant enzymes are believed to aid digestion of proteins, fats, and carbohydrates, facilitating absorption of their nutrients. Therapy is determined by the specific type of anemia. Plant enzymes should not be used alone to treat anemia, and it is important to check for possible interactions with prescribed medications before starting therapy.

- **Physical examination.** General appearance, skin color; vital signs, including temperature; heart and lung sounds; peripheral pulses, capillary refill; abdominal tenderness; obvious bleeding or bruising.

Diagnosis

Anemia affects circulating oxygen levels and tissue oxygenation. Priority nursing diagnoses include the following:

- *Impaired Gas Exchange*
- *Risk for Decreased Cardiac Output*
- *Risk for Ineffective Cerebral Tissue Perfusion*
- *Acute Pain*
- *Fatigue*
- *Activity Intolerance*
- *Self-Neglect.*

(NANDA-I © 2012)

Planning

Treatment goals may include the following:

- The client will report an absence of dyspnea.
- The client will verbalize awareness of signs and symptoms associated with exacerbations of conditions related to anemia.
- The client will describe a plan for balancing activity with rest.
- The client will make appropriate dietary choices to increase iron intake.
- The client will demonstrate appropriate self-administration of supplements.
- The client's RBC count (or hemoglobin) will be maintained within a specified acceptable range.

Implementation

Nursing implementation for the client with anemia is directed toward minimizing the impact of the symptoms while promoting

Clinical Manifestations and Therapies **Anemia**

ETIOLOGY	CLINICAL MANIFESTATIONS	CLINICAL THERAPIES
Iron deficiency anemia ■ Dietary deficiencies: Vegetarian diet Inadequate protein intake ■ Decreased absorption: Partial or total gastrectomy Chronic diarrhea Malabsorption syndromes ■ Increased metabolic requirements: Pregnancy Lactation ■ Blood loss: Gastrointestinal bleeding (especially caused by ulcers or chronic aspirin use) Menorrhagia ■ Chronic hemoglobinuria	■ Onset is usually insidious (manifested slowly over a period of time); early signs and symptoms may include headache, pallor, lethargy, fatigue, shortness of breath, and intolerance of cold temperatures. ■ Late manifestations may include pica, glossitis (inflamed tongue), stomach irritation, and cheilosis (cracks at the corners of the mouth).	■ Increased dietary intake of iron-rich foods ■ Oral or parenteral iron supplements
Vitamin B_{12} deficiency	■ Onset is usually insidious; signs and symptoms include nausea; anorexia; swollen, sore tongue; and skin discoloration (hyperpigmentation) of the hands and knuckles. ■ Neurological symptoms may include diminished reflexes, confusion, memory loss, gait disturbances, and peripheral neuropathy.	■ Increased dietary intake of foods containing vitamin B_{12} (e.g., meats, eggs, and dairy products) ■ Oral or parenteral vitamin B_{12} supplements ■ Parenteral vitamin B_{12} for deficiency caused by malabsorption or lack of IF
Folic acid deficiency	■ Onset is usually insidious; signs and symptoms include pallor, progressive weakness and fatigue, shortness of breath, and heart palpitations, as well as manifestations similar to those associated with vitamin B_{12} anemia, such as glossitis and cheilosis.	■ Increased dietary intake of foods rich in folic acid (folate) ■ Oral folic acid supplements ■ Folic acid supplements are recommended for women who are pregnant or may become pregnant in order to prevent neural tube defects.
Sickle cell disease	■ General symptoms include moderate to severe lethargy and pain (due to vascular occlusion). ■ Reduced tissue oxygenation and blood stagnation can lead to altered levels of consciousness. ■ Sickle cell crisis is marked by trapping of sickled RBCs in the spleen and subsequent splenomegaly; reduced or absent RBC production by bone marrow leading to severe decrease in hemoglobin; and rarely, hyperhemolytic crisis, which manifests as an extreme increase in RBC destruction. ■ Acute chest syndrome leads to an increase in hemoglobin sickling, which exacerbates hypoxia and can be life threatening.	■ Treatment is primarily supportive. ■ Hydroxyurea ■ Sickle cell crisis: Rest Oxygen therapy Narcotic analgesia Vigorous hydration Treatment of precipitating factors ■ Acute chest syndrome: Careful hydration; hemodynamic monitoring Oxygen therapy Transfusion Folic acid supplements ■ Blood transfusions during surgery or pregnancy as necessary ■ Genetic counseling recommended

Clinical Manifestations and Therapies **Anemia** (continued)

ETIOLOGY	CLINICAL MANIFESTATIONS	CLINICAL THERAPIES
Thalassemia	■ Mild to moderate anemia, mild splenomegaly, bronze skin coloring, and bone marrow hyperplasia. ■ Thalassemia major produces severe anemia, heart failure, and liver and spleen enlargement from increased red cell destruction. ■ Fractures of the long bones, ribs, and vertebrae may occur. ■ Accumulation of iron in the heart, liver, and pancreas following repeated transfusions for treatment may eventually cause failure of these organs.	■ Regular blood transfusions ■ Folic acid supplements ■ Possible splenectomy ■ Genetic counseling
Aplastic anemia	■ Onset of manifestations may be insidious or sudden, and include fatigue, pallor, progressive weakness, exertional dyspnea, headache, and ultimately, tachycardia and heart failure. ■ Initial symptoms may include bleeding gums, excessive bruising, and nosebleeds. ■ Deficiency of WBCs increases the risk of infection, causing manifestations such as sore throat and fever.	■ Withdrawal of the causative agent, if known ■ Blood transfusions ■ Bone marrow transplant as indicated

resolution of the condition. While management of life-threatening physiological needs always takes priority over pain management, treatment of pain remains a priority concern. Analgesics should be administered as ordered, preferably using a routine schedule of administration in order to maintain a consistent level of pain control. Client preferences, culture, and specific symptoms must all be considered before implementing care.

Promote Optimal Cardiorespiratory Function

Cardiac output may be affected by acute bleeding and volume loss or by heart failure resulting from severe anemia. Impaired tissue oxygenation leads to an increased respiratory rate and dyspnea.

■ Monitor vital signs, breath sounds, and apical pulse. Increased cardiac workload can affect the blood pressure, heart, and respiratory rates. Increased blood flow can lead to heart murmur or abnormal heart sounds, such as S_3 or S_4. Tachypnea and dyspnea may affect the depth of respirations, alveolar ventilation, and blood and tissue oxygenation.

■ Assess the client for pallor, cyanosis, and dependent edema. Blood is shunted to the vital organs, causing vasoconstriction of skin vessels. This, in addition to lower levels of hemoglobin, causes pallor. Cyanosis, especially of the lips

and nail beds, indicates inadequate oxygenation of blood. Dependent edema occurs in response to right ventricular failure.

■ Closely monitor the client for manifestations of anaphylaxis (e.g., urticaria, erythema or flushing, edema, wheezing, dyspnea, nausea and vomiting, and anxiety) when administering parenteral iron preparations. Anaphylaxis, a systemic type I hypersensitivity (allergic) reaction, can lead to severe cardiopulmonary compromise, necessitating emergency measures to preserve life. Should signs and symptoms of anaphylaxis develop, discontinue administration of the iron and immediately notify the physician. Continuously monitor the client and prepare to administer medications such as diphenhydramine (Benadryl) or epinephrine, as ordered. Institute cardiopulmonary resuscitation measures as necessary.

Promote Balance Between Oxygen Supply and Demand

Anemia causes weakness and shortness of breath on exertion. These symptoms are the result of decreased circulating oxygen levels secondary to low hemoglobin levels. Weakness, fatigue, and/or vertigo may occur even during activities of daily living (ADLs), including those associated with self-care, home life, job performance, and social roles.

- Help identify ways to conserve energy when performing necessary or desired activities. Alternative ways of performing tasks (e.g., sitting when performing hygiene care and kitchen tasks) may reduce oxygen demands. Assistance from others may be necessary to conserve energy and reduce symptoms.
- Help the client and family establish priorities for tasks and activities. Because family members may need to assume responsibility for additional tasks, the plan's success depends on mutually established goals.
- Assist the client to develop a schedule of alternating periods of activity and rest throughout the day. Rest periods decrease oxygen needs, reducing strain on the heart and lungs and allowing restoration of homeostasis before further activities.
- Encourage 8 to 10 hours of sleep at night. Rest decreases oxygen demands and increases available energy for morning activities.
- Monitor vital signs before and after activity. Vital signs provide a measure of activity tolerance. Increased heart and respiratory rates or a change in blood pressure may indicate intolerance of the activity.
- Discontinue activity if any of the following occurs:
  a. Chest pain, breathlessness, or vertigo
  b. Palpitations or tachycardia that does not return to normal within 4 minutes of resting
  c. Bradycardia
  d. Tachypnea or dyspnea
  e. Decreased systolic blood pressure.

  These changes may signify cardiac decompensation resulting from insufficient oxygenation. The intensity, duration, or frequency of the activity needs to be reduced.
- Instruct the client not to smoke. Smoking causes vasoconstriction and increases carbon monoxide levels in the blood, interfering with tissue oxygenation.

Facilitate Enhanced Self-Care

Energy expenditures for ADLs may cause oxygen demands to exceed supply in the client with severe anemia. This can greatly impair the client's ability to maintain self-care. As a result, clients may need assistance with ADLs in order to maintain self-care and self-esteem as well as reduce cardiac workload. Assistance decreases energy expenditures and tissue requirements for oxygen, reducing cardiac workload.

Glossitis, inflammation of the tongue that may cause the tongue and lips to turn red, and cheilosis (fissures or cracks at the corners of the mouth) may occur with nutritional deficiencies of iron, folate, and vitamin B_{12}. Client education should include the following recommendations:

- Monitor the condition of the lips and tongue daily. Glossitis and cheilosis increase the risk for bleeding and infection and may require medical treatment. Pain and discomfort may interfere with oral intake, further worsening the nutritional deficiency.
- Use a mouthwash of saline, saltwater, or half-strength peroxide and water to rinse the mouth every 2–4 hours. This cleanses and soothes oral mucous membranes. Alcohol-based mouthwashes further irritate and dry oral tissues and should be avoided.
- Provide frequent oral hygiene (after each meal and at bedtime) with a soft bristle toothbrush or sponge. A soft toothbrush reduces irritation or bleeding of oral mucosa. Keeping the oral cavity clean also reduces the risk of infection.
- Apply a petroleum-based lubricating jelly or ointment to the lips after oral care to help retain moisture and protect the lips from other drying agents.
- Encourage soft, cool, bland foods to promote comfort and help maintain adequate food and fluid intake. Instruct the client to avoid hot, spicy, or acidic foods. Such foods may further irritate and dry mucous membranes.
- Encourage the client to eat four to six small meals with high protein and vitamin content each day. Small, frequent meals may be better tolerated, increasing intake. Nutrient-rich meals promote healing of the mucous membranes.

Community-Based Care Home Care for the Client With Anemia

When preparing the client and family for home care, include the following topics:

- Nutritional strategies to address deficiencies
- Prescribed medications, vitamins, or mineral supplements and their appropriate use, intended effect, possible adverse effects, and interactions with food or other medications
- Energy conservation strategies
- Other recommended treatment measures and follow-up
- Inheritance patterns of the disorder
- Symptoms of crisis and manifestations to report to the physician if the anemia is genetically transmitted, such as sickle cell disease.

In addition, provide referrals for counseling to facilitate decisions about pregnancy as indicated. Refer for nutritional assistance and teaching, home health care, or assistance with self-care and home maintenance activities as needed. Older adults with nutritional anemias may benefit from community services such as senior meals or Meals-on-Wheels.

SAFETY ALERT
Report signs and symptoms of decreased cardiac output to the physician. Severe anemia can lead to heart failure and may be fatal.

Evaluation

Expected outcomes of nursing care include the following:

- The client's RBC count and hemoglobin level are within normal limits.
- The client and/or family verbalizes understanding of the treatment regimen.
- The client consumes the recommended dietary intake of iron.
- The client is free of side effects of iron therapy.
- The client is active and able to maintain normal activity levels.
- The pediatric client achieves appropriate growth and development milestones.

NURSING CARE PLAN   A Client With Folic Acid Deficiency Anemia

Sheri Matthews is a 76-year-old widow who lives alone. Mrs. Matthews visits her primary care physician for evaluation of her decreased energy level. In particular, Ms. Matthews complains that she does not have "enough energy to clean the house anymore." She also reports shortness of breath when she vacuums. When asked about her current diet, Mrs. Matthews tells Lisa Apana, RN, the nurse in her care provider's office, that she liked to cook when her husband was alive, but preparing an entire meal just for herself seems senseless. She relates that her typical day's menu includes coffee for breakfast; a bologna sandwich and coffee for lunch; and a hot dog or two, a few cookies, and a glass of milk for dinner.

ASSESSMENT

Mrs. Matthews's nursing history includes a 9-kg (20-lb) weight loss since her husband died 8 months ago. She states that she sometimes has heart palpitations and always feels weak. Physical assessment reveals the following: T 98.8°F; P 110 bpm; R 22/min; and BP 90/52 mmHg. Her skin is warm, pale, and dry. Diagnostic tests indicate folic acid deficiency anemia. Mrs. Matthews is started on an oral folic acid supplement and instructed about foods containing folic acid.

DIAGNOSES

- *Activity Intolerance* related to weakness secondary to decreased tissue oxygenation
- *Imbalanced Nutrition: Less Than Body Requirements* related to lack of motivation to cook and understanding of nutritional needs, as manifested by weight loss of 20 lb and folic acid deficiency
- *Deficient Knowledge* related to lack of information about a well-balanced diet and foods containing folic acid

(NANDA-I © 2012)

PLANNING

- The client will verbalize the importance of taking folic acid supplements and eating a balanced diet.
- The client will gain at least 1 lb (0.45 kg) per week.
- The client will return to her previous level of physical energy.
- The client will consume a balanced diet, including foods containing folic acid.

IMPLEMENTATION

- Discuss foods required for a well-balanced diet as well as dietary sources of folic acid.
- Develop a dietary plan with Mrs. Matthews that includes food preferences and foods that are easy and quick to prepare.

- Discuss the importance of taking the folic acid supplement. Advise Mrs. Matthews to continue taking it even after she begins to feel better.
- Help Mrs. Matthews develop a schedule of activities that provides adequate rest and energy for cooking.

EVALUATION

Mrs. Matthews gained 1 lb (0.45 kg) during the first week of treatment. She has met with a nutritionist and has a better understanding of nutritional needs. She states that she can prepare hot meals when she schedules a rest period before and after lunch. Ms. Apana has provided written and verbal information about the folic acid supplement and diet. Mrs. Matthews verbalizes understanding, stating, "I will continue to take the folic acid until the doctor tells me to stop. I'm beginning to enjoy cooking again, now that I have a reason to cook!" Ms. Apana contacts the local senior services representative to determine if Mrs. Matthews is able to participate in the local Meals-on-Wheels program.

CRITICAL THINKING

1. What is the pathophysiological basis for Mrs. Matthews's abnormal vital signs during her initial assessment?
2. Design a week's menu that includes foods high in folic acid.
3. Why was Mrs. Matthews placed on a folic acid supplement in addition to dietary modifications?
4. Why is the older adult at increased risk for developing folic acid deficiency anemia? Consider physiological, economic, and social factors.

REVIEW Anemia

RELATE Link the Concepts and Exemplars

Linking the exemplar of anemia with the concept of development:

1. What effects will anemia have on the development of the school-age child?
2. A young woman is in her fifth month of pregnancy and develops severe anemia. What independent nursing interventions might you initiate to resolve this problem?

Linking the exemplar of anemia with the concept of family:

3. What nursing diagnoses does the nurse create for the mother of three who has anemia?
4. What effect will anemia have on family processes?

READY Go to Companion Skills Manual

REFER Go to Pearson Nursing Student Resources
nursing.pearsonhighered.com

- Additional review materials

REFLECT Case Study

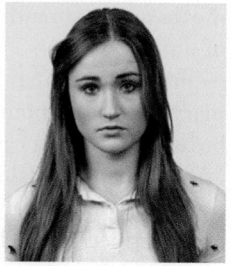

Jessica Riley, 17 years old, is 6 months pregnant with her first child. The father of the baby has ended their relationship. Jessica tried living with her mother but they fought constantly. Jessica moves into her own apartment. She is working as a waitress to try to support herself and has plans to attend cosmetology school.

1. What preventive interventions would you plan for Jessica to reduce her risk of developing anemia?

2. How could the development of anemia impact Jessica and her fetus?

3. What nutrition counseling would you provide Jessica to reduce the risk of anemia?

EXEMPLAR 2.3 Breast Cancer

EXEMPLAR KEY TERMS

Breast cancer, 76
Cachexia, 81
Hormone therapy, 79
Lumpectomy, 79
Lymphedema, 79
Metastasis, 76
Modified radical mastectomy, 79
Radical mastectomy, 79
Segmental mastectomy, 79
Simple mastectomy, 79
Staging, 76

EXEMPLAR LEARNING OUTCOMES

After reading about this exemplar, you will be able to:

1. Describe the pathophysiology, etiology, clinical manifestations, and direct and indirect causes of breast cancer.

2. Identify risk factors and prevention methods associated with breast cancer.

3. Illustrate the nursing process in providing culturally competent care across the life span for individuals with breast cancer.

4. Formulate priority nursing diagnoses appropriate for an individual with breast cancer.

5. Summarize therapies used by interdisciplinary teams in the collaborative care of an individual with breast cancer.

6. Plan evidence-based care for an individual with breast cancer and her family in collaboration with other members of the healthcare team.

7. Evaluate expected outcomes for an individual with breast cancer.

▶ OVERVIEW

Breast cancer is the unregulated growth of abnormal cells in breast tissue. It is the second most commonly occurring cancer in women (with skin cancer being first) and is the second-leading cause of cancer-related death in women in the United States. Every year in the United States, over 200,000 women are diagnosed with breast cancer (ACS, 2013a). The American Cancer Society (2013i) estimated that in this country, more than 232,000 women would be diagnosed with breast cancer in 2013 and approximately 39,000 women would die from it. In the United States, breast cancer is more prevalent among White women than in women of African American/Black, Hispanic/Latina, American Indian/Alaska Native, or Asian/Pacific Islander heritage (NCI, 2013b).

▶ PATHOPHYSIOLOGY AND ETIOLOGY

Cancer of the breast begins as a single, transformed cell and is often hormone dependent. These cancers are classified as noninvasive (in situ) or invasive, depending on the penetration of the tumor into surrounding tissue. Breast cancer may remain a noninvasive disease or an invasive disease without **metastasis** (spreading to other organs) for long periods of time.

Breast cancer may be categorized as carcinoma of the mammary ducts, carcinoma of mammary lobules, or sarcoma of the breast. Most breast cancers are adenocarcinomas and appear to arise in the terminal section of the breast ductal tissue. There are many histological types of breast cancer, and only examples are described here. The most common type is infiltrating duc-

tal carcinoma. Two atypical types of breast cancer are inflammatory carcinoma and Paget disease. Inflammatory carcinoma of the breast, a systemic disease, is the most malignant form of breast cancer. Edema with skin dimpling that resembles an orange peel (peau d'orange) is usually present. Paget disease is a rare type of breast cancer involving infiltration of the nipple epithelium.

Breast cancer can metastasize to other sites through the bloodstream or lymphatic system. The common sites of metastasis of breast cancer are bone, brain, lung, liver, skin, and lymph nodes. **Staging** is a system of classifying cancer according to the size of the tumor, involvement of lymph nodes, and the presence or absence of distant metastasis (**Table 2–7 ●**). The staging of the breast cancer provides important information for making decisions about treatment options and is also used as a basis for prognosis.

Etiology

Possible causes of breast cancer include environmental, hormonal, reproductive, and hereditary factors. Two breast cancer susceptibility genes have been identified: *BRCA1* on chromosome 17 and *BRCA2* on chromosome 13. Both *BRCA1* and *BRCA2* belong to a group of genes known as tumor suppressors (NCI, 2013a). These genes may be responsible for the approximately 10% of women with hereditary breast cancer, with genetic mutations causing up to 80% of breast cancer in women younger than 50 years. Not all mutations of these genes are harmful; however, compared to a woman who does not have an undesirable genetic mutation, a woman with identified harmful mutations in *BRCA1* or *BRCA2* suppression is five times more likely to develop breast cancer and also has an increased risk for ovarian cancer (NCI, 2013a).

TABLE 2–7 Staging of Breast Cancer

STAGE	TUMOR	NODE	METASTASIS
Stage 0	Tis—Carcinoma in situ or Paget disease of the nipple	N0—No regional lymph node metastasis	M0—No evidence of distant metastasis
Stage I	T1—Tumor no larger than 2 cm	N0	M0
Stage IIA	T0—No evidence of primary tumor	N1—Metastasis to movable ipsilateral	M0
	T1	axillary nodes	
	T2—Tumor no larger than 5 cm	N0	M0
Stage IIB	T2	N1	M0
	T3—Tumor larger than 5 cm	N0	M0
Stage IIIA	T0	N2—Metastasis to ipsilateral fixed	M0
	T1	axillary nodes	
	T2		
	T3	N1	M0
		N2	M0
Stage IIIB	T4—Tumor of any size with direct extension to chest wall or skin	Any N	M0
	Any T	N3—Metastasis to ipsilateral internal mammary lymph nodes	M0
Stage IV	Any T	N0 and N1	M1—Distant metastasis

Lifespan Considerations
Older Women With Breast Cancer

- Although the incidence of breast cancer is increasing among premenopausal women, it is still primarily a disease of older women. Despite this, the needs of older women with breast cancer have been inadequately addressed in the professional literature and popular media.

- Women between the ages of 50 and 65 are the group most likely to benefit from annual screening mammography, yet many women in this age group have never had a mammogram.

- For too long, mastectomy was perceived as the only treatment option open to most older women with breast cancer, even those with early-stage disease. Slowly, that perception is changing as breast-conservation treatment gains greater acceptance. The choice of surgical treatment, particularly for older women, is highly individual. Many older women wish to preserve their breasts.

- Although older women with breast cancer may experience coexisting chronic illnesses and impaired physical function, research suggests that they show lower levels of emotional distress compared with younger women. Obviously, the need for services such as personal care, shopping, housekeeping, and transportation increases as the ages of both the woman and the caregiver increase.

Risk Factors

Of the various kinds of risk factors for breast cancer, some can be changed and some cannot. Those that cannot be changed (ACS, 2013i; NCI, 2013b) are as follows:

- *Age and gender.* Women are much more likely to have breast cancer than men, and this risk increases with age.

- *Genetic risk factors.* As previously described.

- *Family history of breast cancer.* Having a first-degree relative (mother, sister, or daughter) with breast cancer increases an individual's risk for development of breast cancer. Having a male family member with breast cancer also poses an increased risk.

- *Personal history of breast cancer.* A woman with cancer in one breast has an increased risk for developing a new cancer in the other breast or in a different part of the same breast.

- *Previous chest irradiation.* Radiation of the chest as a child or young woman for other cancer (e.g., Hodgkin disease) significantly increases the risk.

- *Menstrual history.* Women who begin menstruating before the age of 12 or who have menopause after the age of 55 may be at a higher risk.

Lifestyle factors that are associated with risk for breast cancer include using oral contraceptives, not having children or having them after the age of 30, using hormone replacement therapy for more than 5 years, not breastfeeding, drinking alcohol, obesity, high-fat diets, physical inactivity, and (possibly) environmental pollution. Breastfeeding, moderate or vigorous physical activity, and maintaining a healthy body weight lower an individual's risk for breast cancer.

Prevention

Prevention of breast cancer essentially involves actively limiting exposure to risk factors linked to its development. For example, because alcohol use is a known risk factor, recommendations include limiting alcohol intake to a maximum of one drink per day. Maintaining body weight within normal limits and engaging in physical activity can also reduce the risk for developing breast cancer. Recommendations also include refraining from smoking, avoiding exposure to environmental pollution and radiation, and limiting hormone therapy in terms of both duration and dose (Mayo Clinic, 2012a).

Although early detection cannot prevent breast cancer, it is essential to reducing the client's risk for mortality and promoting positive client outcomes. Early detection begins with monthly breast self-examinations, which women should do 3–5 days after their period starts. Postmenopausal women should conduct self-examinations on the same day each month (MedlinePlus, 2012). The nurse's role in client self-examinations is to assess and encourage clients to do them and to provide instructions as necessary.

⚙ **Stay Current:** *For information on breast self-examinations, go to the National Institute of Health's Web site at* **www.nlm.nih.gov/medlineplus/ency/article/001993.htm***.*

▶ CLINICAL MANIFESTATIONS

The manifestations of breast cancer may include a nontender lump in the breast (most often in the upper outer quadrant, the area with the most glandular tissue), abnormal nipple discharge, a rash around the nipple area, nipple retraction, dimpling of the skin, or a change in the position of the nipple (**Box 2–9 ●**). There may also be nipple pain, scaliness, ulceration, skin irritation, or discharge. Breast cancer is usually painless, but some women report a burning or stinging sensation. Many women with breast cancer have no manifestations, and their tumors are detected by mammography. However, most breast cancers are found by the women themselves during breast self-examination (BSE) or by their partners during sexual activity.

✳ *Go to* **nursing.pearsonhighered.com** *to Appendix B for details about mammography.*

▶ COLLABORATION

Palpation of a mass on self-examination or appearance of a mass on mammography may be the first indicator of breast cancer. Any palpable mass requires evaluation. Clinical examina-

Box 2–9   Signs and Symptoms of Breast Cancer
■ Breast mass or thickening
■ Unusual lump in the underarm or above the collarbone
■ Persistent skin rash near the nipple area
■ Flaking or eruption near the nipple
■ Dimpling, pulling, or retraction in an area of the breast
■ Nipple discharge
■ Change in nipple position
■ Burning, stinging, or pricking sensation

tion and mammography begin the process of diagnosis. Once the diagnosis is made, a number of treatment options are available. The choice of treatment depends on several factors, such as the stage of the cancer, the age of the woman, and the woman's preferences.

Diagnostic Tests

Although clinical examination and mammography both are valuable screening tools, mammography can buy a client precious time. Tumors may be present as many as 8–10 years before they can be detected by palpation, and mammography can detect a tumor up to 2 years before it reaches palpable size.

Although controversy exists about the ability of screening mammography to improve mortality rates for women under the age of 50, the ACS recommends annual mammograms beginning at age 40 and clinical breast examination at least every 3 years for women in their 20s and 30s.

Other diagnostic tests include a percutaneous needle biopsy (to define a cystic mass or fibrocystic changes and provide specimens for cytological examination) and a breast biopsy once a suspicious lump is identified. In aspiration biopsy or fine-needle aspiration biopsy, a needle is used to remove cells or fluid from the breast lesion (**Figure 2–8 ●**). In many facilities, fine-needle aspiration biopsies are performed using a stereotactic

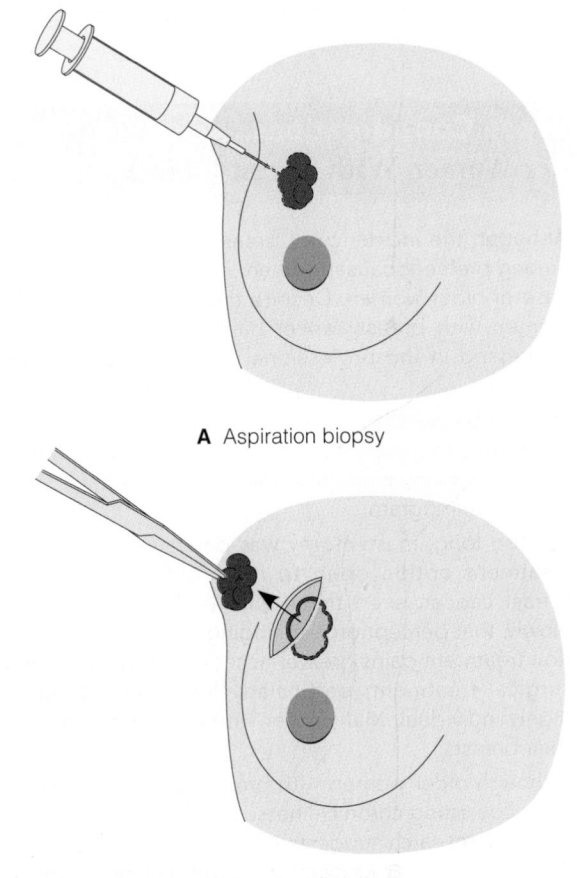

A Aspiration biopsy

B Excisional biopsy

Figure 2–8 ● Types of breast biopsy. *A,* In an aspiration biopsy, a needle is used to aspirate fluid or tissue from the breast. *B,* In an excisional biopsy, tissue from the breast lesion is removed surgically.

biopsy device; mammography and a computer are used to guide the needle.

Surgery

Until recently, the treatment of choice for breast cancer was a radical mastectomy. The trend now is toward more conservative surgery combined with chemotherapy, hormone therapy, or radiation, depending on the stage of the tumor and the age of the woman.

MASTECTOMY Various types of mastectomy surgeries are used to treat breast cancer. **Radical mastectomy** is the removal of the entire affected breast, the underlying chest muscles, and the lymph nodes under the arms. **Simple mastectomy** is the removal of the complete breast only. **Segmental mastectomy** (also referred to as breast conservation surgery or lumpectomy) is the removal of the tumor and the surrounding margin of breast tissues (**Figure 2–9A** ●). **Modified radical mastectomy**

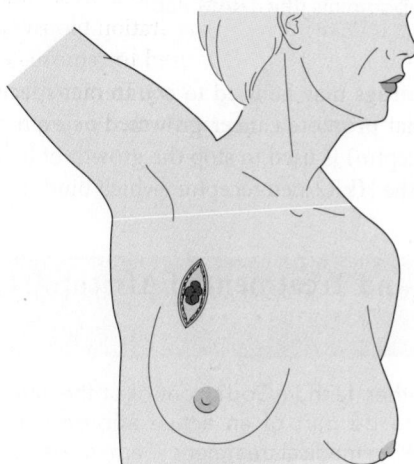

A Lumpectomy

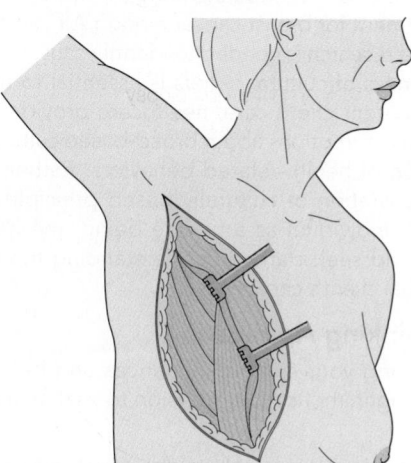

B Modified radical mastectomy

Figure 2–9 ● Types of mastectomy. *A*, In a lumpectomy, only the tumor and a small margin of surrounding tissue are removed. *B*, In a modified radical mastectomy, all breast tissue and the underarm lymph nodes are removed, but the underlying muscles remain.

is the removal of the breast tissue and lymph nodes under the arm (axillary node dissection), leaving the chest wall muscles intact (**Figure 2–9B** ●).

Axillary node dissection is generally performed during surgery for all invasive breast carcinoma to stage the tumor. Because this surgery can cause **lymphedema** (accumulation of fluid in the soft tissues of the arm caused by removal of lymph channels), nerve damage, and adhesions, and because of the role the lymph nodes play in immune system function, nonsurgical methods of detecting lymph node involvement now are being used. A sentinel node biopsy is performed before a node dissection by injecting a radioactive substance or dye into the region of the tumor. The dye is carried to the first (sentinel) lymph node, which is the first node to receive lymph from the tumor and is therefore the most likely to contain cancer cells (if the cancer has metastasized). If the sentinel node is positive, more nodes are removed. If the sentinel node is negative, further node evaluation is usually not indicated.

LUMPECTOMY Breast conservation surgery (**lumpectomy**) may be defined as excision of the primary tumor and adjacent breast tissue followed by radiation therapy. Many women are candidates for this procedure; however, some women, such as those who have multicentric breast neoplasms and those who have large tumors in relation to their breast size, are unsuitable candidates. Selection of women for this procedure is guided by the need for local control of the lesion, cosmetic results, and personal preference.

BREAST RECONSTRUCTION After a mastectomy, some women may choose to have their breast reconstructed. They report that surgical reconstruction of the breast simplifies their lives and restores a sense of body integrity. Other women choose to use a removable breast prosthesis, and some women are comfortable without reconstruction or a prosthesis.

Breast reconstruction may be performed at the time of the mastectomy or at any time thereafter, depending on the woman's preference. A number of procedures may be used to reconstruct a breast (**Figure 2–10** ●). These include placement of a submuscular implant, use of a tissue expander followed by an implant, transposition of muscle and blood supply from the abdomen or back, or (most often) use of a transverse rectus abdominis myocutaneous (TRAM) free-tissue flap.

🟤 **Stay Current:** *Learn about the latest techniques for breast reconstruction at the National Cancer Institute:* **www. cancer.gov/cancertopics/factsheet/Therapy/breast-reconstruction**.

Pharmacologic Therapy

Hormone therapy is often used in the treatment of individuals with breast cancer. One of the most commonly used hormone therapy drugs is tamoxifen citrate (Nolvadex). Tamoxifen is a selective estrogen receptor modulator (SERM). It works by preventing estrogen from attaching to estrogen receptors on the cancer cells, which inhibits tumor growth and ultimately kills

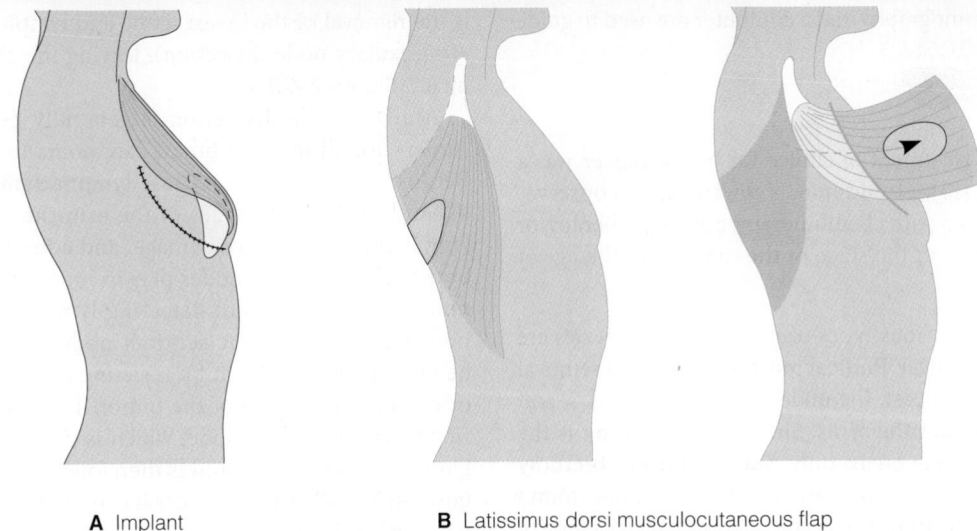

A Implant   **B** Latissimus dorsi musculocutaneous flap

Figure 2–10 ● Types of breast reconstruction surgeries. *A*, A breast implant is inserted under the pectoris muscle. *B*, In an autogenous procedures, a flap of skin, muscle, and fat from the donor site on the woman's body is transferred to the mastectomy site. The most frequently used donor muscle sites are the latissimus dorsi and the rectus abdominis (the TRAM flap).

tumor cells (Mayo Clinic, 2011a). It is used to treat advanced breast cancer, as an adjuvant for early-stage breast cancer, and as a preventive treatment in women at high risk for developing breast cancer.

Targeted drugs may be used to counteract specific genetic mutations that promote cancer growth. For example, trastuzumab (Herceptin) is used to stop the growth of breast tumors that express the HER2/neu receptor (which binds an epidermal

Evidence-Based Practice Spiritual Beliefs and Diagnosis and Treatment of African American Women With Breast Cancer

Problem
African American women die more often from breast cancer than any other group. It is believed that this statistic is the result of African American women's advanced stage of disease at diagnosis, primarily because of a delay in seeking treatment.

Evidence
Of all female ethnic and cultural groups, African American women are most likely to present with a more advanced stage of breast cancer at the time of initial diagnosis (Gullatte et al., 2010). In the context of the well-documented strong association between the African American culture and religiosity/ spirituality (Debnam et al., 2012), some researchers have theorized that the apparent delay in seeking treatment may be related to a cultural tendency among African American women to be fatalistic in their approach to cancer, trusting that the outcome rests in God's hands (Germino et al., 2011). However, in a study of 129 African American women diagnosed with breast cancer, Gullatte et al. (2010) found that research participants, despite being deeply spiritual and religious, were not fatalistic in their views.

Similarly, when Germino et al. (2011) evaluated a group of African American women who survived breast cancer, study findings suggested the high degree of spirituality demonstrated by African American women did not equate to passivity regarding treatment, nor was it indicative of a fatalistic

mentality. Rather, faith in God's control of the situation was considered to be part of an active approach that often included seeking medical treatment (Germino et al., 2011).

Implications
Within the framework of understanding the apparent delay in seeking treatment for breast cancer among African American women, more research is needed to identify causative factors. While awareness of cultural beliefs is essential to the provision of competent client care, healthcare providers should avoid making assumptions about broad-based cultural beliefs and causation of health-related behaviors. Rather, through sensitive exploration of culturally based principles and by viewing each individual as a unique being, the healthcare provider should seek clarity in understanding the basis for each individual client's choices.

Critical Thinking Application
1. Considering your cultural influences and beliefs, what factors might impact your decision to seek treatment for cancer?
2. What additional research might assist with providing greater understanding of the apparent delay in seeking treatment for breast cancer among women of African American heritage?
3. Aside from cultural beliefs, what other factors may impact an individual's decision to seek health care?

Clinical Manifestations and Therapies **Breast Cancer**

ETIOLOGY	CLINICAL MANIFESTATION	CLINICAL THERAPIES
Lymphedema (accumulation of fluid in the soft tissues of the arm) may occur following radical mastectomy secondary to removal of axillary lymph nodes.	■ Swelling of the arm and hand on the side of the mastectomy ■ May be acute, temporary, and mild if occurring immediately postoperative; acute and painful if occurring 4–6 weeks postoperative; or more commonly, chronic and painless if occurring 18–24 months after surgery	■ Exercise ■ Customized compression sleeve ■ Arm pump ■ Diet and weight control ■ Elevation of the arm ■ Prevention of infection ■ Avoidance of invasive procedures on affected arm
Cachexia is physical wasting from weight loss and loss of muscle mass from rapid growth and reproduction of cancer cells and their need for increased nutrients.	■ Weight loss, fatigue, weakness, loss of strength, activity intolerance, and constipation are a few of the possible manifestations.	■ Nutritional counseling ■ Increased caloric intake ■ Periods of rest and activity ■ Monitoring weight ■ Monitoring intake and output
Memory loss and difficulty concentrating may follow treatment with chemotherapy (sometimes referred to as chemo-brain).	■ Memory loss, difficulty focusing on tasks, changes in mood and affect, as well as fatigue ■ Generally lasts for 1–2 years after completing treatment	■ Warning clients in advance of possible occurrence, because it can be very frightening to clients ■ Recommending use of memory aids (e.g., making notes) ■ Providing emotional support to clients

growth factor that contributes to cancer cell growth) on their cell surface. This drug is a recombinant DNA-derived monoclonal antibody that binds to the receptor, inhibiting tumor cell proliferation.

Chemotherapy has become the standard of care for the majority of breast cancer cases with axillary node involvement. In late metastatic disease, chemotherapy becomes the primary treatment to prolong the woman's life. Adjuvant (additional) systemic therapy following primary treatment for early-stage breast cancer refers to the administration of chemotherapy and other pharmacologic agents. This type of therapy has been widely studied; its use reduces both the rate of recurrence and the rate of death from breast cancer. For example, the drug bevacizumab, when combined with chemotherapy to treat metastatic breast cancer, has extended cancer-free survival; letrozole (an aromatase inhibitor) has reduced the risk of recurrence after surgery (in some cases more effectively than tamoxifen).

Radiation Therapy

Radiation therapy typically follows breast cancer surgery to destroy any remaining cancer cells that could cause recurrence or metastasis. If a tumor is unusually large, radiation may be used to shrink the tumor before surgery. Radiation therapy is most commonly used in combination with lumpectomy for early-stage (stage I or II) breast cancer. Palliative radiation therapy is also used to treat chest wall recurrences and some bone metastases to help control pain and prevent fractures. Radiation therapy is administered by means of an external beam or tissue implants.

A new radiation treatment (intraoperative radiotherapy) is provided by a single, concentrated dose of radiation. During surgery, a probe is inserted into the cavity created by the lumpectomy, and radiation equivalent to 6 weeks of doses is emitted for approximately 25 minutes. If this proves successful, the treatment could make lumpectomy available to more women and prevent the client from having 6 weeks of daily radiation treatments following surgery.

■ NURSING PROCESS

Clients diagnosed with breast cancer require holistic care that addresses physical, psychological, social, and spiritual needs. Careful assessment of client response to therapy will improve the care planning process.

Assessment

Collect the following data through the health history and physical examination:

■ *Health history.* Family history of breast cancer, breast changes, nipple discharge, use of hormone replacement therapy, personal history of breast cancer, previous diagnostic tests and treatment for cancer, menstrual history, pregnancies, alcohol intake, physical activity, dietary history

■ *Physical assessment.* Height and weight, breasts, lymph glands.

Further focused assessments are described in the Implementation section that follows.

Diagnosis

Although each client has individual needs, nursing diagnoses relevant to the plan of care for the individual with breast cancer may include the following:

- *Risk for Infection*
- *Risk for Injury*
- *Acute Pain*
- *Anxiety*
- *Decisional Conflict*
- *Grief*
- *Disturbed Body Image*.

(NANDA-I © 2012)

Planning

Goals for treatment may include the following:

- The client will not experience infection.
- The client will make informed treatment decisions.
- The client will express feelings regarding diagnosis, treatment, and prognosis.
- The family and significant others will provide appropriate support for client.

Implementation

Nursing interventions are evidence-based strategies geared toward helping the client meet the goals outlined in the nursing plan of care. As with all elements of the care plan, the selection and implementation of nursing interventions must be individualized and tailored to meet the individual client's needs. While management of life-threatening physiological conditions always takes priority over pain management, in the stable client, treatment of pain remains a priority concern. Analgesics should be administered as ordered; collaboration with the prescribing provider may be needed to achieve a pain management regimen that affords the client consistently acceptable pain relief. In addition to providing effective pain management, examples of nursing interventions that may be appropriate for inclusion in the plan of care for the client with breast cancer follow.

Prevent Infection

Like any surgical client, the client who has breast surgery is at risk for infection. Removal of lymph nodes and the presence of a draining wound increase the risk.

- Assess the surgical dressings for bleeding, drainage, color, and odor every 4 hours for 24 hours, and document your findings. Circle any visible bleeding and drainage on the dressing as a baseline for subsequent assessment. Excessive bleeding or drainage signals postoperative complications that may require emergency attention.
- Observe the incision and IV sites for pain, redness, swelling, and drainage. Assess the drainage system for patency and adequate suction; note the color and amount of drainage. Careful observation for any signs of infection is essential, because client's immune system is compromised. IV catheters should be placed on the uninvolved side only.

- Change dressings and IV tubing using aseptic technique. Moist dressings and IV tubing provide sites for bacterial growth. Routine dressing and IV tubing changes using aseptic technique reduce the risk for infection.
- Encourage a protein-rich diet. Discuss the client's nutritional status with the dietitian, and request a consultation for the client. Adequate nutrition promotes healing and boosts the immune system.
- Teach the client how to care for the drainage system, if present (i.e., clean the site, empty the device, and record the amount, color, and type of drainage). The client is often discharged before removal of the drainage system and dressings and needs teaching to provide self-care.
- At discharge, teach the client to watch for and report to the healthcare provider the manifestations of infection: fever, redness or hardness at the surgical site, or purulent drainage. Any of these manifestations should be reported to the physician/surgeon.
- Explain that the client may experience scaling, flaking, dryness, itching, rash, or dry desquamation of the skin, particularly after radiation therapy. Impaired skin integrity increases the risk of infection.
- Tell the client to avoid deodorants and talcum powder on the affected side until the incision is completely healed. These substances may irritate the skin and impede healing.

Promote Optimal Circulation

Removal of the lymph nodes puts the client at risk for injury and long-term complications, such as lymphedema and infection.

- When obtaining blood pressure and starting IVs, use the nonsurgical side. Compression of the arm on the surgical side may cause lymphedema.
- Elevate the affected arm higher than the shoulder on a pillow, but do not abduct it. The hand should be higher than the elbow. Elevating the arm permits drainage, prevents swelling, and promotes circulation.
- Encourage range-of-motion exercises in the affected arm. Exercise helps develop collateral drainage.
- Explain that lymphedema massage and an elastic compression bandage may help control the swelling after the client has recovered from surgery.

Promote Psychosocial Well-Being

The client with breast cancer is often anxious about the diagnosis, the surgery, the outcome of surgery if nodal involvement is found, and the possible changes in sexual and family relationships. Studies show that young women with breast cancer, a growing population, are particularly vulnerable for anxiety and other psychosocial effects, as are their spouses and their children.

- Explore the client's knowledge base related to breast cancer. Assessing the client's current level of understanding about both the disease and the treatments helps the nurse plan more effective teaching.

Client Teaching Breast Cancer and Reconstructive Surgery

- Controversy exists about the health effects of silicone. While there is no conclusive evidence that silicone implants induce cancer or autoimmune disease, they are associated with hardening and pain caused by contracture of the capsule around the implant. The implant may rupture, releasing silicone gel, or infection may occur. Saline-filled breast implants may be an alternative.

- Reconstruction can be done immediately after a mastectomy or at any time later on. Some surgeons believe that delayed reconstruction offers better cosmetic results.

- Reconstructive surgery can create a natural-looking breast that makes clothes fit better. Since it has no nerve endings, however, the reconstructed breast has no feeling or sensations.

- If a simple mastectomy is done, an implant approximately the same size as the other breast is placed under the pectoral muscle on the operative side. This creates a breast mound that closely resembles the natural breast in shape and softness. If the implant is placed over the pectoral muscle, a high degree of firmness may occur.

- With a simple mastectomy or modified radical mastectomy, a tissue expander may be used to replace the breast. The tissue expander is placed under the pectoral muscle and gradually expanded with saline injections every 2–3 weeks to stretch the overlying skin and create a pocket. After a period of time, usually 1–2 months, the tissue expander is exchanged for a saline implant.

- With more extensive surgery, such as radical mastectomy, a flap of skin, fat, or muscle is transferred from a donor site to the operative area. A new nipple may be created by using tissue from the opposite nipple or from the inner thigh.

- Reconstructive surgery may require multiple surgeries, including all the risks associated with anesthesia. As the complexity of the procedures increases, so does the risk of complications, such as infection.

- To decrease the risk of a fibrous capsule forming around the implant, it is important to perform breast massage as instructed.

- Encourage discussion about resuming life at home and the expected lifestyle changes that must be implemented. Anticipatory guidance can be helpful when planning for and coping with lifestyle and relationship changes.

- Explain the surgical procedure, including information about preoperative medications, anesthesia, and recovery. Knowing what to expect helps decrease anxiety.

- Explain that it is normal to have decreased sensation in the surgical area. Severed or damaged nerves reduce sensation.

- Facilitate a team approach with the surgeon, anesthesiologist, oncologist, plastic surgeon, and other health professionals. Being the client's advocate during this time of anxiety and decision making reduces the stress of coordinating multiple healthcare provider schedules.

Breast surgery, even lumpectomy, alters the appearance of the breast. This loss is expressed through grief. The nurse provides supportive care for the client who is grieving the loss of her breast.

Promote a Healthy Body Image

Breast surgery can change the client's body image. The surgical changes may be compounded by weight gain and other side effects of chemotherapy or hormone therapy. Self-esteem also affects adjustment to a changed body image.

- Assess the client's current body image. Self-image is related to self-esteem. Discuss whether her self-image has changed.

- Explain that redness and swelling in the scar will fade with time. Knowledge that the scar will fade may give the woman a more realistic view of the changes.

- Include the partner and family if possible when discussing the plan of care and ADLs. Request consultation with a psychologist or other professional if the client is interested. Discussion with the partner and family can facilitate the client's emotional healing process.

- Offer pamphlets and suggest books and videos that might increase knowledge about what lies ahead. Knowing what to expect can help the client cope.

- Encourage the client to look at her incision when she feels ready; often, the reality is not as frightening as what the client had imagined. Explain that it is normal to be afraid to look. Reassurance that her behavior is normal decreases anxiety.

- Breast reconstruction options are available for women and men (Ottini et al., 2010). If the client is interested in breast reconstruction, provide written material and encourage discussion with a plastic surgeon and with others who have had reconstruction. It is important for the client to be fully knowledgeable about available options to make an informed decision.

- Offer referral to support groups with clients experiencing similar challenges. Some clients may prefer one-on-one counseling.

Evaluation

Clients are evaluated for expected outcomes based on specific client needs and care planning. Potential outcomes may include the following:

- The client experiences no complications resulting from treatment.
- Side effects from medications are minimized.
- Pain is managed to allow the client to rest and perform essential ADLs.

NURSING CARE PLAN ▸ A Woman With Breast Cancer

Rachel Clemments is a 42-year-old mother of two: Sarah, age 12, and Jennifer, age 18. Because of a family history of breast cancer, she has been closely monitored (annual mammograms and clinical breast examination, monthly BSE, a needle aspiration biopsy with negative findings) for 4 years before her diagnosis. Mrs. Clemments discovers a lump in her left breast during her monthly BSE. An incisional biopsy reveals invasive lobular carcinoma in the left breast. Mrs. Clemments is debating whether to have reconstructive breast surgery. One of her greatest concerns is how her illness will affect her ability to support and care for her daughters. The breast cancer diagnosis seems part of the family legacy. She wonders, "When will it happen to Jennifer? To Sarah?"

ASSESSMENT

During the history, Laura Nelson, RN, the nurse admitting Mrs. Clemments, learns that her mother, two of her aunts, and one sister had been diagnosed with breast cancer. Her mother and one of the aunts died before age 45. Physical assessment findings include temperature 98.5°F oral; pulse 65 bpm; respirations 14/min; and BP 110/62 mmHg. Her weight is 54 kg (120 lb); she is 168 cm (66 in.) tall. Modified radical mastectomy is performed. Histological examination shows a 3-cm tumor; axillary node dissection shows that 4 of 16 lymph nodes are positive.

DIAGNOSES

- *Risk for Infection* related to surgical incision
- *Acute Pain* related to surgery
- *Disturbed Body Image*
- *Decisional Conflict About Treatment* related to concerns about risks and benefits
- *Fear* related to disease process/prognosis

(NANDA-I © 2012)

PLANNING

- The client will remain free of infection.
- The client will experience minimal pain or discomfort during her recovery.
- The client will maintain a positive body image, regardless of her decision about reconstruction.
- The client will evaluate the treatment options in relation to personal values and decide on a course of action.
- The client will identify the sources of her fear and demonstrate behaviors that may reduce fears.

IMPLEMENTATION

- Teach the client about hand hygiene and wound care.
- Assess the client's pain tolerance, and administer analgesics as prescribed.
- Teach the client to use caution when moving the affected arm, to avoid lifting heavy objects, and to wear gloves when gardening.
- Encourage the client to express thoughts and feelings. Refer to appropriate support groups if the client is amenable.

- Assess the client's interest in spiritual/religious support, and refer if appropriate.
- Encourage the client to verbalize fears about her own prognosis and about her daughters' future risks for breast cancer; assess the need/interest for referral to psychological counseling.

EVALUATION

At discharge, Mrs. Clemments has no signs of physical complications and is looking forward to being at home with her daughters as temporary caregivers. Mrs. Clemments met with a Reach to Recovery volunteer who brought her a temporary prosthesis and booklets about postmastectomy exercises, chemotherapy, and breast reconstruction. The volunteer also referred her to a local cancer support group. Mrs. Clemments has talked about her concerns related to breast reconstruction. "I want to avoid anything that would increase the risk of complications. The possibility of recurrence and my fear for my daughters' future health are more than enough to worry about."

CRITICAL THINKING

1. *What role could genetic counseling play in helping Mrs. Clemments and her daughters better understand the daughters' risks for breast cancer?*
2. *Describe the types of mastectomies and their implications for nursing care.*
3. *What medications might help minimize the side effects of chemotherapy?*
4. *Develop a plan of care for Mrs. Clemments for the nursing diagnosis Disturbed Sleep Pattern.*

◤ REVIEW Breast Cancer

RELATE Link the Concepts and Exemplars

Linking the exemplar of breast cancer with the concept of advocacy:

1. How might the nurse advocate for the prevention of breast cancer or its early detection?
2. What role can the nurse play in advocating to make men more aware of the role they can play in breast cancer prevention and early detection?

Linking the exemplar of breast cancer with the concept of sexuality:

3. A client who is preparing for a radical mastectomy says, "My husband says if I only have one breast I am only half a woman." How can you help this woman adapt to the perceived change in her femininity?
4. Is the impact on a client's sexuality completely reversed if she has plastic surgery to repair the appearance of the breast? Is plastic surgery always an option? Explain your answer.

READY Go to Companion Skills Manual

REFER Go to Pearson Nursing Student Resources
nursing.pearsonhighered.com

- Additional review materials

REFLECT Case Study

Judy Franklin, 22 years old, has just graduated from college and is about to start a job as a graphic arts designer in a large marketing company. Judy is also planning her wedding to George 6 months from now. She found a lump in her left breast during self-exam and has come to the physician for an initial consultation. During the assessment, the nurse learns Judy has not told her fiancé about her findings. Judy will not make eye contact with the nurse and appears distracted during the interview.

1. What nursing diagnoses would be appropriate for Judy?
2. How might you assist Judy to inform her fiancé if the lump is determined to be a malignant tumor?
3. What support interventions would you initiate to help Judy as she waits for the results of diagnostic testing to determine the cause of the lump?

EXEMPLAR 2.4   **Colorectal Cancer**

EXEMPLAR KEY TERMS

Colon cancer, 85
Colorectal cancer, 85
Colostomy, 87
Fulguration, 87
Polyps, 85

EXEMPLAR LEARNING OUTCOMES

After reading about this exemplar, you will be able to:

1. Describe the pathophysiology, etiology, clinical manifestations, and direct and indirect causes of colorectal cancer.
2. Identify risk factors and prevention methods associated with colorectal cancer.
3. Illustrate the nursing process in providing culturally competent care across the life span for individuals with colorectal cancer.
4. Formulate priority nursing diagnoses appropriate for an individual with colorectal cancer.
5. Summarize therapies used by interdisciplinary teams in the collaborative care of an individual with colorectal cancer.
6. Plan evidence-based care for an individual with colorectal cancer and his or her family in collaboration with other members of the healthcare team.
7. Evaluate expected outcomes for an individual with colorectal cancer.

▶ OVERVIEW

Colon cancer is cancer of the third segment of the large bowel and may or may not include the anus. **Colorectal cancer** involves both the colon and the rectum. Although the terms are often used interchangeably, they differ in terms of whether the rectum is involved.

Regular colonoscopies can greatly reduce the risk for colorectal cancer by allowing removal of polyps before they become malignant tumors that invade the bowel and metastasize to other areas of the body. The nurse's role focuses on promoting the need for regular screening as well as reporting the early warning signs of the disease in order to reduce occurrence and improve outcomes.

▶ PATHOPHYSIOLOGY AND ETIOLOGY

Nearly all colorectal cancers are adenocarcinomas that begin as adenomatous **polyps** (small vascular growths on the surface of any mucous membrane, referring in this exemplar to growths on the internal surface of the bowel). Most tumors develop in the rectum and sigmoid colon, although any portion of the colon may be affected (**Figure 2–11 ●**).

The tumor typically grows undetected, producing few manifestations. By the time manifestations occur, the disease may have spread into deeper layers of the bowel tissue and adjacent organs. Colorectal cancer spreads by direct extension to involve the entire bowel circumference, the submucosa, and outer bowel wall layers. Neighboring structures, such as the liver, greater curvature of the stomach, duodenum, small intestine, pancreas, spleen, genitourinary tract, and abdominal wall, also may be involved by direct extension.

Metastasis to regional lymph nodes is the most common form of tumor spread. This is not always an orderly process; distal nodes may contain cancer cells while regional nodes

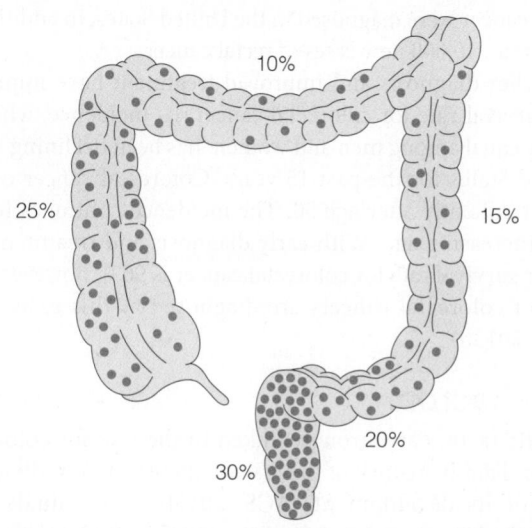

Figure 2–11 ● The distribution and frequency of cancer of the colon and rectum.

TABLE 2–8 The TNM Staging System for Colorectal Cancer

STAGE	PRIMARY TUMOR (T)	REGIONAL LYMPH NODES (N)	DISTANT METASTASIS (M)
	TX—Primary tumor cannot be assessed T0—No evidence of primary tumor	NX—Regional lymph node cannot be assessed	MX—Presence of distant metastasis cannot be assessed
Stage 0	Tis—Carcinoma in situ	N0—No regional lymph node metastasis	M0—No distant metastasis
Stage I	T1—Tumor invades submucosa		
	T2—Tumor invades muscularis propria		
Stage II	T3—Tumor invades through muscularis propria into subserosa or into non-peritonealized pericolic or perirectal tissues		
	T4—Tumor perforates visceral peritoneum or directly invades other organs or structures		
Stage III	Any T	N1—Metastasis in one to three pericolic or perirectal lymph nodes	
		N2—Metastasis in four or more pericolic or perirectal lymph nodes	
		N3—Metastasis in any lymph node along course of a major named vascular trunk	
Stage IV	Any T	Any N	M1—Distant metastasis

remain normal. Cancerous cells from the primary tumor may also spread by way of the lymphatic system or circulatory system to secondary sites, such as the liver, lungs, brain, bones, and kidneys. In addition, "seeding" of the tumor to other areas of the peritoneal cavity can occur when the tumor extends through the serosa or during surgical resection.

Current staging methods primarily use the TNM system, as outlined in **Table 2–8** ●.

Etiology

Colorectal cancer (cancer of the colon or rectum) is the third most common cancer diagnosed in the United States. The ACS (2013b) estimated that in 2013 more than 102,000 new cases of colon cancer were diagnosed in the United States, in addition to more than 40,000 new cases of rectal cancer.

Earlier diagnosis and improved treatment have improved the survival rate for colorectal cancer. Its incidence, which is nearly equal among men and women, has been declining in the United States for the past 15 years. Colorectal cancer occurs most frequently after age 50. The incidence continues to rise with increasing age. With early diagnosis and treatment, the 5-year survival rate for colorectal cancer is 90%; however, only 39% of colorectal cancers are diagnosed at this early stage (ACS, 2013b).

Risk Factors

Genetic factors are strongly linked to the risk for colorectal cancer. Family history of the disease increases an individual's risk for its development (ACS, 2013b). Individuals with familial adenomatous polyposis inevitably will develop colon cancer unless the colon is removed. Hereditary nonpolyposis colorectal cancer (also known as Lynch syndrome) is an autosomal dominant disorder that significantly increases the risk for developing colorectal and other cancers. Tumors associated with Lynch syndrome often affect the ascending colon and tend to occur at an earlier age. Inflammatory bowel diseases also increase the risk of colorectal cancer. Additional risk factors include being over 50 and previous exposure to radiation.

Diet plays a role in the development of colorectal cancer. The disease is prevalent in economically prosperous countries where people consume diets high in calories, meat proteins, and fats. This dietary pattern, common in the United States, is thought to increase the population of anaerobic bacteria in the gut. These anaerobes convert bile acids into carcinogens. Diets high in fruits and vegetables, folic acid, and calcium appear to reduce the risk of colorectal cancer. Cereal fiber, once thought to reduce colorectal cancer risk, now does not appear to play a role either way in its development. Other factors that may reduce the risk of colorectal cancer include regular exercise, taking a daily multivitamin, and the use of aspirin and other nonsteroidal anti-inflammatory drugs.

Prevention

The ACS (2013b) recommends one of the following testing schedules for early detection of colorectal cancer, beginning at age 50. These options are acceptable choices for average-risk adults:

- Yearly fecal occult blood test or fecal immunochemical test (For fecal occult blood test, the take-home, multiple-sample method should be used.)
- Stool DNA test (interval uncertain)
- Flexible sigmoidoscopy every 5 years
- Double-contrast barium enema every 5 years
- Colonoscopy every 10 years
- CT colonography every 5 years.

Clinical Manifestations and Therapies **Colorectal Cancer**

ETIOLOGY	CLINICAL MANIFESTATION	CLINICAL THERAPIES
Rectal bleeding may occur as the cancer cells invade or irritate the bowel mucosa.	■ Dark color to stool, blood may or may not be visible without guaiac testing, classic alteration in smell of stools with frank blood, anemia, decreasing hemoglobin and hematocrit, decreased RBC, often asymptomatic unless guaiac tested	■ Surgical removal of tumor and involved segment of bowel ■ Blood transfusions and hydration if blood loss is significant
Change in bowel habits as cancer cells grow	■ Stools may be pencil thin as the bowel lumen diminishes. ■ Diarrhea or constipation	■ Surgical resection of involved bowel ■ Antidiarrheals may be indicated if diarrhea results ■ Monitor for signs of complete obstruction of bowel, including emesis, acute abdominal pain, or abdominal distention, accompanied by absence of stool for several days.

▶ CLINICAL MANIFESTATIONS

Bowel cancer often produces no manifestations until it is advanced. Because it grows slowly, 5–15 years of growth may occur before manifestations develop. The manifestations depend on its location, type and extent, and complications.

Rectal bleeding is often the initial manifestation that prompts clients to seek medical care. Other common early manifestations include a change in bowel habits, either diarrhea or constipation. Pain, anorexia, and weight loss are characteristic in advanced disease. A palpable abdominal or rectal mass may be present. Occasionally, the client presents with anemia from occult bleeding.

▶ COLLABORATION

The client with a diagnosis of colorectal cancer needs a collaborative approach often requiring intervention from surgeons, nurses specializing in care of ostomies, dietary counselors, radiation therapists, as well as the nurse providing primary care. A holistic approach to the client's care improves both client outcomes and chances for survival.

Diagnostic Tests

Diagnostic and laboratory tests are used for screening, diagnosis, and monitoring purposes. Diagnostic tests include a sigmoidoscopy or colonoscopy as the primary means used to detect and visualize tumors. While flexible sigmoidoscopy can detect 50%–65% of colorectal cancers, many clinicians recommend colonoscopy. Tissue for biopsy is obtained at the time of endoscopy to confirm cancerous tissue and evaluate cell differentiation. Current staging methods primarily use the TNM system, as outlined previously in Table 2–8. Radiological examinations may include a chest x-ray to detect tumor metastasis to the lung, and CT, MRI, or ultrasonic examination may be used to assess tumor depth and involvement of other organs by direct extension or metastasis.

Laboratory tests include a fecal occult blood test (by guaiac or Hemoccult testing) to detect blood in the feces, a CBC to detect anemia resulting from chronic blood loss and tumor growth, and a CEA level, which is a tumor marker that can be detected in the blood of clients with colorectal cancer. CEA levels are used to estimate prognosis, monitor treatment, and detect cancer recurrence.

Surgery

Surgical resection of the tumor, adjacent colon, and regional lymph nodes is the treatment of choice for colorectal cancer. Options for surgical treatment vary from destruction of the tumor by laser photocoagulation performed during endoscopy to abdominoperineal resection with permanent colostomy. When possible, the anal sphincter is preserved and colostomy avoided.

Other surgical treatment options for small, localized tumors include local excision and fulguration. These procedures also may be performed during endoscopy, eliminating the need for abdominal surgery. Local excision may be used to remove a disk of rectum containing a tumor in clients with a small, well-differentiated, mobile polypoid lesion. **Fulguration**, also known as electrocoagulation, is a procedure used to reduce the size of some large tumors for clients who are poor surgical risks. Fulguration requires general anesthesia and may need to be repeated at intervals.

Most clients with colorectal cancer undergo surgical resection of the colon with anastomosis of the remaining bowel as a curative procedure. The distribution of regional lymph nodes determines the extent of resection, because these may contain metastatic lesions. Most tumors of the ascending, transverse, descending, and sigmoid colon can be resected.

Tumors of the rectum usually are treated with an abdominoperineal resection in which the sigmoid colon, rectum, and anus are removed through both abdominal and perineal incisions. A permanent sigmoid colostomy is performed to provide for elimination of feces.

COLOSTOMY   Surgical resection of the bowel may be accompanied by a colostomy for diversion of fecal contents. A **colostomy** is an ostomy made in the colon. It may be created if

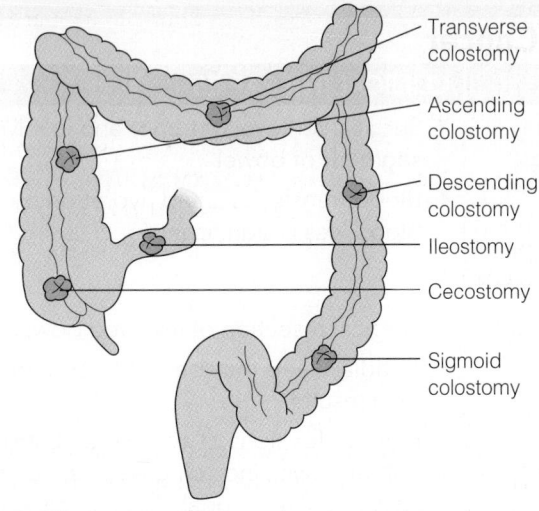

Figure 2–12 ● Various ostomy levels and sites.

the bowel is obstructed by the tumor, as a temporary measure to promote healing of anastomoses, or as a permanent means of fecal evacuation when the distal colon and rectum are removed. Colostomies take the name of the portion of the colon from which they are formed: ascending colostomy, transverse colostomy, descending colostomy, and sigmoid colostomy (Figure 2–12 ●).

A sigmoid colostomy is the most common permanent colostomy, particularly for cancer of the rectum. It is usually created during an abdominoperineal resection. This procedure involves removal of the sigmoid colon, rectum, and anus through abdominal and perineal incisions. The anal canal is closed, and a stoma is formed from the proximal sigmoid colon. The stoma usually is located on the lower left quadrant of the abdomen.

When a double-barrel colostomy is performed, two separate stomas are created (Figure 2–13 ●). The distal colon is not removed, but bypassed. The proximal stoma, which is functional, diverts feces to the abdominal wall. The distal stoma, also called the mucous fistula, expels mucus from the distal colon. It may be pouched or dressed with a 4-in. × 4-in. gauze

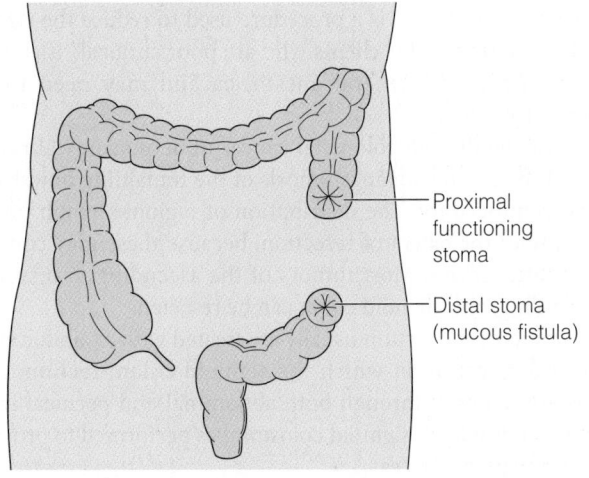

Figure 2–13 ● A double-barrel colostomy. The proximal stoma is the functioning stoma; the distal stoma expels mucus from the distal colon.

dressing. A double-barrel colostomy may be created for cases of trauma, tumor, or inflammation, and it may be temporary or permanent.

An emergency procedure used to relieve an intestinal obstruction or perforation is called a transverse loop colostomy. During this procedure, a loop of the transverse colon is brought out from the abdominal wall and suspended over a plastic rod or bridge, which prevents the loop from slipping back into the abdominal cavity. The loop stoma may be opened at the time of surgery or a few days later at the client's bedside. The bridge may be removed in 1–2 weeks. Transverse loop colostomies are typically temporary.

In a Hartmann procedure, a common temporary colostomy procedure, the distal portion of the colon is left in place and is oversewn for closure. A temporary colostomy may be done to allow bowel rest or healing, such as following tumor resection or inflammation of the bowel. It also may be created following traumatic injury to the colon, such as a gunshot wound. Anastomosis of the severed portions of the colon is delayed, because bacterial colonization of the colon would prevent proper healing of the anastomosis. Approximately 3–6 months following a temporary colostomy, the colostomy is closed, and the colon is reconnected. Clients with temporary colostomies require the same care as clients with permanent colostomies.

LASER PHOTOCOAGULATION   Laser photocoagulation uses a very small, intense beam of light to generate heat in tissues toward which it is directed. The heat generated by the laser beam can be used to destroy small tumors. It is also used for palliative surgery of advanced tumors to remove obstruction. Laser photocoagulation can be performed endoscopically and is useful for clients who cannot tolerate major surgery.

Pharmacologic Therapy

Chemotherapeutic agents, such as IV fluorouracil (5-FU) and folinic acid (leucovorin), are used postoperatively as adjunctive therapy for colorectal cancer. When combined with radiation therapy, chemotherapy reduces the rate of tumor recurrence and prolongs survival for clients with stage II and stage III rectal tumors. The benefit for clients with colon cancer is less clear, but chemotherapy may be used to reduce its spread to the liver and prevent recurrence. Irinotecan (CPT-11) or oxaliplatin also may be used in chemotherapy regimens for colorectal cancer.

Radiation Therapy

Although radiation therapy is not used as a primary treatment for colon cancer, it is used with surgical resection for treating rectal tumors. Small rectal cancers may be treated with intracavitary, external, or implantation radiation. Rectal cancer has a high rate of regional recurrence following complete surgical resection, particularly when the tumor has invaded tissues outside the bowel wall or regional lymph nodes. Pre- or postoperative radiation therapy reduces the recurrence of pelvic tumors, although the effect of radiation therapy on long-term survival is less clear. Radiation therapy also is used preoperatively to shrink large rectal tumors enough to permit surgical removal of the tumor.

NURSING PROCESS

In planning and implementing care, consider both physical care needs and emotional response to the diagnosis. Because colorectal cancer is often advanced at the time of diagnosis, the prognosis, even with treatment, may be poor. Denial and anger are common. Extensive abdominal surgery and a colostomy may be necessary, and the effects of chemotherapy and radiation therapy can leave the client fatigued and discouraged.

Assessment

Collect the following data through the health history and physical examination:

- **Health history.** Usual bowel patterns and any recent changes; weight loss, fatigue, decreased activity tolerance; presence of blood in the stool; pain with defecation, abdominal discomfort, perineal pain; usual diet; family history of colorectal cancer, other specific risk factors, such as inflammatory bowel disease or colon polyps.
- **Physical examination.** General appearance; weight; abdominal shape, contour; bowel sounds, abdominal tenderness; stool Hemoccult or guaiac.

Diagnosis

Nursing diagnoses for the client with colorectal cancer are individualized to each client's needs and may include:

- *Risk for Infection*
- *Acute Pain*
- *Imbalanced Nutrition: Less Than Body Requirements*
- *Anticipatory Grieving*
- *Risk for Ineffective Sexuality Pattern.*

(NANDA-I © 2012)

Planning

The goals for client outcome are determined by the client's condition, prognosis, amount of tissue involved, and staging of the tumor. Suggested goals may include the following:

- The client will not demonstrate evidence of infection.
- Using a predetermined pain rating scale of 0 to 10, with 0 being "no pain" and 10 representing "the worst imaginable pain," the client will consistently rate her pain at 3 or less.
- The client will demonstrate proper ostomy care and management.
- The client will verbalize feelings related to diagnosis and prognosis.
- The family or significant others will provide adequate emotional and physical support for the client upon discharge.
- The client will make an informed choice related to treatment options.

Implementation

Nursing care includes providing emotional support, teaching, and direct care before and after diagnostic procedures and surgery as well as during adjunctive treatments. The risk for sexual dysfunction should be addressed as a nursing diagnosis if a colostomy has been created.

Clients with colorectal cancer are at risk for infection, and nursing care aimed at reducing this is essential. Guidance regarding good hygiene, promoting skin integrity, and avoiding circumstances that elevate risk (e.g., crowds, exposure to individuals who are ill) is part of the nurse's focus. See the exemplar on Cancer for a full discussion of nursing interventions to prevent infection in clients with cancer.

Manage Pain

The client with colorectal cancer may experience pain related to preparatory procedures, diagnostic examinations, and surgery. Following an abdominoperineal resection, "phantom" rectal pain related to the severing of nerves during the wide excision of the rectum may develop. Finally, the primary tumor itself and, potentially, metastatic tumors may impinge on nerves and other organs, causing pain.

In the early postoperative period, an epidural infusion or patient-controlled analgesia often is used to manage pain. Patient-controlled analgesia, routine administration of ordered analgesics, or a continuous analgesia delivery system also may be used for pain management when the tumor is far enough advanced to preclude surgical resection. A detailed discussion of pain medications can be found in the exemplar on Acute and Chronic Pain in the module on Comfort. Use predetermined rating scales to assess client pain levels as described in the exemplar.

- Monitor for adequate pain relief. Use subjective and objective information, including the location, intensity, and character of the pain, as well as nonverbal signs, such as grimacing, muscle tension, apparent dozing, changes in pulse or blood pressure, and rapid, shallow respirations. The client may assume that pain is to be expected or tolerated or may fear becoming addicted to analgesic medications.
- Monitor analgesic effectiveness 30 minutes after administration. Monitor for pain relief and adverse effects. The method of delivery, dosage, or medication itself may need to be adjusted to provide adequate pain relief.
- Assess the incision for inflammation or swelling; assess drainage catheters and tubes for patency. Poorly controlled pain or pain that changes may be related to organ distention from an obstructed nasogastric tube, urinary catheter, or wound drain. It also may indicate an infection.
- Assess the abdomen for distention, tenderness, and bowel sounds. Intra-abdominal bleeding, peritonitis, or paralytic ileus can cause pain that may be confused with incisional pain.
- Administer analgesia before an activity or procedure. Adequate pain relief reduces muscle tension, allowing more comfortable participation in activities.
- Assist with adjunctive comfort measures, such as positioning, diversional activities, management of environmental stimuli, guided imagery, and relaxation techniques. These measures enhance the effects of analgesia by reducing muscle tension.
- Splint incision with a pillow, and teach the client how to self-splint when coughing and deep breathing to prevent respiratory complications related to fear of pain.

Promote Balanced Nutrition

Bowel preparation for diagnostic procedures, surgery, radiation therapy, and chemotherapy place the client with colorectal cancer at risk for nutritional deficiencies. Fluid and electrolyte replacement is provided following surgery, along with possible total parenteral nutrition. Adequate kilocalorie and nutrient intake are necessary for healing after surgery. Additionally, if the tumor is advanced, metabolic needs may be increased and the appetite decreased.

■ Assess nutritional status, using data such as height and weight, skinfold measurements, body mass index, and laboratory data, including serum albumin level. Refer to a dietitian or nutritionist for dietary management. The client who is malnourished before beginning aggressive cancer treatment requires more vigorous nutrition management to promote healing.

■ Assess readiness for resumption of oral intake after surgery or procedures using data such as statements of hunger, presence of bowel sounds, passage of flatus, and minimal abdominal distention. Manipulation of the bowel interrupts peristalsis of the gastrointestinal tract. It is important to ensure that peristalsis has resumed before oral intake begins.

■ Monitor and document food and fluid intake. Documentation helps identify the adequacy of kilocalories and other nutrient intake.

■ Weigh the client daily. Weight fluctuation may indicate adequate or inadequate dietary intake.

■ Maintain total parenteral nutrition and central IV lines as ordered. Parenteral nutrition prevents tissue catabolism and promotes healing when food intake is disrupted for more than 2–3 days.

■ When oral intake resumes, help the client develop a meal plan that incorporates food preferences and considers the client's schedule and environment. Consideration of likes, dislikes, and circumstances in meal planning promotes adequate intake.

Promote Healthy Coping

When a bowel resection is performed for colorectal cancer, the client needs to adjust to the loss of a major body part as well as to the diagnosis of cancer. Even when the prognosis for recovery is good, many people perceive cancer as fatal. Supporting the client and family during the initial stages of grieving can improve physical recovery as well as psychological coping and eventual adaptation.

■ Work to develop a trusting relationship with the client and family. This increases the nurse's effectiveness in helping them work through the grieving process.

■ Listen actively, encouraging the client and family to express their fears and concerns. Assist to identify strengths, past experiences, and support systems:

   a. Demonstrate respect for cultural, spiritual, and religious values and beliefs; encourage use of these resources to cope with losses.

   b. Encourage discussion of the potential impact of loss on individual family members, family structure, and family function. Assist family members to share concerns with one another.

   c. Refer to cancer support groups, social services, or counseling as appropriate.

These resources can be used throughout the grieving process.

Reduce Risk for Sexual Dysfunction

Colorectal cancer and ostomy surgery increase the risk for sexual dysfunction. Physical factors that can lead to sexual dysfunction include disruption of nerves and blood vessels that supply the genitals, radiation therapy, chemotherapy, and other medications prescribed after surgery.

Psychologically, a client with an ostomy experiences an altered body image and may develop low self-esteem. The client may feel undesirable and fear rejection. He or she may be concerned about odors or pouch leakage during sexual activity. This emotional stress can also contribute to sexual dysfunction.

■ Provide opportunities for the client and family to express feelings about the cancer diagnosis, ostomy, and effects of other treatments. Encouraging verbalization provides an opportunity to validate that feelings of anger and depression are normal responses to the diagnosis and change in body function.

■ Provide consistent colostomy care. An accepting attitude and consistent care that provides a secure appliance and controls odor and leakage instill a sense of confidence in the client.

■ Encourage expression of sexual concerns. Provide privacy and caregivers who have established trust with the client and family and are comfortable with discussions about sexual concerns. Sexuality is a very private concern to most people. The client and family are not likely to express their concerns openly unless trust has been established.

■ Reassure the client and significant other that the effect of physical illness and prescribed interventions on sexuality usually is temporary. The client and partner may misinterpret an initial decrease in libido as evidence that sexual activity will not be possible or resume following recovery.

■ Refer the client and partner to social services or a family counselor for further interventions. Clients are often discharged from acute care settings well before concerns about sexual activity surface. Ongoing counseling provides a continuing resource.

■ Arrange for a visit from a member of the United Ostomy Association. People who are living and coping with an ostomy can provide information and support, helping the client with a new ostomy overcome feelings of isolation and rejection.

Evaluation

Client outcome is evaluated based on goals of care. Potential expected outcomes may include the following:

■ The client does not demonstrate any signs or symptoms of infection.

■ The client maintains adequate hydration, as evidenced by urinary output of at least 0.5 mL/kg/hr.

■ Using a predetermined pain rating scale in which 0 represents "no pain" and 10 represents "the worst possible pain," the client consistently rates her pain at a level of 3 or less.

■ The client is able to perform essential daily ADLs.

NURSING CARE PLAN | A Client With Colorectal Cancer

William Cunningham is a 65-year-old retired railroad employee, husband, and father of three grown children. For the past 3 months, Mr. Cunningham has noticed small amounts of blood and occasional mucus in his stools. He has a sensation of pressure in the rectum, and he notices that his stools are smaller in diameter, about the size of pencil. After palpating a mass on digital examination of the rectum, the physician orders a colonoscopy. A large sessile lesion is found in the rectum and biopsied. The pathology report shows the lesion to be adenocarcinoma. Mr. Cunningham is scheduled for an abdominoperineal resection and sigmoid colostomy.

ASSESSMENT	DIAGNOSES	PLANNING
Madonna Hart, RN, completes the admission assessment. Mr. Cunningham states that his bowel habits have recently changed, but he denies pain or other symptoms. Physical assessment findings include temperature 36.9°C (98.4°F); pulse 82 bpm; respirations 18/min; and BP 118/78 mmHg. He is 178 cm (70 in.) tall and weighs 84 kg (185 lb). Laboratory findings are normal except for the previous pathology report of adenocarcinoma of rectal lesion. Mr. Cunningham states, "I really don't want a colostomy, but if that is what it takes to get rid of this, I'm ready to get it over with."	■ *Acute Pain* related to surgical intervention ■ *Risk for Impaired Skin Integrity* (peristomal) related to fecal drainage and pouch adhesive ■ *Risk for Dysfunctional Gastrointestinal Motility* related to effects of surgery on bowel function ■ *Disturbed Body Image* related to colostomy ■ *Risk for Ineffective Sexuality Pattern* related to wide rectal incision, radiation therapy, and colostomy (NANDA-I © 2012)	■ The client will report pain within an acceptable range that allows ease of movement and ambulation. ■ The client will perform colostomy care using correct technique. ■ The client will demonstrate willingness to discuss changes in sexual function. ■ The client will wear clothing to enhance physical and emotional self-esteem.

IMPLEMENTATION

- Provide analgesia as ordered, evaluating its effectiveness.
- Discuss foods that cause odor and gas.
- Teach colostomy care.
- Maintain consistent nursing personnel assignment to facilitate trust.
- Refer to the local United Ostomy Association.
- Provide a list of local medical supply companies that carry ostomy supplies.
- Provide for privacy when teaching and discussing concerns about ostomy.

EVALUATION

On discharge, Mr. Cunningham is able to empty and rinse out his colostomy pouch. He is changing the pouch and caring for surrounding skin appropriately. Ms. Hart has given him verbal and written instructions on colostomy care. He verbalizes understanding of phantom rectal pain and the importance of avoiding rectal suppositories. He expresses an understanding of the need to avoid heavy lifting and the importance of follow-up care. Ms. Hart has referred Mr. Cunningham to a home health agency in his community for further questions and follow-up care.

CRITICAL THINKING

1. *What is the cause of phantom rectal pain?*
2. *Why is it important to discuss dietary concerns with a client with a colostomy, especially odor- and gas-forming foods?*
3. *Outline a plan to teach Mr. Cunningham how to irrigate a colostomy.*
4. *Develop a care plan for Mr. Cunningham for the nursing diagnosis of Disturbed Body Image.*

REVIEW Colorectal Cancer

RELATE Link the Concepts and Exemplars

Linking the exemplar of colorectal cancer with the concept of elimination:

1. What alterations in bowel elimination increase the client's risk for colorectal cancer?

2. What preventive teaching can you provide the client with altered bowel elimination to reduce the risk of colorectal cancer?

Linking the exemplar of colorectal cancer with the concept of self:

3. How might a client's self-concept be altered as the result of treatment for colorectal cancer resulting in a colostomy?

4. You are caring for a client with end-stage colorectal cancer who appears emaciated, is cachectic, and has lost most of her hair as a result of treatment. She refuses visitors because she does not want friends and loved ones to see her looking like this. What nursing interventions can you implement to help her cope with her altered body image and self-concept while promoting socialization?

READY Go to Companion Skills Manual

REFER Go to Pearson Nursing Student Resources
nursing.pearsonhighered.com

- Additional review materials

REFLECT Case Study

Pamela Allen is a 65-year-old female who has been married to Clifford for 40 years. Their only child, 24-year-old Gary, has Down syndrome and lives with them. In the past, Ms. Allen worked as an administrative assistant in a law firm. After Gary was born, Ms. Allen gave up her career to care for Gary.

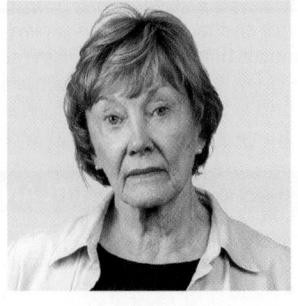

Ms. Allen frequently experiences constipation, and treats this with over-the-counter agents. She considers the constipation more of an annoyance than anything else. The only medical condition she has ever had requiring treatment was endometrial cancer at age 50. The cancer was diagnosed at a very early stage, and she underwent a total hysterectomy and bilateral salpingo-oophorectomy. Because there was no evidence of lymph node involvement, she was considered cured and has been cancer free ever since. Her last examination was 14 months ago.

One day Ms. Allen experiences diarrhea with an odd reddish-brown color and odor. The next day, she is again constipated. She has been straining to have a bowel movement and notes that her stools are thinner than usual. A few weeks later, while still experiencing constipation and odd-shaped stools, she begins to feel a sense of fullness in her rectum and pelvic area, even after defecation. The appearance of the reddish-brown color in her stools has been more regular. She has often been feeling tired lately. On Friday afternoon, she finally makes a decision to call for an appointment with her physician about the symptoms. She is told to come to the office on the following Monday morning. She has a feeling of dread and becomes worried that something serious may be wrong.

1. What specific symptoms described by Ms. Allen would cause you to suspect colorectal cancer?

2. What diagnostic test would you anticipate will be performed in the physician's office on her first visit?

3. Develop a plan of care for Ms. Allen addressing both her physical and psychosocial needs.

EXEMPLAR 2.5   Leukemia

EXEMPLAR KEY TERMS

Acute lymphocytic leukemia (ALL), *94*
Acute myeloid leukemia (AML), *93*
Allogeneic bone marrow transplant, *97*
Autologous bone marrow transplant, *97*
Bone marrow transplant (BMT), *97*
Chronic lymphocytic leukemia (CLL), *95*
Chronic myeloid leukemia (CML), *94*
Leukemia, *92*
Philadelphia chromosome, *94*
Remission, *97*
Stem cell transplant (SCT), *98*

EXEMPLAR LEARNING OUTCOMES

After reading about this exemplar, you will be able to:

1. Describe the pathophysiology, etiology, clinical manifestations, and direct and indirect causes of leukemia.

2. Identify risk factors and prevention methods associated with leukemia.

3. Illustrate the nursing process in providing culturally competent care across the life span for individuals with leukemia.

4. Formulate priority nursing diagnoses appropriate for an individual with leukemia.

5. Summarize therapies used by interdisciplinary teams in the collaborative care of an individual with leukemia.

6. Plan evidence-based care for an individual with leukemia and his or her family in collaboration with other members of the healthcare team.

7. Evaluate expected outcomes for an individual with leukemia.

▶ OVERVIEW

Leukemia (literally, "white blood") is a group of chronic malignant disorders of WBCs and WBC precursors. In leukemia, the usual ratio of RBCs to WBCs is reversed. Leukemias are characterized by replacement of bone marrow by malignant immature WBCs, abnormal immature circulating WBCs, and infiltration of these cells into the liver, spleen, and lymph nodes throughout the body.

▶ PATHOPHYSIOLOGY AND ETIOLOGY

Leukemia occurs when the stem cells in the bone marrow produce immature WBCs that cannot function normally. These cells proliferate rapidly by cloning instead of through normal mitosis, causing the bone marrow to fill with abnormal WBCs. The abnormal cells then spill out into the circulatory system, where they steadily replace the normally functioning WBCs. As this occurs, the protective lymphocytic functions, such as cellular and humoral immunity, are reduced, leaving the body vulnerable to infections.

The malignant WBCs rapidly fill the bone marrow, replacing stem cells that produce erythrocytes (RBCs) and other blood products, such as platelets, thereby decreasing the amount of these products in circulation. The stem cells are replaced by leukemic clones, eventually resulting in anemia. Clients with leukemia commonly experience abnormal bleeding because of the reduced platelet amounts.

Leukemias are classified by their acuity and by the predominant cell type involved. The *acute* leukemias are characterized by an acute onset, rapid disease progression, and immature or undifferentiated blast cells. *Chronic* leukemias, on the other hand, have a gradual onset, prolonged course, and abnormal mature-appearing cells. Lymphocytic (or lymphoblastic) leukemias involve immature lymphocytes and their precursor cells in the bone marrow. Lymphocytic leukemias infiltrate the spleen, lymph nodes, central nervous system, and other tissues. Myeloid (also called myelogenous, myelocytic, or myeloblastic) leukemias involve myeloid stem

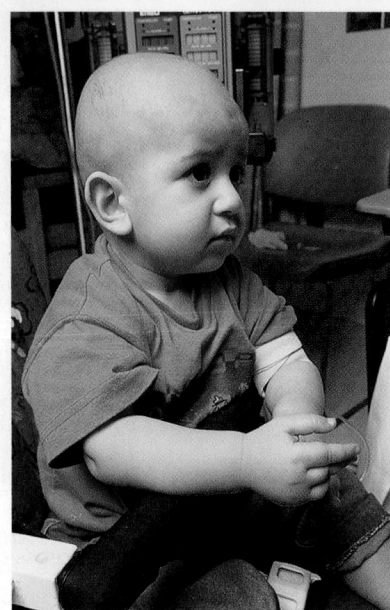

Figure 2–14 ● Acute lymphoblastic leukemia is the most common type of leukemia in children and the most common cancer affecting children under 5 years of age.

cells in the bone marrow, interfering with the maturation of all types of blood cells, including granulocytes, RBCs, and thrombocytes (Porth & Matfin, 2010). Acute lymphocytic (lymphoblastic) leukemia is the most common type of leukemia in children (**Figure 2–14** ●). In adults, acute myeloid leukemia and chronic lymphocytic leukemia are the most

common types (ACS, 2013b). In summary, the general types of leukemia are:

■ Acute lymphocytic (lymphoblastic) leukemia
■ Chronic lymphocytic leukemia
■ Acute myeloid (myeloblastic) leukemia
■ Chronic myeloid (myelogenous) leukemia.

The major types of leukemia are summarized in **Table 2–9** ●. However, this general system of classifying leukemias does not differentiate subtypes of acute leukemias. In the 1970s, the French-American-British (FAB) system for classifying acute leukemias was introduced, which further differentiated acute leukemias by the predominant cell involved and the degree of cell differentiation. Later, the World Health Organization (WHO) designed a similar system of classification; however, the WHO system takes into account factors that affect prognosis, such as genetic mutations and previous exposures to radiation (ACS, 2013f).

Acute Myeloid Leukemia

Acute myeloid leukemia (AML) is characterized by uncontrolled proliferation of myeloblasts (the precursors of granulocytes) and hyperplasia of the bone marrow and spleen (**Figure 2–15** ●). Between 45,000 and 50,000 new cases of all forms of leukemia occur annually. Nearly 90% of leukemia cases involve adults ages 20 years or older. Among adults, AML accounts for 30% of newly diagnosed leukemia cases (ACS, 2013b). However, AML is uncommon in individuals younger than 40 years of age. On average, the individual diagnosed with AML is approximately 67 years old (ACS, 2013f). For

TABLE 2–9   Primary Forms of Leukemia

TYPE AND DESCRIPTION	CLINICAL MANIFESTATIONS	CURATIVE TREATMENT

Acute lymphoblastic leukemia (ALL): abnormal growth of marrow cells that form lymphocytes
    Primarily affects children and young adults; rapid onset and disease progression.
	Weakness, decreased energy, recurrent infections; bleeding; pallor, bone pain, weight loss, sore throat, night sweats
	    Potential CNS manifestations if brain and/or spinal cord is infiltrated include headaches, vomiting, visual disturbances, and seizures
		Chemotherapy; bone marrow transplant (BMT), or stem cell transplant (SCT)

Chronic lymphocytic leukemia (CLL): abnormal growth of marrow cells that form lymphocytes Primarily affects older adults; insidious onset and slow, chronic course.	Fatigue; exercise intolerance; lymphadenopathy and splenomegaly; recurrent infections, pallor, edema, thrombophlebitis	Often requires no treatment, depending on rate of progression; chemotherapy; BMT
Acute myeloid leukemia (AML): abnormal growth of marrow cells that form red blood cells, white blood cells (other than lymphocytes), and platelets Common in older adults, rarely seen in children and young adults.	Fatigue, weakness, fever; anemia; headache; bone and joint pain; abnormal bleeding and bruising; recurrent infection; lymphadenopathy, splenomegaly, and hepatomegaly	Chemotherapy; SCT
Chronic myeloid leukemia (CML): abnormal growth of marrow cells that form red blood cells, white blood cells (other than lymphocytes), and platelets Primarily affects adults; usually associated with Philadelphia chromosome.	Early course slow and stable, progressing to aggressive phase in 3–4 years *Chronic phase:* asymptomatic or very mild, vague symptoms *Accelerated phase:* decreased appetite, weight loss, and fever *Acute phase (blast crisis or blast phase):* progression includes splenomegaly, bone damage, abnormal platelet count	Interferon alpha; chemotherapy with imatinib mesylate (Gleevec), SCT

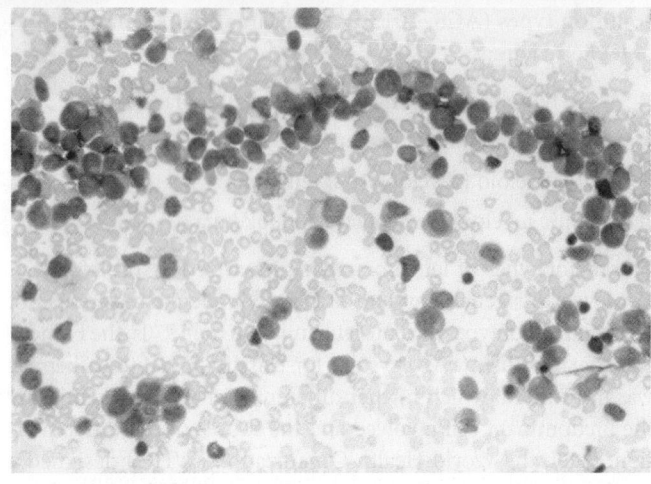

Figure 2–15 ● A blood smear from the bone marrow of a client with acute myeloid leukemia. Note the abnormally large number of myelocyte WBCs (stained purple) among the small RBCs.
Source: Dr. Gopal Murti/Science Source.

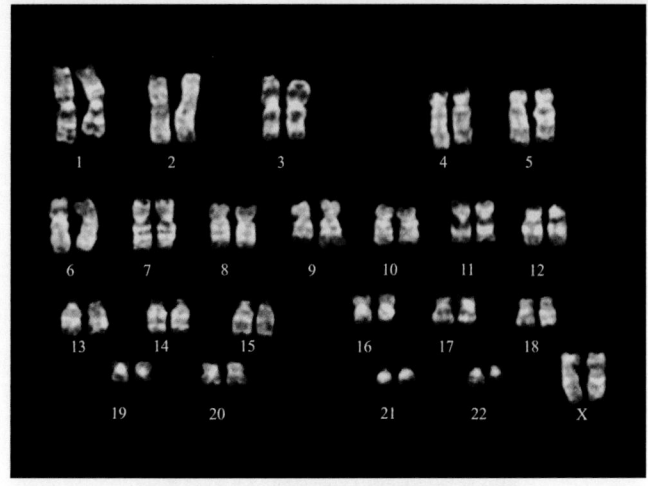

Figure 2–16 ● The Philadelphia chromosome. Note the chromosomes of pairs 9 and 22. In each instance, the left-hand chromosome of the pair is normal, whereas an exchange of material between chromosomes has made the right-hand chromosome 9 larger and the right-hand chromosome 22 smaller. In stem cells within the bone marrow, the chromosome 22 defect leads to chronic myeloid leukemia.
Source: Addenbrookes Hospital/Science Source.

these individuals, the 5-year relative survival rate is approximately 25% (ACS, 2013b).

The manifestations of AML result from neutropenia and thrombocytopenia. Decreased neutrophils lead to recurrent severe infections, such as pneumonia, septicemia, abscesses, and mucous membrane ulceration. The manifestations of thrombocytopenia include petechiae (red or purple spot that looks like a spider caused by a broken capillary), purpura (small areas of subcutaneous bleeding), ecchymoses (bruising), epistaxis (nosebleeds), hematomas, hematuria, and gastrointestinal bleeding. Bone infarctions or subperiosteal infiltrates of leukemic cells may cause bone pain. Anemia is a late manifestation, causing fatigue, headaches, pallor, and dyspnea on exertion. Death usually results from infection or hemorrhage.

Bone marrow aspiration shows a proliferation of immature WBCs. The CBC shows thrombocytopenia and normocytic, normochromic anemia.

Chronic Myeloid Leukemia

Chronic myeloid leukemia (CML) is characterized by abnormal proliferation of all bone marrow elements. This type of leukemia constitutes approximately 15% of adult leukemias. It affects women slightly more frequently than men. The average age of the individual with CML is approximately 65 years and this form of leukemia is very rarely seen in children (ACS, 2013g).

Usually, CML is associated with a chromosome abnormality called the **Philadelphia chromosome**, a balanced translocation of chromosome 22 to chromosome 9 (**Figure 2–16** ●). The fusion gene produced by this translocation, known as *bcr/abl*, is an oncogene capable of initiating a malignancy. Very large doses of ionizing radiation also may induce CML in some clients (ACS, 2013g).

Often, in the early or *chronic phase* of CML, the client is either asymptomatic or demonstrates very mild, vague symptoms. In fact, CML is often diagnosed when a routine blood test reveals abnormal cell counts. In the *accelerated phase,* common symptoms include decreased appetite, weight loss, and fever. During the *acute phase*, also called *blast crisis* or the *blast phase,* blast cells have proliferated and spread beyond the bone

marrow, infiltrating tissues and organs. In addition to decreased appetite, weight loss, and fever, manifestations of the acute phase may include splenomegaly, bone damage, and an extremely high or low platelet count (ACS, 2013g).

Acute Lymphocytic Leukemia

Acute lymphocytic leukemia (ALL) is the most common type of leukemia in children and adolescents. The incidence of ALL decreases after the mid-20s and then gradually increases after about age 50. Genetic factors may play a role in its development, particularly the *bcr/abl* translocation also implicated in CML (ACS, 2013e).

Most (80%) cases of ALL result from malignant transformation of B cells, with the remaining 20% arising from T cells. The malignant cells resemble immature lymphocytes (lymphoblasts); however, they do not mature or function effectively to maintain immunity. These lymphoblasts accumulate in the bone marrow, lymph nodes, and spleen as well as in circulating blood. Some types of lymphoma are thought to represent a later stage of the same disease.

The onset of ALL is usually rapid. Lymphoblasts proliferating in bone marrow and peripheral tissues crowd the growth of normal cells (**Figure 2–17** ●). Normal hematopoiesis is suppressed, leading to thrombocytopenia, leukopenia, and anemia. Manifestations of infections, bleeding, and anemia develop. Lymphadenopathy, liver enlargement, and bone pain resulting from rapid generation of marrow elements are also common. Infiltration of the central nervous system causes headaches, visual disturbances, vomiting, and seizures.

The CBC shows an elevated WBC count with increased lymphocytes on the differential. The RBC and platelet counts are decreased. Bone marrow studies reveal a hypercellular marrow with growth of lymphoblasts. Combination chemotherapy

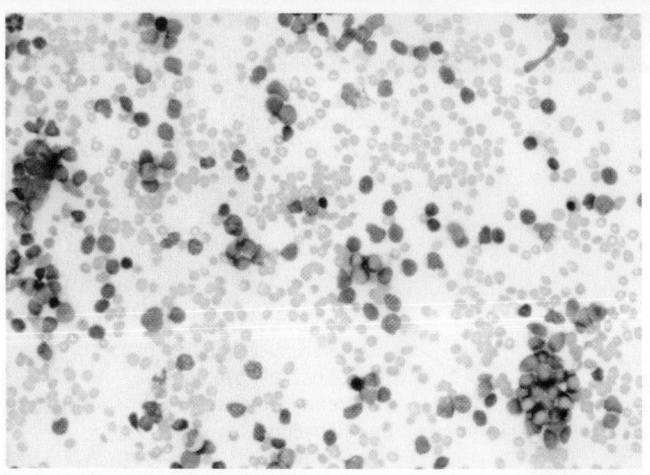

Figure 2–17 ● A blood smear from the bone marrow of a client with acute lymphocytic leukemia. Note the abnormally large number of lymphocytes (stained purple) crowding the bone marrow. As a result, normal production of RBCs, functional WBCs, and platelets is suppressed.
Source: Dr. Gopal Murti/Science Source.

produces complete remission in 80%–90% of adults with ALL. However, because remission is common among adults, the rate of cure for this population is closer to 40% (ACS, 2013e). With treatment, the survival rate among children with ALL is estimated to be more than 85% (ACS, 2012b).

Chronic Lymphocytic Leukemia

Chronic lymphocytic leukemia (CLL) is characterized by proliferation and accumulation of small, abnormal, mature lymphocytes in the bone marrow, peripheral blood, and body tissues. The abnormal cells are usually B lymphocytes that are unable to produce adequate antibodies to maintain normal immune function. Statistically, CLL is the most common form of leukemia diagnosed in adults 20 years of age and older (ACS, 2013b). However, it is rarely seen in children or in adults under the age of 40 years. The average age at the time of diagnosis is 72 years (ACS, 2012d).

Chronic lymphocytic leukemia has a slow onset and is often diagnosed during a routine physical examination. If symptoms are present, they usually include vague complaints of weakness or malaise. Possible clinical findings include anemia, infection, and enlarged lymph nodes, spleen, and liver. As in other leukemias, bone marrow hyperplasia is present. Erythrocyte and platelet counts are reduced. Leukocyte counts may be either elevated or reduced, but abnormal cells are always present. In CLL, years may elapse before treatment is required. The 5-year survival rate for individuals diagnosed with CLL is 82% (ACS, 2013b).

Etiology

Although leukemia is often thought of as a childhood disease, adults ages 20 years or older account for approximately 90% of new diagnoses (ACS, 2013c). In 2013, an estimated 48,610 individuals were newly diagnosed with leukemia, while approximately 23,720 individuals died from leukemia-related complications that same year (ACS, 2013b).

The causes of leukemia are not well understood. Some investigators theorize that exposure to infectious agents can predispose people to leukemia. Genetic factors are also believed to play a role in some types of the disease.

Risk Factors

While the cause of most leukemias is unknown, certain risk factors have been identified. Men are affected more frequently than women. Children with immunodeficiency states, such as ataxia-telangiectasia, congenital hypogammaglobulinemia, and Wiskott-Aldrich syndrome, have an increased risk of ALL. Clients who have undergone treatment for cancer may also have an increased risk. The human T-cell leukemia/lymphoma virus 1, a retrovirus, is known to cause certain leukemias and lymphomas (ACS, 2013d).

People with certain genetic disorders have a higher incidence of leukemia. Children with chromosomal defects, such as Down syndrome, Klinefelter syndrome, Bloom syndrome, and Fanconi anemia, have an increased incidence of ALL. While chromosomal abnormalities are present in many clients with ALL, these mutations are generally believed to have transpired during the individual's lifetime, as opposed to being inherited (ACS, 2013e). In addition, several chromosomal and genetic abnormalities are associated with AML; however, these abnormalities are rarely due to inherited DNA mutations.

Environmental risk factors play a role as well. Risk factors for AML include cigarette smoking and chemicals such as benzene (present in cigarette smoke and gasoline). Exposure to high-dose ionizing radiation, such as from a nuclear reactor or atomic blast, increases the risk for both AML and ALL.

Exposure to high-dose radiation is the only proven risk factor for CML (ACS, 2013g). CLL has no known solid risk factors; what is known is that diet, radiation exposure, smoking, and infection do not appear to be linked to its development (ACS, 2012d).

▶ CLINICAL MANIFESTATIONS

The general manifestations of leukemia (regardless of type) result from anemia, infection, and bleeding. These include pallor, fatigue, tachycardia, malaise, lethargy, and dyspnea on exertion. Infection may cause fever, night sweats, oral ulcerations, and frequent or recurrent respiratory, urinary, integumentary, or other infections. Increased bleeding as a result of thrombocytopenia leads to bruising, petechiae, bleeding gums, and bleeding within specific organs and tissues.

Other manifestations result from leukemic cell infiltration, increased metabolism, and increased leukocyte destruction (see the feature on Multisystem Effects of Leukemia on page 96). Infiltration of the liver, spleen, lymph nodes, and bone marrow causes pain and tissue swelling in the involved areas. Meningeal infiltration may cause manifestations of increased intracranial pressure, such as headache, altered level of consciousness, cranial nerve impairment, and nausea and vomiting. Infiltration of the kidneys may affect renal function, with decreased urine output and increased blood urea nitrogen and creatinine. Increased metabolism causes heat intolerance, weight loss, dyspnea on exertion, and tachycardia. Destruction of large numbers of WBCs releases substantial amounts of uric acid into the circulation; uric acid crystals may obstruct renal tubules, causing renal insufficiency.

Multisystem Effects of Leukemia

Neurologic
- Headache
- Altered LOC
- Cranial nerve impairment

Potential complications
- Subarachnoid hemorrhage
- Retinal hemorrhage
- Seizures, coma

Respiratory
- Dyspnea on exertion
- Pharyngitis, sore throat
- Frequent respiratory infections

Potential complication
- Pulmonary bleeding

Gastrointestinal
- Anorexia, nausea
- Oral ulcerations, infection
- Bleeding gums
- Gingival hyperplasia (gum overgrowth)
- Abdominal pain
- Hepatomegaly
- Occult GI bleeding

Urinary
- Urinary tract infection
- Hematuria

Potential complication
- Renal insufficiency or failure

Musculoskeletal
- Weakness
- Bone tenderness, pain
- Joint pain

Metabolic Processes
- Malaise, lethargy
- Heat intolerance
- Diaphoresis
- Chills, fever
- Night sweats
- Weight loss

Cardiovascular
- Tachycardia, palpitations
- Orthostatic hypotension
- Heart murmurs
- Hematomas
- Edema

Potential complications
- Hemorrhage
- Thrombophlebitis

Hematologic
- Anemia
- Thrombocytopenia
- Leukopenia
- Bleeding (epistaxis)
- Splenomegaly

Potential complication
- DIC

Immunologic
- Frequent or recurrent infections
- Lymphadenopathy

Potential complications
- Abscesses
- Septicemia

Integumentary
- Skin and mucous membrane pallor
- Petechiae
- Bruising, purpura
- Ulcerations
- *Chloromas* (skin infiltrations near bony prominences)

Clinical Manifestations and Therapies **Leukemia**

ETIOLOGY	CLINICAL MANIFESTATIONS	CLINICAL THERAPIES
Anemia may result because when the bone marrow is so busy producing WBCs, inadequate numbers of RBCs are produced.	▪ Pallor, fatigue, tachycardia, malaise, lethargy, and dyspnea on exertion	▪ Improve nutritional status. ▪ Stimulate RBC production with medications (e.g., epoetin). ▪ Perform blood transfusions. ▪ Promote rest. ▪ Monitor vital signs, CBC.
Infection risk increases because of immature WBCs that are ineffective in responding to pathogens.	▪ Fever, night sweats, oral ulcerations, and frequent or recurrent respiratory, urinary, integumentary, or other infections	▪ Teach infection prevention strategies (e.g., hand hygiene, cough etiquette, crowd avoidance). ▪ Teach symptoms to report. ▪ Give antimicrobials as indicated to treat infections. ▪ Monitor vital signs, CBC.
Bleeding may result from reduced coagulation factors, increased fibrinolytic activity, and accelerated intravascular coagulation.	▪ Petechia, bruising, bleeding from gums, hematuria, hematemesis, rectal bleeding	▪ Monitor coagulation studies. ▪ Provide client teaching to reduce injury risk. ▪ Administer platelets, clotting factors. ▪ Replace blood if bleeding occurs.

▶ COLLABORATION

Treatment for leukemia focuses on achieving remission or cure and relieving symptoms. The methods of treatment may include chemotherapy, radiation therapy, and bone marrow or stem cell transplantation. Cure is more often achieved in children with acute leukemia than in adults, although long-term **remission** (a disease-free period with no signs or symptoms) often can be achieved. The nurse's role as a member of the interdisciplinary healthcare team is outlined in the Nursing Process section that follows this section.

Diagnostic Tests

The following diagnostic tests are useful in the diagnosis of leukemia:

- **Complete blood count (CBC) with differential** is done to evaluate cell counts, hemoglobin and hematocrit levels, and the number, distribution, and morphology (size and shape) of WBCs.
- **Platelets** are measured to identify possible thrombocytopenia secondary to the leukemia and the risk of bleeding.
- **Bone marrow examination** provides information about cells within the marrow, the type of erythropoiesis, and the maturity of erythropoietic and leukopoietic cells.

Table 2–10 ● outlines usual diagnostic test results in the various forms of leukemia.

Surgery

Surgical procedures include transplantation of bone marrow or stem cells. Cells may be obtained either from a donor or from the recipient, depending on the procedure.

BONE MARROW TRANSPLANT Bone marrow transplant (BMT) is the treatment of choice for some types of leukemia (see Table 2–9). BMT often is used in conjunction with or following chemotherapy or radiation. There are two major categories of BMT: In allogeneic BMT, the bone marrow of a healthy donor is infused into the client with the illness; in autologous BMT, the client is infused with his or her own bone marrow.

Allogeneic Bone Marrow Transplant Allogeneic bone marrow transplant uses bone marrow cells from a donor (often from a sibling with closely matched tissue antigens; closely matched unrelated donors also may be used). Before allogeneic BMT, high doses of chemotherapy and possibly total body irradiation are used to destroy leukemic cells in the bone marrow. The donor's bone marrow is aspirated (**Figure 2–18** ●) and infused through a central venous line into the recipient. Before BMT and reestablishment of bone marrow function, the client is critically ill and at significant risk for infection and bleeding as a result of the depletion of WBCs and platelets.

Autologous Bone Marrow Transplant Autologous bone marrow transplant uses the client's own bone marrow to restore bone marrow function after chemotherapy or radiation; this procedure is often called bone marrow rescue. In autologous BMT, approximately 1 L of bone marrow is aspirated (usually from the iliac crests) during a period of disease remission. The bone marrow is then frozen and stored for use after treatment. If relapse occurs, lethal doses of chemotherapy or radiation are given to destroy the immune system and malignant cells and to prepare space in the bone marrow for new cells. The filtered bone marrow is then thawed and infused intravenously through a central line. The infused marrow cells slowly become a part of the client's bone marrow, the neutrophil count increases, and normal hematopoiesis takes place.

As in allogeneic BMT, the client is critically ill during the period of bone marrow destruction and immunosuppression.

TABLE 2–10　Diagnostic Findings by Type of Leukemia

TEST	ACUTE MYELOID LEUKEMIA	CHRONIC MYELOID LEUKEMIA	ACUTE LYMPHOCYTIC LEUKEMIA	CHRONIC LYMPHOCYTIC LEUKEMIA
RBC count	Low	Low	Low	Low
Hemoglobin	Low	Low	Low	Low
Hematocrit	Low	Low	Low	Low
Platelet count	Very low	High early, low late	Low	Low
WBC count	Varies	Increased	Varies	Increased
Myeloblasts	Present			
Neutrophils	Decreased	Increased	Decreased	Normal
Lymphocytes		Normal		Increased
Monocytes		Normal/low		
Blasts	Present	Present (crisis)	Present	
Bone marrow	Hypercellular		Hypercellular	
Myeloblasts	Present			
Lymphoblasts			Present	
Lymphocytes				Present

The client is hospitalized in a private room for 6–8 weeks or more. Potential complications include malnutrition, infection, and bleeding.

STEM CELL TRANSPLANT　Allogeneic **stem cell transplant (SCT)** is an alternative to BMT. SCT results in complete and sustained replacement of the recipient's blood cell lines (WBCs, RBCs, and platelets) with cells derived from the donor stem cells. Before SCT, the recipient undergoes treatment similar to that before BMT. The risks for infection and other complications, as well as graft-versus-host disease, are similar as well.

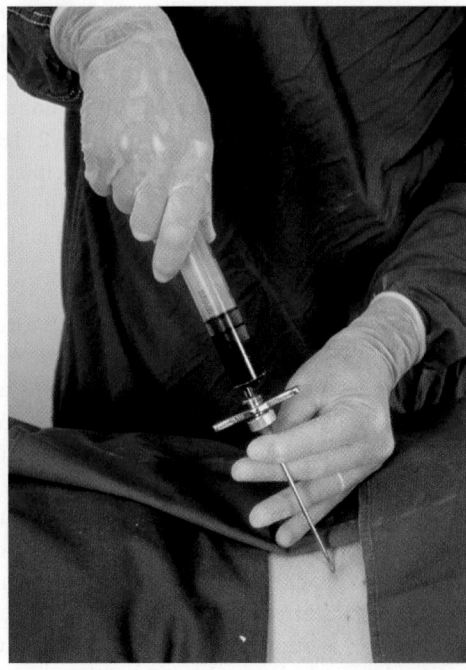

Figure 2–18 ● Allogeneic bone marrow transplant. Bone marrow from the donor is aspirated, then filtered and infused into the recipient.
Source: FRASER, SIMON/Science Source.

Donors must have tissue that is closely matched with that of the recipient. Before harvesting, hematopoietic growth factors, including G-CSF and GM-CSF, are administered to the donor for 4–5 days. This increases the concentration of stem cells in peripheral blood, allowing it to be used for the transplant instead of bone marrow. Peripheral blood is removed, and WBCs are separated from the plasma, then administered via a large central venous catheter. Large concentrations of stem cells also are present in umbilical cord blood. This may be stored and used in some cases (Osborn et al., 2013).

Allogeneic BMT or SCT may precipitate graft-versus-host disease (GVHD), which occurs when immune cells of the donated bone marrow identify the recipient's body tissue as foreign. During GVHD, T lymphocytes in the donated marrow attack the liver, skin, and gastrointestinal tract. Acute GVHD develops within the first 3 months following a transplant and is usually marked by a pruritic, maculopapular rash that begins on the palms and soles of the feet and may extend over the entire body. Additional manifestations of acute GVHD may include jaundice, nausea, vomiting, diarrhea, and dry eyes. Chronic GVHD develops more than 3 months after a transplant procedure. Chronic GVHD may be accompanied by chronic pain, fatigue, weakness, and shortness of breath (MedlinePlus, 2013b). In some cases, chronic GVHD may follow acute GVHD; however, it may also develop in clients with no previous symptoms. GVHD is treated with antibiotics and steroids; immunosuppressant drugs, such as thalidomide and immunotoxin (XomaZyme), may be used if necessary.

Pharmacologic Therapy

Treatment for leukemia, as well as for other forms of cancer, often incorporates two main approaches: killing the cancerous cells and changing the way the body responds to the cancerous cells. Chemotherapy medications have cytotoxic effects. Biological therapies, which alter the body's response to cancer cells, may also be cytotoxic.

TABLE 2–11   Chemotherapeutic Regimens Used to Treat Leukemia

TYPE OF LEUKEMIA	CHEMOTHERAPEUTIC REGIMEN
Acute myeloid leukemia	■ Cytarabine (Cytoxan, an alkylating agent), *with* daunorubicin (Cerubidine, an antitumor antibiotic) *or* idarubicin (Idamycin, an antitumor antibiotic) ■ All-*trans* retinoic acid (ATRA) added for clients with promyelocytic leukemia
Chronic myeloid leukemia	■ Imatinib mesylate (Gleevec), a *bcr/abl* tyrosine kinase (enzyme) inhibitor ■ Hydroxyurea (a DNA inhibitor) *or* homoharringtonine (HHT, a plant alkaloid) if imatinib is not tolerated
Acute lymphocytic leukemia	■ Daunorubicin (Cerubidine, an antitumor antibiotic) *with* vincristine (Oncovin, a plant alkaloid) *with* prednisone *with* asparaginase (Elspar)
Chronic lymphocytic leukemia	■ Fludarabine (Fludara, an antimetabolite) *or* chlorambucil (Chloromycetin, an antitumor antibiotic) ■ Cyclophosphamide (Cytoxan, an alkylating agent), vincristine, and prednisone ■ Cyclophosphamide, doxorubicin (Adriamycin, an antitumor antibiotic), vincristine, and prednisone

CHEMOTHERAPY   Single-agent or combination chemotherapy is the treatment of choice for most types of leukemia, with the goal of eradicating leukemic cells and producing remission. **Table 2–11** ● outlines typical chemotherapeutic regimens for different types of leukemia. Combination chemotherapy reduces drug resistance and toxicity and interrupts cell growth at various stages of the cell cycle, producing a complementary effect of the drugs used.

Chemotherapy for leukemia generally is divided into the induction phase and postremission therapy. During induction, drug doses are high to eradicate leukemic cells from the bone marrow. Often, however, these high doses also damage stem cells and interfere with production of normal blood cells. Circulating mature blood cells are not affected, because they are no longer dividing. The degree of bone marrow suppression is influenced by a number of factors, including age, nutritional status, concurrent chronic diseases (e.g., impaired liver or renal function), the drug and drug dose, and previous treatment.

Once remission has been achieved, postremission chemotherapy is continued to eradicate any additional leukemic cells, prevent relapse, and prolong survival. A single chemotherapeutic agent, combination therapy, or bone marrow transplant may be used for postremission treatment.

BIOLOGICAL THERAPY   Cytokines, such as interferons and interleukins, are biological agents that may be used to treat some leukemias. These agents modify the body's response to cancer cells; in some cases, they are cytotoxic as well. Interferons are a complex group of messenger proteins normally produced in response to antigens such as viruses. They have multiple effects, including moderating immune function and inhibiting abnormal cell proliferation and growth. Interferon alpha may be used to treat some leukemias, particularly CML. Side effects commonly associated with interferon therapy include flulike symptoms, persistent fatigue and lethargy, weight loss, and muscle and joint pain.

Biological response modifiers such as colony-stimulating factors (CSFs), also called hematopoietic growth factors, may be administered to "rescue" the bone marrow following induction chemotherapy. CSFs are cytokines that regulate the growth and differentiation of blood cells. Factors that support neutrophil maturation, granulocyte-macrophage CSF (GM-CSF) and granulocyte CSF (G-CSF) are included among these medications. Bone pain is a common side effect of therapy with these agents. Clients also may experience fevers, chills, anorexia, muscle aches, and lethargy (Wilson, Shannon, & Shields, 2013).

Radiation Therapy

Radiation therapy uses high doses of x-rays or other forms of energy to damage cellular DNA. Although the cell continues to function, it cannot divide and multiply. Cells that divide rapidly, such as bone marrow and cancer cells (radiosensitive cells), respond quickly to radiation therapy. Although normal cells are affected, they are better able to recover from the damage caused by the radiation compared with cancer cells.

Complementary and Alternative Therapy

At present, there are no proven, research-based alternative therapies approved for use in the treatment of cancer (ASCO, 2012a). However, research suggests certain complementary therapies may offer relief from side effects associated with chemotherapy. For example, for some clients, acupuncture may help relieve nausea. Likewise, clinical trials involving clients with leukemia suggest massage may also help to reduce nausea, pain, anxiety, insomnia, and fatigue (Wesa & Cassileth, 2009).

■ NURSING PROCESS

When caring for the client with leukemia, the nurse considers the chronic and life-threatening nature of the disease as well as the effects of treatment in planning care.

Assessment

Focused assessment data related to leukemia include the following:

■ *Health history.* Complaints of fatigue, weakness, dyspnea on exertion, frequent infections, sore throat, night sweats, bleeding gums, or nose bleeds; recent weight loss; exposure to ionizing radiation (multiple x-rays, residence near a site of radiation or atomic testing) or chemicals (occupational); previous treatment for cancer; history of an immune disorder.

■ *Physical examination.* Skin and mucous membranes for bruising, purpura, petechiae, ulcers or lesions; pallor; vital signs, including orthostatic vitals; heart and lung sounds; abdominal examination; stool for occult blood.

Evidence-Based Practice Preparing Childhood Acute Lymphoblastic Leukemia Survivors for Challenges in Adulthood

Problem

In addition to the emotional and psychosocial challenges faced by children with ALL, treatment also requires an immense physical battle. Unfortunately, victory over this disease often sets the stage for future battles that may be equally intense. In adulthood, childhood survivors are at an increased risk for numerous chronic conditions and premature death (Ness et al., 2011).

Evidence

Clients who overcome lymphoma and ALL during childhood demonstrate a much higher incidence of chronic fatigue (CF) in adulthood. For long-term survivors, research suggests that 20 years after diagnosis, the incidence of CF among childhood leukemia/lymphoma survivors (CLSs) is roughly three times higher than in the general population (Hamre et al., 2013). In the past, some researchers linked the development of CF to many potential causes, including previous exposure to viruses associated with specific forms of leukemia. However, current researchers have found that this is not the case (Altera et al., 2012).

Along with increased risk for CF, adult survivors of ALL also face other chronic health challenges. The medications and therapies used in treatment of ALL are associated with lasting effects, including myocardial impairment, growth hormone deficiency, insulin resistance, and peripheral neuropathy.

Researchers theorize that these adverse treatment effects may in part explain the increased incidence of obesity and reduced levels of overall fitness seen among adults who survived ALL as children (Ness et al., 2011).

Implications

While providing the highest quality care to pediatric clients diagnosed with ALL, nurses should also consider the future ramifications of treatment. Remission is the immediate goal. However, promotion of healthy habits and lifestyle choices, such as balanced nutrition and regular exercise, may have far-reaching effects on the quality of life these clients experience in adulthood.

Critical Thinking Application

1. How might emotion-based care of pediatric clients with ALL unintentionally lead to promotion of unhealthy habits by caregivers and family members?

2. Considering the physiological effects of treatments for ALL and the pediatric client's need for rest, in what ways can the nurse still promote physical exercise?

3. Explain how the long-term effects of medications used in the treatment of ALL could influence the activity tolerance, exercise habits, and overall level of fitness of an adult survivor of childhood ALL.

Diagnosis

Nursing diagnoses for the client with leukemia include the following:

- *Risk for Infection*
- *Risk for Bleeding*
- *Imbalanced Nutrition: Less Than Body Requirements*
- *Impaired Oral Mucous Membrane*
- *Anticipatory Grieving.*

(NANDA-I © 2012)

Planning

Goals for client care include the following:

- The client and family members/significant others will describe strategies to reduce risk of infection.
- The client will demonstrate no signs or symptoms of infection.
- The pediatric client will meet developmental milestones.
- The client will express emotions related to his diagnosis.
- The client will receive adequate dietary intake that is sufficient for meeting nutritional needs.
- The client will promptly report symptoms of complications.

Implementation

Nurses play a key role in the long-term multidisciplinary treatment of clients with leukemia. The impact of a diagnosis of leukemia and the long-term nature of treatment can severely stress the coping abilities of both the client and the family. Ongoing psychosocial assessment and emotional support are essential. Referral to support groups and social services may be beneficial. Assist the family in exploration of complementary therapies, such as relaxation, imagery, and nutritional support. Be alert for any interactions that could occur between complementary therapies and the medical regimen. Many clients are treated in an oncology clinic, staying in the hospital only on the day of IV drug administration, and receive oral medications at home. The time at the hospital is used to assess how the family is managing issues such as nutrition, sleep, medication administration, and obtaining psychosocial support. Careful teaching for the family is needed to ensure safe drug administration and identification of issues requiring further care.

Prevent and Manage Adverse Medication Effects

Drug side effects may necessitate infusion of platelets or packed RBCs. Special attention to renal function is needed when the client receives cyclophosphamide. Gross hematuria is a side effect of this drug. Hydration with IV fluids to attain a specific gravity of less than 1.010 prevents or reduces the severity of hematuria. It also prepares the kidneys to manage products of tumor cell breakdown. To achieve this desired specific gravity, the client receives IV fluids at 1.5 times maintenance volume for at least 6–8 hours before and at least 1.5 hours after administration of the drug. Other chemotherapeutic drugs have different infusion times, while some do not require hydration before infusion. Check drug references carefully for recommendations with each drug. Evaluate the infusion site before and frequently during infusion. Although extravasation is not as common with central lines used in cancer treatment as in peripheral lines, it still can occur. Many chemotherapeutic agents are extremely toxic to tissues. In addition, lysis of the cancer cells can produce toxic side effects. Careful monitoring of intake and output is required to record the IV fluids, assess kidney functioning, and monitor excretion of by-products from destroyed tumor cells. Monitor specific gravity every 8 hours as well as before and during administration of the drug and when the IV fluids are reduced to maintenance volume levels. Daily weight measurements are important to assist in planning adequate hydration during chemotherapy as well as to measure nutritional status.

Tumor lysis syndrome (TLS) also is a risk in clients with leukemia who are undergoing their initial treatment with chemotherapy. TLS develops when a large number of malignant cells are destroyed by treatment with chemotherapy or radiation. With cellular lysis, intracellular contents are released into the circulation, causing hyperkalemia, hyperuricemia, and hyperphosphatemia. As a result, the client may experience cardiac arrhythmias, renal failure, and even death. Leukemia is among the conditions most commonly associated with TLS (Bercovitz et al., 2010; Osborn et al., 2013).

Maintain adequate hydration, and administer prescribed medications, such as allopurinol and diuretics, as ordered. Hydration is vital to maintain renal function and promote elimination of tumor lysis by-products. Allopurinol reduces the risk of uric acid crystallization in the kidneys and other tissues (Wilson et al., 2013).

Prevent Infection

Bone marrow suppression necessitates transmission-based precautions. Instruct parents in the prevention of infection, and use nursing care measures to prevent infection as well. Perform careful hand hygiene; take temperature frequently; give mouth care with antibacterial mouthwashes; and inspect the skin, mouth, rectal area, and central line site for any signs of infection.

Changes in WBC function impair the immune and inflammatory responses in the client with leukemia, increasing the risk for infection. WBCs may be immature and ineffective or, in some cases, deficient. Chemotherapy or radiation therapy further depresses bone marrow function and increases the risk for infection. Nursing interventions that target prevention of adverse events related to infection include the following:

- Promptly report manifestations of infection: fever, chills, throat pain, cough, chest pain, burning on urination, purulent drainage, and itching and burning in vaginal or rectal areas. Prompt reporting allows timely intervention to prevent overwhelming infection and sepsis.
- Institute infection protection measures:
  a. Maintain protective isolation as indicated.
  b. Ensure meticulous attention to hand hygiene among all people in contact with the client.
  c. Assist as needed with appropriate hygiene measures.
  d. Restrict visitors with colds, flu, or infections.
  e. Provide oral hygiene after every meal.
  f. Avoid invasive procedures when possible, including injections, IV catheters, catheterizations, and rectal and vaginal procedures. When necessary, use strict aseptic technique for all invasive procedures and monitor carefully for infection.

These precautions minimize exposure to bacterial, viral, and fungal pathogens. Infection is the major cause of death in clients with leukemia. Mucous membranes are especially suscep-

tible to breakdown and infection as a result of tissue damage from chemotherapy or radiation.

- Monitor vital signs, including temperature and oxygen saturation, every 4 hours. Report temperature spikes with chilling, tachypnea, tachycardia, restlessness, change in PaO_2, and hypotension. The inflammatory response may be impaired in leukemia, masking signs of infection until sepsis develops, indicated by manifestations such as those above.
- Monitor neutrophil levels (measured in cubic millimeters) for relative risk for infection: no risk, 2,000–2,500/mm³; minimal risk, 1,000–2,000/mm³; moderate risk, 500–1,000/mm³; severe risk, <500/mm³. Neutrophils are the first line of defense against infection. As levels decrease, the risk for infection increases.
- Explain infection precautions and restrictions and their rationale; explain that these measures are usually temporary. Client and family understanding increases compliance and lowers the risk of infection.

Protect From Injury Related to Bleeding

Bleeding is the second most common cause of leukemia deaths. As platelet counts decrease, the risk of bleeding increases.

- Assess vital signs every 4 hours and body systems every shift for bleeding:
  a. Skin and mucous membranes for petechiae, ecchymoses, and purpura
  b. Gums, nasal membranes, and conjunctiva for bleeding
  c. Vomitus, stool, and urine for visible or occult blood
  d. Vaginal bleeding
  e. Prolonged bleeding from puncture sites
  f. Neurological changes, such as headache, visual changes, altered mentation, decreased level of consciousness, seizures
  g. Abdomen for complaints of epigastric pain, diminished bowel sounds, increasing abdominal girth, rigidity or guarding.

Early identification of bleeding helps prevent significant blood loss and potential shock. Internal hemorrhage may lead to tachycardia, hypotension, pallor, and diaphoresis. Bleeding into the lungs may cause dyspnea; bleeding into the abdomen causes increased girth, pain, and guarding. Intracranial bleeding affects mental status and level of consciousness.

- Avoid invasive procedures, such as rectal temperatures and suppositories, vaginal douches and suppositories, tampons, urinary catheterization, and parenteral injections, if possible. Invasive diagnostic procedures, such as biopsy or lumbar puncture, should not be done if the platelet count is less than 50,000. Invasive procedures can cause tissue trauma and bleeding. Procedures that use large-bore needles should be delayed until the platelet count is increased.
- Apply pressure to injection sites for 3–5 minutes and to arterial punctures for 15–20 minutes. Pressure prevents prolonged bleeding by prompting hemostasis and clot formation.
- Instruct the client to avoid forceful blowing or picking of the nose, forceful coughing or sneezing, and straining to have a bowel movement. These activities can damage mucous membranes, increasing the risk for bleeding.
- Monitor and promptly report abnormal blood levels of electrolytes, uric acid, urea nitrogen, and creatinine or manifestations of tumor lysis syndrome. Significant alterations in

electrolyte levels can lead to complications, such as cardiac dysrhythmias, muscle weakness or tetany, paresthesias, and mental status changes. Excess uric acid can compromise renal function and lead to metabolic acidosis and gout.

Protect Mucous Membrane Integrity

Stomatitis (inflammation and ulceration of the oral mucous membrane) is common in clients with leukemia. Chemotherapy can further impair the integrity of constantly dividing oral tissues.

- Inspect the buccal region, gums, sublingual area, and the throat daily for swelling or lesions. Ask about oral pain or burning. Breakdown of the oral mucous membrane increases the risk of infection and bleeding, causes pain and discomfort with eating and swallowing, and may cause swelling that interferes with the airway.
- Culture any oral lesions. Herpes simplex virus and *Candida* (yeast) are more common in clients with neutropenia. Herpes lesions are usually red, raised, fluid-filled blisters; *Candida* causes a white coating and patches of white plaque.
- Assist with mouth care and oral rinses with saline or a solution of hydrogen peroxide and water (1:1 or 1:3 hydrogen peroxide and water) every 2–4 hours. Apply petroleum jelly to the lips to prevent dryness and cracking. These measures help prevent infection and increase comfort.
- Encourage use of soft-bristle toothbrush or sponge to clean teeth and gums. Toothbrushes with hard bristles may abrade inflamed mucosa, causing bleeding and increasing the risk of infection.
- Administer medications as ordered to treat infection or relieve pain. Topical antifungal agents such as nystatin may be prescribed to treat *Candida* infections. Topical anesthetics such as lidocaine may be prescribed to relieve comfort and facilitate good oral care.
- Instruct the client to avoid alcohol-based mouthwashes, citrus fruit juices, spicy foods, very hot or very cold foods, alcohol, and crusty foods. Suggest bland, cool foods and cool liquids at least every 2 hours. Avoiding mucosa-traumatizing foods and liquids increases comfort; bland, cool foods and liquids cause the least pain. Intake of adequate fluids is necessary to prevent dehydration.

Promote Balanced Nutrition

The client with leukemia may have difficulty meeting nutritional needs because of increased metabolism, fatigue, loss of appetite from radiation, nausea and vomiting from chemotherapy, or painful oral mucous membranes that make chewing and swallowing difficult or painful.

- Weigh regularly, and evaluate weight loss over time to determine degree of malnutrition. A weight loss of 10%–20% may indicate malnutrition. A minimum intake of nutrients is necessary for health and tissue repair; cancer increases metabolic needs over this basal requirement. Weight loss occurs when metabolic requirements are not met. Both the disease process and its treatment can interfere with nutrient intake.
- Address causative or contributing factors to inadequate food and fluid intake:
  a. Provide mouth care before and after meals; use a soft toothbrush or sponges as necessary.
  b. Provide liquids with different textures and tastes.
  c. Increase liquid intake with meals.
  d. Reduce intake of milk and milk products, which make mucus more tenacious.
  e. Assist to a sitting position for eating.
  f. Ensure that the environment is clean and odor free.
  g. Provide medications for pain or nausea 30 minutes before meals, if prescribed.
  h. Provide rest periods before meals.
  i. Offer small, frequent meals, including low-fat, high-kilocalorie foods, throughout the day.
  j. Provide commercial supplements, such as Ensure.
  k. Avoid painful or unpleasant procedures immediately before or after meals.
  l. Suggest measures to improve food tolerance, such as eating dry foods when arising, consuming salty foods if allowed, and avoiding very sweet, rich, or greasy foods.

Anorexia, nausea and vomiting, diarrhea, stomatitis, taste changes, and dysphagia often make eating difficult during cancer treatment when good nutrition is most important. Maintaining nutritional status decreases morbidity and mortality by preventing weight loss, improving the response to treatment, minimizing adverse effects, and improving quality of life. Small, frequent meals, especially high-protein, high-kilocalorie foods, are often better tolerated.

Promote Healthy Grief Response

The diagnosis of a potentially life-threatening cancer causes actual or perceived losses, such as loss of function, independence, normal appearance, friends, self-esteem, and self. Grieving is the emotional response to those losses. The adaptive process of mourning a loss and resolving grief is called grief work; grief work cannot begin until a loss is acknowledged.

- Discuss the roles of the client and family and the ways in which they managed stressful situations in the past. Assess coping strategies and their effectiveness. Help identify sources of strength and support. Discuss changing roles resulting from the leukemia diagnosis and its effect on spiritual, social, and economic status and usual lifestyle. Evaluate cultural or ethnic factors that affect grief reactions.
- Use therapeutic communication skills to facilitate open discussion of losses and provide permission to grieve. Encouraging discussion of the meaning of the loss helps decrease some of the anxiety associated with the loss. This in turn allows the client and family to examine the current situation and compare it with past situations that they have coped with successfully.

Evaluation

Expected outcomes for nursing care of the client with leukemia include the following:

- The client remains free from signs and symptoms of infection.
- The client maintains urinary output of at least 0.5 mL/kg/hr.
- The client is adequately hydrated to allow elimination of drugs and cell components.
- The client's electrolyte values are maintained within normal limits.
- The client rates pain as absent or at a level that is tolerable.
- The client demonstrates adequate knowledge related to the disease process and treatment regimens.

NURSING CARE PLAN   A Client With Acute Myelocytic Leukemia

Catherine Cole is a 37-year-old secretary who lives with her husband, Ray, and teenage daughter, Amy, in an apartment in a large metropolitan area. Approximately 2 months ago, Mrs. Cole began to tire easily and experience night sweats several times a week. She also noted that she was pale, bruised easily, and was having heavier than normal menstrual periods. Blood tests ordered by her primary care provider are abnormal. She is admitted for a bone marrow biopsy.

ASSESSMENT

Mary Losapio, RN, obtains a nursing history and physical assessment for Mrs. Cole. Mrs. Cole tells her, "I'm so tired, and I have these bruises all over me. I'm so afraid of the results of the bone marrow examination. I don't know what we will do if I have cancer." Mrs. Cole clutches her husband's hand and then begins to cry. Physical assessment data include the following: height, 156 cm (64 in.); weight, 48.1 kg (106 lb); and temperature 37.8°C (100°F) oral; pulse 102 bpm; respirations 22/min; and BP 130/82 mmHg.

Numerous petechiae are scattered over the trunk and arms; ecchymoses is noted on lower right arm and right calf. Oral mucosa is red, with several small ulcerations in buccal areas.

Blood count shows reduced RBCs, hemoglobin, and hematocrit levels. The WBC count is high, with myeloblasts seen on differential. The platelet count is very low. A tentative diagnosis of acute myelogenous leukemia is made.

DIAGNOSES

- *Risk for Infection* related to altered WBC production and immune function
- *Risk for Bleeding*
- *Impaired Oral Mucous Membrane* secondary to anemia and reduced platelets
- *Fatigue* related to anemia
- *Anxiety* related to fear of leukemia diagnosis

(NANDA-I © 2012)

PLANNING

- The client will remain free of infection.
- The client will experience no significant bleeding.
- The client will have intact oral mucous membranes.
- The client will manage self-care activities despite fatigue.
- The client will verbalize decreased anxiety.

IMPLEMENTATION

- Place in a private room.
- Limit visitors to immediate family for the present.
- Instruct all staff, the family, and the client to perform carefully hand hygiene. Post a sign over the washbasin in the room as a reminder.
- Record vital signs every 4 hours.
- Avoid invasive procedures unless absolutely necessary.
- Monitor for bleeding every 4 hours, including skin, oral mucosa, abdominal assessment, body fluids, and menstrual pad count.

- Instruct to perform oral hygiene every 2 to 4 hours, using a soft-bristle toothbrush.
- Ask the dietitian to work with Mrs. Cole to identify preferred foods. Instruct to avoid foods that may damage oral mucosa, such as very hot, very cold, or highly acidic or spicy foods.
- Provide for periods of rest alternating with activity.
- Teach about the bone marrow biopsy. Allow time for questions and to verbalize fears.
- Refer to the oncology nurse specialist for further teaching and support.

EVALUATION

The bone marrow biopsy confirms the diagnosis of acute myelogenous leukemia. Mrs. Cole is very upset, but she calms as the physician and the oncology nurse discuss treatment plans and the possibility of remission. She decides to have outpatient chemotherapy. During her hospital stay, Mrs. Cole remained free of infection or further bleeding. She tells Ms. Losapio that her mouth feels better, although it is still painful. During routine assessment, Mrs. Cole remarks, "You know, I was so scared when I came here, but I think I am a little less so now. Sometimes not knowing what is wrong is worse than knowing."

CRITICAL THINKING

1. Describe how alterations in WBCs can increase an individual's susceptibility to infection.
2. List sources of potential infection for the client who is hospitalized.
3. What is the rationale for having the client do her own oral and physical hygiene?
4. Outline a teaching plan for this client and her family for home care to prevent infection.
5. Develop a care plan for Mrs. Cole for the nursing diagnosis of Activity Intolerance.

REVIEW Leukemia

RELATE Link the Concepts and Exemplars

Linking the exemplar of leukemia with the concept of comfort:

1. When caring for a client diagnosed with leukemia, what nursing diagnoses would you implement to address comfort?
2. What interventions would be appropriate for the client receiving chemotherapy who reports fatigue and difficulty meeting self-care needs?

Linking the exemplar of leukemia with the concept of culture:

3. How will you meet the cultural needs of the client who recently moved from Mexico, does not speak English, and has been diagnosed with leukemia?
4. What assessment data will you collect to prioritize nursing diagnoses for a client from India who has been diagnosed with leukemia?

READY Go to Companion Skills Manual

REFER Go to Pearson Nursing Student Resources
nursing.pearsonhighered.com

- Additional review materials

REFLECT Case Study

Johnny is 4 years old and was brought to the clinic by his mother who reports that she can't put her finger on what's wrong but he has not looked well lately. He is pale, has dark circles under his eyes, bruising on his arms and legs, and his mother states that he does not seem to have any energy lately. Johnny tells you that he is very tired all the time.

1. What is your priority when assessing Johnny during this visit?
2. What client teaching will you provide to maintain Johnny's safety?
3. What interventions will you initiate to support Johnny and his family through a new diagnosis of leukemia?

EXEMPLAR 2.6   Lung Cancer

EXEMPLAR KEY TERMS
Brachytherapy, *109*
Bronchogenic carcinomas, *104*
Hemoptysis, *107*
Non-small-cell carcinomas, *104*
Small-cell carcinomas, *104*

EXEMPLAR LEARNING OUTCOMES
After reading about this exemplar, you will be able to:

1. Describe the pathophysiology, etiology, clinical manifestations, and direct and indirect causes of lung cancer.
2. Identify risk factors and prevention methods associated with lung cancer.
3. Illustrate the nursing process in providing culturally competent care across the life span for individuals with lung cancer.
4. Formulate priority nursing diagnoses appropriate for an individual with lung cancer.
5. Summarize therapies used by interdisciplinary teams in the collaborative care of an individual with lung cancer.
6. Plan evidence-based care for an individual with lung cancer and his or her family in collaboration with other members of the healthcare team.
7. Evaluate expected outcomes for an individual with lung cancer.

▶ OVERVIEW

Of all forms of cancer in men and women, lung cancer accounts for the greatest number of deaths. In 2012, an estimated 160,340 deaths (28% of all cancer-related deaths) were due to lung cancer, while an estimated 226,160 individuals were expected to be newly diagnosed with lung cancer that same year (ACS, 2013b). Despite advances in surgical techniques and therapeutic treatments, lung cancer remains a significant health threat with dire consequences.

▶ PATHOPHYSIOLOGY AND ETIOLOGY

The vast majority of primary lung lesions are **bronchogenic carcinomas** (tumors of the airway epithelium). These tumors are further differentiated by cell type: small-cell carcinoma, adenocarcinoma, squamous cell carcinoma, and large-cell carcinoma. For clinical purposes, the latter three cell types frequently are classified together as non-small-cell carcinomas. **Small-cell carcinomas**, which account for approximately 14% of lung cancers, grow rapidly and spread early (ACS, 2013b). These tumors have paraneoplastic properties; that is, they produce manifestations at sites that are not directly affected by the tumor. Small-cell lung carcinomas can synthesize bioactive products and hormones, such as adrenocorticotropic hormones, antidiuretic hormone, a parathormone-like hormone, and gastrin-releasing peptide. **Non-small-cell carcinomas** account for approximately 85% of lung cancers (ACS, 2013b). Each cell type differs in its incidence, presentation, and manner of spread. **Table 2–12** ● outlines the incidence and unique characteristics of each cell type.

Bronchogenic cancer, regardless of cell type, tends to be aggressive, locally invasive, and have widespread metastatic lesions. Tumors begin as mucosal lesions that grow to form masses that obstruct the bronchi or invade adjacent lung tissue. All types frequently spread via the lymph system to nodes and other organs, such as the brain, bones, and liver.

Etiology

Lung cancer develops as damaged bronchial epithelial cells mutate over time to become neoplastic. The genetic abnormality commonly seen is on chromosome 3, with loss of genetic material. Alterations of tumor suppressor genes also are seen in some types of lung cancer.

Risk Factors

The incidence of lung cancer varies from state to state and among nations. The incidence increases with age, occurring most commonly in clients over age 50. Family clusters of lung cancer suggest a genetic predisposition; however, exposure to tobacco smoke may be necessary for expression of the trait. Cigarette smoke contains more than 7,000 chemicals, more than 70 of which are known carcinogens. Among individuals diagnosed with lung cancer, approximately 90% of cases are linked to smoking (CDC, 2013). There is a dose–response relationship between smoking and lung cancer; the more the individual smokes and the longer the individual smokes, the greater the risk. Even former smokers who have abstained for a number of years have a higher risk for developing lung cancer compared with those who have never smoked. Exposure to ionizing radiation and inhaled irritants, asbestos in particular, is also recognized as a risk factor for lung cancer. Exposure to radon, a radioactive gas, is another

TABLE 2–12 Comparison of Lung Cancer Cell Types

	CELL TYPE	PRESENTATION AND ASSOCIATED MANIFESTATIONS	SPREAD
	Small-cell (oat cell) carcinoma	Central lesion with hilar mass common, early mediastinal involvement, no cavitation; syndrome of inappropriate antidiuretic hormone (SIADH), Cushing syndrome, thrombophlebitis	Aggressive tumor; >40% of clients have distant metastasis at time of presentation.
	Adenocarcinoma	Peripheral mass involving bronchi; few local symptoms; hypertrophic pulmonary osteoarthropathy	Early metastasis to central nervous system, skeleton, and adrenal glands
	Squamous cell carcinoma	Central lesion located in large bronchi; client presents with cough, dyspnea, atelectasis, and wheezing; hypercalcemia common	Spreads by local invasion.
	Large-cell carcinoma	Usually peripheral lesion that is larger than associated with adenocarcinoma and tends to cavitate; gynecomastia, thrombophlebitis	Early metastasis

lung cancer risk factor (CDC, 2013). Radon forms as radium, an element present in the earth's crust, disintegrates. Radon tends to accumulate in closed spaces where air circulation is poor, such as caves, mines, and energy-efficient houses.

Prevention

Naturally, in light of the link between lung cancer and smoking, prevention of lung cancer is highly dependent on refraining from or stopping smoking. Despite the increased risk for lung cancer demonstrated among former smokers, there is still good reason to quit. Among smokers who quit before 40 years of age, the risk of death due to conditions associated with continued smoking decreases by approximately 90% (Jha et al., 2013). Aside from avoidance or cessation of smoking, prevention of lung cancer also includes preventing environmental and occupational exposure to known carcinogens, such as radon and asbestos.

▶ CLINICAL MANIFESTATIONS

The manifestations of lung cancer are related to the location and spread of the tumor. Clients may present with symptoms related to the primary tumor, manifestations of metastatic disease, or with systemic symptoms. Initial symptoms often are attributed to smoking or chronic bronchitis. Chronic cough is common, as is hemoptysis. Wheezing and shortness of breath occur as a result of airway obstruction. Dull, aching chest pain occurs as the tumor spreads to the mediastinum; pleuritic pain occurs when the pleura is invaded. Hoarseness and/or dysphagia indicate pressure of the tumor on the trachea or esophagus.

Systemic and paraneoplastic manifestations of lung cancer include weight loss, anorexia, fatigue, and weakness; bone pain, tenderness, and swelling; clubbing of the fingers and toes; and various endocrine, neuromuscular, cardiovascular, and

Multisystem Effects of Lung Cancer

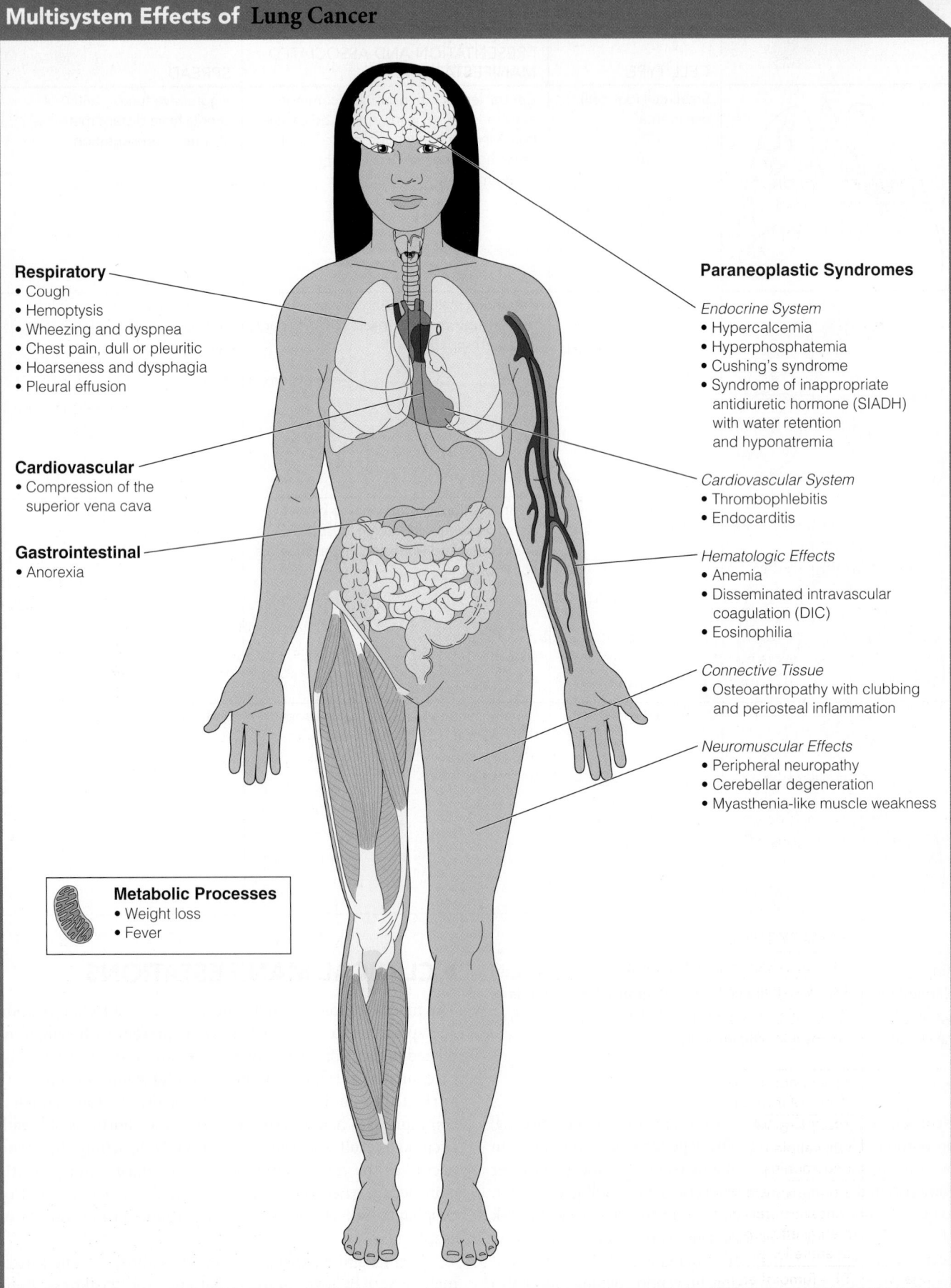

Respiratory
- Cough
- Hemoptysis
- Wheezing and dyspnea
- Chest pain, dull or pleuritic
- Hoarseness and dysphagia
- Pleural effusion

Cardiovascular
- Compression of the
  superior vena cava

Gastrointestinal
- Anorexia

Metabolic Processes
- Weight loss
- Fever

Paraneoplastic Syndromes

Endocrine System
- Hypercalcemia
- Hyperphosphatemia
- Cushing's syndrome
- Syndrome of inappropriate
  antidiuretic hormone (SIADH)
  with water retention
  and hyponatremia

Cardiovascular System
- Thrombophlebitis
- Endocarditis

Hematologic Effects
- Anemia
- Disseminated intravascular
  coagulation (DIC)
- Eosinophilia

Connective Tissue
- Osteoarthropathy with clubbing
  and periosteal inflammation

Neuromuscular Effects
- Peripheral neuropathy
- Cerebellar degeneration
- Myasthenia-like muscle weakness

Clinical Manifestations and Therapies **Lung Cancer**

ETIOLOGY	CLINICAL MANIFESTATIONS	CLINICAL THERAPIES
Hypoxia	■ Shortness of breath, chest pain, reduced oxygen saturation, tachypnea, chronic cough, dyspnea, cyanosis	■ Administer oxygen. ■ Reduce activity level. ■ Position in Fowler's or tripod position.
Paraneoplastic syndrome resulting from growth and metastasis of the tumor	■ Weight loss, anorexia, fatigue, and weakness; bone pain, tenderness, and swelling; clubbing of the fingers and toes; and various endocrine, neuromuscular, cardiovascular, and hematological symptoms	■ Surgical removal of tumor ■ Chemotherapy or radiation therapy to reduce metastasis and tumor size ■ Palliative treatment to reduce symptoms ■ Pain management as indicated
Metastasis to brain	■ Confusion, impaired gait and balance, headache, and personality changes	■ Maintain familiar items in room to promote orientation. ■ Protect from falls and risk for injury. ■ Explain impact of brain metastasis to family in order to prepare them for personality changes.

hematological symptoms. See the Multisystem Effects feature for more information.

Confusion, impaired gait and balance, headache, and personality changes may indicate brain metastasis. Bone metastases cause bone pain, pathological fractures, and possible spinal cord compression, as well as thrombocytopenia and anemia if bone marrow is invaded. When the liver is affected, symptoms of liver dysfunction and biliary obstruction, including jaundice, anorexia, and upper right quadrant pain, are evident.

Lung cancer has both local and systemic effects. Local effects include cough, excess mucus production, shortness of breath or dyspnea, **hemoptysis** (bloody sputum), and chest pain. Systemic effects may include fever, anorexia and malaise, cyanosis, and other manifestations of impaired gas exchange.

▶ COLLABORATION

Because lung cancer typically is advanced when diagnosed and the prognosis generally is poor, prevention of the disease must be a primary goal for all healthcare providers. As stated earlier with 90% of lung cancers related to cigarette smoking, reducing tobacco use can have a significant impact on the death rate from lung cancer—a far greater impact than advances in treatment.

Establishing an accurate diagnosis is the first step in treating lung cancer. Treatment decisions are based on the tumor location, the type of cancer cell, the staging of the tumor, and the client's ability to tolerate treatment. Lung cancer is staged by the tumor size, location, degree of invasion of the primary tumor, and the presence of metastatic disease. Lung cancer staging is summarized in **Table 2–13** ●. Surgery is the treatment of choice for most forms of lung cancer.

TABLE 2–13   The TNM Staging System for Lung Cancer

	PRIMARY TUMOR (T)	REGIONAL LYMPH NODES (N)	DISTANT METASTASIS (M)
	T0—No evidence of primary tumor		
Stage 0	TX—Malignant cells in bronchopulmonary secretions, but no tumor visualized		MX—Presence of distant metastasis cannot be assessed
Stage I	Tis—Carcinoma in situ	N0—No regional lymph node metastasis	M0—No distant metastasis
	T1—Tumor of ≤3 cm in diameter, with no evidence of invasion		
Stage II	T2—Tumor of >3 cm in diameter, or invades visceral pleura, or has associated atelectasis or pneumonitis	N1—Metastasis or direct extension to peribronchial or ipsilateral hilar nodes	
Stage III	T3—Tumor with direct extension into an adjacent structure, or any tumor with associated pleural effusion or atelectasis or pneumonitis of entire lung	N2—Metastasis to ipsilateral mediastinal or subcarinal nodes	
Stage IV	T4—Tumor that invades mediastinum or involves the heart, great vessels, trachea, esophagus, vertebral body, or carina; presence of malignant pleural effusion	N3—Metastasis to contralateral mediastinal, scalene, or supraclavicular nodes	M1—Distant metastasis present

Diagnostic Tests

Diagnostic tests are based on location and size of the tumor along with client condition. Once lung cancer is diagnosed, additional tests may be ordered to rule out possible metastasis. Common diagnostic tests include the following:

- **Chest x-ray** usually provides the first evidence of lung cancer. It is particularly reliable as a diagnostic tool when compared with a previous chest x-ray. In high-risk populations, the chest x-ray may be used as a screening tool for lung cancer.

- **Sputum specimen** is sent for cytological examination to establish the diagnosis of lung cancer. The sputum sample is collected on arising in the morning. If malignant cells are found in the sputum, more expensive and invasive examinations may be unnecessary. However, a sputum sample that is negative for malignant cells does not rule out lung cancer; it may simply indicate that the tumor is not shedding cells into mucous secretions.

- **Bronchoscopy** is frequently done to visualize and obtain a biopsy specimen from the tumor. When a tumor mass or suspicious tissue is identified visually, a cable-activated instrument is used to obtain a tissue specimen. If the tumor cannot be seen, the airways may be flushed with a saline solution (bronchial washing) to obtain cells for cytological examination.

- **Computed tomography (CT)** is used to evaluate and localize tumors, particularly tumors in the lung parenchyma and pleura. It also is done before needle biopsy to localize the tumor. In addition, CT scanning can detect distant tumor metastasis and evaluate tumor response to treatment.

- **Cytological examination and biopsy** involve cells or tissue obtained by aspirating fluid from a pleural effusion, percutaneous needle biopsy, and lymph node biopsy. These procedures may be done in an outpatient or a surgical setting.

- **CBC, liver function studies, and serum electrolytes** including calcium are obtained to evaluate for evidence of metastatic disease or paraneoplastic syndromes.

- **Tuberculin test** is performed to rule out tuberculosis as the cause of symptoms and abnormalities seen on chest x-ray.

- **Pulmonary function tests and arterial blood gases** may be performed before the initiation of treatment if the client has manifestations of respiratory insufficiency (e.g., dyspnea, activity intolerance, and low oxygen saturation levels).

These tests are described in greater detail in Appendix B available online at nursing.pearsonhighered.com.

Surgery

Surgery offers the only real chance for a cure in clients with non-small-cell lung cancer. Unfortunately, most tumors are inoperable or only partially resectable at the time of diagnosis. The type of surgery performed depends on the location and size of the tumor as well as on the client's pulmonary and general health. The goal of surgery is to remove all involved tissue while preserving as much functional lung as possible. **Table 2–14** ● outlines various surgical procedures used to diagnose and treat lung cancer.

Pharmacologic Therapy

Combination chemotherapy (often combined with radiation therapy and/or surgery) is the treatment of choice for small-cell lung cancer because of its rapid growth, dissemination, and sensitivity to cytotoxic drugs. Used in combination, chemotherapeutic drugs allow tumor cells to be attacked at different parts of the cell cycle and in different ways, increasing the effectiveness of therapy. Fifty percent of clients with tumors at early stages achieve complete tumor remission with combination chemotherapy. When a complete tumor response is achieved in the first few cycles of chemotherapy, the chances for long-term survival are much greater.

Combination chemotherapy also is used as an adjunct to surgery or radiation therapy for other types of lung cancer. It may be used to reduce the size of advanced local tumors before surgery and to lengthen survival when distant metastases are present.

Bronchodilators may be prescribed to reduce airway obstruction. Analgesics and pain management strategies are vital when the cancer is advanced. See the module on Comfort for more information about postoperative and cancer pain management.

TABLE 2–14   Types of Surgery for Lung Cancer

PROCEDURE	DESCRIPTION	USED FOR
Laser bronchoscopy	Bronchoscopy-guided laser used to resect tumor	Tumors localized in a main bronchus
Mediastinoscopy	Visualization of the mediastinum using an endoscope passed through a suprasternal incision	Evaluation and biopsy of a mediastinal tumor and lymph nodes
Thoracotomy	Incision into the chest wall	Access the lung and thoracic cavity for surgery
Wedge resection	Removal of a small section (wedge) of peripheral lung tissue	Small, peripheral lung tumors
Segmental resection	Removal of an individual bronchovascular segment of a lobe	Peripheral lung tumor with no evidence of extension to the chest wall or metastasis
Sleeve resection (bronchoplastic reconstruction)	Resection of a section of a major bronchus with reconstruction of remaining normal bronchus	Small lesion of a major bronchus
Lobectomy	Removal of a single lung lobe	Tumors confined to a single lobe
Pneumonectomy	Removal of an entire lung	Tumor widespread throughout the lung, involving the main bronchus, or fixed to the hilum

Radiation Therapy

Radiation therapy is used alone or in combination with surgery or chemotherapy for lung cancer. The goal of treatment may be either cure or symptom relief (palliative). Before surgery, radiation therapy is used to "debulk" tumors. When cancer has spread by direct extension to other thoracic structures and surgery is not feasible, radiation therapy may be the treatment of choice. It also may be used to relieve manifestations such as cough, hemoptysis, pain resulting from bone metastasis, and dyspnea from bronchial obstruction. Complications of lung cancer, such as superior vena cava syndrome, may be treated with radiation. Radiation therapy may be delivered by external beam to the primary tumor site or by intraluminal radiation, or **brachytherapy** with insertion of a radioactive source inside the body near the tumor for more direct effects.

■ NURSING PROCESS

The client with lung cancer is facing invasive treatments with undesirable side effects, possibly surgery, and typically a poor prognosis for long-term survival. Nursing care needs are diverse, related to respiratory status, the cancer itself and possible metastases, and the treatment plan.

Assessment

Nursing assessment related to lung cancer focuses on identifying risk factors for the disease, early manifestations of lung cancer, and respiratory function in the client undergoing treatment. Collect the following data through the health history and physical examination:

- *Health history.* Current symptoms, including chronic cough, shortness of breath, blood-tinged sputum; systemic manifestations such as recent weight loss, fatigue, anorexia, bone pain; smoking history; occupational exposure to carcinogens; chronic diseases such as chronic obstructive pulmonary disease
- *Physical examination.* Assess respiratory function including respiratory rate, depth, breath sounds, and chest excursion. Oxygenation is assessed using pulse oximetry, arterial blood gas results, and pulmonary function studies.

Diagnosis

Priority nursing diagnoses related to respiratory function include the following:

- *Impaired Gas Exchange*
- *Ineffective Breathing Pattern*
- *Risk for Decreased Cardiac Tissue Perfusion secondary to impaired oxygenation*
- *Activity Intolerance*
- *Pain*
- *Anticipatory Grieving.*

(NANDA-I © 2012)

Planning

Goals and identified outcomes are dependent on the specific nursing diagnoses included in the client's plan of care, as well as the individual client. While not intended to be all inclusive, examples of identified outcomes relevant to the plan of care for the client with lung cancer may include the following:

- The client will maintain an oxygen saturation of greater than 90%.
- The client's respiratory rate will range between 12 and 20 breaths per minute.
- The client will deny dyspnea.
- The client's heart rate will be maintained within normal limits.
- The client will demonstrate the ability to make informed decisions regarding all treatments.
- Using a predetermined pain rating scale, the client will report his pain is maintained at a level deemed by him to be tolerable.
- The client will verbalize emotions and concerns related to his diagnosis and treatment.

Implementation

Nurses take a holistic approach to providing care, meeting both the physical and psychosocial needs of the client. Airway and breathing are always the greatest priority, followed by circulation. The client who is hypoxic will be anxious, so reducing anxiety is a priority intervention for that client.

Promote Effective Cardiorespiratory Function

Breathing pattern and ventilation may be affected by the tumor itself or by treatment of the tumor. Thoracic surgery increases the risk caused by the incision and disruption of the muscles of respiration. Maintaining effective lung ventilation is particularly important postoperatively to reexpand remaining lung tissue and prevent surgical complications.

- Suction airway as needed. Suctioning may be required to remove secretions that the client is unable to cough up and expectorate.
- Administer supplemental oxygen as ordered and as needed per protocols.
- Assess and document respiratory rate, depth, and lung sounds at least every 4 hours; evaluate more frequently in the immediate postoperative period or as indicated by condition. Early detection of signs of respiratory compromise or adventitious lung sounds is vital for effective intervention.
- Impaired oxygenation can lead to inadequate perfusion of cardiac tissue, which can cause cardiac complications, including tachycardia and dysrhythmias. For some clients, especially those with compromised respiratory function, continuous EKG monitoring is indicated.
- Elevate the head of the bed to 60 degrees. Elevating the head of the bed reduces pressure on the diaphragm and permits optimal lung expansion.
- Assist the client to turn, cough, and deep breathe and use incentive spirometry. Help splint the chest with a pillow or blanket when coughing. These measures promote airway clearance.
- Provide chest physiotherapy with percussion and postural drainage as needed or ordered. Percussion and postural drainage help maintain airway patency and effective respirations.
- If mechanical ventilation is instituted, work with respiratory therapy and use analgesia or sedation as needed to synchronize respirations with the ventilator. Coordination of the cli-

ent's respiratory effort with ventilator-delivered breaths is important for fully effective mechanical ventilation.

Manage Pain Effectively

Pain is a priority problem in the postoperative period and in the terminal stages of cancer. Poorly managed pain prolongs recovery from surgery. In the client with terminal cancer, chronic and acute pain must be managed effectively to allow a peaceful death.

■ Assess and document pain using a standardized pain scale and objective data. Pain is a subjective experience, best evaluated by the client. Changes in vital signs, guarded movement, or unwillingness to move may indicate unreported pain.

■ Frequently assess and document pain level (using a standard pain scale); provide analgesics as needed. Pain and attempting to avoid chest movement to prevent additional pain can lead to rapid, shallow respirations and ineffective ventilation. Postoperative recovery and restoration of function is facilitated by adequate pain management.

■ For cancer pain, maintain an around-the-clock medication schedule using narcotics, nonsteroidal anti-inflammatory drugs, and other medications as ordered. Addiction is not a concern in the client with terminal cancer; providing adequate pain relief that does not allow "breakthrough" pain is important.

■ Provide or assist with comfort measures, such as massage, positioning, distraction, and relaxation techniques. These techniques promote relaxation and enhance pain relief.

■ Assist the client and family to plan and engage in activities that distract from pain, such as reading, watching television, and engaging in social interactions. Distraction helps the client focus away from the pain.

■ Spend as much time with the client as possible; allow family members to remain with the client. Physical presence of the nurse and family provides emotional support for the client.

Pain management is discussed further in the exemplar on Acute and Chronic Pain in the module on Comfort. Care for the client and the end of life is discussed in the exemplar on End-of-Life Care in the module on Comfort. A discussion of "presencing" can be found in the module on Comfort.

Manage Fatigue and Activity Intolerance

Both resectional lung surgery and inoperable lung cancer reduce the amount of functional lung tissue and surface area for gas diffusion. This can lead to activity intolerance if the oxygen supply is insufficient to meet the body's oxygen demand.

■ Plan rest periods between activities and procedures. Rest periods reduce oxygen demands and fatigue.

■ Assist the postoperative client to increase activities gradually. Increasing activity levels gradually improves exercise tolerance.

■ Teach measures to conserve energy while performing ADLs, such as sitting while showering and dressing and wearing slip-on shoes. These energy-conserving measures reduce oxygen demand and allow the client to remain independent as long as possible.

■ Keep frequently used objects within easy reach. This helps conserve energy.

■ Administer oxygen as prescribed. Teach the client and family about home oxygen use if appropriate. Supplemental oxygen can help improve activity and exercise tolerance.

■ Encourage maintenance of physical activity to tolerance. Maintaining activity levels to the degree possible improves physical and emotional well-being.

■ Allow family members to provide assistance as needed. This helps the client conserve energy and allows the family to retain a sense of usefulness.

■ Provide reassurance and emotional support. These measures help relieve anxiety and promote an effective breathing pattern.

Promote Healthy Grieving

Because lung cancer often is advanced when diagnosed, the client faces the very real prospect of dying from the disease. Grieving for the anticipated loss of life is a normal response as the client and family begin to adapt to the diagnosis. Nursing care goals include promoting expression of feelings and thoughts about the loss and helping the client and family initiate grief work, make decisions, and use appropriate resources and coping mechanisms to deal with the loss. (For detailed discussion of nursing care for the client with terminal illness and his loved ones, refer to the exemplar on Death and Dying in the module on Grief and Loss.) Examples of nursing interventions that promote achievement of these goals include the following:

■ Spend time with the client and family. Time is necessary to develop a trusting, therapeutic relationship.

■ Answer questions honestly; do not deny the probable outcome of the disease. Honesty reinforces reality and provides a sense of control over decisions to be made.

■ Encourage the client and family to express their feelings, fears, and concerns. Open expression of feelings helps promote understanding and acceptance.

■ Discuss advance directives, such as do-not-resuscitate orders, and powers of attorney for health care with the client and family. These documents give the client and family a sense of control over medical care provided if the client is no longer able to express his or her own wishes.

Evaluation

Client response to care is evaluated based on goals of care. Achieved outcomes may include the following:

■ The client maintains an oxygen saturation of greater that 90% at rest and with activity.

■ The client's respiratory rate ranges between 12 and 24 breaths per minute.

■ The client denies dyspnea at rest and during appropriate levels of activity.

■ The client's heart rate is maintained within 10% of the upper and lower limits of his normal range.

■ The client makes informed decisions regarding all treatments.

■ Using a predetermined pain rating scale, the client reports maintenance of his pain at a level deemed by him to be tolerable.

■ The client verbalizes grief and fears related to his diagnosis and treatment.

NURSING CARE PLAN   A Client With Lung Cancer

After coughing up bloody sputum one morning, James Mueller, a 68-year-old retired mill worker, sees his physician. A chest x-ray shows a suspicious density in the central portion of his right lung. Mr. Mueller is admitted to the hospital the following Monday for diagnostic tests.

ASSESSMENT

Anita Sarros, RN, admits Mr. Mueller to the oncology unit and obtains a nursing history. Mr. Mueller is married and has three grown children. He worked in a local paper mill for 35 years before retiring at age 62. He describes himself as "pretty healthy," except for a chronic smoker's cough. He started smoking as a young man in the army. He has a 50-year smoking history, having smoked a pack a day for 50 years, since age 18. Mr. Mueller says he briefly quit smoking following a small heart attack 3 years ago but started again after 4 months. On further questioning, Mr. Mueller says his cough has been productive for the past few months, especially in the morning, and that he is shorter of breath than usual with activity.

Mr. Mueller's vital signs include temperature 98.4°F oral; pulse 78 bpm; respirations 20/min; and BP 162/86 mmHg. His color is good, and his skin is warm and dry. Inspiratory and expiratory wheezes are noted in right chest, but good breath sounds are heard throughout. No other abnormal findings are noted on examination. The physician orders early morning sputum specimens times 3 days for cytological examination and schedules a CT scan of the chest the morning after admission.

Mr. Mueller's CBC shows mild anemia, but remaining routine laboratory tests are essentially normal. Sputum cytology is positive for small-cell bronchogenic cancer. The CT scan shows a central mass approximately 4 cm in diameter with involved mediastinal and subclavicular lymph nodes. A small mass is also noted on the lumbar spine. After conferring with his physician and an oncologist, Mr. Mueller decides to undergo a trial course of chemotherapy.

DIAGNOSES

- *Ineffective Airway Clearance* related to tumor mass
- *Risk for Imbalanced Nutrition: Less Than Body Requirements* related to effects of chemotherapy
- *Risk for Compromised Family Coping* related to new diagnosis of lung cancer
- *Deficient Knowledge* about lung cancer and aids to smoking cessation

(NANDA-I © 2012)

PLANNING

- The client will maintain a patent airway.
- The client will maintain current weight.
- The client will express feelings and concerns about the effect of cancer on the family.
- The client will participate in care.
- The client will contact appropriate support groups.
- The client will verbalize an understanding of the disease, its treatment, and prognosis.
- The client will develop a plan to stop smoking.

IMPLEMENTATION

- Teach coughing, deep breathing, and hydration measures to facilitate airway clearance.
- Discuss symptoms to report to the physician: increased dyspnea or hemoptysis, severe stridor or wheezing, and chest pain.
- Discuss measures to relieve nausea associated with chemotherapy, including premedication with a prescribed antiemetic.
- Have dietitian consult with Mr. and Mrs. Mueller to develop a diet plan for maintaining ideal weight.
- Discuss possible effects of lung cancer with Mr. and Mrs. Mueller.
- Encourage Mr. and Mrs. Mueller to call a family conference to discuss the disease with their children and grandchildren.

- Evaluate family members' knowledge and understanding of lung cancer, correcting misinformation and teaching as needed.
- Have an American Cancer Society volunteer contact the family.
- Refer to local cancer support group.
- Refer to home health department for follow-up and further teaching.
- Work with Mr. Mueller to develop a plan to stop smoking.
- Ask the physician for a prescription for nicotine patches or gum for Mr. Mueller.

EVALUATION

Mr. Mueller had his first chemotherapy treatment in the hospital and was discharged 4 days after admission. After 3 months of chemotherapy, his tumor shows little regression, and a liver scan reveals further metastasis. He and his wife decide to stop chemotherapy, a decision with which the children reluctantly agree. Mr. and Mrs. Mueller are referred to hospice services. With the help of hospice nurses and volunteers, Mr. Mueller is able to remain at home. His pain is managed initially with oral MS Contin, a sustained-release form of morphine sulfate, and later with an intravenous morphine infusion. Mr. Mueller dies at home with his family at his side 9 months after his diagnosis of lung cancer.

CRITICAL THINKING

1. *The oncologist prescribed a chemotherapy regimen of cyclophosphamide, doxorubicin, and vincristine. Describe how each of these drugs works against cancer cells, and discuss the rationale for using this combination.*
2. *Develop a care plan to deal with the specific side effects for the above treatment regimen.*
3. *Mr. Mueller had small-cell (oat cell) cancer. How would his presentation and treatment differ if the diagnosis had been non-small-cell adenocarcinoma, stage T2N2M0?*

▌REVIEW **Lung Cancer**

RELATE Link the Concepts and Exemplars

Linking the exemplar of lung cancer with the concept of acid–base balance:

1. What effect might lung cancer have on the client's acid–base balance?
2. What client teaching will you provide to assist with normalizing acid–base balance?

Linking the exemplar of lung cancer with the concept of infection:

3. What priority client teaching can the nurse provide to reduce the risk of infection in the client diagnosed with lung cancer?
4. When caring for the client with lung cancer, what interventions will you initiate to reduce the risk of infection?

READY Go to Companion Skills Manual

REFER Go to Pearson Nursing Student Resources
nursing.pearsonhighered.com

- Additional review materials

REFLECT Case Study

Michael Harris, 66 years old, has abused alcohol for many years and has smoked two packs of cigarettes a day since age 19. He has been diagnosed with lung cancer. Mr. Harris is divorced and has two children who are grown and live out of town. Mr. Harris lives alone in an apartment and has a girlfriend who also smokes and abuses alcohol. The physician in charge of Mr. Harris's care has told him that he will need a lobectomy of the left lung, radiation therapy, and chemotherapy. Mr. Harris thanks the doctor and says he will get back to him. The nurse remains with Mr. Harris after the doctor leaves the room and overhears him whisper under his breath "Fat chance I'm going to do all that. I'd rather die in peace."

1. How would you respond to this statement?
2. What are the priorities for his care at this time?
3. What interventions can you initiate to help Mr. Harris make the best healthcare and lifestyle decisions?
4. What will your personal feelings and thoughts be if you are caring for Mr. Harris and he decides not to pursue treatment? How might this bias impact your approach to caring for him?

EXEMPLAR 2.7 **Prostate Cancer**

EXEMPLAR KEY TERMS
Androgens, *112*
Orchiectomy, *115*
Prostatectomy, *115*

EXEMPLAR LEARNING OUTCOMES
After reading about this exemplar, you will be able to:

1. Describe the pathophysiology, etiology, clinical manifestations, and direct and indirect causes of prostate cancer.
2. Identify risk factors and prevention methods associated with prostate cancer.

3. Illustrate the nursing process in providing culturally competent care across the life span for individuals with prostate cancer.
4. Formulate priority nursing diagnoses appropriate for an individual with prostate cancer.
5. Summarize therapies used by interdisciplinary teams in the collaborative care of an individual with prostate cancer.
6. Plan evidence-based care for an individual with prostate cancer and his or her family in collaboration with other members of the healthcare team.
7. Evaluate expected outcomes for an individual with prostate cancer.

▶ OVERVIEW

Abnormal growth of prostate tissue may be related to benign prostatic hyperplasia (covered in more detail in the module on Elimination), or it may be an indication of prostate cancer. The diagnosis of prostate cancer is very frightening for most men, who fear death, disfigurement, and loss of sexual function.

When diagnosed early, prostate cancer is curable. When the cancer is confined to the prostate at diagnosis, the 5-year survival rate is 100%. Even when the cancer has spread regionally, approximately 95% of clients are alive after 5 years. More than 75% of prostate cancer diagnoses are made at one of these stages (ACS, 2009).

Many men are found to have prostate cancer on autopsy. Usually, the cancer has produced no manifestations or complications, and these men may have died with no knowledge of the developing disease.

▶ PATHOPHYSIOLOGY AND ETIOLOGY

The prostate gland consists primarily of glandular epithelial cells. The exact etiology of prostate cancer is unknown, although **androgens** (hormones synthesized in the testes, ovaries, and adrenal cortex that promote expression of male sex characteris-

tics) are believed to have a role in its development. Almost all primary prostate cancers are adenocarcinomas, and they develop in the peripheral zones of the prostate gland. This location increases the risk of local spread to the prostatic capsule. Despite its proximity to the rectum, metastasis to the bowel is uncommon, because a tough sheet of tissue, Denonvilliers fascia, acts as an effective physical barrier.

As the tumor enlarges, it may compress the urethra, obstructing urinary flow. The tumor may metastasize and involve the seminal vesicles or bladder by direct extension. Metastasis by lymph and venous channels is common.

Etiology

Cancer of the prostate is the most common type of cancer and the second-leading cause of death among men in North America (ACS, 2013b). It is primarily a disease of older men, increasing in incidence with age, with the majority of cases diagnosed in men older than 65 years. In 2012, researchers anticipated diagnosis of more than 240,000 new cases of prostate cancer and more than 28,000 men were expected to die from this disease that same year (CDC, 2013). Prostate cancer is a major health problem for older men, but the death rate is decreasing as a result of advances in diagnosis and treatment.

Risk Factors

As stated earlier, the greatest risk factor for prostate cancer is age. Among men ages 70 years and older, approximately one in eight will be diagnosed with prostate cancer (ACS, 2013b). In addition to age, race is a significant risk factor for prostate cancer, with African American men being at particularly high risk. According to recent studies, a diet high in dairy foods or processed meat may increase the risk for developing prostate cancer, and obesity may increase the risk for developing an aggressive form of this disease. Some research suggests firefighters may be at increased risk for prostate cancer (ACS, 2013b). Other risk factors being investigated include the following:

- Genetic and hereditary factors, with increased risk in men who have a family history of the disease
- Having a vasectomy, which is believed to increase the levels of circulating free testosterone
- Dietary factors, including a diet high in animal fat and excessive supplemental vitamin A.

Prevention

Prevention of prostate cancer through use of medications has become a prominent research topic. The drugs dutasteride and finasteride, which reduce the amount of certain male hormones, are already being used in the management of symptoms related to benign prostate enlargement. In clinical trials, these medications have been linked to a 25% reduction in the risk for developing prostate cancer. However, side effects such as risk of erectile dysfunction and diminished libido make these drugs less than ideal for use as prophylactic treatments. After analysis of risks and benefits, a 2010 FDA advisory committee recommended against approving both dutasteride and finasteride as preventative treatments for prostate cancer (ACS, 2013b).

Screening recommendations center around the optimal timing for discussion of the benefits and limitations associated with available tests for early prostate cancer detection. Following this discussion between the client and his healthcare provider, the client should be encouraged to consider testing and to make an informed decision that incorporates his individual preferences and values. Guidelines include the following (ACS, 2013b):

- For men at average risk of prostate cancer and whose life expectancy is at least 10 years, this discussion and informed decision should be initiated at 50 years of age.
- For men at high risk for developing prostate cancer, including those whose close relative was diagnosed with prostate cancer prior to age 65 and African Americans, this discussion and informed decision should begin at 45 years of age.
- For men at even higher risk, including those for whom several close relatives have been diagnosed with prostate cancer at an early age, this discussion and informed decision about testing should commence beginning at age 40 years.

▶ CLINICAL MANIFESTATIONS

Men with early-stage prostate cancer are often asymptomatic. Pain from metastasis to bones is often the initial manifestation noted. Urinary manifestations depend on the size and location of the tumor and on the stage of the malignancy; they are often much

Focus on Diversity and Culture
Risk and Incidence of Prostate Cancer

- African Americans have the highest incidence of prostate cancer in the United States and the world, with rates greater than 60% higher than those seen in Whites (CDC, 2013).
- African Americans are more likely to be diagnosed later and to die of prostate cancer, with a mortality rate more than double that of other racial and ethnic groups.
- Asians and Native Americans have the lowest incidence of prostate cancer.

like manifestations of benign prostatic hyperplasia: urgency, frequency, hesitancy, dysuria, and nocturia. The man may also notice hematuria or blood in the ejaculate (Porth & Matfin, 2010). For an overview of manifestations associated with prostate cancer, see the Clinical Manifestations and Therapies feature.

▶ COLLABORATION

Care of the client with prostate cancer focuses on diagnosis, elimination or containment of the cancer, and prevention or treatment of complications. There are currently no clinical strategies to prevent the development of prostate cancer. Therefore, early detection remains the major emphasis for control of this disease.

The treatment of prostate cancer is complex and depends on the grade and stage of the cancer as well as on the age, general health, and preference of the client. In some cases, for example, when the client with a slow-growing tumor is older or has a limited life expectancy, *watchful waiting* is the treatment of choice. Treatments for prostate cancer include surgery, radiation therapy, and hormone manipulation.

Diagnostic Tests

Although an increasing number of clients are now diagnosed with asymptomatic prostate cancer, many clients with prostate cancer have either locally advanced cancer or distant metastasis at the time of diagnosis. The definitive diagnosis can be made only by biopsy; however, other tests may suggest the presence of prostate cancer.

A *digital rectal examination (DRE)* will find the prostate gland nodular and fixed in the client with prostate cancer. Levels of *prostate-specific antigen (PSA)* are used to diagnose and stage prostate cancer and to monitor response to treatment. In addition, the PSA test is used to monitor effects of treatment. Until recently, the National Cancer Institute guidelines included considering a PSA level of 4.0 ng/mL or lower to be normal. However, current research suggests men whose PSA levels meet this criterion may still have prostate cancer. Likewise, an elevated or fluctuating PSA level, which previously was considered to be a relative indication for prostate biopsy, has been known to occur in relation to conditions such as prostatitis and urinary tract infection. For these reasons, PSA levels are now interpreted in conjunction with an individual's health history and, prior to prostate biopsy, additional testing (such as x-rays or cystoscopy) may be warranted to rule out other causative factors (NCI, 2012).

Clinical Manifestations and Therapies Prostate Cancer

ETIOLOGY	CLINICAL MANIFESTATIONS	CLINICAL THERAPIES
Enlarged prostate	■ Dysuria ■ Frequency of urination ■ Reduction in urinary stream ■ Nocturia ■ Hematuria ■ Abnormal prostate on digital rectal examination	■ Surgery ■ Radiation ■ Chemotherapy ■ Hormone therapy
Metastasis of cancer to bones	■ Bone or joint pain ■ Migratory bone pain ■ Back pain	■ Administer analgesics as ordered. ■ Promote balance between rest and activity. ■ Massage
Nerve impingement due to mechanical compression by enlarged prostate	■ Nerve pain ■ Bilateral lower extremity weakness ■ Bowel or bladder dysfunction ■ Muscle spasms	■ Administer analgesics as ordered. ■ Administer muscle relaxants as ordered. ■ Assist with ambulation and institute safety protocols. ■ Provide teaching to optimize patterns of urinary elimination (including instructions for Kegel exercises, if appropriate). ■ As ordered, implement interventions to promote urinary elimination (e.g., insertion of indwelling urinary catheter).
Increased metabolic demands	■ Weight loss ■ Fatigue	■ Encourage balanced nutrition. ■ Offer foods that appeal to the client. ■ Promote balance between activity and rest.

Transrectal ultrasonography may be used when the DRE is abnormal or if the PSA is elevated without otherwise apparent cause. In this test, a small probe is inserted in the rectum. The probe gives off sound waves that create a picture of the prostate on a video screen. Guided by this picture, the physician inserts a narrow needle through the rectal wall into the prostate gland, and the needle removes a sample of tissue for examination. Other tests that may be ordered include a urinalysis or cystoscopy. Bone scan, MRI, or CT may be performed to determine the presence of tumor metastasis.

Grade and stage help determine prognosis and guide treatment decisions. Grade (cancer cell differentiation) is determined by the pathologist. Prostate cancer is staged with a variety of tests. Table 2–15 ● outlines treatment options according to the stage of the cancer.

TABLE 2–15 Prostate Cancer Staging and Treatment

STAGE	DESCRIPTION	TREATMENT
Stage I	Confined to prostate; nonpalpable, focal involvement; well differentiated	■ Observation and follow-up ■ Interstitial or external-beam radiation therapy ■ Prostatectomy
Stage II	Confined to prostate; palpable, involves one or both lobes; poorly differentiated	■ Careful observation in selected clients ■ Prostatectomy ■ Interstitial or external-beam radiation therapy ■ Ultrasound-guided percutaneous cryosurgery
Stage III	Extension of the tumor outside the prostate capsule; possible seminal vesicle involvement	■ External-beam radiation therapy ■ Interstitial radiation ■ Radical prostatectomy ■ Adjunctive hormone therapy ■ Palliative surgery (transurethral prostatectomy or TURP—removal of the prostate through the urethra)
Stage IV	Extension of the tumor into surrounding tissues; lymph node involvement or distant metastasis	■ Hormone therapy ■ External-beam radiation therapy ■ Palliative treatment with radiation therapy and/or TURP ■ Radical prostatectomy with orchiectomy ■ Chemotherapy

TABLE 2–16 Potential Complications Related to Radical Prostatectomy and Radiation Therapy

RADICAL PROSTATECTOMY	RADIATION THERAPY
Erectile dysfunction	Erectile dysfunction[a]
Urethral stricture	Urethral stricture
Fistula/rectal injury	Rectal/anal stricture[a]
Urinary incontinence	Cystitis
Surgical/anesthetic risk	Diarrhea
	Proctitis
	Rectal ulcer
	Bowel obstruction[a]
	Urinary incontinence

[a]Delayed complications; may appear months or years after completion of therapy.

Surgery

Surgery for prostate cancer generally involves **prostatectomy**, or removal of the prostate. For very early disease in older men, cure may be achieved with a simple prostatectomy (e.g., TURP). Types of prostatectomies include the following:

- *Radical prostatectomy* involves removal of the prostate, prostate capsule, seminal vesicles, and a portion of the bladder neck. Many clients experience varying degrees of urinary incontinence and erectile dysfunction (ED) (**Table 2–16 ●**). A fairly new treatment is laparoscopic radical prostatectomy, in which small incisions are made in the abdomen and a laparoscope is inserted and used to remove the prostate. Some surgeons do this from an area other than the operating room by using a robotic interface.

- *Retropubic prostatectomy* may be performed because it allows adequate control of bleeding, visualization of the prostate bed and bladder neck, and access to pelvic lymph nodes.

- *Perineal prostatectomy* is often preferred for older men or those who are poor surgical risks. This approach requires less time, and involves less bleeding.

- *Suprapubic prostatectomy* is rarely used, usually when problems with the bladder are expected. Control of bleeding is more difficult because the surgical approach is through the bladder.

For clients with stage III, locally advanced (beyond the prostatic capsule) cancer, surgery is controversial because of the likelihood of hidden lymph node metastasis and relapse. TURP is not performed as curative therapy, but it may be used to relieve urinary obstruction for men with advanced disease (stage III or IV).

Surgical intervention is now available for men with urinary sphincter insufficiency, which is the major cause of incontinence after prostatectomy. An artificial urinary sphincter is surgically implanted (**Figure 2–19 ●**). To be eligible, the man must be able to manipulate the pump placed in the scrotum and have adequate cognitive function to know when a problem with the appliance occurs.

Pharmacologic Therapy

Androgen deprivation therapy is used to treat advanced prostate cancer. Many cells in the growing tumor are androgen

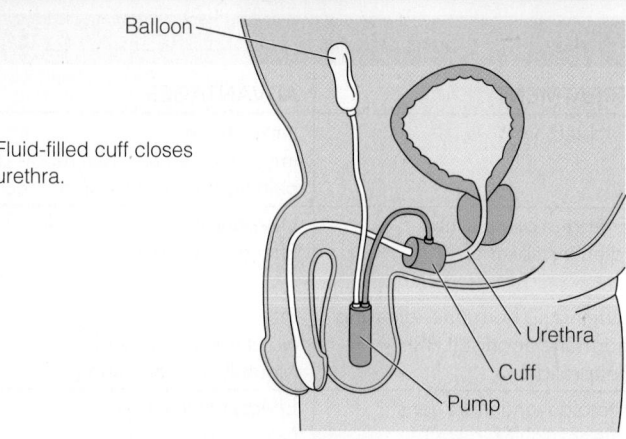

Fluid-filled cuff closes urethra.

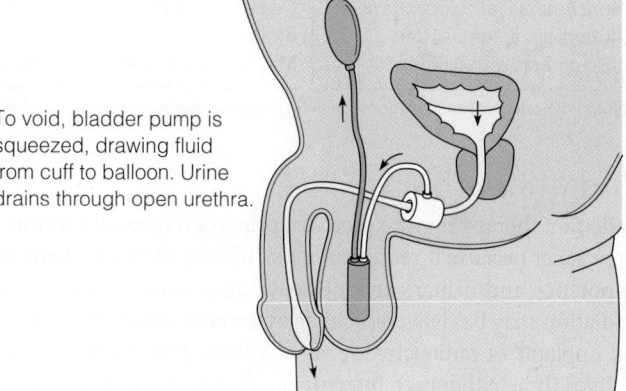

To void, bladder pump is squeezed, drawing fluid from cuff to balloon. Urine drains through open urethra.

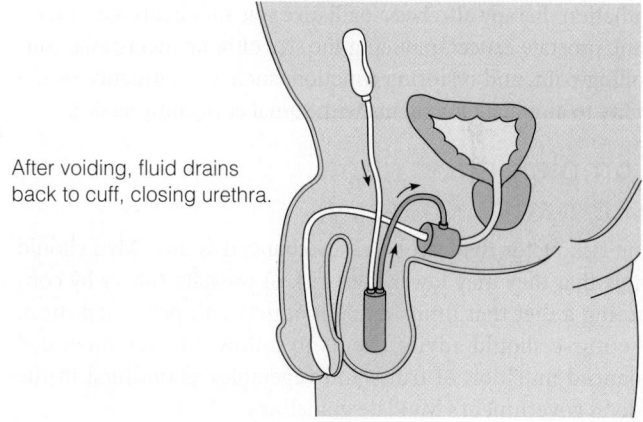

After voiding, fluid drains back to cuff, closing urethra.

Figure 2–19 ● Operation of an artificial urinary sphincter.

dependent and either cease to grow or die if deprived of androgens. Unfortunately, other cancer cells thrive without androgen and are unaffected by therapy to reduce circulating androgens. Therefore, the effects of hormone manipulations vary from complete but temporary regression of the tumor to no response at all.

Strategies to induce androgen deprivation vary from **orchiectomy** (surgical removal of one or both testicles) to oral administration of hormonal agents. **Table 2–17 ●** compares surgical and hormone therapies and the advantages and disadvantages of each. In addition, new drugs are being developed that block the effects of male hormones, and research is being conducted to determine which mix of hormones is best and at what time in the perioperative period they are most effective.

TABLE 2–17   Surgical and Hormone Therapy in the Management of Advanced Prostate Cancer

TREATMENT	ADVANTAGES	DISADVANTAGES
Orchiectomy	Inexpensive Immediate effect; men report diminished pain from metastasis in the recovery room	Body image problems resulting from loss of testicles
Estrogen compounds (diethylstilbestrol)	Inexpensive Effects reversible	Increased risk of cardiovascular problems More likely to cause gynecomastia, hypertrophy of breast tissue
Luteinizing hormone-releasing hormone agonist (LHRH) (leuprolide)	Effects reversible No cardiovascular risk Monthly administration	Very expensive Subcutaneous injection route Slow onset: up to 4 weeks
Steroidal antiandrogens (megestrol [Megace])	Effects reversible No cardiovascular risk Inexpensive	May not drop testosterone levels sufficiently Weight gain
Nonsteroidal antiandrogens (flutamide; often used in conjunction with LHRH)	Does not alter circulating androgens Blocks some side effects of LHRH May be effective if other methods fail	Very expensive

Note: All hormonal manipulations have the potential disadvantage of loss of libido, erectile dysfunction, hot flashes, and gynecomastia.

Radiation Therapy

Radiation therapy may be used as a primary treatment for prostate cancer because it reduces the risk of long-term problems of impotence and urinary incontinence associated with surgery. Radiation may be delivered either by external beam or interstitial implants of radioactive seeds of iodine, gold, palladium, or iridium (brachytherapy). Interstitial radiation has a lower risk of impotence and rectal damage than external-beam radiation. Radiation therapy also has a palliative role for clients with metastatic prostate cancer, reducing the size of bone metastasis, controlling pain, and restoring function, such as continence or the ability to ambulate for clients with spinal cord compression.

Complementary and Alternative Therapy

One risk factor that can be easily changed is diet. Men should know that they may lower their risk of prostate cancer by consuming a diet that limits dairy products and processed meat. The nurse should advise clients to follow the recommended balanced nutrition of fruits and vegetables as outlined in the federal government's MyPlate guidelines.

As a component of wellness promotion, the nurse should emphasize disease prevention, including avoidance of unintentional harm. Natural and over-the-counter therapies and supplements should not be unquestionably presumed to be safe. For example, according to the National Center for Complementary and Alternative Medicine (2011), recent studies demonstrate an increased risk of prostate cancer among men who take vitamin E supplements. Nursing assessment should include interviewing the client as to his use of nutritional supplements and nonprescription therapies. Likewise, clients should be urged to consult their healthcare provider regarding the safety and efficacy of complementary and alternative therapies prior to engaging in their use.

◼ NURSING PROCESS

Nurses plan and implement interventions to help prevent prostate cancer and to facilitate a return to functional health status once prostate cancer is diagnosed. Nurses are in a unique position to increase public awareness about early detection of prostate cancer. Every encounter with men and their families—in clinics, hospital units, or in the home—is an opportunity to provide information about early detection and to identify needs. Several studies have shown a positive correlation between increased awareness of and participation in prostate cancer screening procedures.

◉ *Stay Current:* The National Cancer Institute has free pamphlets about prostate cancer that are useful for educating the public. Download a pamphlet at **www.cancer.gov/cancertopics/wyntk/prostate/page1/AllPages**.

Assessment

Collect the following data through the health history and physical examination:

- ◼ *Health history.* Risk factors, urinary elimination patterns and manifestations, hematuria, pain
- ◼ *Physical assessment.* Digital rectal examination to assess prostate size, symmetry, firmness, and nodules; assess for bladder distention, urinary flow, and urine retention.

Note that a DRE is an advanced nursing assessment.

Diagnosis

Potential nursing diagnoses appropriate for inclusion in the nursing care plan for a client with prostate cancer will vary, depending on the individual client and the medical interventions used. Although not intended to be all inclusive, nursing diagnoses relevant to the care of a client with prostate cancer may include the following:

- ◼ *Impaired Urinary Elimination*
- ◼ *Risk for Urinary Retention*
- ◼ *Risk for Stress Urinary Incontinence*
- ◼ *Sexual Dysfunction*
- ◼ *Pain.*

(NANDA-I © 2012)

Planning

Goals of nursing care may include the following:

- The client will express concerns and emotions related to his diagnosis and the potential effects of treatment.
- The client will demonstrate optimal urinary function, including urine elimination of at least 0.5 mL/kg/hr.
- The client will verbalize awareness of strategies for promoting urinary continence.
- The client will demonstrate the ability to make informed decisions regarding all treatments.
- Using a predetermined pain rating scale, the client will report his pain is maintained at a level deemed by him to be tolerable.

Implementation

Nursing care must be provided with sensitivity because clients are often worried about loss of virility, sexual function, and masculinity, and they may be reluctant to discuss these concerns with the nurse. Holistic care must be provided to meet the client's physical, psychosocial, and spiritual needs.

Promote Urinary Elimination

Urinary incontinence is a disturbing complication following treatment for prostate cancer. Both radical prostatectomy and external-beam radiation therapy can cause incontinence, ranging from passage of a small amount of urine when lifting a heavy object (stress incontinence) to complete and unpredictable loss of control (total incontinence). Older men may experience involuntary passage of urine soon after a strong sense of urgency to void (urge incontinence). For the client, any degree of incontinence may be disturbing. Nursing interventions appropriate for implementation in the promotion of optimal urinary elimination patterns include the following:

- Assess the degree of incontinence and its effects on lifestyle. The nurse needs to determine previous urinary patterns and the type of incontinence currently being experienced to plan appropriate interventions.
- Teach Kegel exercises to help restore continence. Pelvic muscle or Kegel exercises can often either eliminate or improve stress incontinence. (Kegel exercises are discussed in the module on Elimination.)
- Teach methods to control dampness and odor from stress incontinence:
  a. Do not attempt to prevent accidental voiding by restricting fluids. Not only will the man continue to have incontinent episodes, but his urine will become concentrated, exacerbating the problem with odor.
  b. Manage occasional episodes (one to three small-volume accidents per day) with absorbent pads worn inside the underwear and changed as needed. Most pads are made with a polymer gel that controls odor. Appropriate measures help promote good hygiene, decrease anxiety, and increase comfort.
- Refer to physical therapy or a continence specialist for additional measures to promote continence. Special exercises, restricting some types of fluids, and other measures (e.g., bladder training) can help the client deal with incontinence.
- Explore options such as an external collection device (external catheter or Texas catheter) for the man with total incontinence. This device may improve the man's self-esteem and allow resumption of social activities.
- Encourage verbalizing feelings about the impact of incontinence on quality of life. The degree of incontinence does not necessarily correlate with the perceived level of suffering. Listening to these concerns with sensitivity can help the man work through these feelings and may allow him to move toward a healthy adaptation to his disability.

Promote Communication Related to Sexual Function

Surgical treatment for prostate cancer may cause erectile dysfunction and changes in ejaculatory function. Hormone therapy for advanced prostate cancer lowers libido and may also cause erectile dysfunction. The diagnosis of cancer and the body image changes caused by hormone therapy may lower self-esteem, which in turn can diminish sexual desire and willingness to interact sexually with a partner. Most older men are sexually active and fully capable of sustaining an erection. They are likely to fear the effect of treatment on their sexual health. They may allow this concern to guide their decision about the course of treatment, or they may refuse all therapy because of this fear. Reactions vary greatly, and the nurse must maintain a sensitive, nonjudgmental approach to education and support.

- Interview the client about his pretreatment level of sexual function. Knowledge of previous sexual function is necessary to plan appropriate interventions.
- Teach the client about the actual or potential effects of therapy on sexual function. The incidence of erectile dysfunction varies with different therapies for prostate cancer.
- Provide an opportunity for the client and his partner to discuss implications of and concerns about the diagnosis and treatment of sexual function. The treatments for prostate cancer often affect the physiology of erection. The man and his partner need support and counseling during the period of adjustment.
- Discuss medical and surgical treatments for erectile dysfunction. Many men are as devastated by the loss of erectile function as they are by the diagnosis of cancer. Information about achieving erection and maintaining sexual intimacy is essential to quality of life.
- Refer for sexual counseling as appropriate. The man and his partner may require therapy beyond that provided by nurses.

Promote Effective Pain Management

Men with advanced prostate cancer experience many causes of pain. It is not unusual for a client to have three or four distinct pains simultaneously, all from different sources. The most common cause of pain is metastasis to the spinal column, usually the thoracic spine. Other sources of pain include fractures, lymphedema of the lower extremities, and muscle spasms. Because most men with prostate cancer are over the age of 65, many also have pain associated with preexisting conditions, such as osteoarthritis, unrelated to the cancer.

- Assess the intensity, location, and quality of the pain. A cardinal rule of successful pain management is the importance of reducing or eliminating the cause of pain. Appropriate interventions are based on a careful assessment of the client's pain.
- Provide optimal pain relief with prescribed analgesics. It is important for both the client and his family to understand that pain medications should be used on a regular basis to maintain comfort and should not be delayed until pain is severe.
- Teach the client and his family noninvasive methods of pain control. Various modalities can be successful in alleviating pain or reducing its perception, thus enhancing the comfort of the client. For example, some research suggests massage therapy and touch therapy may be useful in reducing cancer-related pain. Clients should always confer with their healthcare provider before undergoing any complementary treatment. In particular, any treatment that requires applying pressure to a tumor is discouraged (NCCAM, 2012a).

Evaluation

Expected outcomes to evaluate client care are based on goals set during the planning stage and may include the following:

- Using a predetermined pain rating scale, the client reports managing pain at a tolerable level.
- The client discusses sexual function without anxiety or discomfort.

Client Teaching Home Care for the Client With Prostate Cancer

Depending on the type of treatment, the following topics should be addressed in preparing the client and his family for home care:

- For the client having a surgical procedure: manifestations of infection and excessive bleeding, catheter care, wound care pain management
- For the client receiving radiation therapy:
  a. Danger of radiation damage to others (sleep in a room alone for a week; avoid close contact with pregnant women, infants, and children)
  b. Condom use during sexual contact (ejaculate may be discolored, distressing sexual partner)
- The importance of keeping appointments with healthcare providers and having yearly PSA and rectal examinations
- If appropriate, community services, such as support groups, home health nurses, and hospice
- Helpful resources:
  a. American Cancer Society (www.cancer.org)
  b. American Urological Association (www.auanet.org)
  c. National Cancer Institute (www.cancer.gov)

- The client lists strategies for managing urinary incontinence.
- The client maintains adequate urine output without complications related to altered urinary elimination.

NURSING CARE PLAN   A Client With Prostate Cancer

William Turner, a 71-year-old African American, lives with his wife in a small retirement community in Florida. His wife had a stroke 2 years ago, and Mr. Turner does all the cooking and housework. He has been in good health for most of his life, having only "a small touch" of osteoarthritis in his knees and hands. He has noticed a gradual onset of urinary urgency and frequency during the past 2 years but has never had incontinence.

During a routine checkup, the nurse practitioner at the local health clinic performs a digital rectal examination and palpates a hard nodule on the surface of Mr. Turner's prostate. After his PSA is found to be elevated, he is referred to a urologist, who diagnoses prostate cancer. Mr. Turner chooses to have surgery, and a radical retropubic prostatectomy and lymph node dissection are performed. The lymph nodes are negative for metastasis. Following surgery, his recovery is uncomplicated. However, the nurse caring for Mr. Turner is concerned about his ability to care for his indwelling catheter because of his arthritis and his wife's physical disabilities from the stroke. The nurse makes a referral to a home health agency to ensure Mr. Turner can manage his care at home. An initial home health assessment is scheduled for the day after Mr. Turner is discharged from the hospital.

ASSESSMENT	DIAGNOSES	PLANNING
The home health nurse notes that the house is clean and neat. Mr. Turner is dressed but still wearing his night urinary drainage bag, although it is 1300. Mr. Turner tells the nurse that his main problem is going to get groceries, because he is embarrassed to be seen with the drainage bag. He says he has not been able to remove the drainage bag and attach the leg bag because of his arthritis. Physical assessment findings include healing of the pelvic incision without signs of infection. There is no tenderness in his calves, chest pain, or shortness of breath. The urine is yellow, without odor. Mr. Turner does state that he sees no need for the pelvic exercises since he is no longer in the hospital. He also expresses the belief that he is cured of cancer and questions the need for follow-up care.	■ *Risk for Stress Urinary Incontinence* related to surgical procedure ■ *Ineffective Health Maintenance* related to inability to care for the urinary drainage system, not understanding need for postoperative exercises, and questions about follow-up care (NANDA-I © 2012)	■ The client will regain urinary continence after catheter removal. ■ The client will change the urinary drainage bag with the appropriate assistance. ■ The client will verbalize the rationale for performing postoperative exercises. ■ The client will verbalize the need for continued follow-up care.

NURSING CARE PLAN (continued)

IMPLEMENTATION

- Discuss the possibility of stress incontinence after the catheter is removed.
- Reinforce the need for Kegel exercises while the catheter is still in place.

- Explore Mr. Turner's support system to identify people who could assist him with catheter care, and arrange a teaching session with them.
- Teach Mr. Turner the importance of follow-up care, relating the care to the history of the disease.

EVALUATION

Good friends from Mr. Turner's church have assisted him with care of his drainage bag and have reminded him to do his Kegel exercises several times a day while the catheter is in place. When the catheter is removed, Mr. Turner has only a small amount of urine leakage after voiding. He understands that it may take several weeks for this to resolve. Efforts to help him understand the need for continued medical care are less successful. Mr. Turner continues to state that he is cured, his wife needs him, and he sees no need to go back to the doctor.

CRITICAL THINKING

1. Outline a teaching plan for Mr. Turner for the nursing diagnosis Risk for Altered Skin Integrity related to urinary incontinence.
2. As a result of Mr. Turner's refusal to have ongoing medical care, he might be labeled as noncompliant. Would you make this nursing diagnosis? Why, or why not?
3. If you were the home health nurse making a home visit and found that Mr. Turner had no urinary drainage for 16 hours, what assessments would you make? How would you handle this problem?

REVIEW Prostate Cancer

RELATE Link the Concepts and Exemplars

Linking the exemplar of prostate cancer with the concept of elimination:

1. What effect might prostate cancer have on the client's ability to urinate if he chooses to treat the cancer by medical, rather than surgical, therapies?

2. How can you promote adequate urinary elimination for this client?

Linking the exemplar of prostate cancer with the concept of tissue integrity:

3. What nursing interventions can promote tissue integrity in the client who recently had surgical removal of the prostate?

4. Write a teaching plan for the client preparing for discharge to home following prostatectomy.

READY Go to Companion Skills Manual

REFER Go to Pearson Nursing Student Resources
nursing.pearsonhighered.com

- Additional review materials

REFLECT Case Study

Maury Blarden is a 45-year-old client who has been diagnosed with prostate cancer. He is married and has a 3-year-old daughter. Mr. Blarden and his wife own a company that offers home renovation and decoration services. Mr. and Mrs. Blarden have been told that surgery is necessary, along with radiation and chemotherapy. Mr. Blarden tells the nurse that he and his wife are trying to have another child, hopefully, a boy. He is not sure that he can take the time away from the business for surgery and therapy. The couple has minimal healthcare coverage and is concerned about the costs of care because they barely make enough to get by.

1. What expected outcomes would be appropriate for this client?

2. Mrs. Blarden asks you, while her husband is out of the room, if the procedure will result in impotence. How will you respond to this question?

3. Will the Blardens be able to have children if he decides to undergo surgery? Explain your answer.

EXEMPLAR 2.8 Sickle Cell Disease

EXEMPLAR KEY TERMS
Alloimmunization, *124*
Hemoglobinopathy, *120*
Hemosiderosis, *123*
Priapism, *121*
Sickle cell anemia, *120*
Sickle cell crisis, *120*
Sickle cell disease (SCD), *120*
Sickle cell trait, *121*
Sickling, *120*
Vaso-occlusive crisis, *120*

EXEMPLAR LEARNING OUTCOMES
After reading about this exemplar, you will be able to:

1. Describe the pathophysiology, etiology, clinical manifestations, and direct and indirect causes of sickle cell disease.

2. Identify risk factors and prevention methods associated with sickle cell disease.

3. Illustrate the nursing process in providing culturally competent care across the life span for individuals with sickle cell disease.

4. Formulate priority nursing diagnoses appropriate for an individual with sickle cell disease.

5. Summarize therapies used by interdisciplinary teams in the collaborative care of an individual with sickle cell disease.

6. Plan evidence-based care for an individual with sickle cell disease and his or her family in collaboration with other members of the healthcare team.

7. Evaluate expected outcomes for an individual with sickle cell disease.

▶ OVERVIEW

Sickle cell disease (SCD) is a hereditary **hemoglobinopathy**, a type of disorder characterized by replacement of normal hemoglobin with abnormal hemoglobin S (Hgb S) in RBCs. **Sickle cell anemia**, a chronic hemolytic anemia, is the most common type of sickle cell disease. (See the exemplar on Anemia within this module and **Table 2–18** ●.)

▶ PATHOPHYSIOLOGY AND ETIOLOGY

When RBCs that contain Hgb S pass through blood vessels, deoxygenation of Hgb S causes the RBCs to become rigid and deformed. As a result of this distortion, the RBCs take on a crescent or sickle shape. Because of the characteristic shape of malformed RBCs associated with this disorder, the process is called **sickling**. Unlike healthy RBCs, sickled RBCs are more rigid and inflexible, and they can occlude small blood vessels, especially capillaries. Vascular occlusion can cause tissue ischemia and organ damage.

Repeated or prolonged ischemia resulting from sickle cell–induced occlusions causes damage to tissues and organs. For example, children with sickle cell disease can experience life-threatening splenic sequestration due to trapping of blood in the spleen. Many children must undergo splenectomy in early childhood, leading to severely compromised immunity. Their infection rate is subsequently high because of impaired immu-

nity, and bacterial infections are the leading cause of death in young children with SCD. Repeated sickling episodes weaken RBC cell membranes and shorten the life span of affected RBCs. Early destruction of RBCs can lead to anemia.

Sickling may be triggered by any condition that increases the body's need for oxygen, including fever, emotional or physical stress, high altitudes, poorly pressurized airplanes, hypoventilation, and vasoconstriction due to cold temperatures. **Sickle cell crisis** (also called **vaso-occlusive crisis**) is the term used to describe painful periods resulting from ischemia due to vascular occlusion. Any condition that increases the body's need for oxygen or alters the transport of oxygen, such as infection or trauma, may result in sickle cell crisis. Although potential causes include those known to trigger sickling, in more than 50% of cases, the exact cause of sickle cell crisis is not identifiable (UMMC, 2009b). Dehydration increases blood viscosity, which can predispose an individual to sickle cell crisis.

Sickled cells can resume a normal shape when rehydrated and reoxygenated. The membrane of these cells becomes more fragile, however, and cell life is shortened to 10–20 days rather than the usual 120 days. In response, bone marrow spaces enlarge to produce more RBCs. In some individuals with SCD, bone marrow ceases to produce new RBCs, leading to aplastic crisis (CDC, 2011b).

Etiology

The disorder is transmitted as an autosomal recessive genetic defect. If both parents have the trait, then with each pregnancy the risk of having a child with the disease is 25%. The Hb S gene changes the structure of the beta chain of the hemoglobin molecule. When hypoxemia develops and Hb S is deoxygenated, it crystallizes into rodlike structures. Clusters of these rods form long chains that deform the erythrocyte into a crescent or sickle shape (**Figure 2–20** ●). The sickled cells tend to clump together and obstruct capillary blood flow, causing ischemia and possible infarction of surrounding tissue.

TABLE 2–18	Forms of Sickle Cell Disease
SICKLE CELL DISEASE	DESCRIPTION
Sickle cell trait HbAS	Most common form of sickle cell disease in the United States
	Heterozygous condition in which the child inherits one sickle cell (Hb S) gene and one normal hemoglobin (Hb A) gene
	Child is carrier of sickle cell disease and rarely has symptoms of the disease.
Sickle cell anemia HbSS	Homozygous condition (child inherits two Hb S genes)
	Child is subject to sickle cell crises.
Sickle cell syndromes HbSC	Variation in which the child inherits a sickle cell gene (Hb S) from one parent and an abnormal hemoglobin gene from the other parent (Hb C). Most often, this produces a less severe form of SCD.
Hb S beta thalassemia	Child inherits a sickle cell gene (Hb S) from one parent and one of two types of genes for beta thalassemia from the other parent.
	Manifestations of SCD can range from mild to severe.

Focus on Diversity and Culture
Cultural Prevalence of Sickle Cell Disease

Sickle cell disease tends to affect people whose origins are in equatorial countries, particularly those in central Africa, the Near East, the Mediterranean region, and parts of India. Hispanics from the Caribbean and Central and South America also may have the Hb S gene. This gene may have originated to protect against lethal forms of malaria, an endemic disease in many equatorial regions.

SCD affects approximately 90,000 to 100,000 individuals in the United States. In African Americans, SCD occurs in 1 out of every 500 births. Among Hispanic Americans, SCD occurs in 1 of every 36,000 births (CDC, 2011c).

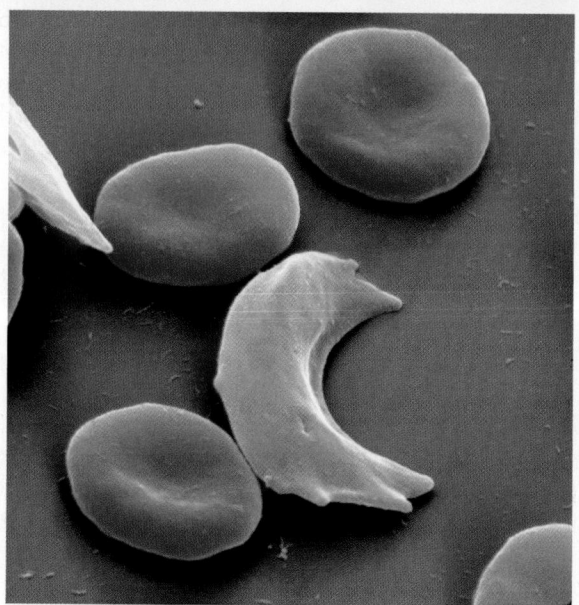

Figure 2–20 ● Blood smear containing normal red blood cells and sickle cells.

Source: Oliver Meckes & Nicole Ottawa/Science Source.

Risk Factors

The disease is most common among people of African descent. In the United States, an estimated 1 in 12 African Americans carries one abnormal hemoglobin (Hb S) gene and thus has **sickle cell trait**. These carriers are likely to remain asymptomatic unless stressed by severe hypoxia. SCD, which requires inheritance of two Hb S genes (one from each parent), occurs in approximately 1 in 500 African American births. Individuals with SCD are at risk for sickle cell crisis.

▶ CLINICAL MANIFESTATIONS

The acute and chronic manifestations of sickle cell anemia arise from episodes of RBC sickling. Sickling causes general manifestations of hemolytic anemia, including pallor, fatigue, jaundice, and irritability. Repeated infarcts associated with sickling can affect the structure and function of nearly every organ system. Clients with SCD may develop an enlarged spleen and liver, renal insufficiency, gallstones, and other manifestations of organ dysfunction. **Priapism** (painful, prolonged penile erection) may develop as well. Abdominal pain may signal infarction of abdominal organs and structures. Skin ulcers may develop as the result of occluded vessels supplying the dermis.

Pain intensity and duration vary depending on the individual and the location. Pain may be transient in a localized area, such as the wrist, to severe, generalized pain that lasts for several days or weeks and may require hospitalization. The pain is often severe enough to require opioid analgesics and the use of a patient-controlled analgesic pump.

Stroke is a significant risk for all clients diagnosed with SCD. Other complications of SCD include aplastic crisis or temporary cessation of bone marrow blood cell production (UMMC, 2009b).

Extensive sickling can precipitate a crisis as a result of occluded circulation, impaired erythropoiesis, or sequestration of large amounts of blood in the liver or spleen (**Table 2–19 ●**).

As previously described, sickle cell crisis occurs when sickled cells obstruct vascular blood flow, which can lead to tissue ischemia and infarction. These excruciating vaso-occlusive crises last an average of 4–6 days. (On a much smaller scale, vaso-occlusion involves tightly wrapping a rubber band around one's finger to the degree that blood flow is obstructed.) For the

TABLE 2–19 Overview of Sickle Cell Crisis

ETIOLOGY	CLINICAL MANIFESTATIONS
Vaso-occlusion (thrombotic)	■ Most common type of crisis; may last for days or weeks. ■ Precipitated by dehydration, exposure to cold, acidosis, or localized hypoxemia. ■ Caused by stasis of blood with clumping of cells in the microcirculation, ischemia, and infarction. ■ Thrombosis and infarction of local tissue may occur if the crisis is not reversed. ■ Cerebral occlusion can result in stroke, manifested by paralysis or other central nervous system complications. ■ Extremely painful; symptoms include fever, tissue engorgement, painful swelling of joints in hands and feet, priapism, and severe abdominal pain.
Splenic sequestration	■ Life-threatening crisis; death can occur within hours. ■ Caused by pooling of blood in the spleen; because the spleen can hold much of the body's blood supply, cardiovascular collapse can result. Most commonly seen in children and adolescents; may be seen in young adults. ■ Clinical manifestations include profound anemia, hypovolemia, and shock.
Aplastic crises	■ Diminished production and increased destruction of red blood cells. ■ Often triggered by human parvovirus B19 viral infection. ■ Signs include profound anemia, pallor, and fatigue.
Acute chest syndrome	■ Common cause of hospitalization for sickle cell disease. ■ Associated with pediatric mortality rate of 2% and adult mortality rate of 4%. ■ Pulmonary infiltrate of abnormal blood cells leads to lower respiratory tract symptoms. ■ Clinical manifestations include fever, cough, chest and back pain, dyspnea, and hypoxemia. ■ Pulmonary infection, infarct, and fat embolism may occur and can lead to pulmonary failure and death.

Source: Data from University of Maryland Medical Center (UMMC). (2009b). *Sickle cell disease—Complications.* Retrieved from http://www.umm.edu/patiented/ articles/what_complications_of_sickle-cell_disease_their_treatments_000058_6.htm; Centers for Disease Control and Prevention. (2011c). *Sickle cell disease (SDC)— Data & statistics.* Retrieved from http://www.cdc.gov/ncbddd/sicklecell/data.html.

individual experiencing the intense vaso-occlusion associated with sickle cell crisis, infarction of small vessels in the extremities causes painful swelling of the hands and feet; large joints also may be affected. Infarction also may affect bone marrow or lead to aseptic necrosis of affected bones resulting in pain from avascular necrosis of the bone marrow and is typically experienced in the back, abdomen, chest, and joints. Acute chest syndrome, a symptom complex that includes fever, chest pain, an increasing WBC count, and pulmonary infiltrates, may develop, as well as other complications, such as pneumonia, pulmonary infarction, pulmonary embolism, and even death (CDC, 2011b; Porth & Matfin, 2010).

Lifespan Considerations

PEDIATRIC CLIENTS Affected children are usually asymptomatic until 4–6 months of age because sickling is inhibited by high levels of fetal hemoglobin. Children with sickle cell disease can also experience chest tightness and shortness of breath, which are diagnostic for acute chest syndrome and medical crisis. Among children with SCD, 10% will experience a stroke, which can result in permanent disabilities, learning impairment, and other neurological outcomes (CDC, 2011b).

Children with sickle cell trait rarely experience sickle cell crisis. However, because they have some abnormal hemoglobin, they may develop symptoms of the disease under conditions of abnormally low oxygen, such as flying in an unpressurized airplane over 7,000 feet or when anesthesia is administered. The most common symptoms experienced by those with sickle cell trait are splenic infarction and hematuria. However, most individuals who carry the trait never have symptoms, even with low oxygen concentrations.

PREGNANT CLIENTS Pregnant women diagnosed with SCD often experience more frequent pain crises, along with more intense symptoms. Additionally, they are at higher risk for complications including miscarriage, premature birth, and low birth weight. With vigilant prenatal care and monitoring, the majority of pregnant women with SCD can expect positive outcomes (CDC, 2011c).

▶ COLLABORATION

Optimal care for the client with sickle cell disease involves coordinated efforts by members of a healthcare team. Neonatal screening, early intervention, prophylactic antibiotics, and parent education have allowed children with sickle cell disease to live into adulthood. A nurse with a specialty in genetics, or a genetics counselor, may be involved in sickle cell gene testing and counseling to identify and inform carriers and children who have the disease.

Diagnostic Tests

In the United States, newborn screening for SCD is mandatory. While prenatal diagnosis of SCD is possible using amniocentesis, the initial diagnosis of SCD in newborns is most often made by testing a few drops of blood obtained by way of a heelstick. For adults, a venous blood sample is usually obtained from the arm. Blood samples are evaluated for the presence of Hb S. Positive samples are further evaluated to identify the number of sickle cell genes present. The presence of two Hb S genes, which correlates with a diagnosis of SCD, warrants further testing (including RBC count) to assess for anemia (Mayo Clinic, 2011b).

For the pediatric client with SCD, additional diagnostic testing may be indicated for prevention of stroke. Beginning at age 2 years, children with SCD should undergo routine ultrasound scanning of the head to assess cerebral blood flow (NHLBI, 2012e).

SAFETY ALERT Neither hot nor cold compresses should be used for pain management in the child with sickle cell disease. Ischemic tissue is fragile and has reduced sensation, increasing the risk of burn injury from hot compresses, whereas cold compresses promote sickling.

Surgery

Bone marrow or hematopoietic stem cell transplantation may be considered. However, a recurrence of the disease is demonstrated in approximately 10% of recipients. For clients experiencing splenic sequestration of RBCs, blood transfusion is the most common treatment; however, in life-threatening instances of splenic RBC sequestration, splenectomy may be necessary (CDC, 2011b).

Pharmacologic Therapy

For the client experiencing complications related to SCD, mainstays of treatment include oxygenation, hydration, and analgesic administration. Oxygen is usually administered to reduce the risk of hypoxemia and associated complications, as well as to promote comfort and minimize dyspnea. Oral and IV fluid replacement also promotes pain relief, since dehydration is often a cause of crisis. Fluids reduce the viscosity of the blood, so adequate hydration is essential. Parenteral analgesics, such as morphine, are generally administered around the clock or via patient-controlled analgesia. Particularly in children, pain medications should not be ordered on an "as needed" basis, because this increases the child's anxiety and delays medication administration.

Treatment with hydroxyurea has been helpful in adults and is now being used more frequently in children. This cytotoxic medication decreases production of abnormal blood cells and leads to a lesser amount of pain being experienced. Additionally, hydroxyurea increases fetal hemoglobin production and red cell mean corpuscular volume (NHLBI, 2012e). Side effects of hydroxyurea include bone marrow suppression, headaches, dizziness, nausea, and vomiting.

For all children between 2 months and 5 years of age who are diagnosed with SCD, treatment often includes daily administration of prophylactic penicillin (NHLBI, 2012e). Children who are functionally asplenic or have had a splenectomy have a resultant decreased capability to fight infection. For this reason,

Clinical Manifestations and Therapies **Sickle Cell Disease**

ETIOLOGY	CLINICAL MANIFESTATIONS	CLINICAL THERAPIES
Dyspnea ■ Due to inadequate delivery of oxygen to cells, tissues, and organs	■ Hypoxia, lethargy, fatigue, shortness of breath, tachypnea, decreased oxygen saturation level	■ Supplemental oxygen ■ Elevate head of bed (HOB) to point of client comfort. ■ Blood transfusions ■ Monitor oxygen saturation level. ■ Auscultate lungs at least every 4 hours and as needed.
Anemia ■ May be due to increased RBC destruction, impaired RBC production, or both.	■ Hypoxia, lethargy, fatigue, pallor, shortness of breath, complaints of dyspnea, tachycardia, decreased RBC and Hgb measurements	■ Blood transfusions ■ BMT or SCT
Impaired circulation ■ Due to impaired flow of sickled RBCs	■ Impaired oxygenation, tachypnea, tachycardia, edema, splenic sequestration of RBCs ■ In pediatric clients (usually in those younger than 4 years old), sickle cells can obstruct small blood vessels in the hands and feet, causing a condition called hand-foot syndrome, which manifests as pain, fever, and swelling.	■ Blood transfusions ■ IV and oral hydration ■ Prevent physical exacerbation and exposure to environments or circumstances that increase oxygen demand. ■ Splenectomy
Risk for infection ■ Due to inadequate circulation	■ Fever, tachypnea, tachycardia, increased WBC count, localized symptoms of infection (e.g., redness, drainage, and swelling at a specific site) ■ Blood cultures positive for infectious organism	■ Administer antibiotics as ordered for prophylactic and acute treatment. ■ Encourage client to adhere to current vaccination recommendations, as well as to receive annual influenza and pneumococcal vaccinations. ■ Adhere to standard precautions and organizational protocols for infection prevention.
Pain ■ Due to vascular occlusion by RBCs	■ Complaints of pain or discomfort ■ Increased blood pressure, pulse, and respiratory rate due to sympathetic nervous system stimulation may or may not be present. ■ Objective indicators of pain, including crying, grimacing, and guarding affected sites	■ Promote oxygenation and vascular flow of blood through hydration and, if indicated, transfusion of RBCs. ■ Administer analgesics as ordered. ■ Administer hydroxyurea as ordered. ■ Massage

infection is a serious condition requiring immediate attention. When an infection is suspected, cultures (blood, urine, and throat) are obtained to identify the source of infection and the offending organism. Aggressive antibiotic therapy is implemented immediately.

Because infection is especially dangerous for the client with SCD, recommendations for clients of all ages include keeping current with vaccinations, plus receiving annual influenza and pneumococcal vaccinations (NHLBI, 2012e).

Stay Current: *To view current Centers for Disease Control and Prevention vaccination schedules, visit* **www.cdc.gov/vaccines/ schedules**.

Nonpharmacologic Therapy

Blood transfusions are also a core component of treatment for the client with SCD. Benefits of transfusions include improved blood and tissue oxygenation, a reduction in sickling, and a temporary suppression of the production of RBCs containing Hb S. Several types of blood transfusion are used.

A complication associated with frequent transfusions is an overload of iron in the body. The iron is stored in tissues and organs (**hemosiderosis**) because the body has no way of excreting it. For this reason, an iron-chelating drug, such as deferoxamine, may be given with vitamin C to promote iron excretion. Another complication of multiple transfusions is the development of alloimmunization to red cell and platelet antigens (Osborn et al., 2013). **Alloimmunization** occurs when the child's immune system reacts against antigens on the donated tissues (e.g., blood and stem cells).

Additionally, chronic transfusions have proven to be an effective treatment for stroke complications related to sickle cell disease. In children who have had strokes from the disease, periodic transfusions (approximately every 3–4 weeks) can reduce the incidence of future strokes (UMMC, 2009c). If administered early in the crisis, blood transfusions may relieve the ischemia caused by vaso-occlusion in major organs and body parts, such as the spleen, lung, kidney, brain, and penis. Exchange transfusion is preferred in order to reduce the potential of fluid volume excess.

Complementary and Alternative Therapy

Research suggests massage effectively reduces pain associated with SCD (NCCAM, 2010). Additional studies are in progress to evaluate the effects of nutritional supplements (i.e., acetyl-L-carnitine and alpha-lipoic acid) on the inflammatory process in clients with SCD (NCCAM, 2012b).

NURSING PROCESS

For the client diagnosed with SCD, a comprehensive physical assessment is essential because any body system can be affected. The nurse focuses on providing care to the client as well as teaching both the client and family how to reduce sickling, provide home care, and symptoms to report to the provider immediately.

Assessment

In clients who are known to have SCD, obtain a detailed history from the client or parents about past crises, precipitating events, medical treatment, and home management. For adult clients, using a pain rating scale, ask the client to rate her chronic or acute pain. For pediatric clients, use age-appropriate pain rating scales and objective (visual) assessment for indicators of pain. (See the module on Comfort for discussion of pain assessment across the life span.) Pain may occur in nearly any body part but most commonly manifests as headache, extremity pain, or abdominal discomfort. Assess the methods of pain management protocols used and ask which interventions have been most effective. Because failure to thrive is common among children with SCD, for pediatric clients, obtain a height and weight for comparison with previous measurements or to serve as a baseline for future comparison.

Fever, neurological changes (e.g., decreased alertness or behavioral changes), and respiratory symptoms are emergency conditions that necessitate prompt treatment. For the client experiencing sickle cell crisis, in addition to assessing for indicators of inflammation or infection, be aware that a crisis can deteriorate into a life-threatening situation. Carefully monitor these clients for signs of shock (hypotension, changes in level of consciousness, dizziness or light-headedness, increased capillary refill time).

SCD is a chronic illness that can interfere with self-concept, level of independent function, and ADLs. Depending on the client's age and developmental stage, disturbed self-concept and body image, guilt about disturbing the family routines, depression, and isolation can occur.

The family of a child with sickle cell disease requires ongoing, thorough psychosocial assessment. If the child is newly diagnosed with the disorder, the family will need assistance to deal with feelings related to the disease's serious, life-threatening nature. Assess parents' understanding of the disease transmission, and ask whether genetic counseling has been obtained. Determine whether the family has adequate healthcare coverage to pay for the child's medical expenses. Ask older children about their knowledge of the disease, and explore their feelings related to the management of a chronic condition. When siblings or other family members are carriers, they should receive periodic counseling during the life span so that they understand the implications for dating, marriage, and having children.

Diagnosis

Using the assessment data, nursing diagnoses are chosen to reflect the needs of the specific client and family members. Examples of nursing diagnoses that may be appropriate for inclusion in the plan of care for a client with sickle cell disease include the following:

- *Impaired Gas Exchange*
- *Risk for Ineffective Breathing Pattern*
- *Risk for Decreased Cardiac Tissue Perfusion*
- *Risk for Imbalanced Fluid Volume*
- *Risk for Ineffective Cerebral Tissue Perfusion*
- *Risk for Infection*
- *Acute Pain*
- *Caregiver Role Strain*
- *Interrupted Family Processes*
- *Delayed Growth and Development*
- *Impaired Physical Mobility.*

(NANDA-I © 2012)

Planning

Identified outcomes are specific to the nursing diagnoses included in the client's plan of care. Examples of identified outcomes and goals appropriate for the client with SCD may include the following:

- The client's oxygen saturation will be maintained at greater than 90%.
- The client's respiratory rate will range between 12 and 20 breaths per minute at rest and with appropriate activity.
- The client will deny shortness of breath and dyspnea at rest and with appropriate activity.
- The client will deny manifestations of acute chest syndrome, including chest pain, adventitious breath sounds, pulmonary infiltrates, and increased WBC count.
- The client will demonstrate no signs or symptoms of stroke.
- The client will demonstrate urine output of at least 0.5 mL/kg/hr.
- The client will demonstrate no signs or symptoms of infection.
- Using a predetermined pain rating scale in which 0 represents "no pain" and 10 represents "the worst possible pain," the adult client will consistently rate his pain at a level of 3 or less.
- Using a predetermined, developmentally appropriate pain rating scale, the pediatric client will consistently rate her pain as being tolerable or absent.
- The client will meet criteria (e.g., height and weight) for normal growth and development.

Implementation

Nursing management for the client in crisis focuses on optimizing tissue perfusion, promoting hydration, controlling pain, preventing infection, ensuring adequate nutrition, preventing complications, and providing emotional support to the child and family.

Promote Optimal Oxygenation and Circulation

Administer oxygen, IV fluids, and blood transfusions as ordered. Because children receive treatment every 3 weeks, nurses commonly insert the intravenous access devices and maintain the lines and infusions used. To prevent hemolysis, the IV fluid administered with a blood transfusion must be saline rather than D₅W. In small children, the blood is usually infused without saline, because they cannot tolerate the additional fluid volume. Monitor for transfusion reactions.

Encourage the client to balance activity and rest. Work with the client and family to identify healthy methods of coping with emotional stress, and plan with the family for the trips to the healthcare facility. Any activities that increase cellular metabolism also increase oxygen demands, so the client or family may need assistance with planning daily activities. For pediatric clients, schedule caregiving activities and play during hospitalizations and clinic visits to allow for optimal rest.

> **SAFETY ALERT**
> Normal saline (0.9% NS) is the only fluid approved for concurrent administration with blood products by the American Association of Blood Banks (Roback, 2011). However, at some institutions lactated Ringer's may be administered with blood products.

Maintain Fluid Volume Balance

For the client with sickle cell disease, dehydration can lead to life-threatening consequences. Administer IV fluids as ordered. Adjust oral intake as necessary to keep the child well hydrated. Calculate the client's fluid maintenance requirements (minimum daily fluid intake), and monitor her oral and IV fluid intake. Teach clients and parents how to monitor intake and output, and provide client teaching regarding fluid management.

Manage Pain

Administer prescribed analgesics around the clock during crises. If patient-controlled analgesia is used, be sure that the constant infusions run as ordered and that the parent or child understands the use of bolus infusions when needed. Reposition the infant and young child carefully, supporting joints and extremities on pillows or special mattresses. Assist the child to assume a comfortable position. Avoid putting stress on painful joints or other body parts. Pain management is important for comfort, healing, and for promoting physical mobility.

Prevent and Manage Infection

Infection makes the client more susceptible to a crisis, and the crisis in turn increases susceptibility to infection. Teach the client or parents how to administer antibiotics for prophylaxis or treatment of infection. Be sure the family has the finances and other resources to obtain and give daily antibiotics. Because infections can be particularly virulent and can cause death in these children, parents should be instructed to obtain immediate care when the child is ill. Encourage the use of the pneumococcal vaccine for all infants and children with the disease. The Hib vaccine series should be started at 2 months of age and continued at recommended ages to prevent another common source of infection.

Client Teaching   The Child With Sickle Cell Disease

- Provide parents with information about SCD and the child's treatment. Even parents of a child previously diagnosed with the disorder may benefit from information about the disease process and its management. Explain the basic effect of tissue hypoxia and the effects of sickling on circulation.

- Teach parents to look for signs of dehydration, such as dry mucous membranes, weight loss, and sunken fontanelles in infants. Give specific instructions about how many ounces of liquid the child needs to drink each day. Emphasize that increased fluid intake is needed to replace the fluids lost from overheating or exposure to hot weather.

- Make sure both the child and family understand the triggers and precipitating factors for sickle cell crises. Encourage them to avoid situations that cause crises. Instruct the child and parents about signs and symptoms of crises that should be reported to their healthcare provider.

- Provide the family with careful instructions about infusion therapy. When regular blood infusions are used, the resulting iron overload is damaging to body organs. Children treated with transfusions need infusion of deferoxamine (Desferal) for iron overload. The medication is usually given by subcutaneous or IV routes over 8–10 hours. Prompt recognition of side effects and careful management of the lengthy infusion process are important. The child needs to be monitored for skin reactions and allergic responses. Have parents demonstrate the infusion technique and state what to do in case of reactions. Pain management is needed during infusion because the site may be tender and uncomfortable.

- Instruct parents that it is important to inform all treating physicians and dentists of the child's medical condition. Special precautions are necessary when the child undergoes surgery of any kind, because hypoxia resulting from anesthesia is a major surgical risk. The child should also wear a medical identification tag or bracelet.

- Family members need ongoing support to deal with the stress of having a child with a chronic condition. Provide resources, respite care for parents, and information as needed for siblings.

- Encourage older children with sickle cell disease to participate in activities with other children between crises but to avoid strenuous physical exertion and contact sports. Play and social interactions that promote learning and development are important.

Facilitate Normal Growth and Development

Emphasize the importance of adequate nutrition and hydration to promote growth. Encourage the child to eat a high-protein, high-calorie diet. Emphasize the importance of folic acid and vitamin C supplements as prescribed. Perform regular growth measurements, and if slow growth is apparent, perform 24-hour diet recalls and other nutritional assessments.

SAFETY ALERT

A priority of nursing care for the client with SCD is the prevention of complications of crises. Observe the child for signs of increasing anemia and shock (mental status change, pallor, vital sign changes). Maintain ongoing monitoring of the child's neurological status for evidence of altered cerebral function. Assess for an enlarged spleen by gentle palpation. Administer blood transfusions and watch the child for any adverse reaction. Assess growth and developmental milestones.

Reduce Risk for Caregiver Role Strain

Sickle cell disease is a chronic disease that is accompanied by life-threatening episodic crises. Family members often need support to help them deal with their feelings about the diagnosis and its implications. Explore resources in the home and community to see if parents will be able to administer medications and fluids and to provide adequate nutrition. Assess their knowledge of signs of infection and of sickle cell crisis and when to seek medical care for the child. Refer the parents for genetic counseling, particularly if they plan to have more children. Encourage adolescents and young adults in the family to receive genetic counseling and testing as well. Referrals to support groups and contact with others with the disease can be helpful.

Collaborate with family members, and provide them with ongoing support to deal with the stress of having a child with a chronic condition. Provide resources, including information about respite care for parents and information as needed for siblings. Sickle cell disease and some other hematological disorders of childhood require that parents provide ongoing monitoring and care for their children with these chronic conditions. Refer parents to support groups or further information.

Stay Current: *Visit the Web site of the Sickle Cell Disease Association of American at* **www.sicklecelldisease.org/index. cfm** *to find resources for families.*

Evaluation

Expected outcomes of nursing care for the client with SCD include the following:

- The client demonstrates no signs or symptoms of hypoxia.
- The client denies dyspnea.
- The client experiences no complications of SCD, including stroke or acute chest syndrome.
- The client demonstrates indicators of adequate hydration, including urine output of at least 0.5 mL/kg/hr and moist mucous membranes.
- The client demonstrates no signs or symptoms of infection.
- The client is current and up to date with all recommended vaccinations.
- The client reports absence of pain or pain at level she finds tolerable.
- Family and healthcare personnel promptly recognize and treat complications of the disease.
- The pediatric client meets normal growth and developmental milestones.
- Parents and other family members are referred for and receive information to manage and understand the disease.
- The family demonstrates adequate knowledge of the disease and treatment regimens.

NURSING CARE PLAN   A Client With Sickle Cell Disease

Mark Gotham is 10 years old. He was diagnosed with sickle cell disease shortly after birth. Both his mother and father carry the trait, but neither has the disease. Mark started fifth grade at a new school last week and was worried the kids would make fun of him because of his small stature and occasional limp. Instead of going to lunch with the other kids, he stayed in the classroom so no one would see how he limps when he walks. He became dehydrated and started to feel severe pain in his right leg. His mother brought him to the emergency department.

ASSESSMENT	DIAGNOSES	PLANNING
Mark is crying in pain and holding his right upper thigh. His vital signs include: temperature 98.4°F oral; pulse 112 bpm; respirations 24/min; and BP 118/65 mmHg. Popliteal, dorsalis pedis, and posterior tibial pulses are palpable in both legs.	■ *Ineffective Tissue Perfusion* related to alteration in hemoglobin ■ *Risk for Deficient Fluid Volume* related to inadequate fluid intake and dehydration ■ *Chronic Pain* related to chronic physical disability and clustering of sickled cells ■ *Risk for Infection* related to chronic disease and splenic malfunction ■ *Deficient Knowledge* (child and parents) related to lack of exposure about cause and treatment of sickle cell disease (NANDA-I © 2012)	■ The child will show no signs and symptoms of acute tissue hypoxia. ■ The child will maintain or be restored to adequate hydration. ■ The child will verbalize that pain is controlled. ■ The child will not develop infection. ■ The child and family will verbalize understanding of risk factors for sickle cell crises and how to minimize them.

NURSING CARE PLAN (continued)

IMPLEMENTATION

- Assess oxygenation status and efficacy of breathing.
- Position client to minimize work of breathing and promote comfort.
- Give oxygen as ordered.
- Administer IV fluids and blood transfusions as ordered.
- Calculate the client's daily fluid requirements and ensure appropriate fluid intake.
- Monitor and record fluid intake and output.
- Assess for signs and symptoms of dehydration.
- Administer analgesics, such as morphine or hydromorphone (Dilaudid), as ordered.
- Isolate the child from possible sources of infection. Instruct parents about signs of infection, and encourage them to seek prompt health care.

- Instruct the child to avoid physical exertion, emotional stress, low-oxygen environments (e.g., airplanes and high altitudes), and known sources of infection.
- Instruct the family to report fever, vomiting, diarrhea, or other signs of fluid imbalance immediately.
- Ask family what pain relief measures are helpful, and integrate them into care for the child.
- Ensure adequate nutrition by providing a high-calorie, high-protein diet. Ensure that the child's immunizations are up to date. Report any signs of infection to the physician immediately.
- Review the basics of sickle cell disease. Teach the child and family about signs and symptoms of crises.
- Arrange for genetic counseling and testing for sickle cell trait for family members if desired.

EVALUATION

- The child demonstrates no shortness of breath and shows no signs of hypoxia.
- The child demonstrates no signs or symptoms of stroke.
- The child shows indicators of adequate hydration, including sufficient urine production.
- Using a predetermined, developmentally appropriate pain rating scale, the client consistently rates his pain as being tolerable or absent.
- The child demonstrates no signs or symptoms of infection.
- The child and parent can verbalize precipitating events of crises.

CRITICAL THINKING

1. What factors in Mark's history may have precipitated sickling?
2. When you admit Mark to the emergency department, what is your priority of care? Explain your answer.
3. What teaching will you provide to reduce the risk of future recurrence of sickling?

REVIEW Sickle Cell Disease

RELATE Link the Concepts and Exemplars

Linking the exemplar of sickle cell disease with the concept of oxygenation:

1. You admit a child in sickle cell crisis. How will you assess oxygenation?

2. How will you promote oxygenation for the client in sickle cell crisis?

Linking the exemplar of sickle cell disease with the concept of infection:

3. What teaching priorities will you provide the parents of a young child who has SCD to reduce the risk of infection?

4. What interventions will you implement during hospitalization for a 9-year-old admitted in sickle cell crisis to reduce the risk of infection?

READY Go to Companion Skills Manual

REFER Go to Pearson Nursing Student Resources
nursing.pearsonhighered.com

- Additional review materials

REFLECT Case Study

Wendell Kozier is a 7-year-old boy with sickle cell disease. Wendell has been held back in school as the result of his many absences secondary to sickle cell crisis and is now in kindergarten. Wendell is very bright, articulate, and inquisitive. He tells the nurse he wants to play hockey when he grows up. Wendell's dad is African American and his mom is Caucasian and African American. Wendell is in the physician's office today for a checkup and immunizations. He was discharged from the hospital following sickle cell crisis 1 month ago.

1. What nursing diagnoses are appropriate for Wendell?

2. How will you respond to Wendell's desire to play hockey? What will you teach his parents about sports and sickle cell crisis?

3. What teaching will you provide to Wendell and his family to help reduce the frequency of sickle cell crisis?

EXEMPLAR 2.9 Skin Cancer

EXEMPLAR KEY TERMS
Actinic keratosis, *131*
Basal cell cancer, *129*
Keratotic basal cell carcinoma, *130*
Melanomas, *128*
Microstaging, *134*

EXEMPLAR LEARNING OUTCOMES

After reading about this exemplar, you will be able to:

1. Describe the pathophysiology, etiology, clinical manifestations, and direct and indirect causes of skin cancer.
2. Identify risk factors and prevention methods associated with skin cancer.
3. Illustrate the nursing process in providing culturally competent care across the life span for individuals with skin cancer.
4. Formulate priority nursing diagnoses appropriate for an individual with skin cancer.
5. Summarize therapies used by interdisciplinary teams in the collaborative care of an individual with skin cancer.
6. Plan evidence-based care for an individual with skin cancer and his or her family in collaboration with other members of the healthcare team.
7. Evaluate expected outcomes for an individual with skin cancer.

▶ OVERVIEW

The skin, despite its ability to protect the internal body from external damage, is a fragile organ and is subject to damage from ultraviolet (UV) radiation and chemicals. Over time, this damage results in alterations in cellular structure and function, leading to malignancies of the skin.

The skin is a common site for malignant lesions. Many of these lesions are found on skin surfaces that have undergone long-term exposure to the sun or the environment. Malignant skin tumors (**melanomas**) are the most common of all cancers. The nonmelanoma skin cancers are basal cell cancer and squamous cell cancer.

▶ PATHOPHYSIOLOGY AND ETIOLOGY

Skin cancer can be classified as melanoma or nonmelanoma in type. Each classification will be considered independently.

Melanoma

Malignant melanomas arise from melanocytes, cells located at or near the basal layer (the deepest epidermal layer). These cells produce melanin, the dark skin pigment. Melanin is made in granules and transferred to keratinocytes (primary cell of the epidermis), where it accumulates on the superficial side of each keratinocyte and forms a shield of pigment over the nucleus as protection against UV rays. Malignant melanomas can develop wherever there is pigment, but about one third of them originate in existing **nevi** (moles).

Almost all malignant melanomas are more than 6 mm in diameter, are asymmetric, and initially develop within the epidermis over a long period. While they are still confined to the epidermis, the lesions (called malignant melanoma in situ) are flat and relatively benign. However, when they penetrate the dermis, they mingle with blood and lymph vessels and are capable of metastasizing. At this latter stage, the tumors develop a raised or nodular appearance and often have smaller nodules, called satellite lesions, around the periphery.

The prognosis for survival among people diagnosed with malignant melanoma is determined by several variables, including tumor thickness, ulceration, metastasis, site, age, and gender. Younger clients and women have a somewhat better chance of survival. Tumors on the hands, feet, and scalp have a poorer prognosis; tumors of the feet and scalp are less visible and may not be diagnosed until they grow into the dermis.

PRECURSOR LESIONS   The three specific precursor lesions for the development of malignant melanoma are congenital nevi, dysplastic nevi, and lentigo maligna. A precursor lesion is also called a premalignant lesion, a name that indicates that the lesion's risk of becoming malignant is greater than normal.

■ *Congenital nevi.* Congenital nevi are present at birth. Some lesions are small; others are large enough to cover an entire body area. Their color can range from brown to black. They are often slightly raised, with an irregular surface and a fairly regular border.

■ *Dysplastic nevi.* Dysplastic nevi are also called atypical moles. Although dysplastic nevi are not present at birth, they appear as normal nevi during childhood and become dysplastic (having abnormal development) after puberty. A client with classic dysplastic nevi has more than 100 nevi, at least one of which is larger than 8 mm in diameter and at least one of which has the characteristics of malignant melanoma (asymmetry, irregular border, color variegation, and a diameter of >6 mm). A familial tendency to dysplastic nevi increases the risk for development of malignant melanoma. However, it is not known whether people with dysplastic nevi and no family history of melanoma face a higher risk for melanoma.

Dysplastic nevi most often appear on the face, trunk, and arms but also are seen on the scalp, female breast, groin, and buttocks. The pigmentation of the nevi is irregular, with mixtures of tan, brown, black, red, and pink. An area of lighter pigmentation is surrounded by a papular area of deeper pigmentation (described as a "fried egg appearance"). The borders of the nevi are irregular.

■ *Lentigo maligna.* Lentigo maligna, also called Hutchinson freckle, is a tan or black patch on the skin that looks like a freckle. It grows slowly, becoming mottled, dark, thick, and nodular. It is usually seen on one side of the face of an older adult who has had a large amount of sun exposure.

CLASSIFICATIONS OF MALIGNANT MELANOMAS
Malignant melanomas are classified into different types. The major types are superficial spreading melanoma, lentigo maligna melanoma, nodular melanoma, and acral lentiginous melanoma. Each of these tumors is characterized by a radial and/or vertical growth phase. During the initial radial phase, which

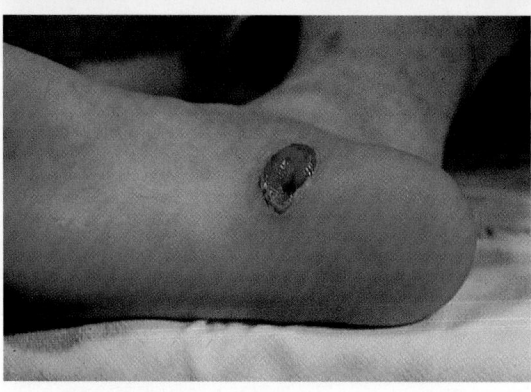

Figure 2–21 ● Malignant melanoma is a serious skin cancer that arises from melanocytes.
Source: L. Solomon/Custom Medical Stock Photo.

may last from 1 to 25 years (depending on the type), the melanoma grows parallel to the skin surface. During this phase, the tumor rarely metastasizes and is often curable by surgical excision. However, during the vertical growth phase, atypical melanocytes rapidly penetrate into the dermis and subcutaneous tissue, greatly increasing the risk for metastasis and death.

■ *Superficial spreading melanoma.* Superficial spreading melanoma is the most common type, comprising approximately 50% of all melanomas (Osborn et al., 2013). The lesions are usually flat and scaly or crusty and are approximately 2 cm in diameter. They often arise from a preexisting nevus. This type of melanoma is found on the trunk and back of men and on the legs of women. Superficial spreading melanomas occur more often in women than in men. The median age of occurrence is the 50s.

The radial growth phase lasts from 1 to 5 or more years. When the lesion enters the vertical growth phase, it grows rapidly, and its color changes from a mixture of tan, brown, and black to a characteristic red, white, and blue. The lesion also develops irregular borders and often has raised nodules and ulcerations (**Figure 2–21 ●**).

■ *Lentigo maligna melanoma.* Lentigo maligna melanoma often arises from the precursor lesion, lentigo maligna. The lesions are large and tan, with different shades of brown. This type of melanoma makes up 15% of malignant melanomas and is the least serious form (Osborn et al., 2013). It occurs on skin that has had long-term sun exposure, such as the face, neck, and sometimes the dorsal surface of the hands and lower extremities. Lentigo maligna melanoma affects women more than men. It is typically diagnosed in people in their 60s and 70s.

Lentigo maligna melanoma is characterized by a proliferation of atypical melanocytes parallel to the basal layer of the epidermis. The radial growth phase may last from 10 to 25 years, with the lesion growing to as large as 10 cm. The lesion becomes malignant as soon as the melanocytes invade the dermis. In the vertical growth phase, raised nodules may appear on the surface of the lesion. The lesion tends to acquire a freckled or mottled appearance.

■ *Nodular melanoma.* Nodular melanoma lesions are raised, dome-shaped, blue-black or red nodules on areas of the head, neck, and trunk that may or may not have been exposed to the sun. The lesions may look like a blood blister, or they may ulcerate and bleed. The lesions arise from unaffected skin rather than from a preexisting lesion. This type makes up 20%–25% of malignant melanomas and is often diagnosed in people in their 50s (Osborn et al., 2013).

Nodular melanoma has only a vertical growth phase, but it grows aggressively during that phase. However, the absence of a radial growth phase makes this type of melanoma more difficult to diagnose before it metastasizes.

■ *Acral lentiginous melanoma.* Acral lentiginous melanoma is the least common form of melanoma, comprising less than 10% of all new cases (Osborn et al., 2013). Also called mucocutaneous melanoma, this condition is less common in people with fair skin and more common in people with dark skin. The lesions progress from tan, brown, or black flat lesions to elevated nodules and are approximately 3 cm in diameter. The radial phase lasts from 2 to 5 years. The nodules are found on the palms of the hands, the soles of the feet, the mucous membranes, and the nail beds. Acral lentiginous melanoma affects men and women equally and is most often diagnosed in people in their 50s and 60s.

Nonmelanoma Skin Cancer

Basal cell cancer and squamous cell cancer arise from epithelial tissue but have different pathophysiologies, classifications, and manifestations.

BASAL CELL CANCER Basal cell cancer is an epithelial tumor believed to originate either from the basal layer of the epidermis or from cells in the surrounding dermal structures. These tumors are characterized by an impaired ability of the basal cells of the epidermis to mature into keratinocytes, with mitotic division beyond the basal layer. This results in a bulky neoplasm that grows by direct extension and destroys surrounding tissue, including healthy skin, nerves, blood vessels, lymphatic tissue, cartilage, and bone. Basal cell cancer is the most common but least aggressive type of skin cancer, rarely metastasizing.

Basal cell cancers tend to recur. Tumors greater than 2 cm in diameter have a high recurrence rate. Predisposing factors for metastasis are the size of the tumor and the client's resistance to treatment with surgery or chemotherapy. Although they rarely metastasize, untreated basal cell cancers invade surrounding tissue and may destroy body parts, such as the nose or eyelid.

Basal cell cancer is classified into different types: nodular, superficial, pigmented, morpheaform, and keratotic. These types are described below and are summarized in **Table 2–20 ●**.

■ **Nodular basal cell carcinoma**, the most common type of basal cell cancer, most often appears on the face, neck, and head. The tumor is made up of masses of cells that resemble epidermal basal cells and grow in a bulky, nodular form from lack of keratinization. In early stages, the tumor is a papule that looks like a smooth pimple. It is often pruritic and continues to grow at a steady rate, doubling in size every 6–12 months. As the tumor grows, the epidermis thins but remains intact. The skin over the tumor is shiny, and either pearly white, pink, or flesh colored. Telangiectasis (red, purple, or blue discoloration under the skin caused by abnormal dila-

TABLE 2–20   Types and Characteristics of Basal Cell Cancers

TYPE	COMMON LOCATION	MANIFESTATION
Nodular	Face, neck, head	Small, firm papule; pearly, white, pink, or flesh colored; telangiectasis; enlarges; may ulcerate
Superficial	Trunk, extremities	Papules or plaque that is flat, erythematous, or scaling; pink color; well-defined borders; may have shallow erosions and surface crusting
Pigmented	Head, neck, face	Dark brown, blue, or black color; border is shiny and well defined
Morpheaform	Head, neck	Looks like a flat scar; ivory or flesh colored
Keratotic	Ear	Small, firm papule; pearly, white, pink, or flesh colored; may ulcerate

tion of a vessel) may be visible over the area of the tumor. As the tumor continues to increase in size, the center or periphery may ulcerate, and the tumor develops well-circumscribed borders. It bleeds easily from mild injury.

■ **Superficial basal cell carcinoma**, found most often on the trunk and extremities, is the second most common type of basal cell cancer. This tumor is a proliferating tissue that attaches to the undersurface of the epithelium. The tumor is a flat papule or plaque, often erythematous, with well-defined borders. The tumor may ulcerate and be covered with crusts or shallow erosions (**Figure 2–22 ●**).

■ **Pigmented basal cell carcinoma**, found on the head, neck, and face, is less common. This tumor concentrates melanin pigment in the center of the basal cancer cells, giving it a dark brown, blue, or black appearance. The border of the tumor is shiny and well defined.

■ **Morpheaform basal cell carcinoma**, the rarest form of basal cell cancer, usually develops on the head and neck. The tumor forms finger-like projections that extend in any direction along dermal tissue planes. The tumor resembles a flat ivory or flesh-colored scar. This form is more likely to extend into and destroy adjacent tissue, especially muscle, nerve, and bone. It is often more difficult to diagnose because of its appearance.

■ **Keratotic basal cell carcinoma** (basosquamous) is found on the preauricular and postauricular groove. It contains both basal cells and squamoid-appearing cells that keratinize. Its appearance is much like that of nodular basal cell cancer. This type of basal cell cancer tends to recur locally and also is the type most likely to metastasize.

SQUAMOUS CELL CANCER   **Squamous cell cancer** is a malignant tumor of the squamous epithelium of the skin or mucous membranes. It occurs most often on areas of skin exposed to UV rays and weather, such as the forehead, helix of the ear, top of the nose, lower lip, and back of the hands. Squamous cell cancer may also arise on skin that has been burned or has chronic inflammation. This is a much more aggressive cancer than basal cell cancer, with a faster growth rate and a much greater potential for metastasis if untreated.

The tumors arise when the keratinizing cells of the squamous epithelium proliferate, producing a growth that eventually fills the epidermis and invades the dermal tissue planes. Keratinization of some cells is present, and the formation of keratin "pearls" is common. The keratin formation diminishes as the tumor grows. As the tumor grows, the tumor cells increase in number and rate of mitosis, forming odd shapes.

Squamous cell cancer begins as a small, firm, red nodule. The tumor may be crusted with keratin products. As it grows, it may ulcerate, bleed, and become painful. As the tumor extends into the surrounding tissue and becomes a nodule, the area around the nodule becomes indurated (hardened) (**Figure 2–23 ●**).

Recurrent squamous cell cancer can be invasive, increasing the risk of metastasis. Invasive squamous cell cancer may arise from preexisting skin lesions, such as scars and actinic keratosis, and extend into the dermis (called intraepidermal squamous cell cancer). This form appears as a slightly raised erythematous plaque with well-defined borders. Metastasis occurs most often via the lymphatics. The degree of risk for metastasis depends on the size and depth of penetration of the tumor.

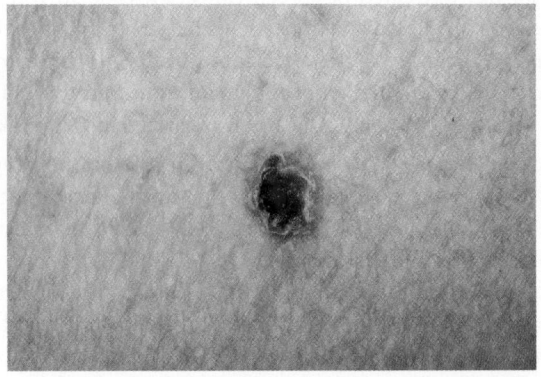

Figure 2–22 ● A superficial basal cell cancer is characterized by erythema, ulcerations, and well-defined borders.
Source: © BSIP SA / Alamy.

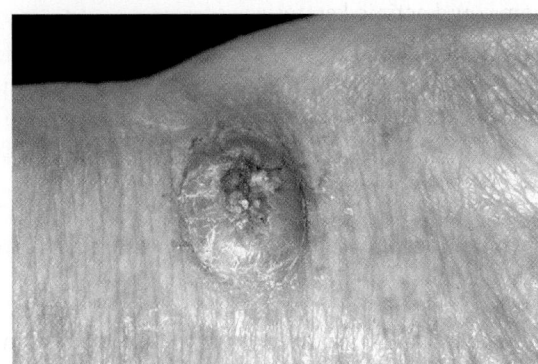

Figure 2–23 ● As a squamous cell cancer grows, it tends to invade surrounding tissue. It also ulcerates, may bleed, and is painful.
Source: © Medical-on-Line/Alamy.

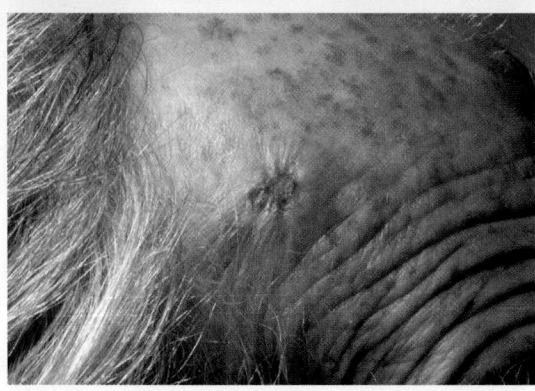

Figure 2–24 ● The effects of long-term sun exposure are illustrated in this epidermal skin lesion, call actinic keratosis.
Source: © Medical-on-Line/Alamy.

Box 2–10   Risk Factors for Melanoma Skin Cancer

- A high number of moles, or large moles
- Fair skin, freckling, blond hair, or blue eyes
- Close relative with the disease
- Men with gene changes from a family history of breast or ovarian cancer
- Treatment with medications that suppress the immune system
- Too much exposure to UV radiation from sunlight, tanning lamps, or tanning booths
- Age older than 50 years
- Xeroderma pigmentosus, a rare, inherited disease in which people are less able to repair damage caused by sunlight
- Past history of melanoma

Actinic Keratosis

Actinic keratosis, also called senile or solar keratosis, is an epidermal skin lesion directly related to chronic sun exposure and photodamage. Actinic keratosis may progress to squamous cell carcinoma. Because of this tendency, the lesions are classified as premalignant.

Actinic keratosis lesions are erythematous, rough macules a few millimeters in diameter. They are often shiny but may be scaly; if the scales are removed, the underlying skin bleeds. They occur in multiple patches, primarily on the face, dorsa of the hands, the forearms, and sometimes, on the upper trunk (**Figure 2–24 ●**). Enlargement or ulceration of the lesions suggests transformation to malignancy.

Etiology

One of the leading causes of skin cancer is exposure to the sun. Research has indicated that tanning beds are among the most dangerous form of UV exposure, and it has been suggested they should be banned because of the high risk of skin cancer that results from their use (Roberts, Hornung, & Polk, 2009). Other factors contributing to etiology includes age, skin type, skin color, and genetic predisposition.

Risk Factors

Risk factors vary according to type of lesion. Melanoma, non-melanoma, and actinic keratosis each have specific considerations related to risk.

MELANOMA SKIN CANCER   Although the exact cause of melanoma is unknown, certain risk factors are associated with the disease. Even a single blistering sunburn during childhood or adolescence more than doubles a child's risk for developing melanoma in later years (Skin Cancer Foundation, n.d.b). The risk factors for melanoma are listed in **Box 2–10 ●**.

NONMELANOMA SKIN CANCER   Multiple etiological factors are involved in the development of nonmelanoma skin cancer, including environmental factors and host factors. Unknown factors may also play a role.

Environmental Factors   The environmental factors implicated in the nonmelanoma skin cancers are UV radiation, pollutants, chemicals, ionizing radiation, viruses, and physical trauma.

Ultraviolet radiation from the sun is believed to be the cause of most nonmelanoma skin cancers. Sunlight contains both short-length rays (UVB) and long-length rays (UVA). UVB rays are absorbed by the top layer of skin and cause sunburn. UVA rays penetrate deeper into the skin layers, causing tissue damage. Both types of rays are believed to cause DNA alterations and also suppress T-cell and B-cell immunity. The amount of UV radiation reaching the earth is increasing, most likely from depletion of the ozone layer surrounding the planet. The U.S. Environmental Protection Agency predicts that for every 1% decrease in the ozone layer, a corresponding 1%–3% increase in cases of nonmelanoma skin cancer per year will occur.

Geographic, environmental, and lifestyle factors affect the amount of exposure to the sun and the risk for nonmelanoma skin cancer. People who live in latitudes close to the equator and those who live at higher altitudes receive greater UV radiation exposure. The amount of clothing worn, the time of day, and the amount of time in the sun also determine the amount of exposure. Exposure to UV radiation in tanning booths has also been implicated in the development of nonmelanoma skin cancer.

Certain chemicals have long been associated with nonmelanoma skin cancer. Polycyclic aromatic hydrocarbons, found in mixtures of coal, tar, asphalt, soot, and mineral oils, have been linked with skin cancers. Psoralens, used in conjunction with UVA for treatment of psoriasis and cutaneous T-cell lymphoma, increase the risk of squamous cell cancer.

Other factors associated with nonmelanoma skin cancer are the use of ionizing radiation, viruses, and physical trauma. X-ray therapy for tinea capitis and the use of radium to treat other malignancies are risk factors. Human papillomavirus is implicated in the development of squamous cell cancer, as is damage to the skin from burns.

Host Factors   Certain host factors increase the risk for nonmelanoma skin cancer. These include skin pigmentation as well as the presence of premalignant lesions.

Skin pigmentation is an important factor in the development of nonmelanoma skin cancer. The amount of melanin pigment produced by the melanocytes determines an individual's skin color. The more melanin, the more the skin is protected from the damage produced by UV rays. Thus, African Americans, Asian Americans, and people of Mediterranean descent have a much lower incidence of nonmelanoma skin cancer than do people who have fair complexions and tend to freckle or sunburn easily, such as people of Irish, Scandinavian, or English ancestry.

Although most people have numerous pigmented lesions on their body, almost all of these are normal. However, a major risk factor in the development of nonmelanoma skin cancer is a change in an existing lesion or the presence of a premalignant lesion, such as actinic keratosis. Organ transplant recipients who undergo immunosuppression to prevent rejection are also at risk for the development of squamous cell cancer.

ACTINIC KERATOSIS   The prevalence of actinic keratosis is highest in people with light-colored skin. These lesions are rare in people with dark skin.

Prevention

Primary prevention includes avoiding prolonged sun exposure and refraining from the use of artificial tanning machines. Recommendations for protection from the sun's harmful rays include daily application of sunscreen that provides a sun protection factor (SPF) of 15 or higher. Prior to extended periods of sun exposure, sunscreen that provides an SPF of 30 or higher should be applied. Sunscreen should be applied 30 minutes before anticipated sun exposure and reapplied every 2 hours, with reapplication immediately after swimming or following periods of

excessive perspiration. Broad-brimmed hats and sunglasses that block UV rays should be worn. Clients should be encouraged to perform head-to-toe skin exams and to seek an annual skin exam from their healthcare provider. Newborns should not be exposed to direct sunlight. For infants 6 months or older, sunscreen should be applied (Skin Cancer Foundation, n.d.a).

SAFETY ALERT
In the prevention of skin cancer, wellness promotion includes educating clients about the risks associated with indoor tanning devices. With just one indoor tanning session, an individual's risk for developing melanoma increases by 20%. With each additional tanning session during the same year, the individual's risk for melanoma increases by nearly an additional 2% (Boniol et al., 2012).

▶ CLINICAL MANIFESTATIONS

The clinical manifestations of each type of skin cancer differ. It is often possible to determine the likelihood of a specific classification based on appearance, although further testing is generally done to confirm the diagnosis. Manifestations of skin cancers are summarized in the Clinical Manifestations and Therapies feature.

Clinical Manifestations and Therapies **Skin Cancer**

ETIOLOGY	CLINICAL MANIFESTATIONS	CLINICAL THERAPIES
Melanomas		
Congenital nevi, precursor to melanoma	■ Range in color from brown to black ■ Often slightly raised, with an irregular surface and fairly regular border ■ Can range in size from small to covering entire body.	■ Surgical excision ■ Chemotherapy ■ Immunotherapy ■ Radiation therapy ■ Regular examinations to assess for recurrence
Dysplastic nevi, precursor to melanoma	■ Have irregular pigmentation with mixtures of tan, brown, black, red, and pink. ■ May have an area of lighter pigmentation surrounded by a papular area of deeper pigmentation. ■ Irregular borders ■ Often appear on the face, trunk, and arms but can be seen on the scalp, female breast, groin, buttocks.	
Lentigo maligna, precursor to melanoma	■ Tan or black patch on the skin that looks like a freckle ■ Grows slowly, becoming mottled, dark, thick, and nodular. ■ Usually seen on one side of the face in an older adult who has had a large amount of sun exposure	
Malignant melanoma	■ Asymmetrical, with an irregular border ■ Color variegation ■ Diameter >6 mm (the size of a pencil eraser)	

Clinical Manifestations and Therapies **Skin Cancer** (continued)

ETIOLOGY	CLINICAL MANIFESTATIONS	CLINICAL THERAPIES
Nonmelanomas		
Nodular basal cell carcinoma	■ Papule that looks like a smooth pimple that grows at a steady rate ■ Skin over the tumor that is shiny and may be pearly white, pink, or flesh colored ■ Chance of visible telangiectasis ■ Tumor that may ulcerate at the center or periphery and bleed easily from mild injury	■ Surgical excision ■ Curettage and electrodesiccation ■ Cryotherapy ■ Radiotherapy ■ Chemotherapy ■ Immunotherapy ■ Radiation therapy ■ Biological therapy ■ Vaccines ■ Regular examinations to assess for recurrence
Superficial basal cell carcinoma	■ Appears as a flat papule or plaque, often erythematous, with well-defined borders. ■ Tumor that may ulcerate and be covered with crusts or shallow erosions ■ Most common on the trunk and extremities	
Pigmented basal cell carcinoma	■ Dark brown, blue, or black, with a shiny surface and well-defined borders ■ Typically found on the head, face, and neck	
Morpheaform basal cell carcinoma	■ Resembles a flat ivory or flesh-colored scar that forms finger-like projections that extend along dermal tissue planes. ■ Usually develops on the head and neck.	
Keratotic basal cell carcinoma	■ Appears similar to nodular basal cell carcinoma.	
Squamous cell cancer	■ Begins as a small, firm, red nodule that may be crusted with keratin products. ■ Tumors that ulcerate, bleed, and become painful as they grow ■ Causes the area around the nodule to harden as the tumor extends into the surrounding tissue and becomes a nodule. ■ Most common on areas of skin exposed to ultraviolet rays and weather, such as the forehead, helix of the ear, top of the nose, lower lip, and back of the hands	
Other Types of Lesions		
Actinic keratosis	■ Erythematous, rough macules a few millimeters in diameter ■ Often shiny but may be scaly; if the scales are removed, the underlying skin bleeds. ■ Occur in multiple patches, primarily on the face, dorsa of the hands, the forearms, and sometimes, on the upper trunk. ■ Enlargement or ulceration of the lesions suggests transformation to malignancy.	■ Cryosurgery ■ Topical creams or gels ■ Shave excision ■ Curettage and electrodesiccation ■ Photodynamic therapy ■ Chemical peels ■ Laser surgery ■ Monitor for changes or abnormalities in lesion(s). (ACS, 2013h)

▶ COLLABORATION

Care of the client with skin cancer requires a collaborative team of healthcare providers in order to promote early detection and prompt intervention and to improve client outcomes. Numerous treatment options may be offered, and the nurse's role is to help the client make an informed decision about the treatment option that is best for his or her needs and circumstances.

Treatment of nonmelanoma skin cancer focuses on removal of all malignant tissue using such methods as surgery, curettage and electrodesiccation, cryotherapy, or radiotherapy. These modalities offer a greater than 90% cure rate. Other methods of treatment are chemotherapy, immunotherapy, and radiation therapy. Biological therapies with interleukin-2 and interferon and therapeutic vaccines containing melanoma antigens are sometimes used. After the malignant tissue is removed, the client should have regular examinations for recurrence.

The management of the client with malignant melanoma begins with identification, diagnosis, and tumor staging. If treatable, the tumor is removed through surgical excision. Malignant melanoma is also treated with chemotherapy, immunotherapy, and radiation therapy.

Diagnostic Tests

Malignant melanoma is most often found on the trunk of men and on the lower extremities of women. Nevertheless, it is important for the client to have a complete physical examination and total skin assessment. A change in the color or size of a nevus is reported in 70% of people diagnosed with a malignant melanoma. The ABCD rule is used to assess suspicious lesions:

Asymmetry (one half of the nevus does not match the other half)
Border irregularity (edges are ragged, blurred, or notched)
Color variation or dark black color
Diameter greater than 6 mm (size of a pencil eraser).

Along with visual examination of all skin surfaces, palpation of regional lymph nodes, the liver, and the spleen is essential to assess for metastasis when a melanoma is suspected or found.

In addition to biopsy of any suspicious lesion, diagnostic tests are conducted to determine whether the tumor has metastasized. Because malignant melanoma may metastasize to any organ or tissue of the body, a variety of tests may be conducted, including the following:

■ Microscopic examination
■ Biopsy
■ Tests for metastasis
   a. Liver function tests
   b. CT of the liver
   c. CBC
   d. Serum blood chemistry profile
   e. Chest x-ray
   f. Bone scan
   g. CT or MRI of the brain.

MICROSTAGING   **Microstaging** describes the assessment of the level of invasion of a malignant melanoma and the maximum tumor thickness. In the Clark system of microstaging,

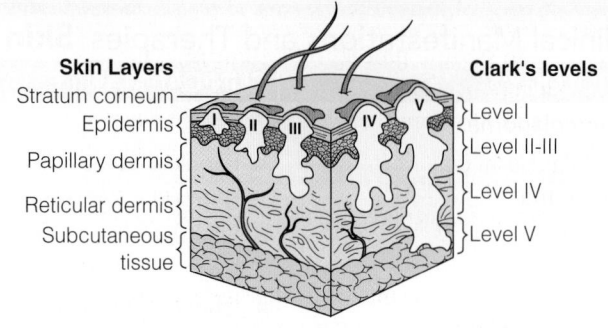

Figure 2–25 ● Clarks' levels for staging measure the invasion of a melanoma from the epidermis to the subcutaneous tissue.

the vertical growth of the lesion is measured from the epidermis to the subcutaneous tissue to determine the level of invasion (**Figure 2–25** ●). However, variations in individual skin thicknesses and different anatomical sites can affect the accuracy of the measurement. In the Breslow system, an adaptation of the Clark system of assessment, the vertical thickness is measured from the granular level of the epidermis to the deepest level of tumor invasion. This determination is important, because as the thickness of the melanoma increases, survival rate decreases.

After the thickness and depth of the tumor are determined, a clinical stage is assigned. The traditional three-stage system is still used, although it does not include tumor thickness. The American Joint Committee on Cancer has adopted a four-stage system that includes tumor thickness, level of invasion, lymph node involvement, and evidence of metastasis.

Surgery

Surgical excision is the preferred treatment for malignant melanoma. If a biopsy identifies the lesion as a melanoma, a wide excision is performed that includes the full thickness of the skin and subcutaneous tissue. Because the risk of local recurrence for thin melanomas (those <0.76 mm) is quite low, margins of 0.5–1.0 cm of normal skin are excised around the tumor. Thick tumors require a 1- to 3-cm margin excision because they are at risk for local recurrence or satellite lesions.

Regional lymph nodes are the most common sites for metastasis of malignant melanoma. Standard surgical treatment for clinically suspicious lymph node involvement includes excision of the primary lesions as well as surgical dissection of the involved lymph nodes. Elective lymph node dissection (ELND) in the treatment of localized malignant melanoma remains controversial. Advocates of ELND believe that the procedure benefits clients with intermediate-thickness tumors, because approximately 20% of people whose lymph nodes were clinically negative at diagnosis show some metastasis on removal of the nodes. Those opposed to ELND believe the risks associated with the procedure are too high for the 80% of people who have no evidence of metastasis after removal of the nodes.

Surgery also is indicated for palliative management of isolated metastasis. Removal of metastatic tumors in the brain, liver, lung, gastrointestinal tract, or subcutaneous tissue may relieve symptoms and prolong life.

Pharmacologic Therapy

In addition to surgical procedures, treatment of the client with melanoma may include immunotherapy. Very sensitive new tests can better detect the spread of melanoma to lymph nodes and can possibly better identify people who could be helped by a treatment such as immunotherapy after surgery. Emerging pharmacologic treatments for these clients include gene therapy and vaccinations.

IMMUNOTHERAPY   Immunotherapy is a relatively new treatment modality for malignant melanoma. The role of the immunological response initially was recognized because of the numerous spontaneous remissions seen in clients with melanoma—a higher occurrence than with any other adult tumor. In addition, researchers have recently identified tumor-specific antigen-antibodies in clients with melanoma. This also has stimulated an interest in immunotherapeutic interventions for the treatment of malignant melanoma.

Agents such as interferons, interleukins, monoclonal antibodies, bacille Calmette-Guérin, levamisole, transfer factors, and tumor vaccines have been used to treat melanoma, with varying response rates. The effectiveness of these agents, used either alone, in combination with chemotherapy, or in combination with each other, is under investigation.

EMERGING TREATMENTS   Melanoma skin cancer research is ongoing and directed toward more specific methods of diagnosis and treatment. Examples of emerging treatments include the following:

- *Gene therapy:* Clinical trials are in progress to test the effectiveness of adding certain genes to the malignant cells.
- *Immune therapy:* Vaccines are being developed to make an individual immune to his or her melanoma cells, or to train the individual's immune cells to fight the cancer.

 Stay Current: Visit the Web site of the National Cancer Institute to stay abreast of current treatment options for melanoma: **www.cancer.gov/cancertopics/pdq/treatment/melanoma/Patient/page4**.

Radiation Therapy

Melanoma responds to higher-dose radiation, especially if the tumor is small. Response rates to radiation therapy depend on the site of the tumor, the thickness of the tumor, the type of melanoma, and the client's general health but may range from 0% to 71%. Radiation frequently is used for palliation of symptoms resulting from metastasis to the brain, bone, lymph nodes, gastrointestinal tract, skin, or subcutaneous tissue. Liver and lung metastases are not treated with radiation therapy, because a loss of organ function may result.

Knowledge of how UV light harms DNA is increasing, providing support for referral to genetic counseling for people with a strong family history of melanoma.

■ NURSING PROCESS

Nursing care of clients diagnosed with any form of skin cancer requires careful assessment and documentation of lesions, monitoring for any change in appearance, and support of the client's physical and emotional needs. Fear of death, altered

Assessment Interview **Skin Cancer**

- Have any members of your family ever been treated for skin cancer?
- Have you had a skin cancer removed from any part of your body?
- Have you noticed any change in the size, shape, or color of a mole, wart, birthmark, or scar?
- Do you have any moles, warts, birthmarks, or scars that itch, are painful, have crusting, or bleed?
- In what parts of the country or world have you lived?
- Have you ever been badly sunburned?
- Do you visit tanning salons?
- Are you exposed to any hazardous chemicals in your job?
- Have you been taught how to examine your skin? If so, how do you do this examination? How often?

body image, and painful treatments often result from the diagnosis, and the nurse needs to provide holistic care that addresses both the physical and emotional needs of the client.

Assessment

Clients with skin cancer should undergo a skin assessment. Specific health history questions are outlined in the Assessment Interview feature.

The physical assessment should include the following:

1. Ask the client to remove all clothing and put on an examination gown. Ensure good light; natural, bright light is best for inspection of lesions. The client may sit, stand, or lie down.
2. Inspect and palpate the skin. Stretching the skin tightly during assessment facilitates assessment of nodular and scaly lesions and lesions in the dermis. Assess for the following:
   a. Obvious lesions
   b. Visible swellings
   c. Alterations in normal contour and borders of nevi
   d. Enlarged lymph glands
   e. Skin or mucosal discolorations
   f. Areas of ulceration, scaling, crusting, or erosion.
3. The order of assessment is as follows:
   a. Head and neck: entire scalp, eyelids, external ear, auditory canals, external surface of the nose, internal surface of the nose, the oral cavity, facial skin, the facial glands (parotid, submaxillary, sublingual)
   b. Thyroid and neck, including lymph glands
   c. Chest and abdomen, with special attention under pendulous breasts, in skinfolds, and in areas covered with hair
   d. Back and buttocks, with special attention to the area between the buttocks
   e. Extremities, with special attention to the axillae, nail beds, webs between the fingers and toes, and soles of the feet
   f. External genitals, with special attention to skinfolds, mucous membranes, and areas covered with hair.
4. Measure and record a description of all skin lesions on an anatomical chart. Take photographs (if possible) of any suspicious lesion, and include them in the client's record for future reference.

Diagnosis

Although many different nursing diagnoses may be appropriate for the client with a malignant melanoma, common responses are the following:

- *Impaired Skin Integrity*
- *Deficient Knowledge related to risk factors for skin cancer*
- *Risk for Infection following surgical procedure or related to open lesion*
- *Hopelessness*
- *Anxiety.*

(NANDA-I © 2012)

Planning

Planning care for the client diagnosed with skin cancer is highly individualized, depending on where the cells are located, the presence of metastasis, the treatment indicated, and the age of the client. Suggested goals for care may include the following:

- The client will describe different treatment options available and the pros and cons of each in order to make an informed decision about treatment.
- The client will demonstrate no signs or symptoms of infection postoperatively.
- The client will conduct skin self-examinations at least once monthly and will report any abnormalities or changes in skin.
- The client will verbalize awareness of measures to prevent skin cancer recurrence, including proper use of sunscreen and clothing and avoidance of artificial tanning machines.
- The client will verbalize emotions and concerns related to diagnosis of skin cancer and the available treatments.

Implementation

In addition to providing client care, nurses play an important role in promoting awareness of skin cancer prevention. Teaching the need for sun protection and avoidance of tanning beds is an important role for the nurse advocate. Additional nursing interventions target preventing infection and facilitating open communication, as well as promoting psychosocial well-being.

Prevent Infection

Malignant melanomas not only destroy skin layers but also invade body structures. Certain types of melanomas may ulcerate before diagnosis, and treatment typically involves some type of surgical biopsy and excision. Any open lesion or incision increases the risk for secondary infection.

- Monitor for manifestations of infection, such as fever, tachycardia, malaise, incisional erythema, swelling, pain, or drainage that increases or becomes purulent. Intact skin is the first line of defense against infection; impaired skin integrity increases the risk for infection. If infection is present, the client may have both systemic and local manifestations.
- Keep the incision line clean and dry by changing dressings as necessary. Moisture increases the risk of infection.
- Follow principles of medical and surgical asepsis when caring for the client's incision. Teach family members and visitors the importance of careful hand washing. Maintain standard precautions if drainage is present. Careful hand washing is essential in preventing the spread of infection. Aseptic techniques are necessary when caring for any surgical incision to prevent infection.
- Encourage and maintain adequate caloric and protein intake in the diet. Suggest a consultation with the dietitian if the client does not want to eat. Adequate kilocalories and protein are necessary for proper healing. The client with cancer has increased metabolic needs; if these needs are not met, nutritional problems that impair healing may result.

Address Feelings of Hopelessness

The diagnosis of malignant melanoma threatens the quality and quantity of life as the client faces the possibility or reality of metastasis; the possibility that the cancer may recur and cause death; and alterations in self-concept, roles, and relationships. Clients with this diagnosis may lose hope, becoming withdrawn, passive, and apathetic. Inspiring hope in clients during this health crisis is a legitimate nursing action.

- Provide an environment that encourages the client to identify and express feelings, concerns, and goals:
    a. Use active listening, ask open-ended questions, and reflect on the client's statements.
    b. Acknowledge and respect feelings of apathy and/or anger as expressions of distress.
    c. Convey an empathetic understanding of fears and concerns.
    d. Provide opportunities to express positive emotions, such as hope, faith, a sense of purpose, and the will to live.
    e. Explore the client's perceptions, and modify or clarify them if necessary by providing information and correcting misconceptions.
    f. Encourage the client to identify support systems and sources of strength and coping in the past.

Verbalizing feelings, concerns, and goals allows others to validate or correct them, promotes a therapeutic nurse–client relationship, and fosters feelings of self-worth. Expressing positive emotions and calling on support systems and sources of strength that were effective in coping with past crises help the individual resolve the crisis and develop hope.

- Encourage active participation in self-care as well as in mutual decision making and goal setting. Meeting self-care needs and making decisions about care increase personal confidence in one's capacity for coping.
- Encourage a focus not only on the present but also on the future: Review past occasions for hope, discuss the client's personal meaning of hope, establish and evaluate short-term goals with the client and family, and encourage them to express hope for the future. The nurse mobilizes the client's resources to strengthen motivation, hope, and the will to live.

Reduce Anxiety

The intensity of anxiety, aroused by a perceived threat, depends on the severity of the present situation and on the client's ability to handle the threat. Anxiety is one of the most common psychosocial responses in clients with cancer. Anxiety increases at the time of diagnosis and remains a constant emotion throughout the course of treatment, regardless of treatment type or setting. Interventions center on helping the client recognize the manifestations of anxiety, determining whether the client

Client Teaching The Client With Malignant Melanoma

Health education for the client and family experiencing the diagnosis and treatment of malignant melanoma involves self-care and ongoing self-monitoring. Education for the client and family is specific to the type of treatment. In addition to wound care, clients who have had a lymph node dissection need instructions on how to protect against bleeding, trauma, and infection. Address the following topics:

- The importance of regular medical checkups every 3 months for the first 2 years, every 6 months for the next 5 years, and yearly thereafter
- How proper self-care combined with regular medical care can help the client lead a fairly normal life
- If assistance for home care is necessary, referrals to a community health agency or a home care agency, as well as referral to a local cancer support group if desired. Other resources in this area include the following:
  a. American Cancer Society (www.cancer.org)
  b. Skin Cancer Foundation (www.skincancer.org).

wishes to do anything about the anxiety, and facilitating coping strategies.

- Provide reassurance and comfort:
  a. Set aside time to sit quietly with the client.
  b. Speak slowly and calmly.
  c. Convey empathetic understanding by touch and supporting coping mechanisms, such as crying and talking.
  d. Do not make demands or expect the client to make decisions.

Coping behaviors differ from situation to situation and from individual to individual. Anxiety at moderate to severe levels narrows perceptions and the ability to function.

- Decrease sensory stimuli by using short, simple sentences; focusing on the here and now; and providing concise information. Higher levels of anxiety result in a focus on the present, inability to concentrate, and difficulty in understanding verbal communications.
- Provide interventions that decrease anxiety levels and increase coping:
  a. Provide accurate information about the illness, treatment, and expected length of recovery.
  b. Encourage discussion of expected physical changes and ways to minimize disfigurement through cosmetics and clothing.
  c. Include family members in teaching sessions.
  d. Encourage participation in care.

Although the prognosis and treatment of melanoma depend on various factors, the prognosis of complete cure is decreased with metastasis. Surgical incisions include excision with wide margins, which may cause disfigurement. Active participation in care gives the client some control over the future and is often an effective means of coping with anxiety.

Evaluation

The efficacy of the nursing care plan is evaluated based on the client's progress in meeting goals of care. Possible expected outcomes used to evaluate care include the following:

- The client demonstrates no signs or symptoms of infection.
- The client's postoperative wound demonstrates signs of adequate healing, including well-approximated wound edges and granulation of tissue.
- Using a predetermined pain rating scale, the client consistently rates his pain at a level he considers to be tolerable or denies pain.
- The client verbalizes awareness of the need to examine all skin lesions for changes or unusual appearance.
- The client describes indications for reporting integumentary changes to his healthcare provider.
- The client makes informed decision regarding treatment options.
- The client avoids unprotected sun exposure and use of tanning bed.
- The client demonstrates healthy methods of coping with alterations in body image.

REVIEW Skin Cancer

RELATE Link the Concepts and Exemplars

Linking the exemplar of skin dancer with the concept of development:

1. What teaching points will you include when teaching a group of teens about skin cancer prevention?
2. How will you respond to an adolescent girl who tells you she has to use the tanning bed or she looks too pale and ugly?

Linking the exemplar of skin cancer with the concept of advocacy:

3. How can you, as a student nurse, advocate for clients to reduce the rate of skin cancer as the result of tanning bed usage?
4. What is the role of the nurse advocate in reducing the rate of skin cancer diagnoses?

READY Go to Companion Skills Manual

REFER Go to Pearson Nursing Student Resources
nursing.pearsonhighered.com

- Additional review materials
- Case Study
- Nursing Care Plan: A Client With Malignant Melanoma

REFLECT Case Study

Roe Jefferson is a nurse on vacation in Hampton Bays, Long Island. Roe has worked in pediatrics for 4 years now and really enjoys her work with parents and children. As she walks along the beach, she sees families with kids swimming and sunning themselves. She notices there are no umbrellas and, when not in the water, the children are not wearing hats and shirts. Several families have infants in car seats sitting in the sun.

1. What interventions would you implement to advocate for the children on the beach if you were Roe?
2. What is the teaching priority for families regarding the use of sunscreen?
3. What safety strategies would you teach families when they plan a day at the beach?

■ REFERENCES

Altera, H. J., Mikovitsb, J. A., Switzerc, W. M., Ruscettid, F. W., Loe, S., Klimasf, N., et al. (2012). A multicenter blinded analysis indicates no association between chronic fatigue syndrome/myalgic encephalomyelitis and either xenotropic murine leukemia virus-related virus or polytropic murine leukemia virus. *mBio, 3*(5), e00266–e00212.

American Cancer Society (ACS). (2009). Prostate cancer. Retrieved from http://www.cancer.org/docroot/CRI/CRI_2_3x.asp?dt=36.

American Cancer Society (ACS). (2011). *Genetic testing: What you need to know.* Retrieved from http://www.cancer.org/cancer/cancercauses/geneticsandcancer/genetictesting/genetic-testing-intro.

American Cancer Society (ACS). (2012a). *Cancer facts & figures 2012.* Retrieved from http://www.cancer.org/acs/groups/content/@epidemiologysurveilance/documents/document/acspc-031941.pdf.

American Cancer Society (ACS). (2012b). *Childhood leukemia overview.* Retrieved from http://www.cancer.org/acs/groups/cid/documents/webcontent/003044-pdf.pdf

American Cancer Society (ACS). (2012c). *Children diagnosed with cancer: Late effects of cancer treatment.* Retrieved from http://www.cancer.org/treatment/childrenandcancer/whenyourchildhascancer/children-diagnosed-with-cancer-late-effects-of-cancer-treatment.

American Cancer Society (ACS). (2012d). *Leukemia—Chronic lymphocytic.* Retrieved from http://www.cancer.org/acs/groups/cid/documents/webcontent/003111-pdf.pdf.

American Cancer Society (ACS). (2012e). *Signs and symptoms of cancer: What are signs and symptoms?* Retrieved from http://www.cancer.org/cancer/cancerbasics/signs-and-symptoms-of-cancer.

American Cancer Society (ACS). (2013a). *Breast cancer—Mammography statistics.* Retrieved from http://www.cancer.org/research/cancerfactsfigures/cancerfactsfigures/breast-cancer-mammography-statistics.

American Cancer Society (ACS). (2013b). *Cancer facts & figures 2013.* Atlanta, GA: American Cancer Society.

American Cancer Society (ACS). (2013c). *Chemotherapy principles: An in-depth discussion of the techniques and its role in cancer treatment.* Retrieved from http://www.cancer.org/acs/groups/cid/documents/webcontent/002995-pdf.pdf.

American Cancer Society (ACS). (2013d). *Infectious agents and cancer.* Retrieved from http://www.cancer.org/acs/groups/cid/documents/webcontent/002782-pdf.pdf.

American Cancer Society (ACS). (2013e). *Leukemia—Acute lymphocytic (adults).* Retrieved from http://www.cancer.org/acs/groups/cid/documents/webcontent/003109-pdf.pdf.

American Cancer Society (ACS). (2013f). *Leukemia—Acute myeloid (myelogenous).* Retrieved from http://www.cancer.org/acs/groups/cid/documents/webcontent/003110-pdf.pdf.

American Cancer Society (ACS). (2013g). *Leukemia—Chronic myeloid (myelogenous) overview.* Retrieved from http://www.cancer.org/acs/groups/cid/documents/webcontent/003057-pdf.pdf.

American Cancer Society (ACS). (2013h). *Treating actinic keratosis.* Retrieved from http://www.cancer.org/cancer/skincancer-basalandsquamouscell/detailedguide/skin-cancer-basal-and-squamous-cell-treating-actinic-keratosis.

American Cancer Society (ACS). (2013i). *What are the key statistics about breast cancer?* Retrieved from http://www.cancer.org/cancer/breastcancer/detailedguide/breast-cancer-key-statistics.

American Society of Clinical Oncology (ASCO). (2012a). *About complementary and alternative medicine.* Retrieved from http://www.cancer.net/all-about-cancer/treating-cancer/complementary-and-alternative-medicine-cam/about-complementary-and-alternative-medicine.

American Society of Clinical Oncology (ASCO). (2012b). *Hypercalcemia.* Retrieved from http://www.cancer.net/all-about-cancer/treating-cancer/managing-side-effects/hypercalcemia.

American Society of Clinical Oncology (ASCO). (2012c). *Understanding chemotherapy.* Retrieved from http://www.cancer.net/all-about-cancer/cancernet-feature-articles/treatments-tests-and-procedures/understanding-chemotherapy.

American Society of Clinical Oncology (ASCO). (2013). *Cancer during pregnancy.* Retrieved from http://www.nlm.nih.gov/medlineplus/cancerandpregnancy.html.

American Society of Hematology. (2011). *Leukemia.* Retrieved from http://www.hematology.org/Patients/Blood-Disorders/Blood-Cancers/5230.aspx.

Bercovitz, R. S., Greffe, B. S., & Hunger, S. P. (2010). Acute tumor lysis syndrome in a 7-month-old with hepatoblastoma. *Current Opinion in Pediatrics, 22*(1), 113–116.

Boniol, M., Autier, P., Boyle, P., & Gandini, S. (2012). Cutaneous melanoma attributable to sunbed use: systematic review and meta-analysis. *BMJ, 345,* e4757.

Bouayed, J., Rammal, H., & Soulimani, R. (2009). Oxidative stress and anxiety: Relationship and cellular pathways. *Oxidative Medicine and Cellular Longevity, 2*(2), 63–67.

Centers for Disease Control and Prevention (CDC). (2011a). *Nutrition for everyone: Iron and iron deficiency.* Retrieved from http://www.cdc.gov/nutrition/everyone/basics/vitamins/iron.html.

Centers for Disease Control and Prevention (CDC). (2011b). *Sickle cell disease (SCD)—Complications and treatments.* Retrieved from http://www.cdc.gov/ncbddd/sicklecell/treatments.html.

Centers for Disease Control and Prevention (CDC). (2011c). *Sickle cell disease (SDC)—Data & statistics.* Retrieved from http://www.cdc.gov/ncbddd/sicklecell/data.html.

Centers for Disease Control and Prevention (CDC). (2012a). *Chronic fatigue syndrome (CFS)—General information.* Retrieved from http://www.cdc.gov/cfs/general/index.html.

Centers for Disease Control and Prevention (CDC). (2012b). *Workplace safety & health topics: Occupational exposure to antineoplastic agents.* Retrieved from http://www.cdc.gov/niosh/topics/antineoplastic.

Centers for Disease Control and Prevention (CDC). (2013). *Lung cancer—Risk factors.* Retrieved from http://www.cdc.gov/cancer/lung/basic_info/risk_factors.htm.

Debnam, K., Holt, C. L., Clark, E. M., Roth, D. L., Foushee, H. R., Crowther, M., et al. (2012). Spiritual health locus of control and health behaviors in African Americans. *American Journal of Health Behavior, 36*(3), 360–372.

Fairchild, A. (2010). Under-treatment of cancer pain. *Current Opinion in Supportive & Palliative Care, 4*(1), 11–15.

Germino, B. B., Mishel, M. H., Alexander, G. R., Jenerette, C., Blyler, D., Baker, C., et al. (2011). Engaging African American breast cancer survivors in an intervention trial: Culture, responsiveness and community. *Journal of Cancer Survivorship, 5*(1), 82–91.

Gullatte, M. M., Brawley, O., Kinney, A., Powe, B., & Mooney, K. (2010). Religiosity, spirituality, and cancer fatalism beliefs on delay in breast cancer diagnosis in African American women. *Journal of Religion and Health, 49*(1), 62–72.

Hall, W., & Degenhardt, L. (2009). Adverse health effects of non-medical cannabis use. *Lancet, 374,* 1383–1391.

Hamre, H., Zeller, B., Kanellopoulos, A., Kiserud, C. E., Aakhus, S., Lund, M. B., et al. (2013). High prevalence of chronic fatigue in adult long-term survivors of acute lymphoblastic leukemia and lymphoma during childhood and adolescence. *Journal of Adolescent and Young Adult Oncology, 2*(1), 2–9.

Henderson, T., Friedman, D. L., & Meadows, A. T. (2010). Childhood cancer survivors: Transition to adult-focused risk-based care. *Pediatrics, 1*(126), 129–136.

Howlader, N., Noone, A. M., Krapcho, M., Neyman, N., Aminou, R., Altekruse, S. F., et al. (Eds.). (2012, April). SEER cancer statistics review, 1975–2009 (vintage 2009 populations). Bethesda, MD: National Cancer Institute. Retrieved from http://seer.cancer.gov/csr/1975_2009_pops09.

Janus, J. J., & Moerschel, S. K. (2010). Evaluation of anemia in children. *American Family Physician, 81*(12), 1462–1471.

Jha, P., Ramasundarahettige, C., Landsman, V., Rostron, B., Thun, M., Anderson, R. N., et al. (2013). 21st-century hazards of smoking and benefits of cessation in the United States. *New England Journal of Medicine, 368*(4), 341–350.

Mayo Clinic. (2011a). *Breast cancer: Treatments and drugs.* Retrieved from http://www.mayoclinic.com/health/breast-cancer/DS00328/DSECTION=treatments-and-drugs.

Mayo Clinic. (2011b). *Sickle cell anemia—Tests and diagnosis.* Retrieved from http://www.mayoclinic.com/health/sickle-cell-anemia/DS00324/DSECTION=tests-and-diagnosis.

Mayo Clinic. (2012a). *Breast cancer prevention: How to reduce your risk.* Retrieved from http://www.mayoclinic.com/health/breast-cancer-prevention/WO00091.

Mayo Clinic. (2012b). *Explore polycythemia vera.* Retrieved from http://www.nhlbi.nih.gov/health/health-topics/topics/poly.

Mayo Clinic. (2012c). *Leukemia.* Retrieved from http://www.mayoclinic.com/health/leukemia/DS00351.

Mayo Clinic. (2012d). *Sickle cell anemia.* Retrieved from http://www.mayoclinic.com/health/sickle-cell-anemia/DS00324.

MedlinePlus. (2012). Breast self exam. Retrieved from http://www.nlm.nih.gov/medlineplus/ency/article/001993.htm.

MedlinePlus. (2013a). *Antioxidants* Retrieved from http://www.nlm.nih.gov/medlineplus/antioxidants.html.

MedlinePlus. (2013b). *Graft-versus-host disease.* Retrieved from http://www.nlm.nih.gov/medlineplus/ency/article/001309.htm.

Muncie, H. L., & Campbell, J. (2009). Alpha and beta thalassemia. *American Family Physician, 80*(4), 339–344.

National Cancer Institute (NCI). (2012). *Prostate-specific antigen (PSA) test.* Retrieved from http://www.cancer.gov/cancertopics/factsheet/detection/PSA.

National Cancer Institute (NCI). (2013a). *BRCA1 and BRCA2: Cancer risk and genetic testing.* Retrieved from http://www.cancer.gov/cancertopics/factsheet/Risk/BRCA.

National Cancer Institute (NCI). (2013b). *Breast cancer risk in American women.* Retrieved from http://www.cancer.gov/cancertopics/factsheet/detection/probability-breast-cancer.

National Cancer Institute (NCI). (2013c). *Cancer genetics overview (PDQ*): Family cancer susceptibility syndromes.* Retrieved from http://www.cancer.gov/cancertopics/pdq/genetics/overview/healthprofessional/page3.

National Cancer Institute (NCI). (2013d). *Psychological stress and cancer.* Retrieved from http://www.cancer.gov/cancertopics/factsheet/Risk/stress.

National Cancer Institute (NCI). (2013e) *Secondhand smoke and cancer.* Retrieved from http://www.cancer.gov/cancertopics/factsheet/Tobacco/ETS.

National Center for Complementary and Alternative Medicine (NCCAM). (2010). *Massage therapy: An introduction.* Retrieved from http://nccam.nih.gov/health/massage/massageintroduction.htm?nav=gsa.

National Center for Complementary and Alternative Medicine (NCCAM). (2011). *Vitamin E supplements increase incidence of prostate cancer, according to SELECT study.* Retrieved from http://nccam.nih.gov/research/results/spotlight/101111.htm?nav=gsa.

National Center for Complementary and Alternative Medicine (NCCAM). (2012b). *Cancer and complementary health practices.* Retrieved from http://nccam.nih.gov/health/cancer/camcancer.htm?nav=gsa.

National Center for Complementary and Alternative Medicine (NCCAM). (2012b). *Get the facts: Antioxidants and health.* Retrieved from http://nccam.nih.gov/sites/nccam.nih.gov/files/Get_The_Facts_Antioxidants_and_Health_12-27-2012.pdf?nav=gsa.

National Heart, Lung, and Blood Institute (NHLBI). (2012a). *Explore aplastic anemia.* Retrieved from http://www.nhlbi.nih.gov/health/health-topics/topics/aplastic/treatment.html.

National Heart, Lung, and Blood Institute (NHLBI). (2012b). *Explore sickle cell anemia.* Retrieved from http://www.nhlbi.nih.gov/health/health-topics/topics/sca.

National Heart, Lung, and Blood Institute (NHLBI). (2012c). *What are thalassemias?* Retrieved from http://www.nhlbi.nih.gov/health/health-topics/topics/thalassemia.

National Heart, Lung, and Blood Institute (NHLBI). (2012d). *What causes aplastic anemia?* Retrieved from http://www.nhlbi.nih.gov/health/health-topics/topics/aplastic/causes.html.

National Heart, Lung, and Blood Institute (NHLBI). (2012e). *What is sickle cell anemia?* Retrieved from http://www.nhlbi.nih.gov/health/health-topics/topics/sca/printall-index.html.

Nelson, R. (2010). Chemotherapy drugs put health care workers at risk. *American Journal of Nursing, 110*(11), 19–21.

Ness, K. K., Kadan-Lottick, N., Armenian, S. H., & Gurney, J. G. (2011). Adverse effects of treatment in childhood acute lymphoblastic leukemia: General overview and implications for long-term cardiac health. *Expert Review of Hematology, 4,* 185–197.

Oncology Nursing Society. (2012). *Oncology Nursing Society position paper on access to quality cancer care.* Retrieved from http://www.ons.org/Publications/Positions/QualityCare.

Osborn, K. S., Wraa, C. E., Watson, A., & Holleran, R. S. (2013). *Medical-surgical nursing: Preparation for practice* (2nd ed.). Upper Saddle River, NJ: Pearson.

Ottini, L., Palli, D., Rizzo, S., Federico, M., Bazan, V., & Russo, A. (2010). Male breast cancer. *Critical Reviews in Oncology/Hematology, 73,* 141–155.

Pack-Mabien A. (2009). A primary care provider's guide to preventive and acute care management of adults and children with sickle cell disease. *Journal of the American Academy of Nurse Practitioners, 21,* 250–257.

Pelosof, L. C., & Gerber, D. E. (2010). Paraneoplastic syndromes: An approach to diagnosis and treatment. *Mayo Clinic Proceedings, 85*(9), 838–854.

Porth, C., & Matfin, G. (2010). *Pathophysiology: Concepts of altered health states* (8th ed.). Philadelphia, PA: Lippincott Williams & Wilkins.

Recklitis, C. J., Diller, L., Li, X., Najita, J., Robison, L. L., & Zeltzer, L. (2010). Suicide ideation in adult survivors of childhood cancer: A report from the childhood survivor study. *Journal of Clinical Oncology, 28*(4), 655–661.

Roback, J. D. (Ed.). (2011). *AABB technical manual* (17th ed.). Bethesda, MD: American Association of Blood Banks.

Roberts, A. (2010). *The complete human body: The definitive visual guide.* New York, NY: DK Publishing.

Roberts, C. K., & Sindhu, K. K. (2009). Oxidative stress and metabolic syndrome. *Life Sciences, 84*(21–22), 705–712.

Roberts, D., Hornung, C., & Polk Jr., H. (2009, July). Another duel in the sun: Weighing the balances between sun protection, tanning beds, and malignant melanoma. *Clinical Pediatrics, 48*(6), 614–622.

Salmela, M., Salantera, S., Ruotsalainen, T., & Aronen, E. T. (2010). Coping strategies for hospital-related fears in pre-school-aged children. *Journal of Paediatrics and Child Health, 46*(3), 108–114.

Selye, H. (1984). *The stress of life* (2nd ed. rev.). New York, NY: McGraw-Hill.

Skin Cancer Foundation. (n.d.a) *Prevention guidelines.* Retrieved from http://www.skincancer.org/prevention.

Skin Cancer Foundation. (n.d.b) *Sunburn.* Retrieved from http://www.skincancer.org/prevention/sunburn.

Stabler, S. P. (2013). Vitamin B_{12} deficiency. *New England Journal of Medicine, 368,* 149–160.

Sung, L., Aplenc, R., Alonzo, T. A., Gerbing, R., & Gamis, A. S. (2012). Predictors and short-term outcomes of hyperleukocytosis in children with acute myeloid leukemia: A report from the Children's Oncology Group. *Haematologica, 97*(11), 1770–1773.

Suskind, D. L. (2009) Nutritional deficiencies during normal growth. *Pediatric Clinics of North America, 56*(5),1035–1053.

Tomlinson, D., & Kline, N. E. (Eds.). (2010). *Pediatric oncology nursing: Advanced clinical handbook* (2nd ed.). Heidelberg, Germany: Springer-Verlag.

Trabert, B., Sigurdson, A. J., Sweeney, A. M., Strom, S. S., & McGlynn, K. A. (2011). Marijuana use and testicular germ cell tumors. *Cancer 117*(4), 848–853.

University of Maryland Medical Center (UMMC). (2009a). *Anemia—Causes.* Retrieved from http://www.umm.edu/patiented/articles/who_becomes_anemic_000057_2.htm.

University of Maryland Medical Center (UMMC). (2009b). *Sickle cell disease—Complications.* Retrieved from http://www.umm.edu/patiented/articles/what_complications_of_sickle-cell_disease_their_treatments_000058_6.htm.

University of Maryland Medical Center (UMMC). (2009c). *Sickle cell disease—Treatment.* Retrieved from http://www.umm.edu/patiented/articles/what_treatments_aimed_at_sickle-cell_disease_itself_000058_7.htm.

U.S. Department of Health and Human Services (2011). *Healthy people 2020: Cancer: Overview.* Retrieved from http://www.healthypeople.gov/2020/topicsobjectives2020/overview.aspx?topicid=5.

Wang, R., Wang, G., Ricard, M. J., Ferris, B., Strulovici-Barel, Y., Salit, J., et al. (2010). Smoking-induced upregulation of AKR1B10 expression in the airway epithelium of healthy individuals. *Chest, 138*(6), 1402–1410.

Wesa, K., & Cassileth, B. R. (2009). Is there a role for complementary therapy in the management of leukemia? *Expert Review of Anticancer Therapy, 9*(9), 1241–1249.

Wilson, B. A., Shannon, M. T., & Shields, K. M. (2013). *Pearson nurse's drug guide.* Upper Saddle River, NJ: Pearson.

Wysowski, D. K., Swartz, L., Borders-Hemphill, V., Goulding, M. R., & Dormitzer, C. (2010). Use of parenteral iron products and serious anaphylactic-type reactions. *Journal of Hematology, 85,* 650–654.

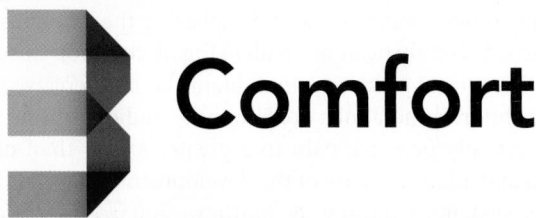 Comfort

◢ THE CONCEPT OF COMFORT

Comfort in health care is defined by Katharine Kolcaba's Comfort Theory as "the immediate state of being strengthened by having the needs for relief, ease, and transcendence addressed in the four contexts of holistic human experience: physical, psychospiritual, sociocultural, and environmental." In this definition, clients achieve *relief* when their needs are met, *ease* is a state of contentment, and *transcendence* allows clients to rise above their problems. In addition, *physical* comfort is related to bodily sensations and homeostatic mechanisms, *psychospiritual* comfort is related to the individual awareness of oneself and one's relationship to a higher being, *sociocultural* comfort is related to family and societal relationships, and *environmental* comfort is related to the external surroundings (Kolcaba, Tilton, & Drouin, 2006).

Increased comfort, reduced stress, and a healing environment are linked to increased client satisfaction and shorter hospital stays (Geimer-Flanders, 2009; HermanMiller, 2010; Seifert & Hickman, 2005). Stressors can include anything from pain to lack of natural lighting to fear of the unknown. Providing a healing environment in which stressors are reduced through adequate comfort measures allows clients to maintain normal vital signs, receive adequate sleep–rest and nutrition, and feel a sense of control over their healing process. **≪**

Concept Learning Outcomes

After reading about this concept, you will be able to:

1. Summarize the physiology of comfort.
2. Examine the relationship between comfort and other concepts/systems.
3. Identify commonly occurring alterations in comfort and their related therapies.
4. Differentiate common assessment procedures used to examine comfort across the life span.
5. Describe diagnostic and laboratory tests to determine the individual's comfort status.
6. Explain management of comfort and prevention of discomfort.
7. Demonstrate the nursing process in providing culturally competent and caring interventions across the life span for individuals with common alterations in comfort.
8. Compare and contrast common independent and collaborative interventions for clients with alterations in comfort.

Concept Key Terms

Acute fatigue, *145*
Acute pain, *143*
Breathing exercises, *150*
Chronic fatigue, *145*
Chronic fatigue syndrome, *145*
Chronic pain, *143*
Comfort, *141*
End-of-life care, *145*
Fatigue, *145*
Fibromyalgia, *145*
Imagery, *150*

Insomnia, *145*
Movement techniques, *151*
Muscle relaxation, *150*
Narcolepsy, *145*
Pain, *143*
Parasomnia, *145*
Polysomnography (PSG), *148*
Restless leg syndrome, *145*
Sleep apnea, *145*
Sleep hygiene, *149*
Sleep loss, *145*
Tender points, *145*

▶ NORMAL PRESENTATION OF COMFORT

Comfort is a relative feeling based on expectations and past experiences. Therefore, a "normal" level of comfort may be different for every client. However, there are some elements of comfort that are common to all individuals.

Physiology Review

An individual experiences comfort when each level of Maslow's hierarchy of needs is fulfilled (**Figure 3–1** ●). The most basic physiological needs of oxygen, shelter, food, water, and sleep are met, and the individual feels safe and free from anxiety, fear, and pain. The individual who experiences true comfort senses love and belonging from family and friends. For individuals seeking health care, comfort also includes participating in a healthy nurse–client relationship. In addition, individuals experience comfort in the areas of self-esteem and self-actualization by giving and receiving respect, feeling confident, and accepting reality.

Because comfort is subjective, the nurse should aim to understand what is "comfortable" or "normal" for the client. Some clients have difficulty articulating this or have such a high tolerance for discomfort that it is difficult to determine an appropriate baseline. For example, a woman who has worked for the Peace Corps in Africa for several years may be unperturbed by an extra day's stay in the hospital, but an Olympic athlete might find the extra day of confinement and rest intolerable.

Signs of comfort can sometimes be determined from client assessment for sympathetic nervous system responses such as heart and respiratory rate, blood pressure, and body and skin temperature. However, "normal" vital signs are not always reliable indicators of comfort. Usually, a number of other criteria are also associated with a client's comfort level, such as the presence or absence of pain; degree of sleep and rest; balance of nutrition and fluids; and sensory perceptions of heat, cold, odor, and noise. Body language, such as grimacing or guarding, is also an important indicator of comfort level.

LIFESPAN CONSIDERATIONS Determining an infant's comfort level is complicated because infants are not yet able to verbalize specific complaints related to discomfort. Infants are likely to respond similarly to pain, fear, hunger, dirty diapers, and many other conditions, and deciphering the true cause of an infant's discomfort can be challenging. A common misconception in medical practice is that infants do not perceive pain as older children and adults do. However, studies indicate that infants actually perceive pain to a greater extent than older children and adults because of the developmental stage of their nervous systems (Mathew & Mathew, 2003; Fitzgerald & Walker, 2009).

Assessment of the older adult's comfort level may also be challenging. Some older adults believe chronic pain and sleep disorders are an inevitable part of the aging process and are therefore reluctant to report discomfort. The misconception that older adults feel less pain than younger adults may lead to undertreatment of pain and discomfort. Although older adults may have a higher pain threshold, their pain tolerance often is lower (Hallingbye, Martin, & Viscomi, 2011). Clients with cognitive impairment, such as Alzheimer disease, are unlikely to express even severe pain verbally, and the nurse must recognize behavioral cues as indicators of pain. Older adults are also more likely to suffer from sleep disorders; approximately 50% of older adults report difficulty sleeping (Neikrug & Ancoli-Israel, 2010). Treatment of sleep disorders and pain in older adults enhances their daytime functioning and quality of life.

Ethnicity is another factor that influences the perception and treatment of discomfort. Some ethnic groups, such as Blacks, tend to be more verbally expressive about their discomfort. While other ethnic groups, such as American Indians, are more likely to endure the discomfort without seeking health care. Regardless of the degree of pain experienced, multiple studies have shown that Blacks and Hispanics are less likely to receive adequate treatment for pain and are more likely than Whites to receive nonopioid analgesics rather than opioid analgesics (Meghani, Byun, & Gallagher, 2012). When caring for clients of different ethnic backgrounds, nurses must be culturally competent in dealing with the client's needs. All clients, regardless of ethnic background, have the right to receive adequate comfort care using pharmacologic and nonpharmacologic methods.

▶ ALTERATIONS TO COMFORT

Very few people meet the criteria for comfort stated by Kolcaba. What aspects of discomfort are most commonly encountered by nurses? This chapter focuses on five common sources of discomfort: pain, end-of-life care, fatigue, fibromyalgia, and sleep–rest disorders. Read Concepts Related to Comfort to see how Comfort is interrelated with other concepts.

Alterations and Manifestations

Pain, fatigue, and sleep–rest disorders are basic alterations in comfort caused by disease, illness, or injury; fibromyalgia is a classic example of a disease characterized by these three types of discomfort. Discomfort is also a reality at the end of life, and nurses must provide comfort for clients and families during end-of-life care. These alterations in comfort will be summarized here and explored in depth in the exemplar sections (also see the Alterations and Therapies feature).

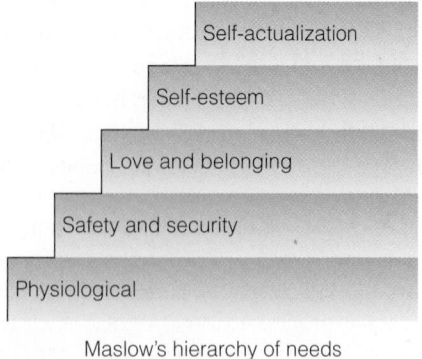

Figure 3–1 ● Maslow's hierarchy of needs.

Concepts Related to **Comfort**

Promotion of comfort is an integral part of nursing care. The exemplars included in this module explore several common manifestations of discomfort, including pain, fatigue, and sleep–rest disorders. However, alterations in comfort are not limited to these specific manifestations. The concept of comfort is interrelated to numerous other physiological and psychosocial concepts. For example, one of the classic symptoms of inflammation is pain. Therefore, nurses can offer comfort to clients with inflammation by administering pain medications as ordered and providing nonpharmacologic comfort measures such as cold therapy. Clients with pain, especially joint pain, lower back pain, or trauma pain, often experience decreased mobility. Nursing interventions for these clients may include ambulation assistance and hygiene care. Impaired tissue integrity is a common cause of discomfort and can

also lead to more serious complications, such as infection. Comfort measures may include assessing the client for infection, providing hygiene care for the wound, and assisting with repositioning for immobile clients.

Promotion of comfort includes both physical and psychosocial wellness. Individuals suffering grief over a lost loved one or lost personal health may need emotional comfort in the form of therapeutic communication or referrals to support groups. Comfort care is also closely tied to ethical issues for many clients, such as individuals with drug addiction who need opioid treatment for severe pain or the family deciding about withdrawing or withholding of life-sustaining treatments for a client at the end of life. The relationship between comfort and the concepts of inflammation, mobility, tissue integrity, grief and loss, and ethics are summarized in the following table.

CONCEPT	RELATIONSHIP TO COMFORT	NURSING IMPLICATIONS
Inflammation		
■ Assessment interview: Inflammation ■ Independent interventions and therapies	Inflammation → pain.	■ Assess pain in clients with inflammation; provide pharmacologic treatments as ordered. ■ Offer comfort measures such as ice or heat; promote adequate sleep and rest.
Mobility		
■ Mobility assessment ■ Assessment interview: Mobility	↓ mobility is often caused by pain, injury, or disease.	■ Assist with ambulation and activities of daily living; encourage adequate sleep and rest. ■ Offer pharmacologic treatments as ordered.
Tissue Integrity		
■ Integumentary assessment ■ Pressure ulcers	↓ tissue integrity = ↑ risk for pain, inflammation, and infection.	■ Assess for skin breakdown; promote mobility. ■ Assist with repositioning as needed; monitor for signs and symptoms of infection.
Grief and Loss		
■ Assessment interview: Grief and loss	Loss or expected loss of a loved one is emotionally distressing.	■ Use therapeutic communication techniques; encourage expression of emotions; facilitate referrals to counselors and support groups.
Ethics		
	Physicians may be reluctant to prescribe opioids based on race, ethnicity, or history of addiction.	■ Advocate for the provision of adequate pain relief to all clients; provide culturally sensitive care; offer nonpharmacologic comfort measures to all clients.

PAIN   Pain is the most common reason individuals seek emergency health care (Bergman, 2012). The International Association for the Study of Pain (2012) has defined **pain** as "an unpleasant sensory and emotional experience associated with actual or potential tissue damage, or described in terms of such damage." Because pain is a perceptual and emotional experience, clients can provide only a subjective description of their pain. Most individuals view pain as a negative, but pain can also be positive in that it provides a warning of injury, illness, and disease. Therefore pain is often called the *fifth vital sign*,

although some physicians object to this classification because pain is subjective, whereas assessment of body temperature, pulse and respiratory rate, and blood pressure is objective.

Pain may be described in terms of location, duration, intensity, quality, and etiology. *Duration* establishes the difference between acute and chronic pain. **Acute pain** is defined as pain that lasts only through the expected recovery period, which is usually 30 days to 6 months. Acute pain typically has a sudden onset related to injury, surgery, or illness. In contrast, **chronic pain** lasts longer than 6 months and persists beyond the expected period of healing.

Alterations and Therapies **Comfort**

ALTERATION	DESCRIPTION/ DEFINITION	MANIFESTATIONS	INTERVENTIONS AND THERAPIES
Acute pain	Pain of varying severity, location, and etiology that lasts fewer than 6 months.	▪ Elevated blood pressure ▪ Increased heart rate ▪ Nausea and vomiting ▪ Sweating ▪ Rapid/shallow respirations ▪ Anxiety ▪ Decreased function in activities of daily living	Pharmacologic pain management: ▪ Opioid analgesics ▪ Nonsteroidal anti-inflammatory drugs (NSAIDs) ▪ Nonopioid analgesics Nonpharmacologic therapy: ▪ Massage ▪ Diversionary therapies (music, involvement in hobbies, aroma therapy) ▪ Application of heat and cold
Chronic pain	Pain of varying severity, location, and etiology that lasts 6 months or more (even if intermittent).	▪ Depression ▪ Irritability ▪ Impaired mobility and/or activity ▪ Sleep disturbance	Pharmacologic pain management: ▪ Nonopioid analgesics ▪ Antidepressants ▪ NSAIDs ▪ Muscle relaxants ▪ Opioid analgesics Nonpharmacologic therapy: ▪ Guided imagery ▪ Massage ▪ Nerve stimulation units ▪ Chiropractic interventions ▪ Physical therapy ▪ Relaxation techniques ▪ Positioning
End-of-life care	Care that takes place when death is imminent	▪ Loss of muscle tone ▪ Slowing of circulation ▪ Change in respirations ▪ Sensory impairments ▪ Impaired metabolic processes	▪ Palliative or aggressive care as chosen by client and family ▪ Maintenance of comfort ▪ Maintenance of hygiene ▪ Psychosocial support for client and family
Fatigue	Lack of energy or motivation with or without drowsiness	▪ Tiredness ▪ Depression ▪ Anxiety ▪ Irritability ▪ Decreased cognition	Pharmacologic therapy: ▪ Sleeping aids ▪ Stimulants ▪ Antidepressants ▪ Pain management Nonpharmacologic therapy: ▪ Improved sleep hygiene ▪ Nutritional supplements ▪ Relaxation techniques ▪ CAM therapies
Fibromyalgia	Widespread muscular and joint pain	▪ Tenderness in the neck, spine, shoulders, and hips ▪ Muscle spasm or stiffness ▪ Chronic fatigue ▪ Sleep disturbances	▪ Warm compresses or heat packs ▪ Massage ▪ Stretching exercises ▪ Fibromyalgia drugs ▪ Good sleep hygiene
Sleep–rest disorders	The inability to fall asleep or stay asleep, or a sleep disturbance that causes lack of adequate rest	▪ Sleep loss ▪ Insomnia ▪ Narcolepsy ▪ Sleep apnea ▪ Parasomnias	▪ Improved sleep hygiene ▪ Pharmacologic therapies ▪ Relaxation techniques ▪ Assistive breathing devices (e.g., CPAP)

According to The Joint Commission (2012), clients in pain have the right to receive adequate assessment and management of their pain. In conjunction with this client right, The Joint Commission has provided pain management standards, including a comprehensive pain assessment when pain is identified, education of healthcare providers about pain assessment and management, policies that allow efficient ordering of pain medications, and education of clients and their families about effective pain management (Berry & Dahl, 2000).

END-OF-LIFE CARE   **End-of-life care** is nursing care given to a client who is near death as well as care provided to the client's family. Although frequently associated with older adults, end-of-life care may be needed by clients of all ages. The National Cancer Institute (2012) states that "end-of-life care provides physical, mental, and emotional comfort, as well as social support, to people who are living with and dying of advanced illness." Nurses contribute to the quality of this care, particularly as it pertains to education, use of evidence-based practices, client advocacy, and evaluation of care. Nursing interventions associated with end-of-life care include helping clients perform daily activities such as bathing and toileting; providing information and emotional and spiritual support to the client and family; and helping the family make ethical decisions about life-sustaining interventions (Hebert, Moore, & Rooney, 2011).

FATIGUE   **Fatigue** is a lack of energy and motivation. Although drowsiness can be associated with fatigue, the two terms are not interchangeable. Fatigue is often accompanied by apathy. Like pain, fatigue can be characterized as acute or chronic. **Acute fatigue** manifests as normal tiredness associated with a single event, such as a poor night's sleep, a stressful experience, or an acute infection. Symptoms of acute fatigue usually begin quickly and are also resolved quickly by adequate sleep–rest and resolution of the underlying cause of fatigue.

In contrast, **chronic fatigue** is more intense and lasts longer than acute fatigue, with a nearly constant state of weariness that diminishes energy and mental capacity (Mayo Clinic, 2010a). Chronic fatigue is often caused by long-term illnesses or medications used to treat chronic disease. Chronic fatigue that lasts more than six months and is accompanied by muscle and joint pain, headaches, and sleep and memory problems may be **chronic fatigue syndrome** (MedlinePlus, 2012). Chronic fatigue syndrome is usually diagnosed after all other causes of fatigue have been ruled out and if the fatigue does not diminish with adequate sleep–rest.

FIBROMYALGIA   **Fibromyalgia** is a disease characterized by widespread musculoskeletal pain, fatigue, sleep disturbances, and decreased cognitive functioning. Widespread pain is defined as pain on both the right and left sides of the body and both above and below the waist (Smith, Harris, & Clauw, 2011). Its existence is often determined by a test of the tenderness at 18 **tender points** located throughout the neck, shoulder, chest, hip, knee and elbow regions. Because no cure for fibromyalgia exists, treatment is symptomatic. According to the National Fibromyalgia Association (n.d.), an estimated 10 million Americans and a total of 3%–6% of the world's population suffer from fibromyalgia.

SLEEP AND REST DISORDERS   According to Maslow, sleep is one of the basic physiological needs of life. Sleep is characterized by a state of unconsciousness and a decreased responsiveness to external stimuli. During sleep, the human body enters a phase of restoration, as manifested by enhanced wound healing, a boost in the immune system, anabolic metabolism, and energy conservation. In infants and children, sleep is also necessary for brain development.

Humans need to spend approximately one third of their lives sleeping. Yet despite the physiological importance of sleep, a recent *Sleep in America* poll (2010) reports that 34%–60% of American adults sleep less than 7 hours on weeknights. In addition, the Institute of Medicine (IOM; 2006) estimates that 50–70 million Americans suffer from disorders of sleep and wakefulness. Sleep deprivation hinders daily functioning and adversely affects health, contributing to diseases such as diabetes, cardiovascular disease, and depression. Sleep deprivation is also linked to an increased risk for motor vehicle crashes (National Sleep Foundation, 2011). The prevalence of sleep disorders and sleep deprivation caused the IOM to make several recommendations, including increasing the awareness of the general public about the problems caused by sleep loss and sleep disturbances and educating and training healthcare professionals about sleep medicine.

The IOM's 2006 report, considered a seminal reference on the subject, focused on the most common sleep disturbances, including sleep loss, sleep-disordered breathing, insomnia, narcolepsy, parasomnias, restless leg syndrome, and several others. **Sleep loss** refers to a duration of sleep shorter than the recommended 7–8 hours per night for adults. Sleep-disordered breathing, or **sleep apnea**, occurs when an individual experiences breathing pauses during sleep. **Insomnia** is characterized by difficulty falling asleep or maintaining sleep or by a short sleep duration even with adequate time spent attempting to sleep. **Narcolepsy** is a condition in which the individual experiences excessive daytime sleepiness even with adequate nighttime sleep, resulting in sleep attacks and cataplexy. **Parasomnias** are unpleasant or undesirable behaviors (such as sleep walking or sleep terrors) that occur at any point during sleep. **Restless leg syndrome (RLS)** is a neurological disorder that results in an irresistible urge to move the legs or other body parts, often resulting in impaired sleep habits.

Genetic Considerations and Nonmodifiable Risk Factors

Genetics plays a major role in an individual's susceptibility to a number of diseases associated with discomfort. For example, cancer, amyotrophic lateral sclerosis (ALS), Marfan syndrome, and sickle cell disease are related to genetic abnormalities. In addition, some genetic mutations directly affect an individual's ability to perceive pain. For example, certain mutations of the *SCN9A* gene are associated with an increased risk for chronic pain disorders such as paroxysmal extreme pain disorder, inherited erythromelalgia (a disease that causes intense burning sensations in the hands and/or feet), and fibromyalgia (Goldberg et al., 2012; Vargas-Alarcon et al., 2012). Conversely, other forms of *SCN9A* mutation cause congenital insensitivity to pain (Cox et al., 2006; National Institutes of Health, 2013). Genetic mutations can also cause sleep disturbances, depression, and anxiety. Genetic mutations are associated with both narcolepsy and fatal familial insomnia (Crocker & Sehgal, 2010). Multiple psychiatric disorders, including autism, anxiety, panic disorder, and other mood disorders are believed to be genetic in origin (Williams et al., 2009).

CASE STUDY \\ PART 1

April Daves is a 34-year-old Black female who was in a severe motor vehicle accident 6 months ago. All of her injuries have healed, but when she continues to have chronic pain in several of her joints and muscles, her primary care physician refers her to an orthopedic specialist. As the nurse at the orthopedic clinic, you are responsible for obtaining Ms. Daves's medical history and making the initial assessment. You learn that Ms. Daves broke her left fibula near the knee, dislocated her left shoulder, and suffered whiplash. She reports almost constant burning pain and stiffness in her left knee, shoulder, and neck, but sometimes she also feels pain in her right knee and in her hips. She figures it is just "sympathy pain," but the combined pain makes movement difficult. She rates her current pain at a 5 on a scale of 0–10, but if she has to move around a lot, it increases to a 7. Her vital signs are temperature 97.2°F oral; pulse 86 bpm; respirations 20/min; and BP 146/82 mmHg. Ms. Daves reports she has been trying to manage her pain with acetaminophen and ibuprofen. However, they aren't always effective, and she often has trouble sleeping at night because of the pain. Her boss is starting to notice a drop in productivity at work because she has trouble staying awake when sitting at her desk.

After the physician reviews Ms. Daves's health history and performs a physical assessment, he sends her for x-rays on her left knee and shoulder. Although the x-rays do not show any obvious abnormalities, he suspects Ms. Daves may have developed osteoarthritis. The physician asks you to schedule Ms. Daves for a CT scan of her left knee and left shoulder. He prescribes meloxicam (Mobic) as an analgesic and recommends that the client return for a follow up visit after her CT scans are completed.

Clinical Reasoning Questions Level I
1. During her client history, what alterations in comfort does Ms. Daves reveal?
2. Based on Ms. Daves's vital signs, what assumptions can you make about her level of discomfort?
3. Why might Ms. Daves's other joints be feeling "sympathy pain," as she describes it?

Clinical Reasoning Questions Level II
4. What nonpharmacologic therapies could you suggest for pain management? Fatigue?

5. What possible conditions could Ms. Daves have other than osteoarthritis?
6. What additional assessments may be beneficial for Ms. Daves's care?

▶ PREVENTION

Prevention of discomfort begins with the client. Personal preferences, lifestyle habits, and culture are all factors in the development of chronic diseases and other contributors to discomfort, and only the client can change behaviors that increase the risk of discomfort. However, nurses provide essential client education that can encourage clients to change their behaviors to decrease the risk of developing a chronic disease or experiencing an acute illness or injury.

Lifestyle habits that predispose individuals to chronic health alterations, such as poor nutrition, smoking, excessive alcohol consumption, and poor sleep hygiene, all increase an individual's risk for experiencing discomfort. Poor nutrition can include both overeating and undernutrition. Eating a healthy diet in combination with good sleep hygiene can help prevent the development of many chronic diseases that lead to symptoms of discomfort.

Smoking, alcohol consumption, and illicit drug use can also lead to alterations in comfort. Because nicotine, alcohol, and illicit drugs are addictive, quitting drug use is associated with withdrawal symptoms. Emotional withdrawal symptoms include anxiety, irritability, insomnia, and depression. Physical withdrawal symptoms include sweating, palpitations, nausea, and difficulty breathing.

Other lifestyle habits that may lead to discomfort are working at a job that requires heavy lifting, long hours, or repetitive movement, which increases the risk of injury and fatigue. Participation in physical activities such as team sports or extreme sports also increases susceptibility to injury and consequent discomfort.

▶ ASSESSMENT

The nursing assessment should explore not only the client's level of discomfort but also the degree to which discomfort is affecting the client's daily life. Some clients may not even realize the extent to which discomfort is impacting their lifestyle and overall well-being.

Nursing Assessment

Every assessment should begin with reviewing the client's health history, followed by interviewing the client regarding any complaints related to discomfort, including pain, fatigue, anxiety, or depression. If the client reports discomfort, the interview and physical examination should be further targeted to address the specific areas of concern. See the Comfort Assessment and Assessment Interview features for a sample client interview and a guide to focused physical assessment of the client experiencing alterations in comfort.

Comfort Assessment

ASSESSMENT/METHOD	NORMAL FINDINGS	ABNORMAL FINDINGS	LIFESPAN OR DEVELOPMENTAL CONSIDERATIONS
Interview Client History			
Client description of symptoms. Pain scale. Depression assessment.	The client should report no signs or symptoms of discomfort.	■ Client reports mild to severe pain. ■ Client reports disrupted sleep patterns. ■ Client reports or displays signs of nausea or vomiting. ■ Client reports lack of appetite or ravenous appetite. ■ Client reports lack of motivation, feelings of despair, or feelings of anxiety.	■ Look for nonverbal signs of discomfort such as crying, shielding an injured area, lack of affect, or withdrawal in nonverbal children and mentally impaired clients. ■ Signs of depression and anxiety in children may indicate abuse, and assessment of the child in the absence of the parent(s) may be warranted. ■ Gastrointestinal discomfort can be a physiological response to disease or it can be a side effect of medication. Check client history for current medications and known drug allergies. ■ Depression and anxiety can be primary or secondary conditions. Be sure to assess the depressed or anxious client for symptoms of chronic conditions.
Physical Assessment			
Vital signs. Visual inspection. Polysomnography (PSG) for identification of suspected sleep disorders. Blood and urine analysis.	Client should have normal vital signs, and no obvious external injuries or infections. Results of all clinical tests should be within normal limits.	■ Severe pain may be accompanied by sympathetic nervous system findings such as increased heart rate, sweating, and nausea. ■ PSG indicates abnormal REM/NREM cycles or severe apnea (Mayo Clinic, 2011a). ■ Client appears depressed, nervous, or confused. ■ Abnormal blood and urine analysis may indicate illness or malnutrition.	■ Children may be fearful of physical assessment. To promote comfort, allow the child to sit on the parent's or guardian's lap during the assessment. ■ Take into consideration biophysical changes that occur in older adults when conducting physical assessment.

Lifespan and Cultural Considerations

Age and developmental stage affect the ability to accurately describe pain and discomfort. Special considerations for assessing discomfort and promoting comfort throughout each developmental stage are described in the Lifespan Considerations feature.

Clients' culture also plays a major role in how they perceive discomfort, as some cultures expect flamboyant descriptions of discomfort while other cultures value stoicism. Cultural differences in expressions of pain are further discussed in the Focus on Diversity and Culture feature on page 161 in the exemplar on Acute and Chronic Pain in this module.

Stay Current: *The Hartford Institute of Geriatric Nursing offers Try This, a site with assessment tools for use on older adults.* **http://hartfordign.org/resources/try_this_series/**

DIAGNOSTIC TESTS Diagnostic tests may be ordered to determine if there is an underlying biological cause of the client's discomfort, as well as to gain additional assessment data. X-rays may be useful for determining whether a physical injury is present. Blood tests may also be conducted. For example, a white blood cell (WBC) count may be useful in identifying infection, and hemoglobin and hematocrit measurements can be used to determine if fatigue is caused by iron-deficiency

Assessment Interview Discomfort (Pain, Depression, Anxiety, Appetite, Sleep Disorder)

Current Problem

- When did your discomfort start?
- How would you describe your discomfort?
- On a scale of 0 to 10, with 0 meaning no pain and 10 meaning the worst pain you can imagine, how would you rate your current pain intensity?
- Which activities make the discomfort better or worse?
- How long have you had this discomfort?
- How does this discomfort affect your activities of daily living?
- What do you do to alleviate your discomfort?
- Are you currently taking any medications to alleviate your discomfort?
- Does your discomfort affect your sleep pattern or your mood?
- Does your discomfort affect your appetite?
- Does eating or drinking make your discomfort better or worse?
- Do you feel that your discomfort is related to another disease or condition?
- Do you feel sad frequently?

- Do you have trouble motivating yourself to participate in daily activities?
- Have you had thoughts of suicide?
- Have you had any changes in daily habits that increased your symptoms of discomfort?

Client History

- Have you had this discomfort in the past?
- How often does this symptom of discomfort occur?
- Have you taken medications for this problem in the past?
- Have you had past experiences that affect the way you view this discomfort?

Lifestyle

- Do you drink alcohol? If so, how much? Do you feel this contributes to your symptoms?
- Do you smoke? If so, how much? Do you feel this contributes to your symptoms?
- Do you exercise? Is your condition related to your participation in physical activity?
- Describe your average daily food and drink intake. Do you feel that your diet contributes to your symptoms?

anemia. **Polysomnographies**, or sleep studies, are often used to diagnose sleep disorders.

CASE STUDY \\ PART 2

Two days before April Daves is scheduled to return to her orthopedic physician, she is awakened by severe pain. Because she is unable to get out of bed, Ms. Daves calls 911. She is transferred to the hospital by ambulance. As her emergency department (ED) nurse, you assess Ms. Daves. Her only complaint is pain, which she rates as a 9 on a scale of 0 to 10. Ms. Daves reports she has been taking her NSAIDs as prescribed. Her heart rate, respiratory rate, and blood pressure are all slightly elevated. Ms. Daves further reports that the pain has prevented her from sleeping more than 3–4 hours each night. Aside from her motor vehicle crash, Ms. Daves has no history of illness or trauma. You report your findings to the ED physician.

After reviewing Ms. Daves's medical history and performing a physical assessment, the physician orders a complete blood count (CBC) and a urinalysis, the results of which are normal. He also obtains the results of Ms. Daves's CT scans, which are normal. The ED physician suspects that Ms. Daves may have fibromyalgia. Using the 2010 fibromyalgia criteria, the ED physician determines that Ms. Daves's widespread pain index is 8 and her symptom severity scale score is 9. The physician diagnoses Ms. Daves with fibromyalgia and prescribes milnacipran (Savella). He instructs her to visit her primary care physician for follow up as soon as possible.

Clinical Reasoning Questions Level I

1. What causes fibromyalgia?
2. What nursing interventions can you implement immediately to help relieve Ms. Daves's pain?
3. For the client with fibromyalgia, what findings would you expect to be revealed by the CBC and urinalysis?

Clinical Reasoning Questions Level II

4. Refer to the exemplar on Fibromyalgia in this module. Based on your knowledge of Ms. Daves's clinical signs and symptoms, what somatic symptoms is she likely to be experiencing?
5. Why did the physician choose milnacipran instead of duloxetine or pregabalin for Ms. Daves's fibromyalgia?
6. What client teaching topics should you review with Ms. Daves before her discharge?

▶ INTERVENTIONS AND THERAPIES

For the client experiencing alterations in comfort, initial interventions are directed at identifying the source of the discomfort. For clients with physical pain, while pain relief is a priority, masking the pain through analgesic administration can make identifying the underlying cause much more difficult. For this reason, especially until the cause of the client's discomfort is identified, interventions to promote comfort may focus on nonpharmacologic measures. These include simple interventions such as applying heat or cold as

Lifespan Considerations Comfort

Infants/Toddlers

■ Infants verbalize discomfort by crying. Ask the parents for descriptions of the infant's manifestations of pain, including suspected location and how the pain influences eating, sleeping, and behavior.

■ Discomfort in otherwise healthy infants may be related to milk components. Bottle-fed infants may need a specialized formula. For breastfed infants, the mother's diet may need to be modified.

■ Infants and toddlers should be comforted by being held, rocking, murmuring soothing words, and rubbing or patting the torso or extremities.

■ Many pain medications have no dosing instructions for children under 2 years old. Warn parents to follow physician's orders for all medications given to infants and toddlers.

Children

■ Involve the child in describing any discomfort, but also ask the parent(s) or guardian about the child's behaviors related to discomfort.

■ Before performing any procedures or tests, explain the procedure to the child to help decrease anxiety. When possible, it may also help to demonstrate the procedure on the parent before performing the procedure on the child.

■ Depending on age and personality, children may be comforted by being held, hugging, holding hands, or receiving a treat like a sucker, sticker, or small toy.

■ If you must perform a painful procedure such as an injection, engage the parent in the child's care by asking the parent to offer comfort or distraction.

Adolescents

■ Adolescents may respond to treatment and comfort better if you interact with them as adults rather than as children.

■ Some adolescents may reject any offer of comfort.

Adults

■ If diagnosed with a chronic or fatal disease, adults may find comfort in knowledge. Take the time to describe the disease and what to expect for tests, medications, and other interventions, and to answer any questions they have.

■ Comfort is a subjective experience, so listen carefully when the client is describing any feelings of discomfort, and care for the client accordingly.

Pregnant Women

■ Pregnant women, especially first-time mothers, may be very anxious about their health and the health of their baby. Take time to explain the expected growth and development of the fetus and expected maternal changes. Answer any questions.

■ Provide tips about self-care, physical activity, and sleeping positions that will help ease discomfort. Encourage adequate nutrition, hydration, and sleep–rest.

Older Adults

■ Older adults are more likely to suffer from chronic conditions such as diabetes, chronic pain, heart disease, cancer, and arthritis. Provide a safe and comfortable environment for regular appointments, and foster a healthy nurse–client relationship to promote comfort.

■ Explain procedures and medications at each visit; some older adult clients have memory deficits. Provide written instructions and explanations. Provide assistance with movement as needed, especially for clients with chronic pain or arthritis.

End of Life

■ Provide adequate pain relief with pharmacologic agents as ordered.

■ Promote psychosocial comfort by offering to arrange a visit from a spiritual leader and/or loved ones.

■ Facilitate referrals for grief counseling for the family and other loved ones.

■ Honor the client's and family's decisions about end-of-life care.

appropriate and providing distractions (e.g., reading material, music, crossword puzzles, humor); client teaching related to sleep hygiene, repatterning thinking, and relaxation therapy; and collaborative interventions including complementary therapy.

Independent

Promotion of comfort includes teaching clients about lifestyle changes that can help decrease their symptoms of pain, depression, or fatigue. Three basic independent categories of teaching include sleep hygiene, psychosocial well-being, and relaxation therapy.

SLEEP HYGIENE Discomfort associated with illness or injury often causes sleep disturbances. Therefore education should include teaching about the importance of sleep hygiene. **Sleep hygiene** refers to a variety of sleep practices that help individuals attain good-quality sleep at night so they can be alert during the day. Good sleep hygiene includes maintaining a regular sleep and awake pattern, performing bedtime rituals, providing a restful environment, and promoting comfort and relaxation. If the client takes medications to promote sleep, teaching should include the appropriate use of pharmacologic agents and their side effects. More details on good sleep hygiene are provided in the Client Teaching feature on page 187 in the exemplar on Fatigue in this module.

For the hospitalized client, sleep disturbances may be related to the hospital environment rather than physical or emotional discomfort. Whenever possible, schedule procedures, medications, meals, and other activities around the client's normal sleep schedule. Nurses should assess the client's individual circadian rhythm, because clients who normally go to sleep late may develop sleep disturbances if forced to attempt sleep before their normal bedtime. In contrast, clients who are early risers may prefer to have physical therapy first thing in the morning.

Once a sleep schedule is identified, bedtime rituals may include assisting the client with hygiene activities such as toileting and a hand and face wash, offering a warm beverage or massage, and retrieving fresh pillows or extra blankets. Reduce environmental distractions such as noise and external light sources, as outlined in **Box 3–1** ●. If good sleep hygiene still does not produce a restful night of sleep, it may be appropriate to request an order for a sedative/hypnotic to help the client sleep.

PSYCHOSOCIAL WELL-BEING   When managing alterations in comfort, clients both in and out of a hospital environment will benefit from the promotion of optimal psychosocial well-being. Laughter helps relieve pain, reduce stress, boost immunity, improve mood, and strengthen relationships (Mayo Clinic, 2010c). A positive attitude can also help ease distress (Mayo Clinic, 2011b). It can decrease depression and stress, increase cardiovascular health, and help the client develop essential coping skills. Clients should be encouraged to participate in enjoyable activities such as gardening, crafting, reading,

or playing games; interacting with a pet; listening to or performing music; spending time in nature; and volunteering to help others (Simon, 2011). Clients who expend energy on enjoyable activities and on helping others tend to focus less on their own discomfort and instead develop a sense of self-worth and purpose in life.

The client's psychosocial well-being may also be enhanced through interacting with family and friends. Family and friends can help lift the burden of an acute or chronic condition by assisting with activities of daily living and by helping clients feel they are not alone. They can encourage the client to persist in following healthcare suggestions and pharmacologic therapies and to seek medical help when needed. A supportive group of family and friends is important not only for clients, it is also essential for caregivers, especially when they are caring for someone with a debilitating disease or at the end of life.

RELAXATION THERAPY   Relaxation techniques reduce stress by slowing the heart and respiratory rates, lowering blood pressure, and increasing blood flow to major muscles. Relaxation techniques can also be used to induce sleep, reduce pain, and calm emotions (Mayo Clinic, 2011c). According to the National Center for Complementary and Alternative Medicine (2011), relaxation techniques are beneficial in the treatment of several symptoms of discomfort, including anxiety, depression, headache, and pain. Some of the major benefits of relaxation therapy are that the techniques can be learned with very little training, are relatively inexpensive to practice, and can be performed without the help of a healthcare provider.

The four major categories of relaxation techniques are breathing, muscle relaxation, imagery, and movement.

■ **Breathing exercises** are used to slow the breathing rate by focusing on taking regular and deep breaths from the diaphragm. This process increases oxygen intake and therefore increases oxygen delivery throughout the body.

■ **Muscle relaxation** involves tightening and then relaxing each muscle group, usually spending between 5–15 seconds in the contraction phase and up to 30 seconds in the relaxation phase. It is most beneficial to relax muscles progressively either from head to toe or from toe to head. This technique helps clients recognize the difference between tension and relaxation, so that they learn to consciously relax muscles that become tense due to stress or discomfort (Mayo Clinic, 2011c).

■ **Imagery**, or guided imagery, involves focusing on pleasant images, such as a beach or garden, to replace negative images, such as pain and darkness. Imagery can be directed by the individual or by a practitioner who uses storytelling or descriptions to guide the client into a more relaxed state. Soothing music or nature sounds may be used to enhance the imagery. Imagery creates a connection between the mind and the body and enhances the client's coping skills. In addition, guided imagery can counteract panic, anger, pain, depression, and insomnia and can decrease recovery time (Cleveland Clinic, n.d.).

Box 3–1   Minimizing Environmental Stimuli in the Hospital Setting

NOISE

■ Place clients in single-bed rooms when possible instead of multiple-bed rooms. If a client must be in a semiprivate or larger room, close the curtains between clients.

■ Keep the client's door closed to reduce hallway noise.

■ Reduce excess noise during evening and early morning hours (e.g., turn off televisions, lower the ringtone of telephones, reduce the volume or discontinue use of the paging system).

■ Minimize noise from staff interactions.

■ Perform only essential activities in the client's room during sleeping hours.

LIGHT

■ Adjust window coverings to block outside lights at night and to allow natural light during the day.

■ At night, use a night-light or turn on bathroom lights instead of overhead lighting.

■ When entering a client's darkened room, use a flashlight instead of turning on the room lights.

Sources: Based on Berman, A., & Snyder, S. J. (2012). Sleep. In Kozier and Erb's fundamentals of nursing: Concepts, process, and practice (p. 1196, Box 45-5). Upper Saddle River, NJ: Pearson Education.; Ulrich, R., Zimring, C., Quan, X., Joseph, A., & Choudhary, R. (2004). Role of the physical environment in the hospital of the 21st century. Retrieved February 4, 2013, from http://www.healthdesign.org/chd/research/role-physical-environment-hospital-21st-century

Medications **Pain**

CLASSIFICATION AND DRUG EXAMPLES	MECHANISM OF ACTION	NURSING CONSIDERATIONS

Nonopioids
 	
Drug examples:
acetaminophen
	Act in the CNS to increase the pain threshold.
	
	May also be used for:
	■ Antipyretic
		Acetaminophen causes hepatotoxicity; intake should be carefully monitored, especially in malnourished individuals or individuals who have consumed alcohol.
		    Acetaminophen is included in many drug mixtures, so be sure the client is not accidentally overdosing.
		    Assess hepatic function for chronic acetaminophen users or in suspected overdose.

NSAIDs
 	
Drug examples:
Aspirin, ibuprofen, naproxen, diclofenac, indomethacin, celecoxib
	Block prostaglandin synthesis by inhibiting COX-1 and/or COX-2.
	
	May also be used for:
	■ Antiplatelet
	■ Anti-inflammatory
	■ Antipyretic
		Aspirin should be used cautiously in children and should never be given to children with chicken pox or flu-like symptoms.
		    NSAIDs may interfere with clinical tests such as pregnancy tests, urine tests, and liver function tests.
		    Clients should be monitored for GI distress and allergic reactions.
		    NSAIDs should be used cautiously in clients receiving anticoagulant therapy.

Opioids
 	
Full agonists
Mixed agonist/antagonist
Partial agonist
 	
Drug examples:
Morphine, fentanyl, oxycodone, methadone
	Activate opioid receptors to decrease the perception of pain.
	
	May also be used for:
	■ Treatment of dyspnea related to acute left ventricular failure (morphine)
	■ Treatment of pulmonary edema and pain of myocardial infarction (morphine)
	■ Narcotics withdrawal symptoms (methadone)
		Monitor clients for respiratory depression.
		    If opioid reversal is indicated, administer incremental doses of the reversal agent (naloxone) until symptoms of overdose are resolved. Opioid reversal may produce withdrawal symptoms.
		    Constipation is one of the most common side effects of opioid use; provide stool softeners or laxatives as needed.

■ **Movement techniques** include yoga and tai chi. Yoga postures stretch specific muscle groups, and tai chi is a series of slow movements that follow a set pattern. Tai chi is said to improve strength, balance, and mental calmness (Vickers, Zollman, & Payne, 2001).

Other forms of relaxation include massage, acupuncture, meditation, and biofeedback. Relaxation techniques can be combined for maximum effectiveness. For example, imagery is often combined with deep breathing exercises. The choice of relaxation techniques depends on the client's individual preferences.

Collaborative

For the client experiencing discomfort, collaborative therapies include both pharmacologic and nonpharmacologic interventions. Pharmacologic interventions involve the administration of medications, examples of which are listed in the Medications feature. Nonpharmacologic therapies may be either alternative therapies, which are used instead of pharmacologic therapies, or complementary therapies, which are used in addition to pharmacologic therapies. Common nonpharmacologic therapies, such as acupuncture and herbal supplements, are discussed in the specific exemplars.

Medications **Sleep**

CLASSIFICATION AND DRUG EXAMPLES	MECHANISM OF ACTION	NURSING CONSIDERATIONS

Hypnotics/Sedatives
 	
■ Benzodiazepines
■ Nonbenzodiazepines
 	
Drug examples:
Temazepam, zolpidem, eszopiclone
	Produces CNS depression by acting on the limbic, thalamic, and hypothalamic regions of the CNS (benzodiazepines).
	    Interacts with GABA receptor (nonbenzodiazepines).
		Monitor older adults for paradoxical reaction.
		    Do not use in depressed, suicidal, or pregnant clients.
		    Tolerance and addiction may result from benzodiazepine use; slowly taper dosage when discontinuing therapy; drugs should not be used for more than 4–6 months.

REVIEW The Concept of Comfort

RELATE Link the Concepts

Linking the concept of comfort with the concept of elimination:

1. How can you help clients with "embarrassing" symptoms such as bowel incontinence feel more comfortable talking about their condition?

2. Describe comfort measures for a client who requires catheterization for treatment of urinary retention.

Linking the concept of comfort with the concept of violence:

3. Explain the psychosocial considerations related to promoting comfort during the care and assessment of a rape victim.

4. When assessing a child who is believed to have been abused, what comfort measures can be used to reduce the child's anxiety and promote trust?

READY Go to Companion Skills Manual

REFER Go to Pearson Student Nursing Resources
nursing.pearsonhighered.com

- Additional review materials

REFLECT Case Study \\ Part 3

Ms. Daves has been visiting her primary care provider as recommended for follow up care. Six months after beginning treatment with milnacipran (Savella), Ms. Daves returns for a regular checkup. As you review her chart, you note that Ms. Daves's physician confirmed the ED physician's diagnoses of fibromyalgia. Upon assessment, Ms. Daves's vital signs are normal, and her pain intensity is a 3 on a scale of 0–10. She also reports that she is sleeping better at night, although she occasionally has insomnia even though the pain is manageable. When you ask how Savella is working for her, she says that it has helped her pain and stiffness but her mouth has been really dry since she started taking it and she sometimes has slight nausea.

Clinical Reasoning Questions Level I

1. What suggestions can you give Ms. Daves to help decrease her dry mouth and nausea?

2. What further assessment should be included to help determine the cause of Ms. Daves's insomnia?

3. Can you suggest other therapies to help decrease Ms. Daves's pain even further?

Clinical Reasoning Questions Level II

4. What nursing interventions can you implement to help prevent future flare-ups of Ms. Daves's fibromyalgia?

5. What information should you give Ms. Daves about milnacipran (Savella) and drug–drug interactions?

6. What coping techniques would be useful for Ms. Daves as she deals with fibromyalgia?

EXEMPLAR 3.1 Acute and Chronic Pain

EXEMPLAR KEY TERMS

Acute pain, *154*
Breakthrough pain, *156*
Central pain, *156*
Chronic pain, *155*
Coanalgesic, *163*
End-of-dose medication failure, *156*
Gate control theory, *154*
Idiopathic pain, *156*
Incident pain, *156*
Narcotics, *164*
Nerve block, *168*
Neuropathic pain, *154*
Nociceptive pain, *154*
Nociceptors, *153*
Opioids, *164*
Pain, *152*
Pain threshold, *159*
Pain tolerance, *158*
Phantom pain, *156*
Psychogenic pain, *156*
Referred pain, *155*
Sensitization, *158*

Somatic pain, *155*
Visceral pain, *155*

EXEMPLAR LEARNING OUTCOMES
After reading about this exemplar, you will be able to:

1. Describe the pathophysiology, etiology, clinical manifestations, and direct and indirect causes of acute and chronic pain.

2. Identify risk factors and prevention methods associated with acute and chronic pain.

3. Illustrate the nursing process in providing culturally competent care across the life span for individuals with acute or chronic pain.

4. Formulate priority nursing diagnoses appropriate for an individual with acute or chronic pain.

5. Summarize therapies used by interdisciplinary teams in the collaborative care of an individual with acute or chronic pain.

6. Plan evidence-based care for an individual with acute or chronic pain and his or her family in collaboration with other members of the healthcare team.

7. Evaluate expected outcomes for an individual with acute or chronic pain.

▶ OVERVIEW

The International Association for the Study of Pain (2012) defines **pain** as "an unpleasant sensory and emotional experience associated with actual or potential tissue damage, or described in terms of such damage." This definition has several implications for nurses. First, pain is both a physical (sensory) experience and an emotional experience. As a physical experience, the degree of pain a client feels depends both on the magnitude of stimuli and on the ability of the individual to transmit neuronal pain signals. As an emotional experience, the degree of pain a client feels depends on the client's mental state; for example, depression makes pain seem more severe, whereas laughter may appear to decrease pain. Second, pain is a result of actual or potential tissue damage. Therefore pain can result from tissue damage that has already happened, such as a fractured bone, or as a warning that tissue damage may occur, such as when touching a hot surface. Third, pain can be described (Berman & Snyder, 2012). This concept is consistent with McCaffery's (1968) classic definition of pain, which states that "pain is whatever the experiencing person says it is, existing whenever he says it does."

Each client's description of pain depends on that individual's perception of that pain. However, some clients will not describe their pain unless asked, which is why a thorough pain assessment is vital to nursing care. The inability to verbalize pain does not necessarily reflect an absence of pain.

Describing Pain

Pain can be described in terms of location, intensity, quality, and duration. Duration was discussed previously, under "The Concept of Comfort," which detailed the difference between acute pain and chronic pain. The other three descriptors of pain are discussed in this section. Medically, pain can also be described based on its etiology, discussed later in the exemplar.

LOCATION   A description of where the pain is located may give a primary indication of the client's underlying problem. For instance, lower back pain often indicates a bulging or herniated disk. Following surgery or traumatic injury, reports of pain in areas other than at the affected site should be thoroughly explored. For example, chest pain after a total joint replacement may indicate a blood clot and should be assessed and treated immediately. Pain may also radiate to other body regions, such as lower back pain that extends to the legs, or it may be referred based on nerve pathways. For example, jaw pain may actually be cardiac in origin.

INTENSITY   Pain intensity is often described as mild, moderate, or severe. Pain can also be rated on visual analog scales, such as the Faces Pain Rating Scale, which is especially useful for young or illiterate clients (**Figure 3–2 ●**), or on a numerical scale from 0 to 10. On a 0–10 pain scale, 0 indicates no pain and 10 indicates the worst possible pain. According to the classic study by Serlin et al. (1995), mild pain correlates with a rating of 1–4,

moderate pain correlates with a rating of 5–6, and severe pain correlates with a rating of 7–10. The intensity of the pain score is often consistent with the degree to which pain interferes with functioning.

QUALITY   The quality of pain can be expressed with common descriptors. A client with sharp pain may say it feels like being stabbed, and a client with burning pain may say it feels like being on fire. Some descriptions of pain provide clues to whether the pain is superficial (e.g., itchy, tingling, cold) or deep (e.g., cramping, aching, dull). Other descriptors include *tender, sensitive, shooting, numb, radiating, throbbing,* and *heavy.* Descriptions of pain quality vary, depending on each client's pain perception, vocabulary, personality, and culture.

▶ PATHOPHYSIOLOGY AND ETIOLOGY

Pain is triggered by the peripheral nervous system, which lies outside the brain and spinal cord. There are two types of neurons in the peripheral nervous system: sensory and motor neurons. **Nociceptors**, or sensory receptors that respond to pain, send a signal along the sensory neurons to the spinal cord, where the signal is transmitted to the brain for interpretation. The brain then sends a signal back to the site of pain via motor neurons, causing the body to respond to the painful stimuli. This process happens so rapidly that the individual may reflexively withdraw from the painful stimuli even before becoming aware of the pain.

Nociceptors (**Figure 3–3 ●**) are specialized pain receptors that are present on all body tissues, with the exception of the brain. Skin and muscles contain many nociceptors, whereas internal organs have relatively few nociceptors. Categories of pain stimuli include biological, chemical, electrical, mechanical, and thermal (**Table 3–1 ●**). The duration of exposure and magnitude of the stimuli determine the intensity of the pain response.

In addition to being stimulated by external factors, cellular injury can trigger the local release of biochemicals that stimulate nociceptors, including prostaglandins, serotonin, bradykinin, and hydrogen ions. These mediators act on ion channels and G protein–coupled receptors to directly or indirectly initiate a pain impulse (Fein, 2012).

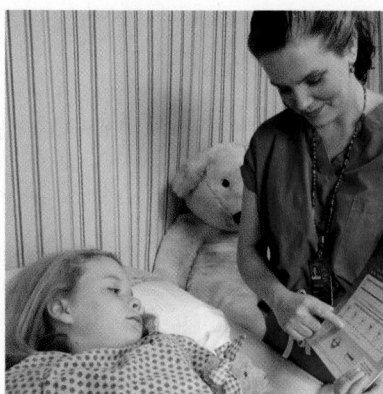

Figure 3–2 ● The nurse is having the child rate her pain by pointing to the face that most closely matches the way she feels. Note her stuffed animals that provide comfort.

TABLE 3–1   Types of Pain Stimuli

CATEGORY	EXAMPLE
Biological	Bacteria Viruses
Mechanical	Shearing forces Fractures
Thermal	Extreme heat (burn) Extreme cold (frostbite)
Electrical	Electrical burn Electrical shock
Chemical	Cleaning solutions Tobacco smoke Acids/bases Radiation

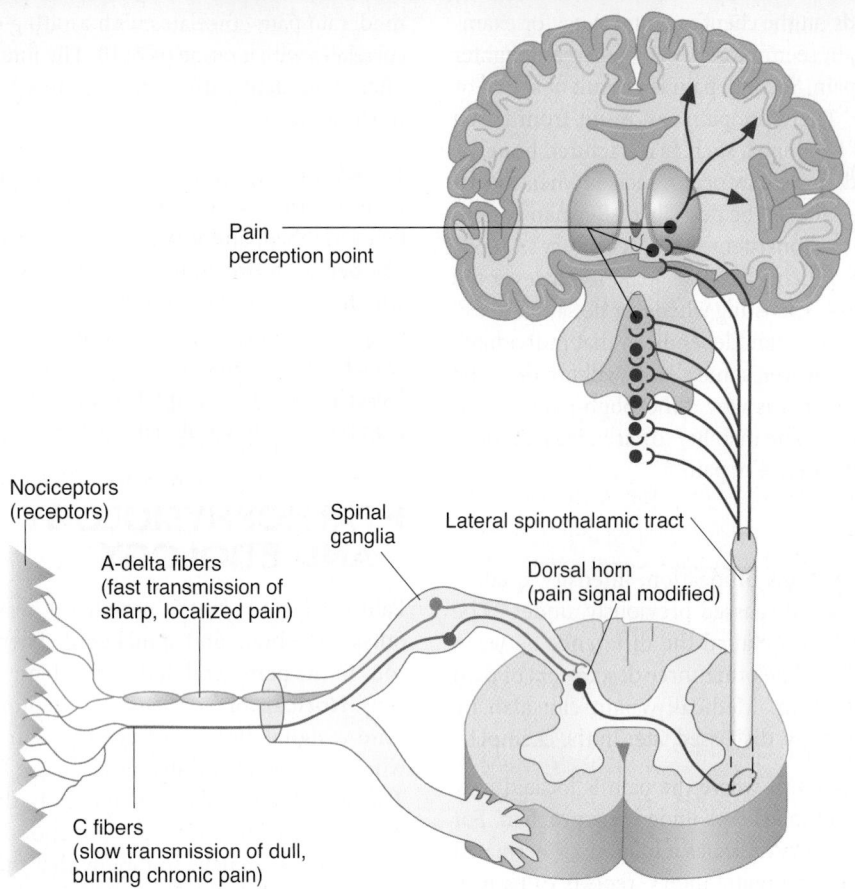

Pain perception point

Nociceptors (receptors)

A-delta fibers (fast transmission of sharp, localized pain)

Spinal ganglia

Lateral spinothalamic tract

Dorsal horn (pain signal modified)

C fibers (slow transmission of dull, burning chronic pain)

Figure 3–3 ● Physiology of pain perception.

Pain Theories

Three theories about pain include the *specificity theory*, the *peripheral pattern theory,* and the *gate control theory*.

■ The *specificity theory* states that pain is a specific sensation that uses sensory neurons separate from other sensations such as heat and touch.

■ The *peripheral pattern theory* states that all sensory nerve fiber endings are the same, and pain is felt only when the fibers are intensely stimulated. It is the responsibility of the brain to decipher differences in signals coming from these nerve fibers.

■ The **gate control theory**, proposed by Melzack and Wall in 1965, is the most widely accepted pain theory to date, although it still does not completely encompass all aspects of pain. The gate theory states that stimulation of small-diameter (pain) fibers causes gates to open, whereas stimulation of large-diameter (heat, cold, mechanical) fibers causes gates to close. The amount of activity in the small fibers versus the large fibers controls the overall perception of pain. Factors that control the gates include physical factors, emotional factors, and behavioral factors.

Etiology

Pain can be classified based on the origin of the pain signal. Pain resulting from external stimuli on an uninjured, fully functional nervous system is called **nociceptive pain**. For example, a sunburn or paper cut will cause pain to warn the individual that tissue damage is present and immediate action is needed to prevent further injury. When the injury is treated or healed, the pain generally resolves. Most nociceptive pain is temporary unless the underlying cause of the pain is not treated. For example, an individual with osteoarthritis may experience nociceptive pain due to contact between bones that are not adequately protected by joint cartilage.

In contrast to nociceptive pain, **neuropathic pain** is caused by nerve malfunction or injuries resulting from trauma, disease, chemicals, infections, and tumors. The consequent spontaneous pain may be due to damage of either peripheral nerves or central nerves (Costigan, Scholz, & Woolf, 2009). Nociceptive pain is often magnified in the presence of neuropathic pain.

TYPES OF PAIN There are several types of pain, the most common classifications being *acute* and *chronic* pain. *Breakthrough, central, phantom,* and *psychogenic* pain are also discussed.

Acute Pain **Acute pain** usually has a sudden onset as a result of an identifiable tissue injury, such as surgery, inflammation, or traumatic injury. The duration of acute pain is short, lasting only until the injury has completely healed. Depending on the type of injury, acute pain could persist for a few minutes up to 6 months. Acute pain initiates the autonomic fight-or-flight response, causing physiological responses such as increased breathing and heart rate, increased blood pressure, sweating, pallor, dilated pupils, and anxiety. The three primary categories of acute pain are somatic pain, visceral pain, and referred pain (Helms & Barone, 2008).

- **Somatic pain** originates from nociceptors located in the skin and musculoskeletal tissues. It is typically localized and described as being sharp. Somatic pain may be accompanied by swelling, cramping, or bleeding, and it usually responds well to mild analgesics. Examples of somatic pain are a cut finger or an overstretched muscle.

- **Visceral pain** originates from internal body organs and the linings of body cavities in the chest, abdomen, and pelvic areas. Because internal organs have relatively few nociceptors, visceral pain is usually described as dull, deep, or aching. In contrast to surface nociceptors, nociceptors on internal organs respond to inflammation, stretching, and ischemic changes rather than to lacerations or extreme temperatures. Visceral pain often manifests as radiating or referred pain, and it responds best to opioid treatment. Examples are myocardial ischemia and urinary colic resulting from renal stones.

- **Referred pain** is sensed in a region other than the site of origin. It occurs when nerve fibers that innervate the injured region and nerve fibers from other regions of the body converge at the same level in the spinal cord (**Figure 3–4 ●**). Examples of referred pain are back pain from pancreatitis and shoulder pain from myocardial ischemia.

Chronic Pain   Chronic pain is pain that lasts beyond the expected time of healing, usually for at least 6 months; it does not always have a known cause. Pain can range from mild to severe, and autonomic responses decrease over time as the body adapts to the persistent pain impulses. However, autonomic responses may be present during severe flare-ups of pain. In addition, pain may evoke hormonal stress responses even in the absence of autonomic responses.

Chronic pain has three main categories.

- *Chronic recurrent pain* is characterized by intense episodes of pain interspersed with periods of no pain. A common example of chronic recurrent pain is migraine headaches.

- *Chronic intractable benign pain* is chronic pain that is always present, although the intensity varies. The most common type of chronic intractable benign pain is lower back pain.

- *Chronic progressive pain* is pain associated with a chronic condition that worsens over time, such as cancer or rheumatoid arthritis.

Many conditions cause chronic pain. For example, arthritis, which develops when cartilage in the joint disintegrates, allowing the bones to rub together, is characterized by inflammation in one or more joints. Cancer usually is associated with chronic pain as a result of the enlarging tumor, which causes nerve compression, visceral expansion, duct obstruction, or bone metastasis. The tumor may also produce biochemicals that stimulate pain, and pain often results from treatments such as chemotherapy and radiation. Neuralgia is a sharp pain that follows the path of a nerve. It is due to nerve damage and is often associated with a disease, trauma, or medication. Common examples of neuralgia include shingles and trigeminal neuralgia.

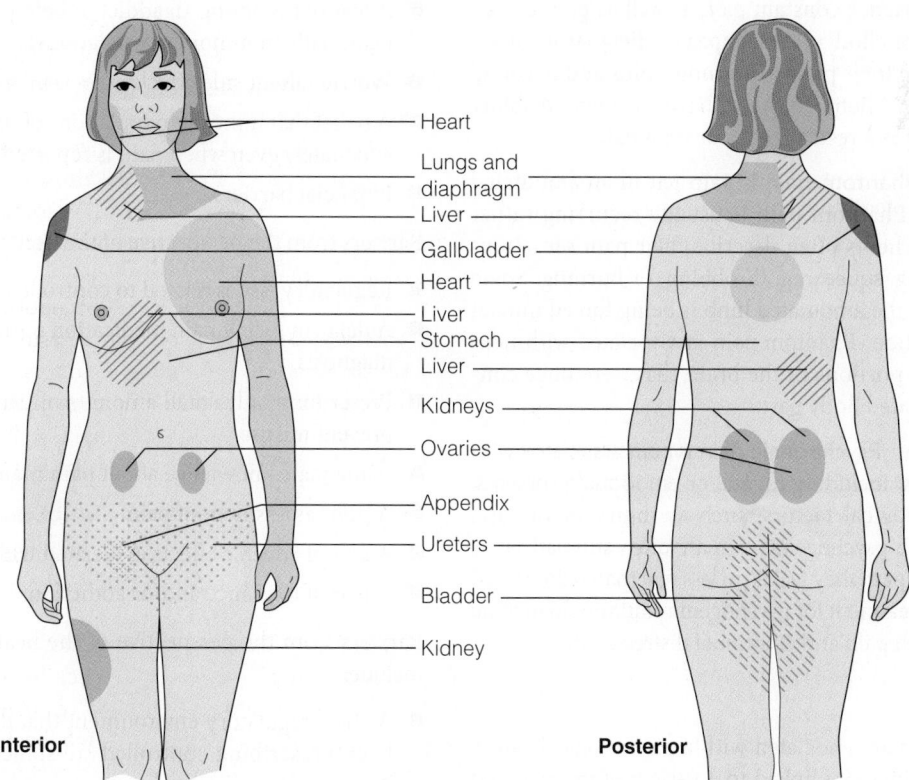

	Heart
	Lungs and diaphragm
	Liver
	Gallbladder
	Heart
	Liver
	Stomach
	Liver
	Kidneys
	Ovaries
	Appendix
	Ureters
	Bladder
	Kidney

Anterior   **Posterior**

Figure 3–4 ● Referred pain is the result of the convergence of sensory nerves from certain areas of the body before they enter the brain for interpretation. For example, a toothache may be felt in the ear, pain from inflammation of the diaphragm may be felt in the shoulder, and pain from ischemia of the heart muscle (angina) may be felt in the left arm.

Breakthrough Pain Breakthrough pain is defined as "a transient exacerbation of pain that occurs either spontaneously, or in relation to a specific predictable or unpredictable trigger, despite relatively stable and adequately controlled background pain" (Davies, Dickman, Reid, Stevens, & Zeppetella, 2009). There are three main types of breakthrough pain: incident pain, idiopathic pain, and end-of-dose medication failure.

- **Incident pain** is short-term, predictable pain that accompanies a movement or activity. It can be caused by voluntary acts such as movement, involuntary acts such as coughing, or procedural events such as changing a wound dressing.

- **Idiopathic pain** is not associated with any known cause. It occurs unpredictably and is therefore harder to treat. Idiopathic pain usually lasts longer than incident pain.

- **End-of-dose medication failure** is pain experienced at the end of one dose of medication before the next dose is scheduled. Although end-of-dose medication failure has traditionally been considered breakthrough pain, some experts now believe that it is not breakthrough pain because it indicates that the background pain is not adequately controlled. End-of-dose medication failure can be prevented by shortening the time between doses or increasing the medication dose.

Central Pain Central pain is caused by damage to nerves in the central nervous system due to stroke, multiple sclerosis, Parkinson disease, or trauma. Central pain may occur shortly after the causative injury, or it may be delayed for weeks or years (NINDS, 2011). Dysfunction of the spinothalamic tract causes abnormal temperature and pain perception, so clients with central pain often experience constant pain as well as pain paroxysms, evoked pain, or allodynia (Haanpaa & Hietaharju, 2010). Clients may describe their pain as burning, "pins and needles," aching, or lacerating. Clients may also have a decreased ability to feel normal touch as a result of the constant pain.

Phantom Pain Phantom pain is pain felt in an amputated limb or body part. Phantom pain is usually recurring rather than constant, and clients often describe their pain sensations as shooting, stabbing, squeezing, throbbing, or burning. Some clients may feel that the amputated limb is being forced into an uncomfortable position. Phantom pain is associated with neurological activity in portions of the brain that were once connected to the amputated body part.

Psychogenic Pain Psychogenic pain is pain associated with psychological factors, including mental or emotional problems, rather than physiological factors, such as injury or disease. Although clients with psychogenic pain are often stigmatized as hypochondriacs, the pain they feel is no less real than pain caused by physical injury. Treatment for psychogenic pain should include interventions for both pain and emotional distress.

Risk Factors

Acute and chronic pain associated with a physiological cause, such as illness or injury, are linked to a variety of internal and external factors and depend on the illness or injury that causes the pain. For example, adolescent boys who perform tricks on bicycles are at higher risk of pain associated with a fractured arm or leg than boys who ride a bicycle without performing

tricks. Similarly, obese individuals are at higher risk of developing type 2 diabetes and associated complications such as diabetic neuropathy than individuals who are not obese.

Preoperative anxiety, younger age, and chronic pain are associated with severe postoperative pain. Clients who are vulnerable to stress and have an impaired cortisol response are more susceptible to persistent pain following a motor vehicle accident. Risk factors related to inadequate pain relief for lower back pain include a previous history of lower back pain, lifting weights, lack of exercise, emotional distress, and dissatisfaction with employment (Bruckenthal, 2008). Age, gender, and genetic polymorphisms also contribute to a client's risk of developing acute or chronic pain conditions.

In addition to risk factors that make clients more susceptible to pain, barriers exist that prevent clients from getting adequate pain relief, including barriers from the perspective of the client, healthcare provider, and healthcare infrastructure (IASP, 2009; McCarberg, 2008; NCI, 2013).

Barriers from the perspective of the client include

- Reluctance to report pain to avoid taking the treatment focus off the primary disease.

- Reluctance to discuss pain because they fear it indicates a progression of their disease.

- A belief that pain is inevitable, so there is nothing that can be done.

- A belief that bearing pain is admirable or beneficial.

- Cultural expectations that demand they not report pain.

- A desire to be seen as a "good" client.

- A fear of becoming an addict or being perceived as an addict (especially in minority populations).

- Worries about side effects associated with pain medications.

- A belief that minority populations do not get treated for pain adequately even when pain is reported.

- Financial barriers.

Barriers from the perspective of the healthcare provider include

- Regulatory issues related to controlled substances (opioids).

- A delay in giving pain medication to the client until after the diagnosis.

- Prescribing only small amounts of drugs upon discharge to prevent misuse.

- Inadequate knowledge about pain management.

- A poor assessment of pain.

- A fear of adverse effects associated with analgesics.

- A fear of tolerance and/or addiction.

Barriers from the perspective of the healthcare infrastructure include:

- A strict regulatory environment that discourages physicians from prescribing controlled substances in the appropriate dosage.

- Lack of availability of controlled substances.

- Low priority given to cancer pain management.

- Inadequate reimbursement for pain treatment.

Prevention

The methods used to prevent pain are as numerous as the causes of pain. For example, external risk factors, such as the risk of injury, can be decreased by safety precautions such as wearing a seatbelt or helmet. Similarly, internal risk factors, such as the risk of developing a chronic disease, can be decreased by living a healthy lifestyle. Unfortunately, many clients live without considering how their lifestyle could contribute to the development of acute or chronic diseases or injuries. Therefore, nurses are responsible for providing pain relief for clients once they are already experiencing pain.

For clients with acute or chronic pain, the best way to prevent future pain is to provide adequate pain relief through pharmacologic and nonpharmacologic therapies. Clients with acute pain should take their pain medications as prescribed until they are completely healed. In addition, clients with chronic pain should take their pain medications on schedule, even in the absence of severe pain. Pain medications are more effective at preventing pain when taken regularly than at reducing pain that has already become severe.

▶ CLINICAL MANIFESTATIONS

Often, the body responds to severe, acute pain by activating the sympathetic nervous system's fight-or-flight response. The sympathetic response causes an increase in blood pressure, pulse, and respiratory rate, diaphoresis, pallor, and dilated pupils. Nurses may also recognize visible symptoms of pain such as crying, grimacing, shielding the site of injury, compensatory posturing, and slow movements. In addition, the client may express anxiety about the condition that is causing acute pain. Some clients may not manifest physiological or behavioral signs of pain even while experiencing moderate to severe pain, and not all clients have the same physiological response to the same intensity of pain.

As the body adapts to pain, visible and physiological symptoms of pain may be harder to detect. The sympathetic response returns to baseline levels unless the client experiences breakthrough pain, and some visible signs of pain, such as crying, cease. Pain fibers may become sensitized, so that the intensity and perception of pain increase over time. Therefore clinical manifestations of chronic pain may include compensatory posturing, muscle spasms or tense muscles, limited mobility, groaning during movements, and clenched teeth. Chronic pain is also often accompanied by psychosocial manifestations, such as depression, withdrawal from previously enjoyable activities, fatigue, and resignation to dealing with constant pain.

Uncontrolled pain has multiple detrimental effects on the body. Compensatory posturing can lead to muscle atrophy, neuropathies, and contractures. To make up for this weakened area, the body overuses another area, occasionally causing pain in that area as well (Tennant, 2008). Possible alterations in insulin and lipid metabolism contribute to the development of atherosclerosis. Changes in the endocrine system may cause immune suppression, increasing the risk of infection and slowing wound healing (Tennant, 2004). Other effects of uncontrolled pain include changes in appetite, sleep disruption, decreased circulating oxygen levels, and increased risk of thrombosis. If allowed to continue, uncontrolled pain will decrease the quality of life for both the client and the client's family.

Lifespan and Cultural Considerations

In each client, a unique set of factors influences how they perceive pain. In addition to physiological factors such as transmission of pain signals, other factors may include the client's developmental stage, ethnic and cultural values, environment, support from family and friends, past experiences with pain, and views on the meaning of pain.

DEVELOPMENTAL STAGE A clients' age and developmental level influence how they express and respond to pain. The influence of age on pain perception and behavior, as well as some related nursing interventions, are described in **Table 3–2 ●**.

CHILDREN AND PAIN Children are less able than adults to accurately describe their pain. However, children as young as 3 years old can give a basic description of the location and intensity of their pain. In addition, most children exhibit specific behaviors in response to pain.

Physiological Considerations for Children in Pain There are several special considerations for children with pain. Compared to adults, children normally have a higher pulse and respiratory rate and lower blood pressure. Take this into consideration when assessing the sympathetic response to pain in children. In addition, a normal sympathetic response to pain is not always present in children, so changes in vital signs may not be a good indicator of pain.

Children tend to experience pain more intensely at the beginning of the painful episode, but the intensity decreases more rapidly than in an adult. Pain brings anxiety and stress to children, who do not understand the purpose of the pain, so providing emotional comfort is a vital part of treating pain in children. In addition, many children do not understand that they can ask for pain relief, so nurses and parents must attempt to gauge the child's level of pain and offer interventions as appropriate. If pain goes untreated in children, physiological consequences may include decreased growth and development, decreased immune function, lack of appetite, hypertension, and increased sensitivity to future pain (Pawar & Garten, 2010).

Children and Behavioral Responses to Pain Children display a variety of behaviors in response to pain. The most common behavioral responses to pain are crying and grimacing. Other common pain behaviors related to age are detailed in Table 3–2 on page 158. Changes in behavior are one of the best indicators of pain in nonverbal children, although verbal children also exhibit behavior changes in response to pain. For example, a child may sit quietly and play with a favorite toy for hours when in pain. Any behavior that is out of the ordinary may be an indicator of pain or discomfort, including both physical and emotional pain.

Children's behavioral responses to pain become more controlled as they age. For example, an infant cries inconsolably when experiencing pain, a school-age child may exhibit a restrained cry or whimper, and an adolescent may not cry at all. Children develop more advanced coping strategies as they age, and they are also less likely to admit needing comfort.

TABLE 3–2   Influence of Age on Pain Perception and Behavior

DEVELOPMENTAL STAGE	RESPONSE TO PAIN	SAMPLE NURSING INTERVENTIONS
Infant	Exhibits body rigidity or thrashing. Exhibits facial expression of pain. Cries inconsolably. Exhibits hypersensitivity or irritability. Has poor oral intake. Is unable to sleep.	Offer a pacifier. Allow the parent to hold the infant. Offer distractions such as music or a small toy.
Toddler and preschooler	May describe pain through basic words or gestures. May be verbally aggressive. May cry intensely. Exhibits physical resistance by pushing away painful stimulus. Guards painful area of body. May see pain as punishment. May request emotional support from parent.	Offer distractions such as toys, books, or treats. Allow the parent to hold the child. Teach the child what to expect when encountering a painful procedure. Encourage the parent to be calm, as children can sense a parent's anxiety.
School-age child	Should be able to accurately describe their pain. Attempts to be brave in response to pain. May exhibit stalling behaviors. Exhibits muscle rigidity and other behaviors in anticipation of pain. May revert to earlier developmental stage with persistent or severe pain.	Simulate/act out the procedure beforehand. Encourage a parent to be present to provide support. Encourage children to express their pain. Give the child a book to read or an activity to do. Encourage cultural practices such as prayer.
Adolescent	May deny pain in the presence of peers. Exhibits changes in sleep patterns or appetite. Exhibits body control. May regress to earlier developmental stage in the presence of a trusted adult.	Discuss pain as with an adult client. Maintain privacy. Encourage distractions such as music or TV to deal with pain.
Adult	May exhibit gender-specific behaviors learned as a child. May ignore pain in order to be a "good" client. May ignore pain to prevent appearing weak. May deny pain based on fear that the condition has worsened.	Discuss the client's misconceptions about pain. Address the client's symptoms of fear and anxiety. Focus on providing adequate pain control based on the client's description of pain intensity.
Older adult	Pain may result from multiple conditions. May view pain as being inherent in aging. May have increased pain threshold compared to younger adults. Manifestations of pain may include decreased energy level, loss of appetite, and general lethargy. May deny pain to prevent becoming dependent on others.	Spend time discussing the client's health status, including pain, with the client. This will give the client self-worth and credibility. Dispel myths related to age and pain. Promote the highest possible level of independence.

Sources: Based on Berman, A., & Snyder, S. J. (2012). Pain management. In A. Berman & S. Snyder (Eds.). *Kozier and Erb's fundamentals of nursing: Concepts, process, and practice* (p. 1212, Table 46-3). Upper Saddle River, NJ: Pearson Education.; Pawar, D., & Garten, L. (2010). Pain management in children. In A. Kopf & N. B. Patel (Eds.), *Guide to pain management in low-resource settings* (pp. 255–268). Seattle, WA: International Association for the Study of Pain; *Pain management across the life span: From pediatrics to geriatrics.* (2009). Retrieved from Sutter Medical Center, Sacramento, CA, http://www.suttermedicalcenter.org/forourphysicians/by-laws_rules/pain-management-module-3.09.pdf

✳ *Go to* **nursing.pearsonhighered.com** *for a minimodule on neonates and pain.*

Children and Pain Memory   Children develop a pain memory that influences how they respond to pain in the future. A child's memory of a painful experience is a better predictor of future pain experiences than is the actual pain reported after a procedure (Noel, Chambers, McGrath, Klein, & Stewart, 2012), and children with pain-related anxiety are more likely to remember experiencing a greater intensity of pain than they

initially reported (Rocha, Marche, & von Baeyer, 2009). Children can undergo **sensitization** (an increased response to pain over time) that causes a lower **pain tolerance** (the maximum amount of pain a client will tolerate), higher levels of stress associated with pain, and an inability to cope with painful experiences. In contrast, other children may develop a higher pain tolerance, such as children with type I diabetes who are subjected to repeated insulin injection.

A child's pain memory and reaction to painful stimuli also are influenced by family and peer experiences. Parents' ability to

TABLE 3–3 Pain in Infants and Children: Common Misconceptions

MYTH	REALITY
Infants and children cannot express pain.	Infants express pain through physiological changes and behavioral responses. Children can accurately point to the area that hurts and rate their pain on a faces pain scale.
The client's report is the only valid method of pain assessment.	Parents are a valid source of information about their child's pain, especially for nonverbal children.
Children in pain do not play.	Children often play to distract themselves from pain.
Children in pain do not sleep well.	Children become exhausted from the mental and physical stress of coping with pain and eventually fall asleep.
Children tolerate pain better than adults.	Pain tolerance typically increases with age.
Children will inform you of their pain.	Children may not tell you they are in pain because they are afraid of what will happen to them, because they feel the need to be brave, or because they do not understand why they have pain.
To prevent drug addictions, administer opioids to children only as a last resort.	Less than 1% of children given opioids for acute pain develop a drug addiction. (Plaisance & Logan, 2006).

cope with their children's pain guides the children to develop their own personal response to pain. Social pressures from peers may influence a child to believe that it is necessary to be brave when facing pain and that admitting pain shows weakness. Past experiences may also lead children to believe that the nurse already knows they are in pain or that if they admit pain, they will be given an injection that will hurt more than the current pain.

Barriers to Pediatric Pain Management Even with more advanced knowledge about how they respond to and perceive pain, children still receive less adequate treatment for pain than adults. Barriers to adequate pain relief in children are related to inadequate pain assessment and a lack of knowledge about how to treat a child's pain safely. Other barriers are related to misconceptions about pain in infants and children (**Table 3–3 ●**). In 2001, the Joint Commission issued standards related to pain assessment and management for clients of all ages (**Box 3–2 ●**).

Box 3–2 The Joint Commission Pain Management Standards

In 1999, The Joint Commission approved pain assessment and management standards for accredited ambulatory care facilities, behavioral healthcare organizations, home care providers, hospitals, office-based surgery practices, and long-term care providers. These standards were implemented in 2001 and remain in effect today. The Joint Commission standards state that clients have the right to appropriate assessment and management of pain. All clients should be screened for pain in the initial assessment and reassessed for pain as required. In addition, the healthcare organization should provide adequate training in pain assessment and management to healthcare providers, and clients with pain and their families should be educated about effective and safe pain management. A new pediatric standard added in 2012 states that pediatric clients should receive both pharmacologic therapy and nonpharmacologic comfort measures before a procedure, to reduce stress and pain related to the procedure.

Sources: Based on The Joint Commission. (2012). *Facts about pain management.* Retrieved from http://www.jointcommission.org/assets/1/18/pain_management.pdf; Joint Commission Standards. (2011). Retrieved from Massachusetts General Hospital Patient Care Services, http://www.mghpcs.org/eed_portal/Documents/Pain/Joint%20Commission%20Standards2011.pdf

Stay Current: *Visit www.childpain.org, the Web site of the Special Interest Group on Pain in Childhood, to learn more on this topic.*

PAIN AND ADULTS Chronic pain is a widespread problem among adults, and conditions associated with chronic pain are more prevalent in women than in men. Approximately 80%–90% of fibromyalgia cases are women, and women are more likely to develop diseases that cause pain, such as osteoarthritis. This disparity may result from the fact that women have a lower **pain threshold** (the point at which pain is initially felt) and a lower pain tolerance than men (IASP, 2007).

Although women are at increased risk for chronic pain conditions, men are not exempt from chronic pain. Men are more likely to experience chronic pain from cluster headaches, coronary heart disease, gout, duodenal ulcer, and pancreatic disease (IASP, 2007).

PAIN AND OLDER ADULTS Estimates suggest that 72.1 million adults will be over age 65 by 2030 (ANA, 2012). As adults age, they develop chronic conditions that are associated with pain (see **Box 3–3 ●**). Over 80% of older adults have at least one chronic condition associated with pain, and approximately 20% of older adults have at least five coexisting chronic conditions (AGS, 2012). This increase in chronic conditions with pain, as well as sources of acute pain such as surgery, causes older adults to be the primary recipients of healthcare services.

Older adults undergo physiological changes that affect how they perceive pain. They have decreased cerebral blood flow, neuronal loss, and a decreased synthesis of neurotransmitters and opioid receptors. These conditions may cause either an increased or a decreased pain response, depending on the client's specific neuronal changes. A decrease in the descending inhibitory signal from the brain produces increased pain sensations, whereas a decrease in excitatory neurotransmitters, receptors, and neurons produces more mild pain sensations (Rastogi & Meek, 2013).

Changes in the gastrointestinal and urinary systems cause decreased drug absorption, metabolism, and excretion.

Box 3–3 Disorders Linked to Pain in Older Adults

- Musculoskeletal pain
  - Low back pain
  - Osteoarthritis
  - Rheumatoid arthritis
  - Joint pain (knees, hips, other)
  - Degenerative disc disease
  - Osteoporosis
  - Contractures
- Neuropathic pain
  - Postherpetic neuralgia
  - Diabetic peripheral neuropathy
- Cancer-related pain (cancer and cancer treatments)
- Nighttime leg pain
- Secondary neuralgia
- Trauma
- Fibromyalgia
- Poststroke pain
- Cardiac disease/angina

Sources: Based on Thomas, D., Flaherty, J., & Morley, J. (2001). The management of chronic pain in long-term care settings. *Supplement to the Annals of Long-Term Care,* November. Newtown Square, PA: MultiMedia Health Care/ Freedom.; International Association for the Study of Pain. (n.d.). *Facts on "Pain in older persons."* Retrieved from http://www.iasp-pain.org/AM/ Template.cfm?Section=2006_2007_Pain_in_Older_Persons1&Template=/ CM/ContentDisplay.cfm&ContentID=3611

Box 3–4 Chronic Pain in the Older Adult

Approximately 25%–50% of all community-dwelling older adults experience significant chronic pain, and approximately 45%–80% of nursing home residents experience substantial pain (AGS Panel, 2002). Older adults with chronic pain often suffer in silence because healthcare providers do not ask if they have pain. However, all individuals, including older adults, have the right to adequate pain assessment and effective pain management, including pharmacologic therapy.

Chronic pain conditions such as fibromyalgia, low back pain, and osteoarthritis are commonly comorbid with depression. These conditions inhibit the treatment of each other, causing faster progression of the disease and increased reliance on a caregiver. Depression is often accompanied by sleep disorders, anxiety, and cognitive impairment (Karp & Reynolds, 2009). Therefore older adults with chronic pain should be assessed for mood disorders in addition to the traditional pain assessment, and nursing care plans should integrate therapies to treat each condition and prevent development of additional comorbidities.

These changes alter the pharmacokinetics of pain medications, producing either a reduced effect (inadequate pain control) or an amplified effect (increased side effects), depending on the unique changes within each client. Drug interactions are also common in older adults who are taking multiple medications, leading to increased pain and discomfort and increased risk of life-threatening outcomes. Therefore, it is essential that nurses and pharmacists know and understand the complete list of drugs each client is taking to prevent drug interactions.

Older adults often face many barriers to effective pain management from both healthcare providers and personal preferences. Healthcare providers may lack the knowledge needed for appropriate assessment, diagnosis, and management of pain in the older population; they may fear that the client will develop opioid dependence or that they will be scrutinized for regulatory reasons; or they may not have time to determine the best course of therapy for each client. Personal barriers include misconceptions about aging, pain, and medication; fear of drug effects; noncompliance; religious beliefs; financial barriers; and comorbidities such as dementia.

Inadequate pain control can dramatically reduce the clients' quality of life, decreasing their ability to perform activities of daily living and increasing their dependence on others. It can cause mood, sleep, and appetite disturbances; decreased mobility; falls; slow rehabilitation; and altered cognitive functioning (AGS Panel, 2009; Rastogi & Meek, 2013). Decreased mobility can lead to deep vein thrombosis, pulmonary embolism, bone fractures, and reduced participation in social activities (Clarke et al., 2012). Altered cognitive functioning is a major contributor to poor pain management, as these clients are harder to assess for pain and are at increased risk for injury and therapeutic noncompliance. Older adults with chronic pain are also at greater risk for mood disorders (**Box 3–4**). Therefore adequate pain management, including client teaching and the provision of effective and safe therapies, is essential in older adults.

EFFECTS OF CULTURAL AND PERSONAL FACTORS ON PAIN Cultural and personal factors that influence an individual's pain experience include ethnic and cultural values, views about the meaning of pain, environment, availability of support, and past pain experiences.

Cultural and Ethnic Influences Clients' ethnic and cultural values play an important role in their perception and description of pain (see the Focus on Diversity and Culture feature). Clients from stoic cultures rarely vocalize pain through groans or crying, and they may avoid showing a behavioral reaction to pain. They may tolerate a higher level of pain without requesting pain relief or even mentioning their pain. In contrast, individuals from expressive cultures routinely moan or scream when faced with pain, and they expect others to care for them to help relieve the pain (David-hizar & Giger, 2004; Narayan, 2010). Despite the variation in verbal and behavioral responses to pain, ethnic or cultural background does not affect the pain threshold (Spear, 1977), so that people of different cultures experience similar pain sensations physiologically. It's simply their response to pain that differs.

Clients' culture also affects how they describe pain. Words may have different connotations in different cultures. For example, individuals from different cultures may use the words *ache, discomfort,* or *sore* rather than *pain.* If the client speaks a different language, some words may not translate correctly into the English word *pain* despite the presence of a competent translator.

Culture may also affect the methods of treatment that a client is willing to undergo. Individuals who believe that pain is

Focus on Diversity and Culture Cultural Differences in Response to Pain

A clients' culture influences their response to and beliefs about pain. Some common cultural differences related to pain are listed here.

Arabs/Muslims

- May not request pain medicine but instead thank Allah for pain if it is the result of a healing medical procedure.
- Pain is considered a test of faith. Therefore Muslim clients must endure pain as a sign of faith in return for forgiveness and mercy. However, Muslims must seek pain relief when necessary because needless pain and suffering are frowned upon.
- Arabs and Muslims prefer to be with family when in pain and may express pain more freely around family.

Asians

- Chinese clients may not ask for medication because they do not want to take the nurse away from a more important task.
- Clients from Asian cultures often value stoicism as a response to pain. A client who complains openly about pain is thought to have poor social skills.
- Filipino clients may not take pain medication because they view pain as being the will of God.
- Indians who follow Hindu practices believe that pain must be endured in preparation for a better life in the next cycle.

Blacks

- Blacks often report higher pain intensity than other cultures.
- They believe suffering and pain are inevitable.

- They believe in prayer and laying on of hands to heal pain and believe that relief is proportional to faith.

Jews

- Jews may be vocal and demanding of assistance.
- They believe that pain must be shared and validated by others.

Hispanics

- Hispanics may believe that pain is a form of punishment and that suffering must be endured if they are to enter heaven.
- They vary widely in their expression of pain: Some are stoic and some are expressive.
- Catholic Hispanics may turn to religious practices to help them endure the pain.

Native Americans

- Native Americans may prefer to receive medications that have been blessed by a tribal shaman They believe such a blessing allows the client to be more at peace with the creator and makes the medicine stronger.
- They tend to be less expressive both verbally and nonverbally.
- They usually tolerate a high level of pain without requesting pain medication.
- They may pick a sacred number when asked to rate pain on a numerical pain scale.

Sources: Based on Munoz, C., & Luckmann, J. (2005). *Transcultural communication in nursing* (2nd ed.). Clifton Park, NY: Delmar Learning; Andrews, M. M., & Boyle, J. S. (2003). *Transcultural concepts in nursing care* (4th ed.). Philadelphia, PA: Lippincott Williams & Wilkins; Al-Atiyyat, N. M. H. (2009). Cultural diversity and cancer pain. *Journal of Hospice and Palliative Nursing, 11*(3), 154–164; Davidhizar, R., & Giger, J. N. (2004). A review of the literature on care of clients in pain who are culturally diverse. *International Nursing Review, 51*(1), 47–55.

punishment or that pain builds character may refuse pain treatment. Clients from stoic cultures are likely to refuse pharmacologic treatments to avoid admitting weakness. Some cultures, such as Eastern cultures, may prefer to treat pain with herbal medicines and complementary and alternative medicine rather than pharmacologic agents.

Because of the critical role culture plays in pain expression and management, nurses must approach each client with cultural competence. Nurses must understand their own cultural beliefs about pain, and they must put aside those beliefs to provide culturally competent care. Discuss culturally acceptable ways of treating pain with the client and the client's family, and suggest ways in which the client can receive pain relief within those parameters.

The Meaning of Pain Depending on a client's cultural beliefs, pain can take on many meanings. For clients who have undergone surgery, pain is a sign that treatment has occurred. Mothers in labor view pain as a temporary inconvenience compared to the precious gift of a new baby. Clients who see pain positively usually have a higher tolerance of pain and are less likely to develop depression and anxiety about their pain.

In contrast, many clients, especially clients with chronic pain, view pain negatively. Unrelenting pain must be endured, leaving feelings of hopelessness, depression, and anxiety. These clients tend to view pain as something that is preventing them from enjoying life. They are more likely to depend on others to care for them and may become angry at the pain for stealing their independence. Clients who give a negative meaning to pain tend to have a lower quality of life physically, emotionally, and socially.

Clients who have strong spiritual beliefs often give a spiritual meaning to pain; pain may be viewed as punishment, a test, or a gift from God. Nurses must respect these beliefs when providing care.

Environmental and Social Support A client's environment can influence the perceived intensity of pain. Clients in a hospital may perceive a greater pain stimulus because of the unfamiliar environment and the numerous sources of disruption. Children can be especially frightened their first time in the hospital, and the fright can intensify pain responses. Providing a more relaxed and welcoming environment will ease anxiety and decrease clients' perception of pain.

Clients who surround themselves with a support network often experience decreased pain sensations. An individual who has no help in dealing with pain may perceive pain as more severe, whereas individuals who have ample family and friends to provide distractions, a positive environment, and a helping hand may tolerate pain better. Family members who are tasked with caregiving responsibilities should be included in client education about pain management.

Previous Experience With Pain   Clients' previous experiences with pain play a major role in their perception of pain. Clients who have undergone a procedure without adequate pain management tend to experience more pain during future procedures even in the presence of adequate pain control. Clients who have seen a loved one suffer severe pain associated with a disease will experience more anxiety and have an exaggerated perception of pain if diagnosed with the same disease compared to clients who have no previous experience with the disease.

Clients' past experience with a treatment plan also influences how they perceive the efficacy of future similar treatments. For example, an individual with severe pain who has tried several drugs or nonpharmacologic remedies unsuccessfully is less likely to believe that new treatments will be effective in managing the pain. When assessing a client for pain, nurses need to ask about past pain experiences and how those experiences might influence the client's current treatment plan.

▶ COLLABORATION

In order to treat pain effectively, nurses collaborate with other healthcare providers. Pharmacologic therapies are nonopioids, NSAIDs, opioids, and coanalgesics. Nonpharmacologic therapies include nerve blocks, spinal cord stimulation, physical therapy, and nutritional supplements, among others. For clients with severe chronic pain, pain clinics offer the expertise needed to discover the right combination of treatments to provide consistent pain relief.

Diagnostic Tests

While laboratory and diagnostic tests may be performed to determine the cause of pain, no laboratory tests are available to directly measure a client's pain level. Instead, pain scales such as a faces pain scale or a numeric pain scale are available to help gauge a client's pain level. Changes in vital signs can also be an indication of pain, although these changes are also seen with other conditions. In addition, the body releases stress hormones in response to pain, which may be detected by blood tests. The most prevalent stress hormones are cortisol and catecholamines.

Surgery

Depending upon the pain's etiology, surgery may be a viable treatment option. For example, surgical repair of a bone fracture may be the first major step toward alleviating severe pain. Recovery from surgery often brings about its own pain, but that pain is usually short-lived compared to the pain that would result from not performing the surgery. In addition, clients may

cope with pain better if they know the surgery was necessary to prevent more severe pain and health risks.

For chronic pain that cannot be managed by pharmacologic or nonpharmacologic therapies, surgery is the last resort. Disrupting pain conduction pathways using surgical procedures is permanent, so it should be used only for intractable pain, such as pain related to cancer. Surgical procedures used to relieve pain vary depending on the source and location of the pain.

Pharmacologic Therapy

Pharmacologic therapies for pain include nonopioids/nonsteroidal anti-inflammatory drugs and opioids (**Box 3–5 ●**).

Box 3–5   Categories and Examples of Analgesics

NONOPIOID ANALGESICS/NSAIDS
- Acetaminophen/paracetamol (Tylenol, many others)
- Aspirin/acetylsalicylic acid (Bayer, many others)
- Celecoxib (Celebrex)
- Choline magnesium trisalicylate (Trilisate)
- Diclofenac sodium (PENNSAID, Voltaren), diclofenac potassium (Cataflam)
- Etodolac
- Ibuprofen (Advil, Motrin)
- Indomethacin (Indocin)
- Ketorolac (Toradol)
- Meloxicam (Mobic)
- Naproxen (Naprosyn), naproxen sodium (Aleve)

WEAK OR PARTIAL OPIOID ANALGESICS
- Buprenorphine hydrochloride (Buprenex)
- Butorphanol tartrate (generic)
- Codeine (Codeine)
- Hydrocodone bitartrate (Vicodin)
- Tramadol hydrochloride (Ultram)

MIXED OPIOID ANALGESICS
- Codeine (Tylenol No. 3, Empirin No. 3)
- Nalbuphine hydrochloride (Nubain)
- Pentazocine hydrochloride (Talwin)

STRONG OPIOID ANALGESICS
- Fentanyl citrate (Actiq, Sublimaze)
- Hydromorphone hydrochloride (Dilaudid)
- Levorphanol tartrate (Levo-Dromoran)
- Meperidine hydrochloride (Demerol)
- Methadone hydrochloride (Dolophine, Methadose)
- Morphine sulfate (Avinza, Roxanol)
- Oxycodone hydrochloride (OxyContin)
- Remifentanil hydrochloride (Ultiva)

COANALGESICS
- Antidepressants (imipramine, milnacipran, nortriptyline)
- Anticonvulsants (gabapentin, pregabalin)
- Antihypertensives (clonidine)
- Antipruritics (hydroxyzine)
- Corticosteroids (prednisone, hydrocortisone)
- Topical local anesthetics (benzocaine, lidocaine)

Source: Wilson, B. A., Shannon, M. T., & Shields, K. M. (2013). *Nurse's drug guide.* Upper Saddle River, NJ: Pearson Education.

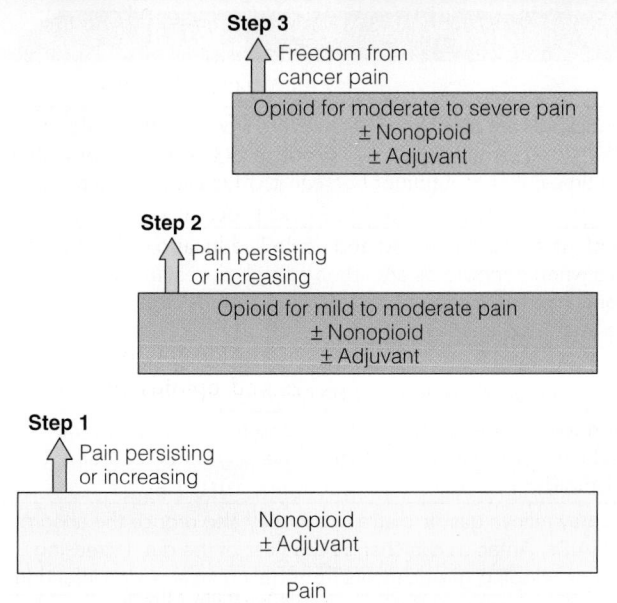

Step 3
Freedom from cancer pain

Opioid for moderate to severe pain
± Nonopioid
± Adjuvant

Step 2
Pain persisting or increasing

Opioid for mild to moderate pain
± Nonopioid
± Adjuvant

Step 1
Pain persisting or increasing

Nonopioid
± Adjuvant

Pain

Figure 3–5 ● The WHO three-step analgesic ladder.

Coanalgesic drugs, or drugs that are used primarily for another purpose but also have some analgesic properties, can also be used to treat pain alone or in combination with other analgesic drugs.

WORLD HEALTH ORGANIZATION (WHO) THREE-STEP APPROACH The World Health Organization has developed a three-step approach to treating pain (WHO, n.d.b; **Figure 3–5** ●). The first step involves administering a nonopioid drug (e.g., aspirin, acetaminophen) with or without a coanalgesic drug and nonpharmacologic interventions. If pain is not adequately controlled with this mild intervention, clients should advance to step 2 and receive a mild opioid (e.g., codeine) in combination with the same or new nonopioid drugs, coanalgesics, and nonpharmacologic therapies. If the client is still experiencing pain, the mild opioid should be replaced with a stronger opioid (e.g., morphine) in step 3. Pain-relieving drugs should be given "by the clock" (every 3–6 hours) rather than on demand to maintain freedom from pain. According to WHO, the three-step approach to administering pain relief is relatively inexpensive and 80%–90% effective.

SAFETY ALERT
If a client is experiencing moderate to severe pain (pain rated 4–10 on a scale of 0–10), it may be appropriate to skip step 1 and proceed directly to step 2 or 3, depending on the condition of the client. For example, a client with severe burns over a large portion of the body will not receive adequate pain control with acetaminophen; in this case, treatment should start at step 3. Starting a client's pain treatment at step 2 or 3 depends on the client's pain report and the judgment of the healthcare provider.

WHO's three-step approach allows the healthcare provider to give increasingly potent combinations of analgesic drugs until the client's pain is managed effectively by a practice that is currently called *rational polypharmacy*. For pain relief, rational polypharmacy is an opioid-sparing approach that combines multiple medications with different mechanisms of action. This combination allows the healthcare provider to use lower doses of opioids and other analgesics to minimize dependence and toxicity (Hahn, 2011). The benefits of combining opioid and nonopioid analgesics are often overlooked. Because these drugs have different mechanisms of action and toxicity profiles, giving a nonopioid drug at the same time as or alternating with an opioid drug creates a synergistic effect with minimal side effects.

SAFETY ALERT
When treating clients with multiple medications, healthcare providers must always be aware of potential drug–drug interactions that may cause additional, and sometimes life-threatening, side effects. In addition, when treating clients with combination drugs, healthcare providers must avoid giving duplicate drugs (e.g., acetaminophen in a combination analgesic plus acetaminophen for fever plus acetaminophen in a cold-and-flu preparation) to prevent an unintentional overdose.

NONOPIOIDS/NSAIDs Nonopioids are analgesic and antipyretic drugs, including acetaminophen and NSAIDs, the most common of which are aspirin, ibuprofen, and naproxen. NSAIDs have anti-inflammatory properties, whereas acetaminophen does not. NSAIDs reduce pain and inflammation by inhibiting cyclooxygenase (COX) signaling pathways, which produce prostaglandins and thromboxane. These inflammatory mediators enhance both the transduction and the transmission of pain signals (Burian & Geisslinger, 2005). NSAIDs carry a "black box" warning from the Food and Drug Administration (FDA) highlighting the risk of serious cardiovascular and gastrointestinal side effects (FDA, 2005).

Nonopioid drugs have a *ceiling effect;* that is, once the client consumes a specific dosage level, consuming more of the drug will not produce a greater analgesic effect but may increase toxic effects. Nonopioid drugs also have a narrow *therapeutic index,* meaning they have a very small efficacy range without being toxic. Given the increased risk for GI bleeding and prolonged bleeding times, repeatedly consuming NSAIDs at doses higher than are recommended could be life-threatening (see Client Teaching feature). **Table 3–4** ● contains a list of common misconceptions related to nonopioid medications and their associated truths.

The mechanism of action and the side effects of acetaminophen differ from those of the NSAIDs. Large doses or long-term use can cause severe liver and kidney toxicity. Acetaminophen is the most common drug associated with drug overdoses, and acetaminophen toxicity is the leading cause of acute liver failure in the Western world. Untreated, acetaminophen-induced acute liver failure can cause death

TABLE 3–4   Misconceptions About Nonopioids

MISCONCEPTION	TRUTH
Over-the-counter (OTC) nonopioids are safe for long-term use.	OTC nonopioids are associated with severe side effects, especially when taken long term. NSAIDs can produce GI toxicity and prolong bleeding times, and acetaminophen can produce liver and kidney toxicity.
OTC nonopioids do not have serious side effects; therefore they can be taken at a higher dose than recommended.	The risk of internal GI bleeding and acute liver failure is significantly increased when nonopioids are taken at high doses. In addition, nonopioids have a ceiling effect, so taking a higher dose will not produce a greater analgesic effect.
A client should not take both a nonopioid and an opioid.	For clients with moderate to severe pain, WHO recommends that both opioid and nonopioid medications be given.
Nonopioids should not be used for severe pain.	While nonopioids are rarely effective alone for severe pain, they may produce a synergistic effect to relieve pain when combined with an opioid.
Gastric distress from NSAIDs should be relieved by antacids.	Antacids may relieve gastric distress, but they also reduce the absorption of NSAIDs. Antacids can change the flora of the gut, increasing the risk of developing gastric ulcers from *Helicobacter pylori* infection.
An NSAID-induced gastric ulcer will always cause gastric distress.	Peptic ulcers caused by NSAIDs are less likely to produce gastric distress than other causes of peptic ulcers.

within days. The maximum recommended dosage of acetaminophen for adults is 4 g per day. If a client consistently takes slightly higher doses (5–6 g per day) or takes one large dose (10–12 g), liver toxicity is likely to occur. The risk for liver toxicity is heightened by alcohol consumption, so clients should be discouraged from drinking alcohol while taking acetaminophen. In addition, clients with liver or kidney disease should take lower doses of acetaminophen (2.5 g per day or less).

When taken in appropriate doses, acetaminophen is well tolerated. Healthcare professionals should not underestimate the effectiveness of acetaminophen and NSAIDs such as aspirin. For example, multiple studies have shown that morphine administration does not provide significantly more pain relief than acetaminophen, especially when both are administered via IV (Bektas et al., 2009; Craig et al., 2012; van Aken et al., 2004). In addition, acetaminophen is associated with fewer adverse events than morphine. Because of the safety profile of acetaminophen, it is included in many over-the-counter combination drugs, especially cold, cough, and allergy preparations, as well as in combination with narcotics for pain relief (**Table 3–5** ●). However, many clients do not realize that their combination medications contain

acetaminophen; the result is inadvertent drug overdose when they take additional medications containing acetaminophen. Nurses and other healthcare professionals must be knowledgeable about the acetaminophen content in each drug and teach clients about acetaminophen content to prevent overdose.

OPIOIDS   **Opioids** are drugs that act on one or more of three opioid receptors: mu, delta, and kappa. Opioids are also commonly referred to as **narcotics**, a term that means they are morphinelike drugs that have potential for abuse. Therefore, they are controlled substances. When activated, opioid receptors in the peripheral and central nervous systems produce an analgesic response (Vallejo, Barkin, & Wang, 2011). Opioid drugs can be classified as weak or partial agonists, full agonists, and mixed agonists.

Weak or Partial Agonists   Weak opioid agonists, such as codeine and hydrocodone, have a low affinity for the opioid receptors (see Box 3–5). Partial agonists have high affinity for the opioid receptors but produce only a partial effect. Both weak and partial agonists have a ceiling effect. Prevention and management of common side effects is outlined in **Box 3–6** ●.

Full Agonists   Full agonists bind with high affinity to mu opioid receptors in the peripheral and central nervous systems and produce a strong analgesic effect. Examples are fentanyl, hydromorphone, methadone, morphine, and oxycodone (see Box 3–5). As the most potent class of pain relievers, they should be used for clients in severe pain or when other medications have failed to control pain. Full opioid agonists do not have a ceiling effect. Therefore, full opioid agonists can be given in increasing doses until pain is relieved or side effects become intolerable. Full agonists are

Client Teaching   NSAID Administration

Clients who routinely take NSAIDs should be taught the concept of the ceiling effect and warned to take only the recommended dosage. To decrease the risk of GI-related side effects, nurses should teach clients to take NSAIDs with food and a full glass of water. Clients who take NSAIDs consistently for more than two weeks should be monitored by a healthcare professional.

TABLE 3–5   Acetaminophen Content in Common Combination Narcotic Medications

DRUG NAME	NARCOTIC	ACETAMINOPHEN CONTENT
Tylenol with Codeine (#1–4)	Codeine (7.5–60 mg/tablet)	300 mg
Capital with Codeine	Codeine (12 mg)	120 mg/5 mL
Anexsia	Hydrocodone (5–7.5 mg)	325–650 mg/tablet
Hydrocet	Hydrocodone (5 mg)	500 mg/capsule
Norco	Hydrocodone (7.5–10 mg)	325 mg/tablet
Vicodin	Hydrocodone (5–10 mg)	500–750 mg/tablet
Percocet	Oxycodone (2.5–10 mg)	325–650 mg/tablet
Roxicet	Oxycodone (5 mg)	325 mg/tablet or 5 mL syrup
Talacen	Pentazocine (25 mg)	625 mg/tablet

Source: Wilson, B. A., Shannon, M. T., & Shields, K. M. (2013). *Nurse's drug guide.* Upper Saddle River, NJ: Pearson Education.

known to produce euphoria, respiratory depression, and tolerance. Euphoria may help the client feel more comfortable even with uncontrolled pain, but respiratory depression may be a life-threatening side effect. Clients who develop tolerance to opioids are likely to experience withdrawal symptoms when the drug is discontinued, so they should be taken off opioids gradually.

Mixed Opioids   There are two types of mixed opioid agonists: mixed agonist–antagonist opioids (e.g., Nubain) and opioids mixed with nonopioids (opioid with acetaminophen, aspirin, ibuprofen, etc.). Mixed agonist–antagonist drugs act as an agonist at one opioid receptor (usually the kappa receptor) and as an antagonist at a different opioid receptor (usually the mu receptor). Because of the antagonist effect on the mu receptor, mixed agonist–antagonist opioids should be given only as the first opioid. If given after another opioid, the antagonist properties of the drug may cause withdrawal symptoms. Mixed agonist–antagonist drugs have a ceiling effect and should not be used for severe pain or in terminally ill clients.

Opioids can be mixed with nonopioid analgesic drugs or with a variety of other drugs, such as cough medicine, caffeine, and muscle relaxers. Codeine is the opioid available in the widest range of combination drugs (see Focus on Diversity and Culture feature). Pain medicines that contain both an opioid and a nonopioid are more efficacious than either drug alone. This greater efficacy allows the client to take a lower dose of each medication, thus decreasing the risk of side effects. When using combination drugs, nurses and other healthcare providers must be aware of the daily dose limits of all ingredients in the combination.

Opioid Side Effects   Of all the side effects associated with opioids, the most life-threatening is severe respiratory depression. Respiratory depression is likely to occur when initial opi-

Box 3–6   Prevention and Management of Common Opioid Side Effects

CONSTIPATION

- Increase fluid intake if client is dehydrated.
- Dietary fiber intake should not increase unless the client is fiber-deficient; opioids cause decreased peristalsis, which could result in bowel obstruction if fiber is increased.
- Daily stool softeners (e.g., Colace) and laxatives (e.g., Dulcolax) may be offered as a prophylactic or treatment for constipation.
- Severe constipation may be treated with suppositories, rectal irrigation, or manual evacuation.

NAUSEA AND VOMITING

- Nausea can be treated with antiemetics such as antipsychotics (e.g., Haldol), prokinetic agents (e.g., Reglan), or serotonin antagonists (e.g., Zofran).

SEDATION

- Clients may be given psychostimulants (e.g., Ritalin) for persistent sedation.
- Sedation may be a sign of respiratory depression, so clients with sedation should be monitored for respiratory rate and pulse oximetry.

PRURITUS

- Apply moisturizers or bathe in tepid water.
- Administer antihistamine medications (e.g., diphenhydramine).

SEXUAL DYSFUNCTION

- Opioid-induced sexual dysfunction may be treated with androgen replacement therapies (i.e., testosterone for men and dehydroepiandrosterone, or DHEA, for women).

Sources: Based on Goodheart, C. R., & Leavitt, S. B. (2006). *Managing opioid-induced constipation in ambulatory-care patients.* Retrieved from Pain Treatment Topics, http://pain-topics.org/pdf/Managing_Opioid-Induced_Constipation.pdf; Manchikanti, L., Abdi, S., Atluri, S., Balog, C. C., Benyamin, R. M., Boswell, M. V., … Wargo, B. W. (2012). American Society of Interventional Pain Physicians (ASIPP) guidelines for responsible opioid prescribing in chronic non-cancer pain: Part 2—Guidance. *Pain Physician, 15*(Suppl. 3), S67–S116.; Swegle, J. M., & Logemann, C. (2006). Management of common opioid-induced adverse effects. *American Family Physician, 74*(8), 1347–1354.

Focus on Diversity and Culture Codeine

Codeine and other opioids are converted to the active form morphine by the CYP2D6 enzyme. Approximately 7%–10% of Caucasians lack the CYP2D6 enzyme, so codeine is ineffective for them. In addition, although 99% of the Chinese population has a functional CYP2D6 enzyme, over 55% of the population contains a polymorphism (i.e., *CYP2D6*10*) that renders it less effective (<30%). Almost 40% of the Japanese population carries the *CYP2D6*10* allele as well. Approximately 20% of African Americans carry the *CYP2D6*17* allele, which also has a decreased effect (80%) compared to the normal CYP2D6 enzyme (Shen et al., 2007). In contrast, 1%–7% of Caucasians and more than 25% of Ethiopians have three or more copies of CYP2D6, causing codeine to be more effective with greater side effects (Gasche et al., 2004).

oid doses are too high or are used in combination with other drugs that also cause respiratory depression (Manchikanti et al., 2012). Respiratory depression is also more common in clients with respiratory disorders such as COPD, asthma, or obstructive sleep apnea (Jarzyna et al., 2011). Clients on opioids must be carefully monitored for respiratory depression. Normally, sedation precedes respiratory depression; therefore, a sedation scale such as the Pasero Opioid-Induced Sedation Scale (POSS) (**Box 3–7** ●) can be used to monitor sedation and guide clinical responses to respiratory depression. Respiratory depression is also accompanied by increased $PaCO_2$, periods of apnea, and confusion.

SAFETY ALERT

All clients on opioids should be monitored for sedation and respiratory depression during the first 24 hours (especially after surgery), during the peak effect, after increasing or decreasing a dose, before additional doses of opioids are given, or when changing opioids or routes of administration. If the respiratory rate falls below 8–10/min, the client should be aroused and naloxone therapy should be considered (Jarzyna et al., 2011).

Common side effects of opioid use are outlined in Box 3–6. Many of these side effects, especially nausea and sedation, will decrease within 3–5 days as the client develops tolerance for the drug. If sedation interferes with quality of life, stimulants can be taken in the morning to counteract daytime sedation. However, stimulants should be used with caution because of potential side effects and lack of usefulness in clinical trials. Tolerance to constipation usually does not develop. Therefore medical interventions will be needed to prevent or treat constipation.

Most opioids are excreted via the kidneys, so a reduction in renal function may increase toxic effects. For this reason, morphine should be used with caution in older adults, and meperidine should not be used at all. Instead, hydromorphone, which has greater potency than morphine and can be used at lower doses, or oxycodone, which is minimally cleared by the kidneys, should be used (Ginsburg, Silver, & Berman, 2009).

Opioid use is often associated with tolerance and addiction, and therefore many physicians are reluctant to prescribe opioids and clients are reluctant to take them even when in severe pain. Tolerance to opioids, in which a higher dose of medication is needed to produce the same analgesic effect, is expected with long-term use. Addiction is different from tolerance in that it can affect the individuals' behavior in addition to their physiological response to the drug. Very few clients exhibit patterns of addiction when opioids are used as recommended. However, if physicians prescribe inadequate doses of opioids because they fear tolerance and addiction, clients may exhibit drug-seeking behaviors simply because their pain medication is ineffective. This situation strains the trust relationship between the client and the healthcare provider. Nurses and other health-

Box 3–7   Pasero Opioid-Induced Sedation Scale (POSS)

S = Sleep, easy to arouse

Acceptable; no action necessary; may increase opioid dose if needed

1 = Awake and alert

Acceptable; no action necessary; may increase opioid dose if needed

2 = Slightly drowsy, easily aroused

Acceptable; no action necessary; may increase opioid dose if needed

3 = **Frequently drowsy, arousable, drifts off to sleep during conversation**

Unacceptable; monitor respiratory status and sedation level closely until sedation level is stable at less than 3 and respiratory status is satisfactory; decrease opioid dose 25%–50% (per opioid analgesic orders or hospital protocol) or notify prescriber (e.g., phy-

sician, nurse practitioner) or anesthesiologist for orders; consider administering a nonsedating, opioid-sparing nonopioid, such as acetaminophen or an NSAID, if not contraindicated.

4 = **Somnolent, minimal or no response to verbal or physical stimulation**

Unacceptable; stop opioid; consider administering naloxone (mix 0.4 mg of naloxone and 10 mL of normal saline in syringe and administer this dilute solution very slowly [0.5 mL over 2 minutes] while observing the patient's response; hospital protocols should include the expectation that a nurse will administer naloxone to any patient suspected of having life-threatening opioid-induced sedation and respiratory depression); notify prescriber or anesthesiologist; monitor respiratory status and sedation level closely until sedation level is stable at less than 3 and respiratory status is satisfactory.

Source: Pasero, C. (2009, June). Assessment of sedation during opioid administration for pain management. *Journal of PeriAnesthesia Nursing, 24*(3), 186–190, Table 1. Retrieved from http://nursing.ucsfmedicalcenter.org/education/classMaterial/203_6.pdf

Box 3–8 Pain Management for the Client with a History of Drug Abuse

According to the National Institute of Drug Abuse (2012), 1.8 million Americans are addicted to prescription pain medications, and another 23 million are addicted to alcohol, marijuana, and other drugs. Therefore, healthcare providers will encounter clients with pain who are addicted to at least one drug. Unfortunately, healthcare providers have a tendency to order nonopioids or lower doses of opioids for clients with a history of abuse; the result is undertreatment and increased drug-seeking behavior. For several reasons, it is critical to provide adequate pain relief in addicted clients, especially clients who are addicted to opioids.

1. Clients who are addicted to opioids have developed drug tolerance. Therefore, they require a *higher* dose to produce an analgesic effect, not a lower dose.
2. Opioid tolerance is often associated with *hyperalgesia*, or an increased physiological response to pain. Therefore, clients with

a history of opioid abuse feel pain more extensively than nonabusers.
3. Abusers whose drug of choice is withheld during their hospital stay will go through withdrawal, which exacerbates pain symptoms, prohibits healing, and increases the length of the hospital stay.

Clients should be given adequate pain control during the acute phase of pain, regardless of their drug abuse history. This should be seen as a medical issue, not an ethical or moral issue. The clients can undergo detoxification after they are no longer in pain. Communication among healthcare providers is critical when treating clients with a history of drug abuse to ensure that increases in dosage are related to pain control and not addictive behavior. Pain levels and a need for prescription opioids should be reassessed frequently throughout treatment.

Sources: Based on Grant, M. S., Cordts, G. A., & Doberman, D. J. (2007). Acute pain management in hospitalized patients with current opioid abuse. *Topics in Advanced Practice Nursing eJournal, 7*(1); National Institute on Drug Abuse. (2012). *DrugFacts: Nationwide trends.* Retrieved from *http://www.drugabuse.gov/publications/drugfacts/nationwide-trends*

care providers must become adept at recognizing behaviors of addiction compared to behaviors associated with inadequate pain control (see **Box 3–8**).

COANALGESICS Coanalgesics are drugs that have analgesic properties, potentiate the effects of pain medications, relieve other discomforts, or reduce the side effects of analgesic drugs. They are especially effective at reducing neuropathic pain. Examples of coanalgesic drugs are antidepressants, anticonvulsants, antihypertensives, antipruritics, corticosteroids, and local anesthetics (see Box 3–5).

- Antidepressants (e.g., imipramine) act to prevent the reuptake of serotonin and norepinephrine, slowing the transmission of pain signals (McDonald & Portenoy, 2006).

- Anticonvulsants (e.g., gabapentin) may produce their analgesic effects through blocking sodium channels and enhancing GABA function.
- Antihypertensives (e.g., clonidine) are α_2-adrenergic receptor agonists that modulate ascending pain sensations.
- Antipruritics (e.g., hydroxyzine) are antihistamines that may relieve pruritus, nausea, and anxiety.
- Corticosteroids (e.g., prednisone) inhibit phospholipase A_2 and COX-2 as well as reduce pain associated with inflammation, and they are effective in treating nausea and vomiting.
- Local anesthetics (e.g., benzocaine, lidocaine) block the transmission of pain signals (Vandermeulen, 2006).

Clinical Manifestations and Therapies **Acute and Chronic Pain**

ETIOLOGY	CLINICAL MANIFESTATIONS	CLINICAL THERAPIES
Acute pain	• Client report of acute pain • Elevated vital signs • Nausea and vomiting • Restlessness and anxiety • Behavioral indications (crying, grimacing, shielding)	• Pharmacologic therapy • Heat/ice • Movement restriction • Distraction • Family support
Chronic pain	• Client report of chronic pain • Normal vital signs • Depression • Irritability • Impaired mobility and/or activity • Sleep disturbances	• Pharmacologic therapy • Injections • Surgery • Massage • Chiropractic interventions • Cognitive-behavioral therapy • Positive attitude • Religious rituals • Support (family, friends, groups)

Nonpharmacologic Therapy

In addition to pharmacologic pain management, many nonpharmacologic therapies can be used to help control pain. These include both invasive and noninvasive therapies.

INVASIVE THERAPIES Invasive therapies include injections, such as nerve blocks or radioablation, or surgeries, such as implantation of electrotherapy devices or interruption of pain conduction pathways. A **nerve block** is an injection of a local anesthetic around nerves to temporarily block nerve activity. Nerve blocks are often associated with dental procedures but may also be used to treat pain associated with musculoskeletal injuries, sciatica, shingles, or cancer. Nerve blocks can be administered through single injections, multiple injections over time, or continuous infusions. Permanent nerve blocks use alcohol or phenol, cryoanalgesia, or radioablation to destroy nerve tissue. Pain may return if nerve fibers regenerate over time.

COMPLEMENTARY AND ALTERNATIVE PAIN CONTROL Numerous complementary and alternative methods for pain control are available for use either alone or in conjunction with pharmacologic therapies. Many complementary therapies for pain are independent nursing interventions, such as repositioning a client to relieve pain or providing client education. Many clients ask about the use of acupuncture for pain. Acupuncture, an integral part of traditional Chinese medicine, involves the stimulation of anatomical points on the body, often by using very thin, metallic needles. Although additional research is needed, the National Center for Complementary and Alternative Therapies reports some evidence that acupuncture can be helpful in treating chronic back pain and pain associated with osteoarthritis (NCCAM, 2010). Some methods are intended to provide physiological pain relief, such as heat or ice, movement restriction, and chiropractic therapy. Some therapies are used to help the mind and spirit overcome the sensations of pain, such as guided imagery, cognitive-behavioral therapy, and religious rituals. Social methods include using support from family and friends, laughter, and a focus on others to help minimize pain. Dietary and herbal supplements can be used as an alternative therapy for pain, but current studies suggest that they may be no better than placebos at providing pain relief (Henrotin, Mobasheri, & Marty, 2012), and they may produce dangerous drug–herb interactions (MedlinePlus, 2011).

▮ NURSING PROCESS

Current studies estimate that 43% of American adults—or approximately 100 million Americans—suffer from chronic pain. This presents an economic burden of $560–$635 billion per year in both healthcare costs and lost work productivity. Because of the overwhelming prevalence of pain, nurses are constantly caring for clients in pain.

Uncontrolled pain can lead to comorbidities such as depression, sleep disturbances, and obesity; changes in the nervous system's response to painful stimuli; accelerated disease progression; and increased length of hospital stay. Proper application of the nursing process provides information needed for appropriate care, attainable and measurable client goals for pain management, effective nursing interventions for pain relief, and evaluation of the client's pain level for potential revision of the nursing care plan.

Assessment

Unless a client's physiological needs require priority attention (e.g., severe burns, complex fracture, gunshot wound), all clients should be asked whether they are experiencing pain. Many clients do not voluntarily complain about pain even when pain is present, and persistent pain can contribute to a poor prognosis.

Client Interview

The client interview should begin with eliciting a description of the client's pain. Ask questions about

- *Location.* "Where does it hurt?"
- *Intensity.* "On a scale of 0 to 10, with 0 representing no pain and 10 representing the worst possible pain, how would you rate the intensity of your pain now?"
- *Duration.* "How long have you had the pain, and how long does it usually last?"
- *Quality.* "Tell me what your pain feels like. Is it burning, throbbing, stabbing?"

Find out when the pain started, and what the client believes caused the pain. Determine if any triggers make the pain worse and what methods help relieve the pain. Find out if the client is taking any medications to relieve the pain. Ask if the client experiences any other symptoms with the pain, such as nausea or dizziness, and if the pain is affecting the activities of daily living. Inquire about use of herbal and dietary supplements.

When you have obtained a thorough description of the client's current pain, the interview should continue with questions about the client's *pain history*. Have the client describe previous diseases or injuries that caused pain, the methods used to control the pain (including the methods that have worked and those that have not), and how others' pain has influenced the client's perception of pain. Find out if the client places any significant meaning on the pain, such as whether it signifies disease progression, causes worry or fear, or impacts the client's relationships. Determine which methods the client uses to cope with pain and if the pain is causing related discomforts such as depression or hopelessness.

As you perform a verbal pain assessment, keep in mind that pain is a subjective experience, and the client is most qualified to describe the pain. Some clients, especially those with pain of an unknown etiology, may have been subjected to disdain and disbelief by others regarding their pain, so it is important to listen openly and nonjudgmentally.

Pain Rating Scales

Pain rating scales are reliable tools for helping clients report the intensity of their pain. There are multiple types of pain scales, including numerical pain scales, faces pain scales, verbal descriptor scales, and observational scales. The type of scale

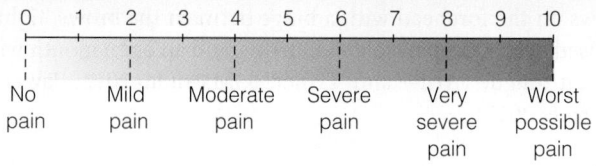

Figure 3–6 ● A universal pain assessment tool with an 11-point numerical pain scale with word modifiers.

chosen will differ with the client, but the same scale should be used for the same client at each assessment to provide consistency throughout the treatment.

- *Numerical pain scales* use an 11-point rating scale (0–10) (**Figure 3–6** ●). They are usually presented horizontally, with 0 on the left and 10 on the right. Numerical pain scales can be combined with other scales, such as the faces scale or the verbal descriptor scale; can be colored, which is helpful for children; or can be presented vertically, which may help clients from Asian cultures who read vertically. To use a numerical pain scale, ask the client to rate the pain on a scale of 0 to 10, with 0 representing no pain and 10 indicating the worst possible pain.

- *Verbal descriptor scales* include words to help describe the pain intensity, such as *mild, moderate,* or *severe.* They are helpful for clients who find it difficult to rate their pain numerically. Verbal descriptor scales may include a description of the extent to which pain interferes with activities of daily living. For example, is the client aware of pain only when paying attention to it (mild pain), or is the client constantly aware of pain that impairs the ability to function (severe pain)? The degree to which pain interferes with functioning is considered a good indication of pain intensity. To use a verbal descriptor scale, read each of the descriptions and ask the client to choose the description that best fits the pain.

- A *faces pain scale* is most commonly used for children starting at age 3. It can also be helpful for clients who do not speak English or who have trouble relating to the numerical pain scales. The most common faces pain scales are the Wong–Baker FACES Rating Scale and the Faces Pain Scale–Revised by the International Association for the Study of Pain (**Figure 3–7** ●). Faces pain scales may include numerical values or verbal descriptions represented by each face. To use a faces pain scale, explain the pain scale using the verbal descriptions while pointing to each of the faces. Then ask the client to point to the face that most represents the level of pain.

- An *observational or behavioral pain scale* is used to determine pain intensity for clients who are unable to provide a verbal report. Observational pain scales include the FLACC (Face, Legs, Activity, Cry, Consolability) scale, CHEOPS (Children's Hospital Eastern Ontario Pain Scale), and BOPS (Behavioral Observational Pain Scale). These pain scales use a numerical scale (usually 0–2 or 0–3) to rate clients for various behaviors, such as facial expression, leg movement, crying, and body position (see the Lifespan Considerations feature). An observational pain scale is also available that is specifically for cognitively impaired clients. It contains areas of assessment similar to those in the pain scales designed for infants, such as facial expression, vocal complaints, and bracing behaviors. To use an observational or behavioral pain scale, the nurse observes the client and rates the client's behavior according to the descriptions provided. In addition, do not assume that cognitively impaired clients are unable to provide a description of pain using numerical, descriptor, or faces pain scales.

- Some pain scales assess more information than pain. For example, the Edmonton Symptom Assessment System uses a 0–10 scale to assess pain, fatigue, drowsiness, nausea, depression, anxiety, feelings of well-being, shortness of breath, and

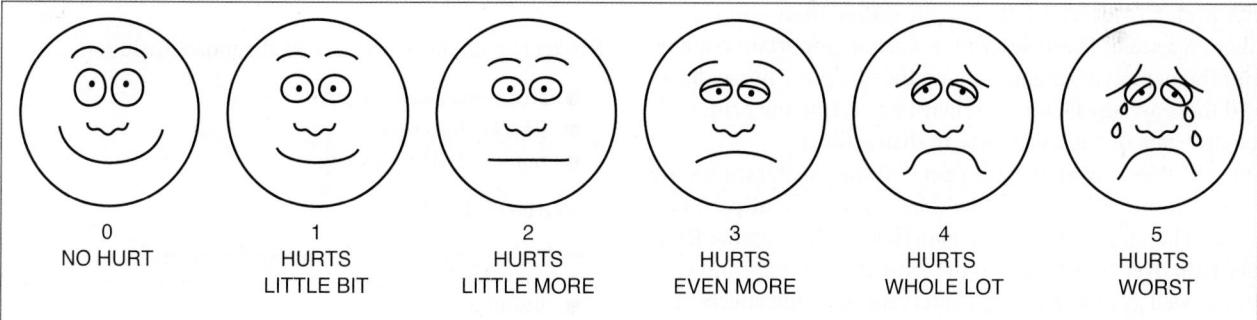

Explain to the person that each face is for a person who feels happy because he has no pain (hurt) or sad because he has some or a lot of pain. Face 0 is very happy because he doesn't hurt at all. Face 1 hurts just a little bit. Face 2 hurts a little more. Face 3 hurts even more. Face 4 hurts a whole lot. Face 5 hurts as much as you can imagine, although you don't have to be crying to feel this bad. Ask the person to choose the face that best describes how he is feeling.

Rating scale is recommended for persons aged 3 years and older.

Brief word instructions: Point to each face using the words to describe the pain intensity. Ask the child to choose the face that best describes own pain and record the appropriate number.

Figure 3–7 ● The Wong–Baker FACES Rating Scale.

Source: From *Wong's Essentials of Pediatric Nursing,* 6th ed. (p. 1301), by D. L. Wong, M. Hockenberry-Eaton, D. Wilson, M. L. Winkelstein, & P. Schwartz. 2001. St. Louis, MO: Mosby. Copyright by Mosby, Inc. Reprinted with permission.

Lifespan Considerations
Neonatal Pain Assessment

Assessing pain in the neonate can be challenging. Symptoms of pain in infants include crying, lethargy, hypertension, hypotension, tachycardia, bradycardia, and apnea. Due to the wide array of symptoms that can indicate pain in the infant, any change in the child's condition should result in the nurse's consideration of a possible relationship to pain.

appetite (Bruera et al., 1991). This scale is particularly useful for clients taking narcotics for chronic pain who may choose to tolerate higher levels of pain to avoid the side effects of chronic opioid use. The Pain Quality Assessment Scale rates several quality descriptors of pain on a scale of 0–10: intense, sharp/dull, heat/cold, sensitive, tender, itchy, radiating, throbbing, and others (Jensen et al., 2006).

When using a pain scale, it is important for clients to understand the pain scale and the importance of accurately rating their pain. The pain intensity described by clients guides the healthcare team in choosing the appropriate interventions to help manage their pain. It also helps nurses track changes in pain even after shift changes, and it helps determine the effectiveness of the interventions. Nurses should remind clients that the goal of most therapeutic interventions is not to reduce pain to 0. Most clients find a reduction of 33%–50% meaningful, even if that reduction corresponds to a decrease of only 1 or 2 points on the numerical pain scale. This decrease in pain intensity usually corresponds to an increase in functioning and a higher quality of life.

In some cases, pain scales do not accurately represent clients' pain experience. Clients in pain may notice changes in pain depending on movement, the time of day, the weather, or the amount of their exertion throughout the day. Therefore, some clients prefer to describe their pain rather than choosing a number on a scale. These descriptions are an important component of the pain assessment, because they help the nurse determine if there are any factors that may be affecting the pain, such as activity, state of consciousness, or distractions.

One effective way to manage pain is to use a pain rating scale in combination with a pain flow sheet to document pain and anticipate changes in pain levels. Pain flow sheets document the clients' pain over time based on the location, intensity, and type of pain as well as pharmacologic interventions, side effects, and sedation level. The use of pain flow sheets has been linked to lower pain intensity scores, suggesting that they can help improve pain management (Faries et al., 1991; Stevens, 1990; Voigt, Paice, & Pouliot, 1995).

✳ Go to **nursing.pearsonhighered.com** for a printable Pain Management Flow Sheet.

Visual Assessment

A visual assessment is the second component of a pain assessment. A visual assessment consists of observing a client's behavior, such as facial expressions, body movement, and posture, to determine if the client is in pain. Visual assessments are particularly important for neonates. Infants in pain have eyebrows that are lowered and drawn together, vertical fur-

rows on the forehead with a bulge between the brows, tightly closed eyes, a deep nasolabial furrow, and an open mouth with a taut tongue (Arif-Rahu, Fisher, & Matsuda, 2012; Pawar & Garten, 2010).

Physical Assessment

A physical assessment includes taking vital signs. Acute pain and exacerbations in chronic pain can manifest in an increased sympathetic response, including increased blood pressure, pulse, and respiratory rate. A physical assessment also includes inspecting for any injuries that could be sources of pain, such as cuts, protruding bones, and ulcers. Any wound that impairs skin integrity is a potential source of pain and infection and should be treated immediately. If the client has specified the location that is producing pain, superficial or deep palpation can pinpoint the exact location of the pain.

Diagnosis

NANDA-I has approved two nursing diagnoses directly related to pain: *Acute Pain* and *Chronic Pain*. The diagnosis should include a statement of the location of the pain (e.g., lower back, left knee, right occipital headache). Pain is often accompanied by physiological and psychological factors that may also be appropriate for nursing diagnoses (NANDA-I, 2012). Nursing diagnoses should include statements of related factors, which are specific for each client.

General nursing diagnoses for clients in acute and chronic pain may include

- *Impaired Physical Mobility*
- *Fatigue*
- *Activity Intolerance*
- *Deficient Knowledge*
- *Anxiety*

(NANDA-I © 2012)

For acute pain, possible nursing diagnoses include

- *Disturbed Sleep Pattern*
- *Risk for Infection*
- *Impaired Skin Integrity*

(NANDA-I © 2012)

For chronic pain, possible nursing diagnoses include

- *Insomnia*
- *Hopelessness*
- *Imbalanced Nutrition: Less/More Than Body Requirements*
- *Social Isolation*
- *Self-Care Deficit*

(NANDA-I © 2012)

For clients who have been prescribed opioids, diagnoses may include

- *Risk for Constipation*
- *Ineffective Breathing Pattern*
- *Fear*
- *Nausea*

(NANDA-I © 2012)

Planning

During the planning phase, the nurse develops client goals and nursing interventions for each nursing diagnosis. Nurses then prioritize the outcomes to determine the order in which to implement nursing interventions. For example, a client with the following nursing diagnoses:

- Acute pain in the right ankle
- Impaired physical mobility related to right ankle pain
- Deficient knowledge about pain management

May have the following expected outcomes:

1. Client will report a 50% reduction in pain.
2. Client will obtain adequate pain relief to allow for mobility.
3. Client will demonstrate skill at using crutches.
4. Client will repeat instructions for managing pain, including elevating ankle, applying ice, and taking pain medication as prescribed.

A client-centered practice involves consulting with clients about their goals, cultural practices, and health beliefs: Client input in the planning process increases clients' motivation to adhere to the care plan and assists in the development of the therapeutic nurse–client relationship.

Implementation

Several interventions are common for clients with acute or chronic pain (also see the Evidence-Based Practice feature):

- Monitor the client's vital signs. Using a pain rating scale, include pain intensity as the fifth vital sign. Observe and document verbal and nonverbal signs of pain and discomfort.
- Listen carefully to the clients' description of their pain, and validate their perception of pain. Advocate on clients' behalf to provide effective pain management.
- Administer analgesics per the instructions of the prescriber. Analgesics should be administered around-the-clock or by self-administration with a client-controlled analgesic (PCA) pump, because analgesics are most effective when given before pain becomes severe. When administering opioids, monitor the client for signs of respiratory depression.

Evidence-Based Practice Overcoming Barriers to Adequate Pain Management

Problem

Pain is a major reason that clients seek health care and take medications, and it accounts for a substantial portion of lost work productivity and disability. However, clients in pain are often underdiagnosed and undertreated, especially racial and ethnic minorities, people of lower socioeconomic status, women, children, older adults, military veterans, surgery and cancer clients, and people at the end of life (IOM, 2011).

Evidence

Pain management remains ineffective due to attitudes and educational deficits of healthcare providers and clients and limitations of pharmacologic agents. Attitudes of healthcare providers can be influenced by both medical evidence and clients' psychosocial influences. In particular, providers are more likely to suggest clients are feigning pain in the absence of medical evidence, and they are less likely to take clients' report of pain into account, if psychosocial influences are present (De Ruddere et al., 2013). Methods of pain management also need to be improved. Using multiple pain medications with different mechanisms of action and side effects will improve efficacy in relieving pain and decrease the incidence of adverse reactions compared to single drug therapies (Sinatra, 2010). In addition, compared to no intervention, physical and psychosocial nonpharmacologic interventions for pain can significantly improve clients' pain level (Park & Hughes, 2012).

Implications

Healthcare professionals need to have a better understanding of pain and pain management. The perception of pain involves both physiological and psychosocial aspects, and pain management should include adequate pharmacologic interventions as well as complementary nonpharmacologic methods to reduce physiological pain and increase psychosocial well-being. Education for healthcare providers should include training programs that offer standardized information about pain, guidelines related to caring for clients in pain, and experience in caring for clients in pain (IOM, 2011). Education should also include information about the proper use of opioids. Opioids, which are the most effective pain medications, are often underprescribed because of prejudices, misconceptions, and fears about their use (Notcutt & Gibbs, 2010). All healthcare providers should be encouraged to keep their knowledge current by participating in continuing education courses, and certification examinations should assess providers' knowledge about pain (IOM, 2011).

Critical Thinking Application

1. Do you have any biases that may hinder your ability to provide adequate pain management for clients? Think about a variety of situations that may present opportunities for bias, including caring for clients of different cultures, clients with drug addiction, young children and older adults, and clients at the end of life.

2. You are caring for a 72-year-old woman with osteoarthritis who is receiving inadequate pain control. How will you act as an advocate to provide better pain management for your client?

3. You are caring for a 19-year-old male who is a known gang member. During a recent altercation, he sustained a stab wound. He is sleeping restlessly and moaning. It is time for his next dose of opioids, but your nurse manager tells you to give him only half the prescribed dose because he is probably a drug addict and you don't want to feed his addiction. What should you do?

4. What are three ways in which you can stay up-to-date on current pain management nursing standards?

Community-Based Care Managing Chronic Pain at Home

Clients with chronic pain have to live at home and care for themselves in spite of their pain. Teaching clients and their family how to administer drugs, watch for side effects, and perform nonpharmacologic interventions will help enhance both the clients' and the caregivers' lives. See **Table 3–6** ● for an overview of medications used for the management of chronic pain. Discussions should include the following topics:

■ Describe the drugs to be taken, including dose, frequency, route of administration, side effects, and potential drug, food, or herbal interactions.

■ Discuss the importance of taking drugs around the clock rather than prn.

■ Dispel any myths or misconceptions about opioid analgesics, including teaching clients that the risk of addiction is very low when pain medications are taken as prescribed.

■ Help clients and their family choose appropriate nonpharmacologic interventions to decrease pain, and teach them how to perform the interventions correctly.

■ Teach clients and their family the importance of adequate sleep and rest and not overusing the area in pain.

■ Provide information about community resources, including support groups, pain clinics, and the American Pain Society.

■ Regularly monitor clients to determine the effectiveness of analgesics and nonpharmacologic interventions as well as to detect adverse reactions to medications. Also educate family members about signs of adverse reactions. If the client exhibits signs of opioid overdose, slowly titrate opioid antagonists (naloxone) to reduce the effects of the opioid agonist. Administer only enough antagonist to reverse adverse effects; administering too much antagonist too quickly leads to significant pain and withdrawal symptoms.

■ Educate the client about nonpharmacologic management of pain, such as sleep hygiene, progressive relaxation, repositioning, and distraction. Combining pharmacologic and nonpharmacologic techniques provides enhanced pain control and increased quality of life. Involving family or friends increases client support and well-being.

■ Help clients with self-care measures, such as bathing, toileting, and oral care. Provide comfort measures, such as offering snacks or drinks; changing bed linens; keeping noise, light, and room temperature at appropriate levels; and giving back massages. Reduce safety hazards, such as cords on the floor or furniture in the walking path.

■ Teach clients with pain and their families about proper medication administration, medication side effects, and nonpharmacologic methods of pain relief. Teach clients with acute pain about the expected time course for healing. Teach clients with chronic pain about resources for home care, financial assistance, support groups, and counseling.

Evaluation

Evaluation of the effectiveness of pain control measures begins with asking clients if they have experienced relief and, if so, to what degree. A consistent pain rating scale should be used throughout the course of care. The nurse should also evaluate behavioral signs of continued pain. The time to onset for pain medication is highly dependent on the route of analgesic administration, the type of nonpharmacologic intervention, and the client's pain level prior to initiation of therapy. Oral medications may take up to an hour to provide relief, while intravenous medications should begin working within minutes. If pain is still present, the nurse must evaluate the care plan, suggest changes to pharmacologic therapy, and implement changes to nonpharmacologic therapy.

TABLE 3–6   Overview of Medications Used in the Management of Chronic Pain

ROUTE	DRUG	NURSING IMPLICATIONS
Oral	Hydromorphone (Exalgo)	To avoid medication errors, be aware that Exalgo is available in both immediate-release and extended-release tablets.
Oral	Methadone (Dolophine)	Evaluate client for continued need of methadone for pain. Methadone has cumulative effects over time, so dosage may be reduced after chronic use.
Oral	Morphine (Kadian, Avinza)	Formulated as extended-release capsules. Do not chew or crush. If client can't swallow the capsule, pellets may be sprinkled over food and swallowed without chewing.
Oral	Oxycodone (OxyContin)	Available in a timed-release formulation for 12-hour dosing. Timed-release formulation must be swallowed whole. Fast-acting formulations (OxyFAST) can be used for breakthrough pain.
Transdermal	Fentanyl (Duragesic)	Patch should be placed on flat surface. Clip, do not shave, hair at site of application. Patch should be changed every 3 days. Slow onset effect (12–24 hours) and slow decay after discontinuation.
Transdermal	Lidocaine (Lidoderm)	Patch used for postherpetic neuralgia. Apply one to three patches on most painful area for up to 12 hours per 24-hour period.
Transmucosal	Fentanyl (Actiq)	A lozenge formulation used for treatment of breakthrough pain. Client should not suck or chew the lozenge. Lozenge should be consumed over 15 minutes.

NURSING CARE PLAN A Client With Chronic Pain

James Grier, age 28, visits the pain clinic with chronic low back pain. He states that he worked in a warehouse three years ago and injured his back while lifting heavy boxes. Although he was treated for the initial injury, he has had chronic back pain since then. During severe flare-ups, he can barely move, and he misses work approximately five days per month because of his back pain.

ASSESSMENT

- In an interview with Kenneth Hill, RN, regarding his pain, Mr. Grier rates his pain as a 7 on a scale of 0–10. Flare-ups usually last about a week before his pain is controlled to a 5. Mr. Grier describes his constant pain as a dull ache, but it throbs during flare-ups with sharp piercing sensations during movement. Nothing seems to relieve the pain except lying completely still, although the pain keeps him from falling asleep. He is currently taking ibuprofen as needed, which is usually 400 mg q4h. In the past, he has taken Vicodin, 5–10 mg q4–6h, with moderate success, although it gives him slight nausea and drowsiness.
- Upon observation, Mr. Hill notes that Mr. Grier has no obvious external sources of pain, but he does have beads of sweat on his forehead. Mr. Hill also notices that Mr. Grier grimaces and holds his breath during movement, and his movements are very slow. A physical assessment indicates a pulse of 92bpm, respiratory rate of 20/min with shallow breaths, blood pressure of 130/84 mmHg, and temperature of 100.8°F.

DIAGNOSES

- *Chronic Pain* related to lower back pain as evidenced by behavioral and sympathetic reactions and the client's report.
- *Impaired Physical Mobility* related to severe lower back pain as evidenced by slow movements and grimacing during movement.
- *Disturbed Sleep Pattern* related to lower back pain as evidenced by client's report.
- *Readiness for Enhanced Knowledge* about pain management.
- *Fear* about potential job loss.

(NANDA-I © 2012)

PLANNING

- After 3 days on the pain medication, the client will report a decrease in pain intensity from a 7 to a 3 or 4 on the numerical scale.
- The client will report increased physical mobility with no increase in pain intensity over baseline during movement.
- The client will demonstrate an understanding of good sleep hygiene and will report receiving adequate sleep.
- The client will demonstrate knowledge about nonpharmacologic methods of pain relief.
- The client will choose three methods of nonpharmacologic pain relief to implement.
- The client will report decreased pain as a result of nonpharmacologic therapies.
- The client will report a decrease in lost workdays as a result of lower back pain.

IMPLEMENTATION

- Consult with a physician about opioid and nonopioid analgesic therapies for Mr. Grier.
- Teach Mr. Grier the importance of taking pain medications around the clock.
- Teach Mr. Grier about nonpharmacologic interventions, including heat, distractions, acupuncture, massage, and mild exercise.

- Encourage Mr. Grier to talk about his pain, and validate his pain experience.
- Provide Mr. Grier with contact information for the pain clinic and encourage him to call the clinic if his prescribed therapies are ineffective.
- Encourage Mr. Grier to set regular follow up appointments to help manage his pain effectively over time.

EVALUATION

Four days after Mr. Grier's appointment, Mr. Hill calls Mr. Grier to assess his pain. Mr. Grier reports that he has been taking his pain medications as prescribed. He is applying heat to his back for 30 minutes three times a day, and he is performing strengthening exercises for his back. When the pain is most severe, he listens to music to help distract him from the pain. Mr. Grier reports that with this new therapy, his pain is now a 4 on a scale of 0–10.

One month after his appointment, Mr. Grier returns to the pain clinic for a follow up appointment. He reports that his pain has been a 2 or 3 for the past week, and he has missed only one day of work in the past month. He continues to take the nonopioid analgesics as instructed and performs strengthening exercises three times a week. His boss has noticed an increase in his work productivity. To maintain pain control without opioids, Mr. Hill recommends alternating acetaminophen and ibuprofen and adding a monthly back massage to Mr. Grier's therapeutic regimen.

CRITICAL THINKING

1. Mr. Grier asks you why he needs to continue the strengthening exercises and include back massages in his therapy. What do you tell him?
2. If Mr. Grier reports excessive nausea in response to his opioid medication, what suggestions will you give him to decrease his nausea and provide comfort?
3. How would you adapt this care plan to a client with knee pain instead of back pain?

REVIEW   Acute and Chronic Pain

RELATE Link the Concepts and Exemplars

Linking the exemplar of acute and chronic pain with the concept of culture and diversity:

1. When you are caring for a client who appears to be in pain but denies it, how might understanding of the client's culture help you interpret the dichotomy between body language and reported pain?

2. How might interpretations and interventions for pain differ among cultures?

Linking the exemplar of acute and chronic pain with the concept of stress and coping:

3. What alterations in stress and coping would you anticipate when a client experiences chronic pain?

4. When caring for a mother with acute pain over the past few weeks, the client relates she has just not had the energy to deal with her children. How is pain impacting this mother's ability to cope with her children's needs?

READY Go to Companion Skills Manual

REFER Go to Pearson Student Nursing Resources
nursing.pearsonhighered.com

- Additional review material
- Chart: Printable pain management flow sheet
- Minimodule: Neonates and Pain

REFLECT Case Study

Mr. Backwater is a 48-year-old Cherokee Indian. His history includes nicotine abuse, lung cancer, arthritis in both knees, and headaches. Mr. Backwater has trouble breathing, especially after exertion. During a routine checkup, the nurse's assessment reveals that Mr. Backwater is experiencing severe pain in his right side when inhaling, and he has painful mouth sores as a result of his chemotherapy treatment. Between the chemotherapy and the mouth sores, Mr. Backwater is losing weight because of inadequate food intake.

1. What cultural influences do you need to consider when assessing Mr. Backwater's pain?

2. Should Mr. Backwater's history of nicotine abuse influence which pharmacologic agents are prescribed for his pain? Why or why not? How can you advocate for Mr. Backwater if inadequate pain medications are prescribed?

3. What cultural practices can you recommend as nonpharmacologic therapy for Mr. Backwater's pain?

EXEMPLAR 3.2   End-of-Life Care

EXEMPLAR KEY TERMS
Advance healthcare directive, *176*
Assisted suicide, *176*
Death anxiety, *183*
Do-not-intubate order (DNI), *176*
Do-not-resuscitate order (DNR), *176*
Durable power of attorney, *176*
End of life, *174*
Euthanasia, *176*
Healthcare proxy, *176*
Hospice care, *177*
Living will, *176*
Palliative care, *177*

EXEMPLAR LEARNING OUTCOMES
After reading about this exemplar, you will be able to:

1. Describe the pathophysiology, etiology, clinical manifestations, and direct and indirect causes of symptoms seen in clients at the end of life.

2. Identify risk factors and prevention methods associated with symptoms seen at the end of life.

3. Illustrate the nursing process in providing culturally competent care for individuals at the end of life.

4. Formulate priority nursing diagnoses appropriate for an individual at the end of life.

5. Summarize therapies used by interdisciplinary teams in the collaborative care of an individual at the end of life.

6. Plan evidence-based care for an individual at the end of life and his or her family in collaboration with other members of the healthcare team.

7. Evaluate expected outcomes for an individual at the end of life.

▶ OVERVIEW

Nurses have a unique responsibility to ensure that individuals at the end of life experience a peaceful death (ICN, 1997; AACN, n.d.). **End of life** refers to the final weeks of life just before death. As skilled clinicians, nurses must understand the technical aspects of managing the physiological changes associated with end-of-life care. As advocates, nurses must ensure that the client is receiving the best possible care by collaborating with other healthcare providers and adjusting the plan of care as needed. As guides, nurses must use communication and intuition to support clients and their families through the dying process (Norlander, 2008).

Box 3–9   Eight Domains of Palliative Care

1. Structure and processes of care
   - Identify clients' and their family's values and goals.
   - Train staff appropriately.
2. Physical aspects of care
   - Administer pain medications as needed to provide comfort.
   - Provide hygiene care (e.g., oral care, skin care, change of bed linens).
3. Psychological and psychiatric aspects of care
   - Promote psychological services for client.
   - Provide grief counseling for family.
4. Social aspects of care
   - Call family to be present at end of life.
   - Refer to social services (e.g., hospice care).
5. Spiritual, religious, and existential aspects of care
   - Facilitate visits with clergy.
   - Allow practice of religious rituals.

6. Cultural aspects of care
   - Hire culturally diverse staff that is representative of surrounding population.
   - Administer care that is culturally competent.
7. Care of the imminently dying clients
   - Communicate signs of impending death to family.
   - Provide comfort to clients and family during last minutes of life.
8. Ethical and legal aspects of care
   - Consider legal and ethical aspects of care, such as advance directives and DNR (do not resuscitate) orders.
   - Discuss ethical decisions with family, such as withdrawal of nutrients.

▶ PATHOPHYSIOLOGY AND ETIOLOGY

According to the Centers for Disease Control and Prevention (CDC, 2012), the top 10 leading causes of death in 2010 and 2011 include: heart disease; malignant neoplasms; chronic lower respiratory disease; cerebrovascular diseases; accidents (unintentional injuries); Alzheimer disease; diabetes mellitus; influenza and pneumonia; nephritis, nephrotic syndrome, and nephrosis; and intentional self-harm (suicide). These 10 causes of death accounted for nearly 75% of all deaths in the United States in 2011. In addition, the top 5 leading causes of infant death in 2011 were congenital malformations, complications related to short gestation and low birth weight, sudden infant death syndrome, maternal complications of pregnancy, and accidents (CDC, 2012).

Etiology

A majority (70%–80%) of Americans claim that they would prefer to die at home. However, only 25% of Americans die at home; approximately 45% die in a hospital or medical center and 22% die in a long-term care facility (CDC, 2005). As people age, they are more likely to die in a long-term care facility (CDC, 2011). Americans age 65 and older have a 40% chance of entering a long-term care facility, and most of those individuals will die either at the long-term care facility or shortly after transfer to a hospital. However, studies indicate that families are less than satisfied with the care their dying loved ones receive, stating concerns about insufficient treatment of symptoms, lack of communication with physicians, inadequate emotional support, and not being treated with respect. These concerns were more likely to occur in hospitals and other institutions than in home hospice care (Teno et al., 2004).

▶ CLINICAL MANIFESTATIONS

Signs of impending death include increased confusion or disorientation, increased periods of sleep, decreased food and liquid intake, changes in respiration (e.g., Cheyne-Stokes breathing, apnea), decreased body temperature and blood pressure, cyanosis, loss of bladder and bowel control, changes in muscle control, and restlessness. Clinical manifestations of dying are discussed in more detail in the exemplar on Death and Dying in the module on Grief and Loss.

When death is inevitable, many clients and families choose palliative care rather than pursuing aggressive treatments aimed at regaining health. During palliative care, the nurse is responsible for caring for clients and their family in eight domains (Box 3–9●) (NCP, 2009).

Nursing Considerations for End-of-Life Care

All clients at the end of life have the right to be treated with dignity, as stated in the Dying Person's Bill of Rights (Box 3–10●). Nursing care for dying clients may take place in a variety of

Box 3–10   The Dying Person's Bill of Rights

- I have the right to be treated as a living human being until I die.
- I have the right to maintain a sense of hopefulness, however changing its focus may be.
- I have the right to express my feelings and emotions about my approaching death in my own way.
- I have the right to participate in decisions concerning my care.
- I have the right to expect continuing medical and nursing attention even though cure goals must be changed to comfort goals.
- I have the right not to die alone.
- I have the right to be free from pain.
- I have the right to have my questions answered honestly.
- I have the right not to be deceived.
- I have the right to have help from and for my family in accepting my death.
- I have the right to die in peace and with dignity.
- I have the right to retain my individuality and not be judged for my decisions which may be contrary to the beliefs of others.
- I have the right to be cared for by caring, sensitive, knowledgeable people who will attempt to understand my needs and will be able to gain some satisfaction in helping me face my death.

Source: From Barbus, A. J. (1975). The Dying Person's Bill of Rights, created at the workshop *The Terminally Ill Patient and the Helping Person.* Lansing, MI: South Western Michigan Inservice Education Council.

settings: a hospital, a long-term care facility, or the clients' home. Regardless of the location, nurses should respect the clients' and family's wishes about death, including any legal and ethical issues.

LEGAL AND ETHICAL ISSUES   When caring for clients at the end of life, nurses are faced with legal and ethical issues, including honoring clients' wishes, finding out who should make medical decisions for the client if the client is unable to make decisions, and deciding how to deal with families that disagree about the course of treatment. Clients who have legal documents specifying their wishes, such as advance directives and DNR orders, have the right to expect care based on these documents. Other ethical issues, such as euthanasia, must follow state and federal laws.

Advance Healthcare Directives   Advance healthcare directives, or advance directives, are legal documents that allow individuals to choose their preferred treatment plan while they are mentally able to ensure that their wishes will be carried out even when they are unable to make decisions themselves. These directives take the form of living wills and durable powers of attorney. All advance directives must be in writing, signed by the client, witnessed, and notarized. For detailed information, refer to the exemplar on Advance Directives in the module on Legal Issues.

A **living will** is a document that describes the client's treatment preferences about life-prolonging procedures, including the use of mechanical breathing, feeding tubes, and resuscitation. It may also indicate if the client wishes to be an organ or tissue donor. This document should be used only when the client is mentally unstable or unable to communicate and only in the case of terminal illness or permanent unconsciousness. It is the nurse's responsibility to determine if the client has a living will and to communicate the client's wishes to other members of the healthcare team.

Most living wills do not cover every possible situation. Therefore some clients select a **durable power of attorney**, which gives the person designated the power to make medical, legal, and financial decisions for the client when the client is no longer able. The durable power of attorney document may designate one individual to make medical decisions, in a document called a **healthcare proxy**, and one individual to make legal and financial decisions. A healthcare agent appointed by a healthcare proxy has the right to speak to physicians and other healthcare providers on behalf of the client to determine the best course of treatment.

Do-Not-Resuscitate Orders   A **do-not-resuscitate order (DNR, or "no-code")** is a medical order written by a physician that states the client's wishes to withhold cardiopulmonary resuscitation (CPR) in the event of respiratory or cardiac arrest. It covers only CPR; it does not pertain to other treatments such as medications or nutrition. The physician will create a DNR order only at the request of the client or the healthcare proxy. A DNR order is different from advance directives in that it is written by a physician, not by the client; but a DNR request can be included in the advance directive. In addition, clients or proxies have the right to request and receive resuscitation even if a DNR order was previously signed. Some facilities may offer an "allow natural death" (AND) order rather than a DNR order.

A **do-not-intubate order (DNI)** prohibits endotracheal intubation in the event of severe respiratory failure or respiratory arrest. The DNI order is separate and distinct from the DNR order, in that the DNI order applies to situations in which the individual is not in cardiopulmonary arrest.

The American Nurses Association (ANA, 2012) has issued a position statement about the impact of DNR and AND decisions on nursing care. The ANA recommends that nurses play an active role in initiating discussions about DNR/AND with clients, families, and healthcare team members to prevent confusion about the clients' and family's wishes about end-of-life care. With this responsibility, nurses have the duty to educate clients and their families about procedures and treatments used at the end of life, to inform clients about advance directives and ensure the documentation and implementation of existing advance directives, to encourage clients to think about their preferences for end-of-life treatment, to communicate clients' end-of-life decisions to the healthcare team, and to advocate for clients' decisions about end-of-life care in spite of differing opinions by the healthcare proxy or physician. Regardless of clients' DNR/AND status, nurses have the responsibility to provide palliative care and other medical treatments for all clients.

A variation of the DNR/AND order is the "comfort measures only" (CMO) order. A CMO order indicates that the client prefers to receive maximum comfort while progressing through the natural dying process. A CMO order is *not* equivalent to a DNR/AND order, although they are often issued simultaneously. Clients with a CMO order should receive effective pain and symptom management, spiritual care, food and fluids as the client is able, and hygiene care.

Euthanasia and Assisted Suicide   Euthanasia and assisted suicide are controversial legal and ethical issues that face nurses caring for clients at the end of life. Both **euthanasia** and **assisted suicide** refer to intentionally ending a life in order to relieve pain and suffering. The difference between the two is who performs the final act that causes death. In euthanasia, the physician or other healthcare provider performs the last act, usually in the form of an intentional drug overdose. In contrast, assisted suicide occurs when the physician or another healthcare team member provides the lethal dose of medication but the client administers the medication to herself or himself. Assisted suicide is legal in Oregon, Washington, and Montana.

There are various terms related to euthanasia, and the ethical and legal ramifications of different types of euthanasia are widely debated. Euthanasia can be voluntary, nonvoluntary, or involuntary, and it can be passive or active. *Voluntary* euthanasia occurs when the client or the client's family gives consent for the actions that will result in death for the client. *Nonvoluntary* refers to euthanasia that occurs when the client and the client's family are unable or unavailable to give consent. *Involuntary* euthanasia is defined as euthanasia performed against the wishes of the client or the client's family. In addition, *passive* euthanasia is performed by the withdrawal or withholding of life-sustaining treatments, whereas *active* euthanasia is performed by the administration of drugs that will cause death.

The American Nurses Association (ANA, 1994) has issued a position statement that nurses should not participate in voluntary, nonvoluntary, or involuntary active euthanasia because it is in direct violation of the *Code for Nurses with Interpretive Statements*. In addition, active euthanasia is illegal in all 50 States. In contrast, passive voluntary euthanasia is considered an acceptable medical practice and occurs often for clients with DNR orders or living wills specifying that the client does not want mechanical breathing, feeding tubes, and other life-prolonging procedures. However, passive nonvoluntary or involuntary euthanasia, which may occur as the result of a "slow code," is ethically questionable and could be grounds for a malpractice suit. A slow code occurs when resuscitation efforts are less vigorous than usual or when the nurse does not hurry to alert the emergency team when a terminally ill client stops breathing.

PALLIATIVE AND HOSPICE CARE According to the World Health Organization (WHO, n.d.a), "**palliative care** improves the quality of life of patients and families who face life-threatening illness by providing pain and symptom relief, spiritual and psychosocial support from diagnosis to the end of life and bereavement." Palliative care should be provided to all clients, especially older adults with an acute life-threatening illness (e.g., stroke, myocardial infarction, trauma) or a chronic progressive illness (e.g., end-stage dementia, liver or kidney failure, terminal cancer). Palliative care for children with a chronic disorder (e.g., cystic fibrosis, hemophilia, muscular dystrophy) should begin at the time of diagnosis. It should provide total care of the child's body, mind, and spirit as well as support for the family (WHO, n.d.a).

Nursing approaches to providing palliative care include relieving pain and other distressing symptoms, affirming life, viewing death as a normal process, integrating psychological and spiritual aspects of care, offering a support system for both clients and their family, and using a team to address the needs of clients and families. Palliative care providers may become more involved as clients near death and cannot perform basic comfort measures, such as hygiene care and nutrition intake, for themselves. This kind of care allows clients to die with dignity, and it assures the family that the client was as comfortable as possible through the dying process.

Most Americans prefer to die at home, free from pain, surrounded by loved ones. Hospice care makes this preference a reality. According to the Hospice Foundation of America (2013), "Hospice is a special concept of care designed to provide comfort and support to patients and their families when a life-limiting illness no longer responds to cure-oriented treatments." Hospice does not seek to lengthen life or hasten death. Instead, **hospice care** provides comfort and dignity for clients' last days by offering care provided by a team-oriented group of trained professionals with a specialized knowledge of pain management. Hospice also provides emotional, social, and spiritual support for clients and their family as well as bereavement and counseling services for the family for one year after the clients' death.

Hospice began in the United States in 1974 with Florence Wald's establishment of the Connecticut Hospice (National Hospice and Palliative Care Organization [NHPCO], 2012). Almost all of the early hospice programs were small, community programs led by volunteers. In 1982, Congress voted to include a hospice benefit for Medicare recipients, and hospice has since grown steadily, to over 5,300 programs in 2011. Care is provided by physicians, nurses, aides, social workers, spiritual caregivers, counselors, therapists, and volunteers. In 2011, over 1.65 million clients used hospice services, 83.3% of those clients being over the age of 65 (NHPCO, 2012). To be eligible for hospice care, clients need to be diagnosed by a physician as having 6 months or less to live. In addition, clients and their family must be comfortable with the clients' receiving only comfort care rather than curative care. Clients can receive hospice care for two 90-day periods and an unlimited number of 60-day periods with continued recertification by a physician or a hospice medical director. In most cases, hospice care is offered through routine visits to the clients' home, although continuous care is available for clients in crisis. Hospice care can also take place in hospice centers, hospitals, nursing homes, and other long-term care facilities. Hospice care also supports the involvement of family in clients' care and is available to help ease the burden of primary caregivers.

Although hospice services were used by approximately 44.6% of individuals who died in 2011 (NHPCO, 2012), there are still many myths about hospice care. When discussing hospice care with clients, it may help to clarify these myths, as stated in the Client Teaching feature.

Lifespan and Cultural Considerations

Facing the death of a child is a life-altering experience. No parents expect to outlive their children, yet 45,000 children died in 2010 in the United States, more than half of them dying under the age of 1 (CDC, 2010). Too often, children who die fail to receive competent and compassionate care that meets their physical, emotional, and spiritual needs (IOM, 2003). Nurses play a vital role in improving care for children facing a life-threatening medical condition.

END-OF-LIFE CARE FOR CHILDREN Children with life-limiting conditions should receive palliative care in much the same way it is provided to adults. However, palliative care is often neglected for infants and very young children. Three main aspects of palliative care for children with terminal illnesses and their families are comfort care, end-of-life decision making, and bereavement support for family members (Guido, 2010c). Nursing care should be based on the best interests of the child, not on the best interests of the parents. However, parents must be involved in the decision making regarding their child's care and should receive complete, timely, understandable information about the diagnosis, prognosis, treatments, and palliative care options for their child. Parents should be allowed to spend as much time as possible with their child, and nursing staff should provide privacy for the family as needed (Guido, 2010c). The basic elements of palliative care for children are stated in **Box 3–11 ●**. **Box 3–12 ●** provides recommendations from the Institute of Medicine on methods nurses can use to improve pediatric palliative and end-of-life care.

Client Teaching Myths and Facts Regarding Hospice

MYTH	FACT
Clients can receive hospice care only for 6 months through Medicare and other insurance policies.	The Medicare hospice program states that terminally ill clients with a life expectancy of 6 months or less may receive hospice care. However, clients who live longer can continue receiving hospice care as long as they meet hospice criteria.
All hospice programs are the same.	All hospice programs must provide certain services, but other services and support may differ. Before selecting or recommending a hospice organization, meet with representatives and learn about the services they provide.
Once clients choose hospice care, they cannot receive curative therapies.	Clients are required to sign an agreement indicating their choice of hospice care instead of curative therapies. However, clients who wish to receive curative treatments can be discharged from hospice and return to traditional medical treatment.
Choosing hospice care means giving up hope. It means that clients will die soon.	Receiving hospice care does not mean that clients give up hope or that death is imminent. It helps stabilize clients' medical condition and helps clients live life fully to the end. It provides opportunities to appreciate personal and spiritual connections, and it allows the family to know that everything possible was done to provide a peaceful death.
Hospice provides 24-hour care.	Hospice teams visit clients intermittently, but they are available 24/7 for support and care. Continuous care is provided only in specific circumstances.
Clients are not permitted to retain their own doctor once they are approved for hospice services.	Hospice reinforces the client-primary physician relationship by advocating office or home visits.
Only clients with cancer qualify for hospice.	In addition to clients who are diagnosed with cancer, a variety of clients qualify for hospice care, including those with diagnoses such as dementia, heart and lung diseases, and HIV/AIDS.
Hospice care benefits only the individual who is sick.	Hospice provides support for the client, the family, and caregivers. Hospice also provides grief services to the community at large.
Hospice is a place.	Hospice care takes place wherever the need exists, usually in the clients' homes or in long-term care facilities.
Hospice is expensive.	Hospice care is often less expensive than conventional care in the last 6 months of life. In addition, Medicare and many traditional insurance policies provide hospice benefits.

Sources: Based on Labyak, M. J. (2001). The experience model. *Home Healthcare Nurse,* 20(3): 48; Naierman, N., & Turner, J. (2009). *Debunking the myths of hospice.* Retrieved from the American Hospice Foundation Web site, http://www.americanhospice.org/articles-mainmenu-8/about-hospice-mainmenu-7/36-debunking-the-myths-of-hospice; Hospice Directory. (n.d.). *Hospice myths and realities.* Retrieved from http://www.hospicedirectory.org/cm/about/choosing/myths_facts; Hospice Foundation of America. (n.d.). *Myths and facts about hospice.* Retrieved from http://www.hospicefoundation.org/hospicemyths

Box 3–11   Principles of Pediatric Palliative Care

- Pediatric palliative care provides care to children and families experiencing a debilitating chronic or life-threatening illness, condition, or injury.
- The uniqueness of each child and family is respected, and the care plan is determined by the goals and preferences of the child and family with guidance from the healthcare team.
- Palliative care ideally begins at the time of diagnosis of a life-threatening or debilitating condition and continues through cure or until death and into the family's bereavement period.
- Palliative care uses a multidimensional assessment to prevent and alleviate physical, psychological, social, and spiritual distress. Care providers should assist children and their families in understanding changes in the child's condition and the implications of these changes as they relate to future care and treatment.
- Palliative care indicates a need for an interdisciplinary care team, including but not limited to physicians, nurses, social workers, chaplains, pharmacists, art therapists, child-life therapists, and speech and language pathologists.
- The primary goal of palliative care is to prevent and relieve suffering, including pain and other symptoms.
- Effective communication includes sharing developmentally appropriate information, listening actively, assisting with medical decision making, and determining goals and preferences.
- Palliative care specialists must be knowledgeable about signs and symptoms of imminent death and the associated care and support of children and their families before and after death.
- Palliative care is appropriate for inclusion in all settings where health care is provided, including hospitals, emergency departments, home care, and schools.
- Palliative care should be provided equally to all children with any life-limiting condition, regardless of race, ethnicity, or ability to pay.
- Palliative care services should be committed to providing excellent and high-quality care based on six aims: timely care, client-centered care, beneficial and/or effective care, accessible and equitable care, knowledge- and evidence-based care, and efficient care.

Source: Based on National Consensus Project for Quality Palliative Care. (2009). *Clinical practice guidelines for quality palliative care,* pp. 9–10. Retrieved February 6, 2013, from http://www.nationalconsensusproject.org/Guideline.pdf

Box 3–12   Improving Pediatric Palliative and End-of-Life Care

In some clinical settings, nurses provide palliative care to infants and children at the end of life. Principles that improve the quality of care provided to infants, children, and their families include the following:

- Palliative care should be designed to care for the child's physical, cognitive, emotional, and spiritual development.
- Appropriate care involves families as part of the care team and respects both the child's and the family's wishes.
- Nurses should provide effective and compassionate care from the time of diagnosis through death and bereavement.
- Nurses should educate themselves and others about the identification and management of the last phase of the child's condition.
- Nurses should advocate within their facility for guidelines aimed at providing consistently excellent palliative, end-of-life, and bereavement care for children and their families.
- Nurses are encouraged to engage in research activities designed to enhance healthcare providers' awareness and understanding of approaches to improving palliative, end-of-life, and bereavement care for children and their families.

Source: Reprinted with permission from "Working Principles for Pediatric Palliative, End-of-Life and Bereavement Care," from "When Children Die: Improving Palliative and End-of-Life Care for Children and Their Families," Summary, p. 7, Box S.1. © 2003 by the National Academy of Sciences. Courtesy of the National Academies Press, Washington, D.C.

Box 3–13   Research: Advance Care Planning

A recent study identified the top three barriers to advance care planning for children as unrealistic parent expectations, differences in the understanding of the child's prognosis between clinicians and client/parents, and lack of parent readiness to have the discussion. Other barriers included ethical considerations, a lack of importance of advance care planning to clinicians, and not knowing what to say. Addressing these barriers may help healthcare providers become more proficient in discussing advance care planning for pediatric clients (Durall, Zurakowski, & Wolfe, 2012).

Palliative care for children should be instituted from the time a child is diagnosed with a life-limiting condition until the time of death. Palliative care is especially important for children who have a disease for which no treatment has been shown to alter progression toward death and medical technology creates a larger burden than benefit for the client (AAP, 2000). In spite of the need for pediatric palliative care, many barriers exist to providing effective care for children with life-limiting conditions and their families. These barriers include (AAP, 2000; IOM, 2003)

- Lack of education and experience of healthcare professionals in providing palliative care to children
- Limited knowledge about caring for children with rare medical conditions
- Ineligibility for hospice care based on the uncertainty of the length of life
- Lack of expertise of hospice programs in caring for children at the end of life
- Financial barriers, including poor reimbursement for time-intensive care, lack of reimbursement for newer therapies that may improve the quality of life, and a general lack of insurance
- Miscommunication and differences in values based on culture or ethnicity
- Misconception that palliative care means that the client can no longer receive curative care

Advance Care Planning   Advance care planning for children is most appropriate early in the course of the child's disease, when the child is not in crisis so rational decisions can be made based on all available options in collaboration with the child, parents, and healthcare team (**Box 3–13** ●). This timing

allows the care plan to be altered to meet the child's individual physical, psychological, and spiritual needs, improving the quality of care and providing satisfaction and relief for the caregivers. If advance care planning begins early, then the care plan can be modified as the child's disease progresses to enhance the child's quality of life (Canadian Paediatric Society [CPS], 2008).

Considerations for Adolescents   Adolescents with a serious medical condition are more capable of making treatment decisions than most teenagers. Although the Patient Self-Determination Act of 1990 limits the legal rights of individuals younger than 18 to make their own healthcare decisions, adolescents have the cognitive skills to participate in discussions regarding their own care. Most adolescents desire autonomy, so all choices for health care, including legal and ethical issues, should be discussed with the client. If the adolescent states a desire to withdraw from or refuse treatment, her parents and healthcare team should discuss the reasons for her decision and help her understand the implications of her decision and any treatment alternatives that may influence her choice. When an adolescent has made a decision based on facts, it may be easier for the parents and healthcare team to accept the decision.

Ethical Issues Surrounding a Child's Death   Making healthcare decisions for dying children can be an emotionally charged experience for both the parents and the healthcare providers. It is common to have misunderstandings and conflicts between the child, the parents, and the clinicians based on differences in clinical understanding, personal and religious preferences, and strong emotions. Sometimes these conflicts lead to ethical issues, including withdrawing or withholding treatments, parental refusal of treatment, and DNR orders.

Withdrawing and withholding treatment have the same meaning ethically and legally. However, it is much harder emotionally for parents and healthcare providers to withdraw a treatment than to withhold a new treatment (IOM, 2003). Nurses and other healthcare providers have the responsibility to accurately portray the child's health condition and the benefits versus the burden of treatment. Some parents may resist the recommendation to withdraw or withhold a treatment, while other parents may refuse a recommended treatment or test. This refusal may be based on religious beliefs (see the Focus on Diversity and Culture feature) or on the belief that children should not be subjected to the side effects of the treatment. Parental refusal of treatment may also be based on the parents' understanding that

Focus on Diversity and Culture
Blood Transfusions

Jehovah's Witnesses believe it is a sin to consume blood, including receiving blood transfusions. Therefore parents who follow the Jehovah's Witness beliefs are likely to refuse blood transfusions for their child, even if that refusal will cause the death of the child. In cases such as these, where parents refuse a treatment that will help the child, healthcare providers must do everything possible to save the child's life while following the wishes of the parents. In extreme circumstances, legal intervention may be needed to overrule the parents' religious wishes in order to provide a life-sustaining treatment for the child.

their child will die in the near future and they want to avoid prolonging the child's suffering and to provide a peaceful death for the child (IOM, 2003).

A physician who feels that withholding a medical treatment based on parental preferences is detrimental to the child's well-being can request legal intervention to remove decision-making rights from the parent on the grounds of child neglect. If the life-saving treatment is urgent, the healthcare team will not be held liable for providing the treatment without a court order and over parental objections. Instead,

withholding a clearly beneficial treatment could lead to prosecution as a criminal offense, even if the decision to withhold treatment was based on parental wishes. In cases such as these, the nurse should provide adequate care for the child while seeking to resolve the conflict with the family.

CULTURAL AND RELIGIOUS CONSIDERATIONS Cultural differences greatly influence what type of care a client or family desires at the end-of-life. Some cultures have very different views on dying, including who should make healthcare decisions, where the client should die, who should be present at the time of death, and what should be done with the body after death. Cultural practices surrounding death also vary. Some cultures prefer that the family be involved in washing the body after death, that certain items be placed with the body, or that the body be taken home before the funeral (Guido, 2010d). Muslims in particular have very strict views about how the body should be treated and positioned after death. Each cultural situation presents a unique opportunity for nurses to communicate with the client and family to determine how to provide culturally competent care for that individual.

In spite of efforts to provide equal care to all clients, minority populations often receive a lower quality of care than Whites. Studies indicate that even after income, insurance status, and age are controlled for, minority populations are less

Evidence-Based Practice Improving the Quality of End-of-Life Care in the Pediatric Intensive Care Unit

Problem

Up to 85% of children's deaths in the pediatric or neonatal intensive care units (PICU, NICU) are results of limited treatment (withdrawing or withholding treatment, DNR orders) (Lee, Tieves, & Scanlon, 2010; Naghib et al., 2010; Weiner et al., 2011). The collaboration of healthcare providers and parents is vital to the perceived quality of care the child receives at the end of life.

Evidence

Healthcare professionals need to play seven major roles when helping parents make end-of-life care decisions for their children: *family supporter* (addresses emotional, spiritual, and informational needs of the family), *family advocate* (helps articulate the family's wishes to the healthcare team), *information giver* (provides parents with medical information and options), *general care coordinator* (facilitates interactions among professionals), *decision maker* (influences the plan of action), *end-of-life care coordinator* (organizes care directly before, during, and after death), and *point person* (develops unique trusting relationship with parents) (Michelson et al., 2013). Having a team of healthcare professionals working together with the parents to provide end-of-life care and help with decision making serves five general functions: facilitating understanding of a complex situation, clarifying and organizing important information and values, serving as a decision-making compass, communicating with others about complex topics, and justifying decisions (Ren-

jilian et al., 2013). When parents have a supportive team around them and share the decision-making process with the healthcare team, they tend to suffer less grief over time than parents who either had no involvement or had the sole burden of making decisions about the care of their child (Caeymaex et al., 2013).

Implications

At a time when anxious and grieving parents feel that everything is uncertain, adequate communication and support from the healthcare team can help reduce their stress and bring them relief. Regular communication from a single familiar individual about the child's condition, options for treatment, and the benefits and burdens of treatment will reduce the risk of receiving conflicting information and help parents make informed decisions that they won't regret years later.

Critical Thinking Application

1. What is the most important role for a nurse to play when caring for a family in which a newborn has only a few hours to live?

2. Suggest two methods of communication other than a face-to-face discussion that may be advantageous to parents with a terminally ill child.

3. Of the seven necessary roles played by healthcare providers, which role would you be most comfortable playing? Which would be least comfortable for you?

likely to receive common medical interventions at the end of life (Searight & Gafford, 2005). In addition, over 82% of all hospice care recipients are White/Caucasian (NHPCO, 2012). Minority populations are also much less likely to have advance directive documents prepared (Searight & Gafford, 2005).

Spiritual and religious beliefs also shape the context of death for many individuals. Clients may feel that death is a punishment, a release from an evil world, or God's will. Spiritual beliefs may cause individuals to feel regret or peace, and religious practices may bring comfort during their last days. Any requests for spiritual support should be quickly fulfilled and respected. If the nurse has conflicting beliefs and feels he cannot assist clients in their spiritual needs, he should find another member of the healthcare team or religious staff to fulfill that role for the client.

▶ COLLABORATION

Collaboration between healthcare providers is essential to providing quality care at the end of life. Nurses interact with clients most frequently, so they are responsible for communicating any changes in the client's condition that would warrant a change in the care plan. This responsibility may involve communicating with physicians about the need for medication changes, religious staff about the need for spiritual support, social workers or psychologists for emotional and social support, and family to determine which care plan to implement based on the clients' condition.

Pharmacologic Therapy

The most common symptom at the end of life is pain, so end-of-life care must include pain management. Other symptoms common at the end of life include anxiety, constipation, delirium, dyspnea, nausea, sleep disturbances, and loss of skin integrity (Guido, 2010a).

PAIN Pain medications are given at low doses initially to minimize discomfort, and then they are gradually increased to provide adequate pain relief 24 hours a day, 7 days a week. The dose of medication should allow the client to function as normally as possible and maintain the desired quality of life. Because the fear of addiction or tolerance is not an issue at the end of life, strong opioid agonists such as morphine should be given continuously for pain, as tolerated by the client, and fast-acting pain medications such as OxyFAST and fentanyl lozenges can be given for breakthrough pain. For clients in a hospital or long-term care facility who are confined to a bed, client-controlled analgesia through IV infusion is a typical method of controlling end-of-life pain.

OTHER SYMPTOMS Palliative care includes the relief of pain and other symptoms, including depression and anxiety, dyspnea, constipation, delirium, nausea, sleep disturbances, and loss of skin integrity. Each of these symptoms should be treated through classical methods as desired by the client and the family. For example, dyspnea can be treated with oxygen, constipation can be relieved with stool softeners and laxatives, and nausea can be treated with antiemetics. Relief of symptoms may also include disease-specific medications, such as digoxin

for congestive heart failure and dialysis for kidney failure. The goal of pharmacologic treatment is to give clients a high quality of life for the time they have left.

Nonpharmacologic Therapy

The use of nonpharmacologic therapies such as feeding tubes, mechanical respiration, and cardiopulmonary resuscitation is common at the end of life. Nurses must communicate clearly with clients and their families about the benefits and burdens of these therapies and discuss the desires of clients and their families to use these life-sustaining interventions.

FEEDING TUBES Clients at the end of life are often unable to take in food and fluids by mouth. Therefore, artificial nutrition and hydration (ANH) often is implemented via a feeding tube for nutrition and IV infusion of fluids for hydration. Withdrawing ANH for clients near death is an ethically controversial issue. Nutrition and hydration are essential to life, and clients, families, and clinicians are often reluctant to withdraw nutrition because they believe that starvation and dehydration are an agonizing way to die. However, clinical evidence suggests that clients who die after ANH withdrawal do not experience feelings of hunger and thirst, and they die peacefully (Slomka, 2003).

Whereas ANH may prolong life, it does not improve the quality of life or the chance of recovery in terminally ill clients (Guido, 2010b). In contrast, it may cause more discomfort for the client, including increasing the client's risk for esophageal perforation, infiltration of formula into the lung, infection, and edema. In clients unable to take in food or drink by mouth, oral care in the form of applying moisture to the mouth and lips is adequate to relieve dry mouth, regardless of the hydration status of the client (Slomka, 2003).

CARDIOPULMONARY RESUSCITATION Cardiopulmonary resuscitation is the provision of artificial ventilation and external cardiac compressions to an individual who demonstrates cardiac and respiratory arrest. Current CPR training incorporates application of an automated external defibrillator (AED) for detection and treatment of certain cardiac dysrhythmias. AEDs are designed to deliver an electrical impulse (shock) to the heart based upon the AED's analysis of the cardiac rhythm. Advanced techniques of CPR include endotracheal intubation, which allows for both manual and mechanical ventilation. In clients with medical conditions such as metastatic cancer, dementia, or renal disease, CPR is often ineffective (Alabi & Haines, 2009). Age is also a predictor of CPR success, clients age 65 or older having a continually decreasing chance of survival to discharge as they age. Clients who are admitted to a hospital from a long-term care facility have a lower chance of survival than any other group (Ehlenbach et al., 2009).

SAFETY ALERT

Clients with frail health are susceptible to damage during CPR, including rib fractures, heart contusions, airway and pulmonary complications, and liver and spleen lacerations.

Complementary and Alternative Therapy Massage and Simple Touch

A small study of 380 advanced cancer clients showed that massage and simple touch are effective in immediately reducing pain and improving mood. Massage had a greater effect on pain and mood than simple touch. However, sim- ple touch therapy (placing both hands on specific parts of the body) can easily be performed at home by a loved one and may be effective in providing symptom relief (Kutner et al., 2008).

For clients without a DNR order, CPR must be adminis- tered by default, even if it is not in the best interest of the cli- ent. Therefore, the desire of the client and family to have CPR performed should be an ongoing discussion as the client's condition changes. The nurse should remind clients and fami- lies that agreeing to a DNR order is not equivalent to con- demning the individual to die, and DNR orders can be reversed at any time.

◼ NURSING PROCESS

Nursing care for clients at the end of life must encompass all facets of the individual. Physical care includes pain and symptom management and hygiene care, emotional care incorporates therapeutic communication, spiritual care makes provisions for a clergy visit or religious rituals, and social care involves encouraging visits from family and friends.

Assessment

End-of-life nursing assessments include: assessing the client's pain level; determining the client's awareness of dying; assess- ing for signs of approaching death (see the Clinical Manifesta- tions and Therapies feature); asking the client and family about a living will, a healthcare proxy, and DNR status; and asking the client and family about any physical, emotional, or spiritual needs.

It may be helpful to interview clients or their families to find out more about the client in order to provide personal- ized means of comfort. Enabling personal preferences related to activities, daily routines, and spiritual practices can bring great comfort to clients and their family members. Encour- age close family members and friends to call or visit as often as possible, and encourage placement of pictures and reminders in the room where the clients can see or hold them.

State of Awareness

Glaser and Strauss (1965) developed an awareness-of-dying model that describes four contexts of clients' awareness of their condition: closed awareness, suspected awareness, mutual pre- tense awareness, and open awareness.

- *Closed awareness.* The client is unaware of his impending death even though the healthcare team and his family have the information. This may be the preference of the client's family or culture, or the healthcare team may believe it will help the client maintain hope. Closed awareness is difficult to maintain for an extended length of time.

Clinical Manifestations and Therapies End-of-Life Care

ETIOLOGY	CLINICAL MANIFESTATIONS	CLINICAL THERAPIES
Muscle control	◾ Decreased food and fluid intake resulting from difficulty swallowing and decreased gastrointestinal activity. ◾ Bladder and bowel incontinence ◾ Increased periods of sleep	◾ Provide nutrients and hydration artificially if requested by the healthcare team and/or client and family. ◾ Provide oral care regularly. ◾ Provide hygiene care as needed.
Circulation	◾ Cyanosis of extremities ◾ Decreased body temperature ◾ Slower and weaker pulse ◾ Decreased blood pressure	◾ Provide warm blankets. ◾ Gently massage to stimulate circulation.
Respiration	◾ Cheyne-Stokes breathing ◾ Noisy breathing (the "death rattle") ◾ Apnea	◾ Administer oxygen through nasal cannula if needed. ◾ Provide mechanical ventilation if needed and desired.
Sensation	◾ Blurred vision ◾ Impaired taste and smell ◾ Increased confusion and disorientation	◾ Provide palliative care. ◾ Maintain client safety

- **Suspected awareness.** No one directly tells the client about her condition, but she begins to suspect that she is near death. Suspected awareness may result in a lack of trust between the client and her healthcare providers.
- **Mutual pretense awareness.** The client, the family, and the healthcare team all know that the client's condition is terminal, but no one discusses it; perhaps, because of the discomfort discussing death or to protect the client or family from emotional distress. Mutual pretense gives the client privacy, but it also prevents the dying individual from confiding in anyone.
- **Open awareness.** The client, family, and healthcare team know about the client's impending death, and it is openly discussed as needed. Open awareness provides the client with the opportunity to participate in finalizing his affairs, and it gives nurses the opportunity to communicate freely with the client and assist in the grieving process.

Diagnosis

Nursing diagnoses that may be appropriate for clients nearing death include

- *Impaired Swallowing*
- *Functional Urinary Incontinence*
- *Bowel Incontinence*
- *Disturbed Sleep Pattern*
- *Risk for Ineffective Peripheral Tissue Perfusion*
- *Acute Confusion*
- *Death Anxiety*
- *Risk for Impaired Skin Integrity*
- *Acute Pain*

(NANDA-I © 2012)

Nursing diagnoses that may be appropriate for family members of clients near death include

- *Hopelessness*
- *Caregiver Role Strain*
- *Compromised Family Coping*
- *Grieving*
- *Decisional Conflict*

(NANDA-I © 2012)

Planning

The nurse collaborates with the client, family, and healthcare team to develop a written care plan based on the client's and family's preferences, the client's advance directives, the decisions of the healthcare proxy, and the client's physical, spiritual, and emotional needs. For clients near death, appropriate outcomes may include

- The nurse will maintain client comfort.
- The nurse will support family members and loved ones as they grieve.
- The nurse will maintain client hygiene.
- The nurse will prevent complications such as loss of skin integrity.

- The nurse will support and comfort the client to reduce fear and anxiety related to death.

Implementation

For the client who requires end-of-life care, interventions incorporate both physiological and psychosocial concerns. In addition to pain management, key interventions address death anxiety and compromised family coping.

Promote Emotional Well-Being

Death anxiety, or anxiety associated with impending death may stem from the client's concerns for self or for others. Likewise, anxiety may be experienced by those close to the one who is dying and who fear that their loved one will suffer. It can also affect healthcare workers who care for dying clients. Interventions to reduce death anxiety include methods to reduce suffering and loneliness, as those are two factors that contribute to death anxiety (Sherman et al., 2010). Implementing pain and symptom management and basic palliative care can reduce suffering. Encouraging family and friends to visit the client can reduce loneliness.

Clients may be encouraged to leave memories for the family. This activity is particularly important for parents who are leaving behind young children. Nurses may suggest leaving notes or videos for the child to open on special occasions such as birthdays and graduations. Nurses may also encourage the client to reminisce about her life, maintain relationships, continue spiritual practices, and complete legal documents (Lehto & Stein, 2009). Simple interventions might include taking time to listen, holding the client's hand, and providing information about the dying process. Providing spiritual support to the client is also vital in reducing death anxiety.

Promote Family Coping

The death of a loved one can be particularly difficult for the spouse, young children who have lost a parent, or parents who have lost a child. Alterations in family coping are especially common when the death is unexpected. Nurses can help families cope with impending or recent death by providing emotional support and information about the client's condition. Interventions may include referring the family to hospice, funeral homes, grief counseling, and support groups. If the family is caring for the client at home, hospice can assist the caregivers by providing respite services. Nurses should refer families with heavy financial burdens to financial counselors.

Evaluation

Client care is evaluated based on the following expected outcomes:

- Client's comfort is maintained throughout the dying process.
- Client is supported by nursing and/or family presence at time of death.
- Family members are informed and prepared for client's dying process.

NURSING CARE PLAN   The Client at the End of Life

ASSESSMENT	DIAGNOSES	PLANNING
Tom Crandall is a 75-year-old man with advanced Alzheimer disease. Three weeks ago, he became very agitated and began having difficulty swallowing. He was transferred from his assisted living facility to a hospital with a psychiatric geron-tology unit. Once transferred, Mr. Crandall experienced a steady decline in health, and he was transferred to the acute care area of the facility after experiencing a major stroke. He is arousable but seems unaware of his surroundings. He is currently receiving oxygen via a face mask and enteral nutrition. The treating physician has called his family and asked them to come to the hospital, advising them that Mr. Crandall is unlikely to live much longer.	■ *Chronic Confusion* ■ *Ineffective Breathing Pattern* ■ *Impaired Swallowing* ■ *Self-Care Deficit* (NANDA-I © 2012)	The nursing plan of care includes the following goals: ■ Maintain client comfort. ■ Support family grieving process. ■ Meet client's hygiene needs. ■ Provide calm and safe environment.

IMPLEMENTATION

The nurses caring for Mr. Crandall implement the following inter-ventions:

- Administer medications, nutrition, and oxygen as ordered.
- Bathe client and change linens as needed to maintain client comfort.

- Provide oral care every 2 hours.
- Encourage family to express feelings about client's terminal condition.
- Prepare family for signs and symptoms of impending death.

EVALUATION

Shortly after the family's arrival, Mr. Crandall died with family members surrounding him. Without regaining consciousness, he died peacefully with a gradual decrease in respirations and heart rate. His family members expressed appreciation that they had had the opportunity to tell him they loved him one last time.

CRITICAL THINKING

1. *What recommendation or request would you make of the provider regarding Mr. Crandall's tube feedings? Explain your answer.*
2. *Mr. Crandall's daughter asks if he will be placed on a mechanical ventilator to support his breathing. How would you respond to this question?*
3. *Would you recommend that Mr. Crandall or his healthcare proxy agree to a DNR order? Why or why not?*

REVIEW End-of-Life Care

RELATE Link the Concepts and Exemplars

Linking the exemplar of end-of-life care with the concept of family:

1. What is the priority nursing diagnosis for the family of the client with a terminal illness requiring end-of-life care?

2. What teaching points would you provide the family of a terminal client regarding end-of-life care?

Linking the exemplar of end-of-life care with the concept of grief and loss:

3. How can the nurse support the family's need to prepare for loss of a family member while meeting the client's need for end-of-life care?

4. Describe your plan of care for helping the family of a termi-nal school-age child provide end-of-life care for the child while meeting its need to grieve.

READY Go to Companion Skills Manual

REFER Go to Pearson Student Nursing Resources
nursing.pearsonhighered.com

- Additional review materials

REFLECT Case Study

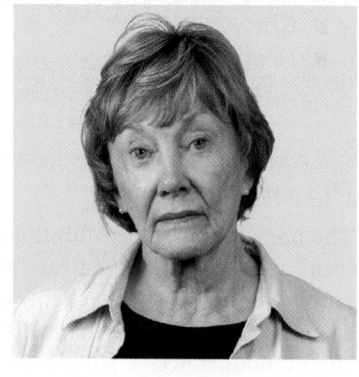

Pam Allen is a middle-aged woman who recently experienced a recurrence of colon cancer. She is dying. Ms. Allen and her husband have elected for her to stay at home. Ms. Allen's healthcare team includes a hospice nurse, a social worker, and her treating physician. Friends and church mem-bers have been bringing food for the Allen family. Mr. Allen has discussed his fears about Ms. Allen's death with the social worker.

Ms. Allen has had very little to eat or drink this week and is rarely urinating. The hospice nurse notices that she has abdominal fullness (ascites) due to the accumulation of fluid in the peritoneal cavity and appears more jaundiced. Her pain continues. She is agitated and has difficulty speaking. At today's visit, the hospice nurse records the following vital signs: T_O 98°F; P 99 bpm; R 30/min (shallow); BP 100/66 mmHg.

1. What is the priority of care for Ms. Allen on this visit?

2. Based on the current assessment, what information would you provide Mr. Allen?

3. Would you consider notifying the physician of your current findings? Why or why not?

EXEMPLAR 3.3 Fatigue

EXEMPLAR KEY TERMS

Acute fatigue, 185
Chronic fatigue, 185
Chronic fatigue syndrome, 187
Fatigue, 185

EXEMPLAR LEARNING OUTCOMES

After reading about this exemplar, you will be able to:

1. Describe the pathophysiology, etiology, clinical manifestations, and direct and indirect causes of fatigue.

2. Identify risk factors and prevention methods associated with fatigue.

3. Illustrate the nursing process in providing culturally sensitive care across the life span for individuals with fatigue.

4. Formulate priority nursing diagnoses appropriate for an individual with fatigue.

5. Summarize therapies used by interdisciplinary teams in the collaborative care of an individual with fatigue.

6. Plan evidence-based care for an individual with fatigue and his or her family in collaboration with other members of the healthcare team.

7. Evaluate expected outcomes for an individual with fatigue.

▶ OVERVIEW

Fatigue is characterized by tiredness, exhaustion, apathy, and lack of motivation. Fatigue is a subjective symptom that points to an underlying cause, such as illness, sleep deprivation, or intense physical or mental exertion. In addition, fatigue may occur because the individual feels the cultural pressure to perform a certain role, such as a mother who works outside the home and was up all night caring for a sick child or a husband who works three jobs to provide for his family. Fatigue usually is relieved by adequate sleep and rest and by treatment of the underlying condition causing the fatigue.

▶ PATHOPHYSIOLOGY AND ETIOLOGY

Fatigue is associated with a decrease in the body's energy reserves that affects all basic body functions, including muscle contraction, neural transmission, and cellular regulation. Any physical condition that requires extracellular energy, such as illness, infection, sleep deprivation, malnutrition, and overexertion, can deplete energy and cause fatigue. Excessive cognitive demands, such as studying for an exam or working long hours, can also deplete energy reserves.

Fatigue associated with a chronic illness may result from a dysregulation of corticotrophin-releasing hormone (CRH) and the hypothalamic-pituitary-adrenal (HPA) axis. The stress response, proinflammatory cytokines, and serotonin and norepinephrine neurotransmitter systems are all linked to CRH and HPA control, so any disruption in these systems can cause fatigue (Jong et al., 2010). Fatigue is also associated with mood disorders such as depression and anxiety, which are also linked to changes in neurotransmitter regulation.

Etiology

According to the U.S. National Library of Medicine (2011), fatigue has many causes, including

- Anemia (including iron deficiency anemia)
- Depression or grief
- Medications such as sedatives or antidepressants
- Persistent pain
- Sleep disorders such as insomnia, obstructive sleep apnea, and narcolepsy
- Hyper- or hypothyroidism
- Regular use of alcohol or illicit drugs
- Chronic diseases such as arthritis, cancer, diabetes, fibromyalgia, and liver or kidney disease

Acute fatigue is mental or physical exhaustion associated with a temporary change in life circumstances, such as acute illness, planning a major event (e.g., a wedding), studying for an exam, starting a new job, or recovering from a natural disaster. Acute fatigue is normally resolved by the completion of the event and a good night of sleep. In contrast, **chronic fatigue** is mental or physical exhaustion associated with a chronic condition or situation that is not resolved quickly, such as a chronic illness or medications taken for a chronic illness, a single mother working to care for her family, or poor lifestyle habits. Caregivers for family members with a chronic or terminal illness are also susceptible to developing chronic fatigue.

Risk Factors

In addition to an acute or chronic illness or condition, other risk factors for fatigue include lifestyle factors (e.g., alcohol abuse, excessive physical activity, inactivity, lack of sleep), medications (e.g., antihistamines, pain medications, heart medications), med-

Box 3–14   Fatigue and Women: Associated Conditions and Lifestyle Factors

- **Anemia.** Deficient iron intake can cause menstruating women to develop anemia and fatigue.
- **Poor nutrition.** Women who go on crash diets or consume high-fat, low-carbohydrate foods are subject to malnutrition, causing lethargy. When poor nutrition is coupled with water pills, hypokalemia can produce fatigue.
- **Endocrine gland function.** Hypothyroidism and loss of adrenal function can both lead to increased fatigue. Approximately 70% of the population with hypothyroidism are women.

- **Depression.** Clinical depression can cause fatigue, and more women than men are diagnosed with depression each year.
- **Heart failure.** Heart failure deprives tissues of oxygen and thus leads to fatigue.
- **Chronic fatigue syndrome.** Chronic fatigue syndrome is characterized by overwhelming fatigue that can last for months or years and doesn't get better with rest.
- **Liver disease.** Fatigue, along with nausea, vomiting, pain, and jaundice, is a symptom of liver disease.

Source: Based on Leider, P. (2009). *When women's fatigue signals danger.* Retrieved February 8, 2013, from http://www.cbsnews.com/2100-500165_162-1259346.html?pageNum=1; Wedro, B. (2013). Fatigue related diseases & conditions. Retrieved from http://www.medicinenet.com/fatigue/related-conditions/index.htm; CDC. (2013). Chronic fatigue syndrome (CFS). Retrieved from http://www.cdc.gov/cfs/

ical procedures (e.g., surgery, chemotherapy), and mood disorders (e.g., depression, grief, stress) (Mayo Clinic, 2010b).

Genetics also plays a role in fatigue. Individuals with alterations in the HPA axis and in neurotransmitter signaling are more susceptible to fatigue (Smith et al., 2006). Women also tend to be highly susceptible to fatigue (**Box 3–14 ●**).

Prevention

Fatigue resulting from lifestyle choices can be prevented by a balanced diet, daily exercise (see the Evidence-Based Practice feature), good sleep hygiene (see the Client Teaching feature), and stress reduction. Eating several small meals each day instead of fewer large meals helps prevent fatigue. Good hydration is also part of a balanced diet (six to eight 8-oz. glasses of water daily). Healthy diets limit refined sugar and fried and processed foods. In addition, avoiding caffeine, alcohol, and tobacco products can also help prevent fatigue.

Practicing good coping techniques is vital to preventing stress-related fatigue. Stressful situations that contribute to fatigue should be identified, and clients should determine ways to reduce or remove those situations. If the cause of stress cannot be removed, relaxation techniques such as deep breathing, meditation, or massage may help reduce feelings of stress. Counseling sessions may also help clients cope with stress.

▶ CLINICAL MANIFESTATIONS

The most common symptoms associated with fatigue are drowsiness, exhaustion, and lack of motivation. Fatigue is also associated with a variety of physical signs and symptoms, including lethargy, muscle weakness, palpitations, dizziness, dyspnea upon mild exertion, loss of appetite, slow movements, and blurry vision. Neurological symptoms of fatigue include

Evidence-Based Practice   Exercise and Fatigue

Problem

Americans often lead a sedentary lifestyle, spending much of their time at a desk or watching TV. This lifestyle can lead to fatigue and other health complications. In addition, many chronic health problems and the treatments they require cause fatigue.

Evidence

In a study of college students who reported persistent fatigue, low-intensity exercise correlated with decreased fatigue after 3–6 weeks of exercise (Dishman et al., 2010). Similarly, mild exercise for 3 weeks reduced mental and physical fatigue in individuals with persistent cancer-related fatigue (Dimeo et al., 2008). Post-therapy mild to moderate exercise has been shown to reduce fatigue in multiple types of cancer, including prostate cancer, breast cancer, and other solid tumors (Cramp & Byron-Daniel, 2012). Exercise also reduces fatigue in other chronic conditions such as obstructive sleep apnea (Kline et al., 2012), multiple sclerosis (Kargarfard et al., 2012; Huisinga, Filipi, & Stergiou, 2011), and fibromyalgia (Hauser et al., 2010). Types of exercise that can improve fatigue include cycling (Dishman et al., 2010), walking (Dimeo et al., 2008), using an elliptical (Huisinga et al., 2011), and aquatic exercises (Cantarero-Villanueva et al., 2013; (Kargarfard et al., 2012).

Implications

Clients who report persistent fatigue should be encouraged to begin a physician-approved mild to moderate exercise regimen. Higher intensity exercise does not appear to produce a greater reduction in fatigue, so clients should be instructed to avoid intense workouts that may increase feelings of fatigue. Specifically, conflicting results of exercise therapy are seen in clients with chronic fatigue syndrome (Twisk & Maes, 2009; White et al., 2011), so these individuals should use exercise therapy with caution.

Critical Thinking Application

1. Physiologically, why does a sedentary lifestyle contribute to fatigue? How does mild activity reverse these physiological changes?
2. For what conditions (other than chronic fatigue syndrome) may an exercise program be contraindicated?
3. Develop a mild exercise program for a client who has recently completed chemotherapy for breast cancer and is experiencing cancer-related fatigue.

Client Teaching   Sleep Hygiene

Fatigue is often the result of inadequate sleep. Nurses should promote and teach good sleep hygiene to all clients with fatigue, sleep–rest disorders, and acute and chronic illnesses that could cause fatigue. Good sleep hygiene includes

- Practicing bedtime rituals that are calming, such as reading, taking a bath, praying, and listening to music.
- Maintaining a restful environment that is free of distractions (e.g., lights and noise), is a comfortable temperature, and has appropriate ventilation.
- Wearing loose-fitting sleepwear.
- Using clean and dry linens.
- Sleeping in a position that aids in muscle relaxation and supports injured areas.

- Scheduling medications to promote sleep (i.e., taking medications that cause alertness in the morning and medications that cause drowsiness at night).
- Avoiding naps during the day.
- Avoiding stimulants such as caffeine and alcohol, especially in the evening; also avoiding heavy meals late in the evening.
- Using the bed for sleep, not other activities such as watching TV.
- Setting consistent times for sleeping and waking, and allowing adequate hours for sleep.
- Exercising in the morning or afternoon rather than the evening.

difficulty concentrating, impaired decision-making abilities, confusion, impaired coordination, and slowed reflexes. In addition, fatigue can be characterized by sleep disturbances, loss of interest in previously pleasurable activities, and a depressed mood.

SAFETY ALERT

Studies have shown that taking short breaks can reduce fatigue and improve performance. Nurses should be vigilant about taking adequate breaks (i.e., 10 minutes every 2 hours, 30 minutes for meals, free of client care responsibilities) to prevent fatigue and errors that may occur because of fatigue (Rogers, 2008).

Chronic fatigue syndrome, also called *myalgic encephalomyelitis*, occurs when an individual experiences severe tiredness that lasts more than 6 months, is not caused by a primary condition (e.g., drug dependence, immune disorders, heart disease, depression, cancer, sleep disorders), and is not relieved by stress reduction. In addition to these conditions, chronic fatigue syndrome is diagnosed only if it is accompanied by at least four of the following symptoms: malaise lasting longer than 24 hours after exercise, feeling unrefreshed after adequate sleep, forgetfulness, confusion, inability to concentrate, joint pain with no swelling, headaches not previously experienced, irritability, mild fever, muscle aches, muscle weakness, sore throat, and sore lymph nodes.

Lifespan and Cultural Considerations

Fatigue in children is generally the result of stress, illness, insufficient sleep, or improper nutrition. Infections and allergies are two common illnesses in children that can cause fatigue, but fatigue can also be a sign of anemia, diabetes, thyroid disorders, depression, sleep apnea, or leukemia. If proper diet and adequate sleep do not correct fatigue in children, nurses should encourage parents to keep a journal of the child's sleep patterns, food intake, and activities that instigate fatigue.

This journal may help a physician diagnose the underlying condition causing fatigue.

Fatigue is extremely common in older adults, 43% of older adults reporting feeling tired most of the time (Hardy & Studenski, 2010). Fatigue tends to increase with age, especially in clients with a chronic illness (Butt et al., 2010). In addition, fatigue is associated with worse health, decreased physical activity, functional decline, and loss of independence. Increased fatigue at baseline is also associated with an increased mortality rate in older adults (Hardy & Studenski, 2008; Moreh, Jacobs, & Stessman, 2010). Therefore, assessment and treatment of fatigue are essential for older adults, especially those with one or more chronic conditions.

Fatigue is also a common occurrence during pregnancy. The body uses large amounts of energy to build the placenta in the first trimester and to support rapid fetal growth in the third trimester. Hormonal changes can also contribute to pregnancy fatigue. In addition, as the baby grows, it increases the mother's physical stress and disrupts sleep, adding to the feelings of fatigue. Pregnant women should be encouraged to rest when they feel tired, allow others to help with everyday tasks, cut out unnecessary commitments, sleep more, consume a healthy diet, take in adequate water, and get regular exercise. If fatigue persists, it may be a sign of iron-deficiency anemia. Expectant mothers should be encouraged to eat more protein, including lean meats and beans, and to take an iron supplement. Vitamin C increases iron absorption, so pregnant women should be encouraged to eat fruits and vegetables that contain high amounts of vitamin C, including citrus fruits, melons, strawberries, tomatoes, broccoli, potatoes, and spinach.

In a country characterized by a melting pot of cultures, another common type of fatigue is culture fatigue or culture shock. Whether moving from a foreign country, a different city within the United States, or back home after being away, changing cultures demands an adjustment period that can cause fatigue. Differences between cultures may include changes in population size, language, nonverbal communication, religions, transportation systems, food, absence of family and friends, and climate. Small changes build over time to cause physical and mental fatigue, which should decrease the

Clinical Manifestations and Therapies **Fatigue**

ETIOLOGY	CLINICAL MANIFESTATION	CLINICAL THERAPIES
Iron-deficiency anemia	■ Mild anemia may be asymptomatic. ■ Moderate anemia may cause fatigue, irritability, headaches, and difficulty concentrating. ■ Severe anemia may cause pale skin, brittle nails, shortness of breath, and light-headedness upon standing.	■ Iron supplements ■ Erythropoietin ■ Monitoring hemoglobin and hematocrit ■ Nutrition counseling
Hypothyroidism	■ Increased sensitivity to cold ■ Hoarseness ■ Unexplained weight gain ■ Muscle weakness/tenderness ■ Joint stiffness ■ Depression	■ Thyroid hormone supplementation (e.g., levothyroxine)
Infection	■ Loss of appetite ■ Fever ■ Coughing ■ Body aches ■ Nausea and vomiting ■ Pain	■ Antiviral agents ■ Antibacterial drugs ■ Antitubercular agents ■ Antifungals

longer the individual lives within the new culture. Nurses should encourage individuals with cultural fatigue to maintain a positive attitude, learn as much as possible about the new culture, and find a friend who can help them adjust to the new culture.

▶ COLLABORATION

Acute fatigue is usually resolved with sufficient sleep and healing of the cause of fatigue. Fatigue associated with an illness is more complicated and requires the support of a healthcare team. For example, fatigue related to a mood disorder such as depression or anxiety may require both pharmacologic treatment and counseling. Some clients may need extensive testing to determine the underlying cause of the fatigue.

Diagnostic Tests

Diagnostic tests are often ordered to find the underlying cause of fatigue. Typical causes of fatigue include anemia; changes in endocrine, kidney, or liver function; and infection. Therefore, initial diagnostic tests may focus on these physiological areas. A sleep study, or polysomnography, may also be ordered to determine if a sleep disorder is the cause of fatigue.

Surgery

If fatigue is related to a change in thyroid function, specifically hyperthyroidism or thyroid cancer, surgery may be scheduled to remove part or all of the thyroid. Fatigue as a sign of cancer may prompt a biopsy and subsequent surgical removal of a solid tumor.

Pharmacologic Therapy

Pharmacologic therapy depends on the cause of fatigue. For example, clients with fatigue related to iron-deficiency anemia should receive iron supplements and/or erythropoietin (e.g., Procrit, Epogen) to stimulate the production of hemoglobin and red blood cells. To be effective, the pharmacologic therapy must be tailored to the client's specific condition.

Nonpharmacologic Therapy

Nonpharmacologic therapies for fatigue include good sleep hygiene, mild to moderate exercise, and cognitive-behavioral therapy. Graded exercise programs may be especially beneficial by helping the client gradually build stamina for exercise. Suggesting activities the client enjoys promotes adherence to the exercise program. Cognitive-behavioral therapy focuses on the client's thoughts and their relationship to the presenting problem. It helps clients identify stressors that contribute to symptoms and to take personal responsibility for change. Nurses can assist clients in minimizing fatigue by determining the client's best time of day and scheduling more challenging activities during that time.

Complementary and Alternative Therapy **Fatigue**

Complementary and alternative therapies for fatigue include acupuncture, massage, and relaxation techniques. Herbal and dietary supplements may include ginseng, NADH, and L-carnitine. However, no complementary or alternative therapy is consistently supported by clinical studies.

NURSING PROCESS

An important component in treating a client with fatigue is determining the underlying cause. Thorough assessment of the client's symptoms, along with measures to promote rest, are priority areas of focus.

Assessment

A nursing assessment for clients with fatigue includes both a health history and a physical examination. The health history should include questions about the duration, timing, and quality of the fatigue; how the fatigue affects activities of daily living and relationships with family members; diet, sleep, and exercise habits; any medications or medical conditions that may contribute to fatigue; and cognitive effects associated with fatigue.

Physical assessment includes assessment of the client's vital signs, mobility, hydration, and muscle strength. Fever and changes in pulse rate may indicate infection or stress. Dyspnea upon exertion is often a sign of fatigue, and decreased muscle strength can be a sign of muscular or nervous system defects. In addition, poor hydration as indicated by poor skin turgor is a source of fatigue. Changes in skin tone, including jaundice and cyanosis, may indicate liver, cardiac, or pulmonary disease.

Diagnosis

Nursing diagnoses related to fatigue may include

- *Insomnia*
- *Sleep Deprivation*
- *Fatigue*
- *Activity Intolerance*
- *Readiness for Enhanced Coping*
- *Stress Overload*

(NANDA-I © 2012)

Clients with chronic fatigue syndrome may have more severe symptoms that indicate other nursing diagnoses, such as

- *Self-Neglect*
- *Ineffective Coping*

(NANDA-I © 2012)

Planning

A plan of care for clients with fatigue may include the following outcomes:

- The client will verbalize an understanding and practice of good sleep hygiene.
- The client will verbalize feelings of increased energy.

- The client will indicate an increased ability to perform activities of daily living.
- The client will participate in a mild exercise program.
- The client will experience increased motivation.
- The client will explain the relationship of fatigue to a disease process and activity level.

It is important to incorporate the client's goals and preferences into the plan of care. Providing client-centered care increases the likelihood that the client will succeed in following the therapeutic regimen.

Implementation

When implementing care to reduce fatigue, it is important to consider the client's cultural and developmental needs regarding sleep rituals. Fatigue is a subjective symptom, so careful attention must be given to clients' assessment of how they are feeling. Interventions may include client teaching related to the importance of adequate rest and sleep, structuring activities to coincide with the client's peak energy level, and assisting the client with self-care activities.

Promote Effective Coping

For clients with chronic conditions, inadequate coping mechanisms may contribute to prolonged feelings of fatigue. Several interventions may enhance clients' ability to cope:

- Assess clients' normal methods of coping and social support network to identify more effective methods of coping.
- Establish rapport with clients' families and significant others and encourage them to participate in establishing the plan of care.
- Encourage clients to be involved in the decision-making process to increase their feelings of self-worth.
- Facilitate the process of setting short-term and long-term goals. Short-term goals provide a sense of accomplishment, and long-term goals help clients adhere to the suggested therapy.

Evaluation

Evaluate clients with fatigue periodically to determine if the medical and nursing interventions are effective. Evaluations should include both subjective and objective data to reveal if the client goals are being met. If the interventions are ineffective, modify the therapy by finding more effective therapies. Further diagnostic tests may also be needed to determine if additional physiological factors are contributing to fatigue.

REVIEW Fatigue

RELATE Link the Concepts and Exemplars

Linking the exemplar of fatigue with the concept of infection:

1. How does infection and/or inflammation put an individual at risk for fatigue?
2. Is fatigue more likely to be acute or chronic as the result of infection?

Linking the exemplar of fatigue with the concept of oxygenation:

3. How does uncontrolled asthma put clients at risk for fatigue?
4. What strategies could asthmatic clients use to decrease their risk for fatigue?

READY Go to Companion Skills Manual

REFER Go to Pearson Student Nursing Resources
nursing.pearsonhighered.com
- Additional review materials

REFLECT Case Study

Mr. Joe Harmon is an 87-year-old Caucasian man. He is a World War II veteran who suffered a massive anteroseptal myocardial infarction (MI) at the age of 57. His MI was secondary to asbestosis. Since the age of 57, he has been hospitalized three times for chronic obstructive pulmonary disease (COPD) and conges-tive heart failure (CHF). His skin color is ruddy, his conjunctiva is pale pink, he walks with a stooped posture, and he experiences dyspnea after walking 100 feet. He states that he feels "OK, just tired most of the time."

1. When obtaining Mr. Harmon's vital signs, what readings would you anticipate?
2. What diagnostic tests do you anticipate might be useful to determine the cause of Mr. Harmon's fatigue?
3. What nursing diagnoses would be appropriate for Mr. Harmon's plan of care?
4. Develop a teaching plan to discuss with Mr. Harmon and his wife.

EXEMPLAR 3.4   Fibromyalgia

EXEMPLAR KEY TERMS
Fibromyalgia, 190
Tender points, 190

EXEMPLAR LEARNING OUTCOMES
After reading about this exemplar, you will be able to:

1. Describe the pathophysiology, etiology, clinical manifesta-tions, and direct and indirect causes of fibromyalgia.
2. Identify risk factors and prevention methods associated with fibromyalgia.
3. Illustrate the nursing process in providing culturally compe-tent care across the life span for individuals with fibromyalgia.
4. Formulate priority nursing diagnoses appropriate for an indi-vidual with fibromyalgia.
5. Summarize therapies used by interdisciplinary teams in the collaborative care of an individual with fibromyalgia.
6. Plan evidence-based care for an individual with fibromyalgia and his or her family in collaboration with other members of the healthcare team.
7. Evaluate expected outcomes for an individual with fibromyalgia.

▶ OVERVIEW

Fibromyalgia is a chronic syndrome characterized by wide-spread musculoskeletal pain, stiffness, fatigue, sleep distur-bances, and difficulty concentrating. Pain usually occurs in specific **tender points** that occur in the neck, spine, shoulders, hips, elbows, and knees. Fibromyalgia affects approximately 10 million Americans, about 75%–90% of whom are women, although men and children can also develop fibromyalgia. Diagnosis of fibromyalgia usually occurs between ages 20 and 50, and the incidence rises with age (National Fibromyalgia Association, n.d.).

▶ PATHOPHYSIOLOGY AND ETIOLOGY

Fibromyalgia is a disorder of pain processing. Pain associated with fibromyalgia results from central amplification of pain sig-nals, including spontaneous nerve activity, enlarged receptive fields, and abnormal levels of neurotransmitters. Hyperalgesia, or an increased response to painful stimuli, is mediated by *N*-methyl-D-aspartate receptors in the dorsal horn. Clients with fibromyalgia also experience *allodynia*, or sensitivity to stimuli that are not normally painful. Descending inhibitory pain pathways are inhibited in fibromyalgia, so that the central amplification is exacerbated (Bellato et al., 2012; Clauw, Arnold, & McCarberg, 2011). Sleep disturbances result from changes in the HPA axis, particularly elevated cortisol levels in the eve-ning. The fourth stage of sleep is the most disrupted as a result of deficiencies in growth hormone and insulin-like growth factor-1 (Bellato et al., 2012; Bradley, 2009).

Etiology

The exact cause of fibromyalgia is unknown; over 70% of cli-ents with fibromyalgia have no precipitating factor for the dis-ease. However, infections such as hepatitis C virus (HCV), HIV, Coxsackie B, and parvovirus may instigate fibromyalgia. Physical trauma (e.g., acute illness, surgery, motor vehicle acci-dents), psychosocial stressors (e.g., chronic stress, abuse), vac-cinations, and chemical substances can all be causative factors (Bellato et al., 2012; Bradley, 2009).

Risk Factors

The overwhelming majority of individuals with fibromyalgia are middle-aged females, so being a female between the ages of 20 and 50 is considered a risk factor for fibromyalgia. Other risk factors include a family history of fibromyalgia, having a psy-chiatric disorder such as attention deficit/hyperactivity disorder (ADHD) or depression, or having a medical disorder such as irritable bowel syndrome or rheumatoid arthritis. Genetic abnormalities may also predispose individuals to fibromyalgia, including polymorphisms in the *5-HTT* and *SCN9A* genes (Bradley, 2009; Vargas-Alarcon et al., 2012).

Prevention

There is no known way to prevent fibromyalgia. However, in the absence of triggering factors and comorbid conditions, maintaining a healthy lifestyle is the best way to decrease the risk of developing fibromyalgia. In addition, prompt diagnosis and treatment of fibromyalgia symptoms can reduce flare-ups and help manage the widespread pain and fatigue characteristic of fibromyalgia.

▶ CLINICAL MANIFESTATIONS

The primary clinical symptoms associated with fibromyalgia are widespread pain and fatigue. Widespread pain is defined as pain above and below the waist and on the right and left sides of the body. Pain is often localized to 18 tender points located in the neck, spine, shoulders, hips, elbows, and knees (**Figure 3–8 ●**). Pain is typically described as deep, gnawing, stabbing, or burning, and it is not the result of inflammation or damage. Clients may also exhibit enhanced sensitivity to heat, cold, and pressure (Bradley, 2009). Pain and stiffness are often worse in the morning or after excessive physical activity.

Fatigue is likely the result of sleep disturbances, especially insomnia. Other sleep disturbances may include nonrestorative sleep, early morning awakening, and poor quality of sleep (Bradley, 2009). Systemic symptoms include mood disorders and cognitive dysfunction (often called *fibro fog*). Other symptoms associated with fibromyalgia include headaches, numbness in the hands and feet, irritable bowel syndrome, restless leg syndrome, and painful menstrual periods.

Lifespan and Cultural Considerations

Although fibromyalgia is most common in middle-aged women, children and adolescents may develop a form of fibromyalgia called *juvenile primary fibromyalgia syndrome* (JPFS). JPFS is most commonly diagnosed in girls between the ages of 13 and 15. Triggers and symptoms of JPFS are similar to those of adult fibromyalgia. Although the majority of adolescents with JPFS continue to experience symptoms into their adult years, approximately 35%–40% of children and adolescents with JPFS no longer report widespread pain within 3–4 years of diagnosis, and a minority (<20%) report being symptom-free (Kashikar-Zuck et al., 2010).

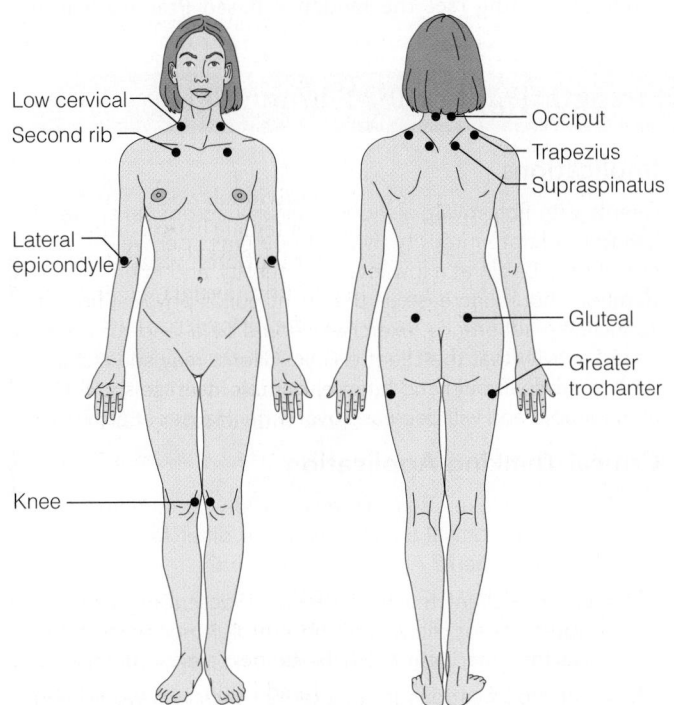

Low cervical
Second rib
Occiput
Trapezius
Supraspinatus
Lateral epicondyle
Gluteal
Greater trochanter
Knee

Figure 3–8 ● Location of 18 paired "tender points" in fibromyalgia.

▶ COLLABORATION

Fibromyalgia is difficult to treat. A combination of pharmacologic and nonpharmacologic therapies is needed to control pain and fatigue. Individuals with fibromyalgia are often referred to a rheumatologist for specialty care. In addition, treatment must address comorbidities such as depression, cognitive impairments, and irritable bowel syndrome.

The underlying cause of fibromyalgia is often unknown, so treatment directed at eliminating the source of pain is limited. A therapy, or group of therapies, that work for one client may not be effective for another client. Therefore consistent evaluation of the client's symptoms and the effectiveness of therapy and revision of the care plan are necessary to provide maximal relief from pain and fatigue associated with fibromyalgia. Clients who are having difficulty finding an effective treatment should be encouraged to keep trying new therapies until they find a treatment that allows them to cope with the disease and maintain an active lifestyle.

Diagnostic Tests

Diagnosis of fibromyalgia is based on criteria set by the American College of Rheumatology. The initial criteria, defined in 1990, stated that the client must have widespread pain in all four quadrants of the body and a painful response to pressure on 11 of 18 tender points (Wolfe et al., 1990). The 2010 updated criteria (**Box 3–15 ●**) define fibromyalgia as a widespread pain index of 7 or more, a symptom severity scale score of 5 or more, the presence of symptoms for at least 3 months, and the absence of a disorder that would otherwise explain the pain (Wolfe et al., 2010).

All laboratory and diagnostic tests are negative for individuals with fibromyalgia. Therefore clients with positive blood tests, abnormal hormone levels, and abnormal imaging scans may have another underlying cause for their pain and fatigue. Symptoms associated with fibromyalgia are common to many diseases. So similar diseases, such as rheumatoid arthritis and hypothyroidism, should be ruled out before fibromyalgia is diagnosed.

Pharmacologic Therapy

Three drugs have been approved by the FDA for the treatment of fibromyalgia: duloxetine (Cymbalta), milnacipran (Savella), and pregabalin (Lyrica). Duloxetine and milnacipran are selective serotonin and norepinephrine reuptake inhibitors (SSNRIs). They are given orally at low doses initially. The drug dosage can then be increased to manage the client's comfort. Common side effects of the drugs are nausea, dry mouth, constipation, dizziness, hot flashes, and insomnia. Both duloxetine and milnacipran interact with many drugs, so carefully survey the client's medications before initiating therapy (Wilson, Shannon, & Shields, 2013). Duloxetine is recommended for clients with significant depression, whereas milnacipran is recommended for clients with significant fatigue or cognitive dysfunction (Bellato et al., 2012).

Pregabalin is a GABA analog with anticonvulsant, analgesic, and anxiolytic properties. To begin therapy, it is given orally at a low dose; the dose can be titrated to a maximum dosage of 450 mg/day. Common side effects are ataxia, dizziness, somnolence, weight gain, and blurry vision (Wilson et al., 2013).

Other pharmacologic therapies for fibromyalgia pain are acetaminophen and NSAIDs. Tricyclic antidepressants such

Box 3–15 2010 Fibromyalgia Diagnostic Criteria

A client who exhibits the following three conditions satisfies the diagnostic criteria for fibromyalgia:

1. Widespread pain index (WPI) ≥7 and symptom severity (SS) scale score ≥5, or WPI 3–6 and SS scale score ≥9
2. Symptoms have been present at a similar level for at least 3 months
3. The absence of a disorder that would otherwise explain the pain.

ASCERTAINMENT

1. WPI: Note the number areas in which the client has had pain over the last week. In how many areas has the client had pain? Score will be between 0 and 19.

Shoulder girdle, left or right	Jaw, left or right
Upper arm, left or right	Chest
Lower arm, left or right	Abdomen
Hip (buttock, trochanter), left or right	Upper or Lower back
Upper leg, left or right	Neck
Lower leg, left or right	

2. SS scale score:

Fatigue
Waking unrefreshed
Cognitive symptoms

For each of the 3 symptoms above, indicate the level of severity over the past week using the following scale:

0 = no problem
1 = slight or mild problems, generally mild or intermittent
2 = moderate, considerable problems, often present and/or at a moderate level
3 = severe: pervasive, continuous, life-disturbing problems

Considering somatic symptoms in general, indicate whether the client has*

0 = no symptoms
1 = few symptoms
2 = a moderate number of symptoms
3 = a great many symptoms

The SS scale score is the sum of severity of the three symptoms (fatigue, waking unrefreshed, and cognitive symptoms) plus the extent (severity) of somatic symptoms in general. The final score is between 0 and 12.

*Somatic symptoms that might be considered: muscle pain, irritable bowel syndrome, fatigue/tiredness, thinking or remembering problem, muscle weakness, headache, pain/cramps in the abdomen, numbness/tingling, dizziness, insomnia, depression, constipation, pain in the upper abdomen, nausea, nervousness, chest pain, blurred vision, fever, diarrhea, dry mouth, itching, wheezing, Raynaud phenomenon, hives/welts, ringing in the ears, vomiting, heartburn, oral ulcers, loss of/change in taste, seizures, dry eyes, shortness of breath, loss of appetite, rash, sun sensitivity, hearing difficulties, easy bruising, hair loss, frequent urination, and bladder spasms.

Source: Wolfe, F., Clauw, D. J., Fitzcharles, M-A., Goldenberg, D. L., Katz, R. S., Mease, P., et al. (2010). The American College of Rheumatology preliminary diagnostic criteria for fibromyalgia and measurement of symptom severity. *Arthritis Care and Research, 62*(5), 600–610. doi:10.1002/acr.20140

as amitriptyline have also been used with some success, although SSNRIs are more commonly used. Tramadol may also be effective in providing pain and sleep relief (Bellato et al., 2012).

Nonpharmacologic Therapy

The two primary nonpharmacologic therapies linked to successful treatment of fibromyalgia are aerobic exercise and strength training (see the Evidence-Based Practice feature).

Evidence-Based Practice   Aerobic Exercise and Strength Training for Fibromyalgia

Problem

Clients with fibromyalgia experience a decrease in physical activity because of pain and fatigue. The combined effects of pain, fatigue, and activity intolerance dramatically reduce clients' quality of life.

Evidence

Aerobic exercise and strength training are effective at reducing pain, fatigue, and depression and increasing health-related quality of life and physical fitness in clients with fibromyalgia (Hauser et al., 2010). Aerobic training improves peak oxygen uptake and decreases pain intensity and fatigue (Dinler et al., 2009; Hooten et al., 2012), and strength training decreased the number of tender points, myalgic score, and Fibromyalgia Impact Questionnaire score (Kingsley, McMillan, & Figueroa, 2010). Land-based and water-based exercises have a similar effect in reducing fibromyalgia symptoms. The intensity of the exercise should be low to moderate (50%–80% of maximum recommended heart rate for age group). In addition, clients should exercise two or three times per week to see clinical benefits (Hauser et al., 2010).

Implications

Clients with fibromyalgia should perform aerobic exercise of low to moderate intensity two or three times per week. Exercise should begin at a low level of intensity, and intensity and duration should increase as the client builds physical fitness. To increase adherence, exercises should be a land- or water-based activity that the client enjoys. Clients may see a short-term increase in pain and fatigue, but this increase should be manageable and will decrease over time (Hauser et al., 2010).

Critical Thinking Application

1. Develop an exercise regimen for a 38-year-old female client with fibromyalgia. How would it differ for a 15-year-old female client? A client with asthma?

2. Prepare a client teaching brochure describing exercise suggestions for clients with fibromyalgia, including references for locations at which the exercise can be performed.

3. What modifications in an exercise program would you recommend to a client who complains of increased joint stiffness after exercise?

Clinical Manifestations and Therapies **Fibromyalgia**

ETIOLOGY	CLINICAL MANIFESTATIONS	CLINICAL THERAPIES
Pain	■ WPI ≥7 and SS scale score ≥5, or WPI 3–6 and SS scale score ≥9 ■ Pain lasting longer than 3 months ■ Pain not associated with any other condition	■ Duloxetine ■ Milnacipran ■ Pregabalin ■ NSAIDs ■ Aerobic exercise ■ Strength training ■ Massage
Fatigue	■ Chronic fatigue ■ Acute fatigue associated with increased activity	■ Milnacipran ■ Good sleep hygiene ■ Relaxation therapy ■ Tai chi
Sleep disruptions	■ Insomnia ■ Restless leg syndrome ■ Nonrestorative sleep ■ Early morning awakening ■ Poor quality of sleep	■ Duloxetine ■ Milnacipran ■ Pregabalin ■ Tramadol ■ Good sleep hygiene

Aquatic exercises may be helpful, and tai chi has been shown to improve symptoms, physical function, quality of sleep, self-efficacy, and mobility. Cognitive-behavioral therapy and relaxation therapy produce a moderate effect in short-term pain reduction and sleep problems compared to other psychological treatments (Bellato et al., 2012). According to the National Center for Complementary and Alternative Medicine, there is insufficient research to support the use of "natural" products, including dietary supplements (NCCAM, 2012).

■ NURSING PROCESS

The primary goals of fibromyalgia treatment are to reduce pain, increase restorative sleep, and improve physical function. Clients require a great deal of support as they seek a diagnosis because fibromyalgia is often diagnosed only after other diagnoses are ruled out.

Assessment

A nursing assessment for clients with symptoms of fibromyalgia includes a client history and a physical assessment. Base the client history on the 2010 criteria shown in Box 3–15 for the diagnosis of fibromyalgia. Also assess the family's history of fibromyalgia and other rheumatic disorders. A physical assessment should include testing the trigger points associated with the widespread pain index.

Diagnosis

Nursing diagnoses that may be appropriate for inclusion in the plan of care for the client with fibromyalgia include

- *Insomnia*
- *Readiness for Enhanced Sleep*
- *Fatigue*

- *Activity Intolerance*
- *Readiness for Enhanced Knowledge*
- *Hopelessness*
- *Anxiety*
- *Ineffective Coping*
- *Chronic Pain*

(NANDA-I © 2012)

Planning

Possible goals of the nursing care plan are

- Client will report decreased pain.
- Client will report fewer sleep disturbances.
- Client will improve activity tolerance.
- Client's score on a symptom severity scale will be less than 5.

Implementation

Nursing interventions for fibromyalgia pertain to pain management, fatigue reduction, and increased activity tolerance. Interventions related to pain management include education about proper use of medications and nonpharmacologic methods to reduce pain, including massage, exercise, distractions, and family support. Interventions to reduce fatigue include encouraging enjoyable but quiet activities such as reading, listening to music, and participating in hobbies. Nurses should also teach clients good sleep hygiene to increase their restorative sleep and to reduce their fatigue. Interventions related to activity intolerance include encouraging the client to alternate periods of activity with periods of rest, delegating responsibilities to other members of the family, and encouraging a mild exercise program to build strength and physical fitness. Nursing interventions should also provide information on coping mechanisms for living with fibromyalgia (see Client Teaching feature).

Client Teaching Coping With Fibromyalgia

Clients often suffer from ineffective coping when diagnosed with fibromyalgia, possibly related to the unknown cause of fibromyalgia, the lack of public knowledge about fibromyalgia, and the lack of outward signs of pain and fatigue. Nurses are instrumental in teaching fibromyalgia clients how to cope with their syndrome. In teaching coping techniques,

- Validate clients' perception of their symptoms.
- Teach clients about the disease, and answer questions.
- Remind clients that the disease is nonprogressive and not life-threatening.
- Emphasize the importance of a positive attitude.
- Recommend a mild to moderate exercise program, or refer clients to a personal trainer.

- Teach clients basic sleep hygiene methods.
- Encourage clients to see a specialist in fibromyalgia.
- Explain the importance of self-efficacy, or the belief that clients can influence the course of the disease by specific behavior that meets health-related goals.
- Identify stressors that make pain and fatigue worse; then develop strategies to avoid those stressors or to minimize symptoms when those stressors occur. Such strategies include distractions, relaxation techniques, a warm bath, or writing in a journal.
- Encourage clients to develop a strong support network of family and friends and to ask for help when needed.
- Refer clients to community resources for more about fibromyalgia or encourage them to join a support group.

Evaluation

The evaluation of client care is based on the following suggested expected outcomes:

- Client is able to reduce pain sufficiently to allow periods of activity and sleep.

- Client voices feelings related to chronic condition.
- Client obtains adequate follow up.
- Client avoids use of narcotics or addictive substances to prevent substance addiction.

REVIEW Fibromyalgia

RELATE Link the Concepts and Exemplars

Linking the exemplar of fibromyalgia with the concept of development:

1. How might the pain of fibromyalgia impact the developmental tasks of the client?
2. What would you expect your findings to be when you perform a developmental assessment of a 32-year-old with fibromyalgia?

Linking the exemplar of fibromyalgia with the concept of addiction:

3. What factors put the client with fibromyalgia at risk for the development of addiction?
4. What would you plan for the client with fibromyalgia to assist in the prevention of addiction?

READY Go to Companion Skills Manual

REFER Go to Pearson Student Nursing Resources
nursing.pearsonhighered.com
- Additional review materials

REFLECT Case Study

Nancy Franklin is a 49-year-old physical therapist with a history of alcoholism. She has not had a drink in 10 years. She was recently in a car accident and sustained whiplash of the shoulders and neck. After 3 months of treatment, Ms. Franklin's pain has not improved, so the physician refers her to a specialist who diagnoses her with fibromyalgia. Ms. Franklin now has trouble getting out of bed in the morning, sleeps most of the morning, and takes naps in the afternoon. The parents of several of the children that she treats have complained because she is chronically late or does not show up for appointments at all. Ms. Franklin is returning to the fibromyalgia clinic today for a follow up visit; she is 30 minutes late.

1. What is your priority nursing diagnosis for Ms. Franklin?
2. What referral might you recommend for Ms. Franklin?
3. What is your plan of care to assist Ms. Franklin in coping with the diagnosis of fibromyalgia?

EXEMPLAR 3.5 Sleep–Rest Disorders

EXEMPLAR KEY TERMS
BiPAP, *198*
Continuous positive airway pressure (CPAP), *196*
Hypersomnia, *195*
Insomnia, *195*
Narcolepsy, *195*

Parasomnias, *195*
Polysomnography (PSG), *197*
Restless leg syndrome, *195*
Sleep apnea, *195*
Sleep loss, *195*

EXEMPLAR LEARNING OUTCOMES

After reading about this exemplar, you will be able to:

1. Describe the pathophysiology, etiology, clinical manifestations, and direct and indirect causes of sleep–rest disorders.

2. Identify risk factors and prevention methods associated with sleep–rest disorders.

3. Illustrate the nursing process in providing culturally competent care across the life span for individuals with sleep–rest disorders.

4. Formulate priority nursing diagnoses appropriate for an individual with sleep–rest disorders.

5. Summarize therapies used by interdisciplinary teams in the collaborative care of an individual with sleep–rest disorders.

6. Plan evidence-based care for an individual with sleep–rest disorders and his or her family in collaboration with other members of the healthcare team.

7. Evaluate expected outcomes for an individual with sleep–rest disorders.

▶ OVERVIEW

Sleep is essential to normal physiological functioning. Adults need 7–9 hours of sleep each night. But, many adults consistently sleep less than 7 hours, with daytime drowsiness and fatigue as a result. Sometimes the causes of this lack of sleep are busy schedules and poor planning. However, a sleep–rest disorder prevents some individuals from getting adequate sleep. A knowledge of common sleep disorders can help nurses to assess clients with drowsiness and fatigue and to develop nursing interventions that may increase sleep effectiveness.

▶ PATHOPHYSIOLOGY AND ETIOLOGY

Sleep is divided into rapid eye movement (REM) sleep and non-REM sleep. Non-REM sleep is divided into four stages, each stage representing a progressively deeper sleep. Each stage of sleep is associated with specific brain wave patterns and eye movements. The physiology of normal sleep is discussed further in the exemplar on Normal Sleep–Rest Patterns in the module on Health, Wellness, and Illness.

Normal sleep patterns can be disrupted by several sleep–rest disorders, including sleep loss, sleep-disordered breathing, insomnia, narcolepsy, and parasomnias such as restless leg syndrome.

- **Sleep loss** occurs when an individual receives fewer than 7–8 hours of sleep each night. A recent Sleep in America poll (National Sleep Foundation, 2010) reported that Americans get an average of less than 7 hours of sleep each weeknight and less than 8 hours of sleep each weekend night, indicating that sleep loss is a major problem in the United States. Even children receive about a half hour less sleep than the minimum hours recommended for them each day (National Sleep Foundation, 2004). The extent of daytime drowsiness and fatigue that accompanies sleep loss depends on the severity of the sleep deprivation. Individuals with chronic sleep loss may develop an inability to concentrate, fall asleep easily when sitting still, and suffer from reduced motivation and reaction time.

- **Insomnia**, the most common sleeping disorder, occurs when an individual has trouble falling asleep or staying asleep. Insomnia can be either a primary disorder or secondary to another condition or to a medication. In addition, insomnia can be acute, lasting a few days to a few weeks, or it can be chronic, lasting for a month or more. Insomnia causes daytime drowsiness, irritability, and fatigue. Severe insomnia may cause cognitive deficits and increase the risk of accidents.

- Sleep-disordered breathing, or **sleep apnea**, is characterized by repetitive periods of complete or partial airway obstruction that cause five or more apneic events (i.e., short pauses in breathing) per hour; more than 30 events per hour characterize severe apnea. Breathing pauses typically last between 10 and 20 seconds and are followed by a loud snore and/or awakening. Decreased oxygenation and repeated awakenings produce nonrestorative sleep and daytime drowsiness. The three types of sleep apnea are obstructive, central, and mixed. Obstructive sleep apnea occurs when the airway is blocked by the soft palate, tongue, and uvula. Snoring is one of the primary signs of obstructive sleep apnea although it does not always indicate apnea. Central sleep apnea occurs when the muscles of the chest and diaphragm fail temporarily. And mixed sleep apnea has characteristics of both obstructive and central sleep apnea.

- In **hypersomnia**, the individual obtains sufficient sleep but still suffers extreme daytime drowsiness. A severe form of hypersomnia is **narcolepsy**, which is characterized by daytime sleep attacks that last from a few seconds to several minutes. Other symptoms of narcolepsy are dreamlike hallucinations, sleep paralysis, and cataplexy. Narcolepsy is a nervous system disorder in which the brain is unable to regulate sleep–wake cycles; in some clients it is linked to a deficiency in hypocretin, a brain neurotransmitter. The onset of symptoms usually occurs between ages 15 and 30.

- **Parasomnias** are abnormal actions that take place during sleep. They often occur between stages of sleep, such as between wakefulness and REM sleep. Examples of parasomnias are sleep-related eating disorders (eating during sleep), somnambulism (sleepwalking), night terrors, sleep paralysis, enuresis (bed wetting), sleep talking, bruxism (grinding teeth), and sexsomnia (sex while sleeping). Many of these parasomnias are potentially harmful. For example, clients with allergies or diabetes and a sleep-related eating disorder may eat something during sleep that causes an allergic reaction or a spike in blood sugar. Similarly, in an episode of somnambulism, clients may walk outside the house and into busy roadways.

- Dyssomnias include restless leg syndrome and periodic limb movement disorder. They are a subset of parasomnias. **Restless leg syndrome** is a neurological sensorimotor disorder that is characterized by an overwhelming urge to move the legs when at rest. Periodic limb movements are repetitive movements that occur every 20–40 seconds and manifest as muscle twitches and jerking movements, usually of the legs.

Etiology

Many factors contribute to sleep disorders, including physical, medical, psychiatric, and environmental factors. Physical factors include injuries, ulcers, aging, and excessive weight; medical factors include conditions such as fibromyalgia, asthma, chronic pain, and genetic polymorphisms; psychiatric factors include depression, anxiety, and life stresses; and environmental factors include alcohol, medications, and extreme temperatures.

Risk Factors

Risk factors for insomnia include being a woman, being over age 60, and having a mental health disorder. The primary risk factor for obstructive sleep apnea is obesity. Other risk factors are a large neck circumference, a narrow airway, being male, and smoking. Hypocretin deficiency is a genetic risk factor for narcolepsy (Nishino et al., 2010). Children are likely to suffer from parasomnias such as sleepwalking. Drug or alcohol abuse contributes to night terrors in adults. Restless leg syndrome occurs more frequently with age and stress and in individuals with chronic conditions such as kidney disease, diabetes, and Parkinson disease.

▶ CLINICAL MANIFESTATIONS

Manifestations of sleep disorders vary from sleeplessness to excessive sleepiness and fatigue to irritability, distractibility, and morning headaches. Because lack of sleep is associated with the onset of a number of chronic conditions, the nurse should thoroughly assess any client reporting frequent difficulty in sleeping or staying awake. A thorough assessment elicits information that may indicate the presence of either a sleep disorder or another developing medical condition.

Lifespan and Cultural Considerations

The prevalence of specific sleep–rest disorders changes over the life course. For example, young children may suffer from enuresis, adolescents from delayed sleep phase syndrome, young parents from sleep loss related to having a newborn, and older adults from insomnia related to chronic health problems.

ADOLESCENTS AND SLEEP   Adolescents experience changes in the body's internal clock associated with puberty. In approximately 7%–16% of adolescents, these changes cause a delay in melatonin release each night; the result is delayed sleep phase syndrome. Signs of delayed sleep phase syndrome include an inability to fall asleep and wake up at the desired time, daytime sleepiness, and behavioral problems. Possible solutions for delayed sleep phase syndrome are practicing good sleep habits, systematically advancing or delaying the internal clock, using bright light therapy in the morning, and taking medications such as melatonin at night (Cleveland Clinic, 2009).

PREGNANT WOMEN AND SLEEP   Pregnant women often develop sleep disorders associated with physical discomfort and changing hormone levels. Insomnia in pregnant women may also be related to emotions and anxiety about labor and delivery, to becoming a mother, and to how the infant will change her relationship with her spouse. Restless leg syndrome and gastroesophageal reflux disease are often worse during pregnancy, and the risk for developing sleep apnea is increased in pregnant women, especially if the woman is obese. Frequent urination can also disrupt sleep. Later in the pregnancy, it is more difficult to find a comfortable position in which to sleep, and decreased lung capacity may contribute to difficulties falling asleep. Because many medications can harm the developing fetus, the best treatment for pregnant women with sleep disorders is practicing good sleep hygiene. **Continuous positive air pressure (CPAP)** is also a safe and effective treatment for pregnant women with obstructive sleep apnea (National Sleep Foundation, n.d.). CPAP is described in the module on Oxygenation.

OLDER ADULTS AND SLEEP   Sleep–rest disorders increase in prevalence with increasing age, especially as older adults develop chronic health problems such as hypertension, depression, and cardiovascular disease. Conversely, individuals with a sleep disorder are at higher risk of developing these chronic diseases (Bloom et al., 2009). Other conditions linked to sleep disorders include menopause, pulmonary disease, arthritis, chronic pain, and Alzheimer dementia. Medications used for chronic medical conditions, such as beta-blockers, corticosteroids, diuretics, and selective serotonin reuptake inhibitors (SSRIs), also can contribute to sleep disturbances. Because sleep disorders are associated with chronic conditions and multiple medications, nurses must conduct a thorough client history to determine if the sleep disorder is a primary condition or related to another medical condition.

Changes in sleep patterns in older adults include long periods of wakefulness, decreased total sleep time, reduced sleep efficiency, and decreased time spent in stages 3 and 4 NREM sleep and in REM sleep. These changes in nighttime sleep patterns are followed by increased daytime napping (Bloom et al., 2009), which may in turn contribute to difficulty sleeping at night. When older adults do not get sufficient sleep, a sleep deficit occurs that results in loss of daytime functioning and decreased quality of life. When daytime activities are limited, older adults lose physical strength; strength loss further disrupts the sleep–wake cycle.

Other physiological changes that may contribute to sleep disorders in older adults are changes in circulation, metabolism, and body tissue density. These changes limit the older adult's ability to generate heat and maintain a comfortable body temperature. Nursing interventions used to promote warmth and sleep for older adults include warming the bed with an electric or prewarmed blanket, using flannel sheets instead of cotton or polyester, encouraging the client to wear warm clothing to bed, and providing extra blankets.

Older adults in long-term care facilities are at increased risk for developing sleep disorders. Similar to community-dwelling older adults, clients in long-term care facilities have precipitating factors such as pain, gastroesophageal reflux, nocturia, dyspnea, and dementia, and they are often taking multiple medications that interfere with sleep. In contrast to community-dwelling adults, individuals in long-term care facilities must also deal with environmental factors that interfere with sleep, such as limited interaction with the community, reduced bright light exposure, physical inactivity, and nighttime noise and sleep disruptions (Bloom et al., 2009).

Focus on Diversity and Culture Ethnicity and Sleep

Studies related to the effects of ethnicity on sleep have determined that Blacks are more likely to suffer from shorter sleep duration, lower sleep efficiency, and higher sleep latency than Whites (Ram et al., 2010). Similarly, a Sleep in America poll (National Sleep Foundation, 2010) found that Whites, Asians, and Hispanics get a comparable number of hours of sleep per night, whereas Blacks reported an average of 30–45 minutes less sleep per night. Whites and Asians were more likely than Blacks or Hispanics to admit that not getting enough sleep impacted their job and family responsibilities. Blacks and Asians were less likely to report taking pills to help them sleep, but were more likely to conduct research and talk to their doctor about their sleep problems. In addition, approximately 44% of Blacks showed excessive sleepiness rates compared to 28% of Whites, based on the Epworth sleepiness scale. Hispanics were less likely than Whites to have heard of several common sleep disorders, including obstructive sleep apnea, restless leg syndrome, and insomnia (Merriman, 2009).

▶ COLLABORATION

The treatment of sleep disorders is complicated by their complex and often unknown etiologies. Therefore sleep disorders are best treated by a team of healthcare professionals, including the client's primary care physician, nurses, sleep specialists, nutritionists, and others, depending on the client's underlying medical conditions.

Diagnostic Tests

The primary diagnostic test for sleep disorders is a **polysomnography (PSG)**, or sleep study. A PSG records the client's blood oxygen levels, heart rate, breathing, and eye and leg movements. An electroencephalogram (EEG) is also conducted to monitor brain waves associated with NREM and REM sleep patterns. The client may also be monitored by video and audio equipment. An analysis of the sleep patterns identifies sleep disorders. Heart rate, breathing, and blood oxygen levels as well as audio monitoring can detect snoring and breathing changes that suggest sleep apnea. The monitoring of leg movements detects periodic limb movement disorder and restless leg syndrome (Mayo Clinic, 2011a). Audio and video equipment can also detect parasomnias such as sleepwalking, sleeptalking, and night terrors.

Surgery

For clients with obstructive sleep apnea, surgery to remove the obstruction may be a treatment option, especially if the obstruction is caused by the tonsils (tonsillectomy) or adenoids (adenoidectomy). An adenotonsillectomy is commonly performed to treat obstructive sleep apnea in children. Partial removal of the soft palate, uvula, and posterior lateral pharyngeal wall (uvulopalatopharyngoplasty, UPPP) may also be a treatment option. Surgery is usually considered only if CPAP therapy is not tolerated.

SAFETY ALERT

Partners of clients with sleep apnea often become aware of apneic episodes because of a pause in snoring. Clients who undergo surgery, such as removing the tonsils, to prevent snoring are at an increased risk for adverse events associated with apnea because there is no warning that apnea is occurring.

Pharmacologic Therapy

The primary pharmacologic agents used to treat sleep–rest disorders are the sedative-hypnotics, including anxiolytics, barbiturates, and benzodiazepines. Antiparkinson drugs, opioids, and anticonvulsants also are occasionally prescribed for sleep–rest disorders. For insomnia drugs, the half-life of the drug is important for determining its effectiveness (see **Table 3–7** ●). Drugs with short half-lives are helpful for clients who have trouble falling asleep but not for clients who have problems staying asleep. In contrast, drugs with longer half-lives are effective for clients who have periods of wakefulness during the night, but they may also produce daytime drowsiness. In addition, many sleep aids produce addiction/tolerance, so the risks of taking a sleep aid should be discussed with the client prior to use.

Several side effects are shared by multiple sleep aids, including headache, dizziness, residual drowsiness, somnolence, and nausea. Other selected side effects include sleep attacks (ropinirole, pramipexole), dyspepsia (ropinirole), tachycardia (eszopiclone, diphenhydramine), and postural hypotension (pramipexole). Side effects are often amplified in older adults, especially dizziness, hallucinations, hypotension, impaired coordination, ataxia, and vertigo. These side effects put older adults at higher risk for injury during ambulation, so safety measures should be implemented and older adults should be supervised if ambulating during the night. In addition, all clients should be warned to avoid driving, handling machinery, or participating in dangerous activities after taking sleep aids. Some sleep aids should not be used by clients with cardiac, respiratory, kidney, or liver disorders or by pregnant or breastfeeding women, so check client history and contraindications before giving sleep aids to clients.

Drug, food, and herbal interactions with sleep aids are also common. The most common drug interactions are with alcohol and other CNS depressants, CYP3A4 inhibitors, and cimetidine. Cimetidine is known to increase plasma levels of multiple sleep aids. Many other drug interactions exist, so nurses and other healthcare team members should carefully review clients' current medications to avoid adverse drug reactions. Common food interactions are grapefruit juice (estazolam, ramelteon), high-fat meals (ramelteon, sodium oxybate), and food in general (zolpidem), all of these interactions decrease absorption of the medication. Common herbal interactions include kava and valerian (benzodiazepines), St. John's wort (eszopiclone), and melatonin (zaleplon), which increase drug levels or produce additional sedative effects.

Sleep aids can induce tolerance, so dosages may need to be increased over time. Some medications, such as chloral hydrate, estazolam, and zolpidem, should be used for only short-term management of insomnia because of tolerance issues. When

TABLE 3–7 Selected Medications Used for Sleep–Rest Disorders

MEDICATION	HALF-LIFE (HOURS)	SLEEP–REST DISORDER	DRUG CLASS
Chloral hydrate (Noctec)	8–11	Short-term for insomnia	Anxiolytic
Clonazepam (Klonopin)	18–40	Restless leg syndrome	Benzodiazepine, anticonvulsant
Diphenhydramine hydrochloride (Benadryl)	8–9	Intractable insomnia	Antiparkinson, antihistamine
Estazolam (Prosom)	10–24	Short-term for insomnia	Anxiolytic, benzodiazepine
Eszopiclone (Lunesta)	5–6	Insomnia	Sedative-hypnotic
Flurazepam (Dalmane)	47–100	Insomnia	Anxiolytic, benzodiazepine
Gabapentin enacarbil (Horizant)	5–6	Restless leg syndrome	Anticonvulsant
Modafinil (Provigil)	15	Narcolepsy, obstructive sleep apnea	CNS stimulant
Pramipexole dihydrochloride (Mirapex)	8–12	Restless leg syndrome	Antiparkinson
Quazepam (Doral)	39	Insomnia	Sedative-hypnotic, anxiolytic, benzodiazepine
Ramelteon (Rozerem)	1–2.5	Insomnia	Melatonin receptor agonist
Ropinirole hydrochloride (Requip)	6	Restless leg syndrome	Antiparkinson
Sodium oxybate (Xyrem)	0.5–1	Cataplexy in clients with narcolepsy	CNS depressant
Temazepam (Restoril)	8–24	Insomnia	Anxiolytic, benzodiazepine
Zaleplon (Sonata)	1	Short-term for insomnia	Sedative-hypnotic, anxiolytic
Zolpidem (Ambien)	1.7–2.5	Short-term for insomnia	Anxiolytic

Source: Wilson, B. A., Shannon, M. T., & Shields, K. M. (2013). *Nurse's drug guide.* Upper Saddle River, NJ: Pearson Education.

treatment with sleep aids is stopped, dosages should be tapered down over a week or more to prevent withdrawal symptoms, including delirium, convulsions, dizziness, GI upset, and parasomnias. Clients should be warned that rebound insomnia may occur after they stop these medications.

Nonpharmacologic Therapy

Nonpharmacologic therapies that may be beneficial in the treatment of sleep–rest disorders include cognitive-behavioral therapy, good sleep hygiene, physical exercise, and relaxation techniques. Nasal strips can also be used to open the nasal passageways and prevent snoring that is not accompanied by airway obstruction.

For obstructive sleep apnea, the most common therapies are weight reduction, avoiding alcohol, avoiding the supine position for sleeping, and using a CPAP or a bilevel positive air pressure (**BiPAP®**) machine to help the airway open (see **Figure 3–9 ●** and the Client Teaching feature). A CPAP or BiPAP machine consists of a generator that produces positive air pressure administered by a close-fitting mask around the mouth and nose. The positive air pressure prevents collapse and obstruction of the airway to relieve apneic episodes. The BiPAP differs from the CPAP in that it produces less pressure during exhalation and more pressure during inhalation, thus causing less resistance to exhalation. The most common side effect of CPAP or BiPAP therapy is a dry mouth and airway, so an in-line or room humidifier is recommended. CPAP can be used for children with obstructive sleep apnea and for clients with surgical contraindications or with persistent apnea after adenotonsillectomy, as often occurs in children with Down syndrome, craniofacial abnormalities, or neuromuscular disorders. Pressure levels may need to be adjusted as the child grows.

Three other common nonpharmacologic therapies for sleep–rest disorders are bright light therapy, stimulus control therapy, and sleep restriction (see the Evidence-Based Practice feature). Bright light therapy uses a light box that provides white light (>2,500–10,000 lux) to increase wakefulness. It can be used in the morning to help clients with delayed sleep phase syndrome wake earlier or in the evening to delay sleep in clients with advanced sleep phase syndrome (Gooley, 2008). Stimulus control therapy involves using the bed only for sleep and sex, not for other activities, such as watching TV, reading, or working. It is the most validated behavioral insomnia treatment and is recommended as standard treatment by the American Academy of Sleep Medicine (Chesson et al., 1999; Schutte-Rodin et al., 2008.)

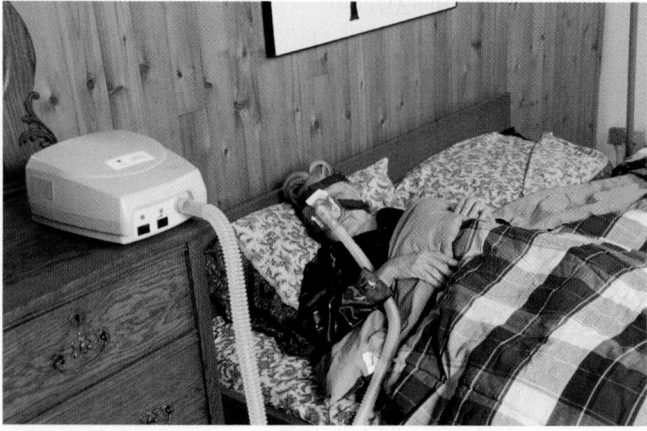

Figure 3–9 ● A client using a nasal mask and CPAP to treat sleep apnea.

Source: Custom Medical Stock Photo, Inc.

Client Teaching   CPAP and BiPAP Machines

Client teaching for a CPAP or BiPAP machine should include:

- Proper fitting of the mask to the face, including wearing the right size mask and keeping the straps tight.
- The importance of getting used to wearing the mask. Step 1: Wear the mask *without* air pressure when awake. Step 2: Wear the mask *with* air pressure when awake. Step 3: Wear the mask *with* air pressure when asleep.
- The method of adjusting the air pressure of the machine to minimize difficulty exhaling.
- The importance of using a humidifier and nasal sprays to minimize dry mouth and nose.
- Relaxation exercises to reduce the claustrophobic feelings caused by wearing the mask.

Evidence-Based Practice   Sleep Restriction

Problem

Insomnia causes individuals to lie in bed for long periods without falling asleep or drifting between stage 1 NREM sleep and drowsy wakefulness. As a result, individuals believe they are getting less sleep than they actually are, and daytime drowsiness then decreases productivity and increases the risk of falling asleep during work or while driving.

Evidence

Research suggests sleep restriction can help reduce primary chronic insomnia. Sleep restriction limits the amount of time in bed to maximize sleep efficiency, then gradually increases the time in bed until the individual is receiving adequate sleep. When sleep restriction therapy begins, time in bed should be close to the estimated time of actual sleep each night but no less than 5 hours. The morning wake time should remain constant throughout therapy. Each week, sleep efficiency is calculated from the total sleep time versus the time spent in bed. When sleep efficiency exceeds 90%, the client should increase time in bed by 15–20 minutes (Harsora & Kessmann, 2009). Sleep restriction reduces the gap between the total sleep time and time in bed by decreasing sleep onset latency and improving total sleep time (Lande & Gragnani, 2010). Combined with sleep hygiene education, sleep restriction helps increase sleep efficiency and decrease hypnotic medication use over time (Taylor et al., 2010). It is noteworthy that sleep restriction is comparable to stimulus control therapy as an effective treatment for primary chronic insomnia in older adults as measured by sleep onset latency, waking after sleep onset, and sleep efficiency (Epstein et al., 2012).

Implications

For clients with chronic insomnia, sleep restriction helps increase sleep efficiency. It may be especially beneficial for older adults who suffer from adverse side effects when using sedative-hypnotic drugs. Clients may be reluctant to try sleep restriction because of the misconception that time spent in bed is the same as receiving adequate sleep. However, time spent in bed not sleeping actually contributes to multiple sleep disturbances. Another barrier to sleep restriction therapy is the need to induce mild sleep deprivation, which may initially cause increased daytime drowsiness and decreased productivity. A sleep log is vital to the success of sleep restriction therapy to methodically reduce the amount of inefficient sleeping (Lande & Gragnani, 2010). This therapy takes 4–8 weeks to achieve maximum effectiveness. Sleep education should also be included as an important part of sleep deprivation therapy.

Critical Thinking Application

1. You meet with a client who wants to quit after 1 week on sleep restriction, because of increased daytime drowsiness. What suggestions would encourage this client to remain on the therapy?
2. How would you explain the importance of sleep efficiency to the client who believes that time spent in bed is equivalent to receiving adequate sleep?
3. What recommendations would you make about timing sleep deprivation therapy for a working adult? A teenager in school? A retired older adult? A single parent?

Complementary and Alternative Therapy   Herbal Supplements for Sleep Disorders

Herbal supplements may be an alternative for individuals who do not tolerate pharmacologic therapy because of side effects. Two herbs that are traditionally used to aid sleep are valerian (*Valeriana officinalis*) and chamomile (*Matricaria recutita*). Valerian usually has to be taken for 2 or 3 weeks before it produces an effect, and clinical trials have not proven its effectiveness. Possible side effects of valerian include indigestion, headache, palpitations, and dizziness. Chamomile, often taken as a tea, has a soothing effect that may induce sleep and decrease restlessness, although this effect has not been proven in clinical studies. It is safe for both adults and children except individuals who are allergic to ragweed or daisies.

Melatonin is a sleep hormone produced by the pineal gland. Synthetic melatonin is sold in many pharmacies and health food stores and may be taken to regulate sleep patterns. It is often helpful for sleep disturbances related to shift work or jet lag. It has been proven effective in treating sleep disorders in children with autism (Rossignol & Frye, 2011) and children with ADHD (Hoebert et al., 2009). It may also be helpful for older adults with insomnia when combined with magnesium and zinc supplements (Rondanelli et al., 2011).

Clinical Manifestations and Therapies **Sleep–Rest Disorders**

ETIOLOGY	CLINICAL MANIFESTATIONS	CLINICAL THERAPIES
Insomnia	■ Inability to fall asleep or remain asleep ■ Drowsiness ■ Fatigue ■ Irritability ■ Cognitive deficits	■ Improved sleep hygiene ■ Stimulus control therapy ■ Sleep restriction therapy ■ Pharmacologic therapy ■ Cognitive-behavioral therapy ■ Exercise therapy ■ Relaxation techniques
Obstructive sleep apnea	■ Snoring ■ Five or more apneic episodes per hour that last 10–20 seconds each ■ Gasping during sleep ■ Frequent nighttime awakenings ■ Daytime drowsiness ■ Morning headache	■ Weight reduction ■ Avoiding alcohol ■ Nasal CPAP or BiPAP ■ Surgery to remove obstruction ■ Modafinil
Narcolepsy	■ Daytime drowsiness ■ Sleep attacks ■ Cataplexy ■ Sleep paralysis ■ Hypocretin deficiency	■ Modafinil ■ Sodium oxybate ■ Antidepressants ■ Good sleep hygiene ■ Counseling and support groups
Sleep loss	■ Sleeping fewer than 7–8 hours per night ■ Fatigue ■ Daytime drowsiness ■ Inability to concentrate ■ Decreased motivation	■ Good sleep hygiene
Restless leg syndrome	■ Overwhelming urge to move the legs ■ Unpleasant sensations in the legs ■ Nighttime leg twitching	■ Pharmacologic therapy ■ Massage ■ Gentle stretching ■ Exercise therapy ■ Good sleep hygiene

■ NURSING PROCESS

Clients experiencing sleep disorders often report a great deal of frustration and annoyance about their sleepless nights. However, sleep disorders are more than just an annoyance: Risks of injury increase dramatically in tired people. In addition to care of clients' sleeplessness, it is important for nurses to promote injury prevention by teaching strategies to reduce risk such as not driving when tired, using caution with potentially dangerous equipment, and preventing fires if clients smoke.

Assessment

A nursing assessment for sleep–rest disorders begins with a client interview, including a sleep history. If the client is married, a spouse may provide additional helpful information about the client's sleep habits. Similarly, parents may provide information about a child's sleep habits. The interview and sleep history may include items such as

■ Do you have trouble falling asleep at night?
■ How often do you wake up during the night? Do you have trouble falling asleep once you have woken up?

■ How do you feel when you wake up in the morning?
■ Describe your normal sleep schedule.
■ Has anyone ever told you that you snore, walk, scream, stop breathing, or jerk in your sleep?
■ Do you suffer from daytime drowsiness? Does it interfere with your daily activities?
■ Do you sleep in strange positions?
■ Does your child wet the bed?
■ Do you experience morning headaches?
■ Does anything unusual happen when you laugh or get angry?
■ Do you drink caffeinated beverages or alcohol or smoke? If so, how often and how much?
■ Has anything happened lately to change your sleep patterns? Medical condition, medications, life stresses?
■ What have you been doing to deal with your sleep problem? Does it help?
■ How do your sleep habits affect your relationships, work, school, and activities?

Assessment tools, such as the Epworth Sleepiness Scale, can help determine if an individual has a sleep–rest disorder (Johns, 1991; University of Maryland Medical Center, 2013). Scores between 0 and 10 are considered normal, and scores between 11 and 24 indicate a sleep disorder. Sleep scales are available that are specific for clients with Parkinson disease, pediatric clients, teachers, women, and others.

A visual and physical assessment also can indicate the presence of fatigue and a possible sleep–rest disorder. Indicators include abnormal vital signs, lack of muscle tone and reflexes, decreased cognitive functioning and coordination, dark circles under the eyes, and irritability. Polysomnography should be conducted for clients with a suspected sleep disorder.

Diagnosis

Nursing diagnoses related to sleep–rest disorders include

- *Insomnia*
- *Sleep Deprivation*
- *Readiness for Enhanced Sleep*
- *Disturbed Sleep Pattern*
- *Fatigue*
- *Wandering* related to somnambulism
- *Ineffective Breathing Pattern* related to sleep apnea
- *Ineffective Coping*
- *Stress Overload*
- *Risk for Injury* related to sedative-hypnotic effects
- *Deficient Knowledge* related to sleep hygiene

(NANDA-I © 2012)

Planning

Appropriate goals for the client with a sleep disturbance include

- The client will sleep through the night.
- The client will use relaxation techniques 30–45 minutes prior to bedtime.
- The client will maintain a consistent bedtime.
- The client will use good sleep hygiene.
- The client will reduce or remove environmental distractions from the bedroom.
- The client will have sufficient energy for normal daily activities.
- The client will report improved quality and quantity of sleep.
- The client's spouse will report decreased snoring.
- The client's spouse will report no apneic episodes.

Implementation

Nursing interventions for sleep–rest disorders should include the client, the client's spouse or parents, and the healthcare team. Possible interventions include

- Educating the client about the factors associated with impaired sleep–rest patterns.
- Instructing the client in the proper use of assistive devices (e.g., BiPAP).
- If a pharmacologic treatment has been prescribed, teaching the client about the proper use of the medication as well as its potential side effects and interactions.
- Teaching the client about the principles of good sleep hygiene.

Evaluation

Evaluation should include data collection about the quality and duration of the client's sleep and how the client feels upon awakening and throughout the day. If outcomes were not achieved, reassess the client to determine if etiological factors were correctly identified, if the client has had any changes in medical conditions or medications, if the client followed the instructions for good sleep hygiene, if the client has avoided daytime napping, and if any pharmacologic or nonpharmacologic therapies have been implemented with success.

NURSING CARE PLAN   A Client With Obstructive Sleep Apnea

ASSESSMENT	DIAGNOSES	PLANNING
Charles Huston visits his primary care physician because his wife, Amy, told him he stops breathing frequently during the night. While speaking with the nurse, Mr. Huston says that he experiences mild drowsiness during the day, and if he sits for too long with no stimulation, he easily falls asleep. His wife reports that Mr. Huston snores heavily, but when he stops snoring he also stops breathing. The condition is worse when he is lying on his back, which Mr. Huston claims is his most comfortable sleeping position.	■ *Ineffective Breathing Pattern* related to airway obstruction ■ *Impaired Gas Exchange* related to apneic episodes ■ *Readiness for Enhanced Sleep* ■ *Imbalanced Nutrition: More than Body Requirements* ■ *Sedentary Lifestyle* ■ *Activity Intolerance* related to obesity (NANDA-I © 2012)	■ Client will breathe consistently through the night. ■ Client will feel refreshed upon awakening. ■ Client will demonstrate understanding of the use of a BiPAP machine. ■ Client will begin a mild exercise program of walking for 30 minutes three times a week, which will increase in intensity as the client loses weight. ■ Client will meet with a nutritionist to develop a healthy eating plan. ■ Client will lose 10 pounds in the next month and 70 pounds in the next year.

Physical Examination
Height: 188 cm (74″)
Weight: 130.2 kg (287 lb)
Temperature: 38.2°C (100.8°F)
Pulse: 88 bpm
Respirations: 16/min
Blood pressure: 149/89 mmHg

Diagnostic Data
A polysomnography reveals an apnea–hypopnea index of 28.

(continued on next page)

NURSING CARE PLAN (continued)

IMPLEMENTATION

- Teach Mr. Huston how to use the BiPAP machine (see Client Teaching feature).
- Instruct Mr. Huston on good sleep hygiene techniques.
- Encourage his verbalization of his feelings, perceptions, and fears.
- Refer Mr. Huston to a nutritionist for a healthy eating plan.

- Refer Mr. Huston to a personal trainer or physical fitness facility for an exercise program.
- Refer Mr. and Ms. Huston to a support group for weight loss.
- Schedule regular follow up appointments to evaluate Mr. Huston's weight loss, fitness, and control of his obstructive sleep apnea.

EVALUATION

Mr. Huston returns for a follow up appointment 1 week after starting the BiPAP machine. He reports regular use of the BiPAP machine and feeling more refreshed during the day. Mr. and Ms. Huston have met with a nutritionist, and Ms. Huston has begun to prepare more healthy meals. Mr. Huston has joined the local YMCA and has met with a personal trainer once. He has lost 2 pounds in the first week. On subsequent follow up appointments, Mr. Huston continues losing weight, but his progress stalls after 6 months at a 40-pound overall weight loss. The care plan is modified to include a more strenuous exercise program and a lower daily calorie intake.

CRITICAL THINKING

1. What suggestions would you make if Mr. Huston complained of a dry mouth, nose, and throat after using his BiPAP machine?
2. Outline two other methods of weight loss that Mr. Huston could incorporate to help him get past his stall in weight loss at 6 months.
3. What other conditions related to Mr. Huston's obesity could increase his daytime drowsiness?

REVIEW Sleep–Rest Disorders

RELATE Link the Concepts and Exemplars

Linking the exemplar of sleep–rest disorders with the concept of development:

1. How do requirements for sleep vary across the developmental stages?
2. What assessment differences might you expect in sleep deprivation across the life span?

Linking the exemplar of sleep–rest disorders with the concept of sexuality:

3. How might sleep–rest disorders impact the client's sexual relationship with a significant other?
4. What interventions would you initiate for the couple when one of the partners has a sleep–rest disorder?

READY Go to Companion Skills Manual

REFER Go to Pearson Student Nursing Resources
nursing.pearsonhighered.com

- Additional review materials

REFLECT Case Study

Jennifer Leno is a 30-year-old nursing student who works 20 hours each week, carries a full-time academic load, and has an 8-year-old child. She begins to drink energy drinks at night to stay awake to study. However, after 2 months of 5 hours of sleep a night and three energy drinks each day, she begins to have problems going to sleep. Her friend Janie offers Ms. Leno zolpidem (Ambien) to help her relax.

1. What might be causing Ms. Leno's insomnia?
2. What is zolpidem, and is it likely to be effective in treating Ms. Leno's symptoms?
3. If you were a friend of Ms. Leno's as well, what advice would you give her?

■ REFERENCES

Administration on Aging. (2012). *A profile of older Americans: 2011.* Retrieved from http://www.aoa.gov/AoARoot/Aging_Statistics/Profile/2011/4.aspx.

Alabi, T. O., & Haines, C. A. (2009). Predicting survival from in-hospital CPR. *Clinical Geriatrics,* 34–36. Retrieved from http://www.clinicalgeriatrics.com/articles/Predicting-Survival-From-In-Hospital-CPR?page=0,0.

American Academy of Pediatrics. (2000). Palliative care for children. *Pediatrics, 106*(2), 351–357. Reaffirmed February 2012, *130*(1), e248.

American Association of Colleges of Nursing. (n.d.). *Peaceful death: Recommended competencies and curricular guidelines for end-of-life nursing care.* Retrieved from http://www.aacn.nche.edu/elnec/publications/peaceful-death.

American Geriatrics Society. (2012). *Geriatrics health professionals leading change. Improving care of older adults.*

Retrieved from http://www.americangeriatrics.org/files/documents/Adv_Resources/PP_Priorities.pdf.

American Geriatrics Society Panel on the Pharmacological Management of Persistent Pain in Older Persons. (2009). Pharmacological management of persistent pain in older persons. *Journal of the American Geriatrics Society, 57*(8), 1331–1346. doi:10.1111/j.1532-5415.2009.02376.x.

American Nurses Association. (1994). *Position statement: Active euthanasia.* Retrieved from the American Nurses Association Web site, http://www.nursingworld.org/MainMenuCategories/Policy-Advocacy/Positions-and-Resolutions/ANAPositionStatements/Position-Statements-Alphabetically/prteteuth14450.html.

American Nurses Association. (2012). *Position statement: Nursing care and do not resuscitate (DNR) and allow natural death (AND) decisions.* Retrieved from http://

nursingworld.org/dnrposition.

Arif-Rahu, M., Fisher, D., & Matsuda, Y. (2012). Biobehavioral measures for pain in the pediatric patient. *Pain Management Nursing, 13*(3), 157–168. doi:10.1016/j.pmn.2010.10.036.

Baetz, M., & Bowen, R. (2008). Chronic pain and fatigue: Associations with religion and spirituality. *Pain Research and Management, 13*(5), 383–388.

Bektas, F., Eken, C., Karadeniz, O., Goksu, E., Cubuk, M., & Cete, Y. (2009). Intravenous paracetamol or morphine for the treatment of renal colic: A randomized, placebo-controlled trial. *Annals of Emergency Medicine, 54*(4), 568–574. doi:10.1016/j.annemergmed.2009.06.501.

Bellato, E., Marini, E., Castoldi, F., Barbasetti, N., Mattei, L., Bonasia, D. E., & Blonna, D. (2012). Fibromyalgia syndrome: Etiology, pathogenesis, diagnosis, and treatment.

Pain Research and Treatment, 2012, 426130.doi:10.1155/2012/426130.

Bergman, C. L. (2012). Emergency nurses' perceived barriers to demonstrating caring when managing adult patients' pain. *Journal of Emergency Nursing, 38*(3), 218–225. doi:10.1016/j.jen.2010.09.017.

Berman, A., & Snyder, S. J. (2012). Pain management. In K. Trakalo (Ed.), *Kozier and Erb's fundamentals of nursing: Concepts, process, and practice* (pp. 1204–1248). Upper Saddle River, NJ: Pearson Education.

Berry, P. H., & Dahl, J. L. (2000). The new JCAHO pain standards: Implications for pain management nurses. *Pain Management Nursing, 1*(1), 3–12. doi:10.1053/jpmn.2000.5833.

Bloom, H. G., Ahmed, I., Alessi, C. A., Ancoli-Israel, S., Buysse, D. J., Kryger, M. H., . . . Zee, P. C. (2009). Evidence-based recommendations for the assessment and management of sleep disorders in older persons. *Journal of the American Geriatrics Society, 57*(5), 761–789.

Bradley, L. A. (2009). Pathophysiology of fibromyalgia. *American Journal of Medicine, 122*(12 Suppl.), S22. doi:10.1016/j.amjmed.2009.09.008.

Bruckenthal, P. (2008). Risk factors associated with the onset of persistent pain. *Medscape Neurology.* Retrieved from http://www.medscape.org/viewarticle/576473.

Bruera, E., Kuehn, N., Miller, M., Selmser, P., & Macmillan, K. (1991). The Edmonton Symptom Assessment Scale (ESAS): A simple method for the assessment of palliative care patients. *Journal of Palliative Care, 7*(2), 6–9.

Burian, M., & Geisslinger, G. (2005). COX-dependent mechanisms involved in the antinociceptive action of NSAIDs at central and peripheral sites. *Pharmacology and Therapeutics, 107*(2), 139–154. doi:10.1016/j.pharmthera.2005.02.004.

Butt, Z., Rao, A. V., Lai, J-S., Abernethy, A. P., Rosenbloom, S. K., & Cella, D. (2010). Age-associated differences in fatigue among patients with cancer. *Journal of Pain Symptom Management, 40*(2), 217–223. doi:10.1016/j.jpainsymman.2009.12.016.

Caeymaex, L., Jousselme, C., Vasilescu, C., Danan, C., Falissard, B., Bourrat, M. M., . . . Speranza, M. (2013). Perceived role in end-of-life decision making in the NICU affects long-term parental grief response. *Archives of Disease in Childhood. Fetal and Neonatal Edition, 98*(1), F26–F31. doi:10.1136/archdischild-2011-301548.

Canadian Paediatric Society. (2008). Advance care planning for paediatric patients. *Paediatric and Child Health, 13*(9), 791–796.

Cantarero-Villanueva, I., Fernandez-Lao, C., Cuesta-Vargas, A. I., Del Moral-Avila, R., Fernandez-de-Las-Penas, C., & Arroyo-Morales, M. (2013). The effectiveness of a deep water aquatic exercise program in cancer-related fatigue in breast cancer survivors: A randomized controlled trial. *Archives of Physical Medicine and Rehabilitation, 94*(2), 221–230. doi:10.1016/j.apmr.2012.09.008.

Centers for Disease Control and Prevention. (2005). *Worktable 309: Deaths by place of death, age, race, and sex: United States, 2005.* Retrieved from http://www.cdc.gov/nchs/data/dvs/Mortfinal2005_worktable_309.pdf.

Centers for Disease Control and Prevention. (2010). *National Vital Statistics Report: Deaths: Final data for 2010.* Retrieved from http://www.cdc.gov/nchs/data/dvs/deaths_2010_release.pdf.

Centers for Disease Control and Prevention. (2011). *QuickStats: Location of death for decedents aged ≥85 years—United States, 2005–2007.* Retrieved from http://www.cdc.gov/mmwr/preview/mmwrhtml/mm6037a9.htm.

Centers for Disease Control and Prevention. (2012). *National Vital Statistics Reports. Deaths: Preliminary data for 2011.* Retrieved from http://www.cdc.gov/nchs/data/nvsr/nvsr61/nvsr61_06.pdf.

Chesson, A. L., Jr., Anderson, W. M., Littner, M., Davila, D., Hartse, K., Johnson, S., . . . Rafecas, J. (1999). Practice parameters for the nonpharmacologic treatment of chronic insomnia. An American Academy of Sleep Medicine report. Standards of Practice Committee of the American Academy of Sleep Medicine. *Sleep, 22*(8), 1128–1133.

Clarke, A., Anthony, G., Gray, D., Jones, D., McNamee, P., Schofield, P., . . . Martin, D. (2012). "I feel so stupid because I can't give a proper answer. . ." How older adults describe chronic pain: A qualitative study. *BMC Geriatrics, 12*, 78. doi:10.1186/1471-2318-12-78.

Clauw, D. J., Arnold, L. M., & McCarberg, B. H. (2011). The science of fibromyalgia. *Mayo Clinic Proceedings, 86*(9), 907–911. doi:10.4065/mcp.2011.0206.

Cleveland Clinic. (n.d.). *Guided imagery.* Retrieved February 4, 2013, from http://my.clevelandclinic.org/departments/integrativemedicine/guided_imagery_facts.aspx.

Cleveland Clinic. (2009). *Delayed sleep phase syndrome.* Retrieved from http://my.clevelandclinic.org/disorders/sleep_disorders/hic_delayed_sleep_phase_syndrome.aspx.

Costigan, M., Scholz, J., & Woolf, C. J. (2009). Neuropathic pain: A maladaptive response of the nervous system to damage. *Annual Review of Neuroscience, 32*, 1–32. doi:10.1146/annurev.neuro.051508.135531.

Cox, J. J., Reimann, F., Nicholas, A. K., Thornton, G., Roberts, E., Springell, K., . . . Woods, C. G. (2006). An *SCN9A* channelopathy causes congenital inability to experience pain. *Nature, 444*, 894–898. doi:10.1038/nature05413.

Craig, M., Jeavons, R., Probert, J., & Benger, J. (2012). Randomised comparison of intravenous paracetamol and intravenous morphine for acute traumatic limb pain in the emergency department. *Emergency Medicine Journal, 29*, 37–39. doi:10.1136/emf.2010.104687.

Cramp, F., & Byron-Daniel, J. (2012). Exercise for the management of cancer-related fatigue in adults. *Cochrane Database of Systematic Reviews*, (11), CD006145. doi:10.1002/14651858.CD006145.pub3.

Crocker, C., & Sehgal, A. (2010). Genetic analysis of sleep. *Genes Dev., 24*(12): 1220–1235.

Davidhizar, R., & Giger, J. N. (2004). A review of the literature on care of clients in pain who are culturally diverse. *International Nursing Review, 51*(1), 47–55.

Davies, A. N., Dickman, A., Reid, C., Stevens, A. M., & Zeppetella, G. (2009). The management of cancer-related breakthrough pain: Recommendations of a task group of the Science Committee of the Association for Palliative Medicine of Great Britain and Ireland. *European Journal of Pain, 13*(4), 331–338. doi:10.1016/j.ejpain.2008.06.014.

De Ruddere, L., Goubert, L., Stevens, M., de C. Williams, A. C., & Crombez, G. (2013). Discounting pain in the absence of medical evidence is explained by negative evaluation of the patient. *Pain* (in press). doi:10.1016/j.pain.2012.12.018.

Dimeo, F., Schwartz, S., Wesel, N., Voigt, A., & Thiel, E. (2008). Effects of an endurance and resistance exercise program on persistent cancer-related fatigue after treatment. *Annals of Oncology, 19*(8), 1495–1499. doi:10.1093/annonc/mdn068.

Dinler, M., Diracoglu, D., Kasikcioglu, E., Sayli, O., Akin, A., Aksoy, C., . . . Berker, E. (2009). Effect of aerobic exercise training on oxygen uptake and kinetics in patients with fibromyalgia. *Rheumatology International, 30*(2), 281–284. doi:10.1007/s00296-009-1126-x.

Dishman, R. K., Thom, N. J., Puetz, T. W., O'Connor, P. J., & Clementz, B. A. (2010). Effects of cycling exercise on vigor, fatigue, and electroencephalographic activity among young adults who report persistent fatigue. *Psychophysiology, 47*(6), 1066–1074. doi:10.1111/j.1469-8986.2010.01014.x.

Durall, A., Zurakowski, D., & Wolfe, J. (2012). Barriers to conducting advance care discussions for children with life-threatening conditions. *Pediatrics, 129*(4), e975–982. doi:10.1542/peds.2011-2695.

Ehlenbach, W. J., Barnato, A. E., Curtis, J. R., Kreuter, W., Koepsell, T. D., Deyo, R. A., & Stapleton, R. D. (2009). Epidemiologic study of in-hospital cardiopulmonary resuscitation in the elderly. *New England Journal of Medicine, 361*, 22–31. doi:10.1056/NEJMoa0810245.

Epstein, D. R., Sidani, S., Bootzin, R. R., & Belvea, M. J. (2012). Dismantling multicomponent behavioral treatment for insomnia in older adults: A randomized controlled trial. *Sleep, 35*(6), 797–805. doi:10.5665/sleep.1878.

Faries, J. E., Mills, D. S., Goldsmith, K. W., Phillips, K. D., & Orr, J. (1991) Systematic pain records and their impact on pain control: A pilot study. *Cancer Nursing, 14*(6), 306–313.

Fein, A. (2012) *Nociceptors and the perception of pain.* Retrieved February 4, 2013, from http://cell.uchc.edu/pdf/fein/nociceptors_fein_2012.pdf.

Fitzgerald, M., & Walker, S. M. (2009). Infant pain management: A developmental neurobiological approach. *Nature Clinical Practice Neurology, 5*(1), 35–50.

Food and Drug Administration. (2005). *COX-2 selective (includes Bextra, Celebrex, and Vioxx) and non-selective non-steroidal anti-inflammatory drugs (NSAIDs).* Retrieved from http://www.fda.gov/drugs/drugsafety/postmarketdrugsafetyinformationforpatientsandproviders/ucm103420.htm.

Gasche, Y., Daali, Y., Fathi, M., Chiappe, A., Cottini, S., Dayer, P., & Desmeules, J. (2004). Codeine intoxication associated with ultrarapid CYP2D6 metabolism. *New England Journal of Medicine, 351*, 2827–2831. doi:10.1056/nejmoa041888.

Geimer-Flanders, J. (2009). Creating a healing environment: Rationale and research overview. *Cleveland Clinic Journal of Medicine, 76*(Suppl. 2), S66–S69. doi:10.3949/ccjm.76.s2.13.

Ginsburg, M., Silver, S., & Berman, H. (2009). Prescribing opioids to older adults: A guide to choosing and switching among them. *Geriatrics and Aging, 12*(1), 48–52.

Glaser, B. G., & Strauss, A. L. (1965). *Awareness of dying.* Chicago, IL: Aldine.

Goldberg, Y. P., Pimstone, S. N., Namdari, R., Price, N., Cohen, C., Sherrington, R. P., & Hayden, M. R. (2012). Human Mendelian pain disorders: A key to discovery and validation of novel analgesics. *Clinical Genetics, 82*(4), 367–373. doi:10.1111/j.1399-0004.2012.01942.x.

Gooley, J. J. (2008). Treatment of circadian rhythm sleep disorders with light. *Annals of the Academy of Medicine (Singapore), 37*(8), 669–676.

Guido, G. W. (2010a). Non-pain symptom management at the end of life. In M. Connor (Ed.), *Nursing care at the end of life* (pp. 81–97). Upper Saddle River, NJ: Pearson Education.

Guido, G. W. (2010b). Hydration and nutrition in terminal care. In M. Connor (Ed.), *Nursing care at the end of life* (pp. 98–107). Upper Saddle River, NJ: Pearson Education.

Guido, G. W. (2010c). Caring for end-of-life patients across the life span. In M. Connor (Ed.), *Nursing care at the end of life* (pp. 108–124). Upper Saddle River, NJ: Pearson Education.

Guido, G. W. (2010d). Cultural and spiritual care at end of life. In M. Connor (Ed.), *Nursing care at the end of life* (pp. 145–154). Upper Saddle River, NJ: Pearson Education.

Haanpaa, M., & Hietaharju, A. (2010). Central neuropathic pain. In A. Kopf & N. B. Patel (Eds.), *Guide to pain management in low-resource settings* (pp. 189–194). Seattle, WA: International Association for the Study of Pain.

Hahn, K. (2011). Rational polypharmacy. *Integrative Pain Practitioner, 21*(4), 38–41.

Hallingbye, T., Martin, J., & Viscomi, C. (2011). Acute postoperative pain management in the older patient. *Aging Health, 7*(6), 813–828.

Hardy, S. E., & Studenski, S. A. (2008). Fatigue predicts mortality in older adults. *Journal of the American*

Geriatrics Society, 56(10), 1910–1914. doi:10.1111/j.1532-5415.2008.01957.x.

Hardy, S. E., & Studenski, S. A. (2010). Qualities of fatigue and associated chronic conditions among older adults. Journal of Pain Symptom Management, 39(6), 1033–1042. doi:10.1016/j.jpainsymman.2009.09.026.

Harsora, P., & Kessmann, J. (2009). Nonpharmacologic management of chronic insomnia. American Family Physician, 79(2), 125–130.

Hauser, W., Klose, P., Langhorst, J., Moradi, B., Steinbach, M., Schiltenwolf, M., & Busch, A. (2010). Efficacy of different types of aerobic exercise in fibromyalgia syndrome: A systematic review and meta-analysis of randomized controlled trials. Arthritis Research and Therapy, 12, R79. doi:10.1186/ar3002.

Hebert, K., Moore, H., & Rooney, J. (2011). The nurse advocate in end-of-life care. Ochsner Journal, 11(4), 325–329.

Helms, J. E., & Barone, C. P. (2008). Physiology and treatment of pain. Critical Care Nurse, 28(6), 38–49.

Henrotin, Y., Mobasheri, A., & Marty, M. (2012). Is there any scientific evidence for the use of glucosamine in the management of human osteoarthritis? Arthritis Research and Therapy, 14(1), 201. doi:10.1186/ar3657.

HermanMiller. (2010). Patient rooms: A changing scene of healing research summary. Retrieved from http://www.hermanmiller.com/MarketFacingTech/hmc/research/research_summaries/assets/wp_Patient_Rooms.pdf.

Hoebert, M., van der Heijden, K. B., van Geijlswijk, I. M., & Smits, M. G. (2009). Long-term follow-up of melatonin treatment in children with ADHD and chronic sleep onset insomnia. Journal of Pineal Research, 47(1), 1–7. doi:10.1111/j.1600-079X.2009.00681.x.

Hooten, W. M., Qu, W., Townsend, C. O., & Judd, J. W. (2012). Effects of strength vs. aerobic exercise on pain severity in adults with fibromyalgia: A randomized equivalence trial. Pain, 153(4), 915–923. doi:10.1016/j.pain.2012.01.020.

Hospice Foundation of America. (2013). What is hospice? Retrieved from http://www.hospicefoundation.org/.

Huisinga, J. M., Filipi, M. L., & Stergiou, N. (2011). Elliptical exercise improves fatigue ratings and quality of life in patients with multiple sclerosis. Journal of Rehabilitation Research and Development, 48(7), 881–890. doi:10.1682/JRRD.2010.08.0152.

Institute of Medicine. (2003). When children die: Improving palliative and end-of-life care for children and their families. Washington, DC: National Academies Press.

Institute of Medicine. (2006). Sleep disorders and sleep deprivation: An unmet public health problem. Washington, DC: National Academies Press.

Institute of Medicine. (2011). Relieving pain in America. Washington, DC: National Academies Press.

International Association for the Study of Pain. (2007). Differences in pain between men and women. Retrieved from http://www.iasp-pain.org/AM/Template.cfm?Section=Real_Women_Real_Pain&Template=/CM/ContentDisplay.cfm&ContentID=4503.

International Association for the Study of Pain. (2009). Barriers to cancer pain treatment. Retrieved from http://www.iasp-pain.org/AM/Template.cfm?Section=Fact_Sheets1&Template=/CM/ContentDisplay.cfm&ContentID=7189.

International Association for the Study of Pain. (2012). IASP taxonomy. Retrieved from http://www.iasp-pain.org/AM/Template.cfm?Section=Pain_Definitions.

International Council of Nurses. (1997). Basic principles of nursing care. Washington, DC: American Nurses Publishing.

Jarzyna, D., Jungquist, C. R., Pasero, C., Willens, J. S., Nisbet, A., Oakes, L., . . . Polomano, R. C. (2011). American Society for Pain Management nursing guidelines on monitoring opioid-induced sedation and respiratory depression. Pain Management Nursing, 12(3), 118–145. doi:10.1016/j.pmn.2011.06.008.

Jensen, M. P., Gammaitoni, A. R., Olaleye, D. O., Oleka, N., Nalamachu, S. R., & Galer, B. S. (2006). The pain quality assessment scale: Assessment of pain quality in carpal tunnel syndrome. Journal of Pain, 7(11), 823–832. doi:10.1016/j.jpain.2006.04.003.

Johns, M.W. (1991). A new method for measuring daytime sleepiness: The Epworth sleepiness scale. Sleep, 14(6), 540–545.

The Joint Commission. (2012). Facts about pain management. Retrieved February 4, 2013, from http://www.jointcommission.org/pain_management/.

Jong, E., Oudhoff, L. A., Epskamp, C., Wagenerd, M. N., van Duijne, M., Fischerg, S., & van Gorp, E. C. (2010). Predictors and treatment strategies of HIV-related fatigue in the combined antiretroviral therapy era. AIDS, 24(10), 1387–1405.

Kargarfard, M., Etemadifar, M., Baker, P., Mehrabi, M., & Hayatbakhsh, R. (2012). Effect of aquatic exercise training on fatigue and health-related quality of life in patients with multiple sclerosis. Archives of Physical Medicine and Rehabilitation, 93(10), 1701–1708. doi:10.1016/j.apmr.2012.05.006.

Kashikar-Zuck, S., Parkins, I. S., Ting, T. V., Verkamp, E., Lynch-Jordan, A., Passo, M., & Graham, T. B. (2010). Controlled follow-up study of physical and psychosocial functioning of adolescents with juvenile primary fibromyalgia syndrome. Rheumatology (Oxford), 49(11), 2204–2209. doi:10.1093/rheumatology/keq254.

Kingsley, J. D., McMillan, V., & Figueroa, A. (2010). The effects of 12 weeks of resistance exercise training on disease severity and autonomic modulation at rest and after acute leg resistance exercise in women with fibromyalgia. Archives of Physical Medicine and Rehabilitation, 91(10), 1551–1557. doi:10.1016/j.apmr.2010.07.003.

Kline, C. E., Ewing, G. B., Burch, J. B., Blair, S. N., Durstine, J. L., Davis, J. M., & Yongstedt, S. D. (2012). Exercise training improves selected aspects of daytime functioning in adults with obstructive sleep apnea. Journal of Clinical Sleep Medicine, 8(4), 357–365. doi:10.5664/jcsm.2022.

Kolcaba, K., Tilton, C., & Drouin, C. (2006). Comfort Theory: A unifying framework to enhance the practice environment. Journal of Nursing Administration, 36(11), 538–544.

Kutner, J. S., Smith, M. C., Corbin, L., Hemphill, L., Benton, K., Mellis, B. K., . . . Fairclough, D. L. (2008). Massage therapy versus simple touch to improve pain and mood in patients with advanced cancer: A randomized trial. Annals of Internal Medicine, 149(6), 369–379.

Lande, R. G., & Gragnani, C. (2010). Nonpharmacologic approaches to the management of insomnia. Journal of the American Osteopathic Association, 110(12), 695–701.

Lee, K. J., Tieves, K., & Scanlon, M. C. (2010). Alterations in end-of-life support in the pediatric intensive care unit. Pediatrics, 126(4), e859–e864. doi:10.1542/peds.2010-0420.

Lehto, R. H., & Stein, K. F. (2009). Death anxiety: An analysis of an evolving concept. Research and Theory for Nursing Practice, 23(1), 23–41. doi:10.1891/1541-6577.23.1.23.

Manchikanti, L., Abdi, S., Atluri, S., Balog, C. C., Benyamin, R. M., Boswell, M. V., . . . Wargo, B. W. (2012). American Society of Interventional Pain Physicians (ASIPP) guidelines for responsible opioid prescribing in chronic non-cancer pain: Part 2—Guidance. Pain Physician, 15(Suppl. 3), S67–S116.

Mathew, P. J., & Mathew, J. L. (2003). Assessment and management of pain in infants. Postgraduate Medical Journal, 79, 438–443. doi:10.1136/pmj.79.934.438.

Mayo Clinic. (2010a). Fatigue. Retrieved February 4, 2013, from http://www.mayoclinic.com/health/fatigue/MY00120.

Mayo Clinic. (2010b). Fatigue causes. Retrieved from http://www.mayoclinic.com/health/fatigue/MY00120/DSECTION=causes.

Mayo Clinic. (2010c). Stress relief from laughter? Yes, no joke. Retrieved February 4, 2013, from http://www.mayoclinic.com/health/stress-relief/SR00034.

Mayo Clinic. (2011a). Polysomnography. Retrieved February 4, 2013, from http://www.mayoclinic.com/health/polysomnography/MY00970/DSECTION=results.

Mayo Clinic. (2011b). Positive thinking: Reduce stress by eliminating negative self-talk. Retrieved February 4, 2013, from http://www.mayoclinic.com/health/positive-thinking/SR00009.

Mayo Clinic. (2011c). Relaxation techniques: Try these steps to reduce stress. Retrieved February 4, 2013, from http://www.mayoclinic.com/health/relaxation-technique/SR00007.

McCaffery, M. (1968). Nursing practice theories related to cognition, bodily pain, and man-environment interactions. Los Angeles: University of California at Los Angeles Students' Store.

McCarberg, B. H. (2008). What are we afraid of? Barriers to providing adequate pain relief. Retrieved from Medscape Neurology, http://www.medscape.org/viewarticle/571671.

McDonald, A. A., & Portenoy, R. K. (2006). How to use antidepressants and anticonvulsants as adjuvant analgesics in the treatment of neuropathic cancer pain. Journal of Supportive Oncology, 4(1), 43–52.

MedlinePlus. (2011). Glucosamine sulfate. Retrieved February 26, 2013, from http://www.nlm.nih.gov/medlineplus/druginfo/natural/807.htm.

MedlinePlus. (2012). Chronic fatigue syndrome. Retrieved February 4, 2013, from http://www.nlm.nih.gov/medlineplus/ency/article/001244.htm.

Meghani, S. H., Byun, E., & Gallagher, R. M. (2012). Time to take stock: A meta-analysis and systematic review of analgesic treatment disparities for pain in the United States. Pain Medicine, 13(2), 150–174. doi:10.1111/j.1526-4637.2011.01310.x.

Melzack, R., & Wall, P. D. (1965). Pain mechanisms: A new theory. Science, 150(3699), 971–979.

Merriman, J. (2009). How does ethnicity affect sleep disorders? Pulmonary Reviews, 14(8), 12–13.

Michelson, K. N., Patel, R., Haber-Barker, N., Emanuel, L., & Frader, J. (2013). End-of-life care decisions in the PICU: Roles professionals play. Pediatric Critical Care Medicine, 14(1), e34–e44. doi:10.1097/PCC.0b013e31826e7408.

Moreh, E., Jacobs, J. M., & Stessman, J. (2010). Fatigue, function, and mortality in older adults. Journals of Gerontology Series A: Biological Sciences and Medical Sciences, 65A(8), 887–895. doi:10.1093/gerona/glq064.

Naghib, S., van der Starre, C., Gischler, S. J., Joosten, K. F., & Tibboel, D. (2010). Mortality in very long-stay pediatric intensive care unit patients and incidence of withdrawal of treatment. Intensive Care Medicine, 36(1), 131–136. doi:10.1007/s00134-009-1693-z.

NANDA-I. (2012). Nursing diagnoses definitions and classifications 2012–2014. West Sussex, UK: Wiley.

Narayan, M. C. (2010). Culture's effects on pain assessment and management. American Journal of Nursing, 110(4), 38–47.

National Cancer Institute. (2012). End-of-life care for people who have cancer. Retrieved February 4, 2013, from http://www.cancer.gov/cancertopics/factsheet/Support/end-of-life-care.

National Cancer Institute. (2013). Pain (PDQ®). Retrieved from http://www.cancer.gov/cancertopics/pdq/supportivecare/pain/HealthProfessional/page1.

National Center for Complementary and Alternative Medicine. (2010). Acupuncture for pain. Retrieved from http://nccam.nih.gov/health/acupuncture/acupuncture-for-pain.htm.

National Center for Complementary and Alternative Medicine. (2011). *Relaxation techniques for health: An introduction.* Retrieved February 4, 2013, from http://nccam.nih.gov/health/stress/relaxation.htm.

National Center for Complementary and Alternative Medicine. (2012). *Fibromyalgia and complementary health approaches.* Retrieved from http://nccam.nih.gov/health/pain/fibromyalgia.htm.

National Consensus Project for Quality Palliative Care. (2009). *Clinical practice guidelines for quality palliative care* (2nd ed.). Pittsburgh, PA: National Consensus Project for Quality Palliative Care.

National Fibromyalgia Association. (n.d.). *Prevalence.* Retrieved February 4, 2013, from http://fmaware.org/PageServera6cc.html?pagename=fibromyalgia_affected.

National Hospice and Palliative Care Organization. (2012). *NHPCO facts and figures: Hospice care in America.* Retrieved from http://www.nhpco.org/sites/default/files/public/Statistics_Research/2012_Facts_Figures.pdf.

National Institute of Neurological Disorders and Stroke. (2011). *Central Pain Syndrome Information Page.* Retrieved from http://www.ninds.nih.gov/disorders/central_pain/central_pain.htm.

National Institute on Drug Abuse. (2012). *DrugFacts: Nationwide trends.* Retrieved from www.drugabuse.gov/publications/drugfacts/nationwide-trends.

National Institutes of Health. (2013). Genetics home reference: SCN9A. Retrieved from http://ghr.nlm.nih.gov/gene/SCN9A.

National Sleep Foundation. (n.d.). *Pregnancy and sleep.* Retrieved February 15, 2013, from http://www.sleepfoundation.org/article/sleep-topics/pregnancy-and-sleep.

National Sleep Foundation. (2004). *2004 Sleep in America poll.* Retrieved from http://www.sleepfoundation.org/sites/default/files/FINAL%20SOF%202004.pdf.

National Sleep Foundation. (2010). *2010 Sleep in America poll.* Retrieved from http://www.sleepfoundation.org/sites/default/files/nsaw/NSF%20Sleep%20in%20%20America%20Poll%20-%20Summary%20of%20Findings%20.pdf.

National Sleep Foundation. (2011). *How much sleep do we really need?* Retrieved from http://www.sleepfoundation.org/article/how-sleep-works/how-much-sleep-do-we-really-need.

Neikrug, A. B., & Ancoli-Israel, S. (2010). Sleep disorders in the older adults—A mini-review. *Gerontology, 56*(2), 181–189. doi:10.1159/000236900.

Nishino, S., Okuro, M., Kotorii, N., Anegawa, E., Ishimaru, Y., Matsumura, M., & Kanbayashi, T. (2010). Hypocretin/orexin and narcolepsy: New basic and clinical insights. *Acta Physiologica (Oxford, England), 198*(3), 209–222. doi:10.1111/j.1748-1716.2009.02012.x.

Noel, M., Chambers, C. T., McGrath, P. J., Klein, R. M., & Stewart, S. H. (2012). The influence of children's pain memories on subsequent pain experience. *Pain, 153*(8), 1563–1572. doi:10.1016/j.pain.2012.02.020.

Norlander, L. (2008). *To comfort always: A nurse's guide to end-of-life care.* Indianapolis, IN: Sigma Theta Tau International.

Notcutt, W., & Gibbs, G. (2010). Inadequate pain management: Myth, stigma and professional fear. *Postgraduate Medical Journal, 86*(1018), 453–458. doi:10.1136/pgmj.2008.077677.

Park, J., & Hughes, A. K. (2012). Nonpharmacological approaches to the management of chronic pain in community-dwelling older adults: A review of empirical evidence. *Journal of the American Geriatric Society, 60*(3), 555–568. doi:10.1111/j.1532-5415.2011.03846.x.

Pawar, D., & Garten, L. (2010). Pain management in children. In A. Kopf & N. B. Patel (Eds.), *Guide to pain management in low-resource settings* (pp. 255–268). Seattle, WA: International Association for the Study of Pain.

Plaisance, L., & Logan, C. (2006). Nursing students' knowledge and attitudes regarding pain. *Pain Management Nursing, 7*(4), 167–175.

Ram, S., Seirawan, H., Kumar, S. K., & Clark, G. T. (2010). Prevalence and impact of sleep disorders and sleep habits in the United States. *Sleep and Breathing, 14*(1), 63–70. doi:10.1007/s11325-009-0281-3.

Rastogi, R., & Meek, B. D. (2013). Management of chronic pain in elderly, frail patients: Finding a suitable, personalized method of control. *Journal of Clinical Interventions in Aging, 8,* 37–46. doi:10.2147/cia.s30165.

Renjilian, C. B., Womer, J. W., Carroll, K. W., Kang, T. I., & Feudtner, C. (2013). Parental explicit heuristics in decision-making for children with life-threatening illnesses. *Pediatrics, 131*(2), e566–e572. doi:10.1542/peds.2012-1957.

Rocha, E. M., Marche, T. A., & von Baeyer, C. L. (2009). Anxiety influences children's memory for procedural pain. *Pain Research and Management, 14*(3), 233–237.

Rogers, A. E. (2008). The effects of fatigue and sleepiness on nurse performance and patient safety. In R. G. Hughes (Ed.), *Patient safety and quality: An evidence-based handbook for nurses* (Chapter 40). Rockville, MD: Agency for Healthcare Research and Quality.

Rondanelli, M., Opizzi, A., Monteferrario, F., Antonielo, N., Manni, R., & Klersy, C. (2011). The effect of melatonin, magnesium, and zinc on primary insomnia in long-term care facility residents in Italy: A double-blind, placebo-controlled clinical trial. *Journal of the American Geriatrics Society, 59*(1), 82–90. doi:10.1111/j.1532-5415.2010.03232.x.

Rossignol, D. A., & Frye, R. E. (2011). Melatonin in autism spectrum disorders: A systematic review and meta-analysis. *Developmental Medicine and Child Neurology, 53*(9), 783–792. doi:10.1111/j.1469-8749.2011.03980.x.

Schutte-Rodin, S., Broch, L., Buysse, D., Dorsey, C., Sateia, M. (2008). Clinical guideline for the evaluation and management of chronic insomnia in adults. *Journal of Clinical Sleep Medicine, 4*(5), 487–504.

Searight, H. R., & Gafford, J. (2005). Cultural diversity at the end of life: Issues and guidelines for family physicians. *American Family Physician, 71*(3), 515–522.

Seifert, P. C., & Hickman, D. S. (2005). Enhancing patient safety in a healing environment. *Topics in Advanced Practice Nursing eJournal, 5.* Retrieved from http://www.medscape.com/viewarticle/499690.

Serlin, R. C., Mendoza, T. R., Nakamura, Y., Edwards, K. R., & Cleeland, C. S. (1995). When is cancer pain mild, moderate, or severe? Grading pain severity by its interference with function. *Pain, 61*(2), 277–284. doi:10.1016/0304-3959(94)00178-H.

Shen, H., He, M. M., Liu, H., Wrighton, S. A., Wang, L., Guo, B., & Li, C. (2007). Comparative metabolic capabilities and inhibitory profiles of CYP2D6.1, CYP2D6.10, and CYP2D6.17. *Drug Metabolism and Disposition, 35*(8), 1292–1300. doi:10.1124/dmd.107.015354.

Sherman, D. W., Norman, R., & McSherry, C. B. (2010). A comparison of death anxiety and quality of life of patients with advanced cancer or AIDS and their family caregivers. *Journal of the Association of Nurses in AIDS Care, 21*(2), 99–112. doi:10.1016/j.jana.2009.07.007.

Simon, N. (2011). 6 ways to feel happier, be healthier. *AARP Bulletin,* May 13.

Sinatra, R. (2010). Causes and consequences of inadequate management of acute pain. *Pain Medicine, 11*(12), 1859–1871. doi:10.1111/j.1526-4637.2010.00983.x.

Slomka, J. (2003). Withholding nutrition at the end of life: Clinical and ethical issues. *Cleveland Clinic Journal of Medicine, 70*(6), 548–552.

Smith, A. K., White, P. D., Aslakson, E., Vollmer-Conna, U., & Rajeevan, M. S. (2006). Polymorphisms in genes regulating the HPA axis associated with empirically delineated classes of unexplained chronic fatigue. *Pharmacogenomics, 7*(3), 387–394. doi:10.2217/14622416.7.3.387.

Smith, H. S., Harris, R., & Clauw, D. (2011). Fibromyalgia: An afferent processing disorder leading to a complex pain generalized syndrome. *Pain Physician, 14,* E217–E245.

Spear, F. G. (1977). Cultural factors in clinical pain assessment. *International Dental Journal, 27*(3), 284–287.

Stevens, B. (1990). Development and testing of a pediatric pain management sheet. *Pediatric Nursing, 16*(6), 543–548.

Taylor, D. J., Schmidt-Nowara, W., Jessop, C. A., & Ahearn, J. (2010). Sleep restriction therapy and hypnotic withdrawal versus sleep hygiene education in hypnotic using patients with insomnia. *Journal of Clinical Sleep Medicine, 6*(2), 169–175.

Tennant, F. (2004). *Complications of uncontrolled, persistent pain.* Retrieved from Practical Pain Management Web site, http://www.practicalpainmanagement.com/pain/other/co-morbidities/complications-uncontrolled-persistent-pain.

Tennant, F. (2008). *Using objective signs of severe pain to guide opioid prescribing.* Retrieved from Pain Treatment Topics, http://pain-topics.org/pdf/Tennant-PainSigns.pdf.

Teno, J. M., Clarridge, B. R., Casey, V., Welch, L. C., Wetle, T., Shield, R., & Mor, V. (2004). Family perspectives on end-of-life care at the last place of care. *Journal of the American Medical Association, 291*(1), 88–93. doi:10.1001/jama.291.1.88.

Twisk, F. N., & Maes, M. (2009). A review on cognitive behavioral therapy (CBT) and graded exercise therapy (GET) in myalgic encephalomyelitis (ME)/chronic fatigue syndrome (CFS): CBT/GET is not only ineffective and not evidence-based, but also potentially harmful for many patients with ME/CFS. *Neuroendocrinology Letters, 30*(3), 284–299.

U.S. National Library of Medicine. (2011). *Fatigue.* Retrieved from http://www.nlm.nih.gov/medlineplus/ency/article/003088.htm.

University of Maryland Medical Center. (2013). *Sleepiness scale.* Retrieved from http://umm.edu/programs/sleep/health/quizzes/sleepiness.

Vallejo, R., Barkin, R. L., & Wang, V. C. (2011). Pharmacology of opioids in the treatment of chronic pain syndromes. *Pain Physician, 14,* e343–e360.

van Aken, H., Thys, L., Veekman, L., & Buerkle, H. (2004). Assessing analgesia in single and repeated administrations of propacetamol for postoperative pain: Comparison with morphine after dental surgery. *Anesthesia and Analgesia, 98*(1), 159–165. doi:10.1213/01.ANE.0000093312.72011.59.

Vandermeulen, E. (2006). Systemic analgesia and co-algesia. *Acta Anaesthesiologica Belgica, 57,* 113–120.

Vargas-Alarcon, G., Alvarez-Leon, E., Fragoso, J. M., Vargas, A., Martinez, A., Vallejo, M., & Martinez-Lavin, M. (2012). A SCN9A gene-encoded dorsal root ganglia sodium channel polymorphism associated with severe fibromyalgia. *BMC Musculoskeletal Disorders, 13,* 23. doi:10.1186/1471-2474-13-23.

Vickers, A., Zollman, C., & Payne, D. K. (2001). Hypnosis and relaxation therapies. *Western Journal of Medicine, 175*(4), 269–272.

Voigt, L., Paice, J. A., & Pouliot, J. (1995). Standardized pain flowsheet: Impact on patient-reported pain experiences after cardiovascular surgery. *American Journal of Critical Care, 4*(4), 308–313.

Weiner, J., Sharma, J., Lantos, J., & Kilbride, H. (2011). How infants die in the neonatal intensive care unit:

Trends from 1999 through 2008. *Archives of Pediatrics and Adolescent Medicine, 165*(7), 630–634. doi:10.1001/archpediatrics.2011.102.

White, P. D., Goldsmith, K. A., Johnson, A. L., Potts, L., Walwyn, R., DeCesare, J. C., . . . Sharpe, M. (2011). Comparison of adaptive pacing therapy, cognitive behavior therapy, graded exercise therapy, and specialist medical care for chronic fatigue syndrome (PACE): A randomized trial. *Lancet, 377*(9768), 823–836. doi:10.1016/S0140-6736(11)60096-2.

Williams, R., IV, Lim, J. E., Harr, B., Wing, C., Walters, R., Distler, M. G., . . . Palmer, A. A. (2009). A common and unstable copy number variant is associated with differences in Glo1 expression and anxiety-like behavior. *PLoS One, 4*(3), e4649. doi:10.1371/journal.pone.0004649.

Wilson, B. A., Shannon, M. T., & Shields, K. M. (2013). *Nurse's drug guide*. Upper Saddle River, NJ: Pearson Education.

Wolfe, F., Clauw, D. J., Fitzcharles, M-A., Goldenberg, D. L., Katz, R. S., Mease, P. . . . Yunus, M. B. (2010). The American College of Rheumatology preliminary diagnostic criteria for fibromyalgia and measurement of symptom severity. *Arthritis Care and Research, 62*(5), 600–610. doi:10.1002/acr.20140.

Wolfe, F., Smythe, H. A., Yunus, M. B., Bennett, R. M., Bombardier, C., Goldenberg, D. L., . . . Sheon, R. P. (1990). The American College of Rheumatology 1990 criteria for the classification of fibromyalgia. *Arthritis and Rheumatism, 33*(2), 160–172. doi:10.1002/art.1780330203.

World Health Organization. (n.d.a). *Palliative care*. Retrieved from http://www.who.int/cancer/palliative/en/.

World Health Organization. (n.d.b). *WHO's pain ladder*. Retrieved from http://www.who.int/cancer/palliative/painladder/en/.

Pearson Nursing Student Resources   Find additional review materials at: **nursing.pearsonhighered.com**

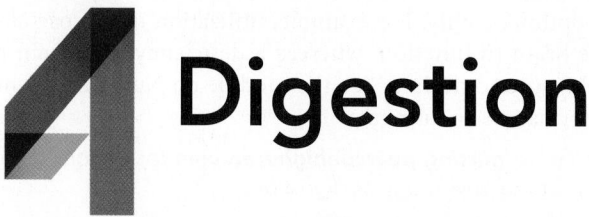# Digestion

◨ THE CONCEPT OF DIGESTION

Digestion refers to the conversion of food into absorbable substances in the gastrointestinal (GI) tract. Digestion occurs through the mechanical and chemical breakdown of food into smaller molecules, with the help of glands located inside and outside the stomach. Digestion is an integrated process that affects the entire human body. Alterations in digestion occur when one or more of the processes that allow the body to break down food and absorb nutrients are impaired. Impairments in digestion may be caused by changes in nutritional status, structural (anatomical) alterations, or as a result of the effects of one or more medications. Because of the prevalence of alterations in digestion, nurses must be knowledgeable about different alterations and their risk factors and be able to assess how alterations in digestion affect other physiological processes. By utilizing critical thinking through the nursing process to make decisions about the care of clients across the life span who are experiencing alterations in digestion, nurses can engage with clients to optimize their health and well-being. **<<**

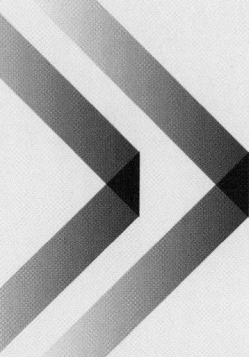

Concept Learning Outcomes

After reading about this concept, you will be able to:

1. Summarize the physiological processes of the gastrointestinal system related to digestion.
2. Examine the relationship between digestion and other systems.
3. Identify commonly occurring alterations in digestion and their related treatments.
4. Differentiate common physical assessment procedures used to examine digestive health across the life span.
5. Describe diagnostic and laboratory tests used to determine the individual's digestion status.
6. Explain management of digestive health and prevention of digestive illnesses.
7. Demonstrate the nursing process in providing culturally competent care across the life span for individuals with common alterations in digestion.
8. Compare and contrast common independent and collaborative interventions for clients with alterations in digestive function.

Concept Key Terms

Absorption, *210*
Acid indigestion, *210*
Anorexia, *210*
Body mass index (BMI), *219*
Digestion, *207*
Enteral nutrition, *222*
Enzymes, *208*
Fluoroscope, *220*
Gastroesophageal reflux disease (GERD), *210*
Heartburn, *210*

Hepatitis, *211*
Malabsorption, *211*
Maldigestion, *211*
Motility, *210*
Nausea, *210*
Nutrients, *208*
Pancreatitis, *211*
Parenteral nutrition (PN), *224*
Pyloric stenosis, *213*
Vomiting, *210*

▶ NORMAL DIGESTION

Physiology Review

The digestive system consists of the mouth, pharynx, esophagus, stomach, small intestine, and large intestine (**Figure 4–1 ●**). Accessory organs such as the liver, gallbladder, and pancreas assist in the normal digestive process. **Nutrients** are substances found in food that are used by the body to promote normal growth, maintenance, and repair. Nutrients include carbohydrates, proteins, fats, vitamins, minerals, and water. The digestive system participates in providing the body with nutrition, balancing fluids and electrolytes, and eliminating waste products. The digestive system works congruently with the metabolic system for secretion of digestive **enzymes**, which assist in digestion of nutrients. Appropriate amounts and proper utilization of nutrients allow the body to function at optimal ability. For example, utilization of glucose allows the brain to function, whereas a deficiency in protein may delay wound healing. See the module on Nutrition for more information on nutrients.

✳ *Go to* **nursing.pearsonhighered.com** *for a more detailed look at the physiology of digestion.*

✺ **Stay Current:** *Nurses must know how to find credible sources of information and be able to direct clients to seek information about good nutrition. Sources of information that may be helpful include the Centers for Disease Control and Prevention's Nutrition for Everyone Web site at* **www.cdc.gov/nutrition/everyone/basics/index.html** *and the USDA's Food and Nutrition Information Center at* **http://fnic.nal.usda.gov**.

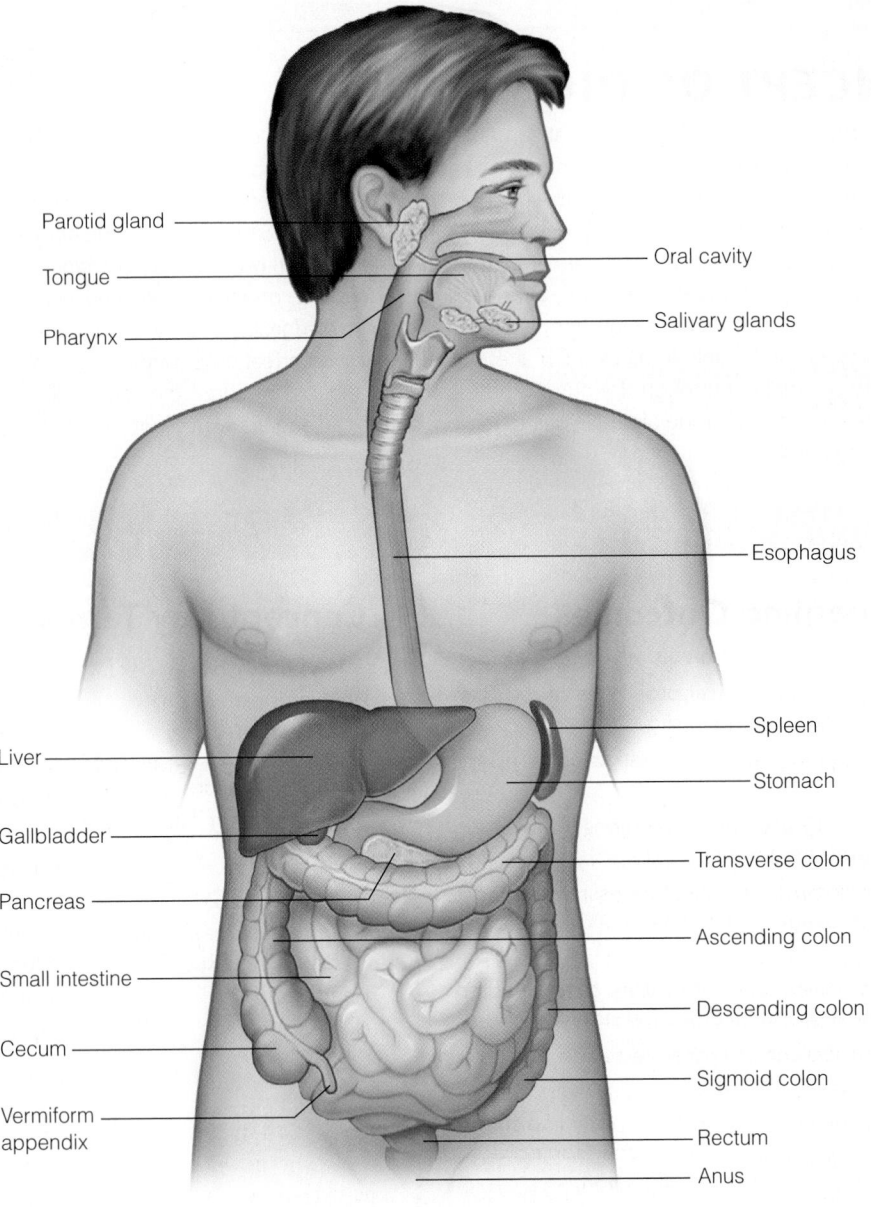

Parotid gland

Tongue

Pharynx

Oral cavity

Salivary glands

Esophagus

Spleen

Stomach

Liver

Gallbladder

Pancreas

Small intestine

Cecum

Vermiform appendix

Transverse colon

Ascending colon

Descending colon

Sigmoid colon

Rectum

Anus

Figure 4–1 ● Organs of the alimentary canal and related accessory organs.

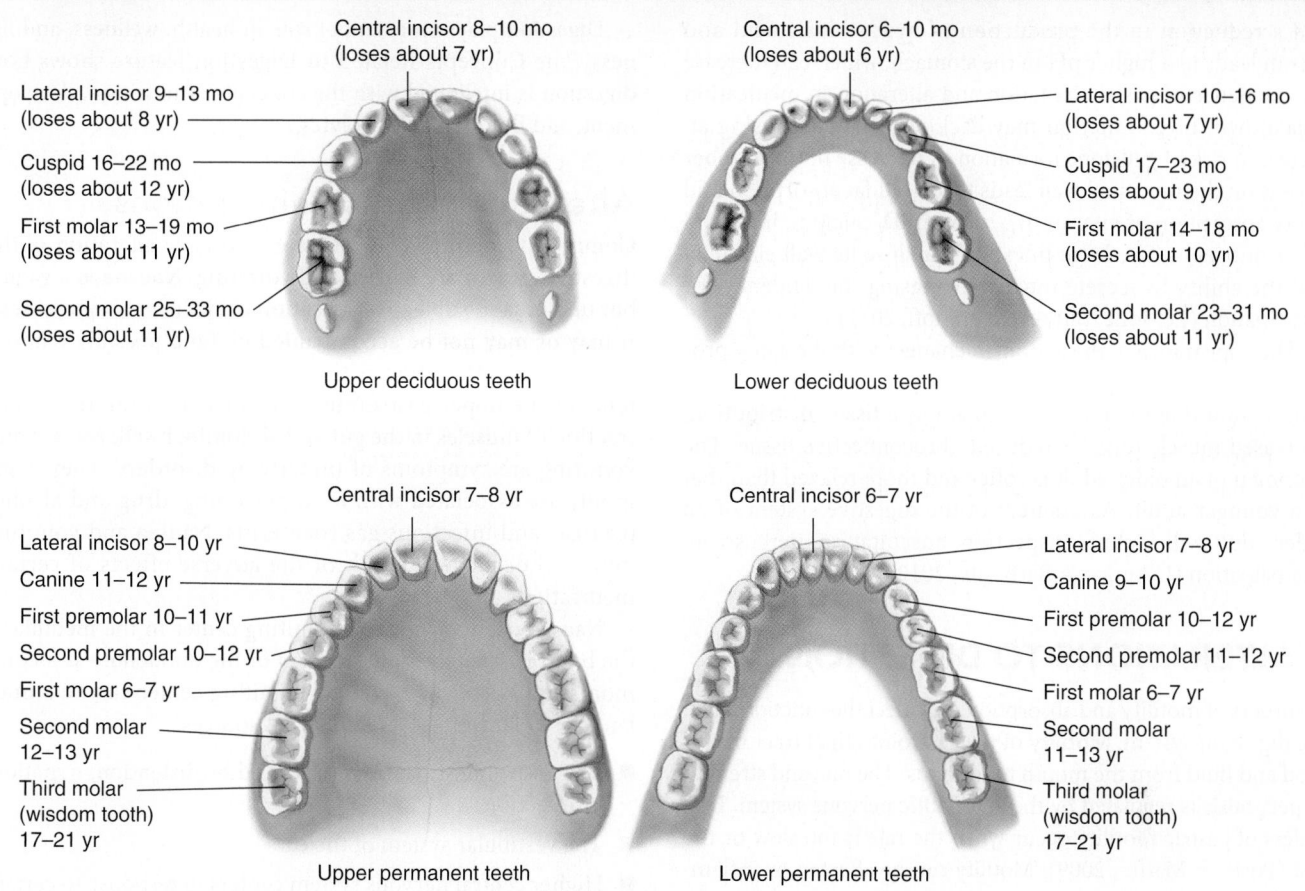

Figure 4–2 ● Typical sequence of tooth eruption for both deciduous and permanent teeth. The bottom deciduous teeth are shed before upper teeth, and bottom permanent teeth erupt first as well.

Genetic and Lifespan Considerations

Variations in the digestive system occur throughout the life span. Growth and development of the individual impacts digestive ability. Age, along with a number of acute and chronic illnesses of the digestive tract, can affect children, pregnant women, developing fetuses, and adults, causing difficulty with absorption of nutrients or motility, thereby affecting overall health. Genetics plays a role in diseases of the digestive system, impacting digestion and absorption of nutrients. Gene and chromosomal alterations in the digestive system can result in Crohn's disease and glucose galactose malabsorption (GGM). The occurrence of Crohn's disease is familial, sparking research to determine genetic abnormalities. The disease has been connected to alterations in chromosome 16, which is responsible for the inflammatory response. The *SGLT1* gene on chromosome 22 is altered in individuals with GGM, resulting in the inability of glucose and galactose to leave the small intestine and the pulling of water into the small intestine causing diarrhea (National Center for Biotechnology Information, 2012).

INFANTS AND CHILDREN The digestive system in a newborn is immature because, until birth, the placenta provides nutrients and removal of waste products. Voluntary control over swallowing does not occur until about 6 weeks of age. The infant's tongue is larger in comparison to the nasal and oral passages. The stomach capacity of a newborn is quite small, holding only 10 to 20 mL at a time, requiring frequent feedings. Teeth

begin to erupt around 6 months of life. By the end of the first year, the infant usually has six to eight teeth (**Figure 4–2 ●**). Most children have a complete set of primary teeth by 3–6 years of age (Raising Children Network, 2013).

Infants have a deficiency of the amylase, lipase, and trypsin enzymes. Enzymes from the pancreas will not be sufficient to aid in digestion until 4–6 months in age. Lack of enzyme production results in frequent abdominal distention and flatulence. Infants have an immature liver. After the first few weeks of life, the infant's liver is able to conjugate bilirubin and excrete bile. Gluconeogenesis, ketone formation, vitamin storage, and myelination remain immature during the first year of life.

By the age of 2, a child's digestive processes generally are complete and he can adapt to a typical schedule of three meals per day. Myelination of the spinal cord allows the child to begin to achieve control over elimination, typically resulting in complete voluntary control by the age of 3.

OLDER ADULTS As the individual ages, many changes occur in the digestive system. Taste can become less acute due to the natural atrophy of the tongue. Tooth enamel can become more brittle, and loss of bone supporting teeth may result in loss of some or all permanent teeth. Saliva production can decrease by as much as one third, which may increase chewing and swallowing time. Esophageal motility may decrease, and a weaker gag reflex can cause discomfort when swallowing, increasing the risk of aspiration. Mucosa in the stomach atrophies, and a reduction in the production of hydrochloric acid and pepsin leads to a higher pH in the stomach, which can increase the incidence of gastric irritation and alteration in medication breakdown. Liver function may decline with age, causing an increased risk of gallstone formation. A decrease in the number of cells on the intestinal wall leads to slowed fat absorption and faulty absorption of vitamin B_{12}, vitamin D, calcium, iron, and other nutrients. The large intestine may lose its wall elasticity and the ability to secrete mucus, increasing the tendency for constipation (LeMone, Burke, & Bauldoff, 2011).

The appearance of the abdomen changes with the aging process. In the older adult, the abdomen may be more rounded and protuberant due to an increase in adipose tissue distribution, decreased muscle tone, or reduced fibroconnective tissue. The abdomen of an older adult is softer and more relaxed than that of a younger adult. Assessment of the digestive system of an older adult will include inspection, auscultation, percussion, and palpation (D'Amico & Barbarito, 2012).

▶ ALTERATIONS TO DIGESTION

Disorders of motility and absorption can affect the functioning of the digestion system. **Motility** of the gastrointestinal tract moves food and fluid from the mouth to the anus. The rate and strength of peristalsis is regulated by the autonomic nervous system. Disorders of gastric motility occur when the rate is too slow or too fast (Porth & Matfin, 2009). Motility can be affected by inflammation, infection, tumors, obstructions, or changes in structure. Direct and indirect factors can influence motility. Food intake and bacteria can affect the number and consistency of stools. Stress and postponement of defecation can influence motility.

Some disorders affecting motility include:

- Gastroesophageal reflux
- Impaired esophageal motility
- Pyloric stenosis
- Diarrhea
- Constipation
- Irritable bowel syndrome
- Encopresis
- Obstructions.

Absorption is defined as "the process of moving nutrients and fluid from the external environment of the gastrointestinal tract to the internal environment" (Porth & Matfin, 2009, p. 600). Absorption occurs through active transport and diffusion. Various medical or surgical conditions can affect absorption of nutrients, resulting in malabsorption. Some disorders affecting absorption include:

- Pernicious anemia
- Lactose intolerance
- Celiac disease
- Crohn's disease
- Gastrectomy
- Acute and chronic pancreatitis
- Liver failure, hepatitis, and cirrhosis.

Digestion plays an essential role in health, wellness, and illness. The Concepts Related to Digestion feature shows how digestion is integrated with the concepts of nutrition, development, and fluids and electrolytes.

Alterations and Manifestations

Common symptoms that indicate a possible alteration of the digestive system are nausea and vomiting. **Nausea** is a vague, but unpleasant, subjective sensation of sickness or queasiness. It may or may not be accompanied by (and possibly relieved by) vomiting. **Vomiting** is the forceful expulsion of the contents of the upper gastrointestinal tract resulting from contraction of muscles in the gut and abdominal wall. Nausea and vomiting are symptoms of underlying disorders. They commonly are associated with food poisoning, drug and alcohol overuse, and infectious gastroenteritis. Nausea and vomiting may also occur as a result of the adverse effects of certain medications.

Nausea occurs when the vomiting center in the medulla of the brain is stimulated. Distention of the duodenum is a common stimulus for nausea. The vomiting center can be stimulated by input from several different sources:

- The gastrointestinal tract produced by distention, irritation, or infection
- The vestibular system of the ear
- Higher central nervous system centers in response to certain sights, smells, or emotional experiences
- Chemoreceptors outside the blood–brain barrier that are stimulated by drugs, chemotherapeutic agents, toxins, systemic disorders, and pregnancy
- Disorders such as acute myocardial infarction and heart failure, which commonly produce nausea and vomiting, possibly due to direct stimulation of the vomiting center by hypoxia
- Increased intracranial pressure (e.g., due to intracranial bleeding or a tumor), which produces vomiting that may or may not be accompanied by nausea.

Anorexia (loss of appetite) commonly precedes nausea, just as nausea frequently precedes vomiting. Vomiting is coordinated by the brainstem. *Emesis* (or *vomitus*) is produced when inspiratory muscles of the thorax (including the diaphragm) and abdomen contract, increasing intrathoracic and intraabdominal pressures. The gastroesophageal sphincter relaxes, and the larynx moves upward to facilitate oral expulsion of gastric contents.

In addition to the subjective sensation of queasiness, nausea frequently is accompanied by autonomic nervous system manifestations such as pallor, sweating, tachycardia, and increased salivation. Vomiting, which stimulates the vagus nerve and parasympathetic nervous system, may be accompanied by dizziness, light-headedness, hypotension, and bradycardia.

In **gastroesophageal reflux disease (GERD)**, stomach contents flow back up into the esophagus. This causes pyrosis or **heartburn**, a burning sensation in the chest or throat. It may also cause **acid indigestion**, which occurs when the individual can taste the stomach acid (National Institutes of Health [NIH], 2011). Treatment ranges from symptom management through

Concepts Related to **Digestion**

Digestion plays an essential role in the body's wellbeing. Nutrition, development, and fluid and electrolytes are directly related to digestion. Digestive processes allow the body to access and absorb nutrients for use. Healthy nutrition is essential for growth and development, with malnutrition increasing the risk for impaired growth and development. Impairments in digestion may result in fluid and electrolyte imbalances, especially impairments that result in vomiting or diarrhea.

CONCEPT	RELATIONSHIP TO DIGESTION	NURSING IMPLICATIONS
Nutrition		
	The ability to digest nutrients provides the body with needed nutrition to maintain normal function.	■ Assess for unplanned weight loss, low body mass index (BMI), infection, and other signs and symptoms of malnutrition. ■ Assess bowel elimination for diarrhea and other malabsorption or digestive problems.
Development		
■ Growth ■ Development	Healthy nutrition and digestion result in normal physical and mental function.	■ Assess height, weight, and mental functioning in developing children. Be alert for children with low height/weight percentages and/or slow mental development. ■ Assess elimination, including diarrhea frequency and other signs indicating digestive abnormalities.
Fluids and Electrolytes		
■ Fluid and electrolyte imbalance	Increased frequency or amount of diarrhea results in fluid and electrolyte imbalances.	■ Assess pattern of bowel elimination. ■ Assess for signs of dehydration including lethargy, poor skin turgor, and low urinary output. ■ Anticipate serum electrolyte tests and electrolyte and fluid supplements.

diet and lifestyle management to pharmacologic therapy and, for some clients, surgery.

Inflammation of the liver is termed **hepatitis**. In hepatitis, the inflammatory process may be triggered by a virus, alcohol, medications, toxins, autoimmune disorder, or other pathogens; the resulting inflammation impacts the liver's ability to function normally. Hepatitis can be acute or chronic. Viral hepatitis is the most common type of hepatitis. Treatment of hepatitis is focused on finding the cause, treating the symptoms, and limiting liver damage.

Malabsorption is a condition in which the intestinal mucosa is unable to absorb nutrients, resulting in nutrients being excreted in the stool. Common systemic manifestations of malabsorption are weight loss, weakness, malaise, muscle cramps, bone pain, abnormal bleeding, and anemia. Selected causes of malabsorption are listed in **Box 4–1** ●.

Maldigestion is a condition in which the preparation of chyme for absorption of nutrients is inadequate, resulting in malabsorption. Selected causes of maldigestion are listed in Box 4–1. See the exemplar on Malabsorption Disorders elsewhere in this module for a discussion of celiac disease, lactase deficiency, and short bowel syndrome.

Pancreatitis, or inflammation of the pancreas, is a condition in which pancreatic cells release pancreatic enzymes into the tissues of the pancreas. Clinical manifestations include abdominal pain, nausea, vomiting, fever, sweating, chills, and fatty stools. Pancreatitis can be acute or chronic.

Acute pancreatitis usually presents with upper abdominal pain. Severe episodes can cause dehydration and low blood

---

Box 4–1   Selected Causes of Malabsorption and Maldigestion

SELECTED CAUSES OF MALABSORPTION	SELECTED CAUSES OF MALDIGESTION
■ Acute enteritis ■ AIDS-related opportunistic infections ■ Celiac disease ■ Crohn's disease ■ Intestinal ischemia or infarction ■ Kaposi sarcoma ■ Scleroderma ■ Short bowel syndrome	■ Biliary obstruction ■ Chronic pancreatitis ■ Cirrhosis or liver failure ■ Cystic fibrosis ■ Gastrectomy ■ Hepatitis ■ Lactose intolerance ■ Pancreatic cancer ■ Zollinger-Ellison syndrome

Alterations and Therapies **Digestion**

ALTERATION	DESCRIPTION	MANIFESTATIONS	THERAPIES
Nausea	Uneasy feeling in the stomach, usually preceding vomiting	Distaste for food May be accompanied by the urge to vomit Abdominal discomfort	▪ Monitor complaints of nausea, remembering that nausea is a subjective sensation best described by the client. ▪ Monitor vital signs, skin turgor and condition, and weight. ▪ Maintain accurate intake and output records. ▪ Monitor amount, color, and specific gravity of urine. ▪ Be aware that nausea can result in dehydration even when not accompanied by vomiting. ▪ Give antiemetics as ordered. ▪ Teach deep breathing to suppress vomiting reflex. ▪ Encourage intake of small quantities of clear fluids and dry foods at separate times to reduce nausea stimulus.

Vomiting	Emptying of stomach contents through the mouth	Expelling stomach contents through the mouth
		Diaphoresis
		Preceding nausea
			▪ Withhold foods initially; give clear liquids in small quantities to prevent dehydration.
			▪ For pediatric clients, administer fluid and electrolyte solution (e.g., Pedialyte). Milk-based infant formula may need to be withheld until symptoms subside.
			▪ Once nausea and vomiting have stopped:
			  • Give clear liquids as tolerated, dry foods (e.g., soda crackers) to reduce nausea and promote comfort.
			  • Introduce bland foods (e.g., rice, applesauce, toast) slowly. Avoid milk products until symptoms disappear.
			  • Reassess need for antiemetic medications.

Gastroesophageal reflux disease (GERD)	Backward flow of stomach contents	Chest discomfort
		Heartburn
		Acid indigestion
			▪ Treatment varies according to severity of the disorder but may include:
			  • Dietary and lifestyle management
			  • Medications
			  • Surgery.

Hepatitis	Inflammation of the liver	Abdominal pain Dark urine Nausea and vomiting Jaundice Fever	▪ Underlying cause and type of hepatitis will dictate treatment. ▪ Acute hepatitis is managed by supportive treatments; chronic hepatitis involves pharmacologic agents that eradicate the virus and prevent further liver damage (Medicine.Net, 2013).

Alterations and Therapies **Digestion** (*continued*)

ALTERATION	DESCRIPTION	MANIFESTATIONS	THERAPIES
Malabsorption disorders	Intestinal mucosa cannot absorb nutrients, which results in the nutrients being excreted in stool.	Diarrhea Weight loss	▪ Underlying cause dictates treatment. In many cases, nutrition management plays an important role in treatment.
Pancreatitis	Inflammation of the pancreas characterized by release of pancreatic enzymes into the pancreatic tissue. May be acute or chronic.	Upper left or midabdominal pain worsening after eating or drinking especially foods with high fat content. Fever Nausea and vomiting Diaphoresis Clay-colored stools if bile duct obstruction occurs	▪ Acute pancreatitis often mild and self-limiting. ▪ Treatment focuses on: • Reducing pancreatic secretions by having the client NPO (nothing by mouth) • Providing supportive care • Eliminating causative factor after resolving inflammation. ▪ Opioid analgesics, fluid replacement and prophylactic antibiotics may be prescribed. ▪ Chronic pancreatitis treatment focuses on managing pain and treating malabsorption and malnutrition: • Opioid analgesics need to be managed carefully to avoid side effects. • Pancreatic enzyme supplements • H_2-blockers and proton pump inhibitors neutralize and reduce gastric secretions.
Pyloric stenosis	Hypertrophic obstruction of the circular muscle of the pyloric canal. Usually diagnosed by 12 weeks of age.	Projectile vomiting Constant hunger Weight loss or inability to gain weight Notable peristaltic wave in abdomen immediately before vomiting occurs.	▪ Restoration of fluid and electrolyte balance followed by surgery to split the pyloric muscle to allow passage of food and fluid.

pressure. Untreated bleeding in the pancreas or organ failure may result. Clients with acute pancreatitis require immediate medical attention (NIH, 2010a). Repeat episodes of acute pancreatitis can lead to chronic pancreatitis.

Chronic pancreatitis presents with upper abdominal pain and chronic weight loss. Common causes of chronic pancreatitis include chronic alcohol abuse, trauma, cystic fibrosis, hyperparathyroidism, and certain medications (e.g., corticosteroids, estrogens, thiazide diuretics). Other conditions can also result in chronic pancreatitis.

Pyloric stenosis is a thickening of the pyloric muscle resulting in a narrowing of the pyloric sphincter between the stomach and small intestine. The condition typically occurs before 6 months of age. Symptoms such as projectile vomiting usually begin around 3 weeks of age, although the onset may vary from 1 week to 5 months of age (NIH, 2013c).

Prevalence

Nausea, vomiting, and diarrhea are common in all age groups. Foods, stress, medications, smells, and tastes are common causes of nausea, vomiting, and diarrhea. Individuals typically avoid foods, tastes, and smells to relieve these symptoms, and many times that is sufficient to resolve the underlying source of distress. Using stress reduction strategies can also relieve nausea, vomiting, and diarrhea. See **Table 4–1** ● for prevalence data about common digestive disorders.

Genetic Considerations and Nonmodifiable Risk Factors

Genetic and nonmodifiable risk factors should be considered when caring for individuals with digestive disorders (**Table 4–2** ●). Early identification of risk factors leads to early intervention

TABLE 4–1   Prevalence of Digestive Disorders

DIGESTIVE DISORDER	PREVALENCE
Gastroesophageal reflux disease	20% of the population exhibit weekly symptoms of acid reflux.*
Viral hepatitis ■ Hepatitis A ■ Hepatitis B ■ Hepatitis C	 17,000 new cases in 2010** 38,000 new cases in 2010; 800,000–1.4 million people living with chronic infection** 17,000 new cases in 2010; 2.7–3.9 million people living with chronic infection
Pancreatitis ■ Acute ■ Chronic	 17 cases/100,000 people* 8.2 cases/100,000 people*

Sources: *National Institutes of Health. (2012). *Digestive diseases statistics for the United States*. Retrieved from http://digestive.niddk.nih.gov/statistics/statistics.aspx.

** Estimated number of new infections in 2010. Centers for Disease Control and Prevention. (2012). *Viral hepatitis statistics & surveillance*. Retrieved from http://www.cdc.gov/hepatitis/Statistics/index.htm.

and disease prevention or lessens the severity of the disease processes. Genetics may play a role in GERD, pyloric stenosis, celiac disease, and pancreatitis.

CASE STUDY \\ PART 1

Jack, a 9-year-old boy, comes home from his afterschool program feeling sick. When his mother asks him what is wrong, he states, "I feel sick to my stomach, I'm tired, and my head hurts." Jack's mother helps him to bed and takes his temperature, which is 102°F. Jack refuses to eat his dinner after a couple of bites. Jack's mother calls you at the health clinic.

Assessment: Jack's parents are Hispanic and came to live in the United States when Jack was 2 years old. Jack and his family travel annually to Mexico to visit grandparents and extended family members. The family returned from Mexico 2 weeks ago. Jack's immunization record is incomplete.

Clinical Reasoning Questions Level I
1. What data points to a possible cause of Jack's illness?
2. What is the priority nursing diagnosis for Jack at this time?

Clinical Reasoning Questions Level II
3. How does Jack's immunization record relate to his signs/symptoms?
4. What independent nursing intervention can you discuss with Jack's mother to help Jack feel more comfortable?
5. What antipyretic medication should you tell Jack's mother to avoid giving to Jack?

▶ PREVENTION

Preventing alterations in digestion involves lifestyle choices and management. Avoiding risk factors in daily life can promote healthy digestion. Identifying causes of a digestive disorder can help determine plans of action to reduce risks. Because digestive disorders have varying etiologies, prevention methods vary. For example, taking steps to prevent conditions leading to pancreatitis, such as gallstones and alcoholism, will prevent pancreatitis (NIH, 2013a). Immunizations (on schedule as recommended for children; before traveling to developing countries for adults) can help to prevent infections with the hepatitis A virus (HAV) and hepatitis B virus (HBV). Collaboration and compliance with health plans to maintain healthy digestion will lessen or prevent complications that can occur with digestive disorders.

Modifiable Risk Factors

Individuals can reduce their risks of developing a digestive disorder through lifestyle choices. Modifiable risk factors can be controlled or altered to reduce the potential for digestive disorders (**Table 4–3 ●**).

Screenings

Individuals suspected of having celiac disease can be screened through blood tests. The primary health care provider may test blood for specific autoantibodies including anti-tissue

TABLE 4–2   Genetic and Nonmodifiable Risk Factors for Digestive Disorders

DIGESTIVE DISORDER	GENETIC FACTORS	NONMODIFIABLE RISK FACTORS
Celiac disease	Approximately 10% of individuals with celiac disease have first-degree family members with the same condition. These family members may wish to be screened (National Digestive Diseases Information Clearinghouse, 2012).	Having a family member with celiac disease
Pancreatitis	A genetic mutation on a gene associated with cystic fibrosis may play a role in pancreatitis. Genetics may play a role in chronic pancreatitis (NIH, 2013a).	Women have a higher incidence of gallstones leading to pancreatitis. African Americans have an increased risk for pancreatitis. Family history of pancreatitis
Pyloric stenosis	Cause is unknown. Genetics may play a role in pyloric stenosis (University of Maryland Medical Center, 2011).	Family history of pyloric stenosis Males have a higher incidence of pyloric stenosis. First-born infants More common in Caucasians (University of Maryland Medical Center, 2011)

TABLE 4–3 Modifiable Risk Factors for Digestive Disorders

DISORDER	MODIFIABLE RISKS
GERD	Obesity, smoking, pregnancy, and alcohol
	Medications including anticholinergics, bronchodilators, and beta-blockers
	Certain foods (e.g., chocolate, caffeine, onions, citrus fruits, and spices) can increase the risk of GERD.
Acute and chronic pancreatitis	Alcohol, hypertriglyceridemia, abdominal injury, and medications such as corticosteroids
Viral hepatitis	Unsafe sexual practices
	Improper hand hygiene
	Sharing of personal items including toothbrush and razor
	Traveling to developing countries without recommended vaccines/immunizations
Pyloric stenosis	Early antibiotics (erythromycin) for whooping cough (Mayo Clinic, 2013b)

transglutaminase antibodies (tTGA) or anti-endomysium antibodies (EMA). Other blood tests may be needed to confirm a celiac disease diagnosis.

Screening in individuals with suspected hepatitis is important for early diagnosis and treatment, prevention of liver damage and other complications, and prevention of spreading of the infection. Individuals who should be screened for hepatitis infection include all pregnant women, individuals born outside of the United States, individuals who use or have used illegal drugs via an injection method, individuals who received clotting factors before 1987, individuals who receive long-term hemodialysis, and healthcare workers after needlestick or mucosal exposure to hepatitis C positive blood (American Association for the Study of Liver Diseases, 2013).

▶ ASSESSMENT

Thorough assessment is necessary to determine the underlying cause of a client's presenting signs and symptoms. Clients presenting with nausea and vomiting require assessment to rule out the possibility of an underlying systemic disease or acute illness that may require immediate care, such as a bowel obstruction. When the cause is known and if there are no other acute symptoms, nursing interventions focus on promoting comfort and preventing complications.

Nursing Assessment

The nurse begins the assessment by explaining the assessment process to the client, inquiring about family or client history of gastrointestinal disorders, and eliciting information about the client's past and current health status and symptoms (see the Assessment Interview: Digestion). Factors to assess include changes in appetite, weight, bowel habits, flatulence, and pain. The nurse listens for cues related to function of the gastrointestinal system, taking into account age, gender, race, culture and cultural practices, environment, health practices, and any current therapies used, both pharmacologic and complementary

Assessment Interview Digestion

Health History
- Describe your current problem.
- Do you currently suffer from difficulty swallowing, nausea, vomiting, constipation, or diarrhea?
- Have you noticed any change in the frequency or the size of your stools?
- Have you noticed bright red blood or black tarry stools?
- Do you drink alcohol?
- Have you ever been diagnosed with digestive problems?
- If so, when? What treatments were prescribed? Were they helpful?
- Has the disease or problem ever recurred? How many times or how often?
- What do you think caused this problem?
- How are you managing this disease or problem now?

Appetite
- How would you describe your appetite?
- Have you experienced any changes in your appetite recently? In the past few months? The past year?
- If you have experienced changes in your appetite, what do you think is causing the changes?
- Have you experienced weight loss or gain in response to your appetite in the past 6 months?

- What (if anything) have you done in response to changes in your appetite?
- Has anything else occurred along with the changes in your appetite?

Symptoms of Abdominal Discomfort
- Are you or have you been experiencing feelings or symptoms of bloating or gas? What do you think may be causing these symptoms?
- What do you do to relieve the symptoms?
- Do you take any antacids or over-the-counter medications to relieve bloating or gas? Any prescription medications? If so, what do you take, and how often?
- How much water do you drink each day?
- How often do you exercise?

Family History
- Is there anyone in your family with a history of digestive problems?
- Which family member, and what disease or problem does he or she have?
- Do you know when it was diagnosed?
- Do you know what treatments were prescribed?

Digestion Assessment

ASSESSMENT	NORMAL FINDINGS	ABNORMAL FINDINGS	LIFESPAN OR DEVELOPMENTAL CONSIDERATIONS
Inspection	The abdomen is symmetrical and contours are flat, rounded, or scaphoid. The abdomen should be free of masses. The umbilicus is centered and may be protruding or inverted. A consistent skin color with macules and moles is considered to be normal (Barbarito & D'Amico, 2012).	■ Asymmetrical contours ■ Marked pulsations ■ Engorged veins ■ Marked distention ■ Cullen's sign ■ Grey Turner's sign	■ Inspection of a pediatric client: a sunken abdomen is abnormal and may indicate dehydration. ■ Assess the midline of the abdomen for depression or bulging, which could indicate separation of the rectus abdominis muscle. As growth occurs, the separation usually becomes less prominent. ■ Infants and children up to age 6 breathe with the diaphragm, causing the abdomen to rise in inspiration and fall with expiration. ■ Abdominal movements such as peristaltic waves are considered abnormal and may indicate intestinal obstruction or pyloric stenosis (Ball, Binder, & Cowen, 2012).
Auscultation	Normal bowel sounds are irregular, high-pitched gurgling sounds that occur 5 to 30 times a minute.	■ Hyperactive bowel sounds may be loud, higher pitched, and rushing. ■ Hypoactive bowel sounds are slow and sluggish. ■ Absent bowel sounds ■ Bruits and venous hums ■ Friction rubs over the liver and spleen	
Percussion	Tympany is a loud hollow sound heard over the abdomen. Dullness is a normal finding upon percussion of the liver, spleen, or other solid organ	■ Dullness in the left lower quadrant can indicate stool in the colon. ■ Dullness over the bladder may indicate distention.	■ Percussion of a pediatric client: different tones, such as dullness, are expected over the liver, spleen, and full bladder. Dullness in the intestinal region could indicate obstruction (Ball et al., 2012).
Palpation	Soft and nontender abdomen Pain-free on palpation	■ Tightness, guarding, or discomfort with palpation ■ Crepitus ■ Irregularities of the abdominal wall such as hernias ■ Tenderness or pain	■ Palpation of a pediatric client should be done last. Check for *tenseness* of the abdomen using light palpation. Use deep palpation to assess for masses and tenderness in the abdomen. Distractions such as toys or pacifiers may help gain the child's cooperation. Monitor the child's face during palpation for grimacing or stiffening, indicating discomfort (London et al., 2011).

or alternative. The nurse should tailor questions related to any changes identified by the client.

Techniques required for physical assessment include inspection, auscultation, percussion, and palpation (see the Digestion Assessment feature).

The nurse should assess for findings of malnutrition throughout the assessment (see the Malnutrition Assessment feature). Position the client supine with a small pillow beneath the head and knees and provide privacy, so that only the abdomen is exposed (**Figure 4–3 ●**). Begin with inspection by look-

ing for abnormalities of the mouth, gums, teeth, abdominal skin color, structures of the abdomen, abdominal contour, symmetry, pulsations, and abdominal movement.

Following inspection, the nurse auscultates the abdomen by listening with the diaphragm of the stethoscope to the bowel sounds in at least four quadrants (**Figure 4–4 ●**). Auscultation of bowel sounds should begin in the right lower quadrant and then proceed through the remaining quadrants (**Figure 4–5 ●**). The nurse should listen for a minimum of 60 seconds to bowel sounds. Hyperactive bowel sounds occur when a client is

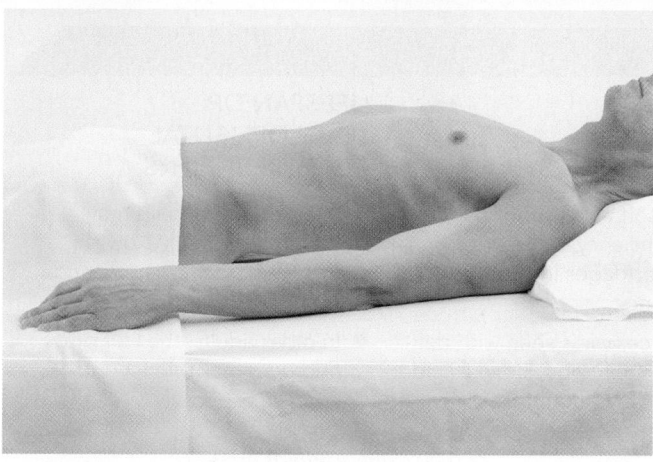

Figure 4–3 ● Client positioned and draped.

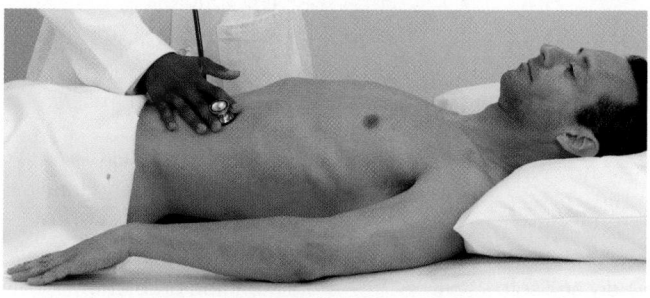

Figure 4–4 ● Auscultating the abdomen for bowel sounds.

suffering from an infection or diarrhea. Hypoactive bowel sounds are common after abdominal surgery or a bowel obstruction. Absent bowel sounds may be indicative of a para-

lytic ileus and should be confirmed by listening over each quadrant for a minimum of 3–5 minutes.

Next, the nurse uses percussion to assess the abdomen, liver, spleen, and gastric bubble. The nurse should tap the client's abdomen as shown in **Figure 4–6** ●. Tympany is a loud, hollow sound heard over the abdomen and is a normal finding. Dullness is often heard over organs such as the liver, spleen, or distended bladder. Dullness in the left lower quadrant can indicate stool in the colon (Barbarito & D'Amico, 2012).

Palpation of the abdomen is useful to determine organ size, placement muscle tone, masses, and presence of fluid. If the client has identified a painful area prior to the assessment, this area should be palpated last. The nurse should follow facility policy regarding whether deep palpation is allowed. If the client experiences muscle tightness or guarding with palpation, this finding could indicate peritonitis. Advise the client to indicate if she experiences any discomfort during the palpation and watch for signs of pain, such as facial expressions or guarding. Palpation of the abdomen requires using both light and deep palpation (**Figure 4–7** ●).

SAFETY ALERT
Palpation is contraindicated in clients suspected of having appendicitis, dissecting aortic aneurysm, or polycystic kidneys; it is also contraindicated in clients who have had an organ transplant.

Lifespan and Cultural Considerations
The nursing assessment of an infant or child begins with inspection, by noting the shape and contour of the abdomen and observing the condition of the umbilicus. A child's abdomen

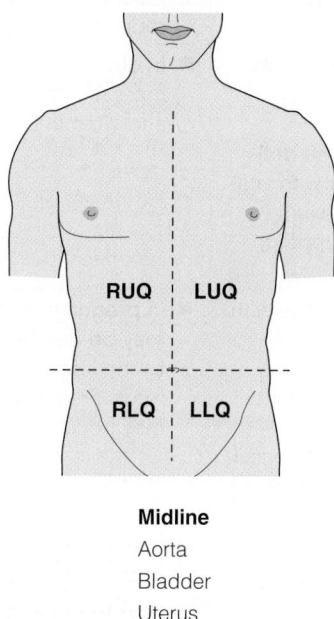

Right Upper Quadrant	**Left Upper Quadrant**
Liver and gallbladder	Left lobe of liver
Pylorus	Spleen
Duodenum	Stomach
Head of pancreas	Body of pancreas
Right adrenal gland	Left adrenal gland
Portion of right kidney	Portion of left kidney
Hepatic flexure of colon	Splenic flexure of colon
Portions of ascending and transverse colon	Portions of transverse and descending colon

Right Lower Quadrant	**Left Lower Quadrant**
Lower pole of right kidney	Lower pole of left kidney
Cecum and appendix	Sigmoid colon
Portion of ascending colon	Portion of descending colon
Bladder (if distended)	Bladder (if distended)
Right ovary and salpinx	Left ovary and salpinx
Right spermatic cord	Uterus (if enlarged)
Right ureter	Left spermatic cord
	Left ureter

Midline
Aorta
Bladder
Uterus

○ = Umbilicus

Figure 4–5 ● The four quadrants of the abdomen.

Malnutrition Assessment

ASSESSMENT	NORMAL FINDINGS	ABNORMAL FINDINGS	LIFESPAN OR DEVELOPMENTAL CONSIDERATIONS
Nails	The nails should be strong and smooth with pink undertones and instant capillary refill.	■ Nails will be soft and spoon shaped when iron deficiency is present. ■ Splinter hemorrhages indicate vitamin C deficiency.	■ In older adults, nails may become thicker, yellowish tinged, harder, opaque, and more brittle.
Hair	Hair should be symmetrical in placement (even distribution) and color with texture being fine to coarse. Hair may be thick, thin, straight, wavy, or curly.	■ Dull, dry, scarce hair is seen with deficiencies of protein, zinc, linoleic acid. ■ Gray patches or asymmetrical graying may indicate protein or copper deficiency.	■ In older adults, the hair grays and becomes thinner and coarser, especially on the face.
Skin	The skin temperature and color should be symmetrical, warm, and moist. The skin should be free from edema and lesions.	■ Flaky, dry skin may indicate deficiency of vitamin A, B, and/or linoleic acid. ■ Niacin deficiency indicated when cracks or hyperpigmentation is observed. ■ Bruising may indicate deficiency of vitamin C or K.	■ Newborns have lanugo, which is replaced within months by vellus hair. ■ Adolescents have increased oil and sweat gland production and development of axillary and pubic hair. ■ In older adults, the skin becomes more thin and fragile (Barbarito & D'Amico, 2012).
Eyes	The eyeball is firm and moist with white sclera and pink conjunctivae. The cornea is clear and symmetrical.	■ Inadequate levels of vitamin A cause eyes to become dry and soft. ■ Pale conjunctivae indicate iron deficiency; red conjunctivae indicate insufficient levels of riboflavin.	■ In pregnant women, dry eyes are a common problem. ■ In older adults, a whitish-yellow color around the cornea indicates fat deposits.
Nervous system	Intact cranial nerves Intact reflexes Congruent mood, language, mental status, and affect	■ Clients deficient in thiamine will present with decreased reflexes and may experience peripheral neuropathies. ■ Irritability and/or disorientation also may be seen with thiamine deficiency.	■ Reflexes in infants include tonic neck reflex and Babinski reflex until age 2. ■ In older adults, reflexes, reflex reactions, and coordination are reduced.
Musculoskeletal system	Smooth movement without pain Steady gait Symmetrical posture Free from tremors, muscle spasms, and pain	■ Muscle wasting is seen with deficits in protein, carbohydrate, and fat metabolism. ■ Calf pain occurs with thiamine deficiency; joint pain may occur with vitamin C deficiency. Low potassium levels can cause muscle cramping, especially in the legs.	■ In older adults, reduced bone mass results from low calcium and vitamin D intake.
Cardiovascular system	Blood pressure within normal range (based on age) +2 peripheral pulses Instant capillary refill Symmetrical color Free from edema	■ Heart size and rate may increase with thiamine deficiency. ■ Diastolic blood pressure may be increased with a high intake of fat. ■ Lowered cardiac output and decreased blood pressure may occur with caloric deficiencies over a long time period.	■ In pregnant women, the heart may be displaced upward and to the left due to the enlarging fetus. Preexisting murmurs may become more prominent.
GI system	Tongue should be smooth, moist, and pink. Membranes should be moist and intact. Swallowing should be intact.	■ Cheilosis (sores at corner of mouth) seen in vitamin B-complex deficiencies, especially riboflavin. ■ Stomatitis and spongy, bleeding gums may also be seen in malnutrition. ■ Gingivitis can be caused by vitamin C deficiency.	■ In the older adult, the gums, buccal mucosa, and lips become more thin and pale in color.

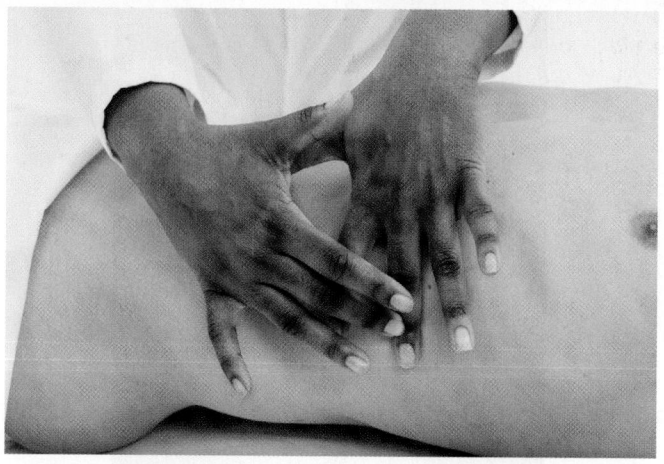

Figure 4–6 ● Percussing the spleen.

is normally symmetric and rounded when the child is lying down. Assessment of children also includes weight, height, head circumference, and calculation of body mass index. **Body mass index (BMI)** is a measurement of a child's weight and height (or length) calculated as kg/m^2 of height. BMI helps determine if the child's weight and height are proportionate.

The nurse uses the diaphragm of the stethoscope to auscultate the digestive system. Bowel sounds normally are heard

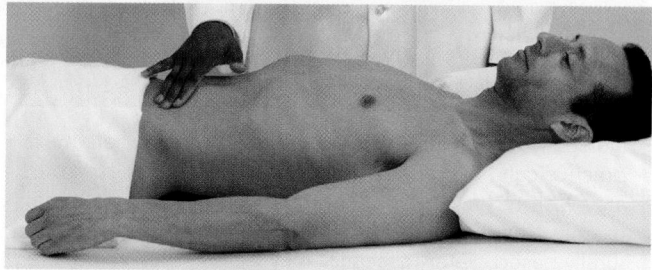

A

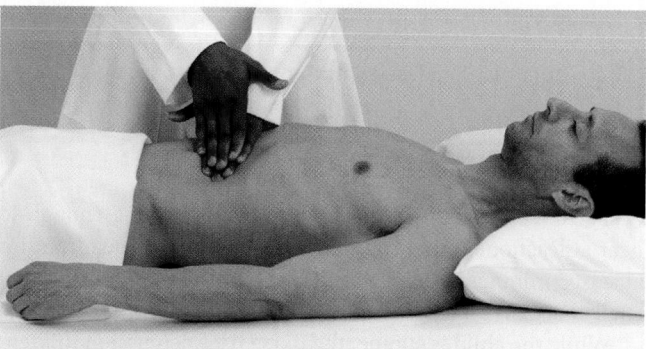

B

Figure 4–7 ● *A,* Light palpation of the abdomen. *B,* Deep palpation of the abdomen.

Lifespan Considerations   Assessment Guidelines for Pediatric Gastrointestinal System

ASSESSMENT FOCUS	ASSESSMENT GUIDELINES
Abdomen—inspection	■ Observe the shape of the abdomen. ■ Note any abdominal distention. ■ Observe the umbilicus for protrusion. ■ Observe for peristaltic waves (visible rhythmic contractions of the intestinal wall smooth muscle).
Abdomen—auscultation	■ Auscultate for bowel sounds in all four quadrants prior to palpation.
Abdomen—palpation	■ Palpate the abdomen and note if it is soft or firm. ■ Palpate the size of the umbilical ring. ■ Does the child complain of pain or tenderness during palpation? Does the infant cry? ■ Describe any masses palpated by location, shape, size, and consistency. ■ Palpate the liver for size and tenderness. ■ Palpate the spleen for size and tenderness.
Mouth and esophagus	■ Note the color of the mucous membranes. ■ Note the presence of increased oral secretions. ■ Note presence of teeth and gums. Is decay or inflammation present? ■ Note the presence of cleft lip or palate.
Nutrition	■ Note weight, height, and head circumference for nutritional status. ■ Note tolerance of feedings, spitting up, emesis, and recurrent respiratory tract infections. ■ Observe amount, color, and frequency of emesis. ■ Note if emesis is associated with feeding and whether it is projectile. ■ Note amount of intake, frequency of feedings, and growth. ■ Note condition of skin and mucous membranes
Stool	■ Observe color, consistency, and size of stool. Note any changes in stool patterns.
Family history	■ Ask about history of gastrointestinal illness with genetic influences such as celiac disease and inflammatory bowel disease.

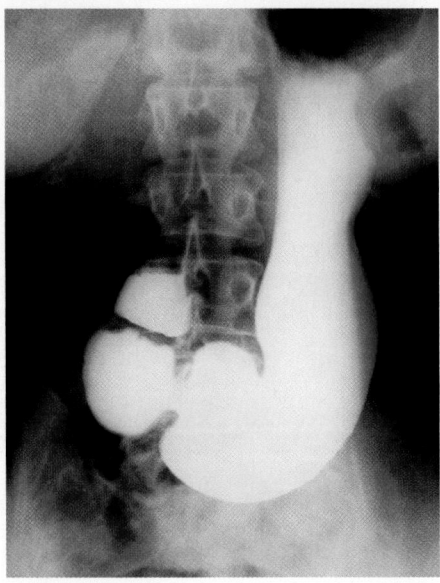

Figure 4–8 ● A barium x-ray of a healthy stomach.
Source: Biophoto Associates/Science Source.

every 10–30 seconds. Listen in each quadrant long enough to hear at least one bowel sound. Auscultate in each quadrant for at least 5 minutes before determining if bowel sounds are absent (Ball et al., 2012).

While the child is supine, the nurse uses percussion to identify the borders of the liver, spleen, bladder, and any masses. Place one fingertip on the abdomen, and with the other hand use one fingertip to gently tap the abdomen.

Palpation of the abdomen should occur last. The assessment should occur when the child is calm and cooperative because the abdominal muscles are more relaxed. Palpate using the edge of the fingers, examining the entire abdomen (London et al., 2011).

Diagnostic Tests

The results of diagnostic tests of nutritional status and GI function are used to support the diagnosis of a specific disease, to provide information to identify or modify the appropriate medication or therapy used to treat the disease, and to help the nurse monitor the client's responses to treatment and nursing care interventions.

UPPER GI SERIES (BARIUM SWALLOW)   Upper GI series are conducted to diagnose esophageal varices, inflammation, ulcerations, hiatal hernia, foreign bodies, polyps, diverticula, and tumors of the esophagus, stomach, and duodenal bulb. The client should have nothing by mouth (NPO) prior to the test. The amount of time the client is NPO will depend on the age of the client. The client drinks 16–20 ounces of liquid barium sulfate or meglumine before the exam. These radiological studies are done by observing movement of a contrast medium with a **fluoroscope (Figure 4–8 ●).**

Nursing interventions for the client experiencing an upper GI series include the following:

■ Instruct the client not to eat or drink fluids or smoke for 8–12 hours for an adult and 4–6 hours for an infant or young child before the test. Tell the client not to take narcotics or anticholinergic medications for 24 hours pretest and not to take any medications for 8 hours pretest.

■ Following the test, ensure the client eliminates the barium by taking laxatives and drinking fluids unless contraindicated.

ENDOSCOPY   An upper GI endoscopy directly visualizes the mucous membrane lining of the esophagus, stomach, and duodenum. A flexible fiberoptic endoscope is used to visualize inflammation, ulcerations, tumors, or varices, and video imaging may illustrate gastric mobility. The endoscopy may also be combined with an ultrasound examination by attaching an ultrasound transducer to the endoscope.

Nursing interventions for clients receiving endoscopy include:

■ Schedule the test at least 2 days after an upper GI series or barium swallow.

■ Remove dentures and eyeglasses.

■ Inform the client not to eat food or drink fluids for 6–8 hours for an adult and 4–6 hours for an infant or young child before the procedure.

■ Explain that the procedure takes 20–30 minutes and that a local anesthetic will be administered to the throat to prevent discomfort. The client may feel some pressure when the scope is placed in the lower esophagus and stomach.

Tell the client to contact the physician after the examination if the client experiences difficulty swallowing; epigastric, substernal, or shoulder pain; fever; or vomiting of blood. After the procedure, keep the client NPO until the gag reflex returns; the client may eat and drink as soon as he or she can swallow safely. Mild bloating, belching, or flatulence may occur.

ABDOMINAL X-RAY   An abdominal x-ray may be ordered for a client to assist in diagnosing obstructions, perforations, and any structural abnormalities. The x-ray is usually performed with two views with the client supine and then standing.

CT SCAN   A computed tomography scan is a noninvasive tool that takes many views of the digestive tract from many different angles to produce cross-sectional images of the organs and soft tissues. CT scan images can provide much more information than x-rays.

SAFETY ALERT
Assess client for allergies to iodine or contrast medium prior to tests that use these chemicals.

AMYLASE   Amylase is a serum blood test that measures the amount of amylase secreted from the pancreas. This test is useful in diagnosing acute pancreatitis. Normal amylase levels for an adult are 60–160 Somogyi units/dL (Osborn et al., 2014). Amylase levels peak in 24 hours of the illness and drop to normal usually in 48–72 hours. No special preparation is needed for this test (LeMone et al., 2011).

LIPASE   Lipase is another serum blood test that measures the secretion of lipase by the pancreas and is useful in diagnosing pancreatitis. The normal lipase level for all age groups is 20–180 International Units/L (Osborn et al., 2014). No special preparation is needed for this test (LeMone et al., 2011).

CASE STUDY \\ PART 2

The next day, you follow up with Jack. You telephone Jack's parents and talk with Jack's father. You ask how Jack is doing. Jack's father states, "His fever is about the same, he hasn't eaten much of anything, and he says his stomach hurts, although it isn't worse than yesterday. His mother said Jack's urine was really dark this morning, but Jack hasn't been drinking." You make an appointment for Jack to see the primary healthcare provider later this afternoon. Before the appointment, you talk with the primary healthcare provider and report Jack's condition, recent trip to Mexico, and Jack's incomplete immunization record. The primary healthcare provider sees Jack in the afternoon and suspects acute viral hepatitis. Jack's blood is drawn to confirm the diagnosis.

Clinical Reasoning Questions Level I

1. What assessment data are of most concern to you?
2. What other questions should you ask about Jack's condition?
3. What specific diagnostic tests would confirm the primary healthcare provider's diagnosis of viral hepatitis?

Clinical Reasoning Questions Level II

4. How does Jack's dark urine relate to a decrease in fluid intake?
5. Why is dark urine significant to the suspected diagnosis of viral hepatitis?
6. What risk factors do Jack and his parents have for viral hepatitis?
7. What measures should be taken at Jack's school or afterschool program or with Jack's family to protect them against viral hepatitis A?

▶ INTERVENTIONS AND THERAPIES

Individuals with digestive disorders require monitoring and early intervention and treatment to prevent potential complications associated with fluid and electrolyte imbalances and nutritional imbalances. The assessment of pain assists in diagnosis of digestive disorders and provides data regarding the efficacy of interventions and treatments. Although interventions and therapies will vary based on the underlying cause of the client's presenting symptoms, promoting fluid and electrolyte balance, nutritional balance, and client comfort are necessary to promote adherence to the treatment plan and prevent complications. In most cases, nausea and vomiting are self-limiting and require no treatment.

Independent

Nurses can be essential in identifying individuals who have digestive concerns and referring them for further evaluation and treatment. Severe vomiting or vomiting in the presence of other symptoms may require acute care to determine the underlying problem and prevent complications.

PROMOTE FLUID AND ELECTROLYTE BALANCE
Encourage clients to restrict intake to small quantities of clear liquids (tea, apple juice, broth, Jell-O) and dry foods such as soda crackers to help reduce nausea and prevent vomiting. Teach clients to avoid food-preparation odors if they produce nausea. Instruct them to restrict fluid intake for 1 hour before and after meals; however, otherwise stress the need to maintain fluid intake to prevent dehydration. Also stress the importance of seeking additional medical help if unable to take in fluids or keep food down. Provide information about electrolyte replacement solutions such as sports drinks and commercially available electrolyte replacement solutions.

PROVIDE CLIENT EDUCATION   Promoting healthy digestion throughout the life span begins at birth. The nurse should teach parents how to position newborns and burping strategies to reduce acid reflux. Encourage sitting upright when eating and maintaining a healthy weight. Discuss the effects of excessive alcohol use on digestion, digestion-related organs, and nutritional status. Discuss foods to help avoid digestion problems. Assess the digestive system beginning with a health history and physical examination, taking into consideration cultural beliefs and values. Interpret lab values and assessment findings for clues to malabsorption, maldigestion, and resulting malnutrition. Lifestyle changes may be needed to reduce symptoms and prevent the long-term effects of the digestive disorder. Involve family and social support systems to help the individual achieve health goals.

SAFETY ALERT
Healthcare providers should use standard precautions and personal protective equipment to prevent the spread of hepatitis if the causative agent is unknown or the individual has chronic hepatitis B or hepatitis C.

Complementary and Alternative Therapy
Nausea and Vomiting

Complementary and alternative therapies may be effective for individuals with nausea and vomiting. The Mayo Clinic (2012a) suggests that individuals experiencing nausea and vomiting try aromatherapy, hypnosis, music therapy, and acupuncture. The use of ginger, an aromatic edible, is a frequent home remedy used for treating nausea. The efficacy of using ginger as a treatment for nausea is still being debated, although it has been effective in some individuals in relieving chemotherapy-related nausea (Mayo Clinic, 2011).

Collaborative

Collaborative care for digestive disorders may include pharmacologic therapies, nutrition and lifestyle management, and surgery. In addition to the primary care provider, other healthcare providers with whom the nurse may collaborate include nutritionists and dietitians, who assist in the nutritional assessment and plan of care for clients, and mental health providers. Mental health providers can provide support to clients with chronic conditions who need assistance with coping skills. They can also assist with alcohol assessment if indicated.

PHARMACOLOGIC THERAPY
A variety of pharmacologic therapies are available to clients with digestive disorders. As with any medications, whether over-the-counter or prescribed, client education focuses on proper administration, potential adverse effects, and when to contact the health care provider if symptoms do not resolve. Common pharmacologic therapies for digestion-associated disorders may include antacids, histamine$_2$-receptor (H$_2$-receptor) agonists, proton pump inhibitors, antiemetics, and a dopamine receptor agonist.

Antacids   Antacids are alkaline substances that are commonly used to relieve simple acid indigestion (Mayo Clinic, 2011). They are available over the counter in compound preparations that include aluminum, magnesium, sodium, or calcium (Wilson, Shannon, & Shields, 2013). Inexpensive and readily available, antacids are an appropriate treatment for infrequent symptoms of heartburn. Although the liquid forms work more quickly, many people prefer to take them in tablet or pill form. Clients with daily symptoms or symptoms that do not resolve with use of antacids should consult with their healthcare provider. Recurring symptoms, painful symptoms, or symptoms accompanied by fever may be an indication of a more serious condition (NIH, 2010b).

H$_2$-Receptor Antagonists   H$_2$-receptor antagonists are useful in the treatment of gastroesophageal reflux disease and peptic ulcer disease because they help suppress volume and acidity of parietal cell secretions (Wilson et al., 2013).

H$_2$-receptor agonists are usually administered twice daily or more often and can be used long term for recurring, mild symptoms. Most H$_2$-receptor antagonists are available over the counter (LeMone et al., 2011). Examples of H$_2$-receptor agonists are famotidine (Pepcid) and ranitidine hydrochloride (Zantac).

Proton Pump Inhibitors   Proton pump inhibitors bind the acid-secreting enzyme (H$^+$,K$^+$-ATPase) that functions as the proton pump, disabling it for up to 24 hours. Proton pump inhibitors are useful in short-term treatment of gastroesophageal reflux, gastric ulcers, and hypersecretory disorders (Wilson et al., 2012). Although it may take several days for clients to see relief, side effects are rare, with headache, diarrhea, abdominal pain, and nausea and vomiting being the most common adverse effects (Wilson et al., 2013). Commonly used proton pump inhibitors include omeprazole (Prilosec) and lansoprazole (Prevacid).

Antiemetics   Unless vomiting is associated with pregnancy, antiemetic medications may be prescribed to prevent or control nausea and vomiting. These drugs fall into a number of different classes, and often are more effective when given in combination with other medications. See the Medications feature on page 223 for more information.

Due to the sedating effect of many antiemetics, nursing considerations focus on client safety. Sedated or drowsy clients may require interventions to prevent risk for falls, and those who are heavily sedated and vomiting may need suction with a nasogastric tube. Antiemetics are contraindicated in those who are comatose, have bone marrow depression, or have a history of hypersensitivity to these drugs (Wilson et al., 2013). Client teaching should include cautioning clients against driving and to report vomiting of blood or severe abdominal pain immediately.

Metoclopramide Hydrochloride   Metoclopramide hydrochloride (Reglan) is a potent dopamine receptor agonist that promotes motility by enhancing esophageal clearance and gastric emptying. It is useful both as an antiemetic for chemotherapy clients and for treating GERD, but long-term use is not recommended because serious adverse effects can occur. Contraindications include sensitivity or intolerance to the drug, lactation, allergy to sulfites, ileus, and mechanical GI obstruction or perforation (Wilson et al., 2013).

NUTRITION THERAPY
Clients who are unable to achieve adequate nutrition through food consumption may require supplementary nutrition. The thought of using enteral and parenteral nutrition can be intimidating for both the client and family. Nurses provide appropriate interventions related to providing enteral and parenteral nutrition and client and family education and support.

Enteral Nutrition   Enteral nutrition, or tube feeding, may be used to meet calorie and protein requirements in clients who are unable to consume enough food to meet the requirements.

Medications **Drugs Used as Antiemetics**

CLASSIFICATION AND DRUG EXAMPLES	MECHANISMS OF ACTION	NURSING CONSIDERATIONS
Antihistamines *Drug examples:* ■ meclizine (Antivert) ■ hydroxyzine (Vistaril, Atarax) ■ dimenhydrinate (Dramamine)	Primarily used to treat nausea and vomiting due to motion sickness.	■ Advise clients to take 30–60 minutes prior to travel. ■ Drowsiness can occur. ■ Monitor for injury and falls. ■ Use with caution for clients with narrow-angle glaucoma, urinary retention, and bowel obstruction.
Serotonin Receptor Agonists *Drug example:* ■ ondansetron (Zofran)	Very effective for clients experiencing nausea and vomiting due to chemotherapy. Effective when given only once or twice a day.	■ Administer orally or intravenously. ■ Headache is a common side effect. ■ If giving frequently, monitor liver function and clotting abilities.
Dopamine Agonists *Drug examples:* ■ prochlorperazine (Compazine) ■ thiethylperazine (Torecan) ■ haloperidol (Haldol) ■ metoclopramide (Reglan)	Effective for clients experiencing nausea and vomiting, but can cause extrapyramidal symptoms, sedation, and hypotension.	■ Can have sedative effects. ■ Monitor older clients closely for adverse effects such as confusion.
Cannabinoids *Drug examples:* ■ dronabinol (Marinol) ■ nabilone (Cesamet)	These drugs are approved to treat the nausea and vomiting associated with chemotherapy, but may produce unpleasant psychiatric effects such as dissociation and dysphoria, and are contraindicated in clients with psychiatric disorders. Tachycardia and hypotension are possible side effects.	■ Change positions slowly to prevent dizziness. ■ Most effective when given 1–3 hours before any nausea-inducing procedures.
Neurokinin Receptor Agonists *Drug example:* ■ aprepitant (Emend)	A new class of antiemetics primarily used to prevent nausea and vomiting associated with chemotherapy.	■ Not for long-term use. ■ Monitor INR levels for clients taking warfarin (Coumadin). ■ Women of childbearing age on birth control should use a second form of birth control. ■ Monitor liver studies.

Tube feeding may be necessary for clients with impairment of the gastrointestinal tract, difficulty swallowing, unresponsiveness, oral or neck surgery or trauma, anorexia, or serious illness. Enteral feedings provide nutrients directly to the stomach or small intestine. Tube feedings may provide all or part of a client's nutritional requirements.

Tube feedings usually are administered through a soft, small-caliber nasogastric or nasoduodenal tube that may have a weighted tip (**Figure 4–9** ●). They also can be administered through a gastrostomy or jejunostomy tube. Small-bore feeding tubes are easily displaced, so tube placement should be checked periodically by aspirating the tube and checking the pH of aspirated contents. A pH < 4 indicates placement in the stomach; pH > 6 indicates the tube is in the jejunum. See **Box 4–2** ●.

Most tube feeding formulas provide 1 kcal/mL with approximately 14% of the calories from protein, 60% from carbohydrates, and 25% to 30% from fat. Administering 1,500 mL per day provides the recommended daily intake of all vitamins and minerals. Formulas that provide more calories per milliliter, more grams of protein, added fiber, or lower fat also are available (**Table 4–4** ●). Commercial products provide instructions for initiating therapy. Enteral feedings may

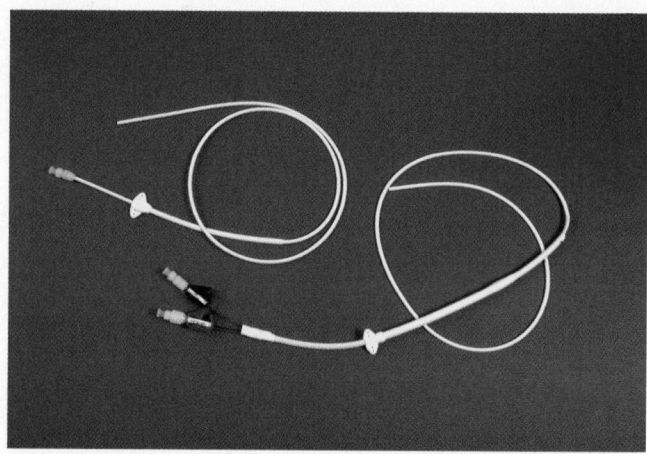

Figure 4–9 ● A nasoduodenal tube and a jejunostomy tube.

Box 4–2 Measures to Verify Feeding Tube Placement

After inserting the feeding tube and verifying appropriate placement through pH of the aspirate and an x-ray, mark the feeding tube position with indelible marker. Prior to each feeding (or every 4 hours if continuous feedings are being administered), assess the abdomen and tube placement before feeding or administering medications. Use the following steps to assess tube placement:

- Assess the abdomen for distention, bowel sounds, and tenderness using the sequence of inspection, auscultation, percussion, and palpation.
- Assess tube condition and placement by verifying that the indelible mark remains at the same position. Ask the client to open the mouth, and inspect the position of the tube in the oropharynx. Do not administer a feeding if the client is having difficulty speaking or is coughing.
- Using a 60-mL syringe, inject 30 mL of air into the feeding tube, then aspirate a small amount of stomach contents and check the pH of the aspirate.

Reassess tube placement if the client vomits or retches, requires oropharyngeal suctioning, complains of discomfort or reflux into the mouth, or develops signs of respiratory distress.

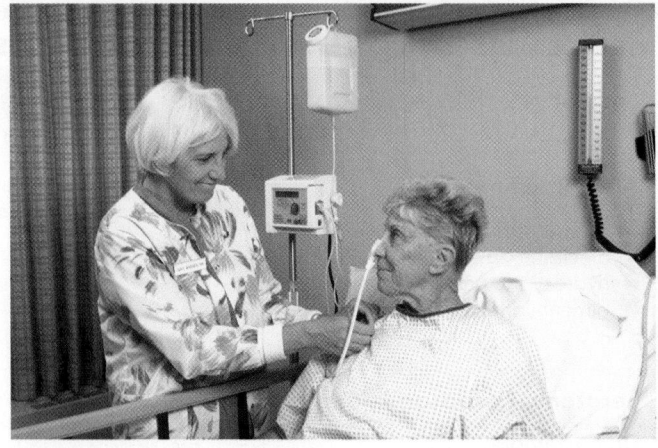

Figure 4–10 ● The nurse secures the feeding tube of a client receiving a continuous enteral feeding.

initially be started with smaller volumes or diluted per physician orders to prevent diarrhea, with the volume gradually increased to provide the required calories for maintenance and healing. Formulas may be administered as a bolus feeding or as a continuous-drip feeding regulated by a feeding pump (**Figure 4–10 ●**).

Aspiration and diarrhea are the most common complications of enteral feedings. Procedures and interventions that reduce the risk for aspiration include:

- Continuous infusion of the formula
- Placing the feeding tube in the jejunum rather than the stomach
- Elevating the head of the bed at least 30 degrees during feeding and for at least 1 hour after feeding
- Dual-lumen tubes that allow gastric suction with simultaneous instillation of an enteral feeding into the jejunum.

Formulas that contain fiber can reduce the incidence of diarrhea. Monitor fluid and electrolyte status carefully and administer additional water as needed.

Parenteral Nutrition Parenteral nutrition (PN) is the intravenous administration of amino acids, often with added carbohydrates, fats, electrolytes, vitamins, and minerals. These hypertonic solutions usually are administered through a central vein, such as the subclavian vein (**Figure 4–11 ●**),

TABLE 4–4 Selected Enteral Feeding Formulas

FORMULA TYPE	CONTAINS	EXAMPLES
Complete—suitable for most clients requiring enteral feedings	<ul><li>1 kcal/mL</li><li>Protein: ~14% total kcal</li><li>Fat: ~30% total kcal</li><li>Carbohydrate: ~60% total kcal</li><li>Recommended daily intake of all minerals and vitamins is 1,500 mL/day.</li></ul>	Compleat, Ensure, Isocal, Nutren, Isolan, Sustacal, Resource
High-calorie complete—appropriate for clients on fluid restriction	As above; provides 1.5–2 kcal/mL.	Ensure Plus, Sustacal HC, Comply, Nutren 1.5, Resource Plus, Isocal HCN, Magnacal, TwoCal HN
Complete lactose-free, high-residue—used to prevent/treat diarrhea, constipation	As above; provides fiber.	Jevity, Profiber, Nutren 1.0 with fiber, Fiberlan, Sustacal with fiber, Ultracal, Ensure with fiber, Fibersource, Accupep HPF, Reabfin, others
Disease-specific formulas:		
Renal failure	Essential amino acids	Amin-Aid, Travasorb Renal, Aminess
Respiratory failure	Fat: >50% total kcal	Pulmocare, NutriVent
Liver failure with hepatic encephalopathy	High amounts of branched-chain amino acids	Hepatic-Acid II, Travasorb Hepatic

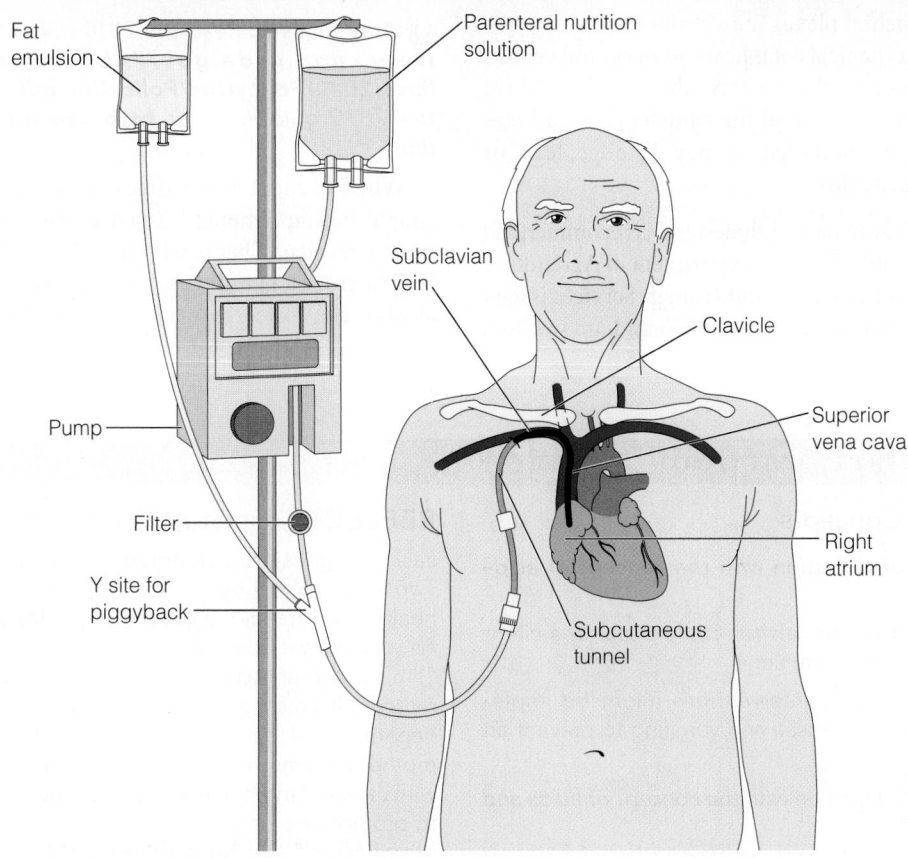

Fat emulsion

Parenteral nutrition solution

Subclavian vein

Clavicle

Superior vena cava

Pump

Right atrium

Filter

Y site for piggyback

Subcutaneous tunnel

Figure 4–11 ● Parenteral nutrition infusing through a catheter in the right subclavian vein.

particularly when therapy may be prolonged. A peripherally inserted central catheter (PICC) line may be used for short-term PN.

PN is initiated when a client's nutritional requirements cannot be met through diet or enteral feedings. Increasingly, PN may be used concurrently with enteral nutrition. Clients who have undergone major surgery or trauma or who are seriously undernourished are often candidates for PN. PN is used for both short- and long-term management of nutritional deficiencies. Many clients are discharged to home with PN and monitored by home health nurses.

To begin therapy, a peripheral or central venous catheter is inserted under aseptic conditions. The location of the catheter tip is confirmed by x-ray. Parenteral nutrition solutions are mixed in the pharmacy using sterile technique under a laminar-flow air hood. Solutions commonly contain 3%–11.4% amino acids (a mixture of essential and nonessential amino acids), 10% or more dextrose, and added electrolytes, minerals, and vitamins. Fat emulsions (lipids) may be added to the solution, although often they are administered separately. The sterility of the solution is maintained, and no medication is added to the solution after it is mixed or to the lumen through which the PN is being administered. When given separately, fat emulsions may be administered either through a peripheral vein or via the same intravenous catheter as PN. PN solutions are always administered with an infusion pump to ensure the correct rate of infusion.

The client receiving parenteral nutrition is at risk for infectious, metabolic, and mechanical complications. Disruption of the skin barrier and administration of a solution high in glucose presents a risk for infection in clients receiving PN. Infection may be local, limited to the insertion site or the catheter itself, or may be systemic. Meticulous sterile technique when inserting the catheter, preparing and administering PN solutions, and during site and catheter care reduces the risk for infection. Using a catheter impregnated with antiseptics and an in-line filter also reduces the risk for infection. The insertion site and the client's temperature are monitored for evidence of infection. Cultures of the solution, catheter, and blood may be obtained if infection is suspected.

Glucose intolerance may develop, particularly early in the course of PN. The concentration of glucose in PN solutions may be gradually increased to reduce this risk. Blood and urine glucose levels are measured every 6 hours until insulin production adjusts to the increased glucose load. Clients with impaired kidney function or liver disease may develop excessively high blood urea nitrogen (BUN) levels or metabolic acidosis. Hyperlipidemia is a common complication of fat infusions; these solutions are given intermittently to allow fats to clear from the blood between infusions. Fluid overload or dehydration may develop, particularly in older adults, therefore, lung sounds and edema should be assessed frequently. In addition, PN formulas can cause electrolyte shifts, with resulting imbalances.

Pneumothorax, brachial plexus injury, and improper positioning are possible mechanical complications of central venous catheter insertion. Once in place, a thrombus (clot) or fibrin sheath may form within or around the catheter. The catheter also can be mechanically occluded, or may dislodge, leak, or break and become an embolus.

Diet A healthy diet low in fat and cholesterol is recommended for optimal digestive health. The U.S. Department of Agriculture and the U.S. Department of Health and Human Services issued new dietary guidelines for Americans in 2010 and are working on updating the guidelines for publication in 2015.

Stay Current: *Read the 2010 USDA dietary guidelines at* **www.cnpp.usda.gov/Publications/DietaryGuide lines/2010/PolicyDoc/PolicyDoc.pdf** *and keep abreast of the 2015 guidelines at* **http://health.gov/dietaryguide lines**.

When a client has a digestive disease, diet modification should be implemented based on the client's symptoms and treatment plan. Clients who have inflammatory diseases often benefit from a bland diet. Nicotine, caffeine, spicy foods, and alcohol can exacerbate a number of digestive disorders and should be avoided.

REVIEW The Concept of Digestion

RELATE Link the Concepts

Linking the concept of digestion with the concept of acid–base balance:

1. What type of acid–base imbalance could occur in a client experiencing nausea and vomiting?

2. What independent caring interventions might be implemented for a client with nausea and vomiting to prevent an acid–base imbalance?

Linking the concept of digestion with the concept of fluids and electrolytes:

3. Healthy individuals are able to balance fluid intake with fluid loss. How does nausea and vomiting impact fluid balance?

4. How can the nurse promote normal fluid and electrolyte balance in the client with digestive abnormalities?

Linking the concept of digestion with the concept of nutrition:

5. How do digestion disorders impact the nutritional status of an individual?

6. What collaborative care strategies could promote healthy digestion to aid in nutritional absorption?

7. Explain how collaborative care strategies, used long term, could have a negative impact on nutrition. (*Hint:* Medications used for GERD.)

READY Go to Companion Skills Manual

REFER Go to Pearson Nursing Student Resources
nursing.pearsonhighered.com

- Additional review materials

REFLECT Case Study \\ Part 3

Jack's diagnosis is confirmed as viral hepatitis type A (HAV). Two days following Jack's appointment with the primary healthcare provider, you follow up with Jack and his parents. As you talk with Jack's mother, she begins to cry. She states, "I'm so worried about Jack. Will he have liver damage?" You reassure his mother that HAV does not typically cause chronic hepatitis or liver damage and that Jack will fully recover. Jack's mother becomes calm and less tearful. You spend time talking with Jack; asking him how he feels and teaching him strategies to promote his health. Jack tells you he is only eating "a couple of bites," but he is drinking. Jack's mother confirms his intake. She states, "His urine is darker and the whites of his eyes look yellowish."

Clinical Reasoning Questions Level I

1. What strategies should Jack and his parents use to prevent spread of HAV?

2. What does "fully recover" mean in terms of the liver?

3. Why are Jack's sclera yellow? How does this phenomenon relate to HAV?

Clinical Reasoning Questions Level II

4. What independent nursing interventions could you teach Jack and his parents in providing skin comfort to Jack?

5. What education should you provide to Jack and his parents about following up with his condition?

EXEMPLAR 4.1 Gastroesophageal Reflux Disease

EXEMPLAR KEY TERM
Gastroesophageal reflux disease (GERD), *227*

EXEMPLAR LEARNING OUTCOMES
After reading about this exemplar, you will be able to:

1. Describe the pathophysiology, etiology, clinical manifestations, and direct and indirect causes of gastroesophageal reflux disease (GERD).

2. Identify risk factors and prevention methods associated with GERD.

3. Illustrate the nursing process in providing culturally competent care across the life span for individuals with GERD.

4. Formulate priority nursing diagnoses appropriate for an individual with GERD.

5. Summarize therapies used by interdisciplinary teams in the collaborative care of an individual with GERD.

6. Plan evidence-based care for an individual with GERD and his or her family in collaboration with other members of the healthcare team.

7. Evaluate expected outcomes for an individual with GERD.

▶ OVERVIEW

Gastroesophageal reflux disease (GERD) is the backward flowing of gastric contents into the esophagus. GERD is a sign of poor digestion that could result in malnutrition. Stomach acid that refluxes into the esophagus is unavailable to digest nutrients such as protein. Undigested protein entering the small intestine does not signal the pancreas to release pancreatic juices to further digest protein. Thus, the body does not digest protein adequately, resulting in a decreased absorption of protein and causing a protein deficiency (Pirtie, 2010).

When gastric contents flow back into the esophagus, the client experiences heartburn. Many people with gastroesophageal reflux have few symptoms, while others develop inflammatory esophagitis as a result of exposure to gastric juices. GERD is a common gastrointestinal disorder, affecting 15%–20% of adults. Up to 7% of people experience daily symptoms such as heartburn, regurgitation, and indigestion. GERD is one of the most common digestive disorders affecting children. Until the age of 12, children with GERD may not experience heartburn; common manifestations may include dry cough, asthma, sore throat, recurrent pneumonia, or difficulty swallowing. Infants and young children may manifest with irritability and arching of the back associated with feedings. As a result of these varying signs and symptoms, GERD may be overlooked initially (Johns Hopkins Children's Center, n.d.). Factors that increase risk for GERD in the pediatric population include premature birth, being male, neurological impairments, trisomy 21, bronchopulmonary dysplasia, and tracheoesophageal fistula (London et al., 2011).

▶ PATHOPHYSIOLOGY AND ETIOLOGY

Normally, the lower esophageal sphincter remains closed except during swallowing. Reflux (backflow) of gastric contents into the esophagus is prevented by pressure differences between the stomach and the lower esophagus. The diaphragm, the lower esophageal sphincter, and the location of the gastroesophageal junction below the diaphragm help maintain this pressure difference (**Figure 4–12 ●**).

Etiology

Gastroesophageal reflux may result from transient relaxation of the lower esophageal sphincter, an incompetent lower esophageal sphincter, or increased pressure within the stomach. Factors contributing to gastroesophageal reflux include increased gastric volume (e.g., after meals), positioning that allows gastric contents to remain close to the gastroesophageal junction (e.g., bending over, lying down), and increased gastric pressure (e.g., obesity or wearing tight clothing). Risk factors for GERD include obesity, excessive alcohol consumption, smoking, hiatal hernia, and pregnancy. Gastric juices contain acid, pepsin, and bile, which are corrosive substances. Esophageal peristalsis and bicarbonate in salivary secretions normally clear and neutralize gastric juices in the esophagus. During sleep, however, and in clients with impaired esophageal peristalsis or decreased salivation, the esophageal mucosa is damaged by gastric juices, causing an inflammatory response (**Figure 4–13 ●**). With prolonged exposure, reflux esophagitis develops. In nonerosive reflux disease, the mucosa remains normal or mildly inflamed. Erosive esophagitis, however, is characterized by red, friable (easily torn) mucosa and superficial ulcers. If untreated, scarring occurs, and esophageal stricture may develop.

Prevention

The prevention of GERD entails behavioral and routine changes associated with eating and lifestyle. Individuals can prevent heartburn or symptoms of GERD by following dietary and lifestyle guidelines:

1. Eat smaller and more frequent meals to prevent increasing pressure in the stomach and on the lower esophageal sphincter associated with larger meals.

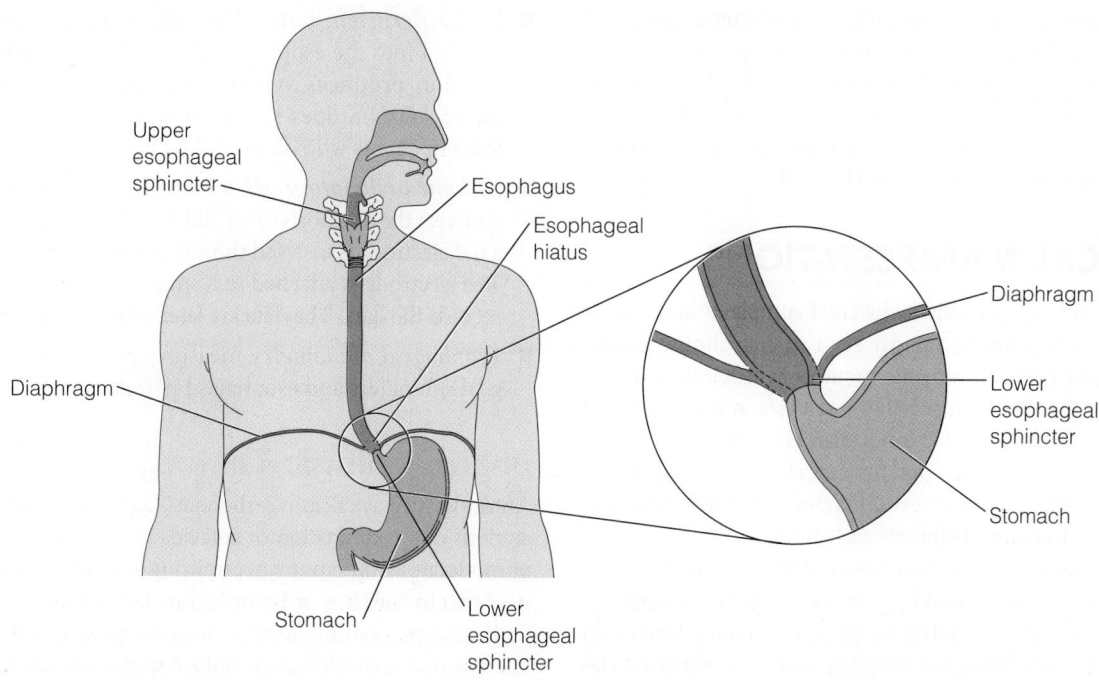

Figure 4–12 ● The esophagus. The inset shows a closer view of the lower esophageal sphincter.

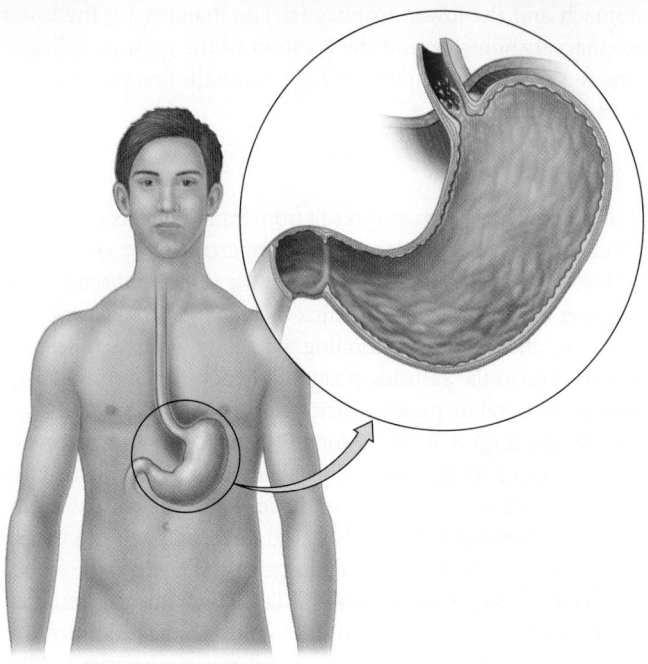

Figure 4–13 ● In gastroesophageal reflux disease, reflux of corrosive gastric secretions into the lower esophagus causes inflammation of esophageal mucosa.

2. Avoid or minimize foods that stimulate acid production in the stomach, such as orange juice, tomatoes, coffee, wine, and chocolate.
3. Avoid eating close to bedtime or naptime to prevent reflux into the esophagus.
4. Elevate the head of the bed to help prevent the stomach from pressing on the lower esophageal sphincter.
5. Avoid wearing tight-fitting clothing or accessories around the abdomen or any area that will squeeze on the stomach, pushing contents upward to the esophagus.
6. Avoid smoking and alcohol consumption because they increase stomach acid. In addition, smoking weakens the lower esophageal sphincter's ability to stay closed.
7. Maintain near or ideal body weight. Obesity increases stomach pressure, causing the lower esophageal sphincter to open and allow stomach contents, including acid, to reflux into the esophagus (NIH, 2013b).

▶ CLINICAL MANIFESTATIONS

In adults, heartburn generally is the chief complaint and usually occurs after meals, when bending over, or when reclining. Regurgitation of sour material into the mouth or difficulty and pain with swallowing may develop. Other manifestations may include atypical chest pain, sore throat, tooth enamel erosion, and hoarseness. Aspiration of gastric contents can also cause respiratory symptoms. GERD may manifest differently in infants and children (see the Lifespan Considerations feature).

Complications include esophageal strictures and Barrett esophagus. Strictures, caused by scar tissue, edema, and spasm, can lead to dysphagia. Barrett esophagus is characterized by changes in the cells lining the esophagus and an increased risk of developing esophageal cancer (Porth & Matfin, 2009).

Lifespan Considerations GERD in Infants and Children

Clinical manifestations of GERD in the pediatric population include coughing, difficulty swallowing, and asthma symptoms. Periods of apnea and frequent upper respiratory infections may occur with pediatric GERD (London et al., 2011).

Infants
- The lower esophageal sphincter (LES) is often immature in the infant.
- The infant with GERD may have small amounts of spit-up or forceful vomiting.

Children
- The child may exhibit poor weight gain, recurrent vomiting, irritability, poor feeding, arching of the back, and respiratory involvement.

▶ COLLABORATION

GERD often is diagnosed based on the client's symptom history and predisposing factors, such as smoking or caffeine use. Collaborative care focuses on diet and lifestyle changes. Pharmacologic therapy may be used for more severe cases. Clients who develop serious complications may require surgery.

Diagnostic Tests

Diagnostic tests that may be ordered for clients with manifestations of GERD include:

- **Barium swallow** to evaluate the esophagus, stomach, and upper small intestine.
- **Upper endoscopy** to permit direct visualization of the esophagus. Tissue may be obtained for biopsy to establish the diagnosis and rule out malignancy.
- In the **Bernstein test**, saline and dilute acid solutions are instilled into the esophagus. In clients with GERD, the acid solution produces symptoms of heartburn, whereas the saline solution does not; neither solution produces symptoms in clients who do not have GERD.
- **24-hour ambulatory pH monitoring** may be performed to establish the diagnosis of GERD. For this test, a small tube with a pH electrode is inserted through the nose into the esophagus. The electrode is attached to a small box worn on the belt that records the data. The data are later analyzed by computer.
- **Esophageal manometry** measures pressures of the esophageal sphincters and esophageal peristalsis.

Pharmacologic Therapy

Antacids, such as calcium carbonate (TUMS) or commercial preparations of a combination of antacids (e.g., Mylanta), relieve mild or moderate symptoms by neutralizing stomach acid and are often tried first by the client at home before the client seeks health care.

Proton pump inhibitors (PPIs) such as omeprazole (Prilosec) and lansoprazole (Prevacid) reduce gastric secretions. PPIs promote healing of erosive esophagitis and also relieve symptoms.

These are available over the counter. Typically an 8-week course of treatment is recommended, although some clients may require 3–6 months of therapy. Relapse is common after PPI therapy is discontinued. Although these drugs have minimal side effects, they may interfere with absorption of calcium and vitamin B_{12}. A study by Khalili and colleagues (2012) indicates that chronic use of PPI therapy is related to an increased risk of hip fractures. The risk was increased especially in women who had a history of smoking.

H_2-receptor blockers reduce gastric acid production and are effective in treating GERD symptoms. When treating GERD, H_2-receptor blockers usually are given twice a day or more frequently for a prolonged period of time. Several H_2-receptor blockers approved by the Food and Drug Administration for the treatment of GERD are available over the counter. A study by Corley and colleagues (2010) shows long-term use (more than 2 years) of H_2-receptor blocker therapy for GERD does increase the risk of hip fracture, although this type of therapy poses a lesser threat than the long-term use of PPI.

A promotility agent, such as metoclopramide (Reglan), may be ordered to enhance esophageal clearance and gastric emptying. Metoclopramide is used to treat clients with regurgitation, symptoms of indigestion, and nighttime symptoms. However, it is not recommended for long-term use. See the Medications feature on page 230 for the nursing considerations to be aware of with drugs used to treat GERD.

Nutrition and Lifestyle Management

Although infants may outgrow GERD once the lower esophageal sphincter matures, in adults GERD often is a chronic condition. Dietary and lifestyle changes help reduce symptoms and long-term effects of the disorder. Topics for client education and health promotion were discussed earlier in the section on prevention.

Surgery

Surgery may be necessary for clients who do not respond to pharmacologic and lifestyle interventions. Antireflux surgeries increase pressure in the lower esophagus, inhibiting gastric content reflux. Laparoscopic fundoplication, a procedure in which the gastric fundus is wrapped around the distal esophagus, narrowing the diameter of the LES, is the treatment of choice for GERD. An open surgical procedure known as Nissen fundoplication also may be done (**Figure 4–14 ●**). Other laparoscopic procedures to tighten the lower esophageal sphincter may include use of an endoscopic suturing system or burning

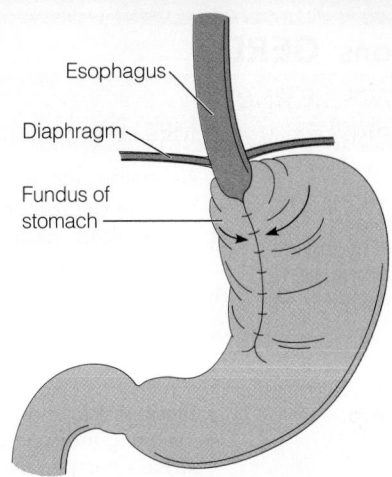

Figure 4–14 ● Nissen fundoplication. The fundus of the stomach is wrapped around the lower esophagus and the edges are sutured together.

spots on the muscle surrounding the sphincter to create scar tissue. Surgery or ablation therapy also is recommended to reduce the risk of esophageal cancer in clients with persistent cell changes in the distal esophagus.

■ NURSING PROCESS

Nursing care for clients with GERD focuses on alleviating symptoms and providing client education regarding nutrition and lifestyle management.

Assessment

The nurse assesses the client's health history, including manifestations such as heartburn, atypical chest pain, and the ability to tolerate acidic, spicy, or fatty foods. Regurgitation of gastric acids, increased symptoms when bending, lying down, or wearing tight clothing, and difficulty swallowing should be assessed. Physical assessment focuses on epigastric tenderness.

Diagnosis

Nursing diagnoses that may be appropriate for the client with gastroesophageal reflux include:

- ■ *Ineffective Health Maintenance*
- ■ *Acute Pain*
- ■ *Readiness for Enhanced Nutrition*
- ■ *Dysfunctional Gastrointestinal Motility.*

(NANDA-I © 2012)

Planning

Relieving the discomfort associated with GERD is the priority of nursing care. Teaching focuses on preventing symptoms and long-term consequences of the disorder.

Implementation

The epigastric pain associated with GERD can be severe, interfering with rest and causing anxiety. Nurses can help clients

---

Lifespan Considerations Feeding Infants With GERD

The infant with GERD should be burped after every 1–2 ounces. An association between GERD and cow's milk allergy has been established, therefore the infant or child should have allergy testing done. Prethickened formulas are available commercially. Formulas such as Pregestimil, Nutramigen, or Alimentum can be used. Positioning the infant or child upright for a minimum of 30 minutes after a feeding can reduce GERD symptoms (London et al., 2011).

Medications **GERD**

CLASSIFICATION AND DRUG EXAMPLES	MECHANISMS OF ACTION	NURSING CONSIDERATIONS
Antacids *Drug examples:* ■ Aluminum hydroxide (Alu-Cap, AlternaGEL)	Neutralize stomach acid secretions. Used for gastroesophageal reflux, peptic ulcers, gastritis.	■ Monitor for metabolic alkalosis and electrolyte imbalances such as hypercalcemia and hypophosphatemia. ■ Antacids reduce the absorption abilities of other medications. Teach the client to take the antacid 1–2 hours before or 1–2 hours after other medications (2 hours for the quinolone antibiotic). ■ Avoid calcium and magnesium-based antacids in clients with renal disease.
Proton Pump Inhibitors *Drug examples:* ■ esomeprazole (Nexium) ■ lansoprazole (Prevacid) ■ omeprazole (Prilosec) ■ pantoprazole (Protonix) ■ rabeprazole (AcipHex)	Block gastric acid secretion by inhibiting the hydrogen-potassium-ATPase pump in the stomach. Proton pump inhibitors are the drugs of choice for severe GERD.	■ Administer 30 minutes before breakfast (and at bedtime if ordered twice a day). ■ Do not crush tablets. ■ Monitor liver function tests for possible abnormal values, including increased AST, ALT, alkaline phosphatase, and bilirubin levels. *Health education for the client and family:* ■ Take as directed for full course of therapy, even if symptoms improve ■ Do not crush, break, or chew tablets. ■ Increase calcium intake because PPIs can interfere with calcium absorption. ■ Avoid cigarette smoking, alcohol, aspirin, and NSAIDs because these substances may interfere with healing. ■ Report black, tarry stools, diarrhea, or abdominal pain to your primary care provider.
H_2-Receptor Blockers *Drug examples:* ■ cimetidine (Tagamet) ■ ranitidine (Zantac) ■ famotidine (Pepcid) ■ nizatidine (Axid)	Block histamine, thus reducing the release of hydrogen ion secretion from the parietal cells, causing the pH to increase in the stomach. Used for acid-related disorders including gastroesophageal reflux and peptic ulcer disease.	■ H_2-receptor blockers are given orally or intravenously. Both prescription and over-the-counter preparations are available. ■ To ensure absorption, do not give an antacid within 1 hour before or after giving an H_2-receptor blocker. ■ When administered intravenously, do not mix with other drugs. Administer in 20–100 mL of solution over 15–30 minutes. Rapid intravenous injection as a bolus may cause dysrhythmias and hypotension. ■ Monitor for interaction with such drugs as oral anticoagulants, beta-blockers, benzodiazepines, and tricyclic antidepressants. H_2-receptor blockers may inhibit the metabolism of other drugs, increasing the risk of toxicity. *Health education for the client and family:* ■ Take the drug as directed, even if pain and gastric discomfort are relieved early in the course of therapy. ■ Take at bedtime if once-a-day dosing is ordered. If spaced through the day, take before meals. Avoid taking antacids for 1 hour before and 1 hour after taking this drug. ■ To promote healing, avoid cigarette smoking (which increases gastric acid secretion) and gastric mucosal irritants such as alcohol, aspirin, and NSAIDs. ■ Long-term use of these drugs can lead to gynecomastia (breast enlargement) and impotence in men and breast tenderness in women. Discontinuing the drug will reverse these effects. ■ Report possible adverse effects such as diarrhea, confusion, rash, fatigue, malaise, or bruising to your primary care provider.
Promotility Agents *Drug examples:* ■ GI stimulate or prokinetic agent ■ metoclopramide (Reglan)	Increase the tone of the lower esophageal sphincter and stomach contractions to move food through the stomach and small intestine. Used for gastroesophageal reflux and gastroparesis. Unlabeled use includes hiccups.	■ Avoid using in clients who have intestinal obstruction or women who are lactating. ■ Teach clients to take 30 minutes before meals and 30 minutes before bedtime. ■ Should be stored in light-resistant bottles. ■ Monitor for common adverse effects including fatigue, extrapyramidal symptoms, diarrhea, and, in rare cases, hypertensive crisis.

Client Teaching GERD

GERD is a lifelong condition that the client and family can manage through a variety of strategies, including dietary changes, remaining upright after meals, and avoiding eating for at least 3 hours before bedtime. Additional strategies that clients may find helpful include:

- Elevating the head of the bed by 6 inches by placing wooden blocks under the legs
- Avoiding tight-fitting garments and belts
- Reducing stress
- Losing weight (if client is overweight) (National Center for Biotechnology Information, 2010b).

reduce pain by providing client education. Instruct clients to eat small, frequent meals to reduce pressure in the stomach, thereby reducing reflux symptoms. Clients who smoke should be referred to a smoking cessation program because cigarette smoking interferes with healing and increases gastric acidity.

H_2-receptor blockers, antacids, and PPIs should be administered as ordered and may relieve pain associated with GERD. Instruct clients using pharmacologic therapy to continue taking medications as prescribed even after symptoms improve. Client education should also include long-term changes in lifestyle, such as limiting intake of fat, acidic foods, alcohol, and coffee in order to promote continued health and manage symptoms over time.

Evaluation

The nurse evaluates the clients' adherence to the plan of care and the extent to which symptoms improve. Appropriate client outcomes may include the following:

- The client expresses freedom from heartburn.
- The client is free from pain.
- The client verbalizes knowledge of GERD and appropriate changes to diet and lifestyle.
- The client demonstrates ability to manage symptoms.

NURSING CARE PLAN A Client With Gastroesophageal Reflux Disease

Taylor Sutton is a 12-year-old boy with trisomy 21. He was diagnosed with GERD at age 2, and has been taking proton pump inhibitors since diagnosis. Taylor's symptoms continue to progress, and he is preparing to receive a laparoscopic Nissen fundoplication.

ASSESSMENT	DIAGNOSES	PLANNING
Taylor has had recurrent episodes of acute respiratory distress and pneumonia from GERD. A dual diagnosis of asthma could not be excluded. His mother, Mrs. Sutton, is present for the preoperative teaching and tells the nurse that Taylor is primarily nonverbal. Mrs. Sutton expresses concern about Taylor's level of pain postoperatively since he is unable to communicate his level of pain. At the time of assessment, his heart is regular, lungs are clear, bowel sounds active. Vital signs are in normal range.	■ *Acute Pain* related to surgical procedure ■ *Impaired Verbal Communication* related to disturbed sensory perception ■ *Anxiety* related to inability to communicate pain (NANDA-I © 2012)	Together the nurse and Taylor's mother develop the following goals for Taylor's plan of care: ■ The client will have no outward symptoms of pain with routine administration of pain medications. ■ The client will use cognitively appropriate communication techniques during hospital stay. ■ The client and caregiver will not exhibit symptoms of anxiety throughout hospital stay.

IMPLEMENTATION

- Administer pain medications when the client begins to demonstrate outward signs of pain.
- Offer alternative forms of pain relief such as an ice pack, repositioning, and distraction.

- Encourage the client and caregiver to use client-appropriate communication techniques when a need arises.
- Encourage the caregiver to express concerns about surgery and pain control to the nurse and healthcare provider.

EVALUATION

In 3 days, Taylor is discharged home. He had little pain during hospitalization, and that was treated promptly with intravenous medication. Taylor was able to tolerate and have a positive response with oral pain medications. Taylor was able to communicate with sign language and one-word requests as needed. His mother stated to the nurse that the procedure and recovery time in the hospital was manageable and she feels comfortable caring for Taylor at home.

CRITICAL THINKING

1. *Individuals of all ages have GERD. How would you adapt the plan of care for a pregnant woman? For a client who is 89 years old?*
2. *What assessment data would you monitor to ensure Taylor's nutritional status is adequate for his growth and development?*

REVIEW **GERD**

RELATE Link the Concepts and Exemplars

Linking the exemplar of GERD with the concept of inflammation:

1. How does the management of GERD impact inflammation in the client?
2. What measures can the client initiate to prevent or reduce inflammation from GERD?

Linking the exemplar of GERD with the concept of nutrition:

3. How does GERD affect the body's ability to absorb nutrients?
4. What nutritional interventions can the nurse provide to the client to improve the client's symptoms of GERD?

READY Go to Companion Skills Manual

REFER Go to Pearson Nursing Student Resources
nursing.pearsonhighered.com

- Additional review materials

REFLECT Case Study

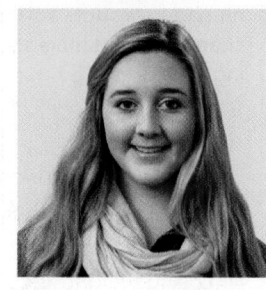

Jenna Riley is a healthy but over-weight 19-year-old girl who lives with her mother and younger brother and attends a local college. Ms. Riley frequently goes out with her friends at night, eating popcorn and pizza and drinking soda. Sometimes they drink beer. She often eats before bed. Her mother comments frequently that she wears clothing that is too tight around the waist.

1. What risk factors for GERD does Ms. Riley exhibit?
2. You are one of Ms. Riley's friends. She asks you what she should do to be healthier. How would you respond?
3. What resources would you recommend Ms. Riley use to assist her in achieving a healthier lifestyle?
4. Create a diet plan for Ms. Riley.

EXEMPLAR 4.2 **Hepatitis**

EXEMPLAR KEY TERM
Hepatitis, 232

EXEMPLAR LEARNING OUTCOMES
After reading about this exemplar, you will be able to:

1. Describe the pathophysiology, etiology, clinical manifestations, and direct and indirect causes of hepatitis.
2. Identify risk factors and prevention methods associated with hepatitis.
3. Illustrate the nursing process in providing culturally competent care across the life span for individuals with hepatitis.

4. Formulate priority nursing diagnoses appropriate for an individual with hepatitis.
5. Summarize therapies used by interdisciplinary teams in the collaborative care of an individual with hepatitis.
6. Plan evidence-based care for an individual with hepatitis and his or her family in collaboration with other members of the healthcare team.
7. Evaluate expected outcomes for an individual with hepatitis.

▶ OVERVIEW

The liver produces bile that helps the body break down and absorb fat. Bile is stored in the gallbladder and is released into the small intestine when needed. The liver also handles and processes nutrients that are carried from the small intestine via the blood. Inflammation of the liver, known as **hepatitis**, impedes the processes or functions of the liver. Hepatitis is a prevalent condition throughout the world that generally results from an underlying infectious agent or virus. It may also result from metabolic and vascular disorders, alcohol or drug abuse, and exposure to toxic substances such as carbon tetrachloride (Thomas, 2011). Hepatitis may be acute or chronic, mild or life threatening: The degree of inflammation and impairment depends on the underlying cause of the inflammation and how quickly it develops.

▶ PATHOPHYSIOLOGY AND ETIOLOGY

Etiology

The inflammatory process of hepatitis, whether caused by a virus, toxin, or other mechanism, damages hepatic cells and disrupts liver function. Cell-mediated immune responses damage hepatocytes and Kupffer cells, leading to hyperplasia, necrosis, and cellular regeneration. The flow of bile through bile canaliculi and into the biliary system can be impaired by the inflammatory process, leading to jaundice (**Figure 4–15 ●**).

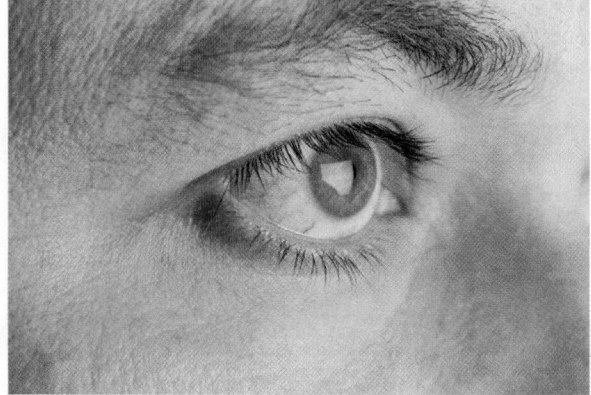

Figure 4–15 ● A client with jaundice.
Source: craftvision/Getty Images.

When the inflammatory process is mild (e.g., hepatitis A), the liver parenchyma is not significantly damaged. The inflammatory processes associated with hepatitis B and hepatitis C, however, can lead to severe liver damage (**Figure 4–16 ●**). The metabolism of nutrients, drugs, alcohol, and toxins and the

① Virus invades parenchymal cells, causing local degeneration and necrosis

② Infiltration by lymphocytes, macrophages, and other white blood cells causes inflammation that blocks drainage

③ Structural changes occur in parenchymal cells, resulting in altered liver function:

Impaired bile excretion | Elevated ALT and alkaline phosphatase levels | Decreased albumin synthesis

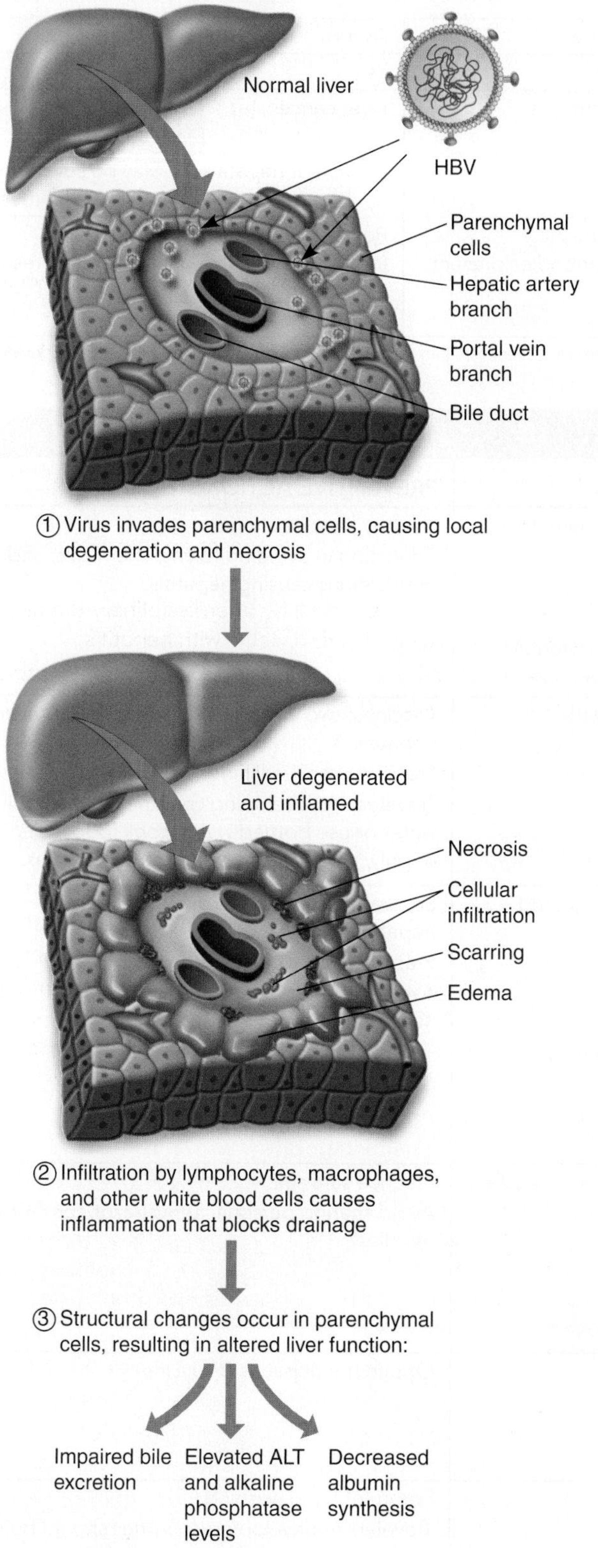

Figure 4–16 ● The hepatitis virus causes degeneration and necrosis of the liver, which result in abnormal liver function and illness.

process of bile elimination are disrupted by the inflammation of hepatitis. Despite the fact that most people associate hepatitis with viral hepatitis, there are many viruses that can cause inflammation of the liver. Because of the diverse functions of the liver, the effects of hepatitis may occur locally throughout the liver or they may occur as a systemic disease. See **Table 4–5 ●** for a comparison of the different types of viral hepatitis, modes or transmissions, onset, carrier state, complications, and laboratory findings.

Risk Factors and Prevention

Risk factors and preventive actions vary according to the cause of hepatitis. See **Table 4–6 ●**.

▶ CLINICAL MANIFESTATIONS

Clinical manifestations of acute and chronic hepatitis generally are similar regardless of the underlying etiology. Acute and chronic hepatitis can manifest with no symptoms or non-specific symptoms to debilitating symptoms (see the Clinical Manifestations and Therapies feature). With acute viral hepatitis, clients usually are asymptomatic during the incubation period. HBeAg in the blood indicates a high degree of HBV infection. As the incubation period progresses, HBsAg (hepatitis B surface antigen) appears. Once the incubation period ends, the course of viral hepatitis involves three phases: the prodromal phase, the icteric phase, and the convalescent phase (recovery).

Prodromal Phase

The prodromal phase of acute hepatitis occurs between exposure to the virus and the appearance of clinical manifestations such as jaundice (yellowing of the skin, mucous membranes, and eyes) resulting from increased levels of bilirubin in the blood. The prodromal phase starts about 2 weeks after exposure to the virus and can be insidious or rapid in onset. Some of the symptoms mimic those of influenza: nausea, vomiting, malaise, and fatigue. Clients may experience frequent episodes of myalgia and arthralgia. Anorexia (loss of appetite) usually occurs early in the prodromal phase. Mild but chronic abdominal pain in the right upper quadrant or epigastrium and a fever below 103°F may be present (Thomas, 2011).

Icteric Phase

The icteric phase begins with the onset of jaundice, approximately 5–10 days after initial symptoms manifest, although some clients will never develop jaundice. The urine may be dark during the icteric phase due to increased levels of conjugated bilirubin, which results from the breakdown of hemoglobin conjugated by hepatocytes and excreted in the bile (Huether, 2010).

Convalescent Phase

The convalescent, or recovery, phase brings an increased sense of well-being, usually following 2–3 weeks of acute illness. Signs of improvement include disappearance of

TABLE 4–5   Comparison of Types of Viral Hepatitis

VIRUS	HEPATITIS A (HAV)	HEPATITIS B (HBV)	HEPATITIS C (HCV)	HEPATITIS D (HDV)	HEPATITIS E (HEV)
Mode of transmission	Fecal–oral	Blood and body fluids; perinatal	Blood and body fluids	Blood and body fluids; perinatal	Fecal–oral
Incubation (in weeks)	2–6	6–24	5–12	3–13	3–6
Onset	Abrupt	Slow	Slow	Abrupt	Abrupt
Carrier state	No	Yes	Yes	Yes	Yes
Possible complications	Rare	Chronic hepatitis	Cirrhosis	Liver cancer	Chronic hepatitis
Cirrhosis	Liver cancer	Chronic hepatitis	Cirrhosis	Fulminant hepatitis	May be severe in pregnant women
Laboratory findings	Anti-HAV antibodies present	Positive HBsAg (HBV surface antigen); anti-HBV antibodies present	Anti-HCV antibodies present	Positive HDVAg (delta antigen) early; anti-HDV antibodies later	Anti-HEV antibodies present

Source: LeMone, P., Burke, K., & Bauldoff, G. (2011). *Medical-surgical nursing: Critical thinking in client care* (5th ed., p. 729). Upper Saddle River, NJ: Pearson Education.

TABLE 4–6   Risk Factors and Preventive Actions for Hepatitis

ETIOLOGY	RISK FACTORS	PREVENTIVE ACTIONS
Nonviral hepatitis	Autoimmune disorders such as systemic lupus erythematous Alcoholism Obesity Diabetes Medications such as high dose of acetaminophen (Tylenol) Toxins including poisonous mushrooms and vinyl chloride	Healthy lifestyle choices Education in avoiding toxins, chemicals, and medications causing hepatitis.
Hepatitis A	Most common: through contaminated food and water Travel in areas with high rates of hepatitis A HIV positive Live with an individual who has hepatitis A Illicit drug use (any form) Man-to-man sexual contact	Vaccines; two vaccines are available to prevent hepatitis A Frequent hand washing Travelers in developing countries should boil water or use bottled water, cook food thoroughly, and peel raw fruits and vegetables.
Hepatitis B	Most common: through sexual contact with contaminated blood or body fluids Multiple sexual partners Man-to-man sexual contact Share needles Live in area that has opportunity for exposure to blood Live with someone infected with hepatitis B Hemodialysis for end-stage renal disease treatment Travel to areas with high rates of hepatitis B	Several vaccines are available to prevent hepatitis B. Practice safe sex. Avoid sharing personal items (razor, toothbrush, needles).
Hepatitis C	Most common: contact with infected blood (sharing of needles) Healthcare worker exposed to infected blood Illicit drug use (injections) History of HIV Body piercing or tattoo with infected equipment Received blood products before 1987	Practice safe sex. Avoid sharing personal items (razor, toothbrush, needles).
Hepatitis D	Illicit drug use (injections) Have the hepatitis B virus Man-to-man sexual contact Multiple blood transfusions	Obtain the hepatitis B vaccine.
Hepatitis E	Drinking contaminated water	Frequent hand washing Travelers in developing countries should boil water or use bottled water, cook food thoroughly, and peel raw fruits and vegetables.

Sources: Based on *Risk factors for hepatitis.* Retrieved from http://adam.about.net/reports/Hepatitis.htm; *Delta agent hepatitis V.* Retrieved from http://www.nlm.nih.gov/medlineplus/ency/article/000216.htm; *Delta agent hepatitis D.* Retrieved from http://www.nlm.nih.gov/medlineplus/ency/article/000216.htm; *Hepatitis C: Risk factors.* Retrieved from http://www.mayoclinic.com/health/hepatitis-c/DS00097/DSECTION=risk-factors; *Hepatitis B: Risk factors.* Retrieved from http://www.mayoclinic.com/health/hepatitis-b/DS00398/DSECTION=risk-factors; *Hepatitis A: Risk factors.* Retrieved from http://www.mayoclinic.com/health/hepatitis-a/DS00397/DSECTION=risk-factors.

Clinical Manifestations and Therapies Hepatitis

ETIOLOGY	CLINICAL MANIFESTATIONS	CLINICAL THERAPIES
Acute hepatitis	■ No symptoms if mild ■ Fever ■ Malaise ■ Fatigue ■ Jaundice ■ Pruritus ■ Abdominal pain in right upper quadrant or epigastrium area ■ Anorexia ■ Nausea/vomiting ■ Myalgia ■ Arthralgia	■ Supportive therapy including rest, nutrition, vitamin supplements, and avoidance of alcohol
Chronic hepatitis	■ No symptoms if mild ■ Fatigue ■ Malaise ■ Arthralgia ■ Right upper quadrant abdominal pain or pressure from the enlarged liver ■ Jaundice	■ Supportive therapy for lifelong management ■ Interferons and antiviral medications ■ Liver transplantation if liver failure occurs

abdominal pain and jaundice as well as increased levels of energy and improved appetite. Complete recovery times vary depending on the type of hepatitis: HAV usually resolves in 9–11 weeks; HBV may require up to 16 weeks to run its course (Thomas, 2011).

▶ COLLABORATION

Collaborative care by an interdisciplinary team that includes nurses, an infectious disease specialist, a gastroenterologist, a nutritionist, and the primary care provider ensures appropriate care for the various challenges that clients with hepatitis face. A social worker may also be helpful in accessing resources for clients. Open communication between clinicians and the client and family is essential in developing and evaluating the client's plan of care. Treatment for hepatitis is primarily supportive, regardless of the cause. Supportive therapy includes rest, proper diet and nutrition, and avoiding alcohol. Increased protein may be necessary depending on the level of functional impairment of the liver. A nutritionist or dietitian helps the client develop a plan that includes low-fat proteins such as egg whites, beans, tofu, and fat-free dairy products.

Client education includes discussions related to prevention and long-term management, including the need to avoid alcohol and substances that are toxic to the liver. Clients who acquire hepatitis as a result of IV drug use will require counseling and additional resources to overcome their addiction. Additional treatment and further assessment may be necessary for clients who acquire hepatitis through sexual activity.

Social services may be helpful in identifying additional resources for clients with a history of drug abuse or sexually risky behaviors. Nurses facilitate client education of these topics as well as education related to pharmacologic management and follow-up care.

Diagnostic Tests

The following diagnostic tests may be used to determine the extent of liver impairment:

■ Alanine aminotransferase (ALT)

■ Alkaline phosphatase (ALP)

■ Lactic dehydrogenase (LDH)

■ Aspartate aminotransferase (AST)

■ Gamma-glutamyltransferase (GGT)

■ Serum bilirubin

■ Liver biopsy.

For a list of specific tests for viral antigens, antibodies, or the virus itself, see **Table 4–7 ●**.

Pharmacologic Therapy

Nearly all people with acute viral hepatitis recover fully without pharmacologic treatment. The Medications feature describes medications that may be used for preventing hepatitis A and hepatitis B, for providing prophylaxis for hepatitis A and hepatitis B (postexposure), and for treating chronic viral hepatitis.

TABLE 4–7 Specific Tests for Viral Hepatitis

Hepatitis A	■ HAV-RNA is viral RNA that is found in stool; RNA is detected in feces up to 2 weeks before symptoms begin. ■ Anti-HAV IgM is found in serum during acute illness, peaking about 1–3 months after exposure and slowly decreasing. It is usually gone by 1 year after exposure. ■ Anti-HAV IgG is found in serum during recovery and indicates immunity to the virus. It remains elevated for years.
Hepatitis B	■ HBV-DNA is viral DNA that is found in serum just before the second month and disappears by the fifth month. ■ HBeAg is a marker for viral replication and appears about 2 months after exposure. ■ HBsAg is the surface antigen on the virus and is usually detected 2 weeks after exposure and 1 week before HBeAg; it usually disappears by the fifth month. Persistent levels indicate either a chronic or a carrier state. ■ Anti-HBc IgM is antibody to HBcAg and is found during acute illness and convalescence but may persist for years. ■ Anti-HBs IgM indicates acute illness and infectivity. ■ Anti-HBs IgG and Anti-HBc IgG both indicate recovery from acute illness.
Hepatitis C	■ HCV-RNA is viral RNA and indicates a replicating virus. ■ Anti-HCV is antibody to the virus but does not indicate immunity.
Hepatitis D	■ HDV-RNA is viral RNA and indicates acute infection. ■ HDAg is hepatitis D antigen and indicates acute infection.
Hepatitis E	■ Anti-HEV is antibody and indicates infection.

Source: Osborn, K. S., Wraa, C. E., Watson, A. B., & Holleran, R. (2014). *Medical-surgical nursing: Preparation for practice* (2nd ed.) Upper Saddle River, NJ: Pearson Education.

■ NURSING PROCESS

As stated earlier, nursing care focuses primarily on supportive measures and client education. Most clients with hepatitis will not require medications and will manage their care at home. Those who do require hospitalization include those with chronic hepatitis that has progressed to cirrhosis, liver cancer, or liver failure, and those clients with fulminant hepatitis.

Assessment

The nurse assesses the client's health history. Physical assessment focuses on abdominal or epigastrium pain, nausea, vomiting, anorexia, fever, joint pain, malaise, and jaundice. Assessment for infection transmission and nutritional status should be conducted.

Diagnosis

Nursing diagnoses that may be appropriate for the individual with hepatitis include:

- *Imbalanced Nutrition*
- *Skin Integrity*
- *Infection*
- *Fatigue*
- *Deficient knowledge*
- *Nausea.*

(NANDA-I © 2012)

Planning

Relieving the discomfort associated with hepatitis and preventing spread of infection are the priorities of nursing care. Teaching focuses on preventing spread of infection and long-term management of hepatitis.

Implementation

Pain associated with hepatitis can interfere with rest and cause anxiety. Educate clients who have abdominal or epigastrium pain about over-the-counter medications to avoid because some medications, such as acetaminophen (Tylenol), aspirin, and ibuprofen (Motrin), may be toxic to the liver. Assess the efficacy of any medications taken to reduce pain and fever.

Encourage the individual with hepatitis to eat a healthy diet and follow recommendations from a nutritionist. Teach clients about food options and praise healthy choices. Adequate nutrition is important for immune function and healing in clients with acute or chronic hepatitis. Help plan a diet of appealing foods that provides a high-kilocalorie intake of approximately 16 carbohydrate kilocalories per kilogram of ideal body weight. Encourage planning of food intake according to symptoms of the disease. Discuss eating smaller meals and using between-meal snacks to maintain nutrient and calorie intake. Instruct to avoid alcohol and diet drinks. Encourage use of nutritional supplements such as Ensure or instant breakfast drinks.

Clients with hepatitis are at increased risk for impaired skin integrity related to pruritus commonly associated with jaundice. Instruct clients to wear cool, lightweight clothes that are not restrictive and to avoid wearing wool. A cool ambient temperature and cool water for bathing may reduce discomfort associated with pruritus (itching). Educate clients about trimming and caring for fingernails to reduce risk for excoriation when scratching. Instruct clients to take antihistamines as ordered to reduce pruritus. An important goal when caring for clients with acute viral hepatitis is preventing spread of the infection. Use standard precautions. Practice meticulous hand hygiene. For clients with HAV or HEV, use standard precautions and contact isolation if fecal incontinence is present. Encourage prophylactic treatment of all members of the client's household and intimate sexual contacts.

Fatigue and possible weakness are common in acute hepatitis. Although bed rest is rarely indicated, adequate rest periods and limitation of activities may be necessary. Many clients with acute hepatitis may be unable to resume normal activity levels for 4 or more weeks. Encourage planned rest periods throughout the day. Assist clients to identify essential activities and those that can be deferred or delegated to others. Suggest using

Medications **Hepatitis**

CLASSIFICATION AND DRUG EXAMPLES	MECHANISMS OF ACTION	NURSING CONSIDERATIONS
Immunizations *Drug examples:* ■ hepatitis A vaccine (Havrix)—two doses ■ recombinant Hepatitis B vaccine (Engerix-B)—three doses OR ■ combined hepatitis A and hepatitis B vaccine (Twinrix)—three doses	Promotes active immunity to hepatitis A and hepatitis B infection (Lilley et al., 2011). Provides active immunity to HBV.	*For hepatitis A vaccine:* ■ Given IM in adults and children (1–18 years of age). ■ Avoid administration to individuals with hypersensitivity to vaccine components or sensitivity to neomycin. *For hepatitis B vaccine:* ■ Given IM in adults and children (1–18 years of age). ■ Avoid administration to individuals with hypersensitivity to vaccine components or sensitivity to yeast.
Postexposure Prophylaxis *Drug examples:* ■ standard immune globulin ■ hepatitis B immune globulin (HBIG) (HepaGam B)	Promotes passive immunity to hepatitis A and hepatitis B infection (Lilley et al., 2011). Provides passive immunity to HBV.	■ *Hepatitis A postexposure:* Standard immune globulin. Must be given within 2 weeks of exposure. Given IM in large muscle mass. ■ *Hepatitis B postexposure:* Hepatitis B immune globulin (HBIG). Must be given within 24 hours of exposure. Given IM in large muscle mass. Begin concurrent hepatitis B vaccine series
Interferon Alfa *Drug examples:* *Conventional interferons:* ■ interferon alfa-2a (Roferon-A) ■ interferon alfa-2b (Intron A) ■ interferon alfacon-1 (Infergen) *Long-lasting interferons:* ■ peginterferon alfa-2a (Pegasys) ■ peginterferon alfa-2b (PEG-Intron)	Human interferons have antiviral, immunosuppressive, and antineoplastic activity. Interferon alpha interferes with viral replication by blocking the virus from entering host cells, inhibiting syntheses of viral RNA and proteins, and viral release from host cells. Conventional interferons have a short half-life and must be administered several times weekly. Long-acting preparations, however, have a higher incidence of adverse effects.	■ Administer by subcutaneous injection. Monitor for manifestations of hypersensitivity (e.g., angioedema or bronchoconstriction); immediately notify physician and administer emergency treatment as needed to maintain cardiorespiratory status. ■ Monitor CBC, platelet count, and renal and liver function studies. Frequently assess mental status. *Health education for the client and family:* ■ This drug may cause flu-like symptoms with fever, fatigue, body aches, headaches, and chills. These symptoms tend to diminish over time with continued use of the drug. If approved by your physician, acetaminophen may be used to promote comfort. Notify your physician immediately if you become severely depressed or develop thoughts of suicide, have severe chest pain or difficulty breathing, notice unusual bleeding or bruising or have bloody diarrhea, notice a change in your vision, develop severe stomach or lower back pain, or notice a new or worsening skin condition. Keep all appointments for lab tests and follow-up visits to your physician. Women: Use a reliable means of birth control and notify your physician immediately if you become pregnant.
Antiretroviral Drugs (Nucleoside/Nucleotide Analogs) *Drug examples:* ■ lamivudine (Epivir-HBV) ■ adefovir (Hepsera) ■ entecavir (Baraclude) ■ tenofovir (Viread) ■ telbivudine (Tyzeka)	These drugs inhibit synthesis of viral DNA. Therapy with antiretroviral drugs may be prolonged as relapse is common when the drug is stopped. Viral resistance to the drug also is a concern. The nucleoside/nucleotide analog antiretroviral drugs were originally developed for treating HIV infection and now also are approved for HBV treatment, although the recommended doses differ for these two uses.	■ Administer PO as ordered. ■ Monitor baseline and periodic renal and liver function tests, CBC with differential, blood chemistries, and serum electrolytes. Notify the physician of significant changes. ■ Lactic acidosis is a risk with these drugs; monitor for manifestations such as hyperventilation, lethargy, and ABG values indicative of metabolic acidosis. Withhold the drug and notify the physician if manifestations of lactic acidosis develop. *Health education for the client and family:* ■ Take the drug as prescribed. Notify your physician if you develop severe abdominal pain, nausea, vomiting, or anorexia or if you become jaundiced. Symptoms of recurrent hepatitis B may develop after you stop taking this drug; notify your physician if this occurs.

Client Teaching Hepatitis

Provide discharge teaching to clients and their families for home care. Include the following:

- Recommended prophylactic treatment
- Infection control measures such as frequent hygiene; not sharing eating utensils; avoiding food handling or preparation activities by the client with hepatitis A; abstaining from sexual relations during acute infection; and using barrier protection if a carrier or from chronic infection
- Managing fatigue and limited activity
- Managing pruritus and maintaining skin integrity; use warm, not hot water when bathing; use mild or no soap; limit duration of baths and showers; pat dry, do not rub; apply an alcohol-free lotion soon after bathing to retain skin moisture; wear loose cotton garments that allow mois-

ture to evaporate from skin; reduce room temperature, especially at night, to prevent overheating; keep fingernails short, and wear cotton mittens or gloves as needed to prevent scratching during sleep.
- Promoting nutrient intake
- Avoiding hepatic toxins such as alcohol, acetaminophen, and selected other drugs; encourage to alert all care providers to presence of infection
- Recommended follow-up
- If chronic hepatitis B or C is being treated with medications, teach how to administer the drug, its dosing schedule, precautions, and management of adverse effects. Stress the importance of keeping follow-up appointments, including recommended laboratory testing.

level of fatigue to determine activity level, with gradual resumption of activities as fatigue and sense of well-being improve.

SAFETY ALERT

If the client diagnosed with hepatitis A is employed as a food handler or child care worker, contact the local health department to report possible exposure of patrons. Maintain confidentiality. Prophylactic treatment of people who may have been exposed to the virus can prevent a local epidemic of the disease.

Evaluation

Outcomes and evaluation parameters include the following:

- The client is free from abdominal or epigastrium pain.
- The client is free from anorexia, nausea, vomiting.
- The client is able to maintain weight.
- The client's skin is intact and without pruritus.
- The client verbalizes knowledge about hepatitis and prevention of spreading the infection
- The client is free from fatigue.

NURSING CARE PLAN   A Client With Hepatitis

Abalonie Gertrush is a 45-year-old male. He presents to the emergency department with right upper quadrant abdominal pain and jaundice. He is diagnosed with alcohol-induced hepatitis.

ASSESSMENT	DIAGNOSES	PLANNING
The nurse conducts a health history, health interview, and physical assessment. The nurse notes the following abnormal assessment data: Yellowish tinge to skin, mucous membranes, and sclera with pruritus Tender and enlarged liver on abdominal palpation Myalgia/arthralgia Temperature 38.3°C (101°F), pulse 84 bpm, respirations 24/min, blood pressure 142/86 mmHg Nausea and anorexia; no vomiting Fatigue Frequent social drinking; up to 6 beers/day	■ *Acute Pain* related to inflammation of the liver ■ *Risk for Impaired Skin Integrity* related to pruritus ■ *Fatigue* related to disease state, nutritional status ■ *Deficient Knowledge* related to new diagnosis of nonviral hepatitis and associated causes (NANDA-I © 2012)	Together the nurse and Mr. Gertrush develop the following goals for his plan of care: ■ The client will express freedom from pain. ■ The client will not experience skin breakdown. ■ The client will use strategies to decrease fatigue. ■ The client will understand relationship between alcohol intake and liver disease.

IMPLEMENTATION

- Teach Mr. Gertrush about pain medication administration when alternative pain reduction measures are unsuccessful.
- Teach Mr. Gertrush strategies to prevent skin breakdown including cool temperature in the environment; use mild or no soap; wear loose-fitting, cotton clothing; and apply moisturizing lotions.

- Teach Mr. Gertrush to alternate activities with rest periods to decrease fatigue and increase tolerance.
- Discuss effects of alcohol intake on liver functioning and impact on daily life.

NURSING CARE PLAN (continued)

EVALUATION

In a follow-up visit to the primary healthcare provider after 3 days, Mr. Gertrush states his pain was better and being relieved with alternative strategies. He is wearing loose-fitting, cotton clothing and has minimal red "scratch" marks on his arms and abdomen without skin breaks. Mr. Gertrush states he is still working on not getting too tired. He is rearranging his schedule to include more rest periods during the day, especially in the late morning and early afternoon time frame. He has begun contacting Alcoholics Anonymous because he wants "to be around for his kids."

CRITICAL THINKING

1. Is Mr. Gertrush's hepatitis contagious to others? Would his family members have to be given prophylactic medications or be taught transmission prevention strategies? Would healthcare providers have to take preventive measures to prevent transmission?
2. How would you handle protecting Mr. Gertrush through a plan to stop alcohol intake?
3. How has Mr. Gertrush's alcohol intake impacted his nutritional status?
4. What complications could occur if Mr. Gertrush continues with his usual alcohol intake?

REVIEW Hepatitis

RELATE Link the Concepts and Exemplars

Linking the exemplar of hepatitis with the concept of digestion:

1. How does hepatitis impact digestion and absorption of nutrients?
2. What dietary changes, if any, should a client with hepatitis make to ensure adequate nutritional balance?
3. What lifestyle changes should the client consider in preventing liver damage in chronic hepatitis?

Linking the exemplar of hepatitis with the concept of family:

4. What actions should the client be taught to prevent the spread of hepatitis to family members and intimate partners?
5. How can the family members promote their health while caring for a member who has hepatitis A, hepatitis B, or hepatitis C?
6. Discuss strategies for teaching young children to prevent spread of infection at day care facilities, schools, and home.

Linking the exemplar of hepatitis with the concept of safety:

7. What actions should healthcare providers implement to ensure workplace safety relating to caring for clients with hepatitis?
8. Discuss strategies needed when reviewing and updating policies and procedures for preventing the spread of infection within healthcare facilities.

READY Go to Companion Skills Manual

REFER Go to Pearson Nursing Students Resources
nursing.pearsonhighered.com

- Additional review materials

REFLECT Case Study

Anna Majewski, a 28-year-old registered nurse, was caring for a client who presented to the emergency department (ED) with a draining abdominal wound sustained from an auto accident 3 weeks ago. The client stated, "I have been treating it like the doctor said, but it is getting worse every day." The ED physician ordered the wound to be irrigated. As Ms. Majewski irrigated the wound, the spray inadvertently squirted over Ms. Majewski's face shield and into her eyes. Ms. Majewski flushed her eyes per agency protocol. The nurse taking the client's medical history elicited that the client has a positive recent history of hepatitis B.

1. What is the next step for Ms. Majewski?
2. How could this situation be prevented from occurring in the future?
3. What are the priority interventions for the client and for Ms. Majewski?
4. Discuss the care needed for the client and for Ms. Majewski in relation to preventing and treating hepatitis.

EXEMPLAR 4.3 Malabsorption Disorders

EXEMPLAR KEY TERMS
Celiac disease, *240*
Lactose intolerance, *243*
Malabsorption, *240*
Short bowel syndrome, *244*

EXEMPLAR LEARNING OUTCOMES
After reading about this exemplar, you will be able to:

1. Describe the pathophysiology, etiology, clinical manifestations, and direct and indirect causes of malabsorption disorders.
2. Identify risk factors and prevention methods associated with malabsorption disorders.

3. Illustrate the nursing process in providing culturally competent care across the life span for individuals with malabsorption disorders.
4. Formulate priority nursing diagnoses appropriate for an individual with malabsorption disorders.
5. Summarize therapies used by interdisciplinary teams in the collaborative care of an individual with malabsorption disorders.
6. Plan evidence-based care for an individual with malabsorption disorders and his or her family in collaboration with other members of the healthcare team.
7. Evaluate expected outcomes for an individual with malabsorption disorders.

TABLE 4–8   Local and Systemic Manifestations of Malabsorption

CATEGORY	MANIFESTATION	CAUSE
Local (GI)	Diarrhea	Disruption of bowel mucosa, which impairs absorption of fluid and electrolytes, leading to excess water in the stool
	Abdominal distention	Gas formation from fermentation of undigested carbohydrates
	Steatorrhea	Impaired fat absorption leading to excess fat in feces
Systemic	Weight loss	Carbohydrate, protein, and fat deficit
	Weakness and malaise	Kilocalorie deficit; impaired absorption of micronutrients (vitamins and minerals) leading to nutrient deficiencies, anemia; fluid and electrolyte losses
	Anemia	Vitamin B_{12}, folic acid, and iron deficits leading to impaired erythropoiesis
	Bone pain	Calcium and vitamin D deficits leading to bone demineralization
	Muscle cramps, paresthesias	Protein wasting, vitamin B_{12} and electrolyte deficits, which impair neuromuscular function
	Easy bruising and bleeding	Vitamin K deficit
	Glossitis, cheilosis	Iron, folic acid, and vitamin B_{12} deficits

▶ EXEMPLAR OVERVIEW

Malabsorption is a condition in which the intestinal mucosa ineffectively absorbs nutrients, resulting in their excretion in the stool. Many bowel disorders can lead to malabsorption. Among the most common are celiac disease, lactase deficiency, and short bowel syndrome.

Regardless of the cause, malabsorption causes common manifestations resulting from impaired absorption of chyme and the nutrients it contains (**Table 4–8** ●). Predominant GI manifestations include anorexia; abdominal bloating; diarrhea with loose, bulky, foul-smelling stools; and steatorrhea (fatty stools). Weight loss, weakness, general malaise, muscle cramps,

Lifespan Considerations
Malabsorption Disorders

Nutrition management is critical for clients with malabsorption disorders, regardless of the root cause or specific disorder. This can be particularly challenging when working with pediatric and older adult clients, who carry a number of risk factors for malnutrition and fluid imbalance. Close monitoring often is necessary until symptoms are controlled successfully and is particularly important for clients who are at increased risk of malnutrition due to malabsorption.

Children may be at increased risk for vitamin D deficiency as a result of malabsorption as evidenced by a review of the literature conducted by O'Malley and Heuberger (2011), who recommend close monitoring for and appropriate treatment of vitamin D deficiency in pediatric clients with gastrointestinal disorders, including those with celiac disease.

A number of factors, including gastrointestinal disease, dementia, side effects of medications, and financial considerations, may increase the older adult's risk for malnutrition, especially during hospital stays. Nurses working with older adults should understand the additional risks these clients carry for malnutrition related to malabsorption. Nurses should intervene early by monitoring older adult clients carefully and working collaboratively with dietitians and healthcare providers to ensure clients' nutritional needs are met (Sullivan, 2011).

bone pain, abnormal bleeding, and anemia are common systemic manifestations of malabsorption. These manifestations result from malnutrition and fluid loss due to poor absorption.

■ CELIAC DISEASE

▶ PATHOPHYSIOLOGY AND ETIOLOGY

Celiac disease, also known as celiac sprue or nontropical sprue, is a chronic immune-mediated disorder of the small intestine in which the absorption of nutrients, particularly fats, is impaired. It is characterized by sensitivity to the gliadin fraction of gluten, a cereal protein. Gluten is found in wheat, rye, barley, and oats. It is also used as a filler in many prepared foods and in medications.

Manifestations of celiac disease often develop in childhood, but may develop at any age. The severity of the disease depends on the extent of mucosal involvement in the intestine and the duration of the disease.

Most absorption of nutrients occurs in the small intestine. The mucosa of the small intestine is arranged in microscopic folds, which in turn contain even smaller finger-like projections called villi. The cells of the villi are covered with microscopic hairs, microvilli, projecting from the cell membrane. The folds, villi, and microvilli of the intestinal mucosa provide a huge surface area for nutrient absorption. Cells of the intestines are specialized to absorb different nutrients. Readily digested nutrients are absorbed in the proximal intestine; others are absorbed more distally in the intestines. Nutrients are absorbed by the processes of simple diffusion (water and small lipids), facilitated diffusion (water-soluble vitamins), and active transport (glucose and amino acids). Once absorbed into the cells of the villi, nutrients enter the blood or lymph for systemic distribution.

Etiology

In celiac disease, the intestinal mucosa is damaged by an immunological response. Gliadin acts as an antigen (a substance that induces the formation of antibodies that interact specifically with it), prompting an inappropriate T-cell–mediated immune response. People with celiac disease have increased antibodies to other antigens as well. The immune response prompts an inflammatory response in the small bowel, resulting in loss of villi and microvilli. The villi shorten and atrophy, resulting in loss of intestinal folds. With the loss of villi, intestinal absorptive surface is lost, and digestive enzyme production, including disaccharidase and particularly lactase, is reduced. The proximal small bowel is affected to the greatest extent, likely due to its greater exposure to dietary gluten.

Risk Factors

The cause of celiac disease is unknown; however, genetic and immune factors are known to play a role in its development. Caucasians of European descent are most commonly affected (Freeman, 2010). Having a first-degree relative with celiac disease significantly increases the risk. High-risk populations have been identified in familial forms of celiac disease including those individuals with iron deficiency anemia, osteopenic bone disease, children who have insulin-dependent diabetes, and genetic disorders, including Down syndrome and Turner syndrome (Freeman, 2010).

▶ CLINICAL MANIFESTATIONS

Local manifestations include abdominal bloating and cramps, diarrhea, and steatorrhea. Systemic manifestations result from the effects of malabsorption and resulting deficiencies. Anemia is common. Clients with celiac disease are often small in stature and may have delayed maturity. Other signs of nutrient deficiencies include tetany, vitamin deficiencies, muscle wasting, and rickets (impaired bone development). When gluten is removed from the diet, the manifestations resolve.

Gastrointestinal malignancies and intestinal lymphoma are potential complications of celiac disease. Other complications include intestinal ulceration and development of refractory disease, or disease that no longer responds to a gluten-free diet.

▶ COLLABORATION

Once celiac disease is confirmed, the focus of client care revolves around the client's adoption of a gluten-free diet. Pharmacologic therapy may be necessary to treat specific deficiencies.

Diagnostic Tests

Laboratory and diagnostic tests are used to make the differential diagnosis for various causes of malabsorption syndromes and to determine the severity of nutrient deficiencies.

An enteroscopy permits direct examination of intestinal mucosa and collection of a tissue specimen for biopsy. Tissue biopsy is necessary to establish the diagnosis of celiac disease. Upper GI series with small-bowel follow-through may be done to evaluate the structures of the upper GI tract. With celiac disease, the typical "feathery" pattern of barium in the small bowel is lost, and the barium may precipitate and clump. Laboratory tests are used to identify pathophysiological effects of the disease. Fecal fat is measured to document the presence of steatorrhea. The fat content of stool is increased in many malabsorptive

disorders, including celiac disease. Serological testing for IgA endomysial antibodies, and IgG and IgA antigliadin antibodies are used to diagnose celiac disease and evaluate compliance with the prescribed gluten-free diet. Serum levels of protein, albumin, cholesterol, electrolytes, and iron may be ordered to evaluate for nutrient deficiencies. The hemoglobin, hematocrit, and RBC indices are used to evaluate anemia. Prothrombin time is increased in vitamin K deficiency.

Pharmacologic Therapy

Clients with severe nutritional deficits may require vitamin and mineral supplements, as well as iron and folic acid to correct anemia. Vitamin K may be administered parenterally if the prothrombin time is prolonged. In clients whose disease fails to respond to dietary management, corticosteroids may be ordered to suppress the inflammatory response.

Nutrition

The client with celiac disease is placed on a gluten-free diet. This treatment generally is successful, as long as the client avoids gluten totally. Gluten is so widely used in prepared foods that this may be no easy task, however, many grocery stores are providing more gluten-free foods. Consultation with a dietitian and detailed dietary instructions are necessary. Clients need to become aware of hidden sources of gluten and to analyze dietary labels.

⚙ **Stay Current:** *A list of common sources of gluten, including foods to be avoided, can be found at* **www.mayoclinic.com/ health/celiac-disease/DS00319/DSECTION=lifestyle-and-home-remedies**.

The prescribed diet is high in calories and protein to correct nutrient deficits. Fat content is restricted to minimize steatorrhea. The diet usually is restricted in lactose as well to compensate for the loss of lactase-containing microvilli. Foods containing lactose may be reintroduced once remission has occurred. Clients with refractory disease may need intravenous nutrition (National Digestive Diseases Information Clearinghouse, 2012).

■ NURSING PROCESS

Nursing care for the client with celiac disease focuses on the effects of the disorder on health and nutrition, as well as the client's ability to manage the disease.

Assessment

In addition to physical examination, nurses assess for the onset, duration, and severity of the manifestations and determine the client's level of understanding of disease, current treatment and diet, and if there is a need for additional client teaching.

Diagnosis

Nursing diagnoses that may be appropriate for clients with celiac disease include the following:

- *Risk for Imbalanced Fluid Volume*
- *Diarrhea*
- *Pain*
- *Risk for Imbalanced Nutrition.*

(NANDA-I © 2012)

Planning

Nursing interventions for the client with celiac disease focus on prevention and management of diarrhea and malnutrition. Involving the client in developing the plan of care is critical to the success of any planned interventions.

Implementation

Steatorrhea and diarrhea typically occur with celiac disease because fat, water, and other nutrients are poorly absorbed, remaining in the bowel to be eliminated in the stool. Diarrhea can interfere with lifestyle, ADLs, skin integrity, and fluid and electrolyte balance. The nurse assesses for fluid balance by weighing daily, monitoring intake and output, and assessing skin and mucous membranes for signs of dehydration. Perianal skin is at risk of breakdown for the client with frequent episodes of steatorrhea and diarrhea. Encourage a liberal fluid intake.

Celiac disease is a chronic condition. With continuing malabsorption, multiple nutrient deficits may occur, resulting in impaired growth and development, impaired healing, muscle wasting, bone disease, and electrolyte imbalances. Maintain accurate dietary intake records to document compliance with the prescribed diet as well as the adequacy of nutrient intake. The nurse monitors laboratory results to confirm nutritional status and guard against development of secondary conditions, such as anemia. Weight should be assessed often, depending on the severity and control of the disease. Arrange for dietary consultation to incorporate food preferences as much as possible.

Provide the prescribed high-kilocalorie, high-protein, low-fat, gluten-free diet. For the client who is unable to absorb enteral nutrients, provide parenteral nutrition as ordered. This will help reverse nutritional deficits and promote weight gain for clients with acute manifestations.

Nursing care for pediatric clients centers on teaching the importance of a gluten-free diet to the child and parents. Reinforce that discontinuing the diet increases the risk for growth retardation and for gastrointestinal cancers in adulthood; lifelong dietary modifications will be necessary and should not be discontinued when symptoms improve. Children and families should see a dietitian several times during childhood, and children's height and weight should be measured often.

Client Teaching   Celiac Disease

The nurse provides a detailed list of foods that contain gluten and need to be eliminated from the diet, as well as foods that are allowed. Client and family teaching includes how to identify gluten-containing commercial products by reading labels and lists of ingredients and encouraging the purchase and use of a gluten-free cookbook. Discuss potential long-term complications of the disorder and manifestations to be reported to the primary care provider. Children and adolescents will require additional teaching about the importance of maintaining their gluten-free diet at school, after school activities, and activities such as birthday parties.

Advise clients and parents to get a dietary prescription, which will enable them to deduct the cost of special ingredients and commercially prepared products as a medical expense. Provide referrals to local support groups available through the American Celiac Society or the Celiac Sprue Association.

If corticosteroids have been prescribed, stress the importance of taking the medication as ordered. Emphasize the need to avoid stopping the medication abruptly and to notify all caregivers that a corticosteroid is part of the client's medication regimen. Instruct to frequently monitor weight. A weight gain of 5 lb (2.3 kg) or more in less than a week usually reflects fluid gain, a possible adverse effect of corticosteroids. Other potential effects include decreased resistance to infection, an impaired inflammatory response, and changes in the metabolism of carbohydrates, proteins, and fats.

Evaluation

An outcome evaluation for an individual with celiac disease includes the following:

- The client is free of abdominal discomfort including bloating, gas, indigestion, nausea, and vomiting.
- The client is able to maintain normal or routine bowel habits.
- The client is able to maintain adequate nutritional status.

Any residual signs of celiac disease should be reported for further treatment.

NURSING CARE PLAN   A Client With Celiac Disease

Spencer Pacey is an 8-month-old boy. He has been eating solid foods for 2 weeks and has had diarrhea since the start of solid food intake. Spencer's parents called for an appointment at the pediatrician's office. Diagnosis of celiac disease is confirmed through fecal fat content and through serum screening tests for transglutaminase and IgA antiendomysial antibodies.

ASSESSMENT	DIAGNOSES	PLANNING
At the time of the appointment, the nurse conducts a health history, health interview, and physical assessment and notes the following abnormal assessment data: Diarrhea since solid food has been introduced Lack of appetite Lack of energy; one parent states, "He is taking two naps instead of his usual one afternoon nap." Abdominal distention	■ *Imbalanced Nutrition: Less Than Body Requirements* related to malabsorption ■ *Deficient Knowledge* related to new diagnosis of celiac disease (NANDA-I © 2012)	Together the nurse and Spencer's parents develop the following goals for Spencer's plan of care: ■ The client's nutritional requirements will be met. ■ The client's parents will acknowledge understanding of celiac disease and nutritional strategies to prevent symptoms.

NURSING CARE PLAN (continued)

IMPLEMENTATION

- Teach Spencer's parents about celiac disease: underlying causes, how it affects nutritional needs of the body and growth and development, dietary treatment.
- Explain to Spencer's parents about lifelong dietary modifications that are needed to prevent symptoms and complications of celiac disease.

- Begin Spencer on a gluten-free diet as ordered.
- Encourage follow-up visits with the pediatrician and dietitian.
- Monitor Spencer's growth and development, naptimes, and energy levels.

EVALUATION

Spencer has been on the gluten-free diet for 2 weeks and has been without diarrhea for the past 7 days. His abdomen is no longer distended. His parents are feeding him gluten-free, solid foods as planned with the dietitian. Spencer's parents state he is a "happier" baby and is more energetic. Spencer's weight and development are on target.

CRITICAL THINKING

1. Why might it be important to include family members in nutrition education for an adult individual with celiac disease?
2. What challenges would the client with celiac disease face when attending school or leaving home to live in a college dorm? What would you include in health teaching for this type of client?
3. If a client with celiac disease requires corticosteroid therapy, why is it important for the client to taper off corticosteroids rather than stop abruptly?

LACTASE DEFICIENCY

▶ PATHOPHYSIOLOGY AND ETIOLOGY

Lactase deficiency occurs when the body is unable to digest and metabolize lactose, or milk sugar. Lactase deficiency is a malabsorption disorder that can result in a great deal of discomfort for the client.

For carbohydrates to be absorbed from the small intestine, they first must be broken down into simple sugars, or monosaccharides. Lactose is the primary carbohydrate in milk and milk products. It is a disaccharide, requiring the enzyme lactase for digestion and absorption. Lactase deficiency can lead to **lactose intolerance** and manifestations of malabsorption. Lactase deficiency usually is genetic in origin, but also occurs secondarily to celiac disease, Crohn's disease, and other disorders affecting the mucosa of the small intestine.

Risk Factors

Risk factors for lactose intolerance include previous radiation therapy for abdominal cancer, history of celiac disease or Crohn's disease, infants born prematurely, and increasing age. Lactose intolerance is not common in young children or in infants. Ethnicity also plays a role in lactose intolerance; it is more common in Native Americans, Asians, Hispanics, and Blacks (Mayo Clinic, 2012b).

▶ CLINICAL MANIFESTATIONS

Many people with lactase deficiency are asymptomatic. Small to moderate amounts of milk (one to two 8-ounce glasses) may be well tolerated. Manifestations of lactose intolerance include lower abdominal cramping, pain, and diarrhea following milk ingestion. Undigested lactose ferments in the intestine, forming gases that contribute to bloating and flatus. Lactic and fatty acids produced by this fermentation irritate the bowel, leading to increased motility and abdominal cramping. The undigested lactose draws water into the intestine, which contributes to increased motility and diarrhea. The diarrhea associated with lactose intolerance may be explosive.

▶ COLLABORATION

The diagnosis of lactase deficiency usually is based on a history of intolerance to milk and milk products and on a trial of a lactose-free diet. If manifestations resolve when lactose intake is eliminated, the diagnosis of lactase deficiency is confirmed.

Diagnostic Tests

The lactose breath test is a noninvasive test that may be used to diagnose lactase deficiency. Expired hydrogen gas (H_2) is measured following oral administration of 50 g of lactose. If lactose is digested and absorbed normally, then little change occurs in the amount of exhaled H_2 between fasting and postlactose administration. With lactose intolerance, exhaled H_2 increases following lactose administration as the sugar ferments in the bowel.

For the lactose tolerance test, 100 g of lactose solution is orally administered, followed by measurement of blood glucose levels at intervals of 30, 60, and 120 minutes. If lactose is digested and absorbed normally, the blood glucose rises more than 20 mg/dL. The expected blood glucose elevation does not occur in lactose intolerance.

Pharmacologic Therapy

Nonprescription lactase enzyme preparations are available to improve milk tolerance. Yogurt containing bacterial lactases may be well tolerated. Calcium supplements are often recommended, particularly for women on a reduced-lactose or lactose-free diet. Supplements for vitamin D, riboflavin, and protein may need to be considered.

Nutrition Management

A lactose-free or reduced lactose diet relieves the manifestations of the disorder. Some clients require total elimination of milk and milk products from the diet. Many can tolerate limited amounts of lactose. Milk pretreated with lactase is readily available.

▶ NURSING CARE

Nursing care for the client with lactose intolerance focuses on providing education and support. Discuss sources of lactose: Milk, ice cream, and cottage cheese are high in lactose; aged cheese and yogurt contain much smaller amounts. Potential hidden sources of lactose include sherbets, desserts made from milk and milk chocolate, sauces and gravies, and cream soups. Suggest a trial of lactase-treated milk or lactase enzyme supplements. Emphasize the importance of obtaining nutrients contained in dairy products from other sources. Proteins may be obtained from meats, eggs, legumes, and grains. Other sources of calcium include sardines, oysters, and salmon, as well as plant sources such as beans, cauliflower, rhubarb, and green leafy vegetables.

▍ SHORT BOWEL SYNDROME

▶ OVERVIEW

The small bowel may be resected due to tumors, infarction of bowel mucosa, incarcerated hernias, Crohn's disease, trauma, and enteropathy resulting from radiation therapy. Resection of significant portions of the small intestine may result in a condition known as **short bowel syndrome**.

▶ PATHOPHYSIOLOGY AND ETIOLOGY

Resection of the small intestine affects the absorption of water, nutrients, vitamins, and minerals. Transit time of ingested foods and fluids is reduced, and digestive processes are impaired. The bowel undergoes an adaptive process in which the remaining villi enlarge and lengthen to increase absorptive surface following resection. For many clients, absorption and bowel function return to preoperative or near-normal levels. Others have continued significant impairment of digestion and absorption, leading to nutrient deficiencies, weight loss, and diarrhea. Short bowel syndrome also is associated with an increased risk for kidney stones and gallstones.

▶ CLINICAL MANIFESTATIONS

The severity of the disorder depends on the total amount of bowel resected, as well as the portions of bowel removed. Removal of the proximal portions, including the duodenum, jejunum, and proximal ileum, and the distal portion of the ileum is associated with more severe malabsorption and manifestations than is resection of midportions of the ileum.

▶ COLLABORATION

Management of short bowel syndrome focuses on alleviating manifestations. Clients often simply require frequent, small, high-kilocalorie, high-protein feedings.

Diagnostic Tests

Laboratory and diagnostic studies are used to evaluate nutrient deficiencies. Total serum proteins and albumin are reduced, as are serum levels of folate, iron, vitamins, minerals, and electrolytes. Anemia and a prolonged prothrombin time (indicative of vitamin K deficiency) may develop.

Pharmacologic Therapy

Multivitamin and mineral supplementation is frequently necessary for the client with short bowel syndrome. Antidiarrheal medications are used to reduce bowel motility, allowing a greater amount of time for nutrient absorption. Some clients are affected by gastric hypersecretion following bowel resection. For these clients, a proton pump inhibitor such as omeprazole (Prilosec) may be ordered.

Nutrition

Clients with severe manifestations of short bowel syndrome may require total parenteral nutrition (TPN). TPN can be very stressful for children. Children with short bowel syndrome often require insertion of multiple central lines over time resulting from either infection or occlusion of the line.

▶ NURSING CARE

Nursing care for the client with short bowel syndrome focuses on the problems of potential fluid volume deficit, malnutrition, and diarrhea.

Fluid losses are generally greatest in the initial periods following surgery, warranting the closest attention at that time. Close monitoring of vital signs, intake and output, daily weights, skin turgor, and condition of mucous membranes is vital. It is important to remember that the risk also is high when other abnormal fluid losses occur through, for example, fever, draining wounds, or excess perspiration.

Lifespan Considerations Short Bowel Syndrome in Children

In addition to helping the parents of a child with short bowel syndrome to monitor and manage their child's condition, nurses working with these clients should arrange for home visits to monitor the child's growth and development. For children on total parenteral nutrition, the nurse also monitors care of the central line and tube feeding site and checks for any side effects, such as fluid and electrolyte imbalance and diarrhea.

Assessment includes documentation of nutritional status, including weight, anthropometric measurements, laboratory values, and kilocalorie intake. Nursing interventions include providing nutritional supplementation with enteral feedings as needed, maintaining central lines and TPN, and using aseptic technique.

For diarrhea, the nurse documents the number and character of stools and administers antidiarrheal medications as ordered. Interventions include limiting intake of milk and milk products for clients who are lactose intolerant and providing good skin care of the perianal region to prevent breakdown from frequent bowel movements. Refer to the discussion of nursing care for the client with celiac disease for other measures for altered nutrition and diarrhea.

Client and family education is critical. Because there is no way to cure or replace the lost bowel at this time, the client must manage the disorder on a day-to-day basis.

Client Teaching Short Bowel Syndrome

Nurses must provide education that includes the following:

- Provide instructions about the recommended diet and medication regimen.
- Stress the importance of maintaining an adequate fluid intake, particularly in hot weather or during strenuous exercise.
- Describe the need for the client to monitor his or her weight frequently and report changes. Include teaching about possible manifestations of dehydration and nutrient deficiencies that should be reported to the physician.
- Refer to a dietitian or counselor, who can help the individual cope with what may be a lifelong problem.

REVIEW Malabsorption Disorders

RELATE Link the Concepts and Exemplars

Linking the exemplar of malabsorption disorders with the concept of elimination:

1. How is bowel function impacted by celiac disease? Lactase deficiency? Short bowel syndrome?
2. When caring for a client with a malabsorption disorder, what precautions must the nurse implement related to bowel elimination?

Linking the exemplar of malabsorption disorders with the concept of development:

3. How does cognitive development impact the treatment of malabsorption disorders?
4. How would you alter the treatment plan of a malabsorption disorder across the life span?

READY Go to Companion Skills Manual

REFER Go to Pearson Nursing Student Resources
nursing.pearsonhighered.com

- Additional review materials

REFLECT Case Study

Chris is a 16-month-old boy who is brought into the clinic by his mother. Chris was born healthy at 6 pounds, 4 ounces. His weight currently is 15 pounds. During the past 3 months, his mother has noticed abdominal distention, irritability, and loose stools. Chris appears pale and slightly lethargic. The child is diagnosed with celiac disease.

1. What assessment data would alert the nurse to a digestive problem?
2. What additional information would the nurse obtain from the mother?
3. Why is Chris pale?
4. What priority nursing diagnosis would you consider for Chris?

EXEMPLAR 4.4 Pancreatitis

EXEMPLAR KEY TERMS
Acute pancreatitis, *246*
Chronic pancreatitis, *246*
Pancreatitis, *245*
Steatorrhea, *247*

EXEMPLAR LEARNING OUTCOMES
After reading about this exemplar, you will be able to:

1. Describe the pathophysiology, etiology, clinical manifestations, and direct and indirect causes of pancreatitis.
2. Identify risk factors and prevention methods associated with pancreatitis.

3. Illustrate the nursing process in providing culturally competent care across the life span for individuals with pancreatitis.
4. Formulate priority nursing diagnoses appropriate for an individual with pancreatitis.
5. Summarize therapies used by interdisciplinary teams in the collaborative care of an individual with pancreatitis.
6. Plan evidence-based care for an individual with pancreatitis and his or her family in collaboration with other members of the healthcare team.
7. Evaluate expected outcomes for an individual with pancreatitis.

▶ OVERVIEW

The normal function of the pancreas involves the release of pancreatic enzymes in the duodenum to assist in the digestion of proteins, starches, and fatty acids. Food entering the small intestine stimulates release of the pancreatic enzymes; however, in **pancreatitis** (inflammation of the pancreas), the pancreatic enzymes are activated early and digest the pancreas and surrounding tissues, a process called autodigestion.

Pancreatitis can be acute or chronic. In the United States, there are 17 newly diagnosed cases of acute pancreatitis for every 100,000 individuals and 100,000 hospitalizations every year. In approximately 20% of individuals who have acute pancreatitis, the severity of the condition requires hospitalization. For chronic pancreatitis, approximately 1.6 to 23 cases occur per 100,000 individuals worldwide (Stevens & Conwell, 2011). This number may not fully represent the population with chronic pancreatitis because many individuals affected by this disorder do not exhibit classic manifestations. Clients with chronic pancreatitis may experience long-term effects of the disease, with chronic changes in enzyme and hormone production (LeMone et al., 2011).

▶ PATHOPHYSIOLOGY AND ETIOLOGY

Knowledge of the normal structure and functions of the exocrine pancreas is important to understand how inflammation affects it and the client. The exocrine pancreas consists of lobules of acinar cells. The acinar cells secrete digestive enzymes and fluids (pancreatic juices) into ducts that empty into the main pancreatic duct (the duct of Wirsung). The pancreatic duct joins the common bile duct and empties into the duodenum through the ampulla of Vater (in some people the main pancreatic duct empties directly into the duodenum). The epithelial lining of the pancreatic ducts secretes water and bicarbonate to modify the composition of the pancreatic secretions. Pancreatic enzymes are secreted primarily in an inactive form and are activated in the intestine, a modification that prevents digestion of pancreatic tissue by its own enzymes (Porth & Matfin, 2009). The pancreatic enzymes, with related functions, are as follows:

- Proteolytic enzymes, including trypsin, chymotrypsin, carboxypolypeptidase, ribonuclease, and deoxyribonuclease, which break down dietary proteins
- Pancreatic amylase, which breaks down starch
- Lipase, which breaks down fats into glycerol and fatty acids.

Acute Pancreatitis

Acute pancreatitis is an inflammatory disorder that involves self-destruction of the pancreas by its own enzymes through autodigestion. The milder form of acute pancreatitis, *interstitial edematous pancreatitis*, leads to inflammation and edema of pancreatic tissue. It often is self-limiting. The more severe form, *necrotizing pancreatitis*, is characterized by inflammation, hemorrhage, and ultimately necrosis of pancreatic tissue.

Acute pancreatitis is more common in middle aged adults. Gallstones and alcoholism account for 80% of the cases of acute pancreatitis in the United States (Stevens & Conwell, 2011). Some clients recover completely, others experience recurring attacks, and still others develop chronic pancreatitis. The mortality and symptoms depend on the severity and type of pancreatitis, as well as the client's age and general health.

Although the exact cause of acute pancreatitis is not known, the following factors may activate pancreatic enzymes within the pancreas, leading to autodigestion, inflammation, edema, and/or necrosis:

- Gallstones may obstruct the pancreatic duct or cause bile reflux, activating pancreatic enzymes in the pancreatic duct system.

- Alcohol causes duodenal edema, and may increase pressure and spasm in the sphincter of Oddi, obstructing pancreatic outflow. It also stimulates pancreatic enzyme production, thus raising pressure within the pancreas.

Other factors associated with acute pancreatitis include tissue ischemia or anoxia, trauma or surgery, pancreatic tumors, third-trimester pregnancy, infectious agents (viral, bacterial, or parasitic), elevated calcium levels, and hyperlipidemia. Some medications have been linked with this disorder, including thiazide diuretics, estrogen, steroids, salicylates, and NSAIDs.

Regardless of the precipitating factor, the pathophysiological process begins with the release of activated pancreatic enzymes into pancreatic tissue. Activated proteolytic enzymes, trypsin in particular, digest pancreatic tissue and activate other enzymes such as phospholipase A, which digests cell membrane phospholipids, and elastase, which digests the elastic tissue of blood vessel walls. This leads to proteolysis, edema, vascular damage and hemorrhage, and necrosis of parenchymal cells. Cellular damage and necrosis release activated enzymes and vasoactive substances that produce vasodilation, increase vascular permeability, and cause edema. A large volume of fluid may shift from circulating blood into the retroperitoneal space, the peripancreatic spaces, and the abdominal cavity. In these cases, acute pancreatitis results in vascular changes, fat and coagulation necrosis, and swelling of the pancreas.

Chronic Pancreatitis

Chronic pancreatitis is characterized by chronic inflammation, fibrosis, and gradual destruction of functional pancreatic tissue. In contrast to acute pancreatitis, which is reversible, chronic pancreatitis is an irreversible process that eventually leads to pancreatic insufficiency. Alcoholism is the primary risk factor for chronic pancreatitis in the United States. Malnutrition is a major worldwide risk factor. About 10%–20% of chronic pancreatitis is idiopathic, with no identified cause. A genetic mutation on a gene associated with cystic fibrosis may play a role in these cases. Children or young adults with cystic fibrosis may develop chronic pancreatitis as well.

In chronic pancreatitis related to alcoholism, pancreatic secretions have an increased concentration of insoluble proteins. These proteins calcify, forming plugs that block pancreatic ducts and the flow of pancreatic juices. This blockage leads to inflammation and fibrosis of pancreatic tissue. In other cases, a stricture or stone may block pancreatic outflow, causing chronic obstructive pancreatitis. In chronic pancreatitis, recurrent episodes of inflammation eventually lead to fibrotic changes in the parenchyma of the pancreas, with loss of exocrine function. This leads to malabsorption from pancreatic insufficiency. If endocrine function is disrupted as well, clinical diabetes mellitus may develop.

Risk Factors and Prevention

Alcoholism and gallstones are the primary risk factors for acute pancreatitis, however, the etiology of about 30% of cases is unclear. Lifestyle choices aimed at managing modifiable risks can prevent acute pancreatitis.

Risk factors for chronic pancreatitis include alcohol abuse, autoimmune disorders, cystic fibrosis, hypertriglyceridemia, hyperparathyroidism, and medications such as estrogens, corticosteroids, and thiazide diuretics (National Center for Biotechnology Information, 2010a). Health promotion strategies in managing lifestyle choices can assist the individual in reducing risk factors for chronic pancreatitis.

▶ CLINICAL MANIFESTATIONS

Acute Pancreatitis

Acute pancreatitis develops suddenly, typically with an abrupt onset of continuous severe epigastric and abdominal pain. This pain commonly radiates to the back and is relieved somewhat by sitting up and leaning forward. The pain often is initiated by a fatty meal or excessive alcohol intake.

Other manifestations include nausea and vomiting; abdominal distention and rigidity; decreased bowel sounds; tachycardia; hypotension; elevated temperature; and cold, clammy skin. Within 24 hours, mild jaundice may appear. Retroperitoneal bleeding may occur 3–6 days after the onset of acute pancreatitis; signs of bleeding include bruising in the flanks (Turner's sign) or around the umbilicus (Cullen's sign). See the Clinical Manifestations and Therapies feature on page 248.

Systemic complications of acute pancreatitis include intravascular volume depletion with shock, acute tubular necrosis and renal failure, and acute respiratory distress syndrome (ARDS). Hypovolemic shock and acute renal failure usually develop within 24 hours after the onset of acute pancreatitis. Manifestations of ARDS may be seen 3–7 days after its onset, particularly in clients who have experienced severe volume depletion.

Localized complications include pancreatic necrosis, abscess, pseudocysts, and pancreatic ascites. Pancreatic necrosis causes an inflammatory mass that may be infected. It may lead to shock and multiple organ failure. Pancreatic pseudocysts, encapsulated collections of fluid, may develop both within the pancreas itself and in the abdominal cavity (**Figure 4–17 ●**). They may impinge on other structures, or may rupture, causing generalized peritonitis. Rupture of a pseudocyst or of the pancreatic duct can lead to pancreatic ascites. An infected pancreatic pseudocyst becomes a pancreatic abscess. A pancreatis abscess may also form as areas in damaged and infected pancreatic tissue become encapsulated (Stevens & Conwell, 2011). Pancreatic ascites is recognized by gradually increasing abdominal girth and persistent elevation of the serum amylase level without abdominal pain.

Chronic Pancreatitis

Chronic pancreatitis typically causes recurrent episodes of epigastric and left upper abdominal pain that radiates to the back. This pain may last for days to weeks. As the disease progresses, the interval between episodes of pain becomes shorter. Other manifestations include anorexia, nausea and vomiting, weight loss, flatulence, constipation, and **steatorrhea** (fatty, frothy, foul-smelling stools caused by a decrease in pancreatic enzyme secretion).

Complications of chronic pancreatitis include malabsorption, malnutrition, and possible peptic ulcer disease. Pancreatic pseudocyst or abscess may form, or stricture of the common bile duct may develop. Diabetes mellitus may develop, and there

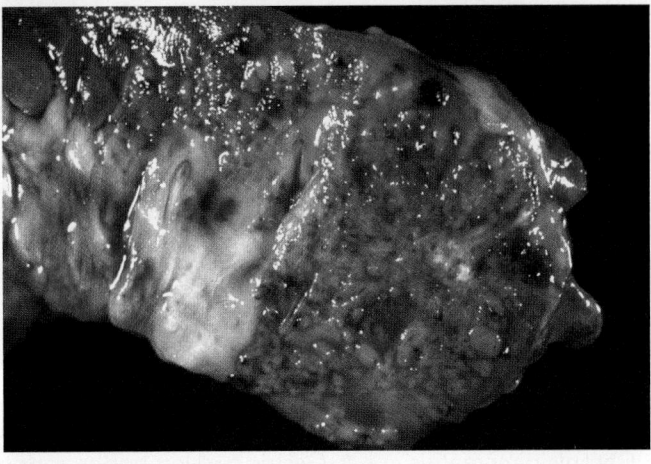

Figure 4–17 ● Acute pancreatitis. Gross clinical specimen of a pancreas affected by acute pancreatitis. A pseudocyst, a pus-filled bleb seen as the yellow area (lower left center), is a potential complication of acute pancreatitis.
Source: CNRI/Science Source.

is an increased risk for pancreatic cancer. Opioid addiction related to frequent, severe pain episodes is common.

▶ COLLABORATION

Because acute pancreatitis often is a mild, self-limiting disease, treatment focuses on reducing pancreatic secretions and providing supportive care. Treatment to eliminate the causative factor is begun after the acute inflammatory process resolves. Severe necrotizing pancreatitis may require intensive care management. Treatment for chronic pancreatitis often focuses on managing pain and treating malabsorption and malnutrition.

Diagnostic Tests

The laboratory tests that may be ordered when pancreatitis is suspected are summarized in **Table 4–9 ●**. Diagnostic studies include the following:

■ *Ultrasonography* can identify gallstones, a pancreatic mass, or pseudocyst.

■ *Endoscopic ultrasonography* can detect changes indicative of chronic pancreatitis in the pancreatic duct and parenchyma.

■ *Contrast-enhanced CT scan* may be ordered to identify pancreatic enlargement, ductal calcifications, fluid collections in or around the pancreas, and perfusion deficits in areas of necrosis.

■ *Magnetic resonance cholangiopancreatography (MRCP)* is a noninvasive test that allows visualization of the bile and pancreatic ducts.

■ *Endoscopic retrograde cholangiopancreatography (ERCP)* may be performed to diagnose chronic pancreatitis and to differentiate inflammation and fibrosis from carcinoma.

■ *Percutaneous fine-needle aspiration biopsy* may be performed to differentiate chronic pancreatitis from cancer of the pancreas; the cells that are aspirated are examined for malignancy.

Clinical Manifestations and Therapies **Pancreatitis**

ETIOLOGY	CLINICAL MANIFESTATIONS	CLINICAL THERAPIES
Acute pancreatitis	■ Severe epigastric and abdominal pain ■ Nausea and vomiting ■ Abdominal distention and rigidity ■ Decreased bowel sounds ■ Tachycardia ■ Hypotension ■ Elevated temperature ■ Cold and clammy skin	■ NPO ■ Intravenous hydration ■ Analgesics ■ Antibiotics
Chronic pancreatitis	■ Gastric and left upper abdominal pain radiating to the back ■ Anorexia ■ Weight loss ■ Nausea and vomiting ■ Constipation ■ Steatorrhea	■ Low-fat diet ■ Abstain from alcohol ■ Surgery to relieve obstruction ■ Pancreatectomy

Pharmacologic Therapy

The treatment of acute pancreatitis is largely supportive. Opioid analgesics such as morphine sulfate or hydromorphone (Dilaudid) may be used to control pain. Prophylactic antibiotics are prescribed for clients with severe or necrotizing pancreatitis to prevent infection.

Clients with chronic pancreatitis may also require analgesics, but must be closely monitored to prevent drug dependence. Pancreatic enzyme supplements are given to manage abdominal pain and reduce steatorrhea (see the Medications feature on page 249). Clients with chronic pancreatitis may need to remain on pancreatic enzyme supplements for life. H_2-blockers such as cimetidine (Tagamet) and ranitidine (Zantac), and proton pump inhibitors such as omeprazole (Prilosec) may be given to neutralize or decrease gastric secretions.

Nutrition

Oral food and fluids generally are withheld during acute episodes of pancreatitis to reduce pancreatic secretions and pro-mote rest of the organ. A nasogastric tube may be inserted and connected to suction. Intravenous fluids are administered to maintain vascular volume, and total parenteral nutrition (TPN) is initiated. Oral food and fluids are begun once the serum amylase levels have returned to normal, bowel sounds are present, and pain disappears. A low-fat diet is ordered, and alcohol intake is strictly prohibited.

Surgery

If the pancreatitis is the result of a gallstone lodged in the sphincter of Oddi, an *endoscopic transduodenal sphincterotomy* may be performed to remove the stone. When cholelithiasis is identified as a causative factor, a cholecystectomy is performed once the acute pancreatitis has resolved. Surgical procedures to promote drainage of pancreatic enzymes into the duodenum or resection of all or part of the pancreas may be done to provide pain relief in clients with chronic pancreatitis. Large pancreatic pseudocysts may be drained endoscopically or surgically.

TABLE 4–9 Laboratory Tests in Exocrine Pancreatic Disorders

TEST	NORMAL VALUE	SIGNIFICANCE
Serum amylase	30–170 units/L 60–160 Somogyi units/dL	Rises within 2–12 hours of onset of acute pancreatitis to two to three times normal. Returns to normal in 3–4 days.
Serum lipase	14–280 units/L 20–180 international units/L	Levels rise in acute pancreatitis; remain elevated for 7–14 days.
Urine amylase	4–37 units/L/2 hr 6.5–48 units/h (SI units)	Urine amylase levels rise in acute pancreatitis.
Serum glucose (fasting)	70–110 mg/dL	May be transient elevation in acute pancreatitis.
Serum bilirubin	0.1–1.0 mg/dL	Compression of the common duct may increase bilirubin levels in acute pancreatitis.
Serum alkaline phosphatase (ALP)	42–136 units/L	Compression of the common duct may increase levels in acute pancreatitis.
Serum calcium	9–11 mg/dL or 4.5–5.5 mEq/L	Hypocalcemia develops in up to 25% of clients with acute pancreatitis.
White blood cells	4,500–10,000/mm^3	Leukocytosis indicates inflammation and is usually present in acute pancreatitis.

Medications **Chronic Pancreatitis**

CLASSIFICATION AND DRUG EXAMPLES	MECHANISMS OF ACTION	NURSING CONSIDERATIONS
Pancreatic Enzyme Replacement *Drug example:* ■ pancrelipase (Lipancreatin)	Pancrelipase enhances the digestion of starches and fats in the gastrointestinal tract by supplying an exogenous source of the enzymes protease, amylase, and lipase. The drug promotes nutrition and decreases the number of bowel movements.	■ Assess for allergy to pork protein. ■ Monitor frequency and consistency of stools. ■ Weigh every other day. Record weights. ■ Give with meals; if not enteric coated, H_2 antagonists or antacids may be given concurrently to prevent destruction of the enzymes by hydrochloric acid. ■ Monitor for side effects: rash, hives, respiratory difficulty, hematuria, hyperuricemia, or joint pain. *Health education for the client and family:* ■ Take with meals or snacks. ■ If medicine is enteric coated, do not crush, chew, or mix with alkaline foods (e.g., milk, ice cream) ■ Be sure to follow prescribed diet. ■ Continue taking this drug until or unless advised by physician that it is no longer necessary.

◼ NURSING PROCESS

In addition to the nursing care discussed in this section, a Nursing Care Plan for a client with acute pancreatitis is provided on page 250.

Assessment

A thorough assessment is necessary and must include bowel sounds, abdominal distention, jaundice, nausea or vomiting, presence of flatus, and last bowel movement. For clients reporting pain, assess the location, nature, duration, and precipitating factors. Inquire about alcohol consumption, dietary intake, and family history of pancreatitis. Assess for previous illnesses, surgery, and current medications (including over-the-counter and CAM therapies).

Diagnosis

The following nursing diagnoses may be appropriate for clients with pancreatitis:

■ *Acute Pain* related to inflammation and edema
■ *Deficient Fluid Volume* related to decreased fluid intake
■ *Nausea* related to irritation of the gastrointestinal system

Complementary and Alternative Therapy
Pancreatitis

Several complementary therapies may be used in conjunction with traditional treatments for clients with acute or chronic pancreatitis. Fasting or use of low-salt, low-fat vegetarian diets may reduce episodes of recurrent pain. Qigong, a system of gentle exercise, meditation, and controlled breathing, is believed to balance the flow of qi (a vital life force) through the body. Qigong lowers the metabolic rate, and may reduce the stimulation of pancreatic enzyme secretion. Magnetic field therapy also may be employed for clients with pancreatitis. All complementary therapies should be prescribed by a trained and competent practitioner.

■ *Imbalanced Nutrition: Less Than Body Requirements* related to decreased intake

(NANDA-I © 2012)

Planning

Nursing care for the client with acute pancreatitis focuses on managing pain, nutrition, and maintaining fluid balance. Careful discharge planning that includes client education and appropriate referrals is necessary to increase the likelihood of the client's return to health.

Implementation

Nursing interventions to manage pain, restore nutritional status, and restore and maintain fluid and electrolyte balance will help reduce the client's risk for a life-threatening event and increase the client's chances for success in meeting and maintaining a healthy lifestyle and therapeutic regimen following discharge.

Manage Pain

Managing pain will include obtaining pain levels using an appropriate pain scale and administering opioid analgesics as ordered. Administering analgesics on schedule rather than waiting for pain to increase will result in better pain management for the client. For clients who are NPO, the nurse offers frequent oral hygiene for client comfort and maintains nasogastric tube patency as ordered.

Restore Nutritional Status

The nurse administers antiemetics as ordered, weighs the client daily, and monitors client intake and output. Ongoing assessment involves monitoring bowel sounds and maintaining a stool chart, noting the frequency, color, odor, and consistency of stools. The nurse also monitors lab values, which reflect nutritional status, including serum albumin, serum transferrin, hemoglobin, and hematocrit. Until oral intake resumes, the nurse administers prescribed intravenous fluids or total

The client with pancreatitis is often acutely ill and, along with family members, needs information about both hospital procedures and self-care at home following discharge. During the acute stage, keep explanations brief and simple.

Prior to discharge, the nurse provides information about the disease and how to prevent further episodes of inflammation to the client and family. The following topics should be covered:

- Alcohol can cause stones to form, blocking pancreatic ducts and the outflow of pancreatic juice. Continued alcohol intake is likely to cause further inflammation and destruction of the pancreas. Avoid alcohol entirely.
- Smoking and stress stimulate the pancreas and should be avoided.
- If pancreatic function has been severely impaired, discuss appropriate use of pancreatic enzymes, including timing, dose, potential side effects, and monitoring of effectiveness.

- A low-fat diet is recommended. Provide a list of high-fat foods to avoid. Crash dieting and binge eating also should be avoided because they may precipitate attacks. Spicy foods, coffee, tea, or colas, and gas-forming foods stimulate gastric and pancreatic secretions and may precipitate pain. Avoid them if this occurs.
- Report symptoms of infection (fever of 38.8°C [102°F] or higher, pain, rapid pulse, malaise) because a pancreatic abscess can develop after initial recovery.

Client referral is an important component of the discharge process. The nurse refers the client and family to a dietitian or nutritionist for diet teaching as needed. Other referrals may be warranted, including referrals to community agencies, such as Alcoholics Anonymous, or to an alcohol treatment program. Provide referrals to community or home health agencies as needed for continued monitoring and teaching at home.

parenteral nutrition. Once the client can resume eating, small, frequent meals are offered.

Meet Fluid and Electrolyte Needs

The client with acute pancreatitis is at risk for a fluid shift from the intravascular space into the abdominal cavity (third spacing). Third spacing of fluid may cause hypovolemic shock, affecting cardiovascular function, respiratory function, renal function, and mental status. For these clients, the nurse assesses cardiovascular status every 4 hours or as indicated, including vital signs, cardiac rhythm, central venous and pulmonary artery pressures, peripheral pulses and capillary refill, and skin color, temperature, moisture, and turgor.

Clients at risk for fluid and electrolyte imbalance also require ongoing monitoring of renal function. The nurse assesses urine output hourly, reporting if less than 30 mL/hr. Monitoring of neurological function, including mental status, level of consciousness, and behavior, is also essential because hypotension and hypoxia may decrease cerebral perfusion. Alcohol withdrawal is a risk for the client with chronic pancreatitis.

SAFETY ALERT
Regularly assess respiratory status (at least every 4–8 hours), including respiratory rate, depth, and pattern; breath sounds; and oxygen saturation and arterial blood gas results. Report tachypnea, adventitious or absent breath sounds, oxygen saturation levels below 92%, PaO_2 < 70 mmHg or $PaCO_2$ > 45 mmHg. Severe abdominal pain causes shallow respirations and hypoventilation, and suppresses cough effectiveness, which can lead to pooling of secretions, atelectasis, and pneumonia.

Evaluation

Outcome and evaluation parameters will include the following:

- The client experiences reduction or elimination of pain.
- The client is able to resume eating.
- The client remains free from alterations in fluid and nutrition status.
- The client is free from nausea.

NURSING CARE PLAN   A Client With Acute Pancreatitis

Constantine Popullia is a 22-year-old female. She presents to the emergency department with severe abdominal pain that is "unrelentless and intense burning" and weight loss. She and her sister have had pancreatitis and multiple episodes have required hospitalization during the past 5 years. Ms. Popullia's serum amylase and lipase are moderately elevated. An ERCP indicated strictures within the biliary bile ducts and inflammation.

ASSESSMENT	DIAGNOSES	PLANNING

The nurse conducts a health history, health interview, and physical assessment and notes the following abnormal assessment findings (in addition to the symptoms listed above):
  Recent weight loss from anorexia and nausea/vomiting
  Steatorrhea
  Tea-colored urine
  Blood pressure 160/92 mmHg, pulse 88 bpm, and respirations 16/min.
	■ *Acute Pain* related to pancreatitis
	■ *Imbalanced Nutrition: Less Than Body Requirements* related to inability to digest and absorb nutrients due to pancreatitis and nausea/vomiting
	
	(NANDA-I © 2012)
		Together the nurse and Ms. Popullia develop the following goals for Ms. Popullia's plan of care:
		
		■ The client will have minimal outward symptoms of pain with routine administration of pain medications.
		■ The client will tolerate IV feedings in meeting body requirements without adverse effects.

NURSING CARE PLAN *(continued)*

IMPLEMENTATION

- Instruct Ms. Popullia on how to use and the purpose of the patient-controlled analgesia (PCA).
- Assess efficacy of the PCA method of pain medication delivery on Ms. Popullia's pain level.
- Offer alternative forms of pain relief such as repositioning (in fetal position) and distraction.

- Begin NPO diet status and TPN therapy as prescribed.
- Monitor laboratory values in relation to nutrition and TPN therapy.

EVALUATION

In 4 days, Ms. Popullia's serum amylase and lipase levels have decreased and she has begun to eat small amounts of food without resulting pain. The PCA has been discontinued; oral analgesics have been prescribed for mild to moderate pain as needed. Plans for discharge are being made including resources for a dietitian to help Ms. Popullia plan a healthy diet to decrease risk of another exacerbation of pancreatitis.

CRITICAL THINKING

1. What connection do serum amylase and serum lipase levels have on nutritional oral intake?
2. How can you demonstrate a nonjudgmental attitude to Ms. Popullia in relation to the most common cause of chronic pancreatitis?
3. What dietary recommendations should you offer Ms. Popullia?
4. Ms. Popullia and her sister have had pancreatitis for more than 5 years. How do you think this interferes with their lifestyles and growth and development?

REVIEW Pancreatitis

RELATE Link the Concepts and Exemplars

Linking the exemplar of pancreatitis with the concept of metabolism:

1. How does pancreatitis influence the normal process of metabolism?
2. What interventions by the client can reduce the long-term effects of pancreatitis?

Linking the exemplar of pancreatitis with the concept of comfort:

3. How can the nurse utilize appropriate pain assessment instruments when caring for a client with pancreatitis?
4. How can the nurse incorporate complementary and alternative practices in the care of a client with pancreatitis?

READY Go to Companion Skills Manual

REFER Go to Pearson Nursing Student Resources
nursing.pearsonhighered.com

- Additional review materials

REFLECT Case Study

Chris Johnson is a 28-year-old male. Recently, Mr. Johnson has been experiencing abdominal pain, but he has not seen his healthcare provider about it. On Saturday night, Mr. Johnson attends a party, staying until almost 2:00 a.m. As Mr. Johnson is driving home, he loses control of his car and the vehicle rolls four times. Mr. Johnson, who is not wearing his seat belt, is ejected from the car. On arrival at the emergency department, Mr. Johnson is highly intoxicated on observation. Mr. Johnson admits to the physician that he has been drinking frequently and has suffered from acute pancreatitis in the past.

1. What additional assessment data would the nurse want to obtain from Mr. Johnson?
2. Mr. Johnson asks the nurse what the difference is between acute and chronic pancreatitis. When and how would you provide education to Mr. Johnson about his diagnosis?
3. What priority interventions would you implement at this time?

EXEMPLAR 4.5 Pyloric Stenosis

EXEMPLAR KEY TERMS
Projectile vomiting, *252*
Pyloric stenosis, *252*

EXEMPLAR LEARNING OUTCOMES
After reading about this exemplar, you will be able to:

1. Describe the pathophysiology, etiology, clinical manifestations, and direct and indirect causes of pyloric stenosis.
2. Identify risk factors and prevention methods associated with pyloric stenosis.
3. Illustrate the nursing process in providing culturally competent care across the life span for individuals with pyloric stenosis.

4. Formulate priority nursing diagnoses appropriate for an individual with pyloric stenosis.
5. Summarize therapies used by interdisciplinary teams in the collaborative care of an individual with pyloric stenosis.
6. Plan evidence-based care for an individual with pyloric stenosis and his or her family in collaboration with other members of the healthcare team.
7. Evaluate expected outcomes for an individual with pyloric stenosis.

▶ OVERVIEW

Pyloric stenosis, narrowing of the pyloric orifice, directly impacts the structure and function of the digestive tract, preventing food within the stomach from passing through the pylorus into the duodenum. This impairs digestion and absorption of food, resulting in dehydration and malnutrition. Pyloric stenosis generally affects infants within the first month of life, causing regurgitation and poor feeding. Rarely is pyloric stenosis seen in adults. When it is, it is as a result of peptic ulcer disease, malignant compression of the gastric outlet, or gas in the bowel wall (pneumatosis intestinalis).

▶ PATHOPHYSIOLOGY AND ETIOLOGY

Etiology

For unknown reasons, the pyloric orifice thickens from inflammation and edema causing a partial or full obstruction between the stomach and duodenum (**Figure 4–18 ●**). As the pyloric orifice narrows, vomiting becomes more forceful. As the obstruction progresses, the infant becomes dehydrated and electrolytes are depleted, resulting in metabolic imbalances.

Risk Factors

Genetics may play a role in pyloric stenosis. Children with parents who had pyloric stenosis are more likely to have the condition (National Center for Biotechnology Information, 2013). Pyloric stenosis is more common in males than females. Antibiotics given in late pregnancy or in the first few weeks of life may be associated with an increased risk of pyloric stenosis (Mayo Clinic, 2013b).

▶ CLINICAL MANIFESTATIONS

Symptoms usually become evident 3–6 weeks after birth. Babies feed normally and then vomit within 30 minutes. As the pyloric stenosis worsens, the vomiting becomes projectile. With

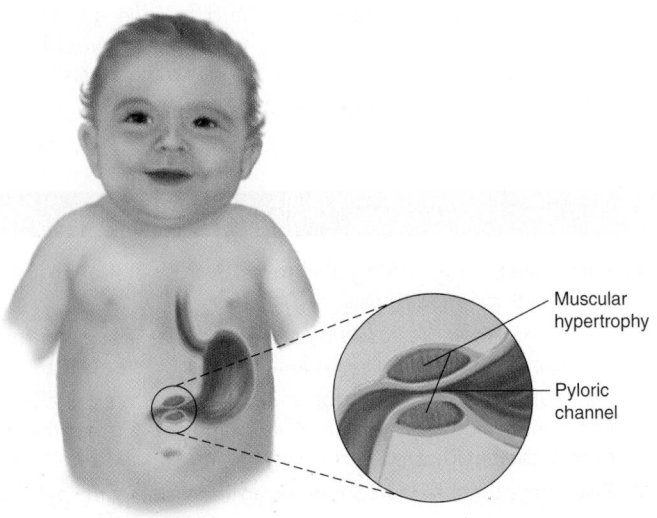

Muscular
hypertrophy

Pyloric
channel

Figure 4–18 ● In pyloric stenosis, the hypertrophied pyloric muscle causes symptoms of projectile vomiting and visible peristalsis.

projectile vomiting, the emesis may be spewed up to 2–3 feet out of the baby's mouth. At times the vomit may contain small amounts of blood. After vomiting, the baby is hungry and may want to feed again. Persistent hunger is a common symptom of pyloric stenosis. Parents may notice a wave-like ripple across the baby's abdomen after feeding and immediately proceeding vomiting. This peristaltic wave is the body's attempt to push the food through the pylorus. Frequent vomiting can easily lead to dehydration and malnutrition. Changes in the stool are common as the baby becomes constipated, and the baby is unable to gain weight or may even lose weight. Parents should contact the primary healthcare provider if the baby exhibits frequent vomiting, projectile vomiting, irritability due to dehydration, or failure to gain weight.

▶ COLLABORATION

Diagnostic Tests

An abdominal ultrasound to determine the diameter and length of the pyloric muscle is usually performed to confirm the diagnosis. An upper gastrointestinal (UGI) study may also be performed, and reveals a narrowing of the pyloric channel, preventing the passage of the contrast medium. Blood tests determine the degree of dehydration, electrolyte imbalance, and anemia. Early diagnosis decreases the severity of electrolyte alterations.

Surgery

Surgery is performed as soon as possible after the infant's fluid and electrolyte balance is restored. Open pyloromyotomy is performed though a periumbilical incision or through a small, transverse upper abdominal incision. Recovery time from a laparoscopic pyloromyotomy is faster than recovery from an open pyloromyotomy (Mayo Clinic, 2013c). With both procedures, the pyloric muscle is split to allow the passage of food and fluid.

The prognosis is good. The infant is usually taking fluids within a few hours following surgery and discharged on full-strength formula within 24 hours after surgery.

■ NURSING PROCESS

Assessment

Observe the infant's abdomen for the presence of peristaltic waves. Then auscultate bowel sounds which are usually hyperactive on auscultation. Palpation reveals an olive-shaped mass in the right upper quadrant of the abdomen.

Assess the infant's history of vomiting, vital signs, weight, and nutritional status. Assess skin turgor, fontanels, mucous membranes, urinary output (weigh diapers), and urine specific gravity to determine whether hydration is adequate. Describe vomiting episodes and estimated emesis amount. Be alert for signs of an electrolyte imbalance, particularly low levels of serum chloride, sodium, and potassium, and an elevated pH. (See the module on Fluids and Electrolytes for a discussion of these electrolyte imbalances.) Assess the parents' level of anxiety related to the child's condition. The child is usually hungry and tries to feed. Crying and general discomfort are frequently observed.

Diagnosis

Among the nursing diagnoses that might be appropriate for the child with pyloric stenosis are:

- *Deficient Fluid Volume* related to inadequate intake and vomiting
- *Imbalanced Nutrition: Less Than Body Requirements* related to vomiting and inability to ingest nutrients
- *Sleep Pattern Disturbance* related to discomfort and hunger
- *Parental Anxiety* related to surgery.

(NANDA-I © 2012)

Planning

The idea of their infant undergoing surgery can be overwhelming for parents. It is critical for the nurse to take time to elicit the parents' input in the plan of care, ensure that parents receive sufficient explanations regarding treatment options, and that informed consent for all procedures, including laboratory tests, is obtained.

Implementation

Nursing care focuses on meeting the infant's fluid and electrolyte needs, minimizing weight loss, promoting rest and comfort, preventing infection, and providing supportive care for parents.

Meet Fluid and Electrolyte Needs

Because projectile vomiting will continue until the obstruction is relieved surgically, withhold oral feedings. Emphasize to the parents the importance of maintaining an NPO status preoperatively. Intravenous fluid therapy is administered to correct fluid and electrolyte imbalances and to maintain adequate hydration. Because gastric fluid is high in potassium, hypokalemia can result. (See the module on Fluids and Electrolytes for a discussion of hypokalemia.) Maintain patency of the nasogastric tube and measure aspirated contents. Inform parents that all diapers will be weighed to measure the infant's output of urine and stool.

Minimize Weight Loss

The infant loses weight because of frequent vomiting. Monitor weight daily both preoperatively and postoperatively. Begin feedings postoperatively according to healthcare provider orders. Some surgeons prefer an NPO period following pyloromyotomy, with slow, incremental increases in volume and strength of feedings once feeding has resumed, while others will implement an earlier postoperative feeding approach.

Promote Rest and Comfort

During the preoperative period the infant is hungry and cries often. The infant is swaddled to maintain warmth and provide comfort. Encourage the parents to hold and cuddle the infant. Provide a pacifier to meet the infant's need to suck.

Postoperatively the infant is uncomfortable because of the surgical incision. Administer analgesics as prescribed to relieve discomfort. Instruct parents to avoid pressure on the incision. When diapering the infant, slide the diaper gently under the buttocks rather than lifting the legs. Swaddling, rocking, and use of a pacifier help to relax the infant. (See the module on Comfort for a discussion of pain management.)

Prevent Infection

Postoperatively the incision is covered with collodion or Steri-Strips and should be kept clean and dry. Inspect the incision site for redness, swelling, or discharge. Monitor the infant's temperature every 4 hours. Auscultate the lungs to assess for any adventitious sounds.

Provide Supportive Care

The need for hospitalization and surgery creates anxiety for parents. Encourage them to participate in the infant's care and to discuss their fears and concerns. Provide simple and clear explanations about the infant's condition and care. Advise parents that occasional vomiting after surgery may occur.

Client Teaching **Home Care Instructions Following Pyloromyotomy**

The infant is generally discharged home the day following surgery. Partner with the family to provide home feeding and care instructions. The following information is provided:

- The infant may be bottle-fed or breastfed.
- An infant may vomit after some feedings following surgery—this does not mean the surgical correction was unsuccessful.
- If the infant vomits, offer a bottle or breast as soon as he or she is interested in feeding again.
- The infant should be burped after every 1–2 ounces during feeding. If breastfeeding, burp the infant every 5–10 minutes.
- After feeding, hold the infant in an upright position for 30 minutes.
- The infant should not play or be rocked for 30 minutes following feedings.

- Administer analgesics as prescribed. Inform the healthcare provider if you believe your infant is not obtaining adequate pain relief.
- Keep the surgical wound area clean and dry. The bandage or strips may fall off, and this is normal. If not, they will be removed at the follow-up visit.
- The infant should be sponge bathed only. Tub baths are not allowed until the wound has healed or as instructed by the healthcare provider.
- Notify the healthcare provider if the infant demonstrates any of the following:
  - Redness, drainage, bleeding, or swelling at the surgical site
  - A fever of 38.1°C (100.5°F) or higher.
  - Is inconsolable.
  - Vomits the majority of two feedings in a row.

Discharge Planning and Home Care Teaching

Instruct parents to observe the incision for redness, swelling, or discharge and to notify the physician immediately if these occur or if the infant develops a fever. To reduce the possibility of infection, advise parents to fold the infant's diaper so that it does not touch the incision. Provide instructions about feeding to ensure the infant's intake.

Evaluation

Expected outcomes of care include pain control, intake of recommended fluid and food with absence of vomiting, and manifestation of normal growth patterns.

NURSING CARE PLAN   A Client With Pyloric Stenosis

Adam Zorkowski is a 2-month-old boy. He presents to the primary healthcare provider with irritability, projectile vomiting, and constipation.

ASSESSMENT

Adam has had recurrent episodes of projectile vomiting. His parents state, "He only vomits once in a while, it comes flying out, and then he wants to eat again." In reviewing the client record, the nurse notes Adam weighs the same as he did at 6 weeks of age. The nurse asks his parents about elimination patterns. They both agree that Adam has required less frequent diaper changes and he seems to be constipated. On abdominal auscultation, Adam has hyperactive bowel sounds and on palpation, an olive-shaped mass in the right upper quadrant of the abdomen is noted. The diagnosis is pyloric stenosis. A laparoscopic pyloromyotomy is performed.

DIAGNOSES

- *Acute Pain* related to surgical procedure
- *Imbalanced Nutrition: Less Than Body Requirements* related to recurrent episodes of vomiting
- *Risk for Aspiration* due to vomiting.

(NANDA-I © 2012)

PLANNING

Together the nurse and Adam's parents develop the following goals for Adam's plan of care:

- The client will have no outward symptoms of pain.
- The client will gain 2.2 lb (1 kg) per month.
- The client will not exhibit signs of aspiration.

IMPLEMENTATION

- Administer pain medications when Adam begins to demonstrate outward signs of pain.
- Following surgery, slowly increase amount of feeding as Adam tolerates. Report any vomiting episodes.

- Encourage the parents to position Adam upright when feeding, keep Adam upright after feeding or lay him on his right side with the head of bed elevated, and avoid overfeeding.

EVALUATION

Following recovery from the laparoscopic pyloromyotomy, Adam is discharged home. He had minimal signs of pain during hospitalization; these were treated effectively with acetaminophen. Adam was able to tolerate full-strength breast milk without vomiting prior to discharge. His parents successfully demonstrated strategies to prevent aspiration when feeding Adam. The nurses taught the parents how to minimize pain when changing diapers and clothing Adam, as well as how to care for the laparoscopic insertion sites. The parents verbalized understanding and demonstrated a diaper change preventing pressure on the laparoscopic sites.

CRITICAL THINKING

1. What assessment data would you monitor to ensure Adam's nutritional status is adequate for his growth and development?
2. Besides weight gain, what other concerns do you have in relation to episodes of vomiting and Adam's growth and development?
3. What strategies promote comfort and minimize acute pain for an infant?
4. What role does the nurse play in pre-, peri-, and postoperative care of an infant versus an adult?

REVIEW Pyloric Stenosis

RELATE Link the Concepts and Exemplars

Linking the exemplar of pyloric stenosis with the concept of acid–base balance:

1. What type of acid-base imbalance can occur with pyloric stenosis?
2. What caring interventions might be implemented in a client with pyloric stenosis to prevent an acid–base imbalance?

Linking the exemplar of pyloric stenosis with the concept of development:

3. How would pyloric stenosis impact an infant's development?
4. How could pyloric stenosis affect cognitive growth in the infant?

READY Go to Companion Skills Manual

REFER Go to Pearson Nursing Student Resources
nursing.pearsonhighered.com

- Additional review materials

REFLECT Case Study

Kanye Long is a 3-week-old male with a history of vomiting for 3 days. Kanye vomits only after being fed. The vomitus resembles partially digested formula without blood or bile. He feeds well, but vomits 1–2 hours following feeding. The emesis is forceful. His mother describes the emesis as being able to project about 30 cm, rather than just dribbling down his mouth. He has already vomited five times today. Kanye has also had two loose stools (no mucus, no blood, not foul). There is no history of irritability, fever, or ill contacts. His birth history is unremarkable.

1. What manifestations does Kanye exhibit to support a diagnosis of pyloric stenosis?

2. How do pyloric stenosis and GERD differ?

3. What are the priority interventions for a client who has had surgery to correct the stenosis?

4. What priority nursing diagnoses would you choose for the preoperative and postoperative period?

■ REFERENCES

American Association for the Study of Liver Diseases. (2013). *Viral hepatitis prevention, screening, and treatment*. Retrieved from http://www.aasld.org/clients/pages/viralhepatitisprevention.aspx#screening.

Ball, J., Bindler, R., & Cowen, K. (2012). *Principles of pediatric nursing: Caring for children* (5th ed.). Upper Saddle River, NJ: Pearson Education.

Barbarito, C., & D'Amico, D. (2012). *Health and physical assessment in nursing* (2nd ed.). Upper Saddle River, NJ: Pearson Education.

Berman, A., & Snyder, S. (2012). *Kozier & Erb's fundamentals of nursing: Concepts, process, and practice* (9th ed.). Upper Saddle River, NJ: Pearson Education.

Centers for Disease Control and Prevention. (2012). *Viral hepatitis statistics & surveillance*. Retrieved from http://www.cdc.gov/hepatitis/Statistics/index.htm.

Corley, D. A., Kubo, A., Zhau, W., & Quesenberry, C. (2010). Proton pump inhibitors and histamine-2 receptor antagonists are associated with hip fractures among at-risk clients. *Gastroenterology, 139*(1). doi:10.1053/j.gastro.2110.03.055.

D'Amico, D., & Barbarito, C. (2012). *Health & physical assessment in nursing* (2nd ed.). Upper Saddle River, NJ: Pearson Education.

Freeman, H. J. (2010). Risk factors in familial forms of celiac disease. *World Journal of Gastroenterology, 16*(15). doi:10.3748/wjg.v16.i15.1828.

Huether, S. E. (2010). Alterations of digestive functions. In K. S. Osborn, C. E. Wraa, A. B. Watson, & R. Holleran (Eds.), *Medical-surgical nursing: Preparation for practice* (2nd ed., pp. 1189–1196). Boston, MA: Pearson Education.

Johns Hopkins Children's Center. (n.d.). *Gastroesophageal reflux disease*. Retrieved from http://www.hopkinschildrens.org/tpl_rlinks_nav1up.aspx?id=5066.

Khalili, H., Huang, E. S., Jacobson, B. C., Camargo, C. A., Feskanich, D., & Chan, A. T. (2012). Use of proton pump inhibitors and risk of hip fracture in relation to dietary and lifestyle factors: A prospective cohort study. *BMJ*. doi:10.1136/bjm.e372.

LeMone, P., Burke, K., & Bauldoff, G. (2011). *Medical-surgical nursing: Critical thinking in client care* (5th ed.). Upper Saddle River, NJ: Pearson Education.

Lilley, L. L., Collins, S. R., Harrington, S., & Snyder, J. S. (2011). *Pharmacology and the nursing process* (6th ed.). Canada: Elsevier.

London, M. L., Ladewig, P. W., Ball, J. W., Bindler, R. C., & Cowen, K. J. (2011). *Maternal & child nursing care* (3rd ed.). Upper Saddle River, NJ: Pearson Education.

Mayo Clinic. (2011). *Antacid: Oral route*. Retrieved from http://www.mayoclinic.com/health/drug-information/DR602357.

Mayo Clinic. (2012a). *Alternate cancer treatments*. Retrieved from http://www.mayoclinic.com/health/cancer-treatment/CM00002.

Mayo Clinic. (2012b). *Lactose intolerance*. Retrieved from http://www.ncbi.nlm.nih.gov/pubmedhealth/PMH0001321.

Mayo Clinic. (2013a). *Pyloric stenosis—Causes*. Retrieved from http://www.mayoclinic.com/health/pyloric-stenosis/DS00815/DSECTION=symptoms.

Mayo Clinic. (2013b). *Pyloric stenosis—Risk factors*. Retrieved from http://www.mayoclinic.com/health/pyloric-stenosis/DS00815/DSECTION=risk-factors.

Mayo Clinic. (2013c). *Pyloric stenosis—Treatment*. Retrieved from http://www.mayoclinic.com/health/pyloric-stenosis/DS00815/DSECTION=treatments-and-drugs.

Medicine.Net. (2013). *Viral hepatitis*. Retrieved from http://www.medicinenet.com/viral_hepatitis/page6.htm#what_is_the_treatment_for_viral_hepatitis.

National Center for Biotechnology Information. (2010a). *Chronic pancreatitis*. Retrieved from http://www.ncbi.nlm.nih.gov/pubmedhealth/PMH0001268.

National Center for Biotechnology Information. (2010b). *Gastroesophageal reflux disease*. Retrieved from http://www.ncbi.nlm.nih.gov/pubmedhealth/PMH0001311.

National Center for Biotechnology Information. (2012). *Glucose galactose malabsorption*. Retrieved from http://www.ncbi.nlm.nih.gov/books/NBK22184.

National Center for Biotechnology Information. (2013). *Pyloric stenosis*. Retrieved from http://www.ncbi.nlm.nih.gov/pubmedhealth/PMH0001965/.

National Digestive Diseases Information Clearinghouse. (2012). *Celiac disease*. Retrieved from http://digestive.niddk.nih.gov/ddiseases/pubs/celiac.

National Institutes of Health [NIH]. (2010a). *Pancreatitis*. Retrieved from http://www.ncbi.nlm.nih.gov/pubmedhealth/PMH0001332.

National Institutes of Health [NIH]. (2010b). *Taking antacids*. Retrieved from http://www.nlm.nih.gov/medlineplus/ency/clientinstructions/000198.htm.

National Institutes of Health [NIH]. (2011). *GERD*. Retrieved from http://www.nlm.nih.gov/medlineplus/gerd.html.

National Institutes of Health [NIH]. (2012). *Digestive diseases statistics for the United States*. Retrieved from http://digestive.niddk.nih.gov/statistics/statistics.aspx.

National Institutes of Health [NIH]. (2013a). *Chronic pancreatitis*. Retrieved from http://www.ncbi.nlm.nih.gov/pubmedhealth/PMH0001268.

National Institutes of Health [NIH]. (2013b). *GERD*. Retrieved from http://www.nlm.nih.gov/medlineplus/gerd.html.

National Institutes of Health [NIH]. (2013c). *Pyloric stenosis*. Retrieved from http://www.ncbi.nlm.nih.gov/pubmedhealth/PMH0001965.

O'Malley, T., & Heuberger, R. (2011). Vitamin D status and supplementation in pediatric gastrointestinal disease. *Journal for Specialists in Pediatric Nursing, 16*(2), 140–150. doi:10.111/j.1744-6155.2011.00280.x.

Osborn, K. S., Wraa, C. E., Watson, A. B., & Holleran, R. (2014). *Medical-surgical nursing: Preparation for practice* (2nd ed.). Upper Saddle River, NJ: Pearson Education.

Pirtie, K. (2010). Acid-reflux—A red flag: A precursor to chronic illness. Retrieved from http://www.westonaprice.org/digestive-disorders/acid-reflux-a-red-flag.

Porth, C. M., & Matfin, G. (2009). *Pathophysiology: Concepts of altered health states* (8th ed.). Philadelphia, PA: Lippincott.

Raising Children Network. (2013). *Dental care for newborns*. Retrieved from http://health.state.tn.us/oral-health/howmanyteeth.html.

Stevens, T., & Conwell, D. L. (2011). *Chronic pancreatitis: Disease management Project—Cleveland Clinic*. Retrieved from https://www.clevelandclinicmeded.com/medicalpubs/diseasemanagement/gastroenterology/chronic-pancreatitis/#cesec4.

Sullivan, J. M. (2011). Caring for older adults after surgery. *Nursing, 41*(4), 48–51. doi:10.1097/01.NURSE.0000394459.56297.85.

Thomas, D. J. (2011). Abdominal problems. In K. S. Osborn, C. E. Wraa, A. B. Watson, & R. Holleran (Eds.), *Medical-surgical nursing: Preparation for practice* (2nd ed., p. 1169). Boston, MA: Pearson Education.

University of Maryland Medical Center (2011). *Pyloric stenosis*. Retrieved from http://www.umm.edu/altmed/articles/pyloric-stenosis-000138.htm.

Wilson, B. A., Shannon, M. T., & Shields, K. M. (2013). *Pearson nurse's drug guide 2013*. Upper Saddle River, NJ: Pearson/Prentice Hall.

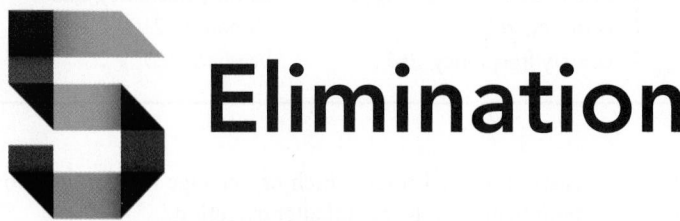

Elimination

◪ THE CONCEPT OF ELIMINATION

Elimination refers to the secretion and excretion of physiological waste products by the kidneys and intestines. Because nurses frequently are the first healthcare professionals to determine that a client is experiencing problems with elimination, nurses must be familiar with the different alterations in elimination, their risk factors, and how these alterations affect other physiological processes. **<<**

Concept Learning Outcomes

After reading about this concept, you will be able to:

1. Summarize the physiology of the renal and gastrointestinal systems related to elimination.

2. Examine the relationship between elimination and other concepts/systems.

3. Identify commonly occurring alterations in elimination and their related therapies.

4. Differentiate common assessment procedures used to examine urinary and gastrointestinal health across the life span.

5. Describe diagnostic and laboratory tests to determine the individual's elimination status.

6. Explain management of urinary and bowel health and prevention of urinary and bowel illness.

7. Demonstrate the nursing process in providing culturally competent and caring interventions across the life span for individuals with common alterations in elimination.

8. Compare and contrast common independent and collaborative interventions for clients with alterations in elimination.

Concept Key Terms

Anuria, 264
Borborygmus, 280
Bowel incontinence, 276
Bruits, 280
Calculi, 271
Constipation, 276
Creatinine clearance, 271
Defecation, 273
Detrusor muscle, 261
Dialysis, 272
Diarrhea, 276
Diuresis, 264
Diuretics, 261
Dysuria, 265
Elimination, 257
Enuresis, 262
Fecal incontinence, 276
Feces, 273
Flatulence, 276
Flatus, 273

Gastrocolic reflex, 275
Glycosuria, 263
Hemodialysis, 272
Hernia, 281
Hyponatremia, 263
Ileus, 274
Laxatives, 274
Meatus, 268
Meconium, 274
Micturition, 260
Neurogenic bladder, 265
Nocturia, 265
Nocturnal
   enuresis, 263
Nocturnal
   frequency, 265
Oliguria, 264
Peristalsis, 273
Peritoneal
   dialysis, 272

(continued on next page)

Elimination processes are an indirect gauge of general health. Alterations in elimination may reflect impaired function of other body systems, side effects from medications, or improper levels of hydration or nutrition (see the Concepts Related to Elimination feature). Alterations that may affect elimination include:

- Changes in neurological function, such as those associated with multiple sclerosis, Parkinson disease, or spinal cord injury, impact innervation of the urinary and gastrointestinal muscles and can lead to absent or inadequate control of the bladder and bowels.

- Increased or decreased food and fluid intake, as well as unhealthy food and drink choices, can alter urine and fecal volume and composition and contribute to elimination problems.

- Changes in respiratory and cardiovascular function can cause alterations in urinary pH, renal blood flow, and glomerular pressure in the kidney, all of which contribute to alterations in urine composition and volume.

- Changes in liver and gallbladder function alter the body's ability to digest fats and utilize nutrients absorbed from the gastrointestinal tract, which can change the composition of both urine and feces and alter excretion.

- Changes in the reproductive system can affect the urinary system; for example, pregnant women have less room for the bladder to expand and must urinate more frequently, and men with an enlarged prostate gland may have one or more problems with urination.

- Changes in musculoskeletal function can impair ambulation; immobility can decrease appetite, slow gastrointestinal motility, and alter bladder function. Immobility also increases the risk of developing urinary calculi and urinary tract infections (Knight, Nigam, & Jones, 2009).

- Disease processes, especially disorders directly related to urinary or gastrointestinal function such as the inflammatory disorders nephritis and inflammatory bowel disease, can alter urinary and bowel function and contribute to elimination problems.

- Many medications used to treat chronic diseases alter urinary and bowel function. For example, opioids frequently cause constipation.

Concepts Related to **Elimination**

CONCEPT	RELATIONSHIP TO ELIMINATION	NURSING IMPLICATIONS
Fluid and Electrolytes		
■ Acute renal failure ■ Chronic renal failure ■ Fluid and electrolyte imbalance	Fluid intake should be directly proportional to fluid output. Excretion of excess electrolytes via urinary elimination helps maintain health.	■ Monitor fluid intake and output for all clients, especially clients with kidney disease, burns, altered mobility, catheters, urinary tract infection, or heart disease. ■ Assess for signs and symptoms of dehydration, including dry mouth and skin, fatigue, thirst, decreased urine output, constipation, headache, dizziness, and tachycardia. ■ Signs of fluid overload include edema, weight gain, shortness of breath, fluid intake greater than output, increased blood pressure. ■ Medications may influence renal sufficiency.
Inflammation		
■ Inflammatory bowel disease ■ Nephritis ■ Peptic ulcer disease	Inflammatory diseases can alter absorption and excretion of fluids, electrolytes, and solids.	■ Monitor urine and feces for blood or infection. ■ Monitor client for edema, fever, discolored urine or stool, hypertension. ■ Client may complain of pain, diarrhea. ■ Clients may be at risk for imbalanced nutrition.

Concepts Related to **Elimination** (continued)

CONCEPT	RELATIONSHIP TO ELIMINATION	NURSING IMPLICATIONS
		■ Be alert for elimination problems in clients with inflammatory disorders of the kidneys, bladder, or GI tract. ■ *Anticipate:* parenteral nutrition; urine, fecal, and blood samples for diagnostic testing; analgesic administration.
Mobility		
■ Fractures ■ Multiple sclerosis ■ Parkinson disease ■ Spinal cord injury	Alterations in mobility influence elimination, especially constipation.	■ Monitor urinary and fecal output for clients with limited mobility, including clients with bone fractures, spinal cord injuries, and Parkinson disease. ■ For clients with limited mobility (especially those who are taking opioids), prophylactic stool softeners or laxatives may be prescribed. ■ Clients with urinary catheters should be monitored for infection; use sterile technique when inserting a catheter, and limit duration of catheterization if possible. ■ Teach clients proper hygiene methods for cleansing the urethral and anal areas to prevent infection and skin breakdown.
Self		
■ Eating disorders	Clients with eating disorders have an altered nutritional status that can affect elimination.	■ Recognize signs and symptoms of eating disorders, including abnormally low body weight, fixation on body image, and unhealthy eating patterns (including severely limited oral intake and binging/purging). ■ Clients with bulimia nervosa may abuse laxatives, diuretics, or enemas to increase urine and fecal elimination. ■ Be aware that abuse of drugs to increase elimination increases the risk of heart failure.
Teaching and Learning		
■ Client/consumer education ■ Staff education	Because elimination problems are often related to a chronic condition, clients will need to learn self-care for discharge home. Elimination problems are common among older adults and hospitalized clients, so staff must be educated about nursing interventions appropriate for these clients.	■ Teach clients proper perineal hygiene methods. ■ Teach clients appropriate care of catheter or fecal pouch. ■ Teach clients bladder and bowel training methods. ■ Teach clients strategies to reduce psychosocial issues related to incontinence. ■ Teach clients proper use of medications for bladder or bowel problems as well as side effects of medications for other conditions that may alter bladder or bowel function. ■ Teach clients to promptly report signs and symptoms of complications to their physician. ■ Utilize proper safety protocols for handling bodily waste. ■ Teach staff members to respect the client's privacy when providing bladder or bowel care.

URINARY ELIMINATION

Urinary elimination serves to control blood volume and composition and to rid the body of excess fluid and electrolytes. Proper regulation of this system is essential to health. If the urinary system is working correctly, urination can be postponed for only so long before the urge becomes too great to control.

▶ NORMAL URINARY ELIMINATION

Through intricate processes, the urinary system filters the blood to remove fluid and electrolytes, reabsorb nutrients to maintain the desired concentration of each, and eliminate the excess. This process helps maintain the concentration of ions needed for neuronal and muscle function, bone strength, and cellular regulation. It also helps maintain homeostatic regulation of blood pressure to ensure adequate circulation of oxygen and nutrients throughout the body.

Physiology Review

Urinary elimination depends on effective functioning of the upper urinary tract (kidneys and ureters) and the lower urinary tract (urinary bladder, urethra, and pelvic floor). **Figure 5–1** ● shows the anatomical structures of the urinary tract.

✴ *Go to nursing.pearsonhighered.com to see a review of the anatomy and physiology of urinary elimination.*

URINATION   **Micturition, voiding,** and **urination** all refer to the process of emptying the urinary bladder. Urine collects in the bladder until pressure stimulates special sensory nerve endings, called *stretch receptors,* in the bladder wall. This stimulation occurs when the adult bladder contains between 250 and 450 mL of urine. In children, a considerably smaller volume (50–200 mL) stimulates these nerves.

The stretch receptors transmit impulses to the spinal cord—specifically to the voiding reflex center located at the level of the second to fourth sacral vertebrae, causing the internal sphincter to relax and stimulating the urge to void. If the time and place are appropriate for urination, the conscious portion of the brain relaxes the external urethral sphincter muscle, and urination takes place. If the time and place are inappropriate, the micturition reflex usually subsides until the bladder becomes more filled and the reflex is stimulated again.

Voluntary control of urination is possible only if the nerves supplying the bladder and urethra, the neural tracts of the cord and the brain, and the motor area of the cerebrum are all intact. The individual must be able to sense that the bladder is full. Injury to any of these parts of the nervous system—for example, by a cerebral hemorrhage or a spinal cord injury above the level

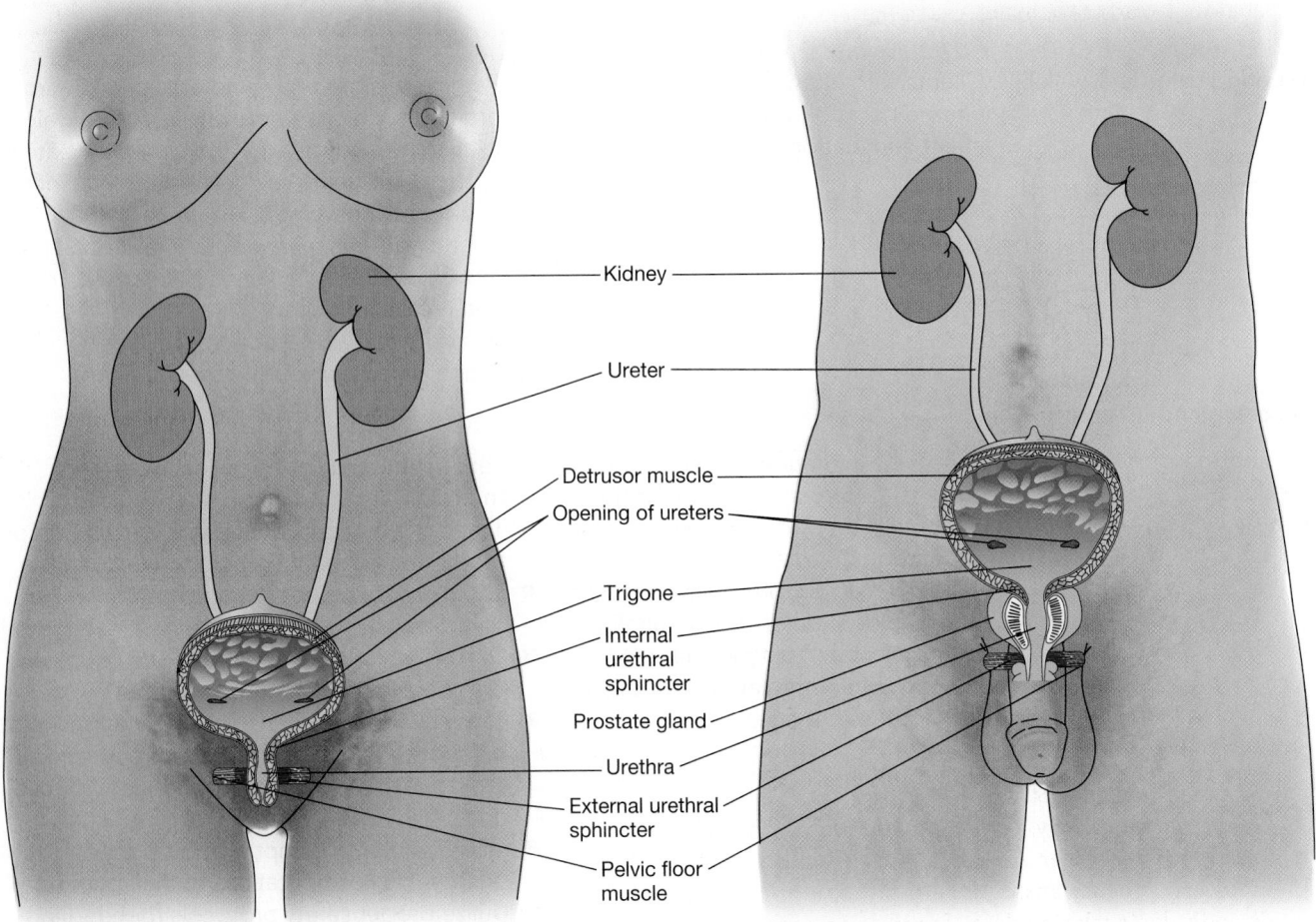

Kidney

Ureter

Detrusor muscle

Opening of ureters

Trigone

Internal urethral sphincter

Prostate gland

Urethra

External urethral sphincter

Pelvic floor muscle

Figure 5–1 ● Female and male urinary bladders and urethras, showing sphincter muscles.
Source: Custom Medical Stock Photo, Inc.

TABLE 5–1   Average Daily Urine Output by Age

AGE	AMOUNT (ML)
1 to 2 days	15–60
3 to 10 days	100–300
10 days to 2 months	250–450
2 months to 1 year	400–500
1 to 3 years	500–600
3 to 5 years	600–700
5 to 8 years	700–1,000
8 to 14 years	800–1,400
14 years through adulthood	1,500
Older adulthood	1,500 or less

of the sacral region—results in intermittent involuntary emptying of the bladder. Older adults whose cognition is impaired may not be aware of the need to urinate or may not be able to respond to this urge appropriately.

Although patterns of urination are highly individual, most people void about five or six times a day. They usually void when they first awaken in the morning, before they go to bed, and around mealtimes. **Table 5–1** ● shows the average urinary output per day at different ages.

FACTORS AFFECTING URINARY ELIMINATION
Numerous factors affect the volume and characteristics of the urine that is produced and the manner in which it is excreted. These factors include fluid and food intake, muscle tone, psychosocial factors, and medical conditions, procedures, and treatments.

Fluid and Food Intake   The healthy body maintains a balance between the amount of fluid ingested and the amount of fluid eliminated. When the amount of fluid intake increases, the fluid output normally increases accordingly. Certain fluids, such as alcohol, increase fluid output by inhibiting the production of antidiuretic hormone (ADH). By contrast, food and fluids high in sodium may cause fluid retention so that the body can maintain the normal concentration of electrolytes. Some foods and fluids change the color of urine. For instance, beets may cause urine to appear red, and foods containing carotene may cause yellow discoloration of the urine.

Muscle Tone   Good muscle tone maintains the elasticity and contractility of the **detrusor muscle**, allowing the bladder to fill adequately and empty completely. Clients who require long-term use of a retention catheter may develop poor bladder muscle tone because continuous drainage of urine prevents the bladder from filling and emptying normally. Pelvic muscle tone also contributes to the ability to store and empty urine.

Psychosocial Factors   Stimulation of the micturition reflex may be affected by privacy, positioning, sufficient time, and, occasionally, running water. Absence of the client's accustomed conditions may produce anxiety and muscle tension that prevent the individual's relaxing the abdominal and perineal muscles and the external urethral sphincter, so voiding is inhibited. Individuals also may voluntarily suppress urination because of perceived time pressures; for example, nurses often ignore the

urge to void until they are able to take a break. This behavior increases the risk of urinary tract infections (UTIs).

Pathological Conditions   Some renal diseases and conditions affect the formation and excretion of urine. Glomerular dysfunction may lead to the presence of abnormal amounts of protein or blood cells in the urine. In some cases, the kidneys cease to produce urine, a condition known as **renal failure**. Heart and circulatory disorders, such as heart failure, shock, or hypertension, affect blood flow to the kidneys, interfering with urine production. When abnormal amounts of fluid are lost through another route (e.g., vomiting or high fever), the kidneys retain water, and urinary output decreases.

Processes that interfere with the flow of urine from the kidneys to the urethra also affect urinary excretion. A urinary stone (calculus) may obstruct a ureter, blocking urine flow from the kidney to the bladder. Hyperplasia of the prostate gland, a common condition affecting older men, may obstruct the urethra, impairing urination and bladder emptying.

Surgical and Diagnostic Procedures   Some surgical and diagnostic procedures affect the passage of urine and even the urine itself. The urethra may swell after cystoscopy (endoscopy of the urinary bladder), and surgical procedures on any part of the urinary tract may result in some postoperative bleeding, which can cause the urine to be tinged red or pink for a time.

Spinal anesthetics can affect the passage of urine because they decrease the client's awareness of the need to void. Swelling in the lower abdomen because of surgery on structures adjacent to the urinary tract (e.g., the uterus) also can affect voiding.

Medications   Many medications, particularly those affecting the autonomic nervous system, interfere with the normal urination process and may cause retention (**Box 5–1** ●). Diuretics (e.g., chlorothiazide and furosemide) increase urine formation by preventing the reabsorption of water and electrolytes from the tubules of the kidney into the bloodstream. Some medications alter the color of the urine. If a medication alters the color of urine, the nurse should warn the client about this side effect to reduce the client's fear and anxiety.

Genetic and Lifespan Considerations
Factors specific to infants, preschoolers, school-age children, older adults, and pregnant women can affect the elimination of urine (see the Lifespan Considerations feature).

Box 5–1   Medications That May Cause Urinary Retention

- Anticholinergic and antispasmodic medications, such as atropine and papaverine
- Antidepressant and antipsychotic agents, such as phenothiazines and monoamine oxidase inhibitors
- Antihistamine preparations, especially those containing pseudoephedrine (e.g., Claritin-D and Sudafed)
- Antihypertensive agents, such as hydralazine (Apresoline) and methyldopate (Aldomet)
- Antiparkinsonism drugs, such as levodopa, trihexyphenidyl (Artane), and benztropine mesylate (Cogentin)
- Beta-adrenergic blockers, such as propranolol (Inderal)
- Opioids, such as hydrocodone (Vicodin)

Lifespan Considerations Changes in Urinary Elimination Through the Life Span

STAGE	VARIATIONS
Fetuses	The fetal kidney begins to excrete urine between the 11th and 12th weeks of development.
Infants	Ability to concentrate urine is minimal; therefore, urine appears light yellow.
	Because of neuromuscular immaturity, voluntary urinary control is absent.
Children	Kidney function reaches maturity between the first and second year of life; urine is concentrated effectively and appears a normal amber color.
	Between 18 and 24 months of age, the child starts to recognize bladder fullness and is able to hold urine beyond the urge to void.
	At approximately 2.5–3 years of age, the child can perceive bladder fullness, hold urine after the urge to void, and communicate the need to urinate.
	Full urinary control usually occurs at 4 or 5 years of age; daytime control is usually achieved by 3 years of age.
	The kidneys grow in proportion to overall body growth.
Adults	The kidneys reach maximum size between 35 and 40 years of age.
	After 50 years, the kidneys begin to diminish in size and function. Most shrinkage occurs in the cortex of the kidney as individual nephrons are lost.
Older adults	An estimated 30% of nephrons are lost by 80 years of age.
	Renal blood flow decreases because of vascular changes and a decrease in cardiac output.
	The ability to concentrate urine declines.
	Bladder muscle tone diminishes, causing increased frequency of urination and nocturia (voiding two or more times at night).
	Diminished bladder muscle tone and contractibility may lead to residual urine in the bladder after voiding, increasing the risk of bacterial growth and infection.
	Urinary incontinence may occur because of mobility problems or neurological impairments.

INFANTS The glomerular filtration rate (GFR) of the newborn's kidney is lower than the adult's. Due to immature function, the newborn's kidney is unable to rapidly excrete excess fluid; as a result, this population is at particular risk for fluid volume overload. Full-term newborns are less able to concentrate urine because the tubules are short and narrow. The limited tubular reabsorption of water and limited excretion of solutes (principally sodium, potassium, chloride, bicarbonate, urea, and phosphate) in the growing newborn also reduce the newborn's ability to concentrate urine, making the effect of excessive insensible water loss or restricted fluid intake unpredictable. The newborn's kidneys also are limited in dilutional capabilities. These limitations regarding concentration and dilution are important considerations in monitoring fluid therapy to prevent dehydration or overhydration. The newborn attains the ability to concentrate urine fully by 3 months of age.

Among healthy newborns, 17% void immediately after birth, 92% void by 24 hours after birth, and 99% void by 48 hours after birth (Walker, 2011). Voiding at birth frequently goes unnoticed, and delivery room nurses must be vigilant to note this urination. Assess a newborn who has not voided within 48 hours following delivery for adequacy of fluid intake, bladder distention, restlessness, and symptoms of pain. Notify the primary healthcare provider as well.

The initial bladder volume is 6–44 mL of urine. Unless edema is present, normal urinary output is limited, and voiding is scanty until fluid intake increases. For the first 2 days after birth, the newborn voids from 2 to 6 times daily, with a urine output of 15 mL/kg per day. The newborn subsequently voids from 5 to 25 times every 24 hours, with a volume of 25 mL/kg per day. Urine output varies according to fluid intake but gradually increases to between 250 and 500 mL per day during the first year.

After the first voiding, the newborn's urine frequently is cloudy (because of mucus content) and has a high specific gravity, which decreases as fluid intake increases. Occasionally, harmless pink stains ("brick dust spots"), which are caused by urates, appear on the diaper. Normally, during early infancy, urine is straw-colored and almost odorless. In these clients, odor can result from certain medications, metabolic disorders, or infection.

PRESCHOOLERS Infants are born without neural urinary control; instead, they void reflexively. As the infant's brain develops, it begins to take control of urination, and a preschooler is able to take responsibility for independent toileting. Most children develop urinary control between 2 and 5 years of age. Control during the daytime normally precedes control during the nighttime. Parents must realize that accidents occur, and the child should never be punished or chastised for a toileting accident. Because children at this age often forget to wash their hands or flush the toilet, they require reminders and appropriate adult modeling. Young children also require instruction in wiping themselves. Girls should be taught to wipe from front to back to prevent fecal contamination of the urinary tract.

SCHOOL-AGE CHILDREN A child's elimination system reaches maturity during early school age. The kidneys double in size between the ages of 5 and 10. During this period, the child urinates six to eight times a day.

Enuresis, the involuntary passing of urine when control should be established (approximately 5 years of age), is a problem for some school-age children. About 10% of 6-year-olds experience difficulty controlling the bladder. Although it is more prevalent in children, adults may also experience enuresis. Diurnal (daytime) enuresis may be persistent and pathological in origin. It affects women and girls more frequently than it does men and boys. The occurrence of enuresis after achieving voluntary bladder control should be reported to the primary care provider.

Nocturnal enuresis, or bed-wetting, is the involuntary passing of urine during sleep. It often occurs because the filling of the small bladder does not awaken the child during the night and instead stimulates an automatic voiding reflex. It is especially prevalent in children who are deep sleepers (Mayo Clinic, 2011a). The incidence of nocturnal enuresis decreases as the child matures, and bed-wetting should not be considered a problem until after 6 years of age. Nocturnal enuresis may be referred to as primary when the child has never achieved nighttime urinary control. Nocturnal enuresis hat appears after the child has achieved nighttime dryness for 6 consecutive months is secondary enuresis. Often, it is related to another problem, such as constipation, stress, or illness, and may resolve when the cause is eliminated. Recent research indicates that nightly nocturnal enuresis is associated with daytime incontinence, encopresis (fecal incontinence), bladder dysfunction, and male gender (Sureshkumar et al., 2009).

OLDER ADULTS Renal function begins to decline around 40 years of age but usually does not create significant issues for an otherwise healthy individual until the ninth decade of life. At that time, decreases in GFR, renal blood flow, maximal urinary concentration, and response to sodium loss are marked. GFR peaks around 140 mL/min/1.73 m^2 in the third decade of life and then declines at a rate of 8 mL/min/1.73 m^2 per decade (Musso & Oreopoulos, 2011). According to a recent study of healthy kidney donors, glomerulosclerosis (periglomerular fibrosis, sclerosis of the glomerular tuft, and collagen deposition in Bowman capsule) increases from a prevalence of 2.7% in 20-year-olds to 73% in 70-year-olds (Rule, Cornell, & Poggio, 2011). In addition, the proportion of sclerotic glomeruli increases from approximately 5% in younger adults to 35% in adults over the age of 80 (Miller, 2009).

Blood flow to the kidney decreases as a result of atrophy in the supplying blood vessels, particularly in the renal cortex. In addition, the proximal tubules decrease in number and length. Compared with a young adult, an older adult usually has a lower creatinine clearance, has urine that is more dilute (having a lower specific gravity), and typically excretes lower levels of glucose, acid, and potassium. As these changes progress, the serum creatinine level and the blood urea nitrogen (BUN) increase (Esposito et al., 2007). In addition, the kidneys of older adults excrete more fluid and electrolytes during the night than during the day, and more urine is formed at night, so it potentially interrupts sleep patterns.

One very important consequence of these changes is impaired excretion of drugs and their metabolites, making older adults extremely susceptible to drug overdose and other adverse effects of medication (even when administered within a normal dose range). This impairment is of particular concern when the individual has multiple health impairments that require several types of pharmacologic therapy. Another consequence of age-related changes is an increased probability of hyperkalemia, particularly when potassium-sparing diuretics, angiotensin-converting enzyme inhibitors, nonsteroidal anti-inflammatory drugs, or beta-blockers are prescribed (Lederer, 2013).

The older adult's decreased ability to concentrate urine results in an increased susceptibility to dehydration, a problem that is further complicated by a deficit in the thirst response; therefore the older individual may not feel thirsty even when significantly dehydrated. In addition, an older adult who has concerns about incontinence may choose not to drink for fear of an incontinence accident. These changes also produce a decline in the ability of older adults to respond to a fluid overload by increasing urine production.

Changes in the bladder and urethra also occur with aging. The bladder becomes more fibrous, with a consequent decrease in capacity and increase in residual urine. The decrease in autonomic regulation of the bladder by the nervous system with aging affects contraction of both the detrusor muscle and the external sphincter. The detrusor muscle becomes less contractile and also somewhat unstable. As a result, the older adult is subject to both an inability to empty the bladder completely and involuntary contractions of the bladder (Miller, 2009). Age-related weakening also occurs in the voluntary pelvic floor muscles, which are important in controlling the release of urine from the urethra. These changes make older adults more likely to have difficulty delaying urination and predispose them to urinary incontinence and UTI. However, it is important for the nurse to remember that even though some anatomical and physiological changes make incontinence more probable with increased age, urinary incontinence is not a normal part of aging.

Older adults tend to have normal to higher basal levels of ADH than younger adults. Although ADH is released as a response to hypotension and hypovolemia (low blood volume), its action is blunted in older adults, and more hormone is required to achieve the desired antidiuretic effect. In addition, the aging kidney is less responsive to circulating ADH, producing urine that is poorly concentrated and rich in sodium and thus putting the older adult at increased risk of **hyponatremia**, an abnormally low concentration of sodium in the blood that can be magnified with the use of diuretics (Blazer & Steffens, 2009).

PREGNANT WOMEN During the first trimester of pregnancy, the enlarging uterus is still a pelvic organ and presses against the bladder, increasing urinary frequency. This symptom decreases during the second trimester, when the uterus becomes an abdominal organ and pressure against the bladder decreases. Urinary frequency reappears during the third trimester, when the presenting part of the uterus descends into the pelvis and again presses on the bladder, thus reducing bladder capacity, contributing to hyperemia, and irritating the bladder. The ureters, especially the right ureter, elongate and dilate above the pelvic brim. The GFR rises by as much as 50% beginning in the second trimester, and it remains elevated until birth. To compensate for this increase, renal tubular reabsorption also increases. However, **glycosuria** (excretion of carbohydrates into the urine) sometimes arises during pregnancy because of the kidneys' inability to reabsorb all the glucose filtered by the glomeruli. Glycosuria may be normal or may indicate gestational diabetes, so it always warrants further testing. The presence of protein, blood, or white cells in the urine is always considered abnormal and should be evaluated.

The postpartum woman has an increased bladder capacity, swelling and bruising of the tissue around the urethra, decreased sensitivity to fluid pressure, and decreased sensation of bladder filling. Consequently, the postpartum woman is at risk for over-distention, incomplete bladder emptying, and buildup of **residual urine** (urine that remains in the bladder after voiding). Women who have had an anesthetic block have inhibited neural functioning of the bladder and are more susceptible to bladder distention, difficulty with voiding, and bladder infections. In addition, immediate postpartum use of oxytocin (to facilitate uterine contractions following expulsion of the placenta) has an antidiuretic effect. After oxytocin is discontinued, the woman experiences rapid bladder filling (Ricci & Kyle, 2009).

Urinary output increases during the early postpartum period (first 12–24 hours) because of puerperal diuresis. The kidneys must eliminate an estimated 2,000–3,000 mL of extra-cellular fluid with a normal pregnancy, causing rapid filling of the bladder. As a result, adequate bladder elimination is an immediate concern. Women with preeclampsia, chronic hypertension, or diabetes experience greater fluid retention than other women, and postpartum diuresis increases accordingly. If urine stasis exists, the chance for a UTI increases because of bacteriuria and the presence of dilated ureters and renal pelves, which persist for approximately 6 weeks after birth. A full bladder also may increase the tendency of the uterus to relax by displacing the uterus and interfering with its contractility, increasing the risk for hemorrhage. In the absence of infection, the dilated ureters and renal pelves return to pre-pregnant size by the end of the sixth week.

▶ ALTERATIONS IN URINATION

Alterations in urination are common throughout the life span due to age-related changes, as well as acute and chronic diseases and their associated treatments. Understanding each alteration and the nursing interventions associated with them will help the nurse provide culturally competent care for each individual client.

Alterations and Manifestations

A number of diseases and processes interfere with the flow of blood to the kidneys or of urine from the kidneys and bladder, interfering, in turn, with the production and elimination of urine.

ALTERED URINE PRODUCTION   **Polyuria** (or **diuresis**) is the production of abnormally large amounts of urine by the kidneys—often several liters more than the client's usual daily output. Polyuria can occur after excessive fluid intake, or it may be associated with diseases such as diabetes mellitus, diabetes insipidus, and chronic nephritis. **Polydipsia,** a medical condition in which extreme thirst leads to compulsive intake of excessive amounts of fluid, is associated with polyuria. Polyuria can cause excessive fluid loss, leading to intense thirst, dehydration, and weight loss.

Anuria is an absence of urine production, whereas **oliguria** is scant urine output, usually less than 500 mL/day or 30 mL/hour for an adult. Although oliguria may result from abnormal fluid losses or a lack of fluid intake, it often indicates impaired blood flow to the kidneys or impending renal failure, and it should be

reported promptly to the primary care provider. Rapid restoration of renal blood flow and urinary output may prevent renal failure.

ALTERED URINARY ELIMINATION   Despite normal production of urine, a number of factors or conditions can affect its elimination. Urinary frequency, nocturia, urgency, and dysuria often are manifestations of underlying conditions such as a UTI. Enuresis, incontinence, retention, and neurogenic bladder may be either a manifestation of an underlying condition or the primary problem affecting elimination of urine. Selected factors associated with altered patterns of urinary elimination are identified in **Table 5–2** ●.

Urinary frequency is voiding at frequent intervals, that is, more than four to six times a day. Increased fluid intake causes some increase in the frequency of voiding. Conditions such as UTI, stress, and pregnancy can cause frequent voiding of small

TABLE 5–2   Selected Factors Associated With Altered Urinary Elimination

PATTERN	SELECTED ASSOCIATED FACTORS
Polyuria	Ingestion of fluids containing caffeine or alcohol Prescribed diuretic Presence of thirst, dehydration, and weight loss History of diabetes mellitus, diabetes insipidus, or kidney disease
Oliguria, anuria	Decrease in fluid intake Signs of dehydration Presence of hypotension, shock, or heart failure History of kidney disease Signs of renal failure, such as elevated BUN and serum creatinine Edema, hypertension
Frequency or nocturia	Pregnancy Increase in fluid intake UTI
Urgency	Presence of psychological stress UTI
Dysuria	Urinary tract inflammation, infection, or injury Hesitancy, hematuria, pyuria (pus in the urine), and frequency
Enuresis	Family history of enuresis Difficult access to toilet facilities Home stresses
Incontinence	Bladder inflammation or other disease Difficulties in independent toileting (mobility impairment) Leakage when coughing, laughing, sneezing Cognitive impairment
Retention	Distended bladder on palpation and percussion Associated signs, such as pubic discomfort, restlessness, frequency, and small urine volume Recent anesthesia Recent perineal surgery Presence of perineal swelling Medications prescribed Lack of privacy or other factors inhibiting micturition

quantities (50–100 mL) of urine. Total fluid intake and output may be normal. **Nocturia** (voiding at night) usually is expressed in terms of the number of times the individual gets out of bed to void, for example, "nocturia ×4."

Urgency is the sudden strong desire to void. Regardless of urine volume, the individual feels a need to void immediately. Urgency, which is an abnormal finding, often accompanies psychological stress and irritation of the trigone and urethra. It also is common in individuals who have poor external sphincter control and unstable bladder contractions.

Dysuria (voiding that is either painful or difficult) can accompany a stricture (decrease in diameter) of the urethra, a UTI, or an injury to the bladder and urethra. Often, clients say that they have to push to void or that burning accompanies or follows voiding. The burning may be described as severe, like a hot poker, or more subdued, like sunburn. **Urinary hesitancy** (a delay and difficulty in initiating voiding) is often associated with dysuria.

Impaired neurological function can interfere with the normal mechanisms of urinary elimination, resulting in a **neurogenic bladder**. The client with a neurogenic bladder does not perceive bladder fullness and is unable to control the urinary sphincters. The bladder may become flaccid and distended, or spastic, with frequent involuntary urination. For additional details, see the Alterations and Therapies feature.

Prevalence

In the United States, urinary dysfunction is common. A study of 17,850 adults age 20 and older found that 51.5% of nonpregnant women and 13.9% of men had experienced urinary incontinence, as defined by a leak in urine at least once over the past 12 months (Markland et al., 2011). Urinary retention is less prevalent than urinary incontinence, but it is common in older men, especially men with benign prostatic hyperplasia (BPH). The prevalence of urinary retention is between 4.5 and 6.8 per 1,000 men; the risk of developing urinary retention increases dramatically with age (Selius & Subedi, 2008). Urinary retention is uncommon in women.

Genetic Considerations and Nonmodifiable Risk Factors

As evidenced by the prevalence of urinary problems, women are at increased risk for urinary incontinence, and men are at increased risk for urinary retention. In women with diabetes, weekly incontinence is highest among non-Hispanic Whites and lowest among African Americans and Asians (Phelan et al., 2009). Disability and a family history of incontinence also increase an individual's risk of developing urinary incontinence. Genetic conditions such as myelomeningocele or spina bifida and conditions associated with aging such as Parkinson disease can also contribute to urinary problems.

Older age is a risk factor for both types of urinary problems. The excretory function of the kidneys diminishes as individuals age, but function usually does not diminish significantly below normal levels unless a disease process intervenes. Arteriosclerosis can reduce blood flow and impair renal function. Conditions that alter normal fluid intake and output, such as influenza or surgery, can compromise the kidney's ability to filter, maintain acid–base balance, and maintain electrolyte balance in older adults. In addi-

tion, the recovery time increases as an individual ages. Decreased kidney function, including extended excretion times, also places older adults at higher risk for medication toxicity.

Among age-related changes, those related to the bladder—especially regarding urgency and frequency—are most noticeable. In men, these changes are often caused by an enlarged prostate gland; in women, they may be caused by weakened muscles supporting the bladder or by weakness of the urethral sphincter. The capacity of the bladder and its ability to empty both decrease with aging. In part, this decrease explains the need for older adults to awaken at night to void (**nocturnal frequency**) and the increase in residual urine retention. The increased retention of residual urine predisposes the older adult to bladder infection.

▶ PREVENTION

Healthy lifestyle habits, such as maintaining a healthy weight, exercising regularly, and using good toileting habits, can prevent or delay the onset of urinary problems. Good toileting habits include avoiding delayed voiding and defecation, avoiding using pelvic floor muscles to force urine flow, and preventing constipation. Eating a diet high in fiber, not smoking, ensuring adequate fluid intake, and avoiding food and drinks that contain bladder irritants (such as alcohol, caffeine, and acid) can help prevent urinary problems. Pregnant women may be encouraged to practice Kegel exercises to help maintain urinary muscle strength and prevent incontinence (Mayo Clinic, 2011d).

Modifiable Risk Factors

Obesity is an independent risk factor for urinary incontinence, especially stress incontinence (Phelan et al., 2009; Subak, Richter, & Hunskaar, 2009), most likely because of the excess force placed on the bladder. Similarly, pregnancy is a risk factor for urinary incontinence because of the weight of the expanding uterus on the bladder. Other risk factors for loss of bladder control include urinary tract infections, increased consumption of bladder irritants, and poor lifestyle habits. Individuals with bowel problems such as constipation are also at higher risk for developing urinary problems.

Medical conditions, procedures, and treatments are also risk factors for urinary problems. Conditions such as diabetes, benign prostatic hyperplasia, arthritis, back problems, multiple sclerosis, Parkinson disease, Alzheimer disease, stroke, and spinal cord injury, increase the individual's risk of developing urinary problems. Medical procedures, especially surgical procedures that require anesthesia, can also influence bladder control. Bladder function can also be modified by pharmacologic treatment of acute or chronic conditions, including opioids for pain, diuretics for hypertension, and muscle relaxants for muscle spasms.

Screening

Currently, there are no standard screening procedures for urinary problems, so many clients with urinary problems are left untreated. Basic verbal screening of all clients, especially older adults, should be included at each regular checkup. Simple questions such as "Do you have difficulty holding your urine?" and "Do you have problems starting your urine stream?" could identify urinary incontinence or retention problems that would

Alterations and Therapies **Urinary Elimination Problems**

ALTERATION	DESCRIPTION/ DEFINITION	MANIFESTATIONS	INTERVENTIONS AND TREATMENTS
Urinary incontinence	Involuntary leakage of urine	Incontinence associated with stress (e.g., coughing, lifting, sneezing) Incontinence related to urgency (i.e., inability to get to a toilet fast enough) Incontinence related to neurological deficits (e.g., after spinal cord injury)	▪ Kegel exercises ▪ Surgery ▪ Bladder training ▪ Pharmacologic agents ▪ Vaginal devices
Urinary retention	Inability to empty bladder completely	Complete lack of voiding Incomplete bladder emptying Overflow incontinence Pain Constant urge to urinate Weak urinary flow	▪ Credé maneuver ▪ Urinary catheter insertion ▪ Discontinuing medications that cause retention ▪ Surgery ▪ Urethral dilation
Prostatic hyperplasia	Enlargement of the prostate—may be benign or malignant	Urinary retention Dribbling at the end of urination Incontinence Nocturnal enuresis Pain	▪ Surgical removal ▪ Medications ▪ Kegel exercises ▪ Scheduled bathroom visits ▪ Limits on alcohol and caffeine
Cancer of the urinary system	Abnormal cellular growth within the organs of the urinary tract	Blood in urine Frequent urination Painful urination Back or pelvic pain	▪ Surgery ▪ Chemotherapy ▪ Radiation therapy
Kidney stones	Formation of calculi within the calyx of the kidney	Mild to severe pain in the side and back, in the abdomen, or during urination Cloudy or foul-smelling urine Frequent urination Nausea and vomiting	▪ Analgesics ▪ Lithotripsy ▪ Dietary alteration to reduce risk of recurrence ▪ Increased fluid intake
Renal failure	Insufficient or absent kidney function	Decreased urine output Fluid retention Shortness of breath Confusion Chest pain or pressure	▪ Administration of diuretics if some kidney function remains ▪ Dialysis (hemodialysis or peritoneal dialysis) ▪ Kidney transplantation
Urinary tract infection	Invasion of the bladder, ureter, or kidney by microorganisms	Persistent urge to urinate Burning sensation during urination Cloudy, red, or strong-smelling urine Pelvic or rectal pain	▪ Administration of antibiotics if infection is caused by bacterium ▪ Increased fluid intake ▪ Cranberry juice to increase urine pH

otherwise be missed during the assessment. Many older adults believe that urinary problems are simply the result of the aging process, but urinary incontinence and retention are never considered normal. They often indicate another medical problem and should be investigated further.

▶ ASSESSMENT

Identification of signs and symptoms related to urinary incontinence or retention is vital to the proper treatment of the client's condition. Physical assessment, a health assessment interview

that collects subjective data, and diagnostic tests are used to assess urinary system function.

Nursing Assessment

A nursing assessment includes conducting a client interview and obtaining a health history (see Assessment Interview feature) as well as performing a physical assessment (see Assessment feature). Documentation of the information obtained during these assessments is a critical part of the nursing process.

Assessment Interview Urinary Elimination

The nurse's assessment interview provides critical information about urinary function. The nurse should be direct but polite, recognizing that discussing urinary function is embarrassing to many clients. Initially, the nurse should ask the client to describe the frequency of urination and any problems with urination. During the remainder of the interview, the nurse should use the vocabulary the client uses (to ensure understanding). In addition to recording the client's answers, the nurse should record any abnormal assessment findings, such as swelling and changes in skin integrity.

Voiding Pattern

- How many times do you urinate during a 24-hour period?
- Has this pattern changed recently?
- Do you need to get out of bed to void at night? How often?

Description of Urine and Any Changes

- How would you describe your urine in terms of color, clarity (clear, transparent, or cloudy), and odor (faint or strong)?

Urinary Elimination Problems

What problems have you had or do you now have with passing your urine?

- Passage of small amounts of urine?
- Voiding at intervals that are more frequent?
- Trouble getting to the bathroom in time or feeling an urgent need to void?
- Painful voiding?
- Difficulty starting urine stream?
- Frequent dribbling of urine or a feeling of bladder fullness associated with voiding small amounts of urine?
- Reduced force of stream?
- Accidental leakage of urine? If so, when does this occur (e.g., when coughing, laughing, or sneezing; at night; during the day)?
- Past urinary tract illness, such as infection of the kidney, bladder, or urethra; urinary calculi; surgery of kidney, ureters, or bladder?

Factors Influencing Urinary Elimination

- *Medications.* Do you take any medications that could increase urinary output or cause urinary retention? Nurses should note the name and specific dosage of all medications because the individual may not be aware that a medication could influence elimination.
- *Fluid intake.* What amount and kind of fluid do you take each day (e.g., six glasses of water, two cups of coffee, three cola drinks with or without caffeine)?
- *Environmental factors.* Do you have any problems with toileting (mobility, removing clothing, toilet seat too low, facility without grab bar)?
- *Stress.* Are you experiencing any major stress? If so, what are the stressors? Do you think these affect your urinary pattern?
- *Disease.* Have you had or do you have any illnesses that may affect urinary function, such as hypertension, heart disease, neurological disease, cancer, prostatic enlargement, or diabetes?
- *Diagnostic procedures and surgery.* Have you recently had a cystoscopy or anesthetic?

Lifespan and Cultural Considerations

Privacy is a major concern during a urinary assessment. This concern may be more evident in adolescents and young adults than in infants and toddlers. Some older adults may also have an increased need for privacy, while others may feel that the urinary assessment is a natural part of the assessment process. When performing a urinary physical assessment, always consider the client's attitude toward the assessment. If desired by the client, have a clinician of the same gender perform the assessment, particularly imperative for certain cultures, including Muslims and Orthodox Jews. Modesty, including covering as much of the body as possible, is especially important for Muslim women. Culturally competent care must be provided to clients of all ages and cultural groups.

Anxiety and embarrassment are also assessment factors that should be considered for clients across the life span. Explain each assessment at an appropriate comprehension level before and as it is performed to help ease anxiety about the procedure. Discussion of other topics may also help distract the client from the assessment, thus decreasing embarrassment, fear, and pain. Incorporating play and parental comfort is especially important for young children. The nurse's presentation of the assessment procedure as a natural process will help the client feel at ease and less reluctant to comply.

When obtaining the nursing history, ask questions using terminology that the individual will understand. For example, a small child may not understand the term *urinate* but may understand *potty* or *pee*. If the client does not speak English well, obtain a translator so communication is clear and accurate.

Diagnostic Tests

Diagnostic tests of urinary system function support the diagnosis of a specific disease, provide information to identify or modify the appropriate medication or therapy for the disease, and help nurses monitor the client's responses to treatment and nursing care interventions.

Go to **nursing.pearsonhighered.com** to see Appendix B for *diagnostic tests to assess the structures and functions of the urinary system.*

Diagnostic tests to assess the structures and functions of the urinary system are summarized in the bulleted list that follows:

- Urine may be tested for characteristics and components through urinalysis, urine culture, postvoiding residual urine, and 24-hour collection for creatinine. Test results may serve as baseline data, support the diagnosis of various health problems, and allow for evaluation of bladder emptying and renal function (**Table 5–3** ●).

Urinary Assessment

ASSESSMENT/METHOD	NORMAL FINDINGS	ABNORMAL FINDINGS	LIFESPAN OR DEVELOPMENTAL CONSIDERATIONS
Skin Assessment			
Inspect the skin and mucous membranes, noting color, turgor, and excretions.	The color of skin and mucous membranes should be even and appropriate to the age and race of the client; skin should be dry with no visible excretions.	■ Pallor of the skin and mucous membranes may indicate kidney disease with resultant anemia. ■ Decreased skin turgor may indicate dehydration. Changes in skin turgor may indicate renal insufficiency with either excess fluid loss or retention. ■ Edema (generalized or in the lower extremities) may indicate fluid volume excess. ■ An accumulation of uric acid crystals, called *uremic frost*, may be seen on the skin of the client with late-stage renal failure.	■ Newborns often have lanugo and vernix present. The hands and feet may be purple or bluish. ■ Individuals with skin conditions such as psoriasis may have altered skin color and texture unrelated to urinary function. ■ Older adults have thinner, drier, more fragile skin with wrinkles; therefore, dehydration may be more difficult to detect in this population. An older individual's perineal skin is more susceptible to breakdown as a result of urinary incontinence. ■ Individuals who smoke or spend a lot of time outdoors may have darker, leathery skin.
Abdominal Assessment			
The client should be in a supine position. Inspect the abdomen, noting size, symmetry, masses or lumps, swelling, distention, glistening, or skin tightness.	The abdomen should be slightly concave, symmetrical, without distention or masses.	■ Enlargements or asymmetry may indicate a hernia or superficial mass. ■ If the urinary bladder is distended, it rises above the symphysis pubis as a rounded mass. ■ Distention, glistening, or skin tightness may be associated with fluid retention. ■ Ascites is an accumulation of fluid in the peritoneal cavity.	■ It is normal for an infant's abdomen to appear swelled and firm, especially if the infant has eaten recently. ■ Young children may mistake an abdominal assessment as tickling; allow the child to "help" with the initial palpation to get used to the sensation. Parents can also help hold the child still and provide reassurance and emotional support. ■ Adolescents may be more comfortable if a nurse of the same gender performs the abdominal assessment. ■ Limit the time older adults with arthritis or cardiovascular problems are in the supine position, which may cause back pain or shortness of breath. Use pillows to prop up the client if needed; propping up may cause the abdomen to appear distended.
Urinary Meatus Assessment			
For the male client: With the client in a sitting or standing position, compress the tip of the glans penis with your gloved hand to open the urinary **meatus**.	The urinary meatus should be midline and free of redness, lesions, or discharge.	■ Increased redness, swelling, or discharge from the urinary meatus may indicate infection or sexually transmitted infection.	■ For pediatric clients, a parent should be present during assessment of the urinary meatus. ■ Explain the procedure thoroughly to clients of all ages, but especially children and adolescents.

Urinary Assessment (*continued*)

ASSESSMENT/METHOD	NORMAL FINDINGS	ABNORMAL FINDINGS	LIFESPAN OR DEVELOPMENTAL CONSIDERATIONS
For the female client: With the client in the dorsal lithotomy position, spread the labia with your gloved hand to expose the urinary meatus.		■ Ulceration of the urinary meatus may indicate a sexually transmitted infection. ■ Hypospadias is displacement of the urinary meatus to the ventral surface of the penis. ■ Epispadias is displacement of the urinary meatus to the dorsal surface of the penis.	■ Adolescents and adults often prefer to have a nurse of the same gender perform this assessment. Be aware of and sensitive to privacy issues. ■ The urinary meatus is usually partially or completely obscured in uncircumcised males and completely visible in circumcised males. Uncircumcised males may be at higher risk for urinary tract infection. ■ Newborn females and postpartum women may have swollen labia. ■ Due to loss of skin elasticity, the urethral meatus may be difficult to distinguish from the clitoris in older women.

Kidney Assessment

Auscultate the renal arteries by placing the bell of the stethoscope lightly in the areas of the renal arteries, located in the left and right upper abdominal quadrants.
   Percuss the kidneys for tenderness or pain.
   Palpate the kidneys. The lower pole of the right kidney may be palpable with deep palpation; the remaining right kidney and the left kidney are normally not palpable.
	Bruits are not normally heard over the renal arteries.
	   No tenderness or pain should be elicited.
	   If palpable, they should be nontender, bilaterally of appropriate size and density, without palpable masses.
		■ Systolic bruits ("whooshing" sounds) may indicate renal artery stenosis.
		■ Tenderness and pain on percussion of the costovertebral angle suggest glomerulonephritis or glomerulonephrosis.
		■ A mass or lump may indicate a tumor or cyst.
		■ Tenderness or pain on palpation may suggest an inflammatory process.
		■ A soft kidney that feels spongy may indicate chronic renal disease.
		■ Bilaterally enlarged kidneys may suggest polycystic kidney disease.
		■ Unequal kidney size may indicate hydronephrosis.
			■ Kidneys may be palpable in a normal newborn.
			■ Kidneys decrease in mass with older age.
			■ Do not palpate kidneys of individuals who have undergone renal transplant or children with Wilms tumor.

Bladder Assessment

Percuss the bladder for tone and position.
   Palpate the bladder (over the symphysis pubis and abdomen) for distention.
	The bladder should be midline without dullness.
	   The bladder is normally not palpable.
		■ A dull percussion tone over the bladder of a client who has just urinated may indicate urinary retention.
		■ A distended bladder may be palpated at any point from the symphysis pubis to the umbilicus and is felt as a firm, rounded organ. It indicates urinary retention.
			■ Palpation of a distended bladder may produce overflow incontinence in older adults.

TABLE 5–3 Normal and Abnormal Findings: Urinalysis

CHARACTERISTIC	NORMAL	ABNORMAL	NURSING CONSIDERATIONS
Amount in 24 hours (adult)	1,200–1,500 mL	<1,200 mL A large amount over intake	Normally, urinary output is approximately equal to fluid intake. Output of less than 30 mL/hr may indicate decreased blood flow to the kidneys and should be reported immediately.
Color	Light straw to amber yellow	Dark amber Dark orange Red or dark brown	Dark yellow to brownish urine is concentrated and may indicate dehydration, fever, or first urination in the morning. Dilute urine may appear almost clear or very pale yellow and may be caused by overhydration, kidney disease, alcohol ingestion, or diabetes insipidus. Red or red brown urine may be caused by sulfisoxazole-phenazopyridine (Azo Gantrisin), phenytoin (Dilantin), cascara, chlorpromazine (Thorazine), docusate calcium and phenolphthalein (Doxidan); and by carrots, rhubarb, and food coloring. Orange urine is caused by fever, urobilin, phenazopyridine (Pyridium), amidopyrine, nitrofurantoin, sulfonamides, carrots, beets, and food coloring. Blue or green urine is caused by Pseudomonas, amitriptyline (Elavil), methylene blue, methocarbamol (Robaxin), and yeast concentrate. Brown or black urine is caused by Lysol poisoning, melanin, bilirubin, methemoglobin, porphyrin, cascara, and injectable iron. Red blood cells in the urine (hematuria) may be evident as pink, bright red, or rusty brown urine. Menstrual bleeding also can color urine but should not be confused with hematuria.
Appearance/clarity	Transparent, clear	Cloudy Mucous plugs, viscid, thick	Hazy or cloudy urine indicates bacteria, pus, RBCs, WBCs, phosphates, prostatic fluid spermatozoa, or urates. Milky urine is the result of fats or pyuria. Yellow foam results from bilirubin, bile, or severe cirrhosis of the liver.
Odor	Faint, aromatic	Offensive	Ammonia smell increases as urine stands outside the body. Urinary tract infection (UTI) causes a foul or unpleasant odor, depending on the causative organism. Asparagus causes a distinctive musty odor. Mousy odors result from phenylketonuria. Sweet or fruity odors occur in starvation and diabetic ketoacidosis (high glucose).
Sterility	No microorganisms present	Microorganisms present	Urine in the bladder is sterile. Urine specimens, however, may be contaminated by bacteria from the perineum during collection.
pH	4.5–8	>8 or <4.5	Freshly voided urine is somewhat acidic. Alkaline urine may indicate a state of alkalosis, a UTI, bacteriuria, antibiotics, sulfonamides, sodium bicarbonate, acetazolamide, potassium citrate, or a diet high in fruits and vegetables. More acidic urine (low pH) is found in starvation, with diarrhea, with a diet high in protein foods or cranberries, in metabolic or respiratory acidosis, and with increased ammonium chloride and mandelic acid concentrations.
Specific gravity	1.005–1.030	>1.030 or <1.005	Concentrated urine has a higher specific gravity; diluted urine has a lower specific gravity. <1.005: diabetes insipidus, overhydration, renal disease, severe potassium deficit >1.030: dehydration, fever, diabetes mellitus, vomiting, diarrhea, contrast media
Protein	2–8 mg/dL	>8 mg/dL	High protein indicates proteinuria, exercise, fever, stress, acute infection, kidney disease, lupus erythematosus, leukemia, multiple myeloma, cardiac disease, preeclampsia, septicemia, lead, mercury, neomycin, barbiturates, sulfonamides.

TABLE 5–3 Normal and Abnormal Findings: Urinalysis (*continued*)

CHARACTERISTIC	NORMAL	ABNORMAL	NURSING CONSIDERATIONS
Glucose	Not present	Present	Glucose in the urine (>15 mg/dL or +4) indicates high blood glucose levels (>180 mg/dL) and may indicate undiagnosed or uncontrolled diabetes mellitus. Also high in stroke, Cushing syndrome, anesthesia, glucose infusions, severe stress, infections, ascorbic acid, aspirin, cephalosporins, and epinephrine.
Ketone bodies (acetone)	Not present	Present	Ketones, the end product of the breakdown of fatty acids, are not normally present in the urine. They may be present (+1 to +3) in the urine of clients who have uncontrolled diabetes mellitus, who are in a state of starvation, or who have ingested excessive amounts of aspirin.
RBCs	None	>2 per low-power field	Blood in urine indicates kidney trauma, kidney diseases, renal calculi, cystitis, excess aspirin, anticoagulants, sulfonamides, menstrual contamination, bleeding from the urinary tract.
WBCs	3–4 per low-power field	>4 per low-power field	High WBCs in urine indicate UTI, fever, strenuous exercise, kidney diseases.
Casts	Occasional hyaline	Fatty, granular, renal tubular epithelial, waxy casts	May indicate fever, kidney diseases, heart failure.

Note: Urine outputs below 30 mL/hr may indicate low blood volume or kidney malfunction. Nurses monitor urine output and should notify the primary provider if urine output averages less than 30 mL/hr over 4 hours.

- Bladder emptying may be evaluated by an ultrasonic bladder scan to examine for residual urine; uroflowmetry to measure the volume of urine voided per second; and cystometrography to evaluate bladder capacity, neuromuscular functions of the bladder, urethral pressures, and causes of bladder dysfunction.

- Radiological examinations include intravenous pyelography (IVP), retrograde pyelography, and renal arteriography or angiography. These examinations are useful in visualizing (via radiographs) the urinary tract to identify abnormal size, shape, and function of the kidneys, kidney pelvis, and ureters, and to detect renal **calculi** (stones), tumors, or cysts.

- A cystoscopy allows direct visualization of the bladder wall and urethra. During this procedure, small stones can be removed, a sample of tissue may be taken for biopsy, and retrograde pyelography may be done. If a contrast dye is instilled in the bladder, then fistulas, tumors, or ruptures can be identified.

- Noninvasive tests include renal ultrasound, CT, MRI, and renal scan. These tests are used to identify and evaluate kidney size and structure as well as renal or perirenal masses and obstructions. In addition, a renal scan may be used to evaluate kidney blood flow, perfusion, and urine production.

- A kidney biopsy is done to obtain tissue for use in diagnosing or monitoring kidney disease.

Regardless of the type of diagnostic test, the nurse is responsible for explaining the procedure and any special preparations needed as well as assessing for medication use that may affect the outcome of the tests. It is critical that the nurse ensure that the client fully understands what conditions the test will be administered under and which preparations the client may need to make in advance (e.g., fasting) for tests to be accurate

and successful. The nurse also supports the client during the examination as necessary, documents the procedures as appropriate, and monitors the results of the tests.

Measurement of blood levels of urea and creatinine is useful for evaluation of renal function. Both substances normally are eliminated by the kidneys through filtration and tubular secretion. Urea, the end product of protein metabolism, is measured as BUN, or blood urea nitrogen. Creatinine is produced in relatively constant quantities by the muscles. The **creatinine clearance** test uses 24-hour urine and serum creatinine levels to determine the GFR, a sensitive indicator of renal function. Other tests related to urinary functions include collection of a urine specimen, measurement of specific gravity, and visualization procedures.

▶ INTERVENTIONS AND THERAPIES

Nursing care of a client with urinary problems includes both independent and collaborative interventions. Independent interventions may include monitoring intake and output, hygiene care, catheter use and care, dialysis, urine collection for diagnostic testing, and client teaching. Collaborative care often includes medication administration and surgical procedures.

Independent

Care of the client with altered urinary elimination depends upon the cause and severity of the problem. Clients with reduced urine output secondary to dehydration require increased fluid intake. Clients with urinary incontinence require determination of the cause, appropriate treatment, and hygiene care. Clients who require catheterization for treatment of urinary retention or because of immobility require catheter care and client teaching about self-catheterization, if appropriate.

Aseptic technique is essential during any procedures that could introduce bacteria into the blood or urinary tract. Washing hands, using sterile gloves, and maintaining a closed urinary collection system decrease the incidence of ascending bladder contamination and subsequent UTI. Maintaining aseptic technique throughout dialysis procedures is necessary to prevent infection in grafts, fistulas, and catheters.

Collaborative

PHARMACOLOGIC THERAPY Pharmacologic therapy for urinary elimination may include diuretics to increase urine production, anticholinergic medications to reduce urinary frequency and treat urinary incontinence, and cholinergic medications to stimulate bladder contractions and promote urination, especially in clients with difficulty voiding. See the Medications feature for additional information.

Diuretics are classified by their mechanism of action. Loop diuretics work in the loop of Henle by blocking reabsorption

of sodium and chloride. Thiazide diuretics act on the distal tubule to block sodium reabsorption and increase potassium and water excretion. Potassium-sparing diuretics work in the distal tubule, allowing sodium to be excreted while inhibiting potassium excretion, thereby preventing the large potassium loss seen with other types of diuretics. Finally, diuretics that cannot be otherwise classified make up a miscellaneous group; this group includes carbonic anhydrase inhibitors and osmotic diuretics.

DIALYSIS For clients with severely reduced or absent renal function, some mechanism of filtering the blood is necessary to prevent illness and death. This filtering is done through renal **dialysis**, a technique by which fluids and molecules pass through a semipermeable membrane according to the rules of osmosis. The two most common methods of dialysis are hemodialysis and peritoneal dialysis. In **hemodialysis**, the client's blood flows through vascular catheters, passes by the dialysis solution in an external machine, and then returns to the client. In **peritoneal dialysis**, the dialysis solution is instilled into the abdominal cavity through a catheter, allowed

Medications **Urinary Elimination**

CLASSIFICATION AND DRUG EXAMPLES	MECHANISM OF ACTION	NURSING CONSIDERATIONS
Anticholinergics *Drug examples:* oxybutynin, tolterodine, darifenacin, solifenacin, trospium, fesoterodine	These reduce urgency and frequency by blocking muscarinic receptors in the detrusor muscle of the bladder, thereby inhibiting contractions and increasing storage capacity. *May also be used for:* —gastrointestinal disorders —respiratory disorders	▪ Anticholinergics are used to relieve symptoms associated with voiding in clients who have neurogenic bladder, reflex neurogenic bladder, or urge urinary incontinence. ▪ Monitor for constipation, dry mouth, urinary retention, blurred vision, and (in older adults) mental confusion. Symptoms may be dose related. ▪ Start with small doses for clients older than 75 years. ▪ Anticholinergics are contraindicated in clients with urinary retention, gastrointestinal (GI) motility problems (partial or complete GI obstruction, paralytic ileus), or uncontrolled narrow-angle glaucoma.
Cholinergic Agents or Parasympathomimetics *Drug examples:* Bethanechol chloride	These medications stimulate bladder contraction and facilitate voiding. *May also be used for:* —GERD —ileus	▪ Do not administer to clients with GI or urinary tract obstructions, asthma, bradycardia, hypotension, or Parkinson disease. ▪ May increase serum aspartate aminotransferase, amylase, and lipase levels. ▪ Effect of medications is antagonized by angel's trumpet, jimson weed, or scopolia. ▪ Overdose is treated with atropine sulfate.
Diuretics ▪ loop ▪ thiazide ▪ potassium-sparing ▪ miscellaneous *Drug examples:* Bumetanide, furosemide, chlorothiazide, metolazone, spironolactone	Each type of diuretic works in a specific place within the nephron to increase fluid excretion and prevent fluid reabsorption. *May also be used for:* —heart failure —edema —polycystic ovary syndrome —diabetes insipidus —female hirsutism —osteoporosis	▪ Monitor hydration and electrolyte balance. ▪ Monitor vital signs, and be alert for signs of hypotension secondary to fluid loss. ▪ Monitor serum BUN, creatinine, electrolyte, and other pertinent laboratory values. ▪ Clients taking potassium-sparing diuretics should avoid salt substitutes.

to rest there while the fluid and molecules exchange, and then removed through the catheter. Both hemodialysis and peritoneal dialysis must be performed at frequent intervals until the client's kidneys can resume the filtering function. For some clients, the nurse is responsible for monitoring the dialysis procedure. Depending upon the type of dialysis indicated, a specially trained nurse may administer the procedure, as well.

CASE STUDY \\ PART 1

Dennis Welborn is a 52-year-old Caucasian male who visits his primary care physician with complaints of severe pain in his back and abdomen and painful urination with blood. As the nurse working at the clinic, you are tasked with taking Mr. Welborn's medical history and preliminary assessment. Mr. Welborn is 6'2" tall and weighs 265 pounds. His vital signs include temperature 100.8°F oral; pulse 95 bpm; respirations 22/min; and BP 140/92 mmHg. Mr. Welborn rates his back and abdominal pain as 9 on a scale of 0–10, and his pain level is a 7 when he is urinating. When asked about his diet, Mr. Welborn admits that as a widower, he often eats out with coworkers for lunch and picks up fast food on the way home from work. He usually drinks three cups of coffee in the morning and diet soda throughout the afternoon and evening. When he gets heartburn, he eats several Tums for relief. An abdominal assessment reveals a distended bladder. Mr. Welborn states he delays urination as long as possible because of the pain. When he does urinate, he has noticed that he has a weak stream and still feels the urge to urinate when he has finished. Per the physician's orders, a blood sample and a urine sample are obtained for analysis, and Mr. Welborn is transferred to the radiology department to have an abdominal x-ray. The x-ray reveals a large stone (1.2 cm) in Mr. Welborn's proximal right ureter, and the urinalysis indicates the presence of small calcium crystals, red blood cells, and bacteria. The blood test also detects high blood calcium levels.

Clinical Reasoning Questions Level I

1. What risk factors does Mr. Welborn have for developing urinary calculi?
2. Other than a distended bladder, what findings might you discover in your assessment of Mr. Welborn?
3. How would the stone in Mr. Welborn's ureter contribute to urinary retention?

Clinical Reasoning Questions Level II

4. What is the priority nursing diagnosis for Mr. Welborn?
5. What nursing interventions can you implement to help manage Mr. Welborn's pain?
6. Refer to the exemplar on Urinary Calculi in this module. What is a likely treatment option to clear the stone from Mr. Welborn's ureter?

BOWEL ELIMINATION

Like urine elimination, formation and expulsion of feces is a complex process that promotes the retention of nutrients and important compounds while ridding the body of waste prod-

ucts. When the digestive system is functioning properly, this process often is taken for granted. However, alterations in bowel elimination can lead to conditions that range in severity from mild to fatal.

▶ NORMAL BOWEL ELIMINATION

Ingested food that is not digestible moves through the gastrointestinal system and is eliminated from the bowel as **feces** or **stool**. **Defecation** is the expulsion of feces from the anus and rectum. It is also called a *bowel movement*. The frequency of defecation is highly individual, varying from several times a day to two or three times a week. Fecal volume also varies.

Physiology Review

The process of wavelike muscular contractions that propels food and digestive products through the digestive tract is called **peristalsis**. Food travels from the mouth to the stomach, where is it broken down into a thick, semifluid mass called *chyme*. Chyme then travels into the duodenum to begin its transport through the small and large intestines via peristaltic waves, and nutrients and water are absorbed into the bloodstream and transported to the liver via the hepatic portal vein for processing. The portion of the chyme that cannot be absorbed continues through the large intestine until it reaches the colon and rectum. The feces are then expelled through the anus.

Normal feces are made up of approximately 75% water and 25% solid materials. They are soft but formed. Very quick propulsion of the feces along the large intestine allow inadequate time for most of the water in the chyme to be reabsorbed, and the feces are more fluid, containing perhaps 95% water. Normal feces require a normal fluid intake; feces that contain less water may be hard and difficult to expel. Feces normally are brown because of the presence of bile and bilirubin, which is a breakdown product of dead red blood cells. Another factor that affects fecal color is the action of bacteria, such as *Escherichia coli* or *Staphylococcus* sp., which normally are present in the large intestine. The action of microorganisms on the chyme is responsible for the odor of feces.

An adult usually forms 7–10 L of **flatus** (gas) in the large intestine every 24 hours. The gases include carbon dioxide, methane, hydrogen, oxygen, and nitrogen. Some are swallowed with food and fluids taken by mouth. Others are formed through the action of bacteria on the chyme in the large intestine. Still other gas diffuses from the blood into the gastrointestinal tract.

FACTORS AFFECTING BOWEL ELIMINATION Many factors affect bowel elimination, including diet, fluid intake and output, activity, defecation habits, medications and medical procedures, pathological conditions, and psychological factors.

Diet Sufficient bulk (cellulose, fiber) in the diet is necessary to provide fecal volume. Bland diets and low-fiber diets lack bulk and therefore create insufficient residue of waste products to stimulate the reflex for defecation. Low-residue foods, such as rice, eggs, and lean meats, move more slowly through the intestinal tract. Increasing fluid intake with such foods increases their rate of movement.

Certain foods are difficult, or even impossible, for some individuals to digest. This difficulty can result in digestive upsets and, in some instances, the passage of watery stools. Irregular eating also can impair regular defecation. Individuals who eat at the same times every day usually have a regularly timed physiological response to the food intake and a regular pattern of peristaltic activity in the colon.

Spicy foods produce diarrhea and flatus in some individuals. Excessive sugar also can cause diarrhea. Other foods that may influence bowel elimination include the following:

- Gas-producing foods, such as cabbage, onions, cauliflower, bananas, and apples
- Laxative-producing foods, such as bran, prunes, figs, chocolate, and alcohol
- Constipation-producing foods, such as cheese, pasta, eggs, and lean meat

Fluid   Healthy fecal elimination usually requires a daily fluid intake of 2,000–3,000 mL, but even when fluid intake is inadequate or output (e.g., urine or vomitus) is excessive, the body continues to reabsorb fluid from the chyme as it passes along the colon. The chyme thus becomes drier than normal, and the result is hard feces. In addition, reduced fluid intake slows the passage of chyme along the intestines, further increasing the reabsorption of fluid from the chyme. If, on the other hand, chyme moves abnormally quickly through the large intestine, the decreased time available for fluid absorption results in soft or even watery feces.

Activity   Activity stimulates peristalsis, facilitating the movement of chyme through the colon. Weak abdominal and pelvic muscles often are ineffective in increasing the intra-abdominal pressure during defecation or in controlling defecation. Weak muscles can result from lack of exercise, immobility, or impaired neurological functioning. Clients confined to bed are often constipated.

Defecation Habits   Early bowel training may establish the habit of defecating at a regular time. Many individuals defecate after breakfast, when the gastrocolic reflex causes mass peristaltic waves in the large intestine. If an individual ignores the urge to defecate, then water continues to be reabsorbed, and the feces become hard and difficult to expel. When the normal defecation reflexes are inhibited or ignored, these conditioned reflexes tend to weaken progressively. When habitually ignored, the urge to defecate ultimately is lost. Adults may ignore these reflexes because of the pressures of time or work. Hospitalized clients may suppress the urge because of embarrassment about using a bedpan, because of lack of privacy, or because defecation is too uncomfortable.

Medications   Some drugs have side effects that interfere with normal elimination. The action on the central nervous system of large doses of certain tranquilizers and repeated administration of morphine or codeine causes constipation by decreasing gastrointestinal activity. Iron tablets, which have an astringent effect, act more locally on the bowel mucosa to cause constipation. A variety of other drugs cause diarrhea.

Some medications directly affect elimination. **Laxatives** are medications that stimulate bowel activity and promote fecal elimination. Stool softeners also facilitate defecation. Certain medications suppress peristaltic activity and may be used to treat diarrhea.

Medications also affect the appearance of the feces. Any drug that causes gastrointestinal bleeding (e.g., aspirin products) can cause the stool to be red or black. Iron salts cause black stool because of the oxidation of the iron. Antibiotics may cause a gray-green discoloration. Antacids can cause a whitish discoloration or white specks in the stool. Pepto-Bismol, a common over-the-counter drug, causes stools to be black.

Diagnostic Procedures   Before certain diagnostic procedures, such as visualization of the colon (colonoscopy or sigmoidoscopy), the client is restricted from ingesting food or fluid. The client also may be given a cleansing enema before the examination. In these instances, normal defecation does not usually occur until eating resumes.

Anesthesia and Surgical Procedures   General anesthetics cause the normal colonic movements to cease or slow by blocking parasympathetic stimulation to the muscles of the colon. Clients who have regional or spinal anesthesia are less likely to experience this problem.

Surgery that involves direct handling of the intestines can cause temporary cessation of intestinal movement. This condition, called **ileus**, usually lasts from 24 to 48 hours. Listening for bowel sounds that reflect intestinal motility is an important nursing assessment following surgery.

Pathological Conditions   Spinal cord injuries and head injuries can reduce the sensory stimulation for defecation. Impaired mobility may limit the client's ability to respond to the urge to defecate, and the client may experience constipation as a result. Alternatively, a client may experience fecal incontinence because of poorly functioning anal sphincters.

Pain   Clients who experience discomfort when defecating (e.g., following hemorrhoid surgery or from an anal fissure) often suppress the urge to defecate to avoid the pain. These clients can experience constipation as a result. Clients taking narcotic analgesics for pain also may experience constipation as a side effect of the medication.

Psychological Factors   Anxiety or anger may lead to increased peristaltic activity and consequent nausea or diarrhea. In contrast, depression may cause slowed intestinal motility, resulting in constipation. An individual's response to these emotional states is the result of variations in the response of the enteric nervous system to vagal stimulation from the brain.

Genetic and Lifespan Considerations

Defecation patterns vary at different stages of life. Altered elimination patterns may occur in newborns and infants, toddlers, children, and older adults.

NEWBORNS AND INFANTS   Term newborns usually pass meconium within 8–24 hours of life and almost always within 48 hours. **Meconium** is formed in utero from the amniotic fluid and its constituents, intestinal secretions, and shed mucosal cells. It can be recognized by its thick, tarry black or dark green appearance (**Figure 5–2A ●**). Transitional (thin brown to green) stools consisting of part meconium and part fecal material are

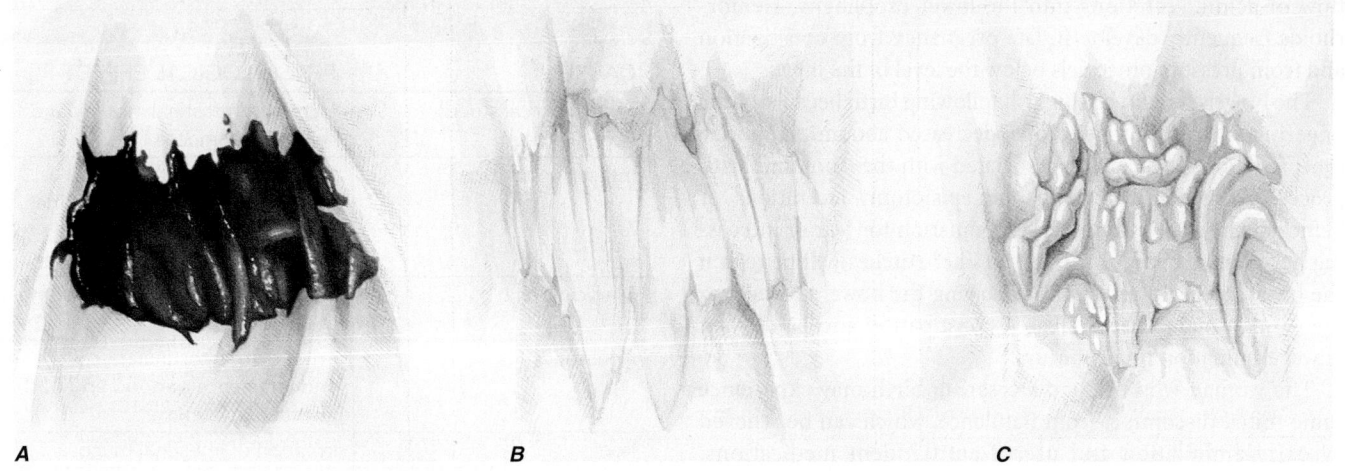

Figure 5–2 ● Newborn stool samples. *A,* Meconium, *B,* Breastfed newborn stool, *C,* Formula-fed newborn stool.

passed for the next day or two, and then the stools become entirely fecal.

Frequency of bowel movement in infants varies but ranges from one every 2 or 3 days to as many as 10 movements daily. Totally breastfed infants may have a bowel movement with every feeding for the first several weeks, then gradually progress to fewer bowel movements. Formula-fed infants also have frequent bowel movements, but not as frequently as breastfed infants, usually 4 or 5 movements per day. Between one and two months of age, the infant's bowel movement pattern changes. Infants may defecate from one or more times a day to once every 1–2 weeks. Mothers should be counseled that the newborn is not constipated as long as the bowel movement remains soft. Formula-fed infants are more likely to experience constipation than breastfed infants.

Because the intestine is immature, water is not well absorbed, and the stool is soft and liquid. Stools from breastfed infants are usually a mustard yellow and may have a seedy appearance (Figure 5–2*B).* Formula-fed infants have stools that range from tan to yellow to green (Figure 5–2*C*). As long as blood is not present, any color is normal. The formula-fed infant has stool that is slightly firmer than that of a breastfed infant.

When the intestine matures, bacterial flora increase. After solid foods are introduced, the stool becomes firmer and less frequent. The odor that accompanies a bowel movement is more offensive once the infant starts to eat solid food.

TODDLERS   Some control of defecation starts between 1.5 and 2 years of age. By this time, children have learned to walk, and their nervous and muscular systems are sufficiently well developed to permit bowel control. A desire to control daytime bowel movements and to use the toilet generally starts when the child becomes aware of the discomfort caused by a soiled diaper and the sensation that indicates the need for a bowel movement. Daytime control typically is attained by 2.5 years of age, after a process of toilet training.

SCHOOL-AGE CHILDREN AND ADOLESCENTS
School-age children and adolescents have bowel habits similar to those of adults. Patterns of defecation vary in frequency, quantity, and consistency. Some school-age children may delay defecation because of an activity such as play.

OLDER ADULTS   Up to half of all older adults suffer from constipation (Toner & Claros, 2012). Some causes are reduced activity levels, inadequate fluid and fiber intake, muscle weakness, and medication side effects. Many older adults believe that "regularity" means a bowel movement every day. Those who do not meet this criterion often seek over-the-counter preparations to relieve what they believe to be constipation. Older adults should be advised that normal patterns of bowel elimination vary considerably, from three times a day to three times a week. Adequate roughage in the diet, adequate exercise, and six to eight glasses of fluid daily are essential measures to prevent constipation. A cup of hot water or tea at a regular time in the morning is also helpful for some. Responding to the **gastrocolic reflex** (increased peristalsis of the colon after food has entered the stomach) is an important consideration as well. For example, toileting is recommended 5–15 minutes after meals—especially after breakfast, when the gastrocolic reflex is strongest (McKay, Fravel, & Scanlon, 2012).

The older adult should be warned that consistent use of laxatives inhibits natural defecation reflexes and is thought to cause, rather than cure, constipation. The habitual user of laxatives eventually requires larger or stronger doses because the effect is progressively reduced with continual use. Laxatives may also interfere with the body's electrolyte balance and reduce the absorption of certain vitamins. The reasons for constipation range from lifestyle habits (e.g., lack of exercise) to serious malignant disorders (e.g., colorectal cancer). The nurse should carefully evaluate any complaints of constipation. A change in bowel habits over several weeks with or without weight loss, pain, or fever should be referred to a primary care provider for a complete medical evaluation.

PREGNANT WOMEN   During pregnancy, elevated progesterone levels cause smooth muscle relaxation, resulting in delayed gastric emptying and decreased peristalsis. As a result, the pregnant woman may complain of bloating and constipation. These symptoms are aggravated as the enlarging uterus displaces the stomach upward and the intestines are moved laterally and posteriorly. The cardiac sphincter also relaxes, and heartburn (pyrosis) may occur as a result of **reflux**, a backward flow of acidic secretions into the lower esophagus. Hemorrhoids frequently develop in late pregnancy from constipation and from pressure on vessels below the level of the uterus.

The bowels tend to be sluggish following birth because of the lingering effects of progesterone, decreased abdominal muscle tone, and bowel evacuation associated with the labor and birth process. A woman who has had an episiotomy, lacerations, or hemorrhoids may tend to delay elimination for fear of increasing her pain or because she believes her stitches will be torn if she bears down. In refusing or delaying the bowel movement, the woman may cause increased constipation and pain when bowel elimination finally occurs.

The woman who has had a cesarean birth may experience some initial discomfort from flatulence, which can be relieved by early ambulation and use of antiflatulent medications. Chamomile or peppermint tea may also be helpful in reducing discomfort from flatulence. It may take a few days for the bowel to regain its tone, especially if general anesthesia was used. The woman who has had a cesarean or a difficult birth may benefit from stool softeners.

▶ ALTERATIONS IN BOWEL ELIMINATION

Impaired peristalsis leads to alterations in bowel elimination. Manifestations may include anal leakage of loose, watery fecal material without stimulation or hardened fecal material that is difficult to expel.

Alterations and Manifestations

Four common problems are related to fecal elimination: diarrhea, flatulence, constipation, and bowel incontinence. Constipation and bowel incontinence are discussed in depth in the exemplar on Bowel Incontinence, Constipation, and Impaction in this module. For more details, see the Alterations and Therapies feature.

DIARRHEA   **Diarrhea**, the passage of liquid feces with increased frequency, results from rapid movement of fecal contents through the large intestine. Rapid passage of chyme reduces the time available for the large intestine to reabsorb water and electrolytes. The individual with diarrhea finds it difficult or impossible to maintain control of the urge to defecate. Often, spasmodic cramps are associated with diarrhea. Bowel sounds usually increase. With persistent diarrhea, irritation of the anal region, extending to the perineum and buttocks, generally results. Fatigue, weakness, malaise, and emaciation are the results of prolonged diarrhea.

Diarrhea is thought to be a protective flushing mechanism caused by irritants in the intestinal tract. It can create serious fluid and electrolyte losses in the body, however, and these losses can develop within frighteningly short periods of time, particularly in infants, small children, and older adults. **Table 5–4** lists some of the major causes of diarrhea and the physiological responses of the body.

The irritating effects of diarrhea stool increase the risk for skin breakdown. The area around the anal region should be kept clean and dry and should be protected with zinc oxide or other ointment. In addition, a fecal collector can be used.

TABLE 5–4   Major Causes of Diarrhea

CAUSE	PHYSIOLOGICAL EFFECT
Psychological stress (e.g., anxiety)	Increased intestinal motility and secretion of mucus
Infection	Overgrowth of pathogenic microorganisms in the intestines, causing inflammation of the mucosa
Medications	Irritation and inflammation of the mucosa
Antibiotics	Irritation of intestinal mucosa and imbalance of good and bad intestinal bacteria
Iron	Irritation of intestinal mucosa
Cathartics	Incomplete digestion of food or fluid
Allergy to food, fluid, drugs	Increased intestinal motility and secretion of mucus
Intolerance of food or fluid	Reduced absorption of fluids
Diseases of the colon (e.g., malabsorption syndrome, Crohn disease)	Inflammation of the mucosa, often leading to ulcer formation

FLATULENCE   Most gases that are swallowed are expelled orally by eructation (belching). Large amounts of gas can accumulate in the stomach, however, resulting in gastric distention. The gases that form in the large intestine are chiefly absorbed through the intestinal capillaries into the circulation. **Flatulence** is the presence of excessive flatus in the intestines that leads to stretching and inflation of the intestines (intestinal distention). Flatus has three primary sources: action of bacteria on the chyme in the large intestine, swallowed air, and gas that diffuses between the bloodstream and the intestine. In addition, flatulence can occur in the colon from a variety of causes, including foods (e.g., cabbage and onions), abdominal surgery, or narcotics. If the gas is propelled by increased colon activity before it can be absorbed, it may be expelled through the anus. If excessive gas cannot be expelled through the anus, it may be necessary to insert a rectal tube to remove it.

CONSTIPATION   **Constipation** is characterized by the passage of fewer than three bowel movements per week or by difficulty in passing stools. Manifestations of this condition may include the absence of stool passage or the passage of dry, hardened stool. In most cases, constipation is due to the slowing of the movement of feces through the large intestine. Constipation may reflect a primary problem or it may indicate an underlying disorder.

BOWEL INCONTINENCE   **Bowel incontinence** or **fecal incontinence** is the inability to voluntarily control the passage of fecal contents and intestinal gas through the anal sphincter. In most cases, fecal incontinence is a manifestation of another disorder. Numerous conditions may cause fecal incontinence, including neurological disorders, traumatic injuries, and inflammatory processes. Psychological alterations, such as depression and confusion, may also contribute to the development of this condition. Episodes of incontinence may be unpredictable, or

Alterations and Therapies **Bowel Elimination**

ALTERATION	DESCRIPTION/ DEFINITION	MANIFESTATIONS	INTERVENTIONS AND THERAPIES
Constipation	Infrequent passage of hard stool	■ Straining with defecation ■ Lumpy or hard stools ■ Sensation of incomplete emptying ■ Fewer than three bowel movements per week	■ Increase fluid and fiber intake. ■ Increase activity level. ■ Administer enema. ■ May require medications (e.g., laxatives, stool softeners, cathartics). ■ Evaluate medication profile for gastrointestinal side effects.
Diarrhea	Passage of liquid stools	■ Frequent, runny stools ■ Hyperactive bowel sounds ■ Bowel incontinence ■ Abdominal cramps ■ Fever ■ Dehydration	■ Increase fluid intake. ■ Administer antidiarrheal medications. ■ Assess for cause (medications, diet, infection).
Bowel incontinence	Inability to control release of feces	■ Leakage of feces from the anus ■ Loss of pelvic muscle control ■ Lack of ability to respond to urge to defecate	■ Administer bowel training. ■ Treat with surgery (sphincter repair and fecal diversion or colostomy). ■ Remove fecal impaction if present. ■ Diet adjustment (e.g., avoid alcohol and caffeine; increase fiber). ■ Administer medications (e.g., laxatives, anti-diarrhea drugs, stool softeners).
Impaction	Mass or collection of hardened feces in the folds of the rectum	■ Constipation ■ Fecal incontinence ■ Abdominal cramping ■ Straining during defecation ■ Small, semi-formed stools ■ Loss of bladder control	■ Manual removal may be necessary. ■ Administer enema as necessary. ■ Increase fluid and fiber intake to prevent recurrence. ■ Evaluate medication profile for gastrointestinal side effects. ■ Improve defecation habits, and reduce constipation.
Bowel cancer	Abnormal growth of cells in the bowel	■ Early cancer: possibly no symptoms ■ Blood in the stool ■ Persistent change in bowel habits ■ Abdominal pain ■ Unexplained weight loss ■ Anemia ■ Bowel obstruction ■ Vomiting	■ Take preventive measures, and make an early diagnosis. ■ Remove surgically. ■ Administer chemotherapy or radiation therapy.
Obstruction	Blockage in the bowel preventing or reducing the passage of fecal material	■ Abdominal distention and cramping ■ Abdominal fullness ■ Constipation or diarrhea ■ Vomiting ■ Inability to pass gas	■ Remove blockage surgically. ■ Nasogastric tube to relieve abdominal pressure.

they may occur at specific intervals, such as following meals. For clients who experience fecal incontinence, embarrassment and shame may lead to social isolation.

Prevalence

The prevalence of bowel problems varies based on etiology. Adults in the United States usually suffer one bout of acute diarrhea each year, on average, whereas children usually suffer two bouts per year (NDDIC, 2012). The prevalence of constipation in adults ranges from 0.7% to 79% (median 16%). Children have a lower prevalence: between 0.7% and 29.6% (median 12%) (Mugie, Benninga, & Di Lorenzo, 2011). In addition, approximately 5.6%–29% of clients admit to fecal incontinence when asked (Alsheik et al., 2012).

Genetic Considerations and Nonmodifiable Risk Factors

Age is a major risk factor for bowel problems. Both young children and older adults are at higher risk for diarrhea, constipation, and fecal incontinence than individuals in other age groups. Women are at higher risk than men for fecal incontinence, especially after pregnancy. Immobility or disability and chronic diseases such as multiple sclerosis and diabetes are major risk factors for constipation.

▶ PREVENTION

Many methods are available for preventing bowel problems. Individuals can prevent diarrhea from infection by washing hands thoroughly, especially after contacting fecal material (e.g., after defecating or changing an infant's diaper). Diarrhea from rotavirus can be prevented by administration of a rotavirus vaccine (RotaTeq, Rotarix). Cooking all food completely and storing and handling food correctly can prevent diarrhea. When traveling to a foreign country, individuals should use only bottled water and should avoid raw fruits, vegetables, and meat.

Being active and consuming adequate fluids and fiber in the diet can prevent constipation and consequent fecal impaction. Clients, such as those taking opioids, who have a high risk of developing constipation may prevent it by taking daily laxatives or stool softeners. Fecal incontinence can also be prevented by the treatment of either constipation or diarrhea, depending on the causative factor.

Modifiable Risk Factors

Consuming a poor diet that is low in fiber and fluids is one of the greatest modifiable risk factors in bowel problems. Another major risk factor is taking medications long term, including antibacterials, proton pump inhibitors, blood pressure medications, opioids, antihistamines, and iron supplements. Almost all medications have diarrhea, constipation, or both as possible side effects. A modifiable risk factor for diarrhea is traveling, especially to developing countries that may have poor sanitation and contaminated food and water. Poor hygiene, especially failing to adequately wash hands after coming into contact with fecal matter, is also a risk factor for diarrhea. Lower socioeconomic status and lower educational level are also risk factors for constipation and diarrhea, most likely because of less access to a healthy diet and clean water and higher exposure to disease.

Screening

A specific screening test for bowel problems, like urinary problems, is uncommon. A verbal interview is the best screening tool; many clients will not mention bowel problems unless asked directly. The nurse caring for clients in the hospital or long-term care facility should include evaluation of clients for bowel movements as a screening procedure to detect bowel problems. In addition, the nurse may encourage clients who are at high risk for colon cancer to have a colon cancer screening. Colon cancer can contribute to bowel problems, especially bowel obstruction.

▶ ASSESSMENT

Assessment of a client with potential bowel elimination problems is vital to understanding the causative factor, its impact on health and wellness, and the treatment options. Assessment takes into consideration the nursing history and physical assessment as well as results from diagnostic tests.

Nursing Assessment

Assessment of fecal elimination includes taking a nursing history; performing a physical examination of the abdomen, rectum, and anus; and inspecting the feces.

> **SAFETY ALERT**
> Never use deep palpation in a client who has had a pulsatile abdominal mass, renal transplant, or polycystic kidneys or who is at risk for hemorrhage.

NURSING HISTORY   A nursing history for fecal elimination helps the nurse to identify the client's normal pattern. The nurse obtains a description of usual feces and any recent changes and collects information about any past or current problems with elimination, presence of an ostomy, and factors influencing the elimination pattern.

Examples of questions to elicit this information can be found in the Assessment Interview. The number of questions to ask is adapted to the individual client, according to the client's responses in the first three categories listed.

When obtaining data about the client's defecation pattern, the nurse needs to understand that the time of defecation and the amount of feces expelled are as individual as the frequency of defecation. Often, the patterns that individuals follow depend largely on early training and convenience.

PHYSICAL EXAMINATION   Physical examination of the abdomen in relation to fecal elimination problems includes inspection, auscultation, percussion, and palpation with specific reference to the intestinal tract (see Bowel Assessment feature). Auscultation precedes palpation, because palpation can alter peristalsis. Examination of the rectum and anus includes inspection and palpation (**Figure 5–3 ●**).

Assessment Interview   Bowel Elimination

Defecation Pattern

■ When do you usually have a bowel movement?

■ Has this pattern changed recently?

Description of Feces and Any Changes

■ Have you noticed any changes in the color, texture (hard, soft, watery), shape, or odor of your stool recently?

Fecal Elimination Problems

■ What problems have you had or do you now have with your bowel movements (constipation, diarrhea, excessive flatulence, seepage, or incontinence)?

■ When and how often do they occur?

■ What do you think causes these problems (food, fluids, exercise, emotions, medications, disease, surgery)?

■ What have you tried to solve the problems, and how effective was it?

Factors Influencing Elimination

■ *Use of elimination aids.* What routines do you follow to maintain your usual defecation pattern? Do you use natural aids such as specific foods or fluids (e.g., a glass of hot lemon juice before breakfast), laxatives, or enemas to maintain elimination?

■ *Diet.* What foods do you believe affect defecation? What foods do you typically eat? What foods do you avoid? Do you take meals at regular times?

■ *Fluid.* What amount and kind of fluid do you take each day (e.g., six glasses of water, two cups of coffee)?

■ *Exercise.* What is your usual daily exercise pattern? (Obtain specifics about exercise rather than asking whether it is sufficient; ideas of what is sufficient vary among individuals.)

■ *Medications.* Have you taken any medications that could affect the intestinal tract (e.g., iron or antibiotics)? (Note the name and specific dosage of all medications because the client may not be aware what medications may affect elimination.)

■ *Stress.* Are you experiencing any stress? Do you think it affects your defecation pattern? If so, how?

Presence and Management of Ostomy

■ What is your usual routine with your colostomy/ileostomy?

■ What type of appliance do you wear, and did you bring a spare with you?

■ What problems, if any, do you have with it?

■ How can the nurses help you manage your colostomy/ileostomy?

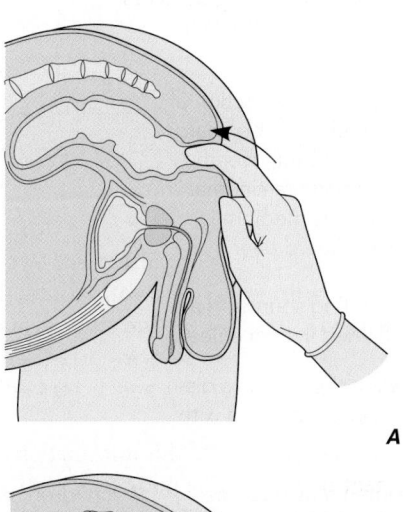

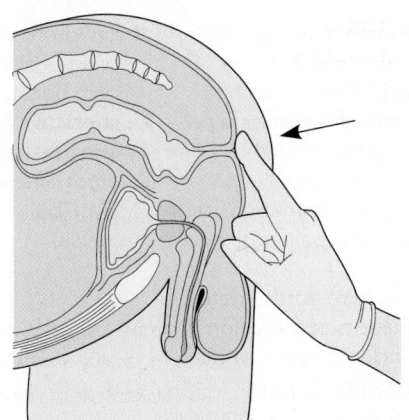

Figure 5–3 ● Digital examination of the *A*, rectum and *B*, anus.

INSPECTING THE FECES   Observe the client's stool for color, consistency, shape, amount, odor, and presence of abnormal constituents.

Lifespan and Cultural Considerations

As in a urinary assessment, privacy and modesty issues must be considered in assessing clients for alterations in bowel elimination. The nurse should explain all procedures in a manner that the client will understand. Individuals (especially children) may use very different terms for a bowel movement. The nurse may need to try several common words before finding one the client understands.

Diagnostic Tests

Diagnostic tests for bowel elimination problems include blood and fecal tests. Blood tests may be used to determine whether bowel problems have a systemic cause for bowel problems, and fecal tests can determine whether the problem is related to infection. A digital rectal exam palpates any abnormalities in the rectum and evaluates the strength of the sphincter muscles. A colonoscopy is often used to visualize the colon and rectum to discover polyps, cysts, or tumors, tissue samples may also be removed for biopsy. A colonoscopy can also detect areas of inflammation or bleeding. X-ray imaging, including barium enema x-ray and defecography, can be performed to visualize the colon and part of the small intestine and to evaluate the completeness of stool elimination. An anorectal manometry procedure is used to evaluate anal sphincter muscle function, and a colorectal transit study is used to determine how food moves through the colon.

Bowel Assessment

ASSESSMENT/METHOD	NORMAL FINDINGS	ABNORMAL FINDINGS	LIFESPAN OR DEVELOPMENTAL CONSIDERATIONS
Abdominal Assessment			
Inspect abdominal contour, skin integrity, venous pattern, and aortic pulsation.	Abdomen should be slightly concave with intact skin. There should not be distended veins or obvious aortic pulsations.	■ Generalized abdominal distention may be seen in gas retention or obesity. ■ Lower abdominal distention is seen in bladder distention or ovarian mass. ■ General distention and an everted umbilicus are seen with ascites and/or tumors. ■ A scaphoid (sunken) abdomen is seen in malnutrition or when fat is replaced with muscle. ■ **Striae** (whitish-silver stretch marks) are seen in obesity. ■ Spider angiomas may be seen in liver disease. ■ Dilated veins are prominent in cirrhosis of the liver, ascites, portal hypertension, or venocaval obstruction. ■ Pulsation is increased in aortic aneurysm.	■ Pregnant women have lower abdominal distention and may have striae and linea nigra. ■ Infants and toddlers may have normal abdominal distention, especially after feeding. ■ Allow young children to sit or lie on a parent's lap during the assessment if needed.
Auscultate all four quadrants of the abdomen with the diaphragm of the stethoscope. Begin in the lower right quadrant, where bowel sounds are almost always present.	Normal bowel sounds (gurgling or clicking) occur every 5–15 seconds. Listen for at least 5 minutes in each of the four quadrants to confirm the absence of bowel sounds.	■ **Borborygmus** (hyperactive high-pitched, tinkling, rushing, or growling bowel sounds) is heard in diarrhea or at the onset of bowel obstruction. ■ Bowel sounds may be absent later in bowel obstruction, with an inflamed peritoneum, and/or following surgery of the abdomen.	■ Pregnant women may have decreased bowel sounds.
Auscultate the abdomen for vascular sounds with the bell of the stethoscope.	No sounds (bruits, venous hum, or friction rub) other than bowel sounds should be auscultated.	■ **Bruits** (blowing sound due to restriction of blood flow through vessels) may be heard over constricted arteries. A bruit over the liver may be heard in hepatic carcinoma. ■ A venous hum (continuous medium-pitched sound) may be heard over a cirrhotic liver. ■ Friction rubs (rough grating sounds) may be heard over an inflamed liver or spleen.	
Percuss the abdomen in all four quadrants.	Normally, tympany is heard over the stomach and gas-filled bowels.	■ Dullness is heard when the bowel is displaced with fluid or tumors or filled with a fecal mass.	
Palpate the abdomen in all four quadrants. Use a circular motion to move the abdominal wall over underlying structures. Feel for masses and note any tenderness or pain the client may have during this part of the exam. Palpate lightly at first (0.5–0.75 inch), then more deeply (1.5–2 inch) with caution. If a mass is palpated, ask the client to raise head and shoulders.	There should be no abdominal masses or pain on palpation.	■ A mass in the abdomen may become more prominent when the head and shoulders are raised, as will a ventral abdominal wall hernia. If the mass is no longer palpable, it is deeper in the abdomen. ■ In cases of peritoneal inflammation, palpation causes abdominal pain and involuntary muscle spasms. ■ Abnormal masses include aortic aneurysms, neoplastic tumors of the colon or uterus, and a distended bladder or distended bowel due to obstruction. ■ A rigid, boardlike abdomen may be palpated when the client has a perforated duodenal ulcer.	■ Children may complain of abdominal pain because of stressful events (e.g., tests) or emotional trauma (e.g., bullying or abuse).

Bowel Assessment (*continued*)

ASSESSMENT/METHOD	NORMAL FINDINGS	ABNORMAL FINDINGS	LIFESPAN OR DEVELOPMENTAL CONSIDERATIONS
Palpate for rebound tenderness. Press the fingers into the abdomen slowly and release the pressure quickly.	Releasing pressure should not cause or increase pain.	■ In peritoneal inflammation, pain occurs when the fingers are withdrawn. ■ Right upper quadrant pain occurs with acute cholecystitis. ■ Upper middle abdominal pain occurs with acute pancreatitis. ■ Right lower quadrant pain at McBurney point occurs with acute appendicitis. ■ Left lower quadrant pain is seen in acute diverticulitis.	

Inguinal Area Assessment

ASSESSMENT/METHOD	NORMAL FINDINGS	ABNORMAL FINDINGS	LIFESPAN OR DEVELOPMENTAL CONSIDERATIONS
Inspect the inguinal area for bulges after asking the client to bear down.	The inguinal area is normally free of bulges.	■ Bulges that appear in the inguinal area when the client bears down may indicate a **hernia** (a defect in the abdominal wall that allows abdominal contents to protrude outward).	■ Inguinal hernias in infants are most obvious when the infant is crying, coughing, or straining during a bowel movement. ■ Males are more likely than females to develop inguinal hernias, regardless of age.
Palpate the inguinal area with the gloved hand. Ask the client to shift weight to the left to palpate the right inguinal area and vice versa. Place your right index finger upward into the inguinal area and ask the client to bear down or cough.	Bulging or masses are normally not palpable.	■ A bulge or mass may indicate a hernia.	

Perianal Assessment

ASSESSMENT/METHOD	NORMAL FINDINGS	ABNORMAL FINDINGS	LIFESPAN OR DEVELOPMENTAL CONSIDERATIONS
Inspect the perianal area. Wearing gloves, spread the client's buttocks apart. Observe the area, and ask client to bear down as if trying to have a bowel movement.	The perianal area should be intact, without obvious lesions.	■ Swollen, painful, longitudinal breaks in the anal area may appear in clients with anal fissures. (These are caused by the passing of large, hard stools or by diarrhea.) ■ Dilated anal veins appear with hemorrhoids. ■ A red mass may appear with prolapsed internal hemorrhoids. ■ Doughnut-shaped red tissue at the anal area may appear with a prolapsed rectum.	■ A parent or guardian should be present during rectal examination of all minors. ■ Some clients prefer to have the examination performed by a clinician of the same gender. ■ Expect the possibility of fecal elimination when the client bears down, especially in older adults with fecal incontinence.

(continued on next page)

Bowel Assessment (continued)

ASSESSMENT/METHOD	NORMAL FINDINGS	ABNORMAL FINDINGS	LIFESPAN OR DEVELOPMENTAL CONSIDERATIONS
Palpate the anus and rectum. Lubricate the gloved index finger and ask the client to bear down. Touch the tip of your finger to the client's anal opening. Flex the index finger, and slowly insert it into the anus, pointing the finger toward the umbilicus (see Figure 5–3). Rotate the finger in both directions to palpate any lesions or masses.	There should be no masses in the anus or rectum.	■ Movable, soft masses may be polyps. ■ Hard, firm, irregular embedded masses may indicate carcinoma.	■ Digital rectal examination is often not tolerated well by children or their parents. It also has limited usefulness in assessing constipation in children. ■ Be aware of skin fragility in older adults when performing a digital rectal examination.
Fecal Assessment			
Inspect the client's feces. After palpating the rectum, withdraw your finger gently. Inspect any feces on the glove. Note color and/or presence of blood. Also use gloved fingers to note consistency.	Stool should be soft with no blood present, either on the stool or as occult blood.		■ Newborn feces are meconium on the first 2–3 days after birth and become yellow, tan, or green after the meconium passes.
Test the feces for occult blood. Use a testing kit such as Occultest or Hemoccult II.	There should be no blood in the feces.	■ A positive occult blood test requires further testing for colon cancer or gastrointestinal bleeding due to peptic ulcers, ulcerative colitis, or diverticulosis.	
Note the odor of the feces.	No distinctly foul odors should be present.	■ Distinctly foul odors may be noted with stools containing blood or extra fat or in cases of colon cancer.	

▶ INTERVENTIONS AND THERAPIES

Clients with bowel elimination problems require sensitive and immediate nursing care. Both independent and collaborative interventions are beneficial for treating clients with diarrhea, constipation, bowel incontinence, and flatulence.

Independent

For clients with constipation, interventions include encouraging increased intake of fluid and fiber, as well as teaching clients about the impact of dietary choices on bowel elimination. Bowel training through interventions such as digital stimulation can be implemented by the nurse or taught to the client to help establish a regular schedule for bowel movements. (For discussion of digital stimulation, see the exemplar on Bowel Incontinence, Constipation, and Impaction in this module.) Kegel exercises and biofeedback can also be used to help the client strengthen rectal muscles. Nurses can also teach clients not to strain too hard when defecating, because straining may close the anal sphincter rather than allowing feces to pass through. For clients with fecal incontinence, nursing care may include providing hygiene care for the client, especially if the client is immobile. Regular assessment of the anal area is also necessary to detect skin breakdown or other problems. If the client has an ostomy pouch, nursing care includes keeping the pouch clean and free of infection.

Collaborative

Many bowel elimination problems are treated in collaboration with physicians and surgeons. Physicians may prescribe medications such as laxatives, antidiarrheal agents, or stool softeners. Medications may be given to promote bowel movement, to promote absorption of excess fluid in the intestine, or to coalesce gas or reduce the production of gas. For details regarding medications, see the Medications feature.

Clients with more acute problems, such as obstruction, ulceration, perforation, or cancer, may require surgical resection of the bowel with or without creation of an ostomy.

Medications **Bowel Elimination**

CLASSIFICATIONS AND DRUG EXAMPLES	MECHANISM OF ACTION	NURSING CONSIDERATIONS
Laxatives ▪ bulk-forming agents ▪ stool softeners ▪ stimulants ▪ saline or osmotic laxatives ▪ herbal agents ▪ miscellaneous agents *Drug examples:* psyllium hydrophilic mucilloid, methylcellulose, docusate sodium, senna, mineral oil, Epsom salts	Promote bowel movement	▪ Contraindicated in clients with nausea, cramps, colic, vomiting, or undiagnosed abdominal pain. Also contraindicated in clients after abdominal surgery. ▪ Should not be used continuously, because they weaken bowel's natural response to fecal distention. ▪ Before administration, assess abdomen for distention, bowel sounds, and bowel patterns. ▪ Teach clients preventive measures for constipation to avoid overdependence on laxatives.
Antidiarrheal Agents *Drug examples:* diphenoxylate with atropine, camphorated opium tincture, difenoxin with atropine, loperamide, bismuth salts, furazolidone	Slow motility of the intestines or promote absorption of excess fluid in the intestine.	▪ Monitor fluid and electrolyte status. ▪ Contraindicated in clients with severe dehydration, electrolyte imbalance, liver and renal disorders, and glaucoma. ▪ Teach clients to seek medical care if diarrhea does not subside in 2 days, fever develops, or dehydration occurs.
Antiflatulent Agents *Drug examples:* simethicone	Coalesce gas bubbles and facilitate passage	▪ Teach clients to seek medical care if symptoms persist or recur. ▪ Side effects include bloating, constipation, diarrhea, gas, and heartburn.

CASE STUDY \\ PART 2

Mr. Welborn's physician consults with a urologist, who suggests that Mr. Welborn be admitted to the hospital for a percutaneous nephrolithotomy. The urologist prescribes IV morphine for pain and schedules the surgery for 8:00 the next morning. The procedure is successful, without complications, and a urinary catheter and nephrostomy tube are put in place during surgery to drain urine. Postoperative pain is again managed with IV morphine, and Mr. Welborn states that his pain is manageable. He is confined to bed until 1 day postsurgery. The day after surgery, Mr. Welborn mentions to you, his nurse, that he did not have his normal morning bowel movement. When he sat on the toilet, he was unable to defecate, and he was afraid to push too hard because of his surgery. He was also unable to have a bowel movement the previous morning because of anxiety about the surgery, and his abdomen is feeling full. Abdominal assessment reveals diminished bowel sounds and dullness to percussion.

Clinical Reasoning Questions Level I

1. What factors may have contributed to Mr. Welborn's constipation?

2. What independent nursing interventions can you implement to help Mr. Welborn eliminate feces?

3. What client teaching can you provide to help Mr. Welborn prevent constipation in the future?

Clinical Reasoning Questions Level II

4. What effects might Mr. Welborn's constipation have on his urinary problems?

5. What complications may develop as a result of Mr. Welborn's constipation? What assessments should you perform to detect these complications?

6. What side effects of the percutaneous nephrolithotomy may Mr. Welborn experience related to his urinary system?

◢ REVIEW **The Concept of Elimination**

RELATE Link the Concepts

Linking the concept of elimination with the concept of infection:

1. What changes in urinary elimination indicate the presence of a urinary tract infection?

2. What effects does viral gastroenteritis have on bowel elimination?

Linking the concept of elimination with the concept of communication:

3. How can therapeutic communication be beneficial when assessing clients with urinary or bowel elimination problems?

4. Describe the importance of accurate documentation when caring for a hospitalized client with urinary or bowel elimination problems.

READY Go to Companion Skills Manual

REFER Go to Pearson Student Nursing Resources
nursing.pearsonhighered.com

- Additional review materials
- MiniModule: Anatomy and Physiology of Urinary Elimination

REFLECT Case Study // Part 3

After 3 days in the hospital, Mr. Welborn is discharged to home. His urinary catheter has been removed, and he states that he can urinate without pain. However, the nephrostomy tube remains in place. In addition, his IV morphine has been discontinued and he now receives acetaminophen (1,000 mg q6h). With consistent ambulation and discontinuation of morphine, Mr. Welborn had two bowel movements before discharge.

Clinical Reasoning Questions Level I

1. What methods can you teach Mr. Welborn to help prevent future renal calculi?

2. Describe the client teaching you will provide Mr. Welborn about caring for his nephrostomy tube.

3. What assessment should be performed on Mr. Welborn before discharge?

Clinical Reasoning Questions Level II

4. What medications might the physician prescribe for Mr. Welborn upon discharge?

5. What follow up appointments should you schedule for Mr. Welborn? Why?

6. How would a referral to a nutritionist benefit Mr. Welborn?

EXEMPLAR 5.1   Benign Prostatic Hyperplasia

EXEMPLAR KEY TERMS
Androgen, *285*
Benign prostatic hyperplasia (BPH), *284*
Continuous bladder irrigation (CBI), *289*
Detrusor muscles, *285*
Digital rectal examination (DRE), *285*
Dihydrotestosterone (DHT), *285*
Diverticula, *285*
Hydronephrosis, *285*
Hydroureter, *285*
Hyperplasia, *284*
Hypertrophy, *285*
Prostate-specific antigen (PSA), *285*
Prostatitis, *284*
Prostatodynia, *284*
Transurethral incision of the prostate (TUIP), *286*
Transurethral needle ablation (TUNA), *286*
Transurethral resection of the prostate (TURP), *286*
TURP syndrome, *289*
Uroflowmetry, *288*

EXEMPLAR LEARNING OUTCOMES
After reading about this exemplar, you will be able to:

1. Describe the pathophysiology, etiology, clinical manifestations, and direct and indirect causes of benign prostatic hyperplasia.

2. Identify risk factors and prevention methods associated with benign prostatic hyperplasia.

3. Illustrate the nursing process in providing culturally competent care across the life span for individuals with benign prostatic hyperplasia.

4. Formulate priority nursing diagnoses appropriate for an individual with benign prostatic hyperplasia.

5. Summarize therapies used by interdisciplinary teams in the collaborative care of an individual with benign prostatic hyperplasia.

6. Plan evidence-based care for an individual with benign prostatic hyperplasia and his family in collaboration with other members of the healthcare team.

7. Evaluate expected outcomes for an individual with benign prostatic hyperplasia.

▶ OVERVIEW

Prostatitis refers to inflammatory disorders of the prostate gland. **Prostatodynia** is a condition in which the client experiences the symptoms of prostatitis but shows no evidence of inflammation or infection. **Benign prostatic hyperplasia (BPH)**, on the other hand, is a nonmalignant enlargement of the prostate gland commonly seen in the aging male.

BPH can be a cause for great anxiety in the aging client who fears loss of his virility and ability to maintain a satisfying sex life. Radical surgeries, which were once the only treatment choice, often left men impotent, and the stories from those days still circulate as current fact. Client education and support play an important role in providing nursing care to clients diagnosed with BPH.

Benign prostatic hyperplasia is the most common benign neoplasm in men. It is characterized by a nonmalignant enlargement of the prostate gland that decreases the outflow of urine by obstructing the urethra, causing difficult urination. Although BPH typically begins in a man's 40s, he may not experience symptoms until much later, depending on how his individual condition progresses. BPH is not considered a precursor to prostate cancer.

▶ PATHOPHYSIOLOGY AND ETIOLOGY

The prostate gland borders the urethra near the lower part of the bladder. About the size of a chestnut (2 cm), it is partially palpable through the front wall of the rectum because it lies just anterior to the rectum. The prostate is composed of glandular structures that continuously secrete a milky alkaline solution. During sexual intercourse, glandular activity increases and the alkaline secretions flow into the urethra. Because sperm motility is reduced in an acidic environment, these secretions aid sperm transport. In addition, the prostate gland produces about one third of all semen.

Benign prostatic hyperplasia begins as small nodules in the periurethral glands, which are the inner layers of the prostate. The nodules are formed from **hyperplasia** (increase in the number of cells) of the stromal and epithelial cells in the prostate gland rather than **hypertrophy** (increase in the size of individual cells). However, the two terms are often used interchangeably for this condition, even by urologists. The hyperplasia of prostatic cells occurs over a long period of time, making BPH more common in older men. The pathophysiological effects result from a combination of factors, including urethral resistance to the effects of BPH, intravesical pressure during voiding, detrusor muscle strength, neurological functioning, and general physical health.

Etiology

The growth of the prostate is influenced by androgens and occurs mostly in the periurethral and transition zones of the prostate gland (Briganti et al., 2009). The androgen that mediates prostatic growth at all ages is **dihydrotestosterone (DHT)**, which is formed in the prostate from testosterone. An **androgen** is a hormone that stimulates the development and maintenance of male sex characteristics. Although androgen levels decrease in aging men, the aging prostate appears to become more sensitive to available DHT. Estrogen, produced in small amounts in men, appears to sensitize the prostate gland to the effects of DHT. Increasing estrogen levels associated with aging or a relative increase in estrogen related to testosterone levels may contribute to prostatic hyperplasia.

Risk Factors

The two main risk factors for developing BPH are age and the presence of testes. Men who have their testes removed before puberty (e.g., testes were removed because of testicular cancer) do not develop BPH, and testes removal later in life results in shrinkage of the prostate gland (Zieve, 2011). In addition, BPH rarely causes symptoms before age 40, and more than half of men in their 60s and 90% of men in their 70s and 80s have some symptoms of BPH. Almost all men develop BPH if they live long enough (NKUDIC, 2012b). Racial background may also play a role in BPH; Black and Hispanic men develop symptoms earlier than White men, and Asian men develop symptoms later than White men.

► CLINICAL MANIFESTATIONS

Although the symptoms of BPH are sometimes referred to as nuisances, they can have a profound effect on daily living. The expanding prostatic tissue compresses the urethra (**Figure 5–4** ●)

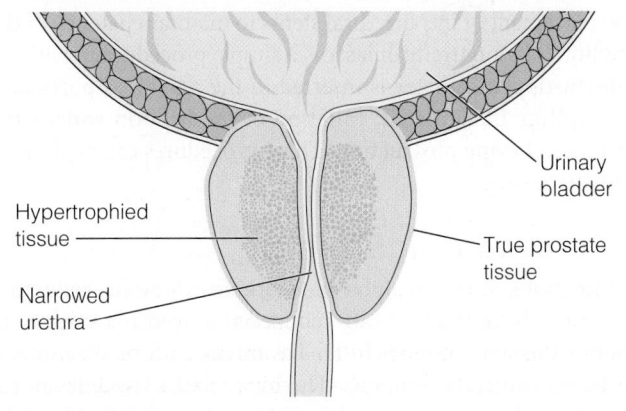

Figure 5–4 ● Benign prostatic hyperplasia.

and causes partial or complete obstruction of the outflow of urine from the urinary bladder. Even though the **detrusor muscles** hypertrophy to compensate for increased resistance to urinary flow, decreased bladder compliance and bladder instability eventually result. These changes manifest as symptoms of voiding (weak urinary stream, increased time to void, hesitancy, incomplete bladder emptying, and postvoid dribbling) and storage (frequency, urgency, incontinence, nocturia, dysuria, and bladder pain). These symptoms are often used to classify BPH. Urinary retention may become chronic, resulting in overflow incontinence with an increase in intra-abdominal pressure. Clients often report sensations of incomplete bladder emptying. There is little correlation between the size of the prostate gland and the urinary manifestations.

SAFETY ALERT
Urinary retention in men with BPH can be precipitated by several classes of medications, including those with anticholinergic properties and over-the-counter medications for the common cold, such as decongestants.

Unless the enlarging mass is reduced, multiple complications may occur. As urine is retained in the bladder, increasing bladder distention occurs. **Diverticula** (saclike projections of mucosa through the muscular layer of the colon) on the bladder wall result from the distention. The distention also may obstruct the ureters. Infection, more common in retained urine and in diverticula, may ascend from the bladder to the kidneys. Possible complications include **hydroureter** (distention of the ureter with urine), **hydronephrosis** (accumulation of urine in the renal pelvis as a result of obstructed outflow), and renal insufficiency.

► COLLABORATION

Care of clients with BPH focuses on diagnosing the disorder, correcting or minimizing the urinary obstruction, and preventing or treating complications. There is no way to reverse BPH. Treatment is often determined by the severity of the manifestations and the presence of complications. Mild cases are often monitored over time and symptoms may remain stable or even improve over time.

Diagnostic Tests

The most common diagnostic test for BPH is a **digital rectal examination (DRE)** (**Figure 5–5** ●): The physician inserts a gloved and lubricated finger into the rectum to palpate the prostate gland and determine its size and condition. Several urine tests may be performed, including a urine flow rate test, a postvoid residual urine test, and a pressure flow study. A urinalysis and urine culture may be done to check for blood or infection. A **prostate-specific antigen (PSA)** test may be performed to rule out prostate cancer. In addition, a cystoscopy may be performed to visualize the bladder and urethra to rule out other causes of urinary symptoms and to visualize the degree of ureter obstruction (NKUDIC, 2012b; Zieve, 2011).

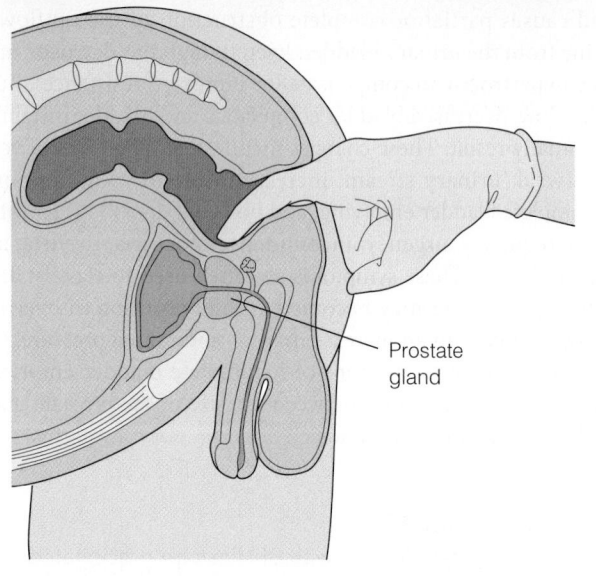

Figure 5–5 ● Digital rectal examination to palpate the prostate gland.

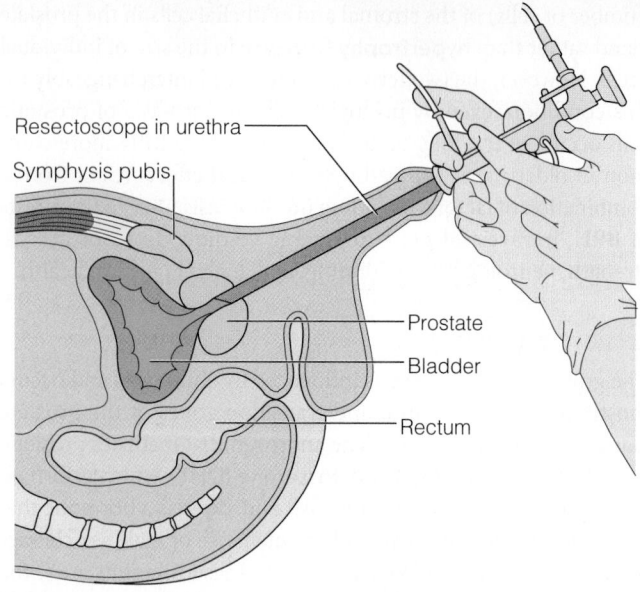

Figure 5–6 ● In a transurethral resection of the prostate, a resectoscope inserted through the urethra is used to remove excess prostate tissue.

Surgery

Men who have urinary retention, recurrent urinary tract infection, hematuria, bladder stones, or renal insufficiency secondary to BPH are candidates for surgical intervention. Surgical treatment may be performed by minimally invasive surgery or through transurethral, open, or laser surgery.

MINIMALLY INVASIVE SURGERY   Not all cases of BPH respond to medications. Therefore a number of procedures that are less invasive than traditional surgery have been developed to relieve the manifestations of BPH. *Transurethral microwave thermotherapy* uses microwaves to heat and destroy excess prostate tissue. During the procedure, a cooling system protects the urinary tract. The procedure takes about an hour and can be performed on an outpatient basis. Although microwave procedures do not cure BPH, they do reduce urinary manifestations. These procedures do not cause impotence or incontinence.

The **transurethral needle ablation (TUNA)** uses low-level radio frequency through twin needles to burn away a region of the enlarged prostate. Shields protect the urethra. TUNA improves the flow of urine through the urethra. It does not cause impotence or incontinence.

TRANSURETHRAL SURGERY   **Transurethral resection of the prostate (TURP)** is the surgical procedure used most often. Obstructing prostate tissue is removed with the wire loop of a resectoscope and electrocautery inserted through the urethra (**Figure 5–6** ●). No external incision is necessary. During the procedure, the surgeon uses the resectoscope to remove obstructing tissue one piece at a time. The tissue is flushed into the bladder with fluid and then flushed out at the end of the operation. This surgery has potential risks, however, including postoperative hemorrhage or clot retention, inability to void, and UTI. Other possible complications are incontinence, impotence, and retrograde ejaculation.

In the **transurethral incision of the prostate (TUIP)**, small incisions are made in the smooth muscle where the prostate is attached to the bladder. The gland is split to reduce pressure on the urethra. No tissue is removed, so this procedure is most appropriate for men with smaller prostate glands. TUIP can be done on an outpatient basis, and it has the additional advantage of lower risk of postoperative retrograde ejaculation than is associated with TURP and other prostatectomy procedures.

OPEN SURGERY   When the prostate gland is very large, an open prostatectomy may be used. This procedure is discussed in the exemplar on Prostate Cancer in the module on Cellular Regulation.

LASER SURGERY   In laser surgery, the surgeon uses a cystoscope to pass the YAG (yttrium-aluminum-garnet) laser fiber through the urethra into the prostate and then vaporizes obstructing prostate tissue with several short bursts of energy. Advantages of laser surgery include decreased blood loss and a more rapid recovery time. However, this method may not be as effective for larger prostates.

NEW TREATMENTS   Newer treatments for BPH include minimally invasive procedures such as balloon urethroplasty and placement of intraurethral stents to maintain patency of the urethra. Balloon urethroplasty is a simple procedure in which a balloon-tipped catheter is inserted in the narrowed portion of the urethra and inflated. Inflation of the balloon widens the urethra, relieving obstruction. These procedures can be done as outpatient surgery.

Pharmacologic Therapy

Medications such as alpha-blockers and 5-alpha reductase inhibitors have dramatically reduced the need for surgery to control the symptoms of BPH. Treatment with medications is based on two considerations: The hyperplastic tissue is androgen-dependent, and smooth muscle contraction within the prostate can exacerbate urinary obstruction (**Table 5–5** ●). The

TABLE 5–5 Agents for Benign Prostatic Hyperplasia

DRUG	ROUTE AND ADULT DOSE (MAXIMUM DOSE WHERE INDICATED)	ADVERSE EFFECTS
Alpha-adrenergic blockers		
doxazosin (Cardura)	po; 1–8 mg/day	*Orthostatic hypotension, headache, dizziness*
prazosin (Minipress)	1 mg qid or bid	<u>First-dose phenomenon</u> (severe hypotension and syncope), tachycardia
tamsulosin (Flomax)	po; 0.4 mg 30 min after a meal (max: 0.8 mg/day)	
terazosin (Hytrin)	po; start with 1 mg at bedtime, then 1–5 mg/day (max: 20 mg/day)	
5-Alpha reductase inhibitors		
dutasteride (Avodart)	po; 0.5 mg/day	*Sexual dysfunction, decreased libido, decreased ejaculate volume*
finasteride (Proscar)	po; 5 mg/day	No serious adverse effects

Italics indicate common adverse effects; underlining indicates serious adverse effects.

first consideration is usually addressed by treatment for mild prostate enlargement with finasteride (Proscar) or dutasteride (Avodart), both of which are 5-alpha reductase inhibitors (antiandrogen agents) that inhibit the conversion of testosterone to DHT and cause the enlarged prostate to shrink in size. Potential side effects include impotence, decreased libido, and decreased volume of ejaculate.

SAFETY ALERT
Pregnant women should not handle crushed tablets of 5-alpha reductase inhibitors because the drug may be absorbed through the skin and can harm a male fetus.

Excessive smooth muscle contraction in BPH may be blocked with alpha-adrenergic antagonists such as terazosin (Hytrin), doxazosin (Cardura), tamsulosin (Flomax), and alfuzosin (Uroxatral). These medications relax the smooth muscle of the prostate and bladder neck to relieve obstruction and increase the flow of urine. They may cause orthostatic hypotension. Client and family teaching includes making position changes slowly to prevent dizziness and accidental falls; taking and recording blood pressure; and checking with the healthcare provider before taking any medication for coughs, colds, or allergies (because these over-the-counter medications may contain an adrenergic agent). Federal research found that using finasteride and doxazosin together is more effective than using each alone to relieve manifestations and prevent the progression of BPH in clients with moderate (25 to less than 40 mL) or enlarged (40 mL or greater) prostate glands (Kaplan et al., 2006).

Certain commonly used medications have been found to worsen symptoms of BPH. Alpha-adrenergic agents, which include decongestants such as pseudoephedrine and phenylephrine, may activate alpha1-adrenergic receptors in the bladder neck, causing restriction of urine flow. Drugs with anticholinergic side effects such as antihistamines, TCAs, and phenothiazines may also adversely affect BPH. Testosterone and other anabolic steroids may increase prostate enlargement, increasing the physical obstruction of the urethra. Older men should avoid drugs that worsen symptoms of BPH.

Nonpharmacologic Therapy

Clients with mild BPH are often treated with "watchful waiting" and lifestyle changes. Mild symptoms clear up with no treatment in as many as one third of men (NKUDIC, 2012b). These men may be scheduled for regular checkups to monitor for early problems. Lifestyle changes that may be appropriate for men with mild BPH include (Zieve, 2011):

- Urinating at the first urge
- Avoiding alcohol and caffeine
- Drinking small amounts of fluids spread throughout the day
- Avoiding drinking fluids within 2 hours of bedtime
- Avoiding over-the-counter cold and sinus medications that contain decongestants or antihistamines
- Exercising regularly, including Kegel exercises
- Reducing stress.

Clinical Manifestations and Therapies **Benign Prostatic Hyperplasia**

ETIOLOGY	CLINICAL MANIFESTATION	CLINICAL THERAPIES
Voiding BPH	Weak or intermittent urinary stream, hesitancy, incomplete emptying, dribbling at the end of urination, straining during urination	▪ Pharmacologic therapy ▪ Lifestyle changes
Storage BPH	Frequency, urgency, incontinence, nocturia, dysuria, bladder pain	▪ Pharmacologic therapy ▪ Lifestyle changes
Urinary retention	Bladder distention, diverticula, ureter obstruction, bladder or kidney infection, hydroureter, hydronephrosis, renal insufficiency	▪ Surgery

NURSING PROCESS

The nurse who is caring for a client with BPH must be sensitive to his concerns and fears and provide education and support. Therapeutic communication helps the nurse obtain a thorough and complete history and assist the client with discussing sensitive topics.

Assessment

Men over the age of 40 should be assessed for possible benign prostatic hyperplasia and, depending upon their health history, should be screened for prostate cancer. Assessment includes a health history, physical assessment, and diagnostic tests. A diagnosis of BPH involves both physical examination and laboratory tests not only to diagnose the disease but also to differentiate it from prostate cancer.

The health history includes risk factors, urinary elimination patterns and manifestations, hematuria, and pain. Symptoms of BPH can be assessed with the International Prostate Symptom Score (IPSS). The IPSS uses a scale of 0 (not at all) to 5 (almost always) to collect data about several subjective factors, including feeling as though the bladder did not empty with urinating; needing to urinate within 2 hours after urinating; starting and stopping the stream several times while urinating; and straining to urinate. This questionnaire also asks how many times during the night the client needs to urinate and how he feels about having the disorder.

Stay Current: To view the IPSS online, visit **http://www.usrf.org/questionnaires/AUA_SymptomScore.html**

The physical examination usually includes a digital rectal examination (DRE) of the external surface of the prostate for size, symmetry, firmness, and nodules; in BPH, it is asymmetrical and enlarged. Note that a DRE is an advanced nursing assessment (see Figure 5–5). Abnormal findings include tenderness, masses, nodules, hardness, or softness. Nodules may be characteristic of prostate cancer, while tenderness indicates prostatitis.

Several diagnostic tests are used in the assessment of BPH. The client's urine is examined for white blood cells (WBCs), red blood cells (RBCs), and bacteria. Urinary function is assessed by measuring residual urine (amount of urine remaining in the bladder after voiding) with ultrasonography or postvoiding catheterization (more than 100 mL is considered high) and through **uroflowmetry**, which measures urine flow rate (normal is greater than 14 mL/sec). A finding of less than 10 mL/sec indicates obstruction. Creatinine levels of the blood are assessed for kidney damage. Prostate-specific antigen levels are obtained to rule out prostate cancer. PSA is a glycoprotein produced only in the cytoplasm of benign and malignant prostate cells; the serum level corresponds with the volume of both benign and malignant prostate tissue.

Diagnosis

Examples of nursing diagnoses that may be considered for clients with BPH include the following:

- *Impaired Urinary Elimination*
- *Risk for Infection* related to urinary retention
- *Overflow Urinary Incontinence* related to sphincter blockage secondary to enlarged prostate
- *Acute Pain* related to bladder distention
- *Deficient Knowledge* related to effect of prostate surgery on sexuality

(NANDA-I © 2012)

Planning

The nursing plan of care should be individualized to meet client needs; every client will require goals specific to his situation. However, commonly created goals may include:

- The client will regain urinary continence after catheter removal.
- The client will verbalize the rationale for performing postoperative exercise.
- The client will verbalize the need for continued follow up care.
- The client will verbalize warning signs of urinary tract infection.
- The client will verbalize proper administration of prescribed medications and adverse affects that should be reported to provider.
- The client will report pain that rates 3 or less on a scale of 0–10.

Implementation

Care of the client with BPH differs based on treatment decisions and need for surgical intervention. If the client does not need surgical intervention, nursing care includes primarily client teaching about topics such as self-care, proper administration of medications, medication side effects to expect, symptoms to report to the physician, and nutrition. Nursing care of all clients involves therapeutic communication, answering the client's questions, and providing emotional support. Clients who need surgical intervention require more in-depth nursing care.

Preoperative Care

Tactful but thorough preoperative care, education, and support are critical to the client's subjective view of the surgery as well as to its objective outcomes. The nurse should assess the client's and family's knowledge about the surgery. Most men are unsure of the function of the prostate gland and even of its exact location, although its relationship to sexual and urinary function is at least generally known. This lack of knowledge, coupled with the growing number of treatment options, is confusing to many men. Clients may be confused about the surgical approach because of the several different methods. Client teaching will help reduce client anxiety related to fear of the unknown.

Understanding the scope of preoperative activities and postoperative conditions increases client cooperation with postoperative care. Men may be anxious about the outcome of their surgery and its potential long-term effects on their sexuality. The nurse communicates willingness to address any concerns or anxiety by maintaining a professional approach and creating a trusting relationship.

Verify that the informed consent form was signed. Explain to the client that he will have a urinary catheter when he returns from surgery and that he may have a drain in his incision, depending on the type of surgery performed. Explain that he also will be wearing sequential pneumatic compression stockings.

Bowel preparation with a 2% neomycin enema may be ordered to cleanse the bowel in the event of a perineal approach.

Postoperative Care

Nursing care of the client after prostate surgery involves pain management, monitoring for complications, implementation of methods to prevent complications, and hygiene care. Monitor vital signs closely for the first 24 hours and regularly thereafter. The client who has had prostate surgery is at risk for hemorrhage and infection. Changes in vital signs are often the earliest manifestations of these complications. Maintain accurate intake and output records, including amounts of irrigating solution used. Frequently assess patency of any catheters and drains. Monitor color and character of urine. Catheters may become occluded by blood clots or kinks, interfering with urinary drainage and increasing the risk of hemorrhage.

Assess and manage the client's pain, which may include incisional pain, bladder spasms, or abdominal cramps due to intestinal gas. Analgesics and nonsteroidal anti-inflammatory drugs (NSAIDs) are administered on a routine and as needed basis to control incisional pain. Bladder spasms may be accompanied by strong urges to void and urine leakage around the catheter. Belladonna and opium (B & O) suppositories may be used to relieve bladder spasms.

Maintain antiembolic stockings and pneumatic compression devices as ordered. Assist with leg exercises and ambulation as ordered. These are important preventive measures because the client who has had prostate surgery is at risk for developing thromboembolism. Encourage him to maintain a liberal fluid intake of 2–3 L a day, and explain that increased fluids reduce burning upon urination after catheter removal, as well as the risk of UTI.

For the first 24–48 hours, a client with a transurethral resection of the prostate (TURP) should be monitored for hemorrhage, evidenced by frankly bloody urinary output, presence of large blood clots, decreased urinary output, increased bladder spasms, decreased hemoglobin and hematocrit, tachycardia, and hypotension. Notify the physician of any of these manifestations. Postoperative hemorrhage may be arterial or venous and may be precipitated by movement, bladder spasms, or obstructed urinary drainage.

Instruct the client with a three-way indwelling catheter with traction to keep his leg straight while the traction is applied. A No. 18–22 Fr three-way catheter with a 30–45 mL balloon usually is inserted following a TURP. The inflated balloon is pulled down into the prostatic fossa, and the catheter tubing is pulled down and taped to the client's leg to apply pressure against the operative site, preventing bleeding.

Pressure on the urethra by the large catheter and on the internal sphincter by the catheter's balloon stimulates the micturition reflex. Explain that the presence of a urinary catheter will cause the sensation of needing to void, but it is important not to strain when trying to void around the catheter or when having a bowel movement. Straining to void or to have a bowel movement may stimulate bladder spasms and increase pain; it also may increase the risk for bleeding. Explain the possibility of bladder spasms, experienced as lower abdominal pressure or pain and a desire to urinate. Ensure that the client expects this possible sensation and knows that medications can help alleviate this discomfort.

Continuous bladder irrigation (CBI) prevents the formation of blood clots, which can obstruct urinary output. If the client has CBI, assess the catheter and the drainage tubing at regular intervals. Maintain the rate of flow of irrigating fluid to keep the output light pink or colorless. Assess the urinary output every 1–2 hours for color, consistency of amount, and presence of blood clots; assess the client for bladder spasms. Bladder distention resulting from output obstruction increases the risk of bleeding. Irrigating fluids are continuously infused and drained at a rate that keeps urine light pink or colorless. Bladder spasms and urine that is frankly bloody, contains many blood clots, or is decreased in amount indicate obstruction and bleeding.

Assess for fluid volume excess and hyponatremia, called **TURP syndrome**, which is manifested by hyponatremia, decreased hematocrit, hypertension, bradycardia, nausea, and confusion. If these manifestations occur, notify the physician. TURP syndrome results from the absorption of irrigating fluids during and after surgery. Untreated, it may result in dysrhythmias and/or seizures.

If the client does not have CBI, follow agency procedure and physician orders for irrigating the indwelling catheter (usually when the urine is frankly bloody or has numerous large blood clots or when bladder spasms increase). In most instances, using sterile technique, gently irrigate the catheter with 50 mL of irrigating solution at a time until the obstruction is relieved or the urine is clear. Ensure equal input and output of irrigating fluid. Intermittent irrigation may be used to prevent obstruction of urinary drainage.

Following catheter removal, assess the amount, color, and consistency of urine. Explain to the client that he may experience burning upon urination, that dribbling after urination is a common experience, and that the urine may contain small blood clots after catheter removal. The CBI and catheter usually are removed in the 24–48 hours following surgery. To improve urinary control, teach the client to start and stop the urine stream several times during each voiding, and have him practice Kegel exercises. Regaining full control may take up to 1 year.

If the client had a retropubic prostatectomy, assess the abdominal incision for the presence of urine or increased or purulent drainage. Because the bladder is not entered during a retropubic prostatectomy, no urine should be found on the dressing.

If the client had a suprapubic prostatectomy, assess urinary output from both the suprapubic and the urethral catheters. The client with a suprapubic prostatectomy often has two separate closed drainage systems: one from the suprapubic incision and one from a urethral catheter. Assess the abdominal dressing for urinary drainage and change saturated dressings frequently. Consult with a skin care specialist if saturated dressing results in skin irritations. Following removal of the urethral catheter (usually 2–4 days after surgery), based on physician orders, clamp the suprapubic catheter and encourage the client to void. Assess residual urine by unclamping the suprapubic catheter and measuring urinary output after voiding. If residual urine is 75 mL or less with several voidings, remove the suprapubic catheter.

The client with a perineal prostatectomy should be assessed for perineal drainage and manifestations of infection. Rectal temperatures and enemas are contraindicated because they may precipitate bleeding. Use a T-binder or padded scrotal support to hold the dressing in place. (The location of the dressing makes application difficult.) Following removal of the dressing and perineal sutures, heat lamps or sitz baths may be used to provide heat and promote healing. Teach the client to perform perineal irrigations with sterile normal saline as ordered and as instructed after each bowel movement. Because of the proximity of the incision to the anus, special wound care is necessary to prevent infection.

Depending on a client's choice of treatment, the procedure may be performed on an outpatient basis. The client having a TURP, although hospitalized for the surgery, may be discharged within 2 days after surgery if there are no complications. Home care often involves care of an indwelling urinary catheter (see Client Teaching feature). Postoperative clients being discharged to home may or may not require temporary assistance from a home health nurse to ensure that they are following postoperative care procedures. For family members of clients who require a great deal of assistance and who choose to recover at home, referral to an agency that provides caregiver respite or home health services may be helpful. The nurse plays an essential role in assessing the postoperative needs of the client and family and in working with them to make sure they are able to manage the recovery process successfully. See **Box 5–2** ● for discharge instructions the nurse should provide the client and family.

Evaluation

A client's individualized plan of care is developed in collaboration with the client and includes outcomes identified with the client's participation. The client's condition is regularly evaluated based on those outcomes. If an outcome is not met, the nurse reviews the plan of care with the client to determine necessary changes. Potential outcomes may include the following:

- The client is continent.
- The client maintains adequate pain control to allow for comfort and performance of ADLs.
- The client is asymptomatic, or symptoms are less severe.
- The client describes symptoms to report to the provider upon occurrence.
- The client lists over-the-counter medications to be avoided.

Client Teaching Caring for Catheters and Drainage Bags

Teaching a client or caregiver how to care for the catheter and drainage bag includes the following information:

- Change from the daytime leg drainage bag to a larger night drainage bag. A larger bag suspended from the bed frame at night permits gravity drainage of urine and prevents reflux of urine into the bladder.
- Avoid strapping on the leg bag too tightly, which can decrease venous return and increase risk for thrombophlebitis (swelling of the veins) and embolic complications such as pulmonary emboli.
- Place a soft cloth between the leg bag and thigh to decrease friction and to absorb dampness under the bag, reducing the risk of skin irritation.
- Empty the leg bag every 3–4 hours during waking hours to prevent overfilling.
- Promptly report to the urologist any unexpected changes in urine color, urine consistency, urine odor, hematuria, evidence of frank bleeding, or large blood clots, as well as a lack of or significant decrease in urine output.

Box 5–2   Discharge Instructions After Prostate Surgery

ACTIVITY

The healing period lasts from 4 to 8 weeks. Avoid strenuous activity and heavy lifting. Except for short rides, do not drive for 2 weeks. Do take long walks; take stairs slowly and carefully. Continue exercises that you did in the hospital to prevent blood clots in the legs. You can take showers, but avoid tub baths while the catheter is in place.

BLEEDING

Bleeding can occur any time after surgery. It is fairly common after a bowel movement, coughing, or increased exercise. If you notice blood in the urine, increase fluids and rest until the urine is clear. If heavy bleeding plugs the channel, call the care provider immediately. Avoid aspirin and NSAIDs for at least 2 weeks.

BOWEL MOVEMENTS

Keep bowel movements regular and soft to prevent pressure on the prostate area. Drink fruit juices and take mild laxatives or stool softeners as ordered.

DIET

Resume your normal diet. Increase fluids to 10 glasses (8 oz) daily. Avoid alcohol unless otherwise advised by your physician.

SEXUAL INTERCOURSE

To prevent bleeding, do not have sex for 6 weeks after surgery. You may still have erections even with the catheter in place. When you resume sex, ejaculate will flow back into the bladder, so you will express little or no semen.

URINATION

After your catheter is removed, you may experience some burning, stinging, or leakage for several weeks, and you may pass small blood clots occasionally. These symptoms will disappear as the area heals. It is best to use pads to control leakage.

WORK

If work is not strenuous, you may return in 4 weeks; otherwise, wait 6–8 weeks.

PLEASE CALL IMMEDIATELY IF:

- You are unable to urinate.
- Bleeding is not controlled by fluids and rest or is excessive.
- You have chills and fever or severe abdominal pain.
- Your scrotum becomes swollen and tender.
- You have pain in one calf, chest pain, or difficulty breathing.

NURSING CARE PLAN	A Man With Benign Prostatic Hyperplasia

William Turner, a 71-year-old African American, lives with his wife in a small retirement community in Florida. His wife had a stroke 2 years ago, and Mr. Turner does all of the cooking and housework. He has been in good health for most of his life, having only a small touch of osteoarthritis in his knees and hands. He has noticed a gradual onset of urinary urgency and frequency over the past 2 years and has found it increasingly difficult to begin his stream. During a routine checkup, the nurse practitioner at the local health clinic performs a DRE and palpates Mr. Turner's prostate, finding it enlarged. After Mr. Turner's PSA is found to be normal, he is referred to a urologist, who diagnoses BPH. Mr. Turner chooses to have surgery, and a TURP is performed. Following surgery, his recovery is uncomplicated. However, the nurse caring for Mr. Turner is concerned about his ability to care for his indwelling catheter because of his arthritis and his wife's physical disabilities from the stroke. The nurse makes a referral to a home health agency to ensure that Mr. Turner can manage his care at home. An initial home health assessment is scheduled for the day after Mr. Turner is discharged from the hospital.

ASSESSMENT

The home health nurse notes that the house is clean and neat. Mr. Turner is still wearing his night urinary drainage bag even though it is 1:00 p.m. Mr. Turner tells the nurse that his main problem is going to get groceries because he is embarrassed to be seen with the drainage bag. He says that he has not been able to remove the drainage bag and attach the leg bag because of his arthritis. Physical assessment reveals no tenderness in his calves, chest pain, or shortness of breath. The urine is yellow, without odor or sedimentation. Mr. Turner states that he sees no need for the pelvic exercises, since he is no longer in the hospital.

DIAGNOSES

- *Stress Urinary Incontinence* related to surgical procedure
- *Ineffective Health Maintenance* related to inability to care for the urinary drainage system, lack of understanding about the need for postoperative exercises, and questions about follow up care
- *Disturbed Body Image* related to wearing drainage bag in public

(NANDA-I © 2012)

PLANNING

Planning care is done in collaboration with Mr. Turner to improve outcomes and include the following goals:
- Mr. Turner will regain urinary continence after catheter removal.
- Mr. Turner will change the urinary drainage bag with the appropriate assistance.
- Mr. Turner will verbalize the rationale for performing postoperative exercise.
- Mr. Turner will verbalize the need for continued follow up care.
- Mr. Turner will verbalize decreased embarrassment about being in public when using the leg bag instead of the drainage bag.

IMPLEMENTATION

- Discuss the possibility of stress incontinence after the catheter is removed.
- Reinforce the need for Kegel exercises while the catheter is still in place.
- Explore Mr. Turner's support system to identify individuals who can assist him with catheter care; arrange a teaching session with them.
- Teach Mr. Turner the importance of follow up care, relating the care to the history of the disease.
- Refer Mr. Turner to a support group for individuals with BPH.

EVALUATION

The nurse evaluates Mr. Turner's care based on the goals of care established during the planning phase. Good friends from Mr. Turner's church have assisted him with care of his drainage bag and have reminded him to do his Kegel exercises several times a day while the catheter is in place. When the catheter is removed, Mr. Turner has only a small amount of leaking of urine after voiding. He understands that it may take several weeks for this leakage to resolve. Efforts to help him understand the need for continued medical care are less successful. Mr. Turner continues to state that he is cured, his wife needs him, and he sees no reason to return to the doctor.

CRITICAL THINKING

1. Outline a teaching plan for Mr. Turner for the risk of altered skin integrity related to urinary incontinence.
2. As a result of Mr. Turner's refusal to have ongoing medical care, he might be labeled noncompliant. Would you make this nursing diagnosis? Why or why not?
3. If you were the home health nurse making a home visit and found that Mr. Turner had had no urinary drainage for 16 hours, what assessments would you make? How would you handle this problem?

REVIEW Benign Prostatic Hyperplasia

RELATE Link the Concepts and Exemplars

Linking the exemplar of benign prostatic hyperplasia with the concept of sexuality:

1. How can you talk with an older man about the impact of BPH on his sexuality without making him uncomfortable?
2. How can you assess his concerns, fears, and knowledge regarding the impact of BPH on his sexuality?

Linking the exemplar of benign prostatic hyperplasia with the concept of infection:

3. What pathophysiology of BPH could increase the risk of UTIs?
4. What nursing interventions will reduce the risk of UTIs?

READY Go to Companion Skills Manual

REFER Go to Pearson Student Nursing Resources
nursing.pearsonhighered.com

- Additional review material

REFLECT Case Study

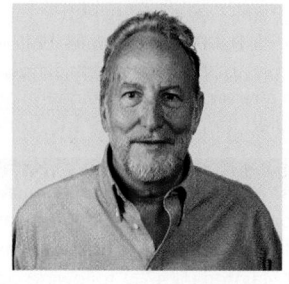

Clifford Allen is a 64-year-old male who has been married to his wife, Pam, for 40 years. They live with their 24-year-old son, Gary, who was born with Down syndrome. Mr. Allen is a middle manager for a small manufacturing company where he has worked for the last 20 years. Overall, Mr. Allen is in good health, although he has been undergoing treatment recently for BPH. He has a history of depression for which he does not seek treatment because he fears the social stigma connected to the diagnosis. Mr. Allen has been considering retiring within the next few years so he and his wife can travel, but mostly to escape his stressful work environment. He enjoys bowling and is involved in activities at church. He and his wife walk each evening after supper.

One evening while bowling, he notices that his bladder feels somewhat full. Mr. Allen calls to make an appointment to see his urologist for a follow up examination. He has been taking finasteride (Proscar) for the last 6 months but does not believe it has been particularly effective. He still has trouble urinating and believes that his symptoms are worse than before he started taking the drug. When he sees the urologist 2 weeks later, he reports that he often feels his bladder is full after voiding, he has difficulty starting his stream, and his stream is weak once started. He gets up frequently at night to void. His score on the American Urological Association Symptom Index is 28, up from 18 six months ago. The urologist confirms that the medication has not been effective and schedules further tests, including a uroflowmetry test, a postvoid residual test, a PSA blood test, and a urinalysis. Results from the uroflowmetry and postvoid residual test show a significant obstruction of urinary flow. The PSA is negative, and the urinalysis is consistent with bladder inflammation. A TURP is recommended in the upcoming weeks.

1. To determine Mr. Allen's understanding of the procedure, what will the nurse want to ask him upon admission to the surgical center?

2. What teaching will the nurse prepare regarding postoperative self-care?

3. Design a nursing plan of care for this client postoperatively.

EXEMPLAR 5.2 **Bladder Incontinence and Retention**

EXEMPLAR KEY TERMS

Bladder training, *295*
Habit training, *295*
Hydronephrosis, *297*
Scheduled toileting, *295*
Urinary incontinence, *292*
Urinary retention, *297*
Vesicoureteral reflux, *297*

EXEMPLAR LEARNING OUTCOMES

After reading about this exemplar, you will be able to:

1. Describe the pathophysiology, etiology, clinical manifestations, and direct and indirect causes of bladder incontinence and retention.

2. Identify risk factors and prevention methods associated with bladder incontinence and retention.

3. Illustrate the nursing process in providing culturally competent care across the life span for individuals with bladder incontinence and retention.

4. Formulate priority nursing diagnoses appropriate for an individual with bladder incontinence or retention.

5. Summarize therapies used by interdisciplinary teams in the collaborative care of an individual with bladder incontinence or retention.

6. Plan evidence-based care for an individual with bladder incontinence or retention and his or her family in collaboration with other members of the healthcare team.

7. Evaluate expected outcomes for an individual with bladder incontinence or retention.

▶ OVERVIEW

When caring for clients with urinary tract disorders, it is important to consider the client's modesty in voiding, possible difficulty in discussing the genitals, embarrassment about being exposed for examination and testing, and fear of changes in body image or function. These psychosocial issues may interfere with the client's willingness to seek help, discuss treatment, and learn about preventive measures. Nursing interventions for clients with urinary tract disorders are directed toward primary prevention, early detection, and management of the disorder through health teaching and nursing care.

URINARY INCONTINENCE

Urinary incontinence, or involuntary urination, is a symptom, not a disease. It is the most common manifestation of impaired bladder control. It can have a significant impact on the client's life, creating physical problems, such as skin breakdown, and leading to psychosocial problems, including embarrassment, isolation, and social withdrawal.

The incidence of urinary incontinence is estimated to be between 10 million and 13 million individuals in the United States and 200 million individuals worldwide. The estimated annual cost of managing urinary incontinence in the United States is $16.3 billion, 75% of which is spent on treating women (Vasavada, 2013). Although urinary incontinence is especially common among older clients, it is not a normal consequence of aging, and it can be treated. An estimated 30% or more of older women living in the community experience urinary incontinence. In long-term care, assisted living, and homebound populations, the incidence is between 50% and 80%. Despite these statistics, the actual prevalence of urinary incontinence is nearly impossible to determine. Embarrassment and the availability of products to protect clothing and prevent detection contribute to clients' not seeking evaluation and treatment of incontinence.

▶ PATHOPHYSIOLOGY AND ETIOLOGY

Urinary continence requires a bladder that is able to expand and contract and sphincters that can maintain a urethral pressure higher than that of the bladder. Incontinence results when the pressure within the urinary bladder exceeds urethral resistance, allowing urine to escape. Any condition causing higher-than-normal bladder pressures or reduced urethral resistance can result in incontinence. Relaxation of the pelvic musculature, disruption of cerebral and nervous system control, and disturbances of the bladder and its musculature are common contributing factors.

Etiology

Incontinence may be an acute, self-limited disorder, or it may be chronic. The causes may be congenital or acquired, reversible or irreversible. Urinary incontinence is acute and reversible if it is associated with partial or complete resolution. Reversible factors include polyuria, exposure to irritants, urinary retention, stool impaction or constipation, restricted mobility or dexterity, psychological conditions, and delirium. Other reversible causes are medications (e.g., diuretics and sedatives), prostatic enlargement, vaginal and urethral atrophy, and UTI. Vaginal childbirth may also contribute to urinary incontinence. Some causes of urinary incontinence, such as acute confusion, may or may not be reversible, depending on the underlying cause of the confusion.

Chronic or irreversible causes of urinary incontinence are often associated with congenital disorders or nervous system disorders. Congenital disorders associated with incontinence include epispadias (absence of the upper wall of the urethra) and meningomyelocele (a neural tube defect in which a portion of the spinal cord and its surrounding meninges protrude through the vertebral column). Central nervous system or spinal cord trauma, stroke, and chronic neurological disorders, such as multiple sclerosis and Parkinson disease, are examples of acquired, irreversible causes of incontinence.

Risk Factors

Age is a primary risk factor for the development of urinary incontinence; older individuals experience more frequent incontinence than younger individuals. In all age groups, women are much more susceptible to urinary incontinence than men, especially women who are homebound or who live in a long-term care facility. Obesity, smoking, diabetes, inactivity, pregnancy, depression, and neurological disorders (e.g., stroke) are all risk factors for urinary incontinence. Individuals who experience two or more UTIs per year or who take certain medications (e.g., medications that affect the adrenergic system, diuretics, and calcium-channel blockers) are also at higher risk for urinary incontinence.

Prevention

Lifestyle modification is the best method of preventing urinary incontinence. Maintaining a healthy weight can help prevent urinary incontinence; this includes weight loss for individuals who are overweight or obese. Eating a diet that is high in fiber can help prevent constipation, which is a risk factor for urinary incontinence. Avoiding bladder irritants such as alcohol, caffeine, and acidic or spicy food can also help prevent urinary incontinence. Drinking adequate fluid is necessary for normal bladder function; individuals should not drink less than six to eight 8 oz glasses of water daily. Similarly, drinking too much water can lead to rapid bladder filling and consequent urinary incontinence. Other prevention methods include exercising regularly, not smoking, reviewing medications for increased risk of urinary incontinence, and reducing physical barriers to toileting for clients at high risk, such as those with mobility or neurological deficits.

▶ CLINICAL MANIFESTATIONS

Symptoms of urinary incontinence include the inability to avoid urinating until a bathroom can be found, increased rate of urination, leakage, uncontrollable wetting, and frequent bladder infections. Incontinence commonly is categorized as stress incontinence, urge incontinence (also known as overactive bladder), reflex urinary incontinence, overflow incontinence, and functional incontinence. **Table 5–6** ● summarizes each type with its physiological cause and associated factors. Mixed incontinence (elements of both stress and urge incontinence) is common. Total incontinence, which may be due to a variety of etiologies, is loss of all voluntary control over urination: Urine loss occurs without stimulus and in all positions. The treatment of total urinary incontinence depends upon the medically diagnosed cause of the condition.

Lifespan and Cultural Considerations

In addition to older adults, two population groups that are highly susceptible to urinary incontinence are children and pregnant women.

CHILDREN   The age at which a child attains urinary continence varies. Therefore diurnal enuresis (daytime incontinence) is not diagnosed until age 5 or 6, and nocturnal enuresis (nighttime incontinence) is not diagnosed until age 7. More than 90% of children are continent during the day by age 5, but nighttime continence takes longer to achieve. About 30% of children at age 4 have nocturnal enuresis, 10% at age 7, 3% at age 12, and 1% at age 18 (NKUDIC, 2012c). Nocturnal enuresis is more common in boys than in girls. Most cases of urinary incontinence in children clear up spontaneously with no treatment.

Causes of nocturnal enuresis in children include maturational delay, uncompleted toilet training, overproduction of urine at night, difficulties in arousal from sleep, conditions that increase urine volume (e.g., diabetes mellitus), constipation, and structural abnormalities (e.g., ectopic ureter). Causes of diurnal enuresis include bladder irritability, weak detrusor muscle, constipation, structural abnormalities, sexual abuse, urinary tract infection, and infrequent voiding (e.g., voluntarily holding urine to avoid using toilets at school or interrupting play) (Figueroa, 2012; NKUDIC, 2012c).

Treatment options for a child who requires treatment for urinary incontinence include bladder training, moisture alarms, and medication (e.g., desmopressin, imipramine, oxybutynin).

TABLE 5–6   Types of Urinary Incontinence

TYPE	DESCRIPTION	PATHOPHYSIOLOGY	CONTRIBUTING FACTORS
Stress	Loss of urine associated with increased intra-abdominal pressure during sneezing, coughing, lifting; usually, small quantity of urine lost	Relaxation of pelvic musculature and weakness of urethra and surrounding muscles and tissues lead to decreased urethral resistance.	■ Multiple pregnancies ■ Decreased estrogen levels ■ Short urethra, change in angle between bladder and urethra ■ Abdominal wall weakness ■ Prostate surgery ■ Increased intra-abdominal pressure caused by tumor, ascites, obesity
Urge	Involuntary loss of urine associated with a strong urge to void	Hypertonic or overactive detrusor muscle leads to increased pressure within bladder and inability to inhibit voiding.	■ Neurological disorders, such as stroke, Parkinson disease, multiple sclerosis; peripheral nervous system disorders ■ Detrusor muscle overactivity associated with bladder outlet obstruction, aging, or disorders such as diabetes
Reflex	Involuntary loss of urine at predictable intervals when a specific bladder volume is reached	Neuronal control of the pontine and/or sacral micturition centers is disrupted.	■ Neurological impairment ■ Tissue damage
Overflow	Inability to empty bladder, resulting in overdistention and frequent loss of small amounts of urine	Outlet obstruction or lack of normal detrusor activity, leading to overfilling of bladder and increased pressure	■ Spinal cord injuries below S_2 ■ Diabetic neuropathy ■ Prostatic hyperplasia ■ Fecal impaction ■ Drugs, especially those with anticholinergic effect
Functional	Incontinence resulting from physical, environmental, or psychosocial causes	Ability to respond to the need to urinate is impaired.	■ Confusion or dementia ■ Physical disability or impaired mobility ■ Therapy or sedation ■ Depression ■ Regression

PREGNANT WOMEN   Pregnant women often experience stress incontinence because of hormonal changes and the excess weight of the growing uterus pressing on the bladder. After delivery, postpartum women are also more likely to experience urinary incontinence because vaginal delivery tends to weaken bladder muscles and damage nerves and supporting structures. This outcome may cause a prolapse of the pelvic floor, which pushes the pelvic organs into the vagina and prevents the urethra from closing completely; the result is incontinence (Mayo Clinic, 2011d; NKUDIC, 2010). Bladder training and Kegel exercises are the best treatments for urinary incontinence in pregnant women.

▶ COLLABORATION

Urinary incontinence is a symptom rather than a disorder, so diagnosis and treatment focus on identifying and treating the underlying cause of incontinence. Diagnosis is based on a nursing history, physical examination, and diagnostic tests. Treatment may include behavioral modifications, medication, or surgery. Diagnosis and treatment are done in collaboration with other healthcare professionals, including physicians, urologists, and surgeons.

Diagnostic Tests

Three common, simple diagnostic tests for clients with urinary incontinence are a bladder diary, urinalysis, and blood tests.

The *bladder diary* is used to record how much the client drinks, when the client urinates and how much urine is produced, whether the client felt the urge to urinate, how many incontinence episodes the client experienced, and what the client was doing at the time of incontinence. The bladder diary can help the healthcare provider to distinguish between stress, urge, reflex, overflow, and functional incontinence and to understand the client's bladder function. A *urinalysis* detects appearance, color, blood, infection, glucose, specific gravity, presence of stones, and other characteristics of urine to identify the underlying cause of incontinence, such as a UTI or calculi. Similarly, a *blood test* identifies potential hormonal or chemical causes of incontinence, such as diabetes mellitus.

Other urine tests that may be used for clients with urinary incontinence are a 24-hour urine sample, postvoid residual measurement, urodynamic testing, and a stress test. The *24-hour urine sample* shows how much urine the client produces in one day and tests kidney and bladder function. The *postvoid residual measurement* shows the amount of residual urine left in the client's bladder after voiding, that is, incomplete emptying and bladder volume. A large postvoid volume may indicate obstruction or nerve or muscle damage. *Urodynamic testing* measures the bladder pressure at rest and while filling. Filling is simulated by the insertion of a catheter and filling the bladder with water. This test measures bladder strength and urinary sphincter health. During a *stress test*, the client is asked to bear down while the physician or nurse watches for urine loss.

Imaging tests may also be performed to reveal the cause of urinary incontinence. A pelvic *ultrasound* is used to visualize structures in the pelvic region and any structural abnormalities. A *cystogram* uses a radioactive dye inserted into the bladder through a catheter to show bladder abnormalities and postvoid volume. In a *cystoscopy*, the physician inserts a cystoscope to visualize the urinary tract, detect abnormalities, and obtain tissue samples (Mayo Clinic, 2011d).

Surgery

Surgery may be used to treat stress incontinence associated with cystocele (prolapsed bladder) or urethrocele (prolapsed urethra) and overflow incontinence associated with an enlarged prostate gland. Suspension of the bladder neck, a technique that brings the angle between the bladder and urethra closer to normal, is effective in treating stress incontinence associated with urethrocele in 80%–95% of clients. A laparoscopic, vaginal, or abdominal approach may be used to perform this surgery.

✳ Go to **nursing.pearsonhighered.com** to see the nursing care for a client undergoing bladder neck suspension.

Prostatectomy, using either the transurethral or the suprapubic approach, is indicated for the male client who is experiencing overflow incontinence as a result of an enlarged prostate gland and urethral obstruction.

Other surgical procedures of potential benefit in the treatment of incontinence are implantation of an artificial sphincter, formation of a urethral sling to elevate and compress the urethra, augmentation of the bladder with bowel segments to increase bladder capacity, implantation of nerve stimulators, and injection of collagen along the urethra to narrow the urinary passageway and support more normal urethral positioning.

Pharmacologic Therapy

Both stress and urge incontinence may improve with drug treatment. Some medications target the underlying cause of urinary incontinence, such as alpha-blockers and 5-alpha reductase inhibitors for men with BPH and antibiotics for individuals with a UTI. Drugs that contract the smooth muscles of the bladder neck may reduce episodes of mild stress incontinence. Imipramine (Tofranil), an antidepressant, is an effective preparation. It can make individuals drowsy, however, so it typically is taken at night. Adverse effects, such as dizziness and irregular heartbeat, and contraindications with a number of other medications may limit its use.

When incontinence is associated with postmenopausal atrophic vaginitis, estrogen therapy may be effective. Options include systemic estrogens and local creams. Clients with urge incontinence may be treated with preparations that increase bladder capacity. The primary drugs used to inhibit detrusor muscle contractions and increase bladder capacity include oxybutynin (Ditropan and the extended-release form, Ditropan XL), an anticholinergic drug, and tolterodine (Detrol and its longer-acting form, Detrol LA), a more specific antimuscarinic agent. These drugs can be taken once or twice a day and have fewer side effects than less-specific anticholinergic drugs. Drugs with anticholinergic effects are contraindicated for the client with acute glaucoma. Urinary retention is a potential side effect that must be considered when these drugs are used.

Nonpharmacologic Therapy

To reduce the incidence of urinary incontinence, the nurse should teach all clients to perform pelvic floor muscle (Kegel) exercises (**Box 5–3** ●) to improve perineal muscle tone. Kegel exercises are most often used for women with urinary incontinence, but they may also benefit men who experience urinary incontinence following prostatectomy for BPH or prostate cancer.

Behavioral modification is another classic method for treating urinary incontinence. Behavioral techniques include scheduled toileting, habit training, and bladder training. **Scheduled toileting** is toileting at regular intervals (e.g., every 2–4 hours). **Habit training** is toileting the client on a schedule that corresponds with the normal pattern. **Bladder training** gradually increases the bladder capacity by increasing the intervals between voidings and resisting the urge to void between scheduled times. Bladder training may also involve double voiding, or voiding once and then voiding a few minutes later to release residual urine; regulating fluid intake; avoiding dietary bladder stimulators; and performing relaxation and distraction techniques to overcome the urge to void (Vasavada, 2013).

Box 5–3 Pelvic Floor Muscle (Kegel) Exercises

■ Identify the pelvic muscles with these techniques:
  a. Stop the flow of urine during voiding, and hold for a few seconds. Clients who have difficulty emptying the bladder completely should not stop urine flow while voiding in order to identify the pelvic floor muscles. Repeated interruption of micturition can interfere with complete bladder emptying and increase the risk for UTI.
  b. Tighten the muscles at the vaginal entrance around a gloved finger or tampon (women).
  c. Tighten the muscles around the anus as though resisting defecation.
■ Perform exercises by tightening pelvic muscles, holding for 3–10 seconds, and then relaxing for 10–15 seconds. Continue the sequence (tighten, hold, relax) for 10 repetitions. Do not perform exercises while urinating other than to initially identify the proper muscle groups.
■ Keep abdominal muscles and breathing relaxed while performing exercises.
■ Initially, exercises should be performed twice a day, working up to four times a day.
■ Encourage exercising at a specific time each day or in conjunction with another daily activity (e.g., bathing or watching the news). Establish a routine, because these exercises should be continued for life.
■ Assistive devices, such as vaginal cones, and biofeedback may be useful for clients who have difficulty identifying appropriate muscle groups.

Children can also benefit from behavioral modification techniques similar to those used for adults. An additional modification technique for children with diurnal enuresis is urgency containment exercises. These exercises include having the child prepare to go to the bathroom when the urge occurs, then sit on the toilet and hold the urine for as long as possible. When starting to urinate, the child is encouraged to start and stop the urine stream to gain control over the pelvic floor muscles and strengthen the sphincters. This process also gives the child confidence to hold the urine until reaching a bathroom, to avoid having an accident (Figueroa, 2012). For children who have nocturnal enuresis, having an adult or sibling wake the child in the middle of the night to urinate may help the child avoid bed-wetting.

Additional nonpharmacologic methods of treating urinary incontinence include using absorbent products such as pads or diapers, inserting a pessary or urethral insert, or using a catheter (Mayo Clinic, 2011d). A pessary is a stiff ring that is inserted into the vagina to hold up the bladder and prevent urine leakage. A urethral insert is a tamponlike device that is inserted into the urethra to act as a plug for leaks. Pessaries are generally used for clients with a prolapsed bladder, whereas urethral inserts are usually used during specific activities that may cause incontinence. Catheters are usually used for clients

Evidence-Based Practice Catheter Care and Infection Prevention

Problem

Urinary incontinence and urinary retention are often managed with insertion of a catheter. The use of a catheter significantly increases the risk of developing a urinary tract infection, and that risk increases with increasing days of use. Nearly 25% of hospitalized clients require catheterization, and 10% of those individuals develop a UTI. Many of these clients do not require a catheter, but the catheter remains because of convenience, misunderstanding of its necessity, and lack of orders for removal (Oman et al., 2012). In nursing homes, over 10% of clients require indwelling catheters, and 50% of those clients develop catheter-associated urinary tract infections (CAUTI) each year (Mody, Saint, Galecki, Chen, & Krein, 2010). Nurses are responsible for using sterile techniques when providing catheter care and for teaching clients to properly care for a catheter at home.

Evidence

The Centers for Disease Control and Prevention (CDC) has issued guidelines for proper catheter use and care based on clinical evidence (Gould et al., 2009). The consistent implementation of these guidelines can help reduce CAUTI. According to these guidelines, catheters should be used only in appropriate situations and only for as long as needed. Duration should be minimal in clients at high risk of mortality from infection, including women, older adults, and clients with impaired immunity. In addition, catheters should not be used in clients or nursing home residents simply to manage incontinence. Alternatives to indwelling catheters should be used when appropriate, including external catheters in male clients without urinary retention or bladder outlet obstruction and intermittent catheterization for clients with long-term catheterization needs (e.g., those with spinal cord injury or neurogenic bladder). The use of a portable ultrasound device to assess urine volume makes catheter insertions unnecessary in clients undergoing intermittent catheterization. Hand hygiene should be performed immediately before and after insertion or manipulation of the catheter, and only individuals with proper training should provide catheter care. Once inserted, an indwelling catheter should be properly secured to prevent movement and urethral traction. A closed drainage system should be maintained at all times, and urine flow should be unobstructed. The collecting bag must be kept below the level of the bladder but not on the floor. Catheters should be changed only on the basis of clinical indications (e.g., infection, obstruction, system compromise) and not at regular intervals. Bladder irrigation is not recommended unless obstruction is anticipated.

A survey of RNs, LPNs, and nurses' aides in nursing homes in Michigan found that although knowledge of some guidelines related to catheter care, such as hand hygiene, was high, knowledge of other guidelines, including practices to maintain closed drainage systems and recommendations for bladder irrigation, was relatively low (Mody et al., 2010). In addition, one hospital that implemented facility-wide education and better product and equipment availability was successful in reducing the number of catheter days (Oman et al., 2012), which is a major risk factor for development of CAUTI. In another hospital, implementation of education about appropriate device utilization and device removal decreased device utilization from 0.5 catheter days/patient days to 0.3 catheter days/patient days and decreased the CAUTI rate from 1.8/1,000 catheter days to 0.7/1,000 catheter days (Revello & Gallo, 2013).

Implications

Nurse education related to catheter use and care is essential to reduce the CAUTI rate. Based on education about indications for catheter use, nurses must learn to analyze each client for the necessity of catheter use and to recognize clients for whom catheter use is not indicated. It is the nurse's responsibility to then approach the physician about removing the catheter in clients who no longer need a catheter. Similarly, it is the nurse's responsibility to implement best practice guidelines related to personal hand hygiene, client perineal hygiene, catheter bag placement, maintenance of a closed urinary system, and other aspects of catheter care. Education regarding these guidelines should be provided regularly, and policies should be put in place to ensure that the guidelines are followed.

Critical Thinking Application

Describe circumstances in which an older woman who has undergone hip replacement surgery would need a urinary catheter before or 1, 7, or 21 days after surgery. Differentiate between conditions that require indwelling or intermittent catheterization and no catheterization. Develop an educational session to provide nurses and other healthcare workers an update on the latest guidelines for catheter use and care in an effort to reduce CAUTI.

Client Teaching Preventing UTIs and Urinary Incontinence

Client teaching is essential for clients who experience problems with urinary incontinence and for their family members. The nurse should discuss the following points with clients to help prevent UTI and urinary incontinence:

- Maintain a generous fluid intake. Reduce or eliminate fluid intake after the evening meal to reduce nocturia.
- Wear comfortable clothing that is easy to remove for toileting.
- Maintain good hygiene, but do not bathe more often than necessary. Frequent bathing and use of feminine hygiene sprays or douches may dry perineal tissues, increasing the risk of UTI or urinary incontinence.
- Perform pelvic muscle (Kegel) exercises several times a day to increase perineal muscle tone.

- Reduce consumption of caffeine-containing beverages (e.g., coffee, tea, and colas), citrus juices, and beverages containing NutraSweet.
- Use behavioral techniques to reduce the frequency of incontinence.
- See your primary care provider regularly for a pelvic or prostate examination.
- For women, discuss possible benefits and risks of hormone replacement therapy, physical therapy, or surgery to treat incontinence.
- Report any change in urine color, odor, or clarity or symptoms such as burning, frequency, or urgency to your primary care provider.

with overflow incontinence due to bladder retention or for clients with neurological damage that affects bladder muscle control. Intermittent self-catheterization is the preferred catheterization method because it significantly decreases the risk of developing a UTI. If the client is unable to perform self-catheterization or has no control of bladder muscles (such as a paraplegic client), an indwelling Foley catheter or suprapubic catheter may be necessary.

SAFETY ALERT
Limiting total fluid intake to less than 1.5–2.0 L per day is not recommended for clients with urinary incontinence. Inadequate fluid increases urine concentration, which leads to bladder wall irritation and possibly increases problems of urge incontinence.

Client teaching is also an essential part of nursing care for clients with urinary incontinence. To learn more about teaching topics, see the Client Teaching feature.

URINARY RETENTION

Urinary retention is the inability to empty the bladder. It is most common in men with BPH, but other factors can contribute to urinary retention as well. Urinary retention can be acute, in which the client is unable to urinate at all, or chronic, in which the bladder constantly contains a small residual volume of urine. Although urinary retention is less common than urinary incontinence, it can become a medical emergency if the client is unable to void.

▶ PATHOPHYSIOLOGY AND ETIOLOGY

When bladder emptying is impaired, urine accumulates and the bladder becomes overdistended. Overdistention causes poor contractility of the detrusor muscle, further impairing urination. If the problem persists, more serious problems, such as **hydronephrosis** (accumulation of urine in the renal pelvis as a

result of obstructed outflow) or **vesicoureteral reflux** (backflow of urine from the bladder to the kidney) can result.

Etiology

Either mechanical obstruction of the bladder outlet or a functional problem can cause urinary retention. Benign prostatic hyperplasia (BPH) is a common cause, with difficulty initiating and maintaining urine flow often being the presenting complaint in men. Acute inflammation associated with infection or trauma of the bladder, urethra, or perineal tissues also may interfere with micturition. Scarring caused by repeated UTIs can lead to urethral stricture and a mechanical obstruction. Bladder calculi also may obstruct the urethral opening from the bladder. Many individuals develop urinary retention after surgery as a result of anesthesia (Baldini et al., 2009), and other medications contribute to urinary retention as well.

Risk Factors

General risk factors for the development of urinary retention include advanced age; male gender; history of previous prostate, bladder, or voiding problems; urinary incontinence; urinary tract infections or prostatitis; cognitive impairment or confusion; diabetes; alcoholic neuropathy; previous transient ischemic attack, stroke, or neurological disease; constipation; abdominal pain; immobility; chronic pain; emotional distress; and drugs (e.g., anticholinergics or opioids) (Johansson et al., 2013). Individuals who have undergone surgery are also at higher risk for urinary retention as a result of anesthesia and limited mobility. Clients who have undergone abdominal or pelvic surgery are at especially high risk if the surgery disrupts the function of the detrusor muscle. Accidents to or infections of the brain or spinal cord can increase a client's risk for urinary retention.

Clients who take medications that interfere with detrusor muscle function are at increased risk of developing urinary retention. Anticholinergic medications, such as atropine, glycopyrrolate (Robinul), propantheline bromide (Pro-Banthine), and scopolamine hydrochloride (Transderm-Scop), can lead to acute urinary retention and bladder distention. Many other drug groups have anticholinergic side effects and may cause urinary retention. Among these are antianxiety agents, such as diazepam (Valium); antidepressant and tricyclic drugs, such as imipramine (Tofranil); antiparkinsonism drugs (L-dopa); antipsychotic agents; and some sedative/hypnotic drugs. In addition, antihistamines, which are common in over-the-counter cough, cold, allergy, and sleep-promoting drugs, have anticholinergic effects and may interfere with bladder emptying. Diphenhydramine (Benadryl) is an example of a nonprescription antihistamine.

Voluntary urinary retention, which is particularly common among nurses, may lead to overfilling of the bladder and a loss of detrusor muscle tone. These individuals are also at increased risk of developing chronic urinary retention.

Prevention

The first step in preventing urinary retention is identifying clients who may be at risk for urinary retention (Johansson et al., 2013). Further diagnostic testing should be done for clients at risk to determine whether the client is currently experiencing previously undetected urinary retention. Behavioral modifications should be implemented for all clients at risk for urinary retention. Timed voiding is especially helpful for clients with cognitive impairment. If needed, clients should be assisted to the toilet, provided with a bedside commode, or taught intermittent self-catheterization to prevent urinary distention and the associated complications. For men with BPH, urinary retention may be prevented by administering 5-alpha reductase inhibitors (Kalejaiye & Speakman, 2009).

▶ CLINICAL MANIFESTATIONS

The client with urinary retention is unable to empty the bladder completely and may feel a resulting discomfort. Urinary retention can be classified as either acute or chronic. Acute retention is the sudden and painful inability to void despite having a full bladder; this is a medical emergency. It may be accompanied by bloating. It is commonly caused by surgical procedures, medications, UTIs, excessive fluid or alcohol intake, or BPH (Kalejaiye & Speakman, 2009; NKUDIC, 2012d).

Chronic retention is painless and is associated with an increase in the residual urine volume. Clients with chronic urinary retention may have difficulty starting and maintaining urination and may be able to produce only a weak flow. They may urinate frequently, feel the urge to urinate but have little success in voiding, or feel they still need to go after urinating (NKUDIC, 2012d). Overflow voiding or incontinence may occur, with 25–50 mL of urine eliminated at frequent intervals.

Assessment of clients with urinary retention reveals a firm, distended bladder that may be displaced to one side of midline. Percussion of the lower abdomen yields a dull tone, reflective of fluid in the bladder. Urinary retention is confirmed with a bladder scan or the insertion of a urinary catheter (if possible) and measurement of the urine output. Use of a bladder scan is preferred to reduce the risk of UTI (Palese et al., 2010).

Severe urinary retention with resulting bladder distention impairs the ability of the vesicoureteral junction to prevent backflow of urine into the ureters (**Figure 5–7 ●**). Reflux of urine from the distended bladder distends the ureters (hydro-

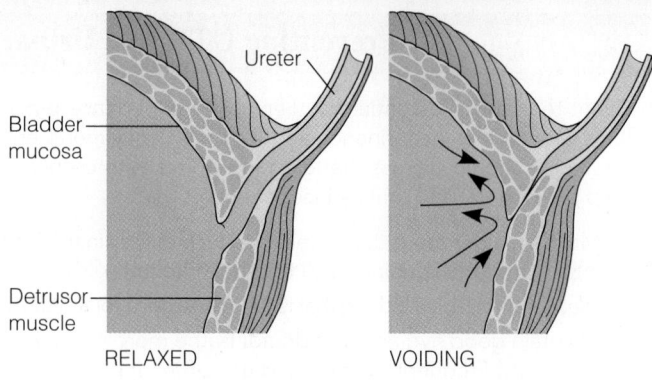

Figure 5–7 ● A competent vesicoureteral junction.

ureter) and kidneys (hydronephrosis). Hydronephrosis impairs renal function, and acute renal failure can result.

▶ COLLABORATION

The nurse can independently perform some treatments for urinary retention, such as catheter care. However, the nurse must collaborate with other healthcare team members for other aspects of care for clients with urinary retention, including diagnostic tests, surgery, and pharmacologic therapy.

Diagnostic Tests

Diagnostic tests for clients with urinary retention are similar to tests for urinary incontinence and include blood and urine tests. Imaging scans such as x-rays, CT scans, bladder scans, and cystoscopy are also used to detect urinary retention. Bladder scans use ultrasound images to detect the amount of residual urine in the bladder. Chronic urinary retention is diagnosed when the individual has more than 100 mL of postvoid residual urine.

Surgery

Mechanical obstructions removed or repaired when possible. Resection of the prostate gland may be done for urinary retention related to BPH. Bladder calculi are removed, and measures to prevent their formation are instituted. Surgery may also be performed to correct a cystocele or rectocele.

Pharmacologic Therapy

Cholinergic medications, such as bethanechol chloride (Urecholine), that promote contraction of the detrusor muscle and emptying of the bladder may be used. A medication with no anticholinergic side effects may be substituted when urinary retention is related to drug therapy.

Nonpharmacologic Therapy

Urinary retention should be immediately treated with complete decompression of the bladder via catheterization. An indwelling urinary catheter or intermittent straight catheterization may be necessary to prevent future urinary retention and overdistention of the bladder until the underlying problem is corrected by surgery or medication or until the client has healed from surgery or other causes of retention.

Clinical Manifestations and Therapies **Urinary Incontinence and Retention**

ETIOLOGY	CLINICAL MANIFESTATIONS	CLINICAL THERAPIES
Stress incontinence	Loss of a small amount of urine when sneezing, coughing, lifting; uncontrollable wetting; weakness of urethra and pelvic muscles; increased pressure on the bladder from pregnancy, obesity, cystocele, or urethrocele	■ Surgery ■ Imipramine ■ Kegel exercises ■ Behavioral modifications ■ Absorbent pads or diapers ■ Pessary ■ Urethral insert
Urge incontinence	Loss of urine associated with a strong urge to void, increased rate of urination, inability to avoid urinating until a bathroom can be found, overactive detrusor muscle, nocturia	■ Oxybutynin ■ Tolterodine ■ Kegel exercises ■ Behavioral modifications ■ Absorbent pads or diapers
Reflex incontinence	Complete emptying of bladder at a predictable bladder volume, neurological deficits, frequency, nocturia, inability to sense full bladder or initiate or inhibit voiding	■ Medication ■ Neuromodulation ■ Surgery ■ Catheterization ■ Absorbent pads or diapers
Overflow incontinence	Loss of urine associated with an overdistended bladder and urinary retention, urinary obstruction, BPH	■ Surgery ■ Catheterization ■ 5-alpha reductase inhibitors ■ Absorbent pads or diapers
Functional incontinence	Loss of urine associated with physical impairments that prevent the client from reaching the toilet in time; mobility impairment; cognitive deficits	■ Catheterization ■ Absorbent pads or diapers ■ Home modifications ■ Physical or occupational therapy ■ Assistive devices ■ Nonrestrictive clothing
Acute urinary retention	Inability to urinate, bladder distention, hydronephrosis, vesicoureteral reflux, pain, abdominal bloating, dull sound upon abdominal percussion	■ Catheterization ■ Change in medication therapy ■ Antibiotics ■ Surgery
Chronic urinary retention	Large postvoid residual volume, bladder distention, urinary obstruction, poor detrusor muscle contractility, urinary inflammation, difficulty starting and maintaining stream, weak flow, frequent urination, little success at voiding, urge to urinate after voiding, overflow incontinence	■ Catheterization ■ Change in medication therapy ■ Surgery ■ Bethanechol

■ NURSING PROCESS

Understanding how to care for clients with urinary incontinence or retention is vital to nursing practice, because clients of any age may experience urinary problems related to physiological changes or medical conditions or treatments. Nursing care of clients with bladder problems involves emptying the bladder, preventing complications, maintaining skin integrity, and providing emotional support.

Assessment

The preliminary assessment and identification of the symptoms of urinary incontinence and retention are truly within the scope of nursing practice. All clients should be asked about their voiding patterns. Clients with mild symptoms may not even realize that they are experiencing a problem. Older adults who are incontinent while in their home or who manage to contain or conceal their incontinence from others do not consider themselves incontinent. Therefore the nurse may need to ask about incontinence in several ways using different terminology to determine if the individual is experiencing incontinence. If incontinence is described, a thorough history and assessment are indicated.

A complete assessment of a client's urinary function includes the following:

- *Health history.* Voiding diary; frequency of urination, amount of urine loss, and activities associated with incontinence; methods used to deal with incontinence; use of Kegel exercises or medications; any chronic diseases, medications, or alternative health therapies, related surgeries, and so on; effects of incontinence or retention on usual activities, including social activities.
- *Physical examination.* Physical and mental status, including any physical limitations or impaired cognition; inspection, palpation, and percussion of abdomen for bladder distention; inspection of perineal tissues for redness, irritation, or tissue breakdown; observation for bulging of bladder into vagina when bearing down; digital rectal examination for prostate size; assessment of pelvic muscle tone as indicated; assessment of hydration status; examination of urine.

Diagnosis

NANDA International (NANDA-I, 2012) includes one general diagnostic label for urinary elimination problems: *Impaired Urinary Elimination.* More specific NANDA-I nursing diagnoses related to urinary elimination include the following:

- *Functional Urinary Incontinence*
- *Overflow Urinary Incontinence*
- *Reflex Urinary Incontinence*
- *Stress Urinary Incontinence*
- *Urge Urinary Incontinence*
- *Risk for Urge Urinary Incontinence*
- *Readiness for Enhanced Urinary Elimination*
- *Toileting Self-Care Deficit*

(NANDA-I © 2012)

Problems of urinary elimination also may become the etiology for other problems the client experiences. Examples include the following:

- Urinary retention and invasive procedures, such as catheterization or cystoscopic examination, can put a client at risk for infection.
- Incontinence is a risk factor for low self-esteem and social isolation because it is considered socially unacceptable and therefore can be physically and emotionally distressing. Often, the client is embarrassed about dribbling or having an accident and may therefore restrict normal activities.
- Incontinence increases risk for impaired skin integrity. Bed linens and clothes saturated with urine irritate and macerate the skin. Prolonged skin dampness leads to dermatitis (inflammation of the skin) and consequent formation of dermal ulcers.

- Functional incontinence is a risk factor for self-care deficits in toileting.
- Impaired urinary function associated with a disease process may put a client at risk for deficient or excess fluid volume.
- A client who has a urinary diversion ostomy may develop a disturbed body image.
- Clients who require new self-care skills to manage (e.g., a new urinary diversion ostomy) may be at risk of deficient knowledge regarding management of their care.
- An incontinent client who is being cared for by a family member for extended periods may be at risk for caregiver role strain as well as for deteriorating family relationships as a result of that strain.

Planning

Goals established for a client depend on the diagnosis and defining characteristics. Examples of overall goals for clients with urinary elimination problems include the following:

- The client will maintain or restore a normal voiding pattern.
- The client will regain normal urine output.
- The client will prevent associated risks, such as infection, skin breakdown, fluid and electrolyte imbalance, and lowered self-esteem.
- The client will perform toilet activities independently, with or without assistive devices.
- The client will contain urine with the appropriate device, catheter, ostomy appliance, or absorbent product.

Implementation

Clients with urinary incontinence or retention may receive primary care in a hospital, in a long-term care facility, or at home. Nursing interventions for each of these clients will depend on the client's type of incontinence or retention, physical mobility status, cognitive status, and location.

Independent nursing interventions for clients with urinary problems may include (a) a behavior-oriented continence training program such as bladder training, habit training, prompted voiding, pelvic muscle exercises, and positive reinforcement; (b) meticulous skin care; and (c) catheter care or client teaching about intermittent self-catheterization. Other interventions include promoting adequate fluid intake, maintaining normal voiding habits, and assisting with toileting. Clients who are receiving home care must be alert and physically able or have caregivers who can assist with implementing the plan of care.

Maintain Normal Voiding Patterns

Prescribed medical therapies often interfere with a client's normal voiding habits. When a client's urinary elimination pattern is adequate, the nurse helps the client adhere to normal voiding habits as much as possible (**Box 5–4 ●**).

Promote Effective Urination

Nursing measures to promote urination include placing the client in normal voiding position and providing privacy. Additional measures include running water, placing the client's hands in warm water, pouring warm water over the perineum, and taking a warm sitz bath.

In acute urinary retention, catheterization may be necessary to relieve bladder distention and prevent hydronephrosis. Use a rela-

Box 5–4 Maintaining Normal Voiding Habits

POSITIONING

■ Assist the client to a normal position for voiding: standing for male clients; for female clients, squatting or leaning slightly forward when sitting. These positions enhance movement of urine through the tract by gravity.

■ If the client is unable to ambulate to the lavatory, use a bedside commode for females and a urinal for males standing at the bedside.

■ If necessary, encourage the client to push over the pubic area with the hands or to lean forward to increase intra-abdominal pressure and external pressure on the bladder.

RELAXATION

■ Provide privacy for the client. Many individuals cannot void in the presence of another individual.

■ Allow the client sufficient time to void.

■ Suggest that the client read or listen to music.

■ Provide sensory stimuli that may help the client relax. Pour warm water over the perineum of a female or have the client sit in a warm bath to promote muscle relaxation. Applying a hot water bottle to the lower abdomen of both men and women may also foster muscle relaxation.

■ Turn on running water within hearing of the client to stimulate the voiding reflex and to mask the sound of voiding for individuals who find it embarrassing.

■ To decrease muscle tension, provide ordered analgesics and emotional support to relieve physical and emotional discomfort.

TIMING

■ Assist clients who have the urge to void immediately. Delays only increase the difficulty in starting to void, and the desire to void may pass.

■ Offer toileting assistance to the client at usual times of voiding, for example, on awakening, before or after meals, and at bedtime.

FOR CLIENTS WHO ARE CONFINED TO BED

■ Warm the bedpan. A cold bedpan may prompt contraction of the perineal muscles and inhibit voiding.

■ Elevate the head of the client's bed to Fowler position, place a small pillow or rolled towel at the small of the back to increase physical support and comfort, and have the client flex the hips and knees. This position simulates the normal voiding position as closely as possible.

---

tively small catheter (16 French for a man, 14 French for a woman). A coudé-tipped catheter is passed more easily in the older man with an enlarged prostate. Using 2% lidocaine gel (10 mL injected into the male urethra, or 6 mL injected into the female urethra) reduces discomfort during catheterization and the risk of catheter-associated infection, and it promotes pelvic muscle relaxation (Bardsley, 2005). Carefully observe the client as the distended bladder drains.

SAFETY ALERT

Some clients experience a vasovagal response, becoming pale, sweaty, and hypotensive if the bladder is rapidly drained. Draining urine in 500 mL increments and clamping the catheter for 5–10 minutes between increments may

prevent this response. Hematuria, the presence of blood in the urine, also may occur with rapid bladder decompression. Promptly notify the physician if hematuria develops.

Assist With Toileting

Clients who are weakened by a disease process or impaired physically may require assistance with toileting. This requirement is common for institutionalized older adults (see Lifespan Considerations). The nurse should assist these clients to the bathroom and remain with them if they are at risk for falling. The bathroom should contain an easily accessible call signal to summon help if needed. Clients also must be encouraged to use handrails placed near the toilet. For clients who are unable to use bathroom facili-

---

Lifespan Considerations The Institutionalized Older Adult and Self-Care Deficit

Functional incontinence may be the predominant problem in an institutionalized older adult. Limited mobility, impaired vision, dementia, lack of access to facilities and privacy, and tight staffing patterns increase the risk for incontinence in previously continent residents. The primary problem in functional incontinence is an outside factor that interferes with the ability to respond normally to the urge to void. An immobilized client may wet the bed if a call light is not within reach; a client with Alzheimer disease may perceive the urge to void but be unable to interpret its meaning or respond by seeking a bathroom. For these clients, self-care deficit in toileting is a primary problem.

To assist clients with self-care, the nurse should do the following:

■ Assess physical and mental abilities and limitations, usual voiding pattern, and ability to assist with toileting. A thorough assessment allows planned interventions to address specific needs and promote independence.

■ Provide assistive devices such as raised toilet seats, grab bars, a bedside commode, or night-lights, as needed to facilitate independence. Fostering independence in toileting bolsters self-concept and maintains a positive body image.

■ Plan a toileting schedule based on the client's normal elimination patterns to achieve a urine output of approximately 300 mL with each voiding. Allowing the bladder to fill to a point at which the urge to void is experienced and then emptying it completely helps to maintain normal bladder capacity and bacteriostatic functions.

■ Position the client for ease of voiding—sitting for females, standing for males—and provide privacy. Normal positioning, usual toileting facilities, and privacy all enhance the ability to void on schedule and empty the bladder completely.

■ Adjust fluid intake so that the majority of fluids are consumed during times of the day when the client is most able to remain continent. Unless fluids are restricted, maintain a fluid intake of at least 1.5–2.0 L per day. An adequate fluid intake is vital to promote hydration and urinary function. Overly concentrated urine can irritate the bladder, increasing incontinence.

■ Assist with clothing that is easily removed (e.g., elastic-waist pants or loose dresses). Velcro and zipper fasteners may be easier to use than snaps and buttons. Clothing that is difficult to remove can increase the risk of incontinence in clients with mobility problems or impaired dexterity.

ties, provide urinary equipment close to the bedside (e.g., urinal, bedpan, or commode) and the necessary assistance to use them.

Maintain Skin Integrity

Skin that is continually moist becomes macerated (softened). Urine that accumulates on the skin is converted to ammonia, which is very irritating to the skin. Because both skin irritation and maceration predispose the client to skin breakdown and ulceration, the incontinent individual requires meticulous skin care. To maintain skin integrity, the nurse washes the client's perineal area with mild soap and water or a commercially prepared no-rinse cleanser after episodes of incontinence, rinses it thoroughly if soap and water were used, dries it gently and thoroughly, and provides clean, dry clothing or bed linen. The nurse applies barrier ointments or creams to protect the skin from contact with urine. If it is necessary to pad the client's clothes for protection, the nurse should use products that absorb wetness and leave a dry surface in contact with the skin. Clients returning home or to a care facility should be instructed in techniques for maintaining skin integrity.

Specially designed incontinence draw sheets, which provide significant advantages over standard draw sheets, may be used for incontinent clients confined to bed. These sheets are like a standard draw sheet but are double layered, with a quilted upper nylon or polyester surface and an absorbent viscose rayon layer below. The rayon soaker layer generally has a waterproof backing on its underside. Fluid (i.e., urine) passes through the upper quilted layer and is absorbed and dispersed by the viscose rayon, leaving the quilted surface dry to the touch. This absorbent sheet helps maintain skin integrity; it does not stick to the skin when wet, decreases the risk of bedsores, and reduces odor.

Plan for Home Care

Successful home care for a client with urinary incontinence involves a combination of the following strategies:

- *Education,* which involves the client, family, and any nonfamily caregivers, including private nursing providers and respite caregivers. The Client Teaching feature addresses the learning needs of the client and family.
- *Bladder training,* which requires that the client postpone voiding, resist or inhibit the sensation of urgency, and void according to a timetable rather than according to the urge to void. The goals are to gradually lengthen the intervals between occasions of urination to correct the client's frequent urination, to stabilize the bladder, and to diminish urgency. This form of training may be used for clients who have bladder instability and urge incontinence. Delayed voiding produces larger voided volumes and longer intervals between instances of voiding. Initially, voiding may be encouraged every 2–3 hours except during sleep, and then every 4–6 hours. A vital component of bladder training is inhibiting the urge-to-void sensation: Every time the client has a premature urge to void, repeat the instruction to practice deep, slow breathing until the urge diminishes or disappears.
- *Habit training* and *scheduled toileting,* which attempt to keep the client dry by voiding on a schedule that corresponds to the client's normal pattern or at regular intervals. With habit training and scheduled toileting, no attempt is made to motivate the client to delay voiding if the urge occurs. Scheduled toileting can be effective for children who are experiencing urinary dysfunction. Biofeedback therapy, in which the child is taught to relax the pelvic floor, also can decrease incidents of wetting (Palmer, 2010).

- *Prompted voiding,* which supplements habit training by encouraging the client to use the toilet (prompting) and reminding the client when to void.
- *Kegel exercises,* which include this technique: Ask the client to think of the perineal muscles as an elevator. When the client relaxes, the elevator is on the first floor. To perform the exercise, contract the perineal muscles, bringing the elevator to the second, third, and fourth floors. Keep the elevator on the fourth floor for a few seconds, and then gradually relax the area. When the exercise is properly performed, contraction of the muscles of the buttocks and thighs is avoided. Kegel exercises can be performed anytime, anywhere, sitting or standing—even when voiding.

Home care for the client with urinary retention varies according to the cause. Some clients may be taught intermittent self-catheterization. Nurses should instruct all clients who have experienced urinary retention to avoid over-the-counter drugs that affect micturition, especially those with an anticholinergic effect (allergy and cold medications, many nonprescription sleep aids). Other home care measures include double-voiding (urinate, remain on the toilet for 2–5 minutes, and then urinate again); scheduled voiding; or when other measures fail, an indwelling catheter. When an indwelling catheter is necessary, teach the client and family to use clean technique when changing from an overnight bag to a leg bag and to report promptly any signs of UTI to the primary care provider.

For hospitalized clients who are being discharged home, the nurse must consider the client's needs for teaching and assistance with care in the home, including assessment of client and family resources and abilities for self-care, available financial resources, and need for referrals and home health services. The Community-Based Care feature on urinary elimination outlines an assessment of home care capabilities related to urinary elimination problems and needs.

Prevent Social Isolation

Urinary incontinence increases the risk for social isolation because of embarrassment, fear of not having ready access to a bathroom, body odor, or other factors. In turn, social isolation can increase problems of incontinence because normal cues and relationships are lost and the need to remain dry becomes less of a concern. To assist clients in the area of social isolation, the nurse should do the following:

- Assess for reasons for and extent of social isolation. Verify the degree of social isolation with the client or significant other. Do not assume that social isolation is related only to urinary incontinence. Other problems frequently associated with aging (e.g., a hearing deficit) may be primary or contributing factors.
- Refer the client for urological examination and incontinence evaluation. Clients who assume that urinary incontinence is a normal part of the aging process may not be aware of treatment options.
- Explore alternative coping strategies with the client, the significant other, staff, and other healthcare team members. Protective pads or shields, good perineal hygiene, scheduled voiding, and clothing that does not interfere with toileting can enhance continence.

Client Teaching Urinary Elimination in the Home Setting

Facilitating Urinary Elimination Self-Care

- Teach the client and family to maintain easy access to toilet facilities, including removing scatter rugs and ensuring that halls and doorways are free of clutter.
- Suggest graduated lighting for nighttime voiding: a dim night-light in the bedroom and low-wattage hallway lighting.
- Advise the client and family to install grab bars and elevated toilet seats as needed.
- Provide for instruction in safe transfer techniques. Contact physical therapy to provide training as needed.
- Suggest clothing that is easily removed for toileting, such as elastic waist pants or Velcro closures.

Promoting Urinary Elimination

- Instruct the client to respond to the urge to void as soon as possible; avoid voluntary urinary retention.
- Teach the client to empty the bladder completely at each voiding.
- Emphasize the importance of drinking eight to ten 8 oz glasses of water daily.
- Teach the client about Kegel exercises to strengthen perineal muscles.
- Inform the client about the relationship between tobacco use and bladder cancer and provide information about smoking cessation programs as indicated.
- Teach the client to promptly report any of the following to the primary care provider: pain or burning on urination, changes in urine color or clarity, malodorous urine, or changes in voiding patterns (e.g., nocturia, frequency, dribbling).

Asepsis

- Teach the client to maintain perineal-genital cleanliness, washing with soap and water daily and cleansing the anal and perineal area after defecating.
- Instruct the female client to wipe from front to back (from the urinary meatus toward the anus) after voiding, and to discard toilet paper after each swipe.
- Provide information about products to protect the skin, clothing, and furniture for the client who is incontinent. Emphasize the importance of cleaning and drying the perineal area after incontinence episodes. Instruct in the use of protective skin barrier products as needed.
- Teach the client with an indwelling catheter and the family about care measures such as cleaning the urinary meatus, managing and emptying the collection device, maintaining a closed system, and bladder irrigation or flushing if ordered.
- For the client with a urinary diversion, teach about care of the stoma, drainage devices, and surrounding skin. For continent diversions, teach the client how to catheterize the stoma to drain urine.
- For the client with an indwelling catheter or urinary diversion, emphasize the importance of maintaining a generous fluid intake (2.5–3 L daily) and of promptly reporting changes in urinary output, signs of urinary retention such as abdominal pain, and manifestations of urinary tract infection such as malodorous urine, abdominal discomfort, fever, or confusion.

Medications

- Emphasize the importance of taking medications as prescribed. Instruct the client to take the full course of antibiotics ordered to treat a urinary tract infection, even though symptoms have been relieved.
- Inform the client and family about any expected changes in urine color or odor associated with prescribed medications.
- For the client with urinary retention, emphasize the need to contact the primary care provider before taking any medication (even over-the-counter medications such as antihistamines) that may exacerbate symptoms.
- For the client taking medications that may damage the kidneys (e.g., aminoglycoside antibiotics), stress the importance of maintaining a generous fluid intake while taking the medication.
- Suggest measures to reduce anticipated side effects of prescribed medications, such as increasing intake of potassium-rich foods when taking a potassium-depleting diuretic such as furosemide.

Dietary Alterations

- Teach the client about dietary changes to promote urinary function, such as consuming cranberry juice and foods that acidify the urine to reduce the risk of repeated urinary tract infections or forming calcium-based urinary stones.
- Instruct the client with stress or urge incontinence to limit the intake of caffeine, alcohol, citrus juices, and artificial sweeteners because these are bladder irritants that may increase incontinence. Also, teach the client to limit evening fluid intake to reduce the risk of nighttime incontinence.

Measures Specific to Urinary Problems

- Provide instructions for clients with specific urinary problems or treatments such as
  a. timed urine specimens.
  b. urinary incontinence.
  c. urinary retention.
  d. retention catheters.

Referrals

- Make appropriate referrals to home health agencies, community agencies, or social services for assistance with resources such as grab bars and raised toilet seats; providing wheelchair access to bathrooms; obtaining toileting aids such as commodes, urinals, or bedpans; and services such as home health aides for assistance with activities of daily living.

Community Agencies and Other Resources

- Provide information about resources for durable medical equipment such as commodes and raised toilet seats, possible financial assistance, and medical supplies such as drainage bags, incontinence briefs, and protective pads.
- Suggest additional sources of information and help such as the National Council of Independent Living, United Ostomy Association, National Association for Continence, and Simon Foundation for Continence.

Community-Based Care Home Care Capabilities Related to Urinary Elimination

Client and Environment

- *Self-care abilities.* Ability to consume adequate fluids, to perceive bladder fullness, to ambulate and get to the toilet, to manipulate clothing for toileting, and to perform hygiene measures after toileting
- *Current level of knowledge.* Fluid and dietary intake modifications to promote normal patterns of urinary elimination, bladder training methods, and specific techniques to promote voiding care for indwelling catheter or ostomy (if appropriate)
- *Assistive devices required.* Ambulatory aids such as walker, cane, or wheelchair; safety devices such as grab bars; toileting aids such as raised toilet seat, urinal, commode, or bedpan; presence of a urinary catheter
- *Physical layout of the toileting facilities.* Presence of mobility aids; toilet at correct height to enable older adults to get up after voiding
- *Home environment factors that interfere with toileting.* Distance to the bathroom from living areas or bedrooms; barriers such as stairways, scatter rugs, clutter, or narrow doorways that interfere with bathroom access; lighting (including night lighting)
- *Urinary elimination problems.* Type of incontinence and precipitating factors; manifestations of urinary tract infection such as dysuria, frequency, urgency; evidence of prostatic hyperplasia and effect on urination; ability to perform self-catheterization and care for other urinary elimination devices such as indwelling catheter, urinary diversion ostomy, or condom drainage

Family

- *Caregiver availability, skills, and responses.* Ability and willingness to assume responsibilities for care, including assisting with toileting, intermittent catheterization, indwelling catheter care, urinary drainage devices or ostomy care; ready access to laundry facilities; access to and willingness to use respite or relief caregivers
- *Family role changes and coping.* Effect on spousal and family roles, sleep/rest patterns, sexuality, and social interactions
- *Financial resources.* Ability to purchase protective pads and garments, supplies for catheterization or ostomy care

Community

- *Environment.* Access to public restrooms and sanitary facilities
- *Current knowledge of and experience with community resources.* Medical and assistive equipment and supply companies, home health agencies, local pharmacies, available financial assistance, support and educational organizations

Encourage Independence

Because urinary incontinence contributes to the institutionalization of many older adults, client and family teaching can have a significant impact on a client's maintaining independence and residence in the community. Address possible causes of incontinence and appropriate treatment measures. Refer for urological examination if one has not already been completed. Discuss fluid intake management, perineal care, and products for clothing protection.

Evaluation

Using the overall goals and desired outcomes identified in the planning stage, the nurse collects data to evaluate the effectiveness of nursing interventions. If the desired outcomes are not achieved, the nurse should explore the reasons before modifying the care plan. The following are examples of questions that must be considered if the outcome "Remains dry between voidings and at night" is not met:

- What is the client's perception of the problem?
- Does the client understand and comply with the healthcare instructions provided?
- Is access to toilet facilities a problem?
- Can the client manipulate clothing for toileting? Can adjustments be made to allow easier disrobing?
- Are scheduled toileting times appropriate?
- Is there adequate lighting for nighttime toileting?
- Are mobility aids (e.g., walker, elevated toilet seat, or grab bar) needed? If these aids are currently used, are they appropriate or adequate? If assistance from a family member or caregiver is needed, is that available and appropriate?
- Is the client performing pelvic floor muscle exercises appropriately as scheduled?
- Is the client's fluid intake adequate? Does the timing of fluid intake require adjustment (e.g., should it be restricted after dinner)?
- Is the client restricting caffeine, citrus juice, carbonated beverages, and artificial sweetener intake?
- Is the client taking a diuretic? If so, when is the medication taken? Do the times require adjustment (e.g., taking second dose no later than 4 p.m.)?
- Should continence aids (e.g., a condom catheter or absorbent pads) be considered or used?

✷ Go to **nursing.pearsonhighered.com** to see a *Nursing Care Plan for a client with impaired urinary elimination.*

REVIEW Bladder Incontinence and Retention

RELATE Link the Concepts and Exemplars

Linking the exemplar of bladder incontinence and retention with the concept of fluids and electrolytes:

The nurse admits an 83-year-old client with a medical diagnosis of congestive heart failure, chronic renal failure, and diabetes mellitus. While the nursing history is being taken, the client says she takes her diuretic in the morning and then spends the next few hours in the bathroom, because if she goes too far away, she ends up wetting her pants and then has to clean up the mess. She says she gets so thirsty in the afternoon that she drinks several glasses of water but stops drinking fluids after 6 p.m. to avoid "wetting the bed." The client's skin turgor is poor, and assessment reveals possible dehydration.

1. What recommendations and client teaching should the nurse provide this client to prevent further dehydration?
2. What lab values should the nurse review to confirm potential dehydration?

Linking the exemplar of bladder incontinence and retention with the concept of self:
A busy 41-year-old executive of a thriving small business informs you that she has been experiencing bladder incontinence when she laughs, coughs, or sneezes and that it is causing her embarrassment at work. She blames it on having had five children.

3. What impact is bladder incontinence having on this client's self-image?
4. What recommendations might you make for this client to reduce her feelings of shame and self-consciousness?

READY Go to Companion Skills Manual

REFER Go to Pearson Student Nursing Resources
nursing.pearsonhighered.com

- Additional review material
- Chart 1: Nursing Care of the Client Undergoing Bladder Neck Suspension
- Nursing Care Plan: A Client with Impaired Urinary Elimination

REFLECT Case Study

Justin Gardner is a 26-year-old man who fractured his third thoracic vertebra when he fell while rock climbing. In preparation for transfer to a rehabilitation center, the doctor orders discontinuation of the client's indwelling urinary catheter and PRN straight catheterization to reduce urinary retention.

1. What assessment data will the nurse collect to determine the presence of urinary retention?
2. What signs and symptoms would the nurse recognize as indicative of the need for straight catheterization?
3. What nursing diagnosis would be appropriate for this client?
4. What client teaching will this client require, related to urinary retention, before discharge if he is to provide safe home care for himself?

EXEMPLAR 5.3 Bowel Incontinence, Constipation, and Impaction

EXEMPLAR KEY TERMS
Constipation, *305*
Encopresis, *312*
Fecal impaction, *307*
Fecal incontinence, *311*
Ulcerative colitis, *306*

EXEMPLAR LEARNING OUTCOMES
After reading about this exemplar, you will be able to:

1. Describe the pathophysiology, etiology, clinical manifestations, and direct and indirect causes of bowel incontinence, constipation, and impaction.
2. Identify risk factors and prevention methods associated with bowel incontinence, constipation, and impaction.

3. Illustrate the nursing process in providing culturally competent care across the life span for individuals with bowel incontinence, constipation, and impaction.
4. Formulate priority nursing diagnoses appropriate for individuals with bowel incontinence, constipation, or impaction.
5. Summarize therapies used by interdisciplinary teams in the collaborative care of individuals with bowel incontinence, constipation, and impaction.
6. Plan evidence-based care for individuals with bowel incontinence, constipation, and impaction and their families in collaboration with other members of the healthcare team.
7. Evaluate expected outcomes for individuals with bowel incontinence, constipation, and impaction.

▶ OVERVIEW

Disorders of intestinal absorption and bowel elimination can affect not only functional elimination status but also other functional health patterns including, but not limited to, health perception and management, nutritional and metabolic patterns, activity and exercise, self-perception and self-concept, and sexuality and reproductive health. Bowel function can be affected by inflammation, infections, tumors, obstructions, or changes in structure.

Clients with intestinal disorders often face extensive diagnostic testing, surgery, and permanent changes in physical appearance and lifestyle. Nursing care is directed toward returning to or maintaining homeostasis, meeting the client's physiological needs, providing emotional support, and educating the client to adapt to changes in lifestyle.

Few body functions respond as readily to internal and external influences as defecation. Factors affecting the gastrointestinal tract directly, such as food intake and bacterial population, affect

the number and consistency of stools. Indirect factors, such as psychological stress or voluntary postponement of defecation, also affect elimination. It is important to evaluate each client's bowel elimination against that client's own normal pattern.

CONSTIPATION

Constipation may be defined as fewer than three bowel movements per week or difficult passage of stools. This term implies either the passage of dry, hard stool or the passage of no stool. It occurs when the movement of feces through the large intestine is slow, allowing time for additional reabsorption of fluid from the large intestine. Difficult evacuation of stool and increased effort or straining of the voluntary muscles of defecation are associated with constipation. The individual also may have a feeling of incomplete stool evacuation after defecation. Careful assessment of a client's habits is necessary before a diagnosis of constipation is made.

▶ PATHOPHYSIOLOGY AND ETIOLOGY

Constipation may be a primary problem or a manifestation of another disease or condition. Acute constipation, a definite change in the bowel elimination pattern, is often caused by an organic process (i.e., anatomical, neuromuscular, metabolic, or endocrine changes). A change in bowel patterns that persists or becomes more frequent or severe may be caused by a tumor or other partial bowel obstruction. With chronic constipation, functional causes that impair storage, transport, and evacuation mechanisms impede the normal passage of stools.

Constipation itself causes health problems for some clients. In children, it often is associated with a UTI. Straining associated with constipation often is accompanied by holding the breath, which can present serious problems for individuals with heart disease, brain injuries, or respiratory disease: Holding one's breath while bearing down increases intrathoracic pressure and vagal tone, slowing the pulse rate (Kowalak, 2009).

Etiology

Psychogenic factors are the most common causes of chronic constipation. These factors include postponing defecation when the urge is felt and the perception of satisfaction with defecation. Clients often use laxatives and enemas to stimulate a bowel movement when they perceive constipation. Overuse of these measures can lead to real intestinal problems that further aggravate the condition. For example, cathartic colon (impaired colonic motility and changes in bowel structure) mimics **ulcerative colitis** (a disease that causes sores in the lining of the rectum and colon) in that the normal pouchlike or saccular appearance of the colon is lost. Melanosis coli is a brownish-black discoloration of the colon mucosa. Long-term laxative use may cause both cathartic colon and melanosis coli. **Table 5–7** ● lists selected causes of constipation.

Risk Factors

Many factors increase a client's risk for constipation, including the following:

- Age older than 65
- Insufficient fiber intake
- Insufficient fluid intake
- Insufficient activity or immobility
- Irregular defecation habits
- Change in daily routine
- Lack of privacy
- Chronic use of laxatives or enemas
- Irritable bowel syndrome
- Pelvic floor dysfunction or muscle damage
- Poor motility or slow transit
- Neurological conditions (e.g., Parkinson disease), stroke, or paralysis
- Emotional disturbances (e.g., depression or mental confusion)
- Medications (e.g., opioids, iron supplements, antihistamines, antacids, and antidepressants).

TABLE 5–7	Selected Causes of Constipation
FACTOR	**RELATED CAUSE**
Activity	Lack of exercise; bed rest
Dietary	Highly refined, low-fiber foods; inadequate fluid intake
Drugs	Antacids containing aluminum or calcium salts; narcotic analgesics; anticholinergic agents; many antidepressants, tranquilizers, and sedatives; antihypertensive agents, such as ganglionic blockers, calcium-channel blockers, beta-adrenergic blockers, and diuretics; iron salts
Large bowel	Diverticular disease, inflammatory disease, tumor, obstruction; changes in rectal or anal structure or function
Psychogenic	Voluntary suppression of urge; perceived need to defecate on schedule; depression
Systemic	Advanced age; pregnancy; neurological conditions (e.g., trauma, multiple sclerosis, tumors, cerebrovascular accident, parkinsonism); endocrine and metabolic disorders (e.g., hypothyroidism, hypercalcemia, uremia, porphyria)
Other	Chronic laxative or enema use

Prevention

Constipation can be prevented through multiple methods. Dietary methods include eating foods high in fiber, limiting foods that are low in fiber, and drinking plenty of fluids. Fiber supplements may also be useful for preventing constipation, but they should be consumed with plenty of water. Behavioral methods include exercising regularly and not ignoring the urge to defecate. Stool can become harder the longer it is in the intestinal tract because water continues to be absorbed, so ignoring the urge to defecate can contribute to constipation. For clients at high risk of acute constipation, stool softeners and laxatives may be used to prevent constipation. However, stimulant laxatives should not be used for an extended time because they can lead to intestinal problems (Mayo Clinic, 2011b).

▶ CLINICAL MANIFESTATIONS

The manifestations of constipation include having bowel movements less often than the usual pattern, frequent flatus, abdominal discomfort, diminished appetite, straining to have a bowel movement, and the passage of hard, dry stools. Upon examination, the abdomen may appear somewhat distended and the client may have reduced bowel sounds.

A group of experts at the International Congress of Gastroenterology in Rome have developed additional criteria for chronic constipation. To be diagnosed with chronic constipation, adults must experience two or more of the following symptoms for at least 12 weeks in the preceding 12 months (McKay et al., 2012):

- Straining with defecation more than 25% of the time
- Lumpy or hard stools more than 25% of the time
- Sensation of incomplete emptying more than 25% of the time

- Manual maneuvers use to facilitate emptying in more than 25% of defecations (e.g., digital evacuation or support of the pelvic floor)
- Fewer than three bowel movements per week

Fecal Impaction

Fecal impaction is a mass or collection of hardened feces in the folds of the rectum. Impaction results from prolonged retention and accumulation of fecal material. In severe impactions, the feces accumulate and extend well up into the sigmoid colon and beyond. Fecal impaction can be recognized by the passage of liquid or foul-smelling fecal seepage (diarrhea) without normal stool, as the liquid portion of the feces seeps out around the impacted mass. Impaction also can be assessed by digital examination of the rectum, during which the hardened mass often can be palpated.

Along with fecal seepage and constipation, symptoms include rectal pain and a frequent but nonproductive desire to defecate. A generalized feeling of illness results: The client becomes anorexic, the abdomen becomes distended, and nausea and vomiting may occur. The client may also experience abdominal cramping and a full sensation in the rectal area.

The causes of fecal impaction usually are poor defecation habits, including long-term dependence on laxatives or enemas, and constipation. Barium used in radiological examinations of the upper and lower gastrointestinal tracts may also be a cause. After these examinations, laxatives or enemas usually are used to ensure removal of the barium.

Digital examination of the impaction through the rectum should be done gently and carefully. Although digital rectal examination is within the scope of nursing practice, some agency policies require a primary care provider's order for manual manipulation and removal of a fecal impaction.

Although fecal impaction generally can be prevented, treatment of impacted feces sometimes is necessary. When fecal impaction is suspected, the client often is given an oil retention enema, a cleansing enema 2–4 hours later, and daily additional cleansing enemas, suppositories, or stool softeners. If these measures fail, manual removal may be necessary.

Lifespan and Cultural Considerations

Constipation is common throughout the life span. Specific developmental and aging changes contribute to constipation in children, older adults, and pregnant women.

CHILDREN Constipation is a common complaint in the pediatric population and accounts for up to 25% of referrals made to pediatric gastroenterologists (Bongers et al., 2010). Because defecation patterns vary among children, identification of an abnormal pattern is sometimes difficult. Infants usually have several bowel movements a day. Breastfed infants may have bowel movements as frequently as every feeding or just one bowel movement every several days. Because of differences in fat digestion and absorption, bottle-fed infants are more prone to hard stools (Infante et al., 2011). For a young child, one bowel movement a day may be normal. As the child grows, however, three to four bowel movements a week may become a normal pattern. According to Rome III criteria, children must have 2 or more of the following symptoms to be diagnosed with functional constipation (Rasquin et al., 2006):

- Two or fewer defecations in the toilet per week
- At least one episode of fecal incontinence per week
- History of retentive posturing or excessive volitional stool retention
- History of painful or hard bowel movements
- Presence of a large fecal mass in the rectum
- History of large diameter stools that may obstruct the toilet

Constipation in children is influenced by a variety of factors. Refer to **Table 5–8** ● for further information.

Constipation during infancy is rare; most often, it is caused by mismanagement of diet. The transition from formula to cow's milk may cause a transient constipation, because the bowel must adjust to the increased protein content of cow's milk.

Constipation occurs most frequently in toddlers and preschoolers. This increased incidence often is associated with learning to control body functions. Many children do not like the sensations of a bowel movement and may begin withholding stool, which accumulates in and dilates the rectum until the next urge to defecate. Withholding can lead to hard stools and painful defecation, causing the child to avoid the experience and start a cycle of withholding and continued constipation (Mayo Clinic, 2011c).

Constipation may occur as a result of limited time for toileting. Busy school-age children may delay toileting, and adolescents participating in sports or other extracurricular activities may have limited time for toileting. Children also may be hesitant to use an unfamiliar bathroom. Encouragement from parents and relaxation of bathroom privileges at school promote regularity and return of previous bowel patterns within a short time. Children and adolescents may need to get up earlier to have breakfast and time for toileting before going to school.

Constipation may follow surgery, especially in children who are immobilized, such as by traction or a body cast. Stool softeners and a diet high in fiber and fluids are given to prevent and treat constipation.

Constipation in the school-age child and adolescent often results in overflow fecal incontinence. Researchers believe overflow fecal incontinence results from fecal impaction, due either to stool leakage as the fecal matter moves toward the anus or to overflow diarrhea (Nurko & Scott, 2011).

OLDER ADULTS Constipation affects older adults more frequently than younger adults. Constipation affects between 24% and 50% of older adults. In this population, 10%–18% of individuals in the community setting use laxatives daily. In the extended care setting, as many as 74% receive daily laxatives (Rao, 2013). Although fecal transit in the large intestine slows with aging, the increased incidence of constipation in older adults is thought to relate more to impaired general health status, increased medication use, and decreased physical activity.

The loss of teeth makes chewing and swallowing food difficult. Ill-fitting, broken, or lost dentures also alter nutritional status. Periodontal disease with subsequent loss of natural teeth is one such factor, because the accompanying inability to chew foods results in a diet of soft, nonfibrous foods. Lack of

TABLE 5–8 Influential Factors in Childhood Constipation

PHYSICAL FACTORS IN INFANCY	PHYSICAL FACTORS IN CHILDREN	PSYCHOLOGICAL FACTORS IN CHILDREN
Familial stool patterns High milk and low fiber intake Cow's milk allergy Early gluten introduction	Anal and rectal disorders (e.g., hypertrophied rectum, anal fissure, anal stenosis, pelvic mass, ectopic anus) Residual stool blockage (fecalith) Overflow fecal soiling around a solid stool	Embarrassment/shame related to soiling or lack of privacy Reluctance to sit on the toilet, especially at school Too early toilet training
Hard stools	Poor rectal sensation	Fear of pain from hard stool
Dehydration	Diseases that influence gastrointestinal or neurological systems (e.g., celiac disease, cerebral palsy, spinal cord lesions)	Being too busy to use the bathroom or having restricted access to a bathroom Parental blame/anger related to soiling and toileting refusal
Perianal group A streptococcal infection, infant botulism	Obesity Stool withholding	
Medications (e.g., diuretics, antihistamines) and analgesia	Metabolic and endocrine syndromes (e.g., hypothyroidism, diabetes insipidus)	
Intestinal or anal conditions (e.g., Hirschsprung disease), cystic fibrosis, anorectal malformations		Teasing and bullying related to incontinence Decreased mobility/activity

Sources: Based on Clayden, G., & Keshtgar, A. S. (2003). Management of childhood constipation. *Postgraduate Medical Journal, 79,* 616–621; Kiefte-de Jong, J. C., Escher, J. C., Arends, L. R., Jaddoe, V. W., Hofman, A., Raat, H., & Moll, H. A. (2010). Infant nutritional factors and functional constipation in childhood: The Generation R study. *American Journal of Gastroenterology, 105*(4), 940–945. doi:10.1038/ajg.2010.96; Rogers, J. (2012). Assessment, prevention and treatment of constipation in children. *Nursing Standard, 26*(29), 46–52; Tabbers, M .M., Boluyt, N., Berger, M. Y., & Benninga, M. A. (2010). Constipation in children. *Clinical Evidence, 2010,* 0303.

fresh fruits and vegetables or other sources of bulk or fiber contributes to the pattern of constipation. The older adult may self-limit daily fluid intake, especially water, to decrease frequency of urination, unintentionally increasing the potential for constipation.

Cultural influences and advertising lead many older adults to believe that a daily bowel movement is important for health. This belief contributes to an increased incidence of perceived constipation in older adults. Because of this perception, the older adult may come to rely on laxatives, suppositories, or enemas to facilitate regular bowel movements. These external aids to defecation can further impair the ability to maintain "normal" bowel habits (a movement of soft stool every 2–3 days).

PREGNANT WOMEN Constipation is a common complaint of pregnant women. In pregnancy, mechanical pressure from the growing uterus contributes to displacement of the small intestine and reduces motility. The increased secretion of progesterone further reduces motility because of decreased gastric tone and increased smooth muscle relaxation; thus the emptying time of the stomach and bowel is prolonged. Hemorrhoids (swollen and inflamed veins in the anus and rectum) frequently develop in late pregnancy from constipation and from pressure on vessels below the level of the uterus, causing the pregnant woman further discomfort.

▶ COLLABORATION

Simple or chronic constipation is treated with education (a daily bowel movement is not necessary for health), modification of diet, and exercise routines. More severe constipation may require diagnostic testing and pharmacologic treatment.

Diagnostic Tests

The initial diagnostic exam for constipation is a digital rectal exam. If constipation is acute or does not resolve, diagnostic examination may be ordered. This may include a barium enema to identify bowel structure, tumors, or diverticula. If the problem is acute, a sigmoidoscopy or colonoscopy may be used for evaluation and biopsy. Rectal muscle contractions and completeness of bowel eliminations can be tested by defecography and anorectal manometry. A colorectal transit study can determine how well food moves through the client's gastrointestinal tract.

Surgery

Most clients with constipation do not require surgery. However, clients who do not respond to medication or who have rectal abnormalities that contribute to constipation (e.g., rectal prolapse, colonic inertia) may undergo surgery to correct the problem or remove the problematic portion of the colon.

Pharmacologic Therapy

Laxative and cathartic preparations are used to promote stool evacuation (see Medications feature). Milder preparations generally are known as laxatives; those known as cathartics have a stronger effect. Most laxatives are appropriate only for short-term use; clients should be encouraged to use over-the-counter constipation remedies no longer than 7 days before consultation with a physician. Cathartics and enemas interfere with normal bowel reflexes and should not be used for simple constipation. Laxatives should never be given to clients with appendicitis, enteritis, ulcerative colitis, diverticulitis, intestinal obstruction, fecal impaction, or undiagnosed abdominal pain (Spratto & Woods, 2012). When the bowel is obstructed, laxatives or cathartics may cause serious mechanical damage and may perforate the bowel.

Medications **Constipation**

CLASSIFICATION AND DRUG EXAMPLES	MECHANISM OF ACTION	NURSING CONSIDERATIONS
Bulk-Forming Laxatives *Drug examples:* Metamucil, Citrucel	Fiber supplements that increase bulk and promote passage of stool. *May also be used for:* —diarrhea	■ These drugs can interfere with the absorption of some medications; bulk-forming laxatives should be taken 2 hours before or after other medications. ■ Always take with sufficient water. ■ May cause increased bloating and abdominal pain in some clients. ■ Sugar-free options are available for diabetic clients. ■ Should not be taken long term. ■ Fiber Gummies (Fleet) may be used for children.
Stimulants (Cathartics) *Drug examples:* Dulcolax, Senokot	Cause rhythmic muscle contractions in the intestines.	■ An ingredient in some stimulants, phenolphthalein, may increase the risk of cancer. ■ Produces a bowel movement in 6–12 hours. ■ Do not use within 1 hour of taking an antacid or milk. ■ May cause stomach discomfort or cramps.
Osmotics *Drug examples:* MiraLAX, sorbitol, Cephulac, PEG-ES	Increase the amount of water in the intestines to soften stools.	■ Often used for clients with idiopathic constipation. ■ Clients with diabetes should be monitored for electrolyte imbalances. ■ Causes a bowel movement within 24–72 hours. ■ PEG-ES is often used to cleanse the bowel before a colonoscopy or barium enema.
Stool Softeners *Drug examples:* Colace, Kaopectate	Moisten the stool and help prevent dehydration.	■ Suggested for use in clients who should avoid straining. ■ Prolonged use may cause an electrolyte imbalance. ■ Generally produces a bowel movement in 12–72 hours. ■ Do not use in the presence of a bowel obstruction.
Lubricants *Drug examples:* mineral oil (Fleet, Zymenol)	Grease the stool, allowing it to move through the intestine more quickly.	■ Typically stimulate a bowel movement within 8 hours. ■ Useful for constipation associated with dry, hard stools. ■ Can be administered orally or rectally. ■ May increase the risk of aspiration and pneumonia in frail older clients.
Saline Laxatives *Drug examples:* Milk of Magnesia, Haley's M-O	Draw water into the colon for easier passage of stool.	■ Used to treat acute constipation if there is no bowel obstruction. ■ Electrolyte imbalance may occur after prolonged use, especially in small children and individuals with renal deficiency. ■ May interfere with some antibiotics. ■ Do not use if pregnant or breastfeeding.
Chloride Channel Activators *Drug examples:* Amitiza	Activate chloride channels to promote fluid release into intestines.	■ Can be safely used for 6–12 months. ■ Used to treat chronic idiopathic constipation. ■ Do not use if bowel obstruction is suspected. ■ May cause fetal harm; do not take during pregnancy. ■ May experience nausea or diarrhea. ■ Causes bowel movement within 24 hours of first dose.
Prokinetic Drugs *Drug examples:* Reglan, Motilium	Increase the weight and frequency of stools by decreasing transit time; activate dopamine receptors in the gut. *May also be used for:* —preventing vomiting in pregnancy —heartburn in GERD	■ May cause tardive dyskinesia, restless leg syndrome, tremor, and other CNS effects; clients should report CNS effects to their physician immediately. ■ Do not take these drugs for longer than 12 weeks. ■ Alcohol can increase the side effects of prokinetic drugs. ■ Take 30 minutes before mealtime.
Enemas *Drug examples:* Fleet, Milk of Magnesia, generic	Liquid saline or medicine is inserted into the rectum to draw water into the colon and promote bowel movement.	■ Body positioning may be embarrassing for many clients; respect the client's privacy at all times. ■ Self-administered enemas are available if desired. ■ Enemas can be used to clear the bowels before colonoscopy if the PEG-ES solution does not empty the bowels completely. ■ Used for significant constipation or fecal impaction on a short-term basis.
Suppositories *Drug examples:* Dulcolax, glycerin	Stimulates muscles in the bowel to promote defecation.	■ Produces a bowel movement in 15 minutes to 1 hour. ■ Only for rectal use; should not be given orally or vaginally.

Evidence-Based Practice   Polyethylene Glycol (PEG) Use in Children

Problem

Constipation and fecal impaction are major problems for many children. However, the relative safety and efficacy of laxatives in children has not been well defined. When treating children with constipation, nurses must understand the clinical data related to laxative use in order to provide accurate information and advice to parents and children.

Evidence

In two studies (101 children), PEG showed an increased number of stools per week compared to placebo. In four studies (338 children), PEG produced significantly more stools per week than lactulose, and children who received PEG were less likely to require additional therapies. In three studies (211 children), stools per week were significantly greater with PEG than with Milk of Magnesia. PEG appeared to have efficacy similar to that of enemas and liquid paraffin (mineral oil; Gordon et al., 2012). One study of 100 children compared PEG plus electrolytes (PEG+E) to a combination of acacia fiber, psyllium fiber, and fructose. Although both treatments were effective at relieving constipation after 8 weeks, PEG+E was better tolerated and more effective than the fiber and fructose mix (Quitadamo et al., 2012). Interestingly, PEG-only was better tolerated than PEG+E in a study of 91 children with constipation and produced more regular soft stool frequency

(Savino et al., 2012). PEG was generally well tolerated by children; adverse effects included flatulence, abdominal pain, nausea, diarrhea, and headache. PEG also appears to be effective in children younger than 3 years of age, although data is scarce (Ahmed, Pai, & Reynolds, 2012).

Implications

Laxatives containing polyethylene glycol are currently the treatment of choice for children with constipation. PEG can be administered with or without additional electrolytes, depending on the child's risk for electrolyte imbalance. Other laxatives can also be used, depending on the child's condition, the effectiveness of PEG in that child, and any adverse experience in the child. Mineral oil may be an equally effective choice for children who do not tolerate PEG. As more studies become available, nurses need to stay abreast of the literature related to safe and effective laxative use in children.

Critical Thinking Application

Explain how an adverse event of PEG such as flatulence would affect a 4-year-old child compared to a 14-year-old adolescent. Determine conditions under which a mild laxative such as lactulose would be preferred over PEG. Develop an educational pamphlet about laxative use in children as a teaching tool for parents of young children with constipation.

When choosing a pharmacologic agent, the healthcare team should consider which agent will be the most effective for evacuating the stool while causing the client the least amount of stress and anxiety. Suppositories and enemas can cause fear in children. Polyethylene glycol electrolyte solution (GoLYTELY) can be administered orally or instilled via a nasogastric tube to promote stool evacuation. More recently, electrolyte-free polyethylene glycol 3350 (MiraLAX) has been used effectively (Portalatin & Winstead, 2012). See the Evidence-Based Practice feature for studies comparing polyethylene glycol to other agents for treatment of constipation in children. Once the stool has been evacuated, methods to prevent reaccumulation of stool in the bowel may be implemented, including eating foods or supplements high in fiber, introducing behavioral methods, and taking stool softeners.

Nonpharmacologic Therapy

Most clients can manage constipation with nonpharmacologic interventions, including education, nutrition, behavioral therapy, and biofeedback. In addition, impacted stool may be manually removed in severe cases.

EDUCATION   Education of the client and family is the first step in treating constipation. A description of the pathophysiology of the condition and nonpharmacologic therapies to prevent constipation is essential. If the client will be treated with pharmacologic therapy, education about the use, therapeutic effects, and side effects of the specific medication should be given. If the client needs treatment by manual removal of stool or surgical correction of the bowel, education involves explaining what to expect before, during, and after the procedure.

NUTRITION   Foods high in fiber are recommended for clients experiencing constipation. Vegetable fiber is largely indigestible and cannot be absorbed, so it increases stool bulk. Fiber also helps draw water into the fecal mass, softening the stool and making defecation easier. Raw fruits and vegetables are good sources of dietary fiber, as is cereal bran. Use 2–3 teaspoons of unprocessed bran with meals (sprinkled on fruit or cereal), or up to one-quarter cup daily, to supply adequate fiber. Removing constipating foods (e.g., bananas, rice, and cheese) from the diet also reduces constipation.

Fluids also are important in maintaining bowel motility and soft stools. The client should drink 6–8 glasses of fluid per day. It is important to advise the client to increase fluid intake when dietary fiber is initially increased to decrease flatus and help maintain softer stools. Constipation in young infants usually can be corrected by increasing the amount of fluids or adding 2 oz of pear or apple juice to daily intake.

BEHAVIOR MANAGEMENT AND BOWEL TRAINING   Behavior modification may prove beneficial in managing constipation. Inactivity is a major contributor to constipation, so encouraging clients to exercise regularly can help decrease constipation and promote defecation. Digital stimulation can also be used to retrain the bowel and trigger a bowel movement. To perform digital stimulation (Dugdale & Longstreth, 2012):

- Insert a lubricated finger into the anus and make a circular motion until the sphincter relaxes.

- Sit in a normal position for a bowel movement, such as on a toilet, bedside commode, or bedpan, depending on the client's mobility. If unable to sit, the client should lie on the left side.

- Try to relax the client as much as possible by providing privacy and a distraction such as reading.
- The client should contract the muscles of the abdomen and bear down while releasing stool. Bending forward increases abdominal pressure and may help empty the bowel.
- If digital stimulation does not produce a bowel movement within 20 minutes, repeat the procedure.
- Perform digital stimulation every day until a regular pattern of bowel movements is established.
- Consistency is essential for bowel retraining. Establish a set time for daily bowel movements, choosing a time that is convenient for the client. The best time for bowel movements is 20–40 minutes after a meal because the gastrocolic reflex helps stimulate bowel activity.

For children, providing rewards for each bowel movement can be effective (NASPGHAN, 2006). These rewards can be simple items, such as stickers on a chart or an afternoon spent with the parent playing a game. For children with psychological issues, child and family psychotherapy may be necessary. In these cases, the family is referred to a child and family counselor.

BIOFEEDBACK Biofeedback uses visual or auditory feedback about a specific body function. In clients with bowel problems, biofeedback is used to strengthen the rectal sphincter and other rectal muscles. A rectal plug monitors the strength of the muscles, and an electrode may be attached to the abdomen. The plug and electrode then record muscle contractions. The client is taught how to squeeze the rectal muscles using the computer display to confirm correct technique, allowing the client to control the muscles more effectively during bowel movements (Dugdale & Longstreth, 2012).

MANUAL REMOVAL OF STOOL Clients with fecal impaction may need to have the hard mass of stool broken up by hand. This procedure involves a healthcare provider such as a trained nurse or physician inserting one or two gloved fingers into the rectum to break up the mass into smaller pieces. Suppositories or an enema is then used to help clear the stool. This

Complementary and Alternative Therapy
Herbal Laxative Use in Children

In some cultures, herbal laxatives are used as complementary therapies. However, their safety and effectiveness are not as well established in children as in adults. One recent study found that psyllium, an ingredient in bulk-forming laxatives, is effective for treatment of constipation in children in combination with acacia fiber and fructose. No clinically significant side effects were found over the 8-week study, but compliance tended to be better for PEG + electrolytes than for psyllium (Quitadamo et al., 2012). Cascara sagrada and senna are stimulant laxatives that have been approved by the U.S. Food and Drug Administration for use to treat constipation in children older than 2 years. Stimulant laxatives should be used with caution in children, however, because they can lead to dependency as well as to abdominal pain. Senna also has been associated with skin problems in children, including diaper rash and blistering (Loo, 2009).

process is done in small steps to prevent injury to the rectum (Dugdale & Longstreth, 2011).

FECAL INCONTINENCE

Fecal incontinence, also called *bowel incontinence*, is the loss of the voluntary control of fecal and gaseous discharges through the anal sphincter. It occurs less frequently than urinary incontinence but is no less distressing to the client. The incontinence may occur at specific times, such as after meals, or it may occur irregularly. Clients often do not reveal fecal incontinence in discussing health concerns, so treatment of this condition is often overlooked. Studies indicate that client reporting of fecal incontinence increases fivefold when the client is asked directly about the issue by the healthcare worker rather than being expected to report incontinence voluntarily (Alsheik et al., 2012). Therefore nurses should be diligent in asking the client about fecal incontinence during the health history interview, especially for older adults and other individuals at high risk for incontinence.

▶ PATHOPHYSIOLOGY AND ETIOLOGY

Fecal incontinence generally is associated with impaired functioning of the anal sphincter or its nerve supply, such as in some neuromuscular diseases, spinal cord trauma, and tumors of the external anal sphincter muscle. Bowel incontinence usually is considered a manifestation of a disorder rather than being a disorder itself. The two types of bowel incontinence are partial and major. Partial incontinence is the inability to control flatus or to prevent minor soiling. Major incontinence is the inability to control feces of normal consistency.

The rate of fecal incontinence among older adults living in the community has been reported to be 7%–17%, compared with 2.6% in the young adult population and 33%–65% in older nursing home residents (Shah, Chokhavatia, & Rose, 2012; Townsend et al., 2012; Whitehead et al., 2009). Fecal incontinence is an emotionally distressing problem that ultimately can lead to social isolation. To minimize the embarrassment associated with soiling, afflicted individuals withdraw into their home or, if in the hospital or nursing home, the confines of their room.

Etiology

Multiple factors, both physiological and psychological, contribute to fecal incontinence (**Box 5–5** ●). The most common causes of fecal incontinence are those that interfere with either sensory or motor control of the rectum and anal sphincters. If the external sphincter is paralyzed as a result of spinal cord injury or disease, defecation occurs automatically when the internal sphincter relaxes with the defecation reflex. If sphincter muscles have been damaged or excessive pelvic floor relaxation has occurred, it may not be possible to override the defecation reflex with voluntary control.

Risk Factors

Individuals with nerve damage, including multiple sclerosis, spinal cord injury, or long-term diabetes, are at greatest risk of

Box 5–5 Selected Causes of Fecal Incontinence

NEUROLOGICAL CAUSES

- Spinal cord injury or disease
- Head injury, stroke, or brain tumor
- Degenerative neurological disease, such as multiple sclerosis, amyotrophic lateral sclerosis, or dementia
- Diabetic neuropathy

LOCAL TRAUMA

- Obstetrical tears
- Anorectal injury
- Anorectal surgery with sphincter damage

INFLAMMATORY PROCESSES

- Infection
- Radiation

OTHER PHYSIOLOGICAL CAUSES

- Diarrhea
- Stool impaction
- Pelvic floor relaxation or loss of sphincter tone
- Tumors

PSYCHOLOGICAL CAUSES

- Depression
- Confusion and disorientation

developing fecal incontinence because they are unable to control the muscles in the bowel and anus. Older age and female gender are also risk factors for fecal incontinence. Age-related changes in anal sphincter tone and response to rectal distention increase the risk for fecal incontinence in older adults. Resting and maximal anal sphincter pressures are decreased, particularly in older women. In addition, less rectal distension is needed to produce sustained relaxation of the anal sphincter in older women.

Dementia and physical disability are also associated with increased fecal incontinence, either because the individual does not comprehend the defecation urge or because the individual is unable to reach the bathroom before defecation occurs.

Prevention

Methods to prevent fecal incontinence involve controlling the cause of incontinence, including constipation and diarrhea. Methods to prevent constipation include increasing physical activity, fiber consumption, and fluid intake. Treating or eliminating the cause of diarrhea, such as an intestinal infection, can help prevent fecal incontinence. In addition, clients should be taught to avoid straining during bowel movements, which can eventually weaken the anal sphincter muscles and cause nerve damage. Kegel exercises can also help strengthen the sphincter muscles to prevent fecal incontinence (Mayo Clinic, 2012a).

▶ CLINICAL MANIFESTATIONS

Fecal incontinence is characterized by the loss of voluntary bowel control, causing stool or mucus to leak out of the anus at unwanted times. This effect can be minor, in which case the client loses only gas or small amounts of liquid fecal material and soils the underwear; or it can be major, in which case the client loses the entire contents of the bowel. It often occurs as a result of nerve or muscle damage that affects control of the rectal muscles. Fecal incontinence may be accompanied by constipation, diarrhea, gas, bloating, abdominal cramping, and urinary incontinence. Emotional distress, including shame and embarrassment, is also common in clients with fecal incontinence.

Encopresis

Encopresis is an abnormal elimination pattern characterized by recurrent soiling or passage of stool at inappropriate times by a child who should have achieved bowel continence. An estimated 1%–2% of children younger than 10 years have encopresis, approximately 80% of those children being boys. In addition, 80%–95% of children with encopresis have a history of constipation (Borowitz, 2013). Children with primary encopresis have never achieved bowel control. Children with secondary encopresis have had bowel continence for several months.

Encopresis usually is associated with voluntary or involuntary retention of stool in the lower bowel and rectum. This leads to constipation, dilation of the lower bowel, and incompetence of the inner sphincter. The retention of stool usually is a result of being "too busy": The child puts off going to the bathroom because leaving the current activities would be an inconvenience. The retention of stool leads to constipation that is untreated and chronic. Loose stool leaks around the hard feces, and the child becomes unaware of a need to eliminate. Soiling may occur during the day or night. Bowel movements are irregular, painful, small, and hard. The child may be ridiculed by peers because of offensive body odor. This rejection leads to withdrawal and behavioral problems, often resulting in altered school performance and attendance. The child continues to hold stool because the passage has become painful. Parents commonly seek health care, believing that the child has diarrhea or constipation.

The underlying constipation that leads to encopresis may be caused by the stress of environmental changes (e.g., birth of a sibling, moving to a new house, attending a new school), issues of anger and control related to bowel training, diet, a full schedule of activities, or a genetic predisposition.

▶ COLLABORATION

Treatment of fecal incontinence and encopresis depends on the underlying cause of the incontinence. Many therapies are similar to the treatment of constipation, because in this case, constipation is a primary cause of incontinence. In addition, a need for psychological treatment may be based on the client's emotional response to the problem. The nurse plays a key role in treatment and management of clients with fecal incontinence through education, implementation of nonpharmacologic therapies, emotional support, and referral to other healthcare workers.

Collaboration for the client with bowel elimination issues frequently involves a nutritionist, who can help support the client in making any needed changes in diet or dietary patterns.

Nurses also may want to consult with the client's pharmacist, who may be able to provide additional information regarding medications and supplements being taken and any related side effects. Physical therapists may offer important points on exercise within the client's range of motion that can promote bowel health and management. Nurses working with children who have problems with bowel elimination should encourage parents to work with teachers and school dieticians to support the child in dietary habits that support healthy bowel elimination.

Diagnostic Tests

The diagnosis of fecal incontinence includes client history and physical examination of the pelvic floor and anus to evaluate muscle tone and rule out a fecal impaction. Impaired sphincter muscles may be palpable on digital examination. Anorectal manometry or a rectal motility test may be used to evaluate the functional ability of the sphincter muscles. In this test, a small, flexible balloon catheter is introduced into the rectum, and pressures are measured in the rectum and internal and external sphincters. Normally, rectal dilation causes the internal sphincter to relax and the external sphincter to contract. Sigmoidoscopy also may be used to examine the rectum and anal canal.

Similarly, a thorough history, physical examination, and diagnostic studies (possibly including barium enema) are necessary to rule out organic causes and anatomical abnormalities related to encopresis. Examination of mental health and cognitive functioning may be indicated. Information about the child's toilet training habits and parents' attitudes concerning those habits is obtained. A dietary history, including eating habits and types of foods eaten, often is helpful as well. Physical examination sometimes reveals a nontender mass in the lower abdomen.

Surgery

When damage to the sphincter or a rectal prolapse (protrusion of rectal mucous membrane through the anus) is the cause of fecal incontinence, surgical repair is the treatment of choice. Surgery also may be indicated when conservative measures have not been effective. Permanent colostomy (the creation of an opening from the large bowel on the abdominal wall) is a last-choice option for some clients, but it can control fecal output when other measures fail.

Pharmacologic Therapy

Management of fecal incontinence is directed toward the identified cause. Medications to relieve diarrhea or constipation may be prescribed (see the Medications feature on page 309). Drugs to control diarrhea include loperamide (Imodium) and bismuth subsalicylate (Kaopectate, Pepto-Bismol). Diarrhea from an infection may also be treated with an appropriate antimicrobial agent. Treatment of encopresis may include the temporary use of lubricants, bulk-forming laxatives, or stool softeners to clear the bowel of impacted stool and encourage normal defecation.

Nonpharmacologic Therapy

Several nonpharmacologic therapies can be used to treat fecal incontinence. A high-fiber diet, ample fluids, and regular exercise are helpful for many clients. Exercises to improve sphincter and pelvic floor muscle tone (Kegel exercises) may be of long-term benefit. Biofeedback therapy may be used for mentally alert clients with intact sphincter muscles but low muscle tone. The nurse may also teach the client self-care techniques that should be used to keep the anal area clean after fecal incontinence.

Treatment of encopresis may include behavior modification techniques, dietary changes, and psychotherapy. Behavior modification programs that reward and reinforce appropriate toileting habits can be successful. Dietary changes include incorporating high-fiber foods, such as fruits, vegetables, and whole-grain cereals, into the diet. Limiting intake of refined and highly processed foods and dairy products also may be helpful. The child should sit on the toilet for several minutes after the morning and evening meals. It takes several months for the bowel to be retrained to respond to sphincter stimulation. Psychotherapy involving the child and family may be indicated in instances of dysfunctional parent–child relationships.

■ NURSING PROCESS

The nurse plays a fundamental role in the care of clients with bowel problems. Assessment, education, administration of medications, hygiene care, monitoring of food and fluid intake, and emotional support are all interventions that the nurse can implement to provide care to clients with constipation, fecal impaction, and fecal incontinence.

Assessment

- ■ *Health history.* The nurse and client discuss the extent, onset, and duration of incontinence; identify contributing factors; history of spinal cord or anorectal injury or surgery; chronic diseases, such as diabetes, multiple sclerosis, or other neurological disorders; medications and use of alternative therapies; nutrition; and hydration patterns.
- ■ *Physical examination.* The nurse palpates and assesses the abdomen for firmness or tenderness as well as for the presence of any mass (retained stool). Bowel sounds should be assessed. If a digital rectal examination is performed, the nurse assesses for the presence of stool in the rectum. The nurse also assesses for hemorrhoids, anal fissures, or other abnormalities of the abdomen or perineum.

Diagnosis

Nursing diagnoses that may be appropriate for inclusion in the plan of care for the client with impaired fecal elimination include the following:

- ■ *Bowel Incontinence*
- ■ *Constipation*
- ■ *Perceived Constipation*
- ■ *Diarrhea*

(NANDA-I © 2012)

Fecal elimination problems may affect many other areas of human functioning and, as a consequence, may be the etiol-

Clinical Manifestations and Therapies **Bowel Elimination**

ETIOLOGY	CLINICAL MANIFESTATIONS	CLINICAL THERAPIES
Acute constipation	Fewer than three bowel movements per week; difficult passage of stools; dry, hard stools; straining; feelings of incomplete evacuation; an abrupt change in bowel elimination patterns; bowel obstruction; UTI; diminished appetite; reduced bowel sounds	■ High-fiber diet or fiber supplements ■ Adequate fluid intake ■ Behavioral modification ■ Pharmacologic therapy ■ Digital stimulation
Chronic constipation	Storage, transport, or evacuation impairment; abdominal discomfort; frequent flatus; straining more than 25% of the time; passage of hard, dry stools more than 25% of the time; abdomen distention; reduced bowel sounds; manual maneuvers needed to facilitate emptying; fewer than three bowel movements per week; symptoms of constipation for at least 12 weeks in the preceding 12 months	■ High-fiber diet or fiber supplements ■ Adequate fluid intake ■ Behavioral modification ■ Pharmacologic therapy ■ Surgery ■ Education ■ Biofeedback ■ Digital stimulation
Fecal impaction	Similar to symptoms of constipation, plus a mass of hardened feces in the rectum and leakage of liquid fecal material around the fecal mass; rectal pain; a frequent nonproductive desire to defecate; distended abdomen; nausea and vomiting; abdominal cramping	■ Manual evacuation of stool ■ Oil retention enema ■ Cleansing enema ■ Suppositories ■ Prevention methods after successful evacuation
Withholding	Most common in children; tightening of the external sphincter and gluteal muscles, squatting, rocking, stiff walking on tiptoes, crossing legs, sitting with heels against the perineum, stretching of the rectum and lower colon, stool retention, soiling by involuntary overflow	■ Polyethylene glycol 3350 with or without electrolytes ■ High-fiber diet or fiber supplements ■ Adequate fluid intake ■ Behavioral modification ■ Education ■ Rewards for defecation ■ Child and family psychotherapy
Partial fecal incontinence	Inability to control flatus; minor soiling; constipation; social isolation; bloating; abdominal cramping; urinary incontinence	■ Treat constipation ■ Kegel exercises ■ Education ■ Surgery to correct bowel defect ■ Behavioral modification ■ Teaching of self-care techniques
Major fecal incontinence	Evacuation of the entire bowel contents at an inappropriate time and place; impaired functioning of the anal sphincter or nerve supply; inability to control feces of normal consistency; diarrhea; gastrointestinal infection; social isolation; urinary incontinence	■ Kegel exercises ■ Colostomy ■ Antidiarrheal drugs ■ Antimicrobial agents ■ Teaching of self-care techniques
Encopresis	Recurrent soiling at inappropriate times by a child who should have achieved bowel continence; constipation; withholding behavior; small, hard, and painful bowel movements; emotional withdrawal	■ Psychological treatment ■ Collaboration with school nurses and teachers ■ Pharmacologic treatment of constipation ■ High-fiber diet ■ Behavioral modification

Client Teaching Fecal Elimination

Facilitating Toileting

To facilitate successful client toileting, nurses should do the following:

- Ensure safe and easy access to the toilet. Make sure lighting is appropriate, scatter rugs are removed or securely fastened, and so on.
- Facilitate instruction as needed about transfer techniques.
- Suggest ways that garments can be adjusted to make disrobing easier for toileting (e.g., Velcro closing on clothing).

Monitoring Bowel Elimination Pattern

- Nurses should instruct the client, if appropriate, to keep a record of time and frequency of stool passage, any associated pain, and color and consistency of the stool.

Dietary Alterations

- Nurses should provide clients with information about required food and fluid alterations to promote defecation or manage diarrhea.

Medications

- Medications should be discussed with the client at each healthcare interaction. Discussions should address problems associated with overuse of laxatives, if appropriate, and the use of alternatives to laxatives, suppositories, and enemas.
- Discuss the addition of a fiber supplement if the client is taking a constipating medication.

Community Agencies and Other Sources of Help

A number of agencies and resources are available for clients who need assistance. Nurses should be informed about what is available in their community and provide the following:

- Appropriate referrals to home care or community care for assistance with resources such as installation of grab bars and raised toilet seats, structural alterations for wheelchair access, homemaker or home health aide services to assist with activities of daily living, and enterostomal therapy nurse for assistance with stoma care and selection of ostomy appliances
- Information about companies from which durable medical equipment (e.g., raised toilet seats, commodes, bedpans, and urinals) can be purchased, rented, or obtained free of charge and supplies (e.g., incontinence pads or ostomy irrigating supplies and appliances) can be obtained
- Additional sources of information and help, such as ostomy self-help and support groups or clubs

---

ogy of other NANDA-I nursing diagnoses. Examples are the following:

- *Risk for Impaired Skin Integrity* related to bowel incontinence or prolonged diarrhea
- *Chronic Low Self-Esteem* related to fecal incontinence and need for assistance with toileting
- *Disturbed Body Image* related to bowel incontinence
- *Deficient Knowledge* (bowel training) related to lack of previous experience
- *Anxiety* related to lack of control of fecal elimination or response of others to fecal incontinence

(NANDA-I © 2012)

Planning

The major goals for clients with fecal elimination problems include the following:

- The client will maintain or restore normal bowel elimination patterns.
- The client will maintain or regain normal stool consistency.
- The client will prevent associated risks, such as fluid and electrolyte imbalance, skin breakdown, abdominal distention, and pain.

Implementation

Caring interventions include promoting regular defecation, perineal skin care, bowel training programs, digital removal of fecal impaction, and use of a fecal incontinence pouch. The Client Teaching Feature also address aspects of fecal elimination.

Promote Regular Defecation

The nurse can help clients achieve regular defecation by attending to the following:

- *Privacy* during defecation is extremely important to most individuals. The nurse should provide as much privacy as possible for such clients but may need to stay with those who are too weak to be left alone. Some clients also prefer to wipe, wash, and dry themselves after defecating. A nurse may need to provide water, a washcloth, and a towel for this purpose.
- *Timing.* A client should be encouraged to defecate when the urge is recognized. To establish regular bowel elimination, the client and nurse can discuss when mass peristalsis normally occurs and provide time for defecation. Many individuals have well-established routines. Other activities, such as bathing and ambulating, should not interfere with the defecation time.
- *Nutrition and fluids.* The diet a client needs for regular, normal elimination varies depending on the kind of feces the client currently has, the frequency of defecation, and the types of foods that the client finds assist with normal defecation.

For constipation, increase the daily fluid intake, and instruct the client to drink hot liquids and fruit juices, especially prune juice. Include fiber in the diet, that is, foods such as raw fruit, bran products, and whole-grain cereals and bread. It is important to advise the client to increase fluid intake when dietary fiber is initially increased to decrease flatus and help maintain softer stools.

For flatulence, limit carbonated beverages, the use of drinking straws, and chewing gum—all of which increase the ingestion of air. Gas-forming foods, such as cabbage, beans, onions, and cauliflower, should be avoided as well.

- **Regular exercise** helps clients to develop a regular defecation pattern. A client with weak abdominal and pelvic muscles, which impede normal defecation, may be able to strengthen them with the following isometric exercises:
    - In a supine position, the client tightens the abdominal muscles as though pulling them inward, holding them for about 10 seconds and then relaxing them. This exercise should be repeated 5–10 times each session and four times a day, depending on the client's health.
    - Again in a supine position, the client can contract the thigh muscles and hold them contracted for about 10 seconds, repeating the exercise 5–10 times each session and four times a day. This exercise helps the client confined to bed gain strength in the thigh muscles that makes it easier to use a bedpan.
- **Positioning.** Although the squatting position best facilitates defecation, the best position on a toilet seat for most individuals seems to be leaning forward.

For clients who have difficulty sitting down and getting up from the toilet, an elevated toilet seat can be attached to a regular toilet. Clients then do not have to lower themselves as far onto the seat or lift themselves as far off the seat. Elevated toilet seats can be purchased for use in the home.

Maintain Skin Integrity

Good skin care is vital for the client with fecal incontinence. Stool contains enzymes and other irritating substances that promote skin breakdown when they are not promptly removed. Skin breakdown can lead to pressure ulcers, particularly when a neurological disorder (e.g., spinal cord injury, dementia, or stroke) impairs mobility.

Good skin care includes the following:

- Clean the skin thoroughly with mild soap and water after each bowel movement. Toilet tissue may be more irritating to the skin and less effective in removing fecal material.
- Apply a skin barrier cream or ointment after each bowel movement. These help protect the skin from irritating substances in the feces.
- If incontinence pads or briefs are used, check frequently for soiling and change when feces are noted. Although these help to protect bedding and clothing from soiling, they can contribute to skin breakdown if they are not checked and changed frequently.

Facilitate Bowel Training Programs

For clients who have chronic constipation, frequent impactions, or fecal incontinence, bowel training programs may be helpful. The program is based on factors within the client's control and is designed to help the client establish normal defecation. Such matters as food and fluid intake, exercise, and defecation habits are all considered. Before beginning such a program, clients must understand it and want to be involved. The major phases of the program are as follows:

- Determine the client's usual bowel habits and factors that help and hinder normal defecation.
- Design a plan with the client that includes the following:
    a. Fluid intake of approximately 2,500–3,000 mL per day
    b. Increase in fiber in the diet
    c. Intake of hot drinks, especially just before the usual defecation time
    d. Increase in exercise
- Maintain the following daily routine for 2–3 weeks:
    a. To stimulate peristalsis, administer a cathartic suppository (e.g., Dulcolax) 30 minutes before the client's defecation time.
    b. When the client experiences the urge to defecate, assist the client to the toilet or commode or onto a bedpan. Note the length of time between the insertion of the suppository and the urge to defecate.
    c. Provide the client with privacy for defecation and a time limit (30–40 minutes usually is sufficient).
    d. Teach the client to lean forward at the hips, to apply pressure on the abdomen with the hands, and to bear down for defecation. These measures increase pressure on the colon. Straining should be avoided because it can cause hemorrhoids.
- Provide positive feedback when the client successfully defecates. Refrain from negative feedback if the client fails to defecate.
- Offer the client encouragement, and convey that patience often is required. Many clients require weeks or months of training to achieve success.
- Provide room odor control with deodorizer tablets, sprays, or other devices. Controlling odor is important to preserve the client's self-esteem.

Provide Manual Removal of Fecal Impaction as Ordered

Digital removal involves breaking up the fecal mass with a finger in the rectum and then removing the mass in portions. Because the bowel mucosa can be injured during this procedure, some agencies restrict and specify the personnel who are permitted to conduct digital disimpaction. Rectal stimulation also is contraindicated for some individuals because it may cause an excessive vagal response, resulting in cardiac arrhythmia. Before disimpaction is performed, an oil retention enema should be given and held for 30 minutes. After a disimpaction, the nurse can use various interventions to remove any remaining feces, such as a cleansing enema or insertion of a suppository.

Because manual removal of an impaction can be painful, the nurse may use, if the agency permits, 1–2 mL of lidocaine (Xylocaine) gel on a gloved finger inserted into the anal canal as far as the nurse can reach. The lidocaine will anesthetize the anal canal and rectum and should be inserted 5 minutes before the disimpaction.

Manual removal of a fecal impaction is described in **Box 5–6** ●.

Box 5–6 Manual Removal of a Fecal Impaction

1. If indicated, obtain assistance from a second individual who can comfort the client during the procedure.
2. Ask the client to assume a left-side-lying position with the knees flexed and the back toward the nurse.
3. Place a bed pad under the client's buttocks and a bedpan nearby to receive stool.
4. Drape the client for comfort and to avoid unnecessary exposure of the body.
5. Put on a pair of clean gloves, and liberally lubricate the index finger to be inserted.
6. Gently insert the index finger into the rectum, and move the finger along the length of the rectum.
7. Loosen and dislodge stool by gently massaging around it. Break up stool by working the finger into the hardened mass, taking care to avoid injury to the mucosa of the rectum.
8. Carefully work stool downward to the end of the rectum and remove it in small pieces. Continue to remove as much fecal material as possible. Periodically assess the client for signs of fatigue, such as facial pallor, diaphoresis, or change in pulse rate. Manual stimulation should be minimal.
9. Following disimpaction, assist the client to clean the anal area and buttocks. Then assist the client onto a bedpan or commode for a short time, because digital stimulation of the rectum often induces the urge to defecate.

Maintain a Fecal Incontinence Pouch

To collect and contain large volumes of liquid feces, the nurse may place a fecal incontinence collector pouch around the anal area. The purpose of the pouch is to prevent progressive perianal skin irritation and breakdown as well as the frequent linen changes necessitated by incontinence. In many agencies, the pouch is replacing the more traditional approach of inserting a large Foley catheter into the client's rectum and inflating the balloon to keep it in place, a practice that may damage the rectal sphincter and rectal mucosa. A rectal catheter also increases peristalsis and incontinence by stimulating sensory nerve fibers in the rectum.

A fecal collector is secured around the anal opening and may or may not be attached to drainage. Pouches are best applied before the perianal skin becomes excoriated. If perianal skin excoriation is present, the nurse either (a) applies a dimethicone-based moisture-barrier cream or an alcohol-free barrier film to the skin to protect it from feces until it heals and then applies the pouch or (b) applies a skin barrier or hydrocolloid barrier underneath the pouch to achieve the best possible seal.

Nursing responsibilities for clients with a rectal pouch include (a) regularly assessing and documenting the perianal skin status, (b) changing the bag every 72 hours or sooner if leakage occurs, (c) maintaining the drainage system, and (d) providing explanations and support to the client and support people.

Some clients (e.g., those who are quadriplegic or paraplegic, or after trauma or stroke) may be treated for fecal incontinence by surgical repair of a damaged sphincter or an artificial bowel sphincter. The artificial sphincter consists of three parts: a cuff around the anal canal, a pressure-regulating balloon, and a pump that inflates the cuff. The cuff is inflated to close the sphincter, maintaining continence. To have a bowel movement, the client deflates the cuff. The cuff automatically reinflates in 10 minutes. Management of this device usually is specific to the model being used; contact the manufacturing company for details. Administering enemas and rectal medications may be harmful with this device in place.

Provide Client Education for Home Care

Managing fecal incontinence is a challenging problem for the client, family, and caregivers. For the client with intact cognition, it can be psychologically devastating. The client may become socially isolated for fear of odor or soiling clothing. The client's self-esteem may suffer from a sense of lost control over body functions and the inability to provide self-care. It is important to stress that incontinence is never normal (i.e., aging alone is not a cause of incontinence) and often is treatable. Encourage the client to seek medical evaluation of the problem.

Topics for client and family education include the following:

- Recommended dietary measures, such as consuming a high-fiber diet and ample fluids to maintain soft, formed stool or maintaining a low-residue diet to reduce the number of stools
- Suggestions for regular exercise to stimulate bowel peristalsis and regular evacuation
- Use of bulk-forming laxatives, such as psyllium seed (Metamucil), to provide stool bulk and reduce the number of small, liquid stools
- Prescribed medications (e.g., loperamide to reduce the number of stools), their appropriate use, and management of adverse effects (e.g., constipation)
- Bowel training program, including techniques for digital anal stimulation, inserting suppositories, or administering enemas as recommended
- The importance of good skin care, particularly if neurological impairment is present
- The potential benefits and associated risks of biofeedback and surgical treatment, if recommended
- Referrals for home care or community health services as indicated

Individualize Care of Pediatric Clients With Encopresis

Children with bowel incontinence require special care based on their developmental level. Nurses should partner with parents to teach toilet training techniques, emphasizing the child's developmental readiness. Encourage parents to praise the child for successes and to avoid punishment and power struggles. Encourage high-fiber diets and regular times for elimination.

Nursing care centers on educating the child and parents about the disorder and its treatment and on providing emotional support. Explain the treatment plan, including dietary changes and use of laxatives or stool softeners. Reassure the child that he or she has a healthy body and, with treatment, will achieve normal functioning. Nurses should monitor the child for at least 6 months to be certain new patterns become established.

Evaluation

The goals established during the planning phase are evaluated according to the specific desired outcomes established during that phase.

If the desired outcomes are not achieved, the nurse should explore the reasons. The nurse might consider some or all of the following questions:

- Were the client's fluid intake and diet appropriate?
- Was the client's activity level appropriate?
- Are prescribed medications or other factors affecting the gastrointestinal function?
- Do the client and family understand the provided instructions well enough to comply with the required therapy?
- Were sufficient physical support and emotional support provided?

REVIEW   Bowel Incontinence, Constipation, and Impaction

RELATE Link the Concepts and Exemplars

Linking the exemplar of bowel incontinence, constipation, and impaction with the concept of mobility:

1. What impact does the concept of mobility have on elimination?
2. How can the nurse promote normal bowel elimination in the client with altered mobility?

Linking the exemplar of bowel incontinence, constipation, and impaction with the concept of metabolism:

3. When caring for a client with liver disease, what special precautions must the nurse implement related to bowel elimination?
4. When caring for a client diagnosed with hypothyroidism, what nursing implementations can be initiated to reduce the impact of this disorder on bowel elimination?

READY Go to Companion Skills Manual

REFER Go to Pearson Student Nursing Resources
nursing.pearsonhighered.com

- Additional review material
- Nursing Care Plan: A Client With Altered Bowel Elimination

REFLECT Case Study

Justin Gardner is a 26-year-old man who fractured his third thoracic vertebra when he fell while rock climbing. He is incontinent of feces secondary to sensory loss and the inability to feel the need to defecate.

1. What nursing interventions can be implemented to promote adequate bowel elimination for this client? Explain your answer.
2. What skin care precautions will the nurse implement to maintain skin integrity?
3. What nursing diagnosis would be appropriate for this client?
4. What client teaching will this client require, related to bowel continence, before discharge if he is to provide effective home care for himself?

EXEMPLAR 5.4   Urinary Calculi

EXEMPLAR KEY TERMS
Calcium oxalate, *319*
Calcium phosphate, *319*
Extracorporeal shock wave lithotripsy (ESWL), *322*
Hydronephrosis, *320*
Lithiasis, *319*
Lithotripsy, *322*
Nephrolithiasis, *319*
Nephrolithotomy, *323*
Nucleation, *319*
Pyelolithotomy, *323*
Renal colic, *320*
Staghorn stones, *319*
Struvite stones, *319*
Ureterolithotomy, *322*
Uric acid stones, *319*
Urinary calculi, *318*
Urolithiasis, *319*

EXEMPLAR LEARNING OUTCOMES
After reading about this exemplar, you will be able to:

1. Describe the pathophysiology, etiology, clinical manifestations, and direct and indirect causes of urinary calculi.
2. Identify risk factors and prevention methods associated with urinary calculi.
3. Illustrate the nursing process in providing culturally competent care across the life span for individuals with urinary calculi.
4. Formulate priority nursing diagnoses appropriate for an individual with urinary calculi.
5. Summarize therapies used by interdisciplinary teams in the collaborative care of an individual with urinary calculi.
6. Plan evidence-based care for an individual with urinary calculi and his or her family in collaboration with other members of the healthcare team.
7. Evaluate expected outcomes for an individual with urinary calculi.

▶ OVERVIEW

Urinary calculi, often referred to as kidney stones, are caused by the development of one or more crystals ranging in size from very small to large enough to fill the renal calyces. These calculi can lodge anywhere in the urinary tract and may cause obstruction and kidney damage. The excruciating pain associated with renal calculi occurs when the multifaceted crystal scrapes against the lining of the ureter, causing extreme irritation. As a

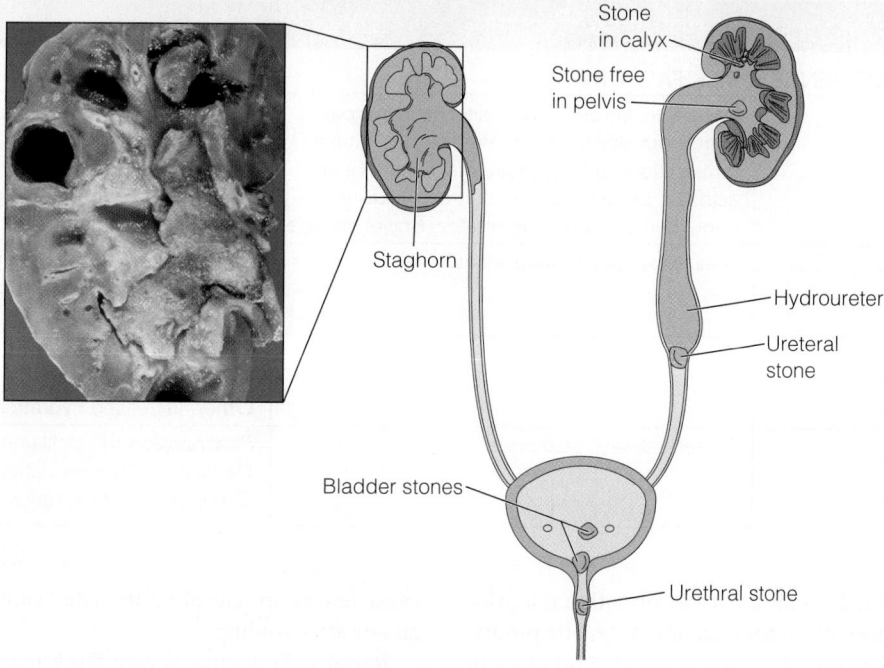

Figure 5–8 ● Development and location of calculi in the urinary tract.
Source: Dr. E. Walker/Science Photo Library/Science Source.

result, pain management is an important consideration in caring for clients with this disorder.

Urinary calculi are the most common cause of upper urinary tract obstruction (Porth & Matfin, 2010). The term **lithiasis** means "stone formation." When the stones form in the kidney, the condition is known as **nephrolithiasis**; when they form elsewhere in the urinary tract (for example, the bladder), the condition is called **urolithiasis**. Stones may form and obstruct the urinary tract at any point (**Figure 5–8 ●**). In the United States and other industrialized countries, renal (or kidney) stones are most common.

▶ PATHOPHYSIOLOGY AND ETIOLOGY

Normally, a balance exists in the kidneys between the need to conserve water and the need to eliminate poorly soluble materials such as calcium salts. This balance is affected by factors such as diet, environmental temperature, and activity. Protective inorganic and organic substances in the urine, such as pyrophosphate, citrate, and glycoproteins, normally inhibit stone formation.

Three factors contribute to urolithiasis: supersaturation, **nucleation** (formation of a crystal from a liquid), and lack of inhibitory substances in the urine. When the concentration of an insoluble salt in the urine is very high (i.e., when the urine is supersaturated), crystals may form (nucleation). Usually, these crystals disperse and are eliminated because the bonds holding them together are weak. However, a nucleus of crystals may develop stable bonds to form a stone. More often, crystals form around an organic matrix, or mucoprotein nucleus, to become a stone. The stimulus required to initiate crystallization in supersaturated urine may be minimal. Things as simple as ingesting a meal high in insoluble salt or decreased fluid intake, as occurs

during sleep, allows the concentration to increase to the point where precipitation occurs and stones form and grow. When fluid intake is adequate, no stone growth occurs. The acidity or alkalinity of the urine and the presence or absence of calculus-inhibiting compounds also affect lithiasis.

Most kidney stones (75%–80%) are calcium stones, composed of **calcium oxalate** and/or **calcium phosphate**. These stones are generally associated with high concentrations of calcium in the blood or urine. **Uric acid stones** develop when the urine concentration of uric acid is high. They are more common in men and may be associated with gout. Genetic factors contribute to the development of uric acid stones and calcium stones. **Struvite stones** are associated with UTI caused by urease-producing bacteria such as *Proteus*. These stones can become very large, filling the renal pelvis and calyces. They are often called **staghorn stones** because of their shape. Cystine stones, which are rare, are associated with a genetic defect. The types of renal calculi, contributing factors, and recommended dietary modifications and other treatments are listed in **Table 5–9 ●**.

Etiology

Most urinary stones form in the renal pelvis and are composed primarily of calcium salts. Urolithiasis affects up to 720,000 individuals annually in the United States (Papadakis & McPhee, 2013). In the United States, the incidence varies by region, with the highest frequency in southern and midwestern states. Males are affected 2 or 3 times more often than females (Porth & Matfin, 2010). Calculi are more common among Whites than Blacks. Most individuals affected are in young or middle adulthood.

Risk Factors

Although the majority of urinary stones are idiopathic (having no demonstrable cause), a number of risk factors have been

TABLE 5–9   Risk Factors and Interventions for Renal Calculi

STONE TYPE AND INCIDENCE	RISK FACTORS	MANAGEMENT
Calcium phosphate and/or oxalate 75%–80%	Hypercalciuria and hypercalcemia: hyperparathyroidism, immobility, bone disease, vitamin D intoxication, multiple myeloma, renal tubular acidosis, prolonged steroid intake, alkaline urine, dehydration, inflammatory bowel disease	*Pharmacology:* Thiazide, diuretics, phosphates, calcium-binding agents *Dietary:* Limited foods high in calcium and oxalate, increased foods that acidify urine *Other:* Increased hydration, exercise
Struvite 15%–20%	UTIs, especially *Proteus* infections	*Pharmacology:* Antibiotic therapy for UTI *Other:* Surgical intervention or lithotripsy to remove stone
Uric acid 5%–10%	Gout, increased purine intake, acid urine	*Pharmacology:* Potassium citrate, allopurinol *Dietary:* Low purine diet *Other:* Increased hydration
Cystine (uncommon)	Genetic defect, acid urine	*Pharmacology:* Penicillamine, sodium bicarbonate *Dietary:* Sodium restriction *Other:* Increase hydration

identified. The greatest risk factor for stone formation is a prior personal or family history of urinary calculi. A genetic predisposition to the accumulation of certain mineral substances in the urine or a congenital lack of protective factors may explain the familial link. Other identified risk factors include dehydration with resultant increased urine concentration; immobility; and excess dietary intake of calcium, oxalate, or proteins. Gout, hyperparathyroidism, and urinary stasis or repeated infections also contribute to calculus formation. Loss of calcium from the bones (e.g., due to immobility) and dehydration are major risk factors for urinary stones.

Prevention

Adequate fluid intake is the most important intervention for preventing all types of kidney stones. In addition, specific measures can be taken to prevent each type of kidney stone. Calcium stones can be prevented by reducing sodium and animal protein intake, getting enough calcium from food, and avoiding foods high in oxalate (e.g., spinach, nuts, wheat bran). Uric acid stones can be prevented by limiting animal protein intake (NKUDIC, 2013). For individuals with a history of kidney stones, medications may help prevent future stone formation. For example, thiazide diuretics are used to prevent calcium stones, allopurinol is used to prevent uric acid stones, and antibiotics may help prevent struvite stones (Mayo Clinic, 2012b).

▶ CLINICAL MANIFESTATIONS

The symptoms caused by urinary calculi vary with their size and location. (See the Clinical Manifestations and Therapies feature.) Manifestations develop from obstructed urine flow resulting in distention and from tissue trauma caused by passage of the rough-edged crystalline stone.

Calculi affecting the kidney calyces and pelvis may cause few symptoms. If the stone has gradually or partially obstructed urinary flow, dull, aching flank pain may be present, but renal calculi often are silent, without symptoms. Bladder calculi may cause few symptoms other than dull suprapubic pain with exercise or after voiding.

Renal colic (acute, severe flank pain on the affected side) develops when a stone obstructs the ureter, causing ureteral spasm. The pain of renal colic may radiate to the suprapubic region, groin, and external genitals (the scrotum or labia). The severity of the pain often causes a sympathetic response with associated nausea; vomiting; pallor; and cool, clammy skin.

Manifestations of UTI, including chills and fever, frequency, urgency, and dysuria, may accompany urinary calculi at any level. Calculi may cause trauma to the urinary tract, resulting in gross or microscopic hematuria. Gross hematuria is often the only sign of bladder stones.

Complications

Urinary stones may obstruct urine flow at any point in the urinary tract, causing complications such as hydronephrosis and urinary stasis with subsequent infection.

OBSTRUCTION   Stones can obstruct the urinary tract at any point, from the calyces of the kidney to the distal urethra, impeding the outflow of urine. If the obstruction develops slowly, there may be few or no symptoms, whereas sudden obstruction (e.g., blockage of a ureter by a passing stone) may cause severe manifestations. Urinary tract obstruction can ultimately lead to renal failure. The degree of obstruction, its location, and the duration of impaired urine flow determine the effect on renal function.

HYDRONEPHROSIS   The kidneys continue to produce urine, causing increased pressure and distention of the urinary tract behind the obstruction. **Hydronephrosis** (accumulation of urine in the renal pelvis as a result of obstructed outflow) and hydroureter (distention of the ureter with urine) are possible results. If the pressure is not relieved, damage to the collecting tubules, proximal tubules, and glomeruli of the kidney are damaged causes a gradual loss of renal function.

Acute hydronephrosis typically causes colicky pain on the affected side. The pain may radiate into the groin. Chronic hydronephrosis develops slowly and may have few manifesta-

Clinical Manifestations and Therapies   **Urinary Calculi**

ETIOLOGY	CLINICAL MANIFESTATIONS	CLINICAL THERAPIES
Acute hydronephrosis caused by the development of a sudden obstruction of urine flow	■ Acute, colicky pain; may radiate into groin ■ Hematuria, pyuria ■ Fever ■ Nausea, vomiting, abdominal pain	■ Lithotripsy or surgical removal of the stone ■ IV therapy ■ Thiazide diuretics if stone is caused by excess calcium ■ Dietary modification ■ Monitoring of BUN and creatinine to determine extent of kidney damage ■ Client teaching to reduce risk factors and prevent recurrence
Chronic hydronephrosis caused by gradual development of obstruction of urine flow	■ Possibly asymptomatic until complete obstruction develops ■ Dull, aching flank pain ■ Hematuria, pyuria ■ Fever ■ Palpable flank mass	■ Lithotripsy or surgical removal of the stone ■ Evaluation of kidney function ■ Dietary modification ■ IV therapy ■ Client teaching to reduce risk of recurrence
Kidney stones	■ Often asymptomatic ■ Dull, aching flank pain ■ Microscopic hematuria ■ Manifestations of UTI	■ Hydration ■ Thiazide diuretics ■ Monitoring of hemoglobin and hematocrit ■ Limits on foods high in calcium ■ Calcium-binding agents
Ureteral stones	■ Renal colic ■ Acute, severe flank pain on affected side ■ Likelihood of pain radiating to suprapubic region, groin, and external genitals ■ Nausea; vomiting; pallor; cool, clammy skin	■ Hydration ■ Monitoring of hemoglobin and hematocrit ■ Limits on foods high in calcium ■ Calcium-binding agents ■ Analgesics for pain (morphine sulfate); NSAIDs (indomethacin) ■ Thiazide diuretics ■ IV fluids
Bladder stones	■ Possibly asymptomatic ■ Dull suprapubic pain, possibly associated with exercise or voiding ■ Gross or microscopic hematuria ■ Manifestations of UTI	If asymptomatic, often no treatment other than increasing hydration and monitoring for hematuria

tions other than dull, aching back or flank pain. When hydronephrosis is significant, a palpable mass may be felt in the flank region. Hematuria and signs of UTI such as pyuria, fever, and discomfort may occur. Gastrointestinal symptoms such as nausea, vomiting, and abdominal pain may accompany hydronephrosis.

INFECTION   The urinary stasis associated with partial or complete obstruction increases the risk of UTI. Upper or lower urinary tract infections may develop. See the exemplar on Urinary Tract Infections in the module on Infection.

Lifespan and Cultural Considerations

Although urinary calculi are most common in middle-aged and older adults, individuals of all ages and races can develop calculi. The incidence of kidney stones in children is increasing. Clinical manifestations include dysuria, hematuria, and pain in the back or lower abdomen. Pain may be short or long in duration and may be accompanied by nausea and vomiting. Some children with small stones may pass the stones with no symptoms. Kidney stones are more likely to develop in children with defects in the urinary tract or with metabolic disorders such as hypercalciuria (NKUDIC, 2012a).

Pregnant women also require special consideration in assessing and treating urinary calculi. Symptoms of urolithiasis are common during pregnancy, and the symptoms are often misdiagnosed as appendicitis, diverticulitis, or placental abruption. If kidney stones do not pass spontaneously, numerous complications can occur, including premature labor, intractable pain, urosepsis, and interruption of normal progression of labor. Treatment of pregnant women is also complicated by the inability to use radiation, anesthesia, and surgery. Renal ultrasonography is the imaging modality of choice for pregnant women, and conservative management, ureteroscopy, or nephrostomy can be used for invasive treatment of larger stones (Wayment, 2012).

Racial differences also contribute to kidney stone formation. Stones are more common in Asians and Whites than in Native Americans, Africans, African Americans, and natives of the Mediterranean region. In addition, individuals who live in hot, dry climates tend to develop stones more frequently than individuals who live in cooler climates (Wolf, 2013).

▶ COLLABORATION

Collaborative care for clients diagnosed with urinary calculi focuses on relieving acute symptoms, destroying or removing stones, and preventing further stone formation. Asymptomatic stones (those not causing pain, infection, or obstruction) are treated conservatively.

Diagnostic Tests

The following laboratory and diagnostic tests may be ordered when urinary calculi are suspected:

- Urinalysis assesses for hematuria and the possible presence of WBCs and crystal fragments. Urine pH is helpful in identifying the type of stone.

- Chemical analysis of any stones passed in the urine determines the type of stone and suggests measures to prevent further stone formation. Retrieving stones or teaching the client to do so is a nursing responsibility. All urine is strained and may be saved. Any visible stones or sediment is sent for analysis.

- Urine calcium, uric acid, and oxalate levels measure the amount of these substances excreted over a 24-hour period and may be assessed to help identify possible causes of lithiasis. Elevated calcium levels occur in hyperparathyroidism, Cushing syndrome, and osteoporosis, all of which may contribute to lithiasis. Uric acid levels may be elevated in clients with gout and those at risk for forming uric acid calculi. Urine oxalate excretion may help to differentiate calcium oxalate from calcium phosphate stones.

- Serum calcium, phosphorus, and uric acid levels may be obtained to help identify factors contributing to calculus formation.

- KUB (kidneys, ureters, and bladder) may be used to identify calculi as opacities in the kidneys, ureters, and bladder.

- Renal ultrasonography may be used to detect stones and evaluate the kidneys for possible hydronephrosis.

- Computed tomography (CT) scan of the kidney, with or without contrast medium, may be used to provide a computer-generated photograph that shows calculi, ureteral obstruction, and other renal disorders.

- Intravenous pyelogram (IVP) may be done to visualize the kidneys, ureters, and bladder after injection of a contrast medium. This procedure is of particular importance when KUB, renal ultrasonography, and CT scan fail to demonstrate clear evidence of urinary calculi.

- Cystoscopy is used to visualize and possibly remove calculi from the urinary bladder and distal ureters.

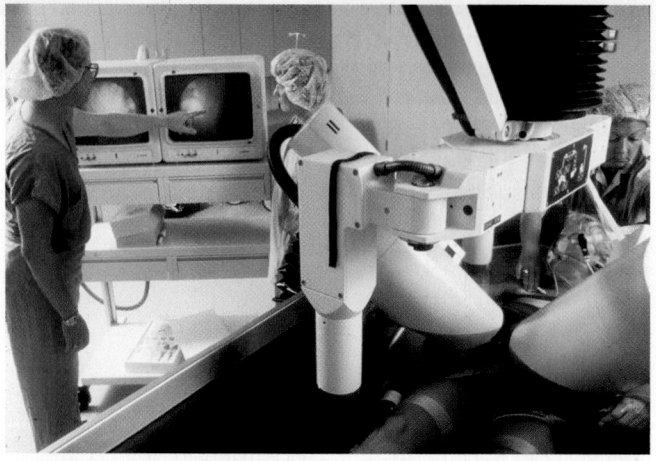

Figure 5–9 ● Extracorporeal shock wave lithotripsy. Acoustic shock waves generated by the shock wave generator travel through soft tissue to shatter the urinary stone into fragments, which are then eliminated in the urine.
Source: SIU BIOMED COMM/Custom Medical Stock Photo.

Surgery

Treatment of existing calculi depends on the location of the stone, extent of obstruction, renal function, presence or absence of UTI, and the client's general state of health. In general, the stone is removed if it is causing severe obstruction, infection, unrelieved pain, or serious bleeding (Johri et al., 2010; Mayo Clinic, 2012b).

Lithotripsy, using sound or shock waves to crush a stone, is the preferred treatment for urinary calculi. Several techniques may be used. **Extracorporeal shock wave lithotripsy (ESWL)** is a noninvasive technique for fragmenting kidney stones by using shock waves generated outside the body. Acoustic shock waves are aimed at the stone under fluoroscopic guidance (**Figure 5–9** ●). These shock waves travel through soft tissue without causing damage and shatter the stone as its greater density stops their progress. Repeated shock waves pulverize the stone into fragments small enough to be eliminated in the urine. The procedure may require 30 minutes to 2 hours to complete. Generally, intravenous sedation is adequate to maintain comfort during the procedure (NKF, 2009).

✳ Go to **nursing.pearsonhighered.com** *for nursing care of the client undergoing a lithotripsy procedure.*

Lithotripsy also may be performed with a percutaneous ultrasonic or laser technique. Percutaneous ultrasonic lithotripsy uses a nephroscope inserted into the kidney pelvis through a small flank incision (**Figure 5–10** ●). A small ultrasonic transducer fragments the stone, and the fragments are removed through the nephroscope. Laser lithotripsy is an alternative to ultrasonic lithotripsy. Laser beams are used to disintegrate the stone without damaging soft tissue. A nephroscope or a ureteroscope (passed up the ureter from the bladder during cystoscopy) is used to guide the laser probe into direct contact with the stone. A double J stent may be inserted into the affected ureter to maintain its patency following ESWL or other lithotripsy procedures.

On rare occasions, surgical intervention is necessary to remove a calculus in the renal pelvis or ureter. **Ureterolithotomy** is an incision made in the affected ureter to remove a calculus.

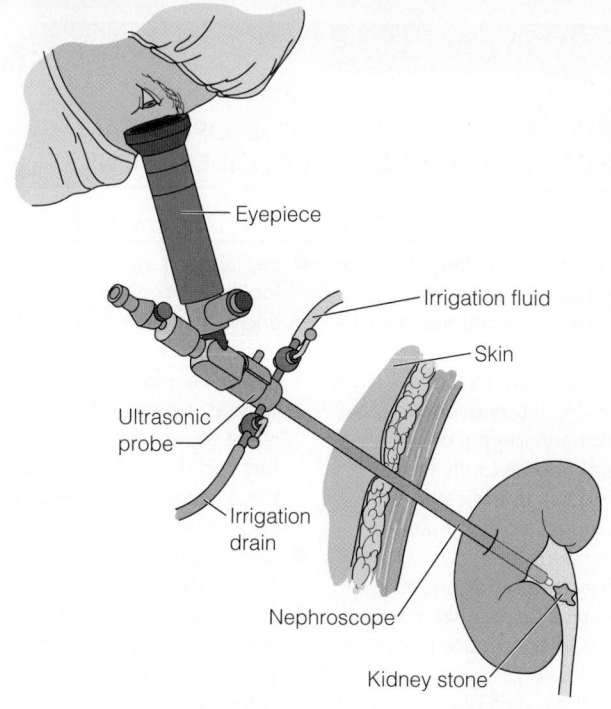

Figure 5–10 ● Percutaneous ultrasonic lithotripsy. A nephroscope is inserted into the renal pelvis, and ultrasonic waves are used to fragment the stone. Then the fragments are removed through the nephroscope.

Pyelolithotomy is an incision into the kidney pelvis and removal of a stone. A staghorn calculus that invades the calyces and renal parenchyma may require a **nephrolithotomy** for removal. Bladder stones may be removed by an instrument passed through a cystoscope to crush the stones. The remaining stone fragments are then irrigated out of the bladder with an acid solution that counteracts the alkalinity that precipitated stone formation.

Pharmacologic Therapy

An acute episode of renal colic is treated with analgesia and hydration. A narcotic analgesic such as morphine sulfate is given, often intravenously, to relieve pain and reduce ureteral spasm. Indomethacin, a nonsteroidal anti-inflammatory drug (NSAID), given as a suppository, may reduce the amount of narcotic analgesia required for acute renal colic. Oral or intravenous fluids reduce the risk of further stone formation and promote urine output.

After analysis of the calculus, various medications may be ordered to inhibit or prevent further lithiasis. A thiazide diuretic, frequently prescribed for calcium calculi, acts to reduce urinary calcium excretion and is very effective in preventing further stones. Potassium citrate alkalinizes urine (raises the pH) and is often prescribed to prevent stones that tend to form in acidic urine (uric acid, cystine, and some forms of calcium stones). See Table 5–9 for other preparations related to types of stones. Nursing responsibilities focus on teaching the client about the prescribed medication, its importance in preventing further stone formation, and potential adverse effects.

Complementary and Alternative Therapy
Urinary Calculi

Many natural remedies have been purported to help dissolve and pass kidney stones, including gravelroot, aloe vera juice, lemon juice, olive oil, apple cider vinegar, dandelion root, celery, and basil. However, few of these remedies have been supported by clinical trials and should therefore be used with caution. The natural remedies that are most supported by clinical trials are the consumption of fruit juices, including orange juice, grapefruit juice, lemon juice, and apple juice. These juices help decrease calcium oxalate crystallization and increase fluid intake to promote the passage of stones (Butterweck & Khan, 2009).

Nonpharmacologic Therapy

Small kidney stones are treated conservatively with increased water intake. The client should be encouraged to drink between 2 and 3 L of water per day. This increases urine production and helps flush out the urinary system. After the stone has passed, dietary changes to prevent recurrence of kidney stones include reduced intake of oxalate-rich foods, salt, and animal protein.

■ NURSING PROCESS

Nursing care for the client with urolithiasis is directed at providing comfort during acute renal colic, assisting with diagnostic procedures, ensuring adequate urinary output, and teaching the client information necessary to prevent future stone formation.

Assessment

Obtain the following subjective and objective assessment data specific to urolithiasis:

- *Health history.* Complaints of flank, back, or abdominal pain; description of radiation, characteristics, timing, aggravating or relieving factors; other symptoms such as nausea and vomiting; possible contributing factors such as dehydration; previous or family history of kidney stones; current or previous treatment measures
- *Physical examination.* General appearance, including position, vital signs, skin color, temperature, moisture, turgor; abdominal, flank, or costovertebral tenderness; amount, color, and characteristics of urine (pH and presence of hematuria, bacteria, pyuria)

Assessment guidelines for percussion and palpation of the kidneys are demonstrated in the Assessment feature. Note that the kidneys of an older client are more difficult to palpate abdominally because the mass of the adrenal cortex decreases with age. The nurse should omit blunt percussion in a frail older individual. Instead, palpation of the costovertebral angles and flanks can be used to reveal any pain or tenderness. In some clinical settings, the primary care provider will perform the kidney assessment.

Kidney Assessment

ASSESSMENT/METHOD	NORMAL FINDINGS	ABNORMAL FINDINGS	LIFESPAN OR DEVELOPMENTAL CONSIDERATIONS
General Survey			

A quick survey of the client enables the nurse to identify any immediate problem as well as the client's ability to participate in the assessment.
1. *Instruct the client.*
2. *Position the client.*
  ■ Begin the examination with the client in a supine position with the abdomen exposed from the nipple line to the pubis (see **Figure 5–11** ●).
3. *Assess the general appearance.*
  ■ Assess general appearance and inspect the client's skin for color, hydration status, scales, masses, indentations, or scars.
4. *Inspect the abdomen for color, contour, symmetry, and distention.*
  ■ It may be helpful to stand at the foot of the exam table and inspect the abdomen from there (see **Figure 5–12** ●).
	The client should not show signs of acute distress and should be mentally alert and oriented.
	
	Normally, the client's abdomen is not distended, is relatively symmetrical, and is free of bruises, masses, and swellings.
	
	In most cases, no sounds are heard upon auscultation of the renal arteries.
		■ Clients with kidney disorders frequently look tired and complain of fatigue. If a kidney disorder is suspected, it is important to look for signs of circulatory overload (pulmonary edema) or peripheral edema (puffy face or fingers), or indications of pruritus (scratch marks on the skin).
		■ Elevated nitrogenous wastes (azotemia) in the blood contribute to mental confusion.
		■ A distended bladder may be visible in the suprapubic area, indicating the need to void and perhaps the inability to do so.
			■ Explain that you will be looking, listening, touching, and tapping on parts of the abdomen. Tell the client you will explain each procedure as it occurs. Tell the client to report any discomfort and that you will stop the examination if the procedure is uncomfortable.
			■ Children may benefit from a demonstration on a doll.
			■ An upper abdominal bruit is occasionally heard in young adults and is considered normal.
			■ On a thin adult, renal artery pulsation may be auscultated.

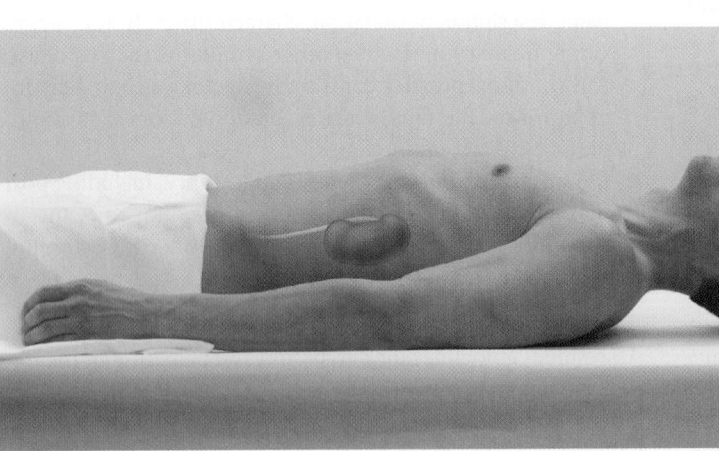

Figure 5–11 ● Position the client.

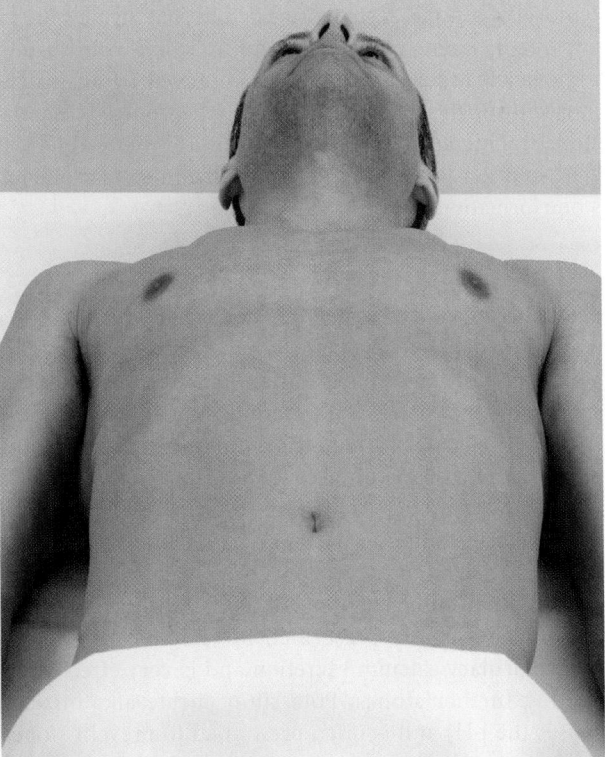

Figure 5–12 ● Inspecting the abdomen from the foot of the bed.

Kidney Assessment (*continued*)

ASSESSMENT/METHOD	NORMAL FINDINGS	ABNORMAL FINDINGS	LIFESPAN OR DEVELOPMENTAL CONSIDERATIONS
5. *Auscultate the right and left renal arteries to assess circulatory sounds.* ■ Gently place the bell of the stethoscope over the extended midclavicular line (MCL) on either side of the abdominal aorta, which is located above the level of the umbilicus (see **Figure 5–13** ●). ■ Be sure to auscultate both the right and left sides, and over the epigastric and umbilical areas.		■ Many diseases contribute to abdominal distention. These include renal conditions such as polycystic kidney disease; enlarged kidneys, as seen in acute pyelonephritis; ascites (accumulation of fluid) due to hepatic disease; and displacement of abdominal organs. Pressure from the abdominal contents on the diaphragm may alter the client's breathing pattern.	

The Kidneys and Flanks

ASSESSMENT/METHOD	NORMAL FINDINGS	ABNORMAL FINDINGS	LIFESPAN OR DEVELOPMENTAL CONSIDERATIONS
1. *Position the client.* ■ Place the client in a sitting position facing away from you with the back exposed. 2. *Inspect the left and right costovertebral angles for color and symmetry.* 3. *Inspect the flanks (the side areas between the hips and the ribs) for color and symmetry.* 4. *Gently palpate the area over the left costovertebral angle (see **Figure 5–14** ●).*	The costovertebral angles and flanks should be symmetrical and even in color; the color should be consistent with the rest of the back. Normally, the client expresses no discomfort upon palpation of the costovertebral angles.	■ A protrusion or elevation over a costovertebral angle occurs when the kidney is grossly enlarged or when a mass is present.	■ Palpation in children can be done over the child's hand if the child resists the assessment.

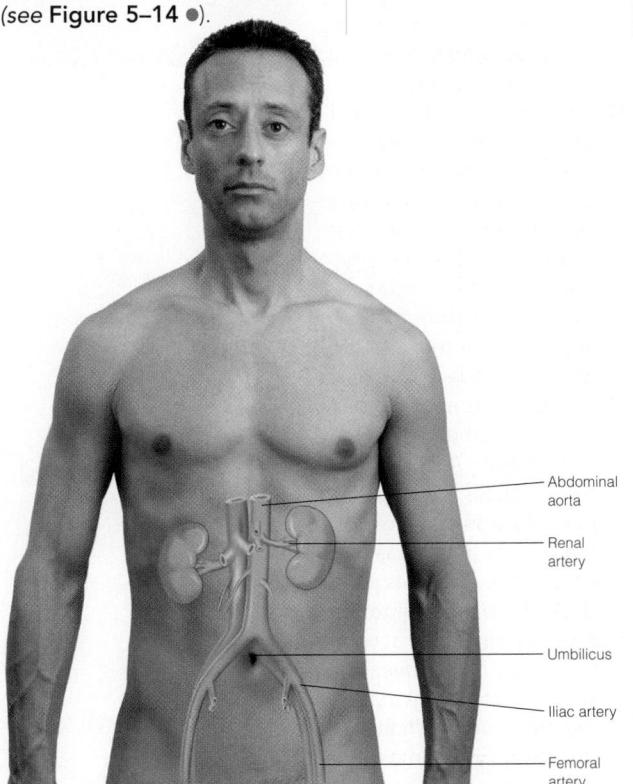

Figure 5–13 ● Auscultating the renal arteries.

Abdominal aorta

Renal artery

Umbilicus

Iliac artery

Femoral artery

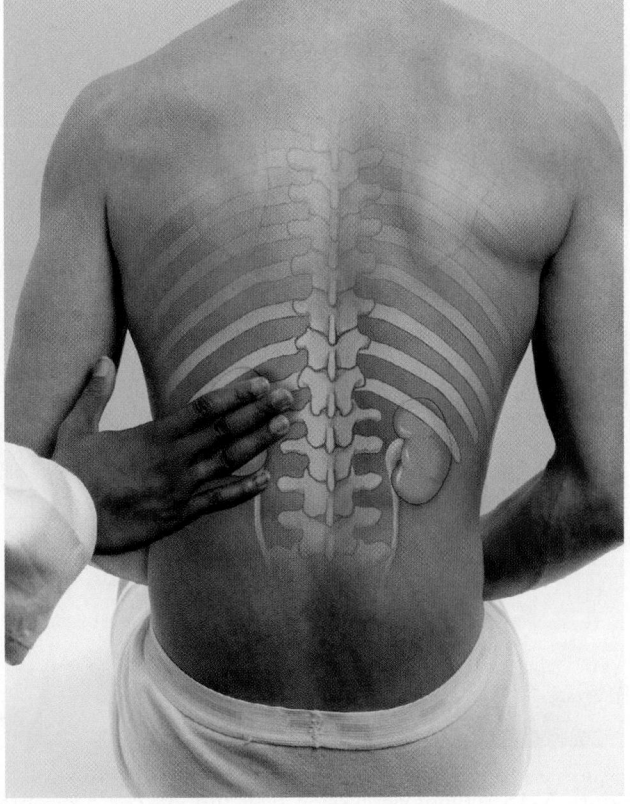

Figure 5–14 ● Palpating the costovertebral angle.

(*continued on next page*)

Kidney Assessment (continued)

ASSESSMENT/METHOD	NORMAL FINDINGS	ABNORMAL FINDINGS	LIFESPAN OR DEVELOPMENTAL CONSIDERATIONS
■ Watch the reaction and ask the client to describe any sensation the palpation causes. 5. *Use blunt or indirect percussion to further assess the kidneys.* ■ Place your left palm flat over the left costovertebral angle. ■ Thump the back of your left hand with the ulnar surface of your right fist, causing a gentle thud over the costovertebral angle (see **Figure 5–15 ●**). ■ Repeat the procedure on the right side. Ask the client to describe the sensation as you examine each side.	The client should feel no pain or tenderness with pressure or percussion.	■ Flank color and symmetry must be carefully correlated to other diagnostic cues as the assessment proceeds. If ecchymosis is present (Grey Turner sign), there may be other signs of trauma, such as blunt, penetrating wounds or lacerations. ■ Pain, discomfort, or tenderness from an enlarged or diseased kidney may occur over the costovertebral angle, flank, and abdomen. When questioned, the client complains of a dull, steady ache. This type of pain is associated with polycystic formation, pyelonephritis, and other disorders that cause kidney enlargement. In the client with polycystic kidney disease, a sharp, sudden, intermittent pain may mean that a cyst in the kidney has ruptured. If the costovertebral angle is tender, red, and warm, and the client is experiencing chills, fever, nausea, and vomiting, the underlying kidney could be inflamed or infected. ■ The pain caused by calculi (stones) in the kidney or upper ureter is unique and different in character, severity, and duration from that caused by kidney enlargement. This pain occurs as calculi travel from the kidney to the ureters and the urinary bladder. ■ Some clients experience no pain, and others feel excruciating pain. A stationary stone causes a dull, aching pain. As stones travel down the urinary tract, spasms occur. These spasms produce sharp, intermittent, colicky pain (often accompanied by chills, fever, nausea, and vomiting) that radiates from the flanks to the lower quadrants of the abdomen and, in some cases, the upper thigh and scrotum or labium.	■ Do not percuss or palpate the client who reports pain or discomfort in the pelvic region. Do not percuss or palpate the kidney if a tumor of the kidney is suspected, such as a neuroblastoma or Wilms tumor. Palpation increases intra-abdominal pressure, which may contribute to intraperitoneal spreading of the neuroblastoma. Deep palpation should be performed only by experienced practitioners.

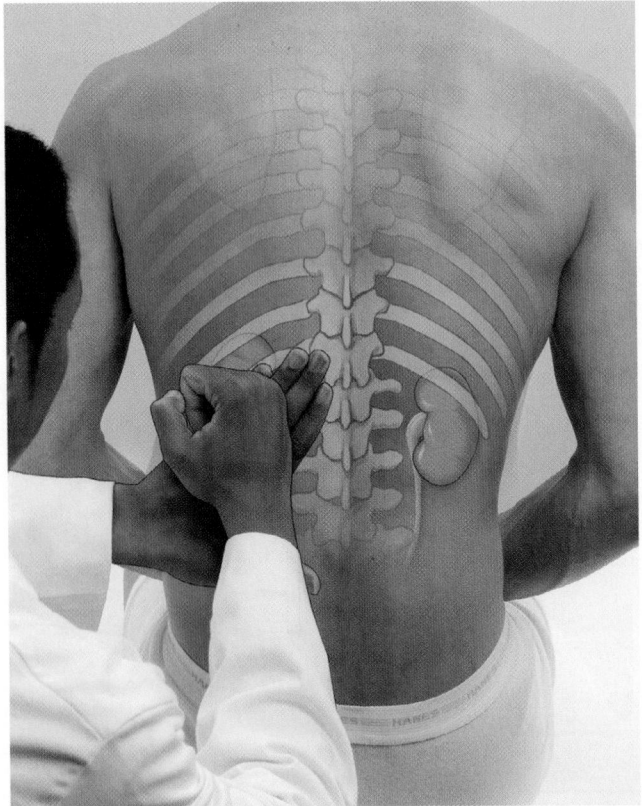

Figure 5–15 ● Blunt percussion over the left costovertebral angle.

Kidney Assessment (continued)

ASSESSMENT/METHOD	NORMAL FINDINGS	ABNORMAL FINDINGS	LIFESPAN OR DEVELOPMENTAL CONSIDERATIONS
		■ If the client reports severe pain, hematuria (blood in the urine) or oliguria (diminished volume of urine), and nausea and vomiting, it is important to be alert for hydroureter, a frequent complication that occurs when a renal calculus moves into the ureter. The calculus blocks and dilates the ureter, causing spasms and severe pain. Hydroureter can lead to shock, infection, and impaired renal function. If the nurse suspects hydroureter or obstruction at any point in the urinary tract, medical collaboration must be sought immediately. ■ Pain or discomfort during and after blunt percussion suggests kidney disease. This finding is correlated with other assessment findings.	

The Left Kidney

1. *Attempt to palpate the lower pole of the left kidney.* ■ Although it is not usually palpable, attempt to palpate the lower pole of the kidney for size, contour, consistency, and sensation. Note that the rib cage obscures the upper poles. ■ Position the client in a supine position. All palpation should be performed from the client's right side. ■ While standing on the client's right side, reach over the client and place your left hand between the posterior rib cage and the iliac crest (the left flank). ■ Place your right hand on the left upper quadrant of the abdomen lateral and parallel to the left rectus muscle just below the costal margin. ■ Instruct the client to take a deep breath. As the client inhales, lift the client's left flank with your left hand and press deeply with your right hand (approximately 4 cm) to	Left kidneys are rarely palpable in healthy individuals. If palpable upon capture, the kidney surface should be rounded, smooth, firm, and nontender.	■ When enlargement occurs in the presence of conditions such as neoplasms and polycystic disease, the kidneys may be palpable. ■ An enlarged palpable kidney could be painful for the client. This suggests tumor, cyst, or hydronephrosis.	■ Because deep kidney palpation can cause tissue trauma, novice nurses should not attempt either deep palpation or capture of the kidney unless supervised by an experienced nurse or nurse practitioner. Deep kidney palpation should not be done in clients who have had a recent kidney transplant or an abdominal aortic aneurysm. ■ Care must be taken not to mistake an enlarged spleen for an enlarged left kidney. An enlarged kidney feels smooth and rounded, whereas an enlarged spleen feels sharper, with a more delineated edge.

(continued on next page)

Kidney Assessment (continued)

ASSESSMENT/METHOD	NORMAL FINDINGS	ABNORMAL FINDINGS	LIFESPAN OR DEVELOPMENTAL CONSIDERATIONS

attempt to palpate the lower pole of the kidney (see **Figure 5–16** ●).

2. *Attempt to capture the left kidney.*
   - Because of its position deep in the retroperitoneal space, the left kidney is not normally palpable. The capture maneuver may enable you to palpate it. This maneuver is possible because the kidneys descend during inspiration and slide back into their normal position during exhalation.
   - Standing on the client's right side, place your left hand under the client's back to elevate the flank as before. Place your right hand on the left upper quadrant of the abdomen lateral and parallel to the left rectus muscle with the fingertips just below the left costal margin. Instruct the client to take a deep breath and hold it. As the client inhales, attempt to capture the kidney between your two hands. Ask the client to exhale slowly and then to briefly hold the breath. At the same time, slowly release the pressure of your fingers.
   - As the client exhales, you will feel the captured kidney move back into its previous position.

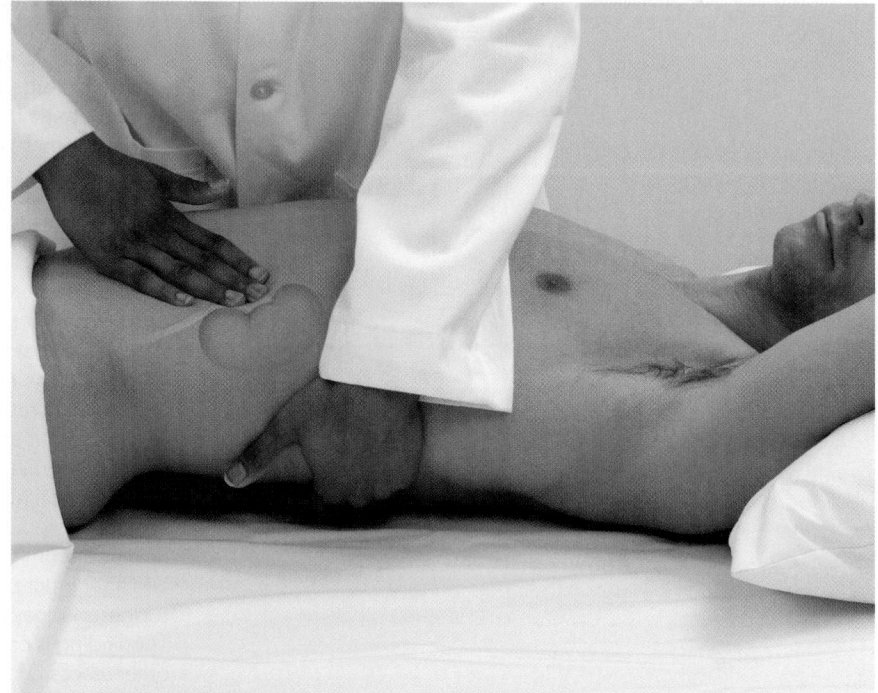

Figure 5–16 ● Palpating the left kidney.

The Right Kidney

1. *Attempt to palpate the lower pole of the right kidney.* ■ Standing on the client's right side, place your left hand under the back parallel to the right twelfth rib (about halfway between the costal margin and iliac crest) with your fingertips reaching for the costovertebral angle. Place your right hand on the right upper quadrant of the abdomen lateral to the right rectus muscle and just below the right costal margin. ■ Instruct the client to take a deep breath. As the client inhales, lift the flank with your left hand and use deep palpation to feel for the lower pole of the kidney.	The kidney surface should be rounded, smooth, firm, and nontender. If palpable, the lower pole of the kidney has a smooth, firm, uninterrupted surface.	■ It is important not to mistake an enlarged liver for an enlarged right kidney. An enlarged kidney feels smooth and rounded, whereas an enlarged liver is closer to the midline and has a more distinct border. Polycystic kidney disease or carcinoma should be suspected when there is gross enlargement of the kidney. The kidneys may be two or three times their normal size in clients with polycystic disease.	■ The lower pole of the right kidney is palpable in some individuals, especially in thin, relaxed females. ■ During the capture maneuver, some clients describe a nonpainful sensation as the kidney slides between the nurse's fingers back into its normal position.

Kidney Assessment (continued)

ASSESSMENT/METHOD	NORMAL FINDINGS	ABNORMAL FINDINGS	LIFESPAN OR DEVELOPMENTAL CONSIDERATIONS
2. Attempt to capture the right kidney. ■ Place your left hand under the client's right flank. ■ Place your right hand on the right upper quadrant of the abdomen with the fingertips lateral and parallel to the right rectus muscle just below the right costal margin. ■ Instruct the client to take a deep breath and hold it. As the client inhales, attempt to capture the kidney between your two hands. ■ Ask the client to exhale slowly and then to briefly hold the breath. At the same time, slowly release the pressure of your fingers. ■ As the client exhales you will feel the captured kidney move back into its previous position.			

Diagnosis

Possible nursing diagnoses for the client with urinary calculi include the following:

■ *Acute Pain*
■ *Impaired Urinary Elimination*
■ *Deficient Knowledge*
■ *Anxiety*
■ *Risk for Imbalanced Nutrition*
■ *Risk for Infection.*

(NANDA-I © 2012)

Planning

Goals appropriate for the client with urinary calculi must be individualized to meet each client's specific needs but may include:

■ The client will request analgesics as needed at onset of pain and report effective pain relief within 20 minutes of parenteral analgesic administration.
■ The client will maintain urine output of 2,500 mL in each 24-hour period without signs of infection or obstruction.
■ The client will verbalize understanding of disease process to include dietary changes that may reduce the risk of recurrence of calculi formation.
■ The client will demonstrate reduced anxiety by nonverbal gestures and return of vital signs to baseline.

Implementation

In collaboration with the healthcare team, the nurse will provide culturally competent interventions to ensure the comfort of the client and promote continuing health following discharge. While treating the client's pain may be the most immediate intervention, client teaching and health promotion help the client maintain urinary health beyond the current need for healthcare intervention.

Manage Pain

Pain is the primary outward manifestation of urolithiasis, particularly when a stone lodges in a ureter, causing acute obstruction and distention. Invasive and noninvasive procedures to remove or crush stones also may be painful. Clients undergoing surgery also experience incisional pain. The intensity of renal colic pain can cause a vasovagal response with resulting hypotension and syncope. Client safety is the first priority.

■ Assess pain using a standard pain scale and its characteristics. Administer analgesia as ordered and monitor its effectiveness. The intensity and type of pain and its responsiveness to analgesia provide valuable clues to its cause. Regularly administering prescribed analgesics controls pain more effectively than waiting until pain becomes intolerable. Administering an ordered NSAID on a routine schedule may significantly reduce the need for narcotic analgesia in clients with renal colic.
■ Unless contraindicated, encourage fluid intake and ambulation in the client with renal colic. Increased fluids and ambulation increase urinary output, facilitating movement of the calculus through the ureter and decreasing pain. Assist with ambulation as needed and closely monitor the client for dizziness or other complications that may increase the risk for impaired mobility.
■ Use nonpharmacologic measures such as positioning, moist heat, relaxation techniques, guided imagery, and diversion as

adjunctive therapy for pain relief. Adjunctive pain relief measures can enhance the effectiveness of analgesics and other prescribed treatment.

- If surgery has been performed, monitor urinary output, catheters, incision, and wound drainage. Pain may be a symptom of proximal distention due to a blocked catheter. Infection or hematoma at the surgical site can increase pain significantly.

Monitor Urinary Output

Obstruction of the urinary tract is the primary problem associated with urolithiasis. A stone that completely obstructs the ureter can lead to hydronephrosis and kidney damage on the affected side. Report symptoms of hydronephrosis, such as dull flank pain or aching and changes in renal function studies (BUN and serum creatinine). Because the other kidney continues to function, urine output may not fall significantly with obstruction of one ureter. A rising BUN and serum creatinine may be early signs of renal failure. Obstruction can ultimately lead to stasis, infection, or irreversible renal damage.

- Monitor amount and character of urine output. If the client is catheterized, measure output hourly. Urine volume reflects possible urinary tract obstruction and adequacy of hydration. Strain all urine for stones, saving any recovered stones for laboratory analysis. Analysis of stones recovered from the urine can direct measures used to prevent further lithiasis. Document any hematuria, dysuria, frequency, urgency, and pyuria. Hematuria, gross or microscopic, is often associated with calculi and with procedures used to remove stones, such as cystoscopy or lithotripsy. A change in the amount of hematuria may indicate stone passage or a complication. Dysuria, frequency, urgency, and cloudy urine are symptoms of UTI, often associated with urolithiasis. Antibiotic therapy may be required.
- Maintain patency and integrity of all catheter systems. Secure catheters well, label as indicated, and use sterile technique for all ordered irrigations or other procedures. A kinked or plugged catheter, particularly a ureteral catheter or nephrostomy tube, may damage the urinary system. Labeling catheters can prevent mistakes such as inappropriate irrigation and clamping. Any catheter increases the risk of infection; aseptic technique in all procedures reduces this risk.

Provide Client Teaching

The client with urolithiasis has multiple learning needs. These include information about the disease and its possible consequences, understanding of any diagnostic or therapeutic procedures performed, and strategies to prevent future lithiasis. The nurse working with a client with urolithiasis should do the following:

- Assess the client's understanding and previous learning. Relating information to previously learned material enhances retention and understanding.
- Present all material in a manner appropriate to the client's knowledge base, developmental and educational levels, and current needs. Learning is an active process that requires the client's participation. Tailoring teaching to the individual increases client involvement and compliance with the care plan.

- Teach about all diagnostic and treatment procedures. Knowing what to expect reduces anxiety, enhances compliance, and hastens recovery.
- If the client will be managed at home or in the community, teach the client to:
  a. Collect and strain all urine, saving any stones.
  b. Report stone passage to the physician and bring in the stone for analysis.
  c. Report to the physician any changes in the amount or character of urine output.

When pain can be managed with oral analgesics, urinary stones are managed at home or in the community. The client needs to know how and why to collect the calculus as well as what the indicators of complications are, such as reduced urine output and cloudy or bloody urine.

- Teach measures to prevent further urolithiasis.
  a. Increase fluid intake to 2,500–3,500 mL per day.
  b. Follow recommended dietary guidelines.
  c. Maintain activity level to prevent urinary stasis and bone resorption (loss).
  d. Take medications as prescribed.

The risk of recurrent lithiasis is approximately 50%; however, this risk can be reduced through measures used to prevent conditions favoring stone formation.

- Teach about the relationship between urinary calculi and UTI, emphasizing preventive measures and the importance of prompt treatment. UTI promotes urolithiasis and thus requires prompt treatment to reduce this risk.

Promote Health and Wellness

Discuss with all clients the importance of maintaining an adequate fluid intake. Stress the need to increase fluid intake during warm weather and strenuous exercise or physical labor. Discuss the relationship between weight-bearing activity and retention of calcium in the bones. Encourage all clients to remain as physically active as possible to prevent bone resorption and possible hypercalciuria.

Instruct clients with known gout to maintain a generous fluid intake so as to produce at least 2 L of urine every day. Discuss the risk of lithiasis with clients who have frequent UTIs and teach measures to reduce the incidence of UTI and the risk for lithiasis.

Prepare the Client for Discharge

The client with urinary calculi needs to know how to manage existing stones and what to do to reduce the risk of future stone formation. Discuss the following topics to prepare the client and family for home care:

- Importance of maintaining a fluid intake adequate to produce 2.0–2.5 L of urine per day
- Prescribed medications, their management, and potential adverse effects
- Dietary recommendations
- Prevention, recognition, and management of UTI
- Any further diagnostic or treatment measures planned (see Client Teaching).

Client Teaching Discharge Instructions for Clients With Urinary Calculi

When the client is to be discharged with dressings, a nephrostomy tube, or a catheter, teach the client and family about the following:

- How to change dressings, maintaining aseptic technique
- How to assess the wound and skin for healing and possible complications such as infection or skin breakdown
- How to manage drainage systems and maintain their patency
- How to empty drainage bags and assess urine output
- When to contact the physician and what the recommendations are for follow up care

Evaluation

The client is evaluated on the basis of the selected outcomes and nursing diagnoses, and the plan of care is amended depending on the client's response to interventions. While straining of the client's urine may indicate that the stone has passed, it is important to assess the client for possible complications such as infection or kidney damage. Expected outcomes include the following:

- The client rates pain at 3 or less on a 0–10 scale and is comfortable enough to perform ADLs.
- The client remains free from signs and symptoms of infection.
- The client chooses appropriate diet to prevent recurrence of renal calculi.
- The client demonstrates adequate fluid intake.

NURSING CARE PLAN A Client With Urinary Calculi

Richard Leton, age 44, owns a small business. He is admitted to the medical unit from the emergency department after awakening at 4 a.m. with severe right-sided pain. His CBC is normal, and urinalysis reveals microscopic hematuria but no protein or bacteria. A renal ultrasound shows a 4–5 mm stone partially obstructing the right ureter.

Stephen Phillips, Mr. Leton's admitting nurse, notes that Mr. Leton is pale, diaphoretic, and very anxious. Mr. Leton complains of nausea and asks for an emesis basin. Mr. Leton received 4 mg of intravenous morphine sulfate shortly after admission to the ED, approximately 2.5 hours ago. He denies pain at this time but says, "I'm scared to death that it'll come back—I couldn't even move, it hurt so bad."

ASSESSMENT

Mr. Leton's history reveals no previous episodes of renal calculi. He felt well until the pain awakened him during the night. He reports that he has been working under a deadline to complete a construction project and that he probably has not been drinking enough fluids "considering how hot it's been." Physical assessment findings include T_O 38.0°C (100.4°F) po, P 98 bpm, R 24/min, and BP 160/86 mmHg. Color is pale to ashen, skin cool and moist. Abdomen firm with moderate tenderness in the right upper outer quadrant. The ED physician orders an IV of 5% dextrose in 1/2 normal saline at 200 mL/h until nausea is relieved, then PO fluids of at least 3,000 mL/24 h; morphine sulfate (MS) 2–10 mg IV prn severe pain; indomethacin (Indocin) 50 mg per rectal suppository q8h; promethazine (Phenergan) 25 mg po or per suppository q6h prn nausea; activity to tolerance; and strain all urine, sending recovered stones for analysis.

DIAGNOSES

- *Anxiety* related to anticipation of recurrent severe pain
- *Risk for Imbalanced Nutrition: Less Than Body Requirements* related to nausea
- *Acute Pain* related to partial obstruction of right ureter by calculus
- *Impaired Urinary Elimination* related to partial obstruction of ureter by calculus
- *Deficient Knowledge* related to lack of information about disease process, contributing factors, and management

(NANDA-I © 2012)

PLANNING

To return to health and achieve expected outcomes, Mr. Leton's goals for care include the following:

- He will demonstrate reduced anxiety by relaxed facial expression, vital signs within his normal range, and ability to rest when not disturbed.
- He will consume at least 50% of diet and 100% of ordered fluids without nausea or vomiting.
- He will request analgesia as needed at onset of pain; he will report effective pain relief.
- He will maintain urine output of 2,500 mL/24 h with no signs of infection or obstruction (such as increased pain, dysuria, pyuria, or hematuria).
- He will relate an understanding of the process of urolithiasis and contributing factors.
- He will verbalize dietary and fluid intake and other measures to reduce risk of future stone formation.

IMPLEMENTATION

The nurse caring for Mr. Leton should do the following:

- Reassure Mr. Leton that measures to prevent further episodes of renal colic are being implemented and that medication is available to relieve pain promptly.
- Assess the effectiveness of analgesia and its adverse effects, especially nausea.
- Maintain IV as ordered until oral fluid intake exceeds 200 mL of fluid per hour while awake.

- Measure and strain all urine. Assess urine for color, clarity, and odor.
- Teach about urolithiasis and its risk factors, especially as they relate to Mr. Leton.
- Teach Mr. Leton the importance of maintaining a high fluid intake, especially when working outdoors in hot weather; recommended dietary modifications and their rationale; ordered medications and their effects; ways to identify and prevent UTI; and symptoms that should be reported to the physician.

(continued on next page)

NURSING CARE PLAN   (continued)

EVALUATION

Mr. Leton's care is evaluated on the basis of the goals of nursing care. Mr. Leton passes the obstructing stone the evening after admission and is discharged the following day. On discharge, he denies pain or nausea, his urine is clear and pale yellow, and urinalysis is normal. Laboratory analysis shows that the calculus was calcium. Mr. Leton is able to state the importance of continuing a high fluid intake. He verbalizes that he will reduce his intake of calcium-rich foods such as milk and milk products and that he will increase his intake of foods to acidify his urine. He is able to list foods to include in his diet. He states, "You'd better believe I'll follow my diet, drink my water, and make sure I don't get an infection. I hope to never feel pain like that again!"

CRITICAL THINKING

1. What factors contributed to the onset and timing of Mr. Leton's ureteral colic?
2. What is the rationale for administering indomethacin, an NSAID, to a client with ureteral colic?
3. Why did Mr. Phillips include a nursing intervention to assess for a relationship between Mr. Leton's nausea, his pain, and the ordered analgesic agent?

REVIEW   Urinary Calculi

RELATE Link the Concepts and Exemplars

Linking the exemplar of urinary calculi with the concept of comfort:

You are caring for a client with urinary calculi who is experiencing severe pain that he rates as an 11 on the 1–10 scale, with 10 being the worst pain he's ever felt.

1. Describe both pharmacologic and nonpharmacologic strategies you would use to relieve the client's pain.
2. What expected outcomes would you assess as indicating that pain management techniques were successful?

Linking the exemplar of urinary calculi with the concept of culture and diversity:

3. How would you respond if a client with urinary calculi informed you of a Web site he looked at last night that recommended increasing magnesium intake to cure kidney stones instead of following the therapy recommended by his provider?
4. A client with urinary calculi has already been seen several times for the same diagnosis. What cultural assessment would you perform to determine whether there is a cultural link to the recurrent diagnosis?

READY Go to Companion Skills Manual

The following skills related to this concept can be found in your skills book:

REFER Go to Pearson Nursing Student Resources
nursing.pearsonhighered.com

- Additional review material
- Chart 2: Nursing Care of the Client Having Lithotripsy

REFLECT Case Study

Guy Markson, age 28, is a business executive with a sedentary lifestyle. His wife says that he is always telling her that he needs to exercise more, but business meetings and job responsibilities seem to get in the way of his plans to work out. Lately, he's been even busier than usual and sometimes forgets to eat lunch or dinner unless he has a business lunch, which is usually red meat and wine.

Mr. Markson called his healthcare provider today, reporting excruciating pain under his rib cage on the left side of his back, saying that when his urine looked bloody, he knew he had to do something. The physician ordered a renal ultrasound, serum laboratory testing (calcium, uric acid, BUN, creatine, phosphorus), and urinalysis to include urine calcium and instructed Mr. Markson to go to the emergency department, which would coordinate the ordered tests and inform him of the results.

When Mr. Markson arrives at the hospital, the nurse administers morphine sulfate for pain and indomethacin by suppository and initiates IV normal saline at 150 mL/hour. A renal ultrasound is performed, and Mr. Markson receives a diagnosis of a 6 mm stone completely obstructing the left ureter, with resulting acute hydronephrosis. Diagnostic tests lead to the suspicion that the stone is a uric acid stone, although further testing will be performed on it when removed. The doctor recommends ESWL as the initial treatment and admits Mr. Markson to the acute care facility.

1. As the nurse admitting this client to the unit, what preparations will you make for the client while awaiting his arrival from the emergency department?
2. What nursing diagnosis would be appropriate for this client?
3. Following successful lithotripsy and confirmation that the stone was composed of uric acid, what discharge teaching will you provide the client and his wife?

■ REFERENCES

Ahmed, M., Pai, B., & Reynolds, T. (2012). Use of polyethylene glycol in children less than 3 years of age. *Journal of the College of Physicians and Surgeons—Pakistan, 22*(4), 267–268. doi:04.2012/JCPSP.267268.

Alsheik, E. H., Coyne, T., Hawes, S. K., Merikhi, L., Naples, S. P., Kanagarajan, N., . . . Ahmad, A. S. (2012). Fecal incontinence: Prevalence, severity, and quality of life data from an outpatient gastroenterology practice.

Gastroenterology Research and Practice, 2012, 947694. doi:10.1155/2012/947694.

Baldini, G., Bagry, H., Aprikian, A., & Carli, F. (2009). Postoperative urinary retention: Anesthetic and perioperative considerations. *Anesthesiology, 110*(5), 1139–1157. doi:10.1097/ALN.0b013e31819f7aea.

Bardsley, A. (2005). Use of lubricant gels in urinary catheterization. *Nursing Standard, 20*(8), 41–46.

Blazer, D. G., & Steffens, D. C. (2009). *The American Psychiatric Publishing textbook of geriatric psychiatry.* Arlington, VA: American Psychiatric Publishing.

Bongers, M E. J., van Wijk, M. P., Reitsma, J. B., & Benninga, M. A. (2010). Long-term prognosis for childhood constipation: Clinical outcomes in adulthood. *Pediatrics, 126*(1), e156–e162. doi:10.1542/peds.2009-1009.

Borowitz, S. (2013). Encopresis. *Medscape Reference.* Retrieved from http://emedicine.medscape.com/article/928795.

Briganti, A., Capitanio, U., Suardi, N., Gallina, A., Salonia, A., Bianchi, M., . . . Montorsi, F. (2009). Benign prostatic hyperplasia and its aetiologies. *European Urology Supplements, 8,* 865–871. doi:10.1016/j.eursup.2009.11.002.

Butterweck, V., & Khan, S. R. (2009). Herbal medicines in the management of urolithiasis: Alternative or complementary? *Planta Medica, 75*(10), 1095–1103. doi:10.1055/s-0029-1185719.

Dugdale, D. C., III, & Longstreth, G. F. (2011). Fecal impaction. *MedlinePlus.* Retrieved from http://www.nlm.nih.gov/medlineplus/ency/article/000230.htm.

Dugdale, D. C., III, & Longstreth, G. F. (2012). Bowel retraining. *MedlinePlus.* Retrieved from http://www.nlm.nih.gov/medlineplus/ency/article/003971.htm.

Esposito, C., Plati, A., Mazzullo, T., Fasoli, G., De Mauri, A., Grosjean, F., . . . Del Canton, A. (2007). Renal function and functional reserve in healthy elderly individuals. *Journal of Nephrology, 20,* 617–625.

Figueroa, T. E. (2012). Urinary incontinence in children. *Merck manual for health care professionals.* Retrieved from http://www.merckmanuals.com/professional/pediatrics/incontinence_in_children/urinary_incontinence_in_children.html.

Gordon, M., Naidoo, K., Akobeng, A. K., & Thomas, A. G. (2012). Osmotic and stimulant laxatives for the management of childhood constipation. *Cochrane database of systematic reviews, 7,* CD009118. doi:10.1002/14651858.CD009118.pub2.

Gould, C. V., Umscheid, C. A., Agarwal, R. K., Kuntz, G., Pegues, D. A. & the Healthcare Infection Control Practices Advisory Committee. (2009). *Guideline for prevention of catheter-associated urinary tract infections 2009,* Centers for Disease Control and Prevention. Retrieved from http://www.cdc.gov/hicpac/pdf/CAUTI/CAUTI-guideline2009final.pdf.

Infante, D. D., Segarra, O. O., Redecillas, S. S., Alvarez, M. M., & Miserachs, M. M. (2011). Modification of stool's water content in constipated infants: Management with an adapted infant formula. *Nutrition Journal, 10,* 55. doi:10.1186/1475-2891-10-55.

Johansson, R-M., Malmvall, B-E., Andersson-Gare, B., Larsson, B., Erlandsson, I., Sund-Levander, M., . . . Christensson, L. (2013). Guidelines for preventing urinary retention and bladder damage during hospital care. *Journal of Clinical Nursing, 22*(3–4), 347–355. doi:10.1111/j.1365-2702.2012.04229.x.

Johri, N., Cooper, B., Robertson, W., Choong, S., Rickards, D., & Unwin, R. (2010). An update and practical guide to renal stone management. *Nephron Clinical Practice, 116*(3), c159–c171. doi:10.1159/000317196.

Kalejaiye, O. & Speakman, M. J. (2009). Management of acute and chronic retention in men. *European Urology Supplements, 8,* 523–529. doi:10.1016/j.eursup.2009.02.002

Kaplan, S. A., McConnell, J. D., Roehrborn, C. G., Meehan, A. G., Lee, M. W., Noble, W. R., . . . Medical Therapy of Prostatic Symptoms Research Group. (2006). Combination therapy with doxazosin and finasteride for benign prostatic hyperplasia in patients with lower urinary tract symptoms and a baseline total prostate volume of 25 ml or greater. *Journal of Urology, 175*(1), 217–221. doi:10.1016/S0022-5347(05)00041-8.

Knight, J., Nigam, Y., & Jones, A. (2009). Effects of bedrest 2: Gastrointestinal, endocrine, renal, reproductive and nervous systems. *Nursing Times, 105*(22).

Kowalak, J. P. (Ed.). (2009). *Lippincott's nursing procedures* (5th ed.). Ambler, PA: Lippincott.

Lederer, E. (2013). Hyperkalemia. *Medscape Reference.* Retrieved from http://emedicine.medscape.com/article/240903-overview.

Loo, M. (2009). *Integrative medicine for children.* St. Louis, MO: Saunders Elsevier.

Markland, A. D., Richter, H. E., Fwu, C-W., Eggers, P., & Kusek, J. W. (2011). Prevalence and trends of urinary incontinence in adults in the United States, 2001 to 2008. *Journal of Urology, 186*(2), 589–593. doi:10.1016/j.juro.2011.03.114.

Mayo Clinic. (2011a). *Bed-wetting.* Retrieved from http://www.mayoclinic.com/health/bed-wetting/DS00611.

Mayo Clinic. (2011b). *Constipation.* Retrieved from http://www.mayoclinic.com/health/constipation/DS00063.

Mayo Clinic. (2011c). *Constipation in children.* Retrieved from http://www.mayoclinic.com/health/constipation-in-children/DS01138.

Mayo Clinic. (2011d). *Urinary incontinence.* Retrieved from http://www.mayoclinic.com/health/urinary-incontinence/DS00404.

Mayo Clinic. (2012a). *Fecal incontinence.* Retrieved from http://www.mayoclinic.com/health/fecal-incontinence/DS00477.

Mayo Clinic. (2012b). *Kidney stones.* Retrieved from http://www.mayoclinic.com/health/kidney-stones/DS00282.

McKay, S. L., Fravel, M., & Scanlon, C. (2012). Management of constipation. *Journal of Gerontological Nursing, 38*(7), 9–15. doi:10.3928/00989134-20120608-01.

Miller, C. A. (2009). *Nursing for wellness in older adults* (5th ed.). Philadelphia, PA: Lippincott.

Mody, L., Saint, S., Galecki, A., Chen, S., & Krein, S. L. (2010). Knowledge of evidence-based urinary catheter care practice recommendations among healthcare workers in nursing homes. *Journal of the American Geriatrics Society, 58*(8), 1532–1537. doi:10.1111/j.1532-5415.2010.02964.x.

Mugie, S. M., Benninga, M. A., & Di Lorenzo, C. (2011). Epidemiology of constipation in children and adults: A systematic review. *Best Practice and Research, Clinical Gastroenterology, 25*(1), 3–18. doi:10.1016/j.bpg.2010.12.010.

Musso, C. G., & Oreopoulos, D. G. (2011). Aging and physiological changes of the kidneys including changes in glomerular filtration rate. *Nephron Physiology, 119*(Suppl 1), P1–P5. doi:10.1159/000328010.

NANDA International. (2012). *NANDA nursing diagnoses: Definitions and classification 2012–2014.* Oxford, UK: Wiley-Blackwell.

National Digestive Diseases Information Clearinghouse. (2012). *Diarrhea.* Retrieved from http://digestive.niddk.nih.gov/ddiseases/pubs/diarrhea/.

National Kidney and Urologic Diseases Information Clearinghouse. (2010). *Urinary incontinence in women.* Retrieved from http://kidney.niddk.nih.gov/kudiseases/pubs/uiwomen/.

National Kidney and Urologic Diseases Information Clearinghouse. (2012a). *Kidney stones in children.* Retrieved from http://kidney.niddk.nih.gov/kudiseases/pubs/stoneschildren/.

National Kidney and Urologic Diseases Information Clearinghouse. (2012b). *Prostate enlargement: Benign prostatic hyperplasia.* Retrieved from http://kidney.niddk.nih.gov/kudiseases/pubs/prostateenlargement/.

National Kidney and Urologic Diseases Information Clearinghouse. (2012c). *Urinary incontinence in children.* Retrieved from http://kidney.niddk.nih.gov/kudiseases/pubs/uichildren/.

National Kidney and Urologic Diseases Information Clearinghouse. (2012d). *Urinary retention.* Retrieved from http://kidney.niddk.nih.gov/kudiseases/pubs/UrinaryRetention/.

National Kidney and Urologic Diseases Information Clearinghouse. (2013). *Diet for kidney stone prevention.* Retrieved from http://kidney.niddk.nih.gov/kudiseases/pubs/kidneystonediet/.

National Kidney Foundation. (2009). *Kidney stone treatment: Shock wave lithotripsy.* Retrieved from http://www.kidney.org/atoz/content/kidneystones_ShockWave.cfm.

North American Society for Pediatric Gastroenterology, Hepatology and Nutrition. (2006). Evaluation and treatment of constipation in infants and children: Recommendations of the North American Society for Pediatric Gastroenterology, Hepatology and Nutrition. *Journal of Pediatric Gastroenterology and Nutrition, 43*(3), e1–e13. doi:10.1097/01.mpg.0000233159.97667.c3.

Nurko, S., & Scott, S. M. (2011). Coexistence of constipation and incontinence in children and adults. *Best Practice & Research: Clinical Gastroenterology, 25*(1), 29–41.

Oman, K. S., Makic, M. B. F., Fink, R., Schraeder, N., Hulett, T., Keech, T., & Wald, H. (2012). Nurse-directed interventions to reduce catheter-associated urinary tract infections. *American Journal of Infection Control, 40*(6), 548–553. doi:10.1016/j.ajic.2011.07.018.

Palese, A., Buchini, S., Deroma, L., & Barbone, F. (2010). The effectiveness of the ultrasound bladder scanner in reducing urinary tract infections: A meta-analysis. *Journal of Clinical Nursing, 19*(21–22), 2970–2979. doi:10.1111/j.1365-2702.2010.03281.x.

Palmer, L. S. (2010). Biofeedback in the management of urinary continence in children. *Current Urology Reports, 11*(2), 122–127.

Papadakis, M. A., & McPhee, S. J. (Eds.). (2013). *Current medical diagnosis and treatment* (52nd ed.). New York, NY: McGraw-Hill.

Phelan, S., Kanaya, A. M., Subak, L. L., Hogan, P. E., Espeland, M. A., Wing, R. R. . . . Brown, J. S. (2009). Prevalence and risk factors for urinary incontinence in overweight and obese diabetic women. *Diabetes Care, 32*(8), 1391–1397. doi:10.2337/dc09-0516.

Portalatin, M., & Winstead, N. (2012). Medical management of constipation. *Clinics in Colon and Rectal Surgery, 25*(1), 12–19. doi:10.1055/s-0032-1301754.

Porth, C. M. (2011). *Essentials of Pathophysiology: Concepts of altered health states* (3rd ed.). Philadelphia, PA: Lippincott.

Porth, C., & Matfin, G. (2010). *Pathophysiology: Concepts of altered health states* (8th ed.). Philadelphia, PA: Lippincott Williams & Wilkins.

Quitadamo, P., Coccorulio, P., Guannetti, E., Romano, C., Chiaro, A., Campanozzi, A., . . . Staiano, A. (2012). A randomized, prospective, comparison study of a mixture of acacia fiber, psyllium fiber, and fructose vs polyethylene glycol 3350 with electrolytes for the treatment of chronic functional constipation in childhood. *Journal of Pediatrics, 161*(4), 710–715. doi:10.1016/j.peds.2012.04.043.

Rao, S. S. C. (2013). *Constipation in the older adult.* Retrieved from http://www.uptodate.com/contents/constipation-in-the-older-adult.

Rasquin, A., Di Lorenzo, C., Forbes, D., Guiraldes, E., Hyams, J. S., Staiano, A., & Walker, L. S. (2006). Childhood functional gastrointestinal disorders: Child/adolescent. *Gastroenterology, 130*(5), 1527–1537.

Revello, K., & Gallo, A-M. (2013). Implementing an evidence-based practice protocol for prevention of catheterized associated urinary tract infections in a progressive care unit. *Journal of Nursing Education and Practice, 3*(1), 99–107. doi:10.5430/jnep.v3n1p99.

Ricci, S. S., & Kyle, T. (2009). *Maternity and pediatric nursing.* Philadelphia, PA: Lippincott.

Rule, A. D., Cornell, L. D., & Poggio, E. D. (2011). Senile nephrosclerosis—Does it explain the decline in glomerular filtration rate with aging? *Nephron Physiology, 119*(Suppl 1), 6–11. doi:10.1159/000328012.

Savino, F., Viola, S., Erasmo, M., Di Nardo, G., Oliva, S., & Cucchiara, S. (2012). Efficacy and tolerability of peg-only laxative on faecal impaction and chronic constipation in children A controlled double blind randomized study vs. a standard peg-electrolyte laxative. *BMC Pediatrics, 12,* 178. doi:10.1186/1471-2431-12-178.

Selius, B. A., & Subedi, R. (2008). Urinary retention in adults: Diagnosis and initial management. *American Family Physician, 77*(5), 643–650.

Shah, B. J., Chokhavatia, S., & Rose, S. (2012). Fecal incontinence in the elderly: FAQ. *American Journal of Gastroenterology, 107*, 1635–1646.doi:10.1038/ajg.2012.284.

Spratto, G. R., & Woods, A. L. (2012). *Delmar nurse's drug handbook*. Clifton Park, NY: Delmar Cengage Learning.

Subak, L. L., Richter, H. E., & Hunskaar, S. (2009). Obesity and urinary incontinence: Epidemiology and clinical research update. *Journal of Urology, 182*(Supple 6), S2–S7. doi:10.1016/j.juro.2009.08.071.

Sureshkumar, P., Jones, M., Caldwell, P. H., & Craig, J. C. (2009). Risk factors for nocturnal enuresis in school-age children. *Journal of Urology, 182*(6), 2893–2899. doi:10.1016/j.juro.2009.08.060.

Toner, F., & Claros, E. (2012). Preventing, assessing, and managing constipation in older adults. *Nursing2012*. Retrieved from http://www.nursingcenter.com/pdf. asp?AID=1467783.

Townsend, M. K., Matthews, C. A., Whitehead, W. E., & Grodstein, F. (2012). Risk factors for fecal incontinence in older women. *American Journal of Gastroenterology, 108*, 113–119. doi:10.1038/ajg.2012.364.

Vasavada, S. P. (2013). Urinary incontinence. *Medscape Reference*. Retrieved from http://emedicine.medscape. com/article/452289.

Walker, M. (2011). *Breastfeeding management for the clinician: Using the evidence*. Sudbury, MA: Jones & Bartlett.

Wayment, R. O. (2012). Pregnancy and urolithiasis. *Medscape Reference*. Retrieved from http://emedicine. medscape.com/article/455830-overview.

Whitehead, W. E., Borrud, L., Goode, P. S., Meikle, S., Mueller, E. R., Tuteja, A., . . . Wen, Y. (2009). Fecal incontinence in US adults: Epidemiology and risk factors. *Gastroenterology, 137*, 512–517. doi:10.1053/j.gastro.2009.04.054.

Wolf, J. S., Jr. (2013). Nephrolithiasis. *Medscape Reference*. Retrieved from http://emedicine.medscape.com/ article/437096-overview.

Zieve, D. (2011). Enlarged prostate. *MedlinePlus*. Retrieved from http://www.nlm.nih.gov/medlineplus/ency/ article/000381.htm.

◢ THE CONCEPT OF FLUIDS AND ELECTROLYTES

The body is largely composed of fluid in many forms. Blood, serum, albumin, urine, bile, hormones, or cerebro-spinal fluid—these are just a few of the fluids required for homeostasis, a part of the delicate balance of fluids and electrolytes that promotes the body's functions.

Within each of these fluids are **electrolytes**, charged ions capable of conducting electricity, in various concentrations and combinations. Learning what fluids contain specific electrolytes can help nurses identify causes of electrolyte imbalances in clients and specifically design care to restore homeostasis.

Homeostasis depends on multiple physiological processes. Fluid and electrolyte balance is critical to maintaining health. Fluid and electrolyte imbalance can result from a variety of conditions, such as dehydration or renal failure, and can also negatively impact both chronic and acute illnesses. In turn, almost every illness has the potential to threaten this crucial balance. Even in the process of daily living, excessive temperatures or vigorous activity can disturb the balance if adequate intake of water and electrolytes is not maintained. Therapeutic measures can also disturb the body's homeostasis unless water and electrolytes are replaced. **<<**

Concept Learning Outcomes

After reading about this concept, you will be able to:

1. Summarize the physiology of the various body systems involved in the maintenance of fluid and electrolyte balance.
2. Examine the relationship between fluid and electrolyte balance and other concepts.
3. Identify commonly occurring alterations in fluid and electrolyte balance and their related therapies.
4. Differentiate common assessment procedures used to examine fluid and electrolyte balance across the life span.
5. Describe diagnostic and laboratory tests to determine the individual's fluid and electrolyte balance.
6. Explain management of fluid and electrolyte balance and prevention of imbalances.
7. Demonstrate the nursing process in providing culturally competent and caring interventions across the life span for individuals with common alterations in fluid and electrolyte balance.
8. Compare and contrast common independent and collaborative interventions for clients with alterations in fluid and electrolyte balance.

Concept Key Terms

Active transport, *338*
Anion, *336*
Body surface area, *343*
Cation, *336*
Colloid, *337*
Colloid osmotic pressure, *338*
Crystalloid, *337*
Dehydration, *339*
Diffusion, *338*
Edema, *338*
Electrolyte, *335*
Extracellular fluid (ECF), *336*
Filtration, *338*
Fluid volume deficit, *350*
Fluid volume excess, *350*
Hematocrit, *351*
Hydrostatic pressure, *338*
Hyperkalemia, *352*
Hypernatremia, *352*
Hypertonic, *337*

Hypodermoclysis, *352*
Hypokalemia, *352*
Hyponatremia, *352*
Hypotonic, *337*
Insensible fluid loss, *340*
Interstitial fluid, *336*
Intracellular fluid (ICF), *336*
Intravascular fluid, *336*
Ions, *336*
Isotonic, *337*
Milliequivalent, *336*
Obligatory losses, *340*
Oncotic pressure, *338*
Osmolality, *337*
Osmosis, *337*
Osmotic pressure, *337*
Saline, *337*
Solutes, *336*
Solvent, *337*
Tonicity, *337*
Transcellular fluid, *336*

▶ NORMAL FLUIDS AND ELECTROLYTES

The proportion of the human body composed of fluid is surprisingly large. Approximately 60% of the average healthy adult's weight is water, the primary body fluid. When an individual is healthy, this volume, reflected in body weight, remains relatively constant and the individual's weight varies by less than 0.2 kg (0.5 lb) in 24 hours, regardless of the amount of fluid ingested.

Water is vital to health and normal cellular functioning, serving as

- a medium for metabolic reactions within cells;
- a transporter for nutrients, waste products, and other substances;
- a lubricant;
- an insulator and shock absorber; and
- one means of regulating and maintaining body temperature.

Distribution and Composition of Body Fluids

The body's fluid is divided into two major compartments, intracellular and extracellular (**Figure 6–1 ●**). Both of these contain oxygen from the lungs, dissolved nutrients from the gastrointestinal tract, excretory products of metabolism such as carbon dioxide, and charged particles called **ions**. The composition of fluids varies from one body compartment to another.

Many salts dissociate in water; that is, they break up into electrically charged ions. The salt sodium chloride breaks up into one ion of sodium (Na^+) and one ion of chloride (Cl^-). These charged particles are called electrolytes because they are capable of conducting electricity. The number of ions that carry a positive charge, called **cations**, and ions that carry a negative charge, called **anions**, should be equal. Examples of cations are sodium (Na^+), potassium (K^+), calcium (Ca^{2+}), and magnesium (Mg^{2+}). Examples of anions are chloride (Cl^-), bicarbonate (HCO_3^-), phosphate (HPO_4^{2-}), and sulfate (SO_4^{2-}).

Electrolytes generally are measured in milliequivalents per liter of water (mEq/L) or milligrams per 100 mL (mg/100 mL). The term **milliequivalent** refers to the chemical combining power of the ion, or the capacity of cations to combine with anions to form molecules. This combining activity is measured in relation to the combining activity of the hydrogen ion (H^+). Thus, 1 mEq of any anion equals 1 mEq of any cation. Clinically, the milliequivalent system is most often used. However, nurses need to be aware that different systems of measurement may be found when interpreting laboratory results. For example, calcium levels frequently are reported in milligrams per deciliter (1 dL = 100 mL) instead of milliequivalents per liter. It also is important to remember that laboratory tests are usually performed using blood plasma, an extracellular fluid. Although these results may reflect what is happening in the intracellular fluid, it generally is not possible to directly measure electrolyte concentrations within the cell.

INTRACELLULAR FLUID Intracellular fluid (ICF) is found within the cells of the body. It constitutes approximately two thirds of the total body fluid in adults. Intracellular fluid is vital to normal cell functioning. It contains **solutes** (substances that dissolve in liquid) such as oxygen, electrolytes, and glucose, and provides a medium in which metabolic processes of the cell take place.

The composition of intracellular fluid differs significantly from that of extracellular fluid. Potassium and magnesium are the primary cations present in ICF, and phosphate and sulfate the major anions. As in extracellular fluid, other electrolytes are present within the cell, but in much smaller concentrations.

EXTRACELLULAR FLUID Extracellular fluid (ECF) is found outside the cells and accounts for about one third of total body fluid. It is subdivided into compartments. The two main compartments of ECF are intravascular and interstitial. **Intravascular fluid**, or plasma, accounts for approximately 20% of the ECF and is found within the vascular system. **Interstitial fluid**, accounting for approximately 75% of the ECF, surrounds the cells. The other compartments of ECF are the lymph and transcellular fluids. Examples of **transcellular fluid** are cerebrospinal, pericardial, pancreatic, pleural, intraocular, biliary, peritoneal, and synovial fluids.

In extracellular fluid, the principal electrolytes are sodium, chloride, and bicarbonate. Other electrolytes (e.g., potassium, calcium, and magnesium) are also present but in much smaller quantities. Plasma and interstitial fluid, the two primary components of ECF, contain essentially the same electrolytes and solutes, with the exception of protein. Plasma is a protein-rich fluid, containing large amounts of albumin; interstitial fluid contains little or no protein. Although extracellular fluid is in the smaller

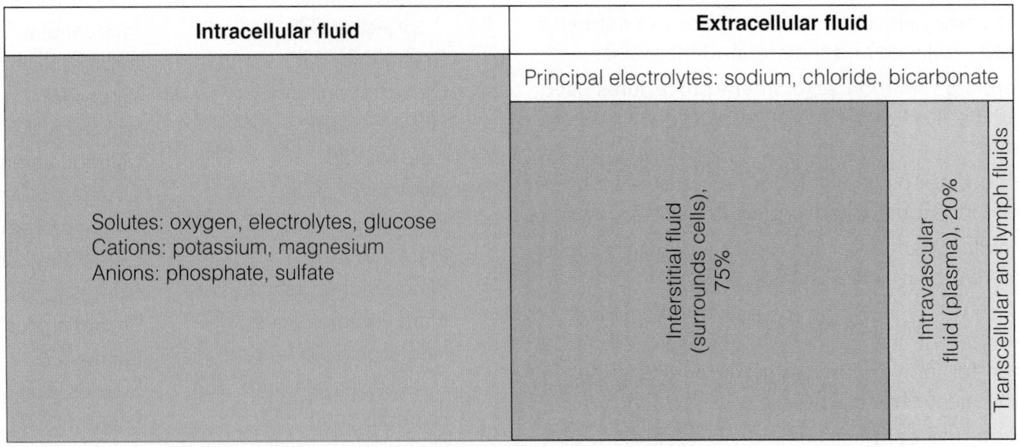

Intracellular fluid	Extracellular fluid
Solutes: oxygen, electrolytes, glucose Cations: potassium, magnesium Anions: phosphate, sulfate	Principal electrolytes: sodium, chloride, bicarbonate Interstitial fluid (surrounds cells), 75% · Intravascular fluid (plasma), 20% · Transcellular and lymph fluids

Figure 6–1 ● Electrolyte composition (cations and anions) of body fluid compartments.

TABLE 6–1   Electrolyte Concentrations in Body Fluid Compartments

| COMPONENTS | EXTRACELLULAR FLUID (ECF) | | INTRACELLULAR FLUID (ICF) |
	VASCULAR	INTERSTITIAL	
Na^+	High	High	Low
K^+	Low	Low	High
Ca^{2+}	Low	Low	Low (higher than ECF)
Mg^{2+}	Low	Low	High
PO_4^-	Low	Low	High
Cl^-	High	High	Low
Proteins	High	Low	High

of the two compartments, it is the transport system that carries nutrients to and waste products from the cells. Interstitial fluid transports wastes from the cells by way of the lymph system as well as directly into the blood plasma through capillaries.

Maintaining a balance of fluid volumes and electrolyte compositions in the fluid compartments of the body is essential to health. Normal and unusual fluid and electrolyte losses must be replaced if homeostasis is to be maintained.

Other body fluids, such as gastric and intestinal secretions, also contain electrolytes. Excessive loss of these fluids from the body (for example, with severe vomiting or diarrhea or when gastric suction removes the gastric secretions) is of particular concern, as fluid and electrolyte imbalances can result. Table 6–1 ● shows electrolyte concentrations in body fluid compartments.

Movement of Body Fluids

The body fluid compartments are separated from one another by cell membranes and the capillary membrane. Whereas these membranes are completely permeable to water, they are considered to be selectively permeable to solutes as substances move across them with varying degrees of ease. Small particles (e.g., ions, oxygen, and carbon dioxide) move easily across these membranes; larger molecules, such as glucose and proteins, have more difficulty moving among fluid compartments. The methods by which electrolytes and other solutes move are osmosis, diffusion, filtration, and active transport.

OSMOSIS   **Osmosis** is the movement of water across cell membranes, from the less concentrated solution to the more concentrated solution (**Figure 6–2** ●). In other words, water moves toward the higher concentration of solute in an attempt to equalize the concentrations on either side of the membrane.

Solutes may be **crystalloids** (salts that dissolve readily into true solutions) or **colloids** (substances such as large protein molecules that do not readily dissolve into true solutions). A **solvent** is the component of a solution that can dissolve a solute. An example of the solute/solvent relationship is sugar added to coffee: Sugar is the solute, and coffee is the solvent.

In the body, water is the solvent; the solutes include electrolytes, oxygen and carbon dioxide, glucose, urea, amino acids, and proteins. Osmosis occurs when the concentration of solutes is higher on one side of a selectively permeable membrane, such as the capillary membrane, than on the other side. For example, a marathon runner loses a significant amount of water through

perspiration, increasing the concentration of solutes in the plasma because of water loss. This higher solute concentration draws water from the interstitial space and cells into the vascular compartment to equalize the concentration of solutes in all fluid compartments. Osmosis is an important mechanism for maintaining homeostasis and fluid balance.

The concentration of solutes in body fluids is usually expressed as the **osmolality**. Osmolality is determined by the total solute concentration within a fluid compartment and is measured as parts of solute per kilogram of water.

Osmolality is reported as milliosmols per kilogram (mOsm/kg). Sodium is by far the greatest determinant of osmolality of extracellular fluids, with glucose and urea also contributing. Potassium, glucose, and urea are the primary contributors to the osmolality of intracellular fluid. The term **tonicity** may be used to refer to the osmolality of a solution. Solutions may be termed isotonic, hypertonic, or hypotonic. An **isotonic** solution has the same osmolality as body fluids. Normal **saline**, 0.9% sodium chloride, is an isotonic solution. **Hypertonic** solutions have a higher osmolality than body fluids; 3% sodium chloride is a hypertonic solution. **Hypotonic** solutions, such as one-half normal saline (0.45% sodium chloride), by contrast, have a lower osmolality than body fluids.

Osmotic pressure is the power of a solution to draw water across a semipermeable membrane. When two solutions of different solute concentrations are separated by a semipermeable membrane, the solution of higher solute concentration exerts a

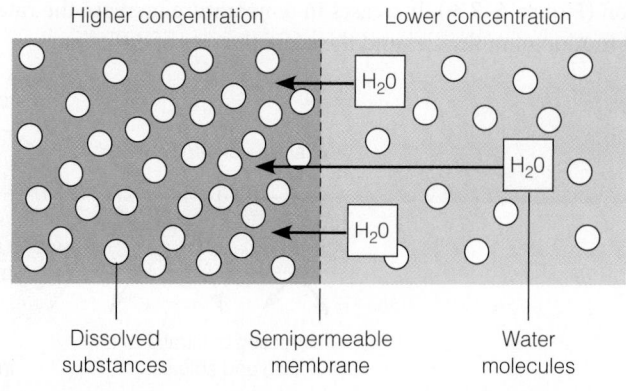

Figure 6–2 ● Osmosis: Water molecules move from the less concentrated area to the more concentrated area in an attempt to equalize the concentration of solutions on two sides of a membrane.

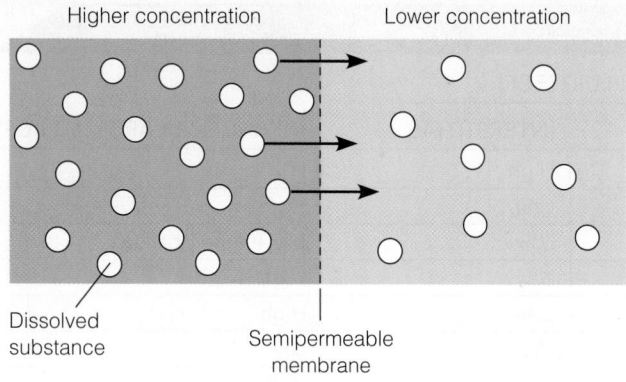

Higher concentration   Lower concentration

Dissolved substance

Semipermeable membrane

Figure 6–3 ● Diffusion: Molecules move through a semipermeable membrane from an area of higher concentration to an area of lower concentration.

higher osmotic pressure, drawing water across the membrane to equalize the concentrations of the solutions. For example, infusing a hypertonic intravenous solution such as 3% sodium chloride will draw fluid out of red blood cells (RBCs), causing them to shrink. On the other hand, a hypotonic solution administered intravenously will cause the RBCs to swell as water is drawn into the cells by their higher osmotic pressure. In the body, plasma proteins exert an osmotic draw called **colloid osmotic pressure** or **oncotic pressure**, pulling water from the interstitial space into the vascular compartment. This is an important mechanism in maintaining vascular volume.

DIFFUSION **Diffusion** is the continual intermingling of molecules in liquids, gases, or solids brought about by the random movement of the molecules. For example, two gases become mixed by the constant motion of their molecules. The process of diffusion occurs even when two substances are separated by a thin membrane. In the body, diffusion of water, electrolytes, and other substances occurs through the "split pores" of capillary membranes.

The rate of diffusion of substances varies according to (a) the size of the molecules, (b) the concentration of the solution, and (c) the temperature of the solution. Larger molecules move less quickly than smaller ones because they require more energy to move about. With diffusion, the molecules move from a solution of higher concentration to a solution of lower concentration (**Figure 6–3** ●). Increases in temperature increase the rate of motion of molecules and therefore the rate of diffusion.

FILTRATION **Filtration** is a process whereby fluid and solutes move together across a membrane from one compartment to another. The movement is from an area of higher pressure to one of lower pressure. An example of filtration is the movement of fluid and nutrients from the capillaries of the arterioles to the interstitial fluid around the cells. The pressure in the compartment that results in the movement of the fluid and substances dissolved in fluid out of the compartment is called filtration pressure. **Hydrostatic pressure** is the pressure a fluid exerts within a closed system on the walls of its container. The hydrostatic pressure of blood is the force blood exerts against the vascular walls (e.g., the artery walls). The principle involved in hydrostatic pressure is that fluids move from the area of greater pressure to the area of lesser pressure. Using the example of the blood vessels, the plasma proteins in the blood exert a colloid osmotic or oncotic pressure (see the earlier section on Osmosis) that opposes the hydrostatic pressure and holds the fluid in the vascular compartment to maintain the vascular volume. When the hydrostatic pressure is greater than the osmotic pressure, the fluid filters out of the blood vessels, which can lead to the development of **edema**, swelling caused by excess fluid trapped in body tissues. The filtration pressure in this example is the difference between the hydrostatic pressure and the osmotic pressure (**Figure 6–4** ●).

ACTIVE TRANSPORT Substances can move across cell membranes from a less concentrated solution to a more concentrated one by **active transport** (**Figure 6–5** ●). This process differs from diffusion and osmosis in that metabolic energy is expended. In active transport, a substance combines with a carrier on the outside surface of the cell membrane, and together they move to the inside surface of the cell membrane. Once inside, they separate, and the substance is released to the inside of the cell. Each substance requires a specific carrier, active transport requires enzymes, and energy is expended.

Active transport is particularly important in maintaining the differences in sodium and potassium ion concentrations of ECF and ICF. Under normal conditions, sodium concentrations are higher in the extracellular fluid, and potassium concentrations are higher inside the cells. To maintain these proportions, the active transport mechanism (the sodium-potassium pump) is activated, moving sodium out of the cells and potassium into the cells.

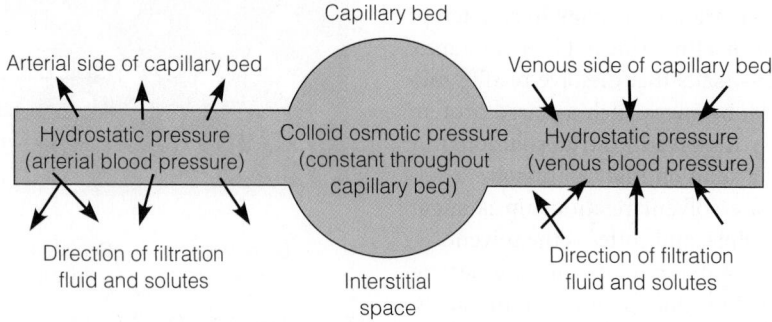

Capillary bed

Arterial side of capillary bed

Venous side of capillary bed

Hydrostatic pressure (arterial blood pressure)

Colloid osmotic pressure (constant throughout capillary bed)

Hydrostatic pressure (venous blood pressure)

Direction of filtration fluid and solutes

Interstitial space

Direction of filtration fluid and solutes

Figure 6–4 ● Schematic of filtration pressure changes within a capillary bed. On the arterial side, arterial blood pressure exceeds colloid osmotic pressure, so that water and dissolved substances move out of the capillary into the interstitial space. On the venous side, venous blood pressure is less than colloid osmotic pressure, so that water and dissolved substances move into the capillary.

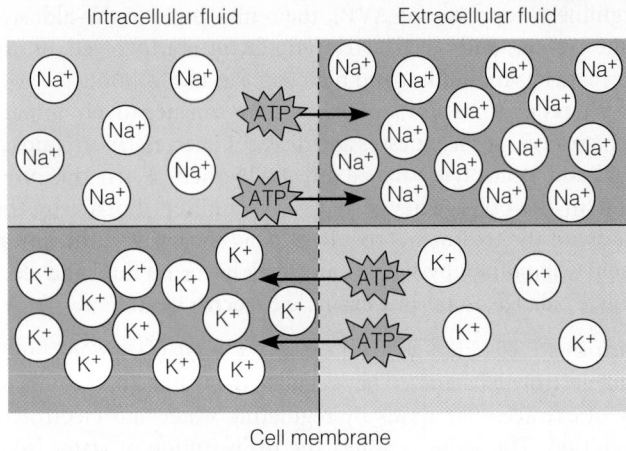

Figure 6–5 ● Active transport: Energy (ATP) is used to move sodium molecules and potassium molecules across a semipermeable membrane against sodium's and potassium's concentration gradients (i.e., from areas of lesser concentration to areas of greater concentration).

Regulating Body Fluids

In a healthy individual, the volumes and chemical composition of the fluid compartments stay within narrow, safe limits. Normally, fluid intake and fluid loss are balanced. Illness can upset this balance so that the body has too little or too much fluid. Fluid imbalance can result in a number of illnesses and conditions. The most common example is **dehydration**, a condition that occurs when a body does not take in as much water as it loses or lacks sufficient reserves to maintain proper function. Edema and hypervolemia occur when the body has excess fluid.

FLUID INTAKE During periods of moderate activity at moderate temperature, the average adult drinks about 1,500 mL per day but needs 2,500 mL per day, an additional 1,000 mL. This added volume is acquired from foods and the oxidation of these foods during metabolic processes. Interestingly, the water content of food is relatively large, contributing about 750 mL per day. The water content of fresh vegetables is approximately 90%, of fresh fruits about 85%, and of lean meats around 60%.

Water as a by-product of food metabolism accounts for most of the remaining fluid volume required. This quantity is approximately 200 mL per day for the average adult (**Table 6–2 ●**).

The thirst mechanism is the primary regulator of fluid intake. The thirst center is located in the hypothalamus of the brain. A number of stimuli trigger this center, including the osmotic pressure of body fluids, vascular volume, and angiotensin (a hormone released in response to decreased blood flow to

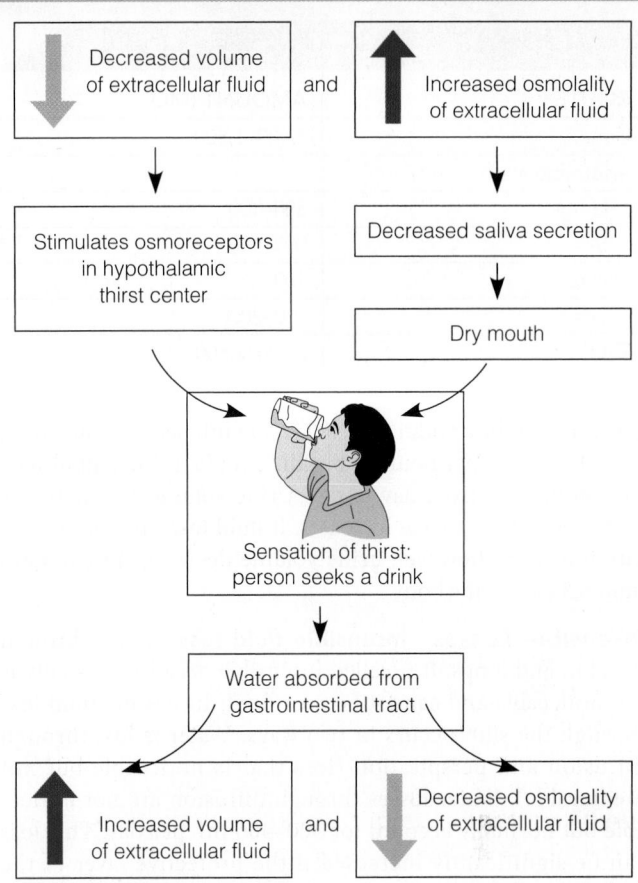

Figure 6–6 ● Factors stimulating water intake through the thirst mechanism.

the kidneys). For example, a long-distance runner loses significant amounts of water through perspiration and rapid breathing during a race, increasing the concentration of solutes and the osmotic pressure of body fluids. This increased osmotic pressure stimulates the thirst center, causing the runner to experience the sensation of thirst and the desire to drink to replace lost fluids.

Thirst is normally relieved immediately after drinking a small amount of fluid, even before the fluid is absorbed in the gastrointestinal tract. However, this relief is only temporary, and thirst returns in about 15 minutes. Thirst is again temporarily relieved after the ingested fluid distends the upper gastrointestinal tract. These mechanisms protect the individual from drinking too much, because it takes from 30 minutes to 1 hour for the fluid to be absorbed and distributed throughout the body. See **Figure 6–6 ●**.

FLUID OUTPUT Fluid losses from the body counterbalance the adult's 2,500-mL average daily intake of fluid, as shown in **Table 6–3 ●**. The four routes of fluid output are:

1. Urine
2. Insensible loss through the skin as perspiration and through the lungs as water vapor in the expired air
3. Noticeable loss through the skin
4. Loss through the intestines in feces.

Urine Urine formed by the kidneys and excreted from the urinary bladder is the major avenue of fluid output. Normal

TABLE 6–2 Average Daily Fluid Intake for an Adult	
SOURCE	AMOUNT (ML)
Oral fluids	1,200–1,500
Water in foods	750
Water as by-product of food metabolism	200
Total	2,150–2,450

TABLE 6–3 Average Daily Fluid Output for an Adult

ROUTE	AMOUNT (ML)
Urine	1,400–1,500
Insensible losses	
Lungs	300–400
Skin	300–400
Sweat	100
Feces	100–200
Total	2,200–2,600

urine output for an adult is 1,400–1,500 mL per 24 hours, or at least 0.5 mL/kg per hour. In healthy people, urine output may vary noticeably from day to day. Urine volume automatically increases as fluid intake increases. If fluid loss through perspiration is large, however, urine volume decreases to maintain fluid balance in the body.

Insensible Losses   Insensible fluid loss occurs through the skin and lungs. It is called insensible because it usually is not noticeable and cannot be measured. Insensible fluid loss through the skin occurs in two ways. Water is lost through diffusion and perspiration (loss that is noticeable but not measurable). Water losses through diffusion are not noticeable but normally account for 300–400 mL per day. This loss can be significantly increased if the protective layer of the skin is lost due to burns or large abrasions. Perspiration varies depending on factors such as environmental temperature and metabolic activity. Fever and exercise increase metabolic activity and heat production, thereby increasing fluid losses through the skin.

Another type of insensible loss is the water in exhaled air. In an adult, this is normally 300–400 mL per day. When the respiratory rate accelerates due to changes such as exercise or an elevated body temperature, this loss can increase.

Feces   The chyme that passes from the small intestine into the large intestine contains water and electrolytes. The volume of chyme entering the large intestine in an adult is normally about 1,500 mL per day. Of this amount, all but about 100 mL is reabsorbed in the proximal half of the large intestine.

Certain fluid losses are required to maintain normal body function. These are known as **obligatory losses**. An adult must excrete approximately 500 mL of fluid through the kidneys each day to eliminate metabolic waste products from the body. Losses of water through respirations, through the skin, and in feces are also obligatory losses, necessary for temperature regulation and elimination of waste products. The total of all these losses is approximately 1,300 mL per day.

MAINTAINING HOMEOSTASIS   The volume and composition of body fluids are regulated through several homeostatic mechanisms. As the kidneys regulate and filter waste, they return electrolytes such as potassium and sodium to the blood for use. The cardiovascular and respiratory systems ensure the body has adequate oxygen to function and use fluids and electrolytes appropriately. The immune system destroys foreign particles and pathogens that can undermine homeostasis. Hormones such as antidiuretic hormone (ADH; also known as

arginine vasopressin or AVP), the renin–angiotensin–aldosterone system, and atrial natriuretic factor are involved, as are mechanisms to monitor and maintain vascular volume.

Illness or injury to any one system can negatively impact homeostasis. Some illnesses and diseases, such as cancer, impact fluid and electrolyte balance directly by their destructive presence in the body. They also have an indirect impact by the nature of the treatments required to rid the body of the illness itself. Chemotherapy, which can wreak havoc on fluid and electrolyte balance, is a prime example of such a treatment.

Kidneys   The kidneys are the primary regulator of body fluids and electrolyte balance. They regulate the volume and osmolality of extracellular fluids by regulating water and electrolyte excretion. The kidneys adjust the reabsorption of water from plasma filtrate and ultimately the amount excreted as urine. Although 135–180 L of plasma per day is normally filtered in an adult, only about 1.5 L of urine is excreted. Electrolyte balance is maintained by selective retention and excretion by the kidneys. The kidneys also play a significant role in acid–base regulation, excreting hydrogen ions (H^+) and retaining bicarbonate.

Antidiuretic Hormone   Antidiuretic hormone, which regulates water excretion from the kidney, is synthesized in the anterior portion of the hypothalamus and acts on the collecting ducts of the nephrons. When serum osmolality rises, ADH is produced, causing the collecting ducts to become more permeable to water. This increased permeability allows more water to be reabsorbed into the blood. As more water is reabsorbed, urine output falls and serum osmolality decreases because the water dilutes body fluids. Conversely, if serum osmolality decreases, ADH is suppressed, the collecting ducts become less permeable to water, and urine output increases. Excess water is excreted, and serum osmolality returns to normal. Other factors also affect the production and release of ADH, including blood volume, temperature, pain, stress, and some drugs such as opiates, barbiturates, and nicotine. (See **Figure 6–7 ●**.)

Renin–Angiotensin–Aldosterone System   Specialized receptors in the juxtaglomerular cells of the kidney nephrons respond to changes in renal perfusion. This initiates the renin–angiotensin–aldosterone system. If blood flow or pressure to the kidney decreases, renin is released. Renin causes the conversion of angiotensinogen to angiotensin I, which is then converted to angiotensin II by angiotensin-converting enzyme (ACE) released from the lungs. Angiotensin II acts directly on the vasculature and promotes vasoconstriction; it also acts on the nephrons to promote sodium and water retention. In addition, it stimulates the release of aldosterone from the adrenal cortex. Aldosterone also promotes sodium retention in the distal nephron. The net effect of the renin–angiotensin–aldosterone system is to restore blood volume (and renal perfusion) through sodium and water retention.

Atrial Natriuretic Factor   Atrial natriuretic factor (ANF) is a peptide hormone released from cells in the atrium of the heart in response to excess blood volume and stretching of the atrial walls. Acting on the nephrons, ANF promotes sodium wasting and acts as a potent diuretic, thus reducing vascular volume. ANF also inhibits thirst, reducing fluid intake.

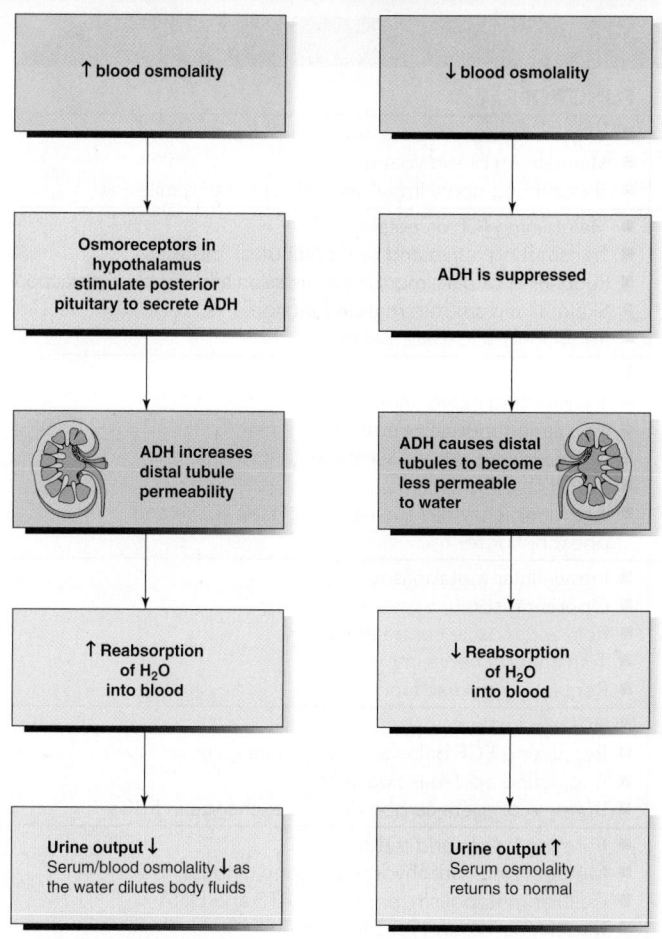

```
↑ blood osmolality                    ↓ blood osmolality
       |                                     |
       ↓                                     ↓
Osmoreceptors in                       ADH is suppressed
hypothalamus
stimulate posterior
pituitary to secrete ADH
       |                                     |
       ↓                                     ↓
ADH increases                          ADH causes distal
distal tubule                          tubules to become
permeability                           less permeable
                                       to water
       |                                     |
       ↓                                     ↓
↑ Reabsorption                         ↓ Reabsorption
of H₂O                                 of H₂O
into blood                             into blood
       |                                     |
       ↓                                     ↓
Urine output ↓                         Urine output ↑
Serum/blood osmolality ↓ as            Serum osmolality
the water dilutes body fluids          returns to normal
```

Figure 6–7 ● Antidiuretic hormone (ADH) regulates water excretion from the kidneys.

Regulating Electrolytes

Electrolytes are present in all body fluids and fluid compartments. Just as maintaining the fluid balance is vital to normal body function, so is maintaining electrolyte balance. Although the concentration of specific electrolytes differs between fluid compartments, a balance of cations (positively charged ions) and anions (negatively charged ions) always exists. Electrolytes are important for the following:

- Maintaining fluid balance
- Contributing to acid–base regulation
- Facilitating enzyme reactions
- Transmitting neuromuscular reactions.

Most electrolytes enter the body through dietary intake and are excreted in the urine. The body does not store some electrolytes, such as sodium and chloride, which must be consumed daily to maintain normal levels. Potassium and calcium, on the other hand, are stored in the cells and bone, respectively. When serum levels drop, ions can shift out of the storage "pool" into the blood to maintain adequate serum levels for normal functioning. The regulatory mechanisms and functions of the major electrolytes are summarized in **Table 6–4** ●.

SODIUM (Na⁺)   Sodium is the most abundant cation in extracellular fluid and a major contributor to serum osmolality.

Normal serum sodium levels are 135–145 mEq/L. Sodium functions largely in controlling and regulating water balance. When sodium is reabsorbed from the kidney tubules, chloride and water are reabsorbed with it, thus maintaining ECF volume. Sodium is found in many foods including bacon, ham, processed and canned foods, processed cheeses, and table salt.

POTASSIUM (K⁺)   Potassium is the major cation in intracellular fluids, with only a small amount found in plasma and interstitial fluid. ICF levels of potassium are usually 125–140 mEq/L, whereas normal serum potassium levels are 3.5–5.3 mEq/L. The ratio of intracellular to extracellular potassium must be maintained for neuromuscular response to stimuli. Potassium is a vital electrolyte for skeletal, cardiac, and smooth muscle activity. It is involved in maintaining acid–base balance as well, and it contributes to intracellular enzyme reactions. Potassium must be ingested daily because the body does not conserve it. Many fruits and vegetables, meat, fish, and other foods contain potassium.

CALCIUM (Ca²⁺)   The vast majority (99%) of calcium in the body is in the skeletal system, with a relatively small amount in extracellular fluid. Although this calcium outside the bones and teeth amounts to only about 1% of the total calcium in the body, it is vital in regulating muscle contraction and relaxation, neuromuscular function, and cardiac function. ECF calcium is regulated by a complex interaction of parathyroid hormone, calcitonin, and calcitriol, a metabolite of vitamin D. When calcium levels in the ECF fall, parathyroid hormone and calcitriol cause calcium to be released from bones into ECF and increase the absorption of calcium in the intestines, thus raising serum calcium levels. Conversely, calcitonin stimulates the deposition of calcium in bone, reducing the concentration of calcium ions in the blood.

With aging, the intestines absorb calcium less effectively and more calcium is excreted via the kidneys. Calcium shifts out of the bone to replace these ECF losses, increasing the risk of osteoporosis and fractures of the wrists, vertebrae, and hips. Lack of weight-bearing exercise (which helps keep calcium in the bones) and vitamin D deficiency (usually due to inadequate exposure to sunlight) contribute to this risk.

Milk and milk products are the richest sources of calcium, with other foods such as dark green leafy vegetables and canned salmon containing smaller amounts. Many clients benefit from calcium supplements.

Calcium levels are often reported in two ways, based on how the calcium circulates in the blood. Approximately 50% of blood calcium circulates in a free, ionized, or unbound form. The other 50% circulates in the blood bound to either plasma proteins or other nonprotein ions. Blood calcium is typically measured from the serum rather than total blood. The normal total serum calcium levels, which range from 9 to 11 mg/dL, represent both bound and unbound calcium. The normal ionized serum calcium, which ranges from 4.25 to 5.25 mg/dL, represents calcium circulating in the free, or unbound, form.

MAGNESIUM (Mg²⁺)   Magnesium is primarily found in the skeleton and intracellular fluid. It is the second most abundant intracellular cation, with normal serum levels of 1.5–2.5 mEq/L. It is important for intracellular metabolism, particularly in the production and use of adenosine triphosphate

TABLE 6–4   Regulation and Functions of Electrolytes

ELECTROLYTE	REGULATION	FUNCTION
Sodium (Na^+)	■ Renal reabsorption or excretion ■ Aldosterone increases Na^+ reabsorption in collecting duct of nephrons	■ Regulating ECF volume and distribution ■ Maintaining blood volume ■ Transmitting nerve impulses and contracting muscles
Potassium (K^+)	■ Renal excretion and conservation ■ Aldosterone increases K^+ excretion ■ Movement into and out of cells ■ Insulin helps move K^+ into cells; tissue damage and acidosis shift K^+ out of cells into ECF	■ Maintaining ICF osmolality ■ Transmitting nerve and other electrical impulses ■ Regulating cardiac impulse transmission and muscle contraction ■ Skeletal and smooth muscle function ■ Regulating acid–base balance
Calcium (Ca^{2+})	■ Redistribution between bones and ECF ■ Parathyroid hormone and calcitriol increase serum Ca^{2+} levels; calcitonin decreases serum levels	■ Forming bones and teeth ■ Transmitting nerve impulses ■ Regulating muscle contractions ■ Maintaining cardiac pacemaker (automaticity) ■ Blood clotting ■ Activating enzymes such as pancreatic lipase and phospholipase
Magnesium (Mg^{2+})	■ Conservation and excretion by kidneys ■ Intestinal absorption increased by vitamin D and parathyroid hormone	■ Intracellular metabolism ■ Operating sodium-potassium pump ■ Relaxing muscle contractions ■ Transmitting nerve impulses ■ Regulating cardiac function
Chloride (Cl^-)	■ Excreted and reabsorbed along with sodium in the kidneys ■ Aldosterone increases chloride reabsorption with sodium	■ HCl production ■ Regulating ECF balance and vascular volume ■ Regulating acid–base balance ■ Buffer in oxygen–carbon dioxide exchange in RBCs
Phosphate (PO_4^-)	■ Excretion and reabsorption by the kidneys ■ Parathyroid hormone decreases serum levels by increasing renal excretion ■ Reciprocal relationship with calcium: increasing serum calcium levels decrease phosphate levels; decreasing serum calcium increases phosphate	■ Forming bones and teeth ■ Metabolizing carbohydrate, protein, and fat ■ Cellular metabolism; producing ATP and DNA ■ Muscle, nerve, and RBC function ■ Regulating acid–base balance ■ Regulating calcium levels
Bicarbonate (HCO_3^-)	■ Excretion and reabsorption by the kidneys ■ Regeneration by kidneys	■ Major body buffer involved in acid–base regulation

(ATP). Magnesium also is necessary for protein and DNA synthesis within the cells. Only about 1% of the body's magnesium is in ECF, where it is involved in regulating neuromuscular and cardiac function. Maintaining and ensuring adequate magnesium levels are an important part of care of clients with cardiac disorders. Cereal grains, nuts, dried fruit, legumes, and green leafy vegetables are good sources of magnesium in the diet, as are dairy products, meat, and fish.

CHLORIDE (Cl^-)   Chloride is the major anion of ECF, and normal serum levels are 95–105 mEq/L. Chloride functions with sodium to regulate serum osmolality and blood volume. The concentration of chloride in ECF is regulated secondarily to sodium; when sodium is reabsorbed in the kidney, chloride usually follows. Chloride is a major component of gastric juice, as hydrochloric acid (HCl), and is involved in regulating acid–base balance. It also acts as a buffer in the exchange of oxygen and carbon dioxide in RBCs. Chloride is found in the same foods as sodium.

PHOSPHATE (PO_4^-)   Phosphate is the major anion of intracellular fluids. It also is found in ECF, bone, skeletal muscle, and nerve tissue. Normal adult serum levels of phosphate range from 2.5 to 4.5 mg/dL. Children have much higher phosphate levels than adults, with that of a newborn nearly twice that of an adult. Higher levels of growth hormone and a faster rate of skeletal growth probably account for this difference. Phosphate is

involved in many chemical actions of the cell; it is essential for functioning of muscles, nerves, and red blood cells. It is also involved in the metabolism of protein, fat, and carbohydrate. Phosphate is absorbed from the intestine and is found in many foods such as meat, fish, poultry, milk products, and legumes.

BICARBONATE (HCO_3^-)   Bicarbonate is present in both intracellular and extracellular fluids. Its primary function is regulating acid–base balance as an essential component of the carbonic acid–bicarbonate buffering system. Extracellular bicarbonate levels are regulated by the kidneys: Bicarbonate is excreted when too much is present; if more is needed, the kidneys both regenerate and reabsorb bicarbonate ions. Unlike other electrolytes that must be consumed in the diet, bicarbonate is produced through metabolic processes in adequate amounts to meet the body's needs.

Genetic and Lifespan Considerations

Age, sex, and body fat affect total body water. Infants have the highest proportion of water, accounting for 70%–80% of their body weight. The proportion of body water decreases with aging. In individuals older than 60 years of age, water represents only about 50% of the total body weight. Women have a lower percentage of body water than men. Women and older adults have reduced body water due to lower muscle mass and a greater

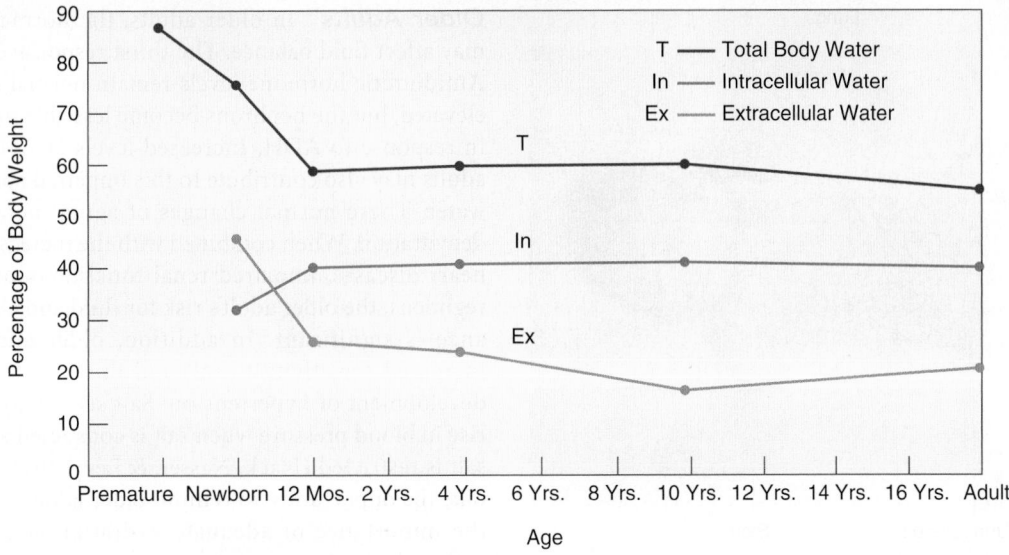

Figure 6–8 ● The major body fluid compartments at various ages. *Extracellular fluid* is composed mainly of vascular fluid (fluid in blood vessels) and interstitial fluid (fluid between the cells and outside the blood and lymphatic vessels.) *Intracellular fluid* is found within cells.

percentage of fat tissue. Fat tissue is essentially free of water, whereas lean tissue contains a significant amount of water.

The ability of the body to adjust fluid and electrolyte balance is influenced by age, gender and body size, and ethnicity.

AGE   Pediatric Differences   Infants and young children differ physiologically from adults in ways that make them vulnerable to fluid and electrolyte imbalances. Infants lose more fluid through the kidneys because immature kidneys are less able to conserve water than are adult kidneys. In addition, infants' respirations are more rapid and their **body surface area** (BSA; relationship between height and weight measured in

square meters) is proportionately greater than that of adults, increasing insensible fluid losses. This greater percentage of BSA also puts them at greater risk when burned.

The percentage of body weight that is composed of water also varies with age (**Figure 6–8** ●). The percentage is highest at birth (and higher in premature than in full-term infants) and decreases with age (**Figure 6–9** ●). Neonates and young infants have a proportionately larger extracellular fluid volume than older children and adults because their brain and skin (both rich in interstitial fluid) constitute a greater proportion of their body weight. Because much of our extracellular fluid is exchanged

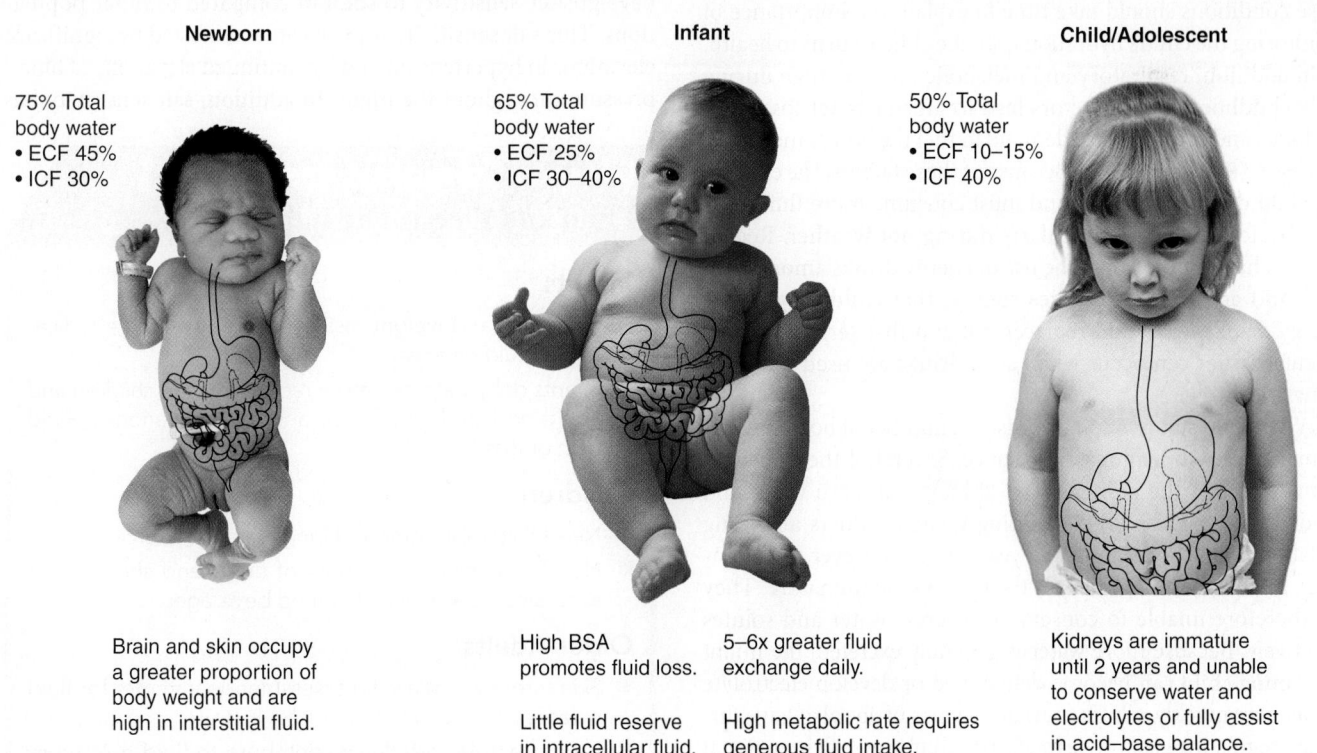

Newborn	Infant	Child/Adolescent
75% Total body water • ECF 45% • ICF 30%	65% Total body water • ECF 25% • ICF 30–40%	50% Total body water • ECF 10–15% • ICF 40%

Brain and skin occupy a greater proportion of body weight and are high in interstitial fluid.

High BSA promotes fluid loss.

Little fluid reserve in intracellular fluid.

5–6x greater fluid exchange daily.

High metabolic rate requires generous fluid intake.

Kidneys are immature until 2 years and unable to conserve water and electrolytes or fully assist in acid–base balance.

Figure 6–9 ● The newborn and infant have a high percentage of body weight comprised of water, especially extracellular fluid, which is lost from the body easily. Note the small stomach size, which limits ability to rehydrate quickly.

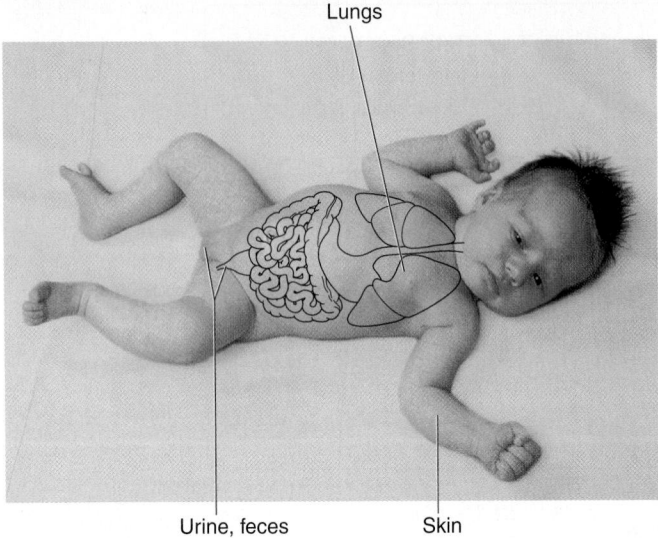

Figure 6–10 ● Normal routes of fluid excretion from infants and children.

each day, infants have a high daily fluid requirement with little fluid volume reserve, making them vulnerable to dehydration. As an infant grows, the proportion of water inside the cells increases, the extracellular amount decreases in comparison, and the risk of fluid imbalance begins to decrease.

Infants and children under 2 years of age lose a greater proportion of fluid each day than do older children and adults and are thus more dependent on adequate intake. Respiratory illnesses, stomach viruses resulting in vomiting or diarrhea, and burns can all result in fluid or electrolyte imbalance in an infant or young child, increasing the risk for serious complications. A nurse working with parents of a young child presenting with these conditions should take time to explain the importance of monitoring the child's hydration until the child returns to health.

In addition, respiratory and metabolic rates are high during early childhood. These factors lead to greater water loss from the lungs and greater water demand to fuel the body's metabolic processes (**Figure 6–10 ●**). Because of these factors, the exercising child dehydrates easily and must consume more fluid during physical activity, particularly during hot weather. Recent concern has emerged over the use of energy drinks among children and adolescents. Studies suggest that children confuse energy drinks with fluid replacement and that serious cardiovascular issues can occur when such drinks are used in excess (Rowland, 2011).

When fluid status is compromised, a number of body mechanisms activate to help restore balance. Several of these mechanisms occur in the kidneys. The kidneys conserve water and needed electrolytes while excreting waste products and drug metabolites. In children under 2 years of age, however, the glomeruli, tubules, and nephrons of the kidneys are immature. They are therefore unable to conserve or excrete water and solutes effectively. Because more water is generally excreted, the infant and young child can become dehydrated or develop electrolyte imbalances quickly. Children under 2 years of age also have difficulty regulating electrolytes such as sodium and calcium. Renal response to high solute loads is slower and less developed, with function improving gradually during the first year of life.

Older Adults In older adults, the normal aging process may affect fluid balance. The thirst response often is blunted. Antidiuretic hormone levels remain normal or may even be elevated, but the nephrons become less able to conserve water in response to ADH. Increased levels of ANF seen in older adults may also contribute to this impaired ability to conserve water. These normal changes of aging increase the risk of dehydration. When combined with the increased likelihood of heart diseases, impaired renal function, and multiple drug regimens, the older adult's risk for fluid and electrolyte imbalance is significant. In addition, older adults experience increased sensitivity to salt and this can be a factor in the development of hypertension. Salt sensitivity is defined as a rise in blood pressure when salt is consumed and a drop when salt is restricted (Flack, Nasser, & Levy, 2011). Nurses should take the opportunity to remind older adults and caregivers of the importance of adequate hydration at each interaction within the healthcare system.

GENDER AND BODY SIZE   Total body water is also affected by gender and body size. Because fat cells contain little or no water, and lean tissue has a high water content, individuals with a higher percentage of body fat have less body fluid. Women have proportionately more body fat and less body water than men. Water accounts for approximately 60% of an adult man's weight, but only 52% for an adult woman. In an individual with obesity, this percentage may be even less, with water being responsible for only 30%–40% of the individual's weight.

ETHNICITY   Suggested sodium intake is 1,500 to 2,300 mg per day or less. According to the Centers for Disease Control and Prevention (CDC) (2013), average sodium intake in the United States was more than 3,400 mg per day. Studies have indicated that certain ethnic groups such as African Americans have greater sensitivity to sodium compared to other populations. This salt sensitivity is primarily manifested by significant elevations in hypertension and by continued elevations of blood pressure throughout the night. In addition, salt sensitivity has

Lifespan Considerations
Fluid and Electrolyte Balance

Infants
- Fontanels and weight loss or gain are valuable indicators of fluid balance.
- Infants dehydrate at a more rapid rate than children and adults and are less tolerant of small fluctuations in fluid gain or loss.

Children
- Need fluid replacement during vigorous exercise.
- Need to consume a variety of fluids and should limit excessive intakes of caffeinated beverages.

Older Adults
- Skin turgor is not a valid assessment parameter for fluid balance.
- Cardiovascular problems contribute to fluid gain more often than an actual fluid and electrolyte imbalance.

Concepts Related to **Fluid and Electrolyte Balance**

Because fluid and electrolyte balance is critical to maintaining homeostasis, it both affects and is affected by other body systems. Throughout the day, the body makes adjustment to changes in temperature through fluid retention or excretion. To illustrate this adjustment, think about an athlete during a basketball game. As the game progresses, more and more sweating occurs. The body is getting rid of excess heat built up by acceleration in metabolism. As more and more heat is lost, and the external temperature rises, the body could respond with hyperthermia, which can be a life-threatening occurrence. (For further discussion, see the module on Thermoregulation.)

Imbalance of fluids and electrolytes can severely affect cognition. Moderate to severe dehydration can result in confusion in the healthiest adult. Fluid and electrolyte imbalance can also be a factor in delirium, and best practice dictates that fluid and electrolyte levels be assessed through diagnostic testing when a client presents with symptoms of delirium. (For further discussion, see the module on Cognition with a focus on confusion.) Similarly, cognitive factors may affect fluid status. Individuals with impaired function due to dementia, other brain disease, or certain drugs that depress the central nervous system may experience impairment of the thirst mechanism, increasing their risk for fluid imbalance.

Clients with an imbalance in fluid and electrolytes, particularly increases in fluid and sodium, can experience overload in the extravascular space, resulting in stress on the cardiovascular system. This is especially important for the client with congestive heart failure. Clients in overload and with resulting perfusion disorders are frequently placed on medications that can cause a fluid or electrolyte imbalance through gains or losses. For information on heart failure, see the module on Perfusion.

Because of the critical relationship between fluid and electrolyte balance and homeostasis, thorough assessment is necessary to determine the underlying cause of any imbalance and prevent or address potential complications.

CONCEPT	RELATIONSHIP TO FLUID AND ELECTROLYTE BALANCE	NURSING IMPLICATIONS
Elimination		
	Certain alterations (e.g., diarrhea) → fluid and electrolyte loss.	■ Be alert for symptoms of sodium and chloride loss. Evaluate client for the degree of dehydration. ■ Children become dehydrated more quickly than adults, so client education and quick response time are essential.
Cellular Regulation		
■ Blood loss	Acute hemorrhage → fluid imbalance manifested by hypovolemia.	■ Be alert to signs and symptoms of blood loss, fatigue, tachycardia, low hemoglobin and hematocrit. ■ Anticipate need for fluid replacement, administration of whole blood, packed cells, or colloids.
Cognition		
■ Mental status assessment	Electrolyte loss or excess can lead to changes in cognition. Confusion and coma may result if loss is severe.	■ Assess mentation. ■ Rule out acute brain trauma before considering other causes.
Thermoregulation		
■ Hyperthermia ■ Hypothermia	Fluid loss can lead to alterations in thermoregulation as the body loses its ability to regulate its heat loss due to hypovolemia.	■ Replace fluids, move client to air conditioning or shade. Consider electrolyte replacement fluid.
Perfusion		
■ Perfusion assessment ■ Medications: perfusion	Fluid loss leads to decreased perfusion.	■ Assess perfusion including pulses, nail beds, color, body position for comfort, orientation. ■ Administer oxygen as ordered. ■ Anticipate need for pharmacotherapy to improve cardiac output.

(continued on next page)

Concepts Related to **Fluid and Electrolyte Balance** (*continued*)

CONCEPT	RELATIONSHIP TO FLUID AND ELECTROLYTE BALANCE	NURSING IMPLICATIONS
Assessment		
	Assists in identifying underlying source of the imbalance and addressing potential complications.	■ Assess vital signs, intake and output, daily weights, skin turgor (except in older adults), and mentation. ■ See the Fluid and Electrolyte Assessment feature on page 349 for more information.

been linked to the need for higher dosages of antihypertensive medications in this population (Cotugna & Wolpert, 2011; Flack et al., 2011).

▶ ALTERATIONS TO FLUIDS AND ELECTROLYTES

Many health conditions cause changes in body fluids that must be regulated and managed. Sometimes management of fluid status in the home or in a short-term ambulatory facility can prevent more serious illness or hospitalization.

Alterations and Manifestations

Examples of conditions that commonly require fluid, electrolyte, or acid–base balance interventions include gastroenteritis, burns, kidney disorders, oral fluid restriction for surgery, anorexia or bulimia, and dehydration and electrolyte imbalances that can result from athletics in hot weather. Common alterations to fluid and electrolyte balance, their manifestations, and interventions and therapies for them are outlined in the Alterations and Therapies feature on page 347.

Compensation

The body continuously attempts to compensate for a fluid and electrolyte imbalance by shifting fluid and electrolytes from one component to another. Therefore, it is rare for only one type of imbalance to occur; the fluid and electrolyte status and symptoms are constantly changing, requiring ongoing assessment and management by the nurse.

Prevalence

Electrolyte disorders are found on a consistent basis among certain populations. Results of a study by Liamis and colleagues (2013) suggest that 15% of those surveyed had at least one electrolyte disorder, with hyponatremia (7.7%) and hypernatremia (3.4%) being most common. The disorders of diabetes mellitus and hypertension were associated with hyponatremia, hypomagnesemia, and hypokalemia. The use of diuretics was independently associated with electrolyte imbalances as were medications such as benzodiazepines. Because even mild electrolyte disorders are associated with significant illness and mortality, the nurse must monitor electrolyte balance on an ongoing basis and discuss discontinuation of problematic drugs.

CASE STUDY \\ PART 1

Hope Balan is a 22-year-old female who presents at the university clinic where you work with complaints of fever, chills, and a sore throat for more than 48 hours. She has been nauseated, and due to the severity of her sore throat has been limiting her fluid intake. Data collected during assessment identifies dry mucous membranes with cracked lips, a very red throat with patches of white, temperature of 102.8°F, pulse 120 bpm, and blood pressure 120/72 mmHg. Her skin is also warm and very dry. She is tired and has not been sleeping well.

Critical Thinking Questions Level I
1. Why is Ms. Balan's pulse rate high?
2. At this time, what are the priorities for care?
3. What additional assessment or diagnostic information would be helpful in planning care for Ms. Balan?

Critical Thinking Questions Level II
4. Would you expect to see an elevation in Ms. Balan's hemoglobin and hematocrit? Why or why not?
5. What would you expect her urine specific gravity to be?
6. What risk factors do college students have for fluid or electrolyte imbalance?

▶ PREVENTION

Lifestyle factors such as fluid intake, diet, exercise, and stress affect fluid and electrolyte balance. The intake of fluids and electrolytes is affected by the diet. Regular weight-bearing physical exercise such as walking, running, or bicycling has a beneficial effect on calcium balance. Individuals who maintain a healthy lifestyle are less likely to experience fluid and electrolyte imbalance.

Modifiable Risk Factors

Stress can increase cellular metabolism, blood glucose concentration, and catecholamine levels. In addition, stress can increase production of ADH, which in turn decreases urine production.

Medications may contribute to fluid and electrolyte imbalance. Diuretics are most often implicated, but clients taking antipsychotic agents are often at risk for alterations in fluid intake

Alterations and Therapies **Fluids and Electrolytes**

ALTERATION	DESCRIPTION	MANIFESTATIONS	INTERVENTIONS AND THERAPIES
Fluid volume deficit (dehydration)	Fluids are lost secondary to diarrhea, vomiting, inability to take in fluids, excessive perspiration, or increased basal metabolic rate due to fever, hyperthyroidism, or medications.	Dry to tenting skin Dry mucous membranes Increased hemoglobin and hematocrit Thirst Decreased urine output Weight loss	▪ Administer fluids via either the oral or intravenous route and treat the underlying cause.
Fluid volume excess	Too much fluid in the body may be caused by excessive fluid intake (intravenous fluid administration, water intoxication) or inadequate fluid excretion (e.g., kidney failure, poor perfusion to the kidneys secondary to congestive heart failure, low cardiac output, hypertension).	Edema Pitting edema Weight gain Ascites Adventitious lung sounds Increased central venous pressure	▪ Administer diuretics to increase fluid excretion, reduce fluid intake, and elevate head of bed if dyspnea results from pulmonary edema.
Elevated electrolyte level	Any electrolyte level may be elevated. Hypernatremia and hyperkalemia are the most common and significant extracellular findings.	Hyperkalemia: fatigue, nausea, muscle weakness, cardiac irregularities Hypernatremia: swelling, irritability, muscle spasms, thirst, confusion, coma Hypercalcemia: nausea and vomiting, excessive thirst, frequent urination, constipation, muscle pain	▪ Limit intake of the elevated electrolyte. ▪ Administer glucose and insulin to lower serum potassium levels by driving potassium from the extracellular space into the intracellular space. ▪ Diuretics will increase potassium and sodium loss but will also remove fluid.
Low electrolyte level	Any electrolyte level can decrease, but hypokalemia (low potassium) is the most common result of diuretics unless a potassium-sparing diuretic is administered.		▪ Administer electrolyte supplement, monitor serum electrolyte levels, monitor for symptoms associated with electrolyte imbalance. For example, low potassium levels can cause cardiac arrhythmias, and client should be placed on cardiorespiratory monitor.
Chronic kidney disease	Damage to the kidney over time causes progressive decline in kidney function; may be caused by diabetes mellitus, hypertension, or cardiac disease.	Confusion Fluid retention	▪ Initially may be treated with diuretics, progresses to need for dialysis or kidney transplant.
Acute renal failure	Rapidly progressive loss of kidney function is characterized by oliguria and fluid and electrolyte imbalances. Can be the result of disturbed blood supply to the kidneys, toxins, or kidney trauma; may be reversible or permanent.	Oliguria Fluid and electrolyte imbalances Fluid retention Drowsiness Dyspnea Fatigue Confusion Nausea	▪ Administer dialysis, monitor fluid and electrolyte balance, transplant kidney, treat the underlying cause.

due to the effect on thirst mechanisms. Clients taking vasoconstrictors, beta-blockers, and certain stimulants are at increased risk of fluid imbalance resulting from heat stroke, as these medications can impair the body's thermoregulation processes.

Heat-Related Illness

In the United States, approximately 6,000 people annually are treated in emergency departments for heat-related illness (CDC, 2011). Individuals with an illness and those participating in strenuous activity are at risk for fluid and electrolyte imbalances when the environmental temperature is high. Fluid losses through sweating increase in hot environments as the body attempts to dissipate heat.

Both salt and water are lost through sweating. When only water is replaced, the individual is at risk for salt depletion. Symptoms include fatigue, weakness, headache, and gastrointestinal symptoms such as loss of appetite and nausea. The risk of adverse effects increases if lost water is not replaced; the individual becomes at risk for heat exhaustion or stroke. Older adults, small children, athletes, laborers, and those who are ill are at greater risk.

Prevention of heat-related illness begins with education. As warmer temperatures approach, nurses can advise clients to (CDC, 2011):

- Limit outdoor activity during the hottest part of the day.
- Take frequent breaks for rest and water.
- Drink water before they begin to feel thirsty.
- Wear lightweight clothes.
- Work or exercise with others when engaging in activity outside.

See the module on Thermoregulation for more information.

▶ ASSESSMENT

Evaluating clients for fluid and electrolyte status is an important nursing care function. Components of the assessment include the nursing history and physical assessment of the client, clinical measurements, and review of laboratory test results.

Nursing Assessment

The nursing history is particularly important for identifying clients who are at risk for fluid and electrolyte imbalances. The current and past medical history reveals conditions such as chronic cardiac disease or diabetes mellitus that can disrupt normal balances. Medications prescribed to treat acute or chronic conditions (e.g., diuretic therapy for hypertension) also may put the client at risk for altered homeostasis. Functional, developmental, and socioeconomic factors must also be considered when assessing the client's risk. Older people and very young children, clients who must depend on others to meet their needs for food and fluid intake, and people who cannot afford or do not have the means to cook food for a balanced diet (e.g., homeless people) are at greater risk for fluid and electrolyte imbalances.

When obtaining the nursing history, the nurse needs not only to recognize risk factors but also to obtain data about the client's food and fluid intake, fluid output, and the presence of signs or symptoms suggesting altered fluid and electrolyte balance. The Assessment Interview provides examples of questions designed to elicit information regarding fluid and electrolyte balance.

Physical assessment to evaluate a client's fluid and electrolyte status focuses on the skin, the oral cavity and mucous membranes, the eyes, the cardiovascular and respiratory systems, and neurological and muscular status. Often, the agency will use a standardized form or computer software to help the nurse make sure that certain elements of physical assessment are conducted consistently between visits and from one client to the next. In addition to these important tools, the nurse should also make note of anything unusual in the client's physical appearance. For example, edema may be readily observed in a client's extremities and recorded during the physical assessment. Data from the physical assessment are used to expand and verify information obtained in the nursing history.

Clinical Measurements

Three simple clinical measurements that the nurse can initiate without a primary care provider's order are daily weights, vital signs, and fluid intake and output.

DAILY WEIGHTS Daily weight measurements provide a relatively accurate assessment of a client's fluid status. Significant changes in weight over a short time (e.g., more than 5 lb in a week or less) indicate acute fluid changes. Each kilogram (2.2 lb) of weight gained or lost is equivalent to 1 L of fluid gained or lost. Such fluid gains or losses indicate changes in total body fluid volume rather than in any specific compartment. Rapid losses or gains of 5%–8% of total body weight indicate moderate to severe fluid volume deficits or excesses. Regular assessment of weight is particularly important for clients in the community and in extended care facilities who are at risk for fluid imbalance. For these clients, measuring intake and output may be impractical because of lifestyle or problems with incontinence. Regular weight measurement, taken daily, every other day, or weekly, provides valuable information about the client's fluid volume status.

VITAL SIGNS Changes in the vital signs may indicate, or in some cases precede, fluid, electrolyte, and acid–base imbalances. For example, elevated body temperature may be a result of dehydration or a cause of increased body fluid losses.

Tachycardia is an early sign of hypovolemia. Pulse volume will decrease if a fluid volume deficit (FVD) is present and increase in the case of a fluid volume excess (FVE). Irregular pulse rates may occur with electrolyte imbalances.

Blood pressure, a sensitive measure to detect blood volume changes, may fall significantly with FVD and hypovolemia or increase with FVE. Postural, or orthostatic, hypotension may also occur with FVD and hypovolemia.

FLUID INTAKE AND OUTPUT The measurement and recording of all fluid intake and output (I&O) during a 24-hour period provides important data about the client's fluid and electrolyte balance.

Most agencies have a form for recording I&O, usually a bedside record on which the nurse lists all items measured and the

Fluid and Electrolyte Assessment

ASSESSMENT/METHOD	NORMAL FINDINGS	ABNORMAL FINDINGS	LIFESPAN OR DEVELOPMENTAL CONSIDERATIONS
Inspection			
View general appearance of skin.	Skin is appropriate color for ethnicity, is dry. Skin is firm, warm, and moist.	■ Flushed, warm, very dry ■ Very moist or diaphoretic or cool and pale	
Turgor: Gently pinch up a fold of skin over the sternum or inner aspect of thigh for adults.	Pinched tissue immediately returns to normal.	■ Skin remains tented for several seconds instead of immediately returning to normal position.	■ Gently pinch up a fold of skin on the abdomen or medial thigh for children. ■ Difficult to assess in very old individuals due to loss of skin elasticity. Use other methods to assess turgor.
Mucous membranes: Assess for dryness and cracking.	Moist in appearance.	■ Dry or cracking	
Edema: Assess for pitting by depressing skin over tibia or on top of foot.	No swelling noted. Depressed skin rebounds immediately.	■ Depression remains when tissue is depressed ("pitting").	
Eyes: Gently palpate eyeball with lid closed.	Eyeball is soft.	■ Eyeball is firm to touch.	
Fontanels: Inspect and gently palpate anterior fontanel.	Fontanel is soft, flush with scalp.	■ Fontanel is bulging. ■ Fontanel is sunken.	
Cardiovascular Assessment			
Heart rate and peripheral pulses	Regular rate, rhythm, pulses equal.	■ Tachycardia, bradycardia ■ Dysrhythmias ■ Weak thready pulse	■ Remember to evaluate vital signs in the normal range for children based on age.
Blood pressure	Normal for age	■ Hypotension, postural hypotension ■ Hypertension	■ Remember to evaluate vital signs in the normal range for children based on age.
Capillary refill: Assess for venous filling.	Quick, less than 2–3 seconds	■ Refill prolonged, sluggish	
Respiratory Assessment			
Assess rate and rhythm, lung sounds.	Rate is normal for age, lungs clear to auscultation.	■ Tachypnea, rales, wheezing, frothy sputum ■ Cyanosis is a late sign.	■ Remember to evaluate vital signs in the normal range for children based on age.
Neurological Assessment			
Assess level of consciousness (LOC), orientation, cognition.	Awake and arousable Alert and oriented to person, place, and time	■ Decreased LOC, lethargy, stupor, or coma ■ Disoriented, confused; difficulty concentrating	
Motor Function Assessment			
Strength and movement	Able to move all extremities as directed, firm grip, 2+ deep tendon reflexes	■ Weakness, decreased motor strength ■ Hyperactive or depressed deep tendon reflexes	
Chvostek sign: Tap over facial nerve about 2 cm anterior to tragus of ear.	No response	■ Facial muscle twitching including eyelids and lips on side of stimulus	
Trousseau sign: Inflate a blood pressure cuff on the upper arm to 20 mmHg greater than the systolic pressure, leave in place for 2–5 minutes.	No response	■ Carpal spasm: contraction of hand and fingers on affected side	

Assessment Interview   Fluid and Electrolyte Balance

Current and Past Medical History

■ Are you currently seeing a healthcare provider for treatment of any chronic diseases such as kidney disease, heart disease, high blood pressure, diabetes insipidus, or thyroid or parathyroid disorders?

■ Have you recently experienced any acute conditions such as gastroenteritis, severe trauma, head injury, or surgery? If so, describe them.

Medications and Treatments

■ Are you currently taking any medications on a regular basis such as diuretics, steroids, potassium supplements, calcium supplements, hormones, salt substitutes, or antacids?

■ Have you recently undergone any treatments such as dialysis, parenteral nutrition, or tube feedings or been on a ventilator? If so, when and why?

Food and Fluid Intake

■ How much and what type of fluids do you drink each day?

■ Describe your diet for a typical day. (Pay particular attention to the client's intake of foods high in sodium and of protein, whole grains, fruits, vegetables.)

■ Have you made any recent changes in your food or fluid intake, for example, as a result of following a weight-loss program?

■ Are you on any type of restricted diet?

■ Has your food or fluid intake recently been affected by changes in appetite, nausea, or other factors such as pain or difficulty breathing?

Fluid Output

■ Have you noticed any recent changes in the frequency or amount of urine output?

■ Have you recently experienced any problems with vomiting, diarrhea, or constipation? If so, when and for how long?

■ Have you noticed any other unusual fluid losses such as excessive sweating?

Fluid and Electrolyte Imbalances

■ Have you gained or lost weight in recent weeks?

■ Have you recently experienced any symptoms such as excessive thirst, dry skin or mucous membranes, dark or concentrated urine, or low urine output?

■ Do you have problems with swelling of your hands, feet, or ankles? Do you ever have difficulty breathing, especially when lying down or at night? How many pillows do you use to sleep?

■ Have you recently experienced any of the following symptoms: difficulty concentrating or confusion; dizziness or feeling faint; muscle weakness, twitching, cramping, or spasm; excessive fatigue; abnormal sensations such as numbness, tingling, burning, or prickling; abdominal cramping or distention; heart palpitations?

Source: Berman, A., Snyder, S. J., Kozier, B., & Erb, G. (2012). *Kozier & Erb's fundamentals of nursing: Concepts, process, and practice* (9th ed., p. 1470). Upper Saddle River, NJ: Pearson Education.

quantities per shift. Some agencies have another form for recording the specifics of intravenous fluids, such as the type of solution, additives, time started, amounts absorbed, and amounts remaining per shift.

It is important to inform clients, family members, and all caregivers that accurate measurements of the client's fluid I&O are required. Explain why and emphasize the need to use a bedpan, urinal, commode, or in-toilet collection device (unless a urinary drainage system is in place). Instruct the client not to put toilet tissue into the container with urine. Clients who wish to be involved in recording fluid intake measurements need to be taught how to compute the values and which foods are considered fluids.

To measure fluid intake, the client or the nurse must record each volume of fluid consumed or provided on the I&O form, specifying the time and type of fluid. All of the following fluids need to be recorded:

■ Oral fluids

■ Ice chips

■ Foods that are or tend to become liquid at room temperature

■ Tube feedings

■ Parenteral fluids

■ Intravenous medications

■ Catheter or tube irrigants.

To measure fluid output, measure the following fluids (remember to observe appropriate infection control precautions):

■ Urinary output

■ Vomitus and liquid feces (The amount and type of fluid and the time of output need to be specified.)

■ Tube drainage, such as gastric or intestinal drainage

■ Wound drainage and draining fistulas.

Fluid intake and output measurements are totaled at intervals pursuant to agency protocol or physician instruction, and the totals are recorded in the client's permanent record.

To determine whether the fluid output is proportional to fluid intake or whether there are any changes in the client's fluid status, the nurse (a) compares the total 24-hour fluid output measurement with the total fluid intake measurement, and (b) compares both to previous measurements. Urinary output is normally equivalent to the amount of fluids ingested; the usual range is 1,500–2,000 mL in 24 hours, or 40–80 mL in 1 hour (0.5 mL/kg per hour). Clients whose output substantially exceeds intake are at risk for **fluid volume deficit**. By contrast, clients whose intake substantially exceeds output are at risk for **fluid volume excess**. In assessing the client's fluid balance, it is important to consider additional factors that may affect intake and output. The client who is extremely diaphoretic or who has rapid, deep respirations has fluid losses that

<table>
<tr><td colspan="2">Box 6–1   Normal Electrolyte Values for Adults*</td></tr>
</table>

Box 6–1   Normal Electrolyte Values for Adults*

VENOUS BLOOD

Sodium	135–145 mEq/L
Potassium	3.5–5.3 mEq/L
Chloride	95–105 mEq/L
Calcium (total)	4.5–5.5 mEq/L or 9–11 mg/dL
(ionized)	50% of the total calcium (4.25–5.25 mg/dL, 2.2–2.5 mEq/L)
Magnesium	1.5–2.5 mEq/L or 1.8–3.0 mg/dL
Phosphate (phosphorus)	1.7–2.6 mEq/L or 2.5–4.5 mg/dL
Serum osmolality	280–300 mOsm/kg water

*Note: Normal laboratory values vary from agency to agency.

cannot be measured but must be considered in evaluating fluid status.

When a significant discrepancy is noticed between intake and output or when fluid intake or output is inadequate (for example, a urine output of less than 500 mL in 24 hours or less than 0.5 mL/kg per hour in an adult), this information should be reported to the charge nurse or primary care provider.

Diagnostic Tests

Many laboratory studies may be conducted to determine the client's fluid and electrolyte status. Some of the more common tests are discussed here.

SERUM ELECTROLYTES   Serum electrolyte levels are often routinely ordered for any client admitted to the hospital as a screening test for electrolyte imbalances. The most commonly ordered serum tests are for sodium, potassium, chloride, magnesium, and bicarbonate ions. Normal values of commonly measured electrolytes are shown in **Box 6–1** ●. Some primary care providers use a diagram format (**Figure 6–11** ●) for keeping track of the client's electrolytes when documenting in their progress notes.

COMPLETE BLOOD COUNT   The complete blood count (CBC), another basic screening test, includes information about the hematocrit (Hct). The **hematocrit** measures the volume (percentage) of whole blood that is composed of RBCs. Because the hematocrit is a measure of the volume of cells in relation to plasma, it is affected by changes in plasma volume. Thus, the hematocrit increases with severe dehydration and decreases

with severe overhydration. Normal hematocrit values are 40%–54% (men) and 36–46% (women).

OSMOLALITY   *Serum osmolality* is a measure of the solute concentration of the blood. The particles included are sodium ions, glucose, and urea (blood urea nitrogen, or BUN). Serum osmolality can be estimated by doubling the serum sodium, because sodium and its associated chloride ions are the major determinants of serum osmolality. Serum osmolality values are used primarily to evaluate fluid balance. Normal values are 280–300 mOsm/kg. An increase in serum osmolality indicates a fluid volume deficit; a decrease reflects a fluid volume excess.

Urine osmolality is a measure of the solute concentration of urine. The particles included are nitrogenous wastes, such as creatinine, urea, and uric acid. Normal values average 200–800 mOsm/kg H_2O in children and adults. An increased urine osmolality indicates a fluid volume deficit; a decreased urine osmolality reflects a fluid volume excess.

URINE SPECIFIC GRAVITY   Specific gravity is an indicator of urine concentration that can be performed quickly and easily by nursing personnel. Normal specific gravity ranges from 1.005 to 1.030 (usually 1.015–1.024). When the concentration of solutes in the urine is high, the specific gravity rises; in very dilute urine with few solutes, it is abnormally low.

CASE STUDY \\ PART 2

It has been 2 weeks since Ms. Balan was seen at the university clinic. She now presents to the emergency department, where you are the admitting nurse. Ms. Balan states she awoke this morning with severe pain in her back, fever, and chills. You note her face, hands, and feet are swollen. When you ask about prior medical history, she tells you she was well until 2 weeks ago when she had to visit the university clinic due to a very sore throat and nausea. She tells you she was diagnosed with strep throat and given amoxicillin clavulanate (Augmentin) to take for 10 days. She says she completed half of her prescription and began to feel better and did not finish the antibiotics. You take her blood pressure and it is 140/100 mmHg and her pulse rate is 92 bpm. Her temperature is 101.2°F. You ask her to provide a urine sample and note her urine is dark in color.

Ms. Balan's lab work reveals blood in her urine. The primary care provider makes a diagnosis of glomerulonephritis.

Critical Thinking Questions Level I
1. What would you expect to be the etiology of Ms. Balan's edema?
2. What is the etiology of hematuria?

Critical Thinking Questions Level II
3. What client teaching is essential for Ms. Balan at this time?
4. What will the treatment plan include to reduce the edema and help Ms. Balan's kidneys heal?

▶ INTERVENTIONS AND THERAPIES

Alterations in fluid and electrolytes may occur as a primary event or as a secondary response to a preexisting disease state or a sudden traumatic event. When alterations of fluid and electrolytes exceed the narrow limits consistent with health, the body needs to adjust quickly.

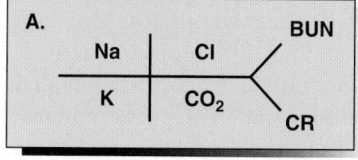

A.

| Na | Cl | BUN |
| K | CO₂ | CR |

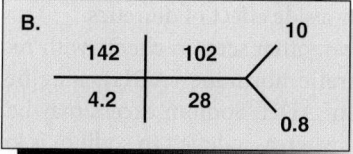

B.

| 142 | 102 | 10 |
| 4.2 | 28 | 0.8 |

Figure 6–11 ● *A*, Format for a diagram of serum electrolyte results. *B*, Example that may be seen in a primary care provider's documentation notes.

Evidence-Based Practice Improving the Documentation of Intake and Output

Problem

Even with the emergence of electronic documentation and record keeping, accurate documentation of client assessment remains problematic in many practice arenas. One of these areas involves the accurate and timely measurement and documentation of intake and output. When an estimate of output is required, discrepancies result when a client spills a drink or omits reporting a voiding occurrence. In many situations, accuracy in measurement is a significant indicator of client response to disease and subsequent response to medical and nursing intervention. The accurate measurement of urine output has been identified to be so significant that, in one critical care setting, it was labeled the "eighth vital sign" (Elliott & Coventry, 2012). Urine output may be the earliest indicator of fluid and electrolyte imbalance.

Evidence

Documentation is a task many nurses find problematic. Court cases acknowledging the lack and inaccuracy of documentation bring further anxiety (Jefferies et al., 2010). One such area of documentation involves the accurate recording of intake and output. A study to establish an evidence-based fluid balance measurement policy occurred in two 31-bed inpatient medical oncology units at a comprehensive cancer center. Findings of the study identified that ordering of intake and output was occurring out of habit rather than based on

client condition. Nurses were estimating intake in a number of situations, for example, when drinks were spilled, when clients failed to void in the specified container, and when meal trays were removed before accurate documentation was performed. A formal plan was developed to ensure accurate fluid balance measurement (Alexander & Allen, 2011).

A standardized plan that included ordering intake and output only when medically indicated was found to be beneficial in standardizing intake and output measurements.

Implications

When physicians and nurses operate from the same plan of care, documentation improves and better client outcomes are identified. In one study, guiding principles were developed that facilitated the process and provided for greater breadth and depth in the documentation process.

Critical Thinking Application

Consider the outcomes that could occur with inaccurate documentation and recording of intake and output. First, underestimates could lead to increased fluids being administered, which could result in fluid overload. Overestimates could lead to fluid restriction, which could result in additional adverse effects. For example, given the cellular intensity of chemotherapeutic agents, fluid restriction could lead to toxicity due to dehydration of the client's extravascular space.

Independent

Interventions for clients experiencing fluid and electrolyte balance typically include the following:

- Monitor intake and output (see the Evidence-Based Practice feature).
- Weigh client daily.
- Engage client in plan of care, particularly with regard to meal planning if clients require dietary modifications.
- Provide client education as indicated, especially with regard to medication regimens and side effects and prevention measures.

Collaborative

The severity of fluid and electrolyte imbalance determines whether treatment will consist of oral replacements or the initiation of intravenous therapy. Intravenous fluids may be ordered for the client with a fluid volume deficit if replacement oral fluids cannot be taken in sufficient quantity. In some clients where intravenous access proves problematic and management of dehydration becomes a concern, **hypodermoclysis**, fluid administered subcutaneously, may be employed as a fluid delivery method, especially among older adults. Electrolyte supplements may be used to replace electrolyte deficits. Diuretics may be ordered to reduce fluid volume excess.

Consult your skills manual for step-by-step descriptions of the following caring interventions related to fluids and electrolytes:

- Initiating intravenous therapy
- Intravenous management

- Monitoring fluid balance
- Medication administration
- Blood transfusions.

PHARMACOLOGIC THERAPY   Pharmacologic therapies are aimed at replacing what has been lost or depleting what may be excessive in order to restore a normal balance to the body's fluid and electrolytes. Fluids are replaced in an attempt to put back what is lost, so blood loss is replaced with blood transfusions, albumins, or other large-molecule protein solutions (colloid). Fluids lost secondary to excessive diuresis, perspiration, inadequate intake, or insensible water losses are replaced using crystalloids.

Electrolyte correction is highly dependent on the specific electrolyte and whether the body is in deficit or in excess. For example, elevated potassium levels (sometimes referred to as **hyperkalemia**) are ultimately corrected by dialysis, but treatments such as administration of glucose and insulin can help to drive potassium back into the cell where elevated levels will create less risk. A deficit in potassium is known as **hypokalemia**, and is frequently a side effect of diuretics.

Sodium excess, often seen in clients with reduced production of antidiuretic hormone (ADH), may be corrected by administration of ADH. Sodium excess may be referred to as **hypernatremia**, whereas a deficit in sodium is known as **hyponatremia**. Sodium deficiency may be treated with oral supplementation or, if the deficiency is severe or life threatening, intravenous supplementation may be administered.

Medications **Fluids and Electrolytes**

CLASSIFICATIONS AND DRUG EXAMPLES	MECHANISMS OF ACTION	NURSING CONSIDERATIONS
Electrolyte Supplements *Drug examples:* ■ sodium chloride (sodium supplement) ■ potassium chloride (potassium supplement)	Replace lost electrolytes and return to homeostasis. Routes may be oral or intravenous.	■ Monitor serum electrolyte levels, intake and output, vital signs.
Colloids *Drug examples:* ■ serum albumin ■ dextran 40	Expand the extracellular fluid volume through replacement of proteins, starches, or other large molecules. Routes are intravenous.	■ Carefully monitor client's condition, laboratory values, and renal function. Fluid overload can occur.
Crystalloids *Drug examples:* ■ 5% dextrose and water ■ normal saline solution ■ lactated Ringer's ■ 5% dextrose and 1/2 normal saline	Intravenous solutions that contain electrolytes and other agents that mimic the body's extracellular fluid are used to replace depleted fluid and promote urine output. They represent different tonicities.	■ Monitor client's fluid and electrolyte status.
Diuretics *Drug examples:* ■ furosemide ■ hydrochlorothiazide ■ spironolactone (Aldactone)	Some block sodium and water reabsorption, and thus promote urine output. Some inhibit aldosterone and inhibit fluid reabsorption. Some deplete potassium, some spare it.	■ Monitor intake and output, daily weight, serum electrolytes, and hydration status. ■ Thiazides are ineffective if the glomerular filtration rate is low.

REVIEW **The Concept of Fluids and Electrolytes**

RELATE Link the Concepts

Linking the concept of fluids and electrolytes with the concept of perfusion:

1. Describe the pathophysiology of fluid and electrolyte balance and how it impacts perfusion.

2. What measures could you implement to promote fluid balance when caring for a client with heart failure?

Linking the concept of fluids and electrolytes with the concept of elimination:

3. Describe the pathophysiology of fluid and electrolyte balance and how it impacts elimination.

4. What assessment findings would you expect to see when a client with benign prostatic hypertrophy experiences an alteration in fluid balance?

Linking the concept of fluids and electrolytes with the concept of tissue integrity:

5. Describe the pathophysiology of fluid and electrolyte balance and how it impacts tissue integrity.

6. What fluid and electrolyte balance assessment findings would you expect to see in a client who has experienced burns over 40% of his body?

READY Go to Companion Skills Manual

REFER Go to Pearson Nursing Student Resources
nursing.pearsonhighered.com

- Additional review materials

REFLECT Case Study \\ Part 3

Ms. Balan is admitted to the hospital because her condition does not improve. Her urinary output has continued to decrease to oliguria, and her edema continues. The nurse also notes the presence of ascites. Ms. Balan's blood pressure is now 148/104 mmHg. Her respiratory rate has increased and she complains of being short of breath. She also complains of a metallic taste in her mouth. The results of urinalysis demonstrate proteinuria. A diagnosis of acute renal failure is made.

Critical Reasoning Questions Level I

1. What type of renal failure does Ms. Balan have: prerenal, intrinsic, or postrenal? Why?

2. What is the etiology of the metallic taste Ms. Balan is experiencing?

3. What additional signs of acute renal failure would the nurse expect to find upon assessment?

Critical Reasoning Questions Level II

4. What is the reason for ascites?

5. What medications would you expect the provider to order?

EXEMPLAR 6.1 Fluid and Electrolyte Imbalance

EXEMPLAR LEARNING OUTCOMES

After reading about this exemplar, you will be able to:

1. Describe the pathophysiology, etiology, clinical manifestations, and direct and indirect causes of fluid and electrolyte imbalance.
2. Identify risk factors and prevention methods associated with fluid and electrolyte imbalance.
3. Illustrate the nursing process in providing culturally competent care across the life span for individuals with fluid and electrolyte imbalance.
4. Formulate priority nursing diagnoses appropriate for an individual with fluid and electrolyte imbalance.
5. Summarize therapies used by interdisciplinary teams in the collaborative care of an individual with fluid and electrolyte imbalance.
6. Plan evidence-based care for an individual with fluid and electrolyte imbalance and his or her family in collaboration with other members of the healthcare team.
7. Evaluate expected outcomes for an individual with fluid and electrolyte imbalance.

▶ EXEMPLAR OVERVIEW

The balance of fluids and electrolytes is delicate and easily disrupted by illness, injury, stress, or strenuous activity. Mild imbalances are resolved quickly by the body, often without any outside intervention. Should intervention be required for a mild fluid or electrolyte imbalance, there is seldom any residual effect. However, more severe imbalances that are complicated by disease processes or that last a significant time can result in both short-term and long-term effects. The body wants and expects a balance, and its chemistry leaves little room for error.

Factors such as illness, trauma, surgery, and medications can affect the body's ability to maintain fluid and electrolytes. The kidneys play a major role in maintaining fluid and electrolyte balance, and renal disease is a significant cause of imbalance. Clients who are confused, experiencing dementia, or unable to communicate their needs are at greater risk for inadequate fluid intake. Vomiting, diarrhea, or nasogastric suction can also lead to fluid and electrolyte imbalance.

Tissue trauma, such as burns or crush injury, causes fluid and electrolytes to be lost from damaged cells. Decreased blood flow to the kidneys as a result of impaired cardiac function stimulates the renin–angiotensin–aldosterone system, causing sodium and water retention. Medications such as diuretics or corticosteroids can result in abnormal losses of electrolytes and in fluid loss or retention. Complications from diabetes, cancer, and head injury also lead to electrolyte imbalances. Fluid and electrolyte imbalances can be classified in terms of fluid volume deficit, fluid volume excess, and electrolyte imbalance.

Fluid imbalances are of two basic types: isotonic and osmolar. **Isotonic imbalances** occur when water and electrolytes are

lost or gained in equal proportions so that the osmolality of body fluids remains constant. **Osmolar imbalances** involve the loss or gain of only water so that the osmolality of the serum is altered. Thus, four categories of fluid imbalances may occur:

1. An isotonic loss of water and electrolytes
2. An isotonic gain of water and electrolytes
3. A hyperosmolar loss of water only
4. A hypo-osmolar gain of water only.

These four imbalances are referred to respectively, as fluid volume deficit, fluid volume excess, dehydration (hyperosmolar imbalance), and overhydration (hypo-osmolar imbalance).

▌ FLUID VOLUME DEFICIT AND DEHYDRATION

▶ OVERVIEW

Fluid volume deficit (FVD) is a decrease in intravascular, interstitial, and/or intracellular fluid in the body. FVD is a relatively common problem that may exist alone or in combination with other electrolyte or acid–base imbalances. **Dehydration** refers to loss of fluid alone, even though it often is used interchangeably with FVD.

▶ PATHOPHYSIOLOGY AND ETIOLOGY

FVD can develop slowly or rapidly, depending on the type of fluid loss. Loss of extracellular fluid volume can lead to hypovolemia (decreased circulating blood volume). Often, electrolytes are lost along with fluid, resulting in an **isotonic fluid volume deficit**. When both water and electrolytes are lost, the serum sodium level remains normal, although levels of other electrolytes, such as potassium, may fall. Fluid is drawn into the vascular compartment from the interstitial spaces as the body attempts to maintain tissue perfusion. This eventually depletes fluid in the intracellular compartment as well.

Hypovolemia stimulates regulatory mechanisms to maintain circulation. The sympathetic nervous system is stimulated, as is the thirst mechanism. Antidiuretic hormone and aldosterone are released, prompting sodium and water retention by the kidneys. Severe fluid loss can lead to cardiovascular collapse.

Another classification of FVD is by location of the deficiency, whether extracellular or intracellular. Extracellular FVD occurs when there is not enough fluid in the extracellular compartment (vascular and interstitial). Depending on the cause of the deficit, sodium may be at a normal, low, or elevated level. Each level is described as a specific type of dehydration:

- **Isotonic dehydration** or *isonatremic dehydration:* This occurs when fluid loss is not balanced by intake and the losses of water and sodium are in proportion. The serum sodium is therefore within normal limits even though the circulating blood volume is lowered. Most of the fluid lost is from the extracellular component. This type of dehydration is commonly manifested through such symptoms as vomiting and diarrhea.

- **Hypotonic dehydration** or *hyponatremic dehydration:* This occurs when fluid loss is characterized by a proportionately greater loss of sodium than of water. Serum sodium is below normal levels. Compensatory fluid shifts occur from the extracellular to intracellular components in an attempt to establish normal proportions, thus leading to even greater extracellular dehydration. Hypotonic dehydration may result from severe and prolonged vomiting and diarrhea, burns, and renal disease. Administering intravenous fluid without electrolytes as treatment for dehydration increases client risk for hypotonic dehydration.

- **Hypertonic dehydration** or *hypernatremic dehydration:* This occurs when sodium loss is proportionately less than water loss. Serum sodium is above normal levels. Compensatory fluid shifts from the intracellular to extracellular components occur as the body attempts to establish normal proportions. The extracellular component therefore remains fairly normal, delaying the onset of signs and symptoms of dehydration until the condition is quite serious. Neurological symptoms reflecting intracellular imbalance may occur simultaneously with more common symptoms of dehydration. The condition may result from health problems, such as diabetes insipidus, or administration of intravenous fluid or tube feedings with high electrolyte levels.

Third Spacing

Fluid and electrolyte balance is essential to supporting vascular function. A shift of fluid from the vascular space into an area where it is not available to support normal physiological processes is known as **third spacing**. The trapped fluid represents a volume loss and is unavailable for normal physiological processes. Fluid may be sequestered in the abdomen or bowel or in other actual or potential body spaces, such as the pleural or peritoneal space. Fluid may also become trapped within soft tissues following trauma or burns.

In many cases, fluid is sequestered in interstitial tissues and unavailable to support cardiovascular function. For example, surgery triggers adaptive stress responses and the release of stress hormones (adrenocorticotropic hormone, cortisol, and catecholamines). These hormones increase blood glucose levels to provide increased fuel for metabolic processes and lead to vasoconstriction that redistributes blood to vital organs (the heart and brain). Renal blood flow falls, stimulating the renin–angiotensin–aldosterone system. This promotes sodium and water retention to maintain intravascular volume. The blood vessel and tissue damage caused by surgery stimulate the release of inflammatory mediators, such as histamine and prostaglandins. These substances lead to local vasodilation and increased capillary permeability, allowing fluid to accumulate in interstitial tissues. Third spacing is difficult to assess because it may not be reflected in measurable data.

Etiology

FVDs may be the result of excessive fluid losses, insufficient fluid intake, or failure of regulatory mechanisms and fluid shifts within the body. The most common cause of FVD is excessive loss of GI fluids, which can result from vomiting, diarrhea, GI suctioning, intestinal fistulas, or intestinal drainage. Other causes of fluid losses include the following:

- Excessive renal losses of water and sodium from diuretic therapy, renal disorders, or endocrine disorders
- Water and sodium losses during sweating from excessive exercise or increased environmental temperature
- Hemorrhage
- Chronic abuse of laxatives and/or enemas.

Inadequate fluid intake may result from lack of access to fluids, inability to request or to swallow fluids, oral trauma, or altered thirst mechanisms. Excessive exercise during very hot weather without sufficient fluid replacement can lead to fluid and electrolyte imbalance. Athletes and those whose jobs require them to expend enormous amounts of energy in hot climates, such as military personnel and ROTC candidates, are frequently at risk for fluid imbalance.

Burns of the skin usually involve a huge loss of body fluids, including water and electrolytes, particularly sodium. Hypotonic dehydration is the type most commonly seen in the initial period after a burn. Because serum proteins are also lost, body fluid is more likely to leak into interstitial spaces, causing edema and further contributing to the fluid deficit. The kidneys decrease urine production because of their decreased blood flow, which leads to lowered urinary output. While the fluid imbalance of burns is therefore very complicated, the first imbalance encountered often is that of dehydration with accompanying hyponatremia.

For burns, gastroenteritis, and other illnesses, initial dehydration in the first 3 days reflects a high loss of extracellular fluid. Approximately 80% of the fluid loss is extracellular and only approximately 20% is intracellular. Over time the relationship begins to change so that in illnesses lasting longer than 3 days, approximately 60% of fluid loss is extracellular while 40% is intracellular. Because the electrolyte composition of extracellular and intracellular fluids differ, electrolyte management needs to be adapted in long-term conditions.

CHILDREN   Children are more likely than adults to experience imbalance from exercise. Because children have a larger body surface area, they can gain more heat from the environment when it is hot and lose more when it is cold (Rowland, 2011). In addition, the high metabolic rate of children is further increased during exercise so that fluid lost in metabolism is significant. Children may not feel thirsty and so fail to drink even when dehydrated (Benelam, 2010).

A number of conditions may contribute to fluid imbalance in pediatric clients. Radiant heat (phototherapy) used to treat hyperbilirubinemia increases insensible water loss through the skin. The increased respiratory rate of pediatric clients increases insensible water loss from the lungs. Children are at increased risk for fever, which increases the metabolic rate and, therefore, the water demands of metabolism (for each degree Celsius increase above 37°C, 0.42 mL/kg/hr of additional fluid is needed). Vomiting and diarrhea also are common causes of fluid imbalance in children. Each year the hospital admission rate for children experiencing fluid and electrolyte imbalance is 400 for each 100,000 (Parkin et al., 2010).

One of the primary causes of gastroenteritis in children is rotavirus. In the United States, it is a major source of morbidity and hospitalization in children younger than 5 years of age. It accounts for approximately 300 deaths, more than 1.5 million outpatient visits, and 200,000 hospitalizations annually (Payne et al., 2013).

Infants may also experience fluid volume deficit through increased water loss in low-birth-weight infants who are kept

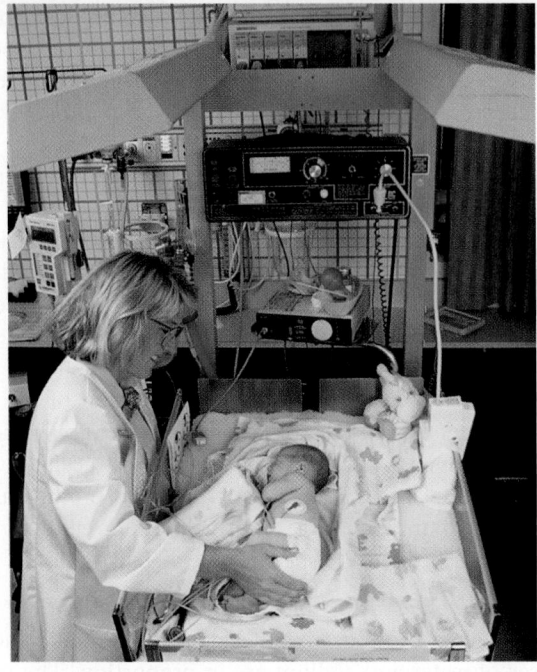

Figure 6–12 ● Use of an overhead warmer or phototherapy with an infant increases insensible fluid excretion through the skin, thus increasing the infant's required fluid intake.

under radiant warmers to maintain heat (**Figure 6–12 ●**). Their high body surface area puts them at risk of dehydration as a result of insensible fluid loss through the skin. Adrenal insufficiency, accumulation of extracellular fluid in a "third space" (e.g., the peritoneal cavity), and overuse of diuretics may also result in FVD in children. Overuse of diuretics is most often seen in adolescents with bulimia.

Lifespan Considerations   Dehydration Risk Factors and Symptoms in the Older Adult

Dehydration Risk Factors

Physical changes of aging:
- ↓ Total body water
- ↓ Lean body mass
- ↓ Thirst from aging, medication, or disease
- Impaired angiotensin production

Lack of free access to fluids:
- Dependency on others
- Cognitive impairment
- Physical impairment

Voluntary fluid restriction to manage:
- Incontinence
- Nocturia
- Diuretic side effect
- Limited physical movement due to mobility or pain issues

Increased insensitive fluid losses:
- Sweating from fever or climate
- ↑ Respiratory rate

- Vomiting
- Diarrhea
- Polyuria
- Exudative wound or fistula

Symptoms of Dehydration

Darkened urine
↓ Urine output
Confusion
Lethargy
Headache
Light-headedness
Sunken eyes
Dry mucous membranes
Dry axillae
Long tongue furrows
Postural changes in pulse and blood pressure

Clinical Manifestations and Therapies **Fluid Volume Deficit and Dehydration**

ETIOLOGY	CLINICAL MANIFESTATIONS	CLINICAL THERAPIES
Decreased cardiac output	■ Hypotension (may be orthostatic or postural initially) ■ Tachycardia ■ Weak pulse ■ Tachypnea ■ Reduced urine output or very concentrated urine with high specific gravity	■ Administer fluid replacement. ■ Administer isotonic intravenous solutions. ■ Monitor vital signs frequently. ■ Monitor intake and output. ■ Assess serum electrolytes and hematocrit. ■ Conduct urine specific gravity and osmolality. ■ Monitor central venous pressure.
Inadequate fluid supply to the tissues	■ Dry, cracked skin ■ Dry mucous membranes ■ Increased hematocrit ■ Poor skin turgor ■ Weight loss	■ Administer isotonic or mildly hypotonic solutions. ■ Measure weight daily. ■ Monitor serum electrolytes and serum osmolality. ■ Monitor hemoglobin and hematocrit.
Third spacing	■ Edema ■ Symptoms of FVD ■ No weight loss	■ Administer hypertonic intravenous fluid.

OLDER ADULTS Older adults have fewer intracellular reserves, contributing to rapid development of dehydration. A blunted thirst perception and altered hormone response also contribute to the development of dehydration in the older adult. Changes in mentation or cognition resulting from altered health status or adverse effects of medications can also increase the risk for an imbalance. Older adults should be informed to drink fluids even though they may not be thirsty (Scales, 2011).

Older adults who live in extended care homes and those who live at home but require assistance with ADLs are particularly vulnerable. Dependence on others, lack of free access to fluids, and voluntary fluid restrictions for fear of incontinence or reliance on others for toileting are factors that can contribute to inadequate fluid intake and chronic dehydration. See the Lifespan Considerations feature on dehydration risk factors and symptoms in the older adult.

PREGNANT WOMEN Pregnancy carries risk for FVD, especially during the first trimester when vomiting from morning sickness or blood loss during a spontaneous abortion (miscarriage) are most likely to occur. During the first prenatal visit, pregnant women should be taught how to avoid dehydration, the proper fluids to consume, and to avoid caffeine, alcohol, and diet drinks.

▶ CLINICAL MANIFESTATIONS

Symptoms of dehydration relate to the severity or degree of the body water deficit. They result from both the decreased fluid (e.g., diminished turgor and mucous membrane moisture) and the body's response to the fluid deficit (e.g., pulse and blood pressure changes). A water loss of as little as 1% to 2% impairs cognition and physical performance. Loss of 7% of body water can lead to circulatory collapse. With a rapid fluid loss (e.g., hemorrhage or uncontrolled vomiting), manifestations of hypovolemia develop rapidly. When the loss of fluid occurs more gradually, the client's fluid volume may become very low before symptoms develop.

Initial symptoms may be as simple as thirst. As fluid loss increases, however, lethargy, dry mucous membranes, reduced urine output, and weakness develop. Manifestations of acute fluid loss are similar to those associated with hypovolemic shock and include hypotension, tachycardia, tachypnea, decreased or absent urine output, and decreased cardiac output. Coma and death may result if treatment is not initiated. See the Multisystem Effects of Fluid Volume Deficit on page 358.

Because rapid weight loss is a good indicator of FVD, it is critical to weigh clients who are at risk for FVD daily. Each liter of body fluid weighs approximately 1 kg (2.2 lb). The severity of the FVD can be estimated by the percentage of rapid weight loss:

■ A loss of 2%–5% of total body weight represents mild FVD.

■ A loss of 6%–9% represents moderate FVD.

■ A loss of 10% or greater represents severe FVD.

Loss of interstitial fluid causes skin turgor (the skin's ability to return to normal shape after being pinched) to diminish. When pinched, the skin of a client with FVD remains elevated. Loss of skin elasticity with aging makes this assessment finding less accurate in older adults. Tongue turgor is not generally affected by age; therefore, assessing the size, dryness, and longitudinal furrows of the tongue may be a more accurate indicator of FVD.

Postural or orthostatic hypotension is a sign of hypovolemia. A drop of more than 15 mmHg in systolic blood pressure when changing from a lying to standing position often indicates loss of intravascular volume. Venous pressure falls as well, causing flat neck veins, even when the client is recumbent. Loss of intravascular fluid causes the hematocrit to increase.

Compensatory mechanisms to conserve water and sodium and maintain circulation account for many of the manifestations of FVD, such as tachycardia, pale, cool skin (vasoconstriction), and decreased urine output. The specific gravity of urine increases as water is reabsorbed in the

Multisystem Effects of Fluid Volume Deficit

Neurologic
- Altered mental status
- Anxiety, restlessness
- Diminished alertness/cognition
- Possible coma (severe FVD)

Mucous Membranes
- Dry; may be sticky
- ↓ tongue size, longitudinal furrows ↑

Integumentary
- Diminished skin turgor
- Dry skin
- Pale, cool extremities

Urinary
- ↓ urine output
- Oliguria (severe FVD)
- ↑ urine specific gravity

Cardiovascular
- Tachycardia
- Orthostatic hypotension (moderate FVD)
- Falling systolic/diastolic pressure (severe FVD)
- Flat neck veins
- ↓ venous filling
- ↓ pulse volume
- ↓ capillary refill
- ↑ hematocrit

Potential Complication
- Hypovolemic shock

Musculoskeletal
- Fatigue

Metabolic Processes
- ↓ body temperature (isotonic FVD)
- ↑ body temperature (dehydration)
- Thirst
- Weight loss
  2–5% mild FVD
  6–9% moderate FVD
  >10% severe FVD

TABLE 6–5   Comparison of Assessment Findings in Clients With Fluid Imbalance

ASSESSMENT	FLUID DEFICIT	FLUID EXCESS
Blood pressure	Decreased systolic blood pressure Postural hypotension	Increased
Heart rate	Increased	Increased
Pulse amplitude	Decreased	Increased
Respirations	Normal	Moist crackles Wheezes
Jugular vein	Flat	Distended
Edema	Rare	Dependent
Skin turgor	Loose, poor turgor	Taut
Output	Low, concentrated	May be low or normal
Urine specific gravity	High	Low
Weight	Loss	Gain

tubules. **Table 6–5** ● compares assessment findings for fluid deficit and fluid excess.

Children

As mentioned, symptoms of dehydration relate to the severity or degree of the body water deficit (**Table 6–6** ●). Mild dehydration is hard to detect in pediatric clients, because children appear alert and have moist mucous membranes. Infants may become irritable, and older children may become thirsty. In moderate dehydration, the child is often lethargic and sleepy. Children, especially infants, may experience periods of restlessness and irritability. Skin turgor is diminished, mucous membranes appear dry, and urine is dark in color and diminished in amount. Pulse rate is usually increased, and blood pressure can be normal or low (**Table 6–7** ●). Severe dehydration is manifested by increasing lethargy or nonresponsiveness, markedly decreased blood pressure, rapid pulse, poor skin turgor, dry

mucous membranes, seizure activity, and markedly decreased or absent urinary output.

Older Adults

Manifestations of FVD may be more difficult to recognize in the older adult. A change in mental status, memory, or attention may be an early sign. Skin turgor is less reliable as an indicator of dehydration, although assessing turgor over the sternum or on the inner aspect of the thigh may be more effective. Dry oral mucous membranes and tongue furrows also are indicative of dehydration. Chronic dehydration may result in dry, itchy skin; dull-appearing, brittle hair; and loss of thirst reflex. Orthostatic, or postural, hypotension may be unrelated to hydration status, and vital signs may not demonstrate typical changes in the dehydrated older adult. Other common signs of dehydration, such as dry oral membranes and upper body weakness, may be better indicators of dehydration in the older adult.

TABLE 6–6   Severity of Clinical Dehydration in Pediatric Clients

CLINICAL ASSESSMENT	MILD	MODERATE	SEVERE
% of body weight lost	≤5% (40–50 mL/kg)	6%–9% (60–90 mL/kg)	≥10% (≥100 mL/kg)
Level of consciousness	Alert, restless, thirsty	Infants and very young children: irritable or lethargic Older children and adolescents: alert, thirsty, restless	Infants and very young children: lethargic to comatose Older children and adolescents: often conscious, apprehensive
Blood pressure	Normal	Normal or low Older children and adolescents: postural hypotension	Low to undetectable
Pulse	Normal	Normal or rapid	Tachycardia or bradycardia
Skin turgor	Normal	Poor	Very poor
Mucous membranes	Moist	Dry	Parched
Urine	May appear normal	Decreased output (<1 mL/kg/hr), dark color; increased specific gravity	Very decreased or absent output
Thirst	Slightly increased	Moderately increased	Greatly increased unless lethargic
Fontanel	Normal	Sunken	Sunken
Extremities	Warm; normal capillary refill	Delayed capillary refill (>2 sec)	Cool, discolored, delayed capillary refill (>3–4 sec)
Respirations	Normal	Normal or rapid	Changing rate and pattern
Eyes	Normal	Slightly sunken, decreased tears	Deeply sunken, absent tears

TABLE 6–7 Clinical Manifestations of Extracellular Fluid Volume Deficit

ETIOLOGY	CLINICAL MANIFESTATIONS
Decreased fluid volume	Weight loss
	Sunken fontanel (infant)
Inadequate circulating blood volume to offset the force of gravity when in upright position	Postural blood pressure drop
Dizziness	Decreased intravascular volume
Increased small-vein filling time	Delayed capillary refill time
	Flat neck veins when supine
Inadequate circulation to the brain	Dizziness, syncope
Inadequate circulation to the kidneys	Oliguria
Cardiac reflex response to decreased intravascular volume	Thready, rapid pulse
Decreased interstitial fluid volume	Decreased skin turgor

▶ **COLLABORATION**

The diagnosis of dehydration is best accomplished by clinical observations. As stated earlier, the major observation that provides clues about the degree of dehydration is the percentage of weight loss. Interdisciplinary care typically is not required in cases of mild impairment. For clients with moderate to severe fluid loss, collaborative care will depend on the underlying cause of the imbalance, presenting symptoms, and assessment of the client's care needs.

Diagnostic Tests

The serum electrolyte panel may be helpful in severe and continuing dehydration that is complicated by electrolyte imbalance or acidosis. The panel includes serum electrolytes, creatinine, and glucose tests. Elevated BUN (5–25 mg/dL) and low serum bicarbonate (<16 mmol/L) are also useful in identifying moderate and severe dehydration (Madati & Bachur, 2008). The results can be used to target the fluid type and amount to best meet the imbalances identified. Urine specific gravity may provide useful information in adults and older children who are dehydrated. However, because of the inability of the child under 2 years of age to concentrate urine effectively, a rising specific gravity may not be seen as definitively in the younger dehydrated child.

Clinical Therapies

Medical management depends on accurate identification of the degree of dehydration. The treatment for extracellular FVD is administration of fluid containing sodium. This may be accomplished by oral rehydration therapy or by intravenous fluids.

ORAL REHYDRATION   Oral rehydration is the safest and most effective treatment for FVD in alert clients who are able to take oral fluids. Adults require a minimum of 1,500 mL of fluid

Evidence-Based Practice Maintaining Oral Hydration in Older Adults

Problem
Abdallah and colleagues (2009) report that dehydration is one of the 10 most common diagnoses responsible for hospitalizing older adults. Older adults are at risk for dehydration due to decreased fluid intake or increased fluid loss. Factors that lead to these decreases in intake are decreased thirst sensation and self-limiting intake to prevent bladder fullness and incontinence. Laboratory findings of dehydration include hypernatremia, elevated BUN, and a BUN-to-creatinine ratio greater than 25:1. Complications of fluid deficit include constipation, infections, renal failure, and death. African Americans, women, people with obesity, and residents of long-term care facilities are particularly at risk.

Evidence
In a qualitative study by Godfrey and colleagues (2012), the authors interviewed 21 older people ages 68 to 96 and 21 staff and family who provided hydration care. The authors evaluated drinking patterns, drink availability, and feelings regarding the pleasures of drinking. Factors identified as positively affecting intake were the pleasures of drinking as social interaction and ease of accessibility, temperature of drinks, and lighting. The more pleasurable the experience, the more the participants were likely to drink. Pinto and Grose (2010) provided additional evidence-based practice guidelines for oral hydration in older adults. The authors identify assessment guidelines and outline what current evidence suggests and what interventions should be implemented about maintaining oral hydration in older adults.

The authors suggested that a contributing factor to the problem of decreased fluid intake in the population is that nurses may lack education specific to the hydration needs of this population. Nurses may fail to realize that older adults may not have access to fluids or may limit their intake of fluids. Nurses may also fail to assess symptoms of dehydration in this population.

Implications
In addition to educating nurses about the hydration needs of older adults and symptoms of dehydration in this population, suggestions for encouraging fluid intake include involving family and friends in oral hydration interventions and assessment, scheduling fluid consumption consistently during waking hours, and providing fluids of different types based on an assessment of client preferences and care needs and serving foods at appropriate temperatures. Godfrey et al. (2012) suggest the use of insulated mugs to keep fluids at the right temperature and providing mugs that can be used by individuals who have less strength and dexterity.

Critical Thinking Application
Why do nurses often overlook fluid needs in clients? What role might medication therapy play in the decreased fluid intake in older adults? What type of fluid administration schedules should be developed to help ensure improved hydration status? How does alteration in taste affect fluid intake? What is the relationship between dysphagia and fluid imbalance?

per day, or approximately 30 mL/kg body weight (ideal body weight is used to calculate fluid requirements for clients who are obese), for maintenance. Fluids are replaced gradually, particularly in older adults, to prevent rapid rehydration of the cells. In general, fluid deficits are replaced at a rate of approximately 30%–50% of the deficit per 24 hours.

With mild fluid deficits, in which the loss of electrolytes has been minimal (e.g., moderate exercise in warm weather), fluid replacement may be accomplished with water alone. When the fluid deficit is more severe, and when electrolytes have also been lost (e.g., FVD caused by vomiting or diarrhea, strenuous exercise for longer than an hour or two), a carbohydrate/electrolyte solution, such as a sports drink, ginger ale, or a rehydrating solution (e.g., Pedialyte or Rehydralyte), is more appropriate. These solutions provide sodium, potassium, chloride, and calories to help meet metabolic needs.

For children with mild to moderate dehydration, oral rehydration therapy is the first intervention, given in frequent, small amounts. A useful guideline for starting oral rehydration is 1 to 3 teaspoons of fluid every 5 to 15 minutes. For the first 2 to 4 hours of treatment, 50 mL of fluid for each kilogram of weight should be the target intake. Hospitalized children and those with severe hydration usually require intravenous fluids following careful assessment of the type of imbalance.

INTRAVENOUS FLUIDS   When the fluid deficit is severe or the client is unable to ingest fluids, the intravenous route is used to administer replacement fluids (**Table 6–8** ●). Isotonic electrolyte solutions (0.9% NaCl or Ringer's solution) are used to expand plasma volume in clients who are hypotensive or to replace abnormal losses, which are usually isotonic in nature. Normal saline (0.9% NaCl) tends to remain in the vascular compartment, increasing blood volume. When administered rapidly, however, this solution can precipitate acid–base imbalances, so balanced electrolyte solutions, such as lactated Ringer's solution, are preferred to expand plasma volume. Often, Ringer's lactate is administered intravenously followed by or accompanied with dilute saline, such as one-half or one-quarter normal saline. This fluid combination replenishes the extracellular fluid volume and adds solutes to return the body fluid to normal.

Five percent dextrose in water or 0.45% NaCl (one-half normal saline) is given to provide water to treat total body water deficits. The D_5W mixture is isotonic (similar in tonicity to the plasma) when administered and thus does not provoke hemolysis of RBCs.

TABLE 6–8   Commonly Administered Intravenous Fluids

	FLUID AND TONICITY	USES
Dextrose in water Solutions	5% dextrose in water (D_5W; Isotonic)	■ Replaces water losses ■ Provides free water necessary for cellular rehydration ■ Lowers serum sodium in hypernatremia
	10% dextrose in water ($D_{10}W$; Hypertonic)	■ Provides free water ■ Provides nutrition (supplies 340 kcal/L)
	20% dextrose in water ($D_{20}W$; Hypertonic)	■ Supplies 680 kcal/L ■ May cause diuresis
	50% dextrose in water ($D_{50}W$; Hypertonic)	■ Supplies 1,700 kcal/L ■ Used to correct hypoglycemia
Saline solutions	0.45% sodium chloride; Hypotonic	■ Provides free water to replace hypotonic fluid losses ■ Maintains levels of plasma sodium and chloride
	0.9% sodium chloride; Isotonic	■ Expands intravascular volume ■ Replaces water lost from extracellular fluid ■ Used with blood transfusions ■ Replaces large sodium losses (as from burns)
	3% sodium chloride; Hypertonic	■ Corrects serious sodium depletion
Combined dextrose and saline solution	5% dextrose and 0.45% sodium chloride; Isotonic	■ Provides free water ■ Provides sodium chloride ■ Maintenance fluid of choice if there are no electrolyte imbalances
Multiple electrolyte solutions	Ringer's solution; Isotonic (electrolyte concentrations of sodium, potassium, chloride, and calcium are similar to plasma levels)	■ Expands the intracellular fluid ■ Replaces extracellular fluid losses
	Lactated Ringer's solution	■ Replaces fluid losses from burns and the lower gastrointestinal tract ■ Fluid of choice for acute blood loss

The dextrose is metabolized to carbon dioxide and water, leaving free water available for tissue needs. Hypotonic saline solution (0.45% NaCl with or without added electrolytes) or 5% dextrose in 0.45% sodium chloride may be used as maintenance solutions. These solutions provide additional electrolytes (e.g., potassium), a buffer (lactate or acetate) as needed, and water. When dextrose is added, they also provide a minimal number of calories.

A fluid challenge (the rapid administration of a designated amount of intravenous fluid) may be performed to evaluate fluid volume when urine output is low and cardiac or renal function is questionable. A fluid challenge helps to prevent fluid volume overload resulting from intravenous fluid therapy when cardiac or renal function is compromised.

In children under 2 years of age, the glomeruli, tubules, and nephrons of the kidneys are immature. They are thus unable to conserve or excrete water and solutes effectively. Because more water is generally excreted, the infant and young child can become dehydrated or develop electrolyte imbalances quickly. In addition, infants have a weaker transport system for ions and bicarbonate, placing them at greater risk for acidosis and acid–base imbalances. Children under 2 years of age also have difficulty regulating electrolytes, such as sodium and calcium. Renal response to high solute loads is slower and less developed, with function improving gradually during the first year of life. As a result, fluid challenge must be administered with caution in young children.

NURSING PROCESS

Nurses are responsible for identifying clients at risk for FVD, initiating and carrying out measures to prevent and treat FVD and reduce the risk of complications, and monitoring the effects of therapy. Health promotion activities focus on teaching clients to prevent FVD, including instructing clients who are ill regarding the importance of maintaining fluid intake, particularly during periods of fever.

Assessment

Carefully monitor clients at risk for abnormal fluid losses through routes such as vomiting, diarrhea, nasogastric suction,

increased urine output, fever, or wounds. Monitor fluid intake in clients with decreased level of consciousness, disorientation, nausea, **anorexia** (loss of appetite), and physical limitations. Assess hydration by looking at skin for dryness, flakiness, or scaling as well as tenting when skin is pinched up (skin turgor). Check oral mucous membranes for dryness.

Collect the following assessment data through the health history interview and physical examination:

- *Health history.* Risk factors, such as medications and acute or chronic renal or endocrine disease; precipitating factors, such as hot weather, extensive exercise, lack of access to fluids, and recent illness (especially if accompanied by fever, vomiting, and/or diarrhea); and onset and duration of symptoms
- *Physical assessment.* Weight; vital signs, including orthostatic blood pressure and pulse; peripheral pulses and capillary refill; jugular neck vein distention; skin color, temperature, and turgor; level of consciousness and mentation; urine output. (See the Lifespan Considerations feature for physical assessment of the older adult.)

Diagnosis

Appropriate nursing diagnoses may include the following:

- *Deficient Fluid Volume*
- *Ineffective Peripheral Tissue Perfusion* related to hypovolemia
- *Risk for Injury* related to postural hypotension
- *Confusion*
- *Activity Intolerance.*

(NANDA-I © 2012)

Planning

Appropriate outcomes, planned together with clients and caregivers, may include the following:

- The client will achieve electrolyte and fluid balance.
- The client will drink 1,500 mL of fluid per day.
- The client will relate the need to replace fluids lost during exercise with sports drinks.
- The client will return to normal hydration status and not develop hypovolemic shock.

For pediatric clients:

- The parents will relate strategies for preventing the child from becoming dehydrated.
- The parents will describe appropriate home management of fluid replacement for diarrhea and vomiting.
- The parents will describe when to seek health care if a child's condition worsens.

Implementation

The focus of care for the client with FVD is on managing the effects of the deficit and preventing complications.

- Record intake and output accurately; occasionally, hourly intake and output may be indicated.
- Weigh the client daily with the same scale and in same or similar clothing (young children should be weighed without clothing). Compare to past weights and calculate weight loss.
- Take vital signs, central venous pressure (CVP), and peripheral pulse volume at least every 4 hours.

Evidence-Based Practice Do Children Participating in Athletics Need Specific Fluid Replacement?

Problem

Fluid loss through simple exercise may be minimal and not require fluid replacement. However, for activities performed for longer durations (especially in warm/hot environments), intake of electrolytes and supplemental carbohydrate can be advantageous for retention of fluid and exercise performance. Does this apply to children?

Evidence

Evidence suggests that there is inequality in fluid intake compared to water loss in children. Results from this correlational study by Williams and Blackwell (2012) demonstrated that fluid losses compared between adults and children were similar, with sodium and chloride loss the greatest. Although evidence was not completely validated due to limited numbers (21) of study participants, outcomes suggested that lack of fluid replacement led to underperformance in children.

Implications

Based on these studies the recommendation from Williams and Blackwell (2012) for fluid replacement in children during exercise should be 13 mL/kg (6 mL/lb) for each hour of exercise. In addition, children needed to be reminded and encouraged to drink fluids. The type of fluid should be based on the likes and dislikes of the child. Carbonated beverages and juices should be avoided because they lead to gastric upset. Nurses must teach those who coach or sponsor children in outside activities to provide hydration breaks and encourage players to drink, even if they are not thirsty.

Critical Thinking Application

How can nurses educate local coaches and children-focused activity centers on the hydration needs of children? Develop a teaching plan that provides information about signs of dehydration in children and provide data about fluid replacement needs.

- Administer and monitor intake of fluids as prescribed.
- Administer intravenous fluid using an electronic infusion pump.
- Monitor laboratory values (electrolytes, BUN, creatinine, osmolality, and urine specific gravity).
- Monitor for changes in level of consciousness and mental status.
- Reposition every 2 hours if client is unable to move independently.
- Initiate safety precautions to avoid falls secondary to dizziness or loss of balance.
- Teach client and family how to reduce orthostatic hypotension:
  a. Move from one position to another in stages; for example, raise the head of the bed before sitting up, and sit for a few minutes before standing.
  b. Avoid prolonged standing.
  c. Rest in a recliner rather than in bed during the day.
  d. Use assistive devices to pick up objects from the floor rather than stooping.
- Teach importance of maintaining adequate fluid intake (at least 1,500 mL/day).
- Teach how to prevent fluid deficit:
  a. Avoid exercising during extreme heat.
  b. Increase fluid intake during hot weather.
  c. If vomiting, take small frequent amounts of ice chips or clear liquids, such as flat cola or ginger ale.
  d. Reduce intake of coffee, tea, and alcohol, which increase urine output and can cause fluid loss (recent studies have called into question the diuretic effects of caffeine).

Sugar facilitates the absorption of sodium in oral rehydration fluids. Teach parents not to give diet beverages for oral rehydration, because they contain no sugar and will not be effectively absorbed. However, if an oral rehydration solution is too concentrated, it can worsen the diarrhea. Juice and cola are highly concentrated and should be diluted to half-strength when given to a child who has diarrhea. Encourage parents to keep an oral rehydration solution in liquid or powder form on hand at all times and to use these solutions rather than juice or soda when the child first develops diarrhea.

Evaluation

Evaluate the client's progress toward meeting the outcomes created in collaboration with the client, and adjust the nursing plan of care as indicated. The client with severe FVD may require evaluation of his or her condition every few minutes to hourly until progress is made.

Expected outcomes of nursing care for the client with dehydration include the following:

- The client has water and electrolytes that are balanced in intracellular and extracellular compartments as measured by serum electrolytes, hematocrit, and assessment findings.
- The client's urinary output is within normal limits.
- The client's fluid intake is adequate to meet maintenance needs.
- The client's vital signs are within normal limits.

FLUID VOLUME EXCESS

▶ OVERVIEW

Fluid volume excess (FVE) results when both water and sodium are retained in the body. FVE may be caused by fluid overload (excess water and sodium intake) or by impairment of the mechanisms that maintain homeostasis leading to excess intravascular fluid (**hypervolemia**) and excess interstitial fluid (edema).

▶ PATHOPHYSIOLOGY AND ETIOLOGY

Extracellular fluid volume excess occurs when there is too much fluid in the extracellular compartment (vascular and interstitial). This imbalance may also be called saline excess or extracellular volume overload. An increase in total body sodium content causes an increase in total body water. Because the increase in sodium and water is isotonic, the serum sodium and osmolality remain normal, and the excess fluid remains in the extracellular space.

Stress responses activated before, during, and immediately after surgery commonly lead to increased antidiuretic hormone and aldosterone levels, leading to sodium and water retention. In the immediate postoperative period, however, this additional fluid tends to be sequestered in interstitial tissues and unavailable to support cardiovascular and renal function (see earlier discussion of third spacing in this module). This sequestered fluid is reabsorbed into the circulation within approximately 48–72 hours after surgery. Although it is then normally eliminated through a process of diuresis, clients with heart or kidney failure are at risk for developing fluid overload.

Interstitial Fluid Volume Excess (Edema)

Interstitial fluid volume excess, or edema, is an abnormal increase in the volume of the interstitial fluid. It may be caused by an extracellular FVE, or it may result from other causes.

The causes of edema are best understood in the context of normal capillary dynamics. Fluid moves between the vascular and interstitial compartments by the process of filtration. Filtration is the net result of forces that tend to move fluid in opposing directions. The strongest forces will determine the direction of fluid movement.

At the capillary level, two forces (blood hydrostatic pressure and interstitial osmotic pressure) tend to move fluid from the capillaries into the interstitial fluid, while two other forces (blood colloid osmotic pressure and interstitial fluid hydrostatic pressure) tend to move fluid in the opposite direction (from the interstitial fluid into the capillaries). The net result of these forces usually moves fluid from the capillaries into the interstitial compartment at the arterial end of the capillaries and fluid from the interstitial compartment back into the capillaries at the venous end of the capillaries. This process brings oxygen and nutrients to the cells and removes carbon dioxide and other waste products.

Edema occurs if the balance of these four forces is altered so that excess fluid either enters or leaves the interstitial compartment. This may occur through increased blood hydrostatic pressure, decreased blood colloid osmotic pressure, increased interstitial fluid osmotic pressure, or blocked lymphatic drainage. Various clinical conditions are associated with these altered forces (**Box 6–2** ●):

1. *Increased blood hydrostatic pressure.* When extracellular FVE occurs, the increased fluid volume in the vascular compartment congests the veins. The pressure against the sides of the capillary is increased, and more fluid then enters the interstitial compartment.

2. *Decreased blood colloid osmotic pressure.* Much of the osmotic pressure that pulls fluid into the capillaries results from the presence of albumin and other plasma proteins made by the liver. The part of the blood osmotic pressure that is caused by plasma proteins is often called **oncotic pressure**, or blood colloid osmotic pressure. Any condition that decreases plasma proteins will decrease blood colloid osmotic pressure and cause edema. For example, if a clinical condition causes large amounts of albumin to leak into the urine, the liver will not be able to make albumin fast enough to replace it. As a result, the plasma protein level will fall, decreasing the blood osmotic pressure. Without this pulling force to return fluid to the capillaries, edema will occur. This is the cause of the edema that occurs in clients who have nephrotic syndrome. Another cause is prolonged surgical procedures with significant blood loss. Intravenous fluids and blood may be infused during surgery to replace these losses, but plasma proteins are lost and not fully restored by infusion, causing edema in the postoperative period.

3. *Increased interstitial fluid osmotic pressure.* Ordinarily, only a few small proteins enter the interstitial fluid,

---

Box 6–2 Clinical Conditions That Cause Edema

EDEMA CAUSED BY INCREASED BLOOD HYDROSTATIC PRESSURE

Increased Capillary Blood Flow
- Inflammation
- Local infection

Venous Congestion
- Extracellular fluid volume excess
- Right heart failure
- Venous thrombosis
- External pressure on vein
- Muscle paralysis

EDEMA CAUSED BY DECREASED BLOOD OSMOTIC PRESSURE

Increased Albumin Excretion
- Nephrotic syndrome (albumin leaks into urine)
- Protein-losing enteropathies (excess albumin in feces)

Decreased Albumin Synthesis
- Kwashiorkor (low-protein, high-carbohydrate starvation diet provides too few amino acids for liver to make albumin)
- Liver cirrhosis (diseased liver unable to make enough albumin)

EDEMA CAUSED BY INCREASED INTERSTITIAL FLUID OSMOTIC PRESSURE

Increased Capillary Permeability
- Inflammation
- Toxins
- Hypersensitivity reactions
- Burns

EDEMA CAUSED BY BLOCKED LYMPHATIC DRAINAGE
- Tumors
- Goiter
- Parasites that obstruct lymph nodes
- Surgery that removes lymph nodes

and the interstitial fluid osmotic pressure is small. If the capillary becomes abnormally permeable to proteins, however, the influx of large amounts of proteins into the interstitial fluid causes a dramatic increase in interstitial fluid osmotic pressure. This increased pulling force keeps an abnormal amount of fluid in the interstitial compartment. This mechanism plays an important part in edema caused by a bee sting or a sprained ankle. It occurs to a greater extent in burns, leading to swelling at the same time that there is a great loss of fluid volume through the burned skin.

4. **Blocked lymphatic drainage.** The lymph vessels normally drain small proteins and excess fluid from the interstitial compartment and return them to the blood vessels. If this process is blocked, fluid accumulates in the interstitial compartment. This may occur when a tumor blocks lymphatic drainage.

Edema causes swelling, which may be localized or generalized. The swelling of tissue may cause pain and restrict motion. Edema that results from extracellular fluid volume excess or right-sided heart failure usually occurs in the dependent portion of the body, often observed in the ankles. In a client who is supine in bed, it is seen in the sacral area or in the scrotal area in men. The skin over an edematous area often appears thin and shiny.

Etiology

Fluid volume excess usually results from conditions that cause retention of both sodium and water. These conditions include heart failure, cirrhosis of the liver, renal failure, adrenal gland disorders, corticosteroid administration, and stress conditions causing the release of antidiuretic hormone and aldosterone. Other causes include an excessive intake of sodium-containing foods, drugs that cause sodium retention, and the administration of excess amounts of sodium-containing intravenous fluids (such as 0.9% NaCl or Ringer's solution). This **iatrogenic** (induced by the effects of treatment) cause of fluid volume excess primarily affects clients with impaired regulatory mechanisms.

Risk Factors

A decrease in cardiovascular reserve or a decrease in cardiac output may result from deconditioning or disease or from the natural aging process. The older adult is at greater risk for fluid volume excess, in part because of natural reductions in kidney function that occur with aging. Additional stressors, such as hypertension, diabetes, or cardiac disease, increase the risk still further.

An increase in fluid volume is anticipated with normal pregnancy, but conditions such as preeclampsia may cause abnormal retention of fluid, resulting in increased stress on the body. Pregnant women with preeclampsia are taught that mild to moderate edema of the lower extremities (dependent edema) is to be anticipated, but edema of the face or hands or severe edema of the lower extremities must be reported to the provider immediately.

Clients with heart disease, kidney dysfunctions, or diabetes with peripheral vascular disease are at increased risk. Any disease that impairs blood flow to the kidney, such as hypertension, can potentially cause fluid volume excess. Any client

receiving intravenous therapy is at risk if careful monitoring of infusion rate and type of solution is not carefully monitored.

CLINICAL MANIFESTATIONS

The following manifestations of fluid volume excess relate to both the excess fluid and its effects on circulation:

- The increase in total body water causes weight gain (>5% of body weight) over a short time period.
- Circulatory overload causes manifestations such as:
  a. A full, bounding pulse
  b. Distended neck and peripheral veins (distended neck veins are difficult to assess in infants)
  c. Increased central venous pressure (>11–12 cm of water)
  d. Cough, **dyspnea** (labored or difficult breathing), and **orthopnea** (difficulty breathing when supine)
  e. Moist crackles (rales) in the lungs or, if severe, pulmonary edema (excess fluid in pulmonary interstitial spaces and alveoli)
  f. **Polyuria** (greatly increased urine output)
  g. **Ascites** (excess fluid in the peritoneal cavity)
  h. Peripheral edema or, if severe, **anasarca** (severe, generalized edema).
- Dilution of plasma by excess fluid causes a decreased hematocrit and BUN.
- Possible cerebral edema (excess water in brain tissues) can lead to altered mental status and anxiety.

Heart failure is not only a potential cause of fluid volume excess, it is also a potential complication of the condition if the heart is unable to increase its workload to handle the excess blood volume. Severe fluid overload and heart failure can lead to pulmonary edema, a medical emergency.

COLLABORATION

Managing fluid volume excess focuses on prevention in clients at risk, treating its manifestations, and correcting the underlying cause. Management includes limiting sodium and water intake and administering diuretics. A consultation with a dietitian or nutritionist may help the client to make appropriate food choices and provide the staff with a better understanding of client food preferences.

Diagnostic Tests

The following laboratory tests may be ordered:

- *Serum electrolytes* and *serum osmolality* are measured. Serum sodium and osmolality usually remain within normal limits.
- *Serum hematocrit* and *hemoglobin* often are decreased because of plasma dilution from excess extracellular fluid.

Additional tests of renal and liver function (e.g., serum creatinine, BUN, and liver enzymes) may be ordered to help determine the cause of fluid volume excess if it is unclear.

Pharmacologic Therapy

Diuretics are commonly used to treat fluid volume excess. They inhibit sodium and water reabsorption, increasing urine out-

Clinical Manifestations and Therapies **Fluid Volume Excess**

ETIOLOGY	CLINICAL MANIFESTATIONS	CLINICAL THERAPIES
Congestive heart failure	■ Dependent edema ■ Distended neck veins ■ Pulmonary edema ■ Tachycardia ■ Dyspnea ■ Hypoxia ■ Respiratory crackles ■ White or pink foamy sputum ■ Liver enlargement ■ Loss of appetite ■ Nausea ■ Weakness ■ Fatigue ■ Decreased activity tolerance ■ Nocturia ■ Paroxysmal nocturnal dyspnea ■ Ascites ■ Cardiogenic shock	■ Diuretics ■ Fluid restrictions ■ Fowler or high–Fowler position ■ Oxygen ■ Medications, including cardiac glycosides, angiotensin-converting enzyme inhibitors, phosphodiesterase inhibitors, and β-adrenergic agonists (particularly dobutamine) ■ Monitoring of lab values: serum electrolytes, brain natriuretic peptide, blood urea nitrogen, creatine, urinalysis, alanine aminotransferase, aspartate aminotransferase, lactate dehydrogenase, bilirubin, total protein, albumin levels, thyroid function tests, and arterial blood gas ■ Chest x-ray ■ Electrocardiography ■ Hemodynamic monitoring ■ Intra-arterial pressure monitoring ■ Central venous pressure monitoring
Liver cirrhosis	■ Weight loss ■ Weakness ■ Anorexia ■ Disrupted bowel function ■ Portal hypertension ■ Bleeding ■ Ascites ■ Jaundice ■ Neurological changes ■ Peripheral edema ■ Anemia ■ Esophageal varices	■ Avoid hepatotoxic drugs. ■ Diuretics ■ Lactulose and neomycin ■ Beta-blocker ■ Ferrous sulfate and folic acid ■ Antacid ■ Antianxiety drugs ■ Low-sodium, low-ammonia diet with vitamin and mineral supplements ■ Paracentesis ■ Hemodynamic monitoring
Adrenal tumor	■ Increased aldosterone production ■ Water and sodium retention ■ Edema ■ Fluid volume excess	■ Removal of the tumor ■ Diuretics ■ Monitoring of serum electrolytes, hemoglobin, and hematocrit ■ Cardiorespiratory monitoring ■ Oxygen
Overadministration of intravenous fluids	■ Edema ■ Pulmonary edema ■ Shortness of breath ■ Orthopnea ■ Hypertension ■ Reduced peripheral perfusion	■ Administration of diuretics ■ Elevate head of bed ■ Cardiorespiratory and oxygen saturation monitoring ■ Administration of oxygen ■ Daily weights ■ Accurate measurement of intake and output ■ Fluid restriction

Box 6–3   Fluid Restriction Guidelines

- Subtract requisite fluids (e.g., ordered intravenous fluids, fluid used to dilute intravenous medications) from total daily allowance.
- Divide remaining fluid allowance:
  a. Day shift: 50% of total
  b. Evening shift: 25% to 33% of total
  c. Night shift: Remainder.
- Explain the fluid restriction to the client and family members.
- Identify preferred fluids and intake pattern of client.
- Place allowed amounts of fluid in small glasses (gives perception of a full glass).
- Offer ice chips (when melted, ice chips are approximately half the frozen volume).
- Provide frequent mouth care.
- Provide sugarless chewing gum (if allowed) to reduce thirst sensation.

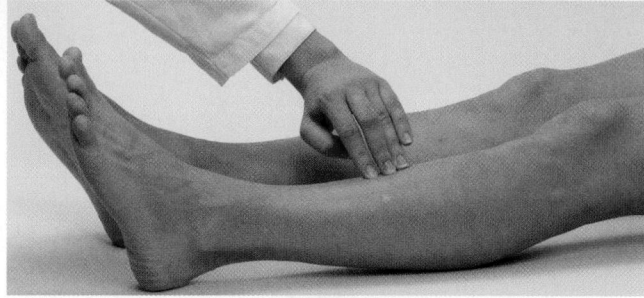

Figure 6–13 ● Palpating for edema over the tibia.

put. The three major classes of diuretics, each of which acts on a different part of the kidney tubule, are as follows:

1. *Loop diuretics*, which act in the ascending loop of Henle
2. *Thiazide-type diuretics*, which act on the distal convoluted tubule
3. *Potassium-sparing diuretics*, which affect the distal nephron.

Fluid Management

Fluid intake may be restricted in clients who have fluid volume excess. The amount of fluid allowed per day is prescribed by the primary care provider. All fluid intake must be calculated, including fluid consumed at meals and that used to administer medications orally or intravenously. Some foods may be higher in fluid content (e.g., watermelon, oranges, and soups) and must be considered as well. **Box 6–3** ● provides guidelines for clients with a fluid restriction.

Dietary Management

Because sodium retention is one of the dietary-related causes of fluid volume excess, a sodium-restricted diet often is prescribed. Americans typically consume more than 4–5 g of sodium every day; recommended sodium intake is 500–2,400 mg/day.

■ NURSING PROCESS

Nursing care focuses on preventing fluid volume excess in clients at risk and on managing problems resulting from its effects. Health promotion related to fluid volume excess focuses on teaching preventive measures to clients who are at risk (e.g., clients who have heart or kidney failure). Discuss the relationship between sodium intake and water retention. Provide guidelines for a low-sodium diet, and teach clients to carefully read food labels to identify "hidden" sodium, particularly in processed foods. Instruct clients who are at risk to weigh themselves on a regular basis, using the same scale, and to notify their primary care provider if they gain more than 5 pounds in a week or less.

Carefully monitor clients receiving intravenous fluids for signs of hypervolemia. Reduce the flow rate and promptly report manifestations of fluid overload to the physician.

Assessment

Collect assessment data through the health history interview and physical examination:

- *Health history.* Risk factors, such as medications, heart failure, and acute or chronic renal or endocrine disease; precipitating factors, such as a recent illness, change in diet, or change in medications; recent weight gain; complaints of persistent cough, shortness of breath, swelling of feet and ankles, or difficulty sleeping when lying down.
- *Physical assessment.* Daily weight, preferably using the same scale and wearing the same or similar clothing; vital signs; peripheral pulses and capillary refill; jugular neck vein distention; edema; lung sounds (crackles or wheezes), dyspnea, cough, and sputum; urine output; and mental status.

A focused assessment includes checking for edema of the legs by pressing the skin for at least 5 seconds over the tibia, behind the medial malleolus, and over the dorsum of each foot (**Figure 6–13** ●). If edema is present, it may be graded on a scale of 1+ mild to 4+ severe (see **Figure 6–14** ●). Assess for periorbital edema, swollen puffy eyelids that may result from crying or fluid volume excess. Men may experience scrotal edema, because the scrotum is in the dependent position when sitting.

Measure the child's intake and output, and weigh the diapers of infants. Sudden weight gain (e.g., 0.5 kg [1 lb] in 1 day) is caused by the accumulation of fluid. A gain of 0.5 kg overnight is caused by retention of approximately 500 mL of saline.

Assess the character of the pulse, and observe for neck vein distention when the client is sitting (usually visible only in adults and older children). Monitor for signs of pulmonary edema (an indication of severe imbalance) by listening to lung sounds in the dependent lung fields (crackles) and assessing for respiratory distress (rapid respiratory rate, use of accessory muscles of respiration). Observe for edema.

The potential for a client (especially a small child) to develop a fluid overload is present whenever an isotonic intravenous solution containing sodium is being administered. Careful assessment of infusion rates is essential to all client care but especially when caring for pediatric clients. Therefore, monitor the infusion rate frequently and carefully, and use a pump when possible to aid in accurate administration.

Diagnosis

Appropriate nursing diagnoses may include the following:

- *Excess Fluid Volume*
- *Risk for Impaired Skin Integrity*

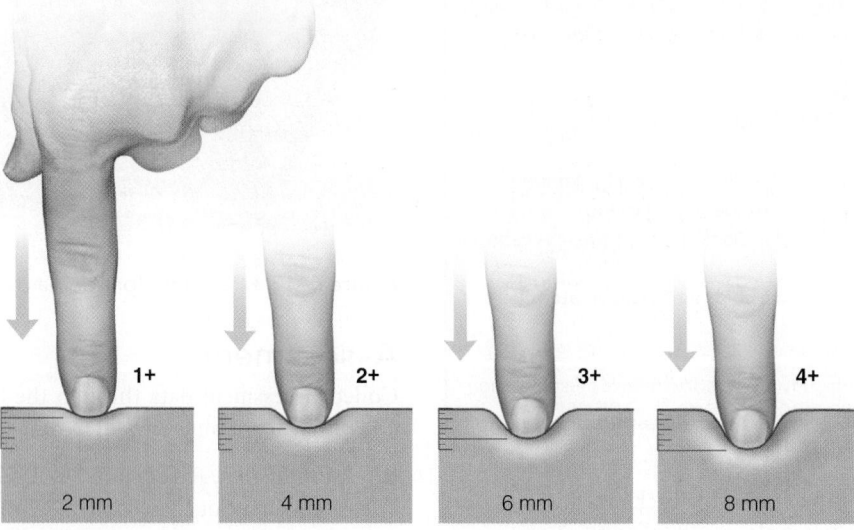

Figure 6–14 ● Grading pitting edema.

- *Risk for Impaired Gas Exchange*
- *Activity Intolerance*
- *Ineffective Health Maintenance.*

(NANDA-I © 2012)

Planning

Outcomes are designed in collaboration with the client and may include the following:

- The client will regain fluid balance.
- The client will have clear lung fields with eupneic breathing.
- The client will maintain skin integrity.
- The client will tolerate increased levels of activity.
- The client will make appropriate food choices to limit sodium.

Focus on Diversity and Culture

Sodium Use

To adapt teaching about low-sodium diets to the cultural practices of a family, ask the family members what types of food they usually eat. Help them to choose low-sodium foods from their diets and to avoid high-sodium foods. This approach is more effective than giving the same list of restricted foods to each family.

For example, some Asians use monosodium glutamate to flavor foods. They should be encouraged to add this at the table for family members who can have extra sodium rather than to use it during cooking. Many Hispanic groups use large amounts of cheese, which contains significant sodium. Encourage them to look for low-sodium cheese and substitute cottage cheese for other types, because it is lower in sodium. Low-sodium milk is available, and is a good option for young children. Canned foods tend to be high in sodium, so teach all families to use fresh or frozen produce rather than canned.

Implementation

Nursing interventions for the client with fluid volume excess may include the following:

- Weigh the client daily.
- Maintain intake and output records.
- Administer oral fluids carefully.
- Perform oral hygiene at least every 2 hours.
- Teach client and significant others about sodium-restricted diet (see the Client Teaching box on low-sodium diet on page 369).
- Administer prescribed diuretics, and monitor response to therapy.
- Report significant changes in serum electrolyte or osmolality.
- Teach client how to safely self-administer diuretics after discharge.
- Reposition client every 2 hours.
- Reduce shearing or friction to skin.
- Provide a low-pressure alternative mattress, foot cradle, heel protectors, and other devices to reduce pressure on tissues.
- Place in Fowler position if dyspnea or orthopnea is present.
- Monitor oxygen saturation and arterial blood gas results.
- Elevate area of edema (if possible) to encourage fluid reabsorption into extracellular fluid compartment.

Evaluation

Evaluate changes in weight, respirations, edema, and activity tolerance to determine the client's response to treatment. To evaluate client understanding of dietary teaching, encourage the client to participate in making appropriate diet choices from the menu. Revise the nursing plan of care as indicated based on client's progress toward meeting outcomes. Expected outcomes may include the following:

- The client maintains fluid balance as evidenced by lack of edema and laboratory diagnostic results.
- The client is able to participate in desired activities.
- The client maintains skin integrity.

Client Teaching   Low-Sodium Diet

- Reducing sodium intake helps the body to excrete excess sodium and water.
- The body needs less than one tenth of a teaspoon of salt per day.
- Approximately one third of sodium intake comes from salt added to foods during cooking and at the table, one fourth to one third comes from processed foods, and the rest comes from food and water naturally high in sodium.
- Sodium compounds are used in foods as preservatives, leavening agents, and flavor enhancers.
- Many nonprescription drugs (e.g., analgesics, cough medicine, laxatives, and antacids), toothpastes, and mouthwashes contain high amounts of sodium.

- Low-sodium salt substitutes are not really sodium free; they may contain half as much sodium as regular salt.
- Use salt substitutes sparingly; larger amounts often taste bitter instead of salty.
- The preference for salt will eventually diminish.
- Salt, monosodium glutamate, baking soda, and baking powder contain substantial amounts of sodium.
- Read labels.
- In place of salt or salt substitutes, use herbs, spices, lemon juice, vinegar, and wine as flavoring when cooking.

NURSING CARE PLAN   A Client With Fluid Volume Excess

Dorothy Rainwater is a 45-year-old Native American woman hospitalized with acute renal failure that developed as a result of acute glomerulonephritis. She is expected to recover, but she has very little urine output. Ms. Rainwater is a single mother of two teenage sons. Until her illness, she was active in caring for her family, her career as a high school principal, and community activities.

ASSESSMENT

Ms. Rainwater's nurse notes that she is in the oliguric phase of acute renal failure and that her urine output for the previous 24 hours was 250 mL; this low output has been constant for the past 8 days. Ms. Rainwater gained 1 lb (0.45 kg) in the past 24 hours. Laboratory test results from that morning are as follows: sodium, 155 mEq/L (normal, 135–145 mEq/L); potassium, 5.6 mEq/L (normal, 3.5–5.3 mEq/L); calcium, 7.6 mg/dL (normal, 9–11 mg/dL), and urine specific gravity, 1.008 (normal, 1.010–1.030). Ms. Rainwater's serum creatinine and blood urea nitrogen are high; however, her arterial blood gases are within normal limits.

The nurse's assessment of Ms. Rainwater yields the following:

- BP 160/92 mmHg; P 102 bpm, with obvious neck vein distention; R 28/min, with crackles and wheezes; head of bed elevated 30°; and T$_O$ 37°C (98.6°F).
- Periorbital and sacral edema present; 3+ pitting bilateral pedal edema; and skin cool, pale, and shiny.
- Alert, oriented, and responds appropriately to questions.
- Client states she is thirsty, slightly nauseated, and extremely tired.

Ms. Rainwater is receiving intravenous furosemide and is on a 24-hr fluid restriction of 500 mL plus the previous day's urine output to manage her fluid volume excess.

DIAGNOSES

- *Excess Fluid Volume* related to acute renal failure
- *Risk for Impaired Skin Integrity* related to fluid retention and edema
- *Risk for Impaired Gas Exchange* related to pulmonary congestion
- *Activity Intolerance* related to fluid volume excess, fatigue, and weakness

(NANDA-I © 2012)

PLANNING

- The client will regain fluid balance, as evidenced by weight loss, decreasing edema, and normal vital signs.
- The client will experience decreased dyspnea.
- The client will maintain intact skin and mucous membranes.
- The client will increase activity levels as prescribed.

IMPLEMENTATION

- Weigh at 6:00 a.m. and 6:00 p.m. daily.
- Assess vital signs and breath sounds every 4 hours.
- Measure intake and output every 4 hours.
- Obtain urine specific gravity every 8 hours.
- Restrict fluids as follows: 350 mL from 7:00 a.m. to 3:00 p.m.; 300 mL from 3:00 p.m. to 11:00 p.m.; and 100 mL from 11:00 p.m. to 7:00 a.m. Client prefers water or apple juice.
- Turn every 2 hours, following schedule posted at head of bed. Inspect and provide skin care as needed; avoid vigorous massage of pressure areas.

- Provide oral care every 2–4 hours (client can brush her own teeth; caution client not to swallow water); use moistened applicators as desired.
- Elevate head of bed to 30°–40°; client prefers to use own pillows.
- Assist to recliner chair at bedside for 20 minutes two or three times a day. Monitor ability to tolerate activity without increasing dyspnea or fatigue.

(continued on next page)

NURSING CARE PLAN (continued)

EVALUATION

At the end of the shift, the nurse evaluates the effectiveness of the plan of care and continues all diagnoses and interventions. Ms. Rainwater gained no weight, and her urinary output during this shift is 170 mL. Her urine specific gravity remains at 1.008. Her vital signs are unchanged, but her crackles and wheezes have decreased slightly. Her skin and mucous membranes are intact. Ms. Rainwater tolerated the bedside chair without dyspnea or fatigue.

CRITICAL THINKING

1. What is the pathophysiological basis for Ms. Rainwater's increased respiratory rate, blood pressure, and pulse?
2. Explain how elevating the head of the bed 30° facilitates respirations.
3. Suppose Ms. Rainwater says, "I would really like to have all my fluids at once instead of spreading them out." How would you reply, and why?
4. Outline a plan for teaching Ms. Rainwater about diuretics.

ELECTROLYTE IMBALANCE

▶ OVERVIEW

All body fluids contain electrolytes in varying concentrations, depending on whether the electrolyte is prominent in the intracellular or extracellular fluid environment. Measurements of serum electrolyte values provide information about the concentration of that electrolyte in the blood. Such measurements reflect the concentration of the electrolyte in other body compartments.

Electrolytes are normally gained and lost in relatively equal amounts, so the body remains in balance. However, when a client has an abnormal route of loss, such as vomiting, wound drainage, diuretic administration, or nasogastric suction, electrolyte balance can be uneven. Monitoring for signs of imbalance is an important part of nursing care for all clients, but especially those at risk.

Signs and symptoms of electrolyte imbalance can be very subtle if the imbalance is minimal. Moderate to severe electrolyte imbalance often produces multisystem effects and can lead to death if not reversed. When caring for clients, it is important to consider the role of electrolytes in maintaining homeostasis and to assess for signs of imbalance. It is often important to assess a client's new symptoms in light of a possible electrolyte imbalance.

Nurses must understand the interactions among electrolytes and that an imbalance rarely occurs with only one electrolyte. For example, if sodium is lost, chloride often accompanies it; fluid volume excess often dilutes other electrolytes, resulting in lower serum levels; and gastric suctioning causing hypokalemia also causes loss of magnesium, sodium, and chloride as well as acid–base imbalance. The content that follows outlines the etiology, manifestation, and indicated interventions for each of the electrolytes and provides information relative to excesses and deficits.

Sodium

Sodium is the most abundant electrolyte in extracellular fluid. Normal serum values for sodium are 135–145 mEq/L. The role of sodium in the body is to assist with maintenance of osmotic pressure and acid–base balance and with the conduction of nerve impulses. The mineralocorticoid aldosterone is the principal mineralocorticoid that assists in regulating serum sodium balance. It does this by stimulating the kidneys to conserve sodium and to excrete potassium when serum sodium levels fall below normal. Water follows the sodium, and blood volume rises. When ECF osmolality increases, antidiuretic hormone is secreted, leading to additional water reabsorption. The atria detect this rise in ECF volume and secrete atrial natriuretic peptide (ANP) to reverse the aldosterone process and promote sodium and water excretion in order to return the ECF to balance.

Sodium balance is also affected by food intake. Most Americans consume far more sodium than is necessary for maintaining sodium balance. This can lead to sodium excess and contribute to health concerns. The primary dietary sources of sodium are foods that are naturally high in sodium and processed foods and condiments (**Box 6–4 ●**).

Education to assist clients and their families with maintaining appropriate sodium intake includes reducing the amount of salt in recipes, avoiding adding salt during meals, and limiting intake of foods that contain high levels of sodium (either naturally or because of processing). In moderate and severely sodium-restricted diets, salt is avoided altogether, as are all foods containing significant amounts of sodium.

HYPERNATREMIA   Hypernatremia occurs when serum sodium levels are greater than 145 mEq/L. Critical values occur at levels greater than 160 mEq/L. Etiologies include the impaired thirst mechanism, profuse sweating, diarrhea, diabetes insipidus, Cushing syndrome, and inappropriate use of oral electrolyte solutions. Hypernatremia is manifested by hyperosmolality of the ECF; cellular dehydration; excessive thirst; elevated temperature; dry, sticky membranes; and restlessness. Management is aimed toward fluid replacement at a rate not to exceed 0.5–1 mEq/hr to prevent intracranial fluid shifts and cerebral edema. Nurses must observe for headache, nausea, and vomiting, increasing blood pressure, and confusion.

HYPONATREMIA   Hyponatremia occurs when serum sodium levels fall below 125 mEq/L. Critical values occur at levels below 115 mEq/L, although new studies suggest 124 mEq/L

Box 6–4   Foods High in Sodium

HIGH IN ADDED SODIUM

Processed Meat and Fish

- Bacon
- Sausage
- Luncheon meat and other cold cuts
- Smoked fish

Selected Dairy Products

- Buttermilk
- Cottage cheese
- Cheeses
- Ice cream

Processed Grains

- Graham crackers
- Most dry cereals

Most Canned Goods

- Meats
- Vegetables
- Soups

Snack Foods

- Salted popcorn
- Nuts
- Potato chips/pretzels
- Gelatin desserts

Condiments and Food Additives

- Barbecue sauce
- Saccharin
- Catsup
- Pickles
- Chili sauce
- Soy sauce
- Meat tenderizers
- Salted margarine
- Worcestershire sauce
- Salad dressings

NATURALLY HIGH IN SODIUM

- Brains
- Oysters
- Kidney
- Shrimp
- Clams
- Dried fruit
- Crab
- Spinach
- Lobster
- Carrots

should be the lowest point (Guarner et al., 2011). Etiology includes diuretic use, renal disease, adrenal insufficiency, vomiting, diarrhea, excessive GI suctioning, irrigation of NG tubes with water rather than saline, repeated tap-water enemas, burns, heart failure, and administration of hypotonic intravenous fluid replacement. Hyponatremia is manifested by edema, muscle cramps, weakness, fatigue, anorexia, nausea and vomiting, and abdominal cramps. At very low levels, symptoms include headache, depression, personality changes, lethargy, hyperreflexia, muscle twitching, and tremors. If levels drop to

below 120 mEq/L, convulsions, coma, and death can occur. Management consists of administration of sodium-containing fluids, increased intake of sodium-rich fluids, and promotion of safety.

Potassium

Potassium is primarily an intracellular cation with 98% of all potassium found within the cell. Potassium plays a role in cellular depolarization and repolarization. As a component of the

Evidence-Based Practice   Sodium Intake—A Focus on Children

Problem

Is there a relationship between sodium intake and hypertension in children and adolescents?

Evidence

In a study of 6,235 U.S. children and adolescents ages 8 to 18 years, daily sodium intake was measured using dietary recall. Acknowledging that reporting in dietary recall is not 100% accurate, these findings suggested these children consumed, on average, 3,387 mg/day of sodium (Yang et al., 2012). In addition, the study outcome suggested that sodium intake increased with age. The presence of overweight or obesity was 39%, and pre–high blood pressure and existing high blood pressure was 14.9%, much of which was attributed to sodium intake. Children with hypertension are predisposed to hypertension in adulthood. The researchers in this study concluded that increased sodium intake was directly related to a rise in systolic blood pressure.

Implications

According to many sources (CDC, 2012), Americans eat too much salt. In addition, there is a direct correlation between sodium intake and increasing blood pressure numbers throughout the United States (Moshfegh et al., 2012). Education of parents and children regarding appropriate salt intake and avoidance of added salt and foods high in sodium may help prevent significant hypertension as children mature into adults.

Critical Thinking Application

1. What foods that children and adolescents typically like are lower in sodium?

2. Design a health promotion activity for adolescents related to sodium intake. Include strategies for ways that adolescents can eat more healthy foods.

potassium pump, it assists in the movement of potassium into the cell while sodium moves outside the cell. It is important to note that both hyperkalemia and hypokalemia can lead to deadly cardiac dysrhythmias.

HYPERKALEMIA Hyperkalemia is a serum potassium of greater than 5.3 mEq/L. Critical values occur at levels around 7.0 mEq/L. Etiologies include renal failure, potassium-sparing diuretics use, excessive potassium intake, adrenal insufficiency, acidosis, severe tissue trauma (including burns), starvation, and medications such as trimethoprim. Hyperkalemia is manifested by tall, peaked T waves and widened QRS, dysrhythmias, cardiac arrest, nausea and vomiting, abdominal cramping, diarrhea, and paresthesias. Management consists of administration of calcium gluconate, administration of insulin and glucose, and sodium polystyrene sulfonate (Kayexalate) orally or by enema. Diuretics may be indicated if renal excretion is normal.

HYPOKALEMIA Hypokalemia is manifested by serum potassium levels of less than 3.5 mEq/L. Critical values occur at levels below 2.5 mEq/L. Etiologies include potassium-depleting diuretics use, corticosteroid use, antibiotics such as amphotericin B, severe vomiting, gastric suctioning, alkalosis, and long-term IV fluid replacement without the addition of potassium. Hypokalemia is manifested by dysrhythmias, flat or inverted T waves, anorexia, decreased bowel sounds, ileus, muscle cramps, increased risk for digoxin toxicity, and suppressed insulin secretion. Management consists of potassium salts replacement.

Chloride

Chloride is most prevalent in the extracellular fluid. It is found with sodium, and together they maintain the electricity of the body in a neutral state. Chloride is also found in combination with hydrogen to form the hydrochloric acid found in the stomach as an aid to digestion. It also plays a role in the maintenance of acid–base balance, especially in the measurement of the anion gap.

HYPERCHLOREMIA **Hyperchloremia** is manifested by a serum chloride greater than 105 mEq/L. Etiologies include diarrhea, renal failure, overactive parathyroid glands, use of carbonic anhydrase inhibitors, metabolic acidosis, and respiratory alkalosis. Manifestations include the presence of Kussmaul respirations, weakness, and increased thirst. Management consists of diuretics, increased intravenous fluids, treatment of the underlying cause, and dialysis.

HYPOCHLOREMIA **Hypochloremia** is manifested by a serum chloride of less than 95 mEq/L. Although it is not a common disorder, when it does occur its etiologies include loss of body fluid, vomiting, and diarrhea. Manifestations include paresthesias of the face and extremities, muscle spasm, and tetany. The abdomen may be distended. Management consists of increased salt in the diet, adding chloride to IV fluids, and treating underlying causes.

Calcium

Calcium has several major functions in the body, including neuromuscular transmission and control of muscle contraction, blood clotting, bone and teeth formation, and cellular membrane functioning. Only 2% of calcium is found in the blood serum. Calcium levels are controlled by vitamin D, calcitonin, and parathyroid hormone.

HYPERCALCEMIA **Hypercalcemia** is manifested by a serum calcium of greater than 11 mg/dL. Etiologies include hyperparathyroidism, bone malignancy, and drug toxicity (e.g., from thiazide diuretics, lithium carbonate, and vitamins A and D). Manifestations include fatigue, weakness, decreased deep tendon reflexes, headache, impaired cognition, anorexia, nausea and vomiting, lethargy, polyuria, renal calculi, anorexia, constipation, cardiac dysrhythmias, muscle weakness, and conjunctival calcifications. Management includes partial parathyroidectomy, discontinuation of thiazide diuretics and vitamin and mineral supplements, and a low-calcium diet.

HYPOCALCEMIA **Hypocalcemia** is manifested by a serum calcium level below 9 mg/dL. Etiologies include transfusion of a large volume of citrated blood, decreased parathyroid hormone, decreased parathyroid hormone, elevated serum phosphorus, decreased magnesium levels, hypoalbuminemia, and alkalosis. Hypocalcemia often occurs through accidental removal of the parathyroid glands during thyroidectomy. Manifestations are based on the speed at which calcium level drops. Bradycardia and hypotension can occur. Clients experience numbness and tingling of the fingers, hyperactive reflexes, muscle cramps, laryngeal spasms, tetany, confusion, and possible seizures. Pathological fractures can occur. Clients also exhibit Trousseau sign and Chvostek sign. When symptoms such as Trousseau and Chvostek sign occur, IV replacement of calcium is indicated. Rates should not exceed 60 mg of elemental calcium per minute.

■ NURSING PROCESS

Almost all body systems are sensitive to changes in fluid and electrolyte balance. Care of the client experiencing an electrolyte imbalance requires the nurse to have a thorough understanding of the etiology, signs and symptoms, and suggested treatment of both excesses and deficiencies in specific electrolytes. Deficiencies can develop quickly and may require immediate intervention. These interventions may include simple replacement of water losses or intricate minute-by-minute monitoring of complex signs and symptoms including laryngeal edema, Chvostek sign, cardiac rhythm, or urine output.

Assessment

Although each electrolyte imbalance has specific assessment components, general assessment of the client with suspected electrolyte imbalance includes a review of the lab data for specific electrolyte excess or deficit, ECG, urinalysis, hemoglobin and hematocrit, and arterial blood gases. These findings should be followed by assessment of subjective data such as abnormal thirst, frequent urination, presence of anorexia or nausea, pain, problems with muscle cramping, and diarrhea. Objective data include vital signs, a mental status exam, deep tendon reflexes, presence of diarrhea or vomiting, heart and lung sounds, and presence of edema. A dietary review should also be performed with emphasis on foods high in sodium or potassium and frequent intake of fluids with added electrolytes.

Diagnosis

Nursing diagnoses applicable to fluid and electrolyte imbalance include:

- *Fluid Volume Deficit*
- *Risk for Electrolyte Imbalance*
- *Decreased Cardiac Output.*

(NANDA-I © 2012)

Planning

Outcomes are designed in collaboration with the client and may include the following:

- The client will maintain electrolyte levels within normal limits as determined by serum electrolyte findings and results of other laboratory diagnostics.
- The client will be free of symptoms of electrolyte or acid–base imbalance.
- The client will maintain regular heart rhythm and output.

Implementation

Nursing interventions to address specific electrolyte imbalances are identified in the discussion of specific electrolyte deficit or excess. General interventions include:

- Monitor sodium, potassium, chloride, and magnesium levels daily; monitor more frequently if levels are significantly elevated or decreased.
- Monitor intake and output as indicated by agency policy.
- Observe for signs and symptoms of dehydration.
- Observe for signs and symptoms of fluid and electrolyte excess or deficiency.

Evaluation

Achievement of expected outcomes for clients with electrolyte imbalance may include:

- The client's electrolyte status returns to appropriate levels as evidenced by normal serum electrolytes, normal urinalysis, and the absence of edema and other symptoms associated with excess or deficit.
- The client maintains appropriate weight for age and height.
- The client maintains equality of intake and output as evidenced by direct measurement (hospital setting) or measurement of intake and documentation of food intake via journals (home setting).

Based on these findings the nurse may revise the nursing care plan as needed based on the client's progress toward meeting outcomes.

REVIEW Fluid and Electrolyte Imbalance

RELATE Link the Concepts and Exemplars

Linking the exemplar of fluid and electrolyte imbalance with the concept of cognition:

1. What impact might the nurse anticipate a fluid and electrolyte imbalance to have on an older client's cognition?

2. What expected outcomes are appropriate for the client with confusion and hyperkalemia?

Linking the exemplar of fluid and electrolyte imbalance with the concept of elimination:

3. You are caring for a client with acute nausea, vomiting, and diarrhea. What impacts do you anticipate these symptoms having on the client's fluid and electrolyte balance? How can you minimize this impact?

4. What focused assessment is a priority for the client with chronic kidney disease who has a potassium level of 5.7?

READY Go to Companion Skills Manual

REFER Go to Pearson Nursing Student Resources
nursing.pearsonhighered.com

- Additional review materials

REFLECT Case Study

Pamela Allen is a 65-year-old woman who has been married to Clifford for 40 years. Their only child, Gary, has Down syn-

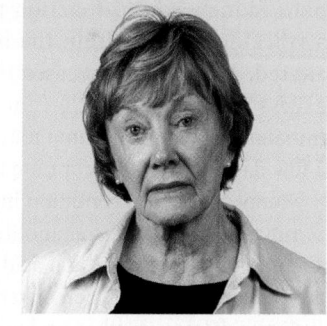

drome and lives with them. Mrs. Allen stopped working after Gary was born to care for him. She has recently been diagnosed with advanced colorectal cancer and had surgery last month (colectomy and colostomy). Because the tumor extended into the perineum and lymph nodes, she has been advised to start radiation and chemotherapy. She previously underwent treatment for endometrial cancer at age 50 but did not receive chemotherapy or radiation at that time.

1. When caring for Mrs. Allen during administration of chemotherapy, what issues might you anticipate could result in fluid and electrolyte imbalance?

2. If Mrs. Allen experiences dehydration following chemotherapy administration, what suggestions could the nurse recommend to improve fluid status?

3. As a result of chemotherapy and radiation causing bowel irritation, Mrs. Allen develops severe acute diarrhea. What changes would you recommend to Mrs. Allen's fluid intake to maintain adequate fluid balance and normal electrolyte levels?

EXEMPLAR 6.2 **Acute Renal Failure**

EXEMPLAR KEY TERMS

EXEMPLAR LEARNING OUTCOMES

After reading about this exemplar, you will be able to:

1. Describe the pathophysiology, etiology, clinical manifestations, and direct and indirect causes of acute renal failure.

2. Identify risk factors and prevention methods associated with acute renal failure.

3. Illustrate the nursing process in providing culturally competent care across the life span for individuals with acute renal failure.

4. Formulate priority nursing diagnoses appropriate for an individual with acute renal failure.

5. Summarize therapies used by interdisciplinary teams in the collaborative care of an individual with acute renal failure.

6. Plan evidence-based care for an individual with acute renal failure and his or her family in collaboration with other members of the healthcare team.

7. Evaluate expected outcomes for an individual with acute renal failure.

▶ OVERVIEW

The kidneys control fluid and electrolyte balance as well as acid–base balance, and they help to control blood pressure, thereby helping to maintain homeostasis. Normally only one functioning kidney is necessary to maintain homeostasis. When both kidneys fail to function properly, fluids accumulate in atypical locations within the body and electrolyte levels are altered. Heart rate increases in an attempt to accommodate excess fluid, and muscle function is affected by electrolyte imbalance. Cerebral edema may occur. Death will result within a few days without appropriate treatment.

Renal failure is a condition in which the kidneys are unable to remove accumulated metabolites from the blood, resulting in altered fluid, electrolyte, and acid–base balance. The cause may be a primary kidney disorder, or renal failure may be secondary to a systemic disease or other urological defects. Renal failure may be either acute or chronic. When acute, renal failure has an abrupt onset and may be reversed with prompt intervention. Chronic kidney disease (formerly known as chronic renal failure) is a silent disease, progressing slowly and with few symptoms until the kidneys are severely damaged and unable to meet the excretory needs of the body. Both acute renal failure and chronic kidney disease are characterized by **azotemia** (increased levels of nitrogenous wastes in the blood). This exemplar discusses the acute form of renal failure.

Acute renal failure (ARF) is a rapid decline in renal function with azotemia and fluid and electrolyte imbalances. The most common causes of ARF are **ischemia** (insufficient blood supply) and exposure to **nephrotoxins** (substances that damage nerves or nerve tissue). The kidneys are particularly vulnerable to both because of the amount of blood that passes through them. A fall in blood pressure or volume can cause ischemia of kidney tissues. Nephrotoxins in the blood damage renal tissue directly.

Recent conversations have suggested the need for a standard by which acute renal failure can be classified. The Acute Dialysis Quality Initiative recommends that a more accurate term for the disease is **acute kidney injury (AKI)**. AKI refers to a sudden decline in kidney function that causes disturbances in fluid, electrolyte, and acid–base balance (Dirkes, 2011). A new classification system, known as RIFLE (risk of injury, injury, failure, loss of function, and end-stage renal failure), establishes AKI diagnostic criteria, as well as outcome and treatment options to reduce kidney injury early. With these new parameters, new biomarkers have been established to identify AKI. These include interleukin 18 (IL-18), neutrophil gelatinase-associate lipocalin (NGAL), and kidney injury molecule-1 (KIM-1) (Dirkes, 2011). Goldstein and Devarajan (2011) suggest that similar problems exist with the diagnosis of AKI in children and report the need for the establishment of a group of similar markers for AKI identification in children.

▶ PATHOPHYSIOLOGY AND ETIOLOGY

The causes and pathophysiology of ARF are commonly categorized as prerenal, intrinsic, and postrenal. Prerenal ARF is the most common, accounting for approximately 55% of cases. In prerenal ARF, **hypoperfusion** (decreased blood flow) leads to ARF without directly affecting the integrity of kidney tissues. Intrinsic (or intrarenal) ARF, caused by direct damage to functional kidney tissue, is responsible for another 40%. Urinary tract obstruction with resulting kidney damage is the precipitating factor for postrenal ARF, the least common form (~5%). **Table 6–9** ● summarizes the causes of ARF, and **Figure 6–15** ● outlines the pathophysiology of ARF.

TABLE 6–9   Causes of Acute Renal Failure

	CAUSE	EXAMPLES
Prerenal	Hypovolemia	Hemorrhage, dehydration, excess fluid loss from gastrointestinal tract, burns, wounds
	Low cardiac output	Heart failure, cardiogenic shock
	Altered vascular resistance	Sepsis, anaphylaxis, vasoactive drugs
Intrarenal	Glomerular/microvascular injury	Glomerulonephritis, disseminated intravascular coagulation, vasculitis, hypertension, toxemia of pregnancy, hemolytic uremic syndrome
	Acute tubular necrosis	Ischemia resulting from conditions associated with prerenal failure; toxins, such as drugs, heavy metals; **hemolysis** (destruction of red blood cells); rhabdomyolysis (muscle cell breakdown)
	Interstitial nephritis	Acute pyelonephritis, toxins, metabolic imbalances, idiopathic
Postrenal	Ureteral obstruction	Calculi, cancer, external compression
	Urethral obstruction	Prostatic enlargement, calculi, cancer, stricture, blood clot

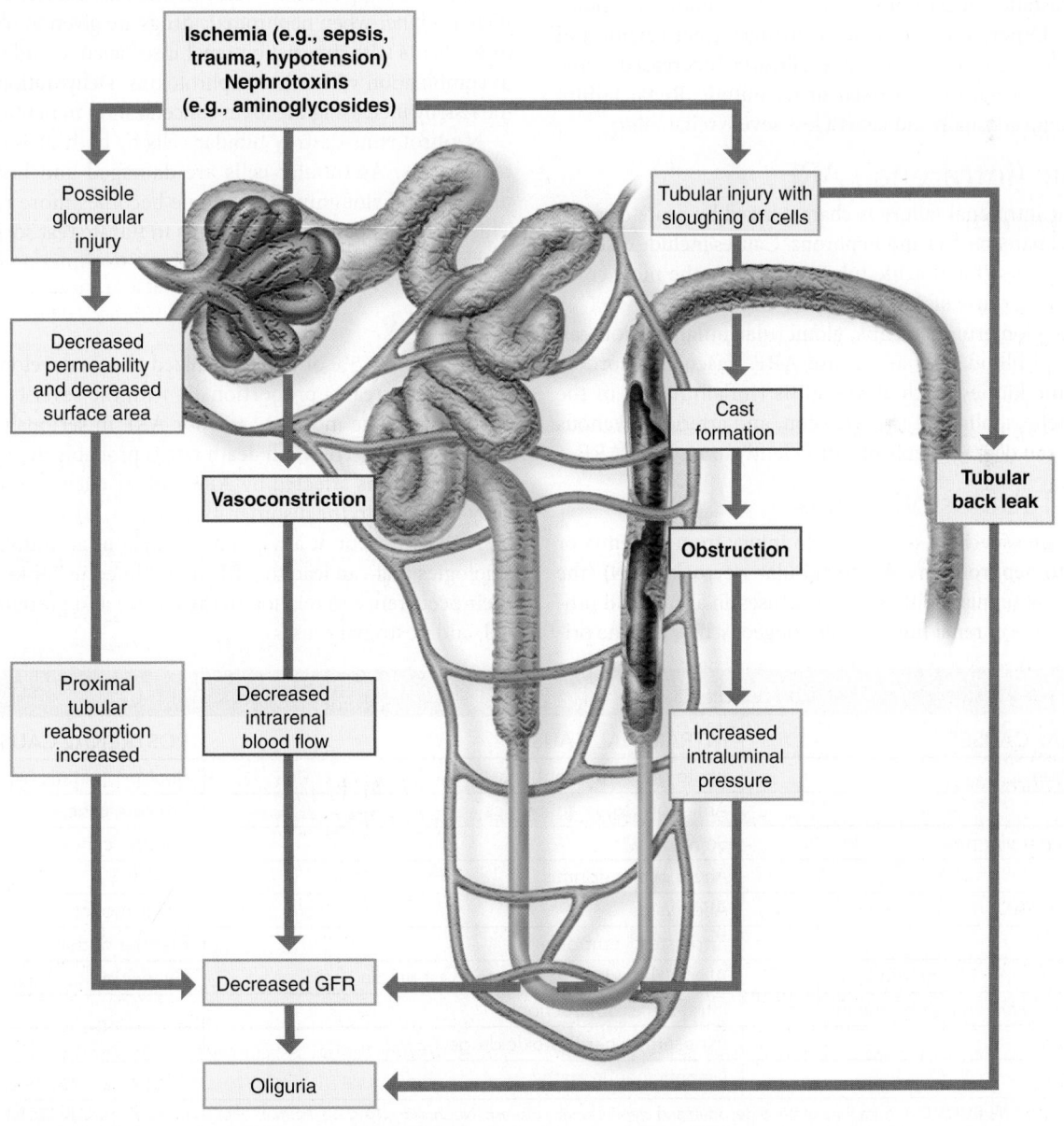

Figure 6–15 ● The pathophysiology of acute renal failure.

Prerenal ARF

Prerenal ARF results from conditions that affect renal blood flow and perfusion. Any disorder that significantly decreases vascular volume, cardiac output, or systemic vascular resistance can affect renal blood flow. Prerenal ARF is common, particularly in trauma, surgery, and critically ill clients. The kidneys normally receive 20%–25% of the cardiac output to maintain the **glomerular filtration rate (GFR)** (the rate at which fluid is filtered through the kidneys). A drop in renal blood flow to less than 20% of normal causes the GFR to fall. As the filtration of substances by the glomeruli is reduced, less reabsorption of substances in the tubule is required. As a result, kidney cells require less energy and oxygen, and their metabolism slows. Prerenal ARF is rapidly reversed when blood flow is restored, and the renal parenchyma remains undamaged. Unresolved ischemia can lead to tubular cell necrosis and significant nephron damage (Porth, 2010). Intrinsic ARF caused by ischemic injury may result.

Postrenal ARF

Obstructive causes of ARF are classified as postrenal. Any condition that prevents urine excretion can lead to postrenal ARF. Benign prostatic hypertrophy is the most common precipitating factor. Others include renal or urinary tract calculi and tumors. Children may experience **oliguria** (decreased urine output) or normal or increased urine output. Renal failure without oliguria usually indicates a less severe renal injury.

Intrinsic (Intrarenal) ARF

Intrinsic or intrarenal failure is characterized by acute damage to the renal parenchyma and nephrons. Causes include diseases of the kidney itself and acute tubular necrosis, the most common intrarenal cause of ARF.

In acute glomerulonephritis, glomerular inflammation can reduce renal blood flow and cause ARF. Vascular disorders affecting the kidney, such as vasculitis (inflammation of the blood vessels), malignant hypertension, and arterial or venous occlusion, can damage nephrons sufficiently to result in ARF.

Acute Tubular Necrosis

Nephrons are especially susceptible to injury from ischemia or exposure to nephrotoxins. **Acute tubular necrosis (ATN)** (the destruction of tubular epithelial cells) causes an abrupt and progressive decline of renal function. Prolonged ischemia is the pri-mary cause of ATN. When ischemia and nephrotoxin exposure occur concurrently, the risk for ATN and tubular dysfunction is especially high. See **Figure 6–16** ● for the pathogenesis of ARF caused by ATN. Risk factors for ischemic ATN include major surgery, severe **hypovolemia** (decreased circulating blood volume), sepsis, trauma, and burns. The impact of ischemia resulting from vasodilation and fluid loss in sepsis, trauma, and burns often is compounded by toxins released by bacteria or from damaged tissue. Injury to the tubule resulting in ATN is the most frequent cause of intrinsic renal failure in children.

Ischemia lasting more than 2 hours causes severe and irreversible damage to kidney tubules, with patchy cellular necrosis and sloughing. The GFR is significantly reduced as a result of ischemia, activation of the renin–angiotensin system, and tubular obstruction by cellular debris, which raises the pressure in the glomerular capsule.

Common nephrotoxins associated with ATN include the aminoglycoside antibiotics and radiological contrast media. Many other drugs (e.g., nonsteroidal anti-inflammatory drugs and some chemotherapeutic drugs), heavy metals (e.g., mercury and gold), and some common chemicals (e.g., ethylene glycol [antifreeze]) also are potentially toxic to the renal tubule. The risk for ATN is higher when nephrotoxic drugs are given to older clients or to clients with preexisting renal insufficiency, and when used in combination with other nephrotoxins. Dehydration increases the risk by increasing the toxin concentration in nephrons.

Nephrotoxins destroy tubular cells by both direct and indirect effects. As tubular cells are damaged and lost through necrosis and sloughing, the tubule becomes more permeable. This increased permeability results in filtrate reabsorption, further reducing the ability of the nephron to eliminate wastes.

Etiology

Approximately 5% of all hospitalized clients develop ARF; the incidence increases proportionally with the severity of the client's illness. The mortality rate for ARF in seriously ill clients may reach 75%. This high death rate is probably more related to the populations affected by ARF—older clients and the critically ill—than to the disorder itself (Porth, 2010).

ARF can occur at any point throughout an individual's life. Etiologies that can lead to ARF are outlined in **Table 6–10** ● by their occurrence in relation to the kidney and prerenal, intrarenal, and postrenal causes.

TABLE 6–10　Etiologies That Can Lead to Acute Renal Failure

PRERENAL CAUSES	INTRARENAL CAUSES	POSTRENAL CAUSES
Dehydration	Acute glomerulonephritis	Benign prostatic hyperplasia
Shock	Aminoglycoside antibiotics	Prostate cancer
Vomiting and diarrhea	Sepsis	Bladder cancer
Surgery	Acute pyelonephritis	Calculi
Cardiac failure	Aneurysms	Fecal impaction
Diuretics	Cholesterol embolus	Bladder outlet obstruction
Nonsteroidal anti-inflammatory drugs	Allergic response to radiocontrast media	Gynecological cancers
Angiotensin-converting enzyme inhibitors	Intratubular obstruction	
Liver failure	Exposure to nephrotoxic drugs	
Hypovolemia	Diabetic nephropathy	

Sources: Elliott, R. W. (2012). Demographics of the older adult and chronic kidney disease. *Nephrology Nursing Journal, 39*(6), 491–496; Porth, C.M. (2010). *Essentials of pathophysiology* (3rd ed.). Philadelphia, PA: Lippincott Williams & Wilkins; and Mayo Clinic. (2012). *Acute kidney failure.* Retrieved from http://www.mayoclinic.com/health/kidney-failure/DS00280/DSECTION=causes.

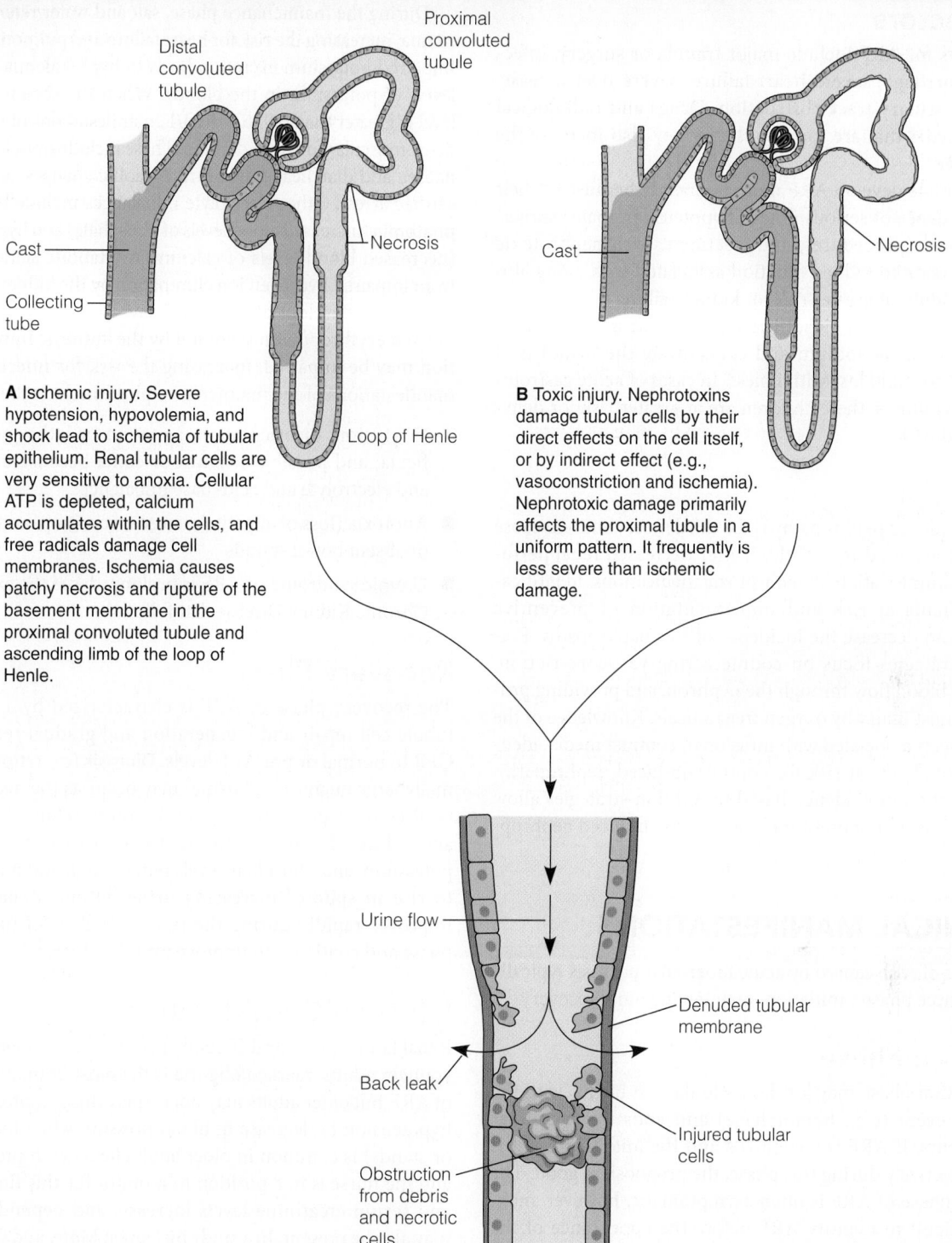

A Ischemic injury. Severe hypotension, hypovolemia, and shock lead to ischemia of tubular epithelium. Renal tubular cells are very sensitive to anoxia. Cellular ATP is depleted, calcium accumulates within the cells, and free radicals damage cell membranes. Ischemia causes patchy necrosis and rupture of the basement membrane in the proximal convoluted tubule and ascending limb of the loop of Henle.

B Toxic injury. Nephrotoxins damage tubular cells by their direct effects on the cell itself, or by indirect effect (e.g., vasoconstriction and ischemia). Nephrotoxic damage primarily affects the proximal tubule in a uniform pattern. It frequently is less severe than ischemic damage.

C Injured tubular cells release intracellular debris, which combines with proteins within the tubules to form casts. These casts, together with sloughed necrotic cells, occlude the tubular lumen, increasing tubular pressure and disrupting the flow of glomerular filtrate. Glomerular filtration slows. The increased pressure pushes filtrate out of the damaged tubule into interstitial tissues (back leak). Renal blood flow and glomerular filtration may be further reduced by intrarenal angiotension II release and vasoconstriction.

Figure 6–16 ● Acute tubular necrosis. In ATN, tubular epithelial cells are destroyed by either ischemic or toxic injury.

ARF or AKI is seen in 4.5% of children cared for in pediatric intensive care units, and up to 8% of infants cared for in neonatal intensive care units (Goldstein & Devarajan, 2011). Potential causes include hemolytic uremic syndrome, acute glomerulonephritis, sepsis, poisoning, hypovolemia, obstructive uropathy, and complication of cardiac surgery. Recently, hematological-oncological complications, bone marrow transplantation, and respiratory failure have become more common causes of ARF. In some cases, a combination of factors leads to the development of ARF. Children who recover from ARF may have residual kidney damage and compromised renal function.

Risk Factors

Risk factors for ARF include major trauma or surgery, infection, hemorrhage, severe heart failure, severe liver disease, and lower urinary tract obstruction. Drugs and radiological contrast media that are toxic to the kidney also increase the risk for ARF.

Older adults develop ARF more frequently because of their higher incidence of serious illness, hypotension, major surgeries, diagnostic procedures, and treatment with nephrotoxic drugs. Decrease in kidney function associated with aging also puts older adults at greater risk for kidney failure.

The child with **renal insufficiency** (decrease in the kidneys' ability to conserve sodium and concentrate the urine) is at greater risk for fluid loss with illness. In cases of acute gastrointestinal (GI) illness, these children are at greater risk for dehydration and ARF.

Prevention

Contrast-induced nephropathy is the third most common cause of hospital-acquired renal failure, after decreased renal perfusion and administration of nephrotoxic medications. Identification of clients at risk and implementation of preventive strategies can decrease the incidence of this nephropathy. Prevention strategies focus on counteracting vasoconstriction, enhancing blood flow through the nephron, and providing protection against injury by oxygen free radicals. Knowledge of the adverse effects associated with infusion of contrast media, identification of clients at risk for contrast-induced nephropathy, and application of evidence-based prevention strategies allow nurses to assist in the prevention of contrast-induced nephropathy (Jorgenson, 2013).

▶ CLINICAL MANIFESTATIONS

The course of ARF caused by acute tubercular necrosis typically includes three phases: initiation, maintenance, and recovery.

Initiation Phase

The initiation phase may last hours to days. It begins with the initiating event (e.g., hemorrhage) and ends when tubular injury occurs. If ARF is recognized and the initiating event is treated effectively during this phase, the prognosis is good. The initiation phase of ARF is often asymptomatic, however, making it difficult to identify ARF before the appearance of the manifestations of the maintenance phase.

Maintenance Phase

The maintenance phase of ARF is characterized by a significant fall in GFR and tubular necrosis. Oliguria may develop, although many clients continue to produce normal or near-normal amounts of urine (nonoliguric ARF). Even though urine may be produced, the kidney cannot efficiently eliminate metabolic wastes, water, electrolytes, and acids from the body during the maintenance phase of ARF. Azotemia, fluid retention, electrolyte imbalances, and metabolic acidosis develop. These abnormalities are more severe in the client with oliguria than in the client without oliguria, leading to a poorer prognosis with oliguria.

During the maintenance phase, salt and water retention cause edema, increasing the risk for heart failure and pulmonary edema. Impaired potassium excretion leads to hyperkalemia (increased levels of potassium in the blood). When the serum potassium level is greater than 6.0–6.5 mEq/L, manifestations of its effect on neuromuscular function develop. These include muscle weakness, nausea and diarrhea, electrocardiographic changes, and possible cardiac arrest. Other electrolyte imbalances include **hyperphosphatemia** (increased blood levels of phosphate) and **hypocalcemia** (decreased blood levels of calcium). Metabolic acidosis results from impaired hydrogen ion elimination by the kidneys.

Anemia develops after several days of ARF because of suppressed erythropoietin secretion by the kidneys. Immune function may be impaired, increasing the risk for infection. Other manifestations of the maintenance phase include the following:

- Confusion, disorientation, agitation or lethargy; hyperreflexia; and possible seizures or coma because of azotemia and electrolyte and acid–base imbalances

- Anorexia (loss of appetite), nausea, vomiting, and decreased or absent bowel sounds

- Uremic syndrome (if ARF is prolonged; see the exemplar on Chronic Kidney Disease that follows).

Recovery Phase

The recovery phase of ARF is characterized by a process of tubule cell repair and regeneration and gradual return of the GFR to normal or pre-ARF levels. **Diuresis** (excretion of abnormally large quantities of urine) may occur as the nephrons and GFR recover, promoting the excretion of retained salt, water, and solutes. Serum creatinine, blood urea nitrogen (BUN), potassium, and phosphate levels remain high and may continue to rise in spite of increasing urine output. Renal function improves rapidly during the first 5–25 days of the recovery phase and continues to improve for up to 1 year.

Lifespan Considerations

Renal failure presents differently in older and younger adults. In younger adults, marked oliguria is the most dramatic symptom of ARF, but older adults may not display this symptom. Postural hypotension (a decrease in blood pressure when the client sits or stands) is common in older adult clients with prerenal ARF, and the nurse is in a position to monitor for this finding. BUN and serum creatinine levels increase, and dependent edema may also be present. In a study by Lanier, Mote, and Clay (2011), the prevalence of orthostatic hypotension was 18% in clients older than 65 years. Ultrasound may demonstrate changes in the size of the kidney, or the presence of calculi, in renal and postrenal causes.

Pediatric manifestations characteristically begin with a healthy child who suddenly becomes ill with nonspecific symptoms that indicate a significant illness or injury. These symptoms may include any combination of the following: nausea, vomiting, lethargy, edema, gross **hematuria** (blood in the urine), oliguria, and hypertension. These manifestations result from electrolyte imbalances (**Table 6–11** ●), uremia (excessive amounts of urea in the blood), and fluid overload. The child appears pale and lethargic.

TABLE 6–11 Electrolyte Imbalances in Acute and Chronic Kidney Disease in Children

ELECTROLYTE IMBALANCE	CAUSE	CLINICAL MANIFESTATIONS
Hyperkalemia (excess potassium in the blood)	Results from inability to adequately excrete potassium derived from diet and catabolized cells. In metabolic acidosis, potassium also moves from intracellular fluid to extracellular fluid.	■ Peaked T waves, widening of QRS waves on electrocardiogram ■ Dysrhythmias: ventricular dysrhythmias, heart block, ventricular fibrillation, cardiac arrest ■ Diarrhea ■ Muscle weakness
Hyponatremia (decreased sodium in the blood)	In the acute oliguric phase, hyponatremia is dilutional, related to the accumulation of fluid in excess of solute.	■ Change in level of consciousness ■ Muscle cramps ■ Anorexia ■ Abdominal reflexes, depressed deep tendon reflexes ■ Cheyne-Stokes respirations ■ Seizures
Hypocalcemia (decreased calcium in the blood)	Phosphate retention (hyperphosphatemia) caused by impaired renal function depresses the serum calcium concentration. Calcium is deposited in injured cells. Hyperkalemia and metabolic acidosis may mask the common clinical manifestations of severe hypocalcemia.	■ Muscle tingling ■ Changes in muscle tone ■ Seizures ■ Muscle cramps and twitching ■ Positive Chvostek sign (contraction of facial muscles after tapping facial nerve just anterior to parotid gland)

Clinical Manifestations and Therapies Acute Renal Failure

ETIOLOGY	CLINICAL MANIFESTATIONS	CLINICAL THERAPIES
Anemia	■ Fatigue ■ Pallor ■ Dizziness, confusion, lethargy ■ Tachycardia, tachypnea, hypotension	■ Iron supplementation ■ Administration of epoetin ■ Blood transfusion ■ Therapies aimed at treating the underlying cause of ARF
Fluid volume excess	■ Dependent **pitting edema** (edema that retains indentation caused by pressure) ■ Respiratory crackles ■ Dyspnea, pulmonary edema, hypoxemia ■ Weight gain ■ Tachycardia ■ Jugular vein distention	■ Fluid restriction ■ Sodium-restricted diet ■ Diuretics ■ Dialysis
Hyperkalemia	■ Ventricular arrhythmias ■ Tall, peaked T waves; widened QRS ■ Cardiac arrest ■ Smooth muscle hyperactivity ■ Nausea and vomiting ■ Abdominal cramping ■ Diarrhea ■ Muscle weakness ■ Paresthesias ■ Flaccid paralysis	■ Removal of all potassium from intravenous solutions ■ Low-potassium diet ■ Administration of glucose and insulin to drive potassium into the cell ■ Potassium-absorbing enema solutions ■ Dialysis

▶ COLLABORATION

Preventing ARF is a goal in caring for all clients, especially those in high-risk groups. Maintaining adequate vascular volume, cardiac output, and blood pressure is vital to preserving kidney perfusion, as is avoiding nephrotoxic drugs whenever possible. When a nephrotoxic drug or substance must be used, the risk of ARF can be reduced by using the minimum effective dose, maintaining hydration, and eliminating other known nephrotoxins from the medication regimen. When discharging a client with instructions to avoid nephrotoxic drugs, the nurse should encourage the client to contact his or her pharmacist. Adding that information to the client's pharmacy history will help the client to avoid nephrotoxic drugs that may be prescribed in the future.

If a client develops ARF, maintaining the fluid and electrolyte balance is a key goal in managing the condition. Other goals in the treatment of ARF include the following:

1. To identify and correct the underlying cause
2. To prevent additional kidney damage
3. To restore the urine output and kidney function
4. To compensate for renal impairment until kidney function is restored.

The complex nature of renal failure makes an interdisciplinary approach critical. The nurse, nephrologist, and nutritionist are essential members of the care team. Consultation with a nephrologist is important in limiting kidney damage and decreasing mortality. Consultation with a cardiologist may be necessary, particularly for clients with a preexisting cardiac condition. In the older adult, nutritional support is especially important. Weight loss of up to 1 lb per day is expected in the older adult with ARF. Any attempt to prevent the weight loss may overtax multiple systems and lead to cardiac failure. For example, the use of nutritional supplements that are high in calories may be contraindicated in the older adult with ARF. Allowing weight loss to occur during this acute phase may better protect the long-term health of the older adult. Dehydration in the older adult is a causative factor in ARF; therefore, fluid restrictions should be modest.

Diagnostic Tests

Diagnostic tests are used to identify the cause of ARF and monitor its effects on homeostasis. These tests include the following:

- *Urinalysis* often shows the following abnormal findings in ARF:
  a. A fixed specific gravity of 1.010 (equal to the specific gravity of plasma), because the tubules are unable to concentrate the filtrate
  b. **Proteinuria** (excess protein in urine) if glomerular damage is the cause of ARF
  c. The presence of RBCs (caused by glomerular dysfunction), white blood cells (WBCs; related to inflammation), and renal tubular epithelial cells (indicating ATN)
  d. Cell casts, which are protein and cellular debris molded in the shape of the tubular lumen (in ARF, RBCs, WBCs, and renal tubular epithelial casts may be present; brownish-pigmented casts and positive tests for occult blood indicate hemoglobinuria or myoglobinuria)
- *Serum creatinine* and *BUN* are used to evaluate renal function. In ARF, serum creatinine levels increase rapidly, within 24–48 hours of onset. Creatinine levels generally peak within 5–10 days. Creatinine and BUN levels tend to increase more slowly when urine output is maintained. The onset of recovery is marked by a halt in the rise of the serum creatinine and BUN.
- *Serum electrolytes* are monitored to evaluate the fluid and electrolyte status. The serum potassium rises at a moderate rate and is often used to indicate the need for dialysis. Hyponatremia is common because of the water excess associated with ARF.
- *Arterial blood gas* studies often show a metabolic acidosis caused by the kidneys' inability to adequately eliminate metabolic wastes and hydrogen ions.
- *Complete blood count (CBC)* shows reduced RBCs, moderate anemia, and a low hematocrit. ARF affects erythropoietin secretion and RBC production. Iron and folate absorption may also be impaired, further contributing to anemia.
- *Renal ultrasonography* is used to identify obstructive causes of renal failure and to differentiate ARF from end-stage chronic kidney disease. In ARF, the kidneys may be enlarged, whereas in chronic kidney disease, they typically appear small and shrunken.
- *Computed tomography* may be done to evaluate kidney size and identify possible obstructions.
- *Intravenous pyelography, retrograde pyelography,* or *antegrade pyelography* may be used to evaluate kidney structure and function. Radiological contrast media are used with extreme caution because of their potential nephrotoxicity. Retrograde pyelography, in which contrast dye is injected into the ureters, and antegrade pyelography, in which the contrast medium is injected percutaneously into the renal pelvis, are preferred, because they have fewer nephrotoxic effects than intravenous pyelography.
- *Renal biopsy* may be necessary to differentiate between acute and chronic kidney disease.
- *Radiographic studies* may be helpful in determining ARF in pediatric clients, because these studies will indicate the size of the kidney. A common cause of ARF in children is **osteodystrophy** (a complex bone disease process of chronic kidney disease in which increased resorption of bone is caused by chronic hyperparathyroidism).

Pharmacologic Therapy

The primary focus in drug management for ARF is to restore and maintain renal perfusion and to eliminate drugs that are nephrotoxic from the treatment regimen. Intravenous fluids and blood volume expanders are given as needed to restore renal perfusion. Dopamine (Intropin), administered in low doses by intravenous infusion, increases renal blood flow. Dopamine is a sympathetic neurotransmitter that improves cardiac output and dilates blood vessels of the mesentery and kidneys when given in low therapeutic doses.

If restoration of renal blood flow does not improve urinary output, a potent loop diuretic, such as furosemide (Lasix), or an osmotic diuretic, such as mannitol, may be given with intravenous fluids. The purpose for giving a potent diuretic is twofold. First, if nephrotoxins are present, the combination of fluids and potent diuretics may, in effect, "wash out" the nephrons, reducing toxin concentration. Second, establishing urine output may

Medications **Acute Renal Failure**

CLASSIFICATION AND DRUG EXAMPLES	MECHANISMS OF ACTION	NURSING CONSIDERATIONS
Loop Diuretics *Drug examples:* ■ bumetanide (Bumex) ■ ethacrynic acid (Edecrin) ■ furosemide (Lasix) ■ torsemide (Demadex)	The loop diuretics, named for their primary site of action in the loop of Henle, are high-ceiling diuretics (the response increases with increasing doses). These are highly effective diuretics used in early ARF to reestablish urine flow and convert oliguric renal failure to nonoliguric renal failure. Loop diuretics may be given with intravenous dopamine to promote renal blood flow. In ATN caused by a nephrotoxin, loop diuretics are used to clear the toxin from the nephrons more rapidly. Loop diuretics cause potassium wasting, which is generally not a concern in ARF because renal failure impairs normal potassium elimination.	■ Assess weight and vital signs for baseline data. ■ Monitor intake and output, daily weight (or more frequently as ordered), vital signs, skin turgor, and other indicators of fluid volume status frequently. ■ Assess for orthostatic hypotension; these potent diuretics can lead to hypovolemia. ■ Monitor laboratory results, especially serum electrolyte, glucose, BUN, and creatinine levels. ■ Administer as ordered: a. Furosemide, undiluted at a rate of no more than 20 mg/min b. Ethacrynic acid, 50 mg diluted with 50 mL of normal saline, at a rate of no more than 10 mg/min c. Bumetanide, undiluted over at least 1 min or diluted in lactated Ringer's solution, normal saline, or 5% dextrose in water for infusion d. Torsemide, undiluted over at least 2 min. ■ Assess response. Urine output typically increases within 10 min after intravenous administration. ■ Monitor hearing and for complaints such as tinnitus. High doses of loop diuretics increase the risk of ototoxicity, especially with ethacrynic acid. These effects may be reversible if they are detected early and the drug is discontinued. ■ Avoid administering concurrently with other ototoxic agents, such as aminoglycoside antibiotics and cisplatin. ■ Health education for the client and family: a. Unless contraindicated, maintain a fluid intake of 2–3 liters per day. b. Rise slowly from lying or sitting positions, because a fall in blood pressure may cause light-headedness. c. Take in the morning and, if ordered twice a day, in the late afternoon to avoid sleep disturbance. d. Take with food or milk to prevent gastric distress. e. Nonsteroidal anti-inflammatory drugs interfere with the effectiveness of loop diuretics and should be avoided.
Osmotic Diuretics *Drug examples:* ■ mannitol (Osmitrol, Isotel) ■ urea (Ureaphil)	The osmotic diuretics act by increasing the osmotic draw in the blood and urine. In the blood, the effect is to pull extracellular water into the vascular system, increasing the GFR. These substances are then freely filtered in the glomerulus and increase the osmotic draw of the urine, inhibiting water reabsorption. The effect is to increase urine volume and flow. In addition, osmotic diuretics dilute waste products in the urine, decreasing the risk of renal damage because of excess concentrations.	■ Assess urine output. Osmotic diuretics are used in early renal failure to maintain urine output but are contraindicated in **anuria** (inability of kidneys to produce urine). A test dose may be administered; urine output of 30 mL/hr following the test dose shows an adequate response. ■ Do not give these diuretics to clients who have heart failure or are severely dehydrated. These drugs increase vascular volume and may worsen heart failure. They are not effective unless extracellular volume is adequate. ■ Administer mannitol intravenously, diluting before use if indicated. Check solution for crystallization. Dissolve crystals by warming the solution slightly. Infuse 15%–25% mannitol solutions through a filter over 30–90 min. ■ Administer urea intravenously, diluting in 100 mL of 5% or 10% dextrose in water for every 30 g of urea. Administer no faster than 4 mL/min through a filter. ■ Monitor vital signs, breath sounds, and urinary output. ■ Discontinue the drug if signs of heart failure or pulmonary edema develop or if renal function continues to decline. ■ Instruct client and family to report shortness of breath, headache, chest pain, or dizziness immediately.

(continued on next page)

Medications **Acute Renal Failure** (continued)

CLASSIFICATION AND DRUG EXAMPLES	MECHANISMS OF ACTION	NURSING CONSIDERATIONS

Electrolytes and Electrolyte Modifiers
 	
Drug examples:
- calcium chloride
- calcium gluconate
- sodium bicarbonate
- sodium polystyrene sulfonate (Kayexalate)
	Calcium chloride or gluconate and sodium bicarbonate are administered intravenously in the initial management of hyperkalemia. Calcium is also administered to correct hypocalcemia and reduce hyperphosphatemia. (Calcium and phosphate have a reciprocal relationship in the body; as the level of one rises, the level of the other falls.) Sodium bicarbonate helps to correct acidosis and move potassium back into the intracellular space. Sodium polystyrene sulfonate is not used to replace an electrolyte but to remove excess potassium from the body by exchanging sodium for potassium in the large intestine.	▪ Assess serum electrolyte levels before and during therapy. Report rapid shifts or adverse responses to the physician.
		▪ Administer as appropriate:
		  a. Intravenous calcium chloride at less than 1 mL/min; intravenous calcium gluconate at 0.5 mL/min. Inject into a large vein through a small-bore needle; avoid infiltration, because extravasation of intravenous solution will cause tissue necrosis.
		  b. Intravenous sodium bicarbonate infusion over 4–8 hr; oral tablets as prescribed.
		  c. Sodium polystyrene sulfonate as an oral solution mixed with sorbitol to prevent constipation, or as a retention enema mixed with warm water. Leave in the bowel for 30–60 min, irrigate using a small tap-water enema.
		▪ Monitor for adverse reactions, such as dysrhythmias, electrolyte imbalances, and metabolic alkalosis.
		▪ Health education for the client and family:
		  a. Intravenous calcium may make you light-headed; remain in bed for at least 30 min after administration.
		  b. Chew sodium bicarbonate tablets and follow with 8 oz of water. Do not take with milk.
		  c. Retain the sodium polystyrene sulfonate enema as long as possible.

prevent oliguria and reduce the degree of azotemia and fluid and electrolyte imbalances. Furosemide also may be used to manage salt and water retention associated with ARF.

Aggressive management of hypertension limits renal injury when ARF is associated with disorders such as toxemia and pregnancy-induced hypertension. Angiotensin-converting enzyme inhibitors or other antihypertensive medications are used to control arterial pressures.

All drugs that are either directly nephrotoxic or that may interfere with renal perfusion (e.g., potent vasoconstrictors) are discontinued. Nonsteroidal anti-inflammatory drugs, nephrotoxic antibiotics, and other potentially harmful drugs are avoided throughout the course of ARF.

The client in ARF has an increased risk of GI bleeding, probably related to the stress response and impaired platelet function. Regular doses of antacids, histamine H_2-receptor antagonists (e.g., famotidine or ranitidine), or a proton-pump inhibitor (e.g., omeprazole [Prilosec]) are often ordered to prevent GI hemorrhage.

Hyperkalemia may require active intervention as well as restricted potassium intake. Serum levels greater than 6.5 mEq/L are treated to prevent the adverse cardiovascular effects of hyperkalemia. With significant hyperkalemia, calcium chloride, bicarbonate, and insulin and glucose may be given intravenously to reduce serum potassium levels by moving potassium into the cells. A potassium-binding exchange resin, such as sodium polystyrene sulfonate (Kayexalate, SPS Suspension), may be given orally or by enema. This agent removes potassium from the body by exchanging sodium for potassium, primarily in the large intestine. When given orally, it is often combined with sorbitol to prevent constipation. Rectally, it is instilled as a retention enema, allowed to remain in the

bowel for approximately 30–60 minutes, and then irrigated out using a tap-water enema.

Aluminum hydroxide (ALternaGEL, Amphojel, Nephrox), an antacid, is used to control hyperphosphatemia in renal failure. It binds with phosphates in the GI tract, which are then excreted in the feces.

Because many drugs are eliminated from the body by the kidney, drug dosages may need to be adjusted. Doses within the usual range can lead to potentially toxic blood levels, because their elimination is slowed and their half-life prolonged. Nursing implications for medications commonly prescribed for the client with ARF are summarized in the Medications feature.

Fluid Management

Once vascular volume and renal perfusion have been restored, fluid intake usually is restricted. The restricted daily fluid intake is calculated by allowing 500 mL for insensible losses (respiration, perspiration, and bowel losses) and adding the amount excreted as urine (or lost in vomitus) during the previous 24 hours. For example, if a client with ARF excretes 325 mL of urine in 24 hours, allow the client a fluid intake (including oral and intravenous fluids) of 825 mL for the next 24 hours. Carefully monitor fluid balance by using accurate weight measurements and the serum sodium as the primary indicators.

Initial emergency treatment of children with fluid depletion focuses on rapid fluid replacement with 20 mL/kg of saline or lactated Ringer's solution given over 5 to 10 minutes and repeated as needed. This ensures renal perfusion and stabilizes blood pressure.

Albumin may also be administered when blood loss is the cause of the client's circulatory depletion. If oliguria persists after restoration of adequate fluid volume, intrinsic renal damage is suspected.

Nutrition

Renal insufficiency and the underlying disease process increase the rate of catabolism and decrease the rate of anabolism (body tissue repair). The client with ARF needs adequate nutrients and calories to prevent catabolism. Proteins are limited to 0.6 g/kg of body weight per day to minimize the degree of azotemia. Dietary proteins should be of high biological value (rich in essential amino acids). Carbohydrates are increased to maintain adequate calorie intake and provide a protein-sparing effect. For additional information refer to the module on Nutrition.

Parenteral nutrition providing amino acids, concentrated carbohydrates, and fats may be instituted when the client cannot consume an adequate diet (e.g., because of nausea, vomiting, or underlying critical illness). The disadvantages of parenteral nutrition in the client with ARF are the high volume of fluid required and the risk for infection through the venous line.

Renal Replacement Therapy

Manifestations of uremia, organ dysfunction caused by accumulated metabolic wastes, severe fluid overload, hyperkalemia, or metabolic acidosis in a client with renal failure indicate a need to replace renal function. **Dialysis** is the diffusion of solute molecules across a semipermeable membrane from an area of higher solute concentration to one of lower concentration according to the rules of osmosis. It is used to remove excess fluid and metabolic waste products in renal failure. Early use of dialysis can reduce the rate of complications. Dialysis may also be used to rapidly remove nephrotoxins in ATN. Although dialysis compensates for lost renal elimination functions, it does not replace lost erythropoietin production. Anemia is a continuing problem for the client receiving dialysis.

In dialysis, blood is separated from a dialysis solution (**dialysate**) by a semipermeable membrane. Either **hemodialysis**, a procedure in which blood flows through vascular catheters, is pumped through the dialyzer unit, and returned to the client, or **peritoneal dialysis**, which uses the peritoneum surrounding the abdominal cavity as the dialyzing membrane, may be used for the client with ARF. **Continuous renal replacement therapy (CRRT)**, in which blood is continuously circulated through a highly porous hemofilter from artery to vein or from vein to vein, is a newer form of dialysis that may be used to treat ARF.

HEMODIALYSIS Hemodialysis uses the principles of diffusion and ultrafiltration to remove electrolytes, waste products, and excess water from the body. Blood is taken from the client via a vascular access and is pumped to the dialyzer (**Figure 6–17 ●**). The porous membranes of the dialyzer unit allow small molecules (e.g., water, glucose, and electrolytes) to pass through but block larger molecules (e.g., serum proteins and blood cells). The dialysate, a solution of approximately the same composition and temperature as normal extracellular fluid, passes along the

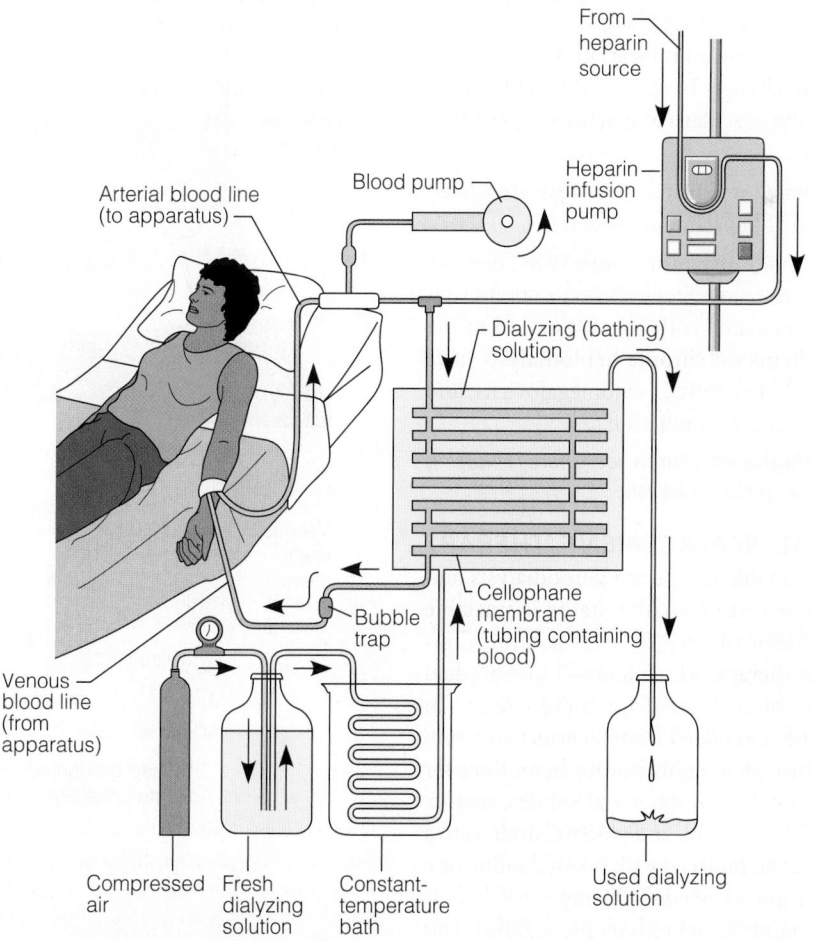

Figure 6–17 ● The components of a hemodialysis system.

TABLE 6–12   Continuous Renal Replacement Therapies

TYPE	INDICATIONS	DESCRIPTION
Continuous arteriovenous hemofiltration (CAVH)	Removes fluid and some solutes.	Arterial blood circulates through a hemofilter, then returns to client through venous line; ultrafiltrate collects in a drainage bag.
Continuous arteriovenous hemodialysis (CAVHD)	Removes fluid and waste products.	Arterial blood circulates through a hemofilter surrounded by dialysate, then returns to client through venous line; ultrafiltrate collects in a drainage bag.
Continuous venovenous hemodialysis (CVVHD)	Removes fluid and waste products.	Venous blood circulates through a hemofilter surrounded by dialysate, then returns to client through double-lumen venous catheter; ultrafiltrate collects in a drainage bag.

other side of the membrane. Small solute molecules move freely across the membrane by diffusion. The direction of movement for any substance is determined by the concentrations of that substance in the blood and the dialysate. Electrolytes and waste products (e.g., urea and creatinine) diffuse from the blood into the dialysate. If it is necessary to add something to the blood, such as calcium to replace depleted stores, it can be added to the dialysate to diffuse into the blood. Excess water is removed by creating a hydrostatic pressure of the blood moving through the dialyzer that is higher than that of the dialysate, which flows in the opposite direction. This process is known as **ultrafiltration**.

Initially, clients with ARF typically undergo daily hemodialysis. As their condition improves, clients may change to three to four sessions per week as indicated. Hemodialysis is not used if the client is hemodynamically unstable (e.g., with hypotension or low cardiac output). The following complications are associated with hemodialysis:

■ Hypotension, the most frequent complication during hemodialysis, may result from changes in serum osmolality, rapid removal of fluid from the vascular compartment, vasodilation, and other factors.

■ Bleeding may result from altered platelet function associated with uremia and the use of heparin during dialysis.

■ Infection (local or systemic) may result from WBC damage and immune system suppression. *Staphylococcus aureus* septicemia is commonly associated with contamination of the vascular access site. Clients on chronic hemodialysis have higher rates of hepatitis B, hepatitis C, cytomegalovirus, and HIV infection than the general population.

✳ Go to **nursing.pearsonhighered.com** to see Chart 1: Nursing Care for the Client Undergoing Hemodialysis.

CONTINUOUS RENAL REPLACEMENT THERAPY

Clients with ARF may be unable to tolerate hemodialysis and rapid fluid removal if their cardiovascular status is unstable (e.g., because of trauma, major surgery, or heart failure). Continuous renal replacement therapy, which allows more gradual fluid and solute removal, often is used for these clients. In CRRT, blood is continuously circulated from an artery to a vein or from a vein to a vein through a highly porous hemofilter for a period of 12 hours or more. Excess water and solutes, such as electrolytes, urea, creatinine, uric acid, and glucose, drain into a collection device. Fluid may be replaced with normal saline or a balanced electrolyte solution as needed during CRRT. This slower process helps to maintain hemodynamic stability and avoid complications associated with rapid changes in composi-

tion of the extracellular fluid. The most common CRRT techniques are outlined in **Table 6–12 ●**.

Typically, CRRT is performed in an intensive care unit or specialized nephrology unit. Both arterial and venous lines are required for some types of CRRT (**Figure 6–18 ●**); for others, a double-lumen venous catheter is used. Strict aseptic technique is vital in caring for vascular access sites to reduce the risk of infection.

VASCULAR ACCESS FOR HEMODIALYSIS AND CONTINUOUS RENAL REPLACEMENT THERAPY   Acute or temporary vascular access for hemodialysis or CRRT usually is gained by inserting a double-lumen catheter into the subclavian,

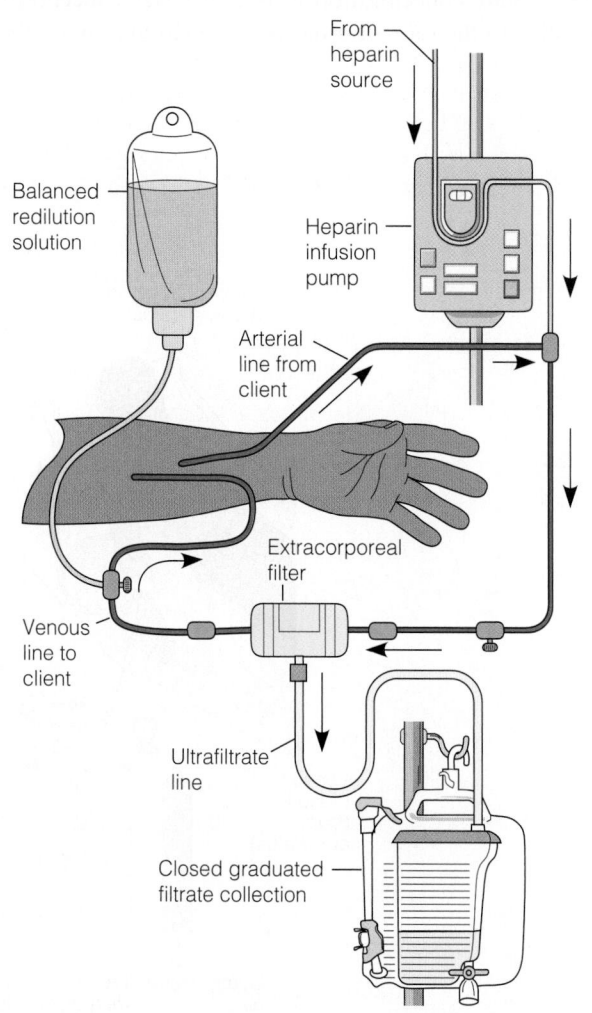

Figure 6–18 ● Continuous arteriovenous hemofiltration.

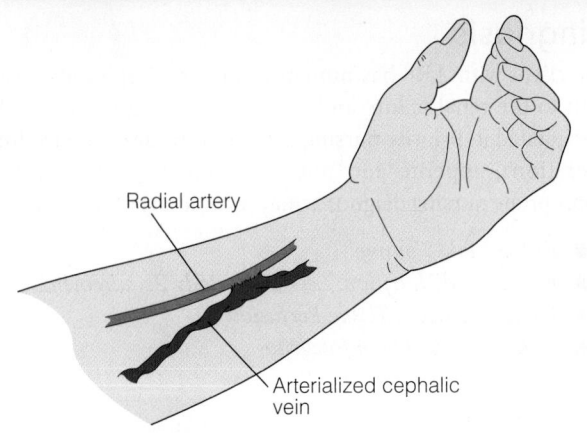

Figure 6–19 ● An arteriovenous fistula.

jugular, or femoral vein. The double-lumen catheter has a central partition separating the blood-withdrawal side of the catheter from the return side. Blood is drawn into the catheter through small openings in the proximal portion of the catheter, and it is returned to the circulation through an opening in the distal end of the catheter to avoid withdrawing the blood that has just been dialyzed.

For longer-term vascular access, an **arteriovenous (AV) fistula** (an artificial connection between a vein and an artery) is created (**Figure 6–19 ●**). In preparation for fistula formation, the nondominant arm is not used for venipuncture or blood pressure measurement during renal failure. The fistula is created by surgical anastomosis of an artery and vein, usually the radial artery and cephalic vein. It takes about a month for the fistula to mature so that it can be used for taking and replacing blood during dialysis. A functional AV fistula has a palpable

pulsation and a bruit on auscultation. Avoid venipunctures and blood pressures on the arm with the fistula.

In chronic kidney disease, an *arteriovenous graft* is most often used for vascular access. The graft, a tube made of Gortex, is surgically implanted and connects the artery and the vein. Blood flows through the graft from the artery to the vein. Occasionally, an *external AV shunt* connecting a peripheral artery with a peripheral vein is used for vascular access. Ideally, an AV fistula or graft is created as soon as the potential need for long-term renal replacement therapies is identified (Dinwiddie, 2004).

The rate of complications and mortality associated with catheter access is higher than with AV fistulas or grafts; however, localized AV fistula, graft, or shunt problems can occur. Infection and clotting or thrombosis are the most common shunt problems. Aneurysms may also develop. Both infection and thrombosis can lead to systemic manifestations, such as septicemia and embolization. These local complications may cause the fistula or graft to fail, necessitating development of a new site. The psychological impact of AV fistula or graft failure is significant, often causing depression and low self-esteem.

PERITONEAL DIALYSIS   In peritoneal dialysis, the highly vascular peritoneal membrane serves as the dialyzing surface (**Figure 6–20 ●**). Warmed, sterile dialysate is instilled into the peritoneal cavity through a catheter inserted into the peritoneal cavity. Metabolic waste products and excess electrolytes diffuse into the dialysate while it remains in the abdomen. Water movement is controlled using dextrose as an osmotic agent to draw it into the dialysate. The fluid is then drained by gravity out of the peritoneal cavity into a sterile bag. This process of dialysate infusion, dwell time of the solution in the abdomen, and drainage is repeated at prescribed intervals.

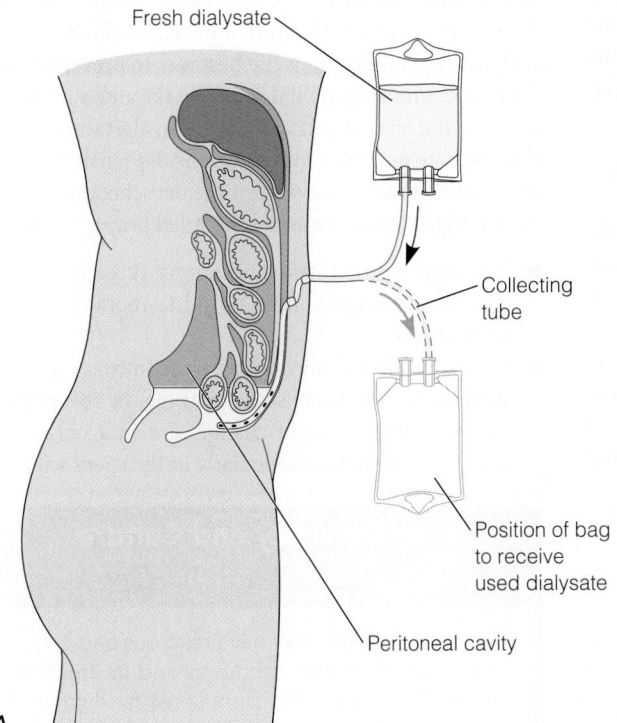

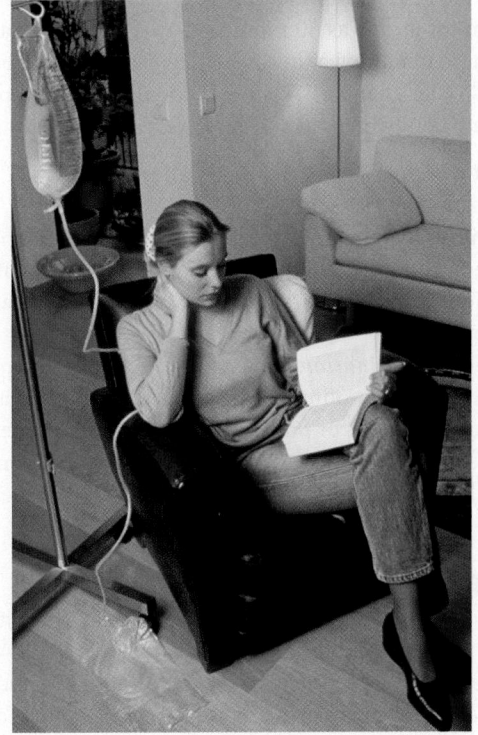

Figure 6–20 ● *A*, Peritoneal dialysis. *B*, Woman receiving peritoneal dialysis.
Source: B, Carolyn A. Mckeone/Science Source.

Because excess fluid and solutes are removed more gradually in peritoneal dialysis, this type of renal replacement therapy poses less risk than other methods for the unstable client; however, this slower rate of metabolite removal can be a disadvantage in clients with ARF. Peritoneal dialysis increases the risk for developing peritonitis, and it is contraindicated for clients who have had recent abdominal surgery, significant lung disease, or peritonitis.

✳ *Go to* **nursing.pearsonhighered.com** *to see Chart 2: Nursing Care for the Client Undergoing Peritoneal Dialysis.*

■ NURSING PROCESS

ARF often can be prevented by measures that maintain fluid volume and cardiac output and that reduce the risk of exposure to nephrotoxins. Carefully monitor critically ill, postoperative, and other at-risk clients for early signs of hypovolemia (low urine output, altered mental status, and changes in vital signs, skin color, or temperature). Promptly report a fall in urine output to less than 30 mL/hr and other evidence of decreased cardiac output. Maintain intravenous fluids as ordered. Alert the physician if the client is receiving more than one nephrotoxic drug or if a nephrotoxic drug is ordered for a client who is dehydrated. Closely observe clients receiving blood or blood cells for early signs of transfusion reaction, and intervene appropriately as needed.

Assessment

Both subjective and objective data are useful when assessing the client with ARF. The client's history and physical assessment can provide clues about the initiating event for ARF. Impaired perfusion for as few as 30 minutes may cause significant renal ischemia, so obtaining a thorough history is essential. For pediatric and older clients, assessments should include input from immediate family members or caregivers.

- *Health history.* Complaints of anorexia, nausea, weight gain, or edema; recent exposure to a nephrotoxin, such as an aminoglycoside antibiotic or radiological procedure using an injected contrast medium; previous transfusion reaction; chronic diseases, such as diabetes, heart failure, or kidney disease
- *Physical examination.* Vital signs, including temperature; urine output (amount, color, clarity, specific gravity, presence of blood cells or protein); weight; skin color; peripheral pulses; presence of edema (periorbital or dependent); lung sounds, heart sounds, and bowel tones

SAFETY ALERT
The unexpected and acute nature of a child's hospitalization creates anxiety for both parents and the child. Assess for feelings of anger, guilt, or fear associated with the hospitalization. Such feelings are likely if ARF developed as a result of dehydration, a preventable injury, or poisoning. Assess coping mechanisms, family support systems, and level of stress.

Diagnosis

The client with ARF has numerous nursing care needs related both to the renal failure and to the underlying condition that precipitated it. Priority nursing care needs relate to fluid volume alterations, appetite and nutrition, and teaching/learning. Appropriate nursing diagnoses may include any of the following:

- *Excess Fluid Volume*
- *Imbalanced Nutrition: Less Than Body Requirements*
- *Ineffective Renal Tissue Perfusion*
- *Risk for Altered Skin Integrity*
- *Risk for Altered Cardiac Perfusion*
- *Risk for Infection*
- *Compromised Family Coping.*

(NANDA-I © 2012)

Planning

Nursing care focuses on preventing complications, maintaining fluid balance, administering medications, meeting nutritional needs, preventing infection, and providing emotional support to the client and family. Possible outcomes, created in collaboration with the client and family, include the following:

- The client's weight will return to baseline measurement.
- The client's urine output will be greater than 30 mL/hr.
- The client's hemoglobin and hematocrit values will be within normal limits.
- The client's serum electrolytes will be within normal limits.
- The client's pulse rate, volume, and rhythm will return to baseline.

Implementation

The care of each client will vary based on the cause of ARF and the specific needs of the individual client. Ensuring compliance with the treatment plan is the best way to prevent complications. Careful monitoring of vital signs, intake and output, serum electrolytes, and level of consciousness can alert the nurse to changes that indicate potential complications. Be sensitive to any cultural or religious practices, even if it means scheduling appointments or nursing activities around scheduled prayer times.

- Maintain hourly intake and output records. Accurate intake and output records help to guide therapy, especially fluid restrictions.
- Weigh the client daily or more frequently as ordered. Use standard technique (same scale, clothing, or coverings) to ensure accuracy. Rapid weight changes are an accurate indicator of fluid volume status, particularly in the client with oliguria.

Focus on Diversity and Culture
Religious and Cultural Preferences

The client with ARF may have religious and cultural preferences that affect the condition and its treatment. Food preferences may put the client at risk for fluid or electrolyte imbalance. Religious practices, such as frequent daily prayers and religious policies against transfusions or dialysis, may impact implementation of care.

- Assess vital signs at least every 4 hours. Hypertension, tachycardia, and tachypnea may indicate excess fluid volume.
- Assess breath and heart sounds, neck veins for distention, and back and extremities for edema; report abnormal findings.
- If not contraindicated, place client in semi-Fowler position to enhance cardiac and respiratory function.
- Report abnormal serum electrolyte values and manifestations of electrolyte imbalance. The client with ARF is at particular risk for the following electrolyte imbalances:
  a. *Hyperkalemia* caused by impaired potassium excretion. Manifestations include irritability, nausea, diarrhea, abdominal cramping, cardiac dysrhythmias, and electrocardiographic changes.
  b. *Hyponatremia* caused by water retention. Manifestations include nausea, vomiting, and headache, with possible central nervous system manifestations of lethargy, confusion, seizures, and coma. If the serum sodium concentration rises and the client's weight falls, insufficient fluids are being administered. If the serum sodium level falls and the client's weight increases, excessive fluids are being administered.
  c. *Hyperphosphatemia* caused by decreased phosphate excretion. Manifestations include hyperreflexia, paresthesias, and possible **tetany** (tonic muscle spasms). ARF impairs electrolyte and water excretion, causing multiple electrolyte imbalances.
- Turn the client frequently, and provide good skin care. Edema decreases tissue perfusion and increases the risk of skin breakdown, especially in the older or debilitated client.
- Restrict fluids as ordered. Provide frequent mouth care, and encourage use of hard candies to decrease thirst. If ice chips are allowed, include the water content (approximately half the total volume) as intake. Fluids are restricted to minimize fluid retention and complications of fluid volume excess.
- Administer medications with meals. Giving oral medications with meals minimizes ingestion of excess fluids.

Address Nutrition Imbalances

Anorexia and nausea associated with renal failure often interfere with food intake and nutrition. In addition, the disease process leading to ARF may contribute to increased nutritional needs for

---

Lifespan Considerations Nutrition and Children With Acute Renal Failure

- Children are at risk for malnutrition because of their high metabolic rate during acute renal failure. Parenteral or enteral feeding may be used initially to minimize protein catabolism.
- The diet is tailored to the individual child's needs for calories, carbohydrates, fats, and amino acids or protein hydrolysates. Depending on the degree of renal failure, sodium, potassium, and phosphorus may be restricted.
- Oral feedings are initiated as soon as tolerated.
- A multidisciplinary team review with a nutritionist may be necessary.

---

healing concurrently with decreased food intake. Interventions for clients experiencing inadequate nutrition include:

- Monitor and record food intake, including the amount and type of food consumed. A detailed intake record helps to guide decisions about nutritional status and necessary supplements.
- Weigh the client daily. Weight changes over time (days to weeks) reflect nutritional status, whereas rapid weight changes are more reflective of fluid volume status. In ARF, weight may remain stable or increase because of fluid retention even though tissue mass is being lost.
- Arrange for consultation with a dietitian. A registered dietitian can assist in planning meals within prescribed limitations that consider the client's food preferences, especially if the client follows cultural or religious mandates regarding foods. Diets restricted in protein, salt, and potassium can be unpalatable; intake and appetite improve when preferred foods are included as allowed.
- Engage the client in planning daily menus. Participation in meal planning increases the client's sense of control and autonomy.
- Allow family members to prepare meals within dietary restrictions. Encourage family members to eat with the client. Familiar foods and social interaction encourage eating and increase enjoyment of meals.

SAFETY ALERT
Remember that acute renal failure requires nutritional intervention. These interventions must take into consideration the increased nutritional needs of children and adolescents brought about by growth and development.

- Provide frequent, small meals or between-meal snacks. These measures promote food intake in the client who is fatigued or anorectic.
- Administer antiemetics as ordered, and provide mouth care before meals. Nausea and a metallic taste in the mouth, common manifestations of uremia, can decrease food intake.
- Administer parenteral nutrition as ordered if the client is unable to eat or tolerate enteral nutrition. Preventing or slowing tissue **catabolism** (the breakdown of body proteins) is important for the client with ARF.

Provide Client Teaching

Client teaching is essential to resolving ARF and preventing any further complications. Prior to providing any information, it is important to assess the client's anxiety level and ability to comprehend instruction; the client with ARF may be critically ill or be experiencing uremic effects that hinder learning. During the initial stages of ARF, it may be necessary to limit information to immediate concerns, such as treatment of the underlying cause of kidney failure. Remember to tailor information and presentation to the client's developmental level as well as physical, mental, and emotional status.

- Assess knowledge and understanding. To enhance understanding and retention, relate the information presented to previous learning.
- Teach client and immediate family about diagnostic tests and therapeutic procedures. Teaching reduces anxiety and improves understanding and cooperation.

- Discuss dietary and fluid restrictions. These measures may be continued after discharge.
- If the client is discharged before the recovery phase of ARF, teach the signs and symptoms of complications, including fluid volume excess or deficit, heart failure, and electrolyte imbalances. Explain to the client that urine output increases as kidney function returns, but that the concentrating ability of the nephrons and electrolyte excretion remain impaired. This impaired function increases the risk of excess fluid loss, possible dehydration, orthostatic hypotension, and electrolyte imbalance.
- Teach client how to monitor weight, blood pressure, and pulse. These are important means of assessing fluid status.
- Instruct client to avoid nephrotoxic drugs and chemicals for up to 1 year following an episode of ARF. During recovery, nephrons are vulnerable to damage by nephrotoxins, such as nonsteroidal anti-inflammatory drugs, some antibiotics, radiological contrast media, and heavy metals. Because alcohol can increase the nephrotoxicity of some materials, discourage alcohol ingestion.

Evaluation

Evaluation of the client with ARF is based on resolution of symptoms and prevention of complications. Data to be evaluated include weight, cardiac rhythm, vital signs, breath sounds, oxygen saturation, serum electrolyte levels, intake and output, and hemoglobin and hematocrit. The client should be evaluated for response to treatment as well as for understanding of the disease process and self-care requirements. Expected outcomes of nursing care include the following:

- The client maintains fluid, electrolyte and acid–base balance as evidenced by absence of signs and symptoms of imbalance.
- The client's nutritional needs are met as evidenced by dietary recall, return to appropriate weight, and absence of signs and symptoms of nutrition imbalance.
- The client acquires no secondary infections.

NURSING CARE PLAN A Client With Acute Renal Failure

Judy Devak is driving home late one evening when she loses control of her car trying to avoid hitting a deer in the road. Her car strikes a tree and rolls into a deep ditch beside the road, out of sight of passing cars. The wreck is not discovered until 2 hours later. On arrival at the accident scene, the paramedics find Ms. Devak hypotensive: BP 90/60 mmHg, pulse 120 bpm, and respirations 24/min. She is alert and in severe pain, with a fractured right femur. After immobilizing Ms. Devak's neck and back and extricating her from the car, the paramedics apply a traction splint to her leg and transport her to the local hospital.

ASSESSMENT	DIAGNOSES	PLANNING
Katie Leaper, RN, obtains a nursing history on Ms. Devak's admission to the intensive care unit (ICU). Ms. Devak indicates that she has been healthy, having experienced only minor illnesses and chickenpox as a child. She has never been hospitalized and has no known allergies to medications. Ms. Devak is not currently taking prescription or nonprescription drugs. Physical assessment findings include temperature 36.3°C (97.4°F) oral, pulse 100 bpm, respirations 18/min, and BP 124/68 mmHg. Ms. Devak's skin is pale, cool, and dry, with multiple scrapes, minor abrasions, and bruises on her face and extremities. Nurse Leaper notes a linear bruise on her chest and abdomen from the seat belt. Ms. Devak's lung sounds are clear, heart tones normal, and abdomen tender but soft to palpation. Right leg alignment is maintained with skeletal traction. One unit of whole blood was infused before ICU admission; a second unit is currently infusing. An indwelling urinary catheter and a nasogastric tube are in place. During the first few hours after admission, Ms. Leaper notes that Ms. Devak's hourly output has dropped from 55 to 45 to 28 mL of clear yellow urine. The physician orders a 500-mL intravenous fluid challenge, STAT urinalysis, BUN, and serum creatinine. The fluid challenge elicits only a slight increase in urine output. Urinalysis results show a specific gravity of 1.010 and the presence of white blood cells, red and white cell casts, and tubular epithelial cells in the sediment. Ms. Devak's BUN is 28 mg/dL; her serum creatinine is 1.5 mg/dL. The physician diagnoses probable ARF and orders a nephrology consultation. In addition, the physician orders aluminum hydroxide, 10 mL every 2 hours via nasogastric tube, and ranitidine, 50 mg intravenously every 8 hours.	■ *Acute Pain* related to injuries sustained in accident ■ *Anxiety* related to being in the ICU ■ *Risk for Excess Fluid Volume* related to impaired renal function ■ *Impaired Physical Mobility* related to skeletal traction ■ *Ineffective Protection* related to injuries and invasive procedures (NANDA-I © 2012)	■ The client will report adequate pain control. ■ The client will verbalize reduced anxiety. ■ The client will maintain stable weight and vital signs within normal range. ■ The client will maintain skin integrity. ■ The client will use the trapeze appropriately to adjust position in bed while maintaining body alignment. ■ The client will remain free of infection, bleeding, or respiratory distress.

NURSING CARE PLAN (continued)

IMPLEMENTATION

- Maintain patient-controlled anesthesia.
- Assess frequently for pain control and response to analgesia.
- Encourage expression of thoughts, feelings, and fears about condition and placement in ICU.
- Document vital signs and heart and lung sounds at least every 4 hours.
- Weigh every 12 hours.
- Document hourly intake and output.

- Restrict fluids as ordered, including diluent for all intravenous medications as intake.
- Assist with mouth care every 3–4 hours; allow frequent rinsing of mouth and ice chips as allowed.
- Assist with position changes at least every 2 hours; teach use of the overhead trapeze.
- Monitor frequently for signs of infection, bleeding, or respiratory distress.

EVALUATION

After just over 3 days of oliguria, Ms. Devak's urine output increases. By the end of the fourth day, she is excreting 60–80 mL/hr of urine. Although her BUN, serum creatinine, and potassium levels remain high, they never reach a critical point, and dialysis is not required. She is transferred from the ICU on the fifth day after admission. When Ms. Devak is able to begin eating, she is placed on a low-potassium diet, restricted to 50 g of protein. Her renal function gradually improves. By discharge, results of her renal function studies, including BUN and serum creatinine, are nearly normal. Ms. Devak verbalizes an understanding of the need to avoid nephrotoxins, such as nonsteroidal anti-inflammatory drugs, until allowed by her physician.

CRITICAL THINKING

1. *What was the most likely specific precipitating factor for Ms. Devak's ARF? Did anything else contribute to her risk?*
2. *Why did the physician prescribe aluminum hydroxide and ranitidine? Consider both the ARF and Ms. Devak's placement in the ICU.*
3. *Ms. Devak is at risk for respiratory distress related to potential fluid volume excess. How does her fractured femur further contribute to risk for respiratory distress?*
4. *Develop a care plan for Ms. Devak for the nursing diagnosis of Deficient Diversional Activity.*

REVIEW Acute Renal Failure

RELATE Link the Concepts and Exemplars

Linking the exemplar of acute renal failure with the concept of elimination:

1. Nurses often are so busy they don't take time to go to the bathroom to urinate until it can no longer be postponed. Explain how this behavior increases the risk of ARF.

2. What would you teach a client who reported this behavior to reduce the client's risk of ARF?

Linking the exemplar of acute renal failure with the concept of acid–base balance:

3. What laboratory results would you review to determine the acid–base balance of the client with ARF?

4. What acid–base finding would you anticipate when caring for a client with ARF?

READY Go to Companion Skills Manual

REFER Go to Pearson Nursing Student Resources
nursing.pearsonhighered.com

- Additional review materials
- Chart 1: Nursing Care of the Client Undergoing Hemodialysis
- Chart 2: Nursing Care of the Client Undergoing Peritoneal Dialysis

REFLECT Case Study

Missy is a healthy 4-year-old who seems to be in perpetual motion. She came home from preschool today and told her mother she was tired and wanted to take a nap. Her mother immediately sensed there was something wrong, because Missy never volunteers to take a nap. Missy's appetite was diminished at dinner, and although she appeared pale, she went to bed that night without complaint.

The following morning, Missy looks very ill, refuses to get out of bed, and hasn't urinated since 8 p.m. the evening before. Missy's mother brings her to the pediatrician's office, where Missy is diagnosed with ATN. Her pediatrician admits Missy to the local acute care facility. You are the nurse admitting Missy to the pediatric unit.

1. What questions would you ask Missy's mother to determine contributory factors to the development of acute tubular necrosis?

2. What orders would you anticipate from the healthcare provider to prevent the development of ARF?

3. What independent nursing orders would you develop to provide holistic, family-centered care for Missy?

4. What nursing diagnosis would be appropriate for Missy's plan of care?

EXEMPLAR 6.3 Chronic Kidney Disease

EXEMPLAR KEY TERMS
Chronic kidney disease (CKD), 390
End-stage renal disease (ESRD), 390
Nephrectomy, 398

Paresthesias, 393
Uremia, 393
Uremic fetor, 393
Uremic frost, 395

EXEMPLAR LEARNING OUTCOMES

After reading about this exemplar, you will be able to:

1. Describe the pathophysiology, etiology, clinical manifestations, and direct and indirect causes of chronic kidney disease.

2. Identify risk factors and prevention methods associated with chronic kidney disease.

3. Illustrate the nursing process in providing culturally competent care across the life span for individuals with chronic kidney disease.

4. Formulate priority nursing diagnoses appropriate for an individual with chronic kidney disease.

5. Summarize therapies used by interdisciplinary teams in the collaborative care of an individual with chronic kidney disease.

6. Plan evidence-based care for an individual with chronic kidney disease and his or her family in collaboration with other members of the healthcare team.

7. Evaluate expected outcomes for an individual with chronic kidney disease.

▶ OVERVIEW

The internal environment of the body normally remains in a relatively constant or homeostatic state. The kidneys help to maintain homeostasis by regulating the composition and volume of extracellular fluid. They excrete excess water and solutes and, when deficits occur, can conserve water and solutes. In addition, the kidneys help to regulate acid–base balance, and they excrete metabolic wastes. Regulation of blood pressure is also a key function of the kidneys.

Both primary kidney disorders (e.g., glomerulonephritis) and systemic diseases (e.g., diabetes mellitus) can affect renal function. In North America, more than 26 million individuals have chronic kidney disease, and 1 in 3 (73 million) is at increased risk for some type of kidney disease (National Kidney Foundation, 2013). Every year, approximately 3.6 of every 1,000 individuals in the United States develop **end-stage renal disease (ESRD)**, the final phase of **chronic kidney disease (CKD)**, in which little or no kidney function remains. Chronic kidney disease is a major cause of lost work time and wages (U.S. Renal Data System, 2012). Ironically, the increased prevalence of chronic kidney disease in recent years is partially related to the success of dialysis and transplantation.

Renal function is dependent on an adequate supply of blood. Blood supports renal cell metabolism and is vital to kidney function, the nephron in particular. Only with sufficient blood supply can the kidney regulate fluid, electrolyte, and acid–base balance and serve as a major organ of excretion. Vascular disorders, therefore, can have a significant impact on renal function. Hypertension causes arteriosclerotic lesions in the afferent (leading into) and efferent (going out of) arterioles and the glomerular capillaries. The GFR declines, and tubular function is affected, resulting in proteinuria and microscopic hematuria. Approximately 10% of deaths attributed to hypertension result from renal failure (Dirkes, 2011).

Although the kidneys usually recover from acute injury, many chronic conditions can lead to progressive renal tissue destruction and loss of function. Nephron units are lost and renal mass decreased, with progressive deterioration of glomerular filtration, tubular secretion, and reabsorption. CKD may progress slowly for many years without being recognized. Eventually, the kidneys are unable to excrete metabolic wastes and to regulate fluid and electrolyte balance adequately—the condition known as ESRD. Because of the increasing prevalence of CKD and ESRD, *Healthy People 2020* selected chronic kidney disease as one of its focus areas (see **Box 6–5** ●).

Box 6–5   *Healthy People 2020:* Chronic and End-Stage Renal Disease (ESRD)

PREVALENCE

- 15.1% of the U.S. population had CKD in 1999–2004. The 2020 target is to reduce that rate to 13.6% (U.S. Department of Health and Human Services, 2013).
- ESRD results from chronic damage to the kidneys over a decade or more.
- Diabetes and hypertension increase the risk for ESRD.
- The number of new cases of ESRD is increasing and correlates to an increase in cases of type 2 diabetes mellitus.
- African Americans are at the highest risk for renal disease.
- American Indians, Native Alaskans, Asians, and Pacific Islanders have higher rates of renal disease than Caucasians.
- Mexicans have a high risk for renal disease related to a higher incidence of type 2 diabetes mellitus.

OBJECTIVES

- Reduce the proportion of U.S. citizens with chronic kidney disease.
- Improve the cardiovascular care of people with chronic kidney disease.
- Reduce the number of deaths among people with chronic kidney disease.
- Reduce the number of new cases of end-stage renal disease.
- Reduce kidney failure related to diabetes.
- Increase the proportion of clients with a chronic disease receiving care from a nephrologist at least 12 months before the start of renal replacement therapy.

ACTIONS

- Early identification of people at risk
- Control of diabetes and hypertension
- Education related to diet and exercise

TABLE 6–13 Pathophysiology of Chronic Kidney Disease

CAUSE	EXAMPLES
Diabetic nephropathy	Initial increases in glomerular flow rate lead to hyperfiltration with eventual glomerular damage, thickening and sclerosis of the glomerular basement membrane and the glomerulus; gradual destruction of nephrons leads to a fall in GFR.
Hypertensive nephrosclerosis	Long-standing hypertension leads to sclerosis and narrowing of renal arterioles and small arteries with subsequent reduction of blood flow. This leads to ischemia, glomerular destruction, and tubular atrophy.
Chronic glomerulonephritis	Chronic interstitial inflammation of renal parenchyma leads to obstruction and damage to the tubules and capillaries that surround them, affecting glomerular filtration and tubular secretion and reabsorption, with gradual loss of entire nephrons.
Chronic pyelonephritis	Chronic infection commonly associated with an obstructive or neurological process and vesicoureteral reflux leads to scarring and deformity of renal calyces and pelvis, resulting in intrarenal reflux and nephropathy.
Polycystic kidney disease	Multiple bilateral cysts gradually compress renal tissue, impairing renal perfusion and leading to ischemia, renal vascular remodeling, and release of inflammatory mediators, which damage and destroy normal kidney tissue.
Systemic lupus erythematosus	Immune complexes form in capillary basement membrane leading to inflammation and sclerosis, with focal, local, or diffuse glomerulonephritis.

▶ PATHOPHYSIOLOGY AND ETIOLOGY

The pathophysiology of CKD varies depending on the underlying disease process and involves a gradual destruction of entire nephron units. In the early stages, as nephrons are lost, remaining functional nephrons hypertrophy (enlarge as a result of an increase in size of the constituent cells). Glomerular capillary flow and pressure increase in these nephrons, and more solute particles are filtered to compensate for lost renal mass. This increased demand predisposes the remaining nephrons to glomerular sclerosis (scarring), resulting in their eventual destruction. Proteinuria resulting from glomerular damage is thought to contribute to tubular injury. This process of continued loss of nephron function may persist even after the initial disease process has resolved (Fauci et al., 2008). **Table 6–13** ● outlines common pathological processes leading to nephron destruction and ESRD.

The course of CKD is variable, progressing over a period of months to many years. In the early stage, known as decreased renal reserve, unaffected nephrons compensate for the lost nephrons. The GFR is approximately 50% of normal, and the client is asymptomatic, with normal BUN and serum creatinine levels. As the disease progresses and the GFR falls further, hypertension and some manifestations of renal insufficiency may be seen. Any further insult to the kidneys (e.g., infection, dehydration, exposure to nephrotoxins, or urinary tract obstruction) at this stage can further reduce function and precipitate the onset of *renal failure* or overt uremia. The serum creatinine and BUN levels rise sharply (**Figure 6–21** ●), the client becomes oliguric, and manifestations of uremia are seen. Finally, in ESRD, the GFR is less than 10%–15% of normal, and renal replacement therapy is necessary to sustain life. **Table 6–14** ● summarizes the stages of CKD.

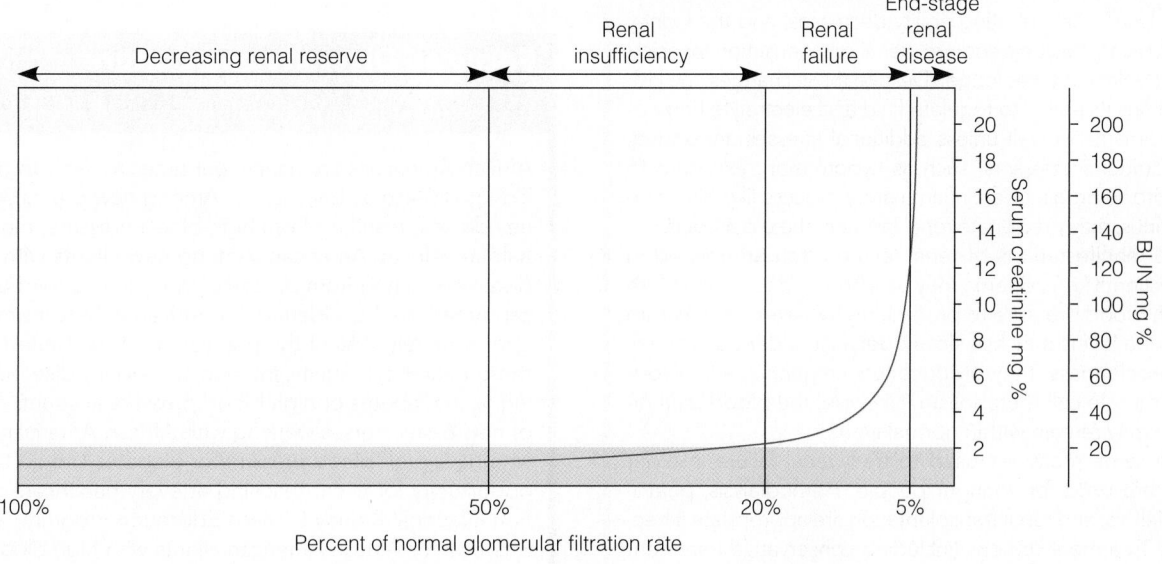

Figure 6–21 ● The relationship of renal function to BUN and serum creatinine values through the course of chronic renal disease.

TABLE 6–14 Stages of Chronic Kidney Disease

STAGE	GLOMERULAR FILTRATION RATE	DESCRIPTION AND MANIFESTATIONS
Stage 1	>90 mL/min/1.73 m^2	Kidney damage with normal or increased GFR
		Asymptomatic; normal BUN and creatinine
Stage 2	60–89 mL/min/1.73 m^2	Mildly decreased GFR
		Asymptomatic, possible hypertension; blood work generally within normal limits
Stage 3	30–59 mL/min/1.73 m^2	Moderate GFR decrease
		Hypertension; possible anemia and fatigue, anorexia, possible malnutrition, bone pain; slight elevation of BUN and serum creatinine
Stage 4	15–29 mL/min/1.73 m^2	Severely decreased GFR
		Hypertension, anemia, malnutrition, altered bone metabolism; edema, metabolic acidosis, hypercalcemia; possible uremia; azotemia with increasing BUN and serum creatinine levels
Stage 5	<15 mL/min/1.73 m^2	End-stage renal disease
		Kidney failure with azotemia and overt uremia

Adapted from National Kidney Foundation. (2002). K/DOQI clinical practice guidelines for chronic kidney disease: Evaluation, classification and stratification. *American Journal of Kidney Disease, 39,* S1–S266. Retrieved from http://www.kdoqi.org.

Etiology

Renal failure is common and costly. At the end of 2009, more than 810,000 people were being treated for ESRD. Between 1980 and 2009, the incidence increased nearly 600%. African Americans are affected at the highest level. The incidence of ESRD is increasing most rapidly in older adults. Although many clients report satisfaction with their quality of life, clients on dialysis are often unable to work, and family structures may disintegrate under the strain of treatment (National Kidney and Urologic Diseases Information Clearinghouse [NKUDIC], 2012).

Lifespan Considerations
Renal Failure in the Older Adult

Structural and functional changes occur in the aging kidney. Structurally, the number of nephrons decreases. Functionally, the GFR decreases, resulting in decreased renal clearance of drugs. Urine-concentrating ability decreases, and the kidney is less able to conserve sodium. Renal compensation for acid–base imbalances takes longer. Despite these changes, the kidney retains its ability to regulate fluid and electrolyte homeostasis remarkably well unless additional stresses are added. Any additional stressors, such as hypotension, exposure to nephrotoxic drugs, or an inflammatory process like glomerulonephritis, may precipitate renal failure in the older adult.

The manifestations of renal failure often are missed in aging clients (e.g., edema may be attributed to heart failure or high blood pressure to preexisting hypertension). Serum creatinine levels may rise slowly. Because older adults have less muscle mass, they produce less creatinine, a by-product of muscle cell metabolism. Likewise, the blood urea nitrogen may remain within normal limits.

The same measures used to treat renal failure in older adults are used for younger people. Hemodialysis, peritoneal dialysis, and renal transplantation are appropriate if necessary. Treatment options (including conservative treatment or no treatment) and their potential benefits and ramifications should be explained clearly to the client and caregivers.

Risk Factors

Conditions causing CKD typically involve diffuse, bilateral disease of the kidneys with progressive destruction and scarring of the entire nephron. Diabetes is the leading cause of ESRD in all population groups in the United States. Hypertension closely follows diabetes as a major cause of ESRD; in many clients, these disorders coexist (U.S. Renal Data System, 2012).

Prevention

According to the National Kidney Foundation (Glasscock, 2010), prevention of ESRD should focus on aggressive management of chronic disease states, especially diabetes and hypertension. In addition, clients should consume diets low in sodium, exercise regularly, keep healthcare provider appointments, avoid smoking, and limit alcohol intake (American Kidney Fund, 2013).

Focus on Diversity and Culture
African Americans and Kidney Disease

African Americans are nearly four times as likely to develop kidney disease as Caucasians. Among new clients with kidney disease resulting from high blood pressure, more than half are African American. Among new clients with kidney disease resulting from diabetes, more than a third are African American. Considering that African Americans make up approximately 12% of the population of the United States, these figures are significant. Because kidney disease resulting from diabetes or high blood pressure accounts for 70% of new cases, nurses working with African American clients who have high blood pressure or diabetes should take the opportunity for client teaching at every healthcare interaction (National Kidney Disease Education Program, 2012). It is critical for African American clients with high blood pressure or diabetes to understand the risk for kidney disease and the importance of following their treatment regimens.

▶ CLINICAL MANIFESTATIONS

CKD often is not identified until its final, uremic stage is reached. **Uremia**, which literally means "urea in the blood," refers to the syndrome or group of symptoms associated with ESRD. In uremia, fluid and electrolyte balance is altered, the regulatory and endocrine functions of the kidney are impaired, and accumulated metabolic waste products affect essentially every other organ system (Porth, 2010). Early manifestations of uremia include nausea, apathy, weakness, and fatigue—symptoms that typically are dismissed as a viral infection or influenza. As the condition progresses, frequent vomiting, increasing weakness, lethargy, and confusion develop (Porth, 2010). See the Multisystem Effects of Uremia on page 394.

Fluid and Electrolyte Effects

Loss of functional kidney tissue impairs the kidneys' ability to regulate fluid, electrolyte, and acid–base balance. In the early stages of CKD, impaired filtration and reabsorption lead to proteinuria, hematuria, and decreased urine-concentrating ability. Salt and water are poorly conserved, and risk for dehydration increases. Polyuria, nocturia, and a fixed specific gravity of 1.008–1.012 are common (Porth, 2010). As the GFR decreases and renal function deteriorates further, sodium and water retention may occur, necessitating salt and water restrictions.

Hyperkalemia develops as renal failure progresses. Manifestations of hyperkalemia, such as muscle weakness, paresthesias, and electrocardiographic changes, are not usually seen until the GFR is less than 5 mL/min. Phosphate excretion is also impaired, leading to hyperphosphatemia and hypocalcemia. Reduced calcium absorption caused by impaired vitamin D activation also contributes to hypocalcemia. Because hypermagnesemia develops with advancing renal failure, clients with renal failure should avoid magnesium-containing antacids.

As renal failure advances, hydrogen ion excretion and buffer production become impaired, leading to metabolic acidosis. Respiratory rate and depth (Kussmaul respirations) increase to compensate for metabolic acidosis. Although metabolic acidosis is often asymptomatic, other possible manifestations include general malaise, weakness, headache, nausea and vomiting, and abdominal pain.

Cardiovascular Effects

Cardiovascular disease resulting from accelerated atherosclerosis is a common cause of death in ESRD. Hypertension, hyperlipidemia, and glucose intolerance all contribute to the process. Cerebral and peripheral vascular manifestations of atherosclerosis are also seen.

Systemic hypertension is a common complication of ESRD. Hypertension results from excess fluid volume, increased renin–angiotensin activity, increased peripheral vascular resistance, and decreased prostaglandins. Increased extracellular fluid volume also can lead to edema and heart failure. Pulmonary edema may result from heart failure and increased permeability of the alveolar capillary membrane.

Retained metabolic toxins can irritate the pericardial sac, causing an inflammatory response and signs of pericarditis. Cardiac tamponade, a potential complication of pericarditis, occurs when inflammatory fluid in the pericardial sac interferes with ventricular filling and cardiac output. Once a common complication of uremia, pericarditis is less common when dialysis is initiated early.

Hematological Effects

Anemia, which is common in clients with uremia, is caused by multiple factors. The kidneys produce erythropoietin, a hormone that controls RBC production. In renal failure, erythropoietin production declines. Retained metabolic toxins further suppress RBC production and contribute to a shortened RBC life span. Nutritional deficiencies (iron and folate) and increased risk for blood loss from the GI tract also contribute to anemia.

Anemia contributes to manifestations such as fatigue, weakness, depression, and impaired cognition. It also affects cardiovascular function, and it may be a major contributing factor to coronary heart disease and heart failure associated with ESRD (Porth, 2010).

Renal failure impairs platelet function, increasing the risk of bleeding disorders, such as epistaxis and GI bleeding. The mechanism of impaired platelet function associated with renal failure is poorly understood.

Immune System Effects

Uremia increases the risk for infection. High levels of urea and retained metabolic wastes impair all aspects of inflammation and immune function. The WBC count declines, humoral and cell-mediated immunity are impaired, and phagocyte function is defective. Both the acute inflammatory response and delayed hypersensitivity responses are affected (Porth, 2010). Fever is suppressed, often delaying the diagnosis of infection.

This increased risk for infection is a growing concern. Recently, the U.S. Renal Data System (2012) found alarming increases in hospitalizations because of infection among clients with ESRD, particularly among those being hospitalized for vascular access infections.

Gastrointestinal Effects

Anorexia, nausea, and vomiting are the most common early symptoms of uremia. Hiccups also are common, as is gastroenteritis. Ulcerations may affect any level of the GI tract and contribute to an increased risk of GI bleeding. Peptic ulcer disease is particularly common in clients with uremia. **Uremic fetor** (a urine-like breath odor often associated with a metallic taste in the mouth) may develop. Uremic fetor can further contribute to anorexia.

Neurological Effects

Uremia alters both central and peripheral nervous system function. Central nervous system manifestations occur early and include changes in cognitive processing, such as difficulty concentrating, fatigue, and insomnia. Psychotic symptoms, seizures, and coma are associated with advanced uremic encephalopathy.

Peripheral neuropathy is also common in advanced uremia. Both the sensory and motor tracts are involved. The lower limbs are initially affected. *Restless leg syndrome*, which involves sensations of crawling, prickling, or itching of the lower legs with frequent leg movement, increases during rest. **Paresthesias** (skin sensations such as prickling or numbing) and sensory loss typically occur in a "stocking-glove" pattern. As uremia progresses,

Multisystem Effects of Uremia

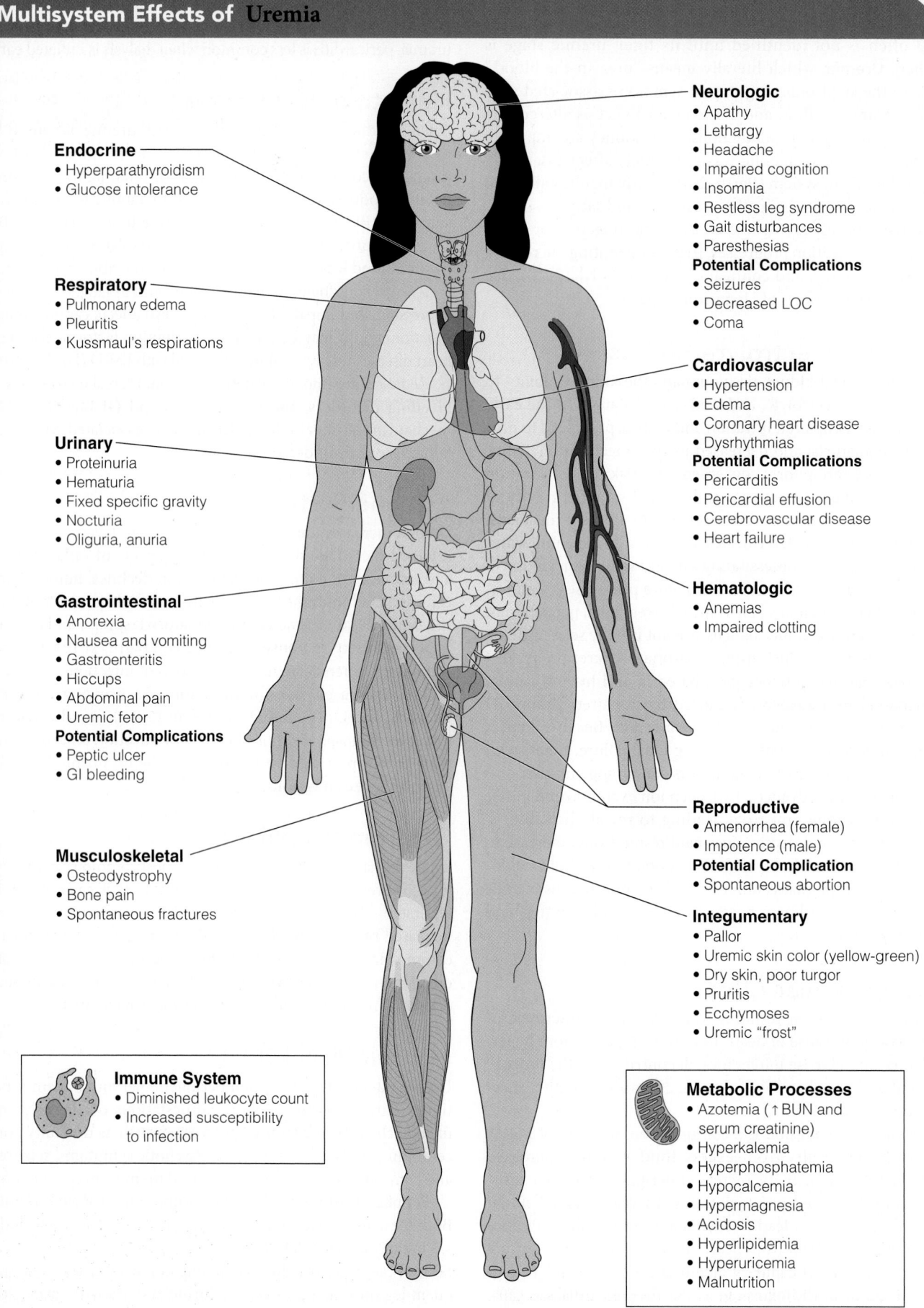

Endocrine
- Hyperparathyroidism
- Glucose intolerance

Respiratory
- Pulmonary edema
- Pleuritis
- Kussmaul's respirations

Urinary
- Proteinuria
- Hematuria
- Fixed specific gravity
- Nocturia
- Oliguria, anuria

Gastrointestinal
- Anorexia
- Nausea and vomiting
- Gastroenteritis
- Hiccups
- Abdominal pain
- Uremic fetor
Potential Complications
- Peptic ulcer
- GI bleeding

Musculoskeletal
- Osteodystrophy
- Bone pain
- Spontaneous fractures

Neurologic
- Apathy
- Lethargy
- Headache
- Impaired cognition
- Insomnia
- Restless leg syndrome
- Gait disturbances
- Paresthesias
Potential Complications
- Seizures
- Decreased LOC
- Coma

Cardiovascular
- Hypertension
- Edema
- Coronary heart disease
- Dysrhythmias
Potential Complications
- Pericarditis
- Pericardial effusion
- Cerebrovascular disease
- Heart failure

Hematologic
- Anemias
- Impaired clotting

Reproductive
- Amenorrhea (female)
- Impotence (male)
Potential Complication
- Spontaneous abortion

Integumentary
- Pallor
- Uremic skin color (yellow-green)
- Dry skin, poor turgor
- Pruritis
- Ecchymoses
- Uremic "frost"

Immune System
- Diminished leukocyte count
- Increased susceptibility to infection

Metabolic Processes
- Azotemia (↑ BUN and serum creatinine)
- Hyperkalemia
- Hyperphosphatemia
- Hypocalcemia
- Hypermagnesia
- Acidosis
- Hyperlipidemia
- Hyperuricemia
- Malnutrition

motor function is also impaired, causing muscle weakness, decreased deep tendon reflexes, and gait disturbances.

Musculoskeletal Effects

Hyperphosphatemia and hypocalcemia associated with uremia stimulate parathyroid hormone secretion. Parathyroid hormone causes increased calcium resorption from bone. In addition, osteoblast (bone-forming) and osteoclast (bone-destroying) cell activity are affected. Combined with decreased vitamin D synthesis and decreased calcium absorption from the GI tract, the resulting bone resorption and remodeling lead to renal osteodystrophy, also known as renal rickets. Osteodystrophy is characterized by osteomalacia (softening of the bones) and osteoporosis (decreased bone mass). Bone cysts may develop. Manifestations of osteodystrophy include bone tenderness, pain, and muscle weakness. The client with osteodystrophy is at increased risk for spontaneous fractures (Porth, 2010).

Endocrine and Metabolic Effects

Accumulated waste products of protein metabolism are a primary factor in the effects and manifestations of uremia. Serum creatinine and BUN levels are significantly elevated. Uric acid levels increase, contributing to an increased risk of gout. Tissues become resistant to the effects of insulin in uremia, leading to glucose intolerance. High blood triglyceride levels and lower-than-normal levels of high-density lipoprotein contribute to the accelerated atherosclerotic process.

CKD affects reproductive function. Pregnancies are rarely carried to term, and menstrual irregularities are common. Reduced testosterone levels, low sperm counts, and impotence affect the male client with ESRD.

Dermatological Effects

Anemia and retained pigmented metabolites cause pallor and a yellowish hue to the skin in clients with uremia. Dry skin with poor turgor, a result of dehydration and sweat gland atrophy, is common. Bruising and excoriations are common as well. Metabolic wastes not eliminated by the kidneys may deposit in the skin, contributing to itching or pruritus. In advanced uremia, high levels of urea in the sweat may result in **uremic frost** (crystallized deposits of urea on the skin).

▶ COLLABORATION

Early management of CKD focuses on eliminating factors that may further decrease renal function and on measures to slow the progression of the disease to ESRD. Treatment goals for clients in all stages of development include the following:

- Maintain nutritional status while minimizing the accumulation of toxic waste products and manifestations of uremia.
- Identify and treat complications of CKD.
- Prepare for renal replacement therapies such as dialysis or renal transplant.

Treatment of CKD should be modified for the older adult. The restrictions on fluid intake and dietary protein should be less stringent, because most older adults have already decreased their protein and sodium intakes as well as their fluid intake.

Constipation, a concern for many older adults, especially those who curb their own fluid intake, may exacerbate the hyperkalemia that accompanies CKD. Nursing and medical management for regularity are important contributions to the treatment plan. Thinning and dry skin is a common concern for all older adults, and the pruritus of CKD can present a real challenge. Careful skin care by the nurse, including moisturizing the skin, will be much appreciated by the older client.

Diagnostic Tests

Diagnostic tests are used both to identify CKD and to monitor kidney function. A number of tests may be performed to determine the underlying renal disorder. Once the diagnosis is established, renal function is monitored primarily through blood levels of metabolic wastes and electrolytes.

- **Urinalysis** is done to measure urine specific gravity and detect abnormal urine components. In CKD, the specific gravity may be fixed at approximately 1.010, equivalent to that of plasma. This fixed specific gravity is the result of impaired tubular secretion, reabsorption, and urine-concentrating ability. Abnormal proteins, blood cells, and cellular casts may also be noted in the urine.

- **Urine culture** is ordered to identify any urinary tract infection that may hasten the progress of CKD.

- **BUN** and **serum creatinine** are obtained to evaluate kidney function in eliminating nitrogenous waste products. Levels of both are monitored to assess the progress of renal failure. A BUN of 20–50 mg/dL signals mild azotemia; levels greater than 100 mg/dL indicate severe renal impairment. Uremic symptoms are seen when the BUN is around 200 mg/dL or higher. Serum creatinine levels of greater than 4 mg/dL indicate serious renal impairment.

- **Creatinine clearance** evaluates the GFR and renal function. In early CKD (renal insufficiency), the GFR is more than 20% of normal, and the creatinine clearance is 30 mL/min or greater. As the disease progresses and the stage of renal failure is reached, the GFR is reduced to less than 20% of normal and the creatinine clearance to 15–29 mL/min. In ESRD, the GFR is less than 10%–15% of normal, and the creatinine clearance is less than 15 mL/min.

- **Serum electrolytes** are monitored throughout the course of CKD. The serum sodium may be within normal limits or low because of water retention. Potassium levels are elevated but usually remain below 6.5 mEq/L. Serum phosphate is elevated, and the calcium level is decreased. Metabolic acidosis is identified by a low pH, low CO_2, and low bicarbonate levels.

- **CBC** reveals moderately severe anemia with a hematocrit of 20%–30% and a low hemoglobin. The number of RBCs and platelets is reduced.

- **Renal ultrasonography** is done to evaluate kidney size. In CKD, kidney size decreases as nephrons are destroyed and kidney mass is reduced.

- **Kidney biopsy** may be done to identify the underlying disease process if this is unclear. It is also used to differentiate acute from chronic kidney disease. Kidney biopsy may be performed in surgery or done percutaneously using needle biopsy.

Clinical Manifestations and Therapies **Chronic Kidney Disease**

ETIOLOGY	CLINICAL MANIFESTATIONS	CLINICAL THERAPIES
Uremia	■ Hyperparathyroidism ■ Glucose intolerance ■ Pulmonary edema ■ Pleuritis ■ Kussmaul inspirations ■ Proteinuria ■ Hematuria ■ Fixed specific gravity ■ Nocturia ■ Oliguria ■ Anorexia, nausea, vomiting, gastroenteritis ■ Hiccups ■ Abdominal pain, peptic ulcer, gastrointestinal bleeding ■ Uremic fetor ■ Osteodystrophy, bone pain, spontaneous fractures ■ Apathy, lethargy, headache, impaired cognition, insomnia, restless leg syndrome, gait disturbances ■ Hypertension, edema, coronary heart disease or failure ■ Anemias, impaired clotting ■ Pallor, uremic skin color, dry skin, poor skin turgor, pruritus	■ Often when uremia develops, the only option is dialysis. ■ Serum electrolytes, BUN, creatine, arterial blood gas (pH), lipid level monitoring ■ Cardiorespiratory monitoring ■ Accurate intake and output ■ Diuretic administration ■ Fluid restriction ■ Dietary consult may be needed to improve nutrition status.
Anemia	■ Fatigue ■ Pallor ■ Dizziness, confusion, lethargy ■ Tachycardia, tachypnea, hypotension	■ Iron supplementation ■ Administration of epoetin ■ Blood transfusion ■ Therapies aimed at treating the underlying cause of renal failure
Fluid volume excess	■ Dependent pitting edema ■ Respiratory crackles ■ Dyspnea, pulmonary edema, hypoxemia ■ Weight gain ■ Tachycardia ■ Jugular vein distention	■ Fluid restriction ■ Sodium-restricted diet ■ Diuretics ■ Dialysis
Hyperkalemia	■ Ventricular arrhythmias ■ Tall, peaked T waves; widened QRS ■ Cardiac arrest ■ Smooth muscle hyperactivity ■ Nausea and vomiting ■ Abdominal cramping ■ Diarrhea ■ Muscle weakness ■ Paresthesias ■ Flaccid paralysis	■ Removal of all potassium from intravenous solutions ■ Low-potassium diet ■ Administration of glucose and insulin to drive potassium into the cell ■ Potassium-absorbing enema solutions ■ Dialysis

Pharmacologic Therapy

CKD affects both the pharmacokinetics and pharmacodynamics of drug therapy. Most medications are excreted primarily by the kidney. The half-life and plasma levels of many drugs increase in CKD. Drug absorption may decrease when phosphate-binding agents are administered concurrently. Proteinuria can significantly reduce plasma protein levels, leading to manifestations of toxicity when highly protein-bound drugs are given. In addition, any potentially nephrotoxic agent should be used with extreme caution. Avoid drugs eliminated by the kidney, such as meperidine, metformin (Glucophage), and other oral hypoglycemic agents.

Furosemide or other loop diuretics may be prescribed to reduce extracellular fluid volume and edema. Diuretic therapy also can reduce hypertension and cause potassium wasting, lowering serum potassium levels. Other antihypertensive agents are used to maintain the blood pressure within normal levels, slow the progress of renal failure, and prevent complications of coronary heart disease and cerebral vascular disease. Angiotensin-converting enzyme inhibitors are preferred, although any class of antihypertensive agent may be prescribed.

Other drugs may be used to manage electrolyte imbalances and acidosis. Sodium bicarbonate or calcium carbonate may be used to correct mild acidosis. Oral phosphorus–binding agents, such as calcium carbonate or calcium acetate, are given to lower serum phosphate levels and normalize serum calcium levels. Aluminum hydroxide may be used in acute treatment of hyperphosphatemia. It is limited to short-term use, however, because of complications such as encephalopathy and osteodystrophy associated with long-term administration of aluminum-containing preparations. Vitamin D supplements may be given to improve calcium absorption.

If the client's serum potassium rises to dangerously high levels, a combination of bicarbonate, insulin, and glucose may be given intravenously to promote potassium movement into the cells. Sodium polystyrene sulfonate (Kayexalate), a potassium-ion exchange resin, can be given either orally or rectally (as an enema).

Folic acid and iron supplements are given to combat anemia associated with CKD. A multiple vitamin preparation is also often prescribed, because anorexia, nausea, and dietary restrictions may limit nutrient intake.

Nutrition and Fluid Management

As renal function declines, the elimination of water, solutes, and metabolic wastes is impaired. Accumulation of these wastes in the body leads to uremic symptoms. Instituted early in the course of CKD, dietary modifications can slow the progress of nephron destruction, reduce uremic symptoms, and help to prevent complications.

Unlike carbohydrates and fats, the body is unable to store excess proteins. Unused dietary proteins are degraded into urea and other nitrogenous wastes, which are then eliminated by the kidneys. Protein-rich foods also contain inorganic ions, such as hydrogen ion, phosphate, and sulfites, that are eliminated by the kidneys. Research has shown that restricting dietary protein intake slows the progression of CKD and reduces uremic symptoms. A daily protein intake of 0.6 g/kg body weight, or approximately 40 g/day for an average male client, provides the amino acids necessary for tissue repair. Proteins should be of high biological value, rich in the essential amino acids. Carbohydrate intake is increased to maintain energy requirements and provide approximately 35 kcal/kg each day.

Water and sodium intake are regulated to maintain the extracellular fluid volume at normal levels. Water intake of 1–2 L/day is generally recommended to maintain water balance. Sodium is restricted to 2 g/day initially. More stringent water and sodium restrictions may be necessary as renal failure progresses. Instruct the client to monitor his or her weight daily and to report any weight gain in excess of 5 pounds over a 2-day period.

In later stages of CKD, potassium and phosphorous intake are also restricted. Potassium intake is limited to less than 60–70 mEq/day (normal intake is ~100 mEq/day). Caution the client and caregivers to avoid using salt substitutes, which typically contain high levels of potassium chloride. Foods high in phosphorus include eggs, dairy products, and meat.

Renal Replacement Therapies

When pharmacologic and dietary management strategies are no longer effective to maintain fluid and electrolyte balance and prevent uremia, dialysis or kidney transplantation is considered. The most common therapies for ESRD in the United States are hemodialysis performed in a dialysis center, followed by peritoneal dialysis and kidney transplant (NKUDIC, 2012). The client's age, concurrent health problems, donor availability, and personal preference influence the choice of renal replacement therapy.

A number of other considerations also affect the choice of long-term treatment. Hemodialysis and peritoneal dialysis each have advantages and disadvantages. Establishing vascular access for hemodialysis may take several months. Planning ahead to develop the access before dialysis is necessary can ease the transition to dialysis. Also, when dialysis treatments will be performed at home, initiating client instruction before the treatments are required can result in more effective learning. If a family member will serve as a dialysis helper, begin training before the onset of uremia.

If transplantation is considered, tissue typing and identification of potential living related donors can be done before the onset of ESRD. To make an informed decision, both the client and the potential donor need to understand the risks, benefits, and options available. If the decision for transplant is made early, dialysis can potentially be avoided.

DIALYSIS Both hemodialysis and peritoneal dialysis can be done in the home, but few clients use home hemodialysis. An important note is that hemodialysis for ESRD is done three times a week for a total of 9–12 hours.

✳ *See Renal Replacement Therapy in the Collaboration section of the earlier exemplar on Acute Renal Failure for more information about dialysis and also Chart 2: Nursing Care of the Client Undergoing Peritoneal Dialysis at* **nursing.pearsonhighered.com** *for more information about nursing care for the client undergoing peritoneal dialysis.*

KIDNEY TRANSPLANT Kidney transplant has become the treatment of choice for many clients with ESRD. Kidneys are the solid organ most commonly transplanted; to date, kidney transplantation is the most successful of transplantation procedures. The first kidney transplant was performed in 1954; the donor and recipient were identical twins. Kidney transplant as a treatment for ESRD is limited primarily by the availability of organs. In 2008, more than 16,000 people received a kidney transplant; however, approximately 80,000 people are currently awaiting a transplant (Organ Procurement and Transplantation Network [OPTN], 2009a).

Kidney transplant improves both survival and quality of life for the client with ESRD. The client on dialysis has a 64.3% probability of surviving after 2 years of dialysis; the transplant recipient has a greater than 90% probability of survival after 2 years. At 5 years, the difference is even greater: 33% for dialysis compared with 80.6% for those who receive a transplant from a deceased donor, and nearly 90% when the donated organ comes from a living donor (NKUDIC, 2012). Quality of life improves dramatically once the client is no longer tethered to a dialysis catheter, machine, or center. Dietary and fluid restrictions are reduced, and the body image is more "whole."

Most transplanted kidneys are obtained from deceased donors; however, transplants from living donors are increasing. In 2009, a total of 41.5% of transplanted kidneys came from living donors, most of whom were related to the recipient (OPTN, 2009a). With both deceased and living donor transplants, a close match between blood and tissue type is desired. Human leukocyte antigens are compared between the donor and recipient; six antigens in common is considered to be a "perfect" match. The success of well-matched living donor transplants is better than that for deceased donor organ transplants, with a 1-year graft survival of 95.1% for living donor transplants compared to 89% for deceased donor transplants (OPTN, 2009b). Close tissue matching probably accounts for the better outcome with living donors. People with normal kidneys who are in good physical health may donate a kidney. Predonation counseling is vital: **Nephrectomy** is major surgery, and the donor faces the risk that trauma or disease may affect the remaining kidney in the future. If the transplant fails, the psychological impact on the donor can be significant.

✳ Go to **nursing.pearsonhighered.com** to see Chart 3: Nursing Care of the Client Having a Nephrectomy.

Deceased donor kidneys are obtained from people who meet the criteria for brain death, are younger than 65 years, and are free of systemic disease, malignancy, or infection, including HIV and hepatitis B or C. Kidneys are removed after brain death has been determined and are preserved by hypothermia or a technique called continuous hypothermic pulsatile perfusion. A kidney preserved by hypothermia must be transplanted within 24 to 48 hours. Continuous hypothermic pulsatile perfusion, however, allows up to 3 days before transplantation.

🌐 **Stay Current:** For more information on how deceased donor kidneys are allocated for transplant, visit the Web site of the United Network for Organ Sharing (UNOS) at **www.unos. org/donation/index.php?topic=organ_allocation**.

The donor kidney is placed in the lower abdominal cavity of the recipient, and the renal artery, vein, and ureter are anastomosed (**Figure 6–22** ●). The renal artery of the donor kidney is connected to the hypogastric artery, and the renal vein is con-

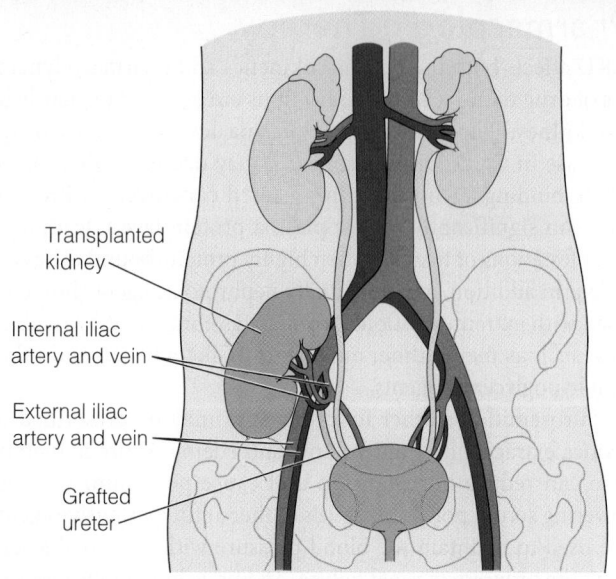

Transplanted kidney

Internal iliac artery and vein

External iliac artery and vein

Grafted ureter

Figure 6–22 ● Placement of a transplanted kidney in the iliac fossa with anastomosis to the hypogastric artery, iliac vein, and bladder.

nected to the iliac vein. The ureter is connected to one of the recipient's ureters or directly to the bladder, using a tunnel technique to prevent reflux.

✳ Go to **nursing.pearsonhighered.com** to see Chart 4: Nursing Care of the Client Having a Kidney Transplant.

Unless the donor and recipient are identical twins, the grafted organ stimulates an immune response to reject the transplanted organ. Immunosuppressive drugs minimize this response. Azathioprine or mycophenolate mofetil are commonly used, often in combination with prednisone, a corticosteroid. Cyclosporine, a potent immunosuppressive, also may be used. These drugs suppress a portion of the immune system and the inflammatory response, increasing the risk for infections and cancers with long-term therapy.

Glucocorticoids such as prednisone and methylprednisolone are used for maintenance immunosuppression and to treat acute rejection episodes. Side effects of long-term corticosteroid use include impaired wound healing, emotional disturbances, osteoporosis, and cushingoid effects on glucose, protein, and fat metabolism.

Azathioprine inhibits both cellular and humoral immunity. Because this drug is rapidly metabolized by the liver, the dose may not need to be altered in the presence of renal failure. Bone marrow suppression, abnormalities of liver function, and alopecia are the primary significant adverse effects of azathioprine. The action of mycophenolate mofetil is similar to that of azathioprine. Its advantages are minimal bone marrow suppression and increased potency in preventing or reversing rejection of the transplanted organ (Fauci et al., 2008).

Cyclosporine primarily affects cellular immunity, the helper T cells in particular. Among its many adverse effects, which include hepatotoxicity and hirsutism, nephrotoxicity is a primary concern for the client having a kidney transplant.

Even with immunosuppressive therapy, however, the transplanted kidney can be rejected at any time. Either acute or chronic rejection may develop. Acute rejection develops within months of the transplant. It is caused by a cellular immune response with T-lymphocyte proliferation (Porth, 2010). Few manifestations may be apparent other than a rise in serum creatinine and possible oliguria. Methylprednisolone, a glucocorticoid, and OKT3 monoclonal antibody are used to manage acute rejection episodes. OKT3 can cause severe systemic reactions, including chills, fever, hypotension, headache, and possible pulmonary edema. Chronic rejection, which may develop months to years following the transplant, is a major cause of graft loss. Both humoral and cellular immune responses are involved in chronic rejection. Chronic rejection does not respond to increased immunosuppression. The presenting manifestations of chronic rejection—progressive azotemia, proteinuria, and hypertension—are those of progressive renal failure.

Hypertension is a possible complication of kidney transplant, resulting from graft rejection, renal artery stenosis, or renal vasoconstriction. Clients may develop glomerular lesions and manifestations of nephrosis. Hypertension and altered blood lipids (increased low-density lipoprotein and decreased high-density lipoprotein levels) increase the risk of death from myocardial infarction and stroke following transplant (Fauci et al., 2008).

Long-term immunosuppression has adverse effects as well. Infection is a continuing threat. Bacterial and viral infections may develop, as well as fungal infections of the blood, lungs, and central nervous system. Tumors are also common, with carcinoma in situ of the cervix, lymphomas, and skin cancers most prevalent. The risk of congenital anomalies is increased in infants whose mothers have undergone immunosuppressive therapy. Corticosteroid use may lead to bone problems, GI disorders (e.g., peptic ulcer disease), and cataract formation.

Complementary and Alternative Therapy

Clients with CKD should avoid herbal supplements, which can contain minerals that may be harmful to the kidneys or contraindicated with one or more medications the client might be taking. Nurses should encourage clients and their caregivers to discuss the use of any over-the-counter or complementary therapies with the physician.

NURSING PROCESS

Measures to reduce the risk of CKD focus on preventing kidney disease and appropriately managing diabetes and hypertension. Nurses promote early and effective treatment of all infections, particularly skin and pharyngeal infections caused by streptococcal bacteria. Discuss measures to reduce the risk for urinary tract infections, and stress the importance of prompt treatment to eradicate the infecting organism. Discuss the relationship among diabetes, hypertension, and kidney disease. Emphasize that maintaining blood glucose levels and blood pressure within the recommended ranges reduces the risk of adverse effects on the kidneys. Ensure that all clients with less-than-optimal renal function are well hydrated, particularly when a nephrotoxic drug is prescribed or anticipated. Finally, encourage the client with ESRD to investigate options for early transplantation to avoid long-term dialysis.

Focus on Diversity and Culture
Jehovah's Witnesses

Some Jehovah's Witnesses are against blood transfusions, but many permit dialysis and organ transplantation if appropriate considerations are made. Organ transplantation for a Jehovah's Witness normally requires removal of all blood from the organ before transplanting it in the Jehovah's Witness. Similarly, dialysis requires banking of the client's own blood to fill the machine if that becomes necessary.

Assessment

Both subjective and objective data are used to assess the client with CKD:

- *Health history*. Complaints of anorexia, nausea, weight gain, or edema; current treatment (if any), including type and frequency of dialysis or previous kidney transplant; chronic diseases, such as diabetes, heart failure, or kidney disease
- *Physical examination*. Mental status; vital signs, including temperature, heart and lung sounds, and peripheral pulses; urine output (if any); weight; skin color, moisture, and condition; presence of edema (periorbital or dependent); bowel tones; and presence and location of an AV fistula, shunt, or graft, or peritoneal catheter.

Diagnosis

Nursing diagnoses for clients with CKD may include the following:

- *Ineffective Tissue Perfusion: Renal*
- *Imbalanced Nutrition: Less Than Body Requirements*
- *Excess Fluid Volume*
- *Impaired Skin Integrity*
- *Risk for Infection*
- *Disturbed Body Image.*

(NANDA-I © 2012)

Planning

The plan of care, made in collaboration with the client, may include the following goals:

- The client will verbalize fluid allotment allowed throughout the day.
- The client's weight will decrease and approach baseline level.
- The client will breathe comfortably, with clear breath sounds.
- The client will remain free of infection.
- The client will share feelings regarding change in body image.

Implementation

Whether the client with ESRD is facing long-term dialysis or renal transplantation, a number of nursing care needs can be identified. This section focuses on nursing care related to impaired renal function, nutritional deficits caused by dietary restrictions and nausea, increased risk for infection, and changes in body image. See the Nursing Care Plan feature that follows for additional potential nursing diagnoses and interventions for the client with CKD.

Promote Effective Tissue Perfusion

Capillaries are an integral part of the nephron. As nephrons are destroyed, kidney perfusion progressively declines. As renal perfusion and nephron function fall, the kidney is less able to maintain fluid and electrolyte balance and to eliminate waste products from the body.

- Monitor intake and output; vital signs, including orthostatic blood pressures; and weight. Weight changes are a more accurate indicator of fluid volume status in the oliguric or anuric client than I&O measurements. These provide important data to identify changes in fluid volume.
- Restrict fluids as ordered. As renal function declines, the ability to eliminate excess fluid is impaired.
- Monitor respiratory status, including lung sounds, every 4 to 8 hours. Fluid volume overload may lead to heart failure and possible pulmonary edema.
- Monitor BUN, serum creatinine, pH, electrolytes, and CBC. Report significant changes. As renal function declines, progressive azotemia with increasing BUN and serum creatinine appears. Metabolic acidosis develops because the kidney is unable to eliminate hydrogen ions and conserve bicarbonate. Hyponatremia, hyperkalemia, hyperphosphatemia, and hypocalcemia are associated with renal failure. The RBC count, hemoglobin, and hematocrit decline because of deficient erythropoietin to stimulate cell production in the bone marrow. An acute fall in hemoglobin and hematocrit may indicate GI bleeding, a risk in clients with ESRD.
- Report manifestations of electrolyte imbalances, such as cardiac dysrhythmias and other electrocardiographic changes.
- Administer antihypertensive medications as ordered. Hypertension management is an important factor in slowing the progression of CKD.
- Time activities and procedures to allow rest periods. The anemia associated with CKD may cause significant fatigue and activity intolerance.

Promote Balanced Nutrition

Anorexia, nausea, and vomiting are common manifestations of ESRD and uremia. The metallic taste associated with uremia combined with a diet restricted in protein and sodium will compound loss of appetite. This increases the risk that food intake will be insufficient to meet metabolic needs. Catabolism exacerbates azotemia and uremia, resulting in muscle tremors and possible tetany, and Kussmaul respirations. Manifestations of electrolyte imbalance may indicate the need for intervention.

- Administer medications to treat electrolyte imbalances as ordered. Carefully monitor for desired and adverse effects. Impaired renal function affects drug elimination and increases the risk for toxic effects. Medications may be prescribed to help maintain electrolyte and acid–base balance and prevent adverse effects of imbalances.
- Monitor food and nutrient intake as well as episodes of vomiting. Careful monitoring helps to determine the adequacy of intake.

- Weigh the client daily before breakfast. This provides the most accurate measurement. Remember that a gain of 2 pounds or more over a 24-hour period is more likely to reflect fluid retention than a gain in body mass.
- Administer antiemetic agents 30–60 minutes before eating. Antiemetics reduce nausea and the risk of vomiting with food intake.
- Assist with mouth care before meals and at bedtime. Mouth care improves taste, stimulates the appetite, and maintains the integrity of oral mucous membranes.
- Serve small meals, and provide between-meal snacks. Small meals are less likely to prompt nausea and help to improve food intake.
- Arrange for a dietary consultation. Provide preferred foods to the extent possible, and involve the client in planning daily menus. Encourage family members to bring food as dietary restrictions allow. Providing preferred foods within restrictions promotes intake.
- Monitor nutritional status by tracking weight; laboratory values, such as serum albumin and BUN; and anthropometric measurements. Indicators of impaired nutrition develop gradually and may be subtle. Careful assessment is important.
- Administer parenteral nutrition as prescribed. Routinely monitor blood glucose levels, and use strict aseptic technique when handling the solution and venous access site. Parenteral nutrition may be necessary to prevent catabolism and increasing azotemia. Hyperglycemia and infection are risks associated with parenteral nutrition. Immune system suppression associated with renal failure further increases the risk for infection.

Reduce Risk for Infection

CKD affects the immune system and leukocyte function, increasing susceptibility to infection. Invasive devices required for hemodialysis or peritoneal dialysis add to this risk. The client who has had a kidney transplant remains on immunosuppressive therapy for life, further depressing the immune system and increasing the risk for infection.

- Use standard precautions and good hand washing technique at all times. Hand washing is a primary means of preventing the transfer of organisms. Clients who are on hemodialysis or who have had multiple blood transfusions to treat anemia have an increased risk for hepatitis B, hepatitis C, and HIV infection.
- Monitor temperature and vital signs at least every 4 hours. A low-grade fever or increased pulse rate may indicate an infection in the client who is immunosuppressed.
- Monitor WBC count and differential. Increased WBCs may indicate a bacterial infection; decreased WBCs may indicate viral infection. A shift in the differential showing more immature WBCs (bands) in circulation is another indicator of infection.
- Culture urine, peritoneal dialysis fluid, and other drainage as indicated. Culture is performed to verify the presence of pathogens.
- Monitor clarity of dialysate return. Dialysate should return clear in the client undergoing peritoneal dialysis. Cloudy dialysate may indicate peritonitis, the most common complication of peritoneal dialysis, and should be reported and cultured.
- Provide good respiratory hygiene, including position changes, coughing, and deep breathing. These measures

improve clearance of respiratory secretions, reducing the risk for infection.

■ Restrict visits from people who are obviously ill. Teach the client and family about the risk for infection and measures to reduce the spread of infection. Because the client's resistance to infection is impaired, extra caution is required to prevent unnecessary exposures.

Promote Healthy Body Image

Chronic disease and impaired kidney function can affect the client's body image. Hemodialysis requires an AV fistula or shunt, and peritoneal dialysis requires a permanent peritoneal catheter. Although kidney transplant can restore an image of wholeness, a visible scar remains, and the organ may be perceived as "foreign."

■ Involve the client in care, including meal planning, dialysis, and catheter, port, or incision care to the extent possible. Involvement improves acceptance and stimulates discussion about the effect of the disease and treatment measures on the client's life.

■ Encourage expression of feelings and concerns, accepting perceptions and feelings without criticism. Self-expression enhances the client's self-worth and acceptance.

■ Include the client in decision making, and encourage self-care. Increased autonomy enhances the client's sense of control, independence, and self-worth.

■ Support positive gains, but do not support denial. The client may have difficulty accepting the renal failure, but adaptation to the loss is important.

■ Help the client to develop and achieve realistic goals. Realistic goals allow the client to see progress.

■ Provide positive reinforcement and feedback. These measures support growth and adaptation.

■ Reinforce effective coping strategies. Reinforcement helps the client to develop positive versus negative strategies for coping.

■ Facilitate contact with a support group or other community members affected by renal failure. The client benefits by providing and receiving support in a group of people going through similar circumstances.

■ Refer for mental health counseling as indicated or desired. Counseling can help the client to develop effective coping and adaptation strategies.

Lifespan Considerations The Child With Chronic Kidney Disease

■ Physical activity is important to help children maintain optimal health and self-esteem.

■ Nurses should encourage children with CKD to participate in developmentally appropriate activities as tolerated.

■ Nurses may partner with children to establish routine plans for physical activity as tolerated that will help to promote strong bones.

■ Nurses should encourage parents to promote children's participation in age-appropriate activities to minimize the psychological consequences of coping with a chronic disease.

Care in the Community

Teaching for home care includes the following topics. See also the Client Teaching feature on assessing for home care.

■ Nature of the kidney disease and renal failure, including expected progression and effects

■ Monitoring weight, vital signs, and temperature

■ Prescribed dietary and fluid restrictions (Involve the client, a dietitian, and the family member usually responsible for cooking. Include strategies to manage nausea and relieve thirst within allowed fluid limits.)

■ How to assess and protect a fistula or shunt for hemodialysis (or the extremity to be used if one is anticipated)

■ Peritoneal catheter care and the procedure for peritoneal dialysis as indicated (Include a family member or significant other, in case the client is unable to perform the procedure independently at some time.)

■ Following kidney transplant, prescribed medications, adverse effects and their management, infection prevention, graft protection, and manifestations of organ rejection.

Refer to a dietitian for diet planning and counseling. If home hemodialysis is planned, refer the designated dialysis helper for formal training. Both the National Kidney Foundation and the

Client Teaching Assessing for Home Care for Clients With Kidney Disease

A number of factors should be considered in assessing the older adult's ability to manage treatment such as dialysis at home:

■ Does the client have reasonable access to a dialysis center or outpatient unit? Is transportation available?

■ Would home hemodialysis be appropriate? Is a caregiver available who can be trained to manage dialysis? Does the client's home have appropriate electrical and plumbing fixtures?

■ Would continuous ambulatory peritoneal dialysis be appropriate? Does the client have the manual dexterity, will, and cognitive ability to manage dialysis infusions? If not, would intermittent peritoneal dialysis using a dialyzing machine be more appropriate?

■ Are family members or other support people available to assist the client as needed?

Resources for Home Care

The following resources may be useful for clients with kidney disease:

■ American Association of Kidney Patients
800-749-2257
813-636-8122
www.aakp.org

■ American Kidney Fund
800-638-8299
866-300-2900 (Spanish help line)
www.kidneyfund.org

■ National Kidney Foundation
800-622-9010
www.kidney.org

American Association of Kidney Patients may be able to provide support and educational materials for the client with ESRD. Local and state chapters of these organizations can provide additional support.

Nurses should assess both fluid and nutritional intake in the older adult. Older clients may consciously or unconsciously decrease fluid intake, due to a blunted thirst mechanism, fear of incontinence or nocturia, or lack of access to beverages due to lack of mobility or other factors. Embarrassment also may be a factor for the older client who needs assistance with toileting. Dehydration may lead to confusion, digestion problems, constipation, and bladder infections. Encourage older adults to drink fluids even when they do not feel thirsty. Educate caregivers to make fluids available throughout the day, and to include the older adult's preferences in providing fluids.

Evaluation

CKD and ESRD are long-term processes that require management by the client. No matter what treatment option the client chooses (hemodialysis, peritoneal dialysis, or renal transplantation), day-to-day management falls to the client and family. When evaluating the client, an important aspect to consider is the client and family's readiness to assume self-care and management. Expected outcomes may include the following:

- The client remains free from infection.
- The client maintains an appropriate weight.
- The client demonstrates ability to participate in self-care, either independently or with assistance.
- The client is able to participate in desired activities.

NURSING CARE PLAN   A Client With End-Stage Renal Disease

Walter Cohen, 45 years old, is the print shop manager at a local community college. He has had type 1 diabetes mellitus since the age of 20 and was diagnosed with diabetic nephropathy 10 years ago. Despite blood pressure control with antihypertensive medications and frequent blood glucose monitoring with insulin coverage, he developed overt proteinuria 5 years ago and has now progressed to end-stage renal disease. He enters the nephrology unit for temporary hemodialysis to relieve uremic symptoms. While there, a continuous ambulatory peritoneal dialysis (CAPD) catheter will be inserted. Mr. Cohen's desire to continue working is the primary factor in his choice of CAPD over hemodialysis.

ASSESSMENT

Richard Gonzalez, Mr. Cohen's care manager, obtains a nursing assessment. Mr. Cohen states that his diabetes has always been difficult to control. He has had numerous hypoglycemic episodes and has been hospitalized "four or five times" for ketoacidosis. Recently, he has developed symptoms of peripheral neuropathy and increasing retinopathy. He attributed his lack of appetite, nausea, vomiting, and fatigue over the past month to "a touch of the flu." His weight remained stable, so he did not worry about not eating much.

Physical assessment findings include temperature 36.5°C (97.8°F) oral, pulse 96 bpm, respirations 20/min, and BP 178/100 mmHg. His skin is cool and dry, with minor excoriations on forearms and lower legs. His breath odor is fetid. Scattered fine rales are noted in bilateral lung bases, and a soft S_3 gallop is noted at cardiac apex. Bilateral pitting edema of lower extremities to just below the knees is observed; fingers and hands are also edematous. Abdominal assessment is essentially normal, with hypoactive bowel sounds. Urinalysis shows a specific gravity of 1.011, gross proteinuria, and multiple cell casts. CBC results are as follows: red blood cells, 2.9 million/mm^3; hemoglobin, 9.4 g/dL; hematocrit, 28%. Blood chemistry abnormalities include the following: BUN, 198 mg/dL; creatinine, 18.5 mg/dL; sodium, 125 mEq/L; potassium, 5.7 mEq/L; calcium, 7.1 mg/dL; and phosphate, 6.8 mg/dL. A temporary jugular venous catheter will be placed for hemodialysis the next day, followed by peritoneal catheter insertion later in the week.

DIAGNOSES

- *Excess Fluid Volume* related to failure of kidneys to eliminate excess body fluid
- *Imbalanced Nutrition: Less Than Body Requirements* related to effects of uremia
- *Impaired Skin Integrity* of lower extremities related to dry skin and itching
- *Risk for Infection* related to invasive catheters and impaired immune function

(NANDA-I © 2012)

PLANNING

- The client will adhere to the prescribed fluid restriction of 750 mL/day.
- The client will demonstrate reduced extracellular fluid volume by weight loss, decreased peripheral edema, clear lung sounds, and normal heart sounds.
- The client will consume and retain 100% of prescribed diet, including snacks.
- The client will demonstrate healing of lower extremity skin lesions.
- The client will remain free of infection.
- The client will demonstrate appropriate peritoneal catheter care and CAPD.

IMPLEMENTATION

- Space fluids, allowing 400 mL from 7 a.m. to 3 p.m., 200 mL from 3 p.m. to 11 p.m., and 100 mL from 11 p.m. to 7 a.m.
- Provide mouth care at least every 4 hours and before every meal.
- Keep sugarless hard candy and ice chips at the bedside; include ice consumed as fluid intake.
- Weigh daily before breakfast; monitor vital signs and heart and lung sounds every 4 hours.
- Document intake and output every 4 hours.

- Arrange dietary consultation for menu planning.
- Administer prescribed antiemetic 1 hour before meals.
- Monitor food intake, noting percentage and types of food consumed.
- Clean lesions on lower extremities every 8 hours and assess healing.
- Teach CAPD procedure and peritoneal catheter care.
- Assist to identify strengths and needs in health regimen management.

NURSING CARE PLAN (continued)

EVALUATION

Mr. Cohen was hospitalized for 2 weeks, undergoing four hemodialysis sessions to reduce uremic symptoms. An arteriovenous fistula has been created in his left arm in case he should need hemodialysis in the future. He begins peritoneal dialysis the second week, and by discharge, he is able to manage the catheter care and dialysis runs with the help of his wife. His heart and lung sounds are normal, and he has minimal peripheral edema on discharge. The excoriations on his legs have healed. His temperature is normal, and no evidence of infection is noted. Mr. Cohen remains anorectic and slightly nauseated but is eating most of his prescribed diet and snacks. He has lost 10 pounds with excess fluid removal by dialysis, but his weight remains stable during the second week. Mr. Cohen and his wife have been introduced to another client who has been on CAPD for several years and promises to help them with problem solving.

CRITICAL THINKING

1. How does diabetes mellitus damage the kidneys and lead to end-stage renal disease? Why is this more significant for a client with type 1 diabetes mellitus than for someone with type 2 diabetes mellitus?
2. Why do high levels of urea in the blood often cause changes in cognition and mental status? What manifestations of encephalopathy would you expect to see?
3. How might Mr. Cohen's insulin dosage and diet need to be changed with the institution of peritoneal dialysis? Why?
4. Develop a care plan for the nursing diagnosis Disturbed Body Image.

REVIEW Chronic Kidney Disease

RELATE Link the Concepts and Exemplars

Linking the exemplar of chronic kidney disease with the concept of perfusion:

1. When providing health promotion education to the community, what information could you provide to improve overall perfusion and, as a result, reduce the risk of kidney damage resulting in CKD?
2. What impact would CKD have on the cardiovascular system of the client? What assessments would indicate the client is experiencing cardiovascular complications?

Linking the exemplar of chronic kidney disease with the concept of development:

3. How does CKD impact a pediatric client's development?
4. What nursing interventions may be helpful in promoting normal development in the pediatric client with CKD?

READY Go to Companion Skills Manual

REFER Go to Pearson Nursing Student Resources
nursing.pearsonhighered.com

- Additional review materials
- Chart 3: Nursing Care of the Client Having a Nephrectomy
- Chart 4: Nursing Care of the Client Having a Kidney Transplant

REFLECT Case Study

Joe Jenkins is a 45-year-old African American who has been a long-distance truck driver for the past 20 years. He is admitted to the hospital with complaints of nausea for several weeks, weakness, fatigue, and loss of appetite. He has been feeling very depressed. He has a past medical history of type 1 diabetes mellitus, hypertension, and diabetic nephropathy. On admission, his vital signs are temperature T_O 37.1°C (98.7°F), P 96 bpm, R 20/min, BP 170/110 mmHg. He has bilateral pitting edema of the lower extremities. His fingers and hands are also edematous. He complains of dry and itching skin. His urine is dark, frothy, and scanty. A specimen is collected for a urinalysis, and blood work is drawn and sent to the laboratory. Urinalysis results show a specific gravity of 1.011, gross hematuria, and 3+ protein. His blood work reveals a BUN of 198 mg/dL and creatinine of 12.5 mg/dL. Based on his past medical history of diabetes, hypertension, and diabetic nephropathy, and on the current findings, a medical diagnosis of CKD is established. Based on Mr. Jenkins's assessment and past medical history, the nursing diagnosis of *Impaired Urinary Elimination* is identified as the highest priority for planning nursing care.

1. What would be the priority nursing interventions when admitting Mr. Jenkins to the acute care facility?
2. What teaching will this client need considering his prediagnosis lifestyle?
3. What alterations will Mr. Jenkins need to make in his life if daily dialysis is required?

REFERENCES

Abdallah, L., Remington, R., Houde, S., Zhan, L., & Melillo, K. D. (2009). Dehydration reduction in community-dwelling older adults. *Research in Gerontological Nursing, 2*(1), 49–57. doi:10.3928/19404921-20090101-01.

Alexander, L., & Allen, D. (2011). Establishing an evidence-based inpatient medical oncology fluid balance measurement policy. *Clinical Journal of Oncology Nursing, 15*(1), 23–25.

American Kidney Fund. (2013). *End stage renal disease.* Retrieved from http://www.kidneyfund.org/kidney-health/kidney-failure/end-stage-renal-disease.html#. Uh9RGxuTgoo.

Benelam, B. (2010). Recognizing the signs of dehydration. *Practice Nursing, 21*(5), 230–234.

Centers for Disease Control and Prevention (CDC). (2011). *Media advisory: Athletes need to take special precautions in hot weather.* Retrieved from http://www.cdc.gov/media/releases/2011/a0808_hot_weather.html.

Centers for Disease Control and Prevention (CDC). (2012). *Where's the sodium: There's too much in many common foods.* Retrieved from http://www.cdc.gov/vitalsigns/Sodium/index.html.

Centers for Disease Control and Prevention (CDC). (2013). *Sodium: the facts.* Retrieved from http://www.cdc.gov/salt/pdfs/sodium_fact_sheet.pdf.

Cotugna, N., & Wolpert, S. (2011). Sodium recommendations for special populations and the resulting implications. *Journal of Community Health, 36*, 874–882.

Dinwiddie, L. C. (2004). Managing catheter dysfunction for better patient outcomes: A team approach. *Nephrology Nursing Journal, 31*(6), 653–660, 661–662, 671.

Dirkes, A. (2011). Acute kidney injury: Not just acute renal failure anymore? *Critical Care Nurse, 31*(1), 37–49.

Elliott, M., & Coventry, A. (2012). Critical care: The eight vital signs of patient monitoring. *British Journal of Nursing, 21*(10), 621–625.

Fauci, A. S., Kasper, D. L., Braunwald, E., Hauser, S. L., Longo, D. L., Jameson, J. L., & Loscalzo, J. (Eds.) (2008). *Harrison's principles of internal medicine* (17th ed.) New York, NY: McGraw Hill.

Flack, J. M., Nasser, S. S., & Levy, P. D. (2011).Therapy of hypertension in African Americans. *American Journal of Cardiovascular Drugs, 11*(2), 83–92.

Friedman, A. (2010). Fluid and electrolyte therapy: A primer. *Pediatric Nephrology, 24*, 843–846.

Glasscock, R. J. (2010). Uremia (end-stage renal disease): How cost effective are preventive strategies? *Journal of Renal Nutrition, 20*(5 Suppl), S131–S134. Retrieved from http://www.ncbi.nlm.nih.gov/pubmed/20797562.

Godfrey, H., Cloete, J., Dymond, E., & Kibgm, A. (2012). An exploration of the hydration care of older people: A qualitative study. *International Journal of Nursing Studies, 49*, 1200–1211.

Goldstein, S. L., & Devarajan, P. (2011). Acute kidney injury in childhood: Should we be worried about progression to CKD? *Pediatric Nephrology, 26*(4), 509–522. doi:10.1007/s00467-010-1653-4.

Guarner, J., Hochman, J., Kurbatova, E., & Mullins, R. (2011). Study of outcomes associated with hyponatremia and hypernatremia in children. *Developmental and Pediatric Pathology, 14*(2), 117–123.

Jeffries, D., Johnson, M., Griffiths, R., Arthurs, K., Beard, D., Chen, T., . . . Zarkos, T. (2010). Engaging clinicians in evidence based policy development. The case of nursing documentation. *Contemporary Nurse, 15*(2), 254–264.

Jorgenson, A. L. (2013). Contrast induced nephropathy: Pathophysiology and preventive strategies. *Critical Care Nurse, 33*(1), 37–47.

Lanier, J. B., Mote, M. B., & Clay, M. C. (2011). Evaluation and management of orthostatic hypotension. *American Family Physician, 84*(5), 527–536.

Liamis, G., Rodenberg, E. M., Hoffman, A., Zietse, R., Stricker, B. H., & Hoorn, E. J. (2013). Electrolyte disorders in community subjects: Prevalence and risk factors. *American Journal of Medicine, 126*(3), 256–263.

Madati, P. J., & Bachur, R. (2008). Development of an emergency department triage tool to predict acidosis among children with gastroenteritis. *Pediatric Emergency Care, 24*(12), 822–830.

Moshfegh, A. J., Holden, J. M., Cogswell, M. E., Kuklina, E. V., Patel, S. M., Gunn, J. P., . . . Galuska, D. A. (2012). Vital signs: Food categories contributing the most to sodium consumption. *Morbidity & Mortality Weekly Report, 61*(5), 92–98.

National Kidney and Urologic Diseases Information Clearinghouse (NKUDIC). (2012, June). *Kidney disease statistics for the United States* (NIH Publication No. 12-3895). Retrieved from http://kidney.niddk.nih.gov/KUDiseases/pubs/kustats/KU_Diseases_Stats_508.pdf.

National Kidney Disease Education Program. (2012). *Identify and manage patients*. Retrieved from http://nkdep.nih.gov/identify-manage.shtml.

National Kidney Foundation. (2013). *About chronic kidney disease*. Retrieved from http://www.kidney.org/kidneydisease/aboutckd.cfm#facts.

Organ Procurement and Transplantation Network (OPTN). (2009a). *Donors recovered in the U.S. by donor type*. Retrieved from http://optn.transplant.hrsa.gov.

Organ Procurement and Transplantation Network (OPTN). (2009b). *Kidney Kaplan-Meyer graft showing survival rates for transplants performed 1997–2004*. Retrieved from http://optn.transplant.hrsa.gov.

Parkin, P., Maccarthur, C., Khambalia, A., Goldman, R., & Friedman, J. (2010). Clinical and laboratory assessment of dehydration severity in children with acute gastroenteritis. *Clinical Pediatrics, 49*(3), 235–239.

Payne, D. C., Vinje, J., Szilagv, P. G., Edwards, K. M., Staat, M. A., Weinberg, G. A., . . . Parashar, U. D. (2013). Norovirus and medically attended gastroenteritis in U.S. children. *New England Journal of Medicine, 366*(12), 1121–1130.

Pinto, S., & Grose, S. (2010). *Hydration: Maintaining oral hydration in older adults*. Glendale, CA: CINAHL Information Systems.

Porth, C. M. (2010). *Pathophysiology: Concepts of altered health states* (7th ed.). Philadelphia, PA: Lippincott Williams & Wilkins.

Rowland, T. (2011). Fluid replacement requirements for child athletes. *Sports Medicine, 41*(4), 279–288.

Scales, K. (2011). Use of hypodermoclysis to manage dehydration. *Nursing Older People, 23*(5), 16–22.

U.S. Department of Health and Human Services. (2011). *Healthy People 2020: Chronic kidney disease*. Retrieved from http://www.healthypeople.gov/2020/topicsobjectives2020/nationaldata.aspx?topicId=6.

U.S. Renal Data System. (2012). *2012 atlas of CKD & ESRD*. Retrieved from http://www.usrds.org/atlas.aspx.

Williams, C. A., & Blackwell, J. (2012). Hydration status, fluid intake and electrolyte loss in youth soccer players. *International Journal of Sports Physiology and Performance, 7*, 367–374.

Yang, Q., Zhang, A., Kuklina, E. V., Fang, J., Ayala, C., Hong, Y., . . . Merrit, R. (2012). Sodium intake and blood pressure among U.S. children and adolescents. *Pediatrics, 120*(4), 611–619.

7 Health, Wellness, and Illness

◢ THE CONCEPT OF HEALTH, WELLNESS, AND ILLNESS

Nurses' understanding of health and wellness largely determines the scope and nature of nursing practice. Clients' health beliefs also influence health practices. Some individuals think of health and wellness (or well-being) as the same thing or, at the very least, as accompanying one another. However, health may not always accompany well-being. An individual who has a terminal illness may have a sense of well-being; conversely, another may lack a sense of well-being, yet be in a state of good health.

For many years the concept of disease was the yardstick by which health was measured. In the late 19th century, the "how" of disease (pathogenesis) was the major concern of health professionals. The 20th century focused on finding cures for diseases. Currently, healthcare providers are increasing their emphasis on promoting health and wellness in individuals, families, and communities. **<<**

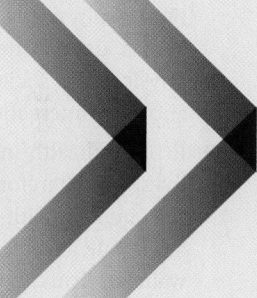

Concept Learning Outcomes

After reading about this concept, you will be able to:

1. Define health, illness, wellness, and disease.
2. Explain the health–illness continuum and the concept of high-level wellness.
3. Define health promotion.
4. Describe the nurse's role in health promotion.
5. Identify characteristics of health, disease, and illness.
6. Differentiate illness from disease and acute illness from chronic illness.
7. Develop and evaluate plans for health promotion across the life span.

Concept Key Terms

Acute illness, *408*
Autonomy, *409*
Chronic illness, *408*
Disease, *408*
Exacerbation, *408*
External locus of control, *415*
Health, *406*
Health beliefs, *415*
Health promotion, *409*
Illness, *408*

Illness behavior, *408*
Internal locus of control, *415*
Lifestyle choices, *415*
Modeling, *418*
Positive reinforcement, *418*
Remission, *408*
Risk factors, *415*
Well-being, *407*
Wellness, *406*

▶ CONCEPTS OF HEALTH, WELLNESS, AND WELL-BEING

Health, wellness, and well-being have many definitions and interpretations. The nurse should be familiar with the most common aspects of these concepts and consider how they may be individualized with specific clients.

Health

Traditionally **health** has been defined in terms of the presence or absence of disease. Nightingale defined health as a state of being well and using every power the individual possesses to the fullest extent (Nightingale, 1859/1969). The World Health Organization (WHO) takes a more holistic view of health. Its constitution defines health as "a state of complete physical, mental, and social well-being, and not merely the absence of disease or infirmity" (WHO, 1948). This definition serves the following purposes:

- It reflects concern for the individual as a total person, functioning physically, psychologically, and socially. Mental processes determine individuals' relationships with their physical and social surroundings, their attitudes about life, and their interaction with others.

- It places health in the context of environment. Individuals' lives, and therefore their health, are affected by everything they interact with—not only environmental influences, such as climate and the availability of food, shelter, clean air, and water to drink, but also other individuals, including family, lovers, employers, coworkers, friends, and associates.

In 1980, the American Nurses Association (ANA) defined health in its social policy statement as "a dynamic state of being in which the developmental and behavioral potential of an individual is realized to the fullest extent possible" (ANA, 1980, p. 5). In this definition, health is more than a state or the absence of disease; it includes striving toward optimal functioning. In 2004, the ANA also stated that health was "an experience that is often expressed in terms of wellness and illness, and may occur in the presence or absence of disease or injury" (2004, p. 48).

PERSONAL DEFINITIONS OF HEALTH Health is a highly individual perception. Consider the following examples of individuals who would probably say they are healthy, even though they have physical impairments that some people would consider illnesses:

- A 15-year-old boy with diabetes takes injectable insulin each morning. He plays on the school soccer team and is editor of the high school newspaper.

- A 32-year-old man is paralyzed from the waist down and needs a wheelchair for mobility. He is taking an accounting class at a nearby college and uses a specially designed automobile for transportation.

- A 72-year-old woman takes antihypertensive medications to treat high blood pressure. She bowls once a week, is a member of the neighborhood golf club, makes handicrafts for a local charity, and travels 2 months each year.

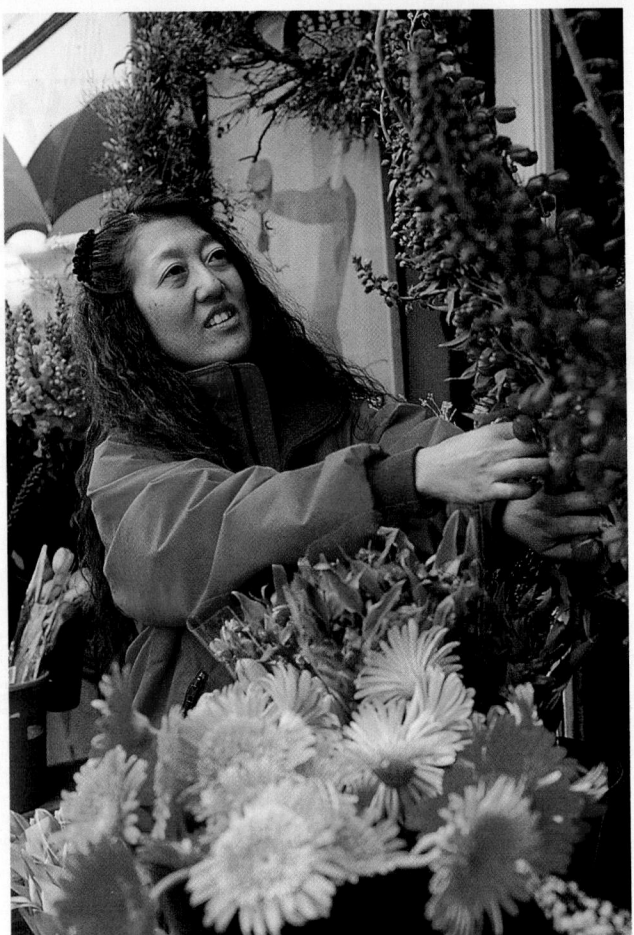

Figure 7–1 ● Satisfaction with work enhances a sense of well-being and contributes to wellness.

Many individuals define and describe health as being free as possible from symptoms of disease and pain, being able to be active and to do what they want or must, and being in good spirits most of the time. These characteristics indicate that health is not something that an individual achieves suddenly at a specific time. It is an ongoing process, a way of life through which an individual develops. Every aspect of the body, mind, and feelings strives to interrelate as harmoniously as possible (**Figure 7–1** ●).

Many factors affect individual definitions of health: the individual's previous experiences, expectations of self, age, and sociocultural influences. Nurses should be aware of their personal definitions of health and appreciate that other individuals also have their own definitions. Individuals' definitions of health influence their behavior related to health and illness. By understanding clients' perceptions of health and illness, nurses can better help them to help regain or attain a state of health. For aid in developing a personal definition of health see **Box 7–1** ●.

Wellness and Well-Being

Wellness is a state of well-being. Basic aspects of wellness include self-responsibility; an ultimate goal; a dynamic, growing process; daily decision making in the areas of nutrition,

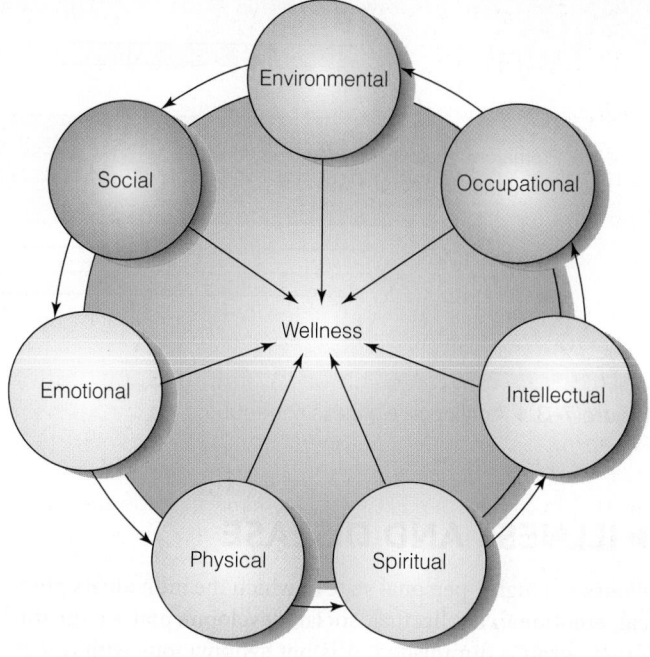

Figure 7–2 ● The seven components of wellness.

Source: Reproduced with permission from Anspaugh, D. J., Hamrick, M. H., & Rosato, F. D. (2010). *Wellness: Concepts and applications* (8th ed.). New York, NY: McGraw-Hill.

stress management, physical fitness, preventive health care, and emotional health; and, most important, the whole being of the individual.

Anspaugh, Hamrick, and Rosato (2010) propose seven components of wellness (**Figure 7–2** ●). To realize optimal health and wellness, individuals must deal with the factors within each component:

1. *The environmental component* involves the ability to promote health measures that improve the standard of living and quality of life in the community and includes influences such as food, water, and air.
2. *The occupational component* is the ability to achieve a balance between work and leisure time. The individual's beliefs about education, employment, and home influence personal satisfaction and relationships with others.
3. *The intellectual component* includes the ability to learn and use information effectively for personal, family, and career development. Intellectual wellness involves striving for continued growth and learning to deal effectively with new challenges.
4. *The spiritual component* is the belief in some force (nature, science, religion, or a higher power) that serves to unite human beings and provide meaning and purpose to life. It includes an individual's own morals, values, and ethics.
5. *The physical component* is the ability to carry out daily tasks, achieve fitness (e.g., pulmonary, cardiovascular, gastrointestinal), maintain adequate nutrition and proper body fat levels, avoid abusing drugs and alcohol or using tobacco products, and generally practice positive lifestyle habits.
6. *The emotional component* is the ability to manage stress and to express emotions appropriately. Emotional wellness involves the ability to recognize, accept, and express feelings and to accept one's limitations.
7. *The social component* is the ability to interact successfully with other individuals and within one's environ-

ment, to develop and maintain intimacy with significant others, and to develop respect and tolerance for those with different opinions and beliefs.

The seven components overlap to some extent, and factors in one component often directly affect factors in another. For example, an individual who learns to control daily stress levels from a physiological perspective is also helping to maintain the emotional stamina needed to cope with a crisis. Wellness involves working on all aspects of the model.

Well-being is a component of health. Hood (2009) describes well-being as "a subjective perception of vitality and feeling well [that] can be described objectively, experienced, and measured. . . . well-being status can be plotted on a continuum" (p. 185).

▶ AN ILLNESS–WELLNESS CONTINUUM

Health and illness or disease can be viewed as the opposite ends of a health continuum. Beginning at a high level of health, an individual can move through good health, normal health, poor health, extremely poor health, and eventually to death. Individuals move back and forth within this continuum day by day. There is no distinct boundary across which individuals move from health to illness or from illness back to health. How individuals perceive themselves and how others see them in terms of health and illness also affect their placement on the continuum. The ranges within which individuals can be thought of as healthy or ill are considerable (**Figure 7–3** ●).

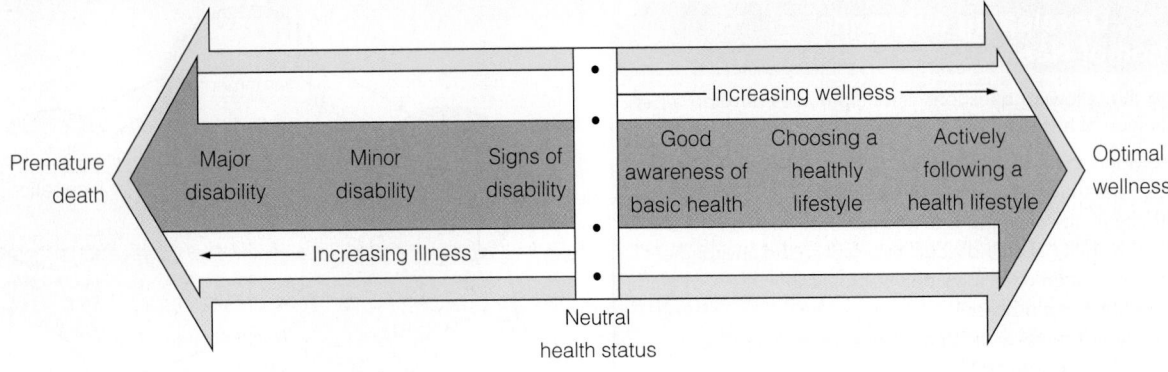

Figure 7–3 ● An illness–wellness continuum.

▶ ILLNESS AND DISEASE

Illness is a highly personal state in which the individual's physical, emotional, intellectual, social, developmental, or spiritual functioning is diminished. It is not synonymous with disease and may or may not be related to disease. One individual can have a disease, such as a growth in the stomach, and not feel ill. Another individual can feel ill—that is, feel uncomfortable—and yet have no discernible disease.

Disease can be described as an alteration in body functions that reduces the capacities or shortens the normal life span. Disease occurs when microorganisms produce a detectable alteration in normal tissue function that results in a reduction of capacities or a shortening of the normal life span. Primitive peoples thought "forces" or spirits caused disease. Later, this belief was replaced by the single-causation theory. Traditionally, the goal of intervention by primary care providers was to eliminate or ameliorate disease processes. Today, multiple factors are considered to interact in causing disease and determining an individual's response to treatment.

Illness and disease can be classified in many ways. The terms *acute* and *chronic* are commonly used. **Acute illness** is typically characterized by severe symptoms of relatively short duration. The symptoms often appear abruptly and subside quickly and, depending upon the cause, may or may not require intervention by healthcare professionals. Some acute illnesses are serious (for example, appendicitis may require surgery). But many acute illnesses, such as colds, subside without medical intervention or with only over-the-counter medications. Following an acute illness, most individuals return to their normal level of wellness.

A **chronic illness** is one that lasts for an extended period, usually 6 months or longer, and often for the duration of the individual's life. Chronic illnesses usually have a slow onset and often have periods of **remission**, when the symptoms disappear, and **exacerbation**, when the symptoms reappear.

Examples of chronic illnesses include arthritis, heart and lung diseases, and diabetes mellitus. Nurses are involved in caring for chronically ill individuals of all ages in all types of settings—homes, nursing homes, hospitals, clinics, and other institutions. Care focuses on promoting the highest possible level of independence, sense of control, and wellness. Clients with chronic illness often need to modify their activities of daily living, social relationships, and perception of self and body image. In addition, many clients must learn how to live with increasing physical limitations and discomfort. Teaching compliance with medications and treatment plans, even when the client feels well, is an essential nursing intervention for individuals with chronic illnesses.

Illness Behaviors

When individuals become ill, they behave in certain ways that sociologists refer to as *illness behavior*. **Illness behavior**, a coping mechanism, involves ways that individuals describe, monitor, and interpret their symptoms, take remedial actions, and use the healthcare system. How people behave when they are ill is highly individualized. It is affected by many variables such as age, sex, occupation, socioeconomic status, religion, ethnic origin, psychological stability, personality, education, and modes of coping.

Effects of Illness on the Client and Family

Illness brings about changes in both the involved individual and the family. The changes depend on the nature, severity, and duration of the illness; attitudes toward the illness by the client and others; the financial costs associated with the illness; the lifestyle changes required; and the adjustments in usual roles.

Clients who are ill may experience behavioral and emotional changes, changes in self-concept and body image, and lifestyle changes. Behavioral and emotional changes associated with short-term illness are generally mild and short-lived. For example, the individual may become irritable and lack the energy or desire for the usual interactions with family members or friends. More acute responses are likely with severe, life-threatening, chronic, or disabling illness. Anxiety, fear, anger, withdrawal, denial, a sense of hopelessness, and feelings of powerlessness are all common responses to severe or disabling illness. For example, a client experiencing a heart attack fears for her life and the financial burden it may place on the family. Another client informed about a diagnosis of cancer or AIDS or crippling neurological disease may, over time, experience episodes of denial, anger, fear, and hopelessness. For a client with a lifelong chronic illness, these feelings can recur with each acute attack of the illness. Repeated acute attacks, the financial expense that they incur, and the resulting emotional strain can greatly stress both the client and the family.

Certain illnesses can also change the client's body image or physical appearance, especially those illnesses that involve severe scarring or loss of a limb or a sense organ. The client's self-esteem and self-concept may also be affected. Many factors play a part in low self-esteem and a disturbance in self-concept, including loss of body parts and function, pain, disfigurement, dependence on others, unemployment, financial problems, inability to participate in social functions, strained relationships with others, and spiritual distress. Nurses must help clients express their thoughts and feelings, as well as provide care that helps the client cope effectively with changes.

Individuals who are ill are vulnerable to loss of **autonomy**, the state of being independent and self-directed without outside control. Family interactions may change so that clients are no longer involved in making family decisions or even in making decisions about their own health care. Nurses must support clients' right to self-determination and autonomy. Clients need sufficient information to participate in decision-making processes and to maintain a feeling of being in control.

Illness often necessitates a change in lifestyle. In addition to participating in treatments and taking medications, the client who is ill may need to change diet, activity and exercise, and rest and sleep patterns.

Nurses can help clients adjust their lifestyle in the following ways:

- Providing explanations about necessary adjustments
- Making arrangements wherever possible to accommodate the client's lifestyle

- Encouraging other health professionals to become aware of the client's lifestyle practices and to support healthy aspects of that lifestyle
- Reinforcing desirable changes in practices with a goal of making them a permanent part of the client's lifestyle.

▶ HEALTH PROMOTION

The vision of **health promotion** was initially expressed in 1979 with the U.S. Surgeon General's report *Healthy People*, which emphasized health promotion and disease prevention. Every decade since then, the Surgeon General has updated the report, establishing benchmarks and monitoring progress. The current *Healthy People 2020: Improving the Health of Americans* (U.S. Department of Health and Human Services, 2010) presents a comprehensive 10-year agenda with four goals:

1. Attain high-quality, longer lives free of preventable disease, disability, injury, and premature death.
2. Achieve health equity, eliminate disparities, and improve the health of all groups.
3. Create social and physical environments that promote good health for all.
4. Promote quality of life, healthy development, and healthy behaviors across all life stages.

To support these goals, *Healthy People 2020* is organized into 42 topic areas with nearly 600 objectives to improve health (**Box 7–2 ●**). *Healthy People 2020* also established a set of 26 leading health indicators, in 12 categories, that reflect the major public health concerns in the United States at the beginning of the 21st century (**Box 7–3 ●**). Each indicator relates to several health objectives. These indicators are expected to help

---

Box 7–2 The 42 Topic Areas in *Healthy People 2020*

1. Access to Health Services
2. Adolescent Health (new for 2020)
3. Arthritis, Osteoporosis, and Chronic Back Conditions
4. Blood Disorders and Blood Safety (new for 2020)
5. Cancer
6. Chronic Kidney Disease
7. Dementias, Including Alzheimer's Disease (new for 2020)
8. Diabetes
9. Disability and Health
10. Early and Middle Childhood (new for 2020)
11. Educational and Community-Based Programs
12. Environmental Health
13. Family Planning
14. Food Safety
15. Genomics (new for 2020)
16. Global Health (new for 2020)
17. Health Communication and Health Information Technology
18. Healthcare-Associated Infections (new for 2020)
19. Health-Related Quality of Life and Well-Being (new for 2020)
20. Hearing and Other Sensory or Communication Disorders
21. Heart Disease and Stroke
22. HIV
23. Immunization and Infectious Diseases

24. Injury and Violence Prevention
25. Lesbian, Gay, Bisexual, and Transgender Health (new for 2020)
26. Maternal, Infant, and Child Health
27. Medical Product Safety
28. Mental Health and Mental Disorders
29. Nutrition and Weight Status
30. Occupational Safety and Health
31. Older Adults (new for 2020)
32. Oral Health
33. Physical Activity
34. Preparedness (new for 2020)
35. Public Health Infrastructure
36. Respiratory Diseases
37. Sexually Transmitted Diseases
38. Sleep Health (new for 2020)
39. Social Determinants of Health (new for 2020)
40. Substance Abuse
41. Tobacco Use
42. Vision

Critical Thinking Questions
1. Which of these topics most interest you?
2. Which do you think are the priorities for your community? For your family? For you?

Box 7–3 The 12 Topics of the Leading Health Indicators in *Healthy People 2020*

1. *Access to health services*

   Strong predictors of access to quality healthcare services include having health insurance (1 in 5 Americans under age 65 do not have that) and a regular primary care provider or other source of ongoing health care (almost 1 in 4 Americans do not have that).

2. *Clinical preventive services*

   Clinical preventive services, such as early prenatal care, and routine disease screening are key to reducing death and disability. Vaccines are among the greatest public health achievements of the 20th century. Immunizations can prevent disability and death from infectious diseases and can help control the spread of infections within communities

3. *Environmental quality*

   An estimated 25% of all deaths and the total disease burden worldwide can be attributed to environmental factors. Nearly 1 in 10 children and 1 in 12 adults in the United States have asthma. That condition is caused, triggered, and exacerbated by air pollution and secondhand smoke.

4. *Injury and violence*

   For Americans age 1–44, injuries are the leading cause of death. Annually, more than 29 million individuals seek emergency department treatment for injuries. More than 180,000 individuals die from injuries each year, and about 51,000 deaths result from violence.

5. *Maternal, infant, and child health*

   The rate of preterm births has risen by more than 20% from 1990 to 2006. That rate is one factor in the high American infant death rate; in 2011, the rate was higher than in 46 other countries.

6. *Mental health*

   Approximately 25% of the adult U.S. population is affected by mental illness during a given year; no one is immune. One in seventeen has been diagnosed with a serious mental illness. Of all mental illnesses, depression and anxiety are the most common. Major depression is the leading cause of disability and is the cause of more than two thirds of suicides each year. Suicide is the 11th leading cause of death in the United States for all age groups. For individuals age 25–34, it is the second leading cause of death.

7. *Nutrition, physical activity, and obesity*

   Regular physical activity throughout life is important for maintaining a healthy body, enhancing psychological well-being, and preventing premature death. A majority of adults (81.6%) and adolescents (81.8%) do not get the recommended amount of physical activity.

   Overweight and obesity are major contributors to many preventable causes of death. On average, higher body weights are associated with higher death rates. The number of overweight children, adolescents, and adults has risen since the 1970s.

   About 1 in 3 adults (34.0%) and 1 in 6 children and adolescents (16.2%) are obese. Obesity-related conditions include heart disease, stroke, and type 2 diabetes.

8. *Oral health*

   Poor oral health, especially gum disease, is linked to chronic diseases such as diabetes, heart disease, and stroke. In pregnant women, poor oral health is associated with preterm births and low birth weight. In 2007, only about half of individuals age 2 and older had seen a dentist in the past year.

9. *Reproductive and sexual health*

   Unintended pregnancies and sexually transmitted diseases (STDs), including infection with the human immunodeficiency virus that causes AIDS, can result from unprotected sexual behaviors. About 19 million new cases of STDs are diagnosed in the United States each year, almost half among young adults age 15–24. Out of every 5 individuals with HIV, 1 is unaware of having it.

10. *Social determinants*

    This new leading indicator recognizes the critical role of the environment in improving health. It focuses attention on the home, school, workplace, neighborhood, and community.

11. *Substance abuse*

    Alcohol and illicit drug use are associated with many of this country's most serious problems, including family disruptions, financial debt, school failure, domestic violence, child abuse, and crime.

12. *Tobacco use*

    Cigarette smoking is the single most preventable cause of disease, disability, and death in the United States. More deaths result from tobacco use than all deaths from HIV, illegal drugs, alcohol, car accidents, suicides, and murders combined.

Source: Based on U.S. DHHS, Office of Disease Prevention. (2010). *Healthy People 2020: Improving the health of Americans.* Retrieved from http://www.healthypeople.gov/2020/.

develop action plans to improve the health of both individuals and communities.

The foundation for *Healthy People 2020* is the belief that individual health is closely linked to community health, and vice versa. For example, community health is affected by the beliefs, attitudes, and behaviors of the individuals who live in the community. As a result, partnerships are important to improving individual and community health. Businesses, local government, and civic, professional, and religious organizations can all participate. Examples include sponsoring a health fair, establishing fitness programs, beginning community recycling, and printing immunization schedules.

Health Promotion, Health Protection, and Disease Prevention

Considerable differences appear in the literature regarding the use of the terms *health promotion, primary prevention, health*

protection, and *illness/disease prevention.* Edelman and Mandle (2009) state, "Prevention, in a narrow sense, means averting the development of disease in the future. In a broad sense, prevention consists of all measures, including definitive therapies, that limit disease progression" (p. 14). Pender, Murdaugh, and Parsons (2010) consider health promotion different from disease prevention or health protection. They define *health promotion* as "behavior motivated by the desire to increase well-being and actualize human health potential," and *disease prevention* or *health protection* as "behavior motivated by a desire to actively avoid illness, detect it early, or maintain functioning within the constraints of illness" (p. 5). The individual's underlying motivation for the behavior is the major difference. **Box 7–4 ●** provides an overview of the differences between health promotion and health protection.

Because an activity may be carried out for numerous reasons, separating the terms *health promotion* and *disease*

Source: Pender, N. J., Murdaugh, C. L., & Parsons, M. A. (2010). *Health promotion in nursing practice* (6th ed.). Upper Saddle River, NJ: Prentice Hall, p. 5. Reprinted with permission.

Box 7–4 Differences Between Health Promotion and Health Protection

HEALTH PROMOTION	HEALTH PROTECTION
■ Not disease oriented	■ Illness or injury specific
■ Motivated by personal, positive "approach" to wellness	■ Motivated by "avoidance" of illness
■ Seeks to expand positive potential for health	■ Seeks to thwart the occurrence of insults to health and well-being

prevention/health protection is difficult. For example, a 40-year-old male may begin a program of walking 3 miles each day. If the goal of his program is to "decrease the risk of cardiovascular disease," then the activity is considered disease prevention or health protection. By contrast, if the motivation for his walking regimen is to "increase his overall health and feeling of well-being," then the activity is considered health promotion. It is most helpful to think of health promotion and health protection as complementary processes because both affect quality of health.

Health promotion can be offered to all clients regardless of their health and illness status or age. For example, weight-control measures can benefit both overweight clients without disease and clients with cardiac or joint disease. See the Lifespan Considerations feature for examples.

The Nurse's Role in Health Promotion

Health promotion is an important component of nursing practice. It is a way of thinking that revolves around a philosophy of wholeness, wellness, and well-being. Since the 1980s, the public has become increasingly aware of and interested in health promotion. Many individuals are aware of the relationship between lifestyle and illness and have begun developing health-promoting habits, such as getting adequate exercise, rest, and relaxation; maintaining good nutrition; and controlling the use of tobacco, alcohol, and other drugs.

Individuals and communities that seek to increase their responsibility for personal health and self-care require health education. The trend toward health promotion has created new opportunities for nurses to strengthen the profession's influence on health promotion. Nurses also have more opportunity to disseminate information that promotes an educated public and to assist individuals and communities to change long-standing health behaviors. Today, nurses serve in a wide variety of organizations and committees.

A variety of programs can be used to promote health, including (a) information dissemination, (b) health risk appraisal and wellness assessment, (c) lifestyle and behavior change, and (d) environmental control programs.

Information dissemination is the most basic type of health promotion program. This kind of program uses a variety of media to offer information to the public about the risk of particular lifestyle choices and personal behavior. It also spells out the specific benefits of changing that behavior and improving the quality of life. Billboards, posters, brochures, newspaper features, books, and health fairs all offer opportunities for disseminating health promotion information. Alcohol and drug abuse, driving under the influence of alcohol or drugs, hypertension, and the need for immunizations are some topics frequently discussed. Information dissemination is a useful strategy for raising individuals' and groups' level of knowledge and awareness about health habits.

When planning information dissemination, it is important to consider factors such as culture, age group, and literacy level. Knowing the best place and method for distributing information increases its effectiveness. For example, churches often provide older adults with social support while serving as a spiritual home, especially in African American communities. The church is often the appropriate place to hold health fairs or even small group discussions on various health topics. It offers a stepping-stone to providing information and suggesting resources for sensitive individual needs—all done in a comfortable, nonthreatening environment.

It is just as critical to know where individuals get misinformation. Sending multiple mailings has become a marketing ploy for advertising "miracle" vitamins, herbs, and food supplements. These are heavily directed toward older adults, who may choose this route to purchase items if they have transportation problems.

Health risk appraisal and wellness assessment programs are used to teach individuals about the risk factors inherent in their lives. This education is meant to motivate them to reduce specific risks and develop positive health habits. Wellness assessment programs are focused on more positive methods of enhancement, in contrast to the risk factor approach used in the health appraisal. A variety of tools are available to facilitate these assessments; some are computer based and can therefore be offered to educational institutions and workplaces at a reasonable cost.

Lifestyle and behavior change programs require the participation of the individual. They are geared toward enhancing the quality of life and extending the life span. Individuals generally consider lifestyle changes after they have been informed of the need to change their health behavior and have become aware of the potential benefits of the process. Many programs are available to the public, on both a group and an individual basis. Topics may include stress management, nutrition awareness, weight control, smoking cessation, and exercise.

Environmental control programs have been developed in response to the continuing increase of contaminants of human origin in our environment. The amount of contaminants already present in our air, food, and water will affect the health of our descendants for several generations. The most common concerns of community groups are toxic and nuclear wastes, nuclear power plants, air and water pollution, and herbicide and pesticide use.

Health promotion activities, such as the variety of programs previously discussed, involve collaborative relationships with both clients and primary care providers. The role of the nurse is to work *with* individuals, not *for* them—that is, to act as a facilitator of the process of assessing, evaluating, and understanding health. The nurse may act as advocate, consultant, teacher, or coordinator of services. For examples of the nurse's role in health promotion, see **Box 7–5** ●.

In these roles, the nurse may work with individuals of all age groups and diverse family units. Alternatively, the nurse may concentrate on a specific population, such as new parents,

Lifespan Considerations   Health Promotion Topics Across the Life Span

Infants
- Infant–parent attachment/bonding
- Breastfeeding
- Sleep patterns
- Playful activity to stimulate development
- Immunizations
- Safety promotion and injury control

Children
- Nutrition
- Dental checkups
- Rest and exercise
- Immunizations
- Safety promotion and injury control

Adolescents
- Communicating with the teen
- Hormonal changes
- Nutrition
- Exercise and rest
- Peer group influences

- Self-concept and body image
- Sexuality
- Safety promotion and accident prevention

Older Adults
- Adequate sleep
- Appropriate use of alcohol
- Dental/oral health
- Drug management
- Exercise
- Foot health
- Health screening recommendations
- Hearing aid use
- Immunizations
- Medication instruction
- Mental health
- Nutrition
- Physical fitness
- Preventive health services
- Safety precautions
- Smoking cessation
- Weight control

school-age children, or older adults. In any case, the nursing process is a basic tool for the nurse in a health promotion role. Although the process is the same, the nurse emphasizes teaching the client (either an individual or a family unit) self-care responsibility. Adult clients decide the goals, determine the health promotion plans, and take responsibility for the success of the plans.

As increasingly knowledgeable healthcare consumers, clients expect and deserve quality care. Whether assisting an individual, a family, or an entire community, quality nursing care seeks to emphasize illness prevention and health promotion. Nurses recognize that a client's state of health and wellness encompasses many dimensions, including social, spiritual, cultural, sexual, environmental, physical, and psychological. Each

Box 7–5   The Nurse's Role in Health Promotion

- Model healthy lifestyle behaviors and attitudes.
- Facilitate client involvement in the assessment, implementation, and evaluation of health goals.
- Teach clients self-care strategies to enhance fitness, improve nutrition, manage stress, and enhance relationships.
- Assist individuals, families, and communities to increase their levels of health.
- Educate clients to be effective healthcare consumers.
- Assist clients, families, and communities to develop and choose health-promoting options.
- Guide clients' development in effective problem solving and decision making.
- Reinforce clients' personal and family health-promoting behaviors.
- Advocate in the community for changes that promote a healthy environment.

client encounter affords the nurse an opportunity to encourage both traditional and innovative health-seeking behaviors.

Assessing and planning the health care of the individual client are enhanced when the nurse understands the concepts of individuality, holism, homeostasis, and human needs. The beliefs and values of each individual and the family's support are reinforced by the community. The reverse is also true: The health of a community is affected by the beliefs, attitudes, and behaviors of the individuals in the community.

▶ VARIABLES INFLUENCING HEALTH

Many variables influence an individual's health status, beliefs, and behaviors or practices. These factors may or may not be under conscious control. Individuals can usually control their health behaviors and can choose healthy or unhealthy activities (external variables). In contrast, individuals have little or no choice of their genetic makeup, age, sex, culture, and sometimes their geographic environment (internal variables).

Internal variables include biological, psychological, and cognitive dimensions. They are often described as nonmodifiable variables because, for the most part, they cannot be changed. Examples include genetic factors, such as race or history of heart disease; presence of mental illness; and disorders of cognition such as autism spectrum disorder. However, when internal variables link to health problems, the nurse and client must work together even more diligently to influence external variables (such as exercise and diet). Regular health exams and appropriate screening for early detection of health problems become even more important. See **Table 7–1 ●** for health screening guidelines across the life span.

TABLE 7–1 Health Screenings and Immunization Guidelines Across the Life Span

AGE GROUP	RECOMMENDED SCREENINGS AND HEALTH PROMOTION
Newborn and infant	■ Screening of newborns for hearing loss; follow up as appropriate (AAP, Joint Committee on Infant Hearing, 2007) ■ Health examinations at 2 weeks and at 2, 4, 6, 9, and 12 months ■ Immunizations: diphtheria, tetanus, acellular pertussis (DTaP), inactivated poliovirus vaccine (IPV), pneumo-coccal (PVC), *Haemophilus influenzae* type b (HIB), hepatitis B (HepB), hepatitis A (HepA), rotavirus, and influenza vaccines as recommended. Varicella and measles-mumps-rubella (MMR) are not given before 12 months of age. ■ Fluoride supplements for infants over 6 months of age if there is inadequate water fluoridation (less than 0.3 parts per million) ■ Screening for tuberculosis ■ Screening for metabolic conditions including phenylketonuria (PKU) ■ Denver Developmental Screening Test (DDST-II) or other developmental screening
Toddler	■ Health examinations at 15 and 18 months and then as recommended by the primary care provider ■ Dental visits starting at age 3 or earlier ■ Immunizations: continuing DTaP, IPV, pneumococcal, MMR, varicella, *Haemophilus influenzae* type b, hepatitis B, hepatitis A, influenza, and meningococcal vaccines as recommended ■ Screenings for tuberculosis and lead poisoning ■ Fluoride supplements if there is inadequate water fluoridation (less than 0.6 parts per million)
Preschool	■ Health examinations every 1–2 years ■ Immunizations: continuing DTaP, IPV, MMR, hepatitis A and B, pneumococcal, influenza, varicella, and other immunizations as recommended ■ Screenings for tuberculosis ■ Vision and hearing screening ■ Regular dental screenings and fluoride treatment if necessary
School-age	■ Annual physical examination or as recommended ■ Immunizations as recommended (e.g., human papilloma virus [HPV], MMR, meningococcal, tetanus-diphtheria [Tdap], influenza) ■ Screening for tuberculosis ■ Periodic vision, speech, and hearing screenings
Adolescent	■ Regular dental screenings and fluoride treatment ■ Health examination as recommended by the primary care provider ■ Immunizations as recommended, such as adult tetanus-diphtheria vaccine, MMR, pneumococcal, HPV, and hepatitis B vaccine ■ Screening for tuberculosis ■ Periodic vision and hearing screenings ■ Regular dental assessments ■ Assessing for mental health status
Young adults	■ Routine physical examination (every 1–3 years for females; every 5 years for males) ■ Immunizations as recommended, such as tetanus-diphtheria boosters every 10 years, meningococcal vaccine if not given in early adolescence, and hepatitis B vaccine ■ HPV vaccine for women up to 26 years old who have not yet received or completed the vaccine series (Knudtson, 2009) ■ Regular dental assessments (every 6 months) ■ Periodic vision and hearing screenings ■ Professional breast examination every 1–3 years for women ■ Papanicolaou smear for women annually within 3 years of onset of sexual activity ■ Testicular examination every year for men ■ Screening for cardiovascular disease (e.g., cholesterol test every 5 years if results are normal; blood pressure to detect hypertension; baseline electrocardiogram at age 35) ■ Tuberculosis skin test every 2 years ■ Smoking: history and counseling, if needed
Middle-aged adults	■ Physical examination (every 3–5 years until age 40, then annually) ■ Immunizations as recommended, such as a tetanus booster every 10 years and current recommendations for influenza vaccine ■ Regular dental assessments (e.g., every 6 months) ■ Tonometry for signs of glaucoma and other eye diseases every 2–3 years or annually if indicated ■ Breast examination for women annually by primary care provider ■ Testicular examination for men annually by primary care provider ■ Screenings for cardiovascular disease (e.g., blood pressure measurement; electrocardiogram and cholesterol test as directed by the primary care provider) ■ Screenings for colorectal, breast, cervical, uterine, and prostate cancer ■ Screening for tuberculosis every 2 years ■ Smoking: history and counseling, if needed

(continued on next page)

TABLE 7–1 Health Screenings and Immunization Guidelines Across the Life Span (*continued*)

AGE GROUP	RECOMMENDED SCREENINGS AND HEALTH PROMOTION
Older adults	■ Total cholesterol and high-density lipoprotein measurement every 3–5 years until age 75 ■ Aspirin, 81 mg, daily, if in high-risk group ■ Diabetes mellitus screen every 3 years, if in high-risk group ■ Smoking cessation ■ Screening mammogram every 1–2 years (women) ■ Clinical breast exam annually (women) ■ Pap smear (women) annually if there is a history of risk factors (exposure to diethylstilbestrol [DES] before birth, weakened immune system from HIV infection, organ transplant, chemotherapy, or chronic steroid use), abnormal smears or previous hysterectomy for malignancy (American Cancer Society, 2009) ■ Note: Women 70 years of age or older who have had three or more normal Pap tests in a row and no abnormal Pap tests in the last 10 years may choose to stop having cervical cancer testing (American Cancer Society, 2009) ■ Annual digital rectal exam ■ Annual prostate-specific antigen (PSA) for men ■ Annual fecal occult blood test (FOBT) ■ Sigmoidoscopy every 5 years; colonoscopy every 10 years ■ Visual acuity screen annually ■ Hearing screen annually ■ Depression screen periodically ■ Family violence screen periodically ■ Height and weight measurements annually ■ Sexually transmitted disease testing, if in high-risk group ■ Annual flu vaccine if over 65 or in high-risk group ■ Pneumococcal vaccine at 65 and every 10 years thereafter ■ Single dose of shingles vaccine for adults 60 years of age or older ■ Tetanus booster every 10 years

Biological Dimension

Genetic makeup, gender, age, and developmental level significantly influence health. *Genetic makeup* influences biological characteristics, innate temperament, activity level, and intellectual potential. It can impact susceptibility to specific diseases, such as diabetes, breast cancer, and ovarian cancer. In some cases, genetic predisposition for health or illness is enhanced when parents are from the same ethnic genetic pool. For example, individuals of African heritage have a higher incidence of sickle cell disease than the general population but may be less susceptible to malaria.

Gender influences the distribution of disease. Certain acquired and genetic diseases are more common in one sex than in the other. Disorders more common among women include osteoporosis and autoimmune diseases such as rheumatoid arthritis. Those more common among men are stomach ulcers, abdominal hernias, and respiratory diseases.

Age is also a significant factor in the distribution of disease. For example, arteriosclerotic heart disease is common in middle-aged men but occurs infrequently in younger individuals; communicable diseases such as whooping cough and measles are common in children but rare in older adults, who have acquired immunity to them.

Developmental level has a major impact on health status. Consider these examples:

■ Because infants lack physiological and psychological maturity, their defenses against disease are lower during the first years of life.

■ Toddlers who are learning to walk are more prone to falls and injury.

■ Adolescents, who need to conform to peers, are more prone to risk-taking behavior and subsequent injury.

■ Declining physical and sensory-perceptual abilities limit older adults' response to environmental hazards and stressors.

Psychological Dimension

Psychological (emotional) factors influencing health include mind–body interactions and self-concept.

Mind–body interactions can affect health status either positively or negatively. Emotional responses to stress affect body function. For example, a student who is extremely anxious before a test may experience urinary frequency or diarrhea. An individual who is worried about the outcome of surgery or about the behavior of a teenager may chain-smoke. Prolonged emotional distress may increase susceptibility to organic disease or precipitate it. Emotional distress may influence the immune system through central nervous system and endocrine alterations. Alterations in the immune system are related to the incidence of infections, cancer, and autoimmune diseases.

Increasing attention is being given to the mind's ability to direct the body's functioning. Relaxation, meditation, and biofeedback techniques are gaining wider recognition among clients and healthcare professionals. For example, women often use relaxation techniques to decrease pain during childbirth. Other individuals may learn biofeedback skills to reduce hypertension.

Emotional reactions also occur in response to body conditions. For example, an individual diagnosed with a terminal illness may experience fear and depression. *Self-concept* is how an individual feels about the self (self-esteem) and perceives the physical self (body image) and her needs, roles, and abilities. Self-concept affects how individuals view and handle situations. Such attitudes can affect health practices, responses to stress and illness, and treatment seeking. An example is the anorexic woman who deprives herself of needed nutrients because she believes she is too fat, even though she is well below an acceptable weight level. Self-perceptions are also associated with an individual's definition of health. For example, a 75-year-old man who can no longer move large objects may need to redefine his concept of health in view of his current abilities.

Cognitive Dimension

Cognitive or intellectual factors influencing health include lifestyle choices and spiritual and religious beliefs. Some clients are better at problem solving and are equipped with better coping skills than others. Nurses must be aware of cognitive and intellectual factors that support or hinder a client's compliance with treatment.

Lifestyle choices refer to an individual's general way of life, including living conditions and individual patterns of behavior, which are influenced by sociocultural factors and personal characteristics. In brief, lifestyle is often considered the behavior and activities over which individuals have control. Lifestyle choices may have positive or negative effects on health. Practices with potentially negative effects on health are often referred to as **risk factors**. For example, overeating, getting insufficient exercise, and being overweight are closely related to the incidence of heart disease, arteriosclerosis, diabetes, and hypertension. Excessive use of tobacco is clearly implicated in lung cancer, emphysema, and cardiovascular diseases. See **Box 7–6** ● for examples of healthy lifestyle choices.

Health beliefs are concepts of about health that individuals believe are true. They may or may not be founded in fact. Some beliefs are influenced by culture, such as the belief that health and wellness are closely associated with the amount and quality of blood in the body. For example, in the American South, some individuals use the phrase "high blood" to mean they have too much blood in the body, causing headaches and dizziness.

Health beliefs can impact whether clients are likely to engage in health promotion or to follow a treatment plan. Social learning theory makes an effort to capture this likelihood through its explanation of locus of control (LOC). Individuals who believe that they can impact their own health and well-being are said to have an **internal locus of control**. These individuals are more likely to take control over their own health, follow therapeutic regimens, and engage in health promotion and prevention activities, including exercise and dietary modifications. Individuals who believe their health is controlled by forces outside their control (e.g., chance, fate, others) are said to have an **external locus of control**. For example, a research study of adults over age 80 studied individuals who attributed their current health status to uncontrollable "old age." Stewart et al.

(2012) found that, compared to the control subjects, those individuals reported more perceived health symptoms, poorer health maintenance behaviors, and a greater likelihood of mortality at 2-year follow up.

Spiritual and religious beliefs can significantly affect health behavior. For example, Jehovah's Witnesses oppose blood transfusions; some fundamentalists believe that a serious illness is a punishment from God; some religious groups are strict vegetarians; and religious Jews perform circumcision on the eighth day of a male baby's life. The influence of spirituality and religion is discussed further in the concept of Spirituality concept.

■ NURSING PROCESS

A thorough assessment of the individual's health status is basic to health promotion. As nurses move toward greater autonomy in client care, expanded assessment skills will provide more meaningful data for health planning.

Assessment

Components of this assessment are the health history and physical examination, physical fitness assessment, lifestyle assessment, spiritual assessment, social support systems review, health risk assessment, health beliefs review, and life stress review.

Health History and Physical Examination

The health history and physical examination provide a means of detecting existing problems. Consider the age of the individual when collecting data. For example, an environmental safety assessment and immunization history must be appropriate to the individual's age. A nutritional assessment is another important part of the health history. The nurse must consider both the age and the body build of the client when gathering information on dietary patterns.

Physical Fitness Assessment

During an evaluation of physical fitness, the nurse assesses several components of the body's physical functioning: muscle endurance, flexibility, body composition, and cardiorespiratory endurance. See the exemplar on Physical Fitness and Exercise in this module.

Lifestyle Assessment

Lifestyle assessment focuses on the personal lifestyle and habits as they affect the client's health. Categories of lifestyle generally assessed include physical activity, nutritional practices, stress management, and habits such as smoking, alcohol consumption, and drug use. Other categories may be included. Several tools are available to assess lifestyle. The goals of lifestyle assessment tools are to provide the following:

- An opportunity for clients to assess the impact of their present lifestyle on their health
- A basis for decisions about desired behavior and lifestyle change
- Consideration of the lifestyles of children and older adults (see the Lifespan Considerations feature).

Box 7–6   Examples of Healthy Lifestyle Choices

- Regular exercise
- Weight control
- Avoidance of saturated fats
- Alcohol and tobacco avoidance
- Seat belt use
- Bike helmet use
- Immunization updates
- Regular dental checkups
- Regular health maintenance visits for screening examinations or tests

Lifespan Considerations Factors Affecting Health Promotion and Illness Prevention in Children and Older Adults

Children

Childhood obesity is a serious health problem. Data collected from 2009 to 2010 by the Centers for Disease Control and Prevention (CDC) show that 18% of American children age 6–11 years are obese and 12% of those age 2–5 years are obese (Ogden et al., 2012). Obesity and overweight in children contribute to long-term health problems such as heart disease and diabetes mellitus.

Specific causes of obesity and strategies to reduce weight vary from child to child. But healthy eating habits and exercise patterns form the overall basis for normal growth and prevention of obesity in children. Parents and caregivers are responsible to provide children with healthy food choices and an environment that makes eating a pleasure. Children are responsible to decide how much and what foods to eat. Adults must be role models for their children, eating well and exercising regularly themselves.

Older Adults

In older adults, health promotion and illness prevention are important. However, an added focus is learning to adapt to and live with increasing changes and limitations. Maximizing strengths continues to be of prime importance in maintaining optimal function and quality of life. Factors that may indicate a need for additional information or resources include the following:

- Increase in physical limitations
- Presence of one or more chronic illnesses
- Change in cognitive status
- Difficulty in accessing healthcare services due to transportation problems
- Inadequacy of support systems
- Need for environmental modifications for safety and maintaining independence
- Attitude of hopelessness and depression, which decreases the motivation to use resources or learn new information

Spiritual Health Assessment

Spiritual health is the ability to develop one's inner being to its fullest potential, including the ability to discover and articulate one's basic purpose in life; to learn how to experience love, joy, peace, and fulfillment; and to help oneself and others achieve their fullest potential (Pender, Murdaugh, & Parsons, 2010, p. 104). Spiritual beliefs can affect an individual's interpretation of life events. Therefore, an assessment of spiritual well-being is a part of evaluating the person's overall health. (See the concept of Spirituality for more information.)

Social Support Systems Review

Understanding the social context in which an individual lives and works is important in health promotion. Individuals and groups, through interpersonal relationships, can provide comfort, assistance, encouragement, and information. Social support fosters successful coping and promotes satisfying and effective living.

Social support systems contribute to health by creating an environment that encourages healthy behaviors, promotes self-esteem and wellness, and provides feedback for actions leading to desirable outcomes. Examples of social support systems are family, peer support groups (including Internet-based support groups), community-organized religious support systems (e.g., churches), and self-help groups (e.g., Mended Hearts, Weight Watchers). The Focus on Diversity and Culture feature addresses aspects of social support within the context of culture.

Life Stress Review

There is abundant research about the impact of stress on mental and physical well-being. A variety of stress-related assessment instruments can be found in the clinical literature.

Stay Current: Visit the following Web sites to see current information about the impact of stress on mental health and physical well-being:

National Institute of Mental Health (NIMH) home page, to search for specific topics, at **http://www.nimh.nih.gov/index.shtml**

NIMH Fact Sheet on Stress, with access at **http://www.nimh.nih.gov/health/publications/stress/fact-sheet-on-stress.shtml**

US National Library of Medicine Medline Plus home page, to search for specific topics, at **http://www.nlm.nih.gov/medlineplus/**

Medline Plus interactive tutorial on Managing Stress, with access at **http://www.nlm.nih.gov/medlineplus/tutorials/managingstress/htm/index.htm**

Focus on Diversity and Culture
Cultural Aspects of Social Support

It is important to understand how various subgroups of American society may define social support.

- African-Americans consider the family and church as major providers of social support.
- Hispanic-Latino Americans and Asian-Americans view the family, which includes close and distant kin, as the core of their social support system.
- Asian-Americans respect older adults and use shame and harmony in giving and receiving support.
- Native Americans live in relational networks that foster mutual assistance and support, with the extended family as a core feature.

Source: Pender, N. J., Murdaugh, C. L., & Parsons, M. A. (2010). *Health promotion in nursing practice* (6th ed.). Upper Saddle River, NJ: Prentice Hall, p. 220. Reprinted with permission.

Medline Plus interactive tutorial on Post-Traumatic Stress Disorder, with access at **http://www.nlm.nih.gov/medlineplus/ tutorials/ptsd/htm/index.htm**

Validating Assessment Data

After collecting assessment data, the nurse and client together review, validate, and summarize the information. During this process, the nurse verbally reviews the current practices and attitudes of the client. This review allows validation of the information by the client, and the conversation may increase the client's awareness of the need for behavior change. The nurse and client need to consider the following:

- Existing health problems
- Perceived degree of control over health status
- Key health beliefs
- Level of physical fitness and nutritional status
- Illnesses for which the client is at risk
- Current positive health practices
- Spirituality
- Sources of life stress and ability to handle stress
- Social support systems
- Information to enhance healthcare practices.

Diagnosis

Nursing diagnoses accepted by NANDA International have generally focused on impaired or imbalanced health patterns or problems. However, the NANDA-I health promotion domain is defined as "the awareness of well-being as normality of function and the strategies used to maintain control of and enhance that well-being or normality of function" (NANDA, 2012, p. 29).

Twenty-five diagnoses within the health promotion domain are particularly useful for healthy clients who require teaching for disease prevention and personal growth. When the nurse and client conclude that the client has positive function in a certain pattern area, such as adequate nutrition or effective coping, the nurse can use this information to help the client reach a higher level of functioning. The following areas are included in the NANDA taxonomy, listed by domain:

- In Domain 1: Health Promotion
  Readiness for Enhanced Immunization Status
  Readiness for Enhanced Self-Health Management
- In Domain 2: Nutrition
  Readiness for Enhanced Nutrition
  Readiness for Enhanced Fluid Balance
- In Domain 3: Elimination and Exchange
  Readiness for Enhanced Urinary Elimination
- In Domain 4: Activity/Rest
  Readiness for Enhanced Sleep
- In Domain 5: Perception/Cognition
  Readiness for Enhanced Knowledge
  Readiness for Enhanced Decision Making
  Readiness for Enhanced Communication
- In Domain 6: Self-Perception
  Readiness for Enhanced Self-Concept
- In Domain 7: Role Relationships
  Readiness for Enhanced Breastfeeding
  Readiness for Enhanced Parenting

Readiness for Enhanced Family Processes
Readiness for Enhanced Relationship
- In Domain 8: Sexuality
  Readiness for Enhanced Childbearing Process
- In Domain 9: Coping/Stress Tolerance
  Readiness for Enhanced Coping
  Readiness for Enhanced Community Coping
  Readiness for Enhanced Family Coping
  Readiness for Enhanced Power
  Readiness for Enhanced Resilience
  Readiness for Enhanced Organized Infant Behavior
- In Domain 10: Life Principles
  Readiness for Enhanced Hope
  Readiness for Enhanced Spiritual Well-Being
  Readiness for Enhanced Religiosity
- In Domain 12: Safety/Protection
  Readiness for Enhanced Comfort

Note: Domain 11: Safety/Protection does not have a health promotion diagnosis.

(NANDA-I © 2012)

These diagnoses provide a clear focus for planning interventions without indicating that a problem exists.

Planning

Health promotion plans are developed according to the needs, desires, and priorities of the client. The client decides on health promotion goals, activities or interventions to achieve those goals, frequency and duration of the activities, and method of evaluation of outcomes. During the planning process, the nurse acts as a resource person, rather than as an adviser or counselor. The nurse provides information when asked, emphasizes the importance of small steps to behavioral change, and reviews the client's goals and plans to make sure they are realistic, measurable, and acceptable to the client.

Steps in Planning

Pender et al. (2010, pp. 122–135) outlined nine steps to develop a joint health promotion–illness prevention plan. These steps actively involve both the nurse and the client from the start:

1. *Review and summarize data from assessment.* The nurse summarizes the data collected from the various assessments (e.g., physical health and fitness status, nutrition, sources of stress, spirituality, health practices).
2. *Emphasize strengths and competencies of the client.* The nurse and the client come to consensus about areas in which the client is doing well and areas that need further development.
3. *Identify health goals and related behavioral change options.* The client selects the top priority personal health goals and selects behavior change options.
4. *Identify behavioral or health outcomes indicating success from the client's perspective.* The focus is on how to achieve the desired outcome. For example, to reduce the risk of cardiovascular disease, the client may need to stop smoking, lose weight, and increase activity level.
5. *Develop a behavior change plan based on client preferences and current knowledge about effective interventions.*

A constructive program of change is based on client "ownership" of those behavior changes selected for implementation within everyday life (Pender et al., 2010, p. 128). Nurses may need to assist clients in examining value–behavior inconsistencies and in selecting the most appealing behavioral change. The client's priorities will reflect personal values, activity preferences, and expectations for success.

6. *Reiterate benefits of change, concentrating on client-approved incentives.* The positive benefits are more likely to be achieved if the client, even if totally to change, is routinely reminded of them. The nurse should encourage the client to keep reminders of the health-related and non-health-related benefits visible to provide motivation.

7. *Address environmental and interpersonal facilitators and barriers to change.* Use environmental and interpersonal factors that support positive change to reinforce the client's efforts to change lifestyle. All individuals experience barriers, some of which can be anticipated and planned for, thereby making change more likely to occur.

8. *Determine a time frame for implementation.* A time frame allows the client to develop appropriate knowledge and skills before a new behavior is implemented. The time frame may be several weeks or months. Scheduling short-term goals and rewards can encourage the client to achieve long-term objectives.

9. *Formalize commitment to behavior change plan goals, and provide needed support.* Previously, commitments to changing behaviors have usually been informal and verbal. Increasingly, formal and written behavior contracts are used to motivate clients to follow through with selected actions. Motivation to follow through is provided by a **positive reinforcement** or reward stated in the contract. Contracting is based on the belief that all individuals have the potential for growth and the right of self-determination.

Explore Available Resources

Another essential aspect of planning is identifying support resources available to the client. These may be community resources, such as a fitness program at a local gymnasium, or educational programs about stress management, breast self-examination, nutrition, or smoking cessation.

Implementation

Implementation is the "doing" part of behavior change. Self-responsibility is emphasized for implementing the plan. Depending on the client's needs, the nursing interventions may include supporting, counseling, facilitating, teaching, consulting, enhancing the behavior change, or modeling.

A major nursing role is to support the client. A vital component of lifestyle change is ongoing nonjudgmental support that focuses on the desired behavior. The nurse can offer support to an individual or in a group setting. The nurse can also facilitate the development of support networks for the client, including family members and friends.

Provide Individual Counseling Sessions

The nurse may schedule counseling sessions as a routine part of the plan or when the client encounters difficulty in carrying out

interventions or meets insurmountable barriers. In a counseling relationship, the nurse and client share ideas. In this sharing relationship, the nurse acts as a facilitator, promoting the client's decision making in regard to the health promotion plan.

Provide Telephone or Internet Counseling

Regular telephone sessions or Internet interaction may help to answer the client's questions, review goals and strategies, and reinforce progress. The nurse may offer to schedule a weekly interaction or invite the client to initiate a call if a problem occurs. The nurse asks the client an open-ended question, such as "How are things going?" If the answer indicates that the original plan is not working, the nurse asks, "What would you like to do?" The client has two choices: continue, or change the plan to a more realistic one. Telephone or Internet support is efficient for the busy client who may not have time for regular in-person sessions.

Offer Group Support

In group sessions, participants learn from the experiences of others in changing their behavior. Group contact gives individuals a renewed commitment to their goals.

Facilitate Social Support

Social networks, such as family and friends, can facilitate or impede efforts directed toward health promotion and illness prevention. The nurse's role is to assist the client to assess, modify, and develop the social support necessary to achieve the desired change. To provide the necessary support, families must communicate effectively, be aware of and support each other's needs and goals, and provide help to achieve those goals. The client may wish the nurse to meet with the family or significant others to enlist their understanding and support.

Provide Health Education

Health education programs can be provided to groups, individuals, or communities. Group programs need to be planned carefully before they are implemented. The decision to establish a health promotion program must be based on an assessment of health needs of the group or groups to be targeted for the health education program. Specific health promotion goals must be set. After the program is implemented, both positive and negative outcomes must be evaluated.

Enhance Behavior Change

Whether individuals will make and maintain changes to improve health or prevent disease depends upon many interrelated factors. To help clients succeed in implementing behavior changes, the nurse needs to understand the stages of change. Then the nurse can choose effective interventions that focus on helping the individual progress through the stages of change. **Figure 7–4** ● and the Client Teaching feature show ways to identify the client's stage of change and suggested strategies relevant to the clients' stage of change.

Provide Modeling

In **modeling**, the client acquires ideas for behavior and coping strategies to be used with specific problems by observing a

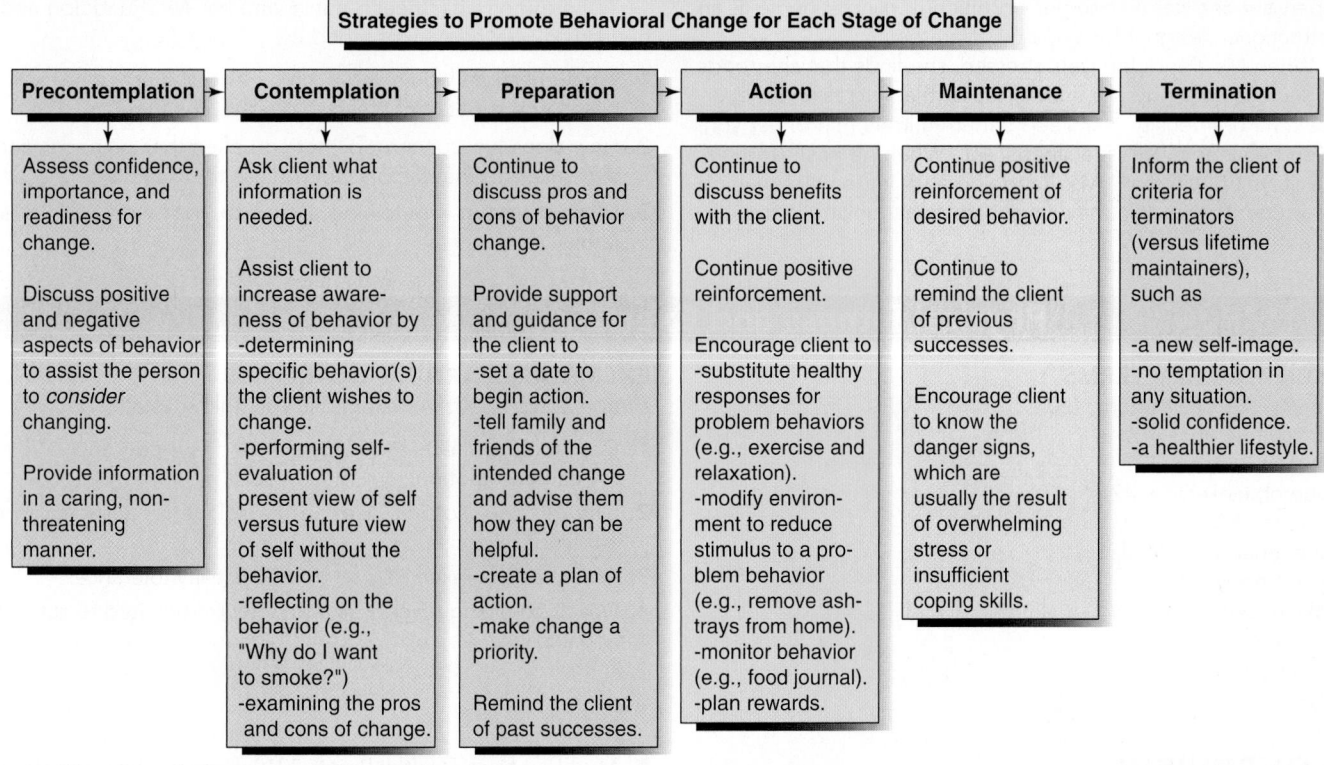

Figure 7–4 ● Strategies to promote behavioral change for each stage of change.

model or role model. The client is not expected to mimic the role model's sequence of actions or behavior patterns, but to modify them to the client's own behaviors. The nurse and client should mutually select models with whom the client can identify, because cultural and ethnic backgrounds and age of the nurse and client can differ. Models should be individuals the client respects. Nurses can also serve as models of wellness. To model effectively, nurses need to adopt a personal philosophy and lifestyle of good health habits.

Evaluation

Evaluation is ongoing, monitoring both short-term goals and long-term goals. Goals are written during the planning phase, and a target date is determined for attaining the specific desired results or behaviors. During evaluation, the client may decide to continue with the plan, reorder priorities, change strategies, or revise the health protection–promotion contract. Evaluation of the plan is a collaborative effort between the nurse and the client.

◢ REVIEW The Concept of Health, Wellness, and Illness

RELATE Link the Concepts

Linking the concept of health, wellness, and illness with the concept of comfort:

1. Your client has a diagnosis of rheumatoid arthritis. What kinds of exercise would you suggest for the days the client experiences severe joint pain?

2. Your client started a yoga class and states that some poses cause her intermittent backache to increase in intensity. The client's attitude is "No pain, no gain." Do you agree? What will you discuss with the client?

Linking the concept of health, wellness, and illness with the concept of stress and coping:

3. Your client with PTSD has difficulty sleeping and complains that he is too tired to exercise. How could you use your knowledge of the stages of change to help him?

4. After her child's epileptic seizure has ended, your client, the mother, states she feels "all beat up." What suggestions do you have for her, after she deals with the immediate crisis?

Linking the concept of health, wellness, and illness with the concept of teaching and learning:

5. You supervise a team of nurses, who share ongoing stresses. You find that they are not taking full advantage of the recreation benefits provided by the organization. How can you educate or mentor them to change?

READY Go to Companion Skills Manual

REFER Go to Pearson Student Nursing Resources
nursing.pearsonhighered.com

- Additional review materials

REFLECT Case Study

Susanna Randolph is a 40-year-old single African American mother, living in a suburban townhouse with her 10-year-old son, Jeff, who has autism. She keeps in regular contact with Jeff's father, who runs a high-tech start-up company. Ms. Randolph pursued a successful career as a medical technologist until her son's diagnosis. After she resigned her post as a laboratory supervisor, she was able to get a position working at home as an instructional designer for a nearby laboratory.

When Ms. Randolph gets stressed, she finds that she tends to decrease her physical activity rather than increase her exercise time or intensity. Her sleep pattern mirrors that of her son; when he sleeps well, she sleeps well. When he has insomnia, she stays up with him. Ms. Randolph and Jeff enjoy brushing their teeth together in their small bathroom, looking in the mirror at their images.

You are the public health nurse who has Ms. Randolph and her son on your home visit schedule.

1. What questions would you ask Ms. Randolph about her wellness routine that might lead to positive changes?

2. How does her concern for her son affect her plans for her own health? What factors can you use to motivate her?

3. What priorities would you assign to your work with this family?

EXEMPLAR 7.1   Physical Fitness and Exercise

EXEMPLAR KEY TERMS

Activity-exercise pattern, 420
Activity tolerance, 421
Aerobic exercise, 421
Anaerobic exercise, 421
Exercise, 421
Functional strength, 421
Hypertrophy, 421
Isokinetic exercise, 421
Isometric exercise, 421
Isotonic exercise, 421
Physical activity, 421

EXEMPLAR LEARNING OUTCOMES

After reading about this exemplar, you will be able to:

1. Describe the effects of exercise on body systems and its role in health promotion.

2. Differentiate isotonic, isometric, isokinetic, aerobic, and anaerobic exercise.

3. Assess activity-exercise pattern and activity tolerance.

4. Develop nursing diagnoses and outcomes related to activity and exercise.

▶ OVERVIEW

The role of physical fitness in health promotion and wellness is gaining both attention and credibility. For example, exercise, in particular walking, is increasingly "prescribed" to clients with Parkinson disease. There is evidence that it combats progression of the condition and that it assist clients to build strength, stability, and endurance (Harvard University, 2012). The Centers for Disease Control and Prevention defines physical fitness as

> the ability to carry out daily tasks with vigor and alertness, without undue fatigue, and with ample energy to enjoy leisure-time pursuits and respond to emergencies. Physical fitness includes a number of components consisting of cardiorespiratory endurance (aerobic power), skeletal muscle endurance, skeletal muscle strength, skeletal muscle power, flexibility, balance, speed of movement, reaction time, and body composition (CDC, 2011).

Benefits of physical activity are many and include (CDC, 2012):

■ Improving mood and overall mental health

■ Reducing the risk for cardiovascular disease

■ Strengthening bone and muscle

■ Reducing the risk of some illnesses, such as type 2 diabetes, and some cancers

■ Improving stability and reducing risk of falling in older adults

Many *Healthy People 2020* objectives pertain to exercise and activity. Following are some of these objectives:

■ Retained from *Healthy People 2010*: Reduce the proportion of adults who engage in no leisure-time physical activity. Increase the proportion of schools that require daily physical education.

■ Modified from *Healthy People 2010*: Increase the proportion of adults and adolescents who engage in aerobic physical activity. Increase the proportion of children and adolescents who do not exceed recommended limits for screen time.

■ New for *Healthy People 2020*: Increase regularly scheduled elementary school recess (President's Council on Fitness, Sports and Nutrition, 2011).

A strong, well-developed body of research evidence supports the role of exercise in improving the health status of individuals with cardiovascular disease, pulmonary dysfunction, disabilities of aging, and depression. Integrating well-researched exercise protocols with conventional nursing and medical approaches results in optimal treatment of these common disorders. Evidence shows that exercise can prevent and even reverse many of the chronic diseases experienced by aging adults. As stated earlier, a growing body of research supports the preventive and therapeutic effects of exercise on a number of conditions, including diabetes, cancer, arthritis, chronic fatigue syndrome, cystic fibrosis, fibromyalgia, menopause, urinary incontinence, Parkinson, Alzheimer, and HIV/AIDS (van de Weert-van Leeuwen et al., 2013; Micozzi, 2011).

An **activity-exercise pattern** refers to an individual's routine of exercise, activity, leisure, and recreation. It includes (a) activities of daily living (ADLs) that require energy expenditure, such as hygiene, dressing, cooking, shopping, eating, working, and home maintenance, and (b) the type, quality, and quantity of exercise, including sports.

Individuals often define their health and physical fitness by their activity. Mental well-being and the effectiveness of body functioning depend largely on mobility status. For example, when an individual is upright, the lungs expand more easily, intestinal activity (peristalsis) is more effective, and the kidneys are able to empty completely. In addition, motion is essential for proper functioning of bones and muscles.

▶ PHYSICAL ACTIVITY AND EXERCISE

The U.S. Department of Health and Human Services defines physical activity and exercise as follows (Edelman & Mandle, 2009, p. 292):

- **Physical activity** is bodily movement produced by skeletal muscle contraction that increases energy expenditure.

- **Exercise** is a type of physical activity defined as a planned, structured, and repetitive bodily movement performed to improve or maintain one or more components of physical fitness.

Individuals participate in exercise programs to decrease risk factors for cardiovascular disease and to increase their health and well-being. **Activity tolerance** is the type and amount of exercise or daily living activities an individual is able to perform without experiencing adverse effects. **Functional strength** is another goal of exercise, and it is defined as the body's ability to perform work.

Types of Exercise

Exercise involves the active contraction and relaxation of muscles. Exercises can be classified according to the type of muscle contraction (isotonic, isometric, or isokinetic) and the source of energy (aerobic or anaerobic).

In **isotonic exercises**, which are dynamic exercises, the muscle shortens to produce muscle contraction and active movement. Most physical conditioning exercises—running, walking, swimming, cycling, and other such activities—are isotonic, as are ADLs and active ROM (range of motion) exercises (those initiated by the client). Examples of isotonic bed exercises are pushing or pulling against a stationary object, using a trapeze to lift the body off the bed, lifting the buttocks off the bed by pushing with the hands against the mattress, and pushing the body to a sitting position.

Isotonic exercises increase muscle tone, mass, and strength and maintain joint flexibility and circulation. During isotonic exercise, both heart rate and cardiac output quicken to increase blood flow to all parts of the body.

In **isometric exercises**, which are static or setting exercises, muscles contract without moving the joint (muscle length does not change). These exercises involve exerting pressure against a solid object and are useful for strengthening abdominal, gluteal, and quadriceps muscles used in ambulation; for maintaining strength in immobilized muscles in casts or traction; and for endurance training. These are often called "quad sets." Isometric exercises produce a mild increase in heart rate and cardiac output, but no appreciable increase in blood flow to other parts of the body.

Isokinetic exercises, which are resistive exercises, involve muscle contraction or tension against resistance; thus they can be either isotonic or isometric. During isokinetic exercises, the individual moves (isotonic) or tenses (isometric) against resistance. Special machines or devices provide the resistance to the movement. These exercises are used in physical conditioning and are often done to build up certain muscle groups. For example, the pectorals (chest muscles) may be increased in size

and strength by weight lifting. An increase in blood pressure and blood flow to muscles occurs with resistance training (Burke & Laramie, 2004).

During **aerobic exercise**, the amount of oxygen taken into the body is greater than that used to perform the activity. Aerobic exercises use large muscle groups that move repetitively. Aerobic exercises improve cardiovascular conditioning and physical fitness and bring more oxygen into the body than is used to perform the activity.

1. *Target heart rate.* The goal is to work up to and sustain a target heart rate during exercise; the target rate is based on the individual's age. To determine target heart rate, first calculate the individual's maximum heart rate by subtracting her current age in years from 220. Then obtain the target heart rate by taking 60%–85% of the maximum. Because heart rates vary among individuals, the talk test is one of several tests that is being used to replace this measure.

2. *Talk test.* This test is easier to implement and keeps most individuals at 60% of maximum heart rate or higher. The test is simple: When exercising, an individual should experience labored breathing, yet still be able to carry on a conversation.

During **anaerobic exercise**, the muscles cannot draw out enough oxygen from the bloodstream, and anaerobic pathways are used to provide additional energy for a short time. This type of exercise, such as weight lifting and sprinting, is used in endurance training for athletes.

Benefits of Exercise

In general, regular exercise is essential for maintaining mental and physical health. **Table 7–2** ● summarizes the benefits of exercise on body systems.

MUSCULOSKELETAL SYSTEM The size, shape, tone, and strength of muscles (including the heart muscle) are maintained with mild exercise and increased with strenuous exercise. With strenuous exercise, muscles **hypertrophy** (enlarge), and the efficiency of muscular contraction increases. Hypertrophy is commonly seen in the arm muscles of a tennis player, the leg muscles of a skater, and the arm and hand muscles of a carpenter.

Joints lack a discrete blood supply. It is through activity that joints receive nourishment. Exercise increases joint flexibility, stability, and range of motion. A growing number of randomized, controlled clinical trials have shown that exercise interventions significantly reduce weakness, frailty, depression, and the risk and incidence of falling in older adults (Burke & Laramie, 2004).

Bone density and strength are maintained through weight bearing. The stress of weight-bearing and high-impact movement maintains a balance between osteoblasts (bone-building cells) and osteoclasts (bone-resorption and breakdown cells). Weight-bearing activity is particularly important for individuals at risk for osteoporosis. Examples of weight-bearing activity are walking, dancing, and weight lifting. Non-weight-bearing exercises offer great benefit for individuals with a variety of health considerations. Examples of non-weight-bearing exercise are swimming and bicycling.

TABLE 7–2 Benefits of Exercise by Body System

BODY SYSTEM	BENEFITS
Musculoskeletal	▪ Increases joint flexibility, stability, and range of motion. ▪ Maintains bone density and strength. ▪ Reduces weakness, frailty, and depression. ▪ Decreases risk and incidence of falling in older adults.
Cardiovascular	▪ Increases strength of heart muscle contraction and blood supply to heart and muscles. ▪ Mediates harmful effects of stress. ▪ Lowers resting heart rate. ▪ Raises HDL level. ▪ Lowers blood pressure. ▪ Improves circulation.
Respiratory	▪ Increases tidal volume. ▪ Increases vital capacity. ▪ Improves gas exchange. ▪ Increases oxygen to the brain. ▪ Improves stamina and immune function.
Gastrointestinal	▪ Facilitates peristalsis. ▪ Relieves constipation. ▪ May improve symptoms of conditions such as IBS.
Metabolic/endocrine	▪ Elevates metabolic rate. ▪ Stabilizes blood sugar.
Urinary	▪ Promotes efficient blood flow and waste excretion.
Psychoneurological	▪ Elevates mood. ▪ Relieves stress and anxiety. ▪ Relieves depressive symptoms.

CARDIOVASCULAR SYSTEM The American Heart Association's collaboration with the American Stroke Association describes the most recent guidelines for primary prevention of stroke and cardiovascular disease, placing great emphasis on physical activity (AHA/ASA, 2011). Adequate moderate-intensity exercise (40%–60% of maximum capacity such as walking a mile in 15–20 minutes) increases the heart rate, the strength of heart muscle contraction, and the blood supply to the heart and muscles through increased cardiac output. In two studies with male participants, levels of "good" (high-density lipoprotein [HDL]) cholesterol were increased through regular endurance (walking/jogging) exercise. Exercise also promotes heart health by mediating the harmful effects of stress. The types of exercise that provide cardiac benefit vary. They include aerobic exercise such as walking and cycling. Recent research supports the benefits of yoga practice in cardiovascular health. Statistically significant effects include lowered systolic and diastolic blood pressure, improved oxygen uptake, improved heart rate variability, improved circulation, and self-reported stress reduction (Fontaine, 2010).

RESPIRATORY SYSTEM Ventilation (air circulating into and out of the lungs) and oxygen intake increase during exercise, thereby improving gas exchange. More toxins are eliminated with deeper breathing, and problem solving and emotional stability are enhanced by increased oxygen to the brain. Adequate exercise also prevents pooling of secretions in the bronchi and bronchioles, decreasing breathing effort and risk of infection. Attention to exercising muscles of respiration (by deep breathing) throughout activity as well as during rest enhances oxygenation (improving stamina) and circulation of lymph (improving immune function). A strong body of evidence supports the use of lower-extremity exercise forms (e.g., walking, treadmill, stationary bike, stair climbing) for treating individuals with chronic obstructive pulmonary disease (COPD). Research reports citing the benefits of yogic breathing and postures for individuals with asthma are increasing in the literature (Fontaine, 2010; Micozzi, 2011).

GASTROINTESTINAL SYSTEM Exercise improves the appetite and increases gastrointestinal tract tone, facilitating peristalsis. Activities such as rowing, swimming, walking, and sit-ups work the abdominal muscles and can help relieve constipation (Fontaine, 2010). Abdominal compressive exercise, such as with twisting and forward bending yoga postures, has been shown to improve symptoms of irritable bowel syndrome (Fontaine, 2010; Micozzi, 2011).

METABOLIC/ENDOCRINE SYSTEM Exercise elevates the metabolic rate, thus increasing the production of body heat, waste products, and calorie use. During strenuous exercise, the metabolic rate can increase to as much as 20 times the normal rate. This elevation lasts after exercise is completed. Exercise increases the use of triglycerides and fatty acids, resulting in a reduced level of serum triglycerides and cholesterol. Weight loss and exercise stabilize blood sugar and make cells more responsive to insulin. The Diabetes Prevention Program, a large 3-year study, showed that even a modest 5% decrease in body weight (about 10 pounds in most participants) achieved through exercise and dietary modification reduced the risk of diabetes by a striking 58%. In those over 60 years of age, the reduction was 71% (Freeman, 2008).

URINARY SYSTEM As adequate exercise promotes efficient blood flow, the body excretes wastes more effectively. In addition, adequate exercise usually prevents stasis (stagnation) of urine in the bladder.

IMMUNE SYSTEM As respiratory and musculoskeletal effort increase with exercise and as gravity is enlisted with postural changes, lymph fluid is more efficiently pumped from tissues into lymph capillaries and vessels throughout the body. Circulation through lymph nodes, where destruction of pathogens and removal of foreign antigens can occur, also improves. Research in older adults has shown benefits of moderate exercise on natural killer cell function, circulating T-cell function, and cytokine production, potentially increasing resistance to viral infections and preventing formation of malignant cells (Freeman, 2008).

While moderate exercise seems to enhance immunity, strenuous exercise may reduce immune function, leaving a window of opportunity for infection during the recovery phase. Adequate rest is important after vigorous training to allow the body to recover (Edelman & Mandle, 2009).

PSYCHONEUROLOGICAL SYSTEM Mental or affective disorders such as depression or chronic stress may affect an individual's desire to move. A client with depression, for example, may lack enthusiasm for taking part in any activity and may even lack energy for usual hygiene practices. Lack of visible energy is seen in a slumped posture with head bowed. Chronic stress can deplete the body's energy reserves to the point that the resulting fatigue discourages the desire to exercise, even though exercise can energize the individual and facilitate coping. By contrast, individuals with eating disorders may exercise excessively in an effort to prevent weight gain.

A strong and growing body of evidence supports the role of exercise in elevating mood and relieving stress and anxiety across the life span. Solid data examining relationships between both aerobic and nonaerobic styles of exercise supports the use of this modality to relieve symptoms of depression. The mechanism of action is thought to be a result of one or more of the following: Exercise increases levels of metabolites for neurotransmitters and serotonin; exercise releases endogenous opioids, thus increasing levels of endorphins; exercise increases levels of oxygen to the brain and other body systems, inducing euphoria; and through muscular exertion (especially with movement modalities such as yoga and t'ai chi) the body releases stored stress associated with accumulated emotional demands. Regular exercise also improves quality of sleep for most individuals. Research has shown the dramatic positive effect that aerobic exercise has on older adults with chronic insomnia (Reid et al., 2010).

COGNITIVE FUNCTION   Current research supports the positive effects of exercise on cognitive functioning, in particular decision making and problem solving , planning, and paying attention. Physical exertion induces cells in the brain to strengthen and build neuronal connections. Recent research indicates that physical exercise also provides positive effects in individuals with Parkinson and Alzheimer diseases (Grazina & Massano, 2013; Brown, Peiffer, & Martins, 2012).

SPIRITUAL HEALTH   Micozzi (2011, p. 127) describes the results of research about the body–spirit connection. The studies have found an association between religious involvement and these effects:

- Lower anxiety
- Fewer psychotic symptoms
- Less substance abuse
- Better coping mechanisms
- Success in aging and end-of-life issues.

Overall, there was an association with longer survival, healthier behavior, and less distress. (For more information, see the module on Spirituality.)

REVIEW   Physical Fitness and Exercise

RELATE Link the Concepts and Exemplars

Linking the exemplar physical fitness and exercise with the concept of metabolism:

1. Identify the benefits of physical activity for a client with type 2 diabetes and osteoporosis.

2. What teaching plan will you implement for the obese client regarding exercise and nutrition?

Linking the exemplar physical fitness and exercise with the concept of mobility:

3. A client with rheumatoid arthritis is interested in beginning a weight-lifting program. What are your teaching priorities for this client?

4. You are caring for a client who normally exercised daily before fracturing his leg. How can you help to meet the client's exercise needs when he is placed in traction for 6 weeks?

Linking the exemplar of physical fitness and exercise with the concept of cognition:

5. How does the presence of a chronic illness or a negative change in cognitive status affect the ability of older adults to engage in exercise? What modifications could the nurse suggest?

6. You are working with the parent of a schizophrenic teenager who has recently gained significant weight. What suggestions could you make to the parent? How could you involve the teenager in the formulation of a care plan?

READY Go to Companion Skills Manual

REFER Go to Pearson Nursing Student Resources
nursing.pearsonhighered.com

- Additional review materials

REFLECT Case Study

Mary Martin is a 75-year-old female who was recently widowed. She has limited income because her husband's pension terminated when he died, so she has moved in with her son, his wife, and their three teenage children. Mary has cataracts and glaucoma, for which she regularly sees an ophthalmologist, but otherwise she is in good health. Mary recently learned she has low bone density.

1. What kind of physical activity and exercise is appropriate for Mary?

2. What are the benefits of these activities on body systems?

3. What are your expected outcomes for Mary?

4. What safety teaching will you provide Mary and her family?

EXEMPLAR 7.2   Oral Health

EXEMPLAR KEY TERMS

Cheilosis, *426*
Dental caries, *424*
Gingiva, *424*
Gingivitis, *426*

Periodontal disease, *424*
Plaque, *425*
Pyorrhea, *426*
Tartar, *426*
Xerostomia, *428*

▶ OVERVIEW

The mouth, also called the *oral* or *buccal cavity*, is lined with mucous membranes and is enclosed by the lips, cheeks, palate, and tongue (**Figure 7–5 ●**).

The lips and cheeks are skeletal muscle covered externally by skin. Their function is to keep food in the mouth during chewing. The palate consists of two regions: the hard palate and the soft palate. The hard palate covers bone in the roof of the mouth and provides a hard surface against which the tongue forces food. The soft palate, extending from the hard palate and ending at the back of the mouth as a fold called the *uvula*, is primarily muscle. When food is swallowed, the soft palate rises as a reflex to close off the oropharynx.

The tongue, composed of skeletal muscle and connective tissue, is located in the floor of the mouth. It contains mucous and serous glands, taste buds, and papillae. The tongue mixes food with saliva during chewing, forms the food into a mass (called a *bolus*), and initiates swallowing. Some papillae provide surface roughness to facilitate licking and moving food; other papillae house the taste buds.

Saliva moistens food so it can be made into a bolus, dissolves food chemicals so they can be tasted, and provides enzymes (such as amylase) that begin the chemical breakdown of starches. Saliva is produced by salivary glands, most of which lie superior or inferior to the mouth and drain into it. The salivary glands include the parotid, the submaxillary, and the sublingual glands.

The teeth chew (masticate) and grind food to break it down into smaller parts. As the food is masticated, it is mixed with saliva.

Each tooth has three parts: the crown, the root, and the pulp cavity. The crown is the exposed part of the tooth, which is outside the gum. It is covered with a hard substance called *enamel*. The ivory-colored internal part of the crown below the enamel is the dentin. The root of a tooth is embedded in the jaw and covered by a bony tissue called *cementum*. The pulp cavity in the center of the tooth contains the blood vessels and nerves.

▶ LIFESPAN CONSIDERATIONS

Teeth usually appear 5–8 months after birth. Baby-bottle syndrome may result in decay of all of the upper teeth and the lower posterior teeth (Pillitteri, 2009). This syndrome occurs when an infant is put to bed with a bottle of sugar water, formula, milk, or fruit juice. The carbohydrates in the solutions cause demineralization of the tooth enamel, which leads to tooth decay.

By the time children are 2 years old, they usually have all 20 of their deciduous (temporary) teeth. At about age 6 or 7, children start losing their deciduous teeth, which are gradually replaced by the 33 permanent teeth. By age 25, most individuals have all of their permanent teeth (**Figure 7–6 ●**).

The incidence of **periodontal disease** (gum disease) increases during pregnancy because the rise in female hormones affects gingival tissue and increases its reaction to bacterial plaque. Many pregnant women experience more bleeding from the gingival sulcus during brushing and increased redness and swelling of the **gingiva** (the gum).

Teeth turn yellowish as a part of the aging process. Teeth are normally off-white. With age, the enamel thins and the yellow-gray color of the inner portion of the teeth begins to show. In addition, coffee drinking and cigarette smoking can stain the teeth. Commercial teeth-whitening products and whitening treatments offered at dental offices are available to consumers who desire whiter teeth for cosmetic reasons.

Lack of fluoridated water and preventive dentistry during their developmental years cause tooth and gum problems in older adults (Edelman & Mandle, 2009). As a result, some older adults may have few permanent teeth left, and some have dentures. Loss of teeth occurs mainly because of periodontal disease rather than **dental caries** (cavities); however, caries are also common in middle-aged adults.

Some receding of the gums and a brownish pigmentation of the gums occur with age. Because saliva production decreases with age, dryness of the oral mucosa is a common finding in older individuals.

■ NURSING PROCESS

Assessment

Assessment of the client's mouth and hygiene practices includes (a) a nursing health history, (b) physical assessment of the mouth, and (c) identification of clients at risk for developing oral problems.

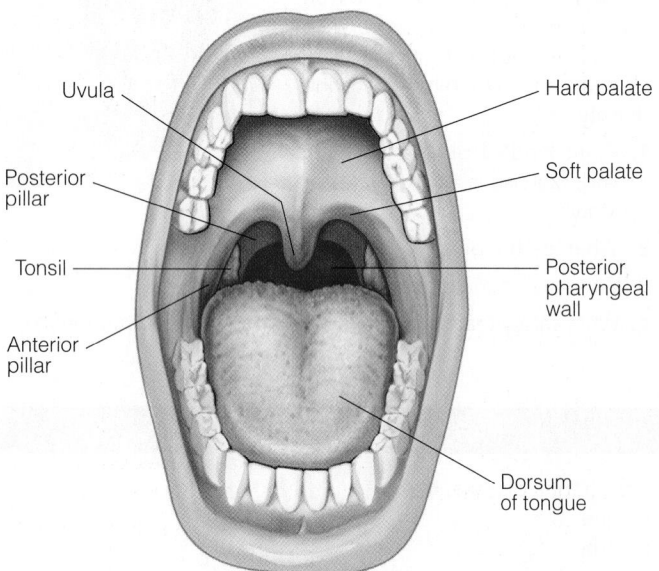

Figure 7–5 ● Oral cavity.

Uvula
Posterior pillar
Tonsil
Anterior pillar
Hard palate
Soft palate
Posterior pharyngeal wall
Dorsum of tongue

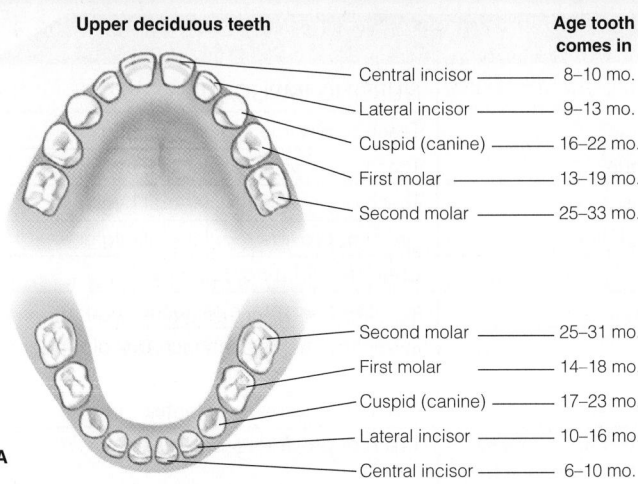

Upper deciduous teeth

	Age tooth comes in
Central incisor	8–10 mo.
Lateral incisor	9–13 mo.
Cuspid (canine)	16–22 mo.
First molar	13–19 mo.
Second molar	25–33 mo.

Second molar	25–31 mo.
First molar	14–18 mo.
Cuspid (canine)	17–23 mo.
Lateral incisor	10–16 mo.
Central incisor	6–10 mo.

A

Lower deciduous teeth

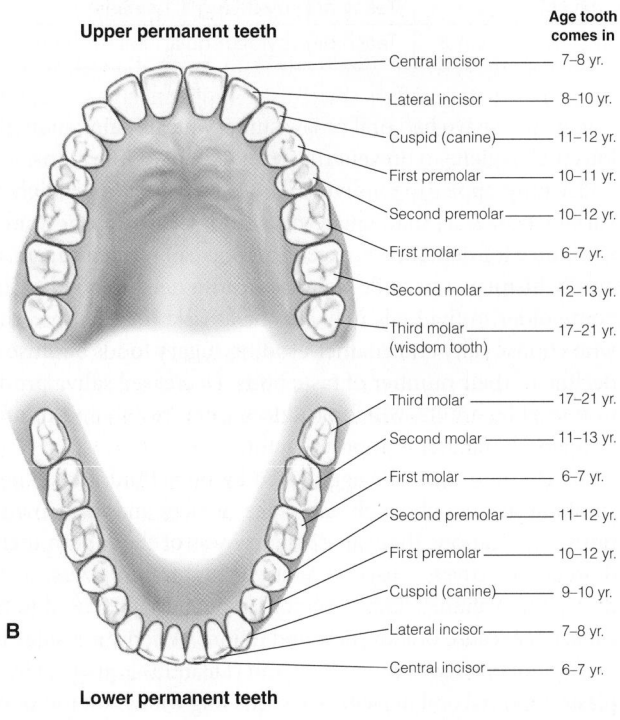

Upper permanent teeth

	Age tooth comes in
Central incisor	7–8 yr.
Lateral incisor	8–10 yr.
Cuspid (canine)	11–12 yr.
First premolar	10–11 yr.
Second premolar	10–12 yr.
First molar	6–7 yr.
Second molar	12–13 yr.
Third molar (wisdom tooth)	17–21 yr.

Third molar	17–21 yr.
Second molar	11–13 yr.
First molar	6–7 yr.
Second premolar	11–12 yr.
First premolar	10–12 yr.
Cuspid (canine)	9–10 yr.
Lateral incisor	7–8 yr.
Central incisor	6–7 yr.

B

Lower permanent teeth

Figure 7–6 ● Deciduous and permanent teeth.

Assessment Interview Oral Hygiene

Oral Hygiene Practices
- What are your usual mouth care and/or denture care practices?
- What oral hygiene products do you routinely use (e.g., mouthwash, type of toothpaste, dental floss, denture cleaner)?
- When was your last dental examination, and how often do you see your dentist?

Self-Care Ability
- Do you have any problems managing your mouth care?

Past or Current Mouth Problems
- Have you had or do you have any problems such as bleeding, swollen or reddened gums, ulcerations, lumps, or tooth pain?

Health History

During the nursing health history, the nurse obtains data about the client's oral hygiene practices, including dental visits, self-care abilities, and past or current mouth problems. Data about the client's oral hygiene helps the nurse determine learning needs and incorporate the client's needs and preferences in the plan of care. Assessment of the client's self-care abilities determines the amount and type of required nursing assistance. Clients whose hand coordination is impaired, whose cognitive function is impaired, whose illness alters energy levels and motivation, or whose therapy imposes restrictions on activities need assistance from the nurse. Information about past or current problems alerts the nurse to specific interventions required or referrals that may be necessary. Questions to elicit this information are shown in the accompanying Assessment Interview. Assessment questions to discuss with parents about their children are shown in the Lifespan Considerations feature.

Physical Assessment

Dental caries and periodontal disease are the two problems that most frequently affect the teeth. Both problems are commonly associated with plaque and tartar deposits. **Plaque** is an invisible soft film that adheres to the enamel surface of teeth; it consists of

Lifespan Considerations Child Oral Hygiene: Assessment Questions for Parents

ASSESSMENT QUESTIONS
1. Do you share spoons, forks and other utensils with your baby?
2. Do you put your young child to bed with a bottle of milk, formula, juice, or other product that contains sugar?
3. Does your local water supply contain fluoride? Do you use bottled water for cooking or drinking?
4. Is your child exposed to cigarette smoke?
5. Do you know whom to contact in case your child knocks out or breaks a tooth?
6. Does your child suck his or her fingers or thumb?

REASONS FOR CONCERN
1. The saliva you may leave on the utensil contains bacteria that can cause tooth decay.
2. The sugar and acid in these liquids can cause tooth decay.
3. Fluoride helps strengthen tooth enamel, which prevents tooth decay.
4. Secondhand smoke can contribute to the development of tooth decay, gum disease and other health issues.
5. The time to consider how to react in a dental emergency is before it happens.
6. Uncontrolled sucking can alter the shape of the mouth.

TABLE 7–3 Common Problems of the Mouth

PROBLEM	DESCRIPTION	NURSING IMPLICATIONS
Halitosis	Bad breath	Teach or provide regular oral hygiene.
Glossitis	Inflammation of the tongue	Teach or provide regular oral hygiene.
Gingivitis	Inflammation of the gums	Teach or provide regular oral hygiene.
Periodontal disease	Gums appear spongy and bleeding	Teach or provide regular oral hygiene.
Reddened or excoriated mucosa		Check for ill-fitting dentures.
Excessive dryness of the buccal mucosa		Increase fluid intake as health permits.
Cheilosis	Cracking of lips	Lubricate lips, use antimicrobial ointment to prevent infection.
Dental caries	Darkened areas on teeth, may be painful	Advise client to see a dentist.
Sordes	Accumulation of foul matter (food, micro-organisms, and epithelial elements) in the mouth	Teach or provide regular cleaning.
Stomatitis	Inflammation of the oral mucosa	Teach or provide regular cleaning.
Parotitis	Inflammation of the parotid salivary glands	Teach or provide regular oral hygiene.

bacteria, molecules of saliva, and remnants of epithelial cells and leukocytes. When plaque is unchecked, tartar (dental calculus) is formed. **Tartar** is a visible, hard deposit of plaque and dead bacteria that forms at the gum lines. Tartar buildup can alter the fibers that attach the teeth to the gum and eventually disrupt bone tissue. Periodontal disease is characterized by **gingivitis** (red, swollen gingiva), bleeding, receding gum lines, and the formation of pockets between the teeth and gums. In **pyorrhea** (advanced periodontal disease), the teeth are loose and pus is evident when the gums are pressed. **Table 7–3** ● lists additional problems of the mouth.

SAFETY ALERT
Always wear gloves when assessing the oral cavity.

To perform an oral health assessment complete the following:

■ Inspect and palpate the lips. Lips should be of normal color for race and without lesions.
■ Inspect and palpate the tongue. Tongue should be pink, smooth, and have good turgor.
■ Inspect and palpate the buccal mucosa. Mucosa should be moist, without lesions, and of appropriate color.
■ Inspect and palpate the teeth. Teeth should be in a state of good hygiene without caries.
■ Inspect and palpate the gums. Gums should be of even color without swelling.
■ Inspect the throat and tonsils. Tonsils (if present) should be of appropriate color and size.
■ Note the client's breath. Breath should not have unusual or foul odors.

Identifying Clients at Risk

Certain clients are prone to oral problems because of lack of knowledge or the inability to maintain oral hygiene. Among these are seriously ill, confused, comatose, depressed, illiterate, and dehydrated clients. In addition, clients with nasogastric tubes and clients receiving oxygen are likely to develop dry oral mucous membranes, especially if they breathe through their mouths.

Clients who have had oral or jaw surgery must maintain meticulous oral hygiene to prevent the development of infections.

Healthy-appearing individuals, too, may be at risk. High-risk variables such as inadequate nutrition, lack of money and/or insurance for dental care, excessive intake of refined sugars, and family history of periodontal disease also need to be identified. Some older individuals may also be at risk, for example, those who choose salty and enamel-eroding sugary foods because of a decline in their number of taste buds. Decreased saliva production in older adults, which produces a dry mouth and thinning of the oral mucosa, is another factor.

A dry mouth can be aggravated by poor fluid intake, heavy smoking, alcohol use, high salt intake, anxiety, and many medications. Medications that can cause dryness of the mouth include diuretics; laxatives, if used excessively; and tranquilizers, such as diazepam (Valium). Some chemotherapeutic agents used to treat cancer also cause oral dryness and lesions. A common side effect of the anticonvulsant drug phenytoin (Dilantin) is gingival hyperplasia. Optimal oral hygiene (e.g., brushing with a soft toothbrush and flossing) is necessary for clients taking these medications.

Clients who are receiving or have received radiation treatments to the head and neck may have permanent damage to salivary glands that results in a very dry mouth and can often be treated with a thick liquid called *artificial saliva*. Some clients prefer to just sip on liquids to moisten their mouth. Radiation can also cause damage to teeth and jaw structure, with actual damage occurring years after the radiation.

Clients in long-term care are at high risk for oral health problems. The nurse must assess the client's oral health and teach the importance of and methods to promote oral hygiene.

Diagnosis

Two nursing diagnoses are related to problems with oral hygiene and the oral cavity:

■ *Bathing Self-Care Deficit in Domain 4: Activity/Rest*
■ *Impaired Oral Mucous Membrane in Domain 11: Safety/Protection*

(NANDA-I © 2012)

The nursing diagnosis *Impaired Oral Mucous Membrane* refers to disruption of the lips and/or soft tissue of the oral cavity. Manifestations include a coated tongue, dry mouth, halitosis, gingivitis, oral pain, discomfort, erythema, oral lesions or ulcers, and dry mouth. These may be the result of ineffective oral hygiene, physical injury or drying effect (e.g., mouth breathing, oxygen therapy, dehydration), mechanical trauma (e.g., oral surgery, braces, or ill-fitting dentures), chemical trauma (e.g., side effects of medications), or radiation therapy.

Planning

In planning care, the nurse and, if appropriate, the client and/or family set outcomes for each nursing diagnosis. The nurse then performs nursing interventions and activities to achieve the client outcomes.

During the planning phase, the nurse also identifies interventions that will help the client achieve these goals. Specific, detailed nursing activities taken by the nurse may include the following:

- Monitor for dryness of the oral mucosa.
- Monitor for signs and symptoms of glossitis (inflammation of the tongue) and stomatitis (inflammation of the mouth).
- Assist dependent clients with oral care.
- Provide special oral hygiene for clients who are debilitated, are unconscious, or have lesions of the mucous membranes or other oral tissues.
- Teach clients about good oral hygiene practices and other measures to prevent tooth decay.
- Educate clients and caregivers about available commercial products (saliva stimulants or saliva replacements) to decrease sense of mouth dryness
- Reinforce the oral hygiene regimen as part of health promotion and discharge teaching.

Implementation

Good oral hygiene includes daily stimulation of the gums, mechanical brushing and flossing of the teeth, and flushing of the mouth. The nurse frequently is in a position to help individuals maintain oral hygiene by helping or teaching them to clean the teeth and oral cavity, by inspecting whether clients (especially children) have done so, or by actually providing mouth care to clients who are ill or incapacitated. The nurse can also identify problems that require the intervention of a dentist or oral surgeon and can arrange a referral.

Promote Oral Health Throughout the Life Span

A major role of the nurse in promoting oral health is teaching clients about specific oral hygienic measures.

Infants and Toddlers   Most dentists recommend that dental hygiene begin when the first tooth erupts and be practiced after each feeding. Cleaning can be accomplished by using a wet washcloth or small gauze moistened with water.

Dental caries occur frequently during the toddler period, often as a result of the excessive intake of sweets or a prolonged use of the bottle during naps and at bedtime. The nurse should

Client Teaching   Dental Health in Very Young Children

Many parents are unaware of the importance of dental health in very young children. They may see their child's teeth as "baby teeth" and think they can put off dental visits until the child begins to lose the primary teeth. Nurses working with parents of very young children may need to help parents learn that care of primary teeth is essential to healthy permanent teeth.

give parents the following instructions to promote and maintain dental health:

- Beginning at about 18 months of age, brush the child's teeth with a soft toothbrush. Use only a toothbrush moistened with water at first and introduce toothpaste later. Use toothpaste that contains fluoride.
- Give a fluoride supplement daily or as recommended by the primary care provider or dentist, unless the drinking water is fluoridated.
- Schedule an initial dental visit for the child at 2 or 3 years of age, as soon as all 20 primary teeth have erupted.
- Some dentists recommend a dental inspection when the child is about 18 months old to provide an early, pleasant introduction to the dental examination.
- Seek professional dental attention for any problems like discoloring of the teeth, chipping, or signs of infection such as redness and swelling.

Preschoolers and School-Age Children   Because deciduous teeth guide the entrance of permanent teeth, dental care is essential to keep these deciduous teeth in good repair and to establish good dental habits early. Abnormally placed or lost deciduous teeth can cause misalignment of permanent teeth. Fluoride remains important at this stage to prevent dental caries. Preschoolers need to be taught to brush their teeth after eating and to limit their intake of refined sugars. Parental supervision may be needed to ensure the completion of these

Client Teaching   Measures to Prevent Tooth Decay

- Brush the teeth thoroughly after meals and at bedtime. Assist children or inspect their mouths to be sure the teeth are clean. If the teeth cannot be brushed after meals, recommend vigorous rinsing of the mouth with water.
- Floss the teeth daily.
- Ensure an adequate intake of nutrients, particularly calcium, phosphorus, fluoride, and vitamins A, C, and D.
- Avoid sweet foods and drinks between meals. Take them in moderation at meals.
- Eat coarse, fibrous foods (cleansing foods), such as fresh fruits and raw vegetables.
- Have topical fluoride applications as prescribed by the dentist.
- Have a checkup by a dentist every 6 months.

self-care activities. Regular dental checkups are required during these years when permanent teeth appear.

Adolescents and Adults Proper diet and tooth and mouth care should be evaluated and reinforced for adolescents and adults. Specific measures to prevent tooth decay and periodontal disease are listed in Client Teaching.

Older Adults About 75% of individuals entering long-term care facilities still retain the majority of their natural teeth (Haumschild & Haumschild, 2009). They are at risk for dental cavities and periodontal disease. Other older adults are at an increased risk because they cannot maintain their oral hygiene practices and/or may not be able to visit the dentist routinely.

Over 100 diseases have oral manifestations, including:

- Cardiovascular disease
- Stroke
- Respiratory infections
- Pancreatic cancer
- Diabetes
- Nutritional problems (Haumschild & Haumschild, 2009)

Oral health problems are more prevalent in older adults but are not caused by aging. Nurses have an important role in promoting optimal geriatric oral health care.

- *Brushing and flossing the teeth.* Thorough brushing of the teeth is important in preventing tooth decay. The mechanical action of brushing removes food particles that can harbor in the teeth and incubate bacteria. It also stimulates circulation in the gums, helping maintain their healthy firmness. One of the techniques recommended for brushing teeth is called the *sulcular technique,* which removes plaque and cleans under the gingival margins. Fluoride toothpaste is often recommended because of its antibacterial protection.
- *Caring for artificial teeth.* Some individuals have artificial teeth in the form of a plate—a complete set of teeth for one jaw. An individual may have a lower plate or an upper plate or both. When only a few artificial teeth are needed, the individual may have a bridge rather than a plate. A bridge may be fixed or removable. Artificial teeth are fitted to the individual and usually will not fit anyone else. Individuals who have dentures or other types of oral prostheses should be encouraged to use them. Ill-fitting dentures or other oral prostheses can cause discomfort and chewing difficulties. They may also contribute to oral problems as well as poor nutrition and lack of enjoyment of food. Those who do not wear their prostheses are prone to shrinkage of the gums, which results in further tooth loss.

  Like natural teeth, artificial dentures collect microorganisms and food. They need to be cleaned regularly, at least once a day. They can be removed from the mouth, scrubbed with a toothbrush, rinsed, and reinserted. Some individuals use a dentifrice for cleaning teeth, and others use commercial cleaning compounds for plates.
- *Assisting clients with oral care.* When providing mouth care for partially or totally dependent clients, the nurse should wear gloves to guard against infections. Other required equipment includes a curved basin that fits snugly under the client's chin (e.g., a kidney basin) to receive the rinse water, as well as a towel to protect the client and the bedclothes.

Lifespan Considerations **Oral Hygiene in Older Adults**

- Oral care may be difficult for certain older adults to perform due to problems with dexterity or problems with dementia.
- Some long-term healthcare facilities have dentists or dental hygienists who come regularly to see clients with special needs.
- Dryness of the oral mucosa is common in older adults. Because it can lead to tooth decay, advise clients to discuss it with their dentist or primary care provider.
- Decay of the tooth root is common among older adults. When the gums recede, the tooth root is more vulnerable to decay.
- Good oral hygiene can have a positive effect on the older adults' ability to eat.

Foam swabs are often used in healthcare agencies to clean the mouths of dependent clients. These swabs are convenient and effective in removing excess debris from the teeth and mouth. The swab, however, is not effective for plaque removal, unless soaked in alcohol-free 0.12% chlorhexidine mouth rinse. All teeth surfaces need to be swabbed with the rinse for at least two minutes (Stein & Henry, 2009, p. 48).

Most individuals prefer privacy when they remove their artificial teeth to clean them. Many do not like to be seen without their teeth; often the first request of many postoperative clients is "May I have my teeth in, please?"

- *Clients with special oral hygiene needs.* For the client who is debilitated or unconscious or who has excessive dryness, sores, or irritations of the mouth, it may be necessary to clean the oral mucosa and tongue in addition to the teeth. Agency practices differ in regard to special mouth care and its frequency. Depending on the health of the client's mouth, special care may be needed every 2–8 hours; see Lifespan Considerations.

Mouth care for unconscious or debilitated individuals is important because they tend to breathe through their mouths rather than their noses. Their mucous membranes therefore become dry, and the result is tooth decay and infections. Dry mouth—also called **xerostomia**—occurs when the supply of saliva is reduced. This condition can be caused by certain medications (e.g., antihistamines, antidepressants, antihypertensives), oxygen therapy, tachypnea, and NPO status, during which the client cannot take fluids by mouth (Berman & Snyder, 2012, p. 780). The result can be irritations of the soft tissues, which can in turn cause inflammation and susceptibility to infection (American Dental Association, n.d.a).

For clients with special oral hygiene needs, the nurse needs to focus on removing plaque and microorganisms, as well as on client comfort. If possible, use a soft-bristled toothbrush, as it provides the best means of removing plaque. The American Dental Association states that the function of toothpaste is to improve a toothbrush's mechanical cleaning power. In addition, fluoride toothpaste strengthens tooth enamel (American Dental Association, n.d.b). If the client cannot tolerate the use of a toothbrush, the nurse can use an oral swab or gauze soaked with saline to swab the teeth and tongue.

Lemon-glycerin swabs are not recommended, as they irritate and dry the oral mucosa and can decalcify teeth. Mouthwashes containing alcohol can irritate the oral mucosa, as well as cause dryness. Mineral oil is contraindicated as a moisturizer for the lips or inside the mouth, because its aspiration can initiate an infection (lipid pneumonia). Saliva substitutes can also help moisturize the oral cavity. Check that they contain carboxymethylcellulose or hydroxyethyl cellulose as active ingredients, such as found in Biotene Oral Balance (Carr, 2010).

Evaluation

Using data collected during care (e.g., status of oral mucosa, lips, tongue, and teeth), the nurse evaluates whether desired outcomes have been achieved.

If outcomes are not achieved, the nurse and client need to explore the reasons before modifying the care plan. Following are examples of questions to consider:

- Did the nurse overestimate the client's functional abilities?
- Is the client's hand coordination or cognitive function impaired?
- Has the client's condition changed?
- Has there been a change in the client's energy level and/or motivation?

REVIEW Oral Health

RELATE Link the Concepts and Exemplars

Linking the exemplar of oral health with the concept of development:

1. What are the different dental concerns of each developmental stage across the life span?

2. Design a teaching plan for a group of young mothers regarding oral health and nutrition for their toddlers.

3. If a client fears visiting a dentist, what possible motivational factors could the nurse point out?

4. You are caring for a 6-year-old child diagnosed with cystic fibrosis. How would you adapt your teaching about oral health to meet this child's needs?

Linking the exemplar of oral health with the concept of comfort:

5. While working as a hospice nurse you are caring for a client requiring end-of-life care. What oral care will be of particular importance to provide this client?

6. What will you teach the client with chronic mouth pain about oral care?

READY Go to Companion Skills Manual

REFER Go to Pearson Nursing Student Resources
nursing.pearsonhighered.com

- Additional review materials

REFLECT Case Study

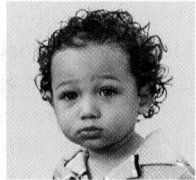

Tyler Martin is a 2-year-old boy. Since he was 4 weeks old, Tyler has been going to various babysitters while his parents work. He and his father have recently moved in with Tyler's grandparents. Tyler loves living at his grandfather's home because of all the attention he gets. Tyler also no longer has to go to day care.

Tyler has generally been in good health; he is of normal weight and has a good appetite. Tyler still loves his bottle, and each night he is given a bottle of milk or juice to help him go to sleep. If he doesn't receive a bottle to sleep with, he screams until someone gives in and brings him one.

1. Are there any concerns in this scenario that require intervention and teaching?

2. What dental visits and tooth care does Tyler require?

3. How would you teach Tyler to brush his teeth? Can he be taught how to floss at this stage? Explain your answer.

EXEMPLAR 7.3 Normal Sleep–Rest Patterns

EXEMPLAR KEY TERMS
Biological rhythms, *430*
Nocturnal emissions, *432*
NREM (non-rapid-eye-movement) sleep, *430*
REM (rapid-eye-movement) sleep, *430*
Sleep, *430*
Sleep architecture, *430*

EXEMPLAR LEARNING OUTCOMES
After reading about this exemplar, you will be able to:

1. Describe the functions and physiology of sleep.
2. Contrast the characteristics of the sleep states.
3. Describe variations in sleep patterns throughout the life span.
4. Plan interventions that promote normal sleep.

▶ OVERVIEW

Sleep is a basic human need; it is a universal biological process common to all individuals. Humans spend about one third of their lives asleep. We require sleep for many reasons: to cope with daily stresses, to prevent fatigue, to conserve energy, to restore the mind and body, and to enjoy life more fully. Sleep enhances daytime functioning. It is vital not only for optimal psychological functioning but also for physiological functioning. Research on obstructive sleep apnea (OSA) has shown that the significant cognitive impairment seen in clients with moderate to severe OSA is associated with brain tissue damage. OSA can also increase brain susceptibility to the effects of aging and other clinical and pathological occurrences (Torelli et al., 2011).

Sleep is an important factor in quality of life, yet sleep disorders and sleep deprivation are an unmet public health problem. Clinical studies have found a clear minimum requirement of sleep continuity to ensure optimal sleep-dependent memory processes (Djonlagic et al., 2012). Numerous *Sleep in America* polls by the National Sleep Foundation show that Americans, from infants to older adults, need more sleep. Over 40 million Americans are undiagnosed, misdiagnosed, or untreated for sleep disorders (Salas et al., 2013).

Furthermore, many members of the general public and health professionals are unaware that sleep disorders are commonly associated with other major medical problems, such as chronic pain, cardiovascular disease, mental illness, dementias, gastrointestinal disorders and diabetes mellitus (Skaer & Sclar, 2010).

See the exemplar on Sleep Disorders in the module on Comfort for more information.

Stay Current: To see the latest information on sleep, visit the National Sleep Foundation at **http://www.sleepfoundation.org/**.

▶ PHYSIOLOGY OF SLEEP

Historically, sleep was considered a state of unconsciousness. More recently, **sleep** has come to be considered an altered state of consciousness in which the individual's perception of and reaction to the immediate environment are decreased. Sleep is characterized by minimal physical activity, variable levels of consciousness, changes in the body's physiological processes, and decreased responsiveness to external stimuli. Some environmental stimuli, such as a smoke detector alarm, will usually awaken a sleeper, whereas many other noises will not. It appears that individuals respond to meaningful stimuli while sleeping and selectively disregard nonmeaningful stimuli. For example, a mother may respond to her own baby's crying but not to the crying of another baby.

The cyclical nature of sleep is controlled by centers located in the lower part of the brain. Neurons within the reticular formation, located in the brainstem, integrate sensory information from the peripheral nervous system and relay the information to the cerebral cortex. The upper part of the reticular formation consists of a network of ascending nerve fibers called the *reticular activating system (RAS)*, which is involved in the sleep–wake cycle. An intact cerebral cortex and reticular formation are necessary for the regulation of sleep and waking states.

Neurotransmitters, located within neurons in the brain, affect the sleep–wake cycle. For example, serotonin is thought to lessen the response to sensory stimulation, and gamma-aminobutyric acid (GABA) is believed to shut off the activity in the neurons of the RAS. Another key factor in sleep is exposure to darkness. Darkness and preparing for sleep cause a decrease in RAS stimulation. During this time, the pineal gland in the brain begins actively to secrete the natural hormone melatonin, and the individual feels less alert. During sleep, the growth hormone is secreted, and cortisol is inhibited.

With the beginning of daylight, melatonin is at its lowest level in the body and the stimulating hormone cortisol is at its highest. Wakefulness is also associated with high levels of acetylcholine, dopamine, and noradrenaline. Acetylcholine is released in the reticular formation, dopamine in the midbrain, and noradrenaline in the pons. These neurotransmitters are localized within the reticular formation and influence cerebral cortical arousal.

Circadian Rhythms

Biological rhythms are daily cycles in many of our physiological functions and activities: sleep, body temperature, alertness, neurotransmitter levels, and so on. They are controlled within the body and are synchronized with environmental factors such as light and darkness. The most familiar biological rhythm is the circadian rhythm. The term *circadian* is from the Latin *circa dies,* meaning "about a day." Although sleep and waking cycles are the best known of the circadian rhythms, body temperature, blood pressure, and many other physiological functions also follow a circadian pattern (Dijk & Archer, 2009).

Sleep is a complex biological rhythm. An individual whose biological clock coincides with the sleep–wake cycle is said to be in circadian synchronization, that is, awake when the body temperature is highest and asleep when the body temperature is lowest. Circadian regularity begins to develop by the sixth week of life, and by 3–6 months most infants have a regular sleep–wake cycle.

Types of Sleep

Sleep architecture refers to the basic organization of normal sleep. There are two types of sleep: **NREM (non-rapid-eye-movement) sleep** and **REM (rapid-eye-movement) sleep**. During sleep, NREM and REM sleep alternate in cycles. Irregular cycling and/or absent sleep stages are associated with sleep disorders (Choudhary & Choudhary, 2009).

NREM SLEEP   NREM sleep occurs when activity in the RAS is inhibited. About 75%–80% of sleep during a night is NREM sleep. NREM sleep is divided into four stages, each associated with distinct brain activity and physiology. Stage I is the stage of very light sleep and lasts only a few minutes. During this stage, the individual feels drowsy and relaxed, the eyes roll from side to side, and the heart and respiratory rates drop slightly. The sleeper can be readily awakened and may deny that she was sleeping.

Stage II is the stage of light sleep during which body processes continue to slow down. The eyes are generally still, the heart and respiratory rates decrease slightly, and body temperature falls. Stage II constitutes 44%–55% of total sleep (Choudhary & Choudhary, 2009). To awaken, an individual requires more intense stimuli in stage II than in stage I.

Stages III and IV are the deepest stages of sleep, differing only in the percentage of delta waves recorded during a 30-second period. During *deep sleep* or *delta sleep,* the sleeper's heart and respiratory rates drop 20%–30% below those exhibited during waking hours. The sleeper is difficult to arouse. The individual is not disturbed by sensory stimuli, the skeletal muscles are very relaxed, reflexes are diminished, and snoring is most likely to occur. Even swallowing and saliva production are reduced during delta sleep (Choudhary & Choudhary, 2009). These stages are essential for restoring energy and releasing important growth hormones (**Box 7–7 ●**).

Box 7–7 Physiological Changes During NREM Sleep

- Arterial blood pressure falls.
- Pulse rate decreases.
- Peripheral blood vessels dilate.
- Cardiac output decreases.
- Skeletal muscles relax.
- Basal metabolic rate decreases 10%–30%.
- Growth hormone levels peak.
- Intracranial pressure decreases.

SAFETY ALERT

In a sleep-deprived client, the loss of NREM sleep causes immunosuppression, slows tissue repair, lowers pain tolerance, triggers profound fatigue, and increases susceptibility to infection (Holshoe, 2009).

REM SLEEP   REM sleep usually recurs about every 90 minutes and lasts 5–30 minutes. Most dreams take place during REM sleep but are usually not be remembered unless the individual arouses briefly at the end of the REM period.

During REM sleep, the brain is highly active, and brain metabolism may increase as much as 20%. For example, during REM sleep, levels of acetylcholine and dopamine increase; the highest levels of acetylcholine release occur during REM sleep. Since both of these neurotransmitters are associated with cortical activation, it makes sense that their levels are high during dreaming sleep. This type of sleep is also called *paradoxical sleep* because electroencephalogram (EEG) activity resembles that of wakefulness. Distinctive eye movements occur, voluntary muscle tone is dramatically decreased, and deep tendon reflexes are absent. In this phase, the sleeper may be difficult to arouse or may wake spontaneously, gastric secretions increase, and heart and respiratory rates often are irregular. It is thought that the regions of the brain used in learning, thinking, and organizing information are stimulated during REM sleep.

Sleep Cycles

During a sleep cycle, individuals typically pass through NREM and REM sleep, with the complete cycle usually lasting about 90–110 minutes in adults. In the first sleep cycle, a sleeper usually passes through all of the first three NREM stages in a total of about 20–30 minutes. Then, stage IV may last about 30 minutes. After stage IV NREM, the sleeper passes back through stages III and II over about 20 minutes. Thereafter the first REM stage occurs, lasting about 10 minutes, completing the first sleep cycle. It is not unusual for the first REM period to be very brief or even skipped entirely. The healthy adult sleeper usually experiences four to six cycles of sleep during 7–8 hours (**Figure 7–7** ●). The sleeper who is awakened during any stage must begin anew at stage I NREM sleep and proceed through all the stages to REM sleep.

The duration of NREM stages and REM sleep varies throughout the sleep period. During the early part of the night, the deep sleep periods are longer. As the night progresses, the sleeper spends less time in stages III and IV of NREM sleep.

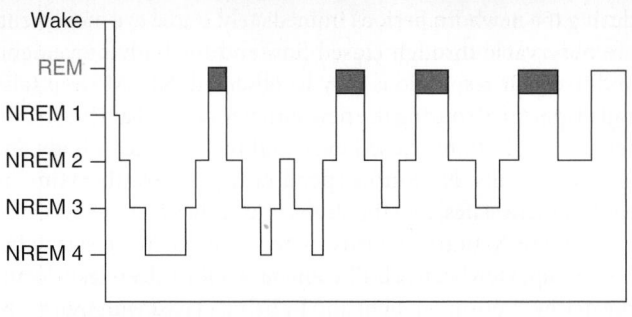

Figure 7–7 ● Time spent by an adult in REM and NREM stages of sleep.

REM sleep increases and dreams tend to lengthen. Before sleep ends, periods of near wakefulness occur, and stages I and II NREM sleep and REM sleep predominate.

▶ FUNCTIONS OF SLEEP

The effects of sleep on the body are not completely understood. Sleep exerts physiological effects on both the nervous system and other body structures. Sleep in some way restores normal levels of activity and normal balance among parts of the nervous system. Sleep is also necessary for protein synthesis, which allows repair processes to occur.

The role of sleep in psychological well-being is best noticed by the deterioration in mental functioning related to sleep loss. Individuals with inadequate amounts of sleep tend to become emotionally irritable, have poor concentration, and experience difficulty making decisions.

NANDA diagnoses for problems with sleep include these three listed in Domain 4: Activity/Rest:

- *Insomnia*
- *Sleep Deprivation*
- *Disturbed Sleep Pattern*

(NANDA-I © 2012)

▶ NORMAL SLEEP PATTERNS AND REQUIREMENTS

Although it used to be believed that maintaining a regular sleep–wake rhythm is more important than the number of hours actually slept, recent research has shown that sleep deprivation is associated with significant cognitive and health problems. Early impairment in cognitive function usually manifests as difficulty with concentration and memory. More significant impairment may manifest in a decreasing ability to perform tasks requiring speed and accuracy (e.g., driving) and in an increasing engagement in risk-taking behaviors. Sleep deprivation has also been found to play a role in obesity, in managing type 2 diabetes, and in cardiovascular health (Stevens, 2011).

Newborns

Newborns sleep 16–18 hours a day, on an irregular schedule with periods of 1–3 hours spent awake. Unlike older children and adults, newborns enter REM sleep (called *active sleep* during the newborn period) immediately. Rapid eye movements are observable through closed lids, and the body movements and irregular respirations may be observed. NREM sleep (also called *quiet sleep* during the newborn period) is characterized by regular respirations, closed eyes, and the absence of body and eye movements. Newborns spend nearly 50% of their time in each of these states, and the sleep cycle is about 50 minutes.

It is best to put newborns to bed when they are sleepy but not asleep. Newborns can be encouraged to sleep less during the day by exposure to light and by being played with more during the day hours. As evening approaches, the environment can be made less bright and quieter, with less activity (National Sleep Foundation, n.d.d).

It is important to teach new parents and caregivers of newborns to put the baby "back to sleep," to make sure the newborn who is lying down while sleeping is sleeping on the back, as babies who sleep on their stomachs are at greater risk for sudden infant death syndrome.

Infants

At first, infants awaken every 3 or 4 hours, eat, and then go back to sleep. Periods of wakefulness gradually increase during the first months. By 6 months, most infants sleep through the night (from midnight to 5 a.m.) and begin to establish a pattern of daytime naps. At the end of the first year, an infant usually takes two naps per day and should get about 14–15 hours of sleep in 24 hours.

About half of the infant's sleep time is spent in light sleep. During light sleep, the infant exhibits a great deal of activity, such as movement, gurgles, and coughing. Parents need to make sure that infants are truly awake before picking them up for feeding and changing. Putting infants to bed when they are drowsy but not asleep helps them to become "self-soothers"; that is, they fall asleep independently, and if they do awake at night, they can put themselves back to sleep. Infants who become used to parental assistance at bedtime may become "signalers" and cry for their parents to help them return to sleep at night (National Sleep Foundation, n.d.d).

Toddlers

Between 12 and 14 hours of sleep are recommended for children 1–3 years of age. Most still need an afternoon nap, but the need for midmorning naps gradually decreases. The toddler may exhibit a great deal of resistance to going to bed and may awaken during the night. Nighttime fears and nightmares are also common. A security object such as a blanket or stuffed animal may help. Parents need assurance that if the child has had adequate attention from them during the day, maintaining a daily sleep schedule and consistent bedtime routine will promote good sleep habits for the entire family (National Sleep Foundation, n.d.d).

Preschoolers

The preschool child (3–5 years of age) requires 11–13 hours of sleep per night, particularly if the child is in preschool. Sleep needs fluctuate in relation to activity and growth spurts. Many children of this age dislike bedtime and resist by requesting another story, game, or television program. The 4- to 5-year-old may become restless and irritable if sleep requirements are not met (National Sleep Foundation, n.d.d).

Parents can help children who resist bedtime by maintaining a regular and consistent sleep schedule. It also helps to have a relaxing bedtime routine that ends in the child's room. Preschool children wake up frequently at night, and they may be afraid of the dark or experience night terrors or nightmares. Often, limiting or eliminating TV reduces the number of nightmares (National Sleep Foundation, n.d.d).

School-Age Children

The school-age child (5–12 years of age) needs 10–11 hours of sleep, but most receive less because of increasing demands (e.g., homework, sports, social activities). They may also be spending more time at the computer and watching TV. Some may be drinking caffeinated beverages. All of these activities can lead to difficulty falling asleep and fewer hours of sleep. Nurses can teach parents and school-age children about healthy sleep habits. A regular and consistent sleep schedule and bedtime routine need to be continued.

Adolescents

Adolescents (12–18 years of age) require 9–10 hours of sleep each night; however, few actually get that much sleep (McKnight-Eily et al., 2009). One research study reported that only 15% of teens slept 8½ hours on school nights. In adolescence, normal biological sleep patterns shift to both sleeping later and waking up later. It is natural not to be able to fall asleep before 11 p.m. (National Sleep Foundation, n.d.e). Many schools, however, start at 7 a.m., a time that is in conflict with the adolescent's sleep patterns and need and contributes to their sleep deprivation (National Sleep Foundation, n.d.a).

Nurses can teach parents to recognize signs and symptoms that their teen is not getting enough sleep (see **Box 7–8** ●).

During adolescence, boys begin to experience **nocturnal emissions** (orgasm and emission of semen during sleep), known as *wet dreams*, several times each month. Boys need to be informed about this normal development to prevent embarrassment and fear.

SAFETY ALERT
Sleep-deprived individuals are as impaired as individuals driving with a blood alcohol content of .08%. Drowsy driving causes over 100,000 crashes each year, resulting in 40,000 injuries and 1,550 deaths (National Highway Traffic Safety Administration, n.d.).

Box 7–8 Sleep Deprivation and Sleep Problems in Teens

The teen:
- Has difficulty waking in the morning for school.
- Falls asleep in class or during quiet times of the day.
- Increases the use of caffeinated beverages such as cola, coffee, and energy drinks.
- Feels tired enough to have trouble initiating or persisting in projects, such as school assignments.
- Is irritable and anxious and angers easily on days after less sleep.
- Sleeps extralong periods of time on the weekend.

Adults

Most healthy adults need 7–9 hours of sleep a night (National Sleep Foundation, n.d.c). However, there is individual variation, as some adults may be able to function well (e.g., without sleepiness or drowsiness) with 6 hours of sleep and others may need 10 hours to function optimally. Signs that indicate a individual may not be getting enough sleep include falling asleep or becoming drowsy during a task that is not fatiguing (e.g., listening to a boring or monotonous presentation), not being able to concentrate or remember information, and being unreasonably irritable.

The National Sleep Foundation (n.d.c) reports that certain adults are particularly vulnerable to getting insufficient sleep: students, shift workers, travelers, and individuals suffering from acute stress, depression, or chronic pain. Adults working long hours or multiple jobs may find their sleep less refreshing. Also, the sleep habits of children have an impact on the adults caring for them. Parents and caregivers whose children get the least amount of sleep are twice as likely to say they sleep less than 6 hours a night (National Sleep Foundation, n.d.c). Parents of infants lose the most sleep—nearly an hour on a typical night. A National Sleep Foundation poll (2009) revealed that women have more difficulty than men falling and staying asleep. Thus women experience more daytime sleepiness. In addition, women may experience more disrupted sleep during pregnancy, menses, and the perimenopausal period.

Nurses need to teach adults the importance of obtaining sufficient sleep and tips on how to promote sleep that result in the client waking up feeling restored or refreshed.

Older Adults

A hallmark change with age is a tendency toward earlier bedtime and wake times. Older adults (65–75 years) usually awaken 1.3 hours earlier and go to bed approximately 1 hour earlier than younger adults (ages 20–30). Older adults may show an increase in disturbed sleep that can create a negative impact on their quality of life, mood, and alertness. Although sleeping becomes more difficult, the need to sleep does not decrease with age (National Sleep Foundation, n.d.b).

The National Sleep Foundation's ongoing research polls looked at the sleep habits of Americans between the ages of 55 and 84. It found that older adults are sleeping 7–9 hours on both weeknights and weekends. Of interest, however, was the striking relationship between the older adult's health and quality of life and the individual's sleep quantity and quality. The poll found that the better the health of older adults, the more likely they are to sleep well. And, conversely, the more diagnosed medical conditions, the more likely they are to report sleep problems (National Sleep Foundation, n.d.b). Older adults who have several medical conditions and complain of having sleeping problems should consult with their primary care provider: They may have a major sleep disorder that is complicating treatment of the other conditions. It is important for the nurse to teach about the connection between sleep, health, and aging.

Some older adult clients with dementia may experience *sundown syndrome*. Although not a sleep disorder directly, it refers to a pattern of symptoms (e.g., agitation, anxiety, aggression, and sometimes delusions) that occur in the late afternoon (thus the name). These symptoms can last throughout the night, further disrupting sleep (National Sleep Foundation, n.d.b).

▶ FACTORS AFFECTING SLEEP

Both the quality and the quantity of sleep are affected by a number of factors. *Sleep quality* is a subjective characteristic and is often determined by whether or not an individual wakes up feeling energetic. *Quantity of sleep* is the total time the individual sleeps.

Following an irregular morning and nighttime schedule can affect sleep. Moderate exercise in the morning or early afternoon usually is conducive to sleep, but exercise late in the day can delay sleep. The individual's ability to relax before retiring is an important factor affecting the ability to fall asleep. It is best, therefore, to avoid doing homework or office work before or after getting into bed.

Night shift workers frequently obtain less sleep than other workers and have difficulty falling asleep after getting off work. Wearing dark wraparound sunglasses during the drive home and light-blocking shades can minimize the alerting effects of exposure to daylight, thus making it easier to fall asleep when body temperature is rising.

Emotional Stress

Most sleep experts consider stress the number one cause of short-term sleeping difficulties (National Sleep Foundation, n.d.c). An individual preoccupied with personal problems (e.g., school- or job-related pressures, financial difficulties, family or marriage problems) may be unable to relax sufficiently to get to sleep. Anxiety increases the norepinephrine blood levels through stimulation of the sympathetic nervous system. This chemical change results in less deep sleep and REM sleep and more stage changes and awakenings.

Stimulants and Alcohol

Caffeine-containing beverages act as stimulants of the central nervous system. Drinking beverages containing caffeine in the afternoon or evening may interfere with sleep. Individuals who drink an excessive amount of alcohol often find their sleep disturbed. Although it may hasten the onset of sleep, alcohol disrupts REM sleep. While making up for lost REM sleep after some of the effects of the alcohol have worn off, individuals often experience nightmares. The alcohol-tolerant individual may be unable to sleep well and become irritable as a result.

Diet

Weight gain has been associated with reduced total sleep time, interrupted sleep, and earlier awakening. Weight loss, on the other hand, seems to be associated with an increase in total sleep time and fewer interruptions of sleep. Dietary L-tryptophan—found, for example, in cheese and milk—may induce sleep, a fact that might explain why warm milk helps some individuals get to sleep.

Smoking

Nicotine has a stimulating effect on the body, and smokers often have more difficulty falling asleep than nonsmokers do.

Smokers are usually easily aroused and often describe themselves as light sleepers. Refraining from smoking after the evening meal usually helps the individual sleeps better; moreover, many former smokers report that their sleeping patterns improved once they stopped smoking.

Motivation

Motivation can increase alertness in some situations (e.g., a tired individual can probably stay alert while attending an interesting concert or surfing the Web late at night). Motivation alone, however, is usually not sufficient to overcome the normal circadian drive to sleep during the night. Nor is motivation sufficient to overcome sleepiness due to insufficient sleep. Boredom alone is not sufficient to cause sleepiness, but when insufficient sleep combines with boredom, sleep is likely to occur.

Medications

Some medications affect the quality of sleep. Most hypnotics can interfere with deep sleep and suppress REM sleep. Beta-blockers have been known to cause insomnia and nightmares. Narcotics such as meperidine hydrochloride (Demerol) and morphine are known to suppress REM sleep and to cause frequent awakenings and drowsiness. Tranquilizers interfere with REM sleep. Although antidepressants suppress REM sleep, this effect is considered a therapeutic action. In fact, selectively depriving a depressed client of REM sleep results in an immediate but transient improvement in mood. Clients accustomed to taking hypnotic medications and antidepressants may experience REM rebound (increased REM sleep) when these medications are discontinued. Warning clients to expect a period of more intense dreams when these medications are discontinued may reduce their anxiety about this symptom.

REVIEW Normal Sleep–Rest Patterns

RELATE Link the Concepts and Exemplars

Linking the exemplar of normal sleep–rest patterns with the concept of cognition:

1. What outcome would you anticipate in the postpartum client's cognition when she is awakened every 2–4 hours by the newborn's cry and need to eat?

2. The daughter of an 80-year-old client who has early dementia complains to the nurse that the client is up and ready to go at 4:30 in the morning. She is concerned that lack of sleep will eventually impact her mother's dementia. What teaching would you provide this client's daughter?

Linking the exemplar of normal sleep–rest patterns with the concept of infection:

3. What is your priority of care for the client with pneumonia who sleeps 4 hours a night?

4. What interventions would you initiate to promote normal sleep patterns for a client with septicemia who is in the ICU?

5. What measures could you suggest to parents of a toddler with an ear infection to promote restful sleep for all of them?

READY Go to Companion Skills Manual

REFER Go to Pearson Nursing Student Resources
nursing.pearsonhighered.com

- Additional review materials

REFLECT Case Study

Ms. Iliana Smith, a 70-year-old Hispanic woman, reports that she is having difficulty falling asleep at night. She enjoys a hearty bedtime snack of chocolate sweets. Her grandson recently gave her a large-screen TV. Sometimes she falls asleep in her recliner, missing the end of the TV show or movie. She says, "I am so tired in the mornings, I can hardly get out of bed."

1. Which assessment tools might be used to determine her problem?

2. Identify lifespan and environmental issues that might be influencing her condition.

3. What will Ms. Smith report if your interventions are successful?

■ REFERENCES

American Academy of Pediatrics, Joint Committee on Infant Hearing. (2007). Year 2007 position statement: Principles and guidelines for early hearing detection and intervention programs. *Pediatrics, 120*, 898–921. doi: 10.1542/peds.2007-2333.

American Cancer Society. (2009). *Cervical cancer: Prevention and early detection.* Retrieved from http://www.cancer.org/cancer/cervicalcancer/moreinformation/cervicalcancerpreventionandearlydetection/cervical-cancer-prevention-and-early-detection-toc.

American Dental Association. (n.d.a.). *Cleaning your teeth and gums (oral hygiene).* Retrieved from http://www.ada.org/public/topics/cleaning_faq.asp.

American Dental Association. (n.d.b.). *Toothpaste.* Retrieved http://www.ada.org/1322.aspx.

American Heart Association/American Stroke Association. (2011). *Guidelines for the prevention of stroke in patients with stroke or transient ischemic attack.* Retrieved from http://stroke.ahajournals.org/content/42/1/227.full.

American Nurses Association. (1980). *Nursing: A social policy statement.* Kansas City, MO: Author.

American Nurses Association. (2004). *Nursing: Scope and standards of practice.* Washington, DC: Author.

Anspaugh, D. J., Hamrick, M. H., & Rosato, F. D. (2010). *Wellness: Concepts and applications* (8th ed.). New York, NY: McGraw-Hill.

Berman, A., & Snyder, S. J. (2012). *Fundamentals of nursing.* Upper Saddle River, NJ: Pearson Education.

Brown, B. M., Peiffer, J. J., & Martins, R. N. (2012). Multiple effects of physical activity on molecular and cognitive signs of brain aging: Can exercise slow neurodegeneration and delay Alzheimer's disease? *Molecular Psychiatry.* doi:10.1038/mp.2012.162.

Burke, M. M., & Laramie, J. A. (2004). *Primary care of the older adult: A multidisciplinary approach* (2nd ed.). Philadelphia, PA: Mosby/Elsevier.

Carr, A. (2010). *Dry mouth.* Retrieved from http://www.mayoclinic.com/health/dry-mouth/an02112.

Centers for Disease Control and Prevention. (2011). *Glossary of terms.* Retrieved from http://www.cdc.gov/physicalactivity/everyone/glossary/.

Centers for Disease Control and Prevention. (2012). *Physical activity.* Retrieved from http://www.cdc.gov/physicalactivity/index.html.

Choudhary, S. S., & Choudhary, S. R. (2009). Sleep effects on breathing and respiratory diseases. *Lung India, 26*, 117–122.

Dijk, D., & Archer, S. N. (2009). Light, sleep and circadian rhythms: Together again. *PLoS Biology, 7*(6), 1–4.

Djonlagic, I., Saboisky, J., Carusona, A., Stickgold, R., & Malhotra, A. (2012). Increased sleep fragmentation leads to impaired off-line consolidation of motor memories in humans. PLoS One, 7(3). doi: 10.1371/journal.pone.0034106.

Edelman, C. L., & Mandle, C. L. (2009). *Health promotion throughout the life span* (7th ed.). St. Louis, MO: Mosby.

Fontaine, K. L. (2010). *Complementary and alternative therapies for nursing practice* (3rd ed.). Upper Saddle River, NJ: Prentice Hall.

Freeman, L. W. (2008). *Mosby's complementary and alternative medicine: A research-based approach* (3rd ed.). Philadelphia, PA: Mosby.

Grazina, R., & Massano, J. (2013). Physical exercise and Parkinson's disease: Influence on symptoms, disease course and prevention. *Reviews in the Neurosciences,* 1–14. doi: 10.1515/revneuro-2012-0087.

Harvard University. (2012). *Another reason to get out there and get moving!* Retrieved from http://www.health.harvard.edu/newsletters/Harvard_Health_Letter/2012/March/another-reason-to-get-out-there-and-get-moving.

Haumschild, M. S., & Haumschild, R. J. (2009). The importance of oral health in long-term care. *Journal of the American Medical Directors Association, 10*(9), 667–671.

Holshoe, J. M. (2009). Antidepressants and sleep: A review. *Perspectives in Psychiatric Care, 45,* 191–197. doi: 10.1111/j.1744-6163.2009.00221.x.

Hood, L. J. (2009). *Leddy and Pepper's conceptual bases of professional nursing* (7th ed.). Philadelphia, PA: Lippincott Williams & Wilkins.

Knudtson, M. (2009). Human papillomavirus and the HPV vaccine: Are the benefits worth the risks? *Nursing Clinics of North America, 44,* 293–299.

McKnight-Eily, L., Liu, Y., Perry, G., Presley-Contrell, L., Strine, T., Lu, H., & Croft, J. (2009). Perceived insufficient rest or sleep among adults—United States, 2008. *MMWR: Morbidity and Mortality Weekly Report, 58,* 1175–1179.

Micozzi, M. S. (2011). *Fundamentals of complementary and alternative medicine* (4th ed.). St. Louis, MO: Saunders.

North American Nursing Diagnosis Association International. (2012). *Nursing diagnoses: Definitions and classification 2012–2014* (9th ed.). Ames, IA: Wiley-Blackwell.

National Highway Traffic Safety Administration. (n.d.) *Research on drowsy driving.* Retrieved from http://www.nhtsa.gov/Driving+Safety/Distracted+Driving/Research+on+Drowsy+Driving.

National Sleep Foundation. (n.d.a). *A look at school start times.* Retrieved from http://www.sleepfoundation.org/alert/look-school-start-times.

National Sleep Foundation. (n.d.b). *Aging and sleep.* Retrieved from http://www.sleepfoundation.org/article/sleep-topics/aging-and-sleep.

National Sleep Foundation. (n.d.c). *Can't sleep? What to know about insomnia.* Retrieved from http://www.sleepfoundation.org/article/sleep-related-problems/insomnia-and-sleep.

National Sleep Foundation. (n.d.d). *Children and sleep.* Retrieved from http://www.sleepfoundation.org/article/sleep-topics/children-and-sleep.

National Sleep Foundation. (n.d.e). *Teens and sleep.* Retrieved from http://www.sleepfoundation.org/article/sleep-topics/teens-and-sleep.

National Sleep Foundation. (2009). *Women and sleep.* Retrieved from http://www.sleepfoundation.org/article/sleep-topics/women-and-sleep.

Nightingale, F. (1859/1969). *Notes on nursing: What it is, and what it is not.* New York, NY: Dover Books.

Ogden, C. L., Carroll, M. D., Kit, B. K., & Flegel, K. M. (2012). *NCHS Data Brief Number 82. Prevalence of obesity in the United States, 2009–2010.* Hyattsville, MD: National Center for Health Statistics.

Pender, N. J., Murdaugh, C. L., & Parsons, M. A. (2010). *Health promotion in nursing practice* (6th ed.). Upper Saddle River, NJ: Prentice Hall.

Pillitteri, A. (2009). *Maternal and child health nursing: Care of the childbearing and childrearing family* (6th ed.). Philadelphia, PA: Lippincott Williams & Wilkins.

President's Council on Fitness, Sports and Nutrition (2011). Retrieved from www.fitness.gov/pdfs/research-digest-june-2011.pdf.

Reid, K. J., Glazer Baron, K., Lu, B., Naylor, E., Wolfe, L., & Zee, P. C. (2010). Aerobic exercise improves self-reported sleep and quality of life in older adults with insomnia. *Sleep Medicine, 11*(9). P. 934-940. doi: 10.1016/j.sleep.2010.04.014.

Salas, R. E., Gamaldo, A., Collop, N. A., Gulyani, S., Hsu, M., David, P. M., … & Gamaldo, C. E. (2013). A step out of the dark: Improving the sleep medicine knowledge of trainees. *Sleep Medicine, 14*(1),105–108. doi: 10.1016/j.sleep.2012.09.013.

Skaer, T. L., & Sclar, D. A. (2010). Economic implications of sleep disorders. *Pharmacoeconomics, 28*(11), 1015–1023. doi: 10.2165/11537390-000000000-00000.

Stein, P. S., & Henry, R. G. (2009). Poor oral hygiene in long-term care. *American Journal of Nursing, 109,* 44–50.

Stevens, M. S. (2011). *Normal sleep, sleep physiology, and sleep deprivation.* Retrieved from http://emedicine.medscape.com/article/1188226-overview#a30.

Stewart, T. L., Chipperfield, J. G., Perry, R. P., & Weiner, B. (2012). Attributing illness to "old age": Consequences of a self-directed stereotype for health and mortality. *Psychology and Health, 27*(8), 881–897.

Torelli, F., Moscufo, N., Garreffa, G., Placidi, F., Romigi, A., Zannino, S., . . . & Guttmann, C. R. (2011). Cognitive profile and brain morphological changes in obstructive sleep apnea. *Neuroimage, 54*(2), 787–793. doi: 10.1016/j.neuroimage.2010.09.065.

U.S. Department of Health and Human Services, Office of Disease Prevention and Health Promotion. (2010). *Healthy people 2020: Improving the health of Americans.* Washington, DC: U.S. Government Printing Office. Also retrieved from www.healthypeople.gov/2020/default.aspx.

van de Weert-van Leeuwen, P. B., Arets, H. G., van der Ent, C. K., & Beekman, J. M. (2013). Infection, inflammation and exercise in cystic fibrosis. *Respiratory Research, 14,* 32. doi: 10.1186/1465-9921-14-32.

World Health Organization. (1948). *Preamble to the constitution of the World Health Organization as adopted by the International Health Conference.* New York, New York, June 19–22, 1946; signed on July 22, 1946, by the representatives of 61 states (Official Records of the World Health Organization, no. 2, p. 100) and entered into force on April 7, 1948.

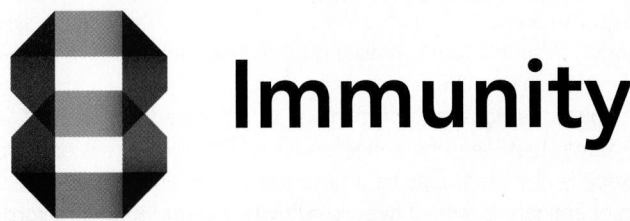

8 Immunity

MODULE AT-A-GLANCE

▼ THE CONCEPT OF IMMUNITY

The human body is continually threatened by foreign substances, infectious agents, and abnormal cells. Recent years have seen the emergence of resistant microorganisms, such as methicillin-resistant *Staphylococcus aureus,* and altered strains of familiar diseases, such as multidrug-resistant tuberculosis. New diseases, such as Lyme disease, *Clostridium difficile,* and human immunodeficiency virus (HIV), also have emerged. The body's major weapon against these threats is the immune system.

The function of the immune system is to protect the body from invasion by foreign **antigens** (foreign substances that trigger the immune response), to identify and destroy potentially harmful cells, and to

(continued on next page)

Concept Learning Outcomes

After reading about this concept, you will be able to:

1. Summarize the physiology of the immune system related to wellness promotion and disease prevention.

2. Examine the relationship between immunity and other concepts/systems.

3. Identify commonly occurring alterations in immunity and their related therapies.

4. Differentiate common assessment procedures used to examine immune health across the life span.

5. Describe diagnostic and laboratory tests to determine the individual's immune status.

6. Explain management of immune health and prevention of infection and disease.

7. Demonstrate the nursing process in providing culturally competent and caring interventions across the life span for individuals with common alterations in immune function.

8. Compare and contrast common independent and collaborative interventions for clients with alterations in immune function.

Concept Key Terms

Acquired immunity, *440*
Acquired immunodeficiency syndrome (AIDS), *438*
Active immunity, *450*
Antibodies, *442*
Antibody-mediated (humoral) immune response, *442*
Antigens, *437*
Autoimmune disorders, *438*
B lymphocytes (B cells), *441*
Cell-mediated (cellular) immune response, *442*
Cytokines, *443*
Eosinophils, *440*
Graft-versus-host disease, *444*
Hypersensitivity, *438*
Immunity, *438*
Immunization, *449*
Immunocompetent, *438*

Immunodeficiency, *438*
Immunoglobulins, *442*
Infection, *438*
Inflammation, *444*
Leukocytes, *438*
Leukocytosis, *438*
Leukopenia, *438*
Lymphocytes, *440*
Macrophages, *440*
Natural killer cells (NK cells, null cells), *441*
Opportunistic infections, *438*
Passive immunity, *450*
Phagocytosis, *443*
Primary immune response, *442*
Secondary immune response, *442*
T lymphocytes (T cells), *441*
Transplacental immunity, *451*
Vaccine, *450*

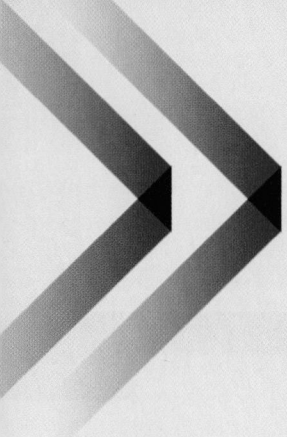

remove cellular debris. Lymphoid organs and specifically designed lymphocytes accomplish these actions through the processes of antibody-mediated immune response and cell-mediated immune response. The immune system recognizes any foreign substances within the body—in simple terms, it distinguishes "nonself" from "self"—and attempts to eliminate foreign substances as efficiently as possible.

Immunity, therefore, is the body's natural or induced response to infection and its associated conditions. Clients who are **immunocompetent** have an immune system that identifies antigens and effectively destroys or removes them. When the immune system functions improperly, the result may be an overreaction or an immunodeficiency. Overreaction of the immune system to an antigen or antigens is termed **hypersensitivity**. In **autoimmune disorders**, for example, the immune system loses the ability to recognize its own tissues and begins to attack them. An **immuno-deficiency** can develop when the immune system is incompetent or unable to respond effectively. **Acquired immunodeficiency syndrome (AIDS)** is an immune system deficit that is induced by infection with HIV and is characterized by **opportunistic infections** (infections that would normally not affect people with intact immune systems).

Our understanding of the components of the immune system and specific immune responses is growing. Having a thorough knowledge of the immune system increases understanding of the local and systemic inflammatory response, resistance to infectious disease, and the importance of immunization. This foundation helps the nurse teach clients and families to follow recommended treatment regimens, to promote and maintain health, and to prevent disease. In addition, the nurse can prescribe appropriate rehabilitative measures, such as increased rest and attention to optimal nutrition. It is vital that today's nurses understand the foundations of the immune system and the immune response. **<<**

▶ NORMAL PRESENTATION

The immune system is a complex and intricate network of specialized cells, tissues, and organs. Cells of the immune system seek out and destroy damaged cells and foreign tissue, yet recognize and preserve host cells (Porth & Matfin, 2010). The immune system performs the following functions:

- Defends and protects the body from **infection** (an invasion of the body tissue by microorganisms).
- Removes and destroys damaged or dead cells.
- Identifies and destroys malignant cells, thereby preventing their further development into tumors.

The immune system is activated by external agents, such as microorganisms; minor injuries, such as small lacerations or bruises; and major injuries, such as burns, surgeries, and systemic diseases (e.g., pneumonia). The response of the immune system may be nonspecific or specific. Nonspecific responses prevent or limit the entry of invaders into the body, thereby limiting the extent of tissue damage and reducing the workload of the immune system. Inflammation is a nonspecific response. When the inflammatory process is unable to destroy invading organisms or toxins, a more specific response, called the *immune response,* is activated.

The effectiveness of the immune system depends on its ability to differentiate normal host tissue from abnormal or foreign tissue. Body cells, tissues, and fluids have unique antigenic properties that the immune system recognizes as "self." External agents, such as microorganisms, cells and tissues from other humans or animals, and some inorganic substances, have antigenic properties that the immune system recognizes as "nonself."

Physiology Review

The immune system consists of molecules, cells, and organs that produce the immune response (**Table 8–1** ●). These com-ponents may be involved in the nonspecific inflammatory response, the specific immunological response, or both.

LEUKOCYTES   **Leukocytes**, or white blood cells (WBCs), are the primary cells involved in both nonspecific and specific immune system responses. Like all blood cells, leukocytes derive from stem cells (hemocytoblasts) in the bone marrow (**Figure 8–1** ●). Unlike red blood cells (RBCs), which are confined to the circulatory system, leukocytes can transport themselves to the site of an inflammatory or immune response. As the mobile units of the immune system, leukocytes detect, attack, and destroy anything that is recognized as "foreign." They are able to move through tissue spaces, where they locate damaged tissue and infection by responding to chemicals released by other leukocytes and damaged tissue.

The normal number of circulating leukocytes is 4,500 to 10,000 cells per cubic millimeter (mm^3) of blood. Many more leukocytes are marginated; that is, they adhere to vascular epithelial cells along the vessel walls, in other tissue spaces, or in the lymph system. In the presence of an attack such as an infection, additional WBCs are released from the bone marrow, and as WBCs move out of the bone marrow into the blood, the bone marrow increases its production of additional leukocytes. This process leads to a WBC count of greater than $10,000/mm^3$, a condition known as **leukocytosis**. A decrease in the number of circulating leukocytes, known as **leukopenia**, occurs when bone marrow activity is suppressed, or when leukocyte destruction increases.

Leukocytes are divided into three major groups: granulocytes, monocytes, and lymphocytes. The granulocytes and monocytes derive from the myeloid stem cells of the bone marrow and are instrumental in the inflammatory response. Lymphocytes derive from the lymphoid stem cells of the bone marrow and are the primary cells involved in the specific immune response. In laboratory tests, the WBC count indicates the total number of circulating leukocytes. The WBC differential identifies the portion of the total represented by each type of leukocyte.

TABLE 8–1   Cells and Tissues of the Immune System

COMPONENT	LOCATION	FUNCTION
Leukocytes		
Granulocytes		
Neutrophils	Circulatory system	Phagocytosis and chemotaxis
Eosinophils	Circulatory system, respiratory tract, and gastrointestinal tract	Phagocytosis Protection against parasites Involvement in allergic response
Basophils	Circulatory system	Release of chemotactic substances
Monocytes and macrophages	Circulatory system (monocytes) and body tissue, such as skin (histiocytes), liver (Kupffer cells), alveoli, spleen, tonsils, lymph nodes, bone marrow, and brain	Trapping and phagocytosis of foreign substances and cellular debris Secretion of interleukin-1 to stimulate lymphocyte growth
Lymphocytes	Circulatory system, lymph system, and tissues	Activation of T and B cells
T cells (mature in thymus gland)		Control of viral infections and destruction of cancer cells Involvement in hypersensitivity reactions and graft tissue rejection
B cells (mature in bone marrow)	Circulatory system and spleen	Production of antibodies (immunoglobulins) to specific antigens
Natural killer (NK) cells	Circulatory system	Cytotoxicity (killing of tumor cells, fungi, viral-infected cells, and foreign tissue)
Lymphoid tissues		
Primary or central lymphoid structures	Bone marrow and thymus gland	Production of immune cells; sites for cell maturation
Secondary or peripheral lymphoid structures	Lymph nodes, spleen, tonsils, intestinal lymphoid tissue, and lymphoid tissue in other organs	Sites for activation of immune cells by antigens

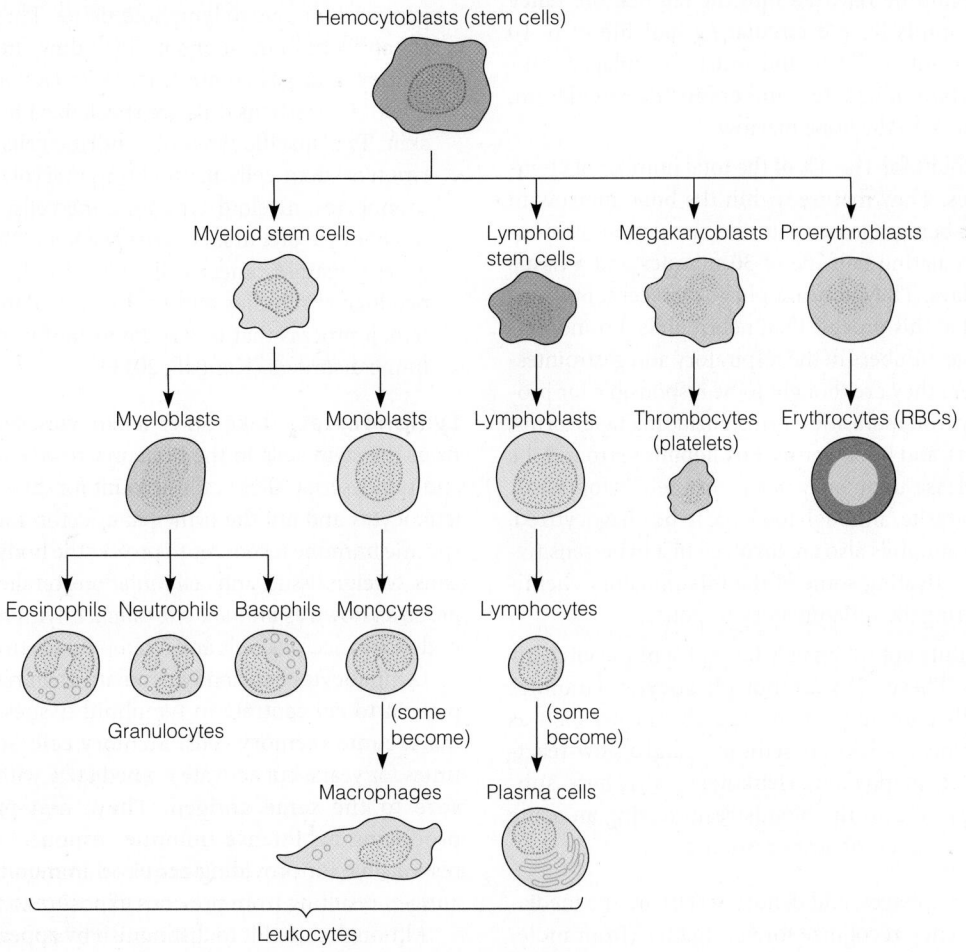

Figure 8–1 ● The development and differentiation of leukocytes from hemocytoblasts.

Granulocytes   Granulocytes constitute 60%–80% of the total number of normal blood leukocytes. Their cytoplasm has a granular appearance, and their nuclei are distinctively multi-lobular (see Figure 8–1). Granulocytes have a short life span, measured in hours to days, compared with the life span of monocytes, which is measured in months to years. Granulocytes play a key role in protecting the body from harmful microorganisms during acute inflammation and infection. There are three types of granulocytes: neutrophils, eosinophils, and basophils.

■ *Neutrophils,* also called *polymorphonuclear leukocytes* (or *polys*), are the most plentiful of the granulocytes, constituting 55%–70% of the total number of circulating leukocytes. Neutrophils are phagocytic cells, responsible for engulfing and destroying foreign agents, particularly bacteria and small particles. Drawn by chemicals released by damaged tissue and invading organisms, neutrophils are the first phagocytic cells to arrive at the site of invasion. Neutrophils are produced in the bone marrow and released into the circulation when they mature. Segmented neutrophils (or segs) are mature forms and usually account for approximately 55% of total leukocytes. Bands are immature neutrophils and usually comprise 5% of leukocytes. As neutrophils mature, their nucleus changes from round to kidney-bean–shaped (banded), and then the nucleus separates into small, attached segments—thus the designations "banded" versus "segmented" neutrophils. A neutrophil takes approximately 10 days to mature and be released into the circulation. Once released, neutrophils have a circulating half-life of 6–10 hours. They cannot replicate and must be replaced constantly to maintain adequate numbers in the circulation. They do not return to the bone marrow.

■ **Eosinophils** account for 1%–4% of the total number of circulating leukocytes. They mature within the bone marrow in 3–6 days before being released into the circulation. Eosinophils have a circulating half-life of 30 minutes and a tissue half-life of 12 days. They, too, are phagocytic cells, but they are less efficient at this process than neutrophils. Eosinophils are found in large numbers in the respiratory and gastrointestinal tracts, where they are thought to be responsible for protecting the body from parasitic worms, including tapeworms, flukes, pinworms, and hookworms. Eosinophils surround the parasite and release toxic enzymes from their cytoplasmic granules. The parasite, although too large to be phagocytized, is destroyed. Eosinophils also are involved in a hypersensitivity response, inactivating some of the inflammatory chemicals released during the inflammatory response.

■ *Basophils* constitute approximately 0.5%–1% of the circulating leukocytes. These cells are not phagocytic. Granules within basophils contain proteins and chemicals, such as heparin, histamine, bradykinin, serotonin, and a slow-reacting substance of anaphylaxis (leukotrienes). These substances are released into the bloodstream during an acute hypersensitivity reaction or stress response.

Monocytes, macrophages, and dendritic cells are the mediators of immunity. They recognize foreign matter (from molecules to cells), initiate immune responses, and are actively phagocytic, with the capacity to phagocytize large foreign particles and cellular debris.

Monocytes   Monocytes are the largest of the leukocytes and constitute 2%–3% of circulating leukocytes. After their release from the bone marrow, monocytes are in circulation for 1–2 days. They then migrate to various tissues throughout the body, attach themselves to the tissues, and remain for months or even years until they are activated. Monocytes activate the immune response against chronic infections such as tuberculosis, viral infections, and certain intracellular parasitic infections.

■ After settling into the tissues, monocytes mature into **macrophages**, which are differentiated by the tissues in which they reside. Histiocytes are tissue macrophages in loose connective tissue, Kupffer cells are found in the liver, alveolar macrophages in the lungs, and microglia in the brain. Tissue macrophages also are found in the spleen, tonsils, lymph nodes, and bone marrow. Once they are in the tissue, macrophages can multiply to encapsulate and trap foreign matter that cannot be phagocytized. Like neutrophils, macrophages are drawn to an inflamed area by chemicals released from damaged tissue, a process known as *chemotaxis*. And like monocytes, macrophages activate the immune response against chronic infections, such as tuberculosis, viral infections, and certain intracellular parasitic infections.

■ *Dendritic cells* are star-shaped cells that originate in both the myeloid and the lymphoid cell lines. These antigen-presenting cells (APCs) have long processes that can capture antigens and migrate to lymphoid tissue. They serve as sentinels for antigens in most organs, including the heart, lungs, liver, kidney, and gastrointestinal tract (Rockefeller University, 2013). Langerhans cells are specialized dendritic cells in the skin. Two specific types of dendritic cells develop from pluripotent stem cells in the bone marrow. DC1s arise from monocytes, myeloid-type immune cells; DC2s derive from lymphocyte precursors (Tripathi et al., 2010). DC1s activate T cells against cancer cells. DC2s assist B lymphocytes to produce antibodies and to downregulate the immune system, a process that is very important in preventing autoimmune disorders (Kimball, 2011).

Lymphocytes   Like other leukocytes, **lymphocytes** derive from the stem cells in the bone marrow (**Figure 8–2 ●**). Small and nondescript, these cells account for 20%–40% of circulating leukocytes and are the principal effector and regulator cells of specific immune responses to protect the body from microorganisms, foreign tissue, and cell mutations or alterations. Through a process known as *immune surveillance*, lymphocytes monitor the body for cancerous cells and attempt to destroy them.

Lymphocytes constantly circulate, then return in a "homing" pattern to concentrate in lymphoid tissues, where they often mature into memory cells. Memory cells stay inactive, sometimes for years, but activate immediately with subsequent exposure to the same antigen. They then proliferate rapidly, producing an intense immune response. Memory cells are responsible for providing **acquired immunity** (resistance to an antigen resulting from previous exposure to that antigen).

Although difficult to distinguish by appearance, lymphocyte types have distinct differences in how and where they mature as

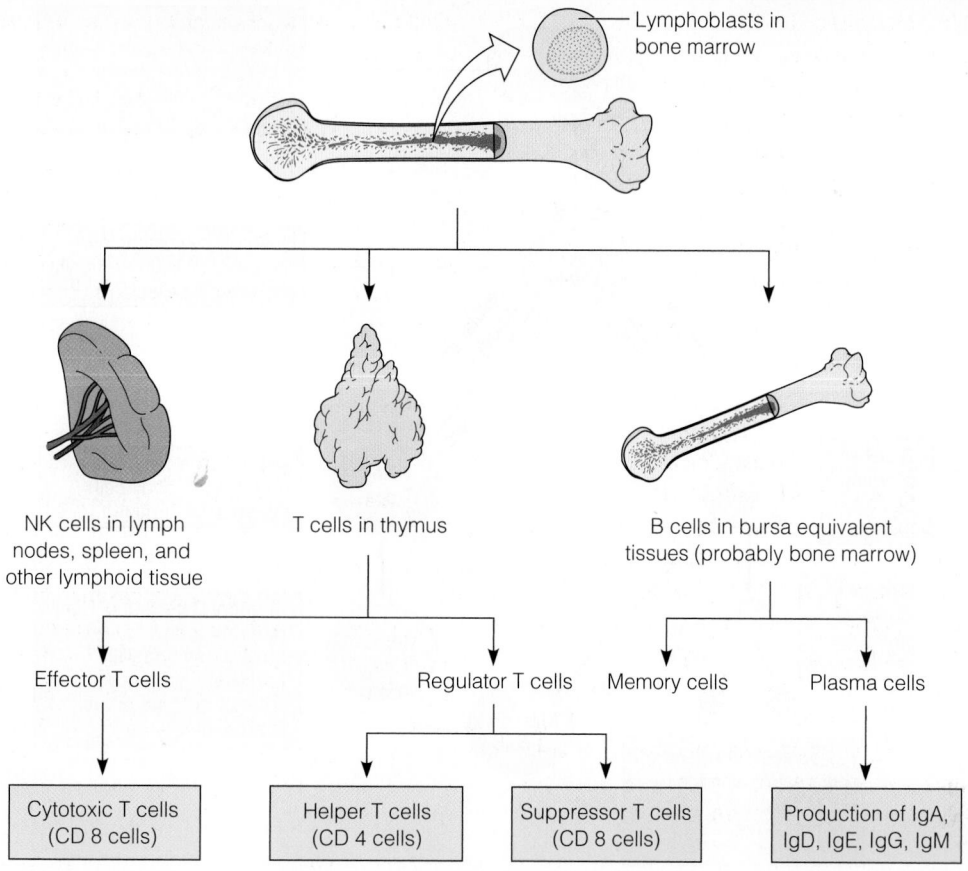

Lymphoblasts in bone marrow

NK cells in lymph nodes, spleen, and other lymphoid tissue

T cells in thymus

B cells in bursa equivalent tissues (probably bone marrow)

Effector T cells

Regulator T cells

Memory cells

Plasma cells

Cytotoxic T cells (CD 8 cells)

Helper T cells (CD 4 cells)

Suppressor T cells (CD 8 cells)

Production of IgA, IgD, IgE, IgG, IgM

Figure 8–2 ● The development and differentiation of lymphocytes from lymphoid stem cells (lymphoblasts).

well as in life cycle, surface characteristics, and function. The three types of lymphocytes are **T lymphocytes (T cells)**, **B lymphocytes (B cells)**, and **natural killer cells (NK cells** or **null cells)**. None of these cells act independently; their functions are closely interrelated.

■ *T cells* mature in the thymus gland and are integral to the specific immune response. On contact with APCs, T lymphocytes mature into active helper T cells, cytotoxic T cells, or memory T cells.

■ *B cells* complete their maturation in the bone marrow and, like T cells, are integral to the specific immune response. On contact with an antigen, B lymphocytes are activated and mature into either plasma cells, which secrete antibodies, or memory cells.

■ *Natural killer cells* are large, granular cells found in the spleen, lymph nodes, bone marrow, and blood. They constitute 15% of circulating lymphocytes. NK cells provide immune surveillance and resistance to infection, and they play an important role in the destruction of early malignant cells. Like B cells and T cells, NK cells are cytotoxic, but unlike T cells, they do not require connection with an APC to become activated and kill cancer cells, virus-infected cells, and cells infected with microbes (Porth & Matfin, 2010). Fortunately, NK cells are inhibited when contact is made with normal host cells.

ANTIGENS Antigens provoke a specific immune response when introduced into the body. Typically, antigens are large

protein molecules, although polysaccharides, polypeptides, and nucleic acids also may be antigenic. Many antigens are proteins found on the cell membrane or cell wall of microorganisms or tissues (e.g., transplanted tissue or organs), incompatible blood cells, vaccines, pollen, egg white, animal dander, and insect or snake venom.

The portion of an antigen that incites a specific immune response is called its *antigenic determinant site* (or *epitope*). Complete antigens (also known as *immunogens*) typically are large molecules with multiple antigenic determinant sites; examples are proteins and certain polysaccharides. Complete antigens have two characteristics:

1. *Immunogenicity*, or the ability to stimulate a specific immune response
2. *Specific reactivity*, or the ability to stimulate specific immune system components

Small molecules that cannot evoke an antigenic response alone (e.g., chemical toxins, drugs, and dust) may link to proteins to function as complete antigens. The proteins to which they link are known as haptens.

When an antigen is encountered in the body, two major groups of cells—lymphocytes and APCs—generate an effective immune response. APCs are recognized by a specific receptor on a lymphocyte, and an immune response is generated by those lymphocytes. Depending on the antigen itself and the type of immune cell activated by contact with the antigen, two separate but overlapping immune responses may occur. The B cell, or

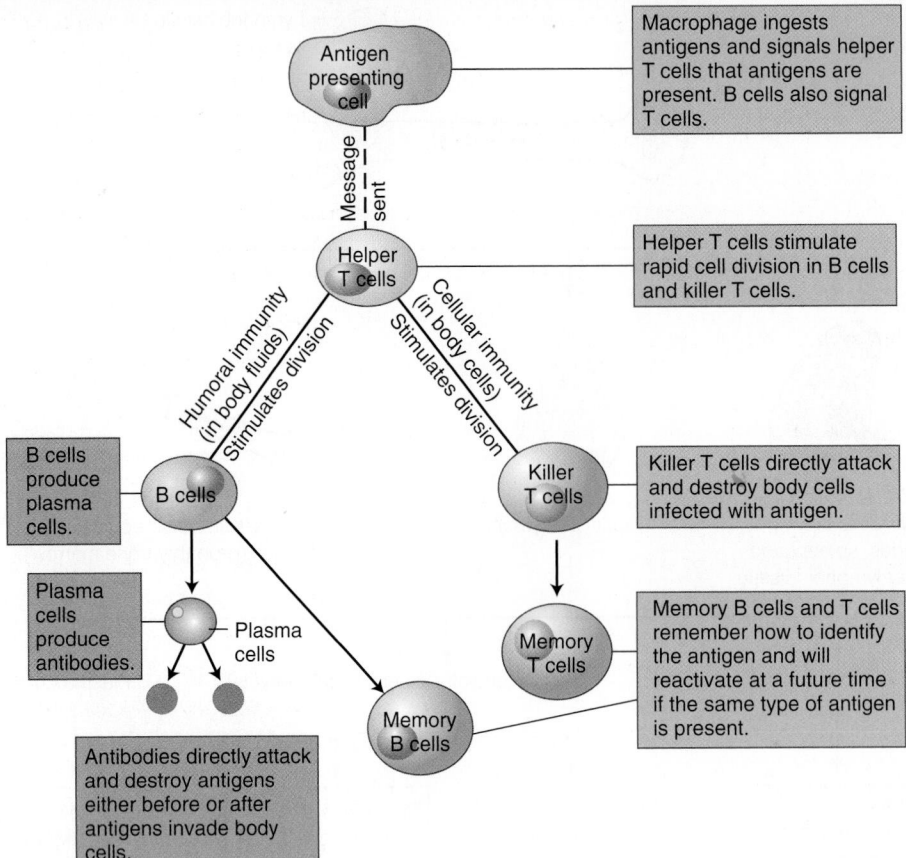

Figure 8–3 ● The primary immune response encompasses a cascade of events that involve humoral immunity and cellular immunity.

humoral branch of the immune system, mainly eliminates extracellular antigens, such as bacteria, bacterial toxins, and free viruses, through the production of **antibodies** (molecules that bind with the antigen and inactivate it). Antibodies are found in serum, body fluids, and certain tissues. When an individual is first exposed to an antigen, the B lymphocyte system begins to produce antibodies that react specifically to that antigen (**Figure 8–3 ●**). It takes approximately 3 days for this process, known as the **primary immune response**, to occur. Subsequent encounters with the antigen trigger memory cells, and the result is a **secondary immune response** within 24 hours.

There are five classes of antibodies, called **immunoglobulins**: IgM, IgG, IgA, IgD, and IgE. Together, these proteins make up the **antibody-mediated (humoral) immune response**. The functions of the five major types of immunoglobulins are as follows:

■ *IgM* antibodies are produced 48–72 hours after an antigen enters the body and are responsible for primary immunity. This immunoglobulin produces antibody activity against rheumatoid factors, gram-negative organisms, and the ABO blood group. IgM activates the complement system by destroying antigenic substances. Because it does not pass the placental barrier, the serum value of IgM is low in newborns; however, it is produced early in life and the level increases after 9 months of age.

■ *IgG* is the major immunoglobulin. IgG results from secondary exposure to the foreign antigen and is responsible for antiviral and antibacterial activity. This antibody passes through the placental barrier and provides early immunity for the newborn. The IgG response is longer and stronger than that of the other immunoglobulins.

■ *IgA* is found in the secretions of the respiratory, gastrointestinal, and genitourinary tracts; tears; and saliva. Its purpose is to protect mucous membranes from invading organisms (viruses, certain bacteria—*Escherichia coli* and *Clostridium tetani*). IgA does not pass the placental barrier. Those having congenital IgA deficiency are prone to autoimmune disease.

■ The role of *IgD* is unknown.

■ *IgE* increases during allergic reactions and anaphylaxis.

Intracellular pathogens, such as viral-infected cells, cancer cells, and foreign tissue, activate T lymphocytes, which are the primary agents of the **cell-mediated (cellular) immune response**. In this immune response, the lymphocytes themselves, in the form of helper T cells, cytotoxic T cells, and NK cells, inactivate the antigen, either directly or indirectly.

Cell-mediated immunity acts at the cellular level by attacking antigens directly and by activating B cells. T lymphocytes comprise the cell-mediated immune response and are subdivided into effector cells and regulator cells. The cytotoxic cell or killer T cell is the primary effector cell. Regulator T cells are divided into two subsets, known as *helper T cells* and *suppressor T cells*.

Helper T cells initiate the immune response, whereas suppressor T cells limit it. Helper T cells accomplish their role by promoting growth of additional T cells, by stimulating proliferation of B cells, and by activating killer T cells. Suppressor

T cells are believed to be important in preventing autoimmune disorders. Proper immune system function depends on the correct balance between helper and suppressor T cells.

Complement is a component of blood serum consisting of 11 protein compounds. It is an inactive enzyme that activates in response to antigen–antibody functions, causing a generalized inflammatory reaction that kills foreign cells. It plays a role in causing some autoimmune disorders as well.

Immune cells also secrete proteins called **cytokines** that carry messages for immune system function. Lymphocytes, monocytes, and macrophages all secrete cytokines that have a variety of effects on the target cells. These effects may include stimulation of growth through cell proliferation, differentiation of cellular actions, production of inflammation, sensitization to pain, and other actions. Interleukins, a type of cytokine, were identified first in WBCs but are present in many cells. Many types of interleukins have been identified, and some are known to influence the function of the immune system.

In addition to destroying viruses and bacteria, cytotoxic T lymphocytes also attack malignant cells. They are responsible for the rejection of transplanted organs and grafted tissues as well.

LYMPHOID SYSTEM   The lymphoid system consists of the lymph nodes, spleen, thymus, tonsils, lymphoid tissue scattered in connective tissues and mucosa, and bone marrow. The thymus and bone marrow, in which T cells and B cells mature, are considered central lymphoid organs. The spleen, lymph nodes, tonsils, and other peripheral lymphoid tissue are considered peripheral lymphoid organs (**Figure 8–4** ●).

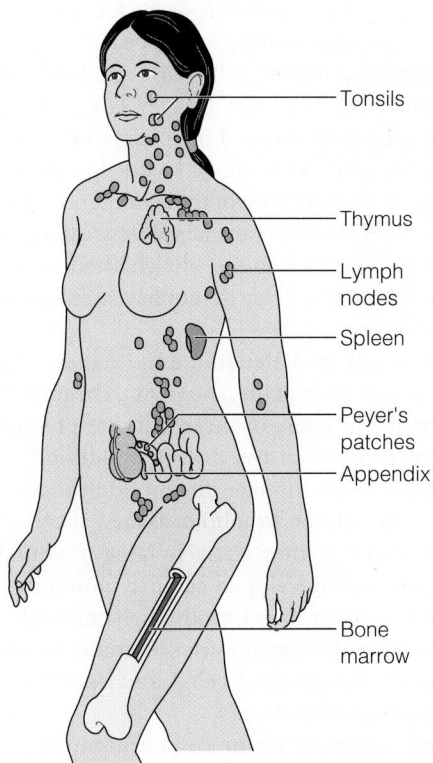

Figure 8–4 ● The lymphoid system, showing the central organs of the thymus and bone marrow and the peripheral organs, including the spleen, tonsils, lymph nodes, and Peyer's patches.

This system exists to recover proteins for the vascular system and to protect the bloodstream from invading organisms. Cells of the immune system, such as neutrophils, macrophages, and dendritic cells, carry antigens from the interstitial space to the lymph nodes for immune surveillance in the lymphatic circulation. Unlike the vascular tree, which has tight epithelial junctions, lymphatic epithelium is replete with open junctions that promote lymphocyte access and effectively protect the bloodstream from antigen entry.

Lymph Nodes   The most numerous elements of the lymphoid system, lymph nodes are small, round, or bean-shaped bodies that are encapsulated and vary in size from 1 mm to 2 cm. Distributed throughout the body, lymph nodes generally occur in groups at the junction of the lymphatic vessels. They can be found in the neck, axillae, abdomen, and groin and have two specific functions:

1. To filter foreign products or antigens from the lymph
2. To house and support proliferation of lymphocytes and macrophages.

Lymph, a clear, protein-containing fluid transported within lymph vessels, enters the node through afferent lymphatic vessels. Inside the node, the lymph flows through sinuses in the cortex of the lymph node (where T lymphocytes, B lymphocytes, and macrophages are abundant) and then through sinuses of the medulla of the lymph node, which contains macrophages and plasma cells. The presence of a foreign antigen stimulates lymphocytes and macrophages to proliferate in the lymph nodes. Macrophages destroy the antigen by **phagocytosis** (engulfing and then digesting the antigen). Immune cells and lymph then leave the lymph node through efferent vessels. An abundant blood supply to the node also facilitates lymphocyte movement.

Spleen   The spleen is the largest lymphoid organ in the body—and the only lymphoid organ that can filter blood. The spleen is located in the upper left quadrant of the abdomen and has two kinds of tissue: white pulp and red pulp. White pulp, in which B cells predominate, is lymphoid tissue that serves as a site for lymphocyte proliferation and immune surveillance. Blood filtration occurs in the red pulp, where phagocytic cells dispose of damaged or aged RBCs and platelets in blood-filled venous sinuses. Other debris and foreign matter, such as bacteria, viruses, and toxins, are removed from the blood as well. The spleen also stores blood and the breakdown products of RBCs for future use. The spleen is not essential for life; if it is removed because of disease or trauma, the liver and bone marrow assume its functions.

Thymus Gland   The thymus gland is located in the superior anterior mediastinal cavity beneath the sternum. During fetal life and childhood, the thymus serves as a site for the maturation and differentiation of thymic lymphoid cells, the T cells. After puberty, the thymus gland begins to atrophy slowly. Thymosin, an immunoregulatory hormone of the thymus, stimulates lymphopoiesis, the formation of lymphocytes or lymphoid tissue.

Bone Marrow   Bone marrow is soft organic tissue found in the hollow cavity of the long bones, particularly the femur and humerus, as well as in the flat bones of the pelvis, ribs, and sternum. Bone marrow produces and stores hematopoietic stem cells, from which all cellular components of the blood are derived (see Figure 8–2).

Lymphoid Tissues Lymphoid tissues are located at key sites of potential invasion by microorganisms: the submucosa of the genitourinary, respiratory, and gastrointestinal tracts and the skin. Plasma cells in these lymphoid tissues defend the body against bacterial invasion at areas exposed to the external environment. In general, these tissues are known as mucosa-associated lymphoid tissue. Diffuse collections of lymphocytes, plasma cells, and phagocytes are scattered throughout the respiratory tract, concentrating at bifurcations of the bronchi and bronchioles. Peyer patches, or gut-associated lymphoid tissue (GALT), comprise the largest collection of immune cells in the body (Neish, 2008). Ingestion and absorption of solid food-stuffs and liquids continually expose the lining of the gut to resident microflora and infectious pathogens. Unlike peripheral lymph nodes, which respond to pathogens with acute inflammatory responses, GALT processes common intestinal antigens without producing acute inflammation. Collections of immune cells make up GALT. Intraepithelial lymphocytes fill the spaces between mucosal epithelial cells. Beneath the basement membrane of gut epithelium lie abundant T cells and mature plasma cells, which are sources of IgA. Peyer patches hold dense collections of lymphocytes in lymphoid nodules. As naive B cells and T cells migrate through Peyer patches, they are sensitized to specific antigens. In mesenteric lymph nodes, these sensitized cells proliferate and circulate throughout the vascular tree, where they produce secretory IgA. Secretory IgA coats mucosal cells and prevents attachment of intraluminal bacteria in the intestine, upper respiratory tract, bronchi, mammary ducts, and salivary glands. Thus, the collection of immune cells in GALT effectively protects mucosa throughout the body that is exposed to resident and foreign pathogens.

Tonsils and Adenoids Tonsils and adenoids protect the body from inhaled or ingested foreign agents. These skin-associated lymphoid tissues contain lymphocytes and dendritic cells, such as Langerhans cells, in the epidermis, which transport antigens to regional lymph nodes for destruction and development of specific immunity to the antigen.

Nonspecific Inflammatory Response

Barrier protection is the body's first line of defense against infection. The skin is the primary barrier; when intact, it prevents invasion by external organisms. The membranes lining the inner surfaces of the body are protected by a barrier of mucus, which traps microorganisms and other foreign substances. These can then be removed by other protective mechanisms, such as ciliary movement or the washing action of tears or urine. In addition, many body fluids contain bactericidal substances that provide barrier protection. These include acid in gastric fluid, zinc in prostatic fluid, and lysozyme in tears, nasal secretions, saliva, and sweat (Porth & Matfin, 2010; Rink & Gabriel, 2000).

When these first-line defenses are breached, the resulting tissue damage or foreign material entering the body induces a nonspecific immune response known as **inflammation**, an adaptive response to what the body sees as harmful. Inflamma-

tion brings fluid, dissolved substances, and blood cells into the interstitial tissues where the invasion or damage has occurred. (The inflammatory response is described in more detail in the module on Inflammation.) The inflammatory response is called a nonspecific response because the same events occur regardless of what causes the inflammatory process. Through the inflammatory reaction, the invader is neutralized and eliminated, destroyed tissue removed, and the process of healing and repair initiated.

Genetic and Lifespan Considerations

Immune function changes across the life span. The developing immune function of infants and children makes them susceptible to infection until their systems reach maturity in late childhood. Conversely, the declining immune function of older adults makes them more prone to infection as well. These developmental processes occur naturally but may be helped or hindered by a number of influencing factors. Genetics ranks among these factors, though its role is difficult to pinpoint outside of infancy.

PEDIATRIC CONSIDERATIONS Immune system development is a complex and multifactorial process. Early in utero experiences, environmental exposures after birth, and other factors influence this important feedback system. While the immune system protects children from harmful diseases, it also can lead to conditions such as asthma, food allergies, or skin atopy.

Infants and children have differing amounts of some immunoglobulins. IgG is the only immunoglobulin that crosses the placenta; as a result, a newborn's levels are similar to those of the mother. This maternal IgG disappears by 6–8 months of age. The infant's IgG level then increases gradually, until mature levels are reached at 7–8 years. IgM levels are low at birth, rise markedly at 1 week of age, and then continue to increase until adult levels are reached at about 1 year. IgA and IgE are not present at birth. Manufacture of these immunoglobulins begins by 2 weeks of age; however, normal values are not achieved until 6–7 years. Thus it is easy to see why children under 6 years of age become ill so often: They do not have a full complement of immunoglobulins.

In contrast, cell-mediated immunity achieves full function early in life. Early in fetal life, the thymus begins producing T cells, and by birth, many of these cells are present. The thymus is large at birth, grows during childhood and adolescence, and decreases in size during adulthood (Nasseri & Eftekhari, 2010). Other lymphoid tissues, such as the spleen and tonsils, also are comparatively large in young children. Because of the well-developed cellular immunity, any blood infused into newborns generally is irradiated to prevent **graft-versus-host disease** (a series of immunologic reactions in response to transplanted cells) as a result of transfused lymphocytes (**Figure 8–5** ●).

Newborns are most prone to development of infection, particularly when born prematurely, because they have lower levels of their own immune protections as well as less IgG obtained from the mother. Specifically, newborns have somewhat lower numbers of NK cells than older children and adults, and this lower number decreases their ability to

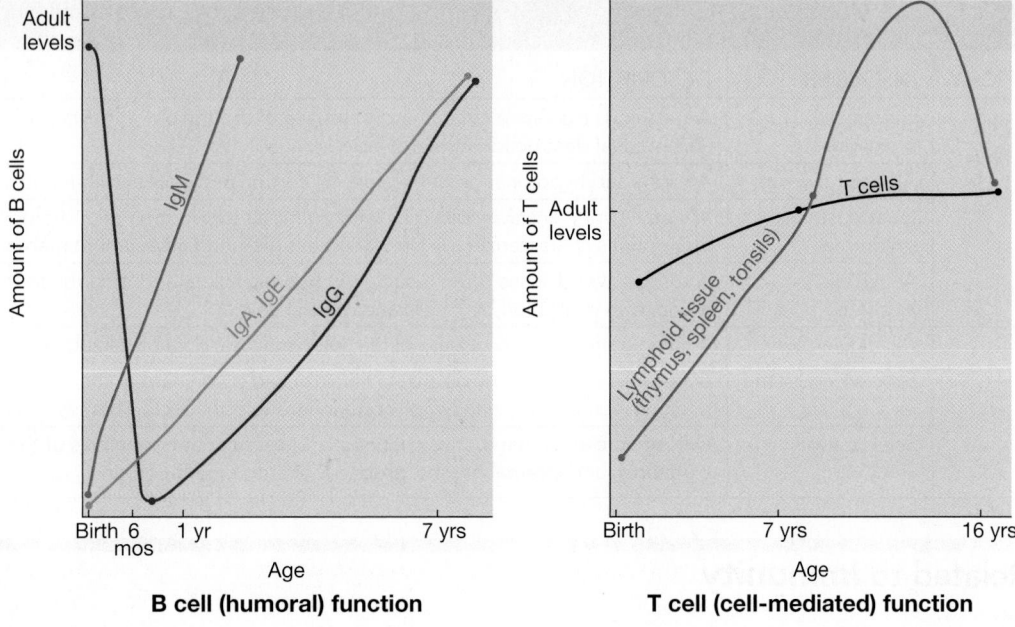

Figure 8–5 ● Different types of immunoglobulins mature at variable times throughout childhood. Children have high levels of some types of immunoglobulins, whereas the levels of other types may be low at certain periods during development.

respond to certain antigens. In addition, the lower levels of some complement proteins in newborns than in older children and adults delay and hamper response to certain infections. Levels of monocytes and macrophages are low as well (Philbin & Levy, 2009). Feeding newborns with human milk protects them against infections, however. Nurses also play an important role by following infection-control practices with newborns and promptly identifying infections in children of all ages.

NORMAL CHANGES ASSOCIATED WITH AGING

Immune function declines with aging, although many of the mechanisms leading to this decline are not clear. External factors, such as nutritional status and the effects of chemical exposure, ultraviolet radiation, and environmental pollution, affect the older adult's immune status. Internal factors, including genetics, the function of the neurological and endocrine systems, chronic and prior illnesses, and individual anatomical and physiological variations, affect it as well. These myriad influences make it difficult to determine the effect of aging on the immune system.

Although in some older adults the immune system is as effective as in younger individuals, normal changes associated with aging demonstrate a decrease in immune response and lowered resistance to infection, with poor response to immunizations. T cells are less responsive to antigens, while B cells produce fewer antibodies. Immune system changes may precipitate insulin resistance, and the hypersensitivity response is reduced or delayed.

Whereas the antibody response to foreign antigens is diminished in older adults, autoantibodies (antibodies that react to the client's own tissues) are more common. Immunological theories of aging propose that a decrease in immune function may result in an increase in autoimmune responses, causing the body to produce antibodies that attack the body itself.

▶ ALTERATIONS TO IMMUNITY

Considering the complexity of the immune system, it is not surprising that abnormal or harmful responses occur. Altered immune system responses include those characterized by hyperresponsiveness of the immune system and those characterized by an impaired immune response. Allergies, autoimmune disorders, and reactions to organ or tissue transplants are all examples of hyperresponsive immune function. AIDS and other immunodeficiency disorders result from impairment of the immune system. **Table 8–2** ● outlines selected autoimmune disorders; other alterations related to the endocrine system but not discussed here are Graves disease, Hashimoto disease, myasthenia gravis, and urticaria. Alterations of the immune system have a number of complications for other systems and impact nursing across the individual, nursing, and healthcare domains (see the Concepts Related to Immunity feature).

Alterations and Manifestations

Allergic reactions, also called *hypersensitivity reactions,* are immune responses that lead to tissue damage. There are four types of allergic reactions:

- *Type I, or immediate hypersensitivity:* Characterized by rapid development of symptoms after exposure to an antigen. Anaphylaxis is the most severe form (Shelton & Shivnan, 2011).

- *Type II, or cytotoxic hypersensitivity:* Involves the rupture of cells targeted by the immune response. A common example is transfusion reactions.

- *Type III, or immune complex reaction:* Includes inflammatory response in the targeted tissues that leads to tissue damage. Autoimmune diseases often involve this type of reaction.

- *Type IV, or delayed-type hypersensitivity:* Characterized by tissue damage at the site of antigen contact 24–48 hours after exposure. Contact dermatitis is an example.

TABLE 8–2   Selected Autoimmune Disorders

ORGAN SPECIFICITY	DISORDER	DESCRIPTION
More organ specific	Hashimoto thyroiditis	A chronic, progressive inflammatory disease of the thyroid, with lymphocyte infiltration and gradual destruction of the gland
	Addison disease	Atrophy and hypofunction of the adrenal cortex, probably autoimmune in origin
	Goodpasture syndrome	A type II hypersensitivity disorder, with pulmonary hemorrhage and progressive glomerulonephritis characterized by circulating antiglomerular basement membrane antibodies
	Active chronic hepatitis	A serious liver disease often resulting in hepatic failure and/or cirrhosis; may be autoimmune, with infiltration by T cells and plasma cells
Less organ specific	Ulcerative colitis	A chronic inflammatory disease of the colon mucosa, possibly of autoimmune origin
	Sjögren syndrome	A systemic inflammatory disorder characterized by dryness of the mouth, eye, and other mucous membranes, with lymphocyte infiltration of affected tissues
	Scleroderma	Diffuse fibrosis, degenerative changes, and vascular abnormalities of the skin, joint structures, and internal organs; probably of autoimmune origin

Concepts Related to **Immunity**

Due to its role in protecting the body, the immune system affects and is affected by a number of other conceptual areas. Three of note are comfort, inflammation, and skin integrity.

The rapid, dramatic nature of immune response can lead to a variety of localized and systemic discomforts. Given the skin's role as the body's primary barrier to foreign bodies and antigens, discomforts of the skin are very common and stem from a variety of sources, including allergic reaction, inflammation, and wound healing.

Inflammation is a reaction of the local circulatory system to an insult, injury, or antigen. It involves movement of fluid and cells out of the bloodstream to the affected tissue in an effort to eliminate infectious agents. Inflammation often resolves itself once the threat is eliminated; it may, however, lead to abscess, scar formation, and persistent inflammation that leads to chronic inflammation.

Tissue integrity has a two-way relationship with immunity: Impaired skin integrity can trigger an immune response, and certain immune responses can lead to impaired skin integrity. Burns, traumatic injuries, and some cancer therapies impair skin integrity, allowing infectious agents to enter the body. Conversely, allergic reactions can result in manifestations such as contact dermatitis. Integrity issues must be treated alongside the underlying problem, and clients must be educated about proper skin care.

CONCEPT	RELATIONSHIP TO IMMUNITY	NURSING IMPLICATIONS
Comfort		
Pain from immune response including: ■ allergic reaction ■ inflammation ■ wound healing	Painful conditions, such as swelling and skin reactions, often occur during immune response.	■ Assess related symptoms, such as edema, rash, malaise, loss of appetite, and trouble sleeping. ■ Be alert to topical and latex allergies that could worsen symptoms. ■ *Anticipate:* Additional assessments, comfort measures
Inflammation		
	Movement of fluid and cells to site of injury or infection cause inflammation during immune response.	■ Assess for fever, skin warmth and redness, edema, and generalized pain. ■ Be alert for abscess formation, purulent exudate, and increased white blood cell count. ■ *Anticipate:* Aspirin, antipyretics, cold packs
Tissue Integrity		
	Impaired skin integrity triggers immune response; some immune responses lead to impaired skin integrity.	■ Important in burns, traumatic injury, cancer therapies, and skin and allergic disorders. ■ *Anticipate:* Antibiotics, medications for pain relief, altered sensation or pain ■ Educate client about care measures for impaired skin.

Alterations and Therapies **Immunity**

ALTERATION	DESCRIPTION	THERAPIES
Hypersensitivity reaction	Hypersensitivity reaction is an altered immune response to an antigen, resulting in harm to the client ranging from an allergy to anaphylactic shock.	▪ Antihistamines for mild reactions ▪ Epinephrine and corticosteroids in life-threatening reactions ▪ Assessment of airway with any hypersensitivity reaction
Rheumatoid arthritis (RA)	Rheumatoid arthritis is a chronic, systemic autoimmune disorder that causes inflammation of connective tissue.	▪ Nonsteroidal anti-inflammatory drugs (NSAIDs) ▪ Low-dose corticosteroids ▪ Antirheumatic drugs, including immunosuppressive and cytotoxic drugs
Human immunodeficiency virus/acquired immunodeficiency syndrome (HIV/AIDS)	AIDS results from a retrovirus (HIV) that is transmitted by direct contact with infected blood and body fluids. HIV infection weakens the immune system, leaving clients vulnerable to opportunistic infections.	▪ Prevention of opportunistic infections ▪ Ensuring adequate respiratory function and perfusion ▪ Stimulating hematopoietic response ▪ Antiviral treatment if CD4 count falls below 200/mm^3 or client exhibits severe disease symptoms
Systemic lupus erythematosus (SLE)	SLE is a chronic inflammatory disease that involves many organ systems.	▪ Dependent on severity of the disease ▪ Aspirin or NSAIDs for arthralgias, arthritis, fever, or fatigue ▪ Antimalarial drugs ▪ High-dose corticosteroids ▪ Immunosuppressive agents

Autoimmune diseases occur when the immune system attacks components of its own body because the immune system loses its ability to distinguish self from other. These disorders have no definitive cause, although bacteria, viruses, and toxins may play a role (AARDA, 2011). Diseases may be localized or generalized, tend to occur more often in females, and often run in families.

Transplant reactions occur when a recipient's body has an immune reaction to newly transplanted organs or tissues. Antigens on the organs or tissues—including the major histocompatibility complex (MHC)—activate the recipient's T cells and stimulate an inflammatory reaction. This reaction can lead to transplant rejection. There are three types of transplant rejection:

▪ *Hyperacute rejection.* Occurs minutes or hours after transplantation. It is characterized by organ swelling, clot formation, and hemorrhage.

▪ *Acute rejection.* Occurs in the weeks following transplantation. In the case of kidney transplant, a decrease in urine output, swelling, pain, and blood and protein in the urine are common.

▪ *Chronic rejection.* Occurs months after transplantation. Slow, insidious organ failure occurs as a result of immune-mediated damage.

Finally, immune deficiencies lead to dysfunction in either the primary or the secondary immune response. Primary immune deficiencies are congenital and may affect T cells, B cells, or both. Defects in white blood cells may also lead to primary immune deficiencies. Acquired later in life, secondary immune deficiencies lead to decreased immune function and increased susceptibility to infection and malignancies. Many types of trauma or stress—including some cancer therapies—can lead to secondary deficiencies, though the best-known example, acquired immunodeficiency syndrome (AIDS), comes from the human immunodeficiency virus (HIV). HIV attacks and depletes helper T cells, causing immune dysfunction. When lymphocyte levels fall below 200, opportunistic infections develop; when this occurs, the client has progressed from HIV to AIDS (Mayo Clinic, 2012).

Prevalence

The prevalence of allergic diseases in the industrialized world has been on the rise for over 50 years. An estimated 40%–50% of schoolchildren worldwide are sensitized to one or more allergens (AAAAI, 2013). In the United States, an estimated 5% of children under 5 and 4% of people age 5 and older have food allergies. This estimate represents an 18% increase over 10 years (NIAID, 2012). Of these children, female non-Hispanic whites under age 5 are most often affected (Branum & Lukacs, 2008). Allergic reactions range from mild to severe, and the severity of one allergic reaction does not predict the severity of subsequent reactions.

Approximately 8% of the U.S. population is affected by autoimmune disease, and nearly 80% of affected individuals are female. In fact, autoimmune diseases are one of the leading causes of death in young and middle-aged women. Lupus is one of the most common autoimmune diseases, affecting 1.5 million Americans; 90% of these individuals are women, with African American, Hispanic, Native American, and Asian women affected more often than White women. Rheumatoid arthritis, multiple sclerosis, and scleroderma are also common and tend to affect more women than men (NIAID, 2012).

Roughly 29,000 organ and tissue transplants are performed in the United States each year; the prevalence of transplant rejection is difficult to determine, however, because rejection can occur long after transplantation (Immune Tolerance Network, 2012). Finding a perfect tissue match is difficult because the odds of two individuals having identical antigens are roughly 1 in 100,000 (NIAID, 2012). As a result, all transplant recipients receive lifelong antirejection therapies in the form of immunosuppressive medications. These drugs work by suppressing the immune system, putting the transplant recipient at risk of serious infections and malignancies. When these drugs are discontinued, organs are at risk of rejection—even years after transplantation.

Primary immune deficiencies affect about 500,000 people in the United States (NIAID, 2012). Secondary immune deficiencies are much more common that primary deficiencies (Chinratanapisit, 2008). This category includes the 1.1 million people in the United States with HIV or AIDS; globally this number exceeds 34 million (NIAID, 2012). Regardless of type, immune deficiencies are debilitating, and morbidity and mortality rates for affected individuals are high.

Genetic Considerations and Nonmodifiable Risk Factors

Genetics is a key component in a number of immune disorders and deficiencies. Evidence suggests that children are at increased likelihood of developing sensitivities to certain allergens if their parents or older siblings are allergic. Children are also more prone to developing allergies in general if one or both of their parents have allergies (AAP, 2012a). Autoimmune diseases are also due—in part—to a genetic predisposition in conjunction with the presence of an environmental trigger (AARDA & NCAPG, 2011). Inherited genetic mutations are the cause of primary immune deficiencies, though secondary immune deficiencies do not have a genetic component (NIAID, 2012). Genetic counseling is recommended for clients with primary immune deficiencies who are considering becoming pregnant.

Gender is also an important factor in immune disease, and a number of conditions are more prevalent in women than in men; this is particularly evident in autoimmune disease. The explanation for this prevalence is unclear, though evidence suggests that estrogen can increase the immune response. Additionally, some autoimmune diseases may be triggered by pregnancy; interestingly, pregnancy can cause some autoimmune diseases to go into remission (AARDA & NCAPG, 2011).

Age is another nonmodifiable risk factor for some immune diseases, most notably secondary immune deficiencies. As individuals age, they are more likely to be exposed to the stress, environmental factors, and bodily insults that lead to these conditions. People over age 55 are also more prone to transplantation problems that can contribute to organ or tissue rejection (Tjang et al., 2008). It also appears that race may play a role in transplantation rejection: African Americans experience higher rejection rates than Whites. Research suggests that this increased rate is linked to a higher B cell count in African Americans (Johns Hopkins Medicine, 2008).

African Americans also exhibit an increased prevalence for the autoimmune diseases SLE and scleroderma compared to people of other races. Interestingly, the prevalence of specific autoimmune diseases varies from race to race across diseases. Studies suggest that these differences are tied to a combination of genetics, metabolism, and environmental risk factors more common to one group than to the others (NIHADCC, 2005).

CASE STUDY \\ PART 1

Marisol Jimenez is a 7-year-old Hispanic American female who was diagnosed with a peanut sensitivity as a toddler. She presents at her pediatrician's office at 8:30 Monday morning after her mother, Luisa, called to report that Marisol had developed urticaria and tightness in her throat Sunday night. As the nurse working with Marisol's pediatrician, you conduct an initial assessment and client interview with Marisol and Ms. Jimenez. Ms. Jimenez reports that Marisol developed a similar rash last year after eating peanut butter cookies at a friend's birthday party; the throat tightness is a new symptom, however. Ms. Jimenez limits Marisol's exposure to peanuts, but Marisol's grandmother recently immigrated from Mexico and speaks little English. Ms. Jimenez is having difficulty getting her to understand Marisol's "peanut problems." As a result, the grandmother served Marisol sopapillas fried in peanut oil at dinner last night. Ms. Jimenez has given Marisol two 12.5 mg doses of diphenhydramine (Benadryl) 6 hours apart, one at 2100 hours last night and the other at 0300 this morning, per the doctor's previous instructions for treating Marisol's sensitivity. In the past, her symptoms cleared up after the second dose, but Marisol tells you that the itchiness "just won't stop" and that her throat "feels like something is squeezing it."

You observe patchy red welts on Marisol's face, some of which are irritated and open due to Marisol's scratching. Her lips appear slightly swollen. On assessment of Marisol's vitals, you note that her blood pressure is slightly decreased and her heart rate is rapid. When you auscultate her lungs, you hear faint stridor. The pediatrician orders a corticosteroid injection and albuterol (4 puffs) via inhaler to Marisol, which you administer. Within 15 minutes after administration of the medications, Marisol's lungs are clear to auscultation and her hives appear to be slightly diminished. The doctor instructs Ms. Jimenez to follow up with an allergist for further evaluation of Marisol's allergies.

Clinical Reasoning Questions Level I

1. What symptoms of hypersensitivity does Marisol have?
2. Why might Marisol's blood pressure be low and her heart rate rapid?
3. What age-appropriate education about peanut allergies can you provide Marisol?

Clinical Reasoning Questions Level II

4. What is the priority nursing diagnosis for Marisol at this time?
5. What independent nursing interventions can you perform to help make Marisol more comfortable while she waits for the corticosteroid injection to provide some relief of her discomfort?
6. Given Marisol's history, what is the significance of her respiratory symptoms?

▶ PREVENTION

In terms of the immune system, two types of prevention must be considered: the prevention of immune disorders themselves and the use of vaccines to prevent infectious diseases. Educating people about modifiable risk factors and encouraging routine vaccination are important prevention initiatives aimed at improving the health of the U.S. population. Guidelines addressing modifiable risk factors are not as well defined as those governing vaccination; they are, however, no less important.

Healthy People 2020 is a nationwide effort to identify and eliminate the most serious preventable threats to health. Reducing the number of preventable childhood illnesses is one of the major goals, and nurses are important partners in this effort. The incidences of the following infectious diseases are targeted for elimination or reduction (U.S. Department of Health and Human Services, Office of Disease Prevention, 2010):

- *Elimination.* Rubella and congenital rubella syndrome, and polio.
- *Reduction.* Pertussis, hepatitis A, hepatitis B, hepatitis C, tuberculosis, varicella, *Haemophilus influenzae* type b, measles, mumps, meningococcal diseases, and pneumococcal infections

To accomplish this goal, an effort to increase the numbers of children protected from vaccine-preventable diseases and to monitor immunization status is a national public health initiative. *Healthy People 2020* states important specific goals for the reduction of vaccine-preventable diseases:

- Adequately immunize 80%–90% of U.S. children by 35 months old.
- Adequately immunize 95% of children in kindergarten.
- Adequately immunize 80%–90% of adolescents.
- Have 95% of children younger than 6 years of age participating in a fully operational, population-based immunization registry. By 2017, the registries should meet 27 functional standards that will ensure appropriate delivery of immunizations and enable states or managed-care organizations to monitor the immunization status of their population (Centers for Disease Control and Prevention [CDC], 2012a; U.S. Department of Health and Human Services, Office of Disease Prevention, 2010).

Modifiable Risk Factors

A number of modifiable factors put people at risk of immune disorders across the life span. Nutrition is of particular interest, especially as it relates to the development of food allergies in children. Unlike food intolerance, which is associated with conditions such as celiac disease and lactose intolerance, food allergies are immune-mediated allergic responses. For the individual with a food allergy, sensitization to proteins in certain foods, such as peanuts, triggers the production of IgE antibodies and may progress to anaphylaxis. Research suggest that early introduction of solid foods decreases the likelihood of food sensitization during early childhood (AAP, 2009). There is, however, some debate about the right age at which to introduce certain foods, such as peanuts, eggs, and cow's milk. This debate centers on the question of whether early exposure increases or decreases the likelihood of sensitivity to these common allergens (American College of Allergy, Asthma and Immunology, 2011). Additionally, balanced nutrition in later childhood and adulthood helps the immune system function optimally. Protein-calorie malnutrition and lipid, vitamin, and mineral deficiencies are all believed to impair the immune response (Percival, 2011).

Weight is a factor closely related to nutrition, and research suggests that being either underweight or overweight can be detrimental to the immune system (Murray, Zentner, & Yakimo, 2009). Individuals who are underweight may suffer the nutritional deficiencies discussed earlier. Individuals who are overweight or obese have increased levels of adipose tissue, which increase the risk of developing inflammatory and autoimmune diseases (Federico et al., 2010). Weight loss measures, including diet and exercise, can improve immune function; interestingly, regular moderate exercise alone positively affects immune function (Murray et al., 2009).

Stress is another modifiable risk factor. Chronic stress leads to heightened endocrine response; this response simultaneously suppresses the immune response, which decreases the immune system's ability to respond to threats (Sizemore, 2012). Stress reduction and relaxation techniques may prove beneficial to the immune system of individuals exposed to prolonged stress (Murray et al., 2009).

Alcohol, drug, and cigarette use can also increase susceptibility to immune diseases. These substances act as toxins in the body; these toxins can, in turn, act as environmental triggers for individuals with genetic predisposition to autoimmune disorders. They can also cause damage or alteration to cells and organs that leads to the development of secondary immune disorders. Furthermore, intravenous drug use is a risk factor for HIV among individuals who share needles.

Unprotected vaginal and anal sex with multiple partners is also a key risk factor for HIV. Intravenous drug use and risky sexual behaviors as modifiable risk factors are explored more thoroughly in the exemplar on Human Immunodeficiency Virus and Acquired Immunodeficiency Syndrome in this module.

Immunizations

One of the great breakthroughs of modern medicine has been the development and widespread availability of vaccines. The average infant born today receives immunizations for 16 diseases during childhood. Diseases for which vaccines are routinely recommended are measles, mumps, rubella, polio, pertussis (whooping cough), diphtheria, tetanus, *Haemophilus influenzae* type b, hepatitis A and B, pneumococcus, varicella (chickenpox), and influenza. In 2006 and 2008, new rotavirus vaccines were approved for administration to infants. In addition, vaccines have been developed recently for older children, adolescents, and adults to protect against pertussis, meningococcus, human papillomavirus, and shingles. Administering these vaccines greatly improves health and reduces the familial burden of caring for ill children and older relatives.

Immunization introduces an antigen into the body and thus allows immunity against a disease to develop naturally. The immunized individual then produces antibodies in response to the antigens. In **active immunity** (which stimulates antibody production without causing clinical disease), an antigen is given in the form of a **vaccine**. Information about each immunization commonly given to children and adults is listed in the Medications feature.

When an individual needs antibodies faster than the body can develop them, **passive immunity** may be induced. In this approach, antibodies are produced in another human or animal host and then given to the child. This approach also is used with at-risk individuals after a single exposure to a disease, in an attempt to prevent the disease from occurring or to reduce its severity. For example, if a child who has never had a tetanus immunization steps on a rusty nail, the child needs immediate protection (passive immunity) from tetanus. Tetanus immunoglobulin is given by injection to combat the tetanus toxin produced when bacterial spores are introduced by the nail. Passive immunity does not confer lasting immunity. So, the tetanus toxoid vaccine also is administered to start the process of antibody development (active immunity).

TYPES OF VACCINES

Types of vaccines used in the United States include the following:

- **Killed virus vaccine.** A vaccine that contains a microorganism that has been killed but is still capable of inducing the human body to produce antibodies (e.g., inactivated poliovirus vaccine).
- **Toxoid.** A toxin that has been treated (by heat or chemical) to weaken its toxic effects but retain its antigenicity (e.g., tetanus toxoid).
- **Live virus vaccine.** A vaccine that contains a microorganism in live but attenuated (weakened) form (e.g., measles and varicella vaccines).
- **Recombinant forms.** An organism that has been genetically altered for use in vaccines (e.g., hepatitis B and acellular pertussis vaccine, which uses proteins from pertussis rather than the whole cell to stimulate the process of active immunity).
- **Conjugated forms.** An altered organism joined with another substance to increase the immune response (e.g., *Haemophilus influenzae* type b vaccine is conjugated with a protein carrier like tetanus toxoid; however, this specific vaccine brand confers no immunity to tetanus).

Improvements in vaccine technology continue to increase the safety and efficacy of immunization against an increasing number of diseases. Today's vaccines often are produced synthetically by means of recombinant DNA technology or genetic engineering.

SAFETY ALERT
Thimerosal, a bacteriostatic agent that contains ethyl mercury, was previously used to prevent contamination of vaccines in multidose vials. Because of the possible association between mercury poisoning and nerve and brain damage, vaccine manufacturers worked to remove thimerosal from vaccines. Many vaccines now have either no thimerosal or only trace amounts (U.S. Food and Drug Administration, 2012).

RESPONSES TO VACCINES Individuals who have received vaccines may have a variety of responses as the body responds to the injected antigen stimulating the immune system. Depending on the specific immunization, up to 50% of vaccine recipients have a local reaction that includes erythema, swelling, pain, and induration at the site of the injection. Systemic reactions that often occur include fever, fussiness or irritability, malaise, and loss of appetite. With some vaccines, other systemic reactions include a rash or arthralgia. The nurse provides guidelines for managing expected mild reactions at home and makes sure clients or their parents have the correct dosage information for the acetaminophen or ibuprofen formulation that is in the home.

Other serious reactions to vaccines occur in rare instances, for which the National Vaccine Injury Compensation Program was established. The range of illnesses and disabilities that may occur include anaphylaxis, encephalopathy, bacterial neuritis, chronic arthritis, thrombocytopenia purpura, and death. Each of these reactions is a reportable event.

Local allergic reactions, such as a wheal and urticaria, can occur in minutes to hours after the injection. A severe local allergic reaction is manifested by warmth, erythema, edema, petechiae, or ulceration occurring 2–8 hours after vaccination. A non-life-threatening systemic allergic reaction, such as generalized urticaria or transient petechiae, may occur within minutes. Anaphylaxis is a life-threatening allergic reaction that may result in shock and death. Its manifestations include hypotension, generalized urticaria, and angioedema. Laryngeal edema has occurred in rare cases with nearly every vaccine.

SAFETY ALERT
Be prepared for potential vaccine anaphylaxis and keep epinephrine (1:1,000) and resuscitation equipment immediately available. The standard dose for epinephrine (aqueous 1:1,000) is 0.01 mg/kg body weight, up to 0.3 mg maximum single dose in children and 0.5 mg maximum single dose in adolescents intramuscularly. The dose can be repeated every 10–15 minutes, up to a total of three doses, until symptoms subside or other emergency care interventions are initiated (Immunization Action Coalition, 2011).

IMMUNIZATION SCHEDULE The recommended schedule for immunization is updated at least annually to reflect new vaccines and the need for repeat immunization. The Advisory Committee on Immunization Practices (ACIP) of the CDC, the American Academy of Pediatrics (AAP), and the American Academy of Family Practitioners (AAFP) collaborate to provide a uniform vaccination schedule. The ACIP publishes vaccination schedules for children, adolescents, and adults in both a technical edition for healthcare professionals and an easy-to-read edition for laypeople. Immunization schedules take the form of charts that show the ages at which common vaccines are recommended.

Stay Current: *To view the most current technical and lay immunization schedules for children and adults, visit the CDC's Web site at* **http://www.cdc.gov/vaccines/schedules/index.html** *and the ACIP Web site at* **http://www.cdc.gov/vaccines/acip/index.html***.*

Children (Birth to 18 Years) Vaccines should be administered to children at specific ages and intervals. The timing for first immunizations is determined by the age at which **transplacental immunity** (passive immunity transferred from mother to infant) decreases or disappears and the age at which the infant or child develops the ability to make antibodies in response to the vaccine. Most vaccines for infants and children are started between the age of 2 and 18 months, depending on the vaccine. If vaccines are not given at the recommended age, catch-up immunizations can be given throughout childhood and into adolescence as needed. Current vaccines specifically recommended to begin in adolescence include papillomavirus vaccine (for both males and females) and meningococcal vaccine (CDC, 2013c).

Scientists also continue to study the duration of protection from vaccines. Some do not confer lifelong immunity. For example, it was determined recently that a second dose of varicella vaccine is necessary for immunity (CDC, 2012b). Many other childhood vaccines require multiple doses as well, including DTaP (diphtheria, tetanus, pertussis), pneumococcal vaccine, MMR (measles, mumps, rubella), and hepatitis A and B vaccines.

Adults Immunization recommendations for adults include boosters of childhood vaccines (e.g., MMR, TDaP), annual vaccines (e.g., influenza), vaccines for older adults (e.g., zoster), and immunizations for individuals at high risk of infection. The CDC recommends that many adult vaccinations, such as HPV and hepatitis A and C, be administered via a multiple-dose series, like in childhood vaccinations. In addition, some immunizations are contraindicated in specific populations, especially during pregnancy or in immunocompromised individuals (CDC, 2013d).

CONTRAINDICATIONS Contraindications for immunizations may include an acute illness with high fever, a hypersensitivity reaction to specific vaccine components, immunoglobulin therapy in the last 3–6 months, cancer treatment, and pregnancy (AAP, 2012b).

PARENT EDUCATION AND INFORMED CONSENT An increasing number of parents are choosing not to immunize their children for philosophical reasons. The following are some of these reasons (Whyte, Whyte, & Cormier, 2011):

- Concerns that overloading the immune system with multiple antigens at a young age is dangerous.
- Doubts about the efficacy of vaccines.
- Lack of confidence in government immunization recommendations and vaccine testing.
- Belief that "herd immunity" of vaccinated children will protect their child.
- Fear that adverse immunization side effects are more likely than contraction of vaccine-preventable diseases.
- Previous negative vaccine reactions in family members or friends.
- Belief that the unnatural immunity provided by vaccines compromises the immune system.

All healthcare providers should be consistent in their message about the value of vaccines and should provide parents with an opportunity to have their questions answered before giving consent for immunization. It is important to understand that parents want to protect their child both from diseases and from any potential harm caused by vaccines. Legislation requiring parental consent for vaccine administration is controlled at the state level and varies from state to state. The federal government, however, requires that Vaccine Information Statements (VISs) be given to parents or guardians prior to the vaccination of a minor (English et al., 2008). These statements explain the benefits and risks of a vaccine.

In most healthcare settings, the nurse is responsible for informing the parents or the child's legal guardian, supplying literature, and obtaining written consent before the vaccine is administered. The nurse has a legal obligation to ensure that consent is obtained from an individual who has the legal authority to give consent. The nurse also has the responsibility to make sure that the most current VIS is provided to the parents about the vaccines to be administered. When teaching about immunizations, make sure that the parents understand the information in the VIS, and answer any questions the parents might have. Identify the vaccines to be given at this visit and on the next visit so that the parents know their child's immunization status. It may save time to give parents the VIS about the next vaccines to take home and review before the next visit.

Discuss vaccine risks and benefits with parents. Parents often hear sensational stories about the consequences of vaccines, so correct information is needed to help them make informed decisions. For example, studies have repeatedly failed to find a relationship between the measles–mumps–rubella vaccine and the development of autism (AAP, 2012b). Other studies have not revealed a relationship between vaccines and disorders such as asthma (Destefano et al., 2002), inflammatory bowel disease (B. Taylor et al., 2002), sudden infant death syndrome (CDC, 2010), and type 1 diabetes mellitus (CDC, 2012c). Despite the lack of evidence, much misinformation has been provided in the media, and parents sometimes come to conclusions about vaccines based on poor information.

Parents have the right to refuse immunizations, but if a disease outbreak occurs, the nonimmunized child must be kept out of child care or school. If the parent chooses not to have the child receive a particular vaccine, document an informed refusal. Forms for documenting refusal to vaccinate can be found online.

▶ ASSESSMENT

Unlike body systems that are composed of a few closely related organs, the immune system is diverse and scattered. Optimal immune function depends on intact skin and mucous membrane barriers, adequate blood cell production and differentiation, a functional system of lymphatics and the spleen, and the ability to differentiate foreign tissue and pathogens from normal body tissue and flora. Because of this diversity of organs and functions, assessment of the immune system often is integrated throughout the health history and physical examination.

Assessment Interview **Immunity**

- When were you last immunized for diphtheria, tetanus, poliomyelitis, rubella, measles, influenza, hepatitis, and pneumococcal pneumonia? Do you have a record of your immunizations?
- When did you last have a tuberculin skin test?
- What infections have you had in the past, and how were these treated?
- Have any of these infections recurred?
- Are you taking any antibiotics; anti-inflammatory medications, such as aspirin or ibuprofen; or medications for cancer?

- Have you had any recent invasive procedures or radiological examinations?
- Do you have any allergies to food, medications, or any other substance, such as latex, bees, or pollen? If so, what happens when you come in contact with this substance?
- On a scale of 1 to 10, how would you rate the stress you have experienced during the last 6 months?
- Do you have any chronic conditions?

Nursing Assessment

Before conducting the interview, the nurse reviews the client's biographical data, including age, sex, race, and ethnic background. This information can provide valuable clues about possible immunological disorders. For example, many autoimmune disorders are more prevalent in women than in men, and epidemiological data show that certain social and racial groups have particular risks for HIV infection. Family history also is important, because the etiology of many disorders affecting the immune system includes a genetic component.

Many interview questions related to the immune system and the disorders that affect it are of a sensitive nature. Be sure to provide privacy for the interview. If family members are present, request that they leave as well. Establish a trusting relationship with the client before asking the most sensitive questions (e.g., those related to the use of illicit drugs or sexual activity).

As with all history taking, the nurse must individualize the specific terms used, the examples given the client, and the teaching techniques used to validate agreement on the meaning of words according to the client's culture, language, and education or intellectual abilities. Cultural competence is necessary for effective communication.

The techniques of inspection and palpation are especially important in assessing a client's immune system:

- Assess the general appearance, and note whether the client's stated and apparent age coincide. Assess height, weight, and body type for apparent weight loss or wasting.
- Check vital signs. An elevated temperature may indicate an infection or inflammatory response.
- Inspect the mucous membranes of the nose and mouth for color and condition. Pale, boggy (edematous) nasal mucosa often is associated with chronic allergies. Petechiae, white patches, or lacy white plaques in the oral mucosa may indicate hemolysis or immunodeficiency.
- Assess skin color, temperature, and moisture. Pale or jaundiced skin may indicate a hemolytic reaction. Pallor also may indicate bone marrow suppression with accompanying immunodeficiency.
- Inspect the skin for evidence of rashes or lesions, such as petechiae, numerous bruises, purple or blue patches or lesions indicative of Kaposi sarcoma, and wounds that are infected, inflamed, or unhealed. Note the location and distribution of any rashes or lesions.
- Inspect and palpate the cervical lymph nodes for evidence of lymphadenopathy (swelling) or tenderness. Palpate the nodes of the axillae and groin as well (**Figure 8–6** ●).

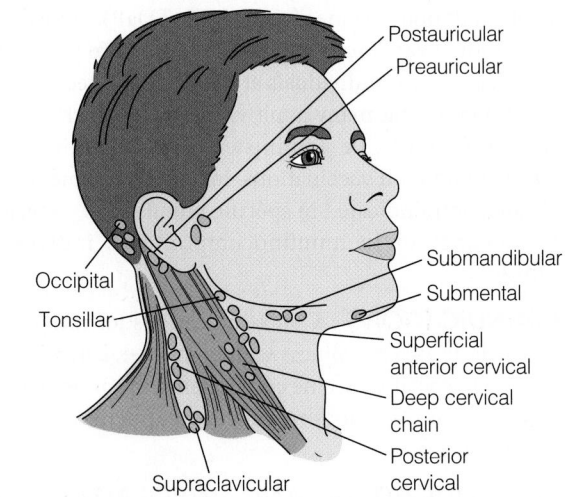

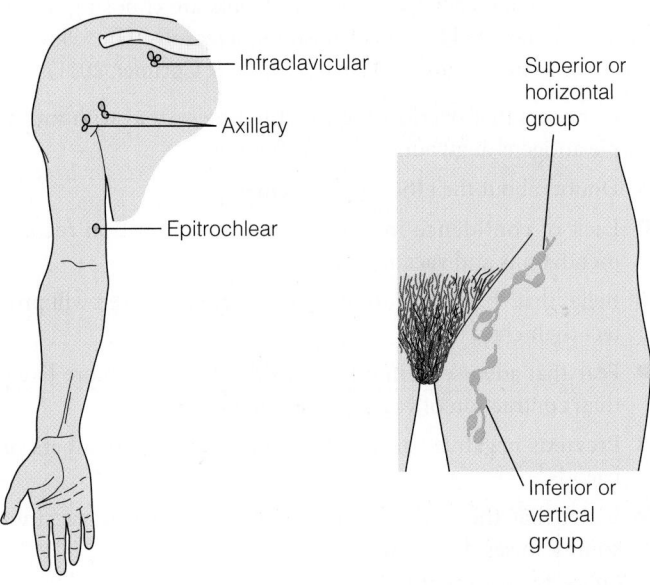

Figure 8–6 ● Lymph nodes that can be assessed by palpation.

Immune System Assessments

ASSESSMENT/METHOD	NORMAL FINDINGS	ABNORMAL FINDINGS	LIFESPAN OR DEVELOPMENTAL CONSIDERATIONS
Family History			
Review history of allergy in family members. Review history of HIV or immune disorder in mother and other family members.	Lack of history eliminates primary immune deficiencies and may also eliminate other disorders that run in families or have a congenital component.	■ Increased likelihood of allergies if parents have allergies. ■ Maternal HIV is indicative of prophylactic treatment in the child.	■ Parents or guardians may provide history for children and adolescents.
Growth and Development (Children)			
Plot height and weight during each visit. Assess appetite and eating habits. Assess achievement of developmental milestones.	Growth and weight gain are steady. Appetite is healthy and normal amounts of food are consumed for age. Development is appropriate for age.	■ Delayed growth ■ Failure to thrive ■ Lack of appetite ■ Lethargy ■ Lack of energy ■ Delayed development	■ Developmental delays in toddlers may be secondary to serious illness.
Skin and Mucous Membranes			
Examine skin and mucous membranes for lesions and other injuries	Skin and mucous membranes are intact. When lesions and injury occur, they heal quickly without additional infection.	■ Frequent and easy bruising ■ Slow healing ■ Frequent infection ■ Frequent allergic response	■ Physiological changes of age increase older adults' susceptibility to skin disorders.
Evidence of Disease			
Assess for frequency and type of infections. Assess respiratory function.	Infection occurs infrequently. When infection does occur, causes are common and easily treatable.	■ Frequent infection ■ Infection caused by unusual or uncommon infectious agents ■ Respiratory infection ■ Untreatable ear infection	■ Ear infections are common among preschool age children.

■ Assess the musculoskeletal system by inspecting and palpating the joints for redness, swelling, tenderness, or deformity. Such changes may indicate an autoimmune disorder, such as rheumatoid arthritis or systemic lupus erythematosus.

■ Check joint range of motion (ROM), including that of the spine. Observe ease of movement, and note any evident stiffness or difficulty moving. Evident fatigue or weakness may indicate acute or chronic illness or immunodeficiency.

Diagnostic Tests

Diagnostic and laboratory tests are ordered specific to the type of immune disorder that is suspected. Possible tests are

■ Enzyme immunoassay and enzyme-linked immunosorbent assay

■ Immunoglobulins

■ Polymerase chain reaction

■ Rapid HIV tests

■ Radioallergosorbent test

■ Skin reactions

■ Western blot test

■ Complete blood count (CBC)

■ Complement.

✳ Go to **nursing.pearsonhighered.com** to see Appendix B for information on diagnostic values and laboratory tests.

CASE STUDY \\ PART 2

Marisol Jimenez recovered from her hypersensitivity reaction quickly. After discharge, several months passed during which she was not exposed to peanuts or peanut products. Then, late in the school year, Marisol's class went on a field trip and the children brought picnic lunches. Marisol was not happy about the turkey sandwich in her lunch, so she traded it with a friend for what she thought was a jelly sandwich. However, the sandwich had both peanut butter and jelly in it. After a couple of bites, Marisol's throat swelled shut and she began gasping for air. Her friend alerted the teacher, who called 911.

Marisol was transported to the emergency department, where you are the admitting nurse. The paramedics give you their field report: 7-year-old female with an anaphylactic reaction to peanut butter. Vital signs include a heart rate of 115; respiratory rate of 29 breaths per minute; blood pressure 85/50 mmHg; and temperature within normal limits. Paramedics administered 0.20 mL (1:1,000) epinephrine intramuscularly and 10 L oxygen by face mask en route to the hospital. Initial pulse oximeter readings were 91% but improved to 95% with oxygen. Marisol is continued on 10 L oxygen by face mask in the ED, and she is given 115 mg of intravenous hydrocortisone. She is aware of her surroundings and resting comfortably, but she is very scared and asking for her mother. You are called away to another client, and you ask a hospital volunteer to sit with Marisol and keep her calm until Ms. Jimenez arrives.

Thirty minutes later, the volunteer calls you back to Marisol's room. Marisol is suddenly having difficulty breathing, her skin has become very pale, and she is confused. You perform a respiratory assessment and note significant stridor. Pulse oximeter readings have fallen to 90%. Because of Marisol's respiratory distress and declining level of consciousness, the physician decides to intubate.

Clinical Reasoning Questions Level I

1. What might be the reason behind the sudden deterioration of Marisol's condition?

2. What independent interventions can you perform to help ease Marisol's fears?

3. Why did the paramedics administer epinephrine to Marisol?

Clinical Reasoning Questions Level II

4. Why is Marisol given hydrocortisone after her arrival at the hospital?

5. *Referring to the concept of acid–base balance:* Would a blood gas analysis be useful in Marisol's case? Why or why not?

6. *Referring to the concept of oxygenation:* What does Marisol's 91% pulse oximeter rating reflect? What is the relationship between Marisol's breath sounds and her pulse oximetry measurements?

▶ INTERVENTIONS AND THERAPIES

The immune system is affected by both physical and psychological factors. These factors inform both independent nursing care and the collaborative efforts of the interdisciplinary healthcare team. While vaccinations and other pharmacologic agents can be crucial to promoting a healthy immune system, lifestyle factors also have a significant impact on immune function.

Independent

Simple as it may sound, proper nutrition, adequate exercise, and a good night's sleep are profoundly important in maintaining an effective immune system. Stress reduction and stress management also play a role. As respiratory and musculoskeletal efforts increase with exercise, and as gravity is enlisted with postural changes, lymph fluid is more efficiently pumped from tissues into lymph capillaries and vessels throughout the body. Circulation through lymph nodes, where destruction of pathogens and removal of foreign antigens can occur, also improves with exercise. Research in older adults has shown benefits of moderate exercise on NK cell function, circulating T-cell function, and cytokine production, potentially increasing resistance

to viral infections and preventing formation of malignant cells (Romeo et al., 2010). While moderate exercise seems to enhance immunity, strenuous exercise may reduce immune function, leaving a window of opportunity for infection during the recovery phase. Adequate rest is important after vigorous training to allow the body to recover (Gleeson & Walsh, 2012). Nursing interventions should include educating the client about how lifestyle can affect immune function. The nurse should also help the client identify and set goals for implementing healthy lifestyle changes.

Collaborative

The goals of medical management are to restore immune function and to prevent further stress on the immune system. Treatment may be supportive for those with only mild manifestations.

PHARMACOLOGIC THERAPY Anti-inflammatories, such as NSAIDs and corticosteroids, are a staple in the management of alterations in immune function, because pain and swelling are frequent manifestations.

Prevention and prompt treatment of infection are essential. Antibiotic therapy is targeted at infectious agents. Antibiotic prophylaxis and specific immunization recommendations for immunodeficiency are needed. Clients with T-cell deficiencies should receive cytomegalovirus-negative, irradiated blood products because of the risk of infection and graft-versus-host disease posed by lymphocytes in donor blood (Ljungman, Hakki, & Boeckh, 2011). Intravenous immunoglobulin may be administered to provide protection until humoral immunity can be established. Hematopoietic stem cell transplantation may be considered if T-cell function cannot be restored by other methods.

NONPHARMACOLOGIC THERAPY Gene transfer appears promising, and long-term observation of clients suggests that this therapy is safe and effective. The majority of clients experience improved immune function and quality of life (Bersenev & Levine, 2012).

COMPLEMENTARY AND ALTERNATIVE THERAPY Many clients with immune disorders have begun trying complementary and alternative medicine to relieve symptoms. The use of acupuncture in alleviating side effects of antiretroviral medicines has become sufficiently popular that in Massachusetts, clients with AIDS can access acupuncture for free (Community Resources Information, Inc., 2009). Johns Hopkins University reports that therapies such as dietary supplements, hydrotherapy, and acupuncture show promise for treating conditions like rheumatoid arthritis, but that relatively few studies have been done (Haaz, 2008).

Alternative therapies designed to bolster the immune system are of particular interest. These therapies seek to increase antibody production or improve other areas of the immune response; this kind of therapy is sometimes referred to as *immune stimulation*. For example, vitamin A, C, D, and E regimens and plant-based therapies have all been studied for their efficacy as immune stimulants and have shown varying degrees of effectiveness in the treatment of asthma and inflammatory diseases (Mainardi, Kapoor, & Bielory, 2009).

Medications **Immunity**

CLASSIFICATION AND DRUG EXAMPLES	MECHANISM OF ACTION	NURSING CONSIDERATIONS
Antibiotics ■ aminoglycosides ■ macrolides ■ tetracyclines ■ cephalosporins ■ penicillins ■ sulfonomides *Drug examples:* cefaclor, erythromycin, penicillin, tobramycin	May be used prophylactically to prevent infection or to treat existing bacterial infection in immunodeficient clients. Specific antibiotics are chosen based on the infection-causing pathogen. *May also be used for:* ■ treatment of *staphylococcus* infections. ■ prophylaxis for ophthalmia neonatorum.	■ Teach clients the importance of taking the entire prescribed amount. ■ Encourage adequate fluid intake. ■ Monitor for signs of allergic reaction. ■ Assess renal and hepatic function and vital signs. ■ Advise against chewing or crushing tablet.
Anti-inflammatories ■ NSAIDs ■ corticosteroids *Drug examples:* aspirin, ibuprofen, naproxen, oxaprozin, prednisone, hydrocortisone, methylprednisolone	May be used to manage pain and swelling common with immune function alterations. NSAIDs block prostaglandin synthesis that leads to inflammation; corticosteroids modify immune response to various stimuli. *May also be used for:* ■ treatment of fever. ■ prophylaxis for stroke and heart attack.	■ Monitor for signs of allergic reaction and renal problems. ■ Encourage clients to take with a full glass of water, milk, or small snack to avoid GI distress. ■ Assess for blood-clotting problems. ■ Advise against abrupt discontinuation of drugs.
Immunizations *Drug examples:* haemophilus b conjugate vaccine, hepatitis A vaccine, meningococcal diphtheria toxoid conjugate, bacillus Calmette-Guérin vaccine, zoster vaccine live	May be used to provide active or passive immunity to clients with a likelihood of contracting certain illnesses due to immunodeficiency. *May also be used for:* ■ prophylaxis against infectious disease in the general population.	Review specific immunization recommendations for immunodeficiency. ■ Assess for hypersensitivity to the vaccine and its components. ■ Evaluate for advanced immunodeficiency. ■ Monitor for vaccine reaction.

Unfortunately, definitive results about vitamin- and plant-based therapies are difficult to come by because recruiting subjects for clinical trials has proven challenging. Public opinion about these therapies is divisive; as a result, subjects tend to come into trials with either very positive or very negative views of the therapies. These views affect the types of positive or negative results the subjects report and their willingness to follow therapy regimens. In addition, some institutions hesitate to approve clinical trials for alternative therapies due to ethical concerns about client well-being when effective conventional therapies exist (Mainardi et al., 2009).

REVIEW   **The Concept of Immunity**

RELATE Link the Concepts

Linking the concept of immunity with the concept of infection:

1. Describe the physiological response of the immune system to a localized bacterial infection (as in a wound). How is this response different from the response to a systemic bacterial infection?

2. How does the body's immune response to the first exposure to an infectious disease differ from its immune response to a second exposure to that disease? What is the reason for this difference?

Linking the concept of immunity with the concept of development:

3. You are caring for a 4-year-old who was just diagnosed with a type I hypersensitivity to shellfish after experiencing an anaphylactic reaction. How can you explain her condition to her in a developmentally appropriate way? How would your explanation be different if she was 8 years old? If she was 12 years old?

4. What aspects of psychological and psychosocial development should you consider when explaining age-related changes in the immune system to a client in his 60s?

READY Go to Companion Skills Manual

REFER Go to Pearson Student Nursing Resources
nursing.pearsonhighered.com

REFLECT Case Study \\ Part 3

Marisol Jimenez has been hospitalized for 2 days. Within 4 hours of receiving IV epinephrine, aerosolized albuterol, and corticosteroids, she was weaned from the ventilator and extubated. She has experienced no further reactions to her exposure, her airways are no longer swollen, and she is maintaining oxygen saturation of 95% without supplemental oxygenation.

You are preparing Marisol and her mother for discharge. Discharge instructions include a self-injectable form of epinephrine, or EpiPen. You explain that the pen should be used immediately to inject epinephrine into Marisol's thigh muscle if she experiences an anaphylactic episode. Marisol should keep the pen with her at all times and should understand how and when to use it. Ms. Jimenez should inform school officials, including Marisol's teachers and the school nurse, about Marisol's allergy and the fact that she has the EpiPen. Marisol will be followed at home by her allergist. She has a follow up appointment scheduled in 1 week.

Clinical Reasoning Questions Level I

1. What additional client education do you anticipate Ms. Jimenez will need at the follow up appointment?

2. Because of her age, what special educational considerations should be made for Marisol? What challenges do you foresee for a child her age managing a food allergy?

3. What are the priorities for Marisol's care that will decrease her risk of having a severe allergic reaction in the future?

Clinical Reasoning Questions Level II

4. Why is the thigh muscle the optimal injection site for the EpiPen?

5. Does Marisol's peanut allergy put her at increased risk for sensitization to other allergens? If so, which ones?

6. What psychosocial impacts might Marisol and Ms. Jimenez experience as a result of Marisol's allergy?

EXEMPLAR 8.1   Human Immunodeficiency Virus and Acquired Immunodeficiency Syndrome

EXEMPLAR KEY TERMS
AIDS dementia complex, 462
Candidiasis, 463
Epidemic, 456
Helper T cells, 457
Highly active antiretroviral therapy (HAART), 456
Human immunodeficiency virus (HIV), 456
Kaposi sarcoma (KS), 464
Opportunistic infections, 463
Pneumocystis jiroveci pneumonia (PCP), 463
Seroconversion, 457
Toxoplasmosis, 463
Vertical transmission, 459
Virions, 457

EXEMPLAR LEARNING OUTCOMES
After reading about this exemplar, you will be able to:

1. Describe the pathophysiology, etiology, clinical manifestations, and direct and indirect causes of human immunodeficiency virus (HIV) and acquired immunodeficiency syndrome (AIDS).

2. Identify risk factors and prevention methods associated with HIV/AIDS.

3. Illustrate the nursing process in providing culturally competent care across the life span for individuals with HIV/AIDS.

4. Formulate priority nursing diagnoses appropriate for an individual with HIV/AIDS.

5. Summarize therapies used by interdisciplinary teams in the collaborative care of an individual with HIV/AIDS.

6. Plan evidence-based care for an individual with HIV/AIDS and his or her family in collaboration with other members of the healthcare team.

7. Evaluate expected outcomes for an individual with HIV/AIDS.

▶ OVERVIEW

In 1981, 5 cases of *Pneumocystis carinii* pneumonia (PCP) and 26 cases of a rare cancer, Kaposi sarcoma, were diagnosed in young, previously healthy gay men in Los Angeles and New York City. The term *acquired immunodeficiency syndrome (AIDS)* was given to this new phenomenon to describe the immune system deficits associated with these opportunistic disorders. Before this time, both PCP and Kaposi sarcoma had been seen only in older adults, debilitated clients, or those with severe immunodeficiency.

Research to identify the cause of this apparently new disease progressed feverishly, and in 1983 a common antibody was identified in clients with AIDS. In 1984, the **human immunodeficiency virus (HIV)**, a retrovirus (meaning that it carries its genetic information in RNA) that is transmitted by direct contact with infected blood and body fluids, was isolated. It then became apparent that the chronic disease known as AIDS was the final, fatal stage of infection with HIV, which was being spread via sexual contact with carriers of the infection.

Human immunodeficiency virus is an example of an emerging infectious agent that jumped from animal to human, probably in the 1950s. Like so many previous **epidemics** (widespread outbreak of infectious disease with many infected people), the HIV/AIDS epidemic began with a few isolated cases and has now become a worldwide concern. (See the accompanying Focus on Diversity and Culture feature.) The virus invaded our lives in ways we never imagined—testing our scientific knowledge, probing our private values, and eluding a vaccine or a cure. The widespread organ involvement associated with the infection has caused much human suffering and death. Progression of HIV-positive status to AIDS has slowed, however, because of the effectiveness of **highly active antiretroviral therapy (HAART)**, which combines the administration of at least three medications that inhibit HIV replication (CDC, 2013a; World Health Organization, 2013a). The change these medications have caused in HIV's progression to AIDS makes monitoring of AIDS less useful as an indicator of infected cases. For this reason, the CDC has developed new surveillance methods based on infection rates in high-risk populations.

Focus on Diversity and Culture HIV/AIDS

An estimated 34 million people are infected with AIDS worldwide, with virtually every country in the world reporting cases of AIDS (WHO, 2013b). The highest incidence is found in the World Health Organization (WHO) regions of Africa, Southeast Asia, the Americas, and Europe. Approximately 69% of all people who are infected with HIV or who have AIDS live in the WHO African region. The most common mode of transmission globally is heterosexual intercourse. The cofactors of general health status, presence of other sexually transmitted diseases, and number of sexual partners correlate with incidence (CDC, 2012e).

▶ PATHOPHYSIOLOGY AND ETIOLOGY

Acquired immunodeficiency syndrome is caused by HIV (specifically, HIV-1). The best example of a primary immunodeficiency disorder, HIV destroys the body's ability to fight infection.

Significant concentrations of the virus are present in blood, semen, vaginal and cervical secretions, and cerebrospinal fluid of infected individuals. The virus also is found in breast milk and saliva. Sexual contact is the primary mode of transmission. However, HIV can be transmitted through contact with infected blood via needle sharing during drug injection. Before mandatory screening of blood and blood products was instituted in 1985, some individuals received HIV through transfusions of infected blood. Today, rigorous testing of the U.S. blood supply has made transmission via transfusion extremely rare (CDC, 2011a).

On entry into the body, the virus infects cells that have the CD4 antigen. Once inside the cell, the virus sheds its protein coat and uses an enzyme called *reverse transcriptase* to convert the viral RNA to DNA (**Figure 8–7 ●**). This viral DNA is then integrated into host cell DNA and duplicated during normal processes of cell division. Within the cell, the virus may remain latent or become activated to produce new RNA and to form **virions** (virus particles that are unable to grow and reproduce outside a host cell). The virus then buds from the cell surface, disrupting its cell membrane and leading to destruction of the host cell.

Although the virus may remain inactive in infected cells for years, antibodies are produced to its proteins, a process known as **seroconversion**. The antibodies usually are detectable 6 weeks to 6 months after the initial infection. Although helper T or CD4 cells are the primary cells infected by HIV, the virus also infects macrophages and certain cells of the central nervous system (CNS). **Helper T cells** play a vital role in normal function of the immune system, recognizing foreign antigens and infected cells and activating antibody-producing B cells. They also direct cell-mediated immune activity and influence the phagocytic activity of monocytes and macrophages. The loss of these helper T cells leads to the immunodeficiencies seen with HIV infection (Porth & Matfin, 2010). **Figure 8–8 ●** illustrates the typical course of HIV infection.

Etiology

HIV carries a significant impact in the United States: The estimated number of people in the United States infected with HIV from 1981 to 2008 was 1.7 million (U.S. Department of Health and Human Services, 2012). In 2010, an estimated 47,129 new cases of HIV/AIDS were diagnosed in the 46 states with confidential name-based reporting. In 2009, a total of 2,223 U.S. children and teens from birth to 19 years of age were diagnosed with HIV/AIDS (Box 8–2) (CDC, 2011b). Men still make up the majority of infected individuals; women account for approximately 23% (CDC, 2013a). The major transmission categories are identified in **Figure 8–9 ●**. Among females, the majority of HIV infections result from heterosexual contact. African American and Hispanic women accounted for 73% of all new female HIV cases in 2009 (CDC, 2011b).

Current trends of which nurses should be aware include the following:

- Among risk groups, the most rapid increases in recent years have been noted in young gay and bisexual men, women, and inner-city injection drug users, especially African Americans and Hispanics (U.S. Department of Health and Human Services, 2012).

- The rapid increase of AIDS cases among women is of special concern; those numbers increased from 7% of cases in 1985 to 23% of newly reported cases in 2009 (CDC, 2011b).

- The rates of infection have slowed dramatically for children under 13 years, thanks to improved interventions during the perinatal period (CDC, 2011). However, the number of cases in children older than 13 remains a concern because of the increasingly early age of sexual initiation, the prevalence of substance abuse, and that age group's general lack of awareness of the risks associated with HIV/AIDS.

- The number of clients age 50 and older with HIV/AIDS has been increasing in recent years. In 2005, the most recent year for which the CDC has statistics, 15% of new HIV/AIDS diagnoses occurred in this age group. Additionally, 24% of people living with AIDS were 50 years old or older, a significant increase from 2001, when only 17% of affected individuals were in this group. One major reason for this increase is the effectiveness of HAART therapy, which has increased the life expectancy of clients with HIV (CDC, 2008c).

- Current research suggests the possibility of developing a "functional cure" for clients with HIV. Theoretically, a functional cure would suppress viral replication to the point where the symptoms go into remission, even without complete eradication of the virus. Additional research is needed to establish the viability of this emerging treatment approach (Vanham & Van Gulck, 2012).

Risk Factors

The risk factors for HIV infection are primarily behavioral. Other risk factors involve hemophilia and blood transfusions,

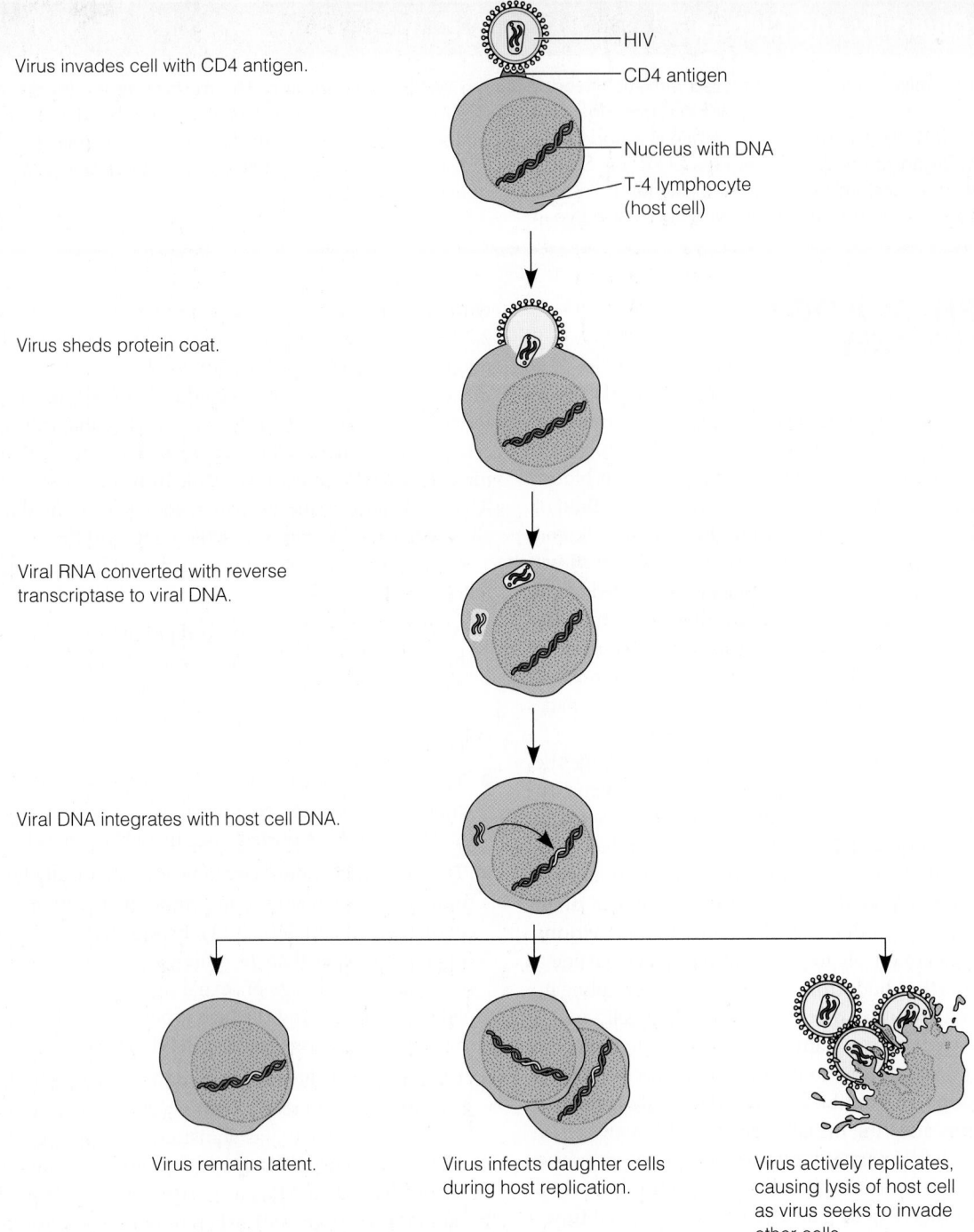

Virus invades cell with CD4 antigen.

HIV
CD4 antigen
Nucleus with DNA
T-4 lymphocyte
(host cell)

Virus sheds protein coat.

Viral RNA converted with reverse
transcriptase to viral DNA.

Viral DNA integrates with host cell DNA.

Virus remains latent.

Virus infects daughter cells
during host replication.

Virus actively replicates,
causing lysis of host cell
as virus seeks to invade
other cells.

Figure 8–7 ● How HIV infects and destroys CD4 cells.

health care as an occupation, poverty, pregnancy and breast-feeding, and older age.

Among adults in the United States, 61% of reported cases are in men who have sex with other men, including gays, bisexuals, and groups such as prison populations. Unprotected anal intercourse is the major route of transmission in these men. Illegal drug use is another risk factor, due to sharing of needles and drug paraphernalia and to the increased likelihood of impaired judgment and risky sexual behaviors while under the influence of drugs (CDC, 2008a). Heterosexual intercourse with an

infected partner and injection drug use are major risk factors for women (CDC, 2011b).

Blood donation poses no risk for the donor of contracting HIV, because only new, sterile equipment is used. In addition, as stated earlier, screening of voluntary blood donors (a process that generally excludes people with high-risk behavior) and of donated blood supplies has reduced the risk for transmission of HIV by transfusion to 1 in 1.5 million (CDC, 2011a).

Current blood-screening methods use antibody testing, and the small risk of HIV transmission through blood supplies

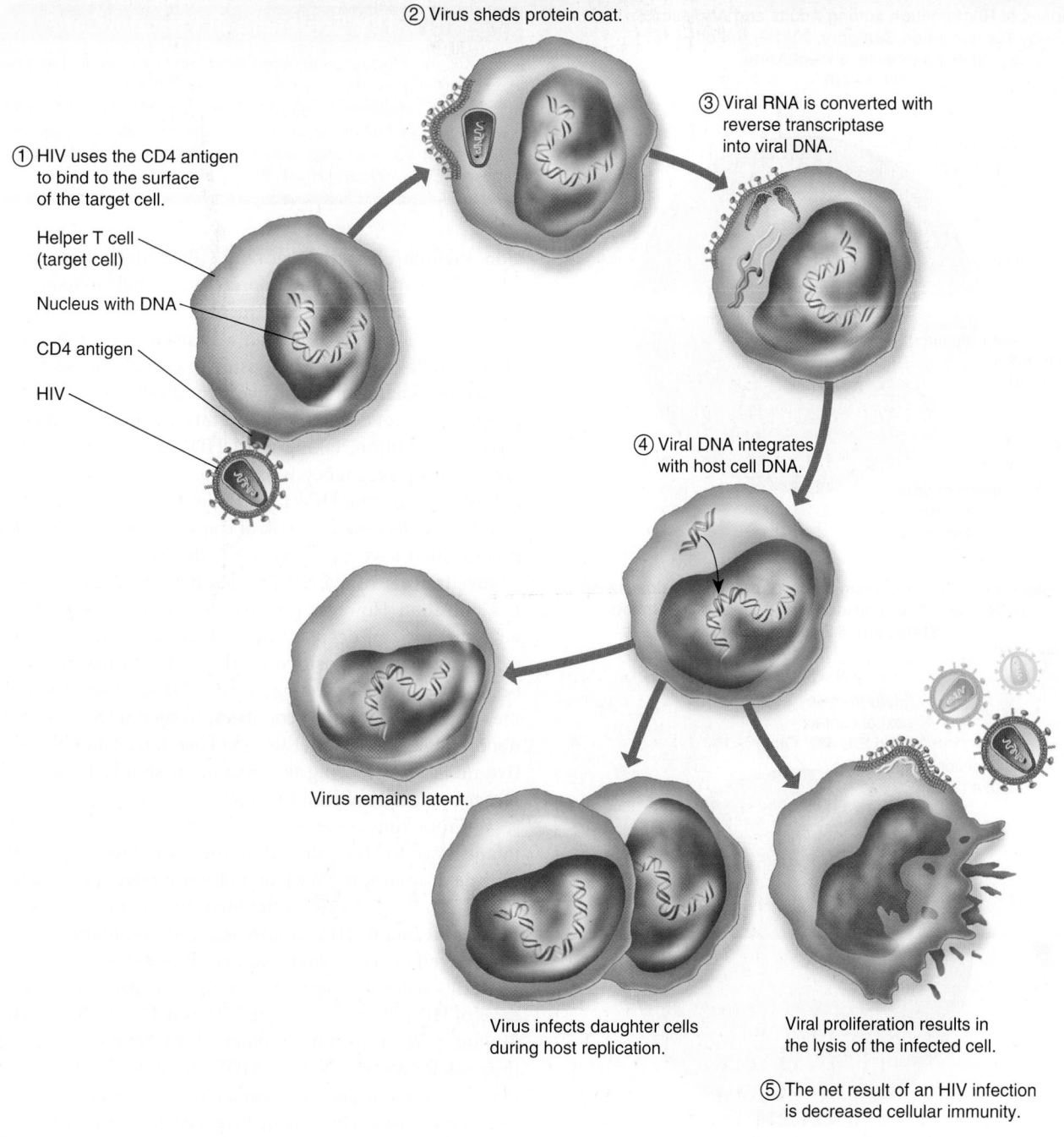

② Virus sheds protein coat.

③ Viral RNA is converted with reverse transcriptase into viral DNA.

① HIV uses the CD4 antigen to bind to the surface of the target cell.

Helper T cell (target cell)

Nucleus with DNA

CD4 antigen

HIV

④ Viral DNA integrates with host cell DNA.

Virus remains latent.

Virus infects daughter cells during host replication.

Viral proliferation results in the lysis of the infected cell.

⑤ The net result of an HIV infection is decreased cellular immunity.

Figure 8–8 ● The HIV virus gains entry into helper T cells, uses the cell DNA to replicate, interferes with normal function of the T cells, and destroys the normal cells.

arises from donors in the so-called window period between contracting the virus and the development of detectable antibodies. This window period usually lasts from 6 weeks to 6 months; rarely, it lasts up to 1 year. Those in the window period are able to transmit HIV to others even though they do not yet test positive for HIV.

A small but real occupational risk exists for healthcare workers. Percutaneous exposure to infected blood or body fluids through a needlestick injury or nonintact skin is the primary route of transmission. Documented evidence indicates that parenteral exposure poses less than a 1% risk of becoming HIV positive (CDC, 2011a). Mucosal exposures, such as splashing in the eyes or mouth, pose a much smaller risk.

Poverty increases an individual's risk for HIV/AIDS. Individuals living in poverty have less access to preventive health care and healthcare education. These individuals also are at risk for illiteracy, making print media and the Internet less effective as health promotion tools. Findings show no significant differences in HIV prevalence by race or ethnicity among low-income urban populations. This finding is surprising considering the racial and ethnic disparities that characterize the U.S. HIV/AIDS epidemic in general (CDC, 2008b).

LIFESPAN CONSIDERATIONS   Infants can acquire HIV by **vertical transmission** from their mothers, either transplacentally or during delivery. Risk factors for perinatal transmis-

Diagnoses of HIV Infection among Adults and Adolescents, by Transmission Category, 2011 — United States and 6 Dependent Areas
N = 50,007

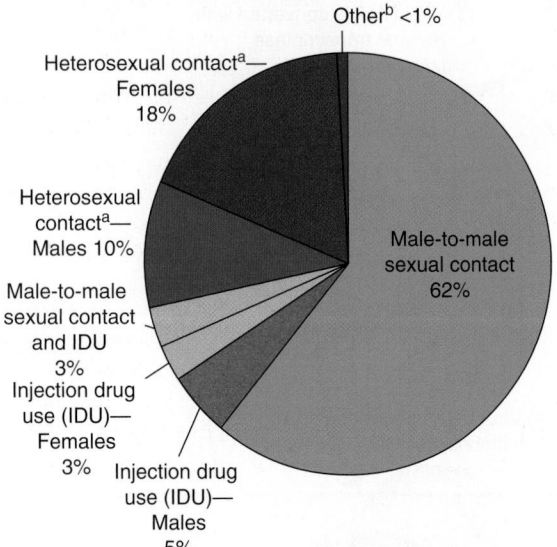

- Other[b] <1%
- Heterosexual contact[a]— Females 18%
- Heterosexual contact[a]— Males 10%
- Male-to-male sexual contact and IDU 3%
- Injection drug use (IDU)— Females 3%
- Injection drug use (IDU)— Males 5%
- Male-to-male sexual contact 62%

Diagnoses of HIV Infection among Adults and Adolescents, by Sex and Transmission Category, 2011 — United States and 6 Dependent Areas
Males
N = 39,495

- Male-to-male sexual contact and IDU 4%
- Injection drug use (IDU) 6%
- Other[b] <1%
- Heterosexual contact[a] 12%
- Male-to-male sexual contact 78%

Females
N = 10,512

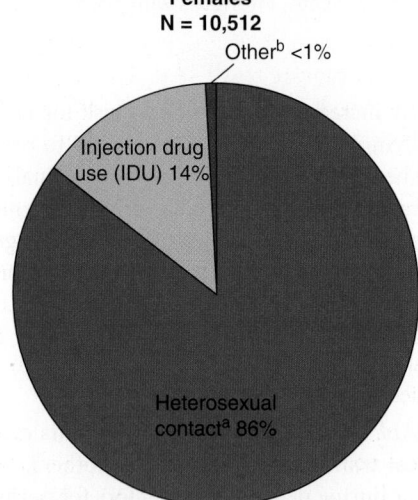

- Other[b] <1%
- Injection drug use (IDU) 14%
- Heterosexual contact[a] 86%

sion include cigarette smoking, illicit drug use, sexually transmitted infections, and unprotected sexual intercourse with multiple partners (U.S. Department of Health and Human Services, 2012). Transmission can also occur during birth from blood, amniotic fluid, and exposure to genital tract secretions.

Asymptomatic pregnant women should be advised that pregnancy is not believed to accelerate the progression of HIV/AIDS. In addition, taking most HIV medications (Retrovir, AZT) during pregnancy is safe and significantly reduces the risk of transmitting HIV-1 to the fetus. Delivery by cesarean section also decreases the risk of transmission. Following birth, infants often have a positive antibody titer, which reflects the passive transfer of maternal antibodies and does not indicate HIV infection. However, prophylactic treatment with antiretroviral therapy can decrease the risk of active infection for all newborns of HIV-positive mothers. Transmission can also occur through breastfeeding (WHO, 2013c). The CDC recommends that in developed countries, women infected with HIV not breastfeed because of this risk. Therefore, if a viable alternative method of feeding is available, it should be used (U.S. Department of Health and Human Services, 2012).

Without these interventions, between 15% and 45% of infants born to HIV-infected mothers are infected perinatally; the rate drops below 2% when mothers receive appropriate care (CDC, 2013b). Because of the high rate of transmission from mother to infant, HIV counseling and voluntary testing are encouraged for all pregnant women (**Box 8–1 ●**).

Adults older than age 50 account for approximately 24% of cases of HIV/AIDS in the United States (CDC, 2008c). Declining immune system function in older adults significantly increases their risk for contracting HIV/AIDS. Older clients who have been in monogamous relationships earlier in their lives often find themselves newly single as a result of divorce or death of a partner; when these clients resume sexual relations, they may not believe they are at risk for HIV and may not take preventive measures, such as using condoms, or may not feel comfortable discussing HIV/AIDS risk or condom use with their new partners. In addition, manifestations of HIV may be overlooked by healthcare professionals or

Figure 8–9 ● Transmission categories of adults and adolescents diagnosed with HIV/AIDS during 2006.
Source: CDC. (2008a). *HIV/AIDS in the United States.* CDC/HIV AIDS Facts. Retrieved from *http://www.cdc.gov/hiv*
Note: Data include persons with a diagnosis of HIV infection regardless of stage of disease at diagnosis. All displayed data have been statistically adjusted to account for reporting delays and missing transmission category, but not for incomplete reporting.
[a]Heterosexual contact with a person known to have, or to be at high risk for, HIV infection.
[b]Includes hemophilia, blood transfusion, perinatal exposure, and risk factor not reported or not identified.

may be attributed to normal age-related physiological changes, an error leading to a delayed diagnosis and increased severity of the disease. As a result of these combined factors, clients in the age group of 50 and over have been called the "invisible population" in terms of HIV prevention (CDC, 2007). Just like their younger counterparts, older clients need to be tested and should know their serostatus and that of their partners. Clients who are uncertain of their risk potential should be counseled to obtain screening.

Prevention

Preventing infection involves preventing new cases of HIV infection, as well as preventing and treating opportunistic infections in clients diagnosed with HIV to prevent the conversion of the virus to AIDS. To date, no safe immunization has been developed to protect against HIV infection. Education, counseling, and behavior modification are the primary tools for AIDS prevention. The benefit of education and behavior modification is evident in the gay male population. The incidence of new HIV infections within this population has declined dramatically in high-prevalence cities. Nurses play a vital role for individuals and communities in providing education about this epidemic and how to prevent infection.

EDUCATION It is important to educate sexually active adolescents and adults about the importance of practicing safe sex and about the ramifications of high-risk sexual behaviors and injecting drugs. In fact, all sexually active individuals need to know how HIV is spread and how to practice safer sex. For guidelines on safer sex, see the exemplar on Responsible Sexual Behaviors in the module on Sexuality. Reducing the number of sexual partners—for example, by entering into and remaining in a long-term, mutually monogamous relationship with an uninfected partner—reduces the risk.

Clients should not engage in unprotected sex, especially if the HIV status of the partner is unknown. Latex condoms have been shown to reduce the risk of transmitting HIV. Their effectiveness is improved when nonoxynol 9, a spermicide, is used for lubrication; however, nonoxynol 9 may cause genital ulcers, which can facilitate HIV transmission. To be effective, condoms must be used with every sexual encounter involving vaginal, oral, or anal intercourse. They also need to be applied and removed properly. A female condom also is available for use. However, the following are the only *totally* safe sex practices:

- No sex
- Long-term, mutually monogamous sexual relations between two uninfected individuals
- Mutual masturbation without direct contact

The most difficult group of high-risk individuals to reach and educate is injection drug users. People in this group should never share needles, syringes, or other drug paraphernalia. Many cities have initiated needle-exchange programs, providing a sterile needle and syringe in return for a used one. A fresh solution of household bleach and water in a 1:10 ratio is effective to clean paraphernalia when sterile supplies are not available. It also is important to teach individuals in this population about safer sex practices, because most heterosexual HIV transmission occurs between injection drug users and their partners.

When possible, nurses provide education regarding the use of autologous transfusion (using the blood clients themselves donate before an anticipated surgery). Seeking donations from family members is not encouraged for several reasons. Family members may have engaged in high-risk behaviors but lie about their risk because of embarrassment or fear of discovery. Furthermore, the family member may have a different blood type or other contraindications to transfusion.

Clients who are HIV positive should refrain from donating blood, organs, or sperm. They should understand the tactics used to avoid exchange of body fluids: not sharing needles or other drug paraphernalia, not sharing razors, and not getting a tattoo. Stress the importance of informing all medical personnel providing direct care (especially anyone performing a dental, surgical, or obstetric procedure) about the diagnosis.

STANDARD PRECAUTIONS Healthcare workers can prevent most exposures to HIV by using standard precautions. Testing to determine HIV status remains voluntary and relies on the use of antibody-screening methods; therefore, it remains impossible to identify every client who is HIV positive. With standard precautions, the healthcare professionals treat all clients alike, eliminating the need to know their HIV status. Treat all high-risk body fluids as if they are infectious, and use barrier precautions to prevent skin, mucous membrane, or percutaneous exposure to these fluids. Also follow standard precautions when caring for newborns of mothers who are HIV positive, as the status of the infant's blood is not known until after discharge. Most institutions recommend that their caregivers wear gloves during all diaper changes and examination of babies. Wear disposable gloves when changing diapers or cleaning the diaper area, especially in the presence of diarrhea, because blood may be in the stool; gloves should be considered part of standard precautions for hospital care (Ball, Bindler, & Cowen, 2012). Table 8–3 ● outlines issues for caregivers of infants who are at risk for HIV/AIDS.

More information about standard precautions can be found in the module on Infection.

POSTEXPOSURE PROPHYLAXIS Healthcare workers exposed to HIV infection or adults who experience a high-risk exposure to HIV may choose postexposure prophylaxis. Risk of exposure for healthcare workers may be through needlesticks or cuts with a sharp object, contact with mucous membrane or nonintact skin, semen, vaginal secretions, and fluids contaminated with visible blood. Other possible risks include cerebrospinal fluid, synovial fluid, and pleural, peritoneal, pericardial, or amniotic fluids.

Some clinicians and facilities recommend prophylactic AZT therapy after exposure by needlestick or splash. However, such therapy must be initiated immediately, and its effectiveness has yet to be established. In 2005, the CDC issued guidelines including recommendations for treatment with HAART, which includes two nucleoside reverse transcriptase inhibitors (NRTIs) for lower risk exposures and the addition of a third drug for higher risk exposure. A 4-week course of treatment is recommended and should be started within 72 hours, but preferably within 2–3 hours of exposure (CDC, 2011a). Counseling and testing are provided to healthcare workers with a documented needlestick exposure.

Stay Current: For up-to-date information on HIV/AIDS prevention, go to the Centers for Disease Control and Prevention at *http://www.cdc.gov/hiv/resources/guidelines/*

TABLE 8–3   Issues for Caregivers of Infants at Risk for HIV/AIDS

Resuscitation	For suctioning use a bulb syringe, mucus extractor, or meconium aspirator with wall suction on low setting. Use masks, goggles, and gloves.
Admission care	To remove blood from baby's skin, as soon as possible after admission give a warm water–mild soap bath using gloves.
Hand washing	Wash hands thoroughly before and after caring for infant. Wash hands immediately if they come in contact with blood or body fluids. Wash hands after removal of gloves.
Gloves	Wear gloves when it is necessary to touch blood or other high-risk fluids. Also wear gloves when handling newborns before and during their initial baths, cord care, eye prophylactics, and vitamin K administration.
Mask, goggle, and gown	These are not routinely needed unless it is necessary to come into contact with placenta or the blood and amniotic fluid on the skin of the newborn.
Needles and syringes	Do not recap or bend used needles; dispose of them in a puncture-resistant plastic container belonging specifically to that baby. After the newborn is discharged discard the container.
Specimens	Double-bag blood and other specimens and/or seal them in an impervious container and label them according to agency protocol.
Equipment and linen	Discard articles contaminated with blood or body fluids or bag them according to isolation or institution protocol.
Body fluid spills	Clean blood and body fluid spills promptly with a solution of 5.25% sodium hypochlorite (household bleach) diluted 1:10 with water. Apply for at least 30 seconds, then wipe after the minimum contact time.
Education and support	Provide education and psychological support for family and staff. Caregivers who avoid contact with a baby at risk or who overdress in unnecessary isolation garb subtly exacerbate an already difficult family situation. Information resources include the National AIDS Hotline (1-800-232-4636).
Exempted personnel	Immunologically compromised staff (pregnant women may be included in this group) and possibly infectious staff members should not care for these infants.

Source: Based on American Academy of Pediatrics, Committee on Pediatric AIDS and Committee on Infectious Diseases. (1999). Issues related to human immuno-deficiency transmission in schools, child care, medical settings, the home, and community. *Pediatrics, 104*(2), 318–324; Mendez, H., & Jule, J. E. (1990). Care of the infant born exposed to AIDS. *Obstetric and Gynecologic Clinics of North America, 17*(3), 637; Krist, A. H., & Crawford-Faucher, A. (2002). Management of newborns exposed to maternal HIV infection. *American Family Physician, 65*(10), 2049–2056.

► CLINICAL MANIFESTATIONS

The clinical manifestations of HIV infection range from no symptoms at all to severe immunodeficiency with multiple opportunistic infections and cancers. It appears that the majority of clients develop an acute, mononucleosis-type illness within days to weeks after contracting the virus. Typical manifestations include fever, sore throat, arthralgias and myalgias, headache, rash, and lymphadenopathy. The client also may experience nausea, vomiting, and abdominal cramping. Clients often attribute this initial manifestation of HIV infection to a common viral illness, such as influenza, upper respiratory infection, or stomach virus. Pathological changes also are noted in the CNS of many infected individuals, although the mechanism of neurological dysfunction is unclear.

Following this acute illness, clients enter a long-lasting, asymptomatic period. Although the virus is present and can be transmitted to others, the infected host has few or no symptoms. The majority of HIV-infected individuals are in this stage of the disease. The length of the asymptomatic period varies widely, but its mean duration is estimated to be 8–10 years.

Some clients with few other symptoms following HIV infection develop persistent generalized lymphadenopathy, defined as enlargement of two or more lymph nodes outside the inguinal chain, with no other illness or condition to account for the lymphadenopathy.

The move from asymptomatic disease or persistent lymphadenopathy to AIDS often is not clearly defined. The client may complain of general malaise, fever, fatigue, night sweats, and involuntary weight loss. Persistent skin dryness and rash may be a problem. Diarrhea is common, as are oral lesions, such as hairy leukoplakia, candidiasis, and gingival inflammation and ulceration. The development of advanced HIV occurs between 10 and 15 years after initial infection; the length of time varies according to the viral load, rate of disease progression, and development of resistance to antiretroviral therapy (World Health Organization, 2013a).

With the development of significant constitutional disease, neurological manifestations, or opportunistic infections or cancers, the client has manifestations that are characteristic of AIDS and a very poor prognosis. HIV/AIDS may be classified with the CDC's case classification system (**Box 8–2 ●**). Under this system, HIV is determined by a positive laboratory test and clinical symptoms that fall into one of four infection stages (stage 1, stage 2, stage 3, and stage unknown). Stages are defined by the severity of infection as determined by T-lymphocyte count, percentage of total lymphocytes, or the presence of an AIDS-defining condition. When T-lymphocyte counts fall below 200/mm^3, T-lymphocyte percentage falls below 14%, or an AIDS-defining condition is documented, the client has stage 3 HIV, or AIDS (CDC, 2008b).

AIDS dementia complex is the most common cause of mental status changes for clients with HIV infection. This dementia results from a direct effect of the virus on the brain and affects cognitive, motor, and behavioral functioning. Fluctuating memory loss, confusion, difficulty concentrating, lethargy, and diminished motor speed are typical manifestations of

Box 8–2   Clinical Staging of Adult HIV Infection

HIV INFECTION, STAGE 1

- Lack of an AIDS-defining condition and either a CD4+ T-lymphocyte count higher than 500/mm^3 or a percentage of total lymphocytes of more than 29%.

HIV INFECTION, STAGE 2

- Lack of an AIDS-defining condition and either CD4+ T-lymphocyte count between 200 and 499/mm^3 or a percentage of total lymphocytes between 14% and 28%.

HIV INFECTION, STAGE 3 (AIDS)

- Presence of an AIDS-defining condition (such as Kaposi sarcoma, PCP, or tuberculosis) or a CD4+ T-lymphocyte count lower than 200/mm^3 or a percentage of total lymphocytes less than 14%.

HIV INFECTION, STAGE UNKNOWN

- No information available about AIDS-defining conditions and no information about CD4+ T-lymphocyte count or percentage.

Source: Based on "Revised surveillance case definitions for HIV infection among adults, adolescents, and children aged <18 months and for HIV infection and AIDS among children aged 18 months to <13 years—United States, 2008. 2008, *MMWR, CDC Recommendations and Reports,* 57(RR 10),* pp. 1–8.

AIDS dementia complex. Clients become apathetic, losing interest in work as well as social and recreational activities. As the complex progresses, the client develops severe dementia with motor disturbances, such as ataxia, tremor, spasticity, incontinence, and paraplegia (Porth & Matfin, 2010).

Infections and lesions that are common in clients with AIDS also may affect the CNS. **Toxoplasmosis** and non-Hodgkin's lymphoma are space-occupying lesions that may cause headache, altered mental status, and neurological deficits. Cryptococcal meningitis and cytomegalovirus infection also are common in people with AIDS. CNS complications have declined with the use of HAART therapy (U.S. Department of Health and Human Services, 2012).

Peripheral nervous system manifestations also are common in clients infected with HIV. Sensory neuropathies with manifestations of numbness, tingling, and pain in the lower extremities affect approximately 30% of clients with AIDS. A Guillain-Barré type of inflammatory demyelinating polyneuropathy can occur as well, resulting in progressive weakness and paralysis.

Opportunistic Infections

Opportunistic infections are the most common manifestations of AIDS and often occur simultaneously. The risk of opportunistic infections is predictable by the T4 or CD4 cell count. The normal CD4 cell count is higher than 1,000/mm^3. When the CD4 count falls below 500/mm^3, manifestations of immunodeficiency develop. With a CD4 count of lower than 200/mm^3, opportunistic infections and cancers are likely.

PNEUMOCYSTIS JIROVECI PNEUMONIA   *Pneumocystis jiroveci* pneumonia (PCP) (previously called *Pneumocystis carinii* pneumonia) is the most common opportunistic infection affecting clients with AIDS and is a common cause of death in clients with AIDS. PCP is caused by a common envi-

ronmental fungus that is not pathogenic in clients with intact immune systems.

The manifestations of PCP are nonspecific and may progress insidiously. Clients often present with fever, cough, dyspnea, tachypnea, and tachycardia. Sputum and complaints of mild chest pain also may be present. Breath sounds initially may be normal. With severe disease, the client may present with cyanosis and significant respiratory distress.

TUBERCULOSIS   Clients with AIDS also may develop tuberculosis. In some clients, active tuberculosis results from reactivation of a previous infection; in others, it is a new, primary disease facilitated by impaired immune function. Rapid progression, diffuse pulmonary infiltrates, and disseminated disease occur more commonly in clients with AIDS.

Clients with pulmonary tuberculosis present with a cough productive of purulent sputum, fever, fatigue, weight loss, and lymphadenopathy. Disseminated disease affects the bone marrow, bone, joints, liver, spleen, cerebrospinal fluid, skin, kidneys, gastrointestinal tract, lymph nodes, brain, and other sites.

CANDIDIASIS   *Candida albicans* infection, or **candidiasis**, is a common, opportunistic fungal infection in clients with AIDS. It usually manifests as oral thrush or esophagitis. Oral thrush presents as white, friable plaques on the buccal mucosa or tongue and, in the client with HIV infection, often is the first indication of progression to AIDS. Clients with esophagitis have difficulty swallowing as well as substernal pain or burning that increases with swallowing. In women with AIDS, vaginal candidiasis is frequent and often recurrent.

MYCOBACTERIUM AVIUM COMPLEX   *Mycobacterium avium* complex (MAC) affects many clients with AIDS and typically occurs late in the course of the disease, when CD4 cell counts are less than 50/mm^3. MAC is more common in women than in men. It is caused by organisms commonly found in food, water, and soil and is a major cause of "wasting syndrome" in individuals with AIDS (**Figure 8–10 ●**).

Manifestations of MAC include chills and fever, weakness, night sweats, abdominal pain and diarrhea, and weight loss. Nearly every organ can be infected, and most people with MAC develop disseminated disease.

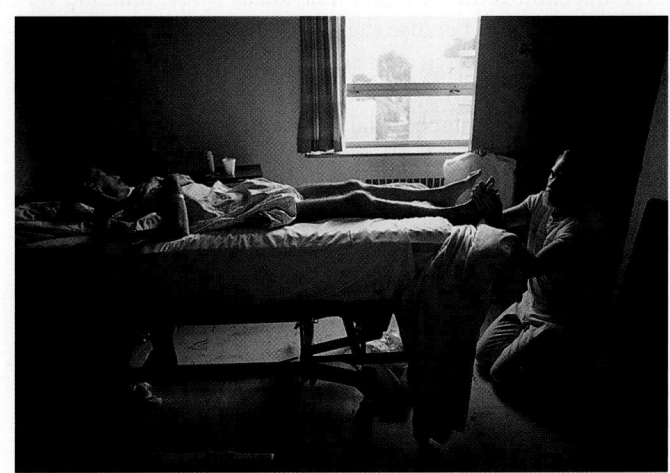

Figure 8–10 ● Wasting syndrome in a client with AIDS.

OTHER INFECTIONS   Herpes virus infections are common in clients with AIDS and may be severe. Cytomegalovirus can affect the retina, gastrointestinal tract, or lungs. Disseminated herpes simplex or herpes zoster infection may occur, although severe mucocutaneous manifestations are more common.

Parasitic infections with *Toxoplasma gondii* and *Cryptococcus neoformans* commonly affect the CNS. Toxoplasmosis occurs as encephalitis or an intracerebral mass lesion. Changes in mental status, focal neurological signs, and seizures may result. *Cryptococcus* infection may present as either meningitis or disseminated disease, primarily affecting the lungs. *Cryptosporidium,* a protozoan affecting the gastrointestinal tract, is an important cause of prolonged diarrhea in clients with AIDS. Bacterial salmonella infections also are a relatively common cause of diarrhea.

Women with AIDS have a high incidence of pelvic inflammatory disease (PID). Although the pathogens appear to be the same as those in PID affecting women who are not infected with HIV, the disease is more severe. Inpatient treatment with intravenous antibiotics often is necessary.

Secondary Cancers

As cell-mediated immune function declines, the risk of malignancy increases. The CDC classification of AIDS currently includes four cancers: Kaposi sarcoma, two lymphomas (non-Hodgkin's lymphoma and primary lymphoma of the brain), and invasive cervical carcinoma.

KAPOSI SARCOMA   Often the presenting symptom of AIDS, **Kaposi sarcoma (KS)** remains the most common cancer associated with the disease. KS may progress slowly or rapidly, and it is an indicator of late-stage HIV disease. The average survival time after diagnosis of KS is 18 months.

Kaposi sarcoma is caused by a virus called the *KS-associated herpesvirus,* also known as *human herpesvirus 8.* This virus appears to be transmitted mainly through sexual contact, although cases have been reported in injection drug users. Men who have sex with men not only have a risk for HIV infection but also have a higher risk for infection with the virus responsible for KS. Women who have sex with these men have a risk for HIV infection and KS as well. Individuals whose immune system is suppressed because they have received an organ transplant also have an increased risk of developing KS (American Cancer Society, 2008).

A tumor of the endothelial cells lining small blood vessels, KS presents as vascular macules, papules, or violet lesions affecting the skin and viscera (**Figure 8–11 ●**). A common site for skin lesions is the face, especially the tip of the nose and pinnae of the ears. Common sites for visceral disease include the gastrointestinal tract, lungs, and lymphatic system.

The lesions of KS usually are painless initially, but they may become painful as the disease progresses. Internally, the tumors may obstruct organ function or cause bleeding. When the lungs are involved, gas exchange may be severely impaired, and the result is pulmonary hemorrhage.

LYMPHOMAS   Lymphomas are malignancies of the lymphoid tissue, including lymphocytes, lymph nodes, and the

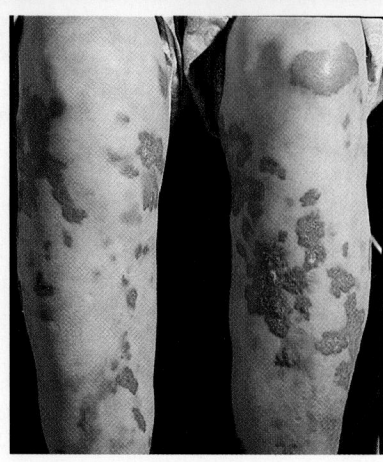

Figure 8–11 ● Kaposi sarcoma lesions.
Source: © Medical-on-Line / Alamy.

lymphoid organs, such as the spleen and bone marrow. In clients with AIDS, two lymphomas are common: non-Hodgkin's lymphoma (including Burkitt lymphoma) and primary lymphoma of the brain. Hodgkin's disease also occurs five times more frequently in clients with HIV infection than in those without. The CNS is the usual site for these lymphomas, but they also may be found in the bone marrow, gastrointestinal tract, liver, skin, and mucous membranes. These malignancies are aggressive tumors that grow and spread rapidly. Headache and changes in mental status are common early symptoms of lymphomas affecting the CNS.

CERVICAL CANCER   Cervical dysplasia is common in women infected with HIV. Cervical cancer develops frequently and tends to be aggressive. Women with concurrent HIV infection and cervical cancer usually die of the cervical cancer, not AIDS. Therefore it is recommended that women with HIV infection have a Papanicolaou (Pap) smear every 6 months and aggressive treatment of cervical dysplasia with colposcopy and conization.

Pediatric Manifestations

The neonate with HIV infection is asymptomatic at birth. The time period for development of opportunistic infections varies; however, the interval from HIV infection to the onset of overt AIDS is shorter in children than in adults. This interval is even shorter in children infected perinatally than in those infected through transfusion.

Opportunistic diseases such as gram-negative sepsis and problems associated with prematurity are the primary causes of mortality in babies infected with HIV. Some infants infected by maternal-fetal transmission suffer from severe immunodeficiency, and HIV disease progresses more rapidly during the first year of life. Many newborns exposed to HIV/AIDS are premature, small for gestational age (SGA), or both and show evidence of failure to thrive during the neonatal and infant periods. They can show signs and symptoms of disease within days of birth. Signs that may be seen during early infancy include enlarged spleen and liver, swollen glands, recurrent respiratory infections, rhinorrhea, interstitial pneumonia (rarely seen in

Clinical Manifestations and Therapies **HIV/AIDS**

ETIOLOGY	CLINICAL MANIFESTATION	CLINICAL THERAPIES
Opportunistic infections result from diminished immune response, including:	Manifestations are dependent on where the infection occurs and on the severity of infection, often related to effectiveness of immune response.	■ Therapy depends on the level of immune function and severity of disease as well as on consideration of comorbid conditions (e.g., liver or kidney disease).
Kaposi sarcoma	Most common AIDS-related cancer, frequently seen in gay and bisexual men, usually manifests as red to purple lesions on the skin but also can be found on internal organs, including the lymph nodes, mouth, GI tract, and lungs. The CDC considers this an AIDS-defining condition.	■ Liposomal daunorubicin, liposomal doxorubicin ■ Recombinant human alpha interferon if CD4 > $200/mm^3$ ■ Radiation therapy
Cytomegalovirus (CMV)	While 50% of adults are infected with CMV, the normal immune system usually can keep it under control. In clients with AIDS and with ineffective immune systems, CMV can infect the eyes, brain, throat, large intestines, stomach, or spinal cord.	■ Preventive therapy or treatment may include administration of cidofovir, ganciclovir, foscarnet, or fomivirsen. ■ Approximately 10% have a strain resistant to ganciclovir.
Candidiasis	The most common HIV-related fungal infection, involving the mucous membranes around the mouth, vagina, esophagus, and skin. Manifests as white bumps, dry mouth, difficulty swallowing, and altered sense of taste. The CDC considers this an AIDS-related complex (ARC) disease.	■ Oral thrush is treated with fluconazole, clotrimazole, ketoconazole, nystatin. ■ Esophageal candidiasis is treated with fluconazole, ketoconazole, itraconazole. ■ Vaginal candidiasis is treated with over-the-counter antifungal remedies, clotrimazole, miconazole.
Aspergillosis	A fungal pathogen found in soil and decaying plant life, more commonly seen in clients with cancer receiving chemotherapy and clients receiving a transplant but may be seen in clients with HIV infection. Manifests with cough, chest pain, shortness of breath, facial pain, fever, and night sweats.	■ Amphotericin B ■ Itraconazole
Histoplasmosis	Infection occurs from inhaling the fungus, infecting the lungs, but can also affect other internal organs. Symptoms include fever, skin lesions, breathing problems, weight loss, and liver enlargement. The CDC considers this an AIDS-defining condition.	■ Clinical trials are under way to study the effect of itraconazole as prophylaxis therapy. ■ Treatment may include amphotericin B or itraconazole and requires long-term maintenance therapy.
Mycobacterium avium complex	In clients who are not HIV positive, this infection normally involves only the lungs, but in clients with HIV infection, the disease usually disseminates and often is seen in those with late-stage AIDS involving the liver, spleen, and bone marrow. Resulting symptoms include night sweats, fevers, unintentional weight loss, diarrhea, low red and white blood cell counts, elevated alkaline phosphate, and painful intestines.	■ Clarithromycin ■ Azithromycin ■ Ethambutol ■ Rifampin ■ Rifabutin ■ Ciprofloxacin ■ Amikacin
Tuberculosis (TB)	Infection occurs from contact with clients who are TB positive and often occurs early in the course of HIV infection, often months or years before other opportunistic infections occur, and may be the first indication of HIV infection. In later stages of HIV infection, TB often infects other organs outside the lungs. Multidrug-resistant TB is of particular concern. Symptoms include cough, fever, night sweats, weight loss, and fatigue.	■ Prophylaxis usually is isoniazid. ■ Treatment may include multiple drugs, including some combination of isoniazid, rifampin, pyrazinamide, and ethambutol.

(continued on next page)

Clinical Manifestations and Therapies **HIV/AIDS** (continued)

ETIOLOGY	CLINICAL MANIFESTATION	CLINICAL THERAPIES
Oral hairy leukoplakia	Often the first opportunistic infection to appear. Symptoms include white lesions on the edges of the tongue caused by Epstein-Barr virus. Occurs almost exclusively in men and indicates serious damage to the immune system. The CDC considers this a category B-defining illness.	■ Acyclovir or topical podophyllin resin
Neurologic disorders seen in some clients diagnosed with HIV/AIDS include:		
AIDS dementia complex	Caused directly by the HIV infection, but the central nervous system also can be damaged by opportunistic infections or toxic effects of drug treatments. Early symptoms include dementia, apathy, and loss of interest in surroundings. Later symptoms involve cognitive and motor problems, resulting in memory loss and mobility issues. The CDC considers HIV encephalopathy an AIDS-defining condition.	■ Zidovudine
Peripheral neuropathy	Severe burning, aching pain in the feet and legs that may prevent walking. Most commonly seen is sensory neuropathy (distal symmetric polyneuropathy). A less frequent but more severe type is acute or chronic inflammatory demyelinating polyneuropathy. Drug-induced or toxic neuropathies can be very painful. CMV-related neurologic syndromes include encephalitis, myelitis, and polyradiculopathy.	■ Acetyl-carnitine from vitamin stores may reduce symptoms.
Gastroesophageal disorders may include:		
Diarrhea	May be caused by infection, lactose intolerance, pancreatic issues, medications, or emotional stress.	■ Avoid diarrhea-causing foods, such as dairy, fatty, or spicy foods and foods high in insoluble fiber. ■ Eat bananas, plain white rice, applesauce, cream of wheat, toasted white bread, crackers, plain pasta, boiled eggs, oatmeal, mashed potatoes, or yogurt. Soluble fiber has been proven to reduce therapy-related diarrhea (Heiser et al., 2004). ■ Over-the-counter products such as l-glutamine, bismuth subsalicylate, attapulgite, or loperamide may help treat the symptoms. Acidophilus capsules, peppermint, ginger, and nutmeg are believed to help with digestive problems. Studies have shown calcium supplements also are helpful.
Malabsorption	Fairly common with advanced AIDS, reduces absorption of nutrients and medications taken orally. Results from gastrointestinal infections and other health problems, causing weight loss, fatigue, anemia, and malnutrition.	■ Careful monitoring of nutritional status, administration of vitamin supplements, increased intake of calories, and administration of IV total parenteral nutrition may help to improve nutritional status.

Source: Adapted from AEGIS. (2006). *Opportunistic infections.* Retrieved from at http://ww1.aegis.org/topics/oi/

Clinical Manifestations and Therapies   Pediatric HIV

ETIOLOGY	CLINICAL MANIFESTATION	CLINICAL THERAPIES
Frequent, chronic, or unusual infections because of poor immune response	Chronic bilateral otitis media Oral candidiasis *Pneumocystis jiroveci* pneumonia Skin disorders Fever	■ Vigorous antimicrobial therapy for treatment of infections ■ Limit exposure to groups of people ■ Obtain recommended immunizations
Poor nutritional intake because of lack of appetite resulting from disease and medications	Failure to thrive (eating disorder of childhood) Weight and body mass index below 10th percentile Chronic diarrhea Skin irritation	■ Monitor growth ■ Supplemental intake such as enteral feedings at night, and total parenteral nutrition (TPN) if needed ■ Meticulous skin care to prevent breakdown
Immune system overgrowth to compensate for lack of proper immune response	Hepatosplenomegaly and lymphadenopathy	■ Assess abdomen frequently. ■ Teach about safe transport to avoid injury to liver and spleen.

adults), recurrent gastrointestinal manifestations (diarrhea and weight loss) and urinary system infections, persistent or recurrent oral candidiasis infections, and loss of achieved developmental milestones (Ball et al., 2012). They also have a high risk of acquiring *Pneumocystis jiroveci* pneumonia.

Most children with AIDS have nonspecific findings, including lymphadenopathy, hepatosplenomegaly, nephropathy, oral candidiasis, failure to thrive and weight loss, diarrhea, chronic eczema and dermatitis, and fever. Specific symptoms often appear within approximately 2 years of infection and include conjunctivitis, ear infections, and tonsillitis.

Bacterial and opportunistic infections, such as *Streptococcus*, *Haemophilus influenzae*, *Salmonella*, and PCP, as well as malignancies, such as lymphoma, frequently occur in children as the disease progresses. Lymphocytic interstitial pneumonitis is a common manifestation of pediatric AIDS, and children often develop encephalopathy, resulting in developmental delay or a deterioration of motor skills and intellectual functioning. Approximately 65% of new cases of HIV in adolescents occur in African Americans, so the teaching of methods to avoid infection must be strongly emphasized in this group (CDC, 2011b).

▶ COLLABORATION

Although multiple research studies are under way to identify a cure for HIV/AIDS, no cure is currently available. This fact and the apparent universally fatal nature of the disease make prevention a vital strategy in HIV care.

The goals of care for the client with HIV disease are as follows:

- Early identification of the infection
- Promotion of health maintenance activities to prolong the asymptomatic period for as long as possible
- Prevention of opportunistic infections
- Treatment of disease complications, such as cancers
- Provision of emotional and psychosocial support

Diagnostic Tests

Diagnostic testing is used to screen and identify HIV infection as well as to monitor the client's disease and immune status. Screening tests should also be administered to women in labor who do not know their HIV status and who received little or no prenatal care. The likelihood that a positive screening test will truly indicate the presence of HIV infection decreases as HIV prevalence in the tested population becomes lower. Therefore, false-positive HIV test results are more likely in settings where the tested population prevalence is lower than in settings where the tested population prevalence is higher. When explaining to clients a positive result from a preliminary rapid diagnostic test, use phrases like "a good chance of being infected" or "very likely infected" to indicate the likelihood of HIV infection, qualified by the HIV prevalence in that particular setting and the client's individual risk.

RAPID DIAGNOSTIC TESTS   Rapid diagnostic tests are widely used because the results can be given immediately (see **Box 8–3** ●). Immediate notification of results is critical, because many clients who are tested for HIV do not return to learn the results. Also, many cannot be located to be given the test results and educated about safe behaviors whether they are positive or negative for HIV. Although confirmation of results requires testing with a second source, such as an enzyme-linked immunosorbent assay or a Western blot test, learning the results immediately gives clients more information to make wise choices about their behaviors and self-care.

Further testing is always required to confirm a reactive or rapid screening test result. The following diagnostic tests may be ordered:

- ***Enzyme-linked immunosorbent assay (ELISA).*** This is the most widely used screening test for HIV infection. ELISA tests for HIV antibodies; it does not detect the virus itself. Therefore, a client may have a negative ELISA test early in

Box 8–3 HIV Testing

Many individuals who are at risk of HIV infection do not have access to regular health care. To reduce barriers to early detection of the virus, rapid HIV tests have been developed. These can be purchased without a prescription over the Internet or through local pharmacies. Specimens are obtained from saliva or fingerstick for a blood sample. Oral fluids are obtained by gently swabbing both the upper and lower outer gum of the mouth. Some options include OraQuick Rapid HIV-1/2 Antibody Test, Reveal Rapid HIV-1 Antibody Test, Uni-Gold Recombigen HIV Test, and Multispot HIV-1/HIV-2 Rapid Test (CDC, 2006d). When these are administered as part of a healthcare interaction, counseling is provided in the same session. Positive results require confirmation through traditional methods. Individuals choosing to test themselves at home are encouraged to follow up with a healthcare provider (U.S. Department of Health and Human Services, 2012).

the course of infection, before detectable antibodies have developed. The test has a sensitivity of 99.5% or higher when performed at least 13 weeks after infection. This means that more than 99.5% of tests performed on blood containing HIV antibodies show a positive result. False-positive results can occur, however; so, an individual who has an initial positive result is always tested repeatedly, and the results are confirmed by use of a different method of antibody detection, usually the Western blot. The enzyme immunoassay (EIA) was developed after the ELISA and works in much the same way as the ELISA. EIA tests that are positive are repeated, and following a second positive test, a Western blot test is performed (Osborn et al., 2013).

- **Western blot antibody testing.** This is more reliable than ELISA but is more time-consuming and more expensive. When it is combined with ELISA, however, a specificity of greater than 99.9% is achieved. Specificity is a measure of the probability that a negative test result indicates no antibodies are present. In this test, the client's serum is mixed with HIV proteins to reveal a reaction. If antibodies to HIV are present, a detectable antigen–antibody response will occur.

- **HIV viral load tests.** These tests measure the amount of actively replicating HIV. Levels correlate with disease progression and with response to antiretroviral medications. Levels higher than 5,000 to 10,000 copies/mL indicate the need for treatment.

- **CBC.** This test is performed to detect anemia, leukopenia, and thrombocytopenia, which often are present in clients with HIV infection. Lymphopenia (low levels of lymphocytes) is especially common in those with this disease.

- **CD4 cell count.** This is the most widely used test to monitor progress of the disease and to guide therapy. The CD4 cell count correlates very closely with the immunodeficiency disorders seen in clients with AIDS. Today, AIDS is defined not only by the presence of opportunistic infections and other diseases indicative of immunodeficiency but also by a CD4 count of less than 200/mm^3 or a percentage of CD4 lymphocytes of less than 14%. CD4 counts are recommended every 3–6 months for all individuals with HIV disease.

OTHER DIAGNOSTIC TESTS In addition to these widely used tests, other tests may be ordered that are both general and specific to the client's manifestations:

- **Tuberculin skin testing** to detect possible tuberculosis infection

- **Magnetic resonance imaging** of the brain to identify lymphomas

- **Specific cultures and serological examinations for opportunistic infections** such as PCP and toxoplasmosis

- **Pap smears** every 6 months for early detection of cervical cancer in women with cervical dysplasia (U.S. Department of Health and Human Services, 2010).

PEDIATRIC TESTING Early identification of babies either with HIV infection or at risk for HIV/AIDS is essential during the newborn period. However, the currently available HIV serological tests (ELISA and Western blot) cannot distinguish between maternal and infant antibodies. It may take up to 18 months for infected infants to form their own antibodies to HIV; therefore these tests are inappropriate for infants before 18 months of age (Ball et al., 2012). HIV DNA polymerase chain reaction (PCR) is the preferred method of testing. A viral culture also may be performed at birth, but this test is more expensive. The first DNA PCR test should be performed on the newborn of a mother with HIV infection during the first 48 hours after birth. However, use of umbilical cord blood for tests can be misleading because HIV-positive umbilical cord blood represents maternal infection. If PCR and viral culture are unavailable, the acid-dissociated p24 antigen may be used to assess HIV infection status in infants older than 1 month (Bernstein, 2007; Cloherty, Eichenwald, & Stark, 2008). A second test should be performed at 1–2 months of age, and a third test is recommended at 2–4 months of age. An infant is considered infected if two separate samples are positive.

When the infant has had two negative tests, testing with ELISA (for HIV antibody) should be done at 12, 15, and 18 months. Most clinicians confirm the absence of HIV infection with a negative HIV antibody assay result at 12–18 months of age (Ball et al., 2012). In addition, a CBC and a CD4 T-cell subset are performed at 3–6 months of age. A quick-response HIV test using saliva is available for use in certain circumstances as well; positive results are checked with blood studies. The CDC considers children under 13 years of age to be infected if their symptoms meet the CDC criteria for AIDS, if they have HIV in their blood or tissues, or if they have antibodies to HIV. The CDC criteria address two issues: the diagnosis of HIV and the clinical classification of children infected with HIV (**Box 8–4 ●**). See the Lifespan Considerations feature for information related to caring for pregnant women with HIV.

Pharmacologic Therapy

As more antiretroviral medications have been developed, a wide array of options has emerged. Highly active antiretroviral therapy (HAART) is a treatment approach that uses a minimum of three antiretroviral agents. It generally includes zidovudine (Retrovir, AZT); an NRTI, plus a second NRTI, such as didanosine or lamivudine; and a nonnucleoside reverse transcriptase

Box 8–4   Clinical Staging of Pediatric HIV Infection

The 1994 Revised HIV Pediatric Classification System remains the standard for determining clinical staging and related treatment for children with HIV. Classifications of children, when infected, are as follows:

- **Category N**—not symptomatic
- **Category A**—mildly symptomatic with two or more of the following:
  - Lymphadenopathy
  - Hepatomegaly
  - Splenomegaly
  - Dermatitis
  - Parotitis
  - Recurrent or persistent upper respiratory infection, sinusitis, or otitis media
- **Category B**—moderately symptomatic with symptoms additional to those previously listed, such as:
  - Anemia
  - Bacterial meningitis, pneumonia, sepsis
  - Candidiasis
  - Cardiomyopathy
  - Cytomegalovirus
  - Diarrhea
  - Hepatitis
  - Herpes simplex virus, herpes zoster
  - Leiomyosarcoma
  - Nephropathy
  - Persistent fever
  - Toxoplasmosis
- **Category C**—severely symptomatic, manifested by:
  - Multiple, recurrent infections
  - Encephalopathy
  - Kaposi sarcoma
  - Lymphoma
  - Wasting syndrome

Source: Adapted from Panel on Antiretroviral Therapy and Medical Management of HIV-Infected Children. *Guidelines for the use of antiretroviral Agents in pediatric HIV infection.* Available at http://aidsinfo.nih.gov/contentfiles/lvguidelines/pediatricguidelines.pdf. Accessed March 26, 2013, pp. E3–E4.

inhibitor (NNRTI), such as nevirapine, or a protease inhibitor (PI), such as indinavir, ritonavir, or saquinavir.

Pharmacologic treatment of HIV disease has four primary foci:

1. To suppress the infection itself, decreasing symptoms and prolonging life
2. To provide prophylaxis of opportunistic infections
3. To stimulate hematopoietic response
4. To treat opportunistic infections and malignancies

SAFETY ALERT

Clients undergoing retroviral therapy are still infectious. Client teaching should include measures to prevent transmission.

Effectiveness of treatment is monitored by viral load and CD4 cell counts; positive results are indicated by a reduction in viral load along with preserving the CD4 count above 350/mm^3. Treatment is recommended when the CD4 count falls below 200/mm^3. Clients with symptoms of severe disease are treated regardless of their CD4 level or viral load, so monitoring these individuals may reveal higher levels of CD4 or lower viral load. Initiating therapy in asymptomatic individuals with higher CD4 levels did not show a protective effect and was thought to perhaps increase viral resistance. Today, in order to help clients adhere to medication administration schedules, the drugs have been combined and the dosing schedules simplified.

Four classes of drugs used in antiretroviral treatment include nucleoside analog reverse-transcriptase inhibitors (NRTIs or NARTIs), nonnucleoside reverse-transcriptase inhibitors (NNRTIs), protease inhibitors (PIs), and entry inhibitors (EIs). HAART combines three or four antiretroviral drugs to reduce the incidence of drug resistance. Combination therapies increase the likelihood of decreasing viral load and symptoms but also burden clients with complicated and expensive medication schedules. Clients beginning the HAART protocol must understand the benefits, risks, costs, and effects on daily life. HAART does not eradicate HIV infection, and the medications are

expensive. Newer triple combinations, such as Trizivir, cost upwards of $1,000 for a 30-day supply of 60 doses, or over $12,000 per year, and this sum does not cover medications to prevent or treat opportunistic infections or cancer. These medications also are scheduled for specific times throughout the day; therefore leading a normal life becomes a challenge. In addition, all HAART medications cause major adverse reactions, leading to less-than-perfect adherence, as with most chronic diseases. In this case, however, the outcome could be fatal.

Each client must be able to adhere to the treatment regimen. It may be preferable to delay therapy until the client can agree to adhere to it, to prevent viral resistance caused by irregular dosing. Some providers gauge client ability to follow the HAART regimen by the client's success with prophylaxis for an opportunistic infection.

Several methods to promote and ensure adherence are being used and studied. One approach uses electronic monitoring devices. Electronic monitoring provides real-time data about the time, date, and frequency of medication dosing. The concept is not new, and there is no guarantee that the medication is actually taken every time the pill container is opened; however, newer generations of the technology have improved the accuracy and usefulness of this kind of tracking. These improved devices include pill box organizers; alarms that alert clients when it is time to take medications; and programmable journals that allow clients to chart medication ingestion, side effects, and symptoms. The transmission of these data to providers via a phone connection makes it easier to detect missed doses and to improve adherence (Haberer et al., 2012).

Some clients undergoing HAART are developing body composition changes and metabolic abnormalities associated with the therapy, especially therapy involving PIs. The body composition changes include increased fat deposition in the midsection, breasts, and neck; atrophy in the face, buttocks, and extremities; and metabolic abnormalities including increased low-density lipoprotein cholesterol and triglycerides as well as insulin resistance. The combination of changes is consistent with metabolic syndrome, which increases the risk of

Medications Antiretroviral Nucleoside Analogues

CLASSIFICATION AND DRUG EXAMPLES	MECHANISM OF ACTION	NURSING CONSIDERATIONS
Zidovudine *Drug examples:* AZT azidothymidine	Zidovudine was the first antiretroviral agent developed to treat HIV infection. It interferes with reverse transcriptase, thus inhibiting replication of the virus. The usual dose is 300 mg twice daily. It is administered orally. Dose-limiting side effects are anemia and neutropenia.	▪ Assess for possible contraindications to therapy, including allergic response or a CD4 count of greater than 350/mm^3. ▪ Administer by mouth, instructing the client to swallow capsules whole. ▪ Assess for adverse effects. Nausea and headache are common. ▪ Assess CBC with differential and creatine phosphokinase. Notify the physician of significant changes. *Health Education for the Client and Family:* ▪ Zidovudine will not cure HIV infection, but it will slow its progress and reduce significant symptoms. ▪ Take the drug at least a half hour before or 1 hour after meals if tolerated. ▪ Notify the physician if signs of an infection or adverse response to zidovudine develop: sore throat, swollen lymph glands, and fever; unusual fatigue or weakness; easy bruising, bleeding gums, or an injury that will not heal; persistent or intractable nausea; and muscle pain or wasting. ▪ Continue all scheduled follow up visits and laboratory studies to monitor for drug toxicity. ▪ Clients should check with the physician before taking any other prescription or over-the-counter drug.
Didanosine *Drug examples:* ddI VIDEX	Like zidovudine, didanosine does not kill HIV; rather, the drug inhibits its replication within the cells. Its activity is similar to that of zidovudine. Didanosine is used alone for clients who are intolerant or resistant to zidovudine. It also is used with zidovudine in combination therapy regimens. Didanosine does not cause the anemia associated with zidovudine, but it may cause neutropenia. Didanosine also is associated with an increased risk of pancreatitis, peripheral neuropathy, and dry mouth.	▪ Assess for possible contraindications, including previous episodes of pancreatitis and impaired renal or liver function. ▪ Administer as directed. ▪ Administer with caution to clients taking vincristine, rifampin, pentamidine, ethambutol, or metronidazole; the action of both drugs may be affected by concurrent administration. Intravenous pentamidine and trimethoprim-sulfamethoxazole taken concurrently may increase the risk of acute and fatal pancreatitis. ▪ Didanosine interferes with the absorption of ketoconazole and dapsone. Doses of these drugs should be scheduled at least 2 hours before or after doses of didanosine. ▪ Evaluate for therapeutic response and possible adverse effects. Notify the physician if manifestations of peripheral neuropathy, diarrhea, depression, or other adverse effects develop. ▪ Stop the drug and notify the physician immediately if the client develops manifestations of pancreatitis or hepatic failure, including nausea and vomiting, severe abdominal pain, elevated bilirubin, or elevated serum enzymes (e.g., amylase, aspartate aminotransferase, and alanine aminotransferase). *Health Education for the Client and Family:* ▪ Take the drug as directed. The prescribed two-tablet dose always must be taken for the amount of antacid required to prevent destruction of the drug by stomach acid. ▪ Take on an empty stomach, at least 1 hour before or 2 hours after meals. ▪ Do not use alcohol while taking didanosine; alcohol may increase the risk of pancreatitis. ▪ Stop the drug and call the doctor immediately if nausea, vomiting, abdominal pain, or diarrhea develops. Any of these may indicate pancreatitis. ▪ Call the doctor if extremity pain, weakness, numbness, or tingling occurs. These side effects usually disappear when didanosine is discontinued. ▪ Other side effects to report to the physician are unusual bleeding or bruising, fatigue, weakness, fever, or persistent sore throat.

Medications **Antiretroviral Nucleoside Analogues** (continued)

CLASSIFICATION AND DRUG EXAMPLES	MECHANISM OF ACTION	NURSING CONSIDERATIONS
Abacavir	Abacavir is a nucleoside analogue that acts against some HIV strains that are resistant to other nucleoside drugs. It is prepared in combination with zidovudine and lamivudine (Trizivir), and one tablet is taken twice daily. This combination drug is composed exclusively of nucleoside analogues; it lacks NNRTIs or PIs. Therefore it is less effective at decreasing viral load and allowing immune system enhancement, but the ease of administration makes it a useful drug for clients who cannot adhere to more complex regimens. The main toxicity is a hypersensitivity response in approximately 5% of clients, which manifests with flulike symptoms. Avoid repeated use in those individuals.	▪ Assess for possible hypersensitivity reactions, anemia, and neutropenia. ▪ Evaluate for desired effect of increased CD4 counts and lower blood levels of p24 antigen. ▪ Notify the physician if the client develops evidence of pancreatitis, impaired hepatic function, or painful peripheral neuropathy. *Health Education for the Client and Family:* ▪ Take without regard to food or water. ▪ Have the client check with the physician before taking any other prescription or over-the-counter medication. ▪ Report all signs and symptoms of hypersensitivity to this drug. ▪ Report to the physician any signs of infection or changes in condition.

cardiovascular disease and diabetes. These conditions commonly are treated with medications.

NUCLEOSIDE REVERSE TRANSCRIPTASE INHIBITORS The NRTIs (also called *nucleoside analogues*) inhibit the action of viral reverse transcriptase, a retroviral enzyme that catalyzes the substrates for converting and copying viral RNA to DNA sequences. This enzyme is necessary for viral integration into cellular DNA and replication. The nucleoside analogues act as a chemical decoy for building blocks in the formation of the DNA copy, preventing the RNA from being copied into DNA. Each drug substitutes for a particular nucleoside base at different points on the chain. See the Medications feature for an overview of this group of drugs.

Zidovudine was the first antiretroviral agent approved for use with HIV infection. It remains in widespread use and has been shown to decrease symptoms and prolong the lives of clients with AIDS. Zidovudine often is given to clients with a CD4 cell count of less than 500/mm^3 because of evidence that it slows the progression to severe disease. Zidovudine also may be used prophylactically following a documented parenteral exposure to HIV. It is used in combination with didanosine, ddC, or 3TC (see the Medications feature).

PROTEASE INHIBITORS Protease is a viral enzyme used in the formation of specific viral protein for viral assembly and maturation. PIs bond chemically with protease to block the function of the enzyme and result in the production of immature, noninfectious viral particles. When combined with other antiviral drugs, these chemicals increase the chance of eliminating the virus by interfering with different stages of its life cycle. Viral resistance occurs rather quickly, however. PIs inhibit and induce metabolism of other drugs, so their use with other medications as well as the dose of those medications must be carefully planned. Some drugs will circulate longer because their metabolism is inhibited; others will be speedily metabolized and eliminated.

Protease inhibitors and nucleoside analogues are associated with serious metabolic derangements. These include elevated cholesterol and triglycerides, insulin resistance and diabetes mellitus, and changes in body fat composition, which are particularly distressing to clients. These body fat changes are primarily abdominal obesity and skeletal wasting; this set of symptoms is referred to as *lipodystrophy* (Robles, 2013). Elevated cholesterol should be treated with pravastatin or atorvastatin. Lovastatin and simvastatin react to PIs, so they should be avoided. Dietary sources of cholesterol should be reduced.

- Saquinavir (Invirase) is used in combination with nucleoside analogues to treat progression of the disease.
- Ritonavir (Norvir) is used in combination with nucleoside analogues to treat progression of the disease.
- Indinavir (Crixivan) is used in combination with nucleoside analogues to treat progression of the disease.
- Nelfinavir (Viracept) is used in clients with failure of or intolerance to other PIs.
- Amprenavir (Agenerase) is the newest PI.
- Lopinavir/ritonavir (Kaletra) is the first combination of PIs active against some HIV strains resistant to other PIs.

NONNUCLEOSIDE REVERSE TRANSCRIPTASE INHIBITORS Nevirapine (Viramune), delavirdine (Rescriptor), and efavirenz (Sustiva) are NNRTIs that may be used in combination with nucleoside analogues and PIs. However, one limitation to NNRTIs is the high incidence of cross-resistance to NRTIs. Some studies have shown that nevirapine and efavirenz may significantly reduce serum levels of the PIs. Only one NNRTI should be used at a time. Nevirapine has a reported risk for liver toxicity and Stevens-Johnson syndrome (Wilson, Shannon, & Shields, 2013).

ENTRY INHIBITORS Entry or fusion inhibitors, such as enfuvirtide (Fuzeon), prevent HIV from entering target cells by binding to the protein envelope that surrounds the virus. When bound to the drug, the virus cannot transform to fit and adhere to cell membranes. The drug's effectiveness is measured by improved CD4 counts and reduced viral loads (Wilson et al., 2013).

TABLE 8–4   Pharmacologic Treatment of Common Opportunistic Infections and Malignancies in HIV Disease

CONDITION	TREATMENT	POTENTIAL ADVERSE EFFECTS
Infections		
Pneumocystis jiroveci pneumonia	trimethoprim/sulfamethoxazole pentamidine	Rash, neutropenia, anemia, thrombocytopenia, and Stevens-Johnson syndrome Hypotension, altered blood glucose levels, hypocalcemia, anemia and leukopenia, liver and renal toxicity, and pancreatitis
Tuberculosis	Combination drug therapy using isoniazid, rifampin, ethambutol, pyrazinamide, or streptomycin	Multiple (see the module on Infection for an exemplar on this diagnosis)
Candidiasis (oral thrush)	clotrimazole troches nystatin suspension	Few toxic responses noted Few toxic responses noted
Esophagitis or recurrent vaginitis	ketoconazole fluconazole amphotericin b	Hepatitis and adrenal insufficiency Hepatitis Bone marrow toxicity, acute renal or hepatic failure, nausea and vomiting, chills, fever, and headache
Mycobacterium avium complex	Combination therapy using: clarithromycin, plus clofazimine ethambutol rifampin ciprofloxacin amikacin	Hepatitis, nausea, diarrhea Diarrhea, nausea and vomiting, skin discoloration, pruritus, and rash Thrombocytopenia, hepatitis, and optic neuritis Bone marrow depression, renal failure, and hepatitis Nausea and rash Bone marrow depression, renal failure, ototoxicity, and hepatitis
Cytomegalovirus	ganciclovir foscarnet combination	Bone marrow depression and fever Renal failure, electrolyte imbalances, and seizures
Herpes simplex or herpes zoster	acyclovir	Nausea and vomiting, diarrhea, central nervous system effects, and renal failure
Toxoplasmosis	pyrimethamine, plus sulfadiazine or clindamycin and folinic acid (leucovorin)	Bone marrow depression, rash, respiratory failure, nausea and vomiting, abdominal pain, and hematuria
Malignancies		
Kaposi sarcoma	Intralesional vinblastine	Inflammation and pain at injection site
Lymphoma	Combination chemotherapy	Nausea and vomiting, bone marrow toxicity, and alopecia

AGENTS USED IN COMBINATION WITH ANTIRETRO-VIRAL THERAPY   Other agents may be administered in combination with antiretroviral therapy. Interferons, which are naturally occurring lymphokines, have been used alone and in combination. Alpha-interferon may be used to treat KS and, in combination with zidovudine, to slow disease progression. Gamma-interferon also is used. As more drugs become available, the burden of choosing the best regimen increases for the healthcare provider. As mentioned, the most important limiting factor in the choice of a regimen is client adherence. Second to that is selecting an effective combination of drugs without overlapping toxicities and without toxicities so debilitating that adherence will be further impaired.

A number of pharmacologic agents are used to prevent and treat opportunistic infections and malignancies in the client with HIV. These agents are outlined in **Table 8–4** ●.

All clients infected with HIV receive pneumococcal, influenza, hepatitis B, and *Haemophilus influenzae* type B vaccines. Individuals with a positive PPD and negative chest x-ray are given prophylactic isoniazid. When the client's CD4 cell count falls to less than 200/mm³, prophylactic treatment for PCP is begun, usually with trimethoprim-sulfamethoxazole. Clients with a CD4 count of less than 100/mm³ are started on prophylactic treatment for MAC.

SAFETY ALERT
Clients may require an implanted venous access device to facilitate blood sampling, intravenous medication administration, transfusions, and parenteral nutrition when frequent intravenous access is needed. However, because of the client's altered immune response, it is of particular importance that strict infection control principles be followed to prevent the introduction of pathogens into the bloodstream.

Nonpharmacologic Therapy

Collaboration among physicians and nurses treating clients with HIV/AIDS is essential. Because of the number of medications that some clients may need to take, regular consultation with a pharmacist will help to ensure a client is not taking any medications that are contraindicated. Nurses should encourage clients with HIV/AIDS to use a single pharmacy to fill prescriptions, so as to decrease further the possibility of taking contraindicated medications.

Lifespan Considerations   Caring for the HIV-Positive Client Who Is Pregnant

Women infected with HIV should be evaluated and treated for other sexually transmitted infections and for conditions occurring more commonly in women with HIV, such as tuberculosis, cytomegalovirus, toxoplasmosis, and cervical dysplasia. Pregnant women infected with HIV and with no history of hepatitis B should receive the hepatitis vaccine, which is not contraindicated prenatally, as well as the pneumococcal vaccine and an annual flu shot. In addition to routine prenatal laboratory tests, a platelet count and a CBC with differential should be obtained at the first prenatal visit and repeated each trimester to identify anemia, thrombocytopenia, and leukopenia, which are associated both with HIV infection and with antiviral therapy.

Pharmacologic Therapy

Testing for HIV antiretroviral drug resistance is recommended before beginning treatment in pregnant women who are infected but who do not require treatment for their own health. When possible, treatment of these women is delayed until after the first trimester. Women who are infected with HIV and are already receiving HAART when they become pregnant are advised to continue their current regimen if it is effective, but they should not receive drugs such as efavirenz (EFV), which have known teratogenic effects (National Institutes of Health Panel on Antiretroviral Therapy and Medical Management of HIV-Infected Children, 2013).

Treatment recommendations also have been developed for the mother and infant for the intrapartum and postpartum periods. The decision about which regimen is most appropriate should be determined following discussion with the woman about the risks and benefits based on her individual HIV status.

Monitoring for Complications

At each prenatal visit, women who are infected with HIV but are asymptomatic are monitored for early signs of complications, such as fever or weight loss during the second or third trimester. Assessment should include:

- Inquiring about signs of vaginal infection
- Inspecting the client's mouth for signs of infections, such as thrush (candidiasis) or hairy leukoplakia
- Auscultating her lungs for signs of pneumonia
- Palpating her lymph nodes, liver, and spleen for signs of enlargement.

In addition, each trimester, the woman should have a visual examination and a funduscopic examination to detect such complications as toxoplasmosis retinitis.

The woman with HIV also should be assessed regularly for serological changes that indicate the disease is progressing. This progression is determined by the absolute CD4 T-lymphocyte count, which provides the number of helper T4 cells. When the CD4 counts fall to $200/mm^3$ or lower, opportunistic infections (e.g., PCP) are more likely to develop.

A pregnancy complicated by HIV infection, even if asymptomatic, is considered high risk, and the fetus is monitored closely. Weekly nonstress testing is begun at 32 weeks' gestation, and serial ultrasounds are done to detect intrauterine growth restriction. Biophysical profiles also are indicated. Invasive procedures such as amniocentesis are avoided when possible to prevent contamination of a noninfected infant. To reduce the risk of perinatal transmission, intrapartum intravenous zidovudine is indicated for all pregnant women regardless of their prenatal therapy regimen.

Intrapartal and Postpartal Care

Scheduled cesarean birth at 38 weeks' gestation and before rupture of the membranes is recommended for women with elevated viral loads (CDC, 2013b). Women who are HIV positive have an increased risk for complications such as intrapartal or postpartal hemorrhage, postpartal infection, poor wound healing, and infections of the genitourinary tract. Thus, they need careful monitoring and appropriate therapy as indicated. Following childbirth, the woman who is HIV positive should be referred to a physician knowledgeable about treating individuals with HIV infection. Because of the profound implications of HIV infection for the woman, her family, the fetus/newborn, and her healthcare providers, screening is recommended for all pregnant women but especially those at increased risk, including women with multiple sexual partners or women who are or have been injection drug users.

In addition, clinics located in areas with a large HIV-positive population may require routine HIV screening of all prenatal clients.

Medical management of the infant begins with prevention of the spread of HIV from mother to newborn. Because of the rapidity of disease progression in perinatally transmitted HIV infection, early identification of infected infants is important to ensure the most effective treatment. Like HIV-positive mothers, their infants should undergo periodic laboratory testing as described previously. All infected mothers should receive oral zidovudine (AZT) after the first trimester of pregnancy and intravenous AZT during labor and delivery. In addition, for term infants of infected mothers, AZT is started prophylactically 2 mg/kg PO every 6 hours (Nash & Smith, 2008). If the infant is confirmed to be HIV positive, AZT is changed to a multidrug antiretroviral regimen.

All infants of infected mothers should start prophylaxis against PCP (a commonly serious or fatal outcome in infants) by 4–6 weeks of age. Prophylaxis should continue to 12 months unless two of the three HIV PCR tests are documented as negative (at 48 hours, 1–2 months, and 2–4 months).

The earlier the child develops AIDS, the poorer the prognosis. Children under the age of 1 are most likely to die of AIDS within 5 years (Collins et al., 2010). Younger children are more likely to die of pulmonary diseases or infection, while children who survive past 10 years of age are more likely to die of cardiac disease, wasting syndrome, encephalopathy, and infection with *Mycobacterium avium* complex. However, as treatment improves, more children are living longer with the disease. Many females infected perinatally are now adolescents or adults who may become pregnant. In spite of the risk of transmission to offspring, these women often intend to become pregnant but have limited knowledge of safe sex practices. In addition, these women are at higher risk for preterm birth, so the risk of complications in the newborn is increased (Badell & Lindsay, 2012).

Nurses may find themselves collaborating with homeless shelter directors and other nonprofits to provide preventive education to communities whose members have an unusually high risk for contracting HIV/AIDS. Counselors and religious leaders can provide support and leadership to clients with HIV infection and their families.

Nurses also may collaborate with day care directors and teachers, school staff, and even camp personnel to ensure the health and safety not only of a child with HIV/AIDS but also of the center's personnel. Nurses should instruct staff in these centers about the use of standard precautions in handling blood and body fluids. Nurses also should assist child care centers in establishing procedures to notify all parents when a child with an infectious disease has been at the center. Parents of immunocompromised children can then take any necessary precautions to minimize the chances of their children becoming ill. Parents of children with HIV infection must be very careful to limit the exposure of their children to infectious diseases.

Complementary and Alternative Therapies

Complementary and alternative medicine has been shown to help decrease side effects of certain medical treatments and to increase client comfort related to acute exacerbations. However, the National Center for Complementary and Alternative Medicine (NCCAM) has issued warnings against the use of garlic supplements with HIV medications. The use of St. John's wort also is contraindicated for clients receiving antiretroviral therapy (NCCAM, 2012). Any client with HIV/AIDS should be encouraged to consult his or her treating physician before beginning any therapy involving complementary and alternative medicine.

▆ NURSING PROCESS

The client with HIV/AIDS has many care needs and requires both physical and psychosocial support (see the Evidence-Based Practice feature that follows). Because no cure or effective treatment currently exists for HIV disease, many of these needs fall within the realm of nursing to promote knowledge and understanding, self-care, comfort, and quality of life. Like the course of many diseases with an ultimately fatal outcome, the course of HIV infection may well be affected by the client's social support systems, control, perceived self-efficacy in management, and coping mechanisms.

As the epidemic continues, nurses are providing care for increasing numbers of clients with HIV infection at various stages of disease. These clients are not only in special care settings but also in general units, maternal–child units, hospices, long-term care facilities, and home settings. As clients with HIV disease live longer, nurses will increasingly encounter those in whom HIV disease is a secondary diagnosis, with another primary diagnosis such as seizures, heart disease, diabetes mellitus, or an operative procedure.

Assessment

Assessment is the basis for differential diagnosis; fitting the correct treatment to the etiology is critical. For example, delirium is an acute confusional state and, unlike dementia, is reversible. Effective nursing interventions are available for such conditions (Coyne, Lyne, & Watson, 2002).

Collect the following data through the health history and physical examination. Further focused assessments are described in the Implementation section that follows.

- *Health history.* Risk factors (transfusion, unprotected sex, and needle exposure), infections (sexually transmitted infections, hepatitis, and tuberculosis), medications, recreational drug use, foreign travel, and pets.
- *Psychosocial assessment.* Assessment of developmental age/ability to understand the diagnosis, coping mechanisms, support systems, access to and availability of resources.
- *Physical assessment.* Height, weight, nutrition, skin and mucous membranes, vision, lymph nodes, breath sounds, abdominal tenderness, motor strength, coordination, cranial nerves, gait, deep tendon reflexes, genitourinary examination, and mental status.

Assessment centers on observation and evaluation of potential sites of infection. The nurse assesses breath sounds, respiratory status, arterial blood gases, level of consciousness, and mental status and reports any evidence of lymphocytic interstitial pneumonitis or neurological abnormalities. Assess the client's height and weight frequently, assess for anemia, and look for *Candida* infections in the mouth. Observe young children for signs of failure to thrive and for *Candida* infections in the diaper area. Note any developmental delays in motor skills or intellectual functioning, which could result from encephalopathy and poor nutrition and can signal an increasing severity in symptom level. These observations should be reported so that further medical evaluation can be carried out.

When conducting the physical assessment, remember that symptoms must be interpreted and reported by the client. Like pain, the client determines and reports the presence and severity of dyspnea.

Diagnosis

Client needs change throughout the course of the disease, so nurses amend plans of care and diagnoses frequently, sometimes with every visit. Possible appropriate nursing diagnoses include the following:

- *Ineffective Coping*
- *Impaired Skin Integrity*
- *Imbalanced Nutrition: Less Than Body Requirements*
- *Risk for Deficient Fluid Volume*
- *Risk for Infection*
- *Anxiety*
- *Fear*
- *Deficient Knowledge.*

(NANDA-I © 2012)

Specific disease-related diagnoses may include the following:

- *Diarrhea* related to gastrointestinal infection, malignancy, or drug reactions
- *Impaired Gas Exchange* related to pulmonary disease
- *Delayed Growth and Development* related to chronic infection and poor nutrition
- *Risk for Compromised Family Coping* related to life-threatening illness

(NANDA-I © 2012)

Evidence-Based Practice Nurses' Willingness to Care for Individuals With AIDS

Clinical Question

As reported by the Centers for Disease Control and Prevention, individuals with AIDS are living longer. As treatment continues to prolong survival, a key challenge will be the increasing number of individuals living with HIV/AIDS—and the additional resources needed for services, treatment, and care. Unfortunately, several studies have found that some professional nurses and students resist caring for clients with AIDS.

Evidence

Sherman's (1996) seminal study examined relationships among moral choices about one's own mortality (death anxiety), spirituality, and social support and nurses' willingness to care for these clients. In a survey of 220 registered nurses employed in eight hospitals in the New York metropolitan area, Sherman found that willingness to care for clients with AIDS was positively correlated with spirituality and perceived social support and was negatively correlated with death anxiety. It is suggested that nurses' willingness to care for individuals with AIDS is related not only to nurses' personal values and beliefs (expressed in spirituality), but also to their professional identity and role expectations.

In their well-known study, nursing educators Valois et al. (2001) addressed nursing reluctance to treat clients with HIV infection and researched the impact of persuasive messages on nursing students' beliefs and attitudes about caring for these clients. Nursing education certainly increases knowledge about and awareness of the science of HIV infection, but it may not modify attitudes or behaviors. The underlying theory of this study was that individuals who receive evidence-based persuasive messages may develop favorable beliefs that will alter their willingness to perform a given behavior. Three main types of beliefs were considered in this study: behavioral belief (related to the expected consequences of adopting a behavior), normative belief (related to perceived social pressures by significant others resulting from adopting a behavior), and control belief (related to resources or barriers that seem to facilitate or hamper adoption of the behavior).

In three sessions, the student nurses in the experimental group were given positive persuasive messages about caring for clients with HIV infection. The persuasive messages were compelling and specific to caring for these clients, and case studies provided opportunities for the students to discuss the elements of the case within the framework of the persuasive messages. Students in the control group studied the science of caring for clients with HIV but did not receive the persuasive messages. When beliefs and attitudes about caring for these clients were compared, the researchers found significantly greater willingness to provide care in the experimental group. Nursing students proved to be well prepared and motivated to receive this information.

Implications

Standards of professional nursing clearly state that nurses will care for individuals with HIV/AIDS. To increase nurses' willingness to do so, students need to be better socialized into their roles and responsibilities. Providing information within an evidence-based framework, analyzing and defining effective nursing care in client cases, and using the standards of professional nursing help to promote the development of positive attitudes among nurses. Discussions within the classroom and clinical settings provide a safe means of bringing fears into the open and sharing experiences. Student groups can serve as support groups, improving communication, decreasing isolation and anxiety, and improving self-esteem and morale. Within the work setting, increased contact with individuals who have HIV/AIDS and perceived support from colleagues and administrators are important factors in making caring a rewarding and positive experience.

Critical Thinking Application

1. These studies were of student nurses and registered nurses and were conducted more than a decade ago. What differences do you think might be found between the two groups today?

2. Carefully consider each of the following clients with AIDS, and write a brief paragraph about how you would feel if you were assigned to care for them:
   a. A heterosexual woman, age 25
   b. A gay man, age 35
   c. A newborn baby girl
   d. A 40-year-old single mother of three teenagers
   e. A 30-year-old homeless drug user
   f. A 17-year-old male client with hemophilia, infected by blood transfusions
   g. A heterosexual male, age 80

Planning

The first step in dealing with HIV infection is prevention. Nurses must be active in evaluating test results and in teaching measures to prevent transmission of HIV to others. Adequate testing, prophylaxis for HIV and PCP, and follow up visits to evaluate the general health of those at risk for the disease are advised. Guidelines from the AAP recommend that pediatricians offer HIV testing and counseling to adolescents who are sexually active or involved in substance abuse (AAP, 2001). Recommendations also have been made for inclusion of HIV/AIDS education in comprehensive health education for children ages 5 and up (UNESCO, 2009) (see the Client Teaching feature on page 476). Nurses can implement these policies and counsel teens about the dangers of and prevention measures for HIV.

Nursing care needs for the client with HIV infection change over the course of the disease. Preventive healthcare measures, health maintenance activities, education, and support of coping mechanisms are important during the early stages of the disease. Counseling the client with a new diagnosis of HIV infection is vital. HIV/AIDS continues to carry a social stigma that may interfere with the client's usual support systems and coping mechanisms. As the disease progresses and the client experiences more physical symptoms, the need for psychosocial support continues, but direct care needs become more important. Acute exacerbation of opportunistic infections

Client Teaching HIV/AIDS Education for Children

The United Nations Educational, Scientific, and Cultural Organization recommends that HIV and AIDS education be part of health education for children ages 5 and above. School nurses should be educated about HIV/AIDS, ethics, testing, and counseling. Nurses can enhance these efforts by doing the following:

- Promote an understanding of the need for HIV/AIDS education.
- Protect the rights of students or staff with HIV infection or AIDS.
- Raise awareness of the sexual health issues affecting children and adolescents.
- Define what HIV/AIDS education is and what it is intended to do.
- Provide guidance to administrators about building support for HIV/AIDS education in the community.
- Prepare teachers to cover sensitive issues of sexuality and infection in class.
- Answer questions about transmission of HIV, symptoms of HIV, and testing for HIV.
- Offer guidance about age-appropriate, socially relevant HIV/AIDS education at all levels.

Source: United Nations Educational, Scientific, and Cultural Organization. (2009). *International technical guidance on sexuality education.* Retrieved from http://unesdoc.unesco.org/images/0018/001832/183281e.pdf; Smith Cox, N. (2003). *School HIV/AIDS policy tool kit.* Wisconsin Department of Public Instruction. Retrieved from http://sspw.dpi.wi.gov/files/sspw/pdf/hivtoolkit.pdf; and New York Statewide School Health Services Center. (n.d.). *Understanding HIV/AIDS.* Retrieved from http://www.schoolhealthservicesny.com/a-zindex.cfm?subpage=182.

may necessitate hospitalization, but typically, the client is managed at home.

SAFETY ALERT

Healthcare workers who come in contact with blood or other body fluids of clients infected with HIV are at risk for exposure to the virus. Use standard precautions in caring for all clients, because HIV status and presence of other infections may not be known.

Implementation

Nursing interventions are directed toward specific nursing diagnoses selected on the basis of client needs. Nurses will find that many clients require interventions to prevent secondary infection, promote adherence to the treatment plan, and promote successful coping.

Prevent Secondary Infections in Those With HIV/AIDS

Bacteria as well as other organisms that are common in the environment infect clients who are immunosuppressed. Nurses should recommend frequent hand washing and limiting exposure to individuals with upper respiratory or other infections to protect the client with HIV from acquiring other infections.

Children with HIV should be immunized as soon as they reach the age recommended for diphtheria, tetanus, and acellular pertussis; inactivated poliovirus; *Haemophilus influenzae* type b; hepatitis B; pneumococcal vaccine; and annual influenza vaccine. Live measles–mumps–rubella vaccine is administered at 12 months of age unless the child is severely immunocompromised, because measles raises the risk of serious outcomes. Live varicella vaccine should be administered if the child has no or mild symptoms of HIV. If the child is exposed to varicella, the parents should notify their healthcare professional, because the child may need varicella zoster immunoglobulin (VZIG) within 96 hours of exposure or if exposed to measles (may need vaccination within 72 hours of exposure). Tuberculosis is more common in children with AIDS, so they should have annual skin tests that are read by health professionals (AAP, 2001). Avoid invasive procedures in the newborn, and encourage the mother to formula-feed the baby rather than breastfeed (CDC, 2013b).

Adolescents and adults with HIV/AIDS require education about how to prevent opportunistic, sexually transmitted, and other infections. The nurse should provide ongoing reinforcement of education as these clients attempt to navigate the world living with HIV/AIDS.

Promote Adherence to Medication Regimen

The treatment regimen of antiretroviral therapies for the client with HIV/AIDS may be complex and time-consuming, presenting an overwhelming challenge to clients and their families. Nonadherence to the prescribed antiretroviral treatment regimen is likely to result in increased morbidity and mortality. Some common reasons for nonadherence are frequent dosing, client lack of confidence in the efficacy of the treatment, and the side effects of the treatment, such as nausea and rashes.

Nonadherence to treatment regimens may be intentional or unintentional. Clients' attitude toward therapy—particularly their belief, or lack of belief, in its effectiveness—has a big impact on adherence. Assessing the clients' readiness for and attitudes toward therapy and preparing them for the effects of HAART may reduce intentional nonadherence. Nurses should also address unintentional nonadherence as best they can.

Nurses' strategies for achieving optimal management of the treatment regimen include educating clients regarding the purpose of the medication, the benefits of adhering to the regimen, and the potential consequences of failing to adhere to the regimen. Behavior modification techniques using positive reinforcement are very effective in promoting adherence. Tailoring the medication regiment to the client's routine promotes adherence. Offer praise and positive reinforcement as clients work to incorporate treatment into their lives.

Ingersoll and Heckman (2005) found that the most effective way providers can foster adherence balances appropriate challenges with support. Clients seem to perceive nonconfrontational providers as giving permission to be less adherent. Although depression, substance use, and financial considerations undoubtedly influence clients' adherence to HAART therapy and need to be addressed, provider–client relationships seem to have the most influence on adherence behavior.

If problems exist in the management of the treatment regimen, carefully listen to the client to help determine the cause.

Collaborate with the client in establishing goals to help meet the prescribed treatment regimen, and consider the effect of cultural beliefs on medication adherence. If further intervention is required, other options include direct observational therapy, home visits, and use of electronic monitoring devices, as described previously in the section on Pharmacologic Therapy.

Promote Effective Coping

On receiving the test results indicating seropositive status, the individual with HIV infection faces multiple issues that only rarely affect other clients. First and foremost, HIV is a disease with no known cure, one that is almost universally thought to be fatal. Social support systems, family relationships, and the ability to obtain and retain useful work and health insurance may be disrupted by the disease. In addition, clients may feel guilty about their lifestyle and how they contracted the disease. As the disease progresses, social isolation, fatigue, changes in body image, medication side effects, and many other issues affect the clients' abilities to cope.

If possible, a primary nurse should be assigned, whether the setting is home health care, hospice, or acute care. Assigning a nurse helps to promote a therapeutic and trusting relationship and provides for continuity of care. Appropriate interventions include the following:

- Assess the client's social support network and usual methods of coping. This assessment will help both the nurse and the client identify individuals and mechanisms that can help the client cope more effectively with the disease.

- Plan for consistent, uninterrupted time with the client. Time and a consistent presence encourage the client to express feelings and work through issues related to HIV infection.

- Interact with the client at every opportunity, including outside nursing care treatments. This purposeful interaction communicates caring and acceptance without fear of HIV disease.

- Support the client's social network. Nontraditional families may offer more support than the traditional family, necessitating a liberal interpretation of the term *family* if unit policy is immediate family only.

- Promote interaction between the client, significant others, and family. The result of hospitalization and manifestations of HIV disease may be isolation from others and a decrease in the client's ability to cope.

- Encourage the client's involvement in making care decisions. This participation in planning gives the client a greater sense of self-worth and more control over the situation and thus increases the client's coping abilities.

- Set and maintain limits on manipulative and other destructive behaviors. The nurse must set limits for the client who is unable to curb inappropriate behaviors.

- Assist the client to accept responsibility for actions without blaming others. Effective coping cannot occur without acceptance of responsibility for one's own actions.

- Support positive coping behaviors, decisions, actions, and achievements. As self-esteem is enhanced, coping improves (Côté & Pepler, 2005).

Because of the stress and social isolation that a family caring for a loved one with HIV/AIDS may face, emotional support for family members is essential. The nurse offers families informa-

tion about support groups, available counseling, and information resources. Current therapeutic information about HIV is available to both healthcare providers and families through the AIDS Clinical Trials Information Service (1-800-448-0440).

Parents of a baby with HIV/AIDS may not bond with the baby or may fail to provide the baby with enough sensory and tactile stimulation. Parents and family members need to be reassured that there are no documented cases of individuals contracting HIV/AIDS from routine care of infected babies. The nurse should encourage family members to hold the baby during feedings, because the infant benefits from frequent gentle touch. Music or tapes of parents' voices will provide auditory stimulation.

Maintain Skin Integrity

Dryness, malnutrition, immobility from fatigue, and skin lesions on pressure sites contribute to impaired integrity of the skin of the client with HIV disease. Maintaining skin integrity is important because of HIV's progressive and debilitating nature. Also, the skin is both the first line of defense against infection in a client with immunosuppression and a site for secondary manifestations (e.g., KS and herpes).

- Monitor the skin frequently for lesions and areas of breakdown. Early identification of impaired skin integrity allows prompt intervention.

- Monitor lesions for signs of infection or impaired healing. Infection or poor tissue perfusion not only impairs healing but also may lead to further skin breakdown.

- Turn the client at least every 2 hours, and more frequently if necessary. Turning decreases unrelieved pressure on bony prominences and improves circulation to the tissues.

- Use pressure-relieving devices, such as pressure and egg-crate mattresses, or sheepskin pads for elbows and heels. These devices provide prophylactic relief of pressure.

- Keep skin clean and dry by using mild, nondrying soaps or oils for cleansing. Night sweats and diarrhea, if present, can cause breakdown and damage to the skin. Frequent cleansing with nondrying products discourages bacterial growth, reducing the risk of infection. Applying protective creams to reddened areas in the rectal area protects skin from the caustic effects of diarrhea.

- Massage around, but not over, affected pressure sites to increase circulation to the surrounding tissue. Massaging over the affected area can cause skin breakdown.

- If you see blisters, leave them intact, and dress them with a hydrocolloid (DuoDERM) dressing. Blisters provide natural sterile coverings for damaged tissue, improving healing and preventing bacterial invasion.

- Caution the client against scratching. If the client is confused, trim his or her fingernails, and use mitts or soft restraints to prevent scratching. If mitts or restraints are used, check the circulation of hands and fingers frequently. Scratching and skin damage allow bacteria to be introduced into lesions, increasing the risk of infection. Tight or restrictive restraints or mitts may compromise circulation.

- Avoid the use of heat or occlusive dressings. Heat can further dry and damage the skin; occlusive dressings may impair circulation and lead to ulceration.

- Prevent skin shearing by using a turnsheet and adequate personnel when repositioning. Shearing causes tissue trauma that can lead to decubitus ulcers.

- Encourage ambulation if possible; if the client is confined to bed, encourage active or passive ROM exercises. Activity increases circulation, decreases pressure and skin breakdown, and helps to maintain muscle tone.

- Monitor nutritional intake and albumin levels. Maintenance of optimal nutrition decreases the risk of tissue breakdown and improves resistance to infection.

Promote Adequate Nutrition

Many factors associated with HIV disease, including manifestations of the disease itself, put the client at risk for altered nutrition and weight loss. Nausea and anorexia may be manifestations of the disease or the result of antiretroviral therapy. Chronic diarrhea is a common manifestation of constitutional HIV disease. Wasting syndrome also is common and is manifested by involuntary weight loss of more than 10%–15% of baseline weight, severe diarrhea, fever, and chronic fatigue and weakness. The exact cause of wasting syndrome is unclear, but the diarrhea and fatigue contribute, as does the increased metabolic rate associated with fever. Oral and esophageal candidiasis and KS of the gastrointestinal tract may cause painful swallowing, making eating difficult and thereby contributing to anorexia. Poor nutritional status in the client with HIV ultimately can result in altered comfort, change in body image, muscle wasting, increased risk for infection, and higher mortality and morbidity.

- Assess nutritional status, including weight, body mass, caloric intake, and laboratory studies, such as total protein and albumin levels, hemoglobin, and hematocrit. The baseline provided by these factors allows a determination of the effectiveness of interventions.

- Identify possible causes of altered nutrition. Identification of causes provides direction for planned interventions.

- Administer prescribed medications for candidiasis and other manifestations as ordered. Eliminating this opportunistic infection improves comfort and facilitates food intake. Topical viscous anesthetic can help to reduce pain and improve oral intake.

- Administer antidiarrheal medications after stools, and administer antiemetics before meals. Provide antipyretics as needed to control fever. Reducing diarrhea improves nutrient absorption; preprandial medication with an antiemetic reduces nausea and improves food intake. Reduction of fever lowers the body's metabolic demands.

- Provide a diet high in protein and kilocalories. A high-protein, high-kilocalorie diet provides the necessary nutrients to meet metabolic needs as well as requirements for tissue healing.

- Offer soft foods, and serve small portions. Soft foods are easily digested. Small portions are more appealing to the anorectic or nauseated client.

- Involve the client in meal planning, and encourage significant others to bring favorite foods from home. The client is more likely to consume adequate amounts of preferred foods. Allowing food choices enhances the client's sense of control.

- Assist with eating as needed. Fatigue and weakness can prevent the client from eating an adequate amount of food.

- Provide supplementary vitamins and enteral feedings, such as Ensure. These improve nutritional status and caloric intake.

- Provide or assist with frequent oral hygiene. Oral hygiene improves comfort and appetite and reduces the risk of mucosal lesions.

- Administer appetite stimulants, such as megestrol (Megace) and dronabinol (Marinol), as ordered. Both drugs may increase appetite and promote weight gain.

Address Ineffective Sexuality Patterns

The diagnosis of HIV infection can significantly alter the client's expressions of sexuality. Guilt over the diagnosis may interfere with libido, and the client may fear spreading the disease to others via sexual relations. The client also may be angry with a significant other or partner who was the probable source of infection.

As the disease progresses, its manifestations can affect body image and self-esteem, again impairing sexuality. Other symptoms, such as nausea, fatigue, and weakness, may interfere with libido and sexual satisfaction as well.

- Examine your own feelings about sexuality, your role in dealing with a client's sexuality, and the client's lifestyle and sexual preferences. To deal effectively with the client's concerns, it is vital that the nurse be comfortable with his or her own feelings of sexuality and be able to accept the client's lifestyle and sexual expression. Referring the client to another nurse or counselor may be in the best interest of the client.

- Establish a trusting, therapeutic relationship through the use of time, active listening, caring, and self-disclosure. Maintain a nonthreatening, nonjudgmental attitude toward the client. Sexuality is a private issue that will be uncomfortable or impossible for the nurse and client to discuss without a mutually trusting relationship.

- Provide factual information about HIV infection and its effects. Facts help the client to separate fears and myths from reality.

- Discuss safer sex practices, including hugging, cuddling, nonsexual contact, use of latex condoms and spermicidal lubricant, and mutual masturbation. Alternative forms of sexual activity and expressing affection can allow the client and significant other to remain close throughout the course of the disease.

- Encourage discussion of fears and concerns with the significant other, if any. Open communication helps a couple to deal with issues related to sexuality.

- For the client without a significant other, stress the need to continue meeting people and developing social relationships while practicing safer sex. The client with HIV infection has a high risk of isolation, and relationships with others help the client to cope with the disease.

- Refer the client and significant other, if any, to local support groups for individuals and partners of people with HIV. Support groups provide a social and support network of people facing the same issues.

Address Knowledge Deficits

Both the client and the significant other have extensive teaching needs. The primary need is current, factual information about the disease, its spread, and its expected course. This information will help them to plan realistically and to combat myths, misperceptions, and prejudices. At the same time, it is important to include information about current research and progress in treating the disease to maintain a sense of hope.

Discuss the following topics with the client and family to prepare for home care:

- Guidelines for safer sex practices
- Nutrition, rest and exercise, stress reduction, lifestyle changes, and maintaining a positive outlook
- Infection prevention and transmission, including hand washing and wearing gloves when handling client's secretions or excretions
- Importance of regular medical follow up and monitoring of immune status
- Signs and symptoms of opportunistic infections and malignancies, as well as other symptoms that should be reported
- Medications and adverse effects
- Use and care of implanted venous access devices, total parenteral nutrition, intravenous pumps and continuous medication delivery systems, and intravenous or aerosolized medications

- Cessation of smoking, alcohol, and recreational or illicit drug use
- Home health services
- Hospice and respite care services
- Community resources, such as support groups, social agencies, and counselors

Evaluation

There are many desired outcomes of care for the client with HIV/AIDS. Expected outcomes of nursing care include the following:

- The client remains free from secondary infection.
- The client has adequate respiratory function and perfusion.
- Nutritional intake of affected clients supports normal nutritional patterns and prevents malnutrition.
- The client demonstrates adequate coping with the stress of chronic disease.
- The child or adolescent with HIV is able to attend school and receive other supports in the educational process.

NURSING CARE PLAN · A Client With HIV Infection

Sara Lu is a 26-year-old elementary school teacher who lives with her parents and two younger sisters. Ms. Lu is very close to her parents and sisters; they share everything with each other.

During the required physical for admission to graduate school, Ms. Lu tells her physician that lately she has felt fatigued. She also states that she has had a persistent sore throat, intermittent bouts of diarrhea, and mild shortness of breath for about a month. She takes no routine medications other than a daily multivitamin and an occasional acetaminophen tablet for a headache. She is active in a drama club in her community, and she jogs 3 miles three to four times a week. She is engaged to be married in 6 months, and her fiancé is the only individual with whom she has had sexual relations. Her sexual activity has been unprotected. Ms. Lu also has a history of open heart surgery 7 years ago to correct a congenital valve defect. She has been physically healthy since that time until about a month or two ago.

The physician orders a mononucleosis test, enzyme-linked immunosorbent assay (ELISA), Western blot analysis, CD4 cell count, a p24 antigen test, and an erythrocyte sedimentation rate (ESR). Ms. Lu is asked to return in 1 week for follow up.

ASSESSMENT

On Ms. Lu's follow up visit, Carole Kee, RN, obtains her health history. Ms. Lu continues to have flulike symptoms but has improved somewhat. She states that she just has not been as active as usual and is worried about her health. Her appetite has decreased because of soreness in her mouth, and she has noted some whitish patches on her tongue and cheeks.

A chest film reveals no abnormality. The results of her laboratory tests are as follows:

- *ELISA:* positive for antibodies against HIV
- *Western blot analysis:* positive for antibodies against HIV
- *p24 antigen test:* positive for circulating HIV antigens
- *ESR:* increased to 25 mm/hr (normal range: women, 15–20 mm/hr; men, 10–15 mm/hr)
- *CD4 cell count:* 599/mm^3 (normal range, 600–1,200 mm^3)

Ms. Lu's physical examination reveals that she has enlarged lymph nodes in her neck and white patches on her oral mucosa. Her skin is warm to the touch. Her vital signs are as follows: T$_O$ 99.9°F (37.7°C), P 84 bpm, R 20 16/min, and BP 120/78 mmHg.

Ms. Lu is told of the results of her laboratory tests and the medical diagnosis of HIV infection. Ms. Lu is obviously distressed and wants to know how this happened, what it means, whether she has infected her loved ones, and whether she will get better.

DIAGNOSES

Nursing diagnoses that may be appropriate for Ms. Lu are the following:

- *Imbalanced Nutrition: Less Than Body Requirements* related to soreness in mouth
- *Risk for Deficient Fluid Volume* related to decreased fluid intake and diarrhea
- *Risk for Infection* related to altered immune protection
- *Anxiety* related to diagnosis and fear
- *Deficient Knowledge* about the HIV disease process

(NANDA-I © 2012)

PLANNING

The goals for care specify that Ms. Lu will:

- Maintain adequate nutrition for optimal body and cellular function.
- Consume at least 2,500 mL of fluid per day.
- Remain free of infections and their complications.
- Verbalize anxiety and use appropriate coping mechanisms.
- Verbalize and demonstrate knowledge of HIV disease.
- Verbalize measures, including safer sex practices, to prevent transmission of HIV to others.

(continued on next page)

NURSING CARE PLAN *(continued)*

IMPLEMENTATION

The following nursing interventions may be appropriate for Ms. Lu:
- Monitor daily weight as well as intake and output.
- Monitor dietary habits and serum albumin levels.
- Teach Ms. Lu the importance of consuming a nutritionally balanced diet and of maintaining adequate fluid intake.
- Suggest strategies for coping with anorexia and nausea.
- Provide referral for dietary consultation.
- Encourage oral care before and after meals.
- Assess bowel sounds, and monitor elimination pattern.
- Administer antiemetic and antimotility medications as ordered.
- Monitor for signs of dehydration, such as poor skin turgor, oliguria, and orthostatic hypotension.
- Increase fluid intake to 2,500 mL daily.

- Use strict aseptic technique for all invasive procedures.
- Teach Ms. Lu to avoid exposure to infection and people with known illnesses.
- Administer antiretroviral medications and antibiotics as prescribed, and monitor response.
- Encourage maintenance of regular physical exercise.
- Provide opportunities for Ms. Lu to verbalize her feelings.
- Avoid false reassurances.
- Provide appropriate and adequate information about HIV/AIDS.
- Teach safer sex practices and other measures to prevent transmission of HIV.
- Teach anxiety-controlling techniques, such as deep breathing and meditation.

EVALUATION

Ms. Lu is eager to learn about her illness and wants her family to come with her for further explanation. She states that she is sure her fiancé will be available as well. Ms. Lu is taking home antifungal medication, diet plans, and a schedule for increased exercise. She will return in 1 week for counseling and in 1 month for a follow up physical.

CRITICAL THINKING

1. How does age affect the body's response to fighting HIV? What other factors affect the risk for HIV infection and its progression?
2. Are the laboratory results for Ms. Lu a true indication that she is HIV positive? What additional tests might be ordered?
3. What is the most likely source of Ms. Lu's infection? What measures could have been used to reduce this risk, and how did she contract HIV? What is another possible source of Ms. Lu's HIV infection?
4. Ms. Lu says that her fiancé would like to have a child. How will you counsel her regarding pregnancy and childbearing?

REVIEW HIV/AIDS

RELATE Link the Concepts

Linking the exemplar of HIV with the concept of stress and coping:

1. How might excessive stress affect the client with HIV and/or AIDS?

2. What nursing interventions could you implement to improve a client's coping methods in order to reduce complications related to HIV infection?

Linking the exemplar of HIV with the concept of grief and loss:

3. You are caring for a client who is newly diagnosed as being HIV positive with no symptoms of AIDS. Why might this client experience grief and loss?

4. What nursing interventions might you initiate to help the client through the grieving process?

Linking the exemplar of HIV with the concept of collaboration:

5. What actions can you take when developing a plan of care for a client with Stage 3 HIV to promote her involvement in her own care and encourage a sense of autonomy and equality with others on her care team?

6. You have been asked to work with the health education teacher at a local high school to create an HIV/AIDS education program suitable for 10th-grade students. What kinds of information and guidance would you need from the teacher? What kinds of information and guidance should you provide to the teacher?

READY Go to Companion Skills Manual

REFER Go to Pearson Nursing Student Resources
nursing.pearsonhighered.com

REFLECT Case Study

Casey Holmes is a physically fit 23-year-old man who had a troubled youth. His parents divorced when he was very young, and he bounced back and forth between them. Both parents remarried. Growing up, he often saw his father hit his stepmother when she made him angry. As an adolescent, Casey was involved with a gang and arrested on a couple of occasions for petty crimes, such as shoplifting and vandalism. He never finished high school and moved out on his own at the age of 18. Since that time, he has held a number of odd jobs and has made an effort to stay out of trouble. He currently works for a landscape contractor. He hates his job because he has to work too hard and is underpaid, but he has not attempted to look for other jobs.

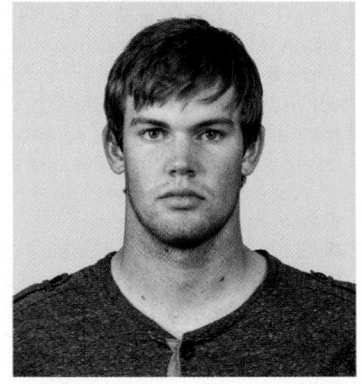

Casey lives with his pregnant girlfriend, Jessica Riley, and her 10-month-old son, Ryan. Casey does not particularly like Ryan and thinks that Jessica spoils him. However, he is very proud of the fact that Jessica is pregnant with his baby. He is controlling of Jessica and does not want anybody else looking at her.

On most days after work and into the evening, Casey drinks beer and smokes marijuana with his buddies. He is irritated that Jessica does not party with him as much as she did when they first met. Casey also uses other drugs when he can afford to buy them. He sometimes worries about the possibility of getting caught in a random drug screen but figures he can always get another job.

1. What factors in Casey's lifestyle place him at risk for HIV infection?

2. What teaching might you provide Casey to help him reduce his risk of HIV infection?

3. What teaching might be indicated for Jessica to reduce her risk of HIV infection related to her relationship with Casey?

EXEMPLAR 8.2   **Hypersensitivity**

EXEMPLAR KEY TERMS

Allergen, 481
Allergy, 481
Anaphylaxis, 482
Antigen, 481
Cell-mediated immune responses, 484
Hypersensitivity, 481
Localized response, 483
Serum sickness, 483
Systemic response, 482
Transfusion reaction, 483

EXEMPLAR LEARNING OUTCOMES

After reading about this exemplar, you will be able to:

1. Describe the pathophysiology, etiology, clinical manifestations, and direct and indirect causes of hypersensitivity.

2. Identify risk factors and prevention methods associated with hypersensitivity.

3. Illustrate the nursing process in providing culturally competent care across the life span for individuals with hypersensitivity.

4. Formulate priority nursing diagnoses appropriate for an individual with hypersensitivity.

5. Summarize therapies used by interdisciplinary teams in the collaborative care of an individual with hypersensitivity.

6. Plan evidence-based care for an individual with hypersensitivity and his or her family in collaboration with other members of the healthcare team.

7. Evaluate expected outcomes for an individual with hypersensitivity.

▶ OVERVIEW

Hypersensitivity is an altered immune response to an **antigen** (a foreign substance triggering the immune response) that results in harm to the client. When the antigen is environmental, or exogenous, the response is called an **allergy**, and the antigen is referred to as an **allergen**. The tissue response to a hypersensitivity reaction may be simply irritating or bothersome, such as a runny nose or itchy eyes, or it may be life-threatening, leading to blood cell hemolysis or laryngospasm.

Hypersensitivity reactions are classified primarily by the type of immune response to contact with the allergen. They are also classified as immediate or delayed hypersensitivity responses. Anaphylaxis and transfusion reactions are examples of immediate hypersensitivity reactions; contact dermatitis is a typical delayed response. The names of allergies sometimes refer to the organ system affected (e.g., allergic rhinitis) or the allergen involved (e.g., hay fever). However, classification by immunological response is the preferred means of categorizing allergies. Although more than one type of reaction may occur simultaneously, it is practical and insightful to study and treat allergy by classified types (King et al., 2005).

▶ PATHOPHYSIOLOGY AND ETIOLOGY

In a hypersensitivity reaction, an antigen–antibody or antigen–lymphocyte interaction causes a response that is damaging to body tissues. Antigen–antibody responses characterize types I, II, and III hypersensitivity, which are also known as *immediate hypersensitivity responses* (**Table 8–5 ●**). Type IV hypersensitivity is an antigen–lymphocyte reaction resulting in a delayed hypersensitivity response.

TABLE 8–5   Types of Hypersensitivity Reactions

TYPE	ETIOLOGY	CLINICAL MANIFESTATIONS	EXAMPLES
Type I: Localized or systemic reactions	Antibodies bind to certain cells, causing release of chemical substances that produce inflammation.	Hypotension, wheezing, gastrointestinal or uterine spasm, stridor, and urticaria.	Extrinsic asthma, allergic rhinitis (hay fever), and food allergies
Type II: Tissue-specific reactions	Antibodies cause activation of a complement system that leads to tissue damage.	Variable; may include dyspnea or fever.	Transfusion reaction, ABO incompatibility, and hemolytic disease of the newborn
Type III: Immune-complex–mediated reactions	Immune complexes are deposited in tissues, where they activate complement; the result is a generalized inflammatory reaction.	Urticaria, fever, and joint pain.	Acute glomerulonephritis and serum sickness
Type IV: Delayed reactions	Antigens stimulate T cells, which release lymphokines that cause inflammation and tissue damage.	Variable; may include fever, erythema, and itching.	Contact dermatitis, tuberculin skin test, and graft-versus-host disease

Type I (IgE-Mediated) Hypersensitivity

Common hypersensitivity reactions, such as allergic asthma, allergic rhinitis (hay fever), allergic conjunctivitis, hives, and anaphylactic shock, are typical of type I or IgE-mediated hypersensitivity. This type of hypersensitivity response is triggered when an allergen interacts with free IgE, causing IgE to bind to mast cells and basophils. This antigen–antibody complex prompts release of histamine and other chemical mediators, complement, acetylcholine, kinins, and chemotactic factors (**Figure 8–12 ●**).

Allergens can be ingested in food, injected as drugs, inhaled through the air, or absorbed through contact with unbroken skin.

When a potent allergen enters the bloodstream and triggers a widespread antibody–antigen reaction and response to these chemical mediators, a **systemic response**, such as anaphylaxis, urticaria, or angioedema, results. Common allergens in children are medications such as penicillin; animal dander; dust mites, mold, and plant pollens; and foods such as nuts, seafood, and egg white.

Anaphylaxis is an acute systemic type I response that may result in shock and death. It occurs in highly sensitive individuals following exposure to a specific antigen, usually through injection or ingestion. The reaction begins within minutes of exposure to the allergen and may be almost instantaneous. The

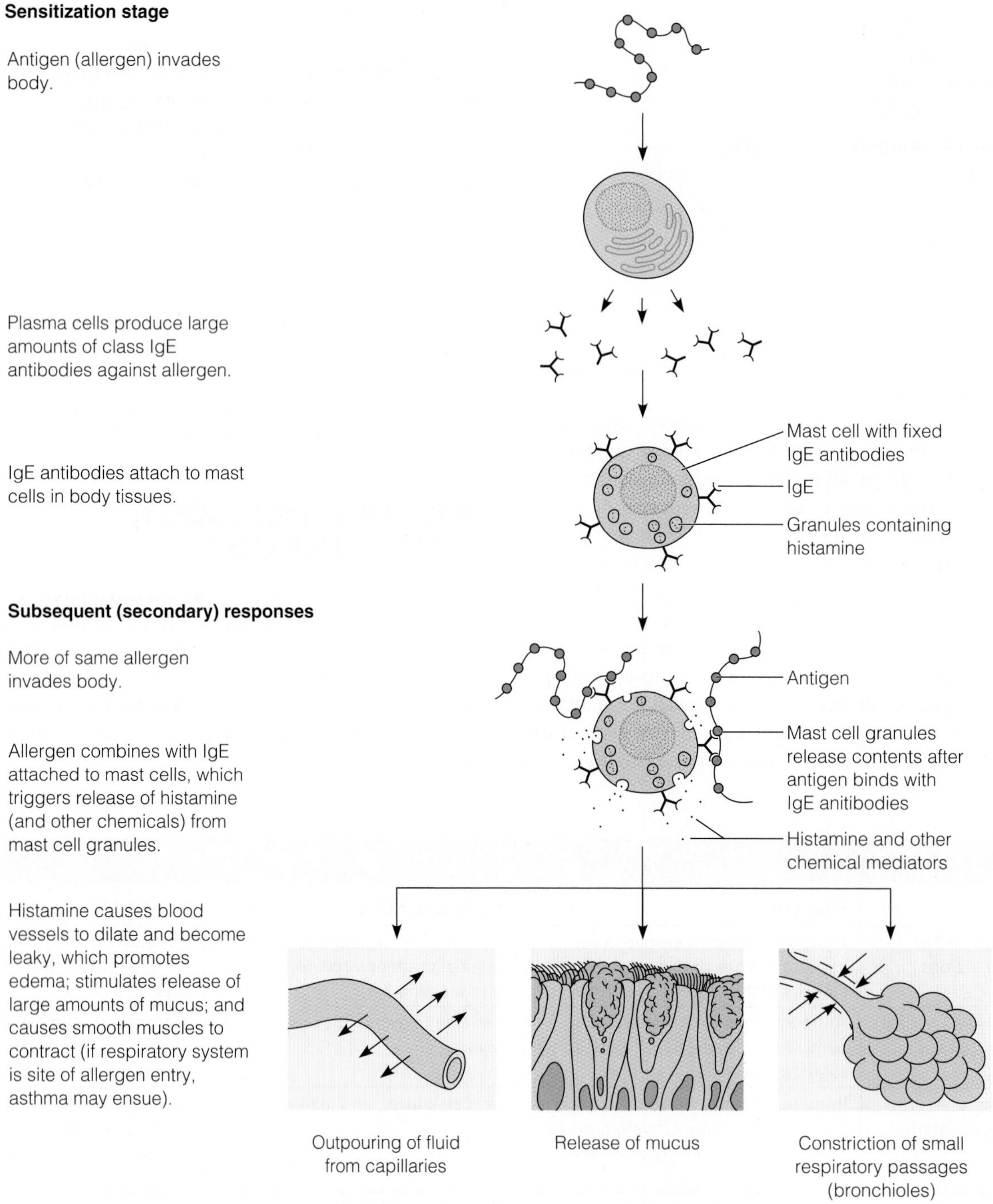

Sensitization stage

Antigen (allergen) invades body.

Plasma cells produce large amounts of class IgE antibodies against allergen.

IgE antibodies attach to mast cells in body tissues.

Subsequent (secondary) responses

More of same allergen invades body.

Allergen combines with IgE attached to mast cells, which triggers release of histamine (and other chemicals) from mast cell granules.

Histamine causes blood vessels to dilate and become leaky, which promotes edema; stimulates release of large amounts of mucus; and causes smooth muscles to contract (if respiratory system is site of allergen entry, asthma may ensue).

- Mast cell with fixed IgE antibodies
- IgE
- Granules containing histamine

- Antigen
- Mast cell granules release contents after antigen binds with IgE antibodies
- Histamine and other chemical mediators

Outpouring of fluid from capillaries

Release of mucus

Constriction of small respiratory passages (bronchioles)

Figure 8–12 ● Type I (IgE-mediated) hypersensitivity response.

Box 8–5 Substances Known to Trigger Anaphylaxis in Sensitized Individuals

HORMONES
- Insulin
- Vasopressin
- Parathormone

ENZYMES
- Trypsin
- Chymotrypsin
- Penicillinase

POLLENS
- Ragweed
- Grass
- Trees

FOODS
- Eggs
- Seafoods
- Nuts and nut by-products
- Grains
- Beans
- Cottonseed oil
- Chocolate

VITAMINS
- Thiamine
- Folic acid

INSECT VENOM
- Yellow jacket
- Hornet
- Paper wasp
- Honey bee

OCCUPATIONAL AGENTS
- Rubber products
- Industrial chemicals (ethylenes)

ANTIBIOTICS
- Penicillins
- Cephalosporins
- Amphotericin b
- Nitrofurantoin

LOCAL ANESTHETICS
- Procaine
- Lidocaine

MEDICAL DIAGNOSTIC AGENTS
- Sodium dehydrocholate
- Sulfobromophthalein

ANTISERUM
- Antilymphocyte gamma globulin

release of histamine and other mediators causes vasodilation and increased capillary permeability, smooth muscle contraction, and bronchial constriction. These chemical mediators cause the client to experience the typical manifestations of anaphylaxis. Initially, a sense of foreboding or uneasiness, light-headedness, and itching palms and scalp may be noted. Hives may develop, along with angioedema (localized tissue swelling) of the eyelids, lips, tongue, hands, feet, and genitals. Swelling also can affect the uvula and larynx, impairing breathing; this response is further complicated by bronchial constriction. The client exhibits air hunger, stridor and wheezing, and a barking cough. These respiratory effects can be lethal if the reaction is severe and intervention is not immediately available. Vasodilation and fluid loss from the vascular system can lead to impaired tissue perfusion and hypotension, a condition known as *anaphylactic shock*. Substances known to trigger anaphylaxis are summarized in **Box 8–5** ●.

A **localized response** is a more common manifestation of type I hypersensitivity. Localized responses typically are atopic responses; that is, they have a strong genetic predisposition. Atopic reactions are the result of localized, rather than systemic, IgE-mediated responses to an allergen. They are prompted by contact of the allergen with IgE in the bronchial tree, the nasal mucosa, and the conjunctival tissues. Chemical mediators are released locally, producing symptoms such as asthma, allergic rhinitis (hay fever), conjunctivitis, or atopic dermatitis. Allergens commonly associated with atopic reactions of this type include pollens, fungal spores, house dust mites, animal dander,

and feathers (Porth & Matfin, 2010). Food allergens also may cause localized responses, such as diarrhea or vomiting. If the gastrointestinal mucosa is altered by a local allergic response, then the allergen may be absorbed, and the resulting reaction maybe systemic. Urticaria (hives) is the most common systemic response to food allergies.

Type II (Cytotoxic) Hypersensitivity

A hemolytic **transfusion reaction** to blood of an incompatible type is characteristic of a type II or cytotoxic hypersensitivity reaction. IgG- or IgM-type antibodies are formed to a cell-bound antigen, such as the ABO or Rh antigen. The binding of these antibodies with the antigen activates the complement cascade, resulting in destruction of the target cell (**Figure 8–13** ●). This type of reaction causes hemolytic disease of the newborn.

Type II reactions may be stimulated by an exogenous antigen, such as foreign tissue or cells, or by a drug reaction, in which the drug forms an antigenic complex on the surface of a blood cell, stimulating the production of antibodies. The resulting antigen–antibody reaction destroys the affected cell; for example, the administration of certain drugs, such as penicillins, may cause a condition known as drug-induced hemolytic anemia. Withdrawal of the drug stops the reaction and cell destruction.

Endogenous antigens (which are produced by the body) also can stimulate a type II reaction, resulting in an autoimmune disorder such as Goodpasture syndrome, in which antigens form to specific tissues in the lungs and kidneys. Hashimoto thyroiditis and autoimmune hemolytic anemia are additional examples of autoimmune type II reactions.

Type III (Immune Complex–Mediated) Hypersensitivity

Type III or immune complex–mediated hypersensitivity reactions result from the formation of IgG or IgM antibody–antigen immune complexes in the circulatory system. When these complexes are deposited in vessel walls and extravascular tissues, complement is activated, and chemical mediators of inflammation, such as histamine, are released. Chemotactic factors attract neutrophils to the site of inflammation. When neutrophils attempt to phagocytize the immune complexes, the lysosomal enzymes released increase tissue damage (**Figure 8–14** ●).

Either systemic or local responses may be seen with type III reactions. For example, **serum sickness**, so named because it was first identified after administration of foreign serum (e.g., horse antitetanus toxin), is a systemic response. Immune complexes are deposited in walls of small blood vessels, the kidneys, and the joints. Manifestations of serum sickness include fever, urticaria or rash, arthralgias, myalgias, and lymphadenopathy. Although foreign serums are no longer administered, serum sickness still occurs in response to some drugs, such as penicillin and sulfonamides.

Localized responses may occur at a number of different sites. As immune complexes accumulate in the glomerular basement membrane of the kidneys—for example, following a streptococcal infection or with systemic lupus erythemato-

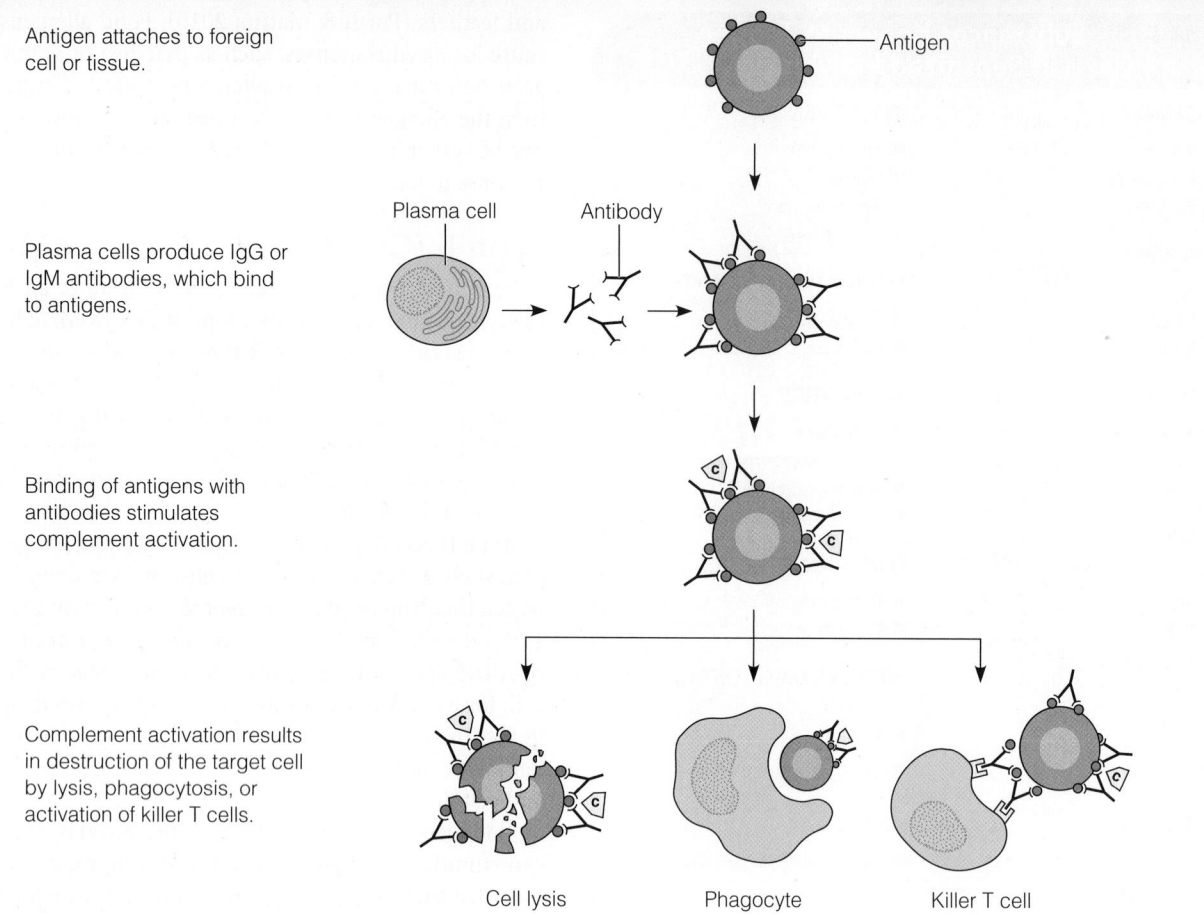

Antigen attaches to foreign cell or tissue.

Plasma cells produce IgG or IgM antibodies, which bind to antigens.

Binding of antigens with antibodies stimulates complement activation.

Complement activation results in destruction of the target cell by lysis, phagocytosis, or activation of killer T cells.

Antigen

Plasma cell   Antibody

Cell lysis   Phagocyte   Killer T cell

Figure 8–13 ● Type II (cytotoxic) hypersensitivity response.

sus—glomerulonephritis develops. When an antigen such as dust from moldy hay is inhaled, an acute alveolar inflammatory response can occur. This condition can develop in agricultural workers.

Type IV (Delayed) Hypersensitivity

Type IV reactions differ from other hypersensitivity responses in two ways. First, they are **cell-mediated immune responses**, not antibody-mediated responses, and involve T cells of the immune system. Second, type IV reactions are delayed rather than immediate, developing 24–48 hours after exposure to the antigen.

Type IV hypersensitivity responses result from an exaggerated interaction between an antigen and normal cell-mediated mechanisms. This exaggerated interaction results in the release of soluble inflammatory and immune mediators (from the lysozymes within the macrophages) and recruitment of killer T cells, causing local tissue destruction (**Figure 8–15 ●**).

CONTACT DERMATITIS   Contact dermatitis is a classic example of a type IV reaction. Intense redness, itching, edema, and thickening affect the skin in the area exposed to the antigen. Fragile vesicles often are present as well. Many antigens can provoke this response; poison ivy is a prime perpetrator. In the healthcare setting, an allergic response to latex also can produce contact dermatitis (see the section titled Latex Allergy that follows). Other

examples of cell-mediated responses are a positive tuberculin test and episodes of graft rejection.

LATEX ALLERGY   Although the repetitive use of latex gloves protects against infection, it also creates a persistent exposure to latex for healthcare workers. When gloves are powdered with cornstarch to facilitate donning and removing them, the cornstarch particles aerosolize when the gloves are removed. The presence of latex particles in the aerosolized cornstarch creates respiratory exposure as well as dermal exposure to latex. In addition, chemicals used in the manufacture of latex products may be irritating. Products such as balloons, condoms, and rubber bands commonly are made of latex.

Sensitivity to latex develops without the user's awareness until a rash appears on the hands. Type IV hypersensitivity (contact dermatitis) can progress to type I systemic allergic reactions without previous symptoms signaling an escalation. It is important to protect the client and the healthcare worker who is allergic to latex. Prevention is aided by employers' selection of products free of latex helps prevent allergic reactions. Nonlatex gloves are recommended for use where there is no contact with infectious materials or blood. Workers should be screened periodically for symptoms of allergy and should be educated about latex sources. Hand washing after using latex products limits exposure (National Institute for Occupational Safety and Health, 2012).

An estimated 8%–12% of healthcare workers are allergic to latex (Occupational Health and Safety Administration, 2008).

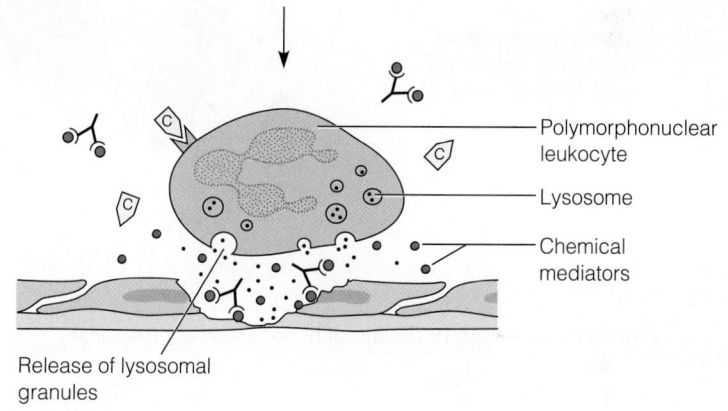

Antigens invade body and bind to antibodies in circulation. Antigen–antibody complexes are formed.

Antigen

Antibody

Antigen–antibody complex

Antigen–antibody complexes are deposited in the basement membrane of vessel walls and other body tissues, activating complement.

Basement membrane

Complement activation leads to release of inflammatory chemical mediators. Infiltration of polymorphonuclear leukocytes (PMNs) is followed by release of lysozymes. Tissue damage may be extensive.

Polymorphonuclear leukocyte

Lysosome

Chemical mediators

Release of lysosomal granules

Figure 8–14 ● Type III (immune complex–mediated) hypersensitivity response.

Among healthcare workers with an allergic reaction to latex, sensitization to gloves is most prevalent (22%), 3.6% report contact urticaria, and 2.3% have asthma or rhinitis (Filon & Radman, 2006).

Latex allergy also is common among clients with certain health conditions. For example, a high percentage of children with spina bifida have historically had latex sensitivities, though studies suggest that use of latex-free prophylaxis with this group has led to a significant drop in this percentage since the late 1990s (Blumchen et al., 2010). The children most at risk for latex allergy include those with spina bifida; congenital urological, gastrointestinal, and tracheoesophageal defects; and a history of atopy. Children who have had five or more surgeries are also more likely to become sensitized to latex. Individuals who are allergic to latex also have a high incidence of allergy to certain foods, including kiwi fruit, bananas, tomatoes, bell peppers, and avocados (Sampathi & Lerman, 2011).

Box 8–6 ● describes measures to protect against latex allergy. **Box 8–7 ●** addresses latex use in the hospital and the home.

Stay Current: *For a list of latex-free medical products, visit the American Latex Allergy Association at* **http:// latexallergyresources.org/medical-products**.

SAFETY ALERT

Starting in September 1998, the Food and Drug Administration (FDA) ordered that medical products with latex carry a warning label that reads: "Caution: This product contains natural rubber latex, which may cause allergic reactions." Check products in your healthcare facility for this label. What products do you expect to need the label? When children have latex allergy, have the family investigate all medical supplies for the warning label.

Etiology

An estimated 50 million people in the United States (or 1 in every 5) are diagnosed with some form of hypersensitivity. The

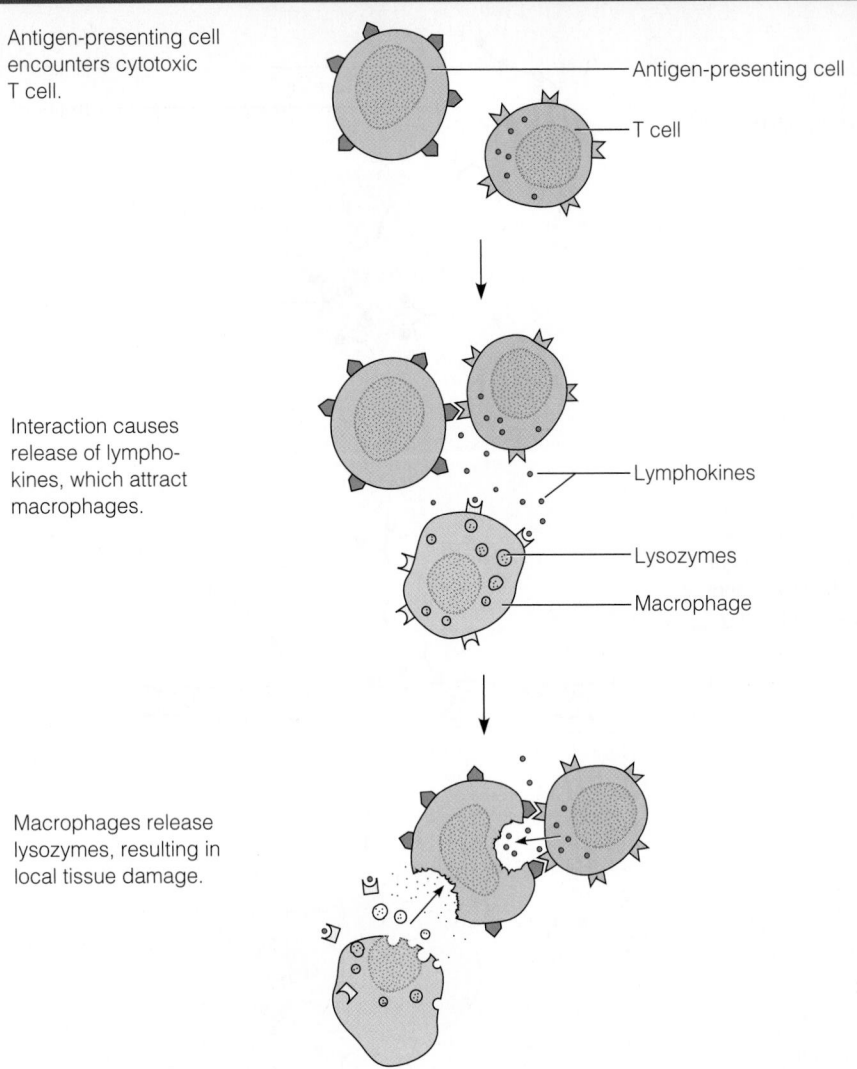

Antigen-presenting cell encounters cytotoxic T cell.

Antigen-presenting cell

T cell

Interaction causes release of lymphokines, which attract macrophages.

Lymphokines

Lysozymes

Macrophage

Macrophages release lysozymes, resulting in local tissue damage.

Figure 8–15 ● Type IV (delayed) hypersensitivity response.

Box 8–6   Measures to Protect Against Latex Allergy

Healthcare personnel are at high risk of developing latex allergy because of intense exposure to products containing latex. An estimated 8%–12% of healthcare workers are latex sensitive.

Nurses can protect themselves by using the following measures:

■ Decrease exposure by using alternative products when available (use synthetic rubbers, polyethylene, nitrile, neoprene, and vinyl gloves).

■ Use powder-free gloves if using latex gloves (the powder has high amounts of latex, which can be inhaled).

■ Avoid use of oil-based hand creams and lotions before putting on latex gloves, because these preparations break down the latex.

■ When symptoms of sensitivity to latex occur on exposure (e.g., rash, hives, nasal congestion, conjunctivitis, cough, or wheeze), contact the employee health department of your facility.

■ If diagnosed as latex-allergic, avoid all contact with latex, and wear a medical identification bracelet.

For more information, contact the National Institute for Occupational Safety and Health (NIOSH) at 1-800-232-4636 or the American Nurses Association at 1-800-274-4262.

---

incidence of hypersensitivity has been noted to be on the increase since the early 1980s. Hypersensitivity is the fifth leading chronic disease in the United States among all age groups and the third most common in children under 18 years of age. Hypersensitivity reactions account for more than 17 million outpatient office visits a year. Each year, nearly 400 people die from penicillin reactions, 200 from food allergies, and 100 from allergies to insects. In 2008, 10 deaths were attributed to latex reactions (Asthma and Allergy Foundation of American, 2009).

Risk Factors

Anyone can have a hypersensitivity reaction. However, risk generally increases with previous exposure, because antigens must be formed with the first exposure before hypersensitivity is likely to occur. Age, sex, concurrent illnesses, and previous reactions to related substances have been identified as having a role in risk for hypersensitivity (Gomes & Demoly, 2005). According to Viale (2009), factors that determine the development and severity of anaphylaxis include the antigen's route of entry, the amount of antigen introduced, the rate of absorption for the antigen, and the individual's degree of hypersensitivity.

Box 8–7 Latex in the Hospital and Home Environment

Any number of products used in both hospital and home environments may contain latex. Nurses must be aware of these products and knowledgeable about the alternatives offered in the settings in which they work. Nurses must also be able to provide appropriate education to clients with latex allergy.

Products in the hospital that frequently contain latex are:

- Band-Aids™
- Anesthesia circuits, bags, and oxygen masks
- Blood pressure cuffs and tubing
- Various types of catheters
- CPR mannequins and training aids
- Some types of dressings
- Earplugs
- Elastic wrap
- Endotracheal tubes, airways
- Gloves
- IV access materials
- Pulse oximeters
- Thermometer probes
- Suction tubing
- Vascular stockings

Products in the home or community that may contain latex are:

- Art supplies
- Balloons
- Balls and toys
- Carpet backing, floor sealant
- Chewing gum
- Elastic in clothing
- Condoms, diaphragms, sponges
- Diapers, rubber pants
- Pacifiers, feeding nipples
- Beach toys and equipment, including sandals
- Gloves used for cleaning or hair coloring

Having a family member with an allergy increases the chance that a child will have an allergy, even to different allergens or by showing different bodily manifestations. If one parent has an allergy of any type, chances are one in three that each child will have an allergy (Asthma and Allergy Foundation of America, 2009).

▶ CLINICAL MANIFESTATIONS

Hypersensitivity can manifest in a number of ways, including anaphylaxis, atopic disease, serum sickness, or contact dermatitis. Therefore symptoms can range from mild to severe or life-threatening and can be either localized or systemic. Characteristic findings in clients with hypersensitivity are summarized in **Table 8–6** ●.

Mild hypersensitivity responses can cause discomfort, fatigue, and even embarrassment to the client. These may last for a few hours to a day or two and normally resolve either by themselves or with over-the-counter treatments. Acute exacerbations of allergic rhinitis or asthma lasting beyond a day or two may result in a localized infection. Localized pain and inflammation, difficulty breathing, and loss of smell, taste, and appetite are associated with moderate to severe respiratory hypersensitivity responses. Moderate hypersensitive responses of the skin include urticaria and atopic and contact dermatitis. Moderate reactions from food allergies include urticaria and gastrointestinal symptoms. Severe reactions, regardless of the antigen's means of entry or the location of the initial reaction, may lead to respiratory distress or death.

Care for clients with allergic responses focuses on minimizing exposure to the allergen, preventing a hypersensitivity response, and providing prompt, effective interventions for allergic responses when they occur. Identifying allergens for the individual to reduce the likelihood of exposure is a key aspect of management. A complete history of the client's allergies is obtained, including medications, foods, animals, plants, and other materials. The type of hypersensitivity response is documented, as is its onset, manifestations, and usual treatment.

When a documented or suspected hypersensitivity reaction occurs, the allergen (e.g., an intravenous medication or a transfusion) is withdrawn immediately. With a type I hypersensitivity response, managing the client's airway takes highest priority, followed by maintaining cardiac output. Type II hypersensitivity responses may necessitate aggressive management of bleeding or renal failure. A type III (immune complex–mediated) reaction is treated by removing the offending antigen and interrupting the inflammatory response.

With a hypersensitivity response, supportive care is important to relieve discomfort. It often involves the administration of selected antihistamine or anti-inflammatory medications. Other therapies, such as plasmapheresis, may be prescribed in selected instances.

TABLE 8–6 Characteristic Findings in Clients with Allergies

SYSTEM	CHARACTERISTIC FINDINGS
Respiratory	Asthma, rhinitis (seasonal and perennial), serous otitis media, cough, pneumonia, croup, and edema of glottis
Gastrointestinal	Abdominal pain and colic, stomatitis, constipation, diarrhea, bloody stools, geographic tongue, and vomiting
Skin	Angioedema, urticaria, eczema, atopic dermatitis, erythema multiforme, purpura, drug and food rashes, and contact dermatitis
Nervous	Headache, tension, fatigue, convulsions, Méniére disease, and tremor
Eye	Conjunctivitis, cataract, ciliary spasm, and iritis
Blood	Thrombocytopenic purpura, hemolytic anemia, leukopenia, and agranulocytosis
Musculoskeletal	Arthralgia, myalgia, rheumatoid arthritis, and torticollis
Genitourinary	Dysuria, vulvovaginitis, and enuresis
Miscellaneous	Anaphylactic shock, serum sickness, and autoimmune disorders

Clinical Manifestations and Therapies **Hypersensitivity**

ETIOLOGY	CLINICAL MANIFESTATION	CLINICAL THERAPIES
Serum sickness is a reaction to proteins in antiserum derived from animals.	Manifestations develop up to 2 weeks after exposure and may include rash, pruritus, arthralgia, fever, lymphadenopathy, hypotension, splenomegaly, glomerulonephritis, or proteinuria.	▪ Often does not require medical intervention. Severe reactions may be treated with corticosteroids, antihistamines, and/or plasmapheresis.
Allergic rhinitis is a seasonal response to pollens of specific plants but also may result from exposure to dust mites, danders, or molds at any time of year.	Rhinorrhea, watery eyes, itchy throat, hives, sore throat, nasal congestion, and headache are common manifestations. Facial edema; if the client does not respond to initial treatment, may result in a severe reaction.	▪ Most effective treatment is reducing exposure to allergen by remaining indoors, showering on entering the house to remove pollen, keeping doors and windows closed, using special filters on air conditioners, and maintaining a clean, dust-free environment. ▪ Pharmacologic therapies include decongestants, antihistamines, antileukotrienes, and immunotherapy. A tapered dose of oral steroids may be necessary to resolve an acute exacerbation.
Graft-versus-host disease results as an immune response to organ, bone marrow, or stem cell transplants.	Acute within the first 3 months after transplant. Manifestations include a skin rash, nausea, vomiting, diarrhea, cramping, abdominal pain, and jaundice. Chronic after the first 3 months. Manifestations include dry eyes and dry mouth, difficulty swallowing, fatigue and muscle weakness, skin reactions, liver disease, shortness of breath, and genitourinary symptoms (Cleveland Clinic, 2011).	▪ Immunosuppressant drugs are the standard therapy. ▪ Careful assessment of clients who have received a transplant. ▪ Education of client regarding symptoms to report immediately.
Allergic asthma.	Characterized by bronchoconstriction and airway inflammation. Clients may complain of having shortness of breath, chest pain, or a feeling like "an elephant is sitting on my chest."	▪ Prevention and treatment are similar to those for allergic rhinitis, with inhaled medications such as albuterol and inhaled corticosteroids being among the most effective treatments. Clients with severe allergic asthma may require antibiotics and oral steroids if an exacerbation continues beyond 2–3 days, trapping mucus and resulting in an infection.

Lifespan and Cultural Considerations

It is not uncommon for people to outgrow certain allergies—particularly food allergies—as they age. Egg, milk, soy, and wheat allergies are among those that many people outgrow; however, it is uncommon to outgrow peanut allergy. Conversely, individuals who develop allergies in adulthood typically have them for the remainder of their lives (NIAID, 2012).

▶ COLLABORATION

Due to technological advances and continued research, a variety of diagnostic tests and treatment protocols are available to clients with suspected or known hypersensitivity. Treatment protocols generally include pharmacotherapy. Individuals with hypersensitivity may need to avoid certain herbal supplements and should be counseled regarding the need to adhere to the care plan in order to decrease the risk for severe reactions.

Diagnostic Tests

To identify possible allergens and hypersensitivity reactions, laboratory tests may be ordered. To determine causes of hypersensitivity reactions, skin tests may be ordered.

LABORATORY TESTING   To identify possible allergens or hypersensitivity reactions, the following laboratory tests may be ordered:

- ■ *White blood cell count with differential.* This test can detect high levels of circulating eosinophils. Normally, eosinophils constitute a very small percentage (1%–4%) of the total of WBCs. Eosinophilia, however, often is present in clients with type I hypersensitivities.

- **Radioallergosorbent test (RAST).** This test measures the amount of IgE directed toward specific allergens. Test results are compared with control values and used to identify hypersensitivities. RAST poses no risk for an anaphylactic reaction. It is particularly useful in detecting allergies to some occupational chemicals and toxic allergens (Goldsby et al., 2003).

- **Blood type and crossmatch.** These tests are ordered before any anticipated transfusions. The client's ABO blood group and Rh status are determined. Two major antigens, designated A and B, may be present on RBCs. Clients with the A antigen are designated as blood type A; those with the B antigen are designated as blood type B. When neither antigen is found on the RBCs, the individual is identified as type O. A third major RBC antigen is the Rh antigen. Individuals with this antigen are called Rh positive; those without are called Rh negative. Because a blood transfusion is actually a transplant of living tissue, antigen matching is vital to prevent significant hypersensitivity reactions. Once blood type is determined, a sample of the client's blood is mixed with a sample of matching donor blood and observed for antigen–antibody reactions in the crossmatch portion of this test. Although this procedure greatly reduces the risk of a hemolytic transfusion reaction (type II hypersensitivity), it does not totally eliminate it.

- **Indirect Coombs test.** This test detects the presence of circulating antibodies (other than ABO antibodies) against RBCs. The client's serum is mixed with the donor's RBCs. If the client's serum contains antibodies to an RBC antigen, agglutination (clumping together) will occur. This is called a positive response. The normal value is negative (no agglutination). This test is also part of the crossmatch of a blood "type and crossmatch."

- **Direct Coombs test.** This test detects antibodies on the client's RBCs that damage and destroy the cells. This test is used following a suspected transfusion reaction, to detect antibodies coating the transfused RBCs. It also can identify hemolytic anemia when the cause is unknown. In the direct Coombs test, the client's RBCs are mixed with Coombs serum, which contains antibodies to IgG and several complement components. Agglutination occurs if the client's RBCs are coated with antibodies; agglutination means the test is positive. As with the indirect Coombs test, the normal test result is negative (no agglutination).

- **Immune complex assays.** These tests may be performed to detect the presence of circulating immune complexes in suspected type III hypersensitivity responses. These assays are particularly useful in diagnosing suspected autoimmune disorders. Nonspecific assays of IgG-, IgM-, and IgA-containing immune complexes, which do not detect specific antibodies, as well as specific antibody assays, may be done. The normal result is a test negative for circulating immune complexes. A negative test does not, however, rule out an immune complex hypersensitivity response. In some cases, a negative result indicates that the disease process has reached a later stage, in which complexes are no longer circulating but have initiated extensive tissue damage, such as glomerulonephritis (Kasper et al., 2005).

- **Complement assay.** This test also is useful in detecting immune complex disorders. In these disorders, complement is, in effect, used up by the development of antigen–antibody complexes. Decreased levels are seen on examination. Both total complement level and amounts of individual components of the complement cascade can be determined.

SKIN TESTING   Skin tests also are used to determine causes of hypersensitivity reactions. These tests identify specific allergens to which an individual may be sensitive. Allergens for testing are selected according to the client's history. Test solutions made from extracts of inhaled, ingested, or injected materials, such as pollens, mites, venoms, and some drugs, are used for the prick test and intradermal testing. Epicutaneous testing (prick testing) generally is done first to avoid a systemic reaction; it is followed by intradermal testing of allergens with a negative response to prick testing (Tierney et al., 2005). Performing the large-dose intradermal test first would place individuals who are highly allergic to a substance at increased risk for an anaphylactic reaction. Substances that cause a reaction to the prick test should not be tested intradermally.

Specific skin tests include the following:

- **Prick (epicutaneous or puncture) test.** A drop of diluted allergenic extract is placed on the skin, and the skin is then pricked or punctured through the drop. A localized pruritic wheal and erythema indicates a positive test. The response is maximal at 15–20 minutes.

- **Intradermal test.** A small amount (just enough to create a wheal) of allergen extract at a 1:500 or 1:1,000 dilution is injected on the forearm or intrascapular area. If several allergens are being tested, injections are spaced 0.25–0.5 cm apart. As control measures, plain diluent (negative control) and histamine (positive control) also are injected. If no response to a particular allergen has occurred at 15–20 minutes, the test is negative. The appearance of a wheal and erythema, with a wheal diameter at least 5 mm greater than that produced by the control, indicates a positive response (**Figure 8–16** ●).

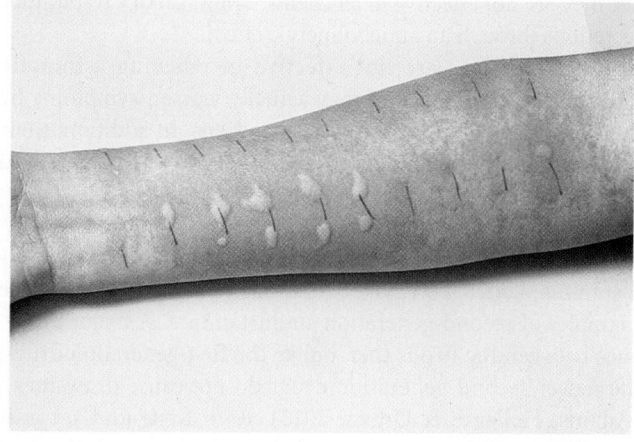

Figure 8–16 ● Skin testing on the forearm, showing induration and erythema typical of a positive response to an antigen.
Source: SUI/Science Source.

■ *Patch test.* A 1-in. patch impregnated with the allergen (e.g., perfume, cosmetics, detergents, or clothing fibers) is applied to the skin for 48 hours. Absence of a response indicates a negative test result. Positive responses are graded from mild (erythema in the exposed area) to severe (erythema, papules, vesicles, or ulceration).

■ *Food allergy test.* This test is performed when a food allergy is suspected but the source or implicated food item has not been clearly identified. Symptoms of a food allergy typically are demonstrated within hours of eating. Initially, the client is asked to keep a diary of foods consumed and any allergic responses for a week. After this period, an elimination diet is prescribed. This diet excludes most common food allergens and all suspected foods for 1 week. Any foods that may contain allergens in combination, such as breads, also are eliminated. If symptoms do not improve, a different variation of the elimination diet is prescribed. If symptoms are relieved, foods are reintroduced to the diet one at a time until the symptoms recur, indicating an allergy to that food.

Pharmacologic Therapy

Pharmacologic treatments are chosen based on the severity of the hypersensitivity reaction and the impact on the client's lifestyle. More severe reactions may require administration via the IV route in order to get the fastest possible action, while mild reactions may be treated with oral medications. A thorough medication history should be collected before the administration of any medication, including medication allergies.

ANTIHISTAMINES
Antihistamines are the major class of drugs used in treating the symptoms of hypersensitivity responses, particularly type I reactions. They also are useful to some extent in relieving manifestations (e.g., urticaria) of some type II and type III reactions.

Antihistamines block H_1-histamine receptors, acting as a competitive antagonist to histamine, but they do not affect the production or release of histamine. The prototype antihistamine is diphenhydramine (Benadryl). It and other antihistamines alleviate the systemic effects of histamine, such as urticaria and angioedema. They also are useful in relieving allergic rhinitis, but they are not effective in all clients. They also dry respiratory secretions through an anticholinergic effect.

Antihistamines are not effective in relieving asthmatic responses to allergens and may actually worsen symptoms by their drying effect on respiratory secretions. In addition, their use is limited by their side effects, especially drowsiness and dry mouth.

Antihistamines can be classified as first- or second-generation. Diphenhydramine is an example of a first-generation antihistamine; cetirizine (Zyrtec) and fexofenadine (Allegra) are examples of second-generation antihistamines. A major difference between the two is that, unlike the first-generation drugs, the newer second-generation drugs do not cause drowsiness. (Adams, Holland, & Urban, 2013). Both first- and second-generation antihistamines are available in both prescription and nonprescription preparations. The preferred route of administration is oral, although diphenhydramine and others can be given parenterally, particularly when immediate action is needed, as in anaphylaxis. Antihistamines often are combined with a sympathomimetic agent, such as pseudoephedrine, to improve their decongestant activity and counteract their sedative effect.

MAST CELL STABILIZERS
Mast cell stabilizers inhibit the release of histamine from sensitized mast cells. Cromolyn sodium (Intal, NasalCrom) is an example and is used to treat allergic rhinitis and asthma. For treatment of hypersensitivity, cromolyn sodium is inhaled or administered intranasally. While it has relatively few side effects and a wide margin of safety, its use has not been studied in children younger than 6 years of age and is not approved for use in that population (Wilson et al., 2013). Other mast cell stabilizers include ketotifen (Zaditor), nedocromil (Alocril), and lodoxamide (Alomide).

LEUKOTRIENE MODIFIERS
Leukotriene modifiers block the action of inflammatory chemicals—known as *leukotrienes*—released by the body in response to allergens. These medications reduce inflammation and nasal congestion associated with allergies and prevent airway constriction associated with asthma. A number of leukotriene modifiers are available for asthma, but only montelukast (Singulair) is approved for management of both allergic rhinitis and asthma. Leukotriene modifiers are available in granules, tablets, and chewable tablets and may take several weeks to achieve full effect. Side effects include fever, nausea, headache, and nasal congestion. Their effects in children under 12 months are not known (Wilson et al., 2013).

CORTICOSTEROIDS
Corticosteroids (glucocorticoids) are used in both systemic and topical forms for many types of hypersensitivity responses. Their anti-inflammatory effects, rather than their immunosuppressive effects, are of most benefit. A short course of corticosteroid therapy often is used for severe asthma, allergic contact dermatitis, and some immune-complex disorders. Corticosteroids in topical forms or delivered by inhaler may be used for longer periods of time with few side effects; however, systemic absorption can occur.

IMMUNOTHERAPY
For clients who receive only minimal benefit from antihistamines and cromolyn sodium, or who require a course of oral steroids more than once a year, immunotherapy may be recommended. Also called *hyposensitization, desensitization,* or *allergy shots,* immunotherapy consists of injecting an extract of the allergen(s) in gradually increasing doses. Immunotherapy is used primarily for allergic rhinitis or asthma related to inhaled allergens. It also has been shown to be effective in preventing anaphylactic responses to insect venom. With weekly or biweekly subcutaneous injections of the allergen, the client develops IgG antibodies to the allergens that appear to effectively block the allergic IgE-mediated response. Once a therapy plateau is reached, injections are continued indefinitely, either monthly or bimonthly. Immunotherapy typically is provided by an allergist or immunologist.

EPINEPHRINE
The immediate treatment for anaphylaxis is parenteral epinephrine, an adrenergic agonist (sympathomimetic) drug that has both vasoconstricting and bronchodilating effects. These qualities, combined with its rapid action, make epinephrine ideal for treating an anaphylactic reaction. For mild

reactions with wheezing, pruritus, urticaria, and angioedema, a subcutaneous injection of 0.3–0.5 mL of 1:1,000 epinephrine generally is sufficient. For clients with an injected toxin such as a bee sting, an additional amount equivalent to half the above may be injected directly into the site of the sting and a tourniquet applied above it to prevent further systemic absorption. Intravenous epinephrine using a 1:100,000 concentration may be used in the client with a more severe anaphylactic reaction.

Clients who have experienced an anaphylactic reaction to insect venom or other potentially unavoidable allergens should carry a kit (commonly called a *bee sting kit* or *EpiPen*) for immediate treatment of future exposures. This kit typically includes a prefilled syringe of epinephrine and an epinephrine nebulizer, allowing prompt self-treatment.

OMALIZUMAB Omalizumab (Xolair) is approved for use by clients with steroid-dependent asthma and high IgE values who have not achieved adequate results with immunotherapy. Xolair inhibits type I hypersensitivity reactions by binding to free-floating IgE, thereby preventing IgE from binding to the mast cell. Since its introduction, Xolair has had wide success for its target client population—so much so that many physicians are trying it on clients with other type I hypersensitivities, including severe allergic dermatitis and severe allergic rhinitis.

Radioallergosorbent testing and approval from the physician, insurance company, and the manufacturer are required before a client can receive Xolair. Administered by subcutaneous injection in a physician's office, clinic, or infusion center, Xolair is an incredibly expensive medication. It also is not an immediate solution: Some clients may not experience improvement in symptoms for several months to a year. The FDA has issued a black box warning that clients who take Xolair may exhibit anaphylactic reactions within 48 hours of receiving the medication, but these episodes are very rare.

Nonpharmacologic Therapy

Other treatments for hypersensitivity generally are dictated by the severity of the response and by the organ system affected. Airway management takes highest priority for the client with an acute anaphylactic reaction. With severe laryngospasm, an emergency tracheostomy or the insertion of an endotracheal tube may be required to maintain airway patency. Because anaphylaxis places the individual at risk for vasomotor collapse and significant hypotension, it is necessary to insert an intravenous line and initiate fluid resuscitation with an isotonic solution, such as Ringer lactate.

Plasmapheresis (removal of harmful components in the plasma) may be used to treat immune complex responses such as glomerulonephritis and Goodpasture syndrome. The client's blood is passed through a blood cell separator, and plasma and the glomerula-damaging antibody–antigen complexes are removed. The RBCs are then returned to the client, along with an equal amount of albumin or human plasma. This procedure usually is done in a series rather than as a one-time treatment. It also is not without risk; informed consent is required. Potential complications of plasmapheresis are those associated with intravenous catheters, shifts in fluid balance, and alteration of blood clotting.

The nurse should refer clients with recurrent moderate and severe hypersensitivity responses to a specialist. Clients with allergic rhinitis, asthma, and atopic dermatitis may be referred to an allergist for further evaluation and testing. Immunologists care for those with other, more complicated immune disorders. Clients with complicated respiratory issues may benefit from working with a respiratory therapist to learn appropriate posturing and breathing techniques. Physical therapists can help clients design an appropriate exercise regimen after surgery or transplantation. Dieticians can help clients with food allergies develop appropriately healthy, tasty recipes and menus.

For children with severe hypersensitivity reactions, nurses at the child's clinic or specialist's office should help the parents design and provide an action plan for the child's school. This plan ensures that teachers, nurses, and other school personnel know how to respond in the event the child has an exacerbation at school. Any medication being kept at school should also accompany the child on field trips. Day care centers and summer camps should receive copies of the child's action plan as well.

Severe allergies in children can be very frightening to the parents. Any parent who has seen a child experience a severe exacerbation or anaphylactic reaction lives in fear that it will happen again—and that the child's life will be at risk. Parents of these clients, as well as clients who are old enough to recognize the manifestations of a hypersensitivity reaction, may benefit from participating in age-appropriate support groups. The nurse should explore available options and offer referrals to hospital, clinic, and community resources.

Stay Current: *The Food Allergy and Anaphylaxis Network* (**http://www.foodallergy.org**) *is a helpful resource for many, as are the Web sites of the American Academy of Allergy, Asthma, and Immunology* (**http://www.aaaai.org**) *and National Jewish Health* (**http://www.nationaljewish.org**), *one of the leading medical research centers in the United States.*

Complementary and Alternative Therapy

Many people with various illnesses find a number of complementary and alternative medicine therapies soothing and comforting. However, clients with type I hypersensitivity should consult their healthcare provider before using herbal remedies, teas, and aromatherapy, because many of these contain substances to which individuals are allergic. Chamomile tea, widely used for its comforting properties, has not been studied thoroughly, but there have been sufficient reports of allergic reactions to chamomile to warrant concern. Like ragweed, chamomile is a member of the daisy family, so individuals with ragweed allergies should avoid using chamomile products (NCCAM, 2012).

Many Asian Americans and Native Americans rely on complementary and alternative medicine because such therapies are a part of their culture. Nurses working with clients from these cultures should ask appropriate questions to determine if the client uses any herbal medicine and should be sensitive to the importance that clients may place on traditional therapies from their cultures of origin.

NURSING PROCESS

Nursing care related to hypersensitivity reactions is directed primarily toward prevention, early identification, and prompt, effective treatment. Nurses are also responsible for teaching clients and families to alert school personnel, coworkers, and all healthcare personnel in hospitals and clinics to the client's allergy or condition.

Health promotion activities include helping clients to identify possible allergens that prompt a hypersensitivity response and discussing possible strategies to avoid these allergens. Anyone with severe food allergies may need assistance from a dietitian to discuss necessary dietary changes and ways to continue meeting nutritional needs. It is important that individuals with hypersensitivities inform healthcare personnel of all allergens. The nurse should advise individuals who experience or are at risk for anaphylactic reactions to wear a medical alert bracelet or tag at all times to identify the substance(s) that provokes this response.

Assessment

The nurse should collect the following data:

- **Health history.** Risk factors; hypersensitivities (e.g., medications, household dust, bee stings); reaction signs and symptoms (rash, hives, difficulty breathing); type of treatment for hypersensitivity reactions; allergy skin testing; history of asthma, hay fever, or dermatitis; use of herbal supplements and over-the-counter and prescription medications.
- **Physical assessment.** Mucous membranes of nose and mouth, skin for lesions or rashes, eyes (tearing and redness), respiratory rate, and adventitious breath sounds.

Further focused assessments are described in the Implementation section that follows.

Diagnosis

Priority nursing diagnoses vary according to the type of hypersensitivity reaction. Because nurses are most likely to see a client experiencing a type I or type II response, this section focuses on diagnoses for these clients.

Airway, breathing, and circulation (the ABCs) are of greatest importance for the client with an anaphylactic reaction. When a hemolytic reaction to an incompatible blood transfusion occurs, the client is at risk for injury. Possibly high-priority nursing diagnoses are the following:

- *Ineffective Airway Clearance*
- *Decreased Cardiac Output*
- *Risk for Injury*
- *Impaired Spontaneous Ventilation*
- *Risk for Shock.*

(NANDA-I © 2012)

Planning

Of key importance in planning nursing care is prevention of hypersensitivity reaction through thorough data collection to help the client avoid exposure to known allergens. Priority goals for the client with hypersensitivity may include the following:

- Client will avoid known substances that provoke hypersensitivity response.
- Client will describe self-care to reduce symptoms of seasonal allergies.

- Client will describe proper self-administration of medications prescribed by the physician.
- Client will help determine substances that cause hypersensitivity by keeping an accurate food journal.

Implementation

Nursing implementations depend on the client's individual needs and the nursing diagnoses selected. Actions in the following section are grouped by nursing diagnosis.

Maintain a Patent Airway

Maintaining a patent airway (or establishing airway clearance in the event of anaphylactic shock) is the highest priority in caring for the client experiencing a hypersensitivity response. Placing the client in Fowler or high Fowler position allows optimal lung expansion and ease of breathing (see Figure 15–11 in the module on Oxygenation).

For mild to moderate reactions, the nurse will do the following:

- Assess respiratory rate and pattern, level of consciousness and anxiety, nasal flaring, use of accessory muscles of respiration, chest wall movement, audible stridor; palpation for respiratory excursion; auscultation of lung sounds and any adventitious sounds, such as wheezes. Extreme anxiety or agitation, nasal flaring, stridor, and diminished lung sounds indicate air hunger and possible airway obstruction, necessitating immediate intervention.

  In anaphylactic reactions, the airway obstruction may be a result of facial angioedema, bronchospasm, or laryngeal edema. In these cases, the nurse will:
- Administer oxygen per nasal cannula at a rate of 2–4 L/min. Apply oxygen emergently, and obtain a physician order for oxygen administration to increase the alveolar oxygen and its availability to cells of the body.
- Insert a nasopharyngeal or oropharyngeal airway, and arrange for immediate intubation as indicated. Ensuring an adequate airway is vital to preserve life.
- Administer subcutaneous epinephrine 1:1,000, 0.3–0.5 mL, as prescribed. This may be repeated in 20–30 minutes if necessary. Also, administer parenteral diphenhydramine (deep intramuscular or intravenous) as prescribed. Epinephrine is a potent vasoconstrictor and bronchodilator, counteracting the effects of histamine. Diphenhydramine is an antihistamine that blocks histamine receptors and their effect. These medications can rapidly reverse manifestations of anaphylaxis (see the Client Teaching feature).
- Provide calm reassurance. Hypoxemia and air hunger terrify the client. Anxiety can impair the client's ability to cooperate with treatment and can increase the respiratory rate, making breathing less effective.

Monitor Cardiac Status

Peripheral vasodilation and increased capillary permeability resulting from the release of histamine can significantly impair cardiac output. In all cases in which a client is exhibiting a hypersensitive reaction, the nurse should:

- Monitor vital signs frequently, noting fall in blood pressure, decreasing pulse pressure, tachycardia, and tachypnea. These changes in vital signs may indicate shock.

Client Teaching Using an EpiPen®

If the client has had a severe or systemic reaction in the past, the nurse ensures that the client and family or caregivers know how to handle an anaphylactic reaction if another one occurs:

- Inform the client that kits with syringes of premeasured epinephrine are available by prescription.
- Ensure that client, family members, and caregivers understand how to use the kit.
- Encourage the client to wear a medical alert bracelet or tag.
- Instruct the client and family on proper storage of the kit, avoiding exposure to sun or high temperature.
- Instruct the client and family to frequently check the expiration date of the EpiPen.
- Emphasize to the client and family that a kit should be readily available in all settings where the client studies, works, or plays, including school, camp, work, and child care. In addition to the client, someone else should always know how to use the kit as well.

- Assess skin color, temperature, capillary refill, edema, and other indicators of peripheral perfusion. As cardiac output falls, peripheral vessels constrict, and tissue perfusion is impaired.
- Monitor level of consciousness. A change in level of consciousness (lethargy, apprehension, or agitation) often is the first indicator of decreased cardiac output.

When cardiac output falls to where tissue perfusion is impaired and hypoxia results, a state of anaphylactic shock exists. In this event, the nurse should:

- Insert one or more large-bore (≥18 gauge) intravenous catheters. It is important to insert intravenous catheters as soon as possible to provide sites for rapid fluid replacement.
- Administer warmed intravenous solutions of lactated Ringer or normal saline as prescribed. These isotonic solutions help to maintain intravascular volume. Solutions are warmed to prevent hypothermia from the rapid administration of large amounts of fluid at room temperature (~70°F [21.1°C]).
- Insert an indwelling catheter, and monitor urinary output frequently. As the cardiac output drops, the glomerular filtration rate falls. With an output of less than 30 mL/hr, the client is at risk for acute renal failure from ischemia.
- Place a tourniquet above the site of an injected venom (e.g., a bee sting), and infiltrate the site with epinephrine as prescribed. Use of a tourniquet and the vasoconstriction resulting from epinephrine infiltration reduce further absorption of the allergen.
- Once breathing is established, place the client flat with the legs elevated. This position enhances perfusion of the central organs, such as the brain, heart, and kidneys.

SAFETY ALERT

Aggressive infusion of intravenous fluids may lead to hypervolemia and pulmonary edema. Assess for shortness of breath and crackles in the lungs.

Reduce Risk for Injury

As noted, the potential for hypersensitivity responses is high in clients subjected to medical treatments. Because a blood transfusion is a transplant of living tissue, the risk for adverse immunological response and injury is particularly significant.

- Obtain and record a thorough history of previous blood transfusions and any reactions experienced, *no matter how mild*. Alert the physician if previous transfusion reactions have occurred. The client who has received prior blood transfusions is at increased risk for a hypersensitivity reaction, because antibody production may have been stimulated by previous exposure to antigens.
- Check for a signed informed consent to administer blood or blood products. It is important to obtain informed consent for such invasive and risky procedures.
- Using two licensed healthcare professionals, double-check client identity, blood type, Rh factor, crossmatch, and expiration date for all blood and blood components received from the blood bank with the client's data. This is an important safety measure to reduce the risk of a hemolytic transfusion reaction as a result of incompatible blood types.
- Take and record vital signs within 15 minutes before initiating the blood infusion. This information provides a baseline for evaluating any changes related to the blood transfusion.
- Administer the prescribed acetaminophen and diphenhydramine prior to beginning a blood transfusion to decrease inflammation and increase client comfort. These medications will not mask serious reactions.
- Infuse blood into a site separate from that of any other intravenous infusion, using a catheter of at least 20 gauge to promote flow. This procedure reduces the risk of damage to the blood cells because of incompatibility with other intravenous solutions or physical trauma.
- Administer blood with normal saline to prime intravenous tubing. When blood is administered with dextrose solutions (e.g., D_5W, D_5NS), blood cell hemolysis and aggregation occur; administration with lactated Ringer can cause agglutination of cells.
- Administer 50 mL of blood during the first 15 minutes of the transfusion. Reactions generally occur within the first 15 minutes.
- During transfusion, monitor for complaints of back or chest pain, increase in the temperature of more than 1.8°F, chills, tachycardia, tachypnea, wheezing, hypotension, hives, rashes, or cyanosis. These signs may indicate an adverse reaction to the blood transfusion.
- Stop the blood transfusion immediately if a reaction occurs, no matter how mild. Remove the blood bag and the tubing with blood in it. Flush new intravenous tubing with normal saline, keeping the intravenous line open. Notify the physician and the blood bank.
- If a reaction is suspected, send the blood and administration set to the laboratory with a freshly drawn blood sample and urine specimen from the client. These will be used to identify the cause of the reaction as well as its effect on the client.
- If no adverse reaction occurs, administer the transfusion over 2–4 hours. This time frame is important to limit the risk of bacterial growth.

Client Teaching   Client and Family Care for Hypersensitivity

- When and how to use an anaphylaxis kit containing epinephrine and antihistamines in injectable, inhaled, and oral forms
- When to seek medical attention
- How to use and look for adverse reactions to prescription and nonprescription antihistamines and decongestants
- What are the advantages of autologous blood transfusion if future surgery is scheduled
- How to prevent an immune complex reaction, such as glomerulonephritis
- What skin care can prevent contact dermatitis, including:
  a. Expose affected areas to air and sun as much as possible.
  b. Avoid direct contact with people who have an infection.

  c. Wear cool, light, nonrestrictive clothing of natural fibers, such as cotton, to avoid irritating affected areas.
  d. Avoid exposure to extremes of heat or cold.
  e. Use bath oils or plain water instead of soaps and detergents.
  f. Take tub baths in cool to lukewarm water rather than showers.
  g. To decrease pruritus, maintain a cool environment and avoid exercising.
  h. Trim fingernails to reduce the risk of skin damage.
- Helpful resources:
  a. American Latex Allergy Association, www.latexallergyresources.org
  b. The Food Allergy and Anaphylaxis Network, www.foodallergy.org

SAFETY ALERT
To reduce bacterial contamination, begin a transfusion of the blood within 30 minutes of its delivery from the blood bank.

Community-Based Care

The vast majority of hypersensitivity responses are appropriately treated by the client or family members, with little or no medical intervention. Therefore teaching is a vital component of care. If the client is at risk for anaphylaxis, involving the family in teaching is essential because the rapidity of the response may keep the client from providing self-care. When teaching the client and family about managing hypersensitivities, include the points in the Client Teaching feature.

Clients with type I hypersensitivities often are misunderstood and even mistreated by their families and community. "Are you really sick, or is it just your allergies?" is not an uncommon response to children returning to school or adults returning to work after being out sick because of an allergic reaction. Sometimes even family members express these negative attitudes. Nurses can help clients who are getting the "it's all in your head" treatment by giving them language, print media, and other resources to help them teach family members, fellow students, and coworkers about this sometimes life-threatening condition.

Evaluation

Clients are evaluated based on their progress in meeting goals set during the planning stage. Potential outcomes may include the following:

- Client exhibits decreased symptoms and decreased frequency of hypersensitivity responses.
- Client demonstrates proper technique when using an EpiPen.
- Client provides accurate and thorough information in food or activity and symptom journal.

REVIEW   Hypersensitivity

RELATE Link the Concepts

Linking the exemplar of hypersensitivity with the concept of oxygenation:

1. You are caring for a client who is having a severe hypersensitivity response. How do you assess the client's oxygenation status?

2. What nursing care can you provide to improve the client's oxygenation status?

Linking the exemplar of hypersensitivity with the concept of comfort:

3. You are caring for a client with seasonal hypersensitivity resulting in rhinorrhea, sore throat, and sinus congestion. What actions will improve the client's comfort?

4. What client teaching would you provide to improve this client's comfort?

Linking the exemplar of hypersensitivity with the concept of teaching and learning:

5. You are working with an adult client who has developed a type I hypersensitivity to insect venom, and who has limited English proficiency. What teaching techniques would be most appropriate for addressing his learning needs? What other resources could you call upon for assistance?

6. What learner characteristics and learning factors would you need to address in order to improve compliance in a 15-year-old female client who experiences contact dermatitis when exposed to sodium lauryl sulfate in cosmetics?

READY Go to Companion Skills Manual

REFER Go to Pearson Nursing Student Resources
nursing.pearsonhighered.com

REFLECT Case Study

Ron Jackson is a 12-month-old, African American child born to Martha Jackson. Ms. Jackson has a history of multiple allergies, including drugs, food, pine pollen, and environmental hypersensitivities. She has brought Ron to the clinic today for a well-baby checkup and to receive his 1-year immunizations. His vital signs are within normal limits, he is meeting developmental milestones, and his growth charts are within the 50th percentile. Ms. Jackson reports that Ron has had several urinary tract infections this spring and that she has been treating them with over-the-counter medications, such as acetaminophen (Tylenol) for fever and discomfort and saline nasal spray to reduce nasal congestion. Ron is currently asymptomatic, bright, and alert.

1. When administering immunizations, what special precautions would you take based on Ron's history?
2. What teaching would you provide to Ms. Jackson regarding his risk for hypersensitivity?
3. What symptoms related to potential hypersensitivity would you teach Ms. Jackson to report?

EXEMPLAR 8.3   **Rheumatoid Arthritis**

EXEMPLAR KEY TERMS

Arthrodesis, *501*
Arthroplasty, *501*
Autoimmune disorder, *495*
Boutonnière deformities, *497*
Immunosuppression, *502*
Juvenile idiopathic arthritis (JIA), *499*
Orthotic devices, *504*
Osteoarthritis, *496*
Pannus, *496*
Pauciarticular arthritis, *499*
Plasmapheresis, *504*
Polyarticular arthritis, *499*
Range of motion (ROM) exercises, *506*
Rheumatoid arthritis (RA), *495*
Swan-neck deformity, *497*
Synovectomy, *501*
Systemic arthritis, *499*
Total lymphoid irradiation, *504*

EXEMPLAR LEARNING OUTCOMES

After reading about this exemplar, you will be able to:

1. Describe the pathophysiology, etiology, clinical manifestations, and direct and indirect causes of rheumatoid arthritis (RA)
2. Identify risk factors and prevention methods associated with RA.
3. Illustrate the nursing process in providing culturally competent care across the life span for individuals with RA.
4. Formulate priority nursing diagnoses appropriate for an individual with RA.
5. Summarize therapies used by interdisciplinary teams in the collaborative care of an individual with RA.
6. Plan evidence-based care for an individual with RA and his or her family in collaboration with other members of the health-care team.
7. Evaluate expected outcomes for an individual with RA.

▶ OVERVIEW

Rheumatoid arthritis (RA) is a chronic systemic **autoimmune disorder** (a disease caused by abnormal, overactive functioning of the immune system that produces a response against the body's own cells and tissues, normally resulting in damage to the tissues). RA causes inflammation of connective tissue, primarily in the joints. The course and severity of the disease are variable. Manifestations of RA may be minimal, with mild inflammation of only a few joints and little structural damage, or relentlessly progressive, with multiple inflamed joints and marked deformity. RA contributes to disability and tends to shorten life expectancy. Most clients exhibit a pattern of symmetric involvement of multiple peripheral joints and periods of remission and exacerbation.

Clients diagnosed with RA must cope with chronic pain, experience alterations in body image, and often require specially modified tools to allow them to perform activities of daily living (ADLs). Holistic care is of particular importance in helping these clients meet physical, psycho-social, and safety needs.

▶ PATHOPHYSIOLOGY AND ETIOLOGY

It is believed that long-term exposure to an unidentified antigen causes an aberrant immune response in a genetically susceptible host. As a result, normal antibodies (immunoglobulins) become autoantibodies and attack host tissues. The transformed antibodies usually present in individuals with RA are called *rheumatoid factors*. The self-produced antibodies bind with their target antigens in blood and synovial membranes, forming immune complexes.

Leukocytes are attracted to the synovial membrane from the circulation, where neutrophils and macrophages ingest the immune complexes and release enzymes that degrade synovial tissue and articular cartilage. Activation of B lymphocytes and T lymphocytes results in increased production of rheumatoid factors and enzymes that, in turn, increase and continue the inflammatory process.

The synovial membrane is damaged by the inflammatory and immune processes. It swells from infiltration of the leukocytes, and it thickens as cells proliferate and enlarge abnormally. The inflammation then spreads and involves synovial blood vessels. Small venules are occluded, and vascular flow to the synovial tissue decreases. As blood flow decreases and metabolic needs increase (because of the increased number and size of cells), hypoxia and metabolic acidosis occur. Acidosis stimulates synovial cells to release hydrolytic enzymes into surrounding tissues, starting erosion of the articular cartilage and inflammation of the supporting ligaments and tendons. The damage to cartilage that occurs in RA results from at least three processes:

1. Neutrophils, T cells, and other synovial fluid cells are activated and degrade the surface layer of the articular cartilage.

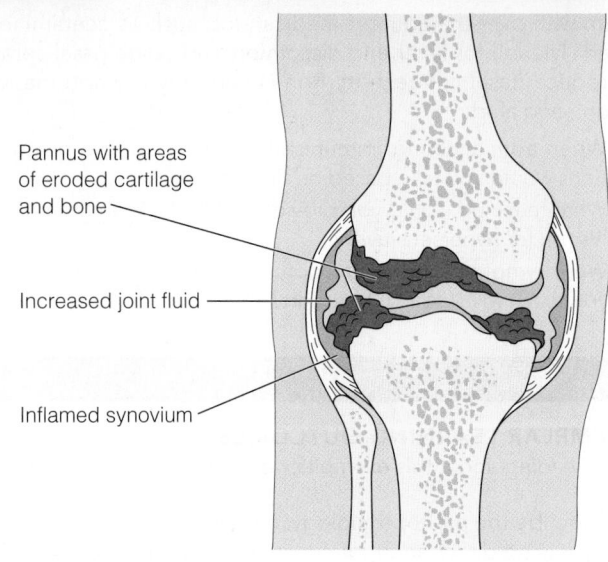

Pannus with areas of eroded cartilage and bone

Increased joint fluid

Inflamed synovium

Figure 8–17 ● Joint inflammation and destruction in rheumatoid arthritis. Note the synovial inflammation with pannus formation and the erosion of cartilage and underlying bone.

2. Cytokines, especially interleukin-1 (IL-1) and tumor necrosis factor alpha (TNF-α), cause the chondrocytes to attack the cartilage.
3. The synovium digests nearby cartilage, releasing inflammatory molecules containing IL-1 and TNF-α.

The inflammation also causes hemorrhage, coagulation, and deposits of fibrin on the synovial membrane, in the intracellular matrix, and in the synovial fluid. **Pannus** tissue, which is an abnormal tissue layer that includes newly formed blood vessels, may develop within the synovial membrane, leading to greater loss of bone and cartilage. (Osborn, Wraa, Watson & Holleran, 2013). The formation of pannus leads to scar tissue formation that immobilizes the joint (**Figure 8–17** ●).

Etiology

Osteoarthritis is the most common form of arthritis in older adults. It is caused by chronic degenerative changes in the cartilage and synovial membranes of the joints. However, RA is the

most common form of autoimmune arthritis, affecting from 1% to 2% of the worldwide population and all races. RA affects three times as many women as men, and while the typical age of onset is between 40 and 60 years, this disease strikes people of all ages (American College of Rheumatology, 2012a). In children under 16 years of age, juvenile idiopathic arthritis (JIA; formerly called *juvenile rheumatoid arthritis*) is the most common form of arthritis (Mayo Clinic, 2012). Remissions are most likely to occur in the first year of the disease: Approximately 10% of clients diagnosed with RA experience long-term remission within 1 year. Following the onset of RA, an estimated 60% of individuals whose disease does not enter remission within approximately 10 years will be disabled to the extent of being unable to maintain employment (Ruffing & Bingham, 2012).

The cause of RA is unknown. A combination of genetic, environmental, hormonal, and reproductive factors are thought to be involved. It is speculated that infectious agents, such as bacteria, mycoplasmas, and viruses (especially Epstein-Barr virus), may play a role in initiating the autoimmune processes in RA. Genetic factors are believed to make a critical contribution to the likelihood of developing RA (Tobón, Youinou, & Saraux, 2010).

Risk Factors

Individuals with a family history of RA may be at increased risk. Several studies have found that heavy smokers are at increased risk for developing RA, but that risk can be reduced if the individual stops smoking. It is important to note that absence of risk factors does not preclude diagnosis of the disease.

▶ CLINICAL MANIFESTATIONS

Although the onset and manifestations of RA are much the same in older and younger clients, differentiating between RA and osteoarthritis in the older adult may be difficult. It is important to establish an accurate diagnosis, however, because the management of these disorders differs significantly. Clinical features distinguishing RA from osteoarthritis are listed in **Table 8–7** ●.

In addition to the characteristic joint deformity commonly seen in RA, signs and symptoms usually include redness, warmth, pain, and swelling at the affected sites. During exacerbations,

TABLE 8–7   Comparison of the Manifestations of Rheumatoid Arthritis and Osteoarthritis

FEATURE	RHEUMATOID ARTHRITIS	OSTEOARTHRITIS
Onset	Usually insidious, may be abrupt	Insidious
Course	Generally progressive, characterized by remissions and exacerbations	Slowly progressive
Pain and stiffness	Predominant on arising, lasting >1 hour; also occurs after prolonged inactivity	Pain with activity; stiffness following periods of immobility, generally relieved within minutes
Affected joints	Appear red, hot, and swollen; "boggy" and tender to palpation; decreased range of motion; weakness	Affected joints may appear swollen; cool and bony hard on palpation; decreased range of motion
	Multiple joints affected in symmetrical pattern; proximal interphalangeal, metacarpophalangeal, wrists, knees, ankles, and toes often involved	One or several joints affected, including hips, knees, lumbar and cervical spine, proximal interphalangeal and distal interphalangeal, wrist, and first metatarsophalangeal joint
Systemic manifestations	Fatigue, weakness, anorexia, weight loss, fever; rheumatoid nodules; anemia	Fatigue

Lifespan Considerations Rheumatoid Arthritis

Children

- JIA typically occurs between ages 3 and 6 and at or around puberty.
- Many children do not complain of pain when symptoms first develop; observable symptoms such as joint swelling and unusual patterns of walking are early key indicators.
- Aspirin is often used to treat JIA because it is fast acting and inexpensive, but it should be discontinued if the child develops chicken pox or flulike symptoms.
- Exercise is important for slowing the progression of JIA; however, joint soreness and discomfort may limit the intensity of exercise (AAP, 2013).

Pregnancy

- Many women diagnosed with RA experience a remission during pregnancy, often followed by a relapse after delivery.
- Anemia may be present as a result of blood loss from salicylate therapy.

- The pregnant woman needs extra rest, particularly to relieve weight-bearing joints, but she should also continue range-of motion exercises.
- During remission, the pregnant woman may stop medication because salicylates may prolong labor and may induce teratogenic effects.
- It is not uncommon for women diagnosed with RA to have prolonged gestations.

Older Adults

- For older adults, RA is managed much as it is for younger individuals.
- Prolonged bed rest or inactivity is not prescribed for acute episodes, however, because it may result in irreversible immobility in the older adult.
- Medications are used with greater caution in older adults because of the increased risk of toxicity.
- In many cases, less emphasis is placed on preventing joint deformity in older adults, and more emphasis is placed on maintaining functional status.

---

when the disease is more active, clients may also experience fever, loss of appetite (anorexia), fatigue, and symmetrical joint deformity. RA may be polyarticular (affecting more than one joint), and in most cases, the hands and feet are affected. However, note that the destruction associated with this disease is not limited to the joints; RA can affect the blood, leading to anemia, as well as potentially damaging all organs of the body (Osborn et al., 2013). See the feature Multisystemic Effects of Rheumatoid Arthritis on page 498.

Over time, the inflammatory process associated with RA produces characteristic joint deformities. Sleep patterns, psychosocial well-being, and overall quality of life are negatively affected as well. In the most severe cases, the progressive, severe effects of RA lead to complete disability and even death.

Joint Manifestations

The onset of RA typically is insidious, although it may be acute (precipitated by a stressor, e.g., infection, surgery, or trauma). Joint manifestations often are preceded by systemic manifestations of inflammation, including fatigue, loss of appetite, weight loss, and nonspecific aching and stiffness. Clients report joint swelling with associated stiffness, warmth, tenderness, and pain.

The pattern of joint involvement typically is polyarticular (involving multiple joints) and symmetrical, but the rate at which joint deformities develop can fluctuate. The proximal interphalangeal (PIP) and metacarpophalangeal (MCP) joints of the fingers, the wrists, the knees, the ankles, and the toes are most frequently involved, although RA can affect any joint. Stiffness is most pronounced in the morning, lasting more than 1 hour. It may also occur with prolonged rest during the day and may be more severe following strenuous activity. Swollen, inflamed joints feel "boggy" or spongelike on palpation because of synovial edema. ROM is limited in affected joints, and weakness may be evident.

The persistent inflammation of RA causes deformities of the joint itself and of the supporting structures, such as ligaments, tendons, and muscles. As the joint is destroyed, ligaments, tendons, and the joint capsule are weakened or destroyed. Joint cartilage and bone also are destroyed. Weakening or destruction of these supporting structures results in lack of opposition to muscle pull, causing deformity.

HANDS AND FINGERS   Characteristic changes in the hands and fingers are ulnar deviation of the fingers and subluxation at the MCP joints. **Swan-neck deformity** is characterized by hyperextension of the PIP joints with compensatory flexion of the distal interphalangeal (DIP) joints. A flexion deformity of the PIP joints with extension of the DIP joints is called a **boutonnière deformity (Figure 8–18 ●)**. The ability to pinch is limited by hyperextension of the interphalangeal joint and flexion of the MCP joint of the thumb.

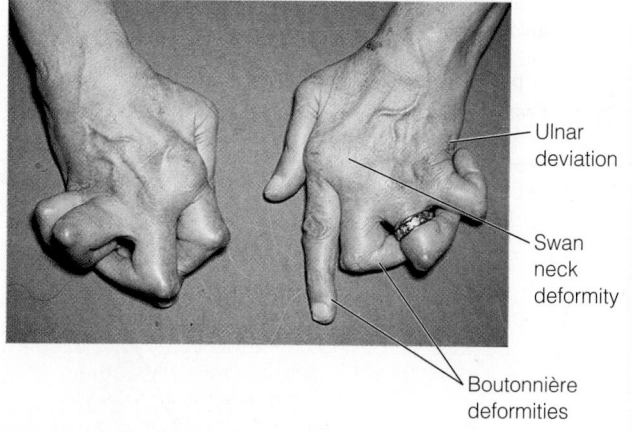

— Ulnar deviation

— Swan neck deformity

— Boutonnière deformities

Figure 8–18 ● Typical hand deformities associated with rheumatoid arthritis.

Source: Biophoto Associates/Science Source.

Multisystemic Effects of Rheumatoid Arthritis

Sensory
- Scleritis
- Episcleritis

Exocrine glands
Sjögren's syndrome
- Dry eyes
- Dry mouth

Respiratory
- Pleural disease
- Interstitial fibrosis
- Pneumonitis

Cardiovascular
- Vasculitis
- Pericarditis

Hematologic
Felty's syndrome
- Splenomegaly
- Neutropenia
- Anemia

Musculoskeletal
General
- Symmetric polyarticular joint swelling
- Joint redness, warmth, pain, tenderness
- Morning stiffness

Spine
- Cervical pain
- Neurologic manifestations

Wrists
- Limited range of motion
- Deformity
- Carpal tunnel syndrome

Hands
- Ulnar deviation
- Swan-neck deformity
- Boutonnière deformity

Knees
- Joint effusion
- Instability

Ankles
- Limited range of motion
- Pain on ambulation

Feet
- Subluxation
- Hallux valgus
- Lateral toe deviation
- Cock-up toe

Integumentary
- Rheumatoid nodules

Metabolic Processes
- Fatigue
- Weakness
- Anorexia
- Weight loss
- Low-grade fever

Multisystemic Effects of Rheumatoid Arthritis

WRISTS AND ELBOWS   Wrist involvement is nearly universal, leading to limited movement, deformity, and carpal tunnel syndrome. Inflammation of the elbows often causes flexion contracture.

KNEES   The knees frequently are affected in RA, and visible swelling often obliterates the normal contours. Instability of the knee joint along with quadriceps atrophy, contractures, and valgus (knock-knee) deformities can lead to significant disability.

ANKLES AND FEET   Ambulation may be limited by pain and deformity when the ankles and feet are involved. Typical deformities of the feet and toes are subluxation, hallux valgus (deviation of the great toe toward the other digits of the foot), lateral deviation of the toes, and cock-up toes (turned-up toes).

SPINE   Spinal involvement usually is limited to the cervical vertebrae. Neck pain is common, and neurological complications can occur.

Extra-Articular Manifestations

RA is a systemic disease with a variety of extra-articular manifestations. These are seen particularly in clients with high levels of circulating rheumatoid factor. As mentioned previously, fatigue, weakness, loss of appetite, weight loss, and low-grade fever are common when the disease is active. In addition, anemia resistant to iron therapy frequently affects clients with RA. Skeletal muscle atrophy also is common, usually being most apparent in the musculature around affected joints.

Rheumatoid nodules may develop, generally in the subcutaneous tissue of areas subject to pressure: on the forearm, in the olecranon bursa, over the MCP joints, and on the toes (**Figure 8–19** ●). Rheumatoid nodules are granulomatous lesions that are firm and either movable or fixed. These nodules also may be found in viscera, including the heart, lungs, intestinal tract, and dura.

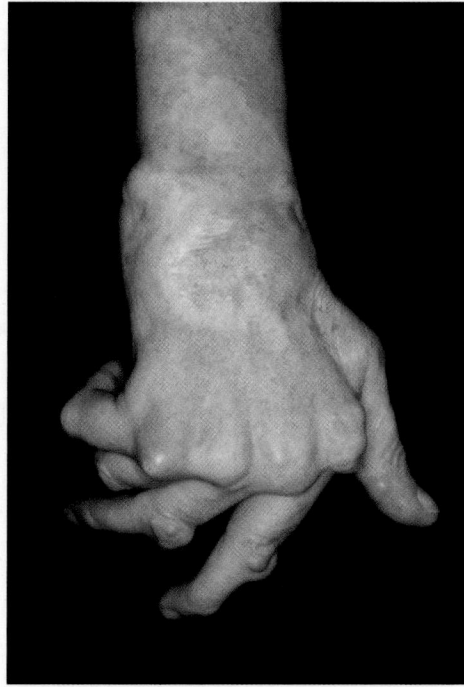

Figure 8–19 ● Rheumatoid nodules.
Source: Princess Margaret Rose Orthopaedic Hospital/Science Source.

Other possible extra-articular manifestations of RA are subcutaneous nodules, pleural effusion, vasculitis, pericarditis, and splenomegaly (enlargement of the spleen).

Increased Risk of Coronary Heart Disease

Individuals with RA have an increased risk of developing coronary heart disease. In turn, coronary heart disease increases the risk for myocardial infarction and death; in fact, RA is associated with a shortened life expectancy (Ruffing & Bingham, 2012). RA affects the heart by:

■ Direct effects on the blood vessels, with measures of C-reactive proteins (inflammatory markers) being more predictive of future cardiovascular disease than levels of low-density lipoprotein.

■ Increased risk for having low high-density lipoprotein level, high cholesterol and triglyceride levels, high blood pressure, and high homocysteine levels—all of which increase the risk for coronary heart disease.

■ The damaging side effects that many medications (e.g., methotrexate and steroids) often have on coronary vessels.

Juvenile Idiopathic Arthritis

Juvenile idiopathic arthritis (JIA) is a chronic inflammatory autoimmune juvenile disorder diagnosed characterized by joint inflammation resulting in decreased mobility, swelling, and pain. It is similar to RA diagnosed in adults. JIA occurs slightly more often in girls than in boys. Although no national studies have been conducted to determine the incidence of JIA in the United States, an estimated 1 in 1,000 children in this country develop some form of juvenile arthritis (CDC, 2011c). Treatment is similar to that provided for adults with RA. JIA may enter remission; occasionally it continues as a chronic disease.

Remission may last for months, years, or a lifetime. JIA affects joints and surrounding tissues in addition to possibly affecting other organs, such as the heart, lungs, liver, and eyes. During the course of this disease, the child may experience pain, impaired mobility, and interference with normal growth and development. However, 70% of children with JIA experience permanent remission by adulthood. In rare cases, the disease is unresponsive to treatment, or the child may suffer lasting impairment, such as bone and joint changes. Children with an early onset of JIA have a better prognosis for complete recovery.

The three types of JIA are pauciarticular, systemic, and polyarticular. **Pauciarticular arthritis** primarily affects the knees, ankles, and elbows, and it occurs more frequently in female clients. **Systemic arthritis** affects male and female clients equally and characteristically manifests as high fever, polyarthritis, and rheumatoid rash. Systemic arthritis also affects internal organs and joints. **Polyarticular arthritis** involves many joints (five or more), particularly the small joints of the hands and fingers. It also may affect the hips, knees, feet, ankles, and neck.

Like the cause of RA, the cause of JIA is unknown, but it is thought to have an autoimmune basis. Inflammation begins

Clinical Manifestations and Therapies **Rheumatoid Arthritis**

ETIOLOGY	CLINICAL MANIFESTATION	CLINICAL THERAPIES
Coronary heart disease (CHD)	Elevated C-reactive protein, low high-density lipoprotein, elevated cholesterol and triglycerides, and high homocysteine Hypertension	▪ Treatment is similar to that of any client with CHD but must include management of rheumatoid arthritis (RA), with additional goal of reducing inflammation that exacerbates risk for worsening CHD.
Pleural effusion (collection of fluid in the pleural space)	Shortness of breath and hypoxia Pain, fever, and heat at the site if fluid becomes infected	▪ Therapeutic aspiration may be sufficient; may require chest tube insertion for continuous drainage. ▪ Chemical or surgical pleurodesis, in which two pleural surfaces are scarred to each other to prevent recurrence of fluid accumulation. ▪ Placement of PleurX catheter with one-way valve for daily drainage of fluid. ▪ Management of inflammatory process resulting from RA can reduce risk of development or reduce reaccumulation of fluid.
Vasculitis (inflammation of veins and/or arteries)	Fever, weight loss, palpable purpura, livedo reticularis, myalgia or myositis, mononeuritis multiplex, stroke, myocardial infarction, hypertension, gangrene, nose bleeds, bloody cough, pulmonary infiltrates, abdominal pain, bloody stools, perforations, and glomerulonephritis	▪ Reducing the inflammatory process. ▪ Immune suppression. ▪ Cortisone. ▪ Specific treatments aimed at the organ system involved.
Pericarditis (inflammation of the pericardium)	Chest pain radiating to the back that is relieved by sitting up and leaning forward and worsened by lying down Dry cough, fever, and anxiety Auscultated friction rub, ST-segment elevation, PR-interval depression in all leads, cardiac tamponade, congestive heart failure, jugular vein distention, and peripheral edema	▪ Pericardiocentesis. ▪ Antibiotics if cause is believed to be infectious (unlikely when associated with RA). ▪ Steroids to reduce inflammation. ▪ Colchicine. ▪ Emergency surgery may be required to restore normal heart function if other treatments fail.
Uveitis (inflammation of the middle layer of the eye; most commonly a complication of juvenile RA)	Redness of the eye, blurred vision, sensitivity to light, dark floating spots along the visual field, and eye pain	▪ Good prognosis if treated promptly. ▪ Glucocorticoid steroids (oral or topical eye drops) after ruling out any corneal ulcers. ▪ Topical cycloplegics to reduce eye swelling. ▪ Antimetabolite medications are used for harder-to-treat or more aggressive cases.

in the joint and leads to pain and swelling. Scar tissue eventually develops, resulting in limited ROM. This may be restricted to a few joints, or it may be systemic, involving multiple joints. Symptoms can include fever, rash, lymphadenopathy, splenomegaly, and hepatomegaly. The child may develop a limp or may obviously favor one extremity over the other. A slow rate of growth or uneven growth of extremities also may be noted. Pain, stiffness, loss of motion, and swelling occur in the large joints, such as the knees. Older children may develop symmetrical involvement of the small joints of the hand. The disease frequently is chronic, extending over several years after an initial manifestation with pain and

other symptoms. However, remissions and exacerbations are characteristic.

Complications such as eye chronic uveitis, which results from chronic inflammation, may occur in children with JIA, especially those with pauciarticular arthritis. Children with polyarticular and systemic JIA should be examined by an ophthalmologist for uveitis every 6 months, and children with pauciarticular arthritis should be examined every 3 months.

As mentioned, interference with normal growth is another potential complication. JIA may result in bone growth disturbance, such as contractures or effusions. Treatment with corticosteroids can inhibit growth as well.

▶ COLLABORATION

The identification of RA depends upon a combination of the client's history, assessment findings, and diagnostic testing. Once the diagnosis of RA has been established, the goals of therapy are to relieve pain, reduce inflammation, slow or stop joint damage, and improve the client's well-being and ability to function. No cure currently exists for RA; the goal of treatment is to relieve its manifestations. An interdisciplinary approach is used, with a balance of rest, exercise, physical therapy, and suppression of the inflammatory processes.

Diagnostic Tests

Diagnostic tests are used to identify RA, as well as to rule out other forms of arthritis and connective tissue disorders. In approximately 25%–35% of clients with RA, the complete blood count reveals a mild anemia. The white blood cell and platelet counts are usually normal; however, the inflammatory response may lead to an increase in both these components. Certain subgroups of clients may also demonstrate a decreased WBC count. More than 70% of clients with RA test positive for rheumatoid factor (RF). However, a more specific marker for this condition is antibodies to cyclic citrullinated peptide (CCP). The anti-CCP test detects these antibodies and may yield positive results even years before RA symptoms emerge. Blood tests also include the erythrocyte sedimentation rate, which typically is elevated with RA, and C-reactive protein (CRP), which is a nonspecific indicator of inflammation ([Ruffing & Bingham, 2012; National Institute of Arthritis and Musculoskeletal Skin Diseases (NIAMS), 2009]).

In the earliest stages of RA, when bone damage is not yet apparent, x-rays are not of great use for diagnosis. Even so, x-rays may help to rule out other potential causes of joint pain and may be useful for monitoring the disease's progression (Ruffing & Bingham, 2012). Examination of the synovial fluid will demonstrate changes associated with inflammation, including increased turbidity (cloudiness), decreased viscosity, and increased protein and WBC levels.

Surgery

Surgical intervention may be employed for the client with RA at a variety of disease stages. Early in the course of the disease, **synovectomy** (excision of synovial membrane) provides temporary relief of inflammation, relieves pain, and slows the destructive process, thus helping to preserve joint function. **Arthrodesis** (joint fusion) may be used to stabilize joints such as cervical vertebrae, wrists, and ankles. **Arthroplasty** (total joint replacement) may be necessary in cases of gross deformity and joint destruction.

Pharmacologic Therapy

The four general approaches used in the pharmacologic management of RA are the following:

- Nonsteroidal anti-inflammatory drugs (NSAIDs) for reduction of inflammation and pain
- Low-dose oral corticosteroids for reduction of inflammation and pain, as well as for slowing disease progression

- Disease-modifying antirheumatic drugs (DMARDs) to relieve disease-related symptoms and to slow disease progression
- Intra-articular steroid injection administration for localized relief of pain and inflammation

NONSTEROIDAL ANTI-INFLAMMATORY DRUGS The NSAIDs include aspirin and numerous other drugs (see the Medications feature on page 502). While a risk for gastrointestinal (GI) toxicity is associated with all NSAIDs, aspirin's incidence of GI toxicity is particularly high. In the treatment of RA, aspirin is also linked to other undesirable characteristics, including the need for multiple doses per day and a narrow therapeutic window, which means that even minor dosage increases can be toxic. For these reasons, other NSAIDs and/or a combination of medications may be preferable to aspirin in the treatment of RA (Ruffing & Bingham, 2012).

Included within the NSAIDs is a special group of drugs called COX-2 inhibitors. These NSAIDs work by selectively blocking the synthesis of prostaglandins generated by way of COX-2 enzymes (Ruffing & Bingham, 2012). In the United States, celecoxib (Celebrex®) is the only available medication in this class. Although the COX-2 inhibitors carry fewer GI-related risks than do traditional NSAIDs, the potential increased risk for stroke and heart attack associated with these drugs has prompted removal of two of them—rofecoxib (Vioxx) and valdecoxib (Bextra)—from the U.S. market.

Most commonly, side effects of NSAIDs involve the GI system and may include stomach lining irritation, erosions, and bleeding ulcers. Taking these medications with food may reduce the symptoms; however, the risk for GI bleeding is not decreased. Concurrent administration of medications known as proton pump inhibitors [e.g., esomeprazole (Nexium), lansoprazol (Prevacid), pantoprazole (Protonix), and rabeprazole (Aciphex)], along with misoprostol (Cytotec), which is believed to have protective effects on the stomach mucosa, may reduce the risk for GI bleeding due to NSAIDs. Diclofenac (Arthrotec) combines both the NSAID and misoprostol (Ruffing & Bingham, 2012). All NSAIDs are potentially nephrotoxic, meaning that they can cause kidney damage. Additionally, they can cause blood pressure alterations that may be particularly dangerous for clients with cardiovascular disorders. NSAIDs may be contraindicated for clients with renal impairment and/or cardiac disease, depending upon the severity of the alteration. The drugs are extensively metabolized in the liver and are contraindicated in clients with liver disease.

In past years, aspirin or other analgesic drugs were the initial treatment of choice for RA, with more powerful medications added to the regimen only when the disease progressed. However, studies have shown that early treatment with more powerful medications (as well as medication combinations) may be more effective in decreasing or preventing the extensive damage associated with RA (NIAMS, 2009).

CORTICOSTEROIDS Systemic corticosteroids can dramatically decrease both inflammation and immune reactions and appear to slow the progression of joint destruction in RA. However, long-term use of corticosteroids is associated with multiple side effects, such as poor wound healing, increased risk of infection, osteoporosis, and gastrointestinal bleeding. Characteristic

Medications NSAIDs Commonly Used to Treat Rheumatoid Arthritis

CLASSIFICATION AND DRUG EXAMPLES	MECHANISM OF ACTION	NURSING CONSIDERATIONS
Nonprescription Aspirin Ibuprofen (Motrin, Advil, Nuprin) Naproxen (Aleve) **Prescription** diclofenac (Arthrotec, Cataflam, Voltaren) diflunisal (Dolobid) etodolac (Lodine) indomethicin (Indocin), ketoprofen (Orudis, Oruvail) meloxicam (Mobic) nabumetone (Relafen) oxaprozin (Daypro) piroxicam (Feldene) sulindac (Clinoril) tolmetin (Tolectin) **COX-2 Inhibitors** celecoxib (Celebrex)	Reduce inflammation and pain by blocking the synthesis of prostaglandins through inhibition of cyclooxygenase enzymes; specifically, COX-1 and COX-2 enzymes. COX-2 inhibitors selectively block prostaglandin synthesis by inhibiting COX-2 enzymes.	■ Monitor for signs and symptoms of GI toxicity, including GI bleeding (e.g., bloody/tarry stools) and gastric distress. ■ Monitor for impaired kidney function, including decreased urine output, unexplained weight gain, and swelling due to fluid retention. ■ If long-term use is indicated, monitor CBC, electrolytes, and kidney and liver function studies.

physical changes associated with long-term use of these drugs may also include weight gain; increased fatty deposits in the face leading to a rounded facial appearance ("moon face"); and development of a humplike growth across the upper back ("buffalo hump"). Ingestion of exogenous steroids can cause a decrease in the body's production of endogenous steroids. Abrupt discontinuation of exogenous steroids may have disastrous consequences and may even be fatal. Clients who discontinue systemic corticosteroids should do so under the direct supervision of a healthcare professional, as tapering (weaning) is required for prevention of the severe physiological effects associated with sudden cessation of exogenous steroid administration. Examples of corticosteroids used in the treatment of RA are prednisone and cortisone. Certain steroids (e.g., methylprednisolone and triamcinolone) may be injected directly into the affected joint.

DISEASE-MODIFYING ANTIRHEUMATIC DRUGS DMARDs are a diverse group of medications including drugs that modify immune and inflammatory responses, such as gold salts, antimalarial agents, and sulfasalazine (see the Medications feature on page 503). However, they share characteristics that make them useful in the treatment of RA. Beneficial effects are not apparent for several weeks or months following the initiation of therapy, but these drugs can produce not only clinical improvement but also evidence of decreased disease activity. Because their anti-inflammatory effect is minimal, NSAIDs are continued during therapy with DMARDS. As many as two-thirds of clients taking these drugs show improvement, although such therapy has not been shown to slow bone erosion or facilitate healing. All of these drugs are fairly toxic, and close monitoring is necessary during the course of therapy.

Immune and Inflammatory Agents Immunosuppression (suppression of the immune response) helps to reduce the body's autoimmune response, thereby limiting the effects of the autoimmune disease process. Immunosuppressive or cytotoxic drugs are increasingly employed in the management of RA. Indeed, many healthcare providers now consider methotrexate the treatment of choice for clients with aggressive RA. Methotrexate may be used along with NSAIDs in the initial treatment plan. A weekly dose can produce a beneficial effect in as few as 2–4 weeks. Gastric irritation and stomatitis are the most frequent side effects associated with methotrexate, but side effects may be better controlled if folic acid is taken at the same time. Alcoholism, diabetes, obesity, advanced age, and renal disease increase the risk of toxic effects (e.g., hepatotoxicity, bone marrow suppression, and interstitial pneumonitis). Other immunosuppressive agents, such as cyclosporine, azathioprine, and monoclonal antibodies, also have been employed in the treatment of clients with severe, progressive, and crippling disease who have failed to respond to other measures.

Tumor necrosis factor (TNF) inhibitors used to treat clients with RA include etanercept (Enbrel), which inhibits the binding of TNF to receptor sites. Infliximab (Remicade) is a biological response modifier and a TNF-α receptor antagonist. Given by intravenous infusion, this drug is administered to reduce infiltration of inflammatory cells and production of TNF-α. Adalimumab (Humira) is a biological response modifier that is given to individuals with RA to reduce the inflammatory events of polyarthritis and to slow the progression of joint damage. Given by subcutaneous injection, the drug cannot be administered if the individual has an acute or chronic infection in any part of the body. Before the drug is initiated, the client should be tested for tuberculosis.

Gold Salts Gold salts may be administered by mouth, but the intramuscular route is more effective. The mode of action of gold is unknown, but it may produce clinical remission in some clients and decrease new bony erosions. Unless toxic reac-

Medications DMARDs Used to Treat Rheumatoid Arthritis

CLASSIFICATION AND DRUG EXAMPLES	MECHANISM OF ACTION	NURSING CONSIDERATIONS
Immunosuppressant/ cytotoxic *Drug examples:* methotrexate azathioprine cyclosporine monoclonal antibodies	Various; for methotrexate, mechanism appears to involve interruption of adenosine and possibly interference with other pathways of inflammation and immunoregulation, as well. Methotrexate inhibits an enzyme (dihydrofolate reductase) needed for metabolism of folic acid.	■ Monitor CBC with differential, platelets, kidney and liver function studies, and chest x-rays. ■ Be alert for indicators of thrombocytopenia, such as unusual bleeding, bruising, and petechiae. ■ Teach client taking methotrexate to avoid supplements that contain folate or its derivatives, as this alters the medication's effects. ■ Clients taking methotrexate should use contraception during and for a minimum of 3 months following therapy.
Sulfasalazine *Drug example:* Azulfidine	Believed to produce anti-inflammatory effects through conversion of intestinal flora. In the GI tract, affects prostaglandins and fluid and electrolyte absorption.	■ Prior to use, clients must be screened for glucose-6-phosphate dehydrogenase (G6PD) deficiency, which may increase risk for RBC destruction hemolysis and anemia. ■ Monitor CBC and liver function studies.
Antimalarials *Drug examples:* chloroquine hydroxychloroquine (Plaquenil)	Unknown	■ Monitor client for visual changes and weakness. ■ Monitor CBC. ■ Administer medication with food or milk to reduce GI distress.
TNF inhibitors *Drug examples:* etanercept (Enbrel) infliximab (Remicade) adalimumab (Humira)	Inhibit tumor necrosis factor (TNF), which is a cytokine that mediates joint damage and destruction.	■ Increased susceptibility to routine and opportunistic infection; monitor for indicators of infection.
Gold salts *Drug examples:* gold sodium auranofin (Ridaura) thiomalate (Myochrysine)	Unknown	■ Monitor for indicators of hypersensitivity, ranging from rash and itching to anaphylaxis. ■ Monitor CBC and urinalysis for indicators of toxicity. ■ Contraindicated in clients with renal disease, hepatic dysfunction, congestive heart failure, and diabetes mellitus.

tions occur, weekly therapy is continued until significant improvement is noted. Clients experiencing benefit from gold therapy may be continued on monthly injections for several years. About one third of clients on gold therapy experience toxic reactions, including dermatitis, stomatitis, bone marrow depression, and proteinuria. Mild skin reactions do not always necessitate discontinuation of therapy.

Antimalarial Agents Hydroxychloroquine (Plaquenil) is an antimalarial agent sometimes employed in the treatment of RA. The desired response requires 3–6 months of therapy, and many clients do not experience significant benefit. Although hydroxychloroquine has a relatively low toxicity, it can cause pigmentary retinitis and vision loss. Because chloroquine is associated with high risk for eye toxicity, this drug is not commonly prescribed (Ruffing & Bingham, 2012). Clients receiving this drug require a thorough vision examination every 6 months.

Sulfasalazine Sulfasalazine, a drug regularly prescribed for chronic inflammatory bowel disease, also may be prescribed for RA.

For clients not responding to the above preparations, penicillamine may be prescribed. Although this agent may be effective in the management of RA, toxic reactions, including bone marrow suppression, proteinuria, and nephrosis, are common and can be severe.

Including the client's pharmacist as a member of the healthcare team helps to ensure that contraindicated medications are not being prescribed and minimizes any potential side effects. Clients with RA should be encouraged to get all their prescriptions filled at a single pharmacy to reduce the chance of contraindicated medications being prescribed by multiple physicians.

Nonpharmacologic Therapy

The primary objectives in treating the client with RA are to reduce pain and inflammation, preserve function, and prevent deformity. Therapies in this area include rest and exercise, physical and occupational therapy, heat and cold, assistive devices and splints, and nutrition, as well as complementary and alternative medicines.

Focus on Diversity and Culture Using Complementary and Alternative Therapy for Rheumatoid Arthritis

Clients of Asian origin may already be taking herbal remedies and using acupuncture to treat symptoms of rheumatoid arthritis by the time they seek assistance from a Western healthcare provider. It is important for the nurse to respect the client's desire to use Eastern medicine.

The nurse working with such clients may want to recommend that they keep a medication and symptom journal that documents the times and dosages of any medications and remedies taken, including herbal teas, as well as the onset of both symptoms and side effects. This journal may assist the client and nurse in determining if a side effect or an improvement in the client's symptoms can be attributed to a specific treatment or a change in a specific treatment, regardless of the treatment's source.

Clients benefit from collaboration among many healthcare providers, including physicians, nurses, physical and occupational therapists, and nutritionists or dieticians. Working together, the healthcare team and the client can find a more effective combination of treatments that will result in minimum discomfort and maximum function for the client.

REST AND EXERCISE A balanced program of rest and exercise is an important component in the management of RA. During an acute exacerbation of the disease, the client may be hospitalized, or a short period of complete bed rest may be prescribed. For most clients, regular rest periods during the day are beneficial to reduce manifestations of the disease. In addition, splinting of inflamed joints reduces unwanted motion and provides local joint rest (see the Orthotic and Assistive Devices section).

Rest must be balanced with a program of physical therapy and exercise to maintain muscle strength and joint mobility. ROM exercises are prescribed to maintain joint function and prevent contractures. Isometric exercises are used to improve muscle strength without increasing joint stress. Isotonic exercises also help to improve muscle strength and preserve function. Low-impact aerobic exercises, such as swimming and walking, have been shown to benefit clients with RA without adversely affecting joint inflammation or prompting acute episodes.

PHYSICAL AND OCCUPATIONAL THERAPY Physical and occupational therapists can design and monitor individualized programs of activity and rest. Physical therapy is aimed at improving mobility and preventing the complications of inactivity. Occupational therapy works to create modifications in practices and tools needed to perform ADLs and promote as normal a lifestyle as possible.

HEAT AND COLD Heat and cold are used for their analgesic and muscle-relaxing effects. Moist heat generally is most effective and can be provided by a tub bath. Some clients relieve joint pain through the application of cold.

ORTHOTIC AND ASSISTIVE DEVICES A variety of **orthotic devices** (orthopedic devices that may include splints or braces applied to reduce strain on a joint) are available to help maintain function. Splints provide joint rest and prevent contractures. Night splints for the hands and/or wrists should maintain the extremity in a position of maximum function. The best "splint" for the hip is lying prone for several hours a day on a firm bed. In general, splints should be applied for the shortest period needed, should be made of lightweight materials, and should be easily removed to perform ROM exercises once or twice a day. Assistive devices, such as canes, walkers, and raised toilet seats, are most useful for clients with significant hip or knee arthritis.

NUTRITION For most clients with RA, an ordinary, well-balanced diet is recommended. Some clients may benefit from substitution of usual dietary fat with omega-3 fatty acids found in certain fish oils. Inactivity can lead to obesity, which places excess strain on the joints and can exacerbate pain. It is important for the client to receive adequate calories and nutrients for health while adapting calorie intake to meet activity levels.

PLASMAPHERESIS AND IRRADIATION Several newer treatments not yet in widespread use may be employed for clients with progressive RA. **Plasmapheresis** has been used to remove circulating antibodies and thereby moderate the autoimmune response. **Total lymphoid irradiation** decreases total lymphocyte levels, although serious adverse effects are associated with this treatment and its continued efficacy has not been established.

Complementary and Alternative Therapy

The client and healthcare team may consider complementary and alternative medicine if the client continues to experience discomfort from RA despite compliance with more traditional therapies. While many clients have reported improvement of pain and swelling with acupuncture or hydrotherapy, these therapies have yet to be proven beneficial clinically. Nutritional supplements such as fish oils may be used if they are not contraindicated. Because a cure is not available and traditional therapies are not always fully effective, the client with RA is vulnerable to quackery. Many nontraditional treatments, including diets, topical preparations, vaccines, hormones, plant extracts, and copper bracelets, have been put forth. These treatments often are costly, and none has been shown to be effective. The nurse should ask the client at each healthcare interaction about any nontraditional therapies being used.

▮ NURSING PROCESS

Clients with chronic, progressive, systemic disorders such as RA have multiple nursing-care needs involving many functional health patterns. Physical manifestations of the disease often result in acute and chronic pain, fatigue, impaired mobil-

Client Teaching Arthritis Self-Management

Individuals with RA can take control of their lives by becoming arthritis self-managers. They can help to prevent deformities and the effects of arthritis by following prescriptions for exercise, rest, weight management, posture, and positioning. The following suggestions for clients with RA are outlined by the Moss Rehab Resource Net (2010):

- Do not attempt any activity you cannot stop immediately if you find you cannot complete it without pain or injury.
- Pain is a sign that you should change your action or way of doing things. Use tools or equipment (e.g., handles, jar openers) as necessary, and alternate periods of activity with rest.
- Use the strongest joints possible to complete tasks. For example, use your palm or the crook of your elbow, not your fingers, to grasp and carry items.
- Avoid activities requiring a tight grip, such as writing with a pen or pencil or screwing/unscrewing objects.

ity, and difficulty performing routine tasks. The disease also has many psychosocial effects. The client has an incurable, chronic disease that may lead to severe crippling. Pain and fatigue can interfere with the client's ability to perform expected roles, such as home maintenance or job responsibilities. Even though the client's hands may appear swollen or deformed, other people may not understand the systemic nature of the disease or realize the difference between RA and osteoarthritis. Information about arthritis self-management is found in the Client Teaching feature, and a Nursing Care Plan for a client with RA is found later in this section.

Assessment

A careful history is important, because the history sometimes is the primary mode of diagnosis. Collect the following data:

- *Health history.* Pain; stiffness; fatigue; joint problems, including location, duration, onset, and effect on function; fever; sleep patterns; past illnesses or surgery; ability to carry out ADLs and self-care activities.
- *Physical assessment.* Height/weight; gait; joints, including symmetry, size, shape, color, appearance, temperature, ROM, and pain; skin, including nodules and purpura; respiratory, including cough and crackles; cardiovascular, including pericardial friction rub, apical bradycardia, and S_3 (third heart sound).

General examination includes assessing for joint swelling and deformities, fever, nodules under the skin, growth delays in children, and enlarged lymph nodes. During the physical examination, examine the hands for swan-neck contractures, which present as hyperextension of the PIP joints with the distal joint in a state of fixed flexion. **Boutonnière deformities**, which present as extreme flexion of the PIP, may also be observed (see Figure 8–18). Painless, hard nodules along the proximal and distal IP joints may be noted as well. Assessment of the lower extremities and feet may reveal nodules or tenderness around the Achilles tendon (Osborn et al., 2014).

Diagnosis

Many nursing diagnoses may be appropriate for the client with RA. Those focusing on predominant manifestations and their effect on the client's life are the following:

- *Chronic Pain*
- *Fatigue*
- *Ineffective Role Performance*
- *Disturbed Body Image*
- *Impaired Physical Mobility*
- *Anxiety*
- *Activity Intolerance*

(NANDA-I © 2012)

The diagnosis of RA is based on the client's history, physical assessment, and diagnostic tests. Diagnostic criteria developed by the American Rheumatism Association are used as well. At least four of the following seven criteria must be present to establish the diagnosis:

1. Morning stiffness lasting for at least 1 hour and persisting for at least 6 weeks
2. Arthritis with swelling or effusion of three or more joints persisting for at least 6 weeks
3. Arthritis of wrist, MCP, or PIP joints persisting for at least 6 weeks
4. Symmetrical arthritis with simultaneous involvement of corresponding joints on both sides of the body
5. Rheumatoid nodules
6. Positive serum rheumatoid factor
7. Characteristic radiological changes of RA noted in hands and wrists

Planning

Outcomes should be created for individualized client needs. These outcomes may include the following:

- Client will report effectiveness of pain management techniques, maintaining pain at tolerable levels by (*specific date*).
- Client will perform ADLs independently (or with minimal assistance, depending on degree of impairment) using tools modified by occupational therapy.
- Client will express feelings about diagnosis of chronic disease and display progression through the grieving process.

Implementation

Nursing care focuses on promoting mobility, encouraging adequate nutrition, and teaching the client and family about the disease and its management (see the Evidence-Based Practice feature). Most care will occur in the community, including physical therapy, with only occasional hospitalizations at the time of an exacerbation of the disease.

Monitor and Treat Chronic Pain

Pain is a constant feature of RA when the disease is active. It accompanies both acute inflammation and lower levels of chronic inflammation. Some clients say the pain in joints and surrounding tissue is like a deep, constant toothache. Pain

Evidence-Based Practice Teaching the Client With Rheumatoid Arthritis

Problem

Rheumatoid arthritis is a disease that can occur at any age, but it is seen most often in older adults. RA causes physical, emotional, and economic difficulties, but appropriate management can do much to reduce pain and disability, increase a sense of control, and improve quality of life. With recent advances in computer technology, the Internet has become a convenient means of providing information to individuals with RA. However, little is known about how many older adults use the computer to gain access to information.

Evidence

In examining the level of acceptance of consumer health information technology (CHIT) among clients, Calvin and Karsh (2009) found older adults to be less likely to accept CHIT. Possible reasons associated with this finding included lack of familiarity with computers, low computer literacy, and perceived lack of control over computer-related technologies. While this population may initially consider the learning of new technological skills an obstacle, research suggests that computer and Internet skills training increases acceptance of this technology by older adults.

Implications

The Internet is a powerful method for providing health information to older adults. Although health history questions rarely contain questions about the client's access to and use of the computer and the Internet, asking about Internet use may be as important as asking about other components of the client's history. If older adults have computers but do not use them, then referral to community resources that provide computer classes can facilitate these clients' success in using the computer and doing online searches for health information. In addition, before recommending an Internet-based health resource, nurses should review the site for content, readability, navigation features, credibility, organization, and graphic appearance.

Critical Thinking Application

1. You are designing an Internet site to teach older adults about RA. What topics would you include? How would your presentation be most effective for this age group?

2. You are conducting a computer-literacy course for older adults with RA at a local library. All of them have computers, but no one has used the Internet to find out about the disease. What sites would you recommend, and why?

3. Develop a plan to include assessment about computers on an agency's health history form. What would you include to convince the agency personnel that this is important?

---

can significantly affect the client's ability to provide self-care and maintain daily activities. It also contributes to the client's fatigue.

- Monitor the pain level and duration of morning stiffness. Pain and morning stiffness are indicators of disease activity. Increased pain may necessitate changes in the therapeutic treatment plan.
- Encourage the client to relate pain to activity level and adjust his or her activities accordingly. Teach the importance of joint and whole-body rest in relieving pain. Pain is an indicator of excess stress on inflamed joints. Increasing pain indicates a need to decrease activity levels.
- Teach the use of heat and cold applications to provide pain relief. The client may apply heat by showering or taking tub baths or by using warm compresses or other local applications, such as paraffin dips. For clients who find that heat increases pain and swelling during periods of acute inflammation, cold packs may be more effective. Both heat and cold have analgesic effects and can help to relieve associated muscle spasms.
- Teach about the use of prescribed anti-inflammatory medications and the relationship of pain and inflammation. Anti-inflammatory agents reduce chemical mediators of inflammation and swelling, relieving pain.
- Encourage the use of nonpharmacologic pain relief measures, such as visualization, distraction, meditation, and progressive relaxation techniques. These techniques can reduce muscle tension and help the client focus away from the pain, decreasing the intensity of the pain experience.

Prevent Fatigue

The pain and chronic inflammatory processes associated with RA lead to fatigue, but other factors contribute as well. Discomfort often disrupts the client's sleep patterns. Anemia, muscle atrophy, oxygenation, and poor nutrition play a role in the development of fatigue. The client with RA also may experience depression or hopelessness, with associated manifestations of fatigue. Interventions to help clients prevent fatigue include:

- Encourage a balance of periods of activity with periods of rest. Both joint rest and whole-body rest are important in reducing the inflammatory response.
- Stress the importance of planned rest periods during the day. Rest is vital during acute exacerbations of the disease and is also important for the client in remission.
- Help the client to prioritize activities, encouraging the performance of the most important ones early in the day. Assigning priorities helps the client to avoid performing relatively unimportant activities at the expense of more meaningful and important ones.
- Encourage regular physical activity in addition to prescribed **range of motion (ROM) exercises** (exercises designed to take each joint through all possible movements to maintain flexibility and movement in the joint). Aerobic exercise promotes a sense of well-being and restful sleep patterns.
- Refer the client to counseling or support groups, which can help in the development of effective coping strategies and in dealing with depression and hopelessness.

Address Ineffective Role Performance

Fatigue, pain, and the crippling effects of RA can interfere with the client's ability to pursue an education or career and to fill other life roles, such as parent, spouse, or homemaker. As the client's role changes, so must the roles of other family members. These role changes contribute to changes in family processes, increased stress in the family, and further difficulty in coping with the effects of the disease. Nursing interventions to promote effective role performance include:

■ Discuss the effects of the disease on the client's career and other life roles. Encourage the client to identify changes brought on by the disease. Discussion helps the client to accept the changes and begin to identify strategies for coping with them.

■ Encourage the client and family to discuss their feelings about role changes and to grieve over lost roles or abilities. Verbalization allows family members to validate and accept feelings about losses and changes, helping them to move into new roles.

■ Listen actively to concerns expressed by the client and family members, and acknowledge the validity of concerns about the disease, the prescribed treatment, and the prognosis. Demonstrating acceptance of these feelings and concerns promotes trust and validates their reality.

■ Help the client and family to identify strengths they can use to cope with role changes. Identifying strengths helps the client and family to consider role changes that maintain self-esteem and dignity.

■ Encourage the client to make decisions and assume personal responsibility for management of the disease. Clients who assume a personal and active role in managing their disease maintain a greater sense of self-control and self-esteem.

Promote a Healthy Body Image

The acute and long-term effects of RA can affect the client's body image and thus lead to feelings of hopelessness and powerlessness, social withdrawal, and difficulty adapting to changes. When inflammation and joint deformity occur despite compliance, the client may have difficulty accepting the need to continue therapeutic measures, particularly those that have side effects or are costly or time-consuming. In addition, unproven alternative treatment strategies and quackery may become increasingly attractive. Nursing interventions to promote a healthy body image include:

■ Demonstrate a caring, accepting attitude toward the client. This attitude helps the client to accept the physical changes brought on by the disease.

■ Encourage the client to talk about the effects of the disease, both the physical effects and the effects on life roles. Verbalization helps the client to identify feelings and gives the nurse an opportunity to validate these feelings.

■ Encourage the client to maintain self-care and usual roles to the extent possible. Discuss the use of clothing and adaptive devices that promote independence. Independence enhances the client's self-esteem.

■ Provide positive feedback for self-care activities and adaptive strategies. Positive reinforcement encourages the client to continue adaptive measures and maintain independence.

■ Refer the client to self-help groups, support groups, and other agencies that provide assistive devices and literature.

These groups and agencies can help the client develop adaptive strategies to cope with the effects of RA, enhancing the client's self-concept, body image, and independence.

■ Encourage children with RA to maintain contact with peers and to attend school when possible. Children require social interaction and education to meet developmental milestones, and changes in body image can make them feel self-conscious or awkward and thus lead to isolation.

Provide Support Related to Impaired Mobility

Physical therapists play an essential role in the client's treatment. The goals of physical therapy are to maintain joint function, strengthen muscles, increase tone, maintain body alignment, and prevent permanent deformities, such as contractures. Range-of-motion exercises, stretching, hydrotherapy, and swimming all help to prevent deformities.

Nurses can help clients with impaired mobility by encouraging them to perform ADLs. Medications may be given to reduce joint swelling and inflammation. In addition, warm or cold compresses applied to involved joints may provide pain relief. Additional interventions include:

■ Promote general health by encouraging a well-balanced diet. Periodically perform dietary and nutritional assessments. Reduced mobility may reduce metabolic needs, and excess weight causes additional muscle strain.

■ For children with JIA, plot growth carefully for children, and watch for changes in growth percentiles. Growth must be carefully monitored for early detection of problems and prevention of long-term complications.

■ Teach the client and family about the condition, prognosis, and importance of optimizing activity levels. It is important the client understand that overexertion may lead to exacerbation of the disease and that activities should be within tolerable limits. Typically, care is provided within the community; hospitalizations are rare.

■ Refer to occupational therapy that can help the client to continue performing ADLs. Tools with larger handles can reduce the pain of gripping, and longer handles on implements reduce reaching. The goal is for the client to maintain independence in performing daily activities.

Evaluation

RA typically is a chronic, progressive disease. As with most diseases of this nature, involvement of the client and family in its management is vital. Evaluation of nursing care is a continuous and ongoing part of meeting the client's needs to determine if the current plan of care is effective. Expected outcomes of nursing care for the client include the following:

■ The client maintains joint mobility.
■ The client expresses comfort and freedom from pain.
■ The client develops or maintains a positive body image.
■ The client is free from infection.
■ Client and family display adequate understanding, support, and management of the therapeutic regimen.

NURSING CARE PLAN A Client With Rheumatoid Arthritis

Janice James is a 42-year-old high school science teacher who began noticing vague joint pain, fatigue, poor appetite, and general malaise, which she initially attributed to a case of the flu. However, her symptoms continued, and she began to notice aching in her hands and wrists, which she attributed to the quilting she loves to do in the evenings. She made an appointment with her family physician when she noticed that her knuckles and finger joints were not just achy but also swollen and hot. She reports feeling very stiff in the mornings, often taking until 10:00 or 11:00 a.m. to begin to feel "normal."

Noting that Ms. James has lost 10 pounds since her last visit and has mild anemia and a significantly elevated erythrocyte sedimentation rate, the physician refers her to the rheumatology clinic for further evaluation. Following examination and laboratory and radiological testing, the rheumatologist establishes a diagnosis of rheumatoid arthritis and initiates a multidisciplinary team conference to plan the management of Ms. James's condition.

ASSESSMENT

Cathy Greenstein, RN, completes an assessment of Ms. James. She notes that Ms. James is well groomed and answers questions readily. However, she appears fatigued and ill. Ms. James relates that her job has been extremely stressful, because teacher layoffs have resulted in larger class sizes and fewer teaching assistants. Despite symptoms, she continues to teach full time but says she feels unable to keep up with all her responsibilities because of her fatigue.

Ms. James states that she is allergic to penicillin. Her past medical history reveals only the usual childhood diseases and three uncomplicated pregnancies, resulting in the births of her children, ages 14, 11, and 9. Physical assessment findings include T_O 37.8°C (100.2°F), P 82 bpm regular, R 18/min, BP 124/78 mmHg. Hands: swelling of the proximal interphalangeal (PIP) and metacarpophalangeal (MCP) joints of both hands; second and third PIP and second MCP joints on right hand are red, shiny, hot, spongy, and tender to palpation; able to extend fingers to 180 degrees but cannot make a complete fist with either hand, with flexion limited to less than 90 degrees; grip strength is weak bilaterally; wrist ROM is limited in all directions. Knees are swollen, and flexion is slightly limited; positive bulge sign in the right knee. Diagnostic findings are an erythrocyte sedimentation rate of 52 mm/hr, a hematocrit of 30%, and positive for rheumatoid factor. Few changes other than soft-tissue swelling are evident on hand and wrist x-rays.

DIAGNOSES

Nursing diagnoses that may be appropriate for Ms. James include the following:

- *Chronic Pain* related to joint inflammation
- *Impaired Home Maintenance* related to fatigue
- *Activity Intolerance* related to the effects of inflammation
- *Deficient Knowledge* regarding her therapeutic regimen

(NANDA-I © 2012)

PLANNING

The expected outcomes for the plan of care specify that Ms. James will:

- Verbalize effective pain management strategies.
- Use assistive devices to minimize joint stress with ADLs.
- Verbalize a plan to reduce responsibilities for home maintenance.
- Express willingness to plan rest breaks during the day.
- Demonstrate understanding of the prescribed therapeutic regimen and its importance for both short- and long-term benefit.

IMPLEMENTATION

The following nursing interventions may be appropriate for Ms. James:

- Teach techniques for relieving pain and morning stiffness, including:
  a. Schedule NSAIDs at equal intervals throughout the day.
  b. Take morning NSAID dose with milk and crackers approximately 30 minutes before rising.
  c. Perform ROM exercises in shower or bathtub.
  d. Apply local heat with paraffin dip or compress; use cold packs as needed.
  e. Learn techniques to minimize joint stress while performing ADLs.

- Provide Arthritis Foundation literature and information.
- Discuss ways to delegate household tasks to other family members.
- Explore ways to incorporate 30-minute rest breaks into work schedule.
- Provide information about the disease process and its manifestations, prescribed medications and their desired and adverse effects, and the importance of balancing rest and activity.

EVALUATION

The initial treatment regimen of aspirin, rest, exercise, and physical therapy succeeded in partially relieving the acute manifestations of rheumatoid arthritis in Ms. James. However, complete remission has not been achieved. She has had difficulty scheduling rest periods at work and has had to struggle to delegate household tasks. "I don't look sick to the kids, and they seem to think housecleaning is a terrible imposition on their time. It's often easier to just do it myself than to fight about it. Besides, that way it gets done right." Ms. James has faithfully followed the prescribed medication regimen and exercise routines, and she has kept her scheduled appointments and maintained contact with the treatment team.

CRITICAL THINKING

1. Ms. James is 42 years old. Would your nursing interventions differ if she were 72 years old? If so, how?
2. Rheumatoid arthritis is a chronic illness. What are the physical, emotional, and economic implications of an illness that results in chronic pain and deformity?
3. Develop a nursing care plan for Ms. James using the nursing diagnosis Ineffective Role Performance.

REVIEW Rheumatoid Arthritis

RELATE Link the Concepts

Linking the exemplar of rheumatoid arthritis with the concept of inflammation:

1. What role does inflammation play in the disease process of RA?

2. What nursing care (independent or collaborative) can you provide that will slow the inflammatory process?

3. What signs and symptoms of RA indicate the inflammatory process?

Linking the exemplar of rheumatoid arthritis with the concept of safety:

4. When caring for a client with RA affecting both knees, what nursing care can you provide to improve the client's safety?

5. What risks for injury would RA in both knees create?

Linking the exemplar of rheumatoid arthritis with the concept of mobility:

6. What are the foreseeable impacts of RA on activities of daily living at different stages in the life span? Why could these be particularly problematic for individuals with JIA?

7. You are caring for a 63-year-old client with RA who recently suffered a broken leg during a car accident. What special considerations should you give to selecting an assistive device to allow her to ambulate while her leg heals?

READY Go to Companion Skills Manual

REFER Go to Pearson Nursing Student Resources
nursing.pearsonhighered.com

REFLECT Case Study

Justine Belamo is a 48-year-old White female who has been married to Gil Belamo for 18 years. Ms. Belamo has a daughter, Majel, from a previous marriage, and she has two teenage children, Mark and Maria, with Gil. Ms. Belamo works as a grocery store clerk. Although she finds her job monotonous, she appreciates the steady income and family health insurance.

Ms. Belamo is overweight and has tried to lose weight most of her adult life. She frequently diets and, in the past, has lost a great deal of weight, but she just can't seem to keep the weight off. She blames menopause for her most recent weight gain.

1. What factors place Ms. Belamo at risk for development of RA?

2. When talking with Ms. Belamo, what interview questions might you ask to determine whether she has any early signs of RA?

3. If Ms. Belamo were to be diagnosed with RA, what teaching might you provide to reduce joint damage?

EXEMPLAR 8.4 Systemic Lupus Erythematosus

EXEMPLAR KEY TERMS

Antigen–antibody complex, *512*
Autoantibodies, *509*
Cellular immune response, *509*
Connective tissue, *509*
Discoid lesions, *510*
Human leukocyte antigen (HLA), *510*
Humoral immune response, *509*
Inflammatory response, *510*
Systemic lupus erythematosus (SLE), *509*

EXEMPLAR LEARNING OUTCOMES

After reading about this exemplar, you will be able to:

1. Describe the pathophysiology, etiology, clinical manifestations, and direct and indirect causes of systemic lupus erythematosus.

2. Identify risk factors and prevention methods associated with systemic lupus erythematosus.

3. Illustrate the nursing process in providing culturally competent care across the life span for individuals with systemic lupus erythematosus.

4. Formulate priority nursing diagnoses appropriate for an individual with systemic lupus erythematosus.

5. Summarize therapies used by interdisciplinary teams in the collaborative care of an individual with systemic lupus erythematosus.

6. Plan evidence-based care for an individual with systemic lupus erythematosus and his or her family in collaboration with other members of the healthcare team.

7. Evaluate expected outcomes for an individual with systemic lupus erythematosus.

▶ OVERVIEW

The generalized disorder known as **systemic lupus erythematosus (SLE)** is a chronic, inflammatory, **connective tissue** disease of unknown origin that affects almost all body systems, including the musculoskeletal system, and is characterized by remissions and exacerbations. It can range from a mild, episodic disorder to a rapidly fatal disease process. Manifestations are widely variable and are thought to result from cell and tissue damage caused by deposition of antigen–antibody complexes in connective tissues. The majority of cases are diagnosed during the teenage and early adult years.

▶ PATHOPHYSIOLOGY AND ETIOLOGY

The pathophysiology of SLE involves production of a large variety of **autoantibodies** (antibodies that react to the client's own tissues) against normal body components, such as nucleic acids, erythrocytes, coagulation proteins, lymphocytes, and platelets. Autoantibody production results from hyperreactivity of B cells (**humoral immune response**) because of disordered T-cell function (**cellular immune response**). The most characteristic autoantibodies in SLE are produced in response to nucleic acids, including DNA, histones, ribonucleoproteins, and other components of the cell nucleus.

The SLE autoantibodies react with their corresponding antigen to form immune complexes, which are then deposited in the connective tissue of blood vessels, lymphatic vessels, and other tissues. These deposits trigger an **inflammatory response** (a chain reaction leading to inflammation described in detail in the module on Inflammation), which leads to local tissue damage. The kidneys are a frequent site of complex deposition and damage; other affected tissues include the musculoskeletal system, brain, heart, spleen, lung, gastrointestinal tract, skin, and peritoneum. The autoantibodies produced and their target tissues determine the manifestations of SLE.

Etiology

Although the exact etiology of SLE is unknown, genetic, environmental, and hormonal factors play a role in its development. Twin studies and a familial pattern of the disease point to a genetic component, as does an increased incidence of other connective tissue diseases in relatives of individuals with SLE. In addition, certain **human leukocyte antigen (HLA)** genes (a major histocompatibility complex) are seen more frequently in individuals with SLE.

Researchers believe that individuals are born with a genetic predisposition for developing lupus. Exposure to environmental factors then triggers manifestation of the disease (Lupus Foundation of America [LFA], 2013a). Environmental factors believed to play a role in activating the pathological mechanisms of SLE include viruses, bacterial antigens, chemicals, drugs, and ultraviolet light.

Sex hormones also are thought to influence the development of SLE. Women with SLE have reduced levels of several active androgens that are known to inhibit antibody responses. In addition, estrogens have been shown to enhance antibody responses and to have an adverse effect in clients with SLE.

Risk Factors

An estimated 244,000 individuals in the United States are diagnosed with SLE, and women comprise 90% of the affected population (NIH, 2011; LFA, 2013b). While SLE can develop at any point in life, it is most common among women of childbearing age. SLE is more common in African Americans, Hispanics, Native Americans, Native Hawaiians, and Asians than it is in Caucasians (LFA, 2013b). Roughly 20% of clients with SLE develop the disease before the age of 20, though it is rare in children younger than 5 years (American College of Rheumatology, 2012b). The number of childhood cases is roughly equal across genders; after puberty, however, significantly more adolescent females are affected than adolescent males (Arthritis Foundation, 2013).

In clients with no other risk factors for the disease, a number of drugs can cause a syndrome that mimics lupus (drug-induced lupus). Procainamide (Procan-SR, Pronestyl) and hydralazine (Apresoline, Hydralyn) are the most commonly implicated drugs, along with isoniazid (INH). Renal and CNS manifestations of SLE rarely occur with drug-induced lupus, but arthritic and other systemic symptoms are common. Manifestations of drug-induced lupus usually resolve when the medication is discontinued.

▶ CLINICAL MANIFESTATIONS

There are three major classifications of SLE. The first, known as *systemic lupus,* involves one or more of the following systems: cardiovascular, central nervous, hematological, kidneys, lungs, and musculoskeletal. The second, known as *drug-induced lupus,* is associated with some antineoplastic drugs, isoniazid (INH), hydralazine (Apresoline), and others. Symptoms of drug-induced lupus generally subside after the drugs are discontinued. The third, known as *discoid lupus,* is limited to the skin.

The course of SLE is mild in most clients, with periods of remission and exacerbation. The number and severity of exacerbations tend to decrease with time. In some clients, however, SLE is a virulent disease, with significant organ system involvement.

Clients with active disease have an increased risk for infections, which often are opportunistic and severe. Infections such as pneumonia and septicemia are the leading cause of death in clients with SLE, followed by the effects of renal or CNS involvement (see the Multisystem Effects feature).

Typical early manifestations of SLE mimic those of rheumatoid arthritis, including systemic manifestations of fever, loss of appetite, malaise, and weight loss, and musculoskeletal manifestations of multiple arthralgias and symmetric polyarthritis. Joint symptoms affect more than 90% of clients with SLE. Although synovitis may be present, the arthritis associated with SLE is rarely deforming.

Most individuals affected by SLE have skin manifestations at some point during their disease. In fact, SLE originally was described as a skin disorder and was named for the characteristic red butterfly rash across the cheeks and bridge of the nose (**Figure 8–20** ●). Many clients with SLE are photosensitive; a diffuse, maculopapular rash on skin exposed to the sun is common. Other cutaneous manifestations include **discoid lesions**

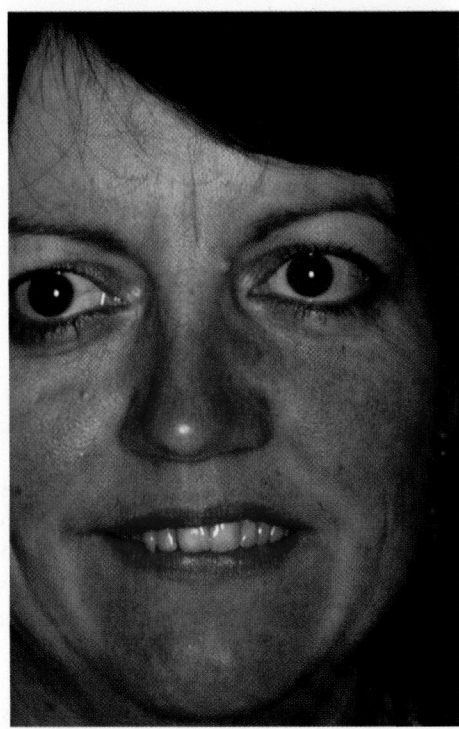

Figure 8–20 ● The butterfly rash of systemic lupus erythematosus.

Multisystem Effects of Systemic Lupus Erythematosus

Integumentary
- Butterfly rash on face
- Photosensitivity
- Maculopapular rash on exposed body surfaces
- Discoid lesions
- Erythematous fingertip lesions
- Splinter hemorrhages
- Alopecia
- Ulcers (lip, mouth, nose)

Endocrine
- Thyroid abnormalities
- Hyperparathyroidism
- Glucose intolerance

Respiratory
- Pleurisy
- Pleural effusion
- Pneumonitis
- Interstitial fibrosis

Urinary
- Proteinuria
- Cellular casts

Potential Complications
- Nephrotic syndrome
- Renal failure

Gastrointestinal
- Anorexia
- Nausea
- Abdominal pain
- Diarrhea
- Hepatomegaly

Musculoskeletal
- Arthralgias
- Symmetric polyarthritis
- Joint swelling and effusion
- Morning stiffness

Neurologic
- Neuropathies (peripheral and central)
- Seizures
- Depression
- Psychosis

Potential Complications
- Stroke
- Organic brain syndrome
  - Intellectual impairment
  - Memory loss
  - Personality changes
  - Disorientation

Sensory
- Conjunctivitis
- Photophobia
- Retinal vasculitis with transient blindness
- Cotton-wool spots on retina

Cardiovascular
- Pericarditis
- Myocarditis
- Endocarditis
- Vasculitis
- Venous or arterial thrombosis

Hematologic
- Anemia
- Leukopenia
- Thrombocytopenia
- Splenomegaly

Reproductive
- Pregnancy-induced hypertension, edema, and proteinuria
- Fetal loss

Metabolic Processes
- Low-grade fever
- Malaise
- Weight loss

Box 8–8   Common Manifestations of Systemic Lupus Erythematosus

- Painful or swollen joints and muscle pain
- Unexplained fever
- Red rash, especially on the face
- Unusual loss of hair
- Pale, cyanotic fingers or toes
- Sensitivity to the sun
- Edema in legs and around eyes
- Ulcers in the mouth
- Enlarged glands
- Extreme fatigue

Approximately 50% of individuals with SLE experience renal manifestations of the disease, including proteinuria, cellular casts, and nephrotic syndrome. Up to 10% develop renal failure as a result of the disease.

Hematological abnormalities, such as anemia, leukopenia, and thrombocytopenia, are common with SLE. Cardiovascular disorders, such as pericarditis, vasculitis, and Raynaud phenomenon, often occur. Less frequently, myocarditis, endocarditis, and venous or arterial thrombosis may develop. Pleurisy, pleural effusions, and lupus pneumonitis are common pulmonary manifestations of SLE.

Many clients with SLE develop transient nervous system involvement, often within the first year of the disease. Manifestations of organic brain syndrome include decline in intellect, memory loss, and disorientation. Other possible neurological manifestations include psychosis, seizures, depression, and stroke. Ocular manifestations of SLE include conjunctivitis, photophobia, and transient blindness due to retinal vasculitis.

Gastrointestinal manifestations of SLE, such as anorexia, nausea, abdominal pain, and diarrhea, may affect up to 45% of clients with the disease. The liver may be enlarged, and liver function tests may yield abnormal results.

Although SLE was once considered a fatal disease, the survival rate has improved through earlier diagnosis and better treatment options. In the 1950s, the 5-year survival rate associated with SLE was approximately 50%. By 2008, the 5-year survival rate for clients diagnosed with SLE had climbed to approximately 96% (Ippolito & Petri, 2008).

Prognosis depends on the severity of the internal organ involvement. Kidney failure is managed by hemodialysis or peritoneal dialysis. Renal transplantation has been very successful for treatment of renal failure secondary to lupus nephritis, a common complication of SLE. See the Lifespan Considerations feature on bottom for a discussion about SLE and pregnancy.

(raised, scaly, circular lesions with an erythematous rim), hives, erythematous fingertip lesions, and splinter hemorrhages. Alopecia is common in clients with SLE, although the hair usually grows back. Painless mucous membrane ulcerations may occur on the lips or in the mouth or nose. Common manifestations of SLE are listed in **Box 8–8** ●.

▶ COLLABORATION

As with rheumatoid arthritis, effective management of SLE requires teamwork, with active participation by both the client and members of the healthcare team. Although currently no cure exists for SLE, the 10-year survival rate is greater than 70% among clients with this disease, which was once considered fatal in most cases. Depending on the severity of a client's manifestations, nurses may want to collaborate with dieticians and physical therapists to help the client develop a nutrition and exercise plan. Referrals to counselors can help clients and caregivers learn to manage stress.

Diagnostic Tests

Because of the diversity of both organ system involvement and manifestations of SLE, diagnosis can be difficult. No one specific test is available to confirm the presence of this disease in all individuals who are suspected of having it. Instead, the diagnosis is based on the client's history and physical assessment, as well as laboratory studies.

The multiple autoantibodies produced in SLE cause a number of abnormalities in laboratory studies. The following tests may be helpful in confirming the presence of SLE:

- *Anti-DNA antibody testing.* This test is a more specific indicator of SLE, because these antibodies rarely are found in any other disorder.
- *Erythrocyte sedimentation rate.* This value typically is elevated, occasionally to 100 mm/hr or greater.
- *Serum complement levels.* These values usually are decreased as complement is consumed or "used up" by the development of **antigen–antibody complexes.**

Lifespan Considerations   SLE and Pregnancy

For women with SLE, all pregnancies are considered high risk. The majority of these pregnancies are not associated with any complications; however, the risk for complications is higher for pregnant women with active SLE than for those whose SLE is in remission. Pregnancy-related complications associated with this disease include preeclampsia, the syndrome known as HELLP (hemolysis, elevated liver function, and low platelets), and a higher rate of spontaneous abortion (LFA, 2013c). During pregnancy, if anti-SSA/Ro antibodies are transferred from mother to fetus through the placenta, neonatal lupus may develop. Neonatal lupus is rare, occurring in only 2% of first-time mothers who test positive for anti-SSA/Ro antibodies. While symptoms seen in infants born with neonatal lupus may be minimal and resolve spontaneously, such as skin rashes or mild liver involvement, the potentially fatal condition of congenital heart block (CHB) may also occur. If indicated, fetal echocardiography may be used to assess for CHB. Usually, this test is performed during the second trimester. The prognosis for CHB varies, depending upon when CHB is detected. With treatment, early CHB may be reversible. However, late CHB may require insertion of a pacemaker at the time of delivery (LFA, 2013d).

Clinical Manifestations and Therapies Systemic Lupus Erythematosus

ETIOLOGY	CLINICAL MANIFESTATIONS	CLINICAL THERAPIES
Organic brain syndrome, resulting from neurological involvement	General term referring to many disorders causing impaired mental function; manifestations include confusion, with impaired memory, judgment, and cognition. Symptoms may include agitation, withdrawal, or depression.	Treatment varies and is aimed at treating the underlying cause of the condition, in this case SLE.
Anemia	Manifestations range from absence of clinical signs and symptoms to more life-threatening, depending on the severity of the condition. Common manifestations include: ■ Weakness ■ Fatigue ■ Poor concentration ■ Shortness of breath ■ Dyspnea ■ Palpitations ■ Intermittent claudication ■ Symptoms of heart failure.	Initial treatment is aimed at restoring normal red blood cell counts as well as treating the underlying cause. Treatment to increase red blood cell count includes: ■ Increased iron intake in diet ■ Iron supplementation ■ Medications to stimulate red cell production, such as erythropoietin. In severe cases blood transfusions may be administered.
Leukopenia	The most common manifestation is frequent infections resulting from inadequate immune response caused by low counts of white blood cells.	Treatment to increase white blood cell count is predominantly aimed at treating the underlying cause of leukopenia. Supportive treatment to resolve infections and prevent further infection may include antibiotics, protective isolation, and strict aseptic technique.
Thrombocytopenia may occur spontaneously but it is more commonly associated with medications used to treat SLE.	Manifestations generally do not arise until platelet count falls to significant levels of less than 50,000. Common manifestations include: ■ Bruising ■ Petechiae ■ Purpura ■ Nosebleeds ■ Bleeding gums.	Treatment is guided by etiology and severity and may include: ■ Corticosteroids ■ IV IgG ■ Splenectomy ■ Administration of IV platelet transfusion.
Pericarditis	■ Chest pain radiating to the back relieved by sitting forward and worsening when lying down ■ Dry cough ■ Fever ■ Fatigue ■ Anxiety ■ Friction rub ■ ST elevation and PR depression	■ Pericardiocentesis to remove fluid produced by inflammatory process, especially if it is restricting function ■ Antibiotics if infectious ■ Corticosteroids to reduce inflammation ■ Colchicine
Renal involvement	■ Proteinuria ■ Cellular casts ■ Nephrotic syndrome ■ Renal failure	Treatment is aimed at correcting the underlying cause and relieving stress on the kidney. Dialysis may be indicated if renal failure results.
Skin involvement is the most common result of SLE.	Photosensitivity with a diffuse maculopapular rash on skin exposed to the sun; discoid lesions, hives, erythematous fingertip lesions, alopecia, and splinter hemorrhages.	■ Avoidance of sunlight ■ Corticosteroids ■ Immunosuppressants ■ Disease-modifying antirheumatic drugs ■ Low-fat, mostly vegetarian, wholesome diet may lessen symptoms.

- *Complete blood count (CBC).* Abnormalities in the CBC include moderate to severe anemia, leukopenia, lymphocytopenia, and possible thrombocytopenia.
- *Urinalysis.* This test shows mild proteinuria, hematuria, and blood cell casts during exacerbations of the disease when the kidneys are involved. Renal function tests including *serum creatinine* and *blood urea nitrogen (BUN)* may also be ordered to evaluate the extent of renal disease.
- *Kidney biopsy.* This test may be performed to assess the severity of renal lesions and to guide therapy.

Surgery

Although there is no surgical treatment for SLE, damage caused by this disease can lead to other conditions that require surgery. The kidneys are particularly vulnerable to injury. Clients with lupus nephritis who progress to develop end-stage renal disease are treated with hemodialysis or peritoneal dialysis and kidney transplantation.

Pharmacologic Therapy

The client with mild or remittent SLE may need little or no therapy other than supportive care. Arthralgias, arthritis, fever, and fatigue often can be managed with aspirin or other NSAIDs. Aspirin is particularly beneficial for clients with SLE, because its antiplatelet effects help to prevent thrombosis. However, it may cause liver toxicity and hepatitis.

Skin and arthritic manifestations of SLE may be treated with antimalarial drugs, such as hydroxychloroquine (Plaquenil). Hydroxychloroquine also has been shown to be effective in reducing the frequency of acute episodes of SLE in individuals with mild or inactive disease. Retinal toxicity and possibly irreversible blindness are the primary concerns with this drug. For this reason, clients taking hydroxychloroquine should undergo an ophthalmological examination every 6 months.

Topical corticosteroids may be used to treat skin lesions. Some physicians recommend avoiding the use of oral contraceptives, because estrogen can trigger an acute episode.

Clients with severe and life-threatening manifestations of SLE (e.g., nephritis, hemolytic anemia, myocarditis, pericarditis, or CNS manifestations) require corticosteroid therapy in high doses. Initially, such clients may need 40–60 mg of prednisone per day. The dosage is then tapered as rapidly as the client's disease allows, although lowering the dosage may precipitate an acute episode. Some clients with SLE require long-term corticosteroid therapy to manage symptoms and prevent major organ damage. These clients are at increased risk for corticosteroid side effects, such as cushingoid effects, weight gain, hypertension, infection, accelerated osteoporosis, and hypokalemia.

Certain cytotoxic or antineoplastic drugs are effective as immunosuppressive agents, and may be used either alone or in combination with corticosteroids to treat clients with active SLE or lupus nephritis. These agents act by decreasing the proliferation of cells within the immune system and are widely used to prevent rejection following a tissue or organ transplant. Usually, they are administered concurrently with corticosteroid therapy, allowing lower doses of both preparations and resulting in fewer side effects. Examples include azathioprine (Imuran), cyclophosphamide (Cytoxan), and cyclosporine (Sandimmune).

When these agents are used in combination, lower, less toxic doses of each drug can be used. The client receiving immunosuppressive agents is at increased risk for infection, malignancy, bone marrow depression, and toxic effects specific to the drug prescribed. Nursing responsibilities for clients on immunosuppressants include:

- Monitor blood count, with particular attention to the WBC and platelet counts. Notify the physician if WBCs fall below 4,000 or platelets below 75,000.
- Monitor renal and liver function studies, including creatinine, blood urea nitrogen, creatinine clearance, and liver enzyme levels. Report abnormal levels to the physician.
- Administer oral preparations with food to minimize gastrointestinal effects.
- Increase fluids to maintain good hydration and urinary output; monitor intake and output.
- Monitor for signs of abnormal bleeding, e.g., bleeding gums, petechiae, joint pain, hematuria, and black or tarry stools.
- Use meticulous hand washing and other appropriate measures to prevent infection; assess for signs of infection.
- Pulmonary fibrosis is a potential adverse effect of cyclophosphamide. Monitor the results of pulmonary function studies, and be alert for dyspnea or cough.

For clients receiving immunosuppressive agents, careful teaching is required to make sure both clients and family members understand appropriate precautions against the threat of infection. Teaching points should include the following:

- Avoid large crowds and situations that increase exposure to infection.
- Report to the physician signs of infection, such as chills, fever, sore throat, fatigue, or malaise.
- Use contraception to prevent pregnancy, as these drugs may increase the risk of birth defects.
- Refrain from taking aspirin or ibuprofen, which may increase the risk of bleeding. Report any signs of bleeding to the physician.
- Women may not experience menstruation while taking cyclophosphamide; menses will resume once the drug is discontinued.
- Report difficulty breathing or cough to the physician if taking cyclophosphamide.

Nonpharmacologic Therapy

Clients with SLE should be counseled to avoid smoking. Among numerous other negative effects, smoking can exacerbate the risks of cardiovascular damage linked to SLE, as well as increasing susceptibility to infection, especially in the lungs. During periods of known or suspected infection, these clients should be advised to consult with their healthcare provider prior to receiving any immunizations. While there is no standard recommended diet for clients with SLE, they should be encouraged to consume a healthy diet that includes oily fish, as omega-3 fatty acids appear to offer protection against cardiovascular disease. Before adding any herb, vitamin, or supplement to the diet, these clients should consult their healthcare provider. Some dietary supplements are associated with known undesirable effects; for example, alfalfa tablets are linked to lupus flares (acute episodes) (LFA, 2013e). Because of the photosensitivity associated with SLE, the client should be cautioned to avoid sun exposure. Clients should use sunscreens with an SPF rating of 15 or higher when outdoors.

NURSING PROCESS

Nursing management focuses on thorough assessments (because of the multitude of systems that can be affected by SLE) and on teaching to enhance general health practices. The client with severe disease, however, has diverse nursing needs that vary according to the organ systems involved. Because of the close link between RA and SLE, many of the nursing diagnoses and interventions identified for the client with arthritis may be appropriate for the client with SLE. The client with lupus nephritis or end-stage renal disease has the nursing care needs outlined in the exemplar on Chronic Renal Failure in the module on Fluids and Electrolytes, and in the exemplar on Nephritis in the module on Inflammation.

Assessment

Assess the client's nutritional status including baseline weight and history of recent weight loss or weight gain. Assess the skin for rashes, ulcers, photosensitivity, ecchymosis, petechiae, cyanosis, and hair loss. Respiratory assessment includes breath sounds and respiratory rate as well as assessment for pleural effusion or pleuritis. Cardiovascular assessment includes vital signs, heart tones, and symptoms of pericarditis or friction rub. Musculoskeletal assessment includes joint pain, joint deformity, pain, weakness, and ability to perform ADLs. Neurological assessment includes changes in affect or cognitive abilities and seizure activity. Gastrointestinal assessment includes splenomegaly.

Because SLE is a chronic disease that affects primarily adolescents, psychosocial assessment is indicated. Assess family interactions, and explore stressful situations, such as divorce or trauma. Treatment-related restrictions and changes in appearance can lead

to withdrawal, depression, and suicidal tendencies. Perform psychological assessments periodically as the client grows and adapts to the disorder or faces new developmental challenges with a chronic disease.

Diagnosis

Nursing diagnoses will depend on the severity of the disease process and organ involvement but are likely to include the following:

- *Risk for Infection*
- *Risk for Imbalanced Fluid Volume*
- *Risk for Imbalanced Nutrition: Less Than Body Requirements*
- *Risk for Ineffective Tissue Perfusion*
- *Risk for Impaired Skin Integrity*
- *Chronic Pain*
- *Risk for Ineffective Management of Therapeutic Regimen*
- *Risk for Activity Intolerance*
- *Risk for Disturbed Body Image*
- *Compromised Family Coping*

(NANDA-I © 2012)

Planning

The goals of nursing care are to assist clients (especially children) to manage and cope with a chronic disease, prevent infection, promote nutrition, facilitate a remission, and recognize and avoid triggers for flares. Goals are created with input from the client based on needs, current status, and severity of disease, including organ involvement. Goals should be specific and contain a time frame for attainment. Goals may include the following:

- Client will be able to verbalize skin care needs to reduce the risk of altered skin integrity at the end of the teaching session.
- Client will demonstrate proper hand hygiene techniques before discharge.
- Client will verbalize the impact of the diagnosis to the healthcare provider.
- Client will verbalize methods for preventing infection, including use of prophylactic antibiotics and home infection control measures.

Implementation

The priority nursing interventions for the client with SLE are focused on problems with impaired skin integrity, ineffective protection, and impaired health maintenance. The Lifespan Considerations feature provides information regarding treatment of children and adolescents with SLE.

Prevent Infection

Infections are a leading cause of death for clients with SLE. Prophylactic antibiotics may be required for dental work and surgical procedures. Instruct the client and family to inform all healthcare providers of the disease in order to plan for prophylactic measures. Educate the client and family on the importance of adhering to the immunization schedule and obtaining a yearly influenza vaccine to prevent infection. Instruct the client on hand hygiene and infection control measures in the home, and warn clients about the dangers of tattooing and body piercing because of the risk of infection.

SLE puts the client at increased risk for infection and multiple organ system problems. In addition, treatment with corticosteroids or immunosuppressive agents further impairs immune responses and the ability to fight infection. The following interventions are appropriate for inclusion in the care of the hospitalized client:

- Wash hands before and after providing direct care. Hand washing removes transient organisms from the skin, reducing the risk of transmission to the client.
- Use strict aseptic technique in caring for intravenous lines and indwelling urinary catheters or in performing any wound care. Aseptic technique offers protection against external and resident host microorganisms.
- Assess the client frequently for infection. Monitor temperature and vital signs every 4 hours. Assess for signs of cellulitis, including tenderness, redness, swelling, and warmth. Report signs of infection to the physician promptly. Therapy can suppress usual responses, such as elevated temperature and inflammation. The fever of infection may be mistaken for the fever commonly associated with SLE. The client receiving immunosuppressive therapy for the disease has an even higher risk for infection.
- Monitor laboratory values, including CBC and tests of organ function; report changes to the physician. An elevation in the WBC count with a shift to the left (increased numbers of immature leukocytes in the blood) may be an early indication of infection. Changes in liver function studies, renal function studies, myocardial enzymes, or other laboratory values may indicate organ system involvement.
- Initiate reverse or protective isolation procedures as indicated by the client's immune status. These procedures provide further protection from infection for clients who are severely immunocompromised.
- Ensure an adequate nutrient intake, offering supplementary feedings as indicated or maintaining parenteral nutrition if necessary. Adequate nutrition is important for healing and immune system function.
- Teach the client the importance of good hand washing after using the bathroom and before eating. Hand washing reduces the risk of infection by endogenous organisms.
- Monitor for potential adverse effects of medications, including thrombocytopenia and possible bleeding, fluid retention

with edema and possible hypertension, loss of bone density, osteoporosis, and possible pathological fractures, renal or hepatic toxicity, and cardiac effects, particularly in the client with fluid retention and hypervolemia. Medications used to treat SLE have many potential adverse effects that can impair normal protective and homeostatic mechanisms.

Maintain Fluid Balance

Because many clients with SLE have renal involvement, it is important for the nurse to monitor intake and output and frequently evaluate fluid and electrolyte status. Renal dysfunction can manifest itself by edema, muscle cramps, diarrhea, tetany, and convulsions.

Promote Adequate Nutrition

Currently, there are no specific dietary plans for the client with SLE; however, the diet may be restricted according to renal involvement, weight gain, weight loss, or other complications. The client is at risk for weight gain associated with treatment involving steroids and a decreased activity level during exacerbations of this disease. Encourage a well-balanced, nutritious diet as well as appropriate fluid intake.

Promote Skin Integrity

Skin lesions are a common manifestation of SLE. A rash or discoid lesion interrupts the integrity of the skin, which is the first line of protection against infection, so the client's already high risk for infection is increased. These lesions, which usually appear on exposed parts of the skin, also can be disfiguring and cause the client emotional distress. The nurse can promote skin integrity through the following interventions:

- Assess the client's knowledge of SLE and its possible effects on the skin. Assessment allows the nurse to base teaching and information on the client's existing knowledge, thereby improving learning and retention.
- Discuss the relationship between sun exposure and disease activity, both dermatological and systemic. It is important for the client to understand that sun exposure may not only cause dermatological manifestations but also trigger an acute episode.
- Teach appropriate strategies for limiting sun exposure, such as avoiding outdoor activity between 10:00 a.m. and 3:00 p.m. and applying sunscreen 30 minutes prior to going out in the sun.
- Encourage the client to keep skin clean and dry and to apply therapeutic creams or ointments to lesions as prescribed. These measures promote healing and reduce the risk of infection.
- Encourage the use of good hygienic measures and a mild soap to prevent infection resulting in stress that can lead to acute exacerbations.
- Recommend limited use of cosmetics. Cosmetics can irritate the skin and increase the risk of integumentary symptoms.
- Recommend the client avoid fluorescent lighting. Exacerbations of SLE have been reported following such exposure (LFA, 2013e).
- Provide instructions on oral care to maintain intact oral mucosa. Alterations in skin integrity, including those in the oral cavity, can increase the risk of acute exacerbations of SLE.
- Provide instructions on the care of the head if alopecia occurs. Alopecia, especially in women, can be very

ore intervening

traumatic, so care of the skin on the head is important because the client cannot wear a wig when skin integrity is affected.

Promote Rest and Comfort

Because of fatigue and joint pain, the client has little energy reserve during acute episodes of the disease. The nurse should encourage frequent rest periods and a nutritious diet to maximize energy stores. A physical therapist can plan a program to encourage mobility and increase muscle strength.

Manage Medication Side Effects

Observe the client for any side effects of medications used for treatment and teach the client and family about these effects. For example, immunosuppressant drugs can promote infection anywhere in the body, and NSAIDs commonly cause gastric distress and bleeding of the gastrointestinal tract. The antimalarial drug hydroxychloroquine can cause serious vision changes; thus frequent eye examinations are needed.

Provide Emotional Support

Adolescents may have an altered body image as a result of rash, alopecia, arthritic changes in the joints, and chronic disease. Referral to a lupus support group, the local department of social services, or counseling may be helpful. The client needs ongoing support and information to deal with the complexity of the disease.

Stay Current: *The American Lupus Society and the Lupus Foundation of America (**http://www.lupus.org**) can provide information to help clients and family members adjust to the disease. The Arthritis Foundation (**http://www.arthritis.org**) also publishes a useful pamphlet: Meeting the Challenge: A Young Person's Guide to Living with Lupus.*

Teach Avoidance of Triggers for Disease Flares

Many clients can recognize the signs of impending flares and the triggers that precede them. Partner with the client and family to implement measures to prevent these triggers. Discuss preventive behaviors, such as avoiding sun exposure and stressors. Clients should be warned that alcohol, smoking, and drugs also pose an increased risk because of the potential to stimulate flares. The nurse may advise female clients who are sexually active to avoid birth control pills that contain the hormone estrogen, because the extra estrogen may exacerbate symptoms. In addition, alternate birth control methods should be discussed.

SAFETY ALERT
Hand washing is essential before and after providing direct care, even if gloves are worn. A decrease in this type of medical asepsis is contributing to the increasing number of hospital-acquired infections that are resistant to antibiotics.

Promote Health Maintenance

As with other chronic diseases, much of the responsibility for maintaining optimal health rests with the client. Disease manifestations such as fatigue, arthralgias, arthritis, and increased risk for infection can interfere with the client's ability to maintain health. Psychosocial issues also can be a significant factor in health maintenance for the client with SLE. These issues may include denial of the significance of the disease, poor coping, lack of financial and other resources, and an inadequate support system.

- Assess the client's ability to maintain optimal health, identifying physical and psychosocial factors that may affect health maintenance. Before intervening to improve the client's

Client Teaching Self-Care of Systemic Lupus Erythematosus

Teaching is a critical factor in preparing clients with SLE for self-care at home. Address the following topics:

- The disease and its potential effects. Promote an optimistic outlook, stressing that the majority of clients do not require long-term corticosteroid therapy and that the disease may improve over time.
- The warning signs of an acute episode (a flare), which include increased fatigue, pain or abdominal discomfort, rash, headache, fever, and dizziness.
- The importance of skin care.
- The importance of avoiding exposure to infection.
- The need to follow the prescribed treatment plan, including rest and exercise, medications, and follow up appointments. Discuss manifestations of an acute episode, and stress the importance of contacting the physician promptly if any of these manifestations occur.
- The significance of wearing a medical alert bracelet or tag that identifies their condition and therapy (e.g., corticosteroids or immunosuppressives).

- Family planning with the client and spouse. The use of oral contraceptives may be contraindicated for the client; if appropriate, provide information about alternative means of birth control. Pregnancy is not contraindicated for most women with SLE. However, the pregnant client requires close monitoring, because acute episodes sometimes accompany pregnancy.
- The need for preventive health care for both men and women with SLE. Women should have gynecological and breast examinations and men should have prostate examinations each year. Both men and women should have regular screenings for cholesterol and blood pressure. Annual influenza vaccinations are important, as are pneumococcal vaccinations for older clients. If clients are taking corticosteroids or antimalarial medications, annual eye examinations should be conducted to screen for and treat any ocular problems.
- Helpful resources:
  a. National Institute of Arthritis and Musculoskeletal and Skin Diseases, http://www.niams.nih.gov/
  b. Lupus Foundation of America, www.lupus.org

health maintenance, the nurse must identify and understand the factors affecting it.

■ Provide care and teaching in a nonjudgmental manner. To intervene effectively, the nurse must accept the client and family as they are.

■ Encourage the client and family members to discuss the effect of the disease on their lives. Open discussion helps the client and the nurse identify barriers to health maintenance and begin exploring alternative strategies.

■ Initiate an interdisciplinary care conference with the client and family. In this care conference, the expression of a number of perspectives will improve the planning of strategies for health maintenance activities.

■ Refer the client and family to counseling as needed. Counseling may help the client and family develop the coping skills necessary to accept and deal with the disease.

■ Refer the client and family to community and social service agencies and to local support groups. These groups and agencies are valuable resources for the client and family.

Evaluation

Successful outcomes of nursing care involve management of this chronic disease. Expected outcomes include the following:

■ Client maintains normal intake and output levels, with demonstrated fluid and electrolyte balance.

■ Client maintains healthy, intact skin.

■ Client maintains a balance of rest and activity to promote health.

■ Client maintains medication regimen to promote health and prevent side effects.

■ Client develops or maintains a positive body image.

REVIEW Systemic Lupus Erythematosus

RELATE Link the Concepts

Link the exemplar of systemic lupus erythematosus with the concept of inflammation:

1. Describe the inflammatory reaction and explain the role this process plays in SLE.

2. What types of treatment for inflammation would also be useful in treating SLE?

Link the exemplar of systemic lupus erythematosus with the concept of health, wellness, and illness:

3. Why would the client with SLE be less likely to have acute exacerbations if he or she made healthy lifestyle choices?

4. Create a teaching plan explaining healthy behaviors that promote fewer acute exacerbations of SLE.

Link the exemplar of systemic lupus erythematosus with the concept of self:

5. How would a diagnosis of SLE affect a client's self-concept? Why might these effects be especially pronounced in male clients with SLE?

6. What interventions would be appropriate for enhancing the self-esteem of an adolescent SLE client?

READY Go to Companion Skills Manual

REFER Go to Pearson Nursing Student Resources
nursing.pearsonhighered.com

REFLECT Case Study

Yvonne Johnson is a 35-year-old African-American woman. She is a single parent to her 15-year-old son, Randall. Ms. Johnson has had relationships with men off and on, but she is not currently involved with anybody. Ms. Johnson completed a bachelor's degree in marketing 5 years ago but has been unable to break into the marketing field locally. Instead, she has been working full time as an administrative assistant for a large company. Her parents and siblings live nearby, and she maintains a close relationship with them.

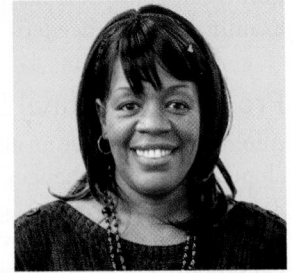

Over the past 4 years, Ms. Johnson has noticed mild swelling in her hands and feet every morning. The symptoms began subtly not long after she graduated from college. She has always attributed the symptom to her sedentary lifestyle and being somewhat overweight. More recently, she has been experiencing pain along with the swelling in her hands and feet.

Ms. Johnson saw her healthcare provider, Dr. Rowe, and told her that she had had pain in her hands for the last several months. When asked about other symptoms, she mentioned the swelling in her hands and feet for the past 4 years. Dr. Rowe thought that the pain was likely occupational (from typing) and suggested that Ms. Johnson take over-the-counter pain relievers, such as ibuprofen. Dr. Rowe noticed that Ms. Johnson's blood pressure was slightly elevated (134/92 mmHg) but attributed this to her race and diet. She suggested that Ms. Johnson lose a little weight and reduce her salt intake.

Ms. Johnson has been trying to follow Dr. Rowe's advice for the past 3 months. Although she has lost approximately 5 pounds, has avoided salty foods, and has been taking ibuprofen three times a day, she continues to have pain in her hands and swelling in her hands and feet. She also wonders whether the symptoms are really associated with her work.

1. What diagnosis do you suspect for Ms. Johnson? Explain the basis of your answer.

2. What diagnostic testing would you anticipate to confirm this diagnosis? Explain your answers.

3. If you are the nurse admitting Ms. Johnson to her provider's office, what specific assessments would you perform to help you confirm the suspected diagnosis?

■ REFERENCES

Adams, M. A., Holland, L. N., & Urban, C. Q. (2013). *Pharmacology for nurses: A pathophysiologic approach* (4th ed.). Upper Saddle River, NJ: Prentice Hall.

American Academy of Allergy Asthma and Immunology. (2013). *Allergy statistics.* Retrieved from http://www. aaaai.org/about-the-aaaai/newsroom/allergy-statistics. aspx.

American Academy of Pediatrics. (2009). *Introduction of solid foods and allergic reactions.* Retrieved from http://www.aap.org/en-us/about-the-aap/aap-press-room/ pages/Introduction-of-Solid-Foods-and-Allergic-Reactions.aspx American Academy of Pediatrics. (2012a). Red book: 2012 Report of the committee on infectious disease (29th ed.). Elk Grove Village, IL: Author.

American Academy of Pediatrics. (2012a). *Health issues: Allergy causes.* Retrieved from http://www.healthychildren.org/English/health-issues/conditions/allergies-asthma/pages/Allergy-Causes.aspx.

American Academy of Pediatrics. (2012b). *MMR Vaccine and Autism.* Retrieved from http://www2.aap.org/immunization/families/mmr.html.

American Academy of Pediatrics. (2013). *Health issues: Juvenile idiopathic arthritis.* Retrieved from http://www.healthychildren.org/English/health-issues/conditions/orthopedic/pages/Juvenile-Idiopathic-Arthritis.aspx?nfstatus=401&nftoken=00000000-0000-0000-0000-000000000000&nfstatusdescription=ERROR%3a+No+local+token.

American Academy of Pediatrics, Committee on Fetus and Newborn and American College of Obstetricians and Gynecologists Committee on Obstetrics. (2007). *Guidelines for perinatal care* (6th ed.). Elk Grove Village, IL: Author.

American Academy of Pediatrics, Committee on Pediatric AIDS. (1998). Human immunodeficiency virus/acquired immunodeficiency syndrome education in schools. *Pediatrics, 101,* 933–935.

American Academy of Pediatrics, Committee on Pediatric AIDS and Committee on Adolescence. (2001). Adolescents and human immunodeficiency virus infection: The role of the pediatrician in prevention and intervention (RE0031). *Pediatrics, 107*(1), 188–190.

American Autoimmune Related Disease Association and National Coalition of Autoimmune Patient Groups. (2011). *The cost burden of autoimmune disease: The latest front in the war on healthcare spending.* Retrieved from http://www.aarda.org/pdf/cbad.pdf.

American Cancer Society. (2008). *Infectious agents and cancer.* Retrieved from http://www.cancer.org/docroot/PED/content/PED_1_3X_Infectious_Agents_and_Cancer.asp?sitearea=PED.

American College of Allergy, Asthma and Immunology. (2011). To feed or not to feed. *AllergyWatch, 13*(4), 1–2.

American College of Rheumatology. (2012a). *Rheumatoid arthritis.* Retrieved from http://www.rheumatology.org/practice/clinical/patients/diseases_and_conditions/ra.asp.

American College of Rheumatology. (2012b). *Systemic lupus erythematosus in children and teens.* Retrieved from http://www.rheumatology.org/practice/clinical/patients/diseases_and_conditions/sle.asp.

Arthritis Foundation. (2013). *Disease center: Systemic lupus erythematosus (lupus) in children and adolescents.* Retrieved from http://www.arthritis.org/conditions-treatments/disease-center/systemic-lupus-erythematosus-lupus-in-children-and-adolescents/.

Asthma and Allergy Foundation of America. (2009). *Allergy facts and figures.* Retrieved from http://www.aafa.org/display.cfm?id=9&sub=30.

Badell, M. L., & Lindsay, M. (2012). Thirty years later: Pregnancies in females perinatally infected with human immunodeficiency virus-1. *AIDS Research and Treatment, 2012,* 418630. doi:10.1155/2012/418630.

Ball, J.W., Bindler, R.C., & Cowen, K.J. (2012). Principles of Pediatric Nursing: Caring for Children (5th ed.). Upper Saddle River, NJ: Pearson.

Bartlett, J. G., & Weber, D. J. (2005). *Management of adults exposed to HIV. Up to Date Online 13.2.* Retrieved from http://222.utdol.com.

Bernstein, H. (2007). Maternal and perinatal infection—Viral. In S. G. Gabbe, J. R. Niebyl, & J. L. Simpson (Eds.), *Obstetrics: Normal and problem pregnancies* (5th ed., pp. 1203–1232). Philadelphia, PA: Churchill Livingstone/Elsevier.

Bersenev, A., & Levine, B. L. (2012). Convergence of gene and cell therapy. *Regenerative Medicine, 7*(6s), 50–56.

Blumchen, K., Bayer, P., Buck, D., Michael, T., Cremer, R., Fricke, C., Henne, T., Peters, H., Hofmann, C., Keil, T., Schlaud, M., Wahn, U. . . ., & Niggemann, B. (2010). Effects of latex avoidance on latex sensitization, atopy and allergic diseases in patients with spina bifida. *Allergy, 65*(12), 1585–1593.

Branum, A. M., & Lukacs, S. L. (2008). Food allergy among U.S. children: Trends in prevalence and hospitalizations. *NCHS Data Brief 10.*

Calvin, K. L, & Karsh, B. A (2009). Systematic review of patient acceptance of consumer health information technology. *Journal of the Medical Informatics Association, 16*(4), 550–560.

Centers for Disease Control and Prevention. (2004). Treating opportunistic infections among HIV-infected adults and adolescents. *MMWR Recommendations and Reports, 53*(RR-15), 1–113.

Centers for Disease Control and Prevention. (2006a). *HIV and its transmission.* Retrieved from http://www.cdc.gov.

Centers for Disease Control and Prevention. (2006b). Preventing tetanus, diphtheria, and pertussis among adolescents: Use of tetanus toxoid, reduced diphtheria toxoid, and acellular pertussis vaccines. *Morbidity and Mortality Weekly Report, 55,* 1–34.

Centers for Disease Control and Prevention. (2006c). Prevention and control of influenza: Recommendations of the Advisory Committee on Immunization Practices. *Morbidity and Mortality Weekly Report, 55,* 1–44.

Centers for Disease Control and Prevention. (2006d). Revised recommendations for HIV testing of adults, adolescents and pregnant women in health-care settings. *Morbidity and Mortality Weekly Report, 55*(RR14), 1–17.

Centers for Disease Control and Prevention. (2007). *HIV/AIDS Surveillance in Women.* Retrieved from http://www.cdc.gov/hiv/topics/surveillance/resources/slides/women/.

Centers for Disease Control and Prevention. (2008a). *HIV and AIDS in the United States: A Picture of Today's Epidemic.* CDC Surveillance Topics. Retrieved from http://www.cdc.gov/hiv/topics/surveillance/united_states.htm.

Centers for Disease Control and Prevention. (2008b). *HIV prevalence estimate—United States, 2006.* Retrieved from http://www.cdc.gov/mmwr/preview/mmwrhtml/mm5739a2.htm.

Centers for Disease Control and Prevention. (2008c). *HIV/AIDS among persons aged 50 and older.* Retrieved from http://www.cdc.gov/flu/professionals/vaccination/vax-summary.htm.

Centers for Disease Control and Prevention. (2008d). *HIV and AIDS in the United States: A picture of today's epidemic.* Retrieved from http://www.cdc.gov.

Centers for Disease Control and Prevention. (2010). *Sudden infant death syndrome (SIDS) and vaccines.* Retrieved from http://www.cdc.gov/vaccinesafety/Concerns/sids_faq.html.

Centers for Disease Control and Prevention. (2011a). *Occupational HIV transmission and prevention among health care workers.* Retrieved from http://www.cdc.gov/hiv/resources/factsheets/hcwprev.htm.

Centers for Disease Control and Prevention. (2011b). *HIV among youth.* Retrieved from http://www.cdc.gov/hiv/youth/index.htm.

Centers for Disease Control and Prevention. (2011c). *Childhood arthritis.* Retrieved from http://www.cdc.gov/arthritis/basics/childhood.htm.

Centers for Disease Control and Prevention. (2012a). *Immunization information system functional standards, 2013–2017.* Retrieved from http://www.cdc.gov/vaccines/programs/iis/func-stds.html.

Centers for Disease Control and Prevention. (2012b). *Varicella vaccine effectiveness and duration of protection.* Retrieved from http://www.cdc.gov/vaccines/vpd-vac/varicella/hcp-effective-duration.htm.

Centers for Disease Control and Prevention. (2012c). *Prevent diabetes.* Retrieved from http://www.cdc.gov/diabetes/consumer/prevent.htm.

Centers for Disease Control and Prevention. (2013a). *Statistics and surveillance.* Retrieved from http://www.cdc.gov/hiv/topics/surveillance/index.htm.

Centers for Disease Control and Prevention. (2013b). *HIV among pregnant women, infants, and children in the United States.* Retrieved from http://www.cdc.gov/hiv/topics/perinatal/index.htm.

Centers for Disease Control and Prevention. (2013c). Advisory Committee on Immunization Practices recommended immunization schedule for persons aged 0 through 18 years—United States, 2013. *Morbidity and Mortality Weekly Report, 62*(1), 2–8.

Centers for Disease Control and Prevention. (2013d). Advisory Committee on Immunization Practices recommended immunization schedule for adults aged 19 years and older—United States, 2013. *Morbidity and Mortality Weekly Report, 62*(1), 9–19.

Chinratanapisit, S. (2008). Disease summaries: Diagnostic approach to the adult with suspected immune deficiency. *World Allergy Organization.* Retrieved from http://www.worldallergy.org/professional/allergic_diseases_center/suspected_immune_deficiency/.

Cleveland Clinic. (2011). *Graft vs. host disease: An overview in bone marrow transplant.* Retrieved from http://my.clevelandclinic.org/services/bone_marrow_transplantation/hic_graft_vs_host_disease_an_overview_in_bone_marrow_transplant.aspx.

Cloherty, J. R., Eichenwald, E. C., & Stark, A. R. (2008). *Manual of neonatal care.* Philadelphia, PA: Lippincott Williams & Wilkins.

Collins, I. J., Jourdain, G., Hansudewechakul, R., Kanjanavanit, S., Hongsiriwon, S., Ngampiyasakul, C., et al. Program for HIV Prevention and Treatment Study Team. (2010). Long-term survival of HIV-infected children receiving antiretroviral therapy in Thailand: A 5-year observational cohort study. *Clinical Infectious Diseases, 51*(12), 1449–1457. doi:10.1086/657401.

Community Resources Information, Inc. (2009). *Acupuncture treatment for HIV/AIDS.* Retrieved from http://www.massresources.org/pages.cfm?contentID=114&pageID=31&subpages=yes&dynamicID=902.

Côté, J. K., & Pepler, C. (2005). Cognitive coping intervention for acutely ill HIV-positive men. *Journal of Clinical Nursing, 14*(3), 321–326.

Coyne, P. J., Lyne, M. E., & Watson, A. C. (2002). Symptom management in people with AIDS. *American Journal of Nursing, 102*(9), 48–57.

DeStefano, F., Gu, D., Kramarz, P., Truman, B. I., Iademarco, M. F., Mullooly, J. P., et al. (2002). Childhood vaccinations and risk of asthma. *Pediatric Infectious Disease Journal, 21*(6), 498–504.

Dilip, S., Wanchub, A., & Bhatnagara, A. (2011). Interaction between oxidative stress and chemokines: Possible pathogenic role in systemic lupus erythematosus and rheumatoid arthritis. *Immunobiology, 216,* 1010–1017.

English, A., Shaw, F. E., McCauley, M. M., & Fishbein, D. R. (2008). Legal basis of consent for health care and vaccination for adolescents. *Pediatrics, 121,* S86. Retrieved from http://pediatrics.aappublications.org/content/121/Supplement_1/S85.full.pdf.

Federico, A., D'Aiuto, E., Borriello, F., Barra, G., Gravina, A. G., Romano, M., & De Palma, R. (2010). Fat: A matter of disturbance for the immune system. *World Journal of Gastroenterology, 16*(38), 4762–4772.

Filon, F. L., & Radman, G. (2006). Latex allergy: A follow up study of 1,040 healthcare workers. *Occupational and Environmental Medicine, 63,* 121–125.

Gleeson, M., & Walsh, N. P. (2012). The BASES expert statement on exercise, immunity, and infection. *Journal of Sports sciences, 30*(3), 321–324.

Gomes, E. R., & Demoly, P. (2005). *Epidemiology of hypersensitivity drug reactions: Risk factors for hypersensitivity drug reactions.* Retrieved from http://www.medscape.com/viewarticle/508375_3.

Haaz, S. (2008). *Complementary and alternative medicine for patients with rheumatoid arthritis.* Retrieved from http://www.hopkinsarthritis.org/patient-corner/disease-management/ra-complementary-alternative-medicine/.

Haberer, J., Kiwanuka, J., Muzoora, D., Nansera, D., Hunt, P., Martin, J., & Bangsberg, D. (2012). Real-time HIV antiretroviral therapy adherence monitoring among adults and children in rural Uganda. Massachusetts

General Hospital. Center for Global Health. Retrieved from http://www.iapac.org/AdherenceConference/presentations/ADH7_80027.pdf.

Haija, A. J., & Schulz, S. W. (2011). The role and effect of complementary and alternative medicine in systemic lupus erythematosus. *Rheumatic Diseases Clinics of North America, 37*(1), 47–62.

Heiser, C. R., Ernst, J. A., Barrett, J. T., French, N., Schultz, M., & Dube, M. P. (2004). Probiotics, soluble fiber, and L-glutamine (GLN) reduce nelfinavir (NFV) or lopinavir/ritonavir (LPV/r) related diarrhea. *Journal of International Associate Physicians AIDS Care (Chic, Ill), 3,* 121–129.

Immune Tolerance Network. (2012). *Immune tolerance in transplantation.* Retrieved from http://www.immunetolerance.org/researchers/clinical-trials/transplantation.

Immunization Action Coalition. (2011). *Medical management of vaccine reactions in children and teens.* Retrieved from http://www.immunize.org/catg.d/p3082a.pdf.

Ingersoll, K. S., & Heckman, C. J. (2005). Patient-clinician relationships and treatment system effects on HIV medication adherence. *AIDS and Behavior, 9*(1), 89–101.

Ippolito, A., & Petri, M. (2008). An update on mortality in systemic lupus erythematosus. *Clinical Experimental Rheumatology, 26*(5), S72–S79.

Johns Hopkins Medicine. (2008). *Study points to one cause of higher rates of transplanted kidney rejection in blacks.* Retrieved from http://www.hopkinsmedicine.org/news/media/releases/Study_Points_to_One_Cause_of_Higher_Rates_of_Transplanted_Kidney_Rejection_in_Blacks.

Kasper, D. L., Braunwald, E., Fauci, A., Hauser, S., Longo, D., & Jameson, J. L. (2005). *Harrison's principles of internal medicine* (16th ed.). New York, NY: McGraw-Hill.

Kimball, J. (2011). *Kimball's biology pages.* Retrieved from http://home.comcast.net/~john.kimball1/BiologyPages/D/DCs.html.

King, H. C., Mabry, R. L., Mabry, C. S., Gordon, B. R., & Marple, B. F. (2005). *Allergy in ENT practice: The basic guide* (2nd ed.). New York, NY: Thieme Medical.

Ljungman, P., Hakki, M., & Michael Boeckh, M. (2011). Cytomegalovirus in hematopoietic stem cell transplant recipients. *Hematology/Oncology Clinics of North America, 25*(1), 151–169.

Lupus Foundation of America. (2013a). *Understanding lupus.* Retrieved from http://www.lupus.org/webmodules/webarticlesnet/templates/new_learnunderstanding.aspx?articleid=2231&zoneid=523.

Lupus Foundation of America. (2013b). *What are the risks for developing lupus.* Retrieved from http://www.lupus.org/webmodules/webarticlesnet/templates/new_learnunderstanding.aspx?articleid=2231&zoneid=523.

Lupus Foundation of America. (2013c). *Pregnancy and lupus.* Retrieved from http://www.lupus.org/webmodules/webarticlesnet/templates/new_learncoping.aspx?articleid=2357&zoneid=528.

Lupus Foundation of America. (2013d). *A clue to congenital heart block.* Retrieved from http://www.lupus.org/webmodules/webarticlesnet/templates/new_researchupdates.aspx?articleid=1688&zoneid=33.

Lupus Foundation of America. (2013e). *Living with lupus.* Retrieved from http://www.lupus.org/webmodules/webarticlesnet/templates/new_learnliving.aspx?articleid=2252&zoneid=527.

Mainardi, T., Kapoor, S., & Bielory, L. (2009). Complementary and alternative medicine: Herbs, phytochemicals and vitamins and their immunologic effects. *Journal of Allergy and Clinical Immunology, 123*(2), 283–294.

Mayo Clinic. (2012). *Juvenile rheumatoid arthritis.* Retrieved from http://www.mayoclinic.com/health/juvenile-rheumatoid-arthritis/DS00018.

Moss Rehab Resource Net. (2010). *Arthritis fact sheet.* Retrieved from http://www.mossresourcenet.org/arthritis.htm#top%20of%20page.

Murray, R. B., Zentner, J. P., & Yakimo, R. (2009). *Health promotion strategies through the life span* (8th ed.). Upper Saddle River, NJ: Pearson Education.

Nash, P., & Smith, J. R. (2008). Common neonatal complications. In K. R. Simpson & P. A. Creehan (Eds.), *AWHONN perinatal nursing* (3rd ed., pp. 612–646). Philadelphia, PA: Lippincott Williams & Wilkins.

Nasseri, F., & Eftekhari, F. (2010). Clinical and radiological review of the normal and abnormal thymus: Pearls and pitfalls. *RadioGraphics, 30*(2), 413–428.

National Center for Complementary and Alternative Medicine. (2012). *Herbs at a glance: Chamomile.* Retrieved from http://nccam.nih.gov/health/chamomile/.

National Institute for Occupational Safety and Health. (2005). *Occupational latex allergies.* Retrieved from http://www.cdc.gov/niosh/topics/latex.

National Institute of Allergy and Infectious Diseases. (2012). *Health and research topics A to Z.* Retrieved from http://www.niaid.nih.gov/topics/foodAllergy/understanding/Pages/quickFacts.aspx.

National Institute of Arthritis and Musculoskeletal Skin Diseases. (2009). *Handout on health: Rheumatoid arthritis.* Retrieved from http://www.niams.nih.gov/Health_Info/Rheumatic_Disease/default.asp.

National Institutes of Health. (2011). *Lupus.* Retrieved from http://report.nih.gov/nihfactsheets/ViewFactSheet.aspx?csid=47.

National Institutes of Health Autoimmune Diseases Coordinating Committee. (2005). *Progress in autoimmune diseases research: Report to Congress.* NIH Publication 05-5140.

National Institutes of Health Panel on Antiretroviral Therapy and Medical Management of HIV-Infected Children. (2013). *Guidelines for the use of antiretroviral agents in pediatric HIV infection.* Retrieved from http://aidsinfo.nih.gov/guidelines.

National Institute of Occupational Safety and Health. (2012). *Home healthcare workers: How to prevent latex allergies.* Publication no. 2012-119. Retrieved from http://www.cdc.gov/niosh/docs/2012-119/pdfs/2012-119.pdf.

Neish, A. S. (2008). Microbes in gastrointestinal health and disease. *Gastroenterology, 136*(1), 65–80.

Occupational Health & Safety Administration. (2008). *Latex allergy.* Retrieved from http://www.osha.gov/SLTC/latexallergy/index.html.

Osborn, K. S., Wraa, C. E., Watson, A., & Holleran, R. S. (2013). *Medical-surgical nursing: Preparation for practice* (2nd ed.). Upper Saddle River, NJ: Pearson.

Percival, S. (2011). Nutrition and immunity: Balancing diet and immune function. *Nutrition Today, 46*(1), 12–17.

Philbin, V. J., & Levy, O. (2009). Developmental biology of the innate immune response: Implications for neonatal and infant vaccine development. *Pediatric Research, 65,* 98R–105R.

Porth, C., & Matfin, G. (2010). *Pathophysiology: Concepts of altered health states* (8th ed.). Philadelphia, PA: Lippincott Williams & Wilkins.

Rink, L., & Gabriel, P. (2000). Zinc and the immune system. *Proceedings of the Nutrition Society, 59*(4), 541–552.

Robles, D.T. (2013). *Lipodystrophy in HIV. Medscape.* Retrieved from http://emedicine.medscape.com/article/1082199-overview.

Rockefeller University. (2013). *Ralph Steinman: Introduction to dendritic cells.* Retrieved from http://lab.rockefeller.edu/steinman/dendritic_intro/.

Romeo, J., Wärnberg, J., Pozo, T., & Marcos, A. (2010). Session 6: Physical activity on immune function; Physical activity, immunity, and infection. *Proceedings of the Nutrition Society, 69*(3), 390–399.

Ruffing, V., & Bingham, C. O. (2012). *Rheumatoid arthritis signs and symptoms.* Retrieved from http://www.hopkinsarthritis.org/arthritis-info/rheumatoid-arthritis/ra-symptoms/.

Sampathi, V., & Lerman, J. (2011). Case scenario: Perioperative latex allergy in children. *Anesthesiology, 114*(3), 673–680.

Shelton, B., & Shivnan, J. C. (2011). Acute hypersensitivity reactions: What nurses need to know. *Johns Hopkins Nursing, 9*(1), 34–36.

Sherman, D. (1996). Nurses' willingness to care for AIDS patients and spirituality, social support, and death anxiety. *Image: Journal of Nursing Scholarship, 28*(3), 205–213.

Sizemore, R. C. (2012). How does stress affect the immune response? *Cell Developmental Biology, 1*(e101).

Taylor, B., Miller, E., Lingram, R., et al. (2002). Measles, mumps, and rubella vaccination and bowel problems or developmental regression in children with autism: Population study. *British Medical Journal, 324,* 393.

Tjang, Y. S., van der Heijden, G., Tenderich, G., Körfer, R., & Grobbee, D. E. (2008). Impact of recipient's age on heart transplantation outcome. *Annals of Thoracic Surgery, 85,* 2051–2055.

Tobón, G. J., Youinou, P., & Saraux, A. (2010). The environment, geo-epidemiology, and auto immune disease: Rheumatoid arthritis. *Journal of Autoimmunity, 35*(1), 10–4.

Tripathi, T., Shahid, M., Sobia, F., Singh, A., Khan, H. M., Khan, R. A., et al. (2010). Immune regulation by various facets of histamine in immunomodulation and allergic disorders. In N. Khardori, R. A. Khan, T. Tripathi, & M. Shahid (Eds.), *Biomedical aspects of histamine: Current perspectives* (pp. 133–147). New York, NY: Springer.

U.S. Department of Health and Human Services, aids.gov. (2012). *U.S. statistics.* Retrieved from http://aids.gov/hiv-aids-basics/hiv-aids-101/statistics/.

U.S. Department of Health and Human Services, Office of Disease Prevention and Promotion. (2010). *Healthy People 2020.* Retrieved from http://www.healthypeople.gov/2020/topicsobjectives2020/objectiveslist.aspx?topicID=23.

U.S. Food and Drug Administration. (2005). *FDA and CDC issue alert on Menactra meningococcal vaccine and Guillain-Barré syndrome.* Retrieved from http://www.fda.gov/bbs/topics/NEWS/2005/NEW1238.htm.

U.S. Food and Drug Administration. (2012). *Thimerosal in vaccines.* Retrieved from http://www.fda.gov/BiologicsBloodVaccines/SafetyAvailability/VaccineSafety/UCM096228.

Valois, P., Turgeon, H., Godin, G., Blondeau, D., & Cote, F. (2001). Influence of a persuasive strategy on nursing students' beliefs and attitudes toward provisions of care to people living with HIV/AIDS. *Journal of Nursing Education, 40*(8), 354–358.

Vanham, G., & Van Gulck, E. (2012). Can immunotherapy be useful as a "functional cure" for infection with human immunodeficiency virus-1? *Retrovirology, 9*(1).

Viale, P. H. (2009). Management of hypersensitivity reactions: A nursing perspective. *Oncology, 23*(21). Retrieved from http://www.cancernetwork.com/supplements/2009/infusion-reactions/display/article/10165/1382802.

Whyte, M. D., Whyte, J, IV, & Cormier, E. (2011). Factors influencing parental decision making when parents choose to deviate from the standard pediatric immunization schedule. *Journal of Community Health Nursing, 28*(4), 201–214.

Wilson, B. A., Shannon, M. T., & Shields, K. M. (2013). *Pearson: Nurse's drug guide, 2013.* Upper Saddle River, NJ: Prentice Hall.

World Health Organization. (2013a). *Antiretroviral therapy.* Retrieved from http://www.who.int/topics/antiretroviral_therapy/en/.

World Health Organization. (2013b). *Global health observator: HIV/AIDS.* Retrieved from http://www.who.int/gho/hiv/en/index.html.

World Health Organization. (2013c). *HIV/AIDS: Mother-to-child transmission of HIV.* Retrieved from http://www.who.int/hiv/topics/mtct/en/index.html.

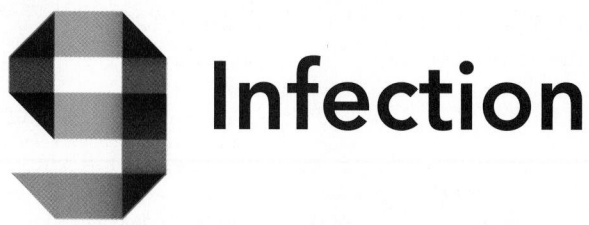

9 Infection

MODULE AT-A-GLANCE

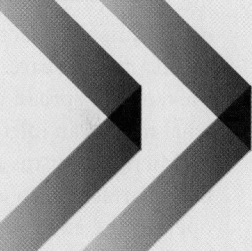

◪ THE CONCEPT OF INFECTION

Infection is the invasion of body tissue by microorganisms with the potential to cause illness or disease. The human body is continually threatened by foreign substances, infectious agents, and abnormal cells. In response to widespread antibiotic use, resistant microorganisms have emerged, such as methicillin-resistant *Staphylococcus aureus* and multidrug-resistant tuberculosis. New diseases have also emerged, including irritable bowel syndrome, anthrax, and Heartland virus. **<<**

Concept Learning Outcomes

After reading about this concept, you will be able to:

1. Summarize the physiology of the immune system related to infection prevention.
2. Examine the relationship between infection and other concepts/systems.
3. Identify commonly occurring alterations in the immune system that increase the risk for or occurrence of infection and their related therapies.
4. Differentiate common assessment procedures used to examine for the presence of infection across the life span.
5. Describe diagnostic and laboratory tests to determine the individual's infection status.
6. Explain management of immune health and prevention of infection.
7. Demonstrate the nursing process in providing culturally competent and caring interventions across the life span for individuals with infection.
8. Compare and contrast common independent and collaborative interventions for clients with infection.

Concept Key Terms

Acute infections, *523*
Airborne precautions, *545*
Antibody, *527*
Antiseptics, *544*
Asepsis, *523*
Bacteremia, *523*
Bacteria, *523*
Bactericidal agent, *544*
Bacteriostatic agent, *544*
Bloodborne pathogens, *545*
Body substance isolation (BSI), *545*
Carrier, *524*
Chronic infection, *523*
Clean, *523*
Colonization, *523*
Communicable disease, *522*
Compromised host, *525*
Contact precautions, *546*
Cultures, *556*
Dirty, *523*

Disease, *522*
Disease surveillance, *532*
Disinfectants, *544*
Droplet nuclei, *524*
Droplet precautions, *546*
Endogenous, *531*
Endotoxins, *528*
Exogenous, *531*
Exotoxins, *528*
Fungi, *523*
Healthcare-associated infections (HAIs), *530*
Iatrogenic infections, *531*
Infection, *521*
Infectious disease, *522*
Isolation, *545*
Local infection, *523*
Medical asepsis, *523*
Occupational exposure, *551*
Opportunistic pathogen, *522*
Parasites, *523*

(continued on next page)

▶ NORMAL PRESENTATION

The immune system is the body's major defense mechanism against infectious organisms and abnormal or damaged cells. Any illness or injury can result in an infection if it is left untreated or if the body's immune system is compromised in some way. More than any other group of healthcare providers, nurses think about infection prevention all the time. They know that if they move from client room to client room with contaminated hands or equipment, they risk infecting everyone they touch. The effectiveness of the other care does not matter if the nurse is not protecting the client against infection. Therefore nurses are directly involved in providing a biologically safe environment. Infection control is central to delivering high-quality nursing care. This concept explains what steps to take to prevent the spread of infection, how infection is shared, and what impact an infection can have on the human body.

Microorganisms exist everywhere: in water, in soil, and on body surfaces such as the skin, intestinal tract, and other areas open to the environment (e.g., mouth, upper respiratory tract, vagina, and lower urinary tract). Most microorganisms are harmless, and some are even beneficial, performing essential functions in the body. Some microorganisms found in the intestines (e.g., enterobacteria) produce substances called *bacteriocins*, which are lethal to related strains of bacteria. Others produce substances that repress the growth of other microorganisms. Some microorganisms are normal resident flora (the collective vegetation in a given area) in one part of the body yet produce infection in another. For example, *Escherichia coli* is a normal inhabitant of the large intestine but a common cause of infection of the urinary tract. **Table 9–1** ● provides a list of common resident microorganisms by body area.

Recall that an infection is an invasion of body tissue by microorganisms. If the microorganisms produce no clinical evidence of disease, the infection is *asymptomatic* or *subclinical*. **Disease** occurs when the microorganisms produce a detectable alteration in normal tissue function. A **communicable disease** is an illness that is directly transmitted from one individual or animal to another by contact with body fluids or indirectly transmitted by contact with contaminated objects, airborne particles, or vectors (e.g., ticks, mosquitoes, other insects). An **infectious disease** is any communicable disease that is caused by microorganisms that are commonly transmitted from one individual or animal to another or from an animal to an individual. Infectious and communicable diseases are a major cause of disease and death in infants and children in the United States. Some subclinical infections can cause considerable damage. For example, cytomegalovirus (CMV) infection in a pregnant woman can lead to significant disease in the unborn child.

Infectious diseases are a major cause of death worldwide. Efforts are made on the international, national, state, commu-nity, and individual levels to control the spread of microorganisms and to protect people from communicable diseases and infections. The World Health Organization (WHO) is the major regulatory agency at the international level. In the United States, the Centers for Disease Control and Prevention (CDC) is the principal public health agency concerned with disease prevention and control at the national level. State and county or city health departments track epidemics and illnesses as reports are made throughout those areas.

Microorganisms vary in **pathogenicity** (ability to produce disease); thus a **pathogen** is a microorganism that causes disease. Many microorganisms that are normally harmless can cause disease under certain circumstances. A "true" pathogen causes disease or infection in a healthy individual, whereas an **opportunistic pathogen** causes disease only in susceptible individuals. Microorganisms also vary in their **virulence**, or

TABLE 9–1   Examples of Common Resident Microorganisms

BODY AREA	RESIDENT MICROORGANISMS
Skin	*Staphylococcus epidermidis*
	Staphylococcus aureus
	Corynebacterium xerosis
	Micrococcus luteus
Nasal passages	*Staphylococcus aureus*
	Staphylococcus epidermidis
Oropharynx	*Streptococcus pneumoniae*
	Streptococcus salivarius
	Neisseria meningitidis
Mouth	*Streptococcus mutans*
	Streptococcus mitis
	Lactobacillus
	Actinomyces
	Spirochetes
Intestine	*Staphylococcus aureus*
	Bacteroides
	Bifidobacterium bifidum
	Eubacterium
	Clostridium
	Lactobacillus
	Escherichia coli
Anterior urethra	*Staphylococcus epidermidis*
	Streptococcus viridians
	Corynebacterium
Vagina	*Lactobacillus*
	Candida albicans

severity of the diseases they produce, and in their degree of communicability. For example, the common cold virus is more readily transmitted than the bacillus that causes leprosy (*Mycobacterium leprae*).

Asepsis is the absence of disease-causing microorganisms. Aseptic technique decreases the possibility of transferring microorganisms from one place to another. There are two basic types of asepsis: medical and surgical. **Medical asepsis** includes all practices intended to confine a specific microorganism to a specific area, thus limiting the number, growth, and transmission of microorganisms. In medical asepsis, objects are referred to as **clean**, which means that almost all microorganisms are absent, or **dirty** (soiled, contaminated), which means that microorganisms are likely to be present, some of which may be capable of causing infection.

Surgical asepsis, or **sterile technique**, refers to practices that keep an area or object free of all microorganisms; it includes practices that destroy all microorganisms and spores (microscopic dormant structures formed by some pathogens that are very hardy and often survive common cleaning techniques). Surgical asepsis is used for all procedures involving sterile areas of the body. **Sepsis** is the whole body inflammatory process, resulting in acute illness; however, the term is often used generally to refer to the state of infection.

Types of Microorganisms Causing Infections

Four major categories of microorganisms cause infection in humans: bacteria, viruses, fungi, and parasites. **Bacteria** are by far the most common infection-causing microorganisms. Several hundred species of bacteria can cause disease in humans and can live and be transported through air, water, food, soil, body tissues and fluids, and inanimate objects. Most of the microorganisms listed in Table 9–1 are bacteria. **Viruses** consist primarily of nucleic acid and therefore must enter living cells to reproduce. Common virus families include the rhinovirus (causes the common cold), hepatitis, herpes, and HIV. **Fungi** include yeasts and molds. *Candida albicans* is a yeast considered normal flora in the human vagina. **Parasites** live on other organisms. They include protozoa, such as the one that causes malaria, helminths (worms), and arthropods (mites, fleas, ticks).

Types of Infections

Colonization is the process by which strains of microorganisms become resident flora. In this state, the microorganisms may grow and multiply, but they do not cause disease. Infection occurs when newly introduced or resident microorganisms succeed in invading a part of the body where the host's defense mechanisms are ineffective, and the pathogen causes tissue damage. The infection becomes a disease when the signs and symptoms of the infection are unique, can be differentiated from other conditions, and alter bodily function or processes.

Infections can be local or systemic. A **local infection** is limited to the specific part of the body where the microorganisms remain. If the microorganisms spread and damage different parts of the body, the result is a **systemic infection**. When a culture of the individual's blood reveals bacteria, the condition is called **bacteremia**. When bacteremia results in systemic

infection, it is referred to as **septicemia**. Unfortunately, these infections have become more common recently.

Infections are also classified as acute or chronic. **Acute infections** generally appear suddenly and last a short time. A **chronic infection** may develop slowly, over a very long period, and often persists for months and sometimes years.

It is important that an individual does not need to have an identified infection to transmit potentially infective microorganisms to another individual. Even microorganisms that are normal for one individual can infect another individual.

Chain of Infection

The chain of infection consists of six links (**Figure 9–1 ●**): the etiological agent, or microorganism; the place where the organism naturally resides (reservoir); a portal of exit from the reservoir; a method (mode) of transmission; a portal of entry into a susceptible host; and a susceptible host.

ETIOLOGICAL AGENT   The extent to which any microorganism is capable of producing an infectious process depends on the number of microorganisms present, the virulence and pathogenicity of the microorganisms, the ability of the microorganisms to enter the body, the susceptibility of the host, and the ability of the microorganisms to live in the host's body.

Some microorganisms, such as the smallpox virus, can infect almost all susceptible people after exposure. By contrast, microorganisms such as *Mycobacterium tuberculosis* infect a relatively small number of the population who are susceptible and exposed. Those at risk are usually people who are poorly nourished or living in crowded conditions, or those whose immune systems are less competent (such as older adults and individuals with HIV or cancer).

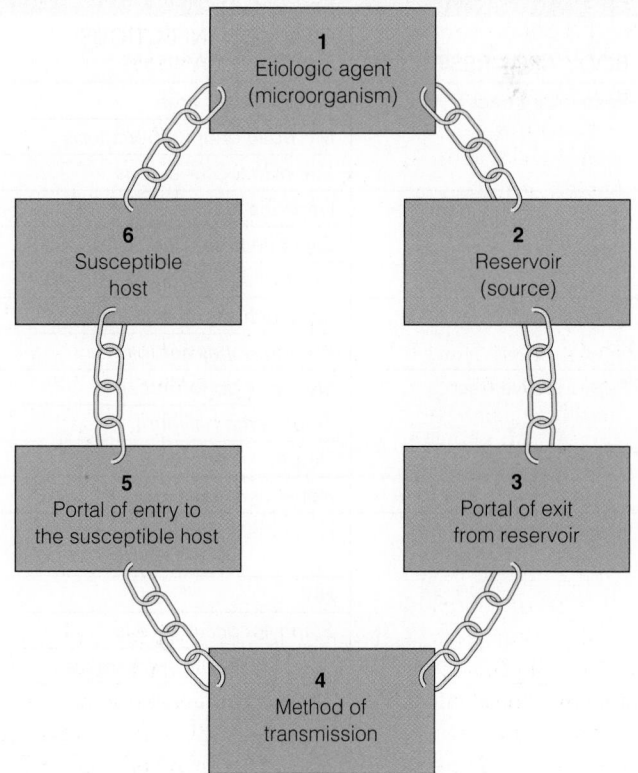

Figure 9–1 ● The chain of infection.

RESERVOIR   There are many **reservoirs**, or sources of microorganisms. Common sources are other humans, the client's own microorganisms, plants, animals, and the general environment. People are the most common source of infection for others and for themselves. For example, an individual with an influenza virus frequently spreads it to others. A **carrier** is a human or animal reservoir of a specific infectious agent that usually does not manifest any clinical signs of disease. For example, the *Anopheles* mosquito reservoir carries the malaria parasite (*Plasmodium* spp.) but is unaffected by it. The carrier state may also exist in individuals with a clinically recognizable disease, such as a dog with rabies. Under either circumstance, the carrier state may be of short duration (temporary or transient carrier) or long duration (chronic carrier). Food, water, and feces can also be reservoirs.

PORTAL OF EXIT FROM RESERVOIR   Before an infection can establish itself in a host, the microorganisms must leave the reservoir. Common human reservoirs and their associated portals of exit are summarized in **Table 9–2** ●.

METHOD OF TRANSMISSION   After a microorganism leaves its source or reservoir, it requires a means of transmission to reach another host through a receptive portal of entry. There are three modes of transmission:

1. ***Direct transmission.*** Direct transmission involves the immediate and direct transfer of microorganisms from one individual to another through touching, biting, kissing, or sexual intercourse. Droplet spread is also a form of direct transmission, but it occurs only if the source and the host are within 3 feet of each other. Sneezing, coughing, spitting, singing, or talking can project droplet spray into the conjunctiva or onto the mucous membranes of the eye, nose, or mouth of another individual.

2. ***Indirect transmission.*** Indirect transmission can be either vehicle-borne or vector-borne.
   a. ***Vehicle-borne transmission.*** A *vehicle* is any substance that serves as an intermediate means to transport and introduce an infectious agent into a susceptible host through a suitable portal of entry. Fomites (inanimate materials or objects), such as handkerchiefs, toys, soiled clothes, cooking or eating utensils, and surgical instruments or dressings, can act as vehicles. Water, food, blood, serum, and plasma are also vehicles. For example, food can become contaminated by a food handler who carries the hepatitis A virus, and the food may then be ingested by a susceptible host.
   b. ***Vector-borne transmission.*** A *vector* is an animal or flying or crawling insect that serves as an intermediate means of transporting the infectious agent. Transmission can occur by injection of salivary fluid during biting or by the deposit of feces or other materials on the skin through the bite wound or a traumatized skin area.

3. ***Airborne transmission.*** Airborne transmission involves droplets or dust. **Droplet nuclei**, the residue of evaporated droplets emitted by an infected host, such as an individual with tuberculosis, can remain in the air for long periods of time. Dust particles containing the infectious agent (e.g., *Clostridium difficile* spores from the soil) can also become airborne. The material is transmitted by air currents to a suitable portal of entry on another individual, usually the respiratory tract.

TABLE 9–2   Human Body Area Reservoirs, Common Infectious Microorganisms, and Portals of Exit

BODY AREA RESERVOIR	COMMON INFECTIOUS MICROORGANISMS	PORTALS OF EXIT
Respiratory tract	Parainfluenza virus	Nose or mouth through sneezing, coughing, breathing, or talking
	Mycobacterium tuberculosis	
	Staphylococcus aureus	
Gastrointestinal tract	Hepatitis A virus	Mouth: saliva, vomitus. Anus: feces; ostomies
	Salmonella species	
	Clostridium difficile	
Urinary tract	*Escherichia coli,* enterococci	Urethral meatus and urinary diversion
	Pseudomonas aeruginosa	
Reproductive tract	*Neisseria gonorrhoeae*	Vagina: vaginal discharge. Urinary meatus: semen, urine
	Treponema pallidum	
	Herpes simplex virus type 2	
	Hepatitis B virus (HBV)	
Blood	Hepatitis B virus	Open wound, needle puncture site, any disruption of intact skin or mucous membrane surfaces
	HIV	
	Staphylococcus aureus	
	Staphylococcus epidermidis	
Tissue	*Staphylococcus aureus*	Drainage from cut or wound
	Escherichia coli	
	Proteus species	
	Streptococcus beta-hemolytic A or B	

PORTAL OF ENTRY TO THE SUSCEPTIBLE HOST

Before an individual can become infected, microorganisms must enter the body. The skin is a barrier to infectious agents; however, any break in the skin can readily serve as a portal of entry. Often, microorganisms enter the body of a host by the same route they used to leave the source. For example, an airborne infection escapes its host or carrier via sneezing or coughing and is transmitted to a new host who inhales the microorganism through the nose or mouth. The mouth, throat, nose, ears, eyes, and genitalia are open to outside exposure and thus are the most frequent portals of entry for microorganisms. Cuts and tears in the skin also provide portals through which microorganisms enter and cause disease.

SUSCEPTIBLE HOST

A susceptible host is any individual who is at risk for infection. Infants and young children are often susceptible hosts. Their immune systems have not fully matured, and they have not yet developed antibodies to many agents. Therefore they cannot defend themselves against infectious and communicable diseases as well as older children and adults can. A **compromised host** is an individual at increased risk, that is, one who, for one or more reasons, is more likely than others to acquire an infection. Impairment of the body's natural defenses and a number of other factors affect susceptibility to infection. Examples are age (the very young or the very old), receiving immune suppression treatment for cancer or chronic illness or following a successful organ transplant, and immune deficiency conditions.

Table 9–3 ● outlines nursing interventions that break the chain of infection, including their rationales.

Physiology Review

Individuals normally have defenses that protect the body from infection. Nonspecific defenses include anatomical and physiological barriers and the inflammatory response. **Specific defenses** involve the immune system when an antigen induces a state of sensitivity and antibodies respond to contain or destroy the antigen.

Intact skin and mucous membranes are the body's first line of defense against invading microorganisms. Unless the skin and mucosa become cracked and broken, they act as an effective barrier against bacteria. Fungi can live on the skin, but they cannot penetrate it. The dryness of the skin also is a deterrent to bacteria. Bacteria are most plentiful in moist areas of the body, such as the perineum and axillae. Resident bacteria of the skin also prevent other bacteria from multiplying. The resident bacteria use up the available nutrients, and the end products of their metabolism inhibit other bacterial growth. Normal secretions make the skin slightly acidic and thus also inhibit bacterial growth.

The nasal passages have a defensive function. As entering air follows the tortuous route of the nasal passages, it comes in contact with moist mucous membranes and cilia. These structures trap microorganisms, dust, and foreign materials. The lungs have alveolar macrophages (large phagocytes) that ingest microorganisms, other cells, and foreign particles.

Each body orifice also has protective mechanisms. The oral cavity regularly sheds mucosal epithelium to rid the mouth of colonizers. The flow of saliva and its partially buffering action help prevent infections. Saliva contains microbial inhibitors, such as lactoferrin, lysozyme, and secretory immunoglobulin A (IgA). The eye is protected from infection by tears, which continually wash microorganisms away and contain inhibiting lysozyme. The vagina also has natural defenses against infection. When a girl reaches puberty, lactobacilli ferment sugars in the vaginal secretions, creating a vaginal pH of 3.5–4.5. This low pH inhibits the growth of many disease-producing microorganisms. The entrance to the urethra normally harbors many microorganisms, including *Staphylococcus epidermidis coagulase* (from the skin) and *Escherichia coli* (from feces). It is believed that the urine flow has a flushing and bacteriostatic action that keeps the bacteria from ascending the urethra. An intact mucosal surface also acts as a barrier.

The gastrointestinal tract also has defenses against infection. The high acidity of the stomach normally prevents microbial growth. The resident flora of the large intestine help prevent the establishment of disease-producing microorganisms. Peristalsis also tends to move microbes out of the body.

Genetic and Lifespan Considerations

A client's susceptibility to infection is affected by age and heredity. Newborns and older adults have reduced defenses against infection. Infections are a major cause of death in newborns, who have immature immune systems and are protected only for the first 2 or 3 months by immunoglobulins passively received from the mother. Infants begin to synthesize their own immunoglobulins between 1 and 3 months of age.

With advancing age, multiple physiological changes cause increased susceptibility to infection. Physiological changes of aging that put older adults at increased risk for infection include the following:

- **Cardiovascular changes:** Decreased cardiac output, loss of capillaries, and decreased tissue perfusion delay inflammatory response and healing.

- **Respiratory system changes:** Decreased mucociliary escalator, decreased elastic recoil, and a diminished cough reflex lead to decreased clearance of respiratory secretions.

- **Genitourinary changes:** Loss of muscle tone, reduced bladder contractility, altered bladder reflexes, and prostatic hypertrophy in men lead to reduced bladder capacity and incomplete emptying.

- **Gastrointestinal system changes:** Impaired swallow reflex, decreased gastric acidity, and delayed gastric emptying increase the risk of aspiration.

- **Skin and subcutaneous tissue changes:** Thinning of skin, decreased cushioning, and decreased sensation lead to increased risk of injury and ulceration.

- **Immune changes:** Decreased phagocytosis, reduced inflammatory response, and slowed or impaired healing processes lead to reduced immunity.

In addition to these physiological changes, the following factors contribute to an older adult's increased risk for infectious disease:

- Decreased activity level related to musculoskeletal, neurological, or balance problems

TABLE 9–3 Nursing Interventions That Break the Chain of Infection

LINK IN CHAIN OF INFECTION	INTERVENTIONS	RATIONALES
Etiological agent (microorganism)	Educate clients and support them and their families in using appropriate methods to clean, disinfect, and sterilize articles.	Knowledge of ways to reduce or eliminate microorganisms reduces the numbers of microorganisms present and the likelihood of transmission.
	Ensure that articles are correctly cleaned and disinfected or sterilized before use.	Correct cleaning, disinfecting, and sterilizing reduce or eliminate microorganisms.
Reservoir (source)	Change dressings and bandages when they are soiled or wet.	Moist dressings are ideal environments for microorganisms to grow and multiply.
	Assist clients to carry out appropriate skin and oral hygiene.	Hygienic measures reduce the numbers of resident and transient microorganisms and the likelihood of infection.
	Dispose of damp, soiled linens appropriately.	Damp, soiled linens harbor more microorganisms than dry linens.
	Dispose of feces and urine in appropriate receptacles.	Urine and feces in particular contain many microorganisms.
	Ensure that all fluid containers, such as bedside water jugs and suction and drainage bottles, are covered or capped.	Prolonged exposure increases the risk of contamination and promotes microbial growth.
	Empty suction and drainage bottles at the end of each shift, before they become full, or according to agency policy.	Drainage harbors microorganisms that, if left for long periods, proliferate and can be transmitted to others.
Portal of exit from the reservoir	Avoid talking, coughing, or sneezing over open wounds and sterile fields, and cover the mouth and nose when coughing and sneezing.	These measures limit the number of microorganisms that escape from the respiratory tract.
Method of transmission	Cleanse hands between client contacts, after touching body substances, and before performing invasive procedures or touching open wounds.	Hand cleansing is an important means of controlling and preventing the transmission of microorganisms.
	Instruct clients and support them and their families in cleansing hands before handling food or eating, after eliminating, and after touching infectious material.	Hand cleansing helps prevent the transfer of microorganisms from one individual to another.
	Wear gloves when handling secretions and excretions.	Gloves and gowns prevent soiling of the hands and clothing.
	Wear gowns if there is danger of soiling clothing with body substances.	
	Place discarded soiled materials in moisture-proof refuse bags.	Moisture-proof bags prevent the spread of microorganisms to others.
	Hold used bedpans steadily to prevent spillage, and dispose of urine and feces in appropriate receptacles.	Urine and feces in particular contain many microorganisms.
	Initiate and implement aseptic precautions for all clients.	All clients harbor potentially infectious microorganisms that can be transmitted to others.
	Wear masks and eye protection when in close contact with clients who have infections transmitted by droplets from the respiratory tract or when sprays of body fluid are possible (e.g., during irrigation procedures).	Masks and eyewear provide protection from airborne droplets and microorganisms in clients' body substances.
Portal of entry to the susceptible host	Use sterile technique for invasive procedures (e.g., injections, catheterizations).	Invasive procedures penetrate the body's natural protective barriers to microorganisms.
	Use sterile technique when exposing open wounds and handling dressings.	Open wounds are vulnerable to microbial infection.
	Place used disposable needles and syringes in puncture-resistant containers for disposal.	Injuries from needles contaminated by blood or body fluids from an infected client or carrier are a primary cause of HBV and HIV transmission to healthcare workers.
	Provide all clients with their own personal care items.	People have less resistance to another individual's microorganisms than to their own.
Susceptible host	Maintain the integrity of the client's skin and mucous membranes.	Intact skin and mucous membranes protect against invasion by microorganisms.
	Ensure that the client receives a balanced diet.	A balanced diet supplies proteins and vitamins necessary to build and maintain body tissues.
	Educate the public about the importance of immunizations.	Immunizations protect people against virulent infectious diseases.

- Poor nutrition and an increased risk of dehydration
- Chronic diseases, such as diabetes mellitus, cardiac disease, and renal disease
- Chronic medication use
- Lack of recent immunizations against preventable infectious diseases
- Altered mental status and dementias
- Hospitalization or residence in a long-term care facility
- Presence of invasive devices, such as indwelling urinary catheters and gastric tubes.

The thymus gland also atrophies, and by age 50–60 years, thymic hormone levels are undetectable. Although the exact relationship of these events to T-cell function is unclear, some T-cell populations decrease or decline in function as the individual ages. The ability of T cells to proliferate following activation also declines with advancing age, and a portion of T cells cannot be activated in older adults (Porth & Matfin, 2010). With these changes, cell-mediated immune function declines, and the client has reduced resistance to antigens, such as *Mycobacterium tuberculosis,* influenza and varicella-zoster viruses, malignant cells, and tissue grafts.

Although immunoglobulin levels remain relatively stable, primary and secondary **antibody** responses decline with aging. This diminished antibody production has clinical implications in that immunizations (single-dose and booster) may not produce the expected protective immune response.

Older adults are not only at increased risk for infection but also may not exhibit the classic manifestations of inflammation and infection. They are likely to take nonsteroidal anti-inflammatory drugs (NSAIDs) and corticosteroids, which interfere with inflammation and healing. The cardinal signs of inflammation—redness, heat, and swelling—tend to be diminished or absent in older adults. The classic signs of infection—fever and chills—may be absent altogether because of age-related changes in the immune system, loss of central temperature control mechanisms, decreased muscle mass, and loss of shivering ability. The older adult may have only subtle signs of sepsis, such as changes in mental status, disorientation, and tachypnea (Porth & Matfin, 2010).

Additional considerations related to infection in children and older adults are further described in the Lifespan Considerations feature.

Heredity also influences the development of infection in that some people have a genetic susceptibility to certain infections. For example, some individuals are deficient in serum immunoglobulins, which play a significant role in the internal defense mechanism of the body. Mutations in inflammatory proteins, such as proteins in the interleukin-12, interleukin-23, and interferon-gamma signaling pathways, can also increase an individual's susceptibility to mycobacterial infection (Chapman & Hill, 2012).

▶ ALTERATIONS

Microorganisms often invade the human body and proliferate when they are undetected, uncontrolled, or not eliminated by the inflammatory and immune responses. In most cases, contact between humans and microorganisms is incidental and may even be beneficial to both organisms. However, many microorganisms are pathogens.

Modern medicine, antibiotic therapy, immunizations, and other public health measures to protect food and water supplies have significantly reduced the prevalence of infectious diseases in many parts of the world. In spite of these advances, many infections, including malaria, typhoid, and tuberculosis, remain prevalent in developing nations. Sexually transmitted infections rage through modern cities and industrialized populations. New varieties and strains of pathogens, such as HIV, evolve to cause disease.

To a certain extent, modern medicine has contributed to the development of infectious diseases caused by antibiotic-resistant strains of microorganisms. For example, tuberculosis is on the rise in the United States, partially because organisms have become resistant to standard therapies. Following organ or tissue transplant and in the treatment of neoplasms, clients receive immunosuppressive therapy, which makes them more susceptible to infection. The implantation of metal and plastic prosthetic devices provides potential sites for colonization of disease-producing organisms (Osmon et al., 2013). Many diseases that were long considered unrelated to microorganisms may also actually be infectious; for example, colonization of the gastric mucosa with *Helicobacter pylori* is the predominant cause of peptic ulcer disease, and oncogenic viruses can transform normal cells into malignant cells.

Poor hygiene behaviors of young children and their caregivers facilitate transmission of infectious diseases in child care settings and other environments, including hospitals, clinics, and physicians' offices. The fecal-oral and respiratory routes are the most common modes of transmission in children. Children often do not wash their hands after toileting unless they are closely supervised. They put toys and their hands in their mouths and then rub their noses and eyes. They often need help in caring for a runny nose. Diapers may leak stool and provide exposure to fecal organisms. In addition, caregivers in child care centers, other people caring for children, and healthcare professionals may not use proper hand hygiene. All of these behaviors promote the transmission of infection.

To see how alterations in other concepts relate to infection, see the Concepts Related to Infection feature on page 529.

Pathogens

Pathogens capable of infecting and causing disease in susceptible hosts include bacteria, viruses, fungi, and parasites, such as protozoa, helminths (worms), and arthropods (**Box 9–1** ●). Each organism causes a different specific reaction in the host.

A number of mechanisms have evolved in pathogens to facilitate their transmission and increase their ability to invade the host and cause disease. Factors influencing the transmission of an organism include its resistance to drying and to variations in environmental temperature. For example, spore-forming organisms are extremely resistant to drying.

Pathogens are often capable of producing toxins or enzymes that alter or destroy the normal function of host cells and promote colonization, proliferation, and invasion by the pathogen. Adhesion factors produced by or incorporated into the cell wall

Lifespan Considerations Infections

Children

Infections are a normal part of childhood, and most children experience some kind of infection from time to time. The majority of these infections are caused by viruses, and for the most part they are transient and relatively benign and can be overcome by the body's natural defenses and supportive care. One example is otitis media, or an ear infection, which is one of the most frequent reasons parents take children to the doctor. In some cases, however, severe and even life-threatening infections occur. Considerations related to children include the following:

- Newborns may not be able to respond to infections due to an underdeveloped immune system. As a result, in the first few months of life, infections may not be associated with typical signs and symptoms (e.g., an infant with an infection may not have a fever).
- Newborns have some naturally acquired immunity that is transferred from the mother across the placenta at birth.
- Breastfed infants enjoy higher levels of immunity against infections than infants fed with formula.
- Fevers of less than 39°C (102.2°F) in children should not be treated, except for comfort of the child (Mayo Clinic, 2013a).
- Children between 6 months and 5 years of age are at higher risk for fever-induced (febrile) seizures. Febrile seizures are not associated with neurological seizure disorders (e.g., epilepsy).
- Children who are immune-compromised (by, e.g., leukemia, HIV) or have a chronic health condition (e.g., cystic fibrosis, sickle cell disease, congenital heart disease) need additional precautions to prevent exposure to infectious agents.
- Hand hygiene, comprehensive immunizations, proper nutrition, adequate hydration, and appropriate rest are essential to preventing and/or treating infections in children.

- Hand washing and good hygiene in day care and schools are important to prevent the spread of infections.
- Adolescents are at high risk for sexually transmitted diseases and should be well educated about how to prevent infections.

Older Adults

Normal aging may predispose older adults to increased risk of infection and delayed healing. As the body ages, changes take place in the skin, respiratory tract, gastrointestinal system, kidneys, and immune system. If unchallenged, these systems work well to maintain the individual's homeostasis, but if compromised by stress, illness, infections, treatments, or surgeries, these defense systems cannot provide adequate protection. Recognizing these changes in older adults is important for the early detection and treatment of infections and delayed healing. Special considerations for older adults include the following:

- Nutrition is often poor in older adults. Certain nutritional components, especially adequate protein, are necessary to build up and maintain the immune system.
- Diabetes mellitus, which occurs frequently in older adults, increases the risk of infection and delayed healing by causing an alteration in nutrition and impaired peripheral circulation, which in turn decrease the oxygen transport to the tissues.
- The immune system reacts slowly to the introduction of an antigen, allowing the antigen to reproduce itself several times before the immune system recognizes it.
- The normal inflammatory response is delayed, and this delay often causes atypical responses to infection, with unusual presentations. Instead of the redness, swelling, and fever that are usually associated with infections, atypical symptoms, such as confusion and disorientation, agitation, incontinence, falls, lethargy, and general fatigue, are often seen first in the older adult.

or membrane of the pathogen improve its ability to attach to and colonize the host. Toxins often increase the disease-producing capability of the pathogen and, in some cases, are totally responsible for it. For example, cholera, tetanus, and botulism result from bacterial toxins, not from the direct effects of the infection. **Exotoxins** are soluble proteins that the microorganisms secrete into surrounding tissue. Exotoxins are highly poisonous, causing cell death or dysfunction. **Endotoxins** are found in the cell wall of gram-negative bacteria and are released only when the cell is disrupted. They have less specific effects than exotoxins but can activate many human regulatory systems, producing fever, inflammation, and potentially clotting, bleeding, or hypotension when released in large quantities. Pathogens may also produce enzymes to enhance their spread to local tissues, chemicals to block specific immune processes or deplete neutrophils and macrophages, or extracellular capsules to discourage phagocytosis.

Stages of the Infectious Process

When infectious disease develops in a host, it typically follows a predictable course, with stages based on the progression and intensity of manifestations. Stages include:

1. Incubation period
2. Prodromal stage
3. Illness stage
4. Convalescent stage

The initial stage is the *incubation period*, during which the pathogen begins active replication but does not yet cause symptoms. Depending on the organism and host factors, the incubation period may last from hours, as with *Salmonella*, to years, as with HIV infection.

In the *prodromal stage*, symptoms begin to appear. At this stage, symptoms are often nonspecific and include general malaise, fever, myalgias, headache, and fatigue.

Maximal impact of the infectious process occurs during the *illness stage* as the pathogen proliferates and disseminates rapidly. Toxic by-products of microorganism metabolism and cell lysis, along with the immune response, produce tissue damage and inflammation during this stage (Porth & Matfin, 2010). Manifestations are more pronounced and specific to the infecting organism and site. Fever and chills may be significant during this phase. However, alcoholic clients and older adults may respond to severe infection by becoming hypothermic. A client in the illness stage

Concepts Related to **Infection**

All individuals develop infections throughout their lifetime; the type of infection determines its clinical manifestations. For example, an infection in the gastrointestinal tract may produce diarrhea, whereas an eye infection is likely to produce purulent drainage. Once an individual becomes infected, the infection may cause an inflammatory response, leading to redness, swelling, and pain. Because of the prevalence of infections in the clinic, hospital, and other healthcare facilities, nursing education is essential to the prevention of infection.

CONCEPT	RELATIONSHIP TO INFECTION	NURSING IMPLICATIONS
Elimination		
■ Bowel retention/ incontinence ■ Bladder retention/ incontinence	GI infection ↑ damage to intestines and a ↓ in absorption, leading to diarrhea. ↑ abnormal gut flora may lead to constipation. UTIs and yeast infections can cause painful and/or frequent urination	■ Be aware of risk for dehydration and imbalanced nutrition: less than requirements, especially in children and older adults. ■ Watch for signs of kidney infection in clients with UTIs. ■ Provide comfort measures related to elimination problems (e.g., hygiene care, pharmacologic interventions, safety interventions). ■ Use proper biohazard precautions when handling urine and feces.
Inflammation		
	↑ infection leads to ↑ inflammation, including pain, swelling, and redness.	■ Provide hygiene care for wounds to prevent infection and inflammation. ■ Provide comfort care (e.g., pain medication, cool compress/ice).
Sexuality		
■ Sexually transmitted infections	↑ sexual partners = ↑ increased risk of STI.	■ Provide client education about STIs, especially for adolescents.
Tissue Integrity		
■ Burns ■ Wound healing ■ Pressure ulcers	↓ tissue integrity = ↑ risk of infection.	■ Provide wound care to prevent infection. ■ Turn bed-ridden clients to prevent pressure ulcers. ■ Cover wounds with antibiotic ointment and sterile gauze.
Teaching and Learning		
■ Client education ■ Staff education	↑ education = ↑ prevention habits = ↓ risk of infection.	■ Attend classes to learn about infection prevention. ■ Teach clients about good hygiene to prevent infection. ■ Teach staff members proper protocols for handling potentially infectious materials.

of infection is often tachycardic and tachypneic because of increased metabolic demands. Localized manifestations include redness, heat, swelling, pain, and impaired function. When the infectious disease affects an internal organ, manifestations are related to inflammatory changes in that organ and surrounding tissue. The client may experience tenderness to palpation over the site or show signs of impaired function, such as the hematuria and proteinuria that are characteristic of renal infections.

If the infectious process is prolonged, manifestations of the continuing immune response may become apparent. Catabolic and anorexic effects of the infection can lead to muscle wasting and loss of body fat. Immune complexes may be deposited at sites other than that of the primary infection, the result being an inflammatory process. Glomerulonephritis (e.g., following strep throat) and vasculitis are possible results. Another possible consequence of prolonged infection and immune response is the triggering of an autoimmune disease process, such as rheumatic cardiomyopathy or celiac disease. Type 1 diabetes mellitus is thought to be the result of such a response (Porth & Matfin, 2010).

As the infection is contained and the pathogen eliminated, the *convalescent stage* of the disease occurs. During this stage, affected tissues are repaired and manifestations resolve. Resolution of the infection is total elimination of the pathogen from the body without residual manifestations.

If a balance between organism and host factors occurs, with neither predominating, chronic disease may develop, or the organism may be driven into a protected site, such as an abscess. A *carrier state* develops when host defenses eliminate the infectious disease, but the organism continues to multiply on mucosal sites (Longo et al., 2012).

Box 9–1   Pathogenic Organisms

BACTERIA

Bacteria are single-celled organisms capable of autonomous reproduction. Bacteria have different characteristics and growth requirements: *Aerobes* require oxygen for survival, whereas *anaerobes* cannot survive in the presence of oxygen; *gram-positive* bacteria stain purple when subjected to crystal violet stain, whereas *gram-negative* bacteria do not stain with crystal violet stain but turn red when subjected to safranin stain, and the colonies formed by replicating bacteria differ from one another.

Mycoplasma

Mycoplasma are very small bacteria that have no cell wall, making them resistant to antibiotics that inhibit cell wall synthesis, such as penicillins.

Rickettsia and Chlamydia

Rickettsia and *Chlamydia* are obligate intracellular parasites with a rigid cell wall; they use vitamins, nutrients, and products of metabolism (e.g., ATP) from the host. *Chlamydia* are transmitted by direct contact, whereas *Rickettsia* infects the cells of arthropods (e.g., fleas, ticks, and lice) and are transmitted from these vectors to humans.

VIRUSES

Viruses are obligate intracellular parasites that are incapable of reproducing outside a living cell. Some viruses are shed continuously from infected cell surfaces; others, after inserting their genetic material into that of the infected cell, remain latent until they are stimulated to replicate. Viruses may or may not cause lysis and death of the host cell during replication. Oncogenic viruses are able to transform normal cells into malignant cells.

FUNGI

Fungi are prevalent throughout the world, but few are capable of causing disease in humans. Most fungal infections are self-limited, affecting the skin and subcutaneous tissue. Some fungi, such as *Pneumocystis jiroveci*, can cause life-threatening opportunistic infections in the immunocompromised host.

PARASITES

The term *parasite* is typically applied to members of the animal kingdom that infect and cause disease in other animals. Protozoa, helminths, and arthropods are considered parasites. Protozoa are single-celled organisms transmitted via direct or indirect contact or by an arthropod vector. Helminths are wormlike parasites. Roundworms, tapeworms, and flukes are examples. They gain entry into humans primarily through ingestion of fertilized eggs or penetration of larvae through the skin or mucous membranes. Arthropod parasites, such as scabies (mites), lice, and fleas, typically infest external body surfaces, causing localized tissue damage and inflammation. Transmission is by direct contact with the arthropod or its eggs.

Source: Data summarized from Porth, C., & Matfin, G. (2010). *Pathophysiology: Concepts of altered health states* (8th ed.). Philadelphia, PA: Lippincott Williams & Wilkins.

Alterations and Manifestations

Infections cause predictable diseases depending on the infecting microorganism, and they often respond predictably to the right treatment. However, complications can occur if the infection spreads to other parts of the body, if the infecting organism develops resistance to treatment, or if the host's immune system is unable to fight off the infection. In addition, infectious agents can be used as biological threats to communities, causing widespread panic and a demand on resources that may prevent adequate treatment.

COMPLICATIONS OF INFECTIOUS DISEASES   Multiple and varied complications are associated with infectious diseases. They are typically specific to the infecting organism and the body system affected.

One life-threatening complication is sepsis, which is a severe reaction to infection. Bacteremia, or the presence of bacteria in the blood, may not have serious effects; however, if the infection becomes severe or if the microorganisms produce toxins, they can cause septicemia. Septicemia may lead to septic shock, a state of life-threateningly low blood pressure caused by overwhelming infection. Unless treated aggressively, septic shock leads to diffuse cell and tissue injury and potentially to organ failure. Older adults are at a higher risk of developing sepsis than younger individuals. Approximately two thirds of the individuals hospitalized for sepsis are over the age of 65, and the rate of septicemia hospitalization is four times higher for clients over the age of 85 than for clients between the ages of 65 and 74 (Hall et al., 2011).

HEALTHCARE-ASSOCIATED INFECTIONS   Healthcare-associated infections (HAIs), also called *hospital-acquired infections* or *nosocomial infections*, are classified as infections that are associated with the delivery of healthcare services in a facility such as a hospital or nursing home. HAIs add hospital days, reduce admissions by occupying available beds, and increase the cost of health care (Scott, 2009). HAIs can either develop during a client's stay in a facility or manifest after discharge. They typically manifest after 48 hours of hospitalization. Infections that manifest during the first 48 hours of hospitalization are attributed to community sources.

Urinary tract infection is the most common type of HAI and the most frequent cause of gram-negative septicemia in hospitalized clients. Surgical site infections and pneumonia are the other two of the top three HAIs. Hospital-acquired pneumonia has a mortality rate of 38%–70% (Laessig, 2010) and is most often associated with mechanical ventilators, tracheostomies, and endotracheal intubation (Porth & Matfin, 2010). Bacteremia is associated with intravascular and urinary catheters. Because of the risk of infection, insertion of central lines and urinary catheters is conducted as a sterile procedure with careful attention to preventing contamination. *Clostridium difficile*–associated diarrhea is a frequently acquired HAI. Associated with antibiotic use, this infection's risk increases with length of hospital stay, especially in an intensive care unit (ICU). Healthcare personnel working in the facility can also acquire HAIs, which can cause significant illness and time lost from work.

HAIs have received increasing attention in recent years. They are believed to involve approximately 1.7 million clients per year, cause 90,000 deaths, and add $28–$33 billion in excess healthcare costs annually (AHRQ, 2009). The Joint Commission (2012), an independent, not-for-profit organization that accredits and certifies healthcare organizations and programs in the United States, included reducing the risk of healthcare-associated infections as one of the 2013 National Patient Safety Goals. The most common settings where HAIs develop are hospital surgical and medical ICUs. The microorganisms that cause HAIs can originate from the clients themselves (an **endogenous** source) or from the hospital environment and hospital personnel (**exogenous** sources). Most HAIs appear to have endogenous sources. *Escherichia coli, Staphylococcus aureus,* and *Enterococci* are the most common infecting microorganisms.

🌐 *Stay Current: Visit The Joint Commission Web site every year to see the latest National Patient Safety Goals:* **http://www.jointcommission.org/standards_information/npsgs.aspx**

A number of factors contribute to HAIs. **Iatrogenic infections** are the direct result of diagnostic or therapeutic procedures. One example of an iatrogenic infection is the bacteremia that results from insertion of an intravascular line. Not all HAIs are iatrogenic, nor are they all preventable.

Another factor that contributes to the development of HAIs is the compromised host, that is, a client whose normal defenses have been lowered by surgery or illness. Clients entering hospitals are often the least able to mount immune defenses to infection. Immunological responses may be compromised and normal defenses impaired in clients with, for example, cancer or chronic diseases, pressure ulcers, or organ transplants (Papadakis & McPhee, 2013). HAIs also occur when antibiotic therapy has altered the body's natural defenses and impaired resistance to harmful microorganisms. Endogenous organisms outside their normal habitats (such as in *E. coli* in the urinary tract) become a threat to the client. Other pharmacologic and therapeutic procedures, such as chemotherapy, the use of corticosteroids, and radiation therapy, also contribute to HAIs. Gram-negative enteric bacteria and gram-positive *S. aureus* are the most common bacteria responsible.

Invasive procedures and altered immune defenses are the main contributors to infection. Urinary catheterization is the number one cause; cardiac catheterization, insertion of peripheral and central intravenous lines, respiratory care procedures such as ventilators, and surgical procedures are also closely linked to HAIs. Consequently, the urinary tract, surgical wounds, the respiratory tract, and invasive catheter sites on the skin are most often affected by hospital-acquired infection. Organisms causing the infection are often resistant to many drugs and may not respond to antibiotics that are usually effective in treating infections acquired outside the hospital. **Table 9–4** ● outlines the most common microorganisms responsible for HAIs and their causes.

Hands are a common vehicle for the spread of microorganisms, and insufficient hand cleansing is an important factor contributing to the spread of HAIs. For routine client care, the WHO (2009b) recommends scrubbing and rinsing for 40–60 seconds using plain granule soap, soap-filled sheets, or liquid soap when hands are visibly soiled, after using the restroom, after removing gloves, before handling invasive devices (such as intravenous tubing), and after contact with medical equipment or furniture. Antimicrobial soaps are usually provided in high-risk areas, such as the newborn nursery, and are frequently supplied in dispensers at the sink. Wearing gloves does not eliminate the need for hand washing.

Soap and water are often inadequate to sufficiently remove pathogens. The CDC recommends use of alcohol-based antiseptic hand rubs (rinses, gels, or foams) before and after direct client contact (CDC, 2002; reaffirmed by WHO, 2009b). Studies have shown that the convenience of antimicrobial foams and

TABLE 9–4 Causes of Healthcare-Associated Infections

MOST COMMON MICROORGANISMS	CAUSES
Urinary tract	
Escherichia coli	Improper catheterization technique
Enterococcus species	Contamination of closed drainage system
Pseudomonas aeruginosa	Inadequate hand cleansing
Surgical sites	
Staphylococcus aureus (including methicillin-resistant strains—MRSA)	Inadequate hand cleansing
Enterococcus species (including vancomycin-resistant strains—VRE)	Improper dressing change technique
Pseudomonas aeruginosa	
Bloodstream	
Coagulase-negative staphylococci	Inadequate hand cleansing
Staphylococcus aureus	Improper intravenous fluid, tubing, and site care technique
Enterococcus species	
Pneumonia	
Staphylococcus aureus	Inadequate hand cleansing
Pseudomonas aeruginosa	Improper suctioning technique
Enterobacter species	

gels, which do not require soap and water, may increase healthcare workers' adherence to hand cleansing. Previous concerns that ready access to antimicrobial foams and gels represented a fire hazard have been addressed in the regulations.

It is important to recognize that performing hand hygiene with either soap or alcohol-based cleansers can damage the skin through the drying effect of the detergents or chemicals. If the nurse develops dermatitis, the client may be at higher risk for infection, because hand washing does not decrease bacterial counts on skin with dermatitis. The nurse is also at higher risk because the normal skin barrier has been broken. The use of hand lotions and creams to replace skin lipids can help prevent and treat dermatitis caused by hand hygiene products (WHO, 2009b).

ANTIBIOTIC-RESISTANT BACTERIA Antibiotic-resistant microorganisms are increasing at an alarming rate, primarily due to the prolonged and inappropriate use of antibiotic therapy. Bacteria with genetic mutations or genes that confer resistance survive antibiotic therapy, and the resulting reproduction of a colony of resistant bacteria can be spread to other organisms. Horizontal gene transfer can also produce resistance in previously susceptible bacteria (Hawkey & Jones, 2009). Other bacteria produce enzymes that inactivate drugs, change drug binding sites, or alter their cell membrane to prevent drug absorption.

Some of the current resistant strains include:

- Methicillin-resistant *S. aureus* (MRSA)
- Multidrug-resistant tuberculosis (MDR-TB)

- Penicillin-resistant *Streptococcus pneumoniae* (PRSP)
- Fluoroquinolone-resistant *Neisseria meningitides*
- Vancomycin-resistant *Enterococcus* (VRE)
- Vancomycin-intermediate or -resistant *S. aureus* (VISA or VRSA) (CDC, 2013a)
- Extended-spectrum beta-lactamase (ESBL)–producing *Enterobacteriaceae*
- Carbapenem-resistant *Enterobacteriaceae* (e.g., *Klebsiella*)
- Multidrug-resistant *Pseudomonas aeruginosa* (Kanj & Kanafani, 2011)

MRSA is becoming more prevalent in community settings in which young people, such as children in day care and amateur and professional athletes, share equipment. MRSA colonizes in the nares and skin. It is transmitted primarily by direct physical contact, not through respiratory droplets (Lin & Hayden, 2010), and healthcare personnel often unknowingly transmit *S. aureus* on their hands. Most *S. aureus* strains resist treatment by methicillin and similar drugs, which are the treatment of choice for *S. aureus* infections. Vancomycin and a semisynthetic derivative, telavancin, are the most uniformly effective drugs for both hospital-acquired and community-acquired MRSA (Rubinstein et al., 2011), although community-acquired MRSA may also be successfully treated by other antibiotics, such as rifampin and clindamycin (Liu et al., 2011). Soft-tissue infections with MRSA may manifest as abscesses, furuncles, or cellulitis and may be mistaken for spider bites.

In 1997, a new form of *S. aureus* emerged with resistance to vancomycin, known as vancomycin-intermediate *S. aureus* (VISA) or vancomycin-resistant *S. aureus* (VRSA). Both VISA and VRSA are resistant to methicillin. Clients with MRSA, VISA, or VRSA are isolated in a private room, and caretakers use contact precautions (which are covered in Box 9-2).

Enterococci are part of the normal flora of the gastrointestinal and female genital tracts. Frequent use of vancomycin causes *Enterococci* to develop resistance, leading to VRE. Direct transmission occurs on the hands of healthcare personnel and from contact with contaminated equipment. In cases of infection, stringent infection control measures are instituted, care is provided with contact precautions, and clients are placed either alone or with other VRE-infected clients.

Streptococcus pneumoniae, the most common cause of community-acquired pneumonia, has developed into its resistant form, penicillin-resistant *S. pneumoniae* (PRSP). Unlike MRSA and VRE, PRSP is transmitted by droplets from the respiratory tract and requires transmission-based droplet precautions (which are covered in Box 9-2).

C. difficile is an organism that has developed very resistant and highly morbid strains associated with frequent use of broad-spectrum antibiotics in hospitals. A common cause of healthcare-associated diarrhea, it is usually treated with metronidazole for mild to moderate cases or vancomycin for severe cases (Cohen et al., 2010). An even more virulent strain has been identified that is resistant to both metronidazole and vancomycin (Warny et al., 2005).

Extended-spectrum beta-lactamase–producing microorganisms are resistant to third-generation cephalosporins and include gram-negative *Klebsiella* and *E. coli*. These organisms colonize indwelling urinary catheters and gastrostomies, as well as mechanical ventilators. They spread by direct and indirect contact.

Universal precautions, the most important being hand washing, and modest use of antibiotics are critical in stopping the spread of antibiotic-resistant bacteria. The nurse should restrict equipment such as stethoscopes, blood pressure cuffs, and thermometers to use with the particular client identified with one of these diseases. Disposing appropriately of used personal protective gear is another important safeguard. Universal precautions are discussed in the section on Prevention.

Certain antibiotics can also induce resistance in some strains of organisms. This resistance has become so widespread that the CDC has created a 12-step Campaign to Prevent Antimicrobial Resistance in Healthcare Settings, which consists of four strategies: preventing infection, diagnosing and treating infection effectively, using antimicrobials wisely, and preventing transmission.

BIOLOGICAL THREAT INFECTIONS Since the terrorist attacks on September 11, 2001, and the anthrax attacks by mail later that year, concern about the possible use of biological weapons has increased in the United States. The most likely pathogens to be used for this purpose are anthrax, smallpox, botulism, pneumonic plague, and viral hemorrhagic fevers.

Stay Current: *For more information about the numerous bioterrorism agents and their associated effects, view the CDC resource available at* **http://emergency.cdc.gov/agent/agentlist.asp**

As with any potential large-scale infectious disease, state public health systems are charged with the responsibility of identifying cases, controlling the spread of infection, and preparing local and state responses for caring for the potentially large numbers of ill adults and children. As a part of this responsibility, public health authorities conduct **disease surveillance**, monitoring patterns of disease occurrence from the cases of infectious and communicable diseases reported by healthcare workers to state health officials. Disease surveillance procedures may be followed for any type of communicable and infectious disease, from *Shigella* to H1N1 influenza to a biological threat infection.

PEDIATRIC INFECTIOUS AND COMMUNICABLE DISEASES Reducing the number of vaccine-preventable diseases is a major national goal in *Healthy People 2020*, and nurses are important partners in this effort. Specific objectives targeted at reducing or eliminating specific infectious diseases (USDHHS, 2013) include:

- *Elimination.* Rubella and congenital rubella syndrome, serogroup A meningitis, and neonatal tetanus.
- *Reduction.* Pertussis, hepatitis B, varicella, measles, and other vaccine-preventable diseases, as well as other illnesses, such as food-borne pathogens and HIV infection. Common preventable infectious diseases are a significant public health problem. The national health objectives reflect the significance of these preventable diseases as a public health problem. **Table 9–5** lists selected infectious and communicable diseases in children.

TABLE 9–5   Selected Infectious and Communicable Diseases in Children

DISEASE	CLINICAL MANIFESTATIONS	CLINICAL THERAPY	NURSING MANAGEMENT
Diphtheria*+			
Causal agent: Corynebacterium diphtheriae *Epidemiology:* Occurs mostly in colder months in unimmunized or partially immunized children and immunized children with waning immunity. Cases of cutaneous and wound diphtheria occur sporadically in the tropics. Maternal immunity lasts up to 6 months after birth. The disease is endemic in areas where immunization is no longer routine, such as Russia. *Transmission:* Contact with nasal or eye discharge or skin lesion, or, less commonly, by indirect contact with contaminated items. Unpasteurized milk has served as a vehicle. *Incubation period:* 2–7 days or longer. *Period of communicability:* Usually 2–4 weeks or until 4 days after antibiotics are started.	Symptoms can be mild or severe with a gradual onset over 1–2 days. Low-grade fever, anorexia, malaise, rhinorrhea (runny nose) with a foul odor, cough, sore throat, hoarseness, stridor or noisy breathing, cervical lymphadenitis, and pharyngitis may be present. In more severe cases, the membranes of the tonsils, pharynx, and larynx are affected. The characteristic membranous lesion is a thick, bluish white to grayish black patch that covers the tonsils. It can spread to cover the soft and hard palates and the posterior portion of the pharynx. Attempts to remove the membrane result in bleeding. *Complications:* Produces an endotoxin that causes myocarditis and peripheral neuropathy (diplopia, slurred speech, difficulty swallowing, or paralysis of the palate) or ascending paralysis similar to Guillain-Barré syndrome.	Diagnostic tests include a culture from any mucosal or cutaneous lesion. Administer IV antitoxin and antibiotics within 3 days of onset of symptoms. The child must be tested for sensitivity to horse serum before being given the antitoxin. When diphtheria is suspected, antibiotic therapy (penicillin G or erythromycin) should be initiated without waiting for laboratory results. Removal of the membrane may be needed to treat airway obstruction. *Prognosis:* With treatment, prognosis is good. If untreated, death can occur due to airway obstruction. *Prevention:* Diphtheria is a vaccine-preventable disease. Booster doses are needed every 10 years after the primary series. This is a reportable disease.	■ Use droplet precautions for pharyngeal disease and contact precautions for cutaneous disease. ■ Monitor closely for signs of increasing respiratory distress, as well as cardiac and neurological complications. Provide humidified oxygen as necessary. ■ Have emergency airway equipment available. ■ Administer antibiotics. Give no medications containing caffeine or other stimulants. ■ Use oral suction gently as necessary. ■ Allow children to use mouthwash if desired. Gargling is not permitted because it can irritate the pharyngeal surfaces. ■ Encourage liquids as tolerated. Intravenous fluids may be necessary. ■ Provide emotional support to the family. ■ Initiate the search for client contacts to give antibiotics and immunization boosters.
Erythema Infectiosum (Fifth Disease)			
Causal agent: Human parvovirus B-19. *Epidemiology:* Occurs worldwide, most often in winter and spring. The disease also occurs in epidemics, with peak activity every 6 years. The incidence is highest in children between the ages of 5 and 14 years. *Transmission:* Respiratory secretions and blood. *Incubation period:* 6–21 days. *Period of communicability:* Believed to be highest the week before symptom onset. 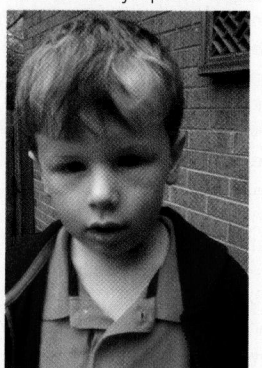 .... **Figure 9–2** ● Lace-like, erythematous, maculopapular rash with erythema infectiosum. *Source:* Christy Millican	Stage 1 begins as a flulike illness (headache, chills, malaise, nausea, body ache) lasting 2–3 days. A symptom-free period of 1–7 days follows. Stage 2 occurs 1 week later with a fiery-red rash on the cheeks, giving a "slapped face" appearance. Circumoral pallor is seen. In 1–4 days a lacelike, symmetric, erythematous, maculopapular rash appears on the trunk and limbs, spreading proximal to distal, but sparing the palms and soles (see **Figure 9–2** ●). Stage 3 lasts 1–3 weeks as the rash fades, but can reappear if the skin is irritated or exposed to sunlight. The rash can be mildly pruritic. *Complications:* Children with hemolytic conditions can have transient aplastic crisis. Arthritis and arthralgia can occur.	Diagnosis is made by physical signs or a serological test for immunoglobulin M (IgM) parvovirus B-19–specific antibody. Medical treatment is supportive, and recovery is usually spontaneous. Children with hemolytic conditions may need blood transfusions if an aplastic crisis occurs. Immunodeficient clients may develop a chronic infection for which IV immune globulin therapy is often effective (Pickering et al., 2012). *Prognosis:* Fetal infection can occur, resulting in fetal hydrops or spontaneous abortion. *Prevention:* Avoid contact with infected individuals.	■ Children with aplastic crisis are often hospitalized. ■ Use standard and droplet precautions. Isolation is needed only for children with aplastic crisis or who are immunosuppressed. ■ Nonaspirin antipyretics may be given to control fever. ■ Use soothing oatmeal or Aveeno baths if the rash is pruritic. Antipruritics may also help to relieve itching. ■ Encourage rest and offer frequent fluids. ■ Keep children out of direct sunlight if possible. Provide protective, light, loose clothing if exposure to sunlight cannot be avoided. ■ Provide quiet diversionary activity. There is no reason to keep the immune-competent child out of school or day care once he or she is no longer infectious. ■ Explain the three stages of rash development to parents.

(continued on next page)

TABLE 9–5 Selected Infectious and Communicable Diseases in Children (*continued*)

DISEASE	CLINICAL MANIFESTATIONS	CLINICAL THERAPY	NURSING MANAGEMENT
Haemophilus Influenzae, Type b⁺			
Causal agent: Coccobacilli *H. influenzae* bacteria, which have several serotypes and may or may not be encapsulated (surrounded by a protective outer covering). *Epidemiology:* Occurs most often in the spring and summer. Most commonly affected are infants and young children in child care centers. Low-birth-weight children and children with chronic illnesses have an increased susceptibility. *Transmission:* Direct contact or droplet inhalation. The organism is frequently asymptomatically colonized in the respiratory tract. *Incubation period:* Unknown. *Period of communicability:* 3 days from onset of symptoms.	Begins with a viral upper respiratory infection. The organism passes through the mucosal barrier to directly invade the bloodstream. It can cause several severe invasive illnesses, including meningitis, epiglottitis, pneumonia, septic arthritis, and cellulitis. It is also a cause of sepsis in infants. Other illnesses include sinusitis, otitis media, bronchitis, and pericarditis. Each disease has very specific clinical manifestations. Invasive disease has decreased 99% since the introduction of the vaccine (Pickering et al., 2012). *Complications:* Illness caused by *H. influenzae* type b responds to antibiotic therapy. If it is left untreated, severe sequelae and death, especially in young infants, can occur from conditions such as meningitis, epiglottitis, sinusitis, pneumonitis, and cellulitis.	Diagnosis is made by culture of blood, cerebrospinal fluid, or middle ear aspirate. Treatment consists of antibiotic therapy. Rifampin may be given to unprotected household contacts (not pregnant women), if another child has not completed immunizations, within 1 week after diagnosis. *Prognosis:* With rapid diagnosis and treatment, recovery is good, but highly dependent on the disease the organism has caused. When treatment is delayed, the prognosis for full recovery becomes much more guarded. *Prevention:* Immunization for *H. influenzae* type b	■ Use droplet precautions until 24 hours after the initiation of antibiotics. ■ Antibiotic therapy is administered intravenously for severe infections. Infections such as otitis media can be managed with oral antibiotics. ■ Unimmunized children under the age of 4 years are at increased risk for developing disease from *H. influenzae*. Specific prophylactic measures for susceptible children may be ordered by the physician. ■ Administer antipyretics to help the child feel more comfortable. ■ Closely monitor IV sites for patency and infiltration. ■ Perform nursing care measures specific to the illness. ■ Inform family members that rifampin turns urine and other body fluids orange, and it will cause stains.
Influenza			
Causal agent: Orthomyxoviridae, types A and B. *Epidemiology:* Prevalent in the United States from October to March, but the virus is active in other parts of the world year-round. During annual epidemics, 10%–40% of healthy children are infected, and 1% are hospitalized (Pickering et al., 2012). *Transmission:* Spreads by aerosolized particles and direct contact with respiratory secretions. *Incubation period:* 1–4 days. *Period of communicability:* 1 day before symptoms until 5 days after onset of illness.	Abrupt onset of fever (38°–40°C), chills, cough, runny nose, sore throat, malaise, aches, headache, and anorexia. Children can have nausea and vomiting, diarrhea, and abdominal pain. Children may also present with croup, bronchiolitis, conjunctivitis, or other nonspecific febrile illness. *Complications:* Otitis media, exacerbations of chronic lung conditions such as asthma and cystic fibrosis. Pneumonia, croup, bronchiolitis, and wheezing can occur in up to 25% of children. Myositis, myocarditis, encephalitis, transverse myelitis, Reye syndrome, and Guillain-Barré syndrome are all potential complications.	Diagnostic tests may include viral culture, rapid antigen testing from throat or nasopharynx, polymerase chain reaction, and immunofluorescence. Treatment is supportive. Antiviral therapy (oseltamivir and zanamivir) may be given to children 1 year of age or older who are at high risk of complications. Zanamivir is approved for children 5 years and older (Food and Drug Administration, 2013). Amantadine and rimantadine should not be used due to viral resistance (Food and Drug Administration, 2013). Follow updated antiviral therapy guidelines on http://www.cdc.gov/flu. When antiviral medication is initiated within 2 days of symptoms, the duration of symptoms may be reduced by 1–1.5 days. *Prevention:* Influenza vaccine is now recommended for infants and children over 6 months of age.	■ Use droplet and contact precautions for hospitalized infants and children. ■ The child is usually cared for at home. Encourage parents to wash hands frequently and to reduce exposure of other family members to the infected child. ■ Provide fluids to keep nasal secretions moist and prevent dehydration. ■ Provide acetaminophen or ibuprofen for fever management and mild pain. ■ If antiviral medications are given, be alert for nausea and vomiting. Zanamivir can exacerbate asthma. ■ Provide rest and quiet diversionary activities. ■ Teach parents to be alert to signs of complications from the viral infection. ■ Nurses should be familiar with pandemic influenza plans for the local area and state (http://www.pandemicflu.gov).

TABLE 9–5 Selected Infectious and Communicable Diseases in Children (*continued*)

DISEASE	CLINICAL MANIFESTATIONS	CLINICAL THERAPY	NURSING MANAGEMENT
Measles (Rubeola)[*][+]			
Causal agent: Morbillivirus, a member of the *Paramyxovirus* group *Epidemiology:* Occurrence peaks in the late winter and early spring. In developed countries, measles occurs mostly in outbreaks among unimmunized children, or possibly those with declining immunity. Spreads by direct contact with droplets or by airborne route. Passive maternal immunity lasts until the infant is age 12–15 months. In developing countries, measles remains an endemic disease and is a significant cause of infant and child morbidity and mortality. *Transmission:* Airborne, respiratory droplets and contact with infected individuals. *Incubation period:* Approximately 8–12 days. *Period of communicability:* Begins 3–5 days before the rash until 4 days after the rash appears. 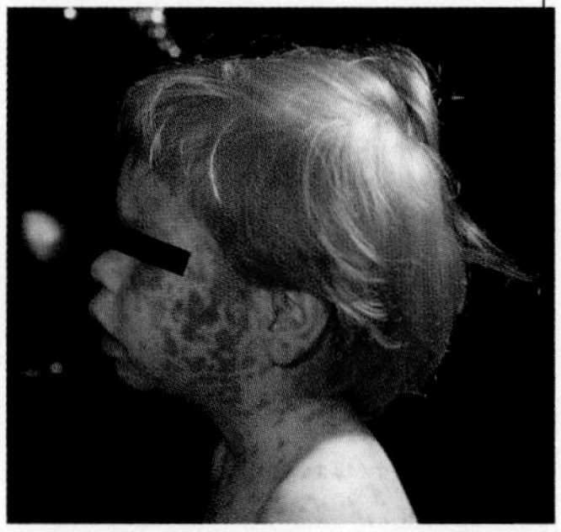	Children are quite ill in the prodromal phase of 3–5 days, with symptoms including high fever, conjunctivitis, coryza, cough, anorexia, and malaise. Koplik spots (small, irregular, bluish white spots on a red background) appear on the buccal mucosa about 2 days before and after the rash appears. The characteristic red, blotchy maculopapular rash that becomes confluent usually appears 2–4 days after onset of prodromal phase. The rash begins on the face and spreads to the trunk and extremities (**Figure 9–3 ●**). Symptoms gradually subside in 4–7 days. Other symptoms include anorexia, malaise, fatigue, and generalized lymphadenopathy. *Complications:* Diarrhea, otitis media, pneumonia, bronchitis, laryngotracheobronchitis, encephalitis, and death. Complications and sequelae occur most often in children who are malnourished, medically fragile, and immunosuppressed. The younger the child, the greater the risk for complications.	Diagnosis can be made by a serological test for IgM measles antibody. Treatment is supportive. No antiviral therapy is available. Antibiotics are used for secondary bacterial infections. *Prognosis:* Recovery is generally good with supportive care. *Prevention:* Measles is a vaccine-preventable disease. Immune globulin, administered up to 6 days after exposure, can be helpful in preventing the disease in susceptible individuals (immunocompromised children, infants less than 1 year of age, pregnant women). All healthcare workers should have documented immunity. This is a reportable disease. A total of 222 cases and 17 outbreaks (defined as an incidence of 3 or more linked cases) were reported in the United States in 2011. Of these cases, 200 were importations from another country (CDC, 2012b).	■ If the child is hospitalized, maintain airborne precautions during the contagious period. ■ Use a cool-mist vaporizer to help clear respiratory passages. ■ Suction nose and oral cavity very gently as necessary. ■ Give nonaspirin antipyretics for fever and antipruritics for itching. ■ Assess lungs carefully, especially in young children in whom pneumonias are a common complication. ■ Antitussives may be ordered to control coughing. ■ Keep lights dim and cover windows if the child has photophobia. ■ Elevate the head of the bed. Keep the room cool with good air circulation. Provide light and nonirritating blankets. ■ Keep skin clean and dry. No soaps should be used. ■ Maintain fluid intake. Offer cool liquids frequently in small amounts. Blended, pureed, and mashed foods are most easily tolerated. ■ Maintain bed rest. Visitors should be immune to measles. ■ Provide diversions such as music, stories, and favorite toys.

Figure 9–3 ● Confluent maculopapular rash with measles.
Source: Center for Disease Control.

Meningococcus			
Causal agent: Neisseria meningitides, a gram-negative diplococcus. *Epidemiology:* Most often in winter or early spring. Spread by respiratory droplets from human carriers. Majority of infections in the United States are caused by serogroups B, C, and Y. Serogroup B infections are most	Abrupt onset of flulike symptoms of fever, chills, malaise, muscle aches, vomiting, and prostration (extreme exhaustion). Neurological meningitis signs include drowsiness, disorientation, hallucinations, and convulsions.	Diagnostic tests include cultures of the blood and cerebrospinal fluid. A Gram stain of petechial skin scrapings may also be done. *Treatment:* Penicillin G is given IV (cefotaxime, ceftriaxone, and ampicillin are alternate antibiotics).	■ The child will be hospitalized. Use standard precautions and droplet precautions until the antibiotic has been administered for 24 hours. ■ Disease onset is abrupt and rapidly progresses to life-threatening. Be alert for development of shock and respiratory compromise. Have emergency equipment available and be prepared to perform resuscitation.

(continued on next page)

TABLE 9–5 Selected Infectious and Communicable Diseases in Children (*continued*)

DISEASE	CLINICAL MANIFESTATIONS	CLINICAL THERAPY	NURSING MANAGEMENT
Meningococcus (continued)			
common in infants younger than 1, while children over 11 and adults are more likely to be infected by C, Y, or W serogroups (Atkinson, Wolfe, & Hamborsky, 2011). Highest rates are in children under 2 years, with incidence of infection dropping drastically after age 2 (Thigpen et al., 2011). African Americans and individuals of low socioeconomic status are at higher risk. Outbreaks have occurred in child care centers, college dormitories, and military recruit camps. *Transmission:* Direct contact with droplet respiratory secretions. *Incubation period:* 1–10 days. *Period of communicability:* Until 24 hours after antibiotic is started.	*Meningococcemia:* An urticarial, maculopapular, or petechial rash also appears that may progress to purpura (**Figure 9–4 ●**). The condition may further deteriorate to shock, hypotension, disseminated intravascular coagulation, and coma. *Complications:* Loss of digits or limbs due to necrosis, hearing loss, arthritis, myocarditis, pericarditis, ataxia, seizures, hemiparesis, cranial nerve palsies, and obstructive hydrocephalus. Up to 10% of children and 25% of adolescents with invasive meningococcal disease die (Pickering et al., 2012). 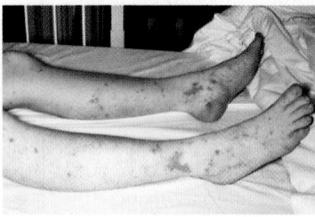 **Figure 9–4 ●** Purpura with meningococcemia. *Source:* John Radcliffe Hospital/Science Source.	Chloramphenicol is used for children allergic to penicillin. The child is managed aggressively in the ICU to maintain the airway, assist ventilation, and manage shock with IV fluids and vasopressors. Plasma, blood, or platelets are used to treat the disseminated intravascular coagulation. *Prevention:* A vaccine has been approved for adolescents 11 years and older. A vaccine is available for children over 2 years old with asplenia and other high-risk conditions. Close contacts are given medication (rifampin, ceftriaxone, or ciprofloxacin) for prophylaxis. Health professionals exposed to oral secretions need prophylaxis (Pickering et al., 2012). This is a reportable disease.	■ When giving IV fluids and blood products, make sure the child does not get overloaded with fluids, and monitor for evidence of increased intracranial pressure. ■ Keep the family informed of the child's status and treatment as the disease progresses. Help the family to mobilize its support system. ■ The child who survives will likely need rehabilitation. Work with the social worker or case manager to transition the child to long-term care. ■ Help identify close contacts who should receive prophylactic antibiotics and educate them about the expected side effects (e.g., orange urine with rifampin). ■ Teach close contacts to be observant for signs of illness and to seek health care promptly if they occur.
Mononucleosis			
Causal agent: Epstein-Barr virus (EBV), a member of the herpesvirus group *Epidemiology:* Occurs worldwide in no seasonal pattern. Infection commonly occurs early in life, and it often spreads among family members. *Transmission:* Direct contact with infected oropharyngeal and genital tract secretions. EBV can survive in saliva for several hours outside the body. EBV can also be transmitted by blood transfusion. *Incubation period:* Estimated to be 30–50 days. *Period of communicability:* Indeterminate, asymptomatic carriage is common (Pickering et al., 2012).	In very young children, mononucleosis can cause irritability but be otherwise asymptomatic. A maculopapular rash may be seen in a few cases. In other children, the disease is characterized by malaise, headache, anorexia, abdominal pain, fatigue, and fever for 2–3 days, followed by lymphadenopathy and a sore throat. Hepatosplenomegaly can occur. Pain from swelling of the tonsils and lymph nodes may be significant. The syndrome typically lasts 2–3 weeks and is self-limited. Weakness and lethargy may continue for several months. *Complications:* Rare side effects include central nervous system symptoms, such as encephalitis, aseptic meningitis, and Guillain-Barré syndrome. Splenic rupture, respiratory failure, and hematological complications such as thrombocytopenia can also occur. In immunodeficient children, fatal infections or lymphomas can develop.	Diagnostic tests include the serological monospot test or a heterophil antibody response test. Greater than 10% atypical lymphocytes and a positive heterophil antibody response test are diagnostic (Pickering et al., 2012). Treatment is supportive. Corticosteroids may be used to control tonsillar swelling and pain when there is impending airway obstruction, massive splenomegaly, myocarditis, or hemolytic anemia. Ampicillin and amoxicillin should be avoided, as a nonallergic rash often develops (Pickering et al., 2012). *Prognosis:* After recovery, the virus remains latent in the lymphoid system. It can be reactivated during periods of immunosuppression. *Prevention:* There is no known prevention.	■ Children are usually treated at home. Standard precautions should be used. ■ Give antipyretics and analgesics for fever and sore throat. Offer warm saltwater for gargling. Offer soft foods and encourage fluids. ■ Maintain bed rest during acute phase. ■ Give adolescents a sense of responsibility by involving them in decisions about care whenever possible. Be sure to include parents and adolescents in discussions. ■ Reassure adolescents who may be worried about keeping up with schoolwork that they can return to school when the fever is gone and swallowing is normal. ■ Teens should avoid kissing until the fever has been gone for several days. ■ Contact sports should be avoided until the liver and spleen are normal, usually in about 4 weeks. ■ If splenomegaly is present, alcohol should be avoided for 3 months after liver function test results return to normal.

TABLE 9–5   Selected Infectious and Communicable Diseases in Children (*continued*)

DISEASE	CLINICAL MANIFESTATIONS	CLINICAL THERAPY	NURSING MANAGEMENT
Mumps (parotitis)[+]			

Causal agent: Rubulavirus in the Paramyxoviridae family *Epidemiology:* Occurs worldwide in unvaccinated children, most often in winter and spring. Infection and vaccination induce lifelong immunity. Maternal antibodies begin to disappear in infants at the age of 12–15 months. *Transmission:* Contact with respiratory tract secretions *Incubation period:* 12–25 days *Period of communicability:* 1–2 days before parotid swelling until 9 days after swelling occurs 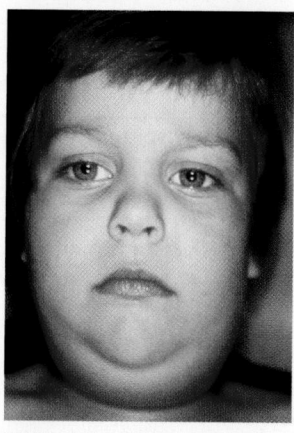 **Figure 9–5** ● Parotid gland swelling with mumps. *Source:* Center for Disease Control.	Malaise, low-grade fever, earache, headache, pain with chewing, and decreased appetite and activity; followed by bilateral or unilateral parotid gland swelling (**Figure 9–5** ●). Swelling peaks around the third day. Meningeal signs (stiff neck, headache, and photophobia) occur in about 15% of clients. *Complications:* Orchitis (inflammation of the epididymis, pain on testicular palpation, and scrotal swelling—most often unilateral) may occur in postpubertal males; sterility is relatively rare (Pickering et al., 2012). Oophoritis, pancreatitis, glomerulonephritis, myocarditis, thrombocytopenia, cerebellar ataxia, and hearing impairment are sometimes seen.	Diagnostic tests include a viral culture from a throat washing, urine, or cerebrospinal fluid. Serum mumps IgM antibody titer may also be performed. Therapy is supportive, focused on symptom relief. *Prognosis:* Mumps is usually self-limiting. *Prevention:* Mumps is a vaccine-preventable disease. This is a reportable disease. In 2009–2010 an outbreak of more than 3,500 cases of mumps occurred in the upper Northeast United States. The infection was originally imported from the United Kingdom (Barskey et al., 2012).	■ Use standard and droplet precautions for hospitalized children while contagious. ■ Children are usually cared for at home. They are generally uncomfortable but are rarely very ill. ■ Avoid exposure to immunocompromised or susceptible individuals. ■ Give nonaspirin analgesics and antipyretics to control fever and pain. ■ Encourage fluid intake. Swallowing and chewing may be painful. Offer soft and blended foods. Avoid foods and beverages that increase salivary flow (citrus, spices, and candies), because they cause pain. ■ Talking may be painful. Provide a bell or other attention-getting device. ■ Apply warm or cool compresses, whichever is preferred, to the parotid area. ■ Be alert for signs of complications. Headache, stiff neck, vomiting, and photophobia may indicate meningeal irritation. ■ Provide scrotal supports if testicular swelling occurs. ■ Reassure children that the facial swelling will go away. ■ Keep children out of school or child care until 9 days after parotid swelling occurs. Encourage diversionary activities.

Pertussis (Whooping Cough)[+]			

Causal agent: Bordetella pertussis *Epidemiology:* Occurs worldwide. Most common in children under 6 months of age. Epidemic cycles occur every 3–4 years. Pertussis can occur in healthcare workers, adolescents, and adults who have waning immunity, and these individuals can spread the disease to unimmunized children. Pertussis immunity may last 10 years following immunization, but there is concern about diminishing efficacy of the vaccine following the last childhood	The onset is insidious. *Catarrhal stage:* The disease begins with nasal congestion, a runny nose, low-grade fever, and a mild nonproductive cough, lasting about 2 weeks. *Paroxysmal stage:* The cough is more severe at night, with coughing spasms when the child attempts to expel a thick mucoid plug. A forceful inspiration through a narrowed glottis and stridor, or "whooping," follows. Young infants may have apnea rather than the "whooping." Sucking on a bottle may trigger the coughing spell. Coughing may be accompanied by flushing;	Diagnostic tests include culture and polymerase chain reaction (PCR) testing. Treatment with macrolide antibiotics (erythromycin, azithromycin, and clarithromycin); corticosteroids, if ordered; and supportive care. *Prognosis:* The disease is most severe in infants under 1 year of age, and most deaths occur in this age group. *Prevention:* Pertussis is a vaccine-preventable disease. Close contacts should be treated with macrolide antibiotics for prophylaxis (Tiwari, Murphy, & Moran, 2005).	■ Use droplet precautions until 5–7 days after antibiotics are initiated. Most hospitalized cases occur in children under the age of 5 years. ■ Use a cardiac monitor and pulse oximetry to continuously assess respirations and oxygen saturation. The smaller the child, the greater the risk for respiratory distress and apnea. ■ Remain with the child during coughing spells, when hypoxic and apneic episodes are most likely. Give oxygen if ordered. Have emergency equipment available. ■ Provide humidification. Gentle suctioning may be necessary.

(*continued on next page*)

TABLE 9–5   Selected Infectious and Communicable Diseases in Children (*continued*)

DISEASE	CLINICAL MANIFESTATIONS	CLINICAL THERAPY	NURSING MANAGEMENT
Pertussis (Whooping Cough) (continued)			
booster (Klein et al., 2012). *Transmission:* Respiratory droplets and direct contact with discharge from the respiratory membranes *Incubation period:* 7–10 days *Period of communicability:* Begins about 1 week after exposure. Communicable for 5–7 days after antibiotic therapy is initiated. The disease is most contagious before the paroxysmal cough stage.	cyanosis; vomiting; and profuse drainage from the nose, eyes, and mouth. Paroxysmal coughing can last 1–6 weeks or more. Dehydration may result from decreased oral intake. *Convalescent stage:* Up to 6 weeks, when paroxysms gradually subside. Adolescents and adults often have symptoms of an upper respiratory infection with persistent coughing spasms lasting longer than 7 days. *Complications:* Pneumonia, atelectasis, otitis media, encephalopathy, seizures, and death. Highest mortality rate and complication rate is in infants under 1 year.	Vaccine protection wanes after 5–10 years. This is a reportable disease. In 2012, more than 41,000 cases of pertussis were reported in the United States (CDC, 2013c).	■ Give nonaspirin antipyretics as needed for fever. ■ Encourage frequent rest periods. ■ Allow the child to eat desired foods in small, frequent feedings. ■ Encourage the child to take fluids. The child may need IV hydration if oral intake is not tolerated. ■ Provide emotional support to parents. ■ Teach parents to watch for signs of respiratory failure and dehydration if the child is managed at home.
Pneumococcal Infection[+]			
Causative agent: Streptococcus pneumoniae, a gram-positive diplococcus *Epidemiology:* The organism is found in the nasopharynx of healthy people. Outbreaks occur in the winter and spring among people in crowded settings. In temperate climates, 8 of 90 serotypes account for most of the invasive pediatric infections. The disease is more common in infants, young children, African Americans, Native Americans, and Alaskan Natives. Of particular concern is the development of penicillin- and multidrug-resistant strains. *Transmission:* Respiratory secretions and droplets *Period of communicability:* Unknown; probably less than 24 hours after beginning effective antibiotic therapy	The signs and symptoms are related to the focal area of infection. The organism causes otitis media, sinusitis, pharyngitis, laryngotracheobronchitis, pneumonia, meningitis, and bacteremia. In otitis media, upper respiratory infection, fever, ear pain, and decreased appetite are seen. In bacteremia, there is unexplained fever and no localized infection site. In pneumonia, fever, chills, chest pain, dyspnea, malaise, and a productive cough are seen. In meningitis, inconsolable crying, increased irritability, lethargy, refusal to eat, nausea, vomiting, diarrhea, myalgia, photophobia, and seizures are seen. *Complications:* Prior to the introduction of a vaccine, it caused 30%–50% of acute otitis media and was a major cause of sinusitis, meningitis, bacteremia, and pneumonia (Durbin, 2004). Other complications include septic arthritis, osteomyelitis, endocarditis, and brain abscess.	Diagnostic tests include bacterial culture from site of infection. Symptomatic care is provided. Antibiotic selection is based on susceptibility of organism to penicillin, macrolides, and other agents. Up to 50% of pneumococcal strains are penicillin-resistant. Third-generation cephalosporins (cefotaxime or ceftriaxone) may be used. Vancomycin and rifampin are used in combination when strains are resistant to the antibiotics listed above (Pickering et al., 2012). *Prevention:* Many serotypes are preventable with immunization. A significant reduction in invasive disease and antibiotic-resistant strains caused by serotypes in the vaccine has occurred since vaccination of infants was initiated (CDC, 2011c).	■ If the child is hospitalized, maintain standard precautions. ■ Provide nonaspirin antipyretics for control of fever and comfort. ■ Encourage fluids, and monitor intake and output. ■ Monitor vital signs and level of consciousness to identify signs of worsening condition. ■ Educate parents about the need for the vaccine, as the unimmunized child could become infected repeatedly with different serotypes. ■ Many children with mild disease are treated at home. Educate parents about the need for proper medication administration and comfort measures for the child and about signs indicating a need to seek additional medical care. ■ Individuals with congenital asplenia or traumatic splenectomy, malignancy, sickle cell disease, and nephrotic syndrome are at higher risk for invasive disease with this organism. ■ Additional factors that increase risk of pneumococcal disease include poverty, crowded housing, homelessness, and exposure to tobacco smoke.

TABLE 9–5   Selected Infectious and Communicable Diseases in Children (*continued*)

DISEASE	CLINICAL MANIFESTATIONS	CLINICAL THERAPY	NURSING MANAGEMENT
Poliomyelitis⁺			
Causal agent: Poliovirus is an enterovirus with three serotypes. *Epidemiology:* Occurs worldwide. Polio primarily affects children and immuno-compromised or unimmunized adults caring for infants who received live poliovirus vaccine. The vaccine induces lifelong immunity. Most cases of polio in the United States are contracted from individuals who were given the oral vaccine in another country. The oral poliovirus vaccine may induce vaccine-associated paralytic polio, but cases are very rare in the United States because the oral vaccine is no longer used. The most recent case of vaccine-associated paralytic polio in the United States occurred in 2009 (CDC, 2011d). *Transmission:* Primarily by the fecal-oral route, but also the respiratory route *Incubation period:* Usually 7–10 days (range 3–21 days) *Period of communicability:* Greatest shortly before and right after clinical symptoms develop when the virus is in the throat; excreted in the feces for several weeks	Affects the central nervous system. Less severe infections may be limited to fever and stiffness in the neck and back, headache, vomiting, and sore throat. In other cases, fever, headache, stiff neck, Kernig or Brudzinski sign, decreased deep tendon reflexes, and progressive weakness occur. With cranial nerve involvement, there may be respiratory tract muscle paralysis. An increased respiratory rate may interfere with the ability to talk, because frequent pauses are needed. Onset of paralysis may be sudden, over hours, or gradual over 3–5 days. Paralysis results from damage to motor neurons. *Complications:* Permanent motor paralysis, respiratory arrest, myocardial failure, aseptic meningitis, and postpolio syndrome.	Diagnosis is made by cell culture from stool or throat swabs. Treatment is supportive. No chemotherapeutic agents that directly kill the poliovirus are available. *Prognosis:* Respiratory complication is life-threatening and involves 5%–10% of all cases. Respiratory paralysis can lead to death, and motor paralysis can result in long-term disability. *Prevention:* Poliomyelitis is a vaccine-preventable disease. This is a reportable disease.	▪ Use standard and contact precautions in the hospital, and keep the child on strict bed rest. ▪ Observe closely for respiratory paralysis (ineffective cough, talking with frequent pauses, shallow and rapid respiratory rate). Have emergency equipment at bedside. Assist ventilations as needed until mechanical ventilation is set up. ▪ Administer sedatives and non-aspirin analgesics as ordered to allow for rest and comfort. Moist hot packs may relieve discomfort. ▪ Encourage fluids. ▪ Position the child to promote body alignment. ▪ Perform range-of-motion exercises to prevent contractures after the acute phase. ▪ Provide emotional support. ▪ Clients are alert and aware. Tell them what is happening to them. ▪ Some children may need long-term orthopedic (physical therapy) support.
Roseola (Exanthem Subitum, Sixth Disease)			
Causal agent: Human herpesvirus type 6 (HHV-6) *Epidemiology:* Occurs worldwide, primarily in children 6–24 months of age (after maternal antibodies decline); no seasonal pattern *Transmission:* Likely to be from respiratory secretions of healthy individuals *Incubation period:* Appears to be 9–10 days *Period of communicability:* Lifelong persistent viral shedding in healthy individuals (Pickering, 2012).	Sudden, high fever up to 40.5°C (105°F) for 3–8 days, during which the child does not appear toxic (normal appetite and behavior). The fever phase is followed by a characteristic pale pink, discrete, maculopapular rash that starts on the trunk and spreads to the face, neck, and extremities. The rash can last for 1–2 days. The child's appetite is normal. *Complications:* Children may have febrile seizures during high fever stage. Encephalopathy can develop in rare cases.	Roseola is self-limiting, and treatment is supportive. *Prognosis:* Roseola is benign in most cases. Nearly all children over 2 years of age have an antibody titer to HHV-6 (Pickering et al., 2012).	▪ Children are rarely hospitalized, but if they are, use standard precautions. ▪ Give nonaspirin antipyretics to control fever. ▪ Observe closely for any seizure activity, especially during the acute febrile periods. ▪ Encourage fluids. ▪ Reassure parents that the rash will disappear in a few days.

(continued on next page)

TABLE 9–5 Selected Infectious and Communicable Diseases in Children (*continued*)

DISEASE	CLINICAL MANIFESTATIONS	CLINICAL THERAPY	NURSING MANAGEMENT
Rotavirus			
Causal agent: Group A, B, and C rotaviruses *Epidemiology:* Occurs during late fall to early spring in yearly diarrhea epidemics in the United States; it is the most common cause of severe diarrhea in children under 5 years. *Transmission:* Fecal-oral route *Incubation period:* 2–4 days *Period of communicability:* Virus is present in stool before onset and may persist up to 21 days after onset of symptoms.	Acute onset of low-grade fever and vomiting followed by watery diarrhea 1–2 days later. Up to 10–20 diarrheal stools a day. Symptoms last 3–8 days. *Complications:* Dehydration and electrolyte disturbances. Death occurs in rare circumstances.	Diagnosis is by enzyme immunoassay or latex agglutination assay to detect (group A rotavirus antigen). Treatment involves adequate fluid and electrolyte replacement with oral rehydration solution. Introducing a regular diet within a few hours of rehydration shortens the duration of the disease (Dennehy, 2005). In severe dehydration, IV fluid resuscitation is performed. No antiviral therapy is available. *Prevention:* Naturally acquired infection protects against reinfection that causes severe diseases. A new vaccine has been approved for infants.	■ Use standard and contact precautions. ■ Hand hygiene with soap and water removes 75% of virus from contaminated hands. Use of alcohol-based hand sanitizers after washing with soap and water increases effectiveness (Dennehy, 2005). ■ Clean contaminated surfaces followed by disinfection with an alcohol-containing disinfectant (Dennehy, 2005). ■ Assess hydration status frequently. ■ Breastfeeding is continued during oral rehydration therapy. Formula feeding can begin 12–24 hours after oral rehydration therapy is started. ■ Older children can be fed complex carbohydrates and lean meats, yogurt, fruits and vegetables 12–24 hours after oral rehydration therapy is started.
Rubella (German Measles)[+]			
Causal agent: An RNA virus, member of the family Togaviridae, genus *Rubivirus* *Epidemiology:* Occurs worldwide and is most prevalent in the winter and spring. Maternal antibodies disappear about 6–9 months after birth. Most U.S. cases occur among foreign-born children and adults from countries that do not have rubella vaccination programs. Congenital rubella syndrome is thought to occur due to lack of immunization. Three cases were reported in 2009 in the United States (NCHS, 2012). *Transmission:* Droplet spread, direct contact with infected individuals, or contact with articles soiled by nasal secretions *Incubation period:* 14–21 days (most commonly 16–18 days) *Period of communicability:* Seven days before until 7 days after the onset of rash. Infants with congenital rubella may shed the virus for months after birth.	Rubella is generally a mild disease with a characteristic pink, nonconfluent, maculopapular rash. The rash appears on the face; progresses to the neck, trunk, and legs; and disappears in the same order. Prodromal symptoms occur 1–5 days before the rash and include low-grade fever, headache, malaise, coryza, sore throat, and anorexia. Forchheimer spots (discrete, erythematous pinpoint or larger lesions on the soft palate) are seen during the prodromal phase. Generalized lymphadenopathy involving the postauricular, suboccipital, and posterior cervical areas is common up to 7 days before the rash. Many cases are asymptomatic. Neonatal signs of congenital rubella syndrome include growth retardation, radiolucent bone disease, hepatosplenomegaly, thrombocytopenia, and purpuric skin lesions (giving a "blueberry muffin" appearance) (**Figure 9–6 ●**). *Complications:* Complications are rare, but include arthritis in adolescents, and encephalitis.	Diagnostic tests include cell culture from a nasal swab and detection of IgM or IgG antibodies. Treatment is supportive. Rubella is generally self-limiting in children. *Prognosis:* Disease is usually mild and benign. Major risk is for fetus if the mother is infected in the first trimester. Congenital rubella syndrome is associated with ophthalmological, cardiac, auditory, and neurological anomalies. *Prevention:* Rubella is a vaccine-preventable disease. Females of childbearing age need to be immunized to reduce the risk for congenital rubella syndrome. All healthcare workers should have documented immunity. 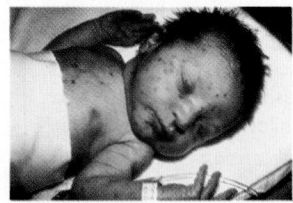 Figure 9–6 ● "Blueberry muffin" appearance in infant with congenital rubella syndrome. *Source:* Center for Disease Control.	■ Maintain standard and droplet precautions for contagious children. ■ Maintain contact precautions for infants with congenital rubella syndrome until 1 year of age unless nasopharyngeal and urine cultures are repeatedly negative after 3 months of age (Pickering, Baker, Kimberlin, & Long, 2012). ■ Children are usually treated at home. They should be isolated from pregnant women. ■ Give nonaspirin analgesics and antipyretics for any pain and fever. ■ Allow children to choose what they would like to eat and drink. Encourage fluids. ■ Provide quiet activities. ■ Exclude children from child care or school for 7 days after onset of rash. School and child care facilities should be notified of the child's illness.

TABLE 9–5 Selected Infectious and Communicable Diseases in Children (*continued*)

DISEASE	CLINICAL MANIFESTATIONS	CLINICAL THERAPY	NURSING MANAGEMENT
Streptococcus A			
Causal agent: Group A streptococci (GAS) *Epidemiology*: The illness is caused by various M-protein groups of group A beta-hemolytic streptococci. Different strains are associated with pharyngeal and pyodermal infections, and also rheumatic fever and acute glomerulonephritis (Pickering et al., 2012). Pharyngeal infections tend to occur more in late fall, winter, and spring. Pyodermal infections tend to occur in warmer seasons because of the association with minor skin trauma and insect bites. *Transmission*: Contact with respiratory secretions for pharyngitis or skin lesions for pyoderma *Incubation period*: Pharyngeal: usually 2–5 days; Pyodermal: usually 7–10 days *Period of communicability*: Four weeks in untreated pharyngeal infections; noncontagious within 24 hours of starting antibiotics 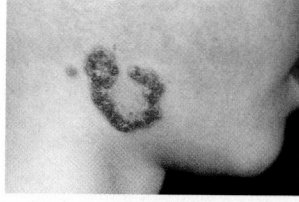 **Figure 9–7 ●** Impetigo. *Source*: © Medical-on-Line/Alamy.	*Pharyngeal*: Abrupt onset with a sore throat, dysphagia, malaise, high fever, chills, headache, abdominal pain, anorexia, and vomiting. A beefy red pharynx with exudate (strep throat) and tender cervical nodes are seen. Palatal petechiae may be seen. Cough and rhinitis are absent in most cases. *GAS respiratory tract infection*: Children under 3 years may develop serous rhinitis and a respiratory illness with moderate fever, irritability, and anorexia rather than pharyngitis. *Scarlet fever*: A characteristic erythematous, "sandpaper" rash that blanches with pressure appears in some cases 12–48 hours after onset of symptoms, concentrates in flexor skin creases, and spares the circumoral area. In 3–4 days, the rash begins to fade, and the tips of the toes and fingers begin to peel. The classic strawberry tongue is seen on days 4–5. *Pyodermal*: Lesions (impetigo) are honey-colored crusts at the site of open lesions (**Figure 9–7 ●**). *Complications*: If untreated, acute otitis media, sinusitis, peritonsillar or retropharyngeal abscess, cervical lymphadenitis, acute rheumatic fever, acute glomerulonephritis occur. Invasive disease with toxic shock syndrome, bacteremia, and necrotizing fasciitis or myositis can be fatal.	Diagnosis can be made by a rapid strep antigen test or culture of secretions from the pharynx and tonsils. Cultures of skin lesions are not indicated (Pickering et al., 2012). Prompt antibiotic treatment is effective. Penicillin V is the drug of choice. Erythromycin is used if the child is allergic to penicillin. Uncomplicated impetigo is treated with mupirocin ointment. Invasive strains causing necrotizing fasciitis or myositis need IV antibiotics and surgical intervention (exploration and debridement of dead tissue). *Prognosis*: Recovery is usually good with antibiotic therapy. It is possible for healthy children to become chronic carriers. *Prevention*: None.	■ Children with uncomplicated infections are usually cared for at home. ■ Promote bed rest during the febrile stage. ■ Give nonaspirin antipyretics to control fever. Teach parents important signs of a worsening condition. ■ For pharyngeal infections, offer warm saltwater for gargling, a soft diet, and nonacidic beverages. Encourage fluids. Provide cool, clear liquids. Swallowing may be difficult. ■ Explain to parents the importance of giving the child the full course of antibiotics. ■ Encourage family members with sore throats to have throat cultures taken. ■ For impetigo, teach the parents to wash the skin, remove crusts, and apply antibiotic ointment. ■ If the child is hospitalized, maintain droplet precautions for pharyngeal infections and contact precautions for skin lesions for 24 hours after beginning antibiotics. Monitor vital signs, especially temperature. Administer antibiotics as ordered. ■ If the child develops invasive streptococcal infection, use standard precautions. The child with toxic shock syndrome will need intensive care to manage shock and fluid and electrolyte imbalances.
Tetanus			
Causal agent: *Clostridium tetani* or tetanus bacillus *Epidemiology*: The bacillus is common and exists as a spore in soil, dust, and animal excretions. The organism produces an endotoxin that affects the central nervous system. *Transmission*: The organism is transmitted to humans through puncture wounds or broken skin. Newborns can acquire tetanus via the umbilical cord if they are born in an unclean area, a contaminated implement is used to cut the cord, or clay is applied to the umbilical cord as a ritual in some Middle Eastern cultures.	Stiffness of the neck and jaw, with painful facial spasms and difficulty chewing and swallowing over a few days, and headache. Noise and sudden movements can stimulate spasms. Spasms of facial muscles may produce a grinning expression (risus sardonicus). Localized prolonged and painful muscle contraction may occur at the site of the wound. Eventually rigidity of the abdomen and trunk produce *opisthotonos* (rigid hyperextension of the entire body). Spasms and fever occur, along with difficulty swallowing the increased oral secretions.	Tetanus immune globulin is given to unimmunized individuals as soon as possible. Tetanus toxoid is given at the same time at a separate site. Medications are provided to treat muscle spasms. Intensive care is provided with cardiorespiratory monitoring, assisted ventilation, IV metronidazole or penicillin G, nutrition, and supportive care. Wound cleansing and debriding are performed. Survival beyond 4 days indicates an increased chance of recovery. Paroxysms become less frequent, and complete recovery may take weeks.	■ Prevent disease by checking immunization records and administering immunizations as necessary. ■ Give immune globulin to unimmunized individuals. ■ Assist with wound debridement. ■ Use standard precautions, as the child with tetanus is hospitalized. ■ Monitor the child's condition. Handle as little as possible. Reduce stimulation by placing the child in a quiet, darkened room. ■ Offer skin and respiratory care. The child may need an endotracheal tube, suctioning, and supplemental oxygen for airway support.

(continued on next page)

TABLE 9–5 Selected Infectious and Communicable Diseases in Children (*continued*)

DISEASE	CLINICAL MANIFESTATIONS	CLINICAL THERAPY	NURSING MANAGEMENT
Tetanus (continued)			
Incubation period: 3 days to 3 weeks (average 8 days) *Period of communicability:* Not communicable to other individuals except through skin wounds	Respiratory muscles can be affected and cause airway obstruction and suffocation. Newborns have difficulty with sucking, progressing to an inability to suck, irritability, and nuchal rigidity. *Complications:* Laryngospasm, respiratory distress, or death	*Prognosis:* 30% mortality; much higher in newborns. Intensive care has improved mortality. *Prevention:* Tetanus is a vaccine-preventable disease. Tetanus boosters are updated every 10 years, or, if a potentially contaminated wound occurs, in 5 years. Proper surgical debridement of wounds decreases the chance of infection.	■ Provide feedings via total parenteral nutrition or feeding tube. ■ Maintain hydration with intravenous fluids and electrolytes. ■ Try to reduce the child's anxiety, as mental status may be unaffected. ■ Prepare the family for a possible poor prognosis.

Note: *Indicates that a vaccine or antitoxin is available for use in high-risk or as-needed situations. +Indicates that the disease has a safe and effective vaccine.

Alterations and Therapies **Infections**

The following summary table covers the infectious illnesses or diseases that a nurse encounters most frequently. Others are, but are not limited to, bacterial meningitis, bacterial endocarditis, giardiasis, chlamydia, tetanus, streptococcus A, *Shigella*, hepatitis, and HIV.

ALTERATION	DESCRIPTION/ DEFINITION	MANIFESTATIONS	INTERVENTIONS AND TREATMENT
Cellulitis	Acute bacterial infection of the dermis and underlying connective tissue	■ Fever ■ Inflammation in area of infection ■ Skin sore or rash	■ Antibiotics ■ Antipyretics ■ Palliative care ■ Fluid administration
Urinary tract infection	Infection of any part of the urinary tract: kidneys, ureters, urinary bladder, or urethra	■ Pain or burning when urinating ■ Fever ■ Urge to urinate often ■ Cloudy or malodorous urine	■ Antibiotics per culture results ■ Antipyretics ■ Fluid management
Viral pneumonia	Infection of the lung, often causing fluid accumulation in one or more lobes	■ Cough with mucus (may be bloody) ■ Fever ■ Chills ■ Chest pain when breathing deeply or coughing ■ Loss of appetite ■ Fatigue	■ Treatment based on symptoms ■ Cough suppressant, expectorant ■ Rest ■ Encouraging breathing ■ Support for respiratory effort, which may include oxygen, Fowler position, respiratory hygiene
Otitis Media	Inflammation of the middle ear	■ Ear pain ■ Redness of the eardrum ■ Pus or fluid in the ear ■ Fever ■ Difficulty hearing	■ Palliative care ■ Antibiotics only if symptoms do not resolve after 48–72 hours
Influenza	Highly contagious viral respiratory disease	■ Fever over 100°F ■ Aching muscles ■ Chills and sweats ■ Dry cough ■ Fatigue and weakness ■ Nasal congestion	■ Antipyretics. ■ Rest. ■ Fluid management. ■ Monitoring for respiratory rate and pattern, and for effective airway clearance. ■ Antiviral medications can reduce duration and severity of symptoms. ■ Prevention through vaccination of at-risk individuals.

Alterations and Therapies **Infections** (continued)

ALTERATION	DESCRIPTION/ DEFINITION	MANIFESTATIONS	INTERVENTIONS AND TREATMENT
Conjunctivitis	Highly contagious inflammation of the conjunctiva	▪ Blurred vision ▪ Crusts that form on eyelids ▪ Eye pain ▪ Redness of the eyes ▪ Sensitivity to light ▪ Increased tears	▪ Antibiotics ▪ Palliative care
Tuberculosis	Chronic, recurrent infectious disease caused by *Mycobacterium tuberculosis*	▪ Cough with mucus (may be bloody) ▪ Fever ▪ Excessive sweating ▪ Fatigue ▪ Breathing difficulty ▪ Fluid around the lungs	▪ Fluid management ▪ monitoring of vital signs, especially temperature ▪ Administering antipyretics and analgesics ▪ Antitubercular medications ▪ Respiratory support as dictated by symptoms ▪ Isolation
Sepsis	Whole body inflammatory process resulting in acute critical illness	▪ Change in mental status ▪ Fast breathing ▪ Fever or hypothermia ▪ Lightheadedness ▪ Tachycardia ▪ Skin rash	▪ Reversal of underlying cause ▪ Protection of respiratory and cardiovascular systems ▪ Fluid management ▪ Monitoring of neurological status, vital signs

Prevalence

Using proper precautions with general medical asepsis, appropriately using personal protective equipment (PPE) (e.g., gloves, masks, gowns, goggles, special resuscitative equipment), and vigilance in the clinical area will place the nurse at significantly less risk for injury. The chance of a healthcare worker's becoming infected from exposure to pathogens varies widely; estimates range from 30% for hepatitis B (nonimmune workers), to 1.8% for hepatitis C, to 0.3% for HIV (CDC, 2011a). The CDC has delineated measures to be taken in cases of possible exposure to these viruses. Hepatitis C, a worldwide epidemic with a higher prevalence than HIV (WHO, 2011; WHO, 2012b), has become a significant concern to all healthcare workers because there is currently no vaccine against the virus and there is no postexposure prophylaxis. Prevention remains the primary goal.

Occupational Safety and Health Administration (OSHA) requires that healthcare employers make the hepatitis B vaccine and vaccination series available to all employees. Other vaccinations may also be made available (e.g., nurses working in an obstetric area should be vaccinated against rubella to protect pregnant clients and their fetuses).

SAFETY ALERT
Nurses should consider in advance whether they would want prophylaxis for HIV exposure, because prophylaxis should optimally begin within 1 hour of exposure.

Genetic Considerations and Nonmodifiable Risk Factors

Some medical therapies may predispose an individual to infection. For example, radiation treatments for cancer destroy not only cancerous cells but also some normal cells, thereby rendering the client more vulnerable to infection. Some diagnostic procedures may also predispose the client to infection, especially when the skin is broken or sterile body cavities are penetrated during the procedure.

Certain medications also increase susceptibility to infection. Antineoplastic (anticancer) medications can depress bone marrow function, the result being a production of white blood cells inadequate to combat infections. Anti-inflammatory medications such as adrenal corticosteroids inhibit the inflammatory response, which is an essential defense against infection. Even some antibiotics used to treat infections can have adverse effects. Antibiotics can kill resident flora, allowing for the proliferation of strains that would not normally grow and multiply in the body. An important example is *C. difficile*–associated disease, an infection of the colon that is almost always caused initially by treatment with an antibiotic for another infection (Fashner et al., 2011).

Any disease that lowers the body's defenses against infection places the client at risk. Examples are chronic pulmonary disease, which impairs ciliary action and weakens the mucous barrier; peripheral vascular disease, which restricts blood flow; burns, which impair skin integrity; chronic or debilitating diseases, which deplete protein reserves; and immune system diseases such as leukemia and aplastic anemia, which alter the production of white blood cells. Diabetes mellitus is a major underlying disease that predisposes clients to infection because compromised peripheral vascular status and increased serum glucose levels increase susceptibility. Older adults who have multiple chronic diseases, particularly individuals over the age of 75 years, are also at greater risk of acquiring an infection than younger people.

Sam Werner is a 58-year-old Black man who comes to the emergency department because he is coughing up blood. As the nurse assigned to care for him, you conduct a client history and preliminary physical assessment. You find that Mr. Werner is undergoing chemotherapy for colorectal cancer, having been diagnosed 4 months ago. He has been having fatigue and sweats, but he attributes these symptoms to side effects of the chemotherapy. However, the fatigue has been worse the past couple days, and he has started coughing as well. His cough has got progressively worse, and today he has started coughing up blood and having chest pains. He also thinks he has a fever, because he is alternately chilled and sweating. Your physical assessment indicates T_O 104.3°F, P 92 bpm, R 20/min, BP 122/74 mmHg . You can hear that his breathing is labored. During your assessment, Mr. Werner has another coughing spell and coughs up more bloody sputum. After conducting his exam, the physician orders a CBC and chest x-ray, which indicate that Mr. Werner has bacterial pneumonia. Because he is immunocompromised from his chemotherapy treatment, Mr. Werner is admitted to the hospital.

Clinical Reasoning Questions Level I

1. What physical symptoms indicate that Mr. Werner has an infection?
2. What nursing interventions can you implement to lessen the effects of the chills and sweating?
3. What safety precautions should you take to clean up the bloody sputum?

Clinical Reasoning Questions Level II

4. What results would you expect from the CBC?
5. What other diagnostic tests could be performed to help diagnose Mr. Werner?
6. *Refer to the exemplar on Pneumonia in this module:* What medication is the physician likely to prescribe?

▶ PREVENTION

Everyone, including healthcare workers and clients, can play a role in preventing infections. techniques, Among the many techniques available to help prevent infection are good hand washing, getting immunizations, preventing airborne droplets from spreading, and taking precautions when handling potentially contaminated materials.

Healthcare Worker Precautions

Prevention of infection is a vital nursing role. Nurses and other healthcare workers can take multiple precautions to prevent infection, both for clients and for themselves.

DISINFECTING AND STERILIZING   The first two links in the chain of infection, the etiological agent and the reservoir, are interrupted by the use of **antiseptics** (agents that inhibit the growth of some microorganisms) and **disinfectants** (agents that destroy pathogens other than spores), and by sterilization.

Disinfecting   A disinfectant is a chemical preparation, such as phenol or iodine compounds, used on inanimate objects. Disinfectants are frequently caustic and toxic to tissues. An antiseptic is a chemical preparation used on skin or tissue. Disinfectants and antiseptics often have similar chemical components, but disinfectants are more concentrated.

Both antiseptics and disinfectants have bactericidal or bacteriostatic properties. A **bactericidal agent** destroys bacteria, whereas a **bacteriostatic agent** prevents the growth and reproduction of some bacteria. Select an agent that is known to be effective against the specific bacteria. For example, spore-forming bacteria such as *C. difficile*, which is a frequent cause of healthcare-associated diarrhea, and *Bacillus anthracis* (anthrax) may be inhibited by only a few of the agents normally effective against other forms of bacteria. Table 9–6 ● lists commonly used antiseptics and disinfectants.

When disinfecting articles, nurses need to follow agency protocol and consider the following factors:

1. *The type and number of infectious organisms.* Some microorganisms are readily destroyed; others require longer contact with the disinfectant.
2. *The recommended concentration of the disinfectant and duration of contact.*
3. *The presence of soap.* Some disinfectants are ineffective in the presence of soap or detergents.
4. *The presence of organic materials.* The presence of saliva, blood, pus, or excretions can readily inactivate many disinfectants.
5. *The surface areas to be treated.* The disinfecting agent must come into contact with all surfaces and areas.

TABLE 9–6 Commonly Used Antiseptics and Disinfectants: Their Effectiveness and Use

| | EFFECTIVE AGAINST | | | | | |
AGENT	BACTERIA	TUBERCULOSIS	SPORES	FUNGI	VIRUSES	USE ON
Isopropyl and ethyl alcohol	X	X		X	X	Hands, vial stoppers
Chlorine (bleach)	X	X	X	X	X	Blood spills
Hydrogen peroxide	X	X	X	X	X	Surfaces
Iodophors	X	X	X	X	X	Equipment, intact skin, and tissues if diluted
Phenol	X	X		X	X	Surfaces
Chlorhexidine gluconate (Hibiclens)	X				X	Hands
Triclosan (Bacti-Stat)	X					Hands, intact skin

Sterilizing **Sterilization** is a process that destroys all microorganisms, including spores and viruses. Four commonly used methods of sterilization are moist heat, gas, boiling water, and radiation.

- ***Moist heat.*** To sterilize with moist heat (such as in an autoclave), steam under pressure is used to attain temperatures higher than the boiling point. It cannot be used for items that can be damaged by heat, moisture, or high pressure, a major disadvantage.

- ***Gas.*** Ethylene oxide gas destroys microorganisms by interfering with their metabolic processes. It is also effective against spores. Its advantages are good penetration and effectiveness for heat-sensitive items. Its major disadvantage is its toxicity to humans.

- ***Boiling water.*** This is the most practical and inexpensive method for sterilizing in the home. The main disadvantage is that this method does not kill spores and some viruses. Boiling for a minimum of 15 minutes is advised to disinfect articles in the home.

- ***Radiation.*** Both ionizing (such as alpha, beta, and x-rays) and nonionizing (ultraviolet light) radiation are used for disinfection and sterilization. The main drawback to ultraviolet light is that the rays do not penetrate deeply. Ionizing radiation is used effectively in industry to sterilize foods, drugs, and other items that are sensitive to heat. Its main advantage is that it is effective for items difficult to sterilize, and its chief disadvantage is that the equipment is very expensive.

ISOLATION PRECAUTIONS

Isolation refers to measures designed to prevent the spread of infection or potentially infectious microorganisms to health personnel, clients, and visitors. Several sets of guidelines have been used in hospitals and other healthcare settings.

Category-specific isolation precautions use seven categories: strict isolation, contact isolation, respiratory isolation, tuberculosis isolation, enteric precautions, drainage/secretions precautions, and blood/body fluid precautions.

Disease-specific isolation precautions do exactly that: provide precautions to protect against a specific disease. These precautions call for use of private rooms with special ventilation, sharing of rooms only with other clients infected with the same organism, and gowning to prevent gross soilage of clothes for specific infectious diseases (Siegel et al., 2007).

Universal precautions (UP) are techniques to be used with all clients to decrease the risk of transmitting unidentified pathogens (Siegel et al., 2007). Universal precautions obstruct the spread of **bloodborne pathogens**, microorganisms carried in blood and body fluids that are capable of infecting other individuals with serious and difficult-to-treat viral infections, namely, hepatitis B virus, hepatitis C virus, and HIV. The CDC recommends not that universal precautions replace disease-specific or category-specific precautions, but that they be used in conjunction with them.

The **body substance isolation (BSI)** system employs generic infection control precautions for all clients, except those with the few diseases transmitted through the air. The BSI system (Gilmore, 2011) is based on three premises:

1. All people have an increased risk for infection from microorganisms entering through mucous membranes and nonintact skin.

Figure 9–8 ● Biohazard alert.

2. All people are likely to have potentially infectious microorganisms in all of their moist body sites and substances.
3. An unknown portion of clients and healthcare workers will always be colonized or infected with potentially infectious microorganisms in their blood and other moist body sites and substances.

The term *body substance* refers to blood, some body fluids, urine, feces, wound drainage, oral secretions, and any other body product or tissue.

In addition to other actions and precautions discussed in this concept, significant emphasis is placed on avoiding injury from sharp instruments, taking measures in cases of exposure to bloodborne pathogens, and communicating information about biohazards to employees. In most cases, federal regulations require that warning labels be affixed to containers of regulated waste and to refrigerators and freezers containing blood or other potentially infectious materials. The labels required are fluorescent orange or orange-red and feature the biohazard legend shown in **Figure 9–8 ●**.

CDC (HICPAC) Isolation Precautions (2007) The Hospital Infection Control Practices Advisory Committee (HICPAC) of the CDC presented updated guidelines for isolation precautions in 2007 (Siegel et al., 2007). These guidelines designate two tiers of precautions:

1. Standard precautions
2. Transmission-based precautions

Standard precautions are used in the care of all hospitalized individuals regardless of their diagnosis or possible infection status. *Transmission-based precautions* are used in addition to standard precautions for clients with known or suspected infections that are spread by contact or by airborne or droplet transmission. The three types of transmission-based precautions may be used alone or in combination but always *in addition to* standard precautions. They encompass all of the conditions or diseases previously listed in the category-specific or disease-specific classifications developed by the CDC in 1983.

Airborne precautions are used for clients who are known to have or suspected of having serious illnesses transmitted by airborne droplet nuclei smaller than 5 microns. Examples of such illnesses are measles (rubeola), varicella (including disseminated zoster), and tuberculosis. The CDC has prepared special guidelines for preventing the transmission of tuberculosis.

🌀 **Stay Current:** *The most current information can be found on the CDC Division of Tuberculosis Elimination Web site:* **http://www.cdc.gov/tb/**

Droplet precautions are used for clients who are known to have or suspected of having serious illnesses transmitted by particle droplets larger than 5 microns. Examples of such illnesses are diphtheria (pharyngeal); *Mycoplasma pneumoniae*; pertussis; mumps; rubella; influenza virus; streptococcal pharyngitis, pneumonia, and scarlet fever in infants and young children; and pneumonic plague.

Contact precautions are used for clients who are known to have or suspected of having serious illnesses that are easily transmitted by direct client contact or by contact with items in the client's environment. According to the CDC (Siegel et al., 2007), such illnesses include gastrointestinal, respiratory, skin, or wound infections or colonization with multidrug-resistant bacteria; specific enteric infections, such as *C. difficile*, enterohemorrhagic *Escherichia coli 0157:H7, Shigella,* and hepatitis A, in diapered or incontinent clients; respiratory syncytial virus, parainfluenza virus, and enteroviral infections in infants and young children; and highly contagious skin infections, such as herpes simplex virus, impetigo, pediculosis, and scabies.

Box 9–2 ● lists recommended isolation precautions for use in hospitals.

ISOLATION PRACTICES   The initiation of practices to prevent the transmission of microorganisms is generally a nursing responsibility that is based on a comprehensive assessment of the client. This assessment takes into account the status of the client's normal defense mechanisms, the client's ability to implement necessary precautions, and the source and mode of transmission of the infectious agent. The nurse decides whether to wear gloves, gown, mask, and protective eyewear. *In all client situations, nurses must cleanse their hands before and after providing care.*

In addition to the precautions cited in this concept, nurses implement aseptic precautions when performing many specific therapies that are described in other modules. The following are examples of aseptic precautions:

■ Use strict aseptic technique when performing any invasive procedure (e.g., inserting an intravenous needle or catheter) and when changing surgical dressings.

■ Change intravenous tubing and solution containers according to hospital policy (e.g., every 48–72 hours).

■ Check all sterile supplies for expiration date and intact packaging.

■ Prevent urinary infections by maintaining a closed urinary drainage system with a downhill flow of urine. Keep the drainage bag and spout off the floor.

■ Implement measures to prevent impaired skin integrity and accumulation of secretions in the lungs (e.g., encourage the client to move, cough, and breathe deeply at least every 2 hours).

PERSONAL PROTECTIVE EQUIPMENT   All healthcare providers must apply clean or sterile gloves, gowns, masks, and protective eyewear according to the risk of exposure to potentially infective materials.

Gloves   Gloves are worn for three reasons:
1. Gloves protect the hands when the nurse is likely to handle any body substances.
2. Gloves reduce the likelihood of nurses' transmitting their own endogenous microorganisms to individuals receiv-

ing care. Nurses who have open sores or cuts on the hands must wear gloves for protection.
3. Gloves reduce the chance that the nurse's hands will transmit microorganisms or a fomite from one client to another client.

In all situations, nurses must change gloves between client contacts. Nurses should clean their hands each time they remove gloves for two primary reasons: The gloves may have imperfections or may have been damaged during wearing, allowing microorganism entry, and the hands may become contaminated during glove removal.

Some of the gloves used in infection control are made of latex, as are various other items used in health care (e.g., catheters, blood pressure cuffs, rubber sheets, intravenous tubing, stockings and binders, adhesive bandages, and dental dams). Because of the frequent use of gloves, healthcare workers and some clients with chronic illnesses have increasingly reported allergic reactions to latex. Latex gloves that are lubricated by powder or cornstarch are particularly allergenic because the latex allergen adheres to the powder, which is aerosolized during glove use or removal of gloves and is then inhaled by the user. Latex gloves that are labeled "hypoallergenic" still contain measurable latex and should not be used by or on individuals with known latex sensitivity. Recent studies show some level of latex allergy in 2.9%–12.1% of healthcare personnel (Occupational Safety and Health Administration, 2008). The individuals at greatest risk for developing latex allergies are those with other allergic conditions and those who have had frequent or long-term exposure to latex. Even though most hospitals have eliminated latex products wherever possible and established a "latex-free environment" goal, clients and healthcare workers should be assessed for possible allergies to latex.

Gowns   The nurse wears a clean or disposable impervious (water-resistant) gown or plastic apron during procedures when the nurse's uniform is likely to become soiled. A sterile gown may be indicated when the nurse changes the dressings of a client with extensive wounds (e.g., burns). *Single-use gown technique* (using a gown only once before it is discarded or laundered) is the usual practice in hospitals. After the gown has been worn, the nurse discards it (if it is paper) or places it in a laundry hamper. Before leaving the client's room, the nurse cleanses his hands.

SAFETY ALERT
Wearing a client hospital gown over your uniform does not serve any infection control purpose.

Face Masks   Masks are worn to reduce the risk of transmitting organisms by the droplet contact and airborne routes, and by splatters of body substances. The CDC (Siegel et al., 2007) recommends that masks be worn by the following individuals:

1. Individuals close to the client if the infection (e.g., measles, mumps, or acute respiratory diseases in children) is transmitted by large-particle aerosols (droplets). Large-particle aerosols are transmitted by close contact and generally travel short distances (about 1 m, or 3 feet).

Box 9–2 Recommended Isolation Precautions in Hospitals

STANDARD PRECAUTIONS

- Designed for all clients in hospital
- Apply to (a) blood; (b) all body fluids, excretions, and secretions except sweat; (c) nonintact (broken) skin; and (d) mucous membranes.
- Designed to reduce the risk of transmission of microorganisms from recognized and unrecognized sources.

1. Perform proper hand hygiene after contact with blood, body fluids, secretions, excretions, and contaminated objects, whether or not gloves are worn.
   a. Perform proper hand hygiene immediately after removing gloves.
   b. Use a nonantimicrobial product for routine hand cleansing.
   c. Use an antimicrobial agent or an antiseptic agent for the control of specific outbreaks of infection.
2. Wear clean gloves when touching blood, body fluids, secretions, excretions, and contaminated items (e.g., soiled gowns).
   a. Clean gloves can be unsterile unless their use is intended to prevent the entrance of microorganisms into the body. (See point b, on sterile gloves.)
   b. Remove gloves before touching noncontaminated items and surfaces.
   c. Perform proper hand hygiene immediately after removing gloves.
3. Wear a mask, eye protection, or a face shield if splashes or sprays of blood, body fluids, secretions, or excretions can be expected.
4. Wear a clean, nonsterile gown if client care is likely to result in splashes or sprays of blood, body fluids, secretions, or excretions. The gown is intended to protect clothing.
   a. Remove a soiled gown carefully to avoid the transfer of microorganisms to other individuals (e.g., clients or other healthcare workers).
   b. Cleanse hands after removing gown.
5. Carefully handle client care equipment that is soiled with blood, body fluids, secretions, or excretions, to prevent the transfer of microorganisms to other individuals and the environment.
   a. Ensure reusable equipment is cleaned and reprocessed correctly.
   b. Dispose of single-use equipment correctly.
6. Handle, transport, and process linen that is soiled with blood, body fluids, secretions, or excretions so as to prevent contamination of clothing and the transfer of microorganisms to other individuals and to the environment.
7. Prevent injuries from used scalpels, needles, and other equipment, and place in puncture-resistant containers.
8. Use respiratory hygiene/cough etiquette.
   a. Educate healthcare facility staff, clients, and visitors.
   b. Post signs in languages appropriate to the population served, with instructions to clients and accompanying family members or friends.
   c. Use source control measures (e.g., covering the mouth/nose with a tissue when coughing, disposing of used tissues promptly, using surgical masks on the coughing individual when tolerated and appropriate).
   d. Use good hand hygiene after contact with respiratory secretions.
   e. Individuals with respiratory infections should be separated from others by at least 3 feet in common waiting areas.
9. Use safe injection practices by using needles only once, especially when obtaining medication from a multiple-dose vial or solution container or when injecting multiple clients.

10. Wear a face mask during catheter placements or when injecting material into the spinal or epidural space.

TRANSMISSION-BASED PRECAUTIONS

Airborne Precautions
Use standard precautions, as well as the following:
1. Place the client in a private room that has negative air pressure, 6–12 air changes per hour, and either discharge of air to the outside or a filtration system for the room air.
2. If a private room is not available, place the client with another client who is infected with the same microorganism.
3. Wear a respiratory device (N95 respirator) when entering the room of a client who is known to have or suspected of having primary tuberculosis.
4. A respiratory protection program should be in place that provides education about the use of respirators, fit-testing, and user seal checks.
5. Susceptible people should not enter the room of a client who has rubeola (measles) or varicella (chickenpox). If they must enter, they should wear a respirator.
6. Limit movement of the client outside the room to essential purposes. Place a surgical mask on the client during transport.

Droplet Precautions
Use standard precautions, as well as the following:
1. Place the client in a private room.
2. If a private room is not available, place the client with another client who is infected with the same microorganism. The curtain should be drawn between client beds.
3. Wear a mask if working within 3 feet of the client.
4. Limit movement of the client outside the room to essential purposes. Place a surgical mask on the client during transport.

Contact Precautions
Use standard precautions, as well as the following:
1. Place the client in a private room.
2. If a private room is not available, consult with infection control personnel to assess the risks associated with other placement options. Beds should be separated by more than 3 feet.
3. Wear gloves as described in standard precautions.
   a. Change gloves after contact with infectious material.
   b. Remove gloves before leaving the client's room.
   c. Cleanse hands immediately after removing gloves, using an antimicrobial agent. *Note:* If the client is infected with *C. difficile*, do *not* use an alcohol-based hand rub, as it may not be effective on these spores. Use soap and water.
   d. After hand cleansing, do not touch possibly contaminated surfaces or items in the room.
4. Wear a gown (see Standard Precautions) when entering a room if there is a possibility of contact with infected surfaces or items or if the client is incontinent or has diarrhea, a colostomy, or wound drainage that is not contained by a dressing.
   a. Remove the gown in the client's room.
   b. Make sure the uniform does not contact possible contaminated surfaces.
5. Limit movement of client outside the room.
6. Dedicate the use of noncritical client care equipment to a single client or to clients with the same infecting microorganisms.

Source: Based on Siegel, J. D., Rhinehart, E., Jackson, M., Chiarello, L., & the Healthcare Infection Control Practices Advisory Committee. (2007). *Guideline for Isolation Precautions: Preventing Transmission of Infectious Agents in Healthcare Settings.* Retrieved from http://www.cdc.gov/hicpac/pdf/isolation/isolation2007.pdf.

2. All individuals entering the room if the infection (e.g., pulmonary tuberculosis and SARS-CoV) is transmitted by small-particle aerosols (droplet nuclei). Small-particle aerosols remain suspended in the air and thus travel greater distances by air. Special masks that provide a tighter face seal and better filtration may be used for these infections.

Various types of masks differ in their filtration effectiveness and fit. Single-use disposable surgical masks are effective for use while the nurse provides care to most clients, but they should be changed if they become wet or soiled. These masks are discarded in the waste container after use. Disposable particulate respirators of different types may be effective for droplet transmission, splatters, and airborne microorganisms. Some respirators now available are effective in preventing inhalation of tuberculin organisms. The National Institute for Occupational Safety and Health (NIOSH) tests and certifies such respirators. Currently, the category N respirator at 95% efficiency (referred to as an *N95 respirator*) meets tuberculosis and SARS control criteria (CDC, 2012m).

During performance of certain techniques requiring surgical asepsis (sterile technique), masks are worn (a) to prevent droplet contact transmission of exhaled microorganisms to the sterile field or to a client's open wound and (b) to protect the nurse from splashes of body substances from the client.

Eyewear Protective eyewear (goggles, glasses, or face shields) and masks are indicated in situations in which body substances may splatter the face. If the nurse wears prescription eyeglasses, goggles must be worn over the glasses to extend around the sides of the glasses.

DISPOSAL OF SOILED EQUIPMENT AND SUPPLIES
Many pieces of equipment are supplied for single use only and disposed of afterward. Some items, however, are reusable. Agencies have specific policies and procedures for handling soiled equipment (e.g., disposal, cleaning, disinfecting, and sterilizing), and nurses need to become familiar with the practices of the employing agency. Appropriate handling of soiled equipment and supplies is essential to prevent inadvertent exposure of healthcare workers and clients to articles contaminated with body substances and to contamination of the environment.

Bagging Articles that are contaminated or likely to have been contaminated with infective material such as pus, blood, body fluids, feces, or respiratory secretions need to be enclosed in a sturdy bag impervious to microorganisms before they are removed from the room of any client. Some agencies use labels or bags of a particular color that designates them as infective wastes.

Linens Soiled linens should be handled as little as possible and with the least agitation possible before being placed in a laundry hamper. This minimal handling prevents gross microbial contamination of the air and of the individuals dealing with the linen. The bag is closed before being sent to the laundry in accordance with agency practice.

Laboratory Specimens Laboratory specimens, if placed in a leakproof container with a secure lid and labeled as a biohazard, need no special precautions. Use care when collecting specimens to avoid contaminating the outside of the container. To prevent personnel from having hand contact with potentially infective material, place containers that are visibly contaminated on the outside in a sealable plastic bag before sending them to the laboratory.

Dishes Dishes require no special precautions. Prevent soiling of dishes by encouraging clients to cleanse their hands before eating. Some agencies use paper dishes for convenience; these are disposed of in the refuse container.

Blood Pressure Equipment Blood pressure equipment needs no special precautions unless it becomes contaminated with infective material. If it does become contaminated, the agency policy should be followed to decontaminate it. Cleaning procedures vary according to whether it is a wall or portable unit. A disposable cuff should be used for clients placed on contact precautions.

Disposable Needles, Syringes, and Sharps Place needles, syringes, and sharps (e.g., lancets, scalpels, broken glass) in a puncture-resistant container. To avoid puncture wounds, use approved safety or needleless systems and do not detach needles from the syringe or recap them before disposal.

Disposable Equipment and Supplies Place garbage and soiled *disposable* equipment, including dressings and tissues, in the plastic bag that lines the waste container. Some agencies separate dry and wet waste material and incinerate dry items, such as paper towels and disposable items. No special precautions are required for disposable equipment that is not contaminated. Federal rules protecting the privacy of personal health information may extend to the client labels placed on disposable supplies such as intravenous fluid containers. Agencies may require that these be returned to the pharmacy so that personal information can be removed before disposal. Check agency policy.

Nondisposable Equipment and Supplies Place *nondisposable* or *reusable* equipment that is visibly soiled in a labeled bag before removing it from the client's room or cubicle, and then send it to a central processing area for decontamination. Some agencies may require that glass bottles or jars and metal items be placed in separate bags from rubber and plastic items. Glass and metal can be sterilized in an autoclave, but rubber and plastic are damaged by this process and must be cleaned by other methods, such as gas sterilization.

TRANSPORTING CLIENTS WITH INFECTION
Avoid transporting clients with infections outside their own rooms unless it is absolutely necessary. If a client must be moved, the nurse follows agency protocol to implement appropriate precautions and measures to prevent soilage of the environment. For example, the nurse ensures that any draining wound is securely covered or that the client who has an airborne infection wears a surgical mask during transport. In addition, the nurse notifies personnel at the receiving area of any infection risk so that they can maintain necessary precautions.

PSYCHOSOCIAL NEEDS OF CLIENTS IN ISOLATION
Clients requiring isolation precautions can develop several problems as a result of the special precautions taken in their care and their separation from other people. Two of the most common are sensory deprivation and decreased self-esteem related to feelings of inferiority. Sensory deprivation occurs when the environment lacks normal stimuli for the client, such

as communication with others. Nurses should be alert to common clinical signs of sensory deprivation, such as boredom, inactivity, slowness of thought, daydreaming, increased sleeping, thought disorganization, anxiety, hallucinations, and panic.

A client's feeling of inferiority can stem from perception of the infection itself or from the required precautions and related isolation. In North America, many people place a high value on cleanliness, and the idea of being "soiled," "contaminated," or "dirty" can make clients feel as if they are at fault and substandard. Although this is obviously not true, infected individuals may feel "not as good" as others and blame themselves. An appropriate nursing diagnosis may be risk for situational low self-esteem.

Nurses need to provide care that prevents or addresses sensory deprivation and feelings of inferiority. Related nursing interventions include:

1. Assess the individual's need for stimulation.
2. Initiate measures to help meet the need for stimulation, including regular communication with the client and diversionary activities, such as toys for a child and books, television, or radio for an adult. Provide a variety of foods to stimulate the client's sense of taste, and stimulate the client's visual sense by providing a view or an activity to watch.
3. Explain the infection and the associated procedures to help clients, their families, and caregivers understand and accept the situation.
4. Demonstrate warm, accepting behavior. Avoid conveying to the client any sense of annoyance about the precautions or any feelings of revulsion about the infection.
5. Do not use stricter precautions than are indicated by the diagnosis or the client's condition.

Sterile Technique

An object is sterile only when it is free of all microorganisms. It is well known that sterile technique is practiced in operating rooms and special diagnostic areas. Less well known, perhaps, is that sterile technique is also employed for many procedures in general care areas, such as administering injections, changing wound dressings, performing urinary catheterizations, and administering intravenous therapy. In these situations, all of the principles of surgical asepsis are applied, as in the operating and delivery rooms; however, not all of the sterile techniques that follow are always required. For example, before an operating room procedure, the scrub nurse generally puts on a mask and cap, performs a surgical hand scrub, and then dons a sterile gown and gloves. In a general care area, the nurse may only perform hand cleansing and don sterile gloves. The basic principles of surgical asepsis and practices that relate to each principle are outlined in **Table 9–7** ●.

STERILE FIELD   A **sterile field** is a microorganism-free area. Nurses often establish a sterile field by using the innermost side of a sterile wrapper or by using a sterile drape. When the field is established, sterile supplies and sterile solutions can be placed on it. Sterile forceps are often used to handle and transfer sterile supplies.

So that sterility can be maintained, supplies may be wrapped in a variety of materials. Commercially prepared items are frequently wrapped in plastic, paper, or glass. Liquids are preferably packaged in amounts adequate for one use only. Any leftover liquid is discarded.

STERILE GLOVES   Latex and latex-free (e.g., nitrile and vinyl) sterile gloves are available to protect nurses from contact with blood and body fluids. Latex and nitrile are more flexible than vinyl, mold to the wearer's hands, allow freedom of movement, and have the added feature of resealing tiny punctures automatically. Therefore, the nurse should wear latex or nitrile gloves when performing tasks that (a) demand flexibility, (b) place stress on the material (e.g., turning stopcocks, handling sharp instruments or tape), and (c) involve a high risk of exposure to pathogens. Vinyl gloves are best for tasks that are unlikely to stress the glove material, require minimal precision, and carry a minimal risk of exposure to pathogens.

Sterile gloves may be donned by the open method or the closed method. The open method is most frequently used outside the operating room because the closed method requires that the nurse wear a sterile gown. Gloves are worn during many procedures to maintain the sterility of equipment and protect a client's wound. Sterile gloves are packaged with a cuff of approximately 5 cm (2 in.) and with the palms facing upward when the package is opened. The package usually indicates the size of the glove (e.g., size 6 or $7\frac{1}{2}$).

STERILE GOWNS   Sterile gowning and closed gloving are carried out chiefly in operating and delivery rooms, where surgical asepsis is necessary. The closed method of gloving can be used only when a sterile gown is worn because the gloves are handled through the sleeves of the gown. Before these procedures, the nurse dons a hair cover and a mask and performs a surgical hand wash.

Preventing Healthcare-Associated Infections

Prevention is the most important control measure for HAIs. The pathogens causing these infections are transmitted primarily by contact with hospital personnel and contaminated inanimate objects (WHO, 2009b). *Effective hand washing is the single most important measure in infection control.* Although infections can also be transmitted by the airborne route, via contaminated equipment, and from the environment, these are less significant routes. Invasive procedures and equipment should be used only when absolutely necessary; for example, it is not appropriate to insert an indwelling catheter when the only indication is incontinence. The use of antimicrobial dressings and antimicrobial venous catheters is central to CDC guidelines for the prevention of HAIs. In addition, a daily audit should be performed to determine whether a central line is necessary or can be removed (O'Grady et al., 2011).

Meticulous use of medical and surgical asepsis is necessary to prevent transport of potentially infectious microorganisms. Many HAIs can be prevented by proper hand hygiene techniques, environmental controls, sterile technique when warranted, and identification and management of clients at risk for infection. Many research studies have investigated the effectiveness of aseptic technique. A number of studies have shown a link between artificial fingernails and infection transmission, especially fungal infections. In addition, skin underneath rings is more highly colonized than other skin, and organisms can remain under the ring for months without proper hand hygiene (WHO, 2009b). In any case, nurses use critical thinking and agency policy in implementing infection control procedures.

TABLE 9–7 Principles and Practices of Surgical Asepsis

PRINCIPLES	PRACTICES
All objects used in a sterile field must be sterile.	■ Before use, all articles are sterilized appropriately by dry or moist heat, chemicals, or radiation. ■ Always check a package containing a sterile object for intactness, dryness, and expiration date. Sterile articles can be stored for only a prescribed time; after that, they are considered unsterile. Any package that appears already open, torn, punctured, or wet is considered unsterile. ■ Storage areas should be clean, dry, off the floor, and away from sinks. ■ Always check chemical indicators of sterilization before using a package. The indicator is often a tape used to fasten the package or contained inside the package. The indicator changes color during sterilization, indicating that the contents have undergone a sterilization procedure. If the color change is not evident, the package is considered unsterile. Commercially prepared sterile packages may not have indicators but may be marked with the word *sterile*.
Sterile objects become unsterile when touched by unsterile objects.	■ Handle sterile objects that will touch open wounds or enter body cavities only with sterile forceps or sterile gloved hands. ■ Discard or resterilize objects that come into contact with unsterile objects. ■ Whenever the sterility of an object is questionable, assume the article is unsterile.
Sterile items that are out of vision or below the waist or table level are considered unsterile.	■ Once left unattended, a sterile field is considered unsterile. ■ Sterile objects are always kept in view. Nurses do not turn their backs on a sterile field. ■ Only the front part of a sterile gown, from shoulder to waist (or table height, whichever is higher), and the cuff of the sleeves to 2 inches above the elbows are considered sterile. ■ Always keep sterile gloved hands in sight and above waist/table level; touch only objects that are sterile. ■ Sterile draped tables in the operating room or elsewhere are considered sterile only at surface level.
Sterile objects can become unsterile by prolonged exposure to airborne microorganisms.	■ Keep doors closed and traffic to a minimum in areas where a sterile procedure is being performed, because moving air can carry dust and microorganisms. ■ Keep areas in which sterile procedures are carried out as clean as possible by frequent damp cleaning with detergent germicides to minimize contaminants in the area. ■ Keep hair clean and keep it short or enclose it in a net to prevent hair from falling on sterile objects. Microorganisms on the hair can make a sterile field unsterile. ■ Wear surgical caps in operating rooms, delivery rooms, and burn units. ■ Refrain from sneezing or coughing over a sterile field. Droplets containing microorganisms from the respiratory tract can travel 1 m (3 feet), making a sterile field unsterile. Some agencies recommend that masks covering the mouth and the nose should be worn by anyone working over a sterile field or an open wound. ■ Nurses with mild upper respiratory tract infections should refrain from carrying out sterile procedures or should wear masks. ■ When working over a sterile field, keep talking to a minimum. Avert the head from the field if talking is necessary. ■ To prevent microorganisms from falling over a sterile field, refrain from reaching over a sterile field unless sterile gloves are worn. Refrain from moving unsterile objects over a sterile field.
Fluids flow in the direction of gravity.	■ Unless gloves are worn, always hold wet forceps with the tips below the handles. When the tips are held higher than the handles, fluid can flow onto the handle and become contaminated by the hands. When the forceps are again pointed downward, the contaminated fluid can flow back down and contaminate the tips. ■ During a surgical hand wash, hold the hands higher than the elbows to prevent contaminants from the forearms from reaching the hands.
Moisture that passes through a sterile object draws microorganisms from unsterile surfaces above or below the sterile surface by capillary action.	■ Sterile, moisture-proof barriers are used beneath sterile objects. Liquids (sterile saline or antiseptics) are frequently poured into containers on a sterile field. If they are spilled onto the sterile field, the barrier keeps the liquid from seeping beneath it. ■ Keep the sterile covers on sterile equipment dry. Damp surfaces can attract microorganisms in the air. ■ Replace sterile drapes that do not have a sterile barrier underneath when they become moist.
The edges of a sterile field are considered unsterile.	■ A 2.5-cm (1-in.) margin at each edge of an opened drape is considered unsterile because the edges are in contact with unsterile surfaces. ■ Place all sterile objects more than 2.5 cm (1 in.) inside the edges of a sterile field. ■ Any article that falls outside the edges of a sterile field is considered unsterile.
The skin cannot be sterilized and is unsterile.	■ Use sterile gloves or sterile forceps to handle sterile items. ■ Prior to a surgical aseptic procedure, cleanse the hands to reduce the number of microorganisms on them.
Conscientiousness, alertness, and honesty are essential qualities in maintaining surgical asepsis.	■ When a sterile object becomes unsterile, it does not necessarily change in appearance. ■ The individual who sees a sterile object become contaminated must correct or report the situation. ■ Do not set up a sterile field ahead of time for future use.

Infection Control for Healthcare Workers

NIOSH is part of the CDC and is a research agency of the U.S. Department of Health and Human Services. It investigates potentially hazardous working conditions and publishes recommendations for preventing workplace illnesses and injuries. For example, in 1999, NIOSH published a study that found that the majority of needlestick injuries in healthcare settings were preventable. This finding, in part, led to the Needlestick Safety and Prevention Act, which went into effect in April 2001.

The Occupational Safety and Health Administration (OSHA), an agency of the U.S. Department of Labor, publishes and enforces regulations to protect healthcare workers from occupational injuries, including exposure to bloodborne pathogens in the workplace. **Occupational exposure** is defined as skin, eye, mucous membrane, or parenteral contact with blood or other potentially infectious materials that may result from the performance of an employee's duties.

There are three major modes of transmission of infectious materials in the clinical setting:

1. Puncture wounds from contaminated needles or other sharps
2. Skin contact, which allows infectious fluids to enter through wounds and broken or damaged skin
3. Mucous membrane contact, which allows infectious fluids to enter through mucous membranes of the eyes, mouth, or nose.

Role of the Infection Control Nurse

All healthcare organizations are required to have interdisciplinary infection control committees that may include representatives from the clinical laboratory, housekeeping, maintenance, dietary, and client care areas. One important member of this committee is the infection control nurse. This nurse is specially trained to be knowledgeable about the latest research and practices in preventing, detecting, and treating infections. All infections are reported to the infection control nurse in a manner that permits recording and analyzing statistics that can assist in improving infection control practices. In addition, the infection control nurse may be involved in employee education and implementation of the control plan for bloodborne pathogen exposure mandated by OSHA.

Client Precautions

Although nursing precautions are a primary source of infection control in the clinic and hospital, clients and their families can also use precautions to prevent infection. These include reducing the presence of modifiable risk factors and getting screenings and immunizations as recommended.

MODIFIABLE RISK FACTORS Individuals are constantly in contact with microorganisms in the environment. Normally an individual's natural defenses ward off the development of an infection. Some individuals are more susceptible to infections than others. Susceptibility is the likelihood of an organism's causing an infection in that individual. The following measures can reduce an individual's susceptibility to infection:

- *Hygiene.* Intact skin and mucous membranes are one barrier against microorganisms entering the body. In addition, good oral care, including flossing the teeth, reduces the likelihood of an oral infection. Regular and thorough bathing and shampooing remove microorganisms and dirt that can result in an infection.

- *Nutrition.* A balanced diet enhances the health of all body tissues, helps keep the skin intact, and promotes the skin's ability to repel microorganisms. Adequate nutrition enables tissues to maintain and rebuild themselves and helps keep the immune system functioning well. In addition, because antibodies are proteins, inadequate nutrition can impair the body's ability to synthesize them, especially when protein reserves are depleted (e.g., as a result of injury, surgery, or debilitating diseases such as cancer). Nurses can teach clients and their families ways to improve the client's nutritional status to help prevent infection.

- *Fluid.* Fluid intake permits fluid output, which flushes out the bladder and urethra, removing microorganisms that could cause an infection.

- *Sleep.* Adequate sleep is essential to maintaining health and renewing energy.

- *Stress.* Excessive stress predisposes people to infections. Nurses can help clients to learn stress-reducing techniques. The nature, number, and duration of physical and emotional stressors can influence susceptibility to infection. Stressors elevate blood cortisone, and the prolonged elevation of blood cortisone decreases anti-inflammatory responses, depletes energy stores, leads to a state of exhaustion, and decreases resistance to infection. For example, an individual recovering from a major operation or injury is more likely to develop an infection than a healthy individual.

IMMUNIZATIONS The use of immunizations has dramatically decreased the incidence of infectious diseases. Immunizations should begin shortly after birth and be completed throughout childhood (except for boosters). Immunizations against diphtheria, tetanus, and pertussis are usually started at 2 months, when the infant's immune system can respond. Immunizations may be given by injection, inhalation, oral solutions, or nasal sprays. They are frequently given in combination to minimize multiple injections. Because of the prevalence of influenza and its potential for causing death, the CDC recommends annual immunization against influenza for all individuals but highly recommends immunization for older adults and individuals with chronic cardiac, respiratory, metabolic, and renal disease. Pneumococcal vaccine is recommended for older adults who were last vaccinated more than 5 years previously and for individuals who are immunocompromised or have risk factors such as chronic pulmonary, liver, or cardiac disease.

Stay Current: CDC recommendations for immunizations change frequently. Updated immunization schedules for all age groups can be found on the CDC Web site at **http://www.cdc. gov/vaccines/schedules/**

- When were you last immunized for diphtheria, tetanus, poliomyelitis, rubella, measles, influenza, hepatitis, and pneumococcal pneumonia?
- When did you last have a tuberculin skin test?
- What infections have you had in the past, and how were these treated?
- Have any of these infections recurred?
- Are you taking any antibiotics, anti-inflammatory medications such as aspirin or ibuprofen, or medications for cancer?
- Have you had any recent diagnostic procedure or therapy that penetrated your skin or a body cavity?
- What past surgeries have you had?
- How would you describe your eating habits? Do you eat a variety of types of foods?
- Do you take vitamins?
- On a scale of 1 to 10, how would you rate the stress you have experienced in the past 6 months?
- Have you experienced any loss of energy, loss of appetite, nausea, headache, or other signs associated with specific body systems (e.g., difficulty urinating, urinary frequency, or a sore throat)?

▶ ASSESSMENT

Assessment of clients for infection is vital to treating the individual as well as preventing the spread of infection. Assessment for infection is also important for clients at risk of infection, such as clients with IV lines, indwelling catheters, and surgical wounds.

Nursing Assessment

During the assessment phase of the nursing process, the nurse obtains the client's history, conducts the physical assessment, and gathers laboratory data.

NURSING HISTORY   During the nursing history, the nurse assesses the degree to which a client is at risk for developing an infection and any client complaints suggesting the presence of an infection. To identify clients at risk, the nurse reviews the client's chart and structures the nursing interview to collect data regarding the factors that influence the development of infection, especially existing disease process, history of recurrent infections, current medications and therapeutic measures, current emotional stressors, nutritional status, and history of immunizations (see the following Assessment Interview feature).

PHYSICAL ASSESSMENT   Signs and symptoms of an infection vary according to the body area involved (see Infection Assessment). For example, sneezing, watery or mucoid discharge from the nose, and nasal stuffiness commonly occur with an infection of the nose and sinuses, and urinary frequency and cloudy or discolored urine often occur with a urinary infec-

tion. Commonly, the skin and mucous membranes are involved in a local infectious process, resulting in:

- Localized swelling
- Localized redness
- Pain or tenderness with palpation or movement
- Palpable heat in the infected area
- Loss of function of the body part affected, depending on the site and extent of involvement.

In addition, open wounds may exude drainage of various colors. Signs of systemic infection include:

- Fever
- Increased pulse and respiratory rate if the fever is high
- Malaise and loss of energy
- Loss of appetite and, in some situations, nausea and vomiting
- Enlargement and tenderness of lymph nodes that drain the area of infection.

Note: As with all history taking, the nurse must individualize the specific terms used, examples given to the client, and teaching techniques used to validate agreement on the meaning of words according to the client's culture, language spoken, and education or intellectual abilities.

Lifespan and Cultural Considerations

Infections manifest in a variety of ways in newborns, infants, and children. See **Table 9–8** ● for a list of the clinical manifestations of infection in infants and children by body system. Infants and children also need special considerations during the assessment. Nurses should make sure that their hands and other instruments are warm before touching a child's bare skin. In addition, nurses should explain procedures before the assessment to children who are old enough to understand. Infants and toddlers may feel more secure if they are held by a parent during the assessment. Distractions such as a pacifier or toy for infants and toys, books, or treats for toddlers and children may calm the child and aid in the assessment process. Nurses may also talk with verbal children about non-assessment-related topics to provide distraction. Other special considerations for specific assessments are provided in the Infection Assessment feature on pages 554–555.

Pregnant women need special considerations if they contract an infection that may cause birth defects, such as rubella, cytomegalovirus, parvovirus, and chicken pox. Cytomegalovirus is the most common infection that causes birth defects. Pregnant women should be educated about the risks of infection and ways to prevent infection during pregnancy. If a pregnant woman has an infection, it can be transmitted to the newborn. Infections that can be transmitted from the mother to the newborn include HIV, group B *Streptococcus*, cytomegalovirus, and listeriosis. Precautions such as antiviral treatment for HIV infections, antibiotics during labor for group B *Streptococcus*, good hygiene techniques, and not eating potentially contaminated foods are all ways to prevent the transmission of the infection to the fetus or newborn.

TABLE 9–8 Clinical Manifestation of Infection in Infants and Children

BODY SYSTEM	INFANTS	CHILDREN	BODY SYSTEM	INFANTS	CHILDREN
Central nervous system	Irritability	Irritability or combativeness	Gastrointestinal system	Vomiting	Nausea and vomiting
	Decreased responsiveness	Stiff neck		Diarrhea	Diarrhea
	Lethargy	Back pain		Abdominal distention	Abdominal discomfort
	Bulging anterior fontanel	Decreased responsiveness		Poor feeding	Abdominal distention
	High-pitched cry	Photophobia		*Additional signs in newborns:*	Poor appetite
	Muscle weakness	Brudzinski sign		Abdominal wall discoloration	
	Additional signs in newborns:	Kernig sign		Paralytic ileus	
	Seizures	Malaise		Bloody stool	
	Subtle changes in muscle tone or hypotonia			Jaundice or hepatosplenomegaly	
Cardiovascular system	Tachycardia	Tachycardia	Renal system	WBCs and bacteria in urine	WBCs and bacteria in urine
	Decreased perfusion	Decreased perfusion		*Additional signs in newborns:*	
	Weak peripheral pulses	Weak peripheral pulses		Decreased urine output	
	Pallor or mottled skin	Pallor or flushed, dry skin		Hematuria, proteinuria	
	Flushed, dry skin	Delayed capillary refill time	Hematopoietic system	Neutropenia	Leukocytosis
	Delayed capillary refill time			Increased immature WBCs (bands) in bacterial infections	Increased immature WBCs (bands) in bacterial infections
	Additional signs in newborns:			Lymphocytosis in viral infections	Lymphocytosis in viral infections
	Cyanosis			*Additional signs in newborns:*	
	Hypotension			Fraction of band cells >0.2	
	Bradycardia			Thrombocytopenia	
Respiratory system	Tachypnea	Tachypnea	Metabolic system	Hyperthermia or hypothermia	Hyperthermia
	Increased work of breathing with retractions, nasal flaring	Dyspnea		Hypoglycemia or hyperglycemia	Chills
	Crackles	Retractions			Hypothermia in septic shock
	Cough	Nasal flaring	Other systems	Rash	Rash
	Stridor	Crackles		Dry mucous membranes	Petechiae and/or purpura
	Decreased oxygen saturation	Cough		Poor skin turgor	Dry mucous membranes
	Irregular breathing	Stridor		Sunken anterior fontanel	Poor skin turgor
	Additional signs in newborns:	Decreased oxygen saturation		Petechiae and/or purpura	
	Apnea (new onset or increased episodes)				
	Increased or new-onset oxygen requirement				
	Grunting				

Infection Assessment

ASSESSMENT/ METHOD	NORMAL FINDINGS	ABNORMAL FINDINGS	LIFESPAN OR DEVELOPMENTAL CONSIDERATIONS
Vital Signs			
	Normal pulse, respiratory rate, temperature, blood pressure	■ Rapid pulse ■ Rapid respiratory rate ■ Fever or hypothermia	■ Infants or toddlers who are sick or in pain may be easier to assess when comforted or held by a parent. ■ Vital signs in children are different than in adults; vital signs should be compared to normal for the client's specific age group.
Ear Assessment			
	Intact ear canal and tympanic membrane, ear canal the same color as complexion, pearly gray tympanic membrane, no fluid or pus, possibly earwax, responsiveness to sound	■ Ruptured tympanic membrane ■ Pus or fluid in ear ■ Ear pain ■ Not responsive to sound, or report that sound is muffled ■ Redness or bulging of the eardrum	■ Infants and children with cleft lip/palate are at an increased risk of developing ear infections. ■ Infants or toddlers with ear pain may resist an ear assessment; distraction with toys or other objects may be helpful. ■ Children's tugging or rubbing the ear(s) may be a sign of otitis media.
Oral Cavity Assessment			
	Mucus membranes pink, smooth, moist, and intact	■ Bleeding or discolored gums ■ Cherry red or dry lips ■ Bright red or enlarged tonsils, white or yellow exudates on the tonsils ■ Bright red throat	■ Tonsils may be removed in some individuals. ■ Demonstrate for children how to open their mouth, stick out their tongue, and say "ah" for the assessment.
Eye Assessment			
	White sclera, normal amount of tears, clear of crusts	■ Red sclera ■ Crusts on eyelids ■ Excessive tears ■ Eye pain or itching	■ Abnormal findings in older adults may be related to glaucoma or other eye disorders rather than infection.
Lymph Node Assessment			
	Cervical nodes less than 1 cm, moveable, soft, and nontender; often nonpalpable	■ Enlarged nodes ■ Asymmetrical nodes ■ Tender nodes	■ Cervical nodes may not be palpable in healthy infants and adolescents; they are often small but palpable in children between the ages of 1 and 11. ■ The frequency of palpable cervical nodes decreases with age.
Respiratory Assessment			
	Normal respiratory rate and breath sounds	■ Rapid breathing ■ Abnormal respiratory sounds (e.g., wheezing, crackles, stridor)	■ Warm your hands and stethoscope before auscultating infants to help prevent resistance to the procedure; a pacifier may also be used. ■ Use a stethoscope with an appropriately sized diaphragm for infants. ■ Clients with lung diseases such as COPD or asthma may have abnormal breath sounds and respiratory rate in the absence of infection.

Infection Assessment (continued)

ASSESSMENT/ METHOD	NORMAL FINDINGS	ABNORMAL FINDINGS	LIFESPAN OR DEVELOPMENTAL CONSIDERATIONS
Skin Assessment			
	Normal complexion depending on race, skin intact, dry, and warm	■ Rash ■ Open wounds with inflammation and/or pus ■ Pallor ■ Redness ■ Increased warmth ■ Sweating ■ Itching or burning	■ Warm your hands before touching bare skin, especially when assessing infants. ■ Individuals with skin conditions such as psoriasis may have abnormal skin findings in the absence of infection. ■ Older adults may have fragile skin that is highly susceptible to infection. ■ Clients with diabetes mellitus may develop neuropathy that decreases sensation and increases the risk of infection; poor circulation may increase the time of healing for skin wounds.
Urinary Assessment			
	Clear or yellow urine with normal smell, no pain or itching	■ Frequent urination ■ Pain or burning during urination ■ Cloudy, bloody, or foul-smelling urine	■ If a urinary sample is needed from infants, a catheter may be used. ■ Children may need help obtaining a clean catch urine sample. ■ UTIs are rare in men, so all cases require further investigation. ■ Be aware of privacy issues, especially for adolescents.

Culture can also play a role in the exposure of individuals to specific infections as well as their beliefs about the cause of disease. In some cultures, infectious diseases are seen as punishment for sin or the result of curses or evil spirits. For example, Native Americans traditionally view illnesses as the result of disharmony with or displeasing the spirits. They may not believe in the germ theory of disease causation.

Diagnostic Tests

To assess the client's response to infection, identify the infecting organism, and monitor the progress of therapy, the following diagnostic tests may be ordered:

■ **WBC count** provides clues about the infecting organism and the body's immune response to it (**Table 9–9** ●).

TABLE 9–9 White Blood Cell Count and Differential for Adults

CELL TYPE AND NORMAL VALUE	INCREASED	DECREASED
Total WBCs: 4,500–10,000 per mm^3	*Leukocytosis:* Infection or inflammation, leukemia, trauma or stress, tissue necrosis	*Leukopenia:* Bone marrow depression, overwhelming infection, viral infections, immunosuppression, autoimmune disease, dietary deficiency
Neutrophils (segs, PMNs, or polys): 50%–70%	*Neutrophilia:* Acute infection or stress response, myelocytic leukemia, inflammatory or metabolic disorders	*Neutropenia:* Bone marrow depression, overwhelming bacterial infection, viral infection, Addison disease
Eosinophils (eos): 1%–3%	*Eosinophilia:* Parasitic infections, hypersensitivity reactions, autoimmune disorders	*Eosinopenia:* Cushing syndrome, autoimmune disorders, stress, certain drugs
Basophils (basos): 0.4%–1%	*Basophilia:* Hypersensitivity responses, chronic myelogenous leukemia, chickenpox or smallpox, splenectomy, hypothyroidism	*Basopenia:* Acute stress or hypersensitivity reactions, hyperthyroidism
Monocytes (monos): 4%–6%	*Monocytosis:* Chronic inflammatory disorders, tuberculosis, viral infections, leukemia, Hodgkin disease, multiple myeloma	*Monocytopenia:* Bone marrow depression, corticosteroid therapy
Lymphocytes (lymphs): 25%–35%	*Lymphocytosis:* Chronic bacterial infection, viral infections, lymphocytic leukemia, pertussis, mononucleosis, tuberculosis	*Lymphopenia:* Bone marrow depression, immunodeficiency, leukemia, Cushing syndrome, Hodgkin disease, renal failure

Source: Based on Corbett, J. V., & Banks, A. D. (2013). *Laboratory tests and diagnostic procedures with nursing diagnoses* (8th ed.). Upper Saddle River, NJ: Pearson Education; Dugdale, D.C., III. (2011). Blood differential. *MedlinePlus.* Retrieved from www.nlm.nih.gov/medlineplus/ency/article/003657.htm; and Pagana, K. D., & Pagana, T. J. (2013). *Diagnostic and laboratory test reference* (11th ed.). St. Louis, MO: Elsevier-Mosby.

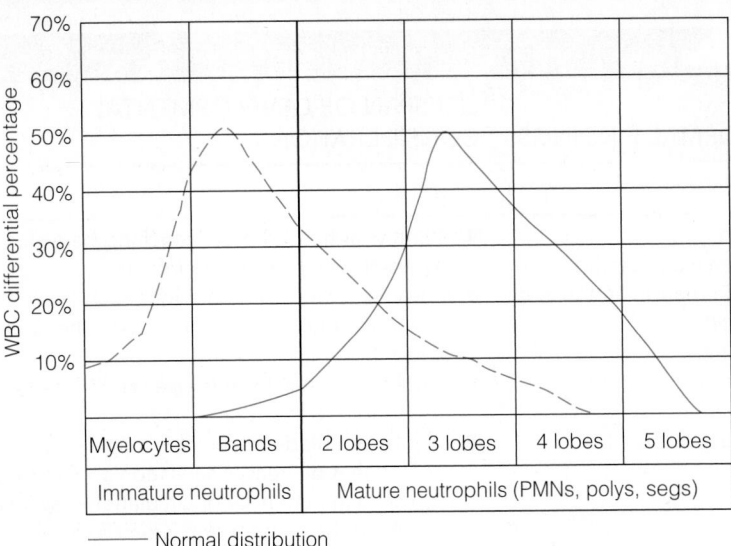

Type of WBC	Normal differential	Shift to left
Myelocytes	0%	Present
Band neutrophils (bands)	3–5%	Increased
Segmented neutrophils (segs, polys, PMNs)	50–65%	May be stable, increased, or decreased

Figure 9–9 ● Neutrophils by stage of maturity and normal distribution in the blood.

- **WBC differential** is also ordered (see Table 9–9). Neutrophilia, or increased numbers of circulating neutrophils (or PMNs), is a common response to infection, as the bone marrow responds to an increased need for phagocytes. Along with neutrophilia, a shift to the left is common in acute infection. This means that there are more immature neutrophils in circulation than normal (**Figure 9–9 ●**), indicating an appropriate bone marrow response.

- **Procalcitonin (CTpr)** is a precursor of the hormone calcitonin. Procalcitonin increases dramatically during infection and sepsis and is accepted as both a marker of sepsis and a harmful mediator in lower respiratory tract and systemic infections (Schuetz, Albrich, & Mueller, 2011).

- **Cultures** *of the wound, blood, or other infected body fluids* are used to identify probable microorganisms by their characteristics, such as shape, growth patterns, and Gram-staining qualities. After the organism is cultured, it is subjected to various antibiotics known to be effective against its particular strain to determine which antibiotic is likely to be most effective. This process is known as sensitivity testing. Generally, 24–48 hours are required to grow the organism, potentially delaying initiation of therapy. Because antibiotics (and possibly oxygen therapy) can alter the ability to culture an organism, obtain specimens before instituting therapy.

- **Serological testing** provides an indirect means of identifying infecting agents by detecting antibodies to the suspected organism. When the antibody titer against a specific organism rises during the acute phase of an infectious disease and begins to fall during convalescence, the diagnosis is supported. Although it is not as accurate as culture, serology is particularly useful for organisms that cannot easily be cultured, such as hepatitis B and HIV (Porth & Matfin, 2010).

- **Direct antigen detection methods** are in the process of being developed. These tests use monoclonal antibodies (see **Box 9–3 ●**), which are purified antibody forms, to

---

Box 9–3 Monoclonal Antibodies

Antigens typically have numerous antigenic determinant sites, each capable of stimulating a different subset of B cells. Each clone secretes a slightly different antibody from the others. The immunoglobulin produced is therefore *polyclonal*, with multiple different antibodies. In 1975, researchers devised a technique for making a single clone of "immortal" B cells that could be maintained indefinitely in a laboratory and would produce a single antibody to a specific antigen. This pure antibody, known as a *monoclonal* antibody, offers the following advantages:

- It can target specific antigens.
- It has a single, constant binding affinity for the antigen.

- It can be diluted to a specific titer or concentration, because it is not mixed with other antibodies.
- It can be purified to avoid adverse responses (McCance & Huether, 2010).

In addition to providing passive protection from disease, monoclonal antibodies are being used in a variety of other ways, including the diagnosis and treatment of cancer, immunosuppression to prevent rejection of transplanted tissue or organs, immune response analysis, imaging techniques for diagnostic uses, and the early detection of viral infections (Lehne, 2010; McCance & Huether, 2010).

detect antigens in specimens from a diseased host (Porth & Matfin, 2010). These tests offer rapid and accurate identification of the offending microorganism.

- **Antibiotic peak and trough levels** monitor therapeutic blood levels of the prescribed medication(s). The therapeutic range—that is, the minimum and maximum blood levels at which the drug is effective—is known for a given drug. By measuring blood levels at the predicted peak (1–2 hours after oral administration, 1 hour after intramuscular administration, and 30 minutes after intravenous administration) and trough (lowest level, usually a few minutes before the next scheduled dose), healthcare personnel can determine whether the client is maintaining a level within the therapeutic range at all times, ensuring maximal effect from the drug. Measuring blood levels of a prescribed medication also helps determine whether the drug is reaching a toxic or harmful level during therapy, an unintended result that can increase the likelihood of adverse effects.

- **Radiological examination of the chest, abdomen, or urinary system** may be ordered to detect organ abnormalities that indicate an inflammatory response or tissue damage.

- **Lumbar puncture** is performed to obtain cerebrospinal fluid (CSF) for examination and culture if a central nervous system (CNS) infection, such as meningitis or encephalitis, is suspected.

- **Ultrasonic examination, such as an echocardiogram or renal ultrasonography,** is a noninvasive diagnostic test used to evaluate organ function.

- **Urinalysis** is a noninvasive test used to assess for the presence of bacteria or blood in the urine.

CASE STUDY \\ PART 2

Mr. Werner is prescribed acetaminophen for his fever and IV fluids to prevent dehydration. His cultures indicated a *Streptococcus pneumonia* infection, so he is placed on high-dose amoxicillin and levofloxacin. He is also placed in a room with humidified air. You begin caring for Mr. Werner on his third day in the hospital. You have been assigned to perform a vital signs and respiratory assessment every 4 hours. Your first assessment indicates that Mr. Werner's pulse and blood pressure are normal, but his breathing rate and temperature are still slightly elevated at 18/min and 101.8°F. Auscultation of his lungs indicates rales in the lower right lobe, and the lower right lobe is dull to percussion. Mr. Werner reports that he still coughs up sputum regularly, but he is no longer coughing up blood.

Clinical Reasoning Questions Level I
1. What is the purpose of the humidified air in Mr. Werner's treatment?
2. What other assessments are important to conduct regularly for someone in Mr. Werner's condition?

3. Mr. Werner will be in the hospital for several more days. What can you do to prevent feelings of isolation and boredom?

Clinical Reasoning Questions Level II
4. Why did the physician not prescribe a cough suppressant?
5. What effect does Mr. Werner's immunocompromised state have on his level of care?
6. What nursing interventions can reduce the risk of the infection spreading to the blood?

▶ INTERVENTIONS AND THERAPIES

The goals of care for the client with an infection are to identify the organ system affected by the infection, identify the causative agent, and achieve a cure by the least toxic, least expensive, and most effective means. Fortunately, most infectious diseases are self-limiting and will resolve with little or no medical care. However, medical treatment may be required for an overwhelming infection or immunocompromised host.

The body part or organ system affected by the infection is often obvious from the client's history and presenting signs and symptoms. Identifying the system allows a narrowing of the range of possible infecting organisms to those known to affect that system. The manner of presentation provides further clues to the diagnosis. For example, pneumococcal pneumonia typically presents with the acute onset of chills, fever, and cough in a previously healthy adult, whereas a client with viral pneumonia relates a gradual onset of symptoms, with systemic manifestations such as muscle aches and headache often predominant. A history of recent activities also provides clues. Family members who all vomit and have diarrhea within 12 hours after a picnic probably do not have the flu.

Once the causative agent has been identified, therapy can be specifically tailored to the client's needs. Treatment of viral infections is often symptomatic and entails supportive care, such as promoting rest and encouraging oral intake of fluids. Skin infections may respond to treatment with a topical agent, which prevents potential adverse effects from one administered systemically.

Independent

All skills and treatments, whether administering medications (see the Medications feature) or preparing a client for discharge, are performed in a manner that prevents possible infection of clients. Some nursing skills are specific to preventing infection, recognizing signs and symptoms of infection, and treating the client who is diagnosed with an infection. Nursing skills used in preventing infection and caring for clients diagnosed with infection include:

- Hand hygiene
- Basic medical asepsis
- Use of standard precautions
- Isolation techniques
- Sterile field
- Use of personal protective equipment and decontamination.

Collaborative

Many interventions for infection must be performed in collaboration with the physician or other healthcare professionals. For example, a physician may order a specimen collection of blood or urine for diagnostic testing. The nurse may be responsible for collecting these specimens from the client and delivering them to the laboratory for testing. The nurse may also be asked to retrieve the laboratory results and inform the physician of them. Once a diagnosis has been made, the nurse may be involved in administering medications ordered by the physician, especially in a hospital setting (see the Medications feature).

SAFETY ALERT

Nurses should encourage clients to take the full regimen of antibiotics as prescribed. Bacterial resistance often results from incomplete antibiotic therapy, which can lead to more serious and resistant infections in the future. Lack of adherence to the antibiotic regimen may also increase the risk of recurrent infections in susceptible hosts, producing further complications. In addition, clients who have leftover antibiotics from one infection may tend to self-medicate using those antibiotics for another infection even if the infection is caused by a different organism. Using antibiotics for non-susceptible organisms is another major cause of bacterial resistance.

Medications **Antimicrobial Agents**

Once the causative agent and affected body system have been identified, specific therapy to cure the infectious disease can begin. The perfect anti-infective agent destroys pathogens while preserving host cells, is effective against many organisms while not promoting the development of resistance, distributes to necessary tissues, and remains in the body for relatively long periods.

Because no available antimicrobial meets all these criteria, physicians look for an agent that is effective, has little toxicity, can be administered with relative convenience, and is cost-effective. In the process of selection, characteristics of both the host and the infecting organism are considered.

CLASSIFICATION	MECHANISM OF ACTION	NURSING CONSIDERATIONS
Antibiotics ■ amino-glycosides ■ macrolides ■ tetracyclines ■ cephalosporins ■ penicillins ■ sulfonamides ■ fluoroquinolones *Drug examples:* cefaclor, erythromycin, penicillin, tobramycin, trimethoprim-sulfamethoxazole	May be used prophylactically to prevent infection or treat existing bacterial infection. Specific antibiotic is chosen based on pathogen causing infection.	■ Teach clients importance of taking the entire prescribed amount. ■ Encourage adequate fluid intake. ■ Monitor for signs of allergic reaction. ■ Assess renal and hepatic function and vital signs.
Antifungal *Drug examples:* amphotericin B, anidulafungin, caspofungin acetate, flucytosine, micafungin, fluconazole, nystatin	Selective for fungal plasma membranes, they inhibit ergosterol synthesis.	■ Carefully monitor client's condition. ■ Use cautiously in clients with renal impairment, severe bone marrow suppression, and pregnancy. ■ Closely monitor kidney function (intake and output, BUN, creatine, daily weights). ■ Monitor serum electrolytes.
Antipyretic, Analgesic *Drug examples:* acetaminophen	Relieves pain and reduces fever.	■ Monitor temperature. ■ Assess pain level. ■ Teach proper administration.
Antipyretic, Analgesic, Anti-inflammatory *Drug examples:* aspirin, ibuprofen	Reduces fever and inflammation, in addition to relieving pain.	■ Monitor temperature. ■ Assess pain level. ■ Teach proper administration.
Antimalaria *Drug examples:* atovaquone, proguanil, chloroquine, hydroxychloroquine sulfate, mefloquine, primaquine phosphate, pyrimethamine, quinine	Interrupts the complex life cycle of plasmodium, with greater success early in the course of the disease.	■ Carefully monitor client's condition. ■ Provide education about prescribed drug treatment. ■ Is contraindicated in clients with hematological disorders or severe skin disorders such as psoriasis, and during pregnancy. ■ Assess lab results (complete blood cell count [CBC], liver and renal function tests, G5PD deficiency). ■ Obtain a baseline electrocardiogram. ■ Monitor for gastrointestinal side effects and changes in cardiac rhythm.

Medications **Antimicrobial Agents** (continued)

CLASSIFICATION	MECHANISM OF ACTION	NURSING CONSIDERATIONS
Antihelminthic *Drug examples:* albendazole, diethyl-carbamazine, ivermectin, mebendazole, praziquantel, pyrantel	Is targeted at killing the parasites locally in the intestine and systemically in the tissues and organs they have invaded.	■ Monitor vital signs, CBC, and liver function studies after obtaining a baseline. ■ Identify specific worm or parasite before initiating therapy. ■ Educate on nature of parasite infestation to prevent future reinfestation. ■ Warn clients if bowel elimination of worm is anticipated. ■ Assess for GI symptoms. ■ Monitor for CNS side effects.
Antiretroviral ■ Nonnucleoside reverse transcriptase inhibitors ■ Nucleoside and nucleotide reverse transcriptase inhibitors ■ Protease inhibitors ■ Fusion and integrase inhibitors *Drug examples:* delavirdine, efavirenz, abacavir, didanosine, amprenavir, atazanavir, darunavir, enfuvirtide, raltegravir, acyclovir, cidofovir, docosanol, idoxuridine, penciclovir	Target specific phases of the HIV replication cycle, requiring multiple drugs taken concurrently.	■ Clients require extensive teaching regarding pharmacotherapy, disease process, and prevention of contaminating others. ■ Psychosocial issues must be addressed to improve compliance with treatment regimen. ■ Use nonjudgmental approach. ■ Assess for side effects that can dramatically affect the client's life. ■ Assess T-cell count and client response to pharmacotherapy.

REVIEW The Concept of Infection

RELATE Link the Concepts

Linking the concept of infection with the concept of metabolism:

1. How does an infection such as hepatitis affect metabolism in the liver?

2. What physiological changes related to obesity increase an individual's risk for infection?

Linking the concept of infection with the concept of reproduction:

3. Describe the links between infection during pregnancy and congenital disorders.

4. Which infections are most likely to occur in neonates in the first few days of life?

READY Go to Companion Skills Manual

REFER Go to Pearson Student Nursing Resources
nursing.pearsonhighered.com

- Additional review materials

REFLECT Case Study \\ Part 3

After one week in the hospital, Mr. Werner is finally going home. His vital signs have stabilized, he is no longer coughing up sputum, and his rales are barely audible. He was able to continue his chemotherapy treatments in the hospital, and he now has only one treatment left. He still feels fatigued from the chemotherapy, but the fatigue is not as severe as during the acute infection. You are providing discharge teaching for Mr. Werner.

Clinical Reasoning Questions Level I

1. What client teaching can you perform to help decrease Mr. Werner's risk of infection while he is still immunocompromised?

2. The physician has prescribed an additional regimen of oral antibiotics. What should you emphasize about the importance of completing the therapeutic regimen?

3. What warning signs should Mr. Werner be watching for that may indicate another infection?

Clinical Reasoning Questions Level II

4. To what other opportunistic infections may Mr. Werner be susceptible?

5. What nursing diagnoses apply to Mr. Werner upon his discharge?

6. What nutritional requirements does Mr. Werner have now that he is going home?

EXEMPLAR 9.1 **Cellulitis**

EXEMPLAR KEY TERMS
Cellulitis, *560*
Erythema, *560*
Inflammation, *560*
Lymphadenopathy, *560*
Lymphangitis, *561*
Tinea pedis, *560*
White blood cells (WBCs), *560*

EXEMPLAR LEARNING OUTCOMES
After reading about this exemplar, you will be able to:

1. Describe the pathophysiology, etiology, clinical manifestations, and direct and indirect causes of cellulitis.

2. Identify the risk factors and prevention methods associated with cellulitis.

3. Illustrate the nursing process in providing culturally competent care across the life span for individuals with cellulitis.
4. Formulate priority nursing diagnoses appropriate for an individual with cellulitis.
5. Summarize therapies used by interdisciplinary teams in the collaborative care of an individual with cellulitis.
6. Plan evidence-based care for an individual with cellulitis and the family in collaboration with other members of the healthcare team.
7. Evaluate expected outcomes for an individual with cellulitis.

▶ OVERVIEW

Infection can occur in a small localized area, affect an entire organ system, or attack the entire body, as in the case of septicemia. Cellulitis is an example of an infection that can be small and well contained, but if not treated promptly, it can develop into a life-threatening septicemia.

Cellulitis is an acute bacterial infection of the dermis and underlying connective tissue. It is characterized by red or lilac, tender, warm, edematous skin with an ill-defined, nonelevated border. Cellulitis usually occurs on the face and lower extremities as a result of trauma or a compromised skin barrier. Its chief symptom is **inflammation**, which includes intense pain, heat, redness, and swelling. It may appear in a localized area as a complication of a wound infection, or it may involve an entire limb. In severe infections, fever may be present, as well as an increase in **white blood cells (WBCs)** and tender lymph nodes (**lymphadenopathy**). Elevated WBCs and fever, though common signs of infection, may not be present in frail, older clients.

▶ PATHOPHYSIOLOGY AND ETIOLOGY

Normal flora gain entry into the dermis through a break in the skin. There, they multiply, causing an inflammatory response with classic signs of inflammation, including **erythema** (redness), pain, warmth at the site, and edema. The wound is generally irregular in shape with well-defined borders. As the organisms grow in number, they can overwhelm the immune response that normally contains and localizes inflammation. This condition allows cellular debris to accumulate, the result being enlarged areas of involvement.

Erysipelas, a superficial cellulitis of the skin caused by group A *Streptococcus*, usually affects the lower extremities or the face (**Figure 9–10 ●**). The involved area is bright red and raised with well-defined borders. If treated promptly, the prognosis is generally very good. Skin infections such as this can predispose the individual to septicemia and septic shock if treatment is delayed. Although antibiotic therapy is effective, the most important method of therapy is prevention.

Etiology

The most common causative organism is *Staphylococcus aureus,* followed by group A *Streptococcus* (Chira & Miller, 2010). Cellulitis can also result from a nearby abscess or sinusitis. Onset is usually rapid.

Risk Factors

Children with cellulitis often have a history of trauma, impetigo, folliculitis, untreated tooth decay, or recent otitis media.

As the skin becomes thinner and less elastic with age, older adults become more susceptible to injury and breakdown of tissue, which can result in cellulitis. Peripheral neuropathy with decreased sensation and circulation can lead to abrasions, burns, and stasis ulcers that can become infected. Reduced physical activity, malnutrition, dehydration, and other systemic illnesses are also predisposing factors. Any interruption of skin integrity can lead to infection, especially with organisms that are part of the normal skin flora.

Other factors that increase the risk for cellulitis include any illness that compromises skin integrity such as diabetes mellitus, obesity, a previous history of cellulitis, peripheral vascular disease, tinea pedis, and a weakened immune system (Mayo Clinic, 2012). Clients with **tinea pedis** (fungal infection of the feet) or lymphatic obstruction are most vulnerable to cellulitis and may experience recurrent infections over time.

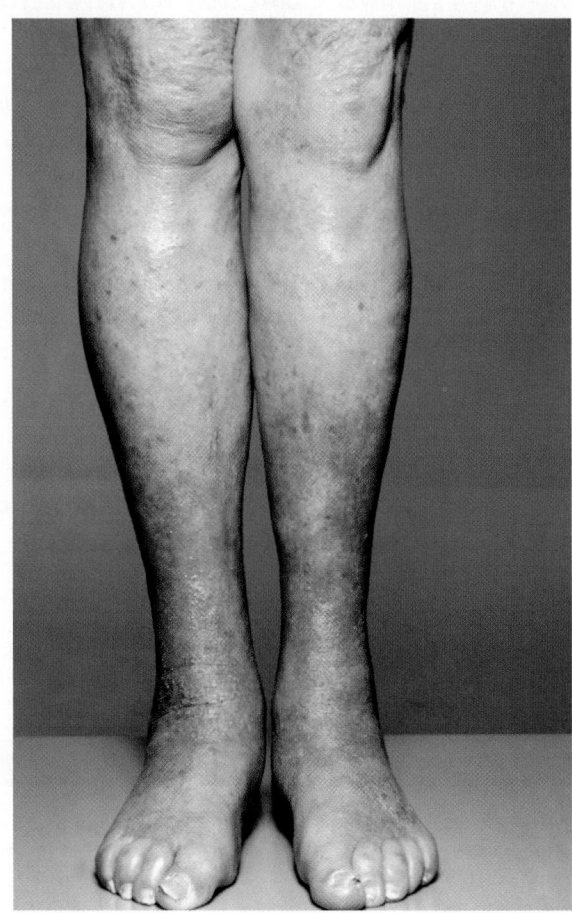

Figure 9–10 ● Erysipelas, a superficial cellulitis of the skin caused by group A streptococcus.

Source: © Wellcome Image Library / Custom Medical Stock Photo.

Evidence-Based Practice Moist Wound Management

Problem

Individuals with open wounds are more susceptible to contracting a skin infection such as cellulitis. Many individuals believe that wounds should be kept dry and should not be covered until a scab forms. However, this slows wound healing and leaves the wound exposed to potential pathogens if the scab comes off.

Evidence

Many studies indicate that keeping a wound moist can promote healing by preventing cell death, improving the rate of re-epithelialization, and protecting the wound from infection. Proper wound moisture management can also reduce pain and improve the cosmetic outcome. In particular, three cleansing techniques can be used individually or in combination to keep the wound moist and help remove any pathogens and debris: compression, pressure irrigation, and soaking. Compression involves pressing excess moisture from a gauze or cloth on the wound and removing the cloth after wound contact, irrigation involves running a steady flow of clean water or saline solution across the wound surface, and soaking involves immersing the wound in clean solution or applying an overhydrated cloth to the wound (Nicks et al., 2010). Proper use of a wound covering is also vital to moist wound management. Many modern wound dressings help maintain a moist environment for nondraining wounds and help remove excess fluid through absorption or evaporation for wounds draining fluid or pus. Wound covering helps maintain a moist healing environment while avoiding maceration and breakdown of adjacent skin, which could lead to infection (Lachenbruch & VanGilder, 2012). An ointment is also an important part of moist wound care. Antibiotic ointments and white petroleum are equally effective at maintaining wound moisture, promoting healing, and preventing infection. For uncomplicated wounds, white petroleum is recommended to prevent the development of resistant organisms (Morton & Phillips, 2012).

Implications

Nurses caring for clients with wounds should implement three methods for keeping a wound moist: cleansing techniques, proper wound covering, and ointment application. These methods of moist wound management promote a healing environment and prevent infections such as cellulitis. Allowing a wound to remain dry or applying a dry wound covering may slow the healing process and increase the risk of infection.

Critical Thinking Application

1. What are the physiological principles that support the need for a moist environment for effective wound healing?
2. How does wound care differ for clients with small acute wounds versus wounds that cover a significant portion of the body, such as a burn?
3. What nursing interventions can you implement when changing a wound dressing and performing irrigation for a toddler who was bitten by a dog?

Prevention

Individuals with a skin wound are at a high risk of developing cellulitis. Good wound care is a vital part of cellulitis prevention. This care includes washing the wound carefully with soap and water and applying an antibiotic cream or ointment daily, covering the wound with a bandage to maintain adequate moisture (see the Evidence-Based Practice feature), and monitoring the wound for signs of infection. Skin protection is also an important part of cellulitis prevention. It is particularly important for individuals at risk for loss of skin integrity or infection, such as individuals with diabetes, HIV, or cancer. Methods of skin protection include keeping the skin moist with lotion, wearing shoes that fit properly, having good nail hygiene, and wearing protective equipment when participating in work or sports (U.S. NLM, 2011; Mayo Clinic, 2012).

SAFETY ALERT

Individuals with diabetes may develop peripheral neuropathy, which decreases sensations in the feet. Therefore, individuals with diabetes are at higher risk for developing skin infections because they do not realize they have been injured. Individuals with diabetes should be taught to check their skin regularly for signs of injury and infection, and superficial skin infections should be treated immediately to prevent complications (Mayo Clinic, 2012).

▶ CLINICAL MANIFESTATIONS

Clients with cellulitis experience a rapid onset and appear ill. Classic signs and symptoms include erythema, edema of the face or infected limb, warmth, and tenderness around the infected site. Other symptoms include fever, chills, malaise, and enlargement and tenderness of regional lymph nodes (also see the Clinical Manifestations and Therapies feature). **Lymphangitis** (inflammation of a lymph vessel) may be present. In some cases, a rapidly progressive lesion can lead to septicemia.

Lifespan and Cultural Considerations

Children with wounds or insect or animal bites often have difficulty not picking at the wounds or scratching bites that itch. Such picking and scratching can increase the risk of developing cellulitis, which is frequently caused by bacteria already present on the skin. Children with wounds or insect bites should be monitored carefully for rapidly progressing inflammation and growing sites of infection, and they should be educated about the risks associated with touching sores. Infants with cellulitis may be more susceptible to sepsis because their immune systems cannot protect them from infection. Facial cellulitis is most common in children under 3 years of age and in adults over age 50. Facial cellulitis may lead to the development of

Clinical Manifestations and Therapies **Cellulitis**

ETIOLOGY	CLINICAL MANIFESTATIONS	CLINICAL THERAPIES
Fever	Tachycardia, tachypnea, elevated temperature, lethargy, chills	▪ Maintain adequate hydration. ▪ Administer antipyretics. ▪ Treat underlying cause.
Skin inflammation	Redness, pain, warmth, edema	▪ Administer antibiotics. ▪ Maintain bed rest. ▪ Provide adequate nutrition to promote healing. ▪ Manage pain using both pharmacologic and non-pharmacologic therapies.
Septicemia	Whole-body inflammation manifested by fever, altered WBC count (may be high or low), and hemodynamic alterations (tachycardia, tachypnea, decreased cardiac output)	▪ Monitor hemodynamic status. ▪ Administer antibiotic therapy. ▪ Provide fluid management. ▪ Provide supportive care based on symptoms. ▪ Measure vital signs frequently.

meningitis, so clients with facial cellulitis should be closely monitored.

Older adults and adults with poor circulation, diabetes, or a weakened immune system may develop cellulitis without loss of skin integrity. These individuals are more likely to develop severe cellulitis with complications than are younger adults with no medical conditions. Older adults and those with poor circulation are also more likely to get recurrent cellulitis. Complications from sinus infections can lead to orbital and periorbital cellulitis, which can lead to loss of vision if not treated aggressively.

Individuals with darker skin tones may have more difficulty identifying the characteristic redness associated with cellulitis. Therefore, presenting symptoms may be focused on fever, pain, and edema of the affected area. Carefully inspect the area to determine the spread of infection.

▶ COLLABORATION

Treatment of cellulitis is aimed at reducing the infection, promoting comfort, and preventing complications such as septicemia. Care is provided in collaboration with family members and other members of the healthcare team. Recovery from an extensive wound that impairs use of an extremity or limb for an extended period of time may require consultation with an occupational or respiratory therapist. If the face is involved, referral to a dentist may be necessary.

Diagnostic Tests

A complete blood count may show an increase in WBCs. Fluid from the affected area may be taken for cultures to identify the causative organism. Blood cultures are taken if the client has a toxic (very ill) appearance.

Client Teaching Infection Control in Clients With Cellulitis

Infection control in clients with cellulitis includes hand hygiene and wound care.

Hand Hygiene

▪ Scrub hands with soap and water for 20 seconds before and after touching the infected area; wash under rings, around cuticles, between fingers, and under fingernails. Dry hands thoroughly after washing.

▪ Do not touch the affected area and then touch another susceptible area such as an uninfected wound or mucus membranes such as the eyes, mouth, or anus

▪ Wash hands before, during, and after handling food, including eating

▪ Wash hands after toileting or changing a child's diaper

▪ Wash hands after touching eyes, nose, or mouth

▪ Wash hands after touching waste products, including household garbage, animal waste, or contaminated materials

Wound Care

▪ Wash the wound with soap and water at least once daily.

▪ Using cleansing techniques, clear away any dead skin or purulent drainage.

▪ Apply an antibiotic ointment and sterile bandage to the wound after washing.

▪ Do not touch the wound unless medically necessary, such as when washing or assessing the wound.

▪ Dispose of all contaminated materials properly.

▪ Monitor the size of the affected area to assess treatment effectiveness.

▪ Keep the wound at a proper moisture; wet or moist wounds heal faster than dry wounds.

Pharmacologic Therapy

Cellulitis on the trunk, limbs, or perianal area is usually treated with oral antibiotics on an outpatient basis. The antibiotic is usually effective against both streptococcal and staphylococcal infections. If the face is involved, antibiotic therapy is administered to prevent serious complications such as periorbital cellulitis. Clients with severe cases or a large affected surface area may be treated with systemic antibiotics and analgesics in the hospital to prevent sepsis. Recovery begins within 48 hours, but therapy should continue for at least 10 days. Untreated cellulitis or cellulitis that does not respond to treatment can lead to osteomyelitis, arthritis, or serious systemic infection.

Nonpharmacologic Therapy

Common nonpharmacologic therapies associated with cellulitis are adequate rest, elevation of the affected area above the heart to reduce swelling, and infection control measures (see the Client Teaching feature). Sterile saline dressings can also be applied to reduce edema and promote drainage.

NURSING PROCESS

The nurse plays an important role in assessing the status of the client and teaching self-care to prevent complications.

Assessment

Assessment centers on recognizing infection, documenting location and related symptoms, and monitoring vital signs. It should also include a health history to determine whether the client has any underlying conditions that may increase susceptibility to cellulitis.

- *Health history.* The health history should include a client interview to determine the cause of any skin wound, such as a cut, bite, or other injury. It is also important to determine whether the wound has been exposed to contaminated water, such as a wound that occurred while swimming in a lake. This may help to determine the causative organism and affect the choice of antibiotic. The health history should also include questions to determine when the client noticed the infection and how rapidly the affected area has spread. During the health history, also assess additional symptoms such as pain, muscle aches, stiffness, and nausea. Note any history of other conditions that may increase susceptibility to infection, such as diabetes, poor circulation, HIV, cancer treatments, and immunosuppression.
- *Physical Examination.* A physical examination should include assessment of vital signs, especially fever, and a thorough assessment of the affected area. The assessment should include observation of redness, swelling, warmth, and size of the affected area. For clients in the hospital, the nurse should assess the affected site frequently (at least every 2 hours), including tracing along the border with a marker so that any change in size can be clearly recognized. In the event of

change, the nurse places a new mark so that future care providers can clearly see if the wound enlarges. Physical assessment may also include observation of lines radiating from the site, indicating involvement of the lymphatic system, and obtaining blood and wound drainage specimens for diagnostic testing.

Diagnosis

Nursing diagnoses that may be appropriate for a client with cellulitis:

- *Impaired Skin Integrity*
- *Acute Pain*
- *Interrupted Family Processes*

(NANDA-I © 2012)

Planning

Planning care for the client with cellulitis is directed at pain management, client teaching related to self-care, and infection resolution without progression to systemic infection. Potential outcomes may include the following:

- Client will report pain of 3 or lower, on a scale of 0 to 10.
- Client will describe situations requiring contact with the provider.
- Client will explain how to take antibiotics and analgesics properly.
- Client will demonstrate understanding of proper wound care and infection control processes.

Implementation

Because of the risk of sepsis, cellulitis is managed carefully. Administer prescribed oral or intravenous antibiotics as scheduled. Supportive care includes warm compresses to the affected area four times daily, elevation of the affected limb, and bed rest. Outpatient follow up is crucial to ensure positive response to therapy.

Advise clients about possible complications, such as abscess formation, and to contact their healthcare provider if any of the following signs develop:

- Spread of the infected area in the 24- to 48-hour period after the start of treatment
- Temperature over 38.3°C (101°F)
- Increased lethargy.

Reinforce to clients and caregivers the importance of compliance with the treatment regimen and the seriousness of the possible complications.

Evaluation

Outcomes developed in collaboration with the client are evaluated to determine the client's progress. The nurse should trace the outer edges of the wound with a black marker to allow better evaluation of changes in the size and area covered by the wound. The provider should be notified if the cellulitis enlarges or spreads.

NURSING CARE PLAN A Client With Cellulitis

Maria Gonzalez is a 74-year-old widow who lives in an assisted living facility in a small town in central Pennsylvania. Her family includes three daughters and two sons who live out of state and a son who lives within 5 miles of Ms. Gonzalez's home. While visiting his mother, he notices a red area on her lower leg and asks her about it. She says it developed earlier today and is very painful. She's been treating it with wet compresses, but that does not seem to be helping much. Her son takes her to the local emergency department, where the nurse admits her to one of the examination rooms.

ASSESSMENT

Ms. Gonzalez speaks Spanish and is able to communicate only minimally in English. Although this arrangement is not ideal, her son acts as an interpreter when necessary. Ms. Gonzalez's history reveals diabetes mellitus with complications of peripheral vascular disease and neuropathy in the right leg, hypertension, coronary artery disease with angina, and cataracts in both eyes. She says she is allergic to penicillin and sulfa drugs. She denies ever having had a similar wound and describes the pain as a 7 on a scale of 0 to 10.

Physical examination of the painful right leg reveals an irregularly shaped, flat area that is red, warm, and painful, extending from just below the knee to mid-shin, and wrapping medially from midline to the back of the leg. The wound measures 6 in. by 5 in. at its widest point. Her vital signs are T 100.8°F oral, P 88 bpm, R 16/min, and BP 122/74 mmHg.

The physician orders laboratory studies that reveal an elevated WBC count. Because of Ms. Gonzalez's age and medical history, the physician orders blood cultures and admits her to the facility for IV antibiotics and monitoring.

DIAGNOSES

- *Impaireded Skin Integrity* related to infectious process
- *Acute Pain* related to the inflammatory process secondary to cellulitis
- *Deficient Knowledge* of the cause of the skin disorder and recommended treatment
- *Anxiety* related to the need to be admitted to the hospital and inability to communicate with staff
- *Impaired Verbal Communication* related to the inability to speak English

(NANDA-I © 2012)

PLANNING

- Skin will heal without evidence of a secondary infection or complication of sepsis.
- Client will obtain relief of pain with the proper use of medications.
- Client will verbalize an understanding of the disease process and participate in the treatment plan.
- Client will describe proper home care, including self-administration of medication after discharge.
- Client anxiety will be reduced after orientation to the hospital environment and speaking with staff members who also speak Spanish.
- Communication will be improved when a Spanish-speaking nurse is assigned and the hospital's translation services are used.

IMPLEMENTATION

- Provide orientation to facility and treatment plan (IV therapy, warm soaks) in Spanish.
- Keep right leg elevated and explain the need to stay in bed.
- Trace outer border of wound with black marker and avoid washing off marks to allow for assessment every 2 hours. Report any increase in size to provider.
- Provide verbal and written instructions (in Spanish) for self-care after discharge, including the following:
  a. Take all antibiotics prescribed until they are gone.
  b. Take medications as prescribed for pain.

  c. Take the antibiotic every 6 hours, even during nighttime hours, for 10 days.
  d. Monitor the size of the wound and notify the physician if there is any increase or if fever returns.
  e. Apply warm, moist heat to wound four times a day.
  f. Wash hands carefully before applying warm, moist compresses.
  g. Reduce activity to bathroom privileges only and keep right leg elevated.
  h. Monitor oral temperature and take two acetaminophen (Tylenol) for temperature higher than 100°F orally.

EVALUATION

Ms. Gonzalez's wound decreased in size over the next 48 hours. She was discharged with a prescription for antibiotics to be taken orally for 10 days and pain medication, although she reported that the pain was almost gone by the time she went home. Her fever subsided within 36 hours of beginning treatment. Ms. Gonzalez will see her physician at the completion of oral antibiotics and says she will call the office sooner if the wound increases in size or her fever returns.

CRITICAL THINKING

1. *Identify barriers to care in this case, including those related to communication. What nursing interventions can be initiated to overcome these barriers?*
2. *What further assessments and interventions might have been indicated if the wound had shown little improvement or the pain had remained severe?*
3. *If Ms. Gonzalez were unable to provide self-care after discharge, what options might the nurse have recommended for her?*

REVIEW Cellulitis

RELATE Link the Concepts and Exemplars

Linking the exemplar of cellulitis with the concept of comfort:

1. What teaching interventions will you provide the client with cellulitis of the leg who is taking a narcotic for pain?
2. What nonpharmacologic interventions will you implement for the client experiencing pain from cellulitis?

Linking the exemplar of cellulitis with the concept of perfusion:

3. How will you assess perfusion in the client with cellulitis of the thigh?
4. What symptoms will you teach the client with cellulitis to report to the provider immediately regarding perfusion?

READY Go to Companion Skills Manual

REFER Go to Pearson Student Nursing Resources
nursing.pearsonhighered.com

- Additional review materials

REFLECT Case Study

Norma James is a 65-year-old widow who lives alone. Although she has lived in the neighborhood for years, she is somewhat socially isolated. She has two adult sons with whom she has limited contact because they live out of state and rarely call. She has only a few individuals she considers friends; she does not particularly like many people and prefers the company of her six cats.

Ms. James has a long history of type 2 diabetes mellitus and hypertension. In more recent years, she has been diagnosed with atrial fibrillation. She has multiple physicians and takes multiple medications, including the following:

- Glucotrol, 10 mg, twice a day
- Captopril, 50 mg, twice a day
- Digoxin, 125 mcg, once a day
- Coumadin, 5 mg, once a day.

Ms. James has a known drug allergy to penicillin.

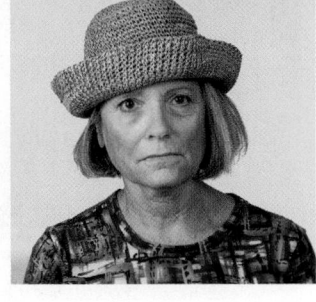

Ms. James does not work; she has very limited savings and relies on Social Security benefits for income. She smokes about half a pack of cigarettes a day and has been a smoker since she was in her 20s. She drinks alcohol "a couple times a year, usually a glass of wine at a special dinner."

She does not drive and relies on her friends, neighbors, or the city bus for transportation. She lives near a grocery store and prides herself on being able to get most things she needs without assistance. She spends most of her time alone at home and occupies herself by watching television, reading, and doing crossword and jigsaw puzzles.

Ms. James noticed a small, tender area on her ankle yesterday and, remembering what the cashier at the convenience store told her, decided to apply butter to the wound.

1. What factors in Ms. James's history put her at risk for cellulitis?
2. What do you suspect the outcome of applying butter to this wound may be?
3. What client teaching would you provide Ms. James?

EXEMPLAR 9.2   **Conjunctivitis**

EXEMPLAR KEY TERMS

Conjunctivitis, 565
Entropion, 567
Photophobia, 567
Trachoma, 567
Uveitis, 567

EXEMPLAR LEARNING OUTCOMES

After reading about this exemplar, you will be able to:

1. Describe the pathophysiology, etiology, clinical manifestations, and direct and indirect causes of conjunctivitis.
2. Identify risk factors and prevention methods associated with conjunctivitis.
3. Illustrate the nursing process in providing culturally competent care across the life span for individuals with conjunctivitis.
4. Formulate priority nursing diagnoses appropriate for an individual with conjunctivitis.
5. Summarize therapies used by interdisciplinary teams in the collaborative care of an individual with conjunctivitis.
6. Plan evidence-based care for an individual with conjunctivitis and the family in collaboration with other members of the healthcare team.
7. Evaluate expected outcomes for an individual with conjunctivitis.

▶ OVERVIEW

The conjunctiva—the thin, transparent membrane that covers the anterior surface of the eye and lines the inner surfaces of the eyelids—is vulnerable to inflammation and infection because of its constant exposure to the environment. **Conjunctivitis** (inflammation of the conjunctiva) is the most common eye disease. It can be caused by bacteria and viruses that are transmitted to the eye by direct contact (e.g., hands, tissues, and towels). Allergens, chemical irritants, and exposure to radiant energy, such as ultraviolet light from the sun or tanning devices, can also lead to this common condition. Its severity can range from mild irritation with redness and tearing to conjunctival edema, hemorrhage, or a severe necrotizing process with tissue destruction.

All neonates born in the United States receive prophylactic treatment to prevent conjunctivitis. By federal law, all infants are given prophylactic eye treatment soon after delivery. The nurse is responsible for administering this eye ointment. Erythromycin is the most common ointment used, but penicillin, tetracycline, or povidone-iodine ointments may also be used.

Sometimes an infant develops chemical conjunctivitis due to the prophylactic eye ointment. A chemical reaction should be considered as a possible cause when conjunctivitis develops within 24–48 hours after instillation of this medication.

▶ PATHOPHYSIOLOGY AND ETIOLOGY

There are several types of conjunctivitis, depending on the cause of inflammation. Bacteria, viruses, allergies, trauma, or irritants cause the conjunctiva to become edematous, inflamed, and reddened, with a yellow or white discharge (**Figure 9–11 ●**). Parents commonly refer to all conjunctivitis as "pink eye."

Conjunctivitis in an infant under 30 days of age is called *ophthalmia neonatorum*. These infections are usually acquired from the mother during vaginal delivery as a result of contact with infected vaginal discharge containing bacterial organisms such as *Chlamydia trachomatis* and *Neisseria gonorrhoeae*. Contact with genital secretions infected with *Gonococcus* species can cause

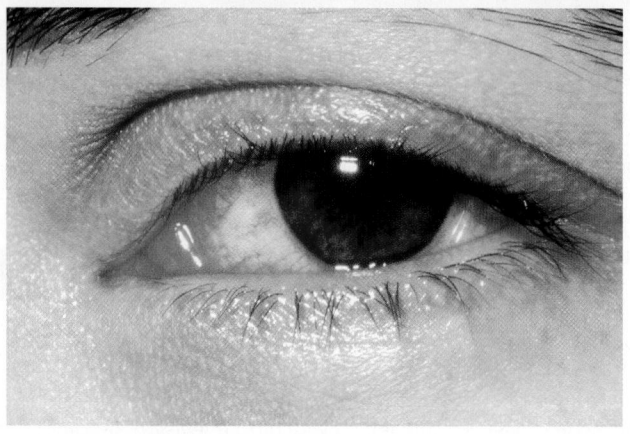

Figure 9–11 ● Acute conjunctivitis. The major difference between bacterial and viral conjunctivitis is that bacterial conjunctivitis has a purulent discharge that may result in crusting, whereas the discharge from viral conjunctivitis is serous (watery). Allergic conjunctivitis produces watery to thick drainage and is characterized by itching.
Source: © Medical-on-Line/Alamy.

gonococcal conjunctivitis, a medical emergency that can lead to corneal perforation. In infants who have frequent tearing and mattering (eyelid discharge that has formed a crust) on awakening, a plugged lacrimal duct may be mimicking conjunctivitis.

Bacterial conjunctivitis is common in older children. It is characterized by edema of the eyelid, reddened conjunctiva, and enlarged preauricular lymph glands. Mucopurulent discharge causes matting and makes the eyes difficult to open upon awakening. Older children with conjunctivitis complain of itching or burning, mild photophobia, and a feeling of scratching under the lids.

Etiology

Redness of the eye may result from various conditions (see **Table 9–10** ●), so do not assume that redness always signals conjunctivitis. Common bacteria that cause conjunctivitis include *Staphylococcus aureus*, *Haemophilus* species, *Streptococcus pneumoniae*, and *Pseudomonas aeruginosa* (CDC, 2012a). Hand-to-eye contact causes most cases. The disease can spread rapidly when groups of youth spend time together, such as young children and adolescents in schools and child care centers and college students in dormitories or on sports teams. The infection can be bilateral but is more commonly unilateral.

Viruses can cause other infections in newborns and children. Viral conjunctivitis is commonly bilateral. Adenovirus is a common cause and spreads hand-to-eye from respiratory adenovirus infection.

Herpes simplex virus (HSV) can also cause infections, either by transfer to a neonate during birth from a mother with herpes infection, or by contact of infants or children of any age with an infected individual. Ophthalmic herpes infection is often accompanied by characteristic vesicular lesions on the skin of the face. A culture of the lesion is performed for diagnosis, and any accompanying conjunctivitis is assumed to be caused by herpes virus. The infection caused by HSV needs prompt and vigorous treatment to prevent eye injury or blindness, which can occur in children with recurrent herpes virus infections as a result of antibody reaction to the viral antigen. Herpes virus infections commonly recur, so periodic treatment and sometime prophylaxis may be needed.

Allergic conjunctivitis is a common cause of eye discomfort (Bielory & Friedlaender, 2008). When conjunctivitis is caused by an allergy, the client complains of intense itching. Examination reveals reddened eyes with watery discharge and conjunctivae with a "cobblestone" appearance. The eyes may also appear edematous.

Risk Factors

Clients who wear contact lenses, especially extended-wear lenses, are at higher risk for conjunctivitis. Others at risk include young children in school and day care settings and clients with compromised immune response. The most common occurrence of viral conjunctivitis is seen in children with viral upper respiratory infections.

Prevention

Bacterial and viral conjunctivitis is highly contagious; therefore infection control strategies are vital to the prevention of conjunctivitis. For individuals who are infected, transmission to others can be decreased by good hand washing techniques, avoiding touching the eyes, washing discharge from the eyes several times daily, washing linens frequently, not sharing towels or other objects that have touched the eyes, and not sharing eye drops dispensers between infected and uninfected eyes. For an individual who is around someone with conjunctivitis, prevention techniques include thorough hand washing, especially

TABLE 9–10	Possible Causes of Acute Red Eye			
	ACUTE CONJUNCTIVITIS	**CORNEAL TRAUMA OR INFECTION**	**ACUTE UVEITIS**	**ACUTE ANGLE-CLOSURE GLAUCOMA**
INCIDENCE	Very common	Common	Common	Rare
PAIN	Mild	Moderate to severe	Moderate	Severe
VISION	Normal	Blurred	Blurred	Markedly blurred
DISCHARGE	May be copious	Watery, may be purulent	None	None
CONJUNCTIVAL ERYTHEMA	Diffuse	Primarily around cornea	Primarily around cornea	Primarily around cornea
CORNEA	Clear	Depends on cause	Usually clear	Cloudy
PUPILS	Normal size, response to light	Normal size, response to light	Small, minimal response to light	Moderately dilated, fixed

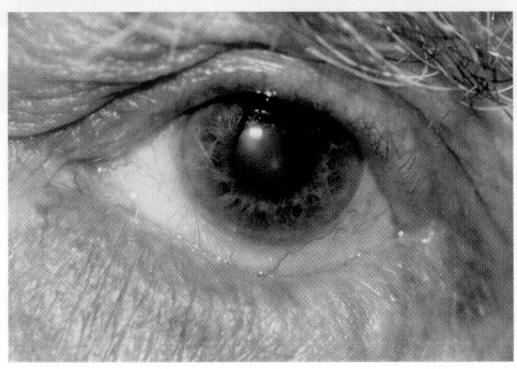

Figure 9–12 ● Entropion.
Source: © SPL/Custom Medical Stock Photo.

after contact with an infected individual, and avoiding sharing with the infected individual any items that touch the face, such as towels, makeup, or pillows (CDC, 2010b).

Although no vaccine is available that protects against all types of conjunctivitis, vaccines are available for conjunctivitis related to rubella, measles, chickenpox, shingles, *Streptococcus pneumoniae* and *Haemophilus influenzae* type b (CDC, 2010b).

▶ CLINICAL MANIFESTATIONS

Redness and itching of the affected eye are common manifestations of acute conjunctivitis. The client may also complain of a scratchy, burning, or gritty sensation. Although pain is not common, **photophobia** (sensitivity to light) may occur. Tearing and discharge accompany the inflammatory process. The discharge may be watery, purulent, or mucoid, depending on the cause of the conjunctivitis. The client may have associated manifestations, such as pharyngitis, fever, malaise, and swollen preauricular lymph nodes.

Early manifestations of **trachoma** include redness, eyelid edema, tearing, and photophobia. Small conjunctival follicles develop on the upper lids. The inflammation also causes superficial corneal vascularization and infiltration with granulation tissue. Scarring of the conjunctival lining of the lid causes **entropion** (inversion of the eyelid) (**Figure 9–12** ●). The lashes then abrade the cornea, eventually causing ulceration and scarring. The opacity of the scarred cornea results in loss of vision (see Focus on Diversity and Culture feature).

Focus on Diversity and Culture
Trachoma

Trachoma, which is a chronic conjunctivitis caused by *Chlamydia trachomatis*, is endemic in poor, undeveloped countries, especially where there are water shortages, numerous flies, and crowded living conditions (WHO, n.d.). Trachoma is rarely seen in the United States except in Native Americans who live in the Southwest. Trachoma is easily transmitted by through contact with eye discharge from infected individuals (on towels, handkerchiefs, fingers) and through transmission by eye-seeking flies. It is the primary cause of preventable blindness worldwide.

▶ COLLABORATION

Collaboration with an ophthalmologist may be indicated if involvement of the cornea is suspected. A nurse in a pediatric practice who observes a number of a children from a single school or day care setting presenting with conjunctivitis may want to contact the school or day care nurse or health coordinator to discuss increased prevention and student education.

Diagnostic Tests

Accurate diagnosis of conjunctivitis is especially important, because other potentially vision-threatening conditions, such as acute **uveitis** (inflammation of the middle layer of the eye, called the *uvea*) or acute angle-closure glaucoma, can also cause a red eye (see Table 9–10). In most cases, a diagnosis of the cause of conjunctivitis is based on the client's history and presenting symptoms.

In severe cases, diagnostic procedures may include the following:

- *Culture and sensitivity* of exudates to determine presence of an infection and identify the infecting organism. Cultures are taken especially in infants or in cases suspected of being an unusual bacterial illness or involving herpes viruses. A Gram stain of discharge and conjunctival scraping for potential *Chlamydia* or herpes is performed. Cultures, if ordered, should be obtained before the start of treatment.

- *Fluorescein stain* with slit-lamp examination to identify possible corneal ulcerations or abrasions, which appear green with staining.

- *Conjunctival scrapings,* which are examined microscopically or cultured to identify the organisms.

Additional laboratory testing, such as blood counts or antibody titers, may be used to identify underlying infectious or autoimmune processes.

Pharmacologic Therapy

Conjunctivitis is treated with antibiotic, antiviral, or anti-inflammatory drugs as appropriate. Topical anti-infectives, applied as either eyedrops or ointment, may include erythromycin, azithromycin, gentamicin, tobramycin, neomycin, ciprofloxacin, ofloxacin, bacitracin, sulfacetamide sodium, amphotericin B, or trifluridine. The fluoroquinolones (e.g., ciprofloxacin, ofloxacin) are broad spectrum antibiotics that are effective against both gram-positive and gram-negative organisms. For severe infections or cellulitis, anti-infectives may be administered orally, by subconjunctival injection, or by systemic intravenous infusion.(See the Medications feature on pages 558–559.)

Viral infections are usually not treated with pharmacologic therapy, except for herpes simplex infections. Individuals with herpes simplex conjunctivitis should be taught how to look for characteristic herpes simplex lesions and to report all lesions immediately.

SAFETY ALERT
Conjunctivitis due to herpes simplex virus infection can cause scarring of the cornea that leads to a permanent loss of vision. Therefore all HSV eye infections should be treated with antiviral medications (e.g., acyclovir) and infection control techniques to prevent the spread of HSV to others.

Clinical Manifestations and Therapies **Conjunctivitis**

ETIOLOGY	CLINICAL MANIFESTATIONS	THERAPIES
Bacterial conjunctivitis	Redness, purulent drainage, burning/irritation, sore throat, photophobia	<ul><li>Antibiotic eyedrops or ointment</li><li>Soaking eyelids with warm cloth</li><li>Eye irrigation to remove discharge</li><li>Avoiding bright lights</li><li>Infection control techniques</li><li>Cool compresses</li></ul>
Viral conjunctivitis	Redness, serous drainage, burning/irritation, sore throat, photophobia	<ul><li>Antiviral drugs (HSV only)</li><li>Cool compresses</li><li>Avoiding bright lights</li><li>Infection control techniques</li><li>Removing discharge with wet cloth</li></ul>

Ceftriaxone is recommended for gonococcal conjunctivitis in newborns because that particular disease is resistant to penicillin. Chlamydial infections are treated with oral erythromycin or tetracycline. Herpes simplex virus infections of the eye are treated promptly by an ophthalmologist, neonatologist, or others who are trained in this serious disease. Neonatal HSV is treated vigorously with parenteral acyclovir for 14 days (or longer if lumbar puncture reveals central nervous system involvement) and with topical ophthalmic medication (trifluridine, iododeoxyuridine, or vidarabine). Careful total evaluation of the newborn with any type of conjunctivitis is important to show any other signs of infection.

Nonpharmacologic Therapies

Frequent eye irrigations may be ordered to remove the copious purulent discharge associated with bacterial conjunctivitis. Soaking the lids with warm saline compresses before cleansing promotes comfort and facilitates the removal of crusts and exudate in conjunctivitis. Viral conjunctivitis may be treated by use of a warm clean cloth to clean drainage away and by avoidance of bright lights and reading. Cool compresses applied to the eyes helps to relieve the feeling of eye irritation.

■ NURSING PROCESS

The nursing role in treating conjunctivitis is primarily one of education to prevent both the disorder itself and its spread when it does occur. Education is a vital strategy for preventing conjunctivitis. Teach all clients about proper eye care, including the importance of not sharing towels, makeup, or contact lenses, as well as avoiding rubbing or scratching the eyes. Instruct clients to avoid using old eye makeup, which can cause eye infections. Teach contact lens users appropriate care (see the Client Teaching feature).

Assessment

Collect the following data through the health history and physical examination of the client with conjunctivitis:

- **Health history.** Presence of redness, discomfort, tearing, photophobia, and drainage; symptom onset; care measures; use of contact lenses; exposure to "pink eye" or recent travel; allergies; previous history of conjunctivitis; and presence of any chronic diseases.

- **Physical assessment.** Visual acuity; inspect eyelids, conjunctiva, sclera, and cornea; vital signs, including temperature, presence and type of discharge (i.e., serous versus purulent).

Diagnosis

Nursing diagnoses relevant to the plan of care for the client with conjunctivitis may include the following:

- *Risk for Infection*
- *Impaired Comfort*
- *Readiness for Enhanced Knowledge*

(NANDA-I © 2012)

Planning

Goals are created on the basis of each client's needs and may include the following:

- The client will demonstrate proper hand hygiene.
- The client will avoid contaminating unaffected eye or other family members.
- The client will experience no visual complications following recovery.

Client Teaching   Contact Lens Care

- Wash hands thoroughly before handling contact lenses.
- Keep storage case clean.
- Remove lenses before sleep, and clean and store the lenses as recommended by the manufacturer.
- Use cleaning and wetting solutions recommended by an eye care professional or the lens manufacturer. Do not use water or homemade solutions for wetting or cleaning lenses.
- If eye redness, tearing, vision loss, discharge, or pain occurs, remove lenses and contact an eye care professional as soon as possible. Using contact lenses during an eye infection can lead to further damage and interfere with healing.
- Do not share contact lenses or allow another individual to "try on" your lenses.

Implementation

Nursing care of the client with conjunctivitis focuses primarily on preventing complications or spread of infection to the other eye or to other individuals in close contact with the client. Individualize care on the basis of specific needs of the client.

Prevent Infection

Acute conjunctivitis is highly contagious. While most clients experience no more than discomfort from the disease, the infection carries a risk for scarring and damage to the delicate cornea of the eye. Preventing the spread of this infection is a vital nursing role.

When conjunctivitis is diagnosed in an infant in the neonatal intensive care unit, the infant is isolated to prevent the spread of the disease to other infants. Typically, however, clients with conjunctivitis are managed in the community, where effective teaching for home care is required to prevent transmission of infection. Bacterial infectious conjunctivitis is extremely contagious.

The nurse can take the following steps to help prevent infection:

- Teach the client to wash hands thoroughly before and after instilling eye medications. Hand washing is the single most important means of preventing transmission of infection.
- Instruct the client to avoid touching or rubbing the eyes to reduce the risk of corneal trauma and spreading the infection. Advise the client to use a new, clean, cotton-tipped swab or cotton ball for cleaning each eye, to prevent cross-contamination.
- Advise the client to avoid sharing towels.
- Teach the client how to instill prescribed eyedrops as ordered. Prescribed medications reduce inflammation and eliminate infection.
- Discuss the importance of avoiding contact lens use until the infection has cleared; discuss the importance of completing the prescribed treatment.

- Tell parents of an infected child that no child should return to child care or school until before taking an antibiotic for 24 hours. Put mittens on a young child to prevent rubbing the eyes.

Promote Comfort

Nursing interventions to promote comfort in clients with conjunctivitis include gently washing drainage from the eyes with a warm cloth; applying a cool compress to reduce itching, burning or other discomforts; and administering pain medications and anti-infective agents as prescribed. If photophobia accompanies conjunctivitis, the nurse can recommend that the client avoid high-acuity activities and use dark sunglasses with UV protection when outdoors or in bright light.

Community-Based Care

Clients with conjunctivitis typically are managed in the community, so they need effective teaching for home care. The nurse should emphasize to the family ways to prevent transmission of infection. If the client is unable to administer eye medications, the nurse should involve the family in teaching, including the following topics:

- Safety and medical asepsis when cleansing the eye
- Instillation of prescribed eyedrops and ointments
- Comfort measures such as reducing lighting intensity and wearing sunglasses
- Avoidance of activities such as excessive reading while the eye is inflamed.

Evaluation

Clients are evaluated on the basis of the outcomes created during the planning process. Resolution of the infection is indicated by return of conjunctiva to a normal white color, absence of drainage, and elimination of symptoms.

REVIEW Conjunctivitis

RELATE Link the Concepts and Exemplars

Linking the exemplar of conjunctivitis with the concept of development:

1. What strategies can you use to stop eye rubbing in children with conjunctivitis who are in different developmental stages?
2. What cognitive developmental issues will the nurse anticipate for a child with recurrent conjunctivitis?

Linking the exemplar of conjunctivitis with the concept of health, wellness, and illness:

3. What strategies could the school nurse teach students to prevent conjunctivitis?
4. When teaching infant care to a group of new parents, what important strategy will you demonstrate to reduce the risk of conjunctivitis?

READY Go to Companion Skills Manual

REFER Go to Pearson Student Nursing Resources
nursing.pearsonhighered.com

- Additional review materials

REFLECT Case Study

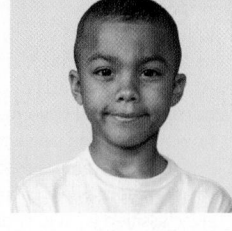

Marcus Young is a typical 6-year-old boy who is enrolled in first grade. He likes his teacher at school and has many friends. He has a stable home life and is close to his parents, Angie and Steve, and his sister, Kelsey. He loves to read and to go to the park and play on the playground equipment. He is very interested in sports and wants to play football and baseball someday. He takes piano lessons but is not interested in this activity at all.

Marcus is normally healthy, is up-to-date on his immunizations, and sees a dentist every 6 months. His mother has brought him to the clinic today because she noticed a white, milky discharge in both eyes this morning, and she says that his eyes were crusted shut when he first woke up. He has had a cold for the past 3 days, with a low-grade fever, rhinorrhea, productive cough, and mild lethargy. You examine the boy's eyes and determine that he has viral conjunctivitis.

1. What client teaching will you provide this family to prevent others from contracting this infection?
2. What teaching will you provide to Mrs. Young regarding how to care for Marcus's conjunctivitis?
3. Develop a nursing plan of care for Marcus.

EXEMPLAR 9.3 Influenza

EXEMPLAR KEY TERMS

Antigenic drift, 570
Antigenic shift, 570
Atelectasis, 574
Avian influenza, 570
Coryza, 570
Epidemic, 570
H1N1 influenza, 570
Influenza, 570
Malaise, 570
Pandemic, 570
Rhinorrhea, 571

EXEMPLAR LEARNING OUTCOMES

After reading about this exemplar, you will be able to:

1. Describe the pathophysiology, etiology, clinical manifestations, and direct and indirect causes of influenza.

2. Identify risk factors and prevention methods associated with influenza.

3. Illustrate the nursing process in providing culturally competent care across the life span for individuals with influenza.

4. Formulate priority nursing diagnoses appropriate for an individual with influenza.

5. Summarize therapies used by interdisciplinary teams in the collaborative care of an individual with influenza.

6. Plan evidence-based care for an individual with influenza and the family in collaboration with other members of the healthcare team.

7. Evaluate expected outcomes for an individual with influenza.

▶ OVERVIEW

Influenza, or "the flu," is a highly contagious, viral respiratory disease characterized by **coryza** (inflammation of the mucous membranes lining the nose, usually associated with nasal discharge), fever, cough, and systemic symptoms, such as headache and **malaise** (a vague feeling of physical discomfort). Influenza tends to be mild and self-limited in healthy adults. Children under the age of 5, older adults, those with compromised immune systems, pregnant women, and people with chronic heart or pulmonary disease, however, have a high incidence of complications (e.g., pneumonia) and a higher risk for mortality related to the disease and its complications (CDC, 2012h).

Influenza usually occurs as an **epidemic** (widespread outbreak of an infectious disease) or a **pandemic** (global epidemic), although sporadic cases do occur. Localized outbreaks of influenza usually occur approximately every 1 to 3 years. The most recent pandemic incidence of influenza occurred in 2009 with the outbreak of H1N1. **H1N1 influenza** (popularly but incorrectly known as "swine flu") is a form of the virus that consists of avian genes, human genes, and genes from flu viruses typically found in pigs from Asia and Europe. H1N1, like all flu viruses, spreads from human to human via airborne droplets (CDC, 2009a).

Avian influenza (bird influenza) has also raised concerns about a potential future pandemic. The avian flu virus have demonstrated limited ability to spread between humans; however, the possibility that it will mutate to allow wider individual-to-individual spread is a concern. This viral strain has a mortality rate of greater than 50% in people who have been infected as a result of close association with infected birds. (See **Box 9–4** ● for more information about avian influenza.)

Box 9–4 Focus on Influenza and Its Potential for Pandemic

Influenza viruses are common in nature and found in wild birds, such as ducks and shore birds, and in some animals, such as pigs. Although wild birds and animals carry the virus, they usually are not harmed by it. Movement of the virus into domesticated animals, however, can be devastating to that animal population.

Three major strains of the virus have been identified as influenza A virus, influenza B virus, and influenza C virus. Type A influenza viruses are subclassified by two proteins found on the surface of the virus: hemagglutinin (HA) and neuraminidase (NA). HA allows the virus to attach to a cell and initiate an infection, whereas NA allows the virus to exit the host cell after replicating. Currently, only three known subtypes of influenza A (H1N1, H1N2, and H3N2) are circulating among humans. The H5N1 virus, commonly called avian influenza, is particularly virulent and is spread by migratory birds. Currently, it is not known to be spread from human to human. However, the H5N1 virus raise fears of a potential human pandemic in the event of individual-to-individual transmission.

Influenza viruses are very changeable, undergoing small, continuous changes as well as occasional large and abrupt changes. **Antigenic drift** is the term for small changes that occur continuously as a virus makes copies of itself. These changes help a virus elude the immune system and necessitate the production of new vaccines every year. Sudden, dramatic changes occur when two different strains of influenza virus (e.g., avian influenza and human influenza) infect the same cell and exchange genetic material. These changes, called **antigenic shift**, create a new subtype of a virus to which people have little or no immunity.

On April 29, 2009, the World Health Organization raised its Influenza Pandemic Alert from Phase 4 to Phase 5 (indicating individual-to-individual contact of the virus in at least two countries of the same region) based on reported instances of H1N1 flu from around the world. By the next week, 23 countries had reported 1,490 cases of H1N1 flu. It is important to note that the cases reported probably represent the most seriously ill people; milder infections may not be reflected in reported numbers. Early symptoms of H1N1 flu include runny nose, fever, cough, headache, muscle and joint pain, and, in some cases, gastrointestinal symptoms, such as diarrhea (WHO, 2009a). The vaccine for H1N1 is now included in the seasonal flu vaccine. An H5N1 vaccine is also available for high-risk clients, but an H5N1 vaccine is not yet available in sufficient quantities should a pandemic occur.

A severe pandemic of any type of influenza could disrupt all aspects of life, not only causing severe illness and death but also overwhelming the healthcare system, impacting social services, and causing significant economic loss. Advance preparations such as those currently being undertaken by the World Health Organization and the United States and other countries can reduce the impact of a pandemic.

Stay Current: Visit the CDC's Web site for updates on flu epidemics at *http://www.cdc.gov/flu/avianflu/h5n1-people.htm*

▶ PATHOPHYSIOLOGY AND ETIOLOGY

The incubation period for influenza is short, only 18–72 hours. The virus infects the respiratory epithelium. It rapidly replicates in infected cells and is released to infect neighboring cells. The resulting inflammation leads to necrosis and shedding of serous and ciliated cells of the respiratory tract, a process that allows extracellular fluid to escape, producing **rhinorrhea** (runny nose). With recovery, serous cells are replaced more rapidly than ciliated cells, and the result is continued cough and coryza. Systemic symptoms of influenza are likely caused by release of inflammatory mediators (Longo et al., 2012) as the influenza infection activates humoral and cell-mediated immune responses.

The respiratory epithelial necrosis caused by influenza increases the risk for secondary bacterial infections. Sinusitis and otitis media are frequent complications of influenza. Tracheobronchitis (inflammation of the trachea and bronchi) may develop. Although tracheobronchitis is not a serious health risk, its manifestations may persist for up to 3 weeks.

Influenza is clearly linked to an increased risk for pneumonia, particularly in young children and older adults. Narrower airways and underdeveloped alveoli increase the risk for pneumonia in young children. Changes in respiratory function associated with aging, including decreased effectiveness of cough and increased residual lung volume (the volume of air remaining in the lung after exhalation), pose little risk in the healthy older adult but greatly increase the risk for pneumonia when associated with influenza. Primary influenza viral pneumonia], while uncommon, is a serious complication that may be fatal. It typically develops within 48 hours of the onset of influenza, often in clients with preexisting heart valve or pulmonary disease. Influenza pneumonia progresses rapidly and can cause hypoxemia and death within a few days. Bacterial pneumonia is more likely to occur in older at-risk adults but also may affect otherwise healthy adults. It usually presents as a relapse of influenza, with a productive cough and evidence of pneumonia on the chest x-ray. (See the exemplar on Pneumonia in this module for more information.) Other respiratory complications of influenza include exacerbation of chronic obstructive pulmonary disease (COPD), chronic bronchitis, or asthma.

Reye syndrome is a rare but potentially fatal complication of influenza. A neurological disease that typically occurs following a viral infection, it is more likely to affect children but also has been identified in older adults. It is associated with administration of aspirin products to children with any viral infection, including influenza. Most often associated with influenza B virus, Reye syndrome develops within 2–3 weeks after the onset of influenza. It has a 30% mortality rate. Hepatic failure and encephalopathy develop rapidly in clients with Reye syndrome.

Other potential complications of influenza, while uncommon, include myositis (inflammation of skeletal muscles), myocarditis (inflammation of the heart muscle), and central nervous system disorders, such as encephalitis and Guillain-Barré syndrome.

Etiology

Influenza virus is transmitted by airborne droplet and direct contact. Influenza A is responsible for most infections and for the most severe outbreaks of influenza. This is primarily a result of its ability to alter its surface antigens, bypassing previously developed immune defenses to the virus. New strains of influenza virus are named according to the strain, geographic origin, and year the strain was identified (e.g., A/Taiwan/89). Surface antigens of the specific virus may be used to further differentiate influenza A viruses. Outbreaks of influenza B virus are generally less extensive and less severe than those caused by influenza A virus. Illness associated with influenza C virus is mild and often goes unrecognized.

Type A influenza viruses are found in birds, pigs, whales, and humans and are believed to have caused four pandemics (in 1918, 1957, 1968, and 2009). Type B influenza viruses are commonly found among humans and often are responsible for influenza outbreaks, but not pandemics. Type C influenza viruses, found in humans, pigs, and dogs, typically cause mild respiratory infections (National Institute of Allergy and Infectious Diseases, 2006).

Risk Factors

People at increased risk of influenza or its complications include infants, young children, and anyone age 50 or older. Residents of nursing homes or other long-term care facilities are at increased risk because of their age as well as the increased risk of exposure from others (residents, visitors, and healthcare providers). Clients with chronic disorders, especially diabetes and cardiac, renal, or pulmonary diseases, are more susceptible as well. Pregnant women, particularly during the second and third trimesters, are also at increased risk of complications. As with any infection, clients with weakened or compromised immune systems, such as those diagnosed with AIDS, receiving treatment for cancer, or taking immunosuppressive medications, are at greatest risk. Healthcare providers who work in a facility where they are likely to be exposed to the influenza virus and day care providers or others who have close contact with infants and young children also face greater risk.

Prevention

Preventing community outbreaks and protecting vulnerable populations (e.g., older adults and people with chronic diseases) are the primary focus for interdisciplinary care related to influenza. Influenza vaccine is recommended for all individuals. The predominant strain of influenza virus varies from year to year. Therefore a new vaccine formulation is prepared yearly, which incorporates antigens of the influenza strains predicted to be the most prevalent for the upcoming flu season (typically the winter months). The vaccine contains egg protein and is not recommended for people who have a severe allergy to eggs or have previously experienced a severe hypersensitivity response to the vaccine. The vaccine is given in the fall, before the annual winter outbreak. Live attenuated vaccine, administered by intranasal spray, is available for healthy people under age 50. The 2012–2013 seasonal flu vaccine, which contained vaccines against two influenza A and one influenza B viruses, was estimated to have a vaccine effectiveness rate of 56%, with effectiveness in the older population (age 65 and older) of only 9% (CDC, 2013b).

Although the CDC has recently changed its recommendations to include all individuals for annual influenza immunization, annual immunization is especially recommended for at-risk clients, including people older than the age of 65, residents of nursing homes, adults and children with chronic cardiopulmonary disorders (e.g., asthma) or chronic metabolic diseases (e.g., diabetes), and healthcare workers who have frequent contact with high-risk clients. Additionally, family members of at-risk clients should be vaccinated to reduce the client's risk of exposure.

Although the vaccine is readily available and inexpensive, not everyone who is at risk will get the vaccine. Many may fear a reaction from the vaccine, even though these vaccines are highly purified and reactions are rare. Approximately 5% of individuals who are vaccinated experience mild symptoms of low-grade fever, malaise, or myalgia for up to 24 hours after vaccination. Serious adverse reactions to influenza vaccine are rare. *Guillain-Barré syndrome*, an acute neurological disorder characterized by muscle weakness and distal sensory loss, has been associated with certain batches of vaccine.

▶ CLINICAL MANIFESTATIONS

Infection with influenza virus produces one of three syndromes:

1. Uncomplicated nasopharyngeal inflammation
2. Viral upper respiratory infection followed by bacterial infection
3. Viral pneumonia.

The onset is rapid; profound malaise may develop in a matter of minutes.

Manifestations of influenza include abrupt onset of chills and fever, malaise, muscle aches, and headache. Respiratory manifestations include cough, sore throat, substernal burning, and coryza. The cough may be severe and either dry and nonproductive or productive. Acute symptoms subside within 2–3 days, although fever may last as long as a week. Along with fatigue and weakness, the cough can persist for days or several weeks.

Individuals who are very young (i.e., less than 5 years old), or older (i.e., older than 65) are at higher risk for developing complications related to influenza infection, including viral and bacterial pneumonia, myositis, Reye syndrome, and exacerbation of chronic respiratory diseases. These complications increase the risk of mortality in these age groups, and mortality increases with age in the older population. Clients should be encouraged to maintain bed rest, drink adequate fluids, and take antiviral and antipyretic medications as prescribed.

Influenza pandemics within the past century have originated in the United States, Asia, and Mexico. Infections that started outside the United States were transported here by infected immigrants and visitors or by U.S. residents who were travelling in infected areas and then returned home. Therefore one aspect of a client history should be a history of recent travel and interaction with potentially infected animals. Testing and documentation of the type of influenza may be necessary to detect emerging strains of influenza virus.

▶ COLLABORATION

Medical treatment of influenza focuses on establishing the diagnosis, providing symptomatic relief, and preventing complications. Collaborative partners include local health departments, hospitals and urgent care centers, primary care and infectious disease clinics, school nurses, and other medical providers.

Diagnostic Tests

The diagnosis of influenza is based on history, clinical findings, and knowledge of an influenza outbreak in the community. A chest x-ray and white blood cell (WBC) count may be done to rule out complications, such as pneumonia. The WBC count is commonly decreased in clients with influenza; bacterial infections usually cause an increased WBC count. If there is a local outbreak of respiratory infections, an influenza rapid diagnostic test can be used to determine whether influenza is the cause of the outbreak or whether influenza is prevalent in a specific client population. Nasal, throat, or nasopharyngeal swabs or washes can be used to obtain specimens for diagnostic testing. Specimens should be obtained as early in the course of disease as possible. Rapid diagnostic tests can produce results in 10–15 minutes (CDC, 2012f).

Pharmacologic Therapy

The CDC (2012b) is currently recommending the use of two antiviral drugs, zanamivir (Relenza) and oseltamivir (Tamiflu), for the treatment and prophylaxis of influenza. These drugs prevent the release of newly formed virus from the surface of infected cells and inhibit the replication of influenza A and B virus (Wilson, Shannon, & Shields, 2013). Zanamivir is given by inhalation, whereas oseltamivir is given orally. Other antiviral drugs that are available include amantadine (Symmetrel), rimantadine (Flumadine), and ribavirin (Virazole).

SAFETY ALERT
Because it is given by inhalation, zanamivir is contraindicated in clients with chronic respiratory conditions such as COPD or asthma.

Antiviral treatment should continue for 5 days; clients with severe illness may be treated longer. For prophylaxis, those who have been exposed to influenza but not vaccinated should receive the vaccine along with the antiviral drug. Antivirals should be administered for 7 days after exposure; in long-term care facilities, treatment should continue for at least 2 weeks or until 1 week after the last case has been identified.

Over-the-counter analgesics, such as aspirin, acetaminophen, and nonsteroidal anti-inflammatory drugs, provide symptomatic relief of fever and muscle ache. However, aspirin should never be given to children because of the risk of Reye syndrome. Antitussives may decrease cough, promoting rest. Antibiotics are not indicated unless secondary bacterial infection occurs.

Nonpharmacologic Therapy

In most clients, influenza is a self-limiting infection. Therefore nonpharmacologic therapy should include bed rest to alleviate fatigue and malaise, boost the immune system, and prevent the spread of infection. Adequate fluid intake in the form of water, juice, warm tea, and soup is essential to prevent dehydration and reduce cough. Hygiene interventions to prevent the spread of infection include adequate hand washing, proper disposal of infected waste materials such as tissues, and covering the nose and mouth when coughing or sneezing.

Clinical Manifestations and Therapies **Influenza**

ETIOLOGY	CLINICAL MANIFESTATION	CLINICAL THERAPIES
Uncomplicated nasopharyngeal inflammation	Dry cough, sore throat, coryza, fever, chills, myalgia, headache, malaise, rhinitis	▪ Rest ▪ Antipyretics ▪ Antivirals ▪ Decongestants ▪ Antitussives at night ▪ Increased fluid intake
Viral upper respiratory infection followed by bacterial infection	Dry cough, fever, myalgia, coryza, sore throat, wheezing, shortness of breath	▪ Rest and fluids ▪ Antivirals ▪ Antibiotics ▪ Antipyretics ▪ Analgesics ▪ Cough expectorant
Viral pneumonia	Fever, productive cough, coryza, myalgia, headache, chest pain, loss of appetite, fatigue, shortness of breath	▪ Rest and fluids ▪ Antivirals ▪ Humidified air ▪ Oxygen
Reye syndrome is linked to children with a virus who are receiving aspirin.	Acute noninflammatory encephalopathy with an altered level of consciousness, hepatic failure with liver biopsy showing fatty metamorphosis, increase in alanine aminotransferase and aspartate aminotransferase, cerebrospinal fluid with white blood cells, and cerebral edema with or without inflammation. Initial symptoms include the following: ▪ Persistent or recurrent vomiting ▪ Listlessness ▪ Personality changes and alteration in level of consciousness ▪ Seizures	▪ Initiate intravenous (IV) therapy with D10/NS. ▪ Maintain patent airway and brain oxygenation. ▪ Monitor cardiorespiratory function; be prepared for potential cardiac arrest. ▪ Assess for hyperventilation to reduce cerebral edema. ▪ Administer osmotic diuretics to reduce intracranial pressure. ▪ Consider possible liver transplantation if extensive liver damage results.
Guillain-Barré syndrome is a possible complication of influenza.	Progressive paralysis of the muscles that may include muscles of respiration.	▪ Provide supportive care to prevent complications such as assistance with activities of daily living, frequent repositioning, and artificial airway with mechanical ventilation to support oxygenation. ▪ Administer IV therapy as ordered. ▪ Provide nasogastric tube to meet nutritional needs if swallowing is impaired. ▪ Provide for rehabilitation after disease recovery to restore baseline functioning.

■ NURSING PROCESS

Stress the importance of yearly influenza vaccination for all clients. Teach about the spread of the disease, including measures to reduce the risk for contracting influenza, such as thorough and timely hand washing and avoiding crowds and people who are ill.

Assessment

Unless there is a known outbreak of influenza in the community, it can be difficult to differentiate the manifestations of influenza from those of other upper respiratory infections. A thorough nursing assessment should provide clues to help determine whether a client's symptoms can be attributed to influenza. The assessment should include the following:

- *Health history.* Known exposure to virus; current symptoms, their onset, and their duration; presence of dyspnea, chest pain, productive cough, and facial pain or pressure in sinus areas; current medications; history of influenza vaccine; chronic diseases, such as heart disease, COPD, or diabetes; and known medication allergies.
- *Physical examination.* General appearance; vital signs, including temperature; skin color; lung sounds; and abdominal exam.

Diagnosis

Nursing diagnoses may differ based on the client's comorbid conditions and any complications that may develop. Suggested nursing diagnoses for clients with influenza include the following:

- *Ineffective Airway Clearance*
- *Ineffective Breathing Pattern*
- *Risk for Infection*
- *Disturbed Sleep Patterns*
- *Fatigue*
- *Deficient Community Health*

(NANDA-I © 2012)

Planning

Outcomes are individualized on the basis of each client's condition and baseline health patterns. Suggested outcomes include the following:

- The client's temperature will remain within normal limits.
- The client will maintain normal fluid balance by increasing fluid intake.
- The client's oxygen saturation will remain within acceptable limits.
- The client will maintain a patent airway.

Implementation

Severe disease or complications of influenza may necessitate hospitalization for respiratory support and management. For these clients, nursing care focuses on maintaining a clear airway, ensuring adequate ventilatory patterns, reducing the risk for infection, and promoting adequate rest.

Maintain Airway Patency

Swelling and congestion of mucous membranes, extracellular fluid exudate, and impaired ciliary action as a result of cell damage increase the risk of impaired airway clearance during influenza. Older adults are at particular risk because of normally reduced ciliary activity and increased lung compliance. The nurse's role in maintaining a patent airway may include the following:

- Assist client to maintain adequate hydration. Assess mucous membranes and skin turgor for evidence of dehydration. Fever and decreased oral fluid intake may lead to dehydration and increased viscosity of secretions. Thick, viscous secretions are more difficult to expectorate.
- Increase the humidity of inspired air with a bedside humidifier. Increasing the water content of inhaled air helps to loosen thick secretions and soothe mucous membranes.

- Teach effective cough techniques. Administer analgesics as ordered. The huff cough (a series of small, low-pressure coughs) is effective to maintain open airways, and it spares energy. Relieving muscle ache increases the ability to cough effectively.

SAFETY ALERT Monitor the effectiveness of the cough and the ability to remove airway secretions. Fatigue and general malaise may impair the ability to cough effectively and mobilize secretions.

Ensure Effective Ventilation

Muscle aches, malaise, and elevated temperature may increase the respiratory rate and alter the depth of respirations, decreasing effective alveolar ventilation. Shallow respirations also increase the risk of **atelectasis** (the collapse of lung tissue affecting all or part of the lung, impacting the exchange of oxygen and carbon dioxide). Interventions that promote respiration and ventilation include:

- Pacing activities to provide for periods of rest. Tachypnea increases the work of breathing, causing fatigue; fatigue, in turn, can further impair ventilation and reduce the effectiveness of coughing.
- Elevating the head of the bed. The upright position improves lung excursion (movement from the resting position) and reduces the work of breathing by lowering the diaphragm, moving abdominal contents downward, creating less resistance to diaphragmatic excursion, and slightly decreasing venous return.

Promote Sleep Hygiene

Airway congestion, malaise, muscle aches, and persistent cough may interfere with rest, increasing fatigue and prolonging recovery. To assist the client in getting enough sleep, the nurse may do the following:

- Assess sleep patterns using subjective and objective information. The client who appears to be sleeping may not be achieving normal sleep patterns because of influenza symptoms. Both subjective and objective data are important to accurately assess sleep.
- Provide antipyretic and analgesic medications to be taken at or shortly before bedtime. These drugs promote comfort by reducing fever and relieving muscle aches.

Prevent Infection

Infection control measures are recommended to prevent individual-to-individual transmission of influenza and to control influenza outbreaks in healthcare facilities.

- Use standard precautions, and encourage all staff and visitors to wash their hands frequently. Hand washing is a primary control measure for infections transmitted via respiratory secretions.
- Instruct clients and visitors to control respiratory secretions by using tissues and to maintain a distance of at least 3 feet from others when coughing or sneezing. Provide masks for clients and visitors who are unable to control secretions. Limiting the spread of aerosolized secretions by covering the nose and mouth and maintaining distance from other people can reduce the spread of the disease to vulnerable populations.

■ Use droplet precautions for clients with suspected or confirmed influenza: private room, masks for caregivers and visitors, and a mask for the client when he or she is being transported within the facility. These measures limit the spread of respiratory secretions.

SAFETY ALERT
If necessary, request a cough suppressant for nighttime use. Cough suppressants are not recommended during the day, because coughing promotes airway clearance. They may, however, be helpful at night to allow rest.

Community-Based Care

Although the symptoms of influenza are distressing, most people with the illness provide self-care and do not contact a healthcare provider. The nurse should encourage appropriate self-care for clients with influenza and discuss the following actions that clients should take related to home care:

■ Increase rest during the acute, febrile phase of the illness.
■ Maintain a liberal fluid intake, even if anorexic.
■ Appropriately use over-the-counter medications for symptom relief.
■ Employ hygiene measures, such as using disposable tissues and frequent hand washing, to reduce spread of the disease.
■ Know the manifestations of potential complications of influenza that should be reported to the primary care provider.

Evaluation

Evaluate the client for airway patency, breathing pattern, oxygenation, and thermoregulation. Consider appropriate alterations to the plan of care if the client is not responding to therapy or develops complications.

REVIEW Influenza

RELATE Link the Concepts and Exemplars

Linking the exemplar of influenza with the concept of oxygenation:

1. Describe the pathophysiology that would cause influenza to diminish the body's ability to meet oxygen demands.

2. Would an older adult with COPD be at any greater risk for complications from influenza? Why, or why not?

Linking the exemplar of influenza with the concept of cognition:

3. Why might the older adult client who develops influenza display alterations in cognition?

4. What caring interventions can the nurse implement to reduce this impact on cognition when working in a long-term care facility with older adults?

READY Go to Companion Skills Manual

REFER Go to Pearson Student Nursing Resources
nursing.pearsonhighered.com

• Additional review materials

REFLECT Case Study

Courtney Hollis is a 34-year-old woman who is married and has three young children ages 6, 3, and 1. She was diagnosed with asthma when she was a child. Ms. Hollis sees her primary care physician with symptoms of a sore throat, fever, malaise, and severe, productive cough. She has been having trouble breathing because of the secretions in her lungs. Her vital signs are temperature 102.1°F oral; pulse 96 bpm; respirations 20/min; and blood pressure 112/78 mmHg. She reports that the flu has been going around her child's school, and her 6-year-old had mild flu symptoms last week. After a client history and physical examination, Ms. Hollis is diagnosed with influenza A and prescribed oseltamivir (Tamiflu).

1. With the task of caring for three young children, Ms. Hollis admits that she will not be able to get bed rest during the day. What client teaching can you provide to help Ms. Hollis rest during the day?

2. On the basis of Ms. Hollis's client and family history, would you recommend that her three children receive the influenza vaccine? Why or why not?

3. What increased risks does Ms. Hollis face because of her history of asthma?

EXEMPLAR 9.4 Otitis Media

EXEMPLAR KEY TERMS
Audiologist, 578
Eustachian tube, 576
Hemotympanum, 577
Labyrinthitis, 576
Middle ear effusion, 576
Myringotomy, 578
Otitis externa, 576
Otitis interna, 576
Otitis media, 576
Otoscope, 578
Tympanic membrane, 576

Tympanocentesis, 579
Tympanogram, 579
Tympanostomy tubes, 579
Vertigo, 577

EXEMPLAR LEARNING OUTCOMES
After reading about this exemplar, you will be able to:

1. Describe the pathophysiology, etiology, clinical manifestations, and direct and indirect causes of otitis media.

2. Identify risk factors and prevention methods associated with otitis media.

3. Illustrate the nursing process in providing culturally compe-tent care across the life span for individuals with otitis media.

4. Formulate priority nursing diagnoses appropriate for an indi-vidual with otitis media.

5. Summarize therapies used by interdisciplinary teams in the collaborative care of an individual with otitis media.

6. Plan evidence-based care for an individual with otitis media and the family in collaboration with other members of the healthcare team.

7. Evaluate expected outcomes for an individual with otitis media.

▶ OVERVIEW

The ear can become infected in any of the three chambers. **Otitis externa** is inflammation of the ear canal (often called *swimmer's ear,* because it is most frequently found in people who spend significant time in the water). **Otitis interna**, also called **labyrinthitis**, is inflammation of the inner ear. **Otitis media**, the topic of this exemplar, is inflammation of the middle ear.

Usually referred to as an "infection," otitis media is one of the most common childhood illnesses and a common reason for office visits, but it is not always accompanied by an actual infection. Although otitis media is very common in children under the age of 5 years, it can occur at any age. Since 2003, an increased number of cases has been observed, and recent changes have been made in recommendations for treatment (American Academy of Pediatrics, Subcommittee on Manage-ment of Acute Otitis Media, 2004; Pelton, 2005).

▶ PATHOPHYSIOLOGY AND ETIOLOGY

The **tympanic membrane** (a thin, tense membrane that sepa-rates the middle ear from the external auditory canal) protects the middle ear from the external environment. However, the **eustachian tube** connects the middle ear with the nasopharynx to help equalize the pressure in the middle ear with the atmo-spheric pressure, and this connecting tube provides a route by which infectious organisms can enter the middle ear from the nose and throat, causing otitis media.

An upper respiratory infection often precedes the develop-ment of otitis media. An estimated 29%-50% of all upper respi-ratory infections lead to acute otitis media (Revai et al., 2007). This infection causes the mucous membranes of the eustachian tube to become edematous. As a result, air that normally flows to the middle ear is blocked, and the air in the middle ear is reabsorbed into the bloodstream. Fluid is pulled from the mucosal lining into the former air space, providing a medium for the rapid growth of pathogens. The tympanic membrane and the fluid behind it become infected.

Types of Otitis Media

The two primary forms of otitis media are serous and acute or suppurative; a chronic form can also develop. Both forms are associated with upper respiratory infection and eustachian tube dysfunction. The eustachian tube is narrow and flat, normally opening only during yawning and swallowing. Allergies or upper respiratory tract infections can cause edema of the tube lining, impairing its function.

SEROUS OTITIS MEDIA   Serous otitis media (also called *oti-tis media with effusion*) occurs when obstruction of the eustachian

tube is prolonged, impairing equalization of air pressure in the middle ear. As the air within the middle ear space is gradually absorbed, the tube obstruction prevents more air from entering the middle ear. The resulting negative pressure in the middle ear causes sterile serous fluid to move from the capillaries into the space, a process that is known as **middle ear effusion**.

ACUTE OTITIS MEDIA   The eustachian tube also provides a route for the entry of pathogens into the normally sterile mid-dle ear, resulting in acute, or suppurative, otitis media. Acute otitis media typically follows an upper respiratory infection. Edema of the eustachian tube impairs drainage of the middle ear, causing mucus and serous fluid to accumulate. This fluid is an excellent environment for the growth of bacteria, which may enter from the oronasopharynx via the eustachian tube.

CHRONIC OTITIS MEDIA   *Chronic otitis media* involves permanent perforation of the tympanic membrane, with or without recurrent pus formation. It usually is the result of recurrent acute otitis media and eustachian tube dysfunction, but it may also result from trauma or other diseases. Changes in the mucosa and bony structures (ossicles) of the middle ear often accompany chronic otitis media.

Marginal perforations, which usually occur in the posterosu-perior portion of the tympanic membrane, are associated with more complications than central perforations. With marginal per-forations, squamous epithelium may migrate from the ear canal into the middle ear, where it begins to desquamate and accumu-late, forming a *cholesteatoma* (a benign and slow-growing cyst or mass filled with epithelial cell debris). The desquamating epithe-lium continues to accumulate until it fills the entire middle ear. It often remains infected, producing collagenases (enzymes) that progressively destroy the ossicles and erode into the inner ear. The inflammatory process impairs the blood supply to the stapes, causing its destruction, which results in conductive hearing loss. Its incidence is highest in children and young adults.

Tympanic membrane perforation can be repaired with a tym-panoplasty to restore sound conduction and the integrity of the middle ear. Delicate surgery may be required to remove a chole-seatoma. If possible, radical mastoidectomy with removal of the tympanic membrane, ossicles, and tumor should be avoided.

Etiology

Approximately 17%–20% of children develop acute otitis media within the first 2 years of life, and one third of children experience six or more episodes before age 7. Peak prevalence of otitis media is between the ages of 6 and 18 months, with a smaller peak at ages 4–5 when entering school. Over 80% of all cases of otitis media occur in children under the age of 6 (Waseem, 2010). Many young children are susceptible to recurrent acute otitis media, which is defined as three or more distinct episodes of acute otitis media within 6 months or four or more episodes within 12 months.

The most common causative organisms of acute otitis media are *Streptococcus pneumoniae*, *Haemophilus influenzae*, and *Moraxella catarrhalis* (Waseem, 2010). Invasion and colonization of the middle ear by bacteria and the resultant migration of WBCs cause pus formation. Accumulated pus can increase middle ear pressure sufficiently to rupture the tympanic membrane. The bacterial infection may also migrate internally, causing mastoiditis, brain abscess, or bacterial meningitis. A more common complication of otitis media is a persistent conductive hearing loss, which typically resolves when the middle ear effusion clears. Viral upper respiratory infection may also predispose the client to acute otitis media, and an upper respiratory infection or allergies (e.g., hay fever) can lead to serous otitis media.

Eustachian tube dysfunction plays a major role in the development of otitis media because fluid cannot drain properly, so infection is allowed to develop. Clients with narrowed or edematous eustachian tubes may also be subject to barotrauma or barotitis media. In these clients, the middle ear cannot adapt to rapid changes in barometric pressure, such as those that occur during air travel or underwater diving.

Risk Factors

Otitis media occurs more frequently among children who attend child care centers, those with allergies, those exposed to tobacco smoke, and those who use pacifiers several hours daily. It is most common during the winter months. Children with conditions such as Down syndrome or cleft lip and palate experience otitis media more often because of eustachian tube dysfunction. To reduce the risk for otitis media, nurses should teach parents to feed infants in an upright position and not to put children to bed with a bottle. Breastfeeding appears to be protective against otitis media. Conditions such as enlarged adenoids or edema from allergic rhinitis can also obstruct the eustachian tube and lead to otitis media. Pacifier use can alter dental structure and promote eustachian tube dysfunction, and it also allows reflux of nasopharyngeal secretions into the middle ear from sucking (Sexton & Natale, 2009). Recurrent otitis media has an increased frequency in children of parents who smoke and in children who attend day care centers (Csakanyi et al., 2012).

Prevention

For infants and children, several practices help reduce the risk of otitis media: breastfeeding for 12 months or more if possible, bottle feeding in the upright position, keeping up to date with immuniza-

Focus on Diversity and Culture

Otitis Media

Native American and Native Alaskan children have a very high rate of otitis media, perhaps related to differences in eustachian tube structure in these individuals (Bluestone & Klein, 2007). These children are seen about three times more frequently in outpatient clinics for otitis media than are other U.S. children (Singleton et al., 2009). Nurses should be alert for the common incidence in these population groups, plan prevention programs, and ensure prompt care and teaching about treatments for families of children affected.

tions, and avoiding air pollution, especially secondhand smoke. Using a small day care or private child care rather than a large day care facility can also decrease the risk of otitis media in children.

▶ CLINICAL MANIFESTATIONS

Typical manifestations of serous otitis media in adults include decreased hearing in the affected ear and complaints of "snapping" or "popping" in the ear. On examination, the tympanic membrane demonstrates decreased mobility and may appear retracted or bulging. Fluid or air bubbles are often visible behind the drum. Severe pressure differences, such as those occurring with barotrauma, may cause acute pain, hemorrhage into the middle ear, rupture of the tympanic membrane, or even rupture of the round window, with sensory hearing loss and severe **vertigo** (a sensation of whirling or rotation). **Hemotympanum** (bleeding into or behind the tympanic membrane, **Figure 9–13** ●) may be observed when examining the ear with an

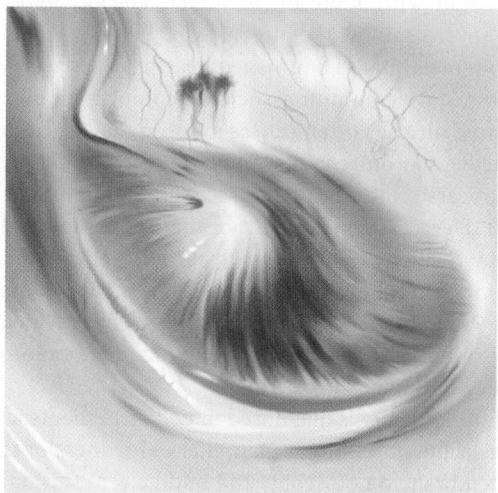

A

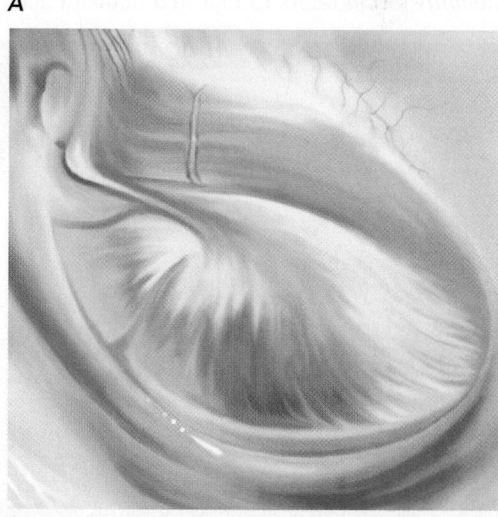

B

Figure 9–13 ● Hemotympanum refers to the presence of blood in the tympanic cavity of the middle ear. This rare condition is characterized by discoloration of the tympanic membrane. *A*, Fresh blood often causes red coloration of the tympanic membrane. *B*, Old blood may produce a black-blue coloration of the tympanic membrane.

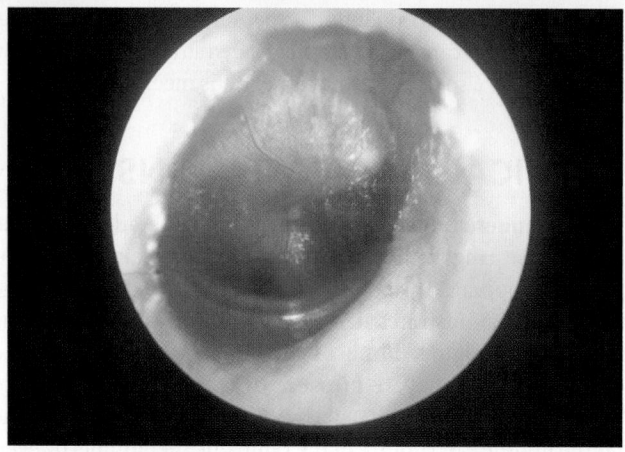

Figure 9–14 ● A red, bulging tympanic membrane of otitis media.
Source: © Medical-on-Line/Alamy.

otoscope (a hand-held instrument with a light and a cone-shaped attachment known as the *ear speculum*).

The client with acute otitis media typically experiences mild to severe pain in the affected ear. The client's temperature is often elevated. Diminished hearing, dizziness, vertigo, and tinnitus are common associated complaints. Pus within the mastoid air cells often causes mastoid tenderness in acute otitis media. On otoscopic examination, the tympanic membrane appears red and inflamed or dull and bulging (**Figure 9–14** ●). Decreased movement of the membrane is demonstrated by tympanometry or air insufflation (blowing air into the ear). Spontaneous rupture of the tympanic membrane (**Figure 9–15** ●) releases a purulent discharge. A **myringotomy** (a surgical incision of the tympanic membrane) may be performed to relieve the pressure.

Acute otitis media is diagnosed in pediatric clients when the child has acute onset of ear pain, marked redness of the tympanic membrane on otoscopy, and middle ear effusion. *Recurrent acute otitis media* refers to repeated bouts of acute otitis

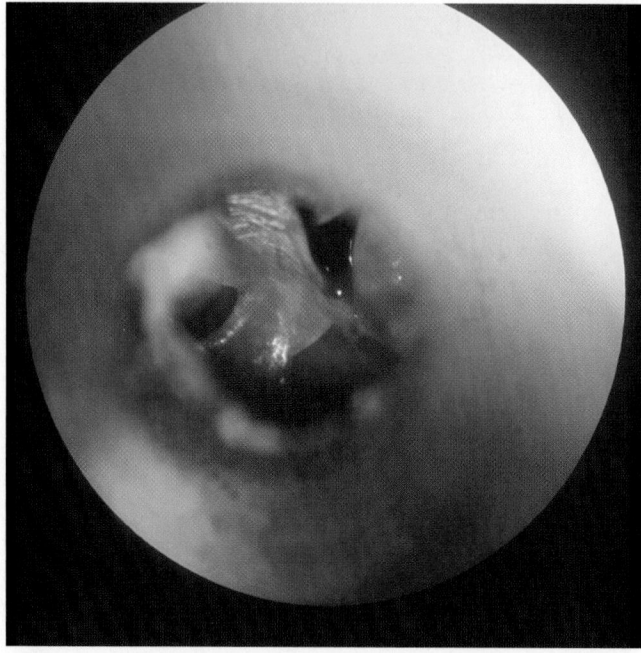

Figure 9–15 ● Perforation of tympanic membrane.
Source: Bo Veisland/Science Source.

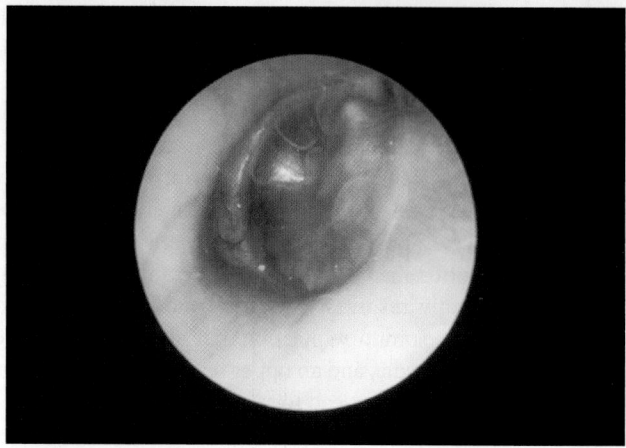

Figure 9–16 ● Otitis media with effusion is noted on otoscopy by fluid line or air bubbles. Pneumatic otoscopy or tympanometry shows a nonmobile tympanic membrane. Note that the light reflex is not in the expected position due to a change in tympanic membrane shape from air bubbles. Where would you expect to see the cone of light?
Source: Southern Illinois University/Getty Images.

media, such as three in 6 months or four in 12 months. *Serous otitis media* is evidenced by fluid in the middle ear without inflammation, as demonstrated in **Figure 9–16** ●. Serous otitis media sometimes becomes chronic (continuing for more than 3 months) and is more commonly associated with hearing loss.

Diarrhea, vomiting, and fever are typical of otitis media. In infants and young children, characteristic behaviors may indicate the presence of otitis media. Pulling at the ear is a sign of ear pain (**Figure 9–17** ●). Irritability and acting out may signal a related hearing impairment. The child with otitis media often awakens crying at night because ear pressure increases when the child is prone or supine.

▶ COLLABORATION

A number of professionals may provide support to a child with recurrent otitis media. Either the nurse or an **audiologist** (a healthcare professional specializing in identifying, diagnosing,

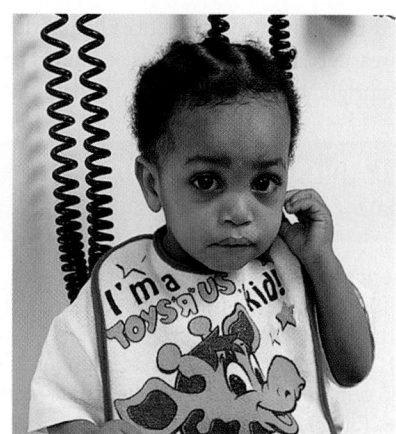

Figure 9–17 ● This young child is pulling at the ear and acting fussy, two important signs of otitis media. Ask the parents about the presence of fever and night awakenings, additional signs that are often observed in children with this condition.

treating, and monitoring disorders of the auditory and vestibular portions of the ear) can conduct a hearing screening. A speech–language pathologist may perform a screening to ensure the child's speech development is age-appropriate. If a child fails a hearing screening, the professional conducting the screening should refer the client to an audiologist for further testing.

Either the nurse, the speech–language pathologist, or the child's classroom teacher can assist the parent with understanding the importance of maintaining verbal communication in the home and reading to the child regularly. If a child does experience hearing or speech loss as a result of recurrent otitis media, the audiologist or speech pathologist can assist the parents and classroom teachers in developing an individual education plan for the child to ameliorate or compensate for any deficit. The audiologist or speech–language pathologist can also assist the parent in accessing any assistive technology the child may require. In some cases, surgery may be required to alleviate pressure in the ear.

The nurse in a pediatrician's office or family practice may collaborate with a child's school nurse (or center director if the child is in day care) about any preventive practices that may need to be emphasized in the child's classroom, such as frequent hand washing, or the need for the child to increase fluid intake or avoid water activities.

Diagnostic Tests

Diagnostic tests that may be conducted in addition to physical examination include the following:

- *Impedance audiometry,* also known as tympanometry, is an accurate diagnostic test for serous otitis media. An audiometer with a sealed probe tip delivers a continuous tone to the tympanic membrane. Compliance of the tympanic membrane and middle ear is measured by a recording of the energy reflected from the membrane surface. With middle ear effusion, compliance is reduced.

- A *complete blood count (CBC)* may be done to assess for an elevated WBC count and increased numbers of immature cells indicative of acute bacterial infection.

- *Tympanocentesis* or *myringotomy* is performed if the tympanic membrane has ruptured. Drainage is cultured to determine the infecting organism.

- *Spectral gradient acoustic reflectometry* measures the condition of the middle ear by introducing a sound and then measuring the response of the tympanic membrane (Windmill & Windmill, 2006). A flat **tympanogram** (a test that provides a graph of the middle ear's ability to transmit sound), indicating absence of normal movement of the tympanic membrane, also suggests otitis media.

- *Culture and sensitivity* may be performed on fluid from the middle ear to determine causative organisms if drainage is noted secondary to rupture of the tympanic membrane. If the tympanic membrane is intact, a tympanocentesis may be done to aspirate some fluid from the middle ear through the tympanic membrane.

- *Audiological testing* may be performed to determine hearing loss if serous otitis media persists for more than 3 months. Children who fail the hearing test should be referred to an audiologist.

Surgery

A myringotomy or tympanocentesis may be performed to relieve excess pressure in the middle ear and prevent spontaneous rupture of the eardrum. To perform a **tympanocentesis**, the physician inserts a 20-gauge spinal needle through the inferior portion of the tympanic membrane, allowing aspiration of fluid and pus from the middle ear to relieve pressure and, if necessary, to obtain a specimen for culture. Myringotomy may be performed to relieve severe pain or when complications of acute otitis media, such as mastoiditis, are present. As soon as the pressure is released, pain subsides and hearing improves.

If infection recurs despite antibiotic treatment for acute otitis media or if serous otitis media continues 4 months or more with persistent hearing loss, myringotomy may be performed, and **tympanostomy tubes** (pressure-equalizing tubes) may be inserted to provide ventilation and drainage of the middle ear during healing. The tube is eventually extruded from the ear, and the tympanic membrane heals. While the tube is in place, it is important to avoid getting any water in the ear canal, because the water may then enter the middle ear space.

Pharmacologic Therapy

Concern in the medical community has grown over the increasing appearance of drug-resistant bacteria as causative agents in otitis media. The American Academy of Pediatrics and the American Academy of Family Physicians joined together to establish recommendations in 2004 (American Academy of Pediatrics, Subcommittee on Management of Acute Otitis Media, 2004). Acute otitis media is now treated with antibiotic therapy for 10 days in children under 6 years of age and for 5–7 days for children 6 years and older. Consistent with current guidelines, in children age 6 months to 2 years with nonsevere illness at presentation and uncertain diagnosis or in children 2 years and older without severe symptoms OR with uncertain diagnosis treatment for acute otitis media is delayed for 48–72 hours after diagnosis.

When an antibiotic is prescribed, the choice of drug depends on the probable organism, ease of administration, cost, previous effectiveness, and any history of allergies. First-line therapy for children is amoxicillin at a dose of 80–90 mg/kg/day. Amoxicillin with clavulanate is a second-line drug. Other available antibiotics include azithromycin, cedfinir, cefpodoxime, ceftriaxone, cefuroximine, clarithromycin, clindamycin, and levofloxacin (Wicker & Mohundro, 2010). Clients who are allergic to penicillin should receive a cephalosporin, trimethoprim-sulfamethoxazole, or macrolides (Waseem, 2010). When the tympanic membrane is intact, topical anesthetic eardrops are sometimes prescribed for several days to provide pain relief.

Acute otitis media in adults is usually treated with antibiotic therapy, especially amoxicillin, trimethoprim-sulfamethoxazole, cefaclor, or azithromycin, for 5–10 days. This course of treatment is long enough to ensure eradication of the infective organism yet short enough to reduce the incidence of bacterial resistance. Analgesics, antipyretics, antihistamines, and local application of heat may provide symptomatic relief. Referral to an audiologist may be necessary if the adult client reports loss of hearing following successful healing of infection.

Complementary and Alternative Therapy Otitis Media

Because many children with otitis media experience ear pain that can disrupt their sleep as well as that of family members, anesthetic eardrops have been used for their analgesic effect on the tympanic membrane. Because some families prefer to use natural remedies for ear pain, a study was conducted to compare Naturopathic Herbal Extract Ear Drops (a naturopathic herbal extract of *Allium sativum*, *Verbascum thapsus*, *Calendula flores*, and *Hypericum perforatum*, lavender, and vitamin E) with a local anesthetic of amethocaine and phenazone. About half of the total of 171 children studied were given the naturopathic pain treatment, the remaining children receiving the anesthetic. Parents rated the children's pain after training with a pain tool. Both treatments were effective in decreasing ear pain over the 3 days of the study. No significant difference was found in the success rates of the two treatments; in fact, the naturopathic agent was as effective as, or even more effective than, the anesthetic at each measurement period. The study concluded that herbal pain control may be very beneficial for treatment of ear pain and can help to decrease the need for antibiotic treatment of otitis media (Sarrell, Cohen, & Kahan, 2003). However, a collective analysis of several studies concluded that insufficient evidence currently exists to describe whether naturopathic treatment is effective for treatment of ear pain in children (Foxlee et al., 2006).

Serous otitis media is not treated with antibiotics, but it is evaluated periodically for the presence of an additional acute otitis media that needs treatment. Children with serous otitis media generally improve within 3 months. Since this type of otitis is more commonly associated with hearing loss and cochlear damage, follow up with audiology is essential. When eustachian tube dysfunction and serous otitis media do not spontaneously resolve, or when they lead to hearing loss, a short course of an anti-inflammatory drug (e.g., oral prednisone for 7 days) is prescribed to reduce mucosal edema of the tube and improve its patency.

Neither decongestants nor antihistamines have been shown to be effective in treating otitis media with or without effusion. Steroids also do not appear to have any long-term beneficial effect.

The *Haemophilus influenzae* type B (Hib) vaccine, which is routinely given to children beginning at 2 months of age, has been influential in reducing the incidence of diseases, such as otitis media, that are caused by *H. influenzae* type B. Another, more recently recommended immunization for pneumococcal disease has also decreased cases of otitis media from that pathogen.

Clinical Manifestations and Therapies Otitis Media

ETIOLOGY	CLINICAL MANIFESTATION	CLINICAL THERAPY
Acute otitis media: Bacterial infection in the middle ear from pathogens transferred from the nasopharynx; most common infectious agents are *Streptococcus pneumoniae*, *Haemophilus influenzae*, and *Moraxella catarrhalis*.	*Behavioral:* Ear pain, pulling at ear, rapid onset, irritability, malaise, and poor feeding	■ Treatment of ear pain with local anesthetic, local herbal pain products, or systemic acetaminophen or ibuprofen
	Examination: Bulging tympanic membrane; air or fluid bubbles present behind tympanic membrane; immobile or poorly mobile tympanic membrane; red tympanic membrane, or other color change (e.g., white, gray, or yellow) as long as bulging is present; and reduced visibility of tympanic membrane landmarks with displaced light reflex	■ Observe child's condition for 48–72 hours; if not improved, treatment with course of antibiotics
Otitis media with effusion: Collection of fluid in the middle ear behind the tympanic membrane, which is not infected with bacteria	*Behavioral:* Difficulty hearing or responding as expected to sounds	■ Symptomatic treatment for pain
	Examination: Signs of acute inflammation NOT present; tympanic membrane retracted or neutral; immobile or partly mobile tympanic membrane; yellow or gray tympanic membrane; opaque or thickened tympanic membrane with visibility of landmarks reduced	■ Careful observation of hearing acuity over several months ■ Speech assessment if loss of hearing acuity occurs ■ Developmental assessment

NURSING PROCESS

Clients with otitis media are commonly treated in outpatient and community settings. The nursing role is primarily one of support and education. Health promotion for otitis media focuses on educating clients about the importance of seeking medical care for prolonged, severe ear pain, with or without drainage, combined with an upper respiratory tract infection. Untreated or repeated attacks of otitis media can progress to a chronic form, to acute mastoiditis, or to eardrum perforation.

Assessment

Collect assessment data through a health history and physical examination. The data collected should include the following:

- *Health history.* Recent upper respiratory infection; presence, intensity, and nature of pain in affected ear; sense of fullness or pressure in the ear; change in hearing; snapping or popping sensation in the affected ear; and presence of vertigo.
- *Physical examination.* Temperature; hearing test; inspect tympanic membrane at each health promotion visit and during examinations for illness; examine the color, transparency, mobility, presence of landmarks, and light reflex; with pediatric clients, ask parents if the child has had a fever, been fussy, or been pulling at the ears; observe for signs of impaired hearing, such as difficulty hearing a whisper or soft sounds.

Physical examination of a young child may be complicated by the child's excessive movement. Parents or other healthcare workers should be enlisted to help hold the child's head steady (**Figure 9–18 ●**). For The nurse should hold the pinna down and back to inspect the auditory canal and tympanic membrane of a child younger than 3 years old. To prevent injury, insert the speculum of the otoscope only 0.25–0.5 in.. To examine adults, pull the pinna up and back to straighten the ear canal. To maximize vision of the ear canal choose the largest diameter speculum that will fit comfortably in the client's ear (Berman & Snyder, 2012). Inspect the tympanic membrane for color, gloss, transparency, mobility, bulging, presence of fluid or blood, perforation, and other abnormalities. A pneumatoscope (an otoscope with a bulb attachment that introduces air into the ear canal) can be used to test mobility of the eardrum (Osborn et al., 2014). Normal tympanic membranes are pearly gray, semitransparent, shiny, and mobile and have a neutral position. Abnormal findings that may indicate otitis media include redness, reduced mobility, presence of fluid or blood, and bulging or retraction of the tympanic membrane. The tympanic membrane is white or yellow in the presence of acute otitis media and otitis media with effusion, whereas an amber-colored tympanic membrane indicates otitis media with effusion (Shaikh et al., 2010).

> **SAFETY ALERT**
> When assessing a client's ears with an otoscope, hold the otoscope with your hand between the otoscope and the client's head, using the client's head to stabilize your hand. This position protects the eardrum and canal from injury if the client moves the head (Berman & Snyder, 2012).

Diagnosis

Nursing diagnoses that may apply to the client with otitis media are the following:

- *Acute Pain*
- *Infection*
- *Risk for Caregiver Role Strain*
- *Deficient Knowledge*
- *Risk for Delayed Growth and Development*
- *Risk for Imbalanced Body Temperature: Hyperthermia*
- *Fatigue*
- *Impaired Verbal Communication*

(NANDA-I © 2012)

Planning

Most clients with otitis media do not require hospitalization; therefore nursing management centers on planning care in the home. Potential outcomes include the following:

- The client or parent will indicate absence of pain.
- The client will be infection-free following the course of treatment.
- Caregivers will manage the child's condition with minimal stress.
- The client or parents will state their understanding of preventive measures.
- The child will have normal hearing.
- The child will have normal motor and language development.

Implementation

Nursing care is individualized based on the diverse needs presented by clients. It focuses on pain management, client and

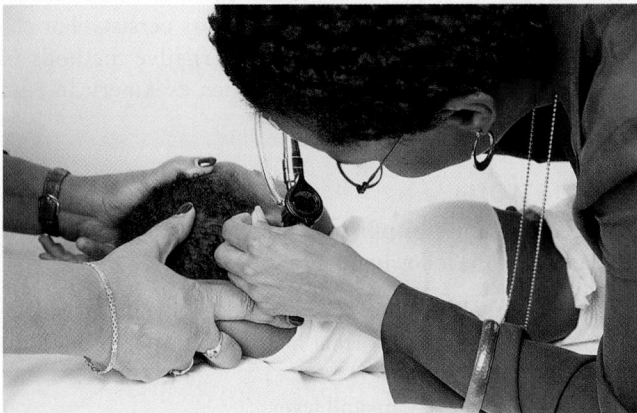

Figure 9–18 ● Parent restraint of a young child during examination of the ear.

family teaching, and preventing recurrence of infection. Screening for potential hearing loss is of particular importance in clients who contract repeated otitis media.

Manage and Control Pain

Tissue edema, effusion of the middle ear, and the resulting inflammatory response can affect the pain-sensitive tissues of the middle ear in otitis media, causing acute discomfort. This discomfort is increased by pressure changes, such as those that occur during air travel or underwater diving. A nurse working with a client who reports pain associated with otitis media should:

- Assess the client's pain for severity, quality, and location. A thorough assessment is important to determine the source of the pain. The pain of otitis media, unlike that of external otitis, is not aggravated by movement of the external ear.
- Encourage the client to use mild analgesics, such as ibuprofen or acetaminophen, as needed to relieve pain and fever. Ibuprofen also has anti-inflammatory properties that may help to relieve inflammation of the ear.
- Advise the client to apply heat to the affected side unless contraindicated. Heat dilates blood vessels, promoting the reabsorption of fluid and reducing swelling.
- Instruct the client to avoid air travel, rapid changes in elevation, or diving. A rapid change in barometric pressure can increase the client's pain significantly.
- Instruct the client to promptly report pain to the primary care provider. Pain that subsides abruptly may indicate spontaneous perforation of the tympanic membrane, which relieves the pressure within the middle ear.

Support Caregivers

The chronic nature of otitis media in some children can create many problems for the family. Parents often become frustrated and disillusioned because the healthcare system is unable to cure the child, and they may fear a permanent hearing impairment. Nursing interventions include the following:

- Reassure parents that as the child grows older, the recurrent infections will eventually cease.
- Teach pain relief techniques, such as correct administration of eardrops, oral administration of acetaminophen, and positioning the baby or child with the head slightly elevated, a position that often decreases pressure and pain.

Provide Age-Appropriate Education to Clients and Family Members

Both the client who has otitis media and the family benefit from learning about the disorder, its causes and prevention, and any specific treatment that is recommended or prescribed. Client teaching typically includes the following:

- Discuss with the client and family the antibiotic therapy (if prescribed) and potential side effects, the importance of completing all ordered doses (if prescribed), the follow up examinations in 2–4 weeks, and, if ventilation tubes are in

place, the importance of avoiding swimming, diving, or submerging the head while bathing.
- Emphasize preventive measures. Exposure to secondhand smoke in the home increases the incidence of otitis media in children; therefore parents who smoke should be encouraged to avoid smoking near the child or in the home. Use of wood burning stoves should also be avoided when possible. Breastfeeding provides some protection from the disease. Pacifier use may increase the incidence of otitis media and should be avoided in the infant with prior infections (Sexton & Natale, 2009).
- If surgical intervention is necessary, teach the client and family members about the surgery and postoperative care. Provide instruction about any special postoperative precautions, such as avoidance of water in the ear canals and of sudden changes in air pressure.
- Inform parents that the child who is having tympanostomy tubes inserted is generally treated in a day surgery setting. Teach the child and parents about what to expect, and provide instructions for safe care upon discharge.
- Explain to parents and clients the problem of developing resistant strains of bacteria. Parents may not understand why the child with a possible infection is not given antibiotics. New research indicates that most children improve after 48–72 hours even without antibiotics, and that overuse of antibiotics contributes to drug resistance.
- Explain to parents of children with serous otitis media that antibiotics, steroids, and antihistamines/decongestants have not been effective and that most children improve in 3 months without medication. Assure parents that if the effusion continues beyond that time, the child will be tested for hearing acuity and, if indicated, for speech development.
- Encourage parents to bring the child back for care if the condition worsens or has not improved in the recommended time.

Facilitate Communication

Nursing interventions for children with decreased hearing or hearing loss related to otitis media include encouraging parents to read and talk frequently with children with decreased hearing to prevent delayed development. Perform hearing and language assessments at regular intervals, and recommend an auditory specialist if hearing loss persists. For clients with permanent hearing loss, alternative methods of communication should be pursued, such as American Sign Language.

Evaluation

Expected outcomes of nursing care for the child with otitis media include the following:

- The child returns to normal sleep and feeding patterns.
- The child maintains normal hearing and speech development.
- The child is free of pain and fever.
- The parents indicate adequate understanding of the treatment regimen.

NURSING CARE PLAN A Client With Otitis Media

Melinda Jeffries is a 2-year-old African American toddler who lives with her mother, father, and 6-year-old sister. Melinda attends child care every day, because both parents work outside the home. The child care center is a large building with multiple classrooms for different age groups. There are approximately 15–20 students in her class on a given day. Melinda's recurrent diagnoses of otitis media include four infections over the course of the winter thus far.

Ms. Jeffries has brought Melinda to the pediatric nurse practitioner's office today because she has an axillary temperature of 102.6°F, has been pulling at her ear, and was awake most of last night crying in pain. The nurse practitioner diagnoses a left acute otitis media, prescribes amoxicillin and corticosteroid eardrops, and instructs the mother to administer ibuprofen every 6 hours for pain and fever control. Ms. Jeffries is concerned that these recurrent ear infections will result in hearing loss and asks about insertion of tubes to prevent further infections. The nurse practitioner explains that the occurrence of ear infections tends to be highest during the winter months; she recommends waiting to see if Melinda improves when the weather gets warmer. Ms. Jeffries agrees, saying that she noticed that pattern with her older child when she was this age.

ASSESSMENT

Melinda is admitted to the provider's office by Sarah McKinney, RN. In her assessment, she finds Melinda irritable and less tolerant of separation from her mother than usual. Examination finds an orange-yellow tympanic membrane with decreased motility, warm dry skin, and vital signs including a temperature 99.8°F axillary, pulse 128 bpm, and respirations 26/min; blood pressure is deferred at this time because of Melinda's age and general good health. Neurological, respiratory, cardiovascular, and abdominal assessments are essentially normal. Auditory examination reveals a slight decrease in hearing, most likely caused by the collection of fluid in the middle ear. Further testing will need to be done when Melinda is asymptomatic.

DIAGNOSES

- *Acute Pain* related to tympanic pressure secondary to fluid accumulation in the middle ear
- *Deficient Knowledge* related to lack of information regarding indications for myringotomy and administration of eardrops
- *Risk for Deficient Fluid Volume* related to hyperthermia
- *Impaired Verbal Communication* related to decreased hearing

(NANDA-I © 2012)

PLANNING

Goals for Melinda's care include:
- Melinda will demonstrate improved hearing with resolution of otitis media.
- Melinda will demonstrate reduced level of pain and increased ability to sleep at night.
- Melinda's mother will be able to describe indications for performing myringotomy and to demonstrate administration of eardrops.
- Melinda will take in fluid adequate to maintain hydration.

IMPLEMENTATION

- Schedule a return visit to retest hearing in 2–3 weeks.
- Encourage Ms. Jeffries to call the office if Melinda shows signs of discomfort uncontrolled by ibuprofen.
- Teach Ms. Jeffries nonpharmacologic pain relief measures, such as application of heat and elevation of the head of the bed at night to promote drainage from the middle ear via the eustachian tube.
- Instruct Ms. Jeffries on the importance of administering the entire dispensed quantity of antibiotics, calling the office if a rash or

other sign of allergic reaction occurs, and encouraging fluid intake.
- Demonstrate the technique for administering eardrops, and then have Ms. Jeffries provide a return demonstration.
- Provide verbal and written instructions about ear care, including scheduled follow up examinations.
- Teach Ms. Jeffries about potential complications, actions to take in response, and when to call the provider.

EVALUATION

Melinda returns in 2 weeks and is found to be infection-free. Her tympanic membrane is normal in appearance, and she is her usual happy self. Hearing tests reveal that her hearing is within the normal range, and consultation with an audiologist is not indicated.

CRITICAL THINKING

1. What are the indications for performance of a myringotomy? Why was this client not a candidate?
2. What other medications might have been prescribed to treat Melinda's ear infection?
3. Had Melinda's hearing not improved after resolution of the infection, what actions could the audiologist have recommended to improve her hearing?
4. Develop a plan of care related to caregiver role strain secondary to Melinda's inability to sleep because of pain.

REVIEW Otitis Media

RELATE Link the Concepts and Exemplars

Linking the exemplar of otitis media with the concept of evidence-based practice:

1. What peer-reviewed research can you find supporting the evidence-based practice of not prescribing antibiotics routinely for all diagnosed otitis media?

2. On the basis of your findings, how would knowledge of this research affect your practice when caring for clients with otitis media?

Linking the exemplar of otitis media with the concept of health policy:

3. How has health policy changed in the treatment of otitis media?

4. Does this change in policy seem reasonable? Why or why not?

READY Go to Companion Skills Manual

REFER Go to Pearson Student Nursing Resources
nursing.pearsonhighered.com

- Additional review material

REFLECT Case Study

Ryan Riley is the 1-year-old son of Jessica Riley. They live in a one-bedroom apartment with Ms. Riley's boyfriend, Casey Miller. Ryan has a history of hospital admission for dehydration, respiratory syncytial virus, and failure to thrive. Because he was found to be underweight and undernourished, social services made arrangements for him to attend Peanut Butter and Jelly day care during the day and to stay with his grandmother, Evelyn Sykes, in the evenings when his mother is working. He is seen for his 12-month immunizations and well-child exam, and his weight is 20 pounds, demonstrating good progress.

Fifteen-month-old Ryan has been running a fever and has a great deal of nasal drainage and congestion. He does not feel well at all. Worried about how ill he was last time he was sick, Ms. Sykes takes him to Neighborhood Pediatrics to be examined. Ryan is diagnosed with an upper respiratory infection. Mrs. Sykes is instructed to give Ryan plenty of fluids and children's Tylenol for the fever.

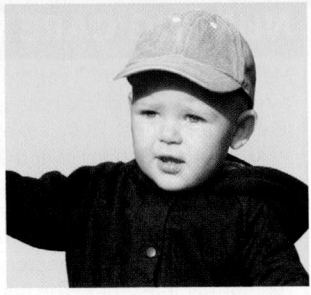

1. What factors place Ryan at risk for developing otitis media?
2. What teaching would you provide Ryan's grandmother to reduce the risk of otitis media?
3. While teaching Ms. Sykes about his care, what symptoms would you tell her need to be reported to the provider should they occur?

EXEMPLAR 9.5   Pneumonia

EXEMPLAR KEY TERMS

Apnea, *590*
Atelectasis, *591*
Bronchiectasis, *588*
Consolidation, *585*
Cyanosis, *588*
Dyspnea, *588*
Empyema, *586*
Hemoptysis, *588*
Hypoxemia, *596*
Lung abscess, *586*
Pleural effusion, *586*
Pleuritic pain, *586*
Pleuritis, *586*
Pneumonia, *584*
Retractions, *590*
Tachypnea, *596*
Thoracentesis, *586*
Unilateral lobar pneumonia, *585*
Virulence, *585*

EXEMPLAR LEARNING OUTCOMES

After reading about this exemplar, you will be able to:

1. Describe the pathophysiology, etiology, clinical manifestations, and direct and indirect causes of pneumonia.
2. Identify risk factors and prevention methods associated with pneumonia.
3. Illustrate the nursing process in providing culturally competent care across the life span for individuals with pneumonia.
4. Formulate priority nursing diagnoses appropriate for an individual with pneumonia.
5. Summarize therapies used by interdisciplinary teams in the collaborative care of an individual with pneumonia.
6. Plan evidence-based care for an individual with pneumonia and the family in collaboration with other members of the healthcare team.
7. Evaluate expected outcomes for an individual with pneumonia.

▶ OVERVIEW

Inflammation of the lung parenchyma (the respiratory bronchioles and alveoli) as a result of infection is known as **pneumonia**. Despite significant advances in antibiotic therapy, pneumonia and influenza together are the eighth leading cause of death in the United States overall and the leading cause of death from infectious disease. In 2011, more than 52,000 deaths in the United States were attributed to pneumonia (CDC, 2012d). Its incidence and mortality rates are highest in older adults and people with debilitating diseases. Pneumonia currently accounts for approximately 3% of adult hospital admissions in the United States (CDC, 2010a).

The respiratory system is constantly open to the possibility of infection. The respiratory tree is exposed to the environment as air moves into and out of the lower respiratory tract. In addition, huge numbers of microorganisms in the oropharynx may be aspirated into the bronchial tree. Both anatomical and physiological defenses help to maintain the sterility of the lower respiratory tract. When these defenses are impaired, the risk for infection increases. For example, drugs, alcohol, or neuromuscular disease may suppress the cough reflex; asthma can both narrow and inflame airways, trapping mucus and impairing oxygenation; and the influenza virus can leave the respiratory epithelium vulnerable to bacterial infection. Even in healthy people, microorganisms and other foreign material occasionally enter the bronchial tree and lung parenchyma.

▶ PATHOPHYSIOLOGY AND ETIOLOGY

Disorders affecting the lower respiratory system (below the larynx) can affect the ability to effectively move air into and out of the lungs (ventilation), exchange oxygen and carbon dioxide across the alveolar-capillary membrane (respiration), and maintain clear and patent airways and ventilate the lungs. Organisms causing such disorders can enter the lung in several ways. The most common means of entry is aspiration of microbe-containing secretions from the oropharynx. Microorganisms may be inhaled following release when an infected

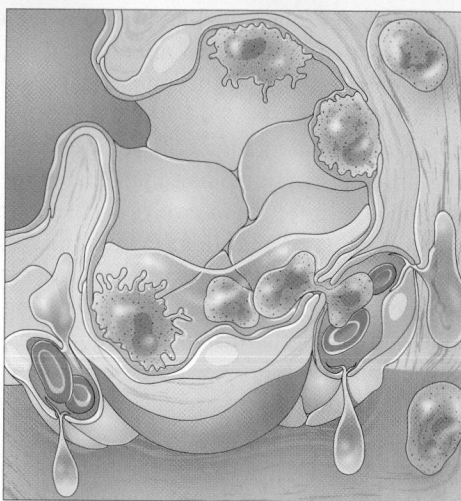

Figure 9–19 ● In pneumonia, the inflammatory response causes fluid to accumulate in the alveoli and edema to form as alveolar capillaries dilate and allow fluid to leak into interstitial tissues.

individual coughs, sneezes, or talks. Inhalation of contaminated aerosolized water can result in viral and some other types of pneumonia. Bacteria also may spread to the lungs through the bloodstream from infection elsewhere in the body. Regardless of the means of entry, host defenses must be overwhelmed either by the number of organisms or by their **virulence** (disease-causing ability) for an infection to develop.

When invading microorganisms colonize the alveoli, they initiate an inflammatory and immune response. The antigen–antibody response and endotoxins released by some organisms damage bronchial and alveolar mucous membranes, causing inflammation with vascular congestion and edema. Infectious debris and exudate can fill alveoli, interfering with ventilation and gas exchange (**Figure 9–19** ●). Pneumonia may develop in any one of four distinct patterns (**Table 9–11** ●):

1. Lobar pneumonia
2. Bronchopneumonia
3. Interstitial pneumonia
4. Miliary pneumonia.

The pathological process, anatomical location, and manifestations of pneumonia vary according to the infective organism. Bacterial and viral pathogens act differently within the lungs:

■ Bacterial pathogens circulate through the bloodstream to the lungs, where they damage cells. Cellular debris and mucus cause airway obstruction. Bacteria tend to be distributed evenly throughout one or more lobes of a single lung, a pattern termed **unilateral lobar pneumonia**.

■ Viruses frequently enter from the upper respiratory tract, infiltrating the alveoli nearest the bronchi of one or both lungs. There, they invade the cells, replicate, and burst out forcefully, killing the cells and sending out cell debris. They rapidly invade adjacent areas, distributing themselves in the scattered, patchy pattern referred to as *bronchopneumonia*.

■ Aspiration of food, emesis, gastric reflux, or hydrocarbons causes a chemical injury and an inflammatory response.

TABLE 9–11 Patterns of Lung Involvement in Pneumonia

PATTERN OF INVOLVEMENT	DESCRIPTION
Lobar pneumonia	Typically involves an entire lobe of a lung. Early in the process, when the immune response is minimal, bacteria spread throughout the affected lobe by rapid accumulation of fluid exudate. As the immune and inflammatory responses develop, red blood cells and neutrophils, damaged epithelial cells, and fibrin accumulate in the alveoli and bronchioles, causing **consolidation** (solidification) of lung tissue. Purulent exudate containing neutrophils and macrophages also forms. The process finally resolves as enzymes destroy the exudate and residual debris is reabsorbed, phagocytized, or coughed out.
Bronchopneumonia	Usually involves dependent portions of lung tissue; characterized by patchy consolidation. Exudate tends to remain primarily in the bronchi and bronchioles, with less edema and congestion of the alveoli than with lobar pneumonia.
Interstitial pneumonia	The inflammatory process primarily involves the interstitium (the alveolar walls and connective tissue supporting the bronchial tree). Involvement may be patchy or diffuse as lymphocytes, macrophages, and plasma cells infiltrate the alveolar septa. While alveoli typically do not contain significant exudates, protein-rich hyaline membranes may line the alveoli, interfering with gas exchange.
Miliary pneumonia	In miliary pneumonia, the spread of the pathogen to the lungs via the bloodstream causes the development of numerous discrete inflammatory lesions. Miliary pneumonia is seen primarily in people who are severely immunocompromised. Because the immune response is poor, damage to pleural tissue may be significant.

Materials with a lower pH cause more inflammation, which sets the stage for bacterial invasion.

Pneumonia may be either infectious or noninfectious. Bacteria, viruses, fungi, protozoa, and other microbes can lead to infectious pneumonia. Noninfectious causes include aspiration of gastric contents and inhalation of toxic or irritating gases. Pneumonias often are classified as community-acquired, healthcare-associated, or opportunistic. Different organisms are implicated in each of these classifications (**Table 9–12** ●). The most common causative organism for community-acquired pneumonia is *Streptococcus pneumoniae* (also called *pneumococcus*), a gram-positive bacterium. This organism causes approximately 50% of the cases of community-acquired pneumonia leading to hospital admission. *Staphylococcus aureus* and gram-negative bacteria are often implicated as healthcare-associated causes of pneumonia. Organisms such as *Pneumocystis jiroveci* generally

TABLE 9–12   Common Organisms Causing Pneumonia in Adults

COMMUNITY-ACQUIRED	HOSPITAL-ASSOCIATED	OPPORTUNISTIC
Streptococcus pneumonia Staphylococcus aureus	Streptococcus pneumoniae Staphylococcus aureus	Pneumocystis jiroveci Mycobacterium tuberculosis
Mycoplasma pneumoniae	Pseudomonas aeruginosa	Cytomegalovirus
Haemophilus influenzae	Haemophilus influenzae	Atypical mycobacteria
Klebsiella pneumoniae	Klebsiella pneumoniae	Fungi
Influenza virus	Escherichia coli	
Chlamydia pneumoniae		
Legionella pneumophila		

cause infections only in individuals who are immunocompromised (opportunistic infections).

Etiology

The several different classifications of pneumonia are based on the infecting organism, including acute bacterial pneumonia, Legionnaires disease, primary atypical pneumonia, viral pneumonia, *Pneumocystis jiroveci* pneumonia, and aspiration pneumonia.

ACUTE BACTERIAL PNEUMONIA   Of the bacterial pneumonias, the pathogenesis of pneumococcal (*Streptococcus pneumoniae*) pneumonia is best understood (**Figure 9–20 ●**). These bacteria reside in the upper respiratory tract of up to 70% of adults. They may be spread by direct individual-to-individual contact via droplets. In many cases, infection results from aspiration of resident bacteria. The typical pattern for pneumo-

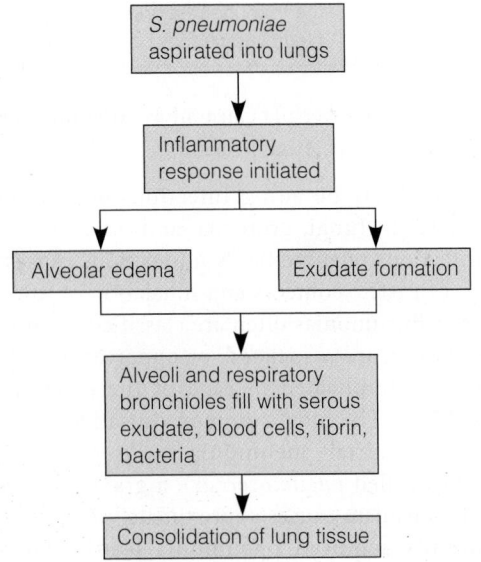

Figure 9–20 ● The pathogenesis of pneumococcal pneumonia.

coccal pneumonia is lobar pneumonia (see Table 9–11), although it may present in a pattern more typical of bronchopneumonia. The lower lobes of the lungs are usually affected because of gravity.

Pneumococcal pneumonia typically resolves uneventfully; normal lung structure is restored on completion of the process. Local extension of the infection to involve the pleura (**pleuritis**) is the most common complication. Pneumonias caused by *Staphylococcus aureus* and gram-negative bacteria often cause extensive parenchymal damage, with necrosis, lung abscess, and empyema, or **pleural effusion** (accumulation of excess fluid in the pleural cavity). Progressive destruction of lung tissue and functional impairment are possible consequences of *Klebsiella* pneumonia.

A **lung abscess** is a local area of necrosis and pus formation within the lung itself and is relatively uncommon. The manifestations of lung abscess develop slowly and include weight loss, malaise, night sweats, fever, and a productive cough. Sputum is foul smelling and tasting. Rupture of the abscess into a larger airway is heralded by production of copious amounts of purulent sputum.

Empyema is accumulation of purulent exudate in the pleural cavity. It is identified by chest x-ray or computed tomography. **Thoracentesis** (insertion of a needle into the pleural space to remove fluid accumulation) may be done, or a chest tube may be inserted to allow continuous drainage of purulent exudates.

The presentation of bacterial pneumonia is usually acute, with rapid onset of shaking chills, fever, and cough that produces rust-colored or purulent sputum. Chest aching or **pleuritic pain** (sharp, localized chest pain that increases with breathing and coughing) is common. Limited breath sounds and fine crackles or rales are heard over the affected area of lung. A pleural friction rub may be audible. If the involved area is large and gas exchange is impaired, dyspnea and cyanosis may be noted.

A more insidious onset with low-grade fever, cough, and scattered crackles is more typical of bronchopneumonia. However, dyspnea is less common with bronchopneumonia. The older adult or debilitated client may have atypical manifestations of pneumonia, with little cough, scant sputum, and minimal evidence of respiratory distress. Fever, tachypnea (rapid respirations), and altered mentation or agitation may be the primary presenting symptoms.

LEGIONNAIRES DISEASE   Legionnaires disease is a form of bronchopneumonia caused by *Legionella pneumophila*, a gram-negative bacterium widely found in water, particularly warm, standing water. Legionnaires disease occurs sporadically and in outbreaks, such as the one that occurred at an American Legion convention in 1976, when the disease was first recognized. Contaminated water-cooled air-conditioning systems and other water sources have been implicated in its spread. Smokers, older adults, and people with chronic diseases or impaired immune defenses are most susceptible to Legionnaires disease.

Symptoms of Legionnaires disease develop gradually, beginning 2–10 days after exposure. Dry cough, dyspnea, general malaise, chills and fever, headache, confusion, diminished appetite and diarrhea, myalgias, and arthralgias are common manifestations. Consolidation of lung tissue is patchy or lobar. Clients who develop Legionnaires disease while in the hospital have a mortality rate close to 50%. Clients who have additional diseases and who are immunocompromised are at higher risk for mortality from Legionnaires disease (Medline-Plus, 2011a).

PRIMARY ATYPICAL PNEUMONIA   Pneumonia caused by *Mycoplasma pneumoniae* is generally classified as *primary atypical pneumonia*, because its presentation and course differ significantly from those of other bacterial pneumonias. Mycoplasma infection often causes pharyngitis or bronchitis. When this type of pneumonia develops, patchy inflammatory changes occur in the alveolar septum and interstitial tissue of the lung. Alveolar exudate and consolidation of lung tissue are not features of atypical pneumonia. Young adults—college students and military recruits in particular—are the primary affected populations.

Primary atypical pneumonia is highly contagious. Its manifestations resemble those of viral pneumonia; systemic manifestations of fever, headache, myalgias, and arthralgias often predominate. The cough associated with atypical pneumonia is dry, hacking, and nonproductive. Because of the typically mild nature and predominant systemic manifestations, mycoplasmal and viral pneumonia are often referred to as *walking pneumonias*.

VIRAL PNEUMONIA   Approximately 10% of pneumonias in adults are viral. Influenza virus and adenovirus are the most common organisms; however, the incidence of cytomegalovirus pneumonia in those who are immunocompromised is on the rise. Other viruses, such as herpes viruses and measles virus, may also cause viral pneumonia. As in primary atypical pneumonia, lung involvement in viral pneumonia is limited to the alveolar septum and interstitial spaces.

Viral pneumonia is typically a mild disease that often affects older adults and people with chronic conditions. It usually occurs in community epidemics. Flulike symptoms of head-

ache, fever, fatigue, malaise, and muscle aching are common, along with a dry cough.

PNEUMOCYSTIS JIROVECI PNEUMONIA   People with AIDS and others who are significantly immunocompromised are at significant risk for developing an opportunistic pneumonia caused by *Pneumocystis jiroveci* (previously known as *P. carinii*), a common parasite found worldwide. Immunity to *P. jiroveci* is nearly universal, except in those who are immunocompromised. Opportunistic infection may develop in people treated with immunosuppressive or cytotoxic drugs for cancer or organ transplant and in people with genetic or acquired immunodeficiency.

Infection with *P. jiroveci* produces patchy involvement throughout the lungs, causing affected alveoli to thicken, become edematous, and fill with foamy, protein-rich fluid. Gas exchange is severely impaired as the disease progresses. *P. jiroveci* pneumonia has an abrupt onset, with fever, tachypnea, shortness of breath, and a dry, nonproductive cough. Respiratory distress can be significant, with intercostal retractions and cyanosis.

Table 9–13 ● compares the manifestations of infectious pneumonias.

ASPIRATION PNEUMONIA   Aspiration of gastric contents into the lungs results in a chemical and bacterial pneumonia known as *aspiration pneumonia*. Major risk factors for aspiration pneumonia include emergency surgery or obstetrical procedures, depressed cough and gag reflexes, and impaired swallowing. Older surgical clients and those with advanced dementia are at significant risk. Enteral nutrition by either nasogastric or gastric tube also increases the risk for aspiration pneumonia. Vomiting is not always apparent; silent regurgitation of gastric contents may occur when the level of consciousness is decreased. Measures to reduce the risk for aspiration pneumonia include minimizing the use of preoperative medications, promoting anesthetic elimination from the body, and preventing nausea and gastric distention.

TABLE 9–13   Manifestations of Infectious Pneumonias

TYPE	ONSET	RESPIRATORY MANIFESTATIONS	SYSTEMIC MANIFESTATIONS
Pneumococcal or lobar pneumonia	Abrupt	Cough productive of purulent or rust-colored sputum; pleuritic or aching chest pain; decreased breath sounds and crackles over affected area; possible dyspnea and cyanosis	Chills and fever
Bronchopneumonia	Gradual	Cough, scattered crackles; minimal dyspnea and respiratory distress; low-grade fever	Fever, tachypnea, altered mental status
Legionnaires disease	Gradual	Dry cough; dyspnea	Chills and fever; general malaise; headache; confusion; diminished appetite and diarrhea; myalgias and arthralgias
Primary atypical pneumonia	Gradual	Dry, hacking, nonproductive cough	Fever, headache, myalgias, and arthralgias predominate
Viral pneumonia	Sudden or gradual	Dry cough	Flulike symptoms
Pneumocystis jiroveci pneumonia	Abrupt	Dry cough; tachypnea and shortness of breath; significant respiratory distress	Fever

The low pH of gastric contents causes a severe inflammatory response when they are aspirated into the respiratory tract. Pulmonary edema and respiratory failure may result. Common complications of aspiration pneumonia are abscesses, **bronchiectasis** (chronic dilation of the bronchi and bronchioles), and gangrene of pulmonary tissue.

Risk Factors

The immature immune systems of infants and young children increase their risk for pneumonia. Older adults are at increased risk because of diminished cough and gag reflexes as well as diminishing immune response. Anyone with a compromised immune system, such as those diagnosed with HIV/AIDS, individuals on medication to prevent rejection of a transplanted organ, and those receiving treatment for cancer such as chemotherapy or radiation therapy, is at increased risk for infection—and for pneumonia in particular. Clients in a debilitated or weakened condition from any cause, including chronic cardiac or respiratory conditions, diabetes mellitus, or alcoholism, also face increased risk. Clients at high risk for pneumonia also face a higher risk for adverse outcomes and complications.

Research indicates a high rate of pneumonia in clients with frequent exposure to cigarette smoke and alcohol or drug abuse. Smoking injures tissues in the airways and decreases the action of cilia. Chemicals in cigarettes have a numbing effect on the cough reflex. All of these actions diminish the lung's natural protective mechanisms. Alcohol interferes with the actions of macrophages, while injection drug users are at risk from infections that originate at the injection site and then spread through the bloodstream to the lungs.

Prevention

Prevention is a key component in managing pneumonia. Identifying vulnerable populations and instituting preventive strategies are measures to reduce the mortality and morbidity associated with the condition. With early identification of the infecting organism, appropriate treatment, and support of respiratory function, most clients recover uneventfully. However, pneumonia remains a serious disease with significant mortality, especially in aged and debilitated populations.

Vaccines offer some degree of protection against the most common bacterial and viral pneumonias. Pneumococcal vaccine, made of antigens from 23 types of pneumococcus, usually imparts lifetime immunity with a single dose. The vaccine is recommended for people who have a high risk of adverse outcome from bacterial pneumonias, including all adults over the age of 65; individuals with chronic diseases such as heart conditions, lung disease, alcoholism, diabetes, and cirrhosis; individuals with chronic renal failure; immunocompromised individuals (e.g., those with malignancy, HIV/AIDS, organ transplant); individuals who smoke or have asthma; and individuals receiving chemotherapy with selected agents, radiation therapy, or long-term steroids. A one-time revaccination is recommended for selected populations, including individuals with immunosuppressive conditions and adults over age 65 who were immunized more than 5 years previously and before age 65 (CDC, 2009b).

> **SAFETY ALERT**
> Annual influenza vaccination helps prevent pneumonia. Inquire about allergic responses to eggs or previous influenza vaccinations before administering influenza vaccine. A significant hypersensitivity response may occur in clients who are allergic to egg protein.

▶ CLINICAL MANIFESTATIONS

Infection of the lower respiratory tract has both local and systemic effects. Local effects include cough, excess mucous production, shortness of breath or **dyspnea** (difficult or labored breathing), **hemoptysis** (bloody sputum), and chest pain. Systemic effects may include fever, diminished appetite and malaise, **cyanosis** (gray to blue or purple skin color caused by deoxygenated hemoglobin), and other manifestations of impaired gas exchange.

Bacteremia can spread the infection to other tissues, leading to meningitis, endocarditis, or peritonitis and increasing the risk of mortality. Entry of the pathogens into the bloodstream can result in septicemia, leading to septic shock.

Lifespan and Cultural Considerations

The populations that are most susceptible to pneumonia include young children and older adults based on increased risk of airway obstruction and on physiological changes in the airway that decrease airway clearance of infecting organisms.

CHILDREN The immature airway of the child makes children more susceptible to the development of pneumonia. The primary physiological aspects of the immature lung that contribute to pneumonia severity are the size of the airways, number of alveoli, differential use of muscles for breathing, and higher oxygen consumption.

A child's airway is shorter and narrower than an adult's. These differences create a greater potential for obstruction (**Figure 9–21 ●**). The infant's airway is approximately 4 mm in diameter, about the width of a drinking straw, in contrast to the adult's airway diameter of 20 mm. The child's little finger offers a good estimate of the child's tracheal diameter and can be used for a quick assessment of airway size.

The trachea increases primarily in length rather than diameter during the first 5 years of life. Also, the tracheal division of the right and left bronchi is higher in a child's airway and at a different angle than in an adult's (**Figure 9–22 ●**). The cartilage that supports the trachea is more flexible and has the potential to compress the airway if the head and neck are not appropriately positioned. The child's narrower airway causes a greater increase in airway resistance (the effort or force needed to move oxygen through the trachea to the lungs) in any condition causing edema of the airway or accumulation of secretions (**Figure 9–23 ●**).

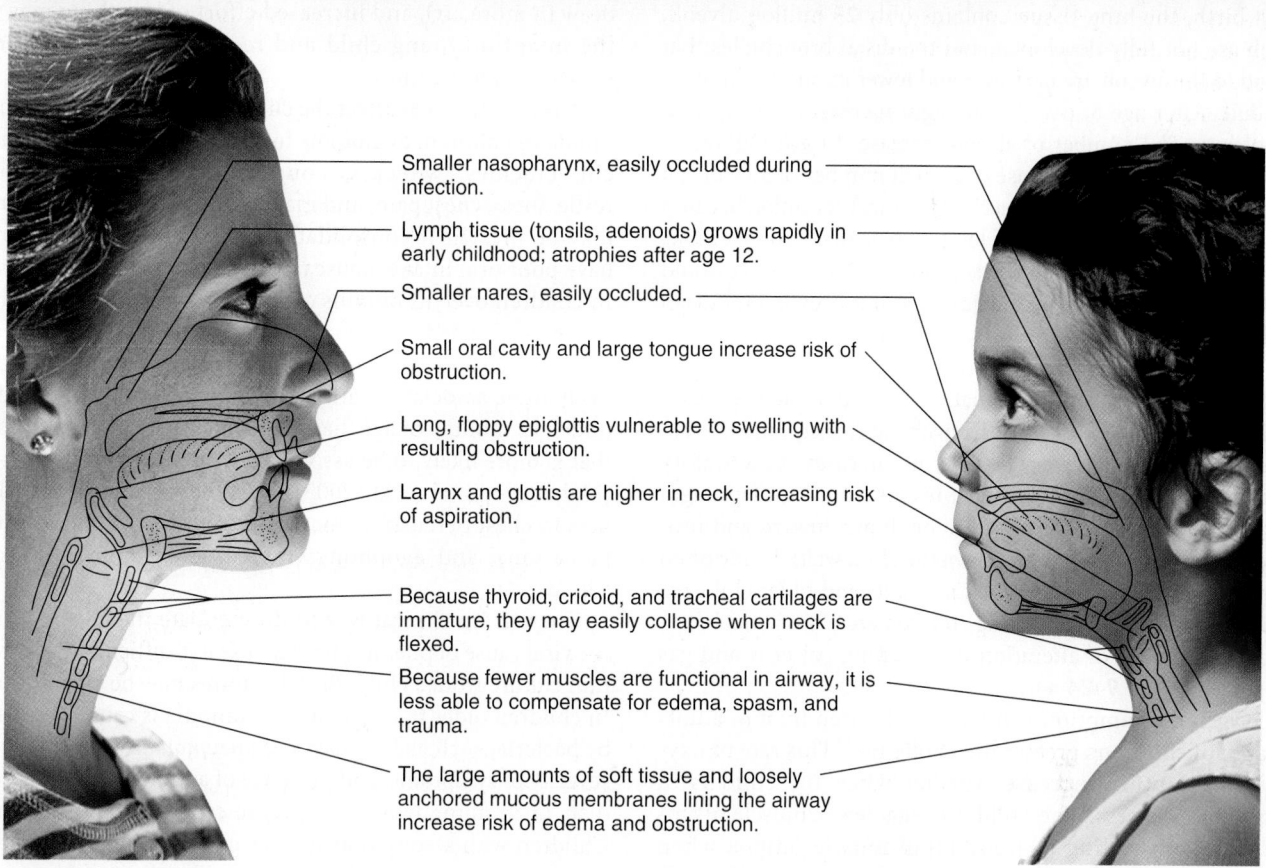

Smaller nasopharynx, easily occluded during infection.

Lymph tissue (tonsils, adenoids) grows rapidly in early childhood; atrophies after age 12.

Smaller nares, easily occluded.

Small oral cavity and large tongue increase risk of obstruction.

Long, floppy epiglottis vulnerable to swelling with resulting obstruction.

Larynx and glottis are higher in neck, increasing risk of aspiration.

Because thyroid, cricoid, and tracheal cartilages are immature, they may easily collapse when neck is flexed.

Because fewer muscles are functional in airway, it is less able to compensate for edema, spasm, and trauma.

The large amounts of soft tissue and loosely anchored mucous membranes lining the airway increase risk of edema and obstruction.

Figure 9–21 ● It is easy to see that a child's airway is smaller and less developed than an adult's, but why is this important? An upper respiratory tract infection, allergic reaction, positioning of the head and neck during sleep, and the small objects children play with can have serious consequences in the child.

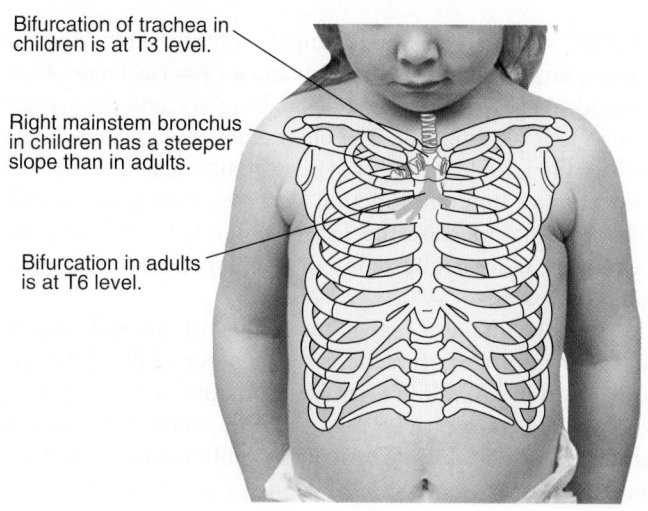

Bifurcation of trachea in children is at T3 level.

Right mainstem bronchus in children has a steeper slope than in adults.

Bifurcation in adults is at T6 level.

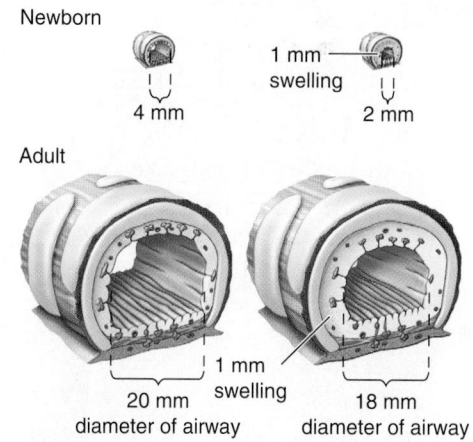

Newborn

1 mm swelling

4 mm

2 mm

Adult

20 mm diameter of airway

1 mm swelling

18 mm diameter of airway

Figure 9–22 ● In children, the trachea is shorter and the angle of the right bronchus at bifurcation is more acute than in the adult. When resuscitating or suctioning, you must allow for the differences. Do you think that this difference is significant in respiratory infection? Why?

Figure 9–23 ● The diameter of an infant's airway is approximately 4 mm, in contrast to an adult's airway diameter of 20 mm. An inflammatory process in the airway causes swelling that narrows the airway, and airway resistance increases. Note that swelling of 1 mm reduces the infant's airway diameter to 2 mm, but the adult's airway diameter is narrowed only to 18 mm. Air must move more quickly in the infant's narrowed airway if the same amount of air is to get to the lungs. The friction of the quickly moving air against the side of the airway increases airway resistance. The infant must use more effort to breathe and must breathe faster to get adequate oxygen.

At birth, the lung tissue contains only 25 million alveoli, which are not fully developed, and the distal bronchioles that extend to the alveoli are narrower and fewer in number than in an adult. After age 8, the alveoli begin increasing in size and complexity. The number of alveoli increases to 300 million by adulthood. As a result, disease of a small number of alveoli can have a much larger impact on a child's clinical condition because of the increased proportion of lung involvement. For example, involvement of 1 million alveoli secondary to pneumonia would be 4% of the lung in a pediatric client but only 0.33% of an adult's lung.

Children under age 6 use the diaphragm to breathe, because the intercostal muscles are immature. By age 6, the child uses the intercostal muscles more effectively. At this age, the ribs are primarily cartilage and very flexible, and in cases of respiratory distress, the negative pressure that results from the diaphragm movement causes the chest wall to be drawn inward and produces **retractions** (visible sinking of the chest wall). While often a late sign of respiratory distress in adults and older children, retractions in infants and young children are often a much earlier manifestation of alteration in breathing patterns and gas exchange (**Figure 9–24 ●**).

Oxygen consumption is higher in children than in adults because of children's greater metabolic rate. This rate of oxygen consumption increases further when the child is in respiratory distress. The child also has fewer muscle glycogen reserves, leading to more rapid muscle fatigue when accessory muscles must be used for breathing (Santillanes & Gausche-Hill, 2008). As a result, children become hypoxic more quickly than adults. Tachypnea, retractions, nasal flaring (opening of the nares on inspiration in an attempt to draw in more air), and increased effort of breathing may tire the infant or young child and result in periods of **apnea** (absence of breathing).

These differences affect the clinical manifestations of pneumonia in children. Symptoms include fever, tachypnea, rhonchi, crackles, wheezes, cough, dyspnea, nasal flaring, restlessness, chest pain, and malaise. Decreased breath sounds may be present if consolidation exists. The child also may have poor oral intake, nausea, vomiting, and abdominal pain. In children over 12 months of age who have clinical manifestations associated with pneumonia, a respiratory rate greater than 50/min and an oxygen saturation of 96% or less are more likely to be associated with a positive chest x-ray. In children under 12 months of age, nasal flaring is an important finding that is more likely to be associated with a positive chest x-ray (Mahabee-Gittens et al., 2005). The older child may have dullness to chest percussion, increased fremitus (vibration felt on palpation), and egophony (increased resonance of voice sounds).

There is no clinical way to differentiate the bacterial from the viral cause of pneumonia, because it is difficult to get a sputum culture from a child. Blood cultures may be taken instead. In children older than 5 years, pneumonia is caused primarily by bacteria, such as *Streptococcus pneumoniae*. The child's age, severity of symptoms, and presence of an underlying lung, cardiac, or immunodeficiency disease create varying responses. Children with a condition such as cystic fibrosis or immunosuppression are susceptible to many other bacterial, parasitic, or fungal infections. Pneumonia in children often resolves much sooner than in adults. The key is early recognition, enabling the child to be managed at home rather than in the hospital.

OLDER ADULTS   Several changes associated with aging and disease affect respiratory function and airway clearance. As an individual ages, the number of cilia decreases, and the gag and cough reflexes diminish. The older adult is at greater risk for dehydration, leading to thick, viscous mucus that is difficult to expectorate. Immune function declines with aging as well. These factors increase the risk of pulmonary infection and reduce the older adult's ability to respond effectively to infectious processes.

Other factors also may increase the risk for and severity of lower respiratory infections in the older adult. These factors include immobility, smoking history, surgical procedures, use of multiple medications, malnutrition, and diseases such as chronic obstructive pulmonary disease and heart disease.

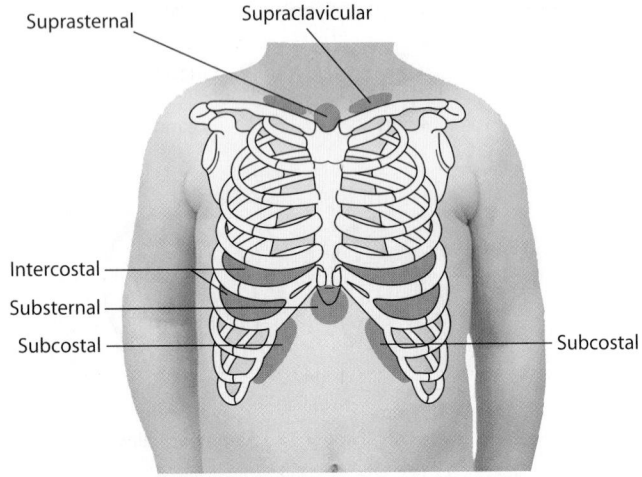

Figure 9–24 ● Retractions may occur in the very young infant in the suprasternal area. In the older infant and child, retractions occur when the airway is severely obstructed, as in croup. The depth and location of retractions are associated with the severity of respiratory distress. Isolated intercostal retractions indicate mild distress. Subcostal, suprasternal, and supraclavicular retractions indicate moderate distress. These retractions accompanied by use of accessory muscles indicate severe distress.

▶ COLLABORATION

Collaboration in caring for an individual with pneumonia may include nurses, doctors, phlebotomists, respiratory therapists, and radiologists. In some cases, consultation with an infectious disease specialist or a pulmonologist may be necessary. Clients who are gravely ill and their families may want the opportunity to talk with the hospital chaplain or their own minister, rabbi, or other spiritual leader.

Diagnostic Tests

The history and physical examination, along with diagnostic testing, are used to establish the diagnosis, determine the extent of lung involvement, and identify the causative organism. Diagnostic tests include the following:

- *Chest x-ray* is obtained to determine the extent and pattern of lung involvement. Fluid, infiltrates, consolidated lung tissue, and **atelectasis** (areas of alveolar collapse) appear as densities on the film.

- *Computed tomography* provides a more detailed image of pulmonary tissue and may be used when the chest x-ray is not diagnostic.

- *Sputum Gram stain* rapidly identifies the infecting organisms as gram-positive or gram-negative bacteria. Antibiotic therapy can then be directed at the predominant type of organism until culture and sensitivity results are obtained.

- *Sputum culture and sensitivity* are ordered to identify the infecting organism and determine the most effective antibiotic therapy. When obtaining sputum for culture, it is important to obtain secretions from the lower respiratory tract, not from the mouth and nasal passages.

- *Complete blood count (CBC) with WBC differential* shows an elevated WBC ($\geq$10,000/mm^3) with increased circulating immature leukocytes (a left shift) in response to the infectious process. WBC changes are minimal in viral and other pneumonias.

- *Serology testing* (blood tests to detect antibodies to respiratory pathogens) may be used to identify the infecting organism when blood and sputum cultures are negative.

- *Pulse oximetry,* a noninvasive method of measuring arterial oxygen saturation (SaO_2), is ordered to continuously monitor gas exchange. The SaO_2 normally is 95% or higher. An SaO_2 of less than 95% may indicate impaired alveolar gas exchange.

- *Arterial blood gas* may be ordered to evaluate gas exchange. Respiratory secretions or pleuritic pain can interfere with alveolar ventilation. Alveolar inflammation can interfere with gas exchange across the alveolar-capillary membrane, especially if exudate or consolidation is present. An arterial partial pressure of oxygen (PaO_2) of less than 75–80 mmHg indicates impaired gas exchange or alveolar ventilation.

- *Fiberoptic bronchoscopy* may be done to obtain a sputum specimen or remove secretions from the bronchial tree.

Pharmacologic Therapy

Medications used to treat pneumonia include antibiotics to eradicate the infection and bronchodilators to reduce bronchospasm and improve ventilation. Initial antibiotic therapy is based on the results of sputum Gram stain and the pattern of lung involvement shown on a chest x-ray. The presence of cardiovascular disease or residence in a long-term care facility is also considered in the initial antibiotic choice. Typically, a broad-spectrum antibiotic, such as a macrolide (e.g., clarithromycin, azithromycin, or erythromycin), a penicillin or a second- or third-generation cephalosporin, or a fluoroquinolone (e.g., ciprofloxacin), is ordered until the results of sputum culture and sensitivity tests are available. **Table 9–14** lists commonly prescribed antibiotics for selected pneumonias.

When an inflammatory response to the infection causes bronchospasm and constriction, bronchodilators may be ordered to improve ventilation and reduce hypoxia. Bronchodilators generally belong to one of two major groups: the sympathomimetic drugs, such as albuterol sulfate (Proventil) and metaproterenol (Alupent), or the methylxanthines, such as theophylline and aminophylline.

TABLE 9–14 Antibiotic Therapy for Selected Pneumonias

CAUSATIVE ORGANISM	ANTIBIOTIC OF CHOICE	ALTERNATIVE ANTIBIOTICS
Streptococcus pneumoniae	penicillin G; amoxicillin	Erythromycin, cephalosporins, doxycycline, fluoroquinolone, clindamycin, vancomycin, trimethoprim-sulfamethoxazole (TMP-SMZ), linezolid
Haemophilus influenzae	Second- or third-generation cephalosporins, doxycycline, azithromycin, TMP-SMZ	Fluoroquinolones, clarithromycin
Staphylococcus aureus	penicillinase-resistant penicillin (e.g., nafcillin); vancomycin for methicillin-resistant organisms	Cephalosporins, vancomycin, clindamycin; ciprofloxacin, fluoroquinolones, TMP-SMZ
Mycoplasma pneumoniae	erythromycin, doxycycline	Clarithromycin, azithromycin, fluoroquinolone
Klebsiella pneumoniae	Third-generation cephalosporin (with aminoglycoside if severe); metronidazole	Aztreonam, imipenem-cilastatin, fluoroquinolone
Legionella pneumophila	macrolide + rifampin; fluoroquinolone	TMP-SMZ, doxycycline + rifampin
Pneumocystis jiroveci	TMP-SMZ, pentamidine + prednisone	Dapsone + trimethoprim, clindamycin + primaquine, trimetrexate + folinic acid
Chlamydia pneumoniae	Doxycycline	Macrolide, fluoroquinolone

An agent may be prescribed to "break up" mucus or reduce its viscosity. Acetylcysteine (Mucomyst), potassium iodide, and guaifenesin (a common ingredient in expectorant cough syrups) help to liquefy mucus, making it easier to expectorate. For many clients, however, increasing fluid intake is an effective means of liquefying mucus.

Oxygen therapy may be indicated for the client who is tachypneic or hypoxemic. Inflammation of the alveolar–capillary membrane interferes with diffusion of gases across the membrane. Diffusion is affected by several other factors, including the partial pressure of gases on each side of the membrane. Increasing the percentage of inspired oxygen above that of room air (21%) increases the partial pressure of oxygen in the alveoli and enhances its diffusion into the capillaries. Supplemental oxygen therefore improves oxygenation of the blood and tissues in clients with pneumonia.

Depending on the degree of hypoxia, oxygen may be administered by either a low-flow or a high-flow system. Low-flow systems include the nasal cannula, simple face mask, partial rebreathing mask, and nonrebreathing mask (**Figure 9–25 ●**).

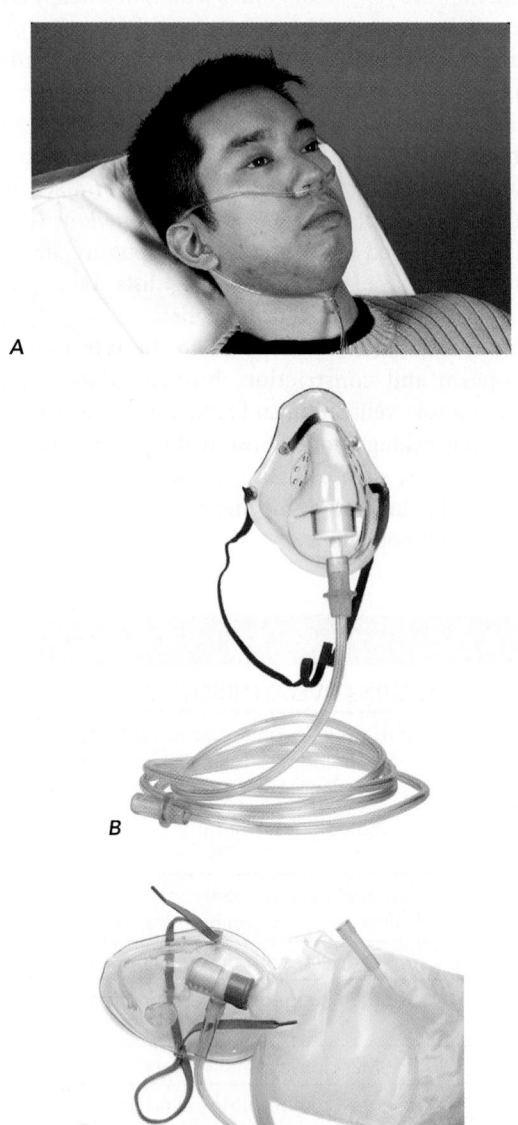

A

B

C

Figure 9–25 ● Low-flow oxygen delivery devices: *A*, nasal cannula; *B*, simple face mask; *C*, nonrebreather mask.
Source: B, Tony McConnell/Science Source.

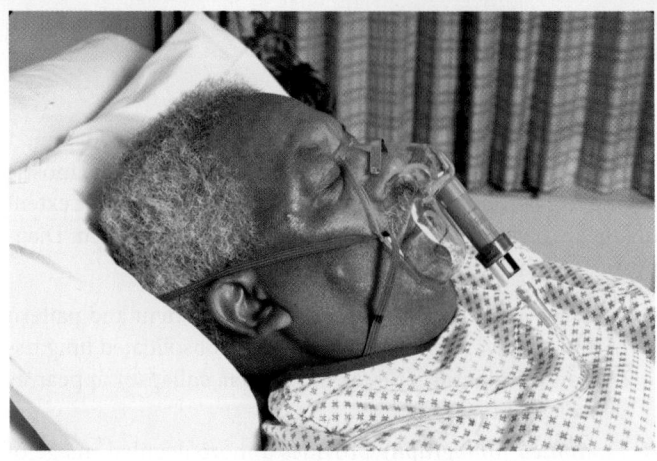

Figure 9–26 ● Venturi mask, a high-flow oxygen delivery system.

A nasal cannula can deliver 24%–45% oxygen concentrations with flow rates of 2–6 L/minute. The nasal cannula is comfortable and does not interfere with eating or talking. A simple face mask delivers 40%–60% oxygen concentrations with flow rates of 5–8 L/minute. Up to 100% oxygen can be delivered by the nonrebreather mask, the highest concentration possible without mechanical ventilation. When the amount of oxygen delivered must be precisely regulated, a high-flow system, such as a Venturi mask, is used (**Figure 9–26 ●**). The Venturi mask regulates the ratio of oxygen to room air, allowing precise regulation of the oxygen percentage delivered, from 24% to 50%. Severe hypoxia may necessitate intubation and mechanical ventilation.

Nonpharmacologic Therapy

Supportive care for all types of pneumonia includes airway management, fluids, and rest. When mucous secretions are thick and viscous, increasing fluid intake to between 2,500 and 3,000 mL/day helps to liquefy secretions, making them easier to cough up and expectorate. If the client is unable to maintain an adequate oral intake, intravenous fluids and nutrition may be required.

Incentive spirometry may be used to promote deep breathing, coughing, and clearance of respiratory secretions. Endotracheal suctioning may be required if the cough is ineffective. On occasion, bronchoscopy is used to perform pulmonary hygiene and remove secretions.

CHEST PHYSIOTHERAPY Chest physiotherapy, including percussion, vibration, and postural drainage, may be performed by a nurse, physiotherapist, respiratory therapist, or trained family member to reduce lung consolidation and prevent atelectasis. Perform *percussion* by rhythmically striking or clapping the chest wall with cupped hands (**Figure 9–27A ●**), using rapid wrist flexion and extension. Cupping traps air between the palm and the client's skin, setting up vibrations through the chest wall that loosen respiratory secretions. The trapped air also provides a cushion, preventing injury. When performed correctly, percussion produces a hollow, popping sound. Percussion may also be done using a mechanical percussion cup. The breasts, sternum, spinal column, and kidney regions are avoided during percussion.

Vibration facilitates the movement of secretions into larger airways. It usually is combined with percussion, although it may be used when percussion is contraindicated

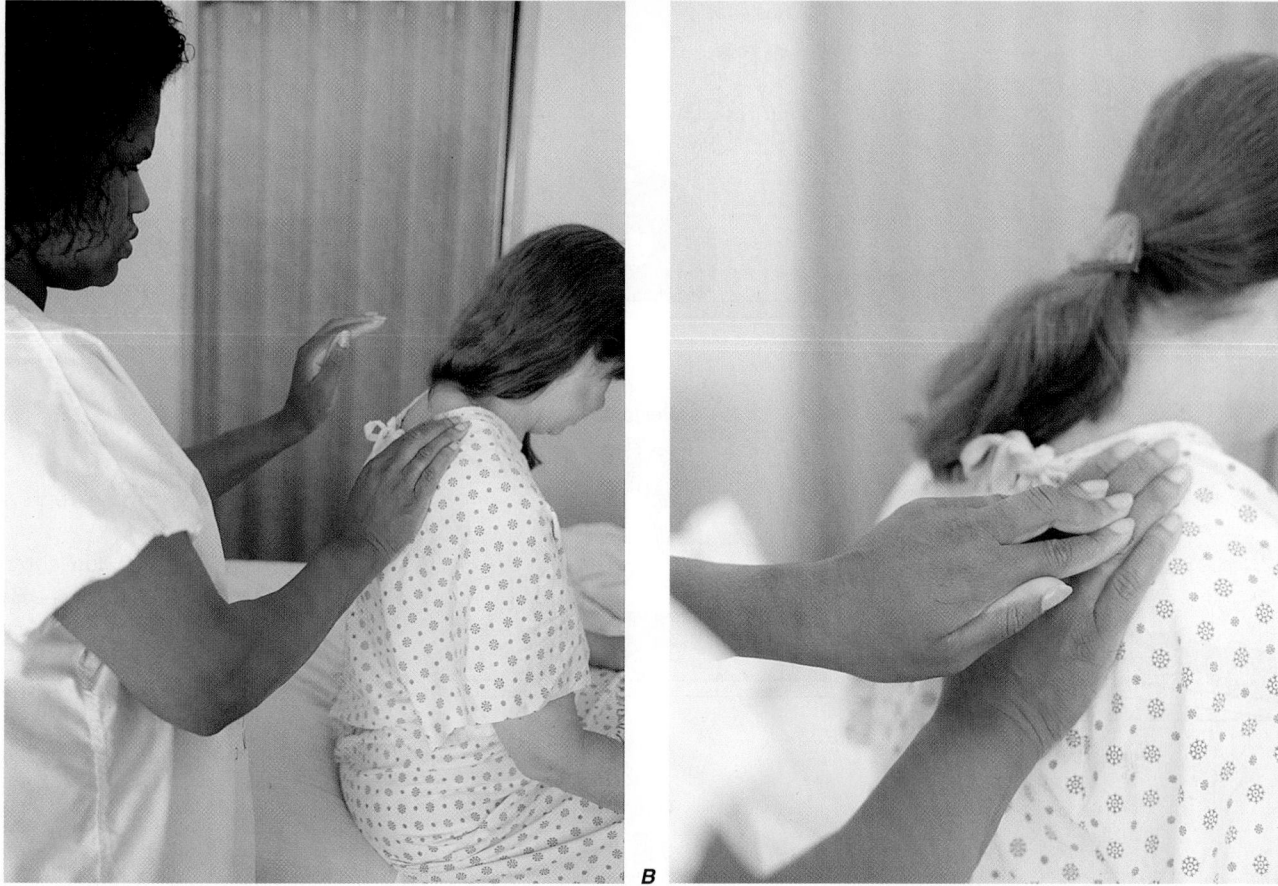

Figure 9–27 ● *A*, Percussing (clapping) the upper posterior chest. Notice the cupped position of the nurse's hands. *B*, Vibrating the upper posterior chest.

or poorly tolerated. Perform vibration by repeatedly tensing the arm and hand muscles while maintaining firm but gentle pressure over the affected area with the flat of the hand (Figure 9–28*B*).

Percussion and vibration are combined with *postural drainage*, which uses gravity to facilitate removal of secretions from a particular lung segment. The client is positioned with the segment to be drained superior to or above the trachea or mainstem bronchus. Drainage of all lung segments requires a variety of positions (**Figure 9–28 ●**); rarely do all segments require drainage. Administer bronchodilators or nebulizer treatments as ordered before postural drainage. It is best to perform postural drainage before meals to avoid nausea and vomiting.

■ NURSING PROCESS

Pneumonia can quickly escalate from minor to severe disease if not treated properly. Adequate assessment and implementation of medical and nursing interventions is vital to the healing process. Frequent pulmonary assessment and aggressive interventions help to prevent problems. Restoring and maintaining mobility improve ventilation and help to mobilize secretions. Promoting adequate fluid intake is necessary,

because fluid helps to liquefy secretions, making them easier to expectorate.

Assessment

Focused assessment of the client with pneumonia includes the following:

- *Health history.* Current symptoms and their duration; presence of shortness of breath or difficulty breathing; chest pain and its relationship to breathing; cough, productive or nonproductive, color and consistency of sputum; other symptoms; recent upper respiratory or other acute illness; chronic diseases, such as diabetes, chronic lung disease, or heart disease; current medications; medication allergies; immunization status.
- *Physical examination.* Presentation; apparent distress; level of consciousness; vital signs, including temperature; skin color and temperature; respiratory excursion, use of accessory muscles of respiration; lung sounds.

Assessment of the pediatric client is different because of children's anatomical and physiological differences, which result in presentation of a different clinical picture. Assessment guidelines for pediatric clients are given in **Table 9–15 ●**).

Ongoing respiratory assessments are important in the care of all clients with pneumonia. Frequency of assessment is determined by

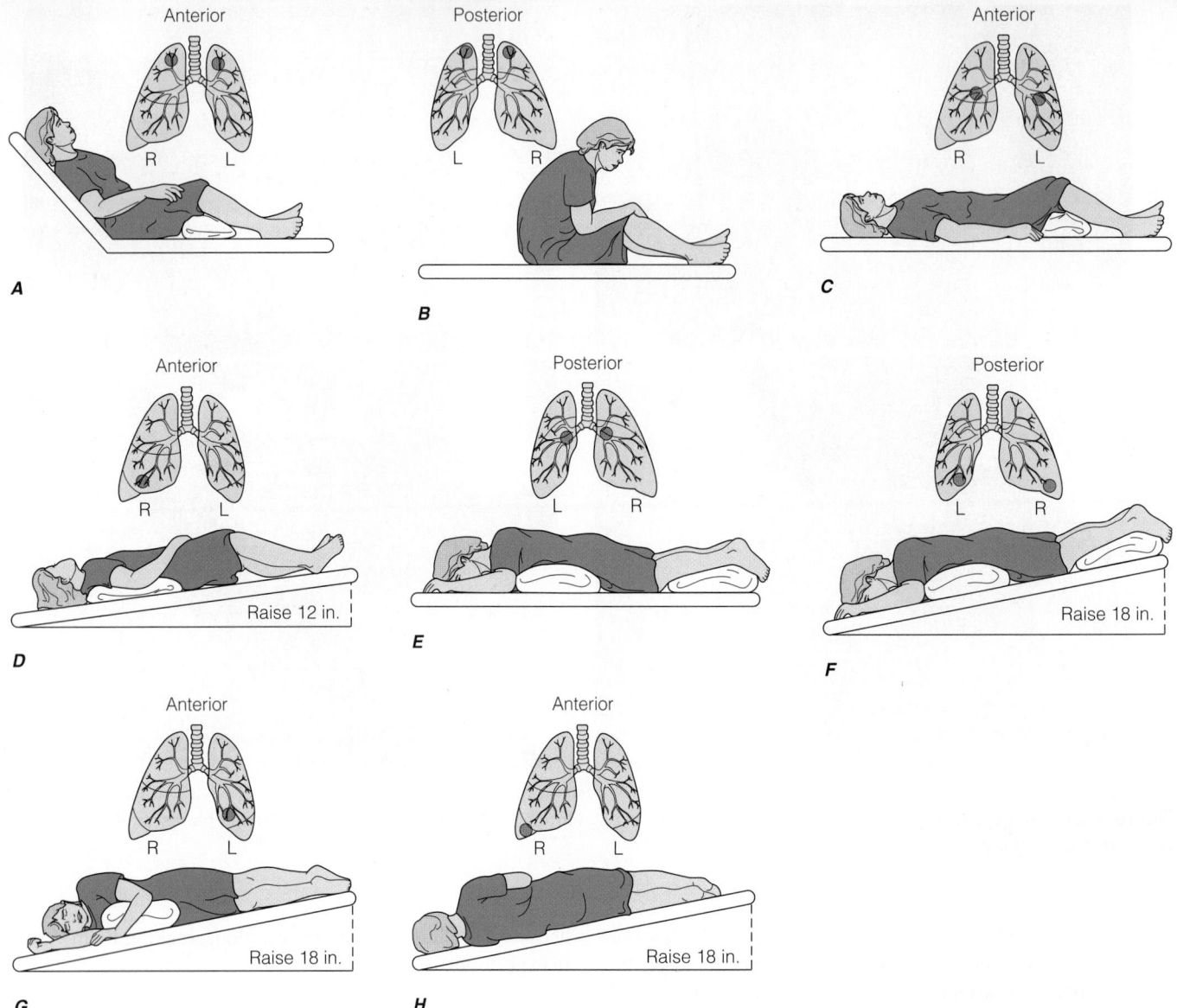

Figure 9–28 ● Positions for postural drainage. *A,* Left and right anterior apical. *B,* Left and right posterior apical. *C,* Left and right anterior upper. *D,* Right middle lobe. *E,* Superior lower lobes. *F,* Left and right lower posterior. *G,* Left lower lateral. *H,* Right lower lateral.

Complementary and Alternative Therapy   Herbal Supplements for Treating Pneumonia

The herb echinacea is widely used to stimulate immune function and treat upper respiratory infections. Because viral upper respiratory infections often precede pneumonia, echinacea may be helpful in preventing pneumonia. Recent research, however, shows mixed results for the effectiveness of echinacea in reducing the duration and severity of an upper respiratory infection (National Center for Complementary and Alternative Medicine [NCCAM], 2012a). Goldenseal, which often is sold in combination with echinacea, is used to treat bacterial, fungal, and protozoal infections of the mucous membranes of the respiratory tract.

Ma huang contains the active ingredient ephedra, which has been used to relieve bronchospasm and ease breathing.

The primary active ingredient in ephedra is epinephrine, a cardiac and central nervous system stimulant. Because of the dangers associated with its use, sale of dietary supplements containing ephedra has been banned. However, this ban does not apply to Chinese herbal remedies or herbal teas (NCCAM, 2012b). If clients inquire about the use of Chinese herbal remedies to reduce pneumonia symptoms, the nurse should inquire whether any of the products contain ma huang or ephedra and advise the client to avoid such products. The nurse should also advise clients who have plant allergies to check with their allergist before taking any kind of herbal supplement.

Clinical Manifestations and Therapies **Pneumonia**

ETIOLOGY	CLINICAL MANIFESTATIONS	CLINICAL THERAPIES
Presence of pathogens causes the hypothalamus to increase the set point of body temperature in an attempt to kill the invader.	Fever	■ Increase fluid intake. ■ Administer antipyretics, such as ibuprofen or acetaminophen. Aspirin may be used in adults but is contraindicated in children because of the risk for Reye syndrome. ■ Minimize clothing and coverings. ■ Monitor temperature frequently. ■ Give a tepid bath if temperature does not respond to other therapies or becomes too high.
Respiratory muscle fatigue	Apnea	■ Use a cardiorespiratory monitor. ■ Measures to reduce the work of breathing include assistance with airway clearance, positioning, and oxygen administration. ■ Recurrent or severe episodes of apnea indicate the need for intubation and mechanical ventilation.
Accumulation of fluid and debris in the airways	Cough	■ Increase fluid intake to liquefy secretions. ■ Frequently change position to prevent atelectasis and help drain different airways. ■ Use chest physiotherapy to promote airway clearance. ■ Use airway suctioning to promote airway clearance if the cough is weak or ineffective. ■ Administer mucolytics to promote sputum expectoration and bronchodilators to open airways, allowing movement of sputum.
Fluid accumulation in the airways impairing gas exchange	Hypoxia	■ Administer oxygen. ■ Encourage coughing and deep breathing to clear airways and promote gas exchange. ■ Monitor vital signs and oxygen saturation. ■ Position to promote airway clearance.

the clinical acuity of the client and the severity of the symptoms displayed. Auscultation of breath sounds, measurement of vital signs and oxygen saturation, and general assessment should be performed at a minimum of every 4 hours for the clinically stable client.

Diagnosis

Clients with lower respiratory disorders such as pneumonia may have multiple nursing care needs, depending on the severity of the illness. Possible nursing diagnoses related to pneumonia include the following:

- *Ineffective Airway Clearance*
- *Ineffective Breathing Pattern*
- *Hyperthermia*
- *Activity Intolerance*
- *Anxiety Related to Hypoxia*
- *Imbalanced Nutrition: Less Than Body Requirements related to altered breathing pattern*
- *Disturbed Sleep Pattern related to orthopnea.*

(NANDA-I © 2012)

Planning

The goal of nursing care is to restore optimal respiratory function. Outcomes are determined in conjunction with client and family and may include the following:

- The client will maintain normal temperature for 24 hours.
- The client will obtain adequate sleep and rest without interruption from coughing or orthopnea.
- The client will maintain adequate fluid and caloric intake.
- The client will demonstrate strong cough sufficient to clear airway.
- The client will maintain oxygen saturation greater than 90%.
- The client will not require supplemental oxygen to maintain oxygen saturations of greater than 90%.

Implementation

In addition to teaching the client to take all antibiotics and other medications exactly as ordered, nursing care focuses on supporting optimal respiratory function, such as maintaining airway patency and an effective breathing pattern and promot-

TABLE 9–15 Assessment Guidelines for the Child With a Respiratory Condition

ASSESSMENT FOCUS	ASSESSMENT GUIDELINES
Position of comfort	■ Is the child comfortable lying down? ■ Does the child prefer to sit up or be in the tripod position (sitting forward with arms on knees for support and extending the neck)?
Vital signs	■ Assess the rate, depth, and ease of respirations. See Table 16–5 in the module on Perfusion for expected respiratory rate ranges by age. ■ Assess the pulse for rate and strength. See Table 16–5 in the module on Perfusion for expected heart rate ranges by age.
Lung auscultation	■ Are breath sounds bilateral, diminished, or absent? ■ Are adventitious sounds (wheezes, crackles, or rhonchi) present?
Respiratory effort (work of breathing)	■ Are there audible inspiratory and expiratory breath sounds or stridor? Is there grunting with expiration? ■ Is breathing labored? ■ Are retractions (visible appearance of the chest being drawn in on inspiration) present, or are accessory muscles used to breathe? ■ Is nasal flaring present? ■ Is **tachypnea** (abnormally rapid rate of respirations) present? ■ Can the child say a full sentence or is a breath needed every few words? Is the cry strong or weak? ■ Do the chest and abdomen rise simultaneously with inspiration, or is paradoxical breathing present in which the chest and abdomen do not rise simultaneously?
Color	■ What is the color of the mucous membranes (pink, pale, mottled, cyanotic)? ■ Does crying improve or worsen the color?
Cough	■ Is the cough dry (nonproductive), wet (productive, mucousy), brassy (noisy, musical), or croupy (barking, seal-like)? ■ Is the coughing effort forceful or weak?
Behavior change	■ Note any sudden behavior changes such as irritability, restlessness, or change in level of responsiveness.
Family history	■ Is there a family history of asthma or cystic fibrosis?

ing rest to reduce metabolic and oxygen needs. Nursing interventions are prioritized on the basis of the most important nursing diagnoses of *Ineffective Airway Clearance, Ineffective Breathing Pattern,* and *Activity Intolerance.*

Maintain Airway Patency

Infections of the lower lungs can generate sputum that hinders respiration, decreasing SaO_2 and making it difficult for the client to breathe. Nursing interventions to help maintain airway patency include the following:

■ Assess the client's respiratory status, including vital signs, breath sounds, SaO_2, and skin color at least every 4 hours. Early identification of respiratory compromise allows intervention before tissue hypoxia is significant.

■ Assess the client's cough and sputum (amount, color, consistency, and possible odor). Assessment of the cough and nature of sputum produced allows evaluation of the effectiveness of respiratory clearance and the response to therapy.

■ Monitor the client's arterial blood gas results; report increasing **hypoxemia** (deficient blood oxygenation) and other abnormal results to the physician. Blood gas changes may be an early indicator of impaired gas exchange caused by airway narrowing or obstruction.

■ Place the client in Fowler or high-Fowler position. Encourage frequent position changes and ambulation as allowed. The upright position promotes lung expansion; position changes and ambulation facilitate the movement of secretions.

■ Assist the client to cough, deep-breathe, and use assistive devices. Provide endotracheal suctioning using aseptic technique as ordered. Coughing, deep breathing, and suctioning help to clear airways.

■ Provide a fluid intake of at least 2,500–3,000 mL/day for the adult client. See **Table 9–16** ● for fluid requirements of the pediatric client. A liberal fluid intake helps to liquefy secretions and facilitate their clearance.

■ Work with the physician and respiratory therapist to provide pulmonary hygiene measures, such as postural drainage, percussion, and vibration. These techniques help to mobilize and clear secretions.

■ Administer prescribed medications as ordered, and monitor their effects. If the infecting organism is resistant to the prescribed antibiotic, little improvement may be seen with treatment. Bronchodilators help to maintain open airways but may have adverse effects such as anxiety and restlessness.

Ensure Effective Ventilation

Chest pain and fatigue associated with a lung infection may cause clients to take shallow breaths, which prevents adequate exhalation of carbon dioxide and inhalation of oxygen. Nursing interventions that promote effective ventilation include:

■ Provide for rest periods. Rest reduces metabolic demands, fatigue, and the work of breathing, promoting a more effective breathing pattern.

TABLE 9–16 Daily Maintenance Fluid Requirements for the Pediatric Client

Standard formula	For the first 10 kg of body weight, administer 100 mL/kg/day	For the second 10 kg of body weight, administer 50 mL/kg/day	For all additional body weight over 20 kg, administer 20 mL/kg/day
Example: For a child weighing 53 lb, which is equal to 24 kg	100 mL/kg/day = 100 mL x 10 kg = 1,000 mL/day	50 mL/kg/day = 50 mL x 10 kg = 500 mL/day	24 kg – 20 kg = 4 kg over 20 kg 4 kg x 20 mL = 80 mL/day
Example total			This 53-lb child requires a total 1,580 mL of fluid to be administered during a 24-hour period.

- Assess the client for pleuritic discomfort. Provide analgesics as ordered. Adequate pain relief minimizes splinting and promotes adequate ventilation. Analgesics, such as ibuprofen or acetaminophen, can have the added benefit of fever control and may aid in sleep.
- Teach the client how to splint the chest by hugging a small pillow, or a teddy bear for the pediatric client, to make coughing less painful. Pain may result from coughing and deep breathing as well as from accessory muscle fatigue.
- Provide reassurance during periods of respiratory distress. Hypoxia and respiratory distress produce high levels of anxiety, which tend to further increase tachypnea and fatigue and decrease ventilation.
- Administer oxygen as ordered. Oxygen therapy increases the alveolar oxygen concentration and facilitates its diffusion across the alveolar–capillary membrane, reducing hypoxia and anxiety.
- Teach the client slow abdominal breathing. This breathing pattern promotes lung expansion.
- Teach the client use of relaxation techniques, such as visualization and meditation. These techniques help to reduce anxiety and slow the breathing pattern.

SAFETY ALERT
Assess respiratory rate, depth, and lung sounds at least every 4 hours. Tachypnea and diminished or adventitious breath sounds may be early indicators of respiratory compromise.

Promote Balance Between Activity and Rest

Clients with pneumonia tire easily because breathing requires increased effort. Activity heightens this fatigue. Therefore periods of activity should be alternated with periods of rest for clients with pneumonia. In the hospital, nurses

- Assess the client's activity tolerance, noting any increase in pulse, respirations, dyspnea, diaphoresis, or cyanosis. These assessment findings may indicate limited or impaired activity tolerance.
- Assist the client with self-care activities, such as bathing. Assistance with activities of daily living reduces energy demands.
- Schedule activities, planning for rest periods. Rest periods minimize fatigue and improve activity tolerance. Minor activities, such as taking vital signs and using the bathroom, may be grouped together. However, major activities, such as chest physiotherapy or showering, should be immediately followed by a period of rest.
- Provide assistive devices, such as an overhead trapeze. These assistive devices facilitate movement and reduce energy demands.

- Enlist the family's help to minimize stress and anxiety levels. Stress and anxiety increase metabolic demands and can decrease activity tolerance.
- Perform active or passive range-of-motion exercises. Exercises help to maintain muscle tone and joint mobility and to prevent contractures if bed rest is prolonged.
- Provide emotional support and reassurance that strength and energy will return to normal when the infectious process has resolved and the balance of oxygen supply and demand is restored. The client may be concerned that activity intolerance will continue to be a problem after the acute infection is resolved.

SAFETY ALERT
Activity intolerance may be an early sign of cardiorespiratory compromise, particularly in the older adult or client with preexisting heart disease. New or worsening manifestations of activity intolerance should be reported to the physician.

Community-Based Care

Many clients with pneumonia will recover at home. Client teaching is an important nursing intervention for these clients. Discuss the following topics when preparing the client and family for home care:

- The importance of completing the prescribed medication regimen as ordered; potential drug side effects and their management, including manifestations that necessitate stopping the drug and notifying the physician
- Recommendations for limiting activities and increasing rest
- The importance of maintaining adequate fluid intake to keep mucus thin for easier expectoration
- Ways to maintain adequate nutritional intake, such as small, frequent, well-balanced meals
- The importance of avoiding smoking or exposure to secondhand smoke to prevent further irritation of the lungs
- Manifestations to report to the physician, such as increasing shortness of breath, difficulty breathing, and increased fever, fatigue, headache, sleepiness, or confusion
- The importance of keeping all follow up appointments to ensure disease cure

Evaluation

Clients with pneumonia are usually treated in the community unless their respiratory status is significantly compromised (e.g., altered mental status, tachypnea, tachycardia, hypotension, hypo- or hyperthermia, and altered blood gases) or if risk factors (e.g., advanced age and/or coexisting heart, kidney, or liver disease) are present. As a result, caregivers must be taught to evaluate the outcome of care and the signs and symptoms requiring immediate consultation with the primary care provider.

NURSING CARE PLAN   A Client With Pneumonia

Mary O'Neal is a 35-year-old executive assistant and part-time college student. On returning home from class one evening, she began to feel chills. She alternated between chills and sweats all night. She stayed home from work the next day and remained in bed most of the day. Her fever continued, and she developed a cough and dull, aching chest pain. When the cough became productive of rust-colored sputum the following day, she decided to seek medical treatment from her family doctor.

ASSESSMENT

Debby Kowalski, RN, the family practice clinic nurse, admits Ms. O'Neal to the clinic and obtains the nursing assessment. Ms. O'Neal denies any previous history of respiratory diseases "other than the usual colds, flu, and such." She also denies any history of smoking or medication allergies. She says her symptoms began abruptly, with an onset of the chills. She describes her chest pain as a dull ache that was initially sub-sternal but now is localized in her lower lateral right chest. The pain increases with deep breathing, coughing, and moving. Her cough is increasing in frequency and severity, and her sputum appears rusty brown. Her vital signs include temperature 101.8°F oral; pulse 104 bpm; respirations 22/min; and blood pressure 116/74 mmHg. Her skin is warm and flushed, with no evidence of cyanosis. Her respirations are shallow and unlabored; respiratory excursion is equal. Breath sounds are diminished in the bases bilaterally, with crackles noted in the right posterior and lateral base.

A STAT CBC shows a WBC of 18,900/mm^3; differential shows increased numbers of neutrophils and immature WBCs (bands). Ms. Kowalski has Ms. O'Neal rinse with an antiseptic mouthwash and then collects a sputum specimen for culture and Gram stain before Ms. O'Neal sees the physician.

The physician orders a chest x-ray after examining Ms. O'Neal. Based on her history, examination, and chest x-ray, he makes the diagnosis of acute bacterial pneumonia, probably pneumococcal. He prescribes oral penicillin V, 500 mg every 6 hours for 10 days. He asks Ms. O'Neal to return for a follow up appointment in 10 days and refers her back to Ms. Kowalski for appropriate teaching.

DIAGNOSES

- *Ineffective Breathing Pattern* related to pleuritic chest pain
- *Hyperthermia* related to inflammatory process
- *Deficient Knowledge* about pneumonia and its treatment

(NANDA-I © 2012)

PLANNING

Goals for Ms. O'Neal's care include:
- The client will maintain normal pulmonary function.
- The client will describe measures to minimize elevations in body temperature.
- The client will identify a schedule for taking her medication that will facilitate compliance with the regimen.
- The client will describe manifestations that should be reported to the physician.

INTERVENTIONS

- Assess knowledge and understanding of pneumonia and its effects.
- Assist to develop a medication schedule that coordinates with normal daily routine.
- Teach client and family about the following:
  a. Importance of avoiding use of a cough suppressant except at night to facilitate rest
  b. Ways to increase fluid intake to reduce fever and maintain thin mucus for easy expectoration
  c. Beneficial effects of rest, especially during the acute phase of her illness
  d. Safe use of aspirin and acetaminophen to reduce fever
  e. Importance of taking all prescribed medication doses as scheduled
  f. Common side effects of penicillin V and their management
  g. Early manifestations of penicillin allergy that necessitate stopping the medication and notifying the physician
  h. Signs of complications or worsening pneumonia to report

EVALUATION

The sputum culture confirms *Streptococcus pneumoniae* as the cause of Ms. O'Neal's pneumonia. When she returns for her follow up appointment, she reports that she began to feel better after 2 days on the penicillin and returned to work the following Monday. Her examination reveals good breath sounds throughout, with no adventitious sounds. The follow up sputum culture is free of pathogens.

CRITICAL THINKING

1. *Do any of the factors identified in the case study increase Ms. O'Neal's risk for acute bacterial pneumonia? If so, which factors?*
2. *Ms. O'Neal's WBC differential showed increased neutrophil and band counts. Describe the reason for and effect of this change.*
3. *Even though Ms. O'Neal has no history of medication allergies, anaphylactic shock remains a potential risk. Describe the sequence of events leading to anaphylactic shock, its initial symptoms, and immediate nursing interventions.*
4. *If Ms. O'Neal had required hospitalization to treat her acute pneumonia, interruption of her usual activities and responsibilities could lead to anxiety. Develop a care plan for this situation, using the nursing diagnosis* Ineffective Role Performance *related to hospitalization.*

REVIEW Pneumonia

RELATE Link the Concepts and Exemplars

Linking the exemplar of pneumonia with the concept of oxygenation:

1. Describe the pathophysiology of pneumonia related to how it impacts oxygenation.

2. What measures could you implement when caring for a client with pneumonia to improve oxygenation?

Linking the exemplar of pneumonia with the concept of development:

3. When caring for a 2-year-old diagnosed with pneumonia requiring use of an oxygen tent, what developmentally appropriate activities might you provide to occupy the child and keep the child in the tent as much as possible?

4. You are caring for a 6-year-old child diagnosed with cystic fibrosis who is hospitalized for recurrent pneumonia diagnoses. How can you promote this child's normal development during hospitalization?

READY Go to Companion Skills Manual

REFER Go to Pearson Student Nursing Resources
nursing.pearsonhighered.com

- Additional review material

REFLECT Case Study

Jimmy Bley is a 78-year-old Caucasian man with moderate emphysema and hearing loss. He is a retired veteran who served as an electronics technician in the army for his entire career. In his retirement, Mr. Bley has taken an interest in computers. He spends most of his time surfing the Internet or playing games on the computer; he also likes to build computers. Mr. Bley has been married for 56 years to his wife, Cecelia. They argue a lot, but they would not know what to do without one another. They have several grown children, grandchildren, and great-grandchildren who live in the same community. Mr. Bley often goes with his wife to the neighborhood senior center for bingo night.

Mr. Bley considers himself healthy. He describes his hearing loss as mild. He has a hearing aid, but he does not like to

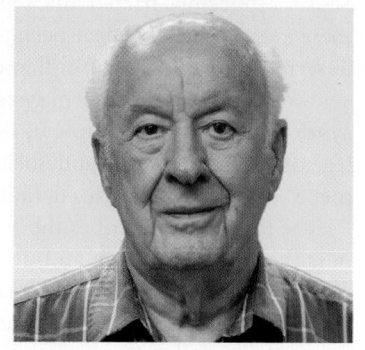

wear it and therefore does not make changing the batteries a priority. He does not perceive his hearing loss to be much of a problem. Likewise, Mr. Bley describes his emphysema as "not that bad." However, he becomes short of breath with most activities; thus it takes time for him to complete tasks. He compensates by taking his time to do most things. He has learned that he must pace himself; if he does not, he becomes exhausted and needs several days to recover. He continues to smoke and knows he should quit, but he just can't seem to get interested in quitting because he enjoys it.

One night, Jimmy is awakened from sleep feeling as though he can't catch his breath. He sits up, and his breathing becomes a little easier and he feels slightly less anxious. However, he also notices that he is hot. When he takes his temperature, he gets a reading of 101.2°F orally. He still feels a little bit short of breath and decides that he will call the clinic in the morning. In the meantime, he goes downstairs, sits in the recliner, and naps fitfully. When Mr. Bley gets to the clinic, the doctor performs a chest x-ray (patchy infiltrates in left lower lobe), CBC with differential (elevated WBC count, with differential showing a shift to the left, indicating a bacterial infection), and arterial blood gas (pH 7.32, PaO_2 52, $PaCO_2$ 48, HCO_3 30) and diagnoses Mr. Bley with pneumonia. Mr. Bley is taken to the local hospital and admitted with orders for intravenous (IV) fluids; a high-calorie, low-salt, low-fat diet; oxygen via nasal cannula at 2 L/min; cefaclor (Keflex, Ceclor), 500 mg IV q8h; aminophylline, 100 mg PO q8h; and Atrovent HFA 2 puffs qid.

1. What factors contributed to the decision to hospitalize Mr. Bley instead of treating him at home?

2. Why would the physician order oxygen at only 2 L/min instead of a 100% mask at 6 L/min? Provide a physiological explanation for this order.

3. Develop a nursing plan of care for this client.

EXEMPLAR 9.6 Sepsis

EXEMPLAR KEY TERMS
Bacteremia, *600*
Ischemia, *603*
Refractory septic shock, *600*
Sepsis, *600*
Septicemia, *600*
Septic shock, *600*
Severe sepsis, *600*
Systemic inflammatory response syndrome (SIRS), *600*

EXEMPLAR LEARNING OUTCOMES
After reading about this exemplar, you will be able to:

1. Describe the pathophysiology, etiology, clinical manifestations, and direct and indirect causes of sepsis.

2. Identify risk factors and prevention methods associated with sepsis.

3. Illustrate the nursing process in providing culturally competent care across the life span for individuals with sepsis.

4. Formulate priority nursing diagnoses appropriate for an individual with sepsis.

5. Summarize therapies used by interdisciplinary teams in the collaborative care of an individual with sepsis.

6. Plan evidence-based care for an individual with sepsis and the family in collaboration with other members of the healthcare team.

7. Evaluate expected outcomes for an individual with sepsis.

▶ OVERVIEW

Sepsis, septicemia, bacteremia, septic shock, blood poisoning—these are all terms that have been used at one time or another to describe the whole-body inflammatory process resulting in acute critical illness. The term **systemic inflammatory response syndrome (SIRS)** was coined in 1992 when the American College of Chest Physicians and Society of Critical Care Medicine met to develop a consensus definition of this critical illness.

The term *SIRS* describes the body's response to a critical illness that can result from an infectious or noninfectious cause (e.g., burns, trauma, and pancreatitis) precipitating a whole-body inflammatory process. Other common terms can be differentiated as follows:

- **Sepsis** is defined as SIRS resulting from an infection.
- **Severe sepsis** is defined as sepsis with acute associated organ failure.
- **Septic shock** is defined as a persistently low mean arterial blood pressure as a result of overwhelming infection despite adequate fluid resuscitation.
- **Refractory septic shock** is a persistently low mean arterial blood pressure despite vasopressor therapy and adequate fluid resuscitation (LaRosa, 2010).

This exemplar explores sepsis that occurs in response to infection-related SIRS.

▶ PATHOPHYSIOLOGY AND ETIOLOGY

Sepsis is the leading cause of death in noncoronary intensive care units and the eleventh leading cause of death in the United States overall (CDC, 2012d). More than 70% of clients with sepsis have comorbidities, and more than 60% of cases occur in people over the age of 65 (LaRosa, 2010). SIRS, which is a precursor to sepsis, can occur as a complication of virtually any infection of any body tissue. In infection-related SIRS, the infection triggers a systemic inflammatory response that leads to a series of adverse events, including vasodilation, increased capillary permeability, and hypercoagulability. SIRS also triggers the activation of certain types of cells that typically help the body during an immune or inflammatory reaction: platelets, neutrophils, macrophages, and endothelial cells. However, during SIRS, the function of these cells is exaggerated, and the uncontrolled cellular release of chemical mediators sparks a system-wide immune and inflammatory response (see the concept of Immunity and the concept of Inflammation).

When the SIRS response is severe, sepsis can develop. Disseminated intravascular coagulation (DIC) is a potential risk associated with sepsis. DIC is characterized by simultaneous bleeding and clotting throughout the vasculature. Sepsis injures blood cells, causing platelet aggregation and decreased blood flow. As a result, blood clots form throughout the microcirculation. The clotting slows circulation further while stimulating excess fibrinolysis. As the body's stores of clotting factors are depleted, generalized bleeding begins. For an illustration of the pathophysiology of sepsis that develops into septic shock, see **Figure 9–29** ●. The progression of sepsis

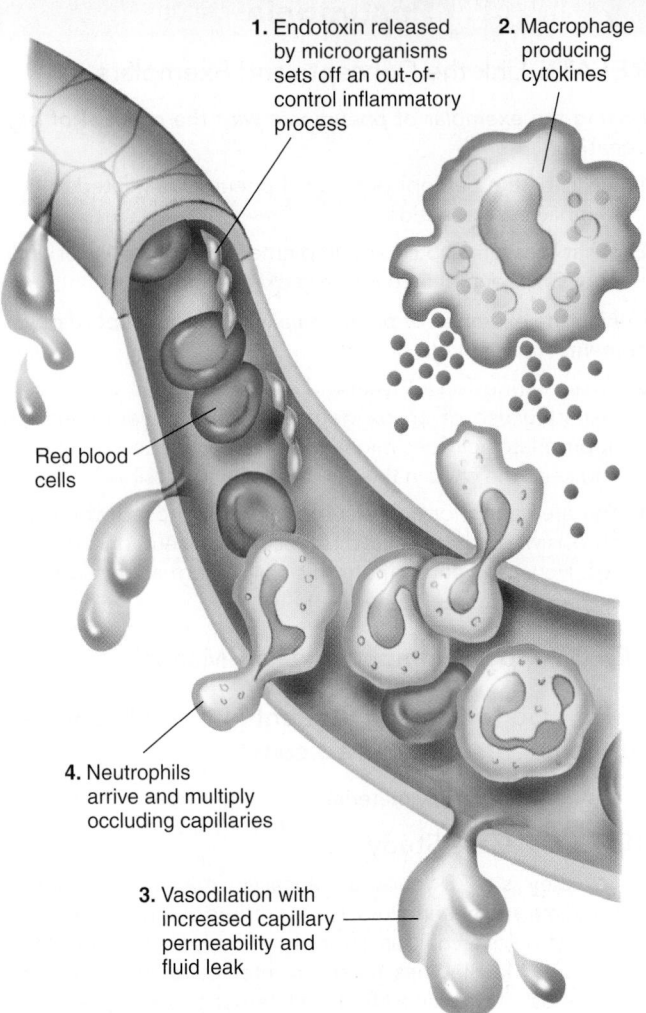

1. Endotoxin released by microorganisms sets off an out-of-control inflammatory process
2. Macrophage producing cytokines
Red blood cells
4. Neutrophils arrive and multiply occluding capillaries
3. Vasodilation with increased capillary permeability and fluid leak

Figure 9–29 ● In septic shock, blood pools in the extremities. Blood flow is sluggish and amounts of oxygen received by the tissues are inadequate for cell metabolism.

may lead to severe sepsis, during which reduced organ perfusion can cause multiple-organ dysfunction syndrome (MODS) and ultimately death.

Clients with sepsis are very ill and require attentive monitoring and rapid intervention in response to sometimes subtle changes in condition. Nurses play a pivotal role in caring for these clients, because they are with the clients constantly and are most competent to monitor their condition.

Etiology

Sepsis due to infection begins with **septicemia** (the presence of pathogens and their toxins in the blood). Sources of infection include bacteria, viruses, and fungi. Rickets and certain types of protozoa may also lead to septic shock (Chulay & Burns, 2010). The presence of bacteria and their toxins in the bloodstream, which is a common cause of sepsis, is called **bacteremia**.

Sepsis is most often the result of gram-positive infections from *Staphylococcus* and *Streptococcus* bacteria but may also follow gram-negative bacterial infections (i.e., *Pseudomonas* sp., *Escherichia coli*, and *Klebsiella* sp.); 6% of cases are related to fungal infections (LaRosa, 2010).

The incidence of gram-negative sepsis has greatly increased since 2003, with a 60% mortality rate despite treatment. The incidence of sepsis is increasing the most in older adults and non-White populations. The reason is believed to be an increase in invasive procedures, immunosuppressive therapy, and anti-microbial resistance (LaRosa, 2010).

Portals of entry for infection that may lead to septic shock are as follows:

- *Urinary system.* Catheterizations, suprapubic tubes, and cystoscopy.
- *Respiratory system.* Suctioning, aspiration, tracheostomy, endo-tracheal tubes, respiratory therapy, and mechanical ventilators.
- *Gastrointestinal system.* Peptic ulcers, ruptured appendix, peritonitis.
- *Integumentary system.* Surgical wounds, intravenous cathe-ters, intra-arterial catheters, invasive monitoring, decubitus ulcers, burns, and trauma.
- *Female reproductive system.* Elective surgical abortion, ascending infections from transmission of bacteria during the intrapartal and postpartal periods, tampon use, and sex-ually transmitted infections.

Risk Factors

Clients at risk for developing infections leading to septic shock include those who are hospitalized, have debilitating chronic ill-nesses, or have poor nutritional status. The risk is heightened after invasive procedures or surgery. Other clients at risk of sep-tic shock include older adults and those who are immunocom-promised.

During periods of immune suppression, the client is vul-nerable to overwhelming infection, which results in circula-tory failure, hypothermia or hyperthermia, tachypnea, mental changes, inadequate tissue perfusion, and hypotension. Fac-tors contributing to massive infection include inadequate neu-trophil production, abnormal granulocytes (that are not able to be actively phagocytic), erosions through normal barriers (e.g., blood vessels and mucous membranes), and altered bone marrow production caused by chemotherapy and some forms of radiation. Such infections must be vigorously treated with antimicrobial therapy and hydration management.

Toxic shock syndrome is an especially virulent form of septic shock and occurs most frequently in menstruating women who use tampons improperly. It is thought that bacterial toxins diffuse from the site of infection in the vagina into the circula-tion. The toxins then trigger a widespread inflammatory response and septic shock. The manifestations of toxic shock syndrome include extreme hypotension, hyperpyrexia, head-ache, myalgia, confusion, skin rash, vomiting, and diarrhea (Porth & Matfin, 2010).

Prevention

Any infant with an infectious process must be watched carefully for early signs of sepsis; thorough teaching of parents and regular caregivers is indicated. Individuals with cancer, especially those undergoing treatment with chemotherapy or radiation therapy, must be carefully monitored for symptoms of sepsis and may be placed on prophylactic antibiotics because their risk is so great.

Because complications from pneumonia are a major cause of sepsis, immunization against organisms that cause pneumonia, such as *H. influenzae* and *S. pneumoniae*, is a primary method of sepsis prevention. Infections from catheter and IV use are also a major cause of sepsis, so aseptic techniques and good hand-washing techniques when inserting, removing, or caring for catheters and IV lines are vital to preventing sepsis.

▶ CLINICAL MANIFESTATIONS

Manifestations of sepsis include fever or hypothermia, tachy-cardia, tachypnea, peripheral vasodilation, septic shock, and mental status changes. Hemodynamic monitoring shows an increase in cardiac output. Lab results show an abnormal CBC (leukocytosis or leukopenia) and alteration in clotting factors (thrombocytosis or thrombopenia), and elevated liver enzyme, C-reactive protein, and creatinine levels are likely. Hypophos-phatemia and positive blood culture are anticipated.

Septic shock has an early phase and a late phase. In early sep-tic shock (sometimes called the *warm phase*), vasodilation results in hypotension due to intense vasodilation and fluid shifts due to increased capillary permeability, weakness, and warm, flushed skin. Septicemia often causes high fever and chills. In late septic shock (sometimes called the *cold phase*), hypovolemia and activity of the compensatory mechanisms result in typical shock manifestations, including cold, moist skin; oliguria; and changes in mental status. Death may result from respiratory failure, cardiac failure, and/or renal failure. Manifestations of septic shock are listed in **Box 9–5** ●.

Lifespan and Cultural Considerations

Manifestations of sepsis in infants include temperature instabil-ity, abdominal distention, poor feeding, lethargy, respiratory dis-tress, hepatomegaly, vomiting, and/or jaundice. Children under 3 months of age with a temperature higher than 38°C (100.4°F) rectally require diagnostic testing to rule out sepsis, because they are at increased risk secondary to immature immune systems and inadequate immune response to infection.

Box 9–5 **Manifestations of Septic Shock**

EARLY (WARM) SEPTIC SHOCK

- *Blood pressure:* normal to hypotension
- *Pulse:* increased, thready
- *Respirations:* rapid and deep
- *Skin:* warm, flushed
- *Mental status:* alert, oriented, anxious
- *Urine output:* normal
- *Other:* increased body temperature; chills; weakness; nausea, vomiting, diarrhea; decreased CVP

LATE (COLD) SEPTIC SHOCK

- *Blood pressure:* hypotension
- *Pulse:* tachycardia, arrhythmias
- *Respirations:* rapid, shallow, dyspneic
- *Skin:* cool, pale, edematous
- *Mental status:* lethargic to comatose
- *Urine output:* oliguria to anuria
- *Other:* normal to decreased body temperature; decreased CVP

In older adults, cardiac changes may include a thickened left ventricular wall, decreased elasticity of the myocardium, and more rigid valves. These changes result in a decreased stroke volume and cardiac output, thus decreasing compensatory responses to septic shock. Decreased arterial wall elasticity and vasomotor tone reduce the older adult's ability to respond to a decrease in oxygenation. Decreased elasticity and turgor of the skin make assessments of skin turgor, and thus dehydration status, more difficult. Decreased immune system response increases the risk of septic shock.

▶ COLLABORATION

Septic shock can be fatal, but early and aggressive therapy improves outcomes (Mayo Clinic, 2013b). Collaborative care of the client with sepsis includes active participation by a number of specialists, such as infectious disease specialists, phlebotomists, and respiratory therapists. Gerontologists and pediatricians may be required for clients in those respective age groups, especially in determining safety and side effects when multiple medications are recommended.

Diagnostic Tests

The following diagnostic tests can help to identify the cause of sepsis and assess the client's physical status:

- *Hemoglobin and hematocrit* are performed, because changes in hematocrit concentrations usually occur in clients with septic shock as fluid leaks from the intravascular to the extravascular spaces. These changes reflect the body's response to endotoxins. In septic shock resulting from intravascular fluid loss, the hemoglobin and hematocrit concentrations are higher than normal.

- *Arterial blood gas* is performed to determine oxygen and carbon dioxide levels and pH. The effects of septic shock and of the body's compensatory mechanisms cause a decrease in pH (indicating acidosis), a decrease in PaO_2 and total oxygen saturation, and an increase in arterial partial pressure of carbon dioxide ($PaCO_2$).

- *Serum electrolytes* are measured to monitor the severity and progression of septic shock. As septic shock progresses, glucose levels decrease, sodium levels decrease, and potassium levels increase.

- *Blood urea nitrogen, serum creatinine levels, urine specific gravity, and osmolality* are obtained to check renal function, which declines as reduced perfusion and microclotting damage the small renal arterioles. As perfusion of the kidneys is decreased and renal function is reduced, the blood urea nitrogen and creatinine levels increase, as does urine specific gravity and osmolality.

- *Blood cultures* are done to identify the causative organism in septic shock and to direct treatment toward destruction of the pathogen.

- *White blood cell (WBC) count and differential* may initially show an increase or decrease in WBCs. As the body attempts to fight the infection, the WBC count may decrease as an increasing number of WBCs are destroyed. Elevated neutrophils indicate acute infection, increased monocytes indicate a bacterial infection, and increased eosinophils indicate an allergic response.

- *Serum enzymes,* such as lactate dehydrogenase, creatine phosphokinase, and serum glutamic-oxaloacetic transaminase, are often elevated in later stages of septic shock as capillaries in the liver are damaged.

- *Hemodynamic monitoring* provides information about preload and cardiac output to direct fluid resuscitation needs. A pulmonary artery catheter may be inserted to monitor cardiac dynamics, fluid balance, and the effects of vasoactive medications.

Other diagnostic tests may be ordered to determine the extent of injury or damage. These tests might include x-ray studies, computed tomography, magnetic resonance imaging, endoscopic examinations, and echocardiograms. Newer diagnostic methods for hypoperfusion include gastric tonometry and sublingual $PaCO_2$. Gastric tonometry measures the partial pressure of carbon dioxide in the gastric lumen. The measurement of sublingual carbon dioxide correlates well with decreased mean arterial pressure (MAP) (Sole, Klein, & Moseley, 2013).

Pharmacologic Therapy

Antimicrobials are a primary pharmacologic treatment if the infection is caused by bacteria or fungi. Generally, broad-spectrum antibiotics are used. The client may be placed on several antibiotics to ensure adequate coverage of the pathogen until culture and sensitivity results return in 72 hours to indicate the best antibiotic of choice. As antibiotics begin to take effect, the client's condition may worsen initially as increasing numbers of toxins are released into the circulating bloodstream because of pathogen destruction, further activating the immune response.

When fluid replacement alone is not sufficient to reverse shock, vasoactive drugs (drugs causing vasoconstriction or vasodilation) and inotropic drugs (drugs improving cardiac contractility) may be administered. When used to treat shock, these drugs increase venous return through vasoconstriction of peripheral vessels; they also improve the pumping ability of the heart by facilitating myocardial contractility and dilating coronary arteries to increase perfusion of the myocardium. More information on pharmacologic treatment for shock can be found in the exemplar on Shock in the module on Perfusion.

OXYGEN THERAPY   Establishing and maintaining a patent airway and ensuring adequate oxygenation are critical interventions in reversing septic shock. All clients in septic shock (even those with adequate respirations) should receive oxygen therapy (usually by mask or nasal cannula) to maintain the PaO_2 at greater than 80 mmHg during the first 4–6 hours of care. If the client's unassisted respiration cannot maintain PaO_2 at this level, endotracheal intubation may be necessary. Care of the client requiring ventilatory assistance is discussed in the module on Oxygenation.

FLUID REPLACEMENT   The most effective treatment for the client in septic shock is the administration of intravenous

Clinical Manifestations and Therapies **Sepsis**

ETIOLOGY	CLINICAL MANIFESTATION	CLINICAL THERAPIES
Disseminated intravascular coagulation may develop as a result of altered coagulation.	Varies from increased tendency to bleed to hemorrhage. Small clots may reduce blood flow to major organs; manifestations will be determined by organs affected. Prolonged clotting times, reduced fibrinogen and platelet levels. Spider angiomas or purpura are often seen on the client's skin if the affected individual is acutely ill.	■ Only effective treatment is to reverse the underlying cause (i.e., sepsis). ■ Platelet transfusions. ■ Fresh-frozen plasma administration. ■ Administration of antithrombin may be considered. ■ Activated protein C is given only in the intensive care unit to clients with severe sepsis.

fluids or blood. Various fluids may be administered alone or in combination as part of fluid replacement therapy. Whole blood or blood products increase the oxygen-carrying capacity of the blood and thus increase the oxygenation of cells. Fluid replacements, such as crystalloid and colloid solutions, increase circulating blood volume and tissue perfusion. Fluid replacements are administered in massive amounts through two large-bore peripheral lines or, most often, through a central line. More information about types of fluids can be found in the module on Fluid and Electrolytes.

> **SAFETY ALERT**
> Optimal fluid balance is +3 L at 12 hours after presentation, with a central venous pressure of <8 mmHg. A higher positive fluid balance and central venous pressure correlates to a greater mortality rate in clients with sepsis (Boyd et al., 2011).

■ NURSING PROCESS

Nursing assessment is critical in reducing the complications associated with sepsis. Identifying clients at risk and performing focused assessments are essential.

Assessment

Sepsis affects the entire body. Client assessment often includes continuous monitoring of vital signs, as well as monitoring of hemodynamic status, if a central venous pressure monitoring device (CVP or central line) or pulmonary artery catheter (PA catheter or Swan-Ganz catheter) is in place. Focused assessments are performed to monitor adequacy of ventilation, perfusion, and renal function.

As septic shock progresses, blood pressure decreases and pulse becomes rapid, weak, and thready. As perfusion of the lungs decreases, crackles, wheezes, and dyspnea are commonly present. Capillary refill is prolonged, and peripheral pulses are weak or nonpalpable. Flattened neck veins that cannot be seen when the client is in the supine position indicate decreased intravascular volume. CVP is very useful in evaluating the fluid balance status of the septic client. While normal CVP typically ranges from 2 to 8 mmHg, CVP will be decreased in clients experiencing septic shock.

Diagnosis

Priority nursing diagnoses for the client with sepsis include the following:

- *Risk for Shock*
- *Impaired Gas Exchange*
- *Risk for Ineffective Renal Perfusion*
- *Ineffective Peripheral Tissue Perfusion*
- *Risk for Imbalanced Fluid Volume*

(NANDA-I © 2012)

Planning

Planning care for the client with sepsis is very fluid, because the client's condition and needs can change very quickly. Because the client is critically ill, reassessment findings will often redirect the plan of care. Potential outcomes that may be appropriate for the client with sepsis include the following:

- The client will maintain oxygen saturation greater than 90% and PaO_2 within normal limits.
- The client will maintain adequate renal perfusion to produce a minimum of 30 mL of urine per hour.
- The client will respond to fluid resuscitation with mean arterial blood pressure that returns to normal range.

Implementation

Diminished tissue perfusion causes **ischemia** (inadequate blood supply) and hypoxia (insufficient oxygen) of major organ systems, with the potential for significant impact on the kidneys, brain, heart, lungs, and gastrointestinal tract. Nurses working with clients who have sepsis should do the following:

- Monitor the client's skin color, temperature, turgor, and moisture. Decreased tissue perfusion is evidenced by the skin becoming pale, cool, and moist; as hemoglobin concentrations decrease, cyanosis occurs.
- Monitor the client's cardiopulmonary function by assessing/monitoring the following:
  a. Blood pressure (by auscultation or hemodynamic monitoring)
  b. Rate and depth of respirations
  c. Lung sounds

d. Pulse oximetry

e. Peripheral pulses (brachial, radial, dorsalis pedis, and posterior tibial); include presence, equality, rate, rhythm, and quality (if unable to palpate pulses, use a device such as a Doppler ultrasound flowmeter to assess peripheral arterial blood flow).

■ Monitor the client's jugular vein distention.

■ Take the client's CVP measurements.

■ Monitor the client's body temperature. An elevated body temperature increases metabolic demands, depleting reserves of bodily energy. It also increases myocardial oxygen demand and may place the client with previous cardiac problems at even greater risk for hypoperfusion.

■ Monitor the client's urinary output per Foley catheter hourly, using a urometer. Urine output is a reliable indicator of renal perfusion.

■ Assess the client's mental status and level of consciousness. The appropriateness of the client's behavior and responses reflects the adequacy of cerebral circulation. Restlessness and anxiety are common early in septic shock; in later stages, the client may become lethargic and progress to a comatose state. Altered levels of consciousness are the result of both cerebral hypoxia and the effects of acidosis on brain cells.

Other nursing interventions appropriate for the client with sepsis can be found in the exemplar on Shock in the module on Perfusion.

Evaluation

Clients with sepsis must be continuously and frequently reevaluated, sometimes as often as every few minutes, because their condition can change quickly. Following fluid administration, the client's blood pressure and perfusion may improve. As fluid leaves the intravascular space, however, the client's condition may decline again. As perfusion declines, renal, cardiac, pulmonary, and neurovascular status may change quickly.

NURSING CARE PLAN   A Client With Septic Shock

Huang Mei Lan is a 43-year-old unmarried woman who lives alone in a major West Coast city. Ms. Huang came to the United States 15 years ago from China and now speaks English well. Her family still lives in China. She worked in a neighborhood sewing shop until 3 years ago, when she was diagnosed with breast cancer. Her treatment included mastectomy of the affected breast and follow up chemotherapy.

Last month, Ms. Huang experienced a recurrence of cancer in the lymph glands of the affected side. Surgery to remove the glands was performed, and chemotherapy was started. Ms. Huang has a central line, a urinary catheter, and a surgical incision. She is underweight, weak, and depressed. Although she has multiple physical problems, she never complains or asks for any kind of medication.

ASSESSMENT

Ms. Huang's primary nurse, Robert O'Brien, enters her room early in the morning to make an initial assessment. He finds Ms. Huang huddled in the middle of the bed, shivering violently. Her vital signs are temperature 104°F oral; pulse 130 bpm; respirations 30/min; and blood pressure 88/42 mmHg. Her skin is hot, dry, and flushed with poor turgor. She is alert and oriented but is restless and appears anxious. Ms. Huang states she is nauseated and suddenly begins vomiting and is incontinent of liquid stool. Laboratory data indicate leukocytosis, respiratory alkalosis, and reduced platelet count. Blood cultures, as well as cultures of Ms. Huang's sputum, urine, and wound drainage, are conducted. She is diagnosed as having septic shock.

Hetastarch is ordered per intravenous line, and intravenous broad-spectrum antibiotics are begun until the organism and its portal of entry can be determined. Despite treatment, Ms. Huang's condition worsens. Her blood pressure continues to drop, her skin becomes cool and cyanotic, and she begins to have periods of disorientation. She is transferred to the critical care unit. As she is being prepared for the transfer, she begins to cry and asks, "Am I going to die?"

DIAGNOSES

■ *Ineffective Breathing Pattern* related to rapid respirations and progression of septic shock
■ *Ineffective Tissue Perfusion* related to progression of septic shock with decreased cardiac output, hypotension, and massive vasodilatation
■ *Deficient Fluid Volume* related to vomiting, diarrhea, high fever, and shift of intravascular volume to interstitial spaces
■ *Anxiety* related to feelings that illness is worsening and is potentially life-threatening and the transfer to the critical care unit

(NANDA-I © 2012)

PLANNING

Goals for Ms. Huang's care include:
■ The client will maintain adequate circulating blood volume.
■ The client will regain and maintain blood gas parameters within normal limits.
■ The client will regain and maintain stable hemodynamic levels.
■ The client will verbalize increased ability to cope with stressors.

INTERVENTIONS

■ Monitor respiratory status, including respiratory rate, rhythm, breath sounds, and oxygen saturation.
■ Monitor cardiovascular status, including arterial blood pressure; rate, rhythm, and quality of pulses; central venous pressure; pulmonary artery pressure; and cardiac output.
■ Monitor urinary output hourly, reporting output of less than 0.5 mg/kg/hr or any sustained decrease in urine production.
■ Monitor neurological status, including mental status and level of consciousness.

■ Monitor color and character of skin.
■ Monitor results of arterial blood gas, blood counts, clotting times, and platelet counts.
■ Monitor body temperature every 2 hours.
■ Explain procedures and provide comfort measures (e.g., oral care, skin care, turning, and positioning).

NURSING CARE PLAN (continued)

EVALUATION

Despite intensive nursing and medical care, Ms. Huang's condition remains critical. The interventions are continued.

CRITICAL THINKING

1. Vasopressors may be used in the treatment of septic shock. Explain the rationale for their use.
2. While monitoring Ms. Huang's arterial blood gas, the nurse notes that her PaO_2 is less than 60 mmHg and her $PaCO_2$ is greater than 50 mmHg. What do these findings indicate, and why have they occurred?
3. Ms. Huang has been given large amounts of colloids intravenously. Hemodynamic monitoring indicates a higher-than-normal CVP and pulmonary artery pressure. What do these findings indicate? What physical assessments would you make to confirm the changes?

REVIEW Sepsis

RELATE Link the Concepts and Exemplars

Linking the exemplar of sepsis with the concept of perfusion:

1. How is perfusion impacted by sepsis?
2. What nursing interventions could you initiate to promote perfusion in the client diagnosed with sepsis?

Linking the exemplar of sepsis with the concept of acid–base balance:

3. When analyzing the arterial blood gas of a client in septic shock, what changes would you anticipate?
4. What interventions (both nursing and collaborative) could you implement to promote acid–base balance in the client diagnosed with sepsis?

READY Go to Companion Skills Manual

REFER Go to Pearson Student Nursing Resources
nursing.pearsonhighered.com

- Additional review material

REFLECT Case Study

Frank Lauer is a 72-year-old man with moderate emphysema and hearing loss. He is a retired veteran who served as a medic in the army for his entire career. In his retirement, Mr. Lauer has taken an interest in electronics. Mr. Lauer has been married for 49 years to his wife, Marie. They have several grown children, grandchildren, and great-grandchildren who live within a few miles. Mr. Lauer occasionally goes with his wife to the senior center for bingo night or to the local movies.

Mr. Lauer's daughter tells him about free flu shots being provided at the local clinic, but he is afraid a flue shot will make him sick, so he declines. A few weeks later, he feels tired and develops a nagging cough. He gets short of breath very easily. His children want him to see the physician immediately, but Mr. Lauer says it's just a cold and he'll feel better in a few days without seeing the doctor. His cough becomes more severe at night, and he begins having trouble breathing but finds that sleeping in the recliner makes him feel better.

A few nights later, Mr. Lauer's cough is so severe that he feels as though he can't catch his breath between coughing episodes. Mrs. Lauer sets up a humidifier next to his chair and encourages him to drink more fluids and see the doctor in the morning. He just laughs and tells her she's a worrier. His breathing improves, and he falls asleep in the chair. In the morning, he feels so weak that he has trouble walking to the bathroom. His temperature is elevated again, his breathing is rapid, and he feels awful. He consents to visiting the doctor, who diagnoses bacterial pneumonia. Blood cultures are drawn and the results indicate septicemia.

1. What factors increased Mr. Lauer's likelihood of being diagnosed with sepsis?
2. How would you explain his condition to both Mr. and Mrs. Lauer?
3. Develop a nursing plan of care listing all potential nursing diagnoses and developing two of them to include goals, interventions, and expected outcomes.

EXEMPLAR 9.7   Tuberculosis

EXEMPLAR KEY TERMS

Anergic, 609
Bacilli, 606
Caseation necrosis, 606
Cavitation, 606
Dormant, 606
Droplet nuclei, 607
Encapsulated, 606
Extrapulmonary tuberculosis, 606
Hematogenous spread, 606
Hemoptysis, 609
Miliary tuberculosis, 606
Mycobacterium tuberculosis, 606
Negative airflow room, 616

Pneumothorax, 609
Purified protein derivative (PPD), 608
Tine test, 608
Tubercle, 606
Tuberculosis, 606

EXEMPLAR LEARNING OUTCOMES

After reading about this exemplar, you will be able to:

1. Describe the pathophysiology, etiology, clinical manifestations, and direct and indirect causes of tuberculosis.
2. Identify risk factors and prevention methods associated with tuberculosis.

3. Illustrate the nursing process in providing culturally competent care across the life span for individuals with tuberculosis.
4. Formulate priority nursing diagnoses appropriate for an individual with tuberculosis.
5. Summarize therapies used by interdisciplinary teams in the collaborative care of an individual with tuberculosis.

6. Plan evidence-based care for an individual with tuberculosis and the family in collaboration with other members of the healthcare team.
7. Evaluate expected outcomes for an individual with tuberculosis.

▶ OVERVIEW

Tuberculosis is a chronic, recurrent, infectious disease caused by *Mycobacterium tuberculosis*, a relatively slow-growing, slender, rod-shaped, acid-fast organism with a waxy outer capsule that increases its resistance to destruction. Because tuberculosis most often affects the lungs, many people think of it as a pulmonary disease, but primary or secondary tuberculosis lesions may affect other body systems, such as the kidneys, genitalia, bone, and brain.

Tuberculosis was a major public health concern early in the 20th century before the development of effective sanitation measures and drug treatment. Although it remains prevalent worldwide, tuberculosis is currently uncommon in the United States, especially among young adults of European descent. However, because of the development of drug-resistant strains, susceptibility of people with HIV/AIDS, and inadequate access to health care for high-risk populations, tuberculosis is still a significant public health threat.

▶ PATHOPHYSIOLOGY AND ETIOLOGY

Minute droplet nuclei containing one to three **bacilli** (rod-shaped bacteria) may elude upper airway defense systems, enter the lungs, and implant in an alveolus or respiratory bronchiole, usually in an upper lobe. As these bacteria multiply, they cause a local inflammatory response. The inflammatory response brings neutrophils and macrophages to the site. These phagocytic cells then surround and engulf the bacilli, isolating them and preventing their spread. The *M. tuberculosis* organisms continue to multiply slowly within the macrophage, however, and some of these bacilli enter the lymphatic system to stimulate a cell-mediated immune response. Neutrophils and macrophages isolate the bacteria but, again, cannot destroy them. A granulomatous lesion called a **tubercle** (a sealed-off colony of bacilli) is formed. Within the tubercle, infected tissue dies, forming a cheeselike center, a process called **caseation necrosis**.

After 2–12 weeks, once the organisms number from 1,000 to 10,000, cellular immune response can be elicited with the tuberculosis skin test. In infants younger than 6 months, however, because of their immature immune system, infection may progress to active tuberculosis even before the skin test becomes reactive (CDC, 2011b). If the immune response is adequate, scar tissue develops around the tubercle, and the bacilli remain **encapsulated** (enclosed). Although these lesions eventually calcify and become visible on x-ray, the client will not develop tuberculosis disease. If the immune response is inadequate to contain the bacilli, the tubercle may rupture, allowing the bacilli to spread; the result is tuberculosis pneumonia. Occasionally, the infection progresses, causing extensive destruction of lung tissue. In *primary tuberculosis*, granulomatous tissue may erode into a bronchus or a blood vessel, allowing the disease to spread throughout the lung or other organs. This severe form of tuberculosis is uncommon in healthy adults (Longo et al., 2012).

A previously healed tuberculosis lesion may be reactivated. *Reactivation tuberculosis* occurs when the immune system is suppressed because of age, disease, or use of immunosuppressive drugs. The extent of lung disease can vary from small lesions to extensive cavitation of lung tissue. Tubercles rupture, spreading bacilli into the airways to form satellite lesions and produce tuberculosis pneumonia. Without treatment, massive lung involvement can lead to death, or a more chronic process of tubercle formation and **cavitation** (formation of a cavity or bubble) may result. People with chronic disease continue to spread *M. tuberculosis* into the environment, potentially infecting others.

✳ Visit **nursing.pearsonhighered.com** to see an illustration of the pathogenesis of tuberculosis.

When primary disease or reactivation allows live bacilli to enter the bronchi, the disease may spread through the blood and lymph system to other organs and become **extrapulmonary tuberculosis**. These distant disease metastases may produce an active lesion, or they may become **dormant** (temporarily inactive but not dead) and reactivate at a later time. Extrapulmonary tuberculosis is especially prevalent in people with HIV/AIDS.

Miliary tuberculosis results from **hematogenous spread** (through the blood) of the bacilli throughout the body. Miliary tuberculosis causes chills and fever, weakness, malaise, and progressive dyspnea. Multiple lesions evenly distributed throughout the lungs are noted on x-ray, but the sputum rarely contains organisms. The bone marrow is usually involved, and the result is anemia, thrombocytopenia, and leukocytosis. Without appropriate treatment, the prognosis is poor.

The kidney and genitourinary tract are common extrapulmonary sites for tuberculosis. The organism spreads to the kidney through the blood, initiating an inflammatory process similar to the one in the lungs. Reactivation can occur years after the original infection. As the lesion then enlarges and caseates, a large portion of the renal parenchyma is destroyed. The infection then can spread to the rest of the urinary tract, including the ureters and bladder. Scarring and strictures commonly result. In men, the prostate, seminal vesicles, and epididymis may be involved. In women, tuberculosis may affect the fallopian tubes and ovaries. Manifestations of genitourinary tuberculosis develop insidiously. Symptoms of a urinary tract infection, including malaise, dysuria, hematuria, and pyuria, develop. Flank pain may be present. Men may develop manifestations of epididymitis or prostatitis: perineal, sacral, or scrotal pain and tenderness; difficulty voiding; and fever. Women may have manifestations of pelvic inflammatory disease, impaired fertility, or ectopic pregnancy.

Tuberculosis meningitis results when tuberculosis spreads to the subarachnoid space. In the United States, this complication most often affects older adults, usually from reactivation of latent disease. Manifestations, which develop gradually, include listlessness, irritability, diminished appetite, and fever. Headache and behavioral changes are common early symptoms in the older adult. As the disease progresses, the headaches increase in intensity, vomiting develops, and the level of consciousness decreases. Convulsions and coma may follow. Without appropriate treatment, neurological effects may become permanent.

Tuberculosis of the bones and joints is most likely to occur during childhood, when bone epiphyses are open and their blood supply is rich. The organisms spread via the blood to vertebrae, the ends of long bones, and joints. Immune and inflammatory processes isolate the bacilli, and the disease often becomes evident years or even decades later. Tuberculous spondylitis usually involves the thoracic vertebrae, eroding vertebral bodies and causing them to collapse. Significant kyphosis (concave curvature of the spinal column) develops, and the spinal cord may be compressed. The large, weight-bearing joints (hips and knees) are most often affected by tuberculous arthritis, although other joints can also be affected, particularly if they have been previously damaged. The involved joint is painful, warm, and tender.

Etiology

Tuberculosis is caused by the organism *M. tuberculosis*. It is transmitted by **droplet nuclei** (airborne droplets produced when an infected individual coughs, sneezes, speaks, or sings). The tiny droplets can remain suspended in air for several hours. Infection may develop when a susceptible host breathes in air containing droplet nuclei and the contaminated particle eludes the normal defenses of the upper respiratory tract to reach the alveoli.

Thanks to improved sanitation, surveillance, and treatment of people with active disease, the incidence of tuberculosis in the United States fell steadily until the mid-1980s. The late 1980s and early 1990s, however, saw a resurgence of the disease, attributed primarily to the HIV/AIDS epidemic, the emergence of multidrug-resistant (MDR) strains of tuberculosis, and social factors, such as immigration, poverty, homelessness, and drug abuse. Today, the number of people affected in the United States continues to decline, with a total of 10,521 cases reported in 2011, the lowest number recorded since national reporting began in 1953 (CDC, 2012i); approximately 6% of new tuberculosis cases are children under the age of 15 (CDC, 2012j). The decline in new cases can be attributed to tuberculosis control programs that emphasize promptly identifying new cases and initiating and completing appropriate therapy.

Worldwide, tuberculosis continues to be a significant health problem, with an estimated 2 billion people (one third of the world's population) infected by *M. tuberculosis*. An estimated 9 million cases of tuberculosis develop annually, and approximately 80% of the reported cases occur in 22 countries, most of which are in Asia and sub-Saharan Africa. In the United States, more than 60% of new cases occur in individuals who are foreign born (CDC, 2012g). Tuberculosis accounted for 1.4 million deaths worldwide in 2011 (WHO, 2013).

Some strains of *M. tuberculosis* have become resistant to the primary drugs used to treat the disease (isoniazid and

Focus on Diversity and Culture
Incidence of Tuberculosis

- The tuberculosis case rate for foreign-born U.S. residents is 12 times higher than for people born in the United States (CDC, 2012i).
- Asians living in the United States have the highest case rates, 25 times higher than that for Whites.
- Case rates for Blacks and Hispanics in the United States are 8 and 7 times greater, respectively, than those for Whites.

rifampin), and the number of MDR cases increased by 10.1% between 2010 and 2011 (CDC, 2012g). Worldwide, approximately 3.7% of new tuberculosis cases and 20% of recurrent cases are MDR, demonstrating resistance to at least isoniazid and rifampin. Of MDR tuberculosis cases identified worldwide, 9% are extensively drug resistant (XDR) (WHO, 2012a). XDR tuberculosis is resistant to isoniazid and rifampin, as well as all fluoroquinones and at least one of three second-line drugs (i.e., amikacin, kanamycin, and capreomycin). The prevalence of MDR and XDR tuberculosis in the United States is lower, with 1.3% of cases reported in 2011 identified as MDR. Only twelve cases of XDR were reported in the United States between 2008 and 2011 (CDC, 2012g).

Risk Factors

Today in the United States, tuberculosis affects primarily immigrants, individuals with HIV/AIDS, and disadvantaged populations. Racial and ethnic minorities, foreign-born individuals, and those with altered immune function are more likely to develop tuberculosis than the White population (CDC, 2012g; see the Focus on Diversity and Culture feature).

Poor urban areas are hit the hardest with tuberculosis, areas that are also affected by the epidemics of injection drug use, homelessness (see the Evidence-Based Practice feature), malnutrition, and poor living conditions. Overcrowded institutions also contribute to spread of the disease. Transmission has been documented in hospitals, homeless shelters, drug treatment centers, prisons, and residential facilities.

The risk for a new infection by *M. tuberculosis* is affected by characteristics of the infectious individual, extent of air contamination, duration of exposure, and susceptibility of the host. The number of microbes in the sputum, frequency and force of coughing, and behaviors such as covering the mouth when coughing affect the production of droplet nuclei. In a small, closed, or poorly ventilated space, droplet nuclei become more concentrated, increasing the risk of exposure. Prolonged contact, such as living in the same household, increases the risk. Less-than-optimal immune function, a problem for people in lower socioeconomic groups, injection drug users, the homeless, and people with alcoholism or HIV infection, increases the susceptibility of the host.

Once infection with *M. tuberculosis* has occurred, clients with HIV/AIDS are at high risk for developing active tuberculosis. HIV infection suppresses cellular immunity, which is vital to limiting the replication and spread of the bacilli.

Evidence-Based Practice Clients With Risk for Tuberculosis Problem

Problem

Homeless people and those living in homeless shelters have several identified risk factors for tuberculosis: a high incidence of drug and alcohol abuse, a high incidence of HIV infection, and crowded living conditions. Access to and participation in tuberculosis screening and completion of pharmacologic therapy, however, are often problematic.

Evidence

In the United States, only 1% of the population experience homelessness in a given year, but more than 5% of people with tuberculosis reported being homeless within the year prior to diagnosis (CDC, 2013d). Studies in specific U.S. populations have indicated that as many as 43% of individuals with tuberculosis had a history of homelessness (Duval County, Florida; CDC, 2012e), and homeless and low-income populations were three times more likely than the general population to be infected with tuberculosis (New York, New York; Kerker et al., 2011). Major outbreaks also tend to cluster in homeless populations, such as an outbreak of 28 cases in Kane County, Illinois, in 2010–2011 all being associated with a specific homeless shelter (CDC, 2012l). Many of these individuals lack access to health care, including both screening and treatment. Of the two major screening tests for tuberculosis, the tuberculin skin test (TST) and the interferon-gamma release assay (IGRA), the TST was more cost effective in the homeless population (Linas et al., 2011). Several states now have recommendations in place to offer free TB screening for individuals living and working at homeless shelters. Many homeless people choose to participate in the screening out of a desire to maintain good health and a recognition that homelessness and shelter life increase their risk of developing tuberculosis. Fear of the results and a desire "not to be bothered" had negative effects on participation. Women with children were least likely to participate in screening, citing fear of a diagnosis resulting in a

loss of child custody (Swigart & Kolb, 2004). Once an individual has been diagnosed with tuberculosis, homelessness is also associated with a risk of not completing the required pharmacologic therapy (Mitruka, Winston, & Navin, 2012), which can lead to recurrent infection and antibiotic resistance.

Implications

Outreach to homeless populations for health services, while difficult, has personal and public health benefits. The homeless often lack access to preventive and health promotion services, instead interacting with healthcare providers only when urgent care is needed. However, a portion of this population desires to maintain good health and is receptive when screening and health promotion services are accessible. Shelter personnel are instrumental in getting individuals to participate in screening. Recruiting the support of these workers can improve resident participation. Regularly scheduling a nurse in a shelter can also improve participation in health promotion activities by allowing trust to develop. This strategy may be particularly important in shelters for women with children—bringing services to the residents to reduce their fear of being perceived as unable to care for their dependent children.

Critical Thinking Application

1. Provide a rationale for the importance of tuberculosis screening and effective treatment for homeless individuals in light of the national goal to eliminate tuberculosis.

2. Develop a client teaching strategy to increase the participation in free tuberculosis screening programs by homeless individuals and to increase medication adherence in those infected with tuberculosis.

3. What can you do personally to help provide tuberculosis screening, treatment, and follow up for the local homeless population?

Prevention

The tuberculin test is used to screen for tuberculosis infection. A cellular, or delayed hypersensitivity, response to *M. tuberculosis* develops within 3–10 weeks after the infection. Injecting a small amount of **purified protein derivative (PPD)** of tuberculin any time thereafter activates this response, attracting macrophages to the area and causing a pronounced local inflammatory response. The amount of induration surrounding the injection site, not the extended area of redness, is used to determine infection (see **Table 9–17** and **Figure 9–30**). It is important to remember that a positive response indicates that infection and a cellular (T-cell) response have developed; however, it does not mean that active disease is present or that the client is infectious to others.

Several methods are currently available for tuberculin testing:

- **Intradermal PPD test (Mantoux test).** Injection of 0.1 mL of PPD (5 tuberculin units) intradermally into the dorsal aspect of the forearm. This test is read within 48–72 hours (the peak reaction period) and recorded as the diameter of induration (raised area, not erythema) in millimeters.

- **Multiple-puncture test (tine test).** A multiple-puncture device is used to introduce tuberculin into the skin. This test

is less accurate than other testing methods. A vesicular reaction is considered positive; any other reaction must be confirmed by a Mantoux test.

Although it is impractical and unnecessary to screen the entire population, the CDC recommends screening people in the following risk groups:

- People with or at high risk for HIV infection

- Close contacts of people who have or are suspected of having infectious tuberculosis

- People with medical risk factors, such as silicosis, chronic malabsorption, end-stage renal failure, diabetes mellitus, immunosuppression, and hematological and other malignancies

- People born in countries with a high prevalence of tuberculosis

- Medically underserved, low-income populations, including racial and ethnic minorities and the homeless

- Individuals with alcoholism and injection drug users

- Residents and staff of long-term residential facilities, such as long-term care facilities, correctional institutions, and mental health facilities

TABLE 9–17	Interpreting Tuberculin Test Results
AREA OF INDURATION	**SIGNIFICANCE**
<5 mm	Negative response; does not rule out infection.
5–9 mm	Positive for people who: ■ Are in close contact with a client who has infectious tuberculosis. ■ Have an abnormal chest x-ray. ■ Have HIV infection or are immunocompromised. ■ Have an organ transplant. Negative for all others.
10–15 mm	Positive for people who have other risk factors: ■ Birth in a high-incidence country ■ Being African American, Hispanic, or Asian American in poverty areas ■ Injection drug use ■ Residence in a long-term care facility, correctional institution, residential care setting, or homeless shelter ■ Medical risk factors (e.g., malnutrition, diabetes).
>15 mm	Positive for all people.

False-negative responses are common in people who are immunosuppressed. A two-step procedure may be necessary to elicit a positive response. If the first test elicits a negative response, a second PPD test is given 1 week later. If the second test also is negative, the client either is free of infection or is **anergic** (unable to react to common antigens). This two-step procedure is recommended for long-term care residents and workers.

Only children who have one or more risk factors, such as close contact with an individual diagnosed with tuberculosis, a compromised immune system, or recent immigration, should have an intradermal tuberculin skin test with PPD (the Mantoux test). Children with a positive PPD should then undergo further diagnostic testing to determine whether active disease is present. Children are more likely than adults to progress rapidly from infection to disease; progression to disease is influenced by age, nutritional and immune status, genetic factors, virulence of the organism, and magnitude of infection. Young age (less than 2 years) and HIV infection are the two greatest risk factors in children for progression to disease (Swaminathan & Rekha, 2010).

If tuberculosis screening tests indicate the presence of tuberculosis infection, clients with latent infection should take precautions to prevent the development of active disease, and clients with active disease should take precautions to prevent the transmission of disease to others. Prophylactic pharmacologic therapy is indicated for treatment of latent disease, and pharmacologic therapy in addition to infection prevention techniques such as staying home during the first several weeks of therapy, covering the mouth and nose when coughing, wearing a mask in public places, and providing adequate room ventilation should be implemented for clients with active disease (Mayo Clinic, 2013c). For clinicians, infection control methods include promptly identifying clients with active disease, using airborne precautions, and effectively treating individuals with suspected or confirmed disease (CDC, 2012k)

▶ CLINICAL MANIFESTATIONS

Initial infection with *M. tuberculosis* causes few symptoms and typically goes unnoticed until the tuberculin test becomes positive or calcified lesions are seen on a chest x-ray. Manifestations of primary progressive or reactivation tuberculosis often develop insidiously and are initially nonspecific. Fatigue, weight loss, diminished appetite, low-grade afternoon fever, and night sweats are common. A dry cough develops, which later becomes productive of purulent and/or blood-tinged sputum (**hemoptysis**). It is often at this stage that the client first seeks medical attention.

Tuberculosis empyema and bronchopleural fistula are the most serious complications of pulmonary tuberculosis. When a tuberculosis lesion ruptures, bacilli may contaminate the pleural space. Rupture also may allow air to enter the pleural space from the lung, causing **pneumothorax** (a partial lung collapse caused by air or gas collecting in the lung or pleural space that surrounds the lungs).

Lifespan and Cultural Considerations

Infants, children, and adolescents with latent tuberculosis have no symptoms. Clinical manifestations of active tuberculosis in infants include a persistent cough, weight loss or failure to gain weight, and low-grade fever. Wheezing and decreased breath sounds may be present. Children with active disease may have fatigue, cough, diminished appetite, weight loss or growth delay, night sweats, chills, a low-grade fever, and enlarged lymph nodes.

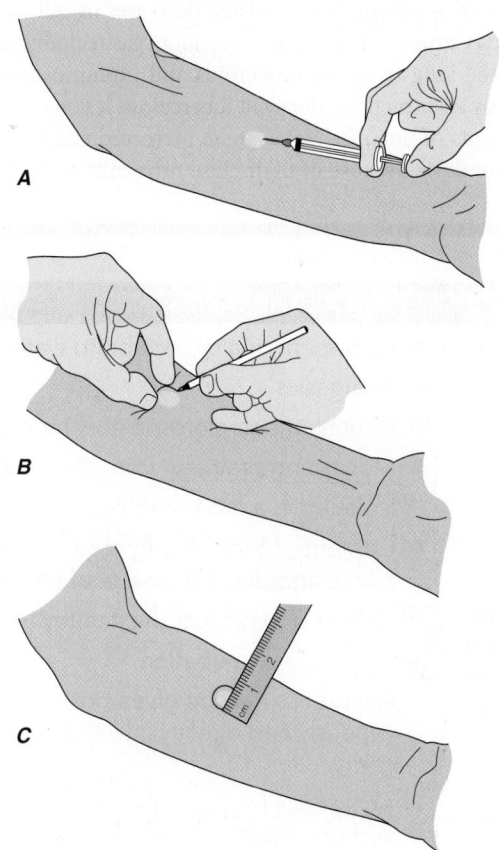

Figure 9–30 ● *A,* Intradermal injection for tuberculin testing. *B,* The injection causes a local inflammatory response (wheal). *C,* Measurement of induration following tuberculin testing.

Community-Based Care Assessment of Community-Dwelling Older Adults for Tuberculosis

Community-dwelling older adults as well as those in care facilities are susceptible to tuberculosis. The older adult with respiratory symptoms often is treated presumptively for pneumonia, without a sputum smear and Gram stain. Older adults living in the community may not have had a tuberculin test or chest x-ray for many years.

Nurses working with these clients typically assess risk factors for tuberculosis, such as the following:

- General health and nutritional status, including intake of specific nutrients, such as vitamin D (lack of vitamin D is associated with a higher risk of developing active tuberculosis)
- Presence of a chronic disease (e.g., silicosis, diabetes, alcoholism, or HIV infection) or past history of a gastrectomy
- Past history of a positive tuberculin test that now has converted to negative
- Medications, such as corticosteroids or other immunosuppressive drugs.

Nurses may also assess living and social situations, such as the following:

- Natural light and ventilation in the home
- Access to clean water, cooking facilities, grocery stores, and other services

- Possible exposure to infected people, such as sharing a household with someone who has active tuberculosis, crowded living facilities, homelessness, frequent participation in activities for older adults, and volunteer work in residential care facilities or other institutional settings
- Access to health care

Tuberculosis is typically treated in the community; hospitalization or institutionalization is rarely necessary or desirable. For the older adult being treated for active tuberculosis in the community, the nurse should assess the following:

- Knowledge and understanding of the disease and the prescribed treatment regimen
- Mental status and ability to follow both the prescribed regimen and precautions to avoid exposing others to the disease
- Transportation and regular access to healthcare services
- Financial resources to complete treatment and follow up care
- Need for home health or social services to ensure adequate treatment

Presenting symptoms of tuberculosis in the older adult are often vague, including coughing, weight loss, diminished appetite, and periodic fevers. These signs and symptoms should not be dismissed as a normal part of aging. The prevalence of active tuberculosis is significantly higher among older adults in the United States than among young adults (Pratt et al., 2011). Among older adults, approximately 90% of cases occur because of reactivation of a dormant bacterium. Older adults are at increased risk for reactivation tuberculosis as a result of age-related decreases in cell-mediated immunity. Chronic illnesses, poor nutrition, gastrectomy, alcoholism, or the long-term use of steroids and immunosuppressive agents may also reactivate dormant tuberculosis lesions.

Residents of nursing homes are at increased risk for acquiring tuberculosis because of their close proximity to each other.

Clinical Manifestations and Therapies Tuberculosis

ETIOLOGY	CLINICAL MANIFESTATION	CLINICAL THERAPIES
Rupture of tuberculosis lesion with contamination of the pleural space resulting in pneumothorax	Shortness of breath, hypoxia, dry cough, cyanosis, chest pain, and subcutaneous emphysema	■ Placement of a chest tube to water-seal ■ Analgesics ■ Continuous cardiorespiratory monitoring ■ Monitoring drainage from chest tube ■ Isolation in a room with negative airflow
Empyema and bronchopleural fistula are the most serious complications of tuberculosis. Empyema is a collection of pus within the pleural space that initiates an inflammatory response, leading to fibrous peel and trapped lung parenchyma. After resection of lung tissue, bronchopleural fistulas may develop because of inadequate healing of the stump, allowing bacteria to move into the pleural space and risking infection of the other lung.	Dyspnea with little exertion, low-grade fever, pleuritic chest pain, chest heaviness on affected side, purulent sputum, decreased breath sounds on involved side of chest, hemithorax, and opacification of the affected side on chest x-ray	■ Computed tomography may be used to locate and direct drainage of the area. ■ Priority is to protect the healthy lung. ■ May require intubation. ■ Antibiotics may be given both intravenously and directly into the infected cavity. ■ Analgesics for pain related to condition and treatment may be required.

Yearly tuberculin skin testing with purified protein derivative (PPD) is often required by state health departments for nursing home residents. If the initial test is negative, a repeat PPD in 1–2 weeks is recommended. This repetition improves sensitivity to the test so that silent cases of tuberculosis are not missed. A chest x-ray and sputum culture for acid-fast bacilli are obtained if the PPD is positive.

▶ COLLABORATION

Interdisciplinary care focuses on the following:

- Early detection
- Accurate diagnosis
- Effective disease treatment
- Preventing the spread of tuberculosis to others

To support the client with active infection, collaboration with an infectious disease specialist may be necessary. A client whose tuberculosis negatively impacts oxygenation may need to see a respiratory therapist, who can serve the client either at home or in an institutional setting. Clients who are homeless may need additional medical care, because the diagnosis and treatment of tuberculosis may lead to the diagnosis of other illnesses that have not been previously identified or for which the client has not been receiving treatment.

Diagnostic Tests

A positive tuberculin test alone does not indicate active disease. Sputum tests for the bacillus and chest x-rays are routinely used to diagnose and evaluate active disease. A series of three consecutive early-morning sputum specimens are typically examined for bacilli. The nurse should use special procedures or personal protective devices when obtaining sputum specimens, including a mask capable of filtering droplet nuclei. If possible, collect specimens in a room equipped with airflow control devices, ultraviolet light, or both. Alternatively, the client should step outside for collection of the specimen. Aerosol therapy, percussion, and postural drainage may help the client to produce sputum. Occasionally, endotracheal suctioning, bronchoscopy, or gastric lavage is necessary to obtain a specimen.

Diagnostic testing often proceeds as follows:

- A *sputum smear* is microscopically examined for acid-fast bacilli. *M. tuberculosis* resists decolorizing chemicals after staining. Therefore *M. tuberculosis* is called *acid fast*. The acid-fast smear provides a rapid indicator of the tubercle bacillus.

- *Sputum culture* that is positive for *M. tuberculosis* provides the definitive diagnosis. However, *M. tuberculosis* is slow growing, requiring 4–8 weeks before it can be detected with traditional culture techniques. Automated radiometric culture systems (e.g., Bactec) allow detection of *M. tuberculosis* in several days.

- *Sensitivity testing* is performed to identify the appropriate drug therapy once the organism is detected.

- A *polymerase chain reaction* permits rapid detection of DNA from *M. tuberculosis*.

- A *chest x-ray* is ordered to diagnose and evaluate tuberculosis. Typical findings in pulmonary tuberculosis include dense lesions in the apical and posterior segments of the upper lobe and possible cavity formation.

Before initiating antituberculosis drug therapy, several additional diagnostic tests may be done to establish baseline data for monitoring potential adverse effects of the drugs:

- *Liver function tests* are obtained before treatment with isoniazid, because this drug is hepatotoxic.

- *A thorough vision examination* is done before treatment with ethambutol, a commonly used antituberculosis medication. Optic neuritis is a potential adverse effect of this drug. Periodic eye examinations are scheduled during the course of therapy.

- *Audiometric testing* is performed before streptomycin therapy is initiated. Ototoxicity is a significant adverse effect of streptomycin and other aminoglycoside antibiotics. Hearing also is evaluated periodically during the course of therapy to detect any hearing loss.

Pharmacologic Therapy

Antibiotics are used both to prevent and to treat tuberculosis infection. Goals of the pharmacologic treatment of tuberculosis are as follows:

- To make the disease noncommunicable to others
- To reduce symptoms of the disease
- To effect a cure in the shortest possible time

PROPHYLAXIS Prophylactic treatment is used to prevent active tuberculosis. Clients with a recent skin test conversion from negative to positive are often started on prophylactic therapy, especially when other risk factors are present. Prophylactic therapy also is used for people in close household contact with an individual whose sputum is positive for bacilli. Single-drug therapy is effective for prophylactic treatment, whereas treatment of active disease always involves two or more chemotherapeutic medications. For adults, isoniazid, 300 mg per day for a period of 6–12 months, is commonly used to prevent active tuberculosis. This therapy may also be used for individuals who are susceptible to tuberculosis infection, such as individuals with HIV.

When isoniazid prophylaxis is contraindicated, Bacille Calmette-Guérin (BCG) vaccine may be prescribed. This vaccine is widely used in developing countries. BCG is made from an attenuated strain of *Mycobacterium bovis*, a closely related bacillus that causes tuberculosis in cattle. In the United States, BCG vaccine is recommended only for foreign-born infants and children as well as infants, children, and healthcare workers with a negative tuberculin test who are repeatedly exposed to untreated or ineffectively treated individuals who have active disease. After vaccination with BCG, a positive reaction to tuberculin testing is common. Periodic chest x-rays may be required for screening purposes.

TREATMENT OF ACTIVE DISEASE The tuberculosis bacillus mutates readily to drug-resistant forms when only one anti-infective agent is used. Active disease is always treated with concurrent use of at least two antibacterial medications to which the organism is sensitive. The primary antituberculosis drugs can prevent development of resistance, because all act by different mechanisms. However, the organism is protected within the tubercle, and 6 or more months of treatment are necessary to eradicate it.

Newly diagnosed tuberculosis is typically treated with an initial regimen of four oral antituberculosis drugs—isoniazid, rifampin, pyrazinamide, and ethambutol daily (or several times per week on a decreasing schedule of frequency)—for the first 2 months of treatment. This initial regimen is followed by at least 4 additional months of therapy with isoniazid and rifampin, given daily, twice per week, or weekly. In the presence of HIV infection, treatment is continued for at least 9 months. The most common antituberculosis drugs and their nursing implications are outlined in Medications feature below. If a drug-resistant strain is suspected, therapy is tailored to the resistance.

SAFETY ALERT
None of the tuberculosis drugs has been proved to be teratogenic. While isoniazid crosses the placenta, most studies show no teratogenic effects. Rifampin crosses the placenta, and the possibility of teratogenic effects is still being studied. However, potential adverse effects on the fetus are weighed against the benefit to the mother before they are prescribed during pregnancy.

ADHERENCE Adherence to the prescribed regimen is evaluated during follow up visits. The urine can be examined for color changes characteristic of rifampin and tested for metabolites of isoniazid. When Adherence is a problem, medications are administered under direct supervision. Twice-weekly therapy is more cost effective in this instance, with a public health nurse watching the client take and swallow the prescribed medication.

Box 9–6 Screening Questions to Identify Risk for Latent Tuberculosis Infection

- Determine client's understanding of tuberculosis.
- Collect demographic information so follow up can be provided if needed.
- Review the client's medical record, including laboratory and radiology findings.
- Question the client's past tuberculosis history and exposure to others diagnosed with tuberculosis.
- Does the client have any symptoms of tuberculosis
- Determine history of present illness and social history
- If the client was previously treated for tuberculosis were they compliant with the treatment regimen
- Was the client born outside the country or traveled outside the country? Have immediate family members recently traveled outside the country?

Source: Based on Centers for Disease Control and Prevention. (2010). *Self-study modules on tuberculosis.* Retrieved from http://www.cdc.gov/tb/education/ssmodules/module8/ss8reading4.htm.

FOLLOW UP Repeat sputum specimens and chest x-rays are used to evaluate the effectiveness of therapy. In most cases, sputum cultures for *M. tuberculosis* are negative within 2 months of therapy; virtually all clients have negative sputum cultures within 3 months. If cultures remain positive at 3 months and beyond, treatment failure and drug resistance are suspected. In this case, cultures of the organism are tested for susceptibility to antituberculosis agents, and two or three previously unused drugs are added to the treatment regimen (Longo et al., 2012). Given adequate treatment, almost all clients are cured of tuberculosis. Nonadherence to the treatment regimen is the greatest barrier to the control of tuberculosis (CDC, 2011b).

Medications **Antituberculosis Drugs**

CLASSIFICATION AND DRUG EXAMPLES	MECHANISM OF ACTION	NURSING CONSIDERATIONS

Isoniazid
 	
Drug examples:
INH
Laniazid
Nydrazid
	Isoniazid (oral, 5 mg/kd/day [max: 300 mg/day]) is the drug of choice for tuberculosis prophylaxis and a first-line drug for treating active disease. It is effective against both intracellular and extracellular organisms. Isoniazid is used alone as a prophylactic medication and in combination with rifampin, ethambutol, or both. A fixed-dose combination form with 150 mg of INH and 300 mg of rifampin (Rifamate) is available as well.	■ Administer on an empty stomach 1 hour before or 2 hours after meals for maximal effect if tolerated; may be given with meals to reduce gastrointestinal effects.
		■ Administer pyridoxine (vitamin B6) concurrently.
		■ Monitor for adverse effects:
		  a. Peripheral neuropathy
		  b Hypersensitivity reactions
		  c. Evidence of anemia, bruising, bleeding, or infection related to agranulocytosis
		■ Isoniazid interferes with the metabolism of diazepam, phenytoin, and carbamazepine. Doses of these drugs may need to be reduced to prevent toxicity.
		
		Health education for the client and family:
		■ Take the medication as prescribed for the entire treatment period to prevent incomplete eradication of the bacteria and development of resistant strains.
		■ Immediately report adverse effects (diminished appetite, nausea, jaundice, allergic reaction) to a healthcare provider immediately.
		■ Take pyridoxine as prescribed to prevent peripheral neuropathy.
		■ Avoid alcohol and other agents that may be harmful to the liver.
		■ Use measures to prevent pregnancy while taking INH; this drug may be harmful to the developing fetus.

Medications **Antituberculosis Drugs** (continued)

CLASSIFICATION AND DRUG EXAMPLES	MECHANISM OF ACTION	NURSING CONSIDERATIONS
Rifampin *Drug examples:* Rifadin Rimactane	Rifampin (oral, 600 mg daily) is commonly used in combination with INH and other antituberculosis drugs. Rifampin stimulates the microsomal enzymes of the liver, increasing the rate of metabolism of many drugs and decreasing their effectiveness.	■ Administer on an empty stomach. ■ Monitor CBC, liver function studies, and renal function studies for evidence of toxicity. ■ Rifampin reduces the effect of oral contraceptives, quinidine, corticosteroids, warfarin, methadone, digoxin, and hypoglycemics. Monitor for the effectiveness of these drugs. *Health education for the client and family:* ■ Rifampin causes body fluids, including sweat, urine, saliva, and tears, to turn red-orange. This effect is not harmful. Avoid wearing soft contact lenses, because they may be permanently stained. ■ Do not miss or skip doses; flulike syndrome and fever occur when drug is resumed. ■ Aspirin may interfere with rifampin absorption and should not be taken concurrently. ■ Fever, flulike symptoms, excessive fatigue, sore throat, or unusual bleeding may indicate an adverse reaction to the drug and should be reported to healthcare provider.
Pyrazinamide *Drug example:* Tebrazid	Pyrazinamide (oral, 15–30 mg/kg/day [max: 3 g/day]) typically is given with INH and rifampin for the first 2 months of tuberculosis treatment. Concurrent use of pyrazinamide allows a shorter course of therapy. Like many of the antituberculosis agents, pyrazinamide is toxic to the liver. Its other principal adverse effect is hyperuricemia. Gout, however, rarely develops.	■ Administer with meals to reduce gastrointestinal side effects. ■ Monitor liver function studies and serum uric acid levels. Notify the physician of any changes. *Health education for the client and family:* ■ Notify healthcare provider of loss of appetite, nausea, vomiting, jaundice, or symptoms of gout (a painful, red, hot, swollen joint, often the great toe or elbow). ■ While taking this drug, avoid using alcohol or other substances that may be harmful to the liver.
Ethambutol *Drug example:* Myambutol	Ethambutol (oral, 15–25 mg/kg/day) is added to the initial treatment regimen or substituted for INH when an INH-resistant strain of tuberculosis is suspected. Ethambutol is a bacteriostatic drug that reduces the development of resistance to the bactericidal first-line agents. Its principal toxic effect is optic neuritis; fortunately, this effect is reversible. Early signs of optic neuritis include decreased visual acuity and loss of red–green discrimination. This drug may be safe for use in pregnancy.	■ Record a baseline visual examination before therapy. Schedule periodic eye exams during the course of treatment. ■ Administer with meals to reduce gastrointestinal side effects. ■ Monitor liver and renal function studies and neurological status while taking this drug. Notify healthcare provider of abnormal findings or significant changes. *Health education for the client and family:* ■ Monitor vision daily by reading newspapers and looking at the same blue object (using usual corrective lenses, if appropriate). Notify healthcare provider of changes in vision or color perception.
Streptomycin	An aminoglycoside antibiotic, streptomycin (intramuscular, 15 mg/kg/day [max: 1 g/day]) is highly effective in treating most mycobacterial infections. Resistance may develop if it is used alone. There are two primary drawbacks to streptomycin: First, it must be administered parenterally, because it is not absorbed in the gastrointestinal tract. Second, it has toxic effects on the kidneys and ears.	■ Administer by deep intramuscular injection into a large muscle mass, rotating sites to minimize tissue trauma. ■ Monitor urine output, weight, and renal function studies (including blood urea nitrogen and serum creatinine) to detect early signs of nephrotoxicity. Report significant changes to the physician. ■ Maintain fluid intake at 2,000–3,000 mL per day to minimize the concentration of drug in the kidney tubules. ■ Assess hearing and balance frequently. Have audiometric testing performed as indicated. *Health education for the client and family:* ■ Maintain a daily fluid intake of at least 2–3 liters. ■ Weigh yourself on the same scale at least twice a week. Report any significant weight gain to healthcare provider. ■ Notify healthcare provider of decreased hearing acuity, ringing or buzzing sensations in the ear, or vertigo.

■ NURSING PROCESS

Nurses play a key role in maintaining public health. Education and tuberculosis screening are major nursing strategies to prevent tuberculosis. Nurses have an important role in identifying individuals with one or more risk factors for infection, such as foreign-born individuals, individuals with HIV, and individuals residing in states with a higher incidence of tuberculosis (California, Texas, New York, and Florida) (CDC, 2012i).

Public health teaching includes increasing awareness of tuberculosis as a reemerging threat. Teach clients in all settings how to reduce the spread of tuberculosis by covering their mouths when coughing or sneezing and disposing of sputum appropriately. Also include in public health education the benefit of screening programs to identify infected (though not necessarily infective) people.

Assessment

Focused assessment for the client with suspected tuberculosis includes the following:

■ *Health history.* Complaints of fatigue, weight loss, night sweats, difficulty breathing, cough (productive or nonproductive), hemoptysis, or chest pain; known exposure to tuberculosis; most recent tuberculin test and results; living circumstances; and alcohol and other recreational drug use
■ *Physical examination.* Vital signs, including temperature; general appearance; respiratory rate and lung sounds; and weight and appearance of malnutrition.

Use screening questions (**Box 9–6** ●) to identify individuals at risk for latent infection. Screen infants and children every 6 months until age 2, and then annually (American Academy of Pediatrics, 2008).

Diagnosis

Nursing diagnoses for the client with the medical diagnosis of tuberculosis may include the following:

■ *Fatigue*
■ *Imbalanced Nutrition: Less Than Body Requirements*
■ *Deficient Knowledge*
■ *Ineffective Therapeutic Regimen Management*
■ *Risk for Infection*
■ *Deficient Community Health*
■ *Social Isolation*

(NANDA-I © 2012)

Planning

Care planning is based on the needs of the client, the resources and support available, the client's general health status, and the client's environment. Suggested outcomes include the following:

■ The client will demonstrate behaviors that reduce the risk of contamination of others.

■ The client will describe required treatment and follow up care required.
■ The client will have adequate resources available to obtain necessary medications and supplies.

Implementation

Nursing care related to tuberculosis focuses primarily on infection control and compliance with prescribed treatment. See the Nursing Care Plan feature.

Provide Client Education

Adequate knowledge and information are necessary to manage the disease and prevent its transmission to others. The client needs to understand the reasons for prolonged drug therapy and the importance of complying with treatment and follow up. Antituberculosis drugs are relatively toxic. The client needs to know how to minimize their toxicity. Interventions to promote the client's understanding of disease transmission and management include the following:

■ Assess the client's knowledge about the disease process, and identify misperceptions and emotional reactions. Teaching based on previous learning enhances understanding and retention of information.
■ Assess the client's ability and interest in learning, developmental level, and obstacles to learning. Assessment allows tailoring the presentation of information to the learning needs and style of the client, promoting learning.
■ Identify the client's support systems, and include significant others in teaching. A knowledgeable significant other provides reinforcement of learning, confirmation of understanding, and encouragement for the client. Including significant others also reduces the risk of inadvertent sabotage of the treatment plan.
■ Establish a relationship of mutual trust with the client and significant others. An atmosphere of trust increases receptiveness to teaching and learning.
■ Develop mutually acceptable learning goals with the client and significant other. Working together to identify learning needs and establish goals increases the client's ownership of and interest in the process.
■ Select appropriate teaching strategies, using learning aids such as literature and visual materials that are appropriate for age, level of education, and intellect. Teaching tailored to the client is more effective and results in better learning.
■ Document your teaching and the level of the client's understanding. Reinforce teaching and learning as needed. Teaching is not complete until the client can demonstrate learning of the information.

Promote Effective Therapeutic Regimen Management

The populations at highest risk for developing active tuberculosis—the homeless and members of lower socioeconomic groups—are also at high risk for being unable to manage its complex treatment regimen. Three or more costly medications

Client Teaching Managing Tuberculosis

Tuberculosis is a chronic disease requiring lengthy treatment with antituberculosis medications. Teaching focuses on treatment and on improving the client's ability to self-manage the disease. A good understanding of the disease, its treatment, and the potential adverse effects of therapy prepares the client to manage care. Teach the client and family about tuberculosis and the prescribed treatment, including:

- Nature of the disease and its spread
- Purpose of treatment and follow up procedures
- Measures to prevent spreading the disease to others
  a. Using disposable tissues to contain respiratory secretions, especially during the first 2 weeks of treatment, when the disease may be transmitted to others
  b. Avoiding exposure to crowds or people with infectious diseases
  c. Ensuring that housemates or others having frequent contact with the client are tested and receive prophylactic treatment if indicated.
- Importance of maintaining good general health by eating a well-balanced, high-protein, high-carbohydrate diet and balancing exercise with rest.
- Names, doses, purposes, and adverse effects of prescribed medications, with emphasis on the importance of taking all medications as prescribed.
- The possible side effects of the prescribed medications and the importance of reporting them to healthcare providers. Possible side effects:

  a. Peripheral neuropathy (numbness, tingling, or a burning sensation of the extremities) may occur with isoniazid (INH). Pyridoxine (vitamin B6) often is prescribed to prevent this adverse effect.
  b. Both INH and rifampin may cause hepatitis. Avoid alcohol while taking these drugs and report any manifestations, such as nausea and diminished appetite, jaundice, a change in urine or stool color, or pain in the upper right quadrant.
  c. Rifampin may cause an orange-red coloration of saliva and urine.
  d. Streptomycin can affect hearing and balance. Promptly report any changes, because they may be irreversible.
  e. Ethambutol may affect red–green color discrimination and visual acuity. Use caution when driving or walking in unfamiliar areas, and promptly report any vision changes.
- Importance of avoiding alcohol and other substances that may damage the liver while taking chemotherapeutic drugs
- Fluid intake needs of 2–3 liters quarts of fluid per day
- Manifestations to report to the healthcare provider: chest pain, hemoptysis, or difficulty breathing; diminished appetite, nausea, or vomiting; yellow tint to skin or sclera; sudden weight gain; swollen feet, ankles, legs, or hands; hearing loss, tinnitus, or vertigo; and change in vision or difficulty discriminating colors.

are prescribed that may have unpleasant or even dangerous side effects. Frequent medical follow up is required. Infectious diseases such as tuberculosis also carry a stigma that may lead to denial of the disease or its seriousness. Individuals with alcoholism and those who use injection drugs need to withdraw from their addiction to be successful in treating the disease, and clients with HIV infection face a potentially fatal disease and costly treatment that may well override their concerns about tuberculosis management. Nursing interventions may include the following:

- Assess the client's self-care abilities and support systems. Assessment is used to help determine the client's ability to follow the prescribed regimen.
- Assess the client's knowledge and understanding of the disease, its complications, treatment, and risks to others. Provide additional teaching and reinforcement as indicated. Lack of understanding is a barrier to compliance with and management of the treatment regimen.
- Work collaboratively to identify barriers or obstacles to managing the prescribed treatment. Working collaboratively with the client and other members of the healthcare team provides insight for overcoming identified barriers to effective treatment.
- Assist the client, significant others (if available), and healthcare team members to develop a plan for managing the pre-

scribed regimen. Including the client in developing a plan to manage care increases the client's sense of control and ownership and helps to ensure that personal, cultural, and lifestyle factors are considered. All of this increases the likelihood of compliance.

- Provide verbal and written instructions that are clear and appropriate for the client's level of literacy, knowledge, and understanding. Clearly written directions provide support and reinforcement.
- Provide active intervention for homeless people, including shelter placement or other housing and ongoing follow up by easily accessed healthcare providers (clinics and public health workers in the neighborhood that do not present transportation or access problems, either real or perceived). Simple referral does not ensure compliance, especially among disenfranchised populations. Active intervention is needed to help ensure treatment compliance.
- Refer clients who are unlikely to comply with the treatment regimen to the public health department for management and follow up. Because tuberculosis presents a significant public health risk, public health follow up is essential. In some cases, it is necessary for nurses to administer medications, observing the client swallow all pills. Direct observation therapy may be needed for children as well as adults.

Reduce Risk for Infection

The spread of tuberculosis is a risk in any facility housing many people. The risk is especially high in residential care facilities for older adults and for people with AIDS. The increasing incidence of tuberculosis among homeless people and members of lower socioeconomic groups increases the risk in hospitals, emergency departments, and public and urgent care clinics. Respiratory precautions are necessary to prevent the spread of the disease to other clients and to healthcare workers via microscopic airborne droplets. The following steps can help to lower the risk of spreading the infection:

■ Place the client in a private room with airflow control that prevents air within the room from circulating into the hallway or other rooms. A **negative airflow room** (a room where air flows out of the room) in which air is diluted by at least six fresh-air exchanges per hour is recommended. A negative flow room and multiple fresh-air exchanges dilute the concentration of droplet nuclei within the room and prevent their spread to adjacent areas.

■ Use standard precautions and tuberculosis isolation techniques as recommended by the CDC, including wearing masks and gowns when caring for clients who do not reliably cover the mouth when coughing. These measures are important to prevent the spread of tuberculosis to others.

■ Discuss with the client the reasons for and importance of respiratory isolation procedures during initial hospitalization. When outpatient treatment is provided, instruct the client to avoid crowds and close physical contact and to maintain ventilation in living facilities, particularly during the first 3 weeks of treatment. These measures help to protect others during initial treatment, when sputum is still likely to contain significant numbers of bacilli.

■ Place a mask on the client during transport to other parts of the facility for diagnostic or treatment procedures. Covering the client's nose and mouth minimizes air contamination and the risk to visitors and personnel.

■ Inform all personnel having contact with the client of the diagnosis. This information allows personnel to take appropriate precautions.

■ Assist visitors to mask before entering the room. Providing visitors with appropriate masks or respirators reduces their risk of infection.

■ Teach the client how to limit transmitting the disease to others:
  a. Always cough and expectorate into tissues.
  b. Dispose of tissues properly, placing them in a closed bag.
  c. Wear a mask if sneezing or unable to control respiratory secretions.
  d. The disease is not spread by touching inanimate objects, so no special precautions are required for eating utensils, clothing, books, or other objects used.

Teaching appropriate precautions helps to prevent the spread of tuberculosis to others while allowing the client as much freedom from restraints as possible.

■ Teach the client how to collect sputum specimens. If necessary, have the client step outside the room when you collect a sputum specimen. This precaution minimizes healthcare personnel's risk of exposure and provides for rapid dilution of any droplet nuclei produced and their exposure to ultraviolet light, which kills the bacteria.

■ Teach the client the importance of complying with the prescribed treatment for the entire course of therapy. Completion of the entire treatment regimen is important to reduce the risk of relapse and the creation of drug-resistant organisms.

SAFETY ALERT

Use personal protective devices to reduce the risk of transmission during client care. The U.S. Occupational Safety and Health Administration (OSHA) requires use of a HEPA-filtered respirator for protection against occupational exposure to tuberculosis. Surgical masks are ineffective in filtering droplet nuclei, so the use of protective devices capable of filtering bacteria and particles smaller than 1 micron is necessary.

The nurse should provide referrals as appropriate:

■ Smoking cessation clinics or support groups
■ Alcohol treatment facilities, Alcoholics Anonymous, and other treatment programs or support groups
■ Drug treatment facilities, Narcotics Anonymous, and other outpatient or inpatient treatment programs or support groups
■ Low-cost community clinics and incentive programs for people with tuberculosis
■ Counseling, support groups, and other community resources that provide additional assistance and support

When caring for a woman who is pregnant or who has recently delivered, the nurse must consider both the woman and the baby. If the new mother is found to have tuberculosis, it is important to prevent direct contact with the newborn until the mother is noninfectious. If maternal tuberculosis is inactive or the mother has been on therapy long enough to prevent infection of the newborn, the mother may breastfeed and care for her baby. Because the newborn has an immature immune response, it is the nurse's responsibility to teach the mother how to reduce the infant's risk of infection.

Evaluation

Compliance with prescribed therapies, resolution of symptoms, and improvement on chest x-ray are all positive evaluation findings. Clients are evaluated on progress toward outcomes, and the plan of care is amended as indicated. Expected outcomes of nursing care include the following:

■ The client with latent infection completes therapy and does not develop active tuberculosis.
■ The client's contacts are evaluated for tuberculosis and those infected are treated.

NURSING CARE PLAN | A Client With Tuberculosis

Harry Facée, age 53, arrives at a metropolitan public health clinic complaining of aching chest pain that has lasted for the past few days. He says that his sputum also is bloody. He is afraid he might have lung cancer, so he came in to see a healthcare provider.

ASSESSMENT

Raj Kamil, RN, the public health nurse at the clinic, obtains an admission history and physical examination of Mr. Facée. Mr. Kamil notes that Mr. Facée is a homeless individual who has lived on the streets and in various shelters for the past "10 years or so." He usually prefers to sleep outdoors, taking refuge in shelters only during very cold or very wet weather. He has a small disability income but usually scrounges for food or eats with other homeless people at soup kitchens. Mr. Facée states that he has had a cough for a long time, which has become worse recently. It is now productive, especially in the mornings. He also admits that he has recently been waking up drenched with sweat in the middle of the night and is more tired than usual.

Although Mr. Facée's clothes are tattered, he is fairly clean. He answers questions appropriately and intelligently. Mr. Kamil does not detect any odor of alcohol on his breath. Mr. Facée is very thin, almost emaciated. His vital signs are temperature 37.8°C (100.2°F), pulse 92 bpm, respirations 20/min, and blood pressure 152/86 mmHg.

Suspecting tuberculosis, Mr. Kamil obtains a sputum specimen for Gram stain and culture, administers a tuberculin test, and sends Mr. Facée for a chest x-ray before he sees the clinic physician. Although the chest x-ray is inconclusive, the Gram stain is positive for acid-fast bacilli. The diagnosis is probable active pulmonary tuberculosis. The physician prescribes daily isoniazid, 300 mg orally; rifampin, 600 mg orally; and pyrazinamide, 1,500 mg orally for 2 months, to be followed by twice-weekly isoniazid, 900 mg orally, and rifampin, 600 mg orally. The physician also orders weekly sputum cultures for the first month.

DIAGNOSES

- *Ineffective Health Maintenance* related to homelessness
- *Risk for Noncompliance* with prescribed treatment related to lack of understanding and resources
- *Imbalanced Nutrition: Less Than Body Requirements* related to increased metabolic needs associated with infection

(NANDA-I © 2012)

PLANNING

Goals for Mr. Facée's care include:
- The client will keep all follow up appointments as scheduled.
- The client will verbalize an understanding of his disease and its treatment.
- The client will follow the prescribed plan of care.
- The client will demonstrate measures to prevent spread of the organism to others.
- The client will gain 1–2 lb of weight per week.
- The client will promptly report symptoms of peripheral neuropathy, including numbness, tingling, or burning sensations.

IMPLEMENTATION

- Teach the client about tuberculosis, and provide a client education pamphlet about the disease.
- Instruct the client about the prescribed medications, potential adverse effects, and importance of completing the entire prescribed regimen.
- Emphasize the importance of continued follow up.

- Teach and demonstrate sputum and droplet control measures.
- Escort the client to the local incentive shelter program for directly observed medical therapy and meals.
- Identify verbally and in writing manifestations to report to the physician.

EVALUATION

Mr. Kamil successfully enrolls Mr. Facée in the local incentive shelter program. In this program, a healthcare worker administers Mr. Facée's medications daily, watching him swallow them. Mr. Facée is assigned a small individual room and can eat three daily meals at the shelter. He still prefers to sleep outside when the weather permits, but he complies with the requirement for supervised medication administration because he "likes the food there." Always a clean individual, Mr. Facée is able to demonstrate appropriate sputum control measures and practices them faithfully. The sputum culture done after 2 months of treatment is negative for tubercle bacilli, and Mr. Facée's chest x-ray indicates no disease progression.

CRITICAL THINKING

1. *Many homeless people have schizophrenia or other mental diseases. How would you adapt the care plan for a homeless client with schizophrenia and active tuberculosis?*
2. *Mr. Kamil was fortunate in having access to an incentive shelter with healthcare workers to supervise medication compliance. Identify available resources in your area for homeless clients infected with tuberculosis.*
3. *Develop a care plan for the nursing diagnosis* Ineffective Airway Clearance *related to mucopurulent sputum and weak cough.*

REVIEW Tuberculosis

RELATE Link the Concepts and Exemplars

Linking the exemplar of tuberculosis with the concept of health policy:

1. What role does the government play in determining policies to mandate tuberculosis testing of those traveling to the United States from other countries, especially those countries with the highest number of cases?

2. What government reporting requirements must be followed when a client is diagnosed with tuberculosis?

Linking the exemplar of tuberculosis with the concept of ethics:

3. You are working in a clinic and read as positive a PPD skin test done 2 days ago. While providing routine teaching, you inform the client of the need to test those who have been in contact with the client, and the client says, "No, I will not tell you who I've been in contact with, and you have no right to share my personal medical information with others, especially the government." What legal rights does this client have regarding privacy of information, and how would you handle this situation?

4. What information can you provide about the necessity for testing and treatment for a parent who is afraid of losing custody of her children if diagnosed with tuberculosis?

READY Go to Companion Skills Manual

REFER Go to Pearson Student Nursing Resources
nursing.pearsonhighered.com

- Additional review materials
- Pathogenesis of Tuberculosis

REFLECT Case Study

Ngong Lee is a 62-year-old female who has been married to Daniel Lee for 42 years. Born and raised in Vietnam, Ms. Lee came to the United States after marrying her husband when she was 20. Their only child, John, died at age 22 in an automobile accident. His death devastated Ms. Lee, but over time, she adequately adjusted and coped with the loss. All of her brothers and sisters have passed away, but she has a few nieces and nephews who still live in Vietnam. She and Mr. Lee have no relatives nearby.

Ms. Lee has noticed a steady weight loss and lack of appetite over the past few weeks, ever since they returned from visiting relatives in Vietnam. At first, she was delighted with her new, slender figure, but as she continued to lose weight, she started to wonder whether she had cancer. This week, she has been waking at night wet with perspiration, and this afternoon, she took her temperature, and she has a slight fever. As she thinks about it, she realizes she's been tired lately and decides that it's time to see a healthcare provider. She makes an appointment at the local clinic and tells the nurse that she has lost 12 pounds in the past 3 weeks and describes her other symptoms. The nurse notices Ms. Lee coughing and asks when the cough started. Ms. Lee looks surprised and says that she hadn't noticed that she'd been coughing. The physician orders a chest x-ray, CBC with differential, PPD, and sputum specimen for culture. The physician advises the nurse to take appropriate precautions, because tuberculosis is the suspected diagnosis.

1. How will the nurse collect the sputum specimen to reduce the spread of infection?

2. When Ms. Lee comes back in 48 hours, her PPD is negative. The chest x-ray ordered by the physician shows dense lesions in the apical and posterior segments of the lung consistent with a diagnosis of tuberculosis. Sputum culture results have not returned yet. What does the nurse anticipate will be ordered for this client?

3. If Ms. Lee is confirmed to have tuberculosis, what teaching will the nurse provide?

4. Ms. Lee's sputum culture returns positive for the presence of bacilli. Why did her PPD come back negative? Will her family in Vietnam need to be tested? How will that testing be arranged? Who else will need to be tested secondary to exposure to Ms. Lee?

EXEMPLAR 9.8 Urinary Tract Infection

EXEMPLAR KEY TERMS
Cystitis, 619
Cystoscopy, 623
Dysuria, 621
Enuresis, 626
Gram stain, 623
Hematuria, 621
Hydronephrosis, 620
Intravenous pyelography (IVP), 623
Neurogenic bladder, 620
Nocturia, 621
Persistent bacteriuria, 627
Pyelonephritis, 619
Pyuria, 621
Reflux, 619
Reinfection, 627
Unresolved bacteriuria, 627
Ureteral stent, 624
Ureteroplasty, 623
Urgency, 621
Urinary drainage system, 619

Vesicoureteral reflux, 619
Voiding cystourethrography, 623

EXEMPLAR LEARNING OUTCOMES
After reading about this exemplar, you will be able to:

1. Describe the pathophysiology, etiology, clinical manifestations, and direct and indirect causes of urinary tract infection.

2. Identify the risk factors and prevention methods associated with urinary tract infection.

3. Illustrate the nursing process in providing culturally competent care across the life span for individuals with urinary tract infection.

4. Formulate priority nursing diagnoses appropriate for an individual with urinary tract infection.

5. Summarize therapies used by interdisciplinary teams in the collaborative care of an individual with urinary tract infection.

6. Plan evidence-based care for an individual with urinary tract infection and the family in collaboration with other members of the healthcare team.

7. Evaluate expected outcomes for an individual with urinary tract infection.

▶ OVERVIEW

The urinary tract includes the kidneys, ureters, urinary bladder, and urethra. Any part of this system can be affected by pathogens. A severe infection may involve multiple components of the urinary tract. Kidney infections can affect urine production and waste elimination and result in renal failure (explained in the Fluids and Electrolytes concept). Infection can interrupt the **urinary drainage system** (the organs required to drain urine from the kidneys, including the ureters, urinary bladder, and urethra), obstructing urine flow and affecting elimination.

- When caring for clients with urinary tract infections, it is important for the nurse to consider the client's modesty in voiding, possible difficulty in discussing the genitals, potential embarrassment about being exposed for examination and testing, and fear of changes in body function. These psychosocial issues can interfere with the client's willingness to seek help, discuss treatment, and learn about preventive measures.

- Nursing interventions for clients with urinary tract infections are directed toward primary prevention, early detection, and management of the disorder through health teaching and nursing care.

- Bacterial infections of the urinary tract are a common reason for seeking health services, second only to upper respiratory infections. More than 8 million people are treated annually for urinary tract infection (UTI) (Porth & Matfin, 2010). Community-acquired UTIs are common in young women but unusual in men under the age of 50.

- Most community-acquired UTIs are caused by *Escherichia coli*, common gram-negative enteral bacteria. Approximately 5%–15% of symptomatic UTIs are caused by *Staphylococcus saprophyticus*, a gram-positive organism. Catheter-associated UTIs often involve other gram-negative bacteria, such as *Proteus*, *Klebsiella*, *Serratia*, and *Pseudomonas*.

▶ PATHOPHYSIOLOGY AND ETIOLOGY

The urinary tract is normally sterile above the urethra. Adequate urine volume, a free flow from the kidneys through the urinary meatus, and complete bladder emptying are the most important mechanisms of maintaining sterility. Pathogens that enter and contaminate the distal urethra are washed out during voiding. Other defenses for maintaining sterile urine include the normal acidity of urine itself and the bacteriostatic properties of the bladder and urethral cells.

The peristaltic activity of the ureters and a competent vesicoureteral junction help to maintain sterility of the upper urinary tract. As the ureter enters the bladder, the distal portion tunnels between the mucosa and muscle layers of the bladder wall (**Figure 9–31** ●). During voiding, increased intravesicular (within the bladder) pressure compresses the ureter, preventing **reflux**, or the backflow of urine toward the kidneys. In males, a long urethra and the antibacterial effect of zinc in prostatic fluid also help prevent contamination of this normally sterile environment.

UTIs can be bacterial, viral, or fungal and may be categorized in several ways. Anatomically, UTIs may affect the lower

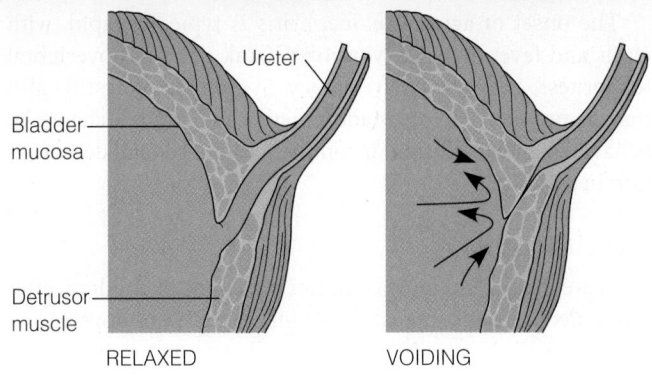

Figure 9–31 ● A competent vesicoureteral junction. Note how increased intravesicular pressure during voiding occludes the distal portion of the ureter, preventing reflux.

or the upper urinary tract. Infections of the lower urinary tract include *urethritis*, inflammation of the urethra; *prostatitis*, inflammation of the prostate gland; and **cystitis**, inflammation of the urinary bladder. The most common upper urinary tract infection is pyelonephritis, inflammation of the kidney and renal pelvis. The infection can involve superficial tissues, such as the bladder mucosa, or invade other tissues, such as prostate or renal tissues.

Epidemiologically, UTIs are identified as community acquired or healthcare associated (often related to catheterization). UTIs can be further categorized as acute or chronic, the latter being either recurrent or persistent.

Cystitis is the most common UTI. This infection tends to remain superficial, involving the bladder mucosa. The mucosa becomes hyperemic (red) and may hemorrhage. The inflammatory response causes pus to form, a process that causes the classic manifestations associated with cystitis.

Pyelonephritis is inflammation of the renal pelvis and parenchyma, the functional kidney tissue. *Acute pyelonephritis* is a bacterial infection of the kidney, and *chronic pyelonephritis* is associated with nonbacterial infections and inflammatory processes that can be metabolic, chemical, or immunological in origin (see the Inflammation concept).

Acute pyelonephritis usually results from an infection that ascends to the kidney from the lower urinary tract. Asymptomatic bacteriuria or cystitis can lead to acute pyelonephritis. Risk factors include pregnancy (due to slowed ureteral peristalsis), urinary tract obstruction, and congenital malformation. Urinary tract trauma, scarring, calculi (stones), kidney disorders such as polycystic or hypertensive kidney disease, and chronic diseases such as diabetes can also contribute to pyelonephritis. **Vesicoureteral reflux**, a condition in which urine moves from the bladder back toward the kidney, is a common risk factor in children who develop pyelonephritis that is also seen in adults when bladder outflow is obstructed.

The infection spreads from the renal pelvis to the renal cortex. The pelvis, calyces, and medulla of the kidney are primarily affected, with WBC infiltration and inflammation. The kidney becomes grossly edematous. Localized abscesses may develop on the cortical surface of the kidney. As with cystitis, *E. coli* is the organism responsible for 85% of the cases of acute pyelonephritis. Other organisms commonly found include *Proteus* and *Klebsiella*, bacteria that normally inhabit the intestinal tract.

The onset of acute pyelonephritis is typically rapid, with chills and fever, malaise, vomiting, flank pain, costovertebral tenderness, and urinary frequency. Symptoms of cystitis also may be present. The older adult may present with a change in behavior, acute confusion, incontinence, or a general deterioration in condition.

Etiology

UTIs are the second most common infections in children, after otitis media. An estimated 8% of girls and 2% of boys have a UTI by age 7 (White, 2011). Most UTIs among newborns and young infants occur in boys, as obstructive structural defects that predispose infants to infection have a higher incidence in males. The incidence of UTIs in older infants and children is higher in girls because the shorter female urethra (2 cm [1 in.] in young girls) has closer proximity to the anus and vagina, increasing the risk of contamination by fecal bacteria.

Pathogens usually enter the urinary tract by ascending from the mucous membranes of the perineal area into the lower urinary tract. Bacteria that have colonized the urethra, vagina, or perineal tissues are the usual source of infection (Porth & Matfin, 2010). From the bladder, bacteria can continue to ascend the urinary tract, eventually infecting the *parenchyma* (functional tissue) of the kidneys (Longo et al., 2012). Hematogenous spread of infection to the urinary tract is rare; infections introduced in this manner are usually associated with previous damage or scarring of the urinary tract. Bacteria introduced into the urinary tract can cause asymptomatic bacteriuria or an inflammatory response with manifestations of UTI.

At least 10%–15% of hospitalized clients with indwelling urinary catheters develop bacteriuria. The longer the catheter remains in place, the greater the risk for infection. Bacteria, including *E. coli, Proteus, Pseudomonas,* and *Klebsiella,* reach the bladder either by migrating through the column of urine within the catheter or moving up the mucous sheath of the urethra outside the catheter (Longo et al., 2012). Bacteria enter the catheter system at the connection between the catheter and the drainage system or through the emptying tube of the drainage bag. Colonization of perineal skin by bowel flora is a common source of infection in catheterized women.

Another cause of UTI is vesicoureteral reflux, the backflow of urine from the bladder into the ureters during voiding. Bacteria in the urine swept up to the kidneys cause pyelonephritis. Vesicoureteral reflux also prevents complete emptying of the bladder, and because urine returns to the bladder, it creates a reservoir for bacterial growth (McCance & Huether, 2010). Vesicoureteral reflux can also result from a structural anomaly in which the ureters insert into the bladder in an abnormal position.

Renal scarring can result from **hydronephrosis** (accumulation of urine in the renal pelvis as a result of obstructed outflow) or pyelonephritis, due to the inflammatory and ischemic effects of the infection. Scars have been associated with hypertension, proteinuria, and kidney failure. The risk of kidney damage increases in the following cases:

- UTI in an infant less than 1 year of age
- Delay in diagnosis and effective antibacterial treatment for an upper UTI

- Anatomical obstruction or nerve supply interruption
- Recurrent episodes of upper UTIs

Risk Factors

A variety of factors can predispose clients to UTI. Some risk factors cannot be changed (e.g., aging and a female's short urethra). Cystitis occurs most frequently in adult females, usually because of colonization of the bladder by bacteria that are normally found in the lower gastrointestinal tract. These bacteria gain entry by ascending the short, straight female urethra. Wiping from back to front after urination can transfer bacteria from the anorectal area to the urethra.

Urinary stasis increases the risk of UTI. Stasis may be caused by abnormal anatomical structures or abnormal function (e.g., a **neurogenic bladder**, in which an interrupted nerve supply from meningomyelocele or a spinal cord trauma impairs the bladder voiding function and leads to incomplete bladder emptying). Children typically void five to six times a day. Infrequent voiding, which is common in school-age children, results in incomplete emptying of the bladder and urinary stasis. Voluntarily suppressing the desire to urinate is a predisposing factor, as retention overdistends the bladder and can lead to an infection.

Congenital and acquired factors that contribute to the risk of infection include urinary tract obstruction by tumors or calculi; structural abnormalities such as strictures, impaired bladder innervation, bowel incontinence, or constipation; and chronic diseases such as diabetes mellitus. Instrumentation of the urinary tract (e.g., catheterization or cystoscopy) is a major risk factor for UTI. Even when performed under strict aseptic conditions, catheterization can result in bladder infection. Research indicates that the risk for catheter-associated UTI is reduced when anesthetic lubricating gels are inserted into the urethra prior to catheter insertion (Bardsley, 2005). The placement of the catheter prevents the flushing action of voiding, and bacteria can ascend to the bladder through the catheter lumen or via exudate between the urethral mucosa and the catheter.

In women, including adolescents, sexual activity (e.g., intercourse, abuse, masturbation) increases the risk for UTI, because bacteria can be introduced into the bladder via the urethra during sexual intercourse. Use of spermicidal compounds with a diaphragm, cervical cap, or condom alters the normal bacterial flora of the vagina and perineal tissues, further increasing the risk for UTI. Diaphragms are not recommended for women with a history of UTIs because pressure from the diaphragm on the urethra can interfere with complete bladder emptying and lead to recurrent UTIs.

Some females lack a normally protective mucosal enzyme, and the resulting decreased levels of cervicovaginal antibodies to enterobacteria further increase their risk. Personal hygiene practices and voluntary urinary retention can contribute to the risk for UTI in women. Up to three UTIs annually are considered within normal limits for sexually active women and do not usually warrant additional diagnostic tests beyond urine culture. A woman who has had a UTI is susceptible to recurrent infection. If a pregnant woman develops an acute UTI, especially with a high temperature, amniotic fluid infection can develop and retard the growth of the placenta.

Asymptomatic bacteriuria (ASB; bacteria in the urine that actively multiply without accompanying clinical symptoms) is a condition that becomes significant if a woman is pregnant, because up to 40% of pregnant women with untreated ASB develop a kidney infection (MedlinePlus, 2012). ASB is almost always caused by a single organism, typically *E. coli*. If more than one type of bacteria is cultured, the possibility of urine-culture contamination must be considered.

The risk for UTI increases during pregnancy, particularly during the second trimester, secondary to the pressure of the fetus, which causes urinary stasis and incomplete bladder emptying. The diagnosis of UTI in the pregnant client carries significant risks for the mother and fetus. UTIs are associated with an increased risk of preeclampsia (Conde-Agudelo, Villar, & Lindheimer, 2008). An increased risk of premature birth and intrauterine growth restriction is associated with acute pyelonephritis, which is often caused by ASB. Although the exact cause is unknown, an increased risk of premature rupture of membranes is associated with UTI. If urine stasis exists, the risk of UTI increases, because of bacteriuria and the presence of dilated ureters and renal pelves, which persist for about 6 weeks after delivery.

The postpartal woman is at increased risk of developing urinary tract problems caused by the normal postpartal diuresis, increased bladder capacity, and decreased bladder sensitivity from stretching or trauma. Possible inhibited neural control of the bladder following the use of general or regional anesthesia and contamination from catheterization also puts the postpartal woman at risk for UTIs. These factors make it essential that the mother empty her bladder completely with each voiding.

UTI in the newborn, which may occur as a result of exposure of the urethra to bacteria in the feces in the diaper, predisposes the neonate to hyperbilirubinemia (elevated serum bilirubin) and bacteremia.

Prostatic hypertrophy and bacterial prostatitis are risk factors among males. Circumcision appears to have a protective effect. Anal intercourse is also a risk factor for men. In healthy adult men, UTIs are unusual and may prompt additional diagnostic testing.

Older clients have an increased incidence of UTI. The greatest increase is seen in men, as the ratio of female-to-male UTI in older adults changes from 50:1 to less than 5:1. Although the bacteriostatic effect of prostatic fluid and a longer urethra provide an effective barrier to bladder infection for adult males, the hypertrophy of the prostate that is commonly associated with aging increases the risk of cystitis in older males. An enlarged prostate can impede urine flow and lead to incomplete bladder emptying and urinary stasis. Because bacteria are not completely flushed with voiding, colonization of the bladder may occur. An increased risk of urinary stasis, chronic disease states (such as diabetes mellitus), and an impaired immune response also contribute to the higher incidence of UTI in older adults. In older women, loss of tissue elasticity and weakening of perineal muscles often contribute to the development of a cystocele or rectocele. Resulting changes in bladder and urethral position increase the risk of incomplete bladder emptying.

> ### Client Teaching Prevention of Urinary Tract Infection
>
> Client teaching is a vital aspect of preventing primary and recurrent urinary tract infections. Nurses should do the following:
>
> ■ Encourage clients to maintain a generous fluid intake of 2.0–2.5 liters per day, increasing intake during hot weather and strenuous activity, which helps clear bacteria from the urinary system.
>
> ■ Discuss the need to avoid voluntary urinary retention by emptying the bladder every 3–4 hours.
>
> ■ Instruct women to cleanse the perineal area from front to back after voiding and defecating, to prevent the transfer of gastrointestinal bacteria to the urethra.
>
> ■ Teach clients to void and wash the perineal area before and after sexual intercourse to flush out bacteria introduced into the urethra and bladder.
>
> ■ Teach measures to maintain the integrity of perineal tissues, such as avoiding bubble baths, feminine hygiene sprays, and vaginal douches, and wearing cotton briefs rather than underwear made from synthetic materials.
>
> ■ Unless contraindicated, suggest the following measures to maintain acid urine: Drink two glasses of low-sugar cranberry juice daily, take ascorbic acid (vitamin C), and avoid excess intake of milk and milk products, other fruit juices, and sodium bicarbonate (baking soda).

Prevention

The primary prevention of urinary tract infections is practice of good personal hygiene. See the Client Teaching feature to learn important ways in which nurses can teach clients to prevent UTIs. Some physicians may recommend prophylactic antibiotic treatment for clients with recurrent UTIs or with asymptomatic bacteriuria (see the Evidence-Based Practice feature).

▶ CLINICAL MANIFESTATIONS

The symptoms of UTI depend on the infection's location as well as the client's age. Symptoms in a newborn tend to be nonspecific: unexplained fever, failure to thrive, poor feeding, vomiting and diarrhea, strong-smelling urine, and irritability. Any child younger than age 2 years with a fever of unknown origin should be tested for a UTI. The more "classic" symptoms of lower UTI, as shown in the following Clinical Manifestations and Therapies feature, are not seen until the toddler years. Approximately 40% of UTIs are asymptomatic.

Typical presenting symptoms of cystitis include **dysuria** (painful or difficult urination), urinary frequency and **urgency** (a sudden, compelling need to urinate), and **nocturia** (voiding two or more times at night). In addition, the urine may have a foul odor and appear cloudy (**pyuria**) or bloody (**hematuria**) because of mucus, excess white cells in the urine, and bleeding of the inflamed bladder wall. Suprapubic pain and tenderness also may be present. Cystitis is usually uncomplicated and readily responds to treatment. When left untreated, the infection

Evidence-Based Practice Vesicoureteral Reflux and Prophylactic Antibiotics

Problem

The presence of vesicoureteral reflux (VUR), the backflow of urine from the bladder to the upper urinary tract, is a risk factor for the development of urinary tract infections. Multiple studies indicate that 18%–35% of children with a UTI also have VUR (Finnell, Carroll, & Downs, 2011).

Evidence

The standard of practice for many years has been to treat children with VUR prophylactically with antibiotics to prevent development of a UTI. Some studies support this practice, antibiotic prophylaxis being associated with lower UTI occurrence in girls with dilating VUR (Brandstrom et al., 2010). However, other studies indicate that the risk of developing recurrent UTI is not significantly different between children with VUR who received prophylactic antimicrobial therapy and those who did not. In addition, children who received antimicrobial prophylaxis were more likely to develop antimicrobial-resistant UTIs (Finnell et al., 2011; Craig et al., 2009). Interestingly, children with VUR on observation therapy were more likely to develop a UTI if they presented with more than one febrile UTI or were older at VUR diagnosis or prophylactic withdrawal (Drzewiecki et al., 2012).

Implications

Children with VUR are at increased risk for developing UTIs; however, prophylactic antibiotic treatment may cause more burden than benefit in some children. Prophylaxis is not consistently associated with a decreased risk of recurrent infection, but it increases the risk of developing resistant infections. Nurses need to conduct a thorough client history of previous UTIs, age of VUR diagnosis, bowel and bladder dysfunction, and bowel and bladder control (i.e., toilet training). Some clients, such as clients with multiple previous UTIs or older age when VUR was diagnosed, may benefit from prophylactic therapy more than younger clients with no history of recurrent UTI.

Critical Thinking Application

1. What symptoms would you teach parents to watch for and report if their child with VUR is on observation therapy?

2. On the basis of evidence presented here and in additional studies, what characteristics of a child with VUR would prompt you to recommend that that child be placed on prophylactic antibiotics?

3. Develop a nursing care plan for a 15-month-old child with VUR and one previous UTI.

---

can ascend to involve the kidneys. Severe or prolonged infection can lead to sloughing of bladder mucosa and ulcer formation. Chronic cystitis can lead to bladder stones.

Lifespan and Cultural Considerations

Urinary tract infection is one of the top two infections in clients in long-term care facilities and is common in both community-dwelling and facility-dwelling older adults. Older clients may not experience the classic symptoms of cystitis. Instead, they often present with nonspecific manifestations, such as nocturia, incontinence, confusion, behavior change, lethargy, loss of appetite, or "just not feeling right." Fever may be present; however, hypothermia also may develop in an older adult. Particu-

larly in a long-term care setting, a change in behavior may be the only indicator of a UTI (MedlinePlus, 2011b). The frustrated the family members and healthcare team may easily suspect any number of other possible causes when an older adult presents with these symptoms.

The symptoms usually seen in younger adults with UTIs—urgency and frequency—are common age-related changes in the older adult and therefore lack diagnostic usefulness. However, if an older adult has not previously experienced urinary urgency and presents with a shortened period of time between the urge to void and actual urination or urinary frequency of more than seven voids per 24-hour period, these symptoms should be thoroughly investigated.

Clinical Manifestations and Therapies **Urinary Tract Infection**

ETIOLOGY	CLINICAL MANIFESTATION	CLINICAL THERAPIES
Lower UTI: cystitis	▪ Frequency, dysuria, urgency, enuresis, strong-smelling urine, cloudy urine, hematuria, abdominal or suprapubic pain	▪ Administer 5- to 7-day course of trimethoprim or sulfamethoxazole or antibiotic matching organism sensitivity; encourage oral fluids; administer analgesic such as acetaminophen or Pyridium.
Upper UTI: pyelonephritis	▪ High fever, chills, abdominal pain, flank pain, costovertebral angle tenderness, persistent vomiting, moderate to severe dehydration ▪ Infants may have nonspecific signs such as poor appetite, failure to thrive, lethargy, irritability. ▪ Older children may have signs of cystitis.	▪ Administer antipyretics and intravenous antibiotics initially; then transition to oral antibiotics matching organism sensitivity for a total of 7–10 days. ▪ Rehydration is essential.

Studies have suggested that adults without catheters in long-term care facilities have a prevalence of 25%–50% for asymptomatic bacteriuria (Beveridge, Davey, Phillips, & McMurdo, 2011), which may also be called *asymptomatic UTI* by some clinicians and researchers. Asymptomatic UTI does not require treatment. In fact, treatment does not improve the morbidity or mortality in affected older adults (Beveridge et al., 2011; Gandhi, 2006; Nicolle et al., 2005). Routine urinalysis for older adults without symptoms is neither appropriate nor cost effective.

Catheter-associated UTIs often are asymptomatic. Gram-negative bacteremia is the most significant complication associated with these UTIs. Most catheter-associated UTIs resolve quickly when the catheter is removed and a short course of antibiotic is administered. Intermittent catheterization carries a lower risk of infection than does an indwelling catheter and is preferred for clients who are unable to empty their bladder by voiding. UTIs in catheterized older adults tend to be polymicrobial and difficult to eradicate. Before an indwelling catheter is used, the potential benefits to the older adult must be carefully weighed against the serious risks posed.

▶ COLLABORATION

Collaborative treatment of UTI focuses on eliminating the causative organism, preventing relapse or reinfection, and identifying and correcting any contributing factors. Drug treatment with antibiotics and urinary anti-infectives is common. In some cases, surgery may be indicated to correct contributing factors.

Diagnostic Tests

- Urinalysis to assess for pyuria, bacteria, and blood cells in the urine. A bacteria count greater than 100,000 (105) per milliliter indicates infection. Rapid tests for bacteria in the urine include using a *nitrite dipstick* (which turns pink in the presence of bacteria) and the *leukocyte esterase test*, an indirect method of detecting bacteria by identifying lysed or intact WBCs in the urine.

- Urine should be a midstream clean-catch specimen; if necessary, use straight catheterization or "mini-cath," with strict aseptic technique. Avoid catheterization if possible to reduce the risk of further infection. Urine from urine collection bags may be used to screen for UTIs in infants, but it cannot be used to confirm a UTI and should not be used for most clients because the specimen collection procedure is not sterile.

SAFETY ALERT
Cleansing with nonsterile gauze moistened with tap water and mild soap is as effective as using a prepackaged sterile towelette and is gentler on the mucus membranes.

- **Gram stain** of the urine may be done to identify the infecting organism by shape and characteristic (gram-positive or gram-negative).

- Urine culture and sensitivity tests may be ordered to identify the infecting organism and the most effective antibiotic. Urine specimens collected for culture must be delivered to the laboratory within 1 hour, or the specimen must be refrigerated to prevent the growth of organisms that occur with prolonged room temperature exposure. Culture requires 24–72 hours, so treatment to eliminate the most common organisms often is initiated without culture. Urine cultures do not distinguish between upper and lower UTIs.

- WBC count with differential may be done to detect the typical changes associated with infection, such as leukocytosis (elevated WBC) and increased numbers of neutrophils.

In clients with recurrent infections or persistent bacteriuria, additional diagnostic testing may be ordered to evaluate for structural abnormalities, renal scarring, and other contributing factors. These tests include the following:

- **Intravenous pyelography (IVP)**, also known as *excretory urography,* is used to evaluate the structure and excretory function of the kidneys, ureters, and bladder. As the kidneys clear an intravenously injected contrast medium from the blood, the size and shape of the kidneys, their calyces and pelves, the ureters, and the bladder can be evaluated, and structural or functional abnormalities, such as vesicoureteral reflux, can be detected.

- **Voiding cystourethrography** involves instilling contrast medium into the bladder, and then using x-rays to assess the bladder and urethra when filled and during voiding. This study can detect structural and functional abnormalities of the bladder and urethral strictures. This test has a lower risk of allergic response to the contrast dye than IVP.

- **Cystoscopy** (direct visualization of the urethra and a bladder through a cystoscope) can be used to diagnose conditions such as prostatic hypertrophy, urethral strictures, bladder calculi, tumors, polyps, diverticula, and congenital abnormalities. A tissue biopsy may be obtained during the procedure, and other interventions may be performed (e.g., stone removal or stricture dilation).

- ***Manual pelvic or prostate examinations*** assess for structural changes of the genitourinary tract, such as prostatic enlargement, cystocele, or rectocele.

- ***Renal and bladder ultrasound and DMSA scintigraphy*** are used to detect pyelonephritis and renal scarring (National Kidney and Urological Diseases Information Clearinghouse [NKUDIC], 2012).

Surgery

Surgery may be indicated for recurrent UTI if diagnostic testing indicates calculi, structural anomalies, or strictures that contribute to the risk of infection. Stones, or *calculi,* in the renal pelvis or bladder are an irritant and provide a matrix for bacterial colonization. Treatment may include surgical removal of a large calculus from the renal pelvis or cystoscopic removal of bladder calculi. *Percutaneous ultrasonic pyelolithotomy* or *extracorporeal shock wave lithotripsy* (see the exemplar on Urinary Calculi in the module on Elimination) may be used instead of surgery to crush and remove stones.

Ureteroplasty, the surgical repair of a ureter, may be indicated for structural abnormality or stricture of a ureter. This may be combined with a ureteral reimplantation if vesicoure-

Box 9–7 Ureteral Stent

Ureteral stents are used to maintain patency and promote healing of the ureters (see **Figure 9–32** ●). A stent may be temporary, used during and after a surgical procedure, or it may be used for longer periods in clients with ureteral obstruction due to tumors, strictures, or other causes.

Stents may be positioned during surgery or cystoscopy. They are made of a nontoxic material such as silicone or polyurethane, with side drainage holes placed along the length of the stent. Stents are radiopaque for easy radiographic identification. One or both ends of the stent may be pigtail or J shaped to prevent migration.

In caring for a client with a ureteral stent, the nurse should do the following:

■ Label all drainage tubes, including stents, for easy identification. Attach each catheter and stent to a separate closed drainage system. Careful labeling allows close monitoring of output from all sources and reservoirs. Separate drainage systems minimize the risk of infection.

■ If the stent has been brought to the surface, secure it and maintain its position. The stent is usually placed in the renal pelvis. It is important to secure it well to prevent trauma to the kidney, inadvertent removal of the stent, and ureter obstruction.

■ Monitor urine output, including color, consistency, and odor. Monitor for signs of infection or bleeding, including fever, tachycardia, pain, hematuria, and cloudy or malodorous urine. The stent facilitates urine flow but can become obstructed by bleeding, calculi, or sediment. Obstruction can result in hydronephrosis and kidney damage. The stent itself is a foreign body in the urinary tract and can increase the risk of UTI.

■ Maintain fluid intake, encouraging fluids that acidify urine, such as low-sugar apple, cranberry, and blueberry juice. The stent can precipitate calculus formation as well as UTI. Increasing fluid intake and acidifying the urine help prevent these complications.

■ For an indwelling stent, stress the need for regular follow up to monitor for and prevent complications such as UTI and calculi. The client with an indwelling stent may tend to forget that the stent is in place and become noncompliant with follow up and preventive measures.

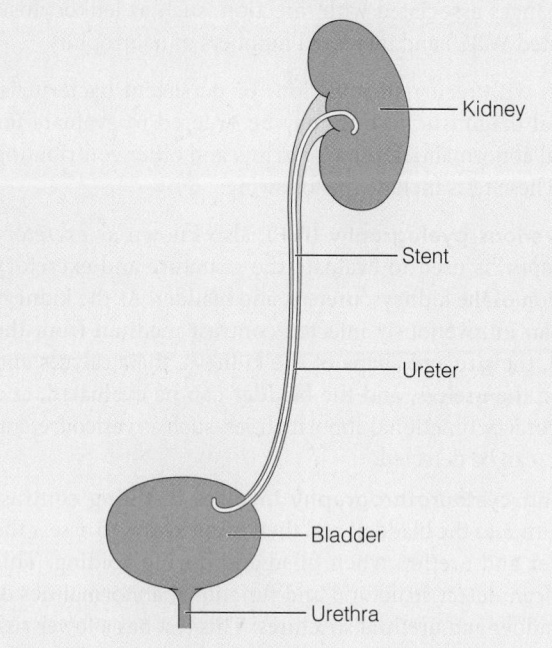

Figure 9–32 ● A ureteral stent.

teral reflux is present. The client returns from these surgeries with an indwelling urinary catheter (Foley or suprapubic) and a **ureteral stent** (a thin catheter inserted into the ureter to provide for urine flow and ureteral support), which remain in place for 3–5 days. **Box 9–7** ● describes nursing care of the client with a ureteral stent in place.

Follow up urine cultures should be obtained according to the frequency specified by agency guidelines. Clients with pyelonephritis may have to repeat urine cultures monthly for 3 months, every 3 months for 6 months, and then annually. Most reinfections occur within 1 year, and subsequent infections may be asymptomatic. Children with renal scarring should have their blood pressure monitored.

Pharmacologic Therapy

Most uncomplicated infections of the lower urinary tract can be treated with a short course of antibiotic therapy. Upper urinary tract infections, in contrast, usually require longer treatment (2 or more weeks) to eradicate the infecting organism. Treatment should be initiated as soon as the UTI is diagnosed.

Antibiotics are selected based on the age of the client, the sensitivity of the cultured organism, renal function, and the client's signs and symptoms. Gender is a consideration in treatment choices, because men require longer periods of treatment than women. The longer urethra in men makes it less likely that bacteria can ascend into the bladder. However, when bacteria do reach the older man's bladder, the infection is considered complicated and requires a longer course of treatment. The antibiotic is changed if necessary after culture sensitivity is determined.

Follow up cultures may be obtained 48–72 hours after drug therapy is started in the pediatric client who is still febrile (White, 2011). Children with pyelonephritis should be maintained on antibiotic prophylaxis until radiological tests are performed to detect any structural defects.

Short-course therapy (either a single antibiotic dose or a 3-day course of treatment) reduces treatment cost, increases compliance, and has a lower rate of side effects. Single-dose therapy is associated with a higher rate of recurrent infection and continued vaginal colonization with *E. coli*, making a 3-day course of treatment the preferred option for uncomplicated cystitis. Oral trimethoprim-sulfamethoxazole (TMP-SMZ), TMP, or a quinolone antibiotic such as ciprofloxacin (Cipro) or enoxacin (Penetrex) may be ordered.

Men and women with pyelonephritis, urinary tract abnormalities or stones, or a history of previous infections with antibiotic-resistant infections require a 7- to 10-day course of TMP-SMZ, ciprofloxacin, ofloxacin (Floxin), or an alternative antibiotic. The client with severe illness may need hospitalization. Intravenous ciprofloxacin, gentamicin, ceftriaxone (Rocephin), or ampicillin may be prescribed for severe illness or sepsis associated with UTI.

Children who appear ill and cannot tolerate oral antibiotics are often hospitalized because they need rehydration and parenteral antibiotic treatment until they have been afebrile for 24 hours. Infants can develop permanent kidney damage or generalized sepsis if the UTI is not treated aggressively. If a structural defect is identified, surgical correction may be necessary to prevent recurrent infections that could lead to renal damage.

Clients who experience frequent symptomatic UTIs may be treated with prophylactic antibiotic therapy. Drugs such as TMP-SMZ, TMP, and nitrofurantoin (Furadantin, Macrodantin, Macrobid) do not achieve effective plasma concentrations at recommended doses, but do reach effective concentrations in the urine. Nitrofurantoin also may be used to treat UTI in pregnant women.

Antibiotics and urinary anti-infectives generally are not recommended to treat asymptomatic bacteriuria in catheterized clients. The preferred treatment for catheter-associated UTI is removal of the indwelling catheter, followed by a 10- to 14-day course of antibiotic therapy to eliminate the infection.

Nonpharmacologic Therapy

Nonpharmacologic therapies can be helpful in treating and preventing urinary tract infection. Drinking adequate fluids will increase urination and flush bacteria out of the urinary system. Drinking cranberry juice in particular is recommended to help fight urinary tract infections. However, fluids that may irritate the bladder, including caffeinated beverages, alcohol, and soft drinks with citrus juices, should be avoided.

◼ NURSING PROCESS

The nursing process for UTI generally focuses on returning the client to maximum health. To maintain optimum urinary health, nurses should be alert for opportunities to provide health promotion, teaching measures to prevent UTI to all clients, particularly to young, sexually active women (see Client Teaching feature in Prevention section).

Assessment

Focused assessment data for the client with a suspected UTI includes the following:

- *Health history.* Current symptoms, including urination frequency and urgency, burning on urination, and number of voidings per night; color, clarity, and odor of urine; other manifestations, such as lower abdominal, back, or flank pain,

nausea or vomiting, or fever; duration of symptoms and any treatment attempted; history of previous UTIs and their frequency; possibility of pregnancy and type of birth control used; chronic diseases such as diabetes; current medications; and any known allergies.
- *Physical examination.* General health; vital signs, including temperature; abdominal shape, contour, and tenderness to palpation (especially suprapubic); and percussing for costovertebral tenderness.

Diagnosis

Nursing diagnoses for clients with UTIs focus on comfort, urinary elimination, and teaching/learning needs and may include the following:

- *Acute Pain*
- *Impaired Urinary Elimination*
- *Deficient Knowledge*
- *Risk for Disproportionate Growth (pediatric clients)*
- *Urinary Retention*
- *Risk for Deficient Fluid Volume*
- *Fear*

(NANDA-I © 2012)

Planning

In planning and implementing nursing care for the client with a UTI, the client's general health, abilities for self-care, and risk factors that may contribute to UTI. Outcomes, developed in collaboration with the client, may include the following:

- describes pain as a 3 or lower on a 1–10 scale.
- regain normal voiding pattern and will produce normal urine without blood, bacteria, or protein.

- verbalize understanding of disease process, proper method of taking medications, and required follow up care.
- strategies for reducing the risk of another UTI.
- client will increase fluid intake and number of voidings each day.
- client will complete the prescribed course of antibiotic therapy.
- client will experience no recurrent UTIs for 1 year.
- client will incorporate preventive self-care measures into daily regimen.

Implementation

Nursing care for the hospitalized client with a complicated UTI focuses on administering prescribed medications, promoting rehydration, assessing renal function, and teaching the client and family how to minimize the risk of future infection.

Manage Pain

Pain is a common manifestation of both lower and upper UTIs. Urinary tract pain is caused primarily by distention and increased pressure within the urinary tract. The severity of the pain is related to the rate at which inflammation and distention develop, not their degree.

> **SAFETY ALERT**
> The older adult with a UTI may not complain of dysuria. Be alert for other manifestations of UTI, such as incontinence or cloudy or malodorous urine. Inflammatory and immune responses tend to diminish with aging, so the irritative symptoms of UTI are reduced.

In cystitis, inflammation causes a sensation of fullness; dull, constant suprapubic pain; and possibly low back pain. The inflamed bladder wall and urethra cause dysuria, pain, and burning on urination. Bladder spasms may develop, causing periodic severe, stabbing discomfort. Pain associated with pyelonephritis is often steady and dull, localized to the outer abdomen or flank region. Urological disorders rarely cause central abdominal pain.

Nursing interventions for the client experiencing pain include the following:

- Assess pain: timing, quality, intensity, location, duration, and aggravating and alleviating factors. A change in the nature, location, or intensity of the pain may indicate an extension of the infection or a related but separate problem.
- Teach or provide comfort measures, such as warm sitz baths, warm packs or heating pads, and balanced rest and activity. Use systemic analgesics, urinary analgesics, or antispasmodic medication as ordered. Warmth relaxes muscles, relieves spasms, and increases local blood supply. Because pain can stimulate a stress response and delay healing, it should be relieved when possible.
- Increase fluid intake unless contraindicated. Increased fluid dilutes urine, reducing irritation of the inflamed bladder and urethral mucosa.
- Instruct the client to notify the primary care provider if pain and discomfort continue or intensify after therapy is initiated. Pain and discomfort in voiding typically are relieved

within 24 hours of initiating antibiotic therapy. Continued discomfort may indicate a complicated UTI or other urinary tract disorder.

Community-Based Care

Because both upper and lower urinary tract infections are usually managed in the community, teaching is the most important nursing intervention. Provide instruction on the following topics:

- Risk factors for UTI and how to minimize or eliminate these factors through increased fluid intake, regular elimination, and personal hygiene measures
- Early manifestations of UTI and the importance of seeking medical intervention promptly
- Maintaining optimal immune system function by attending to physical and psychosocial stressors, such as lack of adequate rest, poor nutrition, and high levels of emotional stress
- The importance of completing the prescribed treatment and keeping follow up appointments
- Minimizing the risk of UTI when an indwelling urinary catheter is necessary:
  a. Use alternatives to an indwelling catheter when possible. For urinary incontinence, try scheduled toileting, incontinence pads or diapers, and external catheters if possible. For urinary retention, teach the client or a family member to perform straight catheterization every 3–4 hours using clean technique.
  b. When an indwelling catheter is necessary, teach care measures such as perineal care, managing and emptying the collection chamber, maintaining a closed system, and bladder irrigation or flushing if ordered.

Facilitate Effective Urinary Elimination

Inflammation of the bladder and urethral mucosa affects the normal process and patterns of voiding, causing frequency, urgency, and burning on urination, as well as nocturia. Urine may be blood tinged, cloudy, and malodorous. The client with short- or long-term urinary retention requires additional measures to assess for and prevent UTI.

> **Lifespan Considerations**
> **Urinary Incontinence in Children**
>
> Because bladder training is such an important milestone for young children, any disorder that affects voiding can have developmental implications. A toddler who has been toilet trained may regress and require diapers temporarily due to incontinence related to the UTI. An older child may develop **enuresis** (the involuntary passage of urine after control has been established) after a prolonged period of being dry at night. A preschooler may perceive the infection as punishment for an imagined wrong, such as masturbation. Reassure parents that this temporary period of urinary incontinence is normal when associated with UTI, and emphasize that they should offer the child support rather than disapproval.

Nursing interventions for clients with impaired urinary elimination include the following:

- Monitor (or instruct the client to monitor) color, clarity, and odor of urine. Urine should return to clear yellow within 48 hours, unless drug therapy causes a change in the color of urine. If clarity does not return, further investigation may be necessary.
- Instruct clients with impaired urinary elimination to avoid caffeinated drinks, including coffee, tea, and cola; citrus juices; drinks containing artificial sweeteners; and alcoholic beverages. Caffeine, citrus juices, and artificial sweeteners irritate bladder mucosa and the detrusor muscle and can increase urgency and bladder spasms.
- Use strict aseptic technique and a closed urinary drainage system when inserting a straight or indwelling urinary catheter. Insert indwelling catheters to the full recommended length (4 inches or more in women and to the bifurcation in men) before inflating the balloon. Bacteria colonizing the perineal tissues or on the nurse's hands can be introduced into the bladder during catheterization. Aseptic technique reduces this risk. Inflating the balloon while it is in the urethra damages urethral tissues and can cause the client significant discomfort.
- When possible, use intermittent straight catheterization to relieve urinary retention. Remove indwelling urinary catheters as soon as possible. Using intermittent straight catheterization allows the bladder to fill and completely empty more normally, maintaining physiological function. The risk of infection associated with an indwelling catheter is about 3%–6% and increases cumulatively with each day (Pellowe, 2009).
- Maintain the closed urinary drainage system, and use aseptic technique when emptying the catheter drainage bag. Maintain gravity flow to prevent reflux of urine into the bladder from the drainage system. Bacteria can enter the drainage system when its integrity is interrupted (e.g., when the catheter is disconnected from the drainage system) or during emptying of the drainage bag. These bacteria can ascend the column of urine to the bladder, causing UTI.
- Provide perineal care regularly and following defecation. Use antiseptic preparations only as ordered. Regular cleansing of perineal tissues reduces the risk of colonization by bowel or other bacteria. Although antiseptic solutions may be ordered for catheter care, they can dry perineal tissues and reduce normal flora, increasing the risk of colonization by pathogens, and they should not be used routinely.

Promote Effective Health Maintenance

Because clients with UTIs are at increased risk for future UTIs, they need to understand the disease process, risk factors, measures to prevent recurrent infection, diagnostic procedures, and best practices for home care. In addition, clients need to understand that, even when the manifestations of UTI are relieved, the treatment plan needs to continue. Failure to complete the full course of therapy and recommended follow up can lead to continued bacteriuria and recurrent infections.

Nurses who work with clients with ineffective health maintenance should do the following:

- Teach clients how to obtain a midstream clean-catch urine specimen. Cleansing of the urinary meatus and perineal area reduces contamination of the specimen by external cells and bacteria; 90% of urethral bacteria are cleared in the first 10 mL of voided urine, so a midstream specimen is representative of urine in the bladder.
- Assess the client's knowledge about the disease process, risk factors, and preventive measures. The client may have little understanding of UTI or its causes and contributing factors.
- Discuss the prescribed treatment plan and the importance of taking all prescribed antibiotics.
- Help the client develop a plan for taking medications, such as taking them with meals (unless contraindicated) or setting out all doses for the day in the morning. Missed doses of antibiotic can result in subtherapeutic blood levels and reduced effectiveness. Taking medication in association with a regular daily activity such as meals helps clients remember doses.
- Instruct clients to keep appointments for follow up and urine culture. Follow up urine culture, often scheduled 7–14 days after completion of antibiotic therapy, is vital to ensure complete eradication of bacteria and prevent relapse or recurrence.
- Teach measures to prevent future UTI, as discussed at the beginning of this exemplar. Keeping urine dilute and acidic and voiding regularly help to flush bacteria out of the bladder and urethra. The proximity of the female urethral meatus to the vagina and anus increases the risk of bacterial contamination, especially during intercourse. Bubble baths, feminine hygiene sprays, synthetic fibers, and douches can dry and irritate perineal tissues, promoting bacterial growth.

Evaluation

The outcome of treatment for UTI may be determined by follow up urinalysis and culture. Cure, as evidenced by the absence of pathogens in the urine, is the desired outcome. When therapy fails to eradicate bacteria in the urine, the condition is known as **unresolved bacteriuria**. **Persistent bacteriuria**, or *relapse*, occurs when a persistent source of infection causes repeated infection after the initial cure. **Reinfection** is the development of a new infection with a different pathogen following successful UTI treatment (Papadakis & McPhee, 2013). Clients are generally required to submit a urinalysis for culture 7–10 days after completing a course of antibiotics to ensure that bacteria have been eliminated.

NURSING CARE PLAN   A Client With Cystitis

Miija Waisanen is a 25-year-old second-year nursing student. She was recently married, and she and her husband live in an apartment near the college she attends. Ms. Waisanen has never been pregnant, and she is using a diaphragm for birth control. She presents at the local urgent care clinic complaining of low back pain, frequency and urgency of urination, and burning on urination, which began yesterday.

ASSESSMENT

Patrice Ramiros, a nurse practitioner, admits Ms. Waisanen to the clinic. Ms. Waisanen denies having had similar symptoms in the past or ever having been diagnosed with a urinary tract infection. She describes her pain as a constant, dull ache that does not change with movement. She feels the need to urinate almost constantly but experiences difficulty in starting her stream and feels burning pain and cramping when voiding. She reports getting up four times last night to urinate. She denies painful intercourse and states that her last menstrual period began only 2 weeks ago. Physical examination reveals pulse 90 beats/minute and regular and blood pressure 112/68 mmHg. She is afebrile. Suprapubic tenderness is noted, but there is no flank or costovertebral angle tenderness. Clean-catch urine specimen shows hematuria, multiple WBCs, and a bacteria count greater than 105 /mL.

Ms. Ramiros prescribes trimethoprim-sulfamethoxazole (TMP-SMZ) 160 mg/800 mg PO two times a day for 3 days, and aspirin or acetaminophen gr × PO every 4 hours as needed for pain. Ms. Waisanen is instructed to return to the clinic in 7 days for a follow up urine culture, or sooner if her symptoms do not improve.

DIAGNOSES

- *Pain* related to infection and inflammatory process in the urinary tract
- *Impaired Urinary Elimination* related to inflammation, as evidenced by frequency, urgency, nocturia, and dysuria
- *Deficient Knowledge* related to lack of information about risk factors for UTI

(NANDA-I © 2012)

PLANNING

- Client will report relief of low back pain and burning on urination.
- Client will report a normal voiding pattern without frequency, urgency, nocturia, and abnormal urine characteristics.
- Client will verbalize understanding of the disease process, related risk factors, follow up instructions, and symptoms of recurrence that indicate the need for medical attention.

IMPLEMENTATION

- Teach comfort measures: warm sitz baths, a heating pad on low heat applied to the lower back or abdomen, rest, increased fluid intake, avoiding caffeinated beverages, and aspirin or acetaminophen as ordered.
- Advise client to refrain from sexual intercourse until infection and inflammation have cleared to avoid further irritation of inflamed tissues.

- Discuss the possible relationship between using a diaphragm for birth control and UTIs in women.
- Discuss dietary and hygiene practices to prevent UTI symptoms.
- Discuss symptoms indicating the need for further intervention and the risks of undertreatment.

EVALUATION

Six months later, Ms. Waisanen rotates through the urgent care clinic for her community-based nursing experience. When Ms. Ramiros asks how she is doing, Ms. Waisanen reports that her symptoms and urine cleared within about a day after she started the antibiotic, and she has had no further problems. She has seen her women's healthcare nurse practitioner to change her birth control to oral contraceptives, increased her intake of fluid and vitamin C, and no longer puts off urinating until she "has time to go."

CRITICAL THINKING

1. What physiological and psychosocial factors put Ms. Waisanen at risk for UTI?
2. Compare the benefits and drawbacks to short-course therapy versus conventional therapy for UTI.
3. Why was it appropriate for the nurse practitioner to use short-course therapy with the advice to return if symptoms did not clear?
4. Develop a care plan for Ms. Waisanen for the nursing diagnosis Ineffective Health Maintenance.

◢ REVIEW Urinary Tract Infection

RELATE Link the Concepts and Exemplars

Linking the exemplar of urinary tract infection with the concept of evidence-based practice:

1. If you were caring for a client with bacteria in the urine who denied any symptoms or problems, how would you explain the decision not to treat this client?
2. What would you tell the client who adamantly demands a prescription for an antibiotic after being informed that taking an antibiotic is not in her best interest?

Linking the exemplar of urinary tract infection with the concept of mobility:

3. What factors put the 90-year-old client who is wheelchair bound at risk for a urinary tract infection?
4. To reduce the risk of urinary tract infections, what preventive measures will you implement for the older client who is confined to bed?

READY Go to Companion Skills Manual

**REFER Go to Pearson Student Nursing Resources
nursing.pearsonhighered.com**

- Additional review materials

REFLECT Case Study

Ms. James, who was introduced in the exemplar on Cellulitis in this module, wakes up one day and does not feel well. She is taken by ambulance to the neighborhood hospital, where a diagnosis of stroke is made. She has a feeding tube and indwelling catheter placed. She later develops a fever and confusion. The urine in the drainage bag is cloudy. A urine specimen is collected and sent to the laboratory for urinalysis and culture and sensitivity. Results confirm the diagnosis of UTI.

1. How will Ms. James's history of diabetes mellitus affect her risk for UTI and her response to treatment?
2. What risk factors does Ms. James have that place her at increased risk for UTI?
3. After Ms. James's indwelling catheter is removed and the UTI is treated with antibiotics for 7 days, urine culture reveals that bacteria remain in the urine. What does the nurse anticipate will be done next if the client still experiences symptoms? How would the treatment differ if the client did not have symptoms?

■ REFERENCES

Agency for Healthcare Research and Quality. (2009). *Fact Sheet: AHRQ's efforts to prevent and reduce healthcare-associated infections.* Retrieved from http://www.ahrq.gov/qual/haiflyer.pdf.

American Academy of Pediatrics. (2008). *Recommendations for preventative pediatric health care.* Retrieved from http://brightfutures.aap.org/pdfs/aap%20bright%20futures%20periodicity%20sched%20101107.pdf.

American Academy of Pediatrics, Subcommittee on Management of Acute Otitis Media. (2004). Diagnosis and management of acute otitis media. *Pediatrics, 113,* 1451–1465.

Atkinson, W., Wolfe, S., & Hamborsky, J. (2011). *Epidemiology and prevention of vaccine-preventable diseases.* Washington, DC: U.S. Department of Health and Human Services.

Bardsley, A. (2005). Use of lubricant gels in urinary catheterization. *Nursing Standard, 20*(8), 41–46.

Barskey, A. E., Schulte, C., Rosen, J. B., Handschur, E. F., Rausch-Phung, E., Doll, M. K., … Gallagher, K. M. (2012). Mumps outbreak in Orthodox Jewish communities in the United States. *New England Journal of Medicine, 367,* 1704–1713. doi:10.1056/NEJMoa1202865.

Berman, A., & Snyder, S. J. (2012). Health assessment. In K. Trakalo (Ed.), *Kozier & Erb's fundamentals of nursing: Concepts, process, and practice* (pp. 574–667). Upper Saddle River, NJ: Pearson Education.

Beveridge, L. A., Davey, P. G., Phillips, G., & McMurdo, M. E. T. (2011). Optimal management of urinary tract infections in older people. *Clinical Interventions in Aging, 6,* 173–180. doi:10.2147/CIA.S13423.

Bielory, L., & Friedlaender, M. H. (2008). Allergic conjunctivitis. *Immunology and allergy clinics of North America, 28*(1), 43–58.

Bluestone, C. D., & Klein, J. O. (2007). *Otitis media in infants and children.* Hamilton, Ontario: BC Decker.

Boyd, J. H., Forbes, J., Nakada, T. A., Walley, K. R., & Russell, J. A. (2011). Fluid resuscitation in septic shock: A positive fluid balance and elevated central venous pressure are associated with increased mortality. *Critical Care Medicine, 39*(2), 259–265. doi:10.1097/CCM.0b013e3181feeb15.

Brandstrom, P., Esbjorner, E., Herthelius, M., Swerkersson, S., Jodal, U., & Hansson, S. (2010). The Swedish reflux trial in children: III. Urinary tract infection pattern. *Journal of Urology, 184*(1), 286–291. doi:10.1016/j.juro.2010.01.061.

Centers for Disease Control and Prevention. (2002). Guidelines for hand hygiene in health-care settings. *Morbidity and Mortality Weekly Report, 51*(RR-16), 1–56.

Centers for Disease Control and Prevention. (2009a). *2009 H1N1 flu ("swine flu") and you.* Retrieved from http://www.cdc.gov/h1n1flu/qa.htm.

Centers for Disease Control and Prevention. (2009b). *Pneumococcal polysaccharide vaccine.* Retrieved from http://www.cdc.gov/vaccines/pubs/vis/downloads/vis-ppv.pdf.

Centers for Disease Control and Prevention. (2010a). *National Hospital Discharge Survey, 2010.* Retrieved from http://www.cdc.gov/nchs/data/nhds/2average/2010ave2_firstlist.pdf.

Centers for Disease Control and Prevention. (2010b). *Preventing the spread of conjunctivitis.* Retrieved from http://www.cdc.gov/conjunctivitis/about/prevention.html.

Centers for Disease Control and Prevention. (2011a). *Bloodborne pathogens—Occupational exposure.* Retrieved from http://www.cdc.gov/oralhealth/infectioncontrol/faq/bloodborne_exposures.htm.

Centers for Disease Control and Prevention. (2011b). *Core curriculum on tuberculosis: What every clinician should know* (5th ed.). Retrieved from http://www.cdc.gov/tb/education/corecurr/pdf/corecurr_all.pdf.

Centers for Disease Control and Prevention. (2011c). *Pneumococcal disease.* Retrieved from http://www.cdc.gov/vaccines/vpd-vac/pneumo/dis-faqs.htm.

Centers for Disease Control and Prevention. (2011d). *Polio disease—Questions and answers.* Retrieved from http://www.cdc.gov/vaccines/vpd-vac/polio/dis-faqs.htm.

Centers for Disease Control and Prevention. (2012a). *Conjunctivitis (Pink Eye).* Retrieved from http://www.cdc.gov/conjunctivitis/clinical.html.

Centers for Disease Control and Prevention. (2012b). *Influenza antiviral medications: Summary for clinicians.* Retrieved from http://www.cdc.gov/flu/professionals/antivirals/summary-clinicians.htm.

Center for Disease Control and Prevention. (2012d). *National Vital Statistics Reports. Deaths: Preliminary data for 2011.* Retrieved from http://www.cdc.gov/nchs/data/nvsr/nvsr61/nvsr61_06.pdf.

Centers for Disease Control and Prevention. (2012e). Notes from the field: Tuberculosis cluster associated with homelessness—Duval County, Florida, 2004–2012. *Morbidity and Mortality Weekly Report, 61*(28); 537-540.

Centers for Disease Control and Prevention. (2012f). *Rapid diagnostic testing for influenza.* Retrieved from http://www.cdc.gov/flu/professionals/diagnosis/rapidlab.htm.

Centers for Disease Control and Prevention. (2012g). *Reported tuberculosis in the United States, 2011.* Atlanta, GA: U.S. Department of Health and Human Services.

Centers for Disease Control and Prevention. (2012h). *Seasonal influenza (flu).* Retrieved from http://www.cdc.gov/flu/about/disease/high_risk.htm.

Centers for Disease Control and Prevention. (2012i). Trends in tuberculosis—United States, 2011. *Morbidity and Mortality Weekly Report, 61*(11), 181–185.

Centers for Disease Control and Prevention. (2012j). *Tuberculosis: Children.* Retrieved from http://www.cdc.gov/tb/topic/populations/TBinChildren/default.htm.

Centers for Disease Control and Prevention. (2012k). *Tuberculosis: Infection control and prevention.* Retrieved from http://www.cdc.gov/tb/topic/infectioncontrol/default.htm.

Centers for Disease Control and Prevention. (2012l). Tuberculosis outbreak associated with a homeless shelter—Kane County, IL, 2007–2011. *Morbidity and Mortality Weekly Report, 61*(11), 186–189.

Centers for Disease Control and Prevention. (2012m). Interim domestic guidance on the use of respirators to prevent transmission of SARS. Retrieved from http://www.cdc.gov/sars/clinical/respirators.html.

Centers for Disease Control and Prevention. (2013a). *Diseases/pathogens associated with antimicrobial resistance: Outbreaks.* Retrieved from http://www.cdc.gov/drugresistance/DiseasesConnectedAR.html.

Centers for Disease Control and Prevention. (2013b). Interim adjusted estimates of seasonal influenza vaccine effectiveness—United States, February 2013. *Morbidity and Mortality Weekly Report, 62*(07); 119–123.

Centers for Disease Control and Prevention. (2013c). *Pertussis (whooping cough): Outbreaks.* Retrieved from http://www.cdc.gov/pertussis/outbreaks.html.

Centers for Disease Control and Prevention. (2013d). *TB in the homeless population.* Retrieved from http://www.cdc.gov/tb/topic/populations/Homelessness/default.htm.

Chapman, S. J., & Hill, A. V. S. (2012). Human genetic susceptibility to infectious disease. *Nature Reviews Genetics, 13,* 175–188. doi:10.1038/nrg3114.

Chira, S., & Miller, L. G. (2010). Staphylococcus aureus is the most common identified cause of cellulitis: A systematic review. *Epidemiology and Infection, 138*(03), 313–317.

Chulay, M., & Burns, S. M. (2010). *AACN Essentials of Critical Care Nursing* (2nd ed.). New York, NY: McGraw-Hill.

Cohen, S. H., Gerding, D. N., Johnson, S., Kelly, C. P., Loo, V. G., McDonald, C., … Wilcox, M. H. (2010). Clinical practice guidelines for *Clostridium difficile* infection in adults: 2010 update by the Society for Healthcare Epidemiology of America (SHEA) and the Infectious Diseases Society of America (IDSA). *Infection Control and Hospital Epidemiology, 31*(5), 431–55. doi:10.1086/651706.

Conde-Agudelo, A., Villar, J., & Lindheimer, M. (2008). Maternal infection and risk of preeclampsia: Systematic review and meta-analysis. *American Journal of Obstetrics and Gynecology, January,* 7–22.

Craig, J. C., Simpson, J. M., Williams, G. J., Lowe, A., Reynolds, G. J., McTaggart, S J., … Roy, L. P. (2009). Antibiotic prophylaxis and recurrent urinary tract infection in children. *New England Journal of Medicine, 361,* 1748–1759. doi:10.1056/NEJMoa0902295.

Csakanyi, Z., Czinner, A., Spangler, J., Rogers, T., & Katona, G. (2012). Relationship of environmental tobacco smoke to otitis media (OM) in children. *International Journal of Pediatric Otorhinolaryngology, 76*(7), 989–993. doi:10.1016/j.ijporl.2012.03.017.

Dennehy, P. H. (2005). Update on a high-morbidity infection: Rotavirus. *Contemporary Pediatrics, 22*(12), 34–40.

Drzewiecki, B. A., Thomas, J. C., Pope, J. C., IV, Adams, M. C., Brock, J. W., III, & Tanaka, S. T. (2012). Observation of patients with vesicoureteral reflux off antibiotic prophylaxis: Physician bias on patient selection and risk factors for recurrent febrile urinary tract infection. *Journal of Urology, 188*(Suppl. 4), 1480–1484. doi:10.1016/j.juro.2012.02.033.

Durbin, W. J. (2004). Pneumococcal infections. *Pediatrics in Review, 25*(12), 418–423.

Fashner, J., Garcia, M., Ribble, L., & Crowell, K. (2011). Clinical inquiry: What risk factors contribute to *C. difficile* diarrhea? *Journal of Family Practice, 60*(9), 545–547.

Finnell, S. M., Carroll, A. E., Downs, S. M., & the Subcommittee on Urinary Tract Infection. (2011). Diagnosis and management of an initial UTI in febrile infants and young children. *Pediatrics, 128*(3), e749–e770. doi:10.1542/peds.2011-1332.

Food and Drug Administration. (2013). *Influenza (flu) antiviral drugs and related information.* Retrieved from http://www.fda.gov/Drugs/DrugSafety/Informationby-DrugClass/ucm100228.htm.

Foxlee, R., Johansson, A., Wejfalk, J., Dawkins, J., Dooley, L., & Del Mar, C. (2006). Topical anesthesia for acute otitis media. *Cochrane Database of Systematic Reviews,* Issue 3. Art. No.: CD005657.DOI:10.1002/14651858. CD005657.pub2.

Gandhi, M. (2006). *Asymptomatic bacteriuria.* Retrieved from http://www.nlm.nih.gov/medlineplus/ency/article/000520.htm.

Gilmore, G. (2011). Isolation precautions. In C. Friedman & W. Newsom (Eds.), *IFIC basic concepts of infection control* (pp. 157–166). Portadown, UK: International Federation of Infection Control.

Hall, M. J., Williams, S. N., DeFrances, C. J., & Golosinskiy, A. (2011). *Inpatient care for septicemia or sepsis: A challenge for patients and hospitals.* Washington, DC: U.S. Department of Health and Human Services, Centers for Disease Control and Prevention, National Center for Health Statistics.

Hawkey, P. M., & Jones, A. M. (2009). The changing epidemiology of resistance. *Journal of Antimicrobial Chemotherapy, 64*(Suppl. 1), i3–i10. doi:10.1093/jac/dkp256.

The Joint Commission. (2012). *National Patient Safety Goals Effective January 1, 2013.* Retrieved from http://www.jointcommission.org/assets/1/18/NPSG_Chapter_Jan2013_HAP.pdf.

Kanj, S. S., & Kanafani, Z. A. (2011). Current concepts in antimicrobial therapy against gram-negative organisms: Extended-spectrum beta-lactamase-producing Enterobacteriaceae, carbapenem-resistant Enterobacteriaceae, and multidrug-resistant *Pseudomonas aeruginosa. Mayo Clinic Proceedings, 86*(3), 250–259. doi:10.4065/mcp.2010.0674.

Kerker, B. D., Bainbridge, J., Kennedy, J., Bennani, Y., Agerton, T., Marder, D., . . . Thorpe, L. E. (2011). A population-based assessment of the health of homeless families in New York City, 2001–2003. *American Journal of Public Health, 101*(3), 546–553. doi:10.2105/AJPH.2010.193102.

Klein, N. P., Bartlett, J., Rowhani-Rahbar, A., Fireman, B., & Baxter, R. (2012). Waning protection after fifth dose of acellular pertussis vaccine in children. *New England Journal of Medicine, 367*(11), 1012–1019.

Lachenbruch, C., & VanGilder, C. (2012). Estimates of evaporation rates from wounds for various dressing/support surface combinations. *Advances in Skin and Wound Care, 25*(1), 29–36. doi:10.1097/01.ASW.0000410688.21987.1d.

Laessig, K. A. (2010). End points in hospital-acquired pneumonia and/or ventilator-associated pneumonia clinical trials: Food and Drug Administration perspective. *Clinical Infectious Diseases, 51*(Suppl. 1), S117–S119. doi:10.1086/653059.

LaRosa, S. P. (2010). *Sepsis.* Retrieved from http://www.clevelandclinicmeded.com/medicalpubs/diseasemanagement/infectious-disease/sepsis/#bib1.

Lehne, R. A. (2010). *Pharmacology for nursing care* (7th ed.). St. Louis, MO: Saunders/Elsevier.

Lin, M. Y., & Hayden, M. K. (2010). Methicillin-resistant *Staphylococcus aureus* and vancomycin-resistant enterococcus: Recognition and prevention in intensive care units. *Critical Care Medicine, 38*(Suppl. 8), S335–S344. doi:10.1097/CCM.0b013e3181e6ab12.

Linas, B. P., Wong, A. Y., Freedberg, K. A., & Horsburgh, C. R. (2011). Priorities for screening and treatment of latent tuberculosis infection in the United States. *American Journal of Respiratory Critical Care Medicine, 184*(5), 590–601. doi:10.1164/rccm.201101-0181OC.

Liu, C., Bayer, A., Cosgrove, S. E., Daum, R. S., Fridkin, S. K., Gorwitz, R. J. … & Chambers, H. F. (2011). Clinical practice guidelines by the Infectious Diseases Society of America for the treatment of methicillin-resistant *Staphylococcus aureus* infections in adults and children. *Clinical Infectious Diseases, 52*(3), e18–e55.

Longo, D. L., Fauci, A. S., Kasper, D. L., Hauser, S. L., Jameson, J. L., & Loscalzo, J. (Eds.). (2012). *Harrison's™ Principles of Internal Medicine* (18th ed.). New York, NY: McGraw-Hill.

Mahabee-Gittens, E. M., Grupp-Phelan, J., Brody, A. S., Donnelly, L. F., Bracey, S. E. A., Duma, E. M., … Slap, G. B. (2005). Identifying children with pneumonia in the emergency department. *Clinical Pediatrics, 44*, 427–435.

Mayo Clinic. (2012). *Cellulitis.* Retrieved from http://www.mayoclinic.com/health/cellulitis/DS00450.

Mayo Clinic. (2013a). *Fever.* Retrieved from http://www.mayoclinic.com/health/fever/ID00052.

Mayo Clinic. (2013b). *Sepsis.* Retrieved from http://www.mayoclinic.com/health/sepsis/DS01004.

Mayo Clinic. (2013c). *Tuberculosis.* Retrieved from http://www.mayoclinic.com/health/tuberculosis/DS00372.

McCance, K. L., & Huether, S. E. (2010). *Pathophysiology: The biologic basis for disease in adults and children* (6th ed.). Maryland Heights, MO: Mosby.

MedlinePlus. (2011a). *Legionnaire's disease.* Retrieved from http://www.nlm.nih.gov/medlineplus/ency/article/000616.htm.

MedlinePlus. (2011b). *Urinary tract infection—Adults.* Retrieved from http://www.nlm.nih.gov/medlineplus/ency/article/000521.htm.

MedlinePlus. (2012). *Asymptomatic bacteriuria.* Retrieved from http://www.nlm.nih.gov/medlineplus/ency/article/000520.htm.

Mitruka, K., Winston, C. A., & Navin, T. R. (2012). Predictors of failure in timely tuberculosis treatment completion, United States. *International Journal of Tuberculosis and Lung Disease, 16*(8), 1075–1082. doi:10.5588/ijtld.11.0814.

Morton, L. M., & Phillips, T. J. (2012). Wound healing update. *Seminars in Cutaneous Medicine and Surgery, 31*, 33–37. doi:10.1016.j.sder.2011.11.007 http://nccam.nih.gov/health/echinacea/ataglance.htm.

National Center for Complementary and Alternative Medicine. (2012b). *Herbs at a glance: Echinacea.* Retrieved from http://nccam.nih.gov/health/echinacea/ataglance.htm?nav=gsa.

National Center for Complementary and Alternative Medicine. (2012b). *Herbs at a glance: Ephedra.* Retrieved from http://nccam.nih.gov/sites/nccam.nih.gov/files/Herbs_At_A_Glance_Ephedra_07-03-2012_0.pdf?nav=gsa.

National Center for Health Statistics. (2012). *Health, United States, 2011: With special features on socioeconomic status and health.* Hyattsville, MD: U.S. Department of Health and Human Services.

National Institute for Occupational Safety and Health. (1999). *Preventing needlestick injuries in health care settings.* (DHHS Publication No. 2000-108) Cincinnati, OH: U.S. Department of Health and Human Services, Public Health Service, Centers for Disease Control and Prevention, National Institute for Occupational Safety and Health.

National Institute of Allergy and Infectious Diseases, National Institutes of Health. (2006). *Focus on the flu.* Retrieved from http://www3.niaid.nih.gov/news/focuson/flu/research/primer/default.htm.

National Kidney and Urological Diseases Information Clearinghouse. (2012). *Pyelonephritis: Kidney infection.* Retrieved from http://kidney.niddk.nih.gov/kudiseases/pubs/pyelonephritis/#7.

Nicks, B. A., Ayello, E. A., Woo, K., Nitzki-George, D., & Sibbald, R. G. (2010). Acute wound management: Revisiting the approach to assessment, irrigation, and closure considerations. *International Journal of Emergency Medicine, 3*(4), 399–407. doi:10.1007/s12245-010-0217-5.

Nicolle, L. E., Bradley, S., Colgan, R., Rice, J.C., Schaeffer, A., & Hooton, T. M. (2005). Infectious Diseases Society of America Guidelines for the diagnosis and treatment of asymptomatic bacteriuria in adults. *Clinical Infectious Diseases, 40*(5), 643–654. doi:10.1086/427507.

Occupational Safety and Health Administration. (2008). Potential for sensitization and possible allergic reaction to natural rubber latex gloves and other natural rubber products. *Safety and Health Information Bulletin* (SHIB 01-28-2008). http://www.osha.gov/dts/shib/shib012808.html.

Osborn, K. S., Wraa, C. E., Watson, A. B., & Holleran, R (2014). Nursing assessment of the patient with sensory disorders. In P. Fuller (Ed.), *Medical-surgical nursing: Preparation for practice* (pp. 1970–1988). Upper Saddle River, NJ: Pearson Education.

Osmon, D. R., Berbari, E. F., Berendt, A. R., Lew, D., Zimmerli, W., Steckelberg, J. M., … Wilson, W. R. (2013). Diagnosis and management of prosthetic joint infection: Clinical practice guidelines by the Infectious Diseases Society of America. *Clinical Infectious Diseases, 56*(1), e1–e25.

Papadakis, M. A., & McPhee, S. J. (Eds.). (2013). *Current medical diagnosis and treatment 2013* (52nd ed.). New York, NY: McGraw-Hill.

Pellowe, C. (2009). Reducing the risk of infection with indwelling urethral catheters. *Nursing Times, 105*(36), 29–30, 32.

Pelton, S. I. (2005). Otitis media: Re-evaluation of diagnosis and treatment in the era of antimicrobial resistance, pneumococcal conjugate vaccine, and evolving morbidity. *Pediatric Clinics of North America, 52*, 711–728.

Pickering, L. K., Baker, C. J., Kimberlin, D. W., & Long, S. S. (Eds.). (2012). *Red Book: 2012 Report of the Committee on Infectious Diseases.* Media, PA: American Academy of Pediatrics.

Porth, C., & Matfin, G. (2010). *Pathophysiology: Concepts of altered health states* (8th ed.). Philadelphia, PA: Lippincott Williams & Wilkins.

Pratt, R. H., Winston, C. A., Kammerer, J. S., & Armstrong, L. R. (2011). Tuberculosis in older adults in the United States, 1993–2008. *Journal of the American Geriatrics Society, 59*(5), 851–857. doi:10.1111/j.1532-5415.2011.03369.x.

Raszka, W. V., & Khan, O. (2005). Pyelonephritis. *Pediatrics in Review, 26*(10), 364–369.

Revai, K., Dobbs, L. A., Nair, S., Patel, J. A., Grady, J. J., & Chonmaitree, T. (2007). Incidence of acute otitis media and sinusitis complicating upper respiratory tract infection: The effect of age. *Pediatrics, 119*, e1408. doi:10.1542/peds.2006-2881.

Rubinstein, E., Lalani, T., Corey, G. R., Kanafani, Z. A., Nannini, E. C., Rocha, M. G., … Stryjewski, M. E. (2011). Telavancin versus vancomycin for hospital-acquired pneumonia due to gram-positive pathogens. *Clinical Infectious Diseases, 52*(1), 31–40.

Santillanes, G., & Gausche-Hill, M. (2008). Pediatric airway management. *Emergency Medicine Clinics of North America, 26,* 961–975. doi:10.1016/j.emc.2008.08.004.

Sarrell, E. M., Cohen, H. A., & Kahan, E. (2003). Naturopathic treatment for ear pain in children. *Pediatrics, 111,* e574–e579.

Schuetz, P., Albrich, W., & Mueller, B. (2011). Procalcitonin for diagnosis of infection and guide to antibiotic decisions: Past, present and future. *BMC Medicine, 9,* 107. doi:10.1186/1741-7015-9-107.

Scott, R. D. (2009). *The direct medical costs of healthcare-associated infections in US hospitals and the benefits of prevention (CS200891-A).* Atlanta, GA: Centers for Disease Control and Prevention.

Sexton, S., & Natale, R. (2009). Risks and benefits of pacifiers. *American Family Physician, 79*(8), 681–685.

Shaikh, N., Hoberman, A., Kaleida, P. H., Ploof, D. L., & Paradise, J. L. (2010). Diagnosing otitis media—Otoscopy and cerumen removal. *New England Journal of Medicine, 362,* e62.

Siegel, J. D., Rhinehart, E., Jackson, M., Chiarello, L., & the Healthcare Infection Control Practices Advisory Committee. (2007). *2007 guideline for isolation precautions: Preventing transmission of infectious agents in healthcare settings.* Retrieved from http://www.cdc.gov/ncidod/dhqp/pdf/isolation2007.pdf.

Singleton, R. J., Holman, R. C., Plant, R., Yorita, K. L., Holve, S., Paisano, E. L., & Cheek, J. E. (2009). Trends in otitis media and myringotomy with tube replacement among American Indian/Alaska native children and the US general population of children. *Pediatric Infectious Disease Journal, 28*(2), 102–107. doi:10.1097/INF.0b013e318188d079.

Sole, M. L., Klein, D. G., & Moseley, M. J. (Eds.). (2013). *Introduction to critical care nursing* (6th ed.). St. Louis, MO: Elsevier.

Swaminathan, S., & Rekha, B. (2010). Pediatric tuberculosis: Global overview and challenges. *Clinical Infectious Diseases, 50*(Suppl. 3), S184–S194. doi:10.1086/651490.

Swigart, V., & Kolb, R. (2004). Homeless persons' decisions to accept or reject public health disease-detection services. *Public Health Nursing, 21*(2), 162–170.

Thigpen, M. C., Whitney, C. G., Messonnier, N. E., Zell, E. R., Lynfield, R., Hadler, J. L., … Schuchat, A. (2011). Bacterial meningitis in the United States, 1998–2007. *New England Journal of Medicine, 364,* 2016–2025.

Tiwari, T., Murphy, T. V., & Moran, J. (2005). Recommended antimicrobial agents for the treatment and postexposure prophylaxis of pertussis: 2005 CDC guidelines. *Morbidity and Mortality Weekly Report, 54* (RR-14), 1–16.

U.S. Department of Health and Human Services. (2011). *CDC global immunization strategic framework 2011–2015.* Retrieved from http://www.cdc.gov/globalhealth/gid/pdf/GID-strat-framewk.pdf.

U.S. Department of Health and Human Services, Office of Disease Prevention and Promotion. (2013). *Healthy People 2020.* Washington, DC. Retrieved from http://www.healthypeople.gov/2020/default.aspx.

U.S. National Library of Medicine. (2011). *Cellulitis.* Retrieved from http://www.ncbi.nlm.nih.gov/pubmedhealth/PMH0001858/.

Warny, M., Pepin, J., Fang, A., Killgore, G., Thompson, A., Brazier, J., Frost, E., & McDonald, L. C. (2005). Toxic production by an emerging strain of *Clostridium difficile* associated with outbreaks of severe disease in North America and Europe. *Lancet, 366,* 1079–1083.

Waseem, M. (2010). Otitis media. *Medscape Reference.* Retrieved from http://emedicine.medscape.com/article/994656-overview.

White, B. (2011). Diagnosis and treatment of urinary tract infections in children. *American Family Physician, 83*(4), 409–415.

Wicker, A. M., & Mohundro, B. L. (2010). Management of pediatric otitis media. *U.S. Pharmacist.* Retrieved from http://www.medscape.com/viewarticle/720085.

Wilson, B. A., Shannon, M. T., & Shields, K. M. (2013). *Nurse's drug guide.* Upper Saddle River, NJ: Pearson Education.

Windmill, S., & Windmill, I. M. (2006). The status of diagnostic testing following referral from universal newborn hearing screening. *Journal of the American Academy of Audiology, 17,* 367–378.

World Health Organization. (n.d.). *Trachoma.* Retrieved from http://www.who.int/topics/trachoma/en/

World Health Organization. (2009a). *Influenza A(H1N1)—Update 5.* Retrieved from http://www.who.int/csr/don/2009_04_29/en/index.html.

World Health Organization. (2009b). *WHO guidelines on hand hygiene in health care.* Geneva, Switzerland: WHO Press.

World Health Organization. (2011). *Key facts on global HIV epidemic and progress in 2010.* Retrieved from http://www.who.int/hiv/pub/progress_report2011/global_facts/en/.

World Health Organization. (2012a). *Global tuberculosis report 2012.* Geneva, Switzerland: WHO Press.

World Health Organization. (2012b). *Hepatitis C.* Retrieved from http://www.who.int/mediacentre/factsheets/fs164/en/.

World Health Organization. (2013). *Tuberculosis.* Retrieved from http://www.who.int/mediacentre/factsheets/fs104/en/.

10 Inflammation

◪ THE CONCEPT OF INFLAMMATION

Inflammation is a nonspecific but complex response to reduce the effects of what the body sees as harmful. Inflammation may result from an injury such as an ankle sprain. It may also result from an underlying infection. Autoimmune diseases frequently cause inflammation sufficient to result in tissue damage. Other harmful agents include pathogens, damaged cells, and irritants such as cigarette smoke.

Under normal circumstances, inflammation acts as a protective process that stimulates healing and prevents further damage or progressive deterioration. The occasional uncomfortable symptoms of normal inflammation usually resolve successfully with palliative care. However, the inflammatory process can escalate and lead to complications such as autoimmune disorders (e.g., rheumatoid arthritis, psoriasis, asthma, and allergies). These conditions may require more aggressive care that includes pharmacotherapy. **<<**

Concept Learning Outcomes

After reading about this concept you will be able to:

1. Summarize the physiology of the inflammatory process.

2. Examine the relationship between inflammation and other concepts/systems.

3. Identify commonly occurring alterations in inflammation and their related therapies.

4. Differentiate common assessment procedures used to examine the inflammatory process across the life span.

5. Describe diagnostic and laboratory tests to determine the individual's inflammatory process status.

6. Explain management of the inflammatory process and prevention of inflammation.

7. Demonstrate the nursing process in providing culturally competent and caring interventions across the life span for individuals with common alterations in the inflammatory process.

8. Compare and contrast common independent and collaborative interventions for clients with alterations in the inflammatory process.

Concept Key Terms

Anaphylaxis, 636
Debridement, 634
Emigration, 634
Exudate, 634
Granulation tissue, 635
H_1 receptor, 635
H_4 receptor, 635
Histamine, 634

Hyperemia, 634
Inflammation, 634
Leukocyte, 634
Leukocytosis, 634
Margination, 634
Mast cell, 635
Regeneration, 634

▶ NORMAL PRESENTATION

Inflammation is an adaptive response to injury or illness that brings fluid (plasma), dissolved substances, and blood cells into the interstitial tissues where the invasion or damage has occurred. This innate immune response is *nonspecific* because the same events occur regardless of the cause of the inflammatory process. Through the inflammatory reaction, the invader is neutralized and eliminated, destroyed tissue is removed, and the process of healing and repair begins. Inflammation is the first phase of the healing process. During the inflammatory process, particulate matter, bacteria, damaged cells, and inflammatory exudate are removed through phagocytosis and a large number of potentially damaging chemicals and microorganisms may be neutralized. This process, called **debridement**, prepares the wound for healing. Adequate nutrition is essential for inflammation and healing to proceed.

Physiology Review

Inflammation is characterized by five signs: (a) pain, (b) swelling, (c) redness, (d) heat, and (e) impaired function of the body part (if the injury is severe). Typically, words with the suffix *-itis* describe an inflammatory process. For example, *appendicitis* means inflammation of the appendix; *gastritis* means inflammation of the stomach.

Injurious agents can be categorized as physical agents, chemical agents, and microorganisms. *Physical agents* include mechanical objects causing trauma to tissues, excessive heat or cold, and radiation. *Chemical agents* include external irritants (e.g., strong acids, alkalis, poisons, and irritating gases) and internal irritants (substances manufactured within the body, such as excessive hydrochloric acid in the stomach). Microorganisms that can cause inflammation are bacteria and viruses.

THE INFLAMMATORY PROCESS Inflammation is a complex response of vascular tissues that is triggered by harmful stimuli. By isolating the damaged area and promoting repair of the surrounding tissue, the inflammatory response protects the body. Without this necessary and beneficial process, wounds and infections would never heal. Inflammation may be classified as either acute or chronic. During acute inflammation, the inflammatory response may occur within minutes of an injury such as a splinter or insect bite. On the other hand, a response to a bacterial infection may take a few hours. It is during the acute inflammatory response that the typical signs of inflammation (redness, swelling, pain, heat, and impaired function) occur. The acute process continues until the trauma or infection is neutralized. When the acute inflammatory response is unable to neutralize the harmful stimuli, the response may become chronic, continuing for months or years. Chronic inflammation ranges from seasonal allergic reactions to pollen to responses that damage healthy tissues in autoimmune diseases.

STAGES OF INFLAMMATION In simplest terms, the complex inflammatory process can be categorized into three stages: vascular and cellular responses, exudate production, and repair.

Vascular and Cellular Responses Immediately after injury or infection, blood vessels temporarily constrict in the surrounding area. The injured tissues release **histamines**, kinins, and prostaglandins in response to the injury or infection. These substances serve as chemical mediators to dilate blood vessels, causing more blood to flow to the injured area. This marked increase in blood supply is referred to as **hyperemia** and is responsible for the characteristic signs of redness and heat that accompany inflammation.

Vascular permeability increases at the site with dilation of the vessels. Fluid, proteins, and **leukocytes** (white blood cells) leak into the interstitial spaces, causing inflammatory swelling (edema) and pain. Pain is caused by the pressure of accumulating fluid on nerve endings and the irritating chemical mediators. Fluid pouring into areas such as the pleural or pericardial cavity can seriously affect organ function. In other areas, such as joints, mobility is impaired by accumulating fluid.

Slowed blood flow in the dilated vessels allows more leukocytes to arrive at the injured tissues. The leukocytes aggregate, or line up, along the inner surface of the blood vessels. This process is known as **margination**. Leukocytes then move through the blood vessel wall into the affected tissue spaces, a process called **emigration**.

In response to the exit of leukocytes from the blood, the bone marrow produces more leukocytes in even larger numbers and releases them into the bloodstream. This process is called **leukocytosis**. A normal leukocyte count of 4,500–10,000 per cubic millimeter of blood can increase to 20,000 or more when inflammation occurs.

All these conditions result in the first stage of inflammation. Often individuals do not seek medical treatment for an acute inflammatory response unless it progresses to the second stage. Typical injuries for which an individual seeks treatment for stage 1 inflammation are sprained ankles and wrists, broken bones, and minor blunt force injuries (e.g., two children running into each other on a playground).

Exudate Production In the second stage of inflammation, inflammatory **exudate** is produced. The term *exudate* comes from the Latin word meaning "to exude" or "to ooze." Exudate consists of fluid that escaped from the blood vessels, dead phagocytic and tissue cells, and the products they release.

The nature and amount of exudate vary according to the tissue involved and the intensity and duration of the inflammation. The major types of exudate are serous, purulent, and hemorrhagic (sanguineous). Serous exudate typically accompanies mild inflammation and presents as clear- or straw-colored with a thin, watery consistency. Purulent exudate is usually opaque, or milky. Commonly referred to as "pus," purulent exudate normally indicates the presence of infection and contains a large quantity of cells and necrotic debris. Because hemorrhagic exudate contains blood from ruptured blood vessels, it is red and thick. This type of exudate leaks from tissue or its capillaries as a result of infection or injury.

Whether the presence of exudate should be reported depends primarily on the underlying cause and the amount and degree of the exudate. A minor cut that exhibits either serous or hemorrhagic exudate may resolve with simple first aid. Exudate that appears over a larger surface or in conjunction with other symptoms, such as fever, warrants a greater degree of medical care.

Reparative Phase The third stage of the inflammatory response involves the repair of injured tissues by regeneration or replacement with fibrous tissue (scar formation). **Regeneration** is the replacement of destroyed tissue cells by cells that are identical or similar in structure and function. Damaged cells are replaced one by one, and new cells are organized so that the architectural pattern and function of the tissue are restored. The ability to regenerate cells varies considerably from one type of tissue to another. For example, epithelial tissues of the skin and the digestive and respiratory tracts have a good regenerative capacity, as long as their underlying support structures are intact. The same is true of osseous, lymphoid, and bone marrow tissues. Tissues that have little regenerative capacity include nervous, muscular, and elastic tissues.

When regeneration is not possible, repair occurs by fibrous (scar) tissue formation. The inflammatory exudate with its interlacing network of fibrin provides the framework for this tissue to develop. Damaged tissues are replaced with the connective tissue elements of collagen, blood capillaries, lymphatics, and other tissue-bound substances. In the early stages of this process, the tissue is called **granulation tissue**. It is a fragile, gelatinous tissue that appears pink or red because of the many newly formed capillaries. Later in the process, the tissue shrinks (the capillaries are constricted, even obliterated) and the collagen fibers contract, leaving a firmer fibrous tissue. This is called a *cicatrix*, or scar tissue.

MEDIATORS OF INFLAMMATION The process of inflammation is initiated by the release of mediators from inflammatory cells such as macrophages and mast cells. **Mast cells** are leukocytes found in most tissues of the body, including the skin, respiratory system, and intestines. They are one of the principal sources of cell-derived mediators of inflammation, including histamine and heparin (**Table 10–1** ●).

In response to injury or contact with an antigen, histamine and heparin work together to increase blood flow to the injured site. Histamine causes the dilation of nearby blood vessels and increases their permeability, while heparin prevents blood clotting. This combined action allows blood to easily enter the affected tissue, resulting in the redness and swelling associated

TABLE 10–1 Chemical Mediators of Inflammation

MEDIATOR	DESCRIPTION
Bradykinin	Causes dilation of vessels; acts with prostaglandins to cause pain; increases vascular permeability; and stimulates histamine release.
Complement	Comprises over 20 proteins; activated sequentially; and is responsible for dilation, permeability, chemotaxis, phagocytosis, and histamine release.
Histamine	Stored and released by mast cells; contributes to early vasodilation and increased permeability; and chemically attracts eosinophils.
Leukotrienes	Stored and released by mast cells and chemically attracts neutrophils and macrophages.
Prostaglandins	Present in most tissues; stored and released by mast cells; and causes vasodilation.

Source: Data from Delves, P. J. (2012). Overview of the immune system. *Merck manual: Health care professionals.* Retrieved from http://www.merckmanuals.com/professional/immunology_allergic_disorders/biology_of_the_immune_system/overview_of_the_immune_system.html

with inflammation. **Figure 10–1** ● illustrates the fundamental steps in acute inflammation.

The four types of histamine receptors are H_1, H_2, H_3, and H_4. Of these the H_1 and H_4 receptors are involved in the inflammatory response. **H_1 receptors** are primarily found on smooth muscle cells, on the endothelium, and in the CNS. Stimulation of these receptors results in vasodilation, bronchoconstriction, pain, itching, and hives. The **H_4 receptors**, located in peripheral white blood cells and mast cells, are also involved in

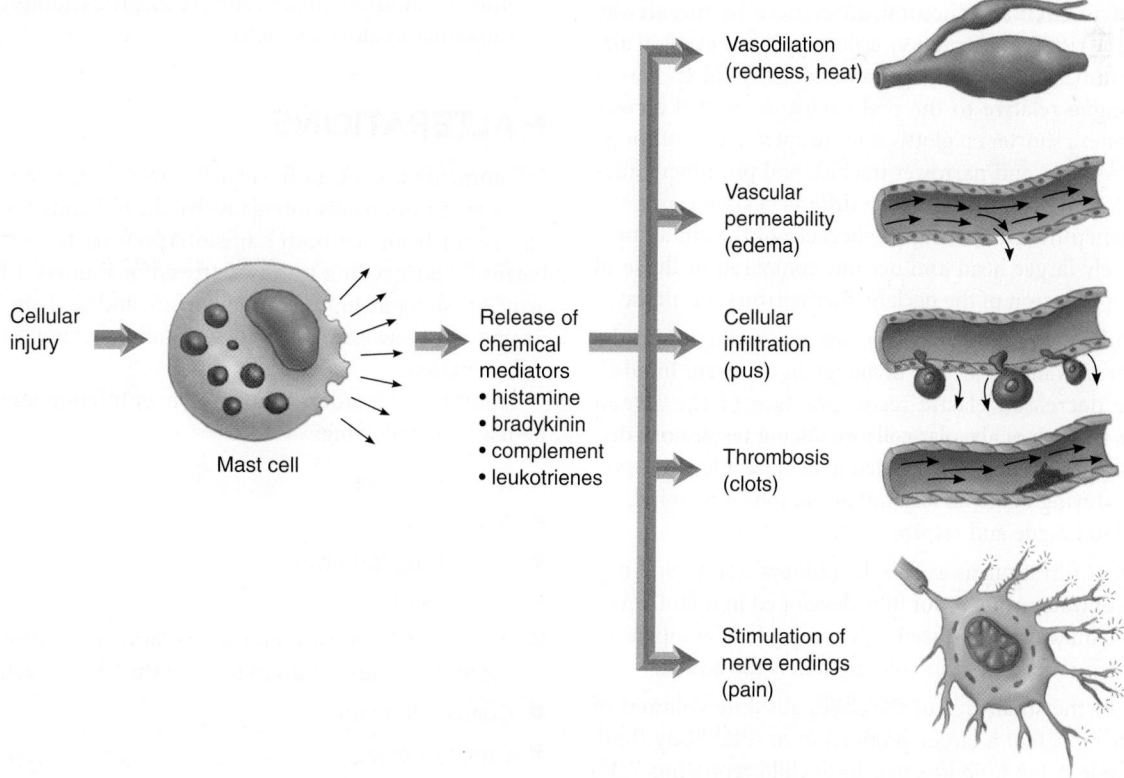

Cellular injury → Mast cell → Release of chemical mediators
• histamine
• bradykinin
• complement
• leukotrienes

→ Vasodilation (redness, heat)

Vascular permeability (edema)

Cellular infiltration (pus)

Thrombosis (clots)

Stimulation of nerve endings (pain)

Figure 10–1 ● Steps in acute inflammation.

Box 10–1   Symptoms and Treatment of Anaphylaxis

Anaphylaxis is a life-threatening allergic reaction that develops extremely rapidly—in seconds to minutes—and requires immediate initiation of the emergency medical system (EMS). Signs and symptoms of anaphylaxis include the following:

- Inflammation of the airways, swelling of the throat (which can become severe enough to block the airway)
- Wheezing, labored breathing
- Abnormal heart rhythm
- Low blood pressure
- Weakness, light-headedness, dizziness
- Nausea, vomiting, or diarrhea
- Cyanosis due to decreased tissue oxygenation or pallor secondary to shock (advanced manifestations)
- Hives, itching.

Epinephrine is the first line of treatment for an anaphylactic reaction. Epinephrine dilates the airways and narrows the blood vessels, essentially counteracting the allergic response. While the intramuscular route is preferred, epinephrine may also be administered subcutaneously or intravenously. For intubated clients in whom no other option is available, epinephrine may be administered via an endotracheal tube (Varon & Acosta, 2010). Some allergic individuals carry self-injectors with epinephrine (e.g., EpiPens) to use in the case of an anaphylactic response. In the event of an anaphylactic reaction, EMS should be called even for clients who carry and use an EpiPen. During and immediately following an anaphylactic response, airway protection is critical, so adjunctive medications may include beta-agonists, antihistamines, and corticosteroids. A severe reaction resulting in laryngeal swelling sufficient to close the airway may require a tracheotomy.

---

immune responses (Bongers, de Esch, & Leurs, 2010). Antihistamines block histamine receptors on tissues, thus reducing the effect of histamine and the resultant allergic symptoms.

When a client is exposed to an allergen that results in a rapid release of inflammatory mediators, anaphylaxis occurs. If left untreated, anaphylaxis may lead to death caused by airway obstruction or vascular collapse (Arnold & Williams, 2011; **Box 10–1** ●). The most common triggers of anaphylaxis are food (including peanuts, shellfish, milk, and egg), insect stings, medications (particularly penicillin, anesthetic agents, and NSAIDs), and latex (Lieberman et al., 2010).

Genetic and Lifespan Considerations

Several differences in anatomy and physiology influence the effects of inflammation on children compared to adults (Kozik & Tweddell, 2006; Schultz et al., 2004; Wheeler, Wong, & Zingarelli, 2011):

- In pediatric clients, structural differences in the airway increase the risk for obstruction, especially in the event of airway inflammation. In comparison to adults, children have a larger tongue relative to the oral cavity, decreased airway muscle tone, a shorter epiglottis, a more anteriorly positioned larynx, a shorter and narrower trachea, and prominent adenoid and lymphoid tissue. These differences are especially evident when the child is supine; because of the child's proportionately larger head and occiput compared to those of adults, hyperflexion of the neck further narrows the airway.

- Fewer and smaller lung alveoli equate to a reduction in the surface area available for gas exchange in children. In addition, the decreased elastic recoil pressure of the alveoli increases the risk of alveolar collapse during respiratory distress. The increased energy needed to achieve adequate oxygenation during acute airway inflammation or anaphylaxis may lead to fatigue and respiratory failure in infants.

- Glomerular filtration, as well as the kidneys' ability to dilute and concentrate urine, is not fully developed in infants. As a result, the infant's renal system is less capable of compensating for fluctuations in fluid volume than is the adult's.

- Because of the small size of the child, absolute volumes of fluid loss represent a larger proportion of total body fluid. For example, a 1-L fluid loss in a 30-lb child represents 7.3% dehydration, whereas the same fluid loss in a 180-lb male represents only 1.2% dehydration.

- Changes in excitation–contraction coupling, left ventricular mass, and the high contractile state of the heart reduce the pediatric client's sympathetic nervous system response to changes in blood volume and stress. While adults typically respond to hypovolemia with a compensatory increase in heart rate, tachycardia often is a late symptom of hypovolemia in children.

- Gastrointestinal inflammation that reduces nutrient absorption affects children more than adults. Children have higher metabolic rates and generally have less stored fat, so decreased absorption of nutrients has more immediate detrimental effects on growth, body weight, energy levels, bone and muscle strength, and overall health.

- The child's immune system response to insult differs significantly from that of the adult. In pediatric clients, macrophages are more responsive to pro-inflammatory molecules, increasing the production of additional inflammatory mediators. In addition, infants are less able than adults to produce anti-inflammatory mediators.

▶ ALTERATIONS

Inflammation can occur in virtually any tissue, organ, or system. Many autoimmune disorders involve the inflammatory response and result from the body's misinterpreting its own tissues as harmful and needing to be destroyed or limited. Rheumatoid arthritis, systemic lupus erythematosus, and Guillain-Barré syndrome are a few examples of autoimmune responses involving inflammation.

Additional disorders that involve an inflammatory component are the following:

- Allergic rhinitis
- Anaphylaxis
- Ankylosing spondylitis
- Appendicitis
- Arthritis (the most common inflammatory disorder—and the leading cause of disability—in the United States)
- Contact dermatitis
- Crohn disease
- Gallbladder disease
- Hashimoto thyroiditis

- Inflammatory bowel disease (affecting 300,000–500,000 Americans each year)
- Nephritis
- Peptic ulcers
- Rheumatoid arthritis
- Systemic lupus erythematosus
- Ulcerative colitis.

Inflammation carries implications for nursing care in a number of areas. Clients with mild alterations (e.g., a sprain) may need simple palliative care, rest, and reminders related to safety and injury prevention. Infection, however, requires treatment, and the resulting acute inflammatory response may cause additional complications for clients. See Concepts Related to Inflammation for a brief overview of inflammation's relationship to a few other systems and concepts.

Alterations and Manifestations

Classic signs of inflammation include redness and swelling. A healthy inflammatory response includes activation and recruitment of WBCs to the affected site. Localized responses are limited in terms of which sites are affected, while generalized responses can affect the entire body. Chronic inflammation of the intestines associated with inflammatory bowel disorders may result in structural changes. For example, Crohn disease results in fibrotic changes to the bowel wall; local obstruction, abscesses, and fistulas may develop. Malabsorption or malnutrition may result. In rheumatoid arthritis (RA), discussed in the module on Immunity, the chronic inflammatory response affects the lining of the joints and can lead to joint deformity. RA is characterized by pain, swelling, and redness of the joint.

Ankylosing spondylitis is a form of arthritis that primarily involves the spine. With this condition, vertebral inflammation leads to severe, chronic pain and discomfort. The sacroiliac (SI) joints, which are located at the base of the spine where the spine joins the pelvis, are affected by disease progression. In severe disease, new bone formation occurs on the spine, causing spinal processes to fuse into a fixed, immobile position, sometimes creating a forward-stooped posture.

For an overview of additional disorders that incorporate an inflammatory component, see the Alterations and Therapies feature.

Prevalence

Millions of adults and children in the United States have inflammatory disorders.

The typical onset of RA occurs in middle age with an increased incidence among older adults. However, RA also occurs in children and young adults. An estimated 1.3 million U.S. adults, or 0.6% of the population, have RA (NIAMS, 2009). (For further discussion of this condition, refer to the exemplar on RA in the module on Immunity.)

Ankylosing spondylitis, which primarily affects the spine and sacroiliac joints, is another debilitating inflammatory disorder. The Centers for Disease Control's NHANES study estimates at least 2.7 million adults in the United States have this form of inflammatory arthritis (SAA, 2012).

A recent estimate of the prevalence of asthma in the United States indicates 8.2% of the population (24.6 million) have this disorder. Asthma is more common among African Americans than Whites and is more often diagnosed in children than adults (CDC, 2011).

Each year in the United States, 80,000 children develop appendicitis. In 50% of pediatric cases, the client has a positive family history of appendicitis. The incidence of ruptured appendix is 30% in children, with a higher incidence in children under 5 years of age (Cleveland Clinic, Children's Hospital, 2009).

Genetic Considerations and Nonmodifiable Risk Factors

Genetic considerations and risk factors vary depending on the nature of the inflammatory disorder. Native and Mexican Americans are at increased risk for gallstones. Family history and female gender are also associated with increased risk. African Americans are more likely than Caucasians to develop nephritis as a complication of systemic lupus erythematosus and tend to develop nephritis earlier in the course of disease (Dooley, 2011). Family history is also associated with peptic ulcer disease, although diet and other modifiable risk factors typically are involved.

Concepts Related to **Inflammation**

When bacteria or a virus enters the body and causes an infection, it triggers the inflammatory response. The normal process of inflammation neutralizes the antigen and initiates healing. Widespread infection prompts a widespread inflammatory response, the manifestations of which include generalized pain and fever. A localized infection results in a limited inflammatory response that causes redness and tenderness at the affected site. An acute inflammatory response usually resolves when the invading pathogen is eradicated. When acute inflammation persists, chronic inflammation may develop. With chronic inflammation, the inflammatory response may be disproportionate to the initial insult and can lead to greater damage than would be expected from the initial cause. Examples of chronic inflammatory disorders include Crohn disease and ulcerative colitis.

Many of the blood cells and components of the inflammatory response are mediated by the immune system, which also protects the body from harm. In autoimmune diseases, inflammation and immune responses are mistakenly initiated against normal healthy tissue. The symptoms of an autoimmune disease depend on the tissue affected. Clients with rheumatoid arthritis experience joint pain, stiffness, and loss of function. If the thyroid is attacked, tiredness and weight gain result.

In asthma, the inflammatory response causes constriction of smooth muscle in the airways to constrict and increased mucus production, resulting in decreased oxygenation. The narrowed airway requires the client to exert more effort to move air in and out of the lungs. Common triggers of this response include pollen, particles from dust mites, and animal dander.

(continued on next page)

Concepts Related to **Inflammation** (*continued*)

CONCEPT	RELATIONSHIP TO INFLAMMATION	NURSING IMPLICATIONS
Infection		
■ Stages of the infectious process	Pathogen triggers activation of inflammatory and immune responses; WBCs are attracted to pathogen with increased WBC production; goal is to destroy invading pathogen.	■ Be alert to signs and symptoms (S/Sx) of hyperthermia, malaise, pain and discomfort, purulent drainage, excess sputum production. ■ Important in clients with altered skin or tissue integrity, chronic respiratory disorders, neuropathy. ■ *Anticipate:* blood test for WBC and differential, culture and serum albumin; treatment includes possible antipyretics and anti-infectives.
Immunity		
■ Hypersensitivity	Foreign substance activates immune response; in abnormal response body perceives normal tissue as a foreign object and initiates an attack against that tissue; inflammation is uncontrollable.	■ Be alert for S/Sx of anaphylaxis: hives, itching, alterations in skin color, airway constriction, weak and rapid pulse, nausea, dizziness. ■ Client c/o joint pain and stiffness, fatigue, shortness of breath. ■ Assess for mentation, patent airway, known allergies. ■ *Anticipate:* administration of epinephrine, oxygen, antihistamines, cortisone, beta-agonists, analgesics; blood tests, x-ray to determine causative factor.
Oxygenation		
■ Oxygenation assessment ■ ARDS ■ Asthma ■ COPD ■ RSV/bronchiolotis	Exposure to allergen or infection (bronchitis, pneumonia) results in abnormal inflammatory response resulting in airway edema, bronchoconstriction, and increased mucus production.	■ Client c/o coughing, wheezing, dyspnea, chest tightness. ■ Be alert for S/Sx of inadequate oxygenation: cyanosis, changes in ABG, labored breathing, abnormal lung sounds, inability to clear sputum. ■ *Anticipate:* administration of epinephrine, bronchodilators, antihistamines, and anti-inflammatory medications. ■ Continuously monitor oxygen saturation using pulse oximetry; administer oxygen as needed. ■ May assess airflow through use of pulmonary function testing.
Teaching and Learning		
■ Client/consumer education	Inflammation may result in temporary or long-term impairment of function. Clients require information related to care and coping.	*Acute inflammation:* ■ Teach clients treatment protocols. ■ Ask client or caregiver for return demonstration of dressing changes. ■ Teach clients about safety precautions, movement restrictions, and nutrition. *Chronic inflammation:* ■ Teach client about the condition, including physiology, treatments, expected course of disease, potential side effects of medications. ■ Assess the client's understanding of the disease, and answer questions. ■ Teach client coping techniques to minimize effects of physical limitations and emotional distress. ■ Teach client disease-appropriate methods to reduce impact of disease on lifestyle.

Alterations and Therapies **Inflammation**

ALTERATION	DESCRIPTION/ DEFINITION	MANIFESTATIONS	INTERVENTIONS/ TREATMENTS
Pain	An unpleasant feeling caused by damaging stimuli; subjective experience described by the client	Acute or chronic pain; onset, location, intensity, etiology, aggravating or alleviating factors described by client or caregiver	▪ Analgesics (acetaminophen, NSAIDs, opioids) ▪ Treatment of underlying cause of pain ▪ Heat/ice, distraction, massage, and relaxation techniques
Edema	Swelling caused by fluid in the body's tissues Peripheral edema: swelling of the limbs Ascites: edema of the abdomen Pulmonary edema: fluid accumulation in the lungs Pleural effusion: edema in the space around the lungs	Swelling or puffiness of skin, stretched skin, shortness of breath (pulmonary edema), decreased mobility, dimple in skin after pressure	▪ Diuretics ▪ Reduced salt intake ▪ Treatment of underlying cause of edema ▪ Assessment of medications for potential adverse effects ▪ Movement ▪ Elevation ▪ Compression
Heat	Increased local or systemic temperature	Elevated body temperature, localized skin warmth and redness	▪ Antipyretics ▪ Application of ice or cool packs
Impaired function	Inability to use the tissue or organ efficiently	Decreased mobility of joint, difficulty breathing, pain during use, altered mental status, decreased peripheral oxygenation, impaired sensory function, impaired nutrition, altered urination, fatigue	▪ Treatment of underlying condition ▪ Physical therapy ▪ Analgesics ▪ Adequate sleep/rest ▪ Administration of oxygen ▪ Administration of parenteral nutrition ▪ Dialysis
Altered oxygenation	Inadequate oxygen intake, decreased ability to expel carbon dioxide, inadequate delivery of oxygen to tissues	Cyanosis, labored breathing, dyspnea, changes in ABG, abnormal lung sounds, chest tightness, inability to clear sputum from lungs, hypotension, heart arrhythmia, fatigue	▪ Treatment of underlying condition (e.g., infection, heart condition, chronic lung disease) ▪ Administration of oxygen, bronchodilators, other medications as prescribed ▪ Encouragement of expectoration ▪ Adequate sleep/rest ▪ Monitoring of ABG, vitals
Infection	Invasion of the body by microorganisms such as bacteria and viruses	Inflammation, pain, mucus production, purulent drainage, hyperthermia, malaise, nausea, vomiting, diarrhea, headache	▪ Antibiotics or antivirals ▪ Antipyretics ▪ Analgesics ▪ Adequate sleep/rest ▪ Adequate fluids/nutrition ▪ Good wound hygiene ▪ Surgical removal of infected part (e.g., appendectomy, tonsillectomy, amputation)

Rheumatoid arthritis occurs among individuals of all races and ethnic groups. Recent research has identified a number of genes that may promote the development of RA in some individuals. Women are 2 to 3 times more likely than men to develop RA (NIAMS, 2009).

In asthma prevalence, differences exist between various population subgroups. Children have higher prevalence than adults, and young males have a higher prevalence than their female counterparts. When adolescence is reached, the trend reverses: Females have a higher prevalence than males. Asthma is more prevalent in Blacks than in Whites and is less prevalent in Asians than in Whites (CDC, 2011).

CASE STUDY \\ PART 1

Ryan Blake is a 29-year-old African American male. He is married with two children under the age of 5. Seven years ago, Mr. Blake was diagnosed with distal colitis characterized by inflammation below the descending colon. Mr. Blake has maintained remission of symptoms with the use of a mesalamine suppository nightly. As the nurse conducting the initial interview and assessment at his gastroenterologist's office, you ascertain that Mr. Blake is experiencing an acute onset of bloody diarrhea and for the past 7 days has experienced an average of five bowel movements per day. Additionally he has rectal urgency, tenesmus (chronic sense of needing to have a bowel movement), and abdominal pain. A CBC revealed an HCT of 39%. Vital signs are temperature 99.8°F oral; pulse 92 bpm; respirations 18/min; and BP 130/78 mmHg. Mr. Blake currently weighs 180 pounds, a loss of 6 pounds in the past 2 weeks.

Mr. Blake is prescribed mesalamine oral tablets in addition to continued use of the mesalamine suppository. Remission is not achieved, so prednisone (60 mg per day) is added until symptoms are controlled; then the dose is tapered to discontinuation. After remission, Mr. Blake will be started on maintenance mesalamine rectally and orally.

Clinical Reasoning Questions Level I

1. Why is a mesalamine suppository used instead of an oral preparation?
2. Why has Mr. Blake lost weight?
3. Why is prednisone prescribed for Mr. Blake?

Clinical Reasoning Questions Level II

4. Identify two nursing diagnoses that are appropriate for inclusion in the nursing plan of care for Mr. Blake.
5. Why has oral mesalamine been added to Mr. Blake's regimen?
6. What adverse effects associated with oral mesalamine should Mr. Blake be made aware of?

▶ PREVENTION

Preventing excessive inflammatory response generally involves avoidance. Individuals with hypersensitivity should avoid known triggers (e.g., dust, pollen, animal dander). Individuals with inflammatory bowel disease or peptic ulcer disease should avoid foods or beverages that trigger inflammation. Hand washing is a primary method of preventing infection that can result in inflammation.

Modifiable Risk Factors

For Crohn disease, ways to lower the risk of triggering a flare-up include a diet low in refined sugars, increased fiber intake, and smoking cessation (NIDDK, 2011). Gallstone formation risk can be lowered by maintaining an appropriate weight, consuming a diet high in fiber and low in fat, and avoiding rapid weight loss (NIDDK, 2012a). There are several risk factors for nephritis, including diabetes mellitus, hypertension, overuse of NSAIDs, and drug abuse. Clients with diabetes or hypertension can reduce their risk by following their treatment protocols, including maintaining a healthy diet.

Screening

Ultimately, the goals of early identification and treatment of inflammatory diseases include reduced mortality and effective management of the disorder. For many acute disorders that have an inflammatory component, such as appendicitis, screening is not possible. However, for some conditions, such as allergic rhinitis, skin testing identifies the allergens that trigger an inflammatory response. Likewise, a thyroid stimulating hormone (TSH) test determines if an asymptomatic client has Hashimoto thyroiditis.

▶ ASSESSMENT

During assessment, the nurse obtains the client's history, conducts the physical assessment, and gathers laboratory data. Assessment for inflammation, which can impact any of the body's tissues, is guided by the area of the body involved. Classic signs and symptoms of inflammation are presented in **Box 10–2** ●.

Nursing Assessment

When taking the client's medical history, the nurse assesses (a) the degree to which a client is at risk of developing inflammation and (b) any client reports that suggest the presence of inflammation. Because inflammation can involve any organ or organ system, a thorough history of the client is required. To identify clients at risk, the nurse reviews the client's chart and structures the nursing interview to collect data regarding the factors influencing the development of inflammation, especially existing conditions. Localized inflammation requires assessment for localized edema, pain or tenderness with palpation or movement, redness or palpable heat at the inflamed area, and reduced or absent function in the body part involved. Conditions causing more widespread inflammation, such as nephritis or allergies, may cause more diverse symptoms.

Box 10–2   Local and Systemic Manifestations of Inflammation

LOCAL MANIFESTATIONS	SYSTEMIC MANIFESTATIONS
■ Erythema	■ Temperature (oral) > 38°C (100.4°F) or < 36°C (96.8°F)
■ Warmth	
■ Pain	■ Pulse > 90 beats/min
■ Edema	■ Respirations > 20/min (tachypnea)
■ Functional impairment	■ WBC > 12,000/mm^3 or >10% bands

Assessment Interview **Inflammation**

- Do you have any pain? If the client reports pain, the nurse should assess the pain for location, intensity, type, severity, current treatments, and effectiveness of treatment.
- Are you taking any anti-inflammatory medications such as aspirin or ibuprofen, or medications for chronic conditions?
- Have you had any recent diagnostic procedure or therapy that penetrated your skin or a body cavity?
- What past surgeries have you had?
- How would you describe your eating habits? Do you eat a variety of types of foods?
- Do you take vitamins or dietary supplements?
- On a scale of 1 to 10, how would you rate the stress you have experienced in the last 6 months?
- Have you experienced any loss of energy, loss of appetite, nausea, headache, or other signs associated with specific body systems (e.g., difficulty urinating, urinary frequency, or a sore throat)?

Note: As with all history taking, the nurse must individualize the specific terms used; give examples to the client; and use teaching techniques to validate agreement on the meaning of words according to the client's culture, language spoken, and education or intellectual abilities.

Lifespan and Cultural Considerations

Inflammatory disorders are often related to internal organs, including the gastrointestinal tract, kidneys, lungs, and gallbladder. Children are often too young to understand the implications of assessment of internal organs, especially as it relates to the discomfort of invasive procedures. For example, assessment of adults with respiratory inflammation often involves bronchoscopy or bronchoalveolar lavage. These procedures are far too invasive and uncomfortable for regular use in children, so less invasive techniques, such as analysis of exhaled breath condensates, should be used if available and appropriate (van de Kant et al., 2009; van de Kant et al., 2012).

Similarly, inflammatory bowel disease (IBD) can be detected in children through sequencing of fecal microbiota rather than the more invasive colonoscopy, which many physicians are reluctant to perform on children (Papa et al., 2012). Fecal calprotectin is also a noninvasive diagnostic test for IBD in children (Canani et al., 2008). Noninvasive techniques for analyzing kidney function include monitoring voiding for volume and frequency as well as analyzing urine for electrolytes, protein, and blood.

If visualization of the inflamed organ is necessary, ultrasound may be a viable option for many disorders rather than endoscopy, especially when used in conjunction with a contrast agent specific for inflammation such as microbubbles (Alzaraa et al., 2012). Other noninvasive imaging tools include x-ray, CT scan, and MRI. Visual examination via inspection is an appropriate option for inflammation of the skin, upper airway, ears, and eyes. Internal inflammation may also be evident upon external inspection based on the presence of edema, swelling, or jaundice.

If less invasive techniques are not available, children may need to undergo local or general anesthesia to allow the physician or nurse to perform the procedure. Anesthesia decreases pain and resistance and increases safety. Parental presence during the assessment or procedure should also be encouraged to limit anxiety for both the child and the parents. Adequate client and parent teaching can also help reduce anxiety and increase compliance, especially in older children.

Assessment of children with inflammation often involves diagnostic tests such as blood tests. Negative blood tests should be interpreted with caution in children with potential inflammatory disorders. Normal blood test results are common for children with inflammatory disorders such as inflammatory bowel disease (Mack et al., 2007) and acute glomerulonephritis (Welch, 2012). False positives may also occur for some laboratory tests, such as an increase in alkaline phosphatase in healthy children and adolescents who are still growing (Shaffer, 2012).

Inflammatory markers (e.g., C-reactive protein, IL-6, TNFα) may be increased in older adults and obese individuals, both of which are associated with a low-grade proinflammatory state. This increase in inflammation may not be linked to a specific disease (e.g., gallbladder disease, asthma, inflammatory bowel disease) but instead is an indicator of poor overall health. These individuals are more susceptible to chronic diseases such as diabetes, heart disease, physical disability, and cognitive decline (Singh & Newman, 2011). African American race is also associated with enhanced baseline inflammation (Carroll et al., 2009).

Diagnostic Tests

A primary laboratory test ordered to detect the presence of inflammation is the erythrocyte sedimentation rate (ESR). ESR measures how far the erythrocyte settles in a tube over a given period of time, usually 1 hour. Normal sedimentation rate is 0–15 mm/h for males and 0–20 mm/h for women. It is not unusual to see the sedimentation rate slightly elevated in older adults. When an inflammatory process is active, the increased proportion of fibrinogen causes red blood cells to stick to one another and settle faster, causing a higher reading.

Another important diagnostic laboratory test is C-reactive protein (CRP). CRP is a protein found in the blood that is produced by the liver and fat cells in response to the inflammatory process. In the absence of liver failure, a rise in CRP levels indicates an inflammatory process somewhere in the body. CRP can also be used to evaluate the effectiveness of treatment for inflammation. Research also indicates that the CRP can be used to assess risk for cardiac disease, as it elevates in response to arterial damage.

Other laboratory tests for inflammation are ordered based on the cause, location, and type of inflammation suspected. A WBC count with differential may be ordered to determine the presence of an infection (**Table 10–2 ●**); serum protein electrophoresis may reveal increased gamma globulin and decreased albumin, indicating systemic lupus erythematosus; and routine chemistry panels may reveal kidney involvement, abnormal liver function, or increased muscle enzymes if the muscle is involved.

TABLE 10–2 The White Blood Cell Count and Differential

Children < 11 Years

Normal ranges vary depending on the age of the child. Nurses should consult the diagnostic values provided by their agency or a current, reliable reference such as the Mayo Medical Laboratory's guide, available at http://a1.mayomedicallaboratories.com/webjc/attachments/110/30a2131-complete-blood-count-normal-pediatric-values.pdf.

Adult and Child > 11 Years

CELL TYPE AND NORMAL VALUE	INCREASED	DECREASED
Total white blood cells (WBCs): 4,000–10,000 ADULT: 4,500–10,000/mm^3	*Leukocytosis:* infection or inflammation, leukemia, trauma or stress	*Leukopenia:* bone marrow depression, viral infections, immunosuppression, autoimmune disease, dietary deficiency
Neutrophils (segs, PMNs, or polys): ADULT: 50%–70%	*Neutrophilia:* acute infection or stress response, myelocytic leukemia, inflammatory or metabolic disorders, tissue necrosis	*Neutropenia:* bone marrow depression, viral infection, Addison disease
Eosinophils (eos): 1%–3%	*Eosinophilia:* parasitic infections, allergic reactions, autoimmune disorders	*Eosinopenia:* stress, certain drugs
Basophils (basos): 0.4%–1%	*Basophilia:* hypersensitivity responses, leukemia, splenectomy, hypothyroidism	*Basopenia:* Because normal levels are low, decreased counts can only be detected by absolute counts. Decreased basophils may indicate allergic reaction or acute infection.
Monocytes (monos): 4%–6%	*Monocytosis:* chronic inflammatory disorders, infections, leukemia, Hodgkin disease	*Monocytopenia:* corticosteroid therapy
Lymphocytes (lymphs): 25%–35%	*Lymphocytosis:* infections, viral infections, lymphocytic leukemia	*Lymphocytopenia:* bone marrow depression, immunodeficiency, Hodgkin disease

Source: Data from VanLeeuwen, A. M., Poelhuis-Leth, D. J., & Bladh, M. L. (2013). *Laboratory diagnostic tests with nursing implications* (5th ed.). Philadelphia, PA: F. A. Davis; Kee, J. L. (2014). *Laboratory and diagnostic tests with nursing implications* (9th ed.). Upper Saddle River, NJ: Prentice Hall.

CASE STUDY \\ PART 2

After experiencing a flare-up of his symptoms, Mr. Blake returns to see his gastroenterologist. Mr. Blake informs you he is averaging several bloody bowel movements daily and complains of abdominal pain. His complaints include severe fatigue and weight loss of 8 pounds. Mr. Blake shows you the large oozing lesions on his lower legs, which were preceded by bruising. He is frustrated by his disease and the negative impact it is having on his quality of life at home and at work. Mr. Blake is fearful his uncontrolled symptoms will interfere with his receiving a promotion at work. Laboratory diagnostic test results include HCT = 29%; K$^+$ = 3.2 mEq/L (range = 3.5–5.3 mEq/L); and albumin 2.8 g/dL (range = 3.5–5.0 dg/L). Vital signs: temperature 100.1°F oral; pulse 95 bpm; respirations 18/min; and BP 132/82 mmHg. Mr. Blake has tried prednisone at home to try to regain remission, but the use of the oral corticosteroid has not helped. The gastroenterologist orders cephalexin for two months for the erythema nodosum. Mr. Blake is admitted to the hospital to receive IV methylprednisolone therapy. After 7 days only partial remission is achieved. Azathioprine is ordered, and remission of symptoms is achieved. Mr. Blake's drug regimen is now mesalamine rectally and oral with azathioprine.

Clinical Reasoning Questions Level I

1. What is the most likely cause of Mr. Blake's low potassium level?
2. What is the goal of adding azathioprine to Mr. Blake's drug regimen?
3. What are other potential sites of extraintestinal manifestations of ulcerative colitis?

Clinical Reasoning Questions Level II

4. What adverse effects associated with azathioprine should you discuss with Mr. Blake?
5. Describe three nursing interventions to address Mr. Blake's psychosocial considerations.

▶ INTERVENTIONS AND THERAPIES

Management of inflammation due to injury generally aims to reduce mobility of the involved area, elevation to reduce edema, antipyretics if fever is involved, and anti-inflammatory medications. Other causes of inflammation necessitate other, more specific treatments. For example, surgery is indicated in most cases of appendicitis and gallbladder disease, antibiotics may be required to treat inflammation caused by infection, and steroids may be indicated for severe systemic inflammation. Review dietary intake with clients to be sure they are receiving adequate nutrients to support healing, including adequate protein, carbohydrates, and vitamins. Vitamins important in cellular repair include vitamin C.

Independent

Nurses working with clients experiencing inflammation should be sure to emphasize the importance of preventing further injury, taking medications as prescribed to treat or prevent illness, and maintaining adequate intake of liquids and nutrients. Family teaching may be necessary if the client needs assistance with changing dressings, preventing exposure of the inflamed area to water while bathing, or any other aspects of daily living until healing occurs. Additional client teaching during the reparative phase may be necessary to ensure that the client does not resume activity too quickly and continues treatment until healing is complete and the client is released by the physician. Other independent interventions include those related to alleviating discomfort and reducing inflammation (e.g., positioning, application of heat or ice) and promoting coping during healing and recovery (acute) or exacerbations (for those with chronic inflammatory conditions).

Collaborative

A chronic inflammatory state is often associated with aging and obesity. These clients may benefit from a balanced diet and exercise, which may require collaboration with a nutritionist and physical therapist. A nutritionist can advise the client on consuming an anti-inflammatory diet that contains omega-3 fatty acids, antioxidant vitamins, and probiotics (Calder et al., 2009), while decreasing consumption of proinflammatory foods that contain saturated fats, cholesterol, and a high glycemic index. A physical therapist can help a client build muscle strength and increase overall physical health by encouraging exercise and physical activity (Addison et al., 2012). Physical therapy can also help clients regain the use of limbs that have been underused because of loss of function related to inflammation.

SURGERY Treatment for many inflammatory conditions involves collaboration with surgeons. For example, clients with appendicitis often require surgical removal of the appendix. Clients with ulcerative colitis may require surgery to remove the colon and rectum. Clients with gallbladder inflammation caused by recurrent gallstones or other conditions may undergo a cholecystectomy. Clients with severe infection and inflammation of extremities may require amputation of the damaged part to avoid life-threatening sepsis. When a client's condition is treated with surgery, the nurse is responsible for pre- and postoperative care and client teaching.

PHARMACOLOGIC THERAPY Pharmacologic therapies are aimed at reducing the inflammatory response and reducing pain associated with the symptoms of inflammation. Common medications include nonsteroidal anti-inflammatory drugs (NSAIDs), which have fewer adverse effects than the more powerful anti-inflammatory corticosteroids. Corticosteroids are normally administered when inflammation is more severe or is life threatening. NSAIDs, in addition to their anti-inflammatory actions, are also analgesics and antipyretics that help not only to reduce inflammation but also to minimize its effects. See the Medications feature for a list of medications used to treat inflammation.

Medications **Inflammatory Diseases**

CLASSIFICATION AND DRUG EXAMPLES	MECHANISM OF ACTION	NURSING CONSIDERATIONS
Nonsteroidal Anti-Inflammatory Drugs *Drug examples:* aspirin, celecoxib, ibuprofen, indomethacin, naproxen	Analgesic, antipyretic, and anti-inflammatory properties act by inhibiting the synthesis of prostaglandin precursors. NSAIDs block inflammation by reversibly inhibiting cyclooxygenase (COX-1 and COX-2), the key enzyme in the biosynthesis of prostaglandins. Also used for colorectal polyps; ankylosing spondylitis; vascular headache; and Paget disease.	■ Administer with food or milk. ■ Pregnancy category C. ■ Contraindicated in clients: a. with peptic ulcer disease b. taking anticoagulants ■ May interact with certain diuretics, causing decreased effectiveness of NSAID. ■ May increase clotting time. ■ Use cautiously in the elderly due to their reduced kidney and liver function.
Glucocorticosteroids *Drug examples:* betamethasone, dexamethasone, hydrocortisone, methylprednisolone, prednisone	Potent anti-inflammatory and immunosuppressant properties. Mimic natural hormones secreted by adrenal cortex; affect almost all body systems. Short- and long-term use indications. Also used for antiemetic in chemotherapy regimens; lupus nephritis; and multiple sclerosis.	■ Contraindicated in clients: a. with a systemic infection (will reduce immune response) b. with systemic fungal infections c. when administered with live virus vaccines ■ Do not discontinue abruptly. ■ Pregnancy category C. ■ If administered IM, give deep IM to avoid possible atrophy or abscess. Avoid deltoid muscle. ■ Monitor blood glucose levels; changes in mood; and signs of Cushing syndrome if used long term. ■ Use with caution in clients with: peptic ulcers; renal disease; hypertension; varicella exposure; or osteoporosis.
Opioid Analgesics *Drug examples:* hydromorphone, fentanyl, morphine, oxycodone	Potent analgesics. Block receptors in brain to achieve analgesia.	■ Take with food if GI upset occurs. ■ Pregnancy category C. ■ Reduce dose for renal impairment. ■ Monitor respiratory rate. See module on Pain for further information about analgesics.
Natural Therapies *Drug examples:* Fish oil, omega-3	Anti-inflammatory activity. Also used for elevated triglyceride levels.	■ Pregnancy category C. ■ Interact with anticoagulants, aspirin, and other NSAIDs. ■ Adverse side effects include potential for bruising and nosebleeds.

Source: Data from Wilson, B. A., Shannon, M. T., & Shields, K. M. (2013). *Pearson: Nurse's drug guide, 2013* (2nd ed.). Upper Saddle River, NJ: Pearson Education; *Drug information handbook: A comprehensive resource for all clinicians and healthcare professionals* (22nd ed.). (2013). Hudson, OH: Lexi-Comp.

| REVIEW | **The Concept of Inflammation** |

RELATE Link the Concepts

Linking the concept of inflammation with the concept immunity:

1. Describe how inflammation affects the immune system.
2. What preventive measures would you recommend to reduce the risk of chronic inflammation?

Linking the concept of inflammation with the concept oxygenation:

3. How does the inflammatory response adversely affect a client's airway?
4. What type of medications would you anticipate administering to reduce inflammation and improve respiratory function?

READY Go to Companion Skills Manual

REFER Go to Pearson Student Nursing Resources
nursing.pearsonhighered.com

- Additional review materials
- Additional case study

REFLECT Case Study \\ Part 3

Review Parts 1 and 2 of the case study. Mr. Blake's condition worsens and he goes to the emergency room. As the triage nurse, you are admitting Mr. Blake. He reports that he is experiencing more than 10 bowel movements daily with continuous bleeding. His abdomen is distended, painful, and tender. Vital signs are temperature 101.1°F oral; pulse 110 bpm; respirations 22/min; and BP 120/60 mmHg. Lab results include HCT 28% and albumin 2.6 g/dL. You note that Mr. Blake is experiencing shortness of breath and his extremities are cool to the touch. Results of an abdominal x-ray indicate 7 cm dilation of his transverse colon. Mr. Blake is admitted with the diagnosis of fulminant UC with toxic megacolon and is scheduled for emergency surgery. Prior to surgery Mr. Blake receives a blood transfusion and IV fluids to replenish electrolytes. Mr. Blake undergoes an ileal pouch–anal anastomosis (IPAA) procedure and recovers without complications.

Clinical Reasoning Questions Level I

1. Which of Mr. Blake's signs and symptoms indicate he will most likely be hospitalized?
2. Why does Mr. Blake have low potassium and albumin levels?

Clinical Reasoning Questions Level II

3. Explain why surgery can potentially cure ulcerative colitis but can offer only symptomatic relief in Crohn disease.
4. What are potential complications from the IPAA surgical procedure?
5. What type and frequency of cancer screening are recommended for clients with ulcerative colitis?

EXEMPLAR 10.1 Appendicitis

EXEMPLAR KEY TERMS
Appendectomy, 646
Appendicitis, 644
Fecalith, 645
Perforation, 644
Peritonitis, 644

EXEMPLAR LEARNING OUTCOMES
After reading about this exemplar, you will be able to:

1. Describe the pathophysiology, etiology, clinical manifestations, and direct and indirect causes of appendicitis.
2. Identify risk factors and prevention methods associated with appendicitis.
3. Illustrate the nursing process in providing culturally competent care across the life span for individuals with appendicitis.
4. Formulate priority nursing diagnoses appropriate for an individual with appendicitis.
5. Summarize therapies used by interdisciplinary teams in the collaborative care of an individual with appendicitis.
6. Plan evidence-based care for an individual with appendicitis and his or her family in collaboration with other members of the healthcare team.
7. Evaluate expected outcomes for an individual with appendicitis.

▶ OVERVIEW

Appendicitis, inflammation of the vermiform appendix, is a common cause of acute abdominal pain. In many cases, appendicitis treatment involves emergency abdominal surgery. Appendicitis affects over 5% of the population; it can occur at any age, but it is more common in adolescents and young adults (Ansari, 2012).

▶ PATHOPHYSIOLOGY AND ETIOLOGY

The appendix is a tubelike pouch attached to the cecum just below the ileocecal valve. It is usually located in the right iliac region, in an area designated as McBurney point (**Figure 10–2A** ●). The function of the appendix is not fully understood, although it is regularly filled with and emptied of digested food.

Obstruction of the proximal lumen of the appendix is apparent in most acutely inflamed appendices. Following obstruction, the appendix becomes distended with fluid secreted by its mucosa. Pressure within the lumen of the appendix increases, impairs its blood supply, and leads to inflammation, edema, ulceration, and infection. The purulent exudate formed causes further distention of the appendix. If treatment is not initiated, tissue necrosis and gangrene result within 24–36 hours, leading to **perforation** (rupture). Perforation allows the contents of the gastrointestinal (GI) tract to flow into the peritoneal space of the abdomen, resulting in **peritonitis**, inflammation and bacterial infection of the entire abdominal area. Appendicitis is classified as simple, gangrenous, or perforated, depending on the stage in the process. In simple appendicitis, the appendix is inflamed but intact. In gangrenous appendicitis, areas of tissue necrosis and

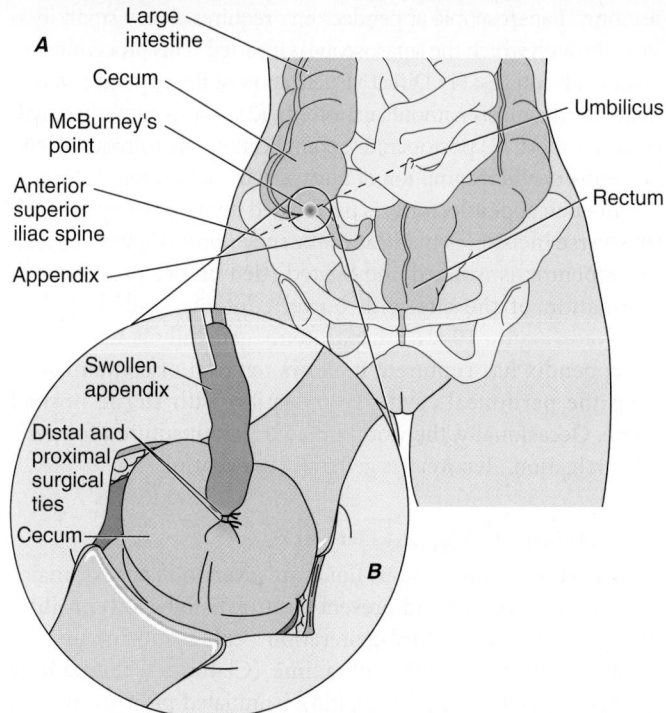

Figure 10–2 ● *A* McBurney point, located midway between the umbilicus and the anterior iliac crest in the right lower quadrant. It is the usual side for localized pain and rebound tenderness due to appendicitis. *B* In an appendectomy, the appendix and cecum are brought through the incision to the surface of the abdomen. The base of the appendix is clamped and ligated; the appendix is then removed.

microscopic perforations are present in the appendix. A perforated appendix shows evidence of gross perforation and contamination of the peritoneal cavity.

Etiology

Appendicitis almost always results from an obstruction in the appendiceal lumen. The obstruction is often caused by a hard mass of feces (**fecalith**). Other obstructive causes include a calculus or stone, parasites (e.g., pinworms), edema of lymphoid tissue, a tumor, or a foreign body. Continued secretion of mucus following acute obstruction of the lumen increases pressure, causing ischemia, inflammation, cellular death, and ulceration.

Risk Factors

Adolescent males are at greatest risk, although fecaliths can occur in both genders at any age. Individuals whose diet is low in fiber or high in carbohydrates are at greater risk for developing fecaliths. GI infections also promote appendicitis.

Prevention

Appendicitis cannot be prevented; however, certain dietary habits may reduce the risk of developing this condition. Eating foods that contain high fiber content, such as fresh fruits and vegetables, decreases the incidence of appendicitis (Cleveland Clinic, 2011).

▶ CLINICAL MANIFESTATIONS

The initial characteristic manifestation of acute appendicitis is continuous, mild, generalized or upper abdominal pain. Over the next 4 hours, the pain intensifies and localizes in the right lower quadrant of the abdomen. Pain associated with appendicitis is aggravated by moving, walking, or coughing. On palpation, localized and rebound tenderness are noted at McBurney point. Rebound tenderness is demonstrated by relief of pain with direct palpation of McBurney point, followed by pain on release of pressure. Extension or internal rotation of the right hip increases the pain. In addition to pain, a low-grade fever, anorexia, nausea, and vomiting are often present.

Because of less acute pain and local tenderness in older adults, the diagnosis is delayed. The course of acute appendicitis is more virulent in older adults, so complications can develop sooner and result in increased mortality (NIAMS, 2013). Pregnant women may develop right lower quadrant, periumbilical, or right subcostal (under the rib cage) pain due to possible displacement of the appendix by the distended uterus. In adolescent and young adult females, symptoms must be differentiated from those associated with ovulation (mittelschmerz), ruptured ectopic pregnancy, and pelvic inflammatory disease.

Possible complications related to acute appendicitis are perforation, peritonitis, and abscess (accumulation of pus). Perforation is manifested by increased pain and a high fever. It can lead to a small, localized abscess; local peritonitis; or significant generalized peritonitis.

A less common disorder is chronic appendicitis, characterized by chronic abdominal pain and recurrent acute attacks at intervals of several months or more. Other conditions, such as inflammatory bowel disease (IBD) and renal disorders, often cause manifestations attributed to chronic appendicitis.

Clinical Manifestations and Therapies **Appendicitis**

ETIOLOGY	CLINICAL MANIFESTATIONS	CLINICAL THERAPIES
Peritonitis resulting from appendix rupture with bowel contents leaking into the abdominal cavity	High fever, acute severe abdominal pain, abdominal distention; resultant death if not treated aggressively and rapidly	▪ Removal of the ruptured appendix ▪ Antibiotics ▪ Fluid resuscitation ▪ Supportive treatment to maintain vital signs
Chronic appendicitis	Chronic recurrent abdominal pain over several months	▪ Appendectomy ▪ Pain management

646   Module 10   Inflammation

Lifespan and Cultural Considerations

It is uncommon for children under the age of 4 to develop appendicitis. However, appendicitis in young children often progresses to rupture because they cannot accurately tell their parents how they feel and where it hurts (Boston Children's Hospital, n.d.). Common manifestations in infants include listlessness, inconsolability, vomiting, and a distended abdomen. Because appendicitis is rare in infants, a differential diagnosis of appendicitis is low on the physician's priority list unless the physician is consistently suspicious of appendicitis. This low diagnostic priority leads to a delay in diagnosis and an increase in rupture, complications, and death in the infant population (Minkes, 2013).

Cultural factors also play a role in the progression of appendicitis in children. A recent study found that the perforation rate for White children was 26.7%; Black children, 35.5%; and Latino children, 36.5%. Only a small percentage of this difference was related to insurance status, income level, and age. The differences between appendicitis perforation rates that was not explained by measurable factors was two thirds for Black children and one third for Latino children compared to White children (Livingston & Fairlie, 2012).

On the other end of the age spectrum, less than 30% of older adults who have appendicitis present with classic symptoms. Almost half of older clients are afebrile, half demonstrate no rebound or involuntary guarding, and one fourth have no lower right quadrant tenderness or pain (Tazkarji, 2008). Instead, older adults are likely to present with confusion (Humes & Simpson, 2011). Approximately 25%–30% of older adults with appendicitis do not seek medical care until 3 or more days after the onset of symptoms.

▶ COLLABORATION

The acutely inflamed appendix can perforate within 24 hours, so rapid diagnosis and treatment are important. Because of this urgency and the low incidence of surgical complications, diagnostic testing and preoperative treatment are limited. The client is admitted to the hospital, and intravenous fluids are initiated. Oral food and fluids are withheld until a diagnosis is confirmed.

Diagnostic Tests

Diagnostic and laboratory tests help confirm the diagnosis and rule out other possible causes for the manifestations. Abdominal ultrasound is the most effective test for diagnosing acute appendicitis. Ultrasound examination has reduced the incidence of exploratory surgery. It is particularly useful with clients who have atypical symptoms (e.g., older adults). Other diagnostic tests used to diagnose appendicitis and rule out other possible conditions include abdominal x-rays, intravenous pyelogram, urinalysis, and pelvic examination. In addition, a white blood cell (WBC) count with differential is obtained. With appendicitis, the total white count is elevated, with an increased number of immature WBCs (bands).

Surgery

The treatment of choice for acute appendicitis is an **appendectomy**, surgical removal of the appendix. Either a laparoscopic approach (insertion of an endoscope to view abdominal contents) or laparotomy (surgical opening of the abdomen) is used for appendectomy. Laparoscopic appendectomy requires a very small incision, through which the laparoscope is inserted. This procedure has several advantages: (1) Direct visualization of the appendix allows definitive diagnosis without laparotomy, (2) postoperative hospitalization is short, (3) postoperative complications are infrequent, and (4) recovery and resumption of normal activities are rapid.

An open appendectomy is performed by laparotomy. A small transverse incision is made at McBurney point (Figure 10–2A); the appendix is isolated and ligated (tied off) to prevent contamination of the site with bowel contents, and it is then removed (Figure 10–2B). Laparotomy generally is used when the appendix has ruptured. It allows removal of contaminants from the peritoneal cavity by irrigation with sterile normal saline. Occasionally, the wound may be left unsutured for periodic irrigation. Recovery is generally uneventful.

Pharmacologic Therapy

Prior to surgery, intravenous fluids are given to restore or maintain vascular volume and prevent electrolyte imbalance. Antibiotic therapy with a third-generation cephalosporin, such as cefoperazone (Cefobid), cefotaxime (Claforan), ceftazidime (Fortaz), or ceftriaxone (Rocephin), is initiated prior to surgery. Third generation cephalosporins are effective against many gram-negative bacteria. Antibiotic administration is repeated during surgery and continued for at least 48 hours postoperatively. The sudden disappearance of pain is an indication that the appendix has ruptured, so administration of strong analgesics is withheld preoperatively during assessment for this indicator. Once the diagnosis is established, an appendectomy is performed and analgesics are administered as ordered to maintain comfort.

■ NURSING PROCESS

Nursing management of the client with appendicitis includes collaborative assessment, preoperative and postoperative care, and prevention of complications. Refer to the module on Perioperative Care for more information on taking care of clients having surgery for appendicitis.

Assessment

Because appendicitis can rapidly progress from inflammation to perforation, prompt assessment is vital. Obtain the following assessment data:

- **Health history.** Current manifestations, including onset, duration, progression, and aggravating or relieving factors; most recent food or fluid intake; known medication or other allergies; current medications; and history of chronic diseases
- **Physical examination.** Vital signs, including temperature; apparent general health; abdominal shape and contour; bowel sounds, tenderness to light palpation.

SAFETY ALERT Keep the client with suspected appendicitis NPO. Do not administer laxatives or enemas, which may cause perforation of the appendix. Do not apply heat to the abdomen, as this may increase circulation to the appendix and also cause perforation.

Diagnosis

The following nursing diagnoses may apply to the client with appendicitis:

- *Risk for Impaired Gas Exchange*
- *Risk for Deficient Fluid Volume*
- *Risk for Infection*
- *Acute Pain*
- *Anxiety*
- *Fear*

(NANDA-I © 2012)

Planning

The plan of care developed in collaboration with the client and family may include the following:

- The client will articulate any concerns about surgery prior to the event.
- The client will articulate an understanding of the procedure, the reasons for it, and any preoperative instructions prior to arrival for surgery.
- The client will verbalize relief from pain following administration of pain management.
- The client will receive appropriate postoperative wound care.
- The client will verbalize instructions for self-care prior to being discharged.

Implementation

Nursing management focuses on promoting comfort, maintaining hydration, providing emotional support, supporting respiratory function, providing care of the surgical site, and monitoring for symptoms of infection.

Promote Effective Respiratory Gas Exchange

General anesthesia during surgery compromises respiratory function.

- It is important for the client to turn, cough, and breathe deeply to prevent atelectasis.
- While the client with uncomplicated appendicitis is usually willing to get out of bed and walk soon after surgery, the client with a ruptured appendix is generally hesitant to move and may need to be repositioned by family or staff. The client must get out of bed as soon as his or her condition allows and walk two or three times a day to decrease recovery time and the risk of pulmonary complications.
- The nurse should encourage the client to splint the incision area with a pillow during coughing to decrease pain.
- Incentive spirometry is frequently ordered for the client. Young children may be resistant to (or too young to understand) this procedure. An effective alternative approach is to give the child bubbles to blow. Giving praise and rewards such as stickers each time the child completes the task is likely to increase compliance with the procedure and decrease the likelihood of complications.

Promote Fluid Volume Balance

- Monitor and continue the intravenous infusion that was initiated preoperatively until bowel function returns after surgery.
- Once bowel sounds return and after the nasogastric tube has been removed (if needed), offer water in small amounts, then other clear fluids.
- After introducing oral fluids, closely monitor the client for nausea.
- Monitor intake and output. If the client had a ruptured appendix and has a nasogastric tube after surgery, accurate assessment of the amount of output from the nasogastric tube is essential. The client may have orders for the amount of fluid lost from the nasogastric tube to be replaced with additional intravenous fluids. The nurse should be alert to an increase in nasogastric drainage postoperatively, as this drainage should decrease over time. Promptly report any concerns to the physician.

Prevent Infection

Preventing complications during the preoperative and postoperative periods is a primary nursing care goal. Perforation and peritonitis are the most likely preoperative complications; postoperative complications include wound infection, abscess, and possible peritonitis.

- Monitor vital signs, including temperature. Tachycardia and rapid, shallow respirations may indicate perforation of the appendix with resulting peritonitis. Fever may develop as well; a decrease in blood pressure may indicate the presence of sepsis.
- Maintain intravenous infusion until oral intake is adequate. Intravenous fluids are given to maintain vascular volume and to provide a route for antibiotic administration.
- Assess wound, abdominal girth, and postoperative pain. Swelling of the wound, increased abdominal girth, or an increase in pain may indicate infection or peritonitis.

Provide Effective Pain Management

The client with appendicitis experiences pain before and after surgery. Analgesia is limited until the diagnosis is established. Postoperative pain is controlled by opioid or nonopioid analgesics.

- Assess pain, including its etiology, location, severity, and duration. Report any unexpected changes in the nature of pain. Both preoperatively and postoperatively, the client's pain provides important clues about the diagnosis and possible complications, such as rupture of the appendix or peritonitis.
- Administer analgesics as ordered. Preoperatively, pain medication can be given after a diagnosis is established. Postoperatively, provide analgesics to maintain comfort and enhance mobility.
- Assess effectiveness of medication 30 minutes after administration. Report unrelieved pain. Pain unrelieved by the prescribed analgesic may indicate a complication or the need for further assessment. For example, continued abdominal discomfort and distention may indicate excess intestinal gas that may be better relieved by ambulation.

SAFETY ALERT
Be alert to the child who does not complain of postoperative pain following surgery for a ruptured appendix. The child who does not verbally complain of pain may cry when approached and resist being moved or refuse to move in the bed. Proper pain management will facilitate the child's recovery and help prevent respiratory complications related to immobilization.

Promote Psychosocial Well-Being

For many clients, hospitalization for appendicitis may be their first and their first experience with healthcare personnel beyond their usual provider. Anxiety may be heightened by the necessarily rapid pace physical examination, diagnostic testing, and preoperative preparation. Preoperative education helps reduce anxiety. In addition, encourage and answer any questions the client or family may have, and provide emotional support as necessary.

Provide Effective Client Teaching

The client whose appendix did not rupture is discharged once bowel function returns and he or she has a bowel movement.

- Give instructions on slowly reestablishing a nutritious diet as tolerated.
- Teach client or parents to recognize the signs and symptoms of infection and to seek early treatment.

If the appendix was ruptured, the client will be hospitalized for several days for intravenous antibiotics. If the wound was left open, it is generally closed after a few days and prior to discharge. Prepare the client and family for this procedure. Sedation or anesthesia is used to decrease the client's anxiety and discomfort. Prior to discharge, the nurse should provide client teaching and ensure that the client (or parents, if the client is a child) can verbalize the following:

- How to care for the wound
- The signs and symptoms of wound infection and when to call the physician
- Method and frequency of taking temperature

Client Teaching
The Client With Appendicitis

Preoperative teaching may be limited by pain and the emergent nature of surgery. Explain why food and fluids are not permitted during this time. If time allows, teach postoperative turning, coughing, deep breathing, and pain management.

The client with uncomplicated appendectomy often is discharged the day of surgery or the day following surgery. Postoperative teaching includes the following:

- Wound or incision care, including hand washing and dressing change procedures as indicated
- Instructions to report to the physician fever, increased abdominal pain, swelling, redness, drainage, bleeding, or warmth of the operative site
- Activity limitations (e.g., lifting, driving), if any
- Return to work if appropriate.

- Activity limitations and restrictions, including when to return to work or school
- Pain management, including medication instructions and possible side effects.

Evaluation

Expected outcomes of nursing care include the following:

- The client demonstrates effective respiratory gas exchange, as evidenced by normal breath sounds, oxygen saturation of greater than or equal to 95%, and no indications of atelectasis.
- The client demonstrates no signs or symptoms of secondary infection.
- Adequate hydration is achieved and maintained, as evidenced by balanced oral intake and output and by no signs or symptoms of fluid overload or dehydration.
- Using a predetermined pain rating scale, the client rates pain at a level that is tolerable.
- The client verbalizes decreased fear and anxiety associated with the hospitalization and procedures.

NURSING CARE PLAN A Client With Acute Appendicitis

Jamie Lynn is a 19-year-old college student majoring in physical therapy. Ms. Lynn arrives at the emergency department at 1 a.m. complaining of general lower abdominal pain that started the previous evening. By midnight, the pain was localized over the right lower quadrant. She also reports nausea and vomiting.

ASSESSMENT	DIAGNOSES	PLANNING
Sue Grady, RN, completes the admission assessment in the emergency department. Ms. Lynn is complaining of nausea and severe abdominal pain, stating, "Walking makes my stomach hurt worse." Physical assessment findings include temperature (oral) 37.8°C (100.2°F), pulse 84 bpm, respirations 16/min, BP 110/70 mmHg; skin warm to touch; abdomen flat and guarded, with marked tenderness in right lower quadrant. Ms. Lynn's complete blood count (CBC) shows WBCs 14,000/mm³; neutrophils 81.1%; lymphocytes 12.5%. The diagnosis is acute appendicitis, and Ms. Lynn is transferred to surgery for a laparoscopic appendectomy.	■ *Risk for Infection* ■ *Impaired Skin Integrity* related to surgical incision ■ *Acute Pain* related to surgical intervention ■ *Anxiety* related to situational crisis (NANDA-I © 2012)	■ Incision will heal without infection or complications. ■ Client will verbalize adequate pain relief. ■ Client will verbalize decreased anxiety. ■ Client will return to preoperative activities.

NURSING CARE PLAN (continued)

IMPLEMENTATION

- Provide analgesics as needed.
- Teach pain management.
- Teach abdominal splinting as needed during coughing, turning, or ambulating.

- Teach home care of incision.
- Discuss activity limitations as ordered.
- Instruct to report fever or warmth, redness, or drainage from the incision.

EVALUATION

On discharge the following evening, Ms. Lynn is fully ambulatory. Her appetite has returned, and she is tolerating food and fluids well. Her temperature is normal. The nurse provides Ms. Lynn with written and verbal information on postoperative care following an appendectomy.

CRITICAL THINKING

1. What is the pathophysiological basis for Ms. Lynn's elevated WBCs?
2. How would Ms. Lynn's postoperative care and teaching differ if she had undergone a laparotomy instead of a laparoscopic appendectomy?
3. Outline a teaching plan to give to clients for home care following an appendectomy.
4. Develop a care plan for Ms. Lynn for the nursing diagnosis Anxiety related to a situational crisis.

REVIEW Appendicitis

RELATE Link the Concepts and Exemplars

Linking the exemplar of appendicitis with the concept of infection:

1. How would you change or anticipate changing your nursing care for a client whose appendix is believed to have ruptured preoperatively?

2. How would the pathophysiology of a client with a ruptured appendix differ from a client whose appendix is removed without rupturing?

Linking the exemplar of appendicitis with the concept of mobility:

3. When caring for a client who required a laparoscopic appendectomy yesterday, what teaching would you provide to stress the importance of mobility?

4. The 14-year-old client who is 1 day postoperative following an appendectomy is reluctant to ambulate for fear of pain. What strategies would you use to encourage ambulation?

READY Go to Companion Skills Manual

REFER Go to Pearson Nursing Student Resources
nursing.pearsonhighered.com

- Additional review material

REFLECT Case Study

Mike Mortimer is a healthy, active 9-year-old boy who lives with his father. His mother died 6 months ago from metastatic breast cancer. At first, everyone at school was really nice to him, but lately they've been teasing him about being a motherless orphan. He's started to wish he didn't have to go to school. This morning he told his dad that he had a stomachache and asked to stay home, but his dad said he didn't have a fever so he needed to get dressed and get going. The school nurse called his father at 11:30 to report that Mike had a fever and was feeling sick to his stomach. The nurse encouraged his dad to take him to the doctor.

When Mike arrives at the doctor's office, he reports severe pain in his lower right quadrant, nausea, and one emesis at school. Vital signs include the following: temperature 100.2°F oral, pulse 96 bpm, respirations 12/min, BP 110/74 mmHg. Rebound tenderness is noted in McBurney point. CBC reveals a WBC count of $11,000/mm^3$, and an ultrasound reveals an inflamed appendix. He is scheduled for surgery and admitted to the local acute care facility.

1. As you admit Mike to the pediatric unit, his father asks you to please give him something for pain. How do you respond?

2. Mike is scheduled to leave the unit for the operating room in 1 hour. What information will you gather to prepare him for surgery?

3. When Mike returns from the operating room, what priority assessments will you perform?

4. What teaching will you provide Mike and his dad prior to discharge?

EXEMPLAR 10.2 Gallbladder Disease

EXEMPLAR KEY TERMS
Biliary colic, 650
Cholangitis, 650
Cholecystitis, 650
Cholelithiasis, 650
Empyema, 650
Gallstone ileus, 650
Laparoscopic cholecystectomy, 652

EXEMPLAR LEARNING OUTCOMES
After reading about this exemplar, you will be able to:

1. Describe the pathophysiology, etiology, clinical manifestations, and direct and indirect causes of gallbladder disease.

2. Identify risk factors and prevention methods associated with gallbladder disease.

3. Illustrate the nursing process in providing culturally competent care across the life span for individuals with gallbladder disease.

4. Formulate priority nursing diagnoses appropriate for an individual with gallbladder disease.

5. Summarize therapies used by interdisciplinary teams in the collaborative care of an individual with gallbladder disease.

6. Plan evidence-based care for an individual with gallbladder disease and his or her family in collaboration with other members of the healthcare team.

7. Evaluate expected outcomes for an individual with gallbladder disease.

▶ OVERVIEW

Altered bile flow through the hepatic, cystic, or common bile duct is a common problem. It often leads to inflammation and other complications. Gallstones are the most common cause of obstructed flow. Tumors and abscesses may also obstruct bile flow.

Cholelithiasis is the formation of stones (*calculi* or *gallstones*) in the gallbladder or biliary duct system. Cholelithiasis is a common problem in the United States, affecting 10%–15% of the U.S. population; approximately 1 million new cases are diagnosed each year (AGA, 2010).

▶ PATHOPHYSIOLOGY AND ETIOLOGY

Most gallstones are formed in the gallbladder. Their migration into the ducts (**Figure 10–3** ●) leads to **cholangitis** (duct inflammation). Although some individuals with cholelithiasis are asymptomatic, many develop manifestations. Early manifestations of gallstones may be vague: epigastric fullness or mild gastric distress after eating a large or fatty meal. Stones that obstruct the cystic duct or common bile duct lead to distention and increased pressure behind the stone, causing **biliary colic**, a severe, steady pain in the epigastric region or right upper quadrant (RUQ) of the abdomen. The pain may radiate to the back, right scapula, or shoulder. The pain often begins suddenly following a meal and may last as long as 5 hours. It is often accompanied by nausea and vomiting.

Obstruction of the common bile duct may cause bile reflux into the liver, leading to jaundice, pain, and possible liver damage. If the common duct is obstructed, pancreatic enzymes are unable to enter the small intestine, and pancreatitis becomes a potential complication.

Cholecystitis is inflammation of the gallbladder. *Acute cholecystitis* usually follows obstruction of the cystic duct by a stone. The resulting increased pressure in the gallbladder leads to ischemia of the gallbladder wall and mucosa. Chemical and

bacterial inflammation often follows. The ischemia can lead to necrosis and perforation of the gallbladder wall.

Acute cholecystitis usually begins with an attack of biliary colic. The pain involves the entire RUQ and may radiate to the back, right scapula, or shoulder. Movement or deep breathing may aggravate the pain. The pain usually lasts longer than biliary colic, continuing for 12–18 hours. Anorexia, nausea, and vomiting are common. Fever is often present and may be accompanied by chills. The RUQ is tender to palpation.

Chronic cholecystitis may result from repeated bouts of acute cholecystitis or from persistent irritation of the gallbladder wall by stones. Bacteria may be present in the bile as well. Chronic cholecystitis often is asymptomatic.

Complications of cholecystitis include **empyema**, a collection of infected fluid in the gallbladder; gangrene and perforation with resulting peritonitis or abscess formation; formation of a fistula into an adjacent organ (such as the duodenum, colon, or stomach); and obstruction of the small intestine by a large gallstone (**gallstone ileus**).

Etiology

Gallstones form when several factors interact: abnormal bile composition, biliary stasis, and inflammation of the gallbladder. Most gallstones (80%) consist primarily of cholesterol; the rest contain a mixture of bile components. Excess cholesterol in bile is associated with obesity, a high-calorie and high-cholesterol diet, and drugs that lower serum cholesterol levels. Bile that is supersaturated with cholesterol can precipitate out to form stones. Biliary stasis, or slowed emptying of the gallbladder, contributes to cholelithiasis. Stones do not form when the gallbladder empties completely in response to hormonal stimulation. Slowed or incomplete emptying allows cholesterol to concentrate and increases the risk of stone formation. Finally, inflammation of the gallbladder allows excess water and bile salt reabsorption, increasing the risk for lithiasis.

Risk Factors

The incidence of gallstones varies among individuals of different ethnic backgrounds and other characteristics: Native Americans

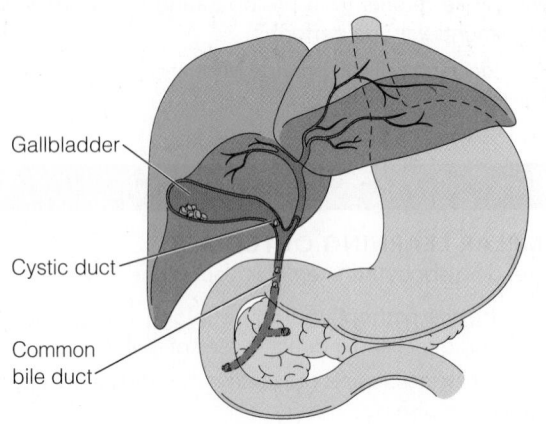

Figure 10–3 ● Common locations of gallstones.

Focus on Diversity and Culture   Gallstones

Native Americans in both the Northern and Southern Hemispheres—and those of the Pima tribe of Arizona in particular—have a higher incidence of gallstones than do Caucasians of American or European heritage. This higher incidence is thought to result from a genetic predisposition to secrete high levels of cholesterol in the bile. Mexican American men and women of all ages also have elevated rates of gallstones (NIDDK, 2012a).

TABLE 10–3 Manifestations and Complications of Cholelithiasis and Cholecystitis

MANIFESTATIONS	CHOLELITHIASIS	CHOLECYSTITIS
Pain	<ul><li>Abrupt onset</li><li>Severe, steady</li><li>Localized to epigastrium and RUQ of abdomen</li><li>May radiate to back, right scapula, and shoulder</li><li>Lasts 30 minutes to 5 hours</li></ul>	<ul><li>Abrupt onset</li><li>Severe, steady</li><li>Generalized in RUQ of abdomen</li><li>May radiate to back, right scapula, and shoulder</li><li>Lasts 12–18 hours</li><li>Aggravated by movement, breathing</li></ul>
Associated symptoms	<ul><li>Nausea, vomiting</li></ul>	<ul><li>Anorexia, nausea, vomiting</li><li>RUQ tenderness and guarding</li><li>Chills and fever</li></ul>
Complications	<ul><li>Cholecystitis</li><li>Common bile duct obstruction with possible jaundice and liver damage</li><li>Common duct obstruction with pancreatitis</li></ul>	<ul><li>Gangrene and perforation with peritonitis</li><li>Chronic cholecystitis</li><li>Empyema</li><li>Fistula formation</li><li>Gallstone ileus</li></ul>

and Hispanics of Mexican origin are at greater risk for gallstones than other populations. Age, family history of gallstones, obesity, rapid weight loss, and being female are all risk factors. Other risk factors include biliary stasis (e.g., pregnancy, fasting, prolonged total parenteral nutrition) and certain diseases or conditions, such as cirrhosis, sickle cell disease, leukemia, hyperlipidemia, ileal disease or resection, and glucose intolerance.

Prevention

The modifiable risk factors that can be controlled or treated to reduce the occurrence of cholelithiasis include obesity, certain medications (estrogen and clofibrate), a high-fat diet, rapid weight loss, and dyslipidemia. Dyslipidemia is identified by a blood test that screens for increased total cholesterol, low-density lipids and triglycerides, or decreased high-density lipids. Risk factors that are nonmodifiable are age, gender, and ethnicity (Zagaria, 2010).

▶ CLINICAL MANIFESTATIONS

Table 10–3 ● compares the manifestations and complications of acute cholelithiasis with those of cholecystitis.

▶ COLLABORATION

Treatment of the client with cholelithiasis or cholecystitis depends on the acuity of the condition and the client's overall health status. When gallstones are present but asymptomatic and the client has a low risk for complications, conservative treatment is indicated. However, when the client experiences frequent symptoms, has acute cholecystitis, or has very large stones, the gallbladder and stones are usually surgically removed.

Diagnostic Tests

Diagnostic tests are ordered to identify the presence and location of stones, identify possible complications, and help differentiate gallbladder disease from other disorders.

- **Serum bilirubin** is measured. Elevated direct (conjugated) bilirubin may indicate obstructed bile flow in the biliary duct system (**Box 10–3** ●).

- **CBC** may indicate infection and inflammation if the WBC count is elevated.

- **Serum amylase and lipase** are measured to identify possible pancreatitis related to common duct obstruction.

- **Abdominal x-ray** (flat plate of the abdomen) may show gallstones that have a high calcium content.

- **Ultrasonography of the gallbladder** is a noninvasive exam that can accurately diagnose cholelithiasis. More accurate than a CT scan, it also can be used to assess emptying of the gallbladder.

- **Oral cholecystogram** is performed with a dye administered orally to assess the gallbladder's ability to concentrate and excrete bile.

- **Gallbladder scan,** such as cholescintigraphy, also known as a *hepatobiliary iminodiacetic acid (HIDA) scan,* uses an intravenous radioactive solution that is rapidly extracted from the blood and excreted into the biliary tree to allow diagnosis of cystic duct obstruction and acute or chronic cholecystitis.

Box 10–3   Sorting Out Total, Direct, and Indirect Bilirubin Levels

When serum bilirubin levels are drawn, the results usually are reported as total bilirubin, direct bilirubin, and indirect bilirubin levels. Most bilirubin is formed from hemoglobin as aging or abnormal red blood cells (RBCs) are removed from circulation and destroyed. Bilirubin is not water-soluble, so it must be bound to albumin before being transported to the liver. This albumin-bound bilirubin is called *indirect* or *unconjugated bilirubin.* Once in the liver, bilirubin is separated from albumin and conjugated to glucuronic acid. This water-soluble form of bilirubin is called *direct* or *conjugated bilirubin.* Conjugated bilirubin is then excreted in the bile.

- Total (serum) bilirubin, the total bilirubin in the blood, includes both indirect and direct forms. In adults, the normal total bilirubin is 0.1–1.2 mg/dL. Total bilirubin levels increase when more is being produced (e.g., by RBC hemolysis) or when its metabolism or excretion are impaired (e.g., by liver disease or biliary obstruction).
- The levels of direct (conjugated) bilirubin, normally 0.1–0.3 mg/dL in adults, rise when its excretion is impaired by obstruction in the liver (e.g., in cirrhosis, hepatitis, exposure to hepatotoxins) or in the biliary system.
- Indirect (unconjugated) bilirubin levels, normally <1.1 mg/dL in adults, rise in RBC hemolysis (e.g., sickle cell disease or transfusion reaction).

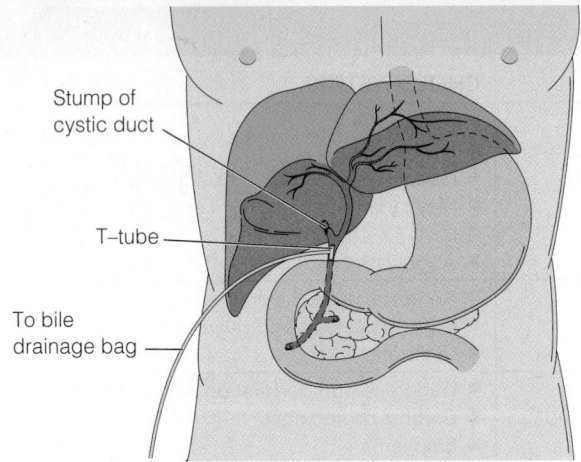

Stump of
cystic duct

T–tube

To bile
drainage bag

Figure 10–4 ● T-tube placement in the common bile duct. Bile fluid flows with gravity into a drainage collection device below the level of the common bile duct.

Surgery

Laparoscopic cholecystectomy (removal of the gallbladder) is the treatment of choice for symptomatic cholelithiasis or cholecystitis (see the Evidence-Based Practice feature). This minimally invasive procedure has a low risk of complications and generally requires a hospital stay of less than 24 hours. Not all clients are candidates for laparoscopic cholecystectomy, however, and there is a risk that a laparoscopic cholecystectomy may be converted to a *laparotomy* (surgical opening into the abdomen) during the procedure.

When stones are lodged in the ducts, a cholecystectomy with common bile duct exploration may be done. A T-tube (**Figure 10–4 ●**) is inserted to maintain patency of the duct and to promote bile passage while the edema decreases. Excess bile is collected in a drainage bag secured below the surgical site. If it is suspected that a stone has been retained following surgery, a postoperative cholangiogram via the T-tube or a direct visualization of the duct with an endoscope may be performed. See **Box 10–4 ●** for nursing care for a client with a T-tube.

Some clients who are poor surgical risks and for whom laparoscopic cholecystectomy is inappropriate may have a *cholecystostomy* to drain the gallbladder or a *choledochostomy* to remove stones and position a T-tube in the common bile duct.

In some cases, shock wave lithotripsy may be used with drug therapy to dissolve large gallstones. In *extracorporeal shock wave lithotripsy,* ultrasound is used to align the stones with the source of shock waves and the computerized lithotripter. Positioning is of prime importance throughout the procedure, which usually takes an hour. Mild sedation may be given during the procedure. Nursing care after the procedure includes monitoring for biliary colic, which can result when the gallbladder contracts to remove stone fragments; nausea; and transient hematuria. *Percutaneous cholecystostomy,* ultrasound-guided drainage of the gallbladder, may be done in high-risk clients to postpone or even eliminate the need for surgery.

Pharmacologic Therapy

Clients who refuse surgery or for whom surgery is inappropriate may be treated with a drug to dissolve the gallstones. Urso-

---

Box 10–4   Nursing Care of the Client With a T-Tube

- Ensure that the T-tube is properly connected to a sterile container; keep the tube below the level of the surgical wound. This position promotes the flow of bile and prevents backflow or seepage of caustic bile onto the skin. The tube itself decreases biliary tree pressure.
- Monitor drainage from the T-tube for color and consistency; record as output. Normally, the tube drains up to 500 mL in the first 24 hours after surgery; drainage decreases to less than 200 mL in 2–3 days and is minimal thereafter. Drainage may be blood-tinged initially, changing to green-brown. Report excessive drainage immediately. (After 48 hours, drainage greater than 500 mL is considered excessive.) Stones or edema and inflammation can obstruct ducts below the tube, requiring treatment.
- Place in Fowler position, which promotes gravity drainage of bile.
- Assess skin for bile leakage during dressing changes. Bile irritates the skin; it may be necessary to apply skin protection with karaya or another barrier product.
- Teach client how to manage the tube when turning, ambulating, and performing activities of daily living. Direct pulling or traction on the tube must be avoided.
- If indicated, teach client how to take care of the T-tube, clamp it, and recognize signs of infection. Clients may be discharged home with the tube in place. Reporting early signs of infection facilitates prompt treatment.

---

diol (Actigall) and chenodiol (Chenix) reduce the cholesterol content of gallstones and lead to their gradual dissolution. These drugs act by reducing cholesterol production in the liver, thus reducing the cholesterol content of bile. Consequently, these drugs are most effective in treating stones with high cholesterol content. They are less effective in treating radiopaque stones with high calcium salt content. Ursodiol is generally well tolerated but can cause diarrhea or constipation, whereas chenodiol has a high incidence of diarrhea at therapeutic doses and may require dose reduction. Chenodiol is also hepatotoxic, so periodic liver function studies are required during therapy. The primary disadvantages of pharmacologic treatment for gallstones are its cost, its long duration (up to 2 years), and the high incidence of recurrent stone formation when treatment is discontinued.

If infection is suspected, antibiotics may be ordered to cure the infection and reduce associated inflammation and edema. Clients with pruritus (itching) due to severe obstructive jaundice and an accumulation of bile salts on the skin may be given cholestyramine (Questran®). This drug binds with bile salts to promote their excretion in the feces. A narcotic analgesic such as morphine may be required for pain relief during an acute attack of cholecystitis.

Nonpharmacologic Therapy

When food intake is eliminated during an acute attack of cholecystitis, a nasogastric tube is inserted to relieve nausea and vomiting. Dietary fat intake may be limited, especially if the client is obese. If bile flow is obstructed, fat-soluble vitamins (A, D, E, and K) and bile salts may need to be administered.

Evidence-Based Practice Pain Management Following Laparoscopic Cholecystectomy

Problem

Following ambulatory surgery procedures such as laparoscopic cholecystectomy, clients must manage their pain after discharge. In a study of analgesic use by ambulatory surgery clients, Older, Carr, and Layzell (2010) found clients were not always compliant with their analgesic regimens.

Evidence

Clients' intentional decision to endure moderate to severe pain by not taking the analgesics was influenced by clients' beliefs concerning pain, their analgesic use, and their previous pain experience. Clients feared the potential unknown side effects of the analgesics and did not believe taking multiple analgesics as part of a multimodal analgesic regimen was safe. The negative perception regarding morphine use was the fear of addiction. A factor that resulted in the clients' ultimately using their analgesic was reaching their pain threshold and no longer tolerating the pain. Additionally, when the healthcare provider encouraged clients to take the analgesic regularly, they increased their compliance with the prescribed analgesic regimen. Client education regarding postoperative pain management and the effective use of analgesics underestimates the role of the client's decision regarding analgesic use (Older et al., 2010).

Implications

Effective pain relief is known to promote healing and immune function following surgery (Stein & Kuchler, 2012). Research reveals a need to carefully prepare clients undergoing ambulatory surgery, including laparoscopic cholecystectomy, for pain management strategies. For example, in combination with additional analgesics, injection of local anesthetics at the surgical site significantly reduces pain following ambulatory surgery (Schug & Chong, 2009). Effective postoperative pain management requires a combination of good preoperative education, discharge planning related to the client's expectations of pain, and compliance of the client with the physician's prescribed analgesic regimen.

Critical Thinking Application

1. Some clients in this study reported purposely not taking their analgesic prescription due to anticipated adverse effects of the drug. How can the nurse intervene to prevent this and to promote effective postoperative pain management?

2. Adjunctive pain relief measures (nonsteroidal anti-inflammatory drugs [NSAIDs], application of heat or cold, etc.) may be recommended to supplement analgesic use. What adjunctive pain relief measures would be appropriate for the nurse to teach clients undergoing laparoscopic cholecystectomy?

3. Some clients in this study did not take the prescribed opioid analgesics because of concern about addiction. How should the nurse respond to a client who expresses this concern?

SAFETY ALERT

The herb goldenseal has been used in treating cholecystitis. However, the evidence is not sufficient to support the safe use of goldenseal, according to the National Center for Complementary and Alternative Medicine (2012). Berberine, one of the active ingredients in goldenseal, stimulates secretion of bile and bilirubin. It also inhibits the growth of many common pathogens, including those known to infect the gallbladder. Goldenseal can stimulate the uterus, so it is contraindicated for use during pregnancy. It also should not be used by nursing mothers.

Clinical Manifestations and Therapies Gallbladder Disease

ETIOLOGY	CLINICAL MANIFESTATIONS	CLINICAL THERAPIES
Biliary colic	■ Severe steady ache in RUQ that begins suddenly and lasts for several hours; may radiate to right scapula or back; nausea/vomiting; fat intolerance	■ Analgesics; adequate rest; adequate nutrition; correction of electrolyte imbalances; antiemetics
Cholecystitis	■ RUQ or epigastric pain that progressively worsens; anorexia; nausea/vomiting; fever/chills; fat intolerance	■ Analgesics; adequate rest; adequate nutrition; IV antibiotic therapy; antiemetics; laparoscopic surgery, which may convert to open surgery with possible T-tube placement; if surgery is contraindicated or chronic, oral dissolution therapy or lithotripsy
Choledocholithiasis	■ RUQ pain, fever, jaundice; pruritus; abdominal tenderness	■ Analgesics; antihistamines; adequate nutrition; IV antibiotic therapy; antiemetics; surgery
Cholangitis	■ RUQ pain; fever; jaundice; pruritus; abdominal tenderness; clay-colored stools; dark urine; low blood pressure; lethargy.	■ Analgesics; antihistamines; adequate nutrition; IV antibiotic therapy; antiemetics; surgery

■ NURSING PROCESS

Nursing care of the client with gallbladder disease is focused on client teaching, pain management, and instruction on healthy nutrition.

Assessment

Assessment data related to cholelithiasis and cholecystitis include the following:

■ *Health history.* Current manifestations, including right upper quadrant pain, its character and relationship to meals, duration, and radiation; nausea and vomiting; other symptoms; duration of symptoms; risk factors or previous history of symptoms; chronic diseases such as diabetes, cirrhosis, or inflammatory bowel disease; current diet; use of oral contraceptives or possibility of pregnancy
■ *Physical assessment.* Current weight; color of skin and sclera; abdominal assessment including light palpation for tenderness; color of urine and stool

Diagnosis

Priority nursing diagnoses for the client with cholelithiasis or cholecystitis often include the following:

■ *Risk for Infection*
■ *Pain*
■ *Imbalanced Nutrition: Less Than Body Requirements.*

(NANDA-I © 2012)

Planning

Goals of nursing care, developed in collaboration with the client, may include the following:

■ Client will demonstrate no signs or symptoms of infection.
■ Client will report adequate pain control.
■ Client will demonstrate understanding of low-fat diet with adequate intake of fat-soluble vitamins.
■ Client will verbalize awareness of symptoms that require immediate notification of the healthcare provider.

Implementation

Nursing interventions for the client who has undergone a laparoscopic or open cholecystectomy are similar to those for other clients who have had abdominal surgery.

Prevent Infection

An acutely inflamed gallbladder may become necrotic and rupture, releasing its contents into the abdominal cavity. While the resulting infection often remains localized, peritonitis can result from chemical irritation and bacterial contamination of the peritoneal cavity.

Following open cholecystectomy (laparotomy), the risk for pulmonary infection is significant due to the high abdominal incision.

■ Monitor vital signs, including temperature, every 4 hours. Promptly report vital sign changes or temperature elevation. Tachycardia, increased respiratory rate, or an elevated temperature may indicate an infectious process.

■ Assess abdomen every 4 hours and as indicated (e.g., when pain level changes abruptly). Increasing abdominal tenderness or a rigid, boardlike abdomen may indicate rupture of the gallbladder, with peritonitis.
■ Assist with coughing and deep breathing or use incentive spirometer every 1–2 hours while client is awake. Splint abdominal incision with a blanket or pillow during coughing. The high abdominal incision of an open cholecystectomy interferes with effective coughing and deep breathing, increasing the risk of atelectasis and respiratory infections such as pneumonia.
■ Place client in Fowler position and encourage ambulation as allowed. Fowler position and ambulation promote lung expansion and airway clearance, reducing the risk of respiratory infections.
■ Administer antibiotics as ordered. Antibiotics may be given preoperatively to reduce the risk of infection from infected gallbladder contents; they may be continued postoperatively to prevent infection.

Provide Effective Pain Management

The pain associated with cholelithiasis can be severe. Sometimes a combination of interventions is indicated:

■ Discuss the relationship between fat intake and pain. Teach ways to reduce fat intake. Fat entering the duodenum initiates gallbladder contractions, causing pain when gallstones are in the ducts.
■ Withhold oral food and fluids during episodes of acute pain. Insert nasogastric tube and connect to low suction if ordered. Emptying the stomach reduces the amount of chyme entering the duodenum and the stimulus for gallbladder contractions, thus reducing pain.
■ For severe pain, administer morphine, meperidine, or another opioid analgesic as ordered. Recent research indicates that morphine is no more likely to cause spasms of the sphincter of Oddi than meperidine.
■ Place in Fowler position. Fowler position decreases pressure on the inflamed gallbladder.

Promote Balanced Nutrition

The client with severe gallbladder disease may develop nutritional imbalances related to anorexia, pain, nausea following meals, and impaired bile flow that alters absorption of fat and fat-soluble vitamins (A, D, E, and K) from the gut.

■ Assess nutritional status, including diet history, height and weight, and skinfold measurements. Clients with gallbladder disease may have an imbalanced diet or may have specific vitamin deficiencies, particularly of the fat-soluble vitamins.
■ Evaluate laboratory results, including serum bilirubin, albumin, glucose, and cholesterol levels. Report abnormal results to the primary care provider. Elevated serum bilirubin may indicate impaired bilirubin excretion due to obstructed bile flow. A low serum albumin may indicate poor nutritional status. Glucose intolerance and hypercholesterolemia are risk factors for cholelithiasis.

Client Teaching The Client With Gallbladder Disease

Client teaching varies depending on the choice of treatment options for cholelithiasis and cholecystitis. If surgery is not an option, teach the client about medications that dissolve stones; their use and adverse effects (diarrhea is a common side effect); and maintenance of a low-fat, low-carbohydrate diet if indicated. Include an explanation about the role of bile and the function of the gallbladder in terms the client and family can understand.

Provide appropriate preoperative teaching for the planned procedure. Discuss the possibility of open cholecystectomy even when a laparoscopic procedure is planned. Teach postoperative self-care measures to manage pain and prevent complications. If the client will be discharged with a T-tube, provide instructions about its care. Discuss manifestations of complications to report to the physician. Stress the importance of follow up appointments.

Following cholecystectomy, a low-fat diet may be recommended initially. Refer the client and food preparer to a dietitian to review low-fat foods. Higher-fat foods may be added to the diet gradually as tolerated.

■ Refer the client to a dietitian or nutritionist for diet counseling to promote healthy weight loss and to reduce pain episodes. A low-carbohydrate, low-fat, higher-protein diet reduces symptoms of cholecystitis. While fasting and very low-calorie diets are contraindicated, a moderate reduction in calorie intake and increased activity levels promote weight loss.
■ Administer vitamin supplements as ordered. Clients who do not absorb fat well due to obstructed bile flow may require supplements of the fat-soluble vitamins.

Evaluation

Client progress toward goals may be evaluated based on the following expected outcomes:

■ Client reports adequate pain control to maintain comfort.
■ Client demonstrates food choices reflecting a diet low in fat and high in fat-soluble vitamins.
■ Client's temperature remains within normal limits, and client displays no symptoms of infection.

NURSING CARE PLAN   A Client With Cholelithiasis

Joyce Red Wing is a 44-year-old married mother of three children. A member of the Chickasaw tribe, she is active in tribal activities and works part time as a cook at a community kitchen. Recently, Ms. Red Wing has noticed a dull pain in her upper abdomen that gets worse after she eats fatty foods; nausea and sometimes vomiting accompany the pain. She had a similar pain after the birth of her last child. She is diagnosed with cholelithiasis and is admitted for a laparoscopic cholecystectomy.

ASSESSMENT

David Corbin, RN, takes Ms. Red Wing's admission history. It includes intolerance of fatty foods and intermittent "stabbing" abdominal pain that radiates to her back. Her usual diet includes tacos or fried bread and biscuits with gravy for breakfast. She reports "not wanting to eat much of anything lately." She states that she has never had surgery before and hopes "everything goes well." Physical assessment includes temperature 37.7°C (100°F) oral, pulse 88 bpm, respirations 20/min, and BP 130/84 mmHg. She has had a recent 5-lb weight loss and currently weighs 59 kg (130 lb). She is 160 cm (63 inches) tall. Abdominal examination elicits tenderness in the right upper abdominal quadrant. She has no jaundice, chills, or evidence of complications.

DIAGNOSES

■ *Risk for Infection* related to potential bacterial contamination of abdominal cavity
■ *Imbalanced Nutrition: Less Than Body Requirements* related to anorexia and recent weight loss
■ *Acute Pain* related to inflamed gallbladder and surgical incisions
■ *Anxiety* related to lack of information about perioperative experience

(NANDA-I © 2012)

PLANNING

■ Client will maintain present weight within 2.3 kg (5 lb) over the next 3 weeks.
■ Client will resume regular diet, decreasing intake of foods high in fat.
■ Client will verbalize adequate pain control after surgery and with activity resumption.
■ Client will remain free of infection.
■ Client will verbalize a decrease in anxiety before surgery.

IMPLEMENTATION

■ Teach about the gallbladder and the function of bile.
■ Discuss pre- and postoperative care, including self-care following discharge.
■ Promote mobility as soon as allowed after surgery.
■ Teach home care of incisions and recognition of signs of infection.

■ Review specific high-fat foods to avoid and ways to maintain her weight.
■ Provide analgesia as needed postoperatively. Teach appropriate analgesic use after discharge.

EVALUATION

Ms. Red Wing is discharged the morning after her surgery. She is afebrile, has no signs of infection, and is able to appropriately care for her incisions. She identifies signs of infection and talks about ways to reduce her fat intake while keeping her weight stable. She verbalizes understanding of initial activity restrictions and resumption of normal activities. Ms. Red Wing states, "It wasn't as bad as I thought it would be at first." She has an appointment to see her surgeon in 1 week.

(continued on next page)

NURSING CARE PLAN (continued)

CRITICAL THINKING

1. What is the rationale for a low-fat diet with cholelithiasis? Discuss nutritional practices as they relate to the medical problem and Ms. Red Wing's culture.
2. How would your discharge teaching for Ms. Red Wing differ if she had had an open cholecystectomy instead of a laparoscopic cholecystectomy?
3. Design a nursing care plan for Ms. Red Wing for the nursing diagnosis Fatigue.

REVIEW Gallbladder Disease

RELATE Link the Concepts and Exemplars

Linking the exemplar of gallbladder disease with the concept of fluids and electrolytes:

1. How might gallbladder disease affect fluid homeostasis?
2. To prevent fluid and electrolyte imbalance, what nursing care might you initiate for the client who reports severe, acute abdominal pain secondary to cholelithiasis?

Linking the exemplar of gallbladder disease with the concept of health, wellness, and illness:

3. What health promotion topics might you teach adults to prevent the development of cholelithiasis?
4. What group would you consider most at risk for development of gallbladder disease?

READY Go to Companion Skills Manual

REFER Go to Pearson Nursing Student Resources
nursing.pearsonhighered.com

- Additional review material

REFLECT Case Study

Helen Martin is a 48-year-old Caucasian female who is married to Gil Martin. They have been married for 18 years. Ms. Martin has a daughter (Tracie) from a previous marriage, and she has two teenage children with Gil (Anthony and Kristina). Ms. Martin works as a teller at a bank. Although she finds her job monotonous, she appreciates the steady income and family health insurance.

Ms. Martin is overweight and has tried to lose weight most of her adult life. She frequently diets and, in fact, has lost a great deal of weight in the past but has been unable to keep the weight off. She blames menopause for her most recent weight gain.

Ms. Martin experiences indigestion following a few meals. Over several weeks, the severity and frequency have increased.

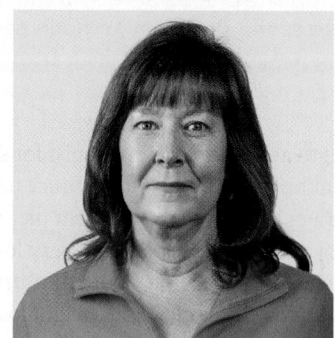

She takes an antacid, believing the problem is just heartburn. The discomfort is usually located in the upper right side of her abdomen, and sometimes it is quite painful. The pain may last up to a couple of hours and then subsides. Occasionally, she feels nauseous as well. After putting up with this for several weeks, she makes an appointment with her physician.

Based on Ms. Martin's symptoms, her physician suspects that she has cholelithiasis and orders an ultrasound scan of her abdomen. The ultrasound confirms the presence of gallstones. The physician tells Ms. Martin that she has two options: (1) conservative therapy that would involve a low-fat, reduced-calorie diet or (2) surgery to remove her gallbladder. Helen decides to try dietary modification.

1. What information would you include in your teaching plan for Ms. Martin about low-fat, low-calorie diets?
2. Based on your own likes and dislikes, design a 1-week diet plan, including all meals and snacks that would meet the low-fat, low-calorie requirements for Ms. Martin.
3. What is the rationale for beginning with conservative treatment rather than immediately initiating surgical intervention?
4. How will you evaluate the effectiveness of conservative treatment for Ms. Martin?

EXEMPLAR 10.3   Inflammatory Bowel Disease

EXEMPLAR KEY TERMS
Colectomy, 662
Crohn disease, 657
Fulminant colitis, 660
Ileostomy, 662
Inflammatory bowel disease (IBD), 657
Stoma, 662
Ulcerative colitis, 657

EXEMPLAR LEARNING OUTCOMES
After reading about this exemplar, you will be able to:

1. Describe the pathophysiology, etiology, clinical manifestations, and direct and indirect causes of inflammatory bowel disease (IBD).

2. Identify risk factors and prevention methods associated with IBD.
3. Illustrate the nursing process in providing culturally competent care across the life span for individuals with IBD.
4. Formulate priority nursing diagnoses appropriate for an individual with IBD.
5. Summarize therapies used by interdisciplinary teams in the collaborative care of an individual with IBD.
6. Plan evidence-based care for an individual with IBD and his or her family in collaboration with other members of the healthcare team.
7. Evaluate expected outcomes for an individual with IBD.

▶ OVERVIEW

Approximately 1.4 million Americans have **inflammatory bowel disease (IBD)**, a collection of chronic inflammatory conditions of the intestines. With both ulcerative colitis (UC) and Crohn disease, the client experiences periods of symptom-free remissions with sporadic periods of active disease (flares). Twice as many individuals develop ulcerative colitis as develop Crohn disease (CCFA, 2011). **Ulcerative colitis** affects the mucosa and submucosa of the colon and rectum.

Classification of IBD is based on the severity of symptoms, primarily the number of bowel movements per day. Clients with mild disease (30% of cases) have fewer than four stools per day, and clients with moderate disease (20%) experience four to six stools per day. UC clients with more than six stools per day (2%) have severe disease. The remaining clients (48%) are in remission (CCFA, 2011).

Crohn disease can affect any portion of the GI tract from the mouth to the anus, but it usually affects the terminal ileum and ascending colon. Areas of disease involvement appear as patches, leaving adjacent areas unaffected. Because any portion of the gastrointestinal tract can be affected, disease activity and severity can fluctuate considerable over time. The extent of the inflammation in Crohn is deep and can extend through the entire bowel wall (CCFA, 2011). A comparison of ulcerative colitis and Crohn disease is found in **Table 10–4** ●.

▶ PATHOPHYSIOLOGY AND ETIOLOGY

The inflammatory process of ulcerative colitis usually begins at the rectosigmoid area of the anal canal and progresses proximally. In most clients, the disease is confined to the rectum and sigmoid colon. It may progress to involve the entire colon, stopping at the ileocecal junction.

Ulcerative colitis begins with inflammation at the base of the crypts of Lieberkühn in the distal large intestine and rectal mucosa. Microscopic, pinpoint mucosal hemorrhages occur, and crypt abscesses develop (**Figure 10–5** ●). These abscesses penetrate the superficial submucosa and spread laterally, leading to necrosis and sloughing of bowel mucosa. Further tissue damage is caused by inflammatory exudates and the release of inflammatory mediators such as prostaglandins and other cytokines. The mucosa becomes red and edematous due to vascular congestion, friable (easily broken), and ulcerated. It bleeds easily, and hemorrhage is common. Edema creates a granular appearance. Pseudopolyps, tonguelike projections of bowel mucosa into the lumen, may develop as the epithelial lining of the bowel regenerates.

TABLE 10–4 Characteristics of Ulcerative Colitis and Crohn Disease

	CHARACTERISTIC	ULCERATIVE COLITIS	CROHN DISEASE
CLINICAL	Gender	Equal	Equal
	Age at onset	Any age, peaks in 15- to 30-year-olds	Any age, peaks in 15- to 30-year-olds
	Course of disease	Chronic disease with periods of remission of symptoms and active disease	Chronic disease with periods of remission of symptoms and active disease
	Diarrhea	5–30 stools per day with blood and mucus	Common, usually less severe than in colitis, with no obvious blood or mucus in stool
	Abdominal pain	Cramping in left lower quadrant; relieved by defecation	Cramping, or steady right lower quadrant or periumbilical pain; tenderness and mass noted in right lower quadrant
	Nutritional deficit	Common, involving anemia, hypoalbuminemia, and weight loss	Common and significant, involving anemia, weight loss, and multiple vitamin and mineral deficits
	Constitutional manifestations	Fever rare; possible associated arthritic, skin, or other organ involvement, such as erythema nodosum or uveitis	Fever, malaise, fatigue; possibly some associated conditions and urinary complications
PATHOLOGICAL	Depth of involvement	Mucosa and submucosa	Transmural (entire bowel wall)
	Portion of bowel involved	Typically rectum and sigmoid colon, possibly extending to entire large bowel	Any portion of GI tract, terminal ileum and ascending colon involvement predominating
	Distribution	Continuous from rectum	Patchy; skip lesions
	Appearance of mucosa	Granular, dull, hyperemic, friable; disease uniform in affected bowel; possibly pseudopolyps	Cobblestone appearance, with areas of normal tissue surrounded by ulceration and fissures
COMPLICATIONS	Acute	Toxic megacolon, perforation, massive hemorrhage	Obstruction, fistulization, abscess formation, malabsorption
	Long term	Colorectal cancer	Colon cancer

Sources: Data from Centers for Disease Control and Prevention. (2012). *Inflammatory bowel disease.* Retrieved from http://www.cdc.gov/ibd; Crohn and Colitis Foundation of America. (2011). *The facts about inflammatory bowel diseases.* Retrieved from http://www.ccfa.org/assets/pdfs/ibdfactbook.pdf

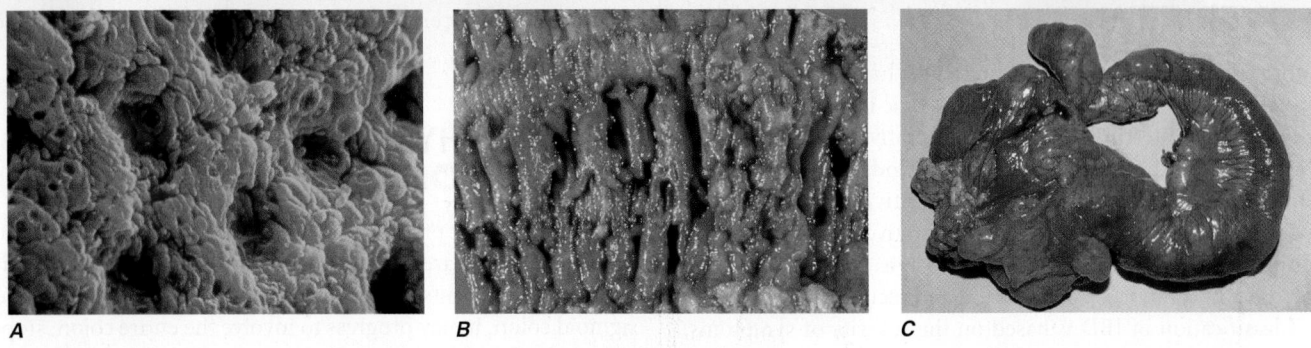

A   B   C

Figure 10–5 ● *A,* Photomicrograph of the mucosa of the large intestine showing the entrances to the crypts of Lieberkühn. The crypts are the focal points for *B,* ulcerative colitis and *C,* Crohn disease.
Source: A, CNRI/Science Source. *B,* Dr. E. Walker/Science Source, *C,* Biophoto Associates/Science Source.

Chronic inflammation leads to atrophy, narrowing, and shortening of the colon, with loss of its normal haustra (small pouches or recesses into which the large intestine is divided).

Crohn disease typically begins as a small inflammatory *aphthoid lesion* (a shallow ulcer with a white base and an elevated margin, similar to a canker sore) of the mucosa and submucosa of the bowel. The initial lesions may regress, or the inflammatory process may progress to involve all layers of the intestinal wall. Deeper ulcerations, granulomatous lesions, and fissures (knifelike clefts that extend deeply into the bowel wall) develop. The inflammatory process involves the entire bowel wall (transmural).

The lumen of the affected bowel assumes a cobblestone appearance as fissures and ulcers surround islands of intact mucosa over edematous submucosa. The inflammatory lesions of Crohn disease are not continuous; rather, they often occur as "skip" lesions with intervening areas of normal-appearing bowel. Some evidence suggests that despite its normal appearance, the entire bowel is affected by this disorder.

As the disease progresses, fibrotic changes in the bowel wall cause it to thicken and lose flexibility, taking on a rubber-hose-like appearance. The inflammation, edema, and fibrosis can lead to local obstruction, the development of abscesses, and the formation of fistulas between loops of bowel or between the bowel and other organs (**Figure 10–6** ●). Fistulas between loops of bowel are known as *enteroenteric fistulas;* fistulas that occur between bowel and bladder are known as *enterovesical fistulas;* and fistulas that occur between bowel and skin are known as *enterocutaneous fistulas.* Perineal fistulas are relatively common, originating in the ileum.

Depending on the severity and extent of the disease, malabsorption and malnutrition may develop as the ulcers prevent absorption of nutrients. When the jejunum and ileum are affected, the absorption of multiple nutrients (including carbohydrates, proteins, fats, vitamins, and folate) may be impaired. Disease in the terminal ileum can lead to vitamin B_{12} malabsorption and bile salt reabsorption. The ulcerations also can lead to protein loss and chronic, slow blood loss with consequent anemia. See the Multisystem Effects of Inflammatory Bowel Disease on page 659.

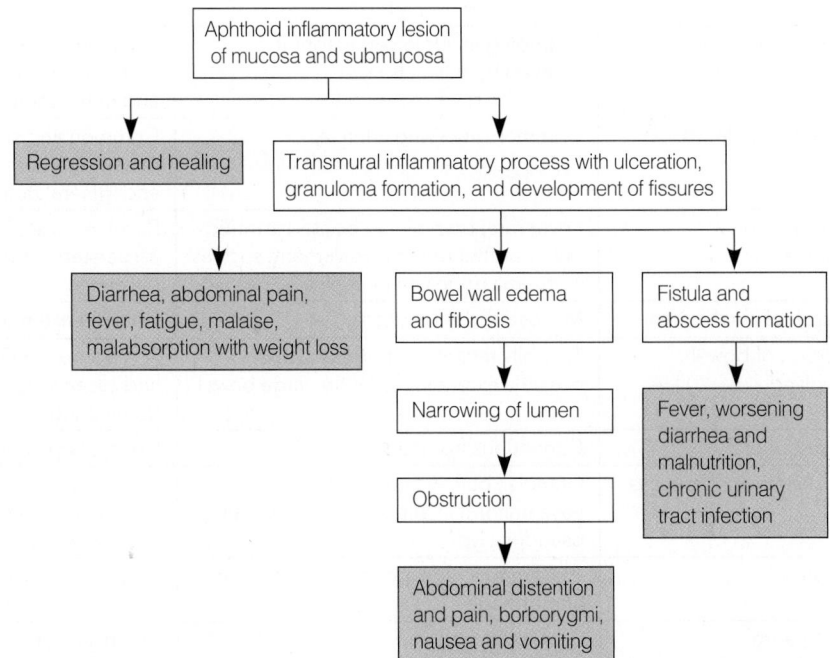

Figure 10–6 ● The progression of Crohn disease.

Multisystem Effects of Inflammatory Bowel Disease

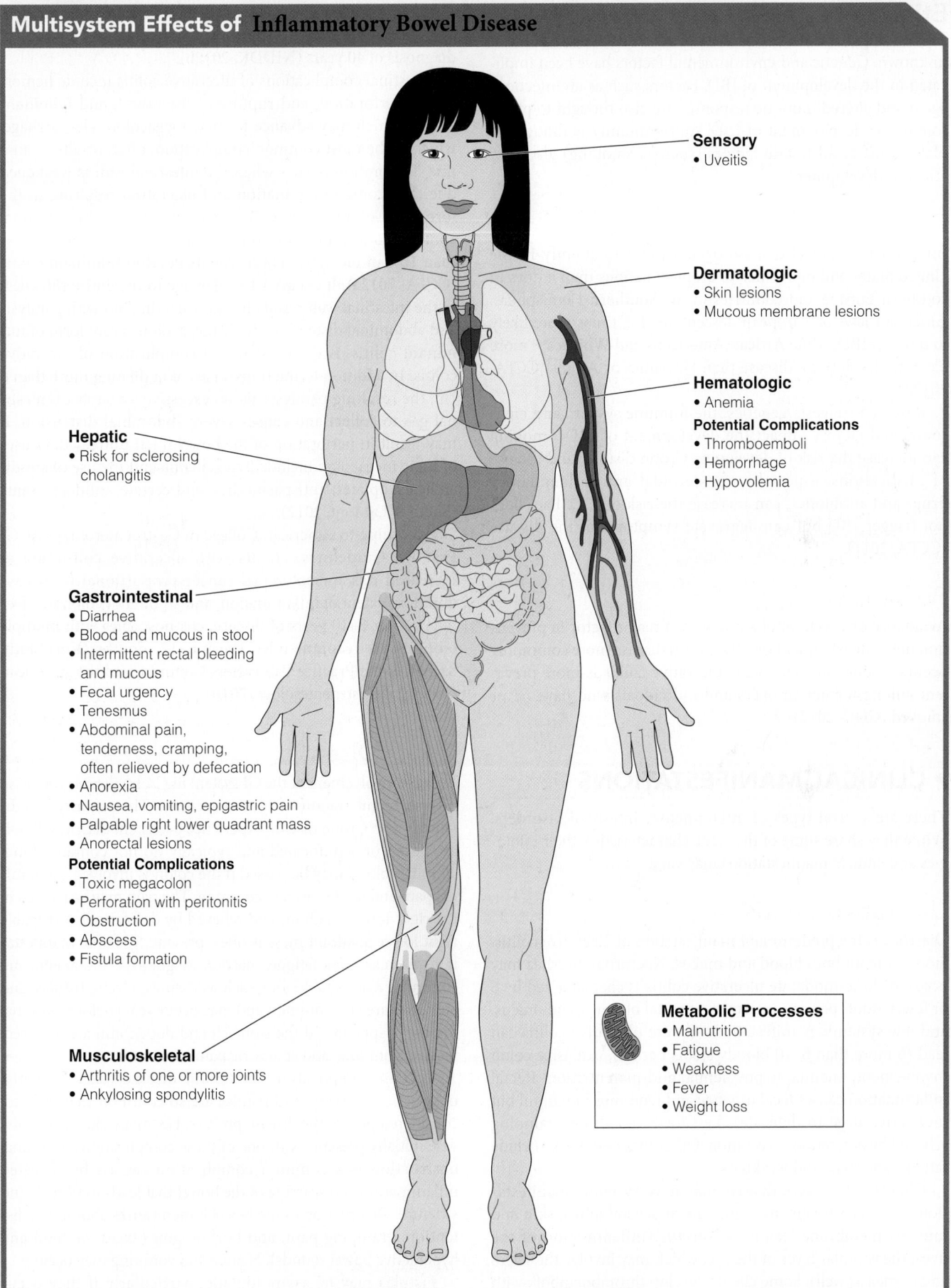

Sensory
• Uveitis

Dermatologic
• Skin lesions
• Mucous membrane lesions

Hematologic
• Anemia
Potential Complications
• Thromboemboli
• Hemorrhage
• Hypovolemia

Hepatic
• Risk for sclerosing cholangitis

Gastrointestinal
• Diarrhea
• Blood and mucous in stool
• Intermittent rectal bleeding and mucous
• Fecal urgency
• Tenesmus
• Abdominal pain, tenderness, cramping, often relieved by defecation
• Anorexia
• Nausea, vomiting, epigastric pain
• Palpable right lower quadrant mass
• Anorectal lesions
Potential Complications
• Toxic megacolon
• Perforation with peritonitis
• Obstruction
• Abscess
• Fistula formation

Musculoskeletal
• Arthritis of one or more joints
• Ankylosing spondylitis

Metabolic Processes
• Malnutrition
• Fatigue
• Weakness
• Fever
• Weight loss

Etiology

The etiology of both ulcerative colitis and Crohn disease is unknown. Genetic and environmental factors have been implicated in the development of IBD. Factors such as an infectious agent and altered immune responses are also thought to play a role in the development of IBD. Autoimmunity is thought to play a role, and lifestyle factors (such as smoking) also may affect its development.

Risk Factors

Inflammatory bowel disease occurs more frequently in the United States and in northern European nations than it does in southern Europe and countries in the Southern Hemisphere. American Jews of European descent are 4–5 times more likely to develop IBD, while African Americans and Whites are more likely to develop the disease than Hispanics or Asians (CCFA, 2012c).

Research suggests genetics, the immune system, and environmental factors impact the development of IBD. Smoking can increase the risk of developing Crohn disease, and the use of medications, especially nonsteroidal anti-inflammatory drugs and antibiotics, can increase the risk of IBD. Diet does not trigger IBD but can aggravate symptoms of the disease (CCFA, 2011).

Prevention

Avoidance or cessation of smoking is a major factor in prevention of the development of IBD. Crohn disease more commonly occurs among smokers, while ulcerative colitis is more prevalent among former smokers and individuals who have never smoked (CDC, 2012).

▶ CLINICAL MANIFESTATIONS

There are several types of inflammatory intestinal disorders. While they share some of the same characteristics, their etiologies and clinical manifestations may vary.

Ulcerative Colitis

Diarrhea is the predominant manifestation of ulcerative colitis. Stools contain both blood and mucus. Nocturnal diarrhea may occur. Mild to moderate ulcerative colitis is characterized by 6 or fewer stools per day, intermittent rectal bleeding and mucus, and few systemic manifestations. Severe ulcerative colitis can lead to more than 6–10 bloody stools per day, extensive colon involvement, anemia, hypovolemia, and malnutrition. Rectal inflammation causes fecal urgency and tenesmus (a painful but ineffective urge to defecate). Left lower quadrant cramping relieved by defecation is common. Other manifestations include fatigue, anorexia, and weakness.

Clients with severe disease may have systemic manifestations such as arthritis involving one or several joints, skin and mucous membrane lesions, or *uveitis* (inflammation of the uvea, the vascular layer of the eye, which may involve the sclera and cornea as well). Some clients develop thromboemboli, with blood vessel obstruction due to clots carried from the site of their formation. Sclerosing cholangitis (inflammation leading

to scarring and narrowing of the bile ducts) may occur; it is more common in men than in women, with an average age of diagnosis of 40 years (NIDDK, 2012b).

Intestinal complications of ulcerative colitis include hemorrhage, perforation, and rupture of the bowel, and **fulminant colitis**, which may advance to toxic megacolon. Hemorrhage, which is the most common complication, often results in anemia. Perforation occurs when the intestinal wall is weakened due to chronic inflammation and ulceration resulting in the formation of an opening. This opening allows the intestinal contents to leak into the abdomen and cause peritonitis. Less than 10% of ulcerative colitis clients develop fulminant colitis (CCFA, 2012a). It occurs when damage to the entire thickness of the intestinal wall results in intestinal dilation with paralysis and abdominal distention. Toxic megacolon, a rare form of fulminant colitis, is the most severe complication of ulcerative colitis. In addition to the transverse colon dilating more than 6 cm, the resulting paralysis allows excessive amounts of intestinal gas to collect and causes severe abdominal distension. It may result in perforation of the bowel if left untreated. Causes of toxic megacolon include hypokalemia and the use of antidiarrheals, opiates, antispasmodics, and certain antidepressants (Sheth & LaMont, 2012).

According to American College of Gastroenterology (ACG) Practice Guidelines, clients with ulcerative colitis are at increased risk for colorectal cancer proportional to disease duration, extent of inflammation, and amount of colon involvement. After 8–10 years of disease, colonoscopies with multiple biopsies are recommended every 6–12 months (Kornbluth, Sachar, & the Practice Parameters Committee of the American College of Gastroenterology, 2010).

Crohn Disease

Because involvement of the GI system in Crohn disease can be so diverse, manifestations vary among clients. The majority of individuals with Crohn disease experience persistent diarrhea. Stools are liquid or semiformed and typically do not contain blood, although blood may be passed if the colon is involved. Abdominal pain and tenderness are common. The pain may be located in the right lower quadrant and relieved by defecation. A palpable right lower quadrant mass is often present. Systemic manifestations such as fever, fatigue, malaise, weight loss, and anemia are common. Anorectal lesions such as fissures, ulcers, fistulas, and abscesses are also common and may occur years before intestinal disease is apparent. If the stomach and duodenum are involved, nausea, vomiting, and epigastric pain may occur.

Certain complications of Crohn disease (e.g., intestinal obstruction, abscess, and fistula) are so common that they are considered part of the disease process. For many clients, the disease initially presents with one of these complications. Intestinal obstruction is a common complication caused by repeated inflammation and scarring of the bowel that leads to fibrosis and stricture. Obstruction of the bowel lumen causes abdominal distention, cramping pain, and borborygmi (excessive loud and hyperactive bowel sounds). Nausea and vomiting may occur.

Fistulas may be asymptomatic, particularly if they occur between loops of small bowel. An abscess caused by fistulization produces chills and fever, a tender abdominal mass, and

Clinical Manifestations and Therapies **Inflammatory Bowel Disease**

ETIOLOGY	CLINICAL MANIFESTATIONS	CLINICAL THERAPIES
Hemorrhage	Pale mucous membranes, thirst, light-headedness, hypotension, reduced urine output	■ Blood transfusions ■ Iron supplements ■ IV fluid ■ Possibly surgery to remove damaged bowel ■ Possibly, vasoconstrictive medications
Megacolon	Fever, tachycardia, hypotension, dehydration, abdominal tenderness and cramping, and a change in the number of stools per day	■ Fecal disimpaction ■ Enemas ■ Suppositories ■ Bowel decompression ■ Colonoscopic decompression ■ Bowel habit retraining ■ Total abdominal colectomy
Diarrhea	Frequent loose stools, abdominal cramping, abdominal tenderness, stool that may or may not contain blood, thirst, dehydration, hypovolemia, malnutrition	■ Monitoring of intake and output ■ IV fluid ■ Antidiarrheal medications (should be avoided in severe ulcerative colitis) ■ Possible guaiac testing
Fistulas	Possibly asymptomatic between bowel loops; between bowel and bladder—frequent UTIs; between bowel and abdominal cavity—abscess, chills and fever, a tender abdominal mass, leukocytosis; between small bowel and colon— weight loss, malnutrition, possible exacerbation of diarrhea	■ Symptomatic treatment: antibiotics, antidiarrheal medication, IV fluid support. ■ Possible dissection of section of bowel with fistula if tissue cannot be repaired

leukocytosis. A fistula between the small bowel and the colon may exacerbate diarrhea, weight loss, and malnutrition. When the bladder is involved, recurrent urinary tract infections (UTIs) occur.

Perforation of the bowel is uncommon but can lead to generalized peritonitis. Massive hemorrhage is also an uncommon complication of Crohn disease. Long-standing Crohn disease increases the risk of colorectal cancer.

Lifespan and Cultural Considerations

Although the occurrence of IBD peaks at 15–30 years of age, it also occurs in the pediatric population. The pediatric etiology differs from that of adult-onset IBD. For example, IBD is more common in males than females in the pediatric population, whereas equal numbers of adult males and females have IBD. In addition, children suffer from Crohn disease more frequently than ulcerative colitis (2.8:1); the opposite is true of adults (0.85:1).

The location of disease is also different in children and adults. Whereas adults with Crohn disease usually present with terminal ileal disease without colonic involvement, the majority of pediatric clients have ileocolonic or colonic disease, increasing the incidence of hematochezia (blood in stool). In addition, children with Crohn disease usually present with inflammatory or nonstricturing, nonpenetrating dis-

ease, whereas adults often present with fistulizing or stricturing disease. Similarly, children with ulcerative colitis usually present with pancolitis, whereas adults more often present with left-sided colitis. Pediatric pancolitis is usually more aggressive, and first surgery often comes earlier for children than for adults (Sauer & Kugathasan, 2009).

An important pediatric consequence of malabsorption of adequate nutrition in this disease is failure to grow. It is not uncommon for children to receive dietary supplements in addition to medications to control their disease. The medications used to treat inflammatory bowel disease in pediatric clients are the same as those used in adults; however, dosage is reduced when they are administered to children. As in adults, the disease in children may progress to the point of requiring surgery to remove a portion of the bowel. Children with IBD can also have lower bone density than children without the disease. Other manifestations of the disease are very similar to those experienced by an adult (CDHNF, 2010).

► COLLABORATION

Interdisciplinary care for inflammatory bowel disease begins by establishing the diagnosis and the extent and severity of the disease. Treatment is supportive, including medications and dietary measures to decrease inflammation, promote intestinal rest and healing, and reduce intestinal motility. Many clients with IBD require surgery at some point to manage the disease or its complications. As a member of the healthcare team, the nurse plays an essential role by providing client teaching about disease management, diagnostic tests, and surgical or other treatments.

Diagnostic Tests

Diagnostic testing establishes the diagnosis of IBD, assesses the extent of the disease, and evaluates the effects of the disorder. A sigmoidoscopy, colonoscopy, or barium upper and lower x-ray series inspect the bowel mucosa for characteristic changes of IBD.

Laboratory tests used to differentiate IBD and to identify effects and complications of the disease include a stool examination for blood and mucus and stool cultures to rule out infectious causes of bowel inflammation and diarrhea. CBC with hemoglobin and hematocrit shows anemia from chronic inflammation, blood loss, and malnutrition, as well as leukocytosis due to inflammation and possible abscess formation. The sedimentation rate is typically elevated during periods of acute inflammation. Serum albumin may decrease because of malabsorption, malnutrition, protein loss through intestinal lesions, and chronic inflammation. Folic acid and serum levels of most vitamins, including A, B complex, C, and the fat-soluble vitamins, often decrease due to malabsorption. Liver function tests may show elevated liver enzymes (such as ALT, alkaline phosphatase, AST, GGTP, and LDH) and bilirubin levels if sclerosing cholangitis is present.

Surgery

Surgical interventions for inflammatory bowel disease differ depending on the primary disease process and the portion of the bowel affected. Generally, surgery is performed only when necessitated by complications of the disease or failure of conservative treatment measures.

Bowel obstruction is the leading indication for surgery in Crohn disease. Other complications that may require surgical intervention are perforation, internal or external fistula, abscess, and perianal complications. The usual treatment is resection of the affected portion of bowel with an end-to-end anastomosis to preserve as much bowel as possible. The disease process tends to recur in other areas following removal of affected bowel segments. The risk of fistula formation increases following surgery. Bowel strictures may be treated with a *strictureplasty*, in which longitudinal incisions are made in the narrowed segment to relieve the stricture while preserving bowel.

COLECTOMY Clients with extensive chronic ulcerative colitis may require a total **colectomy** (surgical resection and removal of the colon) to treat the disease itself; to eliminate complications such as toxic megacolon, perforation, or hemorrhage; or to serve as a prophylactic measure due to the high colon cancer risk associated with extensive ulcerative colitis.

The surgical procedure of choice for extensive ulcerative colitis is a *total colectomy with an ileal pouch-anal anastomosis (IPAA)*. In this procedure, the entire colon and rectum are removed, a pouch is formed from the terminal ileum, and the

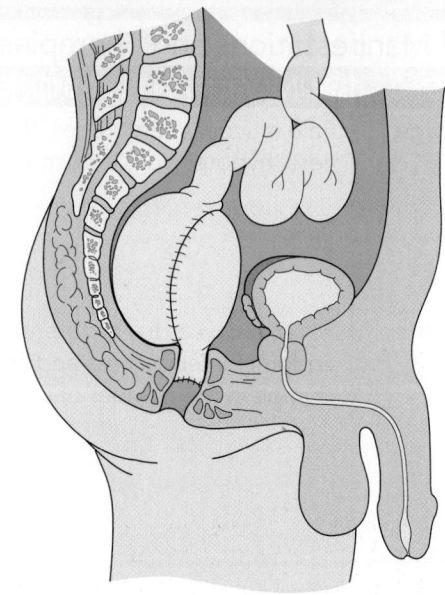

Figure 10–7 ● Ileal pouch–anal anastomosis (IPAA).

pouch is brought into the pelvis and anastomosed (connected) to the anal canal (**Figure 10–7 ●**). A temporary or loop ileostomy (described under the heading Ostomy) is generally performed at the same time and is maintained for 2–3 months to allow the anal anastomosis to heal. When the healing is complete, the ileostomy is closed, and the client has six to eight daily bowel movements through the anus. Advanced age, obesity, and other factors may preclude an IPAA. For these clients, a permanent ileostomy or continent ileostomy may be created.

OSTOMY An intestinal ostomy is a surgically created opening between the intestine and the abdominal wall that allows the passage of fecal material. The surface opening is called a **stoma** (**Figure 10–8 ●**). The precise name of the ostomy depends on the location of the stoma. An **ileostomy** is an ostomy made in the ileum of the small intestine. In an ileostomy, the colon, rectum, and anus are usually completely removed (*total proctocolectomy with permanent ileostomy*). The anal canal is closed, and the end of the terminal ileum is brought to the body surface through the right abdominal wall to form the stoma. A temporary or *loop ileostomy* may be formed to eliminate feces and allow tissue healing for 2–3 months follow-

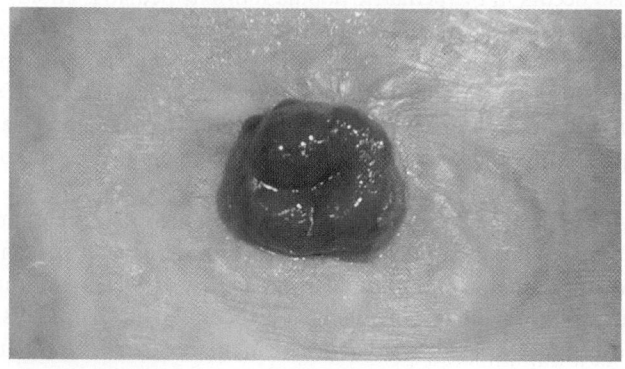

Figure 10–8 ● A healthy-appearing stoma.

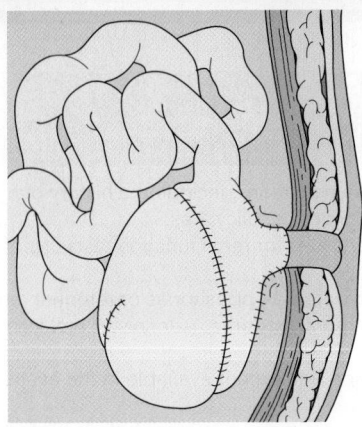

Figure 10–9 ● Continent (Kock) ileostomy.

ing an IPAA. A loop of ileum is brought to the body surface to form a stoma and allow stool drainage into an external pouch. When the ileostomy is no longer necessary, a second surgery is performed to close the stoma and repair the bowel, restoring fecal elimination through the anus.

In a *continent ileostomy* (**Figure 10–9 ●**), an intra-abdominal reservoir is constructed and a nipple valve is formed (the ileum is folded back on itself) from the terminal ileum before it is brought to the surface of the abdominal wall. Stool collects in the internal pouch; the nipple valve prevents it from leaking through the stoma. A catheter is inserted into the pouch to drain the stool.

✻ *See a chart on Nursing Care of the Client Having an Ileostomy at* **nursing.pearsonhighered.com**.

Pharmacologic Therapy

The ultimate goal of care is to terminate acute attacks as quickly as possible and to reduce the incidence of relapse. Drug therapy plays a key role in achieving this goal (see the Medications feature). Locally acting and systemic anti-inflammatory drugs are the primary medications used to manage mild to moderate IBD. Drugs to suppress the immune response may be used to treat clients with severe disease.

Sulfasalazine (Azulfidine) combines a sulfonamide antibiotic that is poorly absorbed from the GI tract with mesalamine, which acts topically on the colonic mucosa to inhibit the inflammatory process. Mesalamine (5-aminosalicylic acid) is also available in preparations that contain not sulfa but other vehicles, such as olsalazine and balsalazide. They have the advantage of causing fewer adverse effects than sulfasalazine.

For acute exacerbations of inflammatory bowel disease, corticosteroids are given to reduce inflammation and induce remission. For ulcerative colitis, the drug may be administered rectally as an enema, a suppository, or foam for its local effect and to minimize systemic effects. Intravenous corticosteroids may be required to treat severe disease; oral preparations are used for less severe manifestations and long-term therapy. Many clients are unable to withdraw from steroid therapy without experiencing relapse and may need chronic low-dose therapy.

Mercaptopurine (6-MP, Purinethol) and other immunosuppressive agents such as azathioprine (Imuran) and cyclosporine (Sandimmune) can be used to treat clients who have not responded to other treatments or who require chronic steroid

therapy. These drugs may allow withdrawal from corticosteroids, maintain remission, and facilitate healing. Long-term therapy may be required to produce a beneficial effect.

Newer treatments for IBD employ other immune response modifiers, such as the monoclonal antibodies infliximab (Remicade) and adalimumab (Humira), to suppress tumor necrosis factor (TNF, an inflammatory mediator substance) in clients with moderate to severe active Crohn disease who have not responded to standard therapies. Only infliximab is approved for use in ulcerative colitis (CCFA, 2011).

Although antibiotic therapy generally is not indicated in IBD, metronidazole (Flagyl) and ciprofloxacin (Cipro) are used when abscesses occur.

Antidiarrheal agents, such as loperamide and diphenoxylate, may be given to slow gastrointestinal motility and reduce diarrhea. These drugs are safe for clients with mild, chronic manifestations, but they are not given during acute attacks because they may precipitate toxic dilation of the colon.

When working with clients who are prescribed pharmacologic therapy for IBD, reinforce the importance of adhering to a strict medication regimen. Emphasize that medications should be continued even when the client is asymptomatic. Discuss the side effects of the drugs and what to do if any of the side effects occur. Teach the client and family members how to recognize and respond to side effects of medications. Because immune status may be altered by steroid use, have the family of a client taking steroids avoid risk of contact with infectious diseases. Instruct them to report any diseases and fevers the client experiences and to report the use of steroids to all healthcare providers. Immunization schedules for pediatric clients may need to be altered.

Nonpharmacologic Therapy

Antigens in the diet may stimulate the immune response in the bowel, exacerbating inflammatory bowel disease. As a result, dietary management for IBD should be individualized. Some clients benefit from eliminating all milk and milk products from the diet. Increased dietary fiber may help reduce diarrhea and relieve rectal manifestations, but it is contraindicated for clients with intestinal strictures caused by repeated inflammation and scarring.

All food may be withheld to promote bowel rest during an acute exacerbation of Crohn disease. Nutritional status during this time is maintained by enteral or total parenteral nutrition (TPN). TPN carries a higher risk of complications than does enteral nutrition. An elemental diet such as Ensure, which contains all essential nutrients in a residue-free formula, may be prescribed. Enteral diets provide essential nutrients to the small intestine to support cell growth, but they are not always palatable.

Complementary and Alternative Therapy

The chronic nature of inflammatory bowel disease and the adverse effects of many prescribed treatments lead many clients with IBD to seek or use complementary and alternative therapies. The lack of research to determine the effectiveness and safety of most alternative therapies in the treatment of IBD, especially herbal supplements, limits the use of these therapies by conventional practitioners (CCFA, 2012b). Additionally, many complementary and alternative therapies used by clients with IBD may interact with prescribed medications. Nurses should instruct the client to discuss all potential therapies with the primary care provider.

Medications Inflammatory Bowel Disease

CLASSIFICATION AND DRUG EXAMPLES	MECHANISM OF ACTION	NURSING CONSIDERATIONS

Sulfasalazine
 	
Drug example:
Azulfidine®
	Sulfasalazine is an anti-inflammatory drug used for its local effect on the intestinal mucosa in IBD. The active part of the drug is mesalamine (5-aminosalicylic acid), which inhibits prostaglandin production in the bowel. Prostaglandin is an important mediator of the inflammatory process; blocking its production reduces inflammation.	■ Assess for contraindications, including a history of hypersensitivity to sulfonamides or salicylates.
		■ Assess baseline values for renal function tests, liver function tests, and CBC.
		■ Administer as ordered. Suppositories or retention enemas are to be administered at bedtime. Administer oral forms with a full glass of water.
		■ Have resuscitation equipment available in the event of anaphylactic response.
		■ Evaluate for therapeutic response, including reduced number of stools, reduced mucus and blood, and improved stool consistency.
		■ Monitor for the following possible adverse responses:
		  a. Skin rash, dermatitis, urticaria, or pruritus
		  b. Evidence of blood dyscrasias such as bleeding, easy bruising, or fever
		  c. Leukopenia, thrombocytopenia, hemolytic anemia, or angranulocytosis
		  d. Changes in urinary output or renal function studies
		  e. Evidence of hepatitis or myocarditis
		
		Health education for the client and family:
		■ Take oral preparations after meals to increase intestinal transit time.
		■ Drink at least 2 quarts of fluid per day to reduce the risk of kidney damage.
		■ Use sunscreen to prevent burns; this drug increases sensitivity to sun.
		■ Avoid use during pregnancy and lactation.
		■ Notify your doctor if you develop skin rash or hives, sore throat or mouth, bleeding gums, joint pain, easy bruising, or fever.

Mesalamine
 	
Drug examples:
Asacol®, Rowasa®
 	
Olsalazine
 	
Drug example:
Dipentum®
	Mesalamine and olsalazine also contain 5-aminosalicylic acid but cause fewer adverse effects than sulfasalazine. Their mechanism of action is the same as that of sulfasalazine. These drugs are available as suppositories, suspension for enema, or oral tablets.	■ Assess for possible contraindications such as pregnancy, lactation, or hypersensitivity.
		■ Administer as ordered. If more than one dose per day is ordered, space doses evenly over the 24-hour period.
		■ Evaluate for desired effects (as for sulfasalazine) and potential adverse effects, including:
		  a. Nausea, diarrhea, abdominal cramps, or flatulence
		  b. CNS effects
		  c. Rash or itching
		  d. Flulike symptoms, general malaise.
		
		Health education for the client and family:
		■ Teach the recommended method of administration, including how to insert rectal suppositories or administer a retention enema.
		■ Shake suspension forms well before using.
		■ Notify your doctor if adverse effects occur. Diarrhea is the most common side effect.

Corticosteroids
 	
Drug examples:
methylprednisolone (Medrol®, Solu-Medrol®)
prednisolone (Delta-Cortef®),
prednisone
	Glucocorticoids are hormones produced by the adrenal cortex. These hormones are necessary for the stress response. Cortisol, the main glucocorticoid, has potent anti-inflammatory effects. Corticosteroids are used to treat acute episodes of IBD. Because of their multiple and significant side effects, they are not used to maintain remission.	■ Contraindicated for clients with peptic ulcer disease, glaucoma or cataracts, diabetes, or psychiatric disorders.
		■ Obtain baseline vital signs and weight; monitor both routinely during therapy.
		■ Monitor for edema.
		■ Administer as ordered. For daily or alternate-day dosing, administer in the morning to reduce adrenal cortisone suppression.
		■ Monitor for desired effects: reduced diarrhea, less blood and mucus in the stool, and less abdominal cramping.
		■ Monitor for adverse effects:
		  a. Increased susceptibility to infection and masking of early signs of infection
		  b. Hyperglycemia
		  c. Hypokalemia
		  d. Edema, hypertension, and signs of heart failure
		  e. Peptic ulcer formation and possible GI hemorrhage

Medications **Inflammatory Bowel Disease** (continued)

CLASSIFICATION AND DRUG EXAMPLES	MECHANISM OF ACTION	NURSING CONSIDERATIONS
		f. Changes in mental status g. With long-term use: Cushingoid effects such as abnormal fat deposits in the face (moon face) and trunk (buffalo hump), muscle wasting and thin extremities, thinning of the skin, and osteoporosis *Health education for the client and family:* ■ Take as prescribed; do not change the dose or time of day. Do not stop the medication abruptly. The dose will be tapered gradually when the drug is discontinued. ■ Notify the physician if adverse or Cushingoid effects occur. ■ Take with food or milk to decrease GI effects. ■ Monitor weight. Notify the physician of a gain of more than 5 pounds. ■ Moderate salt intake and avoid foods and snacks high in sodium. Increase intake of foods high in potassium, such as fruits, vegetables, and lean meats. ■ Carry a card or wear a bracelet or tag at all times identifying corticosteroid use.

■ NURSING PROCESS

Although at this time inflammatory bowel disease cannot be predicted or prevented, effective management may help the client avoid complications of the disease. Stress the importance of complying with the prescribed treatment regimen and promptly reporting manifestations of exacerbations to the physician.

Assessment

A thorough assessment of the client with inflammatory bowel disease should include the following:

- *Health history*. Current manifestations, including onset, duration, severity (number of stools per day, presence of blood or mucus in stool, abdominal pain or cramping, tenesmus); usual diet, ability to maintain weight and nutrition, food intolerances; associated manifestations such as arthralgias, fatigue, malaise; current medications; previous treatment and diagnostic tests
- *Physical examination*. General appearance; weight; vital signs, including orthostatic vitals and temperature; abdominal assessment, including shape, contour, bowel sounds, palpation for tenderness and masses, presence of stoma or scars.

Diagnosis

When planning nursing care for the client with IBD, it is vital to consider the chronic, recurrent nature of the disorder. Potential nursing diagnoses include the following:

- *Risk for Deficient Fluid Volume*
- *Imbalanced Nutrition: Less Than Body Requirements*
- *Constipation*
- *Diarrhea*
- *Acute Pain*
- *Chronic Pain*
- *Disturbed Body Image*

(NANDA-I © 2012)

Planning

In planning care for the client with IBD, many considerations must be reviewed concerning client needs, including severity of disease process, age, frequency of exacerbations, and physical condition. Potential goals of care include the following:

- Client will achieve resolution of discomfort from symptoms such as diarrhea.
- Client will maintain adequate hydration.
- Client will maintain optimal nutritional status.
- Client will demonstrate positive, healthy coping skills.
- Client will describe appropriate home self-care, including administering medication, making dietary choices, and preventing exacerbations.

Implementation

Teaching is a major aspect of care. Diarrhea and disturbed body image are significant problems for the client with IBD. Children and adolescents often have specific needs, especially related to body image and the desire to fit in with peers. With severe disease, impaired nutrition must be considered a priority problem as well.

Monitor Fluid Volume

During an acute exacerbation of IBD, diarrhea can be frequent and painful. The frequency of defecation and associated abdominal pain and cramping may interfere with activities of daily living (ADLs) and increase the risk for fluid volume deficit and impaired skin integrity.

- Use a stool chart to record the frequency, amount, and color of stools. Measure and record liquid stool as output. The severity of diarrhea is an indicator of the severity of the disease and helps determine the need for fluid replacement.

- Monitor vital signs every 4 hours. Tachycardia, tachypnea, and fever may be indicators of fluid volume deficit.
- Weigh daily and record. Rapid weight loss (over days to a week) usually indicates fluid loss, whereas weight loss over weeks to months may indicate malnutrition.
- Assess for other indications of fluid deficit: warm, dry skin; poor skin turgor; dry, shiny mucous membranes; weakness; lethargy; complaints of thirst. The extent of fluid loss may not be readily evident with diarrhea, particularly if the client uses the bathroom without assistance. Systemic manifestations of fluid volume deficit may be the first indicators of the problem.
- Maintain bowel rest by keeping NPO or limiting oral intake to elemental feedings as indicated. Bowel rest during an acute exacerbation of IBD promotes healing and reduces diarrhea and other manifestations.
- Administer prescribed anti-inflammatory and antidiarrheal medications as indicated. Anti-inflammatory medications reduce the extent of bowel inflammation and diarrhea. Unless contraindicated, antidiarrheal medications help reduce fluid loss and increase comfort.
- Maintain fluid intake by mouth or intravenously as indicated. The client with IBD requires fluid to replace ongoing losses, as well as fluid to meet the usual daily needs of the body. If an elemental diet or total parenteral nutrition is prescribed, additional fluids may be required to meet fluid intake needs.
- Provide good skin care. Fluid deficit and tissue dehydration increase the risk for skin excoriations or breakdown.
- Assess perianal area for irritation or denuded skin from the diarrhea. Use gentle cleansing agents such as Peri-Wash or Tucks, diaper wipes, or cotton balls saturated with witch hazel. Apply a protective cream, such as a zinc oxide–based preparation, to protect skin from the irritating effects of diarrheal stool. Digestive enzymes in the stool are very corrosive, increasing the risk of breakdown of the skin when it is exposed to diarrheal stool.

SAFETY ALERT Observe stools for obvious blood and test for occult blood as indicated. Report grossly bloody stools, which may indicate hemorrhage and necessitate emergency surgery.

The intestinal swelling associated with IBD may cause constipation. In addition to promoting adequate fluid intake, instruct the client to take only laxatives recommended by the primary care provider. All laxatives should be avoided during a flare of the disease. Also explain nonpharmacologic interventions to help relieve constipation: These include mild exercise (30-minute walk), abdominal massage, and a warm bath (relaxes the rectal muscles). If these treatments are ineffective and the constipation continues for an extended time, contact the primary care provider. Inform the client to take constipation seriously. In addition to the abdominal discomfort it causes, it may be a symptom of impaction or bowel obstruction.

Promote Healthy Body Image

The client with inflammatory bowel disease may experience frustration at not being able to control, or even predict, fecal elimination, particularly when the disease is severe. Diarrhea can interfere with the ability to complete tasks; maintain employment or engage in social activities; and even meet basic needs such as eating, sleeping, and having sex. Body image can suffer as a result. Treatment of IBD, be it total colectomy with IPAA, ileostomy, or chronic corticosteroid therapy, also can affect the client's self image.

Body image is a major concern for children and adolescents with IBD. Corticosteroid therapy causes growth retardation and delayed sexual maturation. Encourage the client to discuss feelings about these side effects. If a permanent colostomy or ileostomy is required, the nurse can assist the client and family in understanding the need for surgical treatment.

- Accept the client's feelings and self-perception. Negating or denying the reality of the client's perception impairs trust.
- Encourage discussion of physical changes and their consequences as they relate to self-concept. This encouragement demonstrates acceptance and provides an opportunity for the client to describe the personal impact of the disease and its treatment.
- Encourage discussion about concerns regarding the effect of the disease or treatment on close personal relationships. This encouragement demonstrates understanding and provides an opportunity for the client to express feelings about the impact of the disease on relationships and significant others.
- To increase the client's sense of control over the disease and his or her future, encourage the client to make choices and decisions regarding care.
- Discuss possible treatment options and their effects openly and honestly. Open discussion allows for more informed decisions.
- Involve the client in care, teaching and demonstrating as needed. This involvement encourages and facilitates independence and decision making.
- Be accepting and nonjudgmental in providing care. Acceptance of the client despite potential embarrassment about odors or diarrhea enhances self-esteem.
- Arrange for interaction with other clients or groups of individuals with IBD or ostomies. The client may think that no

Lifespan Considerations Psychosocial Considerations for the Pediatric Client With IBD

Provide emotional support and counseling to help the pediatric client adjust to feeling "different" from peers. Inability to compete with peers and frequent absences from school can affect the client's self-esteem. Collaborate with parents in the client's care, and assist them in contacting their child's school to arrange for tutoring or home schooling in the case of extended absences from school.

one who hasn't experienced a similar problem can understand the client's feelings.

- Teach coping strategies (e.g., odor control and dietary modifications) and support their use. These strategies facilitate healthy adaptation to the disease.

Promote Adequate Nutritional Intake

Crohn disease can significantly alter the bowel's ability to absorb nutrients. In both forms of IBD, blood and protein-rich fluid may be lost in diarrheal stools. Malabsorption and continuing nutrient losses may cause multiple nutrient deficits that affect growth and development, healing, muscle mass, bone density, and electrolyte balances.

- Monitor laboratory results, including hemoglobin and hematocrit, serum electrolytes, and total serum protein and albumin levels. These studies provide an indicator of nutritional status.
- Provide the prescribed diet: high-kilocalorie, high-protein, low-fat diet with restricted milk and milk products if lactose intolerance is present. Calories and protein are important to replace lost nutrients. Fat restriction helps reduce diarrhea and nutrient loss, particularly when significant portions of the terminal ileum have been resected.

Client Teaching Dietary Instructions for Children With Inflammatory Bowel Disease

- Provide several small feedings each day, which may be better tolerated than three meals.
- Limit fiber intake to decrease intestine motility and inflammation. Peel fruits and avoid large quantities of whole grains and nuts.
- Offer high-calorie meals if the child is not eating well. If lactose intolerance is not a problem, offer cream soups, milkshakes, puddings, and custards.
- Provide liquid dietary supplements to ensure that protein and caloric requirements are met.
- Watch for foods that cause intestinal problems for the individual child and avoid them.
- Prevent mealtimes from becoming a reason for family strife. Seek help of nurses and dietitians if needed.

- Provide parenteral nutrition as necessary if the client is unable to absorb enteral nutrients. Parenteral nutrition can help reverse nutritional deficits and promote weight gain and healing in the client with acute manifestations.

Community-Based Care Home Care for the Client With IBD

Inflammatory bowel disease is a chronic condition for which the client provides daily self-management. For this reason, teaching is a vital component of care. Clients and family members require instruction for total parenteral nutrition if it is used, as well as information about care of a central venous catheter, including dressing changes and sterile and nonsterile techniques. Instructions should also include how to recognize signs of infection, how to handle infusion pumps and tubing, and how to measure the client's intake and output. Assist clients in obtaining the equipment and supplies necessary for care. During home visits and appointments for health care, have clients or parents demonstrate their mastery of care for the central venous catheter and their understanding of TPN techniques. Teach the client and family about the following topics:

- The type of IBD affecting the client, including the disease process, short- and long-term effects, relationship of stress to disease exacerbations, and manifestations of complications
- Prescribed medications, including drug names, desired effects, schedules for tapering the doses if ordered (as with corticosteroids), and possible side effects or adverse reactions and their management
- Recommended diet and the rationale for any specific restrictions
- Use of nutritional supplements such as Ensure to maintain weight and nutritional status
- Indicators of malabsorption and impaired nutrition; recommendations for self-care and when to seek medical intervention
- If discharged with a central catheter and home parenteral nutrition, written and verbal instructions on catheter care, troubleshooting, and TPN administration (have the

client and a family member demonstrate catheter care and TPN maintenance.)

- Importance of maintaining a fluid intake of at least 2–3 quarts per day, increasing fluid intake during warm weather, exercise, or strenuous work, and when fever is present
- Increased risk for colorectal cancer and importance of regular bowel exams
- Risks and benefits of various treatment options.

If surgery is planned or has been done, include the following topics in home care instructions:

- IPAA or ileostomy care as indicated
- Suppliers from which to obtain ostomy supplies
- Use of nonprescription drugs (e.g., enteric-coated and timed-release capsules) that may not be adequately absorbed before being eliminated through the ileostomy
- Community and national ostomy support groups.

Provide referrals to a dietary consultant or nutritionist, a community healthcare agency, home care services, and home intravenous care services as indicated. In addition, suggest the following resources:

- Crohn and Colitis Foundation of America
- The Israel Foundation for Crohn Disease and Ulcerative Colitis
- United Ostomy Associations of America, Inc.

Providing adequate stress reduction may be helpful in the control of IBD. Teach relaxation techniques such as deep breathing, progressive tensing and relaxing of muscles, and visualization of favorite places. Encourage busy school-age children and teens to have quiet and restful times each day, in addition to periods of physical activity.

- Arrange for dietary consultation. Consider food preferences as allowed. Providing preferred foods in the prescribed diet increases intake and supports nutritional status.
- Provide or administer elemental enteral nutrition and supplements as ordered. Elemental enteral nutritional supplements support healing while providing for bowel rest. They can replace losses and improve nutritional status more rapidly than diet alone.
- Include family members, the primary food preparer in particular, in teaching and dietary discussions. Families can reinforce teaching and help the client maintain the required restrictions or kilocalorie intake.

Evaluation

Expected outcomes of nursing care for the client with IBD include the following:

- The client demonstrates absence of GI distress.
- The client and family demonstrate successful management of medications without side effects.
- The client demonstrates no signs or symptoms of infection.
- The client verbalizes attainment of a positive body image.
- The client demonstrates integration of relaxation techniques into daily life.

NURSING CARE PLAN   A Client With Ulcerative Colitis

Cortez Lewis is a 42-year-old real estate agent and mother of three school-age children. She has had ulcerative colitis for 18 years and has been treated with prednisone and sulfasalazine. Over the past 4 months, she has been having abdominal pain and cramping and frequent bloody diarrhea stools. During the same period, she has lost 9 kg (20 lb), and she has had difficulty maintaining her career. She recently developed several lesions of the lower leg, identified as erythema nodosum. A recent colonoscopy revealed extensive involvement of the entire colon. On admission, Ms. Lewis states, "I'm tired of fighting this disease. I'm a prisoner in my home because of the diarrhea." She is admitted for a total proctocolectomy and IPAA.

ASSESSMENT

Janet Wheeler, RN, completes the admission assessment. Ms. Lewis now weighs 52.2 kg (115 lb). She complains of abdominal cramping, pain, and frequent bloody diarrhea stools. Several reddened lesions are noted on her lower legs. Physical assessment findings include temperature 36.6°C (98°F) oral, pulse 72 bpm, respirations 20/min, and BP 104/72 mmHg. Skin is cool and pale. Abnormal laboratory findings include hemoglobin 7.3 g/dL (normal 12–15 g/dL), hematocrit 23.3% (normal 36%–46%), WBCs 15,580/mm³ (normal 4,500–10,000/mm³), platelet count 995,000/mm³ (normal 150,000–400,000/mm³), serum protein 4.6 g/dL (normal 6–8 g/dL), and serum albumin 2.4 g/dL (normal 3.5–5.0 g/dL). Preparation for surgery is begun.

DIAGNOSES

- *Imbalanced Nutrition: Less Than Body Requirements* related to impaired absorption
- *Diarrhea* related to inflammation of bowel
- *Risk for Deficient Fluid Volume* related to abnormal fluid loss
- *Impaired Tissue Integrity* related to drainage from temporary ileostomy
- *Acute Pain* related to surgical intervention
- *Sexual Dysfunction* related to temporary ileostomy

(NANDA-I © 2012)

PLANNING

- Client will resume prescribed diet within 5 days after surgery.
- Client will demonstrate normal fecal elimination through the temporary ileostomy.
- Client will maintain adequate fluid balance.
- Client will demonstrate appropriate ostomy care prior to discharge.
- Client will report a tolerable level of discomfort.
- Client will verbalize feelings about sexuality and acknowledge importance of discussing sexual issues with husband.

IMPLEMENTATION

- Discuss dietary modifications related to nutritional status and presence of ileostomy. Provide referral to dietitian for diet planning and teaching.
- Teach manifestations of dehydration and importance of maintaining a high fluid intake.
- Teach how to empty and change ostomy pouch of choice.
- Teach stoma and peristomal skin assessment with each pouch change.
- Teach food blockage management.
- Refer to local chapter of the United Ostomy Association.
- Provide list of local medical suppliers for ostomy appliances.

EVALUATION

On discharge, Ms. Lewis is caring for her ileostomy by demonstrating her ability to empty, rinse, and change the pouch. The enterostomal therapy (ET) nurse has provided written and verbal instructions on ileostomy care. Ms. Lewis verbalizes her understanding of the recommended diet and the need to limit high-fiber food intake and avoid enteric-coated and timed-release medications. The ET nurse has discussed sexual aspects of having an ileostomy and has given Ms. Lewis a booklet, "Sex and the Female Ostomate," available through the United Ostomy Association. Ms. Lewis is looking forward to the planned surgery to close the temporary ileostomy.

CRITICAL THINKING

1. *Why is the client with an ileostomy at risk for dehydration? How can Ms. Lewis monitor her fluid status at home?*
2. *Why were Ms. Lewis's hemoglobin and hematocrit low on admission? If her hemoglobin had been low but her hematocrit normal on admission, what might be the explanation?*
3. *Outline a teaching plan that could be given to clients for home care of an ileostomy.*
4. *Develop a care plan for Ms. Lewis for the nursing diagnosis Risk for Impaired Skin Integrity.*

▲ REVIEW **Inflammatory Bowel Disease**

RELATE Link the Concepts and Exemplars

Linking the exemplar of irritable bowel disease with the concept of stress and coping:

1. What stress management techniques might you teach an adolescent diagnosed with IBD?

2. You are caring for a client diagnosed with IBD who was just informed of the need for a colectomy with creation of an ileostomy. The client is very upset and tells the doctor that death is preferable to walking around with "poop coming out of my stomach." What can you do to help this client cope with the idea of an ileostomy?

Linking the exemplar of irritable bowel disease with the concept of elimination:

3. The client with IBD is about to have surgery to create an ileostomy. The client asks, "Will I need to wear a bag all of the time?" How do you respond? Explain your answer.

4. If the client with IBD is to have a colostomy instead of an ileostomy, how do you respond to the same question: "Will I need to wear a bag all of the time?" Explain your answer.

READY Go to Companion Skills Manual

REFER Go to Pearson Nursing Student Resources
nursing.pearsonhighered.com

- Additional review material
- Chart 1: Nursing Care of the Client Having an Ileostomy

REFLECT Case Study

Jodi Thompson is a 17-year-old who is a junior in high school. She is a cheerleader for the school, a member of the debate team, and an honor student. Jodi lives with her mother, Marie, and her two brothers, George (age 10) and Joe (age 8). Jodi's mom works full time, so Jodi is responsible for her brothers' care after school or for arranging care. Jodi's dad died of cirrhosis of the liver when Jodi was 10. Jodi is also responsible for caring for her brothers when her mom works weekends, and she is responsible for getting them off to school in the morning. Jodi is planning to take the SAT exam in a few weeks because she is interested in becoming a dentist. Jodi has come to the clinic today because she has been having abdominal pain and frequent loose stools.

1. What risk factors for inflammatory bowel disease are apparent in Jodi's history?

2. What nutritional teaching will you plan for Jodi?

3. Create a plan of care for Jodi.

EXEMPLAR 10.4   **Nephritis**

EXEMPLAR KEY TERMS
Acute postinfectious glomerulonephritis, *669*
Glomerulonephritis, *669*
Goodpasture syndrome, *670*
Lupus nephritis, *670*
Nephritis, *669*
Plasmapheresis, *673*

EXEMPLAR LEARNING OUTCOMES
After reading about this exemplar, you will be able to:

1. Describe the pathophysiology, etiology, clinical manifestations, and direct and indirect causes of nephritis.

2. Identify risk factors and prevention methods associated with nephritis.

3. Illustrate the nursing process in providing culturally competent care across the life span for individuals with nephritis.

4. Formulate priority nursing diagnoses appropriate for an individual with nephritis.

5. Summarize therapies used by interdisciplinary teams in the collaborative care of an individual with nephritis.

6. Plan evidence-based care for an individual with nephritis and his or her family in collaboration with other members of the healthcare team.

7. Evaluate expected outcomes for an individual with nephritis.

▶ OVERVIEW

Nephritis is an inflammation of the kidneys. The different classifications of nephritis are based on area of involvement or etiology. One example is **glomerulonephritis**, which is an inflammation of the glomerular capillary membrane. Another is **acute postinfectious glomerulonephritis (APIGN)**, which may develop as a response to a group A beta-hemolytic streptococcal infection of the skin (impetigo) or pharynx (strep throat). Other infecting organisms that cause APIGN are *Staphylococcus*, *Pneumococcus*, and *Coxsackie* virus. Clients with systemic lupus erythematosus are also at high risk for developing nephritis (called *lupus nephritis*) as a result of autoimmune attacks on the kidney.

▶ PATHOPHYSIOLOGY AND ETIOLOGY

In *acute proliferative glomerulonephritis*, glomerular damage occurs as a result of an immune complex reaction that localizes on the glomerular capillary wall. The lodging of antibody–antigen complexes in the glomeruli leads to inflammation and obstruction. The glomerular membranes are thickened, and the obstruction of capillaries in the glomeruli by damaged tissue cells leads to a decreased glomerular filtration rate (GFR). Vascular permeability increases allow protein, red blood cells, and red cell casts to be excreted. The retention of sodium and water expands the intravascular and interstitial compartments, resulting in the characteristic finding of edema (**Figure 10–10 ●**).

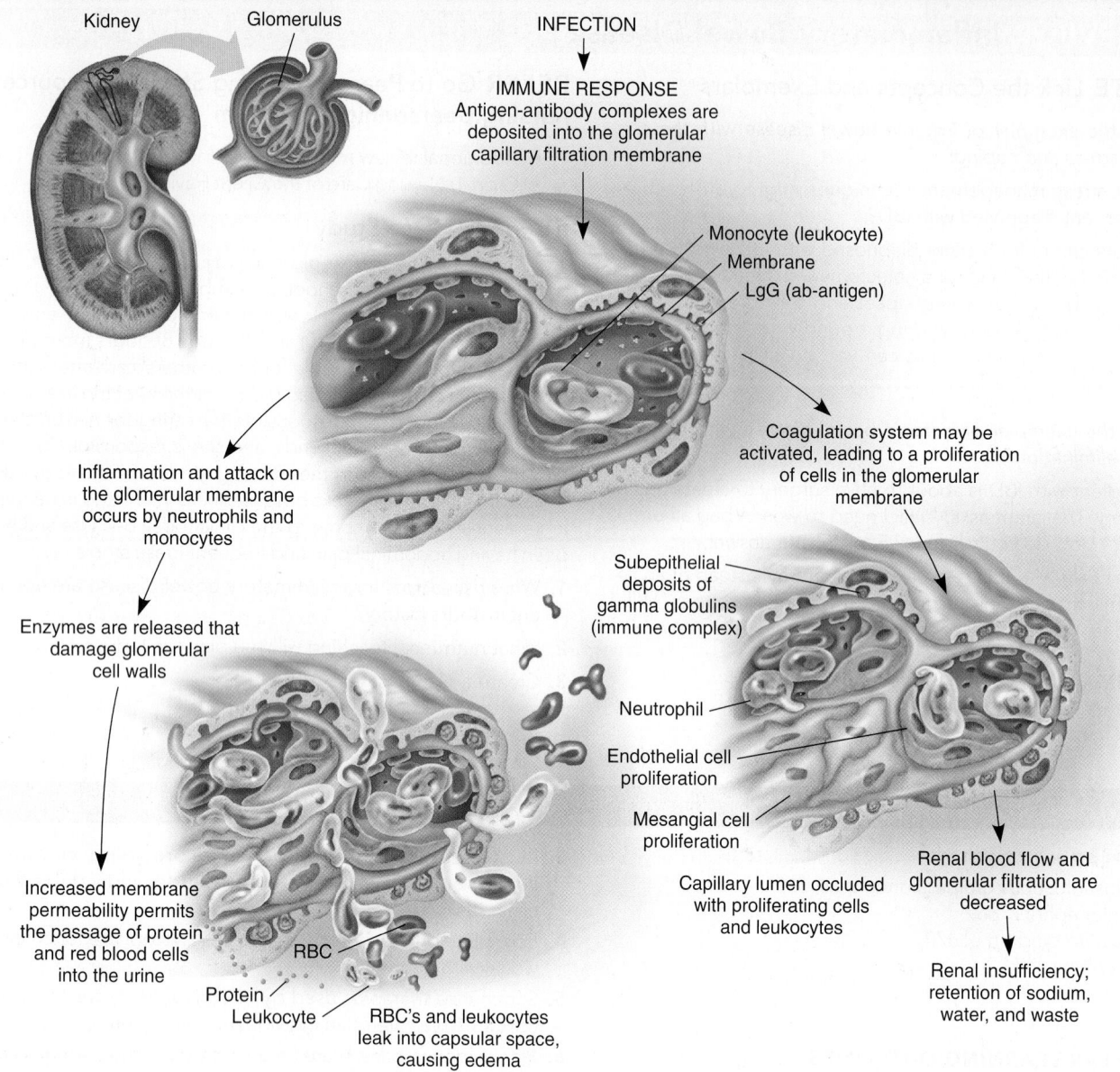

Figure 10–10 ● Infection from group A beta-hemolytic *Streptococcus* leads to an immune response that causes inflammation and damage to glomeruli. Protein and red blood cells are allowed to pass through the glomeruli. Obstruction reduces blood flow to the glomeruli, and damaged cells and renal insufficiency lead to retention of sodium, water, and waste.

Chronic glomerulonephritis is typically the end stage of other glomerular disorders, such as rapidly progressive glomerulonephritis (RPGN), lupus nephritis, and diabetic nephropathy. In many cases, however, no previous glomerular disease has been identified. Slow, progressive destruction of the glomeruli and a gradual decline in renal function are characteristic of chronic glomerulonephritis. The kidneys decrease in size symmetrically, and their surfaces become granular or roughened. Eventually, entire nephrons are lost. Symptoms develop insidiously, and the disease often is not recognized until signs of renal failure develop.

Lupus nephritis is one of the most severe consequences of systemic lupus erythematosus (SLE), an inflammatory autoimmune disorder affecting the connective tissue of the body (see Focus on Diversity and Culture). Approximately 60% of SLE clients develop nephritis, and as many as 22% advance to end stage renal disease. Therefore nephritis is a major cause of mor-

bidity and mortality associated with SLE (Schwartzman-Morris & Putterman, 2012). Immune complexes that form in the glomerular capillary wall are the usual trigger for glomerular injury in SLE. Manifestations of lupus nephritis range from microscopic hematuria to massive proteinuria. Its progression may be slow and chronic or fulminant, with a sudden onset and the rapid development of renal failure.

Goodpasture syndrome is a rare autoimmune disorder of unknown etiology. It is characterized by formation of antibodies to the glomerular basement membrane. These antibodies may also bind to alveolar basement membranes, damaging alveoli and causing pulmonary hemorrhage. Goodpasture syndrome occurs most commonly in clients between the ages of 20 and 30 and again after the age of 60. It affects men more than women and is most prevalent in Whites (NKF, 2009b).

Although the glomeruli may be nearly normal in appearance and function in Goodpasture syndrome, extensive cell proliferation and crescent formation characteristic of RPGN are common. Renal manifestations include hematuria, proteinuria, and edema. Progression to acute renal failure is frequently rapid. Alveolar membrane damage can lead to mild or life-threatening pulmonary hemorrhage. Cough, shortness of breath, and hemoptysis (bloody sputum) are early respiratory manifestations.

Etiology

Each form of nephritis has a distinct etiology. Lupus nephritis is the result of the inflammatory process caused by SLE and is an autoimmune disorder. Glomerulonephritis can result from infection, diabetes mellitus, or SLE. Tubulointerstitial nephritis results from injury to the renal tubules and interstitium, often secondary to glomerular damage (due to drugs, toxins, or radiation) and renovascular disease.

Risk Factors

Clients with diabetes mellitus and/or hypertension are at much higher risk for nephritis secondary to vascular damage to the fragile vessels in the nephron. Infections can travel from the bladder to the kidney or cause scarring that results in urine retention that can damage the nephron. Drug abuse and chronic overuse of over-the-counter painkillers increase risk of nephritis as well.

Nephritis can also result from prematurity, trauma, or family history of kidney disease. Diseases such as SLE, sickle cell anemia, AIDS, and congestive heart failure can damage the kidney, causing nephritis.

Prevention

The exact cause of nephritis is unknown. Preventing viral infections through practicing good hygiene habits, maintaining adequate diabetes and blood pressure control, quitting smoking, and maintaining a healthy body weight reduce the risk of developing this disease (NKF, 2009a).

▶ CLINICAL MANIFESTATIONS

Many clients with acute glomerulonephritis are asymptomatic. The onset is abrupt in other clients, with flank or midabdominal pain, irritability, malaise, and fever. Microscopic hematuria is present in nearly all cases, and gross hematuria, resulting in tea-colored urine, is found in up to 50% of cases and may last for 1–2 weeks. Mild periorbital edema occurs early, along with dependent edema of the feet and ankles. Edema may progress in severity to cause pleural effusion manifested as dyspnea, cough, and crackles (Osborn et al., 2013). Acute hypertension may cause an encephalopathy that includes headache, nausea, vomiting, irritability, lethargy, and seizures. Oliguria may or may not be present.

Acute postinfection glomerulonephritis is characterized by an abrupt onset of hematuria, proteinuria, salt and water retention, and evidence of azotemia (abnormally high levels of nitrogen waste products in the blood) occurring 10–14 days after the initial infection. The urine often appears brown or cola-colored. Salt and water retention increases extracellular fluid volume, leading to hypertension and edema. The edema is noted primarily in the face, particularly around the eyes. Dependent edema, affecting the hands and upper extremities in particular, may also be noted. Other manifestations are fatigue, anorexia, nausea and vomiting, and headache.

The older adult may have fewer apparent symptoms. Nausea, malaise, arthralgias, and proteinuria are common manifestations; hypertension and edema are seen less often. Pulmonary infiltrates may occur early in the disorder, often due to worsening of a preexisting condition such as heart failure.

▶ COLLABORATION

Collaborative care of the client with nephritis may include a nephrologist, primary care provider, nurses, pharmacists, dieticians or nutritionists, and (in the case of school-age children) parents, teachers, and the school nurse. The nurse's role includes client teaching, follow up, and coordination of referral services and communication between members of the healthcare team. Treatment focuses on relief of symptoms and supportive therapy.

Diagnostic Tests

Laboratory and diagnostic testing is valuable for identifying the cause of nephritis and to evaluate kidney function.

The following studies may be ordered to help identify the etiology:

- ***Throat or skin cultures*** detect infection by group A beta hemolytic streptococci. Although poststreptococcal glomerulonephritis typically follows the acute infection by 1–2 weeks, treatment to eradicate any remaining organisms is initiated to minimize antibody production.
- ***Antistreptolysin O (ASO) titer*** and other blood tests detect streptococcal *exoenzymes* (bacterial enzymes that stimulate the immune response in acute postinfection glomerulonephritis). Other titers such as antistreptokinase (ASK) and anti-deoxyribonuclease B (ADNAase B) may be obtained as well.
- ***Erythrocyte sedimentation rate (ESR)*** is a general indicator of inflammatory response. It may be elevated in acute postinfection glomerulonephritis and in lupus nephritis.

Clinical Manifestations and Therapies **Nephritis**

ETIOLOGY	CLINICAL MANIFESTATIONS	CLINICAL THERAPIES
Salt and water retention	■ Hypertension ■ Hematuria ■ Mild to moderate edema	■ Diuretics ■ Antihypertensives ■ Sodium restriction ■ Low protein diet
Severe hypertension	■ Extremely high blood pressure with cerebral dysfunction	■ Emergency care that includes IV diazoxide, hydralazine, or labetalol
Progressive edema, acute inflammatory processes	■ Ascites ■ Pulmonary effusion	■ Immunosuppressive therapy (cyclophosphamide, azathroprine) ■ Corticosteroids ■ Sodium restriction
Encephalopathy resulting from acute hypertension	■ Headache ■ Nausea and vomiting ■ Irritability	■ Antihypertensives ■ Analgesics ■ Additional therapies as warranted
Presence of infection	■ Salt and water retention ■ Fever ■ Malaise ■ Edema	■ Antibiotics ■ Bed rest ■ Sodium restriction ■ Antipyretics

■ *KUB* (kidney, ureter, bladder) *abdominal x-ray* may be done to evaluate kidney size and to rule out other causes of the client's manifestations. The kidneys may be enlarged in acute nephritis, whereas bilateral small kidneys are typical of late chronic glomerulonephritis.

■ *Kidney scan*, a nuclear medicine procedure, allows visualization of the kidney after intravenous administration of a radioisotope. In glomerular diseases, the uptake and excretion of the radioactive material are delayed.

■ *Biopsy,* a microscopic examination of kidney tissue, is essential and the most reliable diagnostic procedure for glomerular disorders. Biopsy helps determine the type of nephritis, the prognosis, and the appropriate treatment. Renal biopsy is usually done percutaneously, by inserting a biopsy needle through the skin into the kidney to obtain a tissue sample. Open biopsy, which requires surgery, may also be done.

The following studies are used to evaluate kidney function:

■ *BUN* measures urea nitrogen, the end product of protein metabolism, which is created by the breakdown and metabolism of both dietary and body proteins. Urea is eliminated from the body by filtration in the glomerulus; minimal amounts are reabsorbed in the renal tubules. Glomerular diseases interfere with filtration and elimination of urea nitrogen, causing blood levels to rise. Increased protein catabolism (destruction), which may occur with GI bleeding or tissue breakdown, can also raise BUN.

✱ *Go to* **nursing.pearsonhighered.com** *for a list of normal BUN values in Appendix B.*

Levels up to 50 mg/dL or 17.7 mmol/L indicate mild azotemia, and levels higher than 100 mg/dL or 35.7 mmol/L indicate severe renal impairment.

■ *Serum creatinine* measures the amount of creatinine in the blood. Creatinine also is a metabolic by-product, produced in relatively constant amounts by skeletal muscles. It is excreted entirely by the kidneys, making serum creatinine a good indicator of kidney function. Normal values are lower in the older adult because of decreased muscle mass. Levels greater than 4 mg/dL indicate serious impairment of renal function.

■ *Urine creatinine* is also an indicator of renal function and the glomerular filtration rate (GFR). Urine creatinine levels decrease when renal function is impaired because creatinine is not effectively eliminated from the body.

■ *Creatinine clearance* is a specific indicator of renal function used to evaluate the GFR. The *clearance,* or amount of blood cleared of creatinine in 1 minute, depends on the amount and pressure of blood being filtered and the filtering ability of the glomeruli. Levels normally decline with age as the GFR decreases in the older adult. Disorders such as nephritis affect glomerular filtration, decreasing the creatinine clearance.

■ *Serum electrolytes* are evaluated because impaired kidney function alters their excretion. Monitoring serum electrolytes is particularly important to prevent complications associated with imbalances.

■ *Urinalysis* often shows RBCs and proteins in the urine of clients with a glomerular disorder. These substances, normally too large to enter glomerular filtrate, escape due to increased porosity of glomerular capillaries in glomerular disorders. A 24-hour urine specimen is used to determine the amount of protein in the urine.

Pharmacologic Therapy

Although no drugs are available to cure glomerular disorders, medications are used to treat underlying disorders, reduce inflammation, and manage the symptoms.

Edema and mild to moderate hypertension should be treated with sodium restriction and a diuretic such as furosemide (Lau & Wyatt, 2005). Immediate emergency care is needed for severe hypertension with cerebral dysfunction; medication such as diazoxide or hydralazine is administered intravenously. Antibiotics are prescribed for the client with acute postinfection glomerulonephritis to eradicate any remaining bacteria, removing the stimulus for antibody production. Nephrotoxic antibiotics, such as the aminoglycoside antibiotics and some cephalosporins, are avoided.

Aggressive immunosuppressive therapy is used to treat acute inflammatory processes such as RPGN, Goodpasture syndrome, and exacerbations of SLE. When begun early, immunosuppressive therapy significantly reduces the risk of end-stage renal disease and renal failure. Prednisone, a glucocorticoid, is prescribed in relatively large doses of 1 mg per kilogram of body weight per day (e.g., a 160-pound man would receive 70–75 mg per day) and tapered according to response. Other immunosuppressive agents such as cyclophosphamide (Cytoxan), azathioprine (Imuran) or mycophenolate (Cellcept) (Fauci et al., 2009) are prescribed in conjunction with corticosteroids. Corticosteroid use in acute postinfection glomerulonephritis may actually worsen the condition, so it is avoided.

ACE inhibitors or angiotensin receptor blockers (ARBs) may be ordered to reduce protein loss associated with nephrotic syndrome. These drugs reduce proteinuria and slow the progression of renal failure. They have a protective effect on the kidney in clients with diabetic nephropathy.

Antihypertensives may be prescribed to maintain blood pressure within normal levels. Blood pressure management is important because systemic and renal hypertension is associated with a poorer prognosis in clients with glomerular disorders.

Nonpharmacologic Therapy

Bed rest may be ordered during acute postinfection glomerulonephritis. Fluid requirements are determined by careful monitoring of urinary output, weight, blood pressure, and serum electrolytes. Initially, only insensible fluid losses are replaced until the status of renal function is known. Dietary restriction of sodium and potassium intake may be necessary; with severe azotemia, protein intake may have to be limited.

When the edema of nephrotic syndrome is significant or the client is hypertensive, sodium intake may be restricted to 1–2 g per day. Dietary protein may be restricted if azotemia is present. When proteins are restricted, those included in the diet should be complete or high-value proteins. Complete proteins supply the essential amino acids required for growth and tissue maintenance; they include milk, eggs, cheese, meats, poultry, fish, and soy. Incomplete proteins either lack one or more essential amino acids or lack adequate proportions. They include breads, cereals and grains, legumes, seeds, and nuts.

Plasma exchange therapy (**plasmapheresis**), a procedure to remove damaging antibodies from the plasma, is used in conjunction with immunosuppressive therapy to treat RPGN and Goodpasture syndrome. Plasma and glomerular-damaging antibodies are removed with a blood cell separator. The RBCs are then returned to the client along with albumin or human plasma to replace the plasma removed. This procedure is usually done in a series of treatments. It is not without risk, and informed consent is required. Potential complications of plasma exchange therapy include those associated with intravenous catheters, fluid volume shifts, and altered coagulation.

◼ NURSING PROCESS

Nursing care is supportive and educational. Monitoring renal function and fluid volume status are key components of care, as is protecting the client from infection. Both manifestations of glomerular disorders and their treatment can interfere with a client's ability to maintain usual roles and responsibilities.

Assessment

Focused assessment data related to glomerular disorders include the following:

- *Health history.* Complaints of facial or peripheral edema or weight gain, fatigue, nausea and vomiting, headache, general malaise, abdominal or flank pain; cough or shortness of breath; changes in amount, color, or character of urine (e.g., frothy urine); history of skin or pharyngeal streptococcal infection, diabetes, SLE, or kidney disease; current medications
- *Physical examination.* General appearance; vital signs; weight; presence of periorbital, facial, or peripheral edema; skin for lesions, infection; throat to obtain culture as indicated; urine specimen for color, character, and odor.

Diagnosis

Nursing diagnoses that may apply to the client with nephritis include the following:

- *Risk for Infection*
- *Excess Fluid Volume*
- *Risk for Impaired Skin Integrity*
- *Imbalanced Nutrition: Less Than Body Requirements*
- *Fatigue*
- *Ineffective Role Performance.*

(NANDA-I © 2012)

Planning

Goals of nursing care should be developmentally appropriate and may include the following:

- Client will demonstrate urinary output of at least 0.5 mL/kg/hr.
- Client will demonstrate dietary intake that adequately meets nutritional and caloric needs.
- Client will demonstrate no signs or symptoms of infection.
- Client will demonstrate no alterations in skin integrity.

For pediatric clients, the following additional goals may be appropriate:

- Client will remain on track to complete educational requirements.
- Client will engage in diversional activities during periods of bed rest and activity restriction.

Implementation

Bed rest is required during the acute phase. Nursing care focuses on monitoring fluid status, preventing infection, preventing skin breakdown, meeting nutritional needs, and providing emotional support to the client and family.

Prevent Infection

Impaired renal function puts the client at risk for infection. Immunosuppressive drugs may mask the presence of infection. Monitor for signs of infection, including fever, increased malaise, and an elevated WBC count, which may be an early indicator of infection.

Avoid or minimize invasive procedures. If catheterization is required, use sterile intermittent straight catheterization or maintain a closed drainage system for an indwelling catheter. Prevent urine reflux from the drainage system to the bladder or the bladder to the kidneys by ensuring a patent gravity flow system.

Instruct the family in good hand hygiene. Limit visitors and screen for upper respiratory infections. Screen family members for the presence of streptococcal infection and, if necessary, refer for treatment.

> **SAFETY ALERT**
> Monitor vital signs, temperature, and mental status every 4 hours. Fever and elevated WBCs are common indicators of infection; anti-inflammatory drugs, however, may moderate this response. Clients taking anti-inflammatory drugs may exhibit tachycardia, increasing lethargy, or confusion as the initial signs of infection.

Protect Skin Integrity

Dependent areas or areas prone to pressure are vulnerable to skin breakdown. Turn the hospitalized client frequently. Pad bony prominences or susceptible areas with sheepskin, or protect skin with a transparent dressing. Make sure the client's bed is free of crumbs. Keep sheets tight and free of wrinkles.

Promote Nutritional Balance

A team approach is often needed to meet the client's nutritional needs. In most cases, the client follows a "no added salt" and low-protein diet. Anorexia presents the greatest challenge to meeting daily nutritional requirements during the acute phase of the disease. To increase the client's appetite, encourage family members to bring the client's favorite foods from home, serve age-appropriate quantities to children, and allow the client to eat with other clients or with family members.

Monitor and Maintain Fluid Volume Balance

Monitor vital signs, fluid and electrolyte status, and intake and output. Hypovolemia can occur as a result of fluid shifting from vascular to interstitial spaces despite the outward clinical signs of excess fluid retention. Monitor the degree of ascites by measuring abdominal girth. Document urine specific gravity.

Maintain fluid restriction as ordered. Offer ice chips (in limited and measured amounts) and frequent mouth care to relieve thirst. Make sure family members and visitors understand the need to limit fluids to prevent excessive intake. Arrange dietary consultation regarding sodium- or protein-restricted diets.

> **SAFETY ALERT**
> Carefully monitor and regulate intravenous infusions; include fluid used to dilute IV medications as intake. Significant "hidden" fluid intake can occur with intravenous medication administration.

Prevent Unnecessary Fatigue

Fatigue is a common manifestation of nephritis. Anemia, loss of plasma proteins, headache, anorexia, and nausea compound this fatigue. The maintenance of usual physical and mental activities may be impaired.

Schedule activities and procedures to provide adequate rest and energy conservation. Assist with ADLs as needed. Reduce energy demands with frequent small meals and short periods of activity. Limit the number of visitors and visit length. Discuss with the client and family the relationship between fatigue and the disease process.

Promote Healthy Self-Esteem

The manifestations and treatment of nephritis can affect the maintenance of usual roles and activities. Fatigue and muscle weakness may limit physical and social activities. Bed rest or activity limitations may be ordered to minimize the degree of proteinuria. If azotemia is present, malaise, nausea, and mental status changes can interfere with role function. Facial and periorbital edema affects the client's self-esteem and may lead to isolation.

Encourage client self-care and participation in decision making. Support coping skills, helping the client identify personal strengths. Discuss the effect of the disease and treatments on roles and relationships, helping the client identify potential changes in roles, relationships, and lifestyle. Help the client and family develop a plan for alternative behaviors and relationships, encouraging the client to maintain usual roles to the extent possible.

Provide accurate and optimistic information about the disorder and its short- and long-term effects. Evaluate the need for additional support and social services for the client and family. Provide referrals as indicated.

Evaluation

Expected outcomes of nursing care include the following:

- The client maintains or regains normal urine output.
- The client develops no areas of redness, abrasions, or skin breakdown over pressure points.
- The client's temperature remains within normal limits, and client is free of secondary infection.
- The client maintains preillness weight and tolerates daily intake that meets nutritional requirements.
- The client takes medications as prescribed.
- The client's sodium and potassium levels reflect adherence to dietary restrictions.

Community-Based Care   Home Care for Clients With Acute Nephritis

Acute postinfectious glomerulonephritis typically resolves following appropriate treatment. Other types of nephritis, however, may be progressive. In either case, the course of the disorder is difficult and may be lengthy, sometimes ranging from months to years. Self-management is essential. Provide instructions for the client and family, including the following topics:

- Information about the disease and the prognosis
- Prescribed treatment, including activity and diet restrictions; the use and potential effects, both beneficial and adverse, of all medications

- Risks, manifestations, prevention, and management of complications such as edema and infection
- Signs, symptoms, and implications of improving or declining renal function
- Measures to prevent further kidney damage, such as avoiding nephrotoxic drugs
- Community resources such as home care providers, support groups, and (for children) home school teachers or tutoring programs

NURSING CARE PLAN   A Client With Acute Nephritis

Jung-Lin Chang is a 23-year-old graduate student in biology. He presents at the university health center with brown and foamy urine. The physician admits him to the infirmary and orders a throat culture, ASO titer, CBC, BUN, serum creatinine, and urinalysis.

ASSESSMENT

Connie King, the nurse admitting Mr. Chang, notes that his history is essentially negative for past kidney or urinary problems. He relates having had a "pretty bad" sore throat a couple of weeks before admission. However, it was during midterms, so he took a few antibiotics he had from a previous bout of strep throat, increased his fluids, and did not see a doctor. The sore throat resolved and he felt well until noticing the change in his urine. He admits that his eyes seemed a little puffy, but he thought this was due to lack of sleep and fatigue. He has eaten little the past 2 days, but was not alarmed because his food intake is irregular most of the time.

Physical assessment findings include temperature 37.1°C (98.8°F) oral, pulse 98 bpm, respirations 18/min, and BP 136/90 mmHg. Weight 75 kg (165 lb), up from his normal of 72.5 kg (160 lb). BUN 42 mg/dL, serum creatinine 2.1 mg/dL. Urinalysis reveals the presence of protein, RBCs, and RBC casts. A subsequent 24-hour urine protein analysis shows 1025 mg of protein (normal 25–150 mg/24 hours).

The physician diagnoses acute postinfection glomerulonephritis and places Mr. Chang on bed rest with bathroom privileges. The physician orders fluid restriction (1200 mL/day) and a restricted sodium and protein diet.

DIAGNOSES

- *Excess Fluid Volume* related to plasma protein deficit and sodium and water retention
- *Imbalanced Nutrition: Less Than Body Requirements* related to anorexia
- *Anxiety* related to prescribed activity restriction
- *Ineffective Therapeutic Regimen Management* related to lack of information about nephritis and treatment

(NANDA-I © 2012)

PLANNING

- Client will maintain blood pressure within normal limits.
- Client will return to usual weight with no evidence of edema.
- Client will consume adequate calories following prescribed dietary limitations.
- Client will verbalize reduced anxiety regarding ability to continue studies.
- Client will demonstrate an understanding of acute nephritis and the prescribed treatment regimen.

IMPLEMENTATION

- Take vital signs every 4 hours; notify physician of significant changes.
- Weigh daily; monitor and record intake and output.
- Schedule fluids, allowing 650 mL on day shift, 450 mL on evening shift, and 100 mL on night shift.
- Arrange dietary consultation to plan a diet that includes preferred foods as allowed.
- Provide small meals with high-carbohydrate between-meal snacks.

- Encourage Mr. Chang to talk about his condition and its potential effects.
- Assist with problem solving and exploring options for maintaining studies.
- Enlist friends and family to listen and provide support.
- Teach Mr. Chang and his family about acute nephritis and the prescribed treatment.
- Instruct in appropriate antibiotic use.

EVALUATION

Mr. Chang is released from the infirmary after 4 days. He decides to return to his parents' home for the 6–12 weeks of convalescence prescribed by his doctor. Mr. Chang's renal function gradually returns to normal with no further azotemia and minimal proteinuria after 4 months. He verbalizes understanding the relationship between the strep throat, his inappropriate use of antibiotics, and the nephritis. He says, "I may not always remember to take every pill on time in the future, but I sure won't save them for the next time again!"

(continued on next page)

NURSING CARE PLAN (continued)

CRITICAL THINKING

1. How did Mr. Chang's use of "a few" previously prescribed antibiotics to treat his sore throat affect his risk for developing acute postinfection glomerulonephritis?
2. What additional risk factors did Mr. Chang have for developing nephritis?
3. The initial manifestations of acute postinfection glomerulonephritis and RPGN are very similar. What diagnostic test would the physician use to make the differential diagnosis? Develop a plan of care for a client undergoing this examination.

REVIEW Nephritis

RELATE Link the Concepts and Exemplars

Linking the exemplar of nephritis with the concept of fluids and electrolytes:

1. If you are caring for a client with nephritis whose kidney function is insufficient to eliminate adequate fluid and waste products from the body, what nursing care might you provide to maintain fluid and electrolyte homeostasis?
2. While caring for a client with acute nephritis and reduced urine output, you review the laboratory studies and find that the client's serum potassium is greater than 6 mg/dL. What are your priorities for care? What orders would you anticipate receiving when you notify the primary provider?

Linking the exemplar of nephritis with the concept of mobility:

3. If the client with nephritis is required to maintain bed rest, how will you promote a return to ambulation when the time comes?
4. To promote future mobility, what nursing care can you provide the client who requires bed rest?

READY Go to Companion Skills Manual

REFER Go to Pearson Nursing Student Resources
nursing.pearsonhighered.com

- Additional review material

REFLECT Case Study

Marina McCullough, 13 years old, comes home from school and tells her mother that she doesn't feel well. She complains of feeling tired, having pain in her left flank, and feeling warm. Her mother goes into the bathroom to get the electronic thermome-

ter to check Marina's temperature and notices that Marina forgot to flush the toilet. When she reaches over to flush the toilet, she notices that the water looks like iced tea. She checks Marina's oral temperature and gets a reading of 100.8°F. She suspects a possible UTI and wonders if Marina is sexually active, but she decides not to approach the subject when Marina isn't feeling well.

Ms. McCullough, Marina's mother, makes an appointment with Marina's pediatrician and takes her in later that afternoon. The nurse admits her, notes mild periorbital edema and +2 pitting edema in both feet, and collects a urine specimen that tests positive for blood and protein. Ms. McCullough administered acetaminophen earlier in the afternoon to treat both the fever and the pain. Marina's vital signs upon arrival at the pediatrician's office are tympanic temperature 99.4°F, pulse 92 bpm, respirations 18/min, and BP 138/86 mmHg. Her weight is 132 lb, which Marina reports is an 8-lb weight gain since she last checked it 3 days ago. Breath sounds reveal mild crackles in bases bilaterally, and the nurse notes a rattling productive cough. Marina reports pain rated 7 in the right flank area, a persistent headache, and nausea and feeling tired.

Marina is diagnosed with nephritis and is admitted to the acute care facility on the adolescent unit. The doctor orders serum electrolytes, CBC with differential, BUN, serum creatinine, creatinine clearance, KUB, urine culture, and kidney scan. Also ordered is fluid restriction to 750 mL per day.

1. How will you ration Marina's fluids throughout a 24-hour day?
2. You are starting a 24-hour urine collection for creatine. How will you instruct the client to begin? What actions will you take to improve accuracy of the 24-hour collection?
3. What priority assessments will you perform when admitting Marina?

EXEMPLAR 10.5 Peptic Ulcer Disease

EXEMPLAR KEY TERMS
Duodenal ulcers, *677*
Gastric outlet obstruction, *678*
Gastric ulcers, *677*
Hemorrhage, *678*
Peptic ulcer disease (PUD), *677*
Peptic ulcers, *677*
Perforation, *678*
Steatorrhea, *679*
Ulcer, *677*
Zollinger-Ellison syndrome, *678*

EXEMPLAR LEARNING OUTCOMES
After reading about this exemplar, you will be able to:

1. Describe the pathophysiology, etiology, clinical manifestations, and direct and indirect causes of peptic ulcer disease.

2. Identify risk factors and prevention methods associated with peptic ulcer disease.
3. Illustrate the nursing process in providing culturally competent care across the life span for individuals with peptic ulcer disease.
4. Formulate priority nursing diagnoses appropriate for an individual with peptic ulcer disease.
5. Summarize therapies used by interdisciplinary teams in the collaborative care of an individual with peptic ulcer disease.
6. Plan evidence-based care for an individual with peptic ulcer disease and his or her family in collaboration with other members of the healthcare team.
7. Evaluate expected outcomes for an individual with peptic ulcer disease.

▶ OVERVIEW

Peptic ulcer disease (PUD), a break in the mucous lining of the GI tract where it comes in contact with gastric juice, is a chronic health problem. PUD affects over 14.5 million individuals in the United States yearly, resulting in 1.4 million ambulatory care visits and approximately 500,000 hospitalizations every year (NIDDK, 2010b).

Peptic ulcers may occur in any area of the GI tract exposed to acid-pepsin secretions, including the esophagus, stomach, and duodenum. The most common are **duodenal ulcers**, which occur in the duodenum. They usually develop between the ages of 30 and 55 and are more common in men than in women. **Gastric ulcers**, which occur in the stomach, more often affect older clients between the ages of 55 and 70. Ulcers are more common in individuals who smoke and who are chronic users of NSAIDs. Alcohol and dietary intake do not seem to cause PUD, and the role of stress is uncertain.

▶ PATHOPHYSIOLOGY AND ETIOLOGY

The innermost layer of the stomach wall, the gastric mucosa, consists of columnar epithelial cells supported by a middle layer of blood vessels and glands and a thin outer layer of smooth muscle. The mucosal barrier of the stomach, a thin coating of mucous gel and bicarbonate, protects the gastric mucosa. The mucosal barrier is maintained by bicarbonate secreted by the epithelial cells, by mucous gel production stimulated by prostaglandins, and by an adequate blood supply to the mucosa. An **ulcer** develops when the mucosal barrier is unable to protect the mucosa from damage by hydrochloric acid and pepsin, the gastric digestive juices.

Helicobacter pylori infection, found in about 70% of individuals who have PUD, is unique in colonizing the stomach. It is spread individual to individual (oral–oral or fecal–oral) and contributes to ulcer formation in several ways. The bacteria produce enzymes that reduce the efficacy of mucous gel in protecting the gastric mucosa. In addition, the host's inflammatory response to *H. pylori* contributes to gastric epithelial cell damage without producing immunity to the infection. Although the gastric mucosa is the usual site for *H. pylori* infection, this infection also contributes to duodenal ulcers. The reason may be increased production of gastric acid associated with *H. pylori* infection.

NSAIDs contribute to PUD through both systemic and topical mechanisms of injury. Prostaglandins are necessary for maintaining the gastric mucosal barrier. NSAIDs interrupt prostaglandin synthesis by disrupting the action of the two cyclooxygenase (COX) enzymes. COX-1 is necessary to maintain the integrity of the gastric mucosa, and COX-2 responds to inflammatory stimulation. The COX-2–selective NSAIDs may be less damaging to the gastric mucosa because they have less effect on the COX-1 enzyme. In addition to their systemic effect, aspirin and many other NSAIDs exert topical injury by crossing the lipid membranes of gastric epithelial cells, damaging the cells themselves.

The ulcers of PUD may affect the esophagus, stomach, or duodenum. They may be superficial or deep, affecting all

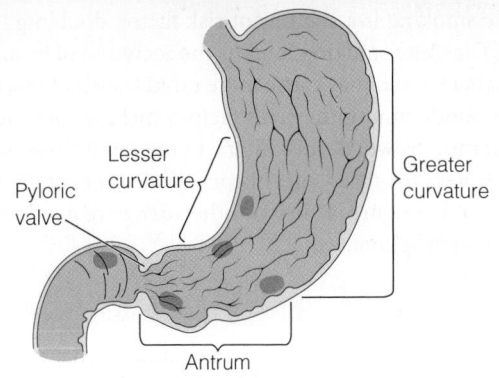

Figure 10–11 ● Common sites affected by peptic ulcer disease.

layers of the mucosa. Duodenal ulcers, the most common, usually develop in the proximal portion of the duodenum, close to the pylorus (**Figure 10–11** ●). They are sharply demarcated and usually less than 1 cm in diameter (**Figure 10–12** ●). Gastric ulcers often are found on the lesser curvature and the area immediately proximal to the pylorus. Gastric ulcers are associated with an increased incidence of gastric cancer.

PUD may be chronic, with spontaneous remissions and exacerbations. Exacerbations of the disease may be associated with trauma, infection, or other physical or psychological stressors.

Etiology

H. pylori infections often occur in several members of a family, especially when the family's water supply is contaminated. Diet is usually not a major factor in the development of peptic ulcers, although caffeine and alcohol consumption may exacerbate the disease.

Risk Factors

Chronic *H. pylori* infection and chronic use of NSAIDs, including aspirin, are the major risk factors for PUD (NIDDK, 2010a). Overall, an estimated 1 in 6 clients infected with *H. pylori* develops PUD. Of the NSAIDs, aspirin is the most ulcerogenic.

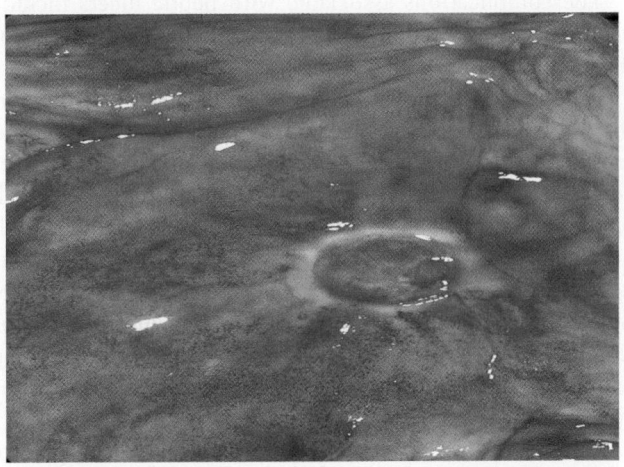

Figure 10–12 ● A superficial peptic ulcer.
Source: SPL/Science Source.

Cigarette smoking is a significant risk factor, doubling the risk of PUD. Cigarette smoking inhibits the secretion of bicarbonate by the pancreas and may cause more rapid transit of gastric acid into the duodenum. Other risk factors include low socioeconomic status; crowded, unsanitary living conditions; unclean food or water; advanced age; history of ulcer or family history of PUD; and concurrent use of other drugs (e.g., glucocorticoids or bisphosphonates).

Prevention

The etiology of the peptic ulcer determines what actions are possible to minimize the risk of developing the disease. Recommendations for prevention of *H. pylori* infection include meticulous hand washing and implementing all recommendations related to food preparation, including ensuring thorough cooking of meat. For clients whose history includes chronic NSAID use, recommendations include adding either a histamine receptor antagonist, proton pump inhibitor, or misoprostol (Cytotec) with the NSAID or changing treatment to a COX-2–selective NSAID to reduce the occurrence of peptic ulcers. It is recommended that all clients started on long-term therapy with nonselective NSAIDs be tested for *H. pylori* regardless of their level of risk (Lanza et al., 2009).

▶ CLINICAL MANIFESTATIONS

Abdominal pain is the classic symptom of peptic ulcer disease. The pain is typically described as gnawing, burning, aching, or hungerlike, and it is experienced in the epigastric region, sometimes radiating to the back. The pain occurs when the stomach is empty (2–3 hours after meals and in the middle of the night) and is relieved by eating, with a classic pain–food–relief pattern. The client may complain of heartburn or regurgitation and may vomit.

The presentation of PUD in the older adult is often less clear, with vague and poorly localized discomfort, perhaps chest pain or dysphagia, weight loss, or anemia. In the older adult, a complication of PUD, such as upper GI hemorrhage or perforation of the stomach or duodenum, may be the presenting symptom.

The complications associated with peptic ulcers include hemorrhage, obstruction, and perforation. See **Box 10–5** ● for the manifestations of these complications.

Among individuals with PUD, 10%–20% experience **hemorrhage** (rapid or excessive bleeding) as a result of ulceration and erosion into the blood vessels of the gastric mucosa. In the older adult, bleeding is the most frequent complication. When small blood vessels erode, blood loss may be slow and insidious, with occult blood in the stool the only initial sign. If bleeding continues, the client becomes anemic and experiences symptoms of weakness, fatigue, dizziness, and orthostatic hypotension. Erosion into a larger vessel can lead to sudden and severe bleeding with hematemesis, melena, or hematochezia and signs of hypovolemic shock.

Gastric outlet obstruction (obstruction of the pyloric region of the stomach and duodenum that impairs gastric outflow) may result from edema surrounding the ulcer, smooth muscle spasm, or scar tissue. Generally, obstruction is a grad-

---

Box 10–5 Manifestations of PUD Complications

HEMORRHAGE
- Occult or obvious blood in the stool
- Hematemesis
- Fatigue
- Weakness, dizziness
- Orthostatic hypotension
- Hypovolemic shock

OBSTRUCTION
- Sensations of epigastric fullness
- Nausea and vomiting
- Electrolyte imbalances
- Metabolic alkalosis

PERFORATION
- Severe upper abdominal pain radiating to the shoulder
- Rigid, boardlike abdomen
- Absence of bowel sounds
- Diaphoresis
- Tachycardia
- Rapid, shallow respirations
- Fever

---

ual rather than an acute process. Symptoms include a feeling of epigastric fullness, accentuated ulcer symptoms, and nausea. If the obstruction becomes complete, vomiting occurs. Hydrochloric acid, sodium, and potassium are lost in vomitus, the potential result being fluid and electrolyte imbalance and metabolic alkalosis.

The most lethal complication of PUD is **perforation**, penetration of the ulcer through the mucosal wall. When perforation occurs, gastric or duodenal contents enter the peritoneum, causing an inflammatory process and peritonitis. Chemical peritonitis from the hydrochloric acid, pepsin, bile, and pancreatic fluid is immediate; within 6–12 hours bacterial peritonitis follows from gastric contaminants entering the normally sterile peritoneal cavity. When an ulcer perforates, the client has immediate, severe upper abdominal pain radiating throughout the abdomen and possibly to the shoulder. The abdomen becomes rigid and boardlike, with absent bowel sounds. Signs of shock may be present and include diaphoresis; tachycardia; and rapid, shallow respirations. Classic symptoms of perforation may not be present in an older adult. Instead, the older adult may present with mental confusion and other nonspecific symptoms. This atypical presentation can lead to delays in diagnosis and treatment, increasing the associated mortality rate.

Zollinger-Ellison Syndrome

Zollinger-Ellison syndrome is a form of peptic ulcer disease caused by a gastrinoma, or gastrin-secreting tumor. Gastrinomas may be benign, although they are usually malignant. Gastrin is a hormone that stimulates the secretion of pepsin and hydrochloric acid. The increased gastrin levels associated with these tumors result in hypersecretion of gastric acid, which in turn causes mucosal ulceration.

Clinical Manifestations and Therapies **Peptic Ulcer Disease**

ETIOLOGY	CLINICAL MANIFESTATIONS	CLINICAL THERAPIES
H. pylori infection	■ Gnawing or burning pain in the epigastric region when stomach is empty ■ Possible heartburn or regurgitation ■ Manifestations in older adults possibly unapparent until complications arise	■ Protein-pump inhibitor (PPI) in combination with 2 antibiotics to eliminate infection OR ■ Bismuth containing product with 2 antibiotics and proton pump inhibitor ■ If retreatment is required, use of different antibiotics (Chey, Wong, & the Practice Parameters Committee of the American College of Gastroenterology, 2007)
NSAIDs	■ Pain in the epigastric region when stomach is empty ■ Possible heartburn or regurgitation ■ Manifestations in older adults possibly unapparent until complications arise	■ Discontinuation or reduction of dose of NSAIDs if possible or change to less ulcerogenic NSAID ■ PPIs, possibly twice-daily doses (Lanza et al., 2009) ■ H_2-receptor agonists ■ Mucosa-protecting agents

The peptic ulcers of Zollinger-Ellison syndrome most often affect the duodenum but may involve the stomach or jejunum. Characteristic ulcerlike pain is common. The high levels of hydrochloric acid entering the duodenum overwhelm the protective buffering mechanism; the result is diarrhea and **steatorrhea** (excess fat in the feces) from impaired fat digestion and absorption. Complications of bleeding and perforation are often seen with Zollinger-Ellison syndrome. Fluid and electrolyte imbalances also may result from persistent diarrhea, with resultant losses of potassium and sodium in particular.

▶ COLLABORATION

Treatment for PUD focuses on treating its cause. Primary treatments include eradicating *H. pylori* infection and treating or preventing ulcers related to use of NSAIDs. The nurse plays an essential role on the healthcare team by providing ongoing assessment and client teaching.

Diagnostic Tests

- ■ *Upper GI series* using barium as a contrast medium can detect 80%–90% of peptic ulcers via x-ray. It commonly is the diagnostic procedure chosen first because it does not require sedation and is less costly and less invasive than gastroscopy. Small or very superficial ulcers may be missed, however.

- ■ *Gastroscopy* allows visualization of the esophageal, gastric, and duodenal mucosa and direct inspection of ulcers. Tissue also can be obtained for biopsy.

- ■ *Biopsy specimens* obtained during a gastroscopy can be tested for the presence of *H. pylori* by several different methods. In the *rapid urease test*, the specimen is placed on a gel containing urea. If urease from *H. pylori* is present, it will convert the urea to ammonia and carbon dioxide, increasing the pH of the gel. This action leads to a color change of the pH indicator in the gel to produce a positive result. Results are obtained within 1 to 24 hours. Biopsy specimen cells also can be microscopically examined or cultured for evidence of

H. pylori. Although these tests are highly specific for *H. pylori* infection, their invasiveness, cost, and lack of availability in some areas limit their usefulness.

- ■ *Noninvasive methods* of detecting *H. pylori* infection include *serological testing* (to detect *H. pylori*–specific IgG antibodies through ELISA), fecal antigen immunoassays (to detect antigens to *H. pylori* in the feces), and the *urea breath test*. In this test, radiolabeled urea is given orally. The urease produced by *H. pylori* bacteria converts the urea to ammonia and radiolabeled carbon dioxide, which can then be measured as the client exhales. This test, as well as fecal antigen testing, can also be used to evaluate the effectiveness of treatment to eradicate *H. pylori*. Treatment with proton pump inhibitors (PPIs) interferes with the urea breath test results, so these drugs should be discontinued for 14 days prior to testing (VanLeeuwen, Poelhuis-Leth, & Bladh, 2013).

- ■ If Zollinger-Ellison syndrome is suspected, *gastric analysis* may be performed to evaluate gastric acid secretion. Stomach contents are aspirated through a nasogastric tube and analyzed. In Zollinger-Ellison syndrome, gastric acid levels are very high.

Surgery

The identification of *H. pylori* infection as the primary cause of PUD and the availability of drugs to effectively treat and heal peptic ulcers have dramatically decreased surgery as a treatment option for PUD. Older clients, however, may have undergone gastric resection surgery for PUD and may have long-term complications related to the surgery.

Pharmacologic Therapy

The medications used to treat PUD include agents to eradicate *H. pylori*, drugs to decrease gastric acid content, and agents that protect the mucosa.

Eradication of *H. pylori* depends on using drug regimens with proven effectiveness. Combination therapies that use two antibiotics with a proton pump inhibitor, known as triple therapy, or a PPI (or histamine receptor antagonist) with bismuth and two antibiotics (quadruple therapy) for 10–14 days are necessary.

Antibiotics used in triple therapy are clarithromycin, amoxicillin, and metronidazole. The quadruple therapy usually utilizes metronidazole and tetracycline. Eradication rates vary by regimen used, duration of therapy (7 vs. 10 vs. 14 days), client compliance, and antibiotic resistance (Chey et al., 2007).

In clients who have NSAID-induced ulcers, the NSAID in use should be discontinued if at all possible. If that is not possible, twice-daily PPIs, histamine receptor antagonists, or sucralfate should be used to promote ulcer healing (Lanza et al., 2009).

Medications that decrease gastric acid content include PPIs and the H_2-receptor antagonists.

- PPIs inhibit the acid-secreting enzyme (H^+/K^+ ATPase) that functions as the proton pump of the parietal cells, disabling it for up to 24 hours. These drugs are very effective, resulting in more than 90% ulcer healing after 4 weeks. Compared to the H_2-receptor blockers, the PPIs provide faster pain relief and more rapid ulcer healing.

- Histamine$_2$-receptor blockers inhibit histamine binding to the receptors on the gastric parietal cells to reduce acid secretion. These drugs are well tolerated and have few serious side effects; however, drug interactions can occur. These drugs must be continued for 8 weeks or longer for ulcer healing.

Agents that protect the mucosa include sucralfate, bismuth, antacids, and prostaglandin analogs.

- Sucralfate binds to proteins in the ulcer base, forming a protective barrier against acid, bile, and pepsin. Sucralfate also stimulates the secretion of mucus, bicarbonate, and prostaglandin.

- Bismuth compounds (Pepto-Bismol®) stimulate mucosal bicarbonate and prostaglandin production to promote ulcer healing. In addition, bismuth suppresses *H. pylori.* There are very few side effects, other than a harmless darkening of stools.

- Antacids stimulate gastric mucosal defenses, thereby aiding in ulcer healing. They provide rapid relief of ulcer symptoms and are often used as needed to supplement other antiulcer medications. Antacids are inexpensive, but clients often have difficulty complying with a long-term regimen because the drugs must be taken frequently and may cause constipation (the aluminum-type antacids) or diarrhea (the magnesium-based antacids). Antacids also interfere with the absorption of iron, digoxin, some antibiotics, and other drugs.

- Prostaglandin analogs (misoprostol) promote ulcer healing by stimulating mucus and bicarbonate secretions and by inhibiting acid secretion. Although not as effective as the other drugs discussed, misoprostol is used to prevent NSAID-induced ulcers. Diarrhea is a common side effect. Because of its uterotropic effect, misoprostol is contraindicated in pregnant women.

Nonpharmacologic Therapy

In addition to pharmacologic treatment, clients are encouraged to maintain good nutrition, consuming balanced meals at regular intervals. It is important to teach clients that bland or restrictive diets are no longer necessary. Mild alcohol intake is not harmful. Smoking is discouraged because it slows the rate of healing and increases the frequency of relapses.

■ NURSING PROCESS

Nurses may identify clients with peptic ulcer disease by looking for the symptoms and noting family history of *H. pylori* infection. Nursing care centers on interventions to promote adequate nutritional intake, promote healing, and prevent recurrences.

Although it is difficult to predict which clients will develop PUD, nurses can promote health by advising clients to avoid risk factors such as excessive aspirin or NSAID use and cigarette smoking. In addition, nurses should encourage clients to seek treatment for manifestations of gastroesophageal reflux disease (GERD) or chronic gastritis, both of which also are associated with *H. pylori* infection.

Assessment

Collect the following subjective and objective data when assessing the client with PUD:

- *Health history.* Complaints of epigastric or left upper quadrant pain, heartburn, or discomfort; its character, severity, timing, and relationship to eating; measures used for relief; nausea or vomiting, presence of bright blood or "coffee-grounds" appearing in vomitus; current medications, including use of aspirin or other NSAIDs; cigarette smoking and use of alcohol or other drugs
- *Physical examination.* General appearance, including height and weight relationship; vital signs, including orthostatic measurements; abdominal examination, including shape and contour, bowel sounds, and tenderness to palpation; presence of obvious or occult blood in vomitus and stool.

Diagnosis

Nursing diagnoses that are frequently appropriate for clients with PUD include the following:

- *Risk for Bleeding*
- *Risk for Deficient Fluid Volume*
- *Imbalanced Nutrition: Less Than Body Requirements*
- *Chronic Pain*
- *Disturbed Sleep Pattern*

(NANDA-I © 2012)

Planning

Goals of treatment are developed in collaboration with the client and may include the following:

- The client will demonstrate no complications related to bleeding.
- The client will demonstrate no signs or symptoms of infection.
- The client will demonstrate fluid volume balance, including maintenance of urine output of at least 0.5 mL/kg/hr.
- The client will demonstrate dietary intake that adequately meets nutritional and caloric needs.
- The client will verbalize risk factors related to PUD exacerbation and recurrence.
- The client will verbalize maintaining pain at a tolerable level.

Box 10–6 Treatment for Complications of Peptic Ulcer Disease

The client hospitalized with a complication of PUD (e.g., bleeding, GI obstruction, or perforation and peritonitis) requires additional interventions to restore homeostasis.

In hemorrhage associated with PUD, initial interventions focus on restoring and maintaining circulation. Normal saline, lactated Ringer, or other balanced electrolyte solutions are administered intravenously to restore intravascular volume if signs of shock (tachycardia, hypotension, pallor, low urine output, and anxiety) are present. Whole blood or packed RBCs may be administered to restore hemoglobin and hematocrit levels. A nasogastric tube is inserted to prevent aspiration of vomited gastric contents.

Gastroscopy with direct injection of a clotting or sclerosing agent into the bleeding vessel may be performed. Laser photocoagulation, which uses light energy, or electrocoagulation, which uses electric current to generate heat, can also be performed via gastroscopy to seal bleeding vessels.

The client is kept NPO until bleeding is controlled. PPIs are administered intravenously [e.g., 40 mg of pantoprazole (Protonix) per intravenous push or admixture daily] to reduce the risk of rebleeding. Surgery may be necessary if medical measures are ineffective in controlling bleeding. Older adults who experience bleeding as a complication of PUD are more likely to rebleed or require surgery to control the hemorrhage.

Repeated inflammation, healing, scarring, edema, and muscle spasm can lead to gastric outlet (pyloric) obstruction. Initial treatment includes gastric decompression with nasogastric suction and administration of intravenous normal saline and potassium chloride to correct fluid and electrolyte imbalance. H_2-receptor blockers are given intravenously as well. Balloon dilation of the gastric outlet may be done via upper endoscopy. If these measures are unsuccessful in relieving obstruction, surgery may be required.

Gastric or duodenal perforation resulting in contamination of the peritoneum with GI contents often requires immediate intervention to restore homeostasis and minimize peritonitis. Intravenous fluids maintain fluid and electrolyte balance. Nasogastric suction removes gastric contents and minimizes peritoneal contamination. Placing the client in Fowler or semi-Fowler position allows peritoneal contaminants to pool in the pelvis. Intravenous antibiotics aggressively treat bacterial infection from intestinal flora. Laparoscopic surgery or an open laparotomy may close the perforation.

Implementation

The priorities of nursing care for the client with PUD include restoring and maintaining fluid volume balance, reducing discomfort, maintaining nutritional status, and preventing or rapidly identifying and intervening for potential complications. Priorities for clients with complications of PUD are described in **Box 10–6** ●.

Restore and Maintain Fluid Volume Balance

Erosion of a blood vessel with resultant hemorrhage is a significant risk for the client with PUD. Acute bleeding can lead to hypovolemia and fluid volume deficit, which can lead to a decrease in cardiac output and impaired tissue perfusion.

■ Monitor stools and gastric drainage for overt and occult blood. Assess gastric drainage (vomitus or drainage from a nasogastric tube) to estimate the amount and rapidity of hemorrhage. Drainage is bright red with possible clots in acute hemorrhage and is dark red or the color of coffee grounds when blood has been in the stomach for a period of time. Hematochezia is present in acute hemorrhage; melena (black, tarry stool) is an indicator of less acute bleeding. When small vessels are disrupted, bleeding may be slow and not overtly evident. With chronic or slow GI bleeding, the risk of a fluid volume deficit is minimal; anemia and activity intolerance are more likely.

■ Maintain intravenous therapy with fluid volume and electrolyte replacement solutions; administer whole blood or packed cells as ordered. Both fluids and electrolytes are lost through vomiting, nasogastric drainage, and diarrhea in an episode of acute bleeding. To prevent shock, it is essential to maintain a blood volume and cardiac output sufficient to perfuse body tissues. Whole blood and packed cells replace both blood volume and RBCs, providing additional oxygen-carrying capacity to meet cell needs.

■ Insert a nasogastric tube and maintain its position and patency. Initially, measure and record gastric output every hour, then every 4–8 hours. Nasogastric suction removes blood from the GI tract, preventing vomiting and possible aspiration. Gastric output is replaced milliliter for milliliter with a balanced electrolyte solution to maintain homeostasis.

■ Monitor hemoglobin and hematocrit, serum electrolytes, BUN, and creatinine values. Report abnormal findings. Hemoglobin and hematocrit are lower than normal with acute or chronic GI bleeding. In acute hemorrhage, initial results may be within normal range because both cells and plasma are lost. Loss of fluids and electrolytes with gastric drainage and diarrhea alters normal levels. Digestion and absorption of blood in the GI tract may result in elevated BUN and creatinine levels.

■ Assess abdomen, including bowel sounds, distention, girth, and tenderness, every 4 hours, and record findings. Borborygmi or hyperactive bowel sounds with abdominal tenderness are common with acute GI bleeding. Increased distention; increasing abdominal girth; absent bowel sounds; or extreme tenderness with a rigid, boardlike abdomen may indicate perforation.

■ Maintain bed rest with the head of the bed elevated. Ensure safety. Loss of blood volume may cause orthostatic hypotension with resultant syncope or dizziness upon standing.

Manage Pain

The pain of PUD is often predictable and preventable. Pain is typically experienced 2–4 hours after eating, as high levels of gastric acid and pepsin irritate the exposed mucosa. Measures to neutralize the acid, minimize its production, or protect the mucosa often relieve this pain, minimizing the need for analgesics.

■ Assess pain, including location, type, severity, frequency, and duration. Assess the relationship of pain to food intake or other contributing factors.

■ Administer PPIs, H_2-receptor antagonists, antacids, or mucosal protective agents as ordered. Monitor for effectiveness and side effects or adverse reactions. The pain associated with PUD is generally caused by the effect of gastric juices on exposed mucosal tissue. These medications reduce pain and promote healing by reducing acid production, neutralizing acid, or providing a barrier for the damaged mucosa.

- Teach relaxation, stress reduction, and lifestyle management techniques. Refer for stress management counseling or classes as indicated. Although there is no clear relationship between stress and PUD, measures to relieve stress and promote physical and emotional rest help reduce the perception of pain and may reduce ulcer genesis.

SAFETY ALERT
Avoid making assumptions about pain. Acute pain may indicate a complication, such as perforation (often manifesting as sudden, severe epigastric pain and a rigid, boardlike abdomen), or it may be totally unrelated to PUD (e.g., angina, gallbladder disease, or pancreatitis).

Facilitate Adequate Rest

Nighttime ulcer pain, which typically occurs between 1 and 3 a.m., may disrupt the sleep cycle and result in inadequate rest. Anticipation of pain may lead to insomnia or other sleep disruptions.

- Emphasize the importance of taking medications as prescribed. The bedtime dose of PPI or H_2-receptor blocker minimizes hydrochloric acid production during the night, reducing nighttime pain.
- Instruct the client to limit food intake after the evening meal, eliminating any bedtime snack. Eating before bedtime can stimulate the production of gastric acid and pepsin, increasing the likelihood of nighttime pain.
- Encourage the use of relaxation techniques and comfort measures such as soft music as needed to promote sleep. Once the pain associated with PUD has been controlled, these measures help reduce anxiety and reestablish a normal sleep pattern.

Promote Balanced Nutrition

In an attempt to avoid discomfort, the client with PUD may gradually reduce food intake, sometimes jeopardizing nutritional status. Anorexia and early satiety are additional problems associated with PUD.

- Assess the client's current diet, including pattern of food intake, eating schedule, and foods that precipitate pain or are being avoided in anticipation of pain. The client may not realize the extent of self-imposed dietary limitations, especially if symptoms are long-standing. Assessment increases awareness and helps the client identify the adequacy of nutrient intake.
- Refer the client to a dietitian for meal planning to minimize PUD symptoms and meet nutritional needs. Consider normal eating patterns and preferences in meal planning. Although no specific diet is recommended for PUD, clients should avoid foods that increase pain. Six small meals per day often help increase food tolerance and decrease postprandial discomfort.
- Monitor for complaints of anorexia, fullness, nausea, and vomiting. Adjust dietary intake or medication schedule as

indicated. PUD and resultant scarring can lead to impaired gastric emptying, necessitating a treatment change.

- Monitor laboratory values for indications of anemia or other nutritional deficits. Monitor for therapeutic effects and side effects of treatment measures such as oral iron replacement. Instruct the client taking oral iron replacement to avoid using an antacid within 1–2 hours of taking the iron preparation. Antacids bind with oral iron preparations, blocking absorption. Anemia can result from poor nutrient absorption or chronic blood loss in clients with PUD. Oral iron supplements may cause GI distress, nausea, and vomiting. If these side effects are intolerable, notify the physician for a possible change of therapy.

SAFETY ALERT
Advise the client to report increasing or persistent symptoms of anorexia, nausea and vomiting, or fullness to the healthcare provider.

Evaluation

Client care may be evaluated for the following expected outcomes:

- Client experiences no complications related to PUD, including uncontrolled or excessive bleeding.
- Client demonstrates balanced oral intake and output, and no signs or symptoms of fluid overload or dehydration.
- Using a predetermined pain rating scale, the client rates pain at a tolerable level (as defined by the client).
- Client verbalizes attainment of adequate rest and sleep.
- Client describes actions that will reduce the risk of recurrence of PUD.

Community-Based Care   Community and Home Care for Clients With PUD

Peptic ulcer disease is managed in home and community-based settings; only its complications typically require treatment in an acute care setting. Provide the following information when preparing the client for home care:

- Prescribed medication regimen, including desired effects and potential adverse effects
- Importance of continuing therapy even when symptoms are relieved
- Relationship between peptic ulcers and factors such as NSAID use and smoking; if indicated, referral to a smoking cessation clinic or program
- Importance of avoiding aspirin and other NSAIDs and the necessity of reading the labels of over-the-counter medications for possible aspirin content
- Manifestations of complications that should be reported to the care provider, including increased abdominal pain or distention, vomiting, black or tarry stools, light-headedness, or fainting
- Stress and lifestyle management techniques that may help prevent exacerbation; referral to resources for stress management, such as classes, counseling, and formal or informal groups

NURSING CARE PLAN   A Client With Peptic Ulcer Disease

Sean O'Donnell is a 47-year-old police officer who lives and works in a metropolitan area. Mr. O'Donnell has had "heartburn" and abdominal discomfort for years but thought they went along with his job. Last year, after becoming weak, light-headed, and short of breath, he was found to be anemic and was diagnosed as having a duodenal ulcer. He took omeprazole (Prilosec®) and ferrous sulfate for 3 months before stopping both, saying he had "never felt better in his life." Mr. O'Donnell has now been admitted to the hospital with active upper GI bleeding.

ASSESSMENT

Rachel Clark is Mr. O'Donnell's admitting nurse and case manager. On initial assessment, Mr. O'Donnell is alert and oriented, although very apprehensive about his condition. His skin is pale and cool. Vital signs include temperature 99.1°F oral; pulse 98 bpm; respirations 20/min; and BP 136/88 mmHg. Mr. O'Donnell's abdomen is distended and tender, with hyperactive bowel sounds; 200 mL bright red blood is obtained on nasogastric tube insertion. Hemoglobin 8.2 g/dL and hematocrit 23% on admission. Mr. O'Donnell is taken to the endoscopy lab, where his bleeding is controlled by laser photocoagulation. On his return to the nursing unit, he receives 2 units of packed RBCs and intravenous fluids to restore blood volume. A 5-day course of high-dose oral omeprazole (40 mg bid) is ordered to prevent rebleeding, and Mr. O'Donnell is allowed to begin a clear liquid diet 24 hours after his endoscopy. Tissue biopsy obtained during endoscopy confirms the presence of *H. pylori* infection.

DIAGNOSES

- *Deficient Fluid Volume* related to acutely bleeding duodenal ulcer
- *Risk for Injury* related to acute blood loss
- *Fear* related to threat to well-being
- *Ineffective Therapeutic Regimen Management* related to lack of knowledge regarding PUD and its treatment

(NANDA-I © 2012)

PLANNING

- Client will maintain normal blood pressure, pulse, and urine output (>30 mL/h).
- Client will remain free of injury.
- Client will seek information to reduce fear.
- Client will identify and use coping strategies to manage fear.
- Client will describe prescribed therapeutic regimen.
- Client will verbalize ability to manage prescribed regimen.

IMPLEMENTATION

- Place call light within reach and encourage client to ask for help when getting up or ambulating. Remind client to rise slowly from lying to sitting and from sitting to standing.
- Discuss situation and provide information about all procedures and treatments.
- Reassure client about the effectiveness of treatment in reducing the risk for further bleeding.

- Discuss current and planned treatment measures; stress the importance of completing the prescribed treatment to reduce the risk of further ulcer development.
- Encourage client to avoid using aspirin or NSAIDs in the future; suggest alternative medications such as acetaminophen.
- Discuss stress reduction techniques and refer for stress reduction counseling or workshops as indicated.

EVALUATION

Mr. O'Donnell is discharged 48 hours after admission. He has had no further evidence of bleeding and has resumed a regular diet. His hemoglobin and hematocrit remain low, and he has a prescription for ferrous sulfate. He will complete the prescribed high-dose omeprazole regimen at home, then begin treatment with omeprazole, amoxicillin, and clarithromycin (Biaxin) to eradicate the *H. pylori* infection detected during endoscopy. After 2 weeks of this regimen, he will continue taking omeprazole at bedtime for 4–8 weeks. He verbalizes a good understanding of his treatment and the importance of completing the entire regimen. Mr. O'Donnell expresses concern about his ability to "keep his cool on the inside" when under stress. Ms. Clark, his case manager, gives him the names of several resources to help with stress management in case he wants help.

CRITICAL THINKING

1. How does *H. pylori* infection contribute to the development of peptic ulcers?
2. Describe the physiological responses to fear and anxiety. Why is it important to alleviate fear and its physical consequences in clients with PUD?
3. What suggestions can you make to help Mr. O'Donnell manage his complex treatment regimen during the next 3 months?
4. Develop a teaching plan that includes stress reduction techniques that Mr. O'Donnell can use while performing his duties as a police officer.

REVIEW Peptic Ulcer Disease

RELATE Link the Concepts and Exemplars

Linking the exemplar of peptic ulcer disease with the concept of addiction:

1. When admitting a client with acute PUD, you learn that the client has a 20+ year history of smoking. How might this behavior contribute to PUD?

2. What teaching would you provide to motivate and support the client to quit smoking?

Linking the exemplar of peptic ulcer disease with the concept of perfusion:

You are caring for a client with acute PUD who has had profuse hemoptysis secondary to ulceration of the stomach lining. The client has had significant blood loss, with approximately 3 L of bloody emesis measured over the past 24 hours. The provider orders iced lavages, which seem to have stopped the bleeding for now.

3. How will you assess this client related to shock?

4. What actions, independent or collaborative, can you take to promote the client's hemovascular stability?

READY Go to Companion Skills Manual

REFER Go to Pearson Nursing Student Resources
nursing.pearsonhighered.com

- Additional review material

REFLECT Case Study

Raymond Combs, 38 years old, owns a chain of neighborhood convenience stores. He is married to his third wife, and they have two children by this marriage and are raising three children from former relationships. Mr. Combs often jokes that he prefers to stay at work because it is less stressful than being at home with the children and his wife.

For the past month, Mr. Combs has been noticing pain in his left upper abdomen approximately 2–3 hours after meals. He describes the pain as a burning, gnawing pain that goes away when he eats. He and his wife make plans to go out for dinner with their next door neighbors. Mr. Combs's wife suggests that he talk to the neighbor, who is a nurse, about the discomfort he's been feeling.

1. You are Mr. Combs's neighbor. When you go out for dinner with Mr. Combs and his wife, he describes the pain and asks what you think is happening. How do you respond?

2. Mr. Combs asks you what he can do to make his problem go away if it is, in fact, an ulcer. How do you respond?

3. Mr. Combs's wife says that she heard that a milk and dairy diet is good for ulcers. How do you respond?

■ REFERENCES

Addison, O., LaStayo, P. C., Dibble, L. E., & Marcus, R. L. (2012). Inflammation, aging, and adiposity: Implications for physical therapists. *Journal of Geriatric Physical Therapy, 35*(2), 86–94. doi:10.1519/JPT.0b013e3182312b14.

Alzaraa, A., Gravante, G., Chung, W. Y., Al-Leswas, D., Bruno, M., Dennison, A. R., & Lloyd, D. M. (2012). Targeted microbubbles in the experimental and clinical setting. *American Journal of Surgery,* i(3), 355–366. doi:10.1016/j.amjsurg.2011.10.024.

American Gastroenterological Association. (2010). *Understanding gallstones.* Retrieved from http://www.gastro.org/patient-center/digestive-conditions/gallstones.

Ansari, P. (2012). Appendicitis. *Merck manual: Health care professionals.* Retrieved from http://www.merckmanuals.com/professional/gastrointestinal_disorders/acute_abdomen_and_surgical_gastroenterology/appendicitis.html.

Arnold, J. J., & Williams, P. M. (2011). Anaphylaxis: Recognition and management. *American Family Physician, 84,* 1111–1118.

Bongers, G., de Esch, I., & Leurs, R. (2010). Molecular pharmacology of the four histamine receptors. In R. L. Thurmond (Ed.), *Histamine in inflammation* (pp. 11–19). New York, NY: Springer Science+Business Media.

Boston Children's Hospital. (n.d.). *Appendicitis.* Retrieved from http://www.childrenshospital.org/az/Site2178/mainpageS2178P1.html.

Calder, P. C., Albers, R., Antione, J. M., Blum, S., Bourdet-Sicard, R., Ferns, G. A., ... Zhao, J. (2009). Inflammatory disease processes and interactions with nutrition. *British Journal of Nutrition, 101*(Suppl. 1), S1–45. doi:10.1017/S0007114509377867.

Canani, R. B., Terrin, G., Rapacciuolo, L., Miele, E., Siani, M. C., Puzone, C., ... Troncone, R. (2008). Faecal calprotectin as reliable non-invasive marker to assess the severity of mucosal inflammation in children with inflammatory bowel disease. *Digestive and Liver Disease, 40*(7), 547–553. doi:10.1016/j.dld.2008.07.017.

Carroll, J. F., Fulda, K. G., Chiapa, A. L., Rodriguez, M., Phelps, D. R., Cardarelli, K. M., ... Cardarelli, R. (2009). Impact of race/ethnicity on the relationship between visceral fat and inflammatory biomarkers. *Obesity (Silver Spring), 17*(7), 1420–1427. doi:10.1038/oby.2008.657.

Centers for Disease Control and Prevention. (2011). *Asthma prevalence, health care use, and mortality: United States, 2005–2009.* Retrieved from http://www.cdc.gov/nchs/data/nhsr/nhsr032.pdf.

Centers for Disease Control and Prevention. (2012). *Inflammatory bowel disease.* Retrieved from http://www.cdc.gov/ibd.

Chey, W. D., Wong, B. C. Y., & the Practice Parameters Committee of the American College of Gastroenterology. (2007). American College of Gastroenterology guideline on the management of *Helicobacter pylori* infection. *American Journal of Gastroenterology. 102,* 1808–1825.

Children's Digestive Health and Nutrition Foundation. (2010). *Pediatric inflammatory bowel disease, evaluation and management.* Retrieved from http://cdhnfsite.wms.cdgsolutions.com/user-assets/Documents/PDF/IBD/IBD7-Final%2015%20%20October%202010.pdf.

Cleveland Clinic. (2011). *Diseases and conditions: Appendicitis.* Accessed from http://my.clevelandclinic.org/disorders/appendicitis/hic_appendicitis.aspx.

Cleveland Clinic, Children's Hospital. (2009). *Appendicitis in children.* Retrieved from http://my.clevelandclinic.org/childrens-hospital/health-info/diseases-conditions/digestive-disorders/hic-appendicitis-in-children.aspx.

Crohn and Colitis Foundation of America. (2011). *The facts about inflammatory bowel diseases.* Retrieved from http://www.ccfa.org/assets/pdfs/ibdfactbook.pdf.

Crohn and Colitis Foundation of America. (2012a). *Intestinal complications.* Retrieved from http://www.ccfa.org/resources/intestinal-complications.html.

Crohn and Colitis Foundation of America. (2012b). *Complementary and alternative medicine.* Retrieved from http://www.ccfa.org/resources/complementary-alternative.html.

Crohn and Colitis Foundation of America. (2012c). *About the epidemiology of IBD.* Retrieved from http://www.ccfa.org/resources/epidemiology.html.

Dooley, M. A. (2011). Clinical manifestations of lupus nephritis. In E. J. Lewis, M .M. Schwartz, S. M. Korbet, & D. T. M. Chan (Eds.), *Lupus nephritis* (pp. 1–34). New York, NY: Oxford University Press.

Fauci, A. S., Braunwald, E., Kasper, D. L., Hauser, S. L., Longo, D. L., Jameson, J. L., & Loscalzo, J. (2009). *Harrison's principles of internal medicine* (17th ed.). New York, NY: McGraw-Hill.

Humes, D. J., & Simpson, J. (2011). Clinical presentation of acute appendicitis: Clinical signs—laboratory findings—clinical scores, Alvarado score and derivate scores. In C. Keyzer & P. A. Gevenois (Eds.), *Imaging of acute appendicitis in adults and children.* Berlin, Germany: Springer-Verlag.

Kornbluth, A., Sachar, D. B., & the Practice Parameters Committee of the American College of Gastroenterology. (2010). Ulcerative colitis practice guidelines in adults: American College of Gastroenterology, Practice Parameters Committee. *American Journal of Gastroenterology, 105,* 501–523.

Kozik, D. J., & Tweddell, J. S. (2006). Characterizing the inflammatory response to cardiopulmonary bypass in children. *Annals of Thoracic Surgery, 81,* S2347–S2354.

Lanza, F. L., Chan, F. K. L., Quigley, M. M., & the Practice Parameters Committee of the American College of Gastroenterology. (2009). Guidelines for prevention of NSAID-related ulcer complications. *American Journal of Gastroenterology, 104,* 728–738.

Lau, K. K., & Wyatt, R. J. (2005). Glomerulonephritis. *Adolescent Medicine Clinics, 16*(1), 67–85.

Lieberman, P., Nicklas, R. A., Oppenheimer, J., Kemp, S. F., & Lang, D. M. (2010). The diagnosis and management of anaphylaxis practice parameter: 2010 update. *Journal of Allergy and Clinical Immunology, 126,* 477–480.e42.

Livingston, E. H., & Fairlie, R. W. (2012). Little effect of insurance status or socioeconomic condition on disparities in minority appendicitis perforation rates. *Archives of Surgery, 147*(1), 11–17. doi:10.1001/archsurg.2011.746.

Mack, D. R., Langton, C., Markowitz, J., LeLeiko, N., Griffiths, A., Bousvaros, A., ... & Hyams, J. (2007). Laboratory values for children with newly diagnosed inflammatory bowel disease. *Pediatrics, 119*(6), 1113-1119.

Minkes, R. K. (2013). Pediatric appendicitis. *Medscape Reference.* Retrieved from http://emedicine.medscape.com/article/926795-overview.

National Center for Complementary and Alternative Medicine. (2012). *Goldseal.* Retrieved from http://nccam.nih.gov/health/goldenseal.

National Institute of Arthritis and Musculoskeletal and Skin Diseases. (2009). *Handout on health: rheumatoid arthritis.* Retrieved from http://www.niams.nih.gov/Health_Info/Rheumatic_Disease/default.asp.

National Institute of Arthritis and Musculoskeletal and Skin Diseases. (2013). *Questions and answers about ankylosing spondylitis.* Retrieved from http://www.niams.nih.gov/Health_Info/Ankylosing_Spondylitis/default.asp.

National Institute of Diabetes and Digestive and Kidney Diseases. (2010a). *H. pylori and peptic ulcers.* Retrieved from http://digestive.niddk.nih.gov/statistics/Digestive_Disease_Stats_508.pdf.

National Institute of Diabetes and Digestive and Kidney Diseases. (2010b). *Digestive diseases statistics for the*

United States. Retrieved from http://digestive.niddk.nih.gov/statistics/Digestive_Disease_Stats_508.pdf.

National Institute of Diabetes and Digestive and Kidney Diseases. (2011). *Crohn disease*. Retrieved from http://digestive.niddk.nih.gov/ddiseases/pubs/crohns/Crohns_508.pdf.

National Institute of Diabetes and Digestive and Kidney Diseases. (2012a). *Gallstones*. Retrieved from http://digestive.niddk.nih.gov/ddiseases/pubs/gallstones/Gallstones_508.pdf.

National Institute of Diabetes and Digestive and Kidney Diseases. (2012b). *Primary sclerosing cholangitis*. Retrieved from http://digestive.niddk.nih.gov/ddiseases/pubs/primarysclerosingcholangitis/Primry_Sclerosing_Cholangitis_508.pdf.

National Kidney Foundation. (2009a). *Glomerulonephritis*. Retrieved from http://www.kidney.org/atoz/content/glomerul.cfm.

National Kidney Foundation. (2009b). *Goodpasture's syndrome*. Retrieved from http://www.kidney.org/atoz/content/goodpasture.cfm.

Older, C. G., Carr, E. C. J., & Layzell, M. (2010). Making sense of patients' use of analgesics following day case surgery. *Journal of Advanced Nursing, 66*, 511–521.

Osborn, K. S., Wraa, C. E., Watson, A. B., & Holleran, R. (2013). *Medical-surgical nursing* (2nd ed.). Upper Saddle River, NJ: Pearson.

Papa, E., Docktor, M., Smillie, C., Weber, S., Preheim, S. P., Gevers, D., . . . Alm, E. J. (2012). Non-invasive mapping of the gastrointestinal microbiota identifies children with inflammatory bowel disease. *PLoS ONE, 7*(6), e39242. doi:10.1371/journal.pone.0039242.

Sauer, C. G., & Kugathasan, S. (2009). Pediatric inflammatory bowel disease: Highlighting pediatric differences in IBD. *Gastroenterology Clinics of North America, 38*, 611–628. doi:10.1016/j.gtc.2009.07.010.

Schug, S., & Chong, C. (2009). Pain management after ambulatory surgery. *Current Opinion in Anaesthesiology, 22*(6), 738–743.

Schultz, C., Temming, P., Bucsky, P., Gopel, W., Strunk, T., & Hartel, C. (2004). Immature anti-inflammatory response in neonates. *Clinical and Experimental Immunology, 135*(1), 130–136. doi:10.1111/j.1365-2249.2004.02313.x

Schwartzman-Morris, J., & Putterman, C. (2012). Gender differences in the pathogenesis and outcome of lupus and of lupus nephritis. *Clinical and Developmental Immunology, 2012*, 9 pages. doi:10.1155/2012/604892.

Shaffer, E. A. (2012). Laboratory tests of the liver and gallbladder. *Merck manual: Health care professionals*. Retrieved from http://www.merckmanuals.com/professional/hepatic_and_biliary_disorders/testing_for_hepatic_and_biliary_disorders/laboratory_tests_of_the_liver_and_gallbladder.html.

Sheth, S. G., & LaMont, J. T. (2012). Toxic megacolon. *Up to date*. Retrieved from http://www.uptodate.com/contents/toxic-megacolon?source=search_result&search=megacolon&selectedTitle=1%7E66#H4.

Singh, T., & Newman, A. B. (2011). Inflammatory markers in population studies of aging. *Ageing Research Reviews, 10*(3), 319–329. doi:10.1016/j.arr.2010.11.002.

Spondylitis Association of America. (2012). *Breaking news: New rate of prevalence of spondyloarthritis*. Retrieved from http://www.spondylitis.org/press/news/542.aspx.

Stein, C., & Kuchler, S. (2012). Non-analgesic effects of opioids: Peripheral opioid effects on inflammation and wound healing. *Current Pharmaceutical Design, 18*(37), 6053–6069.

Tazkarji, M. B. (2008). Abdominal pain among older adults. *Geriatrics and Aging, 11*(7), 410–415.

van de Kant, K. D. G., Klaassen, E. M. M., Jobsis, Q., Nijhuis, A. J., van Schayck, O. C. P., & Dompeling, E. (2009). Early diagnosis of asthma in young children by using non-invasive biomarkers of airway inflammation and early lung function measurements: Study protocol of a case-control study. *BMC Public Health, 9*, 210. doi:10.1186/1471-2459-9-210.

van de Kant, K. D. G., Klaassen, E. M. M., van Aerde, K. J., Damoiseaux, J., Bruggeman, C. A., Stelma, F. F., . . . Dompeling, E. (2012). Impact of bacterial colonization on exhaled inflammatory markers in wheezing preschool children. *Journal of Breath Research, 6*(4), 046001. doi:10.1088/1752-7155/6/4/046001.

VanLeeuwen, A. M., Poelhuis-Leth, D. J., & Bladh, M. L. (2013). *Laboratory diagnostic tests with nursing implications* (5th ed.). Philadelphia, PA: F. A. Davis.

Varon, J. V., & Acosta, P. (2010). *Handbook of critical and intensive care medicine* (2nd ed.). New York, NY: Springer.

Welch, T. R. (2012). An approach to the child with acute glomerulonephritis. *International Journal of Pediatrics, 2012*, 426192. doi:10.1155/2012/426192.

Wheeler, D. S., Wong, H. R., & Zingarelli, B. (2011). "Children are not small adults!" *Open Inflammation Journal, 4*(Suppl. 1-M2), 4–15.

Zagaria, M. E. (2010). Gallstones: Aging and medications increase risk. *US Pharmacist, 32*(12), 21–24.

11 Intracranial Regulation

MODULE AT-A-GLANCE

◪ THE CONCEPT OF INTRACRANIAL REGULATION

Intracranial regulation refers to the processes that affect intracranial compensation and adaptive neurological function. The neurological system regulates and integrates all body functions, muscle movements, senses, cognitive abilities, and emotions. It collects, as sensory input, information from the internal and external environments, processes and interprets the input, and causes responses that are manifested as motor or sensory output. **≪**

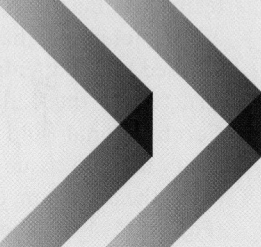

Concept Learning Outcomes

After reading about this concept, you will be able to:

1. Summarize the physiology of the neurological system related to intracranial regulation.

2. Examine the relationship between intracranial regulation and other concepts/systems.

3. Identify commonly occurring alterations in intracranial regulation and their related therapies.

4. Differentiate common assessment techniques used to examine intracranial regulation in clients across the life span.

5. Describe diagnostic and laboratory tests to determine the individual's intracranial regulation.

6. Explain the management of intracranial regulation and prevention of intracranial disease.

7. Demonstrate the nursing process in providing culturally competent and caring interventions across the life span for individuals with alterations in intracranial regulation.

8. Compare and contrast common independent and collaborative interventions for clients with alterations in intracranial regulation.

Concept Key Terms

Aphasia, *698*

Brain death, *694*

Brainstem, *689*

Central nervous system, *688*

Cerebellum, *688*

Cerebrospinal fluid (CSF), *688*

Cerebrum, *688*

Consciousness, *692*

Decerebrate posturing, *691*

Decorticate posturing, *691*

Fasciculations, *701*

Increased intracranial pressure (IICP), *693*

Intracranial regulation, *687*

Kinesthesia, *702*

Locked-in syndrome, *694*

Meninges, *688*

Neuron, *688*

Peripheral nervous system, *688*

Persistent vegetative state, *694*

Reflexes, *689*

Seizures, *694*

Spinal cord, *689*

Tremors, *703*

▶ NORMAL INTRACRANIAL REGULATION

The neurological system is made up of two parts. The **central nervous system**, which consists of the brain and the spinal cord and the **peripheral nervous system**, which is made up of the cranial nerves and the spinal nerves. These systems combine to allow for both voluntary and involuntary activities to occur.

The basic cell of the nervous system is the **neuron**. Neurons are highly specialized cells that send impulses throughout the body. Myelin sheaths that cover many of the larger diameter and long nerves help speed the rate of conduction of nerve impulses.

Physiology Review

CENTRAL NERVOUS SYSTEM   The central nervous system (CNS) consists of the brain and the spinal cord. The brain is the control center of the nervous system, generating thought, emotion, and speech. It is a sensitive organ covered by a protective coating of three connective tissue membranes, known as the **meninges**, that nourish the CNS. In addition to being covered by the meninges, the brain is protected by the bony structure of the skull and cushioned by cerebrospinal fluid. **Cerebrospinal fluid (CSF)** cushions the brain and prevents injury to brain tissue (**Box 11–1** ●). The brain consists of four parts: the cerebrum, cerebellum, brainstem, and diencephalon (**Figure 11–1** ●). The cerebrum is the largest part of the brain; its two hemispheres account for approximately 85% of the brain's weight.

The **cerebrum**, is composed of gray matter and has two hemispheres that are divided into four regions knows as lobes

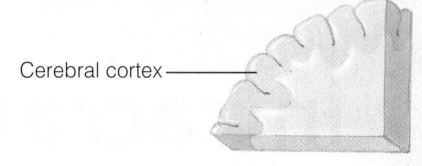
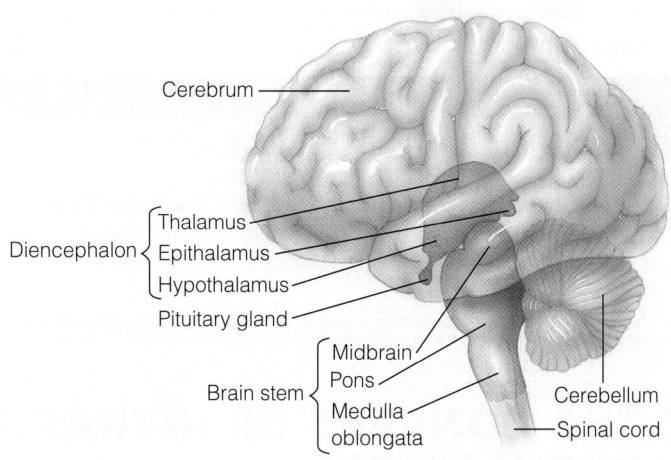

Figure 11–1 ● Regions of the brain.

(**Figure 11–2** ●). The frontal lobe is involved with speech, thought, learning, emotion, and voluntary movement. The prefrontal cortex of the frontal lobe controls more complicated cognitive processes, such as judgment, reasoning, and concern for others. The parietal lobe processes all of the sensory information, including shapes, temperature, pain, and two-point discrimination (e.g., hot vs. cold). The occipital lobe, where the visual cortex is located, processes vision. The last lobe is the temporal lobe, which stores memory and interprets auditory stimuli. The olfactory cortex, which interprets smell, is also located in the temporal lobe.

The cerebellum is the second largest part of the brain. The cerebellum is made up of gray and white matter and is responsible for muscle movement, balance, and control. The cerebellum

Box 11–1   Cerebrospinal Fluid

Cerebrospinal fluid is a clear and colorless liquid formed by the choroid plexus, which is made up of groups of specialized capillaries located in the brain ventricles. Derived from blood plasma, CSF consists of 99% water and contains protein, sodium, chloride, potassium, bicarbonate, and glucose (see below for normal laboratory values for CSF). The usual amount of CSF ranges from 80 to 200 mL and is replaced several times each day. CSF is normally produced and absorbed in equal amounts. CSF circulates from the lateral ventricles of the cerebral hemispheres into the third ventricle, through the midbrain, and into the fourth ventricle. Some CSF flows down the center of the spinal cord as the rest of it circulates into the subarachnoid space and returns to the blood through the arachnoid villi. CSF forms a cushion for the brain tissue, protects the brain and spinal cord from trauma, helps provide nourishment for the brain, and removes the waste products of cerebrospinal cellular metabolism.

COMPONENT	NORMAL VALUE
Appearance	Clear and colorless
pH	7.35
Specific gravity	1.007
White blood cells	0–8 mm^3
Protein	15–45 mg/dL
Glucose	40–80 mg/dL
Chloride	118–132 mEq/L
Pressure	75–175 mmH$_2$O

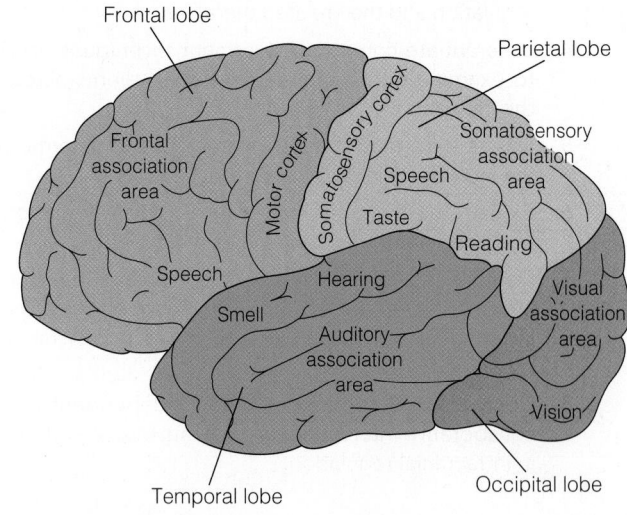

Figure 11–2 ● Lobes of the cerebrum.

coordinates stimuli from the cerebral cortex, transmitting information required for skeletal muscle coordination and smooth movements.

The diencephalon consists of the thalamus, hypothalamus, and epithalamus. The thalamus is the relay center for all signals coming to the brain. The thalamus takes all incoming nerve impulses and sends those signals to the correct region of the brain. The hypothalamus is the autonomic control center, and is involved in regulating activities such as heart rate, blood pressure, respiratory rate and depth, pain, pleasure, and fear. The hypothalamus also controls body temperature, food and water intake and balance, sleep cycles, and digestive motility.

The last part of the brain is the brainstem. The **brainstem** is made up of the midbrain, pons, and medulla oblongata. The brainstem controls reflexes and influences all basic physiological functions including breathing, blood pressure, and heart rate. The brainstem also regulates activities such as vomiting, hiccupping, coughing, and sneezing. Ten of the 12 pairs of cranial nerves originate in the brainstem. The brainstem is also the location of the reticular formation, which contains neurons that integrate sensory information from the peripheral nervous system (see below) and relay the information to the cerebral cortex. The upper part of the reticular formation consists of a network of ascending nerve fibers called the reticular activating system (RAS). The RAS is involved in circadian rhythm.

The brain contains four ventricles, which are chambers filled with CSF. They are linked by ducts that allow the CSF to circulate. One lateral ventricle is located in each hemisphere. These ventricles communicate with the third ventricle through the foramen of Monro. The third ventricle communicates with the fourth ventricle through the cerebral aqueduct that runs through the midbrain. The cerebral aqueduct is continuous with the central canal of the spinal cord.

The **spinal cord** is an extension of the brainstem, specifically the medulla oblongata. In adults, it is 42 cm (16.5 in.) in length and, like the brain, is protected by the meninges and CSF. The bony structure of the spine also provides protection for the spinal cord. The spinal cord transmits impulses to and from the brain.

PERIPHERAL NERVOUS SYSTEM The peripheral nervous system is made up of 12 pairs of cranial nerves and the spinal nerves. The cranial nerves all originate in the brain, with 10 originating in the brainstem and 2 originating in the anterior part of the brain. When assessing and documenting activity related to the cranial nerves, be sure to use the number rather than the name, in order to ensure accurate accounting. Each of the nerves may be either sensory, motor, or mixed nerves. See **Table 11–1** for a summary of the cranial nerves.

The 31 pairs of spinal nerves are named by their location: 8 cervical pairs, 12 thoracic pairs, 5 lumbar pairs, 5 sacral pairs, and a pair of coccygeal nerves (**Figure 11–3**). All spinal nerves produce motor and sensory activities. Each nerve is responsible for a different area of the body. Although each nerve has a specific function, there will always be some overlap between the areas of responsibility.

Reflexes are rapid, involuntary, predictable motor responses to a stimulus. *Somatic reflexes* result in skeletal muscle contraction. *Autonomic reflexes* activate cardiac muscle, smooth muscle, and glands. A reflex occurs over a pathway called a reflex arc.

Genetic and Lifespan Considerations
At birth, babies have what are known as primitive reflexes. These are reflexes that arise in the spinal cord and do not

TABLE 11–1 Cranial Nerves

NAME	NUMBER	FUNCTION	ACTIVITY
Olfactory	I	Sensory	Sense of smell
Optic	II	Sensory	Vision
Oculomotor	III	Motor	Pupillary reflex, extrinsic muscle movement of eye
Trochlear	IV	Motor	Eye–muscle movement
Trigeminal	V	Mixed	*Ophthalmic branch:* sensory impulses from scalp, upper eyelid, nose, cornea, and lacrimal gland *Maxillary branch:* sensory impulses from lower eyelid, nasal cavity, upper teeth, upper lip, alate *Mandibular branch:* sensory impulses from tongue, lower teeth, skin of chin, and lower lip; motor action includes teeth clenching, movement of mandible.
Abducens	VI	Mixed	Extrinsic muscle movement of eye
Facial	VII	Mixed	Taste (anterior two thirds of tongue); facial movements such as smiling, closing of eyes, frowning; production of tears and salivary stimulation
Vestibulocochlear (acoustic)	VIII	Sensory	*Vestibular branch:* sense of balance or equilibrium *Cochlear branch:* sense of hearing
Glossopharyngeal	IX	Mixed	Produces the gag and swallowing reflexes; taste (posterior third of the tongue)
Vagus	X	Mixed	Innervates muscles of throat and mouth for swallowing and talking; other branches responsible for pressoreceptors and chemoreceptor activity
Spinal accessory	XI	Motor	Movement of the trapezius and sternocleidomastoid muscles; some movement of larynx, pharynx, and soft palate
Hypoglossal	XII	Motor	Movement of tongue for swallowing, movement of food during chewing, and speech

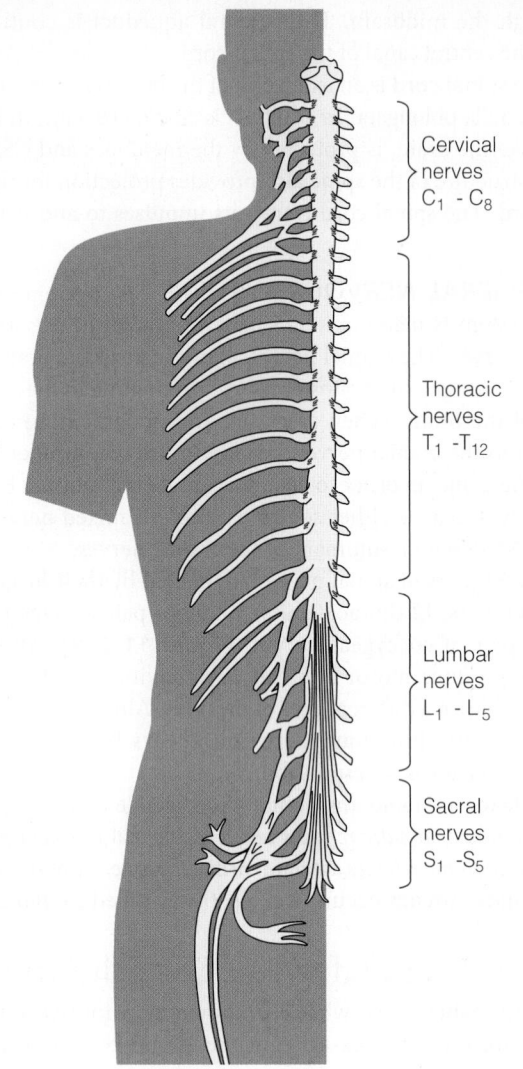

Figure 11–3 ● Spinal nerves.

Cervical nerves C_1 - C_8

Thoracic nerves T_1 -T_{12}

Lumbar nerves L_1 - L_5

Sacral nerves S_1 -S_5

require interpretation by the brain. Several of the common primitive reflexes present at birth are the stepping reflex, the startle reflex, the sucking reflex, and the Babinski reflex (see the module on Reproduction for further discussion). By the end of the first month of age, most of the primitive reflexes have disappeared, although the Babinski reflex is normal in children through the age of 2. The presence of the Babinski reflex from age 2 years and on indicates cerebral damage.

It is important when assessing the newborn to measure the head circumference. The anterior fontanel remains open for a year, the posterior closes at about 2 months. The fontanels are open at birth to accommodate the head passing through the birth canal and then to accommodate on-going brain growth and development. If intracranial edema or bleeding occur, the open fontanels help to accommodate the expansion in the cranium. An abnormally large head circumference is an indicator of increased intracranial pressure, which warrants immediate intervention. Another indicator is the infant's cry: a shrill, "catlike" cry or a weak or absent cry are indicators of cerebral disease.

Neurological changes associated with aging often go unnoticed in the older adult. These include memory loss, a subtle loss of coordination, and slower or diminished reflexes. Sensory changes may occur as well.

Careful assessment of the older adult is recommended, because neurological changes may result from any of a variety of factors, including medications, acute illness (such as infection), and progressive illness (such as Parkinson or Alzheimer disease).

▶ ALTERATIONS TO INTRACRANIAL REGULATION

Alterations of cerebral function may occur due to illness or injury. Assessment of the individual client's patterns of manifestation helps determine the extent of improvement or deterioration of intracranial regulation. Except in the case of direct damage to the brainstem and RAS, brain function deterioration usually follows a predictable progression, that is, a pattern in which higher levels of function are impaired initially, progressing to impairment of

Head in neutral position

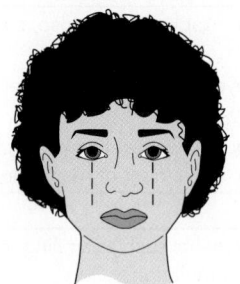

Eyes midline

Head rotated to client's left

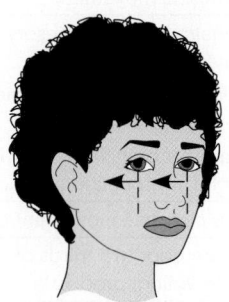

Doll's eyes absent (normal):
Eyes do not follow head movement. Gaze shifts to opposite direction of head movement.

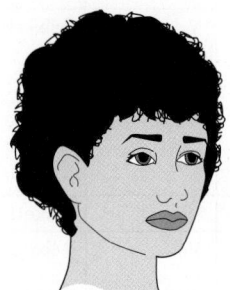

Doll's eyes present (abnormal):
Eyes follow head movement, producing a persistent forward gaze. Eyes do not move in relation to head. Direction of vision follows head to left.

Figure 11–4 ● Doll's eye movements characteristic of altered LOC.

TABLE 11–2   Progression of Deteriorating Brain Function

LEVEL OF CONSCIOUSNESS	PUPILLARY RESPONSE	OCULOMOTOR RESPONSES	MOTOR RESPONSES	BREATHING
Alert; oriented to time, place, and person	Brisk and equal; pupils regular	Eyes move in opposite direction of head movement, Caloric testing (ear irrigation) produces nystagmus.	Purposeful movement; responds to commands	Regular pattern with normal rate, rhythm, and depth
Responds to verbal stimuli; shows decreased concentration; agitation, confusion, lethargy; is disoriented	Small and reactive	Roving eye movements; doll's eyes present (**Figure 11–4 ●**), eye deviation away from cold caloric stimulus and toward warm stimulus	Purposeful movement in response to pain stimulus	Yawning, sighing respirations
Requires continuous stimulation to rouse			**Decorticate posturing** (abnormal posture with the arms flexed at the elbow, adducted, and drawn close to the torso; the wrists and fingers also are flexed; the legs extended and internally rotated; and the feet plantar flexed) with upper extremity flexion (**Figure 11–5A ●**)	Cheyne-Stokes respirations with crescendo–decrescendo pattern in rate and depth followed by period of apnea
Displays reflexive positioning to pain stimulus	Pupils fixed (nonreactive) in midposition	Caloric testing produces nystagmus	**Decerebrate posturing** (abnormal posture with the neck extended; the jaw clenched; arms pronated, extended, and close to the sides; legs extended and feet plantar flexed) with adduction and rigid extension of upper and lower extremities (see **Figure 11–5B ●**)	Central neurogenic hyperventilation with rapid, regular, and deep respirations; apneustic (slow deep breathing holding the breath for 30–90 seconds before rapid exhalation) breathing with prolonged inspiration and pauses at full inspiration and following expiration
Shows no response to stimuli	Fixed pupils in midposition	No spontaneous eye movement or nystagmus	Extension of upper extremities with flexion of lower extremities; flaccidity	Cluster or ataxic breathing with irregular pattern and depth of respirations; gasping respirations or apnea

more primitive functions. Altered level of consciousness (LOC) and behavior changes are early manifestations of the deterioration of the function of the cerebral hemispheres. Structures in the midbrain and brainstem are affected sequentially, with characteristic changes in LOC; patterns of respiration, widening pulse pressure, pupillary, and oculomotor responses; and motor function. Manifestations of progressive deterioration of cerebral function are outlined in **Table 11–2 ●**.

Intracranial regulation has important implications across all body systems and in a variety of areas. The Concepts Related to Intracranial Regulation feature describes some of these relationships.

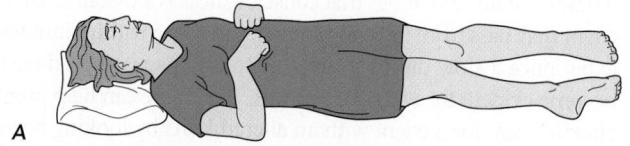
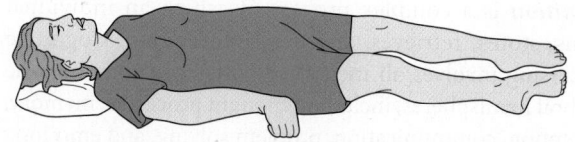

A   B

Figure 11–5 ● A, Decorticate posturing, characterized by rigid flexion, is associated with lesions above the brainstem in the corticospinal tracts. B, Decerebrate posturing, distinguished by rigid extension, is associated with lesions of the brainstem.

Concepts Related to **Intracranial Regulation**

Often the earliest warning signs of alterations to intracranial regulation are alterations in level of consciousness and respirations. The increased CO_2 level associated with respiratory acidosis can result in vasodilation, leading to an increase in intracranial pressure (ICP). Clients with impaired intracranial regulation often experience changes in cognition. This may range from the mild, temporary confusion often associated with a minor fall to the complete unconsciousness associated with traumatic brain injury. Without prompt intervention, increased ICP can lead to herniation and eventual brain death.

CONCEPT	RELATIONSHIP TO INTRACRANIAL REGULATION	NURSING IMPLICATIONS
Acid–Base Balance		
■ Respiratory acidosis	↑ CO_2 → vasodilation → IICP	■ Assess LOC; act immediately to decrease the ICP. ■ Underlying cause determines treatment.
Oxygenation		
■ Oxygenation assessment ■ Collaborative interventions and therapies	↓ LOC may result in ↓ respirations.	■ Assess airway, respirations. ■ *Anticipate:* airway support. An oropharyngeal airway may be sufficient for clients who are drowsy but arousable. Clients with more serious alterations in consciousness may require endotracheal intubation or mechanical ventilation.
Comfort		
■ End-of-life care	↑ ICP → herniation → brain death	■ Provide end-of-life care as appropriate. ■ Assess for advanced directives, including organ donation. ■ Provide psychosocial and spiritual support to family members.
Cognition		
■ Mental assessment ■ Confusion	Alterations in intracranial regulation can impair cognitive function ranging from mild to confusion to lack of consciousness.	■ Assess LOC. ■ Assess vital signs. ■ Underlying cause (e.g., fall, seizure, disease) determines treatment.

Alterations in Level of Consciousness

Consciousness is the state in which the individual is aware of self and environment and is able to respond appropriately to stimuli. Full consciousness requires both normal arousal and full cognition.

■ *Arousal*, or alertness, depends on the reticular activating system (RAS), a diffuse system of neurons in the thalamus and upper brainstem.

■ *Cognition* is a complex process by which an individual learns, stores, retrieves, and uses information. Cognitive processing involves all mental activities controlled by the cerebral hemispheres, including thought processes, memory, perception, communication, problem solving, and emotion.

These two components of consciousness depend on the normal physiological functions of and connections between the arousal mechanisms of the reticular formation and the cognitive functions of the cerebral hemispheres. Because arousal and cognition are independent components of consciousness, each can act separately on stimuli. For example, the RAS reacts to the discomfort of a full bladder by waking the person in the middle of the night. Once the person is awake, however, the frontal cortex alerts the person that the bladder is full and prompts the person to go to the bathroom and empty it.

Conditions that affect either the RAS or the function of the cerebral hemispheres can interfere with the normal LOC. Terms describing altered LOC are listed and defined in **Table 11–3** ●. Nurses should remember that consciousness is a dynamic state: A client may pass from full consciousness to coma within minutes or experience a slow diminishment of consciousness that does not become evident for weeks or months. The nurse can help provide effective care for a client with an altered LOC by looking beyond the diagnostic labels of consciousness and accurately assessing the client's behavior and response to stimuli.

An individual's LOC may be altered by processes that affect the arousal functions of the brainstem, the cognitive functions of the cerebral hemispheres, or both. The major causes of altered

TABLE 11–3 Terms Used to Describe Level of Consciousness

TERM	CHARACTERISTICS OF CLIENT
Full consciousness	Alert; oriented to time, place, and person; comprehends spoken and written words
Confusion	Unable to think rapidly and clearly; easily bewildered, with poor memory and short attention span; misinterprets stimuli; judgment is impaired
Disorientation	Not aware of or not oriented to time, place, or person
Obtundation	Lethargic, somnolent; responsive to verbal or tactile stimuli but quickly drifts back to sleep
Stupor	Generally unresponsive; may be briefly aroused by vigorous, repeated, or painful stimuli; may shrink away from or grab at the source of stimuli
Semicomatose	Does not move spontaneously; unresponsive to stimuli, although vigorous or painful stimuli may result in stirring, moaning, or withdrawal from the stimuli, without actual arousal
Coma	Unarousable; will not stir or moan in response to any stimulus; may exhibit nonpurposeful response (slight movement) of area stimulated but makes no attempt to withdraw
Deep coma	Completely unarousable and unresponsive to any kind of stimulus, including pain; absence of brainstem reflexes, corneal, papillary, and pharyngeal reflexes, and tendon and plantar reflexes

LOC are (1) lesions or injuries that affect the cerebral hemispheres directly and widely or that compress or destroy the neurons of the RAS, (2) metabolic disorders, and (3) medications.

The function of the brain, especially the cerebral hemispheres, depends on continuous blood flow with unimpeded supplies of oxygen and glucose. Processes that disrupt this flow of blood and nutrients may cause widespread damage to the cerebral hemispheres, impairing arousal and cognition. Bilateral hemispheric lesions (such as global ischemia) or metabolic disorders (such as hypoglycemia) are the most common causes of altered LOC related to cerebral dysfunction of the hemispheres. Localized masses that displace normal structures and cause direct or indirect pressure on the opposite hemisphere or brainstem also can affect LOC. Hematoma and cerebral edema are just two examples of such masses. The client who has widespread damage to the cerebral hemispheres but an intact RAS has sleep–wake cycles and may rouse in response to stimuli; the client cannot be said to be alert, however, because cognition is impaired.

DISORDERS AFFECTING LEVEL OF CONSCIOUSNESS
Both localized neurological processes and systemic disorders can alter LOC. Processes occurring in the brain that may directly destroy or compress neurological structures include the following:

- Increased intracranial pressure (IICP)
- Cerebral infarction
- Hematoma
- Hydrocephalus
- Intracranial hemorrhage
- Tumors
- Infections
- Injury from excitatory amino acids
- Demyelinating disorders.

Any systemic condition that affects the delivery of blood, oxygen, and glucose to the brain or that alters cell membranes also may alter LOC. If cerebral blood flow is impaired or the client becomes hypoxic or hypoglycemic, cerebral metabolism is impaired and LOC often declines rapidly. Severe hypoxia

quickly leads to ischemia. Ischemia may be focal (for example, following a stroke) or global (as from cardiac arrest or hypovolemic shock). Clients at particular risk include those with poorly controlled diabetes and those with cardiac or respiratory failure.

Other metabolic alterations that can affect LOC include fluid and electrolyte imbalances, such as hyponatremia (an abnormally low level of sodium in the blood), hyperosmolality (increased osmotic concentration of a solution expressed as osmoles of solute per kilogram of serum water), and acid–base alterations such as hypercapnia (an elevated arterial carbon dioxide level). Accumulated waste products and toxins from liver or renal failure can affect neuronal and neurotransmitter function, altering LOC. Drugs that depress the central nervous system (e.g., alcohol, analgesics, and anesthetics) suppress metabolic and membrane activities in the RAS and cerebral hemispheres, thereby affecting LOC. Glutamate, the main excitatory neurotransmitter in the brain, may accumulate during prolonged ischemia, resulting in acute glutamate toxicity and cell death.

Increased Intracranial Pressure   The normal range for ICP is typically 1–15 mmHg, but can vary based on measurement techniques. Normal ranges across the life span are:

- Infants: 1.5–6 mmHg
- Children: 3–7 mmHg
- Adults: 5–15 mmHg.

Increased intracranial pressure is sustained elevated pressure (15 mmHg or higher in adults) in the cranial cavity (Brosche, 2011; Dunn, 2002). In adults, ICP greater than 20 mmHg warrants immediate treatment interventions.

Like blood pressure, ICP can be affected by routine activities such as sneezing, coughing, or even something as simple as sitting up. The body's compensatory mechanisms control for these minor alterations. However, when ICP rises dramatically or for sustained periods of time, significant tissue ischemia and damage to delicate neural tissue may result. The cranial vault is of a fixed size (except in infants whose suture lines remain open allowing for expansion) and only has room for a prescribed amount of blood, CSF, and brain matter. To compensate for increasing ICP, CSF production decreases, followed by decreasing blood perfusion, resulting in diminished oxygenation of neurons. Because the neurons in the cerebral cortex are the most sensitive to oxygen deficit, changes in cortical function are the earliest manifestations of ICP, demonstrated by personality changes as well as impaired memory and judgment.

Seizures   Seizure activity commonly affects LOC. **Seizures** are periods of abnormal electrical discharges in the brain that may cause involuntary movement and/or behavior and sensory alterations. It appears that the spontaneous, disordered discharge of activity that occurs during a seizure exhausts energy metabolites or produces locally toxic molecules, altering LOC for a time after the seizure. Consciousness returns when the metabolic balance of the neurons is restored.

As the impairment of brain function progresses, more stimuli are required to elicit a response from the client. Initially, the client may rouse to verbal stimuli and respond appropriately to questions, remaining oriented to time, place, and person. With deterioration of neurological function, the client becomes more difficult to rouse and may become agitated and confused when awakened. Orientation to time is lost initially, followed by orientation to place and then to person. Continuous stimulation or vigorous shaking is required to maintain wakefulness as LOC decreases. Eventually, the client does not respond even to deep, painful stimuli.

OUTCOMES OF ALTERED LEVEL OF CONSCIOUSNESS   Possible outcomes of altered LOC and coma include full recovery with no long-term residual effects, recovery with residual damage (e.g., learning deficits, emotional difficulties, or impaired judgment), and more severe consequences such as persistent vegetative state (cerebral death) or brain death.

Persistent Vegetative State   **Persistent vegetative state** (also called *irreversible coma*) is a permanent condition of complete unawareness of self and the environment, and loss of all cognitive functions. Usually the result of severe brain trauma or global ischemia, this condition results from death of the cerebral hemispheres with continued function of the brainstem and cerebellum. Although the homeostatic regulatory functions of the brain continue, the ability to respond meaningfully to the environment is lost.

The client in a persistent vegetative state has sleep–wake cycles and may retain the ability to chew, swallow, and cough but cannot interact with the environment. When the person is awake, the eyes may wander back and forth across the room, but they cannot track an object or an individual. In a minimally conscious state, the client is aware of the environment and can follow simple commands, manipulate objects, gesture or verbalize to indicate yes/no responses, and make meaningful movements (such as blinking or smiling) in response to a stimulus. With appropriate supportive care, the client may remain in this state for years.

Locked-In Syndrome   **Locked-in syndrome** is distinctly different from a persistent vegetative state in that the client is alert and fully aware of the environment and has intact cognitive abilities but is unable to communicate through speech or movement because of blocked efferent pathways from the brain.

Motor paralysis affects all voluntary muscles, although the upper cranial nerves (I through IV) may remain intact, allowing the client to communicate through eye movements and blinking. In essence, the client is "locked" inside a paralyzed body while remaining fully conscious of self and environment.

Infarction or hemorrhage of the pons that disrupts outgoing nerve tracts but spares the RAS is the usual cause of locked-in syndrome. This condition also may result when the corticospinal tracts between the midbrain and pons are interrupted. Disorders of the lower motor neurons or muscles (e.g., acute polyneuritis, myasthenia gravis, and amyotrophic lateral sclerosis) also may paralyze motor responses, leading to locked-in syndrome.

Brain Death   **Brain death** is the cessation and irreversibility of all brain functions, including the brainstem. Although the exact legal criteria for establishing brain death may vary somewhat from state to state, it is generally agreed that brain death has occurred when there is no evidence of cerebral or brainstem function for an extended period (usually 6–24 hours) in a client who has a normal body temperature and is not affected by a depressant drug or alcohol poisoning. Generally recognized criteria are as follows:

- Unresponsive coma with absent motor and reflex movements
- No spontaneous respiration (apnea)
- Pupils fixed (unresponsive to light) and dilated
- Absent ocular responses to head turning and caloric stimulation (Caloric stimulation is performed by irrigating the ear with ice cold water to test the oculovestibular reflex, a reflex controlled by the brainstem. Normally, the cold causes the eyes to move first toward the irrigated side, followed by a return to midline.)
- Flat electroencephalogram (EEG) and no cerebral blood circulation present on angiography (if performed)
- Persistence of these manifestations for 30 minutes to 1 hour and for 6 hours after onset of coma and apnea.

Apnea in the comatose client is determined by the apnea test. The ventilator is removed while oxygenation is maintained by tracheal cannula, allowing the $PaCO_2$ to increase to 60 mmHg or higher. This level of carbon dioxide is high enough to stimulate respiration if the brainstem is functional. The EEG may be used to establish the absence of brain activity when brain death is suspected. A flat (isoelectric) EEG over a period of 6–12 hours in a client who is not hypothermic or under the influence of drugs that depress the CNS is generally accepted as an indicator of brain death.

Prognosis

The prognosis for clients with altered LOC, including coma, varies according to the underlying cause and pathological process. Age and general medical condition also play a role in determining outcome. Young adults may fully recover following deep coma from head injury, drug overdose, or other causes. Recovery of consciousness within 2 weeks is associated with a favorable outcome. In general, the prognosis is poor for clients who lack pupillary reaction or reflex eye movements 6 hours after the onset of coma.

Alterations and Therapies **Intracranial Regulation**

ALTERATION	DESCRIPTION	MANIFESTATIONS	INTERVENTIONS AND THERAPIES
Seizure disorder	Periods of abnormal electrical discharges in the brain	Causes involuntary movement as well as behavior and sensory alterations; can be partial (focal) or generalized.	▪ Maintain airway patency. ▪ Ensure safety. ▪ Administer medications as ordered. ▪ Provide emotional support. ▪ Identify and treat the underlying cause of the disorder. ▪ Realize that surgery may be performed to remove a tumor, lesion, or portion of the brain.
Status epilepticus	A continuous seizure that lasts for more than 30 minutes or a series of seizures during which time consciousness is not regained	Causes involuntary movement as well as behavior and sensory alterations. May cause alterations in breathing, injury, or pain.	▪ Maintain airway patency. ▪ Keep suction equipment at the bedside for excessive secretions. ▪ Give oxygen by mask. ▪ Monitor vital signs and circulation. ▪ Perform neurological assessment. ▪ Establish an intravenous line. ▪ Insert a nasogastric tube. ▪ Ensure safety. ▪ Manage thermoregulation. ▪ Administer medications as ordered; cumulative doses of drugs may produce respiratory depression, so be prepared to assist with ventilations. ▪ Realize that surgery may be performed to remove a tumor, lesion, or portion of the brain.
Increased intracranial pressure (IICP) (also labeled *intracranial hypertension*)	Sustained elevated pressure (15 mmHg or higher) in the cranial cavity	Oxygen deficit causes personality changes as well as impaired memory and judgment. IICP is a medical emergency.	▪ Maintain airway patency. ▪ Monitor neurological status; assessment areas include LOC, behavior, motor/sensory functions, pupillary size and reaction to light, and vital signs. ▪ Monitor IICP monitor or ventilator. ▪ Raise padded bed rails; seizures may occur. ▪ Monitor arterial blood gases. ▪ Elevate head of bed 30 degrees unless otherwise indicated. ▪ Monitor fluid and electrolytes. ▪ Monitor bladder distention and bowel constipation. ▪ Provide emotional support as needed. ▪ Reduce stimuli, coughing, sneezing, and vagal maneuvers that increase ICP. ▪ Identify and treat the underlying cause of the disorder. ▪ Realize that surgery may be performed to remove a tumor, lesion, or portion of the brain.

Box 11–2   Concussion

According to the National Institute of Neurological Disorders and Stroke, a concussion is "a short loss of consciousness in response to a head injury." Concussions are caused by a direct blow to the head or neck or from trauma that causes abrupt acceleration and deceleration forces (Norton et al., 2013). Typically an individual who sustains a concussion will present with signs and symptoms in four categories:

- *Physical:* headache, nausea, vomiting, balance problems, dizziness, visual problems, fatigue, sensitivity to light, numbness/tingling, dazed or stunned
- *Cognitive:* feeling mentally "foggy," feeling slowed down, difficulty concentrating, difficulty remembering, forgetful of recent information, confused about recent events, answers questions slowly, repeats questions
- *Emotional:* irritability, sadness, more emotional, nervousness
- *Sleep:* drowsiness, sleeping less or more than usual, trouble falling asleep (CDC, n.d.).

Nurses can help clients prevent head injury by providing anticipatory guidance related to safe practices, especially wearing protective equipment such as helmets when engaging in sports or activities with a high risk for concussion. School nurses can be particularly helpful by ensuring that coaches, teachers, other staff, and students receive training regarding sports injuries and concussion. This is essential, because between 5% and 10% of athletes will sustain a concussion in any given season. Football carries the greatest risk for concussion among male athletes; soccer carries the greatest risk for female athletes (Sports Concussion Institute, n.d.). As a result of a combination of research and, unfortunately, permanent injuries sustained by players on the field, many states have adopted or are adopting legislation to require schools to engage in a variety of preventive activities, including regulations regarding under what circumstances a player who is injured during a game may return to play.

Stay Current: Nurses need to stay up to date with current practices and be the providers of education for prevention of concussion. Stay current by visiting the CDC's Web site: www.cdc.gov/concussion.

Prevalence

Alterations in intracranial regulation may result from disease processes or from trauma. In particular, traumatic brain injuries (TBIs) are becoming more prevalent. According to the Centers for Disease Control and Prevention (CDC), at least 1.7 million TBIs occur each year. The adolescent and the older adult are the most vulnerable populations, and typically males are at a higher risk than females for TBIs (CDC, 2013).

Falls continue to be the leading cause of TBI (35.2%) in the United States, causing 50% of the TBIs among children ages 0–14 and 61% of all TBIs among adults ages 65 years or older (CDC, 2014). The CDC estimates that concussions, often seen in athletes, occur between 1.6 and 3.8 million times per year (**Box 11–2**) (Sports Concussion Institute, n.d.).

CASE STUDY \\ PART 1

Joshua Thomson is an active 13-year-old who was riding his bike with friends when he fell while attempting to jump over a ditch. His friends helped him home, and his mother has brought him to the urgent care center with complaints of a slight headache and a painful left wrist. As the triage nurse at the clinic, you interview Joshua and his mother. According to Joshua, he was attempting to jump the ditch when his bike tire caught on the curb. He flipped forward over the handle bars of his bike and landed on his back. He does not remember hitting his head on the ground but does remember putting his hands down to brace his fall. His biggest complaint at this moment is the pain he experiences when he moves his left wrist, but he is also nauseated and has a "small headache." Joshua's mother thinks that the headache and nausea may be due to the fact that Joshua has not eaten anything since 7:00 a.m. and it is now 4:00 p.m. The attending physician prescribes an x-ray of Joshua's wrist and acetaminophen (Tylenol) 650 mg for pain.

The x-ray shows that Joshua's left wrist is fractured. He is placed in a cast and given prescriptions for Tylenol for the pain and ondansetron (Zofran) for the nausea and sent home. As the nurse, you give Joshua's mother some discharge instructions for caring for the cast, using both the Tylenol and Zofran, and watching Joshua for any sign of neurological damage.

Clinical Reasoning Questions Level I

1. What neurological alterations would you educate Joshua's mom to watch for?
2. What should Joshua's mother do if she makes any of these observations?

Clinical Reasoning Questions Level II

3. What prevention education should be given to Joshua and his mother?
4. What focused assessment should you perform?
5. Why would the physician prescribe ondansetron (Zofran) for nausea instead of promethazine (Phenergan)?

▶ PREVENTION

Neurological damage usually occurs after a traumatic event. Unfortunately, this does not allow for a great deal of preventive teaching for the client. With all clients, the nurse should stress the importance of wearing protective equipment. Helmets should be used at all times when bicycling, skateboarding, and skating. Sport-specific helmets and equipment are also important when participating in a contact sport. (For more information, see the module on Safety.) For older adults, preventive education to reduce the risk for injury includes client teaching related to fall prevention and to adherence to cautions that accompany prescription medications. Older adults at risk for falls may benefit from a home safety assessment.

▶ ASSESSMENT

A health assessment to determine problems with neurological structure and/or function may be conducted during a health screening, may focus on a chief complaint (such as headaches), or may be part of a total health assessment.

TABLE 11–4   Glasgow Coma Scale for Assessment of Coma in Infants, Children, and Adults

CATEGORY	SCORE	INFANT AND YOUNG CHILD CRITERIA	OLDER CHILD AND ADULT CRITERIA
Eye opening	4	Spontaneous opening	Spontaneous
	3	To loud noise	To verbal stimuli
	2	To pain	To pain
	1	No response	No response
Verbal response	5	Smiles, coos, cries to appropriate stimuli	Oriented to time, place, and person; uses appropriate words and phrases
	4	Irritable; cries	Confused
	3	Inappropriate crying	Inappropriate words or verbal response
	2	Grunts, moans	Incomprehensible words
	1	No response	No response
Motor response	6	Spontaneous movement	Obeys commands
	5	Withdraws to touch	Localizes pain
	4	Withdraws to pain	Withdraws to pain
	3	Abnormal flexion (decorticate)	Flexion to pain (decorticate)
	2	Abnormal extension (decerebrate)	Extension to pain (decerebrate)
	1	No response	No response

Add the score from each category to get the total. The maximum score is 15, indicating the best level of neurological functioning. The minimum is 3, indicating total neurological unresponsiveness.

Source: From Teasdale, G., & Jennett, B. (1974). Assessment of coma and impaired consciousness. *Lancet, 2,* 81–84; and James, H. E. (1986). Neurologic evaluation and support in the child with acute brain insult. *Pediatric Annals, 15*(1), 16–22.

Nursing Assessment

A neurological assessment is important and should be done as soon as possible when working with the client. Some part of a neurological assessment is done with every interaction with the client. The interview is the first step in the assessment process, and many of the answers will guide the nurse to an understanding of the client's problem.

If the client has problems with neurological structure or function, analyze its onset, characteristics, course, severity, precipitating and relieving factors, and any associated symptoms, noting the time and circumstances.

If the client's LOC is altered, the nurse may need to rely on family members for information. The client's LOC can be assessed by using the Glasgow Coma Scale (**Table 11–4 ●**).

Remember that, when beginning the assessment on a child, it is essential to consider the child's developmental age. Simpler interview questions and a shorter assessment may be necessary.

When assessing older adults, the assessment itself does not change, but the length of the assessment may need to be modified: The older adult may tire more easily and require frequent rest breaks. When interviewing older adults, allow time for them to think of an answer and to answer the question. Do not assume that they do not know the answer—allow for sufficient time to answer each question.

Assessment Interview   Neurological Assessment

General Questions

1. Have you ever been diagnosed with a neurological illness?
   - If so, when were you diagnosed?
   - What was the treatment plan?
   - What helped the problem?
   - What made the problem worse?
   - What medications were you prescribed?

2. Do you have a history of fainting or seizures?
   - If so, when was your first episode?
   - Do you experience an aura prior to the seizure?
   - How long does it take you to recover from the seizure?
   - Describe the seizure.
   - What medication do you take to control your seizures?
   - When was your last blood work done?
   - When was your last seizure?

3. Have you noticed any changes in your vision, hearing, or smelling? (See the module on Sensory Perception for specific questions.)

4. Have you noticed a change in your balance and coordination?
   - If so, can you describe these changes?
   - Do you notice tremors?
   - Do you feel that you are "clumsy"?
   - Are you able to bend over without falling over or getting dizzy?

5. Are you having pain?
   - If yes, can you describe the pain?
   - On scale of 0 to 10, with 0 being no pain and 10 being the worst pain you have ever felt, how would you rate your pain?
   - Can you point to one spot where you have the pain?
   - What helps to relieve your pain?
   - What makes the pain worse?

6. Have you noticed any changes in your memory?
   - If yes, can you describe the changes?
   - Do you need to make lists to help you remember things?

Neurological Assessment

ASSESSMENT/ METHOD	NORMAL FINDINGS	ABNORMAL FINDINGS	LIFESPAN OR DEVELOPMENTAL CONSIDERATIONS
Mental Status			
Assess appearance, including dress, hygiene, grooming, gait, and posture.	The client should be appropriately dressed and clean, with normal gait and posture.	■ Unilateral neglect (inattention to one side of body) may occur in some clients who have had a stroke. Poor hygiene and grooming may be seen in clients with dementia. ■ Abnormal gait and posture may be seen in transient ischemic attacks (TIAs), strokes, and Parkinson disease.	■ Infants and children may be lethargic, irritable, difficult to console.
Assess behavior, including actions and affect, content and quality of speech, and LOC. Use the Glasgow Coma Scale (Table 11–4) to document findings.	A score of 15 on the Glasgow Coma Scale indicates that the client is alert and oriented.	■ Emotional swings or changes in personality may be observed in clients who have had a stroke. ■ The face appears masklike (very little expressive movement of facial muscles) in clients experiencing the later stages of Parkinson disease. ■ Apathy is seen in clients with cognitive disorders. ■ **Aphasia** (defective or absent language function) may occur in clients who experience TIAs and strokes. Aphasia is seen in clients with damage to the left cerebral cortex. Aphasia is often seen in clients with strokes of the left hemisphere rather than the right hemisphere. ■ *Dysphonia* (change in the tone of the voice) is common in clients who have had strokes. Dysphonia is seen in clients with paralysis of the vocal cords (cranial nerve X). ■ *Dysarthria* (difficulty speaking) is seen in clients with lesions of upper and lower motor neurons, the cerebellum, and the extrapyramidal tract. ■ Damage to the brainstem and/or cerebral cortex may alter the client's LOC. ■ Drowsiness and decreased LOC may be associated with brain trauma, infections, TIAs, stroke, and brain tumors. ■ Stroke typically produces altered LOC that may range in severity from confusion to coma.	

Neurological Assessment (continued)

ASSESSMENT/ METHOD	NORMAL FINDINGS	ABNORMAL FINDINGS	LIFESPAN OR DEVELOPMENTAL CONSIDERATIONS
Assess cognitive function. Note orientation to time, place, and person. Note attention span and recent and remote memory. Ask the client to: 1. Repeat five to seven numbers. 2. Recall three items after 5 minutes. 3. Recall his or her address, breakfast, or birthday. Assess thought processes (both content and perceptions) by noting responses to questions. Note ability to understand what is said and to express thoughts. Note ability to make logical and safe judgments.	The client should be oriented to time, place, and person; demonstrate attention and ability to remember recent and past events; respond appropriately to questions; and be able to make judgments.	■ Disorientation to time and place may occur in clients with a stroke of the right cerebral hemisphere and in clients with cognitive disorders. ■ Memory deficits are often seen in clients who have had a stroke. ■ Perceptual deficits may be seen in clients who have had strokes. These same deficits may occur after brain trauma and in cognitive disorders. ■ Impaired cognition is often noted in clients with strokes, cerebral trauma, brain tumors, and cognitive disorders.	■ Child's verbal skills and ability to follow directions should be appropriate for age.

Cranial Nerves (CNs)

ASSESSMENT/ METHOD	NORMAL FINDINGS	ABNORMAL FINDINGS	LIFESPAN OR DEVELOPMENTAL CONSIDERATIONS
Test CN I (olfactory). Note client's ability to smell scents (e.g., soap, coffee) with each nostril. This test is usually done only if a problem with the ability to smell is reported.	Sense of smell should be equal in both nostrils.	■ *Anosmia* (inability to smell) may be seen in clients with lesions of the frontal lobe and may occur in clients with impaired blood flow to the middle cerebral artery.	■ *Infants:* Not tested. ■ *Children:* Not routinely tested.
Test CN II (optic). Assess vision in each eye with Snellen chart.	Based on previous ability to see and use of visual aids, client should be able to see with both eyes.	■ Blindness in one eye may be seen in clients with strokes or TIAs. Impaired vision or blindness in one side of both eyes (homonymous hemianopia) is associated with stroke. ■ Impaired vision may occur in clients with strokes and brain tumors. Double vision may be noted in clients with strokes and TIAs.	■ *Infant:* Shine a bright light in the eyes; a quick blink reflex and dorsal head flexion indicate light perception. ■ *Child:* Test vision and visual fields; visual acuity should be appropriate for age.
Test CNs III, IV, and VI (oculomotor, trochlear, and abducens, respectively). Assess extraocular movements by asking the client to follow your finger as you write an *H* in the air. Assess PERRL (pupils equal, round, and reactive to light) by covering one eye at a time and shining a bright light directly into the uncovered eye using a penlight or the ophthalmoscope.	Extraocular movements should be present bilaterally, and pupils should be equal, round, and reactive to light.	■ *Nystagmus* (involuntary eye movement) may be seen in clients with strokes. ■ Constricted pupils are associated with impaired blood flow from a stroke.	■ *Infant:* Shine a penlight in the eyes and move it side to side; infant should be able to focus and track the light. ■ *Child:* Move an object through the six cardinal points of gaze; child should be able to track the object through all fields.

(continued on next page)

Neurological Assessment (continued)

ASSESSMENT/METHOD	NORMAL FINDINGS	ABNORMAL FINDINGS	LIFESPAN OR DEVELOPMENTAL CONSIDERATIONS
Assess for *ptosis* (drooping eyelids).	Eyelids should not droop.	■ Ptosis occurs in clients with strokes, myasthenia gravis, and palsy of CN III.	
Test CN V (trigeminal). Assess ability to feel light, dull, and sharp sensations on the face. With the client's eyes closed, check whether sensation is the same on both sides of the face. Stroke the cheek with a wisp of cotton for light touch, with a closed safety pin for dull touch, and with a tongue depressor for sharp touch. If the sharp point of a safety pin is used to assess sharp touch, avoid scratching the surface of the skin and discard the pin after use. Assess the corneal reflex by touching the corneal surface with a wisp of sterile cotton. The reflex may be absent or decreased in clients who wear contact lenses.	Ability to feel light, dull, and sharp sensations should be intact. Normally the client blinks.	■ Changes in facial sensations are noted with impaired blood flow to the carotid artery. ■ Decreased sensations to the face and cornea on the same side of the body, as well as numbness of the lip and mouth, occur in clients with strokes. ■ Loss of facial sensation or contraction of the masseter and temporal muscles is seen in clients with lesions of CN V. ■ Severe facial pain is seen in clients with trigeminal neuralgia (tic douloureux). ■ The corneal reflex may be impaired in clients with lesions of CN V or VII.	■ *Infant:* Stimulate the rooting and sucking reflex to assess strength and pattern. ■ *Child:* Observe child chewing a cracker to assess bilateral jaw strength. Touch forehead and cheeks with a cotton ball with eyes closed; child should push the cotton ball away.
Test CN VII (facial). Assess ability to taste sweet, sour, and salt on the anterior two thirds of the tongue by asking the client to stick out the tongue and applying a salty, sweet, or sour substance. Assess ability to frown, show teeth, blow out cheeks, raise eyebrows, smile, and close eyes tightly.	Ability to taste sweet, sour, and salt should be intact. Client should be able to frown, show teeth, blow out cheeks, raise eyebrows, smile, and close eyes tightly. Muscle movement should be equal bilaterally.	■ Loss of ability to taste may occur in clients with brain tumors or nerve impairment. ■ Asymmetry or decreased movement of facial muscles is noted in clients with lesions of the upper and lower motor neurons. ■ Paralysis of the lower motor neurons from injury to CN VII results in inability to close eyes, a flat nasolabial fold, paralysis of lower face, and inability to wrinkle forehead. ■ Paralysis of the upper motor neurons from a stroke results in weakness of eyelids and paralysis of lower face. ■ Pain, paralysis, and sagging of facial muscles is seen on the affected side in Bell palsy.	■ *All ages:* Observe facial expressions for bilateral symmetry.
Test CN VIII (acoustic). Assess ability to hear the ticking of a watch and whispered and spoken words.	Client should be able to hear with both ears.	■ Decreased hearing or deafness may occur in clients with strokes and/or tumors of CN VIII.	■ *Infant:* Should blink, move head toward sound, or freeze position on hearing a loud sound. ■ *Child:* Whisper in each ear; child should turn head toward sound and repeat words correctly.

Neurological Assessment (continued)

ASSESSMENT/ METHOD	NORMAL FINDINGS	ABNORMAL FINDINGS	LIFESPAN OR DEVELOPMENTAL CONSIDERATIONS
Test CNs IX and X (glossopharyngeal and vagus, respectively). Assess gag reflex by touching back of client's throat with tongue depressor. If gag reflex is intact, observe client swallowing a small drink of water. Observe for a symmetric rise of soft palate and uvula as the client says "ah." Assess ability to taste salty, sweet, and sour substances on the posterior third of the tongue. (See previous description.)	Client should be able to swallow without difficulty, have symmetrical rise of the soft palate, have intact gag reflex, and taste appropriately.	■ *Dysphagia* (difficulty swallowing) is common in clients with impaired blood flow to the brain. ■ Unilateral loss of the gag reflex occurs in clients with lesions of CNs IX and X.	■ *Infant:* Observe swallowing during feeding. ■ *All ages:* Elicit gag reflex.
Test CN XI (spinal accessory). Assess the client's ability to shrug the shoulders and turn the head against resistance: Ask the client to turn the head to one side against the resistance of your hand; ask the client to shrug the shoulders while you exert downward pressure. Observe symmetry, strength, and size of muscles.	Client should be able to shrug shoulders and turn head against resistance.	■ Muscle weakness is noted in clients with lower motor neuron disease. ■ *Contralateral hemiparesis* (muscle weakness on the side opposite the lesion or trauma) is seen with strokes.	■ *Infants:* Not tested. ■ *Child:* Ask child to raise shoulders and turn head side to side against resistance. Observe for good strength in neck and shoulders.
Test CN XII (hypoglossal). Assess the client's ability to stick out the tongue and move the tongue from side to side against resistance of a tongue depressor. See **Table 11–5** ● for assessment of cranial nerves in the unconscious client.	Client should be able to stick out the tongue and move it from side to side against resistance.	■ Atrophy and **fasciculations** (twitches) of the tongue are seen in clients with lower motor neuron disease. ■ The tongue may deviate toward the involved side of the body.	■ *Infant:* Sucking and swallowing should be coordinated during feeding. ■ *Child:* Use tongue depressor as with adults.

Body Systems

Assess ability to perceive various sensations. Touch both sides of various parts of the body (chest, abdomen, arms, and legs) with one or more of the following: ■ Cotton wisp ■ Sharp object ■ Dull object. Place vibrating tuning fork on bony prominences.	Client can differentiate between soft and sharp and can feel vibrations appropriately.	■ Decreased sensation of pain occurs in clients with injury to the spinothalamic tract. ■ Decreased vibratory sensations are seen in clients with injuries to the posterior column tract. ■ Transient numbness of face, arm, or hand is seen in clients with TIAs. ■ Sensory loss on one side of the body is seen in clients with lesions of higher pathways to the spinal cord.	

(continued on next page)

Neurological Assessment (*continued*)

ASSESSMENT/ METHOD	NORMAL FINDINGS	ABNORMAL FINDINGS	LIFESPAN OR DEVELOPMENTAL CONSIDERATIONS
		■ Bilateral sensory loss is seen in polyneuropathy (a disease in which multiple peripheral nerves are affected, such as Guillain-Barré syndrome and diabetes mellitus). ■ Sensations are impaired in clients with strokes, brain tumors, and spinal cord trauma or compression.	
Assess sense of position (**proprioception**). Move the client's finger or big toe up or down. Ask the client to describe the movement.	Client can accurately describe position of finger or toe when moved up or down.	■ Lesions of the posterior column of the spinal cord may affect sense of position.	
Assess ability to discriminate fine touch. Ask the client to identify: 1. Object in hand, such as a coin or key (tests stereognosis) 2. Number written on hand (tests graphesthesia) (**Figure 11–6 ●**) 3. Two points of simultaneous pinpricks on the hand (tests two-point discrimination) (**Figure 11–7 ●**) 4. Where he or she is being touched (tests localization) 5. How many sensations are felt when the client is touched simultaneously on both sides of the body (tests extinction).	Client can identify and discriminate fine touch.	■ Inability to discriminate fine touch (stereognosis, graphesthesia, two points, point localization, and extinction) may occur in clients with injury to the posterior columns or sensory cortex.	

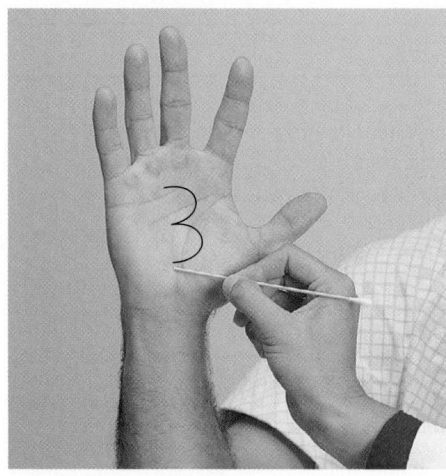
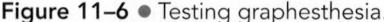

Figure 11–6 ● Testing graphesthesia.

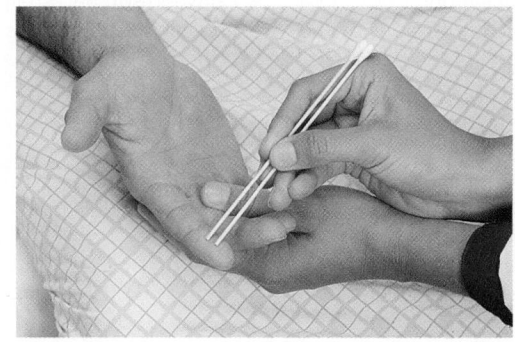

Figure 11–7 ● Testing two-point discrimination.

Neurological Assessment (continued)

ASSESSMENT/ METHOD	NORMAL FINDINGS	ABNORMAL FINDINGS	LIFESPAN OR DEVELOPMENTAL CONSIDERATIONS
Assess bilateral symmetry and size of muscles. Assess for **tremors** (involuntary quivering movements) and fasciculations (irregular movements). Observe movements as client is at rest (not making a purposeful movement) and with activity (making a purposeful movement such as reaching for a glass of water).	Muscles are bilaterally symmetrical and of equal size. Tremors or fasciculations are not present.	■ Atrophy of muscles is seen in clients with disease of the lower motor neurons. ■ Tremors that occur with activity are seen in clients with multiple sclerosis and diseases of the cerebellar system. ■ Tremors that occur at rest and disappear with movement are common in clients with Parkinson disease. ■ Fasciculations occur in clients with disease or trauma to the lower motor neurons, as a side effect of medications, in fever, in sodium deficiency, and in uremia.	
Assess muscle tone.	Muscle tone is appropriate.	■ Muscle tone is decreased (*flaccidity*) in clients with disease or trauma of the lower motor neurons and early stroke. ■ Muscle tone is increased (*spasticity*) in clients with disease of the corticospinal motor tract. ■ Muscles are rigid in clients with disease of the extrapyramidal motor tract. ■ Muscles move in small, regular, jerky movements (known as *cogwheel rigidity*) in clients with Parkinson disease.	■ Children with autism often have low muscle tone.
Assess bilateral muscle strength and movement. Ask the client to: 1. Squeeze your hands. 2. Push feet against the resistance of your hands. 3. Raise both legs off the bed.	Muscle strength and movement are bilaterally equal and strong.	■ Weakness of the arms, legs, or hands is often seen in clients with TIAs. ■ Hemiplegia (paralysis of one half of the body vertically) is noted in clients with strokes. ■ Flaccid paralysis is noted in clients with strokes. ■ Paralysis or decreased movement is seen in clients with multiple sclerosis and myasthenia gravis. ■ There is total loss of motor function below the level of injury in complete spinal cord transection and in injuries to the anterior portion of the spinal cord. ■ Spasticity of muscles may occur as a result of incomplete spinal cord injuries.	

(continued on next page)

Neurological Assessment (continued)

ASSESSMENT/ METHOD	NORMAL FINDINGS	ABNORMAL FINDINGS	LIFESPAN OR DEVELOPMENTAL CONSIDERATIONS
Cerebellar Function			
Assess gait. Ask the client to walk normally, then in a heel-to-toe fashion, then on toes, and finally on heels. Perform the Romberg test: Ask the client to stand with feet together and eyes closed. (Stand close to the client to prevent falling.)	Client has appropriate gait and can walk heel to toe, on toes, and on heels. There should be minimal swaying for up to 20 seconds.	■ *Ataxia* is a lack of coordination and a clumsiness of movements, with staggering, wide-based, and unbalanced gait. Causes of ataxia include stroke and cerebellar tumor. Swaying and falling are seen in clients with cerebellar ataxia. Inability to walk on toes, then heels, may indicate disease of the upper motor neurons. ■ Spastic hemiparesis is often associated with strokes or upper motor neuron disease. The client walks with one leg stiffly dragging while the other leg circles out and forward. One arm is held flexed and close to the side. ■ Steppage gait is noted with disease of the lower motor neurons. The client drags or lifts the foot high, then slaps the foot onto the floor. The client cannot walk on the heels. ■ Sensory ataxia may be associated with polyneuropathy or damage to the posterior columns. The client walks on the heels before bringing down the toes, and the feet are held wide apart. Gait worsens with the eyes closed. ■ Parkinsonian gait is often seen in clients with Parkinson's disease. In Parkinsonian gait, the client stoops over while walking and shuffles the feet. The arms are held close to the side. ■ A positive Romberg test may be seen in clients with cerebellar ataxia.	
Assess coordination. Observe ability to pat knees, alternating front and back of hands and increasing speed. Observe ability to touch each finger of one hand to the thumb. Observe ability to touch the nose, then one of your fingers, then the nose again. Observe ability to run each heel down each shin while in a supine position **(Figure 11–8 ●)**.	Client demonstrates coordinated movements.	■ Ataxic movements are apparent in clients with cerebellar disease.	 **Figure 11–8 ●** Heel-to-shin test.

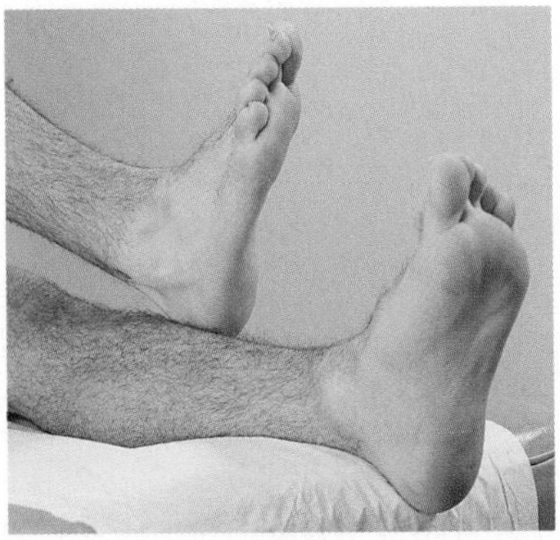

Neurological Assessment *(continued)*

ASSESSMENT/ METHOD	NORMAL FINDINGS	ABNORMAL FINDINGS	LIFESPAN OR DEVELOPMENTAL CONSIDERATIONS
Assess for the Brudzinski sign: With the client supine, flex the client's head to the chest (**Figure 11–9** ●).	There should be no flexion of the hips or knees.	■ Flexion of hips and knees occur in clients with meningeal irritation.	
Assess for the Kernig sign: With the client supine, flex the knees and hips, and then straighten the knee (**Figure 11–10** ●).	There should be no pain or resistance.	■ Excessive pain and/or resistance occurs in clients with meningeal irritation.	
Assess unconscious patients for signs of abnormal posturing.	There should be no abnormal posturing.	■ Observe for decorticate posturing, in which the arms are flexed at the elbow and adducted, drawn close to the torso; wrists and fingers also are flexed; the legs are extended with internal rotation; and the feet are plantar (see Figure 11–5A). ■ Observe for decerebrate posturing, in which the neck is extended, with the jaw clenched; the arms are pronated, extended, and close to the sides; the legs are extended straight out; and the feet are plantar (see Figure 11–5B). ■ Decorticate posturing occurs with lesions of the corticospinal tracts. ■ Decerebrate posturing occurs with lesions of the midbrain, pons, or diencephalons.	

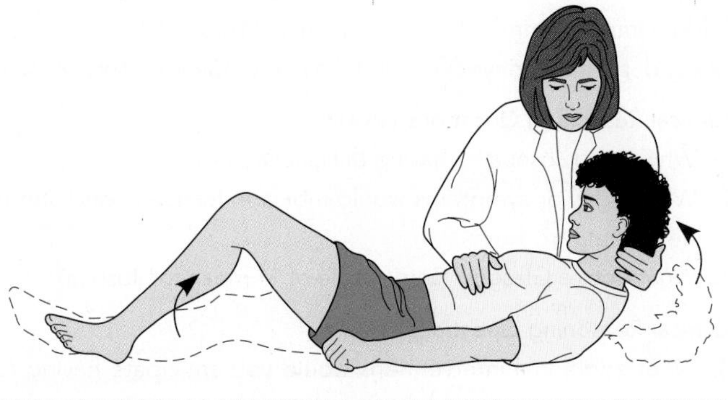

Figure 11–9 ● Assessing the Brudzinski sign.

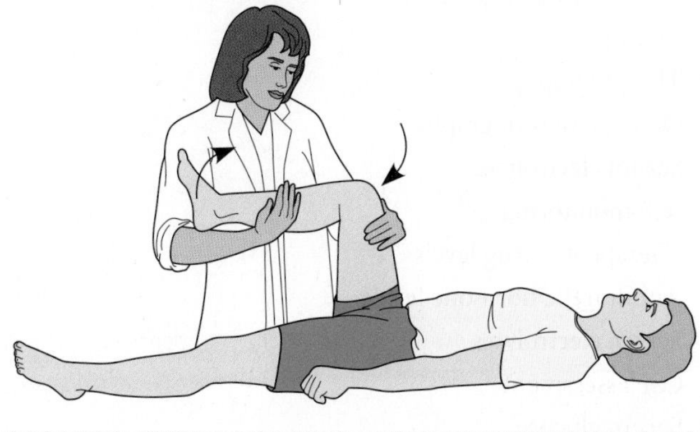

Figure 11–10 ● Assessing the Kernig sign.

Diagnostic Tests

Although a client's history and physical examination may indicate the cause of alterations in LOC, several diagnostic tests may be useful in establishing the diagnosis. The results of diagnostic tests of neurological structure and function are used to support the diagnosis of a specific injury or disease, to provide information to identify or modify the appropriate medications or therapy used to treat the disease, and to help nurses monitor the client's responses to treatment and nursing care interventions.

Prior to any diagnostic testing, the nurse should make sure the client understands the purpose of the test and explain to the client what will take place during testing. The nurse should provide the client with specific instructions, such as fasting and wearing appropriate clothes. Diagnostic tests to assess the

TABLE 11–5 Assessment of Cranial Nerves in the Unconscious Client

CRANIAL NERVES	REFLEX	ASSESSMENT PROCEDURE	NORMAL FINDINGS
II, III	Pupillary	Shine a light source in the eye.	■ Rapid, concentrically constricting pupils indicate intact CNs II and III.
II, IV, VI	Oculocephalic	Should be performed with eyes held open (doll's-eyes) and head turned from side to side. *Precaution:* Cervical spine injury must be ruled out before this assessment is performed.	■ Eyes gazing straight up or lagging slightly behind head motion indicate intact cranial nerves.
III, VIII	Oculovestibular	Place the head in a midline and slightly elevated position. Inject ice water into the ear canal. *Precautions:* Cervical spine injury must be ruled out before this assessment is performed. Tympanic membrane must be intact; otherwise, brain may be filled with bacteria-laden fluid. *Note:* This assessment is usually performed by a physician.	■ Eyes deviating toward the irrigated ear indicate intact CNs III and VIII.
V, VII	Corneal	Cornea is gently swabbed with sterile cotton swab.	■ A blink indicates intact CNs V and VII.
IX, X	Gag	Pharynx is irritated with tongue depressor or cotton swab.	■ Gagging response indicates intact CNs IX and X.

structures and functions of the neurological system include the following:

- Computed tomography (CT) scan of the head with or without contrast
- Magnetic resonance imaging (MRI)
- X-rays
- Echoencephalogram
- EEG
- Ultrasonography of the brain
- Brain echogram
- Cerebral angiography
- Positron emission tomography (PET) scan
- Nerve conduction studies
- Myelogram
- Thermography
- Oculoplethysmography
- Serum electrolytes
- ICP monitoring
- Therapeutic drug levels
- Antidiuretic hormone levels
- Serum electrolytes
- CSF assessment
- Serum glucose
- Serum protein.

✷ *For more details about these diagnostic tests of the neurological system, go to* **nursing.pearsonhighered.com** *and access Appendix B.*

CASE STUDY \\ PART 2

Joshua's mother stops by the pharmacy and picks up the prescriptions. When they arrive home, she makes dinner and then gets Joshua ready for bed. Joshua asks to watch TV before bed, but

complains that the sound is too loud and that he can't see the picture clearly. His mom tells him that he has had a rough day and he should get some sleep. As she tucks him into bed, she kisses him, and Joshua asks what day is tomorrow. She tells Joshua that tomorrow is Sunday and he can sleep in if he wishes.

The next morning, Josh's mother goes in to check on him and he is sleeping peacefully. She goes about her business. At 10:00 a.m., she checks on him again and finds him still asleep. This time she tries to wake him and has difficulty. After shaking him for a minute, Joshua finally opens his eyes. His speech is slurred and he has difficulty keeping his eyes open. Joshua's mom calls 911, and the paramedics take him to the emergency department.

As the nurse on duty, you perform the Glasgow Coma Scale: Joshua arouses to painful stimuli; he localizes pain and is confused; his speech is slurred and he does not recognize his mother. He can follow simple commands. You score him 11 out of 15. The emergency department physician calls for a neurological surgery consult.

Clinical Reasoning Questions Level I

1. Why would Joshua be having difficulty arousing?
2. What signs or symptoms would indicate Joshua's condition is deteriorating?
3. What does a Glasgow Coma Scale of 11 mean for Joshua?

Clinical Reasoning Questions Level II

4. What additional interventions would you anticipate having to administer to Joshua to prevent further increased intracranial pressure?
5. What education would you provide to Joshua's mother?
6. Who would you contact about the possibility of death in this client?

▶ INTERVENTIONS AND THERAPIES

The nurse must be able to recognize a change in the LOC of a client and must provide care for the client immediately. The first step in care is to treat the underlying cause and to prevent

Lifespan Considerations Assessing the Neurological System

Infants

Reflexes commonly tested in newborns include the following:

- *Rooting.* Stroke the side of the face near mouth; infant opens mouth and turns to the side that is stroked.
- *Sucking.* Place nipple or finger 3–4 cm into mouth; infant sucks vigorously.
- *Tonic neck.* Place infant supine, turn head to one side; arm on side to which head is turned extends; on opposite side, arm curls up (fencer's pose).
- *Palmar grasp.* Place finger in infant's palm and press; infant curls fingers around.
- *Stepping.* Hold infant as if weight bearing on surface; infant steps along, one foot at a time.
- *Moro.* Present loud noise or unexpected movement; infant spreads arms and legs, extends fingers, then flexes and brings hands together; may cry.

Most of these reflexes disappear between 4 and 6 months of age.

Children

- Present the procedures as games whenever possible.
- A positive Babinski reflex is abnormal after the child ambulates or at 2 years of age.
- For children under 5 years of age, the Denver Developmental Screening Test II (DDSTII) provides a comprehensive neurological evaluation, particularly for motor function.
- Note the child's ability to understand and follow directions.
- Assess immediate recall or recent memory by using names of cartoon characters. Normal recall in children is the ability to recall a number that is one less than a child's age in years; that is, a 5-year-old child should be able to recall four characters.
- Assess for signs of hyperactivity or abnormally short attention span.
- Children should be able to walk backward by 2 years of age, balance on one foot for 5 seconds by 4 years of age, heel-toe walk by 5 years of age, and heel-toe walk backward by 6 years of age.
- The Romberg test is appropriate for use in children over 3 years of age.

Older Adults

- A full neurological assessment can be lengthy. Conduct the assessment in several sessions if indicated and cease the tests if the client is noticeably fatigued.

- A decline in mental status is not a normal result of aging. Changes are more the result of physical or psychological disorders (e.g., fever, fluid and electrolyte imbalances, medications). Acute, abrupt-onset mental status changes are usually caused by delirium. These changes are often reversible with treatment. Chronic subtle insidious mental health changes are often caused by dementia and are usually irreversible.
- Intelligence and learning ability are unaltered with age. Many factors, however, inhibit learning (e.g., anxiety, illness, pain, cultural barrier).
- Short-term memory is often less efficient. Long-term memory is usually unaltered.
- Because old age is often associated with loss of support, depression is a common disorder. Mood changes, weight loss, anorexia, constipation, and early morning awakening may manifest.
- The stress of being in unfamiliar situations can cause confusion in older adults.
- As an individual ages, reflex responses may become less intense.
- Because older adults tire more easily than younger clients, a total neurological assessment is often done at a different time than the other parts of the physical assessment.
- Although there is a progressive decrease in the number of functioning neurons in the CNS and in the sense organs, older adults usually function well because of abundant reserves in the number of brain cells.
- Impulse transmission and reaction to stimuli are slower.
- Many older adults have some impairment of hearing, vision, smell, temperature and pain sensation, memory, and mental endurance.
- Coordination changes include slower fine finger movements. Standing balance remains intact, and the Romberg test remains negative.
- Reflex responses may slightly increase or decrease. Many show loss of Achilles reflex, and the plantar reflex may be difficult to elicit.
- When testing sensory function, the nurse needs to give older adults time to respond. Normally, older adults have unaltered perception of light touch and superficial pain, decreased perception of deep pain, and decreased perception of temperature stimuli. Many also reveal a decrease or absence of position sense in the large toes.

further deterioration. Primary interventions include maintaining a patent airway and initiating protocols to treat neurological issues. The nurse may need to prepare the client for surgical interventions.

Independent

Specific interventions initiated and performed by the nurse may include the following:

- Ensuring airway patency and adequate ventilation
- Assessing LOC

- Monitoring fluid intake and output
- Reducing environmental stimuli
- Positioning client
- Taking precautions for seizures, including padding side rails
- Monitoring ICP
- Assessing pupils for response to light
- Measuring vital signs

Collaborative

Clients with altered LOC require close monitoring of respiratory status and may require ventilatory assistance. For the client who does not have a gag reflex, insertion of an oral airway may be used to maintain airway patency. More severe alterations in LOC, however, may require endotracheal intubation to maintain a patent airway, particularly if the client's respiratory status is deteriorating. Unless the client has a do-not-resuscitate (DNR) order, the healthcare team should initiate mechanical ventilation even if it is not yet known if the disorder is reversible. Without sufficient support of ventilation, cerebral anoxia develops quickly and may result in brain death. For clients who require ventilatory support, including mechanical ventilation, arterial blood gases should be monitored. Cautious hyperventilation may be ordered to reduce $PaCO_2$ and promote cerebral vasoconstriction to reduce cerebral edema.

FLUID MANAGEMENT   An intravenous catheter is inserted, and fluid balance is maintained using isotonic or slightly hypertonic solutions such as normal saline and lactated Ringer's solution. The nurse should closely monitor the client's response to fluid administration for evidence of increased cerebral edema.

Any underlying fluid and electrolyte imbalance is corrected by administering IV fluid containing appropriate electrolytes. For the client who is hyponatremic and has a low serum osmolality, furosemide (Lasix) or an osmotic diuretic such as mannitol may be administered to promote water excretion, and fluid infusion may be minimized.

NUTRITION   In clients with long-term alterations in consciousness (e.g., persistent vegetative state or locked-in syndrome), the healthcare team initiates measures to maintain nutritional status. Enteral feedings with a gastrostomy tube may be required if the client is unable to tolerate oral administration of food or fluids. In some cases, total parenteral nutrition may be used.

PHARMACOLOGIC THERAPY   Pharmacologic therapy may be necessary to reduce or control seizures. Medications also play a role in the treatment of IICP.

Seizures   Antiepileptic drugs (AEDs) (also called anticonvulsant drugs) can reduce or control most seizure activity. More than 20 drugs are available for use in the treatment of epilepsy. These medications do not cure the disorder; they only manage its manifestations. AEDs generally act in one of two ways: by raising the seizure threshold or by limiting the spread of abnormal activity in the brain.

The goals of medications for epilepsy are to protect the client from harm and to reduce or prevent seizure activity without impairing cognitive function or producing undesirable side effects. Ideally, the lowest possible dose of a single medication that will control the client's seizures is prescribed. Often, however, several medications must be tried before the most effective one is identified, and a combination of drugs may be needed to manage the client's seizures.

Status epilepticus is a life-threatening emergency that requires immediate intervention. Establishing and maintaining the airway are priorities. A solution of 50% dextrose is administered intravenously to prevent hypoglycemia. Diazepam or lorazepam is given intravenously, and the dose is repeated in 10 minutes, if necessary, to stop seizure activity. Phenytoin (Dilantin) is administered intravenously for longer-term control of seizures. Phenobarbital also may be administered to clients in status epilepticus.

Increased Intracranial Pressure   Medications play an important role in the management of IICP. Diuretics, particularly osmotic diuretics, are commonly used to reduce ICP and are the mainstays of pharmacologic treatment. Loop diuretics such as furosemide (Lasix, typically the drug of choice) and ethacrynic acid (Edecrin) may be prescribed for some clients with IICP. Sedation and paralysis are used as chemical restraints to control restlessness and agitation because these movements increase blood pressure, ICP, and cerebral metabolism. Antipyretics such as acetaminophen are used alone or in combination with a hypothermia blanket to treat hyperthermia. (Hyperthermia increases the cerebral metabolic rate and exacerbates an existing increase in ICP.) Anticonvulsants are often required to manage seizure activity associated with brain injury and IICP. Gastrointestinal prophylaxis with intravenous histamine H_2 antagonists or proton pump inhibitors are often used because clients with IICP are at increased risk for developing stress gastritis and ulcers (Tierney, McPhee, & Papadakis, 2005). Corticosteroids may be administered to reduce inflammation.

Intravenous fluids are usually necessary to maintain the client's fluid and electrolyte balance as well as vascular volume. If the client's blood pressure is unstable, vasoactive medications may be administered to maintain the mean arterial pressure (MAP) in a range that supports cerebral perfusion while minimizing increases in ICP. When enteral feeding is not possible, total parenteral nutrition (TPN) may be administered.

REVIEW The Concept of Intracranial Regulation

RELATE Linking the Concepts

Linking the concept of intracranial regulation with the concept of perfusion:

1. What can the nurse do to provide adequate oxygenation to the client?

2. Why is the nurse concerned about the client's mean arterial blood pressure?

Linking the concept of intracranial regulation with the concept of safety:

3. What teaching should the nurse perform when talking with parents and children about sports injuries?

4. Does the teaching change when working with adults only?

Linking the concept of intracranial regulation with the concept of nutrition:

5. Why is it important to maintain the client's nutritional status while the client has increased intracranial pressure?

6. If the client is unconscious, how would the nurse anticipate the client receiving nutrition?

READY Go to Companion Skills Manual

REFER Go to Pearson Nursing Student Resources
nursing.pearsonhighered.com

- Additional review materials

REFLECT Case Study \\ Part 3

Reread Parts 1 and 2 of the Case Study. The neurosurgeon has placed an external ventricular drainage (EVD) system, or ventricular drainage catheter, to allow for drainage of CSF. Joshua's Glasgow Coma Scale score is now 15. Your orders for the day are to clamp the drain and to watch Joshua for signs of deterioration. You performed a focused assessment before clamping the drain and Joshua was oriented times three, and he was watching TV. Four hours after the drain was clamped, you note that Joshua is very sleepy and cannot tell you where he is. You unclamp the drain and inform the neurosurgeon that Joshua has failed the trial.

Clinical Reasoning Questions Level I

1. What other signs and symptoms would show that Joshua was failing the trial?

2. Are there other reasons that Joshua may be tired?

Clinical Reasoning Questions Level II

3. What are the priority nursing diagnoses for Joshua?

4. What are the interventions required when caring for a drain?

5. What other disciplines may need to be involved in providing care to Joshua?

EXEMPLAR 11.1   Increased Intracranial Pressure

EXEMPLAR KEY TERMS
Cerebral perfusion pressure (CPP), *712*
Compliance, *710*
Increased intracranial pressure
   (IICP), *709*
Intracranial hypertension, *709*
Monro-Kellie hypothesis, *709*

EXEMPLAR LEARNING OUTCOMES
After reading about this exemplar, you will be able to:

1. Describe the pathophysiology, etiology, clinical manifestations, and direct and indirect causes of increased intracranial pressure (IICP).

2. Identify risk factors and prevention methods associated with IICP.

3. Illustrate the nursing process in providing culturally competent care across the life span for individuals with IICP.

4. Formulate priority nursing diagnoses appropriate for an individual with IICP.

5. Summarize therapies used by interdisciplinary teams in the collaborative care of an individual with IICP.

6. Plan evidence-based care for an individual with IICP and his or her family in collaboration with other members of the healthcare team.

7. Evaluate expected outcomes for an individual with IICP.

▶ OVERVIEW

Increased intracranial pressure (IICP) (also called **intracranial hypertension**) is sustained elevated pressure (15 mmHg or higher in adults) in the cranial cavity (Brosche, 2011). A client's ICP increases and decreases throughout the day depending on the type of activities in which the client is engaged. Coughing, bending, sneezing, and straining are examples of activities that increase ICP. These typical, brief activities are not harmful; it is only sustained increased pressure that will result in damage to tissue. Cerebral edema is the most frequent cause of sustained increases in ICP. Other causes include head trauma, tumors, abscesses, stroke, inflammation, and hemorrhage.

▶ PATHOPHYSIOLOGY AND ETIOLOGY

In the adult, the rigid cranial cavity created by the skull is normally filled to capacity with three essentially noncompressible elements: the brain (80%), cerebrospinal fluid (8%), and blood (12%). A state of dynamic equilibrium exists; if the volume of any of the three components increases, the volume of the others must decrease to maintain normal pressures in the cranial cavity. This is known as the **Monro-Kellie hypothesis**. The normal ICP is 5–15 mmHg (measured intracranially with a pressure transducer while the client is lying with the head elevated 30 degrees) or 60–180 cm H_2O (measured with a water manometer while the client is lying in a lateral recumbent position).

Cerebral blood flow and perfusion are important concepts for understanding the development and effects of IICP. Whereas blood and CSF contribute nearly equal percentages to normal intracranial volume, vascular factors account for twice the amount of increase in ICP that CSF does. The brain requires a constant supply of oxygen and glucose to meet its metabolic demands; 15%–20% of the resting cardiac output goes to the brain to meet its metabolic needs. Interruption of the cerebral blood flow leads to ischemia and disruption of the cerebral metabolism.

Pressure and chemical autoregulation are compensatory mechanisms in which cerebral arterioles change diameter to maintain cerebral blood flow when ICP increases. In pressure autoregulation, stretch receptors in small blood vessels of the brain cause smooth muscle of the arterioles to contract. Increased arterial pressure stimulates these receptors, leading to vasoconstriction; when arterial pressure is low, stimulation of these receptors decreases, causing relaxation and vasodilation. Chemical, or metabolic, autoregulation works in much the same way as pressure autoregulation. In this case, the stimulus is a buildup of metabolic by-products of cell metabolism, including lactic acid, pyruvic acid, carbonic acid, and carbon dioxide. Carbon dioxide and increased hydrogen ion concentration are potent cerebral vasodilators that may act locally or systemically to increase cerebral blood flow. Conversely, a fall in PaCO$_2$ causes cerebral vasoconstriction. Arterial oxygen tension (PaO$_2$) also affects cerebral blood flow, although it is a less powerful mechanism than that exerted by carbon dioxide and hydrogen ions.

IICP may result from an increase in intracranial contents from a space-occupying lesion, hydrocephalus, cerebral edema (swelling), excess cerebrospinal fluid, or intracranial hemorrhage. Displacement of some CSF to the spinal subarachnoid space and increased CSF absorption are early compensatory mechanisms. The low-pressure venous system is also compressed, and cerebral arteries constrict to reduce blood flow. Brain tissue's ability to accommodate change is relatively restricted. The relationship between the volume of the intracranial components and intracranial pressure is known as **compliance**. When the capacity to compensate for IICP is exceeded, intracranial hypertension develops.

Autoregulatory mechanisms have a limited ability to maintain cerebral blood flow. When autoregulation fails, cerebrovascular tone is reduced and cerebral blood flow becomes dependent on changes in blood pressure. Autoregulation may be lost either locally or globally because of several factors, including increasing ICP, local or diffuse cerebral tissue ischemia or inflammation, prolonged hypotension, and hypercapnia or hypoxia.

Etiology

Increased intracranial pressure may result from head injury, hydrocephalus (**Box 11–3** ●), cerebral edema, excess CSF or intracranial hemorrhage. Head trauma results from different causes throughout the life span. Infants and young children may experience IICP as the result of falling, abuse, or bumping their heads as a result of poor head control or depth perception. Preschool and school-aged children are at risk for bicycle, swimming, or activity-related accidents that cause head trauma. Adolescents and adults are at risk for motor vehicle–related crashes, addiction behavior, and trauma resulting from violence. Older adults are prone to falls that may result in IICP.

Abnormal cellular growth such as intracranial tumors, either benign or malignant, may compete for space in the cranial

---

Box 11–3 Hydrocephalus

Hydrocephalus results from an imbalance between production and absorption of CSF, which results in too much CSF accumulating in the brain, resulting in widening of the ventricles. Hydrocephalus may be congenital or acquired. It may be acquired as a result of head trauma, infection, tumor, or other pathogenic processes. In *communicating hydrocephalus*, the flow of CSF reabsorption is impaired. In *noncommunicating hydrocephalus* (the most frequent type), the CSF is obstructed and cannot enter the subarachnoid space. Two other types of hydrocephalus typically affect adults only: *hydrocephalus ex vacuo*, which may occur as the result of stroke or traumatic brain injury, and *normal pressure hydrocephalus*, most commonly seen in older adults, which may result from trauma, complications from surgery, or an unknown cause (National Institute of Neurological Disorders and Stroke, 2013; Seattle Children's Hospital, 2013).

---

vault, resulting in IICP. Increases in CSF production as seen in hydrocephalus or tissue necrosis as the result of cerebrovascular accidents or aneurysms also may lead to IICP.

Risk Factors

Any factor that increases the client's risk of trauma increases the risk of cerebral trauma resulting in IICP. Risk factors for cerebral trauma are plentiful, but increase when normal safety considerations, such as wearing protective equipment, are ignored. Any trauma to the brain will also change the equilibrium of the Monroe-Kellie hypothesis. Other factors that may influence this equilibrium include medications, poor nutrition, illnesses such as meningitis, and drug and alcohol abuse.

The premature infant is at risk for IICP as a result of intracranial hemorrhage, secondary to the fragile cranial blood vessels. As infants begin to mature, the closing of the fontanels prematurely may result in IICP.

Prevention

Teach the client ways to prevent trauma. As mentioned earlier, provide guidance related to the use of personal protective equipment and other safety measures, including wearing seat belts and avoiding phone use while driving or in motion, to reduce risk for injury. Nurses working with adolescents should emphasize avoidance of recreational drug and alcohol use.

Caution should be taken when caring for the premature infant to avoid rough handling, to provide adequate support of the head, and to avoid hypoxia. Refer to the exemplar on Prematurity in the module on Reproduction for more information on premature infants.

▶ CLINICAL MANIFESTATIONS

With loss of autoregulation, ICP continues to rise and cerebral perfusion falls. Cerebral tissue becomes ischemic, and manifestations of cellular hypoxia appear. Because the neurons of the cerebral cortex are most sensitive to oxygen deficit, changes in cortical function are the earliest manifestations of increasing ICP (Porth & Matfin, 2009). Behavior and personality changes occur; the client may become irritable and agitated. Memory and judgment are impaired, and changes in speech pattern may be noted. Additionally, the client's LOC decreases. As cerebral hypertension and hypoxia progress, LOC continues to decrease in a predictable pattern to coma and unresponsiveness.

Lifespan Considerations

Early signs of IICP in children include headache, nausea and vomiting, dizziness or vertigo, downward deviation of the eyes (called sunsetting), slight change in LOC, and restlessness. In infants, look for these signs and also irritability, bulging fontanel, increased head circumference, and a high-pitched, shrill cry. The infant also will be very sensitive to touch and sound. Late signs of pediatric IICP include significant decrease in level of consciousness, Cushing triad, increased systolic blood pressure and widened pulse pressure, bradycardia, irregular respirations, and fixed and dilated pupils (Ball, Bindler, & Cowen, 2012).

Clinical Manifestations and Therapies **Increased Intracranial Pressure**

ETIOLOGY	CLINICAL MANIFESTATIONS	CLINICAL THERAPIES
Cerebral edema, head trauma, tumors, abscesses, stroke, inflammation, and hemorrhage	■ Decreased LOC: *Early:* Confusion; restlessness, lethargy; disorientation, first to time, then to place and person. *Late:* Comatose with no response to painful stimuli. ■ Pupillary dysfunction: Sluggish response to light, progressing to fixed pupils; with a localized process, pupillary dysfunction is first noted on the ipsilateral side. ■ Oculomotor dysfunction: Inability to move eye(s) upward; ptosis (drooping) of the eyelid. ■ Visual abnormalities: Decreased visual acuity, blurred vision, diplopia. ■ Papilledema (may be late sign). ■ Motor impairment: *Early:* Hemiparesis or hemiplegia of the contralateral side. *Late:* Abnormal responses such as decorticate or decerebrate positioning; flaccidity. ■ Headache: Uncommon but may occur with processes that slowly increase ICP; worse upon rising in the morning and with position changes. ■ Projectile vomiting without nausea. ■ Cushing triad/response: Increased systolic blood pressure, widening pulse pressure, bradycardia. ■ Respirations: Altered respiratory pattern related to level of brain dysfunction. ■ Temperature (may be significantly elevated as compensatory mechanisms fail).	■ Maintain airway patency. ■ Monitor neurological status; assessment areas include LOC, behavior, motor/sensory functions, pupillary size and reaction to light, and vital signs. ■ Monitor IICP monitor or ventilator. ■ Decrease stimuli. ■ Raise pads and bed rails; seizures may occur. ■ Elevate head of bed 30 degrees unless otherwise indicated. ■ Monitor arterial blood gases. ■ Position client as prescribed. ■ Prevent complications associated with immobility. ■ Monitor fluid and electrolytes. ■ Monitor bladder distention and bowel constipation. ■ Provide emotional support as needed. ■ Administer medications as ordered.

▶ COLLABORATION

Management of the client with IICP is directed toward identifying and treating the underlying cause of the disorder and controlling ICP to prevent herniation syndrome. IICP is a medical emergency, and there is little time to complete lengthy diagnostic tests. The diagnosis must be made on the basis of observation and neurological assessment; even subtle changes may be clinically significant. The nurse, who often spends the most time caring for the client, is most likely to assess any subtle changes in condition and must advocate for the client's needs.

Diagnostic Tests

Diagnostic tests are used mainly to determine what might be the cause of IICP. A computed tomography (CT) scan or MRI is generally the initial test used to identify the possible causes of IICP (such as space-occupying lesions or hydrocephalus) and to evaluate therapeutic options. In general, a lumbar puncture is not performed when IICP is suspected because the sudden release of the pressure in the skull may cause cerebral herniation. Serum osmolality and arterial blood gases also are ordered and monitored.

Surgery

Clients with IICP may undergo various intracranial surgical techniques to treat the underlying cause. In addition, infarcted or necrotic tissue may be resected to reduce brain mass. A drainage catheter or shunt may be inserted laterally via a burr hole into a ventricle to drain excess CSF and reduce hydrocephalus. The removal of even a small amount of CSF may dramatically reduce IICP and restore cerebral perfusion pressure.

Pharmacologic Therapy

Medications play an important role in the management of IICP. Diuretics, particularly osmotic diuretics, are commonly used to reduce ICP and are the mainstays of pharmacologic treatment. Loop diuretics such as furosemide (Lasix), the drug of choice, and ethacrynic acid (Edecrin) may be prescribed for some clients with IICP. Antipyretics, such as acetaminophen, are used alone or in combination with a hypothermia blanket to treat hyperthermia. (Hyperthermia increases the cerebral metabolic rate and exacerbates an existing increase in ICP.) Anticonvulsants are often required to manage seizure activity associated with brain injury and IICP. Antihypertensives, in particular beta blockers, may be used if the mean arterial pressure (MAP) is high. Vasopressors may be used if the MAP is low. Gastrointestinal prophylaxis with intravenous histamine H_2 antagonists or proton pump inhibitors are often used because clients with IICP are at increased risk for developing stress gastritis and ulcers.

Intravenous fluids are usually necessary to maintain the client's fluid and electrolyte balance and vascular volume. If the client's blood pressure is unstable, vasoactive medications may be administered to maintain the MAP in a range that supports cerebral perfusion while minimizing increases in ICP. When enteral feeding is not possible, TPN may be administered.

Medications **Increased Intracranial Pressure**

CLASSIFICATION AND DRUG EXAMPLES	MECHANISMS OF ACTION	NURSING CONSIDERATIONS
Osmotic Diuretics *Drug examples:* ▪ mannitol ▪ glucose ▪ urea ▪ glycerol	Osmotic diuretics work by increasing the osmolarity of the blood, thereby drawing water out of edematous brain tissue and into the vascular system for elimination via the kidneys. The effects of these drugs vary with the type of injury.	▪ Monitor vital signs, urinary output, central venous pressure (CVP), and pulmonary artery pressure (PAP) before and every hour throughout administration. ▪ Assess client for manifestations of dehydration. ▪ Assess client for muscle weakness, numbness, tingling, paresthesias, confusion, and excessive thirst. ▪ Monitor neurological status and ICP readings. ▪ Monitor renal function and serum electrolytes throughout therapy. ▪ Do not discontinue medication abruptly. Rebound migraine headaches may occur.
Loop Diuretics *Drug examples:* ▪ furosemide ▪ ethacrynic acid	Loop diuretics inhibit sodium and chloride reabsorption at the ascending loop of Henle. They cause a reduction in the rate of CSF production, thus reducing the ICP.	▪ Monitor vital signs and electrolyte values. ▪ Assess fluid status throughout therapy. ▪ Use infusion pump to ensure accurate fluid administration.

Nonpharmacologic Therapy

Nonpharmacologic therapies for clients may include ICP monitoring and mechanical ventilation. Continuous assessment is necessary to determine and respond to changes in the client's condition.

ICP MONITORING   Critical to preserving brain function and preventing secondary brain damage from IICP are careful assessments and monitoring with ICP monitors, measuring cerebral blood flow and cerebral perfusion pressure, and measuring oxygen levels of brain tissue. ICP monitors facilitate continuous assessment of ICP and the effects of medical therapy and nursing interventions on ICP. In addition, cerebral perfusion pressure (the difference between MAP and ICP) can be calculated, allowing more precise manipulation of therapeutic measures to maintain cerebral perfusion and thereby prevent ischemia. The criteria for ICP monitoring depends on the client's condition, but in general, clients who are comatose and have a Glasgow Coma Scale score of 8 or lower should be monitored.

Basic monitoring systems include an epidural probe, a subarachnoid bolt or screw, and an intraventricular catheter (**Figure 11–11 ●**). Intraventricular fluid-filled catheters are placed in the anterior horn of the lateral ventricle (most often in the right side). Ventricular catheters can drain CSF and measure ICP. The ICP value is measured deep in the brain and is considered most reflective of the whole brain pressure. Subarachnoid devices are placed in the subarachnoid space. A fiberoptic transducer-tipped catheter can be placed in the epidural, subdural, or parenchymal space, with ICP values considered very accurate. Once the intracranial sensor is implanted, it is connected to a transducer that converts the impulses to a signal that the recording device can translate into an oscilloscope tracing, digital value, or graphic recording. Factors that increase the risk for infection during ICP monitoring are listed in **Table 11–6 ●**.

Transcranial blood flow is monitored with transcranial Doppler studies to measure the velocity of blood flow in the cerebral vessels. **Cerebral perfusion pressure (CPP)** is the pressure it takes for the heart to provide the brain with blood

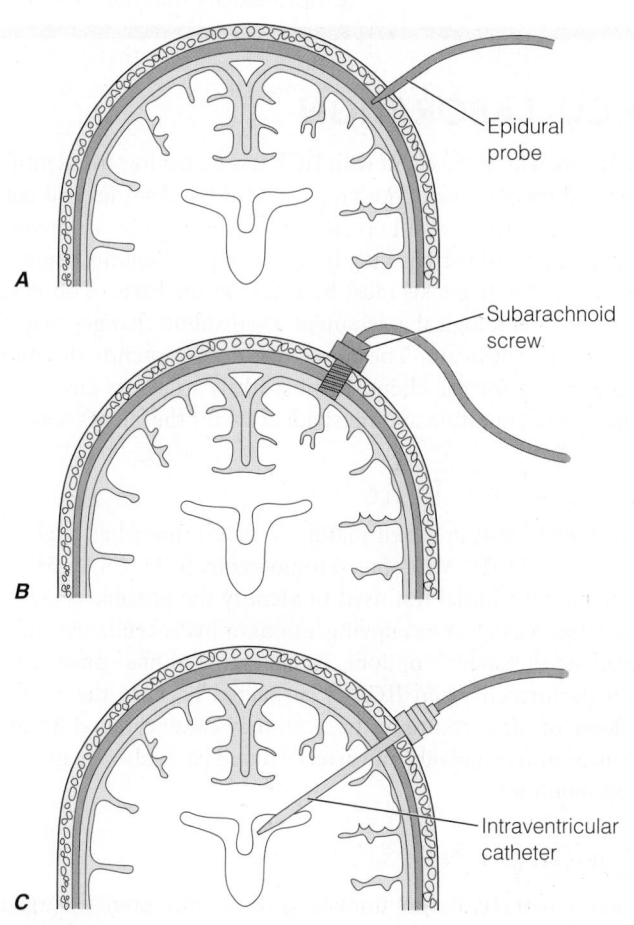

Figure 11–11 ● Types of ICP monitoring. *A*, Epidural probe. *B*, Subarachnoid screw. *C*, Intraventricular catheter.

TABLE 11–6   Risk Factors for Infection With Intracranial Pressure Monitoring

FACTOR	RATIONALE
Intraventricular catheter	Is more invasive than other monitoring devices.
Open head trauma or neurosurgery	Disrupts protective skin and skeletal barriers.
Intracranial hemorrhage	Necessitates frequent flushing of catheter to maintain patency.
Older adult	Tends to have impaired immune defenses.
Monitoring for more than 3–5 days or using open system or frequent irrigation	Offers increased opportunity for pathogens to enter and grow.

and is calculated by subtracting the ICP from the MAP (normal CPP is 70–95 mmHg). Monitoring of brain oxygenation may be conducted using a jugular bulb oxygen saturation (SjO_2) monitor connected to a small fiberoptic catheter inserted into the jugular vein. (Normal SjO_2 is 50%–75%.) Another device used to monitor brain tissue oxygenation is the LICOX system, which includes information about oxygen status and temperature status in the brain tissue itself (Brettler, 2004). In addition, cerebral microdialysis catheters can provide information about the nature of the cerebral interstitial fluid.

MECHANICAL VENTILATION   Clients with IICP often require intubation and are placed on a ventilator for respiratory management. Mechanical ventilation may be used to maintain partial pressure of oxygen and carbon dioxide, thus preventing hypoxemia and hypercapnia, both of which can increase ICP. It is important to maintain adequate oxygenation with a partial pressure of arterial oxygen at about 100 mmHg and a partial pressure of arterial carbon dioxide of about 35 mmHg. The client with IICP and signs of impending herniation may be judiciously hyperventilated to cause cerebral vasoconstriction; however, this also increases cerebral ischemia. Mechanical ventilation is discussed in greater detail in the exemplar on Acute Respiratory Distress Syndrome in the module on Oxygenation.

OTHER THERAPIES   Physical therapy to prevent muscle atrophy may be necessary for a client who is unconscious or bedridden for more than a few days. Respiratory therapy is usually necessary after a client is weaned from a mechanical ventilator. Families of clients who have IICP may benefit from spiritual or psychological counseling. Nurses can provide much needed support by contacting a hospital chaplain or making a referral to an experienced counseling professional.

■ NURSING PROCESS

The nursing care of clients with IICP involves identifying those at risk and managing factors known to increase intracranial pressure. A major focus is protecting the client from sudden increases in ICP or a decrease in cerebral blood flow.

Assessment

Assess for and report manifestations of IICP every 15 minutes to 1 hour and as necessary. Clients with unstable ICP may require continuous or more frequent monitoring. Assessment areas include LOC; behavior; motor/sensory functions; pupillary size and reaction to light; and vital signs, including temperature. Look for trends because vital signs alone do not correlate well with early deterioration. Assessment of neurological status establishes the client's clinical condition and provides a baseline for measuring changes. Sudden changes in neurological signs often indicate deterioration. An elevated temperature with increased oxygen consumption further increases ICP. Pupillary responses mirror the status of the midbrain and pons. Pressure on the brainstem may compromise the function of cranial nerves IX and X and protective mechanisms such as the gag and cough reflexes. The nurse needs to be alert to even the most subtle change as it may indicate early signs of a declining neurological condition.

Monitor pulse oximetry and arterial blood gas measurements. Adequate air exchange to keep oxygen and carbon dioxide levels within normal ranges and maintenance of acid–base balance are critical to reduce the risk of hypoxemia and IICP. If adequate respiratory effort cannot be maintained, mechanical ventilation will be necessary.

SAFETY ALERT
Often the earliest manifestations of a change in ICP are alterations in LOC and respirations.

Diagnosis

Nursing diagnoses for the client with IICP may include the following:

- *Ineffective Airway Clearance*
- *Ineffective Tissue Perfusion: Cerebral*
- *Ineffective Breathing Pattern*
- *Risk for Aspiration*
- *Risk for Infection.*

(NANDA-I © 2012)

Client Teaching   Clients Who Have or Are at Risk for Increased Intracranial Pressure

- Teach the client who is able to follow instructions to avoid coughing, blowing the nose, straining to have a bowel movement, pushing against the bed rails, or performing isometric (muscle-contracting) exercises.
- Advise the client to maintain head and neck alignment when turning in bed and to take rest periods.
- Encourage the family to talk to the client but to maintain a quiet environment with minimal stimuli.
- Inform family members that upsetting the client may increase ICP and that they should avoid discussions that may distress the client.
- For clients unable to make decisions about treatment or sign informed consent, contact the family, who must carry out these functions.

Planning

Planning nursing care for the client with IICP is highly individualized and depends on the cause, treatment, and prognosis. Common goals include the following:

- The client will maintain ICP less than 20 mmHg.
- The client will experience no further complications as a result of IICP.
- The client will not experience infection as the result of ICP monitoring.
- The client will maintain adequate cerebral perfusion to prevent further cellular damage.
- Family members will demonstrate ability to maintain a low-stimuli environment.

Implementation

Nursing interventions include performing neurological assessments, maintaining airway patency, ensuring adequate ventilation, positioning and moving, instituting seizure precautions, and monitoring fluids and electrolytes. Additionally, both client and family need emotional support during this period.

- For the client on a ventilator: Maintain airway patency; preoxygenate with 100% oxygen before suctioning; limit suctioning to 10 seconds because suctioning increases ICP; suction gently. Preoxygenation helps maintain oxygen levels during suctioning. Suctioning stimulates the cough reflex and Valsalva maneuver. Correct suctioning minimizes the risk of hypoxemia.
- Monitor arterial blood gases. They provide a reliable indicator of oxygen and carbon dioxide levels. If oxygen concentration is low, oxygen may be given or increased.
- Elevate the head of the bed to 30 degrees in most cases, as prescribed (if neck trauma is involved the bed may need to be kept flat until x-rays of the cervical spine show no fractures); maintain alignment of the head and neck to avoid hyperextension or exaggerated neck flexion; and avoid the prone position. Keeping the head of the bed elevated facilitates venous drainage from the cerebrum. Obstruction of jugular veins can impede venous drainage from the brain.
- Monitor bladder distention and bowel constipation. Administer stool softeners and use the Credé method (the method of applying pressure to the suprapubic region with the fingers of one or both hands) to empty the bladder. If the Credé method is not effective, evaluate the pros and cons of urinary catheterization if the bladder remains distended. Constipation and bladder distention increase intrathoracic or intra-abdominal pressure and place the client at risk for impaired venous drainage from the brain.
- If the client is alert, assist in moving up in bed. Do not ask the client to push with heels or arms or push against a footboard. Avoid a footboard and restraints. Moving up in bed

requires pushing. Helping the client move prevents initiation of the Valsalva maneuver, which increases ICP.
- Plan nursing care so that activities are not clustered together; avoid turning the client, getting the client on the bedpan, or suctioning within the same time period. Schedule nursing care to provide rest periods between procedures. Multiple procedures, including certain nursing care activities, can increase ICP. Constant stimulation tends to increase ICP. Individualized nursing care ensures optimal spacing of activities and rest.
- Maintain fluid limitations if prescribed. Restricting fluids helps decrease cerebral edema by reducing total body water.
- Reduce stimuli as much as possible by providing a quiet environment and avoiding activities or tasks that jar the client or the bed. Noxious stimuli and emotional upsets cause elevation of ICP, therefore, try to limit situations that may cause emotional upset by maintaining a calm, reassuring manner. Educate family members to refrain from engaging in unpleasant or exciting conversation with and around the client.

Interventions discussed next are for the client with an intracranial monitoring device. Most clinical units have written protocols for managing these systems. The following nursing actions serve only as a general guide.

- Keep dressings over the catheter dry and change dressings on a prescribed basis (usually every 24–48 hours). Wet dressings promote bacterial growth.
- Monitor the insertion site for leaking CSF, drainage, or infection. Monitor for manifestations of infection, including changes in vital signs, chills, increased white blood counts (WBCs), lack of clarity in CSF, or positive cultures of drainage. Close monitoring helps detect the earliest signs of infection and helps prevent major complications. Fever usually is considered the key assessment. However, fever in a client with a neurological disorder may be due to damage to the hypothalamus. Headache, generalized muscle aches, shivering, and chills also may be seen in the client with infection.
- Use strict aseptic technique when in contact with the device. Check drainage system for loose connections. Using aseptic technique and monitoring drainage systems for loose connections help prevent nosocomial infections.

Evaluation

The client is evaluated based on the plan of care developed. Potential expected outcomes may include the following:

- The client's ICP returns to acceptable limits following treatment.
- The client's LOC improves with reduction of ICP.
- The client experiences no infection as the result of ICP monitoring.
- Family describes appropriate outcome expectations related to amount of cellular damage resulting from IICP.

REVIEW Increased Intracranial Pressure

RELATE Linking the Concepts and Exemplars
The nurse is caring for a client who experienced severe head trauma in a motor vehicle crash. The client is placed on a mechanical ventilator set to 28 breaths per minute and is completely non-

responsive to deep, painful stimuli. The client's vital signs are T_O 101.2°F; P 112 bpm; R 28/min; and BP 100/88 mmHg. ICP readings are currently 16 but increase to 34–38 mmHg when touched and 52 mmHg when the endotracheal tube is suctioned.

Linking the exemplar of increased intracranial pressure with the concept of perfusion:

1. What nursing interventions can the nurse perform to optimize brain perfusion?

2. How would you interpret the client's blood pressure and ICP readings to determine brain perfusion?

The family of the client in the preceding scenario is told that if the client survives, he is likely to experience significant neurological losses and may remain in a chronic vegetative state. The client's wife says, "I know him. He's a fighter, and he won't settle for anything less than full recovery." She then relates the story of a television show she saw the other day. The character on the show received this same prognosis and was back to normal within a few weeks.

Linking the exemplar of increased intracranial pressure with the concept of grief and loss:

3. In what stage of the grieving process is this family member?

4. What nursing care can you provide to support this woman's grieving process and to help her accept the likelihood of a less than complete recovery?

READY Go to Companion Skills Manual

REFER Go to Pearson Nursing Student Resources
nursing.pearsonhighered.com

- Additional review materials

REFLECT Case Study

Antwan, 7 years old, was injured when he was struck by a car and thrown several feet into the air. He was unconscious on admission to the emergency department and showed some signs of IICP (dilated and fixed pupils, lack of response to painful stimuli, irregular breathing pattern). Antwan was treated for shock, and his neurological status and vital signs were assessed frequently. The initial evaluation revealed that Antwan had sustained several contusions of the brain but no skull fracture. He was intubated and medicated to manage the airway and IICP. After 7 days in the intensive care unit, he was moved to a general care floor. He is still not fully conscious but quiets when his parents speak to him. He is moving all extremities, but he does not yet follow commands.

1. Describe the neurological nursing assessment that should be performed on Antwan at regular intervals in the general care unit.

2. Identify age-appropriate sensory stimulation strategies that may help promote Antwan's awareness and improvement in LOC.

3. What would you teach Antwan's family to help promote neurological improvement?

4. What changes in Antwan's condition would require immediate notification of the primary provider?

EXEMPLAR 11.2   Seizure Disorders

EXEMPLAR KEY TERMS
Aura, 716
Automatisms, 717
Clonic phase, 716
Epilepsy, 715
Febrile seizures, 716
Focal seizures, 716
Generalized seizures, 716
Intractable seizures, 719
Postictal period, 716
Status epilepticus, 718
Tonic phase, 716

EXEMPLAR LEARNING OUTCOMES
After reading about this exemplar, you will be able to:

1. Describe the pathophysiology, etiology, clinical manifestations, and direct and indirect causes of seizures.

2. Identify risk factors and prevention methods associated with seizures.

3. Illustrate the nursing process in providing culturally competent care across the life span for individuals with seizures.

4. Formulate priority nursing diagnoses appropriate for an individual with seizures.

5. Summarize therapies used by interdisciplinary teams in the collaborative care of an individual with seizures.

6. Plan evidence-based care for an individual with seizures and his or her family in collaboration with other members of the healthcare team.

7. Evaluate expected outcomes for an individual with seizures.

▶ OVERVIEW

Seizures are defined as periods of abnormal electrical discharges in the brain that may cause involuntary movement or behavior or sensory alterations. Seizure disorders affect over 3 million Americans of all ages in the United States. Approximately 2%–4% of children have one or more seizures during childhood from a variety of causes, most often during infancy. **Epilepsy** is a chronic disorder characterized by recurrent, unprovoked seizures secondary to a central nervous system (CNS) disorder.

▶ PATHOPHYSIOLOGY AND ETIOLOGY

Seizures are believed to be the result of abnormal excessive concurrent electrical discharges from the cortical neuronal network of cells on the surface of the brain. Chemical changes in the neurons create an electrical negativity that enables the transfer of information between neurons. When an excessive number of these cells become excited, they discharge abnormally. These cells can be triggered by environmental or physiological stimuli (e.g., emotional stress, anxiety, fatigue, infection, or metabolic disturbances). Acute insults such as a CNS infection, hypoxia, and brain trauma are the most common causes of seizures in children.

Focal seizures (also known as *partial seizures*) are caused by abnormal electrical activity in one hemisphere or in a specific area of the cerebral cortex, most often the temporal, frontal, or parietal lobes. The seizure may spread regionally, and the symptoms are related to the region of the cortex that is affected.

In contrast, **generalized seizures** are the result of diffuse electrical activity that often begins in both hemispheres of the brain simultaneously, then spreads throughout the cortex into the brainstem. As a result, movements and spasms displayed by the client are bilateral and symmetric.

Etiology

Some seizures are idiopathic, that is, not provoked by known stimuli. Genetic factors may lower the seizure threshold by making brain cells more vulnerable to abnormal electrical discharges. Acquired seizures may be caused by underlying pathological conditions such as trauma, infection, hypoglycemia, hypotonic dehydration, electrolyte imbalance, endocrine dysfunction, toxins, tumors, or lesions that may be manifested at any time.

Febrile seizures are generalized seizures that usually occur in children as the result of a rapid temperature rise above 39°C (102°F), usually in association with an acute illness. No evidence of intracranial infection or other defined cause is found. Febrile seizures are usually seen between 3 months and 5 years of age, with a peak incidence between 17 and 24 months of age. There is often a family history of febrile seizures. In addition, children who have one febrile seizure have a 30%–50% greater chance of having future seizures. The lower convulsive threshold of infants may explain this type of seizure. Febrile seizures are generally divided into two types: simple and complex. They affect all ethnic groups, but happen more frequently in some. They occur in 6%–9% of Japanese children, 5%–10% of Indian children, and 2%–5% of children in the United States and Western Europe (Mewasingh, 2010; Waruiru & Appleton, 2004).

Risk Factors

Infants are susceptible to developing epilepsy in the first year of life, with an incidence of 1 per 1,000. The incidence decreases with age. The median age for the development of epilepsy is 5–6 years of age. In the United States, approximately 150,000–325,000 children between 5 and 14 years of age have epilepsy (Epilepsy Foundation, 2012).

Other risk factors include an infant who is small for gestational age, presence of underlying neurological conditions, brain tumors or infections of the brain, stroke, cerebral palsy, autistic disorder, family history, or abuse of drugs. Risk factors and other considerations for older adults are described in the Lifespan Considerations feature.

Prevention

Everyone has a seizure threshold. When this threshold is exceeded, a seizure may occur. Some individuals have abnormally low seizure thresholds, increasing their risk for seizure activity. Others may experience seizures as the result of a pathological process, such as epilepsy. Prevention of seizures is diffi-

Lifespan Considerations
Epilepsy in Older Adults

For years, epilepsy was believed to be a disease that principally affected children. However, some 570,000 adults over the age of 65 suffer from epilepsy. Epilepsy increases risk of falls and broken bones and can threaten the independence of the older adult (Epilepsy Foundation, 2012). These data have important implications for nursing assessments and care.

- The most common cause of epilepsy in older adults is arteriosclerosis of the cerebrovascular system.
- The most common type of seizure in older adults is a complex partial seizure.
- Older adults tend to have longer postseizure manifestations than do younger adults.
- Epilepsy that begins in older adults is often easier to control with antiepileptic drugs (AEDs) than that in younger people. However, some AEDs decrease the effect of statins used to treat arteriosclerosis (the most common cause of epilepsy in older adults).

cult, but there are some steps individuals can take to reduce their risk for seizures or reduce the frequency of seizure activity.

Individuals with epilepsy often experience seizure activity on exposure to a trigger. Triggers may be individualized (e.g., odors, flashing lights). General triggers include fatigue, hypoglycemia, fever, alcohol, hyperventilation, and menstruation. Individuals who are able to identify triggers may succeed in reducing their frequency. Maintaining good self-care (e.g., maintaining the therapeutic regimen, avoiding alcohol, eating properly, and balancing rest and activity) is important for individuals with seizure disorders.

▶ CLINICAL MANIFESTATIONS

The length of a seizure, especially of a generalized seizure, is important because the airway may be compromised during the tonic phase. The initial manifestations of the **tonic phase** of a generalized seizure are unconsciousness and continuous muscular contraction. The basal metabolic rate rises during the peak of seizure activity, increasing the body's demand for oxygen and glucose. The client may become pale or cyanotic as a result of hypoxia. The client also may become hypoglycemic if glucose demand is excessive.

The symptoms of a seizure depend on its type and duration. Seizures are classified into two types: *partial (focal) seizures* and *generalized seizures*. Tonic–clonic seizures are the most common seizure type in children, characterized by alternating repetitive tonic–clonic activity. The tonic phase is followed by the **clonic phase**, characterized by alternating muscular contraction and relaxation. During the **postictal period** following seizure activity, LOC is decreased and the client is often sleepy but arousable. The length of the postictal period varies. An **aura** may provide an early warning sign of a seizure and may be manifest as any type of sensory alteration ranging from odor and taste to vision. When the client recognizes the pattern of an aura, he or she may have time to avoid injury by getting to the floor.

Febrile seizures involve generalized tonic–clonic movements that last less than 15 minutes.

Clinical Manifestations and Therapies **Seizure Disorders**

ETIOLOGY	CLINICAL MANIFESTATIONS	CLINICAL THERAPIES
Simple partial seizures involve activation of only a restricted part of one cerebral hemisphere.	■ No alteration in consciousness occurs. ■ Typically only motor portion of cortex is affected causing recurrent muscle contractions of face or contralateral part of body. Motor movement may be confined to one area. If it spreads sequentially to adjacent parts it is called a Jacksonian march or Jacksonian seizure. ■ If sensory portion is involved, manifestations may include abnormal sensations or hallucinations. ■ Disruption in autonomic nervous system may result in tachycardia, flushing, hypotension, or hypertension. ■ Psychic symptoms such as a sense of déjà vu or inappropriate fear or anger may be experienced.	■ Antiepileptic medications ■ Maintain client safety during seizure. ■ Assess exact manifestations experienced by client and document fully. ■ Vagal nerve stimulation therapy
Complex partial seizures involve activation of only a restricted part of one cerebral hemisphere, usually originating in the temporal lobe.	■ Often proceeded by an aura, which may be visual, auditory, an odd smell, or psychic in nature. ■ Impaired consciousness lasts for several hours before full consciousness is regained. ■ Exhibits repetitive nonpurposeful activity such as lip smacking, aimless walking, or picking at clothing called **automatisms**. ■ Amnesia is common after seizure.	■ Antiepileptic medications ■ Maintain client safety. ■ Vagal nerve stimulation ■ Resection of epileptogenic focus, such as the temporal lobe, may be considered.
Absence seizures (petit mal) involve both hemispheres of the brain as well as deeper structures such as thalamus, basal ganglia, and upper brainstem.	■ Level of consciousness is impaired. ■ Sudden brief cessation of all motor activity is accompanied by blank stare and unresponsiveness. ■ More common in children. ■ Usually lasts 5–10 seconds, sometimes as long as 30 seconds. ■ Vary from occasional to several hundred per day.	■ Antiepileptic medications ■ Maintain client safety.
Tonic–clonic seizures are the most common type seen in adults.	■ Warning aura may proceed seizure activity (visual, gustatory, auditory, visceral, or sense of uneasiness). ■ Sudden loss of consciousness. *Tonic phase:* ■ Sharp tonic muscle contraction forcing air out of the lungs which may cause client to cry out. ■ Loss of postural control causing client to fall in opisthotonic posture. ■ Muscles are rigid with arms and legs extended and jaw clenched. ■ Urinary incontinence is common and may be accompanied by bowel incontinence. ■ Breathing ceases and cyanosis develops. ■ Pupils fixed and dilated. ■ Lasts 15–60 seconds. *Clonic phase follows characterized by:* ■ Alternating contraction and relaxation of muscles in all extremities. ■ Hyperventilation. ■ Eyes roll back. ■ Client froths at the mouth. ■ Varies in duration and subsides gradually generally 60–90 seconds.	■ Antiepileptic medications ■ Maintain client safety. ■ Driving privileges will be suspended until seizure activity is controlled and client is seizure free for a period of time determined by state statutes. ■ Helmets may be recommended to prevent head injury until seizure activity is controlled. ■ Do not restrain client. ■ Pad bed rails. ■ Diazepam, lorazepam, or phenobarbital may be administered during seizure to limit length of seizure.

(continued on next page)

Clinical Manifestations and Therapies **Seizure Disorders** (continued)

ETIOLOGY	CLINICAL MANIFESTATIONS	CLINICAL THERAPIES
	Postictal phase: ■ Client remains unconscious and unresponsive to stimuli. ■ Relaxed and breathes quietly. ■ Regains consciousness gradually and may be confused and disoriented on waking. ■ Headache, muscle ache, fatigue often reported. ■ May sleep for several hours. ■ Amnesia is usual both for the seizure and several minutes before seizure activity.	
Status epilepticus	■ Continuous seizure activity with only very short periods of calm between intense and persistent seizures. ■ Seizures may be any type but most often are generalized tonic–clonic. ■ Client is in great danger of hypoxia, acidosis, hypoglycemia, hyperthermia, and exhaustion if seizure activity is not halted.	■ Provide immediate interventions to preserve life. ■ Establish and maintain an airway. ■ Administer 50% glucose to prevent hypoglycemia. ■ Diazepam or lorazepam is administered IV and repeated every 10 minutes until seizure activity stops. ■ Administer antiepileptics such as phenytoin. ■ Phenobarbital may also be administered.

▶ COLLABORATION

The healthcare team, composed of the nurse, physician, family, and the client, works together to understand care and prevention requirements. In the case of children, the teacher, school nurse, and other adults working with the child are included as extensions of the child's healthcare team to ensure that care and prevention requirements are maintained during school and extracurricular activities. Many seizures are self-limiting and require no emergency intervention.

Diagnostic Tests

Laboratory tests that may be ordered include a complete blood cell count, blood chemistry, urine culture, and lumbar puncture. If the client is taking any anticonvulsants, the serum drug level is monitored regularly. An EEG is often performed at a follow-up visit between seizures. A lead level, toxicology screening, and radiological tests such as a CT scan or MRI and angiography may be performed to identify a cerebral lesion or metabolic disorder in the brain.

Pharmacologic Therapy

Antiepileptic drugs (AEDs), also called *anticonvulsant drugs*, can reduce or control most seizure activity (see Medications: Seizure Disorders). More than 20 drugs are available for use in the treatment of epilepsy. These medications do not cure the disorder; they only manage its manifestations. AEDs generally act in one of two ways: by raising the seizure threshold or by limiting the spread of abnormal activity in the brain.

The goals of medications for epilepsy are to protect the client from harm and to reduce or prevent seizure activity without impairing cognitive function or producing undesirable side effects. Ideally, the lowest possible dose of a single medication that will control the client's seizures is prescribed; often, however, several medications must be tried before the most effective one is identified, and a combination of drugs may be needed to manage the client's seizures.

Status epilepticus is a continuous seizure that lasts for more than 30 minutes or a series of seizures during which time consciousness is not regained. It requires immediate intervention to preserve life. Establishing and maintaining the airway is a priority. A solution of 50% dextrose is administered intravenously to prevent hypoglycemia. Diazepam (Valium) or lorazepam (Ativan) is given intravenously, and if necessary, the dose is repeated in 10 minutes to stop seizure activity. Phenytoin (Dilantin) is administered intravenously for longer-term control of seizures. Phenobarbital also may be administered to clients in status epilepticus.

Clinical Therapies for Children

Children with febrile seizures are usually not treated with an anticonvulsant at the time of the seizure because these seizures typically abate before arrival at the emergency department or clinic. Acetaminophen is given to lower the child's temperature.

Medications **Seizure Disorders**

CLASSIFICATION AND DRUG EXAMPLES	MECHANISMS OF ACTION	NURSING CONSIDERATIONS
Antiepileptic Drugs (AEDs) *Drug examples:* ■ phenytoin (Dilantin) ■ phenobarbital ■ primidone (Mysoline) ■ carbamazepine (Tegretol) ■ valproic acid (Depakene) ■ ethosuximide (Zarontin) ■ clonazepam (Klonopin) ■ gabapentin (Neurontin) ■ lamotrigine (Lamictal) ■ tiagabine HCl (Gabitril)	These drugs act in the motor cortex of the brain to reduce the spread of electrical discharges from the rapidly firing epileptic foci in this area. These agents control seizures without impairing the normal functions of the CNS.	■ Monitor blood pressure, pulse, and respirations. ■ Note evidence of CNS side effects such as blurred vision, dimmed vision, slurred speech, nystagmus, or confusion. Gingival hyperplasia may be noted in clients taking phenytoin. ■ Recognize that if clients are to be on prolonged therapy, they may need a diet rich in vitamin D. ■ Monitor the serum calcium level as ordered; phenytoin can contribute to demineralization of bone. ■ When administering anticonvulsants intravenously, monitor closely for respiratory depression and cardiovascular collapse. ■ Administer gabapentin 2 hours after antacids. ■ Administer tiagabine HCl with food.

Long-term anticonvulsants are not recommended for simple febrile seizures. Diazepam may be ordered for rectal or oral administration at the onset of a child's febrile illness when the parents are severely anxious about a subsequent febrile seizure (American Academy of Pediatrics, 2008).

Any child with a generalized seizure lasting longer than 10 minutes needs to be monitored for electrolytes, glucose, blood gases, increasing fever, and abnormal blood pressure. Most seizure disorders are managed with anticonvulsants, which may be given intravenously or rectally. For children, a single medication (monotherapy) is preferred for seizure control to minimize the potential for adverse effects such as sleepiness and difficulty with speech. An additional antiepileptic may be used only if seizure control is not achieved with the first medication (Raspall-Chaure, Neville, & Scott, 2008). The child should be monitored for continued motor activity and the potential for status epilepticus (a continuous seizure that lasts for more than 30 minutes or a series of seizures during which consciousness is not regained). The postictal period ranges from 30 minutes to 2 hours. Management of status epilepticus is described in **Table 11–7** ●. Serum drug levels are monitored to achieve therapeutic levels or to identify whether toxicity is possible. When tolerated, therapeutic ranges of medications may be exceeded to control seizures. Medication dosage adjustments are often needed in pediatric clients as the child grows.

The physician should provide a seizure action plan for any child with a history of seizure activity who attends school or day care or who is cared for outside the home while the parents work. Nurses can assist parents in making sure that teachers and caregivers understand the action plan and know when and how to use it.

Approximately 25%–30% of children have refractory or **intractable seizures**, seizures that continue to occur even with optimal medical management. These children should be referred to an epilepsy center for other potential treatments, such as a ketogenic diet, vagal nerve stimulation, or evaluation for surgical treatment.

TABLE 11–7 Management of Status Epilepticus

TYPE OF CARE	CLINICAL THERAPY
Emergency assessment and management	■ Maintain a patent airway. Muscle rigidity may compromise the airway. ■ Perform a jaw-thrust maneuver if the airway is obstructed. ■ Keep suction equipment at the bedside in case secretions are excessive. ■ Give oxygen by mask, because increased metabolic demands deplete oxygen stores. ■ Monitor vital signs and circulation with pulse oximeter and cardiorespiratory monitor. ■ Perform neurological assessment.
Ongoing urgent medications	■ Establish an intravenous line to administer any necessary fluids or management. ■ Administer glucose if the child is hypoglycemic; the physical stress of the seizure may result in declining glucose levels. ■ Insert a nasogastric tube. ■ Protect the child from injury. ■ Manage thermoregulation.
Medications	■ Administer benzodiazepines such as diazepam, lorazepam, or midazolam. If there is no response, the dose may be repeated. Phenytoin or phenobarbital may be necessary if seizure activity continues. Cumulative doses of drugs may produce apnea, so be prepared to assist with ventilations.

A ketogenic diet is occasionally used for children under the age of 8 years with myoclonic and absence seizures. This diet involves a high intake of fat (up to 80% of calories), an adequate intake of protein (1 g/kg), and a very low intake of carbohydrates. The medium-chain triglyceride (MCT) ketogenic diet is used extensively for treating refractory childhood epilepsy. This diet increases the plasma levels of medium straight-chain fatty acids (Chang et al., 2013). The child usually begins the diet in the hospital with a fast for 24 hours. The ketosis caused by the diet is believed to produce anticonvulsant effects. The diet is customized to the child to maintain the ideal body weight, maximize ketosis, and achieve optimal seizure control. Motivation must be high for the family to prepare the food and maintain the child on the diet for several years; improved seizure control is directly related to compliance with the diet. The child's urine ketone values are monitored weekly or more frequently. The most common complications are constipation, hyperlipidemia, and kidney stones. Constipation can be treated with MCT oil and increased fluids. Kidney stones are treated by increasing fluid intake and alkalinizing the urine.

A trial of antiepileptic medication withdrawal is often attempted for children who have been seizure free for 2 years, with medications tapered slowly over a period of months (Clore, 2010). Approximately 70% remain seizure free after 2 years; if seizures do recur, they normally do so within the first year after AED withdrawal (Raspall-Chaure et al., 2008).

NURSING PROCESS

Assessment

After the client's first seizure, a thorough history must be taken from the parent, primary caretaker, or witnesses to the event. A description of the seizure and its length should be noted, in addition to whether an aura was present and whether the client lost consciousness. This information helps to identify the type of seizure according to the International Classification of Epileptic Seizures (**Table 11–8**).

Perform a complete physical and neurological examination. Assess and monitor the client's physiological status. Observe the specific seizure activity, LOC, vital signs, and signs of hypoxia. During the postictal period, monitor vital signs, perform neurological checks, and ensure safety. Once the client is stable, a more definitive assessment can be made. LOC is one of the most important indicators of neurological function. Remember that a lack of response may be the result of the postictal state.

To help determine the type of seizure, collect and analyze historical information about the seizure activity, clustering, the aura, the motor activity or changes in muscle tone, automatisms, and any changes in developmental performance.

Assess the family's adaptation to the seizure disorder, including how well the family is coping with the uncertainty of when the next seizure will occur.

Diagnosis

Common nursing diagnoses for an individual with a seizure disorder include the following:

- *Ineffective Breathing Pattern*
- *Ineffective Airway Clearance*

TABLE 11–8 Nursing Assessments Before, During, and After a Seizure

ASSESSMENT	RATIONALE
What was the client's LOC? If consciousness was lost, at what point?	Indicates area of brain involved and type of seizure.
What was the client doing just before the attack?	May suggest precipitating factors.
In what part of the body did the seizure start?	May indicate the site of seizure activity in the brain tissue; for example, if jerking movements were first observed in the right hand, the seizure focus may be in the left motor cortex.
Was there an epileptic cry?	Usually indicates the tonic stage of a generalized tonic–clonic seizure.
Were any automatisms observed, such as eyelid fluttering, chewing, lip smacking, or swallowing?	Often seen in complex, partial, and absence seizures.
How long did movements last? Did the location or character change (tonic to clonic)? Did movements involve both sides of the body or just one side?	Indicates areas in which focal activity originated.
Did the head and/or eyes turn to one side? If so, which side?	Helps localize the focus of the seizure; during the seizure, the head and eyes typically turn away from the side of the epileptogenic focus.
Were there changes in pupillary reactions?	Indicates involvement of the autonomic nervous system.
If the client fell, was the head hit?	Skull x-ray studies may be needed to rule out subdural hematoma or fracture.
Was there foaming or frothing from the mouth?	Usually indicates a tonic–clonic seizure.

Focus on Diversity and Culture
Seizures

Seizures may have a special meaning for some cultural groups. For example, the Hmong believe that the child is experiencing *quag dab peg*, which means the "spirit catches you and you fall down." Hmong view the condition as serious, but there is a sense of pride that the child has the condition. In 1997, Anne Fadiman wrote *The Spirit Catches You and You Fall Down*, a compelling story about the cultural conflict between a Hmong family and healthcare providers over treatment of its daughter's seizures.

- *Risk for Trauma*
- *Chronic Low Self-Esteem*
- *Anxiety*
- *Ineffective Therapeutic Regimen Management*
- *Readiness for Enhanced Family Processes.*

(NANDA-I © 2012)

Planning

Nursing care focuses on maintaining airway patency, ensuring safety, administering medications, and providing emotional support. Both acute care and long-term management are involved. Planning also may include developing a seizure action plan for the client, particularly for children, so that family, close friends, teachers, and other caregivers or even professional colleagues know how to respond appropriately in the event the client has a seizure.

Stay Current: *Sample seizure action plans and other resources can be found at the Epilepsy Foundation's Web site:* **www.epilepsyfoundation.org**.

Implementation

Nursing interventions during seizures include the following:

- Place nothing in the client's mouth during a seizure; loose teeth may be knocked out and aspirated. Position the client on his or her side so secretions can drain. Monitor to ensure adequate oxygenation: Mucous membranes should be pink, the heart rate should be at a normal or slightly elevated rate for age, and the pulse oximetry reading should be greater than 95%. Oxygen is usually administered when the pulse oximetry reading (SpO_2) falls below 95%.
- Protect the client from self-harm during violent seizures (**Figure 11–12 ●**). If the client is in bed, the side rails should be padded to prevent injury. Children who have frequent, recurrent seizures should wear helmets to protect their heads during falls. All clients with seizure disorders should wear some form of medical alert identification. Maintain functioning suction at the bedside to clear the airway as necessary.
- Take special precautions when administering intravenous medications (diazepam, lorazepam, or phenytoin) for the emergency management of status epilepticus. Give these medications very slowly over several minutes to minimize the risk of respiratory or circulatory collapse.

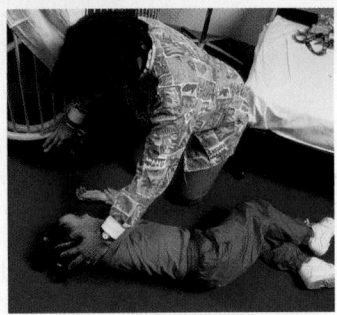

Figure 11–12 ● A client who has a seizure when standing should be gently assisted to the floor and placed in a side-lying position. Clear the area of any objects that might cause harm.

- Give medications for the ongoing management of seizures orally. Crushing pills and mixing them in a teaspoonful of applesauce, pudding, or other soft food make them more palatable and easier for a child or older adult to swallow if the pill is one that may be crushed.
- Understand that the loss of control of body movements and possible loss of consciousness make seizures frightening and difficult to accept. Parents often feel guilty about a child's seizure disorder and compensate by not disciplining or restricting the child appropriately. Stress the need to treat the child as normally as possible. Refer the child and family to support groups and counseling services if indicated.
- Encourage clients and their families to express their fears and anxieties. Answer questions honestly and refer to organizations such as the Epilepsy Foundation of America, where clients and family can get more information about the disorder. Make sure parents know how to administer medications and keep their child safe.

SAFETY ALERT
When the child on a ketogenic diet is hospitalized, it is important to limit glucose and dextrose from all sources. Normal saline intravenous fluid should be used. Medications in elixirs or syrups cannot be used because of the sugar content. Alternatively, medications can be obtained in pill form, crushed, and mixed with an allowable food that has been approved by the pharmacy.

Evaluation

Expected outcomes of nursing management include the following:

- The client achieves good seizure control with medication, ketogenic diet, or surgical intervention.
- The client's self-esteem is enhanced through participation in well-supervised sports and activities.
- The client maintains a patent airway during seizure activity.
- The client's safety is maintained during seizure activity.
- Medication administration reduces the frequency of seizure recurrence.
- An appropriate seizure management plan is created by client and family in conjunction with the healthcare team.

Lifespan Considerations Seizures

Children

- Children and adolescents need to have medications adjusted as they grow and medication plasma levels monitored carefully in order to maintain the level within therapeutic range to obtain optimal effects.
- The child and parents need to be educated about medication regimens. Explain the purpose of each drug, schedule for administration, side effects, and importance of giving all doses. Teaching the older child to take medications without parental intervention gives the child a feeling of control.
- Regular dental care is important because of the effect of phenytoin on the gingiva.
- The parents of children with recurrent febrile seizures should be taught how to administer antipyretics properly. Parents need to know, however, that antipyretics may not prevent a febrile seizure associated with an acute illness. The potential toxicity of an anticonvulsant in a child with febrile seizures is often considered greater than the risk of the seizures, and parents can be reassured that complications from febrile seizures are rare.
- The family should receive help in working with school administrators to develop an Individualized Healthcare Plan so the child can receive needed medications and care during school hours.
- Physical activity and exercise are important for all children. Encourage the child's participation in sports when adequate supervision is provided. Children who are prone to seizures require one-to-one supervision during swimming and water activities.
- The child may be afraid of having a seizure in front of friends. Reassure the child and family that taking medications regularly should control seizures.
- Summer camps for children with seizures can be a safe and comfortable place for the child to enjoy outdoor activities. Talk with parents about communicating with camp administrators and sharing health and action plans as they do with school administers.

Adolescents and Adults

- Depending on state laws, most clients with seizure disorders can drive after they have been seizure free for at least 2 years.
- Adolescent females need to be educated about the potential teratogenicity of some anticonvulsants, such as valproic acid and carbamazepine, which are associated with neural tube defects and heart defects. Until pregnancy is desired, contraception should be used when the adolescent is sexually active.
- Some antiepileptic medications cause a drug interaction with oral contraceptive pills that can lead to contraceptive failure. Effective contraception may require increasing the amount of estrogen in the contraceptive hormones or using medroxyprogesterone injections.
- Families should be taught about safety guidelines. Families of clients with severe seizure disorders need to develop an emergency care plan so that emergency personnel know about the need for care in advance.

NURSING CARE PLAN   A Client With a Seizure Disorder

ASSESSMENT

Janet Carlson is a 19-year-old college student who lives with her parents and one younger sister. Although Ms. Carlson had seizures while she was in grade school, they have been controlled with medication. However, she had a tonic–clonic seizure yesterday and immediately made an appointment with her family physician. She is currently taking phenytoin (Dilantin) 300 mg/day as a maintenance medication to prevent seizures.

Evita Farias, RN, completes a health history for Ms. Carlson. During the history, Ms. Carlson says that she has been under stress because of difficulties in completing her course requirements this semester. She has not been sleeping as many hours at night, and sometimes she forgets to take her medication. Her serum phenytoin level is 8 mcg/mL. Her therapeutic level is 10–20 mcg/mL.

DIAGNOSES

- *Risk for Injury* related to recurrence of generalized tonic–clonic seizure activity and low serum phenytoin levels
- *Deficient Knowledge* of activities that may trigger seizure activity, the effect of stress on seizures, and medication information

(NANDA-I © 2012)

PLANNING

- Verbalize precipitating and triggering factors related to the onset of seizures.
- Verbalize the relationship between emotional and physical stress and seizures.
- Verbalize the importance of taking AEDs.

IMPLEMENTATION

- Teach the client and her family the following:
- Current information about seizures
- Care during and after a seizure
- Medication protocols
- Factors and activities that can trigger seizures
- The importance of follow-up care.
- Refer the client and her family to a local epilepsy support group.
- Recommend that the client purchase and wear a medical ID bracelet.

NURSING CARE PLAN *(continued)*

EVALUATION

Ms. Carlson is instructed to continue taking Dilantin 300 mg/day. Ms. Farias states the importance of nutrition, rest, and measures to reduce stress. She also discusses with Ms. Carlson the importance of maintaining the proper blood levels of her medication, stating that too little or too much of the medication could cause problems. Ms. Carlson understands that the seizures had recurred during a busy time in school when she had forgotten to take her medication. She is now wearing a medical ID bracelet. Ms. Farias provides the Carlsons with the telephone number of the Epilepsy Foundation of America.

CRITICAL THINKING

1. If you were Ms. Carlson's nurse, would your teaching differ if Ms. Carlson were living alone? If so, how? If not, why not?
2. Ms. Carlson tells you that although she knows she should not drive a car, she often drives herself to and from school. What would you say to Ms. Carlson about driving?
3. Ms. Carlson states, "It's embarrassing to wear a medical ID bracelet." How would you respond? What recommendation(s) would you make?

REVIEW Seizure Disorders

RELATE Link the Concepts and Exemplars

Linking the exemplar of seizures with the concept of legal issues:

1. When caring for an adult client newly diagnosed with recurrent seizures, what legal obligation does the nurse have regarding the client's driving privileges versus the obligation to client privacy?
2. If the client says, "You don't have to report this to the DMV—I promise not to drive until I get medical clearance," is it permissible for the nurse to take the client's word for it?

Linking the exemplar of seizures with the concept of thermoregulation:

3. The nurse is caring for a 14-month-old infant with a fever whose mother reports the two older siblings both experienced febrile seizures. What nursing interventions would you initiate with this child?
4. What would differ in your plan of care for a child with a fever if the child had a history of febrile seizures?

READY Go to the Companion Skills Manual
REFER Go to Pearson Nursing Student Resources
nursing.pearsonhighered.com

- Additional review materials

REFLECT Case Study

Joe Hill is a 77-year-old White male admitted with a diagnosis of new-onset seizure. His heart rate is 78 bpm, his blood pressure is 154/90 mmHg, his temperature is 97°F, and his O_2 sat is 99%. He appears confused and is unable to respond to questions. Mr. Hill's wife reports that he has a history of hypertension, but he is otherwise healthy. He is placed on seizure precautions, and his vital signs are monitored.

1. On the basis of this description, what kind of seizure might Mr. Hill have experienced?
2. What factors may have contributed to Mr. Hill's seizure?
3. What will the nurse include in the assessment of this client?
4. What are the priority nursing interventions?

REFERENCES

American Academy of Pediatrics, Steering Committee on Quality Improvement and Management, & Subcommittee on Febrile Seizures. (2008). Febrile seizures: Clinical practice guideline for the long-term management of the child with simple febrile seizures, *Pediatrics, 121*(6), 1281–1286.

Ball, J. W., Bindler, R. C., & Cowen, K. J. (2012). *Principles of pediatric nursing: Caring for children* (5th ed.). Upper Saddle River, NJ: Prentice Hall.

Brettler, S. (2004). Trauma nursing: Traumatic head injury. *RN, 67*(4), 32–38.

Brosche, T. M. (2011). Intracranial pressure and cerebral perfusion ranges. *Critical Care Nurse, 31*(4), 18–19. Retrieved from http://ccn.aacnjournals.org/content/31/4/18.2.full.

Centers for Disease Control and Prevention (CDC). (2013). *Traumatic brain injury.* Retrieved from http://www.cdc.gov/traumaticbraininjury/.

Centers for Disease Control and Prevention (CDC). (2014). *Traumatic brain injury in the United States: Fact sheet.* Retrieved from http://www.cdc.gov/TraumaticBrainInjury/get_the_facts.html.

Centers for Disease Control and Prevention (CDC). (n.d.). *Heads up. Facts for physicians about mild traumatic brain injury.* Retrieved from http://www.cdc.gov/concussion/headsup/pdf/facts_for_physicians_booklet-a.pdf.

Chang, P., Terbach, N., Plant, N., Chen, P. E., Walker, M. C., & Williams, R. S. B. (2013). Seizure control by ketogenic diet-associated medium chain fatty acids. *Neuropharmacology, 69*(100), 105–114. Retrieved from http://www.ncbi.nlm.nih.gov/pmc/articles/PMC3625124.

Clore, E. T. (2010). Seizure precautions for pediatric bedside nurses. *Pediatric Nursing, 36*(4), 191–194.

Dunn, L. T. (2002). Raised intracranial pressure. *Journal of Neurology, Neurosurgery, and Psychiatry, 73*(Suppl I), I23–I27. Retrieved from http://www.ncbi.nlm.nih.gov/pmc/articles/PMC1765599/pdf/v073p00i23.pdf.

Epilepsy Foundation. (2012). *About epilepsy: Epilepsy and seizure statistics.* Retrieved from http://www.epilepsyfoundation.org/aboutepilepsy/index.cfm/statistics.cfm.

Fadiman, A. (1997). *The spirit catches you and you fall down.* New York, NY: Farrar, Strauss, Giroux.

James, H. E. (1986). Neurologic evaluation and support in the child with acute brain insult. *Pediatric Annals, 15*(1), 16–22.

Mewasingh, L. D. (2010). Febrile seizures. *Clinical Evidence, 11*, 324.

National Institute of Neurological Disorders and Stroke. (2013). *Hydrocephalus fact sheet.* Retrieved from http://www.ninds.nih.gov/disorders/hydrocephalus/detail_hydrocephalus.htm.

Norton, C., Feltz, S. J., Brocker, A., & Granitto, M. (2013). Tackling long-term consequences of concussion. *Lippincott's NursingCenter.com.* Retrieved from http://www.nursingcenter.com/lnc/JournalArticle?Article_ID=1484295.

Porth, C. M., & Matfin, G. (2009). *Pathophysiology: Concepts of altered health states* (8th ed.). Philadelphia, PA: Lippincott Williams & Wilkins.

Raspall-Chaure, M., Neville, B. G., & Scott, R. C. (2008). The medical management of the epilepsies in children: Conceptual and practical considerations. *Lancet Neurology, 7*(1): 57–69.

Seattle Children's Hospital. (2013). *Hydrocephalus.* Retrieved from http://www.seattlechildrens.org/ medical-conditions/brain-nervous-system-mental-conditions/hydrocephalus-symptoms/#.

Sports Concussion Institute. (n.d.). *Concussion facts.* Retrieved from http://www.concussiontreatment.com/ concussionfacts.html.

Teasdale, G., & Jennett, B. (1974). Assessment of coma and impaired consciousness. *Lancet, 2,* 81–84.

Tierney, L., McPhee, S., & Papadakis, M. (Eds.). (2005). *Current medical diagnosis & treatment* (44th ed.). New York, NY: McGraw-Hill.

Waruiru, C., & Appleton, R. (2004). Febrile seizures: An update. *Archives of Disease in Childhood, 89*(8),

751–756. Retrieved from http://www.ncbi.nlm.nih.gov/ pubmed/15269077.

Wilson, B. A., Shannon, M. T., & Shields, K. M. (2011). *Pearson nurse's drug guide.* Upper Saddle River, NJ: Pearson.

12 Metabolism

◢ THE CONCEPT OF METABOLISM

After nutrients (carbohydrates, fats, and proteins) have been ingested, digested, absorbed, and transported across cell membranes, they must be metabolized into individual chemicals that the cells can utilize to maintain life. **Metabolism** describes the processes of biochemical reactions occurring in the body's cells that are necessary to produce energy, repair cells, and maintain life. Through the release of hormones, the endocrine system controls the cellular activity that regulates growth and body metabolism. **Hormones** are chemical messengers that are secreted by various glands and exert controlling effects on the cells of the body, regulating such varied functions as growth, reproduction, fluid and electrolyte balance, and gender differentiation. **<<**

Concept Learning Outcomes

After reading about this concept, you will be able to:

1. Summarize the structure and physiology of the body related to metabolism.

2. Examine the relationship between metabolism and other concepts/systems.

3. Identify commonly occurring alterations in metabolism and their related therapies.

4. Differentiate common assessment procedures used to examine metabolism across the life span.

5. Describe diagnostic and laboratory tests to determine an individual's metabolic status.

6. Explain management of metabolic health and prevention of metabolic disorders.

7. Demonstrate the nursing process in providing culturally competent and caring interventions across the life span for individuals with common alterations in metabolism.

8. Compare and contrast common independent and collaborative interventions for clients with alterations in metabolism.

Concept Key Terms

Acromegaly, 735
Carpal spasm, 737
Chvostek sign, 737
Dwarfism, 737
Exophthalmos, 735
Goiter, 735

Hormones, 725
Insulin, 726
Metabolism, 725
Tetany, 737
Trousseau sign, 737

▶ NORMAL METABOLISM

The major endocrine organs are the pituitary gland, thyroid gland, parathyroid glands, adrenal glands, pancreas, and gonads (reproductive glands). The locations of these glands are illustrated in **Figure 12–1** ●. **Table 12–1** ● summarizes the functions of the endocrine organs and their hormones.

✳ Visit **nursing.pearsonhighered.com** to see a minimodule on the anatomy and physiology of the endocrine system.

Genetic and Lifespan Considerations

The endocrine system is responsible for sexual differentiation during fetal development and for stimulating growth and development during childhood and adolescence. Growth hormone, produced by the anterior pituitary gland, is secreted in pulses when the child is in Stage 4 sleep. Growth hormone stimulates the growth of muscles and improves bone mineralization (Grimberg & De León, 2005). Multiple hormones in the endocrine system, including growth hormone, thyroid hormone, adrenal and gonadal androgens, and estrogen, are responsible for skeletal growth and maturation, including the appearance of secondary ossification centers in the bones (Carroll, 2010). Estrogen secretion associated with puberty is a dominant stimulator of

increased skeletal maturity that can be detected by examining the child's bone age (Lee & Kulin, 2005). See **Table 12–2** ● for normal age-related changes to the endocrine system in adults.

▶ ALTERATIONS TO METABOLISM

Disorders of the structure and function of the endocrine glands alter normal hormone levels and the way that body tissues use those hormones. When hormone production increases or decreases, individuals experience alterations in health such as diabetes, obesity, osteoporosis, and glandular disorders.

Individuals with alterations to their metabolism have alterations in other concepts/systems as well. See the Concepts Related to Metabolism for more information.

Alterations and Manifestations

The alterations of metabolism that more commonly occur are diabetes mellitus, obesity, Graves disease, thyroid disorders, osteoporosis, and cirrhosis.

Diabetes is a disorder of metabolism related to the body's production and use of the hormone **insulin**. In type 1 diabetes,

TABLE 12–1   Organs, Hormones, Functions, and Feedback Mechanisms of the Endocrine System

ENDOCRINE ORGAN	HORMONES SECRETED	TARGET ORGANS, FUNCTIONS, AND FEEDBACK MECHANISMS
Thyroid gland	Thyroid hormone: Thyroxine (T_4) is the major hormone secreted by the thyroid gland. It is converted to triiodothyronine (T_3) at the target tissues.	Maintains metabolic rate and growth and development of all tissues. Both T_3 and T_4 are secreted in response to thyroid-stimulating hormone.
	Calcitonin	Maintains blood calcium levels by decreasing bone resorption and decreasing resorption of calcium in the kidneys whenever levels of blood calcium are elevated.
Parathyroid gland	Parathyroid hormone	Maintains blood calcium levels by stimulating bone resorption and formation and by stimulating kidney resorption of calcium in response to falling levels of blood calcium.
Adrenal cortex	Mineralocorticoids (e.g., aldosterone)	Promote kidney tubule reabsorption of sodium and water and excretion of potassium in response to elevated levels of potassium and low levels of sodium, thereby increasing blood pressure and blood volume.
	Glucocorticoids (e.g., cortisol)	Help regulate metabolism of carbohydrates, fats, and proteins. Activate anti-inflammatory responses to stressors. Low cortisol levels stimulate hypothalamic secretion of corticotropin-releasing hormone, which stimulates the anterior pituitary gland to release adrenocorticotropic hormone, which in turn stimulates the adrenal cortex to secrete cortisol.
	Gonadocorticoids (androgens and small amounts of estrogen and progesterone)	Produce a small quantity of sex hormones; Androgens play a role in the secondary development of the reproductive organs.
Adrenal medulla	Catecholamines (epinephrine and norepinephrine)	Stimulate the heart, constrict blood vessels, inhibit visceral muscles, dilate bronchioles, increase respiration and metabolism, and promote hyperglycemia. Secreted in response to physical or psychological stress.
Anterior pituitary (adenohypophysis)	Growth hormone (GH)	Promotes growth of body tissues by enhancing protein synthesis and promoting use of fat for energy, thus conserving glucose. Release is stimulated by GH-releasing hormone in response to low GH levels, hypoglycemia, increased amino acids, low fatty acids, and stress.

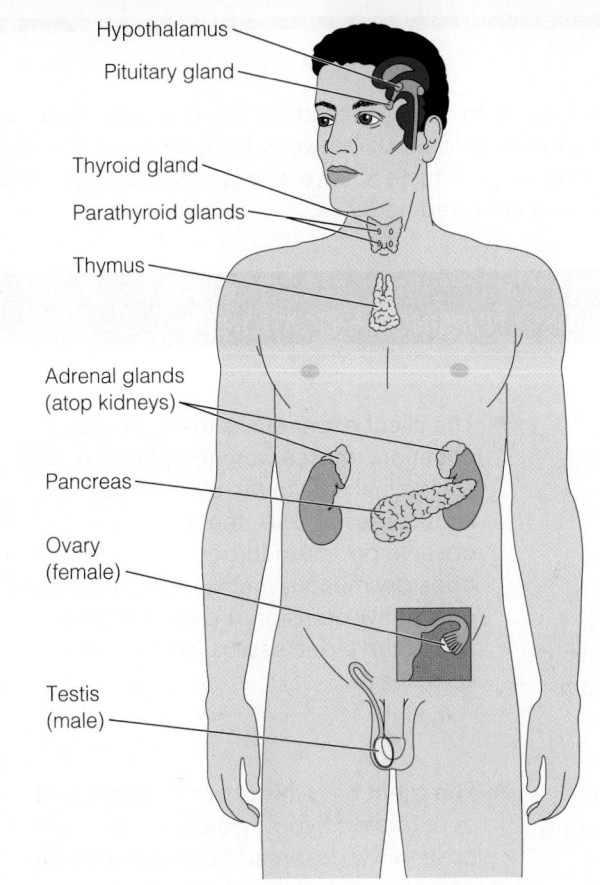

Hypothalamus

Pituitary gland

Thyroid gland

Parathyroid glands

Thymus

Adrenal glands
(atop kidneys)

Pancreas

Ovary
(female)

Testis
(male)

Figure 12–1 ● Location of the major endocrine glands.

there is an absolute deficiency of insulin related to pancreatic beta cell destruction. The client is usually acutely ill at onset and will be hospitalized for treatment of hyperglycemia, diabetic ketoacidosis (DKA), dehydration, and electrolyte disturbances. The symptoms are nausea, vomiting, lethargy, abdominal pain, thirst, fever, blurring vision, and possible alteration in level of consciousness. Therapy includes treatment of the acidosis and

dehydration with fluids. Insulin must be infused to correct the hyperglycemia. The client usually spends several days in the ICU. Prior to discharge, the client and family receives education about diet, medication, and monitoring and should be scheduled for community follow up with either a family doctor or an endocrinologist and diabetes educator.

Type 2 diabetes has a more insidious onset and may develop over several years. There is relative deficiency of insulin, which may be related to insulin resistance and inadequate secretion of insulin to meet body needs. Both of these components are usually present at time of diagnosis. The onset may be acute, with markedly elevated glucose levels resulting in nonketotic hyperglycemia that requires hospitalization for treatment. However, the more common presentation is mildly elevated glucose levels with weight gain and symptoms of hyperglycemia, such as thirst, frequent urination, and increased susceptibility to infections, blurred vision, and fatigue. The mainstays of therapy include diet, glucose monitoring, exercise, and possibly medication. In the early stages, oral medication may not be required. The natural progression of type 2 diabetes is to require medication at some time in the client's future.

Obesity is a state in which excess calories are stored as fat. The Centers for Disease Control (CDC, 2011b) reports that the incidence of obesity has doubled in adults and tripled in youth since 1980. The obesity epidemic increases the risk of hypertension, dyslipidemia, type 2 diabetes, coronary artery disease, stroke, fatty liver and gallbladder disease, sleep disorders, cancers and dementia. BMI (body mass index) is the guideline for evaluating the severity of obesity. Waist circumference is also an important tool used to measure obesity. Obesity usually has no overt symptoms other than those related to the complications already mentioned. Treatment includes exercise, diet, and behavior modifications. Medication may be used in the short term but usually does not sustain weight loss when stopped, and the weight is often gained back. Surgery is also an option for those with the comorbidities related to obesity.

TABLE 12–2   Age-Related Endocrine Changes

AGE-RELATED CHANGE	SIGNIFICANCE
Pituitary: ↓ production of ACTH, TSH, FSH	Decreased secretion of glucocorticoids, 17-ketosteroids, progesterone, androgen, and estrogen (and thus lower levels on diagnostic tests)
Thyroid: ↑ in fibrosis and nodularity, ↓ in gland activity	Lower basal metabolic rate Increased incidence of hypothyroidism Palpable nodules on palpation
Adrenal medulla: ↑ secretion and level of norepinephrine, ↓ beta-adrenergic response to norepinephrine	Decreased response to beta-adrenergic and receptor-blocking medications Possible contribution to increased incidence of hypertension
Pancreas: calcification of blood vessels and distention and dilation of pancreatic ducts	Decreased production of lipase with reduced fat absorption and digestion, leading to intolerance of fatty foods and indigestion Decreased absorption of fat-soluble vitamins
Pancreas: delayed and decreased insulin release; believed to be accompanied by decreased sensitivity to circulating insulin	Decreased ability to metabolize glucose with higher and more prolonged blood glucose levels, possibly contributing to increased incidence of type 2 diabetes mellitus with aging (however, higher-than-normal blood glucose levels are not unusual in older adults without diabetes)

Concepts Related to **Metabolism**

The endocrine system consists of glands and cells that are specialized with chemical transmitters that respond to changes in the body. Together with the central nervous system, the endocrine system regulates and responds to these changes to maintain homeostasis in metabolic pathways of the body. Based on this concept, there are many interrelationships between body systems that may be may be manifested. Several examples of these relationships are listed here.

CONCEPT	RELATIONSHIP TO METABOLISM	NURSING IMPLICATIONS
Acid–base balance		
■ Metabolic acidosis (DKA) in type 1 diabetes	Absolute insulin deficiency: ■ Uptake of glucose by muscles and cells is inadequate. ■ Glucose accumulates in the cells. ■ Energy source comes from protein and fatty acids. ■ Ketones are given off as metabolites and accumulate, causing acidosis, which leads to tissue breakdown, shock, coma, and death.	■ The client experiences thirst, frequent urination, nausea, vomiting, fatigue, and abdominal pain in the early stages. In later stages of DKA, the nurse will observe poor skin turgor, a fruity breath odor, dry mucous membranes, decreased pulses, hypotension, a cool skin temperature, and a decreasing level of consciousness.
Perfusion		
■ Myxedema	Long-standing untreated hypothyroidism: ■ Fluid retention, edema, dyspnea, profound bradycardia, metabolic disorders ■ Cardiovascular collapse	■ The client has a history of undiagnosed or untreated hypothyroidism. The nurse observes widespread edema, especially around the eyes, hands, and feet; impaired mentation; a slow pulse; and decreased blood pressure.
Oxygenation		
■ Ascites	Accumulation of fluid in the abdominal cavity: ■ Pressure on thoracic cavity ■ Inability to expand lungs, causing dyspnea and impaired oxygenation	■ The client has a history of cirrhosis and portal hypertension. A lab review done by the nurse indicates hypoalbuminemia. The nurse's observations note an increased respiratory rate at rest and, on exertion, orthopnea and a positive fluid wave.
Stress and Coping		
■ Feelings of powerlessness and loss related to diabetes	New diagnosis of diabetes or change in severity of an already present disorder can cause feelings of powerlessness as the client confronts changes to lifestyle that will be lifelong.	■ The client may express fear of losing control of his or her body, fear of losing lifestyle choices such as eating and exercising, and fear of hyperglycemia and/or hypoglycemia. The nurse asks open-ended questions that explore the client's feelings. The nurse may also answer questions that arise about the uncertainty of the plan for lifelong health related to diabetes.

Graves disease is a thyroid condition that results in hyperthyroidism. It is an autoimmune disorder that presents with the symptoms of an overactive thyroid such as increased appetite, weight loss, hypermotile bowels, diarrhea, heat intolerance, insomnia, and increased sweating. All symptoms are representative of increased metabolism. Treatment includes pharmacologic therapy with antithyroid drugs, radioactive iodine therapy, or surgery.

Hypothyroidism, which is an underactive thyroid, is the insufficient production of thyroid hormone. Hypothyroidism has numerous causes. In countries other than the United States, iodine deficiency is the leading cause of hypothyroidism. In the United States and Europe, this deficiency is rare and the leading cause of hypothyroidism is autoimmune disease. The presenting symptoms are the opposite of hyperthyroidism and are manifested as slowing of the body's functions. Symptoms include hypothermia, weight gain in the presence of decreased appetite, systemic edema, lethargy, fatigue, constipation, bradycardia, and altered lipid metabolism. Treatment includes daily replacement of the thyroid hormone; if a goiter is present and causing respiratory or neck symptoms, a thyroidectomy may be done.

Osteoporosis is a metabolic bone disorder in which the rate of bone resorption increases and the rate of bone formation decreases. The result is decreased bone mass. It may be a primary disorder or secondary to another disease or medications. The presentation is loss of height with possible increased vertebral curvature, decreased exercise tolerance, and decreased spinal movement. The symptoms may occur over time and not be readily recognized as osteoporosis. Safety from falls is a priority for individuals with this disorder. Treatment includes medications aimed at controlling bone loss, restoring bone formation, and controlling pain. Exercises and supportive devices such as back braces may also be implemented.

Cirrhosis is characterized by widespread destruction of liver cells, which are replaced by less efficient fibrous cells. Cirrhosis has many causes, but all the manifestations are those of a dying liver. Early signs may be vague, such as loss of appetite, indigestion, nausea, vomiting, constipation, diarrhea, and jaundice. The client may report bruising easily. Later symptoms are related to progression of cell damage and may be respiratory problems, central nervous effects, hematological effects, skin effects, renal effects, and hepatic effects. Therapy aims to remove or alleviate the underlying cause, prevent further liver damage, and prevent or treat complications.

Other alterations related to the endocrine system that are not covered as a part of this concept include, but are not limited to, the following:

- Leukodystrophies
- Menkes disease
- Niemann-Pick disease
- Phenylketonuria
- Porphyria
- Tay-Sachs disease
- Zellweger syndrome
- Maple syrup urine disease.

Alterations and therapies for selected endocrine and metabolic disorders are shown in the Alterations and Therapies feature.

Prevalence

Metabolic disorder prevalence is specific to the type of disorder. The most common are diabetes, thyroid disease, lipid metabolism, obesity, metabolic bone disease, and cirrhosis. There are many other metabolism disorders that are less common, such as disorders of the adrenal and pituitary glands, reproductive disorders, disorders of calcium and other electrolytes, and metabolic conditions that cause hypertension, such as pheochromocytoma.

DIABETES   As of 2011, 25.8 million individuals in the United States had been diagnosed with diabetes, and an estimated 7 million had the disease but had not been diagnosed.

Of individuals younger than 20 years of age, 215,000 (0.26% of this age group) had diabetes. Of all individuals age 20 or older, 28.9 million (12.3%) had diabetes; 15.5 million (13.6%) of men and 13.4 million (11.2%) of women in this age group had diabetes (CDC, 2014).

OBESITY   National data on obesity prevalence among U.S. adults, adolescents, and children show that more than 33% of adults and almost 17% of youth were obese in 2009–2010. Differences in prevalence between men and women diminished between 1999–2000 and 2009–2010, with the prevalence of obesity among men reaching the same level as that among women (CDC, 2012b).

THYROID DISORDERS   Thyrotoxicosis occurs in 2% of women and 0.2% of men. In younger individuals, Graves disease is a far more common diagnosis, with peak onset at 20–40 years of age. The overall prevalence of hypothyroidism in women in the United States is 7.5%; in men the prevalence is about 2.8%. It is estimated that 38% of the world's population is affected by hypothyroidism (NIDDK, 2012).

OSTEOPOROSIS   The National Institutes of Health have estimated that 12 million Americans have osteoporosis and 44 million have low bone mass or osteopenia. Approximately 50% of women and 25% of men age 50 or older will have an osteoporosis-related fracture in their lifetime. White and Asian women are at highest risk for an osteoporotic fracture (NIH, 2012).

CIRRHOSIS   Liver cirrhosis is a major cause of death in the United Sates, and its prevalence is related to the cause of the liver disease. The two most common causes are infection with hepatits B or C and alcohol abuse (NIDDK, 2011).

Genetic Considerations and Nonmodifiable Risk Factors

Genetic considerations and nonmodifiable risk factors are also specific to the type of disorder.

TYPE 1 DIABETES   In most cases of type 1 diabetes, the individual must inherit risk factors from both parents. Environmental triggers are also part of the development of type 1 diabetes. Research has suggested that cold weather may be a factor because type 1 diabetes develops more often in the winter months in the colder climates that in the summer. Another trigger may be a virus that has a mild effect on most individuals but triggers type 1 diabetes in others. In many individuals, the development can take many years, as was discovered in a study of the relatives of individuals with type 1 diabetes who later developed the disease. It was found that they had had an antibody in their blood for years. A gene has also been isolated that is found in those with type 1 diabetes: the HLA-DR3 or the HLA-DR4 gene (ADA, 2011b).

TYPE 2 DIABETES   Type 2 diabetes runs in families, in part, because of poor nutritional habits learned in the home environment. In general, children of individuals with type 2 diabetes have a 1 in 7 chance of developing the disease if the parent was diagnosed before age 50 and a 1 in 13 chance if the disease developed in the parent after age 50 (ADA, 2011b).

Alterations and Therapies **Endocrine and Metabolic Disorders**

ALTERATIONS	DESCRIPTION/ DEFINITION	MANIFESTATIONS	INTERVENTIONS AND TREATMENTS
Diabetes mellitus	A disorder of hyperglycemia resulting from defects in insulin secretion, insulin action, or both, leading to abnormalities in carbohydrate, protein, and fat metabolism	Signs of hyperglycemia including thirst, hunger, fatigue, frequent infections, weight gain or loss, blurred vision, parasthesias	▪ Blood glucose monitoring ▪ Nutritional therapy ▪ Physical activity ▪ Pharmacologic therapy ▪ Self-management education
Type 1 diabetes mellitus	Destruction of beta cells, usually leading to absolute deficiency of insulin	Signs of hyperglycemia as above, as well as weight loss, nausea, vomiting, abdominal pain, blurred vision	▪ Insulin administration ▪ Hydration ▪ Dietary management ▪ Self-management education
Type 2 diabetes mellitus	A range from predominantly insulin resistance with relative insulin deficiency to predominantly secretory defect with insulin resistance	Signs of hyperglycemia with possible weight gain, obesity. Cardiac disease may be first presenting disorder.	▪ Exercise ▪ Nutritional and pharmacologic therapy ▪ Weight management
Obesity	Storage of excess calories as fat, resulting from excess energy intake, decreased energy expenditure, or a combination of both. Several hormones are involved in regulating obesity, including thyroid hormone, insulin, and leptin. Genetics may also play a role.	BMI of 30–34.9 with two or more comorbidities (obesity class 1) BMI of 35–39.9 with two or more comorbidities (obesity class 2) BMI of $\geq$40 (obesity class 3)	▪ Individual program of exercise, diet, and behavior modification ▪ Pharmacotherapy ▪ Bariatric surgery for clients who have class 3 obesity or obesity with comorbidities
Graves disease	An autoimmune disorder, the most common cause of hyperthyroidism, occurring when immunoglobulin produced by B lymphocytes stimulate oversecretion of thyroid hormones.	Increased appetite with weight loss, hypermotile bowels, bloating, pain, diarrhea, heat intolerance, insomnia, palpitations, and increased sweating, smooth warm skin, fine hair, and/or hair loss, emotional lability	▪ Pharmacologic therapy ▪ Radioactive iodine therapy ▪ Surgery (subtotal or total thyroidectomy)
Hypothyroidism	Insufficient production of thyroid hormone by the thyroid gland. May be congenital or acquired.	Hypothermia, decreased appetite accompanied by weight gain, systemic edema, lethargy and fatigue, bradycardia, altered lipid metabolism	▪ Pharmacotherapy ▪ Subtotal thyroidectomy (if goiter is large enough to cause respiratory difficulties or dysphagia)
Osteoporosis	Loss of bone mass, increased bone fragility, and increased risk of fracture.	Loss of height, progressive curvature of the spine, low back pain, fractures of forearm, spine, or hip. Often called the silent disease.	▪ Pharmacotherapy including hormonal agents, bisphosphonates, selective estrogen receptor modulators (SERMs) ▪ Weight-bearing exercises
Cirrhosis	In end stage liver disease, gradual destruction of functional liver tissue and replacement by fibrous scar tissue, which forms constrictive bands that disrupt blood flow to liver lobules.	Early stage: enlarged tender liver, dull aching pain in right upper quadrant, weight loss, anorexia, weakness, alternating diarrhea and constipation Later stage: profound weakness, lethargy, altered level of consciousness, ascites, confusion, asterixis, bruising due to clotting disorders	▪ Pharmacotherapy ▪ Paracentesis ▪ Balloon tamponade or interventional surgery for portal hypertension

OBESITY Science shows that genetics plays a role in obesity. Genes can directly cause obesity in disorders such as Bardet-Biedl syndrome and Prader-Willi syndrome. Genes and behavior may both be needed for an individual to be overweight. In some cases, multiple genes increase one's susceptibility to obesity and require outside factors, such as abundant food supply or little physical activity. Currently, genetic tests are not useful for guiding personal diet or physical activity (CDC, 2012b).

OSTEOPOROSIS From family histories, twin studies, and molecular genetics, it is believed that there is a predisposition for osteoporosis that is inherited. Bone health has been found to depend largely on the genes inherited from parents (NOS, 2013).

CIRRHOSIS Cirrhosis is not usually inherited, but some diseases that can result in cirrhosis are genetic in origin. Cystic fibrosis, alpha-1 antitrypsin deficiency, hemochromatosis, Wilson disease, and galactosemia are inherited diseases that interfere with how the liver produces, processes, and stores enzymes, proteins, metals, and other substances needed by the body to function properly. Cirrhosis can result from these conditions (NIDDK, 2012).

CASE STUDY \\ PART 1

Mary Bell is a 65-year-old Caucasian female who comes to the clinic with back and hip pain. Her past medical history includes COPD with intermittent steroid use, hypertension, depression, GERD, and tobacco abuse. Ms. Bell lives alone, cooks for herself, has no family living nearby, and does not exercise. The nurse's observations are that Ms. Bell is a frail, elderly-looking woman who is in moderate pain and moves cautiously. Her gait is unstable.

Clinical Reasoning Questions Level I

1. What risk factors are present (modifiable and unmodifiable) for osteoporosis and possible fracture?
2. Discuss safety risks that are present for Ms. Bell.
3. What further interview questions should the nurse ask?

Clinical Reasoning Questions Level II

4. What are two nursing diagnoses for Ms. Bell at this time?
5. What independent nursing interventions can you perform to help make Ms. Bell more comfortable and safe while in the clinic?
6. What tests do you anticipate will be done for Ms. Bell at this visit?

▶ PREVENTION

The most prevalent metabolic disorders, such as type 2 diabetes, obesity, osteoporosis, and cirrhosis, have modifiable risk factors. The nurse can help the client identify and modify some of these factors with education on healthy lifestyle behaviors that can prevent and or slow down the onset of the disorder and prevent complications.

Although there are no modifiable risk factors for type 1 diabetes, knowledge about the prevalence and symptoms can help family members identify the onset of the disorder and seek further evaluation. If a client already has type 1 diabetes, information about other autoimmune disorders that often occur in individuals with type 1 diabetes can aid the client and family

members to monitor for further development of such diseases as Graves disease, Addison disease, autoimmune hepatitis, celiac sprue, and vitiligo. Blood tests, fecal tests, and physician assessment may detect other related metabolic disorders. In type 2 diabetes, the nurse can help the client by suggesting healthy lifestyle plans of exercise and diet to prevent the onset of type 2 diabetes. Screenings may include those recommended by the American Diabetes Association (ADA), such as lab testing: hemoglobin $A_{1C} > 6.5\%$ indicates diabetes, 5.7%–6% indicates prediabetes and warrants interventions and modification of risk factors. Fasting glucose of >126 mg/dL or a 2 hour postprandial or random glucose over 200 mg/dL may indicate the development of type 2 diabetes. Further blood testing may include serum lipids and serum electrolytes. Other screenings include client history and biophysical measurements such as weight and waist circumference.

In liver disease, alcohol abuse is the leading cause of cirrhosis. The nurse can identify clients at risk during the assessment phase of care by using the **CAGE** questionnaire.

> **C:** Have you ever felt you should **C**ut down on your drinking?
>
> **A:** Have people **A**nnoyed you by criticizing your drinking?
>
> **G:** Have you felt bad or **G**uilty about your drinking?
>
> **E:** Have you ever had a drink first thing in the morning to steady your nerves or change your **E**nergy level?

Obesity has several modifiable risk factors, including excessive food intake and decreased activity. Screenings include biophysical measurements such as weight and waist circumference as well as screening for comorbid conditions such as thyroid disease, diabetes, dyslipidemia, and cardiac disease. A BMI of 25–29.9 kg/m^2 is overweight. BMI 30 kg/m^2 or greater is obesity. A BMI of 40 or greater is extreme or morbid obesity. A waist circumference of 40 inches or greater in men and 35 inches or greater in women is also a measurement of obesity. Obtaining a history of dietary intake and activity can also help screen for a client's risk for obesity. Identifying community resources for the client is a valuable intervention that the nurse can do. Weight Watcher meetings, support groups, and walking trails are effective ways to help a client stay motivated in following a weight loss program.

Osteoporosis has a few modifiable risk factors, such as disordered eating, calcium deficiency, vitamin D deficiency, substance abuse, a sedentary lifestyle, and prolonged use of some medications. The nurse can help the client to identify risk factors and can suggest interventions such as increasing exercise, tobacco cessation, healthy eating behaviors, and adequate intake of calcium and vitamin D. Screening can be done at each office visit to detect any decrease in height, which would suggest osteoporotic changes. DEXA (dual energy x-ray absorptiometry) measures bone density at the spine and hip and is currently the gold standard in screening for osteopenia and osteoporosis. Lab measurements include Vitamin D level and alkaline phosphatase.

Thyroid disorders do not generally have modifiable risk factors but may be related to other autoimmune disorders such as type 1 diabetes. The nurse can educate the client on the risk and encourage the client to be screened routinely for thyroid disease. Physical assessment may detect an enlarged thyroid, and lab testing may detect abnormal thyroid hormone levels.

▶ ASSESSMENT

Endocrine gland functions are assessed with findings from diagnostic tests, a health assessment interview to collect subjective data, and a physical assessment to collect objective data. Because hormones affect all body tissues and organs, manifestations of dysfunction often are nonspecific, sometimes making assessment of endocrine function more difficult than assessment of other body systems.

Nursing Assessment

When conducting a health assessment interview and a physical assessment, it is important for the nurse to consider genetic influences on the health of the adult. During the health assessment interview, ask if any immediate family members have or have had endocrine disorders and, if so, the family member's age of onset and gender. Also ask the client about a family history of such diseases as diabetes mellitus, diabetes insipidus, thyroid disease, growth problems, hypertension, and obesity.

A health assessment interview to determine problems with the endocrine system may be part of a health screening or a total health assessment, or the interview may focus on a chief complaint (e.g., increased urination or changes in energy levels). If the client has a problem with endocrine function, the nurse analyzes its onset, characteristics and course, severity, precipitating and relieving factors, and any associated symptoms, noting the timing and circumstances.

The health history includes information about the client's medical history, family history, and social and personal history. Ask the client about any changes in normal growth and development and in height and weight. The nurse can often detect changes in the size of extremities by asking whether the client has had to have rings enlarged or to buy increasingly larger gloves and shoes. Also identify enlargement of the neck by asking whether the client has difficulty finding shirts or blouses with a collar that fits. Nurses also should explore such changes as difficulty swallowing; increased or decreased thirst, appetite, and/or urination; visual changes; sleep disturbances; altered patterns of hair distribution (e.g., increased facial hair in women); changes in menstruation; changes in memory or ability to concentrate; and changes in hair and skin texture. Ask the client about any blow to the head or previous hospitalizations, chemotherapy, radiation (especially to the neck), and use of medications (especially hormones or steroids).

Ask about the client's occupational and social history as well. Include questions about satisfaction with occupation, personal relationships, and lifestyle. Other areas of assessment include the client's usual means of coping; use of alcohol, smoking, or drugs; diet (including weight gain or loss); exercise patterns; and sleep patterns. Although the client may not recognize changes in behavior, family members may be able to provide important information.

The Assessment Interview feature outlines questions to ask for an endocrine assessment.

During the physical assessment, assess for any manifestations that might indicate a genetic disorder. If findings indicate genetic risk factors or alterations, ask whether the client is willing to undergo genetic testing and, if so, refer for appropriate genetic counseling and evaluation.

Physical assessment of the endocrine system may be performed as part of a total health assessment, or it may be a focused assessment of clients who have known or suspected problems with endocrine function. The only endocrine organ that can be palpated is the thyroid gland; however, other assessments that provide information about endocrine problems include inspection of the skin, hair, nails, facial appearance, reflexes, and musculoskeletal system. Measuring and monitoring trends in height and weight and in vital signs also provide clues to altered function of the endocrine system.

The Endocrine Assessments feature describes the physical assessment, normal and abnormal findings, and lifespan and developmental considerations.

Diagnostic Tests

The results of diagnostic tests support the diagnosis of a specific disease, provide information to identify or modify the appropriate medication or therapy used to treat the disease, and help nurses monitor the client's responses to treatment and nursing care interventions. Specific diagnostic tests to assess the structure and function of the glands of the endocrine system include:

- Hemoglobin A_{1C}
- T_3, T_4, TSH
- Individual hormone levels—parathyroid, catecholamines, estrogen, progesterone, growth hormone, and so on
- Serum electrolytes
- Liver enzymes (AST, ALT, SGOT, LDH)
- Bilirubin
- Serum albumin
- Serum calcium

CASE STUDY \\ PART 2

Ms. Bell's T score is found to be −3.2 in the spine and −3 in the hip. She continues to have pain. Ms. Bell has been started on a bisphosphonate. Her COPD is also exacerbated, and she is started back on steroids. When she comes back to the clinic for a follow up, she is coughing deeply.

Clinical Reasoning Questions Level I

1. What interview questions would be a priority to ask at today's visit?
2. What teaching can be done today to help Ms. Bell understand her diagnosis?

Clinical Reasoning Questions Level II

3. What added risks (related to fracture) are present with Ms. Bell's COPD exacerbation?
4. What type of medications can aggravate Ms. Bell's GERD and why?

Assessment Interview   Endocrine System

General

- Have you had any problems with an endocrine gland (pituitary, thyroid, parathyroid, adrenal, pancreas, ovaries, testes)?
- If you had a problem with any of these glands, how was it treated (medications, surgery, diet, hormone replacement)?
- Does anyone in your family have an endocrine disorder? If so, which family member is affected? At what age did the disorder begin? How does it affect that individual?
- Do you smoke, drink alcohol, or use recreational drugs? If so, how much, what kind, and how often?
- Have you ever been tested for high or low blood sugar?

Nutrition and Metabolism

- Describe what you eat as well as how much (and what type of) fluid you drink in a 24 hour period.
- Do you take any nutritional supplements, herbs, or vitamins?
- Have you noticed any change in your hunger or thirst?
- Has your weight changed? If so, by how many pounds (gain or loss) and over what time period?
- Have you noticed any change in your energy level? If so, explain.
- Have you noticed any change in your ability to tolerate heat or cold?
- Have you noticed any difficulty swallowing? If so, explain.
- Have you noticed any change in the texture of your skin? If so, what were they?
- Have you noticed any change in the color, odor, amount, or frequency of your urination? If so, describe it.
- Describe your physical activities in a usual day.
- Do some activities make you very tired? Explain how you feel.

- How many hours of sleep do you get each night?
- Do you feel nervous and unable to rest?
- Do you sweat at night?
- Have you noticed any change in the color or condition of your skin and hair (color, dryness, oiliness, bruises)?

Cognition and Sensory Perception

- Have you noticed any problem with your memory?
- Do you feel restless, anxious, or confused?
- Have you noticed any change in your voice?
- Have you had any headaches, memory loss, changes in sensation, or depression? If so, describe them.
- Have you noticed any change in your vision? If so, describe it.
- Have you had any heart palpitations?
- Have you had any abdominal pain? If so, what is it like, and where is it located?
- Have you had any pain or stiffness in your muscles and joints?

Stress and Coping

- How does this condition make you feel about yourself?
- How do you feel about taking medications?
- How does this condition affect your relationships with others? Your work?
- Does stress seem to make your condition worse? Explain.
- Describe what you do when you feel stressed.
- Describe any social or community pressures or activities that affect how you care for and feel about this condition.
- Are there any specific treatments that you would not use to treat this condition?

▶ INTERVENTIONS AND THERAPIES

Clients with the disorders discussed in this module—diabetes, liver disease, obesity, osteoporosis, and thyroid disease—require multidisciplinary care for multiple problems. They often face exhausting diagnostic tests, changes in physical appearance and emotional responses, and permanent alterations in lifestyle. Nursing care is directed toward meeting the client's physiological needs, providing education, and ensuring psychological support for the client and family. A holistic approach to the complex needs of clients with metabolic disorders is an essential component of nursing care.

Independent

Following assessment of an individual for metabolic disorders, the nurse can educate the client regarding the diagnostic testing, disease state, and therapies. The nurse can also help the client develop a lifestyle that will limit complications from the disorder. The nurse can aid the client in finding community resources for client support in the quest for health.

When a client is diagnosed with diabetes, the nurse can serve as educator, coach, and advocate to help the client attain optimum health and prevent complications. Education about controlling carbohydrate intake, reducing fat intake, and ensuring adequate protein intake as well as increased exercise will help the client to achieve optimal glycemic control. The nurse may also teach the client about home glucose monitoring and glucose targets that will keep A_{1C} at goal. Controlling complications from diabetes, both acute and chronic, is essential to client well-being, and teaching about complications can be done by the nurse at diagnosis and over time as the disorder progresses. Client education regarding medications is an important adjunct to medical management. The client who is new to insulin needs ongoing support from the nursing team. The nurse may also be an integral part of routine screenings for the public, which may be done by various organizations such as hospital wellness programs, colleges and schools.

In caring for the client with osteoporosis, the nurse can work closely with the family and the client to ensure a safe environment for the client to protect from falls and injury. Nutrition education and informing the client of community resources are an important part of the nursing process.

Endocrine Assessments

ASSESSMENT/METHOD	NORMAL FINDINGS	ABNORMAL FINDINGS	LIFESPAN OR DEVELOPMENTAL CONSIDERATIONS
Skin Assessment			
Inspect the skin color.	Skin color should be even and appropriate to the age and race of the client.	■ Hyperpigmentation may be seen in clients with Addison disease or Cushing syndrome. ■ Hypopigmentation may be seen in clients with diabetes mellitus, hyperthyroidism, or hypothyroidism. ■ A yellowish cast to the skin might indicate hypothyroidism. ■ Purple striae over the abdomen and bruising may be present in clients with Cushing syndrome.	■ Older clients' skin becomes pale due to decreased melanin production and decreased dermal vascularity. ■ In general, children's skin is smoother than the adults' skin because of lack of exposure to the elements and lack of coarse hair.
Palpate the skin, assessing texture, moisture, and the presence of lesions.	Skin should be appropriate to the client's race, smooth, warm, dry, and intact, without abnormal lesions.	■ Rough, dry skin often is seen in clients with hypothyroidism, whereas smooth and flushed skin can be a sign of hyperthyroidism. ■ Lesions (e.g., ulcerations) on the lower extremities might indicate diabetes mellitus.	■ Older clients' skin is drier because of decreased production of sebum. Older clients perspire less because of decreased activity of sweat glands. Older clients may also have a variety of lesions because of aging of the skin, such as senile keratosis and senile lentigines (age or liver spots). ■ In early childhood, sebaceous glands are minimally active, and although exocrine glands function, they produce little sweat.
Nails and Hair Assessment			
Assess texture, distribution, and condition of the nails and hair.	Hair should be of normal texture and appropriately distributed for gender and age; nail surfaces should be smooth, with even color.	■ Increased pigmentation of the nails often is seen in clients with Addison disease. ■ Dry, thick, brittle nails and hair may be apparent in clients with hypothyroidism; thin, brittle nails and thin, soft hair may be apparent in clients with hyperthyroidism. ■ Hirsutism (excessive facial, chest, or abdominal hair) may be seen in women with Cushing syndrome.	■ Older clients' nails may appear thickened and yellow because of decreased circulation to the extremities. Hair feels coarser and drier in the older adult. Dark-skinned clients may have thicker nails. Individuals of Black African descent tend to have very dry scalps and dry, fragile hair. During toddlerhood, hair grows thicker and usually loses curliness. Fine hair becomes visible in distal portions of the upper and lower extremities. Nails are usually pink, convex, and smooth throughout childhood and adolescence.

Endocrine Assessments (*continued*)

ASSESSMENT/METHOD	NORMAL FINDINGS	ABNORMAL FINDINGS	LIFESPAN OR DEVELOPMENTAL CONSIDERATIONS
Facial Assessments			
Inspect the symmetry and form of the face.	The face should be bilaterally symmetrical.	■ Variations of form and structure may indicate growth abnormalities, such as **acromegaly** (continued growth of bone from growth hormone hypersecretion).	■ Older clients may have shrinkage of the lower face and folding in of the mouth because of mandibular resorption of bone due to aging. ■ During toddlerhood, the nasal bridge is low and the mandible and maxilla are small, making the face seem small compared with the skull. In school-age children, the skull seems to grow disproportionately faster than the rest of the cranium.
Inspect position of eyes.	Eyes should be equal in position on both sides of the face. Eyelids should close over the eyes.	■ **Exophthalmos** (protruding eyes) may be seen in clients with hyperthyroidism.	■ Asians and some other groups may have a common variation of epicanthic folds or narrowed palpebral fissures, giving an impression that the upper border of the iris is covered. The palpebral fissures of Asians typically have an upward slant. The eyes of Blacks protrude more than those of Caucasians, and Blacks of both sexes may have eyes protruding beyond the 21 mm standard.
Thyroid Gland Assessment			
Palpate the thyroid gland for size and consistency. Stand behind the client, and place your fingers on either side of the trachea below the thyroid cartilage (**Figure 12–2 ●**). Ask the client to tilt the head to the right. Now ask the client to swallow. As the client swallows, displace the left lobe while palpating the right lobe. Repeat to palpate the left lobe.	The thyroid gland is not usually palpable. If it is, the lobes should feel smooth, rubbery, and free of nodules.	■ The thyroid may be enlarged in clients with Graves disease or a **goiter** (enlarged thyroid gland). ■ Multiple nodules may be seen in clients with metabolic disorders, whereas the presence of only one nodule may indicate a cyst or a benign or malignant tumor. ■ One enlarged nodule suggests malignancy.	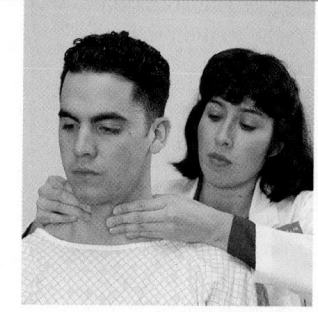 Figure 12–2 ● Palpating the thyroid gland from behind the client. ■ The older client's thyroid may feel more nodular and irregular because of fibrotic changes that occur with aging. It may be palpated lower in the neck because of age-related changes. In children, the isthmus is the only portion of the thyroid that should be palpated. "Shotty" nodes (small, nontender, mobile) are commonly palpated in children between ages 3 and 12.

(*continued on next page*)

Endocrine Assessments (continued)

ASSESSMENT/METHOD	NORMAL FINDINGS	ABNORMAL FINDINGS	LIFESPAN OR DEVELOPMENTAL CONSIDERATIONS
Motor Function Assessment			
Assess the deep tendon reflexes (DTRs). Deep tendon reflexes are assessed with the reflex hammer and include the biceps reflex, brachioradialis reflex, triceps reflex, patellar reflex, and Achilles reflex.	Normal values range from 1+ (present but decreased) to 2+ (normal) to 3+ (increased).	■ Increased reflexes may be seen in clients with hyperthyroidism; decreased reflexes may be seen in those with hypothyroidism.	■ Some older clients may have decreased DTRs because of a decrease in the number of nerve axons and increased demyelination of the nerve axons. There is also a decrease in transmission of impulses along with a delay in reaction time. ■ In children, the nervous system grows rapidly during the postnatal period, reaching 25% of adult capacity at birth, 50% by age 1, 80% by age 3, and 90% by age 7. Development takes place in an orderly fashion, but each child develops at his or her own pace.
Sensory Function Assessment			
Test the client's sensitivity to pain, temperature, vibration, light touch, and stereognosis (the ability to identify an object merely by touch). Ask the client to close his or her eyes. Then, compare symmetrical areas on both sides of the body, and compare the distal to the proximal regions of the extremities: ■ To test pain, use the blunt and sharp ends of a new safety pin. Discard the pin after use. ■ To test temperature, use cups or other containers of cold and hot (not scalding) water. ■ To test vibration, use a tuning fork over one of the client's finger or toe joints. ■ To test light touch, use a cotton wisp. ■ To test stereognosis, place in the client's hand a simple, familiar object, such as a rubber band, cotton ball, or button. Ask the client to identify the object.	Sensory function should be bilaterally intact.	■ Peripheral neuropathy and paresthesias (altered sensations) may occur in clients with diabetes, hypothyroidism, or acromegaly.	■ In some older clients, light touch and pain sensations may be decreased. ■ In children, touch is well developed at birth. Sensitivity to touch and discriminations should be present. The thresholds of touch, pain, and temperature are higher in older children than in infants.

Endocrine Assessments (continued)

ASSESSMENT/METHOD	NORMAL FINDINGS	ABNORMAL FINDINGS	LIFESPAN OR DEVELOPMENTAL CONSIDERATIONS
Musculoskeletal Assessment			
Inspect the size and proportions of the client's body structure.	Size and proportion of the body structure should be bilaterally equal.	■ Extremely short stature may indicate **dwarfism**, which is caused by insufficient growth hormone. ■ Extremely large bones may indicate acromegaly, which is caused by excessive growth hormone.	■ An exaggerated thoracic curve (kyphosis) is common with aging. ■ Growth charts are used to detect deviation from the norm in children and are used from birth to prepubescent adolescence.
Assessing for Hypocalcemic Tetany			
Assess for **Trousseau sign** (spasmodic muscle contractions induced by pressure on the nerves going to those muscles; a test for hypocalcemia) with resulting **tetany** (tonic muscle spasms) by inflating a blood pressure cuff above the antecubital space to a point greater than systolic blood pressure for 2–5 minutes.	A normal finding is no carpal spasm in response to compression of the arm by the blood pressure cuff.	■ Decreased calcium levels cause the client's hand and fingers to contract (**carpal spasm**).	■ Older adults may experience tremors with movement including hands and head, which are not associated with disease. ■ DTRs and superficial reflexes are the same for children and adults although the triceps reflex is absent until age 6.
Assess for **Chvostek sign** (facial grimacing caused by repeated contractions of the facial muscle; a test for hypocalcemia) by tapping your finger in front of the client's ear at the angle of the jaw.	A normal finding is no facial grimacing in response to tapping the client's face in front of the ear.	■ Decreased calcium levels cause the client's lateral facial muscles to contract.	

The client with cirrhosis induced by alcohol abuse will need to know where in the community to go for help with the disorder.

Collaborative

Diagnostic testing can be confusing for clients. When diabetes is diagnosed, tests other than glucose may be done, and the client may not understand why all the extra testing is important. The physician will most likely order more blood tests, such as a full lipid profile, electrolytes and kidney function tests, thyroid and liver function tests, an ECG, and an evaluation of eyes and feet. The client may even be sent to a podiatrist if there is a change in foot architecture or severe neuropathy.

The client who is obese may also need more testing to rule out any comorbidities.

The client with osteoporosis may need lab testing beyond the diagnostic DEXA to monitor therapy and to check Vitamin D levels. Many clients do not realize that ongoing monitoring is required for metabolic disorders.

Medication therapy for clients with diabetes range from oral medications to insulin injections. It is important that the client

be aware that treatment is ongoing and should not stop when levels return to normal. This is also true for those with osteoporosis who feel that one treatment is all they need. The client should be made aware that oral medication and monthly or yearly medications may require regularly scheduled appointments and are important to prevent interruption in therapy. When thyroid replacement therapy is started, it is for life, and the client's physician will monitor hormone levels and adjust medication as needed. The nurse can be part of this team by ensuring that the client knows how important it is to take the medicine regularly and separate it from other medications and food to optimize absorption.

Collaboration with a certified exercise physiologist and certified dietitian may be part of the collaborative team approach to care. A behavioral therapist may be helpful for clients who cannot make changes on their own. The alcoholic who wants to stop drinking to prevent or slow down cirrhosis will benefit from intervention by a specialist in behavioral therapy who works closely with these types of clients. The client who may overeat for psychological reasons may also seek help from a behavioral therapist.

Medications Metabolic and Endocrine Disorders

CLASSIFICATION AND DRUG EXAMPLES	MECHANISM OF ACTION	NURSING CONSIDERATIONS
Insulin *Drug examples:* Short-acting [Humalog(R)] Intermediate-acting (NPH) Long-acting (insulin detemir) forms	Replacement therapy; insulin is an endogenous hormone secreted by the beta cells of the pancreas. It lowers the blood glucose level by stimulating passage of glucose across cell membranes and uptake into the cells. It also promotes the conversion of glucose to glycogen and inhibits the production of hepatic glucose from glycogen.	■ Monitor for and discard vials past the expiration date. ■ Refrigerate, but do not freeze, extra insulin vials not currently in use. ■ Store insulin in a cool place, and avoid exposure to temperature extremes or sunlight. ■ Store compatible mixtures of insulin for no longer than 1 month at room temperature or 3 months at 2–8°C (36–46°F). ■ Discard any vials with discoloration, clumping, granules, or solid deposits on the sides. ■ Insulin pens not in use can be kept in the refrigerator but, while in use, can be kept out of the refrigerator. They should not be exposed to extreme temperatures and should be discarded 30 days after opening (always check package insert for discarding mixed insulin pens).
Antithyroid Agents *Drug examples:* potassium iodide (Thyro-Block) methimazole (Tapazole) propylthiouracil radioactive iodide (I-131, Iodotope)	Inhibit thyroid hormone (TH) synthesis and release.	■ Assess for hypersensitivity to iodine before giving medication (e.g., ask client about allergies to shellfish). ■ Dilute liquid iodine sources in water or orange juice to disguise bitter taste. ■ Monitor for increased bleeding tendencies if the client is also taking anticoagulants (iodine increases their effect). ■ Administer drugs at the same time each day with meals to maintain stable blood levels.
Thyroid Agents *Drug examples:* levothyroxine sodium (T$_4$; Levoxyl, Levothroid, Synthroid) liothyronine sodium (T$_3$; Cytomel) liotrix (T$_3$–T$_4$; Thyrolar)	Increase blood levels of TH, raising the metabolic rate.	■ For best absorption give 1 hour before meals or 2 hours after meals. ■ Thyroid preparations potentiate the effect of anticoagulant drugs. ■ Thyroid medications potentiate the effect of digitalis. ■ The effect of insulin may change as thyroid function increases. ■ During dose adjustment, take the client's pulse before administering the drug. Report a pulse > 100 bpm.
Hormonal Agents *Drug examples:* calcitonin: calcitonin—human (Cibacalcin) calcitonin—salmon (Calciman, Miacalcin) SERMs: raloxifene hydrochloride (Evista) Synthetic parathyroid hormones: teriparatide (Forteo)	Selective estrogen-receptor modulators (SERMs) appear to prevent bone loss by mimicking estrogen's beneficial effects on bone density in postmenopausal women. Synthetic parathyroid hormone, administered subcutaneously, stimulates new bone formation and mass.	■ Parenteral and nasal spray forms may cause an anaphylactic-type allergic response. ■ Alternate nostrils daily when administering calcitonin nasal spray. ■ Observe for side effects. ■ Teach the client the proper technique for handling and injecting the drug at home. ■ Hot flashes are a common side effect.
Bisphosphonates *Drug examples:* alendronate sodium (Fosamax) etidronate disodium (Didronel) ibandronate (Boniva) pamidronate disodium (Aredia) risedronate sodium (Actonel) tiludronate disodium (Skelid)	Bisphosphonates are potent inhibitors of bone resorption that may be used to prevent and treat osteoporosis. They inhibit bone breakdown, preserve bone mass, and increase bone density in the hip and vertebrae.	■ Should not be taken by a woman with a history of blood clots. ■ Take on an empty stomach, first thing in the morning, with water. ■ Remain upright for 30 minutes, and do not eat or drink anything else for 30 minutes to avoid esophagitis. ■ Monitor for pathological fractures and bone pain. ■ Monitor for GI side effects. ■ Monitor calcium lab values. ■ Monitor kidney function, especially creatinine level. ■ Monitor BUN, vitamin D, urinalysis, and serum phosphate and magnesium levels. ■ Monitor dietary habits for adequate intake of vitamin D, calcium, and phosphate.

PHARMACOLOGIC THERAPY The goals of hormone pharmacotherapy vary widely. In many cases, a hormone is administered as replacement therapy for clients who are unable to secrete sufficient quantities of their own endogenous hormones. However, it is important to note that hormone replacement is not the only pharmacologic intervention in endocrine disorders. Medications may also be modulators and inhibitors of endocrine activity when there is an interruption or increase in hormone activity.

An example of replacement therapy is administering thyroid hormone after the thyroid gland has been surgically removed. Replacement therapy supplies the same low-level amounts of the hormone that would normally be present in the body. Conversely, in overactive thyroid disease, antithyroid agents may have to be used to inhibit thyroid hormone synthesis and release. In type 1 diabetes, the hormone insulin is a necessary lifetime replacement, but in type 2 diabetes, it may not be started until later in the progression of the disease. Oral medications that improve insulin sensitivity, those that make the pancreas produce insulin, and those that block incretin degradation or replace the incretin hormone may be used. In osteoporosis, selective serum receptor modulators appear to prevent bone loss by imitating estrogen's effect on bone density. The inhibitory action of bisphosphonates slow bone resorption and preserve bone mass.

REVIEW **The Concept of Metabolism**

RELATE Link the Concepts

Linking the concept of metabolism with the concept of fluids and electrolytes:

1. In type 1 diabetes, the underlying problem of hyperglycemia leads to acidosis. Explain why the client with severe hyperglycemia needs fluid replacement as well as insulin.

2. What age group is at greatest risk for hyperosmolar hyperglycemic nonketotic syndrome (HHNS), and why?

Linking the concept of metabolism with the concept of safety:

3. How can the nurse help the client with osteoporosis prevent falls at home?

4. List some of the mobilization aids that may be used by the client with osteoporosis.

Linking the concept of metabolism with the concept of stress and coping:

5. A client who has had a lifelong battle with obesity feels that everyone is looking at her when she goes to the gym, so she often skips her exercise sessions. What suggestions could you make to help her include exercise in her lifestyle?

6. A client with obesity has given up trying to lose weight because she says that her whole family is large and there is always food around her. What advice can you give her regarding weight loss strategies at home?

READY Go to Companion Skills Manual

REFER Go to Pearson Student Nursing Resources
nursing.pearsonhighered.com

- Additional review material

REFLECT Case Study \\ Part 3

Ms. Bell falls while out grocery shopping and is brought to the emergency room with a fracture of L3 and L4. She is admitted to the medical surgical floor for several days for conservative treatment focusing on alleviating her pain and preventing further injury.

Clinical Reasoning Questions Level I

1. What is the anticipated mortality outcome for a spine fracture versus a hip fracture?

2. In the hospital, what other team members may be called in to help with Ms. Bell's care?

Clinical Reasoning Questions Level II

3. Develop a discharge plan for Ms. Bell that includes safety and medication education.

4. While in the hospital, Ms. Bell is treated with heparin. Comment on the use of long-term heparin therapy for Ms. Bell.

EXEMPLAR 12.1 **Diabetes**

EXEMPLAR KEY TERMS
Dawn phenomenon, *746*
Diabetes mellitus, *740*
Diabetic ketoacidosis (DKA), *746*
Diabetic nephropathy, *749*
Diabetic neuropathies, *749*
Diabetic retinopathy, *749*
Endogenous insulin, *742*
Exogenous insulin, *742*
Glucagon, *740*
Gluconeogenesis, *740*
Glucosuria, *742*
Glycogenolysis, *740*
Hyperglycemia, *741*
Hyperosmolar hyperglycemic state (HHS), *747*
Hypoglycemia, *747*

Insulin, *740*
Insulin reaction, *747*
Ketosis, *741*
Microalbuminuria, *749*
Polydipsia, *742*
Polyphagia, *742*
Polyuria, *742*
Somatostatin, *740*
Somogyi phenomenon, *746*

EXEMPLAR LEARNING OUTCOMES
After reading about this exemplar, you will be able to:

1. Describe the pathophysiology, etiology, clinical manifestations, and direct and indirect causes of diabetes mellitus.

2. Identify risk factors and prevention methods associated with diabetes mellitus.

3. Illustrate the nursing process in providing culturally competent care across the life span for individuals with diabetes mellitus.

4. Formulate priority nursing diagnoses appropriate for an individual with diabetes mellitus.

5. Summarize therapies used by interdisciplinary teams in the collaborative care of an individual with diabetes mellitus.

6. Plan evidence-based care for an individual with diabetes mellitus and his or her family in collaboration with other members of the healthcare team.

7. Evaluate expected outcomes for an individual with diabetes mellitus.

▶ OVERVIEW

Diabetes mellitus (often referred to more simply as *diabetes*) is a disorder of hyperglycemia resulting from defects in insulin secretion, insulin action, or both, leading to abnormalities in carbohydrate, protein, and fat metabolism (American Diabetes Association, 2013). There are four major types of diabetes: type 1 diabetes mellitus (type 1 DM; 5%–10% of diagnosed cases), type 2 diabetes mellitus (type 2 DM; 90%–95% of diagnosed cases), gestational diabetes (2%–5% of all pregnancies), and other specific types of diabetes (1%–2% of diagnosed cases).

Role of Hormones

The endocrine part of the pancreas produces hormones necessary for the metabolism and cellular utilization of carbohydrates, proteins, and fats. The cells that produce these hormones are clustered in groups of cells called the islets of Langerhans. These islets have three different types of cells:

1. Alpha cells produce the hormone **glucagon**, which stimulates the breakdown of glycogen in the liver, the formation of carbohydrates in the liver, and the breakdown of lipids in both the liver and the adipose tissue. The primary function of glucagon is to decrease glucose oxidation and to increase blood glucose levels. Through **glycogenolysis** (the breakdown of liver glycogen) and **gluconeogenesis** (the formation of glucose from fats and proteins), glucagon prevents blood glucose from decreasing below a certain level when the body is fasting or between meals. The action of glucagon is initiated in most individuals when blood glucose falls below approximately 70 mg/dL.

2. Beta cells secrete the hormone **insulin**, which facilitates the movement of glucose across cell membranes into cells, thus decreasing blood glucose levels. Insulin prevents the excessive breakdown of glycogen in the liver and in muscle, facilitates the formation of lipid while inhibiting the breakdown of stored fats, and helps to move amino acids into cells for protein synthesis. After secretion by the beta cells, insulin enters the portal circulation, travels directly to the liver, and is then released into the general circulation. Circulating insulin is rapidly bound to receptor sites on peripheral tissues (especially muscle and fat cells) or is destroyed by the liver or kidneys. Insulin release is regulated by blood glucose: It increases when blood glucose levels increase, and it decreases when blood glucose levels decrease. When an individual eats food, insulin levels begin to rise in minutes, peak in 30–60 minutes, and return to baseline in 2–3 hours.

3. Delta cells produce **somatostatin**, which is believed to be a neurotransmitter that inhibits the production of both glucagon and insulin.

Blood Glucose Homeostasis

All body tissues and organs require a constant supply of glucose; however, not all tissues require insulin for glucose uptake. The brain, liver, intestines, and renal tubules do not require insulin to transfer glucose into their cells. Skeletal muscle, cardiac muscle, and adipose tissue require insulin for glucose movement into the cells.

Normal blood glucose is maintained in healthy individuals primarily through the actions of insulin and glucagon. Increased blood glucose levels, amino acids, and fatty acids stimulate pancreatic beta cells to produce insulin. As the cells of cardiac muscle, skeletal muscle, and adipose tissue take up glucose, the resulting decrease in plasma levels of nutrients suppresses the stimulus to produce insulin. If blood glucose falls, glucagon is released to raise hepatic glucose output, which raises glucose levels. Epinephrine, growth hormone, T_4, and glucocorticoids (often referred to as *glucose counterregulatory hormones*) also stimulate an increase in glucose in times of hypoglycemia, stress, growth, or other increased metabolic demand. The regulation of blood glucose levels by insulin and glucagon is illustrated in **Figure 12–3 ●**.

▌ TYPE 1 DIABETES MELLITUS

Type 1 DM, formerly called *juvenile-onset diabetes* or *insulin-dependent diabetes mellitus*, is the result of pancreatic islet cell destruction and a total deficit of circulating insulin.

▶ PATHOPHYSIOLOGY AND ETIOLOGY

Type 1 DM results from destruction of the beta cells of the islets of Langerhans in the pancreas—the only cells in the body that make insulin. When beta cells are destroyed, insulin is no longer produced. Although type 1 DM may be classified as either an autoimmune or an idiopathic disorder, 90% of the cases are immune mediated. The disorder begins with insulinitis, a chronic inflammatory process that occurs in response to the autoimmune destruction of islet cells. This process, which slowly destroys beta cell production of insulin, usually occurs over a long preclinical period, with the onset of hyperglycemia occurring when 80%–90% of beta cell function is lost. It is believed that both alpha cell and beta cell functions are abnormal, with a lack of insulin and a relative excess of glucagon resulting in hyperglycemia.

Etiology

The onset of type 1 DM most often occurs in childhood and adolescence, but it may occur at any age, even in the 80s and

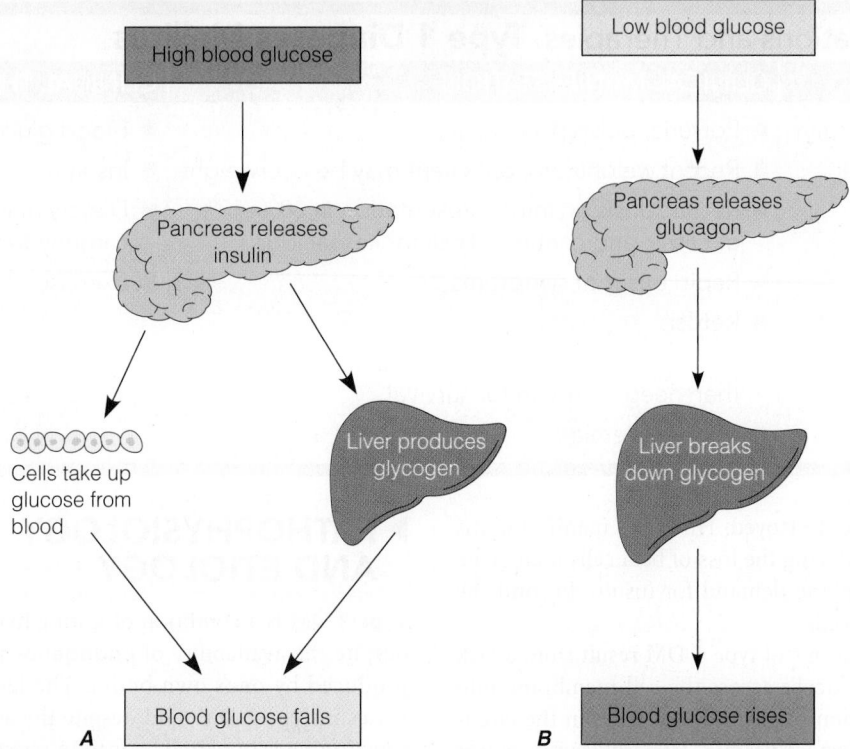

Figure 12–3 ● Regulation (homeostasis) of blood glucose levels by insulin and glucagon. *A,* High blood glucose is lowered by insulin release. *B,* Low blood glucose is raised by glucagon release.

90s. The actual cause and exact sequence are not completely understood.

Genetic predisposition plays a role in the development of type 1 DM (see the Focus on Diversity and Culture feature), and environmental factors are believed to trigger development of the disorder. The trigger can be a viral infection (e.g., mumps, rubella, or coxsackievirus B4) or a chemical toxin (e.g., those found in smoked and cured meats). As a result of exposure to the virus or chemical, an abnormal autoimmune response occurs in which antibodies respond to normal islet beta cells as though they were foreign substances—in other words, by destroying them.

Risk Factors

Although the risk in the general population ranges from 1 in 400 to 1 in 1,000, the child of an individual with diabetes has a

risk of 1 in 20 to 1 in 50. Genetic markers that determine immune responses have been found in 95% of individuals diagnosed with type 1 DM. The presence of these markers does not guarantee that the individual will develop type 1 DM, but it does indicate increased susceptibility. These individuals may also develop other autoimmune disorders such as Graves disease, Addison disease, autoimmune hepatitis, myasthenia gravis, pernicious anemia, celiac sprue, and vitiligo (ADA, 2013).

▶ CLINICAL MANIFESTATIONS

Type 1 DM is characterized by **hyperglycemia** (elevated blood glucose levels), a breakdown of body fats and proteins, and development of **ketosis** (an accumulation of ketone bodies produced during oxidation of fatty acids). As was mentioned earlier, the manifestations of type 1 DM appear when approximately

---

Focus on Diversity and Culture **Risk and Incidence of Diabetes**

- **Non-Hispanic Whites.** 15.7 million (10.8%) of those age 20 years or older have diabetes.

- **Non-Hispanic African Americans.** Of this group, 4.9 million (18.7%) have diabetes. This group is 1.8 times as likely to have diabetes as non-Hispanic Whites of similar age. In addition, African Americans with type 2 diabetes mellitus have higher rates of coronary heart disease, cerebrovascular accident, and end-stage renal disease than do Whites with the disease.

- **Hispanic/Latino Americans.** Of this group, 2.5 million (9.5%) have diabetes. This group is 1.7 times as likely to

have diabetes as non-Hispanic Whites of similar age, and Mexican Americans are twice as likely to have diabetes as non-Hispanic Whites of similar age.

- **American Indians and Alaska Natives.** This group is 2.2 times as likely to have diabetes as non-Hispanic Whites, and diabetes is especially prevalent in American Indians who are of middle age or older. Diabetes is most common among Native Americans of the southern United States (33.5%) and is least common among Alaska natives (5.5%) (Centers for Disease Control and Prevention, 2011b).

Clinical Manifestations and Therapies **Type 1 Diabetes Mellitus**

ETIOLOGY	CLINICAL MANIFESTATION	CLINICAL THERAPIES
Immune-mediated insulin deficiency caused by pancreatic beta-cell destruction	■ Polyuria, polydipsia ■ Recent weight loss, but client may be overweight ■ Ketoacidosis on initial presentation in 30%–40% of cases, and continued risk for ketoacidosis ■ Rapid onset of symptoms ■ Ketosis ■ Initial period of decreased insulin requirement, then need of insulin for survival ■ Hyperglycemia	■ Blood glucose monitoring ■ Insulin ■ Dietary management, balancing carbohydrate intake to insulin ■ Exercise

90% of the beta cells are destroyed. However, manifestations may appear at any time during the loss of beta cells if an acute illness or stress increases the demand for insulin beyond the reserves of the damaged cells.

The clinical manifestations of type 1 DM result from a lack of insulin to transport glucose across the cell membrane into the cells. The accumulation of glucose molecules in the circulating blood results in hyperglycemia. Hyperglycemia causes serum hyperosmolality, drawing water from the intracellular spaces into the general circulation. The increased blood volume increases renal blood flow, and the hyperglycemia acts as an osmotic diuretic. The resulting osmotic diuresis increases urine output (**polyuria**). When the blood glucose level exceeds the renal threshold for glucose—usually approximately 180 mg/dL—glucose is excreted in the urine (**glucosuria**). The decrease in intracellular volume and the increased urinary output cause dehydration. The mouth becomes dry, and the activation of thirst sensors causes the individual to drink increased amounts of fluid (**polydipsia**).

Because glucose cannot enter the cells without insulin, energy production decreases. This decrease in energy stimulates hunger, causing the individual to eat more food (**polyphagia**). Despite increased food intake, the individual loses weight as the body loses water and breaks down proteins and fats in an attempt to restore energy sources. Malaise and fatigue accompany the decrease in energy. Blurred vision also is common, resulting from osmotic effects that cause the lenses of the eyes to swell.

Thus the classic manifestations of type 1 DM are polyuria, polydipsia, and polyphagia, accompanied by weight loss, malaise, and fatigue. Depending on the degree of insulin deficiency, the manifestations vary from slight to severe. Individuals with type 1 DM require **exogenous insulin** (insulin from a source outside the body) to maintain life. See the Clinical Manifestations and Therapies feature for an overview.

TYPE 2 DIABETES MELLITUS

Type 2 DM was formerly labeled *non-insulin-dependent diabetes mellitus* or *adult-onset diabetes*; however, a disturbingly large number of children are being diagnosed with type 2 DM due to the increase in childhood obesity (Mayo Clinic, 2013b). Type 2 DM results from insulin resistance with a defect in compensatory insulin secretion.

▶ PATHOPHYSIOLOGY AND ETIOLOGY

Type 2 DM is a condition of fasting hyperglycemia that occurs despite the availability of **endogenous insulin** (insulin that is produced by one's own body). The level of insulin produced varies in type 2 DM, and despite the availability of insulin, its functioning is impaired by insulin resistance. Insulin resistance exceeds the ability of the pancreas to compensate, and over time the pancreas fails to produce enough insulin to meet body needs (ADA, 2013). Whatever the cause, there is sufficient production of insulin to prevent the breakdown of fats with resultant ketosis; thus type 2 DM is characterized as a nonketotic form of diabetes. However, the amount of insulin available is not sufficient to lower blood glucose levels through the uptake of glucose by muscle and fat cells.

Etiology

Type 2 DM can occur at any age, but it usually is seen in individuals who are of middle age and older. Heredity plays a role in its transmission (see the Focus on Diversity and Culture feature on page 741). In the United States, the incidence of type 2 DM has increased 33% since 2003.

A major factor in the development of type 2 DM is cellular resistance to the effect of insulin. This resistance is increased by obesity, inactivity, illnesses, medications, and increasing age. In obesity, insulin has a decreased ability to influence glucose metabolism and uptake by the liver, skeletal muscles, and adipose tissue. The exact reason is not clear, but weight loss and exercise may improve the mechanism responsible for insulin receptor binding or postreceptor activity (Porth & Matfin, 2009).

Risk Factors

The major risk factors for type 2 DM are as follows:

■ History of diabetes in parents or siblings. Although no HLA linkage has been identified, the children of an individual with type 2 DM have a 15% chance of developing type 2 DM and a 30% risk of developing a glucose intolerance (the inability to metabolize carbohydrate normally).

■ Obesity, defined as being at least 20% over the desired body weight or having a body mass index of at least 27 kg/m^2.

Clinical Manifestations and Therapies **Type 2 Diabetes Mellitus**

ETIOLOGY	CLINICAL MANIFESTATION	CLINICAL THERAPIES
Insulin resistance with relative insulin secretory defect	■ Obesity, little or no weight loss, or possible significant recent weight loss ■ Acanthosis nigricans ■ Slow onset of symptoms ■ Polyuria, polydipsia ■ Glycosuria without ketonuria on initial presentation in 33% of cases ■ Ketoacidosis on initial presentation in 5%–25% of cases ■ Lipid disorders ■ Hypertension ■ Androgen-mediated problems (e.g., acne, hirsutism, menstrual disturbances, polycystic ovary disease) ■ Excessive weight gain and fatigue caused by insulin resistance ■ Hyperglycemia	■ Diet with low-fat foods and decreased calories ■ Decreased sedentary activity time, or increased routine physical activity ■ Blood glucose monitoring ■ Oral medication (metformin) to improve insulin sensitivity

Obesity, especially of the upper body, decreases the number of available insulin receptor sites in cells of skeletal muscles and adipose tissues, a process called *peripheral insulin resistance*. In addition, obesity impairs the ability of the beta cells to release insulin in response to increasing glucose levels.

■ Physical inactivity.

■ Race/ethnicity.

■ In women, a history of gestational diabetes, polycystic ovary syndrome, or delivery of a baby weighing more than 9 lb.

■ Hypertension (≥130/85 mmHg in adults), high-density lipoprotein (HDL) cholesterol of ≥35 mg/dL, and/or a triglyceride level of ≥250 mg/dL.

■ Metabolic syndrome. The National Cholesterol Education Program's Adult Treatment Panel III (NCEP/ATP III) identified metabolic syndrome as a cluster of factors that increase an individual's risk for developing cardiovascular disease. Hypertension, abdominal obesity, dyslipidemia, elevated C-reactive protein, and a fasting blood glucose greater than 100 mg/dL increase the risk of type 2 DM, coronary heart disease, and stroke. Studies have shown that metabolic syndrome is prevalent and increases with age and BMI. Studies also note that the prevalence varies by race and ethnicity, but the pattern is different for males and females (Ervin, 2009).

▶ CLINICAL MANIFESTATIONS

The client with type 2 DM experiences a slow onset of manifestations and often is unaware of the disease until he or she seeks health care for some other problem. Hyperglycemia increases gradually and may exist for a long time before diabetes is diagnosed; as a result, approximately half of those with newly diagnosed type 2 DM already have complications (Mayo Clinic, 2013a).

The hyperglycemia in type 2 DM usually is not as severe as that in type 1, but similar symptoms occur, especially polyuria and polydipsia. Polyphagia is not often seen, and weight loss is uncommon. Other manifestations that result from hyperglycemia are blurred vision, fatigue, paresthesias, and skin infections. If available insulin decreases, especially during times of physical or emotional stress, the individual with type 2 DM may develop diabetic ketoacidosis, but this is uncommon.

Treatment usually begins with prescriptions for weight loss and increased activity. If these changes can be sustained, no further treatment is necessary for many individuals. Hypoglycemic medications are begun when lifestyle changes are insufficient. Often, a combination of insulin and hypoglycemic medication is used to achieve the best glycemic control in the client with type 2 DM. See the Clinical Manifestations and Therapies feature for an overview.

▶ COMPLICATIONS OF DIABETES

The individual with diabetes, regardless of type, is at increased risk for complications involving many body systems. Alterations in blood glucose levels, alterations in the cardiovascular system, neuropathies, increased susceptibility to infection, and periodontal disease are common. In addition, the interaction of several complications can cause problems in the feet. The Multisystem Effects feature shows the progression from cardinal signs to acute and late complications for the client with diabetes. A discussion of each of these complications follows; nursing care and related collaborative care are discussed later in the exemplar.

Acute Complications

The following discussion provides additional information about hyperglycemia and hypoglycemia. **Table 12–3** ● compares diabetic ketoacidosis, hyperosmolar hyperglycemic state, and hypoglycemia.

Multisystem Effects of Diabetes

Early Manifestations
- Type 1 DM
  - Polyuria
  - Polydipsia
  - Polyphagia
  - Weight loss
  - Glycosuria
  - Fatigue
- Type 2 DM
  - Polyuria
  - Polydipsia
  - Blurred vision

Progressive Complications
- Hyperglycemia
  - Diabetic ketoacidosis
  - Hyperglycemic hyperosmolar nonketotic coma
- Hypoglycemia

Late Complications
Neurologic
- Somatic neuropathies
  - Paresthesias
  - Pain
  - Loss of cutaneous sensation
  - Loss of fine motor control
- Visceral neuropathies
  - Sweating dysfunction
  - Pupillary constriction
  - Fixed heart rate
  - Constipation
  - Diarrhea
  - Incomplete bladder emptying
  - Sexual dysfunction

Sensory
- Diabetic retinopathy
- Cataracts
- Glaucoma

Cardiovascular
- Orthostatic hypotension
- Accelerated atherosclerosis
- Cerebrovascular disease (stroke)
- Coronary artery disease (MI)
- Peripheral vascular disease
- Blood viscosity and platelet disorders

Renal
- Hypertension
- Albuminuria
- Edema
- Chronic renal failure

Musculoskeletal
- Joint contractures

Integumentary
- Foot ulcers
- Gangrene of the feet
- Atrophic changes

Immune System
- Impaired healing
- Chronic skin infections
- Periodontal disease
- Urinary tract infections
- Lung infections
- Vaginitis

TABLE 12–3 Comparison of Diabetic Ketoacidosis (DKA), Hyperosmolar Hyperglycemic State (HHS), and Hypoglycemia

		DKA	HHS	HYPOGLYCEMIA
Diabetes type		Primary type 1	Type 2	Both
Onset		Slow	Slow	Rapid
Cause		↓ Insulin	↓ Insulin	↑ Insulin
		Infection	Older age	Omitted meal/snack
				Error in insulin dose
Risk factors		Surgery	Surgery	Surgery
		Trauma	Trauma	Trauma
		Illness	Illness	Illness
		Omitted insulin	Dehydration	Exercise
		Stress	Medications	Medications
			Dialysis	Lipodystrophy
			Hyperalimentation	Renal failure
				Alcohol intake
Assessments	Skin	Flushed, dry, warm	Flushed, dry, warm	Pallid, moist, cool
	Perspiration	None	None	Profuse
	Breath	Fruity	Normal	Normal
	Vital signs	↓ BP	↓ BP	↓ BP
		↑ P	↑ P	↑ P
		R Kussmaul	R normal	R normal
	Mental status	Confused	Lethargic	Anxious; restless
	Thirst	Increased	Increased	Normal
	Fluid intake	Increased	Increased	Normal
	Gastrointestinal effects	Nausea/vomiting	Nausea/vomiting	Hunger
		Abdominal pain	Abdominal pain	
	Fluid loss	Moderate	Profound	Normal
	Level of consciousness	Decreasing	Decreasing	Decreasing
	Energy level	Weak	Weak	Fatigue
	Other	Weight loss	Weight loss	Headache
		Blurred vision	Malaise	Altered vision
			Extreme thirst	Mood changes
			Seizures	Seizures
Laboratory findings	Blood glucose	>300 mg/dL	>600 mg/dL	<50 mg/dL
	Plasma ketones	Increased	Normal	Normal
	Urine glucose	Increased	Increased	Normal
	Urine ketones	Increased	Normal	Normal
	Serum potassium	Abnormal	Abnormal	Normal
	Serum sodium	Abnormal	Abnormal	Normal
	Serum chloride	Abnormal	Abnormal	Normal
	Plasma pH	<7.3	Normal	Normal
	Osmolality	>340 mOsm/L	>340 mOsm/L	Normal
Treatment		Insulin	Insulin	Glucagon
		Intravenous fluids	Intravenous fluids	Rapid-acting carbohydrate
		Electrolytes	Electrolytes	Intravenous solution of 50% glucose

Note: BP = blood pressure; P = pulse; R = respiration.

HYPERGLYCEMIA The major problems resulting from hyperglycemia in the individual with diabetes are diabetic ketoacidosis and hyperosmolar hyperglycemic state. Two other problems are the dawn phenomenon and the Somogyi phenomenon.

Dawn Phenomenon The **dawn phenomenon** is a rise in blood glucose between 4 a.m. and 8 a.m. that is not a response to hypoglycemia. This condition occurs in individuals with both type 1 and type 2 DM. The exact cause is unknown, but it is believed to relate to nocturnal increases in growth hormone, which decrease peripheral uptake of glucose.

Somogyi Phenomenon The **Somogyi phenomenon** is a combination of hypoglycemia during the night with a rebound morning rise in blood glucose to hyperglycemic levels. The hyperglycemia stimulates the counterregulatory hormones, which in turn stimulate gluconeogenesis and glycogenolysis and inhibit peripheral glucose use. This process may cause insulin resistance for 12–48 hours (Cooperman & Griffing, 2011).

Diabetic Ketoacidosis As the pathophysiology of untreated type 1 DM continues, the insulin deficit causes fat stores to break down; the result is continued hyperglycemia and mobilization of fatty acids with a subsequent ketosis. **Diabetic ketoacidosis (DKA)** develops when there is an absolute deficiency of insulin and an increase in the insulin counterregulatory hormones. Glucose production by the liver increases, peripheral glucose use decreases, fat mobilization increases, and ketogenesis (ketone formation) is stimulated. Increased glucagon levels activate the gluconeogenic and ketogenic pathways in the liver. In the presence of insulin deficiency, hepatic overproduction of beta-hydroxybutyrate and acetoacetic acids (ketone bodies) causes increased ketone concentrations and increased release of free fatty acids. Because of a loss of bicarbonate, which occurs when the ketone is formed, bicarbonate buffering does not occur, and a metabolic acidosis—namely, DKA—occurs. Depression of the central nervous system from the accumulation of ketones and the resulting acidosis may cause coma and death if left untreated (Porth & Matfin, 2009). For additional details, see **Figure 12–4** ●.

Diabetic ketoacidosis also may occur in an individual with diagnosed diabetes when energy requirements increase during physical or emotional stress. Stress states initiate the release of gluconeogenic hormones, resulting in the formation of

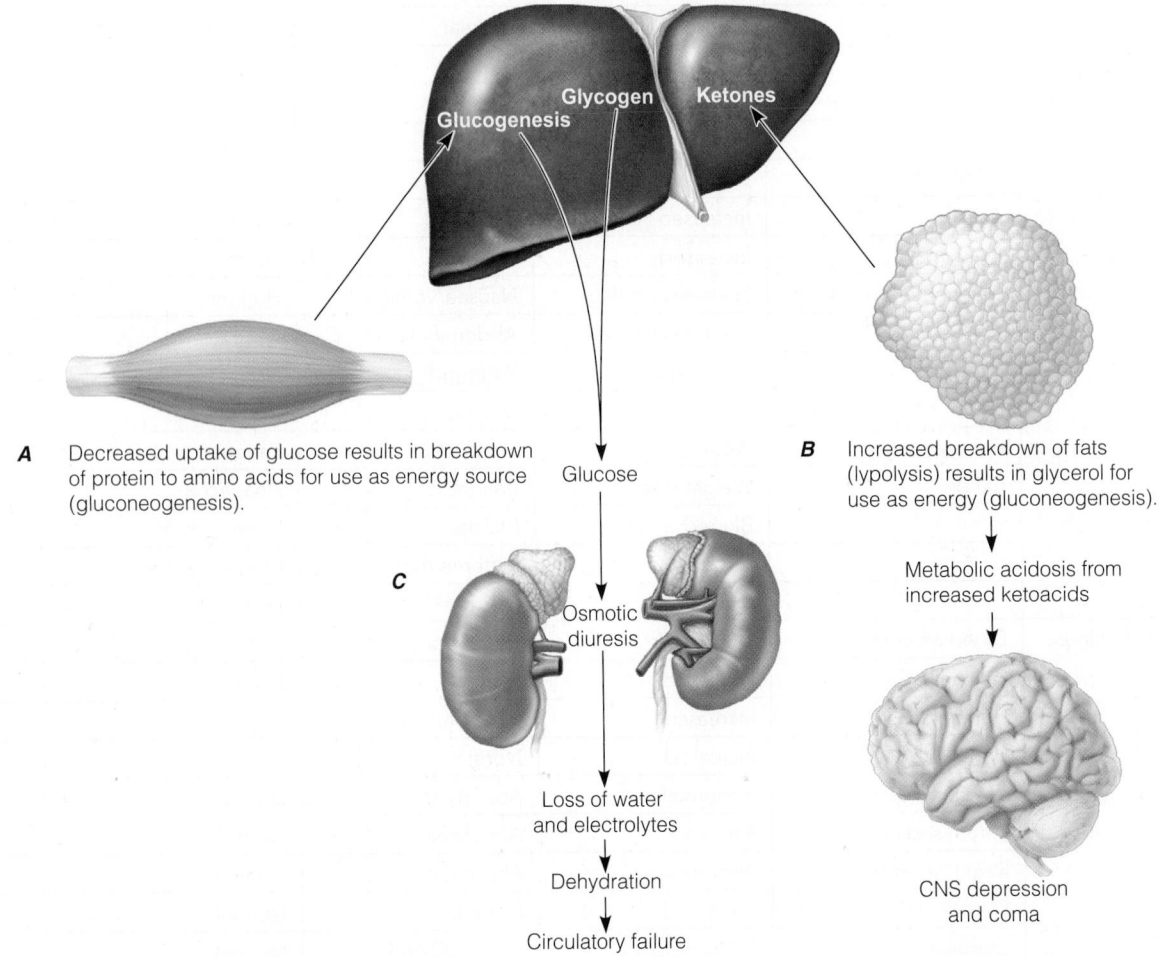

A Decreased uptake of glucose results in breakdown of protein to amino acids for use as energy source (gluconeogenesis).

Glucose

B Increased breakdown of fats (lypolysis) results in glycerol for use as energy (gluconeogenesis).

Glucogenesis Glycogen Ketones

C

Osmotic diuresis

Metabolic acidosis from increased ketoacids

Loss of water and electrolytes

Dehydration

Circulatory failure

CNS depression and coma

Figure 12–4 ● In type 1 diabetes mellitus, without adequate insulin, muscle (*A*), and fat (*B*), cells are metabolized to provide sources of energy. Amino acids from skeletal muscle are converted to glucose in the liver; glycerol from fat cells is converted to glucose and fatty acids (ketoacids), which cause central nervous system (CNS) depression and coma. Increased glucose (*C*) causes osmotic diuresis, leading to dehydration and decreased circulatory volume. These processes create the symptoms of diabetic ketoacidosis. The symptoms can be reversed with intravenous insulin to lower blood glucose. Administration of intravenous fluids raises blood volume to prevent circulatory failure; electrolytes are monitored and corrected.

carbohydrates from protein or fat. The individual who is sick, who has an infection, or who decreases or omits insulin doses is at a greatly increased risk for developing DKA.

Diabetic ketoacidosis involves four metabolic problems:

1. Hyperosmolarity from hyperglycemia and dehydration
2. Metabolic acidosis from an accumulation of ketoacids
3. Extracellular volume depletion from osmotic diuresis
4. Electrolyte imbalances (e.g., loss of potassium and sodium) from osmotic diuresis.

Manifestations of DKA result from severe dehydration and acidosis, and DKA requires immediate medical attention. Admission to the hospital is appropriate when the individual has a blood glucose level greater than 250 mg/dL, a decreasing pH, and ketones in the urine. If the client is alert and conscious, fluids may be replaced orally. In the first 12 hours of treatment, adults usually require 8–10 L of fluid to replace losses from polyuria and vomiting. However, alterations in level of consciousness, vomiting, and acidosis are common, necessitating intravenous fluid replacement. The initial fluid replacement may be accomplished by administering 0.9% saline solution at a rate of 500–1,000 mL/hr. After 2–3 hours (or when blood pressure is returning to normal), administration of 0.45% saline at 200–500 mL/hr may continue for several more hours. When the blood glucose level reaches 250 mg/dL, dextrose is added to prevent rapid decreases; hypoglycemia could result in fatal cerebral edema.

Regular insulin is used in the treatment of DKA and may be given by various routes, depending on the severity of the condition. Mild ketosis may be treated with subcutaneous insulin, whereas severe ketosis requires an intravenous infusion of insulin.

The electrolyte imbalance of primary concern in clients with DKA is depleted body stores of potassium. Initially, serum potassium levels may be normal, but they decrease during treatment. In DKA (and as a result of rehydration), the body loses potassium from increased urinary output, acidosis, catabolic state, and vomiting or diarrhea. Potassium replacement is begun early in the treatment, usually by adding potassium to the rehydration fluids. Replacement is essential for preventing cardiac dysrhythmias secondary to hypokalemia. Cardiac rhythms and potassium levels must be monitored every 2–4 hours.

Hyperosmolar Hyperglycemic State
The metabolic problem called **hyperosmolar hyperglycemic state (HHS)** occurs in individuals who have type 2 DM and is characterized by a plasma osmolarity of 340 mOsm/L or greater (the normal range is 280–300 mOsm/L), greatly elevated blood glucose levels (>600 mg/dL and often as high as 1,000–2,000 mg/dL), and altered levels of consciousness. HHS is a serious, life-threatening medical emergency. Mortality is high—even higher than for DKA—because the metabolic changes are serious and because individuals with diabetes usually are older and have other medical problems that either cause or are caused by HHS.

The precipitating factors associated with HHS include infection, therapeutic agents, therapeutic procedures, acute illness, and chronic illness. The most common precipitating factor is infection. The manifestations of this disorder may be slow to appear, with onset ranging from 24 hours to 2 weeks. The manifestations are initiated by hyperglycemia, which causes increased urine output, and with increased output, plasma volume decreases and glomerular filtration rate drops. As a result, glucose is retained, and water is lost. Glucose and sodium accumulate in the blood and increase serum osmolarity.

Serum hyperosmolarity results in severe dehydration, which reduces intracellular water in all tissues, including the brain. The individual with HHS has dry skin and mucous membranes, extreme thirst, and altered levels of consciousness (progressing from lethargy to coma). Neurological deficits may include hyperthermia, motor and sensory impairment, positive Babinski sign, and seizures. Metabolic acidosis is not part of the pathology; despite elevated blood glucose, sufficient insulin is present to prevent metabolism of fats with the resulting fatty acids and ketones of DKA.

The client admitted to the ICU for treatment of HHS typically manifests blood glucose levels greater than 600 mg/dL, increased serum osmolarity, and altered levels of consciousness or seizures. Treatment is similar to that of DKA: correcting fluid and electrolyte imbalances and providing insulin to lower hyperglycemia. In general, treatment modalities include the following:

- Establish and maintain adequate ventilation.
- Correct shock with adequate intravenous fluids.
- If the client is comatose, institute nasogastric suction to prevent aspiration.
- Maintain fluid volume with intravenous isotonic or colloid solutions, administering potassium intravenously to replace losses.
- Administer insulin to reduce blood glucose, usually until blood glucose levels reach 250 mg/dL (because ketosis is not present, there is no need to continue insulin, as with DKA).

HYPOGLYCEMIA   **Hypoglycemia** (low blood glucose levels) is common in individuals with type 1 DM, and it occasionally occurs in individuals with type 2 DM who are treated with oral hypoglycemic agents. This condition often is called *insulin shock*, **insulin reaction**, or *"the lows"* in clients with type 1 DM. Hypoglycemia results primarily from a mismatch between insulin intake (e.g., an error in insulin dose), physical activity, and carbohydrate availability (e.g., omitting a meal). The intake of alcohol and drugs, such as chloramphenicol (Chloromycetin), sodium warfarin (Coumadin), monoamine oxidase inhibitors, probenecid (Benemid), salicylates, and sulfonamides, also can cause hypoglycemia.

The manifestations of hypoglycemia result from a compensatory autonomic nervous system response and from impaired cerebral function caused by a decrease in the glucose available for use by the brain. The manifestations vary, particularly in older adults (see Table 12–3). The onset is sudden, and blood glucose usually is less than 45–60 mg/dL. Severe hypoglycemia may cause death.

Individuals who have type 1 DM for 4 or 5 years fail to secrete glucagon in response to a decrease in blood glucose. These clients then depend on epinephrine to serve as a counterregulatory response to hypoglycemia. However, this compensatory response can become absent or blunted, and the individual then develops a syndrome called *hypoglycemia unawareness*. In this syndrome, the individual does not experience symptoms of hypoglycemia, even though it is present. Because treatment is not initiated in the absence of symptoms, the individual is likely to have episodes of severe hypoglycemia.

When mild hypoglycemia occurs, immediate treatment is necessary. Individuals experiencing hypoglycemia should take approximately 15 g of a rapid-acting sugar. This amount of sugar is found, for example, in three glucose tablets, half a cup of fruit juice or regular soda, 8 oz of skim milk, five Life Savers candies, three large marshmallows, or 3 tsp of sugar or honey. Sugar should not be added to fruit juice. Adding sugar to the fruit sugar already in the juice could cause a rapid rise in blood glucose, with persistent hyperglycemia.

If the manifestations continue, the 15/15 rule should be followed: Wait 15 minutes, monitor blood glucose, and if the blood glucose is low, eat another 15 g of carbohydrate. This procedure can be repeated until blood glucose levels return to normal (Haire-Joshu, 1996). Individuals with diabetes should have some source of carbohydrate readily available at all times so that hypoglycemic symptoms can be quickly reversed. If hypoglycemia occurs more than two or three times a week, the individual's diabetes management plan should be adjusted.

Clients with diabetes who have severe hypoglycemia often are hospitalized. The criteria for hospitalization are one or more of the following:

- Blood glucose is less than 50 mg/dL, and the prompt treatment of hypoglycemia has not resulted in recovery of sensorium.
- The client has coma, seizures, or altered behavior.
- The hypoglycemia has been treated, but a responsible adult cannot be with the client for the following 12 hours.
- The hypoglycemia was caused by a sulfonylurea drug.

If the client is conscious and alert, 10–15 g of an oral carbohydrate may be given. If the client has altered levels of consciousness, administer parenteral glucose or glucagon.

Glucose is administered intravenously as a 50 mL of 50% (D50) solution, usually at a rate of 10 mL over 1 minute by intravenous push (McPhee & Papadakis, 2009). This is the most rapid method of increasing blood glucose levels.

Glucagon is an antihypoglycemic agent that raises blood glucose by promoting the conversion of hepatic glycogen to glucose. It is used in severe insulin-induced hypoglycemia and may be given in the recommended dose of 1 mg by the subcutaneous, intramuscular, or intravenous route. Glucagon has a short period of action; an oral (if the client is conscious) or intravenous carbohydrate should be administered following the glucagon to prevent a recurrence of hypoglycemia. If the client has been unconscious, glucagon may cause vomiting when consciousness returns.

Chronic Complications

Chronic complications of diabetes include alterations in the cardiovascular system, the peripheral and autonomic nervous systems, and mood as well as increased susceptibility to infection, periodontal disease, and complications involving the feet.

ALTERATIONS IN THE CARDIOVASCULAR SYSTEM
The macrocirculation (large blood vessels) in individuals with diabetes undergoes changes as a result of atherosclerosis; abnor-

malities in platelets, red blood cells, and clotting factors; and changes in arterial walls. Atherosclerosis has an increased incidence and earlier age of onset in individuals with diabetes (although the reason is unknown). Other risk factors that contribute to the development of macrovascular disease of diabetes are hypertension, hyperlipidemia, cigarette smoking, and obesity. Alterations in the vascular system increase the risk of the long-term complications of coronary artery disease, cerebral vascular disease, and peripheral vascular disease.

Alterations in the microcirculation in the individual with diabetes involve structural defects in the basement membrane of smaller blood vessels and capillaries. (The basement membrane is the structure that supports and serves as the boundary around the space occupied by epithelial cells.) These defects cause the capillary basement membrane to thicken; the eventual result is decreased tissue perfusion. Changes in basement membranes are believed to be caused by one or more of the following: presence of increased amounts of sorbitol (a substance formed as an intermediate step in the conversion of glucose to fructose), formation of abnormal glycoproteins, or problems in the release of oxygen from hemoglobin (Porth & Matfin, 2009). The effects of alterations in the microcirculation affect all body tissues but are seen primarily in the eyes and the kidneys.

Coronary Artery Disease   Coronary artery disease is a major risk factor for the development of myocardial infarction in individuals with diabetes, especially the middle-age to older adult with type 2 DM. Individuals with diabetes who have myocardial infarction are more prone to develop congestive heart failure as a complication of the infarction and also are less likely to survive in the period immediately following the infarction. Coronary artery disease is the most common cause of death in individuals with diabetes (National Institutes of Health, 2011).

Hypertension   Hypertension (blood pressure ≥140/80 mmHg) is a common comorbidity of diabetes. It affects 20%–60% of all individuals with diabetes and is a major risk factor for cardiovascular disease and microvascular complications such as retinopathy and nephropathy. Hypertension may be reduced by weight loss, exercise, and decreased sodium intake and alcohol consumption. If these methods are not effective, treatment with antihypertensive medications is necessary.

Stroke (Cerebrovascular Accident)   Individuals with diabetes, especially older adults with type 2 DM, are two to six times more likely to have a stroke. Although the exact relationship between diabetes and cerebral vascular disease is unknown, hypertension (a risk factor for stroke) is a common health problem in those who have diabetes. In addition, atherosclerosis of the cerebral vessels develops at an earlier age and is more extensive in individuals with diabetes (Porth & Matfin, 2009).

The manifestations of impaired cerebral circulation are similar to those of hypoglycemia or HHS, namely, blurred vision, slurred speech, weakness, and dizziness. Individuals with these manifestations have potentially life-threatening health problems and require constant medical attention.

Peripheral Vascular Disease   Peripheral vascular disease of the lower extremities accompanies both types of diabetes, but the incidence is greater in individuals with type 2 DM. Atherosclerosis of vessels in the legs of individuals with diabetes begins at an earlier age, advances more rapidly, and is equally common in men and women. Impaired peripheral vascular circulation leads to peripheral vascular insufficiency with intermittent claudication (pain) in the lower legs and ulcerations of the feet. Occlusion and thrombosis of large vessels and small arteries and arterioles, as well as alterations in neurological function and infection, result in gangrene (necrosis, or the death of tissue). Gangrene from diabetes is the most common cause of nontraumatic amputations of the lower leg. In individuals with diabetes, dry gangrene is most common; it is manifested by cold, dry, shriveled, and black tissues of the toes and feet. The gangrene usually begins in the toes and moves proximally into the foot.

DIABETIC RETINOPATHY

Diabetic retinopathy refers to the changes in the retina that occur in the individual with diabetes. The retinal capillary structure undergoes alterations in blood flow, leading to retinal ischemia and breakdown in the blood–retinal barrier. Diabetic retinopathy is the leading cause of blindness in individuals between 20 and 74 years of age (National Institutes of Health, 2011). Retinopathy has three stages:

1. *Stage I: nonproliferative retinopathy.* Dilated veins, microaneurysms, edema of the macula, and presence of exudates characterize this stage.
2. *Stage II: preproliferative retinopathy.* Retinal ischemia causes infarcts of the nerve fiber layer, with characteristic "cotton wool" patches on the retina. Shunts form between occluded and patent vessels.
3. *Stage III: proliferative retinopathy.* As fibrous tissue and new vessels form in the retina or optic disc, traction on the vitreous humor may cause hemorrhage or retinal detachment.

The prevalence of retinopathy is strongly related to the duration of the diabetes (ADA, 2013). If exudate, edema, hemorrhage, or ischemia occurs near the fovea, the individual experiences visual impairment at any stage. In addition, the individual with diabetes is at increased risk for developing cataracts (opacity of the lens) as a result of increased glucose levels within the lens itself. Screening for retinopathy is important, because laser photocoagulation surgery has proven to be beneficial in preventing loss of vision.

DIABETIC NEPHROPATHY

Diabetic nephropathy is a disease of the kidneys characterized by the presence of albumin in the urine, hypertension, edema, and progressive renal insufficiency. In the United States, this disorder accounts for 44% of new cases of end-stage renal disease requiring dialysis or transplantation. Nephropathy occurs in 20%–40% of individuals with diabetes and is the single leading cause of end-stage renal disease (ADA, 2013).

The exact pathological origin of diabetic nephropathy is unknown. It has been established, however, that thickening of the basement membrane of the glomeruli eventually impairs renal function, and it has been suggested that an increased intracellular concentration of glucose supports the formation of abnormal glycoproteins in the basement membrane and mesangium. The accumulation of these large proteins stimulates glomerulosclerosis (fibrosis of the glomerular tissue). Glomerulosclerosis thickens the basement membrane and simultaneously makes it functionally leaky, allowing large molecules (e.g., proteins) to be lost in the urine. Kimmelstiel-Wilson syndrome is a type of glomerulosclerosis found only in individuals with diabetes. In advanced nephropathy, tubular atrophy occurs, and end-stage renal disease results. (See the module on Fluids and Electrolytes for a discussion of renal failure.)

The first indication of nephropathy is **microalbuminuria** (a low but abnormal level of albumin in the urine). Without specific interventions, individuals with type 1 DM and sustained microalbuminuria develop overt nephropathy, accompanied by hypertension, over a period of 10–15 years. Because type 2 DM may go undetected for years, individuals with this type often have microalbuminuria and overt nephropathy shortly after diagnosis. Microalbuminuria is also a well-established marker of increased cardiovascular disease risk in those with diabetes (ADA, 2013).

Because hypertension accelerates the progress of diabetic nephropathy, aggressive antihypertensive management should be instituted. Management includes control of hypertension with angiotensin-converting enzyme inhibitors (e.g., captopril [Capoten]), weight loss, reduced salt intake, and exercise.

ALTERATIONS IN THE PERIPHERAL AND AUTONOMIC NERVOUS SYSTEMS

Peripheral and visceral neuropathies are disorders of the peripheral nerves and the autonomic nervous system. In individuals with diabetes, these disorders often are called **diabetic neuropathies**. The manifestations depend on the locations of the lesions.

The etiology of diabetic neuropathies involves the following:

- A thickening of the walls of the blood vessels that supply nerves, causing a decrease in nutrients
- Demyelinization of the Schwann cells that surround and insulate nerves, slowing nerve conduction
- Formation and accumulation of sorbitol within the Schwann cells, impairing nerve conduction.

Peripheral Neuropathies The peripheral neuropathies (also called *somatic neuropathies*) include polyneuropathies and mononeuropathies. Polyneuropathies, the most common type of neuropathy associated with diabetes, are bilateral sensory disorders. The manifestations appear first in the toes and feet and then progress upward. The fingers and hands also may be involved, but usually only in later stages of diabetes. The manifestations of polyneuropathy depend on which nerve fibers are involved.

The individual with polyneuropathy commonly has distal paresthesias (a subjective feeling of a change in sensation, e.g., numbness or tingling); pain described as aching, burning, or shooting; and feelings of cold feet. Other manifestations may include impaired sensations of pain, temperature, light touch, two-point discrimination, and vibration. There is no specific treatment for polyneuropathies.

Mononeuropathies are isolated peripheral neuropathies that affect a single nerve. Depending on the nerve involved, manifestations may include the following:

- Palsy of the third cranial (oculomotor) nerve, with headache, eye pain, and inability to move the eye up, down, or medially
- Radiculopathy, with pain over a dermatome and loss of cutaneous sensation, most often located in the chest

- Diabetic femoral neuropathy, with motor and sensory deficits (e.g., pain, weakness, and areflexia) in the anterior thigh and medial calf

- Entrapment or compression of the medial nerve at the wrist, resulting in carpal tunnel syndrome with pain and weakness of the hand; of the ulnar nerve at the elbow, resulting in weakness and loss of sensation over the palmar surface of the fourth and fifth fingers; and of the peroneal nerve at the head of the fibula, resulting in foot drop.

Visceral Neuropathies The visceral neuropathies (also called *autonomic neuropathies*) cause various manifestations, depending on which area of the autonomic nervous system is involved. These neuropathies may include the following:

- Sweating dysfunction, with an absence of sweating (anhydrosis) on the hands and feet and increased sweating on the face or trunk

- Abnormal pupillary function, most commonly seen as constricted pupils that dilate slowly in the dark

- Cardiovascular dysfunction, resulting in such abnormalities as a fixed cardiac rate that does not change with exercise, postural hypotension, and a failure to increase cardiac output or vascular tone with exercise.

- Gastrointestinal dysfunction, with changes in upper gastrointestinal motility (gastroparesis) resulting in dysphagia, loss of appetite, heartburn, nausea and vomiting, and altered blood glucose control. Constipation is one of the most common gastrointestinal symptoms associated with diabetes, possibly as a result of hypomotility of the bowel. Diabetic diarrhea is not as common, but it does occur and often is associated with fecal incontinence during sleep because of a defect in internal sphincter function.

- Genitourinary dysfunction, producing changes in bladder function and sexual function. Changes in bladder function include inability to empty the bladder completely, loss of sensation of bladder fullness, and increased risk of urinary tract infections. Sexual dysfunctions in men include ejaculatory changes and impotence. Sexual dysfunctions in women include changes in arousal patterns, vaginal lubrication, and orgasm. Alterations of sexual function in individuals with diabetes are the result of both neurological and vascular changes.

ALTERATIONS IN MOOD Individuals with DM, both type 1 and type 2, endure the chronic strains of living with complex self-care and are at increased risk for depression and DM-specific emotional distress. A meta analysis of 39 studies demonstrated that 11% of the clients diagnosed with diabetes met the criteria for comorbid MDD (major depressive disorder), and 31% experienced significant depressive symptoms. Depression affects the ability to self-manage DM; depressed clients tend to forget to take their medications, or they run out of medications because they forget to refill their prescriptions in a timely manner. Treating depression has been associated with better control of serum glucose, so screening for depression is an important part of assessing the individual's ability to manage the disease. Tests to identify the scope of depression are available.

Interventions to help clients with depression include antidepressant medications and psychotherapy focused on restoring logical thinking and problem-solving skills. But treating the depression alone does not improve self-management. Stress management programs and education in the self-management of DM are positively correlated with improved self-care. Nurses can assist depressed clients by correcting misconceptions about depression, identifying individual strengths in managing DM, acknowledging negative feelings that are expressed, suggesting problem-solving behaviors to better manage the disease, and referring to appropriate resources (Katon, 2008).

INCREASED SUSCEPTIBILITY TO INFECTION The individual with diabetes has an increased risk of developing infections. The exact relationship between infection and diabetes is not clear, but many dysfunctions that result from diabetic complications predispose the individual to develop an infection. Vascular and neurological impairments, hyperglycemia, and altered neutrophil function are believed to be responsible (Porth & Matfin, 2009).

The individual with diabetes may have sensory deficits that result in inattention to trauma and vascular deficits that decrease circulation to the injured area. In this situation, the normal inflammatory response is diminished, and healing is slowed.

Nephrosclerosis and inadequate bladder emptying with retention of urine predispose the individual with diabetes to pyelonephritis (inflammation of the kidney and its pelvis) and urinary tract infections. Bacterial and fungal infections of the skin, nails, and mucous membranes are common, and tuberculosis is more prevalent in individuals with diabetes than in the general population. Hospitalized clients with a blood glucose greater than 220 mg/dL have higher infection rates (ADA, 2013).

PERIODONTAL DISEASE Although periodontal disease does not occur more often in individuals with diabetes, it does progress more rapidly, especially if the diabetes is poorly controlled. This more rapid progression is believed to be caused by microangiopathy, with changes in vascularization of the gums. As a result, gingivitis (inflammation of the gums) and periodontitis (inflammation of the bone underlying the gums) occur.

COMPLICATIONS INVOLVING THE FEET The high incidence of problems with and amputations of the feet in individuals with diabetes is the result of angiopathy, neuropathy, and infection. Individuals with diabetes are at high risk for amputation of a lower extremity, with an even greater risk in those who have had diabetes for more than 10 years, are male, have poor glucose control, or have cardiovascular, retinal, or renal complications.

Vascular changes in the lower extremities of the individual with diabetes result in arteriosclerosis. Diabetes-induced arteriosclerosis tends to occur at an earlier age, has an equal incidence in men and women, is usually bilateral, and progresses more rapidly. The blood vessels most often affected are located below the knee. Blockages form in the large, medium, and small arteries of the lower legs and feet. Multiple occlusions with decreased blood flow result in the manifestations of peripheral vascular disease (see the exemplar on Peripheral Vascular Disease in the module on Perfusion for more details).

Diabetic neuropathy of the foot produces multiple problems. Because the sense of touch and perception of pain are absent, the individual with diabetes may have some type of foot trauma without being aware of it. This lack of awareness increases the risk for trauma to the tissues of the feet, leading to ulcer development. Infections commonly occur in traumatized or ulcerated tissue.

Despite the many potential sources of foot trauma in the individual with diabetes, the most common are cracks and fissures caused by dry skin or infections (e.g., athlete's foot), blisters caused by improperly fitting shoes, pressure from stockings or shoes, ingrown toenails, and direct trauma (e.g., cuts, bruises, or burns). It is important to remember that the individual with diabetic neuropathy who has lost the perception of pain may not be aware these injuries have occurred. In addition, when a part of the body loses sensation, the individual tends to dissociate from or ignore that part, so an injury may go unattended for days or weeks—or may even be forgotten entirely.

Foot lesions usually begin as a superficial skin ulcer. In time, the ulcer may extend deeper, into muscles and bone and lead to an abscess or osteomyelitis. Gangrene can develop on one or more toes; if untreated, the whole foot eventually becomes gangrenous. (Care of the feet, an essential part of client and family education, is discussed later in this exemplar.)

▶ COLLABORATION

The results of a 10-year DM Control and Complications Trial (DCCT), sponsored by the National Institutes of Health (NIH), have significant implications for the management of type 1 DM. Individuals in the study who kept their blood glucose levels close to normal by frequent monitoring, several daily insulin injections, and lifestyle changes that included exercise and a healthier diet reduced by 60% their risk for the development and progression of complications involving the eyes, the kidneys, and the nervous system. Treatment of the client with DM focuses on maintaining blood glucose at levels as nearly normal as possible through medications, dietary management, and exercise. In order to help the client with diabetes reach the optimal glycemic goal, a team approach that includes collaboration among many sources yields the best outcome for the client. Depending on the available resources and the client's needs, the mutlidiciplinary team may include a certified diabetes educator, a nurse, a family physician, specialists, a dietitian, a podiatrist, and a psychologist and/or psychiatrist, as well as family and friends (Aschner et al., 2010).

Type 2 DM benefits from similar levels of control. Studies of clients with DM who have gastrointestinal surgery for morbid obesity show complete remission of type 2 DM in over three quarters of the cases. Laparoscopic adjustable gastric banding (LAGB) and Roux-en-Y gastric bypass (RYGB) result in remarkable reductions in blood glucose levels and hemoglobin A_{1C}. RYGB, which alters gastrointestinal anatomy, improves insulin sensitivity and is associated with total remission of DM in a significant percentage of clients (Cummings & Flum, 2008; ADA, 2009).

Diagnostic Tests

Diagnostic tests are conducted for screening purposes to diagnose diabetes, and ongoing laboratory tests are conducted to evaluate the effectiveness of diabetic management. Definitions of normal blood glucose levels vary in clinical practice, depending on the laboratory that performs the assay.

DIAGNOSTIC SCREENING Four diagnostic tests may be used to diagnose DM, and each must be confirmed, on a subsequent day, with another of the four tests. The following diagnostic criteria are recommended by the ADA (2013):

1. Hemoglobin $A_{1C} \geq 6.5\%$. This test should be performed in a laboratory using a method that is certified and standardized to the DCCT assay.
2. Symptoms of diabetes plus casual plasma glucose (PG) concentration > 200 mg/dL (11.1 mmol/L). *Casual* is defined as any time of day without regard to time since last meal.
3. Fasting plasma glucose (FPG) > 126 mg/dL (7.0 mmol/L). *Fasting* is defined as no caloric intake for 8 hours.
4. Two-hour PG > 200 mg/dL (11.1 mmol/L) during an oral glucose tolerance test (OGTT). The test should be performed with a glucose load containing the equivalent of 75 g anhydrous glucose dissolved in water.

When using these criteria, the following levels are used for the FPG:

- Normal fasting glucose = 100 mg/dL (6.1 mmol/L)
- Impaired fasting glucose (IFG) > 100 (6.1 mmol/L) and <126 mg/dL (7.0 mmol/L)
- Diagnosis of diabetes > 126 mg/dL (7.0 mmol/L)

When these criteria are used, the following levels are used for the OGTT:

- Normal glucose tolerance = 2-h PG < 140 mg/dL (7.8 mmol/L).
- Impaired glucose tolerance (IGT) = 2-h PG > 140 (7.8 mmol/L) and < 200 mg/dL (11.1 mmol/L).
- Diagnosis of diabetes = 2-h PG > 200 mg/dL (11.1 mmol/L).

Note that although either method may be used to diagnose diabetes, in a clinical setting the FPG is the recommended screening test for nonpregnant adults (ADA, 2013).

PREDIABETES The term *prediabetes* describes individuals who are at increased risk of developing diabetes. Prediabetes is characterized by blood sugar between 100 and 126 mg/dL after fasting overnight, which is high but not high enough to be classified as diabetes. These test results indicate a risk for progression to diabetes, but it is not inevitable. In 2012, an estimated 79 million adults (35%) of adults age 20 and older had prediabetes. Studies suggest that weight loss and increased physical activity among individuals with prediabetes prevent or delay diabetes and may return blood glucose levels to normal. Individuals with prediabetes are already at increased risk for other adverse health outcomes, such as heart disease and stroke (CDC, 2012b).

DIABETES MANAGEMENT MONITORING The following diagnostic tests may be used to monitor diabetes management:

- ***Fasting blood glucose (FBG).*** This test is often ordered, especially if the client is experiencing symptoms of hypoglycemia or hyperglycemia. In most individuals, the normal range is 70–110 mg/dL.
- ***Hemoglobin A_{1C}.*** This test determines the average blood glucose level over approximately the previous 2–3 months. When glucose is elevated or control of glucose is erratic,

glucose attaches to the hemoglobin molecule and remains attached for the life of the hemoglobin, which is about 120 days. The normal level depends on the type of assay done, but values above 7%–9% are considered elevated. The ADA recommends that hemoglobin A_{1C} be performed at the initial assessment, and then at regular intervals, individualized to the medical regimen used.

■ *Urine glucose and ketone levels.* These are not as accurate in monitoring changes in blood glucose as blood levels. The presence of glucose in the urine indicates hyperglycemia. Most individuals have a renal threshold for glucose of 180 mg/dL; that is, when the blood glucose exceeds 180 mg/dL, glucose is not reabsorbed by the kidney and spills over into the urine. This number varies highly, however. Ketonuria (the presence of ketones in the urine) occurs with the breakdown of fats and is an indicator of DKA; however, fat breakdown and ketonuria also occur in states of malnutrition.

■ *Urine test for the presence of albumin (albuminuria).* If albuminuria is present, a 24-hour urine test for creatinine clearance is used to detect the early onset of nephropathy.

■ *Serum cholesterol and triglyceride levels.* These indicate atherosclerosis and an increased risk of cardiovascular impairments. The ADA (2013) recommends treatment goals to lower LDL cholesterol to <100 mg/dL, raise HDL cholesterol to >40 mg/dL in men and >50 mg/dL in women, and lower triglycerides to <150 mg/dL.

■ *Serum electrolytes.* Levels are measured in clients who have DKA or hyperosmolar hyperglycemic state (HHS) to determine imbalances.

Monitoring Blood Glucose

Individuals with DM must monitor their condition daily by testing glucose levels. Two types of tests are available. The first type, long used before the development of devices to directly measure blood glucose, is urine testing for glucose and ketones. Urine testing is less commonly used today. The second type, direct measurement of blood glucose, is widely used in all types of healthcare settings and in the home.

URINE TESTING FOR KETONES AND GLUCOSE
Urine testing for glucose and ketones was at one time the only available method for evaluating the management of DM. An inexpensive, noninvasive, and painless test, it has unpredictable results and cannot be used to detect or measure hypoglycemia. In the healthy state, glucose is not present in the urine because insulin maintains serum glucose below the renal threshold of 180 mg/dL. The accuracy of this measurement is not reliable in DM because the renal threshold may rise with aging or secondary to DM. Urine testing is recommended to monitor hyperglycemia and ketoacidosis in individuals with type 1 DM who have unexplained hyperglycemia during illness or pregnancy. Ketones may be detected through urine testing and reflect the presence of DKA. Individuals who choose not to self-monitor blood glucose by other methods may use urine testing.

SELF-MONITORING OF BLOOD GLUCOSE
Self-monitoring of blood glucose (SMBG) allows the individual with DM to monitor and achieve metabolic control and decrease the

danger of hypoglycemia. The ADA recommends that all clients with DM be taught some method of monitoring glycemic control. The timing of SMBG is highly individualized, depending on the client's diagnosis, general disease control, and physical state. SMBG is recommended three or more times a day for clients with type 1 DM using multiple insulin injections or insulin pump therapy. SMBG by clients with type 2 DM who are not using insulin should provide enough data to help them reach glucose goals. Postprandial blood glucose is often the most useful information for evaluating the level of glycemic control in the client with type 2 DM (ADA, 2009). Clients who check only their fasting glucose would be unaware of the postprandial results.

When adding or modifying therapy, clients with both types of DM should test more often than usual. SMBG is also useful when the individual is ill or pregnant or has manifestations of hypoglycemia or hyperglycemia. Both hypoglycemia and hyperglycemia may contribute to complications and decrease quality of life. With the information assessed with SMBG, clients can alter their diet, their physical activity, and even their medication to reduce the postprandial increases, reduce their risk for complications, and feel better because they no longer experience wide swings in glucose levels (Pearson, 2009).

The ADA annually publishes a comprehensive list of currently available blood glucose-monitoring machines and test strips with approximate prices in *Diabetes Forecast*. Most medical insurance policies cover the cost of these machines, known as *glucose meters*, and the test strips. Many companies provide the meter free of cost. Testing supplies are specific to each glucose meter, so the recipient is obligated to purchase supplies for that particular meter.

Following is the equipment needed for SMBG:

■ A lancet device to perform a finger-stick for obtaining a drop of blood (such as an Autolet, Penlet, or Soft Touch; **Figure 12–5 ●**).

■ A blood glucose monitor (e.g., the Glucometer, the AccuChek, or the One Touch). If the most accurate measurement is desired or recommended, the manufacturer's instructions must be followed carefully. If the timing or

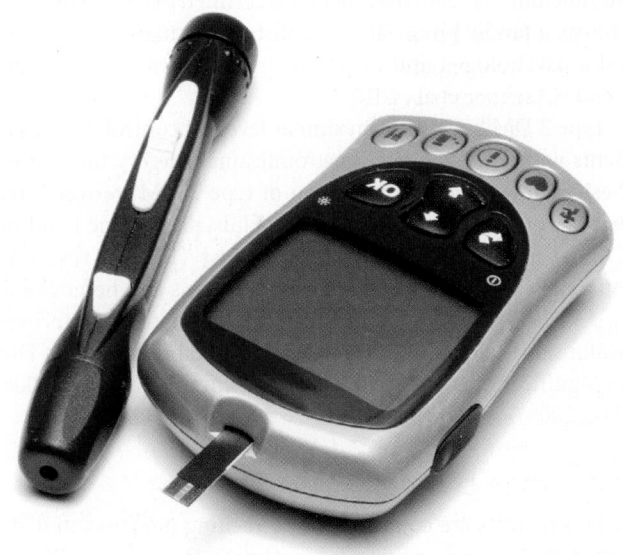

Figure 12–5 ● Lancet and blood glucose monitor for SMBG.
Source: Rob Byron/Shutterstock.

amount of the blood on the strip is not exact, the test will not be accurate. Meters include a memory of previous glucose readings to show a pattern of control. Most of the meters no longer require coding and are simple to use by just placing the strip in the meter and applying a small drop of blood.

A technology for continuous blood glucose monitoring (CGM) has become available in recent years. The CGM has a sensor that is inserted under the skin. This sensor continuously sends data useful as a warning for high or low glucose levels. Fingerstick measurements are required before therapy adjustments are made (McPhee & Papadakis, 2009). The CGM may be used for diagnostic evaluation; clients wear the pump for 3 days under the supervision of physicians and nurses. The data reveals patterns of glycemic control useful for treatment.

A CGM technology currently in development involves a bio-implant that would provide data wirelessly for 1–5 years after being inserted. Noninvasive CGM technologies that are being developed include infrared monitoring and ultrasound (Walsh, 2011).

FACTORS THAT AFFECT GLUCOSE METER PERFORMANCE
According to the U.S. Food and Drug Administration (FDA, 2005), several factors affect the accuracy of blood glucose test results. The quality of the meter and test strips and the client's ability to use the meter correctly contribute to the degree of accuracy. Other factors can create false positive or negative readings.

Hematocrit   Clients with higher hematocrit values usually test falsely low in blood glucose, and clients with lower hematocrit test falsely higher. Anemia and sickle cell anemia are two conditions that can affect hematocrit values.

Other Substances   Overdoses of many medications cause inaccurate results. Glucose meters and supplies vary in sensitivity to medications. Uric acid (a natural substance in the body that can be more concentrated in some individuals with DM), glutathione (an antioxidant also called *GSH*), and ascorbic acid (vitamin C) are known to interfere with accurate results.

Using Correct Supplies and Sample Volume   The test strips must be compatible with the glucose meter, must not be outdated, and must not have been exposed to air and humidity, which can alter strip sensitivity.

Pharmacologic Therapy

The pharmacologic treatment for diabetes mellitus depends on the type of diabetes. Individuals with type 1 DM must have insulin; those with type 2 DM are usually able to control glucose levels with an oral hypoglycemic medication, but they may require insulin if control is inadequate.

INSULIN
The individual with type 1 DM requires a lifelong exogenous source of the insulin hormone to maintain life. Insulin is not a cure for diabetes; rather, it is a means of controlling hyperglycemia. Insulin is also necessary in other situations, such as these:

- An individual with diabetes is unable to control glucose levels with oral antidiabetic drugs and/or diet. The ADA (2013) also states that if a newly diagnosed client with diabetes has

markedly symptomatic and/or increased blood glucose, insulin should be considered at the outset with or without additive agents.

- An individual with diabetes is experiencing physical stress (such as an infection or surgery) or is taking corticosteroids.
- A woman with gestational diabetes is unable to control glucose with diet.
- An individual with diabetes has DKA or HHS.
- An individual with diabetes is receiving high-calorie tube feedings or parenteral nutrition.

Preparations of insulin are derived from animals (pork pancreas) or synthesized in the laboratory from either an alteration of pork insulin or recombinant DNA technology, using strains of *Escherichia coli* to form a biosynthetic human insulin. Insulin analogs have been developed by modification of the amino acid sequence of the insulin molecule. Although different types are prescribed on an individualized basis, it is standard practice to prescribe human insulin.

Insulins are available in rapid-acting, short-acting, intermediate-acting, and long-acting preparations. The trade names and times of onset, peak, and duration of action are listed in **Table 12–4** ●.

Insulin lispro (Humalog) is a human insulin analog that is derived from genetically altered *E. coli* that includes the gene for insulin lispro. It is classified as a rapid-acting or ultra-short-acting insulin. Compared to regular insulin, insulin lispro has a more rapid onset (<15 minutes), an earlier peak of glucose lowering (30–60 minutes), and a shorter duration of activity (3–4 hours). Thus lispro should be administered 15 minutes before a meal, rather than 30–60 minutes before as recommended for regular insulin. Clients with type 1 DM usually also require concurrent use of a longer acting insulin product. Lispro is much less likely than regular insulin to cause tissue changes and may lower the risk of nocturnal hypoglycemia in clients with type 1 DM.

Regular insulin is unmodified crystalline insulin, classified as a short-acting insulin. Regular insulin is clear in appearance and is the only insulin preparation that can be given intravenously; the other types are suspensions and could be harmful if given by this route. Regular insulin is also used to treat DKA, to initiate treatment for newly diagnosed type 1 DM, and in combination with intermediate-acting insulins to provide better glucose control.

The onset and peak and duration of action of insulin can be changed with the addition of acetate buffers and protamine. Zinc and protamine are added to NPH insulins to prolong their action, and they are classified as intermediate- or long-acting insulins. These preparations appear cloudy when properly mixed prior to injection. Protamine and zinc are foreign substances and may cause hypersensitivity reactions. As of July 6, 2005, Lilly discontinued manufacture of pork insulins and Humulin U and Humulin Lente insulin.

Insulin glargine (Lantus) is a 24-hour, long-acting rDNA human insulin analog that is given subcutaneously once or twice a day, usually at bedtime, to treat clients with both type 1 and type 2 diabetes. It has a relatively constant effect (i.e., it does not have a peak time of effect). It is not recommended for use in

TABLE 12–4   Insulin Preparations

	NAME	ONSET (H)	PEAK (H)	DURATION (H)
Rapid acting	lispro (Humalog)	0.25	1–1.5	3–4
	aspart (NovoLog)	0.25	40–50 minutes	3–5
	glulisine (Apidra)	0.25	1–1.5	3–5
Short acting	Regular (Novolin R)	0.5–1.0	2–3	4–6
	Humulin R			
Intermediate acting	NPH (Novolin N)	2	6–8	12–16
	Humulin N			
Long acting	glargine (Lantus)	2 (onset and peak not defined)	16–20	24 +
	detemir (Levemir)	1	6–23	24 +
Combinations	Humalog 50/50	0.5	3	6–12
	Humalog 75/25	0.25	2–4	6–12
	NovoLog 70/30	0.25	1–4	12–24
	Humulin 70/30	0.5	4–8	24
	Novolin 70/30	0.5	4–8	24

pregnancy. Glargine should not be mixed with other insulins; the pH is incompatible (McPhee & Papadakis, 2009). Glargine cannot be used in insulin pumps.

SAFETY ALERT
Glargine (Lantus) and detemir (Levemir) are clear, unlike other intermediate- or long-acting insulins. Do not mistake these for regular insulin. Do not mix them with any other insulins. Do not inject them intravenously, only subcutaneously.

Insulin is dispensed as 100 unit/mL (U-100) and 500 unit/mL (U-500) in the United States. U-100 is the standard insulin concentration used. U-500 insulin is used only in rare cases of insulin resistance when clients require very large doses. U-500 and all the analog insulins require a prescription.

Nursing implications for administering insulin are outlined in **Box 12–1** ●, and instructions for the client are provided in the Client Teaching feature. The considerations for administering insulin include routes of administration, syringe and needle selection, preparing the injection, sites of injection, mixing insulins, and insulin regimens.

All insulins are given parenterally, although current research is investigating the development of a nasal spray and an oral preparation of insulin. Only regular insulin is given by both subcutaneous and intravenous routes; all others are given only subcutaneously. If the intravenous route is not available, regular insulin may also be administered intramuscularly in an emergency situation.

Regular or rapid-acting insulins are used in continuous subcutaneous insulin infusion (CSII) devices, often called *insulin pumps* (e.g., MiniMed). CSII devices have a small pump that holds a syringe of insulin, connected to a subcutaneous needle by tubing. The pump is about the size of a pager and can be worn on a belt or tucked into a pocket. The needle is placed in the skin, usually in the abdomen, and is changed every 3 days. This device delivers a constant amount of programmed insulin throughout each 24-hour period. It also can be used to deliver a bolus of insulin manually (e.g., before meals).

Clients with type 2 diabetes cannot be managed with oral medications during hospitalization because of the risk of hypoglycemia from not eating and the slow response of these medications to correct hyperglycemia. There is growing acceptance of the need to achieve tighter control of blood sugar in individuals

Box 12–1   Medication Administration: Insulin

- Discard vials of insulin that have been open for several weeks or whose expiration date has passed.
- Refrigerate extra insulin vials not currently in use, but do not freeze them.
- Store insulin in a cool place, and avoid exposure to temperature extremes or sunlight.
- Store compatible mixtures of insulin for no longer than 1 month at room temperature or 3 months at 2°–8°C (36°–46°F).
- Discard any vials with discoloration, clumping, granules, or solid deposits on the sides.
- If breakfast is delayed, also delay the administration of rapid-acting insulin.
- Monitor and maintain a record of blood glucose readings 30 minutes before each meal and at bedtime (or as prescribed).

- Monitor food intake, and notify the physician if food is not being consumed.
- Monitor electrolytes (especially potassium), blood urea nitrogen (BUN) levels, and creatinine.
- Observe injection sites for manifestations of hypersensitivity, lipodystrophy, and lipoatrophy.
- If symptoms of hypoglycemia occur, confirm by testing blood glucose level, and administer an oral source of a fast-acting carbohydrate, such as juice, milk, or crackers. Hypoglycemic symptoms may vary but commonly include feelings of shakiness, hunger, and/or nervousness accompanied by sweating, tachycardia, or palpitations.
- If symptoms of hyperglycemia occur, confirm by testing blood glucose level, and notify the physician.

Client Teaching Taking Insulin to Manage Diabetes Mellitus

Self-Administration of Insulin, With a Return Demonstration

1. Wash hands carefully.
2. Have a vial of insulin, the insulin syringe with needle, and alcohol pads ready to use.
3. Remove the cover from the needle.
4. Fill the syringe with an amount of air equal to the number of units of insulin, and insert the needle into the vial.
5. Push air into the vial, invert the vial, and withdraw the prescribed units of insulin.
6. Either carefully replace the cover over the needle or set the syringe down carefully so that the needle does not touch anything.
7. Wipe the selected skin site with alcohol. The injection is less likely to be painful if the alcohol is allowed to dry.
8. Pinch up a fold of skin, and insert the needle into the tissue at the recommended angle.
9. Insert the insulin.
10. Withdraw the needle. Do not rub the injection site. If bleeding occurs, apply light pressure to the injection site with a cotton ball or gauze pad.
11. Do not recap the needle. Dispose of the needle in an appropriate sharps container. Reuse of needles is not recommended.

Using An Insulin Pen for Insulin Delivery

1. Pull the pen cap to remove. Be sure to check insulin for type, expiration date, and appearance.
2. Use an alcohol swab to wipe the rubber seal on the end of the cartridge holder.
3. Remove the paper tab from the outer shield needle.
4. Push the cap needle straight onto the pen. Screw on the needle until secure.
5. Prime the pen by pulling off the outer cover of the needle but do not discard it. Pull off the inner needle shield and throw it away.
6. Dial up 2 units by turning the dose knob.
7. Point the pen up. Tap the cartridge holder to collect air at the top.
8. With the needle pointing upward push the dose knob in until it stops and 0 is seen in the window.

9. Priming is complete when a stream of insulin appears. If a stream of insulin does not appear, repeat up to four times. If the pen still does not prime, change the needles and repeat the priming process.
10. Inject the dose by turning the dose knob to the appropriate amount. If you dial too much, you can dial backward.
11. Prepare the skin for injection using an alcohol pad. Using the thumb on the dose knob and the palm of your hand grasping the pen, inject the insulin until the dose in the window is 0.
12. Count to 5 slowly and then remove the needle.
13. Carefully replace the outer shield and dispose of the cap and needle in the sharps container.

Additional Instructions

- Follow instructions for mixing insulins.
- Always keep an extra vial of insulin available.
- Always have a vial of regular insulin available for emergencies.
- Be aware of the signs of hypersensitivity responses, hypoglycemia, and hyperglycemia.
- Keep candy or a sugar source available at all times to treat hypoglycemia if it occurs. Eat within 15 minutes of injecting rapid-acting insulins.
- Vision may be blurred during the first 6–8 weeks of insulin therapy; this is the result of fluid changes in the eye and should clear up in 8 weeks.
- Avoid alcoholic beverages, which may cause hypoglycemia.

Follow These Guidelines for Sick Days

- Never omit insulin.
- Always monitor blood glucose and/or urine ketones at least every 2–4 hours.
- Always drink plenty of fluids; try to drink at least one glass of water or other calorie-free, caffeine-free liquid each hour.
- Get as much rest as possible.
- Contact the physician if there is persistent fever, vomiting, shortness of breath, severe pain in the abdomen, dehydration, loss of vision, chest pain, persistent diarrhea, blood glucose levels above 250, or ketones in the urine.
- Establish a plan for rotating injection sites, and observe closely for changes in tissues such as hardness, dimpling, or sunken areas.

who are hospitalized with hyperglycemia, whether they are diagnosed with diabetes, have unrecognized diabetes, or have hospital-related diabetes. Although there is no clear evidence for specific goals for the non-critically ill hospitalized client, the ADA (2013) suggests that reasonable targets are less than 140 mg/dL premeal and less than 180 mg/dL random if these targets can be safely achieved.

Maintaining normal blood glucose during hospitalization decreases the risk of postoperative infections and shortens hospital stays. Healing is impaired when hemoglobin is glycosylated (hemoglobin A_{1C}); glycosylated Hgb has increased affinity for oxygen, putting tissues at risk for ischemia (Porth & Matfin, 2009). Further, diabetes leads to small-vessel disease, which impairs circulation and oxygenation of tissue for healing.

Intravenous insulin infusions are preferable for maintaining normal blood glucose during hospitalization, although their use depends on frequent blood glucose monitoring and intensive nursing care. Supplements of regular insulin following sliding-scale prescriptions (relative to monitored blood glucose levels) are ineffective management protocols, risking both hyperglycemia and hypoglycemia. These supplements treat hyperglycemia after it has occurred rather than preventing it. The current trend is to use a basal insulin along with a fixed dose for carbohydrate intake and a correction factor that is geared to the client (ADA, 2013).

Many individuals with diabetes believe the pump allows more normal regulation of blood glucose and provides greater lifestyle flexibility. When recommended procedures are followed, pumps are as safe as multiple-injection therapy. A potential complication is an undetected interruption in insulin delivery, which may result in a rapid onset of DKA. The needle site must be kept clean and changed regularly (usually every 2–3 days) to prevent inflammation and infection.

Other special injection products are available for individuals with physical handicaps. These products include automatic injectors and jet spray injectors. Prefilled syringes are useful for individuals who are visually impaired or traveling. Prefilled syringes are stable for up to 30 days if stored in the refrigerator.

The vial of insulin in use may be kept at room temperature for up to 4 weeks. Stored vials should be kept in the refrigerator and brought to room temperature prior to administration.

Regular insulin does not require mixing. If the solution is cloudy or discolored, the vial should be discarded. The other types of insulin must be mixed to disperse the particles evenly throughout the solution. Mix the vial by gently rolling it between the hands; vigorous shaking causes bubble formation and frothing, which make the dose inaccurate. It is critical that no air bubbles remain in the prepared dose, because even a small bubble can displace several units of insulin.

Although in theory any area of the body with subcutaneous tissue can be used for injections of insulin, certain sites are recommended (**Figure 12–6 ●**). The rate of absorption and peak of action of insulin differ according to the site. The site that allows the most rapid absorption is the abdomen, followed by the deltoid muscle, then the thigh, and then the hip. Because of the rapid absorption, the abdomen is the recommended site. See **Box 12–2 ●** for techniques to minimize painful injections.

Do not massage the site after administering the injection, because massaging may interfere with absorption; however,

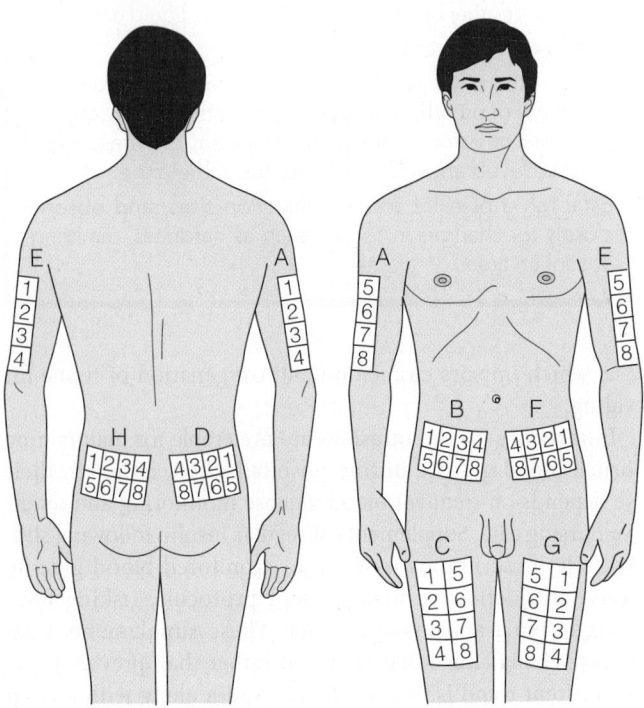

Figure 12–6 ● Sites of insulin injection.

Box 12–2 Techniques to Minimize Painful Injections

- Inject insulin that is at room temperature.
- Make sure no air bubbles remain in the syringe before the injection.
- Wait until alcohol on the skin completely dries before the injection.
- Relax muscles in the injection area.
- Penetrate the skin with the needle quickly.
- Don't change the direction of the needle during insertion or withdrawal.
- Don't reuse dull needles.

Source: Based on AADE (American Association of Diabetes Educators). (2011). *Strategies for insulin injection therapy in diabetes self-management.* Retrieved from www.diabeteseducator.org.

---

pressure may be applied for about 1 minute. Insulin should not be injected into an area to be exercised (such as the thigh before a vigorous walk) or to which heat will be applied; exercise or heat may increase the rate of absorption and cause a more rapid onset and peak of action.

Lipodystrophy (hypertrophy of subcutaneous tissue) or lipoatrophy (atrophy of subcutaneous tissue) may result if the same injection site is used repeatedly, especially with pork and beef insulins. The tissues become hardened and have an orange-peel appearance. The use of refrigerated insulin may trigger the development of tissue atrophy or hypertrophy. These problems rarely occur with the use of human insulins. Lipodystrophy and lipoatrophy alter insulin absorption, delaying its onset or retaining the insulin in the tissue for a period of time instead of allowing it to be absorbed into the body. Lipodystrophy usually resolves if the area is unused for a minimum of 6 months.

HYPOGLYCEMIC AGENTS Hypoglycemic agents are used to treat individuals with type 2 DM. These medications lower blood sugar by stimulating or increasing insulin secretion, preventing breakdown of glycogen to glucose by the liver, and increasing peripheral uptake of glucose by making cells less resistant to insulin. Peripheral uptake is uptake by muscles and fat in the arms and legs rather than in the trunk. Some hypoglycemic agents keep blood sugar low by blocking absorption of carbohydrates in the intestines. The most recent pharmacologic therapy in treating type 2 diabetes includes the incretin effect. Incretin hormones, which are hormones released from the gut endocrine cells during meals, play a significant role in insulin secretion. GLP-1 (glucagon-like peptide) and GIP (glucose-dependent insulinotropic polypeptide or gastric inhibitory polypeptide) may be responsible for as much as 70% of postprandial insulin secretion in healthy individuals. This secretion is greatly reduced or absent in individuals with type 2 diabetes. Byetta (exenatide) and Victoza (liraglutide) are considered GLP-1 agonists and are administered subcutaneously. They help to stimulate insulin and amylin secretion from the pancreatic beta cells, which leads to decreased hepatic gluconeogenesis, slowed gastric emptying, and increased satiety. Another drug related to the incretin effect is the oral preparation of DPP1V inhibitors. These medications work by inhibiting the DPP1V enzyme and therefore preventing the inactivation of endogenous GLP-1. These medications are Januvia (sitagliptin) and Tradjenta (linagliptin). A potential side effect of GLP-1 or DPP1V inhibitors is pancreatitis, and the client must be monitored for this (Inzucchi, Berganstal, & Buse, 2012).

ASPIRIN THERAPY   Individuals with diabetes are up to four times more likely to die from cardiovascular disease. It is recommended that a once-daily dose of 81–325 mg of enteric-coated aspirin be given to reduce atherosclerosis in clients with vascular disease or increased cardiovascular risk factors. Aspirin therapy is contraindicated for clients with aspirin allergy, bleeding tendency, anticoagulant therapy, recent gastrointestinal bleeding, or active liver disease (ADA, 2013).

Nutrition

The management of diabetes requires a careful balance between the intake of nutrients, the expenditure of energy, and the dose and timing of insulin or oral antidiabetic agents. Although everyone has the same need for basic nutrition, the individual with diabetes must eat a more structured diet to prevent hyperglycemia. The goals for dietary management for adults with diabetes, based on guidelines established by the ADA (2013), are as follows:

- Maintain as near normal blood glucose levels as possible by balancing food intake with insulin or oral glucose.
- Achieve optimal serum lipid levels.
- Provide adequate calories to maintain or attain reasonable weights, and to recover from catabolic illness.
- Prevent and treat the acute complications of insulin-treated DM, short-term illnesses, and exercise-related problems, or the long-term complications of diabetes.
- Improve overall health through optimal nutrition, using Dietary Guidelines for Americans and ChooseMyPlate.

The ADA (2008) recommends that carbohydrate intake be individualized to the client's needs, with recommended allowances of 45%–65% of the daily diet. Carbohydrates contain 4 kcal/g and intake should not be restricted to less than 130 g/day. This group of nutrients consists of plant foods (grains, fruits, vegetables), milk, and some dairy products. Carbohydrates can be divided into simple sugars and complex carbohydrates. Glycemic index is the rate at which a food raises blood glucose and, thus, insulin. Proponents of low-carbohydrate diets use glycemic index as the scientific foundation for decreasing intake of foods with a high glycemic index. However, many factors affect the digestion of carbohydrates; to date, research does not support using glycemic index as a basis for therapy. The ADA (2013) does not recommend reliance on glycemic index as a method to treat or prevent diabetes.

The use of sucrose as part of the total carbohydrate content in the diet does not impair blood glucose control in individuals with diabetes. Sucrose and sucrose-containing foods must be substituted for other carbohydrates gram for gram. Dietary fructose (from fruits and vegetables or from fructose-sweetened foods) produces a smaller rise in plasma glucose than sucrose and most starches, so it may offer an advantage as a sweetening agent. However, large amounts of fructose have potentially adverse effects on serum cholesterol and LDL cholesterol, so amounts used should be controlled.

The recommended daily protein intake is 15%–20% of total daily kilocalorie intake. Protein has 4 kcal/g. Sources of protein should be low in fat, low in saturated fat, and low in cholesterol. Although this amount of protein is much less than most individuals normally consume, it is recommended to help prevent or delay renal complications. To help the client accept the decrease in the amount of protein, the nurse may suggest a less severe restriction at diagnosis with a gradual decrease to take place over a period of years.

Dietary fats should be low in saturated fat and cholesterol. Saturated fats should be no higher than 7% of the total kilocalories allowed per day, with dietary cholesterol less than 200 mg/day. Fat has 9 kcal/g. Sources of the different types of fat include:

- *Saturated fat.* Sources are animal meats (meat and butter fats, lard, bacon), cocoa butter, coconut oil, palm oil, and hydrogenated oils.
- *Polyunsaturated fat.* Sources are oils of corn, safflower, sunflower, soybean, sesame seed, and cottonseed.
- *Monosaturated fat.* Sources are peanut oil, olive oil, and canola oil.

Limiting fat and cholesterol intake may help prevent or delay the onset of atherosclerosis, a common complication of diabetes.

Dietary fiber may be helpful in treating or preventing constipation and other gastrointestinal disorders, including colon cancer. It also helps provide a feeling of fullness, and large amounts of soluble fiber may be beneficial to serum lipids. Soluble fiber is found in dried beans, oats, and barley, and in some vegetables and fruits (e.g., peas, corn, zucchini, cauliflower, broccoli, prunes, pears, apples, bananas, oranges). Insoluble fiber, which is found in wheat and corn, and in some vegetables and fruits (e.g., carrots, brussels sprouts, eggplant, green beans, pears, apples, strawberries), does facilitate intestinal motility and give a feeling of fullness.

The ideal level of fiber has not been determined, but an intake of 20–35 g/day is recommended. An increase in fiber may cause nausea, diarrhea or constipation, and increased flatulence, especially if the individual does not also increase fluid intake. Fiber in the diet should therefore be increased gradually.

Although the body requires sodium, most individuals consume much more than is needed each day, especially in processed foods. The recommended daily intake is 1,000 mg of sodium per 1,000 kcal, not to exceed 3,000 mg. The primary concern about sodium is its association with hypertension, a common health problem in individuals with diabetes. It is suggested that table salt (which is 40% sodium) and processed foods high in sodium be avoided in the diabetes meal plan. In normotensive and hypertensive individuals, reduced sodium intake of 2,300 mg per day with a diet high in fruits and vegetables and low in fat lowers blood pressure (ADA, 2011b)

The diet plan for individuals with diabetes restricts the amount of refined sugars. As a result, many individuals use noncaloric sweeteners and foods or drinks made with noncaloric sweeteners. Commercially produced nonnutritive sweeteners are approved for use by the FDA. Although questions have been raised about the safety of these substances in laboratory animal studies, they are considered safe for use by humans. Included in this category of sweeteners are saccharin (Sweet'N Low), aspartame or neotame (Nutrasweet, Equal), sucralose (Splenda), acesulfame potassium (Sunett), and stevia (Truvia).

The nonnutritive sweeteners have negl[e]nt amounts of or no kilocalories, do not produce dental caries, and produce very little or no change in blood glucose levels.

Individuals with diabetes also use nutritive sweeteners, including fructose, agave, honey, sorbitol, and xylitol. The kilocalorie content of these substances is similar to that of table sugar (sucrose), but they cause less elevation in blood glucose. They are often included in foods labeled as "sugar free." Sorbitol may cause flatulence and diarrhea.

Researchers are continuing to study the safety and effectiveness of the sweeteners. In addition, the FDA recommends that the food industry label products with the amount of each ingredient in milligrams per serving and the number of servings per container. When teaching clients about diet, the nurse should include information about the kilocalorie content of sweeteners and the meaning of such phrases as *sugar free* and *dietetic* on labels.

Although drinking alcoholic beverages is not encouraged, neither is it totally prohibited for the client with diabetes. Alcohol consumption may potentiate the hypoglycemic effects of insulin and oral agents. The ADA (2012) recommends that men with diabetes consume no more than two drinks per day and that women with diabetes consume no more than one drink per day. In the following list are guidelines for individuals who include alcohol in their diet plan:

- The signs of intoxication and hypoglycemia are similar; thus the individual with type 1 DM is at increased risk for an insulin reaction.
- Two oral hypoglycemic agents (chlorpropamide and tolbutamide) may interact with the alcohol, causing headache, flushing, and nausea.
- Liqueurs, sweet wines, wine coolers, and sweet mixes contain large amounts of carbohydrate.
- Light beer is the recommended alcoholic drink.
- Alcohol should be consumed with meals and included in the daily food intake. In most instances, the alcohol is substituted for fat in calculating the diet; a drink with 1.5 oz of alcohol is the equivalent of two fat exchanges (90 kcal).

Several systems for meal planning are available to the individual with diabetes. These systems include a consistent-carbohydrate diabetes meal plan, exchange lists, point systems, food groups, carbohydrate counting, and calorie counting. No matter what system is used, however, it must take into account the individual's eating habits, diet history, food values, and special needs. Altering foods and meal patterns is often one of the most difficult parts of diabetes management; careful consideration of individualized preferences enhances compliance with the diet. Although the ADA recommends that a registered dietitian provide the nutrition prescription, nurses must know what is prescribed and be able to reinforce teaching and answer questions.

Sick-Day Management

When the individual with diabetes is sick or has surgery, blood glucose levels increase, even though food intake decreases. The individual often mistakenly alters or omits the insulin dose, causing further problems. The guidelines for dietary management during illness focus on preventing dehydration and providing nutrition for promoting recovery. In general, sick-day management includes the following:

- Monitoring blood glucose at least four times a day throughout an illness
- Testing urine for ketones if blood glucose is greater than 240 mg/dL
- Continuing to take the usual insulin dose or oral hypoglycemic agent
- Sipping 8–12 oz of fluid each hour
- Substituting easily digested liquids or soft foods if solid foods are not tolerated. (The substituted liquids and foods should be carbohydrate equivalents, for example, 1/2 cup sweetened gelatin, 1/2 cup fruit juice, one Popsicle, 1/4 cup sherbet, and 1/2 cup regular soft drink.)
- Calling the healthcare provider if unable to eat for more than 24 hours or if vomiting and diarrhea last for more than 6 hours.

Exercise

The third component of diabetes management is a regular exercise program. The benefits of exercise are the same for everyone, with or without diabetes: improved physical fitness, improved emotional state, weight control, and improved work capacity. In individuals with diabetes, exercise increases the uptake of glucose by muscle cells, potentially reducing the need for insulin. Exercise also decreases cholesterol and triglycerides, reducing the risk of cardiovascular disorders. Individuals with diabetes should consult their primary healthcare provider before beginning or changing an exercise program. The ability to maintain an exercise program is affected by many factors, including fatigue and glucose levels. It is as important to assess the individual's usual lifestyle before establishing an exercise program as it is before planning a diet. Factors to consider include the client's usual exercise habits and living environment, as well as community programs. The exercise that the individual enjoys most is probably the one that he or she will continue (throughout clients should be cautioned to use proper footwear, inspect the feet daily and after exercise, avoid exercise in extreme heat or cold, and avoid exercise during periods of poor glucose control.)

In the individual with type 1 DM, glycemic responses to exercise vary according to the type, intensity, and duration of the exercise. Other factors that influence responses include the timing of exercise in relation to meals and insulin injections and the time of day of the activity. Unless these factors are integrated into the exercise program, the individual with type 1 DM has an increased risk of hypoglycemia and hyperglycemia. Following are general guidelines for an exercise program:

- Individuals who have frequent hyperglycemia or hypoglycemia should avoid prolonged exercise until glucose control improves.
- The risk of exercise-induced hypoglycemia is lowest before breakfast, when free-insulin levels tend to be lower than they are before meals later in the day or at bedtime.
- Low-impact aerobic exercises are encouraged.
- Exercise should be moderate and regular; brief, intense exercise tends to cause mild hyperglycemia, and prolonged exercise can lead to hypoglycemia.

- Exercising at a peak insulin action time may lead to hypoglycemia.

- Self-monitoring of blood glucose levels is essential both before and after exercise.

- Food intake may need to be increased to compensate for the activity.

- Fluid intake, especially water, is essential.

Young adults may continue participating in sports with some modifications in diet and insulin dosage. Blood sugar of less than 100 mg/dL should be treated with a carbohydrate source prior to beginning exercise (ADA, 2013). Athletes should begin training slowly, extend activity over a prolonged period, take a carbohydrate source (such as a drink consisting of 5%–10% carbohydrate) after about 1 hour of exercise, and monitor blood glucose levels for possible adjustments. In addition, a snack should be available after the activity is completed. It may be necessary to omit the usual regular insulin dose prior to an athletic event; even if the athlete is hyperglycemic at the beginning of the event, blood glucose levels will fall to normal after the first 60–90 minutes of exercise. Individuals with type 1 diabetes should avoid exercise in the presence of ketones in the urine.

An exercise program is especially important for the client with type 2 DM. The benefits of regular exercise include weight loss in individuals who are overweight, improved glycemic control, increased well-being, socialization with others, and a reduction of cardiovascular risk factors. A combination of diet, exercise, and weight loss often decreases the need for oral hypoglycemic agents. This decrease is due to an increased sensitivity to insulin, increased kilocalorie expenditure, and increased self-esteem. Regular exercise may prevent type 2 DM in high-risk individuals (ADA, 2009).

Following are general guidelines for an exercise program:

- Before beginning the program, have a medical screening for previously undiagnosed hypertension, neuropathy, retinopathy, and nephropathy.

- Begin the program with mild exercises, and gradually increase intensity and duration.

- Self-monitor blood glucose before and after exercise.

- At least 150 minutes a week of moderate-intensity physical activity is recommended (U.S. Department of Health and Human Services, 2013).

Surgery

Surgical management of diabetes involves replacing or transplanting the pancreas, pancreatic cells, or beta cells. Although it is still in the investigative stage, many researchers believe that transplantation of the tail of the pancreas is the most promising technique for achieving long-term disease control. Islet cell transplantation has had moderate success, and research is continuing. Other research is being conducted in the use of an internally implanted artificial pancreas, or closed-loop artificial beta cells.

Surgery is a stressor that often alters self-management and glycemic control in individuals with diabetes. In response to stress, levels of catecholamines, cortisol, glucagon, and growth hormone increase, as does insulin resistance. Hyperglycemia occurs, and protein stores are decreased. In addition, diet and activity patterns change, and medication types and dosages vary. As a result, surgical clients who have diabetes are at increased risk for postoperative infection, delayed wound healing, fluid and electrolyte imbalances, hypoglycemia, and DKA (Loh-Trivedi & Rothenberg, 2008).

Preoperatively, the client should be in the best possible metabolic state. Screening for complications and regular monitoring of blood glucose are part of preoperative preparation. Oral hypoglycemic agents may be withheld for 1 or 2 days before surgery, and during the perioperative period, regular insulin is often administered to the client with type 2 DM, and to those with hyperglycemia but not diagnosed with DM. All clients with hyperglycemia, whether diagnosed with DM or not, follow a carefully prescribed insulin regimen individualized to specific needs.

The insulin regimen in the perioperative period is individualized. When the client is NPO, short-acting insulin should not be given without intravenous glucose. Clients with type 1 DM and type 2 DM, and clients with hyperglycemia who are critically ill in the perioperative period should receive IV glucose and insulin infusion in an intensive care unit. The target blood glucose level during surgery is between 110 and 140 mg/dL. This level prevents hypoglycemia, which is difficult to detect under anesthesia, and prevents glycosuria, dehydration, and impaired wound healing. IV infusion of glucose, insulin, and added potassium is appropriate for all hyperglycemic clients undergoing surgery (ADA, 2009).

The surgical procedure should be scheduled for as early as possible in the morning to minimize the length of fasting. If there is no food intake after surgery, intravenous dextrose should be administered, accompanied by subcutaneous regular insulin every 6 hours for the noncritically ill surgical client. The dose can be adjusted to blood glucose levels. Although kilocalorie intake is decreased postoperatively, stress can increase insulin requirements. Glucose control is also affected postoperatively by nausea and vomiting, anorexia, and gastrointestinal suction.

During the postoperative period, the client with type 2 DM may continue to require insulin or may resume oral medications, depending on glucose control. The client with type 1 DM may require reduced insulin as healing progresses and stress diminishes. Regular blood glucose monitoring is essential, as are assessments for hypoglycemia.

■ NURSING PROCESS

The responses of clients with diabetes to their illness are often complex and individual, involving multiple body systems. Assessments, planning, and implementation differ for the client with newly diagnosed diabetes, the client with long-term diabetes, and the client with acute complications of diabetes. The plan of care and the content of teaching also differ according to the type of diabetes and the client's age, culture, and intellectual, psychological, and social resources.

Teaching the client (and family) to self-manage diabetes is a nursing responsibility. Even if a formal teaching plan is developed and implemented by an advanced practice nurse, each nurse who interacts with the client must be able to reinforce this knowledge and answer questions. Teaching is necessary for both the individual who is newly diagnosed and for the individual who has had diabetes for years. In fact, the latter may need almost as much teaching as the newly diagnosed client. Products for diabetes care, especially insulins, have changed dramatically, and knowledge about risk reduction to prevent complications has increased.

The American Diabetes Association recommends that teaching be carried out on three levels. The first level focuses on survival skills; the individual learns basic knowledge and skills in diabetes management for the first week or two while adjusting to the idea of having the disease. The second level deals with home management, emphasizing self-reliance and independence in the daily management of diabetes. The third level aims at improving lifestyle and educating the client to individualize self-management of the illness.

Health promotion activities primarily focus on preventing the complications of diabetes. The client should prevent or decrease excess weight, follow a sensible and well-balanced diet, and maintain a regular physical exercise program. These same activities, when combined with medications and self-monitoring, also are beneficial in reducing the onset of complications.

Assessment

The following data is collected through the health history and physical examination:

■ *Health history.* Family history of diabetes; history of hypertension or other cardiovascular problems; history of dizziness, numbness or tingling in hands or feet, and any change in vision (e.g., blurring) or speech; pain when walking; frequent voiding; change in weight, appetite, infections, and healing; problems with gastrointestinal function or urination; or altered sexual function

■ *Physical assessment.* Height/weight ratio, vital signs, visual acuity, cranial nerves, sensory ability in extremities (e.g., touch, hot/cold, and vibration), peripheral pulses, and skin and mucous membranes (e.g., hair loss, appearance, lesions, rash, itching, and vaginal discharge)

Older Adults

When assessing older clients, be aware of normal aging changes in all body systems that may alter interpretation of findings.

Children

Children generally are admitted to the hospital at the time of diagnosis. The nurse assesses the child's physiological status, focusing on vital signs and level of consciousness. The nurse assesses hydration by checking mucous membranes, skin turgor, and urine output. Blood initially is collected hourly to monitor blood gases, glucose, and electrolytes. Once the child is stable, the nurse assesses dietary and caloric intake and the ability of the child or family to manage care.

If parents waited to seek care until the child began to experience symptoms of DKA, they may feel guilty at the time of

diagnosis. The nurse should assess their coping mechanisms, family strengths and resources, and ability to manage the disease, as well as the educational needs of both the child and the parents. It is important to identify family stressors that may cause challenges in the long-term management of diabetes, including access to health insurance and other financial considerations.

Diagnosis

The goals of care are to maintain function, prevent complications, and teach self-management. Although many NANDA nursing diagnoses are appropriate for the individual with diabetes, the following address some of the more common problems:

■ *Knowledge Deficit*
■ *Risk for Impaired Skin Integrity*
■ *Risk for Infection*
■ *Risk for Injury*
■ *Risk for Deficient Fluid Volume*
■ *Sexual Dysfunction*
■ *Ineffective Coping*

(NANDA-I © 2012)

Planning

The nursing plan of care is focused on helping the client learn to provide self-care and reduce the risk of complications. Goals of care include, but are not limited to, the following:

■ The client will describe how to administer medications and respond to side effects appropriately.
■ The client will demonstrate meal planning compliant with the American Diabetic Association diet.
■ The client will demonstrate proper foot care and inspection.
■ The client will demonstrate proper procedure for monitoring blood sugar levels.
■ The client will describe strategies for reducing risk of infection.

Implementation

Nursing care for the client with diabetes is individualized and focuses on teaching the client and family about the disease and its management, planning dietary intake, providing emotional support, and creating strategies for daily management in the community. Some hospitals have developed clinical pathways to streamline and standardize diabetes care. The nurse should include the following when teaching the client and family about care at home:

■ Information about normal metabolism, diabetes, and how diabetes changes metabolism
■ How diet helps keep blood glucose in the normal range; the number of kilocalories required and why; the amount of carbohydrates, meats, and fats allowed and why; and how to calculate the diet while integrating personal food preferences
■ How exercise helps lower blood glucose, the importance of a regular exercise program, types of exercise, integrating personal exercise preferences, and how to handle increased activity

- Self-monitoring of blood glucose, how to care for equipment, and what to do about a high or low blood glucose level
- Medications:
  a. *Insulin: subcutaneous agents.* Type, dosage, mixing instructions (if necessary), times of onset of insulin effect and of peak actions, how to get and care for equipment, how and where to give injections
  b. *Hypoglycemic agents: oral delivery.* Type, dosage, side effects, and interaction with other drugs
- Manifestations of acute complications of hypoglycemia and hyperglycemia, and what to do when they occur
- Hygiene, including skin care, dental care, and foot care
- What to do about food, fluids, and medications when the client is sick
- Helpful resources

Teaching may have to be adapted to the special needs and developmental level of a child or older adult. However, because 40% of all individuals with diabetes are over the age of 65, considering the special needs of the older population is particularly essential. Uncontrolled diabetes in the older adult increases the potential for functional loss, social disengagement, and increased morbidity and mortality. Education for self-care allows the older adult to be more actively involved in diabetes management and decreases the potential for acute and chronic complications from the disease. Considerations for teaching the older adult with diabetes include the following:

- Changes in diet may be difficult to implement for many reasons. Favorite foods are difficult to give up. Balanced meals at regular intervals may not have been part of the client's lifestyle. Purchasing, storing, and preparing foods may be a problem. Dentures may not fit well. Changes in taste sensation often cause the client to increase the use of salt and sugar. (For more information on nutrition and the older adult, see the module on Nutrition.)
- Exercise of any type may not have been part of the activities of daily living. An exercise plan must be individualized for any physical limitations imposed by other chronic illnesses,

Lifespan Considerations Diabetes

Children

- The child's developmental stage and cognitive level influence readiness to take on responsibility for self-care, for example, to obtain and read a blood glucose sample or inject insulin. Children usually can perform some tasks with supervision by 6–8 years of age.
- Caution parents to check the blood glucose level of a toddler who is extremely sleepy or irritable, because these can be signs of hypoglycemia or hyperglycemia.
- The preschool child's need for autonomy and control can be met by allowing the child to choose snacks or pick which finger to stick for glucose testing and to help parents gather the necessary supplies.
- School-age children need to learn how to recognize the signs of hypoglycemia and hyperglycemia and to understand the importance of carrying a rapidly absorbed sugar product.
- Adolescents in particular are present-time oriented and may rebel against the daily regimen of insulin injections, the food plan, and the exercise plan. Adolescence is a time of finding an identity separate from the family and of testing limits. The desire to be like their peers may interfere with their adherence to treatment.
- When the child with diabetes is sick, parents need to be extra attentive to the child's glycemic control.
- Record growth measurements and vital signs in the child's chart. Puberty may be delayed if diabetic control is inadequate.
- The child with type 1 DM may develop circulatory and neurological changes over time. Emphasize the importance of good foot care from an early age.
- The child with diabetes needs an individual health plan (IHP) for management of diabetes while in school or child care. The IHP should include when blood glucose testing needs to be performed, insulin administration and storage instructions, meals and snacks needed, and symptoms and management of hypoglycemia and hyperglycemia.

Older Adults

- The prevalence of diabetes becomes greater with age, increasing from 11.3% with diagnosed diabetes in those age 20 years or older to 26.9% in those age 65 or older (ADA, 2011b).
- Although most older adults with diabetes have type 2 DM, improved survival rates have resulted in an increased number of older adults with type 1 DM. The picture is further complicated by the fact that blood glucose levels increase with age, beginning in the 50s. For this reason, it is more difficult to diagnose diabetes in older adults, because these clients may be mistakenly diagnosed with the disease simply because they exhibit essentially normal age-related changes in glucose. The relationship between normal increases in glucose levels and the presence of diabetes is not yet understood.
- The normal physiological changes of aging may mask manifestations of the onset of diabetes. Signs and symptoms of diabetes in older adults may not include the classic symptoms of polyuria and thirst. Conditions such as orthostatic hypotension, periodontal disease, infections, stroke, gastric hypotony, impotence, neuropathy, confusion, and glaucoma should be considered potential indicators of diabetes. These conditions also may increase the potential for complications from the disease or its treatment (ADA, 2011b).
- The older adult with diabetes has multiple, complex healthcare problems and needs, including risks for polypharmacy, depression, cognitive impairment, urinary incontinence, injurious falls, and persistent pain (ADA, 2013).
- The older adult with diabetes also has a longer recovery period after surgery or serious illness, often requiring insulin to maintain blood glucose levels. The benefits and risks of treatment to maintain glycemic control as well as blood pressure and lipid management must be carefully balanced.

such as arthritis, Parkinson disease, chronic respiratory diseases, and/or cardiovascular diseases.

- Diagnosis of a chronic illness threatens a client's independence and feelings of self-worth. After years of taking care of themselves, older adults with diabetes may now have to depend on others for help in meeting self-care needs. This change of circumstance often leads to withdrawal from social interactions with others.
- Money to purchase medications and supplies often must be taken out of a fixed income.
- Visual deficits may make insulin administration difficult or impossible. Visual deficits also can interfere with blood glucose monitoring, food preparation, exercises, and foot care.

Caring interventions may also focus on the risks for impaired skin integrity, infection, and injury, as well as on sexual dysfunction and ineffective coping. Interventions for each diagnosis are discussed in the following section.

Maintain Skin Integrity

The client with diabetes is at increased risk for altered skin integrity as a result of decreased tissue perfusion from cardiovascular complications, infection, and decreased or absent sensation from neuropathies. In addition, poor vision increases the risk of trauma, and an open lesion is more prone to infection and delayed healing.

Impaired skin and tissue integrity, with resultant gangrene, is especially common in the feet and lower extremities. In fact, individuals with diabetes are at significant risk for lower extremity gangrene. The nurse should conduct baseline and ongoing assessments of the client's feet, including the following:

- Musculoskeletal assessment that includes foot and ankle joint range of motion, bone abnormalities (e.g., bunions, hammertoes, and overlapping digits), gait patterns, use of assistive devices for walking, and abnormal wear patterns on shoes
- Neurological assessment that includes sensations of touch and position, pain, and temperature
- Vascular examination that includes assessment of lower extremity pulses, capillary refill, color and temperature of skin, and edema
- Assessment of hydration status, including dryness or excessive perspiration
- Assessment for lesions, fissures between toes, corns, calluses, plantar warts, ingrown or overgrown toenails, redness over pressure points, blisters, cellulitis, or gangrene

Peripheral neuropathies may result in altered perception of pain, loss of deep tendon reflexes, loss of cutaneous pressure and position sensation, foot drop, changes in the shape of the foot, and changes in bones and joints. Peripheral vascular disease may cause intermittent claudication, absent pulses, delayed venous filling on elevation, dependent rubor, and gangrene. Injuries, lesions, and changes in skin hydration potentiate infections, delayed healing, and tissue loss in the individual with diabetes.

- Teach foot hygiene. The client should wash the feet daily with lukewarm water and mild hand soap; pat them dry and dry well between the toes; and apply a very thin coat of lubricating cream if dryness is present (but not between the toes).

Proper hygiene decreases the chance of infection. The temperature receptors in the client's feet may be impaired, so the water should always be tested before use.

- If the client smokes, discuss the importance of not smoking. Nicotine in tobacco causes vasoconstriction, further decreasing the blood supply to the feet.
- Discuss the importance of maintaining blood glucose levels through prescribed diet, medication, and exercise. Hyperglycemia promotes the growth of microorganisms.
- Conduct foot care teaching sessions (see the Client Teaching feature) as often as necessary. Foot care is a priority in diabetes management to prevent serious problems. Many individuals with diabetes are unaware of lesions or injury until infection and compromised circulation are far advanced. The hows and whys of each component must be included in teaching. A variety of methods may be used, including demonstration, return demonstration, audiovisual aids, and written lists. If the client is wearing shoes and socks, ask him or her to remove them to practice foot care effectively.

Promote Healthy Behaviors

The individual with diabetes is at increased risk for infection. The risk of infection is believed to result from vascular insufficiency that limits the inflammatory response, neurological abnormalities that limit the awareness of trauma, and a predisposition to bacterial and fungal infections. The nurse should do the following:

- Use and teach meticulous hand washing. Hand washing is the single most effective method for preventing the spread of infection.
- Monitor for manifestations of infection: increased temperature, pain, malaise, swelling, redness, discharge, and cough. Early diagnosis and treatment of infections can control their severity and decrease complications.
- Discuss the importance of skin care. Using lukewarm water and mild soap, keep the skin clean and dry. Individuals with diabetes are more prone to develop furuncles and carbuncles; the infection often increases the need for insulin. Clean, intact skin and mucous membranes are the first line of defense against infection.
- Teach dental health measures:
  a. Obtain a dental examination every 4–6 months.
  b. Maintain careful oral hygiene, which includes brushing the teeth with a soft toothbrush and fluoridated toothpaste at least twice a day and flossing as recommended.
  c. Be aware of symptoms requiring dental care: bad breath; unpleasant taste in the mouth; bleeding, red, or sore gums; and tooth pain.
  d. Monitor for the need to make adjustments in insulin if dental surgery is necessary.

All clients with diabetes need to be taught proper oral hygiene, the risk of periodontal disease, and the importance of obtaining dental care for symptoms of oral or dental problems.

- Teach women with diabetes the symptoms and preventive measures for vaginitis caused by *Candida albicans*. The symptoms are an odorless white or yellow cheeselike discharge and itching. Sexual transmission is unlikely, but discomfort may cause the client to avoid sexual activity. Diabetes is a predis-

Client Teaching Foot Care

General Information

- Never go barefoot. Wear slippers when leaving the bed during the night.
- Do not use commercial corn medicines or pads, chemicals (e.g., boric acid, iodine, or hydrogen peroxide), or over-the-counter cortisone medications on the feet.
- Do not put heating pads, hot-water bottles, or ice packs on the feet. If the feet become cold at night, wear socks, or use extra blankets.
- Do not allow the feet to become sunburned.
- Do not put tape on the feet.
- Do not sit with the legs crossed at the knees or ankles.

Buying and Wearing Shoes and Stockings

- Shoes that allow 0.5–0.75 in. of toe room are best; there should be room for toes to spread out and wiggle. The lining and inside stitching should be smooth, and the insole should be soft. The sole should be flexible and cushion the foot. The heel should fit snugly, and good arch support should be present.
- Do not wear open-toed shoes, sandals, high heels, or thongs; these increase the risk of trauma.
- Buy shoes late in the afternoon, when feet are at their largest; always buy shoes that feel comfortable and do not need to be "broken in."
- Shoes made of natural fibers (e.g., leather and canvas) allow perspiration to escape.

- Check the shoes before each wearing for foreign objects, wrinkled insoles, and cracks that might cause lesions.
- Socks or stockings made of wool or cotton allow perspiration to dry.
- Do not wear garters, knee stockings, or pantyhose; these may interfere with circulation.
- Wear insulated boots in the winter.

Inspecting the Feet

- Check the feet daily for red areas, cuts, blisters, corns, calluses, or cracks in the skin. Check between the toes for cracks or reddened areas.
- Check the skin of the feet for dry or damp areas.
- Use a mirror to check each sole and the back of each heel.
- If you are unable to inspect the feet daily, be sure that someone else does.

Care of Toenails

- Cut the toenails after washing, when they are softer and easier to trim.
- Cut the nails straight across with a clipper, and smooth edges and corners with an emery board.
- Do not use razor blades to trim the toenails.
- If you are unable to see your feet well or to reach them easily, have someone else trim the nails. If the nails are very thick or ingrown, if the toes overlap, or if circulation is poor, get professional care from a podiatrist.

---

posing factor for *C. albicans* vaginitis, the most common form of vaginitis. Poor personal hygiene and clothing that keeps the vaginal area warm and moist increase the risk of vaginitis. The infection may spread to the urinary tract and result in urinary tract infections; preventing and treating vaginitis decrease this risk.

Maintain Safety

The client with diabetes is at risk for injury from multiple factors. Neuropathies may alter sensation, gait, and muscle control. Cataracts or retinopathy may cause visual deficits. Hyperglycemia often causes osmotic changes in the lenses of the eye; the result is blurred vision. In addition, changes in blood glucose alter levels of consciousness and may cause seizures. The impaired mobility, sensory deficits, and neurological effects of complications of diabetes increase the risk of accidents, burns, falls, and trauma. To help the client decrease the risk of injury, the nurse can do the following:

- Assess for the presence of contributing or causative factors that increase the risk of injury: blurred vision, cataracts, decreased adaptation to dark, decreased tactile sensitivity, hypoglycemia, hyperglycemia, hypovolemia, joint immobility, and unstable gait. A knowledge base is necessary to develop an individualized plan of care. The risk of injury increases with the number of factors identified.
- Reduce environmental hazards in the healthcare facility, and teach the client about safety in the home and in the community.

- Monitor for and teach the client and family to recognize and seek care for the manifestations of DKA in the client with type 1 DM: hyperglycemia, thirst, headaches, nausea and vomiting, increased urine output, ketonuria, dehydration, and decreasing level of consciousness. Blood glucose levels increase if the need for insulin is unmet or insufficiently met, because the cellular use of fats for fuel results in ketosis. Osmotic diuresis increases urinary output; the result is thirst and dehydration.
- Monitor for and teach the client and family to recognize and seek care for the manifestations of HHS in the client with type 2 DM: extreme hyperglycemia, increased urinary output, thirst, dehydration, hypotension, seizures, and decreasing level of consciousness. HHS is a life-threatening condition requiring recognition and treatment.
- Monitor for and teach the client and family to recognize and treat the manifestations of hypoglycemia: low blood glucose, anxiety, headache, uncoordinated movements, sweating, rapid pulse, drowsiness, and visual changes. Teach client and family to carry some form of rapid-acting sugar source at all times. Severe hypoglycemia causes a decrease in the level of consciousness. The decrease in blood glucose most often results from too much insulin, too little food, or too much exercise.
- Recommend that the client wear a medical alert bracelet or necklace that identifies the client as an individual with diabetes. In case of sudden severe illness or accident, a medical alert bracelet allows immediate medical attention for diabetes.

Maintain Sexual Health

Sexuality is a complex and inseparable part of every individual. It involves not only physical sexual activities but also an individual's self-perception as male or female, roles and relationships, and attractiveness and desirability. Changes in sexual function and sexuality have been identified in both men and women with diabetes.

Alterations in erectile ability occur in approximately 50% of all men with diabetes. The incidence of impotence increases with the duration of the diabetes and often is associated with peripheral neuropathy. Libido usually is unaffected, even when impotence is present.

Women with diabetes may have alterations in sexual function, although the reason is less clear. The problems reported by women involve decreased desire and decreased vaginal lubrication. Women with diabetes are at increased risk for vaginitis as well. These symptoms often make sexual intercourse painful, which may be the source of alterations in libido.

To monitor the client with diabetes for issues involving sexual dysfunction, the nurse should do the following:

■ Include a sexual history as a part of the initial and ongoing assessment of the client with diabetes. A specific history form may be used that addresses sexual development, personal and family values, current sexual practices and concerns, and the changes desired. To elicit information, ask a nonthreatening, open-ended question, such as "Tell me about your experience with sexual function since you have been diagnosed with diabetes." Obtaining accurate information to assess the sexual health of a client is necessary before counseling can begin or referrals can be made.

■ Provide information about the actual and potential physical effects of diabetes on sexual function. Include the effect of poor control of blood glucose on sexual function as part of any teaching plan. Clients benefit from basic information about male and female anatomy, the sexual response cycle, and how diabetes can affect this part of the body. Changes in blood glucose levels not only may cause changes in desire and physical response but also may alter sexual responses as a result of depression, anxiety, and fatigue.

■ Provide counseling or make referrals as appropriate. The nurse is responsible for knowing about sexuality and sexual health throughout the life span and provides information based on knowledge about the effects of illness and treatment on sexual function. The nurse may make specific suggestions to facilitate positive sexual functioning and, as necessary, refer the client to the appropriate healthcare provider for intensive therapy.

Promote Effective Coping

Coping is the process of responding effectively to internal or environmental stressors or potential stressors. When coping responses are ineffective, the stressors exceed the individual's available resources for responding. The client diagnosed with diabetes is faced with lifelong changes. New diet, exercise habits, and medications must be integrated into the lifestyle and carefully controlled. Daily injections may be a reality. Fear of potential complications and of negative effects on the future is common.

If the client is unable to cope successfully with these changes or lacks a strong support system, emotional stress can interfere with glycemic control. In addition, unsuccessful coping often results in noncompliance with prescribed treatments, further impairing glycemic control and increasing the potential for acute and chronic complications.

To help determine how well the client is coping with the diagnosis and illness, the nurse should do the following:

■ Assess the client's psychosocial resources, including emotional resources, support resources, financial resources, lifestyle, and communication skills. Chronic illness affects all dimensions of an individual's life, as well as the lives of family members and significant others. A comprehensive assessment of strengths and weaknesses is the first step in developing an individualized plan of care to facilitate coping.

■ Explore with the client and family the effects (actual and perceived) of the diagnosis and treatment of diabetes on finances, occupation, energy levels, and relationships. Common frustrations associated with diabetes are the disease itself, the treatment modalities, and the healthcare system. Effective coping involves maintaining emotional balance, a healthy self-concept, and satisfying relationships, as well as handling emotional stress.

■ Teach constructive problem-solving techniques. Problem-focused behaviors include setting attainable and realistic goals, learning about all aspects of the problem, learning new procedures or skills that increase self-esteem, and reaching out to others for support.

■ Provide information about support groups and resources such as suppliers of products, journals, books, and cookbooks for individuals with diabetes. Clients who are living on limited incomes or are without health insurance may need assistance in accessing special programs offered by pharmaceutical companies or local clinics to help them pay for their prescriptions. Sharing with others who have similar problems provides opportunities for mutual support and problem solving. Using available resources improves the ability to cope.

Evaluation

Expected outcomes of nursing care of the client with diabetes are individualized on the basis of the nursing care plan and the goals established during the planning phase. These outcomes may include the following:

■ The client demonstrates an age-appropriate understanding of diabetes self-management through medication, diet, exercise, and blood glucose self-monitoring activities.
■ The client's skin integrity remains intact.
■ The client remains free of infection.
■ The client remains free of injury.

NURSING CARE PLAN A Client With Type 1 Diabetes Mellitus

Jim Meligrito, age 24, is a third-year nursing student at a large midwestern university. Mr. Meligrito also works 20 hours a week as a campus student security guard. His working hours are 8 p.m. to midnight, five nights a week. He lives with his father, who also is a student. Neither of the men likes to cook, and they usually eat "whatever is handy." Mr. Meligrito has smoked 8–10 cigarettes a day for 5 years.

Mr. Meligrito was diagnosed with type 1 DM at age 12. Although his insulin dosage has varied, he currently takes a total of 32 U of insulin each day, 10 U of NPH, and 6 U of regular insulin each morning and evening. He monitors his blood glucose about three times a week. He feels that he is too busy for a regular exercise program and that he gets enough exercise in clinicals and in weekend sports activities. He has not seen a healthcare provider for over a year.

One day during a 6-hour clinical laboratory in pediatrics, Mr. Meligrito notices that he is urinating frequently, is thirsty, and has blurred vision. He also is very tired, but he blames all his symptoms on drinking a couple of beers and having had only 4 hours of sleep the night before while studying for an exam, and on the stress he has been under lately from school and work. When he remembers that he forgot to take his insulin that morning, he realizes he must have hyperglycemia but decides that he will be all right until he gets home in the afternoon. Around noon, he begins having abdominal pain, feels weak, has a rapid pulse, and vomits. When he reports his physical symptoms to his clinical instructor, she immediately sends him, accompanied by another student, to the hospital emergency department.

ASSESSMENT

As soon as Mr. Meligrito arrives at the emergency room, his blood glucose level is measured at 300 mg/dL. Urine samples and additional blood samples are sent to the laboratory for analysis. Hemoglobin A_{1C} is 9.5%, urine shows the presence of ketones, electrolytes are normal, and pH is 7.1. His vital signs are as follows: T 37.2°C (99°F), P 140 bpm, R 28/min, and BP 102/52 mmHg. An intravenous infusion of 1,000 mL of normal (0.9%) saline with 40 mEq of KCl is started at a rate of 400 mL/hr. Intravenous regular insulin at 5 U/hr (diluted in 0.9% saline) is begun. Hourly blood glucose monitoring also is initiated. Mr. Meligrito is nauseated and lethargic but remains oriented. Three hours later, he has a blood glucose level of 160 mg/dL, and his pulse and blood pressure are normal. He is dismissed from the emergency department after making an appointment for the next morning with the hospital's diabetes nurse educator. When he meets with the diabetes educator, he says that he no longer feels in control of the diabetes or his future goal of becoming a nurse anesthetist.

DIAGNOSES

Nursing diagnoses that may be appropriate for Mr. Meligrito include the following:

- *Powerlessness* related to a perceived lack of control of diabetes because of present demands on time
- *Deficient Knowledge* of self-management of diabetes
- *Ineffective Role Performance* related to uncertainty about his capacity to achieve the desired role as a registered nurse.

(NANDA-I © 2012)

PLANNING

The expected outcomes for the plan of care specify that Mr. Meligrito will:

- Identify those aspects of diabetes that can be controlled and participate in making decisions about self-managing his care.
- Demonstrate an understanding of diabetes self-management through planned medication, diet, exercise, and blood glucose self-monitoring activities.
- Explore and clarify his perceptions of his role as a student nurse and verbalize his ability to meet his expectations.

IMPLEMENTATION

The following interventions may be appropriate for Mr. Meligrito:

- Mutually establish specific and individualized short-term and long-term goals for self-management to control blood glucose.
- Provide opportunities to express his feelings about himself and his illness.
- Explore perceptions of his own ability to control his illness and his future, and clarify these perceptions by providing information about resources and support groups.

- Facilitate his decision-making abilities in self-managing his prescribed treatment regimen.
- Provide positive reinforcement for increasing his involvement in self-care activities.
- Provide relevant learning activities about insulin administration, dietary management, exercise, self-monitoring of blood glucose, and healthy lifestyle.

EVALUATION

After taking an active part in the weekly educational meetings for 2 months, Mr. Meligrito has greatly enhanced his understanding of and compliance with self-management of his diabetes. He states that he finally understands how insulin, food, and exercise affect his body, having previously thought they were "just things I should do when I wanted to." He decides to perform self-management activities 1 week at a time rather than think too far into (and thereby feel overwhelmed by) the future. Both son and father have developed a workable meal schedule and weekly grocery list, and they have begun eating breakfast and dinner together. Jim and a friend have arranged to walk 2–3 miles three times a week on a community hiking trail. To gain a sense of control over his illness, he has also worked out a schedule that allows time for school, health care, and himself.

CRITICAL THINKING

1. What is the pathophysiological basis for the changes in temperature, pulse, respiration, and blood pressure that were recorded on Mr. Meligrito's admission to the hospital emergency department?
2. How can smoking and poor self-management of diabetes increase the risk of long-term complications?
3. Is powerlessness a common response to a chronic illness? Why, or why not?
4. Consider that you are teaching Mr. Meligrito and another client, Mr. McDaniel (age 75, newly diagnosed with type 2 DM). What components of your teaching plan would be the same, and what components would be different?
5. What does the hemoglobin A_{1C} of 9.5% suggest about Mr. Meligrito's control of his diabetes?

REVIEW Diabetes

RELATE Link the Concepts and Exemplars

Linking the exemplar of diabetes with the concept of development:

1. In consideration of development, how would you approach diabetes teaching for an 8-year-old?

2. Based on developmental level, how would your teaching of a 15-year-old about diabetes differ from your teaching of an adult?

Linking the exemplar of diabetes with the concept of sensory perception:

3. When caring for a client with diabetic neuropathy, what teaching would you provide to reduce the risk of injury?

4. When caring for a client with diabetic retinopathy, what strategies would you teach to facilitate a normal standard of living for the client?

READY Go to Companion Skills Manual

REFER Go to Pearson Nursing Student Resources
nursing.pearsonhighered.com

- Additional review material

REFLECT Case Study

Norma James is a 65-year-old widow who lives alone. She has a long history of type 2 DM and hypertension. Ms. James is not employed; she has very limited savings and relies on Social Security benefits for income. She smokes about half a pack of cigarettes a day and has been a smoker since she was in her 20s.

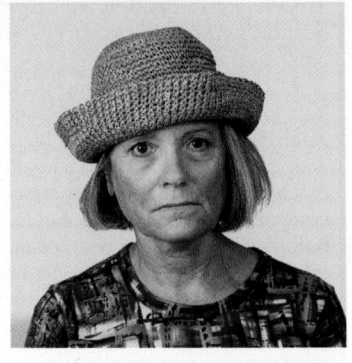

She drinks alcohol "a couple times a year, usually a glass of wine at a special dinner."

Ms. James has a sore on her ankle that she has noticed for the last several months. The sore does not really hurt much, but she has been unable to get it to heal. The cashier at the convenience store tells her that she should use butter to help heal wounds, because the butter keeps the wound moist and helps to enhance healing.

Ms. James decides to follow the cashier's advice and applies butter to her wound for about a week. The wound does not seem to be getting any better; in fact, it looks worse. It now has a yellowish drainage, and the skin around the wound has become red. Her foot also hurts when she walks on it. Ms. James stops the butter treatment and goes to the emergency department.

1. What are the priority nursing diagnoses for Ms. James?

2. What discharge teaching will you provide her?

3. How can you advocate for Ms. James regarding required medical equipment, supplies, and medications and their cost on a limited budget?

4. What expectation would you anticipate for Ms. James regarding follow up care?

EXEMPLAR 12.2 Diabetes in Children

EXEMPLAR KEY TERMS
Acanthosis nigricans, 773
Autoimmune disease, 767
Celiac disease, 771
C peptide, 769
Diabetes mellitus (DM), 766
Euglycemia, 768
Glucagon emergency kit, 778
Individualized education plan (IEP), 768
Maturity onset of diabetes in youth (MODY), 767
Neonatal diabetes mellitus (NDM), 767

EXEMPLAR LEARNING OUTCOMES
After reading about this exemplar, you will be able to:

1. Describe the pathophysiology, etiology, clinical manifestations, and direct and indirect causes of diabetes in children.

2. Identify risk factors and prevention methods associated with diabetes in children.

3. Illustrate the nursing process in providing culturally competent care for children with diabetes.

4. Formulate priority nursing diagnoses appropriate for a child with diabetes.

5. Summarize therapies used by interdisciplinary teams in the collaborative care of a child with diabetes.

6. Plan evidence-based care for a child with diabetes and his or her family in collaboration with other members of the healthcare team.

7. Evaluate expected outcomes for a child with diabetes.

▶ OVERVIEW

Diabetes mellitus (DM) is a disorder of metabolism that results in hyperglycemia due to a defect in insulin secretion, insulin action, or both. Refer to the Concept of Metabolism at the beginning of this module for further discussion of the role of hormones and blood glucose homeostasis in diabetes. Diabetes in children is classified as type 1, type 2, and other (MODY and NDM). Approximately 215,000 individuals in the United States younger than age 20 have DM, either type 1 or type 2. This

number represents 0.26% of all individuals in this age group. Estimates of undiagnosed diabetes are unavailable for this group. Type 1 DM is the leading type of diabetes in children younger than 10. Type 2 DM usually occurs in children and adolescents ages 10–19. MODY and NDM are rare, with an incidence of 1%–5% of all cases of diabetes in young individuals (see **Box 12–3** ●). Whatever its etiology, diabetes remains the leading cause of kidney failure, nontraumatic lower limb amputation, and new cases of blindness in the United States. Diabetes is still considered the major cause of heart disease and stroke; it

Box 12–3 MODY and NDM

Maturity onset diabetes in youth (MODY) and **neonatal diabetes mellitus (NDM)** are considered rare forms of diabetes that come from a mutation of a single gene that results in faulty insulin secretion. They are often referred to as monogenic. Most mutations of monogenic diabetes reduce the body's ability to produce insulin.

NDM is a rare condition in which the infant does not produce enough insulin. NDM occurs in only 1 in 100,000–500,000 live births. MODY usually first occurs during adolescence or early adulthood but sometimes is not diagnosed until later in life. The gene mutations that cause MODY limit the ability of the pancreas to produce insulin. MODY accounts for 1%–5% of cases of diabetes in the United States (National Diabetes Information Clearinghouse, 2007).

The risk factors for MODY and NDM are strongly genetic in origin. Family members of individuals with MODY are at greatly increased risk for developing this type of diabetes (National Diabetes Information Clearinghouse, 2007). In children with the monogenic forms of diabetes, testing includes providing a blood sample from which DNA is isolated. The physician decides if this test is required. A correct diagnosis based on appropriate testing can lead to optimal treatment.

is the seventh leading cause of death in the United States (National Diabetes Information Clearinghouse, 2011). This exemplar discusses diabetes mellitus in children and adolescents; its manifestations, treatment, and implications; and the role that the nurse plays in caring for children and adolescents with diabetes.

TYPE 1 DIABETES MELLITUS IN CHILDREN

Type 1 DM is an **autoimmune disease** (a disease that results from the immune system's failure to recognize itself, resulting in normal host tissues being targeted by immune defenses) in which the pancreatic islet cells are destroyed and there is an absolute deficiency of circulating insulin. The immunological process can occur years before the actual onset of symptoms. The episode of acute onset of hyperglycemia is a result of the destruction of most of the beta cells. New-onset type 1 DM manifests as diabetic ketoacidosis in nearly one third of clients and requires medical intervention when first diagnosed (Rewers et al., 2008).

CASE STUDY \\ PART 1

Lydia Moreland is a 6-year-old female who was diagnosed with type 1 diabetes 3 months ago. She developed nausea and vomiting and complained of thirst. Her mother noted that Lydia was lethargic and sleepy and was frequently going to the bathroom for about 1 week leading up to the acute event. Lydia was admitted to the hospital with new-onset type 1 diabetes and DKA after going to the local urgent care with the listed symptoms.

Clinical Reasoning Questions Level I

1. Discuss the differences between type 1 and type 2 diabetes.
2. What blood tests do you expect will be done on Lydia when she is first admitted to the hospital?
3. What are the priority nursing interventions for Lydia while she has DKA?

▶ RISK FACTORS

The risk factors for type 1 DM are a combination of genetic and environmental factors. A genetic marker has been identified that makes an individual more susceptible to type 1 DM. Other risk factors that have been identified include race, ethnicity, and family history. The one proven environmental trigger of type 1 DM is congenital rubella, although other potential environmental triggers have been identified, such as enteroviral infections, casein, and cereals. Another trigger that is being researched is low levels of vitamin D in early life (Couper & Donaghue, 2009).

CASE STUDY \\ PART 2

Three days later Lydia's DKA is resolved, and she is feeling much better. Her mother is at her bedside and is telling you that she blames herself for Lydia's diabetes. She should have known that it was diabetes because she has type 2 DM. She asks you if it is possible that Lydia got the diabetes from her.

Clinical Reasoning Questions Level II

1. How would you answer Lydia's mother's question?
2. Lydia is a smart 6-year-old and wants to begin checking her own sugars and giving her own injections. How would you go about teaching her? Apply your previous knowledge about child developmental stages to develop the plan for teaching.
3. What glucose targets will you review with Lydia and her mother?

▶ CLINICAL MANIFESTATIONS

The clinical manifestations of all forms of diabetes in children are hyperglycemia, which includes increased thirst, hunger, urination, fatigue, and blurred vision (see **Figure 12–7** ●). Weight loss is an additional symptom in children with type 1 DM. The clinical manifestations of type 1 DM usually appear as an acute event that requires emergency intervention. Some 20%–25% of all diabetic ketoacidosis (DKA) cases are due to new-onset diabetes. DKA is caused by an absolute lack of insulin and, although research studies have found some measurable insulin concentrations, the levels are inadequate to meet the metabolic needs of the child. The clinical hallmarks of DKA are dehydration and electrolyte imbalance.

Speedy diagnosis and treatment are required to prevent further deterioration. Therapy is aimed at correcting the metabolic

Focus on Diversity and Culture
Risk of Diabetes in Children

In the United States, non-Hispanic White youth have the highest rate of new cases of type 1 DM: 24.8 per 100,000 each year among those younger than 10 years old, and 22.6 per 100,000 per year among those ages 10–19.

Type 2 DM rates are greater among youth ages 10–19 than in younger children, with higher rates among U.S. minority populations than in non-Hispanic Whites.

For Asian/Pacific Islander Americans and American Indian youth, the rate of new cases of diabetes is greater for type 2 than for type 1 (National Diabetes Information Clearinghouse, 2011).

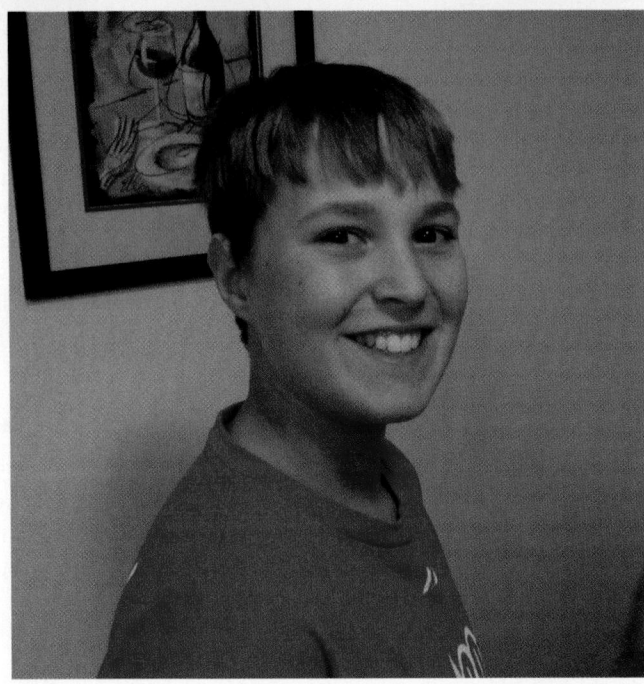
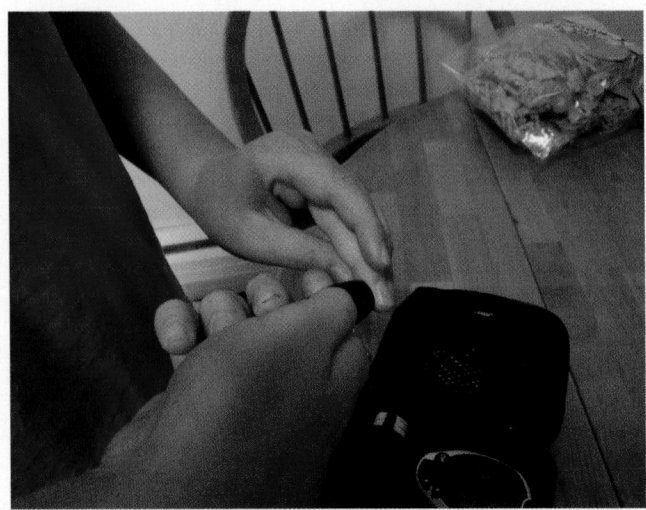

Figure 12–7 ● Six months ago, Ethan, 11 years old, was going for an annual physical, and his grandmother, a retired nurse, noted to his parents that Ethan was often tired and very thirsty; she suggested the family discuss these symptoms with Ethan's pediatrician. By that evening, Ethan was in the emergency department having his blood sugar regulated, and the family spent the next day at a specialized center learning how to manage his newly diagnosed Type 1 diabetes mellitus. Today, Ethan is thriving. He tests his glucose level frequently, and injects himself with insulin four times a day: at breakfast, lunch, and dinner, and at bedtime. He is very careful with his diet and he maintains an active lifestyle. He knows that if his glucose level is high, he needs to drink water and let a responsible adult know.

acidosis, restoring fluid and electrolyte balance, and achieving **euglycemia** (a normal concentration of glucose in the blood). The frequent blood sugar monitoring, IV fluids, and insulin drips required for treatment mandate that the child be cared for in an intensive care environment until stabilized.

▶ COLLABORATION

To achieve optimal glycemic control and prevent acute complications, children with diabetes require a dedicated and knowledgeable team of caretakers. The team consists of a primary care provider (who may be an endocrinologist or a family physician with training in childhood diabetes), a dietitian, a certified diabetes educator, a school nurse, and trained personnel who may be involved in the daily activities of the child in school or day care. The team may also include a social worker or psychologist with education in behavioral modification to address problems that may arise in dealing with a chronic disease in childhood. It is imperative that there be a team approach involving open communication within the group. A plan of care is developed by the primary care provider, the certified diabetes educator, and the parents and child (if appropriate) and is disseminated to the other team members.

Federal laws that protect children with diabetes include Rehabilitation Act of 1973, the Individuals with Disabilities Education Act of 1990 (reauthorized most recently in 2004) and the Americans with Disabilities Act of 1990. Any school or day care that is open to the public must provide for the special needs of the child with diabetes by providing a written **individualized education plan (IEP)** that is developed in partnership with the child's parents and, if the child is old enough, the child.

The child must be allowed to participate in all sports and extracurricular activities that are available at the school or day care (see Section 504 of the Rehabilitation Act of 1973). It is important for parents, school personnel, and the child's treatment team to work together to ensure both the child's health and safety at school and the child's potential for success in the school environment, whether in the class or on the field. A summary of the responsibilities of parents and schools is provided in **Table 12–5** ●. Information on sick-day management is provided in the Concept of Metabolism at the beginning of this module.

Often the nurse is called on to coordinate care for the child with diabetes. It is essential that the nurse be able to work collaboratively with other members of the healthcare team, the family, and an appropriate representative of the child's school. Skilled collaboration and communication on the part of the nurse minimizes risk of harm to the child and ensures that a client-centered plan of care is followed and revised as necessary to support the child's ongoing development and changing interests.

CASE STUDY \\ PART 3

Lydia is discharged at the end of week 1. Her mother is concerned about letting her go back to school, although the doctor has cleared Lydia to return to school. Lydia's mother calls you for advice.

Clinical Reasoning Questions Level II

1. What questions would be important to ask Lydia's mother before offering any advice?

2. What other members of the team could help Lydia's mother cope with the return to school, and how could the nurse facilitate this communication?

TABLE 12–5 Responsibilities of Parents and Schools/Day Care Programs

PARENT /GUARDIAN	SCHOOL OR DAY CARE PROGRAM
Parents are responsible for providing the school with all the information necessary to care for the child during regular and extracurricular activities. Parents should: ■ Create a diabetes management plan with the school. ■ Provide equipment such as glucose meter, insulin, log books, treatment for hypoglycemia (glucagon injection, oral treatment). ■ Maintenance of the supplies ■ Share the individual diabetes medical management plan (IDDMP) signed by the child's personal healthcare team ■ Provide information about diabetes ■ Provide emergency phone numbers ■ Provide a release-of-confidentiality form signed by the legal guardian to facilitate communication of the school personnel with the medical and nursing team	Schools and day care programs are responsible for providing a safe, healthy environment and should: ■ Provide an opportunity for staff to stay informed about diabetes ■ Provide training for school personnel at a level appropriate to their responsibility. ■ Designate trained diabetes personnel ■ Assist students with performing diabetes care tasks ■ Provide accessibility to scheduled insulin at times set out in the student's IDDMP. ■ Provide privacy for checking blood sugars. ■ If appropriate, obtain permission for the child to monitor and treat hypoglycemia independently. ■ Ensure that the school nurse and a backup are trained to intervene for the student in situations such as hypoglycemia or hyperglycemia ■ Give permission as appropriate for the student to carry equipment to self-treat if needed ■ Allow the student to eat snacks in school ■ Allow the child to miss school without consequences for illness or required medical appointments. ■ Give permission for the child to use the restroom and have access to fluids as necessary. ■ Provide an appropriate location for the equipment supplied by the parent or guardian, as well as a plan for safe disposal of sharps. ■ Provide information about the school menu that includes nutrient content.

Source: Based on American Diabetes Association. (2011a). *Diabetes care in the school and day care setting.* Retrieved from http://care.diabetesjournals.org/content/29/suppl_1/s49.full; Centers for Disease Control and Prevention. (2013). Help your child manage diabetes at school. Retrieved from http://www.cdc.gov/Features/DiabetesInSchool/; National Diabetes Education Program. (2012). Helping the students with diabetes succeed: A guide for school personnel. Retrieved from http://ndep.nih.gov/publications/PublicationDetail.aspx?PubId=97#effectivediabetesmanagement; National Diabetes Education Program. (n.d.). School responsibilities under federal laws. Retrieved from http://ndep.nih.gov/media/school-guide-responsibilities-508.pdfl

3. Lydia has been having very high blood sugars every morning even though her blood sugars are in target when she goes to bed. Her mother is very concerned. What appropriate advice could you give Lydia's mother?

Diagnostic Tests

A hemoglobin (A_{1C}) level of 6.5% or higher in combination with a random blood plasma glucose level of 200 mg/dL or higher or a fasting plasma glucose of 126 gm/dL or higher confirms the presence of diabetes. Fasting is defined as no caloric intake for at least 8 hours.

In children with type 1 DM, the diagnosis may be confirmed by the presence of autoantibodies to glutamic acid decarboxylase, pancreatic islet beta cells (tyrosine phosphatase IA-2), and/or insulin. Some forms of type 1 DM have no evidence of autoimmunity and are termed idiopathic. Type 1 DM can also occur in obese children, and documentation of **C peptide** levels (which indicate the activity of the pancreatic beta cells) and the presence or absence of immune markers along with a careful family history and evaluation of presenting symptoms may be useful to the physician in attaining the correct diagnosis. This will be helpful in distinguishing type 1 DM from type 2 DM in children when there is a need (AACE, 2011).

Glucose Monitoring

Children require more frequent glucose monitoring than adults and have different targets due to erratic oral intake and activity. See **Table 12–6** ●.

Insulin

For clients with type 1 DM, exogenous insulin is a lifelong requirement. However, children who are newly diagnosed may go through a partial remission phase when blood sugars are close to normal with smaller amounts of insulin. It is believed that this phenomenon results from activation of the remaining beta cells, and scientists now think that it is important for clients in this honeymoon phase to continue taking insulin by injection to preserve the remaining beta cells for as long as possible (Joslin Diabetes Center, 2011).

Daily insulin dosage for children depends on many factors, including age, weight, stage of puberty, duration and phase of diabetes, state of injection sites, nutritional intake and distribution, exercise patterns, daily routine, results of glucose monitoring, and comorbid illness. See **Table 12–7** ● for recommended doses based on body weight. The correct dose is the dose that achieves the best control for a child without causing hypoglycemia and that at the same time allows healthy progression and growth according to the weight and height charts. For information on how insulin is administered, please see the exemplar on Diabetes in this module. Continuous subcutaneous insulin infusion (CSII) devices (insulin pumps) are fairly popular with young individuals (**Box 12–4** ●).

In addition to the correct daily insulin dosage determined for the child, an additional amount of insulin may need to be administered with a meal based on the child's premeal blood glucose level. This additional amount of insulin is referred to as the *correction factor* and is given to reach the postmeal glucose target (Osborn, Wraa, & Watson, 2014). The healthcare team works with the child to determine the correction factor.

The child and parents also need to learn how to adjust the amount of rapid insulin necessary to cover carbohydrate (CHO)

Evidence-Based Practice Managing Diabetes at School

Problem

Children and adolescents with type 1 diabetes face a number of hurdles in managing their health at school. What is their experience at school and what problems do they face that might benefit from nursing intervention?

Evidence

A study was conducted to evaluate the experience of children and adolescents with type 1 diabetes mellitus in school by surveying clients, parents or guardians, and school personnel. This study was limited to students with type 1 DM. The topics surveyed included overall perceptions of experiences of children and adolescents in the school; time and facility allowance for diabetes self-management; nutritional services; emotional distress of the child; adequacy of school personnel training for diabetes management; school preparedness for emergencies; school policies; and perception of supportiveness of schools in dealing with illnesses and missed school days. The study showed that the majority of children and adolescents surveyed felt that they were treated differently in schools because of their diabetes. It also showed that their perceived experiences and those of the parents were generally good. The researchers state that this is an improvement over earlier surveys. The following ongoing problems were identified:

1. Inadequacy of training for personnel to handle hypoglycemia and emergencies
2. Absence or lack of standardization of individualized diabetes care plans among school systems
3. Inadequate numbers of school nurses

4. Inadequate nutritional information given to parents so they can help the child plan insulin dosing

This study was conducted in Ohio, and the researchers indicated that there are differences from state to state in implementation of the federal regulations regarding the individualized care plan for children with diabetes. They plan to do a national survey using the Children with Diabetes Web site to identify region-specific problems (Schwartz et al., 2010).

Implications

This study highlights the importance of properly trained school personnel, use of diabetes care plans, and adequate information on school meal planning for parents. Nurses working with children with diabetes and their families must ensure that appropriate nutrition education is provided to families and schools and that each child has a care plan for use at school or day care. Nurses can increase the likelihood of properly trained school personnel by advocating for their clients with their schools.

Critical Thinking Application

1. Identify some of the possible barriers to training school personnel regarding care of children with diabetes in the school, and suggest some ways that these obstacles could be overcome.
2. There has been a significant improvement in nutrition in schools over the last five years, but problems remain. Identify some other improvements and possible ways to bring about their implementation that could help children with diabetes and other children have a healthier lifestyle while at school.

TABLE 12–6   Plasma Blood Glucose and Hemoglobin A_{1C} Goals for Type 1 DM by Age Group

	PLASMA BLOOD GLUCOSE GOAL RANGE (MG/DL)		HEMOGLOBIN A_{1C} (%)	RATIONALE
	BEFORE MEALS	BEDTIME/ OVERNIGHT		
Toddlers and preschoolers (0–6 years)	100–180	110–200	<8.5	Vulnerability to hypoglycemia Insulin sensitivity Unpredictability in dietary intake and physical activity A lower goal (<8.0%) is reasonable if it can be achieved without excessive hypoglycemia.
School age (6–12 years)	90–180	100–180	<8	Vulnerability to hypoglycemia A lower goal (<7.5%) is reasonable if it can be achieved without excessive hypoglycemia.
Adolescents and young adults (13–19 years)	90–130	90–150	<7.5	A lower goal (<7.0%) is reasonable if it can be achieved without excessive hypoglycemia.

Key concepts in setting glycemic goals:
- Goals should be individualized and lower goals may be reasonable based on benefit–risk assessment.
- Blood glucose goals should be modified in children with frequent hypoglycemia or hypoglycemia unawareness.
- Postprandial blood glucose values should be measured when there is a discrepancy between preprandial blood glucose values and A_{1C} levels and to help assess glycemia in those on basal/bolus regimens.

Glycemic goals may need to be modified to take into account the fact that most children younger than age 6 or 7 have a form of "hypoglycemic unawareness." They lack the cognitive capacity to recognize and respond to hypoglycemic symptoms and may be at greater risk for hypoglycemia. Children under 5 years of age may be at risk for permanent cognitive impairment after episodes of severe hypoglycemia.

Sources: Based on International Diabetes Federation. (2011). Global IDF/ISPAD Guideline for Diabetes in Childhood and Adolescence. Retrieved from http://www.idf.org/sites/default/files/Diabetes-in-Childhood-and-Adolescence-Guidelines.pdf; National Diabetes Education Program. (2011). *Overview of diabetes in children and adolescents.* Available at http://ndep.nih.gov/media/youth_factsheet.pdf; American Diabetes Association. (2005). Standards of medical care in diabetes. *Diabetes Care, 28*(suppl 1), 54-536; Diabetes Mellitus.

TABLE 12–7   Recommended Insulin Doses for Children with Type 1 DM

During the partial remission phase (honeymoon)	Total daily dose <0.5 Units/kg/day
Prepubertal children (outside partial remission phase)	Total daily dose 0.7–1.0 units/kg/day
Puberty (usually requires substantial increase)	Total daily dose 1–2 units/kg/day

Source: Bangstad, H.-J., Deeb, L. C., Jarosz-Chobot, P., Urakami, T., & Hanas, R. (2009). Insulin treatment in children and adolescents with diabetes. *Pediatric Diabetes, 10*(12), 82–99. doi: 10.1111/j.1399-5448.2009.00578.x.

intake at a meal. The insulin-to-CHO ratio (I:C) may differ according to meal and activity level. The healthcare team or certified diabetes educator works with the child and family to determine appropriate ratios and to teach them how to calculate these ratios for different situations (McDermott, 2010; Osborn, Wraa, & Watson, 2014).

Nutrition Therapy

Dietary recommendations for children with diabetes are based on healthy eating guidelines that are also suitable for all children and adults. (See **Table 12–8** ● for age-specific nutrition recommendations for children with type 1 diabetes.)

Managing Complications

Although the complications of diabetes for adults are very closely related to those for children, a few specific complications are more prevalent in children with diabetes. **Celiac disease**, an immune-mediated disorder characterized by the inability to hydrolyze peptides contained in gluten, occurs with increased frequency in individuals with type 1 DM (1%–16% of individuals compared with 0.3%–1% of the general population). Celiac disease (also called *nontropical sprue*) may be asymptomatic, but general symptoms include poor growth, delayed puberty, nutritional deficiencies, and hypoglycemia. A gluten-free diet is the only accepted treatment for celiac disease (ADA, 2011b).

Box 12–4   Insulin Pumps

Continuous subcutaneous insulin infusion (CSII) devices, often referred to as *insulin pumps*, are widely used among young individuals with diabetes, in part because they have been shown to improve glycemic control in those with type 1 DM (Nimri et al., 2006). The insulin pump is a battery-operated device about the size of a small pager that delivers insulin to the client subcutaneously. It is composed of a pump reservoir (which holds the insulin) that is connected to a tube called an *infusion set*. The tube is connected to a cannula that is inserted into the skin and changed every 2–3 days. Through the infusion set and cannula, insulin is delivered in microliter amounts continuously over 24 hours. Several different companies produce insulin pumps, and the technology is changing rapidly. There are now insulin pumps that communicate with a glucose meter so that the client does not have to enter the blood sugar into the insulin pump to deliver the insulin needed to correct blood glucose. However, the client must enter the carbohydrate amount in grams to deliver the amount of insulin to cover the food eaten. The client still has control over when and what dose to deliver based on preset figures in the pump as determined by the client, family, and healthcare team (McDermott, 2010).

Another autoimmune disorder that occurs with increased frequency in individuals with type 1 diabetes is thyroid disease. It occurs in 17%–30% of clients with type 1 diabetes. The thyroid dysfunction is usually hypothyroidism, but the autoimmune disorder may be expressed as the less common hyperthyroidism.

TABLE 12–8   Age-Specific Nutritional Recommendations

AGE	NUTRITIONAL RECOMMENDATIONS
Infants and toddlers	■ Breastfeeding of infants up to 12 months should be encouraged. ■ Frequent small meals (grazing) may promote better glycemic control. Care must be taken to match the feeding schedule and the insulin. ■ Insulin pump therapy has proven to be effective in infants and toddlers and reduces the trauma of frequent injections. Rapid-acting insulin as a bolus is usually given after the meal so a more accurate estimation of insulin dosing to match food intake can occur. ■ A variety of tastes, colors, and textures of foods should be encouraged while considering personal and cultural preferences. ■ Episodes of food refusal and sickness often cause parental distress. Support from the healthcare team is essential.
School children	■ The focus is on adapting the diabetes regimen to fit the active life of the schoolchild. Advice should be given regarding carbohydrate intake to prevent hypoglycemia and how to adjust insulin and intake when sports activities are involved. ■ Sleepover and party advice should be discussed by the team. ■ Special occasions like birthdays and Halloween should be discussed by the team. ■ Frequent consults with a pediatric nutritionist help in the problem solving in this age group.
Adolescents	■ Weight monitoring is recommended for early recognition of both weight loss and inappropriate weight gain, which may be associated with insulin omission for weight control or may be indicative of an eating disorder. ■ Teach adolescents how to read food labels to help plan carbohydrate intake. ■ Meals and snacks should be eaten at the same time each day. However, erratic eating behavior is not uncommon among adolescents. Parties, vacations, and peer pressure may all contribute. ■ Advise on how to make healthy choices in restaurants. ■ Advice on safe consumption of alcohol and the risk of prolonged hypoglycemia is important.

Source: Based on MedlinePlus. (2013). *Diabetes diet—type 1.* Retrieved from http://www.nlm.nih.gov/medlineplus/ency/article/002440.htm; Smart, C., Aslander-van Vilet, E., & Waldron, S. (2009). Nutritional management in children and adolescents with diabetes. *Pediatric Diabetes, 10*(12), 100–117; KidsHealth. (n.d.). *Eating out when you have diabetes.* Retrieved from http://kidshealth.org/kid/diabetes_basics/diabetes-nutrition/eating_out_diabetes.html?tracking=K_RelatedArticle; Ayling, R. (2012). Nutritional Management of diabetes mellitus in infants and children. In Watson, R.R., Grimble, G., Preedy, V.R., & Zibaldi, S. (Eds). *Nutrition in Infancy.* New York, NY: Springer.

Eating disorders are another possible complication of type 1 and type 2 diabetes in children. When hyperglycemia is present, calories are lost and weight loss occurs; therefore diabetes is unique in that body weight and shape can be altered by stopping insulin. The risks are obvious, but it has been found that insulin omission for weight control occurs in 12%–15% of adolescents. Recognition of this potential disorder by the nurse and reporting to the appropriate caregiver can prevent further deterioration in glycemic control for the adolescent with type 1 diabetes mellitus (Rewers et al., 2009).

Another serious acute complication of diabetes in children is frequent and severe hypoglycemia. Children are at higher risk for hypoglycemia than adults because of children's erratic nutritional intake and increased activity levels and growth spurts. Insulin or oral medication error in dose administration is also implicated as a cause of frequent hypoglycemia. Postexercise hypoglycemia can occur several hours after the activity due to continued uptake of glucose in the muscles in relation to the presence of circulating insulin from the injections. The child and parents must be aware that the adjustment of insulin doses and frequent glucose monitoring prevent profound and unpredictable hypoglycemic events.

In adolescents and young adults, alcohol use and diabetes present a special concern. Alcohol use in combination with oral hypoglycemic medication and/or insulin can result in profound hypoglycemia (see **Box 12–5** ●). This result may occur many hours after alcohol intake due to impaired mobilization of glycogen stores as the liver detoxifies the alcohol and to the impairment of counterregulatory hormones. Clients in these age groups should be cautioned against drinking alcohol, but if they choose to do so, so they should make sure they eat food to accompany the alcohol.

The long-term complications of diabetes remain the same for children as for adults with this lifelong disease. Those living with diabetes are at increased risk for alterations in the cardiovascular system, including coronary artery disease, hypertension, stroke, and peripheral vascular disease. Diabetic retinopathy, diabetic nephropathy, peripheral and visceral neuropathies, and periodontal disease are also concerns. Individuals with diabetes are at increased risk for amputation of a lower extremity, and that risk increases for individuals who have lived with diabetes for more than 10 years. Monitoring blood pressure and lipid levels is essential to lowering long-term risks for children with diabetes. **Table 12–9** ● outlines screening and treatment recommendations.

Box 12–5   Alcohol and Hypoglycemia

There are several reasons why hypoglycemia may occur with alcohol use (ADA, 2013):

- Even small amounts of alcohol may impair someone's ability to detect the onset of hypoglycemia and therefore take appropriate action to correct it.
- Other individuals may mistake hypoglycemia for intoxication.
- Alcohol has been shown to impair the hormonal counterregulatory responses to low blood glucose levels.
- Small amounts of alcohol can augment the cognitive deficits associated with hypoglycemia in individuals with type 1 diabetes.
- Alcohol use may be associated with a delayed effect that increases the risk of next-day hypoglycemia.

Complementary and Alternative Therapy

Regardless of the type of diabetes, the cornerstones for diabetes management in children are diet, exercise, medication (insulin and/or oral medications), and glucose monitoring. However, many individuals have chosen to use complementary and alternative medicine (CAM) to enhance their diabetes management. The 2007 National Health Interview Survey gathered information on CAM use among more than 9,000 children younger than age 18 (National Center for Complementary and Alternative Medicine, 2008). Nearly 12% of the children had used some form of CAM during the past 12 months. CAM use was more prevalent in children whose parents used alternative therapies. Many complementary and alternative therapies have no basis in scientific evidence. A key point to remember in using alternative therapies in children is that, because of their age, children may react to therapies differently than adults. It is important that parents of children who have chosen to use CAM communicate this choice to the physician and diabetes educator to ensure safe and coordinated care. In turn, nurses and healthcare providers should assess the client for use of CAM therapies at each medical interaction.

Some of the more prevalent therapies are dietary supplements such as alpha-lipoic acid, chromium, omega-3 fatty acids, polyphenols, garlic, magnesium, coenzyme Q10, ginseng, and vanadium. Some botanicals have been used, such as prickly pear cactus, gurmar, *Coccinia indica*, aloe vera, fenugreek, and bitter melon, but as with other CAM supplements, there is limited research on their effectiveness in adults and even less information on their use in children (National Center for Complementary and Alternative Medicine, 2013).

Perhaps the most widely studied CAM for diabetes is the use of cinnamon. Abstract cinnamon, the dry bark and twig of *Cinnamomum* species, is a rich botanical source of polyphenols that have been used for centuries in Chinese medicine and have been shown to affect blood glucose and insulin signaling. Although a meta analysis conducted by the University of California–Davis Department of Nutrition yielded positive results regarding the ability of cinnamon to lower blood sugar, the results still remain unclear (P. A. Davis & Yokoyama, 2011). As with all CAM usage, more research is warranted, and any choice to use cinnamon as an alternative or complementary therapy should be made under the guidance of the physician.

TYPE 2 DIABETES MELLITUS IN CHILDREN

Type 2 DM in children is thought to be increasing because of the rise in obesity and inactivity in today's youth. As in adult type 2 DM, insulin resistance leads to pancreatic fatigue as the organ attempts to keep up with insulin production. When the need for insulin can no longer be met, hyperglycemia occurs. Type 2 DM is more common in certain ethnic groups (see the Focus on Diversity and Culture feature).

TABLE 12–9 Screening and Treatment Recommendations for Children With Type 1 Diabetes

	SCREENING RECOMMENDATIONS	TREATMENT RECOMMENDATIONS
Nephropathy	■ At age 10 with diabetes for 5 years: annual screening for microalbuminuria with a random spot sample for albumin-to-creatinine ratio (ACR)	■ Confirmed, persistently elevated ACR on two additional urine specimens from different days can be treated with an ACE inhibitor.
Hypertension	■ Hypertension is defined as an average systolic and diastolic blood pressure greater than the 90th percentile for age, sex, and height measured on at least three separate days. Normal blood pressure for age, sex, and height, with treatment options is available at www.nhlbi.nih.gov/	■ Treatment for high normal blood pressure (above the 90th percentile) should include dietary intervention and exercise. If target blood pressure is not reached within 3–6 months of lifestyle intervention, pharmacologic treatment with ACE inhibitors should be considered. ■ The goal of treatment is to have the blood pressure less than 130/80 or below the 90th percentile for age.
Dyslipidemia	■ Assess for family history of elevated total cholesterol or an early cardiac event. If present or if no family history is known, a fasting lipid profile should be done on children older than age 2. ■ If there is no family concern, the first screening can take place at puberty or approximately 10 years of age. ■ Abnormal lipid profiles should be monitored annually. ■ If lipids are normal, monitor every 5 years.	■ Initial treatment of elevated lipids is the optimization of glucose. ■ After glucose control is achieved, initial treatment of elevated lipid profile includes medical nutrition therapy and following the diet and lifestyle recommendations approved by the American Heart Association (AHA). ■ If the introduction of lifestyle changes fails to correct the problem, statin therapy is reasonable in children over the age of 10 years. ■ The goal is an LDL of less than 100 mg/dL.
Retinopathy recommendations	■ The first ophthalmological exam should occur once the child is 10 years of age and has had diabetes for 3–5 years.	■ Treatment depends on findings and recommendation by the ophthalmologist.
Thyroid disorders	■ Children with type 1 diabetes should be screened for thyroid perioxidase and thyroglobulin antibodies at diagnosis. ■ TSH should be measured after metabolic control is established and then, if normal, rechecked every 1–2 years or if symptoms are present.	■ Treatment depends on findings and symptoms of thyroid disorder.
Celiac disease	■ Children with type 1 diabetes should be screened for celiac disease by measuring transglutaminase or anti-endomysial antibodies with documentation of normal serum IgE levels. ■ Testing should also be done in children with signs and symptoms of celiac disease or in children with frequent unexplained hypoglycemia or deterioration in glucose control.	■ Children with positive antibodies should be referred to a gastroenterologist. ■ Children with biopsy-confirmed celiac disease should be placed on a gluten-free diet, and a dietitian should be consulted who is experienced in dealing with both celiac disease and diabetes.
Psychosocial assessment and care	■ Assessment of psychological and social situation, attitudes about the illness, affect, mood, and psychiatric history should be part of the ongoing care.	■ When glucose management is poor, screening for depression and diabetes-related stress, anxiety, and eating disorders is appropriate.

Source: Adapted from American Diabetes Association (2011b). *Standards of medical care.* Retrieved from http://care.diabetesjournals.org/content/34/Supplement_1/S11.full.pdf+html.

▶ RISK FACTORS

The risk factors for type 2 DM for children are similar to those for adults. Gender (usually female) and being overweight, having a family member who has the disorder, being a member of a high-risk ethnic group, showing signs of insulin resistance, being ages 10–19, and experiencing puberty have all been listed as potential risk factors for type 2 DM in children (Semb, 2008).

Focus on Diversity and Culture
Obesity in Children

In the past 10 years, the rapid increase in obesity among children and teens apparent in the 1980s and 1990s has slowed. However, the heaviest boys are getting heavier, and Hispanic boys and non-Hispanic Black girls are disproportionately affected by obesity (CDC, 2011a).

▶ CLINICAL MANIFESTATIONS

The symptoms of type 2 DM may be less acute than those of type 1 DM, presenting with a range of symptoms that are related to hyperglycemia and that may vary in severity and may include weight gain. Another presenting symptom in children with type 2 DM is the marker of insulin resistance typified by skin changes. **Acanthosis nigricans** is a condition in which the skin is velvety in texture and brownish black in color with hyperkeratotic plaques. Acanthosis nigricans usually appears in the

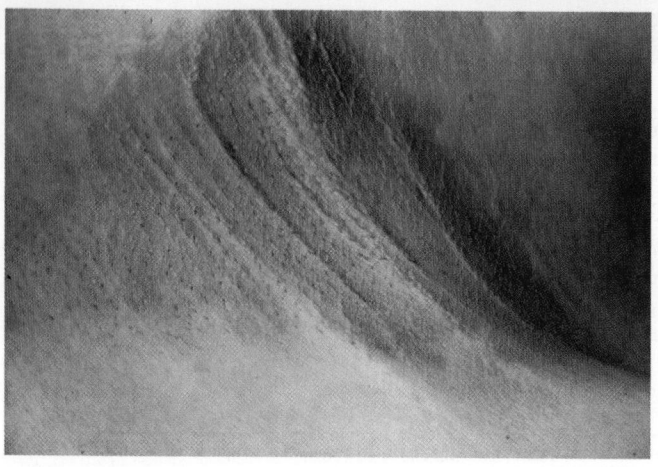

Figure 12–8 ● Acanthosis nigricans.
Source: © Wellcome Image Library/Custom Medical Stock Photo.

folds of the skin, especially in the neck, thigh, axillae, and knuckles (**Figure 12–8 ●**). It is believed to be related to direct and indirect activation of IGF-1 (insulin-like growth factor) receptors that results in proliferation of keratinocytes and fibroblasts. The skin appears dark and thick. There may also be darkening of the mucous membranes, eyelids, and nail beds (Nimblett, 2011).

For many illnesses, there is a major distinction between screening and diagnostic testing. However, for diabetes the same tests are used for both screening and diagnosis (ADA, 2011b). Furthermore, no separate tests are done for children with type 2 diabetes. Children and youth at risk for type 2 DM should be tested in the healthcare setting. Testing for type 2 diabetes in asymptomatic children follows these recommendations from ADA:

- Overweight (BMI >85th percentile for age and sex; weight for height, >85th percentile; or weight >120% of ideal weight for height) plus any two of the following risk factors:
  a. Family history of type 2 diabetes in first- or second-degree relative

b. Race/ethnicity (Native American, African American, Latino, Asian American, Pacific Islander)
c. Signs of insulin resistance or conditions associated with insulin resistance [acanthosis nigricans, hypertension, dyslipidemia, polycystic ovary syndrome (PCOS), or small-for-gestational-age birth weight]
d. Maternal history of diabetes or diabetes during the child's gestation

There are currently no national recommendations for blood glucose targets for children with type 2 DM. It is considered acceptable to use the targets discussed in the section on type 1 DM, adjusting for the individual child.

▶ COLLABORATION

Children and adolescents with type 2 DM require the care of a collaborative team and careful communication among all adults caring for the child in any situation. Nutrition and exercise are the keystones for clinical management of type 2 DM in children and adolescents, even though there is little evidence regarding the nutritional treatment of type 2 DM in children. Therefore the recommendations from pediatric diabetologists are derived from a combination of recommendations for treatment of overweight and obese children, adults with type 2 DM, and children with type 1 DM. The overall goal of therapeutic intervention for children with type 2 DM is to achieve and maintain an age-appropriate BMI. The increase in the number of overweight youth has been associated with increased caloric intake and a sedentary lifestyle. Children with a BMI greater than the 85th percentile for age and sex should be counseled to increase activity and decrease intake of high-calorie foods while adequately meeting the nutrition needs of the growing child. Other goals include optimization of blood glucose and lipid and blood pressure values to prevent the long-term complications of diabetes (Peterson et al., 2007). Nutritional and activity guidelines for children with type 2 DM are found in **Table 12–10 ●**. Evidence-based interventions to reduce incidence of childhood obesity are shown in **Box 12–6 ●**.

TABLE 12–10	Nutritional and Activity Guidelines for Youth With Type 2 Diabetes
TARGET AREAS	**GUIDELINES**
Food modification	■ Individualize food intake based on age, sex and physical activity (should include consultation with dietitian and/or a certified diet educator [CDE]). ■ Limit snack intake (especially snacks with high sugar and fat content, such as potato chips, fast food, desserts). Consumption of sugar-free drinks in place of sweet drinks can be encouraged. ■ Provide a meal plan designed by a dietitian and/or CDE to include high-fiber foods, low-fat foods, and low-concentrated sugar. To prevent or treat hypoglycemia, sweet drinks such as 100% juice with no sugar added can also be included in the diet. ■ Both the child and the family should be included in the teaching regarding blood glucose levels and carbohydrate intake.
Physical activity	■ Physical activity should be at least 30–60 minutes per day most days of the week. ■ Limit sedentary activities such as watching TV and playing video games.
Psychosocial support	■ Encourage peer support groups and family participation in the lifestyle change. Children are not generally worried about long-term complications, so the change in lifestyle must be made attractive to them with exercises and foods that they will accept.

Box 12–6   Evidence-Based Interventions to Reduce Incidence of Childhood Obesity

In the United States, childhood obesity affects approximately 12.5 million children and teens (17% of the population). Changes in obesity prevalence from the 1960s show a rapid increase in the 1980s and 1990s, when prevalence among children and teens tripled. In the short term, obesity in children can lead to both psychological and physiological problems.

Although the prevalence of type 2 DM in teens is low, a recent report estimated that 15% of new diabetes cases among children and adolescents are type 2 DM. In the 1980s, type 2 DM in children was almost unheard of.

Environmental determinants of childhood obesity in the United States include shifts in food consumption, changes in physical activity levels, and higher levels of television viewing with marketing of food to children. The Centers for Disease Control and Prevention (CDC, 2011a) is focusing on using the best available evidence to implement intervention programs. The CDC states that for maximum population impact, the focus should be on strategies that alter food consumption and on physical activity environments where individuals live, learn, work, play and pray.

Examples of these evidence-based interventions include:

■ Encouraging breastfeeding in workplaces to increase the chances of mothers breastfeeding longer

■ Enacting regulations and policies that eliminate availability of high-sugar drinks in child care settings and at school events and after-school programs

■ Increasing activity levels by making it safer for children to bike or walk to school and increasing the quality of school physical education programs

Other changes are also under way and are strengthened by Michelle Obama's initiative to end childhood obesity in a generation with the Let's Move Program.

Critical Thinking Questions

1. What questions would you ask on assessment to determine whether a client consumes sugar-based drinks? What suggestions would you make for changing this habit?

2. What suggestions for increasing physical activity would you make to the family of a child who lives in a neighborhood that experiences a high degree of violence?

3. How can nurses advocate for safer neighborhoods? For changes in policies about menus and availability of sugar-based drinks in schools?

Source: CDC (2011a). Grand rounds: Childhood obesity in the United States. *Mortality and Morbidity Weekly Report, 60*(2).

Hypoglycemic Agents

Hypoglycemic agents are not the first-line therapy for children with type 2 diabetes. Instead, the focus is on decreased insulin sensitivity with advancing sexual maturity, physical growth, and the ability to provide self-management. However, diet and exercise alone are effective for metabolic control in less than 10% of those with type 2 DM, and an oral medication usually is required. Metformin (Glucophage) is an oral hypoglycemic agent approved for use in some children as an adjunct to diet and exercise (Wilson, Shannon, & Shields, 2012). If the onset of symptoms is severe and blood sugar is severely elevated, insulin may be initiated and metformin introduced after stability in glycemic control is achieved. Metformin needs about 4 weeks to take effect (Flint & Arsalian, 2011).

Managing Complications

Those who care for children and adolescents with type 2 diabetes face several potential challenges. Most diabetes training and education materials are designed for children and adolescents with type 1 diabetes. The emphasis on insulin and glucose monitoring may not be appropriate for youth with type 2 diabetes. Most medications used in type 2 diabetes have been tested for safety and efficacy only in individuals older than 18. The American Academy of Pediatrics has recommendations regarding comorbidity screening and management (Copeland, et al., 2013). They present therapeutic recommendations for the following complications: hypertension, dyslipidemia, retinopathy, microalbuminuria, and depression.

■ NURSING PROCESS

The child newly diagnosed with diabetes mellitus requires a nursing assessment of physiological as well as psychosocial, environmental, and developmental needs. On the basis of the assessment findings, the nurse can develop a plan of care that involves the parents and the child at every stage of the nursing process. Ongoing evaluation of interventions will help the child with diabetes to live a healthy and well-adjusted life (see **Table 12–11** ●).

Assessment

The child newly diagnosed with type 1 diabetes mellitus will most likely be seen first in the hospital. The immediate presenting symptoms and pathophysiology involved typically require emergency and possibly critical care intervention as the blood sugars and accompanying electrolyte imbalances are identified and corrected. (See **Box 12–7** ● for assessment and interventions for diabetic ketoacidosis.) As the child stabilizes, the nurse's assessment should focus on skills for survival for discharge, family stress and coping, and follow up. The child and/or parent must be assessed for the ability to administer insulin, identify and treat hypoglycemia, monitor blood sugars, and provide a diet appropriate to the diagnosis. The nurse should assess the family's stress level and make a referral to outside resources, such as counseling, if needed. It is not unusual for parents to blame themselves in the early days of diagnosis, fearing that they could have prevented this disease in some way.

Diagnoses

Many of the nursing diagnoses used for adults are applicable to children (depending on the age of the child). The priority nursing diagnoses for children with diabetes are:

■ *Knowledge Deficit*
■ *Ineffective Coping (family)*
■ *Ineffective Coping (individual)*
■ *Imbalanced Nutrition*
■ *Chronic Pain*
■ *Risk for Injury*
■ *Risk for Infection*
■ *Risk for Unstable Blood Glucose.*

(NANDA-I © 2012)

TABLE 12–11   Provider Schedule for Managing Type 2 Diabetes in Youth

TIME FRAME	TASKS
At diagnosis	■ Establish baseline hemoglobin A_{1C}, lipid profile (repeat every 3–5 years); eye exam. ■ Initiate diabetes education. ■ Administer psychosocial assessment. ■ Establish goals for care and discuss with child (if appropriate) and parents. ■ Evaluate for microalbuminuria. ■ Refer for nutrition therapy, behavioral therapy, and family and community support as needed.
Quarterly	■ Assess injection sites. ■ Assess psychosocial adjustment, self-management skills. ■ Assess dietary needs and physical activity levels. ■ Discuss tobacco, alcohol, and drug use. ■ Measure hemoglobin A_{1C} and fasting glucose levels. ■ Review glucose records.
Annually	■ Administer influenza vaccine. ■ Make physical assessment. ■ Evaluate for microalbuminuria. ■ Make foot assessment. ■ Refer for eye exam (ophthalmologist may recommend frequency).

Source: Adapted from Peterson, K., Silverstein, J., Kaufman, F., & Warren-Boulton, E. (2007). Management of type 2 diabetes in youth: An update. *American Family Physician, 76*(5), 658–664. Retrieved from http://www.aafp.org/afp/2007/0901/p658.html

Planning

Planning for care of children with diabetes depends on the assessment findings. In the acute phase for the newly diagnosed child with type 1 DM, the planning focus is related to the complex pathophysiological alterations in health, such as electrolyte imbalance, fluid deficits, fatigue, and pain. Discharge planning should begin at the time of diagnosis and move forward to prepare the child and the family for self-management of glucose monitoring, insulin and oral medications, and signs and symptoms of hypoglycemia and actions to take. Family involvement is crucial. Developmental stage must be taken into account in planning education for the child. Before discharge, the child and the family are linked to the resources in the community that will support care of the child with diabetes. Possibilities include the following:

■ ADA-certified diabetes education programs
■ Juvenile Diabetes Research Foundation local chapters
■ Insulin pumper support groups (usually sponsored by insulin pump companies).

Implementation

Education in skills for survival can be initiated as early as the family and child feel it is acceptable. Nurses should always assess the child's developmental stage and take that into account when planning teaching and health promotion. For example, the pre-school-age-child who seeks greater control and autonomy may benefit from choosing which snacks to eat. Most school-age children are able to (and need to) learn how to recognize the symptoms of hypoglycemia and hyperglycemia and what to do in the event one of these occurs. Adolescents may exhibit resistance to complying with treatment, as they may find it embarrassing to be singled out as different from their peers or may feel resentful about their illness and the restrictions that it imposes.

The nurse should continually assess barriers to implementing the discharge planning as the teaching proceeds. Health promotion and teaching topics to cover prior to discharge include diet, medication, exercise, glucose monitoring, and pre-

Box 12–7   Diabetic Ketoacidosis

Diabetic ketoacidosis (DKA) is a life-threatening event that occurs when the body lacks sufficient insulin to promote glucose as a fuel source and begins to break down fat for fuel instead. Ketones, the by-products of fat breakdown, build up in the blood and urine. Often the first and acutely presenting sign of type 1 diabetes mellitus, DKA can result from infection or serious illness, injury, surgery, missed doses of insulin, or overwhelming stress (National Center for Biotechnology Information, 2011). Excessive thirst, nausea and vomiting, increased urination, anorexia, abdominal pain, shortness of breath, and fruity-scented breath are common symptoms of DKA. If left untreated, DKA can cause depression of the central nervous system, resulting in coma and even death.

Priority interventions for the child or adolescent with DKA include the following:

■ Assessment of physiological parameters such as vital signs, respiratory status, mental status, and blood sugar is ongoing.

■ Cardiac monitoring is required because of potential hypokalemia, which can result in lethal dysrhythmias. (Insulin in the presence of excess glucose moves potassium into the cells and thus causes serum hypokalemia. There is also loss of total body potassium due to the osmotic diuresis that occurs (Bope, Kellerman, & Rakel, 2011; Rghavan, 2011).

■ Intake and output are monitored hourly.

■ IV fluids are given in boluses of 10–20 mL/kg if hypovolemia is present.

■ Insulin infusions are titrated to bring the blood sugar down slowly, as too rapid a decrease can lead to cerebral complications and neurological changes.

■ Once the acidosis is corrected and the blood sugar is improved, the insulin drip is tapered off, and subcutaneous insulin is initiated.

■ Food is reintroduced when the child is alert and the blood glucose has been stabilized.

Client Teaching Ten Tips for Better Glucose Control

10. *Be persistent.* Parents need to stay involved in the day-to-day management of their child's blood sugar until the child is old enough and mature enough to self-manage responsibly.

9. *Provide structure.* Maintaining daily routines helps keep glucose in control. This step may be a challenge, but sticking as close as possible to a routine usually results in better glucose control.

8. *Support year-round exercise.* To maintain consistent insulin sensitivity, it is best for the child to participate in an activity during the week and on the weekends. Excessive activity at one time with extended periods of inactivity at other times can cause major glucose swings.

7. *Keep accurate, consistent records.* Although glucose meters have memories, the input of information is limited. There is also a psychological effect to writing down blood sugars and food intake. Special notations also help identify a probable cause when blood sugar control is erratic.

6. *Think like a pancreas.* Understanding the underlying basic physiology of the pancreas assists in making correct decisions in relation to food intake and insulin administration. This understanding is not acquired overnight, but with time, experience, and education and support from a trained professional, a child with diabetes gets to know her his own diabetes better than anyone else.

5. *Demand quality from your healthcare team.* Although the decisions regarding diabetes are made by the child and the parents, the diabetes care team has the expertise to support and guide the child through a life with diabetes.

4. *Network with other families.* Support groups and other children with diabetes can be a powerful system to enable the child and the parents.

3. *If it's broken, fix it.* For the child with diabetes, small things can become big things quickly. The child and the parents need to be vigilant for illness and stresses that may cause wide fluctuations in glucose control.

2. *Involve the child.* Children are more apt to follow rules if they have been involved in making the rules. Allowing the child to make decisions gives him the confidence to feel some control over the disease. With young children it can be as simple as allowing the child to pick the finger that will be stuck for glucose measurement.

1. *Let kids be kids.* Sometimes the glucose police need to take a break. Constantly nagging a child to attain perfect numbers results in breakdowns in communication between the child and parent, and the child may give up on even trying to self-manage. The parent should take time for fun and relaxation with and without the child, just as they would if diabetes was not in the picture.

Source: Based on Scheiner, G. (2011). *Ten tips for better glucose control.* Retrieved from http://www.diabetesselfmanagement.com/Articles/Kids-And-Diabetes/top-10-tips-for-better-blood-glucose-control/.

vention, recognition, and intervention for acute complications (see the Client Teaching feature). The family that has difficulty coping may need referral to a counselor who can help deal with the realities of managing diabetes in a child. Prior to discharge, the nurse should review with the family any action plans or instructions to be shared with school or day care personnel.

As the child matures and approaches puberty, special circumstances may occur. The nurse must be ready to assess and implement education strategies to help the adolescent deal with these situations. It is not uncommon for children to go through a period of erratic glucose control as they approach puberty. The reasons may be physiological as well as behavioral. The nurse should be aware of this possibility when a child with previously well-controlled type 1 DM suddenly finds it harder to control her glucose levels.

SAFETY ALERT
Successful maintenance of glycemic control depends in part on frequency of glucose monitoring. Be sure to assess for frequency of monitoring at each client interaction.

The young female with DM must be aware of the possible deleterious effects of hyperglycemia on an unborn fetus. She should be counseled about birth control on reaching puberty.

Other special situations include the adolescent driver, who needs education about the effects of hypoglycemia on safe driving. It is recommended that drivers with DM always check their blood glucose before driving and that they have a source of car-

bohydrate with them at all times. Education regarding onset, peak, and duration of insulin may have to be reviewed before the youth takes on the new responsibility of driving.

Evaluation

Evaluation is specific to the child and depends on the assessment, planning, and interventions. It is particularly important for the nurse to evaluate the child and family for coping mechanisms and knowledge about skills for survival.

Guidelines for postdischarge evaluation of the child with diabetes are as follows:

- The child and the parent should both be present at the interview.
- Skills can be assessed by having the child or parent demonstrate how to deliver the insulin and/or oral medications.
- Asking "How many times a week do you miss your insulin or medication?" is a helpful way to gain accurate information.
- Asking open-ended questions such as "Tell me about the food you are eating" encourages the child to share likes and dislikes and can give the nurse an idea of what the child's daily intake is.
- The nurse should elicit a 24-hour food recall to gain specific information from the child who is not keeping a food log.
- Questions about frequency of hypoglycemia should also address knowledge on actions to take in the case of hypoglycemia.
- The nurse should review the logbook or glucose meter to note trending of glucose control.
- Expectations in the early days postdischarge should be realistic, and support should be given to the child and parent.

Community-Based Care   Children With Diabetes

The child with diabetes should be allowed to participate in the same recreational activities as children who do not have the disease. Overnight trips and school activities that take the child a greater distance from home than usual can be done safely with planning and communication between the child, the parent, and a responsible adult in charge of the activity. Planning should include making sure there are enough supplies, including medications, glucose tablets, monitoring supplies, and a **glucagon emergency kit**, if required. A glucagon kit contains a preparation of purified crystallized glucagon hormone and is used in the treatment of profound hypoglycemia that results in loss of consciousness. These kits usually contain the preparation and a ready-to-use needle and syringe. If a glucagon kit is dispensed, the responsible adult must understand how and when to use it. The child's parents should emphasize to the adults in charge that the child cannot skip meals and that snacks and sugar-free drinks must be readily available and accessible to the child at all times.

Children and teens live in a world where online support for diabetes is available and readily accessible. Parents must be aware of which Web sites and online support are safe and effective for their child. The diabetes care team can help children and parents identify the safest online resources. Communities often have American Diabetes Association Recognized Diabetes Education Programs, which offer classes, individual counseling, and support groups. Another recognized resource for parents and children is the JDRF (Juvenile Diabetes Research Foundation), which has local community groups as well as an extensive online list of resources. Many states also have diabetes camps for children with diabetes. Camps for children with chronic illnesses are in high demand because they provide an opportunity for children to interact with other children who also have a chronic illness. These camps provide age-appropriate fun activities that promote confidence and self-esteem. The campers also learn more about their illness and how to self-manage. The camps are staffed by trained diabetes educators and a medical liaison who is onsite or nearby (Vogt, Chavez, & Schaffner, 2011).

The nurse must realize that there is a period of adjustment as the family and the child learn to live with diabetes. Setting goals at the follow up visit can help the child to fine-tune glucose control to avoid severe highs and lows. Exercise habits should also be assessed to encourage a healthy lifestyle. Evaluation of the child's and parents' knowledge about postexercise hypoglycemia will provide a safe exercise environment for the child. Skills for survival, including actions to take for hyperglycemia, DKA, and sick days, should also be reviewed. The nurse should ensure that the family has a responsible individual trained in the use of a glucagon injection kit and that the medication is readily available.

Nurses work with families to establish specific, measurable, and realistic goals for management. Realistic goals to evaluate at the follow up visit include the following:

- The child remains free of infection and injury.
- The child maintains adequate glucose control while still meeting nutritional needs for growth and development.
- The child and parents recognize early signs of hypoglycemia and hyperglycemia and treat them appropriately, reducing the risk of neurological impairment and/or DKA.

Stay Current: *Visit the Juvenile Diabetes Research Foundation at* **www.jdrf.org** *to learn more about their programs.*

NURSING CARE PLAN   A Pediatric Client With Type 1 Diabetes Mellitus

Michael is a 14-year-old male admitted to ICU with a diagnosis of new-onset type 1 DM. He is in the ninth grade at the local high school. Michael is now living with his mother and has had trouble making the transition from living with his father following his parents' separation and divorce. He was staying at his father's house this weekend when he became ill. His complaints were nausea and vomiting, abdominal pain, frequency of urination, and fatigue. He complained of thirst for several days prior to the acute onset. His father took him to the emergency department, and he was admitted to the ICU this morning. Michael's mother has not been informed yet of his condition, as the relationship between the parents is strained and communication is poor.

ASSESSMENT	DIAGNOSES	PLANNING

Michael's blood glucose is 400 mg/dL, hemoglobin A_{1C} 8.6%, urine positive for ketones, T 99.0°F orally, P 120 bpm, R 26/min deep and labored, BP 98/50 mmHg. Blood work has been done as follows:
 	
 ■ ABG pH 7.21, pCO_2 32, Bicarb 20, pO_2 98%
 ■ Anion gap 18 mEq/L
 ■ BUN 30 mg/dL
 ■ Creat 1.0 mg/dL
 ■ Electrolytes Na 147 mEq/L K 5.2 mEq/L Cl 108 mEq/L
 ■ Hgb 14 g/dL
 ■ Hct 57%
 ■ WBC 11,000
	Nursing diagnoses that may be appropriate for Michael include the following:
	
	 ■ *Risk for Imbalanced Fluid Volume* related to loss of fluid due to osmotic diuresis
	 ■ *Fatigue* related to *Altered Fluid Balance* and *Impaired Gas Exchange*
	 ■ *Decreased Cardiac Output* caused by electrolyte disturbances
	 ■ *Ineffective Coping* (individual) related to *Anxiety* and *Fear* regarding new diagnosis.
		Monitor for signs and symptoms of dehydration.
		
		   Replace fluid volume as ordered by physician.
		
		   Monitor hourly intake and output.
		
		   Monitor for signs and symptoms of hypokalemia as insulin and fluid infusion moves potassium into the cells during rehydration process.

NURSING CARE PLAN *(continued)*

ASSESSMENT

- Urine is 3+ for ketones, serum osmolality is 310 mOsm.
- IV of 0.9% NaCl is infusing at 20 mL/hr pending lab results in 1 hour.
- IV of regular insulin is infusing at 1 unit per hour with hourly glucose finger-sticks and adjustment of insulin per protocol.

Michael is stable 24 hours later and is moved to the diabetes floor on an insulin infusion with orders to start Lantus subcutaneously and stop insulin drip this evening. He will also be on an insulin-to-CHO (I:C) ratio of 1 unit to 15 g CHO using NovoLog insulin via insulin pen and a correction factor of 1 unit for every 30 mg/dL over 150 mg/dL glucose per finger-stick. He is awake and alert. His mother is present and is loudly blaming his father for not taking him to the emergency department sooner. During the assessment, the nurse finds that Michael is quiet and withdrawn and says he does not have diabetes. He just has the flu and will get over it.

DIAGNOSES

- *Ineffective Coping* (family) related to *Anxiety* and already-present family stress.
- *Powerlessness* related to perceived loss of control over independence.
- *Anxiety* related to new diagnosis and breakdown in family unit.
- *Deficient Knowledge* related to lack of information about diagnosis and *Fear* of social stigma associated with a chronic disease.
- *Noncompliance* related to therapeutic regimen due to social support deficit and faulty perceptions of illness seriousness.

(NANDA-I © 2012)

PLANNING

Identify the fears that have the highest priority for the patient. He may fear that he will not be able to participate in school activities or be with his friends as in the past. Lack of knowledge about the disease may leave him with unreasonable fears and anxieties based on misconceptions. Planning for diabetes education will enable him to realize that he can live a normal lifestyle with minimal interruptions.

Because the family unit has changed due to divorce, communication with both parents and the adolescent is important to dispel any misunderstanding about his care. Expected outcomes for the plan of care specify that Michael will:

- Demonstrate how to check his blood glucose level prior to discharge.
- Demonstrate how to draw up and inject insulin doses.
- Articulate survival food guidelines.
- Describe symptoms of hyperglycemia and hypoglycemia.

IMPLEMENTATION

The following nursing interventions may be appropriate:

- In the acute phase of DKA, closely monitor Michael's vital signs, blood glucose, and hydration status.
- With Michael, mutually identify short-term and long-term goals for diabetes self-management with a focus on the skills for survival upon discharge.
- Provide opportunities for Michael to express any fear and anger over the diagnosis and help him to seek positive ways to deal with the changes imposed by diabetes.

- Provide positive reinforcement as Michael learns to manage his diabetes.
- Encourage both parents to be present for diabetes education classes and meetings with the diabetes educator.
- To encourage Michael's independence in decision making, while he is still in the hospital and under the guidance of the nurses he should practice self-injecting his insulin, monitoring his blood sugars, and counting carbohydrates.

EVALUATION

Michael is discharged on his fourth hospital day. He goes home with his mother. He goes to a follow up appointment with the diabetes educator 1 week later. The diabetes educator assesses Michael's logbook and food journal as well as his skills. Michael is doing well, but his mother and father are still having trouble coping with the diagnosis and this difficulty causes Michael much stress. The educator discusses with the family the possibility of meeting with a family counselor. Both parents agree, and another appointment is set up after the family has seen the counselor.

REVIEW Diabetes in Children

RELATE Link the Concepts and Exemplars

Linking the exemplar of diabetes in children with the concept of stress and coping:

1. How might a diagnosis of diabetes increase the stress or anxiety level of a child? A parent?

2. What nursing interventions do you think would help reduce a child's stress level? An adolescent's? A parent's?

Linking the exemplar of diabetes in children with the concept of advocacy:

3. In what ways can the nurse in a pediatric office help parents learn to advocate for their child in the school or day care setting?

4. How can nurses advocate for diabetic clients in their communities?

READY Go to Companion Skills Manual

REFER Go to Pearson Nursing Student Resources
nursing.pearsonhighered.com

- Additional review material MiniModule: Diabetes in Children

REFLECT Case Study A

Mary Wills is a 12-year-old White female who is brought to her healthcare provider by her mother for symptoms related to a cold and sore throat. When the nurse weighs Mary, she notes that Mary is in the 90th percentile for her height and age. Blood work reveals an elevated blood glucose level of 250. Mary says she feels fine and is just a little tired because of her cold. Her mother says that Mary does not play outside very much, preferring to watch TV or read in bed at home. Mary has a few friends, but when they come over, they play computer games or look at books. Mary is not involved in any school activities.

A diet recall with Mary's mother reveals that the family eats takeout food almost every night because both parents work, get home late, and do not feel like cooking. Plenty of snacks are always on hand in case the kids get hungry while waiting for the parents to get home from work. Breakfast is usually a honey bun on the school bus. Mary eats a school lunch and also brings her own snacks. The only family event is going together to get ice cream. Both parents are also obese and sedentary.

Mary's mother has tried some herbs she has seen advertised on TV to help herself and the children lose weight.

1. What can the nurse tell Mary's mother about the risk factors for type 2 DM in children?

2. Develop a teaching plan of care to help Mary and her mother cope with the new diagnosis of type 2 DM (include skills for survival).

3. Mary's mother would like to start using some of the medications she has seen advertised in magazines to treat Mary. She feels that herbs and vitamins are better than prescription drugs. What could the nurse say to Mary's mother regarding the use of dietary supplements and alternative therapies?

REFLECT Case Study B

Tony Chadwick is a 16-year-old African American male admitted to ICU from the urgent care with newly diagnosed type 1 DM with DKA. His mother took him to the local urgent care with a 2-day history of vomiting and abdominal pain. Tony also complained of thirst, blurry vision, and fatigue. His mother smelled a fruity odor on his breath this morning. The nurse at the urgent care clinic found that Tony had a blood glucose level of 520 mg/dL and urine positive for ketones. Tony was immediately transferred to the local hospital, where he was admitted to ICU. He is in the 11th grade and was doing well in school until about 2 weeks ago, when he started to become easily fatigued and irritable. His mother thought that he was just staying up too late and not getting enough sleep. Tony has been well except for an upper respiratory viral infection about 2 months ago that kept him home from school for 3 days.

On arrival in the ICU, Tony is drowsy but wakes to verbal stimuli. He complains of nausea and is vomiting green-colored bile in small amounts. He complains of abdominal pain and a need to urinate.

His mother accompanies him and expresses fear that he will not survive this acute episode. She was told at the urgent care clinic that Tony has diabetes but she does not believe it. She says no one in her family or her husband's has diabetes.

Lab Results:

- A_{1C} 12%
- Anion gap 20
- ABGs pH 7.22
- pCO_2 21
- Bicarb 18
- Electrolytes are pending.
- Chest x-ray is negative.

Physical Assessment:

- Vital signs: T 99.5°F orally; P 120 bpm, thready; R 28/min, deep and labored; BP 90/60 mmHg
- Neuro: As above
- Resp: Lungs clear to auscultation
- CVS: All pulses palpable with radial pulses thready. HS are S_1, S_2.
- Skin: Cool and clammy but skin turgor poor
- Gi: Diminished bowel sounds in all quadrants
- GU: Has not voided
- An IV is started and 0.9% NaCl is infusing. An insulin drip is started per protocol. Tony is connected to a cardiac monitor and exhibits sinus tachycardia. A Foley catheter is inserted and connected to an hourly drainage chamber (for hourly urine output measurement).

1. Tony is a 16-year-old male who is involved in sports. What are some of the fears and anxieties that he may have as he resumes his normal life? How can the nurse help Tony deal with these issues?

2. At the urgent care clinic, Tony's mother said this couldn't be diabetes because no one in the family has ever had it. What could the nurse tell Tony's mother to help her understand the disease and its etiology?

3. Discuss the electrolyte imbalance and blood gas results that occurred on the first day of Tony's admission. How do his vital signs reflect the pathophysiology of DKA?

4. Tony is concerned about being embarrassed when he has to check his blood sugar and take his insulin at school. What interventions could the nurse suggest to help him with privacy?

5. Tony admits to drinking alcohol occasionally. What should the nurse teach Tony about alcohol use and diabetes?

6. List and explain at least four nursing diagnoses for Tony.

EXEMPLAR 12.3   Liver Disease

EXEMPLAR KEY TERMS

Alcoholic cirrhosis, 781
Balloon tamponade, 788
Cirrhosis, 781
Gastric lavage, 788

Hematochezia, 787
Laënnec cirrhosis, 781
Paracentesis, 788
Transjugular intrahepatic portosystemic shunt (TIPS), 788

EXEMPLAR LEARNING OUTCOMES

After reading about this exemplar, you will be able to:

1. Describe the pathophysiology, etiology, clinical manifestations, and direct and indirect causes of liver disease.

2. Identify risk factors and prevention methods associated with liver disease.

3. Illustrate the nursing process in providing culturally competent care across the life span for individuals with liver disease.

4. Formulate priority nursing diagnoses appropriate for an individual with liver disease.

5. Summarize therapies used by interdisciplinary teams in the collaborative care of an individual with liver disease.

6. Plan evidence-based care for an individual with liver disease and his or her family in collaboration with other members of the healthcare team.

7. Evaluate expected outcomes for an individual with liver disease.

▶ OVERVIEW

The liver is a complex organ with multiple metabolic and regulatory functions. Optimal liver function is essential to health. Because of the significant amount of blood in the liver at all times, it is exposed to the effects of pathogens, drugs, toxins, and possibly malignant cells. As a result, liver cells may become inflamed or damaged, or cancerous tumors may develop.

The essential functions of the liver include the metabolism of proteins, carbohydrates, and fats. It also is responsible for the metabolism of steroid hormones and most drugs. It synthesizes essential blood proteins—albumin and clotting factors, in particular. The liver detoxifies alcohol and other toxic substances. Ammonia, a toxic by-product of protein metabolism, is converted to urea in the liver for elimination by the kidneys. The liver produces bile, an essential substance for absorbing fats and eliminating bilirubin from the body. Minerals and fat-soluble vitamins are stored in the liver, as is glycogen (stored carbohydrate for energy reserves). The Kupffer cells that line the sinusoids phagocytize foreign cells and damaged blood cells.

The liver is vital to the digestion and metabolism of nutrients; the production of plasma proteins, including those involved in clotting; and the metabolism and excretion of compounds such as bilirubin, steroid hormones, and ammonia, as well as toxins (such as alcohol) and drugs. Impaired function of liver cells has multiple effects, including:

- Impaired protein metabolism with decreased production of albumin and clotting factors. Low albumin levels contribute to edema in peripheral tissues and *ascites* (accumulation of fluid in the abdomen), as plasma oncotic pressure is reduced. Impaired clotting-factor production increases the risk for bleeding.

- Disrupted glucose metabolism and storage with resulting alterations in blood glucose levels (either hyperglycemia or hypoglycemia).

- Reduced bile production that impairs the absorption of lipids and fat-soluble vitamins. Inadequate vitamin K, a fat-soluble vitamin, affects the production of clotting factors, leading to a bleeding tendency.

- Impaired metabolism of steroid hormones (including estrogen and testosterone) leads to feminization in men and irregular menses in women.

Although many different disorders can disrupt liver function, their manifestations relate to three primary effects: disrupted liver cell function, impaired bilirubin conversion and excretion leading to jaundice, and disrupted blood flow through the liver, with resulting portal hypertension. Cirrhosis of the liver is examined here in more detail because it is the most common cause of liver disease in the United States and demonstrates most of the symptoms commonly found in chronic degenerative liver disease.

Cirrhosis is the end stage of chronic liver disease. It is a progressive, irreversible disorder, eventually leading to liver failure. **Alcoholic cirrhosis** (or **Laënnec cirrhosis**) is the most common type of cirrhosis in North America (University of Maryland Medical Center, 2011). Cirrhosis also may result from chronic hepatitis B or C; prolonged obstruction of the biliary (bile drainage) system; long-term, severe right heart failure; and other, uncommon, liver diseases.

▶ PATHOPHYSIOLOGY AND ETIOLOGY

In cirrhosis, functional liver tissue is gradually destroyed and replaced by fibrous scar tissue. As hepatocytes and liver lobules are destroyed, the metabolic functions of the liver are lost. Structurally abnormal nodules encircled by connective tissue form. This fibrous connective tissue forms constrictive bands that disrupt blood and bile flow within liver lobules. Blood no longer flows freely through the liver to the inferior vena cava. This restricted blood flow leads to portal hypertension (increased pressure in the portal venous system).

Etiology

The incidence and mortality attributable to cirrhosis and chronic liver disease vary significantly among populations.

ALCOHOLIC CIRRHOSIS Alcoholic (or Laënnec) cirrhosis is the end result of alcoholic liver disease. Its development is directly related to alcohol consumption—specifically, the total amount of alcohol consumed, the number of years of excessive alcohol consumption, and blood alcohol levels. Women develop cirrhosis at lower overall levels of alcohol use than men. The reason may be less effective metabolism of alcohol in women, resulting in higher blood alcohol levels (Bruha et al., 2012).

Alcohol causes metabolic changes in the liver: Triglyceride and fatty acid synthesis increases, and a decrease in the formation and release of lipoproteins leads to fatty infiltration of hepatocytes (fatty liver). At this stage, abstinence from alcohol can allow the liver to heal. However, with continued alcohol abuse, the disease continues to progress. Inflammatory cells infiltrate the liver (alcoholic hepatitis), causing necrosis, fibrosis, and destruction of functional liver tissue. In the final stage of alcoholic cirrhosis, regenerative nodules form, and the liver shrinks and develops a nodular appearance. Malnutrition commonly accompanies alcoholic cirrhosis.

■ Although cirrhosis/chronic liver disease is the 12th leading cause of death overall in the United States, it is the 6th leading cause of death for individuals of Native American (including Alaska Natives) and Hispanic (or Latino) origin.

■ Native American men have the highest incidence and mortality rate from cirrhosis and chronic liver disease, followed by Native American women, Hispanic men, and women of Hispanic or Latino origin (CDC, 2012a).

■ At this time, there is no clear explanation for these differences. Contributory factors may include:
   a. Socioeconomic factors that lead to greater stress and alcohol consumption among certain populations
   b. Patterns of alcohol consumption (e.g., consuming alcohol without food calories)
   c. Variations in alcohol metabolism among populations

BILIARY CIRRHOSIS   When bile flow is obstructed within the liver or in the biliary system, the retained bile damages and destroys liver cells close to the interlobular bile ducts. This activity leads to inflammation, fibrosis, and formation of regenerative nodules.

POSTHEPATIC CIRRHOSIS   Advanced progressive liver disease resulting from chronic hepatitis B or C or from an unknown cause is called *posthepatic* or *postnecrotic cirrhosis.* Chronic viral hepatitis appears to be the leading cause of posthepatic cirrhosis in the United States (NIDDK, 2012). In clients with this type of cirrhosis, the liver is shrunken and nodular, with fibrosis and extensive loss of liver cells.

Risk Factors

For most clients, high-risk behaviors are the risk factors for cirrhosis. While many clients tolerate alcohol use in moderation with no adverse effects on the liver, excess alcohol use is the leading cause of cirrhosis. Injection drug use also is a significant risk factor, increasing the risk for contracting bloodborne hepatitis (B, C, or D). These types of viral hepatitis can lead to chronic hepatitis and, ultimately, to cirrhosis.

▶ CLINICAL MANIFESTATIONS

Early in the course of cirrhosis, few manifestations may be present. The liver usually is enlarged and may be tender. A dull, aching pain in the right upper quadrant may be present. Other early signs include weight loss, weakness, and anorexia. Bowel function is disrupted with diarrhea or constipation (Porth & Matfin, 2009).

As the disease progresses, manifestations related to liver cell failure and portal hypertension develop. Impaired metabolism causes such manifestations as bleeding, ascites, gynecomastia (breast enlargement) in men and infertility in women, jaundice, and neurological changes. Portal hypertension accounts for such manifestations as ascites, peripheral edema, anemia, and low white blood cell (WBC) and platelet counts. See the Multisystem Effects of Cirrhosis feature.

Treatment of cirrhosis is supportive and directed at slowing the progression to liver failure and reducing complications. It can include medications to help regulate protein metabolism, maintenance of fluid and electrolyte balance, and supportive therapies, including treatment of underlying problems (e.g., malnutrition, anemia, bleeding, encephalopathy, renal failure, and infections).

Portal Hypertension

Portal hypertension causes blood to be rerouted to adjoining, lower-pressure vessels. This *shunting* of blood involves collateral vessels. Affected veins, which become engorged and congested, are located in the esophagus, rectum, and abdomen. Portal hypertension increases the hydrostatic pressure in vessels of the portal system. Increased hydrostatic pressure in the capillaries pushes fluid out, contributing to ascites formation.

Splenomegaly

Because portal hypertension causes blood to be shunted into the splenic vein, the spleen enlarges (splenomegaly). Splenomegaly increases the rate at which red blood cells (RBCs), WBCs, and platelets are removed from circulation and destroyed. This increased destruction of blood cells leads to anemia (low RBC count), leukopenia (low WBC count), and thrombocytopenia (low platelet count; Porth & Matfin, 2009).

Ascites

Ascites is the accumulation of plasma-rich fluid in the abdominal cavity. Although portal hypertension is the primary cause of ascites, decreased serum proteins and increased aldosterone also contribute to the fluid accumulation. *Hypoalbuminemia* (low serum albumin) decreases the colloidal osmotic pressure of plasma. This pressure normally holds fluid in the intravascular compartment, but when the plasma colloidal osmotic pressure decreases, fluid escapes into extravascular compartments. *Hyperaldosteronism* (an increase in aldosterone) causes sodium and water retention, contributing to ascites and generalized edema.

Esophageal Varices

Esophageal varices are enlarged, thin-walled veins that form in the submucosa of the esophagus. These collateral vessels form when blood is shunted from the portal system because of portal hypertension. The thin-walled varices may rupture and cause massive hemorrhage; even eating high-roughage foods can precipitate bleeding in these clients. Thrombocytopenia, platelet deficiency, and impaired production of clotting factors by the liver contribute to the risk for hemorrhage.

Portal Systemic Encephalopathy

Portal systemic encephalopathy (also known as *hepatic encephalopathy*) results from cerebral edema and the accumulation of neurotoxins in the blood. Ammonia, a by-product of protein metabolism, contributes to hepatic encephalopathy. Ammonium ion is produced as proteins and amino acids are broken down by bacteria in the intestinal tract. Normally, the ammonia produced is then converted by the liver to urea before entering the general circulation. However, as functional liver tissue is destroyed, ammonia can no longer be converted to urea, and it accumulates in the blood. Other

Multisystem Effects of Cirrhosis

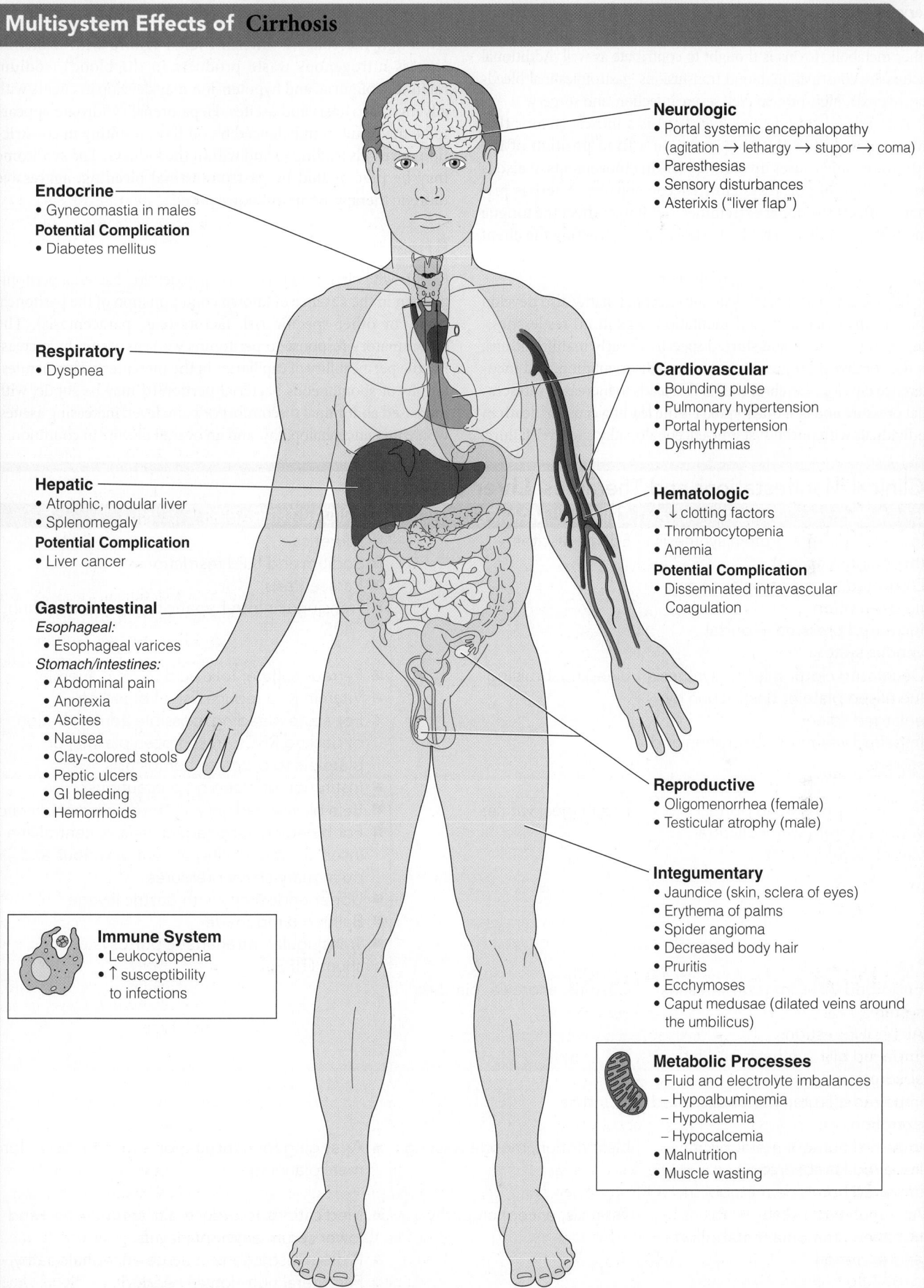

Neurologic
- Portal systemic encephalopathy (agitation → lethargy → stupor → coma)
- Paresthesias
- Sensory disturbances
- Asterixis ("liver flap")

Endocrine
- Gynecomastia in males

Potential Complication
- Diabetes mellitus

Respiratory
- Dyspnea

Cardiovascular
- Bounding pulse
- Pulmonary hypertension
- Portal hypertension
- Dysrhythmias

Hepatic
- Atrophic, nodular liver
- Splenomegaly

Potential Complication
- Liver cancer

Hematologic
- ↓ clotting factors
- Thrombocytopenia
- Anemia

Potential Complication
- Disseminated intravascular Coagulation

Gastrointestinal
Esophageal:
- Esophageal varices

Stomach/intestines:
- Abdominal pain
- Anorexia
- Ascites
- Nausea
- Clay-colored stools
- Peptic ulcers
- GI bleeding
- Hemorrhoids

Reproductive
- Oligomenorrhea (female)
- Testicular atrophy (male)

Integumentary
- Jaundice (skin, sclera of eyes)
- Erythema of palms
- Spider angioma
- Decreased body hair
- Pruritis
- Ecchymoses
- Caput medusae (dilated veins around the umbilicus)

Immune System
- Leukocytopenia
- ↑ susceptibility to infections

Metabolic Processes
- Fluid and electrolyte imbalances
  - Hypoalbuminemia
  - Hypokalemia
  - Hypocalcemia
- Malnutrition
- Muscle wasting

nervous system depressants, such as narcotics and tranquilizers, also may contribute to hepatic encephalopathy. Accumulation of other metabolic toxins is thought to contribute as well. Additional factors are constipation, blood transfusions, gastrointestinal bleeding, hypoxia, high-protein diet, severe infection, and surgery.

Asterixis (also known as liver flap) is a muscle tremor that interferes with the ability to maintain a fixed position of the extremities and causes involuntary jerking movements. It also is an early sign of portal systemic encephalopathy. Asterixis primarily affects the upper extremities, but it may affect the tongue and feet. The nurse may elicit asterixis by instructing the client to extend the arms and dorsiflex the wrists; if present, asterixis causes a downward flapping of the hands.

Individuals with portal systemic encephalopathy also develop changes in personality and mentation. Agitation, restlessness, impaired judgment, and slurred speech are early manifestations; as the condition progresses, confusion, disorientation, and incoherence develop. Cerebral edema that leads to increased intracranial pressure and cerebral hypoxia is the leading cause of death in individuals with portal systemic encephalopathy and liver failure.

Hepatorenal Syndrome

Although the cause is unclear, renal failure with azotemia (excess nitrogenous waste products in the blood), sodium retention, oliguria, and hypotension may develop in clients with advanced cirrhosis and ascites. Hepatorenal syndrome appears to be the result of imbalanced blood flow, resulting in constriction of vessels leading to and within the kidneys. The syndrome may be precipitated by gastrointestinal bleeding, aggressive diuretic therapy, or an unknown cause.

Spontaneous Bacterial Peritonitis

Clients with cirrhosis and ascites may develop bacterial peritonitis even in the absence of known contamination of the peritoneal cavity or other specific risk factors (e.g., paracentesis). The inflammatory response to peritonitis worsens ascites by increasing the permeability of capillaries in the mesentery. The manifestations of spontaneous bacterial peritonitis may be subtle, with increased abdominal discomfort or pain, fever, increasing ascites, worsening encephalopathy, and an overall decline in condition.

Clinical Manifestations and Therapies **Liver Disease**

ETIOLOGY	CLINICAL MANIFESTATION	CLINICAL THERAPIES
Impaired plasma protein synthesis (hypoalbuminemia) Disrupted hormone balance and fluid retention Increased pressure in portal venous system	Edema, ascites	▪ Diuretics ▪ Sodium and fluid restrictions ▪ Paracentesis ▪ Transjugular intrahepatic portosystemic shunt (TIPS)
Decreased clotting factor synthesis Increased platelet destruction by enlarged spleen Impaired vitamin K absorption and storage	Bleeding, bruising	▪ Ferrous sulfate, folic acid to treat anemia ▪ Vitamin K to reduce risk of bleeding ▪ For acute bleeding, possible administration of packed RBCs, fresh frozen plasma, or platelets to promote hemostasis ▪ Institution of bleeding precautions
Increased pressure in portal venous system with collateral vessel development	Esophageal varices	▪ Beta-blocker nadolol with isosorbide mononitrate ▪ For bleeding esophageal varices, central line insertion; monitoring of central venous and pulmonary artery pressures ▪ Upper endoscopy with gastric lavage ▪ Balloon tamponade ▪ Transjugular intrahepatic portosystemic shunt (TIPS)
Engorged veins in gastrointestinal system Alcohol ingestion Impaired bile synthesis and fat absorption	Gastritis, anorexia, diarrhea	
Impaired bilirubin metabolism and excretion	Jaundice	
Impaired nutrient metabolism Impaired fat absorption Impaired hormone metabolism	Malnutrition, muscle wasting	▪ Arranging for consultation with a dietician for meal planning
Accumulated metabolic toxins Impaired ammonia metabolism and excretion	Asterixis, encephalopathy	▪ Medications to reduce nitrogenous load and lower serum ammonia levels ▪ Protein restrictions in acute encephalopathy ▪ Parenteral nutrition as needed

▶ COLLABORATION

Care for the client with cirrhosis is holistic, addressing physiological, psychosocial, and spiritual needs, and the nurse is responsible for coordinating care among providers. The importance of including the family in the plan of care cannot be overemphasized, particularly if alcohol abuse is identified as the cause. Counseling, job coaching, and behavioral therapy may be helpful. Consultation with a nutritionist can help to reinforce any client teaching the nurse has provided as well as give the client an additional resource in this area.

Diagnostic Tests

Studies to confirm the diagnosis of cirrhosis and identify its cause and effects are performed. Diagnostic tests may include the following:

- *Liver function studies.* These include studies of *alanine aminotransferase, aspartate aminotransferase, alkaline phosphatase,* and *gamma-glutamyltransferase.* All four may be elevated in clients with cirrhosis, but usually not as severely as in clients with acute hepatitis. Elevations in these enzymes may not correlate well with the extent of liver damage in cirrhosis.

- *Complete blood count (CBC) with platelets.* A low RBC count, hemoglobin, and hematocrit demonstrate anemia related to bone marrow suppression, increased RBC destruction, bleeding, and deficiencies of folic acid and vitamin B_{12}. Platelet counts are low, related to increased destruction by the spleen. Leukopenia (low WBC count) also relates to splenomegaly.

- *Coagulation studies.* A prolonged prothrombin time results from impaired production of coagulation proteins and lack of vitamin K.

- *Serum electrolytes.* Hyponatremia is common, resulting from hemodilution. Hypokalemia, hypophosphatemia, and hypomagnesemia are also frequently seen, related to malnutrition and altered renal excretion of these electrolytes.

- *Bilirubin.* Both direct (conjugated) and indirect (unconjugated) bilirubin usually are elevated in clients with severe cirrhosis.

- *Serum albumin.* Hypoalbuminemia results from impaired liver production.

- *Serum ammonia.* Levels are elevated, because the liver fails to effectively convert ammonia to urea for renal excretion.

- *Serum glucose and cholesterol.* These levels frequently are abnormal in clients with cirrhosis.

- *Abdominal ultrasound.* This test is performed to evaluate liver size, detect ascites, and identify liver nodules. Ultrasound may be used in conjunction with *Doppler studies* to evaluate blood flow through the liver and spleen (Allan, Kerry, & Phillips, 2010)

- *Esophagoscopy.* Upper endoscopy may be done to determine the presence of esophageal varices.

- *Liver biopsy.* This test is not always necessary to diagnose cirrhosis, but it may be done to distinguish cirrhosis from other forms of liver disease. Biopsy may be deferred if the client's bleeding time is prolonged (e.g., prothrombin time >3 sec over the control).

Pharmacologic Therapy

Medications are used to treat the complications and effects of cirrhosis; they do not reverse or slow the process of cirrhosis itself. Known hepatotoxic drugs and alcohol are avoided, as are drugs metabolized by the liver (e.g., barbiturates, sedatives, hypnotics, and acetaminophen). Several groups of drugs are commonly prescribed:

- Diuretics reduce fluid retention and ascites. Spironolactone (Aldactone) is frequently the drug of first choice, because it addresses increased aldosterone levels, one of the causes of ascites. If additional diuresis is necessary, a loop diuretic, such as furosemide (Lasix), may be added to the regimen.

- Medications are prescribed when the patient develops manifestations associated with hepatic encephalopathy. These drugs reduce the nitrogenous load, and lower serum ammonia levels. Two commonly prescribed medications are lactulose and neomycin. Both exert their effects locally, in the bowel. Lactulose draws ammonia from the blood, to the colon, where it is converted to ammonium ion. This ammonium ion is not absorbable; therefore, it is excreted in the feces. Neomycin sulfate is a locally-acting antibiotic that reduces the number of ammonia-forming bacteria in the bowel.

- The beta-blocker nadolol (Corgard) may be given together with isosorbide mononitrate (Ismo, Imdur, Monoket) to prevent rebleeding of esophageal varices. This drug combination also lowers hepatic venous pressure.

- Ferrous sulfate and folic acid are given as indicated to treat anemia. Vitamin K may be ordered to reduce the risk of bleeding. When bleeding is acute, packed RBCs, fresh frozen plasma, or platelets may be administered to restore blood components and promote hemostasis.

- Antacids are prescribed as indicated. A drug regimen to treat *Helicobacter pylori* infection also may be effective.

- Oxazepam (Serax), a benzodiazepine antianxiety/sedative drug, is not metabolized by the liver and may be used to treat acute agitation.

Nutritional Therapy

Dietary support is an essential part of care for the client with cirrhosis. Dietary needs change as hepatic function fluctuates. Nutritional therapy often involves the following:

- Sodium intake is restricted to less than 2 g/day, and fluids are restricted as necessary to reduce ascites and generalized edema. Fluids often are limited to 1,500 mL/day. Fluid needs are calculated based on response to diuretic therapy, urine output, and serum electrolyte values.

- Unless serum ammonia levels are high, a palatable diet with adequate calories and protein is recommended. Most individuals with mild chronic encephalopathy can tolerate 60–80 g of protein daily. Protein restriction is rarely justified for clients with cirrhosis because they are already in a state of malnutrition. Plant protein is preferred to animal protein. When encephalopathy resolves and serum ammonia levels stabilize, protein intake is allowed as tolerated. The diet is high in calories and includes moderate fat intake to promote healing.

Parenteral nutrition is used as needed to maintain nutritional status when food intake is limited (Wolfe & Katz, 2011).

- Vitamin and mineral supplements are ordered based on laboratory values. Deficiencies in the B-complex vitamins, particularly thiamin, folate, and B_{12}, and in the fat-soluble vitamins A, D, and E, are common. These vitamins may need to be administered in a water-soluble form. Clients with alcohol-induced cirrhosis are at high risk for magnesium deficiency, which requires replacement therapy.

Surgery

Liver transplantation is indicated for some clients with irreversible, progressive cirrhosis. A decline in functional status, increasing bilirubin levels, falling albumin levels, and increasing problems with complications that respond poorly to treatment are indications for liver transplantation. Malignancy, active alcohol or drug abuse, and poor surgical risk are contraindications for the surgery.

■ NURSING PROCESS

Nursing care of clients with cirrhosis is aimed at reducing further liver damage, teaching the client to make healthier lifestyle choices, and minimizing the symptoms of the disease. In addition to the nursing care discussed in this section, see the Nursing Care Plan on page 789.

Assessment

Assessment data related to cirrhosis include the following:

- *Health history.* Current manifestations, including abdominal pain or discomfort, recent weight loss, weakness, and anorexia; altered bowel elimination; excess bleeding or bruising; abdominal distention; jaundice; pruritus (itching); altered libido or impotence; duration of symptoms; history of liver or gallbladder disease; pattern and extent of alcohol or injection drug use; and use of other prescription and nonprescription drugs.
- *Physical assessment.* Vital signs; mental status; color and condition of skin and mucous membranes; peripheral pulses and presence of peripheral edema; and abdominal assessment, including appearance, shape and contour, bowel sounds, abdominal girth, percussion for liver borders, and palpation for tenderness and liver size.

Diagnosis

Nursing care of the client with cirrhosis presents many challenges, because liver function affects all body systems. Many NANDA nursing diagnoses may apply. The diagnoses discussed in this section focus on problems with fluid and electrolyte balance, disturbed thought processes, risk for bleeding, skin integrity, and nutrition; they include the following:

- *Excess Fluid Volume*
- *Risk for Acute Confusion*
- *Ineffective Protection*
- *Impaired Skin Integrity*
- *Imbalanced Nutrition: Less Than Body Requirements*

(NANDA-I © 2012)

Planning

Expected outcomes for a client with cirrhosis may include any of the following:

- The client will maintain proper hydration levels as indicated by urine specific gravity tests.
- The client will maintain appropriate diet.
- The client will report regular bowel elimination pattern.
- The client will be oriented to surroundings, person, and place.
- The client will maintain vital signs within normal limits.
- The client will avoid alcohol.

Implementation

With all clients (including children and young adults), the nurse should stress the relationship between alcohol and drug abuse and liver diseases. Specific interventions deal with excess fluid volume, acute confusion, ineffective protection, impaired skin integrity, and imbalanced nutrition.

Balance Fluid Volume

Cirrhosis affects water and salt regulation because of portal hypertension, hypoalbuminemia, and hyperaldosteronism. Signs of fluid volume overload and portal hypertension may develop, such as ascites, peripheral edema, internal hemorrhoids and varices, and prominent abdominal wall veins. Careful monitoring is necessary, because treatment measures can lead to further fluid and electrolyte imbalances. The nurse's responsibilities may include the following:

- Weigh the client daily. Assess for jugular vein distention, measure abdominal girth daily, check for peripheral edema, and monitor intake and output. Careful assessment to detect fluid shifts is important.
- Assess the client's urine specific gravity. Specific gravity measures the concentration of urine, an indicator of hydration.
- Provide a low-sodium diet (500–2,000 mg/day), and restrict fluids as ordered. Excess sodium leads to water retention and can increase fluid volume, ascites, and portal hypertension.

SAFETY ALERT
Monitor the client with cirrhosis for signs of impaired renal function, such as oliguria, a fixed specific gravity of approximately 1.012, central edema (around the eyes and of the face), and increasing serum creatinine and BUN levels. Such signs may indicate hepatorenal syndrome or acute renal failure from another cause.

Maintain Mental Status

Accumulated nitrogenous waste products and other metabolites affect mental status and thought processes. Effects of hepatic encephalopathy can range from mild confusion to agitation to coma. The nurse's responsibilities include the following:

- Assess neurological status, including level of consciousness and mental status. Observe for signs of early encephalopathy, such as asterixis and changes in handwriting and speech.

Early identification of evidence of encephalopathy allows prompt intervention. Subtle changes in neurological functioning are important.

- Avoid factors that may precipitate hepatic encephalopathy. Avoid hepatotoxic medications and drugs that depress the central nervous system. Cautious use of medications and close monitoring can eliminate iatrogenic causes of encephalopathy.

- Plan for consistent nursing care assignments if possible. Consistent care providers facilitate early identification of subtle neurological changes that indicate hepatic encephalopathy.

- Provide a low-protein diet as prescribed; teach the family the importance of maintaining diet restrictions. Nitrogenous byproducts from dietary protein increase serum ammonia levels.

- Administer medications or enemas as ordered to reduce nitrogenous products. Monitor bowel function, and provide measures to promote regular elimination and prevent constipation. Orally or rectally administered (per enema) medications are ordered to reduce intestinal bacteria and the ammonia they produce. Regular bowel elimination promotes protein and ammonia elimination in the feces.

- Orient the client to surroundings, person, and place; provide simple explanations and reassurance. Modification of verbal interactions to the level of understanding and mental status of the client may reduce anxiety and agitation.

SAFETY ALERT
Closely monitor clients who have experienced gastrointestinal bleeding for signs of hepatic encephalopathy. Blood in the intestinal tract is digested as a protein, which increases serum ammonia levels and the risk for hepatic encephalopathy.

Minimize Bleeding

Impaired coagulation, esophageal varices, and possible acute gastritis place the client with cirrhosis at significant risk for hemorrhage. Clotting is altered by vitamin K deficiency; by impaired manufacture of coagulation factors II, VII, IX, and X; and by increased platelet destruction because of splenomegaly. To prevent or minimize bleeding, the nurse does the following:

- Monitor vital signs, and report tachycardia or hypotension. Increased pulse and decreasing blood pressure may indicate hypovolemia caused by hemorrhage.

- Institute bleeding precautions. Preventive measures can decrease the risk for active bleeding.

- Monitor coagulation studies and platelet count, and report abnormal results. Coagulation studies help to determine the risk for bleeding and the need for treatment.

- Carefully monitor the client who has had bleeding esophageal varices for evidence of rebleeding, such as hematemesis (blood in the vomit), **hematochezia** (bright blood in the stool) or tarry stools, and signs of hypovolemia or shock. Rebleeding is common following variceal hemorrhage, especially within the first week.

SAFETY ALERT
Carefully monitor the respiratory status of the client with a Sengstaken-Blakemore or Minnesota tube, which may be used in the treatment of esophageal varices. Displacement of the tube can obstruct the airway unless an endotracheal tube is in place. The esophageal balloon prevents the client from swallowing oral secretions, increasing the risk for aspiration. Keep the head of the bed elevated 45 degrees to reduce the risk of aspiration and promote gas exchange.

Maintain Skin Integrity

Severe jaundice with bile salt deposits on the skin may cause pruritus. Scratching related to the pruritus damages the skin and impairs its integrity. Malnutrition, particularly protein deficiency, and edema also increase the risk for tissue breakdown and impaired skin integrity. To maintain the client's skin integrity, the nurse should take the following actions:

- Use warm water rather than hot water when bathing the client. Hot water increases pruritus.

- Use measures to prevent dry skin: Apply an emollient or lubricant as needed to keep skin moist, avoid soap or preparations with alcohol, and do not rub the skin. Dry skin contributes to pruritus.

- If indicated, apply mittens to the hands to prevent scratching. Clients with encephalopathy may not understand the need to refrain from scratching.

- Institute measures to prevent skin and tissue breakdown: Turn the client at least every 2 hours, use an alternating-pressure mattress, and frequently assess skin condition. Frequent position changes relieve pressure and promote circulation and tissue oxygenation.

- Administer a prescribed antihistamine (to relieve pruritus) cautiously. Decreased liver function increases the risk for altered drug responses.

Promote Balanced Nutrition

The client with cirrhosis is at risk for malnutrition for a number of reasons. These reasons include possible chronic alcohol use, anorexia, impaired vitamin and mineral absorption, and impaired protein metabolism. In addition, salt and protein restrictions may make the diet less palatable and appealing to the client. To protect the client against malnutrition, the nurse should do the following:

- Weigh the client daily. Instruct the client to weigh self at least weekly at home. Weight is a good indicator of both nutritional status and fluid balance. Short-term weight fluctuations tend to reflect fluid balance, while longer-term weight fluctuations are more reflective of nutritional status.

- Provide small meals with between-meal snacks. A small meal is more appealing for a client with anorexia. Between-meal snacks help the client to maintain adequate calorie and nutrient intake.

- Unless protein is restricted because of impending hepatic encephalopathy, promote protein and nutrient intake by providing nutritional supplements, such as Ensure or instant breakfasts. The sodium and protein content of all meals and snacks must be calculated when these nutrients are restricted.

■ Arrange a consultation with a dietitian for diet planning while the client is hospitalized and when at home. The dietitian can provide detailed instructions, sample menus, and suggestions for improving the palatability of the diet to promote intake.

Manage Complications

Paracentesis (aspiration of fluid from the peritoneal cavity) may be a diagnostic or a therapeutic procedure (to relieve severe ascites that does not respond to diuretic therapy). The goal of paracentesis is to relieve respiratory distress caused by excess fluid in the abdomen. Ascites fluid may be withdrawn in moderate amounts of 500 mL to 1 L daily to reduce the risk of fluid and electrolyte imbalances. Large-volume paracentesis (withdrawal of 4–6 L of fluid at one time) may be used. Albumin often is administered intravenously during large-volume paracentesis to maintain intravascular volume as the pressure of the ascites fluid in the abdomen is relieved.

Bleeding esophageal varices are life-threatening and require intensive care management. Restoration of hemodynamic stability is the first priority. A central line is inserted, and central venous and pulmonary artery pressures are monitored. Blood is given to restore blood volume, and fresh frozen plasma may be administered to restore clotting factors. Somatostatin or octreotide, both of which constrict blood vessels in the gut, is given intravenously to reduce blood flow in the portal venous system. Vasopressin, which produces generalized vasoconstriction, also may be used.

When the client's blood pressure and cardiac output have stabilized, upper endoscopy is performed to evaluate and treat the varices. A large nasogastric tube is inserted before endoscopy, and **gastric lavage** (irrigation of the stomach with large quantities of normal saline) is performed to improve visualization. During endoscopy, the varices may be banded or sclerosed to reduce the risk of recurrent bleeding. In *banding* (*variceal ligation*) small rubber bands are placed on varices to occlude blood flow. *Endoscopic sclerosis* involves injecting a sclerosing agent directly into the varices to induce inflammation and clotting.

Balloon tamponade of bleeding varices may be used if bleeding cannot be controlled through vasoconstriction or if endoscopy is unavailable. A multiple-lumen nasogastric tube (e.g., a Sengstaken-Blakemore or Minnesota tube) is inserted, and the gastric and esophageal balloons are inflated to apply direct pressure on the bleeding varices. Tension is applied to the tube to further compress the varices. Balloon tamponade carries a number of risks, including aspiration, airway obstruction, and tissue ischemia and necrosis. An endotracheal tube is inserted before nasogastric intubation to support the airway and reduce the risk of aspiration. This short-term measure is used only until more definitive treatment can be performed.

SAFETY ALERT
When caring for a client with a multiple-lumen nasogastric tube, always deflate the esophageal balloon before the gastric balloon. This practice prevents the balloon from becoming misplaced and occluding the airway. Always keep an appropriate syringe at the bedside to deflate the esophageal balloon should the client develop respiratory distress.

A **Transjugular intrahepatic portosystemic shunt (TIPS)** is used to relieve portal hypertension and its complications of esoph-

Client Teaching The Client With Cirrhosis of the Liver

Cirrhosis is a chronic, progressive disease. Therefore, the client and family assume major roles in managing the disease and its manifestations and in preventing complications. Teaching topics for home care include the following:

■ The absolute necessity of avoiding alcohol and other hepatotoxic drugs. Suggest inpatient or community-based alcohol treatment programs and Alcoholics Anonymous as indicated.

■ Diet and fluid intake restrictions and recommendations. Include suggestions to promote nutritional intake and increase the flavor of food when sodium is restricted.

■ Prescribed medications. Include their timing, intended and adverse effects, and manifestations to report to the primary care provider.

■ Bleeding precautions.

■ Manifestations of potential complications to be reported to the primary care provider. Stress the importance of promptly reporting evidence of gastrointestinal bleeding for prompt intervention for potential hemorrhage.

■ Skin care techniques to reduce pruritus and the risk of damage.

■ Ways to manage fatigue and conserve energy.

■ Provide referrals for home health services, dietary consultation, social services, and counseling as needed by the client and family. Suggest local support groups where available. If appropriate, suggest hospice services for the client with end-stage liver disease.

ageal varices and ascites. A channel is created through the liver tissue with a needle inserted transcutaneously. An expandable metal stent is inserted into this channel to allow blood to flow directly from the portal vein into the hepatic vein, bypassing the cirrhotic liver. The shunt relieves pressure in esophageal varices and allows better control of fluid retention with diuretic therapy. Stenosis and occlusion of the shunt are frequent complications. TIPS also increases the risk of developing hepatic encephalopathy (because of decreased perfusion of the liver and impaired ammonia metabolism), and it may reduce long-term survival. It generally is used as a short-term measure until a liver transplant can be performed.

Evaluation

The evaluation of the client with cirrhosis includes monitoring laboratory data such as liver function tests (LFTs). Elevated liver enzymes indicate hepatocellular destruction. LFTs should remain stable during the treatment phase of the disease. Other lab tests to monitor are CBC, hematocrit (Hct) and hemoglobin (Hgb), coagulation studies, serum electrolytes, serum albumin, and serum ammonia levels. These values are expected to improve if therapy is successful. Biophysical data expectations include stable vital signs, improvement in level of consciousness, absence of bruising and bleeding, improved appetite, improved mobility, adequate urinary output and bowel elimination, decreasing ascites (as evidenced by decreasing girth measurements), restorative sleep patterns, and decreased discomfort.

NURSING CARE PLAN A Client With Alcoholic Cirrhosis

Richard Wright is a divorced 48-year-old father of two teenagers. He has been admitted to the community hospital with ascites and malnutrition. He has had three previous hospital stays for cirrhosis, the most recent 6 months ago.

ASSESSMENT

Mr. Wright is lethargic but responds appropriately to verbal stimuli. He complains of "spitting up blood the past week or so," and he says, "I'm just not hungry." He has lost 9 kg (20 lb) since his previous admission. He is jaundiced and has petechiae and ecchymoses on his arms and legs. Liz Mowdi, Mr. Wright's nurse, notes pitting pretibial edema. Abdominal assessment reveals a tight, protuberant abdomen with caput medusae. The liver margin is not palpable, and the spleen is enlarged. Vital signs are T 37.7°C (100°F), P 110 bpm, R 24/min, and BP 110/70 mmHg.

Abnormal laboratory results include the following: WBC, 3,700/mm^3 (normal range, 4,500–10,000 µL (mm^3)); RBC, 4.0 million/mm^3 (normal range, 4.6–6.0 million/mm^3); platelets, 75,000/mm^3 (normal range, 150,000–400,000/mm^3); serum ammonia, 105 µm/dL (normal range, 15–45 mcg/dL); total bilirubin, 4.9 mg/dL (normal range, 0.1–1.2 mg/dL); and serum sodium, 150 mEq/L (normal range, 135–145 mEq/L). Potassium, hemoglobin, hematocrit, total protein, and albumin levels are markedly decreased. Hepatic enzymes are elevated. BUN and creatinine levels are marginally elevated. Oxygen saturation is 88% (normal range, 96%–100%) per pulse oximetry.

Endoscopy shows bleeding from a gastric ulcer, and the diagnosis is alcoholic cirrhosis with gastritis. Mr. Wright is started on Aldactone, 25 mg po q8h; Riopan, 30 mL 2 h pc and hs; lactulose, 30 mL qh until onset of diarrhea, then 15 mL tid; a low-protein, 800 mg sodium diet; and fluid restriction of 1,500 mL/day.

DIAGNOSES

Nursing diagnoses that may be appropriate for Mr. Wright include the following:

- *Impaired Gas Exchange* related to pressure of ascites fluid on the diaphragm, manifested in tachypnea and decreased oxygen saturation
- *Excess Fluid Volume* related to electrolyte imbalance and hypoalbuminemia, manifested in ascites and peripheral edema
- *Imbalanced Nutrition: Less Than Body Requirements* related to anorexia and possible alcohol abuse, manifested in weight loss and low serum protein levels
- *Risk for Acute Confusion* related to effects of high ammonia levels as manifested by lethargy
- *Ineffective Protection* related to impaired platelet formation and malnutrition

(NANDA-I © 2012)

PLANNING

The goals for the plan of care for Mr. Wright include the following; he will

- Have a respiratory rate and oxygen saturation within normal limits.
- Have a decrease in abdominal girth of 1–2 cm/day and a decrease in peripheral edema.
- Gain 0.45 kg (1 lb) per week without evidence of increased fluid retention.
- Have serum albumin levels return to normal range.
- Be alert and oriented.
- Have serum ammonia levels within the normal range.
- Demonstrate no further evidence of active bleeding.
- Verbalize willingness to join a community support group.

IMPLEMENTATION

The following nursing interventions may be appropriate for Mr. Wright:

- Weigh daily.
- Provide high-calorie, low-salt, low-protein diet with between-meal snacks.
- Maintain a stool chart.
- Assign the same nurses as much as possible to facilitate evaluation of his mental status and promptly report changes in status or laboratory values.
- Measure abdominal girth every 8 hours, marking level of measurement.
- Institute bleeding precautions.
- Elevate the head of the bed; assist the client to a chair with legs elevated three times a day as tolerated.
- Include significant others in care and teaching, and refer the client to community agencies for discharge follow up.

EVALUATION

A week after admission, Mr. Wright's ascites has decreased, and no further active bleeding is noted. His serum protein levels have increased, and his laboratory values are improving. No further bruising is noted during hospitalization. Although he shows a 5-lb weight loss as excess water is eliminated, he is consuming 100% of his diet. His serum ammonia levels have returned to normal. On discharge, oxygen saturation is 96%; respirations are 18/min. Lactulose will be continued on discharge.

Ms. Mowdi provides both written and verbal information about the medication and cirrhosis, including measures to prevent complications. Mr. Wright and his children express interest in Alcoholics Anonymous and Al-Anon and are referred to those agencies. Before discharge, follow up appointments are made with a psychiatric social worker and a primary caregiver.

CRITICAL THINKING

1. Describe the relationship between portal hypertension, liver dysfunction, and ascites.
2. Outline a 1-day menu for a low-protein, low-sodium, high-calorie diet.
3. What is the pathophysiological basis for hepatic encephalopathy?
4. What are the nursing responsibilities related to lactulose and neomycin?
5. Design a nursing care plan for Mr. Wright for the diagnosis Ineffective Coping.

REVIEW Liver Disease

RELATE Link the Concepts and Exemplars

Linking the exemplar of liver disease with the concept of addiction:

1. What nursing strategies might help the client with alcohol addiction experiencing symptoms of liver disease find the motivation to abstain from alcohol?

2. The family of a client who is addicted to alcohol and has liver disease informs the nurse that the client has relapsed and returned to regular alcohol use after discharge from an alcohol treatment center. What assessment data would the nurse collect from the client?

Linking the exemplar of liver disease with the concept of tissue integrity:

3. When caring for a client with jaundice resulting from liver disease, what specific skin care measures might the nurse initiate to reduce the risk of altered skin integrity?

4. What factors increase the risk of altered skin integrity in the client with chronic or acute liver disease?

READY Go to Companion Skills Manual

REFER Go to Pearson Nursing Student Resources
nursing.pearsonhighered.com

REFLECT Case Study

Saul Mendato is a 60-year-old male whom his wife found unconscious and brought to the emergency department. He has a history of alcohol-induced cirrhosis. The nurse evaluating his laboratory values notes the following: total bilirubin, 4.6 mg/dL; serum ammonia, 95 mcg/dL; platelets, 68,000/mm^3; and RBC, 4.2 million/mm^3.

1. Based on the laboratory reports, Mr. Mendato is at most risk for which complication of cirrhosis?

2. What are the priorities of nursing care?

3. What outcomes would be appropriate for this client?

EXEMPLAR 12.4 Obesity

EXEMPLAR KEY TERMS
Basal metabolic rate (BMR), *790*
Body mass index (BMI), *791*
Lower body obesity, *791*
Metabolic syndrome, *792*
Morbid obesity, *792*
Nutrients, *790*
Obesity, *790*
Satiety, *791*
Triglycerides, *791*
Upper body obesity, *791*
Very-low-calorie diets, *794*

EXEMPLAR LEARNING OUTCOMES
After reading about this exemplar, you will be able to:

1. Describe the pathophysiology, etiology, clinical manifestations, and direct and indirect causes of obesity.

2. Identify risk factors and prevention methods associated with obesity.

3. Illustrate the nursing process in providing culturally competent care across the life span for individuals with obesity.

4. Formulate priority nursing diagnoses appropriate for an individual with obesity.

5. Summarize therapies used by interdisciplinary teams in the collaborative care of an individual with obesity.

6. Plan evidence-based care for an individual with obesity and his or her family in collaboration with other members of the healthcare team.

7. Evaluate expected outcomes for an individual with obesity.

▶ OVERVIEW

Obesity (an excess of adipose tissue) is one of the most prevalent preventable health problems in the United States. Obesity has serious physiological and psychological consequences and is associated with increased morbidity and mortality. It contributes to poor health-related quality of life to a greater extent than smoking, excess alcohol use, or poverty. Obesity is a major public health issue. The most recent national data on obesity prevalence among adults, adolescents, and children shows that 35% of adults and 17% of children and adolescents were obese in 2009–2010 (Ogden et al., 2012).

There was no significant difference in prevalence between men and women at any age. Overall, adults age 60 and over were more likely to be obese than younger adults. Among women 42% of those age 60 and over were obese, compared to 31% of women age 20–39. Ethnicity had a bearing on the statistics. Non-Hispanic

Blacks had the highest age-adjusted rates of obesity (49%); the rate among Mexican Americans was 40% (Ogden et al., 2012).

▶ PATHOPHYSIOLOGY AND ETIOLOGY

All body activities, including activities of daily living and those necessary to maintain cell and tissue function, require energy. **Nutrients** in food (or enteral or parenteral feedings) provide energy and are the building blocks for growth and tissue repair. The body stores excess nutrients and energy (measured as kilocalories) to meet the body's needs when required nutrients are unavailable. This ability to store and release energy is important in maintaining body function. More than 70% of the energy expended each day goes to maintaining the **basal metabolic rate (BMR)**—essentially, the "cost" (in kilocalories) of being alive. Physical activity accounts for only 5%–10% of the energy spent daily.

Energy is stored primarily as fat in adipose tissue. Although mature fat cells (adipocytes) do not multiply, the immature cells in adipose tissue can multiply, particularly when exposed to estrogen during puberty, in late adolescence, during breastfeeding, and in middle age adults who are overweight. Fat cells store excess energy as **triglycerides**, which are formed from dietary fats and carbohydrates. The body breaks down the triglycerides in fat cells when they are needed to provide energy (Porth & Matfin, 2009).

Etiology

Obesity occurs when excess calories are stored as fat. It can result from excess energy intake, decreased energy expenditure, or a combination of both. The etiology of obesity is not, however, as simple as excess kilocalorie intake in relation to energy expenditure. The systems that regulate food intake, energy storage, and energy expenditure are complex and not fully understood.

Appetite, which affects food intake, is regulated by the central nervous system and by emotional factors. The hunger center in the hypothalamus stimulates appetite in response to stimuli such as hypoglycemia. As nutrient levels rise, the satiety center (also in the hypothalamus) sends the message to stop eating. Gastrointestinal filling and hormonal factors also signal **satiety** (a sensation of fullness). Appetite may have little relationship to hunger: Individuals may eat to relieve depression or anxiety.

Several hormones are involved in regulating obesity: thyroid hormone, insulin, and leptin (a peptide produced by fatty tissue that suppresses appetite and increases energy expenditure). Some studies suggest that leptin resistance is a cause of obesity. Insulin is associated with body fat distribution.

Risk Factors

Many factors, including genetic, physiological, psychological, environmental, and sociocultural, contribute to obesity. Heredity may contribute as much as 25%–40% of the risk for obesity. However, it is difficult to separate the role of environment from that of genetic factors. A strong correlation exists between the weight of adopted children and their biological parents. In addition, identical twins tend to have similar body mass indexes, whether they are raised together or apart, providing further evidence of a genetic link to obesity. While several genes that contribute to appetite and fat deposition have been identified, obesity as a purely genetic condition is rare (Bouchard, 2010).

Physical inactivity is probably the most important contributor to obesity. Inactive individuals may consume fewer calories than active individuals and continue to gain weight because of a lack of energy expenditure. Cultural and environmental factors, such as labor-saving devices, reliance on the automobile for transportation, and increased time spent using the computer, contribute to decreased energy expenditure among adults in the United States. Increased time spent watching television is seen as a major contributor to the increase in obesity among children and adolescents (Bouchard, 2010).

Environmental influences, such as an abundant and readily accessible food supply, fast-food restaurants, advertising, and vending machines, contribute to increased food intake. Socio-cultural influences that contribute to obesity include overeating at family meals, rewarding desired behavior with food, religious and family gatherings that promote food intake, and sedentary lifestyles. Socioeconomic status also tends to correlate with the risk for overweight and obesity: In the United States, women with low incomes or low educational levels are more likely to be obese than are those with higher socioeconomic status (Ogden et al., 2012). However, the association between socioeconomic status and obesity is less clear in men. Between 1988–1994 and 2007–2008, the prevalence of obesity increased in adults at all income and education levels (Ogden et al., 2012).

Obesity and extreme obesity among U.S. low-income preschool-age children went down in recent years for the first time. However, obesity in children still remains a public health issue. According to the 2009 Pediatric Nutrition Surveillance System, nearly one third of 3.7 million low-income children age 2–4 were obese or overweight (Ogden et al., 2012).

Psychological factors, such as low self-esteem, also play a role in obesity. Low self-esteem may precipitate unhealthy eating behaviors, and the resulting weight gain may diminish self-esteem even further. An individual may overeat as a result of anxiety, depression, guilt, or boredom; overeating also may be a means of getting attention. Some experts characterize overeating as a food addiction and as a mechanism for coping with stressful life events.

▶ CLINICAL MANIFESTATIONS

While obesity often is defined by weight, it is more accurately defined by the **body mass index (BMI)**, which is an indirect measure of the amount of body fat, or adipose tissue. Adipose tissue is created when energy consumption exceeds energy expenditure. A BMI of 25–29.9 kg/m^2 is classified as *overweight*; a BMI of 30 kg/m^2 or greater is classified as obesity (National Heart, Lung, and Blood Institute, 2013). The terms *overweight* and *obese* are not mutually exclusive; a client who is obese is also overweight (**Table 12–12** ●).

The two major types of body fat distribution are upper body and lower body obesity. **Upper body obesity** (also called *central obesity*) is identified by a waist-to-hip ratio of greater than 1 in men or 0.8 in women. Individuals with upper body obesity tend to have more intra-abdominal fat and higher levels of circulating free fatty acids (Porth & Matfin, 2009). As a result, upper body obesity is associated with a greater risk of complications such as hypertension, abnormal blood lipid levels, heart disease, stroke, and elevated insulin levels. Men tend to have more intra-abdominal fat than women, although women develop a central fat distribution pattern after menopause.

Lower body obesity (also known as *peripheral obesity*) is identified by a waist-to-hip ratio of less than 0.8 and is more commonly seen in women. The risk for hyperinsulinemia, abnormal lipids, and heart disease is lower in individuals with lower body obesity than in those with upper body obesity. Lower body obesity may be more difficult to treat, however.

Because obesity has many contributing factors, its treatment is far more complex than just reducing the amount of food consumed. Treatment is an ongoing process requiring a number of strategies. Most experts recommend an individualized program

TABLE 12–12   Classification of Overweight and Obesity by BMI, Waist Circumference, and Associated Disease Risks

	BMI (KG/M²)	OBESITY CLASS	DISEASE RISK RELATIVE TO NORMAL WEIGHT AND WAIST CIRCUMFERENCE[a]	
			MEN 102 CM (40 IN.) OR LESS, WOMEN 88 CM (35 IN.) OR LESS	MEN > 102 CM (40 IN.), WOMEN > 88 CM (35 IN.)
Underweight	<18.5		—	—
Normal	18.5–24.9		—	—
Overweight	25.0–29.9		Increased	High
Obese	30.0–34.9	I	High	Very high
	35.0–39.9	II	Very high	Very high
Extreme obesity	≥40.0	III	Extremely high	Extremely high

Source: National Heart, Lung, and Blood Institute (2013). *Classification of overweight and obesity by BMI, waist circumference, and associated disease risks.* Retrieved from http://www.nhlbi.nih.gov/health/public/heart/obesity/lose_wt/bmi_dis.htm.

[a]Disease risk for type 2 DM, hypertension, and cardiovascular disease. Increased waist circumference also can be a marker for increased risk even in individuals of normal weight.

of exercise, diet, and behavior modification designed to meet the client's specific needs. Pharmacotherapy usually is recommended only as an adjunct when traditional therapies have been unsuccessful. Surgical treatment (bariatric surgery) generally is limited to clients with **morbid obesity** (BMI ≥ 40 kg/m², or >200% of ideal body weight) who are unable to lose weight through diet and exercise or have serious obesity-related problems, such as metabolic syndrome, hypertension, or heart disease. See the Clinical Manifestations and Therapies feature for more information.

Clinical Manifestations and Therapies
Obesity

CLINICAL MANIFESTATION	CLINICAL THERAPIES
BMI of 25–26.9 with two or more comorbidities	▪ Diet, exercise, and behavior modification
BMI of 27–29.9 with two or more comorbidities	▪ Diet, exercise, and behavior modification ▪ Pharmacotherapy
BMI of 30–34.9 with two or more comorbidities (obesity class I)	▪ Diet, exercise, and behavior modification ▪ Pharmacotherapy ▪ Surgery
BMI of 35–39.9 with two or more comorbidities (obesity class II)	▪ Diet, exercise, and behavior modification ▪ Pharmacotherapy ▪ Surgery
BMI of ≥40 (obesity class III)	▪ Diet, exercise, and behavior modification ▪ Pharmacotherapy ▪ Surgery

Note: Diet, exercise, and behavior modification can be appropriate for clients with hypertension, hyperlipidemia, diabetes, and other obesity-related complications.

▶ COMPLICATIONS OF OBESITY

Obesity is a significant risk factor for cardiovascular disease, including hypertension, coronary heart disease (CHD), and heart failure. The prevalence of hypertension in obese men and women is approximately twice that in individuals with a BMI of less than 25. The increases in blood pressure seen with obesity increase the risk for CHD and stroke. Approximately 60% of individuals with obesity have **metabolic syndrome**, including three or more of the following symptoms: increased waist circumference, hypertension, elevated blood triglycerides and fasting blood glucose, and low HDL cholesterol. Metabolic syndrome is an identified risk factor for atherosclerosis and CHD. The Nurses' Health Study showed that the relative risk for CHD in women increases with a BMI of 25 or more. Obesity also increases the risk for developing heart failure: Left ventricular muscle mass increases, and the ventricle dilates in individuals with obesity, possibly because of increased blood volume and cardiac output. Obesity-associated obstructive sleep apnea also contributes to the risk for heart failure (Endocrine Society, 2008).

Obesity increases the risk of insulin resistance and type 2 DM. Both weight gain in adulthood and abdominal (central) obesity are positively correlated with the risk for developing type 2 DM.

Obesity affects reproductive function in both men and women. Androgen (male sex hormone) levels are reduced in obese men; menstrual irregularities and polycystic ovarian syndrome are more common in obese women. (Polycystic ovarian syndrome is an additional risk factor for hyperinsulinemia and insulin resistance as well; Endocrine Society, 2008).

Increased weight also increases the risk for developing gallstones in both men and women. The risk for developing several types of cancer, including colon, breast, and endometrial, increases in obesity as well. Increased weight places abnormal stress on joints, increasing the prevalence of joint pain and osteoarthritis, particularly in weight-bearing joints (especially the knee joints). Other health-related problems associated with obesity are listed in **Table 12–13** ●.

TABLE 12–13 Health-Related Problems Associated With Obesity

BODY SYSTEM	OBESITY-RELATED PROBLEMS
Cardiovascular	Atherosclerosis, hypercholesterolemia
	Coronary heart disease
	Heart failure
	Hypertension
	Stroke
	Varicosities
	Venous thrombosis
Respiratory	Sleep disorders
	Sleep apnea
Gastrointestinal	Gallbladder disease
	Hiatal hernia
	Colon cancer
Genitourinary	Cancers of the breast, uterus, and prostate
	Complications of pregnancy
	Stress incontinence
Musculoskeletal	Low back pain
	Muscle strains and sprains
	Osteoarthritis
Endocrine and reproductive	Type 2 diabetes mellitus Endometrial cancer
	Polycystic ovarian syndrome
Other	Depression
	Binge-eating disorder
	Postoperative complications

▶ COLLABORATION

Successful treatment of obesity—that is, sustained achievement of normal body weight without adverse consequences—rarely is achieved. Treatment often is interdisciplinary and focuses on reducing the health risks associated with obesity by changing both eating and exercise habits.

Diagnostic Tests

Diagnostic tests that may be part of the physical assessment include the following:

- **Body mass index.** Used to identify excess adipose tissue. The BMI is calculated by dividing the weight (in kg) by the height (in m²). Calculations may not reflect as accurately the extent of adipose tissue in individuals who are highly muscular (e.g., body builders) or in those who have lost muscle mass (e.g., older adults).

- **Anthropometry.** Includes measurements of height, weight, bone size, and skin folds to estimate subcutaneous fat.

- **Underwater weighing (hydrodensitometry).** Considered the most accurate way to determine body fat. This technique involves submerging the whole body and then measuring the amount of displaced water.

- **Bioelectrical impedance.** Uses a low-energy electrical impulse to determine the percentage of body fat by measuring the electrical resistance of the body.

- **Waist circumference.** Measured to determine body fat distribution. Men with a waist measurement of 102 cm (40 in.) or greater and women with a waist measurement of 88 cm (35 in.) or greater have a higher risk for complications of obesity.

Other diagnostic tests may be done to help identify a physiological cause or complications related to obesity. These tests include:

- **Thyroid profile.** Includes a total T_3 and T_3 uptake, free T_4 and total T_4, free T_4 index, and TSH and is done to rule out thyroid disease.

- **Serum glucose.** Measured to identify coexisting diabetes.

- **Serum cholesterol.** Measured to assess for elevated levels.

- **Lipid profile.** HDL levels may be reduced in clients with obesity, whereas low-density lipoprotein (LDL) levels are elevated.

- **Electrocardiography.** Performed to detect effects of obesity on the heart (e.g., rate or rhythm disruptions, myocardial infarction, or heart enlargement).

Pharmacologic Therapy

Many prescription and over-the-counter drugs have been used to help individuals lose weight. When used in combination with diet and exercise, drugs can help to promote weight loss. Their long-term efficacy, however, is questionable; rebound weight gain following the cessation of drug use is common. In addition, tolerance, addiction, and side effects may occur. These products usually are recommended only as an adjunct to therapy and only when traditional therapies have been unsuccessful.

Amphetamines, which have a high potential for abuse, and nonamphetamine appetite suppressants (e.g., phentermine) may be used for a short time to promote weight loss. Phentermine is believed to act directly on the appetite control center in the central nervous system. As with amphetamines, nonamphetamine appetite suppressants stimulate the central nervous system, with resulting increased alertness, nervousness, and insomnia; they reduce fatigue and can interfere with sleep. They are used with caution in clients who have preexisting heart disease, because they can increase blood pressure and heart rate and cause anginal pain.

Sibutramine (Meridia) is an appetite suppressant that acts on the central nervous system. Sibutramine also may increase the metabolic rate, promoting weight loss. It has the additional benefit of lowering cholesterol and triglyceride levels. However, sibutramine increases both pulse rate and blood pressure, potentially limiting its appropriateness for use in clients with hypertension, CHD, or heart failure.

Orlistat (Xenical) has a different mechanism of action: It inhibits fat absorption from the gastrointestinal tract, leading to weight loss. It has the added benefit of lowering blood glucose and cholesterol. The adverse effects of orlistat relate to its inhibition of fat absorption: oily stools, flatulence, and fecal urgency.

These effects tend to diminish, however, when dietary fat intake is limited.

Qsymia and Belviq are the most recent weight loss drugs released. Qsymia is a combination of phentermine and topiramate (an anticonvulsant that has many off-label uses). Belviq acts by stimulating serotonin receptors in the brain and causing feelings of satiety. Qsymia is contraindicated during pregnancy. It may also cause increased heart rate, suicidal thoughts, insomnia, and mood problems and may aggravate hypertension. Side effects of Belviq include depression, migraine, and memory lapses.

Over-the-counter products such as benzocaine and bulk-forming agents also commonly are used in weight management efforts. Methylcellulose and other bulk-forming products may decrease appetite by producing a sensation of fullness. Clients taking these products may experience flatulence or diarrhea and may need to increase fluid intake.

Exercise

Exercise is a critical element in losing weight and keeping it off. Physical activity increases energy consumption and promotes weight loss while preserving lean body mass. Such activity improves physical fitness, decreases appetite, promotes self-esteem, and increases the BMR. Clients may benefit from consulting with a physical therapist or personal trainer who will help them develop an exercise plan that reflects the client's physical condition, interests, lifestyle, and abilities.

If a client is under the care of a physician for another condition, such as asthma or diabetes, the client should consult with the treating physician, but evaluation by a healthcare practitioner is important for any client before beginning an exercise program. The practitioner instructs the client to increase the duration and intensity of activity and to stop exercising and report symptoms if chest pain or shortness of breath occurs. An aerobic exercise program of 30–40 minutes of exercise five or more days a week promotes weight loss while reducing adipose tissue, increasing lean body mass, and promoting long-term weight control. (See the module on Health, Wellness, and Illness for more details.)

Nutrition

Collaboration with a nutritionist helps clients to identify healthy foods that appeal to them and that can make up a diet plan to create a daily 500- to 1,000-kcal deficit. Ideally, the recommended diet should be low in kilocalories and fat, contain adequate nutrients and minerals, and be high in dietary fiber. The client should eat regular meals with small servings. A gradual, slow weight loss of no more than 1–2 lb/week is recommended. For most individuals, this means a diet of 1,000–1,200 kcal/day for most women and 1,200–1,600 kcal/day for men. Fewer than 1,200 kcal each day may lead to loss of lean tissue and nutritional deficiencies. Excessive calorie restrictions also can lead to failure to follow the prescribed diet, feelings of guilt, and overeating.

"Yo-yo" dieting (repeated cycles of weight loss and gain) may lead to a metabolic deficiency that makes subsequent weight loss efforts increasingly difficult. Therefore it is critical that dieters take any weight loss effort seriously and include plans for long-term maintenance. The best approach is to modify dietary intake without severe restrictions, eating a well-balanced, low-fat diet and developing improved eating habits.

Very-low-calorie diets generally are reserved for clients who have a BMI greater than 30 (WIN, 2013b). This type of program offers a protein-sparing modified fast (400–800 kcal/day or less) under close medical supervision. In a typical program, the client consumes 45–70 g of high-quality protein, 30–50 g of carbohydrate, and approximately 2 g of fat per day for 1–2 months. Exercise, nutrition, and behavior modification counseling should accompany the diet. The client generally experiences a dramatic and rapid weight loss while maintaining lean body mass. Suppression of hunger brought on by ketone production associated with fat metabolism is an added benefit of the diet. Complications generally are minor, and benefits include decreased blood pressure, blood glucose, and cholesterol and triglyceride levels along with improved exercise tolerance. Very-low-calorie diets may not be appropriate for use in individuals over age 50 because of normal loss of lean body mass and adverse effects of the diet. Adverse effects generally are minor but can include fatigue, constipation, nausea, diarrhea, and gallstone formation (WIN, 2013b).

Behavior Modification

Behavior modification is a critical component of successful weight management. Strategies such as keeping food records, eliminating cues that precipitate eating, and changing the act of eating often are helpful.

Recording food intake, amount, location of eating, and situations that induce eating often helps the dieter to gain self-control. These strategies generally are most effective when used in combination with other behavior modification approaches.

Researchers have found that for most overweight individuals, eating is regulated by external cues, such as the proximity to food and the time of day. In contrast, hunger and satiety are the cues that regulate eating in adults of normal weight. Strategies to control food cues include keeping food out of view, eliminating snack foods, and eating only in designated areas.

Other behavior modification approaches focus on helping clients to examine factors that affect their eating behaviors. Examining their lifestyle, personality, and environment helps clients to understand eating behaviors and their consequences. The goal is to empower individuals who are stimulated to eat to choose activities that are not related to food.

Social support and group programs such as Weight Watchers, Overeaters Anonymous, and Take Off Pounds Sensibly promote weight loss success through peer support. Most organized programs require participants to pay a fee, which may improve compliance.

Surgery

Surgical treatment of obesity (bariatric surgery) generally is limited to clients who are morbidly obese and unable to lose weight through diet and exercise or have serious obesity-related problems, such as metabolic syndrome, hypertension, or heart disease (WIN, 2013a). In addition, the client must be able to tolerate surgery and be free of addiction to alcohol or other drugs. A thorough psychological evaluation is done before surgery.

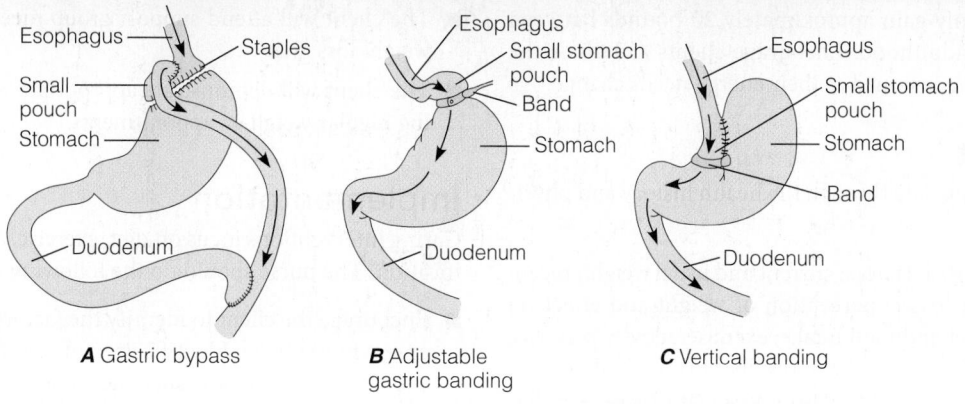

Figure 12–9 ● Types of surgical procedures to treat obesity: *A*, Roux-en-Y gastric bypass surgery; *B*, adjustable gastric banding; and *C*, vertical banded gastroplasty.

The benefits of surgery include major weight loss and improved blood pressure, plus a reduced risk of diabetes, sleep apnea, angina, heart failure, blood lipid levels, and venous disease. Bariatric surgery is not without risk, however, and the decision to undergo surgery is a significant one.

RESTRICTIVE/MALABSORPTIVE PROCEDURES The most commonly used bariatric surgical procedures in the United States are combined restrictive/malabsorptive surgeries. These surgeries restrict stomach capacity, thus limiting food intake, and bypass a portion of the small intestine to restrict the absorption of calories and nutrients. In the Roux-en-Y gastric bypass (**Figure 12–9A** ●), a small stomach pouch is created to restrict food intake. A Y-shaped section of the jejunum is then attached to the pouch to allow food to bypass the lower stomach and duodenum. As a result, calorie and nutrient absorption is limited. A more complex procedure, the biliopancreatic diversion, carries a higher risk of nutritional deficiencies and is used less frequently. In biliopancreatic diversion, a portion of the stomach is removed to reduce its capacity. A bypass of the duodenum and jejunum is created by connecting the ileum either directly to the stomach pouch or just distal to the pyloric valve.

These combined restrictive/malabsorptive surgeries have the advantage of resulting in rapid weight loss that is maintained over time. Many clients maintain a 60%–70% weight loss for 10 years or more following Roux-en-Y gastric bypass surgery (WIN, 2013a). These surgeries also help to improve obesity-associated health problems, such as type 2 DM, hypertension, and sleep apnea. Because these procedures allow food to bypass the duodenum and jejunum, nutrient deficiencies, particularly of iron, calcium, vitamin B_{12}, and, possibly, the fat-soluble vitamins, are common.

RESTRICTIVE PROCEDURES Restrictive procedures, which are safer but generally less effective in the long term, include adjustable gastric banding and the vertical banded gastroplasty. In adjustable gastric banding (Figure 12–9B), a hollow band of silicone rubber is placed around the upper (proximal) portion of the stomach. The band is inflated with saline solution to create a small stomach pouch with a narrow passage to the rest of the stomach. The amount of band inflation can be adjusted with a port implanted under the skin. The vertical banded gastroplasty (Figure 12–9C) uses both a band and staples to create a small stomach pouch. Both procedures

may be performed laparoscopically and can be reversed if necessary. Few nutritional deficiencies are associated with restrictive bariatric procedures. Vomiting is a common postoperative risk with restrictive procedures. The band may slip or break, necessitating a return to surgery. Approximately 15%–20% of clients undergoing vertical banded gastroplasty procedures require a second procedure. For this reason and because of the increased complexity of the vertical banded procedure, it is performed less commonly than adjustable gastric banding (WIN, 2013a). While clients typically lose approximately 50% of their excess body weight within the first year after these procedures, less than one quarter maintain that weight loss over a 10-year period (WIN, 2013a).

COMPLICATIONS OF SURGERY Although the risk for postoperative complications is high, the mortality rate for bariatric procedures is low (<1% for restrictive surgeries and up to 5% for combination procedures). Possible postoperative complications include anastomosis leak with peritonitis, abdominal wall hernia, gallstones, wound infections, deep venous thrombosis, nutritional deficiencies, and gastrointestinal symptoms. Dumping syndrome, which can be precipitated by a meal that is high in simple carbohydrates, may develop following combined bariatric surgeries such as Roux-en-Y gastric bypass and biliopancreatic diversion. In dumping syndrome, stomach contents move rapidly through the small intestine, drawing fluid into the intestine by osmosis. The client experiences nausea, bloating, abdominal pain, weakness, sweating, and possibly syncope.

■ NURSING PROCESS

Maintaining a healthy weight throughout the life span begins in childhood. Obese children and teenagers become obese adults. Promote healthy eating, including a diet rich in whole grains, fruits, and vegetables and low in fat. The U.S. Department of Agriculture's MyPlate and Harvard's Healthy Eating Pyramid provide visual guidance for appropriate food choices to maintain a healthy, well-balanced diet. Encourage all children and adults to maintain an active lifestyle, engaging in at least 30 minutes of aerobic activity daily. Encourage parents to limit the time that children spend watching television, using the computer, and playing video games. Discuss the effects of smoking and excess alcohol use on nutrition and activity.

Adults commonly gain approximately 20 pounds between early and middle adulthood. Encourage clients to reduce the number of calories consumed as their energy needs change.

Assessment

Collect the following data through the health history and physical examination:

- *Health history.* Risk factors; current and usual weight; recent weight gains or losses; perception of weight and effect on health; usual diet and food intake; exercise/activity patterns; previous weight loss efforts and results; current medications; coexisting disorders, such as cardiovascular disease and diabetes; tobacco use; and family history of overweight, diabetes, and weight-related morbidity
- *Physical examination.* Vital signs, weight and height, skinfold measurements, waist-to-hip ratio, and inspection of skin under the breasts and abdominal folds.

SAFETY ALERT
Use of an inappropriate size of sphygmomanometer is a common source of error in measuring blood pressure in clients with obesity. Choose a cuff on which the width of the bladder is 40% of the circumference of the arm and the length of the bladder is sufficient to cover at least 65% of the arm circumference.

Although body weight may be used to identify obesity, measures of body fat are more accurate. Male clients at ideal body weight have 10%–20% body fat, whereas female clients at ideal body weight have 20%–30% body fat.

Diagnosis

Nursing care for clients who are overweight or obese is community based and holistic, focusing on both physiological and psychological responses to weight and appearance. Appropriate NANDA nursing diagnoses may include the following:

- *Imbalanced Nutrition: More Than Body Requirements*
- *Chronic Low Self-Esteem*
- *Noncompliance*
- *Activity Intolerance*

(NANDA-I © 2012)

Planning

Although many factors contribute to obesity, this condition always involves an imbalance of kilocalorie consumption and energy expenditure. Client education includes exercise, diet, and behavior modification. Goals are individualized based on classification of obesity, risk factors, and treatments and may include:

- The client will make sensible dietary choices to plan meals within the caloric limitations chosen by the collaborative team.
- The client will follow an exercise routine planned in collaboration with healthcare team.
- The client will relate strategies to deal with hunger and making unhealthy food choices.

- The client will attend support group meetings to help meet weight loss goals.
- The client will demonstrate appropriate weight loss, attending regular weigh-in appointments.

Implementation

Caring interventions focus on diet, exercise, and behavior modification. The nurse should do the following:

- Encourage the client to identify the factors that contribute to excess food intake. Identification of cues for eating helps the client to eliminate or reduce these cues.
- Establish realistic weight loss goals and exercise/activity objectives. Small, reasonable goals, such as loss of 1–2 lb/ week, increase the likelihood of success.
- Assess the client's knowledge, and discuss well-balanced diet plans. Provide necessary teaching about diet. Knowledge empowers the client to participate and make appropriate diet choices.
- Discuss behavior modification strategies, such as self-monitoring and environmental management. Behavior modification, diet, and exercise are critical to promoting successful long-term weight loss.
- Monitor weight loss, blood pressure, and laboratory data, including blood glucose and lipid levels. Continuing assessment is important not only to evaluate the safety of weight loss strategies but also to reinforce positive benefits of weight loss.

Encourage Exercise

Clients with obesity may experience excess fatigue, tachycardia, and shortness of breath with activity. These symptoms result from the physiological effects of excess weight as well as a sedentary lifestyle. The client may need a medical evaluation before beginning an exercise program. The nurse can assist the client in setting up an exercise program by doing the following:

- Assess the client's current activity level and tolerance of that activity. Assess vital signs. *This assessment provides baseline information to plan an activity program and assess the client's response to that activity.*
- After medical clearance, plan with the client a program of regular, gradually increasing exercise. Consider a consultation with an exercise physiologist. *An individualized exercise program promotes activities within the client's physical capabilities.*

Promote Weight Loss

Most clients who are overweight or obese experience some difficulty integrating all the components of a weight loss program into a daily routine. For a weight loss and maintenance program to be successful, the overweight client must modify dietary intake in a world of daily temptations. There may be many obstacles to exercise, including a busy schedule, activity intolerance, impaired physical mobility, lack of equipment, and the embarrassment of being fat. To assist the client in formulating a successful weight loss program, the nurse can do the following:

- Discuss the client's ability and willingness to incorporate changes into daily patterns of diet, exercise, and lifestyle. This discussion provides data from which to set realistic goals with the client.

- Help the client to identify behavior modification strategies and support systems for weight loss and its maintenance. Weight loss and maintenance are most successful if the client establishes lifestyle patterns that promote interest and motivation and, thus, exercise and diet management. Family and social support is critical for successful adherence to the therapeutic regime.

- Have the client establish strategies for dealing with "stress" eating or interruptions in the therapeutic regime. A sense of failure associated with overeating or lack of exercise can lead to further overeating. Identifying positive strategies to deal with these situations promotes self-acceptance and limits self-punishment through overeating.

Promote Self-Esteem

Although many clients with obesity have accepted their weight and body appearance on some level, most overweight and obese individuals verbalize their experiences of "fat prejudice" in their family, workplace, or community. These clients may have been subjected to ridicule, prejudice, and health problems attributed to being "fat." These experiences, coupled with day-to-day problems such as finding attractive clothing or a chair large enough to sit on, can affect self-esteem. Many clients report that "fat" jokes or comments contribute to their sense of negative self-worth. To help clients deal with these issues, the nurse should do the following:

- Encourage clients to verbalize the experience of being overweight, and validate their experience. This approach provides baseline data to use in developing individualized interventions to address self-esteem issues.

- Set small goals, and offer positive feedback and encouragement. Small goals provide more opportunities for success. Positive feedback and encouragement provide a comfortable environment in which to develop self-esteem.

- Refer clients for counseling as appropriate. Many clients benefit from counseling for issues related to self-esteem.

Evaluation

Expected outcomes of nursing care are individualized based on the nursing care plan. These outcomes may include the following:

- The client identifies and understands factors contributing to weight gain.

- The client understands and applies behavioral modification techniques to reduce weight.

- The client accomplishes the desired weight loss at a rate of 1–2 lb/week.

- The client incorporates physical activity into routines.

NURSING CARE PLAN   A Client With Obesity

Sam Elliott, age 57, has gained 30 lb since retiring 2 years ago. The most active things he does each day are "puttering around" and "walking to the end of the driveway to get the mail." His diet includes juice, oatmeal, a muffin, and coffee with cream for breakfast; donuts and coffee with friends midmorning; a bologna-and-cheese sandwich with chips and a root beer for lunch; and cheese, crackers, and wine before a dinner of meat, potatoes, vegetables, and dessert. He tells the nurse, "I have never had to diet. I just don't know how to get this weight off."

ASSESSMENT

Mr. Elliott is 173 cm (5'8") tall and weighs 91.2 kg (201 lb). His BMI is 30.1 kg/m^2. His cholesterol is 240 mg/dL (normal, 150–200 mg/dL), with an HDL of 37 mg/dL (normal male value, >45 mg/dL) and an LDL of 180 mg/dL (normal, <130 mg/dL). His BP is 138/90 mmHg. His fasting blood glucose is normal at 103 mg/dL. His electrocardiogram shows normal sinus rhythm. He reports fatigue and shortness of breath with activity. His healthcare provider has advised a weight loss of 30 lb and a regular exercise program.

DIAGNOSES

Nursing diagnoses that may be appropriate to Mr. Elliot include the following:

- *Imbalanced Nutrition: More Than Body Requirements* related to food intake in excess of energy expenditure
- *Noncompliance* related to knowledge deficit
- *Activity Intolerance* related to sedentary lifestyle

(NANDA-I © 2012)

PLANNING

The goals for the plan of care specify that Mr. Elliot will:

- Lose 1 lb each week.
- Walk 30 minutes 5 days each week.
- Verbalize an understanding of the relationship between weight loss, weight control, and exercise.
- Identify behavior modification strategies to avoid overeating.
- Identify support systems for behavior modification.

IMPLEMENTATION

The following nursing interventions may be appropriate for Mr. Elliot:

- Assess weight and blood pressure once or twice each week.
- Discuss current eating habits and strategies to reduce fat and calorie intake.
- Discuss cues that promote eating, and identify strategies to eliminate or reduce these cues.

- Teach how to keep a food diary to examine and change eating habits.
- Discuss the role of regular exercise in weight loss and weight control. Instruct to maintain an exercise record to track the intensity and duration of activity.
- Discuss lifestyle and behavior modification strategies to promote successful weight loss and control.

(continued on next page)

NURSING CARE PLAN   (continued)

EVALUATION

Two weeks after changing his diet and beginning to exercise, Mr. Elliott has lost 2 lb. He has maintained a food diary. He has identified boredom as a cue to eating. As a result, he has started volunteering at the local hospital, where he is working with children. He is walking for 30 minutes 5 days a week. He plans to increase his activity periods to 45 minutes. He verbalizes commitment to a lifelong plan of exercising and eating a low-fat diet. His BP has ranged from 132/76 to 136/84 mmHg. He plans to have the employee health nurse at the hospital check his weight and BP each week and to join Weight Watchers for ongoing support.

CRITICAL THINKING

1. What are some possible pathophysiological bases for Mr. Elliott's abnormal cholesterol, HDL, and LDL levels?
2. Develop a teaching plan for a group of overweight men and women.
3. Identify potential barriers to losing weight and strategies to reduce or eliminate these barriers.

REVIEW   Obesity

RELATE Link the Concepts and Exemplars

Linking the exemplar of obesity with the concept of culture and diversity:

1. Research perceptions about obesity and overweight in several cultures, and identify the cultural differences.
2. How would you teach a client from a culture that values obesity as a sign of status to make healthier food choices?

Linking the exemplar of obesity with the concept of health, wellness, and illness:

3. What teaching would you provide an adolescent client who is obese to promote health and reduce the risk of complications in later life?
4. Is it possible to be obese and still maintain optimal health? Explain your answer.

READY Go to Companion Skills Manual

REFER Go to Pearson Nursing Student Resources
nursing.pearsonhighered.com

- Additional review material

Reflect Case Study

Jenna Riley is a healthy but overweight 14-year-old girl who lives with her mother, Evelyn, and her brother, Jason. Her older sister, Jessica, lives a short distance away in her own apartment with her

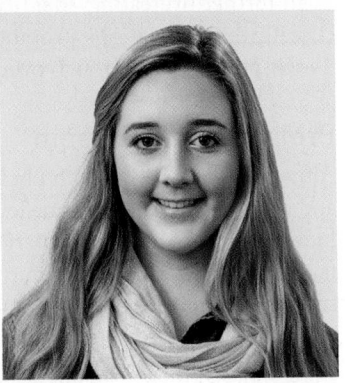

new infant son, Ryan. Jenna misses having her older sister around, and she looks up to Jessica. Jenna has had minimal contact with her father during the last 10 years and does not really even know him. Because her mother works a few evenings a week, Jenna is responsible for her younger brother. She gets along OK with Jason, but she thinks he is such a weirdo.

Jenna is a good student in the eighth grade at the local middle school. She has many friends and spends a great deal of time on the phone or in computer chat rooms talking with them each evening. Jenna is self-conscious about her weight, however. She knows she should try to lose weight, but she doesn't really know how and does not have much discipline when it comes to resisting snacks. She finds it very hard to not join her friends when they eat.

1. What risk factors does Jenna face as a result of obesity?
2. What client teaching will you provide Jenna?
3. What support groups might you recommend for Jenna?
4. Devise a 1-week meal plan for Jenna that reflects healthy eating and promotes sensible weight loss.

EXEMPLAR 12.5   Osteoporosis

EXEMPLAR KEY TERMS
Cancellous bone, 799
Diaphysis, 799
Metaphysis, 799
Osteoporosis, 799

EXEMPLAR LEARNING OUTCOMES
After reading about this exemplar, you will be able to:

1. Describe the pathophysiology, etiology, clinical manifestations, and direct and indirect causes of osteoporosis.
2. Identify risk factors and prevention methods associated with osteoporosis.
3. Illustrate the nursing process in providing culturally competent care across the life span for individuals with osteoporosis.
4. Formulate priority nursing diagnoses appropriate for an individual with osteoporosis.
5. Summarize therapies used by interdisciplinary teams in the collaborative care of an individual with osteoporosis.
6. Plan evidence-based care for an individual with osteoporosis and his or her family in collaboration with other members of the healthcare team.
7. Evaluate expected outcomes for an individual with osteoporosis.

▶ OVERVIEW

Osteoporosis (literally defined as "porous bones") is a metabolic bone disorder characterized by loss of bone mass, increased bone fragility, and increased risk of fractures. The reduced bone mass is caused by an imbalance in the processes that influence bone growth and maintenance. Although osteoporosis may result from an endocrine disorder or malignancy, it most often is associated with aging and is a result of inadequate calcium intake. Children, however, can have osteoporosis related to imbalanced nutrition or other pathological conditions.

▶ PATHOPHYSIOLOGY AND ETIOLOGY

Although the exact pathophysiology of osteoporosis is unclear, it is known to involve an imbalance in the activity of osteoblasts that form new bone and osteoclasts that resorb bone. Until age 35, the time of peak bone mass, formation occurs more rapidly than resorption. After peak bone mass has been achieved, slightly more bone is lost than is gained (about 0.7% per year); this loss is accelerated if the diet is deficient in vitamin D and calcium. In women, bone loss increases after menopause (with loss of estrogen), then slows but does not stop at about age 60. The decline of testosterone levels in men with aging is a more gradual process, and the associated bone loss occurs more slowly.

Osteoporosis affects the **diaphysis** (shaft of the bone) and the **metaphysis** (portion of the bone between the diaphysis and the epiphysis). The diameter of the bone increases, thinning the outer supporting cortex. As osteoporosis progresses, trabeculae are lost from **cancellous bone** (the spongy tissue of bone), and the outer cortex thins to the point where even minimal stress will fracture the bone (Porth & Matfin, 2009).

Etiology

The National Osteoporosis Foundation (2013) has found that osteoporosis is a health threat for an estimated 57 million Americans who have osteoporosis or low bone mass, increasing their risk for the disease. Although osteoporosis can occur at any age and in both men and women, 80% of those with osteoporosis are older women. One in two women and one in four men over age 50 will have an osteoporosis-related fracture in his or her remaining lifetime.

Risk Factors

The risk for developing osteoporosis depends on how much bone mass is achieved between ages 25 and 35 and, afterward, on how much bone mass is lost. Certain diseases, lifestyle habits, and ethnic backgrounds increase the risk of developing osteoporosis. Different variables affect one's risk of osteoporosis. Some of these variables can be modified, but others cannot.

UNMODIFIABLE RISK FACTORS Unmodifiable risk factors include being female, thin, and/or having a small frame. A personal history of fracture after age 50 also is a risk factor. Other unmodifiable risk factors include gender, family history, age, ethnicity, other chronic diseases, and current low bone mass.

Family History Those with a family history of osteoporosis are at increased risk for developing osteoporosis themselves. Those with a history of fracture in a first-degree relative also are at higher risk.

Age and Gender Both men and women are susceptible to osteoporosis as they age, because the osteoblasts and osteoclasts undergo alterations that diminish their activity. Women (especially White and Asian women), however, have a significantly higher risk for the manifestations and complications of osteoporosis, because their peak bone mass is 10%–15% less than that of men. In addition, age-related bone loss begins earlier and proceeds more rapidly in women, beginning in their 30s and accelerating before menopause. Age-related bone loss in men occurs 15–20 years later than in women and at a slower rate. Estrogen in women and testosterone in men appear to help prevent osteoporosis; the decreasing levels of these hormones associated with aging contribute to bone loss.

Ethnicity European Americans and Asians are at a higher risk for osteoporosis than African Americans, who have greater bone density (bone mass positively correlates with the amount of skin pigmentation).

Other Chronic Diseases Clients who have an endocrine disorder, such as hyperthyroidism, hyperparathyroidism, Cushing syndrome, or diabetes, are at high risk for osteoporosis. These disorders affect the metabolism, which in turn affects nutritional status and bone mineralization. Clients with moderate to severe persistent asthma or severe allergies who take steroids frequently also are at greater risk for osteoporosis.

Current Low Bone Mass in Children Children who may show signs of osteoporosis include those with decreased mechanical loading. Children with spina bifida or cerebral palsy that interferes with ambulation have limited pressure on their bones; therefore bones in the affected extremities and the spine have lower mass. Some other conditions associated with lower bone mass include Turner syndrome, growth hormone deficiency, osteogenesis imperfecta, juvenile rheumatoid arthritis, and diabetes. Children who are treated for disorders or injuries with casting and bracing also are at high risk of osteoporosis because of immobilization. Children who are treated for some types of cancer have increased rates of osteoporosis.

MODIFIABLE RISK FACTORS Modifiable risk factors include behaviors that place an individual at risk for developing osteoporosis. These factors also include physical changes (e.g., menopause) for which the contribution to osteoporosis can be modified by preventive strategies.

Female Athletes Female athletes (particularly those who participate in sports that emphasize leanness, such as gymnastics or cross-country running) may be at risk for female athlete triad, a health problem that involves disordered eating, low bone mass, and amenorrhea.

🌐 *Stay Current:* Visit the Web site of the Female Athlete Triad Coalition to learn more about this disorder: **http://www.femaleathletetriad.org/.**

Menopause   With menopause and decreasing estrogen levels, bone loss accelerates in women. Estrogen promotes the activity of osteoblasts, increasing new bone formation. In addition, estrogen enhances calcium absorption and stimulates the thyroid gland to secrete calcitonin, a hormone that suppresses osteoclast activity and increases osteoblast activity.

Calcium Deficiency   Calcium is an essential mineral in the process of bone formation and other significant body functions. When the intake of calcium through the diet is insufficient, the body compensates by removing calcium from the skeleton, weakening the bone tissue. A high intake of diet soda with a high phosphate content also can deplete calcium stores.

Acidosis   Acidosis, which may result from a high-protein diet, contributes to osteoporosis in two ways. First, acidosis may result in calcium being withdrawn from the bone as the kidneys attempt to buffer the excess acid. Second, acidosis may directly stimulate osteoclast function.

Substance Abuse   Both cigarette smoking and excess alcohol intake are risk factors for osteoporosis. Smoking decreases the blood supply to bones, and nicotine slows the production of osteoblasts and impairs the absorption of calcium, contributing to decreased bone density. Alcohol has a direct toxic effect on osteoblast activity, suppressing bone formation during periods of alcohol intoxication. In addition, heavy alcohol use may be associated with nutritional deficiencies that contribute to osteoporosis. Interestingly, moderate alcohol consumption in postmenopausal women actually may increase bone mineral content, possibly by increasing levels of estrogen and calcitonin.

Sedentary Lifestyle   Weight-bearing exercises, such as walking, influence bone metabolism in several ways. The stress of this type of exercise causes an increase in blood flow to bones, which brings growth-producing nutrients to the cells. Walking causes an increase in osteoblast growth and activity.

Medications   Prolonged use of medications that increase calcium excretion, such as aluminum-containing antacids and anticonvulsants, increase the risk of developing osteoporosis. Heparin therapy increases bone resorption, and prolonged use of heparin is associated with osteoporosis. Antiretroviral therapy for individuals with AIDS or HIV infection may cause decreased bone density and osteoporosis (Porth & Matfin, 2009).

Anyone who takes a glucocorticoid medication for more than 3 months is at risk for glucocorticoid-induced osteoporosis. These medications, often prescribed to control many rheumatic diseases, include prednisone (Deltasone, Orasone), prednisolone (Prelone), dexamethasone (Decadron, Hexadrol), and cortisone (Cortisone Acetate). These medications can directly affect bone cells, slowing the rate of bone formation. They also interfere with how the body uses calcium and affect levels of sex hormones, leading to bone loss. The problems that result, such as increased possibility of fractures, can be prevented by a daily regimen of calcium supplements with added vitamin D and one multivitamin (American College of Rheumatology, 2012).

▶ CLINICAL MANIFESTATIONS

The most common manifestations of osteoporosis are loss of height, progressive curvature of the spine, low back pain, and fractures of the forearm, spine, or hip. Osteoporosis often is called the "silent disease," because bone loss occurs without symptoms; the problem may not become apparent until the client has a fracture or radiological studies reveal the condition.

The loss of height occurs as vertebral bodies collapse. Acute episodes generally are painful, with radiation of the pain around the flank into the abdomen. Vertebral collapse can occur with little or no stress; minimal movements, such as bending, lifting, or jumping, may precipitate the pain. In some clients, vertebral collapse may occur slowly, accompanied by little discomfort.

Along with loss of height, characteristic dorsal kyphosis and cervical lordosis develop, accounting for the "dowager's hump" often associated with aging. The abdomen tends to protrude and the knees and hips flex as the body attempts to maintain its center of gravity (**Figure 12–10 ●**).

Fractures are the most common complication of osteoporosis, and the disease is responsible for more than 1.5 million fractures each year. These include 700,000 vertebral compression fractures; 300,000 hip fractures; 250,000 wrist fractures; and 300,000 fractures at other sites (National Osteoporosis Foundation, 2013). There may be no obvious manifestations of osteoporosis until fractures occur. Some fractures are spontaneous; others may result from everyday activities. Wrist and vertebral fractures have not been shown to increase client disability or mortality, but the persistent pain and associated changes in posture may restrict the client's activities or interfere with activities of daily living.

Pharmacotherapy is used for prevention and treatment of osteoporosis. Medications used include hormonal agents, bisphosphonates, and selective estrogen receptor modulators. Estrogen replacement therapy reduces bone loss, increases bone density in the spine and hip, and reduces the risk of fractures in postmenopausal women. It is particularly recommended for women who have undergone surgical menopause before age 50, and it often is prescribed for women with other risk factors. Estrogen therapy alone is associated with an increased risk of endometrial cancer, so it usually is prescribed in combination with progestin (hormone replacement therapy).

▶ COLLABORATION

Care of the client with osteoporosis focuses on stopping or slowing the process, alleviating the symptoms, and preventing complications. Proper nutrition and exercise are important components of the treatment program.

Diagnostic Tests

The manifestations of osteoporosis can mimic those of other bone disorders. Therefore diagnostic tests are needed to differentiate osteoporosis from other problems.

Dual-energy x-ray absorptiometry (DEXA) measures bone density in the lumbar spine or hip and is considered highly accurate. Ultrasound transmits painless sound waves through

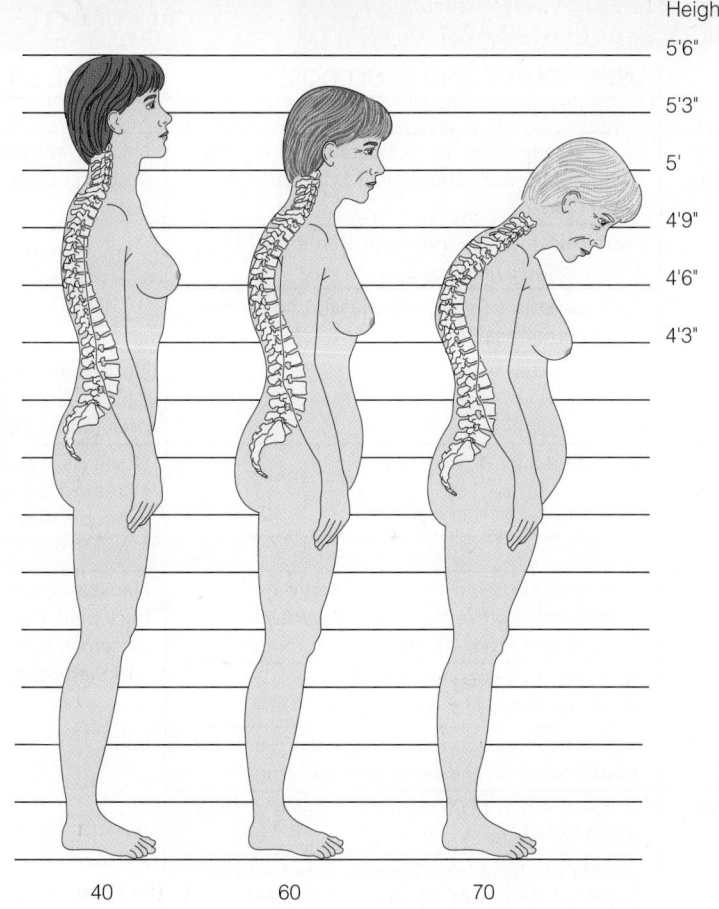

Figure 12–10 ● Spinal changes caused by osteoporosis. As the condition progresses, height can be reduced by as much as 7 in.

the heel of the foot to measure bone density. This 1-minute test is not as sensitive as DEXA, but it is accurate enough for screening purposes.

Laboratory tests include alkaline phosphatase, which may be elevated following a fracture, and serum bone Gla protein (osteocalcin), which can be used as a marker of osteoclastic activity and is therefore an indicator of the rate of bone turnover. This test is most useful to evaluate the effects of treatment rather than to indicate the severity of the disease.

Physical Therapy

Nurses may collaborate with physical therapists to design appropriate exercises for clients with osteoporosis. This collaboration may be particularly helpful for clients who have a comorbid condition that limits exercise, such as chronic obstructive pulmonary disease or asthma. Clients who have problems with balance may benefit from tai chi or yoga, both of which can benefit individuals with osteoporosis. If a nurse working with a female athlete suspects an eating disorder or amenorrhea, the nurse should discuss counseling and nutrition referrals with the client.

Dietary Management

Clients who have osteoporosis or who are at risk for later development of the disease benefit from choosing healthy menu items, particularly those high in calcium and vitamin D. Calcium-rich foods include dairy, vegetables, and beans. Food supplemented with extra calcium includes orange juice, breakfast cereals, and breads. Foods rich in vitamin D include fish. Foods with vitamin D added include milk, cereal, and breads. If inadequate calcium and vitamin D are found in the diet, clients may take supplements to ensure that the body has an adequate supply of these nutrients.

Pharmacologic Therapy

Selected drugs for osteoporosis are listed in **Table 12–14** ●. Calcium gluconate and other calcium compounds are used to treat and prevent osteoporosis. Oral calcium supplements are best taken with meals or within 1 hour following meals. It is recommended that adults 50 years of age and over should obtain at least 1,000–1,200 mg per day of elemental calcium. The most common adverse effects is hypercalcemia caused by taking too much of the supplement. Symptoms include lethargy, drowsiness, weakness, headache, anorexia, nausea and vomiting, increased urination, and thirst. Calcium supplementation is contraindicated in clients with ventricular fibrillation, metastatic bone cancer, renal calculi, or hypercalcemia. Caution should be taken in administering calcium supplements with digoxin, tetracyclines, and calcium channel blockers. The recommended dose of Vitamin D is 800–1,000 international units for adults 50 and older. High-risk clients and older adults may need more (NOF, 2012).

TABLE 12–14   Selected Drugs for Osteoporosis

DRUGS	USES, ROUTES, AND ADULT DOSES	ADVERSE EFFECTS
Hormonal Agents		
calcitonin—human (Cibacalcin) or salmon (Calciman, Miacalcin)	Paget disease: human - subcutaneous, 0.5 mg/day; salmon - subcutaneous/IM, 100 international units/day	Nausea, inflammation at injection site, flushing of face, *anaphylaxis*
	Hypercalcemia: salmon - subcutaneous/IM, 4 international units/kg bid	
	Osteoporosis: salmon - intranasal, 1 spray/day (200 international units)	
raloxifene hydrochloride (Evista)	po, 60 mg/day	Hot flashes, sinusitis, flulike symptoms, nausea, breast pain, vaginal bleeding, pneumonia, chest pain
teriparatide (Forteo)	Subcutaneous, 20 mcg/day	Dizziness, depression, insomnia, vertigo, rhinitis, increased cough, leg cramps, nausea, arthralgia *Syncope, angina*
Bisphosphonates		
alendronate sodium (Fosamax)	Osteoporosis treatment: po; 10 mg/day Osteoporosis prevention: po; 5 mg/day Paget disease: po; 40 mg/day for 6 months	Nausea, dyspepsia, diarrhea, bone pain, back pain, *bone fractures, nephrotoxicity, hypocalcemia, hypophosphatemia, gastric ulcer, esophagitis, dysrhythmias (pamidronate)*
etidronate disodium (Didronel)	po; 5–10 mg/kg/day for 6 months or 11–20 mg/kg/day for 3 months	
ibandronate (Boniva)	po; 2.5 mg/day or one 150 mg tablet per month, taken on the same date each month	
pamidronate disodium (Aredia)	IV; 15–90 mg in 1,000 mL normal saline or D5W over 4–24 hours	
risedronate sodium (Actonel)	po; 30 mg/day at least 30 minutes before the first drink or meal of the day for 2 months	
tiludronate disodium (Skelid)	po; 400 mg/day taken with 6–8 oz of water 2 hours before or after food for 3 months	

Note: Items in *italics* indicate serious adverse effects.

The most common drug class for treating osteoporosis is the bisphosphonates. These drugs are structural analogs of pyrophosphate, a natural substance that inhibits bone resorption. Bisphosphonates inhibit bone resorption by suppressing osteoclast activity, thus increasing bone density and reducing the incidence of fractures by about 50%. Examples are etidronate (Didronel), alendronate (Fosamax), tiludronate (Skelid), and pamidronate (Aredia), which is available as an injectable drug. Adverse effects include GI problems such as nausea, vomiting, abdominal pain, and esophageal irritation. Because these drugs are poorly absorbed, they should be taken on an empty stomach, as tolerated by the client. Recent studies suggest that once-weekly dosing with bisphosphonates may give the same bone density benefits as daily dosing because of the extended duration of drug action.

■ NURSING PROCESS

Osteoporosis is both preventable and treatable; therefore nursing care focuses primarily on planning and implementing interventions to prevent the disease, its manifestations, and the resulting injuries. An important aspect of preventing osteoporosis is educating clients under age 35. Health promotion activities to prevent or slow osteoporosis focus on calcium intake, exercise, and health-related behaviors.

Assessment

The nurse should collect the following data through the health history and physical examination:

■ **Health history.** Age; risk factors; history of fractures; smoking history; alcohol intake; medications; usual diet; menstrual history, including menopause; usual exercise/activity level; low back pain

■ **Physical examination.** Height and spinal curves.

Diagnosis

While there may be some variance regarding appropriate NANDA nursing diagnoses among clients who are at risk for or have osteoporosis, the following should be considered:

■ *Risk for Injury*
■ *Imbalanced Nutrition: Less Than Body Requirements*
■ *Acute Pain*

(NANDA-I © 2012)

Planning

Planning should be structured around self-care strategies that reduce clients' risk for developing osteoporosis and/or minimize its symptoms and effects. Appropriate goals for clients may include the following:

- The client will participate in weight-bearing exercises for approximately 30 minutes a day at least 4 days per week.
- The client's bone density will be evaluated at least every other year.
- The client will get sufficient nutrition, particularly calcium and vitamin D, through diet or diet in combination with dietary supplements.
- The client will be able to discuss risk factors for osteoporosis and how to prevent or minimize them.
- The client with a high risk for injury will modify the home and work environments to minimize risk of falling.

Implementation

Nursing care of clients who have osteoporosis focuses on teaching about the disease process, helping to maintain physical mobility and nutrition, and solving problems associated with pain and injury.

Prevent Injury

Falls that would result in little or no injury in the healthy adult may cause fractures in the client with osteoporosis. Even normal movements, such as twisting, bending, lifting, or rising from bed, can precipitate a vertebral fracture. The nurse should take care to do the following:

- Implement safety precautions as necessary for the client who is hospitalized or in a long-term care facility. Maintain the bed in low position; use side rails if indicated to prevent the client from getting up alone. Provide nighttime lighting to toilet facilities. Most falls are preventable, particularly in hospitals and long-term care facilities.
- Avoid using restraints on the client who is hospitalized or a resident in a long-term care facility if at all possible. Restraints may actually increase the client's risk of falling and the risk of injury associated with a fall.
- Encourage older adults to use assistive devices to maintain independence in activities of daily living. Walking sticks, canes, and other assistive devices encourage client independence and support activities that promote bone growth.
- Teach older clients about safety and fall precautions. An assessment of the client's home for safety and fall risks may reduce the risk of fractures and, in turn, the cost of hospitalization and potential disability and/or death.

Promote Balanced Nutrition

Most Americans do not maintain their recommended daily intake of calcium. Clients therefore must be made aware of the relationship between an adequate calcium intake and maintaining strong bones. Following are steps the nurse can take to help clients ingest adequate calcium:

- Teach adolescents, pregnant or lactating women, and adults through age 35 to eat foods that are high in calcium and to maintain a daily calcium intake of 1,200–1,500 mg, as recommended by the National Institutes of Health.

- Encourage postmenopausal women to maintain a calcium intake of 1,000–1,500 mg daily, through either diet or a calcium supplement. Calcium needs for postmenopausal women vary depending on age.
- Teach clients who are taking calcium supplements about the importance of taking the medication at the proper time and about the possible side effects. Free hydrochloric acid is needed for calcium absorption. Calcium carbonate supplement (e.g., Tums) should be taken 30–60 minutes before meals to allow adequate absorption. Calcium citrate supplements should be taken with meals to prevent gastrointestinal distress. Calcium supplements should be taken in divided doses (two to three times daily) for improved distribution, because the body requires calcium 24 hours per day.
- Inform clients that calcium absorption requires sufficient levels of vitamin D. Clients who are at risk for insufficient levels of vitamin D may need to take a vitamin D supplement in combination with their calcium supplement. The National Institutes of Health recommends 400–800 IU of vitamin D daily for those under 50 years of age and 800–1,000 IU for those age 50 and older.

Relieve Acute Pain

Pain and immobilization can occur in the advanced stages of osteoporosis. Acute pain usually results from a complicating fracture, especially a compression fracture of the vertebrae. For clients experiencing pain, the nurse can do the following:

- Suggest the application of heat to relieve pain. A heating pad may offer temporary pain relief. To avoid the "rebound effect," the heat should be removed every 20–30 minutes.
- Suggest that the client take over-the-counter anti-inflammatory pain medications for treatment of both acute and chronic pain. Clients should be instructed in the dosage and frequency as noted on the manufacturer's label. Continuous administration of ibuprofen or other nonsteroidal anti-inflammatory drugs (NSAIDs) can be useful to provide relief from pain, but clients must be cautioned not to exceed dosage recommendations.

SAFETY ALERT
Teach clients on long-term anti-inflammatory medications to watch for bright red bleeding from the stomach (in vomitus) or dark black bowel movements.

Encourage Exercise

It is important that clients understand the role of physical activity and weight-bearing exercises in preventing and slowing bone loss. The nurse should inform clients that swimming and water aerobic exercises are not as beneficial for maintaining bone density because they are not weight-bearing activities. The nurse should also do the following:

- Before beginning teaching related to exercise, determine the client's preexisting health problems and consult with the client's primary provider to ensure safety in beginning an exercise regime.

- Teach the client who is able to participate in weight-bearing exercises to perform such exercises for a sustained period of 30–40 minutes at least three times a week. The mechanical force of weight-bearing exercises promotes bone growth. Bones weaken and demineralize without exercise. Walking is an easy, low-impact form of exercise. Swimming (including walking on the bottom of the pool) does not require the needed weight bearing.

- Determine the client's interests and help the client to plan an exercise regimen in keeping with the client's preferences.

Promote Healthy Behaviors

Behaviors that help to prevent osteoporosis include not smoking, avoiding excessive alcohol intake, and limiting caffeine intake to two or three cups of coffee each day. The nurse should make sure the client understands the importance of these behaviors.

Evaluation

The nurse should evaluate outcomes when planning with the client at the client's annual checkup. The nurse should ask clients about any pharmacologic therapies at each healthcare visit to ensure that the client is taking the prescribed medications and to provide the opportunity to discuss any possible side effects.

Expected outcomes for the client with osteoporosis include the following:

- The client identifies and implements strategies to change or modify lifestyle factors such as smoking cessation, weight-bearing exercise, and moderation in alcohol use.
- The client achieves adequate calcium intake.
- The client identifies and eliminates safety hazards.
- The client experiences relief from acute pain.

NURSING CARE PLAN   A Client With Osteoporosis

Nancy Bauer is a 53-year-old schoolteacher. She has been married for 36 years and has two children. Ms. Bauer is 65 inches tall. She has smoked one pack of cigarettes a day for 30 years and drinks one to two glasses of wine with dinner each evening. She does not exercise routinely. Ms. Bauer has had symptoms of menopause for 8 years, including hot flashes in the early years and mood swings more recently. She has never been on hormone replacement therapy.

Ms. Bauer is currently seeking medical advice for continuous low back pain. The pain is not relieved with an over-the-counter analgesic, and she frequently wakes up during the night because of the pain. She is diagnosed with osteoporosis.

ASSESSMENT

The nurse practitioner notes that Ms. Bauer's vital signs are within normal limits. She has full range of motion of all extremities and is able to stand and bend over, but she reports discomfort when returning to the upright position. Ms. Bauer has a slightly pronounced "hump" on her upper back and is 1 inch shorter than her stated height on admission. Her muscle strength is symmetrical and strong.

DIAGNOSES

Nursing diagnoses that may be appropriate for Ms. Bauer include the following:
- *Acute Pain* of the lower spine related to vertebral compression
- *Deficient Knowledge* related to osteoporosis and treatment to prevent further damage
- *Imbalanced Nutrition: Less Than Body Requirements* related to inadequate intake of calcium
- *Risk for Injury* related to effects of change in bone structure secondary to osteoporosis.

(NANDA-I © 2012)

PLANNING

The goals for the plan of care specify that Ms. Bauer will:
- Verbalize a decrease in back pain.
- Be able to describe ways to treat her osteoporosis and prevent further complications.
- Verbalize an understanding of the current research and treatment regarding osteoporosis.
- Verbalize how stopping smoking can help to prevent further progression of osteoporosis.
- Seek consultation for supplements and medications to prevent further bone loss.
- Design a program of physical activity to prevent complications of osteoporosis.
- Verbalize safety precautions to prevent fractures resulting from falls.

IMPLEMENTATION

The following nursing interventions may be appropriate for Ms. Bauer:

- Teach back-strengthening exercises.
- Refer to an osteoporosis support group if available.
- Provide realistic, yet optimistic, feedback about loss of height and bone integrity and the potential outcomes of treatment.
- Assess the client's current knowledge base, and correct any misconceptions regarding treatment of osteoporosis.

- Provide current educational literature regarding treatment of osteoporosis.
- Instruct her in dietary and calcium supplements that help to prevent the effects of osteoporosis.
- Discuss physical exercises that help to prevent complications resulting from osteoporosis.
- Review safety and fall precautions, and provide literature regarding how to create a safe home environment.

NURSING CARE PLAN   (continued)

EVALUATION

On her return visit after 6 months, Ms. Bauer reports that she feels much better. She is no longer irritable and does not experience mood swings, because she has been taking her prescribed hormone replacement for 6 months. She is eating products rich in calcium and is taking a twice-daily supplement of calcium with vitamin D. Ms. Bauer has reduced her wine intake to one glass in the evening and now drinks decaffeinated coffee and tea. She also states that since she stopped smoking, she has been walking 30–45 minutes every day.

CRITICAL THINKING

1. What is the rationale for stopping smoking and limiting caffeine and alcohol intake in the treatment of osteoporosis?
2. What foods would you encourage for clients who are at high risk for osteoporosis and whose serum cholesterol and LDL/HDL ratios indicate a high risk for cardiovascular disease?
3. What physical activities would you consider beneficial in helping to prevent the effects of osteoporosis in the female client who is wheelchair bound or has limited mobility?
4. Develop a care plan for Ms. Bauer for the nursing diagnosis Risk for Trauma.

REVIEW Osteoporosis

RELATE Link the Concepts and Exemplars

Linking the exemplar of osteoporosis with the concept of fluids and electrolytes:

1. Create a flowchart diagramming the relationship between calcium and osteoporosis.
2. In addition to calcium, what other electrolytes are required for calcium to be properly metabolized and absorbed into the bone? Explain the physiology involved.

Linking the exemplar of osteoporosis with the concept of safety:

3. What safety issues will the nurse address in caring for a client with osteoporosis? Why?
4. What strategies will the nurse recommend to reduce the risk of fractures for a client with osteoporosis? Why?

READY Go to Companion Skills Manual

REFER: Go to Pearson Nursing Student Resources
nursing.pearsonhighered.com

- Additional review material

REFLECT Case Study

Mary Martin is a 75-year-old female who was recently widowed. She has a limited income because her husband's pension

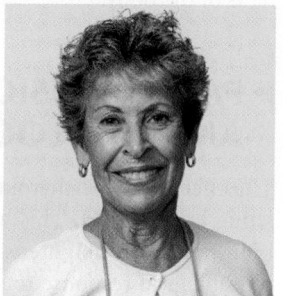

terminated when he died, and she has moved in with her son, his wife, and their three teenage children. Ms. Martin has cataracts and glaucoma, for which she sees an ophthalmologist regularly; otherwise, she is in good health.

Ms. Martin goes to the community health fair with her friend. While at the fair, she has a bone density screening and is told that she needs further evaluation for low bone density, a finding commonly associated with osteoporosis. In a follow up visit with her primary care provider, Ms. Martin is told that her bone scan shows evidence of decreased bone mineral density consistent with osteoporosis. She is told to introduce weight-bearing exercise into her activities, to increase her calcium intake to 1,500 mg/day, and to take vitamin D supplements. She also is given a prescription for alendronate (Fosamax).

1. What teaching will the nurse provide Ms. Martin?
2. What outcomes are appropriate for Ms. Martin?
3. What recommendations will the nurse make to reduce the risk of injury when assessing Ms. Martin's home?

EXEMPLAR 12.6 Thyroid Disease

EXEMPLAR KEY TERMS
Euthyroid, 806
Exophthalmos, 806
Goiter, 806
Graves disease, 806
Hashimoto thyroiditis, 812
Hyperthyroidism, 806
Hypothyroidism, 812
Myxedema, 812
Myxedema coma, 813
Proptosis, 806
Thyroid crisis, 808
Thyroidectomy, 809
Thyroiditis, 808
Thyroid storm, 808
Thyrotoxicosis, 806
Toxic multinodular goiter, 808

EXEMPLAR LEARNING OUTCOMES
After reading about this exemplar, you will be able to:

1. Describe the pathophysiology, etiology, clinical manifestations, and direct and indirect causes of thyroid disease.
2. Identify risk factors and prevention methods associated with thyroid disease.
3. Illustrate the nursing process in providing culturally competent care across the life span for individuals with thyroid disease.
4. Formulate priority nursing diagnoses appropriate for an individual with thyroid disease.
5. Summarize therapies used by interdisciplinary teams in the collaborative care of an individual with thyroid disease.
6. Plan evidence-based care for an individual with thyroid disease and his or her family in collaboration with other members of the healthcare team.
7. Evaluate expected outcomes for an individual with thyroid disease.

▶ OVERVIEW

The thyroid gland is a small saddle-shaped gland that wraps around the anterior portion of the trachea. Altered production or use of thyroid hormone (TH) affects all major organ systems. In the adult, TH changes primarily affect metabolism and cardiovascular, gastrointestinal, and neuromuscular function. Thyroid disorders are among the most common endocrine disorders and, if left untreated, can result in cardiac disease and ultimately death.

▌HYPERTHYROIDISM

Hyperthyroidism (also called **thyrotoxicosis**) is a disorder caused by excessive delivery of TH to the peripheral tissues. Because the primary effect of TH is to increase metabolism and protein synthesis, hyperthyroidism affects all major organ systems of the body.

▶ PATHOPHYSIOLOGY AND ETIOLOGY

The effects of hyperthyroidism are the result of increased circulating levels of TH. This hormonal excess increases the metabolic rate and heightens the sympathetic nervous system's physiological response to stimulation. The sensitizing effect of abnormally elevated TH levels increases the cardiac rate and stroke volume. As a result, cardiac output and peripheral blood flow increase. Elevated TH levels also increase carbohydrate, protein, and lipid metabolism. Lipids are depleted, glucose tolerance decreases, and protein degradation increases; the result is a negative nitrogen balance. Over time, the hypermetabolic effects of excess TH result in caloric and nutritional deficiencies.

Etiology

Hyperthyroidism results from many different factors, including autoimmune stimulation (as in Graves disease), excess secretion of thyroid-stimulating hormone (TSH) by the pituitary gland, thyroiditis, neoplasms (e.g., toxic multinodular goiter), and an excessive intake of thyroid medications. The most common etiologies of hyperthyroidism are Graves disease and toxic multinodular goiter.

Risk Factors

Women are at increased risk for hyperthyroidism, being 10 times more likely than men to develop the condition. Genetic factors, such as a family history of Graves disease, also contribute to increased risk. Other risk factors are increased iodine intake and being between 20 and 40 years in age (National Endocrine and Metabolic Diseases Information Center, 2012).

▶ CLINICAL MANIFESTATIONS

The client with hyperthyroidism typically has an increased appetite yet loses weight and may have hypermotile bowels (characterized by increased peristalsis, bloating, and pain) and diarrhea.

Additional manifestations related to hypermetabolism include heat intolerance, insomnia, palpitations, and increased sweating. The skin is smooth and warm, the hair may become fine, and hair loss in the scalp, eyebrow, axillary, or pubic areas of the body is common. Emotional lability also is common. See the Multisystem Effects of Hyperthyroidism feature.

Treatment of hyperthyroidism focuses on reducing the production of TH by the thyroid gland, thus establishing a **euthyroid** (normal thyroid) state, and preventing or treating complications. Depending on the client's age and physical status, medications, radioactive iodine (RAI) therapy, or surgery may be used.

Graves Disease

Graves disease, the most common cause of hyperthyroidism, is an autoimmune disorder sometimes associated with the presence of other autoimmune disorders, such as myasthenia gravis and pernicious anemia (McPhee & Papadakis, 2009). Clients with Graves disease have an antibody in their serum that binds to TSH receptors in the thyroid follicles and causes the thyroid cells to hyperfunction. When this antibody binds to the TSH receptors on the thyroid gland, it stimulates hormone synthesis and secretion, enlarging the gland. The cause is unknown, but there is a hereditary link. Graves disease is seen eight times more often in women than in men and occurs most frequently between the ages of 20 and 40 (McPhee & Papadakis, 2009).

Clients with Graves disease have an enlarged thyroid gland (**goiter**) and manifestations of hyperthyroidism. The goiter can result from excess TSH stimulation (when the amount of circulating TH is deficient), abnormal growth-stimulating immunoglobulins, or substances that inhibit TH synthesis. A goiter may be present in clients with hyperthyroidism or hypothyroidism.

The ophthalmopathy (disease of the eye) of Graves disease is manifested as proptosis and visual dysfunction. **Proptosis** (forward displacement of the eye) occurs in about one third of cases (Porth & Matfin, 2009). This forward protrusion of the eyeballs (also known as **exophthalmos**) results from an accumulation of inflammation by-products in the retro-orbital tissues. Many times, the sclera is visible above the iris. The upper lids often are retracted, and the individual has a characteristic unblinking stare (**Figure 12–11 ●**). Proptosis usually is bilateral,

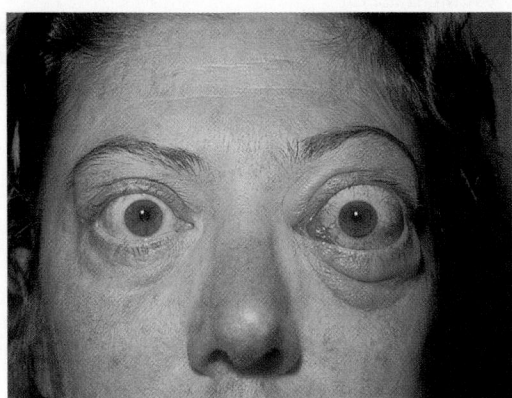

Figure 12–11 ● Exophthalmos in a client with Graves disease. The disease causes edema of fat deposits behind the eyes and inflammation of the extraocular muscles. The accumulating pressure forces the eyes outward from their orbits.
Source: University of Illinois/Custom Medical Stock Photo.

Multisystem Effects of Hyperthyroidism

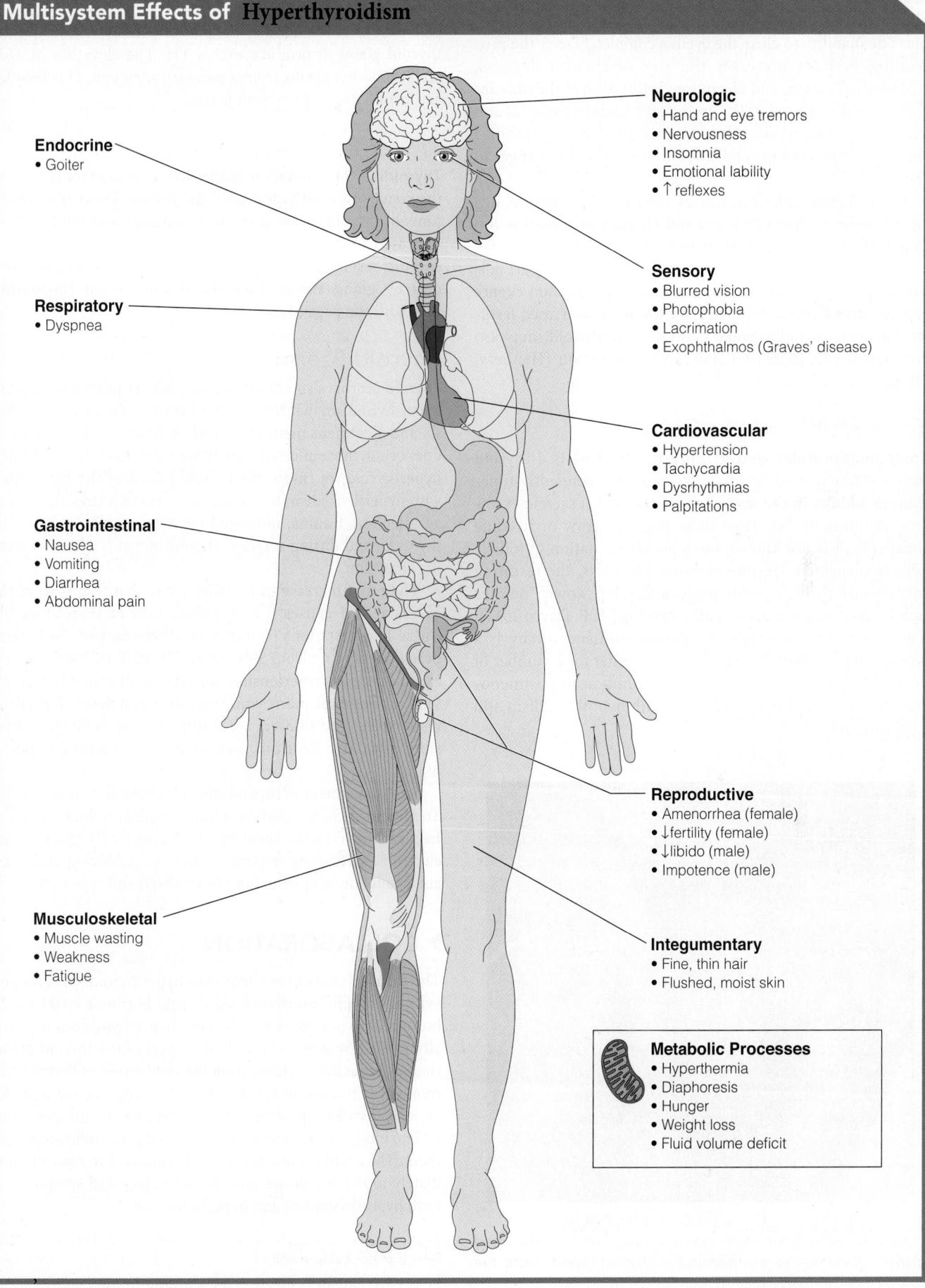

Endocrine
• Goiter

Respiratory
• Dyspnea

Gastrointestinal
• Nausea
• Vomiting
• Diarrhea
• Abdominal pain

Musculoskeletal
• Muscle wasting
• Weakness
• Fatigue

Neurologic
• Hand and eye tremors
• Nervousness
• Insomnia
• Emotional lability
• ↑ reflexes

Sensory
• Blurred vision
• Photophobia
• Lacrimation
• Exophthalmos (Graves' disease)

Cardiovascular
• Hypertension
• Tachycardia
• Dysrhythmias
• Palpitations

Reproductive
• Amenorrhea (female)
• ↓fertility (female)
• ↓libido (male)
• Impotence (male)

Integumentary
• Fine, thin hair
• Flushed, moist skin

Metabolic Processes
• Hyperthermia
• Diaphoresis
• Hunger
• Weight loss
• Fluid volume deficit

but it may involve only one eye. The client may experience blurred vision, diplopia, eye pain, lacrimation, and photophobia. The inability to close the eyelids completely over the protruding eyeballs increases the risk of corneal dryness, irritation, infection, and ulceration. Infiltration of the muscles that move the eye and of the optic nerve leads to paralysis and vision loss. The treatment of Graves disease may stabilize these symptoms but generally does not reverse the changes in the eyes.

Other manifestations of Graves disease include fatigue, difficulty sleeping, hand tremors, and changes in menstruation ranging from decreased flow to amenorrhea. Older clients may present with atrial fibrillation, angina, or congestive heart failure. Hyperthyroidism can also have adverse effects on client's reproductive abilities. Women can experience decreased fertility, amenorrhea, and irregular periods. Hyperthyroidism is also correlated with increased spontaneous abortion (Hanberg, 2008).

Toxic Multinodular Goiter

Toxic multinodular goiter (Figure 12–12 ●) is a thyroid tumor characterized by small, discrete, independently functioning nodules in the thyroid gland tissue that secrete excessive amounts of TH. How these nodules grow or become independent is not known, but a genetic mutation of follicle cells is suspected. Despite elevated TH levels, the resulting manifestations of hyperthyroidism develop slowly; neither ophthalmopathy nor dermopathy develop (A. B. Davis, 2011). The client with this type of hyperthyroidism usually is a woman in her 60s or 70s who has had a goiter for a number of years. Multinodule goiters are most common in postmenopausal women and may present as both hypothyroidism and hyperthyroidism.

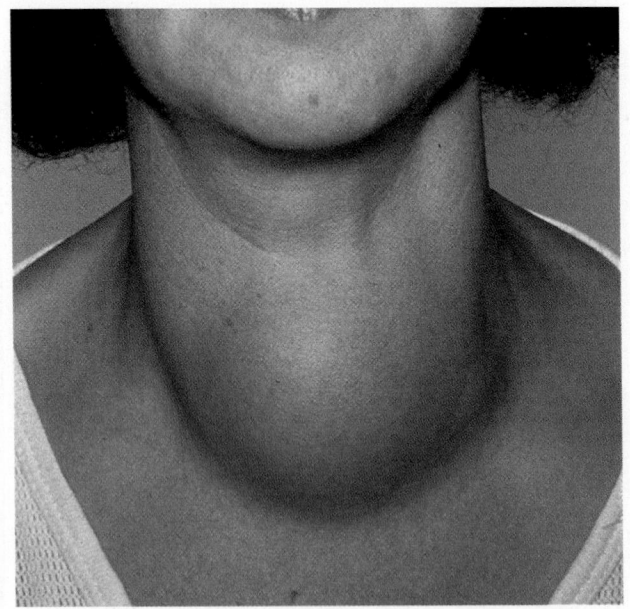

Figure 12–12 ● Toxic multinodular goiter. The formation and growth of numerous nodules in the thyroid gland cause the characteristic massive enlargement of the neck.
Source: Custom Medical Stock Photo.

Excess TSH Stimulation

Overproduction of TSH by the pituitary usually stimulates the thyroid gland to produce excess TH. The elevation in TSH secretion often results from a pituitary adenoma. This secondary form of hyperthyroidism is rare.

Thyroiditis

Thyroiditis (inflammation of the thyroid gland) most often is the result of a viral infection of the thyroid gland. The symptoms of thyroiditis are acute inflammation and the effects of increased TH. Thyroiditis is an acute disorder that may become chronic, resulting in a hypothyroid state as repeated infections destroy gland tissue. (See the discussion of Hashimoto thyroiditis on page 812.)

Thyroid Storm

Thyroid storm (also called **thyroid crisis**) is an extreme state of hyperthyroidism that is rare today because of improved diagnosis and treatment methods (Porth & Matfin, 2009). When it does occur, those affected usually are individuals with untreated hyperthyroidism (most often Graves disease) and individuals with hyperthyroidism who have experienced a stressor, such as an infection, trauma, untreated DKA, or manipulation of the thyroid gland during surgery. Thyroid storm is a life-threatening condition.

The rapid increase in metabolic rate that results from the excessive TH causes the manifestations of thyroid storm. These manifestations include hyperthermia, with body temperatures ranging from 39°C to 41°C (102°F to 106°F); tachycardia; systolic hypertension; and gastrointestinal symptoms (e.g., abdominal pain, vomiting, and diarrhea). Agitation, restlessness, and tremors are common, progressing to confusion, psychosis, delirium, and seizures. The mortality rate is high.

Rapid treatment of thyroid storm is essential to preserve life. Treatment includes cooling without aspirin (which increases free TH) or inducing shivering; replacing fluids, glucose, and electrolytes; relieving respiratory distress; stabilizing cardiovascular function; and reducing TH synthesis and secretion.

▶ COLLABORATION

The focus of care of the client with hyperthyroidism is on preventing complications until the thyroid hormone levels can be brought into normal range. Because hyperthyroidism is generally treated by destruction of all or part of the thyroid gland, thereby reducing or eliminating the production of thyroid hormone, it is important for the client to recognize the need for lifelong thyroid supplementation to replace the hormone that will no longer be produced by the thyroid gland following treatment. The client should understand symptoms to report immediately to the healthcare provider and signs and symptoms of both hyperthyroidism and hypothyroidism.

Diagnostic Tests

Hyperthyroidism is diagnosed according to the manifestations of the specific disorders causing excessive TH and by diagnostic

Clinical Manifestations and Therapies Hyperthyroidism

ETIOLOGY	CLINICAL MANIFESTATIONS	CLINICAL THERAPIES
Autoimmune stimulation (as in Graves disease) Excess secretion of thyroid-stimulating hormone by the pituitary gland Thyroiditis Neoplasms (e.g., toxic multinodular goiter) Excessive intake of thyroid medications.	■ Increased appetite accompanied by weight loss ■ Hypermotile bowels and diarrhea ■ Heat intolerance ■ Insomnia ■ Palpitations ■ Increased sweating ■ Emotional lability	■ Pharmacotherapy ■ Radioactive iodine therapy ■ Surgery (subtotal or total thyroidectomy)

test results (**Table 12–15** ●). Elevated levels of TH (both T_3 and T_4) and increased RAI uptake are diagnostic criteria of hyperthyroidism.

The following diagnostic tests may be ordered:

■ ***Thyroid antibodies (TA) test.*** Serum TA is measured to determine whether a thyroid autoimmune disease is causing the client's symptoms. TA is elevated in Graves disease.

■ ***TSH test (sensitive assay).*** Serum TSH levels are measured and compared with T_4 levels to differentiate pituitary from thyroid dysfunction. The best indicator of primary hyperthyroidism (e.g., in Graves disease) is suppression of TSH below 0.1 mcg/mL. When the sensitive TSH is not suppressed, the hyperthyroidism is caused by a TSH-secreting pituitary tumor.

■ ***T_4 test.*** Serum T_4 levels are measured to determine TH concentration and to test thyroid gland function. T_4 levels are elevated in hyperthyroidism and in acute thyroiditis.

■ ***T_3 test.*** Serum T_3 is measured by radioimmunoassay, which measures bound and free forms of this hormone. This test is effective for the diagnosis of hyperthyroidism. T_3 levels also may be elevated in thyroiditis.

■ ***T_3 uptake test.*** T_3 uptake is measured by an in vitro test in which the client's blood is mixed with radioactive T_3; the results are elevated in hyperthyroidism.

■ ***RAI uptake test.*** An RAI uptake test (thyroid scan) measures the absorption of 131-I or 123-I by the thyroid gland. A calculated dose of RAI is given orally or intravenously, and the thyroid is then scanned (often after 24 hours). The distribution of radioactivity in the gland is recorded (increased uptake of RAI is seen in Graves disease). In addition, the scan reveals the size and shape of the gland.

■ ***Thyroid suppression test.*** RAI and T_4 levels are measured first. The client then takes TH for 7–10 days, after which the tests are repeated. Failure of hormone therapy to suppress RAI and T_4 indicates hyperthyroidism.

Pharmacologic Therapy

Hyperthyroidism is treated by administering antithyroid medications that reduce TH production. Because these drugs do not affect the release or activity of hormone that is already formed, therapeutic effects may not be seen for several weeks. To rapidly decrease the cardiovascular symptoms associated with hyperthyroidism, a beta-blocker, such as propanolol (Inderal), is part of initial treatment.

Radioactive Iodine Therapy

Because the thyroid gland takes up iodine in any form, radioactive iodine (RAI or 131-I) concentrates in the thyroid gland and damages or destroys thyroid cells so that they produce less TH. The RAI is given orally. Results typically occur in 6–8 weeks. In most instances, the client is not hospitalized during treatment and does not require radiation precautions. This type of therapy is contraindicated for pregnant women, because RAI crosses the placenta and can have negative effects on the developing fetal thyroid gland. Because the amount of gland destroyed by RAI therapy is not readily controllable, the client may become hypothyroid and require lifelong TH replacement. Adverse reactions include thyroiditis and cardiac instability caused by liberation of stored TH in the gland (Holcomb, 2006). Clients should be taught to measure their pulse rate and notify the provider if the rate exceeds 100 bpm following therapy until released stores of TH diminish.

Surgery

Some clients with hyperthyroidism have such enlarged thyroid glands that pressure on the esophagus or trachea causes problems with breathing or swallowing. In these clients, a **thyroidectomy** (removal of all or part of the gland) is indicated. A subtotal thyroidectomy usually is performed; this procedure leaves enough of the gland in place to produce an adequate amount of TH.

TABLE 12–15 Laboratory Findings in Hyperthyroidism

TEST	NORMAL VALUES	FINDINGS
Serum TA	Negative to 1:20	Increased
Serum TSH (sensitive assay)	0.35–5.5 mU/mL	Decreased in primary hyperthyroidism
Serum T_4	4.5–11.5 mcg/dL	Increased
Serum T_3	80–200 ng/dL	Increased
T_3 uptake	25–35 relative percentage	Increased
Thyroid suppression		Increased RAI uptake and T_4 levels

A total thyroidectomy is performed to treat cancer of the thyroid; the client then requires lifelong hormone replacement (McPhee & Papadakis, 2009).

Before surgery, the client should be in as nearly a euthyroid state as possible. The client may be given antithyroid drugs to reduce hormone levels and iodine preparations to decrease the vascularity and size of the gland (which also reduces the risk of hemorrhage during and after surgery).

■ NURSING PROCESS

Nursing care of the client with hyperthyroidism is focused on providing client education regarding the disease process, treatment options, and posttreatment self-care. In caring for the client with hyperthyroidism, it is important that the nurse recognize the impact that increased metabolism rates will have on the client's ability to concentrate on information presented by the nurse.

Assessment

The following data are collected through the health history and physical examination:

- **Health history.** Other diseases, family history of thyroid disease, when symptoms began, severity of symptoms, intake of thyroid medications, menstrual history, changes in weight, bowel elimination
- **Physical assessment.** Muscle strength, tremors, vital signs, cardiovascular and peripheral vascular systems, integument, size of thyroid, presence of bruit over thyroid, eyes and vision.

Diagnosis

For the client with hyperthyroidism, the nurse must consider the client's responses to the systemic effects of the disorder. Although each client may have different needs, the NANDA diagnoses discussed in this exemplar focus on the most common problems:

- *Decreased Cardiac Output*
- *Impaired Comfort, Impaired Health Maintenance, and Risk for Infection related to visual changes and visual loss*
- *Imbalanced Nutrition: Less Than Body Requirements*
- *Disturbed Body Image*

(NANDA-I © 2012)

Planning

Care is directed at symptom resolution, client teaching related to self-care, and appropriate treatment modalities. Possible goals include the following:

- The client will report improvement related to manifestations.
- The client will describe situations requiring contact with the provider.
- The client will explain how to take prescribed medications.

Implementation

Hyperthyroidism is often treated on an outpatient basis so it is important that the client understand how to provide self-care, what symptoms to monitor for, and when to call the provider.

Emphasis should be on teaching clients about the importance of taking medications daily and not skipping a dose due to absence of symptoms.

Monitor Cardiac Output

The client with hyperthyroidism is at risk for alterations in cardiac output. Excess TH directly affects the heart, increasing heart rate and stroke volume. Increases in the metabolic demands and oxygen requirements of peripheral tissues increase the demands on the heart, and systolic hypertension, angina, arrhythmias, or cardiac failure may occur. The client often has palpitations and shortness of breath and is easily fatigued. The risk of complications is greater in clients with preexisting cardiovascular disorders. To deal with this risk, the nurse should do the following:

- Monitor blood pressure, pulse rate and rhythm, respiratory rate, and breath sounds. Assess for peripheral edema, jugular vein distention, and increased activity intolerance. Higher TH level increases cardiac rate, stroke volume, and tissue demand for oxygen, causing stress on the heart. This stress may result in hypertension, arrhythmias, tachycardia, and congestive heart failure.

- Suggest keeping the environment as cool and free of distractions as possible. Decrease stress by explaining interventions and by teaching relaxation procedures. A physically comfortable and psychologically calm environment can reduce stimuli and stressors. Stress increases circulating catecholamines, which further increase cardiac workload.

- Encourage the client to balance periods of activity with periods of rest. Rest periods decrease energy expenditure and tissue requirements for oxygen and thus decrease demands on the heart by lowering the cardiac workload.

Promote Visual Health

Visual changes that occur in clients with hyperthyroidism include difficulty in focusing, diplopia (double vision), and visual loss. If the client is unable to close the eyelids because of exophthalmos, the risk of corneal dryness with resultant infection or injury increases. Visual deficits also may result from pressure on the optic nerve from retro-orbital edema and shortening of the eye muscles. Although treatment of hyperthyroidism may stop the progression of eye changes, not all symptoms are reversible. To address the possibility of visual changes, the nurse should do the following:

- Monitor visual acuity, photophobia, integrity of the cornea, and lid closure. The cornea is at risk for dryness, injury, conjunctivitis, and corneal infections. Injury and infection of the cornea can result in further loss of visual acuity.

- Teach measures for protecting the eye from injury and maintaining visual acuity:

  a. Use tinted glasses or shields as protection.
  b. Use artificial tears to moisten the eyes.
  c. Use cool, moist compresses to relieve irritation.
  d. Cover or tape the eyelids shut at night if they do not close.
  e. Elevate the head of the bed to 45° to promote periorbital fluid decrease.
  f. Have the client promptly report any pain or changes in vision.

These measures decrease the risk of injury, provide comfort, decrease periorbital edema that can compromise vision further, and ensure immediate care for problems, thereby minimizing the risk of further visual loss.

Promote Balanced Nutrition

The hypermetabolic state that occurs in hyperthyroidism causes gastrointestinal hypermotility, with nausea, vomiting, diarrhea, and abdominal pain. Although the client may have an increased appetite and eat more than usual, weight loss continues. To help the client maintain adequate nutrition, the nurse should do the following:

- Monitor nutritional status through results of laboratory tests. Serum albumin, transferrin, and total lymphocyte counts commonly are lower than normal in clients with nutritional deficits. A negative nitrogen balance signifies a catabolic state in which protein is lost and metabolic demands are not being met.
- Ask the client to check weight daily (at the same time each day) and to keep a record of results. Regular monitoring detects continued weight loss, which can result from not meeting the body's metabolic demands.
- In collaboration with a dietitian, teach the client about the need for a diet high in carbohydrates and protein that includes between-meal snacks. Six small meals a day may be more desirable than three large meals. Caloric intake may need to be increased to 4,000 kcal/day if weight loss exceeds 10%–17% for height and frame. Increased nutrients are necessary as part of a well-balanced diet and to meet metabolic demands. Clients often are better able to increase food intake by eating frequent, small meals. A 1 lb weight gain requires approximately 3,500 extra kilocalories.

Improve Body Image

Physical changes that are common in hyperthyroidism include exophthalmos, goiter, tremors, hair loss, increased perspiration, loss of strength, fatigue, weight loss, and changes in reproductive and sexual function (amenorrhea in women, impotence in men, and decreased libido in men). In addition, the client often has mood changes and insomnia and is constantly nervous and anxious. There may even be periods of psychosis. These changes are frightening not only for the client but also for family members. To help the client deal with the physical changes and their effects, it is important for the nurse to do the following:

- Establish a trusting relationship, and encourage the client to verbalize feelings about self and to ask questions about the illness and treatment. Provide reliable information, and clarify misconceptions. Establishing trust facilitates open sharing of feelings and perceptions.

Evaluation

Expected outcomes for the client with hyperthyroidism include the following:

- The client's cardiac status stabilizes.
- The client regains or maintains visual acuity.
- The client takes in an appropriate number of calories per day and exhibits no further weight loss.
- The client communicates feelings about changes in body image and verbalizes coping mechanisms.
- The client explains the importance of daily medications and proper self-administration.

NURSING CARE PLAN   A Client With Graves Disease

ASSESSMENT	DIAGNOSES	PLAN
Juanita Manuel is a 33-year-old mother of four small children. She is a second-year student at the local community college and is within one semester of completing the requirements for an associate degree in child care. For the past 3 months, Ms. Manuel has been constantly hungry and has eaten more than usual, but she has still lost 6.8 kg (15 lb). She has repeated bouts of diarrhea and often feels nauseated. Her hands shake, she can feel her heart beating rapidly, and she finds herself laughing or crying for no apparent reason. Ms. Manuel makes an appointment with her family physician. The nurse at the office completes a health history and physical assessment. When asked how she has been feeling, Ms. Manuel replies, "Well, I don't know what's wrong with me—but I keep losing weight and I cry at the drop of a hat. I am also just so hot all the time, and I've never had that problem before. I hope I find out what's wrong and it's nothing serious." The health history indicates that although her appetite has increased, Ms. Manuel has lost 6.8 kg (15 lb). Ms. Manuel states that she has had diarrhea, nausea, palpitations, heat intolerance, and mood changes. Physical assessment findings include the following: T 38.3°C (101°F), P 110 bpm, R 24/min, and BP 162/86 mmHg. Her skin is moist and warm, and her hair is thin and fine. She has visible tremors in her hands. Her eyeballs protrude, and she is unable to close her eyelids completely. Her thyroid is enlarged and palpable. Diagnostic tests reveal the following abnormal results: T_3, 350 ng/dL (normal range: 80–200 ng/dL); T_4, 15.1 mg/dL (normal range: 4.5–11.5 mcg/dL). A thyroid scan demonstrates an enlarged thyroid with increased iodine uptake. After the medical diagnosis of Graves disease, Ms. Manuel is started on the antithyroid medication propylthiouracil at 150 mg orally every 8 hours.	Nursing diagnoses that may be appropriate for Ms. Manuel include the following: - *Imbalanced Nutrition: Less Than Body Requirements* related to weight loss of 6.8 kg (15 lb), with present weight 10% less than normal for height - *Diarrhea* related to increased peristalsis, as evidenced by 8–10 liquid stools per day - *Risk for Infection* related to an inability to close the eyelids completely - *Anxiety* related to a lack of knowledge about the disease process. (NANDA-I © 2012)	The goals for the plan of care specify that Ms. Manuel will: - Gain at least 0.45 kg (1 lb) every 2 weeks. - Regain normal bowel elimination patterns. - Maintain normal vision (with no evidence of corneal damage), and verbalize measures to protect her eyes. - Verbalize medical treatment and self-care needs. - Verbalize a decrease in anxiety.

(continued on next page)

NURSING CARE PLAN   (continued)

IMPLEMENTATION

The following nursing interventions may be appropriate for Ms. Manuel:

- Request that she keep a record of daily weight.
- Discuss adopting a high-kilocalorie diet. Identify her food likes and dislikes, as well as foods that increase diarrhea, before instituting a plan to increase food intake.
- Request that she keep a stool chart, noting the time, type, and precipitating factors for diarrhea stools.

- Teach comfort measures for irritated anal area (clean washcloth and soap, nonirritating ointment).
- Teach how to apply eyedrops (artificial tears).
- Explain the need to elevate the head of the bed to 45° at night and to tape eye shields over the eyes before sleep.
- Teach about Graves disease, the medication's effects and side effects, and the need for continued medical care.

EVALUATION

By her next office visit, Ms. Manuel has gained 0.45 kg (1 lb) and has discussed her dietary needs with her husband and the nurse. She is having diarrhea less often. She has safely applied the eyedrops and states that she uses the eye shields and elevates the head of her bed at night. The office nurse reviews the written and verbal information about Graves disease and the medication prescribed. Ms. Manuel verbalizes her understanding, stating, "I'll always take my medicine—I never want to feel like that again!" She also says that she feels much less anxious now that she understands what has happened.

CRITICAL THINKING

1. What is the pathophysiological basis for Ms. Manuel's abnormal vital signs?
2. What is the rationale for having the client with exophthalmos elevate the head of the bed at night?
3. Outline a teaching plan that could be given to clients for home care following a subtotal thyroidectomy.

HYPOTHYROIDISM

Hypothyroidism is a disorder that results when the thyroid gland produces an insufficient amount of TH.

▶ PATHOPHYSIOLOGY AND ETIOLOGY

When TH production decreases, the thyroid gland enlarges in a compensatory attempt to produce more hormone. The goiter that results is usually a simple or nontoxic form.

The hypothyroid state in adults is sometimes called **myxedema**. The term reflects the characteristic accumulation of nonpitting edema in the connective tissues throughout the body. The edema is the result of water retention in mucoprotein (hydrophilic proteoglycans) deposits in the interstitial spaces. The face of a client with myxedema appears puffy, the tongue is enlarged, and the voice is hoarse and husky (Porth & Matfin, 2009).

Etiology

Hypothyroidism may be either primary or secondary. Primary hypothyroidism, which is more common, may be caused by congenital defects in the gland, loss of thyroid tissue following treatment of hyperthyroidism with surgery or radiation, antithyroid medications, thyroiditis, or endemic iodine deficiency. Secondary hypothyroidism may result from pituitary TSH deficiency or peripheral resistance to TH.

The cardiac drug amiodarone (Cordarone), which contains 75 mg of iodine per 200 mg tablet, is increasingly being implicated in causing thyroid problems (Porth & Matfin, 2009). Clofibrate, estrogens, methadone, amiodarone, and birth control pills increase T_4 measurement; anabolic steroids, androgens, lithium, phenytoin, propanolol, interferon alpha, and

interleukin-2 decrease T_4 measurement in thyroid tests. Of course, the drugs propylthiouracil and methimazole, which are used to treat hyperthyroidism, decrease T_4 measurement as well (McPhee & Papadakis, 2009).

The disorder can occur at any stage of life, but it is common in women between the ages of 30 and 60. The incidence rises after age 50. Therefore careful evaluation of symptoms is important in the older adult, because manifestations of hypothyroidism often are thought to be the result of aging instead of a pathological process.

Risk Factors

Anyone can develop hypothyroidism; however, it is more common among women older than 50 years, among those who have a close relative with an autoimmune condition, and among those who have had thyroid surgery, received radiation to the neck, or been treated with RAI or antithyroid medication. Other factors that result in decreased TH include iodine deficiency and Hashimoto thyroiditis.

IODINE DEFICIENCY   Iodine is necessary for synthesis and secretion of TH. Iodine deficiency may result from certain goitrogenic drugs, which block TH synthesis; lithium carbonate, which is used to treat bipolar mental disorders; and antithyroid drugs. Goitrogenic compounds in foods such as turnips, rutabagas, and soybeans also may block TH synthesis if consumed in sufficient quantities.

In areas of the world where the soil is deficient in iodine, dietary intake of iodine may be inadequate. Individuals living in these areas are more prone to become hypothyroid and to develop simple goiter. In the United States, the use of iodized salt has reduced this risk.

HASHIMOTO THYROIDITIS   **Hashimoto thyroiditis** is the most common cause of goiter and primary hypothyroidism in adults and children. In this autoimmune disorder, antibodies develop that destroy thyroid tissue. Functional thyroid tissue is replaced with fibrous tissue, and TH levels decrease. In addition, decreasing levels of TH during the early stages of the disease prompt the gland to enlarge in an attempt to compensate, causing a goiter. However, as the disease progresses, the thyroid gland becomes smaller. This disorder is more common in women than in men and has a familial link.

▶ CLINICAL MANIFESTATIONS

Hypothyroidism has a slow onset, with manifestations occurring over months or even years. Clients with hypothyroidism characteristically have goiter, fluid retention and edema, decreased appetite, weight gain, constipation, dry skin, dyspnea, pallor, hoarseness, and muscle stiffness. Many clients have a decreased sense of taste and smell, menstrual disorders, anemias, and cardiac enlargement. The pulse typically is slow in clients with hypothyroidism, and sleep apnea is more common. See the Multisystem Effects of Hypothyroidism feature.

Deficient amounts of TH cause abnormalities in lipid metabolism, with elevated serum cholesterol and triglyceride levels. As a result, the client is at increased risk for atherosclerosis and cardiac disorders. Decreased renal blood flow and glomerular filtration rate reduce the kidney's ability to excrete water, which may cause hyponatremia.

Because a decrease in TH levels lowers metabolic rate and heat production, hypothyroidism affects all body systems. Treatment of the client with hypothyroidism focuses on diagnosis, prevention or treatment of complications, and replacement of the deficient TH. With early and continued treatment, the mental and physical symptoms rapidly reverse in clients of all ages, and both appearance and mental function return to normal.

Myxedema Coma

Myxedema coma is a life-threatening complication of long-standing, untreated hypothyroidism usually triggered by an acute illness or trauma. It is characterized by severe metabolic disorders (e.g., hyponatremia, hypoglycemia, and lactic acidosis); hypothermia; a shallow edema, especially around the eyes, hands, and feet; cardiovascular collapse; impaired mentation; and coma. Although rare, myxedema coma most commonly occurs during the winter months in older women with chronic hypothyroidism (Porth & Matfin, 2009).

Myxedema coma may be precipitated by trauma, infection, failure to take thyroid replacement medications, use of central nervous system depressants, and exposure to cold temperatures (Porth & Matfin, 2009). The treatment of myxedema coma addresses the precipitating factors and manifestations and

TABLE 12–16 Laboratory Findings in Hypothyroidism

TEST	NORMAL VALUES	FINDINGS
Serum TA	None to 1:20	Normal
Serum TSH	0.35–5.5 mU/mL (mU = microunit)	Increased in primary hypothyroidism
Serum T_4	4.5–11.5 mcg/dL	Decreased
Serum T_3	80–200 ng/dL	Decreased
T_3 uptake	25–35 relative percentage	Decreased
Thyroid suppression		No change in RAI uptake or T_4 levels

involves maintaining a patent airway; maintaining fluid, electrolyte, and acid–base balance; maintaining cardiovascular status; increasing body temperature; and increasing TH levels. If myxedema coma is left untreated, the mortality rate is high (Shah & Lettieri, 2007).

▶ COLLABORATION

Collaboration with the client's pharmacist will help minimize any side effects and ensure the client is not taking any contraindicated medications prescribed by different doctors. If the client has an existing comorbid condition, collaboration with the client's other physicians' offices may be necessary to ensure optimal care.

Diagnostic Tests

Hypothyroidism is diagnosed by the clinical manifestations and by a decrease in TH, especially T_4 (**Table 12–16 ●**). TSH concentration often is increased, because the negative hormonal feedback from TH is lost. The same laboratory and diagnostic tests used to diagnose hyperthyroidism also are used to diagnose hypothyroidism, with opposite results in most cases.

Pharmacologic Therapy

Hypothyroidism is treated with medications that replace TH. Levothyroxine (T_4) is the treatment of choice. In older clients, an age-related decrease in serum albumin and renal excretion can increase the amount of available drug and cause an exaggerated pharmacologic effect. Therefore the older client may require less thyroid medication than a younger client.

Surgery

If the client with hypothyroidism has a goiter large enough to cause respiratory difficulties or dysphagia, a subtotal thyroidectomy may be performed.

Clinical Manifestations and Therapies **Hypothyroidism**

ETIOLOGY	CLINICAL MANIFESTATION	CLINICAL THERAPIES
Decrease in TH production Possibly primary or secondary	Hypothermia Decreased appetite accompanied by weight gain Systemic edema	■ Pharmacotherapy ■ Subtotal thyroidectomy if goiter is large enough to cause respiratory difficulties or dysphagia

Multisystem Effects of Hypothyroidism

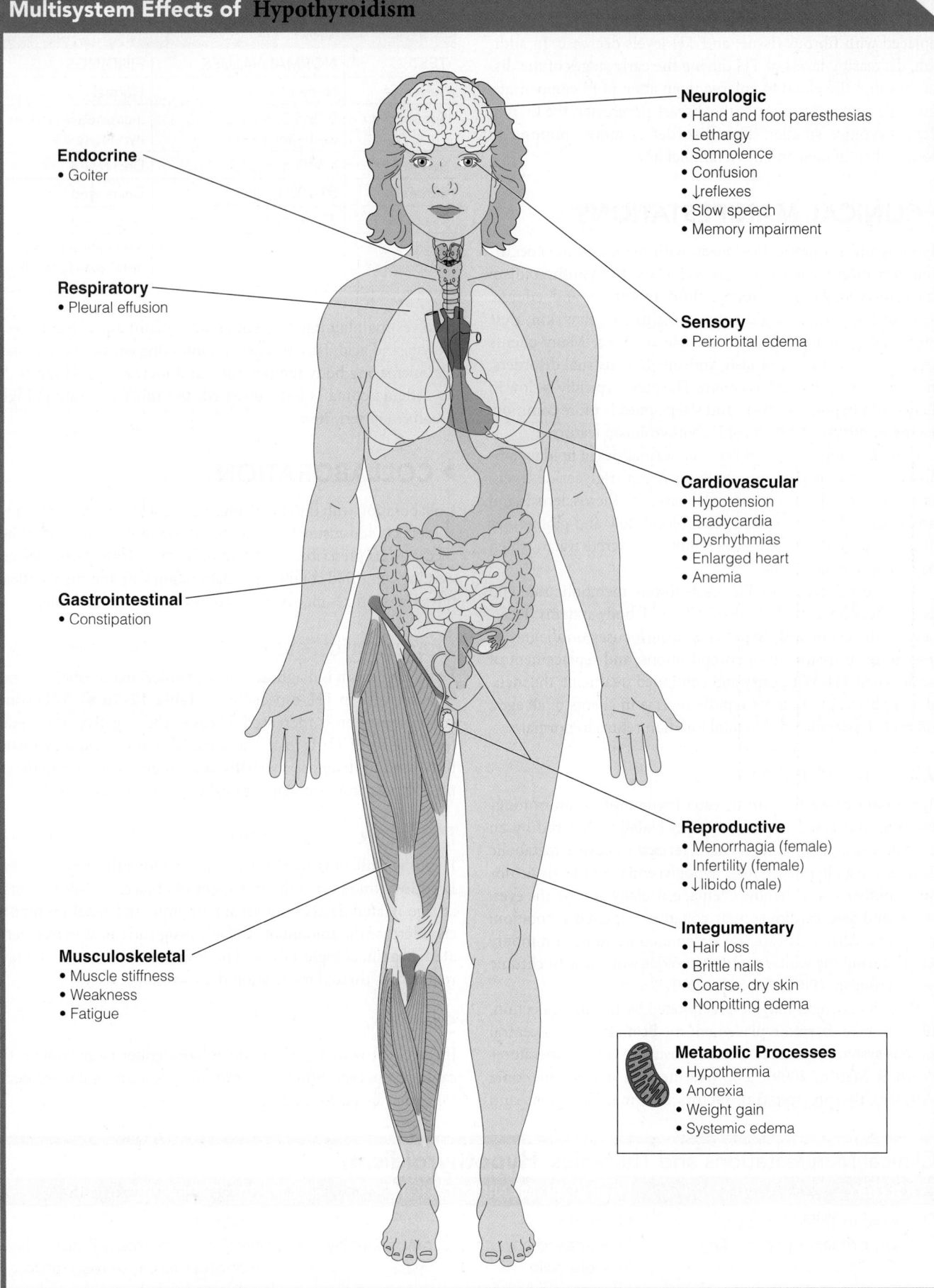

Neurologic
- Hand and foot paresthesias
- Lethargy
- Somnolence
- Confusion
- ↓reflexes
- Slow speech
- Memory impairment

Endocrine
- Goiter

Respiratory
- Pleural effusion

Sensory
- Periorbital edema

Cardiovascular
- Hypotension
- Bradycardia
- Dysrhythmias
- Enlarged heart
- Anemia

Gastrointestinal
- Constipation

Reproductive
- Menorrhagia (female)
- Infertility (female)
- ↓libido (male)

Integumentary
- Hair loss
- Brittle nails
- Coarse, dry skin
- Nonpitting edema

Musculoskeletal
- Muscle stiffness
- Weakness
- Fatigue

Metabolic Processes
- Hypothermia
- Anorexia
- Weight gain
- Systemic edema

NURSING PROCESS

Assessment

Collect the following data through the health history and physical examination. Further focused assessments are described in the Implementation section. When assessing the older client, be aware of normal changes with aging as outlined in the Lifespan Considerations feature.

- *Health history.* Pituitary diseases, when symptoms began, severity of symptoms, treatment of hyperthyroidism with medications or RAI, thyroid surgery, treatment of head or neck cancer with radiation, diet, use of iodized salt, bowel elimination, and respiratory difficulties
- *Physical assessment.* Muscle strength, deep tendon reflexes, vital signs, cardiovascular and peripheral vascular systems, integument, thyroid gland, and weight

Diagnosis

In planning and implementing care for clients with hypothyroidism, the nurse takes into account that the disorder affects all organ systems. Although many nursing diagnoses might be valid, this section focuses on client problems with cardiovascular function, elimination, and skin integrity.

Planning

Goals for the client with hypothyroidism include the following:

- The client's pulse and blood pressure will remain within established limits.
- The client will not exhibit arrhythmias.
- The client's skin will remain warm and dry to touch.
- The client will remain free of edema.
- The client will maintain visual acuity.
- The client will participate in activities without heart rate exceeding or falling below established limits.
- The client's elimination pattern will return to normal.
- The client's skin will remain intact.

Implementation

Care of the client with hypothyroidism is always individualized on the basis of the specific manifestations the client experiences

Lifespan Considerations
Hypothyroidism

Normal Changes With Aging

- The thyroid gland undergoes some degree of atrophy, fibrosis, and nodularity.
- Hair growth decreases.
- Nails are often thick, brittle, and yellow.
- Facial skin sags, and bones become more prominent.
- Deep tendon reflexes decrease.
- Response to questions may be slower.

as well as unique needs. When care is planned, interventions are indicated based on the nursing diagnosis and goals of treatment.

Monitor Cardiac Output

A TH deficit causes a reduction in heart rate and stroke volume, resulting in decreased cardiac output. Fluid may also accumulate in the pericardial sac (from the edema characteristic of hypothyroidism), and coronary artery disease may be present, further compromising cardiac function. The nurse should take the following actions:

- Monitor blood pressure, rate and rhythm of apical and peripheral pulses, respiratory rate, and breath sounds. Hypotension indicates decreasing peripheral blood. Fluid in the pericardial sac restricts cardiac function. Monopolysaccharide deposits in the respiratory system decrease vital capacity and cause hypoventilation.
- Suggest that the client avoid being chilled (e.g., increase room temperature, use additional bed covers, and avoid drafts). Chilling increases metabolic rate and puts increased stress on the heart.
- Explain the need to alternate periods of activity with periods of rest. Ask the client to report any breathing difficulties, chest pain, heart palpitations, or dizziness. Activity increases demands on the heart and should be balanced with rest. Symptoms of cardiac stress include dyspnea, chest pain, palpitations, and dizziness.

Prevent Constipation

The client with hypothyroidism is likely to have a reduced appetite and decreased food intake, a diminished activity level because of muscle aches and weakness, and reduced peristalsis, to the point where fecal impactions may occur. To prevent or minimize constipation, the nurse should do the following:

- Encourage a fluid intake of up to 2,000 mL/day. Discuss preferred liquids and the best times of day to drink fluids. If kilocalorie intake is restricted, ensure that liquids have no kilocalories or are low in kilocalories. *Sufficient fluid intake is necessary to promote proper stool consistency.*
- Discuss ways to maintain a high-fiber diet. *Diets high in fiber and fluid produce soft stools. Fiber that is not digested absorbs water, which adds bulk to the stool and assists in the movement of fecal material through the intestines.*
- Encourage activity as tolerated. *Activity influences bowel elimination by improving muscle tone and stimulating peristalsis.*

Maintain Skin Integrity

The client with hypothyroidism is at risk for impaired skin integrity related to the accumulation of fluid in the interstitial spaces and to dry, rough skin. Decreased peripheral circulation, decreased activity levels, and slow wound healing further increase the risk. The following interventions are for the older client who is hospitalized for surgery or severe hypothyroidism.

To help the client maintain skin integrity, the nurse should do the following:

- Monitor skin surfaces for redness or lesions, especially if the client's activity is greatly reduced. Use a scale for pressure ulcer risk assessment to identify clients at risk. Hypothyroidism causes dry, rough, edematous skin, conditions that increase the risk of skin breakdown.

- Provide measures to promote optimal circulation or teach them to the immobile client:
  a. Use a turning schedule if the client is on bed rest, or teach the client to change position every 2 hours.
  b. Limit the time for sitting in one position; shift weight or lift the body using armrests every 20–30 minutes.
  c. Use pillows, pads, or sheepskin or foam cushions for bed and/or chair.

  Prolonged pressure, especially in clients with edema and circulatory impairment, can occlude capillaries and cause hypoxic tissue damage.

- Teach and implement a schedule of range-of-motion exercises.
- Provide or teach the client measures to maintain skin integrity:
  a. Take baths only as necessary; use warm (not hot) water.
  b. Use gentle motions when washing and drying skin.
  c. Use alcohol-free skin oils and lotions.

  Dry skin and edema increase the risk of skin breakdown. Hot water, rough massage, and alcohol-based preparations may increase skin dryness, further impairing the body's ability to maintain skin integrity.

> **SAFETY ALERT**
> Lift the client up in bed to prevent tissue damage from shearing forces.

Evaluation

Evaluation involves determining whether the client has met expected outcomes and, in the event that outcomes have not been met, modifying outcomes or making changes to the nursing care plan. Any diagnostic tests should be repeated to ensure that medications are at appropriate levels.

NURSING CARE PLAN A Client With Hypothyroidism

ASSESSMENT

Jane Lee is a 60-year-old retired nurse living with her husband and daughter on a farm that has been in the family for four generations. Ms. Lee has gained 4.5 kg (10 lb) in the past few months, even though she is rarely hungry and eats much less than normal. She is always tired and weak—so tired that she has not even been able to help with the chores on the farm or do housework. She is concerned about her appearance and the way she sounds when she talks. Her face is puffy, and her tongue always feels thick. Mr. Lee convinces his wife to make an appointment at a health center in a nearby town.

Brian Henning, RN, completes the health assessment for Ms. Lee at the health center. He finds that she now weighs 68 kg (150 lb), an increase of 4.5 kg (10 lb) over her weight at her last visit 6 months earlier. Ms. Lee states that she always feels cold, tired, and weak. She also states that she is constipated, has difficulty remembering things, and looks different. Physical assessment findings include a palpable and bilaterally enlarged thyroid; dry, yellowish skin; nonpitting edema of the face and lower legs; and slow, slurred speech. Diagnostic tests reveal the following abnormal findings: T_3, 56 ng/dL (normal range, 80–200 ng/dL); T_4, 3.1 mg/dL (normal range, 4.5–11.5 mcg/dL); TSH increased. The medical diagnosis is hypothyroidism, and Ms. Lee is started on levothyroxine at 0.05 mg daily.

DIAGNOSES

Nursing diagnoses that may be appropriate for Ms. Lee include the following:

- *Constipation* related to decreased peristalsis, as evidenced by hard, formed stools every 4 days
- *Impaired Verbal Communication* related to changes in speech patterns and enlarged tongue
- *Situational Low Self-Esteem* related to changes in physical appearance and activity intolerance

(NANDA-I © 2012)

PLANNING

The client goals based on the plan of care for Ms. Lee include that she will:

- Regain normal bowel elimination patterns, having a soft, formed stool at least every other day.
- Experience improvement in verbal communication.
- Regain positive self-esteem as medication reduces physical changes and fatigue.

IMPLEMENTATION

The following nursing interventions may be appropriate for Ms. Lee:

- Teach the client to increase fluids, bulk, and fiber in her diet to help regain a normal bowel elimination pattern of a soft, formed stool every other day.

- Stress that the client must take medication as prescribed and should not expect an immediate reversal of the symptoms affecting her speech.
- Advise the client to plan activities around rest periods. Encourage the client's husband and daughter to help with housecleaning and cooking.

EVALUATION

On return to the health center 2 months later, Ms. Lee reports that she is no longer constipated but is continuing to drink six glasses of water and to eat oatmeal every day. She no longer feels cold, is regaining her normal energy, and even feels well enough to plant her garden. Her speech is clear and easy to understand. As she leaves the examining room, Ms. Lee says, "It's hard to believe that I have changed so much—now I look and feel like the 'old' me!"

NURSING CARE PLAN   (continued)

CRITICAL THINKING

1. *What physical changes that normally occur with aging are similar to the manifestations of hypothyroidism?*
2. *Describe the factors that put Ms. Lee's safety at risk. What alterations in her home environment would you suggest to promote safety until the prescribed medication takes effect?*
3. *The client taking oral thyroid medications may become hyperthyroid. List the manifestations you would include in a teaching plan to signal this condition.*

REVIEW Thyroid Disease

RELATE Link the Concepts and Exemplars

Linking the exemplar of thyroid disease with the concept of mood and affect:

1. What strategies might you employ when teaching a client diagnosed with hypothyroidism and disturbed body image?

2. What impact might hypothyroidism have on the client's mood and affect, and how would this impact alter the nursing plan of care?

Linking the exemplar of thyroid disease with the concept of stress and coping:

3. For what stressors would you assess the client diagnosed with hypothyroidism?

4. The time between initial diagnosis of hyperthyroidism and symptom relief may be several weeks to months as additional diagnostic testing is performed and treatments are decided upon. What teaching might help the client cope with the symptoms of hyperthyroidism?

READY Go to Companion Skills Manual

REFER Go to Pearson Nursing Student Resources
nursing.pearsonhighered.com

- Additional review material

Reflect Case Study

Judy Smith is a 55-year-old female who has recently returned to the United States after a lengthy missionary assignment in South Africa. She arrives at the provider's office today requesting a "head-to-toe" physical examination, including a Pap smear and mammogram. Ms. Smith has been reassigned to serve in the Fiji Islands, where health care is scarce, so she would like a full workup. Vital signs: T_O 99°F, P 112 bpm, R 22/min, BP 134/92 mmHg; weight: 101 lb; height: 5 ft 2 in.; overall physical appearance: thin, looks older than stated age, wispy gray hair in matted bun. You note that Ms. Smith has a visible goiter, and as you question her about it, she says, "Oh, I've had that for a long time. My mother had one, too." She states that she has been going through "the change of life" (for the past 5 years) and is having frequent hot flashes. She has lost 10 lb over the past few years from what she describes as "self-imposed caution" when eating in Third World countries.

As Ms. Smith is talking, you note she has slight tremors as she pushes her hair from her eyes. Her face is flushed, and she is fanning herself throughout the interview. She is anxious and fidgets a lot. Her hair is thin and shiny, and her goiter is palpable, which has caused an enlargement of her neck. She denies sleep apnea but states that she snores.

1. What focused health history would be appropriate to elicit from Ms. Smith?

2. What physical assessment will you perform to obtain a complete picture of Ms. Smith's status?

3. Based on physical assessment, what nursing diagnosis best describes Ms. Smith's health?

■ REFERENCES

American Association of Clinical Endocrinologists. (2011). AACE guidelines. *Endocrine Practice, 17*(2), 23–25.

Allan, R., Kerry, T., & Phillips, M. (2010). Accuracy of ultrasound to identify chronic liver disease. *World Journal of Gastroenterology, 28*, 3510–3520.

American College of Rheumatology. (2012). *Glucocorticoid-induced osteoporosis.* Retrieved from http://www.rheumatology.org/practice/clinical/patients/diseases_and_conditions/gi-osteoporosis.asp.

American Diabetes Association. (2009). Standards of medical care in diabetes—2009. *Diabetes Care, 32*(Suppl 1), S13–S14.

American Diabetes Association. (2011a). *Diabetes care in the school and day care setting.* Retrieved from http://care.diabetesjournals.org/content/29/suppl_1/s49.full.

American Diabetes Association. (2011b). *Standards of medical care.* Retrieved from http://care.diabetesjournals.org/content/34/Supplement_1/S11.full.pdf+html.

American Diabetes Association. (2011c). *Diabetes statistics.* Retrieved from www.diabetes.org/diabetes-basics.

American Diabetes Association. (2012). *Alcohol.* Retrieved from http://www.diabetes.org/food-and-fitness/food/what-can-i-eat/alcohol.html.

American Diabetes Association. (2013). Diagnosis and classification of diabetes mellitus. *Diabetes Care, 36*(S1), S67–S74.

Aschner, P., Horton, E., Leiter, L. A., Munro, N., & Skyler, J. S. (2010). Practical steps to improving the management of type 1 diabetes: Recommendations from the Global Partnership for Effective Diabetes Management. *International Journal of Clinical Practice, 64*(3), 305–315.

Bope, E. T., Kellerman, R., & Rakel, R. (2011). *Conn's current therapy.* Philadelphia, PA: Saunders/Elsevier.

Bouchard, C. (2010). Defining the genetic architecture of the predisposition to obesity: A challenge but not insurmountable task. *American Journal of Clinical Nutrition, 91*(1), 5–6.

Bruha, R., Dvorak, K., & Petrtyl, J. (2012). Alcoholic liver disease. *World Journal of Hepatology, 4*(3), 81–90. Retrieved from http://www.ncbi.nlm.nih.gov/pubmed/22489260.

Carroll, K. L. (2010). Alterations of musculoskeletal function in children. In K. L. McCance & S. E. Huether (Eds.), *Pathophysiology: The biologic basis for disease in adults and children* (6th ed., pp. 1618–1643). Maryland Heights, MO: Mosby Elsevier.

Centers for Disease Control and Prevention. (2011a). Grand rounds: Childhood obesity in the US. *Morbidity and Mortality Weekly Report, 60*(2), 42–45.

Centers for Disease Control and Prevention. (2011b). *National diabetes fact sheet.* Retrieved from http://www.cdc.gov/diabetes/pubs/factsheet05.htm.

Centers for Disease Control and Prevention. (2012a). *The office of minority health.* Retrieved from www.minority-health.hhs.gov.

Centers for Disease Control and Prevention. (2014). *National Diabetes Statistics Report, 2014*. Retrieved from http://www.cdc.gov/diabetes/pdfs/data/2014-report-estimates-of-diabetes-and-its-burden-in-the-united-states.pdf

Cooperman, M., & Griffing, G. (2011). *Somogyi phenomenon*. Retrieved from . http://emedicine.medscape.com/article/125432-overview.

Copeland, K., Silverstein, J., Moore, K., Prazer, G., . . . Flinn, S. (2013). Management of newly diagnosed Type 2 diabetes mellitus in children and adolescents. *Pediatrics 2013, 131*(2), 364–382. doi:10.1542/peds.2012-3494.

Couper, J., & Donaghue, K. (2009). Phases of diabetes in children and adolescents. *Pediatric Diabetes, 10*(Suppl 12), 13–16.

Cummings, D. E., & Flum, D. R. (2008). Gastrointestinal surgery as a treatment for diabetes. *Journal of the American Medical Association, 299*(3), 341–343.

Davis, A. B. (2011). *Toxic nodular goiter*. Retrieved from http://emedicine.medscape.com/article/120497-overview.

Davis, P. A., & Yokoyama, W. (2011). Cinnamon intake lowers fasting blood glucose: Meta-analysis. *Journal of Medicinal Food, 14*(9), 884–889.

Endocrine. NIDDK.GOV (2012). www.endocrine.niddk.nih.gov.

Endocrine Society. (2008). *Disease and Type 2 diabetes in patients at metabolic risk*. Retrieved from www.endo-society.org.

Flint, A., & Arslanian, S. (2011). Treatment of Type 2 diabetes in youth. *Diabetes Care, 34*(Suppl 2), S177–S183.

Grimberg, A., & De León, D. D. (2005). Disorders of growth. In T. M. Moshange (Ed.), *Pediatric endocrinology: The requisites for pediatrics* (pp. 127–167). St. Louis, MO: Elsevier Mosby.

Haire-Joshu, D. (Ed.). (1996). *Management of diabetes mellitus: Perspectives of care across the life span* (2nd ed.). St. Louis, MO: Mosby.

Hanberg, A. (2008). Management of clients with thyroid and parathyroid disorders. *Medical surgical nursing: Clinical management for positive outcomes* (8th ed.). Philadelphia, PA: Saunders.

Holcomb, S. S. (2006). Do the clues add up to Addison's disease? *Nursing, 36*(3), 64hn1–64hn4.

Inzucchi, S., Berganstal, R., & Buse, J. (2012). Management of hyperglycemia in Type 2 diabetes: A patient centered approach. Position Statement of ADA and EASD. *Diabetes Care, 35*(6), 1364–1379.

Joslin Diabetes Center. (2011). *Will diabetes go away?* Retrieved from http://www.joslin.org/info/will_diabetes_go_away.html.

Lee, P. A., & Kulin, H. E. (2005). Normal pubertal development. In T. M. Moshange (Ed.), *Pediatric endocrinology: The requisites for pediatrics* (pp. 63–71). St. Louis, MO: Elsevier Mosby.

Loh-Trivedi, M., & Rothenberg, D. M. (2008). *Perioperative management of the diabetic patient*. Retrieved from http://emedicine.medscape.com/article/284451-overview.

Mayo Clinic. (2013a). *Type 2 diabetes—Complications*. Retrieved from http://www.mayoclinic.com/health/type-2-diabetes/DS00585/DSECTION=complications.

Mayo Clinic. (2013b). *Type 2 diabetes in children*. Retrieved from http://www.mayoclinic.com/health/type-2-diabetes-in-children/DS00946.

McDermott, M. (2010). *Endocrine secrets: Questions you will be asked on rounds, in the clinic, on oral exams* (5th ed.). St. Louis, MO: Mosby.

McPhee, S. J., & Papadakis, M. A. (Eds.). (2009). *Current medical diagnosis and treatment* (48th ed.). New York, NY: Lange Medical Books/McGraw-Hill.

National Center for Biotechnology Information. (2011). *Diabetic ketoacidosis*. Retrieved from http://www.ncbi.nlm.nih.gov/pubmedhealth/PMH0001363/.

National Center for Complementary and Alternative Medicine. (2008). *2007 Statistics on CAM Use in the United States*. Retrieved from http://nccam.nih.gov/news/cam-stats/2007.

National Center for Complementary and Alternative Medicine. (2013). *Children and complementary health approaches*. Retrieved from http://nccam.nih.gov/health/children/.

National Diabetes Education Program. (2011). *Overview of diabetes in children and adolescents*. Retrieved from http://ndep.nih.gov/media/youth_factsheet.pdf.

National Diabetes Information Clearinghouse. (2011). *National diabetes statistics, 2011*. Retrieved from http://diabetes.niddk.nih.gov/DM/PUBS/statistics/.

National Diabetes Information Clearinghouse. (2007). *Monogenic forms of diabetes: neonatal diabetes mellitus and maturity-onset diabetes of the young*. Retrieved from http://diabetes.niddk.nih.gov/dm/pubs/mody/.

National Endocrine and Metabolic Diseases Information Center. (2012). *Hyperthyroidism*. Retrieved from http://www.endocrine.niddk.nih.gov/pubs/hyperthyroidism/index.aspx.

National Heart, Lung, and Blood Institute. (2013). *Classification of overweight and obesity by BMI, waist circumference, and associated disease risks*. Retrieved from http://www.nhlbi.nih.gov/health/public/heart/obesity/lose_wt/bmi_dis.htm.

National Institute of Diabetes and Digestive and Kidney Disease. (2012). *Health information for the public*. Retrieved from http://www2.niddk.nih.gov/.

National Institutes of Health. (2011). *What is osteoporosis?* Retrieved from http://www.niams.nih.gov/Health_Info/Bone/Osteoporosis/osteoporosis_ff.asp.

National Osteoporosis Foundation. (2013). *Are you at risk?* Retrieved from http://www.nof.org/articles/2.

Nimblett, A. (2011) A telltale lesion: Acanthosis nigricans in children can be a precursor of type 2 diabetes. *Advanced Healthcare Network for NPs & PAs*. Retrieved from http://nurse-practitioners-and-physician-assistants.advanceweb.com/Features/Articles/A-Telltale-Lesion.aspx. pp. 45–50.

Nimri, R., Weintrob, H. B., Benzaquen, H., Ofran, R., Fayman, G., & Phillip, M. (2006). Insulin pump therapy in youth with Type 1 diabetes: A retrospective paired study. *Pediatrics, 117*(6), 2126–2131.

Ogden, C., Carroll, M., Kit, B., & Flegal, M. (2012). Prevalence of obesity in the United States, 2009-2010. *NCHS data brief*. No. 82, January 2012. Retrieved from http://www.cdc.gov/nchs/data/databriefs/db82.pdf.

Osborn, K. S., Wraa, C. E., Watson, A. B., & Holleran, R. (2014). *Medical-surgical nursing: Preparation for practice*. (2nd ed.). Upper Saddle River, NJ: Pearson Education.

Pearson, T. L. (2009). *Motivating patients to monitor their blood glucose*. Retrieved from http://www.medscape.com/viewarticle/588565?src=mp&spon=24&uac=116901HG.

Peterson, K., Silverstein, J., Kaufman, F., & Warren-Boulton, E. (2007). Management of type 2 diabetes in youth: An update. *American Family Physician, 76*(5), 658–664.

Porth, C., & Matfin, G. (2009). *Pathophysiology: Concepts of altered health states* (8th ed.). Philadelphia, PA: Lippincott.

Raghavan, V. A. (2011). *Diabetic ketoacidosis*. Retrieved from http://emedicine.medscape.com/article/118361-overview#a0104.

Rewers, A., Klingensmith, G., Davis, C., Petitti, D. B., Pihoker, C., Rodriguez, B., ... Dabelea, D. (2008). Presence of diabetic ketoacidosis at diagnosis of diabetes mellitus in youth: The Search for Diabetes in Youth Study.

Rewers, M., Pihoker, C., Donaghue, K., Hanas, R., Swift, P., & Klingensmith, G. (2009). Assessment and monitoring of glycemic control in children and adolescents with diabetes. *Pediatric Diabetes, 10* (Suppl 12): 71–81.

Roberts, C. K., & Barnard, R. J. (2005). Effects of exercise and diet on chronic disease. *Journal of Applied Physiology, 98*, 3–30.

Schwartz, F., Denham, S., Heh, V., Wapner, A., & Shubrook, J. (2010). Experiences of children and adolescents with type 1 diabetes in school: Survey of children, parents and schools. *Diabetes Spectrum. 23*(1), 47–55.

Semb, S. (2008). Type 2 diabetes in youth: A growing concern. *CME Resource*, Sacramento, CA, pp. 13–15. Retrieved from http://www.netce.com/coursecontent.php?courseid=812.

Shah, A. A., & Lettieri, C. J. (2007). *Endocrine emergencies*. Retrieved from http://www.medscape.org/viewarticle/567307.

U.S. Department of Health and Human Services. (2013). *Physical activity guidelines for Americans*. Retrieved from http://www.health.gov/paguidelines/guidelines/default.aspx.

U.S. Food and Drug Administration. (2005). *Diabetes information: Glucose meters and diabetes management*. Retrieved from http://www.fda.gov/diabetes/glucose.html#8.

U.S. National Library of Medicine and the National Institutes of Health. (2006). *T4 tests*. Retrieved from http://www.nlm.nih.gov/medlineplus/ency/article/003517.htm.

University of Maryland Medical Center. (2011). *Cirrhosis—Causes*. Retrieved from http://www.umm.edu/patiented/articles/what_causes_cirrhosis_000075_2.htm.

Walsh, J. (2011). *Evaluation of insulin pumps and CGMS: Toward an artificial pancreas*. Retrieved from www.diabetesnet.com.

Weight-Control Information Network. (2013a). *Weight loss for life*. Retrieved from http://win.niddk.nih.gov/publications/for_life.htm.

Weight-Control Information Network. (2013b). *Very-low-calorie diets*. Retrieved from http://win.niddk.nih.gov/publications/low_calorie.htm.

Wilson, B. A., Shannon, M. T., & Shields, K. M. (2012). *Pearson nurse's drug guide 2012*. Upper Saddle River, NJ: Prentice Hall, pp. 953–954.

Wolfe, D., & Katz, J. (2012). Cirrhosis. *Medscape*. Retrieved from http://emedicine.medscape.com/article/185856-overview.

13 Mobility

◢ THE CONCEPT OF MOBILITY

The musculoskeletal system is made of the bones and joints of the skeletal system and the muscles, ligaments, tendons, and cartilage of the muscular system. The skeletal and muscular systems work together to support body weight, control movements, and provide stability. Some musculoskeletal structures, such as the rib cage and skull, provide protection for other organs, including the heart, lungs, and brain. The musculoskeletal system allows the performance of gross movement, such as walking, and fine movement, such as writing.

The musculoskeletal system works in tandem with the circulatory and nervous systems. The bones store nutrients and produce white and red blood cells. Subsequently, the blood provides oxygen, calcium, and other nutrients to strengthen bones; it also transports electrolytes that are needed for muscle movement. Similarly, nerves innervate the muscles to provide the electrical stimulus needed to initiate contraction.

Alterations in musculoskeletal integrity have a detrimental effect on the individual's ability to perform activities of daily living (ADLs), communicate, and participate in recreational activities. Impaired mobility is a common source of frustration and pain for clients with musculoskeletal dysfunction or injury. ◀◀

Concept Learning Outcomes

After reading about this concept, you will be able to:

1. Summarize the physiology of the musculoskeletal system related to mobility.
2. Examine the relationship between mobility and other concepts/systems.
3. Identify commonly occurring alterations in mobility and their related therapies.
4. Differentiate common assessment procedures used to examine musculoskeletal health across the life span.
5. Describe diagnostic and laboratory tests to determine the individual's mobility status.
6. Explain management of musculoskeletal health and prevention of immobility.
7. Demonstrate the nursing process in providing culturally competent and caring interventions across the life span for individuals with common alterations in mobility.
8. Compare and contrast common independent and collaborative interventions for clients with alterations in mobility.

Concept Key Terms

5 P's neurovascular assessment, 828
Ambulation, 837
Appendicular skeleton, 820
Atrophy, 821
Axial skeleton, 820
Bradykinesia, 825
Cartilage, 820
Crepitation, 824
Discs, 821
Epiphyseal plate, 820

Kyphosis, 820
Ligaments, 820
Lordosis, 820
Osteoblasts, 820
Osteoclasts, 821
Range of motion, 821
Resorption, 821
Sarcomeres, 820
Sarcopenia, 821
Sprain, 826
Strain, 826
Tendons, 820

▶ NORMAL MOBILITY

Most individuals take mobility for granted until a disease or injury restricts their freedom of movement. Because the musculoskeletal system is interconnected, injury to one structure can impair the function of other structures as well.

Physiology Review

The basic components of the musculoskeletal system include the bones, muscles, joints, tendons, ligaments, and cartilage. The bones provide the framework of the body. Joints are formed between bones, and muscular contraction stimulates movement of bones at the joints. Tendons, ligaments, and cartilage connect bones with either muscles or other bones and provide cushioning during movements.

SKELETON   The human skeleton consists of 206 bones that are divided into the **axial skeleton** (ribs, sternum, vertebral column, and skull) and the **appendicular skeleton** (pectoral girdles, upper limbs, pelvic girdle, and lower limbs). Bones have several functions, including forming the body structure, supporting soft tissues, protecting vital organs, providing a point of attachment for muscles, storing minerals, and forming blood cells.

MUSCLES   The three types of muscle are skeletal muscle, smooth muscle, and cardiac muscle. Skeletal muscle is critical for physical mobility. Skeletal muscles attach to bones via tendons; thus, muscle contraction causes movement of the skeletal bones. The human body contains more than 640 skeletal muscles that are under voluntary control by the nervous system.

JOINTS   Joints are formed where two bones meet; they hold the skeleton together while providing mobility. Structural and functional classifications of joints are generally interrelated. However, some joints, such as the epiphyseal plate in children (cartilaginous/synarthrosis), fall outside this general classification.

LIGAMENTS, TENDONS, AND CARTILAGE   Ligaments, tendons, and cartilage are all connective tissues composed of differing amounts of collagen fibers, proteoglycan matrix, cells such as fibroblasts or chondroblasts, and other structural components. **Ligaments** connect bones to other bones to form a joint. They strengthen and stabilize the joint and may limit the mobility of some joints. **Tendons** connect bones to muscles and carry the contractile forces from the muscle to the bone to cause movement. **Cartilage** is a type of flexible connective tissue found throughout the body. For example, cartilage connects the ribs to the sternum, covers the epiphyses of long bones to cushion the joint, and provides structure for the nose. Cartilage is less flexible than muscle but not as rigid as bones. Of these three types of connective tissue, cartilage is the only one that does not contain blood vessels.

✳ *Go to nursing.pearsonhighered.com for a minimodule that provides a thorough review of the physiology of mobility.*

Genetic and Lifespan Considerations

Bones and muscles adapt as an individual ages. Some bones fuse during infancy, and bones and muscles in children grow in length as the child ages. This growth ability is turned off in adults, so bones begin to undergo remodeling. In older adults, the musculoskeletal system undergoes physiological changes that decrease strength and mobility.

MUSCULOSKELETAL DIFFERENCES IN CHILDREN   A child's musculoskeletal system goes through many important changes as the child grows (**Figure 13–1 ●**). The bones of an infant's skull are not fused at birth, allowing the bones to shift as needed as the head passes through the birth canal. This also provides flexibility of the skull as the infant's head grows, preventing excess pressure on the brain. The spaces between the skull bones form membrane-covered fontanels, or "soft spots." The two largest fontanels are the anterior fontanel (between the frontal and parietal bones) and the posterior fontanel (between the parietal bones and occipital bone). The posterior fontanel usually closes in the first 2–3 months of life, whereas the anterior fontanel remains open until between 7 and 19 months of age (Kaneshiro, 2011).

Long bones of children are also unique in that they contain cartilage between the epiphysis and diaphysis, called the **epiphyseal plate. Osteoblasts** (cells that produce the matrix for bone formation) at the epiphyseal plate work to produce new bone and deposit calcium to increase the length of the bone (secondary ossification), creating a bone that is more porous than adult bone. This is one reason calcium intake is vital for children and adolescents. Adequate calcium intake allows the body to form strong bones to prevent fractures and osteoporosis. The rapid bone growth in children allows fractures to heal more quickly, but it may also produce "growing pains" as the lengthening bones pull on the muscles. When individuals reach skeletal maturity between the ages of 18 and 25, the epiphyseal plates close and leave behind epiphyseal lines.

An infant's spine also adapts as the child develops. At birth, the infant's spinal column is a C-shaped convex curve. As the infant learns to hold up his head, the cervical spine forms a concave curve. Similarly, as the infant starts to crawl and walk, the lumbar spine also forms a concave curve. This gives the spine its characteristic S-shape. This process usually takes about a year to complete. If the spine does not form these curves, the infant may suffer from **kyphosis** (convex curvature) or **lordosis** (concave curvature), both of which can decrease mobility.

Unlike the skeleton, muscles are almost completely formed at birth. Muscle growth occurs as **sarcomeres** (filaments made of actin or myosin) are added and lengthened in the muscle fibers; muscle fibers only increase in circumference and length, not in number. Skeletal muscle increases during childhood from about 25% of body weight at birth to 40%–50% of body weight in adulthood, and boys and girls have equal amounts of muscle until around age 13 to 14. Muscle growth in girls continues until around age 16, with muscle mass peaking at ages 16–20. In contrast, muscles grow rapidly after age 13 and into late adolescence in boys, resulting in a growth period that is twice as long as that of girls, with muscle mass peaking at ages 18–25. Therefore, boys develop much more skeletal muscle than girls (Samour & King, 2013).

BONE REMODELING IN ADULTS   After the skeleton has matured, bone remodeling continues throughout adulthood at

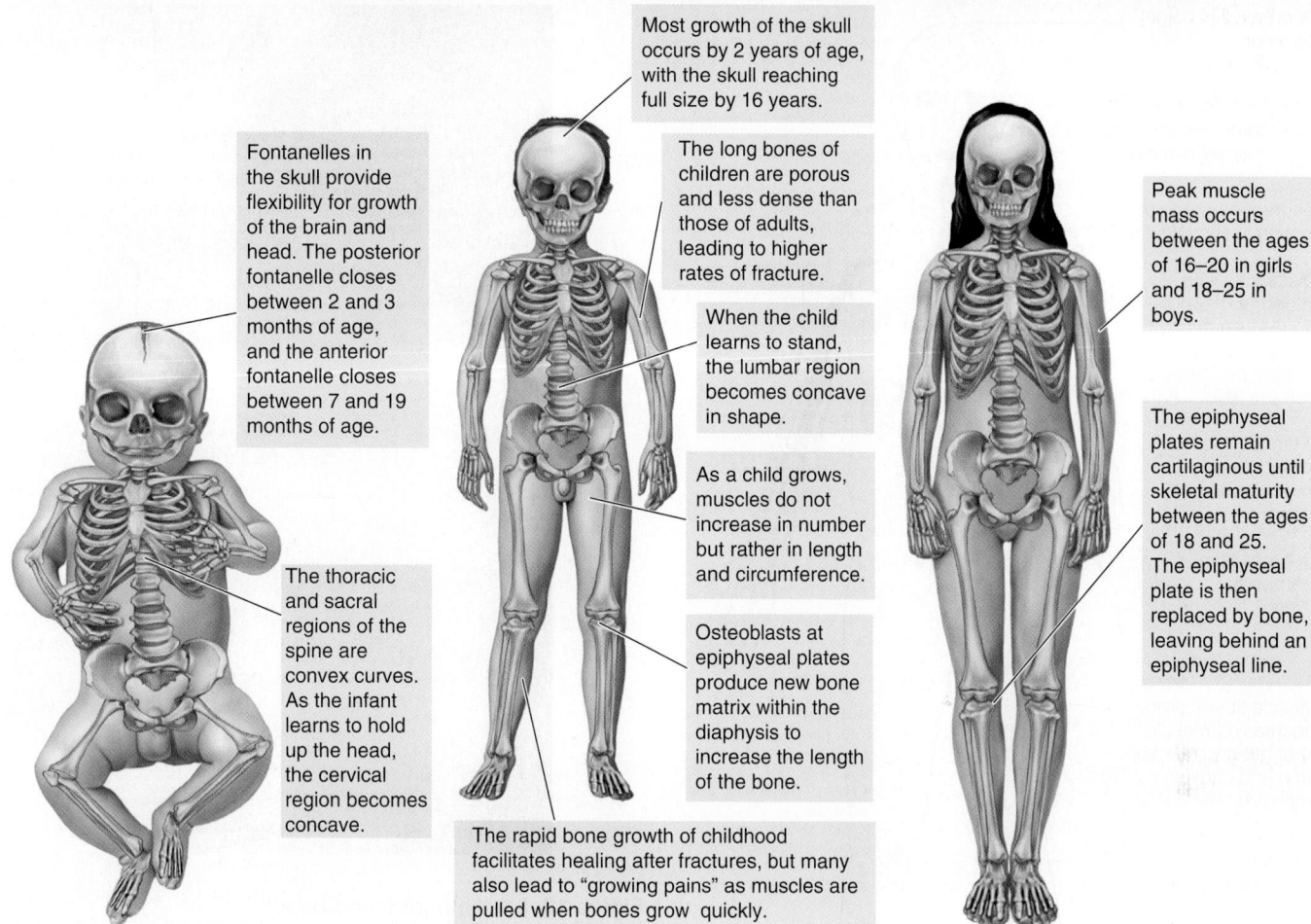

Most growth of the skull occurs by 2 years of age, with the skull reaching full size by 16 years.

Fontanelles in the skull provide flexibility for growth of the brain and head. The posterior fontanelle closes between 2 and 3 months of age, and the anterior fontanelle closes between 7 and 19 months of age.

The long bones of children are porous and less dense than those of adults, leading to higher rates of fracture.

When the child learns to stand, the lumbar region becomes concave in shape.

Peak muscle mass occurs between the ages of 16–20 in girls and 18–25 in boys.

The thoracic and sacral regions of the spine are convex curves. As the infant learns to hold up the head, the cervical region becomes concave.

As a child grows, muscles do not increase in number but rather in length and circumference.

The epiphyseal plates remain cartilaginous until skeletal maturity between the ages of 18 and 25. The epiphyseal plate is then replaced by bone, leaving behind an epiphyseal line.

Osteoblasts at epiphyseal plates produce new bone matrix within the diaphysis to increase the length of the bone.

The rapid bone growth of childhood facilitates healing after fractures, but many also lead to "growing pains" as muscles are pulled when bones grow quickly.

Figure 13–1 ● Skeletal and muscle development throughout childhood.

a much slower rate. Bone **resorption** (the process by which bone is broken down and its minerals released into the blood) occurs when minerals stored in bones are needed for cellular processes, and bone formation (ossification) occurs when excess minerals are available. Bone stress also plays a role in the rate of bone remodeling; bones that are used frequently increase their rate of bone formation, whereas bones that are not used undergo a higher rate of bone resorption. These processes must remain in balance to preserve the structural integrity of the bone. Bone remodeling is also a critical factor in repair of bone injuries.

Hormones that regulate bone remodeling are controlled by blood calcium levels. When blood calcium levels are low, parathyroid hormone is released to stimulate **osteoclast** (cell that breaks down bone tissue) activity and bone resorption to increase blood calcium levels. In contrast, when blood calcium levels are high, calcitonin is released to inhibit osteoclast activity and increase osteoblast activity, thus increasing mineral deposition in bones. Calcium regulation is a vital factor in mobility, because calcium is necessary for not only bone strength but also for transmission of nerve impulses and muscle contraction.

MUSCULOSKELETAL CHANGES IN OLDER ADULTS
Bones, muscles, joints, and connective tissue undergo many physiological changes that decrease mobility in

older adults (**Figure 13–2 ●**). Bone density decreases as bone resorption exceeds bone formation, contributing to bones that are thinner and weaker. This increases the risk of bone fracture from trauma or overuse, especially in women after menopause.

Aging also produces changes in the spinal **discs**, which are located in between the vertebrae. Like ligaments, discs hold the vertebrae together. With their tough outer covering and fluid-filled center, discs serve as shock absorbers. Discs also allow the spine to be mobile. With aging, discs between the vertebrae lose fluid and become thinner. Combined with the decreased bone mass, disc changes lead to spinal column compression, resulting in shorter stature and stooped posture (**Figure 13–3 ●**). Muscle fibers decrease, or **atrophy**, with age in a process called **sarcopenia**. This causes muscles to have less tone and decreased speed and power of contractions, partially as a result of changes in the nervous system, causing decreased muscle strength, slower reaction time, more rapid tiring, and impaired balance (Berman & Snyder, 2012; Dugdale, 2012a).

Tendons and ligaments in joints have decreased elasticity, strength, and hydration, causing stiffness and decreased flexibility and **range of motion** in the joints. Hips and knees may take on a flexed position. Ligaments and tendons tear more easily and heal more slowly. Fluid in the joints may decrease, and cartilage may rub together and erode. This causes pain and inflammation and contributes to slow and unsteady

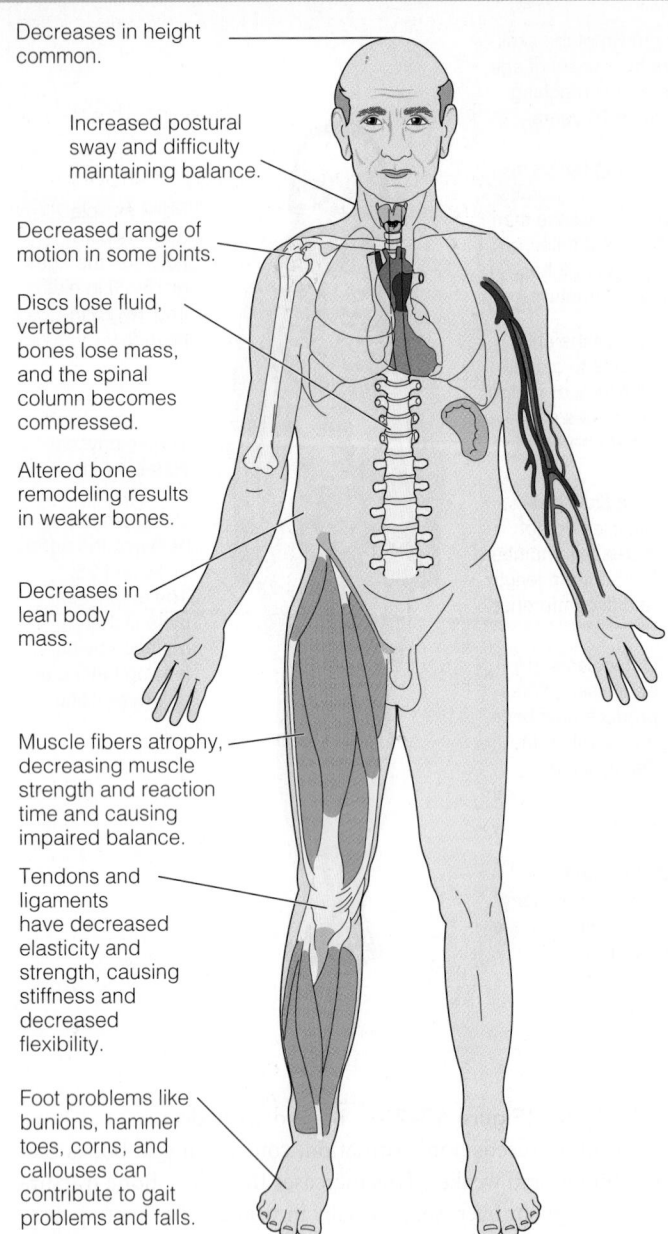

Decreases in height common.

Increased postural sway and difficulty maintaining balance.

Decreased range of motion in some joints.

Discs lose fluid, vertebral bones lose mass, and the spinal column becomes compressed.

Altered bone remodeling results in weaker bones.

Decreases in lean body mass.

Muscle fibers atrophy, decreasing muscle strength and reaction time and causing impaired balance.

Tendons and ligaments have decreased elasticity and strength, causing stiffness and decreased flexibility.

Foot problems like bunions, hammer toes, corns, and callouses can contribute to gait problems and falls.

Figure 13–2 ● Normal changes of aging in the musculoskeletal system.

movements, increasing the risk of falls (Berman & Snyder, 2012; Dugdale, 2012a). These changes decrease activity tolerance in older adults, enhancing the effects of aging in the musculoskeletal system.

▶ ALTERATIONS TO MOBILITY

Changes in the function of the musculoskeletal system affect nearly every aspect of life. Whether the client is healthy and wanting to increase physical fitness or has a medical condition that limits mobility, most clients are distressed when mobility is less than optimal. Alterations in the muscles, bones, and joints are linked to a variety of health problems, including arthritis, fractures, neurological disorders, and traumatic injuries. Regardless of its cause, impaired mobility or immobility can lead to a number of other health alterations (see the Safety Alert). The

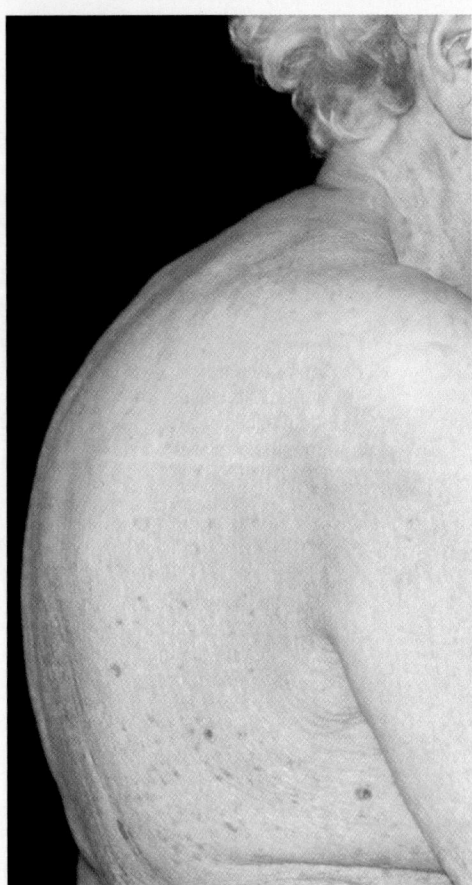

Figure 13–3 ● Kyphosis (hunchback).
Source: Dr. P. Marazzi/Science Source.

exemplars in this module describe some of the most common alterations in mobility and present nursing considerations to keep in mind when caring for clients with limited mobility. The Concepts Related to Mobility feature outlines some of the ways in which mobility is integrated with other concepts.

SAFETY ALERT
Along with exacerbating existing musculoskeletal impairment, immobility can lead to a host of other problems, including atelectasis (collapse of one or more sections of the lungs) and pneumonia; decreased gastrointestinal motility and paralytic ileus; and impaired tissue perfusion, which can predispose the client to developing pressure ulcers. The nurse should encourage and facilitate client activities that safely promote mobility, including frequent turning and repositioning as well as ambulation as ordered by the client's primary care provider.

Alterations and Manifestations

Manifestations of musculoskeletal problems will differ depending on their etiology. For example, a client with a fractured wrist may have trouble writing, whereas a client with osteoarthritis of the knee will have limited walking ability. Common medical conditions that cause alterations in mobility include back problems, fractures, multiple sclerosis, osteoarthritis, Parkinson disease, and spinal cord injuries (see the Alterations and Therapies feature).

Concepts Related to **Mobility**

Conditions that may limit mobility include pain, fatigue, respiratory disorders, cardiovascular disease, nervous system disorders, and musculoskeletal diseases or injuries. Clients with these conditions may benefit from collaborations with a disease specialist, physical or occupational therapist, personal trainer, or nutritional expert to help regain optimal mobility. Clients with a prolonged decrease in mobility may develop an inability to cope, requiring the need for counseling. In addition, increased mobility in children and decreased mobility in older adults is often accompanied by an increased risk of injury, so safety precautions should be taken to limit this risk.

CONCEPT	RELATIONSHIP TO MOBILITY	NURSING IMPLICATIONS
Comfort		
■ Acute and chronic pain ■ End-of-life care ■ Fatigue ■ Fibromyalgia	↑ pain → ↓ activity tolerance → ↑ muscle atrophy and bone resorption ↑ fatigue (especially muscle fatigue) → ↓ muscle control and ↓ balance Clients at end of life often have ↓ mobility in general.	■ Advocate for adequate pain management and give pain medications as prescribed. ■ Encourage mild exercise programs for clients with pain and fatigue to build muscle strength and prevent bone loss. ■ Teach clients the importance of alternating periods of activity with periods of rest. ■ Encourage adequate calcium intake. ■ Assist with mobility for clients in pain or at the end of life. ■ Provide palliative care for clients at the end of life who are immobile.
Health, Wellness, and Illness		
■ Physical fitness and exercise	↑ physical activity → ↑ muscle mass/strength and bone density	■ Encourage physical activity for clients with decreased mobility to help them gain strength. ■ Teach clients the importance of physical activity for maintaining health and wellness.
Stress and Coping		
	↓ mobility → ↑ stress → difficulty coping	■ Teach clients coping methods to counteract the stress of decreased mobility. ■ Encourage clients to adhere to the treatment plan to increase mobility. ■ Teach clients methods to reduce stress.
Collaboration		
	Alterations in mobility require interaction between multiple clinicians to help the client regain full mobility.	■ Refer clients to a personal trainer or nutritionist to help build strong muscles and bones. ■ Refer clients to physical or occupational therapists to increase both gross and fine motor movements. ■ Refer clients to counselors to help with stress and coping.
Safety		
■ Developmental considerations	Infants' learning mobility → ↑ risk of injury (falls, drowning, head injury) Children and adolescents who are involved in sports or other activities are at ↑ risk of injury, causing ↓ mobility. ↓ mobility → ↑ risk of falls and fractures, especially in older adults	■ Teach parents safety precautions for children at different stages of life. ■ Teach children and adults the importance of using safety equipment such as helmets, pads, and seat belts. ■ Assess homes of older clients with decreased mobility for safety hazards to help prevent falls. ■ Teach the proper use of assistive mobility devices such as canes, walkers, and crutches.

Alterations and Therapies **Mobility**

ALTERATION	DESCRIPTION	MANIFESTATIONS	INTERVENTIONS AND THERAPIES
Herniated disc	A spinal disc that slips out of place or ruptures	▪ Back pain that spreads to the buttocks and legs (herniated disc in lower back) or to the shoulders and arms (herniated disc in upper back) ▪ Tingling or numbness ▪ Muscle spasms or weakness ▪ Limited mobility	▪ Rest ▪ Pharmacologic therapy to manage pain and prevent muscle spasms ▪ Physical therapy ▪ Surgery to remove or replace the disc
Scoliosis	A sideways or abnormal S- or C-shaped curve of the spine	▪ Back pain ▪ Uneven hips or shoulders ▪ Obvious abnormal curve of the spine upon inspection ▪ Leaning to one side ▪ Exhaustion of the spine after sitting or standing ▪ Difficulty breathing	▪ Regular checkups ▪ Exercises to improve back strength ▪ Back brace to prevent further curving ▪ Surgery to correct curve ▪ Emotional support
Fractures	A break in the continuity of a bone	▪ Pain from damage to surrounding tissues ▪ Visible fracture on an x-ray ▪ Protrusion of bone out of skin ▪ Limited mobility	▪ Ice packs to limit swelling ▪ Pharmacologic therapy to reduce pain and swelling and prevent infection ▪ Immobilization with splint, brace, cast, or traction ▪ Surgery to stabilize bone or replace fractured bone
Multiple sclerosis	An autoimmune disease that causes damage to the myelin sheath around nerves	▪ Loss of balance/dizziness ▪ Muscle spasms ▪ Numbness or tingling ▪ Problems moving arms or legs ▪ Tremor or weakness in arms or legs ▪ Bowel and bladder problems ▪ Eye, hearing, and speech problems ▪ Cognitive deficits	▪ Pharmacologic therapy to slow the progression of disease and decrease severity of attacks ▪ Physical therapy ▪ Speech therapy ▪ Assistive devices for mobility ▪ Healthy lifestyle (nutrition, activity, rest) ▪ Safety measures to prevent falls ▪ Counseling
Osteoarthritis	Degeneration of cartilage and bone in a joint	▪ Joint pain and swelling ▪ Joint stiffness ▪ Loss of joint flexibility ▪ Bone spurs ▪ Crackling sounds (**crepitation**) during joint movement ▪ Joint tenderness	▪ Pharmacologic therapy to reduce pain and swelling ▪ Physical therapy ▪ Reduction of stress on affected joints ▪ Injections of corticosteroids or hyaluronic acid ▪ Surgery to realign bones or replace joints ▪ Gentle exercises ▪ Weight loss ▪ Application of warm or cold compresses
Parkinson disease	A motor system disorder caused by the loss of dopamine neurons	▪ Tremor in the hands, arms, legs, jaw, and face ▪ Rigidity and stiffness of the limbs and trunk	▪ Pharmacologic therapy to manage symptoms ▪ Deep brain stimulation ▪ Healthy lifestyle

Alterations and Therapies **Mobility** (continued)

ALTERATION	DESCRIPTION	MANIFESTATIONS	INTERVENTIONS AND THERAPIES
		■ **Bradykinesia** (slowness of movement) ■ Impaired balance and coordination ■ Lack of affect ■ Slurred speech	■ Walking carefully ■ Occupational therapy
Spinal cord injury	Direct damage to the spinal cord or indirect damage due to disease of surrounding tissues	■ Weakness or numbness below the injury ■ Muscle spasticity ■ Loss of bladder and bowel control ■ Pain ■ Paralysis ■ Difficulty breathing	■ Immobilization of the spine ■ Pharmacologic treatment to reduce pain and swelling and prevent further damage ■ Surgery to remove tissue, fluid, or objects pressing on the spinal cord ■ Bed rest ■ Spinal traction ■ Physical and occupational therapy

BACK PROBLEMS   Back problems can arise from a variety of causes, including trauma, degenerative disorders, muscle irritation, and pregnancy. Strain over time, poor posture, and improper lifting are common causes of back pain. Being overweight or having poor physical fitness also contributes to back problems. Two common causes of back problems, herniated discs and scoliosis (**Figure 13–4** ●), are discussed in Exemplar 13.1 within this module.

FRACTURES   A fracture is a break in the continuity of a bone. Depending on the location, a fracture can greatly impair mobility and cause excessive pain for the client. Two factors that affect the severity of the fracture are the nature of the event (e.g., a fall) and the strength of the bone. Falls, blunt trauma, motor vehicle crashes, child abuse, and repetitive forces are all common causes of fractures.

A hip fracture, in particular, occurs when the neck, head, or lesser or greater trochanter of the upper femur is fractured. Hip fractures are most common in older female adults, and they are most likely to occur as the result of a fall. Osteoporosis is the greatest risk factor for fractured hips (Mayo Clinic, 2012a). In younger individuals, hip fractures are usually the result of sports injuries or motor vehicle crashes.

MULTIPLE SCLEROSIS   Multiple sclerosis is an autoimmune disorder that destroys the myelin sheath around nerves, disrupting transmission of nerve impulses. This impairs the brain's ability to communicate with the rest of the body, resulting in a variety of symptoms including sensory and motor disturbances and alterations in bowel and bladder control. Symptom attacks vary in location and severity, and they can last for days, weeks, or months. Episodes often alternate with periods of reduced or no symptoms, making multiple sclerosis hard to diagnose (Zieve & Jasmin, 2011).

OSTEOARTHRITIS   Osteoarthritis is characterized by degeneration of cartilage and bone in a joint, sometimes accompanied by bone spurs, or bony growths on normal bone. Osteoarthritis is a normal process of aging due to wear and tear on a

joint. The most commonly affected joints are the knees, hips, hands, and spine. Ankle and foot joints can also be involved, especially if the individual is overweight.

PARKINSON DISEASE   Parkinson disease is a central nervous system disorder caused by degeneration of neurons that

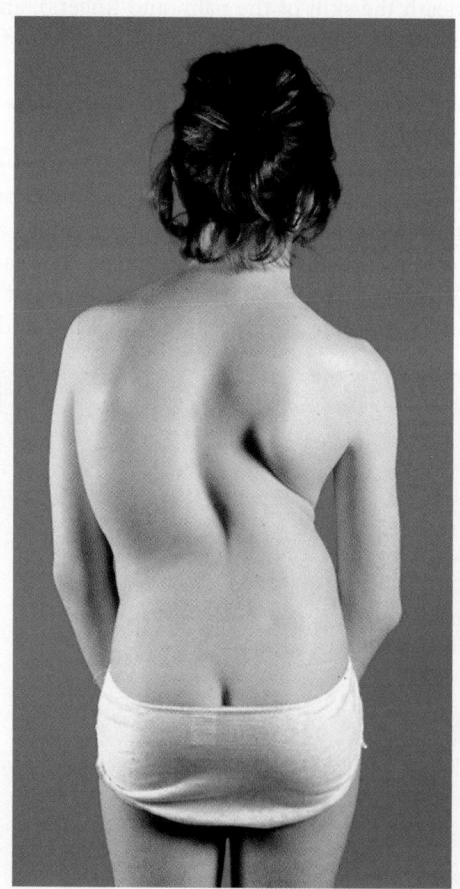

Figure 13–4 ● Scoliosis.
Source: Princess Margaret Rose Orthopaedic Hospital/Science Photo Library/Science Source.

produce the neurotransmitter dopamine. Parkinson disease affects approximately 1% of individuals over the age of 60, and it is more common in men than women (Hauser, 2013). Because Parkinson disease is a progressive disease, early symptoms may not be noticed for several months, and full expression of symptoms may not be seen for many years after diagnosis.

SPINAL CORD INJURIES Spinal cord injuries are medical emergencies that may result in permanent disability or paralysis. Spinal cord trauma often results from motor vehicle crashes, assault, gunshot wounds, sports injuries, and falls. The location of the injury will determine the type and severity of symptoms. Cervical injuries may affect the arms, legs, and trunk of the body. One of the most serious possible effects of cervical injury is paralysis of breathing muscles. Thoracic and lumbar sacral injuries usually affect the legs and may cause loss of bowel and bladder control.

OTHER ALTERATIONS THAT AFFECT MOBILITY Joint disorders are a primary cause of decreased mobility; they can affect one or multiple joints. For example, joint disorders of the head include temporomandibular joint (TMJ) syndrome, which affects chewing and talking. Joint disorders of the elbows and knees may include *tendonitis* (inflammation of a tendon), *synovitis* (inflammation of the synovial membrane; **Figure 13–5** ●), and *bursitis* (inflammation of a bursa). Joint disorders found in the hand and wrist include joint *effusion* (presence of excess fluid), rheumatoid arthritis (**Figure 13–6** ●), Dupuytren's contracture (thickening and contracture of the tissue beneath the skin of the palm and fingers), and carpal tunnel syndrome (**Figure 13–7** ●). Joint disorders of the foot include *gout* (buildup of uric acid; **Figure 13–8** ●), bunions (hallux valgus, a lateral deviation of the great toe; **Figure 13–9** ●), club foot, and hammertoe.

Traumatic injuries are also a source of limited mobility, including sprains, strains, and bruises. A **sprain** is a stretching or tearing of ligaments. The most common sprains are ankle and knee sprains. Sprains are often accompanied by pain, swelling, and bruising. A **strain** is a stretching or tearing of a muscle or tendon. Symptoms include pain, swelling, and muscle

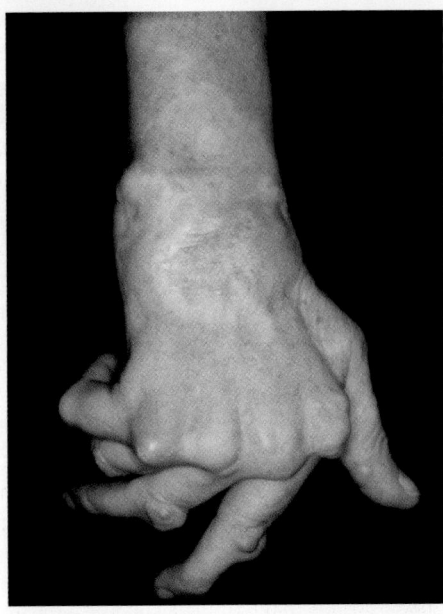

Figure 13–6 ● Rheumatoid arthritis with rheumatoid nodules, ulnar deviation, and swan-neck deformity of fingers.
Source: Princess Margaret Rose Orthopaedic Hospital/Science Source.

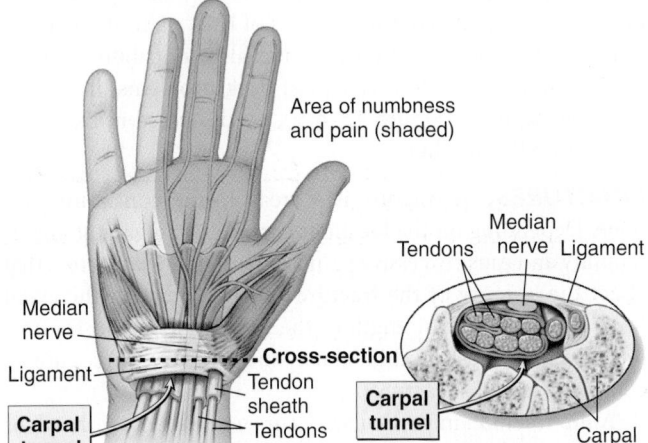

Figure 13–7 ● Carpal tunnel syndrome.

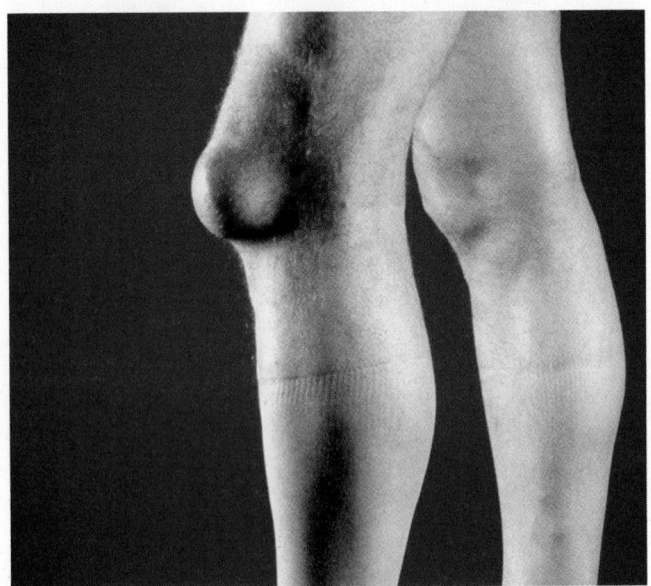

Figure 13–5 ● Synovitis.
Source: Princess Margaret Rose Orthopaedic Hospital/Science Source.

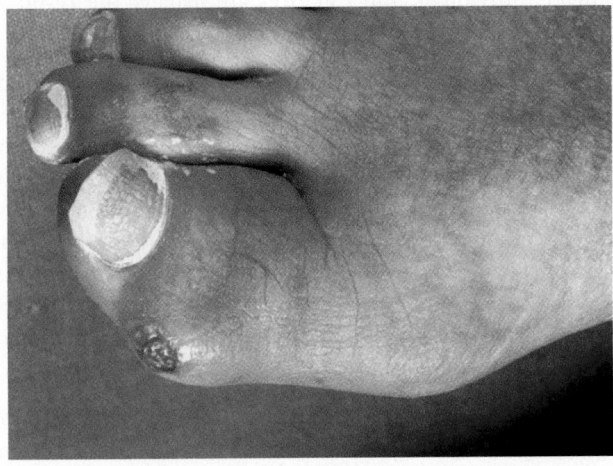

Figure 13–8 ● Gout.
Source: NMSB/Custom Medical Stock.

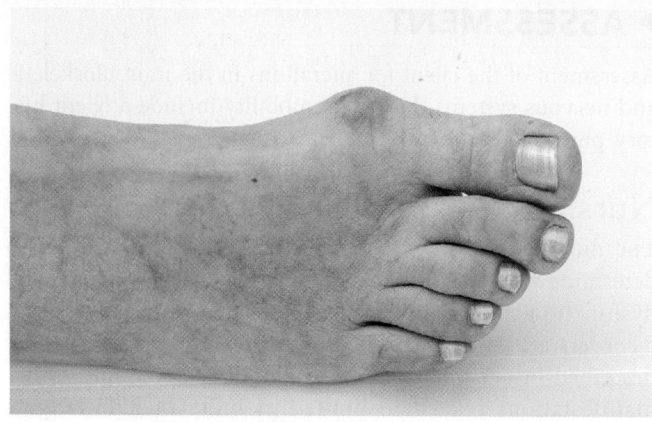

Figure 13–9 ● Bunion (hallux valgus).
Source: Photographee.eu/Shutterstock.

spasms. Strains often occur in the lower back muscles and hamstrings. Muscles strains that cause tearing are often simply called "tears," such as a rotator cuff tear (**Figure 13–10 ●**). Sprains and strains are usually minor and can be treated at home with **RICE** therapy and mild pain relievers. Note that recent evidence suggests that rest and ice may not necessarily be beneficial and that they may actually "delay healing, instead of helping" (Mirkin, 2014).

Rest
Ice
Compression
Elevation

Severe sprains and strains may be treated with surgery, and physical therapy may be needed to regain use of the affected area.

Bruises occur when traumatic force ruptures blood vessels, causing localized pooling of blood. Common symptoms of bruises include skin discoloration ("black-and-blue") and tenderness. Bruises usually heal on their own without further treatment as the body clears away the pooled blood.

Genetic Considerations and Nonmodifiable Risk Factors

One of the primary risk factors for alterations in mobility is aging. Joint problems that decrease mobility, including osteoar-

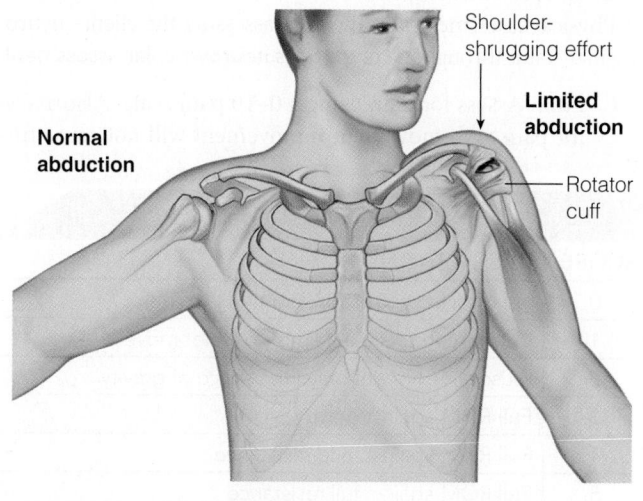

Figure 13–10 ● Rotator cuff tear.

Box 13–1 Genetic Disorders That Affect Mobility

- Muscular dystrophy (MD) is characterized by progressive weakness and degeneration of skeletal muscles. There are more than 30 types of MD, including Duchenne MD and myotonic MD. Duchenne MD is an X-linked disorder, so it primarily affects boys. However, girls can be carriers of the disease. Myotonic MD is the most common type of adult-onset MD. MD is characterized by muscle dysfunction, causing difficulty with advanced motor skills (running, hopping) and progressive difficulty walking. Breathing difficulties and cognitive deficits are also common. Affected muscles eventually atrophy or undergo pseudohypertrophy.
- Marfan syndrome is a disorder of the connective tissues that affects the lungs, heart, blood vessels, eyes, and skeleton. It causes individuals to have long limbs and digits compared to the rest of the body. Deficiencies in the connective tissue lining the brain may cause pain, numbness, and weakness in the legs, and cardiovascular effects may be life threatening.
- Amyotrophic lateral sclerosis (ALS) is a neurological disorder that affects the neurons responsible for voluntary muscle movement. Symptoms include weakness or paralysis in the limbs, slurred speech, trouble swallowing, muscle cramps, and difficulty breathing.
- Ellis–van Creveld syndrome is a rare disorder that affects bone growth. It may cause cleft lip or palate, polydactyly (extra digits), short arms and legs, and tooth abnormalities.
- Other mobility disorders that may have a genetic component include rheumatoid arthritis, gout, developmental dysplasia of the hip, ankylosing spondylitis, and systemic lupus erythematosus.

thritis, gout, kyphosis, lower back pain, and inflammatory disorders, become more common as individuals age. An increased risk of fractures, particularly hip fractures, is associated with osteoporosis in older adults. In addition, some diseases that limit mobility, such as Parkinson disease, primarily affect the older generation.

Genetic factors are also linked to alterations in mobility. Genetic mutations that affect the musculoskeletal or nervous systems will likely affect the individual's mobility (see **Box 13–1 ●**).

CASE STUDY \\ PART 1

Darrell Hayes is a 42-year-old Black male who is experiencing lower back pain. As the nurse at his primary care clinic, you are responsible for obtaining Mr. Hayes's medical history and conducting a preliminary assessment. Mr. Hayes's height is 71″ and his weight is 225 lb (body mass index [BMI] is 31). Mr. Hayes states that his back pain has gradually increased during the past several years because his job on an assembly line requires him to repeatedly bend and twist. Within the past week, his pain has gotten worse, and it now radiates down his left leg into his knee. He rates his pain as a 6 on a scale of 0–10. He adds that his pain is relieved by rest but gets worse when he bends. Mr. Hayes's vital signs include temperature 99.2°F oral; pulse 88 bpm; respirations 18/min; and BP 139/84 mmHg. During the straight-leg-raise test, Mr. Hayes can raise his left leg to approximately 45 degrees before he is in severe pain. He is able to extend and lift his right leg to nearly 90 degrees, but he still experiences moderate pain. After a physical exam by the physician, Mr. Hayes is diagnosed with sciatica and a suspected herniated lumbar disc. He is referred to an orthopedic surgeon for further evaluation.

Clinical Reasoning Questions Level I

1. What factors may contribute to Mr. Hayes's condition?
2. Describe at least three simple tests the physician may perform to identify a potential herniated disc.

Clinical Reasoning Questions Level II

3. What client teaching points will help to prevent exacerbation of Mr. Hayes's back injury?
4. What diagnostic tests can be used to determine the exact location of the herniated disc?
5. What nonpharmacologic nursing interventions might decrease Mr. Hayes's back pain?

▶ PREVENTION

Good lifestyle habits are vital to preventing many bone, muscle, and joint problems. Good nutrition, especially adequate calcium intake, helps maintain strong bones and provide ions for muscle contraction and nerve transmission. In addition, a regular exercise routine stimulates the body to build muscle strength and deposit minerals in bones. Regular exercise also helps maintain flexibility in joints and prevent the development or worsening of some joint disorders, including osteoarthritis and back pain.

Modifiable Risk Factors

Obesity is a major risk factor for mobility problems. Excess weight strains the joints and increases the rate at which cartilage and other protective materials are destroyed, leading to osteoarthritis, back pain, and joint inflammation. Obesity also makes common movements, including climbing stairs, getting in and out of a car, and walking, more difficult. Encouraging clients who are overweight or obese to lose weight is an important nursing intervention to prevent alterations in mobility.

Promotion of mobility begins even before birth. Good maternal nutrition during pregnancy can prevent some disorders that impair mobility. For example, taking folic acid during pregnancy is known to reduce the risk of spina bifida (myelomeningocele), which can cause partial or complete loss of sensation and paralysis of the legs. A well-balanced diet also helps the fetus develop strong bones and muscles and make essential nerve connections.

Screenings

Screenings to prevent musculoskeletal disorders is not a common part of most annual physicals for adults. However, some screening tools are available for clients who have risk factors for specific disorders. For example, older adults may have a bone density scan to detect osteoporosis. Treatment for osteoporosis can strengthen bones and help prevent fractures. Spinal screenings for school-age children can detect scoliosis so observation and treatment can begin early to prevent progression of the disease. Genetic testing can also be done for clients with a family history of muscular dystrophy, Marfan syndrome, Parkinson disease, and others.

▶ ASSESSMENT

Assessment of the client for alterations in the musculoskeletal and nervous systems that affect mobility include a client history, physical assessment, and diagnostic tests.

Nursing Assessment

The nursing assessment includes gathering information to determine whether the client is experiencing musculoskeletal dysfunction; the primary manifestations of musculoskeletal disorders are pain and limited mobility. Pain assessments are described in Exemplar 13.1 elsewhere in this module. Other manifestations related to limited mobility include fatigue, weight changes, and inflammation.

CLIENT HISTORY For the client with alterations in mobility, the nursing assessment should include questions about the client's lifestyle, such as physical activity required at work, ability to perform ADLs, participation in sports or exercise programs, time spent in sedentary activities, and nutritional habits. If the client is in pain, the nurse should ask if the client is taking any medications or performing any interventions to relieve pain. The client history should also include information about the onset, severity, timing, and symptoms associated with the limitations in mobility as well as factors that increase or decrease mobility. In addition, information about past injuries, joint pain, or neurological problems is beneficial when developing nursing diagnoses (see the Assessment Interview feature).

Physical Assessment

Physical assessment of the client with potential musculoskeletal or neurological problems should include inspection and palpation of bones, muscles, and joints for deformities, tenderness, and pain (see the Mobility Assessment feature). A range-of-motion (ROM) assessment should test the client's ability to move the muscle (see **Table 13–1** ● and the Assessment Interview feature). A goniometer should be used to measure ROM (**Figure 13–11** ●). The assessment may require the client to perform actions while standing, sitting, and supine. Joints should be clearly visible during the assessment, while the remainder of the client's body should be draped for privacy. The exam should progress logically from head to toe and proximal to distal.

Physical assessment also includes assessing the client's neurovascular status through use of the **5 P's neurovascular assessment**:

1. *Pain*. Assess for pain using a 0–10 pain scale. Also assess for pain with movement if movement will not cause fur-

TABLE 13–1	Muscle Function Grading Scale
SCORE	**DESCRIPTION**
0	No muscle contraction; paralysis
1	Muscle contracts, but limb does not move
2	Muscle movement only in absence of gravity
3	Full ROM against gravity
4	Full ROM against mild resistance
5	Full ROM against full resistance

Assessment Interview Mobility

History

- Have you ever experienced a bone or muscle injury or problem? If so, describe it.
- Have you ever taken medications to treat a bone or muscle injury or problem? If so, what were they?
- Have you ever received treatments for a bone or muscle injury or problem, such as surgery, physical therapy, or alternative treatments? If so, describe them.
- Has anyone in your family been diagnosed with a musculo-skeletal or nervous disorder?

Current Problem

- Describe the pain you are experiencing (onset, intensity, location, etiology, duration). What relieves the pain or makes it worse?
- Do you have any symptoms accompanying your pain, such as swelling, muscle spasms, cognitive deficits, balance problems, numbness, stiffness, or muscle weakness?
- Do your symptoms limit your ADLs, such as walking, bathing, cooking, or participating in social activities?
- Are you currently taking any medications or other treatments to help decrease your symptoms?

- Do you need to use assistive devices for ambulation or ADLs?
- Does your condition affect your ability to sleep at night?
- Has your condition ever caused you to fall?
- Describe how this condition affects your relationships, your ability to work, or how you feel about yourself.
- Does your condition contribute to feelings of stress? How do you cope with that stress?

Lifestyle

- Describe your typical dietary intake in a 24-hour period, especially your calcium intake.
- Do you take vitamins or other supplements? If so, what type and how often?
- Describe your physical activity in a 24-hour period.
- Do you participate in a regular exercise program?
- Does your job require you to do any physical labor, including lifting, bending, or twisting?
- Do you smoke, drink, or use drugs? Do you feel this is contributing to your condition?

---

ther damage. Determine the location, quality, and etiology of the client's pain.

2. **Pulses.** Compare distal pulses between the injured/affected extremity and the unaffected extremity. Lack of distal pulse may indicate compartment syndrome or arterial compromise.

3. **Pallor.** Observe skin color in the injured/affected extremity and in the skin in general. General pallor may indicate severe loss of blood, whereas pallor and coolness of the injured extremity indicates decreased arterial supply. In contrast, warmth and cyanosis may indicate venous stasis.

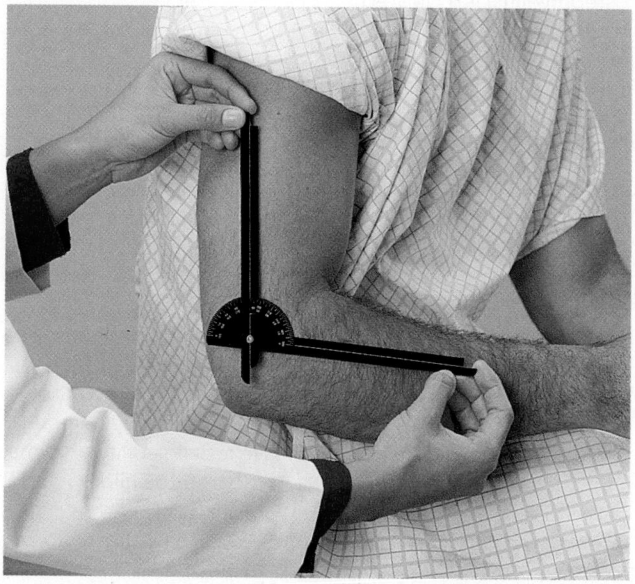

Figure 13–11 ● Using a goniometer to measure joint ROM.

4. **Paresthesia.** Ask the client about changes in sensation, such as burning, tingling, or numbness. The presence of paresthesia indicates neural damage or involvement.

5. **Paralysis/paresis.** For the client with a fracture, assess the client's ability to move body parts distal to the fracture, such as fingers and toes. Inability to move indicates paralysis, whereas muscle weakness indicates paresis. Paralysis or paresis may indicate nerve or tendon damage.

Lifespan and Cultural Considerations

Certain alterations may be more prevalent among clients in specific age groups. For example, infants and children are most likely to have mobility alterations as a result of genetic disorders or congenital malformations. Assessment should be tailored to the specific disorder or malformation. Decreased mobility as a result of trauma from sports injuries, abuse, or motor vehicle crashes is more common in children, adolescents, and young adults. For these clients, assessment should focus on the specific area affected by the traumatic event, as well as the surrounding joints and tissues. Older adults are more likely to present with inflammatory and "wear-and-tear" mobility problems such as arthritis or back pain. Alterations in mobility associated with neurological deficits, such as Parkinson disease, are also more common in older adults. Older clients, clients with obesity, and clients who do not exercise regularly may have decreased ROM and strength or increased pain as a result of decreased muscle tone and stress on the joints. Similarly, pregnant women will likely have decreased ROM and increased back pain. The client interview for pregnant women should include questions to determine if postural changes or other adaptations could increase mobility and decrease pain.

Mobility Assessment

ASSESSMENT/METHOD	NORMAL FINDINGS	ABNORMAL FINDINGS	LIFESPAN OR DEVELOPMENTAL CONSIDERATIONS
Physical Assessment			
■ Inspect for deformities. ■ Palpate for tenderness and pain. ■ Measure extremities for length and circumference. ■ Assess muscle mass and strength.	Client should have no deformities, tenderness, or pain. Extremities should be bilaterally equal in length and circumference. Client should have full ROM against resistance. Dominant side is stronger than nondominant side.	■ Deformities such as scoliosis, bunions, nodules, Boutonnière, and swan-neck ■ Presence of inflammation, tenderness, or pain ■ Unequal bilateral strength, length, or circumference ■ Unable to move against resistance	■ Assessment of older clients, clients in pain, or clients who are weak may take extra time. ■ All procedures and tests should be fully described for clients before they are performed, especially for children who may be frightened.
Gait and Posture Assessment			
■ Inspect body posture and gait. ■ Inspect the spine for curvature.	Body posture should be upright. Gait should be smooth and steady. Cervical and lumbar spine should be concave. Thoracic spine should be convex.	■ Joint problems or muscle weakness may cause changes in gait or posture. ■ Flattened lumbar curve and decreased spinal mobility may be evidence of herniated lumbar disc. ■ Scoliosis is a lateral S-shaped curve of the spine.	■ Lordosis may be seen in clients with obesity or pregnant clients. ■ Kyphosis is common in older adults.
Joint Assessment			
■ Inspect joints for inflammation and deformities. ■ Palpate joints for tenderness, warmth, pain, and crepitus.	There should be no visible inflammation or deformities. Joints should have no tenderness, pain, warmth, or crepitation.	■ Deformities include tissue loss, tissue overgrowth, contractures, and shortening of the muscles and tendons. ■ Edema may cause bulging. ■ Inflammation (arthritis, bursitis, tendonitis, osteomyelitis) is indicated by redness, swelling, warmth, and pain. ■ Crepitation is evidence of lost cartilage.	■ Older adults often have some degree of cartilage loss (osteoarthritis). ■ Athletes who overuse joints may have inflammation from chronic use (e.g., tennis elbow).
Range-of-Motion Assessment			
■ The nurse should provide resistance by pushing in the opposite direction (test both ROM and muscle strength).	Muscles should have full ROM against full resistance. Client opens and closes mouth smoothly with full ROM and no pain or sound. Flexion to 45 degrees Extension to 55 degrees Lateral bending to 40 degrees Rotation to 70 degrees	■ Clicking or popping noises ■ Decreased ROM ■ Pain ■ Swelling ■ Neck pain and limited ROM may indicate herniated cervical disc or cervical spondylosis. ■ Immobile neck with head and neck thrust forward may indicate ankylosing spondylitis.	■ Nonverbal infants and small children may need the nurse to physically perform motions. Individuals with cognitive impairment may need extra guidance or assistance from the nurse. ■ Older adults may naturally have less flexibility of joints compared to children and young adults.

Mobility Assessment (continued)

ASSESSMENT/METHOD	NORMAL FINDINGS	ABNORMAL FINDINGS	LIFESPAN OR DEVELOPMENTAL CONSIDERATIONS
Temporomandibular joint: ■ Palpate the joint while the client opens and closes the mouth (**Figure 13–12 ●**). *Cervical spine:* ■ Flexion: Touch chin to chest. ■ Extension: Look at the ceiling. ■ Lateral bending: Touch ear to shoulder on each side. ■ Rotation: Touch chin to each shoulder.			

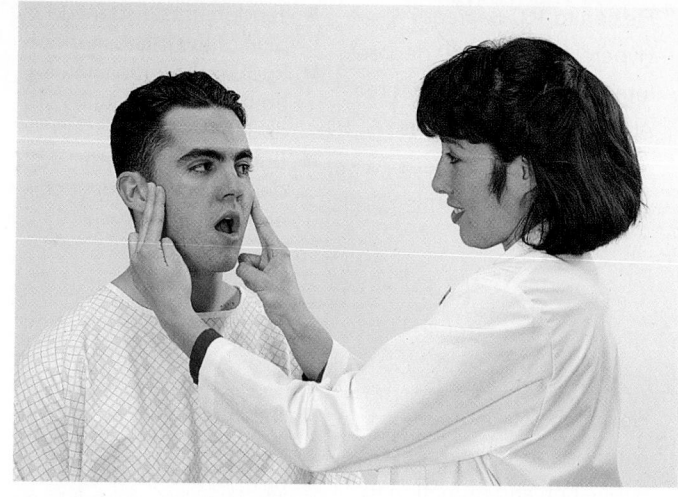

Figure 13–12 ● Palpating the temporomandibular joints.

ASSESSMENT/METHOD	NORMAL FINDINGS	ABNORMAL FINDINGS	LIFESPAN OR DEVELOPMENTAL CONSIDERATIONS
Lumbar spine: ■ Flexion: Touch toes with fingers (**Figure 13–13A ●**). ■ Extension: Bend backward. ■ Lateral bending: Bend right and left (Figure 13–13B). ■ Rotation: Twist shoulders right and left (Figure 13–13C).	Flexion to 90 degrees Extension to 30 degrees Lateral bending to 35 degrees Rotation to 30 degrees	■ Decreased ROM or pain may indicate abnormal curvature, arthritis, herniated disc, or muscle spasm.	

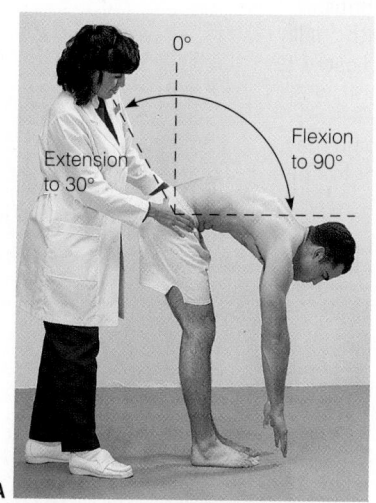 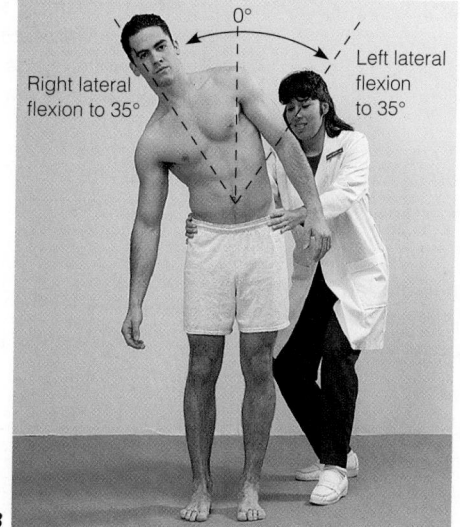 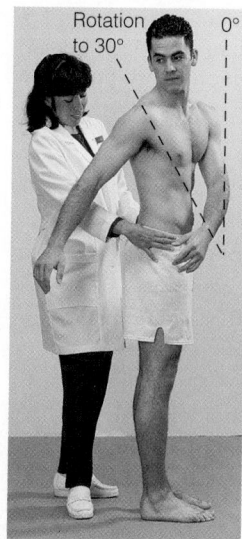

Figure 13–13 ● A, Forward flexion of spine. B, Lateral flexion of spine. C, Rotation of spine.

(continued on next page)

Mobility Assessment *(continued)*

ASSESSMENT/METHOD	NORMAL FINDINGS	ABNORMAL FINDINGS	LIFESPAN OR DEVELOPMENTAL CONSIDERATIONS
Shoulders: ■ Flexion: Slowly raise straight arms from at the side to over the head. ■ Hyperextension: Put straight arms behind the back. ■ Internal rotation: Put forearm behind lower back. ■ Abduction: Raise straight arm out to the side. ■ Adduction: Put straight arm across the chest.	Flexion to 180 degrees Hyperextension to 50 degrees Internal rotation to 90 degrees Abduction to 180 degrees Adduction to 50 degrees	■ Tendonitis is evidenced by pain of the biceps tendon. ■ Ruptured supraspinatus tendon prevents full abduction. ■ Bursitis and calcium deposits limit abduction and cause pain.	
Elbows: ■ Flexion: Touch hands to shoulders. ■ Extension: Straighten elbows. ■ Supination: Bend elbow 90 degrees and turn palm up. ■ Pronation: Bend elbow 90 degrees and turn palm down.	Flexion to 160 degrees Extension to 180 degrees Supination and pronation to 90 degrees	■ Inflammation may indicate arthritis. ■ Pain and tenderness of lateral epicondyle indicate tennis elbow.	
Wrists: ■ Flexion: Bend wrist down. ■ Extension: Bend wrist up. ■ Ulnar deviation: Bend wrist toward little finger. ■ Radial deviation: Bend wrist toward thumb.	Flexion to 90 degrees Extension to 70 degrees Ulnar deviation to 55 degrees Radial deviation to 20 degrees	■ Arthritis causes pain and swelling of the wrist.	
Fingers: ■ Flexion: Make a fist. ■ Extension: Open hand. ■ Abduction: Spread fingers. ■ Adduction: Close fingers.	Client should be able to complete all tasks with full ROM.	■ Flexion and extension are decreased in arthritis. ■ Stiff, painful, swollen finger joints indicate arthritis. ■ Swollen fingers with chalky discharge may indicate gout.	
Hips: (Client should lie down.) Flexion: Bring bent knee up to chest. Hyperextension: Lie on abdomen and lift each leg. Abduction: Move straight leg out to the side. Internal rotation: Bend knee and swing it toward other leg. External rotation: Bend knee and swing it to the side.	Flexion to 120 degrees Hyperextension to 30 degrees Abduction to 45 degrees Internal rotation to 40 degrees External rotation to 45 degrees	■ Limited ROM or pain may indicate arthritis or fracture.	

Mobility Assessment (continued)

ASSESSMENT/METHOD	NORMAL FINDINGS	ABNORMAL FINDINGS	LIFESPAN OR DEVELOPMENTAL CONSIDERATIONS
Knees: ■ Flexion: Do a deep knee bend. ■ Extension: Sit down and hold legs out straight.	Flexion to 130 degrees Extension to 180 degrees	■ Synovitis is common with knee trauma. ■ Swelling may indicate inflammation and excess fluid buildup in the articular capsule or bursitis.	
Ankles: ■ Dorsiflexion: Point foot to ceiling. ■ Plantar flexion: Point foot to floor. ■ Inversion: Walk on outside (lateral portion) of feet (**Figure 13–14 ●**). ■ Eversion: Walk on inside (medial portion) of feet (Figure 13–14).	Dorsiflexion to 20 degrees Plantar flexion to 45 degrees Inversion to 30 degrees Eversion to 20 degrees	■ Contractures or injuries to the Achilles tendon may cause pain and decreased ROM. ■ Arthritis may cause pain or contractures, especially after bed rest.	
Toes: ■ Flexion: Curl toes down. ■ Extension: Straighten toes. ■ Abduction: Spread toes apart. ■ Adduction: Bring toes together.	Flexion to 90 degrees Client is able to perform all tasks.	■ Lateral deviation of great toe is hallux valgus and causes bunions. ■ Swollen, inflamed, and painful toes indicate arthritis or gout. ■ Hyperextension of metatarsophalangeal joint and flexion of proximal interphalangeal joint indicate hammertoe.	

Special Assessments

■ *Phalen's test.* Hold wrists in acute flexion for 60 seconds (**Figure 13–15 ●**).	No tingling, numbness, or pain should be felt.	■ Numbness, tingling, or pain may indicate carpal tunnel syndrome.	

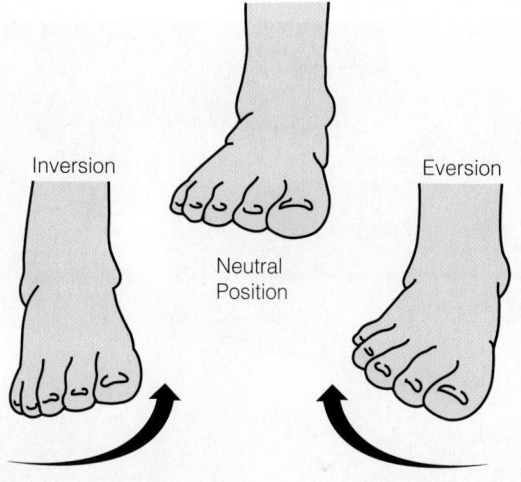

Figure 13–14 ● Inversion and eversion of the ankle and foot.

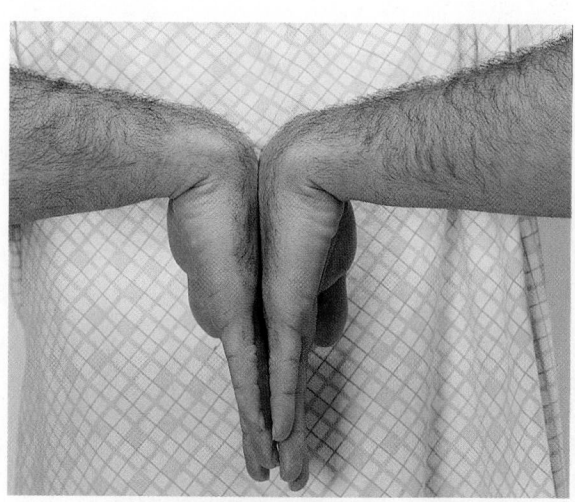

Figure 13–15 ● Phalen's test.

(continued on next page)

Mobility Assessment (*continued*)

ASSESSMENT/METHOD	NORMAL FINDINGS	ABNORMAL FINDINGS	LIFESPAN OR DEVELOPMENTAL CONSIDERATIONS
■ *Bulge test.* Milk upward on the medial knee and tap lateral side of patella (**Figure 13–16 ●**).	No bulge of fluid should appear on the medial knee.	■ Fluid bulge indicates effusion in knee instead of swelling.	
■ *Ballottement test.* Apply downward pressure on knee while pushing patella backward against femur (**Figure 13–17 ●**).	The patella should not move.	■ Increased fluid will cause a tapping sound as the patella displaces the fluid and hits the femur.	
■ *McMurray's test.* When client is lying down, ask client to turn flexed knee toward center of body. Stabilize knee and apply pressure on the lower leg (**Figure 13–18 ●**).	No pain or clicking should be present.	■ Pain, locking, or popping may indicate meniscus injury.	

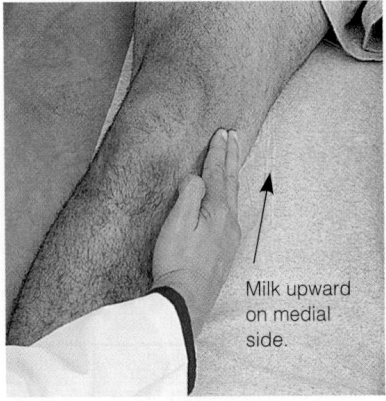
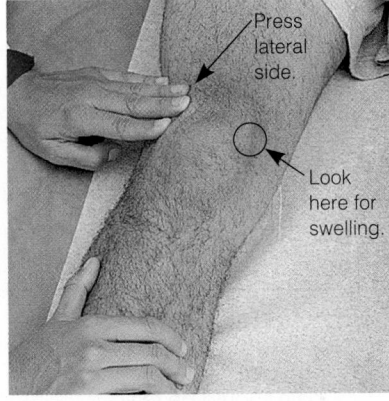

Figure 13–16 ● Checking for the bulge sign.

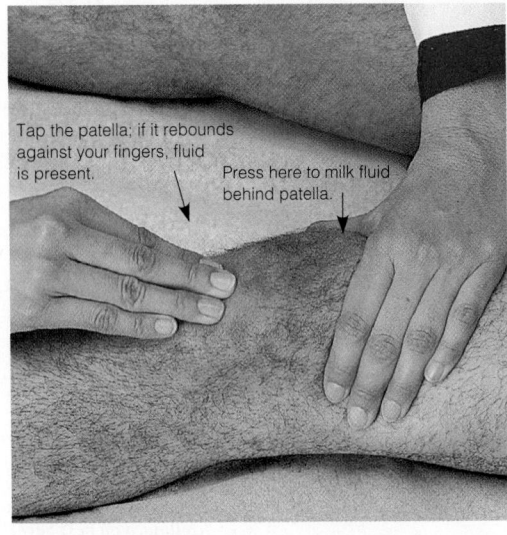

Figure 13–17 ● Checking for ballottement.

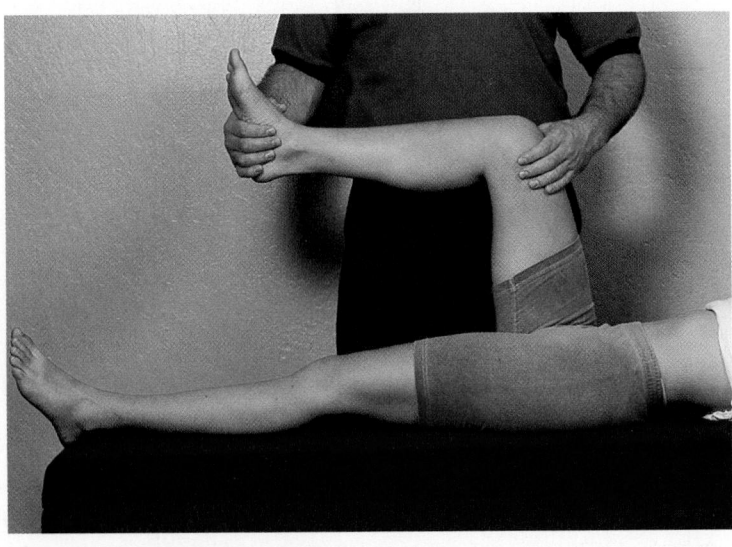

Figure 13–18 ● McMurray's test.

Mobility Assessment (*continued*)

ASSESSMENT/METHOD	NORMAL FINDINGS	ABNORMAL FINDINGS	LIFESPAN OR DEVELOPMENTAL CONSIDERATIONS
■ *Thomas test.* While client is lying down, ask client to extend one leg while bringing opposite leg to the chest (**Figure 13–19 ●**).	Extended leg should not rise off the table.	A hip flexion contracture will cause the extended leg to rise off the table.	

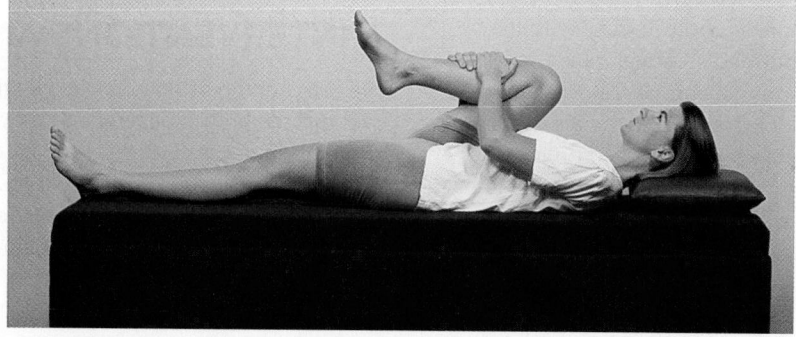

Figure 13–19 ● Thomas test for hip contracture.

Diagnostic Tests

Tests used to detect musculoskeletal and neurological problems that may alter mobility include blood tests (**Table 13–2 ●**), imaging tests, and electrical tests. These tests can be used to support a diagnosis and identify the efficacy of current treatments.

✳ *Selected diagnostic tests are described in Appendix B at* **nursing.pearsonhighered.com***.*

Imaging tests include bone density scans (e.g., dual-photon absorptiometry, dual-energy x-ray absorptiometry, technetium bone scan, peripheral bone density test), computed tomography

TABLE 13–2 Blood Tests for Musculoskeletal Disorders

TEST	FUNCTION
Alkaline phosphatase (ALP)	ALP is produced by bone and other organs. Increased ALP may indicate bone disease, bone fracture, bone tumors, osteomalacia, Paget disease, rickets. Decreased ALP may indicate Wilson disease.
Calcitonin/parathyroid hormone	Calcitonin and parathyroid hormone (PTH) have opposite actions in the regulation of blood calcium levels, which is vital for bone and muscle strength and function. Increased calcitonin may indicate a thyroid tumor. PTH may be increased in osteoporosis that does not respond to therapy. Increased PTH may suggest kidney disease, parathyroid gland tumors, lack of calcium, or vitamin D disorders.
Calcium (Ca)	Increased blood calcium levels could indicate the presence of metastatic bone tumors, Paget disease, bone fractures, or hyperparathyroidism. Decreased blood calcium levels could indicate hypoparathyroidism, osteomalacia, or vitamin D deficiency.
Creatine kinase (CK)	Used to detect muscle damage, muscle inflammation, rhabdomyolysis, polymyositis, and muscular dystrophy. CPK-MM is specific for skeletal muscle.
Growth hormone (GH)	High levels of growth hormone may indicate acromegaly or gigantism. Low levels of growth hormone may result in dwarfism.
Human leukocyte antigen-B27 (HLA-B27)	The presence of HLA-B27 indicates an increased risk for ankylosing spondylitis and arthritis.
Phosphorus (P)	Increased levels may indicate hypoparathyroidism. Decreased levels may indicate hyperparathyroidism or lack of vitamin D, which increases the risk of rickets and osteomalacia.
Rheumatoid factor (RF)	Elevated level may indicate rheumatoid arthritis, scleroderma, lupus erythematosus, and adult Still disease.
Uric acid	Increased uric acid levels may indicate gout, excessive exercise, and a variety of non-musculoskeletal-related disorders.

(CT) scans (e.g., classic CT, discography, quantitative CT), magnetic resonance imaging (MRI), and x-rays (e.g., classic x-rays, arthrography). Many of these tests can be performed with or without specific dyes to detect alterations in bone or connective tissue structures, including joint structures; osteoporosis; unusual bone formation; bone fractures; spinal disc problems; spinal stenosis; and torn muscles, ligaments, and cartilage.

> **SAFETY ALERT**
> Clients with metal implants such as pacemakers; heart valves; brain, eye, or ear implants; and infusion catheters should not undergo MRIs because the strong magnetic field may damage the implants and cause injury to the client. Individuals with embedded shrapnel may also be at risk for injury. Most orthopedic and dental implants are safe for MRIs, but they may distort the image. Clients scheduled to undergo MRI scanning should be screened for potential contraindications.

Other tests include electrical tests such as electromyography (EMG), neurological tests such as a nerve conduction study, and joint aspiration. EMG testing, which is used to analyze the electrical activity of the muscle, can be useful in determining whether nerve compression is present. In conjunction with EMG testing, nerve conduction studies are often conducted to determine if nerves are functioning normally. Nerve conduction studies can be especially useful in the detection of carpal tunnel syndrome or ulnar nerve entrapment. Joint aspiration may be used to remove accumulated fluid from a joint. Through laboratory analysis, the aspirated fluid may be sent for laboratory analysis to detect infection, as well as blood or fat droplets, which may indicate a fracture.

CASE STUDY \\ PART 2

Mr. Hayes is under the care of an orthopedic spine surgeon. After 6 weeks of implementing a regimen including ibuprofen, moist heat packs, and alternating periods of rest and mild activity, Mr. Hayes returns to his surgeon's office. He now complains of numbness and tingling in his left leg. He states that he constantly feels like his leg has "fallen asleep." He has been trying to limit his bending and twisting at work, but he has to move quickly to meet productivity standards on the assembly line. The ibuprofen seems to dull the pain, but the pain often returns before his next dose of medication is scheduled. On the basis of the severity of symptoms, the surgeon decides to refer Mr. Hayes to the pain clinic for an epidural cortisone injection. First, he needs to obtain a myelogram to confirm the exact location of the disc that is causing Mr. Hayes's pain. The myelogram results indicate that Mr. Hayes has a herniated disc at L4–L5. After Mr. Hayes is admitted to the pain clinic, an anesthesiologist administers an epidural cortisone injection in the L4–L5 region and also prescribes the muscle relaxant cyclobenzaprine.

Clinical Reasoning Questions Level I

1. What symptoms indicate that Mr. Hayes's condition is worsening?
2. What nursing interventions should be implemented for Mr. Hayes before, during, and after his myelogram and epidural cortisone injection?

3. Prior to his myelogram and epidural injection, what assessment questions should the nurse ask Mr. Hayes to ensure his safety?

Clinical Reasoning Questions Level II

4. What adverse reactions may occur during the myelogram? How can the nurse assess for adverse effects and complications related to this procedure?
5. What coping strategies might the nurse suggest for Mr. Hayes?
6. What instructions should be included in Mr. Hayes's discharge teaching?

▶ INTERVENTIONS AND THERAPIES

Nursing interventions for clients with alterations in mobility will include both independent and collaborative interventions. In addition to promoting safety and comfort, injury prevention is a main priority for these clients. Client teaching is especially beneficial for individuals who will administer self-care in the home setting and for clients with chronic conditions.

Independent

Primary categories of independent nursing interventions for the client with impaired mobility include education, comfort promotion, and injury prevention. While the specific nursing interventions are dependent on the client and the nature of the impairment, certain considerations within these three categories are applicable to a majority of these clients.

PROVIDING EDUCATION For the ambulatory client or one who will resume ambulation, client teaching should include instruction about body mechanics and proper posture. Even simple modifications in turning, lifting, and bending practices can significantly enhance the client's healing and reduce the risk for further injury. Additionally, because obesity is a risk factor for impaired mobility, clients should be educated as to the importance of regular exercise and good nutrition. Teaching should also incorporate discussion of any medications added to the client's regimen, including safe administration, actions, side effects, and precautions associated with the drugs.

PROMOTING COMFORT During periods of immobility, client positioning and proper padding of joints and bony prominences can prevent discomfort and help prevent skin breakdown. Braces and support devices, such as splints and wrist braces, also help promote comfort by stabilizing weak or injured musculoskeletal structures. The nurse should be knowledgeable in the application of these devices, as well as with regard to the care of clients whose treatment plan includes their use. When a splint or brace is in place, the nurse should routinely assess the surrounding area for signs and symptoms of circulatory impairment, including skin pallor or blanching, weak or absent pulses, and impaired sensation.

PREVENTING INJURY Traumatic injury, certain neurological conditions, and decreased mobility are associated with an increased risk for contractures. The client should be encouraged to perform exercises and stretches, and to utilize braces and splints as prescribed by the client's primary healthcare provider, physical therapist (PT), and occupational therapist (OT) (Vorvick & Zieve, 2012).

The client's environment should be screened for potential hazards, including loose floor coverings, inadequate lighting, and obstructed walkways. Additionally, the nurse should ensure that the client is properly using any assistive devices and provide instruction as needed.

Collaborative

Collaborative interventions include rehabilitative services designed to help the client preserve or regain mobility, as well as pharmacologic interventions. Physical therapy is ordered by the client's primary care provider, and therapeutic exercises are implemented by the PT and the physical therapy assistant (PTA). In some clinical settings, the nurse may also implement portions of the client's physical therapy regimen.

For the client with alterations in mobility, the primary care provider may also order occupational therapy. Exercises and activities implemented by the OT and occupational therapy assistant (OTA) are designed to help the client maintain and optimize skills that are necessary to complete ADLs, such as bathing, housework, and meal preparation. The OT can also help identify necessary modifications to the client's home environment that will allow the client to function as independently as possible.

Preservative interventions are especially important for clients who are confined to bed for prolonged periods. The main types of rehabilitative services include exercise and assisted ambulation. Assisted ambulation includes the use of assistive devices such as crutches, canes, and walkers. These devices can be used during rehabilitation to help clients maintain mobility and prevent further injury. This rehabilitation should begin as early as possible in the client's care.

EXERCISE   Exercise is vital to maintaining muscle strength. Muscles that are not used atrophy and become weak, especially during prolonged bed rest. Specific exercises can be performed to promote strength and range of motion, reduce joint pain and stiffness, and increase flexibility and endurance. Exercise also promotes proper alignment of bones and joints; helps to prevent edema, thrombophlebitis, and pressure ulcers; and stimulates circulation and lung expansion. Exercises can be either passive or active. Passive exercises are administered by the nurse, therapist, or therapy assistant. Active exercises are performed by the client.

- *Range-of-motion exercises* are passive exercises that help the client maintain joint mobility during periods of restricted physical activity. The therapist or nurse moves joints through their full range of motion to maintain or increase strength and flexibility. Before beginning the therapy, the nurse should explain all exercises to the client and determine the client's baseline ROM. If the client experiences pain, ROM exercises should be stopped. As the client heals, he may begin active range-of-motion exercises without the assistance of the healthcare provider.

- *Resistive exercises* are active exercises in which the client works against resistance to increase muscle strength. Resistance can be provided by weights or by the therapist or nurse supplying resistive force.

- *Isometric exercises* are active exercises used to maintain strength when a joint is immobilized. The client is instructed to contract a specific muscle group against another muscle group or immovable object. This prevents overall movement of the body part(s). Isometric exercises are most beneficial for clients who are immobilized while an injury is healing or who experience severe pain during movement.

AMBULATION   **Ambulation** is the ability to walk from place to place independently with or without an assistive device. Clients who are unable to ambulate are at higher risk for thrombophlebitis, osteoporosis, muscle atrophy, constipation, and urinary incontinence and infection. The longer a client is immobile, the harder it is to overcome these effects. In addition to reducing the risk of complications, early ambulation provides several benefits for the client, including strengthening muscles, increasing joint flexibility, stimulating circulation and preventing thrombophlebitis, providing pressure relief, and improving self-esteem.

Safe, effective ambulation requires adequate leg muscle strength. For immobile clients, strengthening exercises should be performed several times daily. When the client is ready to ambulate, she first should sit at the edge of the bed to allow for assessment of vertigo or postural hypotension. Assessment of vital signs, especially blood pressure, may be appropriate. When the client is ready, the nurse should assist the client to a standing position. During ambulation, assistance from a nurse or through use of an assistive device also may be needed. The nurse should encourage the client to verbalize any physical complaints or concerns throughout the activity period. To avoid overexertion and potential injury, short, frequent periods of ambulation are preferable to extended periods of activity.

ASSISTIVE DEVICES   Selection of an assistive device may depend on the client's age and preference (see the Lifespan Considerations feature). Assistive devices are used to provide support and balance for the client and increase confidence in independent ambulation. They reduce the pressure exerted on an injured limb, help to prevent further injury, and assist in healing. Assistive devices include crutches, canes, and walkers.

Lifespan Considerations
Assistive Devices for Ambulation

Clients with injuries to lower limbs may need a device to assist in ambulation. Client preferences for assistive devices may depend on age.

- Toddlers and preschool children may prefer to crawl or scoot, have a parent carry them, or have a walking cast rather than learning how to use an assistive device.

- Active school-age children, adolescents, and young adults will likely choose a walking cast or axillary crutches for ambulation assistance. Clients with long-term assistance needs may prefer Lofstrand crutches rather than axillary crutches.

- Middle-age adults will likely choose crutches or a cane for assistance, depending on the need for weight-bearing or non-weight-bearing assistance.

- Older adults may feel unstable on crutches, so they may instead choose a walker or cane depending on the amount of support needed. Clients who need to avoid putting weight on the injured limb may prefer a wheelchair for mobility.

Crutches commonly feature one of three designs: axillary, Lofstrand, or platform. Axillary crutches are most common for short-term use; body weight is typically supported by the wrists. Lofstrand crutches use a forearm piece for stability. Platform crutches are used for clients who are unable to bear weight on their wrists. Clients can use two crutches for non-weight-bearing ambulation or one crutch for stability and partial weight-bearing ambulation. Crutches must be fitted to the client. If using axillary crutches, the axillary portion should be placed about 2 inches below the underarm, and the handpiece should allow a 20- to 30-degree elbow flexion. Rubber tips should be placed on the bottom of all crutches for safety. Upper body and trunk strength are necessary for proper use of crutches.

Walkers have four legs to provide maximum stability for the client. The client's arms support the majority of the body weight to relieve pressure on the lower extremities. Walkers are generally used for clients with severe injuries such as spinal cord surgery or hip replacement surgery or for clients who are unsteady, such as older adults. Some walkers are available with wheels on the front legs to provide ease of walking while preventing further injury. Walkers without wheels should be used only for clients who are steady enough to stand on their own and bear their full weight for short times while they move the walker forward. All walker legs without wheels have rubber tips to ensure stability. Rubber tips should be replaced if excessive wear is evident. Some walkers have platforms for sitting should the client become weary. Like crutches, walkers should be adjusted to fit the client's height.

Canes are often used by clients who can bear weight but are unsteady or have one weak limb. Many types of canes are available; they can be wooden or metal, have a C-handle or functional grip handle, and have one or four rubber-cushioned feet at the base. Canes should be adjusted for the client's height. Canes are available in a variety of styles to fit the personality of the client if needed for long-term use. Collapsible canes are also available for ease of storage.

PHARMACOLOGIC THERAPY   Pharmacologic treatment of musculoskeletal disorders incorporates a wide variety of medications, including pain relievers (see Exemplar 13.1), muscle relaxants, anti-inflammatory drugs, bone growth stimulators, and neurological drugs (see the Medications feature). Medications used for specific disorders are discussed in more detail in the exemplars in this module.

Collaborative treatment of clients with musculoskeletal disorders may also include nutritional guidance, chiropractic care, support groups, spiritual care, and counseling. For clients with chronic mobility problems, collaborative care should incorporate family members and caregivers.

Medications **Musculoskeletal Disorders**

CLASSIFICATION AND DRUG EXAMPLES	MECHANISMS OF ACTION	NURSING CONSIDERATIONS
Anti-Inflammatory Drugs ■ nonsteroidal anti-inflammatory drugs (NSAIDs) *Drug examples:* ■ ibuprofen ■ aspirin ■ naproxen ■ diclofenac ■ indomethacin ■ celecoxib	Blocks production of inflammatory mediators by inhibiting COX-1 and/or COX-2. *May also be used as an:* —Analgesic —Antipyretic —Antiplatelet	■ Aspirin should never be given to children with infections, particularly influenza. ■ These drugs may interfere with clinical tests such as pregnancy tests, urine tests, and liver function tests. ■ Clients should be monitored for GI distress, bleeding, and allergic reactions.
Antispasmodics ■ Skeletal muscle relaxants *Drug examples:* ■ cyclobenzaprine ■ dantrolene ■ baclofen ■ chlorzoxazone ■ orphenadrine ■ methocarbamol ■ carisoprodol ■ tizanidine	May act in the central nervous system to decrease nervous transmission to skeletal muscles. May interfere with calcium release during muscle stimulation. *May also be used as an:* —Analgesic	■ Clients should be observed carefully for central nervous system (CNS) effects, including confusion, depression, and hallucinations. ■ May cause orthostatic hypotension, loss of spasticity, or dizziness, increasing the risk of falls during ambulation. ■ Clients should not drive or participate in other hazardous activities until they know how these drugs affect them. ■ Effects may be additive with other CNS depressants such as alcohol. ■ Monitor clients for allergic response. ■ Some drugs may discolor urine.
Bone Growth Stimulators ■ bisphosphonates *Drug examples:* ■ alendronate ■ risedronate ■ ibandronate ■ zoledronic acid	Inhibits osteoclast-mediated bone resorption.	■ Use cautiously in clients with renal impairment or liver disease. ■ Hypocalcemia should be corrected before therapy begins; do not administer within 2 hours of consuming calcium.

REVIEW The Concept of Mobility

RELATE Link the Concepts

Linking the concept of mobility with the concept of development:

1. What exercise therapy might be appropriate for a 15-year-old male client with a fractured tibia? How would the exercise regimen change if the client were a 62-year-old male?

2. Describe client teaching that should be provided to a 10-year-old female client with juvenile arthritis.

Linking the concept of mobility with the concept of infection:

3. To which types of infections are clients with limited mobility more susceptible? What nursing interventions can help prevent infection in these clients?

4. When identifying signs and symptoms of infection, describe the elements of the nursing assessment for a client with an open fracture.

READY Go to Companion Skills Manual

REFER Go to Pearson Student Nursing Resources
nursing.pearsonhighered.com

- Additional review materials
- **MiniModule:** The Physiology of Mobility

REFLECT Case Study \\ Part 3

The epidural cortisone injection that Mr. Hayes received for treatment of his herniated disc helped alleviate his numbness and tingling for approximately 3 weeks, but then the neurological effects returned. Due to his severely limited mobility, Mr. Hayes has been unable to work. Within the past 2 days, he also has developed bowel and urinary incontinence. After an emergent office visit, Mr. Hayes's orthopedic spine surgeon diagnoses him with cauda equina syndrome and schedules him for an immediate discectomy, laminectomy, and spinal fusion. His surgery and anesthesia care are uneventful with no reported complications. Twenty-four hours after the surgery, Mr. Hayes's vital signs include temperature 102.1°F oral; pulse 98 bpm; respirations 22/min; and BP 144/82 mmHg. He complains of moderate pain in his back, head, and left leg. His medications include codeine with ibuprofen for pain and inflammation.

Clinical Reasoning Questions Level I

1. What complication might Mr. Hayes's fever indicate? What priority nursing action should be implemented immediately?

2. Describe passive exercises that you can conduct with Mr. Hayes to help him maintain mobility while he is in the hospital.

3. What discharge instructions will you give Mr. Hayes when he is ready to return home?

Clinical Reasoning Questions Level II

4. Under what circumstances should you advocate for Mr. Hayes to receive additional pain medication?

5. What collaborative interventions will be beneficial in helping Mr. Hayes make a full recovery?

6. What independent nursing interventions can be implemented to promote comfort while Mr. Hayes is immobile?

EXEMPLAR 13.1 Back Problems

EXEMPLAR KEY TERMS
Artificial disc surgery, *843*
Cauda equina syndrome (CES), *841*
Cobb angle, *848*
Discectomy, *843*
Electromyogram, *843*
Herniated intervertebral disc, *840*
Laminectomy, *843*
Laminotomy, *843*
Myelogram, *843*
Sciatica, *841*
Scoliometer, *847*
Scoliosis, *845*
Spinal fusion, *843*
Thoracolumbar sacral orthosis (TLSO), *848*
Vertical rotation, *848*

EXEMPLAR LEARNING OUTCOMES
After reading about this exemplar, you will be able to:

1. Describe the pathophysiology, etiology, clinical manifestations, and direct and indirect causes of back problems.

2. Identify risk factors and prevention methods associated with back problems.

3. Illustrate the nursing process in providing culturally competent care across the life span for individuals with back problems.

4. Formulate priority nursing diagnoses appropriate for an individual with back problems.

5. Summarize therapies used by interdisciplinary teams in the collaborative care of an individual with back problems.

6. Plan evidence-based care for an individual with back problems and his or her family in collaboration with other members of the healthcare team.

7. Evaluate expected outcomes for an individual with back problems.

▶ OVERVIEW

Back pain is one of the most common medical problems in the United States. Approximately one out of four adults suffers at least one day of back pain within a 3-month period (National Institute of Arthritis and Musculoskeletal and Skin Diseases [NIAMSD], 2012a). Back problems are associated with a decreased quality of life, including decreased mobility, increased pain and frustration, and loss of work hours. Although clients usually attribute back pain to a specific injury, back problems often result from years of improper bending, lifting, and standing, with one incident acting as "the straw that broke the camel's back."

Back problems are linked to certain lifestyle habits, including bad posture, low fitness level, smoking, athletic injuries, and occupational risk factors. Even children are susceptible to back pain as a result of carrying heavy backpacks (see the Evidence-Based Practice feature). Diseases that contribute to back problems include degenerative disorders (spondylosis, spinal stenosis, osteoporosis), systemic disorders (osteomyelitis, osteoporosis, neoplasms), referred pain (gastrointestinal or genitourinary disorders, abdominal aortic aneurysms, hip pathology), and other disorders such as fibromyalgia. Pregnancy is also a major cause of back pain based on changes in posture to compensate for increasing anterior weight. This exemplar focuses on two common causes of back problems: herniated discs and scoliosis.

HERNIATED DISC

A **herniated intervertebral disc** (also called a ruptured disc, slipped disc, or herniated nucleus pulposus) occurs when a spinal disc ruptures, allowing the fluid in the disc to leak out and irritate nearby nerves (**Figure 13–20** ●). This also causes a decrease in the ability of the disc to cushion the joints of the vertebrae, causing back pain and limiting mobility.

▶ PATHOPHYSIOLOGY AND ETIOLOGY

Intervertebral discs lie between adjacent bones of the vertebral column. The outer annulus fibrosus is composed of strong fibrocartilage, whereas the inner nucleus pulposus contains loose fibers in a mucoprotein gel. These discs provide cushioning, shock absorption, and support for the vertebrae during movement. Herniation occurs when the nucleus pulposus protrudes through a compromised annulus fibrosus. This occurs most often in cervical and lumbar discs, but herniation of thoracic discs can occur as well. Herniation of a thoracic disc is a medical emergency that may result in paralysis.

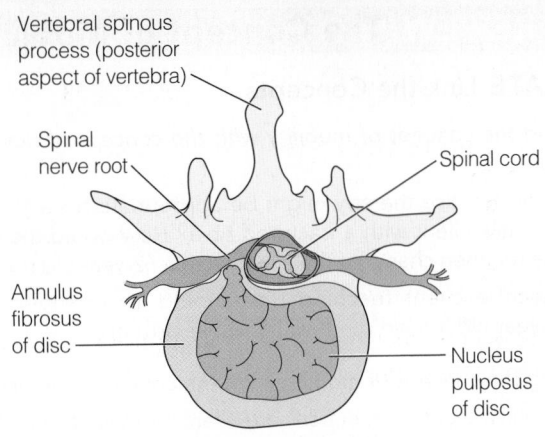

Figure 13–20 ● A herniated intervertebral disc. The herniated nucleus pulposus is applying pressure against the nerve root.

Etiology

Loss of fluid content in the nucleus pulposus and increased susceptibility to tears in the annulus fibrosus occur with aging. This shrinks the disc, decreases its ability to absorb shock, and increases the risk of herniation. Due to the structure of the vertebral column and the pressure of body weight on the spine, herniation occurs most frequently at C5–C6, C6–C7, L4–L5, and L5–S1. Herniation may occur gradually because of degenerative changes such as osteoarthritis or ankylosing spondylitis, or it may occur abruptly as a result of trauma such as lifting a heavy object or a being in a motor vehicle crash. Abrupt herniation is associated with nerve root compression, severe pain, and muscle spasms. Gradual herniation usually results in a slow onset of pain and may be associated with neurological symptoms such as weakness or tingling. If herniation occurs centrally rather than posterolaterally, it can put pressure on the spinal cord.

Evidence-Based Practice Children, Backpack Use, and Back Pain

Problem
Schoolchildren in the United States typically carry backpacks equal to 10%–22% of their body weight (Neuschwander et al., 2010). This may contribute to back, neck, and shoulder pain. Approximately 37% of children report back pain from backpack use, which is associated with heavier backpacks, younger age, female sex, and scoliosis (Skaggs et al., 2006).

Evidence
Heavy backpacks increase the risk of back pain by 50% compared to lighter backpacks (Rodriguez-Oviedo et al., 2012). Backpacks that weigh 15% or more of the child's body weight are associated with alterations in the craniovertebral angle, lumbar disc compression, lumbar asymmetry, lordosis angle, and trunk flexion angle (Bauer & Freivalds, 2009; Brackley, Stevenson, & Selinger, 2009; Kistner, Fiebert, & Roach, 2012; Neuschwander et al., 2010; Ramprasad, Alias, & Raghuveer, 2010). These changes also contributed to increased discomfort or pain, especially after walking (Bauer & Freivalds, 2009; Kistner et al., 2012; Neuschwander et al., 2010). However, changes in craniovertebral angle and lordosis angle were decreased with low load placement in the backpacks (Brackley et al., 2009).

Implications
Multiple studies have linked heavy backpacks with back pain in children. The nurse should discuss the hazards of carrying heavy backpacks with children and their parents. A good time for this discussion may be during back-to-school physicals. Recommendations by the American Academy of Pediatrics (2012) to limit back strain from backpack use include choosing a backpack with wide, padded shoulder straps and a padded back, always using both shoulder straps, and packing heavier items toward the center of the backpack. If possible, backpacks should weigh no more than 10% of the child's body weight. If this is not possible, parents may want to consider purchasing a rolling backpack for their child.

Critical Thinking Application
Describe nursing interventions related to backpack use that may be appropriate for children with scoliosis. Develop a teaching brochure to help students understand the problems that may result from improper backpack use. Explore the possibility of proposing back-strengthening exercises to help children prevent back pain from backpack use.

Client Teaching
Proper Body Mechanics for Lifting

The nurse should teach proper body mechanics to all clients, from school-age children to older adults. Body mechanics are especially important for individuals, including nurses, who regularly perform physical labor such as lifting, bending, and twisting. Guidelines for proper body mechanics for lifting heavy objects include the following:

- Start with the feet in a wide stance to provide balance.
- Bend at the knees, not the back.
- Use the large muscles of the legs and arms rather than the weaker back muscles to lift heavy objects.
- Use a back brace to support the back for frequent heavy lifting.
- If possible, slide, roll, or push an object rather than lift it.
- If the object is too heavy to lift alone, ask for help.

Risk Factors

Herniated discs are most common between the ages of 30 and 50, because discs naturally degenerate with age. Other risk factors for herniated discs include excess weight; regular heavy lifting, bending, and twisting; previous back problems; and smoking (NIAMSD, 2012a). Genetic factors such as male gender, tall height, bone disorders, and degenerative disc disorders also contribute to increased risk of herniated discs.

Prevention

Prevention of herniated discs is primarily associated with good back care. This includes using good posture for sitting and standing, exercising regularly to keep back muscles strong, maintaining a healthy weight to decrease the pressure on the vertebral column, and using proper body mechanics (Mayo Clinic, 2010; see the Client Teaching feature). Using proper body mechanics is especially important for pregnant women, who are highly susceptible to back pain because of the weight of the growing uterus and fetus (Figure 13–21 ●).

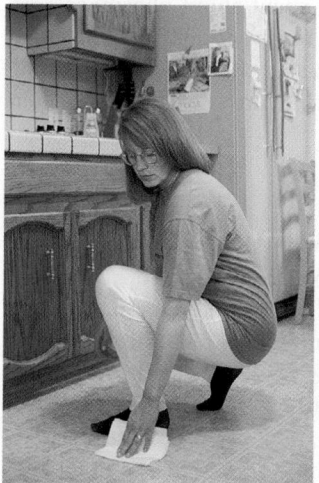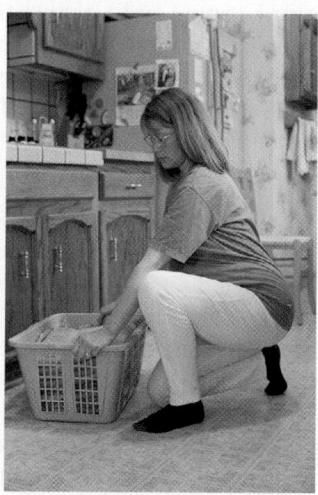

Figure 13–21 ● When picking up objects from floor level or lifting objects, the pregnant woman needs to use proper body mechanics.

▶ CLINICAL MANIFESTATIONS

Clinical manifestations of a herniated disc will depend on the severity and location of the herniation. The most common location of herniated discs is the lumbar region (L4–L5 and L5–S1), followed by the cervical region (C5–C6 and C6–C7).

Lumbar Discs

If the herniated disc is not compressing a nerve, the client may be asymptomatic. If nerve compression is present, clinical manifestations may include pain in the lower back, buttocks, thigh, and leg; numbness or tingling; and muscle weakness. The location of the symptoms depends on the area innervated by the compressed nerve (Mayo Clinic, 2010).

A herniated disc in the lumbar region may cause a condition called sciatica. **Sciatica** occurs when irritation or compression of all or part of the sciatic nerve, which originates in the lower back, produces pain and neurological manifestations. The sciatic nerve is the longest nerve in the body and is made up of branches of the lumbar spinal nerve roots (**Figure 13–22** ●). From its origin point in the lower back, the sciatic nerve divides into two main branches, each of which innervates one side of the lower portion of the body. On each side, one branch of the sciatic nerve travels through the pelvis, deep into the buttock, and then down the leg (University of Maryland Medical Center, 2009). Pressure on one or more of the lumbar nerve roots can also affect the sciatic nerve, leading to pain, burning, tingling, and numbness that radiates from the buttock into the leg and foot. Usually sciatica only affects one side of the body, and it may be more severe when standing, walking, or sitting (American Association of Neurological Surgeons [AANS], 2011). Sciatica may also be aggravated by sneezing or coughing.

Other symptoms associated with lumbar disc herniation include a forward tilt to the trunk when standing and changes in mobility, motor function, and knee and ankle reflexes. Spinal changes may include an absence of normal lumbar lordosis or scoliosis of the lumbar spine. Some clients may experience muscle spasms and problems with sexual function.

The spinal cord does not extend through the entire spinal canal; rather, at approximately L1–L2, it branches into a bundle of free-flowing nerve roots. Because this portion of the spinal cord resembles a horse's tail, it is called the cauda equina, which means "horse's tail" in Latin. Compression of the nerve roots of the cauda equina can lead to **cauda equina syndrome (CES)**, which may result in permanent neurological impairment, including urinary incontinence and paralysis. Causes of CES include massive lumbar disc herniation, spinal stenosis, and trauma (Gardner, Gardner, & Morley, 2011). CES is a medical emergency (Mayo Clinic, 2010). Immediate surgery should be performed to relieve pressure on the nerves. (See the Safety Alert feature.)

SAFETY ALERT
Symptoms of cauda equina syndrome include severe low back pain, bladder or bowel dysfunction, impaired sensation in the genital or saddle region, and sexual dysfunction. Although not always present, unilateral or bilateral sciatica may also occur (Gardner et al., 2011). CES is a medical emergency that requires immediate surgical treatment. Signs and symptoms of CES should be reported to the client's physician immediately.

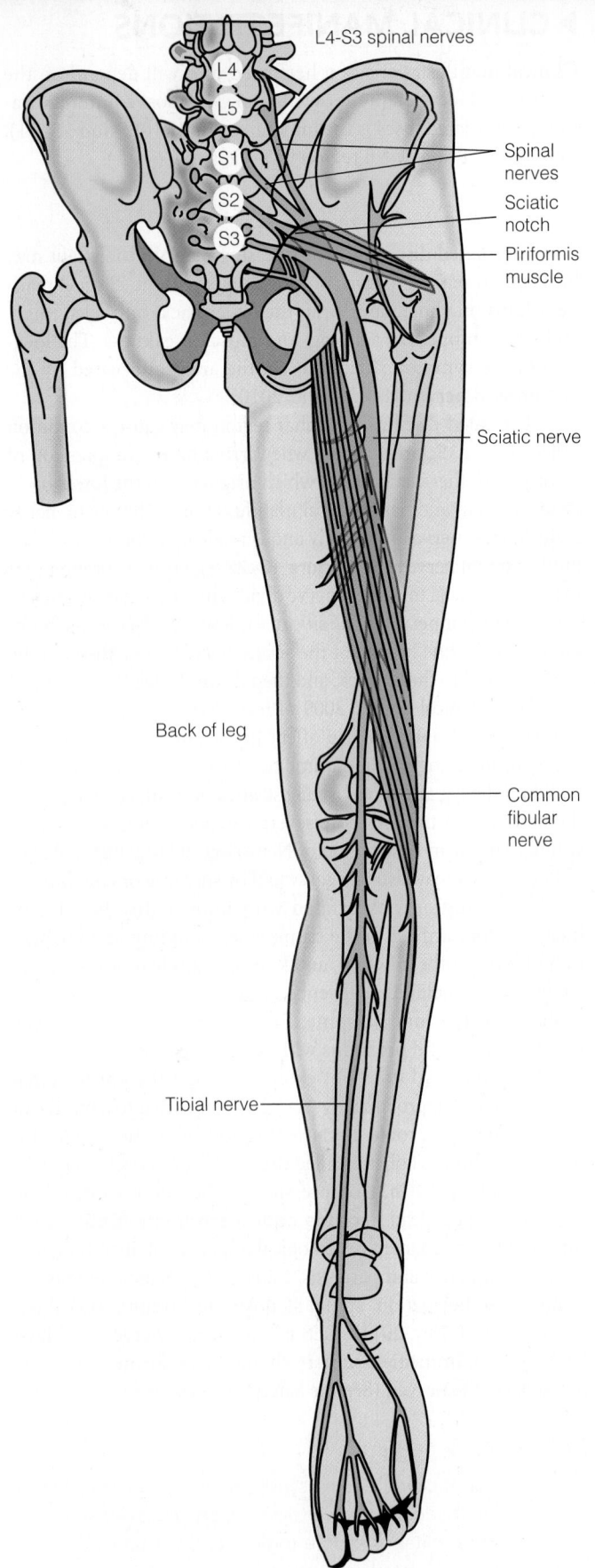

L4-S3 spinal nerves

L4
L5
S1
S2
S3

Spinal nerves

Sciatic notch

Piriformis muscle

Sciatic nerve

Back of leg

Common fibular nerve

Tibial nerve

Figure 13–22 ● The sciatic nerve.

Cervical Discs

Similar to lumbar disc herniation, cervical disc herniation can result in numbness, tingling, muscle spasms, and weakness in the areas serviced by the affected nerves. A stiff neck is also a common feature of cervical disc herniation. In addition, neck and shoulder pain that shoots into the arm or fingers is likely present. The location and intensity of pain may depend on the movement of the neck (AANS, 2011). If a cervical disc compresses the spinal cord instead of a nerve root, symptoms in the lower body may be similar to those seen with lumbar disc herniation.

Lifespan and Cultural Considerations

Herniated discs are rare in children, constituting only 0.5%– 6.8% of all clients hospitalized for lumbar disc herniation. Herniated discs in children are usually the result of trauma or genetic predisposition. A primary clinical symptom of a herniated lumbar disc in children is a positive straight-leg-raise test. During a straight-leg-raise test, the client lies on his back and the clinician raises one leg with the knee straight. If the client experiences sciatic pain when the leg is between 30 and 70 degrees, it is a positive test for a herniated disc at L4–S1. Pain above or below this range indicates other conditions. Children with herniated discs generally have minimal back pain and less numbness and weakness compared to adults (Dang & Liu, 2010). However, sciatica is common in these children.

Older adults are less likely to develop herniated discs than younger adults, because the fluid in the nucleus pulposus is diminished and therefore cannot protrude out as easily. However, if an older adult does develop a herniated disc, recovery after nonsurgical treatment is similar to that for younger adults (Suri et al., 2011).

▶ COLLABORATION

Care of a client with a herniated disc includes identifying the herniated disc and determining a course of treatment. Nursing interventions are aimed at preparing the client for diagnostic testing and teaching the client about pharmacologic, nonpharmacologic, and surgical interventions. The nurse may need to collaborate with physicians, chiropractors, pharmacists, and physical therapists during care of a client with a herniated disc.

Diagnostic Tests

In addition to a health history and physical exam, diagnosis of a herniated disc may include performing one or more diagnostic tests to rule out other causes of back pain. Tests may include mobility tests, imaging tests, and blood tests. Mobility tests include the straight-leg-raise test, gait tests, reflex tests, and muscle strength tests (Ogiela, 2012). These tests can help the physician determine the location, intensity, and cause of pain as well as the associated effects of the herniated disc or other back problems.

A CT scan is the most common imaging test that can conclusively identify a herniated disc, but an MRI may also be needed for more severe cases. A **myelogram**, during which dye is injected into the spinal fluid and visualized by x-ray, may be used to identify areas of pressure on the spinal cord or nerves due to herniated discs (Mayo Clinic, 2010). Diagnostics may also include an **electromyogram**, which measures the electrical activity of the muscles at rest and during contraction. A nerve conduction study may be used to measure the speed and efficacy of nerve impulses, which is useful in identifying nerve damage (AANS, 2011). Several blood tests can be used to test for inflammation, infection, and arthritis, including a complete blood count, erythrocyte sedimentation rate, C-reactive protein, and HLA-B27 (NIAMSD, 2012a).

Surgery

Surgical treatment of a herniated disc is reserved for the most severe cases in which clients do not respond to other therapies. Other indications for spinal surgery include progressive leg weakness or numbness, loss of normal bowel and bladder functions, difficulty standing or walking, and back and leg pain that limits normal activity (AANS, 2011). The type of surgery chosen depends on the location of the disc and the integrity of the spinal column:

- A **laminectomy** is performed to remove the lamina, or the part of the vertebra that covers the spinal canal. This enlarges the spinal canal and relieves pressure on the associated nerves. During a **laminotomy**, which is a similar procedure, only a portion of the lamina is removed. A laminectomy or laminotomy is often performed in conjunction with other procedures, such as a discectomy or spinal fusion.

- A **discectomy** is performed to remove all or part of the herniated disc. Muscles and other tissues are dissected away from the spine to allow for surgical exposure of the ruptured disc. After removal of the disc, surrounding structures are returned to their natural positions. A microdiscectomy may be performed if there is no need for surgical intervention on bones, ligaments, or muscles. Compared to a discectomy, microdiscectomy requires a smaller incision and less disruption of tissues.

- **Spinal fusion** is performed to join two or more vertebrae together using bone grafts, screws, and rods. This prevents motion between the two vertebrae and reduces pain. Bone grafts are usually taken from the hip or pelvis. Tissue rejection may occur if donor bone is used. After spinal fusion, the fused area is immobile. Spinal fusion can be performed on the anterior spine by an incision in the client's abdomen or on the posterior side by an incision in the client's back.

- During an **artificial disc surgery**, a herniated disc is replaced with an artificial disc, similar to a traditional hip or knee replacement. This may be done as an alternative to spinal fusion to maintain flexibility of the spinal joint.

- Newer technology has allowed the use of laser surgery to treat herniated discs. During laser surgery, the surgeon inserts a needle into the disc and delivers laser energy to vaporize the tissue in the disc. This reduces the size of the disc and relieves pressure on the nerves. The usefulness of laser discectomy is still being debated (NIAMSD, 2012a).

Pharmacologic Therapy

First-line therapy for a herniated disc includes nonsteroidal anti-inflammatory drugs (NSAIDs) to reduce pain and swelling. If the client is experiencing neurological problems such as numbness or sciatica, additional medications may include opioids for severe pain and antispasmodics to reduce muscle spasms (see the Medications feature and the exemplar on Acute and Chronic Pain in the module on Comfort). Medications used to treat neuropathic pain, such as gabapentin (Neurontin), pregabalin (Lyrica), and duloxetine (Cymbalta), may also be useful for reducing pain related to nerve damage and have milder side effects compared to opioids. Tramadol (Ultram), which is a centrally acting opiate receptor agonist, may be used to treat mild to moderate pain. Epidural injection of cortisone/corticosteroids or anesthetics may also help reduce pain and inflammation (Mayo Clinic, 2010). Nursing responsibilities include teaching the client about dosing, side effects, and contraindications. If severe pain and neurological symptoms are still present after 1–2 months, surgery may be considered.

Nonpharmacologic Therapy

There are many nonpharmacologic treatment options for individuals with herniated discs. Hot or cold packs can be used individually or alternately to dilate the blood vessels and increase oxygen supply to the area (heat) or to reduce inflammation by decreasing blood flow to the area (cold). Clients with herniated discs should be encouraged to maintain their normal activities. Activity restrictions and strict bed rest are no longer recommended. Mild, low-impact exercise may be helpful to strengthen the back.

> **SAFETY ALERT** Clients with herniated discs should consult a clinician before beginning an exercise regimen. Some exercises, especially those that require bending and twisting, may exacerbate symptoms.

Other forms of nonpharmacologic therapy may require collaboration with a healthcare professional such as a physical therapist or chiropractor. Clients may receive intradiscal electrothermal therapy, in which a needle is inserted into the disc and heated to thicken and seal the disc wall to prevent bulging. Chiropractic therapy uses spinal manipulation to adjust the spine and surrounding tissues, possibly reversing the protrusion of the nucleus pulposus. Massage therapy may benefit clients with herniated discs by relieving muscle tension, stiffness, and spasms and improving joint flexibility and range of motion. The Clinical Manifestations and Therapies feature lists therapies that are used in treating herniated discs at different locations.

Clinical Manifestations and Therapies Herniated Disc

ETIOLOGY	CLINICAL MANIFESTATIONS	CLINICAL THERAPIES
Lumbar herniated disc	■ May have no symptoms if the disc is not pressing on a nerve. If the disc is pressing on a nerve root, manifestations may include pain in the hip, lower back, and lower extremities; sciatica; cauda equina syndrome; limited mobility; muscle spasms; paresthesia of the lower extremities; foot drop; changes in knee and ankle reflexes; inability to walk on toes or sides of the feet.	■ Application of heat or cold ■ NSAIDs or other analgesics ■ Antispasmodics ■ Neuropathic pain medications ■ Epidural cortisone injections ■ Surgery ■ Physical therapy ■ Chiropractic therapy
Sciatica	■ Severe pain that radiates across the buttocks, down the leg, and into the knee or foot; positive straight-leg-raise test	■ NSAIDs or other analgesics ■ Antispasmodics ■ Epidural cortisone injections ■ Surgery ■ Physical therapy
Cauda equina syndrome	■ Bowel and bladder incontinence associated with a herniated lumbar disc; paralysis of lower extremities	■ Emergency surgery to relieve pressure on the cauda equina
Cervical herniated disc	■ May have no symptoms if disc is not pressing on a nerve. If disc is pressing on a nerve root, manifestations may include pain in the neck, shoulders, and upper extremities; paresthesia in the upper extremities; decreased biceps and supinator reflexes; hyperactive triceps reflex. May cause neurological deficits in the lower body if disc is pressing on the spinal cord rather than nerve roots.	■ Application of heat or cold ■ NSAIDs or other analgesics ■ Antispasmodics ■ Nerve pain medications ■ Epidural cortisone injections ■ Surgery ■ Physical therapy ■ Chiropractic therapy

■ NURSING PROCESS

The primary goals of treatment for a client with a herniated disc include relieving pain, healing the involved disc, and regaining mobility. The nurse's role in this process includes assessing the client; providing information about procedures, medications, and therapies; encouraging and supporting the client; and providing proficient nursing care before and after procedures.

Assessment

Nursing assessment begins with interviewing the client regarding her primary complaint and then obtaining a health history. The health history should include the client's description of the pain, previous back injuries or surgeries, current medications, risk factors for back pain, type of employment, and typical recreational activities. A physical assessment may include tests for muscle strength, coordination, gait and posture, sensation, and reflexes. The 5 P's neurovascular assessment may be used to assess neurovascular status. (See the Concept of Mobility portion of this module for discussion of the 5 P's neurovascular assessment.)

Diagnosis

Nursing diagnoses for a client with a herniated disc may include the following:

■ *Risk for Injury* related to altered mobility

■ *Risk for Reflex Urinary Incontinence* related to pressure on cauda equina
■ *Risk for Bowel Incontinence* related to pressure on cauda equina
■ *Impaired Physical Mobility* related to pain
■ *Acute Pain* related to compression of nerve root
■ *Chronic Pain* related to spinal disc degeneration
■ *Disturbed Sleep Pattern* related to severe pain
■ *Activity Intolerance* related to pain associated with movement
■ *Deficient Knowledge* related to treatment options for herniated disc
■ *Ineffective Role Performance* related to inability to perform job
■ *Anxiety* related to surgical procedure.

(NANDA-I © 2012)

Planning

Goals for a client with a herniated disc may include the following:

■ The client will develop no motor deficits.
■ The client will develop no sensory deficits.
■ The client will remain free from infection.
■ The client will demonstrate normal bowel function, including the presence of bowel sounds in all quadrants.

- The client will demonstrate normal urinary function, including urine production at a rate of at least 0.5 mL/kg/hr. The client will report diminished pain to allow performance of ADLs.
- The client will correctly verbalize proper use of medications for pain, inflammation, and muscle spasms.
- The client will verbalize emotions and concerns related to all treatments, including invasive procedures.
- The client will perform job responsibilities without work absences.

Implementation

Nursing interventions for clients with a herniated disc include promoting safety, preventing onset or exacerbation of neurological deficits, providing adequate pain relief, and explaining treatment options. For clients who must undergo surgery, the general principles of nursing care of postsurgical clients apply, in addition to considerations that are specific to clients who undergo spinal surgery. (See also the module on Perioperative Care.)

Prevent Injury

To prevent spinal injury and complications related to disruption of a surgical site, clients should be taught to avoid bending and twisting. Clients should instead be encouraged to maintain body alignment that decreases stress on the vertebral column, such as flexing the hips when in the supine position; placing a small pillow under the knees (lumbar disc) or neck (cervical disc) to decrease pressure on the nerve roots; and using a firm mattress to support the spinal column. Clients with alterations in mobility should be assisted with positioning and ambulation.

Promote Comfort

For clients with pain related to a herniated disc, pain should be assessed on a 0–10 scale, with 0 representing no pain and 10 representing severe pain. The client should be monitored frequently for changes in symptoms that may indicate a worsening of the client's condition, including alterations in mobility and sensation. Pain medications should be administered around the clock or by a patient-controlled analgesic pump. The nurse should teach the client about appropriate administration as well as potential side effects of the medications.

The nurse should also teach the client about coping techniques for pain, including depending on others, alternating rest and activity, and engaging in enjoyable activities. Adequate pain management and effective coping techniques are helpful in promoting adequate sleep–rest patterns. In contrast, inadequate sleep can amplify pain and increase frustration and irritability.

Adequate pain management may require a primary care provider's referral for physical therapy to develop a safe but effective exercise program. Exercise should strengthen muscles and increase mobility without increasing pain. For the client with chronic back pain, counseling referrals may be necessary to treat frustration, depression, and anxiety. Because the client with a herniated disc will receive care from multiple clinicians, adequate documentation is essential for maintaining continuity of care.

Educate the Client About Procedures and Treatments

Multiple procedures may be used to diagnose a herniated disc, including muscle, sensation, and reflex tests and imaging tests. In addition, multiple treatment options are available for herniated discs depending on the severity of symptoms and location of the herniation. All this information may be confusing to a client and, coupled with moderate to severe pain, may increase the client's anxiety. Therefore, a primary nursing responsibility when caring for a client with a herniated disc is explaining diagnostic procedures and treatment options in a way that the client will understand. This is especially important for invasive procedures that require injections (e.g., myelogram, cortisone injection) or surgery (e.g., discectomy, spinal fusion). Clients often feel increased anxiety about spinal procedures because of the risk of unintentional nerve damage and the fear of paralysis. Thoroughly explaining procedures and answering the client's questions will help ease the client's anxiety and increase adherence to the treatment plan.

Provide Preoperative and Postoperative Care to the Surgical Client

Nursing care of clients who require surgical treatment of a herniated disc includes both preoperative teaching and postoperative management of pain and care of the incision site (**Box 13–2 ●**).

Evaluation

The client should be evaluated frequently for progress toward identified outcomes. Satisfactory progress will include a reported decrease in the client's pain, increased mobility, full ROM of joints, normal sensory perception, lack of neurological deficits, and absence of infection and other complications from surgery.

▌SCOLIOSIS

Scoliosis is a lateral, or sideways, curve of the spine; it can be C shaped or S shaped. It is often noticed during the growth spurt just before puberty. Most cases of scoliosis are mild, but severe scoliosis can cause a rotation of the spine, leading to deformities and disability.

▶ PATHOPHYSIOLOGY AND ETIOLOGY

A small degree of sideways curvature is found in many individuals. Scoliosis is diagnosed if the sideways curvature measures more than 10 degrees (**Figure 13–23 ●**) (Mehlman, 2012). Mild scoliosis reflects a curve between 10 and 20 degrees, moderate scoliosis is a curve between 20 and 40 degrees, and severe scoliosis is a curve over 40 degrees. Scoliosis can be classified as either structural or nonstructural. *Nonstructural scoliosis* occurs as the spine bends to compensate for poor posture, differences in leg length, presence of tumors, adaptation to pain, or other physical conditions. Nonstructural scoliosis is usually corrected

Box 13–2 **Nursing Care of Clients Undergoing Surgery for Herniated Disc**

PREOPERATIVE CARE

- *Provide effective pain management* by administering pain medications as prescribed and frequently assessing the client's response to analgesics. Explain that pain is easier to control if pain medications are taken around the clock rather than waiting until pain becomes severe.
- *Demonstrate techniques* that will be performed postoperatively and encourage the client to practice the techniques. *Logrolling*, which maintains neutral alignment of the spine when turning, is performed by the nurse for the first day or two after surgery and then by the client. This technique helps to prevent spinal injury and promotes proper healing of the spine. *Deep breathing* and an *incentive spirometer* are used to prevent respiratory complications, and *leg exercises* should be performed to prevent circulatory complications. A *fracture bedpan* is most comfortable for the client who must remain flat in bed following surgery. *Eating while lying flat* is also a technique that the client may want to practice, as this may be necessary postoperatively.

POSTOPERATIVE CARE

- *Promote wound healing* by positioning the client appropriately and assessing the wound for hematomas, cerebrospinal fluid (CSF) leakage, and infection:
  - The client should be turned every 2 hours using the logrolling technique. The client should not use the side rails to change position because this puts stress on the wound and may change spinal alignment. Neutral body alignment, with no significant flexion or extension of the spine, may be required during the immediate postoperative period. Positions that minimize stress on the surgical site include elevating the head of the bed slightly; placing a small pillow under the neck (cervical surgery) or under the head, knees, or upper leg when the client lies on one side (lumbar surgery); and using a cervical collar to prevent movement of the neck (cervical surgery).
  - Assess the client for hematoma formation at the surgical site. Most hematomas resolve without treatment within several days. However, hematomas may cause incisional pain that is not relieved by analgesics, swelling, decreased motor function, and cauda equina syndrome (Kaner et al., 2009). Hematoma formation should be reported to the physician immediately; surgery may be required to remove the hematoma.
  - Assess the surgical site for CSF leakage, including assessing the wound dressing and bed sheets for moisture. CSF may cause a bulge under the surgical site that can be detected by palpation. A Dextrostix strip can be used to detect the presence of glucose

in the fluid, an indicator of CSF. Leakage of CSF increases the risk of infection of the surgical wound and meninges.
  - Assess the client for signs of infection. Fever should be reported immediately. Signs of infection at the surgical site include redness, purulent drainage, and pain. Clients are also at increased risk for arachnoiditis, or inflammation of the arachnoid membrane, which protects the spinal cord. Arachnoiditis can cause scar tissue and adhesion of the spinal nerves, interfering with nerve function (National Institute of Neurological Disorders and Stroke [NINDS], 2011).

- *Monitor the client for nerve root compression or injury.* Clients should be assessed for hand, arm, and leg strength; the ability to move the fingers and toes and dorsiflex the foot; and the ability to detect touch, as appropriate. Compare bilateral findings and report any muscle weakness or sensory impairment, which could indicate nerve root compression. Following cervical spine surgery, clients should also be assessed for hoarseness and dysphagia (difficulty swallowing), because these alterations may indicate nerve damage and lead to an increased risk for aspiration.

- *Monitor the client for complications* associated with surgery, including pain, urinary retention, respiratory and circulatory complications, and decreased mobility:
  - Pain should be assessed on a scale of 0–10, and analgesics should be administered as prescribed. The surgical incision, edema at the surgical site, and muscle spasms may cause pain similar to pain experienced before the surgery. This pain may persist for several weeks.
  - A common complication of general anesthesia is urinary retention. Clients should void within 8 hours after surgery; males should be allowed to stand to void if possible. The nurse should monitor intake and output and report urinary retention.
  - Encourage deep breathing and use of an incentive spirometer every 2 hours to stimulate respiratory function. Coughing should be discouraged, because this disrupts the healing tissues, especially in clients who have undergone cervical surgery.
  - Decreased mobility can cause respiratory and circulatory problems, including thrombophlebitis. Clients should ambulate as soon as allowed by the physician. Clients will typically sit on the side of the bed the evening after surgery and begin to ambulate on the first or second postoperative day. The nurse can help the client sit up by elevating the head of the bed and helping the client simultaneously swing his legs over the side of the bed and move his upper body to an upright position. The vertebral column should remain in alignment at all times. The nurse should provide stability for ambulating clients until the client is no longer dizzy or weak. Safety is a top priority during ambulation.

by alleviating the underlying cause of the curve. *Structural scoliosis* is a more severe form that involves deformities of the bones in the spinal column.

Etiology

Scoliosis of unknown etiology is called *idiopathic scoliosis*. Idiopathic scoliosis accounts for approximately 80%–85% of scoliosis cases (American Academy of Orthopaedic Surgeons [AAOS], 2011b). Research suggests that idiopathic scoliosis may be the result of abnormal force exerted on the spine by surrounding connective tissues and muscles (Mehlman, 2012). *Congenital scoliosis* occurs when the individual is born with a curved spine. This usually results from incomplete formation or

separation of the vertebrae, and it can be associated with other health issues such as heart and kidney problems. *Neuromuscular scoliosis* occurs when medical conditions that affect the nerves and muscles, such as cerebral palsy, muscular dystrophy, or spinal cord injury, lead to sideways curvature of the spine.

The most common curve pattern is a right thoracic curve (Mehlman, 2012). Left lumbar, right thoracolumbar, and double major curve patterns are also common. The lateral curvature of the spine causes several structural changes to the skeleton. As the curve worsens, the vertebrae rotate, causing a twisting of the spine. The ribs on the inside of the curve are forced closer together, and the ribs on the outside of the curve are spread farther apart (see Figure 13–23). This

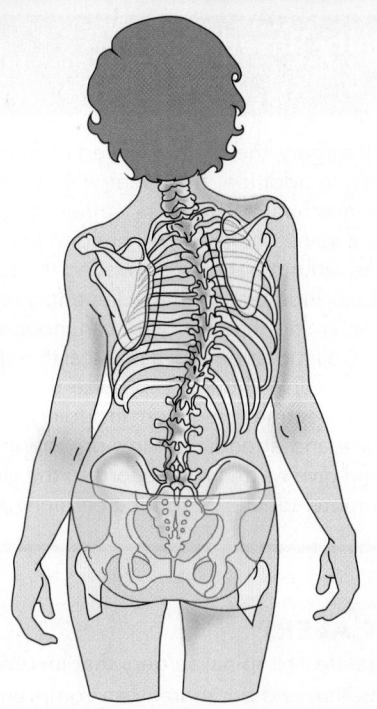

Figure 13–23 ● Scoliosis is diagnosed if the sideways curvature measures more than 10 degrees.

causes formation of the typical rib hump that is most obvious when the individual performs the Adam forward bend test. Similarly, the spinal disc spaces are narrowed on the inside curve and wider on the outside of the curve. This creates an asymmetric vertebral canal that may cause additional complications such as paresthesia.

Risk Factors

Adolescents are at greatest risk of developing scoliosis as they go through a growth spurt just before puberty, usually between the ages of 9 and 15. However, girls are more likely to progress to a greater curvature than boys (Mayo Clinic, 2012e). Other risk factors for developing scoliosis include having a neuromuscular disorder such as cerebral palsy or muscular dystrophy and having a family history of scoliosis.

▶ CLINICAL MANIFESTATIONS

Common manifestations of scoliosis include a spinal curvature to one side, uneven hips or shoulders, differences in leg length, tiredness of the spine, a prominent shoulder blade, and a rib bump. Although not common, back pain may accompany scoliosis. Severe scoliosis may cause heart and lung problems such as difficulty breathing and pneumonia; compression of nerve roots may cause paralysis. Curvature of more than 100 degrees may increase mortality rates.

Mild curves of scoliosis (less than 20 degrees) often do not progress and do not need treatment. Moderate and severe curves (20 degrees to over 100 degrees) will require treatment, especially if the curve continues to progress. Scoliosis curves often worsen as the child grows; progression of curvature dramatically slows when the child stops growing. For girls, this is usually 2 years after the start of menstruation. For boys, growth usually stops in the late teens or early 20s. Curves usually progress only 0.5 to 1 degree per year or less in adults.

Lifespan and Cultural Considerations

Idiopathic scoliosis is classified as one of four types depending on the age of onset. Symptoms and risk factors may vary for each age group (Mehlman, 2012):

- **Infantile idiopathic scoliosis** occurs from birth to 3 years of age. It typically results in a left thoracic curve of the spine and is most commonly seen in boys of European descent. Infantile scoliosis may resolve as the child ages.

- **Juvenile idiopathic scoliosis** occurs in children between 3 and 9 years of age. Symptoms are similar to those of adolescent scoliosis. Children with juvenile idiopathic scoliosis are most likely to have progression of the curve and require surgery.

- **Adolescent idiopathic scoliosis** occurs in children between 10 and 19 years old. This is the most common type of scoliosis; progression of the curvature is seen more frequently in girls. Progression is more likely to occur in younger children with large curves than in older children with small curves.

- **Adult idiopathic scoliosis** may be present from childhood or may develop as a result of aging. Aging causes may be related to degenerative changes of the spine (often called adult degenerative scoliosis), osteoporosis, previous fractures, spondylolisthesis, infections, or tumors. Involvement of the entire spine, including the neck, is more common in adults than in children. Back pain and pain radiating down the legs is also more common in adults (Scoliosis Research Society, n.d.).

▶ COLLABORATION

Nursing care for clients with scoliosis ranges from periodic observation to surgical care. This is often achieved through collaboration with school nurses, physicians, surgeons, physical therapists, and the client's family. The goal of treatment is to limit or stop the progression of the spinal curvature.

Diagnostic Tests

Most schools require scoliosis screenings for children between the ages of 10 and 15 years. One of the primary screening tests for scoliosis is the Adam forward bend test, in which the individual leans forward at the waist with the arms hanging straight down. This allows the clinician to see the spine more clearly. In clients with scoliosis, the Adam test often causes an obvious rib hump, usually on the right side. However, the Adam test may be negative in some clients with scoliosis, so it should never be used as the only diagnostic test. A **scoliometer** can be used to measure the client's rib hump when in the Adam position.

X-rays are the most common imaging test used to definitively diagnose scoliosis. Using an x-ray of the spine, physicians can determine the angle of the curve using the Cobb method (Cobb, 1948). The Cobb method uses lines drawn from the end vertebrae (the vertebrae at the upper and lower limits of the curve that tilt most dramatically toward the apex of the curve) to estimate the degree of curvature. The angle found at the intersection of the two lines is the **Cobb angle**. The degree of **vertical rotation** can be determined with the Nash-Moe method (Nash & Moe, 1969). In this method, a vertebra at the apex of the curve is divided into three equal segments on the half of the vertebra on the convex side of the curve. The location of the pedicle of the vertebra in relation to the segments determines the grade of rotation, with no rotation being the lowest and grade 4 rotation being the highest at over 90 degrees of rotation. Other imaging tests may include MRIs, CT scans, and bone scans.

Surgery

Surgical correction of scoliosis is available for clients with a Cobb angle of greater than 50 degrees. Surgery is usually performed only on clients whose curvature progression is not slowed by bracing and whose bones have stopped growing. If curve progression is severe (at least 45 degrees) before the child has stopped growing, surgeons may insert a rod that can be adjusted in length as the child grows; adjustments usually occur every 6 months (Mayo Clinic, 2012e). Scoliosis surgery involves spinal fusion combined with inserting metal rods on either side of the spine, which are held together by hooks, screws, and wires until the bone heals. Surgery can be done through the back, through the abdomen, or beneath the ribs (Zieve & Ogiela, 2011). Surgery can correct the lateral curvature of the spine, but it often does not correct the abnormal rotation of the spine.

After surgery, most clients will not require long-term therapy or postoperative casting. However, they will need to be on bed rest during the recovery period and may need to wear a brace such as a **thoracolumbar sacral orthosis (TLSO)**, also called the underarm brace or Boston brace, for several months to help support the spine. The TLSO is contoured to conform to the body and is almost invisible under the clothes. In severe cases, halo traction may be used to provide support for the spine (**Figure 13–24 ●**). Complications of surgery may include bleeding, infection, nerve damage, and disc degeneration. The Community-Based Care feature provides more information about postsurgical care.

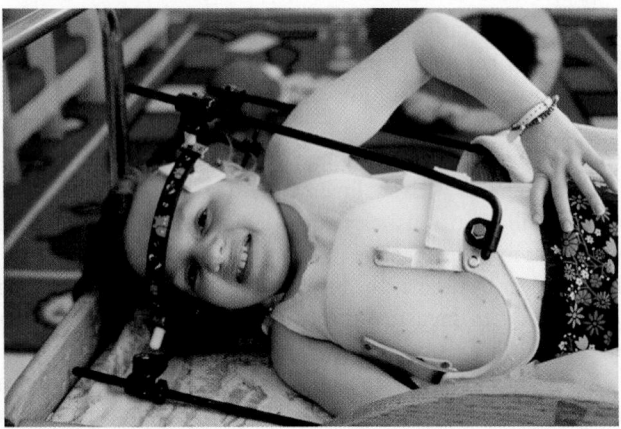

Figure 13–24 ● In severe scoliosis, the child may wear a halo brace, shown here, to hold the body in position after surgery.

Pharmacologic Therapy

Usually, scoliosis is not treated with medication. If needed, clients can take over-the-counter (OTC) analgesics, such as acetaminophen, for mild pain. Pain associated with severe scoliosis or spinal surgery may need stronger pain medications, such as prescription NSAIDs or opioids.

Nonpharmacologic Therapy

Nonpharmacologic therapy will depend on the severity of the spinal curvature. Clients with curvature of less than 20 degrees or clients near the stage of skeletal maturity should be observed for worsening curvature; however, treatment usually is not indicated. These clients should be monitored by a physician every 3–6 months.

For clients with curvatures between 25 and 45 degrees, medical management includes wearing a brace. Braces are intended to prevent further curvature of the spine and work best in clients over the age of 10 who do not have congenital or neuromuscular scoliosis and are still growing (Zieve & Ogiela, 2011).

The choice of brace will depend on the size and location of the curve. The two main types of braces are the TLSO and the Milwaukee brace (full torso brace). The TLSO is the most common type of brace worn both before and after surgery. The Milwaukee brace has a neck ring with rests for the chin and back of the head and wide bars in the front and back. This type of brace is more cumbersome than the TLSO, and compliance is a major problem. Therefore, it is used only when a TLSO is inadequate, such as for curvatures in the cervical spine (Mayo Clinic,

Evidence-Based Practice Adolescent Self-Image and Braces

Problem

Scoliosis is often diagnosed during middle and high school. Adolescents with moderate to severe curves that require surgery or bracing are at risk for disturbed body image.

Evidence

A study of 92 adolescents (ages 11–22) with scoliosis indicated that clients who were under observation had a higher quality of life than clients who wore a brace, even though spine curvature was similar between the two groups. This was most evident for clients with a Cobb angle of less than 20 degrees. Self-image and mental health tended to be negatively correlated with time spent in the brace (Cheung et al., 2007). In another study of 12 adolescents (ages 10–16), clients wearing braces commonly experienced stress, denial, fear, anger, and shame (Sapountzi-Krepia et al., 2006). A third study with 31 adolescents with scoliosis (ages 13–16) indicated that clients with alterations in physical, emotional, and social functioning, vitality, and self-esteem were less likely to be compliant about wearing the brace for the prescribed amount of time each day (Rivett et al., 2009). Importantly, clients receiving brace treatment felt that although they received adequate information from clinicians, they did not receive adequate emotional support and they were not inclined to openly express their feelings to the physician. None of the clients mentioned whether they received support from nurses (Sapountzi-Krepia et al., 2006).

Implications

Adolescents, especially girls, are susceptible to poor self-image when faced with a visible deformity such as scoliosis and the treatment that goes with that diagnosis. Therefore, nurses and other healthcare professionals should create a comfortable atmosphere that encourages clients to share their fears and concerns. Emotional support should be a nursing priority when caring for an adolescent client, and nurses should provide suggestions for ways in which the teen can build self-esteem and confidence.

Critical Thinking Application

Describe how a nurse can play a key role in providing support for clients with scoliosis after diagnosis. Consider ways in which a nurse can build self-esteem and confidence in a male client versus a female client. Identify signs or symptoms of low self-esteem that a nurse should look for in adolescent clients with scoliosis.

2012e). Braces should be worn between 12 and 23 hours per day; brace success increases with increasing time spent wearing the brace each day. This may be a difficult issue for some clients, since adolescents who wear a brace for scoliosis may be at risk for altered self-image (see the Evidence-Based Practice feature).

Multiple studies have shown that alternative therapies such as chiropractic treatment, electrical stimulation, biofeedback, nutritional supplements, and exercise are ineffective in the treatment of scoliosis (Mayo Clinic, 2012e; NIAMSD, 2009).

NURSING PROCESS

Nursing care for a client with scoliosis may include referring the client to a physician for care, teaching the client and family about scoliosis and its treatment options, monitoring curvature progression, providing emotional support, and caring for the client before and after surgery.

Assessment

Assessment of a client with scoliosis includes a health history and physical examination. The health history should include identifying any family history of scoliosis, because individuals with parents or siblings with scoliosis are at higher risk for developing the disorder. It should also include a history of past spinal problems and assessment of other symptoms such as back pain.

A physical examination should include scoliosis screening and referral for diagnostic tests. The initial scoliosis screening is often performed by a school nurse for children in middle school and high school. Girls are often screened twice; boys are usually

Clinical Manifestations and Therapies Scoliosis

ETIOLOGY	CLINICAL MANIFESTATIONS	CLINICAL THERAPIES
Mild scoliosis	■ Spinal curvature with a Cobb angle of less than 20 degrees	■ Observation every 3–6 months
Moderate scoliosis	■ Spinal curvature with a Cobb angle between 25 and 45 degrees; uneven hips or shoulders; differences in leg length; tiredness of the spine	■ Bracing for 12–23 hours per day with a TLSO or Milwaukee brace ■ Counseling or support groups ■ Mild pain medications
Severe scoliosis	■ Spinal curvature with a Cobb angle of greater than 50 degrees; prominent shoulder blade and/or rib bump; back and leg pain; difficulty breathing; nerve root compression	■ Surgical correction of the curve ■ Bracing after surgery with a TLSO brace ■ Nonopioid or opioid analgesics ■ Counseling or support groups ■ Physical therapy

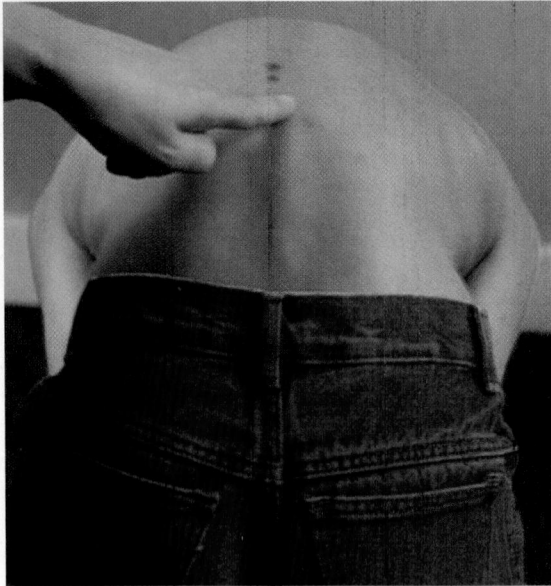

Figure 13–25 ● Inspection of the spine for scoliosis. Ask the child to slowly bend forward at the waist, with arms extended toward the floor. Run your forefinger down the spinal processes, palpating each vertebra for a change in alignment. A lateral curve to the spine or a one-sided rib hump is an indication of scoliosis.
Source: George Dodson/Pearson Education.

screened once. A scoliosis screening includes several visual examinations:

- When the client is standing, the nurse should determine whether the head is centered; whether the hips, shoulders, or rib cage appears uneven; whether one shoulder blade is more prominent; whether the legs are the same length; or whether the body leans to one side. The nurse should also closely assess the spine to determine whether it appears to be straight.

- When the client is in the Adam position, the nurse should assess the spine for obvious curvature, a rib hump, or asymmetry of the back. The physical examination should include palpation of each vertebra to detect abnormal alignment of the spine that may not be visible (**Figure 13–25 ●**). If any abnormalities are detected, the nurse may use a scoliometer to measure the deformity while the client is in the Adam position.

Clients with a spine curvature greater than 10 degrees should be monitored every 6 months for curvature progression. If the curve appears to progress dramatically, the client should be referred to a physician for follow-up.

Diagnosis

Nursing diagnoses related to clients with scoliosis may include the following:

- *Ineffective Breathing Pattern* related to spinal rotation and rib cage deformity
- *Risk for Infection* related to spinal surgery
- *Risk for Impaired Skin Integrity* related to brace wear
- *Impaired Physical Mobility* related to supportive brace

- *Risk for Activity Intolerance* related to spinal deformity
- *Deficient Knowledge* related to treatment options
- *Disturbed Body Image* related to deformity and brace
- *Risk for Chronic Low Self-Esteem* related to inability to discuss deformity with peers
- *Anxiety* related to effectiveness of treatment
- *Ineffective Coping* related to feelings of social isolation and anxiety
- *Noncompliance* related to wearing brace around peers
- *Social Isolation* related to unwillingness to wear brace in public.

(NANDA-I © 2012)

Planning

Expected outcomes for clients with scoliosis may include the following:

- The client will demonstrate effective breathing patterns as evidenced by adequate oxygenation and activity tolerance.
- The client and family will express understanding of treatment options that coincide with severity of spine curvature.
- The client will report compliance with prescribed brace wear.
- The client will state importance of follow-up every 6 months.
- The client will communicate fears and emotions about diagnosis and treatment.
- The client's curvature will not progress during treatment with the brace.

Clients who undergo surgery for scoliosis will have additional outcomes related to surgical procedures:

- The client will demonstrate proficiency with breathing exercises.
- The client will demonstrate no manifestations of neurological impairment.
- The client will demonstrate no signs or symptoms of postoperative infection.
- The client will accurately describe surgical procedure and postoperative expectations.
- The client will verbalize understanding of the importance of limiting activities after surgery.

Implementation

Nursing interventions for clients with scoliosis will depend on the degree of curvature and the proposed treatment. For clients with mild scoliosis who require observation without medical treatment, nursing interventions may include emotional support, teaching about the importance of attending regular follow-up appointments, and teaching proper body mechanics. For clients with moderate scoliosis who require bracing, nursing care will additionally include teaching the client about brace wear and care, emphasizing the importance of wearing the brace for the prescribed amount of time each day, encouraging the client to maintain social interactions, and teaching the client about clothing that can help disguise the presence of the brace. Care of clients who undergo surgery will likely

NURSING CARE PLAN A Child Undergoing Scoliosis Surgery

Frances Bomgardner is an 11-year-old female client who was discovered to have scoliosis during a routine screening at her middle school. Conservative treatment was attempted, although her pediatrician warned that it might not work because of the severity of her curvature. Owing to progression of her scoliosis, Frances is admitted to the local hospital, where she is to undergo spinal fusion. Both Frances and her family are anxious for the procedure to be over, and Frances's mother pulls the nurse aside to ask whether there is any chance that Frances could end up paralyzed as a result of the surgery.

ASSESSMENT

Frances displays a 35-degree lateral curvature with grade 2 vertebral rotation. She is currently wearing a brace, and the skin around and under the brace is intact with no redness, abrasions, or swelling. She and her parents express anxiety related to the upcoming procedure. Frances's vital signs include the following: temperature 97.8°F oral; pulse 86 bpm; respirations 20/min; and BP 102/63 mmHg. Her oxygen saturation is 96%, and her breath sounds are slightly diminished throughout. When asked if she is having difficulty breathing, Frances states, "This brace thing is squeezing me too tight. I can't take a big breath." You immediately notify the physician of Frances's complaint, decreased oxygen saturation, and diminished breath sounds. The physician pages the orthotist, who arrives within 10 minutes. After the orthotist adjusts Frances's brace, her breath sounds are clear and equal throughout, and her oxygen saturation is 99%. Frances reports that she can "breathe normally now."

DIAGNOSES

- *Ineffective Breathing Pattern* related to corrective brace, rib rotation, and anxiety
- *Risk for Ineffective Tissue Perfusion* related to postoperative immobility
- *Risk for Infection* related to surgical procedure
- *Risk for Impaired Skin Integrity* related to brace wear
- *Acute Pain* related to surgical intervention
- *Impaired Physical Mobility* related to movement restriction from brace
- *Deficient Knowledge* related to lack of information about surgery
- *Risk for Situational Low Self-esteem* related to deformity and brace wear
- *Risk for Caregiver Role Strain* related to caring for child after surgery
- *Anxiety* related to unknown outcome of surgery
- *Fear* related to risk of paralysis

(NANDA-I © 2012)

PLANNING

- The client will maintain an oxygen saturation of at least 98% with normal breath sounds.
- The client will deny dyspnea.
- The client will demonstrate adequate peripheral circulation, including no signs or symptoms of thrombophlebitis.
- The client will experience no sensory or motor deficits or impairment, such as numbness, tingling, or permanent loss of mobility.
- The client will verbalize adequate pain control as evidenced by reports of a pain level rating of less than 3 on a scale of 0–10.
- The client and parents will demonstrate knowledge of proper skin care related to brace wear.
- The client will maintain proper body alignment and demonstrate knowledge of activity limits as ordered by the physician.
- The client and parents will verbalize understanding of surgical procedures and postoperative care.
- The client will verbalize feelings about body image related to the disease and its treatment and will utilize recommended counseling services if needed.
- The client's parents will allow family and friends to help care for the child after surgery as needed to reduce stress.
- The client and parents will express satisfaction with the outcome of the surgery and the child's progress toward health and wellness.
- The client and parents will demonstrate knowledge of caring for the surgical incision and potential signs of infection.

IMPLEMENTATION

Preoperative

- Preoperative teaching should be initiated upon the client's admission to the facility. Encourage the client and family members to ask questions. Notify the surgeon if the client or family members have questions or concerns regarding the surgery or expected outcomes.
- Demonstrate procedures that will be required postoperatively, such as logrolling, incentive spirometry, and ROM exercises, and ask the client to perform a return demonstration. In addition, teach the client and family members about applying and caring for the client's supportive brace.

Postoperative

- Continually monitor the client's circulatory and respiratory function through physical assessment and frequent assessment of vital signs, including pulse oximetry. Be alert to the development of respiratory depression, especially following administration of narcotic analgesics. Administer oxygen per protocols and medical orders.
- Complete a postoperative neurovascular assessment every 2 hours during the first 24 hours following surgery, and then every 4 hours for the next 48 hours. Assess and document presence and quality of pedal and distal tibial pulses every

(continued on next page)

NURSING CARE PLAN (continued)

hour for 48 hours. Immediately notify the physician of changes and abnormal findings.

- Use the logroll technique to reposition the client every 2 hours. Pad joints and bony prominences. Prevent flexion or extension of the spine and follow medical orders when using pillows to support the back, knees, and feet.
- Assess the surgical dressing for signs of excessive drainage (including excess fluid or bleeding that causes saturation of the dressing). If a surgical drainage device is in place, monitor and record the color and amount of output collected.
- While the client is immobile, apply antiembolism stockings to reduce the risk of thrombophlebitis. Antiembolism stockings may be removed intermittently per the physician's orders.
- Per the physician's orders, administer passive ROM exercises and supervise the client during active ROM exercises. In some cases, the surgeon will allow the client to sit up between the second and fourth postoperative day. Proceed slowly when transferring the client to a seated position. Ambulation is generally allowed within 3–5 days following sur-

gery. Assist the client with ambulation and encourage the client to report any complaints or concerns, including dizziness.

- Regularly assess the client's pain and administer analgesics per the physician's orders. For clients who receive an epidural block, assess the client's level of sensory and motor blockade and monitor for return to normal sensory perception and motor function. As indicated, use nonpharmacologic pain management strategies.
- Promote independence in completion of daily activities as tolerated by the client. Provide positive reinforcement and encouragement. Offer to facilitate connecting the client and family members with community support groups for clients with scoliosis.
- Reinforce preoperative teaching and repeat instructions as needed. Provide instructions in both oral and written form. Assess the family members' and client's comprehension and encourage questions. Instruct the client and family members to immediately notify the physician of any concerns, including actual or suspected complications.
- Facilitate follow-up appointments and, if indicated, assist the family with appointment scheduling.

EVALUATION

Frances and her parents demonstrate adequate knowledge of scoliosis, the surgical procedure, and postoperative care, substantially reducing their anxiety and fear. Frances's postoperative pain is being managed effectively by medication and distraction techniques. She demonstrates no sensory or motor deficits. Although she appears to be adjusting to her postoperative regimen quite well, Frances has expressed fear that her classmates will ridicule her for wearing a brace when she returns to school. Frances and her parents regularly perform logrolling and passive ROM exercises. Frances has yet to begin ambulating independently on day 4 postsurgery, although she is ambulating with her parents' assistance. The nurse has provided oral and written instructions about brace care, activity limitations, community resources, and follow-up appointments.

CRITICAL THINKING

1. What steps can the nurse take to encourage both Frances and her parents to help Frances ambulate independently?
2. How should the nurse address Frances's concerns about the reaction of her peers when she goes back to school?
3. Develop a care plan for Frances if she develops loss of skin integrity related to bed rest or brace wear.

incorporate the nursing interventions indicated in the care of clients with mild and moderate scoliosis, as well as nursing interventions related to preoperative and postoperative care, as discussed in the Nursing Care Plan feature. For all clients, referral to community support groups or to an individual who has had similar treatment for scoliosis may be beneficial.

Evaluation

Evaluation of the client with scoliosis will include regular assessment of the curvature of the spine as well as assessment of

the skin under the brace to confirm skin integrity. Evaluation should also include interviewing the client about compliance with brace wear and self-image problems. During long-term care of the client with scoliosis, the client's needs will change significantly based on the client's physiological response to care, as well as her ability to cope with the challenges associated with this disorder. The nursing care plan should be revised and updated to reflect the client's current needs, including those within the psychosocial realm.

REVIEW Back Problems

RELATE Link the Concepts and Exemplars

Linking the exemplar of back problems with the concept of addiction:

1. What focused assessment should the nurse implement for a client with chronic back problems who has been taking Percocet for pain?
2. A 46-year-old female client diagnosed with back problems was admitted last evening with an alcohol overdose. What is the priority of nursing care for this client?

Linking the exemplar of back problems with the concept of family:

3. Clients with reduced mobility related to back problems often require care from family members. Describe methods to relieve caregiver role strain for parents caring for a child, a partner caring for a partner, and adult daughters and sons caring for older parents.
4. How can the nurse advocate for a child with scoliosis whose parents do not agree with the treatment plan?

READY Go to Companion Skills Manual

REFER Go to Pearson Student Nursing Resources
nursing.pearsonhighered.com

- Additional review materials

REFLECT Case Study

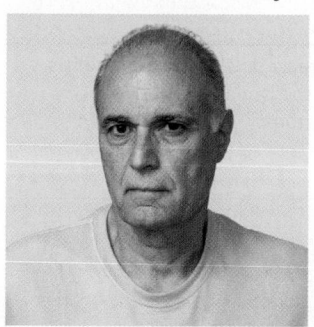

Gilbert Martin is a 53-year-old Hispanic male who is married to Helen Martin. Mr. Martin has a son from a previous marriage and a stepdaughter whom he has raised since she was 3 years old. Mr. Martin's father recently passed away, so he has been helping his mother manage her affairs. Mr. Martin works as a delivery truck driver for a construction company. His job includes assisting with the loading and unloading of construction materials. Mr. Martin considers himself to be in good health with the exception of chronic back pain. Mr. Martin also has hyperlipidemia for which he takes atorvastatin (Lipitor) 20 mg/day. Mr. Martin sees his primary care provider once a year for triglyceride and liver function tests and has been encouraged to follow a low-fat diet.

1. What nonpharmacologic interventions may be implemented to help Mr. Martin reduce his chronic back pain?
2. What factors place Mr. Martin at risk for exacerbation of his back problems?
3. Describe how the stress in Mr. Martin's life may be affecting his chronic low back pain.

EXEMPLAR 13.2 **Fractures**

EXEMPLAR KEY TERMS

Cast, *860*
Closed fracture, *854*
Compartment syndrome, *858*
Deep venous thrombosis (DVT), *858*
Delayed union, *857*
Fat embolism syndrome (FES), *858*
Fracture, *853*
Malunion, *857*
Nonunion, *857*
Open fracture, *854*
Open reduction and internal fixation (ORIF), *860*
Osteomyelitis, *854*
Reduction, *860*
Splint, *862*
Traction, *862*

EXEMPLAR LEARNING OUTCOMES

After reading about this exemplar, you will be able to:

1. Describe the pathophysiology, etiology, clinical manifestations, and direct and indirect causes of fractures.
2. Identify risk factors and prevention methods associated with fractures.
3. Illustrate the nursing process in providing culturally competent care across the life span for individuals with fractures.
4. Formulate priority nursing diagnoses appropriate for an individual with a fracture.
5. Summarize therapies used by interdisciplinary teams in the collaborative care of an individual with a fracture.
6. Plan evidence-based care for an individual with a fracture and his or her family in collaboration with other members of the healthcare team.
7. Evaluate expected outcomes for an individual with a fracture.

▶ OVERVIEW

A bone **fracture** is a break in the continuity of a bone. Fractures are most common in clients who have suffered trauma and in older adults. Fractures vary in type, location, and severity.

▶ PATHOPHYSIOLOGY AND ETIOLOGY

Humans are born with at least 270 bones, some of which fuse together to form the 206 bones found in an adult body. Any of these bones can be fractured. Fractures can be classified according to the break pattern of the bone (**Table 13–3 ●**).

Etiology

Two main factors contribute to development of a fracture: the strength of the force acting against the bone and the strength of the bone. When the force acting on the bone is greater than the bone strength, the bone will fracture. The force acting on the bone may be a direct blow, compression, twisting, trauma such as a fall, or repetitive forces such as running. Single large forces are likely to cause bone fractures at the point of impact (direct force), whereas small repetitive forces are likely to cause fractures at the weakest point of the affected bone (indirect force). The strength of the bone is related to the individual's nutritional status as well as the presence of pathological conditions such as osteoporosis, bone cancer, or Paget disease.

> ### SAFETY ALERT
> When a child presents with a fracture that is uncommon for his age group, abuse should be suspected. However, because a fracture does not always imply abuse, the nurse should tactfully interview the client and caregiver and follow institutional protocols for further investigation when abuse is suspected.

Fracture Healing

Healing of a fractured bone progresses through three stages: inflammatory, reparative, and remodeling (Geris, Schugart, & van Oosterwyck, 2010).

- In the *inflammatory phase*, damage to the bone, blood vessels, and surrounding tissues causes bleeding and the formation of

TABLE 13–3 Common Fractures

FRACTURE TYPE	DESCRIPTION	COMMENTS
Closed	Bone breaks but skin remains intact.	Also called a simple fracture.
Open	Bone breaks and protrudes through the skin.	Client is at increased risk of **osteomyelitis**, or infection of the bone; also called a compound fracture.
Complete	Fracture involves the entire width of the bone.	
Greenstick	Bone fragments are still partially joined.	Also called an incomplete fracture; occurs commonly in children.
Displaced	Broken ends of bones move out of correct anatomical alignment.	Also called an unstable fracture; requires immediate attention to prevent further damage to surrounding tissues.
Nondisplaced	Broken ends of bones remain aligned.	Also called a stable fracture.
Comminuted	Bone fragments into many pieces.	Common in individuals with brittle bones, such as clients with osteogenesis imperfecta.

TABLE 13–3 Common Fractures (*continued*)

FRACTURE TYPE	DESCRIPTION	COMMENTS
Avulsion Avulsion	A fragment of bone is separated from the rest of the bone.	May also involve displacement of surrounding tissues.
Linear	Fracture occurs parallel to the bone's axis.	
Transverse	Fracture occurs at a right angle to the bone's axis.	
Oblique	Fracture occurs diagonal to the bone's axis.	
Spiral	Fracture spirals around the bone.	Occurs as the result of a twisting force; occurs commonly in children as a result of the porous nature of their bones and sports injuries.

(continued on next page)

TABLE 13–3   Common Fractures (*continued*)

FRACTURE TYPE	DESCRIPTION	COMMENTS
Impacted	The two ends of the bone are forced together.	Also called a buckle fracture; this is often seen with children's arm fractures and hip fractures.
Pathologic	Caused by a disease that weakens the bone.	Diseases could include osteoporosis, bone cancer, and osteogenesis imperfecta.
Stress	Caused by small repetitive forces on the bone.	Often caused by participation in sports or exercise.
Compression Compressed	Bone is crushed.	Occurs most commonly in vertebrae; common in clients with osteoporosis.
Depression *	Bone is forced inward.	Occurs commonly in skull fractures.

Source: *Drawings adapted from Marieb, E. N. (1998). *Human anatomy and physiology* (4th ed., p. 180). Menlo Park, CA: Benjamin Cummings.

a hematoma around the injury. Inflammatory cells, mainly macrophages and neutrophils, then enter the wound and degrade debris and bacteria in the area. This phase usually lasts until osteoblasts and endothelial cells begin to proliferate at the fracture site, usually a few days.

- In the *reparative phase*, fibroblasts, osteoblasts, and chondroblasts begin to secrete collagen to form fibrocartilage, which develops into a soft callus that joins the fractured bone. Endothelial cells begin to form blood vessels in the damaged area. Once the soft callus is formed, it is replaced by woven bone through endochondral ossification, which forms a hard callus. This woven bone is immature bone with a random collagen and bone structure. The reparative phase usually lasts 6–8 weeks for relatively simple fractures.

- In the *remodeling phase*, woven bone is replaced by highly organized lamellar bone. Lamellar bone is stronger and more compact with better blood circulation compared to woven bone. Because bones are being continually remodeled, bone fractures usually heal without a scar. However, it may be several years before the bone returns to its original strength.

A bone that fractures and undergoes normal healing is called a union. Multiple factors can influence bone healing (**Table 13–4 ●**). If the bone does not heal properly, it may be classified as a delayed union, nonunion, or malunion. A **nonunion** is a fracture that shows no clinically significant progress toward complete healing for at least 3 months based on x-rays. This may occur at any point along the healing process. A **delayed union** occurs when the healing process takes significantly longer than expected, usually more than 3–6 months (Coulibaly et al., 2010). A **malunion** occurs when the bone fragments join in a position that is not anatomically correct. Nonunions and malunions may need to be surgically corrected.

Risk Factors

The primary risk factors associated with bone fractures are age, presence of bone disease, and poor nutrition. Younger clients are more likely to sustain fractures related to sports injuries, whereas older clients are at higher risk of fractures related to

falls and disease. Bone diseases that decrease the strength of the bone, such as osteoporosis, osteogenesis imperfecta, and bone cancer, increase the client's risk of bone fracture. Inadequate intake of vitamin D, calcium, and phosphorus also contributes to poor bone strength. Lifestyle habits, such as participation in dangerous activities, can also increase the risk of fracture.

Prevention

Fracture prevention begins with education. Children and young adults should be taught the importance of using safety equipment to help prevent fractures, including safety belts, helmets, football and soccer pads, and hard hats. Practicing good lifestyle habits can also increase bone strength and prevent fractures, including consuming adequate calcium, exercising regularly, maintaining a healthy weight, and avoiding smoking and excess alcohol.

Creating a safe living environment is also key to prevention of fractures, including using protective gates at stairways when infants and toddlers are present and removing rugs and electrical cords that may trip older adults who are unsteady. Older adults should also have regular screenings for osteoporosis and risk assessments for falls. Osteoporosis screenings are particularly important for women after menopause, because the loss of estrogen during menopause decreases calcium absorption and increases the risk for osteoporosis. For more teaching points to help older adults prevent falls and fractures, see the Client Teaching feature.

TABLE 13–4 Factors Influencing Bone Healing

LOCATION	POSITIVE FACTORS	NEGATIVE FACTORS
Local	■ Immobilization ■ Timely correction of displacement ■ Application of ice ■ Electrical stimulation	■ Open fracture ■ Delay in correction of displacement ■ Deep bone infection ■ Presence of foreign body in fracture
Systemic	■ Adequate growth hormone, vitamin D, and calcium ■ Adequate blood supply ■ Absence of infection or disease ■ Younger age ■ Moderate activity level prior to injury	■ Malnutrition ■ Immunocompromised status ■ Decreased circulation (as in diabetes and peripheral vascular disease) ■ Advanced age ■ Osteoporosis

---

Client Teaching

Fall Prevention in Older Adults

Several lifestyle changes can help older adults decrease their risk of fractures related to falls. If needed, a nurse can visit the client's home to perform an environmental safety assessment.

- Start a mild or moderate exercise program to help improve balance and strength.

- Wear sensible shoes with nonslip soles and good support both inside and outside the house.

- Walk slowly and carefully in areas that may be slippery, including icy or wet surfaces or polished floors. Use a walker or cane if needed for extra stability. Avoid walking in socks or slippers that lack traction.

- Ask a physician or pharmacist how medications may affect balance and alertness or change bone or muscle strength.

- Make sure hallways and stairways have adequate lighting, even at night. Make room lights, lamps, and flashlights easily accessible.

- Keep rooms free of clutter, including clothing, paper, electric cords, and throw rugs.

- Install hand rails on stairs and around the toilet and bathtub. Also place a rubber mat in the tub or shower.

- Avoid using a step stool if possible. If necessary, use a sturdy step stool with a wide base and hand rail for balance.

- Seek treatment for health conditions that may affect bone or muscle strength, neuronal control of muscles, balance, or vision loss.

▶ CLINICAL MANIFESTATIONS

Clinical manifestations of bone fracture include pain due to tissue trauma and a visible fracture on an x-ray. Pain is generally due to an interruption in the continuity of the bone; damage to ligaments, tendons, and other surrounding tissues; and muscle spasms. Depending on the severity of the fracture, other manifestations may include visible deformity if the bone is displaced, swelling from inflammation, and numbness due to nerve damage. Internal or external loss of blood may result in hypovolemic shock or ecchymosis. If the fractured pieces of bone grate against each other, crepitus may be heard.

Complications

Complications associated with fractures include compartment syndrome, deep venous thrombosis, fat emboli, infection, or loss of sensation. Development of complications depends on the type and severity of fracture and the client's personal factors.

COMPARTMENT SYNDROME Individual muscles are surrounded by fascia, and the muscle tissue, nerves, and blood vessels within the fascia are part of a compartment. Fasciae are designed to hold the muscle in place; therefore, they do not expand, and pressure can build up within the compartment. **Compartment syndrome** occurs when edema and swelling cause increased pressure in a muscle compartment, leading to decreased blood flow and potential muscle and nerve damage (AAOS, 2009a; Vorvick, Ma, & Zieve, 2012a). Decreased blood flow leads to dilation of the blood vessels, causing more edema and stimulating a cycle of continually increasing pressure in the limb. If ischemia to the compartment continues for a significant length of time, the muscles and nerves may die and the limb may need to be amputated.

Symptoms of compartment syndrome include severe pain and tenderness, swelling, paresthesia, pallor, numbness or paralysis, and decreased or absent pulse and poikilothermia (normalization to room temperature) in the distal portion of the affected limb. Compartment syndrome is most common in the lower leg and forearm, but it can also occur in the hand, foot, thigh, and upper arm. It can result from a fracture, muscle bruise, crush injury, or bandage that is too tight, such as a cast. Compartment syndrome is a medical emergency; the first step in treatment is to remove a tight cast. If internal pressure is causing the symptoms, it is generally treated by surgery (i.e., fasciotomy) to relieve pressure (AAOS, 2009a). Clients with a bone fracture in an extremity should be regularly evaluated for swelling, pain, discoloration, and neurovascular function in the fractured limb. Methods to prevent compartment syndrome include elevation and ice to reduce swelling and delaying casting until the swelling is gone.

Compartment syndrome can lead to many complications, including paralysis, the need for amputation, or a Volkmann contracture. A *Volkmann contracture* is a deformity of the wrist, hand, and fingers caused by ischemia to the forearm, usually as a result of compartment syndrome. Ischemia in the forearm causes the nerves and muscles to become scarred and shortened, forcing the joint to be permanently bent (Vorvick et al., 2012b). A Volkmann contracture is common after elbow injuries, especially in children.

DEEP VENOUS THROMBOSIS **Deep venous thrombosis (DVT)** occurs when a blood clot, or thrombus, forms in one of the deep veins, usually in the leg. Symptoms include redness and warmth of the skin, leg pain, cramping, and swelling. If DVT is suspected, the nurse should report the symptoms to a physician immediately. The physician may order a venogram or Doppler ultrasound to visualize the blood clot and confirm diagnosis. DVT is usually treated with bed rest to prevent dislodgement of the clot, anticoagulants such as heparin or warfarin to prevent further clotting, thrombolytics such as tissue plasminogen activator (TPA) to break down the clot, or surgery to insert a filter in the vena cava to prevent blood clots from traveling to vital organs. Measures to prevent DVT include early immobilization of the fracture, regular exercise, prophylactic anticoagulants, and use of compression stockings or boots (Mayo Clinic, 2013a).

If the blood clot dislodges from the leg, it can travel to the brain and cause a cerebrovascular accident (CVA or stroke). In the lungs, a blood clot can cause a pulmonary embolism. In the coronary arteries, a blood clot can lead to myocardial infarction (MI) and other severe damage (Dugdale, 2012b). Risk factors for development of DVT include decreased blood flow, blood vessel injury, and altered blood coagulation (**Table 13–5 ●**). Other risk factors include older age, obesity, poor circulation, inactivity/bed rest, smoking, and cancer. (For more information about DVT, pulmonary embolism, and stroke, see the module on Perfusion.)

FAT EMBOLISM SYNDROME Fat embolism may occur in conjunction with closed long bone or pelvic fractures. Fat emboli released from the bone marrow enter the bloodstream and become trapped in the pulmonary and dermal capillaries. In most clients, release of fat from the bone marrow after a fracture produces no symptoms. However, if a large amount of fat is released, such as in clients with multiple fractures, **fat embolism syndrome (FES)** may occur.

TABLE 13–5 Risk Factors for Deep Venous Thrombosis	
RISK FACTOR	**NURSING IMPLICATIONS FOR CLIENTS WITH FRACTURES**
Blood stasis in a vein	Immobility from casting and bed rest can decrease blood flow in the limb. The nurse should encourage early ambulation, active or passive exercises, and the use of compression stockings or boots to prevent blood stasis.
Blood vessel injury	Blood vessels may be injured by the force that caused the fracture, by movement of the fractured bone, or during surgical repair of the bone, causing clots to form at the site of injury. The nurse should be aware of the location of potential blood vessel injuries so assessments can be targeted to the appropriate location.
Altered blood coagulation	Excess blood loss from injury or surgery may cause the body to increase production of platelets and clotting factors. The presence of tissue debris or fat in the vein may also promote clot formation. The nurse should assess the client for coagulation disorders and monitor use of medications that alter blood clotting.

Classic manifestations of FES are the result of blocked blood flow and the presence of free fatty acids; they usually develop within 12–72 hours after injury and include dyspnea, neurological abnormalities, and petechial rash (Jain et al., 2008). In severe cases, dyspnea may progress to respiratory failure with tachypnea and hypoxia. A syndrome similar to acute respiratory distress syndrome (ARDS) may develop (see the exemplar on ARDS in the module on Oxygenation). Neurological symptoms may include confusion, restlessness, seizures, or coma. A transient petechial rash usually covers the upper anterior trunk, arms, and neck as well as the buccal mucosa and conjunctiva. Other symptoms may include Purtscher retinopathy (sudden loss of vision most often associated with traumatic injury) and mild fever.

Treatment of FES is supportive and includes oxygen administration; approximately one half of clients will require mechanical ventilation. Neurological symptoms usually resolve with adequate oxygenation, and the petechial rash disappears spontaneously within a week. Prophylactic treatment with corticosteroids and early immobilization of the injury may reduce the risk of FES. FES is rarely seen in children under the age of 10.

INFECTION   Impaired skin integrity as a result of an open fracture or surgical correction of a fracture increases the risk of bacterial contamination and development of an infection. Common infecting organisms include *Pseudomonas*, *Staphylococcus*, and *Clostridium*. Clients with greater soft tissue damage or with a compromised immune system are at higher risk of infection. Signs of infection include warmth, redness, pain, swelling, stiffness, fever, chills, and purulent drainage. Treatment includes administration of antibiotics according to the infecting agent and proper hygiene of the infection site. Hygiene care may include debridement, drainage, and culture for identification of the infecting organism. Infection due to fractures can cause cellulitis (see the exemplar on Cellulitis in the module on Infection), osteomyelitis, or gangrene. If the infection is severe or does not respond to antibiotics, tissue death may occur, necessitating amputation.

Lifespan and Cultural Considerations

A client's age plays a role in the type of fracture she is likely to experience. Children often experience long bone fractures as a result of sports and play. Spiral fractures are common in children because of the porous nature of their bones; unexplained midshaft spiral fractures may be an indicator of child abuse. (For more information about abuse, see the exemplar on Abuse in the module on Violence.) Children often recover quickly from fractures because their bones have a rapid growth rate and the epiphyseal plates have not yet been sealed.

Athletes, such as long-distance runners or gymnasts, often experience stress fractures related to repetitive force on specific bones. In addition to repeated stress, adolescents are likely to suffer from stress fractures as a result of imbalanced nutrition. Adults who have finished growing may have a lengthened recovery time because their bones have a slower rate of tissue growth; this is especially true for women after menopause and older adults in general. Older adults with osteoporosis have increased risk of hip fractures and are more likely to develop complications such as DVT and infection.

▶ COLLABORATION

A bone fracture is an emergency situation that often requires the collaboration of multiple healthcare professionals, including nurses, physicians, surgeons, and physical therapists. The nurse's primary roles include assessing the client, maintaining client comfort, assisting with procedures, providing client education, and referring the client to specialists as needed.

Emergency Care

The primary objectives of emergency care of a client with a fracture include immobilizing the fracture and preventing infection. If emergency care is provided outside a medical facility, immobilization should not include trying to reset the bone if it is out of alignment. Instead, the nurse should apply splints above and below the joint to reduce mobility and prevent further damage to the area. Cervical immobilization is essential if a spinal fracture is suspected. If the client is bleeding, the nurse should apply a pressure dressing, and sterile dressings should be applied to all open wounds. Once the client is stabilized and the fracture immobilized, the nurse should assess the extremities for pulses, movement, and sensation. Ice packs may be applied to reduce swelling if needed. Clients may also need to be treated for shock (see the exemplar on Shock in the module on Perfusion).

Diagnostic Tests

The primary diagnostic test for a fractured bone is an x-ray (**Figure 13–26 ●**). Other complementary methods used for

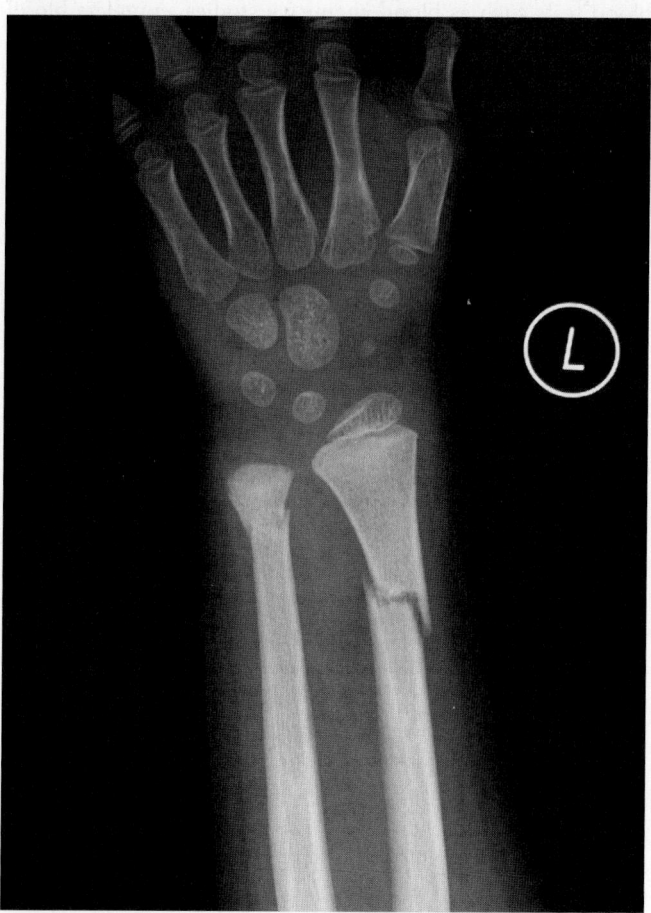

Figure 13–26 ● X-ray of fractured forearm.
Source: kuehdi/Shutterstock.

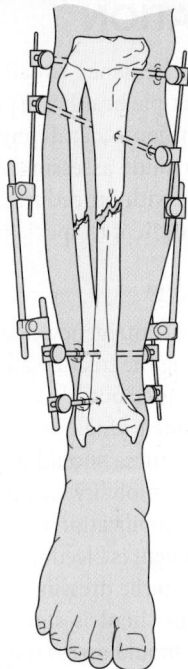

Figure 13–27 ● In external fixation, pins are placed through the bone above and below the fracture site to immobilize the bone. External fixation rods hold the pins in place.

diagnosis include client history; physical assessment; other imaging studies such as bone scans, MRIs, or CT scans; and blood tests such as blood chemistry studies, complete blood count, and coagulation studies.

Surgery

For severe fractures that require direct visualization to repair, such as open fractures and comminuted fractures, the client will undergo surgery. The two main types of surgical repair for bone fractures are external fixation and internal fixation. With external fixation, metal pins and screws are placed into the bone above and below the fracture. The pins and screws are then attached to a metal bar outside the skin (**Figure 13–27 ●**). This is often performed if damage to soft tissues prevents internal fixation. The nurse is responsible for monitoring the client for infection and neurovascular function.

Open reduction and internal fixation (ORIF) is the surgical procedure used to internally repair a bone fracture. During **reduction**, the bone is placed in correct alignment. Nails, screws, pins, wires, plates, or rods are then inserted into the bone to hold the bone in place (**Figure 13–28 ●**). Plates are attached on the outer surface of the bone, whereas rods may be inserted through the marrow space in the center of the bone. Fractures of the long bones are commonly repaired by ORIF; internal fixation allows shorter hospital stays, earlier return to full function, and fewer instances of nonunion and malunion (AAOS, 2007a). Complications of fracture reduction may include infection, neurovascular or vascular injury, and leg length discrepancy. Nursing interventions for clients with internal fixation are found in **Box 13–3 ●**.

Pharmacologic Therapy

Pharmacologic therapy for clients who sustain bone fractures primarily includes analgesics for pain. For severe fractures,

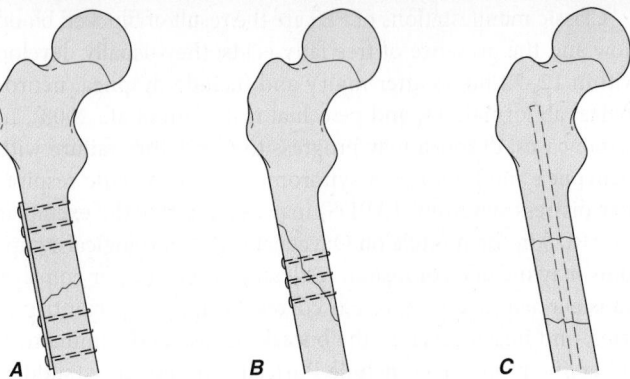

Figure 13–28 ● Internal fixation hardware is entirely within the body. *A,* Fixation of a short oblique fracture using a plate and screws above and below the fracture. *B,* Fixation of a long oblique fracture using screws through the fracture site. *C,* Fixation of segmental fracture using a medullary nail.

opioids or patient-controlled analgesics are prescribed. In addition to opioids, NSAIDs may be administered for both pain and inflammation. See Exemplar 13.1 for a thorough discussion of opioid and nonopioid analgesics, including their side effects and nursing implications. Other common medications for clients with bone fractures include antibiotics to prevent or treat infections and anticoagulants to prevent or treat DVT.

Nonpharmacologic Therapy

The majority of bone fractures are treated with nonpharmacologic therapy, including casts, traction, and pain management. Electrical bone stimulation is an alternative therapy that may also be beneficial (see the Evidence-Based Practice feature).

CASTS AND SPLINTS   A **cast** is a rigid device used to immobilize, support, and protect fractured bones and the surrounding soft tissue (**Figure 13–29 ●**) (AAOS, 2011a). A cast is usually applied to a stable fracture after it has been reduced. Casts are custom made from plaster or fiberglass to exactly fit the injured limb and cannot be easily removed by the client.

Box 13–3   Nursing Interventions for the Client With Internal Fixation

- Assess the client frequently for:
  – Wound drainage
  – Infection
  – Serosanguineous fluid drainage in the Hemovac
  – Bowel sounds
  – Lung sounds
  – Pain
  – Neuromuscular function.
- Administer medications such as analgesics and antibiotics as ordered by the physician.
- Encourage early ambulation if possible. Assist with exercises and ambulation if needed.
- Encourage deep breathing and coughing to prevent lung complications.
- Refer and arrange physical and occupational therapy as ordered.

Evidence-Based Practice Electrical Bone Stimulation

Problem

Bone fractures take extensive time to heal, and occasionally clients have delayed union or nonunion of fractures. Delayed union or nonunion fractures are often treated with an external electrical bone stimulator, which creates a pulsed electromagnetic field by applying electrical current at the fracture site. Several types of electrical stimulators are available, including direct-current, capacitive coupling, and inductive coupling stimulators.

Evidence

Electromagnetic stimulation of the bone at the fracture site mimics the effect of mechanical stress on bone, upregulating extracellular matrix proteins, growth factors, and other factors that enhance cellular repair (Victoria et al., 2009). Osteoblast and osteoclast proliferation and mineral deposition are also enhanced by electrical stimulation. Capacitive coupling and inductive coupling appear to have the greatest effectiveness on nonunions, but clinical studies generally have used small sample sizes and been of variable design, reducing the strength of the results (Griffin & Bayat, 2011). The American Academy of Orthopaedic Surgeons (2007b) recommends the use of electrical stimulation for nonunions from 20 minutes to several hours daily for maximum effectiveness.

Implications

Electrical bone stimulation is an alternative method for healing of bone fractures that have not responded to traditional therapies. Although few well-controlled studies are available, limited evidence suggests that electrical bone stimulation is effective for healing nonunions. Electrical bone stimulation is relatively safe, and the client feels no pain as a result of the electrical pulses. Therefore, electrical bone stimulation may be a good alternative to invasive surgery for clients at high risk for surgical complications or infection. In addition, clients can be taught to administer electrical bone stimulation at home, reducing hospital stays.

Critical Thinking Application

1. What are some contraindications for electrical bone stimulation?

2. Describe ways in which you would encourage clients who are self-administering electrical bone stimulation at home to use the stimulator for the prescribed number of hours each day.

3. Design a high-quality clinical study for electrical bone stimulation.

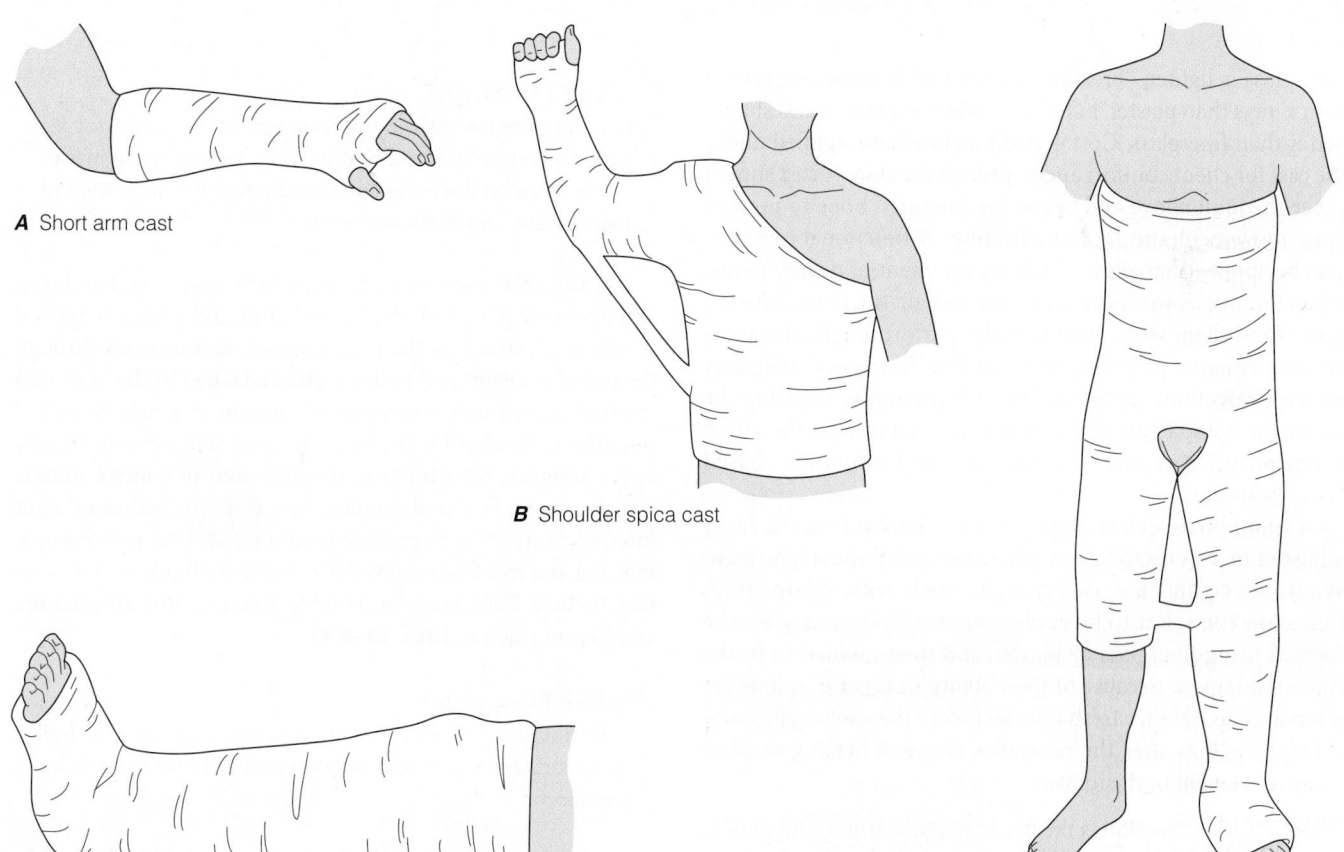

A Short arm cast

B Shoulder spica cast

C Long leg cast

D One-and-one half hip spica cast

Figure 13–29 ● Examples of types of casts used to immobilize fractures.

Community-Based Care Cast Care at Home

Discharge teaching for the client with a cast should include the following instructions:

■ Do not apply pressure to the cast before it is dry, because dents in the cast may cause pressure ulcers. Fiberglass casts dry in less than 1 hour, whereas plaster casts may take up to 48 hours to dry. If the cast becomes damaged, notify a physician.

■ Do not get the cast wet, especially if it is a plaster cast. Use plastic or waterproof shields around the cast while showering or bathing. If a fiberglass cast becomes wet, dry it with a blow dryer on the cool setting.

■ Do not place any objects in the cast. Itching under the cast can be relieved by using a blow dryer on the cool setting.

■ Keep dirt and other irritants away from the inside of the cast.

■ Do not remove any part of the cast, including padding and rough edges.

■ Elevate the injured extremity above the heart as often as possible and apply ice to the cast to prevent swelling under the cast.

■ Regularly assess the injured extremity for symptoms of compartment syndrome, including increased pain and swelling, loss of sensation, coolness, and changes in color. If the client feels the cast is becoming too tight, he should see a physician immediately.

■ Assess the skin around the cast regularly. If the skin becomes raw or looks infected, notify a physician immediately.

■ If using a sling, distribute the weight of the cast evenly around the neck. Ensure that the sling strap remains flat around the neck to prevent impaired circulation.

■ If using crutches, teach the client proper crutch walking or refer the client to a physical therapist. Provide the client with verbal and written instructions regarding the physician's orders for bearing weight on the injured leg.

■ For leg fractures, refer the client to a physical therapist to teach crutch walking, limited weight bearing, transferring, and a home safety inspection.

■ Refer the client to home care agencies for ongoing monitoring of wound healing and local medical equipment sources for crutches, wheelchairs, slings, elevated toilet seats, and other equipment that may facilitate healing or prevent further injury.

■ The physician may order x-rays at follow-up appointments to track the healing progress of the fracture. If the cast needs to be removed for skin or bone assessment or because the cast is too large after swelling is decreased, a cast saw will be used. The cast saw will be noisy and the client will feel vibration, but a guard will prevent the cast saw from cutting the client.

Fiberglass is lighter, "breathes" better, and is more compatible with x-rays than plaster, but plaster is less expensive and shapes better than fiberglass. Cotton padding is usually applied under the cast for client comfort and to protect the skin. A cast should cover the joint above and below the fractured bone to prevent bone movement and facilitate healing. A functional cast may also be applied that allows limited movement of nearby joints; a functional cast works for some, but not all, fractures. Nursing care of the client with a cast includes performing neurovascular assessments, palpating the cast for "hot spots" that may indicate infection, reporting drainage promptly, assessing the client for compartment syndrome, and educating the client about proper cast care at home (see the Community-Based Care feature).

A **splint** provides less support than a cast, but it can be easily adjusted to accommodate swelling and prevent compartment syndrome. Splints are usually ready made with Velcro straps that allow the splint to be easily removed. Splints may also be formed using fiberglass or plaster, and then molded to fit the fractured region. Because of their ability to expand, splints are often used to stabilize fresh injuries before the swelling has subsided, as well as after the reparative phase of healing to allow some movement of the joints.

TRACTION   **Traction** is the use of weights, ropes, and pulleys to apply force to a fractured bone to maintain proper alignment of the bone for healing (**Figure 13–30 ●**). It may also help stretch muscles that have contracted or are producing muscle spasms. The two main types of traction are skin traction and skeletal traction.

SAFETY ALERT
For the client whose injury requires traction, do not let weights rest on the bed or the floor. This will cause inadequate force on the bone and may change the alignment of the fracture, causing a malunion.

During *skin traction*, equipment such as splints, bandages, and boots are placed on the injured limb, and a force is applied to soft tissues such as the skin, muscles, and tendons through the use of a weight and pulley system attached to the bed. Skin traction is used only when a small amount of weight (e.g., 5–7 pounds) is needed for traction, because skin cannot tolerate larger weights. Skin traction is often used to control muscle spasms, to maintain alignment of a fracture before or after internal fixation, or to provide traction if skeletal pins become infected and must be removed. Common methods of skin traction include Buck traction, Dunlop traction, Russell traction, and Bryant traction (**Box 13–4 ●**).

SAFETY ALERT
Skin traction is contraindicated in older adults with frail skin, because it may tear the skin and increase the risk for infection.

Skeletal traction is used when a greater force needs to be applied to the fracture or when skin traction is contraindicated. Skeletal traction may be used in conjunction with skin traction, depending on the location and severity of the fracture. For skeletal traction, pins, wires, or screws are surgically implanted into

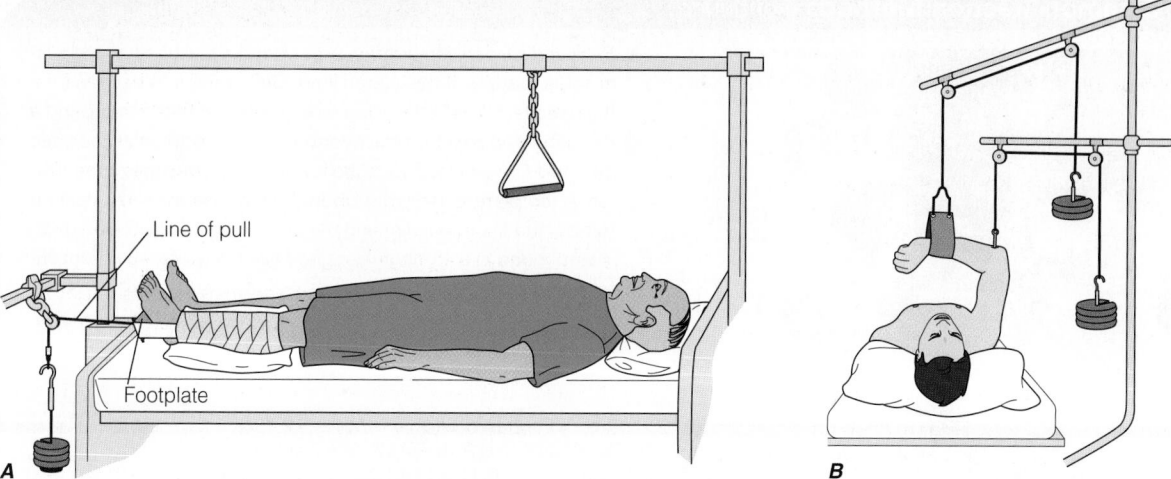

A   *B*

Figure 13–30 ● Traction is the application of a pulling force to maintain bone alignment during fracture healing. Different fractures require different types of traction. *A*, Skin traction applies force to the soft tissues through a pulley system attached to the bed, such as Buck traction shown here for stabilization of the knee and hip. *B*, Skeletal traction applies force directly to the bone, such as the traction used here for a humerus fracture.

Box 13–4   Common Traction Methods

SKIN TRACTION

- *Buck traction* (**Figure 13–31** ●) is the most common orthopedic traction procedure; it is used for fractured or dislocated hips and knee injuries. The foot on the injured side is placed in a foam boot with a small weight (usually 5 lb) attached with a rope and pulley system, and the knee and hip are kept straight. Buck's traction can be unilateral or bilateral.

- *Dunlop traction* (skin or skeletal traction) is used to immobilize a humeral supracondylar fracture in children. The elbow is maintained in a flexed position to prevent circulation and nerve problems.

- *Russell traction* (**Figure 13–32** ●) is used for fractured femurs, hip and knee contractures, and other hip and knee problems. The knee is suspended in a sling, and the knee and lower leg are attached to a series of three pulleys and weights. The angle between the thigh and the bed is approximately 20 degrees, and the hips and knees remain slightly flexed.

- *Bryant traction* (**Figure 13–33** ●) is used to immobilize both lower extremities to treat a fractured femur or developmental dysplasia of the hip in infants and toddlers. The legs are suspended vertically in the air with the hips at a 90-degree angle and the knees slightly flexed. The buttocks are raised slightly off the bed, and the position of the lower body is maintained by weights and pulleys.

SKELETAL TRACTION

- *Skeletal cervical traction* uses Crutchfield, Gardner-Wells, or Vinke tongs inserted into the parietal area of the skull to immobilize the spine after cervical fracture. The tongs are then attached to a pulling device for stabilization.

- *Halo traction* (**Figure 13–34** ●) involves the use of a ring and skull pins attached to a sheepskin jacket and support rods designed to be worn by the client. The screws may need to be tightened periodically to ensure correct alignment of the spine. A halo apparatus is used for fractures of the cervical spine or to correct the alignment of the spine in scoliosis.

- *90–90 traction* (**Figure 13–35** ●) is commonly used in children with a displaced fractured femur. A pin is inserted into the femur close to the knee and attached to a pulley and weight system so the hip and knee are both flexed at a 90-degree angle. The opposite leg may be unrestricted or may be placed in Buck or Russell traction for immobilization.

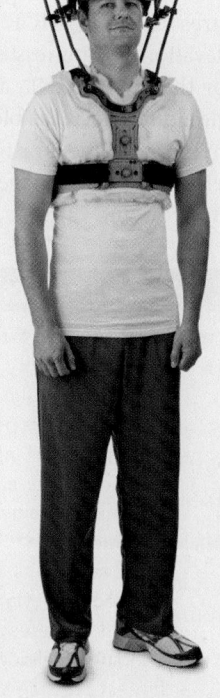

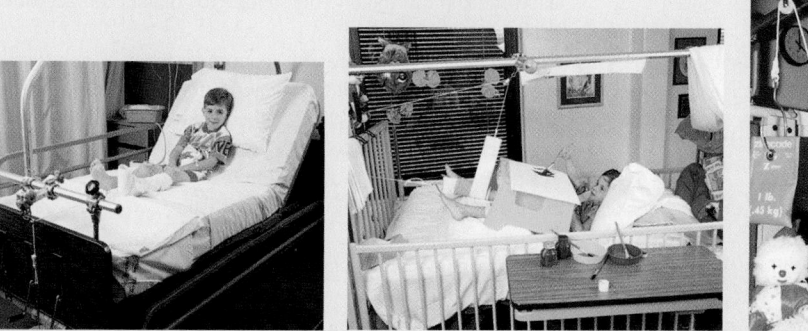

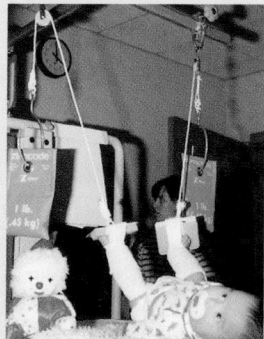

Figure 13–31 ● Buck traction.   **Figure 13–32** ● Russell traction.   **Figure 13–33** ● Bryant traction.   **Figure 13–34** ● Halo traction.

Source: Image courtesy of Ossur, Inc.

(continued on next page)

Box 13–4 Common Traction Methods (continued)

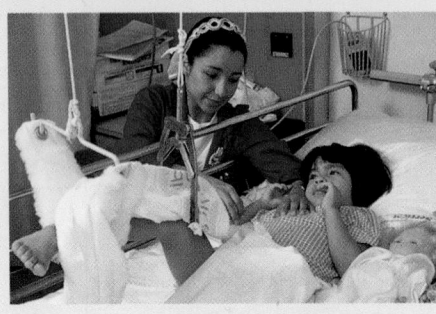

Figure 13–35 ● 90–90 traction.

■ *Balanced suspension traction* uses both skeletal traction and suspension to support the injured limb. One example is traction for a fractured femur. A Thomas leg splint is applied to the thigh, and a Pearson attachment is attached to the Thomas splint at the knee by clamps. A sling supports the lower leg and provides knee flexion. A footplate is used to support the foot. Weights are attached to both the Thomas splint and the Pearson attachment. The thigh is suspended at a 45-degree angle, while the lower leg is horizontal with the bed.

the bone under sterile conditions while the client is under local or general anesthesia. Weights (usually around 25 pounds) are then attached to the implanted hardware in one or more directions to maintain the fracture in correct alignment. The most common types of skeletal traction include Dunlop traction, skeletal cervical traction, halo traction, 90–90 traction, and balanced suspension traction (see Box 13–4). Skeletal pins and other hardware must be cleaned frequently to reduce the risk of infection. If a pin becomes infected, the nurse should notify the client's physician. The pin may need to be removed and placed elsewhere, or the client may need to use skin traction instead of skeletal traction. In addition, the client with a pin infection should be treated with antibiotics. Nursing interventions for clients receiving traction are described in **Box 13–5** ●.

NONPHARMACOLOGIC PAIN MANAGEMENT Nonpharmacologic management of pain for clients with bone fractures includes RICE therapy (rest, ice, compression, and elevation). Compression should be enough to provide support for the injured area, as is provided by a cast or splint, but it should not decrease blood flow to the area and cause compartment syndrome. For nonpharmacologic nursing interventions related to pain management, see **Box 13–6** ● and the exemplar on Acute and Chronic Pain in the module on Comfort.

■ NURSING PROCESS

Nursing care for clients with a fracture includes pain management, client teaching, assessment for complications, and emotional support. Each client's needs will depend on the location and severity of the fracture and the emotional trauma of the situation that caused the fracture.

Assessment

Assessment of a client with a fracture includes obtaining a health history and performing a physical examination. Depending on the severity of the fracture, a physical examination may need to be performed frequently to assess for complications. The health history should include the client's age; a history of chronic illnesses that may increase risk for complications; medications, especially anticoagulants; a history of previous musculoskeletal injuries; the client's normal activity level; and the history of the event that caused the fracture.

Physical assessment should include an assessment of distal pulses in the injured extremity, edema and swelling, skin color and temperature, deformity, range of motion, and sensation. A 5 P's neurovascular assessment should also be conducted, which includes assessment of pain, pulses, pallor, paresthesia, and

Box 13–5 Nursing Interventions for Clients in Traction

■ Teach the client and family about the type and purpose of traction.
■ In skeletal traction:
  – Never remove the weights.
  – Include pin care per policy in frequent skin assessments.
  – Report signs of infection at the pin site, such as redness, drainage, and increased tenderness.
  – Administer analgesics more frequently if needed.
■ In skin traction:
  – Remove weights only when intermittent skin traction has been ordered to alleviate muscle spasm.
  – Frequently assess skin for evidence of pressure, shearing, or pending breakdown.
  – Protect pressure sites with padding and protective dressings as indicated.
■ Maintain the line of pull as follows:
  – Center the client on the bed.
  – Ensure that the weights hang freely and do not touch the floor.

■ Ensure that nothing is lying on or obstructing the ropes. Do not allow the knots at the end of the rope to come in contact with the pulley.
■ For traction to be successful, counter traction is necessary. In most instances, the counter traction is the client's weight. Therefore, do not wedge the client's foot or place it flush with the footboard of the bed.
■ If a problem is detected, assist in repositioning the client. The area of the fracture must be stabilized when the client is repositioned.
■ Perform neurovascular assessments frequently.
■ Encourage the client to perform deep breathing exercises; assess lung function using a peak flow meter or spirometer.
■ Assess for common complications of immobility, including pressure ulcers, renal calculi, DVT, pneumonia, paralytic ileus, and loss of appetite.

Box 13–6   Nursing Interventions for Pain in the Client With a Bone Fracture

Pain associated with a bone fracture is often severe and may slow the healing process or be an indication of a complication such as compartment syndrome or deep venous thrombosis. The location, duration, and etiology of pain should be determined before analgesics are given. After the cause of pain is identified, several nursing interventions may be implemented:

1. Administer analgesics as prescribed. Analgesics may include NSAIDs or opioids, and they may be administered orally, by IV, or through a patient-controlled analgesic pump. Analgesics should be given around the clock for the first 24–48 hours. If medications are given PRN, the nurse should remind the client to request medication before the pain becomes severe. Addiction to opioids is not likely if taken as prescribed for the recommended duration.

2. Elevate the injured area and apply ice packs to decrease swelling.
3. Drain fluids from drainage devices (such as a Hemovac drain) and monitor the drainage for possible hematoma.
4. Encourage the client to move frequently, including changing positions to relieve pressure, wiggling fingers or toes to improve circulation, and ambulating to reduce complications.
5. Teach the client alternative methods of pain management, including relaxation, distraction, imagery, and social interaction.
6. Notify the physician of unrelieved pain, and advocate for increased pharmacologic intervention or assessment for complications such as compartment syndrome.

Clinical Manifestations and Therapies Fractures and Complications

ETIOLOGY	CLINICAL MANIFESTATIONS	CLINICAL THERAPIES
Bone fracture	■ Pain ■ Fracture on x-ray ■ Swelling, deformity, numbness ■ Loss of blood, crepitus	■ Immobilization (casts, traction) ■ Surgical repair ■ Analgesics for pain ■ RICE therapy (rest, ice, compression, elevation)
Compartment syndrome	■ Edema, swelling, ischemia ■ Severe pain, tenderness ■ Paresthesia, numbness, paralysis ■ Absent distal pulse ■ Poikilothermia ■ Skin discoloration (pallor, cyanosis) ■ Renal failure (late symptom)	■ Removal of tight cast ■ Fasciotomy ■ Ice ■ Elevation
Deep venous thrombosis	■ Redness, warmth ■ Leg pain, cramping, swelling ■ Dislodged clots (emboli) may cause stroke, pulmonary embolism, or myocardial infarction.	Treatment: ■ Bed rest ■ Anticoagulants ■ Thrombolytics ■ Surgical insertion of filter Prevention: ■ Early immobilization of the fracture ■ Regular exercise ■ Early ambulation ■ Compression stockings or boots
Fat embolism syndrome	■ Dyspnea, respiratory failure ■ Petechial rash ■ Confusion, seizures, coma ■ Purtscher retinopathy ■ Fever	■ Administer oxygen ■ Mechanical ventilation ■ Corticosteroids ■ Early immobilization of injury
Infection	■ Warmth, redness ■ Pain, swelling, stiffness ■ Fever, chills ■ Purulent drainage	■ Antibiotics ■ Analgesics ■ Antipyretics ■ Wound hygiene ■ Amputation

paralysis/paresis. For further description of the 5 P's assessment, see the Concept of Mobility section within this module.

Diagnosis

Examples of nursing diagnoses for the client with a fracture may include the following:

- *Risk for Peripheral Neurovascular Dysfunction* related to compression of nerves
- *Risk for Ineffective Tissue Perfusion* related to impaired circulation and potential thrombus formation
- *Risk for Infection* related to surgical incision and insertion of hardware
- *Impaired Skin Integrity* related to open bone fracture
- *Acute Pain* related to bone and soft tissue damage
- *Impaired Physical Mobility* related to fractured femur
- *Risk for Disuse Syndrome* related to use of traction to stabilize fracture
- *Deficient Knowledge* related to cast care
- *Disturbed Body Image* related to halo traction
- *Anxiety* related to external fixation.

(NANDA-I © 2012)

Planning

Planning care for the client with a bone fracture will depend on the location and severity of the injury and the prescribed treatment by the physician. For example, a client with a tibia fracture who needs a cast will require very different care from that needed by a client with arm, leg, and spine fractures that need traction or surgery. Common goals for clients with fractures may include the following:

- The client will not demonstrate signs or symptoms of a wound infection from an open fracture, skeletal pins, or surgical incision.
- The client will develop no neurovascular complications related to the fracture or treatment.
- The client will regain full function in the injured extremity.
- The client will describe pain as less than 3 on a scale of 0–10.

Implementation

The primary goals of nursing care for a client with a fracture include managing pain, maintaining proper fracture alignment, promoting mobility, monitoring for neurovascular status, preventing infections, and providing discharge instructions. If surgical treatment is required, the nurse may also prepare the client for hospital admission or transfer to the surgery department. In a community setting, nursing care may involve administering first aid and arranging for transport of the client to an emergency department.

Provide Effective Pain Management

The nurse should regularly assess the client for pain and for muscle spasms and swelling, which may increase pain. Vital signs should be monitored. The nurse should administer pain medications as prescribed and monitor the effectiveness of pain medications to advocate for stronger pain relief if needed. Nursing

interventions to reduce pain include elevating the injured extremity, providing ice to reduce swelling, and using nonpharmacologic methods to reduce pain, such as distraction, deep breathing, and relaxation techniques. When the nurse needs to move the client, movement should be performed gently and slowly to reduce pain and muscle spasms, and the injured extremity should be supported above and below the fracture site to prevent displacement of bony fragments and nerve damage.

Maintain Proper Alignment

Proper alignment of the fractured bones is essential to prevent malunion of the fracture. A splint, a cast, traction, or internal or external fixation will be applied to reduced fractures to immobilize the joints and hold the bones in place. The nurse is responsible for providing verbal and written instructions to the client and family for splint or cast care. When caring for clients in traction, the nurse is responsible for helping the client maintain proper body alignment with the weight and pulley systems as well as ensuring that the weights are always hanging freely. Clients with internal or external fixation will need instructions on weight bearing and care of external pins.

Promote Mobility

Fractures of the hips and lower extremities alter the client's gait and mobility. The nurse is responsible for assisting with ambulation as soon as allowed by the physician. Early ambulation increases circulation and reduces the risk of complications, especially DVT. If ambulation is restricted, such as for clients in traction, the nurse should help the client with passive and active exercises in the uninjured limbs to maintain blood flow and strengthen muscles. The client should also be repositioned every 1 or 2 hours to prevent skin breakdown. Promoting mobility may also include teaching clients how to use assistive devices such as crutches or a walker or referring the client to a physical therapist. Proper use of assistive devices increases client safety and decreases risk of further injury. For clients with a hip or pelvis fracture, client mobility may require a wheelchair or wheeled cart.

Monitor Neurovascular Status

The client's neurovascular status should be monitored using the 5 P's neurovascular assessment (see the Concept of Mobility portion within this module for review of the 5 P's neurovascular assessment). The injured limb should be assessed for swelling, cramping, temperature, hematoma, movement, capillary refill, and sensation to touch. The client should be assessed every 15 minutes for the first 2 hours after a cast is applied and every 1–2 hours thereafter depending on facility policy and the client's condition. Report abnormal findings immediately, because they could indicate a life- or limb-threatening complication such as compartment syndrome or DVT. A cast saw should be readily available for emergent cast removal or bivalving (**Figure 13–36 ●**), which may become necessary in the event of emergent swelling. If compartment syndrome is suspected, the nurse should assist the physician in measuring compartment pressure. Pressure greater than 30 mmHg indicates compartment syndrome, and a fasciotomy may be needed. If DVT is suspected or diagnosed, the nurse should administer anticoagulants as prescribed.

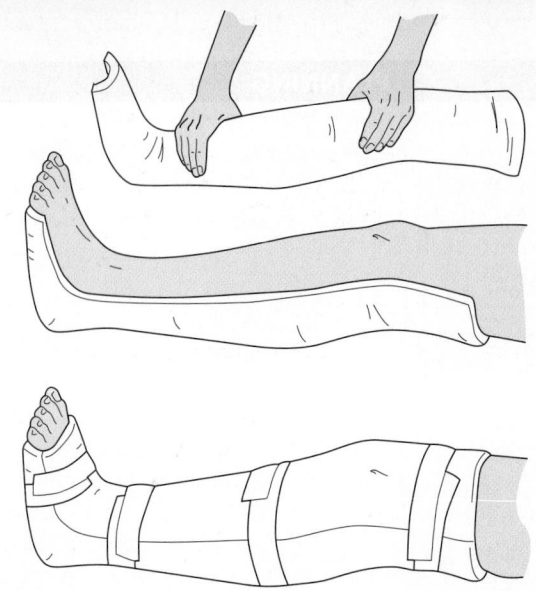

Figure 13–36 ● Bivalving is the process of splitting the cast down both sides to alleviate pressure on or allow visualization of the extremity.

Prevent Infection

Clients with open fractures, surgical repair, or skeletal pins are at increased risk of infection from the wound. Clients with a cast or skin traction and those on bed rest may also be at risk for infection if the skin develops pressure ulcers. For general care of wounds, see the exemplar on Wound Healing in the module on Tissue Integrity. Nursing interventions related to monitoring fracture-related wounds for infection include providing skeletal pin care, drawing blood to monitor white blood cell counts,

obtaining culture samples, checking vital signs, using sterile technique to change dressings, and assessing the wound for signs of infection and drainage. Skeletal pin care will differ based on facility guidelines and physician preference, but may include gently cleansing the pin site daily to weekly with a cleansing solution such as sterile saline or chlorhexidine to remove crusts from the pins. The nurse should administer antibiotics as prescribed. Prophylactic antibiotics may be given for wounds with a high risk of infection, such as wounds related to a motor vehicle crash.

Provide Discharge Instructions

Most clients will receive emergency care for a fracture and return home the same day. Discharge instructions are an important aspect of nursing care for these clients. Teaching topics include cast care, activity restrictions, taking pain medications before pain becomes severe, signs of complications, and injury prevention. Clients with leg fractures who must use stairs may need special instructions for crutches, or they may need a referral to have a temporary or permanent ramp installed. A referral to home health care may be needed for older clients.

Evaluation

Evaluation of the client depends on the location and severity of the fracture as well as the treatment received. Evaluation may include analysis of bone healing with x-rays, assessment of the client's pain and neurovascular status, assessment of the client's range of motion and ability to ambulate independently, and assessment for other complications. Client goals should include full function of the affected body part with no prolonged complications.

NURSING CARE PLAN A Client With an Arm Fracture

Anthony Mandel, a 15-year-old male, enjoys mountain biking with his friends on park trails. Today, while attempting to jump a hill while cycling, Anthony lost control of his bike and flipped forward over the handle bars, landing on his extended left arm. He felt and heard a bone snap, and he could see bone through a wound in his left arm. His friends called Anthony's mother, who rushed to the scene and transported Anthony to the emergency department (ED).

ASSESSMENT	DIAGNOSES	PLANNING
Upon admission to the ED, the dorsal aspect of Anthony's left distal forearm reveals a 4-inch laceration with obvious deformity. Fractured bone is visible. He denies hitting his head, losing consciousness, or any other injuries. Anthony is pale, anxious, and complaining of pain. The digits on his left hand are warm and pink, and radial pulses are strong and equal bilaterally. Anthony denies numbness or tingling in his left arm or hand, but he continues to complain of pain, which he rates as 10 on a scale of 0–10, with 10 being the worst. Anthony's vital signs include temperature 98.9°F oral; pulse 102 bpm; respirations 20/min; and BP 119/68 mmHg. An x-ray reveals a fractured left distal radius. The ED nurse inserts an intravenous access device in	■ *Risk for Infection* related to compound fracture ■ *Risk for Ineffective Peripheral Tissue Perfusion* related to bone fracture and splint ■ *Impaired Skin Integrity* related to open fracture of left distal radius ■ *Acute Pain* related to left distal radius fracture ■ *Fear* related to unknown diagnosis and treatment ■ *Deficient Knowledge* related to manifestations of complications related to bone fracture (NANDA-I © 2012)	■ The client will maintain normal distal pulse, capillary refill, and sensation in fingers. ■ The client's wound will demonstrate no signs or symptoms of infection ■ The client will verbalize a pain intensity of less than 3 on a scale of 0–10. ■ The client and mother will demonstrate knowledge of signs and symptoms to report to the physician immediately. ■ The client and mother will verbalize understanding of cast care. ■ The client's fear will be diminished after diagnosis and treatment. ■ The client and mother will demonstrate knowledge of and practice good wound hygiene.

(continued on next page)

NURSING CARE PLAN (continued)

ASSESSMENT	DIAGNOSES	PLANNING
Anthony's right hand, and he is sedated with midazolam (Versed) 1 mg IV and given fentanyl 50 mcg IV for analgesia. After requesting a consultation by the on-call orthopedic surgeon, the ED physician irrigates Anthony's wound and realigns the fractured bone. The ED physician then applies a sterile dressing to the wound. For stabilization and to prevent further injury to surrounding tissues, the ED physician places a splint on Anthony's left arm. After obtaining consent for surgery from Anthony's mother, the orthopedic physician orders that Anthony be scheduled for emergent ORIF of the left distal radius. Anthony's fracture is surgically repaired without incident and the surgeon applies a splint to Anthony's left forearm. He is discharged to home that evening.		

IMPLEMENTATION

- Routinely assess the client for signs and symptoms of impaired circulation in the left arm, including pallor, diminished or absent pulses, and reports of numbness or tingling.
- Protect the client's splint from contamination.
- Administer preoperative antibiotics as ordered.
- Elevate the client's injured limb above the level of his heart.

- Administer pain medication as prescribed by the physician.
- Explain the surgical admission process to the client and his mother and encourage them to ask questions.
- Teach client and mother signs and symptoms of complications related to bone fractures, including compartment syndrome and infection.

EVALUATION

Five days postoperatively, Anthony's mother transports him to the orthopedic surgeon's office for a follow-up visit. He denies complaints and reports that he is having "just a little bit of pain, maybe a one on a zero-to-ten scale." Anthony's left hand is warm, his fingers are pink and mobile, and his left radial pulse is strong. Anthony's mother reports that Anthony is taking his prophylactic antibiotic as prescribed. Anthony is scheduled for another follow-up visit in 2 weeks, at which time he remains free from complications and has no complaints. Four weeks following his injury, Anthony's cast is removed, and he begins a short course of physical therapy to regain full mobility in his injured arm.

CRITICAL THINKING

1. Why did the physicians apply a splint to Anthony's fractured arm instead of a cast?
2. Describe methods of wound cleansing that must be implemented to remove dirt and debris from the laceration on Anthony's left arm.
3. Develop a list of written discharge instructions the nurse would provide to Anthony and his mother.

REVIEW Fractures

RELATE Link the Concepts and Exemplars

Linking the exemplar on fractures with the concept of safety:

1. What safety principles can you teach children to decrease their risk for sustaining a bone fracture? Adolescents? Older adults?

2. What safety principles should you teach clients with a leg fracture? Arm fracture? Spine fracture?

Linking the exemplar on fractures with the concept of perfusion:

3. What nursing interventions will reduce the risk of deep venous thrombosis in the client in traction with a broken femur?

4. What are the nursing priorities for clients with decreased perfusion to fingers or toes?

READY Go to Companion Skills Manual

REFER Go to Pearson Student Nursing Resources
nursing.pearsonhighered.com

- Additional review materials

REFLECT Case Study

Saul Genmar is a 21-year-old man who has graduated from Harvard and is working as a car salesman. He is engaged to Joanne Bolit, who is a 19-year-old sophomore at Smith College. Ms. Bolit lives at home when she is not in school, and Mr. Genmar has an apartment with three friends. The previous night, Mr. Genmar and his friends met at a local tavern to watch a football game and drink beer. While traveling home, Mr. Genmar was involved in a one-car motor vehicle crash, during which he drove off the road in a residential area and struck a tree. Mr. Genmar's injuries were limited to his right leg, and no one else was injured. Mr. Genmar has a compound fracture of his right tibia and has returned from surgery with an external fixation device and is in traction. Ms. Bolit came to visit and is lying on the bed next to Mr. Genmar.

1. What is your priority of care for Mr. Genmar as you begin your shift?

2. How will you address the client and his girlfriend when you enter the room to deliver care?

3. What teaching interventions will you initiate for both Mr. Genmar and Ms. Bolit?

EXEMPLAR 13.3 Hip Fractures

EXEMPLAR KEY TERMS

Arthroplasty, *871*
Avascular necrosis, *869*
Extracapsular hip fracture, *869*
Hemiarthroplasty, *871*
Intracapsular hip fracture, *869*
Revision surgery, *872*

EXEMPLAR LEARNING OUTCOMES

After reading about this exemplar, you will be able to:

1. Describe the pathophysiology, etiology, clinical manifestations, and direct and indirect causes of hip fractures.

2. Identify risk factors and prevention methods associated with hip fractures.

3. Illustrate the nursing process in providing culturally competent care across the life span for individuals with hip fractures.

4. Formulate priority nursing diagnoses appropriate for an individual with a hip fracture.

5. Summarize therapies used by interdisciplinary teams in the collaborative care of an individual with a hip fracture.

6. Plan evidence-based care for an individual with a hip fracture and his or her family in collaboration with other members of the healthcare team.

7. Evaluate expected outcomes for an individual with a hip fracture.

▶ OVERVIEW

A hip fracture is a break in the neck, head, or trochanter region of the upper femur (**Figure 13–37** ●). Although hip fractures are most often associated with older adults, they can occur at any age as a result of trauma. Hip fractures often result in long-term functional impairment in older adults.

▶ PATHOPHYSIOLOGY AND ETIOLOGY

There are two types of hip fractures: intracapsular and extracapsular. Extracapsular fractures can be further divided into intertrochanteric or subtrochanteric. **Intracapsular hip fractures** occur at the head or neck of the femur within the capsule of the hip joint. **Extracapsular hip fractures** occur within the trochanter region, which is between the neck and diaphysis of the femur. *Intertrochanteric fractures* take place between the neck and the lesser or greater trochanter, whereas *subtrochanteric fractures* occur immediately below the lesser trochanter (AAOS, 2009b). In children, hip fractures may also include pelvic bones (Millis, 2011).

Hip fractures to the neck and intertrochanteric regions are the most common. Fractures of the neck are especially dangerous because the fracture often cuts off the blood supply to the head and neck of the femur, causing **avascular necrosis** (death of bone tissue due to lack of blood supply; also called osteonecrosis). This may also prevent cartilage and supporting bone from receiving adequate blood, leading to arthritis (AAOS,

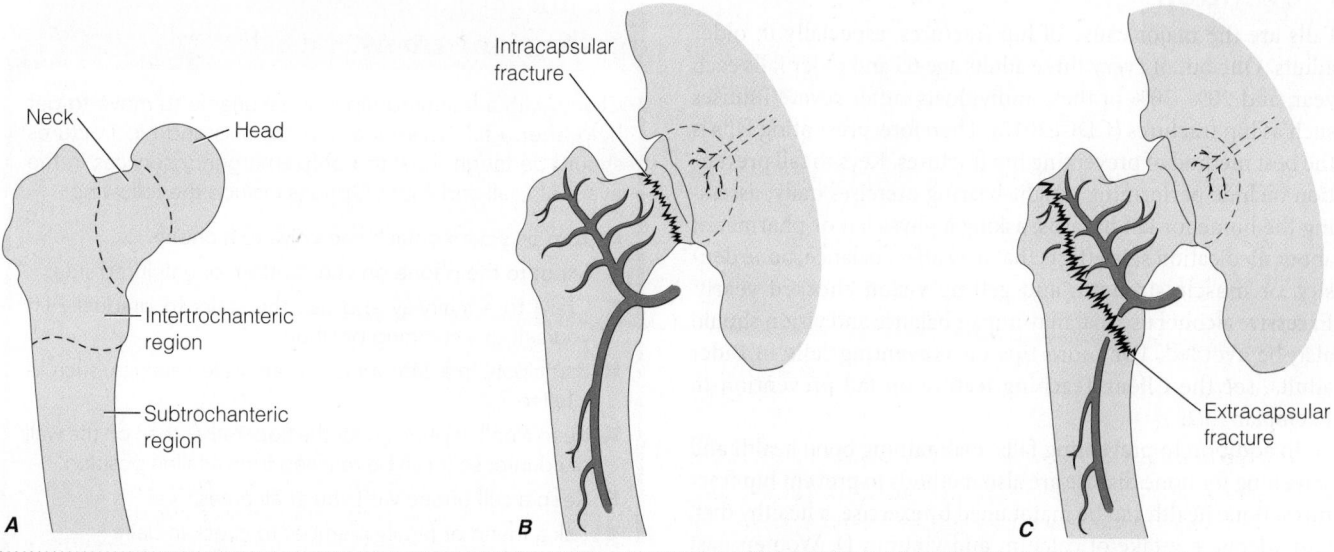

Figure 13–37 ● Regions where hip fractures may occur: *A,* The head of the femur, the neck of the femur, and the trochanteric regions of the femur. *B,* Intracapsular fractures occur across the head or neck of the femur. *C,* Extracapsular fractures occur across the trochanteric regions.

2009b). Extracapsular hip fractures are less likely to develop avascular necrosis due to a more diverse blood supply.

Etiology

Hip fractures are usually the result of trauma, such as a fall or motor vehicle crash. In older adults, a hip fracture is most often the result of falling sideways from a standing height onto the hip. Individuals with weak bones may suffer a hip fracture from simply standing on the leg and twisting (AAOS, 2009b; Mayo Clinic, 2012a). The most common causes of hip fractures in children are car and bike crashes, whereas teens are likely to suffer hip fractures due to sports injuries (Millis, 2011). Adults may fracture a hip as the result of a car crash, a fall from a great height, or other severe trauma.

Risk Factors

The greatest risk factors for a hip fracture are old age and osteoporosis. Hip fracture rates increase exponentially with age; adults ages 85 and older are 10–15 times more likely to sustain a hip fracture than adults ages 60–65 (Centers for Disease Control and Prevention [CDC], 2010). Older age is associated with osteoporosis, decreased muscle mass, vision and balance problems, and a slower reaction time. Osteoporosis occurs when new bone is not formed as quickly as the old bone is removed, causing bones to become brittle and less dense. Women after menopause are at an increased risk of developing osteoporosis. Women sustain approximately 75% of all hip fractures, and White women are more likely to sustain a hip fracture than Black or Asian women (CDC, 2010).

Other risk factors for hip fractures include chronic medical conditions that cause fragile bones, such as endocrine disorders, intestinal disorders, or cancer; some medications that weaken bone or cause dizziness; nutritional problems such as eating disorders or lack of calcium or vitamin D; physical inactivity, especially lack of weight-bearing exercise; and tobacco and alcohol use (Mayo Clinic, 2012a).

Prevention

Falls are the major cause of hip fractures, especially in older adults. One out of every three adults age 65 and older falls each year, and 20%–30% of these individuals suffer severe injuries such as hip fractures (CDC, 2012). Therefore, preventing falls is the best method of preventing hip fractures. Keys to fall prevention include performing weight-bearing exercises daily; assessing the home for fall hazards; asking a physician or pharmacist about medication side effects that may affect balance, bone density, or muscle strength; and getting vision checked yearly. Excessive alcohol use that may impair balance and vision should also be avoided. For more tips on preventing falls in older adults, see the Client Teaching feature on fall prevention in Exemplar 13.2.

In addition to preventing falls, maintaining bone health and screening for bone disease are also methods to prevent hip fractures. Bone health can be maintained by exercise, a healthy diet, and adequate intake of calcium and vitamin D. Women past menopause who are not taking estrogen should consume 1,500 mg of calcium daily; all other adults should consume 1,000 mg of calcium daily. The U.S. Preventive Services Task Force (2011)

recommends osteoporosis screenings for all women ages 65 and older and for women younger than age 65 who are at high risk for osteoporosis. Tests to screen for osteoporosis include dual-energy x-ray absorptiometry of the hip and lumbar spine and quantitative ultrasonography of the calcaneus.

A mobility assessment is essential to assessing an older adult's risk of falls. This should include assessing the client's gait, balance, and ability to change position. For example, the nurse should monitor the client's ability to get up from a chair, turn while walking, raise the foot completely off the floor, and sit down. Difficulty with any of these tasks increases the client's risk for falls. The World Health Organization provides the Fracture Risk Assessment (FRAX®) tool to help estimate a client's risk of fracture, including hip fracture, at www.shef.ac.uk/FRAX/index.aspx.

▶ CLINICAL MANIFESTATIONS

Clients with a hip fracture will experience severe pain in the hip, upper thigh, groin, or lower back, especially when attempting to flex or rotate the hip. They may be unable to move, stand, or walk (see the Client Teaching feature). The client may feel stiffness as well as bruising and swelling in the hip area. The leg on the side of the injured hip may appear shorter than the uninjured leg and may turn outward. In severe injuries, bone may be visible through the skin.

Hip fractures are usually the result of trauma. Therefore, other injuries may also be present, such as additional bone fractures, head injuries, or damage to the intestines, bladder, or reproductive organs.

Complications

Complications associated with a hip fracture are the result of a major loss of mobility and include deep venous thrombosis, pressure ulcers, urinary tract infections (UTIs), pneumonia,

Client Teaching
Calling for Help After a Fall

Clients with a fractured hip may be unable to move to get help after a fall. Clients at risk for falls and hip fractures should be taught how to notify emergency services in the event of a fall and injury. Options include the following:

- Turn on your stomach and crawl to a phone.
- Scoot to the phone on your bottom or uninjured side.
- Crawl to a stairway and use the stairs to gradually lift yourself to a standing position.
- Participate in a 24-hour emergency alert service, such as Lifeline.
- Keep a bell or phone near the floor rather than on the wall or counter so it can be reached from a fallen position.
- Keep a cell phone with you at all times.
- Ask a friend or family member to check in daily.
- Cover up with a blanket and try to stay warm until help arrives.

and muscle atrophy. Other complications include postoperative infection, mental deterioration, avascular necrosis, and non-union or malunion of the bone.

Most older adults with a hip fracture lose their ability to live independently for at least a year after the injury, and some will remain in a long-term care facility for the rest of their lives. It is estimated that only one in four individuals will fully recover from a hip fracture. Hip fracture increases the risk of death approximately threefold; about 20%–27% of older adults with a hip fracture will die within a year of their injury. Although men are less likely to sustain a hip fracture than women, a higher percentage of men die as a result of hip fracture complications (CDC, 2010; Panula et al., 2011).

Lifespan and Cultural Considerations

Hip fractures in children, adolescents, and young adults are often due to sports injuries or motor vehicle crashes. Children's bones heal more quickly than adults' and therefore need prompt medical attention to set the fracture and immobilize the joint. Hip fractures in children may involve the epiphyseal plate, which lies between the head and neck of the femur; physicians must account for epiphyseal plates in bones when performing treatment. Treatment for hip fractures in children often involves casting or repair surgery rather than hip replacement surgery.

▶ COLLABORATION

Collaborative care team members for a client with a hip fracture may include nurses, treating physicians (e.g., orthopedic surgeon and the client's primary care physician), pharmacists, and physical and occupational therapists. The nurse should also collaborate with any specialists the client may consult for specific conditions, especially respiratory and cardiac conditions. If the client needs rehabilitative care after discharge from an acute care facility, the nurse may refer the client to social services.

Diagnostic Tests

Diagnosis of a fractured hip is based on a physical exam and imaging tests. A fractured hip is usually evident based on the abnormal position of the leg and hip. X-rays are the primary imaging tool used to diagnose hip fractures and determine the location of the fracture. CT scans and MRIs can also be used to detect hairline fractures that are not visible by x-ray.

Surgery

The first-line treatment for a hip fracture is surgery. Surgery should take place as soon as possible after the fracture; ideally, the client should be taken to a healthcare facility that offers 24-hour surgical care. The type of surgery will depend on the condition of the client and the location and severity of the fracture. The goal of surgery is to reduce pain, stabilize the fracture, and return the client to a normal activity level. The three basic types of surgery are repair with hardware, partial hip replacement, and total hip replacement.

Repair of an intracapsular fracture often involves using individual screws (percutaneous pinning) or a single larger screw (compression hip screw) that slides within the barrel of a plate.

If the fracture is displaced, open reduction and internal fixation surgery will be conducted to realign the fracture. If damage is only to the head of the femur, the goal of surgery is to repair the cartilage that has been injured. If the acetabulum, or socket of the hip, is fractured, it may require surgical repair as well.

Repair of an extracapsular fracture involves the use of a compression hip screw similar to an intracapsular fracture or the insertion of an intramedullary nail into the marrow canal of the bone through an opening made in the greater trochanter. The nail is secured in place by screws at the top and bottom of the nail. Alternatively, a plate may be used on the outside of the bone to immobilize the fracture (AAOS, 2009b).

In older clients with avascular necrosis, severe fracture, or other underlying bone conditions, hip replacement may be the best treatment option. Hip replacement can involve replacement of the ball, or head, of the femur (**hemiarthroplasty**), or replacement of the ball and socket, or head and acetabulum (total hip replacement, or **arthroplasty**). Total hip replacement is often the best option for clients with previous joint damage from arthritis.

Several hardware options are available for hip replacements. Some prostheses for head replacement are made from a single casting, such as the Austin-Moore prosthesis (**Figure 13–38 ●**). More modern prostheses are modular, allowing different combinations of stem, neck length, and head (**Figure 13–39 ●**). This allows an individualized fit of the prosthesis. In addition, the prosthesis can be cemented or uncemented during surgery. Uncemented prostheses are placed into a medullary canal that has been shaped for a snug fit of the prosthesis. It often contains a porous surface that promotes bony ingrowth to stabilize the prosthesis. Alternately, a smaller prosthesis can be used and cemented into the larger canal with methyl-methacrylate cement (Raaymakers et al., 2010). Uncemented prostheses generally have a longer recovery time because it takes a long time for the natural bone to grow and attach to the prosthesis; they

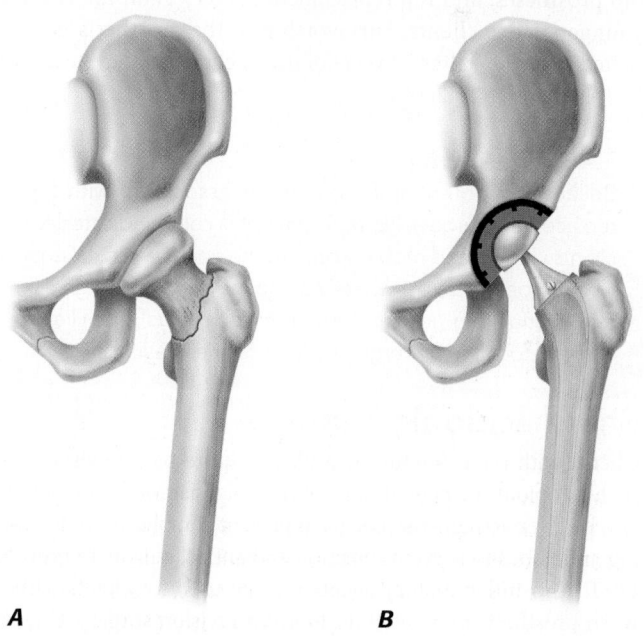

Figure 13–38 ● *A*, A hip fracture and *B*, repair with an Austin-Moore prosthesis.

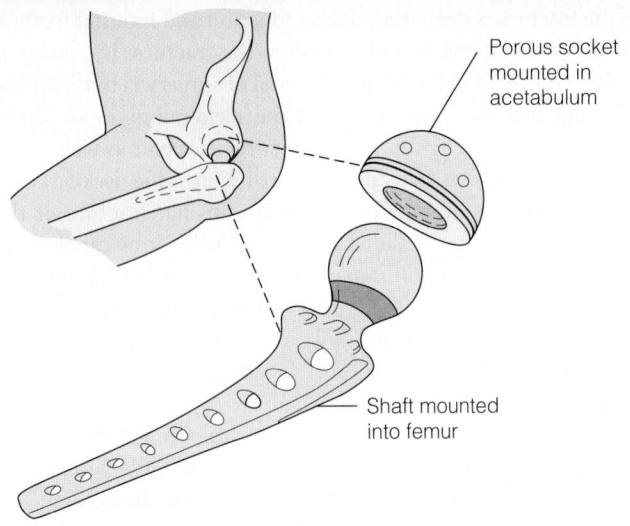

Porous socket
mounted in
acetabulum

Shaft mounted
into femur

Figure 13–39 ● Total hip prosthesis.

are often used for younger, more active clients with good bone growth rates (NIAMSD, 2012b).

Complications associated with hip replacement include dislocation of the prosthesis, infection, and delayed healing. Hip dislocation occurs because the artificial ball and socket are smaller than the original bone, allowing the ball to become dislodged in certain positions, such as when the knee is pulled up to the chest. In addition, failure of the prosthesis may occur. Over time, particles wear off the joint surfaces, causing inflammation and loosening of the prosthesis. After 10 or more years of wear, this may create a need for **revision surgery**, or replacement of the artificial joint. Revision surgery carries greater risk than the original hip replacement surgery (NIAMSD, 2012b). For this reason, internal fixation or casting of the fractured hip is traditionally preferred over hip replacement in younger clients. However, newer technology is increasing the longevity of hip prostheses, and hip replacement surgery is on the rise for younger, active clients. Survivorship of the prosthesis is estimated to be 90% after 20 years of use in clients under the age of 55 (Aldinger et al., 2009).

SAFETY ALERT
Because of potential complications associated with hip replacement surgery, hip replacement is contraindicated for clients with limited mobility prior to the fracture (e.g., clients who are bedridden or wheelchair bound), clients at high risk for infection (e.g., immunocompromised clients), and clients who are too ill to undergo any form of anesthesia.

Pharmacologic Therapy

Clients with a hip fracture will likely require pain medications, such as opioids or patient-controlled analgesia. Medications may also be given to high-risk clients to prevent complications, including antibiotics to prevent infection and anticoagulants to prevent DVT. Anti-inflammatory agents may be used for clients with a worn prosthesis in an attempt to avoid revision surgery. Clients may also receive bone density enhancers (e.g., bisphosphonates) to help stimulate bone growth, especially if a noncemented prosthesis is implanted or if the client is at risk for a second hip fracture.

Nonpharmacologic Therapy

For clients who cannot undergo surgery or who have a stable hip fracture, a hip fracture will be managed by nonsurgical methods, including bed rest, traction, or casting. Traction will likely include either Buck or Russell traction (see Box 13–4). Traction may also be used briefly for clients awaiting surgery. Casting will likely involve a hip spica cast, such as the one-and-one half hip spica cast shown in Figure 13–29. Treatment will also involve prevention of complications, including exercise and compression stockings to prevent muscle stiffness and DVT and respiratory exercises to prevent pneumonia.

After surgery, nonpharmacologic therapy will include rehabilitation such as physical and occupational therapy. Early mobility is encouraged; many clients will begin ambulation on the day after surgery. Physical therapy will include ROM and strengthening exercises, and occupational therapy will help the client gain independence in ADLs and may include learning how to use a wheelchair or walker.

■ NURSING PROCESS

Nursing care for the client with a hip fracture includes managing pain, promoting mobility, and preventing complications such as infection and DVT. Nursing care may also involve referring the client to physical or occupational therapists, home health care, or assistive device supply stores. In addition, nurses should provide emotional support and encouragement for the client, who likely faces a long and complicated recovery.

Assessment

A preoperative nursing assessment of the client with a hip fracture begins by obtaining vital signs and performing a physical assessment of the injured hip, looking for shortening and external rotation of the leg, mobility status, and loss of skin integrity related to a compound fracture or skin abrasions from the fall or accident. The nurse should assess the client for degree of injury (including hematoma, inflammation, and swelling), cognitive function, and pain level. The client's neurovascular status should be assessed by using the 5 P's, comparing neurovascular responses in the injured limb to the uninjured limb (see Exemplar 13.2 elsewhere in this module).

SAFETY ALERT
Paralysis is a sign of severe nerve damage and should be reported to the physician immediately.

The nurse should obtain a medical history, including a history of the current traumatic event and a past history of osteoporosis or other conditions that affect strength, mobility, balance, and coordination. Because hip fractures often occur in older clients and clients are at higher risk for developing complications as they age, obtaining the client's age is a vital part of the nursing assessment. A history of other medical conditions or medications that may affect the client's treatment should also be noted. To complete the nursing assessment, the nurse may be responsible for arranging and transporting the client to imaging procedures such as an x-ray.

Clinical Manifestations and Therapies **Hip Fracture**

ETIOLOGY	CLINICAL MANIFESTATIONS	CLINICAL THERAPIES
Intracapsular hip fracture	■ Fracture to the head or neck of femur ■ Pain in the hip region ■ Inability to move or stand, outward turn of the leg, shorter leg on injured side	■ Repaired with individual screws or compression hip screw with plate ■ Repair of damaged cartilage ■ Hemiarthroplasty or arthroplasty ■ Analgesics ■ Prophylactic antibiotics or anticoagulants ■ Bisphosphonates ■ Traction or casting ■ Physical and occupational therapy
Extracapsular hip fracture	■ Fracture to the trochanter region of the femur ■ Pain in the hip region ■ Inability to move or stand, outward turn of the leg, shorter leg on injured side	■ Repaired with compression hip screw or intramedullary nail in marrow canal or plate on outside of bone ■ Analgesics ■ Prophylactic antibiotics or anticoagulants ■ Bisphosphonates ■ Traction or casting ■ Physical or occupational therapy

Postoperative assessment of the client with a hip fracture involves many of the same assessments that were conducted preoperatively, including vital signs, pain intensity, cognitive dysfunction, and the 5 P's neurovascular assessment. (See the Concept of Mobility portion of this module for a review of the 5 P's neurovascular assessment.) In addition, assessment should include the client's ability to ambulate, oxygenation status, presence of infection of the surgical incision, urinary or bowel complications associated with anesthesia and immobility, and signs of DVT.

Diagnosis

Examples of nursing diagnoses that may be appropriate for inclusion in the plan of care for the client with a hip fracture may include the following:

- *Risk for Infection* related to surgical incision
- *Acute Pain* related to fractured hip
- *Impaired Physical Mobility* related to inability to move hip joint
- *Impaired Skin Integrity* related to skin abrasions
- *Risk for Falls* related to insufficient strength and balance
- *Acute Confusion* related to traumatic event
- *Anxiety* related to lengthy rehabilitation process
- *Deficient Knowledge* related to treatment options for fractured hip
- *Stress Overload* related to multiple severe injuries and their treatment
- *Caregiver Role Strain* related to caring for an individual with limited mobility.

(NANDA-I © 2012)

Planning

Goals for the client with a hip fracture may include the following:

- The client will achieve adequate pain control, as evidenced by reports of pain that rate no higher than 3 on a scale of 0–10.

- The client will ambulate independently after surgery and rehabilitation.
- The client will have adequate wound healing of skin abrasions.
- The client will not develop an infection from wounds or surgical incisions.
- The client will demonstrate increased muscle strength and balance.
- The client will be oriented to time, location, and environment.
- The client will verbalize decreased anxiety with understanding of the rehabilitation process.
- The client will verbalize an understanding of treatment options for a hip fracture.
- The client will implement nonpharmacologic methods to reduce stress.
- The client's caregiver will ask for help when needed to provide relief from caregiver responsibilities.

Implementation

Nursing interventions for clients with a hip fracture are similar to general recommendations for clients with other types of bone fractures, including managing pain, maintaining proper alignment, promoting mobility, monitoring the client's neurovascular status, and monitoring for infection (see Exemplar 13.2). Other nursing interventions include pre- and postoperative interventions, emotional care, and instructions for home care.

Plan Effective Preoperative and Postoperative Care

The majority of clients with a hip fracture will undergo surgery to repair or replace the injured hip. Preoperative interventions include pain management, immobilization of the hip with traction or other restraints, and providing information about the treatment plan. Preoperative care may also include administering prescribed prophylactic antibiotics and transporting the client to surgery.

Postoperative nursing interventions are aimed at managing pain, promoting mobility, and preventing complications. The client should be taught about correct positioning of the hip to prevent hip displacement after arthroplasty. The nurse should help the client with passive and active exercises, assist with ambulation as soon as prescribed by the physician, and teach the client about signs and symptoms of DVT. Anticoagulants should be administered as prescribed to prevent DVT. Clients who are bedridden should perform respiratory exercises to maintain lung function and should be monitored for signs of pneumonia and other respiratory complications. Bedridden clients and clients with limited mobility should be turned frequently to prevent pressure ulcers. Good wound hygiene should be used for the surgical incision and any other skin wounds; infections should be treated promptly with antibiotics.

Promote Psychosocial Wellness

Although physical care of the client is important for recovery after a hip fracture, emotional and mental care of the client is also a major nursing intervention needed for clients with a hip fracture. Whether the client is younger and has experienced a traumatic motor vehicle crash or sports injury or is older and experienced a fall in the home, a hip fracture causes emotional distress related to the traumatic event. Most clients will experience anxiety or fear related to extreme pain, an unknown diagnosis and treatment plan, or a poor prognosis. Older clients may experience confusion as a result of the trauma or surgery, and they also may feel despair over their loss of independence.

Nursing interventions may include the following:

- Encourage the client and family to share their feelings about the traumatic event as well as treatment and long-term care options.
- Provide information about the client's condition and explain the treatment plan.
- Provide verbal and written instructions for care.

- Orient the client to the time, day, place, and situation.
- Refer the client and family to a home health agency, rehabilitation center, or long-term care facility.
- Promote a trusting relationship so the client can express concerns and ask questions about her condition or treatment plan.
- Support the use of coping mechanisms to decrease stress, including the use of family, friends, and support services.

Provide Thorough Discharge Instructions

The client who has had surgery for a hip fracture will need extensive care after leaving the hospital. This may be provided at home or in a rehabilitation or long-term care facility. Clients who will be cared for at home and their caregivers will need proper training to ensure maximal healing. Topics for instruction include the following:

- Proper use of an abduction pillow while resting or sleeping to maintain proper hip alignment.
- Proper sitting and bending techniques, including sitting on a high chair and using a high toilet seat to prevent excess flexion of the hip.
- Proper use of a walker or cane.
- Explanation of weight-bearing limitations as prescribed by the physician.
- Explanation of all medications, including dosage, schedule, and potential side effects.
- Referral to physical therapists, home care agencies, or local medical equipment sources as needed.

Evaluation

The client should be evaluated for return of mobility, absence of neurological complications, a decrease in pain, and complications from the fracture and from surgery. Evaluation should also include assessment of the client's emotional state as he progresses throughout treatment. Participation in physical therapy and other rehabilitation programs should be evaluated to determine if the client is benefiting from the exercise and returning to full function.

NURSING CARE PLAN   Presurgical Care of a Client With a Hip Fracture

Giorgina Mancini is a 68-year-old Italian American with a history of osteoarthritis and osteoporosis. She has lived alone since her husband died 3 years ago, but she is well known in her neighborhood for providing delicious food made from scratch to anyone who stops by at mealtime. While carrying groceries up the front steps to her porch, Mrs. Mancini falls and lands on her right hip. Her neighbor, who witnesses the fall, calls 911 and Mrs. Mancini is transported by ambulance to the local emergency department.

ASSESSMENT	DIAGNOSES	PLANNING
The nurse conducting Mrs. Mancini's initial assessment finds that her right leg is externally rotated and shortened. Mrs. Mancini complains of severe pain with an intensity of 8 on a 0–10 pain scale. Her legs and feet are warm with strong pedal pulses bilaterally. She denies numbness or tingling. Mrs. Mancini is able to move the toes on her	■ *Risk for Ineffective Peripheral Tissue Perfusion* related to fractured right hip and soft tissue damage ■ *Acute Pain* related to fractured right hip and soft tissue damage ■ *Impaired Physical Mobility* related to fractured right femur and application of traction	■ The client will develop no complications related to impaired peripheral circulation. ■ The client will verbalize a decrease in pain to a 4 or less on a scale of 0–10. ■ The client will participate in passive ROM exercises.

NURSING CARE PLAN (continued)

ASSESSMENT	DIAGNOSES	PLANNING
right foot, and she has full range of motion in her left leg. Her vital signs include temperature 97.8°F oral; pulse 80 bpm; respirations 22/min; and BP 112/63 mmHg. Diagnostic tests include CBC, serum electrolytes, and x-ray studies of the right hip and pelvis. The CBC reveals a hemoglobin of 10.4 g/dL, which is slightly decreased from normal. The physician orders type and crossmatch for two units of blood. All other blood tests are within normal limits. The x-ray reveals a fracture in the right lesser trochanter region. Mrs. Mancini is admitted to the hospital with an order for 10 lb of straight leg traction. Surgery to repair the fracture with an intramedullary nail in the marrow canal is scheduled for the next morning.	■ *Impaired Skin Integrity* related to abrasions sustained during a fall ■ *Risk for Infection* related to contaminated skin wounds ■ *Impaired Social Interaction* related to not being home to provide food for visitors (NANDA-I © 2012)	■ The client will allow proper care of abrasions, including cleansing and application of a sterile bandage. ■ The client will not develop an infection of the abrasions. ■ The client will provide a phone number of a close friend or family member to be present in the hospital as needed during her recovery.

IMPLEMENTATION

■ Administer pain medications and traction as prescribed by physician.
■ Turn the client every 2 hours to prevent pressure ulcers.
■ Apply compression stockings to client's legs.
■ Conduct passive ROM exercises on the client's left leg and both arms every 4 hours while awake to enhance circulation.

■ Assess the client every 2–4 hours for neurovascular status of the right leg.
■ Clean abrasions with sterile solution and apply a sterile bandage.
■ Provide client teaching about traction and hip repair surgery.
■ Call a close friend or family member to encourage visitation of the client as tolerated.

EVALUATION

The client expressed a decrease in pain from 8 to 5 after pain medication and a further reduction to 3 after traction. The client's abrasions from the fall were cleaned and appeared minor. A sterile bandage and antibiotic ointment were applied to each abrasion. The nurse conducted passive ROM exercises for the client twice in the evening and once in the morning before surgery. Compression stockings were applied. Neurovascular checks revealed no complications. The client was prepped for surgery, including receiving preoperative teaching and prophylactic antibiotics. Several friends have visited and waited at the hospital during the surgery. A new care plan reflecting postoperative interventions will be developed.

CRITICAL THINKING

1. Prepare a document explaining the process of traction and its necessity while waiting for surgery.
2. Why is it important for Mrs. Mancini to feel connected to friends and family members during her hospital stay?
3. Develop a postoperative care plan for Mrs. Mancini.

REVIEW Hip Fractures

RELATE Link the Concepts and Exemplars

Linking the exemplar of hip fractures with the concept of health, wellness, and illness:

1. Describe the modifiable risk factors and teaching interventions for clients at risk for hip fractures.

2. In an older female client, what findings from a nutritional screening would indicate an increased risk for hip fractures? What teaching could the nurse provide to lower this risk?

Linking the exemplar of hip fractures with the concept of elimination:

3. What nursing interventions can be implemented for a client with a hip fracture who is taking opioids for pain management and has developed constipation?

4. Develop a care plan for a client with urinary retention after hip replacement surgery.

READY Go to Companion Skills Manual

REFER Go to Pearson Student Nursing Resources
nursing.pearsonhighered.com

• Additional review materials

REFLECT Case Study

Maria Haley is 65 years old and lives alone in her two-story house. Her husband Del passed away 2 years ago but left her financially comfortable if she is careful. Mrs. Haley has two grown children who are both married, but she has no grandchildren yet. Her children both live in another state. Mrs. Haley is active at the senior center in town, is an avid bridge player, and enjoys relatively good health. She is taking simvastatin 20 mg/day for a slightly elevated cholesterol level. Mrs. Haley also takes 10 mg of lisinopril once a day for borderline hypertension with good control. Because Mrs. Haley lives alone, she doesn't bother to cook much and fixes frozen dinners or soup for her meals at night. As active as Mrs. Haley is, she does not do much exercising and weighs 140 pounds, which is a 10-pound increase over last year's weight. Mrs. Haley drives but admits to the nurse that things seem blurry at night.

1. What factors put Mrs. Haley at risk for hip fracture?

2. During her annual checkup, what safety teaching regarding risks for hip fracture will you address with Mrs. Haley?

3. What nutritional suggestions might you implement to help with the prevention of hip fractures?

4. What recommendations regarding exercise will you make to Mrs. Haley?

EXEMPLAR 13.4 Multiple Sclerosis

EXEMPLAR KEY TERMS

Axon, 876
Demyelination, 876
Exacerbation, 877
Lesions, 876
Multiple sclerosis (MS), 876
Myelin, 876
Oligodendrocytes, 876
Plaques, 876
Pseudoexacerbation, 877
Remyelination, 877

EXEMPLAR LEARNING OUTCOMES

After reading about this exemplar, you will be able to:

1. Describe the pathophysiology, etiology, clinical manifestations, and direct and indirect causes of multiple sclerosis.

2. Identify risk factors and prevention methods associated with multiple sclerosis.

3. Illustrate the nursing process in providing culturally competent care across the life span for individuals with multiple sclerosis.

4. Formulate priority nursing diagnoses appropriate for an individual with multiple sclerosis.

5. Summarize therapies used by interdisciplinary teams in the collaborative care of an individual with multiple sclerosis.

6. Plan evidence-based care for an individual with multiple sclerosis and his or her family in collaboration with other members of the healthcare team.

7. Evaluate expected outcomes for an individual with multiple sclerosis.

▶ OVERVIEW

Multiple sclerosis (MS) is an immune-mediated disorder of the central nervous system (CNS) in which immune cells attack the myelin sheath around nerve cells, causing decreased transmission of nervous signals. **Myelin** forms a fatty insulating layer around nerve cells to increase the speed of electrical transmission along the nerve. Symptoms of MS often go into remission after the initial manifestation of the disease, making MS difficult to diagnose. Each individual affected by MS will experience a different set of symptoms and a range of severity of symptoms depending on the nerves that are affected.

▶ PATHOPHYSIOLOGY AND ETIOLOGY

The CNS consists of the brain, spinal cord, and optic nerves. Each **axon**, or nerve fiber, in the CNS is covered by a myelin sheath to protect the nerve and increase the efficiency of electrical impulses along the neuron membranes. In some individuals, cells of the immune system, such as lymphocytes and macrophages, cross the blood–brain barrier and attack and destroy the myelin sheath in a process called **demyelination**. This causes inflammation and leads to the formation of **lesions** (areas of inflammation and damage) in the surrounding area.

In addition to the myelin sheath, the underlying axon as well as **oligodendrocytes** (cells that produce myelin) may be damaged by the immune system. Unlike damage to the myelin sheath, which can be repaired by oligodendrocytes over time, damage to the axons is not reversible. However, repeated attacks on the myelin may stimulate the formation of scar tissue, or **plaques**, causing permanent damage. Axon damage and a lack of myelin disrupts nerve impulses in the CNS, causing neurological symptoms such as muscle weakness, visual disturbances,

and balance and coordination problems (Multiple Sclerosis Association of America [MSAA], 2013). The pattern of inflammation, damage, and repair causes MS to manifest in one of four patterns (**Box 13–7 ●**).

Etiology

MS is generally characterized as an autoimmune disease. However, because the exact antigen is unknown, many scientists prefer to call MS an immune-mediated process. The events that trigger the immune response against the myelin sheath are unknown, but links have been found to environmental, infectious, and genetic factors. Environmental factors may include geography, sunlight, and environmental toxins. Individuals who live farther from the equator and are exposed to less sunlight are more likely to develop MS, causing some scientists to believe that vitamin D plays a protective role (Munger & Ascherio, 2011).

Multiple studies have attempted to link viruses to the development of MS, including measles virus, herpes virus, rubella virus, HTLV-1, and Epstein-Barr virus. Environmental studies indicate that individuals must encounter a factor such as a virus before the age of 15 to develop MS later in life (Multiple Sclerosis Foundation [MSF], 2009). Although the links between many viruses and MS are unsubstantiated, several studies have linked increased antibody titers to the Epstein-Barr virus with an increased risk of developing MS (Lindsey, Hatfield, & Vu, 2010; Munger et al., 2011). However, this issue remains controversial.

Genetic factors may also play a role in the development of MS. MS is not hereditary, but individuals with a first-degree relative such as a parent or sibling with MS have an increased risk of developing MS. The risk of developing MS is approximately 0.1% for the general population. For first-degree relatives, this risk increases to 3%–5%, whereas the risk is 31% for identical twins (MSAA, 2013). Some scientists believe that MS develops

Box 13–7 Classifications of Multiple Sclerosis

The four main classifications of MS are relapsing-remitting MS, primary-progressive MS, secondary-progressive MS, and progressive-relapsing MS (MSAA, 2013; National Multiple Sclerosis Society [NMSS], 2012).

- *Relapsing-remitting MS* is the most common form of MS at the time of diagnosis, affecting approximately 85% of clients with MS. Individuals with relapsing-remitting MS experience clearly defined flare-ups with worsening neurological function followed by periods of partial or complete remission with few or no symptoms. Remission is thought to occur when oligodendrocytes repair the damaged myelin sheath (**remyelination**). Clients can experience periods of relapse that last for days or months and periods of remission that last from weeks to months to years.
- *Primary-progressive MS* affects approximately 10% of clients with MS. These individuals experience a slow but nearly continuous worsening of their disease from the time of onset with no distinct

remissions. The rate of progression may vary over time, from temporary minor improvements to plateaus to obvious worsening of symptoms.
- *Secondary-progressive MS* develops within 10 years of diagnosis in about half of the clients with relapsing-remitting MS who are not receiving treatment. Individuals with secondary-progressive MS experience an initial period of relapsing-remitting MS followed by a progressive form of the disease with or without occasional flare-ups and minor remissions. This form of MS may develop as a result of the eventual destruction of oligodendrocytes, preventing the body from repairing the myelin sheath.
- *Progressive-relapsing MS* is relatively rare, occurring in only 5% of individuals with MS. These individuals experience a steady worsening of disease with acute relapses. In contrast to relapsing-remitting MS, the periods between relapses are characterized by continued progression of the disease rather than remission of symptoms.

---

in a genetically susceptible individual after exposure to an environmental factor such as an infectious agent (MSF, 2009).

Risk Factors

In addition to the environmental, infectious, and genetic risk factors described above, several other risk factors have been linked to the development of MS. Multiple sclerosis is usually diagnosed in individuals between the ages of 20 and 40, although individuals as young as 2 and as old as 75 have been diagnosed with MS. Women are twice as likely as men to develop MS, and individuals of European descent are more likely to develop MS compared to individuals of Asian, African, or Native American descent (Mayo Clinic, 2012b). Smoking also increases the risk of developing MS, and individuals with MS who smoke are at greater risk for escalation of disease symptoms (MSAA, 2013). As the Focus on Diversity and Culture feature explains, individuals in certain countries may also be at more risk.

▶ CLINICAL MANIFESTATIONS

Clinical manifestations of multiple sclerosis depend on the location and severity of damage in the CNS. No two clients will present with the same set of symptoms, and many symptoms are common in other diseases as well, making diagnosis difficult. Symptoms may be persistent, may go into remission, or may become exacerbated depending on the immune process causing them. Individuals suffering from exacerbation may

experience one or more symptoms that last from days to months, and symptoms can be different during distinct exacerbations. A true **exacerbation** must last at least 24 hours and must be separated from the previous attack by at least 30 days. Symptoms that last for less than 24 hours are termed paroxysmal attacks.

Common symptoms of MS include fatigue, paresthesia (numbness, tingling, burning), lack of coordination and balance, unsteady gait, tremors, bladder and bowel dysfunction, visual disturbances (unilateral loss of vision, optic neuritis, double vision, blurred vision, oscillopsia, red-green color distortion), dizziness, sexual dysfunction (impotence, dyspareunia, anorgasmia), pain (headache, Lhermitte sign, trigeminal neuralgia, allodynia), cognitive dysfunction (lack of concentration, memory loss, reasoning problems, poor judgment), depression, anxiety, and muscle spasticity or weakness in one or more limbs (see the Multisystem Effects feature). Less common symptoms include speech disorders, swallowing problems, hearing loss, seizures, breathing problems, itching, "MS hug" (a sensation of a tight band around the abdomen), and partial or complete paralysis.

Although there is no common trigger for relapse, several factors may influence a relapse. Many clients cite stress and fatigue as contributors to flare-ups. Some clients experience heat sensitivity, or a relapse of symptoms associated with increases in body temperature (e.g., fever caused by infection). Infection and increased body temperature may cause a **pseudoexacerbation**, or a temporary aggravation of symptoms that is directly related to a trigger and subsides as soon as the trigger is removed.

The primary symptoms of MS that result from demyelination may lead to secondary and tertiary symptoms as well. Secondary symptoms result from chronic primary symptoms. For example, individuals with urinary retention may develop urinary tract infections, individuals with muscle weakness in the legs may develop muscle atrophy and pressure sores from immobility, and individuals with balance problems and an unsteady gait may fall and fracture a bone. Tertiary symptoms relate to psychosocial problems, such as relationship difficulties, loss of a job because of decreased performance, or hopelessness. Tertiary symptoms often occur as a result of symptom exacerbation and lack of coping skills.

Focus on Diversity and Culture Parasites

Parasites tend to weaken the immune response. Therefore, individuals with an increased likelihood for parasitic infection, such as those who live in developing countries, are less likely to be diagnosed with MS, which is triggered by a strong immune response. With improved sanitation and decreased exposure to parasites, the diagnosis of MS is on the rise in these countries (MSAA, 2013).

Multisystem Effects of Multiple Sclerosis

Neurologic
- Emotional lability
  (euphoria or depression)
- Forgetfulness
- Apathy
- Scanning speech
- Impaired judgment
- Irritability

Potential Complications
- Convulsive seizures
- Dementia

Sensory
Visual
- Blurred vision
- Diplopia
- Nystagmus
- Visual field defects (blind spots)
- Eye pain

Auditory
- Vertigo
- Nausea

Tactile (especially hands or legs)
- Numbness
- Paresthesias (tingling,
  burning sensation)
- Diminished sense of temperature
- Pain with spasms
- Loss of proprioception

Potential Complication
Visual
- Blindness

Respiratory
- Diminished cough reflex

Potential Complication
- Respiratory infections

Urinary
- Hesitancy
- Frequency
- Retention
- Reflex bladder emptying

Potential Complications
- Recurring UTIs
- Incontinence

Gastrointestinal
Oral/esophageal
- Difficulty chewing
- Dysphagia

Upper/lower GI
- Decreased or absent
  sphincter control
- Bowel incontinence
- Constipation

Musculoskeletal
- Fatigue
- Limb weakness
- Ataxic movements
  (shaky, irregular, uncoordinated)
- Intention tremors
- Spasticity
- Muscular atrophy
- Dragging of foot and foot drop
- Dysarthria with slurred speech

Reproductive
- Impotence (male)
- Loss of genital sensation

Lifespan and Cultural Considerations

Studies suggest that 2%–5% of individuals with MS experience symptoms before the age of 18. Diagnosis is more challenging in children than adults because of the multitude of other childhood disorders with symptoms similar to MS. In addition to symptoms experienced by adults, children with MS often experience seizures and mental status changes that are not common in adults, and children have a higher rate of relapse. Children with MS may suffer from reduced academic performance, difficulty in family and peer relationships, and distorted self-image. MS usually progresses more slowly in children, but because of the early onset of symptoms, disability may accumulate at a younger age compared to clients with adult-onset MS (NMSS, n.d.b).

Because MS most commonly affects women of childbearing age, women with MS must decide whether they want to become pregnant. Evidence suggests that pregnancy does not influence the overall course of disease, and MS does not affect a woman's ability to become pregnant. However, pharmacologic treatment of MS involves drugs that may be harmful to a fetus. Interestingly, pregnant women are usually protected from exacerbations during the second and third trimester, but they have a 20%–40% risk of developing a flare-up in the first 6 months postpartum. Women who experience gait difficulties before pregnancy may experience an exacerbation of these symptoms, especially during the third trimester when the woman's center of gravity naturally shifts. Bladder problems and fatigue may also be intensified in pregnant women with MS compared to pregnant women without MS (NMSS, n.d.c). Pregnant women with MS may experience decreased pain during labor as a result of sensory deficits.

Cultural differences have also been observed in clients with MS. Although Whites are more susceptible to developing MS, Blacks with MS tend to be older and have more symptoms at the time of diagnosis. These symptoms are usually limited to the optic nerve and spinal cord, making Blacks more susceptible to vision and mobility problems. They also tend to have more progressive disease that responds less to current disease-modifying therapies. In contrast, Hispanics are usually younger than Whites at diagnosis, and they tend to have fewer mobility problems and bladder and bowel dysfunction than Whites. However, they may experience more depression and have less access to services needed to treat MS (MSAA, 2013).

Evidence-Based Practice Aging Clients With Multiple Sclerosis

Problem

Multiple sclerosis does not shorten the affected individual's life span, so clients may require treatment for 20 or more years following diagnosis. These clients are not only suffering from cumulative loss of function from MS, they are also dealing with the loss of function related to the normal aging process.

Evidence

Older individuals with MS feel that work and social engagement, accessibility to effective health care, maintaining independence, financial flexibility, and cognitive and mental health are vital to maintaining a good quality of life (Ploughman et al., 2012). However, these areas often represent unmet needs for clients who are aging with MS. Compared to younger individuals with MS, older individuals with MS are more likely to have progressive disease, are more physically disabled, have more bladder and bowel problems, have a greater loss of balance, and have an increased need for support while walking. Physical limitations greatly limit daily activities and independence, preventing older clients with MS from feeling productive (DiLorenzo, 2011). These physical disabilities cause older individuals with MS to feel they have less freedom and need more assistance than their peers without MS. Having less freedom as a result of physical disability and financial restrictions means that travel and social opportunities are limited and they are less able to be spontaneous. They need more assistance from family and friends at an earlier age than their peers in areas such as housework, shopping, bathing, dressing, and meal preparation. Needing help in these areas causes older clients with MS to feel they are a burden on their caregivers (Finlayson, van Denend, & Hudson, 2004).

Implications

Nursing care for aging clients with MS should focus on helping the client meet needs that increase their quality of life, including independence, social interaction, and adequate health care. The nurse can encourage clients to use assistive devices to increase mobility and independence and allow them to participate in social activities. Referring clients to home care or assisted living facilities will help them maintain independence while relieving the burden of daily activities for the client and her caregivers. Interdisciplinary health care is essential for older clients with MS. The nurse should make sure the client is aware of appropriate healthcare services, such as physical therapy, eye physicians, support groups, and wellness promotion programs. The nurse should assess older individuals with MS for mental health problems, and clients with emotional or mood problems should be referred to a counselor for professional assistance. The nurse should also assist older clients with MS by teaching coping methods, such as pacing themselves, planning and prioritizing activities, and participating in the community (DiLorenzo, 2011).

Critical Thinking Application

1. You are caring for a 64-year-old woman who has had MS for 32 years and is confined to a wheelchair. She expresses feelings of loneliness because she feels limited in her ability to participate in social activities. What teaching should you give this client to help her increase her social interactions?

2. While you are making a home visit to a 59-year-old woman who has had MS for 28 years, she reveals that she has bladder control problems associated with MS and soils herself at least 3 times per week. This makes her reluctant to leave the house. What can you do to help her resolve this problem?

3. During a routine follow-up appointment, a 73-year-old man with MS suggests that he is a burden on his family and they would all be better off without him. What nursing interventions are a priority for this client?

▶ COLLABORATION

The variety of symptoms associated with MS increases the need for collaboration among multiple clinicians, including nurses, neurologists, immunologists, urologists, ophthalmologists, obstetricians, pulmonologists, cardiologists, primary care providers, therapists (physical, occupational, speech, psychological), nutritionists, and home health agencies. In particular, nursing care will focus on symptom management, client teaching, emotional support, and referrals to other healthcare services, depending on the client's disease manifestations.

Diagnostic Tests

No single test can be used to definitively diagnose MS. Instead, the medical history, physical examination, and several diagnostic tests are used to diagnose MS. Diagnostic tests include an MRI, lumbar puncture, evoked potential test, and blood tests (Mayo Clinic, 2012b; MSAA, 2013; NMSS, n.d.a). Using these tests, the client must meet three criteria to be diagnosed with MS: lesions in at least two separate areas of the CNS, evidence that the two areas of damage occurred at least 1 month apart, and rule out all other possible diagnoses.

- An *MRI* uses powerful magnets and radio waves to produce detailed images of the brain and spinal cord. An MRI is able to detect the presence of lesions in the CNS that may indicate demyelination and MS. Gadolinium may also be injected to help detect areas of current disease activity.

- A *lumbar puncture*, or spinal tap, is used to obtain a sample of cerebrospinal fluid (CSF). The CSF is then tested for the presence of elevated immunoglobulins (IgG), oligoclonal bands, and myelin breakdown products, all of which are indicative of MS.

- *Evoked potential tests* measure the electrical activity of the brain in response to stimulation of sensory nerve pathways, specifically visual evoked potentials, brainstem auditory evoked potentials, and sensory evoked potentials. These tests are able to detect the slowing of electrical conduction that is caused by demyelination of the nerves. Evoked potential tests are often useful for identifying a second demyelinating event that causes no clinical symptoms and did not create a lesion that is detectable by MRI.

- *Blood tests* are used to rule out other infectious or inflammatory diseases that may mimic the symptoms of MS.

Surgery

Surgery is not a common treatment for clients with MS. However, clients with specific symptoms may require surgery. For example, clients with severe pain may undergo a rhizotomy, which selectively destroys problematic nerve roots in the spinal cord. Similarly, clients with spasticity may undergo musculoskeletal surgery to lengthen or transfer a tendon or muscle to reduce tension. Surgery may also be indicated to allow for placement of a pump that administers intrathecal baclofen (ITB) therapy.

Pharmacologic Therapy

Pharmacologic therapy is the mainstay of treatment for clients with MS. Since 1993, 10 disease-modifying therapies have been approved for the treatment of relapsing-remitting MS; the primary result of taking these medications is a decrease in the number of relapses.

- The beta interferons (Avonex, Betaseron, Extavia, Rebif) reduce the number of inflammatory cells that cross the blood–brain barrier, leading to a reduction of neuronal inflammation. Beta interferons can slow the progression of disease and decrease the severity of attacks. Side effects may include reactions at the injection area, liver damage, and mood changes. Nursing responsibilities include assessing liver function and CBC for baseline parameters and every 3 months to test side effects, assessing the injection site, and monitoring changes in the client's condition and function to assess for efficacy.

- Glatiramer acetate (Copaxone) blocks the immune system's attack on myelin. Side effects may include flushing, chest pain, or heart palpitations.

- Fingolimod (Gilenya) traps immune cells in the lymph nodes, making them unable to access the CNS. Side effects include bradycardia, diarrhea, cough, and headache.

- Natalizumab (Tysabri) interferes with the movement of immune cells across the blood–brain barrier; it is used only in clients who cannot tolerate other treatments because it increases the risk of developing a fatal brain infection (multifocal leukoencephalopathy).

- Mitoxantrone (Novantrone) is an immunosuppressant that is only used to treat advanced MS because of cardiovascular and other serious side effects.

- Teriflunomide (Aubagio) is a pyrimidine synthesis inhibitor that inhibits the function of lymphocytes. It may cause serious liver damage.

- Dimethyl fumarate (Tecfidera) is thought to inhibit immune cells and have antioxidant properties that protect the nerves from damage. Side effects may include flushing and gastrointestinal events.

- Baclofen (Lioresal) is administered to reduce spasticity in clients with a variety of disorders, including cerebral palsy, traumatic spinal cord injury, and multiple sclerosis. For clients with certain conditions, including multiple sclerosis, when oral baclofen fails to adequately reduce spasticity, ITB may be considered.

SAFETY ALERT
Disease-modifying therapies may cause damage to a fetus. Therefore, they are not approved for women who are pregnant. Women who want to become pregnant should discontinue their MS medications before attempting to conceive. These drugs are also not recommended during breastfeeding.

Disease-modifying therapies are not approved for the treatment of progressive forms of MS. Therefore, clients with MS are often treated with medications that are specific for their symptoms (**Table 13–6 ●**). When a new medication is added to the regimen of a client with MS, the nurse is responsible for reviewing with the client the dosage and schedule for taking the medication and teaching the client and family about side effects they should report to the physician.

TABLE 13–6 Medications for Symptoms of Multiple Sclerosis

SYMPTOM	MEDICATION EXAMPLES
Acute exacerbations	dexamethasone, methylprednisolone, adreno-corticotropic hormone (ACTH), prednisone
Fatigue	amantadine, fluoxetine, modafinil
Spasticity	baclofen, dantrolene, diazepam, tizanidine
Constipation	bisacodyl, docusate, glycerin, magnesium hydroxide
Pain	carbamazepine, clonazepam, gabapentin, phenytoin
Erectile dysfunction	alprostadil, sildenafil, tadalafil, vardenafil
Depression	bupropion, citalopram, duloxetine, paroxetine, sertraline
Urinary tract infection	ciprofloxacin, methenamine, sulfamethoxazole + trimethoprim
Bladder dysfunction	imipramine, desmopressin, oxybutynin, prazosin, tamsulosin
Tremor	Isoniazid, buspirone, propranolol
Walking	Dalfampridine

Sources: Data from Mayo Clinic. (2012c). *Multiple sclerosis: Treatments and drugs.* Retrieved from http://www.mayoclinic.com/health/multiple-sclerosis/DS00188/DSECTION=treatments-and-drugs; National Institute of Neurological Disorders and Stroke. (2012a). *Multiple sclerosis: Hope through research.* Retrieved from http://www.ninds.nih.gov/disorders/multiple_sclerosis/detail_multiple_sclerosis.htm#210833215; Reitman, N., & Kalb, R. (2012). *Multiple sclerosis: The nursing perspective* (6th ed.). New York, NY: National Multiple Sclerosis Society.

Some medications may require tests for adverse side effects. For example, clients taking corticosteroid therapy for exacerbations should be monitored for glucose intolerance, osteoporosis, and cataract formation. Clients taking muscle relaxants for spasticity should be monitored for hepatotoxicity, dizziness, and skeletal muscle activity. Some muscle relaxants may produce withdrawal symptoms if not tapered during discontinuation. The nurse should be familiar with the potential adverse effects of each drug and conduct tests to monitor the client's condition as prescribed by the physician.

Nonpharmacologic Therapy

The progressive, lifelong nature of MS requires that clients not only take medications as needed for symptoms but also participate in nonpharmacologic therapies to reduce symptoms and regain functionality. This could include rehabilitation, proper nutrition and fluids, and good lifestyle habits. Rehabilitation includes the following (NMSS, n.d.d):

- Physical therapy emphasizes walking, strength, and balance by encouraging stretching, ROM exercises, strength training, gait training, and training in the use of assistive devices. The goal of physical therapy is to maintain optimal functioning and prevent complications.

- Occupational therapy is used to enhance independence, productivity, and safety for activities related to personal care, leisure, and employment.

- Speech/language therapy is used for clients with speech or swallowing problems related to MS to enhance clarity of speech and promote safe swallowing and overall health.

- Cognitive therapy is used to help treat changes in the client's ability to think, reason, concentrate, and remember.

- Vocational rehabilitation offers job training, job placement assistance, mobility training, and assistive technology assessments in an effort to help clients maintain their current employment or find new employment that accepts their limitations.

Maintaining a healthy lifestyle is essential for clients with MS to reduce complications and exacerbations. In addition to rehabilitation, clients should participate in a regular mild exercise program such as walking, swimming, and weight training to increase muscle strength and balance. Fatigue is a common symptom of MS, so clients should get plenty of rest. Symptoms may be exacerbated by increased body temperature, so the client should be encouraged to avoid excessive heat, and to keep cool by staying in air-conditioned areas and drinking cold beverages. Eating a balanced diet and maintaining adequate hydration will help the client maintain a healthy weight and maintain bone and muscle health. The client's diet may need to be adapted to accommodate changes in the client's ability to chew and swallow as well as movement limitations such as tremor and muscle weakness. The nurse may also teach clients methods to reduce stress, such as tai chi, massage, deep breathing, or distraction techniques (Mayo Clinic, 2012b). Some other alternative therapies may be helpful for the client with MS; others may be risky (see the Complementary and Alternative Therapy feature).

NURSING PROCESS

Individuals who are diagnosed with MS are often in their prime of life. The physical, emotional, and cognitive effects of MS can affect every area of the individual's life, including relationships,

Complementary and Alternative Therapy
Multiple Sclerosis

Complementary and alternative therapy is commonly used by clients with MS. However, many of these therapies are unsubstantiated by clinical trials, so clients should be cautioned in their use of these types of therapies. The effectiveness of many therapies is greatly exaggerated by companies selling the products. Many therapies, such as acupuncture, aromatherapy, therapeutic horseback riding, electromagnetic therapy, massage, and prayer have low risk and may be beneficial for some symptoms. Other therapies, such as hyperbaric oxygen, marijuana, and bee venom therapy, carry more risk than benefit. Herbal remedies may benefit specific symptoms, such as valerian for insomnia or cranberry for prevention of UTIs, but others may irritate the urinary tract, interact with steroid medications, or stimulate the immune system (Reitman & Kalb, 2012). Low-dose naltrexone has also been suggested as an alternative therapy, and studies indicate that it improves the client's quality of life but has no impact on physical symptoms (Cree, Kornyeyeva, & Goodin, 2010).

Clinical Manifestations and Therapies **Multiple Sclerosis**

ETIOLOGY	CLINICAL MANIFESTATIONS	CLINICAL THERAPIES
Primary symptoms (result from demyelination)	■ Sensory disturbances (visual, hearing, speech, balance, pain) ■ Motor disturbances (weakness, paresthesias, bowel and bladder function, unsteady gait, spasticity, breathing problems) ■ Cognitive dysfunction (concentration, memory, reasoning, judgment, depression)	■ Disease-modifying therapies ■ Symptom-specific medications ■ Corticosteroids to treat exacerbations ■ Assistive devices ■ Physical therapy/rehabilitation
Secondary symptoms (result from prolonged primary symptoms)	■ Pressure sores ■ Osteoporosis ■ Aspiration pneumonia ■ Urinary tract infections ■ Back or hip pain ■ Muscle atrophy, poor postural alignment ■ Bone fractures	■ Antibiotics ■ Analgesics ■ Bisphosphonates ■ Physical therapy ■ Immobilization of fractures ■ Nutrition and fluids
Tertiary symptoms (psychosocial complications)	■ Social problems (partner, family, friends, social isolation) ■ Vocation problems (loss of job, loss of transportation) ■ Emotional problems (depression, irritability, hopelessness)	■ Psychological counseling ■ Antidepressants ■ Referral to home care, transportation assistance ■ Encourage social interaction ■ Client teaching to minimize isolation ■ Caregiver support ■ Vocational rehabilitation

work, and self-image. The individual's relationship with her partner may become strained because of the extra care needed and the inability to perform normal household roles during exacerbations or when the disease causes immobility. The individual's work often suffers because of physical and cognitive limitations, sometimes leading to job loss and financial problems. The individual's self-image may be disturbed, which can lead to social isolation, depression, inadequate coping, and lack of desire to perform ADLs.

The nurse plays a major role in the health care of individuals with MS. Nurses have the most contact with the client and therefore have the responsibility to follow and document the progression of the client's disease course and treatment. Continued assessment of the timing and severity of exacerbations, effectiveness of medications, and the client's functional status are integral to good nursing care. The nurse is in a unique position to listen to the client, offer emotional and physical support, teach the client about the disease and how to prevent exacerbations, and refer the client to the needed services.

Assessment

Nursing assessment of the client with diagnosed or suspected MS should include a medical history and physical examination. Collection and documentation of these data allow for effective treatment evaluation of disease progression over time. A thorough medical history includes onset, type, intensity, and pattern of symptoms; factors that affect symptoms; ongoing medical problems and medications; past history of surgery, trauma, or infection; health history of family members; and exposure to environmental hazards. The nurse should also interview the client as to how his symptoms affect his everyday life.

A physical examination begins by observing the client's ability to move and walk, affect, balance and coordination, hygiene, and speech. The Expanded Disability Status Scale (EDSS; Kurtzke, 1983) is frequently used to assess neurological impairment in clients with multiple sclerosis. This scale combines a general Disability Status Scale with a Functional System grade. The Functional System is divided into pyramidal, cerebellar, brainstem, sensory, bowel and bladder, visual, cerebral, and other. Using the 0–10 EDSS scale, clients with a score of 1–2.5 have minimal disability with ambulation, clients with a score of 3–6.5 have moderate disability and ambulate with an assistive device, and clients with a score of 7–10 have severe disability and are confined to a wheelchair or bed. In addition, an EDSS score of 4 marks the transition from relapsing-remitting MS to secondary-progressive MS (Hutchinson, 2009).

An MS Functional Composite (MSFC) scale can also be used to assess specific physical function using three tests. A nine-hole peg test is used to assess arm function, a timed 25-foot walk test assesses leg function, and the MS Symptom Checklist (MSSC) assesses the presence of 26 common MS symptoms in the areas of motor function, sensory disturbance, mental and emotional concerns, bowel and bladder elimination, and brainstem symptoms.

Other tests that may be included in the physical assessment include a cranial nerve assessment, which tests the function of each of the 12 cranial nerves; assessment of motor symptoms, including ROM and muscle strength (see Table 13–1), and assessment of reflexes (Thompson & Mauk, 2011).

Diagnosis

Clients with MS may have a variety of nursing diagnoses that could be related to any of the 12 domains depending on the location of myelin damage and resulting symptoms. A sample of relevant nursing diagnoses includes the following:

- *Impaired Physical Mobility* related to motor nerve dysfunction
- *Functional Urinary Incontinence* related to ineffective nerve transmission to the bladder
- *Constipation* related to damage to nerves that regulate peristalsis
- *Fatigue* related to disease process
- *Bathing Self-Care Deficit* related to lack of coordination
- *Hopelessness* related to lack of cure for disease
- *Disturbed Body Image* related to changes in physical functioning
- *Caregiver Role Strain* related to caring for an individual with a disability
- *Ineffective Role Performance* related to loss of physical functioning
- *Sexual Dysfunction* related to damaged sensory nerves
- *Ineffective Coping* related to lack of knowledge about disease process.

(NANDA-I © 2012)

Planning

Just as a variety of nursing diagnoses may be appropriate for inclusion in the plan of care for a client with MS, numerous client goals are relevant to these nursing diagnoses. For example, client goals related to the previously described nursing diagnoses may include the following:

- The client will participate in physical and occupational therapy and an exercise program to maintain independent physical mobility.
- The client will state methods to reduce urinary incontinence and how to discreetly deal with urinary incontinence when outside the home.
- The client will verbalize understanding of methods to prevent and treat constipation.
- The client will receive 8 hours of sleep per night and rest as needed during the day to decrease fatigue.
- The client will demonstrate maximum independence during ADLs, such as personal care and bathing.
- The client will receive psychological counseling as needed.
- The client will accept and adapt to debilitating symptoms and participate in programs to regain maximal function.
- The client's caregiver will receive help from home health agencies, family, and friends to provide relief from caregiver duties.
- The client will participate in vocational rehabilitation and find a job that accommodates individuals with disabilities.
- The client and partner will verbalize awareness of means by which to achieve satisfaction and sexual intimacy through techniques other than sexual intercourse.
- The client will verbalize an understanding of coping techniques.

Implementation

Nursing interventions for many symptoms related to MS can be found in other exemplars throughout this textbook. See Table

Client Teaching | Multiple Sclerosis

Multiple sclerosis is often diagnosed at a young age, and the client will live with the disease for many years. Therefore, it is essential that the client fully understand the disease and its implications. Teaching topics may include the following:

- The overall pathophysiology of the disease
- A projected disease course and disease classifications
- Symptoms commonly experienced by clients with MS
- Medications used to treat MS and its symptoms, including dosing, schedule, side effects, and drug–drug interactions
- Mechanisms to prevent exacerbations, such as managing fatigue and stress and avoiding cold and heat extremes, high humidity, physical overexertion, and infections
- Mechanisms to avoid complications, including pressure sores, infections, and bone fractures
- Cautions for women who want to become pregnant or are pregnant or breastfeeding
- Safety modifications for the home
- Community resources, such as the National Multiple Sclerosis Society.

13–6 for medications used to manage symptoms related to MS. Nursing interventions for symptoms specific to MS and mobility are discussed here. In addition, one primary nursing intervention is client teaching on a variety of topics (see the Client Teaching feature).

Promote Independent Mobility

Clients should be assessed for ambulation ability at each appointment. Nursing interventions should aim to help the client remain independently mobile for as long as possible. The nurse should advocate for clients who may benefit from medications to reduce spasticity and increase walking ability. Clients with ambulation problems should be encouraged to begin an exercise program and physical therapy. The nurse may also need to assess the client's home for safety to prevent falls for clients with an unsteady gait or muscle weakness.

Many clients resist using an assistive device for walking because of impaired self-image. The nurse plays an important role in teaching clients the advantages of assistive devices, including independence and increased safety. This may also include providing emotional support for the client to maintain a positive self-image while using an assistive device. Participation in physical therapy is essential for clients who need training in the use of ambulation devices. Clients may need multiple assistive devices depending on the activity. For example, a client may use a cane at home for short distances but a walker or wheelchair in public when longer distances are involved.

For clients who are confined to a wheelchair, the nurse should provide information about motorized wheelchairs, handicap-accessible transportation services, and home modifications that will increase the client's ability to move around the home or town. Methods to prevent complications such as pressure sores and urinary retention should also be discussed.

Promote Self-Care

Clients with motor deficits such as tremor, walking difficulties, ataxia, muscle weakness, or spasticity may have trouble performing self-care, including bathing, eating, toileting, dressing, transferring, and hygiene care. The ability of the client to perform ADLs should be a guide to determine how much assistance the client needs in all areas of life. Clients who need assistance with ADLs are usually still able to make adequate decisions about self-care even if they cannot physically perform the activities. Therefore, caregivers should be encouraged to consult clients about their preferences for self-care. Maintaining some control over basic activities is essential to the client's emotional well-being and should be incorporated into each nursing intervention.

Helping the client maintain independence in ADLs is essential for promoting a positive self-image and encouraging participation in social activities. Nursing interventions could include encouraging the client to wear arm or wrist braces to provide stability during self-care activities; teaching the client to perform self-care activities when energy levels are high; using assistive devices while eating, such as plate guards and modified utensils; modifying the consistency of foods to make eating easier; and receiving assistance from others for meal preparation. The nurse can also teach clients techniques for bowel and bladder control, including adequate fluid intake, scheduling regular voiding, self-catheterization, bowel training, and exercise to maintain muscle strength. Clients with self-care deficits may also benefit from occupational therapy.

Assess Emotional Status

Clients with MS may have an altered emotional status either as a primary symptom of the disease or a tertiary symptom related to inadequate coping. The nurse should assess the client's emotional status at every appointment, including:

- Depression, anxiety, and hopelessness
- Use and effectiveness of coping mechanisms
- Stress levels
- Interference of symptoms with relationships, especially with partner and children
- Adequate social interaction
- Feelings of adequacy in performing home and work responsibilities

- Changes in self-image related to symptoms of MS
- Feelings of being a burden to caregivers.

If the client is experiencing any emotional problems, the nurse may need to advocate for medication such as antidepressants or refer the client to a psychologist or psychiatrist. The nurse may also provide information on coping mechanisms and methods of reducing stress. Nursing care for individuals who avoid social interaction because of symptoms may include techniques to promote social interactions, such as managing symptoms, planning for and prioritizing social activities outside the home, and encouraging social interaction inside the home.

Facilitate Referrals for Collaborative Care

In addition to a neurologist, clients with MS will need integrated care from multiple healthcare workers. For example, a client with urinary incontinence or retention or chronic urinary tract infections should be referred to a urologist. Clients who want to become pregnant should be referred to an obstetrician. Clients with motor deficits should be referred to a physical or occupational therapist. Clients with mood disorders such as depression or anxiety need to receive counseling and treatment from a psychologist or psychiatrist. Clients with swallowing difficulties should see a nutritionist to find a diet with adequate nutrition that is easy to swallow as well as a speech/language therapist to maintain swallowing function. Clients with visual disturbances should be referred to an ophthalmologist. Each client will need an individualized healthcare team to help maintain optimal functioning.

Evaluation

Evaluation of clients with MS should include assessing for disease exacerbation as well as for progression from relapsing-remitting MS to secondary-progressive MS. Type and severity of symptoms should also be evaluated, and medications related to each symptom should be reevaluated for necessity and effectiveness. The presence of complications such as infection should be continually evaluated, because complications may lead to an exacerbation. Other points of evaluation include mobility and the need for assistive devices, emotional stability of the client, and areas of deficient knowledge. MS is an ever-changing disease that requires constant evaluation and revision of the care plan to meet the current needs of the client.

NURSING CARE PLAN   A Client With Multiple Sclerosis

Holly West, a 42-year-old female client who grew up in Canada, was diagnosed with MS approximately 7 years ago, although she has had mild symptoms for 12 years. She works as a grocery manager at a store near her home. She lives with her husband and two children, ages 14 and 17. Recently, Mrs. West has experienced worsening urinary incontinence, fatigue, weakness, and mobility issues due to spasticity in her leg muscles. She also has a fever, chest congestion, and a productive cough. After evaluation at her local hospital's emergency department, she is admitted to the hospital for evaluation and treatment of pneumonia and exacerbation of her MS.

ASSESSMENT	DIAGNOSES	PLANNING
Carl Kartler, RN, is assigned to care for Mrs. West. Her primary complaint is congestion and the inability to cough up sputum. She also states, "I'm so tired of missing work. My husband has to take care of me like I'm a baby." Vital signs include temperature 101.0°F oral; pulse 92 bpm; respirations 28/min; and BP 112/62 mmHg. Auscultation	■ *Ineffective Airway Clearance* related to excessive mucus production ■ *Ineffective Breathing Pattern* related to presence of sputum in the airways ■ *Functional Urinary Incontinence* related to damaged nerves that control bladder function	■ The client will maintain a patent airway. ■ The client will freely expectorate sputum. ■ The client's lung sounds will be clear to auscultation. ■ The client's oxygen saturation will remain above 95% on room air. ■ The client will demonstrate knowledge of bladder training.

NURSING CARE PLAN *(continued)*

ASSESSMENT	DIAGNOSES	PLANNING
of Mrs. West's lungs reveals scattered rhonchi throughout and her oxygen saturation is 96% on room air. She is pale, but her skin is warm and dry. The physician orders a stat respiratory treatment of aerosolized albuterol for Mrs. West, after which her breath sounds are improved; rhonchi are diminished. Her course of therapy also will include ACTH (adrenocorticotropic hormone) and intravenous antibiotics.	■ *Impaired Physical Mobility* related to weakness and spasticity of leg muscles ■ *Fatigue* related to infection and multiple sclerosis ■ *Ineffective Role Performance* related to inability to perform home and work roles ■ *Bathing Self-Care Deficit* related to muscle weakness ■ *Hyperthermia* related to infectious process (NANDA-I © 2012)	■ The client will be free from infection. ■ The client will demonstrate knowledge of bladder training. ■ The client will participate in physical therapy to increase muscle strength and balance. ■ The client will rest as needed during the day to prevent fatigue. ■ The client will verbalize an ability to adapt work and self-care to level of energy.

IMPLEMENTATION

- Encourage coughing, deep breathing, and expectoration of sputum.
- Administer respiratory treatments as ordered.
- Assess breath sounds every 4 hours and as needed.
- Assess oxygen saturation every 4 hours and as needed.
- Administer oxygen as needed per medical orders and hospital protocol.
- Administer antibiotic therapy as ordered.
- Administer ACTH as ordered.
- Teach client bladder training techniques, including Kegel exercises, delayed urination, and scheduled urination.

- Facilitate client referral to a urologist as ordered for bladder incontinence and risk for urinary tract infection.
- Facilitate client referral to physical and occupational therapists as ordered to increase muscle strength and ability to perform ADLs as well as assistive device training if needed.
- Teach client the importance of performing activities during peak energy levels.
- Teach client the importance of resting throughout the day.
- Encourage independence with mobility and self-care. Assist with ADLs as needed based on the client's fatigue levels.
- Offer and facilitate client referral to a MS support group.

EVALUATION

After 5 days in the hospital, the client is ready for discharge. She denies dyspnea, and her lungs are clear to auscultation. Her oxygen saturation is 99% on room air. The client is given an additional 10-day prescription of antibiotics and verbalizes an understanding of the importance of completing the course of antibiotics. The client demonstrates good pulmonary hygiene techniques and has been referred to physical and occupational therapists. After attending physical therapy and receiving instruction on cane use, the client has increased independence for ambulation. Occupational therapy has increased the client's ability to perform ADLs, and she understands the importance of performing strenuous activities during times of peak energy. She does still require some help with eating in the evening when she is most fatigued. The client has been referred to a urologist and has verbalized understanding of bladder training techniques.

CRITICAL THINKING

1. *How would you change the care plan for Mrs. West if she were confined to a wheelchair?*
2. *What teaching points should you provide for Mrs. West's husband about helping with self-care activities?*
3. *Develop a care plan for the nursing diagnosis Deficient Knowledge related to prevention of infection.*

REVIEW Multiple Sclerosis

RELATE Link the Concepts and Exemplars

Linking the exemplar of multiple sclerosis with the concept of sensory perception:

1. What assessment findings would you anticipate for a client with multiple sclerosis regarding alterations in visual acuity?

2. If the demyelination from multiple sclerosis is affecting the client's brainstem, what physical assessment data is a priority for the nurse to gather related to sensory perception?

Linking the exemplar of multiple sclerosis with the concept of mood and affect:

3. How will the administration of interferon beta-1a put the client at risk for alterations in mood and affect?

4. What mental health data is a priority for the nurse to assess before planning care for the client with MS?

READY Go to Companion Skills Manual

REFER Go to Pearson Student Nursing Resources
nursing.pearsonhighered.com

- Additional review materials

REFLECT Case Study

Elena Jones is a 48-year-old charge nurse who works in a busy pediatric ICU. She works 3 days a week doing 12-hour shifts and attends management and committee meetings on her days off. Mrs. Jones lives with her husband Brett and their three children: Debbie, 16; Jason, 11; and Ryan, 8. Debbie is busy visiting colleges that are interested in recruiting her because she is a star soccer player. She has been sneaking out of the house at night to visit her boyfriend. Jason has been in trouble in school for sassing teachers and has mild ADHD. Ryan has just discovered an interest in playing football after school. Brett is a remodeler who runs his business out of the home.

Mrs. Jones began having symptoms of neck pain and blurred vision. She has consulted a number of physicians but did not receive a satisfactory diagnosis until she saw a neurologist who ordered an MRI and diagnosed her with multiple sclerosis. Following her initial treatment, she quickly entered a period of remission that lasted for a few weeks. From that time on, she has experienced three to four exacerbations per year. She has had to

quit her job because she is unable to walk and has blurred vision that precludes driving. Her physician begins prednisone infusions five times a week for 1 week during flare-ups of MS.

1. What role might stress be playing in exacerbating her MS? What strategies can you promote to reduce stress?

2. How might you guide Mrs. Jones's family to contribute to improving her condition?

3. What are your expected outcomes for Mrs. Jones's care?

EXEMPLAR 13.5   Osteoarthritis

EXEMPLAR KEY TERMS
Arthroplasty, 888
Arthroscopy, 888
Bouchard nodes, 886
Debridement, 888
Heberden nodes, 886
Joint fusion, 888
Joint irrigation, 888
Joint resurfacing, 888
Osteoarthritis (OA), 886
Osteophytes, 886
Osteotomy, 888
Viscosupplementation, 890

EXEMPLAR LEARNING OUTCOMES
After reading about this exemplar, you will be able to:

1. Describe the pathophysiology, etiology, clinical manifestations, and direct and indirect causes of osteoarthritis.

2. Identify risk factors and prevention methods associated with osteoarthritis.

3. Illustrate the nursing process in providing culturally competent care across the life span for individuals with osteoarthritis.

4. Formulate priority nursing diagnoses appropriate for an individual with osteoarthritis.

5. Summarize therapies used by interdisciplinary teams in the collaborative care of an individual with osteoarthritis.

6. Plan evidence-based care for an individual with osteoarthritis and his or her family in collaboration with other members of the healthcare team.

7. Evaluate expected outcomes for an individual with osteoarthritis.

▶ OVERVIEW

Osteoarthritis (OA) is the most common form of arthritis, affecting over 50 million American adults (American College of Rheumatology [ACR], 2012). OA develops as wear and tear on the joints breaks down the cartilage in the joint, causing bone to rub on bone. It is the most common cause of disability in older adults and can affect any joint in the body, especially the hands, knees, and hips. Treatment aims to reduce pain, improve function of the affected joint, and slow disease progression.

▶ PATHOPHYSIOLOGY AND ETIOLOGY

In healthy joints, articular cartilage covers the ends of bones to allow the bones to glide over each other without friction during movement of the joint. Cartilage also absorbs shock from physical movement. As an individual ages, the cartilage begins to break down and wear away, allowing the bones to rub against each other. Particles that break off the joint irritate the synovial tissue, causing the pain, stiffness, inflammation, and swelling characteristic of OA (**Figure 13–40 ●**).

Small deposits of bone, called bone spurs or **osteophytes**, may also grow at the edges of the joint, changing the shape of the joint (NIAMSD, 2010). If these bony lumps occur in the digits, they are called **Bouchard nodes** (middle joint of the digit) or **Heberden nodes** (end joint of the digit). As changes to the joint occur, the joint no longer moves smoothly, causing mobility problems. OA typically involves the weight-bearing

joints of the hips and knees, the digits of the hands and big toe, and the cervical and lumbar spine. (See the Focus on Diversity and Culture feature for information on ethnic differences in location of OA.) Approximately 46% of individuals will develop OA of the knee within their lifetime (ACR, 2012).

Etiology
Osteoarthritis can be classified as either idiopathic or secondary. Idiopathic OA has no identifiable cause, but most scientists

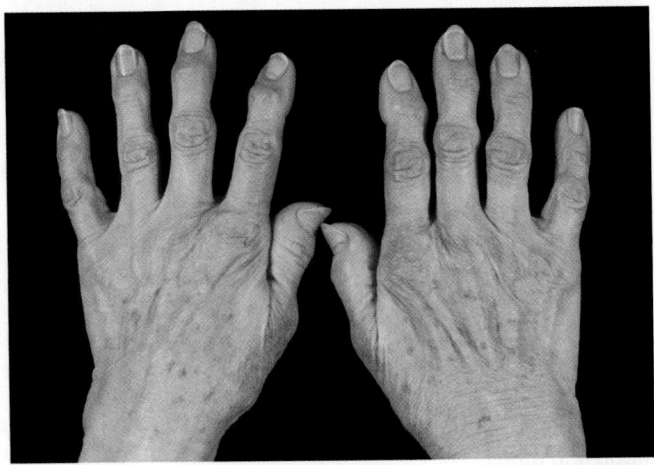

Figure 13–40 ● Typical interphalangeal joint changes associated with osteoarthritis.
Source: L. Samsuri/Custom Medical Stock.

In the United States (Allen, 2010):

- Knee OA is more common in Blacks than Whites.
- Knee OA is more common in Chinese women than White women.
- Hip and hand OA is less common in Chinese than Whites.
- Self-reported OA is less common in Hispanics than Whites.
- Blacks report greater pain and functional limitations compared to Whites for knee OA.

believe it is caused by both mechanical and molecular factors. Idiopathic OA can be further divided into localized or generalized, with localized OA affecting one or two joints and generalized OA affecting three or more joints. Secondary OA is caused by an underlying condition, such as injury; congenital malformation; metabolic, endocrine, or neuropathic disease; or other medical cause.

Risk Factors

The greatest risk factor for OA is older age. OA rarely occurs in individuals under the age of 40, but at least 80% of individuals over age 55 have some x-ray evidence of the disorder. Before age 45, more men than women have OA, but after age 45, women are two to three times more likely to develop OA than men (Kalunian, 2013; NIAMSD, 2010). Men often develop OA in the hip, knees, and spine, whereas women usually develop OA in the hip, knees, and hands. Jobs that require hard labor, heavy lifting, bending, or repetitive motion are linked to increased rates of OA. Obesity also increases the risk of developing OA, because the added weight increases stress on weight-bearing joints, causing the joint to wear down more quickly.

Certain medical conditions may increase an individual's risk of developing OA. For example, individuals born with malformed joints (bow legs, unequal leg length) or defective cartilage have an increased risk of developing OA. In addition, diseases such as diabetes, hypothyroid, gout, and Paget disease increase the risk of developing OA. Joint injuries from sports, accidents, or repetitive use also increase the risk of OA (Mayo Clinic, 2013b).

Prevention

Two of the most important guidelines to prevent OA are to maintain an ideal body weight and participate regularly in a moderate exercise program. Weight-bearing joints endure three to six times the individual's body weight in force while walking. Therefore, being overweight magnifies the force on the joint and leads to rapid degeneration of the cartilage. Both inactivity and excessive exercise can lead to premature breakdown of the joint cartilage; a moderate exercise program that involves walking, jogging, cycling, or swimming provides the most benefit for keeping bones, muscles, and joints strong and functioning properly.

Other important guidelines for maintaining good joint health include using good posture and proper body mechanics, avoiding repetitive stress on joints, stopping an activity when the joint becomes painful, and avoiding injury to the joints. If an injury does occur, the client should be encouraged to seek treatment immediately.

CLINICAL MANIFESTATIONS

Osteoarthritis begins with mild symptoms and progressively worsens over time. Symptoms of OA vary depending on the joint affected and individual factors. Some clients with visible joint degeneration on x-ray have no associated symptoms in the affected joint. However, many clients with OA develop pain associated with joint degeneration; this pain is usually worsened by activity and relieved by rest. Pain and stiffness is also associated with prolonged inactivity, such as sleeping at night or taking a long car ride. Other symptoms include tenderness to the touch, swelling related to excess fluid in the joint (effusion), crackling or grating of the joint (crepitus) due to rough surfaces rubbing against each other, and bone spurs that contribute to joint swelling. This joint damage typically causes the joint to have a decreased range of motion.

Complications

Osteoarthritis can lead to a host of complications as the severity of the condition worsens. Joint pain and degeneration, stiffness, an unsteady gait, and effects of medications all increase the risk of falling, causing fractures and additional mobility limitations. As physical limitations increase, the client may experience a decreased ability to perform ADLs. As the individual is less able to perform work responsibilities, she may develop financial difficulties related to the cost of treatment and lost wages. As the disability persists, the individual may develop anxiety, depression, and feelings of helplessness. Both the physical disability and the associated mood disorder may lead the individual to have difficulty participating in social and family activities.

COLLABORATION

Treatment of OA requires multidisciplinary care from nurses, primary care physicians, rheumatologists, physical and occupational therapists, and many others. There is currently no cure

Lifespan Considerations
Juvenile Osteoarthritis

Children can develop juvenile osteoarthritis, which is usually secondary OA related to a congenital abnormality, genetic condition, or joint injury. Juvenile OA typically occurs only in the one or two joints affected by the abnormality or injury. Children with OA are less likely to become disabled and may outgrow the condition as they age. However, children and adolescents with joint abnormalities or injuries who do not develop OA during childhood are at increased risk of developing OA later in life.

for OA, so treatment aims to relieve pain and maintain function of the joint. Helping clients learn how to cope with a chronic disease is also a vital part of nursing care for clients with OA. According to *Healthy People 2020* (U.S. Department of Health and Human Services, 2013), interventions that can reduce arthritis pain and functional limitations include increased physical activity, self-management education, and weight loss among adults who are overweight/obese.

Diagnostic Tests

In addition to a medical history and physical examination, several tests can be used to help diagnose OA and track the disease's course. The most commonly used diagnostic test is an x-ray of the affected joint, but other tests may include an MRI, ultrasound, blood tests, and joint fluid analysis. An x-ray can reveal a narrowing of the space between bones in the joint, indicating a lack of cartilage. However, x-rays may not show signs of OA until significant cartilage loss has occurred. An x-ray may also show bone spurs or other bone damage. MRI and ultrasound produce more detailed images of the bone and soft tissues, including cartilage, ligaments, and tendons. This is a more sensitive way to determine the extent of joint damage.

Although there is no blood test available that can conclusively identify OA, other blood tests can help rule out other causes of joint pain, such as rheumatoid arthritis. Current research is also investigating the usefulness of serum hyaluronic acid as a prognostic marker for clients with knee osteoarthritis. Joint fluid analysis is used to detect inflammation and the presence of bacteria (infection) or uric acid crystals (gout).

Surgery

Clients with severe arthritis that is not managed by medication and nonpharmacologic interventions may be good candidates for surgery. Depending on the joint and extent of damage, several options are available for surgery, including arthroscopy, joint resurfacing, joint irrigation, osteotomy, joint fusion, and arthroplasty. The purpose of surgery is to remove damage, relieve pain, and restore function of the joint.

ARTHROSCOPY   In the procedure known as **arthroscopy**, a small arthroscope consisting of a small fiberoptic light source, magnifying lens, and camera is inserted into the joint to visualize the joint structures. Small surgical instruments may also be inserted into the joint to remove or trim structures that may be causing pain (**debridement**). Arthroscopy is often combined with **joint irrigation**, in which a fluid is injected into the joint to allow the surgeon to visualize joint structures more easily and to help remove debris and infection in the joint. Arthroscopic surgery for clients with OA is unpredictable, because this surgery is not designed to repair cartilage that is worn from the ends of bones. However, arthroscopic surgery does relieve pain in some clients with OA, and it can be used to treat OA in clients who have little success with other treatments (Johns Hopkins Medicine, n.d.). Arthroscopy can also be used to explore the extent of damage in the joint in preparation for future surgery.

JOINT RESURFACING   In **joint resurfacing**, a small amount of bone is removed at the articulating surface of the joint and a metal replacement is fitted over the end of the bone. Joint resurfacing is often performed instead of total joint replacement in younger clients in the early stages of arthritis. Artificial joints often wear out and need to be replaced within 15–20 years, and the amount of bone removed during arthroplasty makes revision complicated. Joint resurfacing removes less bone than arthroplasty, allowing younger clients to experience more successful total joint replacement later in life when the metal component has become worn. Joint resurfacing is often performed for hip and shoulder joints.

OSTEOTOMY   **Osteotomy** is a procedure that entails surgical removal of a wedge of bone above or below the joint to realign the joint and shift the weight away from the damaged portion of the joint. To further help redistribute weight, the tibia and femur are reshaped. Surgical staples or screws are inserted to stabilize the repositioned bones. This procedure is usually performed instead of joint replacement surgery if there is damage to only one side of the joint in healthy, younger adults. After an osteotomy, the client should be able to participate in any physical activity that he enjoyed before the surgery, even high-impact exercise. Osteotomies are commonly performed on the knee and hip, but can be used for other joints as well.

JOINT FUSION   **Joint fusion**, also known as arthrodesis, is used to permanently fuse two or more bones together at a joint using pins, plates, screws, and rods. A bone graft may also be used to stimulate bone growth at the site of fusion. Joint fusion is often recommended for badly damaged smaller joints, such as the spine, wrist, ankle, finger, or toe.

ARTHROPLASTY   A total joint replacement is known as **arthroplasty**. In an arthroplasty, the surgeon removes the damaged joint surfaces and replaces them with plastic, metal, or ceramic prostheses. Prostheses may be joined to bone surfaces with cement, or they may contain porous surfaces that stimulate bone growth to hold the prosthesis in place. More information about cement versus porous surfaces for prostheses as well as total hip replacement can be found in Exemplar 13.3 within this module.

Because of advances in technology, the surgeon can choose the type of prosthesis based on the client's weight, sex, age, activity level, and general health. Artificial joints usually last about 15–20 years, so the best candidates for arthroplasty are older adults. Hip and knee arthroplasties (**Figure 13–41 ●**) are the most common, but other joints can also be replaced, including shoulders, elbows, ankles, wrists, fingers, and toes. Total recovery time after joint replacement of a major joint (hip, knee) is 4–6 weeks short term (independent function) and around 6 months long term (full function). The greatest risks after arthroplasty include infection, blood clots, and long-term breakdown of the artificial joint.

Pharmacologic Therapy

Many OTC medications are effective for treatment of mild to moderate osteoarthritis pain. Acetaminophen (Tylenol) is usually suggested as a first-line therapy because most clients tolerate it well. However, acetaminophen can produce liver toxicity if taken in high doses or in clients with chronic liver disease or

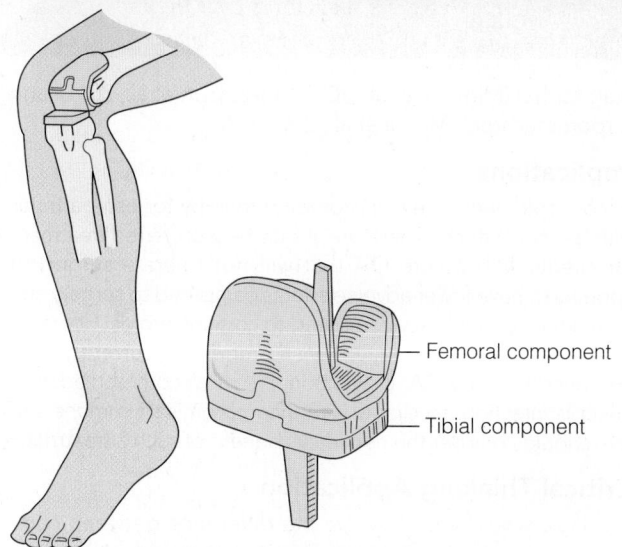

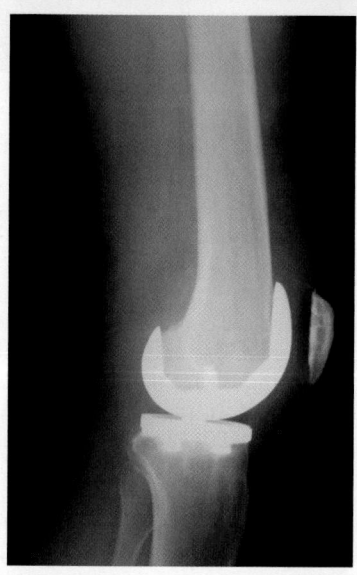

Figure 13–41 ● Total knee replacement.
Source: David Frazier/Getty Images.

excess alcohol intake (see the Safety Alert feature). Ibuprofen (Advil, Motrin) and naproxen (Aleve) are NSAIDs that treat both pain and inflammation. Stronger NSAIDs are available by prescription, including the COX-2 inhibitor celecoxib (Celebrex). NSAIDs are generally well tolerated, but they can produce cardiovascular and gastrointestinal effects. For clients with severe OA pain, opioid analgesics such as codeine, tramadol, or hydrocodone may be prescribed. However, opioids carry the risk of tolerance and addiction, so they should be prescribed as a last resort. For more information about analgesics, see the exemplar on Acute and Chronic Pain in the module on Comfort.

SAFETY ALERT

At present, the U.S. Food and Drug Administration (FDA) (2011) adult guidelines for acetaminophen administration include not exceeding a dosage of 4,000 mg/day. The maker of Tylenol, McNeil Consumer Healthcare, recommends a maximum adult dose of no more than 3,000 mg/day (Johnson & Johnson, 2011). In all cases, clients should be aware of the potential for unintentionally exceeding the maximum acetaminophen dosage due to simultaneously taking more than one medication that contains acetaminophen. Likewise, clients with impaired liver function may be at risk for toxicity-related injury, even when following the guidelines. Acetaminophen toxicity may cause severe liver damage, liver failure, and death (FDA, 2011).

Topical analgesic creams, rubs, and sprays may also be prescribed for clients with OA. These drugs are applied directly to the skin surrounding the joint. They work by stimulating nerve endings, depleting substance P, or blocking prostaglandins to decrease pain signals received by the brain. Examples include capsaicin cream (Capzasin, Zostrix), diclofenac gel (Voltaren), salicylates (Aspercreme, Bengay), and menthol (Icy Hot, Biofreeze). The nurse should teach clients to keep these topical medications away from the eyes, nose, and mouth and to discontinue use if irritation occurs.

Cortisone injections may also be administered for treatment of OA pain. The corticosteroid medication is injected directly into the joint to reduce inflammation and pain. Because frequent use of corticosteroids can cause joint damage, cortisone injections are limited to three to four injections per year for weight-bearing joints. A relatively new option for OA treatment by injection is hyaluronic acid (see the Evidence-Based Practice feature).

Nonpharmacologic Therapy

Osteoarthritis is a progressive disease, so early treatment can significantly improve outcomes and quality of life. In addition to treating pain with analgesics, nonpharmacologic treatment for OA includes heat and cold application, use of assistive technology, weight reduction, rest, and education about the disease, exercise, and coping techniques (see the Community-Based Care feature).

Heat can be applied to painful joints to decrease pain and improve flexibility. Heat application can include warm towels, hot packs, heating pads, or warm showers or baths. Cold in the form of ice packs or cold packs can be applied to reduce pain and swelling. Mild cold should be used for swelling, and deeper cold should be used for pain.

SAFETY ALERT

To avoid skin injury, application of hot packs should not exceed 20 minutes and cold packs should be applied for no more than 10–30 minutes.

Assistive technology can be used to help minimize stress placed on the affected joint. Canes, crutches, and walkers can be used to protect joints of the lower limbs, and devices such as grippers, reachers, dressing aids, and enlarged pens can reduce stress on the spine and upper limbs. Orthotics such as braces or shoe inserts may be beneficial to help maintain proper alignment of the joints. Many assistive devices can be bought commercially or custom made to meet the specific needs of the client. The nurse may need to refer the client to a physical or occupational therapist for instruction about proper use of the assistive device.

Evidence-Based Practice Hyaluronic Acid Injections

Problem

Hyaluronic acid (HA) is a normal component of synovial fluid, where it acts as a lubricant and shock absorber. During osteoarthritis, HA is degraded, leading to pain and reduced movement of the joint (Iannitti, Lodi, & Palmieri, 2011).

Evidence

Multiple studies have indicated that HA injections (**viscosupplementation**) are effective for the treatment of knee OA. HA works by restoring the elastic and viscous properties of the synovial fluid, reducing pain, and improving function (Navarro-Sarabia et al., 2011). HA also appears to preserve cartilage when used long term (Wang et al., 2011). HA is normally given in a series of three to five weekly injections, and the series of injections can be given every 6–12 months. HA is more effective for pain compared to corticosteroid injections starting at 4 weeks postinjection (Bannuru et al., 2009). In a large, multiple-center, double-blinded, randomized clinical trial for clients with knee OA, clients with HA injections showed significant improvement in the areas of pain, function, and global assessment during a series of four sets of five injections over 40 months. No significant safety problems were noted during the course of treatment (Navarro-Sarabia et al., 2011). Although viscosupplementation is currently approved only for knee OA, it is showing promise in clinical trials for hip (Migliore et al., 2009), ankle (Sun et al., 2011), and carpometacarpal (Mandl et al., 2009) OA.

Implications

Viscosupplementation is a promising therapy for osteoarthritis with few side effects. Therefore, it may be a preferred treatment for clients with severe OA that will not tolerate surgery. It appears to have fewer adverse effects compared to surgery and more long-term efficacy compared to corticosteroids. However, HA injections are more expensive and are currently only approved for knee OA. In addition, the most common adverse effect is infection, so clients with a compromised immune system should consider the risk versus benefit of such a treatment.

Critical Thinking Application

1. How would you describe the difference between cortisone and hyaluronic acid injections to an older client with mild cognitive deficits (administration, mechanism of action, side effects, duration of effect, follow-up)?

2. Viscosupplementation is a relatively new therapy. What would you say to a client who is skeptical of the long-term side effects of this treatment?

3. If you were asked to develop a brochure stating the pros and cons of hyaluronic acid injections, what information would you include?

Obesity is a major contributor to osteoarthritis development, because excess weight dramatically increases the force on weight-bearing joints. Therefore, the nurse should encourage clients who are overweight or obese and who have OA of the knee, hip, or ankle to begin a weight loss program. Weight-bearing joints withstand three to six times the force of the total body weight when the individual walks, so even a small reduction in weight can greatly reduce the force on the affected joint.

Clients with OA should be encouraged to get adequate sleep and rest. Arthritis pain may interfere with nighttime sleep, so the nurse should teach the client good sleep hygiene (see the exemplar on Sleep–Rest Disorders in the module on Comfort) and nonpharmacologic methods to reduce pain (see the exemplar on Acute and Chronic Pain in the module on Comfort). Clients should be encouraged to get adequate rest throughout the day to prevent overstressing the affected joints. Rest should be done for short periods with the joint in correct alignment. In addition, if the arthritic joint is in use and develops increased pain, the client should be instructed to stop the activity immediately and rest the joint for 12–24 hours. Resting the joint should result in decreased pain and swelling. If possible, the nurse should encourage the client to find activities that do not require repetitive use of the injured joint. Assistive devices may be beneficial to promote rest of the injured joint.

Community-Based Care Home Care for Clients With Osteoarthritis

Clients with osteoarthritis need to manage their condition while living at home. Several techniques can help clients cope with their disease and maintain function as the disease progresses. Modifications the client can make include the following:

- Make home safety improvements, such as removing throw rugs and clutter, installing hand rails, and placing commonly used items within easy reach.
- Learn about osteoarthritis, including the disease process and treatments.
- Begin an exercise program to gain strength and range of motion.
- Avoid excessive or repetitive use of joints and overstretching of the muscles associated with the affected joint.
- Practice good posture and avoid soft furniture that requires excess effort to stand.
- Use pharmacologic and nonpharmacologic pain management techniques.

Participating in a mild exercise program is an important treatment for OA. Exercises such as walking, biking, or swimming are best for clients with OA. The amount and type of exercise will depend on the joints involved and the extent of joint damage (see the Client Teaching feature for exercise guidelines). The nurse should teach clients to stop exercising if they experience new pain. In addition, daily ROM exercises can strengthen muscles to provide support for the damaged joint. Physical therapy and other rehabilitation programs can help clients determine which exercises are best for their specific condition; rehabilitation is especially important after joint replacement surgery.

Client Teaching Exercise Guidelines for Clients With Osteoarthritis

Exercise is an important aspect of nursing care for clients with osteoarthritis. Exercise can increase flexibility, improve blood flow, help the client lose weight, and improve mood. Types of exercises include the following:

- *Stretching* of all muscle groups for 10 minutes daily. Clients should avoid overstretching, because this can cause muscle damage.
- Active *range-of-motion* exercises daily for all joints. These exercises help keep joints limber.
- *Balance* and *agility* exercises can help maintain daily living skills.
- Low-intensity *isometric* exercises, or static exercises, can strengthen muscles without moving painful joints.
- *Isotonic*, or strengthening, exercises, in which a fixed weight is carried through the range of motion, should start with small weights or a resistance band and a partial range of motion. Resistance and range should be increased gradually.
- Low-impact *aerobic* exercises, such as walking, cycling, or swimming, are well tolerated by clients with OA. These exercises improve cardiovascular health, strengthen muscles, and improve balance and gait. Water exercises are especially beneficial for clients with OA of the weight-bearing joints, because water buoyancy helps decrease force on the joints.

Some clients will not respond to traditional treatments for osteoarthritis and will look for alternative ways to relieve pain. The Complementary and Alternative Therapy feature provides further information on alternative treatments.

NURSING PROCESS

Osteoarthritis is a progressive, incurable disease. Nursing care for clients with OA focuses on reducing pain, maintaining mobility and function, and helping clients learn how to use assistive devices. If OA becomes severe, clients may also need pre- and postoperative nursing care. For clients who are overweight or obese, the nurse should encourage the client to begin a weight loss program to reduce force on weight-bearing joints.

Complementary and Alternative Therapy
Osteoarthritis

Alternative therapies for OA include acupuncture, massage, and gentle exercises (tai chi and yoga). The use of glucosamine and chondroitin for OA has shown mixed results in clinical trials, with most indicating that these nutritional supplements are no better than placebo but may increase the risk of bleeding (Mayo Clinic, 2013b). Stem cell therapy using autologous mesenchymal stem cells is currently under investigation for use in clients with knee OA (Centeno et al., 2008; Emadedin et al., 2012).

Assessment

A nursing assessment for clients with OA includes a health history and physical examination. The health history should include a family history of OA, description of symptoms (onset, location, intensity, modifying factors), physical activity (exercise, occupation, recreation), mobility, and ability to perform ADLs. A physical assessment should include height and weight and assessment of the affected joint, including appearance, temperature, pain, crepitus, ROM, deformities, and Heberden or Bouchard nodes. As part of the assessment, the physician may also order diagnostic tests; the nurse may be responsible for transporting the client to the appropriate location for testing.

Diagnosis

Nursing diagnoses related to osteoarthritis may include the following:

- *Chronic Pain* related to loss of joint cartilage
- *Impaired Physical Mobility* related to cartilage degradation and pain
- *Sedentary Lifestyle* related to joint pain during movement
- *Imbalanced Nutrition: More Than Body Requirements* related to overeating and lack of exercise
- *Dressing Self-Care Deficit* related to decreased range of motion of fingers.

(NANDA-I © 2012)

Planning

Client goals for the individual with OA may include the following:

- The client will verbalize understanding of the indications for and effects of analgesic medications.
- The client will demonstrate knowledge of nonpharmacologic pain management techniques.
- The client will verbalize an understanding of the need to rest when pain worsens during physical activity.
- The client will perform ROM exercises daily.
- The client will demonstrate increased ROM of the affected joint.
- The client will begin a mild exercise program based on a physical therapist's recommendations.
- The client will enroll in nutritional counseling or a weight loss program.
- The client will independently perform dressing self-care with the use of assistive devices.

Implementation

Nursing interventions for clients with OA should aim to decrease pain, promote mobility through exercise, teach clients how to use assistive devices for ADLs and self-care, and encourage weight loss in clients who are overweight or obese.

Promote Comfort

Pain as a result of joint degeneration is the most common symptom of OA, and it influences the client's ability to ambulate and perform ADLs. Therefore, pain management is the primary nursing

Clinical Manifestations and Therapies **Osteoarthritis**

ETIOLOGY	CLINICAL MANIFESTATIONS	CLINICAL THERAPIES
Knee	■ Pain, effusion ■ Crepitus ■ Instability ■ Deformity ■ Osteophytes ■ Stiffness, unsteady gait, limited movement	■ Rest/heat/ice ■ OTC analgesics ■ Assistive devices ■ Weight loss ■ Corticosteroid injections ■ Viscosupplementation ■ Osteotomy ■ Arthroplasty ■ Physical therapy/exercise
Hip	■ Referred pain to inguinal region, buttock, thigh, or knee ■ Limited ROM ■ Unsteady gait, stiffness	■ Rest/heat/ice ■ Physical therapy/exercise ■ Assistive devices ■ OTC analgesics ■ Weight loss ■ Corticosteroid injections ■ Joint resurfacing ■ Osteotomy ■ Arthroplasty
Shoulder	■ Pain ■ Stiffness ■ Thickened joint capsule ■ Loss of ROM ■ Crepitus	■ Physical therapy/exercise ■ OTC analgesics ■ Corticosteroid injections ■ Arthroscopic debridement ■ Joint resurfacing ■ Arthroplasty ■ Rest/heat/ice
Spine	■ Radiating pain ■ Stiffness, muscle spasm ■ Limited ROM ■ Nerve root compression, weakness, numbness	■ Rest/heat/ice ■ OTC analgesics ■ Weight loss ■ Spinal fusion ■ Back-strengthening exercises
Elbow	■ Pain ■ Loss of ROM ■ Grating or locking sensation ■ Swelling, numbness in fingers	■ OTC analgesics ■ Corticosteroid injections ■ Physical therapy/exercise ■ Arthroscopy ■ Osteotomy ■ Arthroplasty
Ankle	■ Pain, swelling, inflammation ■ Stiffness, difficulty walking ■ Limited ROM ■ Deformities	■ OTC analgesics ■ Orthotics ■ Physical therapy/exercise ■ Weight loss ■ Corticosteroid injections ■ Arthroscopic debridement ■ Joint fusion ■ Arthroscopy
Wrist	■ Pain, swelling ■ Stiffness, weakness ■ Limited ROM ■ Crepitus	■ Rest/heat/ice ■ OTC analgesics ■ Bracing ■ Corticosteroid injection ■ Joint fusion ■ Arthroplasty ■ Physical therapy/exercise

Clinical Manifestations and Therapies Osteoarthritis (continued)

ETIOLOGY	CLINICAL MANIFESTATIONS	CLINICAL THERAPIES
Fingers	■ Pain ■ Heberden nodes, Bouchard nodes ■ Crepitus ■ Swelling, tenderness ■ Decreased ROM ■ Cysts	■ Rest/heat/ice ■ OTC analgesics ■ Assistive devices ■ Splinting ■ Corticosteroid injection ■ Joint fusion ■ Arthroplasty
Toes	■ Pain ■ Heberden nodes, Bouchard nodes ■ Decreased ROM ■ Swelling	■ Rest/heat/ice ■ OTC analgesics ■ Corticosteroid injection ■ Joint fusion ■ Arthroplasty

intervention needed for clients with OA. The nurse should obtain a pain description and monitor pain levels with each client interaction. Pain from OA is often managed by mild analgesics, which should be taken on a regular schedule before pain becomes severe. The nurse should also teach the client nonpharmacologic pain management techniques, including good body mechanics, heat/ice, distraction techniques, guided imagery, and relaxation.

Pain associated with OA is cyclical: Joints stiffen with prolonged rest, causing pain when the client begins movement. As movement warms and lubricates the joints, pain subsides. However, with excessive movement, the client will begin to feel pain again, which is relieved by rest. Because of this cycle, the nurse should teach clients the importance of alternating rest and activity. Short periods of rest can help relieve joint stress while avoiding stiffness, and short periods of activity can prevent pain from overuse. Moderation of both rest and activity are key to maintaining mobility and reducing pain for clients with osteoarthritis.

Optimize Physical Mobility

Clients with osteoarthritis benefit greatly from performing mild exercise (see the Client Teaching feature). Exercise can increase the ROM of affected joints, strengthen muscles to provide support for the joint, and promote general health. Exercise can also help clients with OA in weight-bearing joints increase balance, coordination, and strength to promote independent ambulation. The nurse should assess clients with newly diagnosed OA for ROM of the affected joints as a baseline for future comparison, and ROM should be assessed with each subsequent nurse–client interaction. The nurse should also perform a mobility assessment to determine whether the client has problems walking, sitting, rising, or climbing stairs. These assessments can help guide the nurse in suggesting appropriate exercises and assistive devices for the client. The nurse should also teach the client a variety of exercises to promote mobility or should refer the client to a physical or occupational therapist for teaching and rehabilitation.

Clients will need to learn how to perform ADLs while suffering from a progressive disorder that causes pain, stiffness, and decreased mobility of joints. Assistive devices play a key role in helping clients maintain independence in performing ADLs. Assistive devices can also help reduce stress on affected joints, which may help slow the progression of disease.

The nurse should perform a functional assessment to determine which devices may provide the most benefit for the client; the assistive device needed will likely depend on the location of the OA. For example, a client with knee arthritis may benefit from the use of a cane or walker. Safety devices such as hand rails and shower chairs may be beneficial for clients with hip OA. A client with shoulder or spine arthritis may benefit from the use of a reacher device, which can be used to grab objects over the head or on the floor. A client with osteoarthritis of the hand may need to use button or zipper hooks, toothbrushes or eating utensils with large handles, or electric can openers. The list of possible assistive devices is endless and can be tailored to the specific needs of the client. Once the client has chosen the appropriate assistive devices, the nurse should provide training or referrals for training in the proper use of each device.

Promote Balanced Nutrition

Obesity is a major risk factor for the development of osteoarthritis; excess weight can also contribute to the progression of OA. Therefore, clients who are overweight or obese will decrease their risk of disease progression if they begin a weight loss program. Weight loss promotes general health and wellness and decreases the risk of a myriad of other chronic diseases. A weight loss program should include both decreased caloric intake (balanced diet) and increased caloric expenditure (exercise). Many clients will benefit from a weight loss support group or accountability program such as Weight Watchers or Curves. The nurse should provide referrals to community weight loss programs as appropriate.

Evaluation

The client with osteoarthritis should be evaluated in several areas with each follow-up appointment, including assessments for pain, ROM of the affected joint, ability to ambulate smoothly and independently, ability to independently perform ADLs, interference of the OA with the client's preferred lifestyle, and adequate sleep and rest. Diagnostic tests such as x-rays should also be performed periodically to monitor joint space and osteophyte formation, especially if the client reports increased pain or decreased ROM. Changes in the client's condition necessitate a change in the nursing care plan.

NURSING CARE PLAN A Client With Osteoarthritis of the Knee

Gloria Kirsch is a 63-year-old grade school teacher who has suffered from knee osteoarthritis for the past 8 years. She lives at home with her husband of 44 years. During the past year, the pain in her right knee has become progressively more severe, and she is no longer able to keep up with the kids in her classroom. Therefore, Mrs. Kirsch visits her primary care physician for treatment.

ASSESSMENT

Courtney Whitmore, RN, completes a health history and physical examination of Mrs. Kirsch upon admission. Ms. Whitmore finds that Mrs. Kirsch has a BMI of 31 (H 64", W 182 lb). Her client history indicates that Mrs. Kirsch is on atorvastatin for high cholesterol and losartan for hypertension. Her vital signs include temperature 99.4°F oral; pulse 66 bpm; respirations 17/min; and BP 132/85 mmHg. A physical examination reveals that Mrs. Kirsch has full ROM of the wrists, elbows, and ankles; slightly reduced ROM of the shoulders and hips; and minimal ROM in the knees. In particular, flexion of her right knee is limited to 105°, and extension is limited to 35°. Her left knee also has reduced ROM, with flexion to 140° and extension to 10°. Mrs. Kirsch walks with a limp, favoring her right knee. Diagnostic x-rays show a joint space grade of 3 on a 0–3 scale (0 = normal, 3 = bone-to-bone contact) for the right knee and 2 for the left knee. Osteophytes are also prominent on the distal femur and proximal tibia of the right knee. The physician recommends that Mrs. Kirsch undergo knee replacement surgery for her right knee, which is scheduled for the next week.

DIAGNOSES (POSTOPERATIVE)

- *Risk for Infection* related to surgical procedure
- *Risk for Injury* related to alteration in mobility
- *Risk for Impaired Skin Integrity* related to decreased mobility in the postoperative period
- *Acute Pain* related to surgical incision and hip surgery
- *Impaired Physical Mobility* related to weight-bearing restrictions
- *Imbalanced Nutrition: More Than Body Requirements* related to diet and lack of exercise
- *Ineffective Role Performance* related to inability to keep up with children at work
- *Anxiety* related to lack of mobility after surgery

(NANDA-I © 2012)

PLANNING

- The client will remain free from infection.
- The client will remain free from postoperative complications, including bleeding or impairment of the surgical wound.
- The client will remain free from injury.
- The client will demonstrate no skin breakdown or ulcerations.
- The client will report that pain is tolerable, with a rating of no greater than 3 on a scale of 0–10.
- The client will demonstrate right knee mobility within limitations.
- The client will perform ROM exercises to maintain muscle strength.
- The client will ambulate with assistance on postsurgery day 1.
- The client will ambulate independently with an assistive device on postsurgery day 3.
- The client will lose 3 pounds by her 4-week follow-up appointment.
- The client will participate in a mild exercise program to increase strength and stability of the knee as well as help lose weight.
- The client will express decreased anxiety related to recovery from knee arthroplasty.

IMPLEMENTATION

- Assess the surgical site frequently; report signs of bleeding or infection.
- Administer antibiotics as ordered.
- Use standard precautions per protocol during all client care.
- Assess pain at least hourly for the first 24 hours postoperatively and as needed thereafter.
- Administer pain medications as prescribed.
- Teach client nonpharmacologic pain management techniques, including heat/ice, distraction, and relaxation.
- Teach client ROM exercises for each joint, and help client perform passive ROM exercises with each shift.

- Help client change positions every 2 hours to prevent pressure sores and stimulate blood flow.
- Assist client with ambulation at least three times daily starting on day 1 postsurgery.
- Teach the client how to properly use a walker and cane.
- Facilitate referrals to dietary specialists and weight loss support groups.
- Teach the client about the normal progression of healing after a knee arthroplasty.

EVALUATION

Mrs. Kirsch returns to her primary care physician for follow-up 4 weeks after surgery. She is experiencing decreased pain and increased ROM in her right knee. However, her left knee is experiencing increased pain, likely because of compensatory posturing during healing from her right knee replacement. She is ambulating independently with no assistive device at home, but she takes a cane with her when she needs to walk longer distances. Her surgical incision healed properly with no signs of bleeding or infection. Mrs. Kirsch proudly reports that she has joined Weight Watchers and the local YMCA, and she has lost 10 pounds since being released from the hospital. She feels more confident about returning to work, knowing that she can once again keep up with her students.

CRITICAL THINKING

1. In addition to infection, a potential complication of knee replacement surgery is deep venous thrombosis. Describe nursing interventions to help prevent DVT.
2. What nursing interventions could the nurse implement if Mrs. Kirsch refused to attempt ambulation on day 1 postsurgery?
3. Develop a list of discharge instructions for Mrs. Kirsch and her husband.

REVIEW Osteoarthritis

RELATE Link the Concepts and Exemplars

Linking the exemplar of osteoarthritis with the concept of comfort:

1. What assessment data will you gather to help plan for chronic pain relief in the client with osteoarthritis?

2. Compare and contrast the various complementary and alternative therapies for pain relief for the client with osteoarthritis.

Linking the exemplar of osteoarthritis with the concept of safety:

3. Create a safety plan for the client with severe osteoarthritis in both hands who lives alone.

4. What teaching interventions will you initiate for the client with osteoarthritis of the knees who is learning to use a walker?

READY Go to Companion Skills Manual

REFER Go to Pearson Student Nursing Resources
nursing.pearsonhighered.com

- Additional review materials

REFLECT Case Study

Maureen Murphy is a 68-year-old woman who has recently been diagnosed with osteoarthritis in her right hip. Mrs. Murphy lives with her husband Marty, who is 75 and has been diagnosed with early dementia. Mr. Murphy has a descending aortic aneurysm that required surgery 5 months ago. He has not recovered as well as expected and is frequently confused and forgetful as well as weak. Mrs. Murphy is retired and carries good health insurance for herself and her husband. Each has an IRA as well as Social Security benefits. Mrs. Murphy is extremely well organized, pays attention to detail, and gets very agitated when her routine is interrupted. Mr. and Mrs. Murphy belong to a small community church and have many caring friends and neighbors.

Mrs. Murphy's healthcare provider recommends hip replacement, to which she readily agrees. She has been limping and in pain, which is causing problems as she attempts to care for her husband. The physician has told Mrs. Murphy that she will be in the hospital for 1 week after surgery and then 2 weeks at a rehabilitation hospital. Before surgery, Mrs. Murphy is trying to arrange for her husband's care as well as her own.

1. What priorities of care do you see for Mrs. Murphy prior to surgery?

2. What safety concerns do you anticipate for Mrs. Murphy and her husband when Mrs. Murphy is discharged from rehabilitation?

3. What resources will you recommend for Mrs. Murphy's home care after discharge from rehabilitation?

EXEMPLAR 13.6 **Parkinson Disease**

EXEMPLAR KEY TERMS

Bradykinesia, *895*
Cognitive deficits, *897*
Deep brain stimulation (DBS), *898*
Dopamine, *895*
Festination, *897*
Freezing, *897*
Hypophonia, *897*
Lewy bodies, *896*
"On–off" effect, *898*
Parkinsonian gait, *897*
Parkinsonism, *897*
Parkinson disease (PD), *895*
Pill-rolling, *897*
Postural instability, *897*
Retropulsion, *897*
Rigidity, *897*
Tremor, *896*

EXEMPLAR LEARNING OUTCOMES

After reading about this exemplar, you will be able to:

1. Describe the pathophysiology, etiology, clinical manifestations, and direct and indirect causes of Parkinson disease.

2. Identify risk factors and prevention methods associated with Parkinson disease.

3. Illustrate the nursing process in providing culturally competent care across the life span for individuals with Parkinson disease.

4. Formulate priority nursing diagnoses appropriate for an individual with Parkinson disease.

5. Summarize therapies used by interdisciplinary teams in the collaborative care of an individual with Parkinson disease.

6. Plan evidence-based care for an individual with Parkinson disease and his or her family in collaboration with other members of the healthcare team.

7. Evaluate expected outcomes for an individual with Parkinson disease.

▶ OVERVIEW

Parkinson disease (PD) is a progressive neurological disorder that primarily affects movement. It was first described in 1817 by James Parkinson, a British physician who called it the "shaking palsy." It is usually characterized initially by unilateral hand tremors, but progresses to include bilateral tremors, rigidity, **bradykinesia** (slow movements), and postural instability. These symptoms decrease the client's quality of life and increases dependence on others. It is estimated that at least 500,000 individuals in the United States currently have PD, with approximately 50,000 new cases each year. The cost of care for these individuals is estimated at more than $6 billion annually (NINDS, 2013).

▶ PATHOPHYSIOLOGY AND ETIOLOGY

Dopamine is a brain neurotransmitter that regulates voluntary movement, reward-seeking behavior, memory and learning, attention, sleep, affect, and many other functions. Dopamine receptors are expressed throughout the brain, including the substantia nigra (Beaulieu & Gainetdinov, 2011). Individuals with Parkinson disease have motor deficits that result from the progressive loss of dopaminergic neurons in the substantia nigra and other areas of the brain; motor deficits begin to appear when 60%–80% of the dopamine is lost. Dopaminergic cell death is a result of oxidative stress, impaired mitochondrial function, and protein misfolding and aggregation (Hindle, 2010). PD is also characterized by the presence of **Lewy bodies** in neurons, which are abnormal aggregates of proteins, including alpha-synuclein. The purpose of Lewy bodies, including whether they are helpful or harmful, is still under investigation.

Loss of dopaminergic neurons that connect the substantia nigra to the cholinergic neurons in the corpus striatum results in abnormal nerve-firing patterns that cause impaired movement (National Institutes of Health [NIH], 2012). Dopamine and acetylcholine must be balanced to produce smooth movement. When dopamine neurons are degenerated, acetylcholine signaling is increased, causing an imbalance that contributes to the clinical manifestations of Parkinson disease.

Etiology

The cause of Parkinson disease is unknown, but many researchers believe it results from a combination of genetic susceptibility and exposure to environmental factors or toxins, and some cases of PD appear to be hereditary. Most cases of PD are sporadic, which means the disease occurs randomly with no apparent genetic link.

Risk Factors

Age is the primary risk factor for developing PD. The average age of onset is 60 years, and the risk increases with advancing age. Men are also at higher risk, with 50% more men than women developing PD. Some studies indicate that individuals who live in rural areas or work in certain professions are at higher risk, providing an environmental link for the development of PD. In a few individuals, PD is inherited; approximately 15%–25% of individuals with PD have a relative with PD. Genetic mutation of several genes has been linked to PD, including *SNCA* (alpha-synuclein), *LRRK2*, and *PARK2* (NIH, 2012). Individuals with early-onset or juvenile PD are more likely to have a genetic mutation than individuals with late-onset PD.

Prevention

Because the cause of PD is unknown, there is no definitive way to prevent the development of the disease. However, several prevention techniques have been suggested by experts, including consuming a healthy diet that is high in fruits and vegetables, avoiding herbicides and pesticides, and consuming moderate amounts of caffeine and green tea. Consumption of nutritional supplements may also help prevent PD, including vitamins C, D, and E, coenzyme Q10, creatine, and stilbenes (Chao et al., 2012).

▶ CLINICAL MANIFESTATIONS

Symptoms of Parkinson disease are mild at the beginning of the disease and progressively worsen over time. The clinical manifestations of Parkinson disease can be divided into motor and

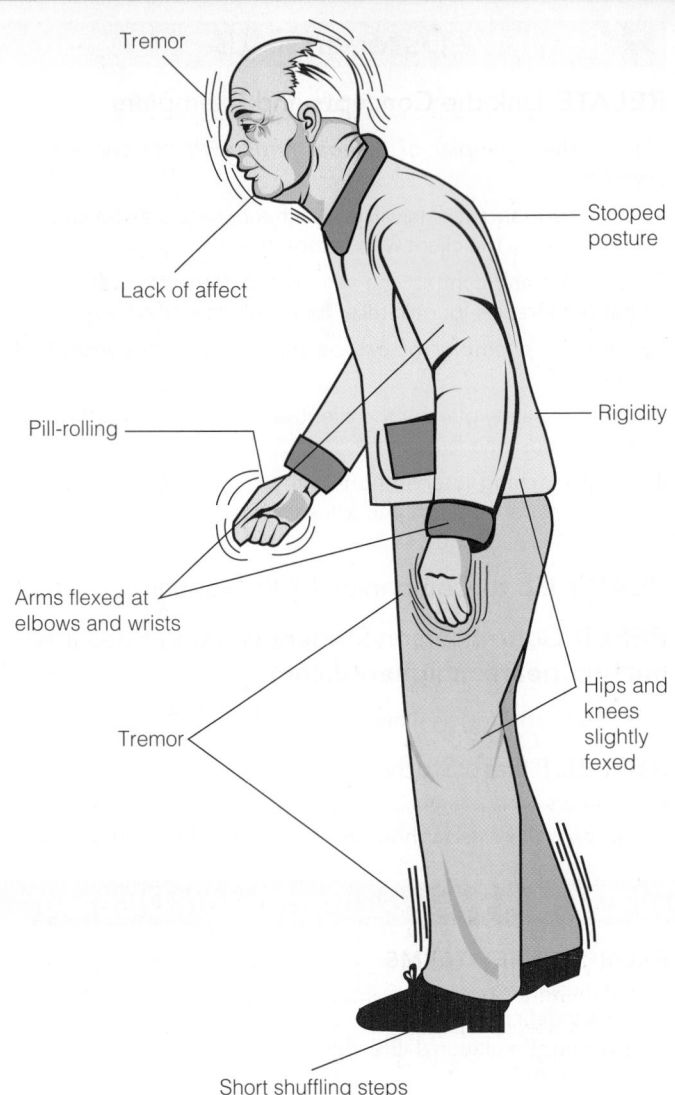

Figure 13–42 ● The classic motor symptoms of Parkinson disease include tremor, rigidity, bradykinesia, lack of affect, and postural instability. Many clients also exhibit a Parkinsonian gait.

nonmotor symptoms. Motor symptoms include the four classic symptoms of PD: tremor, rigidity, bradykinesia, and postural instability (**Figure 13–42 ●**). Nonmotor symptoms include cognitive deficits, emotional changes, and sleep problems. Clients with PD may experience these and many other symptoms during the progression of the disease (**Table 13–7 ●**).

Motor Symptoms

Motor symptoms associated with PD often begin unilaterally. With progression of the disease, motor symptoms begin to affect the client bilaterally, but the side affected initially will continue to display more prominent deficits in motor function. Two of the three symptoms of tremor, rigidity, and bradykinesia are required for a diagnosis of PD. Postural instability generally develops later in the course of the disease.

Tremor, or trembling, of one hand is an early sign of PD; some individuals develop tremor in the foot or jaw before the hand. Tremor is most prominent when the individual is at rest,

TABLE 13–7 Manifestations of Parkinson Disease

MOTOR SYMPTOMS	NONMOTOR SYMPTOMS
■ Tremor ■ Rigidity ■ Bradykinesia ■ Postural instability ■ Small, cramped writing (micrographia) ■ Lack of affect ■ Muscle cramps ■ Dystonia (twisting and repetitive movements) ■ Oculogyric crisis	■ Cognitive deficits ■ Emotional changes ■ Sleep problems ■ Constipation ■ Bladder problems (hesitation or frequency) ■ Sexual dysfunction ■ Skin problems (seborrhea, hyperhidrosis) ■ Anosmia (decreased ability to smell) ■ Orthostatic hypotension ■ Pain/discomfort

and it generally abates with movement. Tremor may be accompanied by a "**pill-rolling**" motion in which the thumb and fingers gently rub together. Trembling of both hands, arms, legs, jaw, and face may occur as the disease progresses. Trembling may interfere with ADLs, including eating, dressing, bathing, walking, and talking. Tremor can be exacerbated by stress or excitement. Tremor is generally the symptom that causes the individual to seek medical help.

Rigidity, or resistance to movement, occurs because of the involuntary contraction of all skeletal muscles. Muscles remain contracted when they should relax, upsetting the balance of opposing muscles and preventing movement. This may lead to muscle aches or weakness. Muscle stiffness of the trunk and limbs can limit the range of motion of joints and cause pain. For clinicians, rigidity is most obvious when another individual tries to move the client's arm, which will move only in short, jerky movements known as "cogwheel" rigidity (NINDS, 2013).

Bradykinesia, or slowed movement, affects both voluntary and automatic movements. Bradykinesia of voluntary movements causes the performance of ADLs, such as bathing and dressing, to take several hours. This can lead to frustration for the client. Bradykinesia can also affect the ability of the client to stand from a seated position. Steps may become shorter during walking, and the arms may not swing automatically. The client may also have a decreased blink rate. Another common effect of bradykinesia is difficulty with speech, swallowing, and chewing. This manifests itself in excessive drooling, difficulty eating, slurred speech, lengthy pauses during speech, and a lower voice volume (**hypophonia**).

Postural instability may develop later in the course of the disease, along with a **parkinsonian gait**. **Postural instability** is characterized by a stooped posture that leads to balance problems and falls. It may lead to **retropulsion**, or the tendency to topple backwards when bumped or when rising, standing, or turning. A parkinsonian gait is characterized by small, shuffling steps. The steps may be characterized by bradykinesia, or they may be rapid, as if the individual is trying to run (**festination**). When walking, the whole foot generally strikes the ground simultaneously, or the toe strikes first, which differs from the normal gait of the heel striking first. The individual may also experience **freezing**, in which it feels as though her feet are stuck to the floor. This usually occurs on the first step or when pivoting, walking through a doorway, or crossing the street. Freezing may increase the risk of falling forward.

Nonmotor Symptoms

Some nonmotor symptoms appear early in the disease and include fatigue, irritability, and loss of sense of smell. Other nonmotor symptoms, such as dementia, occur later in the disease progression. These nonmotor symptoms can be just as debilitating to the individual as the motor symptoms.

Cognitive deficits usually begin with slowed thinking. Clients may also develop confusion and memory loss. Later in the course of disease, dementia may affect social interactions, language, reasoning, and other mental skills. This is normally referred to as Parkinson dementia; symptoms of Parkinson dementia are similar to Alzheimer dementia.

EMOTIONAL CHANGES Emotional changes associated with PD may include depression, which can occur at any time throughout the course of the disease. Other forms of emotional changes include fear, anxiety, and panic attacks. An inability to cope may lead to social withdrawal and apathy.

SLEEP PROBLEMS Sleep problems are common among clients with PD and may be an early indicator of the disease. Fatigue may or may not be linked to sleep disturbances. Sleep disorders common to individuals with PD include insomnia, daytime sleep attacks, restless leg syndrome, parasomnias, and rapid eye movement sleep behavior disorders. Frequent awakening during the night may be linked to lack of automatic muscle movement, forcing the individual to wake up to change positions during the night.

Parkinsonism

Individuals with the combination of motor symptoms typically seen in Parkinson disease are said to have **parkinsonism**. Not everyone who has parkinsonism has Parkinson disease. Parkinsonism can result from medications, head trauma, and other neurodegenerative disorders. Clients with tremor, bradykinesia, and rigidity that do not respond to dopaminergic drugs are usually classified as having parkinsonism rather than Parkinson disease.

Lifespan and Cultural Considerations

Approximately 5%–10% of individuals with Parkinson disease have "early-onset" or "young-onset" PD, which begins before the age of 50. Early-onset PD shares many clinical manifestations with older-onset PD. However, clients with early-onset PD generally have a slower disease progression and a lower rate of dementia. They are more likely to have dystonia at onset and dyskinesias (involuntary movements, such as a tic or spasm) in response to levodopa treatment. Early-onset PD is often inherited, though it may be idiopathic (National Parkinson Foundation [NPF], n.d.b).

Even rarer than early-onset PD is juvenile PD, which is diagnosed in individuals before the age of 20. Juvenile PD usually begins with dystonia and bradykinesia, and symptoms respond well to levodopa. Juvenile PD is most commonly seen in Japan and often runs in families (NIH, 2012). It is primarily linked to the presence of mutated *PARK2*, which is normally involved in ubiquitination and degradation of unwanted or damaged proteins (Shimura et al., 2001).

▶ COLLABORATION

Like many chronic disorders, Parkinson disease is best treated by a team of physicians, nurses, therapists, and others. There is no cure for PD, so treatment is designed to help control symptoms and teach the client how to live with the disease. Nursing care should also include support for the caregiver, especially as the disease progresses.

Diagnostic Tests

The FDA has recently approved an imaging technique called DaTscan for clients with symptoms of PD. DaTscan involves the injection of radioactive Ioflupane I-123, which binds to dopamine transporters (DaT) in the brain. This allows visualization of dopaminergic neurons using single photon emission computed tomography (SPECT). Clients with degeneration of dopamine neurons will show less uptake of Ioflupane I-123, which can be evaluated by a trained neurologist. Clients should have the thyroid blocked before injection of Ioflupane I-123 to prevent accumulation of radioactive iodine in the thyroid, and clients should drink plenty of water after the test to promote excretion of the iodine. DaTscan is helpful for differentiating between essential tremor and tremor due to parkinsonian syndromes, but it does not distinguish among Parkinson disease and other dopamine degenerative disorders such as multiple system atrophy (MSA) or progressive supranuclear palsy (PSP) (GE Healthcare, 2011).

Other diagnostic tests for individuals with PD may include an MRI or blood tests to help rule out other causes of the client's symptoms. A client with PD will have normal results from an MRI or CT scan. In addition to ruling out other conditions, diagnosis of PD is based on the client's medical history and a neurological and physical examination.

Surgery

Surgical treatment of PD is reserved for clients with advanced disease. The most common surgical procedure is deep brain stimulation. Pallidotomy or thalamotomy may also be used.

DEEP BRAIN STIMULATION **Deep brain stimulation (DBS)** is a procedure in which a neurostimulator is implanted into the individual to send electrical signals to one of three brain regions: the subthalamic nucleus, the globus pallidus, or the thalamus. The subthalamic nucleus is the most common target and gives the best response. Stimulation of the globus pallidus or subthalamic nucleus reduces tremor, bradykinesia, and rigidity, whereas stimulation of the thalamus primarily reduces tremor. Clients may have DBS on one or both sides of the brain; stimulation will affect symptoms on the opposite side of the body (NINDS, 2013). The DBS apparatus consists of three parts: the lead (electrode), which is placed in the brain; the neurostimulator, which is usually placed near the collarbone; and a thin, insulated wire, which connects the stimulator and the lead (Jasmin, 2012).

DBS often allows clients to decrease their dosage of levodopa, which can decrease side effects such as dyskinesias. Clients will need frequent follow-up for several months after surgery to adjust the neurostimulator settings and set a new medication dosage. Complications of DBS include hemorrhage, infection, misplacement or dislodging of the leads, component failure, and stimulation-related adverse effects (Machado, Deogaonkar, & Cooper, 2012).

PALLIDOTOMY AND THALAMOTOMY These procedures may be performed to reduce symptoms and improve mobility. A *pallidotomy* involves destroying a portion of the basal ganglia called the globus pallidus, which is involved in the regulation of voluntary movement. A pallidotomy improves symptoms of tremor, rigidity, and bradykinesia and may also improve gait and balance. A *thalamotomy* involves destroying part of the brain's thalamus, which may help reduce tremor (NINDS, 2013). Treatment is performed on the opposite side of the worst symptoms; complete destruction of the thalamus may increase the risk of speech and cognitive problems (NPF, n.d.b). Pallidotomies and thalamotomies have largely been replaced by deep brain stimulation, because DBS can be turned off or reversed if adverse events occur.

Pharmacologic Therapy

No pharmacologic cure is available for Parkinson disease. However, many medications are effective at reducing the severity of symptoms. The goals of pharmacologic treatment for clients with PD are to improve the quality of life, reduce disability, and maintain the ability to work. The medications chosen by the physician will depend on the client's age, symptoms, and response to the drug. Information about medications used to treat Parkinson disease is found throughout the following section and in the Medications feature.

LEVODOPA The symptoms of PD result from a lack of dopamine in the brain. Therefore, the best way to treat PD is to increase brain dopamine levels. The primary drug used for this purpose is levodopa, which is the mainstay of PD treatment. Levodopa is effective at reducing tremor, bradykinesia, and rigidity, but problems with balance and nonmotor symptoms may not be relieved.

Levodopa is a natural chemical that can cross the blood–brain barrier and be converted directly to dopamine in the brain. Levodopa can also be converted to dopamine outside the brain, which leads to the most common side effects of nausea and orthostatic hypotension. Therefore, levodopa is almost always given in combination with carbidopa, which prevents levodopa from converting to dopamine until it reaches the brain.

As the client continues to take levodopa, its effectiveness diminishes. This causes the client to experience an **"on–off" effect** characterized by a sudden lack of symptom control and unexpected dyskinesias. With increasing doses and long-term exposure, levodopa usually causes dyskinesia, which may become less tolerable for the client than the symptoms of PD. Therefore, many physicians hesitate to prescribe levodopa to clients too early in the course of the disease.

> **SAFETY ALERT**
> Although the FDA requires generic drugs to show an "essential similarity" to the correlating brand name drug, generic substitutions may have different levels of efficacy and side effects in comparison to brand name counterparts. Clients should be cautioned to consult their primary care provider before switching to a generic drug. The client should also report any differences in effectiveness and side effects after switching medications.

Medications **Parkinson Disease Motor Symptoms**

CLASSIFICATION AND DRUG EXAMPLES	MECHANISMS OF ACTION	NURSING CONSIDERATIONS
Levodopa *Drug examples:* ■ levodopa ■ levodopa/carbidopa	Metabolic precursor to dopamine; restores dopamine levels in the brain. *May also be used for:* —Parkinsonism —Pain relief for shingles, bone pain	■ Cornerstone therapy for Parkinson disease ■ Effective dosage must be titrated, which may take several weeks to avoid adverse effects. ■ Long-term use of high doses causes dyskinesia. ■ Effectiveness may become less predictable over time; may produce "wearing-off" or "on–off" effects. ■ A high-protein diet may interfere with levodopa absorption from the GI tract; clients should avoid protein-rich meals when taking levodopa. ■ Do not take vitamin products containing vitamin B_6 if taking levodopa without carbidopa. ■ Should be used cautiously in clients with heart, kidney, liver, or endocrine disease. ■ May interfere with several laboratory tests and other drugs; clients should be monitored for interactions. ■ A metabolite of levodopa may cause urine and sweat to be dark colored. ■ Psychological side effects may be more common in older adults.
Dopamine Agonists *Drug examples:* ■ pramipexole ■ ropinirole ■ apomorphine ■ rotigotine ■ bromocriptine	Mimic the role of dopamine in the brain. *May also be used for:* —Restless leg syndrome —Reducing prolactin levels (bromocriptine)	■ May cause compulsive behaviors such as gambling, overeating, compulsive shopping, or hypersexuality; clients should be warned to report behaviors that are out of character to their physician. ■ Side effects are similar to levodopa and include nausea, hallucinations, sleep attacks, orthostatic hypotension. ■ Apomorphine is an injectable, short-acting agonist used for quick relief of symptoms in clients who are experiencing "wearing-off" or "on–off" effects; can be used up to five times daily. ■ Rotigotine is a transdermal patch that is replaced once per day; clients should rotate the placement of the patch. ■ Bromocriptine may produce fibrosis in the heart or chest cavity (pleuropulmonary fibrosis); rarely prescribed for PD.
MAO-B Inhibitors *Drug examples:* ■ selegiline ■ rasagiline	Prevents the breakdown of brain dopamine by inhibiting monoamine oxidase-B and interferes with dopamine reuptake in synapses. *May also be used for:* —Depression —ADHD	■ Can increase the risk of hallucinations if taken with levodopa/carbidopa. ■ Do not use in combination with most antidepressants and certain narcotics and decongestants. ■ Selegiline is available in an orally disintegrating formula for clients who have difficulty swallowing. ■ If levodopa-induced side effects occur when taking MAO-B inhibitors, the dose of levodopa should be reduced.
COMT Inhibitors *Drug examples:* ■ entacapone ■ tolcapone	Prolongs the actions of levodopa by blocking an enzyme that breaks down levodopa.	■ Side effects are related to increased levodopa effect. ■ Tolcapone is rarely prescribed due to risk for liver failure; clients on tolcapone need regular monitoring of liver function. ■ COMT inhibitors are only effective in combination with levodopa. ■ Formulations of entacapone combined with levodopa/carbidopa are available in a single tablet. ■ Taper dose when discontinuing COMT inhibitors. ■ May cause urine to be brownish-orange. ■ Should not be given with nonselective MAOIs.
Anticholinergics *Drug examples:* ■ benztropine ■ trihexyphenidyl	Decrease activity of acetylcholine. *May also be used for:* —Drug-induced extrapyramidal symptoms	■ Effective in only approximately half of clients for a brief period. ■ Cause significant antimuscarinic effects, including confusion, dry mouth, urinary retention, blurred vision, and constipation, especially in older adults. ■ Intake and output should be monitored regularly. ■ May increase susceptibility to heat stroke if client exercises vigorously in hot weather.
Amantadine	Exact mechanism is unknown; may be related to an increased release of dopamine from neuronal storage sites. *May also be used for:* —Treatment and prophylaxis of influenza A	■ Clients should be taught to watch for side effects, including mottled skin (livedo reticularis), edema, agitation, and hallucinations. ■ Dosage should be reduced in clients with renal insufficiency. ■ Maximum effect occurs in 2 weeks to 3 months; effectiveness may wane after 6–8 weeks of treatment; clients should be instructed to notify the physician when drug is no longer effective. ■ Abrupt discontinuation of amantadine may produce parkinsonian crisis.

Sources: Data from Mayo Clinic. (2012d). *Parkinson's disease.* Retrieved from http://www.mayoclinic.com/health/parkinsons-disease/DS00295; National Institute of Neurological Disorders and Stroke [NINDS]. (2013). *Parkinson's disease: Hope through research.* Retrieved from http://www.ninds.nih.gov/disorders/parkinsons_ disease/detail_parkinsons_disease.htm; Stacy, M., Davis, T. L., Heath, S., Isaacson, S. H., Tarsy, D., Williams, M., & Moore, A. P. (2009). The clinicians' and nurses' guide to Parkinson's disease. *Medscape Education.* Retrieved from http://www.medscape.org/viewarticle/701955; Wilson, B. A., Shannon, M. T., & Shields, K. M. (2013). *Nurse's drug guide.* Upper Saddle River, NJ: Pearson Education.

DOPAMINE AGONISTS Dopamine agonists are not converted directly to dopamine; instead, they act similarly to dopamine in the brain by activating dopamine receptors. Dopamine agonists are not as effective as levodopa, so they are often used alone early in the course of disease when symptoms are minor. Dopamine agonists have a longer duration of action compared to levodopa, so they may also be used later in the disease with levodopa to prevent the "on–off" effect. In addition to the side effects seen with levodopa, dopamine agonists may also produce hallucinations, swelling, drowsiness, and compulsive behaviors such as gambling and overeating.

DOPAMINE MODIFIERS Dopamine modifiers are used to extend the action of dopamine in the brain; they include the MAO-B (monoamine oxidase-B) inhibitors and the COMT (catechol-o-methyltransferase) inhibitors. MAO-B inhibitors may be given as monotherapy early in the course of disease to delay the need for levodopa therapy by a year or more. When given with levodopa, MAO-B inhibitors can enhance and prolong the response to levodopa and reduce wearing-off effects. COMT inhibitors reduce the breakdown of levodopa to an inactive intermediate product, thus increasing the availability of levodopa in the brain. When taken with levodopa, COMT inhibitors can decrease the duration of "off" periods and reduce the required dose of levodopa.

Complementary and Alternative Therapy
Coenzyme Q10

Coenzyme Q10 is necessary for cellular processes, especially mitochondrial function. One study found that coenzyme Q10 is superior to placebo at slowing the progression of Parkinson disease if taken at 1,200 mg/day, but not at lower doses (Shults et al., 2002). However, coenzyme Q10 does not modify existing symptoms (Storch et al., 2007). The most recent study conducted by the Parkinson Study Group was stopped in 2011 by the National Institute for Neurological Disease and Stroke because of a lack of efficacy of coenzyme Q10 in slowing the progression of the disease and relieving symptoms (Parkinson Study Group, 2011). Coenzyme Q10 is available as a nutritional supplement, but the cost of the high dosage required makes it cost prohibitive for many clients.

OTHER MEDICATIONS Anticholinergics were the first class of drugs used to treat PD. They reduce tremor and rigidity by decreasing acetylcholine and restoring the balance of acetylcholine and dopamine in the brain. Because of side effects in older adults and limited usefulness for most PD symptoms,

Client Teaching — Strategies to Minimize Symptoms and Complications of Parkinson Disease

Strategies to minimize the effects of PD:

- Take medications on time, every time.
- Consume a varied and balanced diet; high-protein meals should be discouraged because protein can decrease the transport of levodopa across the blood–brain barrier.
- Use a proper walking technique: Place the heel on the ground before the toe, stand up straight, look ahead instead of down, and do not move too quickly. Use an assistive device for balance if needed.
- Maintain a strong voice by taking a breath before speaking, expressing ideas in short sentences, drinking plenty of liquids, speaking louder than necessary, reducing throat clearing and coughing, and resting the voice when it is tired.
- Stop smoking and cut back on caffeine and alcohol consumption if they increase tremor or balance problems.
- Allow plenty of time for ADLs. Sit down to perform activities to conserve energy and use assistive devices such as items with large handles, footstools, electric toothbrushes, and others. See an occupational therapist for techniques to make ADLs easier.
- If bladder incontinence is a problem, try a regular schedule for going to the bathroom or use a protective pad for accidents. If pain is experienced during urination, a urinary tract infection may be present and should be treated by a physician.
- Practice good sleep hygiene.

Strategies to prevent complications associated with PD:

- See a speech/language pathologist to prevent or treat swallowing and speech problems.
- Discuss medications with a physician or pharmacist to prevent drug–drug and food–drug interactions.
- Increase fiber and fluid intake to prevent constipation.
- Maintain balance to prevent falls: Do not pivot the body before the feet, do not lean or reach, do not carry things while walking, avoid walking backward, remove obstacles and throw rugs, install hand rails, and install adequate lighting that is easy to turn on and off.
- Participate in a support group to increase social interaction and prevent depression.
- Participate in an exercise program to maintain muscle strength and improve mobility, flexibility, balance, posture, and emotional well-being (see Evidence-Based Practice).
- Be cautious when driving. PD can affect the client's ability to drive safely because of changes in perception, mental clarity, tremor, and medication side effects. Consider taking public transportation or arrange for a safety assessment through the local DMV.

*Stay Current: Additional tips are available at the Web site of the National Parkinson Foundation: **www.parkinson.org/Parkinson-s-Disease/Living-Well**.*

Sources: Based on Mayo Clinic. (2012d). *Parkinson's disease.* Retrieved from http://www.mayoclinic.com/health/parkinsons-disease/DS00295; National Institutes of Health (NIH). (2012). Parkinson's disease. *NIHSeniorHealth.* Retrieved from https://nihseniorhealth.gov/parkinsonsdisease/whatisparkinsonsdisease/01.html; National Parkinson Foundation (NPF). (n.d.a). *Parkinson's disease: Living well.* Retrieved from http://www.parkinson.org/Parkinson-s-Disease/Living-Well; Stacy, M., Davis, T. L., Heath, S., Isaacson, S. H., Tarsy, D., Williams, M., & Moore, A. P. (2009). The clinicians' and nurses' guide to Parkinson's disease. *Medscape Education.* Retrieved from http://www.medscape.org/viewarticle/701955.

anticholinergics are only prescribed to younger clients whose primary symptom is tremor.

Amantadine is an antiviral medication that can provide short-term relief of mild symptoms of Parkinson disease. It may also be used in addition to levodopa to help control dyskinesia for clients in the later stages of PD.

DRUGS FOR NONMOTOR SYMPTOMS Clients with Parkinson disease often experience many nonmotor symptoms. Classic medications for PD do not treat these symptoms, so additional medications are often prescribed, including antidepressants (amitriptyline, fluoxetine), anxiolytics (benzodiazepines), and atypical antipsychotics. The antipsychotics quetiapine and clozapine may be prescribed at bedtime to reduce frightening dreams or to treat psychosis; clients on clozapine should have their blood monitored frequently for agranulocytosis. Olanzapine and risperidone may be given to treat hallucinations, but like traditional antipsychotics, they may worsen PD motor symptoms.

Orthostatic hypotension may be treated with fludrocortisone, and sildenafil may be used to treat erectile dysfunction. Oxybutynin is often prescribed for clients with bladder dysfunction. Seborrheic dermatitis can be treated with ketoconazole. Rivastigmine can be used to treat dementia in PD.

Nonpharmacologic Therapy

Nonpharmacologic therapy is an essential aspect of treatment for clients with Parkinson disease. In spite of regular medication usage, clients with PD still develop progressively worsening symptoms. Medications have limited effectiveness over time and frequently produce side effects. Therefore, nonpharmacologic therapies are used as an adjunct to help clients prolong the early, mild stage of disease and delay disability. Several techniques can be used by the client to help minimize symptoms and prevent complications. The nurse plays a vital role in educating clients with PD about these preventive strategies (see the Client Teaching feature).

Exercise is the most important nonpharmacologic therapy for clients with PD (see the Evidence-Based Practice feature). The nurse should encourage clients to participate in an exercise program, especially a combination of walking and strength training. However, any type of exercise is beneficial for clients with PD; tai chi, yoga, and Alexander techniques may all provide some improvement in flexibility, balance, muscle strength, and posture.

Participation in physical, occupational, and speech therapy can play an essential role in the ability of a client with PD to remain mobile. *Physical therapy* often focuses on lower body strength and mobility to improve walking and prevent contractures and falls. Physical therapy may also help the client become more proficient at transfers. *Occupational therapy* often focuses on the upper extremities, especially finger function, to improve the client's ability to independently perform ADLs, such as cooking and grooming. Occupational therapy can also help a client maintain the ability to perform work functions, allowing the client to keep her job longer. *Speech therapists* help the client with speech and swallowing, which can enhance the client's daily functioning in the areas of communication and nutrition. Therapists are also responsible for helping clients learn how to use assistive devices that are within their area of expertise (PT: walkers, canes; OT: button hooks, electric razor; ST: pen grips, "magic slate").

Evidence-Based Practice Exercise for Clients With Parkinson Disease

Problem

Clients with Parkinson disease develop motor problems that cause changes in gait, muscle strength and coordination, and balance. These symptoms decrease the client's mobility and ability to perform ADLs and increase the risk for falls and other complications.

Evidence

Exercise, including stretching, aerobic exercise, and strength training, can help clients with PD increase their mobility and strength. A Cochrane review of eight trials (203 participants) indicated that treadmill training improved gait speed, stride length, and walking distance for individuals with PD in a variety of clinical trials. In addition, treadmill training was not significantly associated with adverse events or client dropout (Mehrholz et al., 2010). Another study of 67 individuals with PD compared high-intensity treadmill exercise, low-intensity treadmill exercise, and stretching and resistance exercises for gait speed, cardiovascular fitness, and muscle strength. All three types of exercise improved distance on the 6-minute walk test, with the low-intensity treadmill group showing the most improvement. Both treadmill exercises improved cardiovascular fitness, whereas stretching and resistance improved muscle strength (Shulman et al., 2013). A third study of 121 individuals with PD indicated that individuals who participated in flexibility/balance/function exercises had improved overall physical function and ADLs scores, whereas individuals who performed aerobic exercises showed improvement in walking economy (oxygen uptake) (Schenkman et al., 2012).

Implications

It is important for clients to participate in both aerobic activity and strength training for maximum benefit. Exercises do not appear to stop disease progression, but they may improve body strength so the individual is less disabled compared to clients who do not exercise. Exercise improves balance, minimizes gait problems, and strengthens muscles to increase physical functioning. Both structured exercise programs and general physical activity (walking, gardening, swimming, dancing) are beneficial for clients with PD (NINDS, 2013).

Critical Thinking Application

1. How would you explain the importance of exercise to a client with mild PD who is skeptical of its beneficial effects?

2. What special considerations would you have when suggesting an exercise program for an older client with severe bilateral tremors in his legs and who requires a walker for ambulation?

3. Develop an exercise program for a 67-year-old male client with a gait speed of 1.2 m/s, stride length of 0.79 m, cadence of 115 steps/min, and 6-minute walk distance of 472 m.

Clinical Manifestations and Therapies Parkinson Disease

ETIOLOGY	CLINICAL MANIFESTATIONS	CLINICAL THERAPIES
Lower limb and trunk motor deficits	<ul><li>Tremors</li><li>Rigidity</li><li>Bradykinesia</li><li>Postural instability</li><li>Muscle cramps</li><li>Dystonia</li><li>Parkinsonian gait</li><li>Balance problems</li><li>Immobility, freezing</li><li>Stooped posture, retropulsion, festination</li></ul>	<ul><li>Levodopa</li><li>Dopamine- or levodopa-modifying drugs</li><li>Deep brain stimulation</li><li>Walking and balance training</li><li>Exercise program</li><li>Physical therapy</li><li>Environment modification to reduce risk of falls</li><li>Mobility devices</li></ul>
Upper limb motor deficits	<ul><li>Tremors (with "pill-rolling")</li><li>Rigidity (especially "cogwheel" rigidity)</li><li>Bradykinesia</li><li>Micrographia</li><li>Muscle cramps</li><li>Dystonia</li><li>Uncoordinated hand movements</li><li>Inability to perform ADLs</li></ul>	<ul><li>Levodopa</li><li>Dopamine- or levodopa-modifying drugs</li><li>Deep brain stimulation</li><li>Allow adequate time for ADLs</li><li>Exercise program</li><li>Occupational therapy</li><li>Assistive devices</li></ul>
Head and neck motor deficits	<ul><li>Tremors</li><li>Rigidity</li><li>Bradykinesia</li><li>Lack of affect</li><li>Dystonia</li><li>Oculogyric crisis</li><li>Difficulty chewing and swallowing, drooling</li><li>Speech deficits (slurred speech, lengthy pauses, hypophonia)</li></ul>	<ul><li>Levodopa</li><li>Dopamine- or levodopa-modifying drugs</li><li>Deep brain stimulation</li><li>Speech therapy</li><li>Provide soft foods</li></ul>
Cognitive effects	<ul><li>Confusion</li><li>Slowed thinking</li><li>Memory loss</li><li>Dementia</li></ul>	<ul><li>Rivastigmine</li><li>Promote reorientation</li><li>Provide support to caregivers</li></ul>
Emotional effects	<ul><li>Anxiety</li><li>Fear, panic attacks</li><li>Depression, social withdrawal, apathy</li></ul>	<ul><li>Antidepressants</li><li>Anxiolytics</li><li>Support group</li></ul>
Sleep problems	<ul><li>Fatigue</li><li>Irritability</li><li>Restless leg syndrome</li><li>Sleep attacks, insomnia, parasomnias, rem sleep behavior disorders</li></ul>	<ul><li>Atypical antipsychotics</li><li>Good sleep hygiene</li></ul>
Bowel and bladder effects	<ul><li>Constipation</li><li>Urinary hesitancy or frequency</li></ul>	<ul><li>Oxybutynin</li><li>High-fiber diet</li><li>Laxatives/stool softeners</li><li>Adequate fluids</li><li>Bladder or bowel training</li></ul>
Other	<ul><li>Sexual dysfunction</li><li>Seborrhea</li><li>Hyperhidrosis</li><li>Anosmia</li><li>Orthostatic hypotension</li><li>Pain</li></ul>	<ul><li>Fludrocortisone</li><li>Sildenafil</li><li>Ketoconazole</li><li>Teach client to change positions slowly.</li></ul>

NURSING PROCESS

Nurses are essential for evaluating the progression of the client's Parkinson disease, monitoring the client's ability to perform ADLs and ambulate independently, and providing client teaching and emotional support. Nurses also play a key role in performing client assessments for changes in symptoms, effectiveness of medications, and new client concerns. Documentation of this information is critical for current and future care of the client.

Assessment

Assessment of clients with Parkinson disease involves collecting a health history and performing a physical assessment. A general health history should include a history of brain disorders or trauma, exposure to environmental toxins, medication and drug use, and family history of PD. A PD-specific health history should include the client's description of symptoms, including onset, duration, severity, aggravating or alleviating factors, response to medication, interference with mobility or ADLs, interference with work or relationships, "on–off" or "wearing-off" effects, and use of assistive devices. The nurse may need to ask specifically about nonmotor symptoms, because many clients do not associate these symptoms with PD. Nonmotor symptoms include cognitive deficits, emotional changes, sleep problems, bladder and bowel changes, orthostatic hypotension, sexual dysfunction, and others.

Physical assessment often follows the Unified Parkinson's Disease Rating Scale (UPDRS), which rates clients in 42 different areas in the categories of mentation, behavior, and mood; ADLs; motor examination; and complications of therapy (Fahn, Elton, & Members of the UPDRS Development Committee, 1987):

- The mentation, behavior, and mood assessment includes intellectual impairment, thought disorder, depression, and motivation.
- The ADL assessment includes speech, swallowing, hand-writing, hygiene, walking, tremor, and others.
- The motor examination assessment includes facial expression, tremor at rest, finger taps, hand movements, rapid alternating movement of hands, leg agility, ability to rise from a chair, posture, gait, bradykinesia, and others.
- Complications included in the assessment are dyskinesias, "on–off" periods, sleep disturbances, and others.
- The modified Hoehn and Yahr Staging scale and Schwab and England Activities of Daily Living Scale are also included as part of the UPDRS.

In 2007, the Movement Disorder Society sponsored a revision of the UPDRS, called the MDS-UPDRS, which is divided into four parts: nonmotor experiences of daily living, motor experiences of daily living, motor examination, and motor complications (Goetz et al., 2007). This revised scale was made available in 2008.

Diagnosis

Nursing diagnoses related to Parkinson disease may include, but are not limited to, the following:

- *Risk for Falls* related to lack of balance and coordination
- *Impaired Physical Mobility* related to rigidity of leg muscles and bradykinesia

- *Feeding Self-Care Deficit* related to tremor
- *Impaired Swallowing* related to bradykinesia of throat muscles
- *Disturbed Sleep Pattern* related to lack of automatic muscle movement
- *Impaired Verbal Communication* related to lower voice volume
- *Impaired Urinary Elimination* related to loss of control of bladder muscles
- *Constipation* related to ineffective bowel contractions
- *Fear* related to freezing of muscles
- *Impaired Memory* related to neuron degeneration
- *Caregiver Role Strain* related to caring for immobile individual.

(NANDA-I © 2012)

Planning

Client goals for individuals with Parkinson disease are specific to the nursing diagnoses included in the plan of care, and will be tailored to the client. Examples include the following:

- The client will remain free from injury.
- The client will demonstrate progressive improvement in scores for the 6-minute walk test.
- The client will participate in a daily exercise program that includes walking and strength training.
- The client will participate in occupational therapy to gain knowledge of assistive devices for feeding and will obtain kitchen utensils to aid in feeding self-care.
- The client will participate in speech therapy for training in swallowing and enhanced verbal communication.
- The client will verbalize an understanding of good sleep hygiene.
- The client will participate in physical therapy to improve walking and balance.
- The client will verbalize an understanding of bladder training techniques.
- The client will demonstrate normal bowel elimination patterns, including one bowel movement daily.
- The client will report episodes of freezing and demonstrate an understanding of techniques to overcome freezing.
- The client will use techniques to augment memory, including writing down important information.
- The client's caregiver will utilize help from friends, family, and healthcare agencies to provide relief from daily tasks.

Implementation

For most clients with Parkinson disease, early implementation of strategies to maintain mobility and independently perform ADLs will provide the most benefit throughout the course of the disease. These interventions may need to be adjusted as the disease progresses, but many therapies implemented early during the course of treatment will prolong the mild stage of the disease and provide muscle strength and coordination in the later stages of disease.

Prevent Injury

Safety is a priority for helping clients with walking difficulties maintain their mobility. Modifications such as using lift chairs, elevating the back legs of chairs, and installing a raised toilet seat can help clients with PD rise from a seated position more easily. Installing hand rails for stability and removing floor hazards such as clutter, cords, and rugs are all important safety modifications for clients with PD. These modifications can help the client be more confident while ambulating and may help prevent falls and other accidents.

Optimize Mobility

The best strategy for mobility that a nurse can provide for clients with PD is to encourage the client to walk daily and participate in an exercise program. Aerobic exercise and strength training increases muscle strength, balance, and coordination to counteract the effects of tremor, rigidity, bradykinesia, and postural instability. Range-of-motion exercises can help with joint mobility and function and help prevent contractures. Treadmill walking can help increase stride length, gait, and cardiovascular health to help clients overcome the parkinsonian gait and maintain general physical fitness. For clients who cannot ambulate independently, a caregiver should be encouraged to help the client ambulate several times daily.

Techniques for proper walking, including intentionally picking up the feet instead of shuffling and placing the heel on the floor first, can easily be provided to clients through oral and written instructions. The nurse can also teach tricks to overcome freezing, such as stepping over an imaginary line. Methods to maintain balance when walking, including standing upright and not carrying anything, are also beneficial for clients with PD. Understanding and implementing these techniques early in the course of disease will help clients naturally integrate these practices later in the disease when symptoms are more severe.

Participation in physical and occupational therapy is also vital for helping clients with PD maintain mobility as long as possible. The nurse is essential for referring clients to the proper therapy, providing clients with information about what to expect during therapy, and following up with clients to ensure that they are attending therapy sessions and that the therapy sessions are beneficial. Clients who require assistive devices for walking may receive training during physical therapy sessions, or the nurse may provide this training if needed.

When helping clients learn ambulation strategies, the nurse must also provide encouragement and emotional support. As the client's disability increases, the client will be more susceptible to fear, anxiety, and depression. The nurse can help the client overcome these barriers by listening to the client's fears, providing resources for support and mobility training, and helping the client celebrate small victories related to the client's mobility and physical functioning.

Promote Independence

In addition to difficulty ambulating, deficits in performing ADLs constitute a major burden for clients with PD and their caregivers. ADLs include cooking and eating, performing hygiene acts (bathing, dressing, grooming, brushing teeth, toileting), and maintaining a house (housework, laundry, driving, shopping, using the phone, managing finances). The nurse can promote independence in ADLs by encouraging the client to take adequate time to perform each task. This takes planning on the part of the client, especially if the client is getting ready for an appointment or social activity, but it also requires patience from both the client and caregiver.

The use of assistive devices is key to helping clients maintain their independence in performing ADLs. Assistive devices for cooking and eating include electric can openers, food processors, mixers, utensils with large handles, finger guards, sloped plates, and many others. Clients with severe hand tremors have difficulty transporting food from the plate to the mouth. The nurse can teach clients techniques to reduce tremor while eating, such as holding a piece of bread in the opposite hand or using purposeful movement. Swallowing is often a problem for clients with PD, so the nurse can encourage the client to prepare soft foods, to cut food into small pieces or puree food, and to eat smaller meals more frequently. Speech therapy can help clients learn swallowing techniques to prevent choking and aspiration, and occupational therapy can help clients learn techniques to reduce tremor, grasp objects, and increase safety.

SAFETY ALERT Individuals with PD who have difficulty swallowing may aspirate foods that have a thin consistency, such as juice or broth. Aspiration can lead to life-threatening complications, including pneumonia.

Assistive devices are often helpful for hygiene activities. Devices such as shower seats, retractable shower heads, button hooks, zipper pulls, long shoe horns, electric razors and toothbrushes, elevated toilet seats, and hand rails can help clients maintain independence in performing personal hygiene. A nurse can provide suggestions for assistive devices, referrals for equipment suppliers, and training in the use of assistive devices. The nurse may also provide training to caregivers about assisting the client with hygiene care and helping the client overcome privacy or embarrassment issues when assistance is needed. An occupational therapist can also provide tools and techniques to aid the client in performing hygiene acts independently.

Clients with PD may also use assistive devices when maintaining a house. Magnifying glasses can help with anything that requires reading, such as reading mail, managing finances, or looking at the newspaper. Phones with sound amplifiers and large buttons can ease difficulties with phone use. Clients may be encouraged to use public transportation if available for running errands or going to appointments. Housework can be aided by devices such as a shopping and laundry carts, shopping bag carriers, reachers and grippers, and scrub brushes with large or telescopic handles. Similar to other assistive devices, the nurse can provide suggestions, referrals, and training, and the client can participate in occupational therapy to learn more about maintaining independence in these activities. Clients with advanced disability may consider hiring a friend, family member, or company to provide assistance with housework.

Other ADLs that may be affected by Parkinson disease are communication and sleep. The nurse can help the client overcome these problems by providing oral and written information about vocal training and good sleep hygiene. Vocal training may include teaching clients to speak louder than they think is necessary, take a deep breath before speaking, and express thoughts in short sentences. Referral to a speech therapist is also an essential aspect of treatment for clients with voice changes. If writing is a problem, the nurse can encourage the client to use writing tools with large handles or nonslip grips, type messages, or use a recording device to make note of important information. An occupational therapist can also provide training in writing techniques for the client with PD. If sleep problems are severe and are not resolved by good sleep hygiene or a change in medication, the nurse may also recommend pharmacologic therapy.

Each client with PD will have a unique set of difficulties in performing ADLs. The roles of the nurse are to determine which ADLs are causing the most difficulty and to provide insight into techniques, devices, and therapies that may help clients maintain independence in each area.

Evaluation

Evaluation of clients with PD includes regular assessment using the UPDRS to determine the client's level of disability. Significant changes in the UPDRS score may indicate a need for a modification of pharmacologic, nonpharmacologic, or surgical therapy. Evaluation should also include an assessment of the client's emotional status, because this can change frequently.

NURSING CARE PLAN A Client With Parkinson Disease

Benjamin Tinsley, age 86, was diagnosed with Parkinson disease at age 74. Mr. Tinsley lives at home with his second wife, age 80, and he has a son who lives in the same city. Mr. Tinsley visited his primary care physician for routine follow-up.

ASSESSMENT

Client history indicates that Mr. Tinsley has had PD for 12 years. Initial pharmacologic therapy was pramipexole for 2 years, then levodopa/carbidopa for 7 years. Mr. Tinsley has been on levodopa/carbidopa plus entacapone for the past 3 years. Primary complaints include severe right-hand tremor, parkinsonian gait (requires assistive device when walking), low voice volume, difficulty rising from a seated position, and constipation. The right-hand tremor interferes with eating, hygiene care, and other ADLs, and Mr. Tinsley has lost 10 pounds in the past 2 months. The parkinsonian gait and postural instability make walking and standing difficult, and Mrs. Tinsley states that Mr. Tinsley falls at least once per day, which is often associated with freezing. The nurse completes Mr. Tinsley's physcial assessment using the UPDRS and the Schwab and England ADL scale.

DIAGNOSES

- *Risk for Injury* related to altered mobility
- *Impaired Walking* related to parkinsonian gait
- *Impaired Transfer Ability* related to inability to rise from a seated position
- *Imbalance Nutrition: Less Than Body Requirements* related to right-hand tremor and difficulty self-feeding
- *Self-Care Deficit: Bathing, Dressing, Feeding, Toileting* related to right-hand tremor and postural instability
- *Constipation* related to inadequate physical activity and decreased food intake
- *Impaired Verbal Communication* related to low voice volume

(NANDA-I © 2012)

PLANNING

- The client will sustain no injuries.
- The client will participate in treadmill training during physical therapy.
- The client will acquire a chair lift and an elevated toilet seat with hand rails and demonstrate understanding of how to use these assistive devices.
- The client will use purposeful movement to reduce tremor while eating.
- The client will purchase a shower chair and assistive devices for dressing.
- The client will ambulate at least four times daily and eat a diet high in fiber and fluids.
- The client will intentionally take a deep breath before speaking and speak louder than normal.
- The client will have hand rails installed throughout his home.

IMPLEMENTATION

- Facilitate referral of client to physical therapy for the purpose of treadmill training and strength and balance training.
- Facilitate referral of client to occupational therapy for assistance with eating and hygiene care.
- Facilitate referral of client to speech therapy for vocal training.
- Refer the client to equipment suppliers to purchase assistive and safety devices.
- Provide client teaching in the use of assistive devices.

- Discuss the importance of consuming a balanced diet that is easy for the client to eat.
- Provide training to the caregiver in the areas of hygiene care, assistance with standing and walking, removal of safety hazards, and proper meal preparation.
- Encourage the client and caregiver to be patient when performing ADLs to help the client maintain independence as long as possible.

EVALUATION

Mr. Tinsley returns to his primary care provider in 3 months for a follow-up appointment. He reports that he has been attending PT, OT, and ST regularly, and with proper training on assistive devices, he is able to independently perform ADLs more frequently than before his previous appointment. He is still very slow in performing ADLs, but he is thankful that he can be independent. Mrs. Tinsley reports that this has helped lift some of her burden of caregiving as well. Mr. Tinsley has made slight improvement on his 6-minute walk distance (302 m to 387 m), and he is better able to feed himself by using larger utensils and practicing purposeful movements. As a result, he has gained 3 pounds since his last appointment. Mr. Tinsley reports that he still has difficulty rising from a seated position, and his constipation has not improved much.

CRITICAL THINKING

1. What additional nursing interventions can be implemented for improvement of Mr. Tinsley's constipation?
2. Describe the components of a focused nursing assessment to determine the severity of Mr. Tinsley's difficulty rising from a seated position.
3. Develop a nursing care plan for Mr. Tinsley that reflects the development of dysphagia (difficulty swallowing).

REVIEW Parkinson Disease

RELATE Link the Concepts and Exemplars

Linking the exemplar of Parkinson disease with the concept of cognition:

1. Describe the impact of Parkinson disease on cognition.

2. What safety measures can the nurse initiate for the client with Parkinson disease who has alterations in cognition?

Linking the exemplar of Parkinson disease with the concept of elimination:

3. What factors associated with Parkinson disease put the client at risk for constipation?

4. What nursing interventions might be appropriate for implementation when caring for the client with Parkinson disease who is at risk for developing urinary retention?

READY Go to Companion Skills Manual

REFER Go to Pearson Student Nursing Resources
nursing.pearsonhighered.com

- Additional review material

REFLECT Case Study

Kody Manuel is a 65-year-old male who was diagnosed with Parkinson disease 1 year ago. Mr. Manuel is retired from the railroad where he worked in management. He lives with his daughter Susan Ransone and her husband Val. They both work outside the home, and they have one infant daughter, Isabelle. Mr. Manuel has been able to care for himself at home while his daughter and son-in-law work. Isabelle is taken to a day care center in the morning by Mrs. Ransone, and Mr. Ransone picks her up in the evening.

Mr. Manuel was started on levodopa 1 month ago. He has been reading about Parkinson disease online and is very disturbed by what he has learned. He doesn't think the levodopa is working for him, and he tells his daughter and son-in-law that he needs to move out in order to prevent disruption of their home as the disease progresses. While visiting the physician today, he tells the nurse about his plans to move.

1. What data should be obtained from Mr. Manuel before continuing the discussion about his decision to move out of his daughter's home?

2. What potential psychosocial concerns can the nurse identify, based on Mr. Manuel's statements?

3. How should the nurse respond to Mr. Manuel's report that the levodopa is not working for him?

EXEMPLAR 13.7 Spinal Cord Injury

EXEMPLAR KEY TERMS
Autonomic dysreflexia, *911*
Complete SCI, *910*
Compression, *908*
Hyperextension, *908*
Hyperflexion, *908*
Incomplete SCI, *910*
Level of injury, *909*
Paraplegia, *911*
Rotational injury, *908*
Spinal cord injury (SCI), *906*
Spinal shock, *909*
Tetraplegia, *911*
Transection, *908*

EXEMPLAR LEARNING OUTCOMES
After reading about this exemplar, you will be able to:

1. Describe the pathophysiology, etiology, clinical manifestations, and direct and indirect causes of spinal cord injury.

2. Identify risk factors and prevention methods associated with spinal cord injury.

3. Illustrate the nursing process in providing culturally competent care across the life span for individuals with a spinal cord injury.

4. Formulate priority nursing diagnoses appropriate for an individual with a spinal cord injury.

5. Summarize therapies used by interdisciplinary teams in the collaborative care of an individual with a spinal cord injury.

6. Plan evidence-based care for an individual with a spinal cord injury and his or her family in collaboration with other members of the healthcare team.

7. Evaluate expected outcomes for an individual with a spinal cord injury.

▶ OVERVIEW

Spinal cord injury (SCI) is often the result of trauma from, for example, a motor vehicle crash, a fall, or a gunshot wound. SCI occurs when vertebrae or other objects are forced against the spinal cord, damaging nerve cells and preventing transmission of nerve impulses between the body and the brain. Depending on the extent and location of nerve damage, SCI can lead to anything from slight muscle weakness in a few muscles to complete loss of sensory and motor function. Approximately 12,000 new cases of SCI occur each year in the United States (National SCI Statistical Center [NSCISC], 2013).

▶ PATHOPHYSIOLOGY AND ETIOLOGY

The brain and spinal cord are the two major components of the central nervous system. The spinal cord transports sensory signals from the body to the brain and motor signals from the brain to the body. The spinal cord consists of an H-shaped core of gray matter, which is made of neurons, support cells called glia, and blood vessels, and a surrounding area of white matter, which is made of myelin-coated axons (**Figure 13–43 ●**). The gray matter is divided into four regions: interneurons of the dorsal horn that connect to visceral and somatic sensory neu-

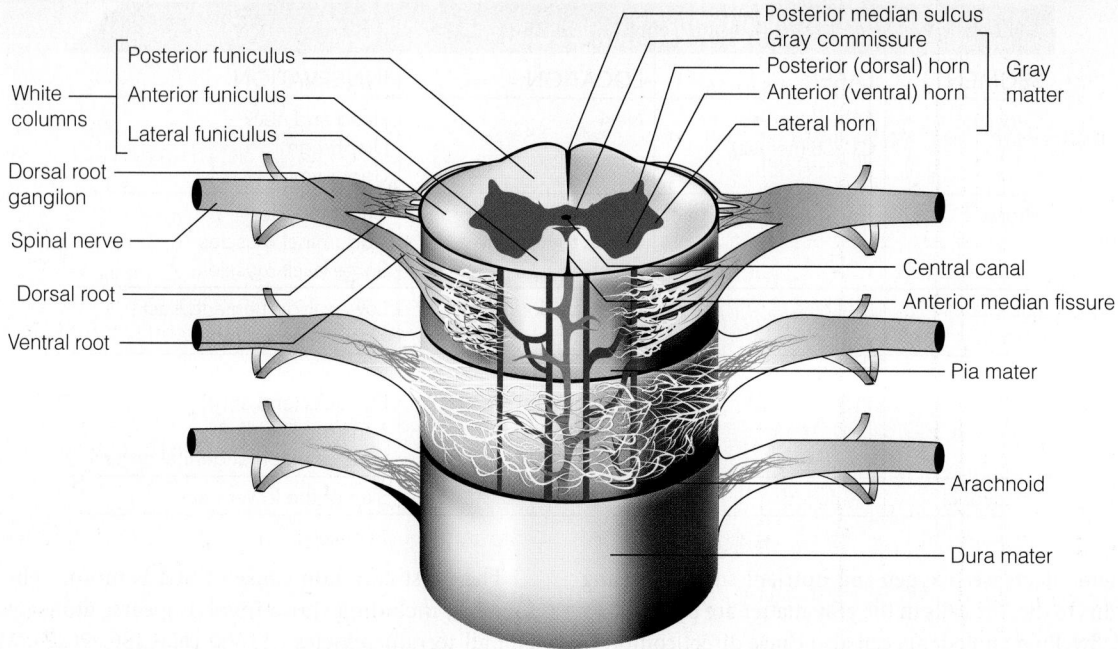

Figure 13–43 ● The structure of the spinal cord.

rons in the dorsal root, and visceral and somatic motor neurons of the ventral horn that combine to form the ventral root. The dorsal and ventral roots then join together on each side of the body to form the spinal nerve. The axons of the white matter make up the descending and ascending pathways. Descending pathways carry signals from the brain to control the motor neurons, and ascending pathways carry signals from the sensory neurons to the brain. Axons in the white matter travel from the brain along the entire length of the spinal cord until it connects with the desired spinal nerve.

The 33 bones of the vertebral column encase and protect the spinal cord. The vertebral column is divided into five segments, and the spinal nerves protrude from each of these segments to innervate specific areas of the body (see **Figure 13–44** ● and **Table 13–8** ●) (NINDS, 2012b).

Between the bones of the vertebral column are spinal discs that provide cushioning during movement, and spinal nerves protrude from the spinal column between the vertebrae near the spinal discs. The spinal cord is more susceptible to direct injury by lesser or repetitive forces at the location of the spinal discs because of their soft nature, whereas damage to the portion of the spinal cord that is surrounded by hard vertebral bones requires greater force.

Most damage to the spinal cord occurs due to a sudden, traumatic force that distorts the normal structure of the vertebral column. When displaced bone fragments, disc material, or ligaments connecting the vertebrae come into contact with the spinal cord, the result is bruising or tearing of the nerves. The force may also cause damage to blood vessels in the gray matter, causing bleeding that can spread to the white matter and nearby segments of the spinal cord.

The initial physical trauma produces a series of events that kills neurons, demyelinates axons, and triggers an inflammatory response. Reduction in blood flow due to damage, swell-

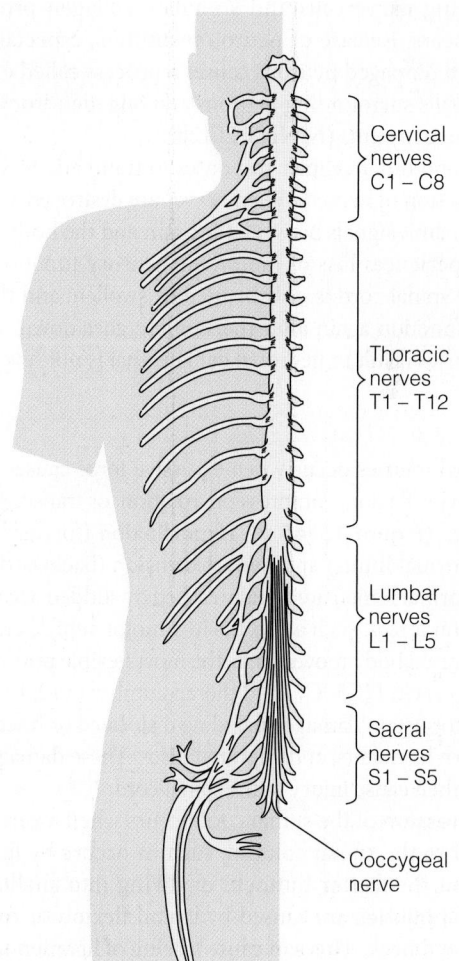

Figure 13–44 ● The vertebral column and spinal cord are divided into five segments, and spinal nerves protrude from each segment to innervate the body.

TABLE 13–8 Vertebral Column and Spinal Nerves

SEGMENT	LABEL	LOCATION	INNERVATION
Cervical	C1–C7 (vertebrae) C1–C8 (nerves)	Neck	Head and neck Diaphragm Upper limbs
Thoracic	T1–T12	Upper back; vertebrae attach to rib cage	Chest muscles Abdominal muscles Some back muscles
Lumbar	L1–L5	Lower back	Lower abdomen and back Parts of lower limbs
Sacral	S1–S5	Hip area	Bowels and bladder Buttocks (and anus) Parts of lower limbs Parts of external genital organs
Coccygeal	1–4 fused	Tailbone	Skin of the lower back

ing, and edema decreases oxygen and nutrient supply, causing many neurons to die; the cells in the gray matter are particularly susceptible. Swelling and edema can also cause direct compression of the nerves. Immune cells that are normally trapped in the blood vessels are able to leak into the spinal cord where they cause an inflammatory response, scavenge debris, and fight infection. They may also secrete cytokines that cause damage to surrounding nerve cells and stimulate collagen production, forming scars. Release of neurotransmitters, especially glutamate, from damaged neurons causes a process called excitotoxicity that kills surrounding neurons and oligodendrocytes (cells that produce myelin) (NINDS, 2012b).

These and other cellular responses to traumatic SCI result in the destruction of nerves. When nerves are destroyed and can no longer transmit signals between the brain and the body, the individual experiences loss of motor and sensory function. Sometimes, the spinal cord is only bruised or swollen, and the nerves begin to function again after the swelling goes down. However, many injuries result in neuronal damage that is not reversible.

Etiology

Spinal cord injuries occur when excessive force causes hyperextension, hyperflexion, compression, rotation, or transection of the spinal cord (**Figure 13–45 ●**). **Hyperflexion** (forward bending beyond normal limits) and **hyperextension** (backward bending beyond normal limits) are usually caused by sudden acceleration–deceleration forces, such as occurs in a motor vehicle crash. During these rapid body movements, the most flexible portions of the spine, the cervical (C5–C7) and thoracolumbar (T12, L1) regions, are likely to sustain damage, including dislocated or fractured vertebrae, torn ligaments, and ruptured discs. These damaged structures can then cause injury to the spinal cord.

Compression of the spinal cord occurs when a vertical force is applied to the spinal column, such as occurs by falling and landing on the feet or buttocks or diving into shallow water. **Rotational injuries** are caused by lateral flexion or twisting of the head and neck. This can cause tearing of ligaments or dislocation or fracture of the vertebrae and an unstable spinal injury. **Transection** of the spinal cord occurs when the individual is injured by a gunshot, stabbing, or similar force that partially or completely severs the spinal cord.

The most common cause of SCI is motor vehicle crashes (36.5%), including those involving cars, motorcycles, bikes, and all-terrain vehicles (ATVs) (NSCISC, 2013). Motor vehicle crashes can cause any one or a combination of the five types of forces and may involve both passengers and pedestrians. Falling is the second most common cause (28.5%), usually resulting in compression injuries. Violence (14.3%), especially gunshot wounds, typically results in transection of the spinal cord. SCIs associated with sports (9.2%) often result from football and diving. Alcohol is a factor in about 25% of SCIs (Mayo Clinic, 2011).

Risk Factors

Males are four times more likely to sustain a spinal cord injury than females, and nearly half of all SCIs occur in individuals between the ages of 16 and 30 years. Individuals who engage in risky behavior, such as diving into a too-shallow pool, playing sports without protective gear, or driving ATVs or motorcycles at high speed over rough terrain, are also at higher risk for SCIs. Not surprisingly, it is often single, young adult males who engage in risky behavior, which combines to give this group of individuals the highest risk for SCIs. Race and ethnicity can also contribute to the risk for SCIs: Among individuals who have sustained a spinal cord injury since 2010, 67.0% are Caucasian, 24.4% are African American, 2.1% are Asian, and 0.8% are Native American; 7.9% of individuals with a SCI are of Hispanic origin (NSCISC, 2013). Older adults are more likely to sustain a SCI from a fall, especially if the individual also has arthritis or osteoporosis.

Prevention

An individual can implement many precautions to prevent a spinal cord injury. The first precaution is to drive safely. Always drive defensively, because it is impossible to control other drivers. Wear a seat belt at all times, and make sure every child in the vehicle is appropriately placed in a child safety seat with a seat belt. Do not drink and drive, do not ride with a driver who is intoxicated, and be aware of medications that should not be taken if intending to drive.

Diving into water that is too shallow is a common cause of compression injuries. Always check water depth before diving,

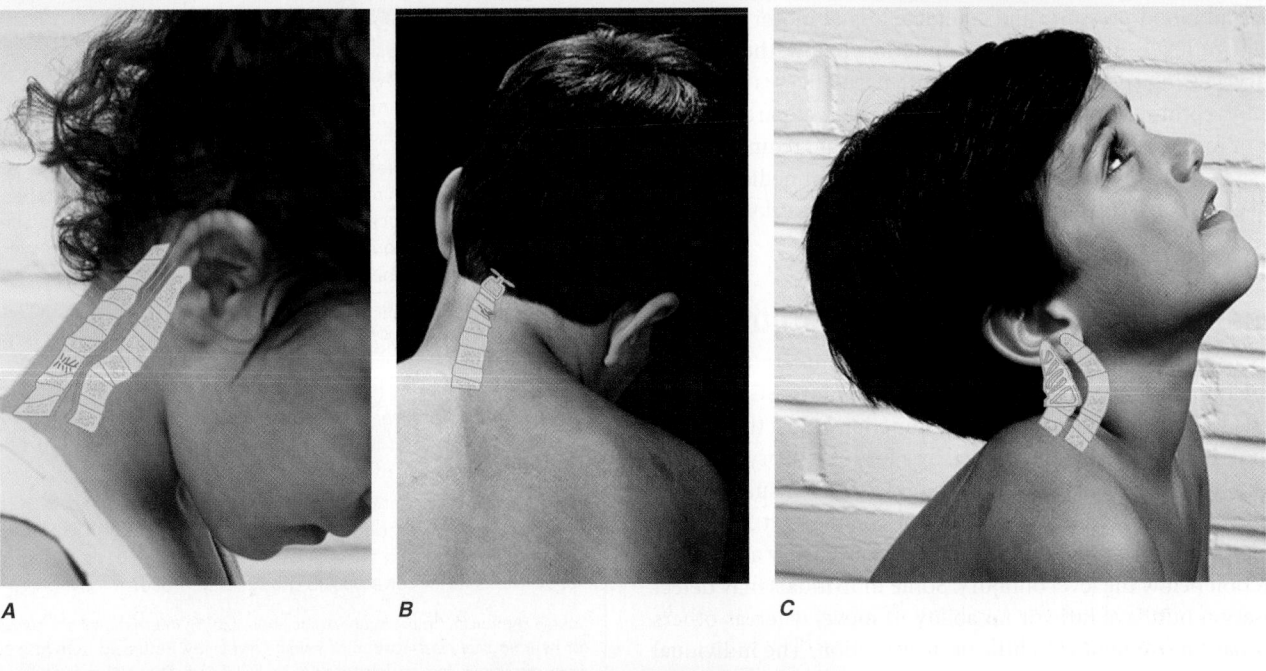

A   *B*   *C*

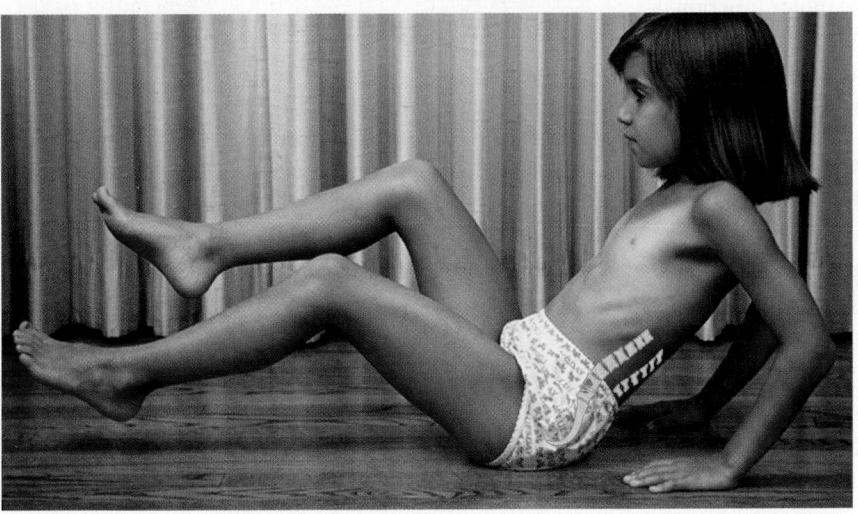

D

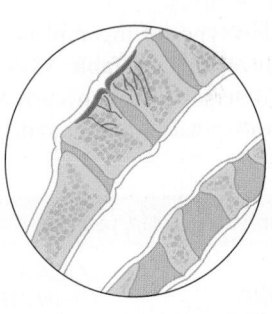

Figure 13–45 ● Mechanics of injury to the spinal cord: *A,* Hyperflexion often due to diving and frontal motor vehicle crashes. *B,* Rotation in which the head and neck are twisted. *C,* Hyperextension often due to rear-end motor vehicle crashes and falls. *D,* Compression due to falls that put vertical pressure on the spinal column. Infants and young children are at higher risk for injury to the brain and spinal cord because of developing bones and muscles.

and never dive into an aboveground pool. In addition, individuals who play sports should wear the proper safety gear. Avoid leading with the head (e.g., sliding headfirst in baseball or tackling in football).

Individuals, especially toddlers and older adults, should take precautions to prevent falls that may cause a SCI. All individuals can decrease their risk of SCI by avoiding areas with high crime rates.

▶ CLINICAL MANIFESTATIONS

Both the vertical location of the injury along the spinal column (called the **level of injury**) and the specific area of the spinal cord or spinal nerve that is damaged will determine the extent and type of physical manifestations the client experiences after

injury. All systems below the level of injury will be affected by damage to the spinal cord, so the higher the level of injury, the greater the extent of motor and sensory deficits. For example, a client who experiences damage at the C3 level will experience more widespread effects than an individual with an injury at the T11 level.

Emergency signs and symptoms that may indicate a spinal cord injury include extreme pain or pressure in the neck or back; weakness, paralysis, or lack of sensation in any part of the body; loss of bladder or bowel control; impaired breathing after injury; or an oddly positioned or twisted neck or back. Muscle spasms may also occur (Mayo Clinic, 2011).

Half of the individuals with a SCI develop **spinal shock**, which is characterized by spinal cord swelling; decreased blood flow and blood pressure; and complete loss of motor function, spinal reflexes, and autonomic function below the level of injury. During spinal shock, even undamaged nerves may have trouble communicating with the brain, causing paralysis and loss of reflexes and sensations in the limbs that are unrelated to the site of injury. Spinal shock usually occurs immediately after injury and can last from several hours to several weeks (NINDS, 2012b).

Classification of Spinal Cord Injury

SCIs can be classified as complete or incomplete using the ASIA Impairment Scale (**Box 13–8** ●). **Complete SCIs** involve a total loss of all sensory and motor function below the level of the injury. It is usually determined by a loss of sensory function in the S4–S5 area, or anal area. Complete SCIs usually cause irreversible damage. If the SCI is not complete, it is termed **incomplete**, involving only a partial loss of sensory and motor function below the level of injury. Some individuals may detect sensation but have little or no ability to move, whereas others may have movement with little or no sensation. The individual has a better chance of recovering sensory and motor function if the injury is incomplete (National Spinal Cord Injury Association [NSCIA], 2012).

Four main types of incomplete syndromes are associated with spinal cord injury (**Table 13–9** ●). In addition, posterior cord syndrome, a very rare occurrence in which the posterior portion of the spinal cord is injured, is characterized by a loss of

---

Box 13–8 **American Spinal Injury Association (ASIA) Impairment Scale (AIS)**

A = Complete. No sensory or motor function is preserved in the sacral segments S4–S5.

B = Sensory incomplete. Sensory but not motor function is preserved below the neurological level and includes the sacral segments S4–S5 (light touch, pin prick at S4–S5, or deep anal pressure), AND no motor function is preserved more than three levels below the motor level on either side of the body.

C = Motor incomplete. Motor function is preserved below the neurological level, and more than half of key muscle functions below the single neurological level of injury (NLI) have a muscle grade of less than 3 (grades 0–2).

D = Motor incomplete. Motor function is preserved below the neurological level, and at least half (or more) of key muscle functions below the NLI have a muscle grade ≥ 3.

E = Normal. If sensation and motor function as tested with the ISNCSCI exam are graded as normal in all segments, and the client had prior deficits, then the AIS grade is E. Someone without an initial SCI does not receive an AIS grade.

Source: American Spinal Injury Association. (2011). *International standards for neurological classification of spinal cord injury.* Retrieved from http://www.asia-spinalinjury.org/elearning/ISNCSCI_Exam_Sheet_r4.pdf.

---

proprioceptive and vibration sense below the level of injury with preservation of muscle strength, temperature, and pain sensation. Posterior cord syndrome has recently been omitted from the ASIA international standards for classification of SCI (McKinley et al., 2007). Cauda equina syndrome (CES), which

---

TABLE 13–9 Syndromes Associated With Incomplete Spinal Cord Injury

SYNDROME	LOCATION AND CAUSE OF INJURY	SYMPTOMS	PROGNOSIS
Central cord syndrome	Hyperextension of the neck, especially from falls and motor vehicle crashes; damage to the center of the spinal cord	More severe motor loss of the upper extremities than the lower extremities, bladder dysfunction (usually urinary retention), varying degrees of sensory loss below the level of injury	Almost all clients will have some degree of neurological recovery, starting in the lower extremities and moving upward. However, some will have sustained functional loss. Younger clients have a higher recovery rate than older clients.
Anterior cord syndrome	Injury to the anterior two thirds of the spinal cord, especially the anterior spinal artery	Paraplegia below the level of injury (or tetraplegia for injuries higher than C7), bilateral loss of pain and temperature sensations with preservation of proprioception and vibratory senses below the level of injury	Clients with anterior cord syndrome have the worst prognosis for recovery of neurological function and require long periods of rehabilitation. Only 10%–20% of clients experience motor recovery.
Brown-Sequard syndrome	Hemisection of the spinal cord, usually caused by a penetrating trauma (gunshot, knife)	Ipsilateral (same side) motor paralysis and loss of proprioception and vibratory sense below the level of injury Contralateral (opposite side) loss of pain and temperature sensation below the level of injury	Best prognosis of all incomplete SCI syndromes; approximately 75%–90% will recover functional motor strength and ability to ambulate independently.
Conus medullaris syndrome	Injury to the conus medullaris, which is the tapered inferior end of the spinal cord; located at the L1 level	Symmetrical pattern of upper and lower motor neuron dysfunction, saddle anesthesia, variable degrees of lower extremity weakness, areflexic bladder and bowel	Prognosis for recovery of bowel and bladder function is poor.

Sources: Based on Chin, L. S. (2013). Spinal cord injuries. *Medscape Reference.* Retrieved from http://emedicine.medscape.com/article/793582-overview; Fehlings, M. G., Vaccaro, A. R., Boakye, M., Rossignol, S., Ditunno, J. F., Jr., & Burns, A. S. (2013). *Essentials of spinal cord injury: Basic research to clinical practice.* New York, NY: Thieme Medical Publishers, Inc.; McKinley, W., Santos, K., Meade, M., & Brooke, K. (2007). Incidence and outcomes of spinal cord injury clinical syndromes. *Journal of Spinal Cord Medicine, 30*(3), 215–224.

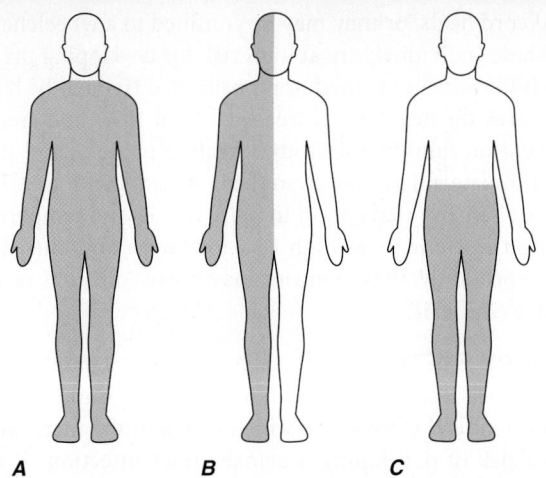

Figure 13–46 ● Types of paralysis. *A,* Complete quadriplegia or partial paralysis of the upper extremities and complete paralysis of the lower part of the body. *B,* Hemiplegia is paralysis of one half of the body when it is divided along the median sagittal plane. *C,* Paraplegia is paralysis of the lower part of the body.

is characterized by injury to the nerve roots emanating from the conus medullaris, is not a true SCI. It is characterized by bladder and bowel retention and should be treated by surgical decompression within 48 hours (Fehlings et al., 2013). (See Exemplar 13.1 for further discussion of CES.)

Effects of Spinal Cord Injury Throughout the Body

A spinal cord injury has many effects on the rest of the body. Individuals with SCI often experience paraplegia or tetraplegia depending on the level of injury (**Figure 13–46 ●**). **Tetraplegia** (also called quadriplegia) is paralysis of the upper and lower limbs and trunk; it is usually associated with a cervical injury. **Paraplegia** is paralysis of all or part of the trunk, legs, and pelvic organs; it is usually associated with spinal cord damage in the thoracic or lumbar regions. Incomplete tetraplegia (40.6%) is the most common neurological category at discharge, followed by incomplete paraplegia (18.7%), complete paraplegia (18.0%), and complete tetraplegia (11.6%) (NSCISC, 2013). Hemiplegia can also occur, in which one half of the body is paralyzed when divided along the median sagittal plane.

Other common symptoms that occur due to spinal cord injury include pain, bladder and bowel problems, respiratory and cardiovascular problems, and reproductive problems. *Pain* can be due to either neurogenic pain resulting from damage to nerves in the spinal cord or physiological pain resulting from compensatory use of muscle groups (e.g., pain in shoulder muscles from pushing a wheelchair).

Urinary and *bowel* problems occur when nerves that innervate the muscles that control the urinary system or bowel no longer transmit signals properly. Muscles in the bladder, urethra, and sphincters no longer work together effectively, causing the bladder to empty without warning, become distended, or force urine back into the kidneys due to uncoordinated release of the bladder and urethral sphincter. Similarly, if the anal sphincter remains tight, bowel movements occur randomly when the bowel is full; however, if it is permanently relaxed ("flaccid bowel"), the individual is unable to have a bowel movement (NINDS, 2012b).

Individuals with complete thoracic or cervical injuries often lose control of *respiratory* muscles, including the diaphragm, intercostal muscles, neck muscles, and abdominal muscles. The higher the level of injury, the greater the loss of muscle control. For example, an individual with a SCI at level C3 or higher loses control of all four muscle groups needed for breathing. These individuals require immediate ventilator support. The diaphragm is controlled by spinal nerves in the C3–C5 region, and nerves in the T1–T12 region control the intercostal and abdominal muscles; injuries in these regions will affect all muscles below the injury (NSCIA, 2012). Any injury below the C5 level conserves diaphragm function, but breathing tends to be rapid and shallow and the individual cannot clear secretions from the lungs because of weak thoracic muscles (NINDS, 2012b).

Cardiovascular problems can occur for individuals with cervical injuries. Blood pressure instability, particularly hypotension, often occurs due to loss of tone in blood vessels and blood pooling in distal arteries. Damage to the cardiac accelerator nerves can cause bradycardia (slow heart rate) or arrhythmias in which the heart beats rapidly and irregularly. Arrhythmias usually appear in the first 2 weeks after injury (NINDS, 2012b).

Spinal cord injuries can also cause *reproductive* problems for men and women. Many men with SCI are capable of having an erection, but the erection may not be hard enough or last long enough for intercourse. Men may also face fertility issues due to an inability to ejaculate or retrograde ejaculation, in which semen is deposited in the bladder instead of the urethra. Women often have no change in fertility, but they may have less satisfaction from intercourse. Women with an SCI who desire to become pregnant should discuss options with an obstetrician and other members of the healthcare team who are familiar with SCIs (NSCIA, 2012).

Complications

With each detrimental effect of a spinal cord injury comes the potential for complications. The most common complications affect the cardiovascular system, respiratory system, integumentary system, and urinary system. In addition, clients may suffer emotional changes due to the reality of their new situation.

CARDIOVASCULAR SYSTEM   One of the most common and life-threatening complications of SCI is autonomic dysreflexia. **Autonomic dysreflexia** is the abrupt onset of excessively high blood pressure as the result of an overactive autonomic nervous system (ANS); it usually occurs in clients who have injuries above T5 (NSCIA, 2012). Autonomic dysreflexia is triggered by an irritation, pain, or other stimulus below the level of injury, such as an urge to urinate or defecate, pressure sores, burns, or pressure from tight clothing. An overdistended bladder is the most common cause. When the irritated area tries to send a signal to the brain, the signal is blocked by the injury, causing a reflex action that stimulates the ANS to contract blood vessels, causing a rapid increase in blood pressure. Symptoms of autonomic dysreflexia include flushing, sweating, a pounding headache, bradycardia, sudden hypertension

Avoiding Autonomic Dysreflexia

Autonomic dysreflexia is caused by irritation or pain below the level of injury. Methods to avoid irritation include the following:

- Regularly empty the bladder and bowels.
- If using an indwelling catheter, keep the tubing free of kinks and keep the drainage bag and tubes clean and empty.
- Treat urinary tract infections promptly.
- Consume adequate fluid and fiber to prevent constipation.
- Change positions frequently.
- Regularly assess the skin for impaired integrity, including pressure sores and ingrown toenails.
- Avoid burns, including sunburns.
- Do not wear clothing that is too tight.
- Take medications as prescribed to prevent pain and other complications that may initiate autonomic dysreflexia.
- Do not become overstimulated during sexual activity.

(<200/100), vision changes, and goosebumps. Treatment should be immediate and may include changing positions, emptying the bladder or bowels, or removing tight clothing (NINDS, 2012b). If not treated immediately, autonomic dysreflexia can lead to seizures, stroke, myocardial infarction, and death. Methods to avoid autonomic dysreflexia are outlined in the Client Teaching feature.

Another common complication of spinal cord injury is deep venous thrombosis, especially for clients with little to no mobility. Individuals with a SCI are at three times the risk for developing blood clots in comparison to other individuals with limited mobility. If blood clots become dislodged, they may travel throughout the body and cause stroke or pulmonary embolism, both of which are life-threatening complications. Anticoagulant therapy may be provided as a preventive measure.

RESPIRATORY SYSTEM   If innervation of respiratory muscles is affected by a SCI, multiple respiratory complications can occur in addition to difficulty breathing. Any loss of respiratory muscle control decreases lung capacity, increases respiratory congestion, and makes coughing difficult. If the client is unable to draw enough air into the lungs, atelectasis (collapsed lung) may occur. An inability to clear secretions and use of mechanical ventilation increases the client's risk for pneumonia. Individuals on mechanical ventilation increase their risk of developing complications by 1%–3% per day of intubation. More than 25% of all deaths associated with SCI are related to ventilator-associated pneumonia (NINDS, 2012b). Symptoms of pneumonia include shortness of breath, pale skin, fever, a "heavy" chest, and increased congestion (NSCIA, 2012). Individuals with pneumonia should be treated immediately with antibiotics.

INTEGUMENTARY SYSTEM   Spinal cord injuries are associated with a temporary or permanent loss of mobility. Many individuals are confined to a bed for weeks while the spinal cord heals, or they may be confined to a wheelchair for life. These individuals are at high risk for developing pressure sores if they are not turned or repositioned frequently. If pressure sores do develop, decreased blood flow and nervous intervention inhibits the wound healing process, and it may also stimulate autonomic dysreflexia. Clients with a SCI may also lose sensory perception to pain, touch, and temperature, putting these clients at high risk for burns and cuts. If not treated promptly, these injuries may cause infection or autonomic dysreflexia.

URINARY SYSTEM   Every SCI has the potential to cause urinary problems. Many clients must undergo indwelling or intermittent catheterization, which dramatically increases the client's risk of developing a urinary tract infection. If urine backs up into the kidneys, it could cause a serious kidney infection. Kidney or bladder stones may also develop. For more information about urinary tract infections, see the exemplar on Urinary Tract Infections in the module on Infection. For more information on other bladder and bowel problems, see the module on Elimination.

EMOTIONAL CHANGES   Spinal cord injuries cause a plethora of physical changes instantly. Clients often go through a process of grief upon the loss of mobility and independence. Some clients will progress through the grief process and eventually accept their new condition. These clients have the best chance of having a good quality of life. Others, however, may be unable to accept their new condition and fight anger and depression for many years. These clients may need additional psychological care, including medications and counseling.

Lifespan and Cultural Considerations

Although spinal cord injury in the pediatric population is not as common as in adults, it can have significant physiological and psychological consequences. Both the location and common mechanisms of injury are different for children than for adults. For cervical injuries, preteens are more likely to be injured in the C2 region, whereas teens suffer C4 injuries and adults suffer C4–C5 injuries. The most common causes of injury are motor vehicle crashes for younger children and sports injuries (especially football) for adolescents. Injuries related to violence, especially gunshots, and ATVs were more common in children than in adults (Parent et al., 2011).

Children tend to have better neurological recovery after a SCI compared to adults. Incomplete injuries have the best prognosis, but even severe complete injuries can show improvement over time in children. However, children who sustain a SCI in their preteen years have a significantly increased risk of developing scoliosis. More than 95% of children who have a SCI before their adolescent growth spurt develop scoliosis, compared to just over 50% of children who have a SCI after the growth spurt (Parent et al., 2011).

Pregnant women with a SCI also need special care. Women with SCI are considered to be "high risk" during pregnancy, but that does not mean pregnancy should be avoided. Instead, the woman will need to work closely with a team of healthcare professionals, including an obstetrician, neurologist, respiratory therapist, physiatrist, nurse, and others to prevent complications and prepare for pregnancy, labor, and delivery. Pregnant women are at higher risk for autonomic dysreflexia (especially during labor and delivery), changes in bowel and bladder function, urinary tract infections, pressure sores, respiratory complications, muscle spasms, and swelling in the lower limbs. The woman may not be able to continue taking prescribed medications during pregnancy, so alternative therapies may be needed to manage symptoms.

Pregnant women with decreased sensation in the lower trunk may not feel the typical pains of labor, so they should be taught the common signs of labor such as changes in breathing, abdominal tightening, and backache. New mothers must also consider the effects of her SCI on breastfeeding; muscle spasticity may increase during breastfeeding, and women with limited sensation in their breasts may have reduced milk production (NSCIA, 2012).

▶ COLLABORATION

Care of an individual with actual or suspected SCI begins with emergency care at the moment of injury and often continues throughout the remainder of the individual's life. Emergency care, surgical repair, and pharmacologic and nonpharmacologic therapies are all required for adequate treatment of an individual with a SCI.

Emergency Care

Spinal cord injury is not always obvious. All individuals who have trauma to the head or are unconscious should be treated as if they have a SCI. Individuals with penetrating injuries near the spine and individuals who have suffered from a fall or motor vehicle crash should also be suspected of having a SCI. Initial care should focus on maintaining the client's ability to breathe, preventing movement that could cause more damage, and preventing shock. About one third of clients will need respiratory support via intubation, particularly those with high cervical injuries. Immediate medical attention is necessary to immobilize the spine with a neck collar and backboard and transport the client from the scene of the accident to the hospital. At the hospital, the client should be transferred from the stretcher to the bed with the backboard still in place. The spine should be realigned using a rigid brace or axial traction as soon as possible after arrival at the hospital.

Diagnostic Tests

Diagnostic tests for SCI should include imaging tests such as x-rays, myelograms, CT scans, or MRIs. X-rays can reveal major vertebral fractures and other bone problems; x-rays must adequately show all regions of the spinal column so that no injuries, especially noncontiguous fractures (spinal fractures separated by at least one normal vertebra), are overlooked. Injecting a contrast dye during a myelogram allows the radiologist to directly view damage to the spinal cord and surrounding tissues. CT scans and MRIs are more sensitive than simple x-rays at detecting abnormalities, especially damage to soft tissue and small fractures. Imaging tests are useful for determining both the location of the injury and if the spinal cord is being compressed.

Somatosensory evoked potentials or magnetic evoked potentials can be used to detect neural response to physiological, electrical, or magnetic stimulation. Common sites for stimulation include the median nerve at the wrist, the common peroneal nerve at the knee, and the posterior tibial nerve (Chawla, 2012). Arterial blood gases (ABGs) should be monitored regularly to evaluate oxygenation and ventilation, and hemoglobin and hematocrit should be measured to detect major blood loss.

Surgery

The timing of surgical treatment for a spinal cord injury is a controversial issue. Some studies indicate that early decompression (removal of debris that is compressing the spinal cord) results in a better recovery compared to late decompression, whereas other studies indicate that there is no difference in neurological recovery between early and late decompression. A recent large study of six hospitals throughout North America compared outcomes between early decompression (less than 24 hours after injury) and late decompression (more than 24 hours after injury). This study found that the odds of at least a two-grade AIS improvement were 2.8 times higher in clients who underwent early decompression compared to late decompression (Fehlings et al., 2012). Spinal decompression surgery is most often performed in clients with progressive neurological deterioration, facet dislocation (displacement of one vertebra on another), spinal nerve compression, and extradural lesions (Chin, 2013).

After a SCI, surgery may also be needed to stabilize the spine. Spine stabilization may involve realigning the spine and using instrumentation such as rods and screws to internally immobilize the spine. A bone graft from the client or bone bank is often added to promote fusion of the vertebrae. Surgery can also be performed to set up spinal traction using Gardner-Wells tongs or other traction devices (**Figure 13–47** ●) or external fixation with a halo brace (**Figure 13–48** ●). A halo brace is often used for clients with cervical fractures without major cord damage. The client may be in traction or external fixation for several weeks or months.

Pharmacologic Therapy

Pharmacologic therapy for clients with a SCI is primarily symptomatic. Symptoms that may require treatment include pain,

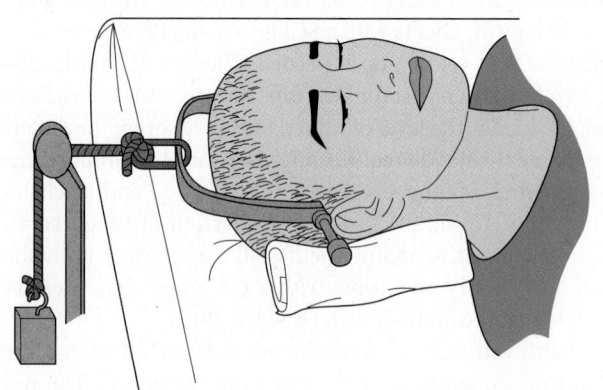

Figure 13–47 ● Cervical traction may be applied by any of several methods, including the Gardner-Wells method.

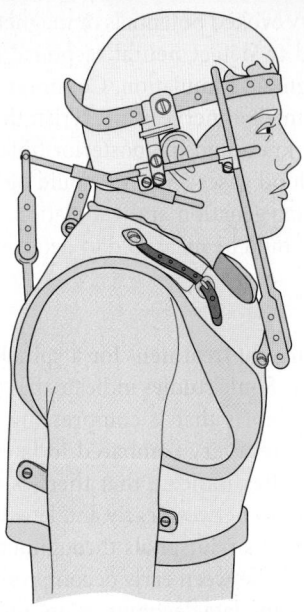

Figure 13–48 ● The halo external fixation device.

constipation, infections, hypotension, and muscle spasticity. Medications to treat these symptoms are discussed elsewhere in this textbook. Most clients will receive high-dose methylprednisone within 8 hours after injury to improve neurological recovery. Methylprednisone appears to decrease inflammation and reduce damage to surrounding nerve cells. Adverse effects are usually minor. Prophylactic anticoagulation therapy (e.g., heparin, Coumadin) may be given to help prevent DVT and pulmonary embolism. Infections, especially pneumonia, should be treated promptly with appropriate antibiotics; pain can be treated with opioids, NSAIDs, and other analgesics as needed.

Nonpharmacologic Therapy

Clients with a spinal cord injury will require extensive nursing care. Immediate nursing care involves maintaining an airway, assisting with ventilation, and immobilizing the client. Nursing care also includes preventing complications such as urinary or bowel problems, pressure sores, and infection. During the healing process, the nurse will also play a role in the client's rehabilitation and client teaching for home care.

PROMOTE EFFECTIVE VENTILATION   The most important therapy for clients with a SCI is to maintain a patent airway and assist with ventilation as needed. Clients with injuries above T12 will experience some decrease in respiratory muscle control; the higher the level of injury, the more severe the deficiencies. Some clients will require only insertion of an oropharyngeal airway, whereas others will require intubation and mechanical ventilation (Chin, 2013). During insertion of tubes, cervical alignment must be maintained at all times. Most individuals with a C4 injury and some with a C3 injury may eventually learn to breathe on their own (NSCIA, 2012).

Clients with decreased respiratory muscle control also have a hard time coughing and clearing lung secretions. The nurse should help the client with cough assist treatments and encourage the client to drink water if possible to keep secretions from becoming thick. The nurse may also teach the client breathing

exercises, such as incentive spirometry. Keeping the airway clear of secretions is important both for ease of breathing and to prevent the development of pneumonia.

PREVENT COMPLICATIONS   Many primary complications related to the injury and secondary complications related to immobility can affect clients with a SCI. Primary complications include urinary, bowel, and gastrointestinal problems. Most SCIs affect bladder and bowel control because of a disruption of nervous transmission to the muscles that control these organs. Individuals with bladder dysfunction often use intermittent or indwelling catheters to empty their bladders. Individuals with bowel dysfunction should implement a scheduled bowel program; if constipation is severe, the client may need manual removal of stool to prevent fecal impaction. Gastrointestinal problems usually involve decreased peristalsis (ileus) and difficulty swallowing. Some clients will need a nasogastric tube to remove stomach contents (nasogastric decompression) to prevent aspiration pneumonia. Food or medicine can also be administered through the nasogastric tube as needed throughout recovery for clients with swallowing problems.

Secondary complications are often related to immobility. Clients with a SCI may be on bed rest for an extended period, or they may be confined to a wheelchair for the rest of their lives. Both the injury and immobility cause decreased blood flow, which can lead to complications such as pressure sores, DVT, and infection. Nonpharmacologic interventions to prevent pressure sores include turning the client every 1–2 hours, providing good skin care, observing the client's skin for damaged areas, padding hard surfaces (both exterior surfaces such as bed railings and interior surfaces such as bony prominences), removing items that may cause compression of blood vessels (e.g., keys, belts, cell phones), performing passive and active ROM exercises, and ambulating if possible. For clients with severe pressure sores, nonpharmacologic treatment may include covering the wound with a sterile dressing and eating foods high in protein to promote healing. In addition to many of these same interventions, compression stockings or boots can stimulate circulation in the legs to prevent DVT.

Individuals with a SCI are at high risk for infection from additional bone fractures and skin wounds from the traumatic event, surgical incisions, traction or external fixation pins, pressure sores, decreased airway clearance, and catheterization. Each of these types of infection requires different nonpharmacologic interventions. For example, skin wounds should be gently cleansed, covered with sterile gauze, and monitored for drainage and other signs of infection. Pneumonia can be prevented by keeping the airway clear of secretions, and urinary tract infections can be prevented by keeping the bladder empty and using sterile technique during catheterization.

FACILITATE REHABILITATIVE AND HOME-BASED CARE   When the initial traumatic injuries have been treated and the client is stabilized, the client faces a long road of recovery to regain maximal function. Rehabilitation is a core component of this recovery. Rehabilitation team members may include a physical therapist, occupational therapist, rehabilitation nurse, recreation therapist, and physiatrist. Therapists emphasize strengthening existing muscle function, redeveloping fine

Community-Based Care Home Care for a Client With a Spinal Cord Injury

Clients with a SCI require months of rehabilitation. During this time, the client may be moved from intensive care to rehabilitation to assistive care to home care. The nurse must interact with the client at every stage of the rehabilitation process to prevent complications and provide client teaching to promote independence. Information for home care may include the following:

- Techniques to perform self-care activities
- Use of mobility and assistive devices

- Home adaptations, especially related to wheelchair access and safety
- Community resources such as Lifeline, support groups, counseling, and foundations (National Spinal Cord Injury Association, American Paralysis Association)
- Coping skills for the client and caregiver
- Referrals to home health agencies and therapists.

motor skills to perform ADLs, and learning new technology to increase independence (Mayo Clinic, 2011). Rehabilitation will include learning how to use assistive devices such as a wheelchair, walker, or Lofstrand crutches as well as devices to aid with ADLs. Another vital component of rehabilitation is preparing clients to return home and live independently (see the Community-Based Care feature).

Rehabilitation for clients with partial lower limb function may include gait training. Gait training involves using mechanical or human assistance to help the client walk on a treadmill. In addition to providing cardiovascular and respiratory benefits, gait training helps the client gain joint stability, retrain the muscles to walk, increase walking speed, and gain independence. Secondary complications are also decreased. Gait training often uses a

harness system to provide support and safety for the client (NSCIA, 2012).

■ NURSING PROCESS

A spinal cord injury is a serious medical condition that requires collaboration between experts in a variety of fields. The nurse is an important part of this team. Nursing care of clients with a SCI can be divided into emergency care, acute care of a stabilized client, and rehabilitation. The nurse focuses on stabilizing the client, preventing and treating complications, promoting self-care, and educating the client and family. The nurse also plays a major role in the community to prevent SCI by promoting safety.

Clinical Manifestations and Therapies Spinal Cord Injury

ETIOLOGY	CLINICAL MANIFESTATIONS	CLINICAL THERAPIES
Spinal cord injury (general)	■ Pain ■ Loss of sensation ■ Loss of bladder or bowel control ■ Paralysis ■ Muscle spasms ■ Spinal shock ■ DVT ■ Reproductive problems	■ Immobilization ■ Spinal decompression surgery ■ Methylprednisolone ■ Analgesics ■ Antispasmodics ■ Catheterization ■ Skin care ■ ROM exercises ■ Rehabilitation
Cervical injury	*In addition to symptoms for general SCI:* ■ Tetraplegia ■ Oddly twisted neck ■ Weakness, loss of respiratory muscle control ■ Hypotension ■ Bradycardia, arrhythmias ■ Autonomic dysreflexia ■ Decreased peristalsis	*In addition to therapies for general SCI:* ■ Airway patency ■ External fixation or traction ■ Nasogastric decompression
Thoracic injury	*In addition to symptoms for general SCI:* ■ Paraplegia ■ Impaired breathing ■ Autonomic dysreflexia	*In addition to therapies for general SCI:* ■ Airway patency
Lumbar/sacral injury	*In addition to symptoms for general SCI:* ■ Paraplegia ■ Cauda equina syndrome	*In addition to therapies for general SCI:* ■ Surgery to relieve pressure on cauda equina

Assessment

Nursing assessment of the client with a SCI includes obtaining a health history and performing ongoing physical assessments. The health history should include questions about the client's overall health before the traumatic event, an accounting of the traumatic event (time, location, and type of event), any medications the client is taking, and any symptoms the client is experiencing, including pain, numbness, and difficulty breathing.

The physical examination of a client with a SCI includes assessing vital signs regularly, assessing the client's respiratory status, maintaining a patent airway, and assisting with breathing if needed. A neurological examination should follow the ASIA International Standards for Neurological Classification of Spinal Cord Injury. This includes testing key muscles for strength using the muscle function grading scale (see Table 13–1), testing areas of innervation for each spinal nerve for sensation of light touch and pin prick, and scoring the client on the ASIA Impairment Scale (see Box 13–8). The nurse should also assess the client for reflexes, bowel sounds, bladder distention, pain, ABGs, and other injuries from the event.

Diagnosis

Nursing diagnoses will vary with the level and extent of injury. Some nursing diagnoses that may apply to clients with a spinal cord injury include the following:

- *Ineffective Airway Clearance* related to impaired gag reflex
- *Risk for Aspiration* related to impaired gag reflex and gastrointestinal motility
- *Ineffective Breathing Pattern* related to impaired diaphragmatic innervation
- *Risk for Autonomic Dysreflexia* related to C7 spinal cord injury
- *Impaired Physical Mobility* related to T5 spinal cord injury
- *Acute Pain* related to injuries from motor vehicle crash
- *Urinary Retention* related to flaccid bladder
- *Bowel Incontinence* related to defecation reflex
- *Self-Care Deficit: Bathing, Dressing, Feeding, Toileting* related to upper limb paralysis
- *Risk for Post-Trauma Syndrome* related to traumatic event with life-changing injuries.

(NANDA-I © 2012)

Planning

Client goals related to a spinal cord injury may include the following:

- The client will maintain a patent airway.
- The client will participate in speech and occupational therapy as ordered to optimize control of muscles used for swallowing.
- The client will maintain clear breath sounds and oxygen saturation of greater than 95% on room air.
- The client will deny dyspnea.
- The client will verbalize understanding of potential triggers of autonomic dysreflexia and will avoid these triggers.
- The client will participate in physical and occupational therapy to regain as much mobility as possible.

- The client will verbalize adequate pain control, as evidenced by reporting pain as tolerable and that rates no higher than 3 on a scale of 0–10.
- The client will demonstrate safe, effective self-catheterization.
- The client will develop techniques for using assistive devices to help with ADLs.
- The client and caregiver will contact a home health agency to assist with ADLs.
- The client will attend counseling sessions to overcome emotional trauma.

Implementation

The nursing interventions needed for clients with a spinal cord injury will depend on the level, severity, and classification of the injury. Immediate care will include assistance with ventilation, immobilization, care of wounds, and bladder and bowel control. Interventions during the recovery phase will include assistance with mobility, exercise, and self-care activities and prevention of complications. Rehabilitation interventions will include assistance with ambulation, training for ADLs, and referral to rehabilitation therapy.

Manage Emergent and Urgent Problems

Nursing interventions that need to be implemented immediately after injury will focus on immobilizing the spine and providing an adequate airway. This may involve assisting the physician in applying a cervical brace and other immobilization devices and inserting an oropharyngeal airway, intubation tube, or nasogastric tube. This may also involve providing support to the client while the client is being moved from the transport bed to a hospital bed. The nurse will also be responsible for monitoring vital signs, ABGs, and machines used to stabilize the client, such as a mechanical ventilator. Abnormal reports should be immediately reported to a physician, because they may indicate additional complications.

When the client's status has stabilized, the nurse can begin to provide care for non-life-threatening injuries, such as skin wounds, bone fractures, and loss of bladder and bowel control. Nursing care involves cleansing skin wounds and applying an antibiotic ointment and sterile bandage. The client may need an indwelling catheter and fecal incontinence pouch until the client is able to perform self-catheterization, ambulate to the toilet, or participate in bowel and bladder training. If the client is constipated, nursing care may include encouraging increased intake of fluids and fiber or manually removing impacted feces.

Provide Assistance With ADLs

Clients with a SCI will be hospitalized, potentially for several weeks. During this time, nursing care includes assisting the client with self-care activities (bathing, eating), monitoring vital signs every 4 hours, assessing the client for complications (DVT, infection, pressure sores, excess sputum, autonomic dysreflexia, distended bladder), and providing client education and emotional support. The nurse should perform respiratory and neurological assessments regularly, because worsening symptoms may require immediate intervention. Nursing interventions to help prevent complications include helping the client perform ROM exercises, turning the client every 2 hours, keeping the catheter and fecal pouch clean and empty, providing pin care for clients in traction or external fixation, helping the client cough to clear sputum every 2 hours, and applying compression stockings or boots. The client may also begin physical or occupational therapy during this time; the nurse may be responsible for providing referrals for therapy or transporting the client to therapy sessions.

SAFETY ALERT

Compression stockings or boots are necessary to help immobile clients stimulate blood flow and to prevent deep venous thrombosis. However, they may also trigger autonomic dysreflexia in clients with a SCI. If the client develops autonomic dysreflexia, compression stockings or boots should be immediately removed. In addition, compression stockings or boots can be removed for 30–60 minutes several times daily to provide relief for the client.

Facilitate Rehabilitation

When the client's injuries have healed as much as possible, the client is ready to begin aggressive rehabilitation. The client may be in the hospital, in an extended care facility, or at home during this time. Nursing care may include referring the client to a rehabilitation facility, providing emotional support, performing periodic neurological assessments, teaching the client to use assistive devices, and training the client or caregiver to perform catheterization. Providing bowel and bladder training for the client may also be the responsibility of the nurse.

Evaluation

Evaluation of clients with a spinal cord injury involves monitoring vital signs, performing neurological assessments, and assessing the client for signs and symptoms of complications that may range in severity from life threatening to minor. The client's emotional status should also be monitored; anger, frustration, anxiety, and depression are common emotions for clients with a spinal cord injury. The goal of nursing care is to return the client to as close to maximal physical health as possible.

NURSING CARE PLAN A Client With a Cervical Spinal Cord Injury

Caleb Peralta, a 20-year-old college junior, is admitted to the hospital by ambulance following a diving accident. He was socializing at a lake with friends, and on diving into the lake, he struck his head on a concealed rock formation.

ASSESSMENT	DIAGNOSES	PLANNING
When Mr. Peralta is admitted to the emergency department, he has flaccid paralysis involving all extremities. Below the clavicle, he has no sensation; he cannot feel or move his arms and legs. His bladder is distended, and bowel sounds are absent. Mr. Peralta was apneic at the scene; a friend performed rescue breathing for the client until the ambulance crew arrived. Mr. Peralta was intubated by emergency medical personnel and manually ventilated while en route to the ED. Upon ED arrival, mechanical ventilation was initiated. Mr. Peralta's vital signs include temperature 96.8°F oral; pulse 57 bpm; respirations controlled at 16/min; and BP 92/61 mmHg. ABG results include pH 7.36, PaO_2 54, $PaCO_2$ 41, and SaO_2 96%. A CT scan indicates a fracture and spinal cord injury at the C5 level; halo traction is applied. A Foley catheter is inserted into his bladder, with immediate returns of 100 mL clear yellow urine. A nasogastric tube is inserted and attached to low-pressure continuous suction.	■ *Risk for Ineffective Airway Clearance* related to C5 spinal cord injury and tracheal intubation ■ *Risk for Aspiration* related to neurological injury, tracheal intubation, and decreased peristalsis ■ *Impaired Swallowing* related to C5 spinal cord injury ■ *Ineffective Breathing Pattern* related to C5 spinal cord injury ■ *Impaired Gas Exchange* related to paralysis of respiratory muscles ■ *Impaired Physical Mobility* related to C5 spinal cord injury ■ *Urinary Retention* related to flaccid bladder ■ *Dysfunctional Gastrointestinal Motility* related to spinal cord injury ■ *Self-Care Deficit: Bathing, Dressing, Feeding, Toileting* related to upper extremity paralysis ■ *Risk for Impaired Skin Integrity* related to immobility (NANDA-I © 2012)	■ The client will maintain a patent airway. ■ The client will demonstrate no signs or symptoms of aspiration. ■ The client will demonstrate effective ventilation, as manifested by oxygen saturation of greater than 95%, absence of cyanosis, and ABGs within normal limits. ■ The client will demonstrate no signs or symptoms of autonomic dysreflexia. ■ The client will demonstrate no signs or symptoms of deep venous thrombosis. ■ The client will demonstrate production of at least 0.5 mL/kg/hr of urine. ■ The client will demonstrate no signs or symptoms of urinary tract infection. ■ The client will demonstrate adequate bowel elimination patterns, including passage of at least one stool daily. ■ The client's skin will remain intact and free from impairment, including skin breakdown or ulceration.

IMPLEMENTATION

■ Monitor the client's endotracheal tube placement and tube patency; administer tracheal suctioning as ordered and as needed to prevent obstruction.

■ Routinely assess the client's respiratory status, including breath sounds, continuous oxygen saturation monitoring, and ABG results as ordered.

■ Avoid exposing the client to triggers for autonomic dysreflexia, including bladder or bowel distention, constrictive garments, or development of pressure sores.

■ Monitor for signs and symptoms of autonomic dysreflexia and immediately report any suspected manifestations to the physician.

(continued on next page)

NURSING CARE PLAN (continued)

- Administer intravenous fluid as ordered; monitor for signs and symptoms of fluid volume overload.
- Insert a Foley catheter per the physician's order and monitor and record fluid intake and output.
- Report decreased or inadequate urine output to the client's physician.
- Routinely assess the client's halo pins and clean the sites per the physician's orders.
- Monitor and document nasogastric output.
- Turn the client every 2 hours. Inspect the skin for breakdown or injury and report any alterations to the client's physician.

- Provide urinary hygiene care and catheter care as needed to prevent infection.
- Place and monitor a fecal incontinence pouch; empty pouch as needed and report abnormalities or decreased stool production to the physician.
- Apply compression stockings or boots as needed to prevent DVT. Remove stockings during ROM exercises.
- Perform passive ROM exercises on the client's extremities every 4 hours.

EVALUATION

After 2 weeks, Mr. Peralta is moved from the intensive care unit to the neurosurgical unit for continuing care. Because he is hospitalized in the city where he attends college, several hundred miles from home, his family (father, mother, and sister) have been able to visit only one weekend a month. His parents have requested that he be transferred to a rehabilitation hospital in his home town when he is able to travel. His vital signs have stabilized and are within normal limits. Mr. Peralta is still receiving oxygen by nasal cannula, but he is able to breathe without assistance. He has not regained sensation below the neck. One night, as his nurse is repositioning him and inspecting his back for indications of skin breakdown, he states, "I wish I had died when I hit my head. I can't even scratch my own nose. I'm useless."

CRITICAL THINKING

1. How should Mr. Peralta's care plan be modified based on his statement to the nurse?
2. If Mr. Peralta remains a tetraplegic with no control of his bowel or bladder, develop a training session to educate his parents about how to care for him.
3. What types of rehabilitation therapy will be most beneficial for Mr. Peralta?

REVIEW   Spinal Cord Injury

RELATE Link the Concepts and Exemplars

Linking the exemplar of spinal cord injury with the concept of ethics:

1. What is the healthcare team's ethical responsibility to a tetraplegic client who wants to remove the ventilator and be allowed to die?
2. A client with a drug abuse problem has sustained a gunshot wound to the spinal cord and is in severe pain. How should you respond if the physician will not prescribe opioids?

Linking the exemplar of spinal cord injury with the concept of acid-base balance:

3. An unconscious client with a T5 spinal cord injury has just been intubated and is being manually ventilated at a rate of 28 respirations per minute. The ED physician orders an ABG analysis. Presuming the client's ABG results reflect hyperventilation, would the nurse expect the client's $PaCO_2$ to be increased or decreased? What effect would uncompensated hyperventilation have on the client's blood pH?
4. What nursing interventions should be implemented for a client with a SCI who develops respiratory acidosis?

READY Go to Companion Skills Manual

REFER Go to Pearson Student Nursing Resources
nursing.pearsonhighered.com

- Additional review materials

REFLECT Case Study

Robert Morris is a 25-year-old male who is in rehabilitation following a spinal cord injury that resulted from falling from his parents' roof while cleaning gutters. He lost his balance and fell two stories to the ground, fracturing his L1 vertebrae. Mr. Morris had a job in the marketing department of a large department store in a town 15 miles away, but he doesn't think he'll be able to remain in the job following his injury. He is currently taking a medical leave of absence.

Mr. Morris is engaged to Laura Knecht, 25 years old, who is a newly graduated occupational therapist employed by a local hospital. They have dated since high school and always planned to marry. Ms. Knecht has been very supportive of Mr. Morris during his convalescence, but he has been noticeably cool and withdrawn toward her. Mr. Morris plans to live with his parents when he is discharged. They are concerned about Mr. Morris's treatment of Ms. Knecht, whom they love very much. His 18-year-old sister has been giving Mr. Morris a hard time about how he is treating his fiancée.

Mr. Morris is paralyzed from the waist down, and the physicians do not seem to be sure whether the paralysis is permanent or not. Mr. Morris spent 4 weeks in a rehabilitation hospital and is planning for discharge, after which he will receive physical therapy in the home. You are the home health nurse visiting Mr. Morris in the rehabilitation center to obtain a current assessment and begin developing his plan of care.

1. How should you respond to Mr. Morris if he confides his concerns that he will never be able to hold a decent job or have a family?
2. Why might Mr. Morris be attempting to distance himself from his fiancée? How should you address this issue?
3. Design Mr. Morris's initial plan of care for his first week at home.

■ REFERENCES

Aldinger, P. R., Jung, A. W., Pritsch, M., Breusch, S., Thomsen, M., Ewerbeck, V., & Parsch, D. (2009). Uncemented grit-blasted straight tapered titanium stems in patients younger than fifty-five years of age: Fifteen to twenty-year results. *Journal of Bone & Joint Surgery, 91*(6), 1432–1439. doi:10.2106/JBJS.H.00297.

Aleissa, S., Parsons, D., Grant, J., Harder, J., & Howard, J. (2011). Deep wound infection following pediatric scoliosis surgery: Incidence and analysis of risk factors. *Canadian Journal of Surgery, 54*(4), 263–269. doi:10.1503/cjs.008210.

Allen, K. D. (2010). Racial and ethnic disparities in osteoarthritis phenotypes. *Current Opinions in Rheumatology, 22*(5), 528–532. doi:10.1097/BOR.0b013e32833b1b6f.

American Academy of Orthopaedic Surgeons (AAOS). (2007a). *Internal fixation for fractures.* Retrieved from http://orthoinfo.aaos.org/topic.cfm?topic=A00196.

American Academy of Orthopaedic Surgeons (AAOS). (2007b). *Nonunions.* Retrieved from http://orthoinfo. aaos.org/topic.cfm?topic=A00374.

American Academy of Orthopaedic Surgeons (AAOS). (2009a). *Compartment syndrome.* Retrieved from http://orthoinfo.aaos.org/topic.cfm?topic=a00204.

American Academy of Orthopaedic Surgeons (AAOS). (2009b). *Hip fractures.* Retrieved from http://orthoinfo. aaos.org/topic.cfm?topic=a00392.

American Academy of Orthopaedic Surgeons (AAOS). (2011a). *Care of casts and splints.* Retrieved from http://orthoinfo.aaos.org/topic.cfm?topic=A00095.

American Academy of Orthopaedic Surgeons (AAOS). (2011b). *Introduction to scoliosis.* Retrieved from http://orthoinfo.aaos.org/topic.cfm?topic=A00633.

American Academy of Pediatrics. (2012). *Back to school tips.* Retrieved from http://www.aap.org/en-us/about-the-aap/aap-press-room/news-features-and-safety-tips/pages/Back-to-School-Tips.aspx.

American Association of Neurological Surgeons (AANS). (2011). *Herniated disc.* Retrieved from http://www.aans.org/Patient%20Information/Conditions%20and%20Treatments/Herniated%20Disc.aspx.

American College of Rheumatology (ACR). (2012). *Osteoarthritis.* Retrieved from http://www.rheumatology.org/practice/clinical/patients/diseases_and_conditions/osteoarthritis.asp.

American Spinal Injury Association. (2011). *International standards for neurological classification of spinal cord injury.* Retrieved from http://www.asia-spinalinjury.org/elearning/ISNCSCI_Exam_Sheet_r4.pdf.

Bannuru, R. R., Natov, N. S., Obadan, I. E., Price, L. L., Schmid, C. H., & McAldindon, T. E. (2009). Therapeutic trajectory of hyaluronic acid versus corticosteroids in the treatment of knee osteoarthritis: A systematic review and meta-analysis. *Arthritis and Rheumatism, 61*(12), 1704–1711. doi:10.1002/art.24925.

Bauer, D. H., & Freivalds, A. (2009). Backpack load limit recommendation for middle school students based on physiological and psychophysical measurements. *Work, 32*(3), 339–350. doi:10.3233/WOR-2009-0832.

Beaulieu, J.-M., & Gainetdinov, R. R. (2011). The physiology, signaling, and pharmacology of dopamine receptors. *Pharmacological Reviews, 63*(1), 182–217. doi:10.1124/pr.110.002642.

Berman, A., & Snyder, S. J. (2012). Promoting health in older adults. In K. Trakalo (Ed.), *Kozier & Erb's fundamentals of nursing: Concepts, process, & practice* (pp. 411–433). Upper Saddle River, NJ: Pearson Education.

Brackley, H. M., Stevenson, J. M., & Selinger, J. C. (2009). Effect of backpack load placement on posture and spinal curvature in prepubescent children. *Work, 32*(3), 351–360. doi:10.3233/WOR-2009-0833.

Centeno, C. J., Busse, D., Kisiday, J., Keohan, C., Freeman, M., & Karli, D. (2008). Increased knee cartilage volume in degenerative joint disease using percutaneously implanted, autologous mesenchymal stem cells. *Pain Physician, 11*(3), 343–353.

Centers for Disease Control and Prevention (CDC). (2010). *Hip fractures among older adults.* Retrieved from http://www.cdc.gov/homeandrecreationalsafety/falls/adulthipfx.html.

Centers for Disease Control and Prevention (CDC). (2012). *Falls among older adults: An overview.* Retrieved http://www.cdc.gov/homeandrecreationalsafety/falls/adultfalls.html.

Chao, J., Leung, Y., Wang, M., & Chang, R. C. (2012). Nutraceuticals and their preventive or potential therapeutic value in Parkinson's disease. *Nutrition Reviews, 70*(7), 373–386. doi:10.1111/j.1753-4887.2012.00484.x.

Chawla, J. (2012). Clinical applications of somatosensory evoked potentials. *Medscape Reference.* Retrieved from http://emedicine.medscape.com/article/1139393-overview#a1.

Cheung, K. M. C., Cheng, E. Y. L., Chan, S. C. W., Yeung, K. W. K., & Luk, K. D. K. (2007). Outcome assessment of bracing in adolescent idiopathic scoliosis by the use of the SRS-22 questionnaire. *International Orthopaedics, 31*(4), 507–511. doi:10.1007/s00264-006-0209-5.

Chin, L. S. (2013). Spinal cord injuries. *Medscape Reference.* Retrieved from http://emedicine.medscape.com/article/793582-overview#showall.

Cobb, J. R. (1948). Outline for the study of scoliosis. In J. W. Edwards (Ed.), *AAOS, Instructional Course Lectures* (Vol. 5, pp. 261–275). Ann Arbor, MI: American Academy of Orthopaedic Surgeons.

Coulibaly, M. O., Sietsema, D. L., Burgers, T. A., Mason, J., Williams, B. O., & Jones, C. B. (2010). Recent advances in the use of serological bone formation markers to monitor callus development and fracture healing. *Critical Reviews in Eukaryotic Gene Expression, 20*(2), 105–127.

Cree, B. A. C., Kornyeyeva, E., & Goodin, D. S. (2010). Pilot trial of low-dose naltrexone and quality of life in multiple sclerosis. *Annals of Neurology, 68*(2), 145–150. doi:10.1002/ana.22006.

Dang, L., & Liu, Z. (2010). A review of current treatment for lumbar disc herniation in children and adolescents. *European Spine Journal, 19*(2), 205–214. doi:10.1007/s00586-009-1202-7.

DiLorenzo, T. (2011). Aging with multiple sclerosis. *Clinical Bulletin: Information for Health Professionals.* New York, NY: National Multiple Sclerosis Society.

Dugdale, D. C., III. (2012a). Aging changes in the bones—muscles—joints. *MedlinePlus.* Retrieved from http://www.nlm.nih.gov/medlineplus/ency/article/004015.htm.

Dugdale, D. C., III. (2012b). Deep venous thrombosis. *MedlinePlus.* Retrieved from http://www.nlm.nih.gov/medlineplus/ency/article/000156.htm.

Emadedin, M., Aghdami, N., Taghiyar, L., Fazeli, R., Modhadasali, R., Jahangir, S., . . . Bahaban Eslaminejad, M. (2012). Intra-articular injection of autologous mesenchymal stem cells in six patients with knee osteoarthritis. *Archives of Iranian Medicine, 15*(7), 422–428. doi:023268/AIM.0010.

Fahn, S., Elton, R., & Members of the UPDRS Development Committee. (1987). Unified Parkinson's Disease Rating Scale. In: S. Fahn, C. D. Marsden, D. B. Calne, & M. Goldstein, (Eds.), *Recent developments in Parkinson's disease* (Vol. 2, pp. 153–163, 293–304). Florham Park, NJ: Macmillan Health Care Information.

Fehlings, M. G., Vaccaro, A. R., Boakye, M., Rossignol, S., Ditunno, J. F., Jr., & Burns, A. S. (2013). *Essentials of spinal cord injury: Basic research to clinical practice.* New York, NY: Thieme Medical Publishers.

Fehlings, M. G., Vaccaro, A., Wilson, J. R., Singh, A., Cadotte, D. W., Harrop, J. S., . . . Rampersaud, R. (2012). Early versus delayed decompression for traumatic cervical spinal cord injury: Results of the Surgical Timing in Acute Spinal Cord Injury Study (STASCIS). *PLoS ONE, 7*(2), e32037. doi:10.1371/journal.pone.0032037.

Finlayson, M., van Denend, T., & Hudson, E. (2004). Aging with multiple sclerosis. *Journal of Neuroscience Nursing, 36*(5).

Gardner, A., Gardner, E., & Morley, T. (2011). Cauda equina syndrome: A review of the current clinical and medico-legal position. *European Spine Journal, 20*(5), 690–697.

GE Healthcare. (2011). *DaTscan Ioflupane I123 injection.* Retrieved from http://us.datscan.com.

Geris, L., Schugart, R., & van Oosterwyck, H. (2010). *In silico* design of treatment strategies in wound healing and bone fracture healing. *Philosophical Transactions of the Royal Society A, 368*(1920), 2683–2706. doi:10.1098/rsta.2010.0056.

Goetz, C. G., Fahn, S., Martinez-Martin, P., Poewe, W., Sampaio, C., Stebbins, G. T., . . . LaPelle, N. (2007). Movement Disorder Society–sponsored revision of the Unified Parkinson's Disease Rating Scale (MDS-UPDRS): Process, format, and clinimetric testing plan. *Movement Disorders, 22*(1), 41–47. doi:10.1002/mds.21198.

Griffin, M., & Bayat, A. (2011). Electrical stimulation in bone healing: Critical analysis by evaluating levels of evidence. *ePlasty, 11*, e34.

Hauser, R. A. (2013). Parkinson disease. *Medscape Reference.* Retrieved from http://emedicine.medscape.com/article/1831191-overview.

Hindle, J. V. (2010). Ageing, neurodegeneration, and Parkinson's disease. *Age and Ageing, 39*(2), 156–161. doi:10.1093/ageing/afp223.

Hutchinson, M. (2009). Predicting and preventing the future: Actively managing multiple sclerosis. *Practical Neurology, 9*, 133–143. doi:10.1136/jnnp.2009.177212.

Iannitti, T., Lodi, D., & Palmieri, B. (2011). Intra-articular injections for the treatment of osteoarthritis: Focus on the clinical use of hyaluronic acid. *Drugs in R&D, 11*(1), 13–27. doi:10.2165/11539760-000000000-00000.

Jain, S., Mittal, M., Kansal, A., Singh, Y., Kolar, P. R., & Saigal, R. (2008). Fat embolism syndrome. *Journal of the Association of Physicians of India, 56*, 245–249.

Jasmin, L. (2012). Deep brain stimulation. *MedlinePlus.* Retrieved from http://www.nlm.nih.gov/medlineplus/ency/article/007453.htm.

Johns Hopkins Medicine. (n.d.). *Johns Hopkins sports medicine patient guide to knee arthroscopy.* Retrieved from http://www.hopkinsortho.org/knee_arthroscopy.html.

Johnson & Johnson. (2011). *McNeil consumer healthcare announces plans for new dosing instructions for Tylenol® products.* Retrieved from http://www.jnj.com//news/all/mcneil-consumer-healthcare-announces-plans-for-new-dosing-instructions-for-tylenol-products.

Kalunian, K. C. (2013). Patient information: Osteoarthritis symptoms and diagnosis (beyond the basics). *Wolters Kluwer Health UpToDate.* Retrieved from http://www.uptodate.com/contents/osteoarthritis-symptoms-and-diagnosis-beyond-the-basics.

Kaner, T., Sasani, M., Oktenoglu, T., Cirak, B., & Ozer, A. F. (2009). Postoperative spinal epidural hematoma resulting in cauda equina syndrome: A case report and review of the literature. *Cases Journal, 2*, 8584. doi:10.4076/1757-1626-2-8584.

Kaneshiro, N. K. (2011). Fontanelles—Bulging. *MedlinePlus.* Retrieved from http://www.nlm.nih.gov/medlineplus/ency/article/003310.htm.

Kistner, F., Fiebert, I., & Roach, K. (2012). Effect of backpack load carriage on cervical posture in primary schoolchildren. *Work, 41*(1), 99–108. doi:10.3233/WOR-2012-1289.

Kurtzke, J. F. (1983). Rating neurologic impairment in multiple sclerosis: An expanded disability status scale (EDSS). *Neurology, 33*(11), 1444–1452.

Lindsey, J. W., Hatfield, L. M., & Vu, T. (2010). Epstein-Barr virus neutralizing and early antigen antibodies in multiple sclerosis. *European Journal of Neurology, 17*(10), 1263–1269. doi:10.1111/j.1468-1331.2010.03005.x.

Machado, A. G., Deogaonkar, M., & Cooper, S. (2012). Deep brain stimulation for movement disorders: Patient selection and technical options. *Cleveland Clinic Journal of Medicine, 79*(Suppl. 2), S19–S24. doi:10.3949/ccjm.79.s2a.04.

Mandl, L. A., Hotchkiss, R. N., Adler, R. S., Lyman, S., Daluiski, A., Wolfe, S. W., & Katz, J. N. (2009). Injectable hyaluronan for the treatment of carpometacarpal osteoarthritis: Open label pilot trial. *Current Medical Research and Opinion, 25*(9), 2103–2108. doi:10.1185/03007990903084016.

Marieb, E. N. (1998). *Human anatomy and physiology* (4th ed., p. 180). Menlo Park, CA: Benjamin Cummings.

Mayo Clinic. (2010). *Herniated disc.* Retrieved from http://www.mayoclinic.com/health/herniated-disc/DS00893.

Mayo Clinic. (2011). *Spinal cord injury.* Retrieved from http://www.mayoclinic.com/health/spinal-cord-injury/DS00460.

Mayo Clinic. (2012a). *Hip fractures.* Retrieved from http://www.mayoclinic.com/health/hip-fracture/DS00185.

Mayo Clinic. (2012b). *Multiple sclerosis.* Retrieved from http://www.mayoclinic.com/health/multiple-sclerosis/DS00188.

Mayo Clinic. (2012c). *Multiple sclerosis: Treatments and drugs.* Retrieved from http://www.mayoclinic.com/health/multiple-sclerosis/DS00188/DSECTION=treatments-and-drugs.

Mayo Clinic. (2012d). *Parkinson's disease.* Retrieved from http://www.mayoclinic.com/health/parkinsons-disease/DS00295.

Mayo Clinic. (2012e). *Scoliosis.* Retrieved from http://www.mayoclinic.com/health/scoliosis/DS00194.

Mayo Clinic. (2013a). *Deep vein thrombosis (DVT).* Retrieved from http://www.mayoclinic.com/health/deep-vein-thrombosis/DS01005.

Mayo Clinic. (2013b). *Osteoarthritis.* Retrieved from http://www.mayoclinic.com/health/osteoarthritis/DS00019.

McKinley, W., Santos, K., Meade, M., & Brooke, K. (2007). Incidence and outcomes of spinal cord injury clinical syndromes. *Journal of Spinal Cord Medicine, 30*(3), 215–224.

Mehlman, C. T. (2012). Idiopathic scoliosis. *Medscape Reference.* Retrieved from http://emedicine.medscape.com/article/1265794-overview.

Mehrholz, J., Friis, R., Kugler, J., Twork, S., Storch, A., & Pohl, M. (2010). Treadmill training for patients with Parkinson's disease. *Cochrane Database of Systematic Reviews,* Issue 2. Art. No.: CD007830. doi:10.1002/14651858.CD007830.pub2.

Migliore, A., Massafra, U., Bizzi, E., Vacca, F., Martin-Martin, S., Granata, M., . . . Tormenta, S. (2009). Comparative, double-blind, controlled study of intra-articular hyaluronic acid (Hyalubrix) injections versus local anesthetic in osteoarthritis of the hip. *Arthritis Research & Therapy, 11*(6), R183. doi:10.1186/ar2875.

Millis, M. B. (2011). Hip fracture. *Boston Children's Hospital.* Retrieved from http://www.childrenshospital.org/az/Site453/mainpageS453P0.html.

Mirkin, G. (2014). Why ice delays recovery. Retrieved from http://drmirkin.com/fitness/why-ice-delays-recovery.html.

Multiple Sclerosis Association of America (MSAA). (2013). *MS overview.* Retrieved from http://mymsaa.org/about-ms/overview.

Multiple Sclerosis Foundation (MSF). (2009). *What causes multiple sclerosis?* Retrieved from http://www.msfocus.org/causes-multiple-sclerosis.aspx.

Munger, K. L., & Ascherio, A. (2011). Prevention and treatment of MS: Studying the effects of vitamin D. *Multiple Sclerosis, 17*(12), 1405–1411. doi:10.1177/1352458511425366.

Munger, K. L., Levin, L. I., O'Reilly, E. J., Falk, K. I., & Ascherio, A. (2011). Anti-Epstein-Barr virus antibodies as serological markers of multiple sclerosis: A prospective study among United States military personnel. *Multiple Sclerosis, 17*(10), 1185–1193. doi:10.1177/1352458511408991.

Nash, C. L., Jr., & Moe, J. H. (1969). A study of vertebral rotation. *Journal of Bone & Joint Surgery, 51*(2), 223–229.

National Institute of Arthritis and Musculoskeletal and Skin Diseases (NIAMSD). (2009). *Scoliosis.* Retrieved from http://www.niams.nih.gov/Health_Info/Scoliosis/scoliosis_ff.asp.

National Institute of Arthritis and Musculoskeletal and Skin Diseases (NIAMSD). (2010). *Handout on health: Osteoarthritis.* Retrieved from http://www.niams.nih.gov/Health_Info/Osteoarthritis.

National Institute of Arthritis and Musculoskeletal and Skin Diseases (NIAMSD). (2012a). *Handout on health: Back pain.* Retrieved from http://www.niams.nih.gov/health_info/Back_Pain.

National Institute of Arthritis and Musculoskeletal and Skin Diseases (NIAMSD). (2012b). *Hip replacement.* Retrieved from http://www.niams.nih.gov/Health_Info/Hip_Replacement.

National Institute of Neurological Disorders and Stroke (NINDS). (2011). *NINDS arachnoiditis information page.* Retrieved from http://www.ninds.nih.gov/disorders/arachnoiditis/arachnoiditis.htm.

National Institute of Neurological Disorders and Stroke (NINDS). (2012a). *Multiple sclerosis: Hope through research.* Retrieved from http://www.ninds.nih.gov/disorders/multiple_sclerosis/detail_multiple_sclerosis.htm#210833215.

National Institute of Neurological Disorders and Stroke (NINDS). (2012b). *Spinal cord injury: Hope through research.* Retrieved from http://www.ninds.nih.gov/disorders/sci/detail_sci.htm#186383233.

National Institute of Neurological Disorders and Stroke (NINDS). (2013). *Parkinson's disease: Hope through research.* Retrieved from http://www.ninds.nih.gov/disorders/parkinsons_disease/detail_parkinsons_disease.htm.

National Institutes of Health (NIH). (2012). Parkinson's disease. *NIHSeniorHealth.* Retrieved from https://nihseniorhealth.gov/parkinsonsdisease/whatisparkinsonsdisease/01.html.

National Multiple Sclerosis Society (NMSS). (2012). *Multiple sclerosis: Just the facts. General information.* Washington, DC: National Multiple Sclerosis Society.

National Multiple Sclerosis Society (NMSS). (n.d.a). *Diagnosing MS.* Retrieved from http://www.nationalmssociety.org/about-multiple-sclerosis/what-we-know-about-ms/diagnosing-ms/index.aspx.

National Multiple Sclerosis Society (NMSS). (n.d.b). *Pediatric (child) MS.* Retrieved from http://www.nationalmssociety.org/about-multiple-sclerosis/pediatric-ms/index.aspx.

National Multiple Sclerosis Society (NMSS). (n.d.c). *Pregnancy and reproductive issues.* Retrieved from http://www.nationalmssociety.org/living-with-multiple-sclerosis/healthy-living/pregnancy/index.aspx.

National Multiple Sclerosis Society (NMSS). (n.d.d). *Rehabilitation.* Retrieved from http://www.nationalmssociety.org/about-multiple-sclerosis/what-we-know-about-ms/treatments/rehabilitation/index.aspx.

National Parkinson Foundation (NPF). (n.d.a). *Parkinson's disease: Living well.* Retrieved from http://www.parkinson.org/Parkinson-s-Disease/Living-Well.

National Parkinson Foundation (NPF). (n.d.b). *Parkinson's disease overview.* Retrieved from http://www.parkinson.org/parkinson-s-disease.aspx.

National SCI Statistical Center. (2013). *Spinal cord injury facts and figures at a glance.* Birmingham, AL: University of Alabama at Birmingham.

National Spinal Cord Injury Association (NSCIA). (2012). *Introduction to spinal cord injury.* Retrieved from http://www.spinalcord.org/resource-center/askus/index.php?pg=kb.book&id=56.

Navarro-Sarabia, F., Coronel, P., Collantes, E., Navarro, F. J., Rodriguez de la Serna, A., Naranjo, A., . . . AMELIA study group. (2011). A 40-month multicentre, randomized placebo-controlled study to assess the efficacy and carry-over effect of repeated intra-articular injections of hyaluronic acid in knee osteoarthritis: The AMELIA project. *Annals of the Rheumatic Diseases, 70*(11), 1957–1962. doi:10.1136/ard.2011.152017.

Neuschwander, T. B., Cutrone, J., Macias, B. R., Cutrone, S., Murthy, G., Chambers, H., & Hargens, A. R. (2010). The effect of backpacks on the lumbar spine in children: A standing magnetic resonance imaging study. *Spine, 35*(1), 83–88. doi:10.1097/BRS.0b013e3181b21a5d.

Ogiela, D. (2012). Herniated disc. *MedlinePlus.* Retrieved from http://www.nlm.nih.gov/medlineplus/ency/article/000442.htm.

Panula, J., Pihlajamaki, H., Mattila, V. M., Jaatinen, P., Vahlberg, T., Aarnio, P., & Kivela, S.-L. (2011). Mortality and cause of death in hip fracture patients aged 65 or older—A population-based study. *BMC Musculoskeletal Disorders, 12*, 105. doi:10.1186/1471-2474-12-105.

Parent, S., Mac-Thiong, J.-M., Roy-Beaudry, M., Sosa, J. F., & Labelle, H. (2011). Spinal cord injury in the pediatric population: A systematic review of the literature. *Journal of Neurotrauma, 28*(8), 1515–1524. doi:10.1089/neu.2009.1153.

Parkinson Study Group. (2011). *Termination of QE3 study.* Retrieved from http://parkinson-study-group.org/docs/Clinical_Trials_in_Progress/QE3_Final_PSG_Post_May_27_2011_2.pdf.

Ploughman, M., Austin, M. W., Murdoch, M., Kearney, A., Fisk, J. D., Godwin, M., & Stefanelli, M. (2012). Factors influencing healthy aging with multiple sclerosis: A qualitative study. *Disability and Rehabilitation, 34*(1), 26–33. doi:10.3109/09638288.2011.585212.

Raaymakers, E., Schipper, I., Simmermacher, R., & van der Werken, C. (2010). Proximal femur 31-B3 arthroplasty. *AO Foundation.* Retrieved from https://www2.aofoundation.org/wps/portal/surgery?showPage=redfix&bone=Femur&segment=Proximal&classification=31-B3&treatment=&method=Arthroplasty&implantstype=&approach=&redfix_url=1284974569031&Language=en.

Ramprasad, M., Alias, J., & Raghuveer, A. K. (2010). Effect of backpack weight on postural angles in preadolescent children. *Indian Pediatrics, 47*(7), 575–580.

Reitman, N., & Kalb, R. (2012). *Multiple sclerosis: The nursing perspective* (6th ed.). New York, NY: National Multiple Sclerosis Society.

Rivett, L., Rothberg, A., Stewart, A., & Berkowitz, R. (2009). The relationship between quality of life and compliance to a brace protocol in adolescents with idiopathic scoliosis: A comparative study. *BMC Musculoskeletal Disorders, 10*, 5. doi:10.1186/1471-2474-10-5.

Rodriguez-Oviedo, P., Ruano-Ravina, A., Perez-Rios, M., Garcia, F. B., Gomez-Fernandez, D., Fernandez-Alonso, A., . . . Turiso, J. (2012). School children's backpacks, back pain and back pathologies. *Archives of Disease in Childhood, 97*(8), 730–732. doi:10.1136/archdischild-2011-301253.

Samour, P. Q., & King, K. (2013). *Essentials of pediatric nutrition.* Burlington, MA: Jones & Bartlett.

Sapountzi-Krepia, D., Psychogiou, M., Peterson, D., Zafiri, V., Iordanopoulou, E., Michailidou, F., & Cristodoulou, A. (2006). The experience of brace treatment in children/adolescents with scoliosis. *Scoliosis, 1*, 8. doi:10.1186/1748-7161-1-8.

Schenkman, M., Hall, D. A., Baron, A. E., Schwartz, R. S., Mettler, P., & Kohrt, W. M. (2012). Exercise for people in early- or mid-stage Parkinson disease: A 16-month randomized controlled trial. *Physical Therapy, 92*(11), 1395–1410. doi:10.2522/ptj.20110472.

Scoliosis Research Society. (n.d.). *Idiopathic scoliosis: Adult.* Retrieved from http://www.srs.org/patient_and_family/scoliosis/idiopathic/adults.

Shimura, H., Schlossmacher, M. G., Hatton, N., Frosch, M. P., Trockenbacher, A., Schneider, R., . . . Selkoe, D. J. (2001). Ubiquitination of a new form of alpha-synuclein by parkin from human brain: Implications for Parkinson's disease. *Science, 293*(5528), 263–269.

Shulman, L. M., Katzel, L. I., Ivey, F. M., Sorkin, J. D., Favors, K., Anderson, K. E., . . . Macko, R. F. (2013). Randomized clinical trial of 3 types of physical exercise for patients with Parkinson disease. *JAMA Neurology, 70*(2), 183–190. doi:10.1001/jamaneurol.2013.646.

Shults, C. W., Oakes, D., Keiburtz, K., Beal, M. F., Haas, R., Plumb, S., . . . Parkinson Study Group. (2002). Effects of coenzyme Q10 in early Parkinson disease: Evidence of slowing of the functional decline. *Archives of Neurology, 59*(10), 1541–1550.

Skaggs, D. L., Early, S. D., D'Ambra, P., Tolo, V. T., & Kay, R. M. (2006). Back pain and backpacks in school children. *Journal of Pediatric Orthopedics, 26*(3), 358–363.

Stacy, M., Davis, T. L., Heath, S., Isaacson, S. H., Tarsy, D., Williams, M., & Moore, A. P. (2009). The clinicians' and nurses' guide to Parkinson's disease. *Medscape Education.* Retrieved from http://www.medscape.org/viewarticle/701955.

Storch, A., Jost, W. H., Vieregge, P., Spiegel, J., Greulich, W., Durner, J., . . . German Coenzyme Q(10) Study Group. (2007). Randomized, double-blind, placebo-controlled trial on symptomatic effects of coenzyme Q(10) in Parkinson's disease. *Archives of Neurology, 64*(7), 938–944.

Sun, S. F., Hsu, C. W., Sun, H. P., Chou, Y. J., Li, H. J., & Wang, J. L. (2011). The effect of three weekly intra-articular injections of hyaluronate on pain, function, and balance in patients with unilateral ankle arthritis. *Journal of Bone and Joint Surgery, American Volume, 93*(18), 1720–1726. doi:10.2106/JBJS.J.00315.

Suri, P., Hunter, D. J., Jouve, C., Hartigan, C., Limke, J., Pena, E., . . . Rainville, J. (2011). Nonsurgical treatment of lumbar disc herniation: Are outcomes different in older adults? *Journal of the American Geriatrics Society, 59*(3), 423–429. doi:10.1111/j.1532-5415.2011.03316.x.

Thompson, H. J., & Mauk, K. L. (2011). *Nursing management of the patient with multiple sclerosis: AANN, ARN, and IOMSN clinical practice guideline series.* Glenview, IL: American Association of Neuroscience Nurses, Association of Rehabilitation Nurses, and International Organization of Multiple Sclerosis Nurses.

University of Maryland Medical Center. (2009). *Back pain and sciatica—Symptoms and causes.* Retrieved from http://www.umm.edu/patiented/articles/what_causes_pain_low_back_pain_or_sciatica_000054_2.htm.

U.S. Department of Health and Human Services. (2013). *Healthy People 2020: Arthritis, osteoporosis, and chronic back conditions.* Retrieved from http://www.healthypeople.gov/2020/topicsobjectives2020/overview.aspx?topicId=3.

U.S. Food and Drug Administration (FDA). (2011). *Questions and answers about oral prescription acetaminophen products to be limited to 325 mg per dosage unit.* Retrieved from http://www.fda.gov/Drugs/DrugSafety/InformationbyDrugClass/ucm239871.htm.

U.S. Preventive Services Task Force. (2011). Screening for osteoporosis: U.S. Preventive Services Task Force recommendation statement. *Annals of Internal Medicine, 154*(5), 356–364.

Victoria, G., Petrisor, B., Drew, B., & Dick, D. (2009). Bone stimulation for fracture healing: What's all the fuss? *Indian Journal of Orthopaedics, 43*(2), 117–120. doi:10.4103/0019-5413.50844.

Vorvick, L. J., Ma, C. B., & Zieve, D. (2012a). Compartment syndrome. *PubMed Health.* Retrieved from http://www.ncbi.nlm.nih.gov/pubmedhealth/PMH0002204/.

Vorvick, L. J., Ma, C. B., & Zieve, D. (2012b). Volkmann's ischemic contracture. *PubMed Health.* Retrieved from http://www.ncbi.nlm.nih.gov/pubmedhealth/PMH0002201/.

Vorvick, L. J., & Zieve, D. (2012). Contracture deformity. *MedlinePlus.* Retrieved from http://www.nlm.nih.gov/medlineplus/ency/article/003185.htm.

Wang, Y., Hall, S., Hanna, F., Wluka, A. E., Grant, G., Marks, P., . . . Cicuttini, F. M. (2011). Effects of Hylan G-F 20 supplementation on cartilage preservation detected by magnetic resonance imaging in osteoarthritis of the knee: A two-year single-blind clinical trial. *BMC Musculoskeletal Disorders, 12*, 195. doi:10.1186/1471-2474-12-195.

Wilson, B. A., Shannon, M. T., & Shields, K. M. (2013). *Nurse's drug guide.* Upper Saddle River, NJ: Pearson Education.

Zieve, D., & Jasmin, L. (2011). Multiple sclerosis. *PubMed Health.* Retrieved from http://www.ncbi.nlm.nih.gov/pubmedhealth/PMH0001747/.

Zieve, D., & Ogiela, D. (2011). Scoliosis. *MedlinePlus.* Retrieved from http://www.nlm.nih.gov/medlineplus/ency/article/001241.htm.

14 Nutrition

◢ THE CONCEPT OF NUTRITION

Just as the body must have oxygen to sustain itself, nutritional intake is essential to ongoing health and physical well-being. In addition, the intake of food is often considered enjoyable and contributes to the emotional stability of individuals by providing opportunities for social interaction and communication. **Nutrition** is the science of the intake of nutrients and their actions in body functioning. ≪

Concept Learning Outcomes

After reading about this concept, you will be able to:

1. Summarize the physiology of the gastrointestinal system related to nutrient metabolism.

2. Examine the relationship between nutrition and other concepts/systems.

3. Identify commonly occurring alterations in nutrition and their related therapies.

4. Differentiate common assessment procedures used to examine nutritional health across the life span.

5. Describe diagnostic and laboratory tests to determine the individual's nutritional status.

6. Explain management of nutritional health and prevention of illness.

7. Demonstrate the nursing process in providing culturally competent and caring interventions across the life span for individuals with common alterations in nutrition.

8. Compare and contrast common independent and collaborative interventions for clients with alterations in nutrition.

Concept Key Terms

Absorption, 926
Anthropometric measurements, 940
Carbohydrate, 927
Chyme, 931
Dietary Reference Intakes (DRIs), 927
Enteral nutrition, 947
Essential nutrient, 927
Fiber, 928
Food choices, 924
Food insecurity, 927
Food security, 927
Hunger, 924
Kilocalorie, 929
Lacto-ovo-vegetarian, 926
Lacto-vegetarian, 926
Lipids, 929
Macronutrient, 927

Micronutrient, 927
Mineral, 930
MyPlate, 927
Nutrient density, 927
Nutrients, 927
Nutrition, 923
Overnutrition, 936
Parenteral nutrition (PN), 948
Protein, 929
Satiety, 927
Saturated fat, 929
Sphincter, 931
Undernutrition, 936
Unsaturated fat, 929
Vegan, 926
Vitamin, 930
Water, 931

▶ NORMAL NUTRITION

Nutritional intake happens several times a day. One of the reasons individuals eat is because they are hungry (**Figure 14–1 ●**). **Hunger** is a bothersome feeling that makes individuals think of food and encourages them to satisfy this feeling by eating. It is theorized that hunger is a response to chemical mediators in the hypothalamus that promote food-seeking behaviors. Although hunger may initiate the process of intake of various nutrients, it is the choices that individuals make that determine if nutritional intake is appropriate to meet the body's various needs or if the choices become a contributing factor to disease. Thus, food choice is a contributing factor to wellness and to illness.

Food Choice

Individuals base **food choices** on a number of factors (**Table 14–1 ●**). The factor that most directly affects food choice is taste. Although it may be an unconscious process, individuals compare the taste of a given food item to how it tasted in previous experiences with the same or similar food items. The same food prepared by one method may be appealing, but when prepared in an alternative format that is unfamiliar, it may be rejected. This is especially the case with children.

Taste can be negatively affected by the intake of certain drugs, by the aging process, and by the presence of illness. Many antibiotics alter the taste of food or lead to the sensation of nausea, resulting in the avoidance of food. Because the aging process affects the number and type of taste buds, older adults often overseason their food to compensate for these changes. Health-related diet changes directly affect choice as individuals eliminate certain foods from the diet to meet the recommendations of their healthcare provider.

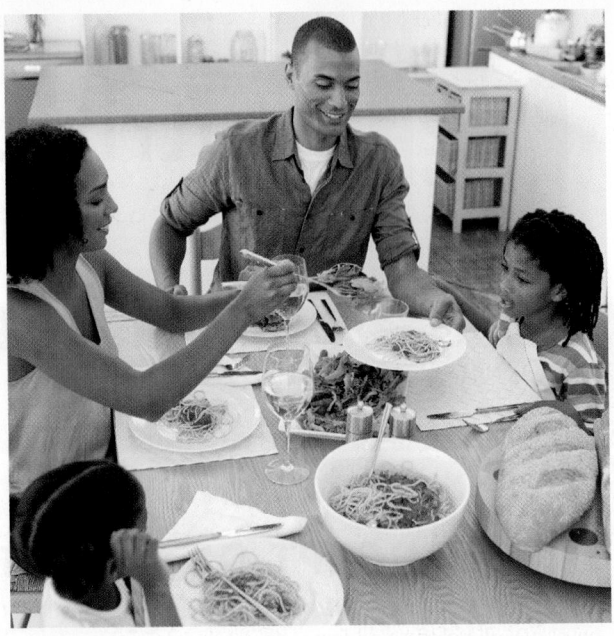

Figure 14–1 ● Individuals eat because they are hungry, but the food choices they make are contributing factors to wellness and illness.

Source: wavebreakmedia/Shutterstock.

Other factors affecting food choice include food smell, food habits, convenience, availability, and cost. Smell affects choice in both positive and negative ways. When a food smells pleasing, its aroma can initiate the hunger reflex. The opposite is also true: When food smells bad, people will avoid it. Bragulat et al. (2010) suggest that food odors are powerful appetite cues and that these cues affect a food's flavor. Food odors also may be determinants of intake and can even facilitate overeating.

Food habits also affect choice. For example, if a family never prepares or serves certain foods, the family members may avoid these foods in other settings due to unfamiliarity. Toddlers often have food habits called *food jags*. For instance, they may eat the same food item for several days in a row and refuse suggestions for alternatives.

Convenience is a factor in choice. The increase in the availability of easy-to-prepare meals, complete meals prepared as frozen foods, and take-out meals has often made such meals the first choice of busy families. Many times, however, the most convenient foods are not the healthiest foods. For some older adults the availability of food may be altered. This is especially true of those who may not have transportation. In addition, many older adults may have grown their own food and simply walked to the garden to make a food choice and now no longer have this option. Older adults often eat cereal for at least one meal a day due to its convenience. One study suggests that ready-to-eat cereal consumption may contribute to nutritional quality in the older adult population (Albertson, Wold, & Joshi, 2012).

The attractiveness of a food's packaging was the strongest predictor of food selection in a study by Van der Laan et al. (2012). These authors suggest that if healthy food were packaged in a more appealing format, it would be chosen more frequently. Cost is another significant factor in food choice. Food prices have continued to increase, and a report on the state of hunger in the world from the Food and Agriculture Organization of the

TABLE 14–1	Factors Affecting Food Choice
FACTOR	CONSIDERATIONS
Taste	Previous experiences Preparation/cooking methods Medication side effects Aging (loss of taste buds)
Smell	Pleasing aromas initiate hunger reflex Bad smells diminish interest Lack of familiarity
Habits	People eat what is familiar Toddlers get food jags
Convenience	Time Transportation Ease of preparation
Packaging	Attractive packaging influences choice Appearance of food overall
Emotion	Social experience, reinforcement Loneliness may impact food choice, intake
Body image	Choices that promote appropriate weight Food restriction to lose weight
Health benefits	Foods that meet specific health needs Foods that cause a hypersensitivity reaction or intolerance Foods that promote appropriate overall good health

United Nations (2012) suggests that it is the price of food, rather than the availability of food, that contributes to hunger in the United States and the world. The price of a healthy diet is greater than that of a less healthy diet, and a healthy diet may be unaffordable for low- and average-income families (Harrison et al., 2010). Increases in food cost have been associated with a significant loss of weight, decreased waist circumference, decreased body mass index, an increase in obesity, and insulin resistance (Lee, Ralston, & Truby, 2011).

Emotion also plays a role in food choice with foods associated with happy times or positive memories likely to be chosen first. Eating with others directly affects food choice. Children especially may select foods they normally decline at home as their food of choice when eating with others. Researchers suggest that some portion of food choice is unconscious, and that these choices are associated with the pleasure that food brings (Jacquier et al., 2012). This may explain the decrease in food intake and increase in undernutrition and unintentional weight loss often seen in older adults who experience loss of a spouse or alterations in living arrangements (**Figure 14–2** ●) (Callen, 2010; Stajkovic, Aitken, & Holroyd-Leduc, 2011). With 18% of seniors living alone and 43% reporting that they feel lonely on a regular basis, many older adults may be at risk for inadequate nutrition intake related to feelings of loneliness and depression.

Body image, amounts and types of food available, health benefits, advertising, and religious preferences also impact food choice. Body image may be a factor in limiting food intake in some populations. Body image is a significant factor in the etiology of eating disorders (Torres-McGehee et al., 2012). However, some studies suggest that overnutrition and obesity have less of a negative impact on self-esteem, the desire to lose weight, and concerns over body image in African American adolescents as compared to their Caucasian peers (Chen & Wang, 2011).

Perceived health benefits of food consumed, adequacy of dentition, and health status are additional factors that affect food choice (Hammond, Chapman, & Barr, 2010). Proximity of food is also a factor. A study by Davis and Carpenter (2009) found that the proximity of fast-food restaurants to local schools led to adolescent consumption of fast food, and this consumption had a direct effect on adolescent obesity. Fast food consumption by adolescents has increased fivefold during the past two decades. It is interesting to note that despite many fast-food restaurants now posting the calories in each meal, this effort did not have an effect on adolescent or adult food choice (Eibel, Gyamfi, & Kersh, 2011).

Portion size influences food choice. Many individuals are taught to eat what is placed before them without having a true understanding of the volume of food they consume. Americans have become accustomed to serving sizes that exceed recommended portion size and at many restaurants they can have their order "super-sized." In many instances these larger sized portions have become the norm. **Figure 14–3** ● illustrates the increases in

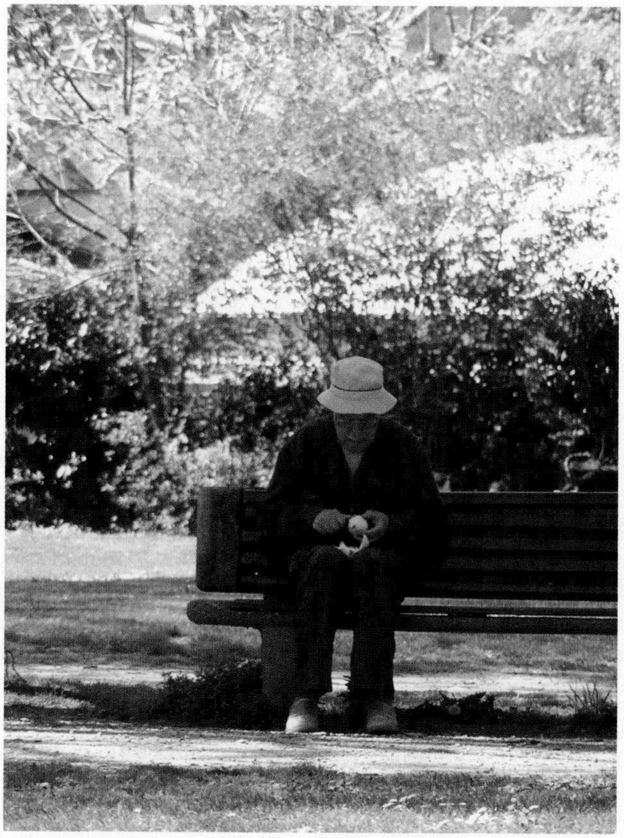

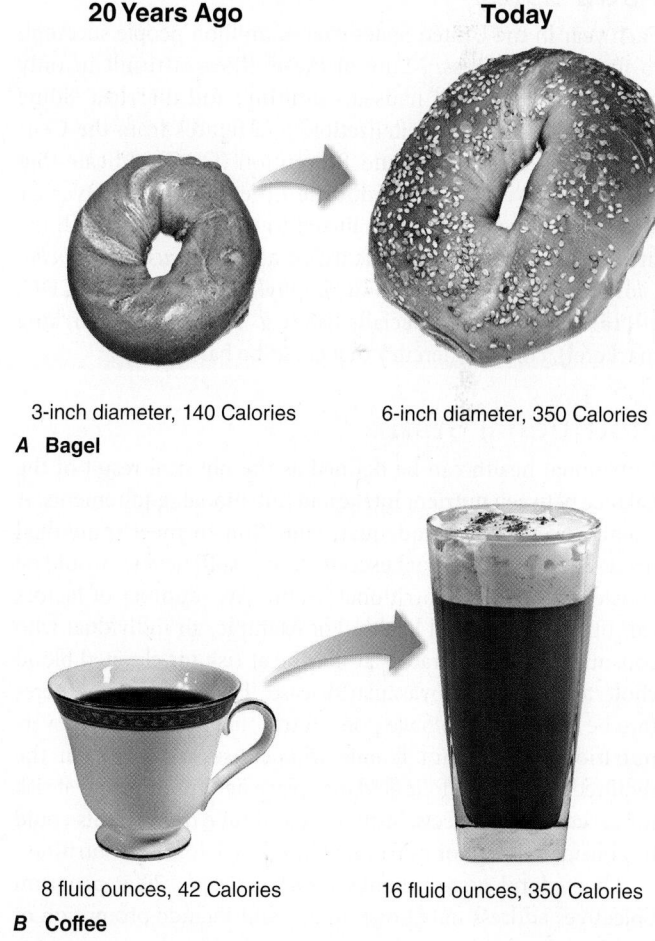

20 Years Ago   **Today**

3-inch diameter, 140 Calories   6-inch diameter, 350 Calories

A **Bagel**

8 fluid ounces, 42 Calories   16 fluid ounces, 350 Calories

B **Coffee**

Figure 14–3 ● Example of the increase in portion sizes over the past 20 years. *A,* A bagel has increased in diameter from 3 inches to 6 inches. *B,* A cup of coffee has increased from 8 fl oz to 16 fl oz and now commonly contains calorie-dense flavored syrup as well as steamed whole milk.

Figure 14–2 ● Many older adults live alone, which can lead to a decrease in food intake.
Source: Pierdelune/Shutterstock.

food portions during the past 20 years. A bagel has increased in diameter from 3 inches to 6 inches and a cup of coffee has increased from 8 fluid ounces to 16 fluid ounces and now often contains calorie-dense flavored syrup and whole milk.

The outcome of studies on the effect of portion size suggests this increase in size contributes to overnutrition and resultant obesity. Large portion sizes make children eat more than they would if serving sizes were smaller. Many organizations provide aids that assist individuals to visualize and better identify appropriate portion sizes. The American Diabetes Association (www.diabetesselfmanagement.com) offers these tips:

- A 3- to 4-ounce meat serving is equivalent to the size of your palm and the thickness of your little finger.
- One-half cup of vegetables is equivalent to the amount that would fit into two cupped hands.
- A 1-cup (8-ounce) serving of food is equivalent to the size of your fist.
- One fruit serving is equivalent to the size of your fist.
- One ounce of cheese is equivalent to the size of your thumb.
- One ounce of nuts is about one handful.

Food Safety

Each year in the United States over 48 million people succumb to foodborne illness. Many of these illnesses result in only minor discomforts of nausea, vomiting, and diarrhea. Some individuals require hospitalization, and figures from the Centers for Disease Control and Prevention (CDC) indicate that 3,000 people die from foodborne illness annually. Over 31 known pathogens have been linked to these illnesses, with the most common pathogens identified as *Norovirus, Salmonella, Clostridium perfringens,* and *Staphylococcus aureus* (CDC, 2011a). Some foods, especially fish (e.g., shark, swordfish, king mackerel), contain mercury that could be harmful.

Nutritional Status

Nutritional health can be defined as the physical result of the balance between nutrient intake and nutritional requirements. A client who consumes adequate nutrition to meet individual needs and avoids habitual excesses and insufficiencies would be considered in good nutritional health. Any number of factors can impair nutritional health. For example, an individual who consumes excess saturated fat may be at risk for elevated blood cholesterol and cardiovascular disease. This person may therefore be considered to have poor nutritional health due to overnutrition. A pregnant female who consumes less than the required amounts of folic acid may place her unborn child at risk for certain birth defects, such as neural tube defects; this could be considered in poor nutritional health due to undernutrition.

The federal government's *Healthy People 2020* program objectives address nutritional intake and include promotion of health and reduction of the risk of developing chronic diseases by encouraging Americans to consume healthful diets and to achieve and maintain healthy body weights. Emphasis is on modifying individual behavior patterns and habits, and creating policies and environments that will support these behaviors in various settings, such as schools and local community-based

organizations (U.S. Department of Health and Human Services [USDHHS], 2013a).

Healthy People 2020 goals include the following key recommendations:

- Consume a variety of nutrient-dense foods within and across the food groups, especially whole grains, fruits, vegetables, low-fat or fat-free milk or milk products, and lean meats and other protein sources.
- Limit the intake of saturated fat and trans fats, cholesterol, added sugars, sodium (salt), and alcohol.
- Limit caloric intake to meet caloric needs as identified by the USDHHS.
- The goals also include a reduction in the consumption of calories from solid fat and added sugar (SoFAS) foods in the population ages 2 years and older. A diet high in SoFAS contributes to excessive weight gain and poor health. Added sugars provide no nutritional value to foods. Excessive fat and sugar intake promotes tooth decay, obesity, type 2 diabetes, unhealthy cholesterol levels, and heart disease. Being overweight increases susceptibility for developing high blood pressure, diabetes, cardiovascular diseases, and certain types of cancer. The evidence is clear that many chronic diseases are linked to unhealthy dietary patterns. Excessive consumption of SoFAS, in combination with a failure to consume plant-based foods, may contribute to higher rates of developing chronic diseases (USDHHS, 2013a).

These statistics on nutritional health disparities and resultant goals illustrate the importance of nutritional screening and assessment as the first step toward reaching these important goals.

A growing number of clients are adopting vegetarian diet plans. For some, this choice is rooted in an increased awareness of the relationship between dietary intake and heart disease. In general, these plans are far lower in fat than plans that include meat. Some choose vegetarian or vegan diets out of a personal respect for animals and distress over the conditions in which animals raised for meat live. The **lacto-vegetarian** eats milk, cheese, and dairy foods but avoids meat, fish, poultry, and eggs. The **lacto-ovo-vegetarian** includes eggs, and the **vegan** eats only foods of plant origin. Some plans allow the inclusion of fish as well.

Vegan diet plans can lead to deficiencies in certain nutrients: calcium, omega-3 fatty acids, iron, zinc, and vitamin B_{12}. The lack of vitamin B_{12} can lead to the development of pernicious anemia. These clients should include a daily source of vitamin B_{12} in their diets, such as a fortified breakfast cereal, fortified soy beverage, or meat substitute. All vegetarians should ensure that they get adequate amounts of calcium, iron, zinc, and vitamin D through foods such as tofu, lentils, and Swiss chard. To facilitate the **absorption** (intake) of iron into the body from the alimentary canal, vitamin C should also be plentiful in the diet.

Stay Current: *The U.S. Department of Agriculture's National Agriculture Library (**www.nal.usda.gov**) publishes various resources that provide research information about vegetarian diets and staying healthy.*

Clients can experience food allergies or food intolerance. A food allergy is manifested by urticaria, angioedema, rhinoconjunctivitis, asthma, gastrointestinal disorders, and anaphylaxis (Mansoor & Sharma, 2011). An estimated 5% of children and

4% of adults have allergies to food. Milk is the most frequent allergy followed by eggs and peanuts (National Institute of Allergy and Infectious Diseases, 2011). An example of food intolerance is lactose intolerance. Lactose is a sugar found in milk and milk products. Lactose intolerance is caused by a deficiency of the enzyme lactase, which is produced by the cells lining the small intestine, and results in distressing gastrointestinal symptoms including nausea, abdominal pain, and diarrhea. Lactose intolerance is discussed in detail in the exemplar on Malabsorption Disorders in the module on Digestion.

SATIETY **Satiety** is the feeling of fullness and satisfaction that should inhibit eating until the next meal. Results of studies suggest that when protein replaced fat in meals containing the same number of calories, satiety was significantly increased. Whole grains may function in a similar manner. When considering the health risks associated with obesity and the importance of decreasing calorie intake, food choices that increase satiety may be beneficial (Giacco et al., 2011).

FOOD INSECURITY According to an economic research report for the U.S. Department of Agriculture (USDA), 85.1% of American households were food secure throughout the entire year of 2011; of the remaining numbers, 5.7% had very minimal **food security**; that is, the members of the household had just sufficient resources to access appropriate quantities and variety of food. A lack of food security, **food insecurity**, by definition, means that one or more members of a household must reduce their eating patterns due to a lack of money or lack of resources to access appropriate amounts and variety of food (Coleman-Jensen et al., 2012). These numbers are up over previous years. Black, non-Hispanic households had the highest rates of food insecurity, with approximately one out of every four households experiencing food insecurity. Adults with food insecurity report poor quality of life and conditions such as weight loss, compromised immune systems, and osteomalacia (Kregg-Byers & Schlenk, 2010).

Stay Current: To learn more about food insecurity, visit the USDA Web site at **www.ers.usda.gov/topics/food-nutrition-assistance/food-security-in-the-us.aspx**. In addition, screening tools and information about food insecurity specific to the pediatric population can be found at the No Kid Hungry Web site: **www.nokidhungry.org/?gclid=CI29yPzt67YCFdCZ4AodjggA0A**.

According to Feeding America (2011), 16.7 million children lived in food-insecure households in 2011. The percentage of children living in food-insecure households in 2011 was essentially unchanged from 2010 (22%) and remained higher than the 17% observed in 2007. These households were unable at times during the year to provide adequate, nutritious food for their children (Coleman-Jensen et al., 2012). These children often present with conditions such as underweight, wasting, growth effects, and rickets (Kregg-Byers & Schlenk, 2010). Parents often may go hungry to ensure their children have adequate food to eat. Food insecurity among children may be higher in the summer months, when children are unable to access meals at school.

Nutrients

Food contains all of the nutrients the body needs to maintain its health. **Nutrients** are substances found in food that the body needs for growth as well as for maintenance and repair. To eat a

balanced and appropriate diet, experts suggest the inclusion of foods that are nutrient dense. **Nutrient density** refers to the ratio of good nutrients to the calories a food contains (American Dietetic Association, 2011; USDA & USDHHS, 2010). The most nutrient-dense foods contain an abundance of vitamins, minerals, fiber, and other key nutrients with a decreased amount of calories. At the negative end of the nutrient density scale are foods such as candy, which is full of calories but has no essential nutrients.

The major nutrients are carbohydrates, proteins, lipids (fats), vitamins, minerals, and water. Nutrients are classified according to their work in the body. Carbohydrates, proteins, and fats supply energy and are termed **macronutrients** because the body needs them in large amounts to maintain health and well-being. Vitamins and minerals are considered **micronutrients** because they are needed in smaller amounts. This does not mean, however, that their role in the body is less important. Water is an **essential nutrient** needed for body survival. Adequate water intake contributes to fluid balance. It also plays an important role in nerve and muscle functioning and in the transport of nutrients to all body systems. Nutrient use by the body is presented in **Figure 14–4 ●**.

The USDA publishes the *Dietary Guidelines for Americans* every 3–5 years. They include recommended intake for sodium, moderation of alcohol use, safety in preparing meals, and age-specific nutrition needs.

Stay Current: The USDA's dietary guidelines for 2015 are in process. Visit **www.health.gov/dietaryguidelines/2015.asp** for the latest information on the 2015 guidelines.

Many organizations provide information regarding suggested nutrient intake and supporting a healthy diet. **Dietary reference intakes (DRIs)** provide a standard for identifying needed amounts of each nutrient.

Stay Current: For a review of the DRI guidelines and as a basis for a client teaching, visit **www.iom.edu/Activities/Nutrition/SummaryDRIs/~/media/Files/Activity%20Files/Nutrition/DRIs/5_Summary%20Table%20Tables%201-4.pdf**.

Another guide to nutrient intake is the USDA's **MyPlate** plan, which outlines suggested food intake by food groups (e.g., bread and meat daily). The ChooseMyPlate Web site provides valuable information to individuals and families regarding the five food groups that help build a healthy diet. The MyPlate plan illustrates the five food groups (fruits, vegetables, grains, protein, and dairy foods) that are the building blocks for a healthy diet using a place setting for a meal (**Figure 14–5 ●**). The individual is invited to think about what goes on the plate or in the cup or bowl. Nurses can also access these sites and receive information to assist in client teaching for food intake to maintain health.

Stay Current: Visit **www.choosemyplate.gov** for the latest information from the USDA.

CARBOHYDRATES **Carbohydrates** are organic components of food that supply energy in the form of calories to the body. The primary sources of carbohydrates are plant foods. These foods contain sugars and starches. The simple sugars, called monosaccharides, are glucose, fructose, and galactose,

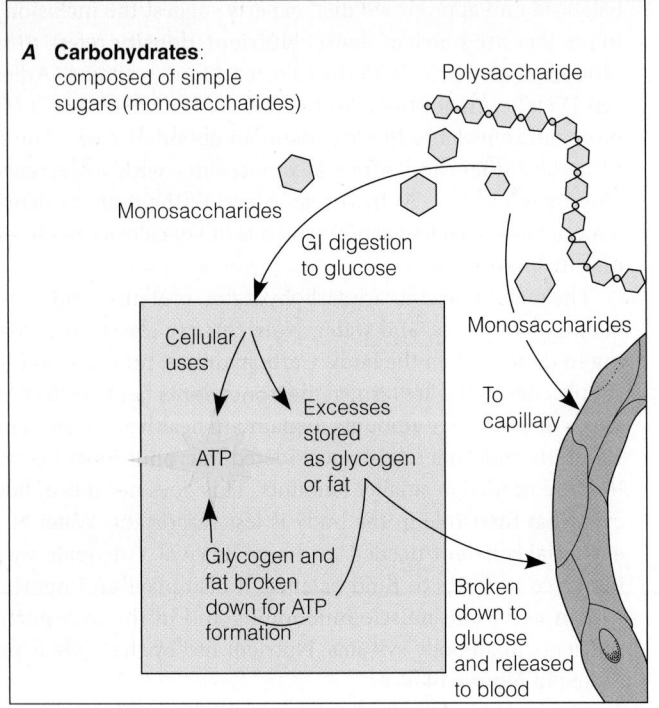

A **Carbohydrates**:
composed of simple
sugars (monosaccharides)

Polysaccharide

Monosaccharides

GI digestion
to glucose

Monosaccharides

To
capillary

Cellular
uses

ATP

Excesses
stored
as glycogen
or fat

Glycogen and
fat broken
down for ATP
formation

Broken
down to
glucose
and released
to blood

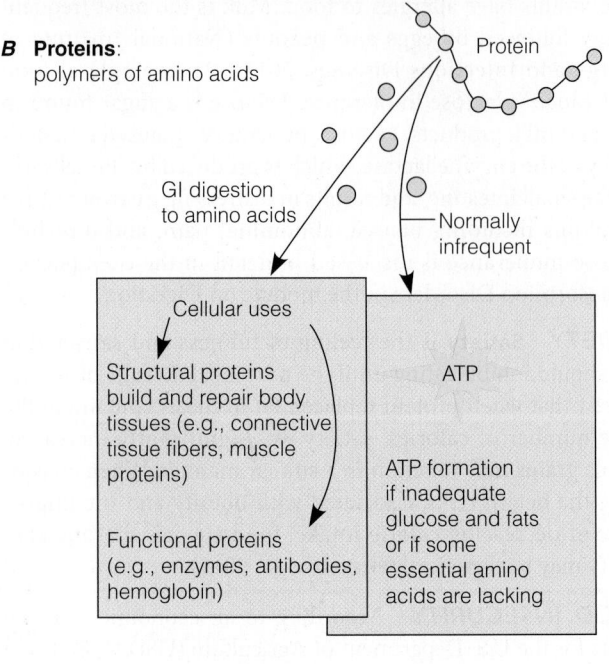

B **Proteins**:
polymers of amino acids

Protein

GI digestion
to amino acids

Normally
infrequent

Cellular uses

Structural proteins
build and repair body
tissues (e.g., connective
tissue fibers, muscle
proteins)

Functional proteins
(e.g., enzymes, antibodies,
hemoglobin)

ATP

ATP formation
if inadequate
glucose and fats
or if some
essential amino
acids are lacking

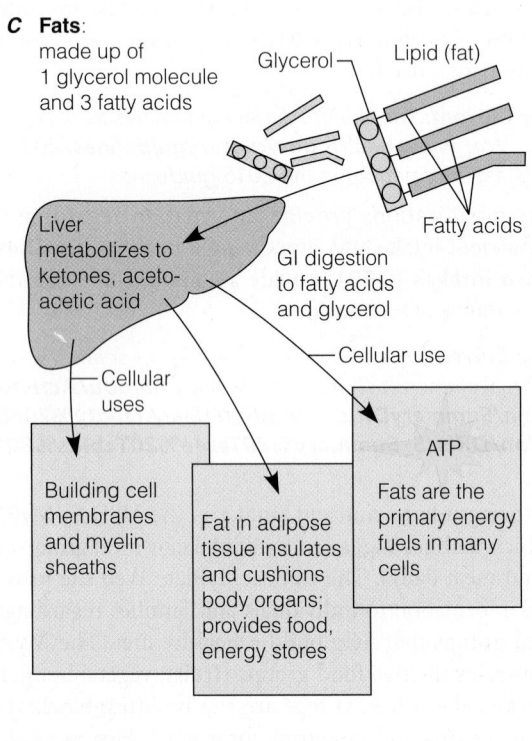

C **Fats**:
made up of
1 glycerol molecule
and 3 fatty acids

Glycerol

Lipid (fat)

Fatty acids

Liver
metabolizes to
ketones, aceto-
acetic acid

GI digestion
to fatty acids
and glycerol

Cellular use

Cellular
uses

ATP

Building cell
membranes
and myelin
sheaths

Fat in adipose
tissue insulates
and cushions
body organs;
provides food,
energy stores

Fats are the
primary energy
fuels in many
cells

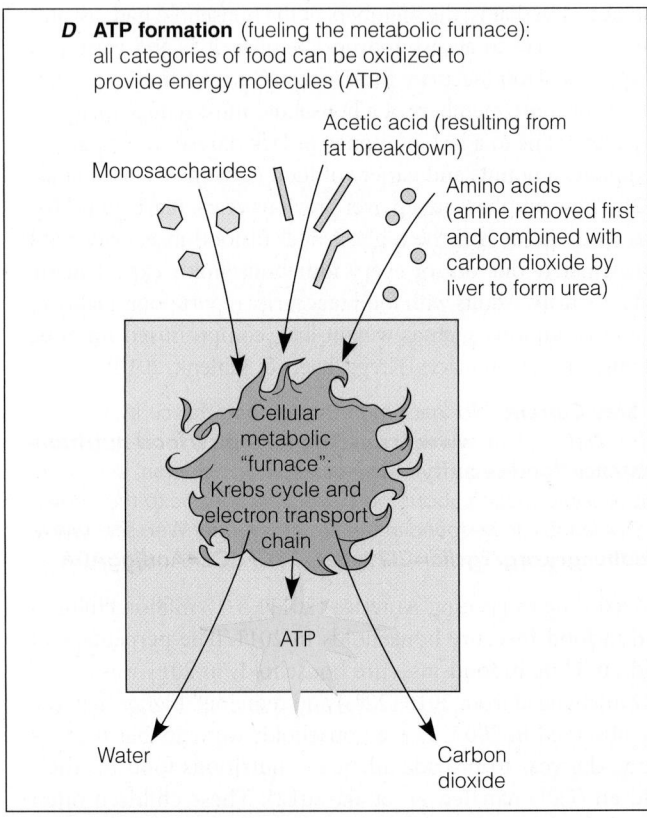

D **ATP formation** (fueling the metabolic furnace):
all categories of food can be oxidized to
provide energy molecules (ATP)

Acetic acid (resulting from
fat breakdown)

Monosaccharides

Amino acids
(amine removed first
and combined with
carbon dioxide by
liver to form urea)

Cellular
metabolic
"furnace":
Krebs cycle and
electron transport
chain

ATP

Water

Carbon
dioxide

Figure 14–4 ● A schematic overview of nutrient use by body cells: *A,* carbohydrates; *B,* proteins; *C,* fats; and *D,* ATP formation.

which are quickly absorbed from the bloodstream. The disaccharides are sucrose, lactose, and maltose. These two saccharides are found in milk, sugar cane, sugar beets, honey, and fruits. The polysaccharides are complex carbohydrates and are found in grains, legumes, and root vegetables. The polysaccharides break down more slowly than monosaccharides and disaccharides, and they supply energy for longer periods of time.

Lastly, dietary **fiber** is a polysaccharide carbohydrate and contributes to disease prevention, especially in the gastrointestinal tract and the cardiovascular system.

Once ingested and metabolized, carbohydrates are converted primarily to glucose. All sugars must be converted to glucose because glucose is the only molecule body cells can use to make adenosine triphosphate (ATP), which transports energy in cells.

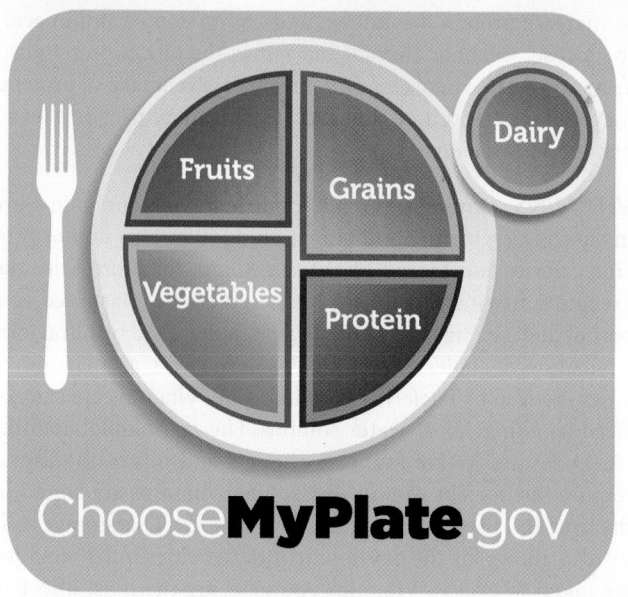

Figure 14–5 ● The MyPlate schematic from the USDA.

Kilocalorie (also *Kcalorie*; abbreviation: *kcal*) is a term that identifies the energy-producing ability of nutrients. Kilocalories are calculated according to the amount of heat required to raise the temperature of 1 kilogram of water by 1 degree at 1 atmosphere of pressure. Carbohydrates supply 4 kcal per gram. The minimum necessary daily carbohydrate intake is unknown, but the recommended daily intake is 125–175 g, most of which should be comprised of complex carbohydrates.

Because carbohydrates are not stored on a significant basis, individuals must eat carbohydrates throughout the day. When eaten in excess, the body converts the excess glucose to glycogen or fat. Glycogen is stored in the liver and muscles; fat is stored as adipose tissue. Excess intake of carbohydrates over time can result in obesity, dental caries, and elevated plasma triglycerides. Over extended periods of time, carbohydrate deficiencies lead to tissue wasting from protein breakdown and metabolic acidosis from an excess of ketones as a by-product of fat breakdown.

Both the Institute of Medicine and the USDA's *Dietary Guidelines for Americans* suggest the carbohydrates should come from the consumption of foods high in fiber and low in added sugars. At least half of the grains consumed should be whole grains, and fruits and vegetables should complete the carbohydrate intake.

LIPIDS   **Lipids**, also known as fats, are substances that dissolve in alcohol but not in water. They contain carbon, hydrogen and oxygen. They serve as a secondary source of fuel for the body. Lipids are divided into three categories: triglycerides, phospholipids, and sterols. Most individuals use the term *fats* instead of *lipids*. Fats provide most of the energy for the body's work, supplying 9 kcal per gram of food eaten, twice that of the carbohydrates. Fat is also the storage form of excess energy intake from food eaten.

In addition to supplying energy, fat is useful in body protection. Fat surrounds vital organs, protects portions of our bony skeleton from shock, and aids in insulation and temperature management. Fat also aids in the absorption of the fat-soluble vitamins and assists in the feeling of fullness (satiety) after a meal.

The triglycerides are the most abundant fats, accounting for approximately 90%–95% of fats consumed. They are composed of fatty acids that are classified based on their length. They are further defined according to the level of saturation and whether they are essential or nonessential. **Saturated fats** contain all the material they are capable of holding (i.e., they hold all the hydrogen ions they can). If fats do not contain all of the material they are capable of holding and, thus, have a place where hydrogen ions are missing, they are **unsaturated fats**. If only one set place is missing, the fat is termed *monounsaturated*. If two or more are missing, the fat is termed *polyunsaturated*. Research suggests that unsaturated fats are more heart healthy and that consumption of some unsaturated fats such as olive oil can even be heart protective.

Some fat is essential for the digestion, absorption, and transportation of the fat-soluble vitamins (vitamins A, D, E, and K). In this sense, *essential* means the body cannot make the nutrient, so it must be taken into the body as food. Fat also contains the essential fatty acids, linoleic and linolenic acid. The primary role of these two acids in the body is the formation of prostaglandins. Prostaglandins are responsible for muscle activity, blood vessel response, blood clotting, and the immune system response of inflammation. Other functions of fats in the body include:

- Storage form for energy
- Padding
- Insulation
- Cell membrane integrity.

Two other groups of fats also play a vital role in body performance. These are phospholipids and sterols. The phospholipid lecithin plays a role in fat transport. Sterols, such as cholesterol, provide the bile necessary for digestion. Excessive cholesterol intake also plays a significant role in heart disease as discussed in the module on Perfusion.

PROTEINS   **Proteins** are naturally occurring substances that consist of amino acids. Proteins are essential components of all living organisms. They are the last of the macronutrients. Proteins vary from the other macronutrients in that they also contain nitrogen, which fats and carbohydrates do not. In addition to playing a significant role in muscle function, proteins are also a critical component of all tissues of the human body, including our bones and blood. Proteins can also serve as an energy source, supplying 4 kcal per gram. Proteins are classified as essential or not essential and as either complete or incomplete. As with the fatty acids, essential amino acids are those that the body cannot supply, so they must be eaten.

Complete proteins contain all nine of the essential amino acids and are found in animal products such as meat, poultry, fish, milk, eggs, and cheese. Incomplete proteins do not contain all essential amino acids in the quantities necessary to support growth and development. Incomplete proteins are found in legumes, nuts, grains, cereals, and vegetables. Incomplete proteins can be combined in the diet or augmented by complementary food items to equal a complete protein. For example, rice contains small amounts of specific essential amino acids; however, these same essential amino acids are found in greater amounts in dry beans. Similarly, dry beans contain smaller amounts of certain essential amino acids that can be found in larger amounts in rice. Together, these two foods can provide all of the essential amino acids the body needs. For many years it was thought that these foods needed to be consumed at the same time, but new research suggests they only need to be consumed within the same day (CDC, 2011b).

Proteins perform many essential functions in the body. They continuously build new tissues including muscles and red blood cells, they function as enzymes and antibodies, and they respond to injury to help prevent blood loss by clotting of the blood. In addition they form hormones and help maintain fluid and electrolyte and acid–base balance.

The recommended daily intake of protein is 56 g for men and 45 g for women. Healthy people with adequate caloric intake have an equal rate of protein synthesis and protein breakdown and loss, reflected as nitrogen balance. If the breakdown and loss of proteins exceed intake, a negative nitrogen balance results, which can lead to metabolic complications. Excessive breakdown or loss may occur with burns, major illnesses, or altered emotional states. Protein deficits are manifested by weight loss, tissue wasting, edema, and anemia. Edema occurs as a cell membrane loses it integrity. Anemia occurs due to the inability to reproduce cells. When protein deficiency is severe, two disease states most commonly manifested in children can develop: marasmus and kwashiorkor. **Box 14–1** ● compares these two disorders.

When protein intake exceeds breakdown, a positive nitrogen balance occurs. This is normal during growth, tissue repair, and pregnancy. Abnormal rates of protein use may result during times of stress, when the body releases adrenal corticosteroids to increase protein breakdown and conversion of amino acids to glucose. Anabolic steroids may affect the rate of protein use, as may excessive intake of proteins. Excessive intake of proteins may lead to obesity and can have a significant impact on a number of body systems.

VITAMINS   **Vitamins** are micronutrient compounds that are involved in regulating body functioning. Vitamins do not provide calories and cannot be manufactured; therefore, with the exception of vitamins D and K, they must be consumed as a part of dietary intake. Vitamin D is manufactured by ultraviolet irradiation of cholesterol molecules in the skin, and vitamin K is synthesized by bacteria in the intestine. Vitamins are categorized as either fat or water soluble. The fat-soluble vitamins (A, D, E, and K) are found in the fats and oils of foods and require bile for absorption. Fat-soluble vitamins are stored in the liver and tissues until needed by the body. This storage ability also allows for the development of toxicities if the vitamins are taken in excess. Vitamins A and D are the most affected. Any interruption in fat absorption can directly affect levels of fat-soluble vitamins.

Vitamin A is essential for function of the eye. Vitamin D plays a role in calcium absorption and transport. Vitamin E is an antioxidant and reduces formation of dangerous radicals that would adversely affect body tissues and functioning. Vitamin K is a functioning part of the coagulation cascade.

The water-soluble vitamins, B complex and C, are absorbed with water in the GI tract. However, vitamin B_{12} must become attached to intrinsic factor to be absorbed. Unlike the fat-soluble vitamins, water-soluble vitamins consumed in excess of body requirements are excreted in the urine. Each of the B vitamins plays a role in cellular functioning throughout the body. Vitamin C plays a significant role in tissue healing

Stay Current: *The most current information for the source, function, and minimum daily recommended intake levels for all of the vitamins is provided at* **http://ods.od.nih.gov/factsheets/list-VitaminsMinerals**.

A number of new studies have suggested that the recommendations for vitamin D may be insufficient, especially for individuals who do not get adequate sunlight, infants who are breastfed, and older adults. **Table 14–2** ● outlines new recommendations.

MINERALS   In the body **minerals** are salts dissolved in water and in this state they carry an electrical charge and are referred to as electrolytes. Minerals work with other nutrients to maintain fluid balance with a proper amount of fluid and electrolytes in each body compartment. The role of minerals in maintaining fluid and electrolyte balance is reviewed in detail in the module on Fluids and Electrolytes. In addition, minerals play a role in acid–base balance, which is further discussed in the module on Acid–Base Balance.

The most abundant mineral in the body is calcium. The majority of calcium exists in the bones and teeth. A very small amount of calcium exists in the blood where it helps regulate metabolic functions. On a constant basis calcium moves into and out of the bone as the body's demand for calcium dictates. Many older adults do not consume adequate amounts of calcium (Garriguel, 2011). Phosphorus plays a role in energy production

Box 14–1   Comparison of Marasmus and Kwashiorkor

MARASMUS	KWASHIORKOR
■ Wasting and weakening of muscles, including the heart ■ Delayed brain development, learning impairment ■ Depressed metabolism and loss of insulation from body fat, leading to significantly low body temperature ■ Delayed physical growth and development ■ Deterioration of the intestinal lining, inhibiting absorption of nutrients ■ Anemia ■ Weakened immune system ■ Fluid and electrolyte imbalances	■ Some weight loss and muscle wasting, with some retention of body fat ■ Retarded growth and development but less severe than that seen with marasmus ■ Edema, leading to ascites ■ Fatty degeneration of the liver ■ Anorexia ■ Emotional lability ■ Sores and skin eruptions, pigmentation changes ■ Dry, brittle hair that changes color, straightens; alopecia

Sources: Based on Ramirez Prada, D., Delgado, G., Hidalgo Patino, C. A., Perez-Navero, J., & Gil Campos, M. (2011). Using of WHO guidelines for the management of severe malnutrition to cases of marasmus and kwashiorkor in a Colombia children's hospital. *Nutricion Hospitalaria, 26*(5), 977–983; Scrimshaw, N. S., & Viteri, F. E. (2010). INCAP studies of kwashiorkor and marasmus. *Food and Nutrition Reviews, 11*(1), 34–41; UNICEF. (2013). *Clinical forms of acute malnutrition: Marasmus and kwashiorkor.* Retrieved from http://www.unicef.org/nutrition/training/2.3/12.html; and National Center for Biotechnology Information. (2012). Kwashiorkor. *Pub Med Health.* Retrieved from http://www.ncbi.nlm.nih.gov/pubmedhealth/PMH0002571.

TABLE 14–2   Recommended Dietary Allowances (RDAs) for Vitamin D

AGE	MALE (INTERNATIONAL UNITS)	FEMALE (INTERNATIONAL UNITS)	PREGNANCY (INTERNATIONAL UNITS)	LACTATION (INTERNATIONAL UNITS)
0–12 months*	400 (10 mcg)	400 (10 mcg)		
1–13 years	600 (15 mcg)	600 (15 mcg)		
14–18 years	600 (15 mcg)	600 (15 mcg)	600 (15 mcg)	600 (15 mcg)
19–50 years	600 (15 mcg)	600 (15 mcg)	600 (15 mcg)	600 (15 mcg)
51–70 years	600 (15 mcg)	600 (15 mcg)		
>70 years	800 (20 mcg)	800 (20 mcg)		

*Adequate intake (AI).

Source: Office of Dietary Supplements. (2011). *Vitamin D.* Retrieved from http://ods.od.nih.gov/factsheets/VitaminD-HealthProfessional.

and participates in the buffer system. Magnesium also plays a role in energy production and neuromuscular transmission and activity. Iron plays a role in red cell formation, and deficiency is most often manifested as iron deficiency anemia. Zinc is essential to normal central nervous system function. Fluoride is beneficial for tooth enamel, but is not considered an essential mineral. Iodine deficiency is seldom seen in the United States; it is mentioned here for its need in the synthesis of thyroid hormone, and in some parts of the world, its deficiency is noteworthy and is seen in the development of goiter leading to thyroid gland dysfunction.

Stay Current: *Information about the role of each mineral in the body and recommended intake can be found at* **http://ods.od.nih.gov/factsheets/list-VitaminsMinerals.**

WATER **Water** comprises about 60% of an adult's body weight and about 75% of an infant's body weight. Obesity decreases the percentage of body weight from water. Estimates are that adults should drink at least 64 ounces of water per day and with added exercise, even more.

Water provides the following functions in the body:

- Transports nutrient and wastes.
- Regulates metabolic processes.
- Serves as a solvent for vitamins, minerals, glucose, and amino acids.
- Acts as a lubricant.
- Acts as a cushion.
- Regulates body temperature.
- Maintains blood volume.
- Assists in maintaining a healthy weight.

Water is considered an essential nutrient. Without water an individual can live only a few days. When adequate water is not provided, the body will pull water from other sources leading to increased blood viscosity, retention of toxicities and waste, and an increased risk for health interruption (Popkin, D'Anci, & Rosenberg, 2010).

Digestion and Metabolism

THE DIGESTIVE PROCESS   The digestive process begins in the mouth. Food is mechanically broken down by the teeth, and the salivary enzymes begin the chemical processes of digestion. The food bolus then moves down the esophagus where no diges-

tion takes place. The bolus moves through various **sphincters** (circular bands of muscle) that keep the bolus moving in one direction. The bolus then empties into the stomach where food is stored and digestive enzymes further aid digestion and prepare the food to move into the small intestine. Minimal absorption occurs in the stomach, but the food bolus is further broken down by the chemical action of digestive enzymes. **Table 14–3** outlines the role of the various enzymes on nutrient digestion.

The bolus then changes its name to **chyme**, a mass comprised of the food bolus, water, and digestive enzymes. It takes approximately 4 hours for the chyme to leave the stomach and enter the small intestine. The cells in the small intestine are individual and recognize the various nutrients needed for absorption. The cells are selective and they can recognize and absorb all of the nutrients needed by the body. They are transported to cells either via the lymph system or small capillaries. Depending on their type, nutrients are absorbed all along the tract with some, such as carbohydrates, absorbed quickly and others, such as fats and proteins, absorbed farther down the tract. The colon has the same

TABLE 14–3   Selected Digestive Enzymes and Their Actions

SITE OF PRODUCTION	ENZYME	PRIMARY ACTION
Mouth	Salivary amylase	Digests carbohydrates in the mouth.
Stomach	Gastric lipase	Digests lipids in the stomach.
	Pepsin	Digests proteins in the stomach.
Pancreas	Pancreatic amylase	Digests carbohydrates in the small intestine.
	Pancreatic lipase	Digests lipids in the small intestine.
	Proteases	Digests proteins in the small intestine.
Small intestine	Lactase	Digests lactose in the small intestine.
	Lipase	Digests lipids in the small intestine.
	Maltase	Digests maltose in the small intestine.
	Sucrase	Digests sucrose in the small intestine.
	Various peptidases	Digest proteins in the small intestine.

type of action and is primarily responsible for the absorption of fluid.

✳ *For more information on digestion, see the module on Digestion and the Physiology Review of Digestion minimodule at* **nursing.pearsonhighered.com**.

METABOLISM Metabolism is the chemical process that enables the body to use the energy extracted from ingested food. The type of metabolism that occurs is related to the type of cells undergoing metabolism. The liver is the organ primarily responsible for metabolic processes. Following digestion the liver begins the metabolic processing of the various macronutrients. For carbohydrates, the liver converts complex sugars to glucose. It converts glucose to energy and it converts glucose to fatty acids. For proteins, the liver removes ammonia from the blood and converts it to urea. It also makes plasma proteins such as the components of the coagulation cascade. For lipids, the liver manufactures bile and sends it to the gallbladder to aid in digestion. It also breaks down fatty acids for energy when needed. The liver also detoxifies alcohol and is responsible for the metabolism of all oral drugs.

Genetic and Lifespan Considerations

Genetic factors play a role in nutritional status and nutrient intake, not only in health and disease, but also in the food we consume. Genetically engineered crops such as soybeans, maize, canola, rice, and potatoes are already available. Researchers suggest that just as we study the effect of genetics on factors such as lipids in heart disease, gastrointestinal disorders, and obesity, the effect of engineered food on humans should also be reviewed (Magaña-Gómez & Calderón de la Barca, 2009).

As mentioned previously, genetics plays a role in the nutritionally related disorders of lactose intolerance and hypercholesteremia. Additional information relative to these disorders can be found in the exemplar on Malabsorption Disorders in the module on Digestion and in the exemplar on Coronary Artery Disease in the module on Perfusion.

Studies are being conducted to identify the relationship among genetic variation, nutrient metabolism, and energy balance and the relationship of these to disease states such as heart disease (Kalupahana & Moustaid-Moussa, 2011). The use of the systems genetics was suggested as the researchers reviewed nutrient–gene interactions and their effect on diet intervention in disease states. The researchers hope data gained from these studies will explain why some clients respond to dietary intervention and others do not.

NUTRITION FOR INFANTS AND CHILDREN Infants and children have unique nutritional requirements due to the rapid physical and functional changes associated with growth and development. In their first year of life, children triple their birth weight. During this time period infants must learn to eat solid foods, to feed themselves, and to make transitions to eating new foods. Adequate nutrient intake is essential for bone formation, teeth development, and the additional increase in metabolism that marks the years of rapid growth.

Nurses should encourage breastfeeding for all infants. The American Academy of Pediatrics (AAP) (2012) recommends exclusive breastfeeding for the first 6 months, followed by continued breastfeeding as foods are introduced for the first full year of life. Not only does breastfeeding provide positive nutritional balance, but it also provides promotion of gastrointestinal functioning, enhancement of immune function, and psychological benefits (**Figure 14–6** ●) (Ball, Bindler, & Cowen, 2012). Exclusive breastfeeding reduced the incidence of otitis media by 50% and any breastfeeding reduced the incidence of gastrointestinal disorders by 64%. Breastfeeding was also associated with a reduction in the incidence of sudden infant death syndrome (AAP, 2012). For premature infants breastfeeding may be even more important (Ahmed, 2010). Support programs for breastfeeding mothers are available from the AAP and other organizations. For mothers who are unable to breastfeed, several ready-to-feed formulas are available that are nutritionally adequate to meet the needs of babies throughout the first year.

🌐 **Stay Current:** *The KidsHealth Web site at* **http://kidshealth. org/parent/centers/fitness_nutrition_center.html** *provides updated information on nutrition in children, as well as interactive games to teach nutrition to children and parents.*

NUTRITION FOR ADOLESCENTS Adolescence is a time of rapid growth physically, emotionally, and socially. Nutritional needs increase, especially for protein, calcium, iron, and

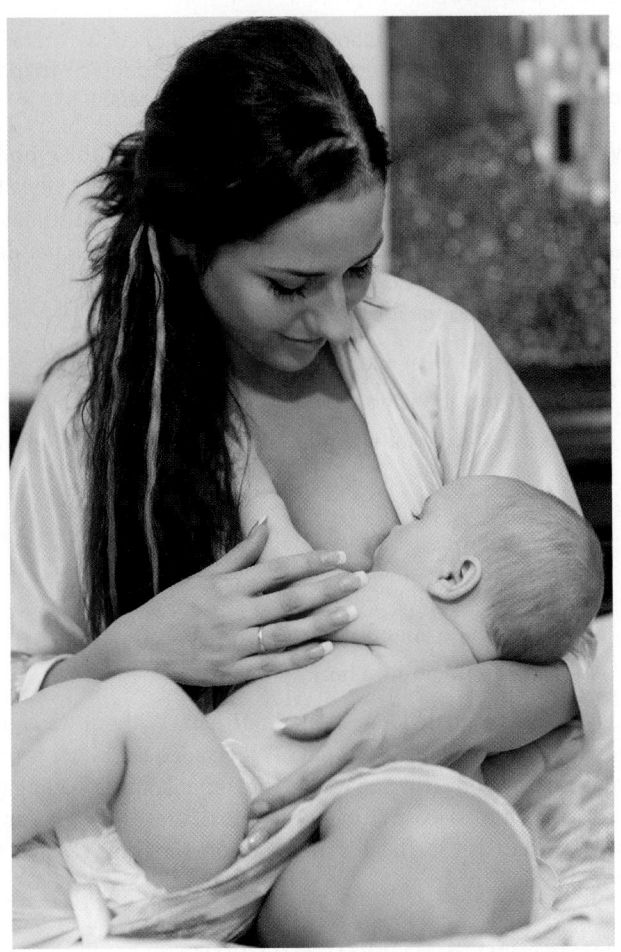

Figure 14–6 ● Breastfeeding provides positive nutritional balance, promotes gastrointestinal functioning, enhances immune function, and provides psychological benefits.
Source: Dmitry Melnikov/Shutterstock.

overall caloric intake. Calcium intake is especially important, with one estimate suggesting that 26% of adult calcium deposition is established in early adolescence with peak rates of calcium deposition occurring at 12.5 years for females and 14.0 years for males (Donaldson & Gordon, 2013). With inappropriate intake, precursors to osteoporosis may appear during adolescence.

Bone health in adulthood depends on bone density acquired during adolescence. The identification of risk factors associated with poor bone health early in adolescence and the provision of nutrition education, exercise, and lifestyle counseling can help teenagers maximize bone mass before their skeletal growth is completed, thus improving bone health into adulthood and beyond (Donaldson & Gordon, 2013).

Adolescents experience periods of "growth spurts" during which their nutritional and caloric needs increase significantly. Females experience a change in fat disposition and males experience an increase in muscle mass and lean body tissue. Females may have reached close to their adult height prior to adolescence and males may experience significant skeletal growth (Thompson, Manore, & Vaughan, 2013). Appropriate food choices are essential for proper growth.

Struggles about adolescents' food choices and food intake occur frequently throughout all households in all parts of the world. Adolescence is a time of identity formation, and adolescents align with peers in regard to food selection. Adolescents pay as little attention to calorie and nutrient information as their adult counterparts, which at times, is significantly lacking. One factor that continues to provide a strong impact on food choice is parental food choices (Williams & Mummery, 2012). At times this factor is negative, with adolescents moving away from family traditions; at other times, it is positive with food choices being made based on a food's familiarity and comfort. Studies on food consumption suggest caloric information or nutrient content is not a major consideration in choice among adolescents (Williams & Mummery, 2012). As is common with older adults, taste, hunger, and appearance impact the food choices of adolescents. Ease of preparation (microwavable) and location were identified as the most important factor—even more so than food prices—in one study (Back, 2011).

Females experience social pressure, both during adolescence and young adulthood, to be thin, significantly limiting dietary intake. Extreme dieting is particularly dangerous in the adolescent years because poor intake affects calcium and other nutrient levels and also causes a loss of estrogen. Eating disorders lead to complications such as cardiac dysthymias, electrolyte imbalances, and even death. The reverse is often seen in the male population as males are pressured to gain muscle mass. This too puts pressure on the bones (Haines et al., 2011).

Throughout the globe, overnutrition and obesity are a concern in the adolescent population (Musaiger et al., 2012; Nguyen et al., 2013; Remesh, 2012; et al., 2012). Obesity has been associated with depression (Merikangas et al., 2012), hypertension (Sarry El-Din et al., 2012), and type 2 diabetes (Sweat et al., 2012). Contributing factors include a sedentary lifestyle, fast-food and empty-calorie eating, and an overconsumption of sugar-laden drinks (Elbel, Gyamfi, & Kersh, 2011; Peters et al., 2011). Overweight and obesity can have a negative impact on self-esteem. Chen and Wang (2011) report that the incidence of obesity is greater in the African American population, but the impact of obesity on self-esteem is less in the African American population compared to Caucasians.

One of the objectives of the *Healthy People 2020* program is to increase the proportion of schools that offer nutritious foods and beverages outside of school meals (USDHHS, 2013a). Interventions aimed at improving the nutritional status of adolescents should begin in the school systems and include healthier food choice options, healthy eating campaigns, increased activity opportunities during and after school, and the inclusion of nutrition education (Kong et al., 2012). Interventions for obesity include such programs as the Banishing Obesity and Diabetes in Youth (BODY) project for students who have been identified as being at risk for overweight and obesity. At-risk students were identified through anthropometric measurements and blood studies (cholesterol and blood sugar) assessed during required gym classes. Students identified as overweight or obese were asked to participate (with parental permission) in a study. Participants were encouraged to exercise and maintain appropriate intake to promote weight loss and promote reduction of identified risks. Participants were given a personalized report detailing their results along with specific recommendations on how to improve their health. The researchers suggest the study is easily replicable and had great success. Other schools are following similar community-based obesity intervention programs within high schools (Mobley et al., 2012). Magee, Everts, and Jamison (2012) note that obesity prevention and management can be an important part of the practice of advanced practice nurses because their role enables them to take the time necessary to collaborate with clients and their families. Family functioning is an important factor in the success of nutrition programs (Van Ryzin & Nowicka, 2013).

Another *Healthy People 2020* goal is to reduce the proportion of children and adolescents who are considered obese (USDHHS, 2013a). Extreme obesity (i.e., BMI >99th percentile) has reached 4% in the United States. Obesity in childhood and adolescence promotes risk factors in adulthood. Weight loss treatment strategies, although effective, achieve only modest losses. In cases where obesity is significantly life threatening (BMI >60 kg/m^2), in-hospital weight loss regimens are recommended prior to surgical intervention (Koeck et al., 2013). Adolescents who are severely obese demonstrated anxiety, depression, anger, disruptive behavior, and poor-self-concept. Psychological counseling before and following a surgical procedure is essential for the adolescent who must deal with ongoing changes in body image (Jarvholm et al., 2012). Although not always considered first-line treatment, bariatric surgery must remain an option for those adolescents who are significantly overweight and is often an underused intervention (Oyetunji et al., 2012).

NUTRITION FOR ADULTS The *Dietary Guidelines for Americans 2010* reports that 34% of Americans were classified as obese in 2008 (USDA & USDHHS, 2010). Food choices directly affect weight, with the greatest impact occurring due to the number of calories consumed. Adult men require more calories than women with the suggested healthy range for men at 2,400 to 3,000 calories per day, depending on age and activity level. Women typically need 1,600 to 2,400 calories per day, also depending on activity with greater calories needed with increased activity. Calorie needs generally decrease as a result of a decrease in the metabolic rate that occurs around the age of 50. For females of childbearing age, the USDA dietary guidelines suggest that women should consume foods that supply heme iron and add vitamin C–rich food to facilitate iron absorption. Women should also add 400 mcg per day of synthetic folic acid from fortified foods supplements.

Food choice in the adult population is similar to that of the older adult counterparts. Socioeconomic status, knowledge of nutrients, and beliefs and perceptions about nutrition as it relates to health and accessibility all have an effect on adult food choice (Beydoun & Wang, 2008). Health-related knowledge has a positive effect on healthy food purchasing. Individuals with low socioeconomic status purchased fewer fruits and vegetables, less milk, and fewer meat products, and adults with higher socioeconomic status had healthier eating indices (Wang & Chen, 2011).

NUTRITION FOR OLDER ADULTS   The older adult experiences unique nutritional requirements due to the physical and functional changes that occur with aging. Although many older adults experience a decline in physical activity level and have lower calorie needs, there is not a concurrent need for a decreased intake of most vitamins and minerals. In fact, the dietary requirement for some nutrients increases with age. For example, the daily recommended intake for the general adult population and the older adult population is the same with the exception of vitamin D, calcium, vitamin B_{12}, and vitamin B_6, all of which require increases. Obtaining a well-balanced diet while consuming fewer calories overall can present a challenge to many older adults.

A variety of factors place the nutritional well-being of older adults at risk. Physiological changes can affect food choices and consumption and place the older adult at risk for undernutrition. These changes include the following:

- Xerostomia (decreased salivation due to decreased function of salivary glands) decreases the taste of food, impairs chewing, and leads to avoidance of certain foods (Quandt et al., 2011; Wilkie, 2012).

- Loss of teeth, dental caries, and ill-fitting dentures lead to decreased protein and fruit and vegetable intake due to chewing difficulties.

- Thirst dysregulation, in which an older adult may not realize he is thirsty, results in failure to consume adequate water throughout the day. This can contribute to the additional problem of constipation. Lack of thirst recognition is a specific problem among older adults with dementia, and caregivers much be cognizant of the need to offer liquids repeatedly throughout the day (Quandt et al., 2011).

- A decreased number of taste buds leads to decreased interest in foods, lack of desire to eat, and decreased intake leading to appetite dysregulation. Some sources would classify this decreased intake as "anorexia of the elderly" (Donini et al., 2013). The loss of taste buds also results in increased use of additional amounts of spices such as salt, which may impact overall health, especially in the older adult with hypertension.

- Cognitive impairment with dementia leads to decreased nutrient and overall food intake. Individuals with dementia are unable to feed themselves; they may hold food in the mouth, refuse to open the mouth, and turn the head away in a direct refusal to eat. In addition the client with dementia may refuse to sit and wanders continuously.

- Constipation is a frequent complaint in the older adult population. Its etiology includes decreased fluid intake; lack of exercise; normal, age-related decreases in peristalsis; decreased fiber intake (related to lack of or ill-fitting dentition); decreased metabolism; and the misconception that a bowel movement needs to occur daily. Medications may also contribute to constipation in this population (Gallegos-Orozco et al., 2012).

- Polypharmacy is the use of different medications by an individual who has one or more health alterations (Heuberger & Caudell, 2011). Just one medication can affect food taste, promote nausea and vomiting, cause dry mouth, and suppress appetite. With the use of multiple medications, the impact is even greater. In addition, interactions occur between nutrients and drugs that can affect expected pharmacokinetics and pharmacodynamics. Lastly, the aging process may lead to accidental overdose or omission of drugs due to forgetfulness or repeated dosing (Heuberger & Caudell, 2011).

Obesity is also a concern among the older adult population. Concepts that promote undernutrition can also lead to overnutrition. These include decreased metabolic rate, lack of exercise, high carbohydrate intake, hormonal changes in women, and polypharmacy. Obesity places the older adult at risk for cardiovascular disease, diabetes, and musculoskeletal disruption (Singh & Kaur, 2012).

One of the goals of *Healthy People 2020* is to improve the health, function, and quality of life of older adults (USDHHS, 2013a). The federal government acknowledges that nutritional intake in this population remains a concern. Funding has been awarded through the Older Americans Act (OAA) to provide nutrition services to this population. The OAA provides congregate nutrition services, which include meals served at group sites such as senior centers, schools, churches, or senior housing complexes; home-delivered nutrition services; and family caregiver support. Nutrition services received $816 million in fiscal year 2012 (Napili & Colello, 2013).

Stay Current: *An excellent Web site that can assist older adults in understanding nutritional status and choice is MyPlate for Older Adults, created by Tufts University (**http://hnrca.tufts.edu/my-plate-for-older-adults**). The Web site can also be used by nurses for nutritional guidance.*

► ALTERATIONS TO NUTRITION

Alterations to nutrition take many forms. Overnutrition and undernutrition are major concerns throughout all populations and all ages and have direct effects on physical and emotional well-being. Appropriate food intake is essential to normal growth and development throughout the life span. Appropriate

Concepts Related to **Nutrition**

Many illnesses and disorders are treated by limitations of intake of certain food products that place clients at risk for exacerbations of these health interruptions. For example, clients with coronary artery disease need to limit their intake of cholesterol and saturated fat because these further contribute to artery blockage. The nurse needs to be prepared to teach clients about food that should be included or avoided on these diet plans. Additional information is found in the module on Perfusion. The relationships between nutrition and the concepts of fluid and electrolyte balance, tissue integrity, elimination, mobility, and perfusion are summarized below.

CONCEPT	RELATIONSHIP TO NUTRITION	NURSING IMPLICATIONS
Fluids and Electrolytes		
■ Chronic renal failure	Normal levels of protein intake lead to increased workload in poorly performing kidneys.	■ Protein-restricted diets are often implemented in the client with chronic renal failure.
Tissue Integrity		
■ Wound healing	Deficiency in protein intake leads to delayed wound healing.	■ Lack of protein intake leads to lack of cellular integrity that is manifested by edema. Clients recovering from major surgery, burns, or severe trauma may need additional protein intake to help provide for tissue healing.
Elimination		
■ Constipation	Decreased fiber intake leads to slowed peristalsis.	■ Fiber in the diet promotes bulk and draws fluid into the bowel, which aids in fecal elimination. Intake of fiber can reduce the need for laxatives in the treatment of constipation.
Mobility		
■ Fractures	When the intake of calcium and vitamin D is insufficient, bone loss can occur, leading to osteoporosis and fractures.	■ Clients need to be encouraged to maintain intake of calcium-rich and vitamin D–rich foods and to safely spend time in the sun for appropriate intervals.
Perfusion		
■ Hypertension	Regular (in special populations) or increased sodium intake leads to fluid retention and can increase blood pressure.	■ Increased sodium intake, especially in salt-sensitive clients, can lead to increased blood pressure. Nurses must teach clients how to read labels and provide lists of low-sodium foods. Nurses must also be familiar with the DASH diet plan (http://dashdiet.org).

food choice is also foundational to disease management and intervention. Weight affects one's body image, self-concept, and overall self-efficacy (Olander et al., 2013). In addition, eating is a social event and affects individual and family interactions at all levels.

Promotion of appropriate food intake is an essential part of nursing care. Food is often thought of as a form of comfort for clients and when its intake is interrupted, an individual's physiological and psychological well-being are also impacted.

During times of acute illness or surgery of the gastrointestinal track, traditional nutritional intake is often avoided. The client may have a nasogastric tube and have nothing by mouth, or alterations in the esophagus or stomach could lead to the need for enteral administration of nutritional products. The inability to eat in a normal manner can produce psychological discomfort, so the nurse must be ready to assist the client in coping with these changes. The module on Comfort discusses interventions for coping.

Alterations and Manifestations

UNDERNUTRITION According to the Child Health Now Fact Sheet, **undernutrition** is the underlying cause of 3.5 million preventable maternal and child deaths worldwide each year and it plays a significant role in approximately 35% of the diseases seen in children under the age of 5. In some discussions, the terms *malnutrition* and *undernutrition* are used interchangeably. Based on the most current literature review, undernutrition is the more accurate term and is representative of insufficient food intake and being hungry. According to the 2012 World Hunger and Poverty Facts and Statistics, 13.1%, or almost one in seven people in the world are hungry. Children are the most visible victims of undernutrition. Children who are undernourished suffer over 150 days of illness annually. Child undernutrition can begin in utero: Undernutrition in pregnant women can result in children with low birth weight, learning disabilities, mental retardation, poor health, blindness, or premature death (Vanderslice, 2012).

According to the USDA, 16.7 million children under age 18 in the United States live in households where they are unable to consistently access enough of the nutritious food necessary for a healthy life. In 1993, Feeding America launched the national Kids Cafe program, which provides free meals and snacks to low-income children through a variety of community locations where children already congregate during the afterschool hours, such as Boys and Girls Clubs, churches, and public schools. In addition to providing meals to kids, some Kids Cafe programs also offer a safe place, where under the supervision of trustworthy staff, a child can get involved in educational, recreational, and social activities. All Kids Cafe programs also offer nutrition education throughout the school year. In addition to the Kids Cafe, the Feeding America Backpack Program has been helping children get the nutritious and easy-to-prepare food they need over the course of the weekend when school meals are unavailable. Bags of food assembled at more than 150 local food banks are distributed at the end of the week to nearly 230,000 children every year.

Stay Current: *For more information, visit the Feeding America Web site at www.feedingamerica.org.*

Undernutrition increases the risk of the development of infections in children due to a decrease in the immune response. Undernutrition leads to slower bone development, and children experiencing undernutrition may be short for their developmental age. This is referred to as *stunting* and may be seen in as many as 20% of children worldwide. Hungry children may also experience learning disabilities due to lack of specific nutrients such as iodine.

Undernutrition is less common than overnutrition in the United States, but it can have devastating physical health consequences when protein-calorie malnutrition or other nutrient deficiencies develop. Adolescents and younger adults experience problems similar to their younger family members because undernutrition can lead to growth failure, compromised immune status, poor wound healing, muscle loss, and physical and functional decline in these members of the populations. Generally, individuals at risk for undernutrition include those who have a chronic illness or who are poor, older, hospitalized, impose self-enforced restrictive eating, or have an alcohol abuse problem. See the Multisystem Effects of Undernutrition feature.

One specific form of undernutrition in childhood is failure to thrive. Failure to thrive is due to inadequate calorie intake and absorption or overexpenditure of calories. Failure to thrive occurs in 5%–10% of the children seen in primary care settings (Cole & Lanham, 2011). Data suggestive of failure to thrive include BMI at less than the 5th percentile, length for age less than the 5th percentile, and weight decline (Cole & Lanham, 2011). See the exemplar on Failure to Thrive in the module on Development for more information.

OVERNUTRITION The worldwide transition toward refined foods and the increased intake of animal protein and of fats are resulting in a significant increase in diseases directly linked to **overnutrition** such as obesity, diabetes, and cardiovascular diseases. Researchers further suggest that the problem of overnutrition is increasing even in countries where hunger is considered endemic. Across the world people are consuming increased levels of refined sugar; fat and sugar account for more than half of caloric intake and refined grains have replaced whole grains (Chopra, Galbraith, & Darnton-Hill, 2002). Overnutrition in the form of excess dietary intake of fat, especially saturated fat, has been associated with an increased risk of atherosclerosis. Overweight and obesity are linked to increased risk for hypertension, cardiovascular disease, type 2 diabetes, some cancers, degenerative joint disease, and other conditions. Additionally, excess body weight has been shown to increase the risk of all-cause mortality in adults 30–74 years of age. In the United States, 63% of males and 55% of females 20–74 years of age are considered overweight or obese, a statistic that has increased by 25% during the past 30 years.

The prevalence of obesity and overweight has doubled in children and adolescents in the past 30 years to 13% and 14%, respectively. For additional information, see the exemplar on Obesity in the module on Metabolism. Addressing the problem will require a multidisciplinary approach that includes information about obesity, its complications, and treatment options and the presentation of this information as part of the traditional school curriculum. Part of this school curriculum includes physical recreation activities and the involvement of students in computer-driven programs. The developers of the curriculum suggest that families be involved both directly and indirectly in as many activities as possible (Ayliffe & Glanville, 2010).

Prevalence

Data from the CDC outline the following statistics for the United States related to obesity:

- More than one third of U.S. adults (35.7%) are obese.
- Obesity-related conditions include heart disease, stroke, type 2 diabetes, and certain types of cancer, which are some of the leading causes of preventable death.
- In 2008, medical costs associated with obesity were estimated at $147 billion; the medical costs for people who are obese were $1,429 higher than those for people of normal weight.
- Obesity now affects 17% of all children and adolescents in the United States—triple the rate from just one generation ago.

Multisystem Effects of Undernutrition

Neurologic
- ↓Cognition
- ↓Consciousness (drowsiness, lethargy)
- Tremors
- Paresthesias
- Impaired coordination

Endocrine
- ↓Thyroid hormones
- ↓Testosterone (male)
- ↓Estrogen (female)

Integumentary
- Hair: brittle, dull, dry, loss of color
- Nails: fragile, brittle, spoon-shaped
- Petechiae
- Poor wound healing

Respiratory
- ↓Respiratory rate
- ↓Vital capacity

Hepatic
- Hepatomegaly
- ↓Bile synthesis

Cardiovascular
- Dysrythmias and conduction disturbances
- ↓HR
- ↓BP
- Enlarged heart

Potential Complication
- Heart failure

Gastrointestinal

Oral/esophageal:
- Cheilosis
- Glossitis
- Gingivitis

Stomach/intestines:
- Ascites
- Constipation
- Intestinal atrophy
- Steatorrhea
- ↓Gastric and pancreatic secretions

Potential Complication
- Malabsorption syndrome

Reproductive
- Amenorrhea

Metabolic Processes
- ↓Weight
- ↓Core body temperature
- Edema

Musculoskeletal
- Muscle wasting
- Tenderness
- Impaired strength

Immune System
- ↓Cell-mediated and humoral immunity
- ↑Susceptibility to infections

Alterations and Therapies **Nutrition**

ALTERATION	DESCRIPTION	MANIFESTATIONS	INTERVENTIONS AND THERAPIES
Carbohydrate deficiency and excess	Excess occurs when carbohydrate intake exceeds the recommended intake. Deficiency occurs when intake is less than recommended.	■ With excess carbohydrate intake, weight gain may be seen as well as elevated blood glucose and storage of excess intake as fat. ■ With deficiency the body may use protein and fat for energy leading to weight and muscle mass loss and ketonuria.	■ Provide clients with the suggested intake for carbohydrates and provide education regarding weight management and appropriate exercise.
Protein deficiency and excess	Excess occurs when protein intake exceeds the recommended intake. Deficiency occurs when protein intake is less than recommended.	■ In the client with normal kidney function, protein excess or deficiency does not require nursing intervention. ■ With illness, protein deficiency can lead to poor wound healing, lack of tissue integrity, and adverse effects on blood components.	■ Clients who are vegetarians may need assistance in maintaining adequate protein intake. ■ Individuals with critical illnesses who are receiving alternative nutrition may need protein replacement therapy.
Mineral deficiencies and excess	Excessive levels occur when intake of minerals such as calcium exceeds the recommended amount. Deficiency occurs when mineral intake is insufficient.	■ Excessive intake of calcium can lead to hypercalcemia and can place clients at risk for renal calculi. ■ Insufficient intake of calcium places clients at risk for osteoporosis.	■ Provide clients with lists of foods high in calcium. Teach the relationship between vitamin D and calcium absorption.
Vitamin deficiencies	Excessive levels occur when vitamin intake exceeds the recommended amount. Deficiencies occur when intake of vitamins is insufficient.	■ Deficiency of vitamin C can lead to scurvy. Toxicity is rare. Vitamin C functions as an antioxidant. ■ Deficiency of thiamin can lead to beriberi. ■ Deficiency of niacin can lead to pellagra. Toxicity produces a flushing-like feeling; the client becomes very red and hot. ■ Deficiency of vitamin B_6 can lead to convulsions and nerve damage. Toxicity is rare. ■ Deficiency of vitamin B_{12} can lead to pernicious anemia. Toxicity is rare. ■ Vitamin A deficiency is a worldwide concern and leads to increased risk for infections, night blindness, and keratinization. Toxicity is rare, but can cause dry skin, headache, fatigue, and dizziness. Significant overdoses can lead to hepatotoxicity. ■ Vitamin D deficiency causes rickets in children and osteomalacia in older adults. Toxicity is rare. ■ Vitamin E toxicity is rare, as is deficiency except in premature infants, in whom it can lead to erythrocyte hemolysis. ■ Vitamin K deficiency is rare except in newborns.	■ Vitamin K is administered to newborns due to their immature liver function and to aid in coagulation. ■ Encourage intake of foods rich in each of the vitamins. ■ Teach that exposure to sunlight assists in vitamin D formation.

■ According to the World Health Organization (WHO), obesity is also a worldwide problem; it has nearly doubled since 1980, and worldwide more than 40 million children under the age of 5 were overweight in 2011.

Both the CDC and the WHO agree that obesity is a significant health risk and, more importantly, that it is preventable. One of the primary roles nurses can play regarding intervention and prevention of obesity is education. The first step is providing information about appropriate food choice and portion size. Nutrition education can occur in a variety of settings from preschools to high schools to college dorms and senior citizen centers. Many senior citizen centers provide congregate meals, and participants are ready audiences.

The National Association of Anorexia Nervosa and Associated Disorders (ANAD) (2013) provides the following information about the prevalence of feeding and eating disorders:

■ Almost 50% of people with feeding and eating disorders meet the criteria for depression.

■ Only 1 in 10 men and women with feeding and eating disorders receive treatment. Only 35% of people who receive treatment for eating disorders get treatment at a specialized facility for eating disorders.

■ In the United States, up to 24 million people of all ages and genders have a feeding and eating disorder (anorexia, bulimia, and binge eating disorder).

■ Feeding and eating disorders have the highest mortality rate of any mental illness.

For additional information on eating disorders refer to the exemplar on Feeding and Eating Disorders in the module on Self.

Genetic Considerations and Nonmodifiable Risk Factors

Although it may not be the client's first option, many health interruptions respond positively to changes in food intake. For example, in clients with elevated cholesterol, dietary modifications impact total cholesterol and also the amount of low-density lipoproteins. This leads to decreased coronary artery disease risk. These choices are voluntary and are considered modifiable.

Some factors associated with food choice that clients cannot modify include allergies to specific food products, especially peanuts, eggs, and fruit; lactose intolerance and the need to avoid milk and milk products; and adjustment of carbohydrate intake in the client with diabetes. In many cases, these factors have a genetic link.

Some researchers consider age to be a nonmodifiable risk factor for obesity. According to Garko (2011) as people age, hormone levels change and when these changes are associated with a sedentary lifestyle, body fat begins to accumulate and muscle mass begins to decrease. The loss in muscle tissue accompanied by a declining metabolic rate contributes to the increased risk of becoming overweight or obese.

CASE STUDY \\ PART 1

Stacy Carpenter is a 9-year-old Hispanic female who is seen in the pediatric clinic today for a well-child checkup because she wants to play softball in the fall. Stacy weighs 120 pounds, which places her at the 120th percentile for weight. She is 55 inches tall. Stacy's blood pressure is 130/90 mmHg and her heart rate is 90 bpm at rest. Stacy's mother is visibly overweight. Stacy's mother knows that obesity is a problem in many school-aged children today and asks for help in changing Stacy's diet, lifestyle, and weight loss strategies. The nurse asks Stacy to do a quick 24-hour food recall. Stacy identifies the following:

■ Breakfast: two Pop Tarts, glass of chocolate milk, and one glazed donut

■ Lunch: two slices of pepperoni pizza and two breadsticks, one serving of canned peaches, a bottle of fruit juice, and a sugar cookie for dessert.

■ Supper: three chicken enchiladas, Mexican rice, refried beans, chips and salsa, and two sopapillas.

When the nurse asks about exercise, Stacy says she really does not do any exercising except for recess at school.

Clinical Reasoning Questions Level I

1. In evaluating Stacy's diet, what findings would concern the nurse the most?

2. Why might Stacy's blood pressure be high?

3. What role, if any, does Stacy's ethnicity play in her weight problems?

Clinical Reasoning Questions Level II

4. What could be the cause of the elevation of Stacy's blood pressure?

5. Should Stacy's mom be concerned and what should the nurse teach her at this point?

▶ PREVENTION

Modifiable Risk Factors

Nutritional intake is a modifiable risk factor for atherosclerotic vascular disease (Mahe et al., 2011), osteoporosis, age-related macular degeneration (Cimberele, 2010), hypertension, and some cancers. Nutritional intake is also directly related to life expectancy differences around the world.

Screenings

Screenings identify the need for further evaluation. In many school systems across the country, nutrition screening is performed using body mass index (BMI) and is considered a required screening in the same manner as scoliosis screening. Screening tools are discussed in the following section on assessment.

▶ ASSESSMENT

Many factors can influence nutritional health. When gathering data for a nutritional assessment, it is important to know the common risk factors for poor nutritional status. Several screening tools are available to assist in determining nutritional status. Evaluation of nutritional status is an important part of total client assessment and includes:

■ Review of the nutritional history

■ Food and fluid intake record

- Laboratory data
- Food–drug interactions
- Health history and physical assessment
- Anthropometric measurements
- Psychosocial assessment.

Nursing Assessment

An initial nutrition screening provides an inexpensive, quick way of determining which clients need more extensive nutritional assessment by the healthcare team. The Joint Commission's patient care standards require that a nutritional screening occur within 24 hours of a client's hospital admission. "The standards for nutritional and functional screening clearly state that these are performed when warranted by the patient's needs or condition. Your organization would define in writing the criteria that identify when these screenings and more in-depth assessment are performed. When applicable for the patient's condition, these screenings must be completed within 24 hours after inpatient admission" (Joint Commission, 2012). When clients are in the hospital for more than a week, nutritional assessment should be part of the daily plan of care.

The initial assessment of nutritional status includes inspection of the body overall for signs of malnutrition, measurement of height and weight with comparisons to identified norms, weight history (loss or gain), usual eating habits, ability to chew and swallow, and any recent changes in appetite or food intake. One internationally recognized tool for a guide to a quick assessment is the Mini Nutritional Assessment (MNA), a two-part tool that has been tested extensively. The MNA provides a reliable, rapid assessment for clients in the community and in any healthcare setting. It is available in a number of languages. The first part of the screening asks about food intake, mobility, and BMI. It also screens for weight loss, acute illness, and psychological health problems. If the client scores 11 points or less, the *second* part (G-R) of the MNA is completed, for an additional 12 questions. The entire assessment takes less than 15 minutes. Although the tool provides information about overall status and potential for risk, it does lack specificity (Neelemaat et al., 2011). A shorter version of the MNA with just six questions is also available (see **Figure 14–7** ●). It provides initial information as to risk that can be followed up by using the full MNA or other comprehensive tools.

Stay Current: *The Mini Nutritional Assessment Short Form (MNA®-SF) is available as a free iPhone app through iTunes.*

Assessment of nutritional status also involves a review of the client's historical information, anthropometric data, and a review of systems and laboratory results. Socioeconomic factors are also reviewed with an emphasis on the client's ability to purchase food, access to food sources, and food preparation abilities.

HISTORY The Assessment Interview feature outlines questions to be asked during the history. A major component of a client's nutritional status is a review of foods eaten. Tools to collect this data include a 24-hour diet recall or the keeping of a diet diary for 3 days or a week or longer. To get as accurate a picture as possible, the client should follow his or her standard typical intake. Portion sizes should also be included. The diets

Assessment Interview **Nutrition**

Current Nutritional Intake

- Do you follow a special diet? Why? Do you eat meat? Eggs?
- Have you noticed any weight gain or weight loss greater than 5 pounds during the past month?
- Have your eating habits changed during the past month? If so, how?
- Are you able to obtain food when you choose to do so? Where do you obtain your food?
- What is an example of a typical day of food intake?
- Do you modify your diet based on a disease or health interruption? If so, how?
- Do you take any nutritional supplements? If so, how often?
- Do you have enough money to buy food?
- Do you use any special food preparation techniques?
- Do you count calories?
- Do you eat three meals per day?
- Describe a typical 24-hour diet.

Lifestyle

- Do you eat out often? How many times a week?
- What type of restaurants do you frequent?

Physical

- Have you been diagnosed with a nutrition-related anemia?
- Do you have any physical problems that limit or affect your food intake, for example, dentition problems, trouble swallowing?
- Do you have any digestive problems, such as lactose intolerance, ulcers, constipation diarrhea?

can then be evaluated for nutrient intakes and compared to standard guidelines such as the DRIs. Diet analysis software is available or items can be evaluated through nutrient food charts. This is a time-consuming procedure. When combined with other portions of the assessment, adequacy of nutritional status is indicated and possible problem areas can emerge.

ANTHROPOMETRIC DATA Specific **anthropometric measurements** include height and weight (length in babies), body mass index, waist-to-hip circumference, and skinfold thickness. Data from these measures can help the nurse identify individuals who are at risk for undernutrition or overnutrition. Obtain height and weight first. Height should be measured specifically as individuals are often inaccurate when reporting height. Determine the height using the measuring stick of a scale. The client should stand erect, look straight ahead, and position the heels together with the arms at the sides. If the client cannot stand, height estimates can be obtained using a knee height caliper. This device uses the distance between the client's patella and heel to estimate height (Perry, 2009). Weight should be obtained at the same time each day, on the same scale, and with the client wearing similar clothing. It is important for the scale to be calibrated. Findings are then compared with identified standards for gender and age.

Mini Nutritional Assessment
MNA®

Nestlé
NutritionInstitute

Last name:	First name:

Sex:	Age:	Weight, kg:	Height, cm:	Date:

Complete the screen by filling in the boxes with the appropriate numbers. Total the numbers for the final screening score.

Screening

A Has food intake declined over the past 3 months due to loss of appetite, digestive problems, chewing or swallowing difficulties?
0 = severe decrease in food intake
1 = moderate decrease in food intake
2 = no decrease in food intake ☐

B Weight loss during the last 3 months
0 = weight loss greater than 3 kg (6.6 lbs)
1 = does not know
2 = weight loss between 1 and 3 kg (2.2 and 6.6 lbs)
3 = no weight loss ☐

C Mobility
0 = bed or chair bound
1 = able to get out of bed/chair but does not go out
2 = goes out ☐

D Has suffered psychological stress or acute disease in the past 3 months?
0 = yes   2 = no ☐

E Neuropsychological problems
0 = severe dementia or depression
1 = mild dementia
2 = no psychological problems ☐

F1 Body Mass Index (BMI) (weight in kg)/(height in m^2)
0 = BMI less than 19
1 = BMI 19 to less than 21
2 = BMI 21 to less than 23
3 = BMI 23 or greater ☐

IF BMI IS NOT AVAILABLE, REPLACE QUESTION F1 WITH QUESTION F2.
DO NOT ANSWER QUESTION F2 IF QUESTION F1 IS ALREADY COMPLETED.

F2 Calf circumference (CC) in cm
0 = CC less than 31
3 = CC 31 or greater ☐

Screening score
(max. 14 points) ☐☐

12–14 points:	Normal nutritional status
8–11 points:	At risk of malnutrition
0–7 points:	Malnourished

Ref. Vellas B, Villars H, Abellan G, et al. *Overview of the MNA® - Its History and Challenges.* J Nutr Health Aging 2006;10:456-465. Rubenstein LZ, Harker JO, Salva A, Guigoz Y, Vellas B. *Screening for Undernutrition in Geriatric Practice: Developing the Short-Form Mini Nutritional Assessment (MNA-SF).* J. Geront 2001;56A: M366-377.

Guigoz Y. *The Mini-Nutritional Assessment (MNA®) Review of the Literature - What does it tell us?* J Nutr Health Aging 2006; 10:466-487. Kaiser MJ, Bauer JM, Ramsch C, et al. *Validation of the Mini Nutritional Assessment Short-Form (MNA®-SF): A practical tool for identification of nutritional status.* J Nutr Health Aging 2009; 13:782-788.

® Société des Produits Nestlé, S.A., Vevey, Switzerland, Trademark Owners

© Nestlé, 1994, Revision 2009. N67200 12/99 10M

For more information: www.mna-elderly.com

Figure 14–7 ● Mini Nutritional Assessment (MNA®).
Source: Nestlé Nutrition Institute. (2013). *Mini nutritional assessment.* Retrieved from http://www.mna-elderly.com/forms/mini/mna_mini_english.pdf.

TABLE 14–4 Body Mass Index Calculations

MEASUREMENT UNITS	FORMULA AND CALCULATION
Kilograms and meters (or centimeters)	Formula: weight (kg)/[height (m)]^2 With the metric system, the formula for BMI is weight in kilograms divided by height in meters squared. Since height is commonly measured in centimeters, divide height in centimeters by 100 to obtain height in meters. Example: Weight = 68 kg, height = 165 cm (1.65 m) Calculation: 68 ÷ (1.65)^2 = 24.98
Pounds and inches	Formula: weight (lb)/[height (in.)]^2 × 703 Calculate BMI by dividing weight in pounds (lbs) by height in inches (in.) squared and multiplying by a conversion factor of 703. Example: Weight = 150 lbs, height = 5′5″ (65″) Calculation: [150 ÷ (65)^2] × 703 = 24.96

SAFETY ALERT
Weight scales should be calibrated twice yearly to ensure accurate readings.

Body mass index is calculated from height and weight data. The formula for calculating BMI is same for both adults and children. The calculation is based on the formulas shown in **Table 14–4** ●. BMI can also be determined using a chart that is linked with height and weight or with a BMI calculator.

Stay Current: *Go to the CDC Web site to use the BMI calculators for adults (**www.cdc.gov/healthyweight/assessing/bmi/adult_BMI/english_bmi_calculator/bmi_calculator.html**) and for children and teens (**http://apps.nccd.cdc.gov/dnpabmi/**).*

Tables 14–5 ● and 14–6 ● list interpretations of BMI results (CDC, 2011b). The calculated BMI number for children and teens is plotted on the gender-specific CDC BMI-for-age growth charts and a percentile ranking is noted. Percentiles are the most commonly used indicator to assess the size and growth patterns of children in the United States. The percentile suggests a child's BMI among children of the same sex and age. For adults, the least risk for malnutrition is associated with scores between 18.5 and 25 and for children less risk is associated with numbers between the 5th and 85th percentile. BMI values above and below these numbers are associated with increased health risks (CDC, 2011b). Although opinions differ as to the usefulness of BMI measures and its calculation formula, several studies indicate its usefulness in the early identification of obe-

TABLE 14–5 BMI Ranges for Adults

BMI	WEIGHT STATUS
Below 18.5	Underweight
18.5–24.9	Normal
25.0–29.9	Overweight
30.0–34.9	Obese, class I
35.0–39.9	Obese, class II
40.0 and above	Extreme obesity, class III

TABLE 14–6 BMI Ranges for Children and Teens

PERCENTILE RANGE	WEIGHT STATUS
Less than 5th percentile	Underweight
5th percentile to less than 85th percentile	Normal
85th percentile to less than 95th percentile	Overweight
Equal to or greater than 95th percentile	Obese

sity risk and subsequent health problems (Metcalf et al., 2011). In addition, the American Heart Association recently endorsed both BMI and waist circumference as appropriate tools in assessing obesity (Cornier et al., 2011).

Waist-to-height ratio also provides data about nutritional status and health risk. Various online sites provide calculations for this measurement. Measure waist circumference at a horizontal line 1 inch above the belly button. Then enter the circumference and the height. If the measurements indicate the body is higher than normal range of upper-body fat, the client is at increased risk for chronic diseases, such as type 2 diabetes, heart disease, and high blood pressure.

Stay Current: *Calculations for waist-to-height ratio can be obtained at **www.health-calc.com/body-composition/waist-to-height-ratio**.*

Nurses need to remember that information from these data are only a general indicator of nutritional status and do not provide any information regarding nutrient deficiency or excess. Relationships have been identified between increased waist circumference and elevated blood pressure. In a study by Chen and Li (2011) increased BMI and waist circumference values demonstrated significant correlations with elevated systolic and diastolic blood pressure in preschool children with obesity. Chen and Li recommend the use of these two anthropometric measures in screening children for hypertension.

PHYSICAL EXAMINATION All body systems are impacted by nutritional intake (refer back to the Multisystem Effects of Undernutrition feature on page 937). The physical examination should include the assessments outlined in the Nutrition Assessment feature.

Lifespan and Cultural Considerations

As stated earlier, nutrition needs change across the life span. During assessment, remember to take the client's age into consideration. See the Lifespan Considerations feature.

Obesity disproportionally affects minorities as well as low socioeconomic groups. Heart disease is the number one cause of death for all Americans, and stroke is the fourth. The risk of these diseases is significantly higher for African Americans. According to the American Heart Association, African Americans can adjust these odds through prevention by understanding the risks and taking simple steps to address them (American Heart Association, 2013). These steps include visiting their healthcare providers and working with them on specific risk factors. Many African Americans are salt sensitive and decreasing salt intake is one easy step toward better health. African Americans are nearly twice as likely to have diabetes as non-Hispanic Whites. About 15% of all African Americans ages 20 and older have the disease. Prevention is first step with this disorder and includes obesity management and implementation of exercise programs.

Nutrition Assessment

ASSESSMENT/ METHOD	NORMAL FINDINGS	ABNORMAL FINDINGS	LIFESPAN OR DEVELOPMENTAL CONSIDERATIONS
Height and Weight			
	Normal weights for adult men and women are available from several reference standards, including Health Check Systems (www.healthchecksystems.com/heightweightchart.htm) and the revised Metropolitan Life tables.	■ Weight and/or height outside the outlined parameters, indicating either under- or overnutrition	■ Muscle mass weighs more, so individuals with significant muscle mass and decreased body fat may need to use more refined methods such as DEXA scanning to determine over- or underweight. DEXA uses a very low dose x-ray for measurement of body composition and body fat. ■ Specific height and weight tables based on percentiles are useful in infants and children.
Body Mass Index (BMI)			
Using a formula, compare height to weight.	Formula: **English BMI Formula** BMI = [Weight in Pounds/ (Height in inches × Height in inches)] × 703 **Metric BMI Formula** BMI = [Weight in Kilograms/ (Height in Meters × Height in Meters)] (www.bmi-calculator.net/bmi-formula.php) Norms: 18.5–24.9	■ See Table 14–5. When compared to chart, low BMI suggests underweight/undernutrition; high BMI suggests overweight or obesity.	■ BMI is calculated for individuals ages 20 and older. ■ Growth percentile charts reflect height and weight more accurately in infants, children, and teens (see Table 14–6).
Waist-to-Height Ratio			
	Online calculator will indicate whether client is underweight, at appropriate weight, or overweight.	■ Those with higher than normal range of upper-body fat are at risk for chronic diseases.	■ Indicates risk for certain disorders. ■ May be less than accurate in the very old.
Food Diary			
	Review of specific nutrient intake over a designated period of time.	■ Documented lack of intake of specific nutrients and indications for over- or undernutrition.	■ Foods should be recorded at the time eaten. Especially helpful in the older adult who may eat the same food items every day, or who may eat simple meals such as cold cereal. ■ Used as an adjunct to other nutritional screenings. ■ Especially helpful for mothers who question foods eaten by young children.
Nutrient Assessment/Food Frequency Questionnaires			
	Perform 24-hour recall and evaluate diet for equivalency to recommended intake of various nutrients. Food frequency questionnaires ask participants to report the frequency of consumption and portion size of approximately 125 line items over a defined period of time.	■ Deficits and excesses are identified.	■ Teach about replacement of changes in food choice. ■ Identifies deficiencies and excesses in the diet.
Six-Item Mini-Nutritional Assessment			
	This six-item tool provides a general review of the nutritional status of older adults.	■ Early problem identification	■ Allows teaching about possible areas of deficiency.

Lifespan Considerations Nutrition

Infants

- A mother's intake during pregnancy may provide insight into an infant's nutritional status.
- Height and weight percentiles evaluate nutritional status compared with standard norms.
- Infant formulas are developed to meet the needs of specific age groups.
- Breastfeeding is recommended for the first 6 months.
- Infant formula and cereal are often iron fortified.
- Foods are introduced in a specific method beginning at around age 4–6 months.

Children

- Toddlers often eat food in a repetitive format.
- Teach clients about choking hazards and the size of food.
- Toddlers often eat on the run, so finger foods are appropriate.
- Children can be iron deficient and may need supplements.
- School lunch programs may be the child's best option for appropriate food intake.
- Some programs offer food for the weekend when children may be at risk for undernutrition due to lack of family resources.

Adolescents

- Fast-food consumption is associated with higher total calorie intake and poorer diet quality (Powell & Nguyen, 2013).
- Body image may affect food choice.
- Adolescents experience eating disorders.
- Consumption of food is often a social interaction.
- Peers significantly influence adolescent food intake.
- Up to 30% of adolescents in the United States are obese as defined by BMI.
- Obese adolescents are more likely to have risk factors for cardiovascular disease.
- Obese adolescents are more likely to have prediabetes, and are at a greater risk for bone and joint problems, sleep apnea, and social and psychological problems (CDC, 2013).
- Obese adolescents are more likely to become obese adults.
- Appropriate nutrition and fluids are necessary to fuel the body for sports and activities.

- Most adolescents do not meet the recommendations for eating 2½ cups to 6½ cups of fruits and vegetables each day, placing them at risk for vitamin deficiency.
- Most do not eat the minimum recommended amounts of whole grains (2–3 ounces each day).
- Most eat more than the recommended maximum daily intake of sodium (1,500–2,300 mg each day) placing them at risk for prehypertension (CDC, 2013).

Adults

- Typically these are years of wellness.
- Research demonstrates that adults seek appropriate nutritional information and intake.
- Adults read labels.
- Childbearing and family rearing years focus on wellness, family interaction.
- Adults often participate in exercise plans.
- They experience few health interruptions.

Older Adults

- Dentition and swallowing are frequent problems and are direct factors in food choice.
- Access to food and socioeconomic factors play a significant role in food choices.
- Dry mouth, decreased thirst sensation, and taste and smell diminish with age.
- Loneliness and/or depression occur due to loss of spouse and/or friends.
- Polypharmacy may contribute to alterations in taste.
- Some older adults prepare food and consume it for several days in a row.
- Congregate and Meals-on-Wheels programs may provide the most nutrient-dense meal of the day.
- Constipation is reported.
- Muscle mass declines.
- Chronic disease may adversely affect meal planning and food choices.
- Adults with limited mobility may restrict food intake due to embarrassment in requesting help with toileting.
- Depression affects 15%–19% of Americans ages 65 and older (Cahoon, 2012).

Stay Current: *Ethnic/cultural food pyramids are also available for various populations from the USDA at* **http://fnic.nal. usda.gov/dietary-guidance/myplatefood-pyramid-resources/ ethniccultural-food-pyramids**.

Culture can impact food choices, and many cultures recognize both acceptable and prohibited food choices. These choices are based on location, tradition, religious beliefs, and food availability in the culture of origin (Sobal & Bisogni, 2009). For example, alligators exist in many parts of the world, but they are unacceptable as a food choice by many groups. Likewise, horses, turtles, and dogs are eaten (and even considered a delicacy) in some cultures, though they are unacceptable food sources in other cultures.

Culture also impacts food preparation and consumption. For example, African and Caribbean clients usually will consume

foods that contain many types of meats and an increased amount of wheat and rice. When nurses understand the relationships among culture, ethnicity, and food choices, they are better able to provide the education necessary in disease management. For more information, see the Focus on Diversity and Culture feature.

Diagnostic Tests

Tests used to assist in the diagnosis of nutritional deficiencies include lipids, a complete blood count, serum glucose, serum albumin, and total protein. Low hematocrit levels may indicate anemia such as iron deficiency anemia or could indicate blood loss. A low serum albumin may provide additional information as to the etiology of a client's edema. Total protein pro-

Focus on Diversity and Culture Nutrition

Overweight and obesity

- The prevalence of obesity has increased in the White, Black, and Hispanic racial and ethnic groups.
- The prevalence of overweight is highest among Mexican American males.
- The prevalence of obesity is highest among Mexican American females.
- Hypertension, a comorbid condition of overweight and obesity, affects one out of three adults in the United States.
- The prevalence of hypertension is highest among Black persons.
- Adults of low socioeconomic status have twice the rate of overweight or obesity than those of medium and high socioeconomic status.

Undernutrition

- Undernutrition can contribute to growth retardation. By definition, 5% of children would be expected to be at the 5th percentile for height. However, up to 15% of Black children have growth retardation in the first year of life, and 11% of Asian and Pacific Islander children have growth retardation during the second year.
- Five percent of older adults live in dependent care facilities and of this number more than 50% are malnourished.
- Pregnant Mexican American females are more likely than those of other ethnic groups to have iron deficiency and low folic acid levels. Females of lower economic status and those with less education are also more likely to have inadequate folic acid or iron status.
- Black women and adolescents under age 15 years are more likely to have insufficient gestational weight gain and deliver low-birth-weight babies than women of other populations.

Poverty and Food Insecurity

- Poverty is a major risk factor for food insecurity and malnutrition. Public programs such as Women, Infants and Children (WIC) and the Supplemental Nutrition Assistance Program (SNAP; formerly the Food Stamp program) assist families in poverty with accessing healthy food for their children.
- Among Americans, the prevalence of poverty was 15.1% in 2011.
- Children under age 18 experience a 22% poverty rate, although this rate is higher in some states.
- The prevalence of poverty is highest among Black and Hispanic populations.

Religion

- Some religions support days of fasting
- Certain foods are omitted from food choices in certain religions, for examples, types of meats or no meats.

Sources: U.S. Department of Health and Human Services (USDHHS). (2013b). *Healthy People 2020: Nutrition and weight status—Overview*. Retrieved from http://www.healthypeople.gov/2020/topicsobjectives2020/overview.aspx?topicId=29; National Center for Children in Poverty. (2013). *Topics: Child poverty*. Retrieved from http://www.nccp.org/topics/childpoverty.html; and U.S. Bureau of the Census, https://www.census.gov/newsroom/releases/archives/facts_for_features_special_editions/cb10-ff06.html.

---

vides information about globulin as well. Elevated glucose levels could be an early indicator of prediabetes. Prealbumin (PAB), also called transthyretin (TTHY), is a hepatic protein found in the serum that provides a sensitive indication of protein deficiency because of its short half-life of 2 days. Depending on the laboratory test used, the normal PAB range is 15–36 mg/dL or 150–360 mg/L (SI units). PAB can also assess improvement in nutritional status with parenteral or enteral feeding; levels can increase by 1 mg/dL daily with adequate nutritional support.

Cholesterol levels normally range between 160 and 200 mg/dL in adult men and women. A cholesterol level below 160 mg/dL has been identified as a possible indicator of malnutrition. In addition, serum levels of each of the vitamins and minerals can provide additional information about certain disease states, for example, in the diagnosis of anemias such as vitamin B_{12} or iron deficiency anemia.

CASE STUDY \\ PART 2

Stacy returns to the clinic 6 months later with complaints of feeling tired and having a sore throat. Stacy's weight remains at the 120th percentile, and her mother relates that Stacy is also being followed for elevated blood sugar. Her blood pressure is 136/92 mmHg. Stacy and her mom report that Stacy has not really changed her diet and that she is exercising some, but she really enjoys her video games and staying inside. She was not successful at her athletic events because she "could not run fast enough." A diet history is similar to that reported in her first visit.

Clinical Reasoning Questions Level I

1. What are the priorities for care for Stacy at this time?
2. What interventions might be appropriate for Stacy?

Clinical Reasoning Questions Level II

3. What risks, if any, does Stacy's blood pressure have on her overall health?
4. What laboratory tests would you expect the practitioner to order?
5. What resources are available to help Stacy's mom with meal planning and food selection?

▶ INTERVENTIONS AND THERAPIES

The opportunities for nursing intervention in the area of nutrition occur on a daily basis. As nurses assist clients with eating and evaluate what they have eaten, nurses can play a pivotal role in education regarding the relationship between food choices and health promotion and food choices and the management of illness and disease. Many of these interventions occur through the natural process of nurse–client communication and should

Evidence-Based Practice　Intervention in Preventing Childhood Obesity

Problem

The prevalence of childhood obesity increases with each decade and is one of the greatest problems facing the United States (Murray & Anzeljc, 2011). Data collected by the National Health and Examination Survey (NHANES) through 2008 revealed that among all U.S. youth, 32% are overweight and nearly 18% are obese (above the 95th percentile BMI) (Murray & Anzeljc, 2011). Obesity in childhood predisposes children to multiple physical and psychosocial problems both now and in the future and can be a contributing factor to early mortality. During the past three decades, the number of overweight children has doubled among 2- to 5-year-olds (Seal & Broome, 2011). Major contributing factors were determined to be intake of sugar-sweetened beverages, the availability of high-carbohydrate food choices, and the use of food as a reward. In addition, the highest risk factors for childhood obesity were parental obesity and unhealthy food choices in the home environment (Murray & Anzeljc, 2011).

Evidence

Significant health and social consequences are associated with childhood obesity (Seal & Broome, 2011). Research suggests that genetics, home, school, and community factors all contribute to the problem (Agency for Healthcare Research and Quality, 2011). The White House Task Force on Childhood Obesity (Barnes, 2010) has released guidelines for the prevention, identification, and treatment of childhood obesity. The guidelines include creating a healthier start on life for children from pregnancy to early childhood, serving healthier food in schools, ensuring access to healthy, affordable food, and increasing the opportunities for physical activity. Additional interventions identified from research include breastfeeding only for the first 6 months of life, eating breakfast daily, eating with family, limiting sugar-sweetened beverages, and

participating in at least 60 minutes of physical activity a day (Clabaugh & Neuberger, 2011; Murray & Anzeljc, 2011). Findings identified parental involvement as a key indicator and recommended parents praise children for positive intake, avoid using food as a reward, offer healthy food choices, significantly limit high-calorie food and drinks in the home, and model healthy behaviors (Seal & Broome, 2011).

Implications

Nurses in the community, especially in local school systems, are strategically placed to provide education to children about appropriate food choices and the factors that lead to childhood obesity (Clabaugh & Neuberger, 2011). Nurses should advocate for the removal of sugar-sweetened beverages from school cafeterias and vending machines. Most researchers suggest that the problem is not only food intake but also lack of exercise; nurses can provide opportunities and suggestions for constructive play and share this information with teachers and parents (Rabbitt & Coyne, 2012).

A new evidence-based strategy for addressing childhood obesity, the ToyBox, has been developed in Europe. Comprised of researchers, epidemiologists, public health experts, psychologists, pediatricians, and others, the ToyBox program will make recommendations for addressing physical activity and healthy eating in this population because the belief is that obesity is a multifactorial problem (Manios et al., 2012; Summerbell et al., 2012).

Critical Thinking Application

Given the significant picture of childhood obesity, what role can the nurse play in its prevention? What role should parents play? What role should schools play? What role should primary care providers play?

---

play a significant part in discharge teaching especially in the area of food and medication interaction.

Independent

Nurses function as educators as they interact with clients and discuss the impact of a client's nutritional status on overall health. Appropriate nutritional intake begins with appropriate food choices of the correct type and volume. Many health interruptions can find their etiology in inappropriate food choices or the lack of inclusion of certain foods in the diet. In addition, the amount of food eaten is an important teaching point. Portion size alone has significantly increased during the recent past. One of the goals of *Healthy People 2020* is for healthcare providers to give clients more comprehensive information regarding weight status and health outcomes. Nurses can assist with this by providing weekly opportunities for weight and diet evaluation. In addition, nurses can provide nutritional counseling for individuals who are over- or underweight and recommend various online resources or community programs that assist with weight management and healthy eating behavior. See the Evidence-Based Practice feature for evidence of nurses' potential impact on obesity in children.

Collaborative

Several collaborative interventions are available for the management of nutrition. Most acute care centers employ a dietitian and nurses can consult with this professional or schedule teaching opportunities for nutritionally related disorders or those disorders that require the client to be placed on a modified diet. For disease-specific disorders such as diabetes or those with advanced cardiovascular risks, clients should be referred to diabetic nurse educators or cardiac rehabilitation centers. Most public health departments and long-term or assisted care facilities employ dietitians who can provide nutritional information from weight loss management to weight gain to intervention for constipation or eating disorders. Weight loss clinics and personal trainers and other support personnel such as occupational and physical therapists can also be included as a part of healthcare teams to treat the problem of obesity. Hopkins and Elliott (2011) suggest that primary care providers need to play a larger role in initiating and intervening in the prevention and treatment of childhood obesity.

Other collaborative interventions include surgery and other invasive treatments. For people with morbid obesity, bariatric or lap band surgery is an option. Although rare, bariatric surgery is considered in adolescents in severe cases of obesity that meet certain

Medications **Nutrition**

CLASSIFICATION AND DRUG EXAMPLES	MECHANISMS OF ACTION	NURSING CONSIDERATIONS
Vitamin Supplements *Examples:* ■ Multiple vitamins ■ Niacin ■ Vitamin B$_6$ ■ Vitamin B$_{12}$ ■ Vitamin C ■ Vitamin D	Supplements replace vitamins removed from food by cooking and/or correct deficiencies in the food consumed in the diet. Niacin can be taken for treatment of elevated cholesterol. Vitamin B$_6$ is used as a supplement to isoniazid (INH) therapy in the treatment of tuberculosis to prevent side effects of paresthesia and other neurological discomforts. Vitamin B$_{12}$ is administered to clients with pernicious anemia who are unable to absorb vitamin B$_{12}$. Vitamin C assists with the absorption of iron in the treatment of anemia and aids in wound healing. Vitamin D assists with the absorption of calcium and is administered to those who have insufficient intake as a component of osteoporosis treatment.	■ Teach clients importance of taking vitamins as recommended by the company. Remind them that fat-soluble vitamins are stored in the body and excess consumption can occur and can lead to toxicity. ■ In some preparations, niacin can lead to significant flushing. ■ Vitamin B$_6$ must be taken continuously during the treatment of INH. ■ Remind clients that vitamin B$_{12}$ replacement will likely be lifelong. ■ Provide information relative to the role of vitamin C in promotion of wound healing. Note that the role of vitamin C in facilitating the absorption of iron is such that they should be taken at the same time. ■ Vitamin D is present in fortified cereals and included in the same formulation for treatment of osteoporosis or osteopenia (e.g., Fosamax D). It is also essential in the prevention of rickets.
Mineral Supplements *Examples:* ■ Iron ■ Calcium ■ Folic acid	Used to treat iron deficiency anemia and anemia due to blood loss. Replaces lost calcium, especially in postmenopausal women. Used in the prevention of open neural cords.	■ Provide information about foods high in iron and calcium. ■ Remind clients that iron may turn feces black and may lead to constipation; provide suggestions for increasing fiber in diet and increased fluid intake. ■ If iron is prepared in a liquid format, client needs to use straw because iron can stain teeth. For children, iron should be placed to the back of the mouth to avoid teeth. ■ Adolescents may often be deficient in iron due to blood loss during menses, the increased metabolic rate of growth, and poor nutrition intake. ■ Calcium is prepared in a variety of different forms including tablets and gummies. Needs to be taken consistently. ■ Calcium interferes with absorption of antibiotics such as tetracycline so these meds must be taken several hours apart. ■ Cereals and breads are often calcium fortified and could be added to the diet plan. ■ Encourage intake of prenatal vitamins, especially folic acid. Folic acid levels are low in adolescents due to poor and inconsistent intake.
Protein and Nutrient Supplements *Examples:* ■ Ensure ■ Boost ■ Nutrition bars	Provide needed protein and nutrient replacement for individuals who are unable to consume enough through traditional dietary intake.	■ Helpful in the older adult population who may have dentition or appetite problems and fail to consume adequate amounts of nutrients. ■ For each of these, watch calorie intake, especially in clients with diabetes.
■ Intravenous administration of albumin, total parenteral nutrition (TPN)	Replace lost protein due to burns, major trauma, and significant surgical intervention or in situations in which the person cannot eat orally.	■ Follow dosage scheduling; may need separate line or tubing, requires monitoring of infusion and timing of administration. Often requires separate IV line. ■ Monitor serum albumin levels throughout administration time frame.

parameters of weight loss attempts and bone growth (Zeltner et al., 2011). See the exemplar on Obesity in the module on Metabolism for more information on pharmacologic therapy, behavior modification, and bariatric surgery for clients with obesity.

Some individuals find themselves unable to consume food orally. This may be due to impairment of the gastrointestinal tract, temporary considerations following surgery, or other factors. These individuals may require nutrition therapy in the form of enteral or parenteral nutrition. **Enteral nutrition**, or tube feeding, may be used to meet calorie and protein requirements in clients who are unable to consume enough food to meet the requirements. Tube feeding may be necessary for clients with impairment of the gastrointestinal tract, difficulty swallowing, unresponsiveness, oral or neck surgery or trauma, anorexia, or serious illness. Enteral feedings provide nutrients directly to the stomach or small intestine. **Parenteral nutrition (PN)** is the intravenous administration of amino acids, often with added carbohydrates, fats, electrolytes, vitamins and minerals. PN is initiated when a client's nutritional requirements cannot be met through diet or enteral feedings. Increasingly, PN may be used concurrently with enteral nutrition. Clients who have undergone major surgery or trauma or who are seriously undernourished are often candidates for PN. PN is used for both short- and long-term management of nutritional deficiencies. Many clients are discharged to home with PN and monitored by home health nurses. Enteral and parenteral nutrition are discussed further in the module on Digestion.

PHARMACOLOGIC THERAPY   Many of the pharmacologic agents specific to nutrition can be purchased over the counter. Vitamins can be purchased in the form of a multivitamin, which typically contains the recommended intakes of most vitamins and minerals needed on a daily basis. Vitamins can also be purchased individually. In many preparations iron is included in the multivitamin. Minerals can also be purchased individually. Multiple claims are made about the health benefits of vitamin and mineral supplementation; some of these are supported by research, many are not. Examples include folic acid supplementation during pregnancy and the prevention of open neural cords (American Academy of Pediatrics, 2013; Czeizel et al., 2011), vitamin C and facilitation of increased iron absorption (CDC, 2011b), and increased tissue healing and calcium replacement in the prevention of osteoporosis (Garriguel, 2011). Nurses must be familiar with the possible negative effects of misuse of these agents and be able to teach clients accordingly. See the Medications feature for more information.

SAFETY ALERT
Some vitamins when taken in excess, especially the fat-soluble vitamins, can lead to significant toxicity. An example of this is vitamin D. When taken in excess, it can cause bone destruction, rather than contributing to bone formation.

SURGERY   Many gastrointestinal surgeries will affect a client's nutritional status. For example, clients with Crohn disease or ulcerative colitis may lose a portion of their bowel and this would affect absorption. For additional information of inflammatory disorders of the bowel, refer to the exemplar on Inflammatory Bowel Disease in the module on Inflammation. Clients undergoing gastric resection may experience vitamin B_{12} deficiency. Bariatric surgery is an option for people with morbid obesity. For additional information, see the exemplar on Obesity in the module on Metabolism. Children can experience blockage of the outlet to the duodenum from the stomach and experience projectile vomiting due to the disorder of pyloric stenosis. This surgery is usually curative and, once repaired, the infant is able to retain feedings. See the exemplar on Pyloric Stenosis in the module on Digestion for more information. Other pediatric disorders that affect nutritional intake are intussusception and megacolon.

NONPHARMACOLOGIC THERAPY   Nutrition intervention is a major topic today for many individuals as they seek intervention for weight loss, dietary changes, health maintenance, and nutritional replacement or enhancement. Athletes who wish to add muscle mass may choose additional protein intake. Many clients take additional calcium for bone strength. Excess vitamin intake and supplements may place clients at risk. Nurses must be able to participate in client teaching and provide accurate and up-to-date information about these types of intervention and their strengths, weaknesses, and concerns.

Stay Current: *Various intervention groups are available to assist clients with nutritional concerns. These include Overeaters Anonymous (**www.overeatersanonymous.org**), TOPS clubs (**www.tops.org/default.aspx**), and Weight Watchers (**www.weightwatchers.com**).*

For a clinical application of independent and collaborative interventions for a client with alterations in nutrition, see the Nursing Care Plan.

NURSING CARE PLAN   A Client With Undernutrition

ASSESSMENT	DIAGNOSES	PLANNING
Joe Calhoun is a 72-year-old White male who is seen at the clinic today for his annual physical exam. Mr. Calhoun is 6 feet tall and weighs 155 pounds. In a quick review of his history the nurse notes that since his last visit 6 months ago, he has lost 15 pounds. After an initial head–to-toe exam that is within the expected norms for his age, the nurse also notes that Mr. Calhoun's mucous membranes are pale and that his pulse is slightly elevated at 90 bpm. His blood pressure is 120/70 mmHg. Previous vital signs for Mr. Calhoun were a pulse of 70 bpm and a blood pressure of 140/80 mmHg. His current medications include losartan (Avapro) 150 mg for blood pressure, Simvastatin for cholesterol, and an 81-mg aspirin daily. He takes no other prescription or over-the-counter medications except for Advil as needed for headache. The nurse questions Mr. Calhoun about changes in his life and nutritional intake during the past 6 months. The nurse also asks Mr. Calhoun to do a 24-hour dietary recall. Mr. Calhoun tells the nurse that his	■ *Imbalanced Nutrition: Less Than Body Requirements* ■ *Decreased Cardiac Output* related to anemia ■ *Social Isolation* related to loneliness. (NANDA-I © 2012)	Goals for Mr. Calhoun's care include: ■ The client will increase intake of protein to at least 3 ounces per day. ■ The client will increase intake of fresh vegetables to at least one meal per day. ■ The client will increase calorie intake by 300–500 calories per day. ■ The client will gain 2 pounds by next visit (1 month). ■ The client will socialize at least once a week with friends from church.

NURSING CARE PLAN (continued)

ASSESSMENT	DIAGNOSES	PLANNING
wife Irene died 6 months ago and that he has been "sad" and has difficulty cooking for himself. He is able to drive and does go to the grocery store each week. His daughter checks on him daily but she lives in another state. His friends from church check on him too and used to bring him casseroles but that has not happened recently. His dietary recall was as follows: "I eat cereal for breakfast and dinner and go to the senior citizen's center for lunch." He also states the food he cooks does not taste like his wife's cooking and that "It's hard to cook for one." Mr. Calhoun denies having any difficulty chewing and has his own teeth. He denies constipation. He states he has no problem swallowing. The nurse calculates that at best Mr. Calhoun is consuming 900 calories each day and many of these are empty calories. His complete blood count report identifies a red blood cell count of 3.9/mcL and a hemoglobin and hematocrit of 13 g/dL and 37%, respectively.		

IMPLEMENTATION

- Instruct client to take one multivitamin daily.
- Refer client to dietitian.
- Teach client to weigh self first thing every Saturday to note weight loss or gain; record the weights in a diary.
- Encourage client to add one high-protein drink to diet daily.

- In coordination with dietitian, teach client how to perform a 3-day diet history for evaluation.
- Reinforce consumption of high-density foods.
- Encourage client to continue going to the senior citizen's center or to weekly lunch with church friends.
- Refer client for psychological counseling.

EVALUATION

At his follow-up appointment 1 month later, Mr. Calhoun has gained 2 pounds. He continues to meet with the dietitian weekly and is consuming 200–300 more calories a day. He looks less pale although his CBC demonstrates that he is still slightly anemic. His RBC count, hemoglobin, and hematocrit have increased some. He is taking his vitamins and protein drink daily. He relates that cooking for himself is still difficult and that at times he has to "make himself eat." He has been meeting with friends from church at least once a week and sometimes more often, and he says "It has helped me a lot. They understand how much I miss Irene."

CRITICAL THINKING

1. What resources (e.g., congregate meal centers, senior citizen centers) are available in your community to help senior citizens who are living alone? What is the nurse's role in assisting clients to find resources once they have been dismissed from care?
2. What intervention would you suggest if this client, in addition to his losses, demonstrated early stages of dementia?
3. With the expected increase in the senior citizen population and the likelihood that there will be many more men in Mr. Calhoun's situation, what proactive intervention can nurses implement to help prepare to care for these individuals?

REVIEW The Concept of Nutrition

RELATE Link the Concepts

Linking the concept of nutrition with the concept of metabolism:

1. Describe the relationship among calcium, vitamin D, and the treatment of osteoporosis.
2. What foods would be included to provide additional calcium and vitamin D in a client's diet?

Linking the concept of nutrition with the concept of development:

3. What are the symptoms of failure to thrive and what factors place a 1-year-old infant at greatest risk for the disorder?
4. What type of teaching plan should be developed to assist a mother with food choices for a 1-year-old to treat failure to thrive?

Linking the concept of nutrition with the concept of healthcare systems:

5. Develop at least four strategies to assist an 86-year-old woman who does not drive to access her local food store on a weekly basis.
6. What normal physiological changes of aging might affect this client's nutritional well-being?

READY Go to Companion Skills Manual

REFER Go to Pearson Nursing Student Resources
nursing.pearsonhighered.com

- Additional review materials

REFLECT Case Study \\ Part 3

Stacy comes to see the nurse in the clinic at her school. She tells the nurse about her feelings about her weight and her need to exercise. She has lost 7 pounds, but cannot seem to "lose any more." She asks the nurse to help her develop a diet plan for 3 days considering she eats breakfast and lunch at school.

Clinical Reasoning Questions Level I

1. How would you follow up with Stacy?

2. How would you encourage exercise?

3. What role should the school play in providing options for food choices?

Clinical Reasoning Questions Level II

4. What plan would you develop for Stacy?

5. What teaching would you perform at this time?

6. Would you include Stacy's peers and if so, how would you involve them?

■ REFERENCES

Agency for Healthcare Research and Quality. (2011, December 20). *Evidence-Based Practice Center systematic review protocol: Childhood obesity preventions programs—A comparative effectiveness review and meta-analysis.* Retrieved from http://www.effectivehealthcare.ahrq.gov/ehc/products/330/902/Childhood-Obesity_Protocol_20111220.pdf.

Ahmed, A. H. (2010). Role of the pediatric nurse practitioner in promoting breastfeeding for late preterm infants in primary care settings *Journal of Pediatric Health Care, 24*(2), 116–122.

Albertson, A. M., Wold, A. C., & Joshi, N. (2012). Ready-to-eat cereal consumption patterns: The relationship to nutrient intake, whole grain intake and body mass index in an older American population. *Journal of Aging Research, 2012,* pp. 1–8.

American Academy of Pediatrics (AAP). (2012). Policy statement: Breastfeeding and the use of human milk. *American Academy of Pediatrics, 129*(3), 600–603. Retrieved from http://pediatrics.aappublications.org/content/129/3/e827.full.html.

American Academy of Pediatrics (AAP). (2013). *Where we stand: Folic acid.* Retrieved from http://www.healthychildren.org/English/ages-stages/prenatal/pages/Where-We-Stand-Folic-Acid.aspx.

American Heart Association. (2013). *African Americans: Heart disease and stroke.* Retrieved from http://www.heart.org/HEARTORG/Conditions/More/MyHeartandStrokeNews/African-Americans-and-Heart-Disease_UCM_444863_Article.jsp.

Ayliffe, B., & Glanville, T. (2010). Achieve health body weight in teenagers: Evidence-based practice guideline for community nutrition interventions. *Canadian Journal of Dietetic Practice and Research, 71*(4), e78–e86.

Back, E. A. (2011). Effects of parental relations and upbringing in trouble adolescent eating behaviors. *Eating Disorders, 19*(40), 403–424.

Ball, J., Bindler, R., & Cowen, K. (2012). *Principles of pediatric nursing* (5th ed.). Boston, MA: Pearson.

Barnes, M. (2010). *White House Task Force on Childhood Obesity report to the president: Solving the problem of childhood obesity within a generation.* Retrieved from http://www.letsmove.gov/white-house-task-force-childhood-obesity-report-president.

Beydoun, M. A., & Wang, Y. (2008). Do nutrition knowledge and beliefs modify the association of socio-economic factors and dietary quality among U.S. adults? *Preventive Medicine, 46,* 145–153.

Bragulat, V., Dzemidzic, M., Bruno, C., Cox, C. A., Talavage, T. A., Considine, R. V., & Kareken, D. A. (2010). Food-related odor probes of brain reward circuits during hunger: A pilot fMRI. *Obesity, 18,* 1566–1571.

Callen, B. (2010). Nutritional screen in community dwelling older adults. *International Journal of Older People Nursing, 6*(4), 272–281.

Centers for Disease Control and Prevention (CDC). (2011a). *Estimates of foodborne illness in the United States.* Retrieved from http://www.cdc.gov/foodborneburden.

Centers for Disease Control and Prevention (CDC). (2011b). *Nutrition for everyone: Vitamins and minerals.* Retrieved from http://www.cdc.gov/nutrition/everyone/basics/vitamins.

Centers for Disease Control and Prevention (CDC). (2013). *Childhood obesity facts.* Retrieved from http://www.cdc.gov/healthyyouth/obesity/facts.htm.

Chen, B., & Li, H. (2011). Waist circumference as an indicator of high blood pressure in preschool obese children. *Asia Pacific Journal of Clinical Nutrition, 20*(4), 557–562.

Chen, X., & Wang, Y. (2011). Is ideal body image related to obesity and lifestyle behaviours in African American adolescents? *Child: Care, Health and Development, 38*(2), 219–228.

Chopra, M., Galbraith, S., & Darnton-Hill, I. (2002). A global response to a global problem: The epidemic of overnutrition. *Bulletin of the World Health Organization, 80,* 952–958.

Cimberele, M. (2010). Awareness of modifiable risk factors in addressing age-related eye diseases. *Ocular Surgery News, 28*(22), 9–13.

Clabaugh, K., & Neuberger, G. B. (2011). Research evidence for reducing sugar sweetened beverages in children. *Issues in Comprehensive Pediatric Nursing, 34,* 119–130.

Cole, S. Z., & Lanham, J. S. (2011). Failure to thrive: An update. *American Family Physician, 83*(7), 829–834.

Coleman-Jensen, A., Nord, M., Andrews, M., & Carlson, S. (2012, September). Household food security in the United States. *USDA Economic Research Report, No. 141.*

Cornier, M. A., Després, J. P., Davis, N., Grossniklaus, D. A., Klein, S., Lamarche, B., … & Poirier, P. (2011). Assessing adiposity: A scientific statement from the American Heart Association. *Circulation, 2011*(124), 1996–2019.

Czeizel, A. E., Dudas, I., Paput, L., & Banhidy, F. (2011). Prevention of neural-tube defects with periconceptional folic acid, methylfolate, or multivitamins? *Annals of Nutrition and Metabolism, 58,* 263–271.

Davis, B., & Carpenter, C. (2009). Proximity of fast-food restaurants to schools and adolescent obesity. *American Journal of Public Health, 99*(3), 505–510.

Donaldson, A. B., & Gordon, C. M. (2013, April). Bone health in adolescents. *Contemporary Pediatrics,* pp. 14–20.

Donini, L. M., Poggiogalle, E., Piredda, M., Pinto, A., Barbagallo, M., Cucinotta, D., & Sergi, G. (2013). Anorexia and eating patterns in the elderly. *PLoS One, 8*(5), e63539. doi:10.1371/journal.pone.0063539.

Elbel, B., Gyamfi, J., & Kersh, R. (2011). Child and adolescent fast-food choice and the influence of calorie labeling: A natural experiment. *International Journal of Obesity, 35,* 493–500.

Feeding America. (2011). *Hunger in America.* Retrieved from http://feedingamerica.org/hunger-in-america/hunger-facts/hunger-and-poverty-statistics.aspx.

Food and Agriculture Organization of the United Nations. (2012). *The state of food insecurity in the world 2012: Economic growth is necessary but not sufficient to accelerate reduction of hunger and malnutrition.* Retrieved from http://www.fao.org/docrep/016/i3027e/i3027e.pdf.

Gallegos-Orozco, J. F., Foxx-Orenstein, A. E., Sterler, S. M., & Stoa, J. M. (2012). Chronic constipation in the elderly. *American Journal of Gastroenterology, 107*(1), 18–25.

Garko, M. G. (2011, January). Overweight and obesity epidemic in America—Part IV: What risk factors and causes are and why it is important to know about them. *Health and Wellbeing Monthly,* pp. 1–5. Retrieved from http://letstalknutrition.com/overweight-and-obesity-epidemic-in-america_part_iv.

Garriguel, D. (2011). Bone health: Osteoporosis, calcium and vitamin D. *Health Reports, 22*(3), 1–8.

Giacco, R., Della, P. G., Luongo, D., & Riccardi, G. (2011). Whole grain intake in relation to bodyweight: From epidemiological evidence to clinical trials. *Nutrition, Metabolism and Cardiovascular Diseases, 21*(12), 901–908.

Haines, J., Ziyadeh, N. J., Franko, D. L., McDonald, J., Mond, J. M., & Austin, S. B. (2011). Screening high school students for eating disorders: Validity of brief behavioral and attitudinal measures. *Journal of School Health, 81*(9), 530–535.

Hammond, G. K., Chapman, G. E., & Barr, S. I. (2010). Healthy midlife Canadian women: How bone health is considered in their food choice systems. *Journal of Human Nutrition and Dietetics, 24,* 61–67.

Harrison, M., Lee, A., Findlay, M., Nicholls, R., Leonard, D., & Martin, C. (2010). The increasing cost of healthy food. *Australian and New Zealand Journal of Public Health, 34*(2), 179–186.

Hopkins, K. F., & Elliott, L. (2011). How can primary care providers manage pediatric obesity in the real world? *Journal of the American Academy of Nurse Practitioners, 23,* 278–288.

Hueberger, R. A., & Caudell, K. (2011). Polypharmacy and nutritional status in older adults: A cross-sectional study. *Drugs & Aging, 28*(4), 314–323.

Jacquier, C., Bonthoux, F., Baciu, M., & Ruffieux, B. (2012). Improving the effectiveness of nutritional information policies: Assessment of unconscious pleasure mechanisms involved in food-choice decisions. *Nutrition Reviews, 70*(2), 118–131.

Jarvholm, K., Olbers, T., Marcus, C., Marlid, S., Gronowitz, E., Friberg, P. … & Flodmark, C.-E. (2012). Short-term psychological outcomes in severely obese adolescents after bariatric surgery. *Obesity, 20,* 318–323.

Joint Commission. (2012). *Nutritional, functional, and pain assessments and screens.* Retrieved from http://www.jointcommission.org/mobile/standards_information/jcfaqdetails.aspx?StandardsFAQId=471&StandardsFAQChapterId=78.

Kalupahana, N. S., & Moustaid-Moussa, N. (2011). Overview of symposium "Systems genetics in nutrition and obesity research." *Journal of Nutrition and Obesity Research, 141*(3), 512–514.

Koeck, E., Davenport, K., Barefoot, L. C., Quireshi, F. G., Davidow, D., & Nadler, E. P. (2013). Inpatient weight loss as a precursor to bariatric surgery for adolescents with extreme obesity: Optimizing bariatric surgery. *Clinical Pediatrics, 52*(7), 608–611.

Kong, A. S., Farnsworth, S., Canaca, J. A., Harris, A., Palley, G., & Sussman, A. L. (2012). An adaptive community-based participatory approach to formative assessment high schools for obesity intervention. *Journal of School Health, 82*(3), 147–154.

Kregg-Byers, C. M., & Schlenk, K. A. (2010). Implications of food insecurity on global health policy and nursing practice. *Journal of Nursing Scholarship, 42*(3), 278–285.

Lee, J. H., Ralston, R. A., & Truby, H. (2011). Influence of food cost on diet quality and risk factors for chronic disease: A systematic review. *Nutrition & Dietetics, 68*, 248–261.

Mahe, G., Carsin, M., Zeeny, M., & De Bosschere, J. P. (2011). Dietary pattern, a modifiable risk factor that can be easily assessed for atherosclerosis vascular disease prevention in clinical practice. *Public Health Nutrition, 14*(2), 319–326.

Magaña-Gómez, J. A., & Calderón de la Barca, A. M. (2009). Risk assessment of genetically modified crops for nutrition and health. *Nutrition Reviews, 67*(1), 1–16.

Magee, S. D., Everts, C., & Jamison, M. (2012). Increased body mass index interventions: A provider comparison study. *Kansas Nurse, 87*(6), 15–18.

Manios, Y., Grammatikaki, E., Androustsos, O., Chinapaw, M. J., Gibson, E. L., Buijs, G., … & de Bourdeaudhuij, I. (2012). A systematic approach for the development of a kindergarten-based intervention for the prevention of obesity in preschool age children: The ToyBox study. *Obesity Reviews, 13*(Suppl. 1), 3–12.

Mansoor, D. K., & Sharma, H. P. (2011). Clinical presentation of food allergy. *Pediatric Clinics of North America, 58*(2), 315–326.

Merikangas, A. K., Mendola, P., Pastor, P. N., Reuben, C. A., & Cleary, S. D. (2012). The association between major depressive disorder and obesity in U.S. adolescents: Results from the 2001–2004 National Health and Nutrition Examination Survey. *Journal of Behavioral Medicine, 35*, 149–154.

Metcalf, B. S., Hosking, J., Fremeaux, A. E., Jeffrey, A. N., Voss, J. D., & Wilkin, T. J. (2011). BMI was right all along: Taller children really are fatter (implications of making childhood BMI independent of height). *International Journal of Obesity, 35*, 541–547.

Mobley, C. C., Stadler, D. D., Staten, M. A., El Ghormli, L., Gillis, B., Hartstein, J., … & Virus, A. (2012). Effect of nutrition changes on foods selected by students in a middle school-based diabetes prevention intervention program: The HEALTHY experience. *Journal of School Health, 82*(2), 82–90.

Murray, R. D., & Anzeljc, S. (2011). Childhood obesity in practice. *Primary Care Reports, 17*(4), 37–47.

Musaiger, A. O., Abdulrahman, O., Al-Mannai, M., Tayyem, R., Al-Lalla, O., Ali, E. Y. H. … & Chirane, M. (2012). Prevalence of overweight and obesity among adolescents in seven Arab countries: A cross-cultural study. *Journal of Obesity, 2012*, 1–5.

Napili, A., & Colello, K. J. (2013). Funding for the Older Americans Act and other aging services programs. *Congressional Research Service.* Retrieved from http://www.fas.org/sgp/crs/misc/RL33880.pdf.

National Association of Anorexia Nervosa and Associated Disorders (ANAD). (2013). *Eating disorder statistics.* Retrieved from http://www.anad.org/get-information/about-eating-disorders/eating-disorders-statistics.

National Center for Biotechnology Information. (2012). Kwashiorkor. *PubMed Health.* Retrieved from http://www.ncbi.nlm.nih.gov/pubmedhealth/PMH0002571.

National Center for Children in Poverty. (2013). *Topics: Child poverty.* Retrieved from http://www.nccp.org/topics/childpoverty.html.

National Institute of Allergy and Infectious Diseases. (2011). *Guidelines for diagnosis and management of food allergy in the United States.* Washington, DC: U.S. Department of Health and Human Services.

Neelemaat, F., Meijers, J., Kruizenga, H., van Ballengooigen, H., & Bokhorst-de van der Schueren, M. (2011). Comparison of five malnutrition screening tools in one hospital inpatient sample. *Journal of Clinical Nursing, 20*, 2144–2152.

Nestlé Nutrition Institute. (2013). *Mini nutritional assessment.* Retrieved from http://www.mna-elderly.com/forms/mini/mna_mini_english.pdf.

Nguyen, V. N., Phuong, H. T. K., Hoang, T., Nguyen, D., & Robert, A. R. (2013). High prevalence of overweight among adolescents in Ho Chi Minh City, Vietnam. *BMC Public Health, 13*(1), 1–7.

Office of Dietary Supplements. (2011). *Vitamin D.* Retrieved from http://ods.od.nih.gov/factsheets/VitaminD-HealthProfessional.

Olander, E. K., Fletcher, H., Williams, S., Atkinson, L., Turner, A., & French, D. P. (2013). What are the most effective techniques in changing obese individuals' physical activity self-efficacy and behavior: A systematic review and meta-analysis. *International Journal of Behavioral Nutrition and Physical Activity, 10*, 29. doi:10.1186/1479-5868-10-29.

Oyetunji, T. A., Franklin, A. L., Ortega, G., Akolkar, N., Qureshi, F. G., Abdulla, F. … & Fullum, T. M. (2012). Revisiting childhood obesity: Persistent underutilization of surgical intervention. *American Surgeon, 78*(7), 788–793.

Perry, L. (2009). Using height, weight and other body measurements in nutritional assessments. *NursingTimes.net.* Retrieved from http://www.nursingtimes.net/using-height-weight-and-other-body-measurements-in-nutritional-assessments/1958313.article.

Peters, B. S. E., Verly, E., Marchioni, D. M. L., Fisberg, M., & Martini, L. A. (2011). The influence of breakfast and dairy products on dietary calcium and vitamin D intake in postpubertal adolescents and young adults. *Journal of Human Nutrition and Dietetics, 24*, 69–74.

Popkin, B. M., D'Anci, K. E., & Rosenberg, I. H. (2010). Water, hydration and health. *Nutrition Reviews, 68*(8), 438–458.

Powell, L. M., & Nguyen, B. T. (2013). Fast-food and full-service restaurant consumption among children and adolescents: Effect on energy, beverage, and nutrient intake. *JAMA Pediatrics, 167*(1), 14–20.

Quandt, S. A., Savoca, M. R., Leng, X., Chen, H., Bell, R. A., Gilbert, G. H., … Arcury, T. A. (2011). Dry mouth and dietary quality in older adults in North Carolina. *Journal of the American Geriatrics Society, 59*(3), 439–445.

Rabbitt, A., & Coyne, I. (2012). Childhood obesity: Nurses' role in addressing the epidemic. *British Journal of Nursing, 21*(12), 731–735.

Ramirez Prada, D., Delgado, G., Hidalgo Patino, C. A., Perez-Navero, J., & Gil Campos, M. (2011). Using of WHO guidelines for the management of severe malnutrition to cases of marasmus and kwashiorkor in a Colombia children's hospital. *Nutricion Hospitalaria, 26*(5), 977–983.

Remesh, A. (2012). Prevalence of adolescent obesity among high school students of Kerala, South India. *Archives of Pharmacology Practice, 3*(4), 289–292.

Sarry El-Din, A. M., Erfan, M., Kandeel, W. A., Kamal, S., El-Shafy El Banna, R. A., & Fouad, W. A. (2012). Prevalence of pre-hypertension and hypertension in a sample of Egyptian adults and its relation to obesity. *Australian Journal of Basic and Applied Sciences, 6*(13), 481–489.

Scrimshaw, N. S., & Viteri, F. E. (2010). INCAP studies of kwashiorkor and marasmus. *Food and Nutrition Reviews, 11*(1), 34–41.

Seal, N., & Broome, M. (2011). Evidence-based interventions for pediatric weight control. *Journal for Nurse Practitioners, 7*(4), 293–302.

Singh, S., & Kaur, K. (2012). Association of age with obesity related variables and blood pressure among women. *Annals of Biological Research, 3*(7), 3633–3637.

Sirma, E., Dallar Bilge, Y., Önen, S., & Engiz, Ö. (2012). Prevalence of obesity and associated risk factors among adolescents in Ankara, Turkey. *Journal of Clinical Research in Pediatric Endocrinology.* Retrieved from http://www.jcrpe.org/eng/makale/377/43/Full-Text.

Sobal, J., & Bisogni, C. A. (2009). Constructing food choices decisions. *Annals of Behavioral Medicine, 39*(Suppl. 1), 37–46.

Stajkovic, S., Aitken, E. M., & Holroyd-Leduc, J. (2011). Unintentional weight loss in older adults. *Canadian Medical Association Journal, 183*(4), 443–449.

Summerbell, C. D., Moore, H. J., Vogele, C., Kreichauf, S., Wildgruber, A., Manios, Y., … & Gibson, E. L. (2012). Evidence-based recommendations for the development of obesity prevention program targeted at preschool children. *Obesity Review, 13*(Suppl. 1), 129–132.

Sweat, V., Bruzzese, J.-M., Albert, S., Pinero, D. J., Fierman, A., & Convit, A. (2012). The Banishing Obesity and Diabetes in Youth (BODY) project: Description and feasibility of a program to halt obesity-associated disease among urban high school students. *Journal of Community Health, 37*, 365–371.

Thompson, J., Manore, M., & Vaughan, L. (2014). *The science of nutrition* (3rd ed.). Glenview, IL: Pearson.

Torres-McGehee, T. M., Monsma, E. V., Dompier, T. P., & Washburn, S. A. (2012). Eating disorder risk and the role of clothing in collegiate cheerleaders' body images. *Journal of Athletic Training, 47*(5), 541–548.

UNICEF. (2013). *Clinical forms of acute malnutrition: Marasmus and kwashiorkor.* Retrieved from http://www.unicef.org/nutrition/training/2.3/12.html.

U.S. Department of Agriculture (USDA) & U.S. Department of Health and Human Services (USDHHS). (2010, December). *Dietary guidelines for Americans 2010* (7th ed.). Washington, DC: U.S. Government Printing Office.

U.S. Department of Health and Human Services (USDHHS). (2013a). *Healthy People 2020: Nutrition and weight status—Objectives.* Retrieved from http://www.healthypeople.gov/2020/topicsobjectives2020/objectiveslist.aspx?topicId=29.

U.S. Department of Health and Human Services (USDHHS). (2013b). *Healthy People 2020: Nutrition and weight status—Overview.* Retrieved from http://www.healthypeople.gov/2020/topicsobjectives2020/overview.aspx?topicId=29.

Van der Laan, L. N., De Ridder, D. T., Viergever, M. A., & Smeets, P. A. (2012). Appearance matters: Neural correlates of food choice and packaging aesthetics. *Plus One, 7*(7), 1–11.

Van Ryzin, M. J., & Nowicka, P. (2013). Direct and indirect effects of a family-based intervention in early adolescence on parent–youth relationship quality, late adolescent health, and early adult obesity. *Journal of Family Psychology, 27*(1), 106–116.

Vanderslice, L. (2012). Hunger notes. *World Hunger Education Service.* Retrieved from http://www.worldhunger.org/about.htm.

Wang, Y., & Chen, X. (2011). How much of racial/ethnic disparities in dietary intakes, exercise, and weight status can be explained by nutrition- and health-related psychosocial factors and socioeconomic status among US adults? *Journal of the American Dietetic Association, 111*(12), 1904–1911.

Wilkie, S. (2012). Xerostomia. *Utah Department of Health.* Retrieved from http://health.utah.gov/oralhealth/resources/Xerostomia_Presentation_2012.pdf.

Williams, S. L., & Mummery, W. K. (2012). Associations between adolescent nutrition behaviours and adolescent and parent characteristics. *Nutrition & Dietetics, 69*, 85–101.

Zeller, M. H., Guilfoyle, S. M., Reiter-Purtill, J., Ratcliff, M. B., Inge, T. H., & Long, J. D. (2011). Adolescent bariatric surgery: Caregiver and family functioning across the first postoperative year. *Surgery for Obesity and Related Diseases, 7*, 143–150.

15 Oxygenation

◢ THE CONCEPT OF OXYGENATION

Oxygenation can be defined as the mechanism that facilitates the body's ability to supply oxygen to all cells of the body. The function of the respiratory system is to obtain oxygen from atmospheric air, transport this air through the respiratory tract into the alveoli, and ultimately diffuse oxygen into the blood to carry oxygen to all the cells of the body. The respiratory system achieves all this through **ventilation**, the processes of **inspiration** (inhaling) and **expiration** (exhaling). These processes transport oxygen to the alveoli so that oxygen can be exchanged for carbon dioxide, which is then expelled from the body. The actual exchange of oxygen and carbon dioxide is called **respiration**. Breathing, often an unnoticed activity, contributes to vital oxygenation of the cells and tissues. When oxygen status changes, breathing usually compensates to bring more air into the lungs. Changes in breathing patterns should be taken seriously and addressed promptly because alterations in oxygen delivery can cause serious consequences. **◀◀**

Concept Learning Outcomes

After reading about this concept, you will be able to:

1. Summarize the physiology of the respiratory system related to oxygenation.
2. Examine the relationship between oxygenation and other concepts/systems.
3. Identify commonly occurring alterations in oxygenation and their related therapies.
4. Differentiate common assessment procedures used to examine respiratory health across the life span.
5. Describe diagnostic and laboratory tests to determine the individual's oxygenation status.
6. Explain management of respiratory health and prevention of alterations in oxygenation.
7. Demonstrate the nursing process in providing culturally competent and caring interventions across the life span for individuals with common alterations in oxygenation.
8. Compare and contrast common independent and collaborative interventions for clients with alterations in oxygenation.

Concept Key Terms

Apnea, *959*
Arterial blood gas
  (ABG), *965*
Atelectasis, *963*
Auscultation, *954*
Bradypnea, *959*
Bronchoscopy, *966*
Bronchovesicular, *955*
Chest x-ray (CXR), *966*
Chronic obstructive
  pulmonary disease
  (COPD), *957*
Crackles, *963*
Cyanosis, *957*
Dyspnea, *959*
Eupnea, *954*
Expiration, *953*
Hypercarbia, *957*
Hypoxemia, *957*

Incentive spirometry, *966*
Inspiration, *953*
Orthopnea, *959*
Oxygenation, *953*
Palpation, *962*
Patent airway, *956*
Peak expiratory flow
  rate (PEFR), *966*
Percussion, *962*
Pneumothorax, *959*
Pulmonary function
  tests (PFTs), *966*
Pulse oximetry, *966*
Respiration, *953*
Rhonchi, *963*
Stridor, *963*
Suctioning, *969*
Surfactant, *955*
Symmetry, *962*

(continued on next page)

▶ NORMAL OXYGENATION

Physiology Review

Adequate oxygenation of the body depends on a healthy, intact respiratory system. The respiratory system obtains oxygen from the air and transports it into the alveoli, where oxygen diffuses into capillaries and is carried by the blood to all cells of the body. The respiratory system also passes carbon dioxide from the body.

The upper respiratory system is the inlet for air into the body. The nose is the typical inlet. The nose is divided into two nares, which are moist, pink, mucosa-lined passageways. Nares warm, humidify, and filter air as it is breathed into the nose. The upper respiratory tract has two protective mechanisms to prevent foreign matter from entering the lower respiratory tract: sneezing and cilia. Foreign matter that enters the nose irritates the nasal passages and induces sneezing. Sneezing is a reflexive action that clears the upper airway. This reflexive action is active even in the neonatal period. Cilia are microscopic fine hairs within the posterior portion of the nares that trap small particles of foreign matter to prevent their entry into the lower respiratory tract. The cilia propel foreign matter into the pharynx to be coughed out or swallowed.

Breathing also happens through the mouth, which allows air to enter the respiratory system through the pharyngeal cavity. The respiratory system shares this cavity with the gastrointestinal system, providing passage for air during breathing and for food or drink during swallowing.

A protective mechanism within the pharyngeal cavity prevents food or drink from entering the lower respiratory tract. The glottis is the opening into the lower respiratory tract. The epiglottis is pendulous tissue that covers the tracheal opening during swallowing or any time foreign matter contacts the glottis. The closure of the epiglottis is a reflexive response.

The lower respiratory tract is enclosed in the musculoskeletal structures of the neck and thoracic cavity. The trachea, which sits midline in the neck, is the entrance for air into the lungs. During normal breathing, the muscular structures of the neck are relaxed and the larynx easily rises and falls with each swallow. The chest wall effortlessly and symmetrically rises and falls with each equally spaced breath. Inspiration is half the rate of expiration. **Eupnea** describes breathing within the expected respiratory rates. **Auscultation**, listening to the body's sounds with a stethoscope, is an important diagnostic tool. When airways are clear and functioning, auscultation of the trachea will reveal a **tubular** sound of air movement, as if produced through a tube.

The trachea bifurcates (divides in two) into two bronchi to access the right and left lungs (**Figures 15–1** ● and **15–2** ●). The right bronchus is shorter and wider than the left. Each bronchus further divides into bronchioles that terminate in the alveoli sacs. These passageways for air dilate and contract. The trachea and larger bronchi are supported by C-shaped cartilage rings, as well as by smooth muscle. The smaller bronchioles are supported by smooth muscles only. Bronchioles deliver air to the alveoli. These

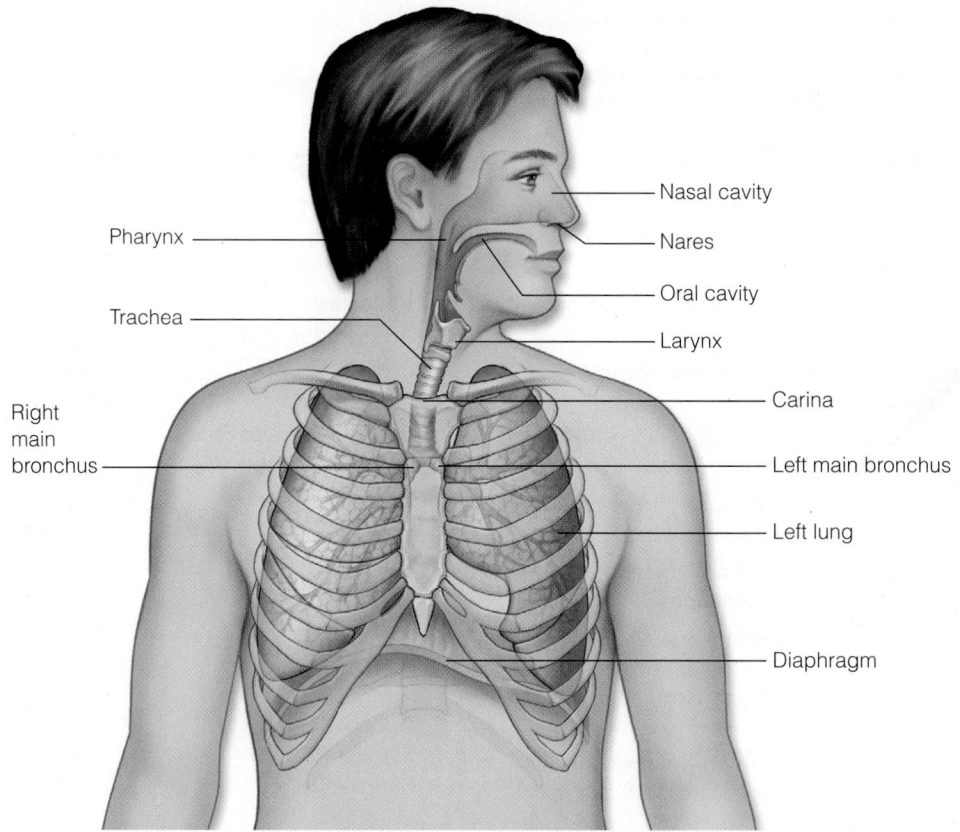

Labels:
- Nasal cavity
- Nares
- Oral cavity
- Larynx
- Carina
- Left main bronchus
- Left lung
- Diaphragm
- Pharynx
- Trachea
- Right main bronchus

Figure 15–1 ● Anatomy of the respiratory system.

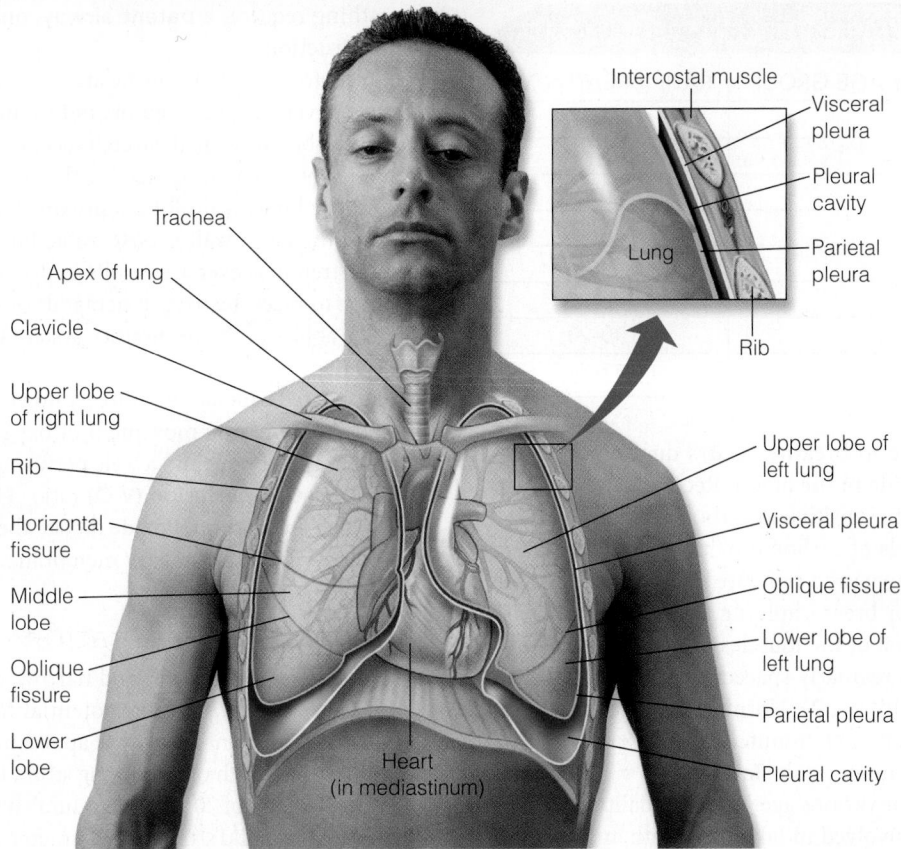

Figure 15–2 ● Anterior view of thorax and lungs.

air passageways dilate and contract as the autonomic nervous system regulates the smooth muscles supporting them. The movement of air within the bronchial tree creates a mixture of sounds of air flowing through a tube and the breeziness of the open alveolar lung fields. This is termed **bronchovesicular** sound.

The lungs are also described in terms of their lobes. The lobes lie obliquely in the thoracic cavity. The right lung has three lobes; the left lung has two lobes. The inferior lobes are the largest. Most of the inferior lobes lie in the posterior thoracic cavity. Each lung has a pleural lining to aid respiration and separate it from the other lung. The pleural lining has two layers, and a minute amount of fluid between the layers allows the structures to glide across one another during respiration.

The final portion of the lower respiratory system is the air sacs. The outcroppings of the air sacs are called alveoli. The alveoli are the portion of the lungs that fulfills the function of the respiratory system. Alveoli are not directly connected to a specific bronchiole, but are interconnected to the terminal airways and to each other (**Figure 15–3** ●). This facilitates the filling of each alveoli with air. The sounds of air moving into and out of the lobes at the alveolar level are soft and breezy, defined as **vesicular**.

The alveoli have specialized cells that produce surfactant. **Surfactant** controls surface tension and keeps the alveoli from collapsing and sticking to themselves. Surfactant is produced only with adequate oxygenation. Alveolar macrophages keep the alveoli region free of microbes and are swept upward from the alveolar region by cilia in the airway passages. Macrophages are large cells of the immune system that remove waste and harmful microorganisms from the alveoli and from other areas of the body. Mast cells in the alveoli mediate the immune response within the airways.

Alveoli have a simple squamous epithelial lining and basement membrane that interface with the basement membrane and epithelial lining of pulmonary capillaries. This interface is where oxygen and carbon dioxide diffusion occurs. The concentration of oxygen is greater in the alveoli than in the blood in the capillaries, so oxygen diffuses across the membranes into the blood. The concentration of carbon dioxide is greater in the blood, so it diffuses into the alveoli.

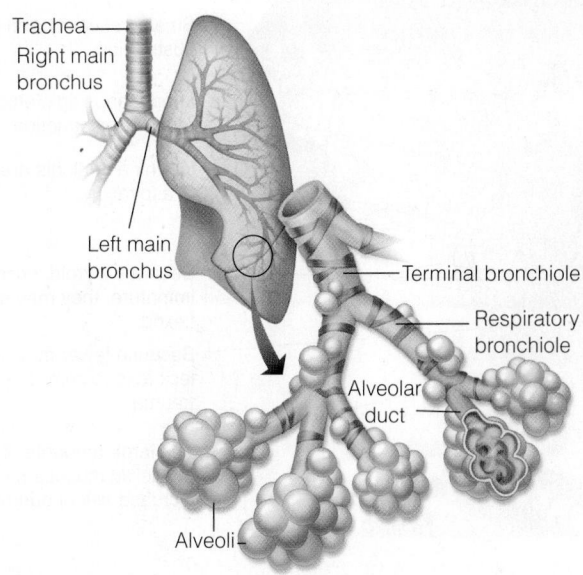

Figure 15–3 ● Respiratory bronchioles, alveolar ducts, and alveoli.

TABLE 15-1 Respirations Throughout the Life Span

VALUE RANGES BY AGE GROUP	RATE (BREATHS/MIN)
Newborns	30–60
Infants	20–40
Preschoolers	20–30
6 years	16–22
10 years	16–20
Adolescence	12–20
Adults	10–20
Older adults	12–24

The typical drive to breathe occurs due to an increased level of carbon dioxide in the blood. Receptor sites within the medulla and pons are sensitive to carbon dioxide levels in the blood. Elevated levels of carbon dioxide induce inhalation of air into the lungs. Yawns and sighs are induced after periods of shallow breathing or breath holding. Exhalation is a passive response to relaxation of the muscles of respiration. The typical breathing rate is regularly spaced, with inspiration half as long as expiration (I:E = 1:2). Normal respiratory rates range from 30 to 60 breaths per minute in newborns to 10 to 20 breaths per minute in an adult. **Table 15-1 ●** shows normal respiratory ranges for various age groups. Quality of breathing refers to the effort involved in taking a breath and the sounds that may occur with inspiration or expiration. Quality of

breathing requires a **patent airway**, one that is open and free of obstruction.

Receptor sites in the aortic arch and carotid arteries monitor oxygen levels. These receptors induce inspiration when oxygen levels fall below normal. Stretch receptors within the lungs control the volume of air inhaled with each breath. During relaxed states, the lungs will fill to approximately 500 mL. The expansion of the chest wall is observable but is neither shallow nor great. Strenuous exercise results in deeper breaths of increasing volume to meet the oxygen demands of skeletal muscles.

The ability of the respiratory system to deliver oxygen to the blood depends on an inflated and well-oxygenated alveolus and an associated capillary with freely flowing blood at an adequate blood pressure. The movement of oxygen across the alveolar–capillary membrane into a well-perfusing capillary is defined as the **ventilation-perfusion (V-Q)** ratio. The concentration levels of oxygen and carbon dioxide dictate the movement of each gas across the alveolar–capillary membrane.

Lifespan Considerations

A child's airway is shorter and narrower than an adult's. These differences create a greater potential for obstruction (**Figure 15-4 ●**). The infant's airway is approximately 4 mm in diameter, about the width of a drinking straw, in contrast to the adult's airway diameter of 20 mm. The child's little finger is a good estimate for the child's tracheal diameter and can be used for a quick assessment of airway size.

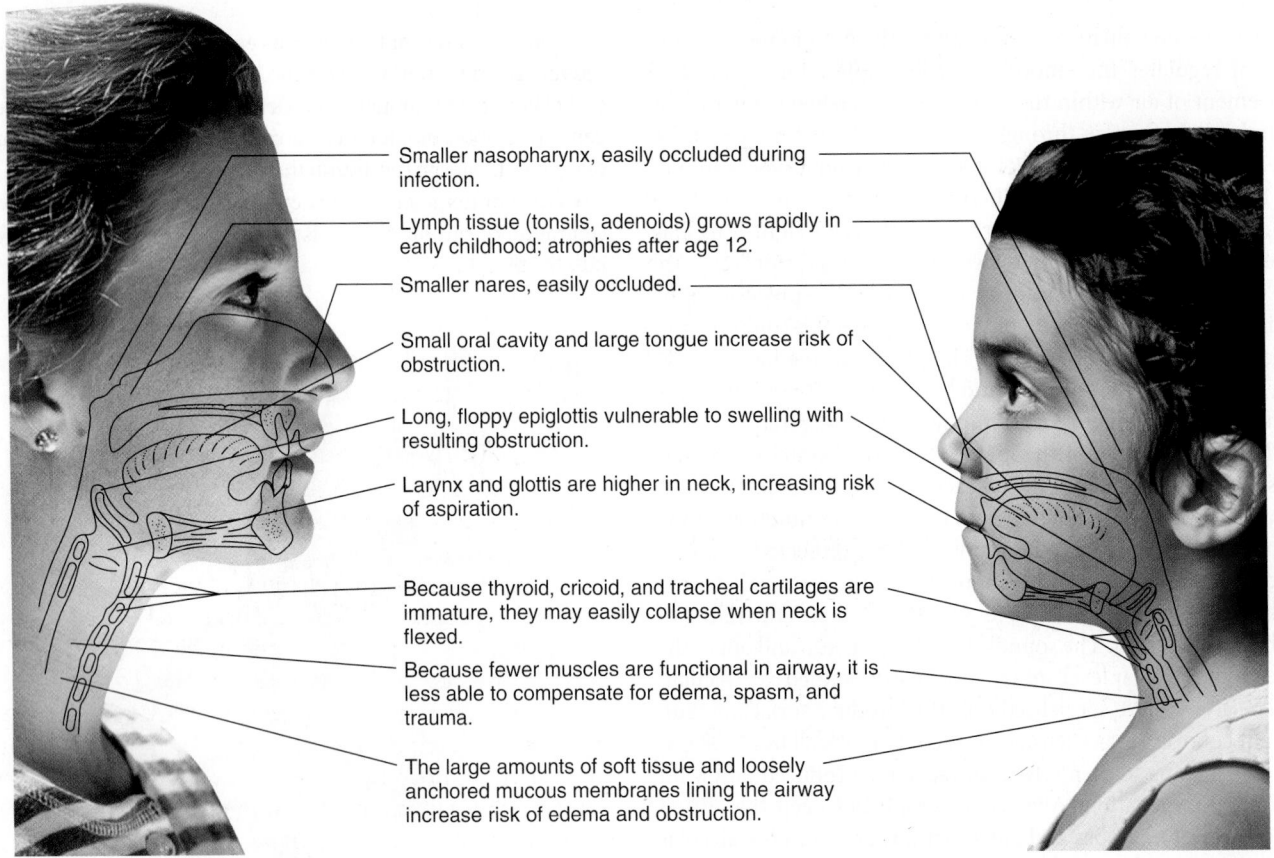

Smaller nasopharynx, easily occluded during infection.

Lymph tissue (tonsils, adenoids) grows rapidly in early childhood; atrophies after age 12.

Smaller nares, easily occluded.

Small oral cavity and large tongue increase risk of obstruction.

Long, floppy epiglottis vulnerable to swelling with resulting obstruction.

Larynx and glottis are higher in neck, increasing risk of aspiration.

Because thyroid, cricoid, and tracheal cartilages are immature, they may easily collapse when neck is flexed.

Because fewer muscles are functional in airway, it is less able to compensate for edema, spasm, and trauma.

The large amounts of soft tissue and loosely anchored mucous membranes lining the airway increase risk of edema and obstruction.

Figure 15-4 ● Children's airways are smaller and less developed than adults' airways. An upper respiratory tract infection, allergic reaction, positioning of the head and neck during sleep, and the small objects children play with can have serious consequences in children.

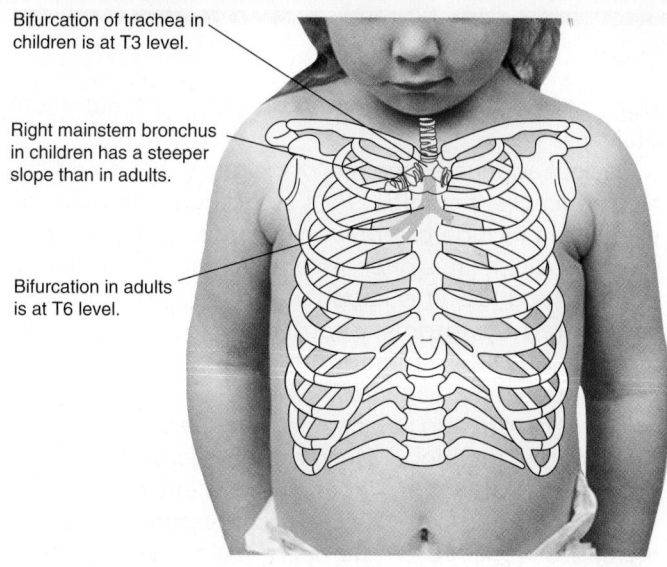

Bifurcation of trachea in children is at T3 level.

Right mainstem bronchus in children has a steeper slope than in adults.

Bifurcation in adults is at T6 level.

Figure 15–5 ● In children, the trachea is shorter and the angle of the right bronchus at bifurcation is more acute than in the adult. When you are resuscitating or suctioning, you must allow for the differences.

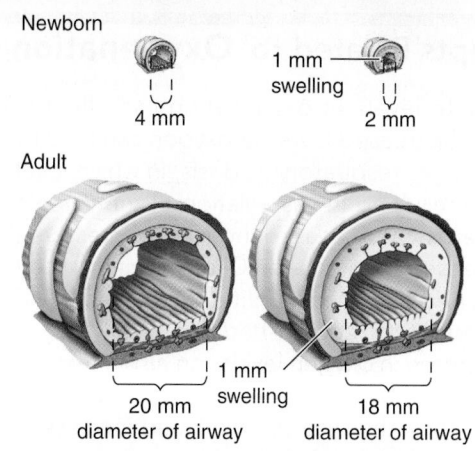

Newborn

1 mm swelling

4 mm

2 mm

Adult

20 mm diameter of airway

1 mm swelling

18 mm diameter of airway

Figure 15–6 ● The diameter of an infant's airway is approximately 4 mm, in contrast to an adult's airway diameter of 20 mm. An inflammatory process in the airway causes swelling that narrows the airway, and airway resistance increases. Note that swelling of 1 mm reduces the infant's airway diameter to 2 mm, but the adult's airway diameter is only narrowed to 18 mm. Air must move more quickly in the infant's narrowed airway to get the same amount of air to the lungs. The friction of the quickly moving air against the side of the airway increases airway resistance. The infant must use more effort to breathe and breathe faster to get adequate oxygen.

The trachea primarily increases in length rather than diameter during the first 5 years of life. Also, the tracheal division of the right and left bronchi is higher in a child's airway and at a different angle than in an adult's (**Figure 15–5** ●). The cartilage that supports the trachea is more flexible and has the potential to compress the airway if the head and neck are not appropriately positioned. The child's narrower airway causes a greater increase in airway resistance (the effort or force needed to move oxygen through the trachea to the lungs) in any condition causing edema of the airway or accumulation of secretions (**Figure 15–6** ●).

At birth, the lung tissue contains only 25 million alveoli, which are not fully developed, and the distal bronchioles that extend to the alveoli are narrow and fewer in number than in an adult. After 8 years of age, the alveoli begin increasing in size and complexity. The number of alveoli increases to 300 million by adulthood (Brashers, 2010). As a result, disease of a small number of alveoli can have a much larger impact on a child's clinical condition because of the increased proportion of lung involvement. For example, involvement of 1 million alveoli secondary to pneumonia would be 4% of the lung in a pediatric client but only 0.33% of an adult's lung.

▶ ALTERATIONS TO OXYGENATION

Mild impairments in oxygenation can cause fatigue, irritability, and discomfort. More severe alterations in oxygenation can result in tissue hypoxia, depleting the body's ability to transmit oxygen to vital systems and, without intervention, may quickly become life threatening. The Concepts Related to Oxygenation feature provides a brief overview of the relationship of oxygenation to acid–base balance, cellular regulation, cognition, comfort, and perfusion.

Alterations and Manifestations

Alterations in oxygenation can be described in relation to changes in breathing patterns, patency of airway, or interference with gas exchange. Damage to the supporting thoracic structure, either by injury or disease, can interfere with effective respiration. Irritation or inflammation of the respiratory mucosa also affects the ability of the respiratory system to obtain adequate oxygenation for the cells within the body.

Although physiologically elevated levels of carbon dioxide drive respiration, if the carbon dioxide levels are abnormally increased, a condition known as **hypercarbia**, the body loses its ability to respond appropriately to increased levels of carbon dioxide. When this happens, instead of increased carbon dioxide levels initiating the breathing response, decreased levels of oxygen initiate the drive to breathe. This is commonly seen in individuals with **chronic obstructive pulmonary disease (COPD)** resulting from prolonged cigarette smoking, because smoking is a common cause of prolonged elevated levels of carbon dioxide.

Hypoxemia is defined as a decreased level of oxygen. Chest wall in-drawing is an early indicator of hypoxemia. **Cyanosis** is a late sign of hypoxemia and is seen as a blue tinge to the skin in fair individuals. In individuals with darker pigmentation, cyanosis may present as gray coloration of the skin. An indicator of chronic hypoxemia is clubbed nail beds. Clubbed nail beds have an angle of 180° or greater, depending on the duration of time an individual has had hypoxemia.

The airway of an infant is very small in diameter. It can be occluded with minimal amounts of sputum or swelling from inflammation. Infants are obligatory nose breathers; therefore, even stuffy noses can interfere with the infant's breathing process. Children, especially infants and toddlers, learn about their world by placing things into their mouths and noses. Small objects may become caught in their airways, interfering with breathing.

Concepts Related to **Oxygenation**

Inadequate levels of oxygenation can affect acid–base balance. Decreased levels of oxygen can lead to a condition known as respiratory acidosis, in which levels of CO_2 increase, resulting in vasodilation of the vessels. The client experiences increased intracranial pressure (ICP) and an increased heart rate. Clinical manifestations can include headache, irritability, decreased level of consciousness (LOC), and flushed skin.

A decrease in oxygen levels can also affect cellular regulation. When oxygen is decreased, as seen with anemia or blood loss, the systemic workload increases, shunting blood from the periphery to the vital organs. Manifestations include fatigue, pallor, jaundice, and tachycardia.

Clients with impaired oxygenation may also experience cognitive impairment. The client may exhibit memory loss, slurred speech, or may appear incoherent. It is essential for the nurse to carefully assess a client with signs of impaired cognition in order to rule out acute brain injury.

Lack of adequate amounts of oxygen in the blood can also affect client comfort. Pain associated with ischemic events can include cerebral pain, cardiac pain, and pulmonary pain. Pain is often associated with shock due to severe blood loss. It is important for the nurse to assess for related symptoms when this occurs, especially increased pulse, respirations, blood pressure, restlessness, anxiety, and diaphoresis (sweating).

Perfusion can also be affected by inadequate amounts of oxygen in the blood. Decreased tissue perfusion creates oxygen deficit to organs. The client may exhibit changes in pulse rate and blood pressure due to an increased workload on the heart. Color, capillary refill, and orientation may be affected due to decreased oxygenation to the tissues.

CONCEPT	RELATIONSHIP TO OXYGENATION	NURSING IMPLICATIONS
Acid–Base Balance		
■ Respiratory acidosis	↑CO_2 →vasodilation → ↑ICP and pulse rate.	■ Client c/o headache, irritability, ↓LOC, flushed skin. ■ Important in chest trauma, aspiration, pneumonia, OD. ■ Be alert in clients with problems r/t airway clearance, limited ambulation, anxiety or signs/symptoms of ↓O_2.
Cellular Regulation		
Anemias: ■ Blood loss ■ Glucose-6-phosphate dehydrogenase (G6PD) deficiency ■ Aplastic	↓O_2 increases systemic workload and shunts blood from periphery to vital organs.	■ Be alert to signs/symptoms of fatigue, pallor, jaundice, tachycardia. ■ Anticipate need for vitamin supplements, blood transfusions, dietary changes. ■ Consider activity intolerance.
Cognition		
	↓O_2 to brain can cause changes in cognition.	■ Assess mentation. Rule out acute brain trauma before considering other causes.
Comfort		

Pain from ischemic events including:
■ Cerebral
■ Cardiac
  • Pediatric congenital issues such as heart defects
  • Adult infarcts, congestive failure, valvular issues, cardiomyopathy
■ Shock states
■ Pulmonary
	↓O_2 to tissues manifests as pain.	■ Assess related symptoms such as ↑pulse, respirations, BP, restlessness, anxiety, diaphoresis; client reports of discomfort.
		■ Anticipate need for additional assessments, medications for pain relief, diversional therapies.

Concepts Related to **Oxygenation** (continued)

CONCEPT	RELATIONSHIP TO OXYGENATION	NURSING IMPLICATIONS
Perfusion		
	↓ tissue perfusion creates oxygen deficit to organs.	■ Assess perfusion including pulses, nail beds, color, body position for comfort, orientation. ■ Administer oxygen. ■ Anticipate need for pharmacotherapy to improve cardiac output. ■ Surgery to correct defect. ■ Monitor arterial blood gases.

Adults also may be at risk of catching a foreign object in their airways. Large bites of improperly chewed and swallowed food can become lodged in the throat, interfering with the passage of air into the lungs. Older adults are at even greater risk of choking on food because their cough reflex response is decreased. The incidence of gastroesophageal reflux increases with age, increasing the risk of aspiration of food into the lower respiratory tract.

Loss of airway patency can result from increased sputum production from upper and lower respiratory infection or irritation. Thick sputum secretions are of special concern in relation to blocking large and small airways. Inflammation of airways due to infections or irritants narrows airways, decreasing the movement of air through the respiratory system.

Respiratory rate, rhythm, depth, and quality determine adequate oxygenation to the cells. A respiratory rate greater than 20 breaths per minute in adults is called **tachypnea**. Anxiety or stress may cause an individual to breathe very rapidly, inhaling and exhaling deeply. Hyperventilation is rapid and deep inhalation and exhalation of air from the lungs. In hypoventilation, a reduced amount of air enters the alveoli, resulting in a decrease of oxygen and an increase of carbon dioxide. A respiratory rate of less than 10 breaths per minute in adults is called **bradypnea**. **Apnea** is the absence of breathing. Continuous apnea is termed *respiratory arrest* and is life threatening.

Dyspnea, labored breathing or shortness of breath that is uncomfortable or painful, also occurs when breathing is insufficient to meet oxygen demand. Exertional dyspnea occurs with activity. **Orthopnea** is difficulty breathing when an individual is supine. The nurse's ability to differentiate changes in respiratory rate is critical when working with any individual but particularly critical when working with older adult clients, because pulmonary function declines with age. Chest walls and airways lose their elasticity, becoming more rigid; musculoskeletal strength decreases; and the effort to breathe increases.

Several breathing patterns with irregular rates, rhythms, depth, and quality indicate abnormalities within other body systems. Kussmaul breathing occurs in the presence of metabolic acidosis and results in very deep and rapid breaths. These deep, rapid exhalations rid the body of large amounts of carbon dioxide, which affects the acid–base balance. Cheyne-Stokes respirations exhibit

as deep, rapid breathing and slow, shallow breathing with periods of apnea. Cheyne-Stokes respirations are seen in individuals with congestive heart failure, increased intracranial pressure, and drug overdoses. Biot respirations are seen in individuals with central nervous system disorders. Biot respirations present as shallow breathing with periods of apnea. Benzodiazepines, barbiturates, and opioids may cause decreased depth and rate of breathing due to their oxygenation-compromising central nervous system effects.

Abnormalities within the alveolar–capillary bed system alter V-Q ratios. Airflow in an alveolus blocked by sputum, inflammation with its complementary swelling, atelectasis, or fluid volume excesses can cause decreased ventilation. Blood clots, plaque buildup, and emphysemic alveoli interfere with capillary blood flow. Each of these V-Q mismatches results in inadequate oxygenation of body cells. Any and all of these types of V-Q mismatch may occur simultaneously (**Figure 15–7 ●**).

Any alteration that impairs the oxygenation process can be life threatening. In addition to determining and then treating the presenting alteration, it is critical to determine its cause. A mild case of exercise-induced asthma may only require administration of an albuterol inhaler prior to the individual participating in exercise or sports activities. By contrast, COPD is much more difficult to treat.

In addition to the exemplars detailed in this module, other diseases and some injuries, such as a fractured pleural rib, can cause impairment in oxygenation. One disease that presents multiple problems for clients and their physicians is sickle cell disease. An inherited blood disorder, sickle cell disease impairs the transport of oxygen through the blood. Sickle cell can cause a variety of complications, including organ failure. For more information, see the exemplar on Sickle Cell Disease in the module on Cellular Regulation.

Pneumothorax, or a partial lung collapse resulting from air or gas collecting in the lung or in the pleural space that surrounds the lungs, is a respiratory emergency. A pneumothorax that appears without any known cause is termed a *spontaneous pneumothorax*. Risk factors for this type of pneumothorax include emphysema, cystic fibrosis, and tuberculosis. A tension pneumothorax results from injury (e.g., a fractured rib) or as a result of a progressive lung disease, such as asthma or emphysema. Tension pneumothorax is more difficult to treat than pneumothorax and

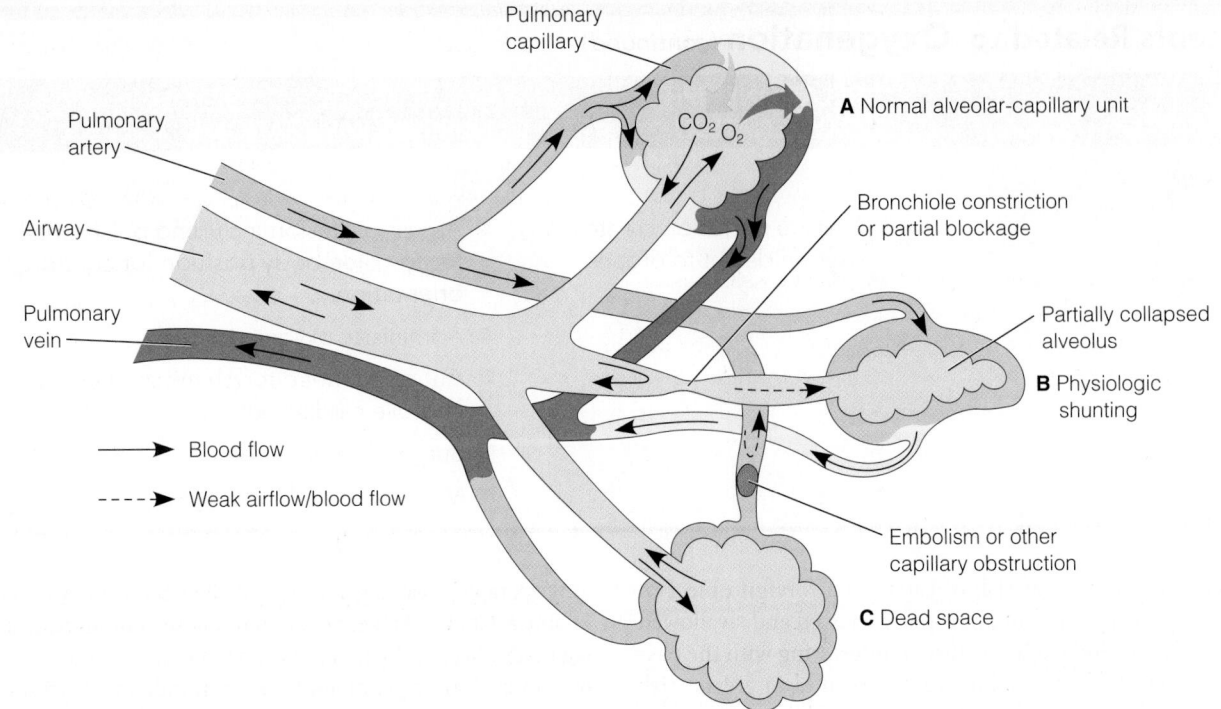

Figure 15–7 ● Ventilation-perfusion relationships. *A*, Normal alveolar–capillary unit with an ideal match of ventilation and blood flow. Maximum gas exchange occurs between alveolus and blood. *B*, Physiological shunting: a unit with adequate perfusion but inadequate ventilation. *C*, Dead space: a unit with adequate ventilation but inadequate perfusion. In the latter two cases, gas exchange is impaired.

Alterations and Therapies **Oxygenation**

ALTERATION	DESCRIPTION	MANIFESTATIONS	INTERVENTIONS AND THERAPIES
Hypoxemia	Decreased level of oxygen	▪ Early manifestations include chest wall in-drawing. ▪ Late manifestation = cyanosis.	▪ Administer oxygen if O_2 falls below 90. ▪ Identify and treat underlying cause.
Dyspnea	Labored breathing or shortness of breath	▪ Clearly audible, labored breathing; anxiety. ▪ Distressed facial expression. ▪ Nasal flaring.	▪ Identify and treat the underlying cause. ▪ Administer oxygen if O_2 falls below 90.
Apnea	Absence of breathing	▪ Lack of respiratory effort that can lead to respiratory arrest.	▪ Identify and treat underlying cause. ▪ Administer respiratory stimulants, as appropriate.
Tachypnea	A respiratory rate greater than 20 breaths per minute for children and adults; 60 breaths per minute for an infant	▪ Excessive rapid breathing. ▪ Rapid breathing at rest. ▪ Shallow breathing.	▪ Identify and treat underlying cause.
Orthopnea	Difficulty breathing when lying down	▪ Dyspnea while lying down.	▪ Identify and treat underlying cause ▪ Elevate the head, neck, and chest while sleeping.
Pneumothorax	Partial lung collapse	▪ Chest pain. ▪ Shortness of breath.	▪ Identify and treat underlying cause. ▪ Observation ▪ Needle or chest tube insertion ▪ Surgery

can result in heart failure. Signs and symptoms of a pneumothorax include sudden sharp pleuritic pain, worsened by movement such as breathing and coughing; asymmetrical chest wall movement; shortness of breath; and cyanosis.

Prevalence

The inability to oxygenate properly can occur at any point during the life span. The very young (less than 1 year of age) and older adults (over the age of 65) are at increased risk for alterations in oxygenation. Very young children are more susceptible to respiratory disorders that affect oxygenation. Older adults carry an increased risk of developing a variety of health impairments (e.g., respiratory ailments, cardiovascular issues) that can affect oxygenation.

Genetic Considerations and Nonmodifiable Risk Factors

A genetic link seems to be associated with alterations in oxygenation. Studies have examined the genetic effect of hemoglobin and hematocrit. There appears to be a significant inherited pattern of variation in hemoglobin concentration, whereas the hematocrit shows a lower genetic effect. Differences in hemoglobin concentration and hematocrit between the genders add to the evidence of genetic control of these variables and, therefore, the ability to oxygenate. Women typically have lower concentrations of hemoglobin and hematocrit compared to males (Kravitz & Robergs, 2013).

CASE STUDY \\ PART 1

Melissa Dawson is a 30-year-old Caucasian female who was diagnosed with severe persistent asthma as a young child. She presents at her pulmonologist's office at 0900 on Thursday after calling and requesting to be worked in because she is not "getting enough air." As the nurse working with Ms. Dawson's pulmonologist, you conduct her client interview and initial assessment when she comes to the clinic. It takes a little time to get through the client interview; Ms. Dawson can only speak a few words at a time and appears short of breath. Ms. Dawson reports that she came down with bronchitis over the holiday weekend and went to an urgent care clinic to get an antibiotic. The P.A. at the clinic prescribed a Z-pack (azithromycin). Ms. Dawson states she has been on 40 mg prednisone since Monday for asthma symptoms and has been using her rescue inhaler 4 times daily in addition to her Flovent Diskus (fluticasone) inhaler. Ms. Dawson tells you that she woke up in the middle of the night unable to get enough air, and that her nail beds were blue. She used her rescue inhaler and her symptoms improved enough that she decided not to go the emergency department but to wait and call the office first thing this morning.

You observe that Ms. Dawson is holding back tears. She is sitting on the exam table leaning forward with her hands on her knees. Her voice is hoarse. Her face is pale and she has dark rings around her eyes. Ms. Dawson tells you her voice only gets hoarse when she is very, very sick. On taking her vitals, you note that Ms. Dawson's blood pressure is elevated and her respirations are 32. Her oxygen saturation (SaO_2) is 91% on room air. When you auscultate her lungs, you hear decreased breath sounds. The pulmonologist puts her on 4 LPM oxygen by nasal cannula.

Clinical Reasoning Questions Level I

1. What symptoms of altered oxygenation does Ms. Dawson have?
2. Why might Ms. Dawson's blood pressure be high?
3. Why might Ms. Dawson be close to tears?

Clinical Reasoning Questions Level II

4. What is the priority nursing diagnosis for Ms. Dawson at this time?
5. What independent nursing interventions can you perform to help make Ms. Dawson more comfortable while she waits for the specialist?
6. *Refer to the exemplar on Asthma in this module:* What additional interventions should the nurse anticipate implementing as part of Ms. Dawson's immediate care?

▶ PREVENTION

A number of factors affect a healthy respiratory system. Exposure to airborne irritants (e.g., cigarette smoke, pollen, chemicals, pollution) may produce an inflammatory response within the airways. Infectious illnesses of the respiratory tract and hemoglobin disorders such as sickle cell disease interfere with effective respiratory function. Lifestyle behaviors may affect respiratory health. Some medications affect respiratory rate and depth. Generally, inflammation, infection, sputum production, and compromised airflow contribute to alterations in respiratory health. *Healthy People 2020* has several directives related to maintaining or attaining respiratory health. These include the following:

- Management of environmental air quality to decrease the concentration of respiratory irritants affecting asthma and COPD in the United States. Environmental air quality includes interior and external air sources. A decrease in the use of tobacco products is necessary to stop the unnecessary damage to the health of tobacco users and those exposed secondhand to tobacco smoke. Exposure to polluted air in homes and workplaces and to tobacco smoke exacerbates COPD, asthma, and respiratory syncytial virus; it also is associated with sudden infant death syndrome.
- Vaccination is encouraged to decrease transmission of preventable diseases, many of which are transmitted by respiratory secretions. Many illnesses historically seen in children now are prevented by immunization. Immunization for influenza and pneumonia protects adults from serious respiratory illness.

Modifiable Risk Factors

Several modifiable risk factors are associated with alterations in oxygenation. Any alteration that affects the heart's ability to pump and circulate blood throughout the body, such as hypertension or atherosclerosis, can cause alterations in oxygenation as the blood carries and circulates oxygen. Other modifiable risk factors that affect the body's ability to oxygenate properly include obesity, type 2 diabetes, smoking, and stress and anxiety. Taking control of these variables can decrease the risk a client has for developing alterations in oxygenation.

Assessment Interview Oxygenation

Current Respiratory Problems

- Have you noticed any changes in your breathing pattern (e.g., shortness of breath, difficulty breathing, need to be in upright position to breathe, or rapid and shallow breathing)?
- If so, which of your activities might cause these symptoms to occur?
- How many pillows do you use to sleep at night?

History of Respiratory Disease

- Have you had colds, allergies, asthma, tuberculosis, bronchitis, pneumonia, or emphysema?
- How frequently have these occurred? How long did they last? And how were they treated?
- Have you been exposed to any pollutants?

Lifestyle

- Do you smoke? If so, how much? If not, did you smoke previously, and when did you stop?
- Does any member of your family smoke?
- Is there cigarette smoke or other pollutants (e.g., fumes, dust, coal, asbestos) in your workplace?
- Do you drink alcohol? If so, how many drinks (mixed drinks, glasses of wine, or beers) do you usually have per day or per week?
- Describe your exercise patterns. How often do you exercise and for how long?

Presence of Cough

- How often and how much do you cough?
- Is it productive, that is, accompanied by sputum, or nonproductive, that is, dry?
- Does the cough occur during a certain activity or at certain times of the day?

Description of Sputum

- When is the sputum produced?
- What is the amount, color, thickness, and odor of the sputum?
- Is it ever tinged with blood?

Presence of Chest Pain

- How does going outside in the heat or the cold affect you?
- Do you experience any pain with breathing or activity?
- Where is the pain located?
- Describe the pain. How does it feel?
- Does it occur when you breathe in or out?
- How long does it last, and how does it affect your breathing?
- Do you experience any other symptoms when the pain occurs (e.g., nausea, shortness of breath or difficulty breathing, light-headedness, palpitations)?
- What activities precede your pain?
- What do you do to relieve the pain?

Presence of Risk Factors

- Do you have a family history of lung cancer, cardiovascular disease (including strokes), or tuberculosis?
- The nurse should also note the client's weight, activity pattern, and dietary assessment. Risk factors include obesity, sedentary lifestyle, and diet high in saturated fats.

Medication History

- Have you taken or do you take any over-the-counter or prescription medications for breathing (e.g., bronchodilator, inhalant, narcotic)?
- If so, which ones? And what are the dosages, times taken, and results, including side effects? Are you taking them exactly as directed?

▶ ASSESSMENT

Assessment of a client's respiratory system includes both subjective and objective data obtained through physical assessment and taking the client's health history. Physical assessment begins with simple observation during the initial interaction with the client. During the health history, the nurse elicits information on lifestyle behaviors, any current trouble breathing, presence of cough or sputum, and any risk factors (e.g., occupational exposure to chemicals, allergies, recent illness, cigarette smoking). See the Assessment Interview: Oxygenation.

Nursing Assessment

The assessment of any body system requires a systematic approach using all five senses to ensure that nothing is missed. The nurse uses her eyes to observe expected and unexpected findings, a process called *inspection*. The nurse uses **palpation** to feel the areas related to the body system for **symmetry**, equality of the size, shape, or condition of opposite sides of the body. Next, the nurse uses **percussion**, a method of tapping the chest or back to assess underlying structures; tones heard during per-

cussion determine solid-filled or air-filled spaces at the area percussed. Finally, the nurse uses auscultation to hear the sounds within the respiratory system (**Box 15–1** ●). Use of a stethoscope facilitates the hearing of sounds within the body. Any assessment is best supported by obtaining a full set of vital sign measurements with pulse oximetry.

The client presenting with breathing problems may provide a number of objective and subjective indicators that confirm the report. Self-posturing (leaning forward or against a table or wall to breathe) may be evident. A client may have difficulty speaking, taking breaths in the middle of sentences. The individual's voice may be raspy. In the absence of a productive cough, repeated throat clearing may indicate the presence of phlegm. Individuals who cannot breathe well often become frustrated when answering questions because the effort to answer further impairs breathing, and the effort to breathe quickly brings on fatigue. When working with any individual, as well as with someone with impaired breathing, the nurse should be patient and sympathetic. A pulse oximetry reading above 90% may not be a true indicator of the level of respiratory distress if the client has used an albuterol inhaler within 30–60 minutes of presenting

Box 15–1   Adventitious Breathing Sounds

A number of adventitious sounds can be heard while auscultating the lower respiratory tract:

- **Stridor** is a high-pitched sound within the trachea and larynx that suggests narrowing of the tracheal passage.
- **Crackles** are high-pitched popping sounds, much like when one pours milk over crisped rice cereal. Crackles are heard on inspiration and are caused by fluid associated with or resulting from inflammation, or exudates, within the lung fields or localized atelectasis. **Atelectasis** is the collapse of lung tissue affecting all or part a lung, impacting the exchange of oxygen and carbon dioxide. The primary cause of atelectasis is the obstruction of the bronchus serving the affected area.

- **Rhonchi** is a long, low-pitched sound that continues throughout inspiration. Rhonchi suggests blockage of large airway passages, which can sometimes be cleared with coughing.
- **Wheezing** is a high-pitched whistling sound most often heard on expiration and caused by the narrowing of bronchi, but wheezes can also be heard on inspiration.
- When inflamed pleural surfaces rub together, they can make a low-pitched, grating sound. This occurs more during inspiration, but can also occur during expiration.

Oxygenation Assessment

ASSESSMENT/ METHOD	NORMAL FINDINGS	ABNORMAL FINDINGS	LIFESPAN OR DEVELOPMENTAL CONSIDERATIONS
Nasal Assessment			
Inspect the nose symmetry.	The nose should be midline and symmetrical.	- Asymmetry indicates trauma or surgery.	- Nasal flaring in the neonate may be indicative of respiratory compromise.
Inspect the nasal cavity using a flashlight.	The septum should fall midline and be intact. The mucosa of the nares is pink and moist without drainage. Both nares should be patent.	- Redness and/or swelling is observed. - Deviated septum narrows or occludes one naris. - Foreign bodies may be found in the nares, especially of infants, toddlers, and preschoolers. - Purulent drainage occurs. - Watery nasal drainage occurs. - Pale turbinates are seen.	- Nasal passages of neonates and small children are smaller than those of adults. Ensuring a clear nasal cavity may decrease risk for respiratory compromise as neonates and infants are nasal breathers.
Respiratory Rate Assessment			
Count respiratory rate for one full minute, counting one inspiration and one expiration as one breath.	Normal respiratory rate is eupnea (see Table 15–1 for development impact on rate).	- Bradypnea - Tachypnea - Apnea - Cheyne-Stokes respirations	- A child's respiratory rate is higher than that of an adult's. Rely on both sight and touch to obtain an accurate respiratory rate. Neonates are sporadic breathers so short periods of apnea (less than 15 seconds) are expected.
Assess quality of breathing: determine regularity in timing. Assess depth of inspiration. Observe effort to breathe.	The I:E ratio is normally 1:2. The cycle of inspiration and expiration should be followed by a resting period in which the sensors of the respiratory system will initiate the next cycle. Normal breathing is referred to as eupnea.	- Shortness of breath - Dyspnea - Orthopnea	- Infants and children have softer chest walls and depend more heavily on the diaphragm to breathe. Therefore, they exhibit what is known as "seesaw" breathing. - In older adults, lifestyle choices such as smoking can affect the quality of breathing, as can the development of respiratory diseases.
Inspection of Thoracic Cavity			
Anteroposterior diameter is half the transverse diameter.	Normal ratio is 1:2. (See **Figures 15–8** ● and **15–9** ●)	- Anteroposterior equals transverse thoracic diameter measurements, called a barrel chest.	- Rapid growth early in life, the plateau in young adulthood, and decline in later life can affect normal ratios.

(continued on next page)

Oxygenation Assessment (*continued*)

ASSESSMENT/ METHOD	NORMAL FINDINGS	ABNORMAL FINDINGS	LIFESPAN OR DEVELOPMENTAL CONSIDERATIONS
Inspection of the Muscles of Breathing			
	The chest wall gently rises and falls with each breath. The muscles in the neck are relaxed. The trachea is mid-line. The intercostal muscles raise the chest upward and outward with inhalation, then calmly relax with exhalation.	■ Retraction of the intercostals occurs. ■ Sternocleidomastoid muscles of the neck contract. ■ Posturing occurs.	■ Infants and children are more likely than adults to experience retractions and posturing with respiratory ailments. The adult client is more likely to compensate in other ways.
Inspection and Palpation of the Thoracic Wall for Symmetry			
	Symmetrical movement of the hands is observed with sym-metrical hand placement on the chest wall. The trachea is midline.	■ Asymmetry of movement occurs. ■ Decreased expansion occurs. ■ The trachea shifts from mid-line.	■ Rapid growth early in life, the plateau in young adulthood, and decline in later life can affect normal symmetry. Respiratory ailments can also affect thoracic wall symmetry.
Skin Assessment in Relation to the Respiratory System			
Assess color of skin	Skin color should be normal for race or ethnicity.	Cyanosis is a blue tinge to the skin in fair individuals and gray coloration of the skin in darker pigmented individuals.	■ Acrocyanosis is a normal finding for neonates/newborns. Cyano-sis at any other stage of devel-opment is considered an abnormal finding.
Assess nail beds	Nail beds are an extension of the finger and are normally curved with a 160° angle of the nail bed to the finger.	Clubbed nail beds have an angle of 180° or greater, depending on the duration of time an individ-ual has had hypoxemia.	■ Clubbing of the nails can occur with chronic cardiovascular or respiratory disease. Knowledge of the client's baseline is essential to the assessment process.

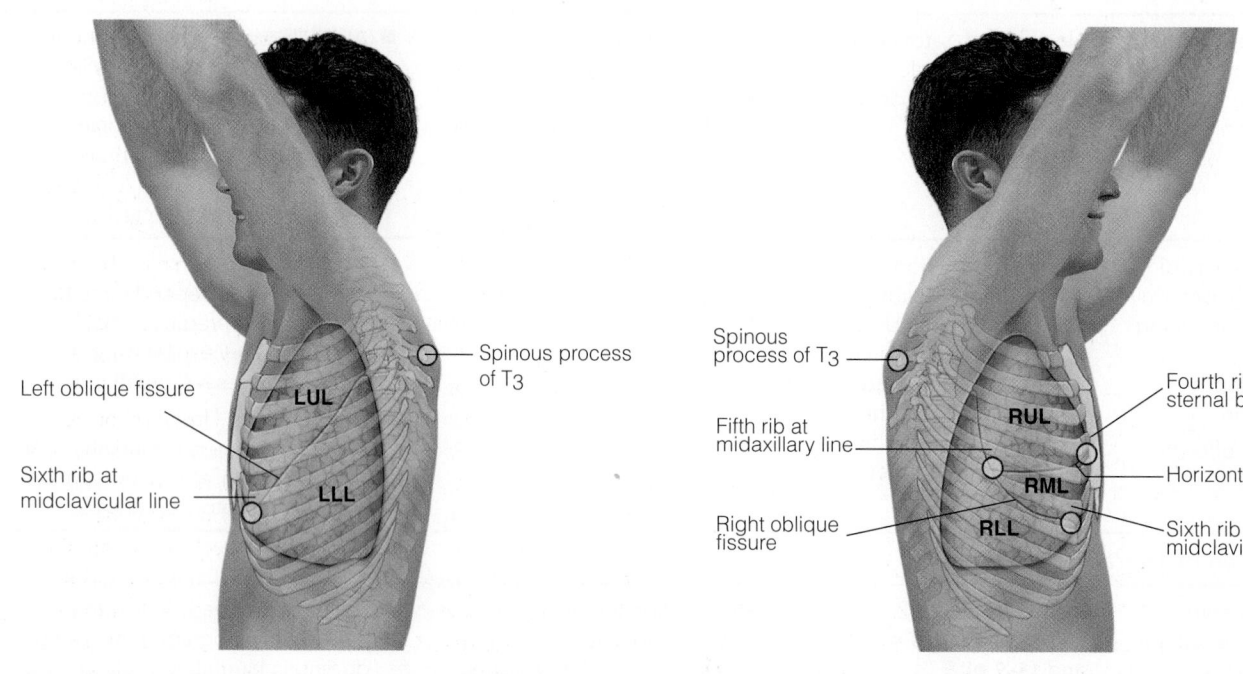

Figure 15–8 ● Lateral view of lobes of the left lung.

Figure 15–9 ● Lateral view of lobes of the right lung.

Lifespan Considerations Respiratory Development

Infants

■ Respiratory rates are highest and most variable in new-borns. The respiratory rate of a neonate or newborn is 30–60 breaths per minute.

■ Infant respiratory rates average about 30 breaths per minute.

■ Because of the structure of the ribcage, infants rely almost exclusively on diaphragmatic movement for breathing. This is seen as abdominal breathing, as the abdomen rises and falls with each breath.

Children

■ The respiratory rate gradually decreases, averaging around 25 breaths per minute in the preschooler and reaching the adult rate of 12–18 breaths per minute by late adolescence.

■ During infancy and childhood, upper respiratory infections are common but usually not serious. Infants and pre-schoolers also are at risk for airway obstruction by foreign objects, such as coins and small toys. Cystic fibrosis, a chronic disease usually identified in early childhood, is a congenital disorder that affects the lungs, causing them to

become congested with thick, tenacious (sticky) mucus. Asthma is another chronic disease often identified in child-hood. The airways of the asthmatic child react to stimuli such as allergens, exercise, or cold air by constricting, becoming edematous, and producing excessive mucus. Airflow is impaired, and the child may wheeze as air moves through narrowed air passages.

Older Adults

■ Older adults are at increased risk for acute respiratory dis-eases such as pneumonia and chronic diseases such as emphysema and chronic bronchitis. Nursing assessment of older adults with difficulty breathing includes assessing for possible infection.

■ Pneumonia may not present with the usual symptom of a fever, but may present with atypical symptoms, such as confusion, weakness, loss of appetite, and increased heart rate and respiration.

■ In assessing adults with chronic illness, it is important to assess for any changes in medication (including compli-ance with the therapeutic regimen), fluid and nutrition sta-tus, and cognition.

at the clinic or emergency department. Increased frequency of use of albuterol inhalers or nebulizer treatments indicates a severe respiratory episode. See the Oxygenation Assessment for an outline of the assessment procedure.

Clients who present with impairment at or near respiratory failure will not be able to respond to questions. Assessment questions should be tailored and asked of any family member or friend accompanying the client to the emergency depart-ment. The client's physician should be notified immediately on the client's arrival at the hospital. The immediate concern is to return respiratory status as near to normal as possible. Adrena-line may be given in the case of respiratory failure related to anaphylaxis or allergic reaction. Chest tubes and ventilators may be necessary. Support for family is also important at this time, as is an understanding of the client's religious and cul-tural preferences. An example of religious practice is having prayers said over those who are very sick that may bring com-fort to the family when the client is diagnosed with a critical respiratory illness.

Lifespan and Cultural Considerations

Variability in respiratory rates and susceptibility to illness impact assessment of clients at different points on the lifespan (see the Lifespan Considerations feature). For clients who are pregnant, assessment considerations include the following:

■ Assess for rhinitis of pregnancy (nasal stuffiness) and epistaxis (nosebleeds). Pregnant woman often experience nasal stuffi-ness and nosebleeds due to increased amounts of estrogen.

■ Assess for emphysema, asthma, or chronic obstructive pul-monary disease due to an increased anterior-posterior (AP) diameter.

■ Assess for tactile fremitus due to respiratory disease.

■ Assess for low-pitched resonance of moderate intensity due to high diaphragm.

■ Assess vesicular breath sounds with a longer inspiratory phase (3:1) (Davidson, London, & Ladewig, 2011).

Diagnostic Tests

Specific diagnostic tests are used to assess for abnormalities of the respiratory system and to monitor for changes in individuals with chronic oxygenation impairment. Tests are used to determine the presence of inflammation or infection, detect changes in acid-base balance, and view thoracic structures.

A sputum specimen may be used to identify the presence of microbes, metabolites of inflammation, and immunoglobulins. A sputum culture is used to identify specific microbes within the lower respiratory tract. Sputum is expectorant matter that may contain all or some mucus, cellular debris, blood, microorgan-isms, and purulent matter from the respiratory tract. It is impor-tant to ensure that the liquid obtained from an individual is from the lung fields and not from spit from his or her mouth. The proper identification of the microbe facilitates the selection of the appropriate antibiotic, antiviral, or antifungal agents to treat the inflammation. Excessive use of antibiotics for inflammatory processes that do not respond to the prescribed antibiotic has contributed to the emergence of drug-resistant microbes.

Arterial blood gas (ABG) provides a direct indication of oxy-gen and carbon dioxide exchange and the acid–base balance within the blood. The major chemical components monitored by ABG are hydrogen ions (pH), carbon dioxide (CO_2), oxygen (O_2), and bicarbonate (HCO_3^-). See **Table 15–2** for normal ABG laboratory values. Each ABG component is reviewed in turn.

TABLE 15–2 Arterial Blood Gas Values

pH	7.35–7.45
$PaCO_2$	35–45 mm Hg
PaO_2	75–100 mm Hg
HCO_3^-	24–28 mEq/l

Initial assessment focuses on the oxygen values of the ABG. The oxygen value is defined by the amount of oxygen bound to hemoglobin (SaO_2) and the amount of oxygen dissolved in blood serum (PaO_2). An oxygen saturation value (SaO_2) in a healthy individual without any respiratory abnormalities is greater than 95%. The values of oxygen dissolved in blood serum (PaO_2) range from 75 to 100 mmHg. Oxygen levels that indicate hypoxemia should be treated by administering oxygen. Mild hypoxemia ranges from 60 to 79 mmHg, moderate hypoxemia ranges from 40 to 59 mmHg, and severe hypoxemia is less than 40 mmHg (Pruitt, 2010).

The pH level is then assessed. The normal pH range is narrow, from 7.35 to 7.45; pH values less than 7.35 indicate acidosis and values greater than 7.45 indicate alkalosis (Kee, 2014).

Carbon dioxide values are assessed. Carbon dioxide is an acid expired from the lungs; changes in carbon dioxide levels are regulated by respiratory patterns. Carbon dioxide values range from 35 to 45 mmHg; values less than 35 mmHg indicate alkalosis and values greater than 45 mmHg indicate acidosis (Kee, 2014).

Bicarbonate (HCO_3^-) is a base excreted via the kidneys; changes in bicarbonate levels are metabolic responses of the kidneys. Bicarbonate values range from 24 to 28 mEq/L. Values less than 24 mEq/L indicate acidosis and values greater than 28 mEq/L indicate alkalosis (Kee, 2014).

The body's natural inclination is to maintain a homeostatic balance. In relation to ABGs or acid–base balance, this means that the body will alter the carbon dioxide and bicarbonate levels to return the pH level to within normal range. Altering the individual components within acid–base balance is called *compensation*. A blood gas that has a pH less than 7.35 indicates acidosis. If the same blood gas has a carbon dioxide greater than 45 mmHg, respiratory acidosis is present. The next value to be assessed is the bicarbonate level. If the value is in the normal range, the blood gas has not compensated. If the bicarbonate level is elevated and the pH remains elevated, the blood gas is partially compensated. A compensated blood gas will have carbon dioxide levels and bicarbonate levels that cause the pH to be in its normal range (Pruitt & Jacobs, 2004). A pH within normal range allows the body to achieve homeostasis.

Pulse oximetry is a noninvasive method of assessing arterial blood oxygenation. A clip or adhesive device with an infrared probe analyzes blood as it perfuses past the view of the two opposing sensors of the probe. Expected SaO_2 values in a healthy individual (one who has no alterations in pulmonary function) are greater than 95%.

Individuals who respond poorly to bronchodilators or who have poor oxygenation may benefit from assessment of their pulmonary function. Diagnosis and differentiation of reactive airway diseases necessitate the use of **pulmonary function tests (PFTs)**. PFTs demonstrate changes in pulmonary health related to ventilation airflow, lung volume and capacity, and the diffusion of gas. They also incorporate spirometry, peak flow meters, and the body plethysmograph. PFTs include measurement of inspired and expired air as well as the diffusion ability of the alveolar–capillary membrane. A spirometer is used to measure airflow and lung volumes. **Incentive spirometry** measures the forced emptying of alveolar gas. Simply put, spirometry measures air exhaled from the lungs. Spirometry tests may be carried out in a primary care provider's office or clinic. Levels for forced expiratory volume over 1 second (FEV_1) and the ratio of FEV_1 to forced vital capacity (FEV_1/FCV) are used to screen for pulmonary function deficits. **Box 15–2 ●** diagrams all the pulmonary function tests. Results outside the anticipated range for the individual's age, gender, height, and weight may indicate the need to alter care interventions.

Peak expiratory flow rate (PEFR) is used to monitor the ability of an individual to exhale a specific volume of air related to the individual's age, gender, height, and weight. PEFR allows individuals with asthma to monitor the reactivity of their lungs and adjust asthma treatments according to the plan developed by the primary care provider and the individual. PEFR is not diagnostic for reactive airway diseases such as asthma and COPD.

An anterior-posterior **chest x-ray (CXR)** allows for two-dimensional visualization of the contents of the thoracic cavity. Chest x-rays reveal the presence of fluids, exudates, or masses within the thoracic cavity. CT scans and MRIs provide more information about the structures within the thoracic cavity. Thoracic computed tomography (CT) produces cross-sectional images of the contents of the chest. Thoracic CT may be used with dye to determine the presence of pulmonary embolism. Magnetic resonance imaging (MRI) allows for assessment of pulmonary embolism without the use of dye and is best for visualizing soft tissue and vascular structures. MRI is contraindicated in the individual who has implanted metal devices.

Pulmonary angiography and pulmonary V-Q scans demonstrate the ventilation and perfusion activities of the respiratory system. A pulmonary angiogram is used to identify structural changes in the pulmonary vasculature. Structural changes that cause occlusions may include blood clots, tumors, aneurysms, and overinflated alveoli. A pulmonary ventilation-perfusion scan (V-Q scan) uses radioactive isotopes to identify defects of ventilation and perfusion. Injected radioactive albumin helps identify defects of perfusion, whereas inhaled radioactive gas identifies defects of ventilation.

Bronchoscopy, a procedure that allows direct visualization of the lungs, is usually performed by a pulmonologist but may be performed by a primary care or emergency care physician. A bronchoscope is inserted orally into the trachea and advanced to the bronchi bifurcation. Bronchoscopy may be used for direct visualization and photography of pulmonary structures, suctioning of mucous plugs from larger bronchioles, and collection of lung tissue biopsy specimens. Sedation is necessary for client comfort.

Thoracentesis is both an intervention and a test. Thoracentesis is performed to drain excessive pleural fluid from between the pleural linings. The fluid drained is often analyzed for blood, fiber, and microbe content.

Box 15–2 Pulmonary Function Tests

Pulmonary function tests (PFTs) are performed in a pulmonary function laboratory. After preparing the client, a nose clip is applied and the unsedated client breathes into a spirometer or body plethysmograph, a device for measuring and recording lung volume in liters versus time in seconds. The client is instructed on how to breathe for specific tests; for example, to inhale as deeply as possible and then exhale to the maximal extent possible. Using measured lung volumes, respiratory capacities are calculated to assess pulmonary status. The specific values determined by PFT and illustrated in **Figure 15–10** ● include the following:

- *Total lung capacity (TLC)* is the total volume of the lungs at their maximum inflation. Four values are used to calculate TLC:
  a. *Total volume (TV)*, the volume inhaled and exhaled with normal quiet breathing (also called tidal volume)
  b. *Inspiratory reserve volume (IRV)*, the maximum amount that can be inhaled over and above a normal inspiration
  c. *Expiratory reserve volume (ERV)*, the maximum amount that can be exhaled following a normal exhalation
  d. *Residual volume (RV)*, the amount of air remaining in the lungs after maximal exhalation
- *Vital capacity (VC)* is the total amount of air that can be exhaled after a maximal inspiration. It is calculated by adding together the TV, IRV, and ERV.

- *Inspiratory capacity (IC)* is the total amount of air that can be inhaled following a normal quiet exhalation. It is calculated by adding the TV and IRV.
- *Functional residual capacity (FRC)* is the volume of air left in the lungs after a normal exhalation. The ERV and RV are added to determine the FRC.
- *Forced expiratory volume (FEV1)* is the amount of air that can be exhaled in 1 second.
- *Forced vital capacity (FVC)* is the amount of air that can be exhaled forcefully and rapidly after maximum air intake.
- *Minute volume (MV)* is the total amount or volume of air breathed in 1 minute.

In older clients, residual capacity is increased, and vital capacity is decreased. These age-related changes result from the following:

- Calcification of the costal cartilage and weakening of the intercostal muscles, which reduce movement of the chest wall
- Vertebral osteoporosis, which decreases spinal flexibility and increases the degree of kyphosis, further increasing the anterior-posterior diameter of the chest
- Diaphragmatic flattening and loss of elasticity.

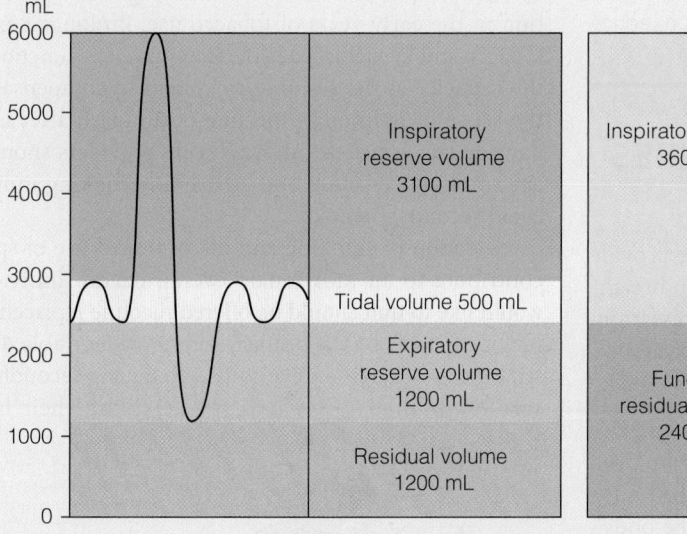
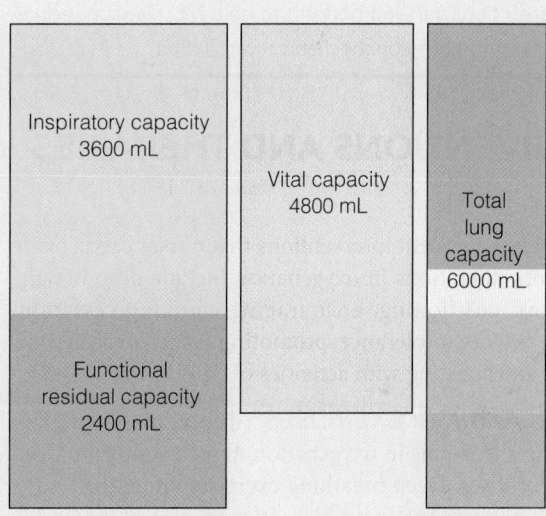

Figure 15–10 ● The relationship of lung volumes and capacities. Volumes (in milliliters) shown are for an average adult male.

CASE STUDY \\ PART 2

Ms. Dawson is prescribed Advair Diskus (fluticasone and salmeterol) to replace her Flovent Diskus and has a follow-up appointment in 7 days. She fills her prescription for Advair and begins it later that evening. Upon trying to go to sleep, Ms. Dawson experiences difficulty breathing when lying down. She takes two puffs of her rescue inhaler and props herself up with three pillows and feels more comfortable. She falls asleep without difficulty.

At 0400 the next morning, Ms. Dawson awakens coughing. She gets up for a drink of water and continues to cough and has trouble catching her breath. She is sweating profusely and begins to feel dizzy. Ms. Dawson is able to make it back to her bed and calls her mother, but she is unable to explain her symptoms before passing out. Ms. Dawson's mother is concerned when her daugh-

ter does not respond. Aware of Ms. Dawson's recent exacerbation, she calls 911.

Ms. Dawson is transported to the emergency department. You are the admitting nurse in the emergency department (ED). The paramedics give you their field report: 30-year-old female found unconscious in her home. Vital signs upon initial assessment include a heart rate of 100; respiratory rate of 28 breaths per minute; blood pressure elevated at 140/92; and temperature within normal limits. Paramedics report that initial pulse oximeter readings were 85% but they improved to 90% with oxygen administration—8 LPM by face mask. Ms. Dawson is continued on 8 LPM oxygen by face mask in the ED. She is now alert and oriented but says she still feels like she cannot catch her breath. Current pulse oximeter reading is 93%. The physician on call orders a blood gas analysis, which is drawn per protocol.

Blood gas results reveal severe respiratory acidosis. You perform a follow-up respiratory assessment and you note that breath sounds are significantly decreased and she appears cyanotic. Pulse oximeter readings have fallen to 90% despite increasing her oxygen to 10 LPM by face mask. Ms. Dawson is admitted to the hospital for further treatment.

Clinical Reasoning Questions Level I

1. Why would Ms. Dawson experience easier breathing with the use of pillows at bedtime?

2. Why does Ms. Dawson feel dizzy and pass out?

3. What does a pulse oximeter measure? Is this an accurate way to measure oxygenation?

4. Ms. Dawson's blood gas results "reveal severe respiratory acidosis." Based on this, what would you expect her ABG results to be?

Clinical Reasoning Questions Level II

5. Why did the pulmonologist add Advair to the current treatment regimen?

6. Why is the finding of significantly decreased breath sounds important?

7. *Refer to the exemplar on ARDS in this module.* What independent interventions can you perform to help Ms. Dawson reduce her anxiety while she is on mechanical ventilation?

▶ INTERVENTIONS AND THERAPIES

Independent

Examples of independent interventions that nurses can provide to clients with alterations in oxygenation include deep breathing exercises, positioning, encouraging smoking cessation, monitoring activity intolerance, promoting secretion clearance, suctioning, and assisting with activities of daily living (ADLs).

DEEP BREATHING EXERCISES Individuals who are experiencing alterations in oxygenation may benefit from deep breathing exercises. Deep breathing exercises affect the body's sympathetic nervous system, which, in turn, affects the body's respiratory system. Controlling respiratory effort can ultimately improve oxygenation.

Deep breathing exercises are known as diaphragmatic, or abdominal, breathing. The diaphragm is a large muscle that is located between the chest and the abdomen. When the diaphragm contracts, it is forced down, causing the abdomen to expand. This expansion causes negative pressure within the chest and forces air into the lung while also pulling blood into the chest and, therefore, improving venous return to the heart.

Individuals can be taught deep breathing exercises by using the following steps:

1. Instruct the individual to place one hand on the chest and another hand on the abdomen while taking a deep breath. The hand on the abdomen should rise higher than the hand on the chest. This ensures the diaphragm is pulling air into the base of each lung.

2. Instruct the individual to exhale through the mouth while depressing the abdomen. This ensures that all air is being expelled.

This exercise should be repeated several times a day in order to train the body in the technique of deep breathing.

POSITIONING Optimal positioning can have a positive effect on oxygenation. Individuals experiencing alterations in oxygenation benefit from being placed in the Fowler position (**Figure 15–11** ●). Fowler position allows for improved breathing because it decreases the compression of the chest due to gravity.

Fowler position has several variations. High-Fowler position elevates the client's head 80 to 90 degrees; Fowler position elevates the client's head 45 to 60 degrees; and semi-Fowler position elevates the client's head 30 to 45 degrees. High-Fowler position may be used to feed a client on feeding precautions or to deliver a breathing treatment. Fowler position may be used to increase comfort during eating and other activities. Semi-Fowler may be used for clients receiving tube feedings to decrease the risk for aspiration.

ENCOURAGING SMOKING CESSATION Tobacco smoke exposure causes increased mucous production and reduced cilia action within the airway passages. Individuals who smoke present with a chronic cough and sputum production in the early years of tobacco use. Prolonged exposure to tobacco smoke yields a decline in pulmonary function. Because the capacity of the respiratory system to compensate is great, the sense of pulmonary decline occurs well after irreversible damage has occurred. All healthcare providers should encourage smoking cessation and advise nonsmoking individuals to avoid secondary smoke.

Cessation of smoking and discontinued use of spit tobacco contribute to an individual's overall health. Individuals who would like to quit should be offered nicotine replacement therapies, as ordered by the primary care provider. **Table 15–3** ● lists strategies to decrease tobacco use. Reducing secondhand exposure of children to tobacco smoke within their homes and

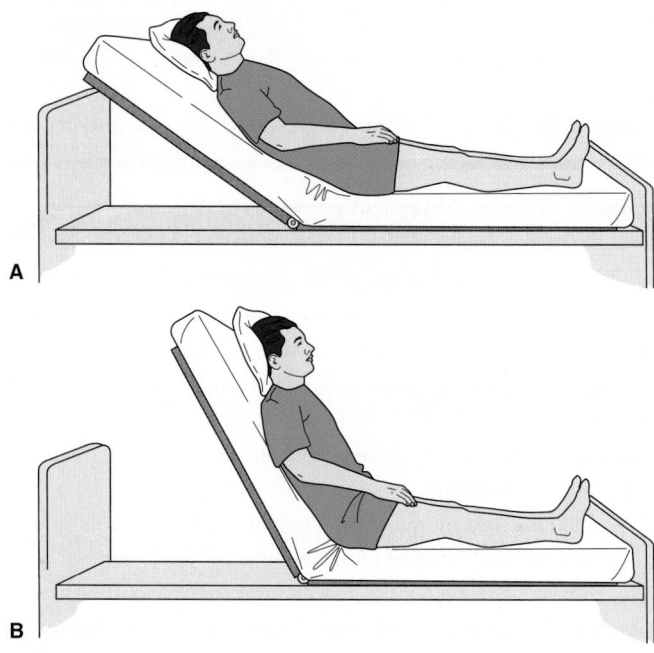

Figure 15–11 ● *A,* Fowler position. *B,* High-Fowler position.

TABLE 15–3   Interventions for Tobacco Cessation

ASK	ADVISE	ASSESS	ASSIST	ARRANGE
Identify and document tobacco use status for every individual at every healthcare interaction.	Urge every tobacco user to quit in a clear, strong, and personalized manner.	Determine if the tobacco user is willing to attempt to quit tobacco use at this time.	Request tobacco cessation medication order from primary care provider. Provide resources for counseling and support groups for the individual willing to attempt to quit tobacco use.	Establish a plan for follow-up contact for the individual willing to attempt to quit tobacco use within 1 week of quit date. Continue to ask tobacco users about quitting tobacco use at each visit.
Nurses document tobacco use with admission history and physical assessment.	Nurses provide tobacco cessation publications and teach about physiological consequences of tobacco use with daily care interactions such as taking vital signs.	Nurses ask if individuals have attempted quitting tobacco before, what was effective, what did not work, and encourage trying with present visit.	Nurses seek nicotine replacement during hospitalizations and suggest to individuals who have had nicotine replacement during hospitalization that they are on their way to quitting.	Nurses collaborate with individuals who desire to quit to arrange tobacco cessation support group contacts and request in-hospital tobacco cessation teaching.

Source: Adapted from the Tobacco Cessation Clinical Practice Guidelines as established by the U.S. Department of Health and Human Services. Used with permission.

decreasing the exposure to secondhand smoke in public buildings will diminish the detrimental effects of tobacco for non-smoking individuals.

For more information on cessation of smoking, see the exemplar on Nicotine Use in the module on Addiction.

MONITORING ACTIVITY TOLERANCE   Alterations in the respiratory system can affect an individual's activity levels. An individual may have insufficient physiological or psychological energy to endure or complete required or desired daily activities. For the client with poor oxygenation, fatigue or weakness can occur from scheduling too many activities too close together. Dyspnea or shortness of breath occurs at varying points in an exercise program, depending on the individual's endurance level. Nurses may need to adapt schedules for clients who are hospitalized in order to space periods of activity with periods of rest. For clients who manage their treatment at home, the nurse may need to provide education related to activity tolerance.

PROMOTING SECRETION CLEARANCE   Lung sounds that indicate the presence of fluids or exudates will benefit from deep breaths and coughing to clear pulmonary secretions. Clients unable to clear their own secretions will require suction. Individuals who are producing sputum with a cough may require the collection of a sputum specimen. They may benefit from postural drainage to clear secretions from various lung fields. (See *Companion Skills Manual* text for these skills.)

SUCTIONING   When clients have difficulty handling their secretions or an airway is in place, suctioning may be necessary to clear air passages. **Suctioning** is aspirating secretions through a catheter connected to a suction machine or wall suction outlet. Even though the upper airways (the oropharynx and nasopharynx) are not sterile, sterile technique is recommended for all suctioning to avoid introducing pathogens into the airways.

Suction catheters may be either open tipped or whistle tipped (**Figure 15–12 ●**). The whistle-tipped catheter is less irritating to respiratory tissues, although the open-tipped catheter may be more effective for removing thick mucous plugs. An oral suction tube, or Yankauer device, is used to suction the oral cavity (**Figure 15–13 ●**). Most suction catheters have a thumb port on the side to control the suction. The catheter is connected to suction tubing, which in turn is connected to a collection chamber and suction control gauge.

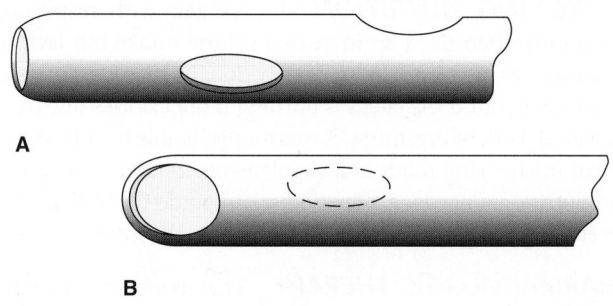

A

B

Figure 15–12 ● Types of suction catheters. *A,* Open tipped. *B,* Whistle tipped.

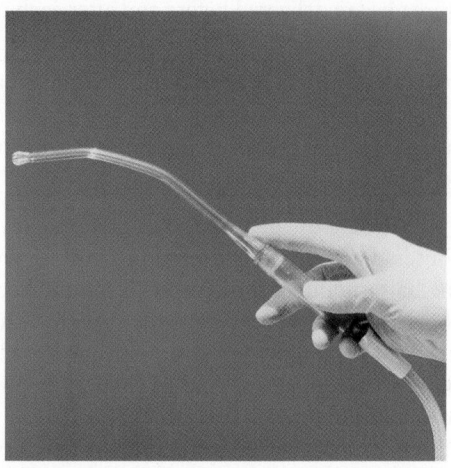

Figure 15–13 ● Oral (Yankauer) suction tube.

Infants

- A bulb syringe is used to remove secretions from an infant's nose or mouth. Care needs to be taken to avoid stimulating the gag reflex.

Children

- A catheter is used to remove secretions from an older child's mouth or nose.

Older Adults

- Older clients may have cardiac and/or pulmonary disease, increasing their susceptibility to hypoxemia related to suctioning. Watch closely for signs of hypoxemia. If noted, stop suctioning and hyperoxygenate.

The nurse decides when suctioning is needed by assessing the client for signs of respiratory distress or evidence that the client is unable to cough up and expectorate secretions. Dyspnea, bubbling or rattling breath sounds, poor skin color (cyanosis), or decreased oxygen saturation (also called O$_2$ sat) levels may indicate the need for suctioning. Good nursing judgment is necessary, because suctioning irritates mucous membranes and can increase secretions if performed too frequently. In other words, suctioning is based on clinical need, not a fixed schedule.

Oral and oropharyngeal suctioning removes secretions from the upper respiratory tract. Nasopharyngeal and nasotracheal suctioning provides closer access to the trachea and requires sterile technique.

Following endotracheal intubation or a tracheostomy, the trachea and surrounding respiratory tissues are irritated and react by producing excessive secretions. Sterile suctioning is necessary to remove these secretions from the trachea and bronchi to maintain a patent airway. The frequency of suctioning depends on the client's health and how recently the intubation was done. Additionally, suctioning may be necessary in clients who have increased secretions because of pneumonia or inability to clear secretions because of altered level of consciousness (LOC).

Suctioning is associated with several complications: hypoxemia, trauma to the airway, nosocomial infection, and cardiac dysrhythmia, which is related to the hypoxemia. The following techniques are used to minimize or decrease these complications:

- **Hyperinflation.** This involves giving the client breaths that are 1–1.5 times the tidal volume set on the ventilator through the ventilator circuit or via a manual resuscitation bag. Three to five breaths are delivered before and after each pass of the suction catheter.
- **Hyperoxygenation.** This can be done with a manual resuscitation bag or through the ventilator and is performed by increasing the oxygen flow (usually to 100%) before suctioning and between suction attempts.

When administering tracheostomy and endotracheal suctioning, the outer diameter of the suction catheter should not exceed one half the internal diameter of the tracheostomy or endotracheal tube to prevent hypoxia (Higgins, 2009). The nurse uses sterile techniques to prevent infection of the respiratory tract. The traditional method of suctioning an endotracheal tube or tracheostomy is sometimes referred to as the *open method*. If a client is connected to a ventilator, the nurse disconnects the client from the ventilator, suctions the airway, reconnects the client to the ventilator, and discards the suction catheter. Drawbacks to the open airway suction system include

the nurse needing to wear personal protective equipment (e.g., goggles or face shield and a gown) to avoid exposure to the client's sputum and the potential cost of one-time catheter use, especially if the client requires frequent suctioning.

With the *closed airway/tracheal suction system* (in-line suctioning) (**Figure 15–14** ●), the suction catheter attaches to the ventilator tubing and the client does not need to be disconnected from the ventilator. The nurse is not exposed to any secretions, because the suction catheter is enclosed in a plastic sheath. The catheter can be reused as many times as necessary until the system is changed. The nurse needs to inquire about the agency's policy for changing the closed suction system.

ASSISTING WITH ACTIVITIES OF DAILY LIVING Individuals who are too weak to provide their own care may need assistance with activities of daily living (ADLs). An individual with compromised oxygenation may have very poor endurance for activities. Personal care must be provided for individuals too weak or too fatigued to carry out their own ADLs. The family and the healthcare team must collaborate to provide sufficient support to the individual with compromised oxygenation, while encouraging the individual to do as much as possible to maintain appropriate physical strength and prevent deteriorating mental condition.

Collaborative

Collaborative interventions and therapies are those interventions that require a medical order or are implemented by other healthcare professionals. A primary example of a collaborative intervention that is used to alleviate alterations in oxygenation is improved nutrition. Other collaborative interventions that may be used for clients with impaired oxygenation include pharmacologic therapies, administration of oxygen, and use of a thoracic catheter.

IMPROVING NUTRITION Individuals with respiratory alterations often need an increased calorie intake but lack the endurance to consume adequate nutrition. Increased calories are necessary because the client is burning more calories due to the increased work of breathing. A nutritionist is able to aid the individual in choosing foods and supplements to meet daily caloric and nutritional needs. A nutritionist can guide the individual in developing menus consisting of frequent, small, nutritious meals.

PHARMACOLOGIC THERAPY Therapeutic management related to maintaining or attaining the health of the respiratory system focuses on the individual's ability to maintain a patent airway through the automatic protective mechanisms in the upper and lower respiratory tracts. The ability of the individual

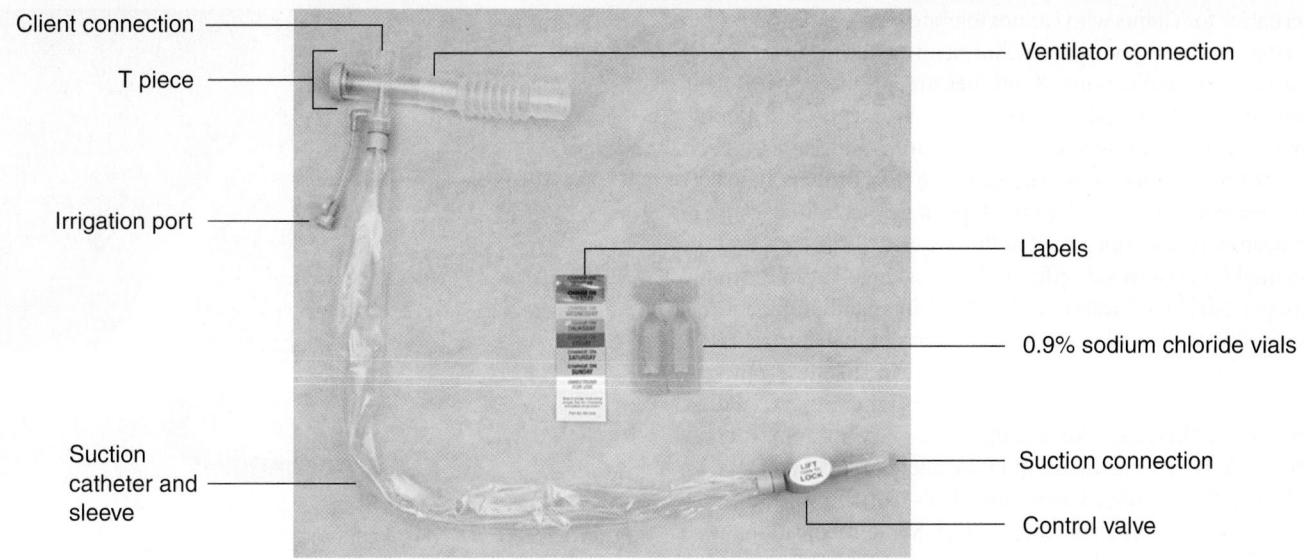

Client connection

T piece

Irrigation port

Suction catheter and sleeve

Ventilator connection

Labels

0.9% sodium chloride vials

Suction connection

Control valve

Figure 15–14 ● A closed airway suction (in-line) system.

to maintain breathing patterns within the acceptable rates and quality for his particular age group is also assessed. Inspiration and expiration must provide adequate ventilation of the lung fields (**Figure 15–15** ●). Individuals also must demonstrate an ability to breathe easily without the use of positioning or accessory muscles. An individual's respiratory pattern should be adequate to maintain adequate gas exchange. A collaborative assessment with the healthcare team helps support the indication of excessive increases or decreases in oxygen or carbon dioxide levels.

A client whose lung sounds indicate narrowing of the airways will benefit from a bronchodilator and possibly an anti-inflammatory agent to improve airway patency. The administration of bronchodilators, as ordered by the primary care provider, relaxes the muscles around the airway, improving airflow. Common bronchodilators of short duration (short-acting beta-agonists, or SABAs) are levalbuterol (Xopenex) and albuterol (Proventil, Ventolin). Inflammation of the airways also contributes to impaired oxygenation. The administration of corticosteroids (various adrenal cortex steroids, such as prednisone) in the presence of inflammation, as ordered by the primary care provider, aids in opening the air passageways by reducing

the inflammation. Because oral steroids have a number of side effects, they are usually administered for a short period of time. Dosages are tapered, with the individual slowly decreasing the amount taken over the course of the prescription.

Individuals with chronic respiratory problems such as COPD and asthma usually benefit from use of a long-acting beta-agonist (LABA) in combination with an inhaled corticosteroid (ICS). Commonly prescribed preparations include Symbicort and Advair. Because LABAs may be contraindicated in some individuals, inhaled corticosteroids are available without the addition of the LABA; common examples are budesonide (Pulmicort) and mometasone furoate (Asmanex).

Short-acting beta-agonists and corticosteroids can be administered through a nebulizer. Nebulizers aerosolize a solution of medication so that it can be directly inhaled by the client via a mouthpiece or mask.

Anticholinergic medications relax the smooth muscles of the airways and decrease mucous secretions by blocking the parasympathetic effect. The most commonly prescribed anticholinergic agent for impaired respiratory function is an ipratropium bromide inhaler (e.g., Atrovent). Inhaled anticholinergics are a good

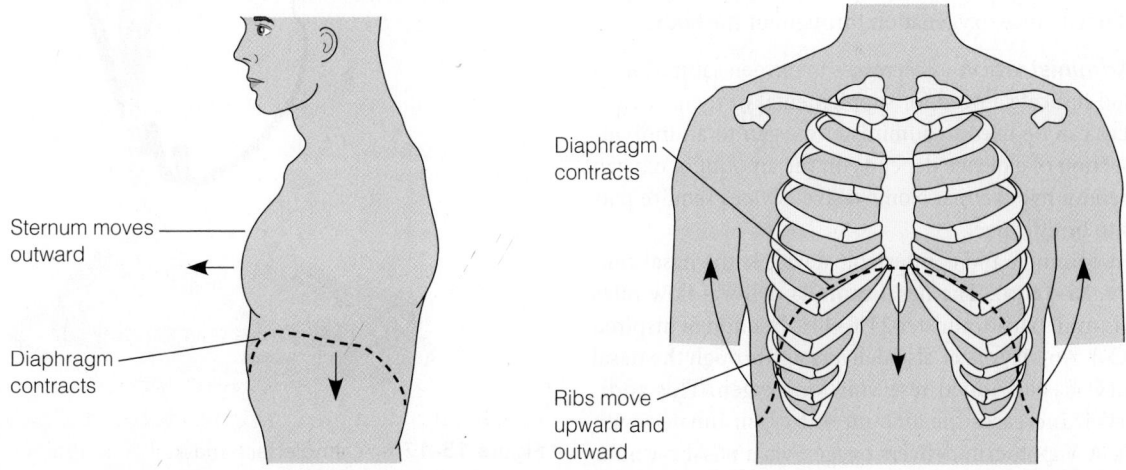

Sternum moves outward

Diaphragm contracts

Diaphragm contracts

Ribs move upward and outward

Figure 15–15 ● Respiratory inspiration: lateral and anterior views. Note the volume expansion of the thorax as the diaphragm flattens.

alternative for clients who cannot tolerate beta-agonists, and can be effective in relieving bronchospasm resulting from use of beta-blocker medications. Xanthines are another type of drug sometimes used to treat asthma, chronic bronchitis, and emphysema. Xanthines cause small airway dilation and increase heart rate and renal blood flow. Theophylline (Slo-Bid) is one of the more generic names used for this type of medication. Because of the narrow therapeutic range of this type of medication and the potential for serious side effects, clients taking xanthines should have periodic blood tests to ensure they are maintaining optimal therapeutic levels and to guard against risk of toxicity.

Additional medications may be prescribed. These can vary depending on the nature of the respiratory impairment. Allergic asthmatic individuals, for example, may take immunotherapy (allergy shots) or other medications for allergies to prevent attacks.

Medication compliance in individuals with chronic or recurrent respiratory impairment is critical. Some medications used for treating respiratory diseases are fairly expensive. Although albuterol and corticosteroids are reasonably inexpensive, LABAs usually are more expensive and are associated with higher insurance copayments. For individuals who require multiple prescription medications to maintain respiratory health, the combined costs of these medications may be overwhelming. Most pharmaceutical companies have programs to assist clients who lack health insurance or whose standard of living is at or close to the poverty level. Most free clinics are able to provide free medication to qualifying individuals. Usually, individuals are not required to see the doctor at the free clinic to receive free medication; a prescription from the treating physician is sufficient.

Teenagers often do not take medications as prescribed, either because they are embarrassed to be seen taking medication or because their hectic schedules do not make it possible for them to be home at certain times to take medication. Additional client teaching may be necessary when working with teenagers.

Older adults may be at risk for accidental noncompliance with medication administration schedules. A nurse working with an older adult exhibiting signs of confusion or early dementia should consult with the client or family members to determine whether additional support is available regarding medication administration.

NONPHARMACOLOGIC THERAPY   Nonpharmacologic therapies for alterations in oxygenation include oxygen administration and thoracic catheter insertion. Each of these therapies can be used to enhance oxygenation throughout the body.

Oxygen Administration   Decreases in oxygen saturation in arterial blood indicate a need for supplemental oxygen. A variety of devices can be used to administer oxygen to an individual. The selection of a device depends on the amount of oxygen needed to relieve hypoxemia. Noninvasive devices require patent airways to be effective.

The most common and comfortable device is the nasal cannula (**Figure 15–16 ●**). The nasal cannula delivers flow rates from 2 to 6 L/min that administer 24%–44% fraction of inspired oxygen (FiO_2). An Oxymizer also delivers air through the nasal passage, but it has an added reservoir for oxygen. This additional reservoir increases the amount of oxygen inhaled with each breath. A Vapotherm delivers oxygen via a nasal cannula, but it warms and filters oxygen and increases the positive end-

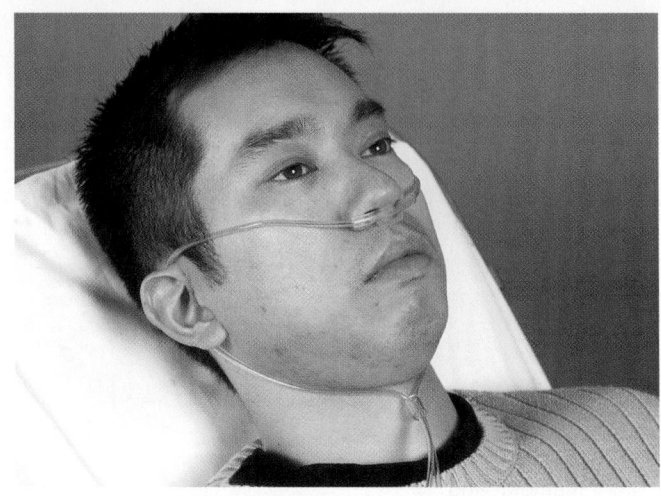

Figure 15–16 ● A nasal cannula.

expiratory pressure of oxygen delivery via the cannula. Vapotherms are used in neonatal intensive care units. Another common device is a simple mask that covers the mouth and nose. It is fitted to the individual's face size. The mask itself provides an additional gas reservoir to that provided by the nasopharynx alone (**Figure 15–17 ●**). Flow rates may be set from 5 to 10 L/min. The FiO_2 delivered is from 30% to 50%. To attain FiO_2 levels of 60% or more, masks that have an attached reservoir are necessary to provide adequate oxygen. The nonrebreather mask has a one-way valve between the attached reservoir and the face mask (**Figure 15–18 ●**). This ensures that appropriate levels of oxygen are inhaled, with no carbon dioxide from exhaled gases. Oxygen delivery at a specified flow rate requires the use of a venturi mask (**Figure 15–19 ●**). Venturi masks are set with a specific oxygen flow rate and specific jet adapter device. Flow rates of 24%–40% may be set with the venturi mask. **Table 15–4 ●** summarizes the types of oxygen devices, along with flow rates and oxygen delivery amounts.

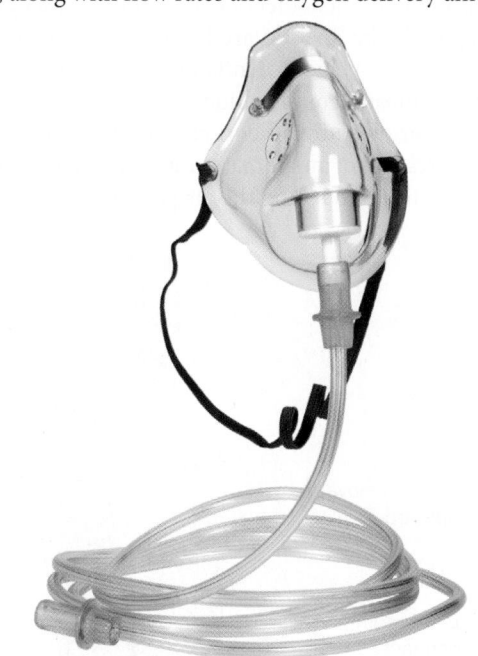

Figure 15–17 ● A simple face mask.
Source: imagedb.com/Shutterstock.

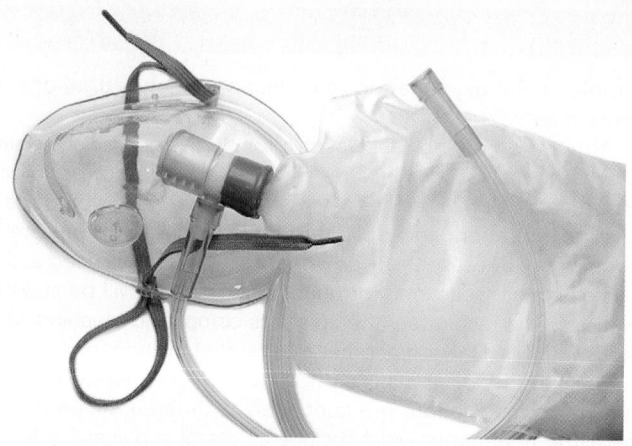

Figure 15–18 ● A nonrebreather mask.
Source: © 72/Fotolia.

DEVICE	FLOW RATE SETTING	OXYGEN CONCENTRATION (FIO$_2$)
Nasal cannula	1–6 L/min	24%–44%
Oxymizer	1–6 L/min	24%–88%
Vapotherm	1–40 L/min	24%–100%
Face mask	5–10 L/min	30%–50%
Nonrebreather	10–15 L/min	Greater than 60%
Venturi mask	Set with jet adapter for flow rate and FiO$_2$	

TABLE 15–4   Oxygen Delivery Systems

> **SAFETY ALERT**
> No one should smoke in a room where supplemental oxygen is being used. Recommend putting a "NO SMOKING" sign in every room where supplemental oxygen is used.

Nursing care for the client receiving supplemental oxygen includes ensuring that flow is sufficient as required, that the client is reasonably comfortable with the manner of oxygen administration, and that indwelling catheters (lines) remain clear. For the client being discharged to home with supplemental oxygen, both the nurse and the respiratory therapist delivering the oxygen to the home must teach the client how to use the devices properly, the importance of checking oxygen levels in tanks, the need for a portable device for trips outside of the house, and the need to maintain the lines and keep them clear of obstruction.

Clients who are prescribed supplemental oxygen may feel they have lost their quality of life. The nurse can assist the client in understanding that supplemental oxygen will help the client maintain quality of life, and that the client can still participate in any number of activities. The nurse should be alert to any possible signs of depression in a client whose oxygen impairment is sufficient to warrant supplemental oxygen. Frustration, rising medical costs, and other issues can contribute to depression in a client with respiratory impairment.

Thoracic Catheter Use   A chest tube, or thoracic catheter, is used to treat conditions in which fluid enters the pleural cavity, causing lung collapse. Inserted under emergency conditions, and treated as a surgical procedure, a chest tube will typically remain in place for 2–5 days until the client's x-rays indicate that all fluid from the pleural cavity has been removed.

There are many nursing considerations when working with a client who has a thoracic catheter, some of which will be specific to the underlying cause of the lung collapse. Typically, however, the nurse will need to do the following:

■ Ensure oxygen therapy is immediately available at all times, if not already ordered and in place.

■ Monitor dressings for drainage and air leakage; follow agency protocol for replacing or securing dressings.

■ Monitor tubing to make sure it is free of kinks or other impediments.

■ Monitor and record client vital signs as ordered.

■ Monitor for and report any decrease in oxygen saturation, any changes in breath sounds, or any tympany or hollow sound with chest percussion.

■ Assess for pain; administer pain medications as needed (PRN), notifying physician of any increase in client restlessness or anxiety.

■ Monitor and report any changes in respiration or any excessive bleeding.

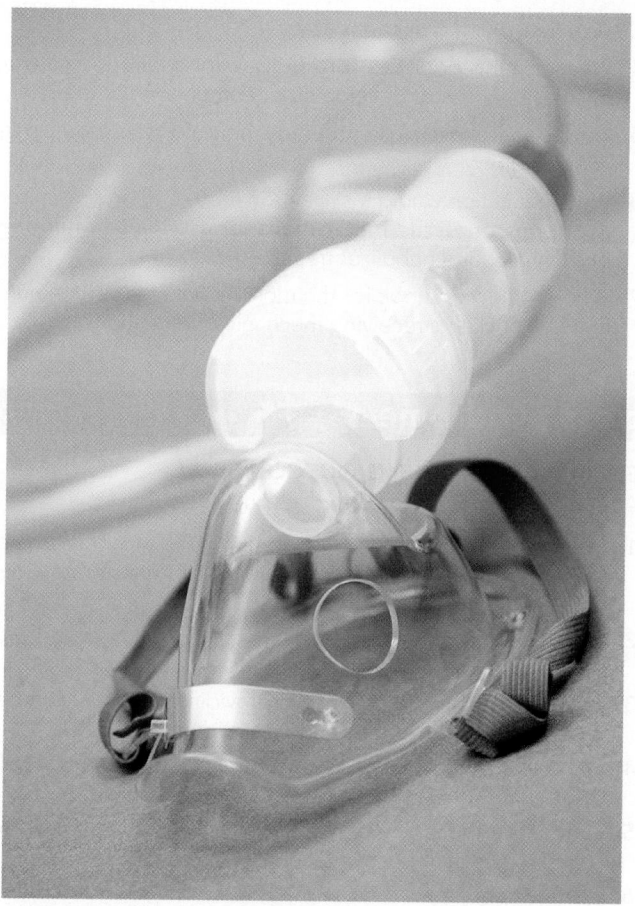

Figure 15–19 ● A venturi mask.
Source: © Eva Vargyasi/Fotolia.

REVIEW The Concept of Oxygenation

RELATE Link the Concepts

Linking the concept of oxygenation with the concept of infection:

1. Why would alterations in oxygenation lead to an increased risk of certain infections?

2. What are some ways to decrease the risk of infections caused by alterations in oxygenation?

Linking the concept of oxygenation with the concept of mobility:

3. How might alterations in oxygenation affect mobility?

4. What are some nursing interventions that can decrease the risk of altered mobility for clients with alterations in oxygenation?

Linking the concept of oxygenation with the concept of perfusion:

5. How are the concepts of oxygenation and perfusion related?

6. What disease processes related to oxygenation can affect the body's ability to perfuse adequately?

Linking the concept of oxygenation with the concept of cognition:

7. How might an alteration in oxygenation impact an individual's orientation?

8. How might lack of oxygenation to the brain be detected?

READY Go to Companion Skills Manual

REFER Go to Pearson Nursing Student Resources
nursing.pearsonhighered.com

- Additional review materials

REFLECT Case Study \\ Part 3

Ms. Dawson has been hospitalized for 10 days. During the course of her care, she required tracheal intubation and mechanical ventilation. Further examination of her symptoms including chest x-rays and blood cultures revealed pneumonia was the culprit for her sudden asthma exacerbation. Within 24 hours of beginning IV antibiotics, Ms. Dawson was weaned from the ventilator and extubated. She has completed a 10-day course of IV antibiotics and no longer requires

supplemental oxygenation to maintain oxygen saturations of more than 93%.

You are preparing Ms. Dawson for discharge to her home. Discharge instructions include self-administration of nebulizer treatments 3 or 4 times per day as needed, as well as chest percussion, vibration, and postural drainage (PVD) for persistent congestion. Because she lives alone, Ms. Dawson will need assistance with her self-care. Fortunately, her mother will be staying with her. The respiratory therapist has completed teaching sessions with Ms. Dawson and her mother that include how to perform chest PVD, as well as how to use the nebulizer. Her admission medications are continued, with the addition of the nebulizer treatments, which include albuterol and acetylcysteine (Mucomyst). You have completed Ms. Dawson's teaching about the safe administration and effects of her newly added medications. Ms. Dawson's continued care includes a follow up appointment with her pulmonologist in 3 days, as well as instructions to return to the emergency department immediately should she experience difficulty breathing or any other problems.

Clinical Reasoning Questions Level I

1. What additional client education do you anticipate Ms. Dawson will need at her follow-up appointment?

2. When Ms. Dawson goes to the pulmonologist's office for her follow-up, what will the nurse's assessment include?

3. For healthy clients without respiratory disorders, what is the normal oxygen saturation level (SaO_2)?

Clinical Reasoning Questions Level II

4. What are the priorities for Ms. Dawson's care in order to decrease her risk of developing pneumonia in the future?

5. How does chest physiotherapy help to decrease chest congestion?

6. What education would Ms. Dawson require when prescribed two forms of rescue medications for asthma (albuterol by both inhaler and nebulizer treatment)?

7. Where would you look for the most recent research on nursing care of clients receiving mechanical ventilation?

EXEMPLAR 15.1 Acute Respiratory Distress Syndrome

EXEMPLAR KEY TERMS

Acute respiratory distress syndrome (ARDS), 975
Barotrauma, 982
Bilevel ventilator (BiPAP), 980
Continuous positive airway pressure (CPAP), 980
Negative pressure ventilator, 979
Noninvasive ventilation (NIV), 979
Pneumomediastinum, 982
Pneumopericardium, 982
Positive end-expiratory pressure (PEEP), 980
Positive-pressure ventilators, 979
Refractory hypoxemia, 975
Terminal weaning, 983
Weaning, 982

EXEMPLAR LEARNING OUTCOMES

After reading about this exemplar, you will be able to:

1. Describe the pathophysiology, etiology, clinical manifestations, and direct and indirect causes of acute respiratory distress syndrome (ARDS).

2. Identify risk factors and prevention methods associated with ARDS.

3. Illustrate the nursing process in providing culturally competent care across the life span for individuals with ARDS.

4. Formulate priority nursing diagnoses appropriate for an individual with ARDS.

5. Summarize therapies used by interdisciplinary teams in the collaborative care of an individual with ARDS.

6. Plan evidence-based care for an individual with ARDS and his or her family in collaboration with other members of the healthcare team.

7. Evaluate expected outcomes for an individual with ARDS.

▶ OVERVIEW

Acute respiratory distress syndrome (ARDS) is a disorder with rapid onset characterized by noncardiac pulmonary edema and progressive **refractory hypoxemia** (the decrease of arterial oxygen despite administration of oxygen at high flow rates). ARDS is widely recognized as a severe form of acute respiratory failure. The mortality rate associated with acute respiratory distress syndrome remains around 30%–40% (American Lung Association [ALA], 2013a).

Extensive lung tissue inflammation and small blood vessel injury occur, with malfunction of other organs following. The onset of ARDS is rapid, with an arterial blood gas (ABG) showing respiratory failure. The initial admitting diagnoses of individuals who develop ARDS are varied, with most individuals presenting to the hospital with another critical event, such as a drug overdose or exposure to a toxic inhalant, and being admitted to intensive care. Both direct and indirect injuries to the body can result in ARDS. **Table 15–5** ● features some of the conditions commonly associated with the development of ARDS.

▶ PATHOPHYSIOLOGY AND ETIOLOGY

The underlying pathology in ARDS is acute lung injury resulting from an unregulated systemic inflammatory response to acute injury or inflammation. Inflammatory cellular responses and biochemical mediators damage the alveolar–capillary membrane. This damage develops rapidly, often within 90 minutes of the systemic inflammatory response and within 24 hours of the initial insult.

Damaged capillary membranes allow plasma and blood cells to escape into the interstitial space. Increased interstitial pressure and damage to the alveolar membrane allow fluid to enter the alveoli. Within the alveoli, the fluid dilutes and inactivates surfactant. The inflammatory process damages surfactant-producing cells, leading to a deficit of surfactant, increased alveolar surface tension, and alveolar collapse with atelectasis. The lungs become less compliant, and gas exchange is impaired. As the syndrome progresses, hyaline membranes form, further reducing gas exchange and compliance. Finally, fibrotic changes occur in the lungs. Intra-alveolar septa thicken, and alveolar surface area for gas exchange is reduced. Hypoxemia becomes refractory or resistant to improvement with supplemental oxygen, and the $PaCO_2$ rises as diffusion is further impaired.

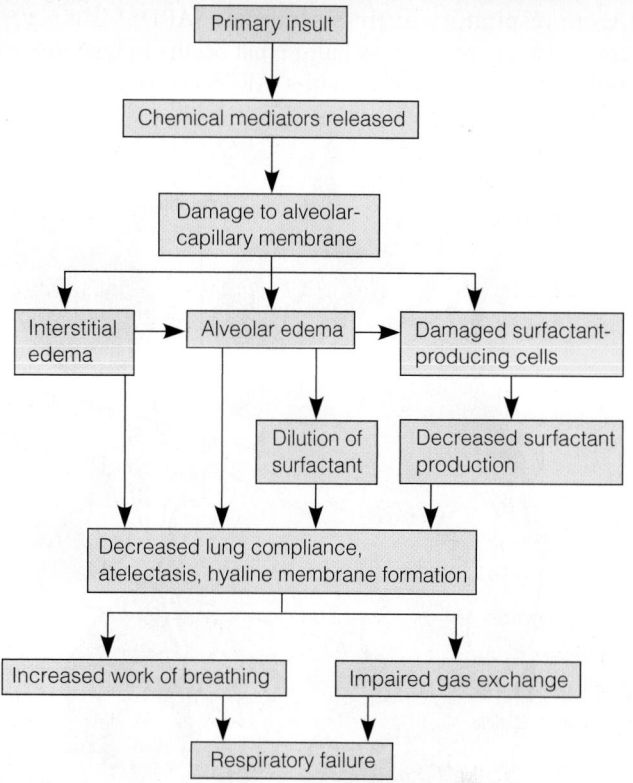

Figure 15–20 ● Pathogenesis of acute respiratory distress syndrome.

Figures 15–20 ● and **15–21** ● illustrate the pathogenesis and pathophysiology of ARDS. As ARDS progresses, tissue hypoxia becomes significant, and metabolic acidosis develops. Carbon dioxide exchange is impaired, as is oxygen exchange, leading to combined respiratory and metabolic acidosis. Sepsis and multiple organ system dysfunction of the kidneys, liver, gastrointestinal tract, central nervous system, and cardiovascular system are the leading causes of death in ARDS. If the process is halted before sepsis or organ system dysfunction occurs, the long-term prognosis for recovery is good.

Etiology

Approximately 190,000 Americans are affected by ARDS each year. ARDS affects all ages (ALA, 2013a; National Heart, Lung, and Blood Institute [NHLBI], 2012a). The mortality rate ranges from 25% to 45%. Men and African Americans have a greater risk of dying of ARDS compared to women and people from

TABLE 15–5   Conditions Associated With Development of Acute Respiratory Distress Syndrome

CONDITIONS	EXAMPLES
Shock	Hemorrhagic shock, septic shock
Inhalation injuries	Aspiration of gastric contents, smoke and toxic gases, near-drowning, oxygen toxicity
Infections	Gram-negative sepsis, viral pneumonias, *Pneumocystis jiroveci* pneumonia, miliary tuberculosis
Drug overdose	Heroin, methadone, propoxyphene, aspirin
Trauma	Burns, head injury, lung contusion, fat emboli
Other	Disseminated intravascular coagulation, pancreatitis, uremia, amniotic fluid and air emboli, multiple transfusions, open heart surgery with cardiopulmonary bypass

Acute respiratory distress syndrome (ARDS) is a severe form of acute respiratory failure that occurs in response to pulmonary or systemic insults. ARDS is characterized by noncardiogenic pulmonary edema resulting from inflammatory damage to alveolar and capillary walls. Many disorders may precipitate ARDS, although sepsis is the most common.

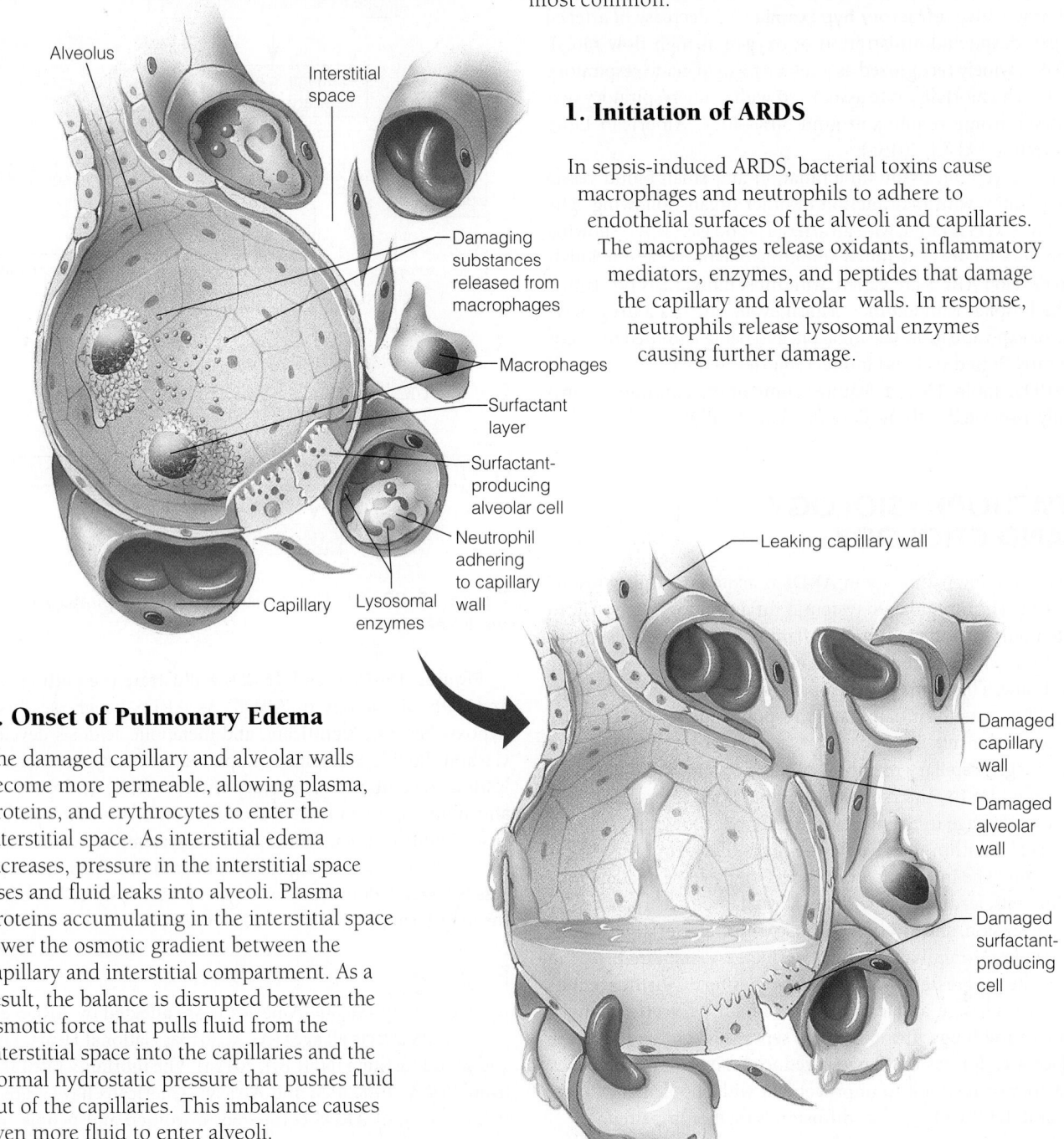

1. Initiation of ARDS

In sepsis-induced ARDS, bacterial toxins cause macrophages and neutrophils to adhere to endothelial surfaces of the alveoli and capillaries. The macrophages release oxidants, inflammatory mediators, enzymes, and peptides that damage the capillary and alveolar walls. In response, neutrophils release lysosomal enzymes causing further damage.

2. Onset of Pulmonary Edema

The damaged capillary and alveolar walls become more permeable, allowing plasma, proteins, and erythrocytes to enter the interstitial space. As interstitial edema increases, pressure in the interstitial space rises and fluid leaks into alveoli. Plasma proteins accumulating in the interstitial space lower the osmotic gradient between the capillary and interstitial compartment. As a result, the balance is disrupted between the osmotic force that pulls fluid from the interstitial space into the capillaries and the normal hydrostatic pressure that pushes fluid out of the capillaries. This imbalance causes even more fluid to enter alveoli.

Figure 15–21 ● Pathophysiology of acute respiratory distress syndrome.

4. End-Stage ARDS

Fibrin and cell debris from necrotic cells combine to form hyaline membranes, which line the interior of the alveoli and further reduce alveolar compliance and gas exchange. Because CO_2 cannot diffuse across hyaline membranes, $PaCO_2$ levels now begin to rise while PaO_2 levels continue to fall. Rising $PaCO_2$ levels can lead to respiratory acidosis. Without respiratory support, respiratory failure will develop.
Even with aggressive treatment, almost 50% of clients with ARDS die.

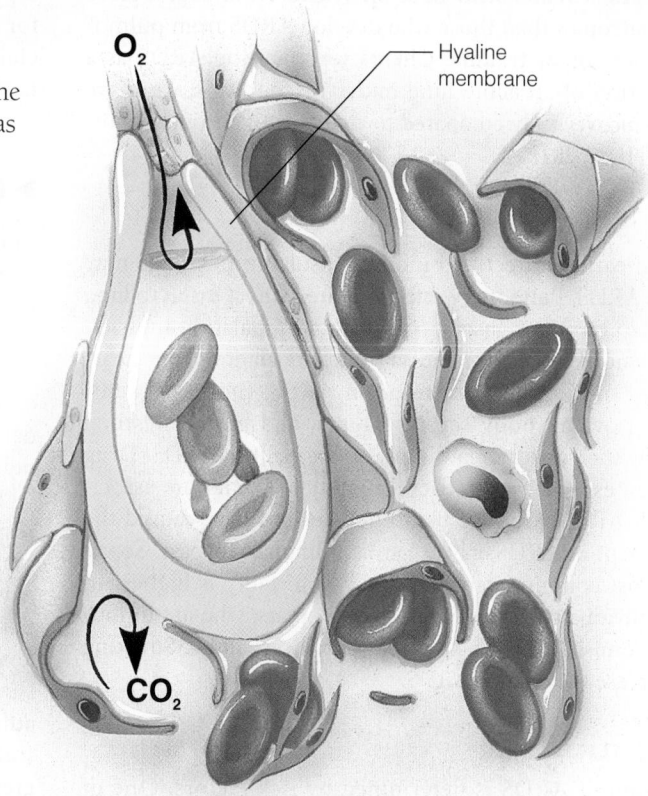

3. Alveolar Collapse

Protein-rich fluid accumulates in the alveoli, inactivating surfactant and damaging type II alveolar cells that produce surfactant. (Surfactant is important in maintaining alveolar compliance—the ability of tissue to stretch or distend.) As active surfactant is lost, the alveoli stiffen and collapse, leading to atelectasis, which increases breathing effort.

Decreased alveolar compliance, atelectasis, and fluid-filled alveoli interfere with gas exchange across the alveolar-capillary membrane. Blood oxygen (PaO_2) levels fall. Because carbon dioxide diffuses more readily than oxygen, however, blood carbon dioxide ($PaCO_2$) levels also fall initially as tachypnea causes more CO_2 to be expired.

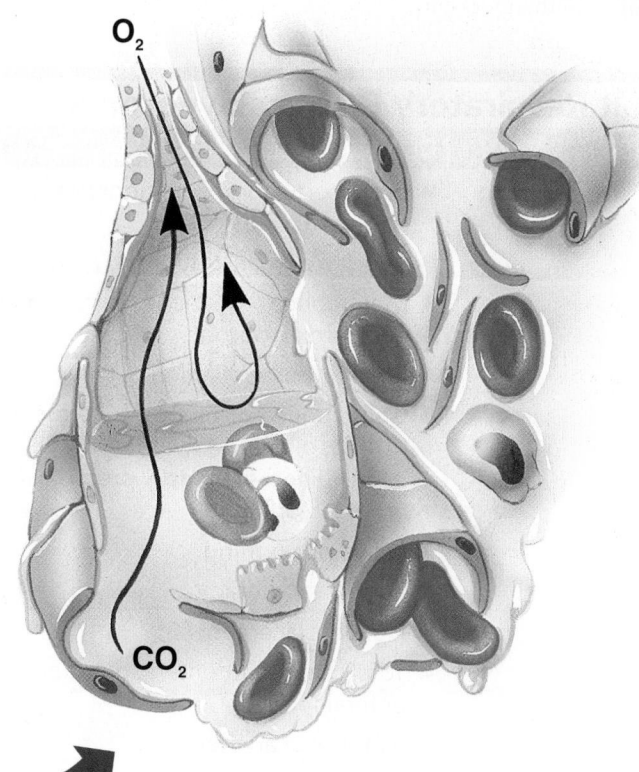

Figure 15–21 ● Pathophysiology of acute respiratory distress syndrome. (*continued*)

other races. Clients who develop ARDS from sepsis have poorer outcomes than those who develop ARDS from pulmonary infections or trauma. Clients who develop ARDS as a complication of an acute lung injury or condition are more likely to recover fully compared to clients with chronic conditions (NHLBI, 2012a).

Risk Factors

As stated earlier, direct and indirect insults to the lungs may result in ARDS. Pulmonary infections are a direct insult to lung tissue. Aspiration of gastric contents and inhalation injuries, such as smoke inhalation and saltwater inhalation from near-drowning in saltwater, can result in ARDS. Indirect insults, including overall body sepsis, trauma, and gastrointestinal infections such as pancreatitis, also may result in ARDS. Drug overdoses, especially with tricyclic antidepressants, are associated with ARDS. Multiple blood transfusions have caused the development of ARDS, as has cardiopulmonary bypass. Sepsis is the most common cause of ARDS. Mortality is highest in those individuals who are older than 70 years, who are immunocompromised, and who have chronic liver failure. Smoking may increase the risk for ARDS.

Prevention

Prevention of ARDS is determined by risk factors. One of the greatest risk factors for ARDS is aspiration. The risk of aspiration can be decreased by elevating the head of the bed for individuals experiencing respiratory infections, especially while ingesting food either by mouth or through a nasogastric tube.

▶ CLINICAL MANIFESTATIONS

Initial manifestations of ARDS typically develop 24–48 hours after the initial insult. Dyspnea and tachypnea are early manifestations. Laboratory findings are consistent with the presenting illness. ABG values may be within the normal range. Chest x-ray (CXR) will often be clear of infiltrates, with the exception of direct pulmonary illness. Baseline laboratory data as well as diagnostic tests aid in identifying the change in pulmonary status.

Progressive respiratory distress develops, with increasing respiratory rate, intercostal retractions, and use of accessory muscles of respiration. Tachycardia occurs as the demands for oxygen to the cells of the body increase. CXR will show interstitial changes with patchy infiltrates. Pulse oximetry and ABG levels may demonstrate hypoxemia refractory to oxygen administration. Cyanosis develops that may not improve with oxygen administration. Breath sounds are initially clear, but crackles (rales) and rhonchi develop later. As respiratory failure progresses, mental status changes, such as agitation, confusion, and lethargy, occur.

Clinical Manifestations and Therapies   Adult Respiratory Distress Syndrome

ETIOLOGY	CLINICAL MANIFESTATIONS	CLINICAL THERAPIES
Hypoxia	■ Dyspnea ■ Tachypnea ■ Intercostal retractions ■ Tachycardia ■ Cyanosis ■ Atelectasis	■ Bronchodilators, beta-agonists, corticosteroids ■ Oxygen administration ■ Monitoring of pulmonary artery pressures and cardiac output ■ Mechanical ventilation ■ Continuous positive airway pressure (CPAP), bilevel ventilator (BiPAP), or positive end-expiratory pressure (PEEP) as necessary ■ Prone positioning ■ Surfactant therapy
Nutritional imbalance	■ Confusion ■ Fluid/electrolyte imbalance ■ Weakness or fatigue	■ Fluid replacement ■ Total parenteral/enteral nutrition or enteral feedings ■ Nutritional analysis
Activity intolerance	■ Irritability ■ Fatigue ■ Confusion ■ Lethargy ■ Inability to maintain activities of daily living	■ Care may need to be split to prevent overtaxing the client. ■ Assess level of consciousness as indicated. ■ Severe activity intolerance resulting from significant hypoxia may require administration of paralytics and sedation to reduce oxygen demands.

▶ COLLABORATION

Clients with ARDS are seriously ill and require contributions from many members of the healthcare team. In addition to nurses, respiratory therapists, dietitians, physical therapists, and physicians may all play a significant role in the provision of healthcare services to the client. The role of the nurse is to constantly monitor the client's condition, respond to subtle cues indicating a change, and intervene appropriately. The focus of nursing care is discussed in more detail in the Nursing Process section.

Diagnostic Tests

Several diagnostic tests can be used to diagnose ARDS. These tests include:

- Arterial blood gas analysis to determine low levels of oxygen in the blood
- Chest radiography (chest x-ray or chest computed tomography [CT]) to determine fluid in the lungs
- Blood tests such as a complete blood count, blood chemistries, and blood cultures. These tests help find the cause of ARDS, such as an infection.
- Sputum culture to determine exact cause of infection (National Institutes of Health [NIH], 2012a).

Pharmacologic Therapy

Although no definitive drug therapy currently exists for ARDS, a number of medications may be used. Inhaled nitric oxide reduces intrapulmonary shunting and improves oxygenation by dilating blood vessels in better ventilated areas of the lungs. Surfactant therapy may be prescribed due to the decrease in surfactant production that is often associated with ARDS.

Interventions to block the inflammatory response, such as using nonsteroidal anti-inflammatory agents and corticosteroids, are under investigation. Corticosteroids may be used late in the course of ARDS to improve oxygenation and lung mechanics when fibrotic changes occur.

Nonpharmacologic Therapy

Nonpharmacologic management for ARDS includes several different types of treatment modalities, such as mechanical ventilation, the use of artificial airways, proper nutrition and adequate amounts of fluids, suctioning (discussed earlier in this module), and other clinical therapies.

MECHANICAL VENTILATION The mainstay of ARDS management is endotracheal intubation and mechanical ventilation. With ARDS, it is rarely possible to maintain adequate tissue oxygenation with oxygen therapy alone.

With mechanical ventilation, the FiO_2 (fraction of inspired oxygen—the percentage of oxygen administered) is set at the lowest possible level to maintain a PaO_2 higher than 60 mmHg and oxygen saturation of approximately 90%. When the PaO_2 cannot be maintained with less than 50% inspired oxygen, there is a risk that oxygen toxicity will accentuate ARDS. It is often necessary to add positive end-expiratory pressure (PEEP) to

mechanical ventilator settings in order to prevent collapse of alveoli and promote oxygenation. The client who does not require intubation but needs additional respiratory support may receive bilevel ventilation (BiPAP) or continuous positive airway pressure (CPAP). Maintaining open airways and alveoli enhances gas diffusion and reduces V-Q mismatch. PEEP increases intrathoracic pressure resulting in a decrease in cardiac output while increasing the risk of barotrauma which can result in long-term pulmonary complications. Either assist-control or synchronized intermittent mandatory ventilation may be used along with PEEP in treating the client with ARDS. It is important to remember that mechanical ventilation does not cure ARDS; it simply supports respiratory function while the underlying problem is identified and treated.

Types of Ventilators Two broad, general classifications of mechanical ventilators are available. **Negative-pressure ventilators** create negative (subatmospheric) pressure externally to draw the chest outward and air into the lungs, mimicking spontaneous breathing. The iron lung, cuirass ventilator, and PulmoWrap are examples of negative-pressure ventilators. Negative-pressure ventilators are primarily used by clients with neuromuscular disorders (e.g., postpolio syndrome and amyotrophic lateral sclerosis) that interfere with the ability to maintain adequate ventilation. They also may be used by clients who primarily require ventilator support during sleep.

Positive-pressure ventilators are used more often than negative-pressure ones, especially in treating clients with acute respiratory failure. These ventilators push air into the lungs rather than drawing it in like negative-pressure ventilators. The amount of air delivered with each breath can be delivered in milliliters (volume ventilator) or until a specific pressure is reached (pressure ventilators). Either invasive ventilation using an endotracheal tube or tracheostomy or noninvasive positive-pressure ventilation can be used. Increasingly, noninvasive techniques, which use a nasal or face mask, nasal plugs, or an oral mouthpiece, are being used (Fenstermacher & Hong, 2004).

Noninvasive ventilation (NIV) provides ventilator support using a tight-fitting face mask, thus avoiding intubation. Its primary use is to support clients with obstructive sleep apnea, neuromuscular disease, or impending respiratory failure (e.g., advanced COPD). NIV also may be used for clients in respiratory failure who refuse intubation. The degree of success varies and is primarily limited by client intolerance as a result of the physical and psychological discomfort of wearing a mask when dyspneic (Fishman et al., 2008). NIV tends to be more successful in clients without significant underlying lung disease (e.g., respiratory failure related to neuromuscular disease).

Several variables are used to trigger, cycle, and limit airflow with positive-pressure ventilators. The trigger prompts the ventilator to deliver a breath. The client's inspiratory effort triggers ventilator-assisted breaths. Ventilator-controlled breaths usually are triggered by a preset time interval (e.g., a breath is delivered every 5 sec for a rate of 12 breaths/minute). The ventilator cycle, or duration of inspiration, can be limited by volume, pressure, flow, or time. Volume-cycled ventilators deliver air until a preset volume is delivered. Pressure-cycled ventilators cycle off when a preset pressure is achieved within the airways. Flow-cycled ventilators are cycled by a preset inspiratory flow rate, and time-cycled ventilators deliver air for a set time interval. Airflow delivered by the ventilator also can be limited by factors such as airway pressure (e.g., a volume-cycled ventilator can be set to immediately stop inspiratory flow if airway pressure exceeds a preset value).

Modes of Ventilation   A number of different modes or patterns of ventilation may be used with positive-pressure ventilators. The mode determines whether a breath is initiated by the client or the ventilator and the pattern of airway support provided by the ventilator. CPAP, bilevel airway pressure support, assist-control mode ventilation, synchronized intermittent mandatory ventilation, PEEP, pressure-support ventilation, and pressure-control ventilation are common modes of ventilation in use today (**Table 15–6 ●**).

- *Continuous positive airway pressure.* **Continuous positive airway pressure (CPAP)** applies positive pressure to the airways of a client who is breathing spontaneously. CPAP may be used with either endotracheal intubation or a tight-fitting face mask. All breathing is spontaneous (client triggered) and pressure controlled. CPAP is used to help maintain open airways and alveoli, decreasing the work of breathing.

- *Bilevel ventilators.* A **bilevel ventilator (BiPAP)** provides inspiratory positive airway pressure as well as airway support during expiration. Bilevel ventilation is primarily used at night with a tight-fitting mask (nasal, facial, or oral). Three modes of ventilation can be used with BiPAP: (a) spontaneous breathing (S); (b) timed mode (T), in which pressure-supported breaths are delivered at a predetermined rate; and (c) spontaneous/timed (S/T), in which the ventilator switches to timed mode if spontaneous breathing falls below a preset rate (International Ventilator Users Network, 2009).

- *Assist-control mode ventilation.* **Assist-control mode ventilation (ACMV)** is frequently used to initiate mechanical ventilation and when the client is at risk for respiratory arrest (e.g., overdose or head injury). Assisted breaths are triggered by inspiratory effort; however, if the respiratory rate falls below a preset number (e.g., 14 breaths/minute), ventilator-controlled breaths are delivered. All breaths, assisted and controlled, are delivered at a specific tidal volume or pressure and inspiratory flow rate.

- *Synchronized intermittent mandatory ventilation.* **Synchronized intermittent mandatory ventilation (SIMV)** allows the client to breathe spontaneously, without ventilator assistance, between delivered ventilator breaths. Mandatory or ventilator-controlled breaths are delivered at a preset rate, volume, and/or pressure, coordinated with the client's inspiratory efforts. This mode of ventilation is used to support ventilation, to exercise respiratory muscles between ventilator-assisted breaths, and during the weaning process (Fishman et al., 2008).

- *Positive end-expiratory pressure.* **Positive end-expiratory pressure (PEEP)** requires intubation and can be applied to any of the previously described ventilator modes. With PEEP, a positive pressure is maintained in the airways during exhalation and between breaths. Keeping alveoli open between breaths improves V-Q relationships and diffusion across the alveolar–capillary membrane. This reduces hypoxemia and allows use of lower percentages of inspired oxygen. PEEP is particularly useful for treating the client with ARDS.

- *Pressure-support ventilation.* **Pressure-support ventilation (PSV)** delivers ventilator-assisted breaths when the client initiates an inspiratory effort. The cycle is flow limited; inspiration is terminated when inspiratory airflow falls below a preset rate. This mode decreases the work of breathing. It can be used in combination with SIMV when the respiratory drive is depressed. Ventilator support can be gradually withdrawn during weaning.

- *Pressure-control ventilation.* **Pressure-control ventilation** controls pressure within the airways to reduce the risk of airway trauma (e.g., following thoracic surgery). Ventilation is time triggered and time cycled, but pressure is limited. The ventilator maintains a preset airway pressure throughout inspiration. Because all breaths are controlled by the ventilator, heavy sedation may be required to prevent competition between inspiratory effort and ventilator control.

Ventilator Settings   In addition to choosing the mode of ventilation, other parameters are set to meet individual client needs when positive-pressure ventilation is used (**Table 15–7 ●**). The most important of these parameters are rate, tidal volume, and oxygen concentration.

For most adult clients, the rate is initially set between 12 and 15 ventilator breaths per minute. With ACMV or SIMV, the client's respiratory rate often is higher than the ventilator setting because of spontaneous breathing. Exhaled carbon dioxide ($ETCO_2$) or the $PaCO_2$ may be used to determine the rate. A $PaCO_2$ of less than 38 mmHg indicates hyperventilation and respiratory alkalosis; the set rate is reduced. A $PaCO_2$ above 42 mmHg or an $ETCO_2$ greater than 45 mmHg indicates hypoventilation and a need to increase the rate.

The tidal volume setting controls the amount of gas delivered with each ventilator breath. The normal adult tidal volume at rest is approximately 7 mL/kg body weight, or 400–550 mL. The tidal volume delivered by mechanical ventilation is slightly higher (500–750 mL) to compensate for tubing dead space. Higher tidal volumes can cause lung tissue trauma.

The percentage of oxygen delivered with ventilator breaths is adjusted to maintain the oxygen saturation and PaO_2 within acceptable ranges. Because prolonged delivery of high oxygen concentrations increases the risk of oxygen toxicity and pulmonary fibrosis, the FiO_2 is set at the lowest possible level for adequate tissue oxygenation. For most clients, the goal is to maintain an oxygen saturation of greater than 90%. Lower oxygen saturation levels may be appropriate for clients with long-standing COPD.

Complications   Although endotracheal intubation and mechanical ventilation can be lifesaving in respiratory failure, they are not without risk. Improper endotracheal tube placement or advancement of the tube into a mainstem bronchus can result in ventilation of one lung only. The inflated lung becomes overdistended and traumatized, and the uninflated lung develops atelectasis. In NIV, associated complications include gastric dilation, aspiration, facial skin necrosis, drying of the eyes and mucous membranes, stress, and claustrophobia (Fishman et al., 2008).

TABLE 15–6   Modes of Positive-Pressure Ventilator Operation

MODE	DESCRIPTION	PATTERN
Spontaneous breathing	Client has full control of rate, tidal volume, pressures.	
Assist-control mode ventilation (ACMV)	Client can trigger ventilator to deliver breaths at preset volume or pressure and inspiratory flow rate; breaths will be delivered at preset rate if client does not initiate.	
Synchronized intermittent mandatory ventilation (SIMV)	Mandatory breaths delivered by ventilator are synchronized with client's inspiratory effort.	
Continuous positive airway pressure (CPAP)	Positive pressure is maintained in airways; all breaths are spontaneous.	
Positive end-expiratory pressure (PEEP)	Used in conjunction with other ventilator modes; positive airway pressure is maintained throughout respiratory cycle.	
Pressure support ventilation (PSV)	Pressurized inspiratory flow supports the client's inspiratory effort, decreasing the work of breathing.	

TABLE 15–7   Ventilator Settings

PARAMETER	DESCRIPTION
Rate (f)	Number of ventilator breaths per minute: usually 12–15 in adults using assist-control mode ventilation; may be lower in synchronized intermittent mandatory ventilation
Tidal volume (V_l)	Amount of gas delivered with each ventilator breath; usually 8–10 mL/kg body weight
Oxygen concentration (FiO_2)	Percentage of oxygen delivered with ventilator breaths; can be set between 21% (room air) and 100%
I:E ratio	Duration of inspiration to expiration: usually 1:2–1:1.5
Flow rate	Speed at which air is delivered
Sensitivity	Effort required by client to initiate ventilator-assisted breath
Pressure limit	Maximal pressure within airways that will terminate a ventilator breath

■ *Hospital-acquired pneumonia (HAP).* Infection is a significant risk associated with intubation and mechanical ventilation. Normal upper respiratory tract defense mechanisms are bypassed, with loss of air humidification and trapping of pathogens. Oral secretions and gastric contents can enter the respiratory tree through the open epiglottis. Frequent, meticulous oral hygiene is vital in preventing HAP (also called ventilator-associated pneumonia). Often, the cough reflex is inhibited or impaired by the underlying disease process and the continued presence of the endotracheal tube. Even when strict asepsis is used for suctioning and other respiratory procedures, the lower airways are contaminated within 24 hours of intubation. Secretions often become thick and tenacious, increasing the risk of atelectasis.

■ *Barotrauma.* Barotrauma (also called volutrauma) is lung injury caused by alveolar overdistention. Both the volume of delivered gas and the pressures under which it is delivered can contribute to barotraumas. As a result, overdistended alveoli rupture, allowing air to escape into the pulmonary interstitial spaces and the mediastinum, pleural space, and other tissues. Subcutaneous emphysema, pneumothorax, and pneumomediastinum are possible results of barotrauma. Subcutaneous emphysema, or air in the subcutaneous tissue, causes tissue swelling of the chest, neck, and face. A "crackling" or air bubble popping sensation is felt on palpation of subcutaneous emphysema. Swelling may be massive. Once the cause is corrected, the air is gradually reabsorbed.

■ *Pneumothorax.* Pneumothorax is identified by signs of unequal chest expansion, a sudden loss or significant decrease in breath sounds on the affected side, and a hyperresonant percussion tone. Rapid chest tube insertion is necessary to prevent tension pneumothorax and cardiovascular compromise. **Pneumomediastinum** is the presence of air in the mediastinum (the space between the lungs that contains the heart, great vessels, trachea, and esophagus). Air in the mediastinal space can interfere with the function of all of these organs and lead to such complications as **pneumopericardium** (air in the pericardial sac). Pneumomediastinum may have few manifestations, but the CXR shows widening of the mediastinal space.

■ *Cardiovascular effects.* Positive-pressure ventilation increases intrathoracic pressure, which can interfere with venous return to the heart and ventricular filling. As a result, cardiac output falls. Use of PEEP increases the effects of mechanical ventilation on cardiac output. The decreased cardiac output can affect liver and kidney function secondarily.

■ *Gastrointestinal effects.* Gastrointestinal complications are commonly associated with prolonged mechanical ventilation. Stress ulcers (erosive gastritis) may develop, leading to painless gastrointestinal hemorrhage. Histamine H_2-receptor blockers or sucralfate are often used to prevent stress ulcers. Air leaks around the endotracheal tube can cause gastric distention; a nasogastric tube often is inserted to prevent vomiting. Sedation and other medications used during mechanical ventilation can slow intestinal motility, leading to constipation.

Weaning From Ventilator Support   The process of removing ventilator support and reestablishing spontaneous, independent respirations is called **weaning**. Weaning begins only after the underlying process causing respiratory failure has been corrected or stabilized. The process and time required for weaning depend on factors such as preexisting lung condition, duration of mechanical ventilation, and the client's general condition, both physical and psychological. In all cases, the vital signs, respiratory rate, extent of dyspnea, blood gases, and clinical status are used to evaluate weaning and its progress.

Following a brief period of mechanical ventilation, a T-piece unit or CPAP may be used for weaning. In T-piece weaning, the ventilator is removed for brief periods during which oxygen is delivered using a T-piece (**Figure 15–22 ●**). The duration of periods off the ventilator is gradually increased until the client can maintain adequate independent respirations for several hours. Vital signs, oxygen saturation, $ETCO_2$, and PaO_2 are

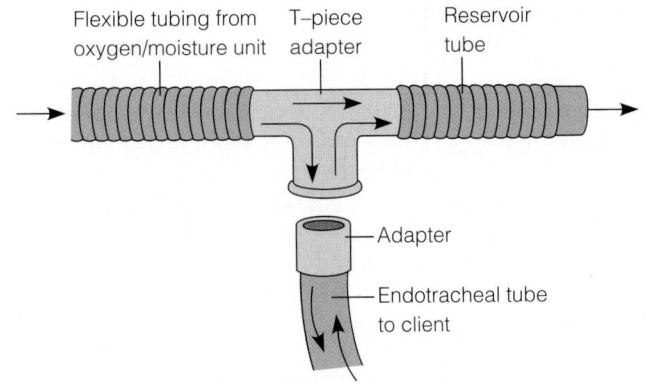

Figure 15–22 ● A T-piece, or "blow-by," unit for weaning from mechanical ventilation.

carefully monitored during the process. If signs of respiratory distress develop, the client is placed back on the ventilator at previous settings. When mechanical ventilation is no longer needed, the endotracheal tube is removed. CPAP weaning follows a similar process, with trials of spontaneous breathing supported by the ventilator in CPAP mode.

Both SIMV and PSV are used for weaning when the duration of mechanical ventilation has been longer and reconditioning of respiratory muscles is needed. When SIMV is used, the number of mandatory ventilator-assisted breaths is gradually decreased as ABG, ETCO$_2$, and the respiratory rate are monitored. When the client is able to tolerate SIMV at 4 breaths per minute without rest periods of greater ventilatory support, CPAP or T-piece weaning is attempted before extubation (Fishman et al., 2008).

Weaning is the primary use for PSV. Initially, PSV is set slightly below the peak inspiratory pressures required during volume-cycled ventilation. Pressure support levels are gradually decreased, often in a cyclic pattern of periods of minimal support alternating with periods of higher support to recondition respiratory muscles. When the PSV level is just enough to overcome endotracheal tube resistance, support is discontinued and the client is extubated (Fishman et al., 2008).

When an illness is terminal or irreversible with a poor prognosis, terminal weaning may be requested by the client or family. **Terminal weaning** is the gradual withdrawal of mechanical ventilation when survival without assisted ventilation is not expected. Unlike weaning when recovery is expected, which usually occurs in an intensive care unit, the client is moved to a quiet medical–surgical room, a hospice room, or even the client's home before terminal weaning is initiated. Family members are encouraged to remain with the client throughout the process. If possible, decisions about sedation and analgesia before and during weaning are made with the client, as are decisions about hydration and nutritional support following weaning. Ventilator support is gradually withdrawn using the same modes described earlier (SIMV or PSV). Analgesia and sedation are given to promote comfort during weaning.

ARTIFICIAL AIRWAYS

Artificial airways are inserted to maintain a patent air passage for a client whose airway has become or may become obstructed. A patent airway is necessary so that air can flow to and from the lungs. Four of the more common types of airways are oropharyngeal, nasopharyngeal, endotracheal, and tracheostomies.

Oropharyngeal and Nasopharyngeal Airways

Oropharyngeal and nasopharyngeal airways are used to keep the upper air passages open when they may become obstructed by secretions or by the tongue. These airway devices are easy to insert and have a low risk of complications. Sizes vary and should be appropriate to the size and age of the client. The airway device should be well lubricated with water-soluble gel before insertion.

Oropharyngeal airways (**Figure 15–23 ●**) stimulate the gag reflex and are used only for clients with altered levels of consciousness (e.g., because of general anesthesia, overdose, or head injury). Nasopharyngeal airways are tolerated better by alert clients and are inserted through the nares, terminating in the oropharynx (**Figure 15–24 ●**). When caring for a client with a nasopharyngeal airway, provide frequent oral and nares

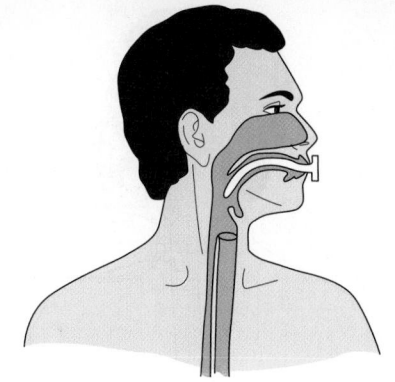

Figure 15–23 ● An oropharyngeal airway in place.

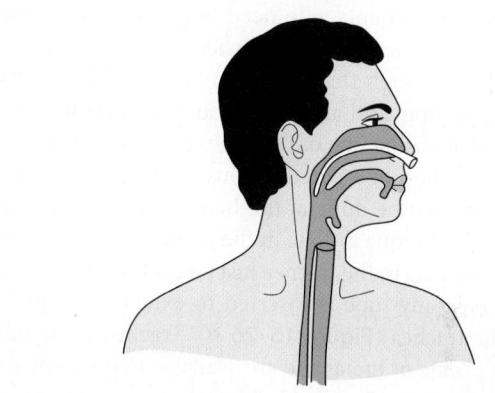

Figure 15–24 ● A nasopharyngeal airway in place.

care, repositioning the airway in the other naris every 8 hours or as ordered to prevent necrosis of the mucosa.

Endotracheal Tubes

Endotracheal tubes are most commonly inserted in clients who have had general anesthetics or who are in emergency situations where mechanical ventilation is required. An endotracheal tube is inserted by the primary care provider, nurse, or respiratory therapist with specialized education. It is inserted through the mouth or the nose and into the trachea with the guide of a laryngoscope (**Figure 15–25 ●**). The tube terminates just superior to the bifurcation of the trachea into the bronchi. The tube may have an air-filled cuff to prevent air leakage around it. Because an endotracheal tube passes through the epiglottis and glottis, the client is unable to speak while the tube is in place.

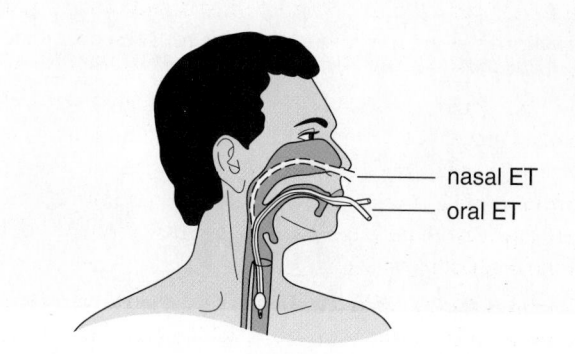

nasal ET
oral ET

Figure 15–25 ● An endotracheal tube.

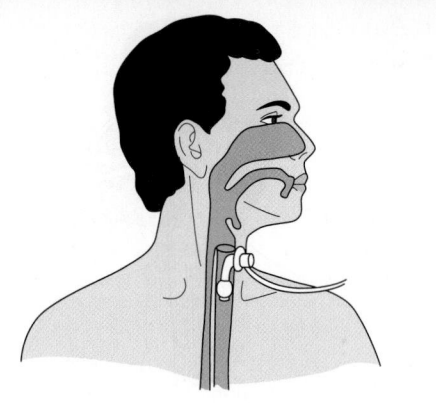

Figure 15–26 ● A tracheostomy tube in place.

Tracheostomies Clients who need long-term airway support may have a tracheostomy. A tracheostomy is an opening into the trachea through the neck. A tube is usually inserted through this opening, and an artificial airway is created. Tracheostomy is done using one of two techniques: the traditional open surgical method or a percutaneous insertion. The percutaneous method can be done at the bedside in a critical care unit. The open technique is done in the operating room: A surgical incision is made in the trachea just below the larynx, and a curved tracheostomy tube is inserted to extend through the stoma into the trachea (**Figure 15–26** ●). Tracheostomy tubes can be either plastic or metal and are available in different sizes with and without cuffs (**Figure 15–27** ●). Fenestrated tracheostomy tubes are available to allow the client to speak with the tube in place.

Tracheostomy tubes have an outer cannula that is inserted into the trachea and a flange that rests against the neck and allows the tube to be secured in place with tape or ties. All tubes also have an obturator, which is used to insert the outer cannula and is then removed. The obturator is kept at the client's bedside in case the tube becomes dislodged and needs to be reinserted. Some tracheostomy tubes have an inner cannula that may be removed for periodic cleaning.

Cuffed tracheostomy tubes are surrounded by an inflatable cuff that produces an airtight seal between the tube and the trachea. This seal prevents aspiration of oropharyngeal secretions

and air leakage between the tube and the trachea. Cuffed tubes are often used immediately after a tracheostomy and are essential when ventilating a client with a tracheostomy using a mechanical ventilator. Children do not require cuffed tubes, because their tracheas are resilient enough to seal the air space around the tube.

Low-pressure cuffs (**Figure 15–28** ●) are commonly used to distribute a low, even pressure against the trachea, thus decreasing the risk of tracheal tissue necrosis. They do not need to be deflated periodically to reduce pressure on the tracheal wall. Foam-cuffed tracheostomy tubes do not require injected air; instead, when the port is opened, ambient air enters the balloon, which then conforms to the client's trachea. Air is removed from the cuff before insertion or removal of the tube.

The nurse provides tracheostomy care for the client with a new or recent tracheostomy to maintain patency of the tube and reduce the risk of infection. Initially a tracheostomy may need to be suctioned (see the section on suctioning that follows) and cleaned as often as every 1–2 hours. After the initial inflammatory response subsides, tracheostomy care may only need to be done once or twice a day, depending on the client.

When the client breathes through a tracheostomy, air is no longer filtered and humidified as it is when passing through the upper airways; therefore, special precautions are necessary. Humidity may be provided with a mist collar. Clients with long-term tracheostomies may wear a light scarf or a 4-in. × 4-in. gauze held in place with a cotton tie over the stoma to filter air as it enters the tracheostomy.

NUTRITION AND FLUIDS The client on mechanical ventilation requires close monitoring of fluid and electrolyte status as well as adequate nutrition. Mechanical ventilation promotes sodium and water retention as a result of its effects on cardiac output. Renal perfusion is decreased, stimulating the renin–angiotensin–aldosterone system to retain sodium and water. A Swan-Ganz catheter is often inserted to monitor pulmonary artery pressures and cardiac output. An arterial line allows repeated blood gas analysis and continuous arterial pressure monitoring. Serum electrolytes are drawn frequently, and intake, output, and daily weight are carefully monitored. Enteral or parenteral nutrition is provided during mechanical ventilation

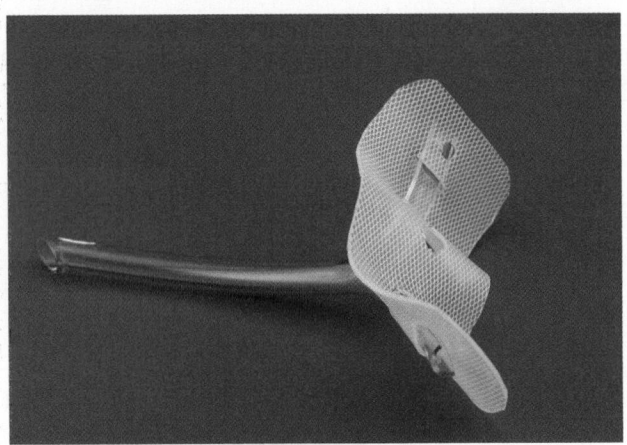

Figure 15–27 ● An uncuffed tracheostomy tube.
Source: © C. Childs/Custom Medical Stock Photo–All rights reserved.

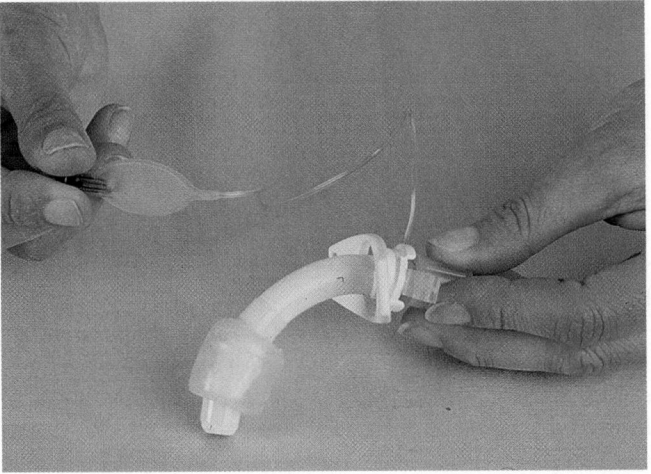

Figure 15–28 ● A tracheostomy tube with a low-pressure cuff.

because the endotracheal tube prohibits eating. A nasogastric, gastrostomy, or jejunostomy feeding tube is placed for enteral nutrition. A jejunostomy tube may be used to reduce the risk of regurgitation and aspiration.

OTHER CLINICAL THERAPIES   Atelectasis frequently occurs in dependent lung regions in clients with ARDS. Prone positioning in conjunction with mechanical ventilation reduces the pressure of surrounding tissue on dependent regions and improves oxygenation.

Other management strategies include treatment of any infection and correction of the underlying condition. Infections are treated with intravenous antibiotic therapy tailored to the causative organism. Low-molecular-weight heparin may be ordered to prevent thrombophlebitis and possible pulmonary embolus or disseminated intravascular coagulation, a possible complication of ARDS.

■ NURSING PROCESS

Caring for the client with ARDS requires careful and continuous monitoring of airway, breathing, and circulation. Changes in level of consciousness, oxygenation, or perfusion require rapid nursing interventions to maintain life. The focus of nursing care is on meeting these essential client needs.

Assessment

Collect assessment data through the health history and physical assessment:

- *Health history.* Previous respiratory alterations, previous illnesses and surgeries, and any illness or direct or indirect injury in the previous 3–4 days.
- *Physical assessment.* Respiratory rate and rhythm; auscultation of the lungs; level of consciousness, including orientation; baseline vital signs, peripheral perfusion.

Confusion, agitation, or anxiety are early signs of hypoxemia, especially in older clients. Changes from baseline vital signs alert the nurse to subtle changes in cardiac or respiratory status. Individuals developing ARDS may express desperate anxiety because of the inability to get enough air to relieve their shortness of breath.

Diagnosis

Any combination of the following NANDA diagnoses may be appropriate for the individual with ARDS:

- *Risk for Acute Confusion*
- *Ineffective Airway Clearance*
- *Ineffective Breathing Pattern*
- *Impaired Spontaneous Ventilation*
- *Impaired Gas Exchange*
- *Decreased Cardiac Output*
- *Dysfunctional Ventilatory Weaning Response*
- *Risk for Imbalanced Fluid Volume*
- *Imbalanced Nutrition: Less Than Body Requirements*
- *Risk for Infection*
- *Acute Pain*
- *Anxiety.*

(NANDA-I © 2012)

Additional NANDA diagnoses may be appropriate depending on the underlying condition causing the acute respiratory distress.

Planning

The goal of care for individuals with ARDS is to protect the lungs from fibrotic damage while providing adequate oxygenation to the body systems. Expected outcomes may include the following:

- The client will be oriented to name, place, and time with each healthcare personnel individual interaction.
- The client will receive adequate ventilatory support to maintain oxygenation of body cells.
- The client will be free of pulmonary tissue damage.
- The client will maintain patent airways.
- The client will maintain cardiac output adequate to perfuse all body systems.
- The client will receive adequate nutrition to maintain body processes.
- The client will be free of any sign or symptom of infection.
- The client will not develop thrombosis.
- The client will manage pain successfully.
- The client will cope with or be free from anxiety.

Implementation

All body systems are at risk of failure caused by poor oxygenation and alterations in perfusion. The healthcare team will identify and treat the causative agent, as this is critical to returning the client to normal health. Common interventions for the client with ARDS include the following:

- Conduct CBC, chemistry panel, ABG, blood cultures, sputum cultures, and gastric and stool cultures as indicated by symptoms.
- Monitor vital signs at least hourly. Continual monitoring may be required.
- Monitor oxygenation status with ABG and pulse oximetry.
- Monitor neurological status, including orientation and LOC.
- Auscultate lung and heart sounds.
- Provide analgesia, anxiolytics, and sedation medications as ordered.
- Provide beta-agonist to maintain patent airways as ordered.
- Maintain head of bed at 30° or higher.
- Position the individual prone for 30 minutes to an hour as tolerated three or four times a day. This position may facilitate oxygenation of the posterior alveoli and posterior drainage.
- Suction airways as needed.
- Monitor hemodynamic status with central venous catheters or pulmonary artery catheter as ordered.
- Monitor renal function by intake and output as well as blood urea nitrogen and creatinine levels.
- Place Foley catheter.
- Administer intravenous fluids as needed, but avoid fluid overload.
- Monitor glucose levels, and maintain levels within normal limits.
- Assess peripheral pulses.

Maintain a Patent Airway

Ineffective airway clearance may either cause respiratory failure or occur as a result of interventions. Impaired ventilation frequently leads to acute respiratory failure. Although intubation and mechanical ventilation can be lifesaving measures, they also increase the risk of respiratory infection and ineffective secretion management.

- Suction as needed to maintain a patent airway. Indicators for suctioning include crackles and rhonchi on auscultation, frequent coughing or setting off of the high-pressure alarm, and increasing restlessness or anxiety. Although clients with a tracheostomy can usually cough up secretions, the length and diameter of endotracheal tubes makes this extremely difficult. Even with humidification, secretions often become thick and tenacious, further inhibiting their removal.
- Obtain sputum for culture if it appears purulent or is odorous. Culture is necessary to identify pathogens and guide antibiotic therapy.
- Perform percussion, vibration, and postural drainage as ordered. These techniques help loosen secretions and move them into larger airways for removal by coughing or suctioning.
- Firmly secure the endotracheal or tracheostomy tube. Provide adequate slack on ventilator tubing to prevent tension on the tube when turning, positioning, or transferring the client to a chair or stretcher. If necessary, loosely restrain hands. These measures are important to ensure proper airway placement and prevent its inadvertent removal.
- Assess fluid balance, and maintain adequate hydration. Adequate hydration helps liquefy secretions.

Promote Spontaneous Ventilation

In ARDS, the client's ability to maintain adequate ventilation is impaired. This is a concern both before initiation of mechanical ventilation and during the weaning process.

- Assess and document respiratory rate, vital signs, and oxygen saturation every 15–30 minutes. Close monitoring is vital to detect early signs of increasing respiratory distress and inability to sustain adequate breathing.
- Promptly report worsening ABG and oxygen saturation levels. Close assessment of these values allows timely intervention as needed.

- Administer oxygen as ordered, monitoring response. Observe closely for respiratory depression, especially in the client with COPD. Oxygen administration reduces the hypoxemic respiratory drive. Chronically high $PaCO_2$ levels depress the respiratory center; hypoxemia may provide the only respiratory drive.
- Place in Fowler or high-Fowler position. Sitting positions decrease pressure on the diaphragm and chest, improving lung ventilation and decreasing the work of breathing.
- Minimize activities and energy expenditures by assisting with ADLs, spacing procedures and activities, and by allowing uninterrupted periods of rest. Rest is vital to reduce oxygen and energy demands.

Enhance Cardiac Output

With positive-pressure ventilation, increased intrathoracic pressure decreases cardiac output. When PEEP is applied, intrathoracic pressure increases further; this can significantly decrease venous return, ventricular filling, stroke volume, and cardiac output. Manifestations of decreased cardiac output include hypotension and compensatory tachycardia as the heart attempts to maintain cardiac output despite decreased stroke volume. In the client who is already hypoxic because of ARDS, this drop in cardiac output can increase tissue damage. Urine output falls, and dysrhythmias may develop.

- Monitor and record vital signs, including apical pulse, at least every 2 hours (more frequently immediately following initiation of mechanical ventilation or addition of PEEP). Frequent assessment is vital to detect early signs of decreased cardiac output.
- Assess LOC at least every 4 hours. Altered LOC, confusion, and restlessness are early signs of cerebral hypoxia resulting from decreased cardiac output.
- Monitor pulmonary artery pressures, central venous pressure, and cardiac output readings every 1–4 hours. Changes in these measurements may indicate worsening cardiac status.
- Assess heart and lung sounds frequently. Increasing crackles or abnormal heart sounds may indicate heart failure.
- Weigh daily at the same time. Accurate daily weights are the best indicator of fluid volume status.
- Provide frequent skin care, keeping skin clean and dry and protecting pressure points. Tissue hypoxia increases the risk of skin breakdown, which in turn increases the risk of infection and sepsis.
- Maintain intravenous fluids as ordered. Intravenous fluids are given to maintain vascular volume and prevent dehydration.
- Administer analgesics, sedatives, and neuromuscular blockers as needed. These medications may be prescribed to decrease cardiac workload.

Monitor for Dysfunctional Ventilatory Weaning Response

Assessment findings indicative of dysfunctional weaning include the following:

- Dyspnea, apprehension, or agitation
- Decreasing oxygen saturation level
- Cyanosis or pallor, diaphoresis
- Increased blood pressure, pulse, and respiratory rate
- Diminished or adventitious breath sounds, use of accessory muscles
- Decreased LOC
- Deteriorating ABG values
- Shallow, gasping breaths or paradoxic abdominal breathing.

The client with dysfunctional ventilatory weaning response has difficulty adjusting to reduced mechanical ventilator support, prolonging the weaning process. Airway congestion, inadequate rest or nutrition, pain, anxiety, and a nonsupportive environment are factors that can contribute to difficulty weaning. With ARDS, the pathological processes of the disease and its effects on gas exchange may be responsible for a prolonged or ineffective weaning process.

- Assess vital signs every 15–30 minutes following changes in ventilator settings and during T-piece trials. Vital signs (heart and respiratory rates in particular) can provide early signs of hypoxemia and poor tolerance of the weaning process.
- Place in Fowler or high-Fowler position. Fowler position facilitates lung expansion and reduces the work of breathing.
- Fully explain all weaning procedures, along with expected changes in breathing. Adequate explanations help reduce anxiety and improve cooperation.
- Remain with the client during initial periods following changes of ventilator settings or T-piece trials. This provides reassurance and allows close monitoring of the response.
- Limit procedures and activities during weaning periods. Reducing energy expenditures and cardiac work facilitates the weaning process.
- Provide diversion, such as television or radio. Diversion helps distract the focus from breathing.
- Begin weaning procedures in the morning, when the client is well rested and alert; weaning may be discontinued overnight to provide rest. The work of breathing increases during the weaning process; adequate rest is important.

- When SIMV is used for weaning, decrease the SIMV rate by increments of two breaths per minute. Slow reduction of ventilator support allows respiratory muscle reconditioning and gradual resumption of the work of breathing.
- Avoid administering drugs that may depress respirations during the weaning process (except as ordered at night to facilitate rest when ventilator support is provided). Sedatives or analgesics that depress respirations can impair the weaning process.
- Keep oxygen at the bedside following weaning and extubation. Supplemental oxygen may be necessary to maintain adequate blood and tissue oxygenation.
- Provide pulmonary hygiene with percussion and postural drainage. Maintaining patent airways and adequate alveolar ventilation is vital during the weaning process.

Relieve Anxiety

Critical illness creates anxiety for any client. In ARDS, this anxiety is compounded by the presence of an endotracheal tube or tracheostomy, mechanical ventilator, numerous monitors and equipment, and potentially, neuromuscular blockade and paralysis of voluntary muscles. Fear of continued dependence on the mechanical ventilator and inability to return to a normal life may compound this anxiety.

- Explain all monitors, procedures, unusual sounds, and machinery. Understanding the environment and the various sounds and alarms reduces anxiety. Have patience with multiple requests for explanation from clients or family members; they are under extreme stress during this time and may not initially remember explanations.
- Provide a simple means of communication, such as a whiteboard or iPad, or use methods such as looking to the right for "yes" and to the left for "no." Reassure that endotracheal tube removal restores the ability to speak. The inability to speak and call out for help is frightening for the client. Providing an alternate means of communication helps reduce anxiety.
- Encourage frequent family visits, especially if the time of visitations is being limited. Encourage family participation in care. Family visits help reduce anxiety and feelings of abandonment. Allowing family members to participate in care helps reduce their anxiety as well.
- Explain to the family that the client can hear and understand. Emphasize the importance of talking to the client, not over or about the client. The family may not understand that the client may be mentally alert although unable to respond. Talking to the client about everyday things reduces the client's sense of isolation and fear.
- Provide distraction with radio or television if allowed. Distraction helps reduce the focus on machines and unusual sounds of monitors and alarms.

Evidence-Based Practice   The Client Who Is Intubated

Problem

Endotracheal intubation is a common procedure in the neonatal intensive care unit (NICU) and other intensive care environments. Several studies have evaluated the success rate of neonatal endotracheal intubations. These studies indicate that successful intubation frequently requires more than one attempt and is rarely accomplished within the recommended time frame.

Alleviating pain in neonates should be the goal of all healthcare workers providing care because painful experiences have the potential for severe consequences (Kumar, Denson, & Mancuso, 2010).

Evidence

A consensus statement from the International Evidence-Based Group for Neonatal Pain recommends that analgesia or sedation should be used for all tracheal intubation unless it is being performed for resuscitation in labor and delivery or in life-threatening situations where intravenous access is unavailable. The American Academy of Pediatrics (AAP) also recommends implementation of an effective pain prevention program that includes the use of both pharmacologic and nonpharmacologic therapies to prevent pain that is associated with any procedure, including endotracheal intubation (Kumar et al., 2010).

Implications

There is considerable variation in the use of premedication prior to intubation. Reasons for the lack of appropriate use of medication include the potential for adverse reactions, inadequate time for medication administration, and the belief that risk/benefit ratios are worsened as a result of the medications. Current evidence and recommendations, however, emphasize the benefits of premedication for intubation and attempt to identify knowledge gaps and provide guidance in making decisions regarding the use of premedication with endotracheal intubation in the neonate (Kuman et al., 2010).

Critical Thinking Application

1. What tools are available to assist the nurse in evaluating the newborn or young client's subjective perception of pain?
2. What factors might contribute to pain in the client who is intubated and mechanically ventilated?
3. Identify five nonpharmacologic measures the nurse could implement to reduce or relieve pain in clients who are intubated and mechanically ventilated.

■ Attend to physical needs promptly and completely. This provides reassurance that needs will be met even though the client is unable to ask for assistance.

■ Reassure client that intubation and mechanical ventilation are temporary measures to allow the lungs to rest and heal. Reinforce that the client will be able to breathe independently again. The client may fear continued dependence on mechanical ventilation.

SAFETY ALERT

Frequently monitor anxiety level. High levels of anxiety increase oxygen use and often interfere with the ability to work with the respirator. This can increase hypoxemia and further increase anxiety; intervention is necessary to break this cycle. See the accompanying Evidence-Based Practice feature for information about assessing and managing pain in neonates who are intubated.

Prepare for Discharge

Provide referrals to home health and respiratory care services as indicated, as well as for occupational therapy and counseling as needed. When preparing the client who has recovered from ARDS and the family for home care, discuss the topics outlined in the Community-Based Care box.

Evaluation

The client's response to nursing care is evaluated often and nursing care is adjusted accordingly. Expected outcomes for the client with ARDS often include:

■ Client maintains oxygen saturation greater than 90%.
■ Vital signs remain within acceptable limits.
■ Client's airway remains clear.
■ Client experiences no complications secondary to hypoxia.
■ Arterial blood gas results indicate acid–base balance is maintained.

Community-Based Care   ARDS

■ ARDS developed as a consequence of serious illness, not as a consequence of client or family action or inaction. Provide factual information about ARDS.

■ Maximal respiratory function following ARDS is usually achieved within 6 months, although respiratory function may remain significantly impaired. This may necessitate changes in occupation, lifestyle, and family roles.

■ Avoid smoking and exposure to secondhand smoke and environmental pollutants in order to prevent further lung damage.

■ Obtain immunization for pneumococcal pneumonia and annual influenza immunizations to prevent further episodes of serious respiratory disease.

NURSING CARE PLAN   A Client With Acute Respiratory Distress Syndrome

Peggy Adamson is a 36-year-old, single woman admitted to the hospital following a near-drowning in a local lake. On admission to the emergency department, Ms. Adamson is alert and oriented, having been rescued and resuscitated within 2 minutes of submersion. Rescuers report that she seemed to have aspirated "a lot" of water. She was water-skiing when the accident occurred. She is admitted to the intensive care unit for observation. Oxygen is started per nasal cannula at 6 L/min, intravenous fluids are administered to correct electrolyte imbalances, and 40 mg of furosemide (Lasix) are given intravenously for hypervolemia.

ASSESSMENT

Throughout her admission, Ms. Adamson has remained alert and oriented, with stable vital signs. Her respiratory rate has been 20–24 breaths/min with scattered crackles, oxygen saturations of around 94%, and a PaO_2 of 75–80 mmHg on 6 L/min of oxygen. Her pulse has been 96–100 bpm and regular. Tonight, Ms. Adamson seems apprehensive and anxious. Although her blood pressure is 116/74 mmHg, unchanged from previous levels, her heart rate is up to 106 bpm, and her respiratory rate is 28/minute. Her lungs have scattered crackles but good breath sounds throughout, unchanged from previous assessments. Ms. Adamson's oxygen saturation has dropped to 84%. The provider orders an ABG and increases the oxygen to 8 L/mine. ABG results show the following: pH, 7.48; PaO_2, 65 mmHg; $PaCO_2$, 32 mmHg. Portable chest x-ray reveals scattered infiltrates and a normal heart size. The physician orders a nonrebreather mask at 8 L/min and repeat ABGs in 1 hour. Ms. Adamson's oxygen saturation continues to fall, and subsequent blood gases show a PaO_2 of 55 mmHg. The attending physician diagnoses probable ARDS and orders nasotracheal intubation and mechanical ventilation.

DIAGNOSES

- *Ineffective Breathing Pattern* related to hypoxia
- *Impaired Gas Exchange* related to effects of near-drowning
- *Anxiety* related to hypoxemia
- *Risk for Decreased Cardiac Output* related to mechanical ventilation
- *Risk for Infection* related to endotracheal intubation

(NANDA-I © 2012)

PLANNING

- Client will breathe effectively with the mechanical ventilator.
- Client will demonstrate improved oxygen saturation, ETCO₂, and ABG values.
- Client will express fears related to intubation and mechanical ventilation.
- Client will demonstrate reduced anxiety levels.
- Client will maintain adequate cardiac output and tissue perfusion.
- Client will tolerate endotracheal intubation and mechanical ventilation without evidence of infection or barotrauma.

IMPLEMENTATION

- Obtain all necessary supplies and notify respiratory therapy and radiology in preparation for intubation and mechanical ventilation.
- Explain the purpose and procedure of intubation.
- Provide an opportunity to express fears related to intubation and mechanical ventilation. Answer questions, and provide reassurance.
- Discuss communication strategies while intubated; obtain a whiteboard, iPad, or other writing device.
- Administer analgesics and/or sedatives as ordered.
- Monitor oxygen saturation and ETCO₂ levels continuously initially after instituting mechanical ventilation; report changes to the physician.
- Obtain ABG as ordered or indicated; monitor and report results.
- Perform suction via endotracheal tube as needed to maintain clear airway.

- Allow periods of uninterrupted rest.
- Monitor vital signs at a minimum of every 1–2 hours.
- Assess skin color, capillary refill, and extremity pulses every 4 hours.
- Monitor urine output hourly; report output of less than 30 mL/hour.
- Assess for the presence of edema every 4 hours.
- Promote client communication through use of signals or writing device.
- Assess lung sounds and chest excursion at a minimum of every 1–2 hours.
- Perform continuous cardiorespiratory monitoring while requiring mechanical ventilation and until condition stabilizes after extubation.

EVALUATION

Ms. Adamson is intubated and placed on a volume-cycled ventilator at 50% FiO₂ and a tidal volume of 700 mL in the assist-control mode at 16 breaths per minute. She has difficulty working with the ventilator initially, so a fentanyl drip is ordered to reduce her anxiety.

Ms. Adamson's oxygen saturation, ETCO₂, and ABG results do not begin to improve until 5 mmHg of PEEP is added to ventilator settings. After 3 days of mechanical ventilation with PEEP and aggressive fluid and diuretic therapy, Ms. Adamson begins to improve. She is placed on SIMV, and over the course of another 3 days, she is gradually weaned off the ventilator to a face mask with CPAP. She eventually recovers fully, with minimal apparent long-term effects.

CRITICAL THINKING

1. *Endotracheal intubation and mechanical ventilation were effective in supporting Ms. Adamson's respiratory status as she recovered from ARDS. Discuss a possible sequence of events had it not been possible to wean her from the ventilator.*
2. *How might the presentation and management of an acute episode of respiratory failure caused by ARDS differ from respiratory failure related to COPD?*
3. *What measures can nurses take to prevent the development of ARDS?*
4. *Develop a nursing care plan for Ms. Adamson for the nursing diagnosis* Risk for Powerlessness *related to tracheal intubation and mechanical ventilation.*

REVIEW Acute Respiratory Distress Syndrome

RELATE Link the Concepts and Exemplars

Linking the exemplar of acute respiratory distress syndrome with the concept of acid–base balance:

1. What impact will ARDS likely have on acid–base balance, and how can the nurse intervene to promote normal balance?

2. Are the symptoms of ARDS entirely the result of acid–base imbalance, or are other factors involved? Explain your answer.

Linking the exemplar of acute respiratory distress syndrome with the concept of grief and loss:

3. When caring for a client with ARDS who is not responding to treatments as anticipated, what nursing care might the family require as it deals with the possibility of the client's death?

4. How might you, as the nurse, help to support the family in this process?

Linking the exemplar of acute respiratory distress syndrome with the concept of comfort:

5. When caring for a client with ARDS, what symptoms might the client exhibit that may signal the client is in discomfort?

6. What treatments or diversional activities may be appropriate for this client?

READY Go to Companion Skills Manual

REFER Go to Pearson Nursing Student Resources
nursing.pearsonhighered.com

- Additional review material

REFLECT Case Study

Mr. Robert Michaels is a 75-year-old man with emphysema, asthma, high blood pressure, and almost complete hearing loss. A lifelong smoker, he quit smoking a few years ago when he was diagnosed with emphysema. For some time, he has been on oxygen therapy at night. He takes several medications daily, including 10 mg of prednisone, a corticosteroid inhaler, albuterol by nebulizer, and high blood pressure medication with a diuretic.

Two days ago, Mr. Michaels felt sick and was running a temperature. Mrs. Michaels, his wife, took him to his primary care provider's office where he was diagnosed with an upper respiratory infection and sent home with an oral antibiotic. Mr. Michaels woke up in the middle of the night in respiratory distress. Mrs. Michaels called 911, and her husband was transported by ambulance to the emergency department, where he was diagnosed with pneumonia and acute respiratory distress syndrome. Mr. Michaels was placed on mechanical ventilation and admitted to the critical care unit.

1. What are the nursing priorities for Mr. Michaels?

2. What considerations need to be given to Mr. Michaels' hearing loss?

3. What factors are likely to exacerbate his respiratory function?

4. How can you promote oxygenation for this client?

EXEMPLAR 15.2   Asthma

EXEMPLAR KEY TERMS
Airway remodeling, 990
Airway resistance, 991
Asthma, 990
Edema, 990
Hyperresponsiveness, 991
Hyperventilation, 991
Orthopneic position, 1002
Retractions, 992
Status asthmaticus, 991

EXEMPLAR LEARNING OUTCOMES
After reading about this exemplar, you will be able to:

1. Describe the pathophysiology, etiology, clinical manifestations, and direct and indirect causes of asthma.

2. Identify risk factors and prevention methods associated with asthma.

3. Illustrate the nursing process in providing culturally competent care across the life span for individuals with asthma.

4. Formulate priority nursing diagnoses appropriate for an individual with asthma.

5. Summarize therapies used by interdisciplinary teams in the collaborative care of an individual with asthma.

6. Plan evidence-based care for an individual with asthma and his or her family in collaboration with other members of the healthcare team.

7. Evaluate expected outcomes for an individual with asthma.

▶ OVERVIEW

Asthma is a chronic inflammatory disease of the lungs characterized by recurrent episodes of wheezing, breathlessness, chest tightness, and coughing. While most episodes or asthma "attacks" are relatively brief, some clients with asthma may experience longer episodes with some degree of airway impairment daily. Mild, brief episodes may resolve spontaneously, but most asthma attacks require treatment. Asthma in early life may lead to an irreversible decline of pulmonary function in adulthood as a result of permanent, structural changes called **airway remodeling**. These changes can lead to progressive or permanent loss of lung function.

▶ PATHOPHYSIOLOGY AND ETIOLOGY

In asthma, the airways are in a persistent state of inflammation. During symptom-free periods, airway inflammation in asthma is subacute or quiet. Even during these periods, however, inflammatory cells, such as eosinophils, neutrophils, and lymphocytes, may be found in airway tissues, and **edema** (swelling caused by excess fluid in bodily tissue) may be present.

An acute inflammatory response, during which resident inflammatory cells interact with inflammatory mediators, cytokines, and additional infiltrating inflammatory cells, may be triggered by a variety of factors. Common triggers for an acute asthma attack include exposure to allergens, respiratory tract infection, exercise, inhaled irritants, and emotional upsets. The inflammatory response resulting from exposure to one of these triggers leads to bronchoconstriction, airway edema, and impaired clearance of secretions. Airway narrowing impedes airflow and increases the work of breathing; trapped air mixes with inhaled air, impairing gas exchange.

When a trigger such as inhalation of an allergen or irritant occurs, an acute or early response develops in the airways. The airways of clients with asthma are hyperreactive and predisposed to bronchospasm. Sensitized mast cells in the bronchial mucosa release inflammatory mediators, such as histamine, prostaglandins, and leukotrienes. Resident and infiltrating inflammatory cells also produce inflammatory mediators, such as cytokines, bradykinin, and growth factors. These mediators stimulate parasympathetic receptors and bronchial smooth muscle to produce bronchoconstriction. They also increase capillary permeability, which allows plasma to escape and leads to mucosal edema. Production of mucus is stimulated; excess mucus collects in the narrowed airways.

The asthma attack is prolonged by the late-phase response, which develops 4–12 hours after exposure to the trigger. Inflammatory cells, such as basophils and eosinophils, are activated, and they damage airway epithelium, produce mucosal edema, impair mucociliary clearance, and produce or prolong bronchoconstriction. The degree of hyperreactivity depends on the extent of inflammation. Together, bronchoconstriction, edema, and mucous secretion narrow the airway. Airway resistance increases, limiting airflow and increasing the work of breathing (Figure 15–29 ●).

If an asthma attack goes untreated, limited expiratory airflow traps air distal to the spastic, narrowed airways. Trapped air mixes with inspired air in the alveoli, reducing oxygen ten-

sion and gas exchange across the alveolar–capillary membrane. Blood flow is reduced, further affecting gas exchange. As a result, hypoxemia develops. Hypoxemia and increased lung volume caused by trapping stimulate the respiratory rate. **Hyperventilation** (unusually fast respiration, or overbreathing) causes the $PaCO_2$ (the amount of pressure exerted by dissolved carbon dioxide) to fall, leading to respiratory alkalosis. (See the Acid–Base Balance module for more information about acid–base imbalances.)

To summarize, in an acute asthma attack, inflammatory mediators are released from sensitized airways, causing activation of inflammatory cells. This progression leads to bronchoconstriction, airway edema, and impaired mucociliary clearance. Airway narrowing limits airflow and increases the work of breathing; trapped air mixes with inhaled air, impairing gas exchange.

Etiology

Asthma triggered by allergies accounts for up to 50% of asthma attacks in the United States. Common allergens that can cause airway inflammation include pollens, weeds, molds, dust mites, and animal dander. Allergic asthma is an alteration of type I hypersensitivity, which is explained in more detail in the module on Immunity.

Asthma also may occur from exposure to aspirin and other nonsteroidal drugs. It may result from exercise, cold or hot air, viral infections, and even stress. Genetic involvement seems to be a component, but the role played by genetics in asthma is not clear. Occupational asthma arises from exposure to respiratory irritants in the workplace.

In an individual with asthma, any combination of these stimuli may result in airway **hyperresponsiveness** (an exaggerated bronchoconstrictor response) and airway obstruction from overproduction of mucus and edema of the airway mucosa (Figure 15–30 ●). **Status asthmaticus** is a severe, prolonged form of asthma that is difficult to treat. Untreated asthma or asthma that is unresponsive to treatment is a medical emergency that can result in respiratory failure.

According to the American Academy of Allergy, Asthma, and Immunology (AAAAI, 2013b) asthma affects 10% of children in the United States, making it the most common serious chronic childhood illness. Overall, asthma affects some 25 million Americans, resulting in millions of lost workdays each year, either for adult clients with asthma or for parents staying home with asthmatic children (AAAAI, 2013a, 2013b).

PEDIATRIC DIFFERENCES The child's narrower airway causes a greater increase in **airway resistance** (the effort or force needed to move oxygen through the trachea to the lungs). As air moves from the child's nares down the trachea to the distal airways (alveoli), it must flow through a relatively small area. Friction and increasing resistance are generated as air passes through the airway. When edema and swelling of the trachea occur in response to a virus, bacterium, or other irritant, the airway is further narrowed, and air is inspired more quickly to maintain oxygenation status (see Figure 15–6). The resulting negative pressure in the airway draws tissues closer together, further narrowing the airway and increasing airway resistance.

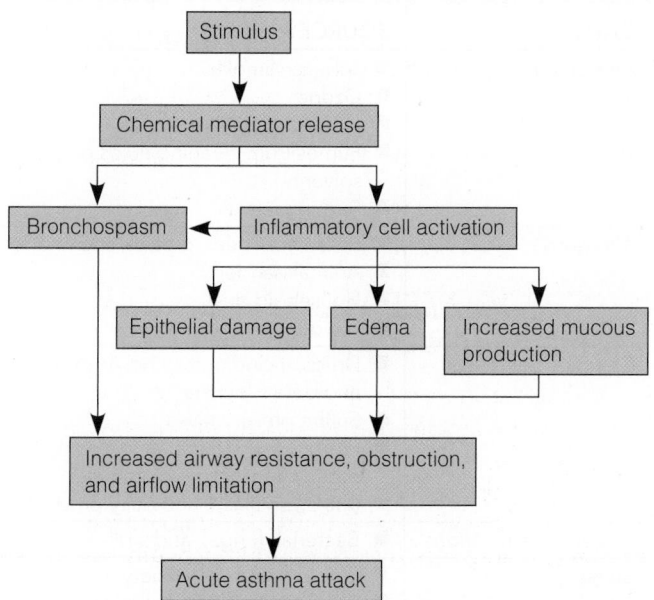

Figure 15–29 ● Pathogenesis of an acute episode of asthma.

NORMAL BRONCHIOLE

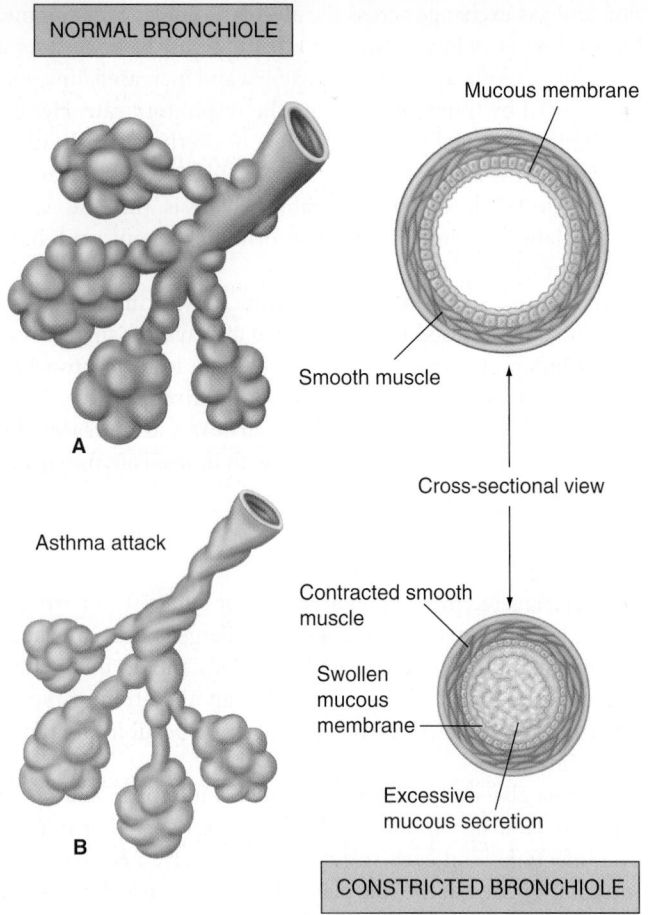

Mucous membrane

Smooth muscle

Cross-sectional view

A

Asthma attack

Contracted smooth muscle

Swollen mucous membrane

Excessive mucous secretion

B

CONSTRICTED BRONCHIOLE

Figure 15–30 ● Changes in bronchioles during an asthma attack. *A*, Normal bronchiole. *B*, In asthma attack.

Children under 6 years of age use the diaphragm to breathe, because the intercostal muscles are immature. By 6 years of age, the child uses the intercostal muscles more effectively. The ribs are primarily cartilage and very flexible. In cases of respiratory distress, the negative pressure caused by movement of the diaphragm draws the chest wall inward, causing **retractions** (sunken areas seen between the ribs during inspiration). See **Figure 15–31** ● for sites of retractions associated with respiratory distress.

Oxygen consumption is higher in children than in adults because of their greater metabolic rate. This rate of oxygen consumption increases when the child is in respiratory distress. The child also has fewer muscle glycogen reserves, leading to more rapid muscle fatigue when accessory muscles must be used for breathing (Froh, 2006).

Risk Factors

Risk factors include genetic factors, exposure to certain infections early in life, air pollution, and allergies (**Table 15–8** ●). Early childhood exposure to respiratory syncytial virus (RSV), parainfluenza virus, adenovirus, mycoplasma, and chlamydia has been associated with the development of asthma. Atmospheric air can be polluted by ozone, industrial gaseous wastes,

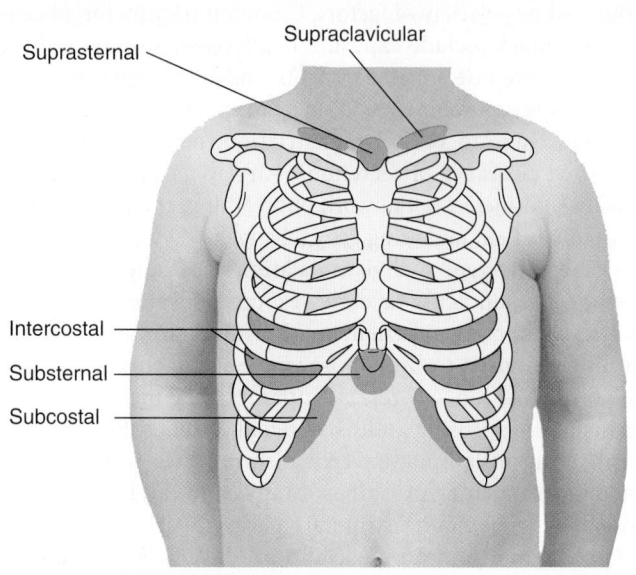

Suprasternal   Supraclavicular

Intercostal

Substernal

Subcostal

Figure 15–31 ● Retraction sites.

and particulate matter, such as pollens or tobacco smoke. Obesity, maternal smoking, and premature birth also increase the risk for asthma.

Prevention

Asthma attacks often can be prevented by avoiding allergens and environmental triggers. Modifying the home environment by controlling dust, removing carpets, covering mattresses and pillows to reduce dust mite populations, and installing air-filtering systems may be useful. Pets may need to be removed from the household. Stuffed animals provide wonderful living spaces for dust mites and should be removed from bedrooms.

TABLE 15–8	Common Causes of Asthma
CAUSE	**SOURCES**
Air pollutants	■ Tobacco smoke ■ Ozone ■ Nitrous and sulfur oxides ■ Fumes from cleaning fluids or solvents ■ Burning leaves
Allergens	■ Pollen from trees, grasses, and weeds ■ Animal dander ■ Household dust ■ Mold
Chemicals and food	■ Drugs, including aspirin, ibuprofen, and beta-blockers ■ Sulfite preservatives ■ Food and condiments, including nuts, monosodium glutamate (MSG), shellfish, and dairy products
Respiratory infections	■ Bacterial, fungal, and viral
Stress	■ Emotional stress/anxiety ■ Exercise in dry, cold climates

Eliminating all tobacco smoke in the house is vital. Wearing a mask that retains humidity and warm air while exercising in cold weather may help prevent attacks of exercise-induced or cold-triggered asthma. Early treatment of respiratory infections is vital to prevent exacerbations.

The client with moderate or severe asthma who is prescribed controller medications to prevent asthma attacks must take these daily in order for the medicine to be effective. Compliance with medication regimens varies greatly among those with asthma, as some will stop taking the medication once symptoms improve, which only increases the likelihood of another asthma attack. Client teaching about prevention must include the issue of compliance with medication regimens.

▶ CLINICAL MANIFESTATIONS

Clinical manifestations of asthma include coughing, wheezing, shortness of breath, chest tightness, tachypnea and tachycardia, and anxiety and apprehension. Asthma is defined by severity and control as well as by the frequency of exacerbations. Asthma that is not well controlled is evident by daytime symptoms, nocturnal awakenings because of symptoms, frequent use of a short-acting beta-agonist (SABA), and inability or difficulty performing normal activities, including exercise.

The onset of symptoms may be either abrupt or insidious, and an attack may subside rapidly or persist for hours or days. During an attack, tachycardia, tachypnea, and prolonged expiration are common. Diffuse wheezing may be heard on auscultation. With more severe attacks, use of accessory muscles for respirations, retractions, loud wheezing, and distant breaths sounds may be noted. Fatigue, anxiety, apprehension, and severe dyspnea that allow only one or two words to be spoken between breaths may occur with persistent severe episodes. The onset of respiratory failure is marked by inaudible breath sounds with reduced wheezing and an ineffective cough. Without careful assessment, this apparent relief of symptoms can be misinterpreted as improvement.

The frequency of attacks and the severity of symptoms vary greatly from person to person. Although some people have infrequent, mild episodes, or flares, others have nearly continuous manifestations.

Certain audible manifestations may offer a clue as to the location of airway obstruction. Examples include the following:

- Snoring may indicate a nasopharyngeal obstruction, enlarged tonsils, or adenoids.

- Inspiratory strider is a clinical manifestation of a partially obstructed upper airway.

- Expiratory stridor or wheeze, and/or a croupy or low-pitched cough is indicative of obstruction of the mid to lower trachea and central bronchus.

- Inspiratory and expiratory stridor signals a fixed obstruction at the larynx or subglottic space.

- Hoarseness indicates obstructed vocal chords.

Disease Monitoring

Severity of asthma symptoms can be difficult for the client to describe and for the nurse to assess. A peak expiratory flow reading (PEFR) provides an objective measure of lung function that allows clients to monitor symptoms and communicate their severity to others. Using small, inexpensive PEFR meters, clients take readings at varying times of day over several weeks to establish their personal best or normal PEFR. This value is then used to evaluate the severity of the airway obstruction. Traffic colors are used for simplicity: Green (80–100% of personal best) indicates asthma that is under control; yellow (50–80%) means caution, indicating a need for medication or treatment; and red (≤50%) signals an immediate need for a bronchodilator and further medical treatment if the level does not return to the yellow range immediately following administration of the bronchodilator.

Asthma in Children

An asthma attack can be frightening for both the child and the parent. Asthma interferes with a child's ability to sleep, concentrate in school, and play, causing multiple frustrations for both the child and the family. It is critical for parents to understand how, when, and why to give children their medications. Inappropriate use of medication can increase the child's risk for another attack. The nurse plays an essential role by taking time to understand the parents' understanding of their child's asthma management and by providing important client teaching regarding use of asthma medications and avoidance of triggers. The nurse should assess the parents' understanding at each healthcare interaction and provide additional teaching as necessary.

Children with asthma should have written asthma action plans that both parents and caregivers (including classroom teachers) can follow. Action plans ensure that medications are given in a timely manner without risk of overdose, and they ensure successful outcomes for the child and family.

If someone in the family smokes, the nurse provides education on the danger that secondhand smoke poses to those with asthma. The nurse also provides parents and caregivers with information about smoking cessation programs and therapies available in their area.

🔅 *Stay Current: Additional resources for parents can be found at the following Web sites:*

- American Academy of Allergy, Asthma, and Immunology: ***www.aaaai.org***

- Allergy and Asthma Network: Mothers of Asthmatics: ***www.aanma.org***

Asthma and Pregnancy

Asthma is the most common respiratory disease found in pregnancy; it affects 8% of all women in their childbearing years (American College of Allergy, Asthma, and Immunology [ACAAI], 2010). One third of clients with asthma experience improvement in their asthma during pregnancy; one third experience little or no change; and the remaining third of clients experience worsening of their asthma during pregnancy.

Clinical Manifestations and Therapies **Asthma**

SEVERITY	CLINICAL MANIFESTATIONS	CLINICAL THERAPIES
Mild intermittent	■ Daytime symptoms occur no more than twice a week. ■ Nighttime symptoms occur no more than twice per month. ■ Peak flow rates between attacks are normal. ■ Attacks (or flares) last hours to a few days. ■ Typical symptoms include shortness of breath, labored breathing, and fatigue.	■ Bronchodilator or beta-agonist, usually via inhaler or nebulizer. Beta-agonist usually prescribed for use before anticipated exposure (e.g., exercise). ■ A short course of oral corticosteroids may be prescribed if attack lasts beyond 1 day or is related to infection or other disease process that may extend recovery time. Inhaled corticosteroids usually take a few days to work and may not be prescribed for intermittent asthma except during periods of exposure to known triggers (e.g., ragweed). ■ If triggers include allergens, oral antihistamine may be prescribed.
Mild persistent	■ Daytime symptoms occur more than twice a week but less than once per day. ■ Nighttime symptoms occur more than twice a month. ■ Exacerbations may affect activity. ■ Typical symptoms include shortness of breath, labored breathing, and fatigue.	■ Bronchodilator or beta-agonist. Long-acting beta-agonist (LABA) may be prescribed for daily use regardless of whether the client is symptomatic. ■ Inhaled corticosteroids are prescribed for daily use to prevent symptoms during likely periods of exacerbation. ■ If triggers include allergens, antileukotrienes may be prescribed.
Moderate persistent	■ Symptoms occur daily. ■ A short-acting bronchodilator (e.g., albuterol inhaler) is used daily. ■ Nighttime symptoms occur more than once a week. ■ Exacerbations may last for days. ■ Exacerbations affect activity. ■ Symptoms of exacerbations include shortness of breath, labored and painful breathing, and chest tightness; may include coughing, wheezing, tachypnea, tachycardia, and fatigue.	■ Medications include LABAs, inhaled corticosteroids, antileukotrienes (if allergens are triggers). ■ Immunotherapy may be tried if triggers include allergens. ■ Cromolyn sodium or theophylline (long-acting bronchodilators) may be prescribed. ■ A nebulizer may be prescribed for use during exacerbations. ■ Oral corticosteroids may be prescribed for use during exacerbations lasting more than 1–2 days.
Severe persistent	■ Continuous symptoms occur with frequent exacerbations. ■ Physical activity is limited. ■ Symptoms include shortness of breath, labored and painful breathing, chest tightness, coughing, wheezing, tachypnea, tachycardia, difficulty speaking without pausing for breathing, and extreme fatigue.	■ Medications include LABA inhalers, inhaled corticosteroids, antileukotriene (if allergens are triggers). ■ Immunotherapy may be tried if triggers include allergens. ■ Cromolyn sodium or theophylline (long-acting bronchodilators) may be prescribed. ■ Oral corticosteroids may be prescribed for use during exacerbations lasting more than 1–2 days. ■ Steroids and beta-agonists delivered via nebulizer may be prescribed and used daily. ■ Steroid-dependent individuals with asthma and high IgE scores who do not receive relief from immunotherapy may be prescribed omalizumab (Xolair).

Evidence-Based Practice Improving Asthma Management in Adolescence

Problem

When children reach adolescence, they often find it more difficult to manage chronic illnesses such as asthma. Primary interventions for this age group typically involve education related to adherence with the therapeutic regimen and school asthma plans. Given that adolescents are particularly vulnerable to peer pressure, especially related to lifestyle choices, what effect might interventions that include peer participation and support have on health outcomes for adolescents with asthma?

Evidence

Asthma control often relies more on lifestyle management than on medication management. Kyngas and Rissanen (2001) found that adolescents are twice as likely to adhere to medical treatment for chronic conditions when they experience peer support. Rhee, Ciurzynski, and Yoos (2008) evaluated a peer-led asthma self-management program conducted in a camp setting. They found that peer-led interventions can be effective (to the extent of nearly eliminating the need for adult support during the sessions) when peer leaders receive proper training and when other variables (such as transportation to/from the sessions) are addressed. Yang, Sylva, and Lunt (2010) examined whether early adolescent healthy lifestyle for asthma management is associated with the social support that is received by both parents and peers. Researchers found that social support and peer acceptance are impor-

tant to maintaining a healthy lifestyle that supports asthma management in early adolescence and that interventions to promote peer support and provide peer education may assist in promoting healthy lifestyle management among early adolescents with asthma.

Implications

The evidence suggests the need to include questions related to peer support when assessing lifestyle management and adherence to treatment plans with adolescents who have asthma. Adolescents who feel supported by their peers may find it easier to make choices that are likely to improve their health outcomes and overall quality of life. Collaboration with school personnel (e.g., school nurses, coaches, teachers) may be necessary to inform the assessment and provide additional support in the school setting.

Critical Thinking Application

Consider the possible perceptions and beliefs of adolescents with asthma in your practice setting.

1. How would you assess these perceptions and beliefs?
2. How would you assess the role that peers play in an adolescent's lifestyle choices and asthma management?
3. Develop an education program for adolescents that explains asthma and discusses how adolescents can help their friends who have asthma stay healthy and safe.

The highest incidence of asthma exacerbation in clients who are pregnant occurs between 24 and 36 weeks of gestation. Asthma is often dormant during labor and birth, but PEFR should be monitored to detect changes in maternal respiratory status (ACAAI, 2010).

Prematurity and low birth weight are more common among infants of women who have asthma (ACAAI, 2010). Asthma has also been linked with higher rates of hyperemesis gravidarum, preeclampsia, uterine hemorrhage, and perinatal mortality. The goal of therapy is to prevent maternal exacerbations, because even a mild exacerbation can cause severe hypoxia-related complications in the fetus. If an exacerbation occurs, it should be managed in the same way as for a woman who is not pregnant, because the asthma drugs used are less of a threat to the fetus than a serious asthma attack (ACAAI, 2010).

Caring for a woman who is pregnant and has asthma calls for a multidisciplinary effort. If the client is not already in the

care of a pulmonologist, the nurse should make a referral. The nurse should encourage the client to talk with the pulmonologist about a stepwise action plan so that the client knows what to do in the event of an exacerbation. The nurse should encourage the client to use her peak flow meter daily as a method of monitoring her condition.

▶ COLLABORATION

Clients with asthma may benefit from a collaborative effort that includes a number of healthcare providers, including a respiratory therapist. The role of the nurse is discussed in more detail in the Nursing Process section.

Diagnostic Tests

An important diagnostic tool for a client with persistent asthma is the peak expiratory flow reading (PEFR). Nurses

---

Focus on Diversity and Culture Asthma Management

Asthma occurs in all racial and ethnic groups, but these groups differ in the use of preventive medications for asthma. Research indicates that differences in health beliefs, fear of steroids, or communication issues rather than financial barriers may play a role in the use of preventive asthma medications (ACAAI, 2010). Learning about the

family's cultural beliefs and practices, including nutrition habits, will help the nurse assess risks for asthma exacerbation that may be hidden within family cultural beliefs or habits. For example, families with specific food preferences may require additional education when a child has identified food allergies.

Lifespan Considerations
Children With Asthma

Growing children will have gradually increasing peak flow readings as their lungs grow and they exhale larger volumes of air with each breath. Daily use of peak flow monitors is particularly important in pediatric clients in order to track baseline or "normal" expiratory flow. Baseline should be reestablished as recommended by the physician.

should encourage all clients to use their peak flow meters daily and to keep a record of their readings, even on days when they are in the green zone (80%–100% of personal best). Nurses should remind clients with persistent asthma of the importance of using their peak flow meters at each healthcare interaction.

For clients who are suspected of having allergic asthma, scratch or patch testing and IgE testing allow the physician to determine the severity of the client's allergies as well as specific triggers to which the client reacts. Allergy testing normally is available only through an allergist or immunologist and is described in more detail in the module on Immunity.

Other diagnostic tests that may be useful for the client with asthma include the following:

- CBC with differential if infection is suspected
- ABG to monitor acid–base balance
- Pulmonary function studies
- Chest x-ray
- Oxygen saturation monitoring
- Transcutaneous oxygen and carbon dioxide monitoring.

✳ *Go to* **nursing.pearsonhighered.com** *to see Appendix B for information on diagnostic tests that may be useful for the client with asthma.*

Pharmacologic Therapy

Medications are used to prevent and control asthma symptoms, reduce the frequency and severity of exacerbations, and reverse airway obstruction. Drugs used for long-term control of asthma are taken daily to maintain control of the disease. The primary drugs in this group are anti-inflammatory agents, short-acting and long-acting bronchodilators, and leukotriene modifiers. Quick-relief medications provide prompt relief of bronchoconstriction and airflow obstruction with associated wheezing, cough, and chest tightness. Short-acting adrenergic stimulants (rapid-acting bronchodilators), anticholinergic drugs, and methylxanthines fall into this category.

A stepwise approach for managing asthma is recommended. This approach is based on the severity of disease (**Table 15–9** ●). For all clients, an inhaled SABA is recommended for quick relief of acute symptoms. Up to three treatments at 20-minute intervals or a single nebulizer treatment may be used as needed. Strategies for long-term control may need to be modified if a short-acting bronchodilator is needed more than twice a week (NHLBI, 2012b).

Many of the drugs used for continued asthma management and relief of an acute attack can be administered by a metered-dose inhaler (MDI), dry powder inhaler (DPI), or nebulizer. The advantages of administering medications locally by inhalation include rapid onset and reduced systemic effects. In an MDI, a chemical propellant is used to deliver the medication when the canister is depressed. In contrast, a DPI contains no propellant. Instead, the medication is released by inhaling rapidly through the mouthpiece.

BRONCHODILATORS   Most clients with asthma need bronchodilator therapy to relieve bronchoconstriction by relaxing the smooth muscles of the airway. Inhalation of nebulized medication is the preferred means of administration.

The primary bronchodilators used include adrenergic stimulants, methylxanthines, and anticholinergic agents. These drugs often are administered in combination with an anti-inflammatory agent. Adrenergic stimulants (beta$_2$-agonists) affect receptors on smooth muscle cells of the respiratory tract, causing smooth muscle relaxation and bronchodilation. Long-acting adrenergic stimulants, such as inhaled salmeterol and oral sustained-release albuterol, are used in conjunction with anti-inflammatory drugs to control symptoms but are not appropriate to treat an acute episode of asthma. Inhaled SABAs, such as albuterol, bitolterol, pir-

TABLE 15–9   Stepwise Approach to Asthma Management for Adults

STEP/DISEASE SEVERITY	PREFERRED TREATMENT	ALTERNATE OR AS NEEDED TREATMENT
Step 1: mild intermittent	No daily medication needed	Systemic corticosteroids for severe exacerbations; inhaled short-acting beta agonists (SABAs)
Step 2: mild persistent	Low-dose inhaled corticosteroids	Cromolyn, leukotriene modifier, nedocromil, or sustained-release theophylline; inhaled short-acting beta agonists (SABAs)
Step 3: moderate persistent	Low- to moderate-dose inhaled corticosteroids *and* long-acting inhaled β$_2$-agonist	Increase inhaled corticosteroid dose *or* combine inhaled corticosteroid with leukotriene modifier or theophylline; inhaled short-acting beta agonists (SABAs)
Step 4: severe persistent	High-dose inhaled corticosteroid *and* long-acting inhaled β$_2$-agonist	Add systemic corticosteroid; inhaled short-acting beta agonists (SABAs)

Source: National Institutes of Health. (2012). *Asthma.* Retrieved from http://www.nhlbi.nih.gov/health/health-topics/topics/asthma.

Client Teaching Using a Metered-Dose or Dry Powder Inhaler

- Firmly insert a charged metered-dose inhaler canister into the mouthpiece unit or spacer (if used).
- Remove mouthpiece cap. Shake canister vigorously for 3–5 seconds.
- Exhale slowly and completely.
- Holding the canister upside down, place the mouthpiece in the mouth, closing lips around it if a spacer is being used. When no spacer is used, hold the mouthpiece directly in front of the mouth.
- Press and hold the canister down while inhaling deeply and slowly for 3–5 seconds (see **Figure 15–32** ●).
- Hold breath for 10 seconds, release pressure on the container, remove from mouth, and exhale. Wait 20–30 seconds before repeating the procedure for a second puff.
- Rinse the mouth after using the inhaler to minimize systemic absorption and drying of the mucous membranes.
- Rinse the inhaler mouthpiece and spacer after use; store in a clean location.

Dry Powder Inhaler

- Keep the inhaler and medication in a clean, dry location. Do not refrigerate or store in a humid place (for example, the bathroom).
- Remove the cap and hold the inhaler upright. Inspect to be sure that the mechanism is clean and the mouthpiece is clear.
- If necessary, load the dose into the inhaler, following manufacturer's directions.
- Hold the inhaler level with the mouthpiece end facing down.
- Breathe out slowly and completely. Tilt your head back slightly.
- Place the mouthpiece in your mouth with your teeth over the mouthpiece. Seal your lips around the mouthpiece. Do not block the inhaler with your tongue.

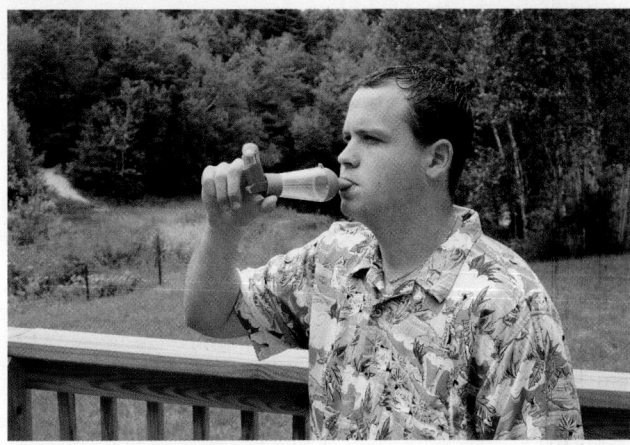

Figure 15–32 ● Proper use of a metered-dose inhaler with spacer.

- Breathe in rapidly and deeply through your mouth over 2–3 seconds to activate the flow of medication.
- Remove the inhaler from your mouth and hold your breath for 10 seconds.
- Exhale slowly through pursed lips to allow the medication to enter distal airways. Never exhale into the inhaler mouthpiece to prevent clogging.
- Rinse your mouth or brush your teeth after using the inhaler to avoid a bad taste from the medication and to prevent a yeast infection (if a corticosteroid medication is being used).
- Store the inhaler in a clean, sealed plastic bag; do not wash the inhaler unless so directed by the manufacturer. The mouthpiece should be cleaned weekly using a dry cloth.

buterol, and terbutaline, administered by MDI or DPI, are the treatment of choice for quick relief. They act within minutes, but their duration generally is short, lasting only 4–6 hours. Tachycardia and muscle tremors (common side effects of adrenergic agonists) are minimal with inhalation therapy.

Anticholinergic medications prevent bronchoconstriction by blocking parasympathetic input to bronchial smooth muscle. Ipratropium bromide, an anticholinergic drug administered by MDI, is useful when asthma symptoms are poorly controlled by adrenergic stimulants alone. Anticholinergic drugs act more slowly than adrenergic stimulants, requiring as much as 60–90 minutes to achieve maximal effect.

Theophylline is a methylxanthine used as adjunctive treatment for asthma. It relaxes bronchial smooth muscle and may also inhibit the release of chemical mediators of the inflammatory response. Regular monitoring of serum theophylline levels is necessary because of wide individual variations in metabolism and elimination of the drug and its toxic effects. Serum levels of 10–20 mcg/mL or lower are recommended. Theophylline may be used as a long-term bronchodilator, given once or twice daily. A related drug, aminophylline, may

be administered intravenously to treat an acute, severe exacerbation of the disease.

CORTICOSTEROIDS AND NSAIDS Corticosteroids and two nonsteroidal anti-inflammatory agents, cromolyn sodium and nedocromil, are used to suppress airway inflammation and reduce asthma symptoms. Corticosteroids block the late response to inhaled allergens and reduce edema and bronchial hyperresponsiveness. The preferred route of administration is by MDI or DPI to minimize systemic absorption and reduce the many adverse effects of prolonged steroid use (cushingoid effects). For a severe acute attack, corticosteroids may be given systemically to alleviate symptoms and induce remission.

Cromolyn sodium and nedocromil are anti-inflammatory agents used to prevent acute episodes of asthma. They reduce airway hyperreactivity and inhibit the release of mediator substances. These drugs are used for long-term control of asthma, not quick relief. Cromolyn sodium and nedocromil have a wide margin of safety and few side effects (see **Box 15–3** ●).

LEUKOTRIENE MODIFIERS The leukotriene modifiers montelukast (Singulair), zafirlukast (Accolate), and zileuton

Medications Asthma

CLASSIFICATION AND DRUG EXAMPLES	MECHANISMS OF ACTION	NURSING CONSIDERATIONS
Adrenergic Stimulants *Drug examples:* epinephrine isoproterenol (Isuprel) metaproterenol (Alupent, Metaprel) terbutaline (Brethaire, Brethine) isoetharine (Bronkosol, Bronkometer) albuterol (Proventil, Ventolin) bitolterol (Tornalate) pirbuterol (Maxair) salmeterol (Serevent) formoterol (Foradil) *Combination products:* albuterol/ipratropium (Combivent) salmeterol/fluticasone (Advair)	Adrenergic stimulants affect sympathetic receptors in the respiratory tract. Administered by metered-dose inhalers or dry powder inhalers, these drugs are the treatment of choice for acute bronchial asthma. Nearly all of the drugs in this class (epinephrine and isoproterenol being the exceptions) selectively activate β_2-receptors at the doses typically used to treat asthma. β_2-receptor activation results in smooth muscle relaxation and bronchodilation. Formoterol and salmeterol are highly selective to β_2-receptors, resulting in fewer adverse effects. Formoterol and salmeterol have been shown to increase the risk of serious asthma exacerbations and death, however. These drugs should only be used when the disease cannot be adequately controlled with other medications. Oral forms of adrenergic agonists may be used for prophylaxis but are not effective in treating an acute attack because of their slow onset. When administered orally or parenterally, their effect on sympathetic nervous system receptors can produce undesirable side effects such as nervousness, irritability, tachycardia, and cardiac dysrhythmias.	▪ Use with caution in clients with hypertension, cardiovascular disease or dysrhythmias, hyperthyroidism, or diabetes. ▪ When given to a client who is hypoxemic and acidotic, these drugs may cause potentially dangerous cardiac stimulation. ▪ When given by MDI, wait 1–2 minutes between puffs to allow airways to dilate, permitting the second dose to reach distal airways. ▪ Observe for desired effect of reduced dyspnea and wheezing. Central nervous system stimulation (anxiety, irritability, and insomnia) and tremor are common side effects. Health Education for the Client and Family ▪ Use the prescribed inhaler or nebulizer as directed. ▪ If you are taking a bronchodilator along with another medication by inhalation, use the bronchodilator first to open airways and enhance the effectiveness of the second medication. ▪ Rinse the mouth after using inhalers to reduce systemic absorption of the medication. ▪ Keep a log to track your bronchodilator use. If the drug becomes less effective, or if you need a higher dosage or more frequent doses than prescribed, contact your physician. ▪ Report palpitations, irregular pulse, and other side effects to the physician.
Methylxanthines *Drug examples:* theophylline (Bronkotabs, Quibron, Slo-Phyllin Theolair, Theo-Dur, others) aminophylline (Somophyllin)	The methylxanthines are central nervous system (CNS) stimulants chemically related to caffeine. These drugs produce bronchodilation through relaxation of bronchial smooth muscle. As CNS stimulants, they produce adverse effects such as nervousness, insomnia, and tremors. When administered in large doses, convulsions may result. Once the drugs of choice for preventing and treating asthma attacks, they are now used primarily to prevent nocturnal asthma in affected adult clients. Theophylline has a narrow margin of safety and high potential for toxicity. Because the metabolism and excretion of theophylline vary significantly from person to person—affected by such factors as age, smoking, genetic factors, alcoholism, and other chronic diseases—monitoring of serum levels is vital.	▪ The therapeutic blood level for theophylline is *Adult:* 5–20 mcg/mL, *Elderly:* 5–18 mcg/mL. ▪ Monitor for manifestations of toxicity. Anorexia, nausea, vomiting, restlessness, insomnia, cardiac dysrhythmias, and seizures are early manifestations. Other manifestations include epigastric pain, hematemesis, diarrhea, headache, irritability, muscle twitching, palpitations, tachycardia, flushing, and circulatory failure. ▪ Administer with meals or a full glass of water or milk to minimize gastric irritation. ▪ Monitor effect closely when administering concurrently with other medications such as barbiturates, anticonvulsants, thyroid hormone, beta-blockers, bronchodilators, and others. ▪ Aminophylline is incompatible with many other intravenous drugs. Use a separate line or flush the line with normal saline before and after administering any other preparation. Health Education for the Client and Family ▪ Oral methylxanthines are ineffective to treat an acute asthma attack; do not delay other treatment by using these drugs. ▪ Check with the physician before taking any over-the-counter medications or other prescription drugs while on theophylline. ▪ Do not smoke while using this drug. ▪ Report adverse effects to the physician.

Medications **Asthma** (continued)

CLASSIFICATION AND DRUG EXAMPLES	MECHANISMS OF ACTION	NURSING CONSIDERATIONS
Anticholinergics *Drug examples:* atropine ipratropium bromide (Atrovent) tiotropium bromide (Spiriva) *Combination products:* albuterol/ipratropium (Combivent)	Anticholinergics are potent bronchodilators, blocking muscarinic receptors of the parasympathetic nervous system. Activation of muscarinic receptors produces smooth muscle contraction and bronchoconstriction; blockade of these receptors facilitates smooth muscle relaxation and bronchodilation. Atropine is used infrequently because of its tendency to dry secretions of the mucous membranes and other side effects. Ipratropium and tiotropium bromide are available as inhalers and have fewer side effects than atropine.	■ Assess for possible contraindications to the drug, including hypersensitivity, glaucoma, prostatic hypertrophy, or bladder-neck obstruction. ■ Assess for desired and/or adverse effects: improving or worsening symptoms; nausea, vomiting, abdominal cramping, anxiety, dizziness; headache. ■ Provide ice chips, fluids, or hard candy to relieve dry mouth. Health Education for the Client and Family ■ To prevent overdose, take no more than the prescribed number of doses per day. ■ If the drug becomes less effective over time, notify the physician; an adjustment in dosage may be needed.
Corticosteroids *Drug examples:* beclomethasone dipropionate (Vanceril, Beclovent) triamcinolone acetonide (Azmacort) flunisolide (AeroBid) fluticasone propionate (Flovent) dexamethasone sodium phosphate (Decadron Phosphate Respihaler) *Combination products:* salmeterol/fluticasone (Advair)	The anti-inflammatory effect of corticosteroids helps both prevent and treat acute episodes. Corticosteroids are used to reduce the frequency and severity of asthma attacks and allow reduced dosages of other drugs. The beneficial effects of corticosteroids for asthma result from their ability to decrease the synthesis and release of inflammatory mediators (such as histamine and leukotrienes), reduce inflammatory cell activation and infiltration, and decrease airway edema. Corticosteroids also decrease mucous production in the airways and increase the number and receptivity of β_2-receptors. The cushingoid side effects of corticosteroids, always a major concern with their use, are minimized when they are inhaled. Note that the combination product salmeterol/fluticasone is associated with an increased risk of serious asthma exacerbations and death. It is recommended for use only when asthma is inadequately controlled using other medications or for clients who clearly require both a bronchodilator and an inhaled corticosteroid for managing their asthma (Adams, Holland & Urban, 2014).	■ Administer inhaler doses after bronchodilators to facilitate transport of the medication to distal airways. ■ Assess for common side effects: sore throat; hoarseness; and oropharyngeal or laryngeal *Candida albicans* infection. ■ Administer antifungal medications or gargles as ordered. Health Education for the Client and Family ■ Rinse the mouth after using the inhaler and maintain good oral hygiene to reduce the risk of fungal infections. ■ These medications should not be used to alleviate the symptoms of an acute attack. ■ Several weeks of continued therapy may be required before a beneficial effect is noticed. ■ Notify the physician if you develop weight gain, fluid retention, muscle weakness, redistribution of fat, or mood changes.
Mast Cell Stabilizers *Drug examples:* cromolyn sodium (Intal, NasalCrom) nedocromil (Tilade)	Cromolyn sodium and nedocromil inhibit inflammatory cells in the airway, blocking early and late responses to inhaled antigens. Both drugs also prevent bronchoconstriction in response to inhaling cold air. These drugs act primarily by stabilizing the cytoplasmic membrane of mast cells, preventing the cells from releasing inflammatory mediators such as histamine. These drugs are used only for preventing asthma attacks, not to treat an acute attack. They are administered by metered-dose inhaler, and have a wide margin of safety. Clients using nedocromil may complain of an unpleasant taste.	■ Evaluate for potential adverse effects of wheezing and bronchoconstriction. Health Education for the Client and Family ■ Gargling or sipping water can decrease the throat irritation associated with nebulizer treatment. ■ Use appropriate technique. Inhale deeply with head tipped back to open airways, hold breath, and then exhale. Repeat until all of the drug has been inhaled. ■ These drugs are used only to prevent asthma attacks; they are not effective in treating an acute attack. ■ Several weeks may be required before a beneficial effect is noted.
Leukotriene Modifiers *Drug examples:* montelukast (Singulair) zafirlukast (Accolate) zileuton (Zyflo)	Leukotriene modifiers interfere with the inflammatory process in the airways by suppressing the effects of leukotrienes, a group of inflammatory mediators. Leukotrienes are powerful bronchoconstrictors and vasodilators; blocking their synthesis or their receptors improves airflow, decreases symptoms, and reduces the need for short-acting bronchodilators. They are used for maintenance therapy in adults and children over the age of 12 as an alternative to inhaled corticosteroid therapy. They are not used to treat an acute attack.	■ Administer at least 1 hour before or 2 hours after meals. ■ These drugs inhibit some liver enzymes, affecting the metabolism of warfarin and possibly terfenadine and theophylline. Monitor prothrombin times and theophylline blood levels. ■ Monitor liver enzymes, because these drugs may be toxic to the liver. Health Education for the Client and Family ■ Take the drugs as prescribed on an empty stomach. ■ Notify the physician if a change in color of stools or urine is noted or if jaundiced.

Lifespan Considerations Medication Administration in Children With Asthma

Typically, inhalation is the preferred method of administration for asthma medication, because it rapidly delivers the medication to the lungs for prompt onset of action. Other benefits are reduced risk of adverse effects and lower dosing compared to the oral route. However, inhalers are relatively inefficient and have special challenges for infants and young children. Effective medication delivery to the lung is affected by respiratory rate, degree of airflow obstruction, the medication being administered, and the device being used. Many devices require cooperation, coordination, and appropriate technique.

- Children older than 5 years of age are usually able to use a metered-dose inhaler (MDI), coordinating medication release and inspiration; however, they may prefer to use a holding chamber or spacer with a valve. Spacers help enhance the amount of the drug that reaches the lungs. They also trap larger particles, preventing them from reaching the mouth and being swallowed, which can cause local and systemic side effects (Zagaria, 2010). Valves prevent the escape of medication during use. The plastic spacer should be washed with a household detergent and permitted to air-dry. When teaching the child to use an MDI without a spacer, let the child learn to breathe in slowly with straws.

- Spacers have a mouthpiece or mask attachment. When selecting a spacer for infants and children up to 4 years of age, choose one with a mask, because children in this age range tend to be nasal breathers. Choose a mask size that fits the child's face and that has a flexible seal to prevent air from leaking around the facial features. When the young child is uncooperative, it may still be difficult to maintain a seal. Crying leads to prolonged exhalation and short inspiratory efforts, which reduce lung deposition. Use play or distraction to help improve cooperation for medication

delivery. Many manufacturers now offer child-friendly masks that resemble cartoon characters or super heroes, which may help children find the masks more appealing.

- Some inhaler and spacer brands have a whistle on inhalation that indicates a breath is too fast or too shallow; in others, the whistle signifies an adequate breath has been taken. When teaching the child and family about inhaler use, make sure you know what the whistle means.

- With nebulizers, no coordination of breathing is required, making them easier for young children to use. A mask or mouthpiece is used. The humidification provided during treatment provides an additional benefit. While nebulizers are not more effective than MDIs with a spacer, they may lead to better outcomes, because the child only needs to breathe in and out normally. Nebulizers should not be used with the mouthpiece held away from the mouth, because lung deposition of the medication is significantly reduced and because this increases the risk of depositing some medication in the eyes. Nebulizers are expensive, need a power source, and take 8–10 minutes to complete the treatment. Infants and young children may have difficulty cooperating for the duration of the nebulizer treatment. Crying and a face mask that is too large for the child's face can further decrease delivery of the medication to the lower airways.

- Dry powder inhalers (DPIs) are activated when the client takes a breath, so puffs do not need to be coordinated with inhalation. No spacer is required, and no propellant is used. DPIs can be used by children ages 5 and older. Delivery to the lower airway varies between 15% and 30%, depending on the type of inhaler. Children with severe asthma may not be able to produce enough airflow to get an adequate dose of medication.

Sources: Data from Zagaria, M. A. E. (2010). Inhalant agents for asthma, bronchospasm, and COPD: Focus on delivery devices and inhalation technique. *American Journal for Nurse Practitioners, 14*(3), 21–25; Sleath, B., Ayala, G. X., Gillette, C., Williams, D., Davis, S., Tudor, G., et al. (2011). Provider demonstration and assessment of child device technique during pediatric asthma visits. *Pediatrics, 127*(4), 642–648; Asthma Initiative of Michigan for Healthy Lungs. (2011). *How to use a metered-dose inhaler the right way.* Retrieved from http://www.getasthmahelp.org/inhalers_main.asp.

Box 15–3 Side Effects of Corticosteroids

Corticosteroids carry a risk of side effects that can be severe and even life threatening. The side effects vary depending on whether the corticosteroid is administered orally or by inhalation. Duration of therapy also is a factor.

Side effects of corticosteroids given orally as short-term therapy (and which typically resolve once therapy concludes) include:

- Glaucoma (elevated pressure in the eyes)
- Fluid retention, which causes swelling in the lower legs
- Hypertension
- Mood swings
- Weight gain (fat deposits in the abdomen, face, and the back of the neck).

Side effects of corticosteroids given by mouth for long-term treatment include:

- Cataracts (clouding of the lens in one or both eyes)
- Hyperglycemia

- Increased risk of infections
- Osteoporosis
- Increased risk of fractures
- Suppression of adrenal gland hormone production
- Bruising, thin skin
- Delayed wound healing
- Growth suppression in children.

Side effects of long-term steroid use may take additional time and adjunctive therapies to resolve. Some adverse effects, such as growth suppression and osteoporosis, may not resolve.

Oral thrush and hoarseness may result from use of inhaled and nebulized corticosteroids. These can be avoided easily by rinsing and gargling with water following medication administration.

Source: Based on Cleveland Clinic. (2013). *Corticosteroids.* Retrieved from http://my.clevelandclinic.org/drugs/corticosteroids/hic_corticosteroids.aspx; Mayo Clinic. (2010). *Corticosteroids.* Retrieved from http://www.mayoclinic.com/health/drug-information/DR602333; Wilson, B. A., Shannon, M. T., & Shields., K. M. (2012). *Pearson nurse's drug guide 2012.* Upper Saddle River, NJ: Pearson Education.

(Zyflo Filmtab) are oral medications that reduce the inflammatory response in clients with asthma. They appear to improve lung function, diminish symptoms, and reduce the need for short-acting bronchodilators. These drugs affect the metabolism and excretion of other medications, such as warfarin and theophylline, and they may cause liver toxicity. Nursing implications for medications used to treat asthma are outlined in the Medication feature.

Complementary and Alternative Therapy

A number of herbal preparations and other complementary therapies have been shown to be helpful in treating asthma. The National Center for Complementary and Alternative Medicine (NCCAM) reports that asthma ranks in the top 15 conditions for which individuals turn to complementary therapy. Although there is renewed evidence and interest in use of deep breathing and relaxation techniques to manage asthma, there is a substantial lack of evidence to support the use of complementary therapies as alternatives to the use of pharmacology combined with trigger avoidance (NCCAM, 2012). Nurses working with clients with asthma should assess for use of complementary and alternative therapies and encourage clients to discuss these with their primary care provider.

Herbal preparations that include *Atropa belladonna* (the natural form of atropine) or ephedra (also called *ma huang*), an herb that contains ephedrine, should not be used, as they can interact with prescribed medications. Because of the dangers associated with its use, sale of herbal products containing ephedra has been banned (NCCAM, 2012). Advise clients asking about the use of Chinese herbal remedies to treat asthma to inquire if any recommended product contains ma huang or ephedra—and to avoid such products. Capsaicin also may relieve acute asthma symptoms. Other herbal preparations include quercetin and grape seed extract. Refer clients interested in using natural preparations to a qualified herbalist, and emphasize the importance of talking to the physician before using these preparations along with conventional treatment.

In addition to herbals, other complementary therapies, such as biofeedback, yoga, breathing techniques, acupuncture, homeopathy, and massage, have been found to alleviate or help control asthma symptoms.

■ NURSING PROCESS

The immediate priority for nursing care is to help the client maintain oxygenation and a patent airway. The long-term goal of care is to improve an individual's ability to function, ability to participate in ADLs and exercise, and ultimately, quality of life.

Assessment

Assessment of the client experiencing an acute asthma attack must be very focused and timely. For clients with persistent asthma, assessment should focus on concerns and symptoms at each healthcare interaction, but also on the client's overall quality of life. Clients who live with chronic illness may be at increased risk for depression, and nurses should be alert for the need to assess symptoms of mood or anxiety (Bruce, 2009).

- *Health history.* Current symptoms, including chest tightness, shortness of breath, dyspnea; duration of current attack; measures used to relieve symptoms and their effect; identified precipitating factors for the attack; frequency of attacks; current medications; and known allergies
- *Physical examination.* Apparent level of distress; color; vital signs; respiratory rate and excursion; breath sounds throughout lung fields; apical pulse.

During the physical examination, the nurse also auscultates lung sounds, inspects and palpates the chest for symmetry, and assesses for use of accessory muscles, which indicates an increased need for oxygen at the alveolar level. In addition, the nurse assesses for the presence and nature of pulmonary secretions (thinned secretions are easier to expectorate than thick mucus) and for tobacco use. The nurse also observes the position or posturing of the individual. Self-posturing (e.g., a tripod stance) may indicate respiratory distress.

During the health history, the nurse also assesses how effectively asthma is being controlled. This includes assessment of how often symptoms require use of short-acting beta-agonists, how often the client wakes with symptoms, and how often the client requires primary or emergency care to address asthma management. A history of symptom and control issues for the previous few weeks may help the nurse understand how asthma affects the client. Monitoring PEFR and keeping a daily log should be encouraged to help the client recognize and respond to changes in oxygenation status earlier, which may help reduce the extent of exacerbations. A daily log may also help identify triggers or exposures that aggravate asthma symptoms.

Diagnosis

The age and developmental level of the client, the severity of the client's asthma and its etiology, and the presence of comorbid conditions (if any) will impact nursing diagnosis of the client. The following diagnoses may be appropriate for clients with asthma:

- *Ineffective Breathing Pattern*
- *Ineffective Airway Clearance*
- *Impaired Gas Exchange*
- *Activity Intolerance*
- *Anxiety*
- *Ineffective Therapeutic Regimen Management.*

(NANDA-I © 2012)

Planning

The planning process is informed by the assessment of the client's current condition and the client's goals for the future.

Together, the nurse and client will develop a plan of care that may include the following goals:

- The client will experience improved asthma control as evidenced by fewer and less severe exacerbations.
- The client will require fewer healthcare visits to maintain asthma control.
- The client will reduce exposure to irritants that aggravate asthma symptoms.
- The client will experience improved quality of life (as evidenced by fewer days missed from school or work, greater ease and comfort, and ability to participate in health promotion activities).

Implementation

Asthmatic clients require careful monitoring and rapid intervention during exacerbations in order to prevent hypoxia and promote oxygenation. Because of the chronic nature of the disorder, clients are often the best source of information regarding the implementations that work best for them, and they should be consulted when planning and implementing care.

> **SAFETY ALERT**
> The following signs and symptoms signal hypoxia:
> - Increasing restlessness, irritability, or unexplained sudden confusion
> - Rapid heart rate accompanied by a rapid respiratory rate.

Promote Effective Gas Exchange

Bronchospasm and bronchoconstriction, increased mucous secretion, and airway edema narrow the airways and impair airflow during an acute attack of asthma. Both inspiratory and expiratory volume are affected, decreasing the oxygen available at the alveolus for the process of respiration. Narrowed air passages increase the work of breathing, increasing the metabolic rate and tissue demand for oxygen.

- Monitor skin color and temperature and LOC. Cyanosis, cool clammy skin, and changes in LOC (e.g., agitation, lethargy, and confusion) indicate worsening hypoxia.
- Assess ABG results and pulse oximetry readings; notify the physician of abnormal values or changes in status. These values provide information about gas exchange and the adequacy of alveolar ventilation. A fall in oxygen saturation levels is an early indicator of impaired gas exchange.
- Place in Fowler, high-Fowler, or **orthopneic position** (with head and arms supported on the overbed table) to facilitate breathing and lung expansion. These positions reduce the work of breathing and increase lung expansion, especially of basilar areas.
- Administer oxygen as ordered. If a mask is used, monitor closely for feelings of claustrophobia or suffocation. Supplemental oxygen reduces hypoxemia. Small children may require use of a pediatric tent. Oxygen therapy via mask or tent can be frightening; monitor client for anxiety during administration.
- Administer nebulizer treatments and provide humidification as ordered. Nebulizer treatments are used to administer

bronchodilators and other medications; humidity helps loosen secretions.
- Increase fluid intake. Increasing fluids helps keep secretions thin.

> **SAFETY ALERT**
> Frequently assess respiratory status (at least every 1–2 hours): respiratory rate and depth, chest movement or excursion, breath sounds, and PEFR. Respiratory status can change rapidly during an acute asthma attack and its treatment. Decreasing PEFR readings indicate worsening airflow restriction. Slowed, shallow respirations with significantly diminished breath sounds and decreased wheezing may indicate exhaustion and impending respiratory failure. Immediate intervention is necessary.

Enhance Breathing Pattern

The physiological changes in lung ventilation that occur during an acute asthma attack impair both lung expansion and emptying. Hypoxia and dyspnea can also cause anxiety, compounding the problem by increasing the respiratory rate. Collaborative and nursing interventions can help restore a more normal breathing pattern and adequate lung ventilation.

- Monitor vital signs and laboratory results. Tachypnea, tachycardia, elevated blood pressure, and increasing hypoxemia and hypercapnia are signs of compromised respiratory status.
- Assist with ADLs as needed. This conserves client energy and reduces fatigue.
- Provide rest periods between scheduled activities and treatments. Scheduled rest is important to prevent fatigue and reduce oxygen demands.
- Administer medications, including bronchodilators and anti-inflammatory drugs, as ordered. Monitor for desired and possible adverse effects. Medications are used to improve airway status and facilitate breathing.

> **SAFETY ALERT**
> Frequently assess respiratory rate, pattern, and breath sounds. Note manifestations of ineffective breathing, including rapid rate, shallow respirations, nasal flaring, use of accessory muscles, intercostal retractions, and diminished or absent breath sounds. Early identification of ineffective respirations allows timely initiation of interventions to prevent a decline in condition resulting in more severe complications.

Help Relieve Anxiety

Acute exacerbations of asthma can produce significant anxiety. Fear of being unable to breathe and feelings of suffocation associated with acute asthma are significant. Financial or other concerns may cause the client to want to avoid hospitalization. Increasingly frequent and severe episodes may cause fear for the future. Hypoxia contributes to anxiety as well, stimulating the sympathetic nervous system and the fight-or-flight response.

- Assess level of anxiety. Interventions for severe anxiety or panic differ from those for mild or moderate anxiety.

Lifespan Considerations Life-Threatening Total Airway Obstruction in Children

When a life-threatening total airway obstruction occurs, efforts to clear the obstruction include back blows and chest thrusts in an infant or abdominal thrusts in older children. In the emergency department, oxygen is administered. Efforts are made to visualize the foreign body with a laryngoscope and remove it with Magill forceps. Whenever possible, the child is taken to the operating room so that optimal conditions exist to protect and maintain the child's airway during removal of the foreign body. When a partial airway obstruction exists, fluoroscopy and fiberoptic bronchoscopy may be used to identify, locate, and extract the foreign body.

Following removal of the foreign body, the child is stabilized and observed for a few hours in a short-stay unit. Depending on the type of object, location of the object, and degree of obstruction, surgical removal and hospitalization may be required.

In some cases, children are initially treated for the complication or for asthma without recognizing that a foreign body was the cause of the respiratory distress. This occurs more often when the airway foreign body is not visualized on an x-ray. When the child is nonresponsive to medications, further diagnostic testing may reveal the foreign body (Srivastava, 2010).

- Assist the client to identify coping skills that have been successful in the past. Successful coping helps the client regain control of the situation, reducing anxiety.
- Listen actively to concerns; do not deny or negate the fear of dying or of being unable to breathe. Active listening promotes trust and helps the client express concerns.
- Include the client in care planning and decisions as appropriate, without making excessive demands. Participating in decision making increases the client's sense of control. Because high levels of anxiety interfere with the ability to make decisions, it is important to avoid placing demands on the client that may further increase the level of anxiety.
- Reduce excessive environmental stimuli, and maintain a calm demeanor. This promotes rest.
- Allow supportive family members to remain with the client. Significant others provide additional support and can help reduce anxiety.
- Assist in the use of relaxation techniques, such as guided imagery, muscle relaxation, and meditation. These techniques help restore psychological balance and reduce sympathetic stimulation and responses.

Promote Adherence to Therapeutic Regimen

Once acute asthma is under control and effective respirations have been reestablished, it is important to ensure the client understands the importance of adhering to the treatment plan in order to prevent recurring attacks.

- Assess the client's level of understanding about asthma and the prescribed treatment regimen. Provide additional information and teaching as indicated. Assessment helps identify and clarify misperceptions and difficulties with disease management.
- Discuss the client's perception of the illness and its effect on his or her lifestyle. Open discussion can help identify conflicts between lifestyle and the treatment regimen.
- Assist the client and significant others to identify problems or difficulties integrating the treatment regimen into their lifestyle. Asthma and its management may necessitate lifestyle modifications to prevent acute exacerbations, which can significantly impact family members. Examples include eliminating cigarette smoking or pets from the household, removing carpets, or daily damp-dusting to remove dust mites.

- Assess knowledge and understanding of prescribed medications, use of over-the-counter preparations, and use of complementary or alternative therapies. This is important to determine misperceptions or possible misuse of medications.
- Provide verbal and written instructions at the client's level of understanding. Written instructions reinforce teaching and allow future reference.
- Refer to counseling, support groups, or self-help organizations. Counseling, support groups, and self-help organizations can help the client and family adapt to living with asthma and the treatment regimen.

Provide Education Regarding Activity Intolerance

Clients with mild asthma may not experience any activity intolerance except during and immediately following a flare. For the client with moderate to severe asthma, however, activity intolerance can greatly limit quality of life.

- Teach the client how to monitor cardiopulmonary response to activity by taking his or her own pulse and blood pressure.
- Teach the client how to monitor and record peak flow rates before and after activities.
- Help the client assess his or her capacity to sustain activities and determine activities and exercises in which the client can participate.
- Assess the need for short-acting bronchodilators before activity or exercise.
- Teach the client to space periods of activity with periods of rest.
- Assist the client with ADLs as needed.

Evaluation

The nurse evaluates the client's response to treatment, which may be compared to the following common expected outcomes:

- Client maintains oxygen saturation greater than 90%.
- Client demonstrates proper use of medications.
- Client lists common triggers for asthmatic exacerbation and strategies to avoid triggers.
- Client and family members list symptoms requiring immediate notification of primary provider.
- Client responds appropriately to asthma flare-up.
- Client maintains optimal nutrition to promote health.
- Client describes appropriate follow-up care to control condition.

NURSING CARE PLAN · A Client With Asthma

Sarah Mitchell is a 35-year-old working mother with moderate persistent asthma. Her known triggers are allergies to dust mites, cockroach feces, grass and tree pollens, and some molds. She takes immunotherapy once a week and takes maintenance medications daily. She works as a full-time preschool teacher.

Mrs. Mitchell calls her allergist's office asking to be seen because she is having a bad asthma flare. She reports having to use her rescue inhaler every 3–4 hours, that her chest is very tight, and that she is having trouble breathing. She has used her home peak flow meter three times since late yesterday and has been in the yellow zone each time. She did not sleep last night because of her asthma symptoms.

ASSESSMENT

The nurse, Clancy O'Hara, admits Mrs. Mitchell when she arrives at the allergist's office. During the health history Mrs. Mitchell confirms she is compliant with her medication regimen. She takes a LABA in combination with a low-dose corticosteroid, a daily antihistamine, and montelukast. In checking Mrs. Mitchell's medical record, Clancy notes that the client is maintaining her scheduled immunotherapy appointments. Mrs. Mitchell reports that she is not aware of any unusual allergy exposure but says that several of her students have a cold this week.

On physical examination, Clancy notes that Mrs. Mitchell's vital signs are as follows: T_O 37°C (98.6°F), P 96 bpm, R 36/min, BP 128/86 mmHg. Other assessment data include needing to pause frequently while speaking, use of accessory muscles for respirations, and scattered wheezes audible over both lung fields with stethoscope. ABG results are pH 7.32, PaO_2, 88; $PaCO_2$, 47; and HCO_3, 38. Pulses are strong and equal bilaterally, and the client expectorates small amount of white mucus into a tissue.

DIAGNOSES

- *Ineffective Breathing Pattern* related to exacerbation of asthma
- *Impaired Gas Exchange* related to bronchoconstriction and mucus in airways
- *Fatigue* related to ineffective sleep pattern
- *Activity Intolerance* related to inadequate oxygenation

(NANDA-I © 2012)

PLANNING

Together Clancy and Mrs. Mitchell agree on the following outcomes:
- Mrs. Mitchell's breathing will return to the green zone within 24 hours.
- Mrs. Mitchell's need for her rescue inhaler will decline within 3 days and return to baseline within 1 week.
- Mrs. Mitchell will maintain baseline respiratory rate and pattern sufficient to meet her ADLs within 72 hours.

IMPLEMENTATION

Mrs. Mitchell's provider prescribes a higher-dose inhaled steroid to use 10–15 minutes after she uses her LABA. The provider also gives Mrs. Mitchell a short, tapered course of prednisone. Clancy initiates the following implementations:

- Teaches Mrs. Mitchell how to properly self-administer medications and about possible side effects associated with steroid use, including those that should be reported immediately.
- Explains the importance of taking the steroid as ordered and not stopping the medication suddenly.
- Provides strategies for managing fatigue, including a handout with written instructions.

- Teaches Mrs. Mitchell the importance of proper nutrition and hydration in asthma management.
- Observes Mrs. Mitchell's technique when measuring peak flow.
- Reviews signs and symptoms indicating worsening condition, and instructs Mrs. Mitchell to call the provider if these occur.
- Schedules Mrs. Mitchell to return in 6 weeks for a further evaluation, but tells her to call the office if her symptoms worsen or if she sees no meaningful improvement in 3–4 days.

EVALUATION

Mrs. Mitchell returns in 6 weeks for her follow-up appointment and reports improvement of symptoms and no further recurrence. She expresses a desire to continue on the higher-dose steroid until school is out. Clancy assesses that Mrs. Mitchell's breathing rate and pattern have returned to baseline. Peak flow measurements indicate Mrs. Mitchell's breathing is within her green zone, and breath sounds are clear and equal bilaterally.

CRITICAL THINKING

1. *Why is the prescription of the short, tapered course of oral prednisone appropriate for Mrs. Mitchell? Why is the continued use of the higher-dose inhaled corticosteroid appropriate? What special teaching will the client taking steroids require?*
2. *What should the nurse teach Mrs. Mitchell about the importance of nutrition and hydration to asthma management?*
3. *What signs and symptoms would you want Mrs. Mitchell to report to the provider immediately?*

REVIEW Asthma

RELATE Link the Concepts and Exemplars

The client has a history of severe persistent asthma, taking a daily LABA in combination with an inhaled corticosteroid, montelukast, and albuterol in both oral, inhaler, and nebulizer form for emergencies. Oral prednisone is prescribed approximately twice a year for severe flare-ups.

Linking the exemplar of asthma with the concept of metabolism:

1. What risk factors does this client have for osteoporosis? Explain the rationale for your answer.

2. What risk factors does this client have for diabetes and obesity? Explain the rationale for your answer.

Linking the exemplar of asthma with the concept of acid–base balance:

3. When caring for a client in status asthmaticus, what would you anticipate finding when analyzing ABG results? Explain the pathophysiology resulting in these findings.

4. What nursing interventions could be initiated to promote acid–base balance?

Linking the exemplar of asthma with the concept of cognition:

5. How could asthma affect an individual's ability to comprehend? Explain your answer with appropriate rationales.

6. What nursing interventions could be initiated to promote cognition?

READY Go to Companion Skills Manual

REFER Go to Pearson Nursing Student Resources
nursing.pearsonhighered.com

- Additional review materials

REFLECT Case Study

Hannah McGregor, a 9-year-old with asthma, lives at home with her parents and two brothers, who are 6 and 4 years old. Hannah developed asthma at approximately 5 years of age and has had wheezing episodes that were generally controlled by rescue medications. Two weeks ago, Hannah had a severe episode of asthma that started at school and was possibly associated with the paint or glue used on a project. She did not have any quick-relief medications at school, and she delayed going to the school nurse so that she could finish her project. By the time her mother arrived to pick her up, Hannah was in respiratory distress. After receiving treatment in the emergency department, Hannah was admitted to the pediatric intensive care unit.

Hannah and her mother are in the health center to meet with the provider to learn more about asthma management. At today's visit, Hannah's lungs are clear to auscultation, and her peak expiratory flow reading is in the green zone. Mrs. McGregor reports that she has given all prescribed medications since the hospitalization. Both Hannah and her mother are motivated to prevent a future hospital admission if possible. The nurse uses a model to show Hannah how asthma narrows her airway and makes it difficult to breathe. The nurse then works with Mrs. McGregor and Hannah to develop a plan for asthma control with daily medications.

1. What are the current recommendations for managing Hannah's asthma and to help prevent asthma episodes?

2. How should Hannah handle future episodes that start at school?

3. What arrangements are needed for Hannah to have access to her medications at school?

EXEMPLAR 15.3 **Chronic Obstructive Pulmonary Disease**

EXEMPLAR KEY TERMS

Air trapping, *1006*
Barrel chest, *1009*
Bronchitis, *1006*
Chronic bronchitis, *1006*
Chronic obstructive pulmonary disease (COPD), *1005*
Emphysema, *1006*
Expectorate, *1014*
Forced expiratory volume in 1 second (FEV_1), *1008*
Percussion, *1011*
Postural drainage, *1011*
Pursed-lip breathing, *1009*
Sputum, *1005*
Tripod position, *1009*
Vibration, *1011*

EXEMPLAR LEARNING OUTCOMES

After reading about this exemplar, you will be able to:

1. Describe the pathophysiology, etiology, clinical manifestations, and direct and indirect causes of chronic obstructive pulmonary disease (COPD).

2. Identify risk factors and prevention methods associated with COPD.

3. Illustrate the nursing process in providing culturally competent care across the life span for individuals with COPD.

4. Formulate priority nursing diagnoses appropriate for an individual with COPD.

5. Summarize therapies used by interdisciplinary teams in the collaborative care of an individual with COPD.

6. Plan evidence-based care for an individual with COPD and his or her family in collaboration with other members of the healthcare team.

7. Evaluate expected outcomes for an individual with COPD.

▶ OVERVIEW

Obstructive pulmonary diseases are those that cause obstruction of the airways, usually through a combination of bronchoconstriction and inflammation. These include bronchitis (chronic or acute) and emphysema.

The term **chronic obstructive pulmonary disease (COPD)** is used to describe a specific progressive disorder that slowly alters the structures of the respiratory system over time, irreversibly affecting lung function. The disease is one of periodic exacerbations, often related to respiratory infection, with increased symptoms of dyspnea and **sputum** (mucus or mucopurulent matter

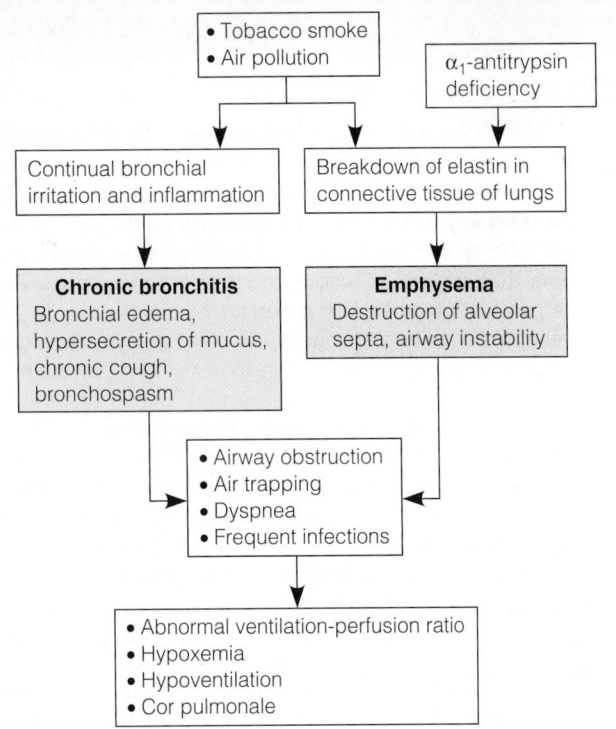

Figure 15–33 ● Pathogenesis of chronic obstructive pulmonary disease.

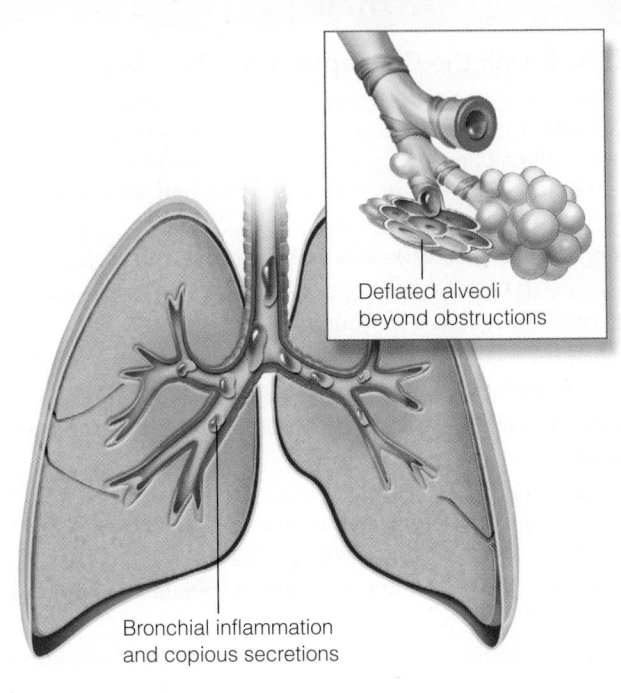

Figure 15–34 ● Chronic bronchitis.

expectorated from the lungs) production. Unlike acute processes in which lung tissues recover, airways and lung parenchyma do not return to normal following an exacerbation; instead, they demonstrate progressive destructive changes. COPD is not curable, but it can be managed (and sometimes prevented) with appropriate medical interventions and lifestyle choices.

Although one or the other may dominate, COPD typically includes components of both chronic bronchitis and emphysema, two distinctly different processes. Small airways disease, narrowing of small bronchioles, is also part of the COPD complex. Through different mechanisms, these processes cause airways to narrow, resistance to airflow to increase, and expiration to become slow or difficult (**Figure 15–33 ●**). The result is a mismatch between alveolar ventilation and blood flow or perfusion, leading to impaired gas exchange.

▶ PATHOPHYSIOLOGY AND ETIOLOGY

Chronic obstructive pulmonary disease results from repeated exposure to respiratory irritants that begin to damage the structures of the respiratory system. Damage to the large and small airway passages causes increased mucous production, causing arrest in cilia action. Excessive amounts of fluid accumulate with the lung mucosal cells, causing edema. In turn, edema causes narrowing of airway passages, resulting in airflow limitation, **air trapping** (decreased airflow with exhalation), and ultimately, hyperinflation of the lungs. This process leads to **bronchitis** (best defined as inflammation of the mucous membranes of the bronchial tubes).

Chronic bronchitis is a disorder of excessive bronchial mucous secretion (**Figure 15–34 ●**). It is characterized by a productive cough lasting 3 or more months in 2 consecutive years (ALA, 2013b). Cigarette smoke is the major factor implicated in the development of chronic bronchitis. Inhaled irritants lead to a chronic inflammatory process with vasodilation, congestion, and edema of the bronchial mucosa. Goblet cells increase in size and number, and mucous glands enlarge. Thick, tenacious mucus is produced in increased amounts. Changes in bronchial squamous cells impair the ability to clear mucus (Fishman et al., 2008). Narrowed airways and excess secretions obstruct airflow; expiration is affected first, then inspiration. Because ciliary function is impaired, normal defense mechanisms are unable to clear the mucus and any inhaled pathogens. Recurrent infection is common in chronic bronchitis.

Emphysema is characterized by destruction of the walls of the alveoli, with resulting enlargement of abnormal air spaces (**Figure 15–35 ●**). Deficiency of α_1-antitrypsin, an enzyme that normally inhibits the activity of proteolytic enzymes and tissue destruction in the lungs, contributes to the development of emphysema in some individuals, especially when combined with exposure to cigarette smoke. Inflammatory cells that collect in distal airway tissues appear to lead to destruction of elastic fibers in the respiratory bronchioles and alveolar ducts. Alveolar wall destruction causes alveoli and air spaces to enlarge, with loss of corresponding portions of the pulmonary capillary bed. As a result, the surface area for alveolar–capillary diffusion is reduced, affecting gas exchange. Elastic recoil is lost, reducing the volume of air that is passively expired. The loss of support tissue also affects airways, increasing the risk of expiratory collapse and further air trapping. Anatomically, either respiratory bronchioles or alveoli may be the primary tissue involved. As in chronic bronchitis, cigarette smoking is strongly implicated as a causative factor in most cases of emphysema.

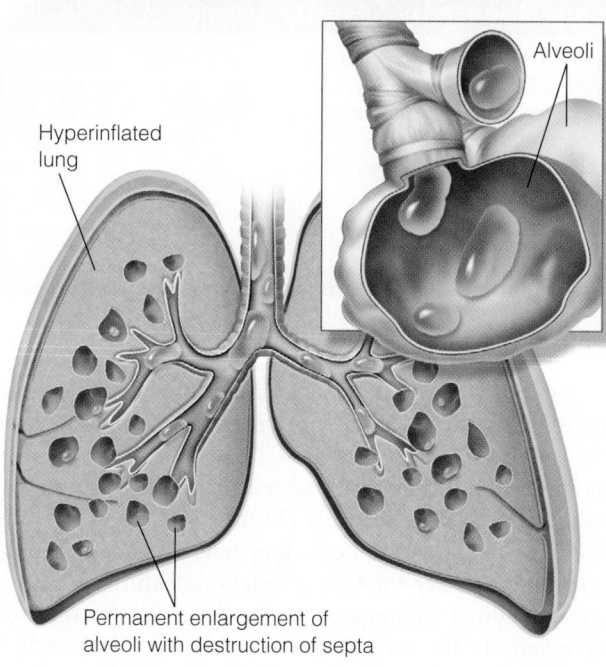

Figure 15-35 ● Emphysema.

Asthma often exists as a comorbid disease in the client with COPD. Clients who have lived with moderate to severe persistent asthma for most of their lives may develop COPD as a result of airway remodeling and damage to alveoli over time. Asthma is discussed in detail in the exemplar on Asthma in this module.

To summarize, COPD is a progressive, nonreversible process of airway narrowing and loss of supporting tissue. Three separate processes typically are involved:

1. Chronic bronchitis with persistent airway edema, excessive mucous production, and impaired airway clearance
2. Emphysema with loss of interstitial membranes and airway support tissue, resulting in airway collapse and loss of alveolar surface area for gas exchange
3. Small airway disease with bronchoconstriction.

The result of these processes and their combined effects is increased work of breathing, impaired expiration with air trapping, and impaired gas exchange.

Etiology

Chronic obstructive pulmonary disease is a leading cause of death, illness, and disability in the United States. COPD is often thought to be a disease that affects older adults, but 70% of individuals with COPD are under 65 years of age. Mortality rates are nearly equal for women and men, though rates for women have significantly increased since 1970. The direct costs of care in the United States are $18 billion annually, and indirect costs related to disability and loss of productive work are estimated at $14.4 billion annually. Although COPD is not curable, the symptoms of the disease can be managed (Centers for Disease Control and Prevention [CDC], 2009; Global Initiative for COPD, 2013).

Cigarette smoking is the greatest risk factor for COPD in the United States and other developed nations, accounting for

approximately 80% of cases. Other causes that have contributory effects of COPD on the lungs include exposures to occupational respiratory irritants and air pollution (both indoors and outdoors) in industrialized nations. The use of wood, coal, or animal dung for cooking fires in close quarters in less-developed nations increases the risk of COPD in women from those countries. Accounting for less than 1% of the population with COPD are those with α_1-antitrypsin deficiency (a lack of a protein produced by the liver that protects the integrity of lung tissue). This lack of protein synthesis is genetic and most commonly seen in individuals of northern European origin. α_1-Antitrypsin deficiency causes individuals to develop COPD at earlier ages than those who develop the disease from chronic airway irritations (CDC, 2012; Global Initiative for COPD, 2013).

Risk Factors

Smoking is the greatest risk factor for COPD: The more an individual smokes, the greater the risk of acquiring the disease. Frequent exposure to smoke also increases an individual's risk for COPD. Long-term exposure to chemical irritants in the workplace or through a hobby also increases risk for COPD. Some evidence indicates that clients with asthma are more likely to develop COPD compared with the general population.

While short-term exposure to respiratory irritants normally does not pose a risk for COPD, there are indications that short-term exposure to high levels of highly irritating substances can result in impairment of lung function, leading to COPD and other respiratory disorders. A longitudinal study of first responders and workers at the World Trade Center following the terrorist attacks of September 11, 2001, found that these individuals experienced significantly decreased lung function within the first year following the attacks. The exposure-related decrease in lung function of the study participants within that year was equivalent to 12 years of aging-related decline in lung function (Banauch et al., 2006).

Prevention

The key to preventing COPD is not engaging in behaviors that have been linked with the etiology of the disease. It is essential

Focus on Diversity and Culture
Smoking and the U.S. Hispanic Population

Among the U.S. Hispanic population, tobacco use is the leading preventable cause of death. Issues associated with this high rate of tobacco use appear to include acculturation, education levels, and alcohol and substance abuse (Rodríguez-Esquivel et al., 2009). A 2007 study found that Hispanic clients with COPD do not receive referral to smoking cessation classes as frequently as clients of other ethnicities (Adams et al., 2008). Nurses working with Hispanic clients who exhibit chronic cough and sputum or who are diagnosed with COPD should inquire about nicotine and alcohol use and provide client teaching and appropriate referrals in these areas. Nurses should also be able to provide referrals to mental health resources that serve Spanish-speaking clients. Materials about COPD and about smoking cessation should also be provided in Spanish wherever Hispanic clients are being served.

Box 15–4 Classification of Chronic Obstructive Pulmonary Disease by Severity

Stage I: Mild. Usually, but not always, chronic cough and sputum production. Mild airflow limitation; FEV_1/forced vital capacity (FVC) < 70%; FEV_1 of >80% predicted

Stage II: Moderate. Usually worse symptoms, with shortness of breath typically developing on exertion; FEV_1/FVC < 70%; FEV_1 of between 80% and 50% predicted

Stage III: Severe. Worse symptoms, with noticeable shortness of breath; FEV_1/FVC < 70%; FEV_1 of between 50% and 30% predicted

Stage IV: Very severe. Severe symptoms; FEV_1/FVC < 70%; FEV_1 of <30% predicted or FEV_1 of <50% predicted plus respiratory failure or clinical signs of right heart failure.

Source: Global Initiative for COPD. (2013). *Global initiative for chronic obstructive lung disease.* Retrieved from http://www.goldcopd.org/Guidelines/guidelines-resources.html.

that clients not smoke or quit smoking, if possible. It is also important to decrease exposure to secondhand smoke, occupational respiratory irritants, and air pollutants. This is especially important for the Hispanic population as they have an increased risk of developing COPD. For more information please refer to Focus on Diversity and Culture: Smoking and the U.S. Hispanic Population.

▶ CLINICAL MANIFESTATIONS

The clinical presentation of COPD varies from simple chronic bronchitis without disability to chronic respiratory failure and severe disability. **Forced expiratory volume in 1 second (FEV_1)** is the amount of air that can be exhaled in 1 second as measured by a spirometer. A client's FEV_1 reading combined with symptom manifestations determines the client's level of COPD severity. **Box 15–4 ●** outlines the classifications of COPD severity.

Manifestations are typically absent or minor early in the disease. Initial symptoms are a chronic cough and sputum production, which tend to begin long before changes in pulmonary function. See the Client Teaching feature regarding effective coughing techniques. No incidence of shortness of breath occurs in the early stages of pulmonary decline as a result of COPD. When the client finally seeks care, chronic productive cough, dyspnea, and exercise intolerance often have been present for as long as 10 years. The cough typically occurs in the mornings and often is attributed to "smoker's cough." Initially, dyspnea occurs only on extreme exertion; as

Client Teaching Effective Coughing Techniques

Several coughing techniques may be useful. For controlled cough technique, teach the client as follows:

1. Following prescribed bronchodilator treatment, inhale deeply, and hold breath briefly.
2. Cough twice, the first time to loosen mucus and the second to expel secretions.
3. Inhale by sniffing to prevent mucus from moving back into deep airways.
4. Rest. Avoid prolonged coughing to prevent fatigue and hypoxemia.

For huff coughing, teach the client to:

1. Inhale deeply while leaning forward.
2. Exhale sharply with a "huff" sound to help keep airways open while mobilizing secretions.

In addition, include the following topics when teaching for home care:

- Maintain adequate fluid intake (at least 2.0–2.5 quarts of fluid daily).
- Avoid respiratory irritants, including cigarette smoke (both primary and secondary), other smoke sources, dust, aerosol sprays, air pollution, and very cold, dry air.
- Prevent exposure to infection, especially upper respiratory infections.
- Stress importance of pneumococcal vaccine and annual influenza immunization.
- Follow prescribed exercise program, maintain activities of daily living, and balance rest and exercise.

- Maintain nutrient intake (e.g., eating small, frequent meals and using nutritional supplements to provide adequate calories).
- Suggest ways to reduce sodium intake if prescribed.
- Identify early signs of an infection or exacerbation, and the importance of seeking medical attention for the following: fever, increased sputum production, purulent (green or yellow) sputum, upper respiratory infection, increased shortness of breath or difficulty breathing, decreased activity tolerance or appetite, and increased need for oxygen.
- Teach about prescribed medications, including purpose, proper use, and expected effects.
- Avoid use of over-the-counter medications unless approved by the physician.
- Discuss other prescribed therapies, such as use of home oxygen, percussion, postural drainage, and nebulizer treatments.
- Describe use, cleaning, and maintenance of any required special equipment.
- Discuss importance of wearing an identification band and carrying a list of medications at all times in case of an emergency.

Provide referrals to home care services, such as home health, assistance with activities of daily living as needed, home maintenance services, respiratory therapy and home oxygen services, and other agencies such as Meals-on-Wheels and senior services as indicated.

the disease progresses, dyspnea becomes more severe and accompanies mild activity. Manifestations characteristic of chronic bronchitis and emphysema develop. Manifestations of chronic bronchitis include a cough that produces copious amounts of thick, tenacious sputum; cyanosis; and evidence of right-sided heart failure, including distended neck veins, edema, liver engorgement, and an enlarged heart. Adventitious lung sounds, including loud rhonchi, and possible wheezes are prominent on auscultation.

SAFETY ALERT
Chronic cough and sputum are not normal occurrences. An individual experiencing chronic cough and sputum beyond 3–4 days should consult with a healthcare professional. Individuals with a smoking history as well as chronic cough and sputum production should have PFTs to determine lung function.

Emphysema is insidious in onset. Dyspnea is the first symptom. Initially occurring only with exertion, dyspnea may progress to become severe even at rest. Cough is minimal or absent. Air trapping and hyperinflation increase the anteroposterior chest diameter, a condition called **barrel chest**. The client often is thin, is tachypneic, uses accessory muscles of respiration, and often assumes a **tripod position** (a position of sitting and leaning forward) (**Figure 15–36 ●**). On auscultation, breath sounds are diminished, and the percussion tone is hyperresonant. The client may utilize **pursed-lip breathing**. Pursed-lip breathing involves exhaling through a narrow opening between the lips to prolong the expiratory phase in an effort to promote more alveolar emptying while maintaining open alveoli.

Prolonged impairment of gas exchange as a result of COPD eventually results in cardiac dysfunction. Chest pain and hypertension may be the earliest manifestations, indicating that the heart is having to work harder to provide oxygen through the bloodstream. Eventually, congestive heart failure may result. Clients with COPD should be seen by their specialist or primary care provider at least every 6 months in order for their disease progression to be evaluated and therapies to be modified or added.

The work of breathing requires calories. Caloric demand increases as the effort to breathe increases. Tachypnea makes eating more difficult. Increased caloric demand with decreased caloric intake often occurs in the latter stages of COPD, often resulting in weight loss and possibly anemia.

Anxiety related to increasing periods of dyspnea occurs with exacerbations in moderate and severe COPD. Severe COPD can result in impairment of other body systems because of insufficient airflow, further restricting quality of life.

▶ COLLABORATION

Nurses will find it helpful to collaborate with physical therapists, nutritionists, pharmacists, family members, and sometimes counselors to help clients achieve outcomes and improve their quality of life. In particular, nurses should be aware of who is caring for the client with COPD who continues to live at home and should discuss with the client and

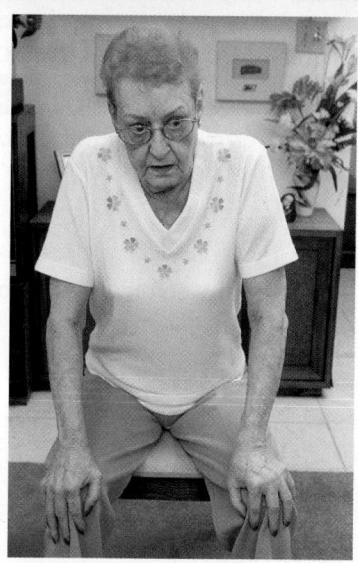

Figure 15–36 ● Typical appearance of a client with emphysema. Note the client's anxious expression and assumption of the tripod position, leaning forward with the hands on the knees.

family the need for those individuals to have sufficient information and training so they can provide care that meets best practice guidelines.

Diagnostic Tests

Diagnostic tests are used to help establish the diagnosis of COPD and identify the predominant component, emphysema or chronic bronchitis. These procedures also are used to assess respiratory status and monitor treatment effectiveness.

✳ Go to **nursing.pearsonhighered.com** to see Appendix B for more detailed information about related diagnostic tests.

PULMONARY FUNCTION TESTING Pulmonary function testing is performed to establish the diagnosis and evaluate the extent and progression of COPD. Results are based on calculated norms for each person by age, height, sex, and weight; note these as well as all current medications on the requisition. In clients with COPD, the total lung capacity and residual volume typically are increased. The FEV_1 and FVC are decreased as a result of narrowed airways and resistance to airflow.

VENTILATION-PERFUSION SCANNING Ventilation-perfusion scanning may be performed to determine the extent of V-Q mismatch—that is, the extent to which lung tissue is ventilated but not perfused (dead space), or perfused but inadequately ventilated (physiological shunting). A radioisotope is injected or inhaled to illustrate areas of shunting and absent capillaries.

SERUM α_1-ANTITRYPSIN LEVELS Serum α_1-antitrypsin levels may be drawn to screen for deficiency, particularly in clients with a family history of obstructive airway disease, those with an early onset, women, and those who do not smoke. Normal adult serum α_1-antitrypsin levels range from 80 to 260 mg/dL. Fasting is not required before this test.

Clinical Manifestations and Therapies **Chronic Obstructive Pulmonary Disease**

ETIOLOGY	CLINICAL MANIFESTATIONS	CLINICAL THERAPIES
Bronchitis	■ Chronic cough with mucous production ■ Dyspnea ■ Tachycardia ■ Narrowed airway passages ■ Wheezing ■ Air trapping	■ Smoking cessation ■ Bronchodilators ■ Corticosteroids ■ Fluids to thin secretions ■ Elevate the head of the bed ■ Low-flow oxygen ■ Monitoring of arterial blood gases and oxygen ■ Mechanical ventilation may be necessary if client cannot meet oxygen demands.
Emphysema	■ Air trapping ■ Possible wheezing ■ Dyspnea ■ Barrel chest ■ Pursed-lip breathing ■ Posturing	■ Oxygen administration as needed ■ Pursed-lip breathing technique ■ Teach posture changes to improve ventilation. ■ Low-flow oxygen ■ Monitoring of arterial blood gases and oxygen ■ Mechanical ventilation may be necessary if client cannot meet oxygen demands. ■ Nutritional assessment and increased calorie intake

Cardiac dysfunction	■ Chest pain
	■ Poor perfusion
	■ Arrhythmias, particularly premature ventricular contractions
	■ Hypertension
	■ Cardiac hypertrophy
	■ Congestive heart failure
		■ Medications:
		  a. Positive inotropics
		  b. Calcium blockers
		  c. Antiarrhythmic medications
		  d. Diuretics
		  e. Nitrites
		  f. Antihypertensives
		■ Monitoring of exercise tolerance
		■ Holter monitoring
		■ Antiembolism stockings to improve venous return
		■ Fluid restrictions may be necessary if not medically managed.

ARTERIAL BLOOD GAS Arterial blood gas values are used to evaluate gas exchange, particularly during acute exacerbations of COPD. Clients with emphysema as the predominant component often have mild hypoxemia and normal or low carbon dioxide tension. Respiratory alkalosis may be present as a result of an increased respiratory rate. Clients with chronic bronchitis and airway obstruction as the predominant component may have marked hypoxemia and hypercapnia with respiratory acidosis. Oxygen saturation levels are low because of marked hypoxemia.

SAFETY ALERT
Hypercapnia (elevated $PaCO_2$ levels) often is chronic in clients with COPD (CO_2 retainers). In these clients, administering oxygen can actually increase the $PaCO_2$, leading to somnolence and acute respiratory failure. While oxygen is the drug of choice for treating clients with COPD, close monitoring is necessary during oxygen therapy.

PULSE OXIMETRY Pulse oximetry is used to monitor oxygen saturation of the blood. Marked airway obstruction and hypoxemia often cause oxygen saturation levels of less than 95%. Pulse oximetry may be continuously monitored to assess the need for supplemental oxygen.

EXHALED CARBON DIOXIDE Exhaled carbon dioxide (capnogram or $ETCO_2$) may be measured to evaluate alveolar ventilation. The normal $ETCO_2$ reading is 35–45 mmHg; it is elevated when ventilation is inadequate and decreased when pulmonary perfusion is impaired. $ETCO_2$ monitoring can reduce the frequency of ABG determinations.

COMPLETE BLOOD COUNT WITH WHITE BLOOD CELL DIFFERENTIAL Complete blood count with white blood cell (WBC) differential often shows increased red blood cells and hematocrit (erythrocytosis) as chronic hypoxia stimulates increased erythropoiesis to improve the oxygen-carrying capacity of the blood. Polycythemia (increased numbers of all blood cells) may be evident. Increased WBC count and a higher percentage of immature WBCs (bands) are often indicative of bacterial infection.

CHEST X-RAY Chest x-rays of a client with COPD will show small white patches indicative of the hyperinflated alveolar sacs filled with secretions that are common in emphysema. Clients with more advanced chronic bronchitis will have long fields with larger areas of white, indicating the secretions. A CXR also may show flattening of the diaphragm because of hyperinflation and evidence of pulmonary infection if present.

Surgery

When medical therapy is no longer effective, lung transplantation may be an option. Both single and bilateral transplants have been performed successfully, with a 2-year survival rate of 75%. Lung reduction surgery is an experimental surgical intervention for advanced diffuse emphysema and lung hyperinflation. The procedure reduces the overall volume of the lung, reshapes it, and improves elastic recoil. As a result, pulmonary function and exercise tolerance improve, and dyspnea is reduced.

Pharmacologic Therapy

Immunization against pneumococcal pneumonia and a yearly influenza vaccine are recommended to reduce the risk of respiratory infections. A broad-spectrum antibiotic may be prescribed if infection is suspected. Recent studies indicate that clients with purulent sputum and increased dyspnea will likely benefit from antibiotic therapy, even if no other signs of infection are present. Current recommendations are to prescribe antibiotics only if known infection is present (Rennard, 2012).

Bronchodilators improve airflow and reduce air trapping in clients with COPD, resulting in improved dyspnea and exercise tolerance. These agents accomplish this by relaxing bronchial smooth muscle, thus widening the airway and making breathing easier for the client; they have no anti-inflammatory properties. Bronchodilators may be given by MDI, DPI, nebulizer, or orally. Oral administration may promote adherence but is associated with much higher rates of adverse effects. A spacer or holding chamber may facilitate effective use of an MDI. Ipratropium bromide, an anticholinergic agent administered by MDI, is frequently prescribed. It has a longer duration of action than the short-acting beta$_2$-adrenergic stimulant bronchodilators and few side effects. Salmeterol, a LABA, may be used in combination therapy. Oral theophylline, a methylxanthine, is a weak bronchodilator and has a narrow therapeutic range, but it often is prescribed for its other effects. Theophylline stimulates the respiratory drive, strengthens diaphragmatic contractions, and improves cardiac output. As a result, dyspnea, exercise tolerance, and quality of life improve for the client with COPD. Bronchodilators are discussed in further detail, including their nursing implications, in the exemplar on asthma in this module.

Corticosteroid therapy may be used when asthma is a major component of COPD. It also improves symptoms and exercise tolerance and may reduce the severity of exacerbations and the need for hospitalization. Oral corticosteroids, such as prednisone, are used initially. If a beneficial response occurs, the amount is reduced to the lowest effective dose. Every-other-day dosing or administration by inhaler is preferred to minimize steroid side effects, such as cushingoid effects, mood swings, and increased risk for osteoporosis and vertebral fractures.

New research indicates that the use of statins may result in significant improvement for the client with COPD. Data indicate that statins are associated with a decrease in all-cause mortality as well as a reduction in the rate of respiratory-related emergency care. Furthermore, it appears that in addition to targeting systemic inflammation, statins may also target airway inflammation (Reuters Health Information, 2009).

Oxygen Therapy

Long-term oxygen therapy is used for severe and progressive hypoxemia. Oxygen therapy improves exercise tolerance, mental functioning, and quality of life in clients with advanced COPD. It also reduces the rate of hospitalization and increases the length of survival. Oxygen may be used intermittently, at night, or continuously. Clients with severe hypoxemia see the greatest benefit with continuous oxygen. Home oxygen may be supplied as liquid oxygen, compressed gas cylinders, or oxygen concentrators. An acute exacerbation of COPD may necessitate oxygenation and inspiratory positive-pressure assistance with a face mask or intubation and mechanical ventilation. Oxygen administered without intubation and mechanical ventilation requires caution: Administering oxygen to clients with chronic elevated carbon dioxide levels in the blood can actually increase the $PaCO_2$, leading to increased somnolence and even respiratory failure. Close monitoring of LOC and ABG values during oxygen therapy is vital (Simmons & Simmons, 2004).

Percussion, Vibration, and Postural Drainage

Percussion, vibration, and postural drainage (PVD) are dependent nursing functions performed according to a primary care provider's order. **Percussion**, sometimes called *clapping*, is forceful striking of the skin with cupped hands. Mechanical percussion cups and vibrators are also available. When the hands are used, the fingers and thumb are held together and flexed slightly to form a cup, as one would to scoop up water. Percussion over congested lung areas can mechanically dislodge tenacious secretions from the bronchial walls. Cupped hands trap the air against the chest, and the trapped air sets up vibrations through the chest wall to the secretions. When done correctly, the percussion action should produce a hollow, popping sound. Percussion is avoided over the breasts, sternum, spinal column, and kidneys.

Vibration is a series of vigorous quiverings produced by hands that are placed flat against the client's chest wall. Vibration is used after percussion to increase the turbulence of the exhaled air and thus loosen thick secretions. It is often done alternately with percussion.

Postural drainage is the drainage by gravity of secretions from various lung segments. Secretions that remain in the lungs or respiratory airways promote bacterial growth and subsequent infection. They also can obstruct the smaller airways and cause atelectasis. Secretions in the major airways, such as the trachea and the right and left main bronchi, are usually coughed into the pharynx, where they can be expectorated, swallowed, or effectively removed by suctioning.

A wide variety of positions is necessary to drain all segments of the lungs, but not all positions are required for every client. Only those positions that drain specific affected areas are used. The lower lobes require drainage most frequently, because the upper lobes drain by gravity. Before postural drainage, the client may be given a bronchodilator medication or nebulization therapy to loosen secretions. Postural drainage treatments are scheduled two or three times daily, depending on the degree of lung congestion. The best times include before breakfast, before lunch, in the late afternoon, and before bedtime. It is best to avoid hours shortly after meals, because postural drainage at these times can be tiring and may induce vomiting.

The nurse needs to evaluate the client's tolerance of postural drainage by assessing the stability of the client's vital signs, particularly the pulse and respiratory rates, and by noting signs of intolerance, such as pallor, diaphoresis, dyspnea, nausea, and fatigue. Some clients do not react well to certain drainage positions, and the nurse must make appropriate adjustments. For example, some become dyspneic in Trendelenburg's position and require only a moderate tilt or a shorter time in that position.

The sequence for postural drainage treatment is usually as follows: positioning, percussion, vibration, and removal of secretions by coughing or suction. Each position is usually assumed for 10–15 minutes, although beginning treatments may start with shorter times and gradually increase.

Following postural drainage treatments, the nurse should auscultate the client's lungs, compare the findings to the baseline data, and document the amount, color, and character of expectorated secretions.

Other Interventions

Smoking cessation not only can prevent COPD from developing but also can improve lung function once the disease has been diagnosed. With smoking cessation, FEV_1 improves, and survival is prolonged, largely because of lower rates of lung cancer and heart disease. Sustained quitting is difficult; only 4% to 7% of smokers succeed in long-term abstinence from smoking (American Cancer Society, 2013). Use of nicotine patches or gum and an antidepressant, such as bupropion (Wellbutrin, Zyban), improves the chances of success. More information about nicotine abuse can be found in the Nicotine Use exemplar in the Addiction module.

In addition to refraining from smoking, exposure to other airway irritants and allergens should be avoided. The client should remain indoors during periods of significant air pollution to prevent exacerbations of the disease. Air-filtering systems or air conditioning may be useful.

Pulmonary hygiene measures, including hydration, effective coughing, percussion, and postural drainage, are used to improve clearance of airway secretions. Cough suppressants are usually ineffective, and sedatives are generally avoided because they may cause retention of secretions.

EXERCISE   Unless disabling cardiac disease is present, a regular exercise program is beneficial for:

- Improving exercise tolerance
- Enhancing ability to perform ADLs
- Preventing deterioration of physical condition.

A program of regular aerobic exercise (e.g., walking for 20 minutes at least three times weekly) designed to gradually increase exercise tolerance is recommended. Activities that strengthen the muscles used for breathing and ADLs, such as swimming and golf, are also beneficial. Breathing exercises are used to slow the respiratory rate and relieve accessory muscle fatigue. Pursed-lip breathing slows the respiratory rate and helps maintain open airways during exhalation by keeping positive pressure in the airways. Abdominal breathing relieves the work of accessory muscles of respiration.

HYDRATION   Adequate hydration maintains the moisture of the respiratory mucous membranes. Normally, respiratory tract secretions are thin and therefore are moved readily by ciliary action. However, when the client is dehydrated or the environment has a low humidity, the respiratory secretions can become thick and tenacious. Fluid intake should be as great as the client can tolerate.

Humidifiers are devices that add water vapor to inspired air. Room humidifiers provide cool mist to room air. Nebulizers are used to deliver humidity and medications. They may be used with oxygen delivery systems to provide moistened air directly to the client. Humidifiers prevent mucous membranes from drying and becoming irritated and loosen secretions for easier expectoration.

Complementary and Alternative Therapy

Complementary therapies may be useful to help manage symptoms of COPD. Dietary measures, such as minimizing intake of dairy products and salt, may help reduce mucous production and keep mucus more liquefied. Be sure to recommend measures to replace the protein and calcium in dairy products to help maintain nutritional balance. Hot herbal teas made with peppermint may act as expectorants to help relieve chest congestion.

Clients may be interested in trying complementary therapies to assist them in quitting smoking. Acupuncture, hypnotherapy, and guided imagery are some popular complementary therapies that clients may want to pursue, but the evidence of their effectiveness is questionable. A recent review of randomized controlled studies of hypnotherapy determined that there is insufficient evidence regarding the effectiveness of hypnotherapy as a therapy for smoking cessation (Barnes et al., 2010).

■ NURSING PROCESS

Nursing care is focused on promoting oxygenation. Health promotion activities include smoking cessation, reducing the risk of infection, and maintaining client safety. Because of the chronic nature of this disease process, teaching the client how to maximize self-care while knowing when to notify the healthcare team is another important role of the nurse.

Assessment

Focused assessment for the client with COPD includes collecting the following data:

- *Health history.* Current symptoms, including cough, sputum production, shortness of breath or dyspnea, activity tolerance; frequency of respiratory infections, and most recent episode; previous diagnosis of emphysema, chronic bronchitis, or asthma; current medications; smoking history in pack-years (packs per day times number of years smoked); and history of exposure to secondhand smoke and to occupational or other pollutants.

- **Physical examination.** General appearance, weight for height, mental status; vital signs, including temperature; skin color and temperature; anteroposterior:lateral chest diameter; use of accessory muscles, nasal flaring, or pursed-lip breathing; respiratory excursion and diaphragmatic excursion; percussion tone; breath sounds throughout; neck veins, apical pulse and heart sounds, peripheral pulses, and edema.

Auscultation of the chest may yield very little information to aid in establishing the diagnosis of COPD. Often, lung sounds are distant or reduced, although occasionally, wheezes or inspiratory crackles may be heard. However, these sounds are also associated with other diagnoses. Heart sounds may be difficult to hear if the client has a barrel chest. Auscultation over the xiphoid process (the lowest portion of the sternum) makes it easier to hear heart tones.

The nurse inspects and palpates the chest for symmetry. Increased anteroposterior diameter indicates chronic respiratory effort. The use of accessory muscles during breathing is also assessed. The position of the individual is observed. Upright posturing is an effective aid for ease of breathing. Self-posturing may indicate respiratory distress. An individual with COPD may sit upright with support of an overbed table.

Because COPD is a progressive and deteriorating illness, many clients with COPD reach the point at which they can no longer continue to live successfully at home. The nurse working with the client with COPD at home may want to use a home care assessment for oxygenation for clients with COPD (**Box 15–5** ●).

Diagnosis

Clients with COPD have multiple nursing care needs. Because of the obstructive nature of the disease, airway clearance is a high priority. Nutritional deficit is common, particularly when emphysema is predominant. Because this chronic disease affects all functional health patterns, psychosocial issues are also of concern in planning nursing care. NANDA diagnoses appropriate for the client with COPD include the following:

- *Ineffective Breathing Pattern*
- *Ineffective Airway Clearance*
- *Activity Intolerance*
- *Imbalanced Nutrition: Less Than Body Requirements*
- *Compromised Family Coping*
- *Decisional Conflict: Smoking.*

(NANDA-I © 2012)

Planning

Nursing care of the client with COPD, especially in later stages, requires careful planning in order to meet the client's oxygenation demands. Possible outcomes for this client may include the following:

- The client will adapt breathing patterns to meet oxygenation demands adequately.
- The client will experience ease of respirations with the use of positioning and pursed-lip breathing.
- The client will maintain a patent airway, allowing adequate oxygenation.
- The client will maintain oxygen saturation levels above 90%.
- The client will tolerate activity levels, allowing completion of ADLs.

Implementation

The highest priorities of nursing implementation are aimed at promoting oxygenation, which includes monitoring and promoting airway clearance and effective breathing patterns.

Box 15–5 Home Care Assessment: Oxygenation

CLIENT

- *Self-care abilities.* Ability to ambulate and perform activities of daily living (ADLs) independently
- *Exercise and activity pattern.* Type and regularity of usual exercise, perceived and actual energy for desired and required leisure activities
- *Assistive devices required.* Supplemental oxygen, humidifier, nebulizer treatments, or inhalers; walker, cane, or wheelchair; grab bars, shower chair, and other devices to promote safety and minimize energy expenditure; scale to monitor weight on a regular basis
- *Home environment.* Factors that impair airway clearance, gas exchange, or activity tolerance; indoor pollutants, such as cigarette smoke, dust, and allergens (e.g., pets); lack of humidity in the air; barriers, such as stairs
- *Current level of knowledge.* Importance of avoiding smoking and other pollutants; dietary salt and other restrictions if appropriate; recommended activities; medications; need to limit exposure to respiratory infections; use of prescribed nebulizer, multidose inhaler, powdered dose inhaler, or home oxygen; activity level

FAMILY

- *Caregiver availability, skills, and responses.* Ability and willingness to provide care as needed (help with ADLs, providing meals, assisting with transportation and shopping, caring for dependents, and performing treatments, such as percussion and postural drainage)
- *Family role changes and coping.* Effect on financial status, parenting and spousal roles, sexuality, social roles
- *Alternate potential primary or respite caregivers.* Other family members, volunteers, church members, paid caregivers or housekeeping services, and available community respite care (e.g., adult day care or senior centers)

COMMUNITY

- *Environment.* Usual temperature and humidity; presence of air pollutants, such as automobile exhaust, industrial smoke and pollutants, and smoke from field burning
- *Current knowledge of and experience with community resources.* Medical and assistive equipment and supply companies, respiratory and physical therapy services, home health agencies, local pharmacies, available financial assistance, and support and educational organizations, such as the local lung association and COPD support groups

Ongoing reassessment to determine effectiveness of interventions will help guide the nursing plan of care.

Promote Airway Clearance

Both chronic bronchitis and emphysema affect the ability to maintain open airways. In chronic bronchitis, copious amounts of thick, tenacious mucus impair ciliary action, making it difficult to clear mucus from the airways. The loss of supporting tissue caused by emphysema increases the risk for airway collapse. In both cases, air is trapped distally, and less oxygen is available to the alveoli for diffusion. Normal respiratory defense mechanisms are impaired, and mucous-plugged airways provide an ideal environment for bacterial growth. Respiratory infection further impairs airway clearance and is often the cause of an acute exacerbation.

- Assess respiratory status every 1–2 hours or as indicated. Assess rate and pattern; cough and secretions (color, amount, consistency, and odor); and breath sounds, both normal and adventitious. Frequent assessment is vital to monitor current status and response to treatment. Adventitious sounds should decrease with effective intervention. Diminished or absent breath sounds may indicate increasing airway obstruction and possible atelectasis.
- Monitor ABG results. Increasing hypoxemia, hypercapnia, and respiratory acidosis may indicate increasing airway obstruction.
- Weigh daily, monitor intake and output, and assess mucous membranes and skin turgor. Dehydration causes respiratory secretions to become thicker, more tenacious, and difficult to **expectorate** (expel or spit out); fluid overload can further compromise respiratory status.
- Encourage a fluid intake of at least 2,000–2,500 mL/day unless contraindicated. Adequate fluid intake helps keep mucous secretions thin.
- Place in Fowler, high-Fowler, or orthopneic position (with head and arms supported on the overbed table); encourage movement and activity to tolerance. Upright positions improve ventilation and reduce the work of breathing. Activity helps mobilize secretions and prevent them from pooling.
- Assist with coughing and deep breathing at least every 2 hours while awake. Position the client seated upright and leaning forward during coughing. The upright position promotes chest expansion, increasing the effectiveness of coughing and reducing the work involved.
- Provide tissues and a paper bag to dispose of expectorated sputum. This important infection control measure reduces the spread of respiratory organisms to other people.
- Refer to a respiratory therapist, and assist with or perform percussion and postural drainage as needed. Percussion helps loosen secretions in airways; postural drainage facilitates movement of these secretions out of the respiratory tract.
- Administer expectorant and bronchodilator medications as ordered. Correlate timing with respiratory treatments. Using expectorants and bronchodilators before coughing, percussion, and postural drainage increases their effectiveness in clearing airways.
- Provide supplemental oxygen as ordered. Supplemental oxygen helps maintain adequate blood and tissue oxygenation.

SAFETY ALERT Promptly report changes in oxygen saturation, skin color, or mental status. A drop in oxygen saturation levels, increasing cyanosis, or altered LOC indicates hypoxemia, possibly related to airway obstruction. Provide endotracheal, oral, or nasopharyngeal suctioning as necessary to stimulate cough and help clear secretions.

Enhance Breathing Patterns

- Monitor vital signs and laboratory results. Tachypnea, tachycardia, an elevated blood pressure, and increasing hypoxemia and hypercapnia are signs of compromised respiratory status.
- Assist with ADLs as needed. This conserves client energy and reduces fatigue.
- Provide rest periods between scheduled activities and treatments. Scheduled rest is important to prevent fatigue and reduce oxygen demands.
- Teach and assist with techniques to control breathing pattern:
  a. Pursed-lip breathing
  b. Abdominal breathing
  c. Relaxation techniques including visualization and meditation.

Breathing exercises are frequently indicated for clients with restricted chest expansion, such as people with COPD or clients recovering from thoracic surgery. Pursed-lip breathing helps keep airways open by maintaining positive pressure, and abdominal breathing improves lung expansion. Relaxation techniques reduce anxiety and its effect on the respiratory rate.

- Administer medications, including bronchodilators and anti-inflammatory drugs, as ordered. Monitor for desired and possible adverse effects. Medications are used to improve airway status and facilitate breathing.

SAFETY ALERT Prepare for intubation and mechanical ventilation if respiratory status deteriorates (increasing hypoxemia and hypercapnia, decreased LOC, cyanosis, or worsening airway obstruction). Respiratory failure is a possible complication of an acute exacerbation of COPD and requires immediate intervention to preserve life.

Promote Activity

Clients with COPD, especially the more advanced stages, are at high risk for activity intolerance, especially if they do not intake sufficient fluids and nutrition.

- Assess at each healthcare interaction how the client is meeting ADLs.
- Discuss the importance of spacing periods of activity with periods of rest as well as other strategies, including trying to accomplish more important tasks early in the day.
- Design, together with the physician, physical therapist, and client, an exercise plan that meets the client's current level of performance but also helps build the client's stamina and strength. Regular exercise is critical to the maintenance of lung function and quality of life.

Evidence-Based Practice Physical Activity in Clients With COPD

Problem

The correlation between physical activity and performance of essential activities of daily living, quality of life, and higher-level functioning is well established. This is particularly true for older adults and for people with disease-related impairment in physical abilities. Physical inactivity is both a cause and an effect of declining physical function in older adults as well as in clients with chronic obstructive pulmonary disease.

Evidence

Pulmonary rehabilitation is an effective therapy for clients who have COPD. It consists of exercise training combined with education and instruction in how clients can manage their COPD. Evidence suggests that pulmonary rehabilitation decreases dyspnea while increasing functional exercise capacity and improving quality of life. Therefore, pulmonary rehabilitation is recommended in guidelines for COPD management around the world. Research indicates that pulmonary rehabilitation is a highly effective intervention whose benefits can be extended to new populations. These populations include clients during or immediately following an acute exacerbation of COPD and those with other chronic lung diseases (Holland & Hill, 2011). The researchers advocate that new models of pulmonary rehabilitation should be explored.

Models that incorporate rapid intake of clients following acute exacerbation, appropriate exercise programs, and home-based interventions that promote cost effectiveness may enhance the quality of life for clients with COPD.

Implications

Nurses working with a client with COPD may need to collaborate with the client's primary care provider or pulmonologist to initiate referrals for pulmonary rehabilitation services early in the care plan. Pulmonary rehabilitation can promote exercise and stamina in this client population and assist in providing essential client education related to disease management and health promotion.

Critical Thinking Application

1. For older adult clients with COPD, how might physical inactivity represent both a cause and an effect of declining physical function?

2. Use the physiological and psychological effects of regular exercise to explain the correlation of exercise with improved symptoms in the client with COPD.

3. Consider the age of most clients with COPD. What other physical or psychosocial factors commonly limit physical activity in this population? How can you use this information in designing an appropriate exercise program?

Promote Balanced Nutrition

With advanced COPD, minimal activity, including eating, can cause fatigue and dyspnea. The client may be unable to consume a full meal without resting. At the same time, the increased work of breathing increases metabolic demands, and more calories are required. The client may appear cachectic (thin and wasted). Poor nutritional status further impairs immune function and increases the risk of a complicating infection.

- Assess nutritional status, including diet history, appropriate weight for height (use reference tables of desired weights), and anthropometric (skinfold) measurements. It is important to differentiate nutritional status from body type rather than assume a nutritional impairment.
- Observe and document food intake, including types, amounts, and caloric intake. This information can provide direction for supplementation if needed.
- Monitor laboratory values, including serum albumin and electrolyte levels. These values provide information about the adequacy of nutritional intake, including protein.
- Consult with a dietitian to plan meals and nutritional supplements that meet caloric needs. More concentrated sources of high-energy foods may be required to maintain caloric intake without excess fatigue. A diet high in proteins and fats without excess carbohydrates is recommended to minimize carbon dioxide production during metabolism (carbohydrates are metabolized to form CO_2 and water).
- Provide frequent, small feedings with between-meal supplements. Frequent, small meals help maintain intake and reduce fatigue associated with eating.

- Place the client in a seated or high-Fowler position for meals. An upright position promotes lung expansion and reduces dyspnea.
- Assist client with choosing preferred foods from the menu; encourage family members to bring food from home if allowed. Providing preferred foods encourages eating.
- Keep snacks at the bedside. Snacks provide additional caloric intake.
- Provide mouth care before meals. This helps enhance the appetite.
- If unable to maintain oral intake, consult with the physician about enteral or parenteral feedings. Maintenance of caloric and nutrient intake is vital to prevent catabolism.

Promote Family Coping

Chronic illness affects the entire family structure. Roles and relationships change; additional demands are placed on the family. Family members may blame the client for causing the illness or have distorted perceptions about it, even denying its existence. They may refuse to assist or participate in care. The client may develop an attitude of helplessness or dependence or may demonstrate anger, hostility, or aggression.

- Assess interactions between client and family. Assessment helps identify desired and potential destructive behaviors.
- Assess the effect of the illness on the family. Assessment of family interactions, roles, and relationships assists in planning appropriate interventions.

- Provide information and teaching about COPD. Education helps the family gain an understanding of the client's condition and needs.
- Help family members recognize behaviors and attitudes that may hinder effective treatment, such as continuing to smoke in the house. Family members may be unaware of the effect of their behavior on the client's ability to change habits and cope with a disabling disease.
- Initiate a care conference involving the client, family, and healthcare team members from a variety of disciplines. A wide range of perspectives and areas of expertise aids in problem solving and facilitates communication.
- Refer the client and family to support groups and pulmonary rehabilitation programs as available. Support groups and structured rehabilitation programs enhance coping abilities.
- Refer to community agencies or services such as home health, homemaker services, or Meals-on-Wheels as appropriate. Agencies or community services can provide additional support beyond the family's means or capabilities.

Encourage Smoking Cessation

Smoking is more than a habit; it is an addiction. The client who must quit is facing a significant loss, not only of nicotine but also of a lifestyle. Although the client may fully comprehend the consequences of continuing to smoke, the decision to give up a part of his or her life is not easy. This fear may be expressed in such concerns as "I'll gain weight" or "What will I do with my hands?" In addition to providing practical information, a plan, and assistance with nicotine withdrawal, the nurse must support the client's decision-making process to comply with a physician's order to stop smoking.

- Assess the client's knowledge and understanding of the choices involved and the possible consequences of each. The decision to quit smoking ultimately belongs to the client. He or she needs a full understanding of the consequences of quitting or continuing to smoke.
- Acknowledge concerns, values, and beliefs; listen without making judgments. The nurse needs to avoid imposing his or her values and beliefs about smoking on the client.
- Spend time with the client, encouraging expression of feelings. This demonstrates acceptance of the client and his or her right to make the decision.
- Help plan a course of action for quitting smoking, and adapt it as necessary. When the client develops the plan, he or she has more ownership in it and interest in making it work.
- Demonstrate respect for decisions and the right to choose. Respect supports self-esteem and the ability to cope.
- Provide referral to a counselor or other professional as needed. Counselors or other people trained to assist with smoking cessation can help with decision making.

Evaluation

Observe and record the client's breathing and vital signs, focusing on trends and patterns. Compare the client's actual respiration and breathing patterns to the outcome goal established. Some interventions may require time before progress is observed. For example, improving the ease of breathing may occur readily with a change in medications, but quitting smoking may take weeks or months.

Potential outcomes to evaluate the effectiveness of care may include:

- The client consistently maintains oxygen saturation greater than 90%.
- The client modifies ADLs to reduce fatigue related to activity intolerance.
- The client demonstrates appropriate use of medications, for example, inhalers.

NURSING CARE PLAN A Client With Chronic Obstructive Pulmonary Disease

Anna Mercurio, known as "Happy" to all her friends, is an 83-year-old widow who lives with her two adult sons. During the past 15 years, Mrs. Mercurio has become increasingly short of breath while gardening and walking, two of her favorite activities. She also has developed a chronic cough that is particularly bad in the mornings. Ten years ago, her family physician told her that she had emphysema. She is admitted to the hospital with possible pneumonia and acute exacerbation of COPD.

ASSESSMENT

Jeff Harris, RN, admits Mrs. Mercurio to the medical unit. In the nursing history, Mr. Harris notes that she denies ever smoking but says that her husband and two sons have been smokers "for practically their whole lives." She says she lived an active life before developing lung disease, but her breathing and coughing have progressed, so that she now must rest after just a few minutes of housework or other activity. Her cough is productive of moderate to large amounts of sputum, particularly in the mornings. She developed increasing shortness of breath and sputum 2 days ago. This morning, she could not complete her morning activities without resting, so she contacted her doctor.

DIAGNOSES

- *Ineffective Airway Clearance* related to pneumonia and COPD
- *Impaired Gas Exchange* related to acute and chronic lung disease
- *Risk for Impaired Spontaneous Ventilation* related to loss of hypoxemic respiratory drive and respiratory muscle fatigue
- *Impaired Home Maintenance* related to activity intolerance

(NANDA-I © 2012)

PLANNING

- The client expectorates secretions effectively.
- The client returns to the level of pulmonary function prior to acute exacerbation.
- The client demonstrates improved ABG and oxygen saturation values.
- The client maintains spontaneous respirations without excess fatigue.
- The client verbalizes willingness to allow sons or a housekeeper to assist with daily household tasks.

NURSING CARE PLAN (continued)

ASSESSMENT	DIAGNOSES	PLANNING
On physical examination, Mr. Harris notes the following: skin very warm and dry, color dusky. Pauses frequently while speaking to breathe. Respirations 36/minute, fairly shallow; coughs frequently, producing large amounts of thick, tenacious green sputum. Other vital signs: pulse 115 bpm and irregular, BP 186/60 mmHg, temperature 39°C (102.4°F). Appears very thin; weight 43.6 kg (96 lb), height 160 cm (63 in.). Anteroposterior: lateral chest diameter approximately 1:1; moderate kyphosis noted. Chest hyperresonant to percussion. Auscultation reveals distant breath sounds with scattered wheezes and rhonchi throughout lung fields. Chest x-ray shows flattening of diaphragm, slight cardiac enlargement, prominent vascular and bronchial markings, and patchy infiltrates. Initial laboratory work reveals moderate erythrocytosis, leukocytosis, and low serum albumin. ABG results: pH 7.19; PaO_2, 54 mmHg; $PaCO_2$, 59 mmHg; HCO_3, 30 mg/dL; and oxygen saturation, 88%. Admitting orders include sputum specimen for culture; intravenous penicillin G, 2 million units every 4 hours; albuterol/ipratropium (Combivent) inhaler, two puffs every 6 hours; salmeterol/fluticasone (Advair) dry powder inhaler, twice a day; bed rest with bathroom privileges; oxygen per nasal cannula at 2 L/min continuously; and regular diet.		

IMPLEMENTATION

- Assess respiratory status and LOC every 1–2 hours until stable, then at least every 4 hours.
- Closely monitor response to oxygen therapy, including skin color, oxygen saturation, sputum consistency, and respiratory drive.
- Increase fluid intake to at least 2,500 mL/day, and provide a bedside humidifier.
- Elevate head of bed to at least 30° at all times.
- Teach "huff" coughing technique.
- Administer medications as ordered, providing ipratropium inhaler before fluticasone inhaler. Provide mouth care after inhalers.

- Contact respiratory therapy for percussion and postural drainage following inhaler treatments.
- Provide uninterrupted rest periods following treatments and procedures.
- Meet with Mrs. Mercurio and her sons to develop a postdischarge care plan.
- Refer to home health department for nursing follow-up.
- Refer to social services for possible assistance with home maintenance.

EVALUATION

After the first day in the hospital, Mrs. Mercurio's condition begins to improve slowly. On discharge 6 days later, she is able to provide self-care with less fatigue and dyspnea. She is using oxygen at night only, admitting that it is just for security. Although a few scattered wheezes and rhonchi are still present in her lungs, Mrs. Mercurio's sputum is thinner, white, and easily expectorated. She will continue taking oral penicillin V for an additional 10 days at home. She will also continue using the Advair and Combivent inhalers as prescribed at home. Although Mrs. Mercurio's sons admit they will probably never be able to quit smoking, they have agreed to smoke only in the garage or outside. A home health nurse will initially evaluate Mrs. Mercurio's progress three times weekly. Arrangements have been made for a housekeeper to come twice a week for cleaning and laundry. Mrs. Mercurio is glad to be returning home and grateful for the arrangements that have been made.

CRITICAL THINKING

1. Mrs. Mercurio has never been a smoker but has had long-term exposure to secondhand smoke. How does secondhand smoke contribute to lung diseases in adults and children?
2. The client with an acute exacerbation of COPD is at risk for respiratory failure. What changes in Mrs. Mercurio's assessment findings could indicate this complication may be developing?
3. Develop a nursing care plan for Mrs. Mercurio for the nursing diagnosis Risk for Infection related to secondhand smoke exposure.

REVIEW **Chronic Obstructive Pulmonary Disease**

RELATE Link the Concepts and Exemplars

Linking the exemplar of chronic obstructive pulmonary disease with the concept of fluids and electrolytes:

1. Why is it important for the client with COPD to drink sufficient fluids?

2. Why might a bedridden client with COPD choose to drink less and how can the nurse promote hydration in this client?

Linking the exemplar of chronic obstructive pulmonary disease with the concept of safety:

3. Why is it important for the nurse to assess the client with COPD for risk for injury related to the use of oxygen?

4. What teaching would you provide a client who is to be discharged with home oxygen therapy for the first time?

Linking the exemplar of chronic obstructive pulmonary disease with the concept of infection:

5. Why is the client with COPD at a greater risk for developing respiratory infections?

6. What therapies could be used to decrease the risk of infection in the client with COPD?

READY Go to Companion Skills Manual

REFER Go to Pearson Nursing Student Resources
nursing.pearsonhighered.com

- Additional review materials

REFLECT Case Study

James Winston is a 58-year-old White man living in North Carolina. Before retiring this past fall, he worked on a heavy-machinery production line most of his adult life. He served in the Marines during the Vietnam War. Throughout his work years, he was a weekend gardener. He has smoked a pack of cigarettes every day since high school, and he has increased to two packs a day since retirement. "I have been lying around the house waiting for spring so I can garden," he says.

Now that spring has arrived, trees are blooming, grass is again in need of mowing, and Mr. Winston is admitted to the medical unit with shortness of breath. The initial assessment demonstrates an afebrile man with vital signs as follows: temperature 98.9°F, pulse 88 bpm, respirations 32/min, BP 164/96 mmHg, and pulse oximetry reading of 89%. Mr. Winston is tachypneic, sitting upright and forward with his hands on his knees. He has removed his oxygen face mask because "it smothers me," he says.

1. What other assessment data are needed before providing care for this client?

2. What are the priority interventions for Mr. Winston? Why do these take priority?

3. What diagnostic examination would confirm this is COPD?

4. What interventions may be necessary for Mr. Winston to resume the healthy behaviors in his life?

EXEMPLAR 15.4 Respiratory Syncytial Virus/Bronchiolitis

EXEMPLAR KEY TERMS
Apnea, *1019*
Atelectasis, *1019*
Bronchiolitis, *1018*
Comorbidity, *1019*
Play therapist, *1020*
Respiratory syncytial virus (RSV), *1018*
Rhinorrhea, *1019*

EXEMPLAR LEARNING OUTCOMES
After reading about this exemplar, you will be able to:

1. Describe the pathophysiology, etiology, clinical manifestations, and direct and indirect causes of respiratory syncytial virus (RSV)/bronchiolitis.

2. Identify risk factors and prevention methods associated with RSV/bronchiolitis.

3. Illustrate the nursing process in providing culturally competent care across the life span for individuals with RSV/bronchiolitis.

4. Formulate priority nursing diagnoses appropriate for an individual with RSV/bronchiolitis.

5. Summarize therapies used by interdisciplinary teams in the collaborative care of an individual with RSV/bronchiolitis.

6. Plan evidence-based care for an individual with RSV/bronchiolitis and his or her family in collaboration with other members of the healthcare team.

7. Evaluate expected outcomes for an individual with RSV/bronchiolitis.

▶ OVERVIEW

Respiratory syncytial virus (RSV) is a highly contagious respiratory infection that affects almost all children before 2 years of age. While persons of any age can contract the disease, in those older than 2 years it is likely to present as a simple cold or be asymptomatic. Only those 2 years old and younger will normally experience the more severe form of the disease. Older adults who are already at risk for impaired oxygenation may also be at risk for acquiring the more severe form of RSV, although they are at lower risk than young children. Because acquired immunity to the virus is weak, individuals may have repeated infections of RSV throughout their life span, although the symptoms tend to be less severe with repeated exposure.

Bronchiolitis is a lower respiratory tract illness that occurs when an infecting agent (virus or bacterium) causes inflammation and obstruction of the small airways (the bronchioles).

At least 1 in 7 infants develops bronchiolitis during the first year of life (Alverson & Ralston, 2011). Children with bronchiolitis have an increased risk for wheezing and asthma later in childhood (Sorce, 2009).

The most common cause of bronchiolitis is infection with RSV. Adenovirus, parainfluenza virus, influenza virus, and human meta pneumovirus are other potential causes. RSV occurs in annual epidemics from October to March. It is transmitted through direct contact with respiratory secretions or indirectly through contaminated surfaces. The virus is shed by the infected child for 3–8 days, and the incubation period is 2–8 days. Nearly all children have been infected with RSV by 2 years of age, and reinfection (via siblings or close family contacts) throughout life is common. RSV is a common cause of lower respiratory tract infections in infants and children. Infants at risk for severe infection with RSV include those under 24 months of age with chronic lung disease who have required medical therapy within 6 months of RSV season onset, those with significant congenital heart disease, and preterm infants under 35 weeks of gestation (Healthy Children.org, 2012).

▶ PATHOPHYSIOLOGY AND ETIOLOGY

Respiratory syncytial virus infects the squamous epithelial cells of the bronchioles and alveoli. Infected cells merge with adjacent cells, creating large masses of cells, or *syncytia*, that subsequently burst and die. The resulting debris clogs the minute airways of the lower respiratory tract, irritating the airway and resulting in edema and mucosal secretions. Partial airway obstruction and bronchospasms follow.

The cycle is repeated throughout both lungs as the airway cells are invaded by the virus. The partially obstructed airways allow air in, but the mucus and airway swelling block expulsion of the air. This creates wheezing and crackles in the airways. Acute rhinorrhea also appears. **Atelectasis** (collapse of alveoli or section of alveoli) occurs in some areas, and air trapping and hyperinflation in others. Hypoxemia results because of the V-Q mismatch. The client with RSV is therefore at risk for respiratory failure as the oxygen level decreases and the carbon dioxide level increases. **Apnea** (absence of respirations) and pulmonary edema may occur.

This highly contagious viral infection is spread by direct physical contact with respiratory secretions or an infected individual. Virus droplets have also been detected in air as many as 22 feet from the infected individual.

Etiology

Respiratory syncytial virus is a primary cause of respiratory infections among both children younger than 2 years and older adults. Between 75,000 and 125,000 children are hospitalized each year because of RSV. Worldwide, RSV affects some 64 million people and causes more than 150,000 deaths each year (CDC, 2010b). Approximately 14,000 high-risk adults and older adults die from RSV infections annually, with more than 170,000 adults being infected by the virus each year, at a cost of over $1 billion dollars (CDC, 2010b). There are approximately 149,000 hospitalizations per year, with the frequency much higher for children younger than 1 year, males, and non-Whites.

Risk Factors

The risk of infection with RSV is higher for infants and toddlers who are not breastfed or who live in homes with secondary cigarette exposure, attend daycare, live in crowded conditions, or are socioeconomically disadvantaged (CDC, 2010b).

Risk of infection is higher when the parent or caregiver smokes. Tobacco smoke increases mucous production and reduces the action of cilia within the airway passages. Exposure to secondhand smoke is thought to alter maturation of the respiratory epithelium.

Infants and toddlers who have a history of prematurity, chronic lung disease, acyanotic congenital heart disease, or reduced immunity are at greater risk for complications from RSV and may require hospitalized care. As mentioned, all children under the age of 2 have smaller airways, so they are at risk for serious complications from RSV/bronchiolitis compared with older children and adults. In adults, high-risk populations include the older adults, those with chronic pulmonary disease, and those with congestive heart failure.

Prevention

The best way to prevent RSV is through good hand hygiene and infection control measures. This can be accomplished through frequent washing of hands with soap and water and avoiding sharing items such as food, cups, or utensils with infected individuals. Using hand disinfectants will also kill the virus (CDC, 2010b).

Infants who are at a high risk for serious RSV infections and associated complications may be given a medication known as palivizumab (Synagis). This medication is given to these infants each month during RSV season because it only offers protection for a 30-day period (NIH, 2012b).

▶ CLINICAL MANIFESTATIONS

The typical clinical presentation in otherwise healthy children begins 3–5 days after exposure to the virus. The early signs of a mild infection include **rhinorrhea** (drainage of mucus from the nose), cough, irritability, and a low-grade fever for 1–3 days. Copious mucous secretions occur in the lung fields and nasal passages and are usually green in color. The fever can lead to dehydration.

Signs and symptoms of a more serious infection may occur even in infants and toddlers with no history of **comorbidity** (the presence of one or more additional disease processes). These signs and symptoms, which call for medical care, include increased irritability, excessive coughing, and wheezing.

Focus on Diversity and Culture
Alaskan Native Infants

RSV is a major cause of hospitalization among Alaskan Native infants and is responsible for one third of hospitalizations of children younger than 3 years in Alaska. Alaskan children hospitalized with RSV at any age are at a high risk for rehospitalization as a result of respiratory infection. Alaskan Native children living in rural areas have a higher rate of chronic lung disease; however, the relationship between RSV and chronic lung disease remains unclear (National Center for Preparedness, Detection, and Control of Infectious Diseases, 2009).

Clinical Manifestations and Therapies **RSV/Bronchiolitis**

ETIOLOGY	CLINICAL MANIFESTATIONS	CLINICAL THERAPIES
Increased airway secretions	▪ Rhinorrhea ▪ Cough ▪ Shortness of breath	Treatment at home may include: ▪ Fluids ▪ Rest ▪ Antipyretics ▪ Nasal suctioning using bulb syringe in children too young to clear their own airway.
Partial airway obstruction caused by increased secretions and resulting edema	▪ Wheezing and crackles ▪ Fever ▪ Irritability ▪ Anorexia ▪ Poor fluid intake ▪ Tachypnea ▪ Grunting ▪ Retractions	Evaluation by primary provider; treatment may include: ▪ Increase fluid intake ▪ Antipyretics ▪ Suctioning the airway to relieve obstructions ▪ Positioning to optimize oxygenation ▪ Administration of oxygen via oxygen tent or oxyhood.
Hypoxia	▪ Apnea ▪ Tachypnea ▪ Marked retractions of the ribcage ▪ Use of accessory muscles ▪ Listlessness ▪ Cyanosis ▪ Respiratory acidosis	Treatment at the emergency department may include: ▪ Hydration with intravenous or oral fluids to prevent insensible fluid loss ▪ Humidified oxygen therapy ▪ Bronchodilators, steroids, beta-agonists ▪ Suctioning to remove excess secretions if child cannot cough or swallow ▪ Cardiopulmonary monitoring and pulse oximetry ▪ Intubation and mechanical ventilation.

Of even more concern are marked retractions of the ribcage, nasal flaring, rapid respiratory rate, blue skin, listlessness, and, most importantly, periods without breathing. The emergency medical system should be called to provide transport to the hospital when a child presents with these symptoms.

▶ COLLABORATION

Infants who demonstrate signs of respiratory distress while infected with RSV will require hospitalization. The plan of care includes monitoring breathing patterns, maintaining patent airways, maintaining adequate fluid and caloric intake, and supporting appropriate developmental behaviors. The respiratory therapist and nurse collaborate to monitor breathing patterns and keep airways clear of secretions. Infants who need endotracheal intubation will be closely cared for by the respiratory therapist.

Rapid breathing rates may require delivery of fluids and nutrition via an intravenous line. A nutritionist collaborates with the healthcare team to ensure caloric intake meets the needs of the infant with RSV. A **play therapist** (a therapist edu-

cated in recreational activities related to the various age groups of people) is available in larger healthcare facilities to induce age-appropriate activities for children's play needs.

Diagnostic Tests

Laboratory tests that are used to identify the virus causing bronchiolitis include immunofluorescent or enzyme immunoassay techniques from a posterior nasopharyngeal specimen

Lifespan Considerations
Diagnostic Tests for RSV Infection

Antigen detection tests and cultures are generally reliable in young children. They are less reliable in older children and adults, however, because of the lower viral loads in their respiratory specimens. Real-time polymerase chain reaction assays are more useful in these populations, because these tests are able to multiply the existing DNA/RNA so that it can be detected more easily (CDC, 2010a).

(CDC, 2010a). Viral cell culture and/or antigen detection tests may also be performed. CXRs show hyperinflation, patchy atelectasis, and other signs of inflammation. Arterial blood gases indicate effectiveness of gas exchange.

Pharmacologic Therapy

Few medications are prescribed for RSV infection and bronchiolitis. Use of nebulized epinephrine in combination with systemic corticosteroids has been found to result in some reduction in hospitalizations (Selden & Scarfone, 2009). Bronchodilators can be offered to see if a clinical response occurs. Antipyretics may be used. Unless the child also has a bacterial infection, antibiotics will not be used.

Ribavirin is an antiviral drug specifically available for treatment of RSV infection. Its use remains controversial, however, because it has only marginal benefit. It is expensive, requires a cumbersome delivery, and has potential health risks for caregivers. Its use is reserved for cases of severe disease, such as infants with complicated congenital heart disease or who are immunocompromised (AAP Subcommittee on Diagnosis and Management of Bronchiolitis, 2006).

Nonpharmacologic Therapy

No effective therapy for RSV infection and bronchiolitis exists. Hospitalized children are isolated, roomed together, or placed on the same unit to minimize the spread of the virus to other hospitalized children. Humidified oxygen using a hood, face tent, mask, or nasal cannula is provided to maintain pulse oximetry oxygen saturation readings at greater than 90% (Ball, Bindler, & Cowen, 2012). The delivery method chosen is based on the desired concentration of oxygen, degree of humidity, and the child's response. Other supportive care includes hydration with oral or intravenous fluids and nasal suctioning to facilitate breathing. The child with apnea or respiratory failure will be cared for in the critical care unit, usually intubated and ventilated when too fatigued to breathe effectively.

■ NURSING PROCESS

Nursing management focuses on maintaining respiratory function, supporting overall physiological function and hydration, reducing the child's and the family's anxiety, and preparing the family for home care. Prevent the transmission of RSV and other organisms by using airborne and standard precautions.

Assessment

Assessment allows the nurse to determine the severity of symptoms. Collect assessment data through the health history and physical assessment:

- *Health history.* Symptoms and behaviors for the previous 2 weeks, eating habits, fluid intake, any previous breathing problems or illnesses, birth history, and a list of those who provide care for the child other than the parents (e.g., grandparents, day care providers, and baby sitters).

- *Physical examination.* Breathing pattern, including rate, rhythm, and quality; inspection and palpation of the chest; use of accessory muscles when breathing, which indicates an increased need for oxygen; self-posturing.

Most children continue to play despite illness. Increased fatigue levels will interfere with play. Lack of play is an indication of severe illness in children.

Infants who are premature, have cardiac or respiratory disorders, or are immunocompromised have the greatest risk of severe RSV requiring hospital care. Assess for a more pronounced cough, wheezing, fevers to 102°F, and poor feeding. Also assess for signs of increased respiratory effort: marked retractions with nasal flaring, rapid respiratory rate, cyanosis, listlessness, and apnea.

Teach the parents or caregiver how to assess breathing patterns at home. Use of accessory muscles when breathing indicates an increased need for oxygen. A tripod stance, in which the client leans forward, resting arms on a table or on his or her knees, indicates respiratory distress.

SAFETY ALERT
Signs of life-threatening illness in the infant with bronchiolitis include central cyanosis, respiratory rate greater than 70 breaths per minute, listlessness, and apneic episodes. The chest is hyperinflated, and air exchange is so poor that breath sounds are very diminished on auscultation.

Diagnosis

Likely NANDA diagnoses for the infant at or child with RSV infection include the following:

- *Ineffective Breathing Pattern*
- *Ineffective Airway Clearance*
- *Impaired Gas Exchange*
- *Fluid and Electrolyte Imbalance: Less Than Body Requirements*
- *Impaired Nutrition: Less Than Body Requirements*
- *Activity Intolerance.*

(NANDA-I © 2012)

Planning

Care of the infant with RSV infection requires collaboration between the parents and the healthcare team. Goals often include the following:

- The client's breathing patterns will remain at or return to regular rate, rhythm, and quality for the individual's age group.
- The client's airways will remain clear of secretions; swelling of mucosal linings will decrease to normal for the individual's age group.
- The client's fluid intake will meet daily requirements for the individual's age group.
- The client's daily nutritional needs will be met as required for the individual's age group.
- If a child, the client will return to play activities as expected for the individual's age group.

Client Teaching Caring for the Child With RSV/Bronchiolitis

Parents of a child with RSV/bronchiolitis require some specific instructions in order to care for their child at home and prevent the need for hospitalization. Teaching points include the following:

- Clearing oral and nasal passages with a bulb syringe.
- When to return the child to the primary care provider or hospital. Signs and symptoms that indicate additional care

is required include increasing irritability, wheeze, cough, and visible retractions of the ribcage.

- When to initiate the emergency medical system. Manifestations that require emergent care include rapid respiratory rate, blue coloring of the skin, listlessness, marked retractions with nasal flaring, and apnea.
- Not smoking around infants and children.

Implementation

The priority of nursing care is maintaining a clear airway and promoting oxygenation. Parents of children requiring hospitalization are normally very anxious and protective. Including them in providing care and teaching the importance of interventions may help reduce that anxiety and allow them a measure of control in their child's life.

Promote Airway Clearance

The nurse working with a client who cannot clear the airway effectively should:

- Monitor temperature, pulse, respiration, blood pressure, and pulse oximetry.
- Auscultate lung sounds.
- Encourage oral fluids to maintain thinned pulmonary secretions. Thinned secretions are easier to expectorate than thick, tenacious mucus. Intravenous fluids may be needed for the child with respiratory rates too great to safely feed orally or for the child who is too weak to consume adequate fluid volumes.
- Suction the mouth and nose to maintain a patent airway.
- Provide client teaching to the parents related to airway clearance and when to return to the primary care provider or the hospital (see Client Teaching: Caring for the Client with RSV/Bronchiolitis).
- Administer medications as ordered.

Promote Effective Breathing Pattern

The nurse working with a client with an ineffective breathing pattern should:

- Continue to monitor breathing pattern, including rate, rhythm, and quality.
- Teach the parents or caregiver how to observe breathing patterns. Observable retractions of the ribcage indicate respiratory distress. If these are observed, the child should be taken to the hospital.
- Inspect and palpate chest for use of accessory muscles. Use of accessory muscles may indicate an increased need for oxygen.
- Assess for self-posturing. A tripod stance indicates respiratory distress.
- Administer bronchodilators and oxygen therapy as ordered.

Promote Adequate Nutrition

Children with RSV and bronchiolitis are at risk for impaired nutrition and require additional interventions:

- Monitor dietary intake. Adequate calories support healing.
- Take daily weight measurements, if in hospital setting.
- Offer foods that the client prefers.
- Offer small, frequent feedings.
- Encourage parents to continue to feed the child and provide liquids as normal. The child should not be forced to eat. If not eating or drinking as much as normal, the child may need more frequent feedings.

Monitor Fluid Balance

Nursing interventions related to the child's risk for fluid volume deficit due to fever and poor oral intake include the following:

- Assess for poor skin elasticity, dry mucous membranes, and decreased urinary output.
- Record intake and output.
- Weigh each diaper for accurate output.
- Teach parents to count diapers per day.
- Encourage oral intake.
- Monitor intravenous fluid rate if such fluids are ordered.

Reduce Fatigue

Nursing interventions to reduce fatigue associated with activity intolerance include the following:

- Assess capacity to play. Even children who are ill play. Children who do not exert themselves to play may be experiencing increased fatigue levels. Increased levels of fatigue may indicate the disease is more severe. Follow-up with the primary care provider may be indicated.
- Organize care to allow for rest periods.

Evaluation

When caring for a child with RSV or bronchiolitis, the child must be evaluated after treatment. Observe and record the rate, rhythm, and quality of breathing patterns, focusing on the changes in vital signs and breathing patterns. Airway patency should remain clear either through suctioning or by the child's ability to cough and clear the airway. Monitor fluid and caloric intake to ensure the child's needs are met. Children should resume or continue play as appropriate for their developmental stage.

NURSING CARE PLAN A Client With Respiratory Syncytial Virus

Deborah Coley brings her 14-month-old son, Tyshawn, to the emergency department. Ms. Coley reports that Tyshawn has had a runny nose and a slight fever for 3 or 4 days and that he woke up coughing and crying during the night with a fever of 102°F. She says that she gave him some more children's Motrin and some juice and that she was able to stop him crying, but also that he is "not breathing right." She says that he had a slightly wet diaper this morning, but not as bad as it usually is.

ASSESSMENT	DIAGNOSES	PLANNING
Nurse Williams notices that Tyshawn has marked retractions of his ribcage. He is secreting green mucus from his nose, and he coughs frequently. His respiratory rate is 42/min, and his oxygen saturation is 78%. Tyshawn is irritable, not wanting to comply with the initial physical examination. The attending physician suspects infection with RSV and prescribes a bronchodilator via nebulizer and oxygen therapy using a pediatric tent, after which Tyshawn's symptoms will be reassessed. His nasal secretions are sent to the lab to confirm the presence of RSV.	■ *Ineffective Breathing Pattern* related to lung infection ■ *Impaired Gas Exchange* related to damaged alveoli ■ *Ineffective Airway Clearance* related to large amounts of mucus and client's young age ■ *Anxiety* related to child's difficulty breathing (NANDA-I © 2012)	■ The client will return to normal breathing rate and pattern. ■ The client will maintain adequate oxygenation. ■ The client will experience no further complications from the disease process. ■ The client will meet his nutritional needs. ■ The client will expectorate mucus and allow suctioning as needed.. ■ The client's mother will express relief at the client's improved status.

IMPLEMENTATION

■ The nurse administers a bronchodilator via nebulizer as ordered by the attending physician, then sets up the pediatric tent to provide oxygen therapy.

■ The nurse reevaluates Tyshawn's oxygenation saturation levels and respiratory rate following the nebulizer treatment and again following the oxygen therapy.

■ The nurse provides client teaching to Mrs. Coley related to RSV and the possibilities of recurrence.

EVALUATION

During administration of the oxygen therapy, Tyshawn falls asleep. After the oxygen therapy, his respiratory rate is 32/min, and his oxygen saturation is at 92%. He is breathing through his mouth, indicating his nose is still stuffy.

CRITICAL THINKING

1. *What was the purpose of administering a bronchodilator to Tyshawn?*
2. *If Tyshawn's oxygen saturation did not improve following therapy, what other pharmacologic interventions could the nurse anticipate the physician might add to his treatment regimen?*
3. *How would treatment with antibiotics most likely affect Tyshawn's outcomes?*

REVIEW Respiratory Syncytial Virus/Bronchiolitis

RELATE Link the Concepts and Exemplars

Linking the exemplar of respiratory syncytial virus/bronchiolitis with the concept of comfort:

1. What can you do to help a 3-month-old baby with RSV infection feel more comfortable?

2. What would you do differently to provide comfort to a 2-year-old with RSV infection?

Linking the exemplar of respiratory syncytial virus/bronchiolitis with the concept of stress and coping:

3. How can you help parents to cope with the fear and anxiety related to hospitalization of their child?

4. When assessing the parents of a hospitalized child, how can you determine if they are coping in a healthy manner?

Linking the exemplar of respiratory syncytial virus/bronchiolitis with the concept of infection:

5. What treatment methods are most effective for an infant who is experiencing complications associated with RSV?

6. How can the spread of RSV be reduced?

READY Go to Companion Skills Manual

REFER Go to Pearson Nursing Student Resources
nursing.pearsonhighered.com

• Additional review materials

REFLECT Case Study

Ryan Riley is 9 months old. He has been sick off and on for the past week with a cold. He is not interested in eating or playing

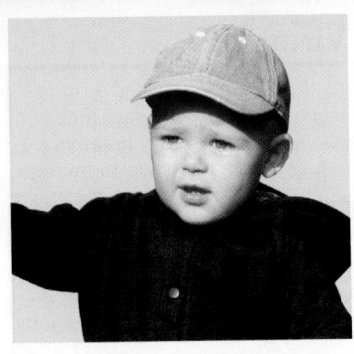

and has no energy. Ryan's mother, Jessica, leaves him in the care of her boyfriend, Casey, while she goes to work. Casey puts Ryan in his crib and leaves him alone all evening. During the course of the evening, Ryan gets worse and has nothing to drink. When Jessica comes home later that evening, Ryan feels very sick and is having problems breathing. Jessica immediately takes him to the hospital.

At the emergency department, Dr. Gordon asks Jessica how long Ryan has been sick, how many wet diapers he had in the past day, and when he last ate. Jessica tells Dr. Gordon that Ryan has had a cold for a week or so, but got sick just today. She admits that she doesn't know when he last ate or the number of wet diapers he has had. She tells Dr. Gordon that she has been working a lot of hours during the past several days. Dr. Gordon diagnoses Ryan with RSV infection and dehydration.

1. What signs and symptoms are priorities for the nursing assessment?
2. What are likely NANDA diagnoses for Ryan?
3. What are the priority nursing interventions for Ryan?
4. What tests or therapies is Dr. Gordon likely to order for Ryan?

EXEMPLAR 15.5   Sudden Infant Death Syndrome

EXEMPLAR KEY TERMS
Prone, *1024*
Sudden infant death syndrome (SIDS), *1024*
Supine, *1024*

EXEMPLAR LEARNING OUTCOMES
After reading about this exemplar, you will be able to:

1. Describe the pathophysiology, etiology, and direct and indirect contributing factors related to sudden infant death syndrome (SIDS).
2. Identify risk factors and prevention methods associated with SIDS.
3. Illustrate the nursing process in providing culturally competent care for infants, parents, and caregivers to reduce the risk of SIDS.
4. Formulate priority nursing diagnoses appropriate for an infant at risk for SIDS.
5. Summarize therapies used by interdisciplinary teams in the collaborative care of an infant at risk for SIDS.
6. Plan evidence-based care for the family who loses an infant to SIDS.
7. Evaluate expected outcomes for an individual with an infant at risk for SIDS.

▶ OVERVIEW

Sudden infant death syndrome (SIDS) is the sudden death of an apparently healthy infant that remains unexplained after other possible causes have been ruled out through autopsy, death scene investigation, and review of the medical history. SIDS is the third leading cause of infant mortality in the United States, accounting for 7.7% of all infant deaths; most SIDS deaths occur in infants between 2 and 4 months of age (CDC, 2013). It is currently unpredictable and, in some cases, unpreventable.

▶ PATHOPHYSIOLOGY AND ETIOLOGY

There is no confirmed causative factor or pathophysiology for SIDS; it can be diagnosed only after a review of the child's clinical history, examination of the scene of death, and an autopsy that fails to find a cause of death. Sudden and unexplained infant deaths are investigated for cause. The CDC tabulates data to determine trends and similarities in relation to infant deaths. Nurses must be aware that data related to infant deaths are gathered and reported for research purposes and must know the procedures for gathering and reporting such data in the clinic or hospital where they work.

Etiology

Sudden infant death syndrome is referred to as a syndrome because of the many and varied autopsy and clinical findings that characterize most children who die of the disorder. The autopsy does not identify a disease process that caused the death.

In SIDS, three factors occur simultaneously and lead to the sudden unexpected death of the infant. First, the infant has a vulnerability, a brainstem abnormality that controls respiratory and autonomic responses to stressors during sleep. Second, significant stressors contributing to SIDS are prone or side sleeping, face-down sleeping, and bed sharing. Infants in the prone or side-lying positions are vulnerable because the brainstem abnormality compromises their protective reflexes, such as arousal and head turning, when experiencing asphyxia. Third, infants are in a critical developmental period within the first 6 months of life. It is important to note that SIDS has not been found to be associated with newborn apnea or immunizations (AAP Task Force on Sudden Infant Death Syndrome, 2011).

Risk Factors

Some infant and maternal risk factors have been associated with an increased incidence of SIDS. These are summarized in **Box 15–6 ●**.

Infants placed **prone** (face-down) to sleep are at greatest risk. Infants should always be placed **supine** (on the back). The side-lying position also increases risk. Risk increases if a baby who has consistently been placed supine is placed prone for a nap or nighttime sleep. This often occurs when a caregiver other than a parent cares for the child. Grandparents, child care workers, and healthcare workers should be told to consistently place infants supine.

Maternal smoking during pregnancy and exposure to secondhand smoke during infancy have been correlated with an increased incidence of SIDS. The death rate from SIDS is nearly

Box 15–6   Risk Factors for Sudden Infant Death Syndrome

- Preterm and low birth weight
- Race (in decreasing order of frequency): most common in American Indians and Alaska Natives, followed by non-Hispanic Blacks, non-Hispanic Whites, Asian or Pacific Islanders, and Hispanics
- Gender: more common in males than in females
- Age: most common in infants between 2 and 4 months of age
- Sleeping in a prone or side-lying position
- Exposure to environmental tobacco smoke or mother who smoked during pregnancy
- Overheating (e.g., overdressing or too many bed covers)
- Bed sharing, especially with people who smoke or are under the influence of alcohol or drugs
- Loose bedding: use of pillows, comforters, quilts, and blankets
- Sleeping on soft surfaces: waterbed, sofa, pillows, with stuffed toys

Source: Based on Centers for Disease Control and Prevention. (2013). *SIDS.* Retrieved from http://www.cdc.gov/sids.

twice that for babies who are exposed to smoke compared to those who are not (CDC, 2013). Smoking outside, away from babies, does not decrease the risk, because smoky hair and clothes also affect babies' respiratory status.

A previous case of SIDS in the family increases the risk for SIDS recurrence. Other risk factors associated with SIDS involve infant sleeping environments. Babies placed on soft sleeping surfaces with loose bedding are at increased risk, as are babies who are overheated or who share a bed with adults or other children. Sleeping with a baby on the couch, a recliner chair, or soft bedding places the baby at risk. Although bed sharing appears to be harmful, babies who sleep in the same room or in a separate co-sleeper that facilitates breastfeeding have a lower incidence of SIDS. Infants who are dressed in sleeper pajamas instead of being covered with blankets have less risk. Babies who sleep in bedrooms that are heated to the comfort level of typical adults also have less incidence of SIDS.

Breastfeeding appears to be protective, perhaps because breastfed babies are more easily aroused from sleep than formula-fed babies. Offering a pacifier at sleep times appears to support ease of arousal from sleeping and is considered to be protective.

▶ CLINICAL MANIFESTATIONS

There are no warning signs or early clinical manifestations to indicate that a baby will die of SIDS. The first symptom is cardiopulmonary arrest. Clinical findings after the death include evidence of a struggle or change in position and the presence of frothy, blood-tinged secretions from the mouth and nares. Most deaths are unobserved. Typically, parents find the infant dead in the crib in the morning or after a nap, and they report having heard no cries or disturbances during the sleep interval.

▶ COLLABORATION

All members of the healthcare team must work together to promote safety for the infant in order to reduce the occurrence of SIDS. All new parents should be taught the importance of "back to sleep" for their infants. Clients who purchase used older cribs and linens need to be taught how to assess them for safety because guidelines at the time of manufacture were different than those for bedding designed today. Infants at increased risk should be identified as early as possible to initiate precautions.

Modeling Protective Behaviors

Members of the healthcare team are in a perfect position to teach new families to care for their baby. Protective behaviors should be modeled as well as taught. All members of the healthcare team need to place the newborn on its back for sleep. Because many nurses and physicians were educated that the appropriate sleep position for babies was prone, some healthcare providers may find it difficult to alter behaviors from what they learned to the positioning that is now supported by research. Supine positioning for sleeping has been found to be even more protective of SIDS for the premature infant. Neonatal healthcare workers, nursery, and pediatric healthcare personnel need to be conscious of their positioning behaviors, particularly since parents observe positioning behaviors of healthcare workers and then copy those behaviors.

Addressing the Psychosocial Needs of the Family

Sudden infant death may occur despite following all the precautions. The sudden, unexpected nature of the infant's death is confirmed in the emergency department. Nurses are part of

Focus on Diversity and Culture   Sudden Infant Death Syndrome

Rates of SIDS are highest for African Americans and American Indians and lowest for Asians and Hispanics. In 2008, the rate of SIDS among African Americans was more than twice that of Caucasians, and the rate among American Indians was more than three times greater than that among Caucasians (Health Resources Services Administration, 2008).

To promote the use of the supine sleeping position for African American babies, the Back to Sleep campaign joined with the National Black Child Development Institute and other historically Black organizations to develop materials for a new initiative to reduce SIDS in African American communities. The CJ Foundation for SIDS offers culturally competent materials in both English and Spanish as well as materials developed as part of an effort to reduce deaths due to SIDS among Native Americans. These resources can be accessed at www.cjsids.org/resource-center/education-and-outreach/educational-materials.html.

an interdisciplinary team that supports the family through their grief.

The nurse's role is to be empathetic and provide support during one of the greatest crises a family must face. The focus is on supporting the family during the acute grieving period. Guidelines for the support of families experiencing SIDS should include baptism services, religious support, grief counseling, assistance with funeral arrangements, and counseling on cessation of breastfeeding when appropriate. A spiritual leader of the family's particular belief system is asked to come to the family's aid in coping with grief. Other healthcare providers involved with the infant's care may also provide emotional support during the family's time of grief; some healthcare providers attend the funeral services to emotionally support the grieving family.

Reassure the parents that they are not responsible for the infant's death, and assist them in contacting other family members and mobilizing support. Giving parents information about the potential reactions of siblings can help them respond to their needs. Older children may need reassurance that SIDS will not happen to them. They may also believe that bad thoughts or wishes about their baby brother or sister caused the death.

Nurses in perinatal or pediatric care as well as social workers may direct the family to a support group for those who have suffered the death of a child. Support groups can help parents, siblings, and other family members express these fears and work through their feelings about the infant's death. Local hospice organizations also provide supportive services to families grieving the loss of a child. Parents may need extra support at a later time with the birth of a subsequent newborn.

Refer to the module on Grief and Loss for more information.

Stay Current: *The First Candle organization at* **www.first-candle.org** *can help families locate a support group in their geographic area.*

When a Death Occurs

The assessment carried out after the death of an infant in the home is completed by a medical examiner and law enforcement agents. Other potential causes have to be ruled out. Sudden, unexplained infant deaths may be the result of homicide, undiagnosed genetic disorders, accidents, or other cardiopulmonary pathologies. Investigative questions are utilized to establish the cause and manner of the death or to support investigator's findings in court.

Families who have suddenly lost a baby are interviewed. The purpose of the interview is to determine any cause, clinical or accidental, and to rule out homicide. The CDC stresses balancing investigation with supporting a grieving family. Often, the investigation has the positive effect of demonstrating the family's innocence to friends and neighbors.

The physical address of the location where the death occurred is recorded. An assessment of the scene, including orientation of fixtures and body placement as well as body appearance, is completed. A health history of the infant, including diet, metabolic disorders, birth defects, and maternal pregnancy history, is recorded. A pathologist summarizes the findings from the autopsy and investigation reports to determine the cause of death.

This process can be intimidating to family members who may resent these intrusions during the time of grief and who may reject findings that they do not understand or with which they do not agree. Collaborative care for these families may include grief counselors, chaplains and religious leaders, nurses (including school nurses working with older children who lose a sibling), and psychotherapists. In particular, the parents' grief will be acute, and they should receive a psychosocial assessment at each healthcare interaction.

■ NURSING PROCESS

Nursing care is focused on prevention. When caring for the family who lost an infant to SIDS, the priority of care is to support the parents in the grieving process, reduce feelings of guilt, provide referrals to support groups, and help them cope with their loss.

Assessment

Nurses who provide care during pregnancy and early infancy should assess for risk for SIDS and not hesitate to ask appropriate questions. Collect assessment data through the health history and physical assessment:

- **Health history.** Does the mother or any other member of the household smoke? How and where does the mother put the child to sleep? What other caregivers put the child to sleep? What are the child's breathing patterns? Will the mother breastfeed or use formula? Has there been a previous death of an infant within the family?
- **Physical examination.** Respiratory rate and patterns.

Diagnosis

The following NANDA diagnoses are appropriate for the infant at risk for SIDS and immediate family members:

- *Risk for SIDS*
- *Knowledge Deficit* related to risk factors associated with SIDS
- *Enhanced Parenting* related to preventive measures associated with SIDS.

(NANDA-I © 2012)

The following NANDA diagnoses may be appropriate for those families who have just lost a baby to SIDS:

- *Grieving*
- *Compromised Family Coping*
- *Risk for Spiritual Distress.*

(NANDA-I © 2012)

Planning

Nurses collaborate with families and prospective family to design appropriate outcomes with the goal of decreasing an infant's risk for SIDS. These outcomes may include the following:

- Parents and other adults living in the household will describe appropriate habits to lower the risk for SIDS, including putting the infant on his back to sleep.
- Any adult in the household who smokes will participate in a smoking cessation program.
- Parents who lose a baby to SIDS will participate in grief counseling or a support group.

Evidence-Based Practice Infant Sleep Positioning

Problem

Following the AAP recommendation that infants be placed to sleep in a nonprone position, there was a decline in the amount of deaths due to SIDS, but this decline has plateaued in recent years. Other causes of sudden unexpected infant death that occur during sleep, including suffocation, asphyxia, and entrapment, have increased in incidence (AAP Task Force on Sudden Infant Death Syndrome, 2011).

Evidence

The AAP is expanding its recommendations from focusing only on SIDS to focusing on safe sleep environments that can reduce the risk of all sleep-related infant deaths. These recommendations include supine positioning during sleep, using a firm sleep surface, breastfeeding, room sharing without bed sharing, routine immunizations, and the use of a pacifier. Items that should be avoided include soft bedding, overheating, and exposure to secondhand smoke, alcohol, and illicit drugs (AAP Task Force on Sudden Infant Death Syndrome, 2011).

Implications

Nurses, healthcare providers, and child care professionals should endorse the recommendations for reducing SIDS-related deaths. This means NICU and nursery staff should model and implement all SIDS risk reduction recommendations as soon as the infant is clinically stable and before the anticipated discharge. Nurses working with parents of newborns must provide additional client teaching and follow-up and ensure parents are able to demonstrate the teaching. All child care providers should also receive education on safe infant sleep practices, incorporating these as written policies (AAP Task Force on Sudden Infant Death Syndrome, 2011).

Critical Thinking Application

1. Identify methods to increase education of the public regarding safe sleep environments for newborns and infants to decrease the risk of sleep-associated deaths.

2. Develop a teaching plan about preferred infant sleeping routines for a group of child care providers.

Parents who lose a baby may not feel ready to participate in counseling or support groups. The nurse should encourage, not push, parents to seek help, offering referral sources and calling to check on the parents at appropriate intervals following the death. The nurse on duty when the baby is brought to the emergency department should determine if the family has spiritual support and notify the hospital chaplain or offer to call the family's spiritual leader.

Implementation

Client teaching is an important nursing intervention. By educating parents of newborns on preventive strategies, it is possible to continue to reduce the number of SIDS deaths occurring annually.

Reduce Risk for SIDS

Caring interventions focus on teaching parents how to reduce risks. For caring interventions related to loss, see the Grief and Loss module.

The most important teaching can be summed up by the phrase "Back to sleep, tummy to play." "Back to sleep" should be applied to all sleeping sessions, whether a nap or at night. Protective behaviors should be modeled as well as taught.

Specifically, nurses will model and teach:

- "Back to sleep"
- Tummy for play time while awake
- Cuddle time for loving, upright position on lap or chest
- Cease smoking during pregnancy and around infants
- Use bedding that is firm
- Crib or co-sleeper in parents' room
- Sleeper or warm pajamas
- Blankets secured lower than infant's chest
- Avoid overheating sleeping room
- Parents need to tell caregivers "Back to sleep only."

Stay Current: Visit the NICHD Web site at **www.nichd.nih.gov/SIDS/Pages/sidsnursesce.aspx** to learn about their continuing education program for nurses on SIDS risk reduction.

Client Teaching The Safe to Sleep Campaign

The single most important method of preventing SIDS is putting the infant to sleep on the back. The Back to Sleep campaign was launched in June 1994 to increase parents' and caregivers' understanding of this crucial issue. The campaign was redesigned and debuted in 2012 as Safe to Sleep. Based on new guidelines from the American Academy of Pediatrics, Safe to Sleep includes strategies for reducing the risk of SIDS and other sleep-related causes of infant death such as suffocation and strangulation. These strategies include emphasizing Back to Sleep for *every* sleep time; using firm (not soft) sleeping surfaces covered by a fitted sheet; and keeping soft objects, toys, and loose bedding out of the sleep area.

The original Back to Sleep campaign is credited with widespread success: As of 2006, the National Center for Health Statistics reported a more than 50% drop in SIDS death rates (National Institute of Child Health and Human Development, 2013). This campaign saturates hospitals, pediatricians' offices, clinics, child care programs, local health departments, and other agencies serving mothers with young children with resources that demonstrate the importance of putting babies to sleep on their backs.

Evaluation

Nurses evaluate understanding of infant care to protect against risk for SIDS by discussion during follow-up visits and during perinatal care. Nurses determine if families understand the importance of supine sleeping and nonsmoking behaviors. Nurses ask if the sleeping arrangements for an infant include a separate, firm surface and whether dressing and heating arrangements provide for adequate warmth without overheating. A final evaluation may be related to SIDS occurring despite families following all the precautions. Nurses are part of an interdisciplinary team that supports the family through their grief.

REVIEW Sudden Infant Death Syndrome

RELATE Link the Concepts and Exemplars

The parents of an infant who has died of SIDS ask the emergency department nurse for ideas on how they can tell the 2-year-old sibling that the baby has died.

Linking the exemplar of sudden infant death syndrome with the concept of development:

1. Based on the typical developmental stages of a 2-year-old's language, what suggestions might the nurse make?

2. How would the nurse's suggestions differ if the family asks for ideas for how to tell a 10-year-old sibling what has happened?

Linking the exemplar of sudden infant death syndrome with the concept of family:

3. What resources could you recommend to the family of an infant who died of SIDS in your community?

4. What strategies might you suggest to help the family members of an infant who died from SIDS who are displaying unhealthy coping strategies?

Linking the exemplar of sudden infant death syndrome with the concept of grief and loss:

5. What interventions can the nurse implement to help a family who has lost an infant due to SIDS?

6. How can the nurse help the family respond to a sibling's response to loss?

READY Go to Companion Skills Manual

REFER Go to Pearson Nursing Student Resources
nursing.pearsonhighered.com

- Additional review materials

REFLECT Case Study

Susan Miller is a 24-year-old, gravida 2 para 2 woman in the postpartum unit. Her son died at the age of 4 months because of SIDS. Mrs. Miller expresses fear that her newborn daughter, Grace, could also die from SIDS. She has heard that if SIDS occurs in a family, the likelihood of recurrence is greater.

1. What are possible nursing diagnoses for Mrs. Miller? For Grace?

2. Create a teaching plan that includes typical infant care, stressing behaviors that can reduce the risk of SIDS for this mother and child.

3. What coping strategies might you suggest to Mrs. Miller to help her reduce her anxiety related to a reoccurrence of SIDS with her new daughter?

■ REFERENCES

Adams, P. A., Holland, L. N., & Urban, C. Q. (2014). *Pharmacology for nurses: A pathophysiologic approach* (4th ed.). Upper Saddle River, NJ: Pearson Education.

Adams, S. G., Hospenthal, A. C., Baillargeon, G. M., Kazis, L. E., Pugh, J. A., & Anzueto, A. (2008). Hispanic patients with chronic obstructive pulmonary disease did not receive referral to smoking cessation courses as commonly as patients of other ethnicities. *American Journal of Respiratory and Critical Care Medicine, 177*(5) 473–478.

Alverson, B., & Ralston, S. L. (2011). Management of bronchiolitis: Focus on hypertonic saline. *Contemporary Pediatrics, 28*(2), 30–38.

American Academy of Allergy, Asthma, and Immunology (AAAAI). (2013a). *Diseases 101: Adult asthma.* Retrieved from http://www.aaaai.org/patients/gallery/adultasthma.asp.

American Academy of Allergy, Asthma, and Immunology (AAAAI). (2013b). *Tips to remember: Childhood asthma.* Retrieved from http://www.aaaai.org/patients/publicedmat/tips/childhoodasthma.stm.

American Academy of Pediatrics (AAP) Subcommittee on Diagnosis and Management of Bronchiolitis. (2006). *Diagnosis and management of bronchiolitis.* Retrieved from http://www.pediatrics.org/cdl/10.1542/peds.2006-2223.

American Academy of Pediatrics (AAP) Task Force on Sudden Infant Death Syndrome. (2011). SIDS and other sleep related infant deaths: Expansion of recommendations for a safe infant sleeping environment. *Pediatrics, 128*(5), 1030–1039.

American Cancer Society. (2013). *Tobacco related cancers fact sheet.* Retrieved from http://www.cancer.org/cancer/cancercauses/tobaccocancer/tobacco-related-cancer-fact-sheet.

American College of Allergy, Asthma, and Immunology (ACAAI). (2010). *Asthma and pregnancy.* Retrieved from http://www.acaai.org/allergist/liv_man/pregnancy/pages/default.aspx.

American Lung Association (ALA). (2013a). Acute respiratory distress syndrome (ARDS). In *Lung disease data: 2012.* Retrieved from http://www.lungusa.org.

American Lung Association (ALA). (2013b). *Lung disease data: 2012.* Retrieved from http://www.lungusa.org.

Asthma Initiative of Michigan for Healthy Lungs. (2011). *How to use a metered-dose inhaler the right way.* Retrieved from http://www.getasthmahelp.org/inhalers_main.asp.

Ball, J. W., Bindler, R. C., & Cowen, K. (2012). *Principles of pediatric nursing: Caring for children* (5th ed.). Upper Saddle River, NJ: Pearson Prentice Hall.

Banauch, G. I., Hall, C., Weiden, M., Cohen, H. W., Aldrich, T. K., Christodoulou, V., et al. (2006). Pulmonary function after exposure to the World Trade Center collapse in the New York City Fire Department. *American Journal of Respiratory Care and Critical Care Medicine, 174*, 312–319.

Barnes, J., Dong, C. Y., McRobbie, H., Walker, N., Mehta, M., & Stead, L. F. (2010). Hypnotherapy for smoking cessation. Retrieved from http://onlinelibrary.wiley.com/doi/10.1002/14651858.CD001008.pub2/abstract.

Brashers, V. L. (2010). Alterations in pulmonary function. In K. L. McCance, S. E. Heuther, V. L. Brashers, & N. R. Rote, *Pathophysiology: The biological basis for disease in adults and children* (6th ed., pp. 1266–1304). St. Louis, MO: Mosby Elsevier.

Bruce, D. (2009). *Asthma and depression: People with asthma have twice the risk of developing mood and anxiety disorders.* Retrieved from http://www.webmd.com/asthma/features/asthma-depression.

Centers for Disease Control and Prevention (CDC). (2009). *Facts about chronic obstructive pulmonary disease.* Retrieved from http://www.cdc.gov/copd/copdfaq.htm.

Centers for Disease Control and Prevention (CDC). (2010a). *Respiratory syncytial virus: Laboratory testing.* Retrieved from http://www.cdc.gov/rsv/clinical/labtesting.html.

Centers for Disease Control and Prevention (CDC). (2010b). *Respiratory syncytial virus: Transmission and prevention.* Retrieved from http://www.cdc.gov/rsv/about/transmission.html.

Centers for Disease Control and Prevention (CDC). (2012). Respiratory diseases: Chronic obstructive pulmonary disease. *Healthy people 2020.* Retrieved from http://www.healthypeople.gov/Document/HTML/Volume2/24Respiratory.htm#_Toc489704826.

Centers for Disease Control and Prevention (CDC). (2013). *SIDS (sudden infant death syndrome).* Retrieved from http://www.cdc.gov/sids.

Cleveland Clinic. (2013). *Corticosteroids.* Retrieved from http://my.clevelandclinic.org/drugs/corticosteroids/hic_corticosteroids.aspx.

Davidson, M. R., London, M. L., & Ladewig, P. A. (2011). *Olds' maternal–newborn nursing & women's health across the lifespan* (9th ed.). Upper Saddle River, NJ: Pearson Prentice Hall.

Fenstermacher, D., & Hong, D. (2004). Mechanical ventilation: What have we learned? *Critical Care Nursing Quarterly, 27*(3), 256–294.

Fishman, A. P., Elias, J. A., Fishman, J. A., Grippi, M. A., Senior, S. M., & Pack, A. J. (2008). *Fishman's pulmonary diseases and disorders* (4th ed.). New York, NY: McGraw-Hill.

Froh, D. K. (2006). Alterations in pulmonary function in children. In K. L. McNance & S. E. Heuther (Eds.), *Pathophysiology: The biologic basis for disease in adults and children* (5th ed., pp. 1249–1278). St. Louis, MO: Elsevier Mosby.

Global Initiative for COPD. (2013). *Global initiative for chronic obstructive lung disease.* Retrieved from http://www.goldcopd.org/Guidelines/guidelines-resources.html.

Health Resources Services Administration, U. S. Department of Health and Human Services. (2008). *SIDS deaths by race and ethnicity 1995–2001.* Vienna, VA: National Sudden Infant Death Resource Center.

HealthyChildren.org. (2012). *Bronchiolitis.* Retrieved from http://www.healthychildren.org/English/health-issues/conditions/chest-lungs/Pages/Bronchiolitis.aspx?

Higgins, D. (2009). Tracheostomy care: Part 1–Using suction to remove respiratory secretions via a tracheostomy tube. *Nursing Times, 105*(4), 16–17.

Holland, A., & Hill, C. (2011). New horizons for pulmonary rehabilitation. *Physical Therapy Review, 16*(1), 3–9.

International Ventilator Users Network. (2009). *Home ventilator guide.* Retrieved from http://www.ventusers.org/edu/HomeVentGuide.pdf.

Kee, J. L. (2014). *Laboratory and diagnostic tests with nursing implications* (9th ed.). Upper Saddle River, NJ: Pearson Education.

Kravitz, L., & Robergs, R. (2013). Is it genetic? Retrieved from http://www.unm.edu/~lkravitz/Article%20folder/genetics.html.

Kumar, P., Denson, S., & Mancuso, T. (2010). Premedication for non-emergency endotracheal intubation in the neonate. *Pediatrics, 125*(3), 608–615.

Kyngas, H., & Rissanen, M. (2001). Support as a crucial predictor of good compliance of adolescents with a chronic disease. *Journal of Clinical Nursing, 10,* 767–774.

Mayo Clinic (2010). *Corticosteroids.* Retrieved from http://www.mayoclinic.com/health/drug-information/DR602333.

National Center for Complementary and Alternative Medicine. (2012). *Asthma and complementary health practices.* Retrieved from http://nccam.nih.gov/health/asthma/facts.

National Center for Preparedness, Detection, and Control of Infectious Diseases. (2009). *RSV in Alaskan children.* Retrieved from http://www.cdc.gov/ncidod/aip/research/rsv.html#rsv_ak.

National Heart, Lung, and Blood Institute (NHLBI). (2012a). *ARDS.* Retrieved from http://www.nhlbi.nih.gov/health/health-topics/topics/ards.

National Heart, Lung, and Blood Institute (NHLBI). (2012b). *Asthma.* Retrieved from http://www.nhlbi.nih.gov/health/health-topics/topics/asthma.

National Institutes of Health. (2012a). *Acute respiratory distress syndrome (ARDS).* Retrieved from http://www.nhlbi.nih.gov/health/health-topics/topics/ards.

National Institute of Child Health and Human Development. (2013). *Safe to sleep education campaign.* Retrieved from http://www.nichd.nih.gov/SIDS/Pages/sids.aspx.

National Institutes of Health (2012b). *Respiratory syncytial virus.* Retrieved from http://www.nlm.nih.gov/medlineplus/ency/article/001564.htm.

Pruitt, B. (2010). Interpreting ABGs. *Nursing, 40*(7), 31–36.

Pruitt, W. C., & Jacobs, M. (2004). Interpreting arterial blood gases: Easy as A B C. *Nursing, 34*(8), 50–53.

Rennard, S. I. (2012). Patient information: Chronic obstructive pulmonary disease (COPD) treatments (beyond the basics). UpToDate. Retrieved from http://www.uptodate.com/contents/chronic-obstructive-pulmonary-disease-copd-treatments-beyond-the-basics.

Reuters Health Information. (2009). COPD patients may derive significant benefit from statin therapy. Retrieved from http://cme.medscape.com/viewarticle/706421?src=cmenews.

Rhee, H., Ciurzynski, S. M., & Yoos, H. L. (2008). Pearls and pitfalls of community-based group interventions for adolescents: Lessons learned from an adolescent asthma camp study. *Issues in Comprehensive Pediatric Nursing, 31,* 122–135. doi:10.1080/01460860802272888.

Rodríguez-Esquivel, D., Cooper, T. V., Blow, J., & Resor, M. (2009). Characteristics associated with smoking in a Hispanic sample. *Addictive Behaviors, 34,* 593–598.

Selden, J. A., & Scarfone, R. J. (2009). Bronchiolitis: An evidence-based approach to management. *Clinical Pediatric Emergency Medicine, 10,* 75–81.

Simmons, P., & Simmons, M. (2004). Informed nursing practice: The administration of oxygen to patients with COPD. *Medsurg Nursing, 13*(2), 82–85.

Smyth, R. L., & Openshaw, P. J. M. (2006). Bronchiolitis. *Lancet, 368,* 312–322.

Sorce, L. R. (2009). Respiratory syncytial virus: From primary care to critical care. *Journal of Pediatric Healthcare, 23*(2), 101–108.

Srivastava, G. (2010). Airway foreign bodies in children. *Clinical Pediatric Emergency Medicine, 11*(2), 67–72.

Yang, T., Sylva, K., & Lunt, I. (2010). Parent support, peer support, and peer acceptance in healthy lifestyle for asthma management among early adolescents. *Journal of Specialists in Pediatric Nursing, 15*(4), 272–281. doi:10.1111/j.1744-6155.2010.00247.x.

Zagaria, M. A. E. (2010). Inhalant agents for asthma, bronchospasm, and COPD: Focus on delivery devices and inhalation technique. *American Journal for Nurse Practitioners, 14*(3), 21–25.

16 Perfusion

◨ THE CONCEPT OF PERFUSION

The essential function of the cardiovascular and pulmonary systems is to provide a continuous supply of oxygenated blood to every cell in the body. The physiological process of perfusion requires the heart to transport and distribute blood throughout the body. Changes in perfusion affect all human functions, including self-care, comfort, mobility, fluid volume status, respiration, and tissue integrity. Impaired perfusion may also affect self-concept and role performance. «

Concept Learning Outcomes

After reading about this concept, you will be able to:

1. Summarize the physiology of the cardiovascular system related to perfusion.
2. Examine the relationship between perfusion and other concepts/systems.
3. Identify commonly occurring alterations in perfusion and their related therapies.
4. Differentiate common assessment procedures used to examine cardiovascular health across the life span.
5. Describe diagnostic and laboratory tests to determine the individual's perfusion status.
6. Explain management of cardiovascular health and prevention of cardiovascular illness.
7. Demonstrate the nursing process in providing culturally competent and caring interventions across the life span for individuals with common alterations in perfusion.
8. Compare and contrast common independent and collaborative interventions for clients with alterations in perfusion.

Concept Key Terms

Action potential, *1043*
Afterload, *1042*
Apical-radial pulse, *1064*
Arterial blood pressure, *1045*
Arteriosclerosis, *1045*
Atrial gallop, *1035*
Bradycardia, *1063*
Cardiac cycle, *1040*
Cardiac index, *1042*
Cardiac output (CO), *1040*
Cardiac reserve, *1041*
Clotting, *1049*
Compliance, *1044*
Contractility, *1042*
Coronary circulation, *1036*
Depolarization, *1043*

Desaturated blood, *1046*
Diastole, *1034*
Diastolic blood pressure, *1045*
Dysrhythmia (arrhythmia), *1063*
Ectopic, *1073*
Ejection fraction, *1040*
Elasticity of the arterial wall, *1063*
Electrocardiogram (ECG), *1071*
Electrocardiography, *1043*
First heart sound (S_1), *1034*
Foramen ovale, *1040*
Fourth heart sound (S_4), *1034*

(continued on next page)

▶ NORMAL PERFUSION

The heart is a hollow, cone-shaped organ, approximately the size of an adult's fist and weighing less than 1 lb. It is located in the mediastinum of the thoracic cavity, between the vertebral column and the sternum, and is flanked laterally by the lungs. Two thirds of the heart mass lies to the left of the sternum; the upper base lies beneath the second rib, and the pointed apex is approximate with the fifth intercostal space (ICS), midpoint to the clavicle (**Figure 16–1** ●).

The Pericardium

The heart is covered by the **pericardium**, a double layer of fibro-serous membrane (**Figure 16–2** ●). The pericardium encases the heart and anchors it to surrounding structures, forming the pericardial sac. The snug fit of the pericardium prevents the heart from overfilling with blood. The outermost layer is the parietal pericardium. The visceral pericardium (or epicardium) adheres to the heart surface. The small space between the visceral and parietal layers of the pericardium is called the pericardial cavity. A serous lubricating fluid produced in this space cushions the heart as it contracts.

Layers of the Heart Wall

The heart wall consists of three layers of tissue: the epicardium, the myocardium, and the endocardium (see Figure 16–2). The epicardium covers the entire heart and great vessels, and then folds over to form the parietal layer lining the pericardium and adheres to the heart surface. The myocardium, the middle layer of the heart wall, consists of specialized cardiac muscle cells (myofibrils). These cells provide the bulk of the contractile heart muscle. The endocardium, which is the innermost layer,

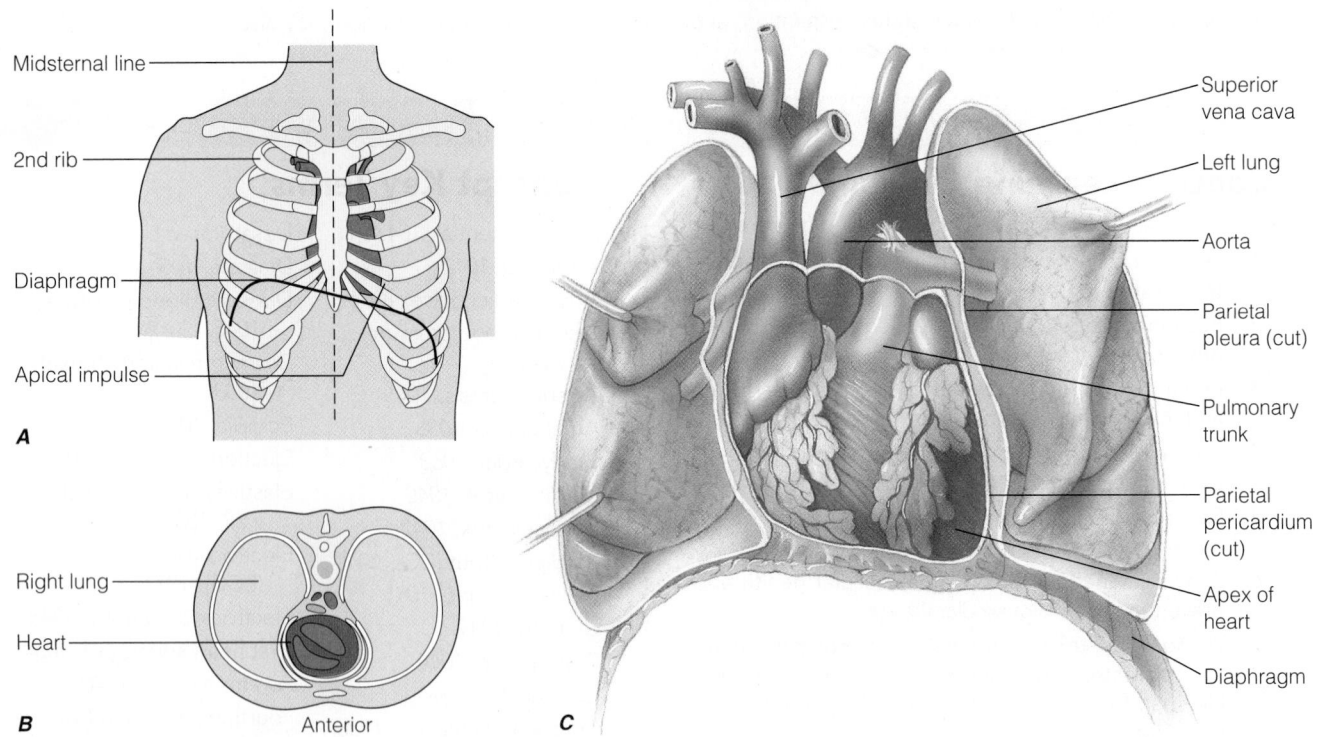

Figure 16–1 ● Location of the heart in the mediastinum of the thorax. *A*, Relationship of the heart to the sternum, ribs, and diaphragm. *B*, Cross-sectional view showing relative position of the heart in the thorax. *C*, Relationship of the heart and great vessels to the lungs.

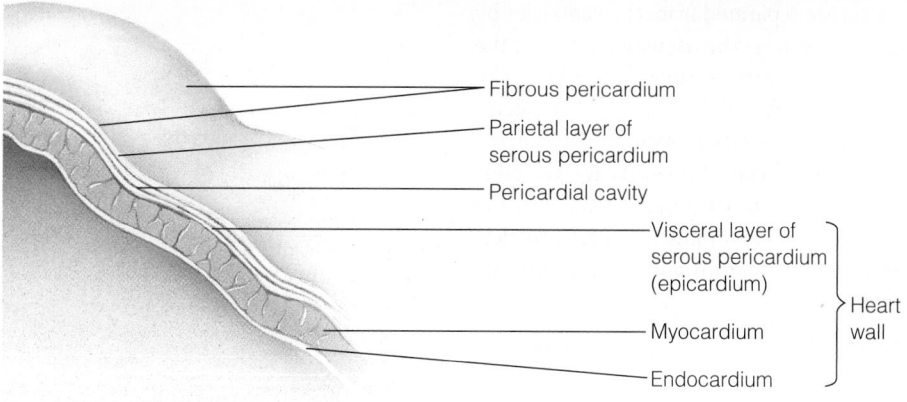

Figure 16–2 ● Coverings and layers of the heart.

is a thin membrane composed of three layers; the innermost layer is made up of smooth endothelial cells that line the inside of the heart's chambers and great vessels. The myocardium is the muscular layer of the heart that contracts during each heartbeat. The outermost layer of the heart is the epicardium.

Chambers and Valves of the Heart

The heart has four hollow chambers, two atria (a left and a right) and two ventricles (also a left and a right). They are separated longitudinally by the interventricular septum (**Figure 16–3 ●**).

The right atrium receives deoxygenated blood from the veins of the body: The superior vena cava returns blood from the head, neck, arm, and chest areas; the inferior vena cava returns blood from the lower body; and the coronary sinus drains blood from the heart. The left atrium receives freshly oxygenated blood from the lungs through the pulmonary veins.

The right ventricle receives deoxygenated blood from the right atrium and pumps it through the pulmonary artery to the pulmonary capillary bed for oxygenation. The newly oxygenated blood then travels through the pulmonary veins to the left atrium. Blood enters the left atrium and crosses the mitral (bicuspid) valve into the left ventricle. Blood is then pumped out of the aorta to the arterial circulation.

Each chamber of the heart is separated by a valve that allows unidirectional blood flow to the next chamber or great vessel

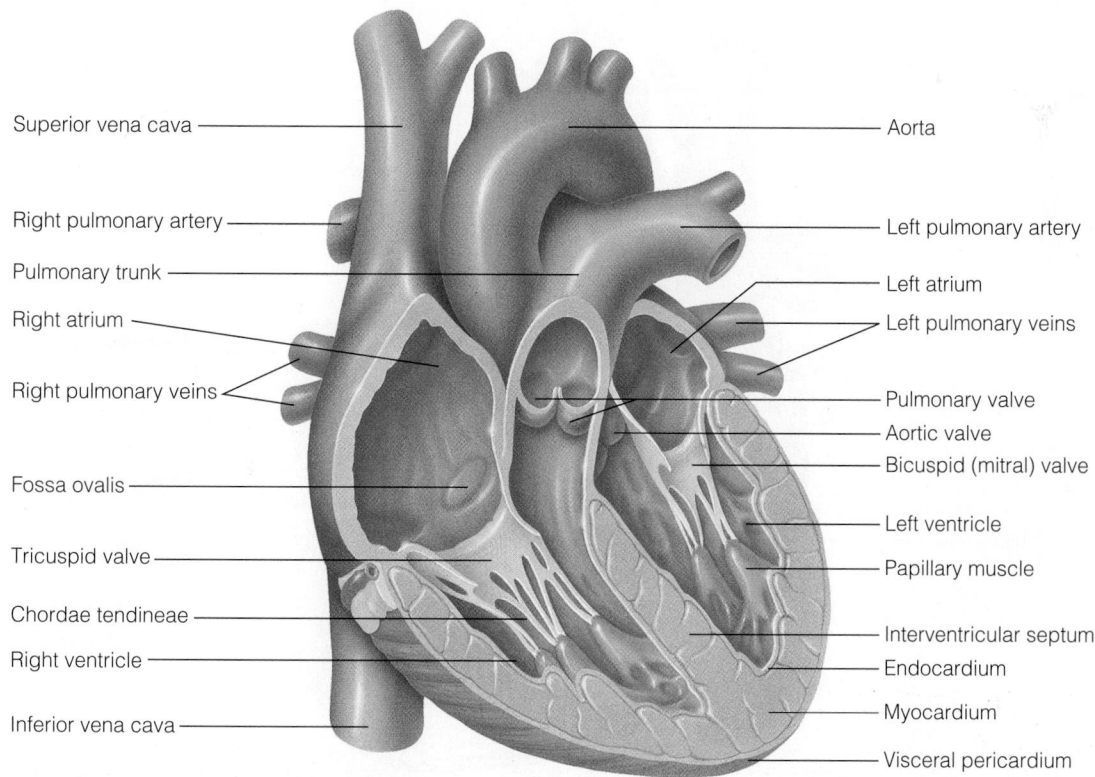

Figure 16–3 ● The internal anatomy of the heart, frontal section.

(see Figure 16–3). The atria are separated from the ventricles by the two atrioventricular (AV) valves: the tricuspid valve on the right side, and the bicuspid (or mitral) valve on the left. The chordae tendineae anchor the flaps of the valves to the papillary muscles. These structures control the movement of the AV valves to prevent backflow of blood. The ventricles are connected to their great vessels by the semilunar valves. On the right, the pulmonary (pulmonic) valve joins the right ventricle with the pulmonary artery. On the left, the aortic valve joins the left ventricle to the aorta.

NORMAL HEART SOUNDS   Heart sounds originate from closure of the heart valves (**Figure 16–4** ●). These are heard as the "lub-dub" of the heart when auscultated over the precordium (the area of the chest that lies over the heart). Closure of the AV valves produces the **first heart sound (S_1)**, which is characterized by the syllable "lub." The AV valves close when the ventricles fill. Closure of the semilunar valves produces the **second heart sound (S_2)**, which is characterized by the syllable "dub." The semilunar valves close when the ventricles empty blood into the aorta and pulmonary arteries.

The heart sounds are associated with the contraction and relaxation phases of the heart. **Systole** refers to the phase of ventricular contraction. In the systolic phase, the ventricles are filled and then contract to expel blood into the aorta and pulmonary arteries. Systole begins with the closure of the AV valves (S_1) and ends with the closure of the aortic and pulmonic valves (S_2). **Diastole** refers to the phase of ventricular relaxation. In the diastolic phase, the ventricles relax and are filled during atrial contraction. Diastole begins with the closure of the aortic and pulmonic valves (S_2) and ends with the closure of the AV valves (S_1) (**Figure 16–5** ●).

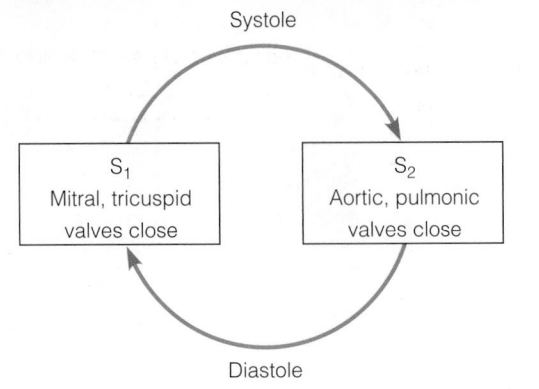

Figure 16–5 ● Heart sounds in systole and diastole.

Splitting of S_2 may occur in some individuals toward the end of inspiration. This results from a slight difference in the time that it takes the semilunar valves to close. The increase in intrathoracic pressure during inspiration is considered a normal splitting of S_2. The aortic valve closes just slightly earlier than the pulmonic valve. As a result, a split sound is heard (instead of "dub," one hears "t-dub"). The valves close at the same time during expiration, and the sound of S_2 is "dub."

Two other heart sounds may be present in some healthy individuals. The **third heart sound (S_3)** may be heard in children, in young adults, or in pregnant females during the third trimester. It is heard after S_2 and is termed a **ventricular gallop**. When the AV valves open, blood flow into the ventricles may cause vibrations. These vibrations create the S_3 sound during diastole. The **fourth heart sound (S_4)** may be heard in children, well-conditioned athletes, and even healthy older adults

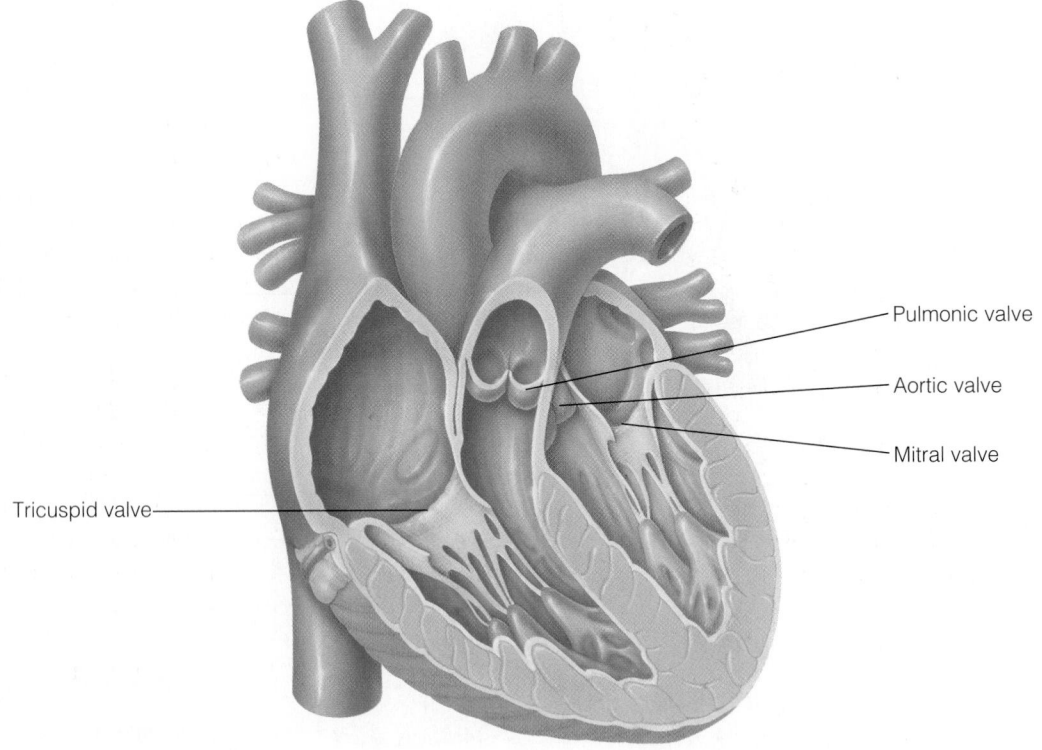

Figure 16–4 ● Valves of the heart.

without cardiac disease. The S_4 sound is caused by atrial contraction and ejection of blood into the ventricles in late diastole. It is heard before S_1 and is termed an **atrial gallop**. The S_3 and S_4 sounds may be associated with pathological conditions such as myocardial infarction or heart failure.

Heart sounds are interpreted according to the characteristics of pitch, duration, intensity, phase, and location on the precordium. **Table 16–1** ● provides information about the characteristics of heart sounds.

ADDITIONAL HEART SOUNDS The valves of the heart open silently unless the tissue has been damaged. Clicks and snaps may be heard in clients with valvular disease. An opening snap may be heard in mitral stenosis. Ejection clicks occur in

TABLE 16–1 Characteristics of Heart Sounds

HEART SOUNDS	CARDIAC CYCLE TIMING	AUSCULTATION SITE	POSITION	PITCH
S_1 — LUB dub	Start of systole	Apex with diaphragm	Position does not affect the sound	High
S_2 — lub DUB	End of systole	Both at second intercostal space (ICS); pulmonary component best at left sternal border (LSB); aortic component best at right sternal border (RSB) with diaphragm	Sitting or supine	High
Split S_1	Beginning of systole	If normal, at second ICS, LSB; abnormal if heard at apex	Best heard in the supine position	High
Fixed split S_2	End of systole	Both at second ICS; pulmonary component best at LSB; aortic component best at RSB with diaphragm	Best heard in the supine position	High
Paradoxic split S_2	End of systole	Both at second ICS; pulmonary component best at LSB; aortic component best at RSB with diaphragm	Best heard in the supine position	High
Wide split S_2	End of systole	Both at second ICS; pulmonary component best at LSB; aortic component best at RSB with diaphragm	Best heard in the supine position	High
S_3	Early diastole right after S_2	Apex with the bell	Auscultated best in left lateral position or supine	Low
S_4	Late diastole right before S_1	Apex with the bell	Auscultated best in left lateral position or supine	Low

TABLE 16–2   Additional Heart Sounds

CLICKS	HEART SOUNDS	CARDIAC CYCLE TIMING	AUSCULTATION SITE	POSITION	PITCH
	Aortic click	Early systole	Second ICS, RSB for aortic click and apex with diaphragm	Sitting or supine position may increase sound	High
	Pulmonic	Early systole	Second ICS, LSB for pulmonic click with diaphragm	Sitting	High
	Opening snap	Early diastole	Third to fourth ICS, LSB with diaphragm	Sitting or supine position may increase the sound	High
	Friction rub	Can occur at any time	Best heard with the diaphragm; location variable	May be heard in any position, but is heard best when the client sits forward	High, harsh in sound, grating

damaged pulmonic and aortic valves, and nonejection clicks are heard in prolapse of the mitral valve.

Friction rubs result from inflammation of the pericardial sac. When this occurs, the surfaces of the parietal and visceral layers of the pericardium cannot slide smoothly and produce a rubbing or grating sound. **Table 16–2** ● provides information regarding interpretation of additional heart sounds.

Heart murmurs are harsh, blowing sounds caused by disruption of blood flow into the heart, between the chambers of the heart, or from the heart into the pulmonary or aortic systems. Methods to distinguish murmurs and the classification of heart murmurs are provided in **Tables 16–3** ● and **16–4** ●, respectively.

Pulmonary, Systemic, and Coronary Circulation

Because each side of the heart receives and ejects blood, the heart is often described as a double pump. Blood enters the right atrium and moves to the pulmonary bed at almost the exact same time that blood is entering the left atrium. The circulatory system has two parts: the pulmonary circulation and the systemic circulation. Pulmonary circulation moves blood through the capillary bed surrounding the lungs to link with the gas exchange system of the lungs. The systemic circulation supplies blood to all other body tissues. In addition, the heart muscle is supplied with blood via the coronary circulation.

PULMONARY CIRCULATION   The **pulmonary circulation** consists of the right side of the heart, the pulmonary artery, the

pulmonary capillaries, and the pulmonary vein. Because it is located in the thorax near the heart, the pulmonary circulation is a low-pressure system. Pulmonary circulation begins with the right side of the heart. Deoxygenated blood from the venous system enters the right atrium through the superior and inferior vena cava and is transported to the lungs via the pulmonary artery and its branches (**Figure 16–6** ●). After oxygen and carbon dioxide are exchanged in the pulmonary capillaries, oxygen-rich blood returns to the left atrium through several pulmonary veins. Blood is then pumped out of the left ventricle through the aorta and its major branches to supply all body tissues. This second circuit of blood flow is called the systemic circulation.

SYSTEMIC CIRCULATION   The **systemic circulation** consists of the left side of the heart, the aorta and its branches, the capillaries that supply the brain and peripheral tissues, the systemic venous system, and the vena cava. The systemic system is a high-pressure system responsible for moving blood to peripheral areas of the body.

CORONARY CIRCULATION   The **coronary circulation** is a network of vessels that supply the heart muscle. The left and right coronary arteries originate at the base of the aorta and branch out to encircle the myocardium (**Figure 16–7A** ●). These arteries supply blood, oxygen, and nutrients to the myocardium. The left main coronary artery divides to form the anterior descending and circumflex arteries. The anterior descending artery supplies the anterior interventricular septum

TABLE 16–3 Distinguishing Heart Murmurs

ASK YOURSELF	INFORMATION
1. How loud is the murmur?	Murmurs are graded on a scale of 1–6: ■ *Grade 1:* Barely audible with stethoscope; often considered physiological, not pathological. Requires concentration and a quiet environment. ■ *Grade 2:* Very soft but distinctly audible. ■ *Grade 3:* Moderately loud; no thrill or thrusting motion is associated with the murmur. ■ *Grade 4:* Distinctly loud, in addition to a palpable thrill. ■ *Grade 5:* Very loud, can actually hear with part of the diaphragm of the stethoscope off the chest; palpable thrust and thrill are present. ■ *Grade 6:* Loudest, can hear with the diaphragm off the chest; visible thrill and thrust.
2. Where does it occur in the cardiac cycle: systole, diastole, or both?	Location in cardiac cycle: ■ Systole: early systole, midsystole, late systole ■ Diastole: early diastole, mid-diastole, late diastole ■ Both
3a. Is the sound continuous throughout systole, diastole, or only heard for part of the cycle?	Duration of murmur: ■ Continuous through systole only ■ Continuous through diastole only ■ Continuous through systole and diastole. Systolic murmurs may be of two types: ■ Midsystolic: Murmur is heard after S_1 and stops before S_2. ■ Pansystolic/holosystolic: Murmur begins with S_1 and stops at S_2. Diastolic murmurs may be one of three types: ■ Early diastolic: Murmur auscultated immediately after S_2 and then stops. There is a gap between where this murmur stops and S_1 is heard. ■ Mid-diastolic: Murmur begins a short time after S_2 and stops well before S_1 is auscultated. ■ Late diastolic: This murmur starts well after S_2 and stops immediately before S_1 is heard.

3b. What does the configuration of the sound look like?

Potential configurations:

4. What is the quality of the sound of the murmur?	■ Blowing ■ Harsh ■ Musical ■ Raspy ■ Rumbling
5. What is the pitch or frequency of the sound?	■ Low ■ Medium ■ High
6. In which landmark(s) do you best hear the murmur?	Use the five landmarks for auscultation: ■ Pulmonic areas 1 and 2 ■ Aortic area ■ Tricuspid area ■ Mitral area ■ Apex

(continued on next page)

TABLE 16–3   Distinguishing Heart Murmurs (*continued*)

ASK YOURSELF	INFORMATION
7. Does it radiate?	■ To the throat, neck, or back? ■ To the axilla or arm?
8. Is there any change in pattern with respirations?	■ Increases/decreases with inspiration. ■ Increases/decreases with expiration.
9. Is it associated with variations in heart sounds?	■ Associated with split S_1? ■ Associated with split S_2? ■ Associated with S_3? ■ Associated with S_4? ■ Associated with a click or ejection sound?
10. Does the intensity of the murmur change with position?	■ Increases/decreases with squatting? ■ Increases/decreases with client in the left lateral position? (Do not have the client perform the Valsalva maneuver or any abrupt position changes because some clients do not tolerate position changes well.)

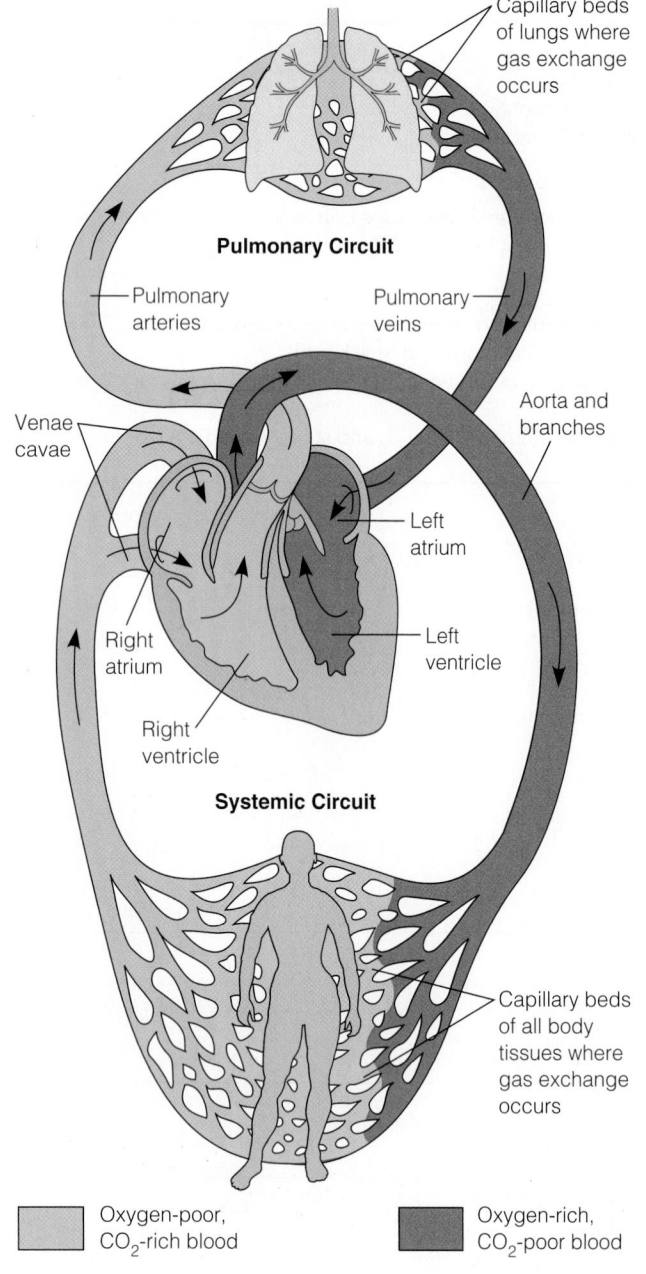

Oxygen-poor, CO_2-rich blood

Oxygen-rich, CO_2-poor blood

Figure 16–6 ● Pulmonary and systemic circulations.

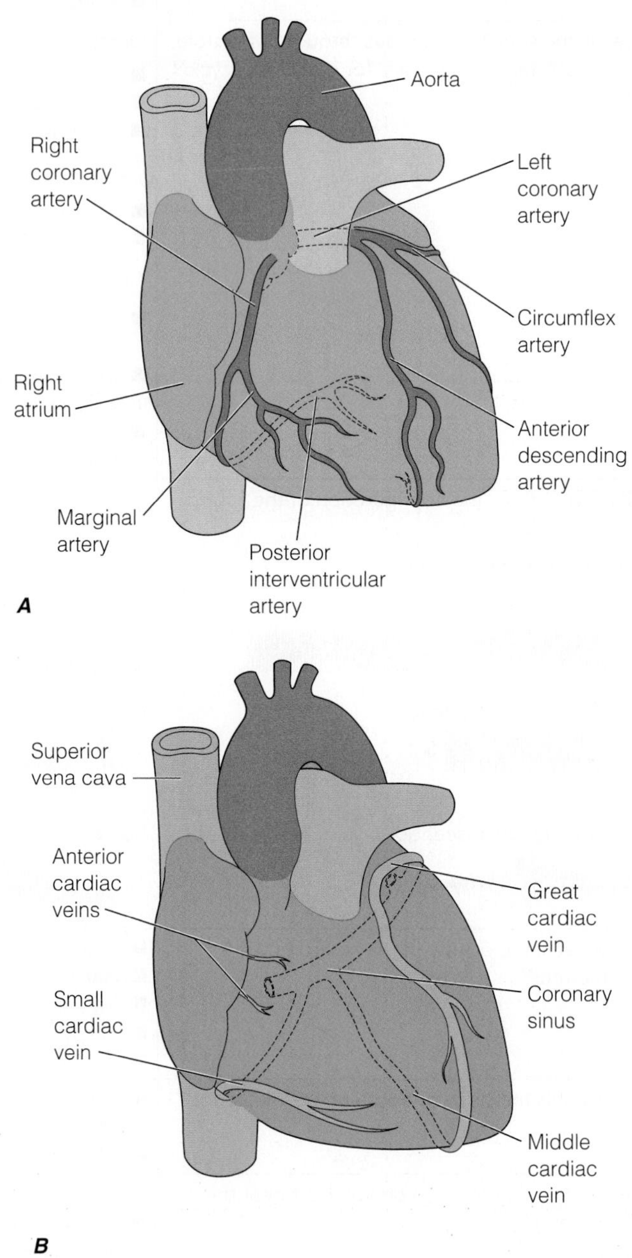

Figure 16–7 ● Coronary circulation. *A,* Coronary arteries. *B,* Coronary veins.

TABLE 16–4   Classifications of Heart Murmurs

MURMUR	CARDIAC CYCLE TIMING	AUSCULTATION SITE	CONFIGURATION OF SOUND	CONTINUITY
Aortic stenosis	Midsystolic	RSB, second ICS	S_1 ... S_2	Crescendo–decrescendo, continuous
Pulmonary stenosis	Midsystolic	LSB, second to third ICS	S_1 ... S_2	Crescendo–decrescendo, continuous
Mitral regurgitation	Systole	Apex	S_1 ... S_2	Holosystolic, continuous
Tricuspid regurgitation	Systole	Fourth ICS, LSB	S_1 ... S_2	Holosystolic, continuous
Mitral stenosis	Diastole	Apical	S_2 ... S_1	Rumble sound that becomes louder toward the end, continuous
Tricuspid stenosis	Diastole	Lower LSB	S_2 ... S_1	Rumble sound that becomes louder toward the end, continuous
Ventricular septal defect (left-to-right shunt)	Systole	Third to fifth ICS, LSB	S_1 ... S_2	Holosystolic, continuous
Aortic regurgitation	Diastole (early)	Third ICS, LSB	S_2 ... S_1	Decrescendo, continuous
Pulmonic regurgitation	Diastole (early)	Third ICS, LSB	S_2 ... S_1	Decrescendo, continuous

MURMUR	QUALITY	PITCH	RADIATION	CHANGES WITH RESPIRATIONS
Aortic stenosis	Usually harsh, coarse	Medium	Most commonly into neck, into carotid area, and down LSB, possibly apex	Expiration may intensify the sound of the murmur
Pulmonary stenosis	Usually harsh	Medium	Toward the left upper neck and shoulder areas	Inspiration may intensify sound of the murmur
Mitral regurgitation	Blowing, can be harsh in sound quality	High	Usually to left axilla, LSB, and base	Expiration may intensify the sound of the murmur
Tricuspid regurgitation	Blowing	High	May radiate to LSB and midclavicular line but not to axilla	Inspiration may intensify the sound of the murmur
Mitral stenosis	Rumbling	Low, best heard with bell	Rare	Expiration may intensify the sound of the murmur
Tricuspid stenosis	Rumbling	Low	Rare	Inspiration may intensify the sound of the murmur
Ventricular septal defect (left-to-right shunt)	Harsh	High	May radiate across precordium but not to axilla	Expiration may intensify the sound of the murmur

(continued on next page)

TABLE 16–4 Classifications of Heart Murmurs (*continued*)

MURMUR	QUALITY	PITCH	RADIATION	CHANGES WITH RESPIRATIONS
Aortic regurgitation	Blowing	High, best auscultated with diaphragm unless client is sitting up and leaning forward	May radiate to second ICS, RSB, and may proceed to apex	Expiration may intensify the sound of the murmur if the client leans forward and sits up
Pulmonic regurgitation	Blowing	High, best auscultated with diaphragm	May radiate to second ICS, RSB, and may proceed to apex	Inspiration may intensify the sound of the murmur

and the left ventricle. The circumflex branch supplies the left lateral wall of the left ventricle. The right coronary artery supplies the right ventricle and forms the posterior descending artery. The posterior descending artery supplies the posterior portion of the heart. Ventricular contraction delivers blood through the pulmonary circulation and the systemic circulation. However, it is during ventricular relaxation that the coronary arteries fill with oxygen-rich blood. After the blood perfuses the heart muscle, the cardiac veins drain the blood into the coronary sinus, which empties into the right atrium of the heart (Figure 16–7*B*).

Blood flow through the coronary arteries is regulated by several factors. Aortic pressure is the primary factor. Other factors include the heart rate (most flow occurs during diastole, when the muscle is relaxed), metabolic activity of the heart, and blood vessel tone (constriction).

Transition From Fetal to Pulmonary Circulation

Blood flows from the placenta to the fetus through the umbilical vein to the ductus venosus (the fetal vascular channel between the umbilical vein and the inferior vena cava) and into the right atrium of the heart. The **foramen ovale** (an opening between the atria of the fetal heart) allows blood to flow from the right atrium to the left atrium and then into the left ventricle. Blood is then pumped into the aorta and systemic circulation. Some blood returns from the head and upper extremities to the superior vena cava and right atrium, and some blood travels to the right ventricle, where it is pumped into the pulmonary artery. The majority of the blood from the pulmonary artery passes through the ductus arteriosus, the vascular channel between the pulmonary artery and the aorta, and into the systemic circulation. A small amount of the blood from the pulmonary artery goes to the lungs. Blood eventually returns to the placenta by way of the umbilical arteries.

After the umbilical cord has been cut, the newborn must quickly adapt to receiving oxygen from the lungs. The transition from fetal to pulmonary circulation occurs in just a few hours. The first breath expands the lungs. Blood that previously flowed through the ductus arteriosus to the aorta begins flowing to the lungs. Increased pulmonary blood flow and decreased **pulmonary vascular resistance** (pressure within the pulmonary blood vessels that must be overcome in order for blood to flow through the vessel) result. Pressure in the left atrium increases as increased blood flow is returned from the lungs through the pulmonary veins.

The force or resistance of the blood in the body's blood vessels that helps return blood to the heart is called **systemic vascular resistance**. Systemic vascular resistance increases and right atrial pressure falls after the umbilical cord is cut. Increased pressure in the left atrium stimulates closure of the foramen ovale. The flaps of the foramen ovale close, and fibrin deposits permanently seal the opening, unless there is excess pressure on the right side of the heart. In response to higher oxygen saturation, the ductus arteriosus normally constricts and closes within 18 hours after birth. Permanent closure occurs 2 to 3 weeks after birth, unless oxygen saturation remains low. Because fetal tissues have adapted to low oxygen saturation, newborns with cyanotic heart disease may appear relatively comfortable even when the arterial partial pressure of oxygen (PaO_2) is between 20 and 25 mmHg. In contrast, healthy newborns typically have a PaO_2 between 50 and 70 mmHg. Older children and adults would rapidly develop acidosis and cerebral anoxia with such a low PaO_2. **Figure 16–8** ● compares fetal and postnatal circulation through the heart.

The Cardiac Cycle and Cardiac Output

The contraction and relaxation of the heart constitute one heartbeat, and this process is called the **cardiac cycle** (**Figure 16–9** ●). As mentioned, ventricular filling is followed by ventricular systole, a phase during which the ventricles contract and eject blood into the pulmonary and systemic circuits. Systole is followed by a relaxation phase known as diastole. During diastole, the ventricles refill, the atria contract, and the myocardium is perfused. Normally, the complete cardiac cycle occurs approximately 70–80 times per minute. This is recorded as the heart rate.

During diastole, the volume in the ventricles increases to approximately 120 mL (the end-diastolic volume) and at the end of systole, approximately 50 mL of blood remains in the ventricles (the end-systolic volume). The difference between the end-diastolic volume and the end-systolic volume is called the **stroke volume (SV)**. Stroke volume ranges from 60 to 100 mL/beat and averages approximately 70 mL/beat in an adult. **Cardiac output (CO)** is referred to as the amount of blood pumped by the ventricles into the pulmonary and systemic circulations in 1 minute. Multiplying the stroke volume (SV) by the heart rate (HR) determines the cardiac output (CO):

$$HR \times SV = CO$$

The **ejection fraction** is the stroke volume divided by the end-diastolic volume and represents the fraction or percent of

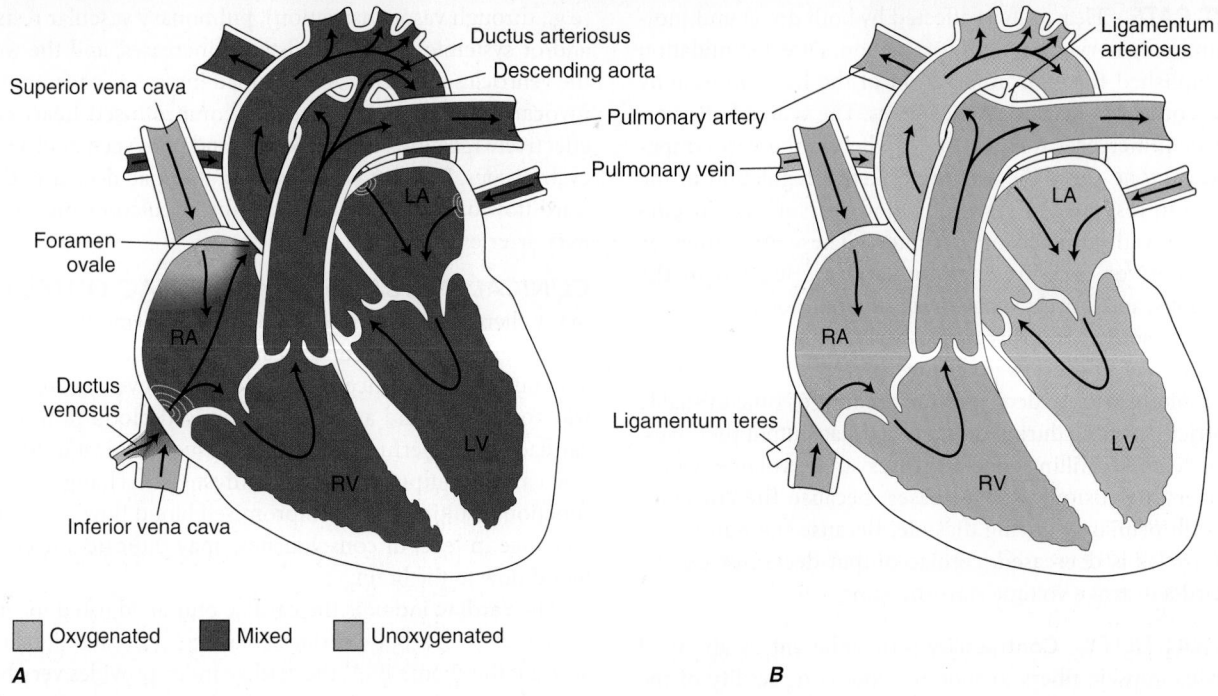

Figure 16–8 ● The arrows indicate the flow of blood through the heart while the color indicates level of oxygen saturation in the blood. *A,* Fetal circulation. *B,* Pulmonary circulation. LA, left atrium; LV, left ventricle; RA, right atrium; RV, right ventricle.

the diastolic volume that is ejected from the heart during systole. For example, a stroke volume of 80 mL divided by an end diastolic-volume of 120 ml equals an ejection fraction of 66%. The normal ejection fraction ranges from 50% to 70% (approximately 60%).

The average adult cardiac output ranges from 4 to 8 L/min. Cardiac output is an indicator of the heart's ability to function as a pump. If the heart cannot pump effectively, cardiac output and tissue perfusion are decreased. Body tissues that do not receive enough blood and oxygen (carried in the blood on hemoglobin) become **ischemic** (deprived of oxygen). If the tissues do not receive enough blood flow to maintain the functions of the cells, the cells die (cellular death results in necrosis or infarction).

Activity level, metabolic rate, physiological and psychological stress responses, age, and body size all influence cardiac output. In addition, cardiac output is determined by the interaction of four major factors:

1. Heart rate
2. Preload
3. Afterload
4. Contractility.

Changes in each of these variables influence cardiac output intrinsically, and each variable can be manipulated to affect cardiac output. The heart's ability to respond to an increase in strenuous activity and adjust its cardiac output is called **cardiac reserve**.

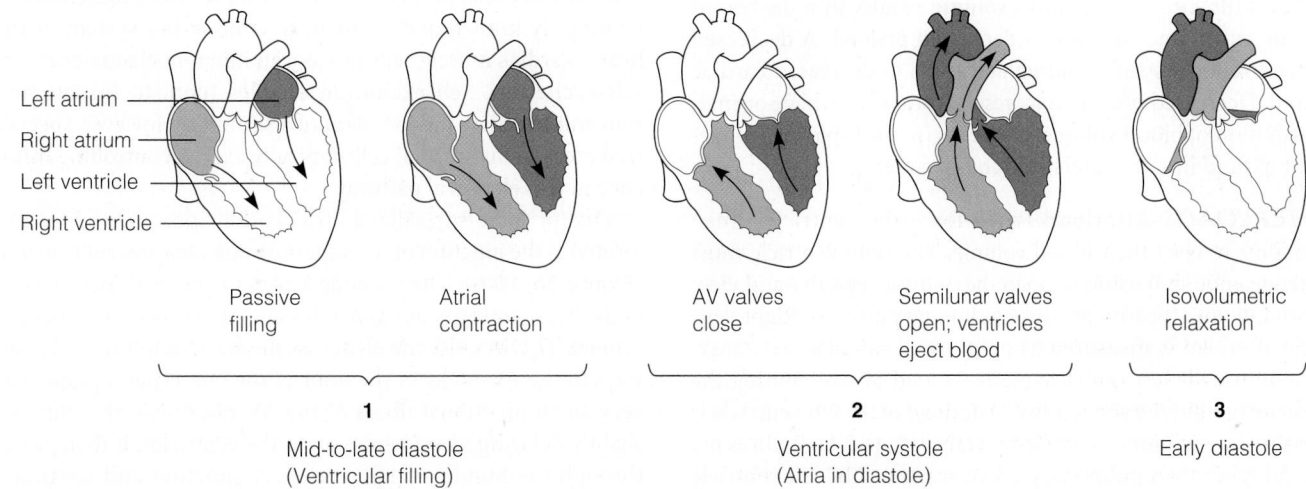

Figure 16–9 ● The cardiac cycle has three events: (1) ventricular filling in mid-to-late diastole, (2) ventricular systole, and (3) isovolumetric relaxation in early diastole.

HEART RATE Heart rate is affected by both direct and indirect autonomic nervous system stimulation. Direct stimulation is accomplished through innervation of the heart muscle by sympathetic and parasympathetic nerves. The sympathetic nervous system increases the heart rate, whereas the parasympathetic vagal tone slows the heart rate. Reflex regulation of the heart rate in response to systemic blood pressure also occurs through activation of sensory receptors. These are known as baroreceptors or pressure receptors and are located in the carotid sinus, aortic arch, venae cavae, and pulmonary veins.

With an increase in heart rate, cardiac output increases (up to a point) even if there is no change in stroke volume. However, a rapid heart rate decreases the amount of time available for ventricular filling during diastole. Cardiac output then falls, because decreased filling time decreases stroke volume. Coronary artery perfusion also decreases, because the coronary arteries fill primarily during diastole. Because the number of cardiac cycles is decreased, cardiac output decreases during bradycardia if stroke volume stays the same.

CONTRACTILITY Contractility is the inherent capability of the cardiac muscle fibers to shorten. Poor contractility of the heart muscle reduces the forward flow of blood from the heart, increases the ventricular pressures from accumulation of blood volume, and reduces cardiac output. Increased contractility may stress the heart.

PRELOAD Preload is the amount of cardiac muscle fiber tension, or stretch, that exists at the end of diastole, just before contraction of the ventricles. Preload is influenced by venous return and the compliance of the ventricles. The relationship between cardiac muscle fiber length (stretch) and the force with which the fibers contract to accomplish emptying is referred to as Starling's law of the heart.

This mechanism has a physiological limit. Just as continuous overstretching of a rubber band causes the band to relax and lose its ability to recoil, overstretching of the cardiac muscle fibers eventually results in ineffective contraction. Disorders such as renal disease and congestive heart failure result in sodium and water retention and increased preload. Vasoconstriction increases venous return and preload.

Too little circulating blood volume results in a decreased venous return and therefore a decreased preload. A decreased preload reduces stroke volume and leads to decreased cardiac output. Decreased preload may result from hemorrhage or maldistribution of blood volume, as occurs in third spacing (movement of fluid into the interstitial compartment).

AFTERLOAD Afterload is the force the ventricles must overcome to eject their blood volume. The right ventricle must generate enough tension to open the pulmonary valve and eject its volume into the low-pressure pulmonary arteries. Right ventricle afterload is measured as pulmonary vascular resistance. In contrast, the left ventricle ejects its load by overcoming the pressure behind the aortic valve. Afterload of the left ventricle is measured as systemic vascular resistance. Arterial pressures are much higher than pulmonary pressures; thus, the left ventricle has to work much harder than the right ventricle.

Alterations in vascular tone affect afterload and ventricular work. As the pulmonary or arterial blood pressure increases (e.g., through vasoconstriction), pulmonary vascular resistance and/or systemic vascular resistance increases, and the work of the ventricles increases. As workload increases, consumption of myocardial oxygen increases. A compromised heart cannot effectively meet this increased demand of oxygen, and a vicious cycle ensues. By contrast, a very low afterload decreases the forward flow of blood into the systemic circulation and the coronary arteries.

CLINICAL INDICATORS OF CARDIAC OUTPUT For many clients who are critically ill, invasive hemodynamic monitoring catheters are used to measure cardiac output in quantifiable numbers. Advanced technology, however, is not the only way to identify and assess compromised blood flow. Because cardiac output perfuses the body's tissues, clinical indicators of low cardiac output may be manifested by changes in organ function resulting from compromised blood flow. For example, a change in level of consciousness may indicate a decrease in blood flow to the brain.

The **cardiac index** is the cardiac output adjusted for the client's body size or body surface area (BSA). Because it takes into account the client's BSA, the cardiac index provides very beneficial data regarding the heart's ability to perfuse the tissues. Cardiac index is an accurate indicator of the effectiveness of the circulation.

The BSA is stated in square meters (m^2), and the cardiac index is calculated as the cardiac output divided by the BSA. Cardiac measurements are considered adequate if they fall within the range of 2.5–4.2 $L/min/m^2$. For example, two clients are determined to have a cardiac output of 4 L/min. This parameter is within normal limits. However, one client is 157 cm (5 feet, 2 inches) tall and weighs 54.5 kg (120 lb), with a BSA of 1.54 m^2. This client's cardiac index is 4 ÷ 1.54, or 2.6 $L/min/m^2$. The second client is 188 cm (6 feet, 2 inches) tall and weighs 81.7 kg (280 lb), with a BSA of 2.52 m^2. This client's cardiac index is 4 ÷ 2.52, or 1.6 $L/min/m^2$. The cardiac index results show that the same cardiac output of 4 L/min is adequate for the first client but grossly inadequate for the second.

The Conduction System of the Heart

The cardiac cycle, perpetuated by a complex electrical circuit, is commonly known as the intrinsic conduction system of the heart. Cardiac muscle cells possess an inherent characteristic of self-excitation. Self-excitation enables them to initiate and transmit impulses independent of a stimulus. However, specialized areas of myocardial cells typically exert a controlling influence in this electrical pathway.

One of these specialized areas is the sinoatrial (SA) node, located at the junction of the superior vena cava and right atrium (**Figure 16–10 ●**). The SA node acts as the normal "pacemaker" of the heart and typically generates an impulse 60–100 times per minute. This impulse travels across the atria via internodal pathways to the AV node, in the floor of the interatrial septum. The very small junctional fibers of the AV node slow the impulse, slightly delaying its transmission to the ventricles. It then passes through the bundle of His at the AV junction and continues down the interventricular septum through the right and left bundle branches and out to the Purkinje fibers in the ventricular muscle walls.

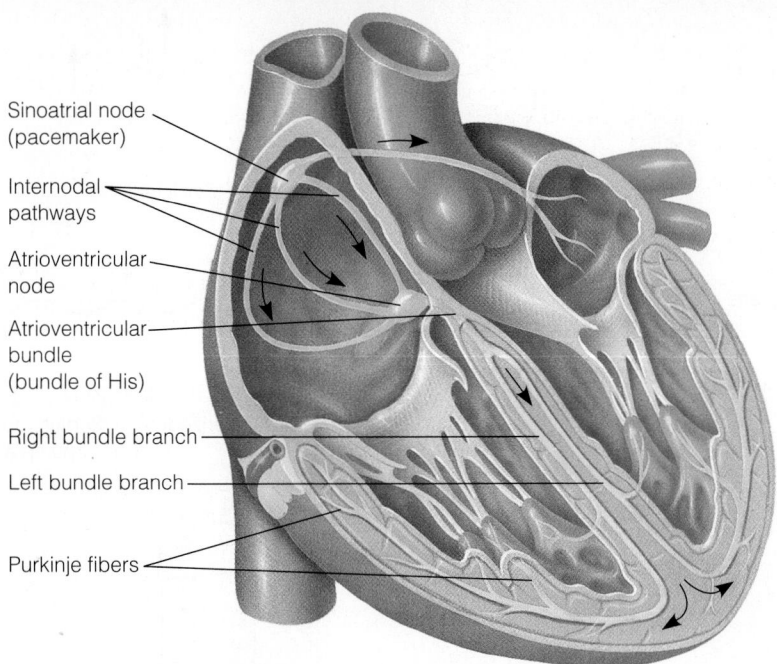

Sinoatrial node
(pacemaker)

Internodal
pathways

Atrioventricular
node

Atrioventricular
bundle
(bundle of His)

Right bundle branch

Left bundle branch

Purkinje fibers

Figure 16–10 ● The intrinsic conduction system of the heart.

This path of electrical transmission produces a series of changes in ion concentration across the membrane of each cardiac muscle cell. The electrical stimulus increases the permeability of the cell membrane, creating an action potential (electrical potential). The result is an exchange of sodium, potassium, and calcium ions across the cell membrane. This changes the intracellular electrical charge to a positive state. The process of depolarization results in myocardial contraction. As the ion exchange reverses and the cell returns to its resting state of electronegativity, the cell is repolarized, and the cardiac muscle relaxes. The cellular action potential serves as the basis for **electrocardiography** (a diagnostic test of cardiac function).

THE ACTION POTENTIAL   Movement of ions across cell membranes causes an electrical impulse that stimulates muscle contraction. This electrical activity, called the **action potential**, produces the waveforms represented on electrocardiogram (ECG) strips.

In the resting state, positive and negative ions align on either side of the cell membrane, producing a relatively negative charge within the cell and a positive extracellular charge (**Figure 16–11** ●). The cell is said to be polarized. The negative resting membrane potential is maintained at approximately −90 mV by the sodium–potassium pump in the cell membrane.

Depolarization   **Depolarization** is the phase when the heart contracts, resulting from ion channel functions. Two types of ion channels function to produce the electrical changes that occur during the depolarization phase: the fast sodium channels and the slow calcium channels. A fast action potential occurs in atrial and ventricular muscle cells and the Purkinje conduction system, and it uses the fast sodium channels. A slow action potential occurs in the SA and AV nodes, which use the slow calcium channels. The action potential for contraction of

the heart is initiated in the SA node. When a resting cell is stimulated by an electrical charge from a neighboring cell or spontaneous event, its cell membrane permeability changes. Sodium ions enter the cell, and the membrane becomes less permeable to potassium ions. Addition of positively charged ions to intracellular fluid changes the membrane potential from negative to slightly positive, at +20 to +30 mV.

As the cell becomes more positive, it reaches a point called the **threshold potential** (the point at which an action potential is capable of being generated). The response to the action potential in the myocardial muscle cells causes a chemical reaction of calcium within the cell. This in turn causes actin and myosin filaments to slide together, producing cardiac muscle contraction. The action potential then spreads to surrounding cells, causing a coordinated muscle contraction. As soon as the myocardium is completely depolarized, repolarization begins.

Repolarization   **Repolarization** is the process that returns the cell to its resting, polarized state. During rapid repolarization, fast sodium channels close abruptly, and the cell begins to regain its negative charge. During the plateau phase, muscle contraction is prolonged as slow calcium–sodium channels remain open. When these channels close, the sodium–potassium pump restores ion concentration to normal resting levels. The cell membrane is then polarized, ready for the cycle to start again. Each heartbeat represents one cardiac cycle, with one depolarization and repolarization cycle and one complete cardiac muscle contraction and relaxation (systole and diastole).

Normally, only pacemaker cells demonstrate automaticity (the ability to generate an electrical impulse). Pacemaker cells have a resting potential that is much less negative (−70 to −50 mV) than that of other cardiac muscle cells. Their thresh-

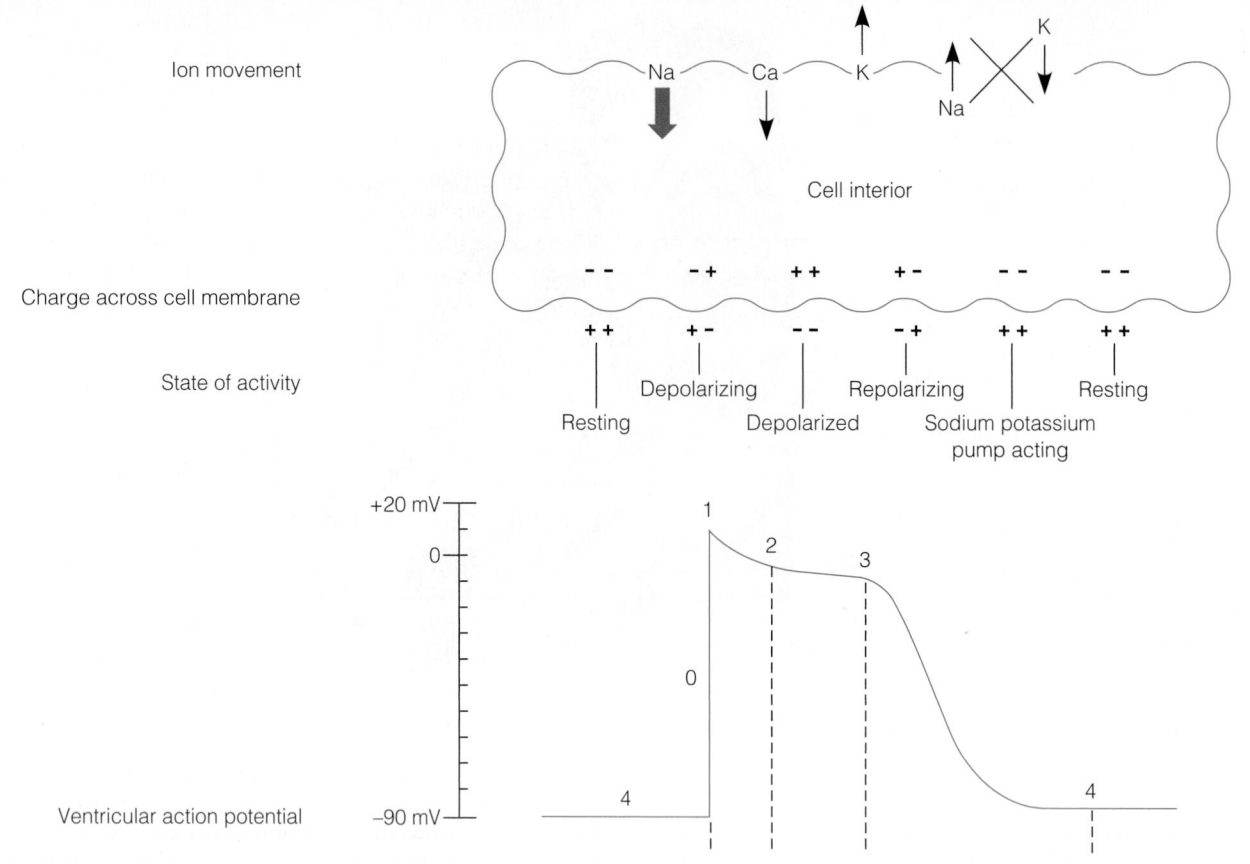

Figure 16–11 ● Action potential of a cardiac muscle cell. In the resting state (phase 4), the cell membrane is polarized; the cell's interior has a negative charge compared to that of extracellular fluid. On depolarization (phase 0), sodium ions diffuse rapidly across the cell membrane into the cell, and calcium channels open. In the fully depolarized state (phase 1), the cell's interior has a net positive charge compared to its exterior. During the plateau period (phase 2), calcium moves into the cell and potassium diffusion slows, prolonging the action potential. In phase 3, calcium channels close, the sodium–potassium pump removes sodium from the cell, and the cell membrane again becomes polarized with a net negative charge.

old potential is lower than that of other myocardial cells. These differences result from constant leakage of sodium and potassium ions into the cell.

Myocardial cells have a unique protective property, known as the **refractory period**. During the refractory period, they resist stimulation. This property protects cardiac muscle from spasm and tetany. During the absolute refractory period, depolarization will not occur, regardless of cell stimulation. The absolute refractory period is followed by the relative refractory period. During the relative refractory period, a greater-than-normal stimulus is required to generate another action potential. During the supernormal period that follows, a mild stimulus will cause depolarization. Many cardiac dysrhythmias are triggered during the relative refractory and supernormal periods.

Pulse

The **pulse** is a wave of blood created by contraction of the left ventricle of the heart. Generally the pulse wave represents the stroke volume output or the amount of blood that enters the arteries with each ventricular contraction. **Compliance** of the arteries refers to their ability to contract and expand. When an individual's arteries become less compliant, as can happen during the process of aging, greater pressure is required to pump the blood into the arteries.

In a healthy individual, the pulse reflects the heartbeat. The pulse rate is the same as the rate of the ventricular contractions of the heart. However, in some types of cardiovascular disease, the heartbeat and pulse rates can differ. For example, a client's heart may produce very weak or small pulse waves that are not detectable in a peripheral pulse far from the heart. In these instances, the nurse should assess the heartbeat and the peripheral pulse. A **peripheral pulse** is a pulse located away from the heart, for example, in the foot or wrist. In contrast, the apical pulse is a central pulse. It is located at the apex of the heart and is referred to as the **point of maximal impulse (PMI)**.

FACTORS AFFECTING THE PULSE The rate of the pulse is expressed in beats per minute (bpm). A pulse rate varies according to a number of factors. The nurse should consider each of the following factors when assessing a client's pulse:

- *Age.* As age increases, the pulse rate gradually decreases overall. See **Table 16–5** ● for specific variations in pulse rates from birth to adulthood.
- *Gender.* After puberty, the average male's pulse rate is slightly lower than the female's.
- *Exercise.* The pulse rate normally increases with activity. The rate of increase in the professional athlete is often less than in the average individual because of greater cardiac size, strength, and efficiency.

TABLE 16–5 Variations in Pulse and Respirations by Age

AGE	AVERAGE PULSE (AND RANGES)	AVERAGE RESPIRATIONS (AND RANGES)
Newborn	130 (80–180)	35 (30–80)
1 year	120 (80–140)	30 (20–40)
5–8 years	100 (75–120)	20 (15–25)
10 years	70 (50–90)	19 (15–25)
Teen	75 (50–90)	18 (15–20)
Adult	80 (60–100)	16 (12–20)
Older adult	70 (60–100)	16 (15–20)

- *Fever.* The pulse rate increases (a) in response to the lowered blood pressure that results from peripheral vasodilation associated with elevated body temperature and (b) because of the increased metabolic rate.
- *Medications.* Some medications decrease the pulse rate, and others increase it. For example, cardiotonics (e.g., digitalis preparations) decrease the heart rate, whereas epinephrine increases it.
- *Hypovolemia.* Loss of blood from the vascular system normally increases pulse rate. In adults the loss of circulating volume results in an adjustment of the heart rate to increase blood pressure as the body compensates for the lost blood volume. Adults can usually lose up to 10% of their normal circulating volume without adverse effects.
- *Stress.* In response to stress, sympathetic nervous stimulation increases the overall activity of the heart. Stress increases the rate as well as the force of the heartbeat. Fear and anxiety as well as the perception of severe pain stimulate the sympathetic system.
- *Position changes.* When an individual is sitting or standing, blood usually pools in dependent vessels of the venous system. Pooling results in a transient decrease in the venous blood return to the heart and a subsequent reduction in blood pressure and increase in heart rate.
- *Pathology.* Certain diseases such as some heart conditions or those that impair oxygenation can alter the resting pulse rate.

Blood Pressure

Arterial blood pressure is a measure of the pressure exerted by the blood as it flows through the arteries. Because the blood moves in waves, two types of blood pressure are measured. The **systolic blood pressure** is the pressure of the blood as a result of contraction of the ventricles, that is, the pressure of the height of the blood wave. The **diastolic blood pressure** is the pressure when the ventricles are at rest. Diastolic pressure is the lower pressure and is present at all times within the arteries. The difference between the diastolic and the systolic pressures is called the **pulse pressure**. A normal pulse pressure is about 40 mmHg but can be as high as 100 mmHg during exercise. A consistently elevated pulse pressure occurs in arteriosclerosis. A low pulse pressure (e.g., less than 25 mmHg) occurs in conditions such as severe heart failure.

Blood pressure is measured in millimeters of mercury (mmHg) and recorded as a fraction: systolic pressure over the diastolic pressure. A typical blood pressure for a healthy adult is 120/80 mmHg (pulse pressure of 40). A number of conditions are reflected by changes in blood pressure. Because blood pressure can vary considerably among individuals, it is important for the nurse to know a specific client's baseline blood pressure. For example, if a client's usual blood pressure is 180/100 mmHg, and it is assessed following surgery to be 120/80 mmHg, this significant drop in pressure may indicate complications and must be reported to the primary care provider.

DETERMINANTS OF BLOOD PRESSURE Arterial blood pressure is the result of several factors: the pumping action of the heart, the peripheral vascular resistance (the resistance supplied by the blood vessels through which the blood flows), and the blood volume and viscosity.

Pumping Action of the Heart When the pumping action of the heart is weak, less blood is pumped into arteries (lower cardiac output), and the blood pressure decreases. When the heart's pumping action is strong and the volume of blood pumped into the circulation increases (higher cardiac output), the blood pressure increases.

Peripheral Vascular Resistance Peripheral resistance can increase blood pressure. The diastolic pressure especially is affected. Some factors that create resistance in the arterial system are the capacity of the arterioles and capillaries, the compliance of the arteries, and the viscosity of the blood.

The internal diameter or capacity of the arterioles and the capillaries determines in great part the peripheral resistance to the blood in the body. The smaller the space within a vessel, the greater the resistance. Normally, the arterioles are in a state of partial constriction. Increased vasoconstriction, such as occurs with smoking, raises the blood pressure, whereas decreased vasoconstriction lowers the blood pressure.

If the elastic and muscular tissues of the arteries are replaced with fibrous tissue, the arteries lose much of their ability to constrict and dilate. This condition, most common in middle-aged and older adults, is known as **arteriosclerosis**.

Blood Volume When the blood volume decreases (for example, as a result of a hemorrhage or dehydration), the blood pressure decreases because of decreased fluid in the arteries. Conversely, when the volume increases (for example, as a result of a rapid intravenous infusion), the blood pressure increases because of the greater fluid volume within the circulatory system.

Blood Viscosity Blood pressure is higher when the blood is highly **viscous** (thick), that is, when the proportion of red blood cells to the blood plasma is high. This proportion is referred to as the **hematocrit**. The viscosity increases markedly when the hematocrit is more than 60%–65%.

FACTORS AFFECTING BLOOD PRESSURE Among the factors influencing blood pressure are age, exercise, stress, race, gender, medications, obesity, diurnal variations, and disease processes.

- *Age.* Newborns have a mean systolic pressure of about 75 mmHg. The pressure rises with age, reaching a peak at the onset of puberty, and then tends to decline somewhat. In older adults, elasticity of the arteries is decreased—the arteries are more rigid and less yielding to the pressure of the blood. This produces an elevated systolic pressure. Because the walls no longer retract as flexibly with decreased pressure, the diastolic pressure may also be high.

■ *Exercise.* Physical activity increases the cardiac output and hence the blood pressure; thus 20–30 minutes of rest following exercise is indicated before the resting blood pressure can be reliably assessed.

■ *Stress.* Stimulation of the sympathetic nervous system increases cardiac output and vasoconstriction of the arterioles, thus increasing the blood pressure reading; however, severe pain can decrease blood pressure greatly by inhibiting the vasomotor center and producing vasodilation.

■ *Race.* African American males over 35 years of age have higher blood pressures than European American males of the same age.

■ *Gender.* After puberty, females usually have lower blood pressures than males of the same age; this difference is thought to be due to hormonal variations. After menopause, women generally have higher blood pressures than before.

■ *Medications.* Many medications, including caffeine, may increase or decrease the blood pressure.

■ *Obesity.* Both childhood and adult obesity predispose to hypertension.

■ *Diurnal variations.* Pressure is usually lowest early in the morning, when the metabolic rate is lowest, then rises throughout the day and peaks in the late afternoon or early evening.

■ *Disease process.* Any condition affecting the cardiac output, blood volume, blood viscosity, and/or compliance of the arteries has a direct effect on the blood pressure.

Genetic and Lifespan Considerations

The risk for heart disease in women increases after menopause due to the drop in estrogen production. Women who experience menopause early double their risk of developing heart disease. In contrast, age typically becomes a risk factor for women at 55 years old. Women are more likely to experience angina than men. Heart disease tends to run in families.

Clients whose parents or siblings develop heart disease at a young age are more likely to develop it themselves. If a father or brother had a heart attack before age 55, or if a mother or sister had a heart attack before age 65, an individual will most likely develop heart disease. Men are more likely to have heart attacks earlier in life than women.

DEVELOPMENTAL ASPECTS OF NORMAL CARDIAC FUNCTIONING
It is important for nurses who care for children to understand the differences in pediatric cardiology. These differences impact not only how children respond to cardiac alterations but also their response to therapy.

Cardiac Functioning Infants have a greater risk of heart failure than older children because the immature heart is more sen-

sitive to volume or pressure overload. After birth, the placenta separates and a sudden change in blood pressure occurs, causing a shift in circulation and the closing of key heart valves. The heart then begins to pump blood to the lungs and the baby breathes independently.

A newborn's heart beats about 120 times per minute due to the demand for oxygen-rich blood. During infancy, the heart's muscle fibers are less developed and less organized, resulting in limited functional capacity. Stroke volume does not increase substantially until the heart muscle is fully developed at 5 years of age. As the child's heart grows and develops, the systolic blood pressure rises, reaching adult levels by puberty. The infant's metabolic rate and oxygen requirements double at birth. This results in a higher neonatal heart rate—one that can maintain a high cardiac output and adequate oxygen transport. The heart rate gradually slows throughout childhood and settles around 70 beats per minute by the late teen years. Factor influencing neonatal and heart rate include physical/emotional stress, exercise, fever, and respiratory distress. As infants experience tachycardia, cardiac output is increased. There is little cardiac reserve capacity until oxygen demands begin to decrease.

Oxygenation Hematocrit and hemoglobin concentrations appropriate for the child's age are necessary for adequate oxygen transport. The oxygen arterial saturation is the amount of oxygen that can potentially be delivered to the tissues. **Desaturated blood** results when oxygenated and deoxygenated blood mix because of a congenital heart defect. Cyanosis, which indicates **hypoxemia** (lower-than-normal amounts of oxygen in the blood), results from a concentration of 5 or more grams of deoxygenated hemoglobin per 100 mL of blood or from arterial saturations of less than 85%.

The child's bone marrow responds to chronic hypoxemia by producing more red blood cells in an effort to increase the amount of hemoglobin available for oxygenation. This increase is known as **polycythemia**. A hematocrit value of 50% or higher is common in children with cyanotic heart defects.

Children respond to severe hypoxemia with bradycardia. Cardiac arrest in children generally results from prolonged hypoxemia related to respiratory failure or shock rather than from a primary cardiac insult (as in adults). Bradycardia is therefore a significant warning sign of cardiac arrest. Appropriate management of hypoxemia often reverses bradycardia and prevents cardiac arrest.

Alterations in cardiovascular function may be the result of a congenital defect, acquired infection, or injury. Congenital heart disease is the leading cause of death, excluding prematurity, during the first year of life. Congenital heart defects cause more deaths in the first year of life than any other birth defect. Although, heart defects may be genetic or part of a chromosome syndrome, many children do not have other types of birth defects. Rapid advances in the treatment of congenital heart defects have allowed children to undergo surgery at younger ages. As a result, nursing care required to identify and manage infants and children with heart disease has become more challenging.

CARDIOVASCULAR CHANGES IN PREGNANCY
During pregnancy, blood flow increases to organ systems with an

increased workload. Thus, blood flow increases to the uterus, placenta, and breasts, whereas blood flow to the liver and brain remains unchanged. Cardiac output begins to increase early in pregnancy, and at 25–30 weeks of gestation it peaks at 30%–50% above prepregnancy levels. It generally remains elevated during the third trimester.

The pulse may increase by as many as 10–15 bpm at term. The blood pressure decreases slightly, reaching its lowest point during the second trimester, then gradually increases to near prepregnancy levels by the end of the third trimester.

The enlarging uterus puts pressure on pelvic and femoral vessels, interfering with returning blood flow and causing stasis of blood in the lower extremities. This condition may lead to dependent edema and varicosity of the veins in the legs, vulva, and rectum (hemorrhoids) during late pregnancy. This increased blood volume in the lower legs may also make the woman who is pregnant prone to postural hypotension.

When the woman lies supine, the enlarging uterus may press on the vena cava, thus reducing blood flow to the right atrium, lowering blood pressure, and causing dizziness, pallor, and clamminess. Research indicates that the enlarging uterus may also press on the aorta and its collateral circulation (Cunningham et al., 2014). This condition is called supine hypotensive syndrome; it may also be referred to as vena caval syndrome or aortocaval compression (**Figure 16–12 ●**). It can be corrected by having the woman lie on her left side or by placing a pillow or wedge under the woman's right hip as she lies in a supine position.

Blood volume progressively increases beginning in the first trimester, increases rapidly until about 30–34 weeks of gestation, and then plateaus until birth at approximately 40%–50% above prepregnancy levels. This increase occurs because of increases in both erythrocytes and plasma (Gordon, 2012).

The total erythrocyte (red blood cell) volume increases by approximately 30% in women who receive iron supplementation (but only by ~18% without iron supplementation). This increase in erythrocytes is necessary to transport the additional oxygen required during pregnancy. However, the

increase in plasma volume during pregnancy averages approximately 50%. Because the plasma volume increase (50%) is greater than the erythrocyte increase (30%), the hematocrit, which measures the concentration of red blood cells in the plasma, decreases slightly (Gordon, 2012). This decrease is referred to as the **physiological anemia of pregnancy** (pseudoanemia).

Iron is necessary for hemoglobin formation, and hemoglobin is the oxygen-carrying component of erythrocytes. Thus, the increase in erythrocyte levels results in an increased need for iron by the woman who is pregnant. Even though the gastrointestinal absorption of iron is moderately increased during pregnancy, it is usually necessary to add supplemental iron to the diet to meet the expanded red blood cell and fetal needs.

Leukocyte production increases slightly to an average of 8,500/mm^3, with a range of 5,600 to 12,200/mm^3. During labor and the early postpartum period, these levels may reach 20,000–30,000/mm^3. Because of this normal increase in white blood cells, the result should not be used clinically to diagnose the presence of infection (Gordon, 2012).

Both the fibrin and plasma fibrinogen levels increase during pregnancy. Although the blood-clotting time of the woman who is pregnant does not differ significantly from that of the woman who is not, clotting factors VII, VIII, IX, and X increase; thus, pregnancy is a somewhat hypercoagulable state. These changes, coupled with venous stasis in late pregnancy, increase the woman's risk of developing venous thrombosis during pregnancy.

NORMAL CHANGES OF AGING A wide range of changes occur with aging, but it is often difficult to distinguish between disease processes and the natural consequences of aging. A decrease in cardiovascular reserve or in cardiac output may be the result of deconditioning or disease and not the result of natural aging processes. Differences in cardiovascular functioning also exist from one individual to another. An older individual with a good family history and healthy lifestyle can enjoy much greater cardiac function than a middle-aged individual with a family history of cardiovascular problems or a history of smoking. Older people should not expect to become debilitated from aging alone.

It is important to remember the concept of compensation in cardiovascular function. Changes such as decreased renal functioning may occur with aging, and this causes a change in other systems in order to try to improve functioning. Sometimes, these compensatory changes cause problems of their own. For example, kidneys that are poorly perfused as a result of decreased cardiac output produce renin, which eventually increases blood pressure and sodium retention. These gradual compensatory changes are initially benign but can lead to decreased cardiac and renal function and to fluid overload. See **Figure 16–13 ●** for normal changes of aging in the cardiovascular system.

How an individual ages is determined by genetic factors as well as by physical and social environments. Aging changes are gradual and may not be noticed by the individual or by members of the family. Different body systems age at different rates. Many cardiovascular functions also involve

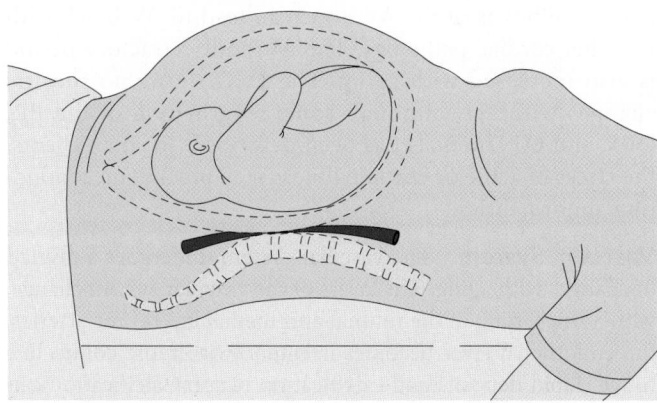

Figure 16–12 ● Vena caval syndrome. The gravid uterus compresses the vena cava when the woman is supine. This reduces the blood flow returning to the heart and may cause maternal hypotension.

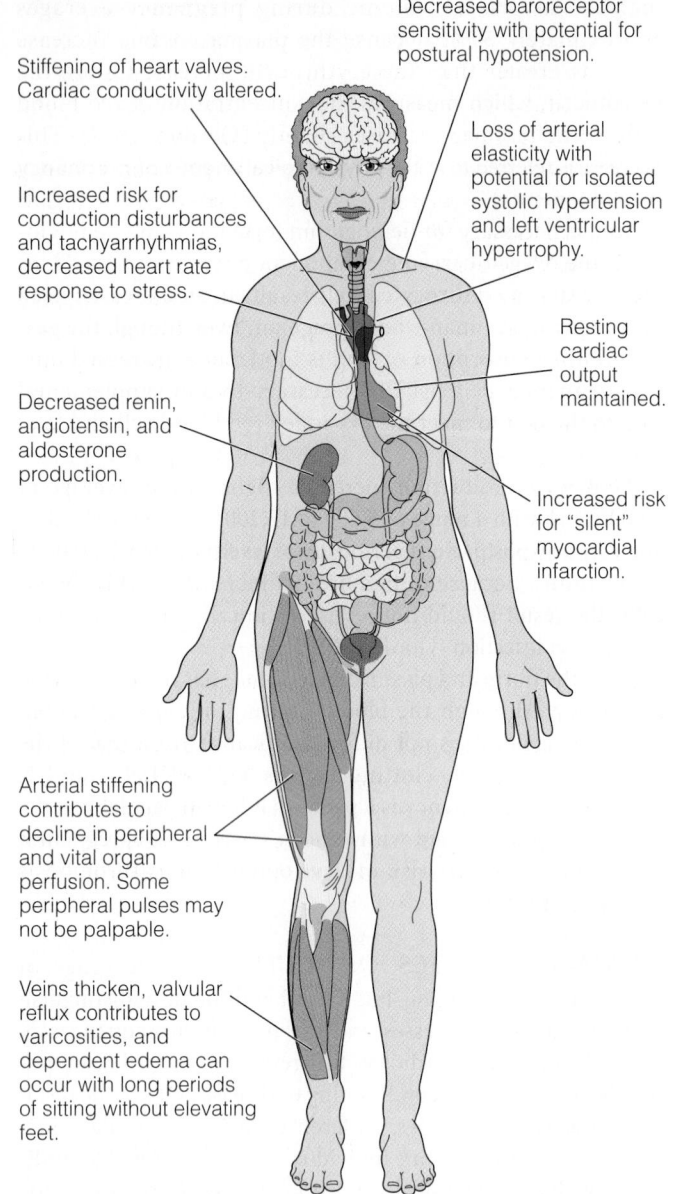

Stiffening of heart valves. Cardiac conductivity altered.

Decreased baroreceptor sensitivity with potential for postural hypotension.

Increased risk for conduction disturbances and tachyarrhythmias, decreased heart rate response to stress.

Loss of arterial elasticity with potential for isolated systolic hypertension and left ventricular hypertrophy.

Resting cardiac output maintained.

Decreased renin, angiotensin, and aldosterone production.

Increased risk for "silent" myocardial infarction.

Arterial stiffening contributes to decline in peripheral and vital organ perfusion. Some peripheral pulses may not be palpable.

Veins thicken, valvular reflux contributes to varicosities, and dependent edema can occur with long periods of sitting without elevating feet.

Figure 16–13 ● Normal changes of aging in the cardiovascular system.

neurological or endocrine systems, and these interrelated processes are vulnerable to aging. A change in one system can affect the functioning of many others. Physical or emotional stress may cause a more pronounced response and require a longer time for recovery. Taking a trip or getting the flu can cause much greater stress and negative changes for a frail older individual.

Another feature of aging is the atypical presentation of disease in an older individual. For example, a middle-aged individual experiencing a myocardial infarction will most likely complain of the typical substernal chest pain with radiation down the left arm; however, the older individual may complain of heartburn, nausea and vomiting, or excessive fatigue. Complaints of fatigue, decreased activity, sleep disturbance, or pain are not normal and should be investigated. The older individual has a decreased capacity to adapt to stress to the

cardiovascular system and may need medical or nursing interventions. Therefore, nurses should be alert to possible problems and include a wide range of diagnostic possibilities in any given situation. Mental status changes should not be assumed to be the result of dementia. Mental status changes, in addition to agitation and falls, may be the first sign of cardiac problems in the older individual. The nurse should conduct a thorough assessment of any older adult client complaining of or exhibiting changes in mental status.

Cardiovascular System Specific changes in the cardiovascular system with aging include **myocardial hypertrophy** (an increase in the size of muscle cells of the myocardium). This will change the function of the left ventricular wall and the ventricular septum. The left ventricular wall is 25% thicker in the average 80-year-old compared to that in the average 30-year-old. Inside individual cardiac cells, lipofuscin and amyloid deposits accumulate, and the structure of the myocardium shows increased collagen and connective tissue (McCance & Huether, 2010). Heart valves become stiff with aging as the result of fibrosis and calcification. In addition, changes in the valve rings can contribute to stenosis or incompetence resulting in changes in the heart muscle and its chambers.

Resting heart rate is relatively unchanged with normal aging, and in the absence of disease, cardiac output is not much changed. However, a slight decline in cardiac output does occur after age 20. The average man with a cardiac output of 5.0 L/min at age 20 will likely have a cardiac output of 3.5 L/min at age 75. This cardiac output is sufficient to maintain normal adult functioning. The heart has the ability to increase its rate in response to stress.

Electrical activity of the heart is affected in aging, with a decrease in the number of normal pacemaker cells in the SA node. By age 75, only 10% of the original pacemaker cells are still functional, but under normal circumstances, this number can still support cardiac function. Similarly, the number of cells in the AV node and in the left bundle branch is lower for the older individual. Similar changes have been demonstrated that show a decrease in cells in the bundle of His at age 40 and a decrease in right bundle branch cells by age 50. Other studies show an increase in fat and collagen in these regions. Fibrosis of the AV node can lead to AV block with no other cardiac pathology. The AV node refractory period is also increased with aging. The ECG shows no specific changes with age, although some lengthening of the PR, QRS, and QT intervals has been described. In some clients, the stress of acute or chronic illness may precipitate conduction abnormalities.

Vascular System The vascular system undergoes a myriad of changes with aging. The layers of the vascular system change, with a thickening of the intimal and medial layers. For arteries, the endothelial layer becomes irregular, with more connective tissue. Lipid deposits and calcification occur. Calcification can extend to the medial layer with increased collagen deposits. These changes can all lead to decreased elasticity or "hardening" of the arterial walls. Blood pressure elevation frequently occurs with aging, although it is not considered a normal variant. Isolated systolic hypertension (systolic blood pressure > 140 mmHg) is frequently seen in the older individual. Normally, the arterial wall diameter is controlled by a balance of systems including the autonomic nervous system and beta-adrenergic stimulation. However, decreased responsiveness to beta-adrenergic stimulation may be noted in older clients.

Pulmonary System   Pulmonary changes that occur with aging can affect cardiovascular function. Decreased chest wall compliance is the result of decreased elasticity of lung tissue and stiffness of thoracic and spinal joints. An increase in anteroposterior diameter is seen with aging. This can lead to higher residual volumes. Airway closure in dependent lung areas can occur at higher volumes. This removes portions of the lung from exchange functions. A combination of early airway closure, decreased diffusing capacity, increased lung volumes, and changes in alveolar structure can lead to lower arterial oxygen tension (PaO_2). Because carbon dioxide is diffused more readily, no change in $PaCO_2$ (arterial carbon dioxide tension) is noted with aging. Elevated $PaCO_2$ would indicate pathology. Age-related changes that increase susceptibility to pneumonia and other infections include decreased ciliary functioning and suppression of the immune system.

Renal System   Renal function declines with age, and the kidneys decrease in size and weight. By the ninth decade of life, the weight of the kidney is 25% less than the weight of the young adult kidney. Functional decline is also the result of decreased renal blood flow and decreased glomerular filtration. By age 80, the glomerular filtration rate is reduced 30%–50% compared with that of the 30-year-old. Because of a concomitant decrease in muscle mass, serum creatinine levels are not elevated. However, the clearance rate for creatinine and other chemicals, including many medications, is reduced. This results in a longer half-life for drugs administered to the older individual. With aging, decreased levels of renin and aldosterone are found in the plasma. This leads to an increased sensitivity to dietary sodium consumption. Decreased ability to clear sodium from the blood can lead to body water overload. This increased preload can tax the myocardium. Additionally, an antidiuretic hormone is less able to be suppressed when serum osmolality is low, and this results in further retention of body water. A decreased ability to concentrate urine can result in dehydration. In addition to monitoring for fluid volume depletion, older clients should be monitored for fluid volume excess because they have a decreased ability to adapt to sudden increases in intravascular volume.

▶ ALTERATIONS TO PERFUSION

Nurses care for many clients with alterations in cardiac function secondary to the prevalence of cardiac disease. Clients may present with cardiac disease as a primary diagnosis or they may be seen for a variety of other problems complicated by a secondary diagnosis of cardiac disease. Clients with alterations to perfusion will likely have alterations to other concepts as well. Acid–base imbalance is of particular concern when working with clients with altered perfusion. Acute respiratory acidosis exists when an acute ventilation failure occurs. This may result from depression of the central respiratory center. Common causes include drug-induced respiratory depression, inadequate ventilation due to neuromuscular disease or paralysis, and airway obstruction. Chronic respiratory acidosis is usually secondary to other medical conditions, such as chronic obstructive pulmonary disease (COPD), neuromuscular disorders, severe restrictive ventilator defects, and thoracic skeletal deformities.

Clients developing CO_2 retention have a high work of breathing. Some clients with ventilation-perfusion inequalities increase ventilation and some do not. Acute respiratory acidosis produces little change in the bicarbonate concentration and the pH falls and PCO_2 rises. Clients with chronic respiratory acidosis experience a smaller fall in pH due to the retention of bicarbonate by the kidneys, and ventilation is not on pace to provide adequate perfusion. A decrease in alveolar oxygen levels leads to a decrease in arterial oxygen levels.

Causes of metabolic acidosis are categorized by increases in plasma acidity. Identification of underlying disease processes should be considered for clients in metabolic acidosis in order to begin treatment. The clinical symptoms of metabolic acidosis can be life threatening if left untreated. Pulmonary vasoconstriction and increased pulmonary vascular pressures leading to right ventricular failure may result. Generalized myocardial depression occurs with a pH of less than 7.2. Respiratory muscle fatigue may result in clients who have underlying lung disease.

Disorders of **clotting** (the process of coagulation where blood is converted from a liquid to a gel), can result in impairments of excessive bleeding (as discussed in the exemplar on DIC) or excessive clotting (as discussed in the exemplar on DVT).

Alterations and Manifestations

ALTERATIONS TO PEDIATRIC CARDIOLOGY   Most pediatric disorders are related to congenital cardiac defects. With the recent advances in pediatric cardiology, children who would not have survived to their first birthday are now entering adolescence. As a result, nurses may care for clients with profound alterations in cardiac anatomy requiring special considerations when planning care. Cardiac congenital anomalies are discussed in more detail in Exemplar 16.2 within this module.

COMMON CARDIOVASCULAR ILLNESSES OF ADULTHOOD   Coronary artery disease (CAD) is the leading cause of death in the United States. CAD occurs when the arteries supplying the heart muscle harden and become narrow. The buildup, called atherosclerosis, is a result of cholesterol and other materials. As the arteries become narrower, the diameter of the arteries decreases. The heart muscle does not receive a sufficient amount of blood or oxygen. Clients with CAD may experience angina (chest pain) or a myocardial infarction (heart attack). CAD can weaken the heart muscle and may contribute to arrhythmias and heart failure.

Myocardial infarctions occur when the flow of oxygenated blood to a section of heart muscle is blocked. Blockages need immediate treatment or the heart muscle begins to die. Necrotic tissue is replaced with scar tissue, which may result in long-term cardiac illnesses.

Concepts Related to **Perfusion**

In addition to acid–base balance, a number of concepts and systems affect and are affected by adequate (or impaired) perfusion including, but not limited to, cognition, comfort, fluids and electrolytes, intracranial regulation, and oxygenation.

Cognition. Due to autoregulation, the brain has the ability to maintain relatively constant blood flow despite changes in perfusion pressure. Clinical signs or symptoms of ischemia can be seen when cerebral perfusion pressure drops below the lower limit of autoregulation. Altered mental status is an early symptom of decreased cerebral blood flow.

Comfort. The heart generates sufficient cardiac output to transport and distribute blood to the body's tissues. Impaired tissue perfusion results when the blood supply available to the site of injury is present but decreased. Pain is a common symptom.

Fluids and Electrolytes. Inadequate fluid resuscitation may lead to multiple-organ failure and death. Hypovolemia causes a decrease in extracellular fluid. In severe cases, inadequate tissue perfusion may occur. A loss of volume causes an inappropriate redistribution of body fluids.

Intracranial Regulation. Without adequate cerebral blood flow, energy-dependent brain processes cease, leading to irreversible brain injury. Adequate cerebral blood flow must be maintained to ensure adequate cerebral perfusion pressure (CPP). CPP is the difference between the mean arterial blood pressure and the mean cerebral venous pressure.

Oxygenation. Respiratory gases are transported with the assistance of red blood cells. Ventilation, diffusion, and perfusion are essential for gas exchange to occur. The process of perfusion pumps bloods from the cardiovascular system to the lungs.

CONCEPT	RELATIONSHIP TO PERFUSION	NURSING IMPLICATIONS
Acid–Base Balance		
■ Respiratory acidosis ■ Metabolic acidosis	■ Retention of CO_2 ■ Low pH, low or normal $PaCO_2$	■ Evaluate client's respiratory drive and function. Treat underlying problem. Reestablish effective ventilation. ■ Assess for lactic acidosis and acute renal failure.
Cellular Regulation		
■ Collaborative interventions and therapies	Heart may not provide tissues with enough blood to meet metabolic needs.	■ Client may experience S/Sx of heart failure. Evaluate mental status, noting development of confusion. Monitor VS. Apply supplemental O_2 as needed.
Cognition		
■ Mental assessment	Hypoxemia can cause altered mental state.	■ Assess mental status. Rule out acute brain injury.
Comfort		
■ Comfort assessment ■ Acute and chronic pain	↓ perfusion of tissues may manifest itself as pain.	■ Note abdominal pain, chest pain, changes in extremity temperature, pain in extremities, ↑ BP, resp, restlessness, anxiety. ■ Monitor VS, pain scale, redness, swelling in extremities. Administer O_2 as needed. Administer meds as ordered.
Fluids and Electrolytes		
■ Fluid and electrolyte assessment ■ Regulating body fluids	Fluid volume excess may result in hypervolemia, impaired gas exchange, and other life-threatening alterations.	■ Decrease work of breathing, administer supplemental O_2 as needed, maintain perfusion pressure, monitor pulse ox and ABGs, administer meds as ordered. ■ Balance fluids. Ensure bed rest. Conduct a focused pulmonary assessment. Assess for jugular venous distention (JVD). Assess for chest pain, N/V, SOB.

Concepts Related to **Perfusion** (continued)

CONCEPT	RELATIONSHIP TO PERFUSION	NURSING IMPLICATIONS
Intracranial Regulation		
■ Neurological assessment ■ Glasgow Coma Scale ■ Increased intracranial pressure	Cerebral blood flow (CBF)	■ Regulate to meet brain's metabolic needs. ↑ CBF can ↑ ICP. ↓ CBF may result in cerebral ischemia. ■ Monitor VS. Observe pupils and LOC. Assess using the Glasgow Coma Scale. Maintain correct body positioning. Observe for S/Sx of ↑ ICP.
Oxygenation		
■ Oxygenation assessment ■ Independent interventions and therapies	Factors affecting transport of respiratory gases to the tissues	■ Client may experience ↓ energy, restlessness, tachypnea, tachycardia, hypertension, confusion. ■ Monitor vital signs. Use high-Fowler positioning, if able. Encourage deep breathing. Administer O_2. Provide for periods of rest between activities.

Another cause of myocardial infarction is severe spasms of a coronary artery, resulting in an interrupted blood supply to a section of the heart. These spasms may occur without the presence of atherosclerosis. Prompt, rapid medical treatment significantly improves the client's outcome. It is estimated that 50% of those who die as a result of myocardial infarction do so within the first 60 minutes of the first symptom.

COMMON CARDIOVASCULAR ILLNESSES OF AGING Cardiovascular disease can have a slow onset with progressive deterioration of other organ systems such as the kidney and lung. Some common conditions, such as hypertension or hyperlipidemia, are risk factors for developing more serious conditions at any age. These conditions require ongoing assessment and treatment at any age (**Table 16–6 ●**).

TABLE 16–6   Age-Related Cardiac Changes

AGE-RELATED CHANGE	SIGNIFICANCE
Myocardium: ↓ efficiency and contractibility. *Sinoatrial node:* ↑ in thickness of shell surrounding the node and ↓ in number of pacemaker cells.	■ Decreased cardiac output when under physiological stress, with resulting tachycardia that lasts longer than in younger people. The individual may require rest time between physical activities.
Left ventricle: Slight hypertrophy, prolonged isometric contraction phase and relaxation time; ↑ time for diastolic filling and systolic emptying cycle.	■ Stroke volume may increase to compensate for tachycardia, leading to increased blood pressure.
Valves and blood vessels: Aorta is elongated and dilated, valves are thicker and more rigid, and resistance to peripheral blood flow increases by 1% per year.	■ Blood pressure increases to compensate for increased peripheral resistance and decreased cardiac output.

Prevalence

High blood pressure affects 29% (70 million) of American adults. More than 360,000 deaths in 2013 were attributed to high blood pressure as the primary cause. Of people who have a first heart attack, 69% have high blood pressure, as do 77% of people who have a first stroke, and 74% of people with chronic heart failure. Only about half of people who have high blood pressure (52%) have it under control (Centers for Disease Control and Prevention [CDC], 2015).

Heart disease is the leading cause of death for both men and women. One of every four deaths in the United States is attributed to heart disease, and approximately 610,000 people die of heart disease in the United States every year. Coronary heart disease is the most common, killing 370,000 people annually. Every year, about 525,000 Americans have a first heart attack, and 210,000 have a repeat attack (CDC, 2015).

About 5.1 million people in the United States have heart failure, which is the primary cause of death in 55,000 people each year, and a contributing cause of death in 280,000 people. About half of people with heart failure die within 5 years of diagnosis (CDC, 2013b).

Every year, more than 795,000 Americans have a stroke, and about 610,000 of them are first strokes. Stroke kills almost 130,000 Americans each year, which is 1 in every 20 deaths. Stroke is the leading cause of long-term disability.

Genetic Considerations and Nonmodifiable Risk Factors

Risk factors for perfusion abnormalities may be identified as nonmodifiable or modifiable. Nonmodifiable risk factors are not affected by changes in client behavior. They include age, gender, race, family history, and personal health history.

It is important for the nurse to consider genetic influences on the health of the adult. During the client interview, ask about

Alterations and Therapies **Perfusion**

ALTERATION	DESCRIPTION	MANIFESTATIONS	INTERVENTIONS AND THERAPIES
Coronary artery disease: rapid, irregular heart rate	As plaque builds within the coronary artery, the diameter of the artery decreases. This reduces blood flow to the cardiac muscle until a myocardial infarction occurs. Necrosis of the heart muscle may occur as a result of decreased perfusion.	▪ Pain or discomfort in chest. May also include atypical locations such as arm, left shoulder, back, neck, or jaw. ▪ SOB ▪ Cold, clammy skin ▪ Feeling of indigestion or fullness ▪ Dizziness, anxiety ▪ Rapid, irregular heart rate	▪ Administration of oxygen ▪ Administration of nitrates for vasodilatory effects ▪ Telemetry monitoring ▪ Tissue plasminogen activator, streptokinase, or other medication to eliminate clots, preventing perfusion of cardiac muscle (Review client's current and past medical history prior to administration.) ▪ Antiarrhythmic medications ▪ Bed rest ▪ Anxiety reduction measures ▪ Possible prep for coronary artery bypass grafting
Cardiomyopathy	Inflammation of the cardiac muscle, resulting in an increase in heart size and reduced cardiac function. May be classified as primary (no known cause) or secondary (results from hypertension, valvular disease, artery disease, congenital heart defects, or another known cause) and as dilated, hypertrophic, and restrictive.	▪ S/Sx may not present until later in the disease. ▪ SOB, especially with physical exertion, may include CP. ▪ Fatigue ▪ Lower extremity edema ▪ Arrhythmias ▪ Heart murmur	▪ Medications (calcium-channel blockers, beta-blockers, antidysrhythmics) ▪ Monitoring of VS, including pulse ox ▪ Focused cardiac/respiratory assessment for detection of crackles or dry cough, murmurs or extra heart sounds ▪ Monitoring of I/O. ▪ Assessment of capillary refill time ▪ Instruct to avoid nitrates because they lower BP, and digoxin because it increases the force of contractions. ▪ Antibiotics to reduce the risk for bacterial endocarditis ▪ Septal myectomy, ethanol ablation, implantable cardioverter–defibrillator ▪ Heart failure management ▪ Fluid and sodium restriction ▪ Regular follow-up care
Dysrhythmia	Irregular electrical pattern seen on an ECG. May result from new or existing coronary artery disease, serum electrolyte imbalances, injury, congenital defect, myocardial infarction, or malfunction of conduction system.	▪ Irregular heart rate	▪ Cardiac monitoring. Notify physician of changes in heart rate or rhythm. ▪ Administration of antidysrhythmic medications, as ordered ▪ Supplemental O_2 as needed ▪ Structure activities of daily living to provide for adequate rest periods. ▪ Monitoring of lab values

Alterations and Therapies **Perfusion** (*continued*)

ALTERATION	DESCRIPTION	MANIFESTATIONS	INTERVENTIONS AND THERAPIES
Valvular heart disease	May be acquired or congenital. May be caused by valvular stenosis or valvular insufficiency	▪ SOB ▪ Weakness or lightheadedness ▪ Chest discomfort ▪ Edema of lower extremities ▪ Palpitations ▪ Rapid weight gain (2–3 lb per day)	▪ Client teaching to include diet, lifestyle changes, signs and symptoms of heart failure ▪ Medications may include diuretics, antidysrhythmics, vasodilators, angiotensin-converting enzyme inhibitors, beta-blockers, and/or anticoagulants. May also include antibiotics to prevent bacterial endocarditis.
Cardiogenic shock	Inadequate perfusion of the tissues as a result of blood loss, infection, destruction of or inadequate production of blood cells, reduced cardiac output caused by cardiac disease, or systemic vasodilation.	▪ Confusion ▪ Loss of consciousness ▪ Sudden, rapid heartbeat ▪ Diaphoresis ▪ Tachypnea ▪ Decreased urine output ▪ Extremities cool to touch	▪ Administer fluids and, depending on cause, blood transfusions or volume expanders. ▪ Medications may include vasoconstrictors and those needed to treat the underlying cause. ▪ Monitor and assess cardiorespiratory function and oxygen saturation. ▪ Administer oxygen as indicated. ▪ Assess level of consciousness, and report significant deviations from baseline. ▪ Those in acute shock may require mechanical ventilation.
Hypertension	Pressure in the arterial blood vessels is elevated, causing the heart to pump with much more force in order to overcome higher pressures. Causes may be primary (no known cause; most often diagnosed) or secondary (result of another disease process, e.g., diabetes mellitus, pheochromocytoma, or arteriosclerosis).	▪ Clients are often asymptomatic until hypertension becomes significant. ▪ Clients may present with headaches (particularly in the a.m.), dizziness, nausea, nosebleeds, fatigue and difficulty sleeping.	▪ Assess cardiovascular risk status. ▪ Encourage lifestyle changes. ▪ Conduct a nutritional assessment. ▪ Encourage smoking cessation. ▪ Obtain detailed family history.
Pregnancy-induced hypertension	Blood pressure elevates, causing damage to nephrons with leakage of protein into the urine. As BP continues to rise, can result in fetal demise, seizures, stroke, and death.	▪ Proteinuria, headache, edema of hands and lower extremities	▪ Instruct client to reduce sodium intake. ▪ Monitor BP. ▪ Elevate extremities. ▪ If BP exceeds acceptable limits, client will be admitted and intravenous magnesium sulfate administered. ▪ If unable to control BP with magnesium sulfate, the only option is to deliver the baby, which will resolve the problem and gradually return BP to normal limits.

- Familial hypercholesterolemia is a single-gene disorder that results in atherosclerosis and coronary artery disease, which may occur at an earlier age than in the general population (i.e., before age 55 in men and age 65 in women). However, increased cholesterol levels may also be inherited and are a risk factor for coronary artery disease in both men and women.
- Marfan syndrome is an autosomal-dominant inherited disorder that affects the skeleton, eyes, and cardiovascular system. The cardiovascular effects are a dilation of the proximal aorta and aortic dissection associated with degeneration of the elastic fibers in the tunica media of the aorta. Thoracic aortic aneurysms may also be present.
- Supraventricular aortic stenosis is a genetic vascular disorder resulting in an hourglass-shaped stenosis of the ascending aorta. It may also affect other major arteries, including the pulmonary, carotid, cerebral, renal, and coronary arteries.
- Hypertropic cardiomyopathy, a disease of sarcomere proteins, has a genetic transmission.
- Williams syndrome is a rare genetic disorder characterized by characteristic "elfin-like" features and heart and blood vessel problems (as well as other physical problems).
- Long QT syndrome is an inherited genetic disorder that results from structural abnormalities of the potassium channels in the heart, leading to dysrhythmias. This can result in unconsciousness and may cause sudden cardiac death in teenagers and young adults when exposed to stressors ranging from exercise to loud sounds.

family members with health problems affecting cardiac function or a family history of high cholesterol levels or early-onset coronary artery disease. During the physical assessment, assess for any manifestations that might indicate a genetic disorder (**Box 16–1 ●**). If data are found to indicate genetic risk factors or alterations, ask about genetic testing and refer for appropriate genetic counseling and evaluation.

CASE STUDY \\ PART 1

During your shift, Mr. Bill Evans, a 64-year-old African American male client presents to the emergency department after collapsing at home. His wife states that just before losing consciousness, the client seemed confused and complained of numbness and tingling in the left arm and double vision. She also states that his speech was slurred and the left side of his face drooped. He has a history of CAD, HTN, CHF, atrial fibrillation, and diabetes. Current vitals are T 98.9°F; P 91 bpm; R 24/min; and BP 182/98 mmHg. Mr. Evans has regained consciousness and is aware of his surroundings but demonstrates right-sided weakness, slurred speech, and difficulty forming words.

Clinical Reasoning Questions Level I

1. What symptoms of alterations in perfusion does Mr. Evans demonstrate?
2. Identify three nonmodifiable risk factors related to alterations in perfusion.

3. Describe the pathophysiology of a cerebrovascular accident (CVA).

Clinical Reasoning Questions Level II

4. Would you expect that Mr. Evans experienced a hemorrhagic or ischemic CVA? Why?
5. What issues can you identify as priorities in caring for this client?
6. What are some potential complications that the nurse needs to be aware of?

▶ PREVENTION

Modifiable Risk Factors

Modifiable risk factors include smoking, high blood pressure, high blood cholesterol, obesity, physical inactivity, and diabetes, all of which can be controlled by lifestyle changes or medication. Secondary risk factors that can contribute to an individual's risk for developing heart disease include stress and alcohol intake.

Screenings

Clients first symptom of a perfusion alteration may present as myocardial infarction or sudden death. A client may not experience preceding chest pain. Because of this, screening tests may be performed to detect signs of coronary artery disease before serious events occur. Screening tests are of particular benefit to those with risk factors for CAD.

An ECG may be ordered to detect electrical changes, such as ST depressions or Q waves that suggest CAD or signs of a previous myocardial infarction. Results of the ECG may indicate the need for further testing. Another type of screening is a stress test. These screenings place the heart under controlled stress and are able to detect the presence of blockages that may limit flow. There are two types of basic stress testing. Exercise cardiac stress testing involves exercising the client under controlled conditions to stress the heart. The second basic type of stress testing is physiological stress testing, which involves chemically stressing the heart to mimic the effects of exercise. Commonly administered medications are dobutamine and adenosine. This type of testing may be considered for clients with limited mobility.

If either of these methods produces inconclusive results, the physician may order a radionuclide stress test. This involves the injection of a radioactive isotope (usually thallium or Cardiolite) into the client's vein. Once the isotope has been absorbed by normal heart muscle, an image of the heart becomes visible. The nuclear images are viewed with the client at rest and then again after exercise. The two sets of images are then compared. If present, blockages will be evident on the images taken after exercise. They may be referred to as "cold spots" on the images.

Stress echocardiography may be used to supplement screenings for CAD. An echocardiogram produces sound waves that are used to produce images of the heart at rest and at the peak of exercise. In hearts with normal blood flow, the left ventricle demonstrates stronger contractions of the heart muscle during peak exercise. In clients with CAD, a left ventricle segment not receiving adequate blood flow will exhibit reduced contractions of heart muscle. Stress echocardiography may be used in clients with false-positive stress tests.

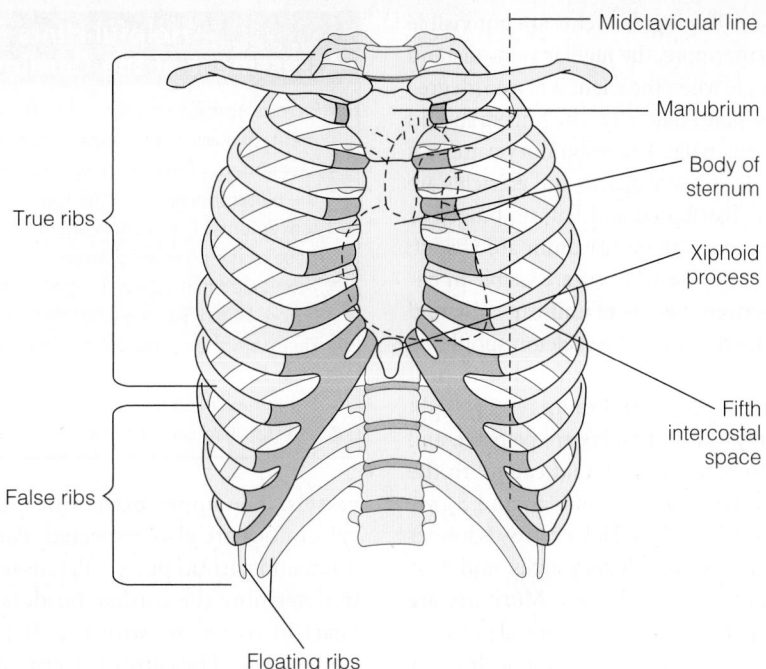

Figure 16–14 ● Landmarks for cardiovascular assessment.

Electron beam computerized tomography offers new technology for CAD screening. This test can identify calcium blockages as mild as 10%–20%. With mild blockages the recommended treatment is risk factor modification. Calcium scoring may be used to persuade those at risk to engage in lifestyle modifications. Scores range from zero (no evidence of CAD) to over 400 (extensive evidence of CAD). Not all insurance plans cover calcium scoring at this time.

▶ ASSESSMENT

Nursing assessment, including assessment of pulse and blood pressure, and the collection of subjective data are essential to designing the nursing plan of care. Symptoms such as pain, fatigue, and shortness of breath are assessed by careful questioning of the client.

Nursing Assessment

Physical assessment of the cardiovascular system requires the use of inspection, palpation, percussion, and auscultation. During each of the procedures, the nurse is gathering objective data related to the function of the heart as determined by the heart rate and the quality and characteristics of the heart sounds. In addition, the nurse observes for signs of appropriate cardiac function, in relation to oxygen perfusion, by assessing skin color and temperature, abnormal pulsations, and the characteristics of the client's respiratory effort. Knowledge of normal parameters and expected findings is essential in determining the meaning of the data during a physical health assessment.

ANATOMICAL LANDMARKS FOR CARDIOVASCULAR ASSESSMENT   Anatomical landmarks for assessing the cardiovascular system include the sternum, clavicles, and ribs. By correlating assessment findings with the overlying body landmarks, the nurse can gain vital information concerning underlying pathological mechanisms. Many landmarks identified during the respiratory assessment are utilized when performing a cardiac assessment. These include, but are not limited to, the sternum and the second intercostal space through the fifth intercostal space (ICS).

The sternum is the flat, narrow center bone of the upper anterior chest (**Figure 16–14** ●). The adult sternum has three parts. The upper sternum is called the manubrium, the middle part is called the body, and the inferior piece is called the xiphoid process. The average sternal length in an adult is 18 cm (7 in.). During cardiovascular assessment, the sternum is used as a vertical landmark. The angle of Louis is used to locate the second ICS.

The clavicles are bones that attach at the top of the manubrium of the sternum above the first rib. The midclavicular line is used as a landmark for cardiovascular assessment (see Figure 16–14).

The ribs are flat, arched bones that form the thoracic cage. There are 12 pairs of ribs. Between each rib is an ICS. The first ICS lies between the first and the second rib, and each remaining ICS is numbered successively (see Figure 16–14). The intercostal spaces, horizontal landmarks for cardiac assessment, are used to locate the base of the heart and the apex of the heart and to auscultate the valvular sounds. The second ICS is located by feeling the angle of Louis, sliding the finger laterally to the second rib, and then sliding the finger down below the rib to the ICS. Each succeeding ICS is located by sliding the finger over the rib into the ICS.

INSPECTION   Adults normally have uniform skin color on the face, trunk, and extremities. The eyes are symmetric. The periorbital area is flat, and the eyes do not bulge. The sclera of the eye should be white, the cornea clear, and the conjunctiva pink. The lips should be smooth and noncyanotic. The head should be steady and the skull proportional to the face. The earlobe should be smooth and without creases. The jugular veins are not visible when the chest is upright. Furthermore, the jugular veins distend only 3 cm above the sternal angle when the client is at a 45-degree angle. Carotid pulsations are visible bilaterally. The fingers should be round and even, with flat, pink nails. The respiratory pattern is even, regular, and unlabored. Intercostal spaces and clavicles are visible; chest veins are evenly distributed and flat; no bulges or masses are visible. Pulsations over the pericardium are absent; however, aortic pulsations in the epigastric area are visible in clients who are thin. The lower extremities are of uniform color and temperature, with even hair distribution. The skeleton should be free of deformity, and the neck and extremities should be in proportion to the torso. Palpation over the pericardium reveals slight vibration at the apical area only. Carotid pulses are palpable and equal in intensity. Dullness to percussion should extend to the midclavicular line at the fifth ICS. Heart sounds S_1 and S_2 are heard equally at Erb's point (third left ICS). However, S_2 is louder than S_1 at the aortic and pulmonic auscultatory areas, and S_1 is louder than S_2 at the tricuspid and apical areas. Murmurs are absent. The carotid pulse is synchronous with the apical pulse.

Physical assessment of the cardiovascular system follows an organized pattern. It begins with inspection of the client's head and neck, including eyes, ears, lips, face, skull, and neck

vessels. The upper extremities, chest, abdomen, and lower extremities are also inspected. Palpation includes the precordium and carotid pulses. Percussion of the chest is conducted to determine the cardiac borders. Auscultation includes the heart in five areas with the diaphragm and the bell of the stethoscope. The carotid arteries and the apical pulse are auscultated. Helpful hints for the physical assessment are listed in **Box 16–2** ●.

Perfusion Assessment

ASSESSMENT/METHOD	NORMAL FINDINGS	ABNORMAL FINDINGS	LIFESPAN OR DEVELOPMENTAL CONSIDERATIONS
Apical Impulse Assessment			
First using the palmar surface and then repeating with finger pads, palpate the precordium for symmetry of movement and the apical impulse for location, size, amplitude, and duration. The sequence for palpation is shown in **Figure 16–15** ●. To locate the apical impulse, ask the client to assume a left lateral recumbent position. Simultaneous palpation of the carotid pulse may also be helpful.	The apical impulse is not palpable in all clients but may be palpated in the mitral area and has only a brief, small amplitude.	■ An enlarged or displaced heart is associated with an apical impulse lateral to the midclavicular line or below the fifth left ICS.	■ The apical impulse is often not visible in older and pediatric clients. Assessment remains the same as in the adult population.

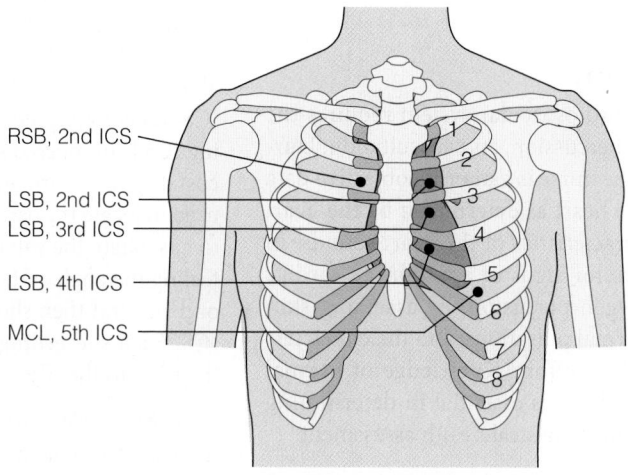

RSB, 2nd ICS
LSB, 2nd ICS
LSB, 3rd ICS
LSB, 4th ICS
MCL, 5th ICS

Figure 16–15 ● Areas for inspection and palpation of the precordium, indicating the sequence for palpation.

Perfusion Assessment (*continued*)

ASSESSMENT/METHOD	NORMAL FINDINGS	ABNORMAL FINDINGS	LIFESPAN OR DEVELOPMENTAL CONSIDERATIONS
		■ Increased size, amplitude, and duration of the apical impulse are associated with left ventricular volume overload (increased afterload) in conditions such as hypertension (HTN) and aortic stenosis and with pressure overload (increased preload) in conditions such as aortic or mitral regurgitation. ■ Increased amplitude alone may occur with hyperkinetic states, such as anxiety, hyperthyroidism, and anemia. ■ Decreased amplitude is associated with a dilated heart in cardiomyopathy. ■ Displacement alone may also occur with dextrocardia, diaphragmatic hernia, gastric distention, or chronic lung disease. ■ A **thrill** (a palpable vibration over the precordium or an artery) may accompany severe valve stenosis. ■ A marked increase in amplitude of the apical impulse at the right ventricular area occurs with right ventricular volume overload in atrial septal defect. ■ An increase in amplitude and duration occurs with right ventricular pressure overload in pulmonic stenosis and pulmonary hypertension. A lift or heave may also be seen in these conditions and in chronic lung disease.	■ When assessing a pediatric client, it may be more beneficial to auscultate the apical pulse in the area of the left nipple.

(*continued on next page*)

Perfusion Assessment (*continued*)

ASSESSMENT/METHOD	NORMAL FINDINGS	ABNORMAL FINDINGS	LIFESPAN OR DEVELOPMENTAL CONSIDERATIONS
		■ A palpable thrill in this area occurs with ventricular septal defect. ■ Right ventricular enlargement may produce a downward pulsation against the fingertips. ■ An accentuated pulsation at the pulmonary area may be present in hyperkinetic states. ■ A prominent pulsation reflects increased flow or dilation of the pulmonary artery. ■ A thrill may be associated with aortic or pulmonary stenosis, aortic stenosis, pulmonary HTN, or atrial septal defect. ■ Increased pulsation at the aortic area may suggest aortic aneurysm. ■ A palpable S_2 may be noted with systemic HTN.	
Palpate the subxiphoid area with the index and middle finger.	Diastolic movements of S_3 and S_4 may be felt.	■ Right ventricular enlargement may produce a downward pulsation against the fingertips. ■ An accentuated pulsation at the pulmonary area may be present in hyperkinetic states. ■ A prominent pulsation reflects increased flow or dilation of the pulmonary artery. ■ A thrill may be associated with aortic or pulmonary stenosis, aortic stenosis, pulmonary HTN, or atrial septal defect. ■ Increased pulsation at the aortic area may suggest aortic aneurysm. ■ A palpable S_2 may be noted with systemic HTN.	■ Useful in clients with an increased AP diameter. ■ Useful in infants because respiratory excursions may interfere with parasternal palpation.

Perfusion Assessment (*continued*)

ASSESSMENT/METHOD	NORMAL FINDINGS	ABNORMAL FINDINGS	LIFESPAN OR DEVELOPMENTAL CONSIDERATIONS
Cardiac Rate and Rhythm Assessment			
Auscultate heart rate.	The heart rate should be 60–100 bpm, with regular rhythm.	■ A heart rate of >100 bpm is tachycardia. A heart rate of <60 bpm is bradycardia.	■ Consider using a pediatric chest piece when auscultating heart sounds on a pediatric client or very thin adult.
Simultaneously palpate the radial pulse while listening to the apical pulse.	The radial and apical pulses should be equal.	■ If the radial pulse falls behind the apical rate, the client has a **pulse deficit**, indicating weak, ineffective contractions of the left ventricle.	
Auscultate heart rhythm.	The heart rhythm should be regular.	■ Dysrhythmias (abnormal heart rate or rhythms) may be regular or irregular in rhythm; their rates may be slow or fast. Irregular rhythms may occur in a pattern (e.g., an early beat every second beat, called bigeminy), sporadically, or with frequency and disorganization (e.g., atrial fibrillation). A pattern of gradual increase and decrease in heart rate that is within the normal range and that correlates with inspiration and expiration is called sinus arrhythmia.	
Heart Sounds Assessment			
See guidelines for cardiac auscultation in **Box 16–3** ●. Identify S_1, and note its intensity. At each auscultatory area, listen for several cardiac cycles. See Figure 16–16 for auscultation areas.	S_1 is loudest at the apex of the heart.	■ An accentuated S_1 occurs with tachycardia, states in which cardiac output is high (e.g., fever, anxiety, exercise, anemia, stress, and hyperthyroidism), complete heart block, and mitral stenosis. ■ A diminished S_1 occurs with first-degree heart block, mitral regurgitation, congestive heart failure (CHF), coronary	■ Review history for presence of pacemaker. ■ Presence of asymptomatic bradycardia may not be of importance in older adults.

(continued on next page)

Perfusion Assessment (*continued*)

ASSESSMENT/METHOD	NORMAL FINDINGS	ABNORMAL FINDINGS	LIFESPAN OR DEVELOPMENTAL CONSIDERATIONS
		artery disease, and pulmonary or systemic HTN. The intensity is also decreased with obesity, emphysema, and pericardial effusion. Varying intensity of S_1 occurs with complete heart block and grossly irregular rhythms.	
Listen for splitting of S_1.	Splitting of S_1 may occur during inspiration.	■ Abnormal splitting of S_1 may be heard with right bundle branch block and premature ventricular contractions.	
Identify S_2, and note its intensity.	S_2 immediately follows S_1 and is loudest at the base of the heart.	■ An accentuated S_2 may be heard with HTN, exercise, excitement, and conditions of pulmonary HTN, such as CHF and cor pulmonale. ■ A diminished S_2 occurs with aortic stenosis, a fall in systolic blood pressure (shock), and increased anteroposterior chest diameter.	
Listen for splitting of S_2.	No splitting of S_2 should be heard.	■ Wide splitting of S_2 is associated with delayed emptying of the right ventricle, resulting in delayed pulmonary valve closure (e.g., mitral regurgitation, pulmonary stenosis, and right bundle branch block). ■ Fixed splitting occurs when right ventricular output is greater than left ventricular output and pulmonary valve closure is delayed (e.g., with atrial septal defect and right ventricular failure). ■ Paradoxic splitting occurs when closure of the aortic valve is delayed (e.g., left bundle branch block).	

Perfusion Assessment (*continued*)

ASSESSMENT/METHOD	NORMAL FINDINGS	ABNORMAL FINDINGS	LIFESPAN OR DEVELOPMENTAL CONSIDERATIONS
Identify extra heart sounds in systole.	No extra heart sounds should be heard.	■ Ejection sounds (or clicks) result from the opening of deformed semilunar valves (e.g., aortic and pulmonary stenosis). ■ A midsystolic click is heard with mitral valve prolapse.	■ A fourth heart sound is commonly present in older adults without evidence of a cardiovascular event.
Identify the presence of extra heart sounds in diastole.	No extra heart sounds should be heard.	■ An opening snap results from the opening sound of a stenotic mitral valve. ■ A pathological S_3 (a third heart sound that immediately follows S_2, called a ventricular gallop) results from myocardial failure and ventricular volume overload (e.g., CHF and mitral or tricuspid regurgitation). ■ An S_4 (a fourth heart sound that immediately precedes S_1, called an atrial gallop) results from increased resistance to ventricular filling after atrial contraction (e.g., HTN, coronary artery disease, aortic stenosis, and cardiomyopathy). ■ A combined S_3 and S_4 is called a summation gallop and occurs with severe CHF.	■ Considered abnormal in clients of any age.
Identify extra heart sounds in both systole and diastole.	No extra heart sounds should be heard during systole and diastole.	■ A pericardial friction rub results from inflammation of the pericardial sac, as with pericarditis.	
Murmur Assessment			
Identify any murmurs. Note location, timing, presence during systole or diastole, and intensity.	No murmurs should be heard.	■ Midsystolic murmurs are heard with semilunar valve disease (e.g., aortic and pulmonary stenosis) and with hypertrophic cardiomyopathy.	■ Innocent murmurs do not need treatment.

(continued on next page)

Perfusion Assessment *(continued)*

ASSESSMENT/METHOD	NORMAL FINDINGS	ABNORMAL FINDINGS	LIFESPAN OR DEVELOPMENTAL CONSIDERATIONS
Use the following scale to grade murmurs: I = Barely heard II = Quietly heard III = Clearly heard IV = Loud V = Very loud VI = Loudest; may be heard with stethoscope off the chest. (A thrill may accompany murmurs of grade IV to grade VI.) Note pitch (low, medium, or high), and quality (harsh, blowing, or musical). Note pattern/shape, crescendo, decrescendo, and radiation/transmission (to axilla or neck).		■ Pansystolic (holosystolic) murmurs are heard with atrioventricular valve disease (e.g., mitral and tricuspid regurgitation, ventricular septal defect). ■ A late systolic murmur is heard with mitral valve prolapse. ■ Early diastolic murmurs occur with regurgitant flow across incompetent semilunar valves (e.g., aortic regurgitation). ■ Mid-diastolic and pre-systolic murmurs, such as with mitral stenosis, occur with turbulent flow across the atrioventricular valves. ■ Continuous murmurs throughout systole and all or part of diastole occur with patent ductus arteriosus.	■ Pulmonary flow murmurs, Still murmur, and venous hums are often seen in children as a normal part of development. They do not require treatment.

ASSESSING THE PULSE A pulse is commonly assessed by palpation (feeling) or auscultation (hearing). The middle three fingertips are used for palpating all pulse sites except the apex of the heart. A stethoscope is used for assessing apical pulses. A Doppler ultrasound stethoscope (DUS; see

Box 16–3 Guidelines for Cardiac Auscultation

1. Locate the major auscultatory areas on the precordium (see **Figure 16–16 ●**).
2. Choose a sequence of listening. Either begin from the apex and move upward along the sternal border to the base, or begin at the base and move downward to the apex. One suggested sequence is shown in Figure 16–16.
3. Listen first with the client in the sitting or supine position. Then, ask the client to lie on his or her left side, and focus on the apex. Finally, ask the client to sit up and lean forward. These position changes bring the heart closer to the chest wall and enhance auscultation. Carry out the following steps when the client assumes each of these positions:
   a. First, auscultate each area with the diaphragm of the stethoscope to listen for high-pitched sounds (S₁, S₂, murmurs, and pericardial friction rubs).
   b. Next, auscultate each area with the bell of the stethoscope to listen for lower-pitched sounds (S₃, S₄, and murmurs).
   c. Listen for the effect of respirations on each sound. While the client is sitting up and leaning forward, ask the client to exhale and hold the breath while you listen to heart sounds.

Figure 16–17 ●) is used for pulses that are difficult to assess. The DUS headset has earpieces similar to standard stethoscope earpieces, but it has a long cord attached to a volume-controlled audio unit and an ultrasound transducer. The DUS detects movement of red blood cells through a blood vessel. In contrast to the conventional stethoscope, it excludes environmental sounds.

A pulse is normally palpated by applying moderate pressure with the three middle fingers of the hand. The pads on the most

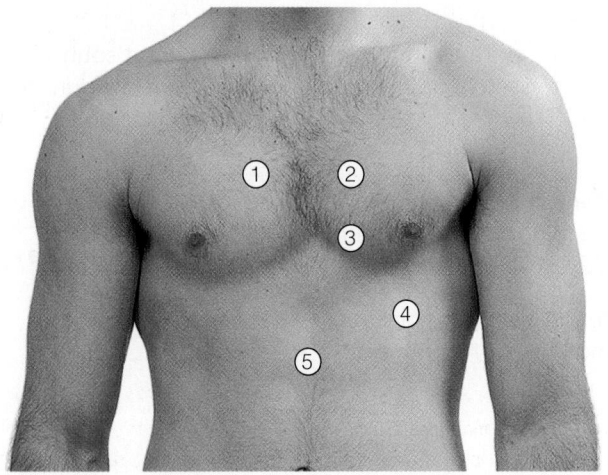

Figure 16–16 ● Areas for auscultation of the heart.

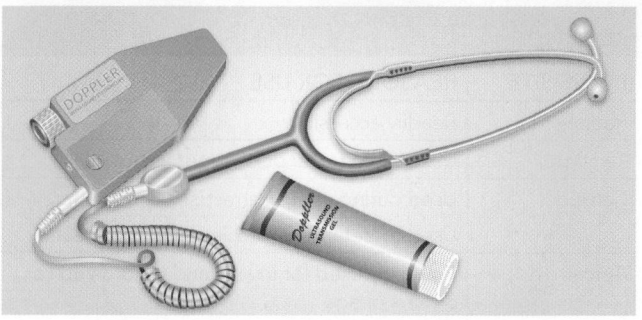

Figure 16–17 ● A Doppler ultrasound stethoscope (DUS).

distal aspects of the finger are the most sensitive areas for detecting a pulse. With excessive pressure one can obliterate a pulse, whereas with too little pressure one may not be able to detect it. Before the nurse assesses the resting pulse, the client should assume a comfortable position. The nurse should also be aware of the following:

- Any medication that could affect the heart rate.
- Whether the client has been physically active. If so, wait 10–15 minutes until the client has rested and the pulse has slowed to its usual rate.
- Any baseline data about the normal heart rate for the client. For example, a physically fit athlete may have a heart rate below 60 bpm.
- Whether the client should assume a particular position (e.g., sitting). In some clients, the rate changes with the position because of changes in blood flow volume and autonomic nervous system activity.

When assessing the pulse, the nurse collects the following data: the rate, rhythm, volume, arterial wall elasticity, and presence or absence of bilateral equality. An excessively fast heart rate (e.g., over 100 bpm in an adult) is referred to as **tachycardia**. A heart rate in an adult of less than 60 bpm is called **bradycardia**. If a client has either tachycardia or bradycardia, the apical pulse should be assessed.

The **pulse rhythm** is the pattern of the beats and the intervals between the beats. Equal time elapses between beats of a normal pulse. A pulse with an irregular rhythm is referred to as a **dysrhythmia** or **arrhythmia**. It may consist of random, irregular beats or a predictable pattern of irregular beats (documented as "regularly irregular"). When a dysrhythmia is detected, the apical pulse should be assessed. An ECG is necessary to define the dysrhythmia further.

Pulse volume, also called the pulse strength or amplitude, refers to the force of blood with each beat. Usually, the pulse volume is the same with each beat. It can range from absent to bounding. A normal pulse can be felt with moderate pressure of the fingers and can be obliterated with greater pressure. A forceful or full blood volume that is obliterated only with difficulty is called a full or bounding pulse. A pulse that is readily obliterated with pressure from the fingers is referred to as weak, feeble, or thready.

The **elasticity of the arterial wall** reflects its expansibility or its deformities. A healthy, normal artery feels straight, smooth, soft, and pliable. Older adults often have inelastic arteries that feel twisted (tortuous) and irregular upon palpation.

When assessing a peripheral pulse to determine the adequacy of blood flow to a particular area of the body (perfusion),

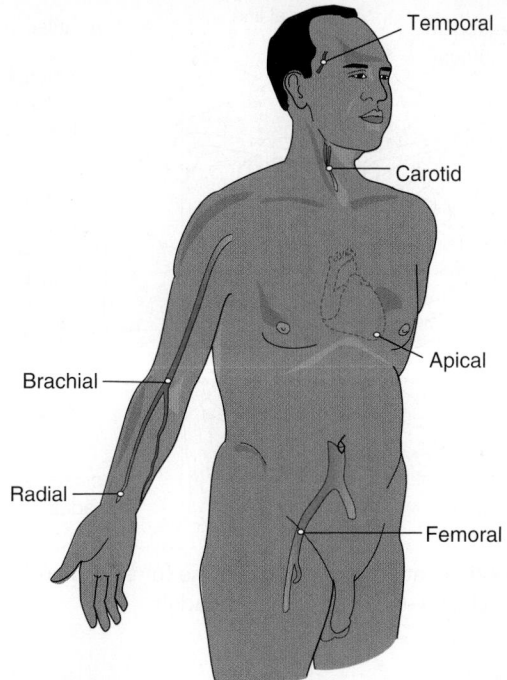

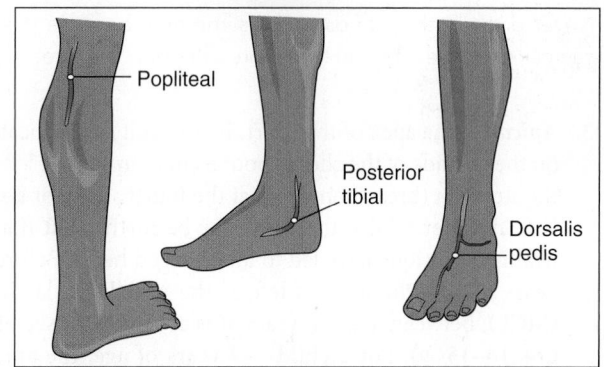

Figure 16–18 ● Nine sites for assessing pulse.

the nurse should also assess the corresponding pulse on the other side of the body. The second assessment gives the nurse data with which to compare the pulses. For example, when assessing the blood flow to the right foot, the nurse assesses the right dorsalis pedis pulse and then the left dorsalis pedis pulse. If the client's right and left pulses are the same, the client's dorsalis pedis pulses are bilaterally equal. The pulse rate does not need to be counted when assessing for perfusion and equality.

When a peripheral pulse is located, it indicates that pulses more proximal to that location will also be present. For example, if the dorsalis pedis, the most distal pulse of the lower extremity, cannot be felt, the nurse next palpates for the posterior tibial pulse. If it is not felt, the popliteal pulse must be assessed. If the popliteal pulse is found, it is not necessary to assess the femoral pulse since it must also be present in order for the more distal pulse to exist.

Pulse Sites   A pulse may be measured in nine sites (see **Figure 16–18** ●).

1. *Temporal*, where the temporal artery passes over the temporal bone of the head. The site is superior (above) and lateral to (away from the midline of) the eye.
2. *Carotid*, at the side of the neck where the carotid artery runs between the trachea and the sternocleidomastoid muscle.

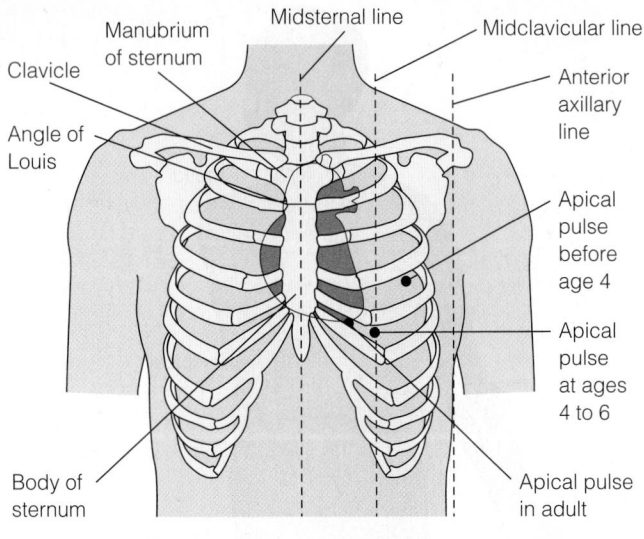

Figure 16–19 ● Location of the apical pulse for a child under 4 years old, a child 4–6 years old, and an adult.

SAFETY ALERT
Never press both carotids at the same time because this can cause a reflex drop in blood pressure or pulse rate.

---

3. **Apical**, at the apex of the heart. In an adult this is located on the left side of the chest, about 8 cm (3 in.) to the left of the sternum (breastbone) and at the fourth, fifth, or sixth ICS. In older adults, the apex may be further left if any health conditions have led to an enlarged heart. Before 4 years of age, the apex is left of the midclavicular line (MCL); between 4 and 6 years, it is at the MCL (see **Figure 16–19** ●). For a child 7–9 years of age, the apical pulse is located at the fourth or fifth intercostal space.
4. **Brachial**, at the inner aspect of the biceps muscle of the arm or medially in the antecubital space.
5. **Radial**, where the radial artery runs along the radial bone, on the thumb side of the inner aspect of the wrist.
6. **Femoral**, where the femoral artery passes alongside the inguinal ligament.
7. **Popliteal**, where the popliteal artery passes behind the knee.
8. **Posterior tibial**, on the medial surface of the ankle where the posterior tibial artery passes behind the medial malleolus.
9. **Pedal (dorsalis pedis)**, where the dorsalis pedis artery passes over the bones of the foot, on an imaginary line drawn from the middle of the ankle to the space between the big and second toes. The radial site is most commonly used in adults. It is easily found in most people and readily accessible. Some reasons for use of each site are given in **Table 16–7** ●.

Apical Pulse Assessment Assessment of the apical pulse is indicated for clients whose peripheral pulse is irregular or unavailable as well as for clients with known cardiovascular, pulmonary, and renal diseases. It is commonly assessed prior to administering medications that affect heart rate. The apical site is also used to assess the pulse for newborns, infants, and children 2–3 years old.

TABLE 16–7 Reasons for Using Specific Pulse Site

PULSE SITE	REASONS FOR USE
Radial	Readily accessible
Temporal	Used when radial pulse is not accessible
Carotid	Used during cardiac arrest/shock in adults
	Used to determine circulation to the brain
Apical	Routinely used for infants and children up to 3 years of age
	Used to determine discrepancies with radial pulse
	Used in conjunction with some medications
Brachial	Used to measure blood pressure
	Used during cardiac arrest for infants
Femoral	Used in cases of cardiac arrest/shock
	Used to determine circulation to a leg
Popliteal	Used to determine circulation to the lower leg
Posterior tibial	Used to determine circulation to the foot
Pedal	Used to determine circulation to the foot

Apical-Radial Pulse Assessment An **apical-radial pulse** may need to be assessed for clients with certain cardiovascular disorders. Normally, the apical and radial rates are identical. An apical pulse rate greater than a radial pulse rate can indicate that the thrust of the blood from the heart is too weak for the wave to be felt at the peripheral pulse site, or it can indicate that vascular disease is preventing impulses from being transmitted. Any discrepancy between the two pulse rates is called a pulse deficit and needs to be reported promptly. In no instance is the radial pulse greater than the apical pulse.

ASSESSING BLOOD PRESSURE Blood pressure is measured with a blood pressure cuff, a sphygmomanometer, and a stethoscope. The blood pressure cuff consists of a rubber bag (a bladder; see **Figure 16–20** ●) that can be inflated with air. It is covered with cloth and has two tubes attached to it. One tube connects to a rubber bulb that inflates the bladder. A small valve on the side of this bulb traps and releases the air in the bladder.

The other tube is attached to a sphygmomanometer. The sphygmomanometer indicates the pressure of the air within the bladder. The two types of sphygmomanometers are aneroid and digital. The aneroid sphygmomanometer is a calibrated dial with a needle that points to the calibrations (**Figure 16–21** ●).

Community-Based Care
Monitoring Pulse in the Home

■ Assist in obtaining and using an electronic pulse device if indicated.

■ Teach the client to monitor the pulse prior to taking medications that affect the heart rate. Tell the client to report any notable changes in heart rate or rhythm (regularity) to the healthcare provider.

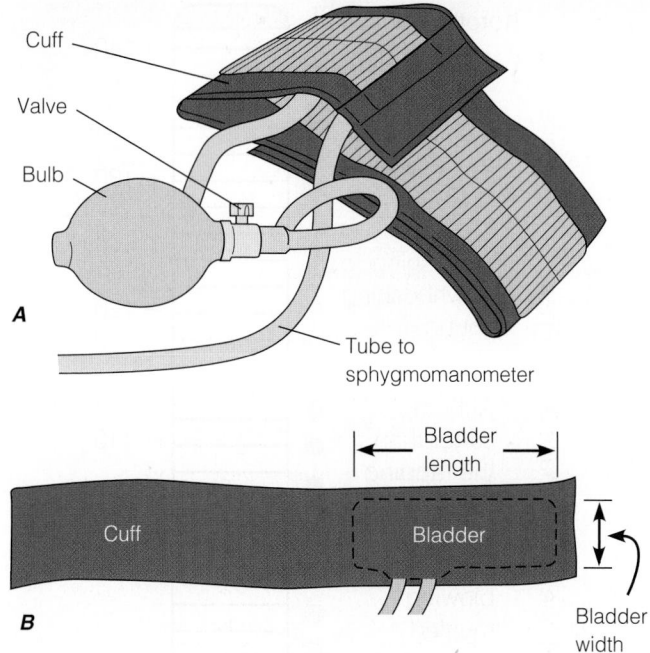

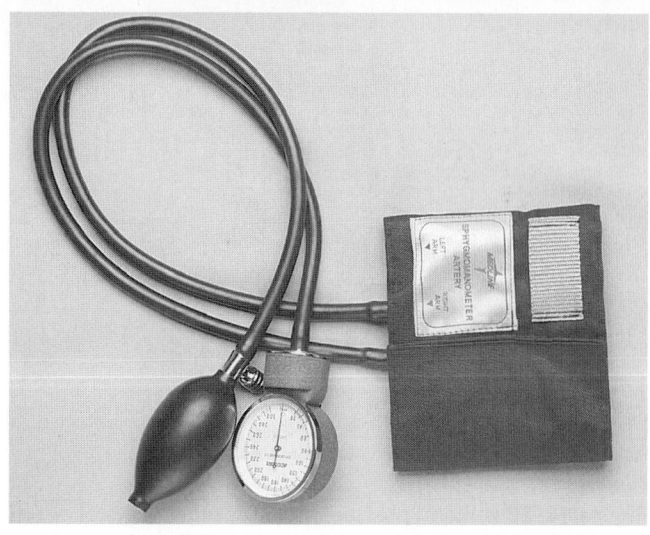

Figure 16–21 ● An aneroid sphygmomanometer and cuff.

Figure 16–20 ● A, A blood pressure cuff and bulb. B, The bladder inside the cuff.

Many agencies use digital (electronic) sphygmomanometers (**Figure 16–22 ●**), which eliminate the need to listen for the sounds of the client's systolic and diastolic blood pressures through a stethoscope. Electronic blood pressure devices should be calibrated periodically to check accuracy. All healthcare facilities should have manual blood pressure equipment available as backup.

Doppler ultrasound stethoscopes are also used to assess blood pressure (see Figure 16–17 earlier in the module). These are of particular value when blood pressure sounds are difficult to hear, such as in infants, clients with obesity, and clients in shock. Systolic pressure may be the only blood pressure obtainable with some ultrasound models.

Lifespan Considerations   Assessing the Pulse

Infants

■ Use the apical pulse for the heart rate of newborns, infants, and children 2–3 years old to establish baseline data for subsequent evaluation, to determine whether the cardiac rate is within normal range, and to determine if the rhythm is regular.

■ Place a baby in the supine position, and offer a pacifier if the baby is crying or restless. Crying and physical activity will increase the pulse rate. For this reason, take the apical pulse rate of infants and small children before assessing body temperatures.

■ Locate the apical pulse in the fourth intercostal space, lateral to the MCL during infancy.

■ Brachial, popliteal, and femoral pulses may be palpated. Due to a normally low blood pressure and rapid heart rate, infants' other distal pulses may be hard to feel.

■ Newborn infants may have heart murmurs that are not pathological, but reflect functional incomplete closure of fetal heart structures (ductus arteriosus or foramen ovale).

Children

■ To take a peripheral pulse, position the child comfortably in the adult's arms, or have the adult remain close by. This may decrease anxiety and yield more accurate results.

■ To assess the apical pulse, assist a young child to a comfortable supine or sitting position.

■ Demonstrate the procedure to the child using a stuffed animal or doll, and allow the child to handle the stethoscope before beginning the procedure. This will decrease anxiety and promote cooperation.

■ The apex of the heart is normally located in the fourth intercostal space in young children; in the fifth intercostal space in children 7 years of age and over.

■ Locate the apical impulse along the fourth intercostal space, between the MCL and the anterior axillary line (see Figure 16–19).

■ Count the pulse prior to other uncomfortable procedures so that the rate is not artificially elevated by the discomfort.

Older Adults

■ If the client has severe hand or arm tremors, the radial pulse may be difficult to count.

■ Cardiac changes in older adults, such as decrease in cardiac output, sclerotic changes to heart valves, and dysrhythmias, often indicate that obtaining an apical pulse will be more accurate.

■ Older adults often have decreased peripheral circulation, so pedal pulses should also be checked for regularity, volume, and symmetry.

■ The pulse returns to baseline after exercise more slowly than with other age groups.

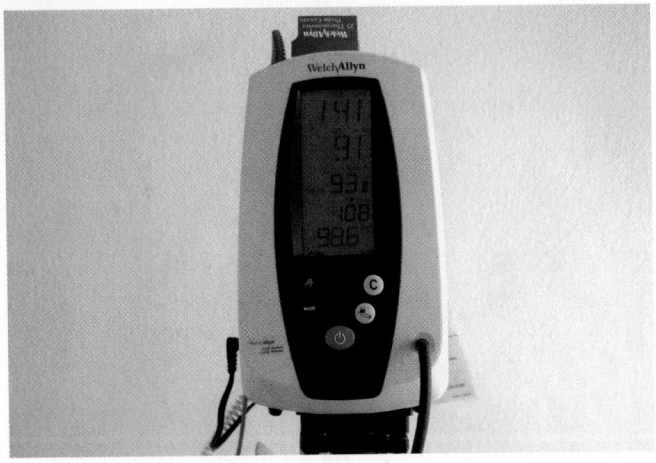

Figure 16–22 ● Blood pressure monitors register systolic and diastolic blood pressures and often other vital signs.

Blood Pressure Sites

The blood pressure is typically assessed in the client's upper arm using the brachial artery and a standard stethoscope. Assessing the blood pressure on a client's thigh may be indicated in these situations:

- The blood pressure cannot be measured on either arm (e.g., because of burns or other trauma).

- The blood pressure in one thigh is to be compared with the blood pressure in the other thigh.

Blood pressure is not measured on a particular client's limb in the following situations:

- The shoulder, arm, or hand (or the hip, knee, or ankle) is injured or diseased.

- A cast or bulky bandage is on any part of the limb.

- The client has had surgical removal of axilla (or hip) lymph nodes on that side, such as for cancer.

- The client has an intravenous infusion in that limb.

- The client has an arteriovenous fistula (e.g., for renal dialysis) in that limb.

Methods

Blood pressure can be assessed directly or indirectly. Direct (invasive monitoring) measurement involves the insertion of a catheter into the brachial, radial, or femoral artery. Arterial pressure is represented as wavelike forms displayed on a monitor. With correct placement, this pressure reading is highly accurate.

Two noninvasive methods of measuring blood pressure are the auscultatory and palpatory methods. The auscultatory method is most commonly used in hospitals, clinics, and homes. Required equipment is a sphygmomanometer, a cuff, and a stethoscope. When carried out correctly, the auscultatory method is relatively accurate.

When taking a blood pressure using a stethoscope, the nurse identifies phases in the series of sounds called **Korotkoff sounds (Figure 16–23 ●)**. First the nurse pumps the cuff up to about 30 mmHg above the point where the pulse is no longer felt, which is identified as the point when the blood flow in the artery is stopped. The pressure is then slowly released (2–3

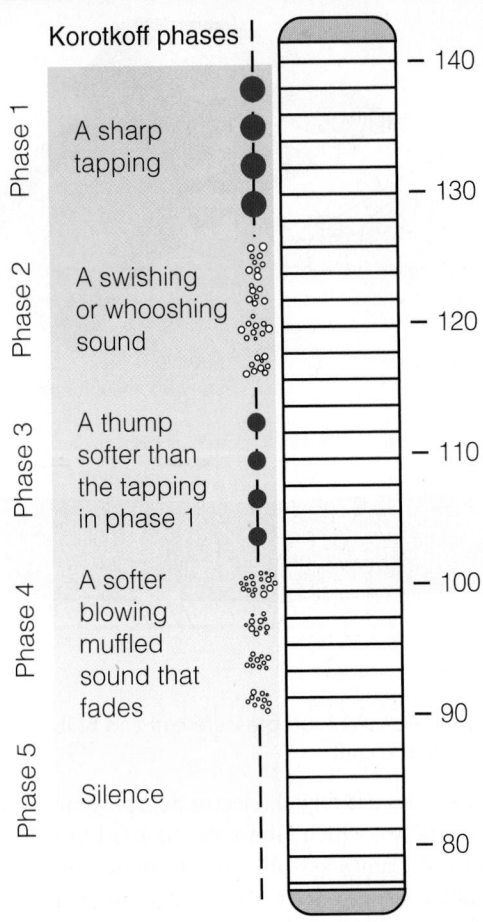

Figure 16–23 ● Korotkoff sounds can be differentiated into five phases. In the illustration, the blood pressure is 138/90 or 138/102/90 mmHg.

mmHg per second) while the nurse observes the readings on the manometer and relates them to the sounds heard through the stethoscope. Five phases occur but may not always be audible (see **Box 16–4 ●**).

The palpatory method may be used if the Korotkoff sounds cannot be heard and electronic equipment to amplify the sounds is not available. It may also be used to prevent misdirection from the presence of an auscultatory gap. An *auscultatory gap*, which occurs particularly in hypertensive clients, is the temporary disappearance of sounds normally heard over the brachial artery when the cuff pressure is high followed by the reappearance of the sounds at a lower level. This temporary disappearance of sounds occurs in the latter part of phase 1 and phase 2 and may cover a range of 40 mmHg. If a palpated estimation of the systolic pressure is not made prior to auscultation, the nurse may begin listening in the middle of this range and underestimate the systolic pressure. In the palpatory method of blood pressure determination, instead of listening for the blood flow sounds, the nurse uses light to moderate pressure to palpate the pulsations of the artery as the pressure in the cuff is released. The pressure is read from the sphygmomanometer when the first pulsation is felt.

Common Errors in Assessing Blood Pressure

The importance of the accuracy of blood pressure assessments can-

Box 16–4   Korotkoff Sounds

■ *Phase 1:* The pressure level at which the first faint, clear tapping or thumping sounds are heard. These sounds gradually become more intense. To ensure that they are not extraneous sounds, the nurse should identify at least two consecutive tapping sounds. The first tapping sound heard during deflation of the cuff is the systolic blood pressure.

■ *Phase 2:* The period during deflation when the sounds have a muffled, whooshing, or swishing quality.

■ *Phase 3:* The period during which the blood flows freely through an increasingly open artery and the sounds become crisper and more intense and again assume a thumping quality but softer than in phase 1.

■ *Phase 4:* The time when the sounds become muffled and have a soft, blowing quality.

■ *Phase 5:* T.he pressure level when the last sound is heard. This is followed by a period of silence. The pressure at which the last sound is heard is the diastolic blood pressure in adults.*

*In agencies where the fourth phase is considered the diastolic pressure, three measures are recommended (systolic pressure, diastolic pressure, and phase 5). These may be referred to as systolic, first diastolic, and second diastolic pressures. The phase 5 (second diastolic pressure) reading may be zero; that is, the muffled sounds are heard even when there is no air pressure in the blood pressure cuff. In some instances, muffled sounds may not be heard. In this case, a dash is inserted where the reading would normally be recorded (e.g., –/–/110 mmHg).

---

not be overemphasized. Many assessments about a client's health are made on the basis of blood pressure. They are an important indicator of the client's condition and are used as a basis for identifying nursing interventions. Two possible reasons for blood pressure errors are haste on the part of the nurse and subconscious bias. For example, a nurse may be influenced by the client's previous blood pressure measurements or diagnosis and "hear" a value consonant with the practitioner's expectations. Some reasons for erroneous blood pressure readings are given in **Table 16–8** ●.

SAFETY ALERT

Electronic/automatic blood pressure cuffs can be left in place for many hours. Remove the cuff and check skin condition periodically.

Hypotension   Hypotension is a below normal blood pressure reading—one that is consistently between 85 and 110 mmHg in an individual whose baseline blood pressure is typically higher. **Orthostatic hypotension** is a blood pressure that

Lifespan Considerations   Blood Pressure

Infants

■ Use a pediatric stethoscope with a small diaphragm.

■ The lower edge of the blood pressure cuff can be closer to the antecubital space of an infant.

■ Use the palpation method if auscultation with a stethoscope or DUS is unsuccessful.

■ Arm and thigh pressures are equivalent in children under 1 year of age.

■ One quick way to determine the normal systolic blood pressure of a child is to use the following formula:

Normal systolic BP = 80 + (2 × child's age in years)

Children

■ Blood pressure should be measured in all children over 3 years of age and in children under 3 years of age with certain medical conditions (e.g., congenital heart disease, renal malformation, medications that affect blood pressure).

■ Explain each step of the process and what it will feel like. Demonstrate on a doll.

■ Use the palpation technique for children under 3 years old.

■ Cuff bladder width should be 40% and length should be 80%–100% of the arm circumference (**Figure 16–24** ●).

■ Take the blood pressure prior to other uncomfortable procedures so that the blood pressure is not artificially elevated by the discomfort.

■ In children, the diastolic pressure is considered to be the onset of phase 4, where the sounds become muffled.

■ In children, the thigh pressure is about 10 mmHg higher than the arm pressure.

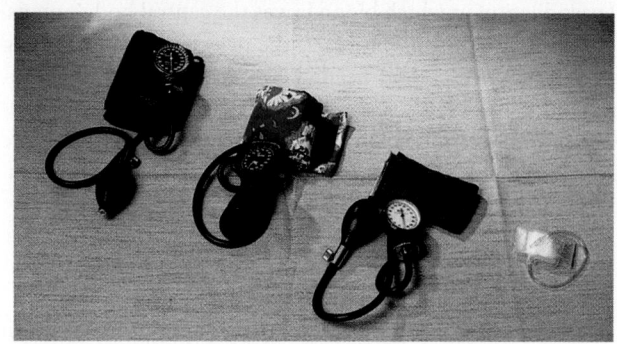

Figure 16–24 ● Pediatric blood pressure cuffs (with manometers).

Older Adults

■ Skin may be very fragile. Do not allow cuff pressure to remain high any longer than necessary.

■ Determine if the client is taking antihypertensives and, if so, when the last dose was taken.

■ Medications that cause vasodilation (antihypertensive medications) along with the loss of baroreceptor efficiency in older adults place them at increased risk for having orthostatic hypotension. Measuring blood pressure while the client is in the lying, sitting, and standing positions, and noting any changes can determine this.

■ If the client has arm contractures, assess the blood pressure by palpation, with the arm in a relaxed position. If this is not possible, take a thigh blood pressure.

TABLE 16–8 Selected Sources of Error in Blood Pressure Assessment

ERROR	EFFECT
Bladder cuff too narrow	Erroneously high
Bladder cuff too wide	Erroneously low
Arm unsupported	Erroneously high
Insufficient rest before the assessment	Erroneously high
Repeating assessment too quickly	Erroneously high systolic or low diastolic readings
Cuff wrapped too loosely or unevenly	Erroneously high
Deflating cuff too quickly	Erroneously low systolic and high diastolic readings
Deflating cuff too slowly	Erroneously high diastolic reading
Failure to use the same arm consistently	Inconsistent measurements
Arm above level of the heart	Erroneously low
Assessing immediately after a meal or while client smokes or has pain	Erroneously high
Failure to identify auscultatory gap	Erroneously low systolic pressure and erroneously low diastolic pressure

falls when the client sits or stands. It usually results from peripheral vasodilation in which blood leaves the central body organs, especially the brain, and moves to the periphery, often causing the individual to feel light-headed or faint. Causes of hypotension include dehydration, bleeding, severe burns, and analgesics such as meperidine hydrochloride (Demerol). Hypotensive clients should be carefully monitored for fall risks. When assessing for orthostatic hypotension:

- Place the client in a supine position for 10 minutes.
- Record the client's pulse and blood pressure.
- Assist the client to slowly sit or stand. Support the client in case of faintness.

Community-Based Care Taking Blood Pressure Readings in the Home

- If a client takes blood pressure readings at home, use the same equipment or calibrate it against a system known to be accurate.
- Observe the client or family member taking the blood pressure and provide feedback if further instruction is needed.
- The client may monitor blood pressures at home to establish a baseline or pattern of abnormal readings not seen in the physician's office or clinic.
- If the client is in a chair or low bed, position yourself so that you maintain the client's arm at heart level and you can read the sphygmomanometer at eye level.

- Immediately recheck the pulse and blood pressure in the same sites as previously.
- Repeat the pulse and blood pressure after 3 minutes.
- Record the results. A rise in pulse of 15–30 beats per minute or a drop in blood pressure of 20 mmHg systolic or 10 mmHg diastolic indicates orthostatic hypotension (Mayo Clinic, 2014).

HEALTH ASSESSMENT INTERVIEW A health assessment interview to determine problems with cardiac structure and function may be conducted during a health screening, may focus on a chief complaint (e.g., chest pain), or may be part of a total health assessment. If the client has a problem with cardiac function, analyze its onset, characteristics, course, severity, precipitating and relieving factors, and any associated symptoms, noting the timing and circumstances. For example, ask the client the following:

- What is the location of the chest pain you experienced? Did it move up to your jaw or into your left arm?
- Describe the type of activity that brings on your chest pain.
- Have you noticed any changes in your energy level?
- Have you felt light-headed during the times your heart is racing?

The interview begins by exploring the client's chief complaint (e.g., chest pain, palpitations, or shortness of breath). For the client with chest pain, assess in terms of location, quality or character, timing, setting or precipitating factors, severity, aggravating and relieving factors, and associated symptoms (Table 16–9 ●).

Explore the client's history for heart disorders, such as angina, heart attack, congestive heart failure, hypertension, and

TABLE 16–9 Assessing Chest Pain

CHARACTERISTIC	EXAMPLES
Location	Substernal, precordial, jaw, back; Localized or diffuse; Radiation to neck, jaw, shoulder, arm
Character/quality	Pressure; tightness; crushing, burning, or aching quality; heaviness; dullness; "heartburn" or indigestion
Timing	Onset: Sudden or gradual? Duration: How many minutes does the pain last? Frequency: Is the pain continuous or periodic?
Setting/precipitating factors	Awake, at rest, sleep interrupted? With activity? With eating, exertion, exercise, elimination, emotional upset?
Intensity/severity	Can range from 0 (no pain) to 10 (worst pain ever felt)
Aggravating factors	Activity, breathing, temperature
Relieving factors	Medication (nitroglycerin, antacid), rest; there may be no relieving factors
Associated symptoms	Fatigue, shortness of breath, palpitations, nausea and vomiting, sweating, anxiety, light-headedness, dizziness

Assessment Interview Perfusion

Current and Past Medical History

- Have you ever had any problems with your heart, such as angina (pain), heart attack, or disease of the valves? If so, describe. How were these problems treated?
- Have you been diagnosed with high blood pressure? If so, how is it treated?
- Do you have a history of rheumatic fever, scarlet fever, or strep throat infections? If so, describe them and their treatment.
- Have you had your cholesterol checked recently? If so, what is it? If you have high cholesterol, how is it treated?
- Have you ever had tests to check the function of your heart? If so, describe them.
- Do you take any medications to make your heart function more effectively, such as aspirin, those to control heart rate, anticoagulants, or diuretics? If so, how often do you take them?
- Do you have a pacemaker? If so, at what age did you receive it, and for what problem? How do you check the batteries?

Lifestyle

- Do you smoke, chew tobacco, or use snuff? If so, how often and how much?
- Do you drink alcohol? If so, what type, how much, and for how long?
- Are you able to manage your activities of daily living and work independently? Explain.
- Describe your food and liquid intake during a 24-hour period. How often do you eat fried foods, fast foods, or meat?
- How much salt do you use on food?
- Do you eat high-fiber foods? If so, what are they, and how often do you eat them?

Signs and Symptoms

- Have you had a recent weight gain or loss? Explain.
- Have you noticed any change in the color of your skin (e.g., pale or dusky or flushed)? If so, do you know what causes this?
- Have you had any swelling in your feet or legs? If so, where and how much? What do you do to relieve it?
- Describe any chest pain you have experienced. When did it occur? Where was it located? On a scale of 0–10, with 10 being the worst pain you have ever had, rate the pain and describe it (e.g., burning, crushing, stabbing, squeezing, heavy, or tight).
- What were you doing when the pain began (e.g., were you working or resting)? Did it begin suddenly or gradually? How long did it last?

- Did you have any other symptoms with the pain, such as nausea or vomiting, sweating, racing heart, pale skin, palpitations?
- What made the pain worse? What did you do to try to relieve the pain? Did that work?
- Describe any cough you have had. Was it dry or wet? Do you cough up mucus? If so, what color is it? How long have you had the cough?
- Have you experienced any numbness or tingling, dizziness or light-headedness, or palpitations? If so, describe.
- Have you ever used oxygen?

Sleep and Rest

- How long do you sleep each night? Do you feel rested after you sleep?
- Does your heart problem interfere with your ability to sleep and rest? Explain.
- How many pillows do you use at night?
- Where do you sleep at night (e.g., in a recliner to breathe more easily)?
- Do you ever feel short of breath while you are resting or sleeping? If so, does this wake you up? Explain.

Self

- How does having this condition make you feel about yourself?
- How does this condition affect your relationships with others?
- Has having this condition interfered with your ability to work? Explain.
- Has this condition interfered with your usual sexual activity?
- Have you ever had chest pain during sexual activity? What do you do for it?
- Do you use a slower pace or different positions that are less stressful for you during sexual activities? Does this help?

Stress and Coping

- Has having this condition created stress for you?
- Have you experienced any kind of stress that makes this condition worse? Explain.
- Describe what you do when you feel stressed.
- Describe how specific relationships or activities help you cope with this problem.
- Describe specific cultural beliefs or practices that affect how you care for and feel about this problem.
- Are there any specific treatments that you would not use to treat this problem?

---

valvular disease. Ask the client about previous heart surgery or illnesses, such as rheumatic fever, scarlet fever, or recurrent streptococcal throat infections. Also ask about the presence and treatment of other chronic illnesses, such as diabetes mellitus, bleeding disorders, or endocrine disorders. Review the client's family history for coronary artery disease, hypertension, stroke, hyperlipidemia, diabetes, congenital heart disease, or sudden death. See the Assessment Interview for interview questions and leading statements.

Ask the client about past or present occurrence of various cardiac symptoms, such as chest pain, shortness of breath, difficulty breathing, cough, palpitations, fatigue, light-headedness or dizziness, fainting, heart murmur, blood clots, or swelling. Because cardiac function affects all other body systems, a full history may need to explore other related systems, such as respiratory function and/or peripheral vascular function.

Review the client's personal habits and nutritional history, including body weight; eating patterns; dietary intake of fats, salt, and fluids; dietary restrictions; hypersensitivities or intolerances to food or medication; and use of caffeine and alcohol. If the client uses tobacco products, ask about type (e.g., cigarettes, pipe, cigars, or snuff), duration, amount, and efforts to quit. If the client uses street drugs, ask about type, method of intake (e.g., inhaled or injected), duration of use, and efforts to quit. Include questions about the client's activity level and tolerance, recreational activities, and relaxation habits. Assess the client's sleep patterns for interruptions in sleep caused by dyspnea, cough, discomfort, urination, or stress. Ask how many pillows the client uses when sleeping.

Also consider psychosocial factors that may affect the client's stress level: What is the client's marital status, family composition, and role within the family? Have there been any changes? What is the client's occupation, level of education, and socioeconomic level? Are resources for support available? What is the client's emotional disposition and personality type? How does the client perceive his or her state of health or illness, and how able is the client to comply with treatment?

Diagnostic Tests

The results of diagnostic tests of cardiac function are used to support the diagnosis of a specific disease, to provide information to identify or modify the appropriate medications or therapy used to treat the disease, and to help nurses monitor the client's responses to treatment and nursing care interventions. Diagnostic tests appropriate for determining cardiac function may include the following:

- Serum cholesterol, triglycerides, and lipids
- Stress/exercise tests
- X-ray, magnetic resonance imaging (MRI), computed tomography (CT), or positron-emission tomography test
- Echocardiogram
- A transesophageal echocardiogram
- Cardiac catheterization with either coronary angiography or coronary arteriography
- Pericardiocentesis
- Electrocardiography (see **Boxes 16–5** ● and **16–6** ●)
- Troponin, MB isoenzyme of creatine kinase.

Regardless of the type of diagnostic test, the nurse is responsible for explaining the procedure and any special preparation needed, assessing for medication use that may affect the outcome of the tests, supporting the client during the examination as necessary, documenting the procedures as appropriate, and monitoring the results of the tests.

CASE STUDY \\ PART 2

Mr. Evans is transferred to the ICU and placed on cardiac monitoring. A CVA care path is initiated. A CT scan confirms an ischemic stroke of the right parietal/temporal region and he continues to

have trouble managing his secretions. His work of breathing is increasing. Supplemental O_2 is now being delivered via nonrebreather mask. His O_2 sats are in the high 80s. VS are now T 99.8°F; P 94 bpm; R 26/min; and BP 120/76 mmHg.

Thirty-six hours after admission, you notice bilateral crackles in the lungs. Upon auscultation, you note they are worse on the right side. Mr. Evans has pitting edema in his lower extremities and his urine output has significantly decreased. He is difficult to arouse and is oriented to person only. Physician and respiratory therapy have been called to assess the need for possible mechanical ventilation.

Clinical Reasoning Questions Level I

1. Describe the pathophysiology of an ischemic stroke.
2. Why might Mr. Evans's urine output be decreasing?
3. If you were going to ask the off-going nurse three questions, what would they be? Why?

Clinical Reasoning Questions Level II

4. Identify two potential alterations in perfusion that may arise as complications of the CVA.
5. What signs/symptoms are indicative of increased intracranial pressure (ICP)?
6. How does increased ICP affect cerebral perfusion pressure?

▶ INTERVENTIONS AND THERAPIES

Independent

Nursing interventions are aimed at supporting, improving, and promoting perfusion adequate to meet the client's oxygenation needs and prevent tissue damage. Depending on the disease process involved, this may include caring interventions to reduce stress on the heart, decrease cardiac workload, increase the efficacy of cardiac contractions, and meet fluid needs.

Nurses also provide teaching at a primary level to reduce the risk of cardiac disease in later life. Lifestyle modifications, such as reducing fat intake, aerobic exercise adequate to attain optimal heart rate, and eating a well-balanced diet, are influential in reducing the risk of coronary artery disease.

Once an initial assessment of a client for alterations in perfusion has been made, the nurse develops a plan of care and prioritizes nursing interventions. Interventions for circulatory problems usually fall into three broad categories: inputs, outputs, and pressure supports. Inputs include arterial lines, venous lines, fluids, drug regimens, transfusions, and blood component therapies. Outputs include suctioning with specialized equipment such as a Hemovac and chest tubes and procedures such as thoracentesis. Pressure supports include dressings, direct compression, tourniquets, and cardiopulmonary resuscitation. An evaluation of the planned actions, based on the client's response, should be continuous and modified as the client's condition dictates.

In coping with alterations in perfusion, care should be directed toward promoting, maintaining, or regaining the best possible cardiopulmonary function. The design for nursing management is to assess the situation and client for stressors. The client should be interviewed, observed, and examined to identify actual and/or potential circulatory problems. The client's responses are determined to be appropriate, deficient, or excessive, and interventions

Box 16–5   The Electrocardiogram

The **electrocardiogram (ECG)** is a graphic record of the heart's activity. Electrodes applied to the body surface are used to obtain a graphic representation of cardiac electrical activity. These electrodes detect the magnitude and direction of electrical currents produced in the heart. They attach to the electrocardiograph by an insulated wire called a **lead**. The electrocardiograph converts the electrical impulses it receives into a series of waveforms that represent cardiac depolarization and repolarization. Placement of electrodes on different parts of the body allows different views of this electrical activity, much like turning the head while holding a camera provides different views of the scenery. ECG waveforms and patterns are examined to detect dysrhythmias as well as myocardial damage, effects of drugs, and electrolyte imbalances.

The ECG waveforms reflect the direction of electrical flow in relation to a positive electrode. Current flowing toward the positive electrode produces an upward (positive) waveform; current flowing away from the positive electrode produces a downward (negative) waveform. Current flowing perpendicular to the positive pole produces a biphasic (both positive and negative) waveform. Absence of electrical activity is represented by a straight line, referred to as the **isoelectric line**.

The ECG waveforms are recorded by a heated stylus and reproduced on heat-sensitive paper. The paper is marked at standard intervals representing time and voltage or amplitude (**Figure 16–25** ●). Each small box is 1 mm². The recording speed of the standard ECG is 25 mm/second, so each small box represents 0.04 second. Five small boxes horizontally and vertically make one large box, equivalent to 0.20 second. Five large boxes represent 1 full second. Measured vertically, each small box represents 0.1 mV.

Both bipolar and unipolar leads are used in recording the ECG. A bipolar lead uses two electrodes of opposite polarity (negative and positive). A unipolar lead uses one positive electrode and a negative reference point at the center of the heart. The electrical potential between the two monitoring points is graphically recorded as the ECG waveform.

The heart can be viewed from both the frontal plane and the horizontal plane (**Figure 16–26** ●). Each plane provides a unique perspective of the heart muscle. The frontal plane is an imaginary cut through the body that views the heart from top to bottom (superior to inferior) and side to side (right to left). This perspective of the heart is analogous to a paper doll cutout. It provides information about the inferior and lateral walls of the heart. The horizontal plane is a cross-sectional view of the heart from front to back (anterior to posterior) and side to side (right to left). Information regarding the

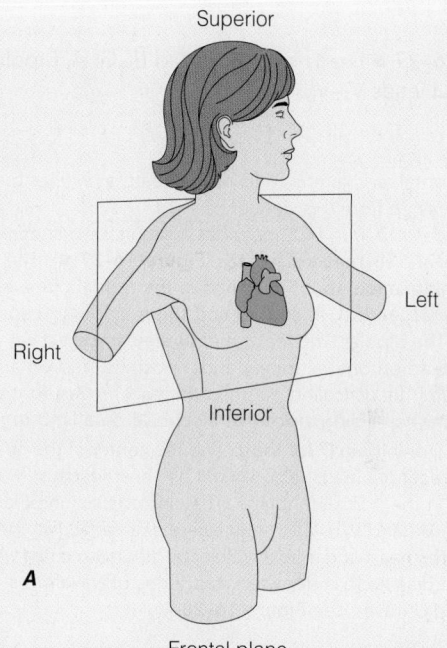

A

Frontal plane

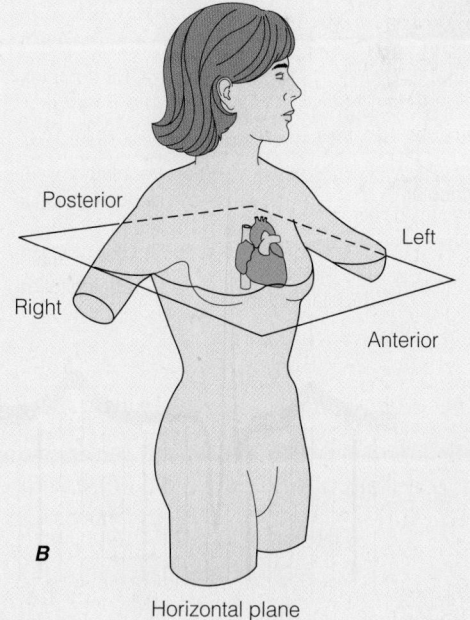

B

Horizontal plane

1 large box or 5 mm = 0.5 mV

1 large box or 5 mm = 0.20 Second

1 small box or 1 mm = 0.04 Second

1 mm = 0.1 mV

Figure 16–25 ● Time and voltage measurements on ECG paper at a recording speed of 25 mm/second.

Figure 16–26 ● Planes of the heart. *A*, Frontal plane. *B*, Horizontal plane.

(continued on next page)

Box 16–5 **The Electrocardiogram** (*continued*)

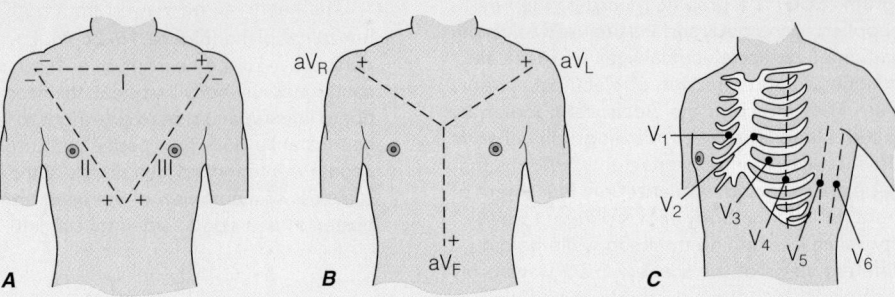

Figure 16–27 ● Leads of the 12-lead ECG. *A*, Bipolar limb leads I, II, III. *B*, Unipolar limb leads aV$_R$, aV$_L$, aV$_F$. *C*, Unipolar precordial leads V$_1$–V$_6$.

anterior, septal, and lateral walls of the heart, as well as the posterior wall, is obtained from this view.

A standard 12-lead ECG provides a simultaneous recording of six limb leads and six precordial leads (**Figure 16–27 ●**). The limb leads provide information about the heart in the frontal plane and include three bipolar leads (I, II, and III) and three unipolar leads (aV$_R$, aV$_L$, and aV$_F$). The bipolar limb leads measure electrical activity between a negative lead on one extremity and a positive lead on another. The unipolar limb leads (called augmented leads) measure the electrical activity between a single positive electrode on a limb (right arm [R], left arm [L], or left leg [F for foot]), and the center of the heart.

The precordial leads, also known as chest leads or V leads, view the heart in the horizontal plane. They include six unipolar leads (V$_1$, V$_2$, V$_3$, V$_4$, V$_5$, and V$_6$), which measure electrical activity between the center of the heart and a positive electrode on the chest wall.

The cardiac cycle is depicted as a series of waveforms, the P, Q, R, S, T, and U waves (see **Figure 16–28 ●**):

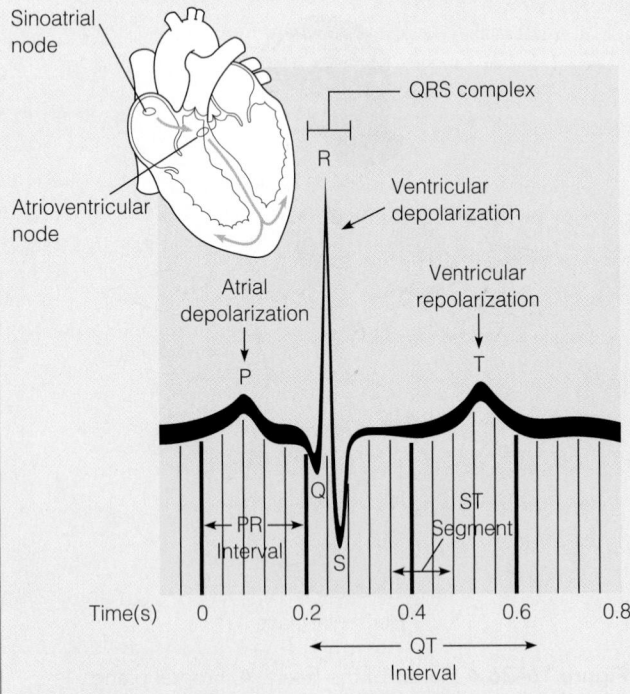

Figure 16–28 ● Normal ECG waveform and intervals.

■ The *P wave* represents atrial depolarization and contraction. The impulse is from the sinoatrial node. The P wave precedes the QRS complex and is normally smooth, round, and upright. P waves may be absent when the SA node is not acting as the pacemaker. Atrial repolarization occurs during ventricular depolarization and usually is not seen on the ECG.

■ The *PR interval* represents the time required for the sinus impulse to travel to the AV node and into the Purkinje fibers. This interval is measured from the beginning of the P wave to the beginning of the QRS complex. If no Q wave is seen, the beginning of the R wave is used. The PR interval is normally 0.12–0.20 second (up to 0.24 second is considered normal in clients over age 65). PR intervals greater than 0.20 second indicate a delay in conduction from the SA node to the ventricles.

■ The *QRS complex* represents ventricular depolarization and contraction. The QRS complex includes three separate waves: The Q wave is the first negative deflection, the R wave is the positive or upright deflection, and the S wave is the first negative deflection after the R wave. All three waves may not be present in every QRS but the name remains unchanged. The normal duration of a QRS complex is from 0.06 to 0.10 second. QRS complexes of greater than 0.10 second indicate delays in transmitting the impulse through the ventricular conduction system.

■ The *ST segment* signifies the beginning of ventricular repolarization. The ST segment, which is the period from the end of the QRS complex to the beginning of the T wave, should be isoelectric. An abnormal ST segment is displaced (elevated or depressed) from the isoelectric line.

■ The *T wave* represents ventricular repolarization. It normally has a smooth, rounded shape that is usually less than 10 mm tall. It usually points in the same direction as the QRS complex. Abnormalities of the T wave may indicate myocardial ischemia or injury or electrolyte imbalances.

■ The *QT interval* is measured from the beginning of the QRS complex to the end of the T wave. It represents the total time of ventricular depolarization and repolarization. Its duration varies with gender, age, and heart rate; usually, it is 0.32–0.44 second long. Prolonged QT intervals indicate a prolonged relative refractory period and a greater risk of dysrhythmias. Shortened QT intervals may result from medications or electrolyte imbalances.

■ The *U wave* is not normally seen. It is thought to signify repolarization of the terminal Purkinje fibers. If present, the U wave follows the same direction as the T wave. It is most commonly seen in hypokalemia.

Box 16–6   Interpreting an Electrocardiogram

Interpreting an electrocardiogram strip to determine the cardiac rhythm is a skill that takes practice to learn and master. Many methods are used to analyze ECGs, and it is important to use a consistent method for such analysis. Identifying and interpreting complex dysrhythmias require advanced skills and knowledge obtained through further training. One method for analyzing an ECG strip is the following:

■ *Step 1: Determine rate.* Assess heart rate. Use P waves to determine the atrial rate and R waves for the ventricular rate. Several approaches can determine the heart rate:

  a. Count the number of complexes in a 6-second rhythm strip (the top margin of ECG paper is marked at 3-second intervals), and multiply by 10. This provides an estimate of the rate and is particularly valuable if rhythms are irregular.

  b. Count the number of large boxes between two consecutive complexes, and divide 300 (the number of large boxes in 1 min) by this number. For example, there are 6 large boxes between two R waves; 300 divided by 6 equals a ventricular rate of 50 bpm. Memorize the following sequence for rapid rate determination: 300, 150, 100, 75, 60, 50, 43. One large box between complexes equals a rate of 300; two large boxes, a rate of 150; three, a rate of 100; and so on.

  c. Count the number of small boxes between two consecutive complexes, and divide 1,500 (the number of small boxes in 1 min) by this number. For example, there are 19 small boxes between two R waves; 1,500 divided by 19 equals a ventricular rate of 79 bpm. This is the most precise measurement of heart rate.

■ *Step 2: Determine regularity.* Regularity is the consistency with which the P waves or QRS complexes occur. In a regular rhythm, all waves occur at a consistent rate. Rhythm regularity is determined by measuring the interval between consecutive waves. Place one point of an ECG caliper (a measuring device) on the peak of the P wave (for atrial rhythm) or the R wave (for ventricular rhythm). Adjust the other point to the peak of the next wave, P to P or R to R (**Figure 16–29 ●**). Keeping the calipers set at this distance, evaluate the intervals between consecutive waves. The rhythm is regular if all caliper points fall on succeeding wave peaks. Alternately, use a strip of blank paper on top of the ECG strip, and mark the peaks of two or three consecutive waves. Then, move the paper along the strip to consecutive waves. Wave peaks that vary by more than one to three small boxes (depending on the rate) are irregular. Irregular rhythms may be irregularly irregular (if the intervals have no pattern) or regularly irregular (if a consistent pattern to the irregularity can be identified).

■ *Step 3: Assess P waves.* The presence or absence of P waves helps determine the origin of the rhythm. All the P waves should be alike in size and shape (morphology). If P waves are not seen

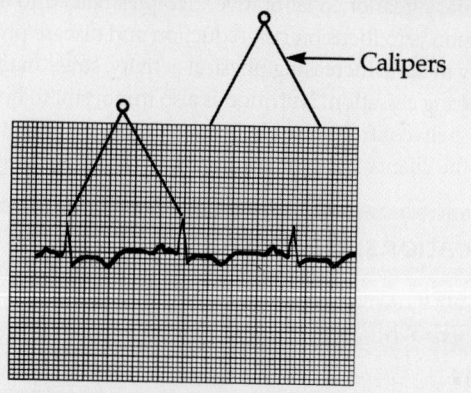

Figure 16–29 ● Using calipers to evaluate intervals between consecutive waves.

or if they differ in shape, the rhythm may not originate in the sinoatrial node.

■ *Step 4: Assess the P to QRS relationship.* Determine the relationship between P waves and QRS complexes. There should be one—and only one—P wave for every QRS complex, because the normal stimulus for ventricular contraction originates in the sinoatrial node.

■ *Step 5: Determine interval durations.* To evaluate impulse transmission through the cardiac conduction system, measure the PR interval, QRS duration, and QT interval. To measure, count the number of small boxes from the beginning of the interval to the end, and multiply by 0.04 second. Then, determine whether the interval duration is within its normal limits. For example, assume the PR interval is 3.5 small boxes wide, or 0.14 second. This is within the normal limits of 0.12–0.20 second. This interval should be consistent, not varying from beat to beat. A PR interval of greater than 0.20 second or one that varies from beat to beat is abnormal.

The QRS complex duration is normally between 0.06 and 0.10 second. A QRS complex of greater than 0.12 second indicates delayed ventricular conduction.

The QT interval is normally 0.32–0.44 second. It varies inversely with the heart rate: The faster the heart rate, the shorter the QT interval. As a general rule, the QT interval should be no more than half the previous R–R interval. A prolonged QT interval indicates a prolonged relative refractory period of the heart.

■ *Step 6: Identify abnormalities.* Note the presence and frequency of **ectopic** (extra) beats, deviation of the ST segment above or below the baseline, and abnormalities in waveform shape and duration.

---

are planned accordingly. The nurse attempts to reduce client stress, support adaptive behaviors, replace deficiencies, modify or remove excessive responses, and prevent injury and complications. As a priority, the nurse should assist in the evaluation of planned actions, report client responses, and assist in modifying the interventions as indicated.

Skills used to care for the client with perfusion-related problems include the following:

■ Assessing pulses

■ Recording and interpreting an ECG

■ Administering cardiopulmonary resuscitation

■ Achieving defibrillation

■ Measuring for and application of elastic compression stockings

■ Fetal monitoring

■ Applying sequential compression devices

■ Applying continuous cardiorespiratory monitoring

■ Obtaining capillary wedge pressures

■ Measuring cardiac output

■ Reading central and peripheral blood pressures

■ Caring for the client with an arterial pressure monitor.

Collaborative

The primary goal of collaborative therapies related to alterations in perfusion is to focus on risk reduction and disease progression. This may include increasing physical activity, stress management, and smoking cessation. Nutrition is also important to heart health and may help control some CAD risk factors. Treatment is dependent on the client's symptoms and severity of underlying disease.

PHARMACOLOGIC THERAPY Many of the medications administered by nurses have an impact on perfusion. Beta-blockers, antihypertensives, cardiac glycosides, and even some narcotics, such as morphine sulfate, have a profound impact on cardiac functioning and perfusion. The Medications feature describes some of the more commonly prescribed medications.

Medications **Perfusion**

CLASSIFICATION AND DRUG EXAMPLES	MECHANISMS OF ACTION	NURSING CONSIDERATIONS
Statins *Drug examples:* ▪ atorvastatin ▪ fluvastatin ▪ lovastatin ▪ pravastatin	Inhibit 3-hydroxy-3-methylglutaryl coenzyme (HMG-CoA), a reductase, which results in less cholesterol biosynthesis.	▪ Assess triglyceride, total cholesterol, low-density lipoprotein, and high-density lipoprotein levels. ▪ Avoid in clients who are or may become pregnant or are nursing. ▪ Monitor liver function tests. ▪ Avoid in clients with liver disease or heavy alcohol consumption. ▪ Teach client to avoid alcohol while taking. ▪ Assess for muscle pain, tenderness, or weakness.
Antihypertensives *Diuretics* *Drug examples:* ▪ furosemide ▪ hydrochlorothiazide ▪ bumetanide ▪ triamterene ▪ spironolactone ▪ metolazone	Reduce fluid volume in the vessels.	▪ Monitor serum electrolyte levels. ▪ Obtain client's weight daily. ▪ Teach client importance of compliance with the medication regimen. ▪ Assess hydration status. ▪ Monitor breath sounds for fluid volume excess.
Angiotensin-converting enzyme (ACE) inhibitors and angiotensin II receptor blockers *Drug examples:* ▪ benazepril ▪ captopril ▪ lisinopril ▪ losartan ▪ valsartan	Angiotensin II is a potent natural vasoconstrictor; its actions are blocked by ACE inhibitors and angiotensin inhibitors.	▪ Follow vital sign changes. ▪ First dose may cause severe hypotension, so monitor BP carefully. ▪ The first dose is best administered at bedtime. ▪ Monitor BP carefully if given intravenously (IV), and with subsequent alteration in level of consciousness if this occurs. ▪ Assess for angioedema, which can be life threatening. ▪ Monitor complete blood count for neutropenia or agranulocytosis.
Combination Drugs *Drug examples:* ▪ Combines hydrochlorothiazide with propranolol, metoprolol, timolol, or bisoprolol	These contain a diuretic, usually a potassium-sparing diuretic, and another class of drugs, such as adrenergic agents or ACE inhibitors.	▪ Monitor serum electrolyte levels. ▪ Obtain client's weight daily. ▪ Teach client importance of compliance with the medication regimen. ▪ Assess hydration status. ▪ Monitor breath sounds for fluid volume excess.
Vasodilators *Drug examples:* ▪ diazoxide ▪ hydralazine ▪ minoxidil ▪ nitroprusside	These cause dilation of blood vessels.	▪ These may produce reflex tachycardia. ▪ These may produce angina in clients with coronary artery disease. ▪ Monitor for sodium and water retention. ▪ IV nitroprusside is the drug of choice for treating hypertensive emergency, but care must be taken not to drop BP too quickly. Metabolizes to cyanide, so careful monitoring is required.
Adrenergic Antagonists *Drug examples:* ▪ beta-blockers (atenolol, metoprolol) ▪ alpha$_1$-antagonists (doxazosin, prazosin) ▪ alpha$_2$-agonists (clonidine, methyldopa) ▪ alpha$_1$- and beta-blocker (labetalol) ▪ adrenergic neuron blockers (guanadrel, reserpine)	These reduce autonomic nervous system effects by blocking beta$_1$-adrenergic receptor sites in the heart, blocking alpha$_1$-adrenergic receptors in arterioles, stimulating alpha$_2$ receptors in the brainstem, and/or blocking peripheral adrenergic neurons.	▪ Monitor vital signs. ▪ Hold medication if heart rate is <60 bpm or if BP is <90/60 mmHg. ▪ Use care when ambulating, monitoring for potential orthostatic hypotension. ▪ Monitor clients with diabetes for hypoglycemia.

Medications **Perfusion** (*continued*)

CLASSIFICATION AND DRUG EXAMPLES	MECHANISMS OF ACTION	NURSING CONSIDERATIONS
Calcium-Channel Blockers *Drug examples:* ▪ nifedipine ▪ verapamil ▪ diltiazem	Treats angina, dysrhythmias, and hypertension, reducing available calcium, muscular contractility, peripheral vascular resistance, and BP.	▪ Obtain baseline ECG, heart rate, and BP before beginning therapy. ▪ Teach client to maintain a daily BP log and about the need for compliance with the medication regimen. ▪ Contraindicated in clients with third-degree block of sick sinus syndrome. ▪ Monitor for tachycardia and hypotension if administered IV. ▪ Teach client to avoid grapefruit juice.
Cardiac Glycosides *Drug example:* ▪ digoxin	Causes the heart to beat more forcefully and more slowly, improving cardiac output (positive inotropic affect).	▪ Monitor serum potassium. ▪ Administer with caution to older adults and to those post–myocardial infarction or with incomplete heart block or renal insufficiency. ▪ Side effects such as drowsiness, fatigue, dizziness, visual disturbances, anorexia, nausea, or vomiting may indicate toxic levels. ▪ Follow serum drug levels in order to maintain therapeutic levels.
Phosphodiesterase Inhibitors *Drug example:* ▪ milrinone	Block the enzyme phosphodiesterase in cardiac and smooth muscle, increasing the amount of calcium available for myocardial contraction, which results in positive inotropic actions and vasodilation.	▪ Assess serum potassium levels. ▪ Monitor for dysrhythmia. ▪ During IV administration, monitor for ventricular dysrhythmias.
Nitrates *Drug examples:* ▪ amyl nitrite ▪ isosorbide dinitrate ▪ nitroglycerin	Potent vasodilators that dilate both arterial and venous smooth muscle. Dilation of veins reduces preload.	▪ Monitor BP frequently for hypotension. ▪ To prevent falls, reduce dizziness, and reduce the oxygen demands on the heart, have client lie down when taking this medication for chest pain. ▪ Teach client how to take medication when having chest pain and how often it may be repeated before calling 911. ▪ Contraindicated in clients with cardiac tamponade and pericarditis or clients with head injury, shock, and increased intracranial pressure. ▪ Teach client to avoid alcohol consumption, which can lead to severe hypotension and cardiovascular collapse.
Thrombolytics *Drug examples:* ▪ reteplase ▪ tissue plasminogen activator (t-PA) ▪ alteplase ▪ streptokinase ▪ urokinase	Administered to dissolve clots resulting in myocardial infarction or stroke, with quick restoration of circulation.	▪ Must be administered within 12 hours of symptom onset; best if given within 4 hours. ▪ Research suggests clients older than 75 years do not experience reduced mortality from these drugs. ▪ Monitor clients carefully for bleeding, because all clots, even those formed as the result of venipuncture, are dissolved. ▪ In clients who may be receiving thrombolytics, attempt to minimize invasive procedures in order to avoid future bleeding sites. ▪ Do not administer to clients who have recently (within the past 2 weeks) fallen, been involved in a motor vehicle crash, or experienced any form of trauma. ▪ Closely monitor cardiac rhythm, because return of perfusion to the blocked vessel often results in reperfusion arrhythmias that may include ventricular tachycardia.

REVIEW The Concept of Perfusion

RELATE Link the Concepts

Linking the concept of perfusion with the concept of inflammation:

1. Why does tissue become swollen and red around the site of injury?
2. How is the process of tissue repair affected by alterations in perfusion?

Linking the concept of perfusion with the concept of cognition:

3. Describe the cognitive impairments a nurse might observe in a client with elevated intracranial pressure.
4. Describe the pathophysiology of hypoxia as it relates to perfusion and cognitive impairments.

Linking the concept of perfusion with the concept of elimination:

5. Describe the link between cardiac output and renal failure.
6. Define renal autoregulation.
7. What class of drugs may be administered to improve renal perfusion pressure?

READY Go to Companion Skills Manual

REFER Go to Pearson Nursing Student Resources
nursing.pearsonhighered.com

- Additional review materials
- Additional case study

REFLECT Case Study \\ Part 3

On day 4 of admission, you go into Mr. Evans's room to perform the morning assessment and find that his blood pressure is 258/128 mmHg and pulse is 112 bpm. He was placed on mechanical ventilation 2 days ago. During the prescribed sedation vacation, you note that he is minimally responsive and grimaces as if in pain. Upon auscultation, you note that his lungs have crackles throughout and you are suctioning pink frothy sputum via the closed suctioning system.

Clinical Reasoning Questions Level I

1. What do you think may have caused this complication?
2. What additional assessments are needed?
3. What lab/diagnostic test do you expect the physician to order?

Clinical Reasoning Questions Level II

4. Utilize the SBAR format to provide this new information to the physician.
5. What medications do you expect to be found on the client's medication administration record?
6. What is the priority nursing intervention at this time?

EXEMPLAR 16.1   Cardiomyopathy

EXEMPLAR KEY TERMS
Cardiomyopathy, *1076*
Dilated cardiomyopathy, *1077*
Hypertrophic cardiomyopathy, *1078*
Peripartum cardiomyopathy, *1078*
Restrictive cardiomyopathy, *1078*
Syncope, *1079*

EXEMPLAR LEARNING OUTCOMES
After reading about this exemplar, you will be able to:

1. Describe the pathophysiology, etiology, clinical manifestations, and direct and indirect causes of cardiomyopathy.
2. Identify risk factors associated with cardiomyopathy.
3. Illustrate the nursing process in providing culturally competent care across the life span for individuals with cardiomyopathy.
4. Formulate priority nursing diagnoses appropriate for an individual with cardiomyopathy.
5. Summarize therapies used by interdisciplinary teams in the collaborative care of an individual with cardiomyopathy.
6. Plan evidence-based care for an individual with cardiomyopathy and his or her family in collaboration with other members of the healthcare team.
7. Evaluate expected outcomes for an individual with cardiomyopathy.

▶ OVERVIEW

The term **cardiomyopathy** refers to diseases that affect the heart muscle and its ability to pump effectively. The American Heart Association (AHA) (2013a) classifies cardiomyopathies as either primary or secondary. Causes of primary cardiomyopathies are those usually affecting the heart alone and causes of secondary myopathies result from an underlying condition or illness. Examples of secondary cardiomyopathies include ischemia, infectious diseases, exposure to toxins, connective tissue disorders, metabolic disorders, and nutritional deficiencies.

Cardiomyopathies may also be classified as intrinsic or extrinsic. Intrinsic cardiomyopathies result from abnormalities originating in the heart muscle cell. Extrinsic abnormalities result from diseases not unique to heart muscle cell abnormalities. In clients with cardiomyopathy, the heart becomes enlarged, thick, or rigid (AHA, 2013a). In rare instances, sections of the heart muscle may be replaced with scar tissue. Eventually, the heart becomes weaker and is less able to pump blood throughout the body. This inability to function normally can lead to heart failure, arrhythmias, and disorders of one or more heart valves.

▶ PATHOPHYSIOLOGY AND ETIOLOGY

Cardiomyopathies are categorized by their pathophysiology and presentation into five types: dilated, hypertrophic, restrictive, arrhythmogenic right ventricular dysplasia, and unclassified cardiomyopathies (AHA, 2013a). Table 16–10 ● compares the causes, pathophysiology, manifestations, and management of the cardiomyopathies.

TABLE 16–10 Classifications of Cardiomyopathy

	DILATED	HYPERTROPHIC	RESTRICTIVE	ARRHYTHMO-GENIC RIGHT VENTRICULAR DYSPLASIA	UNCLASSIFIED
CAUSES	Usually idiopathic; may be secondary to chronic alcoholism or myocarditis.	Hereditary; may be secondary to chronic hypertension.	Usually secondary to amyloidosis, radiation, or myocardial fibrosis.	Inherited cause of sudden death in young people and athletes. Rare in children younger than 10 years of age and older than 40 years of age.	Congenital, family history.
PATHOPHYSIOLOGY	Scarring and atrophy of myocardial cells. Thickening of ventricular wall. Dilation of heart chambers. Impaired ventricular pumping. Increased end-diastolic and end-systolic volumes. Mural thrombi common.	Hypertrophy of ventricular muscle mass. Small left ventricular volume. Septal hypertrophy may obstruct left ventricular outflow. Left atrial dilation.	Excess rigidity of ventricular walls restricts filling. Myocardial contractility remains relatively normal.	Genetically determined myocardial dystrophy. Evidence of fibro-fatty replacement of right ventricle and subepicardial regions of left ventricle.	May progress to dilated or restrictive cardiomyopathies.
MANIFESTATIONS	Heart failure. Cardiomegaly. Dysrhythmias, S_3 and S_4 gallop; murmur of mitral regurgitation.	Left ventricular hypertrophy. Dysrhythmias. Loud S_4. Sudden death. Dyspnea, anginal pain, syncope.	Dyspnea, fatigue. Right-sided heart failure. Mild to moderate cardiomegaly. S_3 and S_4 gallop. Mitral regurgitation murmur.	Ventricular tachyarrhythmias. High risk of sudden death.	Symptoms of heart failure, chest pain, dysrhythmias, progression to heart failure and/or death. Clients may be asymptomatic with detection during routine screenings or postmortem.
MANAGEMENT	Management of heart failure. Implantable cardioverter–defibrillator (ICD) as needed. Cardiac transplantation.	Beta-blockers. Antidysrhythmic agents. Calcium-channel blockers. ICD, dual-chamber pacing. Surgical excision of part of the ventricular septum.	Management of heart failure. Exercise restriction.	Antiarrhythmics and implantation of defibrillators. Prescreening for sport eligibility has shown effectiveness in detecting asymptomatic clients.	Treatment specific to type of cardiomyopathy. Treatment may mirror same as that for heart failure. Monitor lab values as predictors of poor outcomes.

Dilated Cardiomyopathy

Dilated cardiomyopathy is the most common type of cardiomyopathy, accounting for 87% of all cases of cardiomyopathy. Dilated cardiomyopathy is a common cause of heart failure. It is estimated that as many as one third of those diagnosed with dilated cardiomyopathy inherit the disease from their parents (AHA, 2013a). Dilated cardiomyopathy most commonly occurs between the ages of 20 and 60. Men are more likely than women to be diagnosed (AHA, 2013a).

With dilated cardiomyopathy, the heart's ventricles and atria are affected as a result of the inability to pump efficiently. Both end-diastolic and end-systolic volumes increase, reducing the left ventricular ejection fraction and thus decreasing cardiac output. As the heart muscle begins to dilate and become thinner, the inside of the left ventricular chamber enlarges, leading the way for progression into the right ventricle and atria. Over time, due to the heart's inability to pump efficiently, the muscle becomes weaker and heart failure can occur. Clinical manifestations of dilated cardiomyopathy include shortness of breath, fatigue, swelling of the lower extremities and abdomen, and jugular venous distention. Disorders of the heart valve, arrhythmias, and blood clots may occur with disease progression.

A form of dilated cardiomyopathy, **peripartum cardiomyopathy** is a relatively rare but serious dysfunction of the left ventricle that may occur in the last month of pregnancy or the first 5 months postpartum in a woman with no previous history of heart disease. As the heart function decreases, the lungs, liver, and other body systems are affected. The heart dysfunction is usually reversible, but may progress and may necessitate heart transplantation. A heart biopsy may be indicated to determine the underlying cause. Subsequent pregnancy poses a high risk for complications, especially for those where the heart remains enlarged. Family planning is highly encouraged for these individuals (Medline Plus, 2012).

Hypertrophic Cardiomyopathy

Hypertrophic cardiomyopathy is characterized by decreased compliance of the left ventricle and hypertrophy of the ventricular muscle mass. In hypertrophic cardiomyopathy, the heart muscle becomes abnormally thick, which decreases the heart's ability to pump blood. Ventricular filling is impaired, leading to small end-diastolic volumes and low cardiac output. The heart's conduction system may also be affected, leading to an increased risk for life-threatening arrhythmias.

The pattern of left ventricular hypertrophy is unique in that the muscle may not hypertrophy equally. This is known as asymmetric septal hypertrophy. In a majority of clients, the interventricular septal mass, especially the upper portion, increases to a greater extent than the free wall of the ventricle. The enlarged upper septum narrows the passageway of blood into the aorta, impairing ventricular outflow.

Restrictive Cardiomyopathy

Restrictive cardiomyopathy is characterized by rigid ventricular walls. This classification of myopathy results in restriction of the heart to stretch and fill with blood properly. Decreased ventricular compliance reduces blood flow and may result in diastolic dysfunction and then heart failure. Contractility is unaffected, and the ejection fraction is normal. Limited therapies are available for restrictive cardiomyopathy; they consist of symptomatic, supportive, and pharmaceutical interventions.

Arrhythmogenic Right Ventricular Dysplasia

Clients diagnosed with arrhythmogenic right ventricular dyplasia (ARVD) are at high risk for ventricular tachyarrhythmias and sudden death. The heart muscle becomes thickened and ARVD may range in classification from mild to severe. ARVD results as the client's body progressively replaces the muscle of the right ventricle with fatty and fibrous tissue. Both men and women are affected, and ARVD accounts for up to one fifth of sudden cardiac deaths in individuals under age 35 (Framingham Heart Study, 2013). ARVD is commonly associated with sudden cardiac death in athletes. Treatment modalities range from no treatment to medications and surgery. Most cases of ARVD are hereditary. Family members of clients with ARVD should be closely screened for sign and symptoms of the illness.

Etiology

The cause of dilated cardiomyopathy is unknown, although it is commonly associated with exposure to toxins, metabolic conditions, and infections. Reversible dilated cardiomyopathy may develop as a result of alcohol and cocaine abuse, chemotherapeutic drugs, pregnancy, and systemic hypertension. About one third of cases are a result of inheriting mutations in certain genes (Trelogan, 2011). Several genes appear to cause dilated cardiomyopathy but only one has been isolated. The dystrophin gene is found in muscle fibers and is also responsible for certain types of muscular dystrophy.

Causes of restrictive cardiomyopathy include scarring of the heart from an unknown cause or amyloidosis. Restrictive cardiomyopathy may occur after heart transplantation. Fibrosis of the myocardium and endocardium causes excessive stiffness and rigidity of either or both ventricles.

The cause of peripartum cardiomyopathy is unknown. However, systolic dysfunction and pulmonary edema should be ruled out. Nutritional disorders have been suggested but not validated (Carson, 2013). The left ventricle may not demonstrate dilation but the ejection fraction is typically reduced below 45% (Sliwa et al., 2010).

Hypertrophic cardiomyopathy is usually inherited. About one half of children of those diagnosed with this type of cardiomyopathy will inherit the genetic mutation for the disease. Siblings and close relatives are urged to discuss screenings for the myopathy with their healthcare provider.

Risk Factors

Risk factors for cardiomyopathies include a family history of cardiomyopathy, heart failure, sudden cardiac arrest, endocrine and metabolic diseases, alcoholism, and hypertension. Many forms of cardiomyopathy are idiopathic, with no known cause or risk factors, and often result in death.

▶ CLINICAL MANIFESTATIONS

Each form of cardiomyopathy has subtle differences in symptoms. Manifestations of dilated cardiomyopathy develop gradually. Some clients may be asymptomatic or develop minor symptoms with very little impact on activities of daily living (ADLs). Heart failure often presents years after the onset of dilation and pump failure. Both right- and left-sided failure may be accompanied by dyspnea on exertion, orthopnea, paroxysmal nocturnal dyspnea, weakness, fatigue, peripheral edema, and ascites. Both S_3 and S_4 are commonly heard, as well as an AV regurgitation murmur. As the cardiomyopathy progresses, clients begin to suffer from arrhythmias. Clients with ventricular arrhythmias are at a higher risk for sudden death.

Peripartum cardiomyopathy usually presents with anemia and infection. Consequently, treatment focuses on underlying abnormalities. Peripartum cardiomyopathy may resolve with bed rest as the heart gradually returns to normal size. Clients diagnosed with hypertrophic cardiomyopathy may be asymptomatic for many years. Symptomatic clients may experience shortness of breath (dyspnea), angina, **syncope** (transient loss of consciousness and muscle tone after exercise or activity), and heart palpitations. Symptoms develop as physical activity and oxygen demand increase, commonly during and after exercise. In children and young adults, sudden cardiac death may be the first sign of the disorder. Hypertrophic cardiomyopathy is a sudden cause of cardiac arrest in young people, including young athletes (AHA, 2013a).

Individuals who are diagnosed with hypertrophic cardiomyopathy may experience angina. This angina may result from ischemia caused by overgrowth of the ventricular muscle, coronary artery abnormalities, or decreased coronary artery perfusion. Syncope results when the outflow tract obstruction severely decreases cardiac output and cerebral blood flow. Ventricular dysrhythmias and atrial fibrillation are common. Other manifestations of hypertrophic cardiomyopathy include fatigue, dizziness, and palpitations. A harsh, systolic ejection murmur of variable intensity, heard best at the lower left sternal border and apex, is characteristic in hypertrophic cardiomyopathy. An S_4 murmur may also be noted on auscultation and palpation.

Clients with restrictive cardiomyopathy may live a normal life and present as asymptomatic or with very few symptoms of illness. Others develop symptoms that progress and worsen as heart function decreases. Less common are fainting and chest pain or pressure occurring during exercise or during periods of rest (exercise intolerance). Jugular venous pressure is elevated, and S_3 and S_4 are common.

Arrhythmogenic right ventricular dysplasia (ARVD) is usually diagnosed in clients younger than 40 years of age and may cause sudden death in athletes. ARVD can occur in clients with no family history. However, genetic causes and congenital malformations have been identified.

Unclassified cardiomyopathies do not fit into a specific category but are identified as primary diseases of the heart muscle and result in cardiac dysfunction.

▶ COLLABORATION

The overall goals of treatment of cardiomyopathies are to manage the signs and symptoms, delay disease progression, and reduce the risk for complications. The healthcare provider's prescriptive plan may include pharmacologic interventions, surgically implanted devices, or a combination of both. Treatment of hypertrophic cardiomyopathy and ARVD focuses on reducing contractility and preventing sudden cardiac death. Strenuous physical exertion is restricted, because it may precipitate dysrhythmias or sudden cardiac death. Dietary and sodium restrictions may help diminish the manifestations. Peripartum cardiomyopathy may resolve during the postpartum period if the heart returns to its normal size. Future pregnancies may result in heart failure.

Diagnostic Tests

Diagnosis begins with a thorough history and physical assessment. Commonly explored is information regarding signs and symptoms of illness and family history of cardiomyopathy, heart failure, or sudden cardiac arrest. Other diagnostic tests include:

- Echocardiography
- Electrocardiography and ambulatory ECG monitoring
- Chest x-ray
- Hemodynamic studies
- Cardiac stress testing
- Radionuclear scans
- Cardiac catheterization and coronary angiography
- Myocardial biopsy
- Genetic testing.

Pharmacologic Therapy

ACE inhibitors, angiotensin II receptor blockers, and calcium-channel blockers may be prescribed to lower blood pressure. Beta-blockers, calcium-channel blockers, and digoxin are medicines commonly used to slow the heart rate. Beta-blockers may also be prescribed, in clients with hypertrophic cardiomyopathy, to relax the heart, stabilize the rhythm, and slow the pumping action of the heart. They should be used with caution in clients with dilated cardiomyopathy. Diuretics may be added to the regimen to aid in the treatment of heart failure. Anticoagulants are given to reduce the risk of thrombus formation and embolization. Abnormal electrolyte imbalances should be corrected because they may be a sign of dehydration, heart failure, high blood pressure, or other illnesses. Aldosterone blockers may be used to correct the imbalances. Antidysrhythmics may be administered to help prevent abnormal heart rhythms but are used with caution due to significant side effects.

Surgery

Cardiac transplantation is the definitive treatment for dilated cardiomyopathy. However, organ rejection is a lifelong risk

Clinical Manifestations and Therapies **Cardiomyopathy**

ETIOLOGY	CLINICAL MANIFESTATIONS	CLINICAL THERAPIES
Heart failure (both left and right sided) often develops as the result of reduced cardiac output.	■ Dyspnea on exertion, orthopnea, paroxysmal nocturnal dyspnea ■ Weakness, fatigue ■ Peripheral edema ■ Ascites	■ Treatment of underlying cause ■ Medications to include diuretics, vasodilators, beta-blockers, and calcium-channel blockers ■ Daily monitoring of client's weight and client's intake and output ■ Elastic stockings to improve venous return ■ Abdominocentesis to reduce ascites ■ Sleeping in semi-Fowler position ■ Periods of activity followed by periods of rest
Dysrhythmias are common because of dilation of the heart muscle that damages conduction pathways and leads to the formation of alternate paths.	■ Electrocardiogram may show supraventricular tachycardias, atrial fibrillation, and complex ventricular tachycardias.	■ Treatment of underlying cause ■ Medications to include antidysrhythmics, nitrates, and beta-blockers ■ May potentially require implanted cardiac defibrillator ■ Client teaching regarding awareness of pulse rate and rhythm and when to interact with healthcare team
Angina may result from ischemia caused by overgrowth of the ventricular muscle, coronary artery abnormalities, or decreased coronary artery perfusion.	■ Chest pain radiating to the jaw, back, or left arm ■ Shortness of breath ■ Activity intolerance ■ Intermittent claudication ■ Nausea or vomiting	■ Treatment of underlying cause ■ Medications to include nitrates and beta-blockers ■ Client teaching regarding how to respond to symptoms and when to call 911 ■ Surgery may be required to repair damaged coronary arteries
Syncope may occur when the outflow tract obstruction severely decreases cardiac output and blood flow to the brain.	■ Dizziness, light-headedness, fainting (sudden loss of consciousness) ■ Nausea	■ Treatment of underlying cause ■ Medications to include beta-blockers ■ Client teaching about the importance of sitting down as soon as symptoms start in order to prevent injuries from falls

for the recipient. With restrictive cardiomyopathies, transplantation is not a viable option because the underlying process causing fibrosis is not eliminated, and eventually, the transplanted organ is affected as well. (See Exemplar 16.6 for more information about cardiac transplantation.) Left ventricular assist devices (LVADs) may be used to support cardiac output until a donor heart is available. The LVAD is an electronic pump surgically implanted into the abdominal cavity that aids in the perfusion of blood throughout the body.

Surgical ventricular remodeling is an alternative to heart transplantation. During the procedure the size of the left ventricle is reduced to improve the function of the heart and reduce the overall size of the muscle. The surgeon either removes a section of the heart muscle or makes a tuck in the existing muscle.

An implantable cardioverter–defibrillator is often inserted to help maintain a stable heart rhythm. When needed, the pacemaker will send an electrical impulse to stimulate the heart to contract. The most common type of pacemaker

attaches to the heart in two different places, allowing the healthcare provider to alter the sequence of contractions within the heart muscle.

NURSING PROCESS

Nursing assessment and care for clients diagnosed with cardiomyopathies is similar to those for clients with heart failure. Client and family education regarding the disease process and its management is vital. Understanding and recognizing the symptoms of cardiomyopathy are keys to learning how to manage the illness. Some degree of activity restriction is often necessary. The client should be taught to conserve energy while performing ADLs. Rest periods between activities should be encouraged. Strong support systems are beneficial as the client adapts to required lifestyle changes. Important lifestyle modifications include limiting salt, fat, and fluids in the diet; regular exercise; maintenance of an appropriate weight; smoking cessation; limiting or eliminating alcohol; and stress reduction.

The client with hypertrophic cardiomyopathy requires care similar to that provided for the client with myocardial ischemia. Nitrates and other vasodilators are avoided. If surgery is performed, nursing care is similar to that for any client undergoing open heart surgery or cardiac transplantation. Genetic counseling should be initiated to identify those at familial risk.

The client undergoing cardiac transplantation and other surgical interventions requires pre- and postoperative care.

Assessment

The nurse should obtain both subjective and objective data when assessing the client with cardiomyopathy:

- **Health history.** Complaints of increasing shortness of breath, dyspnea with exertion, decreasing activity tolerance, or paroxysmal nocturnal dyspnea. Also note the number of pillows used for sleeping, recent weight gain, presence of a cough, chest or abdominal pain, anorexia or nausea, history of cardiac disease, previous episodes of heart failure. Client history of hypertension or diabetes should be considered. Current medications, usual diet and activity, as well as any recent changes are important diagnostic factors.
- **Physical examination.** General appearance; work of breathing, ease of conversation, position changes; apparent anxiety; vital signs, including apical pulse; color of skin and mucous membranes; jugular venous distention, peripheral pulses, capillary refill, presence and degree of edema; heart and breath sounds; abdominal contour, bowel sounds, tenderness; right upper abdominal tenderness, and liver enlargement.

Diagnosis

Appropriate nursing diagnoses for clients with cardiomyopathy include the following:

- *Cardiac Output, Decreased* related to impaired left ventricular filling, contractility, or outflow obstruction
- *Fatigue* related to decreased cardiac output
- *Fluid Volume: Excess* related to compensatory mechanisms
- *Activity Intolerance* related to decreasing cardiac function
- *Knowledge, Deficient* related to the importance of a low-sodium diet
- *Grieving* related to uncertain or poor prognosis.

(NANDA-I © 2015)

Planning

The plan of care will be based on the type and severity of cardiomyopathy. The individual needs of the client are essential to treatment adherence. Goals may include the following:

- The client will maintain blood pressure within specified limits.
- The client will alter his or her lifestyle to demonstrate adjustment to alterations in activity level caused by the disease process.

- The client will modify his or her diet to support long-term management of the condition.

Implementation

When providing care for the client with alterations in perfusion, it is important for the nurse to monitor for subtle changes in vital signs and level of consciousness. Alterations in peripheral capillary refill time, pulse rate or volume, and level of consciousness may be early warning signs of decreased perfusion.

Monitor Cardiac Output

As the heart fails as a pump, stroke volume and tissue perfusion decrease. Nursing interventions include:

- Monitor vital signs and oxygen saturation as indicated. Decreased cardiac output stimulates the sympathetic nervous system to increase the heart rate in an attempt to restore cardiac output. Tachycardia at rest is common. Diastolic blood pressure may initially be elevated because of vasoconstriction. In late stages, compensatory mechanisms fail, and blood pressure falls. Oxygen saturation levels are beneficial in providing a measure of gas exchange and tissue perfusion.
- Monitor BNP (B-type natriuretic peptide) levels, and report trends. BNP levels indicate the severity of heart failure: As the cardiac index decreases and left ventricular pressures increase, BNP levels increase. Identifying trends provides additional information regarding cardiac output and the effectiveness of the cardiac pump.
- Auscultate heart and breath sounds regularly. The S_1 and S_2 sounds may be diminished if cardiac function is poor. A ventricular gallop (S_3) is an early sign of heart failure; an atrial gallop (S_4) may also be present. Crackles are often heard in the lung bases; increasing crackles, dyspnea, and shortness of breath indicate worsening heart failure.
- Administer supplemental oxygen as needed. This decreases the effects of hypoxia and ischemia and results in increased oxygenation and perfusion.
- Administer prescribed medications as ordered. Medications are used to decrease the cardiac workload and increase the effectiveness of contractions.
- Encourage periods of rest throughout the day. Elevate the head of the bed to reduce the work of breathing. Provide a bedside commode, and assist with ADLs. Instruct the client to avoid the Valsalva maneuver. These interventions reduce cardiac workload.

Monitor Fluid Volume

As cardiac output falls, compensatory mechanisms cause salt and water retention, thereby increasing blood volume. Increased fluid volume places additional stress on the failing ventricles, making them work harder to shift the fluid load. The nurse should do the following:

- Assess respiratory status and auscultate lung sounds at least every 4 hours. Notify the healthcare provider of significant changes in condition. Declining respiratory status indicates worsening left heart failure.

Client Teaching **Cardiomyopathy**

Cardiomyopathies are chronic, progressive disorders generally managed in the home and community care settings unless surgery or transplant is planned or end-stage heart failure develops. When educating the client and family about home care, the nurse should include the following topics:

- Activity restrictions and dietary changes to reduce manifestations and prevent complications
- Prescribed drug regimen, its rationale, and its intended and possible adverse effects
- Disease process, the expected outcomes, and treatment options
- Cardiac transplantation, including the procedure, the need for lifetime immunosuppression to prevent transplant rejection, and the risks of postoperative infection and long-term immunosuppression
- Symptoms to report to the healthcare provider or for which immediate care is needed
- Cardiopulmonary resuscitation procedures and available training sites
- Referrals to home and social services and counseling as indicated
- Availability of community resources regarding support groups and respite care.

- Monitor intake and output. Notify the healthcare provider if urine output is less than 30 mL/hr. Diuretics may reduce circulating volume, producing hypovolemia despite persistent peripheral edema. A fall in urine output may indicate significantly reduced cardiac output and renal ischemia.
- Weigh the client daily. Weight is an objective measure of fluid status: 1 L of fluid is equal to 2.2 lb of weight. Significant weight gain may indicate worsening heart failure.
- Record abdominal girth every shift. Note complaints of a loss of appetite, abdominal discomfort, or nausea. Venous congestion can lead to ascites and may affect gastrointestinal function and nutritional status.
- Monitor and record hemodynamic measurements. Report significant changes and negative trends. Hemodynamic measurements provide a means of monitoring condition and response to treatment.
- Restrict fluids as ordered. Allow choices of fluid type and timing of intake, scheduling most fluid intake during morning and afternoon hours. Offer ice chips and frequent mouth care; provide hard candies if allowed. Providing choices increases the client's sense of control. Ice chips, hard candies, and mouth care help relieve dry mouth and thirst.

Monitor Activity

Clients with heart failure have little or no cardiac reserve to meet increased oxygen demands. As the disease progresses and cardiac function is compromised, activity intolerance increases. Low cardiac output and the inability to participate in activities may impede self-care. The nurse should do the following:

- Organize nursing care to allow rest periods. The grouping of care activities allows adequate time to "recharge."
- Assist with ADLs as needed. Encourage independence when possible. Assisting with ADLs helps ensure that care needs are met while reducing cardiac workload. Involving the client promotes a sense of control and reduces a sense of helplessness.
- Plan and implement progressive activities. Use passive and active range-of-motion (ROM) exercises as appropriate. Consult with a physical therapist on an activity plan. Progressive activity slowly increases exercise capacity by strengthening and improving cardiac function without strain. Activity also helps prevent skeletal muscle atrophy. ROM exercises prevent complications of immobility in severely compromised clients.
- Provide written and verbal information regarding expected activity level on discharge. Written information provides a reference for important information. Verbal information allows clarification and validation of the material.

Provide Low-Sodium Diet

Diet is an important part of long-term management of heart failure. It also contributes to reducing fluid retention. The nurse should do the following:

- Discuss the rationale for sodium restrictions. Understanding fosters adherence with the prescribed diet.
- Consult with a dietitian to plan and review a low-sodium and, if necessary for weight control, low-kilocalorie diet. Give the client a list of high-sodium, high-fat, high-cholesterol foods to avoid. Dietary planning and teaching increase the client's sense of control and participation in disease management. Food lists are useful memory aids. Introduce the client to available printed and electronic media sources for diet information.

Evaluation

The effectiveness of nursing care and collaborative treatment, will be evaluated using nursing diagnoses and anticipated outcomes or goals:

- The client will verbalize symptoms that need to be immediately reported to the healthcare provider.
- The client will maintain blood pressure within acceptable range as a means of demonstrating adequate tissue perfusion.
- The client identifies activity tolerance strategies important for maintaining as normal a lifestyle as possible.
- The client articulates the need for a low-sodium diet.

> ## REVIEW **Cardiomyopathy**

RELATE Link the Concepts and Exemplars

Linking the exemplar of cardiomyopathy with the concept of oxygenation:

1. What physical assessment findings related to oxygenation would you anticipate for the client with cardiomyopathy?

2. What are the priority interventions for the client who presents to the emergency department with dyspnea and a history of cardiomyopathy?

Linking the exemplar of cardiomyopathy with the concept of comfort:

3. The client with cardiomyopathy reports fatigue that is interfering with ADLs. What strategies might you recommend to help this client improve independence in performing ADLs?

4. What techniques would be beneficial for the client with cardiomyopathy to improve sleep and rest at home?

READY Go to Companion Skills Manual

REFER Go to Pearson Nursing Student Resources
nursing.pearsonhighered.com

- Additional review materials

REFLECT Case Study

Deshawn Jones is a 28-year-old African American male who plays professional basketball. He is 6 feet 2 inches tall and weighs 180 pounds. Mr. Jones's wife, Sylvia, owns a popular local restaurant. Mr. and Mrs. Jones have a 2-year-old son, Pete. Mr. Jones is away much of the winter for out-of-town games. The Joneses have a strong family support system nearby to assist with care of the children.

Mr. Jones's father died suddenly at the age of 30 while running track. After an autopsy, he was diagnosed with hypertrophic cardiomyopathy. Mr. Jones's mother is alive and healthy, helps Mrs. Jones at the restaurant, and cares for Pete when needed. Mr. Jones's younger sister, April, is away at college.

Mr. Jones has had occasional twinges of chest pain when practicing basketball. He has decided to see a family healthcare provider for a full physical.

1. What factor in Mr. Jones's history puts him at greater risk for cardiomyopathy?

2. What assessment data will you obtain when examining Mr. Jones?

3. How will you respond to Mr. Jones when he tells you that he is afraid he will die suddenly at a young age, like his father?

EXEMPLAR 16.2 **Congenital Heart Defects**

EXEMPLAR KEY TERMS

Aortic stenosis, *1092*
Atrial septal defect (ASD), *1084*
Atrioventricular (AV) canal, *1086*
Coarctation of the aorta, *1092*
Congenital heart defect, *1083*
Endocardial cushion defect, *1086*
Heaving, *1101*
Holosystolic, *1086*
Hypercyanotic episode, *1087*
Hypoplastic left heart syndrome (HLHS), *1093*
Palliative procedure, *1096*
Patent ductus arteriosus, *1084*
Preload, *1087*
Pulmonary atresia, *1088*
Septal defect, *1084*
Shunt, *1094*
Stenosis, *1087*
Syncope, *1092*
Tetralogy of Fallot, *1088*
Total anomalous pulmonary venous return, *1091*
Transposition of the great arteries (TGA), *1090*
Tricuspid atresia, *1088*

Truncus arteriosus, *1090*
Ventricular septal defect (VSD), *1085*

EXEMPLAR LEARNING OUTCOMES
After reading about this exemplar, you will be able to:

1. Describe the pathophysiology, etiology, clinical manifestations, and direct and indirect causes of congenital heart defects.

2. Identify risk factors associated with congenital heart defects.

3. Illustrate the nursing process in providing culturally competent care across the life span for individuals with congenital heart defects.

4. Formulate priority nursing diagnoses appropriate for an individual with a congenital heart defect.

5. Summarize therapies used by interdisciplinary teams in the collaborative care of an individual with a congenital heart defect.

6. Plan evidence-based care for an individual with a congenital heart defect and his or her family in collaboration with other members of the healthcare team.

7. Evaluate expected outcomes for an individual with a congenital heart defect.

▶ OVERVIEW

The term **congenital heart defect** refers to a defect in the heart or great vessels resulting from an alteration in normal fetal development or persistence of a fetal structure that does not convert to extrauterine anatomy after birth. It is estimated that 8 infants per 1,000 live births are diagnosed with a congenital heart defect. Many congenital heart defects have no known

cause. Others may be hereditary or occur as a result of the mother taking medications while pregnant. Defects have been linked to antiseizure medications and the acne medication isotretinoin (Accutane). The diagnosis and treatment of congenital heart defects have dramatically improved during the past few decades. The majority of children with congenital heart defects now survive to adulthood and can live active, productive lives.

▶ PATHOPHYSIOLOGY AND ETIOLOGY

Congenital heart defects were previously categorized as cyanotic or acyanotic. Current standards of practice categorize them by pathophysiology and hemodynamics. These categories include the following:

■ Heart defects that increase pulmonary blood flow
■ Heart defects that decrease pulmonary blood flow
■ Heart defects that result in obstructed systemic blood flow (AHA, 2013b).
■ Mixed defects

Defects that Increase Pulmonary Blood Flow

The most common congenital heart defects result from a miscommunication between the left and right sides of the heart (**septal defect**) or between the great arteries (**patent ductus arteriosus**). Such defects allow blood to flow between the left and right sides of the heart. The pressures on the left side of the heart are higher than the pressures on the right side. This results in blood shunting from the left side to the right side of the heart and increases the amount of blood pumped to the lungs. The size of the connection and volume of blood flow through the septum determine how quickly the child becomes asymptomatic. The increased blood flow to the lungs causes increased pulmonary vascular resistance (constriction of the pulmonary vascular bed, in an effort to reduce the blood flow) and pulmonary artery hypertension. Right ventricular hypertrophy develops to compensate for increasing pulmonary vascular resistance and delivers the blood to the lungs.

Table 16–11 ● describes the pathophysiology, clinical manifestations, and clinical therapy for heart defects that increase pulmonary blood flow.

TABLE 16–11 Pathophysiology, Clinical Manifestations, and Clinical Therapy for Heart Defects That Increase Pulmonary Blood Flow

DEFECT PATHOPHYSIOLOGY, CLINICAL MANIFESTATIONS, AND CLINICAL THERAPY	ANATOMY
Patent Ductus Arteriosus (PDA)	
This is a common congenital defect in the fetus. When pulmonary circulation is established and systemic vascular resistance increases at birth, pressures in the aorta become greater than pressures in the pulmonary arteries. Blood is shunted from the aorta to the pulmonary arteries, increasing circulation to the pulmonary system. In cases in which the passageway between the blood vessels does not close, some blood returns to the lungs. PDA is often seen in premature infants. The ductus arteriosus in the preterm newborn is not as responsive to the increased oxygen content with the conversion to pulmonary circulation, and it is less likely to close. **Clinical Manifestations** Dyspnea; tachypnea; tachycardia; full, bounding pulses; widened pulse pressure; hypotension may be noted when cardiac output is low. Congestive heart failure (CHF), intercostal retractions, hepatomegaly, and growth failure with a large PDA. A continuous "machinery" murmur during systole and diastole and a thrill in the pulmonic area. High risk for frequent respiratory infections, pneumonia, and infective endocarditis. **Diagnostic Procedures** Chest x-ray and electrocardiogram (ECG) demonstrate left ventricular hypertrophy. Upon echocardiogram, the PDA is visible and a left-to-right shunt can be measured on echocardiogram. **Clinical Therapy** Intravenous indomethacin often stimulates closure of the ductus arteriosus and may be given to some newborns. Transcatheter occlusion is the least invasive surgical option and has become the treatment of choice. Surgical ligation of the ductus arteriosus is another option. Prophylaxis for infective endocarditis may be necessary until the PDA is closed. **Prognosis** No long-term sequelae occur if the PDA is treated before pulmonary vascular disease develops. If it is not treated, the child's life span is shortened as pulmonary hypertension and pulmonary vascular obstructive disease develop. Clients undergoing treatment should live healthy lives after appetite, growth, and activity levels return to normal.	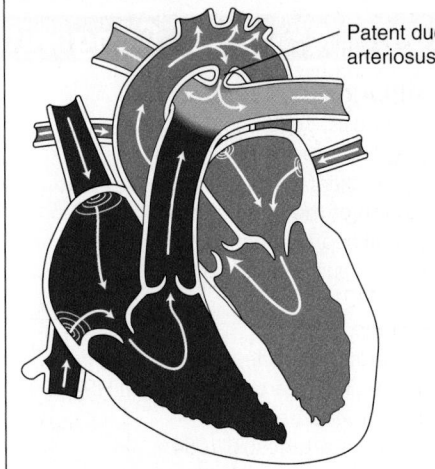 Patent ductus arteriosus ◼ Mix of oxygenated and unoxygenated blood
Atrial Septal Defect (ASD)	
An **atrial septal defect (ASD)** occurs when there is an opening in the atrial septum permitting left-to-right shunting of blood. ASD is commonly recognized in adulthood. Subtle physical examination findings and minimal symptoms during the first two to three decades of life often contribute to a delay in diagnosis. Approximately 70% of atrial septal defects are detected in the fifth decade of life (Markham, Cribbs, & Willis, 2011). The disease sequelae depend on the size of the defect, size of the shunt, and associated abnormalities.	

TABLE 16–11 Pathophysiology, Clinical Manifestations, and Clinical Therapy for Heart Defects That Increase Pulmonary Blood Flow *(continued)*

DEFECT PATHOPHYSIOLOGY, CLINICAL MANIFESTATIONS, AND CLINICAL THERAPY	ANATOMY

Clinical Manifestations

Infants and young children usually have no symptoms. Small and moderate-size ASDs may not be diagnosed until the preschool years or later. Often considered after a heart murmur is detected on routine examination.

Abnormal findings on chest x-ray or ECG.

Presenting symptoms include pulmonary arterial hypertension, atrial arrhythmias, exercise intolerance, and congestive heart failure.

Heart sound S_1 may be split, reflecting forceful right ventricular contraction and delayed closure of the tricuspid leaflets (Markham et al., 2011).

A soft systolic ejection murmur occurs in the pulmonic area with wide splitting of the second heart sound (S_2). The split S_2 is fixed because of reduced respiratory variation. Occurs only if pulmonary artery pressure is normal and pulmonary vascular resistance is low.

Midsystolic murmur at lower left sternal border, due to increased blood flow across the tricuspid valve.

Mitral valve regurgitation may be present in clients with an ostium primum defect and an associated cleft of the mitral valve.

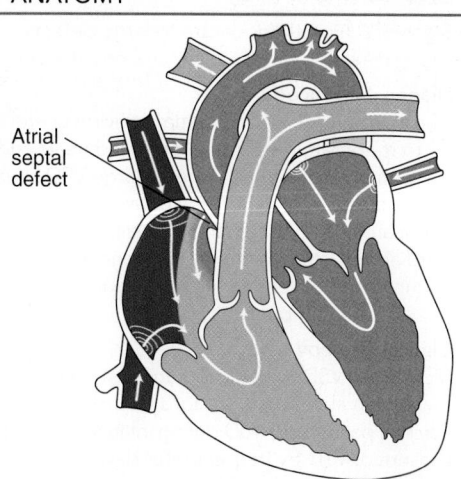

Atrial septal defect

Diagnostic Procedures

Transthoracic echocardiography may clarify an uncertain diagnosis by providing direct nonvisualization of most ASDs.

Chest x-ray often demonstrates cardiomegaly in clients presenting with a clinically significant left-to-right shunt.

MRI has been used successfully to identify the size and position of larger ASDs but is limited for small defects.

ECG reveals little information unless the ASD is large, has excessive shunting, or right ventricular hypertrophy is present.

Clinical Therapy

Spontaneous closure of some ASDs occurs within the first 4 years of life. No activity limitations are needed.

Surgery to close or patch the ASD is performed when significant increased pulmonary blood flow causes CHF or when spontaneous closure has not occurred by 4 years of age. Minimally invasive approaches have increased in recent years.

Prognosis

The mortality rate of surgical repair of an ASD is less than 1% for clients younger than 45 years of age without heart failure and who have systolic pulmonary artery pressure less than 60 mmHg (Markham et al., 2011). Many clients with uncorrected small and moderate-size ASDs live to middle age without symptoms. CHF, pulmonary hypertension, and atrial arrhythmias are likely to develop by the sixth decade in untreated adults.

Ventricular Septal Defect (VSD)

A **ventricular septal defect (VSD)** consists of one or more holes in the septum and results in increased pulmonary blood flow. Blood is shunted from the left ventricle directly across the open septum into the pulmonary artery. A VSD occurs in approximately 2–6 of every 1,000 live births (Ramaswamy & Srinivasan, 2011). VSDs may occur as primary anomalies or as single components of intracardiac anomalies including tetralogy of Fallot, complete atrioventricular canal defects, transposition of the great arteries, and correct transpositions (Ramaswamy & Srinivasan, 2011). Second to bicuspid aortic valves, VSDs are the most common congenital heart defect.

Clinical Manifestations

Symptoms of a VSD depend on the size of the defect and degree of left-to-right shunt. Adults usually present with small to moderate defects because larger ones would have been identified earlier in life.

A murmur may be detected on routine examination in infants with small defects.

Excessive sweating during feedings may be observed in infants with moderate defects as a result of increased sympathetic tone.

Fatigue with feedings due to increased cardiac output. Similar presentation to exercise intolerance.

Lack of adequate growth due to increased caloric need.

Frequent respiratory infections.

Lack of adequate growth.

A systolic murmur is auscultated at the third or fourth left intercostal space at the sternal border.

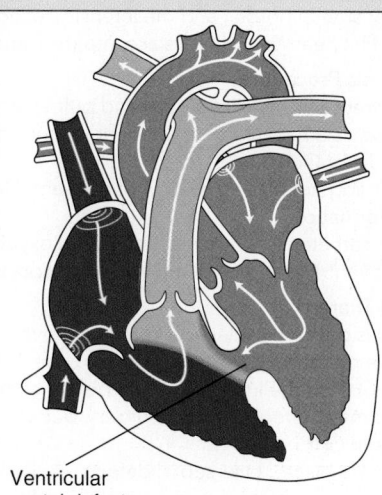

Ventricular septal defect

(continued on next page)

TABLE 16–11   Pathophysiology, Clinical Manifestations, and Clinical Therapy for Heart Defects That Increase Pulmonary Blood Flow (*continued*)

DEFECT PATHOPHYSIOLOGY, CLINICAL MANIFESTATIONS, AND CLINICAL THERAPY	ANATOMY
Signs of CHF with moderate to large defects. Tachypnea only with exercise and not at rest (Eisenmenger syndrome). **Diagnostic Procedures** Chest x-ray, MRI, and ECG may provide useful but inconclusive information with small to moderate defects. An enlarged heart and pulmonary vascular markings may be seen on a chest x-ray when a large VSD causes shunting. Right and left ventricular hypertrophy may be seen on an ECG. Echocardiogram establishes the diagnosis when shunting is present. Cardiac catheterization may be beneficial prior to surgery. Findings usually reveal increased oxygen in the right ventricle and increased systolic pressure in the right ventricle and pulmonary artery. **Clinical Therapy** Most small VSDs close spontaneously within the first 6 months of life. Treatment is conservative when no signs of CHF or pulmonary artery hypertension are present. Surgical patching of VSD during infancy is typically performed when poor growth is noted. Closure of VSD by transcatheter device (i.e., Rashkind device) during cardiac catheterization may be used to repair some defects. Prophylaxis for infective endocarditis may be required. **Prognosis** Highest risk associated with surgical repair is in the first few months of life. Children typically respond well to surgery and experience substantial catch-up growth. Tachyarrhythmias and right bundle branch block are possible complications.	
Atrioventricular (AV) Canal (Endocardial Cushion Defect)	
Atrioventricular (AV) canal, also known as **endocardial cushion defect**, refers to a combination of defects in the atrial and ventricular septa and portions of tricuspid and mitral valves. As a result, blood moves freely among the four heart chambers, mixing oxygen-rich and oxygen-poor blood. The amount of blood flowing from the heart to the lungs increases. This extra blood flow is commonly the cause of symptoms seen in children. AV canal is estimated to occur in 2 out of 10,000 live births. This defect is seen in approximately 20% of children with Down syndrome. Most complex AV canal defects result in AV valve and large septal defects between both atria and ventricles. **Clinical Manifestations** Severity of symptoms depends on the amount of mitral regurgitation and the left-to-right shunting of blood across the septum. Infants may present with CHF, tachypnea, tachycardia, failure to gain weight and grow, frequent pneumonia, pallor, sweating, cyanosis, and trouble breathing, especially during feedings. A **holosystolic** (heard during the entire phase of systole) murmur is loudest at the left lower sternal border, and the intensity reflects the amount of mitral regurgitation. The first heart sound (S$_1$) is accentuated, and S$_2$ is split. **Diagnostic Procedures** Chest x-ray shows cardiomegaly and pulmonary vascular markings. ECG reveals atrial enlargement, right ventricular hypertrophy, and an incomplete right bundle branch block. Echocardiogram reveals dilation of the ventricles, septal defects, and details of valve malformation. Cardiac catheterization reveals increased oxygen in the right atrium and increased right ventricle and/or pulmonary artery pressure. **Clinical Therapy** Surgery is performed during infancy to prevent pulmonary vascular disease. Palliative pulmonary artery banding may be used to reduce blood flow to the lungs and CHF so the infant can grow before corrective surgery. Oxygen may be required until surgery, but it may increase pulmonary blood flow and worsen CHF. Patches are placed over septal defects, and valve tissue is used to form functioning valves. The mitral valve may be replaced. Prophylaxis for infective endocarditis is required. **Prognosis** Information regarding long-term survival following successful surgery is lacking. Arrhythmias and mitral valve insufficiency occur postoperatively. There is no difference in short-term survival rates between infants with and without Down syndrome.	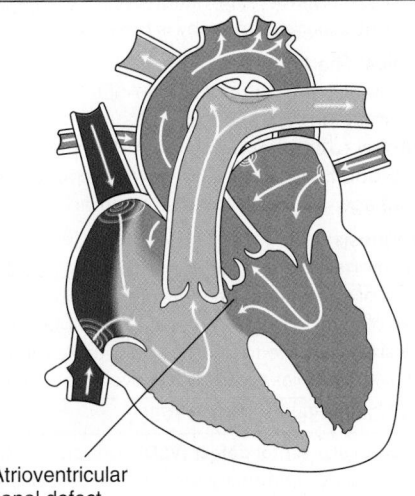 Atrioventricular canal defect

Defects That Decrease Pulmonary Blood Flow

Defects that obstruct the pulmonary blood flow result in little or no blood reaching the lungs to be oxygenated. If an atrial or ventricular septal opening exists between the left and right side of the heart, the right-sided pressures exceed those on the left, resulting in right-to-left shunting. In this case, cyanosis often results.

The bone marrow is stimulated to produce more red blood cells to increase the hemoglobin available to carry oxygen. Polycythemia may result and place the child at risk for thromboembolism. Over time, platelet survival is reduced and clotting factors are impaired, increasing the infant's risk of bleeding with surgery. Brain abscesses are also more common in children with cyanotic heart defects.

When infants and children with cyanosis rise in the morning, they may experience an abrupt decrease in systemic resistance and pulmonary blood flow. This physiological change can trigger a **hypercyanotic episode** (also known as a hypoxic or "tet" episode) when combined with the sudden increase in cardiac output and venous return associated with crying, feeding, exercise, a warm bath, and straining with defecation. The partial pressure of oxygen (PO_2) is lowered, and the partial pressure of carbon dioxide (PCO_2) rises. Hypoxemia becomes progressively worse as the respiratory center in the brain overreacts, increasing the respiratory effort. The extra respiratory effort further increases the cardiac output and contributes to a life-threatening decline unless rapid intervention is successful.

Table 16–12 ● describes the pathophysiology, clinical manifestations, and clinical therapy for heart defects that decrease pulmonary blood flow.

TABLE 16–12 Pathophysiology, Clinical Manifestations, and Clinical Therapy for Heart Defects That Decrease Pulmonary Blood Flow

DEFECT PATHOPHYSIOLOGY, CLINICAL MANIFESTATIONS, AND CLINICAL THERAPY	ANATOMY
Pulmonary Stenosis (PS)	
Stenosis, or abnormal narrowing of the valve blood flow into the pulmonary artery, increases **preload** (the volume of blood in the ventricle at the end of diastole that stretches the heart muscle before contraction) and results in right ventricular hypertrophy. Pulmonary stenosis accounts for 8%–12% of congenital heart defects and can sometimes be seen to progress during the last 12 weeks of pregnancy (Guy, 2012). It is often seen in children with Noonan syndrome. Noonan syndrome is an autosomal dominant congenital disorder that affects both males and females. Children with Noonan syndrome typically present with distinct facial characteristics, including a webbed neck and flat-bridge nose. **Clinical Manifestations** Pulmonary stenosis is often present without symptoms. Dyspnea and fatigue may occur on exertion. Signs of CHF and hepatosplenomegaly are rare but may result from chronic pressure overload. Chest pain on exertion may occur in severe cases. A loud systolic ejection murmur, with a widely split second heart sound (S_2), and a thrill may be found with maximal intensity at the left upper sternal border. A pulmonic ejection click usually denotes a mild to moderate degree of stenosis. With severe stenosis, it may become buried in the first heart sound. **Diagnostic Procedures** Chest x-ray may show an enlarged pulmonary artery with normal heart size and normal pulmonary vascularity. ECG may show right atrial enlargement and right ventricular hypertrophy. Echocardiogram provides information about the pressure gradient across the valve and size of valve ring. Cardiac catheterization findings include increased right ventricular pressure and a normal to slightly lowered pulmonary artery pressure. **Clinical Therapy** Dilation by balloon valvuloplasty, performed during cardiac catheterization, treats simple pulmonic stenosis. Surgical valvotomy may be used when other defects such as VSD are present. Surgical resection may be needed for narrowing above the valve area. Pulmonary regurgitation may result but typically does not present as a significant problem. **Prognosis** Pulmonic stenosis does not typically increase in severity. Lifelong infective endocarditis prophylaxis is recommended.	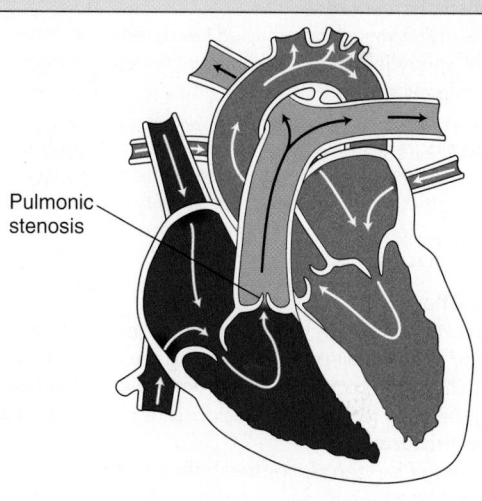 Pulmonic stenosis ■ Decreased unoxygenated blood flow

(continued on next page)

TABLE 16–12 Pathophysiology, Clinical Manifestations, and Clinical Therapy for Heart Defects That Decrease Pulmonary Blood Flow (*continued*)

DEFECT PATHOPHYSIOLOGY, CLINICAL MANIFESTATIONS, AND CLINICAL THERAPY	ANATOMY

Tetralogy of Fallot (TOF)

Tetralogy of Fallot consists of four defects—pulmonic stenosis, right ventricular hypertrophy, VSD, and an overriding aorta (aorta positioned directly over a VSD). Some children have a fifth defect, an open foramen ovale or ASD. TOF is classified as a rare disease affecting fewer than 200,000 people in the United States. With TOF, elevated pressures in the right side of the heart cause a right-to-left shunt.

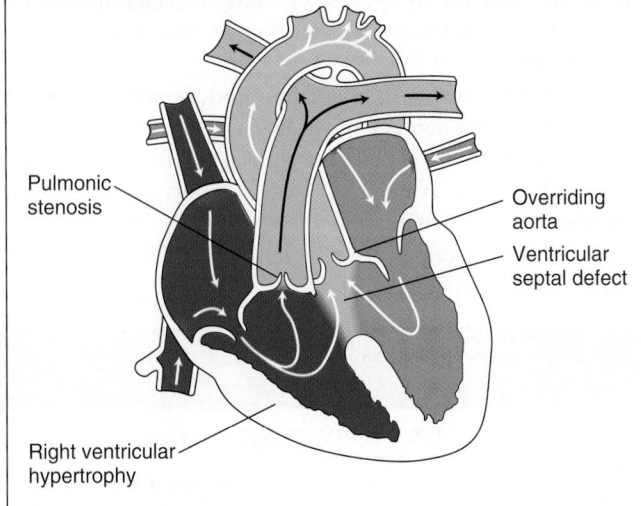

Clinical Manifestations
The infant becomes hypoxic and cyanotic as the ductus arteriosus closes. The degree of pulmonary stenosis determines the severity of symptoms.

A systolic murmur is heard in the pulmonic area and is transmitted to the suprasternal notch. A thrill may be palpated in the pulmonic area.

Polycythemia, hypoxic episodes, metabolic acidosis, poor growth, clubbing of the fingers, and exercise intolerance may develop.

Toddlers with uncorrected defects instinctively squat (assume a knee–chest position) to decrease the return of systemic venous blood to the heart.

Diagnostic Procedures
Chest x-ray shows a boot-shaped heart, resulting from the large right ventricle, decreased pulmonary vascular markings, and a prominent aorta.

ECG shows right ventricular hypertrophy.

Echocardiogram shows the VSD, obstruction of pulmonary outflow, an overriding aorta, and the size of the pulmonary arteries.

Cardiac catheterization reveals the severity of the anatomical defects.

Blood tests demonstrate an elevated hematocrit and hemoglobin and an increased clotting time.

Clinical Therapy
Management of hypercyanotic episodes includes placing the infant in the knee–chest position, calming the child, giving oxygen, and administering morphine and propranolol intravenously. Monitoring the child for metabolic acidosis or prolonged unconsciousness is critical.

A total repair is often performed before 6 months of age when the infant has a hypercyanotic episode. A palliative shunt procedure (e.g., Blalock–Taussig) may be performed.

Prognosis
Not all children benefit from surgery, but most have improved longevity and prolonged quality of life. Junctional tachycardia may occur and may require treatment with medication or use of a temporary pacemaker.

Pulmonary Atresia and Tricuspid Atresia

Pulmonary atresia is the absence of communication between the right ventricle and the pulmonary artery occurring at the site of the pulmonary valve or in the main pulmonary artery. It occurs in fewer than 1% of children with congenital heart defects. In **tricuspid atresia**, the tricuspid valve is absent. Blood flows to the left side of the heart through the foramen ovale. The PDA provides the only flow of blood to the pulmonary arteries. A VSD or transposition of the great arteries is often present.

Clinical Manifestations
Cyanosis is present at birth.

Tachypnea, CHF, pulmonary edema, hepatomegaly, acidosis, hypoxic episodes, clubbing, polycythemia, and growth delays occur.

A continuous murmur from the PDA is heard in the pulmonic area. A single S_2 is heard in the aortic area, and a harsh systolic murmur may be heard in the tricuspid area.

TABLE 16–12 Pathophysiology, Clinical Manifestations, and Clinical Therapy for Heart Defects That Decrease Pulmonary Blood Flow (*continued*)

DEFECT PATHOPHYSIOLOGY, CLINICAL MANIFESTATIONS, AND CLINICAL THERAPY	ANATOMY
Diagnostic Procedures Chest x-ray may reveal a normal size or slightly enlarged sized heart. ECG may reveal right atrial hypertrophy. Echocardiogram shows a small hypoplastic right ventricular cavity and tricuspid valve, an absent right ventricular outflow tract, a dilated right atrium, and right-to-left shunting across the atrial septum. **Clinical Therapy** Prostaglandin E_1 is given immediately to maintain a PDA. Digoxin and diuretics are also used. Rastelli balloon atrial septostomy is performed to increase the atrial opening (refer to Table 16–17 on pages 1099–1100). Rastelli or modified Fontan procedure results in improved survival. **Prognosis** Outcome depends on the size of the pulmonary outflow tract developed by surgery and the fibrosis in the right ventricle. The child has increased risk for arrhythmia and right ventricular dysfunction.	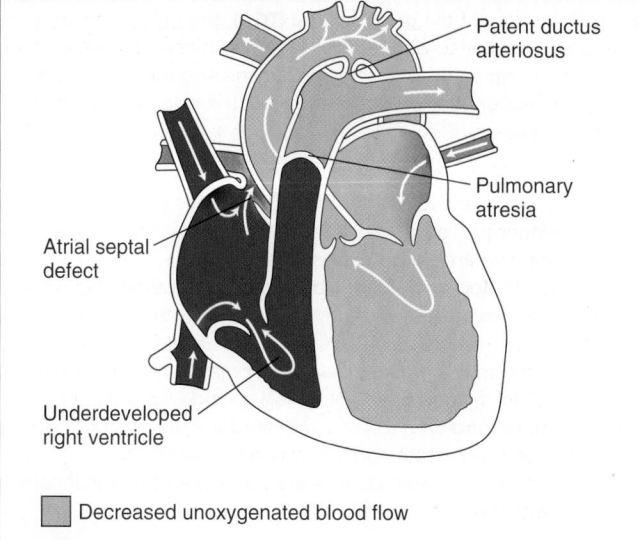

Mixed Defects

Many complex congenital heart defects involve a combination of defects that make the newborn dependent on mixing pulmonary and systemic circulations for survival during the postnatal period. This mixing of oxygen-rich blood with oxygen poor-blood results in a general, desaturated systemic blood flow and cyanosis. Pulmonary congestion may occur because of increased pulmonary blood flow and obstruction of systemic flow.

The pathophysiology, clinical manifestations, and clinical therapy for mixed heart defects are shown in **Table 16–13** ●.

Defects That Obstruct Systemic Blood Flow

An anatomical stenosis of the aorta causes obstruction of blood flow and results in a pressure load on the left ventricle and decreased cardiac output. The greater the narrowing, the more obstructed the blood flow to the circulation. This results in higher pressure in the ventricle and decreased cardiac output. Neonates with severe left outflow obstruction or left ventricular dysfunction may develop decreased cardiac output and shock.

The pathophysiology, clinical manifestations, and clinical therapy for heart defects that obstruct the systemic blood flow are shown in **Table 16–14** ●.

Etiology

Most congenital heart defects develop during the first 8 weeks of gestation. They usually result from a combined or interactive effect of genetic and environmental factors, such as the following:

- Fetal exposure to drugs (e.g., phenytoin, lithium, warfarin, and valporic acid).
- Maternal viral infections (e.g., rubella and coxsackie B5).
- Maternal metabolic disorders (e.g., phenylketonuria, diabetes mellitus, and hypercalcemia).
- Maternal complications of pregnancy (e.g., increased age and antepartal bleeding).
- Genetic factors (family recurrence patterns). Chromosomal abnormalities have been identified related to numerical excesses or deficiencies and structural abnormalities among family members.
- Chromosomal abnormalities (e.g., Turner syndrome, Noonan syndrome, DiGeorge syndrome, *cri du chat* syndrome, Down syndrome, and trisomy syndromes 13, 18, and 21). Congenital heart defects are commonly seen in Down syndrome clients.

Deletion of chromosome 22q11 is associated with congenital heart disease, particularly tetralogy of Fallot, interrupted aortic arch, ventricular septal defect, and truncus arteriosus (McDonald-McGinn, Emanuel, & Zacai, 2013). Other disease characteristics include defects in the palate, learning disabilities, mild differences in facial features, and recurrent infections. Knowledge about other chromosome deletions or mutations associated with cardiovascular defects is emerging. Because of the genetic component, the incidence of congenital heart defects is expected to slowly increase as clients live longer and begin families of their own. Depending on the type of defect, signs and symptoms may be present at birth or develop later.

TABLE 16–13 Pathophysiology, Clinical Manifestations, and Clinical Therapy for Mixed Heart Defects

DEFECT PATHOPHYSIOLOGY, CLINICAL MANIFESTATIONS, AND CLINICAL THERAPY	ANATOMY
Transposition of the Great Arteries (TGA)	

In **transposition of the great arteries (TGA)**, the pulmonary artery and the aorta are transposed. TGA is life threatening at birth with initial survival initially depending on an open ductus arteriosus and foramen ovale. TGA is estimated to occur in approximately 5% of the population. An ASD or VSD may also be present.

Clinical Manifestations

Cyanosis, apparent soon after birth, progresses to hypoxia and acidosis. Cyanosis does not improve with oxygen administration. Cyanosis may be less prevalent when a large VSD is present.

CHF may develop immediately or over days or weeks. Tachypnea (60 breaths/min) is often present without retractions or other signs of dyspnea.

A systolic murmur is present if a VSD is present; no other murmur is generally heard. The second heart sound (S_2) is loud.

Infants take a long time to feed and need frequent rest periods because of rapid respiratory rate and increasing fatigue.

Growth failure may be evident as early as 2 weeks of age if corrective surgery is not performed.

Diagnostic Procedures

Chest x-ray may reveal a classic egg-shaped heart on a string (narrow superior mediastinum) with enlarged ventricles and increased pulmonary vascular markings.

ECG reveals right ventricular hypertrophy.

Echocardiogram often shows the abnormal position of the great arteries rising from ventricles.

Hyperoxitest confirms a cyanotic congenital heart defect.

Cardiac catheterization shows increased right ventricular pressure, and the catheter can enter the aorta through the right ventricle.

Blood tests reveal an increased hematocrit and hemoglobin or polycythemia.

Clinical Therapy

Prostaglandin E_1 is ordered to maintain a patent ductus arteriosus until a palliative procedure can be performed. Oxygen is administered for severe hypoxemia.

Balloon atrial septostomy may be performed during cardiac catheterization in newborns as a first stage. The defect may also be corrected surgically. Other defects may be repaired in stages as the infant grows.

Corrective surgery (arterial switch) is usually performed before 1 week of age.

Prognosis

Survival without surgery is impossible. The 10-year survival rate following an arterial switch is approximately 90% (Gorler et al., 2011). Arrhythmias, decreased right ventricular function, pulmonary vascular disease, and sudden death are long-term complications after the Mustard and Senning procedures. Follow-up every 6–12 months is recommended. Other complications of surgical repair include pulmonary artery or aortic stenosis, coronary artery obstruction, and mitral regurgitation. Infective endocarditis prophylaxis may be necessary.

Labels: Patent ductus arteriosus; Pulmonary artery; Aorta

Truncus Arteriosus	

In **truncus arteriosus**, a single large vessel empties both ventricles and provides circulation for the pulmonary, systemic, and coronary circulations. A VSD is usually present. Truncus arteriosus is an uncommon congenital heart defect characterized by a single semilunar valve. Additionally, the pulmonary arteries originate from the common arterial trunk distal to the coronary arteries and proximal to the first brachiocephalic branch of the aortic arch (McElhinney & Wernovsky, 2012).

TABLE 16–13 Pathophysiology, Clinical Manifestations, and Clinical Therapy for Mixed Heart Defects (*continued*)

DEFECT PATHOPHYSIOLOGY, CLINICAL MANIFESTATIONS, AND CLINICAL THERAPY	ANATOMY

Clinical Manifestations

Cyanosis develops soon after birth; however, this is also a condition of increased pulmonary blood flow. Severe CHF, dyspnea, retractions, fatigue, poor feeding, poor growth, polycythemia, clubbing, increased pulse pressure, bounding peripheral pulses, a widened pulse pressure, frequent respiratory infections, and cardiomegaly occur.

The VSD produces a harsh systolic murmur in the lower sternal border. A systolic click may be heard in the apex and pulmonic area.

Diagnostic Procedures

Chest x-ray shows cardiomegaly, a large aorta, and increased pulmonary vascular markings.

ECG reveals right and left ventricular hypertrophy.

Echocardiogram shows the absence of two semilunar valves.

Cardiac catheterization documents a left-to-right shunt at the level of the ventricle, pressure that is equal in the ventricles, the truncus, and pulmonary arteries.

Clinical Therapy

The Rastelli procedure is performed to close the VSD and create a passage to pulmonary arteries. Repeated surgery is necessary to enlarge the pulmonary artery conduit.

Digoxin and diuretics are given.

Prognosis

Survival is improved, but truncal valve stenosis and regurgitation result. The long-term prognosis is unknown. The child should not participate in competitive sports.

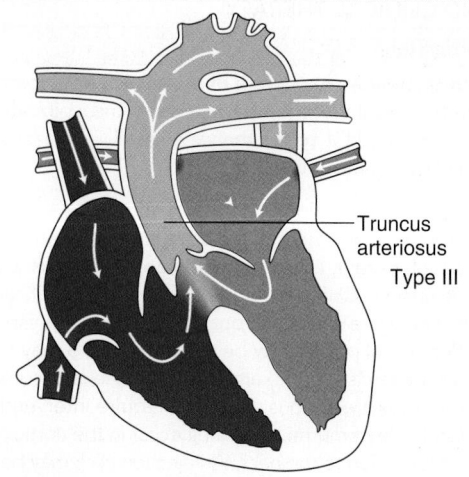

Truncus arteriosus Type III

■ Mixed oxygenated and unoxygenated blood

Total Anomalous Pulmonary Venous Return

In **total anomalous pulmonary venous return**, the pulmonary veins empty into the right atrium, or into veins leading to the right atrium, rather than into the left atrium. The foramen ovale must remain patent for mixed blood from the right atrium to pass to the systemic circulation. Any obstruction of the pulmonary veins increases the condition's severity. Total anomalous pulmonary venous return is rare, occurring in approximately 1% of the population.

Clinical Manifestations

Mild cyanosis and frequent respiratory infections occur. Increased cyanosis may occur with feedings as the filled esophagus compresses the common pulmonary vein.

If the pulmonary veins are obstructed in any way, cyanosis will be increased. Increased pulmonary blood flow will result in signs of CHF.

A precordial bulge may be palpated. Heart sound S_2 has a wide, fixed split when there is no pulmonary vein obstruction. An ejection murmur and gallop rhythm may be heard in the pulmonic area.

Diagnostic Procedures

Chest x-ray shows cardiac enlargement, a large pulmonary artery, and increased pulmonary blood flow.

ECG reveals hypertrophy of the right atrium and ventricle.

Echocardiogram shows enlargement of the right atrium, a patent foramen ovale, and lack of connection between the pulmonary veins and left atrium.

Cardiac catheterization shows a higher oxygen level in the right atrium and the abnormal circulation.

Clinical Therapy

Prostaglandin E_1 is given to maintain a patent ductus arteriosus.

Hypoxemia and CHF are treated.

Balloon atrial septostomy may be performed to promote better mixing of blood so surgery can be delayed until the infant is stabilized.

Surgery to reconnect or baffle the pulmonary veins to the left atrium is performed.

Prognosis

Prognosis is good when the defect is caught and repaired early and if there is no obstruction of the pulmonary veins at the new connection to the heart. Left untreated, the heart will continue to enlarge, resulting in heart failure.

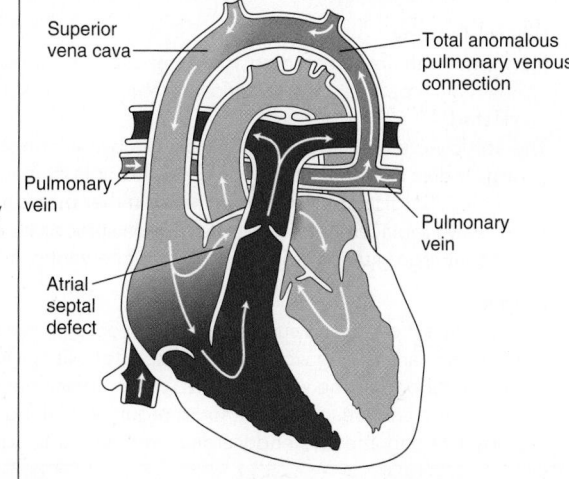

Superior vena cava

Total anomalous pulmonary venous connection

Pulmonary vein

Pulmonary vein

Atrial septal defect

TABLE 16–14   Pathophysiology, Clinical Manifestations, and Clinical Therapy for Heart Defects That Obstruct the Systemic Blood Flow

DEFECT PATHOPHYSIOLOGY, CLINICAL MANIFESTATIONS, AND CLINICAL THERAPY	ANATOMY

Aortic Stenosis (AS)

In **aortic stenosis**, narrowing of the aortic valve obstructs blood flow to systemic circulation. The valve is often bicuspid rather than tricuspid. The pressure gradient across the valve usually increases as the child grows and cardiac output increases.

Clinical Manifestations
Most infants and children are asymptomatic, with normal growth and development. Life-threatening aortic stenosis is detected in some newborns. CHF develops in infants with significant stenosis.
Blood pressure is normal, but a narrow pulse pressure may be noted. Peripheral pulses may be weak. The child may complain of chest pain after exercise, but exercise intolerance is uncommon. Syncope and dizziness are serious signs that require intervention.
A systolic heart murmur and thrill occur in the aortic or pulmonic areas with transmission to the neck. An ejection click may be heard. Splitting of the second heart sound (S$_2$) may be noted with severe aortic stenosis.

Diagnostic Procedures
Chest x-ray is usually normal but may reveal a slight prominence of the left ventricle and aorta with increased severity.
ECG is usually normal in mild cases but with increased severity may show mild left ventricular hypertrophy and inverted T waves.
Echocardiogram reveals the number of the valve cusps, pressure gradient across the valve, and size of the aorta.
Stress testing may be used in asymptomatic children to determine the amount of obstruction present with exercise.

Clinical Therapy
Newborns with life-threatening aortic stenosis need prostaglandin E$_1$ to maintain a patent ductus arteriosus until the aortic valve can be dilated.
The aortic valve may be successfully dilated by balloon valvuloplasty during cardiac catheterization. Surgical valvuloplasty may also be performed. Surgical treatment is palliative rather than curative.
Aortic valve replacement is performed when stenosis is severe or if significant regurgitation results from other interventions.

Prognosis
Chest pain, syncope, and sudden death can occur in symptomatic children, particularly during vigorous exercise. Stenosis is usually progressive during childhood as the valve calcifies. Valve replacement may be necessary once the child reaches adulthood, requiring lifelong anticoagulant therapy. Lifelong infective endocarditis prophylaxis is required.

Aortic stenosis

☐ Decreased oxygenated blood flow
☐ Mixed oxygenated and unoxygenated blood

Coarctation of the Aorta (COA)

In **coarctation of the aorta**, narrowing or constriction in the descending aorta, often near the ductus arteriosus or left subclavian artery, obstructs the systemic blood outflow. When this occurs, the heart must pump harder to force blood through the narrow part of the aorta.
    Coarctation of the aorta is usually congenital and may range from mild to severe. However, it might not be diagnosed until adulthood. It often occurs with other heart defects and requires careful follow-up. Coarctation of the aorta is commonly seen in clients with certain genetic disorders, such as Turner syndrome. Turner syndrome is a chromosomal abnormality occurring only in females.

Clinical Manifestations
Symptoms are dependent on the rate of blood flow through the artery but constriction is progressive. Infants may present with symptoms during the first few days of life; others may not present until adolescence.

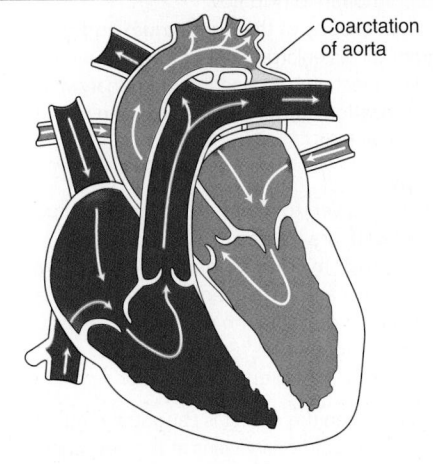
Coarctation of aorta

TABLE 16–14 Pathophysiology, Clinical Manifestations, and Clinical Therapy for Heart Defects That Obstruct the Systemic Blood Flow (*continued*)

DEFECT PATHOPHYSIOLOGY, CLINICAL MANIFESTATIONS, AND CLINICAL THERAPY	ANATOMY
Back pressure of blood and congestion of the lungs that progresses to heart failure. Symptoms include dyspnea, coughing, fatigue, and swelling of feet and legs. A distinguishing clinical feature is a difference between the femoral and carotid pulses. A distinctive harsh murmur may be heard when a stethoscope is placed over the client's back. **Diagnostic Procedures** Chest x-ray may reveal cardiomegaly, pulmonary venous congestion, and indentation of the descending aorta. Rib notching may be seen but is rare in clients younger than 10 years of age. Magnetic resonance imaging shows the site of coarctation. ECG shows left ventricular hypertrophy; right ventricular hypertrophy may be seen in severe cases. Echocardiogram shows the size of the aorta, the actual coarctation, and the function of the aortic valve and left ventricle. **Clinical Therapy** Angioplasty occurs during cardiac catheterization for initial relief and recurrence. A catheter, via the groin, with a balloon on the end of it is threaded into the aorta through the blood vessels. Once the catheter reaches the coarctation, the physician inflates the balloon to expand the aorta. When the aorta is fully expanded, the balloon and catheter are removed. Surgical resection with end-to-end anastomosis or with patching using the subclavian artery may be performed. Repair in the first year of life is recommended to decrease exposure to hypertension. **Prognosis** Prognosis depends on the severity of the defect and success of treatment.	

Hypoplastic Left Heart Syndrome (HLHS)

Hypoplastic left heart syndrome (HLHS) is one of the most severe congenital heart defects. In HLHS, the left side of the heart does not form correctly during fetal growth, resulting in underdeveloped heart structures (CDC, 2013c). In clients with an absence of or stenosis of mitral and aortic valves, an abnormally small left ventricle, a small aorta, and aortic or mitral stenosis or atresia develops. Current evidence demonstrated that HLHS accounts for 2%–3% of congenital heart defects. Most causes of heart defects are unknown but genetic and environmental risk factors are considered. **Clinical Manifestations** Once closure of the ductus arteriosus occurs, the newborn may have progressive cyanosis, tachycardia, tachypnea, dyspnea, retractions, and decreased peripheral pulses. A systolic murmur may be present or absent. Poor peripheral perfusion, pulmonary edema, and CHF can lead to shock, acidosis, and death. **Diagnostic Procedures** Chest x-ray shows cardiomegaly and increased pulmonary vascularity. Echocardiogram shows the small left ventricle. Diagnosis may occur prenatally during routine ultrasound scans. Cardiac catheterization may be performed in preparation for surgical intervention. An atrial septostomy may be considered to promote homogeneity of the blood. **Clinical Therapy** An infusion of prostaglandin is usually begun to promote an open pathway for the blood to enter circulation from the right ventricle. The medication prevents closure of the patent ductus arteriosus. Supplemental oxygen is avoided because it tends to promote blood flow to the lungs, which may decrease blood flow to the body and place excessive demands on the stressed right ventricle.	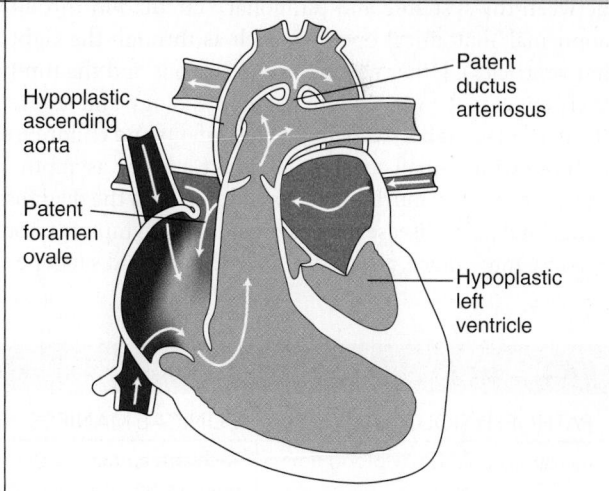

(*continued on next page*)

TABLE 16–14 Pathophysiology, Clinical Manifestations, and Clinical Therapy for Heart Defects That Obstruct the Systemic Blood Flow (*continued*)

DEFECT PATHOPHYSIOLOGY, CLINICAL MANIFESTATIONS, AND CLINICAL THERAPY	ANATOMY
Treatment options include comfort or palliative care, the Norwood procedure, and heart transplantation. Heart transplantation is limited by the scarcity of newborn organs and a lifelong need for antirejection therapy. However, the incidence of rejection does continue to be lower in clients who received transplants as newborns. The Norwood procedure has become a more common intervention as outcomes have improved. Surgery is performed in three stages. The Norwood procedure is performed in the first week of life, followed by the Glenn procedure at approximately 3–8 months of age, and then the Fontan procedure (see Table 16–17 on page 1099) at between 18 months and 3 years of age.	
Prognosis Once considered fatal within the first month of life, HLHS now has a survival rate around 60% for children 3–5 years of age. Treatment decisions may be difficult because the parents must consider the potential for distress associated with multiples surgeries and the high medical costs. Children are restricted from competitive sports and very demanding physical activities but otherwise have a good quality of life. If failure of the single ventricle occurs, the child may require a heart transplant during adolescence or adulthood.	

▶ CLINICAL MANIFESTATIONS

The presence of a heart murmur is often the first indication of a congenital heart defect. A loud murmur indicates blood is flowing with higher-than-normal pressure to get through a narrowed valve or vessel, or through a **shunt** (movement of blood between the systemic and pulmonary circulation through an abnormal anatomical opening, such as through the right and left ventricles). Other clinical manifestations and the timing of their appearance vary by the pathophysiology and severity of the defect (see **Table 16–15** ●). Some infants and children, such as those with a small atrial septal defect, may be asymptomatic except for a heart murmur. Older children with the diagnosis of congenital heart disease may have additional symptoms, such as exercise intolerance, chest pain, arrhythmias, and syncope.

Defects That Increase Pulmonary Blood Flow

An infant's heart rate, respiratory rate, and metabolic rate are increased when the pulmonary blood flow increases. Sucking breast milk or formula takes energy, and diaphoresis often occurs with feeding. The infant may be unable to take in enough calories to support the metabolic rate and growth, resulting in poor weight gain. If CHF develops, signs include dyspnea, tachypnea, intercostal retractions, and periorbital edema. Frequent respiratory infections occur as the moist environment in the lungs supports bacterial growth. See Table 16–15 for the pathophysiology, clinical manifestations, and clinical therapy for specific congenital heart defects with increased pulmonary blood flow.

TABLE 16–15 Clinical Manifestations of Heart Defects by Pathophysiology

PATHOPHYSIOLOGY	CLINICAL MANIFESTATIONS	TYPES OF DEFECTS
Increased pulmonary blood flow	Tachypnea, tachycardia, murmur, congestive heart failure, poor weight gain, diaphoresis, periorbital edema, frequent respiratory infections	Patent ductus arteriosus, atrial septal defect, ventricular septal defect, atrioventricular canal defect (endocardial cushion defect), truncus arteriosus, total anomalous pulmonary venous return
Decreased pulmonary blood flow	Cyanosis, hypercyanotic episodes, poor weight gain, polycythemia	Pulmonic stenosis, tetralogy of Fallot, pulmonary atresia, tricuspid atresia, transposition of the great arteries
Mixed defects—postnatal survival depends on mixing of systemic and pulmonary blood	Cyanosis, poor weight gain, pulmonary congestion, or congestive heart failure may occur with increased shunting	Transposition of great arteries, total anomalous pulmonary venous connection, truncus arteriosus, double outlet right ventricle
Obstructed systemic blood flow	Diminished pulses, poor color, delayed capillary refill time, decreased urine output, congestive heart failure with pulmonary edema	Coarctation of aorta, aortic stenosis, hypoplastic left heart syndrome, mitral stenosis, interrupted aortic arch

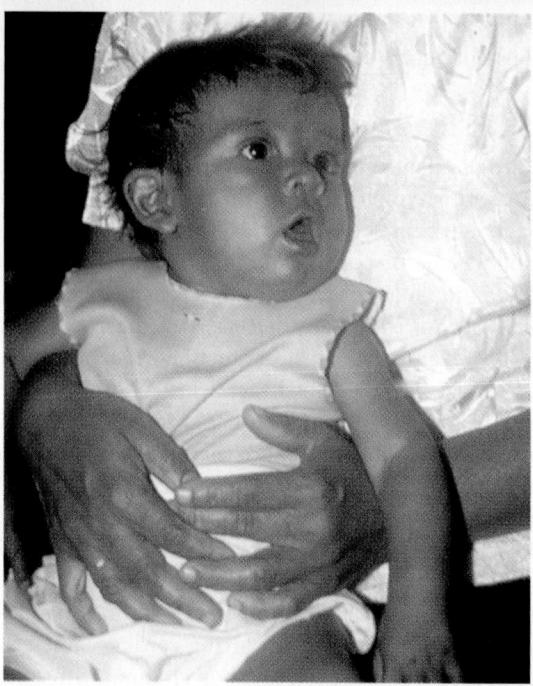

Figure 16–30 ● The infant is cyanotic due to a heart defect that reduces pulmonary blood flow.

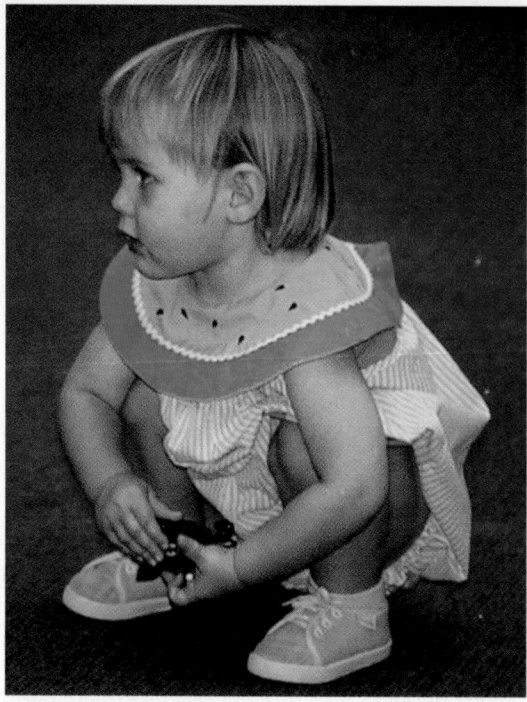

Figure 16–31 ● A young child with an uncorrected or partially corrected defect that reduces pulmonary blood flow may squat (assume a knee–chest position) to reduce systemic blood flow return to the heart.

Defects That Decrease Pulmonary Blood Flow

Initially, clinical manifestations in infants include cyanosis shortly after birth, dyspnea, and a loud murmur. The skin may be ruddy or mottled before cyanosis is observed. Cyanosis that does not respond as expected to oxygen is a classic sign (**Figure 16–30** ●). Signs and symptoms of chronic hypoxemia include fatigue, clubbing of the fingers and toes, exertional dyspnea, and delayed developmental milestones. The infant may need to stop sucking periodically during feedings to breathe, and diaphoresis may be seen with the increased work of feeding. These infants have a higher metabolic rate, and inadequate calories may be consumed, resulting in poor weight gain. See Table 16–15 for the pathophysiology, clinical manifestations, and clinical therapy for these defects.

When the infant or child has severe obstruction to pulmonary blood flow, hypercyanotic episodes can develop suddenly. Hypercyanotic episodes usually appear between 2 months and 2 years of age. Signs include increased rate and depth of respirations; increased heart rate; increased cyanosis, pallor, and poor tissue perfusion; diaphoresis; irritability and crying; and seizures and loss of consciousness. Toddlers with uncorrected cyanotic heart disease often squat to relieve dyspnea (**Figure 16–31** ●). The knee–chest position reduces the cardiac output by decreasing the venous return from the lower extremities and by increasing the systemic vascular resistance.

Older children may have additional symptoms, such as exercise-induced dizziness and syncope. These are serious signs indicating a need for medical evaluation.

Mixed Defects

These complex congenital heart defects demonstrate varying degrees of cyanosis and congestive heart failure. When the pulmonary vascular resistance is lower than systemic resistance, pulmonary congestion develops, followed by congestive heart failure. With decreased pulmonary blood flow, the infant will most likely present with severe cyanosis and polycythemia. See Table 16–15 for the pathophysiology and clinical manifestations of heart defects.

Defects That Obstruct Systemic Blood Flow

Low cardiac output is responsible for diminished pulses, poor color, delayed capillary refill time, and decreased urinary output. The blood cannot move past the obstruction, so it backs up into the left atrium and then the lungs, causing congestive heart failure and pulmonary edema. Children with mild obstruction may have leg cramps, cooler feet than hands, and stronger pulses and higher blood pressure in the upper extremities than in the lower extremities. Decreased blood supply to the gastrointestinal tract may lead to necrotizing enterocolitis. See Table 16–15.

▶ COLLABORATION

Regular, ongoing follow-up with a primary healthcare provider and cardiologist is important for clients diagnosed with a congenital heart defect. Even with advances in medical treatment, not all clients are cured. Further surgeries may be needed after initial childhood surgeries. Diet and nutrition are important for those with feeding and weight gain issues. Many clients may also be placed on lifelong medications to improve heart function and help lower blood pressure. Activity level should be discussed with the healthcare provider prior to beginning any new physical exercise programs. Women considering pregnancy should discuss those plans with a healthcare provider prior to becoming pregnant. Genetic counseling is beneficial in women with congenital heart defects because the baby may also be at risk for developing the condition.

Diagnostic Tests

Diagnostic procedures and laboratory tests used in the evaluation of congenital cardiac conditions are described in **Table 16–16** ●.

Pharmacologic Therapy

Medications administered to children with congenital heart defects may include any of those discussed in the Pharmacologic Therapy section in the Concept part of this module. In addition, prostaglandin may be administered to maintain fetal circulation, specifically to maintain a patent ductus arteriosus, which allows blood to pass through the ductus and perfuse the

rest of the body. Prostaglandin is used only for defects that rely on the patent ductus arteriosus.

Clinical Interventions

One third of infants born with congenital heart defects develop life-threatening symptoms in the first few days of life. Treatment for congenital heart defects depends on the severity of symptoms and whether the condition is imminently life threatening.

Interventional catheterization or surgical correction is the treatment of choice for many defects. Many heart defects can be completely repaired, with restoration of normal hemodynamics and physiology. For complex heart defects, however, treatment may only be a **palliative procedure**, a surgical or interventional cardiac catheterization procedure that does not create normal anatomical or hemodynamic results but allows adequate blood flow to oxygenate the tissues. A palliative procedure may be used for children with a potentially fatal or lethal condition or as an initial procedure while the infant is small and before definitive corrective surgery can be performed. **Table 16–17** ● lists the types of interventions during cardiac catheterization and surgical procedures performed on children with congenital heart defects.

Evidence-Based Practice   Neurodevelopmental Outcomes in Children With Complex Congenital Heart Disease

Problem

Infants with serious congenital heart defects are exposed to pathophysiology (prolonged hypoxemia, profound acidosis, and low cardiac output) because of the timing of surgical interventions. In addition, nutrition may be less than adequate for their metabolic rate and brain growth. With the rising potential for children with complex congenital heart defects to have developmental and cognitive problems, parents and school officials need information to evaluate and plan for educational supports as necessary.

Evidence

A longitudinal study of 131 infants with complex congenital heart defects explored neurological and developmental outcomes. It specifically excluded infants who were expected to have neurological problems prior to surgical intervention (e.g., prematurity, chromosomal abnormalities, and radiographic evidence of brain malformation). Infants were assessed prior to surgery, and 56% had abnormalities on the neurological examination; similar findings were found on the postoperative examination. Upon follow-up of 94 children at school entry, 28.4% had neurological abnormalities and 5% had severe impairments. Mean intelligence quotient (IQ) scores were found to be in the low-normal range (in the 90s). Approximately 20% of the children had cognitive difficulties. Behavior problems (e.g., withdrawal, anxiety, sadness, somatic symptoms) were common in this population. A majority of parents (75%) expressed concerns about their child's development. Education supports were provided to 22% of the children and 23% were receiving rehabilitation services. This study revealed that a large percentage of children with complex congenital heart defects have neurodevelopmental abnormalities prior to surgery (Majnemer et al., 2008, 2009).

Another study evaluated the neurocognitive functioning of 45 European children between ages 6 and 16 years scheduled for elective open heart surgery compared with 41 healthy peers. Children diagnosed with genetic syndromes, cognitive impairment (IQ < 70), and severe learning disabilities were excluded. Results revealed that the children with scheduled cardiac surgery demonstrated neurocognitive deficits in motor planning and visual memory when compared with the control group. This finding was true in clients scheduled for their first surgery as well as those scheduled for follow-up surgery. It was speculated that these deficits may be associated with the cardiac disease rather than cardiac surgery (Van der Rijken et al., 2009).

Implications

These studies suggest that children with congenital defects are at greater risk for neurological and cognitive impairments as well as for behavior problems. Nurses working with children with congenital heart defects should be sure to include neurological assessment as part of the child's holistic assessment at each healthcare interaction. In addition, nurses should include assessment of parent coping and the need for education related to both their child's heart condition and to cognitive functioning and behavioral concerns.

Critical Thinking Application

1. What implications does this information have for nurses working with children in primary care clinics?

2. What implications does this information have for nurses working in early childhood intervention and school settings?

3. What resources are available in your community for children younger than 5 years old who have cognitive impairments? Behavior problems? For children 5 years old and older?

TABLE 16–16 Diagnostic Procedures and Laboratory Tests Used to Evaluate Cardiac Conditions

DIAGNOSTIC PROCEDURE	PURPOSE	NURSING IMPLICATIONS
Cardiac catheterization	An invasive medical procedure used in the diagnosis and treatment of various conditions. A flexible tube or catheter is inserted into a blood vessel in the arm, groin, or neck and threaded until it reaches the heart. Practitioners may place dye in the catheter to assist in the visualization of blood flow, perform ultrasound during catheterization, or perform heart muscle biopsies. The practitioner can also use cardiac catheterization to view the overall flow of blood between the heart chambers and arteries.	■ Client should be NPO 6–8 hr prior to procedure. ■ Check orders related to the administration of routine, scheduled medications. ■ Blood thinners and antiplatelet medications will most likely be placed on hold. ■ Ensure any lab work ordered specific to the procedure has been reviewed and placed on the medical record. ■ Prep client for procedure, as ordered. *Postprocedure:* ■ After sheath removal, apply consistent pressure to the access site for 20–30 min. Monitor client vital signs per order. ■ Assess access site frequently. Palpate and assess temperature, color, pulses, and client discomfort. ■ After stabilization of access site, elevate head of bed to 30 degrees. ■ Document access site assessment, including hematoma size, hematoma characteristics, skin color, skin temperature, and the presence of pedal pulses, bruits, or both. ■ Provide client education regarding common complications and methods to prevent bleeding. Clear instructions should emphasize when to seek medical assistance.
Chest x-ray	A radiographic exam of the chest, lungs, heart, large arteries, ribs, and diaphragm. It reveals the size and contour of the heart and characteristics of pulmonary vascular markings.	■ Explain the procedure to the client to alleviate stress and anxiety. Two images are usually taken from different angles. ■ Explain that equipment used today limits radiation as much as possible. ■ Explain to the child that the tech may ask him or her to inhale and exhale deep breaths.
Echocardiography	This noninvasive test uses sound waves to create a moving picture of the heart. It allows the practitioner to see a clear picture of how the heart is formed. This test is important for diagnosing CHD and its progression over time.	■ Decrease anxiety by reassuring the client that the exam is painless.
Electrocardiography (ECG)	This noninvasive test records the electrical activity of the heart. An ECG demonstrates the rate and rhythm of the heart and also records the strength and timing of electrical signals as they pass through the heart.	■ Document current medications. ■ Reassure the child that the procedure is painless. ■ Explain to the parent and child the need to remain still during the recording.
Exercise testing	This test is typically performed on a treadmill or stationary bicycle to evaluate controlled increases in activity. The child is usually connected to ECG leads, a blood pressure cuff, and pulse oximetry monitor. Once the test begins, the acceleration and pitch of the machine are increased in intervals. The test is concluded when the child demonstrates noticeable fatigue or a predetermined stopping point is reached. The test is beneficial for identifying cardiac compensation or inadequate cardiac output.	■ Educate the child and parent about the procedure. ■ Reassure the child that the test can be stopped at any point. ■ Instruct the child (in age appropriate terms) to report dizziness, shortness of breath, chest pain, and excessive fatigue. ■ Assess vital signs prior to, during, and after the exam.

(continued on next page)

TABLE 16-16 Diagnostic Procedures and Laboratory Tests Used to Evaluate Cardiac Conditions (*continued*)

DIAGNOSTIC PROCEDURE	PURPOSE	NURSING IMPLICATIONS
Holter monitor (ambulatory ECG)	Used when a 24- to 48-hr recording of the heart's electrical activity is ordered. An ECG demonstrates the rate and rhythm of the heart and also records the strength and timing of electrical signals as they pass through the heart.	■ Normal daily activity is typically not limited. ■ Remind the parent and child to avoid submersing the electrodes in water. Swimming and bathing are not allowed until the test is completed. ■ Ask the parent to keep a daily log of activities and sleeping and eating habits.
Hyperoxitest	Most sensitive tool for differentiating primary pulmonary and cyanotic congenital heart disease. If cyanosis is respiratory in nature, PCO_2 should greatly improve with 100% O_2 supplementation.	■ Administer oxygen through a plastic hood for at least 10 min to replace all alveolar air with oxygen.
Magnetic resonance imaging (MRI)	An imaging test that uses powerful magnets and radio waves to create images of the heart's myocardium, structure, valve function, blood vessels, and other soft tissues.	■ Verify that child has no metal implants. ■ Reduce anxiety by discussing the shape, size, and sounds of the machine. ■ Administer sedation, as ordered. ■ Monitor vital signs and level of consciousness as appropriate.
LABORATORY TEST	PURPOSE	NURSING IMPLICATIONS
Arterial blood gas	A sample of arterial blood is drawn and analyzed to help determine the status of pulmonary gas exchange and acid–base balance. Blood is drawn from either a direct arterial puncture or arterial line.	■ If ordered, a topical agent may be used to decrease pain associated with the needlestick. ■ After collecting the sample, place pressure on the puncture site for 5–10 min to decrease chances of hematoma formation.
Complete blood count	Venous blood is collected and analyzed to assess the status of red blood cells, white blood cells, hemoglobin, hematocrit, and platelets.	■ Educate the parent and child about the procedure. ■ Follow hospital policy regarding skin preparation. ■ Apply light pressure and bandage to site after puncture.
Serum digoxin level	A venous sample of blood is drawn to assess serum digoxin levels of clients receiving the medication.	■ Collect amount of blood recommended for procedure. ■ Educate the parent and child about the procedure. ■ Document last dosage and time of medication.
Antistreptolysin O antibody titer	This test detects previous infection by group A streptococcus.	■ Educate the parent and child about the procedure. ■ Follow hospital policy regarding skin preparation.
Erythrocyte sedimentation rate (ESR)	This test detects the rate at which red blood cells coagulate. The ESR increases with inflammation and assists in detecting acute illness.	■ Educate the parent and child about the procedure. ■ Follow hospital policy regarding skin preparation.
C-reactive protein (CRP)	This test detects the level of C-reactive protein produced by the liver. The CRP rises when there is inflammation in the body.	■ Educate the parent and child about the procedure. ■ Follow hospital policy regarding skin preparation.
Serum lipid panel	This test is used to measure total cholesterol, HDL, LDL, and triglycerides.	■ Follow orders regarding the need to fast.

Sources: Based on Morton, P. G., & Fontaine, D. K. (2013). *Critical care nursing: A holistic approach.* New York, NY: Wolters Kluwer/Lippincott Williams & Wilkins; National Heart, Lung, and Blood Institute. (2012). *What is cardiac catheterization?* Retrieved from http://www.nhlbi.nih.gov/health/health-topics/topics/cath; and National Heart, Lung, and Blood Institute. (2013). *How are congenital heart defects diagnosed?* Retrieved from http://www.nhlbi.nih.gov/health/health-topics/topics/chd/diagnosis.html.

TABLE 16–17 Clinical Interventions for Congenital Heart Defects

HEART CATHETERIZATION PROCEDURE	DESCRIPTION OF INTERVENTION	THERAPEUTIC USE AND DEFECT TREATED
Balloon angioplasty and valvuloplasty	A deflated balloon is threaded up to the coronary arteries to widen blocked areas where blood flow is reduced or completely obstructed.	Used as a primary or adjunctive treatment for pulmonary stenosis, aortic stenosis, and coarctation of the aorta.
Patent ductus arteriosus (PDA) closure	Catheters are inserted in the groin and advanced to the aorta. A coil or plug may be placed, via the catheter, to occlude the defect.	Used to correct PDA.
Rashkind balloon atrial septostomy	Balloon catheter is used to increase oxygen saturation and enlarge a defect.	Used in the treatment of transposition of the great arteries (TGA).
Transcatheter closure	Procedure used to push an umbrella or clamshell shaped device to plug a septum defect.	Used to correct atrial and ventral septal defects.

SURGICAL PROCEDURE	DESCRIPTION OF INTERVENTION	THERAPEUTIC USE AND DEFECT TREATED
Aorta resection with end-to-end anastomosis	Aortic isthmus and ductal tissues are resected along with the inferior and lower lateral side of the aorta.	Used to correct coarctation of the aorta.
Blalock–Taussig shunt	A Gore-Tex tube is placed from the innominate artery to the pulmonary artery.	Used as a palliative treatment for tetralogy of Fallot (TOF), pulmonary atresia, tricuspid atresia, and other defects affecting blood supply to the lungs. In most cases, final repair will need to be done at a later time.
Brock procedure	Excision of fibromuscular obstruction in the right ventricle. The excision is completed using a surgical instrument inserted through the right ventricle.	Used as a palliative procedure to increase pulmonary blood flow and reduce right-to-left shunting in tetralogy of Fallot.
Damus–Kaye–Stansel procedure	Aorta and pulmonary artery are joined using a patch.	Used as a corrective procedure for TGA and complex single-ventricle defects.
Fontan procedure	This operation results in the flow of systemic venous blood to the lungs without passing through a ventricle.	Performed to treat some complex congenital heart defects including tricuspid atresia, pulmonary atresia, hypoplastic left heart syndrome (HLHS), and a double-inlet ventricle.
Glenn procedure	Involves connecting superior vena cava to the right pulmonary artery and detaching it from the right atrium.	Used in clients with HLHS and other conditions requiring the redirection of blood flow.
Jatene procedure	Involves switching the main pulmonary artery and the aorta and relocating the ostia of the coronary arteries to the new aorta.	Used as a corrective procedure for TGA.
Mustard or Senning procedure	Restores circulation but reverses the direction of blood flow in the heart. Blood is pumped to the lungs via the left ventricle and pumped throughout the body via the right ventricle.	Used in clients diagnosed with TGA.
Norwood procedure	Reroutes the blood flow around some of the defective areas of the heart by creating new pathways for blood circulation to and from the lungs.	Used in clients with HLHS. Variations for the procedure may be used to treat conditions in which one of both of the lower chambers of the heart are defective.
Norwood procedure with Sano modification	Gore-Tex tube graft connects the right ventricle and pulmonary arteries, provides pulmonary blood flow, and replaces the Blalock–Taussig shunt used in the Norwood procedure.	Used to treat HLHS.
Patch aortoplasty	This surgery widens the narrowing section of the descending aorta. A synthetic patch is used.	Used to correct coarctation of the aorta.

(continued on next page)

TABLE 16–17   Clinical Interventions for Congenital Heart Defects (*continued*)

SURGICAL PROCEDURE	DESCRIPTION OF INTERVENTION	THERAPEUTIC USE AND DEFECT TREATED
Pulmonary artery banding	Creates a narrowing of the main pulmonary artery that decreases blood flow to the branch pulmonary arteries and reduces pulmonary blood flow.	Used in clients with pulmonary overcirculation and left-to-right shunting who require pulmonary blood flow reduction and those diagnosed with TGA.
Rastelli procedure	Excision of right ventricular muscle with large intraventricular baffle sutured into place. This results in closure of the ventricular septal defect and redirection of left ventricular outflow to the aortic valve. A conduit is used to achieve right ventricular to pulmonary artery continuity.	Used to repair TGA with ventricular septal defect and pulmonary stenosis.
Ross procedure	Client's diseased aortic valve is replaced with his or her own pulmonary valve, or the pulmonary valve is replaced with a cadaver pulmonary valve.	Used as a treatment for aortic stenosis.
Subclavian flap aortoplasty	Lengthwise incision is made along coarctation to create a flap that enlarges the constricted area. A benefit of this procedure is the possibility that the anastomosis may grow as the child ages.	Used as a corrective treatment for coarctation of the aorta.
Transplantation	Client's diseased heart is replaced with viable donor heart.	Used in cases of severe heart failure or when a badly damaged or defective heart cannot be made to function adequately through medical or surgical treatment.

NURSING PROCESS

Nursing care of pediatric clients with a congenital anomaly should address the family's needs as well as those of the pediatric client. Parents and grandparents often are overwhelmed by the complexity of the child's medical condition, worried the infant will die, and confused by the decisions they are asked to make. Siblings are often frightened as a result of the anxiety they sense from the adults in their life and also need support.

Assessment

Frequently, the first assessment finding in a child with a congenital heart defect is a heart murmur. The location and sound of the murmur can provide significant detail regarding the type of defect the child has. Assessing heart murmurs is a very specialized skill that requires practice.

When caring for a child with a congenital heart defect, it is important to gather data regarding the mother's prenatal and antepartum experience. Family history of heart defects or other congenital anomalies should also be documented.

Performing a nursing assessment of the child with a potential or actual cardiac condition involves a careful review of the signs and symptoms in many body systems and an analysis of their relationship to cardiac functioning. Use the guidelines in **Table 16–18** ● to perform a comprehensive nursing assessment of the cardiovascular system.

Physiological Assessment

Before surgery, the nurse sees the infant or child regularly to assess growth and to detect signs of worsening congestive heart failure. Many infants with a small defect will have no problems with growth. Failure to gain weight is an indication of an increased metabolic rate and an inability to consume adequate calories for both metabolic function and growth. Assessment of length and head circumference helps determine the full impact of the condition on growth.

Psychosocial Assessment

The nurse should assess the parents' ability to cope with the child's diagnosis. Parents may initially be in shock and feel guilty or anxious. They need opportunities to express their feelings and to learn to cope with the child's illness. The initial period of diagnosis, hospitalization, and early care of the infant at home is very stressful. Parents need special support if their infant has a life-threatening heart defect.

Diagnosis

Potential nursing diagnoses for the child with a congenital heart defect that increases pulmonary blood flow include the following:

- *Fluid Volume: Excess* related to heart failure and pulmonary vasculature overload
- *Infant Feeding Pattern, Ineffective* related to shortness of breath and fatigue
- *Infection, Risk for* related to pulmonary vascular congestion and chronic illness
- *Family Processes, Interrupted* related to crisis of child's serious illness.

(NANDA-I © 2015)

TABLE 16–18 Assessment Guidelines for the Child With a Cardiac Condition

ASSESSMENT FOCUS	ASSESSMENT GUIDELINES
Respirations	■ Inspect the rate, depth, and respiratory effort. ■ Is a cough present? ■ Identify the signs of increased respiratory effort: tachypnea (rapid rate of respirations), dyspnea, retractions, nasal flaring, and expiratory grunting. ■ Auscultate breath sounds for adventitious sounds (wheezes, crackles).
Pulses	■ Assess the pulse rate, rhythm, and quality. ■ Compare the apical, brachial, and radial pulse rates. ■ Compare the brachial and femoral pulses for strength.
Blood pressure	■ Compare the blood pressure to expected value for age, sex, and height percentiles. ■ Compare blood pressure values between upper and lower extremities.
Color	■ Observe overall color; note pallor, dusky color, or cyanosis. ■ Contrast color in peripheral and central locations (e.g., nail beds to mucous membranes). Note whether crying improves or worsens color.
Heart	■ Inspect the anterior chest for bulging or **heaving** (lifting of the chest wall during contraction). ■ Palpate the chest wall for pulsations, heaves, or vibrations. ■ Locate the point of maximum intensity. ■ Auscultate the heart for the heart sounds and their quality (loud versus weak, distinct versus muffled). Muffled or indistinct sounds are associated with congestive heart failure or a heart defect. ■ Are extra heart sounds or murmurs present? Describe murmurs by intensity, location, radiation, timing, and quality. ■ Auscultate the heart with the child in sitting and reclining positions to detect differences in heart sounds.
Fluid status	■ Observe for signs of periorbital, facial, or peripheral edema. ■ Observe for abdominal distention. ■ Palpate the liver to detect hepatomegaly. ■ Observe for signs of dehydration with acute illnesses.
Activity and behavior	■ Is exercise intolerance present? ■ Does the child tire with feeding? ■ Identify changes in activity level or behavior.
General	■ Assess growth. ■ Note presence of diaphoresis and when it occurs.

Examples of nursing diagnoses that may apply to a child with a congenital heart defect that decreases pulmonary blood flow include the following:

■ *Cardiac Output, Decreased* related to ventricular restriction and an obstructed outflow tract
■ *Infection, Risk for* related to unfiltered bacteria in the blood and sites of blood shunting that promote bacterial growth
■ *Caregiver Role Strain* related to care of a child with chronic illness
■ *Activity Intolerance* related to cyanosis and dyspnea on exertion

(NANDA-I © 2015)

Examples of nursing diagnoses for a child following cardiac surgery include the following:

■ *Breathing Pattern, Ineffective* related to respiratory muscle fatigue
■ *Pain, Acute* related to surgical incision and expansion of chest with coughing and deep breathing exercises
■ *Fluid Volume: Imbalanced, Risk for* related to impact of surgery on heart's pumping action
■ *Infection, Risk for* related to surgery and chronic disease status.

(NANDA-I © 2015)

Planning

The goal in caring for children with congenital heart defects is to ensure that the children will live long, healthy lives. To maintain optimal health, the treatment plan should include interventions aimed at supporting perfusion throughout the body that are adequate for sustaining life. Other treatment goals include the following:

■ The parents and family will verbalize concerns and fears related to the child's diagnosis.
■ The parents and family will articulate resources available in the community, such as support groups and financial assistance agencies.
■ The parents will articulate an understanding of the child's diagnosis and participate in the treatment plan.
■ The child will maintain heart rate and oxygenation levels consistent with cardiac output specific to heart defect.
■ The child will maintain adequate energy levels by engaging in activities appropriate to capabilities.

Implementation

Participate with members of the cardiology team to provide information to and educate the family about the child's condition. Information may include the following:

■ General information about the congenital heart defect, including a description of the heart's anatomy and physiology and of the defect itself

- Information about genetic and environmental influences associated with the congenital heart defect
- Overview of the child's prognosis and timing of medical and surgical interventions
- Interventions for congestive heart failure if it develops.

Provide Psychosocial Support

Parents often need support for anxiety about an uncertain surgical outcome. Determine if parents have a support system as they learn about the child's diagnosis and make difficult decisions about the child's surgery. If the parents do not have adequate support systems, identify some resources for support, such as social services, pastoral services, or a parent of a child with a similar heart defect. Some parents may be concerned that signing consent for surgery places the child in even more danger of illness or even death.

Parents should be offered genetic counseling if planning a future pregnancy.

Teach Presurgical Home Care

Children are often managed at home until surgery. Parents should encourage feeding to promote growth, and recognize the infant may take longer to eat. Breastfeeding is encouraged because of its beneficial effects for the infant. A high-calorie formula may be used if the infant does not gain enough weight. Feedings through a nasogastric or gastrostomy tube may also be given at night or 24 hours a day to ensure that adequate calories are ingested. Even when nasogastric or gastrostomy feedings are used, encourage the infant to take some formula orally to provide positive oral stimulation.

> **SAFETY ALERT**
> Babies with congenital heart defects typically do best when fed on demand. More frequent feedings work well because these children tend to tire easily during longer feedings. Keep in mind that children with congenital heart defects may not grow and gain weight as rapidly as other infants of the same age.

Efforts should be made to reduce the child's exposure to infectious diseases. Nurses, parents, family members, and caregivers should wash their hands frequently. Respiratory infections make hypoxemia worse in children with cyanosis. Fever increases the metabolic rates and oxygen demands. Disturbances in the electrolyte balance may lead to vomiting, diarrhea, and certain drug toxicities. The healthcare provider should be notified regarding any of the following: fever, poor feeding, vomiting, and diarrhea.

Routine health maintenance and promotion visits are important. The nurse should give immunizations according to the recommended schedule and provide prophylaxis for respiratory syncytial virus during the peak season.

Prepare for Surgery

When the child is preschool age or older, preparation for hospitalization and scheduled surgeries is essential to help alleviate the child's fear and anxiety. If an infant or toddler is having surgery, the nurse should provide parents with information about how the child will look, the equipment that will be used, and what care will be provided during the immediate postoperative period.

Provide Postoperative Care

In the immediate postoperative period, the child will be cared for in the intensive care unit. When the child returns to the general nursing unit, assessment focuses on signs of surgical complications, such as infection, arrhythmias, and impaired tissue perfusion.

The nurse should monitor the vital signs, including blood pressure and the fifth vital sign—pain. The child may not be on a cardiac monitor, so auscultate the apical pulse to detect an irregular heart rate or bradycardia, which are both signs of reduced cardiac output that require immediate intervention. Assess the respiratory system for breath sounds, respiratory effort, and signs of distress that may indicate pneumonia or fluid in the pleural space. Check pulse oximetry, capillary refill, extremity warmth, pedal pulses, level of consciousness, and urine output to assess impaired tissue perfusion. Reduced urine output is another sign of decreased cardiac output.

Monitor the child's temperature, and inspect the surgical incision site. Fever, excessive incisional pain, spreading erythema around the incision, and wound drainage beginning 3–4 days postoperatively may be early signs of infection.

Manage Pain

Pain management with 24-hour intravenous opioids should be provided for several days postoperatively until the child is taking fluids. Once the child is taking oral fluids and foods, oral analgesics may be given around the clock. The nurse should teach parents and caregivers to lift and move the child carefully and avoid stress on the incision to reduce potential pain.

> **SAFETY ALERT**
> Holding a pillow or stuffed animal against the chest reduces the pain from coughing and deep breathing.

Promote Respiratory Function

The nurse should encourage the child to take deep breaths and cough or to perform spirometry exercises regularly to promote full lung expansion. Chest physiotherapy may be performed in children under 3 years of age.

Manage Fluids and Nutrition

The nurse should encourage the infant or child to begin oral fluids and nutrition when permitted. Although oral fluids are rarely limited, intake and output should be carefully assessed. Parents may be encouraged to bring in favorite foods for the child when they can be tolerated. The nurse should administer antibiotics as ordered. If intravenous antibiotics are continued after the child's oral intake is normal, the line can be converted to a heparin or saline lock.

Promote Activity

The nurse should encourage the child to increase activity gradually, with longer periods out of bed every day, but ensure adequate rest periods to promote healing. Provide diversional activities and opportunities for therapeutic play so the child can better manage the stresses associated with pain and frightening procedures (**Box 16–7** ●).

Box 16-7 Posttraumatic Stress Disorder and Heart Surgery

Children between 5 and 12 years of age were evaluated for symptoms of posttraumatic stress disorder (PTSD) 1–3 days before and 4–8 weeks after undergoing heart surgery. No children had PTSD at the preoperative assessment, even though 18 (42%) had had prior cardiac surgery. Results indicated that the number of PTSD symptoms increased in children who spent 48 hours or more in the intensive care unit. No significant relationship was found in PTSD scores for children with prior cardiac surgery or chronological age (Connolly et al., 2004).

Not surprisingly, another study focusing on parents of children undergoing cardiac surgery requiring cardiopulmonary bypass found that as many as 16.4% of mothers and 13.3% of fathers met full criteria for PTSD at time of discharge, with another 15.7% of mothers and 13.3% of fathers meeting partial criteria (Helfricht et al., 2008). These studies indicate that both children and parents experience heart surgery as a traumatic event and suggest that nurses need to include psychosocial assessment as part of the ongoing assessment process for these children and their families. See the module on Stress and Coping for more information about PTSD.

Plan Discharge and Postsurgical Home Care

Infants and children may be discharged from the hospital within a few days of surgery. Parents need information spread over several days to prepare for care of the child at home. The nurse should encourage a nutritious diet and snacks so the infant or child has an opportunity to catch up from previous growth deficits. Acetaminophen or ibuprofen may be used for pain management after discharge.

The nurse should prepare parents for potential behavior problems of young children that may result from the stress of hospitalization, such as nightmares, separation anxiety, and overdependence on parents. Encourage parents to reassure children about their security and to promote play and other means to deal with their feelings. If the child's symptoms continue for several weeks, a referral for psychological evaluation and care may be needed.

Complementary and Alternative Therapy
Congenital Heart Defects

Caution parents of children with congenital heart defects to avoid using complementary therapies, such as herbal products, that may interfere with the prescribed medications. Products containing ginkgo are known to interact with warfarin, which is of particular concern for any child on anticoagulant therapy. The adverse effects of herbal remedies have not been fully identified.

Reassure parents of children with a complete correction of the cardiac defect that there should be no further cardiovascular problems. Provide parents with full information about the child's defect and the surgery performed to share with the child's current and future healthcare providers. Encourage parents to allow the child to live a normal and active life.

Children are at risk for infective endocarditis, especially within the first 6 months after surgery. Prophylactic antibiotics are indicated for invasive procedures. Any unexplained fever or malaise seen in the 2 months following surgical repair or after dental work may be a sign of infection. The child should be examined for petechiae and splenomegaly and evaluated for infective endocarditis.

Evaluation

Examples of expected outcomes of nursing care include the following:

- The child's pain is managed effectively.
- Full lung expansion is maintained with incentive spirometry exercises or chest physiotherapy.
- The child's incision heals without infection.

NURSING CARE PLAN A Client With Ventricular Septal Defect

Baby Girl Polasani is born to Theresa and Jason Polasani. She is their third child; they have a 4-year-old girl and a 6-year-old boy at home.

ASSESSMENT	DIAGNOSES	PLANNING
Upon admission to the newborn nursery, the baby is weighed (4,000 g), measured (chest, 33 cm; height, 53.34 cm), and found by exam to be at 39 weeks of gestation. Vital signs are as follows: T_{AX} 98.0°F; P 148 bpm; R 52/min; BP 68/44 mmHg. When performing a complete assessment, the nurse finds nothing abnormal until assessing heart sounds, when a loud systolic murmur is heard. An echocardiogram is ordered, which demonstrates a large ventricular septal defect (VSD). The pediatrician recommends monitoring Baby Girl Polasani's condition and allowing her to remain in the normal nursery and spend time with her mother as long as she remains stable. Two days later, her weight has increased to 4,400 g, she is edematous, and she has course crackles throughout the lung fields. She is tachypneic, and her oxygen saturation is 88% on room air. She is lethargic, and vital signs are as follows: temperature, 98°F axillary; pulse 188 bpm; respirations 76/min; BP 54/36 mmHg. The pediatrician diagnoses her with congestive heart failure secondary to her VSD, and she is transferred to the neonatal intensive care unit.	■ *Cardiac Output, Decreased* related to cardiac anomaly (VSD) ■ *Fluid Volume: Excess* related to heart failure ■ *Skin Integrity, Risk for Impaired* related to altered fluid status ■ *Nutrition: Imbalanced, Less than Body Requirements* related to increased metabolic needs and rapid tiring during feedings ■ *Coping: Family, Compromised* related to situational crisis with child's health problems (NANDA-I © 2015)	Goals of care include the following: ■ The newborn's cardiac output will be sufficient to meet the body's metabolic demands. ■ The newborn will manifest adequate oxygenation. ■ The newborn's peripheral and central edema will decrease. ■ The newborn's intake and output will be balanced once excess fluid is excreted. ■ The newborn will demonstrate expected weight gain for age.

(continued on next page)

NURSING CARE PLAN (continued)

IMPLEMENTATION

- Administer digoxin as ordered.
- Take apical pulse, and listen to heart sounds regularly, especially before each dose of digoxin. Record apical pulse with each recorded dose of digoxin.
- Place newborn on a cardiorespiratory monitor.
- Prevent injury by monitoring for digoxin side effects and serum potassium level.
- Stagger care to provide for rest periods.
- Place newborn in semi-Fowler position.
- Evaluate respiratory rate and sounds.
- Take pulse oximetry readings to determine oxygen saturation.
- Provide oxygen and humidification if ordered. Observe for diaphoresis, a sign of increased respiratory effort.
- Administer diuretics as ordered.
- Weigh daily. Measure abdominal girth daily. Observe for peripheral edema.
- Measure intake and output carefully by weighing diapers.
- Maintain fluid restrictions as ordered.
- Monitor electrolytes.

- Provide skin care for edematous body parts, and elevate extremities.
- Change newborn's position frequently.
- Inspect skin frequently for redness and skin breakdown over pressure points.
- Hold newborn at a 45-degree angle for feeding.
- Give frequent small feedings with rest periods in between, or insert a feeding tube per order.
- Use high-calorie formula.
- Transition to supplemental nasogastric feeding if the newborn is not able to gain weight.
- Encourage parents to room-in or visit newborn frequently.
- Explain procedures and treatment.
- Involve parents in care as much as possible.
- Have parents hold the child often.
- At discharge, provide clear instructions and information about what to do in an emergency as well as whom and where to call with questions.
- Allow parents to verbalize questions, concerns, and feelings.
- Refer parents to support groups or other resources as needed.

EVALUATION

Expected outcomes used to evaluate the child's response to care include the following:
- The child's cardiac output is sufficient, as indicated by increased energy, adequate feeding intake, and decreased edema.
- The child maintains normal serum levels of potassium and therapeutic levels of digoxin.
- The child has adequate energy to eat.
- The child has normal respiratory rate for age, with no evidence of adventitious sounds or diaphoresis.
- The child's intake and output are proportional, and electrolyte levels remain within normal ranges.
- The child has no skin breakdown after edema resolves.
- The child gains recommended weight according to growth grids, with all dietary requirements met.
- The parents participate in developing and implementing the treatment plan and in providing care to the child.

CRITICAL THINKING

1. How would you explain the child's congenital defect and a rationale for why she developed congestive heart failure?
2. Why would this baby have an increased metabolic rate and need for increased calories?
3. How will this child's care needs change as she grows if surgery is delayed until she is older?

REVIEW Congenital Heart Defects

RELATE Link the Concepts and Exemplars

Linking the exemplar of congenital heart defects with the concept of family:

1. What is the priority of care for the family of a newborn diagnosed with a cyanotic heart defect?

2. How might you support the family of a child who requires extensive and numerous open heart surgeries?

Linking the exemplar of congenital heart defects with the concept of development:

3. Why might the child with a significant unrepaired congenital defect fail to meet developmental milestones?

4. What interventions would the nurse initiate for the family whose infant is not meeting developmental milestones due to a congenital heart defect?

READY Go to Companion Skills Manual

REFER Go to Pearson Nursing Student Resources
nursing.pearsonhighered.com

- Additional review materials

REFLECT Case Study

Billy Sexton is a few hours old; he was born at 32 weeks' gestation to Mr. and Mrs. Sexton. Mr. Sexton, age 26, is in law school, and Mrs. Sexton, age 25, teaches first grade at the local elementary school. Billy is their first child. Billy is taken to the neonatal intensive care unit (NICU) where he is examined and diagnosed with tetralogy of Fallot following a cardiac echocardiogram.

Mr. and Mrs. Sexton leave the NICU in a state of shock and don't even know what questions to ask the neonatologist. The practitioner has told them that Billy will require open heart surgery when he is older and has adequate weight gain. Until that time, Billy will be treated medically. The idea of taking him home with such a serious heart problem is truly frightening to the mother. Mr. Sexton finds himself wondering whether his son will survive and, if he does, whether he will ever be able to act like a normal child.

1. How will you help the parents understand the pathophysiology of Billy's heart defect?
2. What is your priority nursing diagnosis for Billy?
3. Create a teaching plan for the family to prepare them for Billy's discharge from the hospital.

EXEMPLAR 16.3   Coronary Artery Disease

EXEMPLAR KEY TERMS

Acute coronary syndrome (ACS), *1105*
Acute myocardial infarction (AMI), *1105*
Angina pectoris, *1105*
Arrhythmogenic, *1112*
Atherosclerosis, *1106*
Bradydysrhythmia, *1112*
Cardiac markers, *1114*
Cardiac rehabilitation, *1123*
Cardiogenic shock, *1113*
CK-MB, *1115*
Collateral channels, *1106*
Coronary artery disease (CAD), *1105*
Dermatome, *1107*
Dysrhythmias, *1112*
Homocysteine, *1110*
Ischemia, *1106*
Metabolic syndrome, *1110*
Pericarditis, *1113*
Regurgitation, *1113*
Troponins, *1115*
Ventricular aneurysm, *1113*

EXEMPLAR LEARNING OUTCOMES

After reading about this exemplar, you will be able to:

1. Describe the pathophysiology, etiology, clinical manifestations, and direct and indirect causes of coronary artery disease.
2. Identify risk factors and prevention methods associated with coronary artery disease.
3. Illustrate the nursing process in providing culturally competent care across the life span for individuals with coronary artery disease.
4. Formulate priority nursing diagnoses appropriate for an individual with coronary artery disease.
5. Summarize therapies used by interdisciplinary teams in the collaborative care of an individual with coronary artery disease.
6. Plan evidence-based care for an individual with coronary artery disease and his or her family in collaboration with other members of the healthcare team.
7. Evaluate expected outcomes for an individual with coronary artery disease.

▶ OVERVIEW

Coronary artery disease (CAD) is the most common type of heart disease and the number one cause of death for both men and women (National Heart, Lung, and Blood Institute [NHLBI], 2013a). CAD is caused by impaired blood flow to the myocardium. Accumulation of atherosclerotic plaque in the coronary arteries is the usual cause. CAD may be asymptomatic, or it may lead to angina pectoris, acute coronary syndrome, myocardial infarction (MI) or heart attack, dysrhythmias, heart failure, and even sudden death.

Angina pectoris (or angina) is chest pain resulting from reduced coronary blood flow, which causes a temporary imbalance between myocardial blood supply and demand. The imbalance may be caused by CAD, atherosclerosis, or vessel constriction that impairs the myocardial blood supply. Hypermetabolic conditions, such as exercise, thyrotoxicosis, stimulant abuse (e.g., cocaine), hyperthyroidism, and emotional stress, can increase myocardial oxygen demand, precipitating angina. Anemia, heart failure, ventricular hypertrophy, or pulmonary diseases may affect blood and oxygen supplies as well, causing angina.

Acute coronary syndrome (ACS) refers to any condition that develops as a result of sudden, reduced blood flow to the heart. ACS includes unstable angina and acute myocardial ischemia with or without significant injury of myocardial tissue.

An **acute myocardial infarction (AMI)**, which refers to necrosis (death) of myocardial cells, is a life-threatening event. It occurs when blood flow to a portion of the cardiac muscle is blocked. If circulation to the affected myocardium is not promptly restored, loss of functional myocardium affects the heart's ability to maintain an effective cardiac output. This may ultimately lead to cardiogenic shock and death.

Heart disease remains the leading cause of death in the United States. Of the major heart diseases, MI, or *heart attack*, as well as other forms of ischemic heart disease cause the majority of deaths. Approximately, 1.5 million cases of myocardial infarction occur in the United States annually (Zafari et al., 2013).

The majority of deaths from MI occur during the initial period after symptoms begin: approximately 60% within the first hour, and 40% before hospitalization. Heightening public awareness of the manifestations of MI, the importance of seeking immediate medical assistance, and training in cardiopulmonary resuscitation (CPR) techniques are vital to decreasing the number of MI-related deaths.

▶ PATHOPHYSIOLOGY AND ETIOLOGY

The two main coronary arteries, the left and the right, supply blood, oxygen, and nutrients to the myocardium. They originate in the root of the aorta, just outside the aortic valve. The left main coronary artery divides to form the anterior descending and circumflex arteries. The anterior descending artery supplies the anterior interventricular septum and the left ventricle, including the apex of the heart. The circumflex branch supplies the lateral wall of the left ventricle. The right coronary artery supplies the right ventricle and forms the posterior descending artery. The posterior interventricular artery supplies the posterior portion of the heart (see Figure 16–7 in the Concept section).

Blood flow through the coronary arteries is regulated by several factors. Aortic pressure is the primary factor. Other factors include heart rate (most of the flow occurs during diastole, when the muscle is relaxed), metabolic activity of the heart, blood vessel tone (constriction), and collateral circulation. Although no connections occur between the large coronary arteries, small arteries are joined by **collateral channels** (sometimes called collateral circulation; these are small blood vessels that develop to connect small arteries). Should larger vessels of the heart become occluded, collateral channels may provide alternative routes for blood flow.

Coronary atherosclerosis is the most common cause of reduced coronary blood flow. **Atherosclerosis** is a progressive disease characterized by atheroma (plaque) formation, which affects the intimal and medial layers of large and midsized arteries. Atherosclerosis is initiated by unknown precipitating factors that cause lipoproteins and fibrous tissue to accumulate in the arterial wall. Although the precise mechanisms are unknown, abnormal lipid metabolism and injury to, or inflammation of, endothelial cells lining the artery appear to be key to its development.

In the bloodstream, lipids are transported while attached to proteins called apoproteins. High levels of certain lipoproteins (a type of apoprotein) increase the risk of atherosclerosis. Low-density lipoproteins (LDLs), which are high in cholesterol, carry cholesterol to peripheral tissues, where some of it is released to be taken up and incorporated into cells for use in producing energy. Very-low-density lipoproteins (VLDLs), which are large molecules composed primarily of triglycerides and cholesterol, carry triglycerides to muscle and fat cells. When the triglycerides are released into these tissues, the remainder of the molecule is an LDL. High-density lipoproteins (HDLs), in contrast, attract cholesterol, returning it from peripheral tissues to the liver.

Hyperlipidemia itself may damage arterial endothelium. Other potential mechanisms of vessel injury include hypertension, environmental toxins, infections, and inflammatory processes. Endothelial dysfunction is involved in the lesion formation accompanying atherosclerosis and can be an independent predictor of cardiac events damage promotes platelet adhesion and aggregation, and also attracts leukocytes.

At the site of injury, atherogenic (atherosclerosis-promoting) lipoproteins collect in the intimal lining of the artery. These lipoproteins appear to actually bind with the extracellular portion of the vessel endothelium. Macrophages migrate to the injured site as part of the inflammatory process. Contact with platelets, cholesterol, and other blood components stimulates smooth muscle cells and connective tissue within the vessel wall to proliferate abnormally. Although blood flow is not affected at this stage, the early lesion appears as a yellowish, fatty streak on the inner lining of the artery. Fibrous plaque develops as smooth muscle cells

enlarge, collagen fibers proliferate, and blood lipids accumulate. The lesion protrudes into the arterial lumen and is fixed to the inner wall of the intima. It may invade the muscular media layer of the vessel as well. The developing plaque not only gradually occludes the vessel lumen but also impairs the vessel's ability to dilate in response to increased oxygen demands. Fibrous plaque lesions often develop at arterial bifurcations or curves or in areas of narrowing. As the plaque expands, it can produce severe stenosis or total occlusion of the artery.

The final stage of the process is the development of atheromas, which are complex lesions consisting of lipids, fibrous tissue, collagen, calcium, cellular debris, and capillaries. These calcified lesions can ulcerate or rupture, stimulating thrombosis. The vessel lumen may be rapidly occluded by the thrombus (clot), or it may embolize to occlude a distal vessel.

Plaque formation may be eccentric (located in a specific, asymmetric region of the vessel wall) or concentric (involving the entire vessel circumference). Manifestations of the process usually do not appear until approximately 75% of the arterial lumen has been occluded.

Atherosclerosis tends to develop where arteries bifurcate or branch. Certain vessels have a higher likelihood of being affected, including the coronary arteries (the left anterior descending artery in particular), the renal arteries, the bifurcation of the carotid arteries, and the branching sections of peripheral arteries. In addition to obstructing or occluding blood flow, atherosclerosis weakens arterial walls and is a major cause of aneurysm in vessels such as the aorta and iliac arteries.

Ischemia

As a result of declining artery circumference, blood supply to the cardiac tissue is reduced, and the imbalance between myocardial blood supply and demand causes temporary and reversible myocardial ischemia. **Ischemia** results when the oxygen supply is inadequate to meet metabolic demands. The critical factors in meeting the metabolic demands of cardiac cells are coronary perfusion and myocardial workload. Coronary perfusion can be affected by several different mechanisms:

- One or more vessels may be partially occluded by large, stable areas of plaque.
- Platelets can aggregate in narrowed vessels, forming a thrombus.
- Normal or already narrowed vessels may spasm.
- A drop in blood pressure may lead to inadequate flow through coronary vessels.
- Normal coronary autoregulation mechanisms may be interrupted as coronary blood flow becomes pressure dependent.

Workload is affected by heart rate, myocardial contractility, preload (the amount of blood in the ventricles just prior to systole), and afterload (the peripheral pressure that must be overcome to move blood out of the heart into the circulation). The oxygen content of the blood and hematocrit are contributing factors to myocardial ischemia. **Table 16–19** ● lists factors that may lead to myocardial ischemia.

Cellular processes are compromised as adenosine triphosphate stores are depleted in ischemic tissue. Reduced oxygen

TABLE 16-19   Causes of Myocardial Ischemia

CONDITION	EFFECT ON MYOCARDIAL WORKLOAD
Atherosclerosis	■ Restricts blood flow.
Thrombosis	■ Causes sudden, severe myocardial ischemia and possible heart attack.
Coronary artery spasm	■ Decreases or prevents blood flow to part of the heart muscle.
Severe illness	■ Metabolic demands of the heart increase and blood pressure may decrease with infection, bleeding, or other severe illness.

causes cells to switch from aerobic metabolism to anaerobic metabolism. Anaerobic metabolism causes lactic acid to build up in the cells. It also affects cell membrane permeability, releasing substances such as histamine, kinins, and specific enzymes that stimulate terminal nerve fibers in the cardiac muscle and send pain impulses to the central nervous system. The pain radiates to the upper body because the heart shares the same **dermatome** (an area supplied with afferent nerve fibers by a single posterior spinal root) as this region. Therapeutic strategies to reduce injury include the reestablishment of myocardial perfusion before irreversible damage occurs. It is estimated that each 30-minute delay from onset of symptoms to primary intervention results in an 8% increase in the relative risk of 1-year mortality.

Angina results from ischemia and can be a one-time event or a chronic condition. Angina is categorized into three types:

1. *Stable angina* is the most common and predictable form of angina. It occurs with a predictable amount of activity or stress and is a common manifestation of CAD. Stable angina usually occurs when the work of the heart is increased by physical exertion, exposure to cold, or stress. Stable angina is relieved by rest and nitrates.
2. *Prinzmetal (variant) angina* is atypical angina that occurs unpredictably (unrelated to activity) and often at night. It is caused by coronary artery spasm with or without an atherosclerotic lesion. The exact mechanism of coronary artery spasm is unknown. It may result from hyperactive sympathetic nervous system responses, altered calcium flow in smooth muscle, or reduced prostaglandins that promote vasodilation.
3. *Unstable angina* occurs with increasing frequency, severity, and duration. Pain is unpredictable, occurs with decreasing levels of activity or stress, and may occur at rest. Clients with unstable angina are at risk for MI. (Unstable angina is discussed below in the Acute Coronary Syndrome section.)

Silent myocardial ischemia, or asymptomatic ischemia, is a major component of the total number of clients experiencing ischemic heart disease. Clients at risk for silent ischemia include those with stable angina, unstable angina, postinfarction angina, or variant angina. Other risk factors include clients who have survived a cardiac arrest or have had a heart transplant or percutaneous coronary intervention or cardiac bypass surgery and clients who have diabetes. Silent ischemia often occurs with exercise and is associated with a higher relative risk of serious or fatal cardiac events.

Acute Coronary Syndrome

Acute coronary syndrome is a dynamic state in which coronary blood flow is acutely reduced but not fully occluded. Myocardial cells are injured by the acute ischemia that results. Most people affected by ACS have significant stenosis of one or more coronary arteries.

Acute coronary syndrome may be precipitated by one or more of the following:

1. Rupture or erosion of atherosclerotic plaque, with formation of a thrombosis. When the artery is not completely occluded, an episode of chest pain at rest may occur.
2. Coronary artery spasm (e.g., Prinzmetal angina).
3. Progressive vessel obstruction by atherosclerotic plaque or restenosis following a percutaneous revascularization procedure.
4. Inflammation of a coronary artery.
5. An increase in myocardial oxygen demand and/or a decrease in supply (i.e. acute blood loss or anemia).

Coronary artery disease is commonly due to atherosclerotic occlusion of the coronary arteries. Plaque rupture often is triggered by hemodynamic factors, such as increased heart rate, blood flow, and blood pressure in response to a surge of sympathetic nervous system activity. Sympathetic hyperactivity has been shown to impair the autonomic nervous system control of the cardiovascular system, and acute mental stress has been shown to be a risk factor for atherosclerosis (Chumaeva et al., 2010).

When atherosclerotic plaque ruptures or erodes, the exposed lipid core of the plaque stimulates platelet aggregation and the extrinsic clotting pathway. Thrombin is generated and fibrin is deposited, forming a clot that severely impairs or obstructs blood flow to tissue distal to the area of plaque rupture. As a result, these cells become ischemic.

Injured myocardial cells contract less effectively, potentially reducing cardiac output if a large area of myocardium is affected. Lactic acid released from ischemic cells stimulates pain receptors, causing chest pain. Ischemia and injury affect electrical impulse conduction, producing inversion of the T wave and possibly elevation of the ST segment on an ECG.

Acute Myocardial Infarction

Atherosclerotic plaque may form stable or unstable lesions. Stable lesions progress by gradually occluding the vessel lumen, whereas unstable (or complicated) lesions are prone to rupture and thrombus formation. Stable lesions often cause angina; unstable lesions often lead to ACS or acute ischemic heart diseases.

Myocardial infarction occurs when blood flow to a portion of cardiac muscle is completely blocked, resulting in prolonged tissue ischemia and irreversible cell damage. Coronary occlusion is usually caused by ulceration or rupture of a complicated atherosclerotic lesion. When an atherosclerotic lesion ruptures or ulcerates, substances are released that stimulate platelet aggregation, thrombin generation, and local vasomotor tone. As a result, the vessel constricts and a thrombus forms, occluding the vessel and interrupting blood flow to the myocardium distal to the obstruction.

Cellular injury occurs when the cells are denied adequate oxygen and nutrients. When ischemia is prolonged, lasting more than 20–45 minutes, irreversible hypoxemic damage causes cellular death and tissue necrosis. Oxygen, glycogen, and adenosine triphosphate (ATP) stores of ischemic cells are rapidly depleted. Cellular metabolism shifts to an anaerobic process, producing hydrogen ions and lactic acid. Cellular acidosis increases the vulnerability of cells to further damage. Intracellular enzymes are released through damaged cell membranes into interstitial spaces.

Cellular acidosis, electrolyte imbalances, and hormones released in response to cellular ischemia affect impulse conduction and myocardial contractility. The risk for dysrhythmias increases, and myocardial contractility decreases, reducing stroke volume, cardiac output, blood pressure, and tissue perfusion.

The subendocardium suffers the initial damage, within 20 minutes of injury, because this area is the most susceptible to changes in coronary blood flow. If blood flow is restored at this point, the infarction is limited to subendocardial tissue (a subendocardial or non-Q-wave infarction). If blood flow is not restored, the damage progresses to the epicardium within 1–6 hours. When all layers of the myocardium are affected, it is known as a transmural infarction. A significant Q wave develops with a transmural infarction, indicating the client suffered a Q-wave MI. Complications such as heart failure are more frequently associated with Q-wave MIs. Clients with non-Q-wave MIs may experience favorable early prognosis. However, late complications include recurrent angina, transmural myocardial infarction, and sudden death.

The necrotic or infarcted muscle is surrounded by regions of injured and ischemic tissues. Tissue in this ischemic area is potentially viable; restoration of blood flow minimizes the amount of tissue lost. The surrounding tissue also undergoes metabolic changes. It may be stunned (its contractility impaired for hours or days following reperfusion) or hibernating (a process that protects myocytes until perfusion is restored). Myocardial remodeling may occur, with cellular hypertrophy and loss of contractility in regions distant from the infarction. These changes are dependent on the rate at which blood flow is restored to the site of injury.

When a larger artery is compromised, collateral vessels connecting smaller arteries in the coronary system dilate to maintain blood flow to the cardiac muscle. The degree of collateral circulation helps determine the extent of myocardial damage from ischemia. Acute occlusion of a coronary artery without any collateral flow results in massive tissue damage and may result in death. Progressive narrowing of the larger coronary arteries allows collateral vessels to develop and enlarge, meeting the demand for blood flow. Good collateral circulation can limit the size of an MI.

Myocardial infarctions are described by reference to the damaged area of the heart. The coronary artery that is occluded determines the area of damage. MI usually affects the left ventricle, because it is the major "workhorse" of the heart; its muscle mass is greater, as are its oxygen demands. Occlusion of the left anterior descending artery affects blood flow to the anterior wall of the left ventricle (an *anterior* MI) and part of the interventricular septum. Occlusion of the left circumflex artery causes a *lateral* MI. Right ventricular, inferior, and posterior infarcts involve occlusions of the right coronary artery and posterior descending artery. Occlusion of the left main coronary artery is the most devastating, causing ischemia of the entire left ventricle and a grave prognosis. Identifying the infarct site helps predict possible complications and determine appropriate therapy.

Acute myocardial infarction may also develop as a result of cocaine intoxication. Cocaine increases sympathetic nervous system activity by both increasing the release of catecholamines from central and peripheral stores and interfering with the reuptake of catecholamines. This increased catecholamine concentration stimulates the heart rate and increases its contractility, increases the automaticity of cardiac tissues and the risk of dysrhythmias, and causes vasoconstriction and hypertension. The client with cocaine-induced MI may present with an altered level of consciousness, confusion and restlessness, seizure activity, tachycardia, hypotension, increased respiratory rate, and respiratory crackles. (Further information about the effects of cocaine can be found in the module on Addiction.)

Etiology

The underlying cause of atherosclerosis and related disease is unknown. An individual's tendency to develop cardiovascular disease may be inherited. Lifestyle habits such as diet, smoking, and physical activity also play a role.

Risk Factors

The causes of atherosclerosis are not known, but certain risk factors have been linked with the development of atherosclerotic plaques. The Framingham Heart Study provided vital research into the relationship between risk factors and the development of heart disease (see the Evidence-Based Practice feature that follows). Research into CAD is ongoing, looking at causative factors, manifestations, and protective measures for many populations. Risk factors for CAD are frequently classified as nonmodifiable (factors that cannot be changed) and modifiable (factors that can be changed). **Table 16–20** ● lists risk factors for coronary artery disease.

TABLE 16–20 Risk Factors for Coronary Artery Disease

NONMODIFIABLE	MODIFIABLE	
	Pathophysiological	Lifestyle

Age
  Men ≥45 years old
  Women ≥55 years old
Gender
Family history of CAD
Race
	Hyperlipidemia
	  Elevated LDL
	  Reduced HDL
	High blood pressure
	Diabetes mellitus
	Stress
	Kidney disease
		Cigarette smoking
		Obesity
		Physical inactivity
		Atherogenic diet
		Use of oral contraceptives (women only)
		Hormone replacement therapy
		(women only)

Evidence-Based Practice The Framingham Heart Study

Problem

What role do genetics and lifestyle play in cardiovascular disease?

Evidence

The Framingham Heart Study (FHS) has been committed to identifying the common factors or characteristics contributing to cardiovascular disease since 1948 (FHS, 2013). The first cohort of the study included 5,209 participants from the town of Framingham, Massachusetts. These participants had not yet developed obvious symptoms of cardiovascular disease or suffered a heart attack or stroke. Careful monitoring of each study cohort has resulted in valuable information identifying risk factors associated with cardiovascular disease.

Data collected from the study participants has been key in identifying risk factors associated with cardiovascular disease. Of particular interest have been components of the American lifestyle linked to high rates of disease and disability. The researchers discovered that at-risk lifestyles include an unhealthy diet, physical inactivity, and obesity. The effects of cigarette smoking were not demonstrated to be hazardous until soon after the study began. A major implication of the overall research findings is the value of practicing primary preventive education. Many national awareness campaigns have been formed as a means of better educating the American public. Education about the effects of lifestyle on the cardiovascular system must also be fostered in young children and reinforced throughout childhood and into the teen and young adult years. As healthy choices become habits, cardiac disease will be reduced.

The Framingham Heart Study has also been beneficial in lending insight into genetic influences and their role in assessing cardiovascular risk. Future implications include how to best to manage information regarding cardiovascular disease and multifactorial patterns of inheritance (Ebomoyi, 2010). Genetic defects have also been linked to congenital heart defects and other structural abnormalities.

Implications

Findings from the Framingham Heart Study support the need for nurses to be vigilant regarding the need to provide education related to lifestyle modifications for clients at risk for or diagnosed with coronary heart disease, and in particular for clients with a family history of cardiovascular illness.

Critical Thinking Application

1. What kinds of strategies can be used in elementary school settings to teach cardiovascular health in a fun, informative manner?

2. Identify three possible health implications related to the role of genetics and increased cardiovascular risk.

3. What changes do you need to make in your lifestyle to role model heart-healthy living?

The development of CAD is the primary risk factor for angina and MI. Although ischemic heart disease can result from trauma, stimulant drug use (cocaine, amphetamines), or other causes, these are not common.

NONMODIFIABLE RISK FACTORS Age is a nonmodifiable risk factor for CAD. More than 50% of those who experience a heart attack are age 65 or older; 80% of deaths caused by MI occur in this age group. Gender and genetic factors also are nonmodifiable risk factors for CAD. Men are diagnosed with CAD at an earlier age than women. Family history of early heart disease is considered an early risk factor in clients with a father or brother diagnosed before 55 years of age and in a mother or sister diagnosed before 65 years of age.

MODIFIABLE RISK FACTORS Modifiable risk factors include lifestyle factors and pathological conditions that predispose the client to developing CAD. Behavioral or lifestyle factors can be controlled or completely eliminated. Lifestyle changes require significant commitment by the client; ongoing support from the healthcare team is vital for success.

Disease conditions that contribute to CAD include hypertension, diabetes mellitus, and hyperlipidemia. Although these conditions are not a matter of choice, they are modifiable risk factors that can often be controlled through medication, weight control, diet, and exercise.

Hypertension Hypertension is consistent blood pressure readings of greater than 140 mmHg systolic or 90 mmHg diastolic. Hypertension is common, affecting more than one third of people over age 50 in the United States. Its prevalence is higher in African Americans than in Hispanics and is higher in Hispanics than in White Americans. Hypertension damages the endothelial cells of arteries, possibly by excess pressure and altered characteristics of blood flow. This damage can stimulate the development of atherosclerotic plaque.

Diabetes Mellitus Diabetes mellitus contributes to CAD in several ways. Diabetes is associated with higher blood lipid levels, a higher incidence of hypertension, and obesity—all risk factors in their own right. In addition, diabetes affects the endothelium of blood vessels, contributing to the process of atherosclerosis. Hyperglycemia and hyperinsulinemia, altered platelet function, elevated fibrinogen levels, and inflammation also are thought to play a role in the development of atherosclerosis in people with diabetes.

Hyperlipidemia Hyperlipidemia is an abnormally high level of blood lipids and lipoproteins. Lipoproteins carry cholesterol in the blood. Low-density lipids (LDLs) are the primary carriers of cholesterol. High levels of LDL (memory cue: LDLs = **l**ess **d**esirable **l**ipoproteins) promote atherosclerosis, because LDL deposits cholesterol on artery walls. **Table 16–21** ● lists desirable and high-risk levels for total and LDL cholesterol. In contrast, high-density lipids (HDLs) (memory cue: HDLs = **h**ighly **d**esirable **l**ipoproteins) help clear cholesterol from the arteries, transporting it to the liver for excretion. HDL levels of greater than 35 mg/dL have a protective effect, reducing the risk of CAD; in contrast, HDL levels of lower than 35 mg/dL are associated with an increased risk for CAD. Triglycerides (compounds of fatty acids bound to glycerol and used for fat storage by the body) are carried on VLDL molecules. Elevated triglycerides also contribute to the risk for CAD.

TABLE 16–21   Classification of Serum Cholesterol and Triglyceride Values

	TOTAL CHOLESTEROL (mg/dL)	LOW-DENSITY LIPOPROTEIN CHOLESTEROL (mg/dL)	TRIGLYCERIDE (mg/dL)
Optimal		<100	
Desirable	<200	100–129	<150
Borderline high	200–239	130–159	150–199
High	≥240	160–189	200–499
Very high		190 mg/dL and above	500 mg/dL and above

Note: As defined by the American Heart Association.

Cigarette Smoking   Cigarette smoking, an independent risk factor for CAD, is responsible for more deaths from CAD than from lung cancer or pulmonary disease (Woods et al., 2010). The effects of smoking on the cardiovascular system are dose dependent. The male cigarette smoker has two to three times the risk for developing heart disease compared with the nonsmoker; the female smoker has up to four times the risk. For both men and women who stop smoking, the risk of mortality from CAD is reduced by one half. (National Cholesterol Education Program [NCEP], 2002).

Tobacco smoke promotes CAD in several ways. Carbon monoxide damages vascular endothelium, promoting cholesterol deposition. Nicotine stimulates catecholamine release, increasing blood pressure, heart rate, and myocardial oxygen use. Nicotine also constricts arteries, limiting tissue perfusion (blood flow and oxygen delivery). Furthermore, nicotine reduces HDL levels and increases platelet aggregation, increasing the risk of thrombus formation.

Obesity   Obesity (excess adipose tissue) is generally defined as a body mass index of 30 kg/m^2 or greater and affects the risk for CAD. People who are obese have higher rates of hypertension, diabetes, and hyperlipidemia. In the Framingham Heart Study, men over age 50 who were obese had twice the incidence of CAD and AMI of those who were within 10% of their ideal weight.

Fat distribution also affects the risk for CAD. Central obesity, or intra-abdominal fat, is associated with an increased risk. The best indicator of central obesity is the waist circumference. A waist-to-hip ratio of greater than 0.8 (women) or 0.9 (men) increases the risk for CAD.

Physical Inactivity   Physical inactivity is associated with a higher risk for CAD. Research data indicate that people who maintain a regular program of physical activity are less prone to developing CAD than sedentary people. Cardiovascular benefits of exercise include increased availability of oxygen to the heart muscle, decreased oxygen demand and cardiac workload, and increased myocardial function and electrical stability. Other positive effects of regular physical activity include decreased blood pressure, blood lipids, insulin levels, platelet aggregation, and weight.

Diet   Diet is a risk factor for CAD, independent of fat and cholesterol intake. Diets high in fruits, vegetables, whole grains, and unsaturated fatty acids appear to have a protective effect.

EMERGING RISK FACTORS   Research demonstrates a link between elevated serum levels of **homocysteine** (an amino acid that is a homologue of cysteine) and CAD. Until menopause, women have lower homocysteine levels than men, which may partially explain premenopausal women's lower risk for CAD.

Homocysteine levels are negatively correlated with serum folate and dietary folate intake; that is, increasing folate intake lowers homocysteine levels.

Based on evidence that aspirin and antiplatelet therapies reduce the risk for MI, clot-promoting factors are identified as risk factors for CAD. Inflammation also has recently been identified as a risk factor. Inflammatory processes may increase the development of atherosclerotic plaque, and they are implicated in plaque rupture (NCEP, 2013). Inflammation also promotes clot formation at the site of ruptured plaque. It is not generally recommended that clients routinely be tested for these factors.

The **metabolic syndrome** is a group of metabolic risk factors occurring in an individual that create a highly elevated risk for CAD (**Box 16–8** ●). In fact, metabolic syndrome has emerged as a risk factor for premature CAD that is equal to cigarette smoking. Three underlying causes of metabolic syndrome have been identified: overweight/obesity, physical inactivity, and genetic factors. Metabolic syndrome is closely associated with insulin resistance (impaired tissue responses to insulin). Genetics, abdominal obesity, and physical inactivity also play a role in causing metabolic syndrome.

RISK FACTORS UNIQUE TO WOMEN   Risk factors unique to women include premature menopause, oral contraceptive use, and hormone replacement therapy (HRT). At menopause, serum HDL levels drop and LDL levels rise, increasing the risk for CAD. Early menopause (natural or surgically induced) increases the risk for CAD and MI. Women who have bilateral oophorectomy without hormone replacement before age 35 are eight times more likely to have an MI than women experiencing natural menopause. Estrogen replacement therapy reduces the risk for CAD and MI in these women. Oral contraceptives, by contrast, have been demonstrated to increase the risk for CAD if associated with genetic predisposition, smoking, hypertension, and obesity. This increased risk is caused by the tendency of oral contraceptives to raise low-density lipoprotein and lower high-density lipoprotein. The risk is greater if the female is older than 35 years of age and smokes.

Box 16–8   Risk Factors for Metabolic Syndrome

- Large waistline
- High triglyceride level
- Low HDL levels
- Hypertension
- Elevated fasting blood glucose
- Clotting tendency
- Inflammatory factors

▶ CLINICAL MANIFESTATIONS

Although the clinical manifestations of angina and MI are similar initially, important differences exist. Differentiating between ischemic causes of chest pain and other causes can be subtle and complex; chest pain should be assessed by an experienced healthcare professional.

Angina

The cardinal manifestation of angina is chest pain. The pain typically is precipitated by an identifiable event, such as physical activity, strong emotion, stress, eating a heavy meal, or exposure to cold. The classic sequence of angina is activity–pain, rest–relief. The client may describe the pain as a tight, squeezing, heavy pressure or a constricting sensation. It characteristically begins beneath the sternum and may radiate to the jaw, neck, shoulder, or arm. Less characteristically, the pain may be felt in the jaw, epigastric region, or back. Anginal pain usually occurs in a crescendo–decrescendo pattern (increasing to a peak, then gradually decreasing) and typically lasts 2–5 minutes. It generally is relieved by rest. Additional manifestations of angina include dyspnea, pallor, tachycardia, and great anxiety and fear.

Women frequently present with atypical symptoms of angina, including indigestion or nausea, vomiting, fatigue, and upper back pain. The manifestations of angina are summarized in **Box 16–9** ●.

The severity of angina can be graded by the degree to which it limits the client's activities. Class I angina does not occur with ordinary physical activities. It is prompted by strenuous, rapid, or prolonged physical exertion. Class II angina may develop with rapid or prolonged walking or stair climbing, whereas Class III angina significantly limits ordinary physical activities. The client with Class IV angina may have angina with any level of exertion, primarily at rest.

Acute Coronary Syndrome

The cardinal manifestation of ACS is chest pain, usually substernal or epigastric. The pain often radiates to the neck, left shoulder, and/or left arm. The pain may occur at rest, and it typically lasts longer than 10–20 minutes. In ACS, the chest pain is more severe and prolonged than that previously experienced by the client. It may be a new onset of pain, or it may represent a pattern of increasing frequency and severity of anginal pain. Dyspnea, diaphoresis, pallor, and cool skin may be present. Tachycardia and hypotension may occur. The client may be nauseated or feel light-headed.

Acute Myocardial Infarction

Pain is a classic manifestation of MI. Chest pain resulting from MI is more severe than anginal pain. However, it is not the intensity of the chest pain that distinguishes MI from angina or ACS but its duration and its continuous nature. The onset of pain is sudden and usually is not associated with activity. In fact, most MIs occur in the early morning. Clients with a history of angina may have more frequent anginal attacks in the days or weeks before an MI (unstable angina or ACS). Chest pain may be described as crushing and severe; as pressure, heaviness, or a squeezing sensation; or as chest tightness or burning. The pain often begins in the center of the chest (substernal) and may radiate to the shoulders, neck, jaw, or arms. It lasts more than 15–20 minutes and is not relieved by rest or nitroglycerin.

Women and older adults often experience atypical chest pain, presenting with complaints of indigestion, heartburn, nausea, and vomiting (see the Lifespan Considerations feature). Women have traditionally had worse outcomes related to diagnosis and treatment when compared to men. Women may tend to ignore chest pain as they have historically been the caregivers and not the recipients of care.

Box 16–9   Manifestations of Angina

- *Chest pain:* substernal or precordial (across the chest wall); may radiate to neck, arms, shoulders, or jaw
- *Quality:* tight, squeezing, constricting, or heavy sensation; may also be described as burning, aching, choking, dull, or constant
- *Associated manifestations:* dyspnea, pallor, tachycardia, anxiety, and fear
- *Atypical manifestations:* indigestion, nausea, vomiting, upper back pain
- *Precipitating factors:* exercise or activity, strong emotion, stress, cold, heavy meal
- *Relieving factors:* rest, position change; nitroglycerin

Lifespan Considerations Recognizing Acute Myocardial Infarction in Women and Older Adults

Women and older adults often present with manifestations of myocardial infarction (MI) different from those of younger and middle-aged men. However, heart disease is the number one cause of death in both groups, making early recognition and aggressive treatment vital.

Women are more likely than men to have a "silent" or unrecognized heart attack or to present in cardiac arrest or with cardiogenic shock. Women often experience epigastric pain and nausea, causing them to blame their discomfort on heartburn. Shortness of breath is common, as are fatigue and weakness of the shoulders and upper arms.

Older people often seek treatment for vague complaints of difficulty breathing, confusion, fainting, dizziness, abdominal pain, or cough. They often attribute their symptoms to a stroke. The prevalence of silent ischemia is greater in older adults.

It is important for healthcare providers to stress the importance of quickly seeking medical help for atypical manifestations of MI. Prompt diagnosis and intervention reduce the mortality and morbidity of MI in women and older adults, just as it does in men. Despite this fact, both women and older adults are more likely to delay seeking treatment and are less likely to be accurately diagnosed and aggressively treated for cardiac heart disease (CHD). The incidence of CHD continues to increase in younger women indicating a need for continued support for this age group.

Box 16–10   Manifestations of Acute Myocardial Infarction

- Chest pain: substernal or precordial (across the entire chest wall); may radiate to neck, jaw, shoulder(s), or left arm
- Tachycardia, tachypnea
- Dyspnea, shortness of breath
- Nausea and vomiting
- Anxiety, sense of impending doom
- Diaphoresis or sweating
- Cool, mottled skin; diminished peripheral pulses
- Hypotension or hypertension
- Palpitations, dysrhythmias
- Signs of left heart failure
- Decreased level of consciousness

Compensatory mechanisms cause many of the other symptoms of MI. Sympathetic nervous system stimulation causes anxiety, tachycardia, and vasoconstriction. This results in cool, clammy, mottled skin. Pain and blood chemistry changes stimulate the respiratory center, causing tachypnea. The client often has a sense of impending doom and death. Tissue necrosis causes an inflammatory reaction that increases the white blood cell count and elevates the temperature. Serum cardiac enzyme levels rise as enzymes are released from necrotic cardiac cells.

Other manifestations may vary, depending on the location and amount of infarcted tissue. Hypertension, hypotension, or signs of heart failure may develop. Vagal stimulation may cause nausea and vomiting, bradycardia, and hypotension. Hiccuping may develop as a result of diaphragmatic irritation. If a large vessel is occluded, the first sign of MI may be sudden death. Typical manifestations of MI are listed in Box 16–10 ●.

It is not uncommon for someone experiencing chest pain for the first time to attribute it to indigestion. It is important for healthcare providers to ensure that clients understand the possible implications of such pain in order to promote rapid notification of the emergency medical system, because the first hour following the beginning of chest pain is a time of increased risk for sudden death. If thrombolytics (also called fibrinolytics) are considered for treatment (discussed below in the Collaboration section), it is vitally important for the client to be seen in the emergency department as soon as possible after ischemia occurs.

COMPLICATIONS   The risk for complications associated with MI is related to the size and location of the MI.

Dysrhythmias   Infarcted tissue is **arrhythmogenic**—that is, it affects the generation and conduction of electrical impulses in the heart. This increases the risk for disturbances or irregularities of heart rhythm (**dysrhythmias**), which are the most frequent complication of MI.

Premature ventricular contractions are common following an MI, developing in more than 90% of clients with an acute MI. Premature ventricular contractions may be predictive of more dangerous dysrhythmias, such as ventricular tachycardia or ventricular fibrillation. The risk of ventricular fibrillation is greatest the first hour after MI; it is a frequent cause of sudden cardiac death associated with acute MI. Its incidence declines with time.

If the infarct affects a conduction pathway, electrical conduction may be affected. Any degree of AV block may occur following MI, especially when the anterior wall is infarcted. First-degree and Mobitz I (Wenckebach) blocks are most common, although complete heart block may develop. **Bradydysrhythmia** (abnormal slow rhythms) also may develop, particularly when the inferior wall of the ventricle is affected.

Clinical Manifestations and Therapies Coronary Artery Disease

ETIOLOGY	CLINICAL MANIFESTATIONS	CLINICAL THERAPIES
Damage to cardiac cells as well as anaerobic metabolism, increasing the risk of dysrhythmias	<ul><li>Premature ventricular contractions, tachycardia, heart block, with increased risk for ventricular fibrillation</li><li>Pulse rate irregularities; may be weak</li></ul>	<ul><li>Antidysrhythmic medications</li><li>Oxygen administration</li><li>Nitrates to restore cardiac perfusion</li><li>Placement of stent in coronary artery to restore cardiac perfusion</li><li>Continuous cardiac monitoring</li></ul>
Increased quantities of lactic acid, causing pain	<ul><li>Feeling of pressure or banding around the chest, with reports of acute and severe pain that may be stabbing or burning and with radiation to the left arm, jaw, back, or neck</li></ul>	<ul><li>Administration of an analgesic, often morphine sulfate, which causes coronary vasodilation in addition to pain control</li><li>Administration of nitrates and oxygen to reduce ischemia</li><li>Continuous cardiac monitoring</li></ul>
Reduced cardiac output and sympathetic nervous system stimulation, causing tachypnea	<ul><li>Skin color may be gray or pale, capillary refill time may be delayed if output is significantly reduced, hypotension, symptoms of shock, altered level of consciousness</li></ul>	<ul><li>Reduction of the cardiac workload</li><li>Administration of oxygen</li><li>Administration of vasoconstricting medications to improve blood pressure as indicated</li></ul>

Pump Failure Myocardial infarction reduces myocardial contractility, ventricular wall motion, and compliance. Impaired contractility and filling may produce pump failure. The risk of heart failure is greatest when large portions of the left ventricle are infarcted. Heart failure may be more severe with an anterior infarction. Loss of 20%–30% of the left ventricular muscle mass may cause manifestations of left-sided heart failure, including dyspnea, fatigue, weakness, and respiratory crackles on auscultation. Inferior or right ventricular MI may lead to right-sided heart failure, with manifestations such as neck vein distention and peripheral edema. Hemodynamic monitoring is often initiated for clients with evidence of heart failure.

Cardiogenic Shock Cardiogenic shock (impaired tissue perfusion resulting from pump failure) results when functioning myocardial muscle mass decreases by more than 40%. The heart is unable to pump enough blood to meet the needs of the body and maintain organ function. Low cardiac output resulting from cardiogenic shock also impairs perfusion of the coronary arteries and myocardium, further increasing tissue damage. Mortality from cardiogenic shock is greater than 70%, although this can be reduced by prompt intervention with revascularization procedures.

Infarct Extension Approximately 10% of clients experience extension or reinfarction in the area of the original infarction during the first 10–14 days after an MI. Extension of the MI is characterized by increased myocardial necrosis from continued impairment of blood flow and ongoing injury. Expansion of the MI is described as a permanent expansion of the infarcted area from thinning and dilation of the muscle. Infarct extension and expansion may cause manifestations such as continuing chest pain, hemodynamic compromise, and worsening heart failure.

Structural Defects Necrotic muscle is replaced by scar tissue that is thinner than the ventricular muscle mass. This can lead to such complications as ventricular aneurysm, rupture of the interventricular septum or papillary muscle, and myocardial rupture.

A **ventricular aneurysm** is an outpouching of the ventricular wall. It may develop when a large section of the ventricle is replaced by scar tissue. Because it does not contract during systole, stroke volume decreases. Blood may pool within the aneurysm, causing clots to form.

Ischemia of the papillary muscle or chordae tendineae may cause structural damage leading to papillary muscle dysfunction or rupture. This affects AV valve function (usually the mitral valve), causing **regurgitation** (backflow of blood into the atria during systole). The interventricular septum may perforate or rupture as a result of ischemia and infarction.

Myocardial rupture is a risk between days 4 and 7 after MI, when the injured tissue is soft and weak. This potential complication of MI is often fatal.

Pericarditis Tissue necrosis prompts an inflammatory response. **Pericarditis** (inflammation of the pericardial tissue surrounding the heart) may complicate AMI, usually within 2–3 days. Pericarditis causes chest pain that may be aching or sharp and stabbing, and aggravated by movement or deep breathing. A pericardial friction rub may be heard on auscultation of heart sounds.

Dressler syndrome, which is thought to be a hypersensitivity response to necrotic tissue or an autoimmune disorder, may develop days to weeks after AMI. It is a symptom complex characterized by fever, chest pain, and dyspnea. Dressler syndrome may spontaneously resolve or recur over several months, causing significant discomfort and distress.

▶ COLLABORATION

Care of clients with CAD focuses on aggressive risk factor management to slow the atherosclerotic process and maintain myocardial perfusion. Until manifestations of chronic or acute ischemia are experienced, the diagnosis often is presumptive, based on history and the presence of risk factors.

The management of stable angina focuses on maintaining coronary blood flow and cardiac function. Stable angina often can be managed by medical therapy. As for CAD, risk factor management is a vital component of care for the client with angina.

Immediate treatment goals for the MI client are as follows:

- Relieve chest pain.
- Reduce the extent of myocardial damage.
- Maintain cardiovascular stability.
- Decrease cardiac workload.
- Prevent complications.

Slowing the process of CAD and reducing the risk of future MI is a major long-term management goal for the client.

Rapid assessment and early diagnosis is important in treating AMI. "Time is muscle" is a medical truism for the client with AMI. The evolution of an AMI is dynamic: The quicker the artery is reopened (medically, surgically, or spontaneously), the more myocardium can be salvaged. Survival and long-term outcomes following AMI are improved by the rate at which circulation is restored to the infarcted heart muscle. Reestablishing blood flood reduces myocardial oxygen demand. The AHA recommends initiation of percutaneous coronary intervention (PCI) within 60 minutes from medical contact.

A major problem interfering with timely reperfusion is delay in seeking medical care following the onset of symptoms. Potential delays to treatment have been identified to occur during three intervals: from onset of symptoms to client recognition, during prehospital transport, and during emergency department evaluation (O'Connor et al., 2010).

Up to 44% of clients with symptoms of chest discomfort or pain wait more than 4 hours before seeking treatment. Many factors are cited as reasons for treatment delay, including advanced age, perception that the symptoms are not serious, denial, limited access to medical care, unavailability of an emergency response system, and in-hospital delays. Immediate evaluation of the client presenting with manifestations of MI is essential to early diagnosis and treatment.

Diagnostic Tests

Laboratory testing is used to assess for risk factors such as an abnormal blood lipid profile (elevated triglyceride and LDL levels and decreased HDL levels). Total serum cholesterol is elevated in hyperlipidemia. A lipid profile also includes triglyceride, HDL, and LDL levels and enables calculation of the ratio of HDL to total cholesterol. The ratio should be at least 1:5, with 1:3 being the ideal ratio. Elevated lipid levels are associated with an increased risk of atherosclerosis (see Table 16–21). In clients with a strong family history of premature CAD or familial hypercholesterolemia, lipoprotein(a) also may be measured. Elevated levels of lipoprotein(a) may independently increase the risk of CAD. Other subsets of blood lipids may also be measured in selected clients.

Diagnostic tests to identify subclinical (asymptomatic) CAD may be indicated when multiple risk factors are present. Relevant diagnostic tests include the following:

■ *C-reactive protein* is a serum protein associated with inflammatory processes. Recent evidence suggests that elevated blood levels of this protein may be predictive of CAD.

■ *Ankle–brachial blood pressure index (ABI)* is an inexpensive, noninvasive test for peripheral vascular disease that may be predictive of CAD. The systolic blood pressure in the brachial, posterior tibial, and dorsalis pedis arteries is measured by Doppler. An ABI of less than 0.9 in either leg indicates the presence of peripheral arterial disease and a significant risk for CAD.

■ *Exercise ECG testing* may be performed. ECGs are used to assess the response to increased cardiac workload induced by exercise. The test is considered "positive" for CAD if myocardial ischemia is detected on the ECG (depression of the ST segment by >3 mm; **Figure 16–32** ●), the client develops chest pain, or the test is stopped because of excess fatigue, dysrhythmias, or other symptoms before the predicted maximal heart rate is achieved.

■ *Electron beam computed tomography* creates a three-dimensional image of the heart and coronary arteries that can reveal plaque and other abnormalities. This noninvasive test requires no special preparation and can identify clients at risk for developing myocardial ischemia.

■ *Myocardial perfusion imaging* may be used to evaluate myocardial blood flow and perfusion, both at rest and during stress testing (exercise or mental stress). Perfusion imaging studies are costly, however, and therefore are not recommended for routine CAD risk assessment.

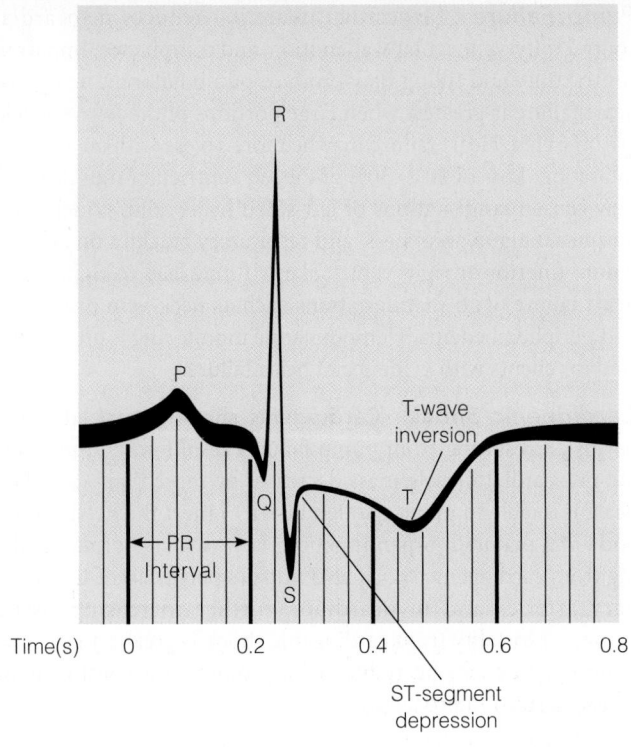

Figure 16–32 ● ECG changes during an episode of angina. Note characteristic T-wave inversion and ST-segment depression of myocardial ischemia.

Diagnostic testing to establish the diagnosis of AMI involves serum levels of **cardiac markers** (proteins released from necrotic heart muscle). These tests are ordered on admission and for 3 succeeding days. Serial blood levels help establish the diagnosis and determine the extent of myocardial damage. The proteins most specific for diagnosis of MI are creatine kinase (CK), or creatine phosphokinase (CPK), and cardiac-specific troponins (**Table 16–22** ●):

■ *Creatine kinase (CK)* is an important enzyme for cellular function found principally in cardiac and skeletal muscle and the brain. CK levels rise rapidly with damage to these tissues, appearing in the serum 4–6 hours after AMI, peaking within

TABLE 16–22 Cardiac Markers

				CHANGES OCCURRING WITH MI		
MARKER	NORMAL LEVEL	PRIMARY TISSUE LOCATION	SIGNIFICANCE OF ELEVATION	APPEARS	PEAKS	DURATION
CK (CPK)	Male: 12-80 units/L	Cardiac muscle, skeletal muscle, brain	Injury to muscle cells	3–6 hr	12–24 hr	24–48 hr
	Female: 10-70 units/L					
CK-MB	0% -3% of total CK	Cardiac muscle	MI, cardiac ischemia, myocarditis, cardiac contusion, defibrillation	4–8 hr	18–24 hr	72 hr
cT_nT	< 0.2 mcg/L	Cardiac muscle	Acute MI, unstable angina	2–4 hr	24–36 hr	10–14 days
cT_nl	< 3.1 mcg/L	Cardiac muscle	Acute MI, unstable angina	2–4 hr	24–36 hr	7–10 days

Note: CK = creatine kinase; CPK = creatine phosphokinase; CK-MB = MB isoenzyme of creatine kinase; cT_nl = cardiac-specific troponin I; cT_nT = cardiac-specific troponin T.

12–24 hours, and then declining over the next 48–72 hours. The CK level correlates with the size of the infarction: The greater the amount of infarcted tissue, the higher the serum CK level.

■ **CK-MB** (also called MB-bands) is a subset of CK specific to cardiac muscle. This isoenzyme of CK is considered the most sensitive indicator of MI. Elevated CK alone is not specific for MI; however, elevated CK-MB of greater than 5% is considered a positive indicator of MI. CK-MB levels do not normally rise with chest pain from angina or causes other than MI.

■ *Cardiac muscle* **troponins**, *cardiac-specific troponin T (cT_nT), and cardiac-specific troponin I (cT_nI)* are proteins released during MI that are sensitive indicators of myocardial damage. These proteins are part of the actin–myosin unit in cardiac muscle and normally are not detectable in the blood. With necrosis of cardiac muscle, troponins are released and blood levels rise. The specificity of cT_nT and cT_nI to cardiac muscle necrosis makes these markers particularly useful when skeletal muscle trauma contributes to elevated CK levels (e.g., when CPR has been performed or traumatic injury occurred at the time of the MI). They are sensitive enough to detect very small infarctions that do not cause significant CK elevation. Both cT_nT and cT_nI remain in the blood for 10–14 days after an MI, making them useful to diagnose MI when medical treatment is delayed.

Other laboratory tests may include the following:

■ *Myoglobin* is one of the first cardiac markers to be detectable in the blood after an MI. Myoglobin is released within a few hours of symptom onset. It may be used in assessing reperfusion after thrombolysis.

■ *Complete blood count* shows an elevated white blood cell count resulting from inflammation of the injured myocardium. The erythrocyte sedimentation rate also rises because of inflammation.

■ *Arterial blood gas* may be ordered to assess blood oxygen levels and acid–base balance.

Electrocardiography, echocardiography, and myocardial nuclear scans are the most common diagnostic tests performed when AMI is suspected. With the exception of the ECG, the timing of these tests depends on the client's immediate condition. Hemodynamic monitoring may be initiated in the unstable client following MI. Specifically consider the following:

■ The ECG reflects changes in conduction resulting from myocardial ischemia and necrosis. Classic ECG changes seen in AMI include T-wave inversion, ST-segment elevation, and formation of a Q wave. Ischemic changes in the heart are seen as depression of the ST segment or inversion of the T wave (see Figure 16–32). With myocardial injury, elevation of the ST segment occurs (**Figure 16–33A ●**). Significant Q-wave development (Figure 16–33B) indicates a transmural, or full-thickness, infarction. Myocardial damage can be localized using the 12-lead ECG.

■ For the client with CAD, diagnostic testing may include stress electrocardiography (exercise stress test), which uses ECGs to monitor the cardiac response to an increased workload during progressive exercise.

■ *Echocardiography* is done to evaluate cardiac wall motion and left ventricular function. Stunned and infarcted tissue does not contract as effectively (if at all) as healthy myocardium.

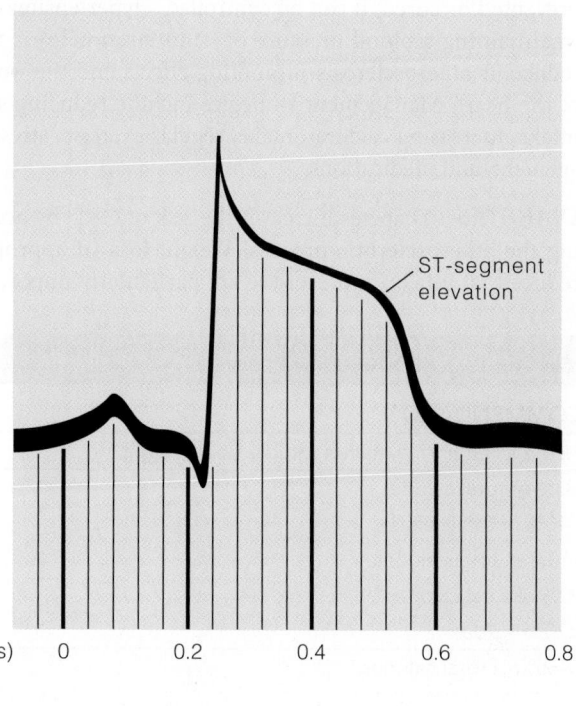

A

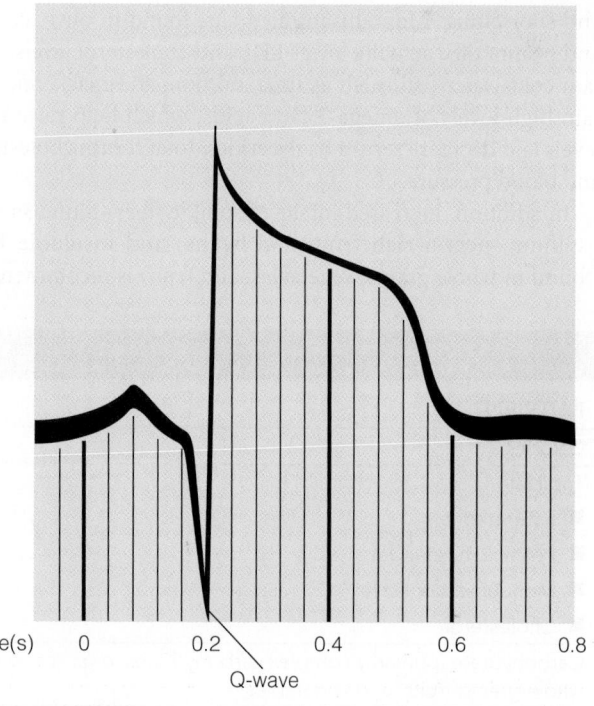

B

Figure 16–33 ● ECG changes characteristic of MI. *A*, ST-segment elevation characteristic of myocardial injury. *B*, Clinically significant Q-wave characteristic of a transmural infarction.

- *Radionuclide imaging* may be done to evaluate myocardial perfusion. These studies cannot differentiate between an acute MI and old scar tissue but do help identify the specific area of myocardial ischemia and damage.
- *Hemodynamic monitoring* may be initiated when AMI significantly affects cardiac output and hemodynamic status.

Conservative Management

Conservative management of CAD focuses on risk factor modification, including smoking, diet, exercise, and management of contributing conditions, such as hypertension and diabetes.

SMOKING Smoking cessation reduces the risk for CAD within months after quitting and improves cardiovascular status. People who quit reduce their risk by 50%, regardless of how long they smoked before quitting. For women, the risk becomes equivalent to that for a nonsmoker within 3–5 years of smoking cessation (Woods et al., 2010). In addition, stopping smoking improves HDL levels, lowers LDL levels, and reduces blood viscosity. Advise clients who have CAD regarding smoking cessation. Health promotion activities focus on preventing children, teenagers, and adults from starting to smoke.

DIET Dietary recommendations include reducing the consumption of saturated fat and cholesterol as well as developing strategies to lower LDL levels (**Table 16–23** ●). Most fats are a mixture of saturated and unsaturated fatty acids. The highest proportions of saturated fat are found in whole-milk products, red meats, and coconut oil. Nonfat dairy products, fish, and poultry as primary protein sources are recommended. Solidified vegetable fats (e.g., margarine and shortening) contain *trans* fatty acids, which behave more like saturated fats. Soft margarines and vegetable oil spreads contain low levels of *trans* fatty acids and should be used instead of butter, stick margarine, and shortening. Monounsaturated fats, found in olive, canola, and peanut oils, actually lower LDL and cholesterol levels. Certain cold-water fish, such as tuna, salmon, and mackerel, contain high levels of omega-3 fatty acids, which help raise HDL levels and decrease serum triglycerides, total serum cholesterol, and blood pressure.

In addition, increased intake of soluble fiber (found in oats, psyllium, pectin-rich fruit, and beans) and insoluble fiber (found in whole grains, vegetables, and fruit) is recommended.

Folic acid and vitamins B_6 and B_{12} affect homocysteine metabolism, reducing serum levels. Leafy green vegetables (e.g., spinach and broccoli) and legumes (e.g., black-eyed peas, dried beans, and lentils) are rich sources of folate. Meat, fish, and poultry are rich in vitamins B_6 and B_{12}. Vitamin B_6 also is found in soy products; vitamin B_{12} is in fortified cereals. Increased intake of antioxidant nutrients (vitamin E, in particular) and foods rich in antioxidants (fruits and vegetables) appears to increase HDL levels and have a protective effect against CAD.

Moderate alcohol consumption may provide some health benefits, particularly in middle-aged and older adults. Alcohol consumption should be limited to no more than two drinks per day for men or one drink per day for women. A drink is 5 ounces of wine, 12 ounces of beer, or 1.5 ounces of whiskey. The health benefits for individuals who drink versus those who abstain have not been fully investigated.

Clients being treated for CAD who are overweight or obese are encouraged to lose weight via a combination of healthy eating (maintaining a nutritionally sound diet) and increased exercise. High-protein, high-fat weight loss programs are not recommended for weight reduction.

EXERCISE Regular physical exercise reduces the risk for CAD in several ways. It lowers VLDL, LDL, and triglyceride levels, and it raises HDL levels. Regular exercise reduces blood pressure and insulin resistance. Unless contraindicated, all clients are encouraged to participate in at least 30 minutes of moderate-intensity physical activity 5 to 6 days each week. To achieve weight loss and prevent weight gain, 60 to 90 minutes of moderate intensity exercise daily is recommended. Exact physical activity requirements vary from person to person and may need to be increased to obtain maximum weight loss goals (CDC, 2011).

HYPERTENSION Although hypertension often cannot be prevented or cured, it can be controlled. Hypertension control (maintaining a blood pressure of <140/90 mmHg) is vital to reduce its atherosclerosis-promoting effects and the workload of the heart. Management strategies include reducing sodium intake, increasing calcium intake, regular exercise, stress management, and medications.

DIABETES Diabetes increases the risk of CAD by accelerating the atherosclerotic process. Weight loss (if appropriate), reduced fat intake, and exercise are particularly important for

TABLE 16–23 Dietary Recommendations From the National Cholesterol Education Program

NUTRIENT	RECOMMENDATION
Calories	Adjusted to attain/maintain desirable body weight
Total fat	20–35% of total calories
■ Saturated fats	■ <10% of total calories
■ Polyunsaturated fat	■ ≤10% of total calories
■ Monounsaturated fat	■ 20% of total calories
■ Cholesterol	■ <200 mg/day
Carbohydrate (primarily complex carbohydrates; e.g., whole grains, fruits, and vegetables)	45%–65% of total calories
Dietary fiber	20–30 g/day
Protein	About 10%–35% of total calories

Source: Compiled from National Cholesterol Education Program (NCEP). (2013). *Program description.* Retrieved from www.nhlbi.nih.gov/about/ncep/ncep_pd.htm.

Medications **Cholesterol-Lowering Drugs**

CLASSIFICATION AND DRUG EXAMPLES	MECHANISMS OF ACTION	NURSING CONSIDERATIONS
Statins *Drug examples:* ▪ lovastatin (Mevacor) ▪ pravastatin (Pravachol) ▪ simvastatin (Zocor) ▪ fluvastatin (Lescol) ▪ atorvastatin (Lipitor)	Statins inhibit the enzyme 3-hydroxy-3-methylglutaryl coenzyme A reductase in the liver, lowering LDL synthesis and serum levels. The statins are first-line treatment for elevated LDL and are used in conjunction with diet and lifestyle changes. Although their side effects are minimal, they may cause increased serum liver enzyme levels and myopathy.	▪ Monitor the client's serum cholesterol and liver enzyme levels before and during therapy. Report elevated liver enzyme levels. ▪ Assess the client for muscle pain and tenderness. Monitor the client's creatine phosphokinase level if present. ▪ If the client is taking digoxin concurrently, monitor for and report digoxin toxicity. *Health education for the client and family:* ▪ The client should promptly report muscle pain, tenderness, or weakness; skin rash, hives, or changes in skin color; abdominal pain, nausea, or vomiting. ▪ The client should not use these drugs if pregnant or planning to become pregnant. ▪ The client should inform the healthcare provider if the client is taking any other medications concurrently.
Bile Acid Sequestrants *Drug examples:* ▪ cholestyramine (Questran) ▪ colestipol (Colestid) ▪ colesevelam (Welchol)	Bile acid sequestrants lower LDL levels by binding bile acids in the intestine and by reducing their reabsorption and cholesterol production in the liver. These medications are used in combination therapy regimens and for women who are considering pregnancy. Their primary disadvantages are inconvenience of administration (because of bulk) and gastrointestinal side effects (e.g., constipation).	▪ Mix cholestyramine and colestipol powders with 4–6 oz of water or juice; administer once or twice a day as ordered with meals. ▪ Store in a tightly closed container. *Health education for the client and family:* ▪ The client should promptly report constipation, severe gastric distress with nausea and vomiting, unexplained weight loss, black or bloody stools, or sudden back pain. ▪ Drinking ample amounts of fluid while taking these drugs reduces problems of constipation and bloating. ▪ The client should not omit doses, because this may affect the absorption of other drugs the client is taking.
Nicotinic Acid *Drug examples:* ▪ niacin (Nicobid, Nicolar, Niaspan, others)	Nicotinic acid in both prescription and nonprescription forms lowers total and LDL cholesterol and triglyceride levels. The crystalline form and Niaspan, a prescription extended-release tablet, also raise HDL levels. Because the doses required to achieve significant cholesterol-lowering effects are associated with multiple side effects, nicotinic acid generally is used in combination therapy, particularly with the statin drugs.	▪ Give oral preparations with meals accompanied by a cold beverage to minimize gastrointestinal effects. ▪ Administer with caution to clients who have active liver disease, peptic ulcer disease, gout, or type 2 diabetes. ▪ Monitor blood glucose, uric acid levels, and liver function tests during treatment. *Health education for the client and family:* ▪ Flushing of the face, neck, and ears may occur within 2 hours following dose; these effects generally subside as treatment continues. Alcohol use during nicotinic acid therapy may worsen this effect. ▪ The client should report weakness or dizziness with changes in posture (lying to sitting; sitting to standing). The client should change positions slowly to reduce the risk of injury.
Fibric Acid Derivatives *Drug examples:* ▪ gemfibrozil (Lopid) ▪ fenofibrate (TriCor) ▪ clofibrate (Atromid-S)	The fibrates are used to lower serum triglyceride levels; they have only a slight to modest effect on LDL. They affect lipid regulation by blocking triglyceride synthesis. They are used to treat very high triglyceride levels and may be used in combination with statins.	▪ Monitor serum LDL and VLDL levels, electrolytes, glucose, liver enzymes, renal function tests, and complete blood count during therapy. Report abnormal values. ▪ Up to 2 months of treatment may be required to achieve a therapeutic effect; rebound, with decreasing benefit, may occur in the second or third month of treatment. *Health education for the client and family:* ▪ The client should take with meals if the drug causes gastric distress. ▪ The client should promptly report flulike symptoms (e.g., fatigue, muscle aching, soreness, or weakness). ▪ The client should not use this drug if pregnant or planning to become pregnant. The client should use reliable birth control measures while taking this drug. ▪ The client should contact the healthcare provider before stopping this drug and before taking any over-the-counter preparations.

the client with diabetes. Because hyperglycemia apparently also contributes to atherosclerosis, consistent blood glucose management is vital.

Pharmacologic Therapy

Medications are used extensively in both treatment of existing cardiac disease and prevention of potential cardiac disease. A number of drug groups are useful.

DRUGS USED TO LOWER CHOLESTEROL   Drug therapy to lower total serum cholesterol and LDL levels and to raise HDL levels now is an integral part of CAD management (see the Medications feature). This therapy is used in conjunction with diet and other lifestyle changes and is based on the client's overall risk for CAD.

Drugs used to treat hyperlipidemia act specifically by lowering LDL levels. The goal of treatment is to achieve an LDL level of less than 130 mg/dL (NCEP, 2013). Medications to treat hyperlipidemia are expensive; the cost–benefit ratio needs to be considered, because long-term treatment may be required. The four major classes of cholesterol-lowering drugs are statins, bile acid sequestrants, nicotinic acid, and fibrates.

The statins, including lovastatin (Mevacor), pravastatin (Pravachol), simvastatin (Zocor), and others, are first-line drugs for treating hyperlipidemia. They effectively lower LDL levels and may also increase HDL levels. The statins can cause myopathy; all clients are instructed to report muscle pain and weakness or brown urine. Liver function tests are monitored during therapy, because these drugs may increase liver enzyme levels.

The other cholesterol-lowering drugs, such as the bile acid sequestrants, nicotinic acid, and fibrates, are primarily used when combination therapy is required to effectively lower serum cholesterol levels. They also may be used for selected clients, such as younger adults and women who wish to become pregnant, or to specifically lower triglyceride levels.

Clients at high risk for MI are often started on prophylactic low-dose aspirin therapy. Aspirin inhibits the aggregation of platelets, thereby decreasing the risk of blood clots. Aspirin is contraindicated for clients with a history of aspirin sensitivity, bleeding disorders, or active peptic ulcer disease. Clients on long-term aspirin therapy should be screened for aspirin resistance. Angiotensin-converting enzyme inhibitors or angiotensin receptor blockers may also be prescribed for high-risk clients, including those with diabetes or those with other CAD risk factors.

DRUGS USED TO TREAT ANGINA   Drugs may be used for both acute and long-term relief of angina. The goal of drug treatment is to reduce oxygen demand and increase oxygen supply to the myocardium. Three main classes of drugs are used to treat angina: nitrates, beta-blockers, and calcium-channel blockers.

Nitrates   Nitrates, including nitroglycerin and longer-acting nitrate preparations, are used to treat acute anginal attacks and prevent angina.

Sublingual nitroglycerin is the drug of choice to treat acute angina. It acts within 1–2 minutes, decreasing myocardial work and oxygen demand through venous and arterial dilation, which in turn reduce preload and afterload. It may also improve myocardial oxygen supply by dilating collateral blood vessels and reducing stenosis. Rapid-acting nitroglycerin is also avail-

able as a buccal spray in a metered system. For some clients, this may be easier to handle than small nitroglycerin tablets.

Longer-acting nitroglycerin preparations (oral tablets, ointment, or transdermal patches) are used to prevent attacks of angina, not to treat an acute attack. The primary problem with long-term nitrate use is the development of tolerance (a decreasing effect from the same dose of medication). Tolerance can be limited by a dosing schedule that allows a nitrate-free period of at least 8–10 hours daily. This is usually scheduled at night, when angina is less likely to occur.

Headache is a common side effect of nitrates and may limit their usefulness. Nausea, dizziness, and hypotension are also common effects of therapy.

Beta-Blockers   Beta-blockers, including propranolol, metoprolol, nadolol, and atenolol, are considered first-line drugs to treat stable angina. They block the cardiac-stimulating effects of norepinephrine and epinephrine, preventing anginal attacks by reducing heart rate, myocardial contractility, and blood pressure, thus reducing myocardial oxygen demand. Beta-blockers may be used alone or with other medications to prevent angina.

Beta-blockers are contraindicated for clients with asthma or severe chronic obstructive pulmonary disease, because they may cause severe bronchospasm. They are not used in clients with significant bradycardia or AV conduction blocks, and they are used cautiously in clients with heart failure. Beta-blockers are not used to treat Prinzmetal angina, because they may make it worse.

Calcium-Channel Blockers   Calcium-channel blockers reduce myocardial oxygen demand and increase myocardial blood and oxygen supply. These drugs (which include verapamil, diltiazem, and nifedipine) lower blood pressure, reduce myocardial contractility, and in some cases, lower heart rate, decreasing myocardial oxygen demand. They are also potent coronary vasodilators, effectively increasing oxygen supply. Like beta-blockers, calcium-channel blockers act too slowly to effectively treat an acute attack of angina; they are used for long-term prophylaxis. However, because they may actually increase ischemia and mortality in clients with heart failure or left ventricular dysfunction, these drugs are not usually prescribed in the initial treatment of angina. They are used cautiously in clients with dysrhythmias, heart failure, or hypotension.

Aspirin   The client with angina, particularly unstable angina, is at risk for MI because of significant narrowing of the coronary arteries. Low-dose aspirin (80–325 mg/day) is often prescribed to reduce the risk of platelet aggregation and thrombus formation.

DRUGS USED TO TREAT MYOCARDIAL INFARCTION
Fibrinolytic, analgesic, and antidysrhythmic agents are among the principal classes of drugs used in treating AMI. In addition, aspirin, a platelet inhibitor, is now considered an essential part of treating AMI. A 160- to 325-mg aspirin tablet is given by emergency personnel, with the instruction that it is to be chewed (for buccal absorption). This initial dose is followed by a daily oral dose of 160–325 mg.

Analgesics   Pain relief is vital in treating the client with AMI. Pain stimulates the sympathetic nervous system, increasing the heart rate and blood pressure and, in turn, the myocardial workload. Sublingual nitroglycerin may be given (up to three 0.4-mg doses at 5-minute intervals). Intravenous nitroglycerin may be continued for the first 24–48 hours to reduce myocardial work. In addition to pain relief, nitroglycerin decreases myocardial oxygen demand and may increase the supply of oxygen to the myocardium. Nitroglycerin is a peripheral and arterial vasodilator that reduces afterload. It dilates coronary arteries and collateral channels in the heart, increasing coronary blood flow to save myocardial tissue at risk. Nitrates may, however, cause reflex tachycardia or excessive hypotension, so close monitoring by the nurse is necessary during administration. It also is important to ask the client about use of sildenafil (Viagra) within the 24 hours before administering nitroglycerin, because the combination can precipitate a significant drop in blood pressure.

Morphine sulfate is the drug of choice for pain unrelieved by nitroglycerin and for sedation. Following an initial intravenous dose of 4–8 mg, small doses (2–4 mg) may be repeated intravenously every 5 minutes until pain is relieved. It is important for the nurse to assess the client frequently for pain relief and possible adverse effects of analgesia, such as excessive sedation. Pain unrelieved by expected or usual doses should be reported to the healthcare provider, because it may indicate a complication such as extension of the infarct. Antianxiety agents such as diazepam (Valium) may also be administered to promote rest.

Fibrinolytics   Fibrinolytic agents, which are drugs that dissolve or break up blood clots, are first-line drugs used to treat acute MI when access to a cardiac catheterization lab for revascularization procedures is not immediately available. Fibrinolytic drugs activate the fibrinolytic system to lyse (destroy) the clot, restoring blood flow to the obstructed artery. Early fibrinolytic administration (within the first 6 hours of MI onset) limits infarct size, reduces heart damage, and improves outcomes. Activation of the fibrinolytic system can cause multiple complications; approximately 0.5%–5% of clients receiving fibrinolytic drugs experience serious bleeding complications. In addition, not every client is a candidate for fibrinolytic therapy. For example, it is contraindicated in clients with known bleeding disorders, active peptic ulcer disease, a hemorrhagic ophthalmic condition, or history of severe hypertension; those who are concurrently on anticoagulant therapy; those who have had a recent invasive or surgical procedure; and those who are pregnant.

Several fibrinolytic agents are commonly used today. Among these, little difference in effectiveness has been demonstrated; there are, however, big differences in cost. Streptokinase, a biological agent derived from group C *Streptococcus* organisms, is the least expensive of the drugs. Its primary drawback is the risk for a severe hypersensitivity reaction, including anaphylaxis. Streptokinase is administered by intravenous infusion. Anisoylated plasminogen streptokinase activator complex (APSAC) is a related drug that can be administered by bolus over 2–5 minutes. It has many of the same effects as streptokinase but is considerably more expensive. Tissue plasminogen activator, tenecteplase, and reteplase are more effective in reestablishing myocardial perfusion, especially when the pain developed more than 3 hours previously. These drugs, however, are the most expensive.

Antidysrhythmics   Dysrhythmias are a common complication of AMI, particularly in the first 12–24 hours. Antidysrhythmic medications are used as needed to treat dysrhythmias.

They also may be given prophylactically to prevent dysrhythmias. Ventricular dysrhythmias are treated with a class I or class III antidysrhythmic. Symptomatic bradycardia (bradycardia with associated hypotension and other signs of low cardiac output) is treated with intravenous atropine, 0.5–1 mg. Intravenous verapamil or the short-acting beta-blocker esmolol (Brevibloc) may be ordered to treat atrial fibrillation or other supraventricular tachydysrhythmias.

Other Medications   Beta-blockers such as propranolol (Inderal), atenolol (Tenormin), and metoprolol (Lopressor) reduce pain, limit infarct size, and decrease the incidence of serious ventricular dysrhythmias in AMI. These drugs decrease the heart rate, reducing cardiac work and myocardial oxygen demand. Initial doses are given intravenously. Oral beta-blocker therapy has been shown to suggest lower mortality and reinfarction rates.

Angiotensin-converting enzyme (ACE) inhibitors also reduce mortality associated with AMI. These drugs reduce ventricular remodeling following an MI, reducing the risk for subsequent heart failure. It is not known whether ACE inhibitors will prevent ischemic events, but they have been demonstrated to decrease the risk of stroke or heart attack.

Anticoagulants and antiplatelet medications are often prescribed to maintain coronary artery patency following thrombolysis or a revascularization procedure. Abciximab (ReoPro) suppresses platelet aggregation and reduces the risk of reocclusion following angioplasty. It also improves vessel opening with fibrinolytic therapy, permitting lower doses of fibrinolytic drugs to be used. Standard or low-molecular-weight (LMW) heparin preparations often are given to clients with AMI. Heparin helps establish and maintain patency of the affected coronary artery. It also is used, along with long-term warfarin, to prevent systemic or pulmonary embolism in clients with significant left ventricular impairment or atrial fibrillation following AMI. See the Medications feature for the nursing implications of antiplatelet drugs.

Clients with pump failure and hypotension may receive intravenous dopamine, a vasopressor. At low doses (<5 mg/kg/min), dopamine improves blood flow to the kidneys, preventing renal ischemia and possible acute renal failure. With increasing doses, dopamine increases myocardial contractility and causes vasoconstriction, improving blood pressure and cardiac output.

Antilipemic agents are used for the client with hyperlipidemia. A stool softener, such as docusate sodium, is prescribed to maintain normal bowel function and reduce straining.

Clinical Therapy

The client with a suspected or confirmed MI is monitored continuously. Care is provided in the intensive coronary care unit for the first 24–48 hours, after which time less intensive monitoring (e.g., telemetry) may be required. An intravenous line is established to allow rapid administration of emergency medications.

Bed rest is prescribed for the first 12 hours to reduce the cardiac workload. A bedside commode is allowed, because it generally provides a less stressful experience than using a bedpan. If the client's condition is stable, sitting in a chair at the bedside is permitted after 12 hours. Activities are gradually increased as tolerated. A quiet, calm environment with limited outside stimuli is preferred. Visitors are limited to promote rest. Oxygen is

Medications **Antiplatelet Drugs**

CLASSIFICATION AND DRUG EXAMPLES	MECHANISMS OF ACTION	NURSING CONSIDERATIONS
Oral Antiplatelet Drugs *Drug examples:* ■ aspirin ■ clopidogrel (Plavix)	Antiplatelet drugs suppress platelet aggregation in arteries, preventing the development of an arterial thrombus. Aspirin and clopidogrel block different platelet activation pathways to inhibit platelet aggregation and clot formation. The dose of aspirin given to achieve antiplatelet effects is low, typically 80 mg/day.	■ Inquire about a history of intracranial hemorrhage, upper gastrointestinal bleeding, peptic ulcer disease, or known bleeding tendency. ■ Observe for and report increased bruising, petechiae, purpura, and apparent or occult bleeding (e.g., melena and hematemesis). ■ Do not administer concurrently with warfarin (Coumadin). *Health education for the client and family:* ■ Take as directed. Take aspirin with food or milk; clopidogrel may be taken at any time of day. ■ Do not use nonsteroidal anti-inflammatory drugs (NSAIDs) or other over-the-counter drugs that may contain aspirin or an NSAID unless prescribed by your healthcare provider. ■ Check with your healthcare provider before using any herbal remedies, such as evening primrose oil, feverfew, garlic, ginkgo biloba, or grapeseed extract, while taking these medications. ■ Report unusual bruising or excessive bleeding. ■ Inform all care providers (including dental professionals) about use of these drugs.
Intravenous Antiplatelet Drugs *Drug examples:* ■ abciximab (ReoPro) ■ eptifibatide (Integrilin) ■ tirofiban (Aggrastat)	The intravenously administered antiplatelet drugs abciximab, eptifibatide, and tirofiban block the final common pathway of platelet activation and thus are more effective than the orally administered antiplatelet drugs. However, the risk of bleeding is greater than with the orally administered antiplatelet drugs.	■ Determine history of bleeding disorders, intracranial hemorrhage, or recent trauma or surgery. ■ Inquire about recent use of oral antiplatelet or anticoagulant drugs. ■ Monitor complete blood count, including hemoglobin, hematocrit, and platelet count; clotting studies, including prothrombin time, International Normalized Ratio (INR), partial thromboplastin time; vital signs; and electrocardiogram during therapy. ■ Maintain separate intravenous lines for blood draws and for administration of other drugs during infusion. ■ Closely observe for and immediately report anaphylaxis or bleeding uncontrolled by pressure. Keep resuscitation equipment readily available. ■ Maintain bed rest during infusion. *Health education for the client and family:* ■ This drug is given to reduce the risk of clotting and myocardial infarction. It helps maintain blood flow through the affected vessel following angioplasty and stent placement. ■ Immediately report any chest tightness, difficulty breathing, shortness of breath, or itching that develops during the infusion. ■ Your risk of bleeding should return to normal within about 2 days following the infusion. ■ Immediately report any unusual bruising or bleeding.

administered by nasal cannula at 2–5 L/min to improve oxygenation of the myocardium and other tissues.

A liquid diet may be prescribed for the first 4–12 hours to reduce gastric distention and myocardial work. Following that, a low-fat, low-cholesterol, reduced-sodium diet is allowed. Sodium restrictions may be lifted after 2–3 days if no evidence of heart failure is present. Small, frequent feedings are often recommended. Drinks containing caffeine, as well as very hot and cold foods, may also be limited.

REVASCULARIZATION PROCEDURES Several procedures may be used to restore blood flow and oxygen to ischemic tissue. Nonsurgical techniques include transluminal coronary angioplasty, laser angioplasty, coronary atherectomy, and intracoronary stents. Coronary artery bypass grafting (CABG) is a surgical procedure that may be used.

Percutaneous Coronary Revascularization Percutaneous coronary revascularization (PCR) procedures are used to restore blood flow to the ischemic myocardium in clients with CAD. Approximately 600,000 PCR procedures are done annually in the United States. Factors that may influence the choice of revascularization strategy include:

■ Diabetes mellitus

■ Chronic kidney disease

- Complete of revascularization
- Systolic dysfunction
- Previous history of CABG
- Type of MI.

The PCR procedures are similar to the procedure used for coronary angiography. A catheter introduced into the arterial circulation is guided into the opening of the narrowed coronary artery. A flexible guidewire is inserted through the catheter lumen into the affected vessel. The guidewire is then used to thread an angioplasty balloon, arterial stent, or other therapeutic device into the narrowed segment of the artery. The procedure is performed in the cardiac catheterization laboratory using local anesthesia. The hospital stay is short (1–2 days), minimizing costs.

In a percutaneous transluminal coronary angioplasty (PTCA), a balloon-tipped catheter is threaded over the guidewire, with the balloon positioned across the area of narrowing (**Figure 16–34** ●). The balloon is inflated in a step-by-step fashion for approximately 30 seconds to 2 minutes to compress the plaque against the arterial wall, with a goal of reducing the vessel obstruction to less than 50% of the arterial lumen. Percutaneous transluminal coronary angioplasty typically is accompanied by placement of a stent. Intracoronary stents are metallic scaffolds used to maintain an open arterial lumen. Stents have been shown to reduce the rate of restenosis by approximately one-third. The majority of clients having angioplasty today are treated with stents. The stent is placed over a balloon catheter, guided into position, and expanded as the balloon is inflated. It then remains in the artery as a prop after the balloon is removed. Endothelial cells will completely line the inner wall of the stent to produce a smooth inner lining. Antiplatelet medications (aspirin and ticlopidine) are given following stent insertion to reduce the risk of thrombus formation at the site.

✳ Go to *nursing.pearsonhighered.com* to see nursing care of the client having a PCR.

In contrast to stent procedures, which enlarge the artery by displacing plaque, atherectomy procedures remove plaque from the identified lesion. The directional atherectomy catheter shaves the plaque off vessel walls using a rotary cutting head, retaining the fragments in its housing and removing them from the vessel. Rotational atherectomy catheters pulverize plaque into particles small enough to pass through the coronary microcirculation. Laser atherectomy devices use laser energy to remove plaque.

Complications following PCR procedures include hematoma at the catheter insertion site, pseudoaneurysm, embolism, hypersensitivity to contrast dye, dysrhythmias, bleeding, vessel perforation, and restenosis or reocclusion of the treated vessel.

Coronary Artery Bypass Grafting Surgery for CAD involves using a section of a vein or an artery to create a connection, or bypass, between the aorta and the coronary artery beyond the obstruction (**Figure 16–35** ●). This allows blood to perfuse the ischemic portion of the heart. The internal mammary artery (IMA) in the chest and the saphenous vein from the leg are the vessels most commonly used for CABG.

Bypass grafts are safe and effective. Angina is totally relieved or significantly reduced in 90% of clients who undergo complete revascularization. While anginal pain may recur after surgery, CABG surgery improves or completely relieves angina symptoms in most clients, CABG is a viable option for blockages that cannot be treated with angioplasty. Many people remain symptom free for as long as 10–15 years.

A median sternotomy commonly is used to access the heart. The heart is usually stopped during surgery. A cardiopulmonary bypass (CPB) pump is used to maintain perfusion to the rest of the organs during open heart surgery. Venous blood is removed from the body through a cannula placed in the right atrium or the superior and inferior venae cavae. Blood then circulates through the CPB pump, where it is oxygenated, has its temperature regulated, and is filtered. Oxygenated blood is returned to the body through a cannula in the ascending aorta (**Figure 16–36** ●). CPB enables surgeons to operate on a quiet heart and a relatively bloodless field. Hypothermia can be maintained to reduce the metabolic rate and decrease oxygen demand during surgery.

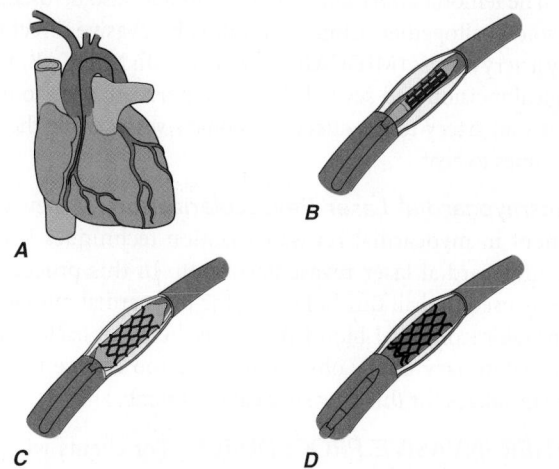

Figure 16–34 ● Percutaneous coronary revascularization. *A,* The balloon catheter with the stent is threaded into the affected coronary artery. *B, C,* The stent is positioned across the blockage and expanded. The balloon is deflated and removed, leaving the stent in place.

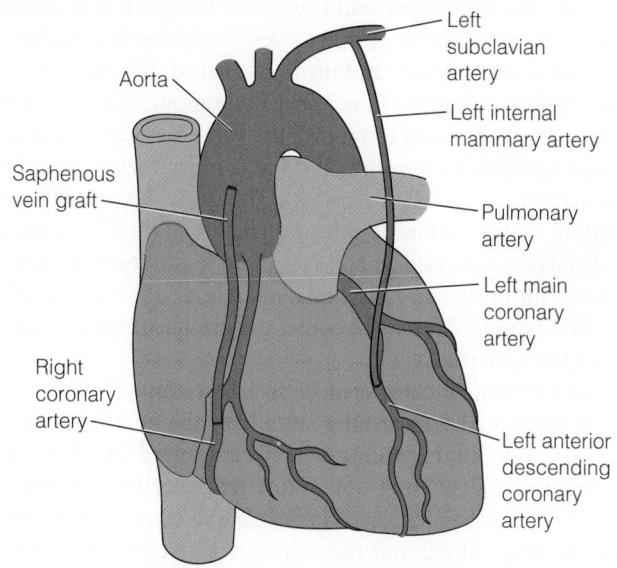

Figure 16–35 ● Coronary artery bypass grafting using the internal mammary artery and a saphenous vein graft.

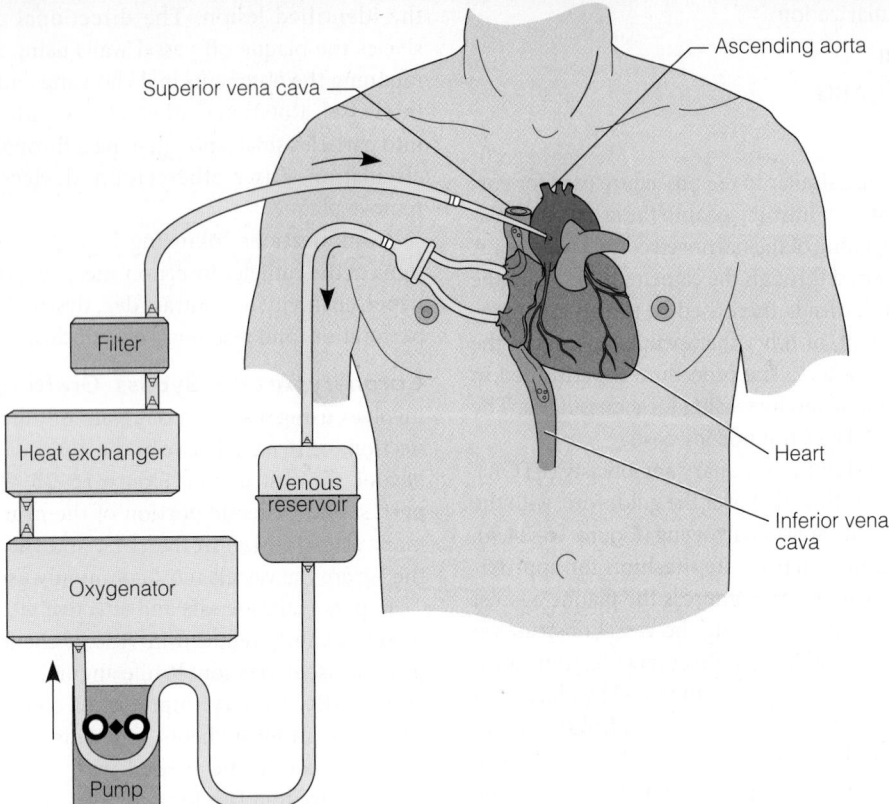

Figure 16–36 ● A diagrammatic representation of cardiopulmonary bypass. A cannula in the superior and inferior venae cavae removes venous blood, which is then pumped through an oxygenator and heat exchanger. After filtering, oxygenated blood is returned to the ascending aorta.

Newer techniques have been developed that allow surgeons to perform CABG without cardioplegia (stopping the heart) and CPB. Off-pump coronary artery bypass (OPCAB) allows use of a smaller incision for access. Although CPB is employed for the majority of coronary artery bypass procedures, OPCAB is a promising alternative. Lower mortality and morbidity rates as well as faster recovery rates have been demonstrated for clients undergoing OPCAB as compared to CABG.

When the saphenous vein is used for the graft, it is excised from its normal attachments in the leg, flushed with a cold heparinized saline solution, and then reversed so that its valves do not interfere with blood flow. When appropriate, a laparoscopic approach may be used to remove the vein. The vein is anastomosed (grafted) to the aorta and the coronary artery, distal to the occlusion (see Figure 16–35). This provides a bridge, or conduit, for blood flow past the obstruction. If the IMA is used, its distal end is excised and anastomosed to the coronary artery distal to the obstruction. The IMA often is used to revascularize the left coronary artery because of the greater oxygen demand of the left ventricle.

Once grafting is completed, CPB is discontinued and the client is rewarmed. Rewarming stimulates the heart to resume beating. Temporary pacing wires are sutured in place and passed through the chest wall in case temporary pacing is necessary. Chest tubes are placed in the pleural space and mediastinum to drain blood and reestablish negative pressure in the thoracic cavity. The sternum is closed using heavy wires and bone wax. The skin is closed with sutures or staples, and sterile dressings are applied over sternal and leg incisions.

✳ Go to *nursing.pearsonhighered.com* to see nursing care of the client having a CABG.

Minimally Invasive Coronary Artery Surgery   Minimally invasive coronary artery surgery is a potential future alternative to CABG. Two approaches may be used: Port-access coronary artery bypass uses several small holes, or "ports," in the chest wall to access vessels for connection to the CPB pump and the surgical site. The femoral artery and femoral vein may also be used. CPB is avoided altogether using the minimally invasive direct coronary artery bypass (MIDCAB) approach. With MIDCAB, a small surgical incision and several chest wall ports are used to graft a chest wall artery to the affected coronary vessel while the heart continues to beat.

Transmyocardial Laser Revascularization   A new development in myocardial revascularization techniques is called transmyocardial laser revascularization. In this procedure, a laser is used to drill tiny holes into the myocardial muscle itself to provide collateral blood flow to ischemic muscle. Clients whose coronary artery obstructions are too diffuse to bypass are candidates for this new surgical treatment.

OTHER INVASIVE PROCEDURES   For clients with large MIs and evidence of pump failure, invasive devices may be used to temporarily take over the function of the heart, allowing the injured myocardium to heal. The intra-aortic balloon pump is widely used to augment cardiac output. Ventricular assist devices are indicated for clients requiring more or longer-term artificial support than the intra-aortic balloon pump provides.

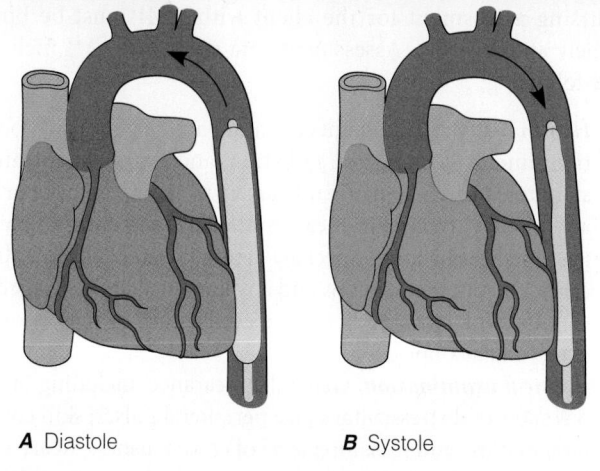

A Diastole   **B** Systole

Figure 16–37 ● The intra-aortic balloon pump. *A,* When inflated during diastole, the balloon supports cerebral, renal, and coronary artery perfusion. *B,* The balloon deflates during systole, so cardiac output is unimpeded.

Intra-Aortic Balloon Pump   The intra-aortic balloon pump (IABP), also called intra-aortic balloon counterpulsation, is a mechanical circulatory support device that may be used after cardiac surgery or to treat cardiogenic shock following AMI. The IABP temporarily supports cardiac function, allowing the heart to recover gradually by decreasing myocardial workload and oxygen demand and increasing perfusion of the coronary arteries.

A catheter with a 30- to 40-mL balloon is introduced into the aorta, usually via the femoral artery. The balloon catheter is connected to a console that regulates the inflation and deflation of the balloon. The IABP catheter inflates during diastole, increasing perfusion of the coronary and renal arteries, and deflates just before systole, decreasing afterload and cardiac workload (**Figure 16–37** ●). The inflation–deflation sequence is triggered by the ECG pattern. During the most acute period, the balloon inflates and deflates with each heartbeat (1:1 ratio), providing maximal assistance to the heart. As the client's condition improves, the IABP is weaned to inflate–deflate at varying intervals (e.g., 1:2, 1:4, and 1:8). This provides a continually decreasing amount of support as the heart muscle recovers. When mechanical assistance is no longer required, the IABP catheter is removed.

Ventricular Assist Devices   Use of ventricular assist devices (VADs) to aid the failing heart is becoming more common as technology advances. Whereas the IABP can supplement cardiac output by approximately 10%–15%, the VAD temporarily takes partial or complete control of cardiac function, depending on the type of device used. VADs may be used as temporarily or completely in AMI and cardiogenic shock when there is a chance for recovery of normal heart function after a period of cardiac rest. The device also may be used as a bridge to heart transplant. Nursing care for the client with a VAD is supportive and includes assessing hemodynamic status and for complications associated with the device. Clients with a VAD are at considerable risk for infection; strict aseptic technique is used with all invasive catheters and dressing changes. Pneumonia also is a risk because of immobility and ventilatory support. Mechanical failure of the VAD is life threatening and requires immediate medical attention.

Cardiac Rehabilitation

Cardiac rehabilitation is a medically supervised program designed to aid people with their recovery from heart attacks, heart surgeries, and percutaneous coronary interventions. Cardiac rehabilitation begins with admission for a cardiac event such as an AMI or a revascularization procedure. Phase 1 of the program is the inpatient phase. A thorough assessment of the client's history, current status, risk factors, and motivation is obtained. During this phase, activity progresses from bed rest to independent performance of ADLs and ambulation within the facility. Both subjective and objective responses to increasing activity levels are evaluated. Excess fatigue, shortness of breath, chest pain, tachypnea, tachycardia, or cool, clammy skin indicates activity intolerance. Phase 2, immediate outpatient cardiac rehabilitation, begins within 3 weeks of the cardiac event. The goals for the outpatient program are to increase activity level, participation, and capacity; improve psychosocial status and treat anxiety or depression; and provide education and support for risk factor reduction. Phase 3, a continuation program, is directed at providing a transition to independent exercise and exercise maintenance. During the final phase, the time between visits may be increased as the client is provided with opportunities to implement modifications discussed in the rehabilitation program.

Complementary and Alternative Therapy

Diet and exercise programs that emphasize physical conditioning and a low-fat diet rich in antioxidants have been shown to be effective in managing CAD. Supplements of vitamins C, E, B_6, and B_{12}, as well as folic acid, may be beneficial. Other potentially helpful complementary therapies include red wine or grape juice, foods containing bioflavonoids, green tea, nuts, and herbals and garlic (effective only for hypertension). The nurse should emphasize the need for clients to talk to their healthcare providers before taking any herbal preparations, because interactions with prescribed drugs are common. Behavioral therapies of benefit for clients with CAD include relaxation and stress management, guided imagery, treatment of depression, anger/hostility management, meditation, tai chi, and yoga.

Complementary and Alternative Therapy
Diet for CHD

Two diet programs have been shown to have a beneficial effect on CHD: the Pritikin diet and the Ornish diet.

The Pritikin diet is basically vegetarian, high in complex carbohydrates and fiber, low in cholesterol, and extremely low in fat (<10% of daily calories). Egg whites and limited amounts of nonfat dairy or soy products are allowed. The Pritikin program requires 45 minutes of walking daily and recommends multivitamin supplements, including vitamins C and E and folate.

The Ornish diet also is vegetarian, although egg whites and a cup of nonfat milk or yogurt per day are allowed. No oil or fat is permitted, even for cooking. Two ounces of alcohol a day are permitted. The Ornish program also calls for stress reduction, emotional–social support systems, daily stretching, and walking for 1 hour three times a week.

■ NURSING PROCESS

The focus of nursing care for clients with angina is similar to the interdisciplinary care focus—that is, to reduce myocardial oxygen demand and improve the oxygen supply. Angina usually is treated in community settings; the primary nursing focus is education.

Nursing care of the client with an AMI focuses on reducing cardiac work, identifying and treating complications in a timely manner, and preparing the client for rehabilitation.

Nurses are instrumental in educating adults about their risk for CAD, promoting participation in screening programs to identify that risk, and teaching all clients measures to reduce their risk for CAD. Present information about healthy lifestyle habits to community and religious groups, schoolchildren (grades K–12), and through the print media. In promoting healthy lifestyle habits, nurses can positively affect the incidence, morbidity, and mortality from CAD.

The nurse should strongly encourage all clients to avoid smoking in the first place and to stop all forms of tobacco use. Discuss the adverse effects of smoking and the benefits of quitting. Provide information about dietary recommendations to maintain a healthy weight and optimal cholesterol levels. Discuss the benefits and importance of regular exercise. Finally, encourage clients with cardiovascular risk factors to undergo regular screening for hypertension, diabetes, and abnormal blood lipids.

In addition to health promotion measures identified for CAD, emphasize the importance of actively managing CAD risk factors to slow progression of the disease. As mentioned, encourage clients to stop smoking. Discuss the use of cholesterol-lowering drug therapy with clients who have hypercholesterolemia. Encourage regular aerobic exercise and a diet based on AHA or NCEP guidelines.

Assessment

Nursing assessment for CAD focuses on identifying risk factors. Obtain the following data when assessing the client:

- *Health history.* Current manifestations, such as chest pain or heaviness, shortness of breath, and weakness; current diet, exercise patterns, and medications; smoking history and pattern of alcohol intake; history of heart disease, hypertension, or diabetes; and family history of CAD or other cardiac problems
- *Physical examination.* Current weight and its appropriateness for height; body mass index; waist-to-hip ratio; blood pressure; and strength and equality of peripheral pulses.

Focused assessment data for the client with angina include the following:

- *Health history.* Chest pain, including type, intensity, duration, frequency, aggravating factors, and relief measures; associated symptoms; history of other cardiovascular disorders, peripheral vascular disease, or stroke; current medications and treatment; usual diet, exercise, and alcohol intake patterns; smoking history; and use of other recreational drugs
- *Physical assessment.* Vital signs and heart sounds; strength and equality of peripheral pulses; skin color and temperature (central and peripheral); and physical appearance during pain episode (e.g., shortness of breath, apparent anxiety, color, and diaphoresis).

Nursing assessment for the client with AMI must be both timely and ongoing. Assessment data related to AMI include the following:

- *Health history.* Complaints of chest pain, including its location, intensity, character, radiation, and timing; associated symptoms, such as nausea, heartburn, shortness of breath, and anxiety; treatment measures taken since onset of pain; past medical history, especially cardiac related; chronic diseases; current medications and any known allergies to medications; and smoking history as well as use of recreational drugs and alcohol
- *Physical examination.* General appearance, including obvious signs of distress; vital signs; peripheral pulses; skin color, temperature, and moisture; level of consciousness; heart and breath sounds; cardiac rhythm (on bedside monitor); and bowel sounds and abdominal tenderness.

Diagnosis

Nursing diagnoses that may apply to the client with CAD include the following:

- *Obesity*
- *Ineffective Health Maintenance.*

(NANDA-I © 2015)

Nursing diagnoses appropriate for a client with angina include the following:

- *Tissue Perfusion: Cardiac, Risk for Decreased*
- *Self-Health Management, Ineffective.*

(NANDA-I © 2015)

Specific nursing diagnoses for a client with AMI include the following:

- *Pain, Acute*
- *Tissue Perfusion: Peripheral, Ineffective*
- *Coping, Ineffective*
- *Fear.*

(NANDA-I © 2015)

Planning

Planning care for the client at risk for CAD may include the following goals:

- The client will verbalize modifiable risk factors.
- The client will describe dietary changes to reduce the risk for CAD.
- The client will alter lifestyle to include increasing activity, quitting smoking, or changing diet.

Planning care for the client with symptomatic CAD may include the following goals:

- The client will describe lifestyle choices that may worsen CAD.
- The client will prevent cardiac muscle damage by adhering with the treatment regimen.
- The client will control blood pressure through the proper administration of medications, making dietary changes, and exercising as tolerated.

Planning care for the client with ineffective tissue perfusion may include the following:

- The client will understand how to take medications and what symptoms to report to the healthcare provider.
- The client will reduce activity as needed to maintain optimal tissue perfusion.
- The client will describe emergency actions to take when experiencing chest pain.

Implementation

The focus of nursing care is on improving cardiac output, reducing cardiac workload, maximizing function, and teaching the client how to care for self at home while reducing the risk of further cardiac damage. It is important to treat the client holistically, dealing with the client's psychosocial, spiritual, and cultural needs as well as the client's physical needs. Learning of a diagnosis that affects the heart is very frightening to clients, and they often require assistance in coping with fear and anxiety.

Promote Balanced Nutrition

This nursing diagnosis may be appropriate for clients who are obese, who have a waist-to-hip ratio of greater than 0.8 (female) or 0.9 (male), or whose diet history or serum cholesterol levels indicate a need to reduce fat and cholesterol intake. The nurse should do the following:

- Encourage assessment of food intake and eating patterns to help identify areas that can be improved. Clients often are unaware of their fat and cholesterol intake, particularly when they eat many meals away from home. Careful assessment increases awareness and allows the client to make conscious changes.
- Discuss AHA and therapeutic lifestyle change dietary recommendations, emphasizing the role of diet in heart disease. Provide guidance regarding specific food choices, with healthy alternatives. Specific diet information and suggestions help the client make better food choices.
- Refer the client to a clinical dietitian for diet planning and further teaching. Suggest cookbooks that offer low-fat recipes to encourage healthier eating, and provide AHA and American Cancer Society recipe pamphlets and information on low-fat eating. These resources provide tools for the client to use as eating patterns change.
- Encourage gradual but progressive dietary changes. Drastic changes in eating patterns may cause frustration and discourage the client from maintaining a healthy diet over the long term.
- Discourage the use of high-fat, low-carbohydrate, or other fad diets for weight loss. These diets may adversely affect serum cholesterol and triglyceride levels, and they often are too drastic to maintain over the long term.
- Encourage reasonable goals for weight loss (e.g., 1.0–1.5 lb per week and a 10% weight loss over 6 months). Provide information about weight loss programs and support groups, such as Weight Watchers and Take Off Pounds Sensibly (TOPS). Gradual but steady weight loss is more likely to be sustained. Recognized programs that emphasize healthy eating provide support and incentive for making lifetime dietary changes.

Promote Effective Health Maintenance

Clients with risk factors for CAD may be unable to identify or independently manage their risk factors. The nurse should do the following:

- Discuss risk factors for CAD, stressing how changing or managing those factors that can be modified reduces the client's overall risk for the disease. Clients with significant non-modifiable risk factors may be discouraged, reducing their ability to eliminate or control modifiable risk factors.
- Discuss the immediate benefits of smoking cessation. Provide resource materials from the AHA, the American Lung Association, and the American Cancer Society. Refer to a structured smoking cessation program to increase the likelihood of success in quitting. Long-time smokers may assume that the damage from smoking has already been done and that quitting would not be "worth the price."
- Help the client identify specific sources of psychosocial and physical support for smoking cessation, dietary, and lifestyle changes. Supportive individuals, support groups, and aids such as nicotine patches help the client achieve success and provide encouragement during difficult times (e.g., during withdrawal symptoms).
- Discuss the benefits of regular exercise for cardiovascular health and weight loss. Help the client to identify favorite forms of exercise or physical activity. Encourage planning for 30 minutes of continuous aerobic activity (e.g., walking, running, bicycling, or swimming) four to five times a week. Encourage identification of an "exercise buddy" to help maintain motivation. Engaging in preferred activities with a partner maintains motivation and increases the likelihood of maintaining an exercise program. Encourage continuation of the plan, even when days are missed. Exercise is cumulative, so increasing the duration of exercise on subsequent days can "make up" for a lost day.
- Provide information and teaching about prescribed medications, such as cholesterol-lowering drugs. Discuss the relationship between hypertension, diabetes, and CAD. Teaching is important to promote understanding of and adherence with the prescribed drug regimen.

Manage Acute Pain

Chest pain occurs when the oxygen supply to the heart muscle does not meet the demand. Myocardial ischemia and infarction cause pain, as does reperfusion of an ischemic area following fibrinolytic therapy or emergent percutaneous transluminal coronary angioplasty. Pain stimulates the sympathetic nervous system, increasing cardiac work. Pain relief is a priority of care for the client with AMI. Appropriate nursing interventions include the following:

- Assess the client for verbal and nonverbal signs of pain. Document the characteristics and intensity of the pain, using a standard pain scale. Verify nonverbal indicators of pain with the client. Frequent, careful pain assessment allows early intervention to reduce the risk of further damage. Pain is a subjective experience; its expression may vary with location and intensity, previous experiences, and cultural and social background. Pain scales provide an objective tool for measuring pain and a way to assess pain relief or reduction.

- Administer oxygen at 2–5 L/min via nasal cannula. Supplemental oxygen increases oxygen supply to the myocardium, decreasing ischemia and pain.
- Promote physical and psychological rest. Provide information and emotional support. Rest decreases cardiac workload and sympathetic nervous system stimulation, promoting comfort. Information and emotional support help decrease anxiety and provide psychological rest.
- Titrate intravenous nitroglycerin as ordered to relieve chest pain, maintaining a systolic blood pressure of greater than 100 mmHg. Nitroglycerin decreases chest pain by dilating peripheral vessels, reducing cardiac work, and dilating coronary vessels, including collateral channels, thus improving blood flow to ischemic tissue.
- Administer 2–4 mg of morphine by intravenous push for chest pain as needed. Morphine is an effective narcotic analgesic for chest pain. It decreases pain and anxiety, acts as a venodilator, and decreases the respiratory rate. The resulting reduction in preload and sympathetic nervous system stimulation reduces cardiac work and oxygen consumption.

Monitor Tissue Perfusion

Cardiac muscle damage affects compliance, contractility, and cardiac output. The extent of the effect on tissue perfusion depends on the location and amount of damage. Anterior wall infarcts have a greater effect on cardiac output than do right ventricular infarcts. Infarcted muscle also increases the risk for cardiac dysrhythmias, which can also affect the delivery of blood and oxygen to the tissues. The nurse should do the following:

- Assess and document vital signs. Report increases in heart rate and changes in rhythm, blood pressure, and respiratory rate. Decreased cardiac output activates compensatory mechanisms that may cause tachycardia and vasoconstriction, increasing cardiac work.
- Assess the client for changes in level of consciousness; decreased urine output; moist, cool, pale, mottled, or cyanotic skin; dusky or cyanotic mucous membranes and nail beds; diminished to absent peripheral pulses; and delayed capillary refill. These are manifestations of impaired tissue perfusion. A change in level of consciousness is often the first manifestation of altered perfusion, because brain tissue and cerebral function depend on a continuous supply of oxygen.
- Auscultate heart and breath sounds. Note abnormal heart sounds (e.g., an S_3 or S_4 gallop or a murmur) or adventitious lung sounds. Abnormal heart sounds or adventitious lung sounds may indicate impaired cardiac filling or output, increasing the risk for decreased tissue perfusion.
- Monitor the client's ECG rhythm continuously. Dysrhythmias can further impair cardiac output and tissue perfusion.
- Monitor the client's oxygen saturation levels. Administer oxygen as ordered. Obtain and assess arterial blood gas (ABG) levels as indicated. Oxygen saturation is an indicator of gas exchange, tissue perfusion, and the effectiveness of oxygen administration. ABG levels provide a more precise measurement of blood oxygen levels and allow assessment of acid–base balance.

- Administer antidysrhythmic medications as needed. Dysrhythmias affect tissue perfusion by altering cardiac output.
- Obtain serial CK, isoenzyme, and troponin levels as ordered. Levels of cardiac markers, CK isoenzymes in particular, correlate with the extent of myocardial damage.
- Plan for invasive hemodynamic monitoring. Hemodynamic monitoring facilitates AMI management and treatment evaluation by providing a means of assessing pressures in the systemic and pulmonary arteries, the relationship between oxygen supply and demand, cardiac output, and cardiac index.

Promote Effective Coping

Coping mechanisms help an individual deal with a life-threatening event or with acute changes in health. However, certain coping mechanisms may be detrimental to restoring health, particularly if the client relies on them for a prolonged period. Denial, for example, is a common coping mechanism among clients after an MI. During the initial stages, denial can reduce anxiety. Continued denial, however, can interfere with both learning and treatment adherence. Appropriate interventions include the following:

- Establish an environment of caring and trust. Encourage the client to express feelings. A trusting nurse–client relationship provides a safe environment for the client to discuss feelings of helplessness, powerlessness, anxiety, and hopelessness. The nurse may then be able to provide additional resources to meet the client's needs.
- Accept denial as a coping mechanism, but do not reinforce it. Denial may initially help by diminishing the psychological threat to health, decreasing anxiety. However, its prolonged use can interfere with acceptance of reality and cooperation, possibly delaying treatment and hindering recovery.
- Note aggressive behaviors, hostility, or anger. Document any failure to comply with treatments. These signs may indicate anxiety and denial.
- Help the client identify positive coping skills used in the past (e.g., problem-solving skills, verbalization of feelings, asking for help, or prayer). Reinforce use of positive coping behaviors. Coping behaviors that have been successful in the past can help the client deal with the current situation. These familiar methods can decrease feelings of powerlessness.
- Provide opportunities, as possible, for the client to make decisions about the plan of care. This promotes self-confidence and independence. Participating in care planning gives the client a sense of control and the opportunity to use positive coping skills.
- Provide privacy for the client and family members to share their questions and concerns. Privacy provides an opportunity for the client and family members to share their feelings and fears, offer support and encouragement to one another, relieve anxiety, and establish effective coping methods.

Manage Fear

The fear of death and disability can be a paralyzing emotion that adversely affects the client's recovery from AMI. The nurse should do the following:

- Identify the client's level of fear, noting verbal and nonverbal signs. This information enables the nurse to plan appropriate interventions. Clients may not voice concerns; attention to nonverbal indicators is important. Controlling fear helps decrease sympathetic nervous system responses and catecholamine release that may increase feelings of fear and anxiety.

- Acknowledge the client's perception of the situation. Allow the client to verbalize concerns. A sudden change in health status causes anxiety and fear of the unknown. Verbalizing these fears may help the client cope with change and allow the healthcare team to provide information and correct misconceptions.
- Encourage questions, and provide consistent, factual answers. Repeat information as needed. Accurate and consistent information can reduce fear. Honest explanations help strengthen the client–nurse relationship and help the client develop realistic expectations. Anxiety and fear decrease the ability to concentrate and retain information; therefore, information may need to be repeated.
- Encourage self-care. Allow the client to make decisions regarding the plan of care. This promotes personal responsibility for health and allows some control over the situation. Clients' confidence increases as their dependence decreases.
- Administer antianxiety medications as ordered. These medications promote rest and relaxation and decrease feelings of anxiety, which may act as barriers to health restoration.
- Teach nonpharmacologic methods of stress reduction (e.g., relaxation techniques, mental imagery, music therapy, breathing exercises, meditation, and massage). Stress management techniques can help reduce tension and anxiety, provide a sense of control, and enhance coping skills.

Promote Effective Cardiac Perfusion

The pain of angina results from impaired blood flow and oxygen supply to the myocardium. Nursing interventions that may prevent ischemia and shorten the duration of pain include the following:

- Instruct the client to keep prescribed nitroglycerin tablets always on hand so one can be taken at the onset of pain. Anginal pain indicates myocardial ischemia. Nitroglycerin reduces cardiac work and may improve myocardial blood flow, relieving ischemia and pain.
- Start oxygen at 4–6 L/min via nasal cannula or as prescribed. Supplemental oxygen reduces myocardial hypoxia.
- Space activities to allow rest between them. Activity increases cardiac work and may precipitate angina. Spacing of activities allows the heart to recover.
- Teach the client about prescribed medications to maintain myocardial perfusion and reduce cardiac work. Emphasize that long-acting nitrates, beta-blockers, and calcium-channel blockers are used to *prevent* anginal attacks, not to *treat* an acute attack. It is important for the client to understand the purpose and use of prescribed drugs to maintain optimal myocardial perfusion.
- Instruct the client to take sublingual nitroglycerin before engaging in activities that precipitate angina (e.g., climbing stairs or sexual intercourse). This prophylactic dose of nitroglycerin helps maintain cardiac perfusion when increased work is anticipated, preventing ischemia and chest pain.
- Encourage the client to implement and maintain a progressive exercise program under the supervision of the primary

care provider or a cardiac rehabilitation professional. Exercise slows the atherosclerotic process and helps develop collateral circulation to the heart muscle.
- Refer the client to a smoking cessation program as indicated. Nicotine causes vasoconstriction and increases the heart rate, decreasing myocardial perfusion and increasing cardiac workload.

Promote Effective Therapeutic Regimen Management

Denial may be strong in clients with angina pectoris. Because many people think of the heart as the locus of life itself, problems such as angina remind people of their mortality, an uncomfortable fact. Denial may lead to "forgetting" to take prescribed medications or attempting activities that will precipitate angina. Some clients, by contrast, are afraid to engage in any activities because of the fear of chest pain. Their inactivity may actually hasten the atherosclerotic process and inhibit collateral circulation development, worsening angina.

- Assess the client's knowledge and understanding of angina. Assessment allows tailoring of teaching and interventions to the needs of the client.
- Teach about angina and atherosclerosis as needed, building on the client's current knowledge base. This can help the client understand that angina is a manageable disease and that pain can usually be controlled and progression of the disease slowed.
- Provide written and verbal instructions about prescribed medications and their use. Written instructions reinforce teaching and are available to the client for future reference.
- Stress the importance of taking chest pains seriously while maintaining a positive attitude. Although it is vital for the client to recognize the significance of chest pain and deal with it appropriately, it is also important to maintain a positive outlook.
- Refer the client to a cardiac rehabilitation program or other organized activities and support groups for clients with CAD. Programs such as these help the client develop risk factor management strategies, maintain a program of supervised activity, and gain coping skills. See the Client Teaching feature for more information.

Evaluation

Client care is evaluated on the basis of the client's progress toward goals and may be based on the following expected outcomes:

- The client demonstrates adequate circulation as evidenced by PaO_2 and $PaCO_2$ within normal limits.
- The client maintains systolic blood pressure, pulse pressure, mean blood pressure, central venous pressure, and/or pulmonary wedge pressures within the normal range.
- The client reduces anginal events and demonstrates proper actions when angina begins.
- The client shows an absence of complications resulting from CAD.

Client Teaching   Cardiac Rehabilitation

Cardiac rehabilitation begins with admission to the healthcare facility and continues through the inpatient stay and after discharge into the rehabilitative period. The emphasis is on realistic application of information to maintain lifestyle changes.

Assessing the client's readiness to learn is an important first step in preparing for home care. The client in strong denial may not identify any relevance to the information being taught. Evaluate the client's ability to learn, assessing physiological and psychological health, beliefs regarding personal responsibility for health, and expectations of the healthcare system. Also assess the client's developmental level, ability to perform psychomotor skills, cognitive function, learning disabilities, existing knowledge base, and the influence of previous learning experiences. Provide written material to supplement teaching and encourage questions.

Include the following topics in teaching for home care:

- The normal anatomy and physiology of the heart, and the specific area of heart damage

- The process of CAD and implications of MI
- Purposes and side effects of prescribed medications
- The importance of adhering with the medical regimen and cardiac rehabilitation program and of keeping follow-up appointments
- Information about community resources, such as the local chapter of the AHA.

After discharge, follow up by telephone within 1 week and periodically thereafter during the recovery period. Provide telephone numbers of resource personnel who are available to respond to questions and concerns after discharge. Motivational and social support may be helpful to clients in adopting healthier behaviors after AMI.

Because the client who has had an MI is at high risk for sudden cardiac death, encourage family members to learn CPR and provide information about community resources for CPR training.

NURSING CARE PLAN   A Client With Acute Myocardial Infarction

Betty Williams, a 62-year-old psychologist, is admitted to the emergency department with complaints of severe substernal chest pain. Mrs. Williams states that the pain began after lunch, about 4 hours ago. She initially attributed the pain to indigestion. She described the pain, which now radiates to her jaw and left arm, as "really severe heartburn." It is accompanied by a "choking feeling," severe shortness of breath, and diaphoresis. The pain is unrelieved by rest, antacids, or three sublingual nitroglycerin tablets (0.4 mg).

Oxygen is started via nasal cannula at 5 L/min. Central and peripheral intravenous lines are inserted. A 12-lead electrocardiogram (ECG) and the following lab work are obtained: cardiac troponins, CK and CK isoenzymes, ABG levels, complete blood count, and a chemistry panel. Morphine sulfate relieves Mrs. Williams's pain.

Mrs. Williams's medical history includes type 2 diabetes, angina, and hypertension. She has a 45-year history of cigarette smoking, averaging 1.5–2 packs per day. Family history reveals that Mrs. Williams's father died at age 42 of AMI, and her paternal grandfather died at age 65 of AMI. Mrs. Williams is taking the following medications: tolbutamide (Orinase), hydrochlorothiazide, and isosorbide (Isordil).

Based on ECG changes and cardiac markers, an acute anterior MI is diagnosed. Mrs. Williams has no contraindications to fibrinolytic therapy and is deemed a good candidate. Intravenous alteplase (Activase) is given by bolus, followed by intravenous infusions of alteplase and heparin. She is transferred to the coronary care unit.

ASSESSMENT

Dan Morales, RN, is Mrs. Williams's primary care nurse. Mrs. Williams is alert and oriented to person, place, and time. Vital signs are as follows: temperature 99.6°F (37.5°C); pulse 118 bpm; respirations 24/min with adequate depth; blood pressure 172/92 mmHg. Auscultation reveals a fourth heart sound (S_4) and fine crackles in the bases of both lungs. The ECG shows sinus tachycardia with occasional premature ventricular contractions (PVCs). Her skin is cool and slightly diaphoretic. Capillary refill is less than 3 seconds, and peripheral pulses are strong and equal. Her nail beds are pink.

A triple-lumen central line is in place. Nitroglycerin is infusing at 200 mcg/min in the distal lumen. The alteplase infusion is in the middle lumen, and a heparin infusion is in the proximal lumen. The peripheral intravenous line has a saline lock. Mrs. Williams states, "The pain is better since the nurse in the ER gave me a shot. But it has been coming and going. I would rate it a four right now, but it was terrible before. The physician told me that this drug I'm getting will quickly open up the artery that is blocked. I hope it works! Do many people get this drug?"

DIAGNOSES

- *Pain, Acute* related to ischemic myocardial tissue
- *Anxiety* and *Fear* related to change in health status
- *Protection, Ineffective* related to the risk of bleeding secondary to fibrinolytic therapy
- *Cardiac Output, Decreased, Risk for* related to altered cardiac rate and rhythm

(NANDA-I © 2015)

PLANNING

Goals of care include the following:

- The client will rate chest pain as 2 or lower on a pain scale of 0–10.
- The client will verbalize reduced anxiety and fear.
- The client will demonstrate no signs of internal or external bleeding.
- The client will maintain an adequate cardiac output during and following reperfusion therapy.

NURSING CARE PLAN (continued)

IMPLEMENTATION

- Instruct the client to report all chest pain. Monitor and evaluate pain using a scale of 0–10. Titrate intravenous nitroglycerin infusion for chest pain; stop infusion if systolic blood pressure is below 100 mmHg. Administer 2–4 mg of morphine intravenously for chest pain unrelieved by nitroglycerin infusion.

- Encourage the client to verbalize fears and concerns. Respond honestly, and correct misconceptions about the disease, therapeutic interventions, or prognosis.

- Assess the client's knowledge of CAD. Explain the purpose of fibrinolytic therapy to dissolve the fresh clot and reperfuse the heart muscle, limiting heart damage.

- Explain the need for frequent monitoring of vital signs and potential bleeding.

- Assess the client for manifestations of internal or intracranial bleeding: complaints of back or abdominal pain, headache, decreased level of consciousness, dizziness, bloody secretions or excretions, or pallor. Test all stools, urine, and vomitus for occult blood. Notify the healthcare provider immediately of any abnormal findings.

- Monitor the client for signs of reperfusion: decreased chest pain, return of ST segment to baseline, and reperfusion dysrhythmias (e.g., PVCs, bradycardia, and heart block).

- Continuously monitor the ECG for changes in cardiac rate, rhythm, and conduction. Assess vital signs.

- Treat dangerous dysrhythmias or other cardiac events per protocol. Notify the healthcare provider.

- Discuss continuing cardiac care and rehabilitation with the client.

EVALUATION

The initial morphine dose reduces Mrs. Williams's chest pain from a rating of 8 to 4. The nitroglycerin infusion and fibrinolytic therapy further reduce her pain to 2. The nitroglycerin infusion is gradually discontinued after 24 hours. As her pain subsides, Mrs. Williams states that she feels "much better now that the pain is gone. I was afraid it would just get worse." She verbalizes an understanding of fibrinolytic therapy to limit myocardial damage. No indication of bleeding problems are noted. Reperfusion is indicated by relief of chest pain, return of the ST segment to baseline on the ECG, early peaking of CK levels, and increased frequency of PVCs but no significant dysrhythmias. Mrs. Williams remains in coronary care unit for 36 hours and is then transferred to the floor.

CRITICAL THINKING

1. How would the initial plan of care have changed if Mrs. Williams were not a candidate for fibrinolytic therapy?
2. Two days after her initial therapy, Mrs. Williams complains of palpitations. You notice frequent PVCs on the ECG monitor. What do you do?
3. What health promotion topics would you teach Mrs. Williams before discharge?
4. Mrs. Williams states, "I've been smoking for over 45 years, and I'm not going to stop now! Besides, it calms me down when I'm anxious." How would you respond to this statement?

◢ REVIEW **Coronary Artery Disease**

RELATE Link the Concepts and Exemplars

Linking the exemplar of coronary artery disease with the concept of health, wellness, and illness:

1. What nutritional recommendations will you teach the client with, or at risk for, CAD?

2. What will you teach the client about physical fitness and exercise in regards to reducing the risk of CAD?

Linking the exemplar of coronary artery disease with the concept of metabolism:

3. What role does obesity play with regard to risk for CAD? Explain the physiology of this impact.

4. What teaching would you provide a client with type 2 diabetes mellitus to reduce the risk of CAD?

READY Go to Companion Skills Manual

REFER Go to Pearson Nursing Student Resources
nursing.pearsonhighered.com

- Additional review materials
- Chart 1: Nursing Care of the Client Having Percutaneous Coronary Revascularization
- Chart 2: Nursing Care of the Client Having a Coronary Artery Bypass Graft

REFLECT Case Study

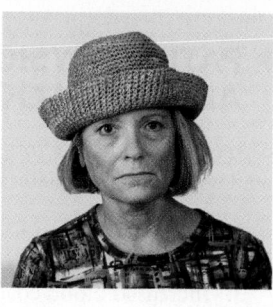

Norma James is a 65-year-old widow who lives alone. Although she has lived in the neighborhood for years, she is somewhat socially isolated. She has two adult sons with whom she has limited contact; they live out of the state and rarely call. She has only a few individuals whom she considers friends; she does not particularly like people and prefers the company of her six cats.

Mrs. James has a long history of type 2 diabetes mellitus and hypertension. In more recent years, she has been diagnosed with atrial fibrillation. She has multiple healthcare providers and takes multiple medications including:

- Glucotrol, 10 mg, twice a day
- Captopril, 50 mg, twice a day
- Digoxin, 125 mcg, once a day
- Coumadin, 5 mg, once a day.

Mrs. James has a known drug allergy to penicillin.

Mrs. James does not work outside the home and has very limited savings; she relies on Social Security benefits for income. She smokes about 1/2 pack of cigarettes a day and has been a smoker since she was in her 20s. She drinks alcohol "a couple times a year, usually a glass of wine at a special dinner."

She does not drive and relies on her friends, neighbors, or the city bus for transportation. She lives near a grocery store and prides herself on being able to get most things she needs without any assistance. She spends most of her time alone at home and occupies herself by watching television, reading, and doing crossword and jigsaw puzzles.

1. According to Mrs. James's history, what are her risks for developing coronary artery disease?
2. What lifestyle changes would you discuss with Mrs. James to reduce this risk?
3. Create a teaching plan to help Mrs. James understand the risks associated with her lifestyle behaviors that are increasing her risk of developing CAD.

EXEMPLAR 16.4 Deep Venous Thrombosis

EXEMPLAR KEY TERMS
Venous thrombectomy, 1134
Venous thrombosis, 1130
Virchow triad, 1130

EXEMPLAR LEARNING OUTCOMES
After reading about this exemplar, you will be able to:

1. Describe the pathophysiology, etiology, clinical manifestations, and direct and indirect causes of deep venous thrombosis.
2. Identify risk factors and prevention methods associated with deep venous thrombosis.

3. Illustrate the nursing process in providing culturally competent care across the life span for individuals with deep venous thrombosis.
4. Formulate priority nursing diagnoses appropriate for an individual with deep venous thrombosis.
5. Summarize therapies used by interdisciplinary teams in the collaborative care of an individual with deep venous thrombosis.
6. Plan evidence-based care for an individual with deep venous thrombosis and his or her family in collaboration with other members of the healthcare team.
7. Evaluate expected outcomes for an individual with deep venous thrombosis.

▶ OVERVIEW

Venous thrombosis (also known as thrombophlebitis) is a condition in which a blood clot (thrombus) forms on the wall of a vein and is accompanied by inflammation of the vein wall and some degree of obstructed venous blood flow. As the name implies, deep venous thrombosis (DVT) occurs when the thrombosis is located in a deep vein of the body. Prevention of venous thrombosis is an important nursing action in caring for the immobilized, postoperative, or postpartum client.

▶ PATHOPHYSIOLOGY AND ETIOLOGY

Three pathological factors, called the **Virchow triad**, are associated with thrombophlebitis:

1. Stasis of blood
2. Vessel damage
3. Increased blood coagulability.

Vessel trauma stimulates the clotting cascade. Platelets aggregate at the site, particularly when venous stasis is present. Platelets and fibrin form the initial clot. Red blood cells are trapped in the fibrin meshwork, and the thrombus propagates (grows) in the direction of blood flow. The inflammatory response is triggered, causing tenderness, swelling, and erythema in the area of the thrombus.

Initially, the thrombus floats within the vein. Pieces of the thrombus may break loose and travel through the circulation as emboli. Fibroblasts eventually invade the thrombus, scarring the vein wall and destroying venous valves. Permanent valve damage may occur even if valve patency is restored. The valve damage will most likely affect directional flow.

Deep venous thrombi occur in the body's deep veins, those leading to the vena cava. Locations of the deep veins include the pelvis, thigh, or calf. Although less common, DVT can occur in the arm, chest and other location. The deep veins of the legs, primarily in the calf, and of the pelvis provide the most hospitable environment for venous thrombosis (**Figure 16–38 ●**). Approximately one half of DVTs are asymptomatic. The symptoms that do present depend on the location and size of the blood clot.

Etiology

Thrombi can be either venous or arterial. Venous thrombi tend to occur at sites where the vein may be normal but blood flow is low. Arterial thrombi tend to occur at sites of arterial plaque rupture. DVT is a common complication of hospitalization, surgery, and immobilization. Other significant risk factors for venous thrombosis include abdominal or thoracic surgery, certain cancers, trauma, pregnancy, and use of oral contraceptives or hormone replacement therapy (Clinical Guidelines Committee of the American College of Physicians, 2011) (**Box 16–11 ●**).

Box 16–11 Factors Associated With Venous Thrombosis

- Immobilization: myocardial infarction, heart failure, stroke, postoperative
- Surgery: orthopedic, thoracic, abdominal, genitourinary
- Cancer: pancreatic, lung, ovary, testes, urinary tract, breast, stomach
- Trauma: fractures of the spine, pelvis, femur, tibia; spinal cord injury
- Pregnancy and delivery
- Hormone therapy: oral contraceptives, hormone replacement therapy
- Coagulation disorders

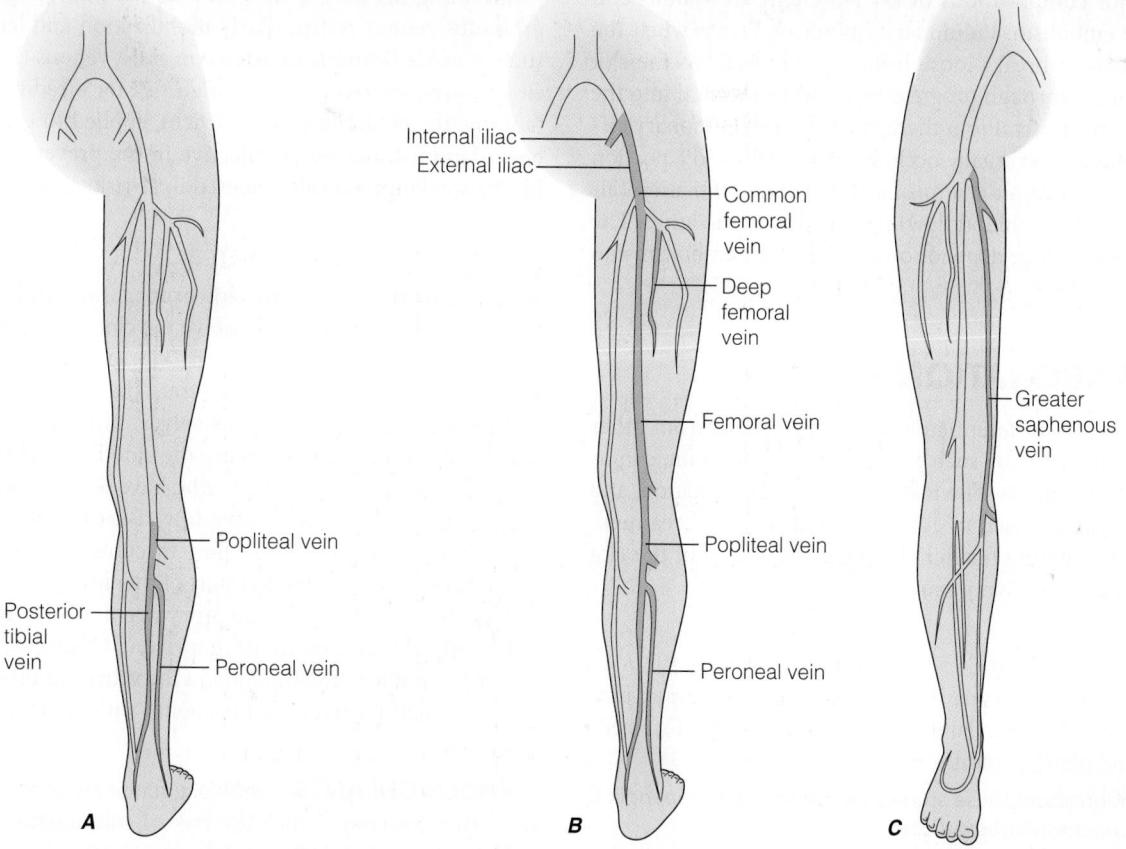

Figure 16–38 ● Common locations of venous thrombosis. *A*, The most common sites of DVT. *B*, DVT extending from the calf to the iliac veins. *C*, Superficial venous thrombosis.

Risk Factors

Individual preventive approaches minimize the risk factors that can predispose individuals to DVT. Specific conditions warranting prevention include the following:

- *Orthopedic procedures.* Examples include total hip replacement, traumatic hip fracture, and total knee replacement. For total hip replacement, the incidence of DVT without prophylaxis is 25%; for traumatic hip fracture, approximately 50%; and for total knee replacement, as high as 60%.
- *Atrial fibrillation.* Individuals with atrial fibrillation can form thrombi within the atria that can enter the general circulation and cause stroke. Transesophageal echocardiography identifies clients at risk for thromboembolism.
- *Acute myocardial infarction.* The risk of DVT in clients who have had an MI approaches 20%. Older clients with heart failure, recurrent angina, or ventricular arrhythmias are most at risk.
- *Ischemic stroke.* In clients with stroke and paralyzed lower extremities, the incidence of DVT is 40%.

Women in the childbearing years have a higher risk of DVT than men. Unique factors placing women at risk include use of birth control pills that contain estrogen and progestin. These oral contraceptives increase a woman's risk of blood clot by 2–8 times. Progestin-only contraceptives do not appear to place women at increased risk. Pregnancy increases

the blood volume and stresses the blood vessels due to hormonal changes. During pregnancy and the first few months during the postnatal period, the risk of DVT or pulmonary embolus is increased to 4 times higher than that of a nonpregnant female.

▶ CLINICAL MANIFESTATIONS

When present, the manifestations of DVT are primarily caused by the inflammatory process accompanying the thrombus. Calf pain, which may be described as tightness or a dull, aching pain in the affected extremity, particularly upon walking, is the most common symptom. Tenderness, swelling, warmth, and erythema may be noted along the course of involved veins. The affected extremity may be cyanotic and often is edematous. Rarely, a cord may be palpated over the affected vein. See **Box 16–12** ● for a summary of the manifestations of DVT.

Box 16–12   Manifestations of Deep Venous Thrombosis

- Usually asymptomatic
- Dull, aching pain in affected extremity, especially when walking
- Possible tenderness, warmth, erythema along affected vein
- Cyanosis of affected extremity
- Edema of affected extremity

The major complications of DVT are chronic venous and pulmonary embolism. Pulmonary embolism occurs when the clot fragments or breaks loose from the vein wall. As the clot travels, it moves through progressively larger veins and into the right side of the heart. From there, it enters the pulmonary circulation, where it eventually occludes arterial flow to a portion of the lungs. The result is a mismatch between ventilation (air flow) and perfusion (blood flow) in a portion of the lungs. The effect on gas exchange depends on the size of the embolism and the vessel it occludes.

▶ COLLABORATION

It is important to differentiate venous thrombosis from other causes of extremity pain, such as cellulitis, muscle strain, contusion, and lymphedema. The history, physical examination, and diagnostic tests are used to establish the diagnosis. Treatment focuses on preventing further clotting or extension of the clot and addressing underlying causes.

Diagnostic Tests

Laboratory studies that may be ordered include D-dimer, prothrombin time (PT), partial thromboplastin time (PTT), bleeding time, and platelet count.

✳ Information about these studies can be found in Appendix B at *nursing.pearsonhighered.com.*

Diagnostic tests for DVT include the following:

- *Duplex venous ultrasonography* is a noninvasive test used to visualize the vein and measure the velocity of blood flow in the veins. Although the clot often cannot be visualized directly, its presence can be inferred by an inability to compress the vein during the examination.

- *Plethysmography* is a noninvasive test that measures changes in blood flow through the veins. It is often used in conjunction with Doppler ultrasonography. Plethysmography is most valuable in diagnosing thromboses of larger or more superficial veins.

- *Magnetic resonance imaging (MRI)* is another noninvasive means of detecting DVT. It is particularly useful when thrombosis of the venae cavae or pelvic veins is suspected.

- *Ascending contrast venography* uses an injected contrast medium to assess the location and extent of venous thrombosis. Although invasive, expensive, and uncomfortable, contrast venography is the most accurate diagnostic tool for venous thrombosis. It is used when the results of less invasive tests leave the diagnosis unclear (Tierney, McPhee, & Papadakis, 2005).

Prophylaxis

Medications and other measures are used to prevent venous thrombosis when the risk is high. Low-molecular-weight heparins prevent DVT in clients who are undergoing general or orthopedic surgery, experiencing acute medical illness, or on prolonged bed rest. Oral anticoagulation also may be used as a prophylactic measure in clients with fractures or those who are undergoing orthopedic surgery.

Elevating the foot of the bed with the knees slightly flexed promotes venous return. Early mobilization and leg exercises such as ankle flexion and extension assist venous flow by muscle compression. For clients at high risk for bleeding, intermittent pneumatic compression devices, applied to the legs, have been demonstrated to be effective in the prevention of DVT. Elastic stockings may also be used in at-risk clients.

Pharmacologic Therapy

Anticoagulants to prevent clot propagation and enable the body's own lytic system to dissolve the clot are the mainstay of treatment for venous thrombosis. Fibrinolytic drugs such as streptokinase or t-PA may accelerate the process of clot lysis and prevent damage to venous valves. Thrombolytic therapy may be recommended to dissolve the blood clot. This therapy is most likely to be used in clients who have serious complications related to DVT and who have low risk of serious bleeding. Thrombolytic outcomes are best in cases with a short time frame between diagnosis and start of therapy.

Nonsteroidal anti-inflammatory agents (NSAIDs) such as indomethacin (Indocin) or naproxen (Naprosyn) may be ordered to reduce inflammation in the veins and provide symptomatic relief, particularly for clients with superficial venous thrombosis.

ANTICOAGULANTS Anticoagulants are given to prevent clot extension and reduce the risk of subsequent pulmonary embolism. See the Medications feature for the nursing implications for anticoagulant therapy.

Anticoagulation is initiated with unfractionated heparin or LMW heparin. Following an initial intravenous bolus of 7,500–10,000 units of unfractionated heparin, a continuous heparin infusion of 1,000 to 1,500 International Units per hour is started. The dosage is calculated to maintain the aPTT at approximately twice the control or normal value. An infusion pump is used to deliver the prescribed dosage. Frequent monitoring of the infusion is an important nursing responsibility. Subcutaneous heparin injections may be used as an alternative to intravenous infusion in some instances.

LMW heparins are increasingly used to prevent and treat venous thrombosis. They do not require the close laboratory monitoring of unfractionated heparins. LMW heparin is administered subcutaneously in fixed doses once or twice daily, allowing the option of outpatient treatment. LMW heparins have additional advantages, in that they are more effective and carry lower risks for bleeding and thrombocytopenia than conventional, unfractionated heparins.

Oral anticoagulation with warfarin may be initiated concurrently with heparin therapy. Overlapping heparin and warfarin therapy for 4–5 days is important because the full anticoagulant effect of warfarin is delayed, and warfarin may actually promote clotting during the first few days of therapy (Tierney et al., 2005). Warfarin doses are adjusted to maintain the INR at 2–3 (Kasper et al., 2005).

Once this level has been achieved, the heparin is discontinued and a maintenance dose of warfarin is prescribed to prevent recurrent thrombosis. Anticoagulation generally is continued for at least 3 months. When DVT recurs or risk factors such as altered coagulability or cancer are present, anticoagulant therapy

Medications **Anticoagulants**

CLASSIFICATION AND DRUG EXAMPLES	MECHANISMS OF ACTION	NURSING CONSIDERATIONS
Heparin	Heparin interferes with the clotting cascade by inhibiting the effects of thrombin and preventing the conversion of fibrinogen to fibrin. This prevents the formation of a stable fibrin clot. At therapeutic levels, heparin prolongs the thrombin time, clotting time, and activated partial thromboplastin time (aPTT). When given intravenously, its effect is immediate. Given subcutaneously, its onset of action is within 1 hr. Heparin has a short biological half-life and should be given frequently or via continuous infusion. *Heparin-induced thrombocytopenia (HIT)* is a potential complication of therapy with unfractionated heparin.	■ Assess for history of unexplained or active bleeding. Assess laboratory results for abnormal clotting profile or evidence of active bleeding. ■ Give a test dose as indicated to clients with a history of multiple allergies or a history of asthma. ■ Administer by deep subcutaneous injection; abdominal sites are preferred. Avoid injecting within 2 in. of the umbilicus. Rotate sites. Do not aspirate prior to injecting or massage after the injection. ■ Intravenous solutions may be diluted with dextrose, normal saline, or Ringer's solution. Use an infusion pump. ■ Keep protamine sulfate, a heparin antagonist, available to treat excessive bleeding. ■ Monitor and report abnormal laboratory results and aPTT values outside the desired range. ■ Promptly report evidence of bleeding such as hematemesis, hematuria, bleeding gums, or unexplained abdominal or back pain. *Health education for the client and family:* ■ Report unusual bleeding or excessive menstrual flow. ■ Use an electric razor and a soft-bristle toothbrush; prevent injury by clearing pathways, using a nightlight, and other measures. Do not consume alcohol. ■ Avoid contact sports while on anticoagulant therapy. ■ Do not consume large amounts of food rich in vitamin K (yellow and dark green vegetables). ■ Do not use aspirin or NSAIDs while on heparin therapy unless advised to do so by your healthcare provider. ■ Wear a medical alert tag and advise all healthcare providers (including dentists and podiatrists) of therapy.
Low-Molecular-Weight (LMW) Heparins *Drug examples:* ■ ardeparin (Normiflo) ■ dalteparin (Fragmin) ■ enoxaparin (Lovenox) ■ tinzaparin (Innohep)	LMW heparins are the most bioavailable fraction of heparin. They provide a more precise and predictable anticoagulant effect than unfractionated heparins. Like unfractionated heparin, LMW heparin prevents conversion of prothrombin to thrombin, liberation of thromboplastin from platelets, and formation of a stable clot. LMW heparins cannot be used interchangeably with each other or with unfractionated heparin. Although the risk of heparin-induced thrombocytopenia (HIT) is significantly lower with LMW heparin, clients who were previously treated with unfractionated heparin may develop HIT when treated with LMW heparin.	■ Assess for evidence of active bleeding, a history of bleeding disorders or thrombocytopenia, or sensitivity to heparin, sulfites or pork products. ■ Monitor for unusual or masked bleeding. PT and aPTT levels may be within normal levels even in the presence of hemorrhage. ■ Administer by deep subcutaneous injection into abdominal wall, thigh, or buttocks. Rotate sites. Do not aspirate or massage. *Health education for the client and family:* ■ Subcutaneous self-administration technique, timing of doses, and site rotation. Do not rub site after administering to minimize bruising. ■ Do not take aspirin, NSAIDs, or other over-the-counter drugs unless recommended by your healthcare provider. ■ Promptly report excessive bruising or bleeding, chest pain, difficulty breathing, itching, rash, or swelling to your healthcare provider. ■ Keep follow-up appointments as scheduled.
Oral Anticoagulant *Drug example:* ■ warfarin (Coumadin)	Warfarin interferes with synthesis of vitamin K–dependent clotting factors by the liver, leading to depletion of these factors. It has no effect on already circulating clotting factors or on existing clots. Warfarin inhibits extension of existing thrombi and the formation of new clots. Its action is cumulative and more prolonged than that of heparin.	■ Assess laboratory results and history for evidence of abnormal bleeding. ■ Multiple drugs affect the metabolism and protein binding of warfarin; note all medications and assess for interactions with warfarin. ■ Do not give during pregnancy because warfarin may cause congenital malformations. ■ Oral tablets may be crushed and given without regard to meals.

(continued on next page)

Medications **Anticoagulants** (continued)

CLASSIFICATION AND DRUG EXAMPLES	MECHANISMS OF ACTION	NURSING CONSIDERATIONS
		■ Dilute intravenous warfarin with supplied diluent; administer within 4 hr by direct intravenous injection at a rate of 25 mg/min. ■ Keep vitamin K available to reverse effects of warfarin in the event of excessive bleeding or hemorrhage. ■ Monitor PT or INR; report values outside the desired range. *Health education for the client and family:* ■ If bleeding occurs (hematemesis, bright red or black tarry feces, hematuria, bleeding gums, excessive bruising, etc.), do not take the prescribed dose and notify the healthcare provider immediately. Report rash or manifestations of hepatitis (dark urine, malaise, yellow skin or sclera). ■ Take warfarin at the same time every day; do not change brands because their effects may differ. ■ Menstrual bleeding may be slightly increased; contact the healthcare provider if it increases significantly. Use reliable birth control to prevent pregnancy while taking warfarin. Immediately contact the healthcare provider if you think you may be pregnant. ■ Take precautions to prevent injury and bleeding: Use a soft-bristle toothbrush and electric razor, wear shoes, and use a night-light. Avoid participating in contact sports. ■ Do not smoke, use alcohol, or take any over-the-counter drugs unless specifically recommended by the healthcare provider. Notify all healthcare providers, including dentists and podiatrists, of therapy. Wear a medical alert tag. ■ Obtain lab tests as scheduled and keep all scheduled follow-up appointments.

may be prolonged. Regular follow-up is necessary to be sure prothrombin times (INR) remain within the desirable range for anticoagulation.

Surgery

Venous thrombosis is typically treated with conservative measures and anticoagulation. In some cases, however, surgery is required to remove the thrombus, prevent its extension into deep veins, or prevent the effects of embolization.

Venous thrombectomy is done when thrombi lodge in the femoral vein and their removal is necessary to prevent pulmonary embolism or gangrene. Successful thrombus removal rapidly improves venous circulation. The duration of this effect varies.

When venous thrombosis is recurrent and anticoagulant therapy is contraindicated, a filter may be inserted into the vena cava to capture emboli from the pelvis and lower extremities, preventing pulmonary embolism. Several different filters are available (**Figure 16–39** ●). The Greenfield filter is widely used for its ability to trap emboli within its apex while maintaining patency of the vena cava. The filter can be inserted under fluoroscopy with local anesthesia. Mortality and morbidity associated with the filter are very low.

Extensive thrombosis of the saphenous vein may necessitate ligation and division of the saphenous vein where it joins the femoral vein to prevent clot extension into the deep venous system. The vein affected by septic venous thrombosis is excised to control the infection. Antibiotic therapy also is initiated.

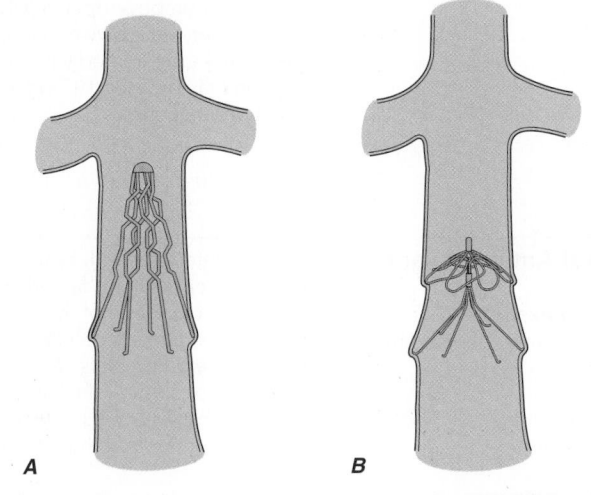

A   *B*

Figure 16–39 ● Venal caval filters. *A,* Greenfield filter. *B,* Nitinol filter.

Clinical Therapy

Treatment of venous thrombosis also includes measures to relieve symptoms and reduce inflammation. With superficial venous thrombosis, applying warm, moist compresses over the affected vein, extremity rest, and anti-inflammatory agents usually provide relief of symptoms.

Bed rest may be ordered for clients with DVT. The duration of bed rest typically is determined by the extent of leg edema. The legs are elevated 15–20 degrees, with the knees slightly flexed, above the level of the heart to promote venous return and discourage venous pooling. Elastic antiembolism stockings or pneumatic compression devices are contraindicated in clients with known DVT, but are frequently ordered by physicians for use in the prevention of DVTs. These devices stimulate the muscle-pumping mechanism to promote the return of blood to the heart. When permitted, walking is encouraged, as is avoiding prolonged standing or sitting. Crossing the legs also is avoided, as are tight-fitting garments or stockings that bind.

■ NURSING PROCESS

Prevention of venous thrombosis is an important component of nursing care for all at-risk clients. To promote venous blood flow from the lower extremities, the nurse should position clients with the feet elevated and the knees slightly bent. Avoid placing pillows under the knees and positions in which the hips and knees are sharply flexed. Use a recliner chair or footstool when sitting. Ambulate clients as soon as possible, and maintain a regular schedule of ambulation throughout the day. Teach ankle flexion and extension exercises, and frequently remind clients to perform them. Apply elastic hose and pneumatic compression devices when appropriate. Instruct clients to avoid crossing the legs when in bed or sitting. Inquire about possible prophylactic heparin or warfarin therapy for clients undergoing orthopedic surgery or other high-risk procedures. Frequently assess intravenous sites. Change the site and catheter as dictated by agency protocol and if evidence of local inflammation is noted.

Assessment

Assess clients at risk for venous thrombosis for manifestations and risk factors, and obtain the following information:

- *Health history.* Complaints of leg or calf pain, its duration and characteristics, and the effect walking on the pain; history of venous thrombosis or other clotting disorders; current medications
- *Physical examination.* Redness and edema of the affected extremity; tenderness, warmth, and cordlike structures on palpation; body temperature.

Diagnosis

Nursing diagnoses that apply to the client with DVT include the following:

- *Pain*
- *Ineffective Tissue Perfusion: Peripheral*
- *Protection, Ineffective*

- *Mobility: Physical, Impaired*
- *Tissue Perfusion: Peripheral, Risk for Ineffective*

(NANDA-I © 2015)

Planning

Goals of nursing care include the following:

- The client will have pain control sufficient to allow rest and comfort.
- The client will not experience complications resulting from embolization of the thrombus.
- The client will have adequate tissue perfusion to prevent cellular damage.

Implementation

In addition to preventive measures, priority nursing diagnoses for the client with venous thrombosis relate to pain, maintenance of tissue perfusion and integrity, and the potential adverse effects of prescribed treatments.

Manage Pain

The pain associated with venous thrombosis results from inflammation of the involved vein. It may be aggravated by use of the involved extremity. Associated edema and swelling may contribute to discomfort. Measures to reduce the inflammation often help relieve the pain. The nurse should do the following:

- Regularly assess pain location, characteristics, and level using a standardized pain scale. Report increasing pain or changes in its location or characteristics. Tissue substances released during the inflammatory process can stimulate pain receptors. In addition, localized swelling presses on pain-sensitive structures in the area of the inflammation, contributing to discomfort. As inflammation and swelling are reduced, pain should abate. Continued or increasing pain may indicate extension of the thrombosis. Sudden chest pain may indicate a pulmonary embolism, necessitating immediate intervention.
- Measure calf and thigh diameter of the affected extremity on admission and daily thereafter. Report increases promptly. The inflammatory process causes vasodilation and increases vessel permeability, in turn causing edema of the affected extremity. Baseline and subsequent measurements provide a measure of treatment effectiveness.
- Apply warm, moist heat to the affected extremity at least four times daily, using warm, moist compresses or an aqua-K pad. Moist heat penetrates tissues to a greater depth. Warmth promotes vasodilation, allowing reabsorption of excess fluid into the circulation. Vasodilation also reduces resistance within the affected vessel, reducing pain. As edema subsides, pressure on the surrounding tissues is relieved, thereby reducing pain.
- Maintain bed rest as ordered. Using leg muscles during walking exacerbates the inflammatory process and increases edema. This, in turn, increases venous compression and pain.

Promote Effective Peripheral Perfusion

As thrombi develop, they occlude the lumen of the vein and obstruct blood flow. In addition, the accompanying inflammatory response may precipitate vessel spasms, further impairing arterial and venous blood flow as well as tissue perfusion. Impaired tissue perfusion in turn deprives tissues of nutrients and oxygen. As a result, distal tissues of the affected extremity are at risk for ulceration and infection. Nursing interventions include the following:

■ Assess the skin of the affected lower leg and foot at least every 8 hours, or more often as indicated. Frequent assessment is important to rapidly detect early signs of tissue breakdown and implementation of measures to protect vulnerable tissues. Early intervention allows healing and restoration of tissue integrity; if allowed to continue, the process can lead to necrosis and potential gangrene.

■ Elevate the client's extremities at all times, keeping knees slightly flexed and legs above the level of the heart. Elevation of the extremities promotes venous return and reduces peripheral edema. Knee flexion promotes muscle relaxation.

■ Use mild soaps, solutions, and lotions to clean the affected leg and foot daily. Pat dry after washing, and apply a non-alcohol-based lotion or moisturizing cream. Daily hygiene with nondrying soaps and solutions removes potential pathogens from the skin surface and maintains skin integrity and the first line of defense against infection. Caustic or harsh soaps or solutions can dry and crack the skin. Dry, cracked skin permits bacteria and other microorganisms to enter and infect the tissue, potentially leading to ulceration and venous gangrene.

■ Use an egg-crate mattress or sheepskin on the bed as needed. Egg-crate mattresses and sheepskins distribute weight more evenly, preventing excess pressure on affected tissues.

■ Encourage frequent position changes (at least every 2 hours) while awake. Frequent position changes reduce pressure on bony prominences and edematous tissue, reducing the risk of tissue breakdown.

Promote Effective Protection

Anticoagulant therapy interferes with the body's normal clotting mechanisms, increasing the risk for bleeding and hemorrhage. The nurse should do the following:

■ Monitor laboratory results, including the INR (prothrombin time), aPTT, hemoglobin, and hematocrit as indicated. Report values outside the normal or desired range. Coagulation studies are used to monitor the effect of anticoagulant medications. Values within the desired range prevent further clot development while carrying a low risk for bleeding and hemorrhage. A fall in the hemoglobin and hematocrit may indicate undetected bleeding.

Encourage Physical Mobility

Although prolonged bed rest rarely is required, it is associated with many problems, including constipation, joint contractures, muscle atrophy, and boredom. Nursing care goals include maintaining joint range of motion (ROM), minimizing muscle atrophy, and reducing boredom. Interventions appropriate to assists clients in meeting these goals include the following:

■ Encourage active ROM exercises at least every 8 hours. Provide passive ROM as needed. ROM exercises maintain joint

mobility and prevent contractures. Active ROM (performed by the client) also helps prevent muscle atrophy and preserve function. While passive ROM exercises do not prevent muscle atrophy, they do maintain joint mobility.

■ Encourage frequent position changes, deep breathing, and coughing. Prolonged immobility can lead to impaired airway clearance and respiratory complications, such as atelectasis or pneumonia. Turning, coughing, and deep breathing facilitate expulsion of secretions from the respiratory tract, airway clearance, and alveolar ventilation.

■ Encourage increased fluid and dietary fiber intake. Constipation is a frequent complication of immobility that results from decreased gastrointestinal motility and loss of abdominal muscle strength. Increasing fluid and fiber intake helps maintain soft, easily expelled stools.

■ Assist the client with and encourage ambulation as allowed. Ambulation promotes venous blood flow, helps maintain muscle tone and joint mobility, and increases the sense of well-being.

■ Encourage diversional activities, such as reading, television or video games, and socializing. Boredom may lead to dozing and inertia, with little physical movement or mental stimulation, increasing the risk for complications of immobility.

Promote Effective Cardiopulmonary Perfusion

A thrombus that forms in the deep veins of the legs or pelvis may break loose or fragment, becoming an embolism. Emboli that originate in the venous system usually become trapped in the pulmonary circulation (pulmonary embolism). Gas exchange in the affected area is impaired as blood flow ceases or is reduced to an area of the lungs that is well ventilated. The nurse should do the following:

■ Frequently assess the client's respiratory status, including rate, depth, ease, and oxygen saturation levels. A mismatch of ventilation and perfusion can significantly affect gas exchange, leading to rapid and shallow respirations, dyspnea and air hunger, and a fall in oxygen saturation levels.

■ Initiate oxygen therapy, elevate the head of the bed, and reassure the client who is experiencing manifestations of pulmonary embolism. Oxygen therapy and elevating the head of the bed promote ventilation and gas exchange in those alveoli that are well perfused, helping maintain tissue oxygenation. Reassurance helps reduce anxiety and slow the respiratory rate, promoting greater respiratory depth and alveolar ventilation.

Evaluation

Client outcomes are evaluated based on their progress in meeting established goals and may include the following:

■ The client identifies warning sign of DVT.
■ No long-term complications are identified.
■ The client vocalizes the risks associated with decreased mobility.
■ The client and nurse collaborate with the interdisciplinary team to identify DVT recurrence strategies.

Client Teaching   Home Care for Deep Venous Thrombosis

Treatment measures for venous thrombosis may be initiated and carried out on an outpatient basis or continued for an extended period of time following hospital discharge. The nurse should include the following topics when teaching for home care:

- Explanation of the disease process
- Treatment measures, including laboratory tests and their purposes as well as medications and adverse effects that should be reported

- Appropriate methods of heat application
- Prescribed activity restrictions
- Measures to prevent future episodes of venous thrombosis
- The importance of follow-up visits and laboratory tests as scheduled.

Refer clients to community nursing services for continued assessment and reinforcement of teaching. Provide referrals for assistance with ADLs and home maintenance services as indicated. Consider referral for physical therapy if needed.

NURSING CARE PLAN   A Client With Deep Venous Thrombosis

ASSESSMENT

Mrs. Opal Hipps, age 75, lives alone with her dog, Chester, in her family home in the suburbs. She retired from her job as a postal clerk 10 years ago and now spends a lot of time reading and watching television. During the past week, she has developed a vague, aching pain in her right leg. She ignored the pain until last night, when it developed into a much more severe pain in her right calf. She noticed that her right lower leg seemed larger than the left, and it was very tender to the touch. After seeing her healthcare provider and undergoing Doppler ultrasound studies, Mrs. Hipps is admitted to the hospital with the diagnosis of deep venous thrombosis in the right leg. She is placed on bed rest and intravenous heparin. Michael Cookson, RN, is assigned to admit and care for Mrs. Hipps.

Mr. Cookson notices that Mrs. Hipps was admitted 14 months ago for repair of a fractured femur. Mrs. Hipps says, "This business about a blood clot really has me worried." She also tells Mr. Cookson that she is worried about who will care for her dog while she is in the hospital. Physical findings include the following: height, 157 cm (62 in.); weight, 68 kg (149 lb); temperature, 37.3°C (99.2°F); vital signs within normal limits otherwise. Her left leg is warm and pink, with strong peripheral pulses and good capillary refill. Her right calf is dark red, very warm, and dry to the touch. It is tender to palpation. The right femoral and popliteal pulses are strong, but the pedal and posterior tibial pulses are difficult to locate. The right calf diameter is 1.27 cm (0.5 in.) larger than the left.

DIAGNOSES

- *Pain* related to inflammatory response in affected vein
- *Anxiety* related to unexpected hospitalization and uncertainty about the seriousness of her illness
- *Tissue Perfusion: Peripheral, Ineffective* related to decreased venous circulation in the right leg
- *Skin Integrity: Impaired, Risk for* related to pooling of venous blood in the right leg

(NANDA-I © 2015)

PLANNING

Goals of care include the following:

- The client will verbalize relief of right leg pain by the day of discharge.
- The client will verbalize reduced anxiety by the second day of hospitalization.
- The client will demonstrate reduced right leg diameter by 0.25 in. (0.64 cm) by the fifth day of hospitalization.
- The client will maintain intact skin in the right foot throughout the hospital stay.

IMPLEMENTATION

- Elevate legs, maintaining slight knee flexion, while in bed.
- Apply warm, moist compresses to right leg using a 2-hours-on, 2-hours-off schedule around the clock.
- Administer prescribed analgesics, and evaluate their effectiveness.
- Spend time with Mrs. Hipps to explain venous thrombosis and its treatment.

- Arrange for a friend or neighbor to care for Mrs. Hipps's dog.
- Apply antiembolism stockings as ordered; remove for 30 minutes every 8 hours.
- Monitor laboratory values to assess effect of anticoagulant therapy; report values outside the desired range.
- Assist with progressive ambulation when allowed.
- Inspect legs and feet, and record findings, every 8 hours.

EVALUATION

Seven days after admission, the pain in Mrs. Hipps's right leg has subsided and the diameter of her right calf is equal to that of her left calf. Mrs. Hipps admits to Mr. Cookson that her fears really relate to a cousin who was hospitalized for a similar problem and had his leg amputated. After Mr. Cookson talks with her about her condition and the steps she can take to prevent its recurrence, Mrs. Hipps is much less anxious. Before discharge, Mr. Cookson reviews instructions for antiembolism stockings, daily walking, warfarin schedule, and scheduled follow-up appointment. Mrs. Hipps's neighbor, Kate, comes to pick her up. As Mr. Cookson is helping Mrs. Hipps into the car, Kate hands her a small brown dog and says, "I took good care of Chester for you, but he's missed you." Mrs. Hipps smiles, and assures Mr. Cookson that she will call the number he provided if she has any questions.

CRITICAL THINKING

1. Describe the pathophysiological reasons for the pain in Mrs. Hipps's right leg.
2. How would you respond if Mrs. Hipps tells you she does not have the money to buy the prescribed anticoagulant when she goes home?
3. How would you change your teaching and discharge planning if Mrs. Hipps had difficulty caring for herself?
4. Design a plan of care for Mrs. Hipps for the nursing diagnosis of Activity Intolerance.

REVIEW **Deep Venous Thrombosis**

RELATE Link the Concepts and Exemplars

Linking the exemplar of deep venous thrombosis with the concept of mobility:

1. What strategies can you implement to reduce the risk of DVT in the client who is confined to bed?

2. Develop a teaching plan aimed at reducing the risk of DVT in an older client who has limited mobility.

Linking the exemplar of deep venous thrombosis with the concept of reproduction:

3. Why is the pregnant client at increased risk for DVT?

4. Explain the specific factors that increase the risk for DVT at each stage of pregnancy (prenatal, antenatal, and postpartum).

READY Go to Companion Skills Manual

REFER Go to Pearson Nursing Student Resources
nursing.pearsonhighered.com

- Additional review materials

REFLECT Case Study

Jennifer Walker is a 20-year-old college student majoring in business. She lives with her boyfriend, Sam Hough, age 21, in an off-campus apartment. They enjoy walking around the campus with their dog, Shelby, and playing tennis and golf. Sam's parents are both physicians and Ms. Walker's mother is a nurse.

At her examination several months ago, Ms. Walker obtained a prescription for oral contraceptives. She has been taking them daily. Recently, she began to notice pain in her left leg when she walks. She ignored it for several days thinking she had just pulled a muscle while playing tennis but the pain got worse. Today she is unable to put any pressure on the leg. She also notes a red area on the calf of her leg that is hot to the touch and very tender. She calls the campus clinic and makes an appointment to be seen today.

1. What factors in Ms. Walker's history put her at risk for developing a DVT?

2. What is your priority nursing diagnosis for Ms. Walker?

3. What teaching will you provide Ms. Walker during her visit to the campus clinic?

EXEMPLAR 16.5 Disseminated Intravascular Coagulation

EXEMPLAR KEY TERMS
Disseminated intravascular coagulation (DIC), *1138*
Fibrin degradation products, *1138*
Schistocytes, *1140*

EXEMPLAR LEARNING OUTCOMES
After reading about this exemplar, you will be able to:

1. Describe the pathophysiology, etiology, clinical manifestations, and direct and indirect causes of disseminated intravascular coagulation.

2. Identify risk factors associated with disseminated intravascular coagulation.

3. Illustrate the nursing process in providing culturally competent care across the life span for individuals with disseminated intravascular coagulation.

4. Formulate priority nursing diagnoses appropriate for an individual with disseminated intravascular coagulation.

5. Summarize therapies used by interdisciplinary teams in the collaborative care of an individual with disseminated intravascular coagulation.

6. Plan evidence-based care for an individual with disseminated intravascular coagulation and his or her family in collaboration with other members of the healthcare team.

7. Evaluate expected outcomes for an individual with disseminated intravascular coagulation.

▶ OVERVIEW

Disseminated intravascular coagulation (DIC) is a disruption of hemostasis characterized by widespread intravascular clotting and bleeding. It may be acute and life threatening, or it may be relatively mild.

▶ PATHOPHYSIOLOGY AND ETIOLOGY

Disseminated intravascular coagulation is triggered by endothelial damage, release of tissue factors into the circulation, or inappropriate activation of the clotting cascade by an endotoxin or products of microorganisms. Although it can occur as a complication of any condition that causes endothelia damage or the release of tissue factors, DIC most commonly presents in severe sepsis and septic shock. Although both gram-negative and gram-positive organisms are most commonly associated with DIC, viruses, fungi, and parasitic infections may also cause DIC (Levi & Schmaier, 2012).

Both the intrinsic and the extrinsic clotting cascades may be activated, although activation of the extrinsic cascade is more common. The widespread clotting in the microvasculature consumes clotting factors (prothrombin, platelets, factor V, and factor VIII in particular) and activates fibrinolytic processes with anticoagulant production. As a result, hemorrhage occurs (**Figure 16–40 ●**). Clients may experience problems related to both clotting and bleeding. Organ dysfunction may result from damage to the microvasculature.

The sequence of DIC is as follows:

1. Endothelial damage, tissue factors, or toxins stimulate the clotting cascade.

2. Excess thrombin within the circulation overwhelms naturally occurring anticoagulants.

3. Widespread clotting occurs within the microvasculature.

4. Thrombi and emboli impair tissue perfusion, leading to ischemia, infarction, and necrosis.

5. Clotting factors and platelets are consumed faster than they can be replaced.

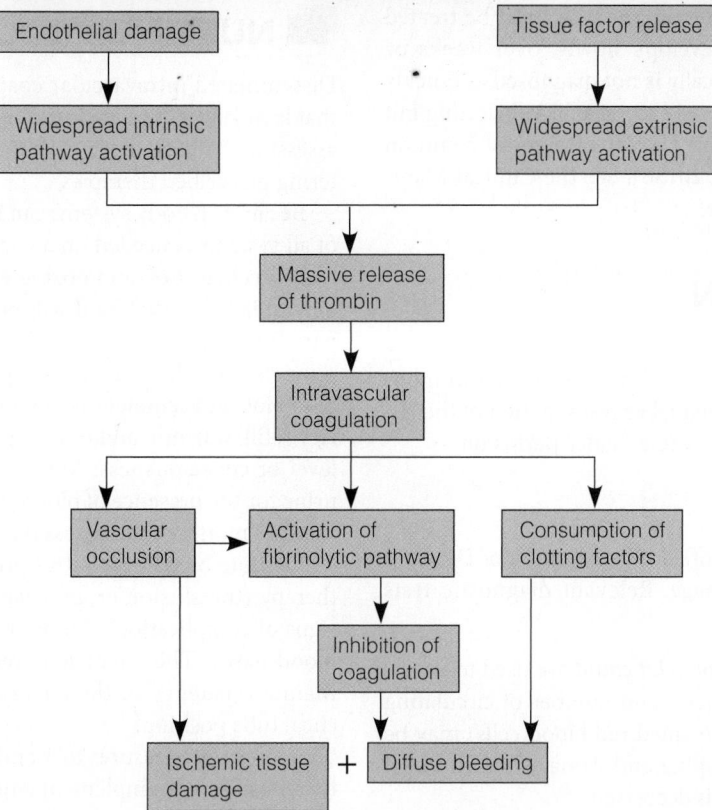

Figure 16–40 ● Disseminated intravascular coagulation (DIC). Endothelial cell injury or release of tissue factors activates the intrinsic or extrinsic clotting pathway (or both). As a result, numerous microthrombi form throughout the vasculature, causing ischemic tissue damage. Simultaneously, rapid consumption of clotting factors and activation of fibrinolytic mechanisms trigger widespread bleeding.

6. Clotting activates fibrinolytic processes, which begin to break down clots.
7. **Fibrin degradation products** (potent anticoagulants) are released, contributing to bleeding.
8. Clotting factors are depleted, the ability to form clots is lost, and hemorrhage occurs.

It is estimated that DIC occurs in as many as 1% of all hospitalized clients (Levi & Schmaier, 2012). DIC is a complication or an effect of the progression of an illness, not a specific illness itself. It occurs secondary to an underlying condition and is typically associated with other clinical conditions (**Box 16–13** ●).

Risk Factors

Acute DIC can occur in pregnant clients, most often with pregnancies complicated by preeclampsia, placental abruption, fetal demise, amniotic fluid embolism, and septic abortion. It is suggested that the degree of placental separation in abruptions correlates with the severity of DIC, suggesting that leakage of thromboplastin-like material from the placental system is responsible for the occurrence of DIC (Levi & Schmaier, 2012). DIC also occurs in some clients affected by HELLP (hemolysis, elevated liver enzymes, low platelet counts) syndrome. HELLP syndrome is thought to be a variant of preeclampsia but may be seen without a diagnosis of preeclampsia. HELLP syndrome is thought to occur in 0.2%–0.6% of all pregnancies.

Box 16–13 Conditions That May Precipitate Disseminated Intravascular Coagulation

TISSUE DAMAGE
- Trauma: burns, gunshot wounds, frostbite, head injury
- Obstetric complications: septic abortion, abruptio placentae, amniotic fluid embolus, retained dead fetus
- Neoplasms: acute leukemia, adenocarcinomas
- Hemolysis
- Fat embolism

VESSEL DAMAGE
- Aortic aneurysm
- Acute glomerulonephritis
- Hemolytic uremic syndrome

INFECTIONS
- Bacterial infection or sepsis
- Viral or mycotic infections
- Malaria

▶ CLINICAL MANIFESTATIONS

The manifestations of DIC result from both clotting and bleeding, although bleeding is more obvious, especially in acute DIC. Bleeding may be internal or external and range from oozing blood following an injection to frank hemorrhage from every body orifice. The two types of DIC are acute and chronic. Acute

DIC develops rapidly over hours or days and must be treated immediately. Chronic DIC develops slowly, over weeks or months. It lasts longer and typically is not diagnosed as quickly as acute DIC. Chronic DIC causes excessive blood clotting but usually does not lead to bleeding. Cancer is the most common cause of chronic DIC (NHLBI, 2013b). See the Clinical Manifestations and Therapies feature.

▶ COLLABORATION

Treatment of DIC is directed toward treating the underlying disorder and preventing further bleeding or massive thrombosis. Supportive measures are essential as resuscitation of the client's circulatory system is primary to enhance perfusion.

Diagnostic Tests

Diagnostic tests are used to confirm the diagnosis of DIC and evaluate the risk for hemorrhage. Relevant diagnostic tests include the following:

- *Complete blood count and platelet count* are used to evaluate the hemoglobin, hematocrit, and number of circulating platelets. **Schistocytes** (fragmented red blood cells) may be noted as a result of cell trapping and damage within fibrin thrombi. The platelet count is decreased.
- *Coagulation studies* show prolonged prothrombin time, partial thromboplastin time, and thrombin time as well as a low fibrinogen level caused by depletion of clotting factors. A declining fibrinogen level on two consecutive readings can help make the diagnosis of DIC.
- *Fibrin degradation products or fibrin split products* are increased as a result of the fibrinolysis that occurs with DIC.
- *Fibrinogen levels* may be decreased or normal in circumstances where elevated levels are expected..
- *D-dimer* is elevated in both acute and chronic DIC.

Clinical Therapy

When bleeding is the major manifestation of DIC, fresh frozen plasma, cryoprecipitate, and platelet concentrates are given to restore clotting factors and platelets. Heparin, although controversial because it may exacerbate bleeding in addition to preventing further clotting, may be administered. Heparin interferes with the clotting cascade and may prevent further clotting factor consumption as a result of uncontrolled thrombosis. It is used when bleeding is not controlled by plasma and platelets as well as when the client has manifestations of thrombotic problems, such as acrocyanosis (cyanotic, or blue, color in the hands and/or feet) and possible gangrene. Long-term heparin therapy (administered by injection or continuous infusion using a portable pump) may be necessary for clients with chronic DIC.

In severe cases of DIC, supportive care is essential to maintain life. Intracranial bleeding may result in altered levels of consciousness, damage to the respiratory center, and increased intracranial pressure. Supportive care may include mechanical ventilation and control of organ damage caused by reduced perfusion.

■ NURSING PROCESS

Disseminated intravascular coagulation is a complex disorder that is managed by a critical care team. Nursing care focuses on assessing the bleeding, preventing further injury, and administering prescribed therapies.

Because all body systems can be involved, careful assessment of all systems is needed on a continual basis. Observe for petechiae, ecchymoses, and oozing every 1–2 hours. Check dependent areas because blood will pool there. Intravenous sites are particularly prone to oozing and should be assessed every 15 minutes. Examine stool for the presence of blood, and measure blood loss as accurately as possible. Assess extremities for capillary refill, warmth, and pulses. Frequently assess vital signs and level of consciousness. Measure intake and output. Monitor urine for the presence of blood. Blood urea nitrogen and creatinine are monitored to assess renal function.

Institute bleeding-control precautions, monitor prescribed therapy (transfusion or anticoagulant therapy), and report any signs of complications. Monitor oxygen saturation and arterial blood gases. The client may require mechanical ventilation. Maintain patency of the airway, and ensure correct endotracheal tube position.

Implement measures to maintain skin integrity, such as gentle repositioning. Implement a nutritional plan of tube feedings or total parenteral nutrition. Identify the family members' coping strategies and support system to facilitate their ability to manage this life-threatening crisis.

Assessment

Focused nursing assessment for DIC includes obtaining the following information:

- *Health history.* Recent abortion (spontaneous or therapeutic) or current pregnancy; recent blood transfusion; trauma; symptoms of or exposure to infectious diseases; presence of a known malignant tumor; history of abnormal bleeding episodes or a hematological disorder
- *Physical examination.* Bleeding from puncture wounds (e.g., injections), intravenous sites, or incisions; hematuria, obvious or occult blood in emesis or stool, nosebleeds, or other abnormal bleeding; vital signs; heart and breath sounds; abdominal assessment, including girth, contour, bowel sounds, tenderness, or guarding to palpation; color, temperature, and skin condition of hands, feet, and digits; petechiae or purpura of skin or mucous membranes.

Diagnosis

Clients with acute DIC often are critically ill, with multiple nursing care needs. As mentioned, septic shock may precipitate DIC; hemorrhagic shock may occur as a complication of DIC. Priority nursing diagnoses discussed in this section include the following:

- *Ineffective Tissue Perfusion*
- *Impaired Gas Exchange*
- *Pain*
- *Fear.*

(NANDA-I © 2015)

Clinical Manifestations and Therapies **Disseminated Intravascular Coagulation**

ETIOLOGY	CLINICAL MANIFESTATIONS	CLINICAL THERAPIES
Cardiovascular System		
Tachycardia Hypotension Circulatory collapse Major vessel thrombosis	■ Decreased perfusion ■ Shock ■ Inappropriate clotting ■ Tissue necrosis and gangrene ■ Oozing from wounds, IV sites, and mucous membranes	■ Administer fluids as ordered. ■ Monitor intake and output. ■ Monitor vital signs. ■ Maintain bedrest.
Respiratory System		
Tachypnea Decreased breath sounds	■ Impaired gas exchange resulting from microclots in the pulmonary vasculature	■ Monitor respiratory status. ■ Maintain ventilatory support if required.
Central Nervous System		
Confusion Coma Seizures	■ Impaired cerebral perfusion	■ Conduct neurological assessment every 2 hr during critical period, then every 4 hr until stabilized.
Urinary System		
Oliguria Anuria Renal failure Hematuria	■ Impaired renal perfusion ■ Impaired clotting mechanism leading to bleeding	■ Monitor urine output hourly. ■ Maintain patent urinary catheter. ■ Monitor urine for blood.
Gastrointestinal System		
Gastrointestinal bleeding Abdominal distention Bleeding from mucous membranes Occult blood in stool or emesis	■ Impaired clotting mechanisms leading to bleeding	■ Monitor for occult blood in stools and emesis. ■ Monitor for overt signs of bleeding from gums. ■ Measure abdominal girth every 4 hr.
Integumentary System		
Petechiae Purpura Ecchymosis Bleeding or oozing from wounds or intravenous access site Pallor Cool extremities Cyanosis of extremities	■ Impaired clotting mechanism leading to bleeding ■ Impaired tissue perfusion	■ Monitor skin for evidence of bleeding. ■ Protect from injury. ■ Monitor distal pulses, temperature, and capillary refill.

Planning

Goals of nursing care may include the following:

- The client will have increased vacular volume as evidenced by hemodynamic stability and adequate urine output.

- The client will maintain adequate gas exchange, related to mechanical ventilation, as evidenced by arterial blood gas results and oxygen saturation monitoring within normal limits.
- The client will experience adequate pain control, as evidenced by the ability to rest comfortably.

- The client will show early recognition of illness progression by frequently monitoring vital signs after discharge and reporting abnormal results to the healthcare provider.

Implementation

Care of the client diagnosed with DIC often requires specialized nursing in critical care. Continuous monitoring for inadequate oxygenation, altered perfusion, and bleeding are priorities of nursing care.

Promote Effective Tissue Perfusion

Thrombi and emboli forming throughout the microcirculation affect the perfusion of multiple organs and tissues. Additionally, bleeding as a result of clotting factor consumption affects cardiac output and blood flow to these tissues. Appropriate interventions include the following:

- Assess extremity pulses, warmth, and capillary refill. Monitor the client's level of consciousness and mental status. Monitoring central and peripheral tissue perfusion facilitates early treatment of impaired perfusion.
- Carefully reposition the client at least every 2 hours. Position changes facilitate circulation and tissue perfusion and provide an opportunity to assess for purpura, pallor, and bleeding.
- Discourage the client from crossing the legs, and do not elevate the knees on the bed or with a pillow. These positions may impair arterial and venous flow to the lower legs and feet, increasing vascular stasis and the risk for thrombosis.
- Minimize use of tape on the skin; instead use binders, nonadhesive dressings, and other devices as needed. Preventing skin trauma reduces the risk for bleeding and potential infection.

Monitor Gas Exchange

Microclots in the pulmonary vasculature are likely to interfere with gas exchange in the client with DIC. The nurse should do the following:

- Monitor the client's oxygen saturation continuously. Administer oxygen as ordered. Oxygen saturation levels are a noninvasive means of assessing gas exchange. Supplemental oxygen promotes gas exchange and reduces cardiac work, relieving dyspnea.
- Place the client in the Fowler or high-Fowler position as tolerated. Elevating the head of the bed improves diaphragmatic excursion and alveolar ventilation.
- Maintain bed rest. Bed rest reduces oxygen demands and cardiac work.
- Encourage deep breathing and effective coughing. Increased respiratory depth and clearance of secretions from airways improves alveolar ventilation and oxygenation.
- Institute cautious nasotracheal suctioning if cough is ineffective or an endotracheal tube is in place. Removal of secretions facilitates ventilation and oxygenation. However, care must be used to minimize suction-induced hypoxia and airway trauma.
- Administer analgesics and antianxiety drugs as needed to control pain and anxiety. Provide reassurance and comfort

measures. Pain and anxiety increase the respiratory rate and decrease the depth of respirations, reducing effective ventilation and gas exchange.

Manage Pain

Both the underlying cause of DIC and the tissue ischemia from microvascular clots can cause pain. Identifying the etiology of pain is important to identify potential complications or harmful effects of DIC and institute effective treatment. Nursing interventions to minimize pain include the following:

- Use a standard pain scale to evaluate and monitor pain and analgesic effectiveness. Monitoring pain and response to medication facilitates development of an appropriate and effective treatment plan.
- Handle extremities gently. Gentle handling reduces the risk of further injury to and pain in ischemic tissues.
- Apply cool compresses to painful joints. Application of cold decreases pain through the gate-control mechanism, inhibiting the dorsal horn of the spinal cord and reducing the sensation of pain.

Manage Fear

The underlying serious illness and a complication such as DIC result in an uncertain prognosis, often accompanied by fear. Nursing interventions to reduce fear include the following:

- Encourage the client and family to verbalize concerns. This helps the client and family identify their concerns and frame questions.
- Answer questions truthfully. Providing honest answers is vital to developing a therapeutic nurse–client relationship. Accurate responses allow the client and family to set priorities as they plan for an uncertain future.
- Help the client and family identify coping strategies to manage this significant situational stressor. Implementing previously effective coping methods may provide the skills to manage the current crisis.
- Provide emotional support. The presence of a caring nurse helps reduce the fear and anxiety associated with a crisis.

Client Teaching Disseminated Intravascular Coagulation

Although the immediate crisis of acute DIC is resolved before discharge, the client may have some continuing effects of the disorder, such as impaired tissue integrity of distal extremities. Teach the client and family about specific care needs, such as foot care or dressing changes. Provide instruction about any continuing medications and follow-up care.

Clients with chronic DIC may require continuing heparin therapy, using either intermittent subcutaneous injections or a portable infusion pump. Teach the client and family members how to administer the injection or manage the infusion pump. Provide a referral to home health care or a home intravenous management service for assistance. Discuss the manifestations of excessive bleeding or recurrent clotting that need to be reported to the healthcare provider.

- Maintain a calm environment. A calm environment provides reassurance that the situation is in control, reduces anxiety, and promotes rest.
- Respond promptly when the client calls for help. Prompt response to expressed needs helps develop a trusting relationship and a sense of security that assistance is readily available.
- Teach relaxation techniques. Relaxation techniques can reduce muscle tension and other signs of anxiety. Gaining control over physical responses can help the client gain a sense of control over the situation.

Evaluation

The client's response to nursing care may be evaluated using the following expected outcomes:

- The client experiences no long-term complications from DIC.
- The family demonstrates effective coping techniques to deal with severity of client's illness.
- The client's bleeding is controlled.
- The client's body systems are capable of meeting needs of oxygenation and perfusion to prevent tissue destruction.

NURSING CARE PLAN A Client With Disseminated Intravascular Coagulation

Addy McMannis, 19 years old, is admitted to the hospital with toxic shock syndrome believed to have resulted from improper use of tampons. She has intravenous fluids infusing at 125 mL/hr and is receiving broad-spectrum antibiotics. She reports feeling very weak and fatigued and says all she wants to do is sleep. Two days later, she is diagnosed with disseminated intravascular coagulation.

ASSESSMENT

Petechiae and small bruises are noted over all of Ms. McMannis's extremities. She also reports bleeding from the gums during oral care. Hematuria is noted. Laboratory studies are as follows: platelet count, 71,000; hematocrit, 28%; prolonged prothrombin time, partial thromboplastin time, and thrombin time; low fibrinogen level; elevated white blood cell count. Vital signs are as follows: temperature 100.2°F oral; pulse 108 bpm; respirations 24/min; blood pressure 104/60 mmHg.

DIAGNOSES

- *Ineffective Tissue Perfusion*
- *Fatigue*
- *Risk for Injury*

(NANDA-I © 2015)

PLANNING

Goals of care includes the following:

- Client's status will improve as evidenced by decreased bleeding and increased platelet count.
- Client's vital signs will stabilize within 24–48 hr of administration of ordered therapies.
- Client will use a sponge for oral care to reduce the risk for bleeding.
- Client will follow up with primary care provider following discharge.
- Client will verbalize appropriate use of tampons prior to discharge.
- Client will verbalize and demonstrate ability to follow discharge instructions related to deep breathing, bed rest, and other interventions.
- Client will verbalize signs and symptoms that require notifying the healthcare provider as well as those requiring emergent care.

IMPLEMENTATION

- Assess pulses, warmth, and capillary refill in extremities. Monitor level of consciousness.
- Teach client to use a sponge for oral care to reduce risk of gum trauma and only an electric razor when shaving.
- Administer medications as indicated.
- Support oxygenation, which may include mechanical ventilation.
- Monitor the client for bleeding (stools, venipunctures, open wounds, and emesis).
- Encourage gentle repositioning frequently to prevent loss of skin integrity.

- Discourage crossing of the legs or elevation of the knees to promote circulation to the feet.
- Minimize use of tape on the client's skin to prevent altered skin integrity.
- Schedule care to allow periods of uninterrupted sleep and prevent overtiring.
- Provide emotional support to the client and family.
- Monitor respiratory pattern, breath sounds, and oxygenation.

EVALUATION

Ms. McMannis continues to receive antibiotics to treat toxic shock syndrome and is also given fresh frozen plasma and platelet concentrates, which control bleeding. Her platelet count decreases initially but eventually returns to near normal, and she is discharged a week later with instructions to follow up with her primary care provider and immediately report any signs of bleeding or bruising.

CRITICAL THINKING

1. Why, if the disease is caused by small clots forming, do clients experience bleeding with this disease?
2. What effect does the administration of platelet concentrate have on platelet production?
3. Was the diagnosis of toxic shock syndrome related to the occurrence of disseminated intravascular coagulation? Explain your answer.

▲ **REVIEW** **Disseminated Intravascular Coagulation**

RELATE Link the Concepts and Exemplars

Linking the exemplar of disseminated intravascular coagulation with the concept of elimination:

1. What pathophysiology places the client with DIC at increased risk for renal failure?

2. Prioritize care for the client diagnosed with DIC who experiences acute renal failure as a result.

Linking the exemplar of disseminated intravascular coagulation with the concept of intracranial regulation:

3. What assessment findings would indicate possible increased intracranial pressure in the client diagnosed with DIC?

4. What is your priority nursing intervention if signs of increased intracranial pressure are found in the client with DIC?

READY Go to Companion Skills Manual

REFER Go to Pearson Nursing Student Resources
nursing.pearsonhighered.com

- Additional review materials

REFLECT Case Study

Rhonda Fischer, 29 years old, has just delivered her fourth child by emergency cesarean section at 39 weeks' gestation for fetal intolerance of labor after attempted induction of labor for prolonged rupture of membranes and chorioamnionitis.

Ms. Fischer was placed on IV antibiotics prior to surgery and is now on the postpartum unit. During a focused assessment, the nurse notes that Ms. Fischer is having frank bleeding from her incision and is oozing blood from around her IV site. Her vital signs include TO 99.7°F; P 96 bpm; R 28/min; BP 100/65 mmHg.

1. What are the first laboratory data you will want to review on Ms. Fischer's medical record?

2. What nursing diagnosis will you add to Ms. Fischer's plan of care based on these assessment findings?

3. What nursing interventions will you initiate for Ms. Fischer?

4. What client teaching will you provide Mr. and Ms. Fischer to explain the diagnosis of DIC made by the obstetrician?

EXEMPLAR 16.6 Heart Failure

EXEMPLAR KEY TERMS
Cardiac tamponade, *1157*
Decompensation, *1145*
Exercise intolerance, *1157*
Frank–Starling mechanism, *1145*
Heart failure, *1144*
Hemodynamics, *1151*
Mean arterial pressure (MAP), *1152*
Nocturia, *1149*
Orthopnea, *1148*
Paroxysmal nocturnal dyspnea, *1149*
Pulmonary edema, *1145*

EXEMPLAR LEARNING OUTCOMES
After reading about this exemplar, you will be able to:

1. Describe the pathophysiology, etiology, clinical manifestations, and direct and indirect causes of heart failure.

2. Identify risk factors associated with heart failure.

3. Illustrate the nursing process in providing culturally competent care across the life span for individuals with heart failure.

4. Formulate priority nursing diagnoses appropriate for an individual with heart failure.

5. Summarize therapies used by interdisciplinary teams in the collaborative care of an individual with heart failure.

6. Plan evidence-based care for an individual with heart failure and his or her family in collaboration with other members of the healthcare team.

7. Evaluate expected outcomes for an individual with heart failure.

▶ OVERVIEW

Heart failure is a condition in which the heart is unable to pump enough blood into circulation to meet the body's needs (NHLBI, 2013a). This inability to pump is due to the inability of the heart to fill with enough blood or the inability of the heart to pump with enough force to meet the metabolic demands. Heart failure may result from a combination of the two.

Heart failure is a progressive condition, developing over time as the heart muscle becomes weaker. Frequently, it is a long-term effect of coronary heart disease and MI when left ventricular damage is extensive enough to impair cardiac output. Other diseases of the heart, including structural and inflammatory disorders, also may cause heart failure. In normal hearts, failure can result from excessive demands placed on the heart. Heart failure may be acute or chronic.

Heart failure develops when the heart cannot effectively fill or contract with adequate strength to function as a pump to meet the needs of the body. As a result, cardiac output falls, leading to decreased tissue perfusion. The body initially adjusts to reduced cardiac output by activating compensatory mechanisms to restore tissue perfusion. These compensatory mechanisms may result in vascular congestion—hence, the commonly used term *congestive heart failure*. As these mechanisms are exhausted, heart failure ensues, with increased morbidity and mortality.

Heart failure is a disorder of cardiac function. It frequently is the result of impaired myocardial contraction, which may result from coronary heart disease and myocardial ischemia or infarct or from a primary cardiac muscle disorder, such as cardiomyopathy or myocarditis. Structural cardiac disorders, such as valve disorders or congenital heart defects, and hypertension also can lead to heart failure when the heart muscle is damaged by the long-standing excessive workload associated with these conditions. Other clients without a primary abnormality of myocardial function may present with manifestations

TABLE 16–24 Selected Causes of Heart Failure

IMPAIRED MYOCARDIAL FUNCTION	INCREASED CARDIAC WORKLOAD	ACUTE NONCARDIAC CONDITIONS
■ Coronary heart disease	■ Hypertension	■ Volume overload
■ Cardiomyopathies	■ Valve disorders	■ Hyperthyroidism
■ Rheumatic fever	■ Anemias	■ Fever, infection
■ Infective endocarditis	■ Congenital heart defects	■ Massive pulmonary embolus

of heart failure as a result of acute excess demands placed on the myocardium, such as volume overload, hyperthyroidism, and massive pulmonary embolus (**Table 16–24** ●).

Pulmonary edema is an abnormal accumulation of fluid in the interstitial tissue and alveoli of the lung. Both cardiac and noncardiac disorders can cause pulmonary edema. Cardiac causes include AMI, acute heart failure, and valvular disease. Cardiogenic pulmonary edema, the focus of this section, is a sign of severe cardiac **decompensation** (the loss of effective compensation). Noncardiac causes of pulmonary edema include primary pulmonary disorders, such as acute respiratory distress syndrome, trauma, sepsis, drug overdose, preeclampsia, or neurological events.

Pulmonary edema is a medical emergency: The client is literally drowning in the fluid in the alveolar and interstitial pulmonary spaces. Its onset may be acute or gradual, progressing to severe respiratory distress. Immediate treatment is necessary.

▶ PATHOPHYSIOLOGY AND ETIOLOGY

The mechanical pumping action of cardiac muscle propels the blood it receives to the pulmonary and systemic vascular systems for reoxygenation and delivery to the tissues. Cardiac output is the amount of blood pumped from the ventricles in 1 minute. Cardiac output is used to assess cardiac performance, especially left ventricular function. Effective cardiac output depends on adequate functional muscle mass and the ability of the ventricles to work together. Cardiac output normally is regulated by the oxygen needs of the body: As oxygen use increases, cardiac output increases to maintain cellular function. Cardiac reserve is the ability of the heart to increase cardiac output to meet metabolic demand. Ventricular damage reduces the cardiac reserve.

Cardiac output (CO) is a product of heart rate (HR) and stroke volume (SV). Heart rate affects cardiac output by controlling the number of ventricular contractions per minute. It is influenced by the autonomic nervous system, catecholamines, and thyroid hormones. Activation of a stress response (e.g., hypovolemia or fear) stimulates the sympathetic nervous system (SNS), increasing the heart rate and its contractility. Elevated heart rates increase cardiac output. Very rapid heart rates, however, shorten ventricular filling time (diastole), reducing stroke volume and cardiac output. On the other hand, a slow heart rate reduces cardiac output simply because of fewer cardiac cycles.

Stroke volume (the volume of blood ejected with each heartbeat) is determined by preload, afterload, and myocardial contractility. Preload is the volume of blood in the ventricles at end diastole (just before contraction). The blood in the ventricles exerts pressure on the ventricle walls, stretching muscle fibers. The greater the blood volume, the greater the force with which the ventricle contracts to expel the blood. End-diastolic volume depends on the amount of blood returning to the ven-

tricles (venous return) and on the distensibility or stiffness of the ventricles (compliance).

Afterload is the force needed to eject blood into the circulation. This force must be great enough to overcome arterial pressures within the pulmonary and systemic vascular systems. The right ventricle must generate enough force to open the pulmonary valve and eject its blood into the pulmonary artery. The left ventricle ejects its blood into the systemic circulation by overcoming the arterial resistance behind the aortic valve. Increased systemic vascular resistance (e.g., hypertension) increases afterload, impairing stroke volume and increasing myocardial work.

Contractility is the natural ability of cardiac muscle fibers to shorten during systole. Contractility is necessary to overcome arterial pressures and eject blood during systole. Impaired contractility affects cardiac output by reducing stroke volume. The ejection fraction is the percentage of blood in the ventricle that is ejected during systole. A normal ejection fraction is 50%–70%.

When the heart begins to fail, mechanisms are activated to compensate for the impaired function and maintain the cardiac output. The primary compensatory mechanisms are as follows:

1. The Frank–Starling mechanism
2. Neuroendocrine responses, including activation of the sympathetic nervous system (SNS) and the renin–angiotensin system
3. Myocardial hypertrophy.

These mechanisms and their effects are summarized in **Table 16–25** ●.

Decreased cardiac output initially stimulates aortic baroreceptors, which in turn stimulate the SNS. Stimulation of the SNS produces both cardiac and vascular responses through the release of norepinephrine. Norepinephrine increases heart rate and contractility by stimulating cardiac beta-receptors. Cardiac output improves as both heart rate and stroke volume increase. Norepinephrine also causes arterial and venous vasoconstriction, increasing venous return to the heart. Increased venous return increases ventricular filling and myocardial stretch, increasing the force of contraction (the **Frank–Starling mechanism**). Overstretching the muscle fibers past their physiological limit results in an ineffective contraction.

Blood flow is redistributed to the brain and the heart to maintain perfusion of these vital organs. Decreased renal perfusion causes renin to be released from the kidneys. Activation of the renin–angiotensin system produces additional vasoconstriction and stimulates the adrenal cortex to produce aldosterone and the posterior pituitary to release antidiuretic hormone (ADH). Aldosterone stimulates sodium reabsorption in renal tubules, promoting water retention. ADH acts on the distal tubule to inhibit water excretion, and it also causes vasoconstriction. The effect of these hormones is significant vasocon-

TABLE 16–25 Compensatory Mechanisms Activated in Heart Failure

MECHANISM	PHYSIOLOGY	EFFECT ON BODY SYSTEMS	COMPLICATIONS
Frank–Starling mechanism	The greater the stretch of cardiac muscle fibers, the greater the force of contraction.	■ Increased contractile force leading to increased CO	■ Increased myocardial oxygen demand ■ Limited by overstretching
Neuroendocrine response	Decreased CO stimulates the SNS and catecholamine release.	■ Increased heart rate, blood pressure, and contractility ■ Increased vascular resistance ■ Increased venous return	■ Increased vascular resistance ■ Tachycardia, with decreased filling time and decreased CO ■ Increased myocardial work and oxygen demand

	Decreased CO and decreased renal perfusion stimulate the renin–angiotensin system.
	  Angiotensin stimulates aldosterone release from the adrenal cortex.
	  Antidiuretic hormone is released from the posterior pituitary.
	  Atrial natriuretic peptide and brain natriuretic peptide are released.
	  Blood flow is redistributed to vital organs (heart and brain).
		■ Vasoconstriction and increased blood pressure
		■ Salt and water retention by the kidneys
		■ Increased vascular volume
		■ Water excretion inhibited
		■ Increased sodium excretion
		■ Diuresis
		■ Vasodilation
		■ Decreased perfusion of other organ systems
		■ Decreased perfusion of skin and muscles
			■ Increased myocardial work
			■ Renal vasoconstriction and decreased renal perfusion
			■ Increased preload and afterload
			■ Pulmonary congestion
			■ Fluid retention and increased preload and afterload
			■ Pulmonary congestion
			■ Renal failure
			■ Anaerobic metabolism and lactic acidosis

Ventricular hypertrophy	Increased cardiac workload causes myocardial muscle to hypertrophy and ventricles to dilate.	■ Increased contractile force to maintain CO	■ Increased myocardial oxygen demand ■ Cellular enlargement

striction as well as salt and water retention, with a resulting increase in vascular volume. Increased ventricular filling increases the force of contraction, improving cardiac output.

The effects of the renin–angiotensin–aldosterone system and ADH release are counterbalanced to a certain extent by two additional hormones. The increased vascular volume and venous return prompted by vasoconstriction and sodium and water retention increase the volume and pressures in the heart. Stimulation of stretch receptors in the atria and ventricles leads to the release of atrial natriuretic peptide (ANP) and brain natriuretic peptide (BNP) from stores in the atria (ANP and BNP) and ventricles (BNP). These hormones promote sodium and water excretion and inhibit the release of norepinephrine, renin, and ADH, with resulting vasodilation. Although beneficial, the effects of these hormones are too weak to completely counteract the vasoconstriction and the sodium and water retention that occurs in heart failure.

Ventricular remodeling occurs as the heart chambers and myocardium adapt to fluid volume and pressure increases. The chambers dilate to accommodate excess fluid resulting from increased vascular volume and incomplete emptying. Initially, this additional stretch causes more effective contractions. Ventricular hypertrophy occurs as existing cardiac muscle cells enlarge, increasing their contractile elements (actin and myosin) and force of contraction.

Although these responses may help in the short-term regulation of cardiac output, it is now recognized that they also hasten the deterioration of cardiac function. The onset of heart failure is heralded by decompensation. Heart failure progresses as a result of the very mechanisms that initially maintained circulatory stability.

The rapid heart rate shortens diastolic filling time, compromises coronary artery perfusion, and increases myocardial oxy-

gen demand. Resulting ischemia further impairs cardiac output. Beta-receptors in the heart become less sensitive to continued SNS stimulation, thus decreasing heart rate and contractility. As the beta-receptors become less sensitive, norepinephrine stores in the cardiac muscle become depleted. In contrast, alpha-receptors on peripheral blood vessels become increasingly sensitive to persistent stimulation, promoting vasoconstriction and increasing afterload and cardiac work.

As mentioned, ventricular hypertrophy and dilation initially increase cardiac output, but chronic distention eventually causes the ventricular wall to thin and degenerate. The purpose of hypertrophy is thus defeated. In addition, chronic overloading of the dilated ventricle eventually stretches the fibers beyond the optimal point for effective contraction. The ventricles continue to dilate to accommodate the excess fluid, but the heart loses the ability to contract forcefully. The heart muscle may eventually become so large that the coronary blood supply is inadequate, causing ischemia.

Chronic distention exhausts stores of ANP and BNP. The effects of norepinephrine, renin, and ADH prevail, and the renin–angiotensin pathway is continually stimulated. This mechanism ultimately raises the hemodynamic stress on the heart by increasing both preload and afterload. As heart function deteriorates, less blood is delivered to the tissues and to the heart itself. Ischemia and necrosis of the myocardium further weaken the already failing heart, and the cycle repeats.

In normal hearts, the cardiac reserve allows the heart to adjust its output to meet the metabolic needs of the body, increasing the cardiac output by up to five times the basal level during exercise. Clients with heart failure have minimal to no cardiac reserve. At rest, they may be unaffected; however, any stressor (e.g., exercise, illness) taxes their ability to meet the demand for oxygen and nutrients. Manifestations of activity intolerance when the individual is at rest indicate a critical level of cardiac decompensation.

Classifications

Heart failure is commonly classified in several different ways, depending on the underlying pathology. Classifications include systolic versus diastolic failure, left-sided versus right-sided failure, low-output versus high-output failure, or acute versus chronic failure.

SYSTOLIC VERSUS DIASTOLIC FAILURE   Systolic failure occurs when the ventricle fails to contract adequately to eject a sufficient volume of blood into the arterial system. Systolic function is affected by loss of myocardial cells as a result of ischemia and infarction, cardiomyopathy, or inflammation.

Diastolic failure results when the heart cannot completely relax in diastole, disrupting normal filling. Passive diastolic filling decreases, increasing the importance of atrial contraction to preload. Diastolic dysfunction results from decreased ventricular compliance caused by hypertrophic and cellular changes and impaired relaxation of the heart muscle.

LEFT-SIDED VERSUS RIGHT-SIDED FAILURE   Depending on the pathophysiology involved, either the left or the right ventricle may be primarily affected. In chronic heart failure, however, both ventricles typically are impaired to some degree.

Coronary heart disease and hypertension are common causes of left-sided heart failure, whereas right-sided heart failure often is caused by conditions that restrict blood flow to the lungs, such as acute or chronic pulmonary disease. Left-sided heart failure also can lead to right-sided failure as pressures in the pulmonary vascular system increase with congestion behind the failing left ventricle.

As left ventricular function fails, cardiac output falls. Pressures in the left ventricle and atrium increase as the amount of blood remaining in the ventricle after systole increases. These increased pressures impair filling, causing congestion and increased pressures in the pulmonary vascular system. Increased pressures in this normally low-pressure system increase fluid movement from the blood vessels into interstitial tissues and the alveoli (**Figure 16–41** ●). The manifestations of left-sided heart failure result from pulmonary congestion (backward effects) and decreased cardiac output (forward effects).

In right-sided heart failure, increased pressures in the pulmonary vasculature or right ventricular muscle damage impair the right ventricle's ability to pump blood into the pulmonary circulation. The right ventricle and atrium become distended, and blood accumulates in the systemic venous system. Increased venous pressures cause abdominal organs to become congested and peripheral tissue edema to develop (**Figure 16–42** ●). Dependent tissues tend to be affected because of the effects of gravity.

LOW-OUTPUT VERSUS HIGH-OUTPUT FAILURE
Clients with heart failure resulting from coronary heart disease, hypertension, cardiomyopathy, and other primary cardiac disorders develop low-output failure and manifestations such as those previously described. Clients in hypermetabolic states (e.g., hyperthyroidism, infection, anemia, or pregnancy) require increased cardiac output to maintain blood flow and oxygen to the tissues. If the increased blood flow cannot meet the oxygen

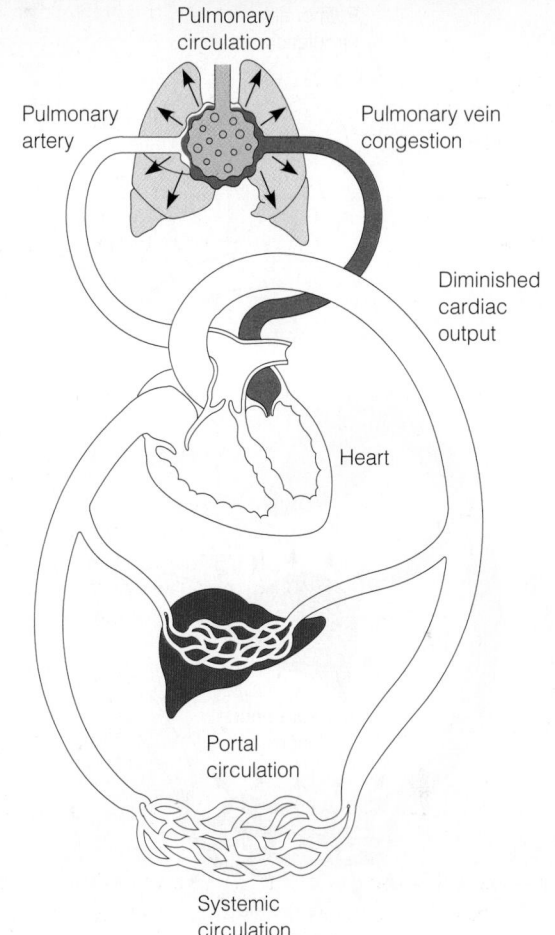

Figure 16–41 ● The hemodynamic effects of left-sided heart failure.

demands of the tissues, compensatory mechanisms are activated to further increase cardiac output, which in turn further increases oxygen demand. Thus, even though cardiac output is high, the heart is unable to meet increased oxygen demands. This condition is known as high-output failure.

ACUTE VERSUS CHRONIC FAILURE   Acute failure is the abrupt onset of a myocardial injury (e.g., a massive MI) resulting in suddenly decreased cardiac function and signs of decreased cardiac output. Chronic failure is a progressive deterioration of the heart muscle as a result of cardiomyopathies, valvular disease, or coronary heart disease.

PULMONARY EDEMA   In cardiogenic pulmonary edema, the contractility of the left ventricle is severely impaired. The ejection fraction falls because the ventricle is unable to eject the blood that enters it, causing a sharp rise in end-diastolic volume and pressure. Pulmonary hydrostatic pressures rise, ultimately exceeding the osmotic pressure of the blood. As a result, fluid leaking from the pulmonary capillaries congests interstitial spaces in the tissues, decreasing lung compliance and interfering with gas exchange. As capillary and interstitial pressures increase further, the tight junctions of the alveolar walls are disrupted, and the fluid enters the alveoli, along with large red blood cells and protein molecules. Ventilation and gas exchange are severely disrupted, and hypoxia worsens.

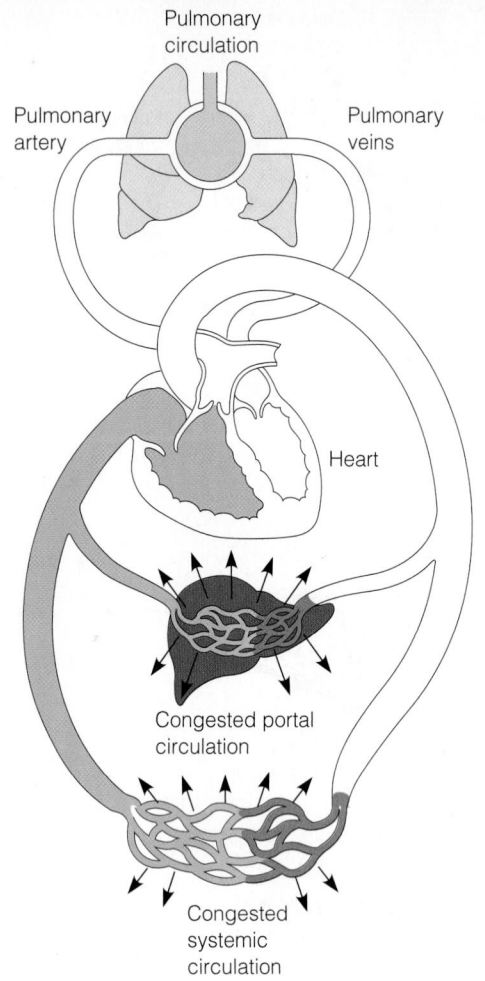

Figure 16–42 ● The hemodynamic effects of right-sided heart failure.

Etiology

The NHLBI (2013c) estimates that 5.8 million people in the United States have heart failure. At-risk populations include those 65 years of age and older, African Americans, overweight clients, clients with history of myocardial infarction, and men.

The prognosis for a client with heart failure depends on the underlying cause of the heart failure and how effectively the precipitating factors can be treated. Children diagnosed with congenital heart defects can also develop heart failure. Congenital heart defects cause the heart to work harder, weakening the heart muscle, which can lead to heart failure. Fewer than 50% of clients diagnosed with heart failure are living 5 years after the initial diagnosis with fewer than 25% alive at 10 years (Heart Failure Society of America, 2013). Clients with heart failure have an increased risk for sudden cardiac death.

Risk Factors

The most prevalent risk factors for heart failure are coronary artery disease, cigarette smoking, obesity, substance abuse, hypertension, and diabetes (NHLBI, 2013a). Other causes include cardiomyopathy, heart valve disease, arrhythmias, and

congenital heart defects. Clients who have had heart attacks are also at an increased risk of heart failure. The infarcted heart muscle dies, or becomes necrotic, which weakens the heart's ability to pump effectively. Those suffering from severe lung disease have an increased oxygenation demand placed on the heart. This places an increased workload on the heart and may result in progressive heart failure. Sleep apnea is now considered an important risk factor for developing hypertension and has been linked to heart failure, diabetes, and stroke.

Heart failure in children is most commonly a result of an overcirculation failure or pump failure. In overcirculation failure, an overload blood flow pattern occurs in one or more of the sections of the heart leading to an interruption in the normal blood flood. As a result, the heart becomes an inefficient pump. Pump failure can occur as a result of infection or a congenital defect. Often one of the heart valves does not function properly, causing pressure to back up inside the heart chambers. On rare occasions, severe chest trauma may result in pump failure.

▶ CLINICAL MANIFESTATIONS

The manifestations of systolic failure are those of decreased cardiac output: weakness, fatigue, and decreased exercise tolerance. The manifestations of diastolic failure include shortness of breath, tachypnea, and respiratory crackles if the left ventricle is affected; distended neck veins, liver enlargement, anorexia, and nausea if the right ventricle is affected. Many clients have components of both systolic and diastolic failure (see the Multisystem Effects of Heart Failure feature).

Left-Sided Failure

Fatigue and activity intolerance are common early manifestations of left-sided heart failure. Dizziness and syncope also may result from decreased cardiac output. Pulmonary congestion causes dyspnea, shortness of breath, and cough. The client may develop **orthopnea** (difficulty breathing when supine), prompting use of two or three pillows or a recliner for sleeping. Cyanosis from impaired gas exchange may be noted. On auscultation of the lungs, inspiratory crackles (rales) and wheezes may be heard in lung bases. An S_3 gallop may be present, reflecting the heart's attempts to fill an already distended ventricle.

Right-Sided Failure

In right-sided heart failure, edema develops in the feet and legs or, if the client is bedridden, in the sacrum. Congestion of gastrointestinal tract vessels causes anorexia and nausea. Right upper quadrant pain may result from liver engorgement. Neck veins distend and become visible, even when the client is upright, because of increased venous pressure.

Other Manifestations

In addition to the previous manifestations for the various classifications of heart failure, other signs and symptoms commonly are seen. A fall in cardiac output activates mechanisms that cause increased salt and water retention. This causes weight gain and further increases pressures in the capillaries, resulting in edema. **Nocturia** (voiding two or more times at night) develops as edema fluid from dependent tissues is reabsorbed while the client is supine. **Paroxysmal nocturnal dyspnea**, a frightening condition in which the client awakens at night acutely short of breath, also may develop. Paroxysmal nocturnal dyspnea occurs when edema fluid that has accumulated during the day is reabsorbed into the circulation at night, causing fluid overload and pulmonary congestion. Severe heart failure may cause dyspnea at rest as well as with activity, signifying little or no cardiac reserve. Both an S_3 and an S_4 gallop may be heard on auscultation.

Complications

The compensatory mechanisms initiated in heart failure can lead to complications in other body systems. Congestive hepatomegaly and splenomegaly caused by engorgement of the portal venous system result in increased abdominal pressure, ascites, and gastrointestinal problems. With prolonged right-sided heart failure, liver function may be impaired. Myocardial distention can precipitate dysrhythmias, further impairing cardiac output. Pleural effusions and other pulmonary problems may develop. Major complications of severe heart failure are cardiogenic.

The client with acute pulmonary edema presents with classic manifestations (**Box 16–14** ●). Dyspnea, shortness of breath, and labored respirations are acute and severe, accompanied by orthopnea. Cyanosis is present, and the skin is cool, clammy, and diaphoretic. A productive cough with pink, frothy sputum develops as a result of fluid, red blood cells, and plasma proteins in the alveoli and airways. Crackles are heard throughout the lung fields on auscultation. As the condition worsens, lung sounds become harsher. The client often is restless and highly anxious, although severe hypoxia may cause confusion or lethargy.

Box 16–14 Manifestations of Pulmonary Edema

RESPIRATORY
- Tachypnea
- Paroxysmal nocturnal dyspnea
- Labored respirations
- Cough productive of frothy, pink sputum
- Dyspnea
- Crackles, wheezes
- Orthopnea

CARDIOVASCULAR
- Tachycardia
- Cool, clammy skin
- Hypotension
- Hypoxemia
- Cyanosis
- Ventricular gallop

NEUROLOGICAL
- Restlessness
- Feeling of impending doom
- Anxiety

As noted earlier, pulmonary edema is a medical emergency. Without rapid and effective intervention, severe tissue hypoxia and acidosis will lead to organ system failure and death.

▶ COLLABORATION

The main goals for care of the client with heart failure are to slow its progression, reduce cardiac workload, improve cardiac function, and control fluid retention. Treatment strategies are based on the evolution and progression of heart failure (**Table 16–26** ●).

TABLE 16–26 Stages of Heart Failure

STAGE	DESCRIPTION	RECOMMENDED INTERVENTIONS
I (mild)	No limitation of physical activity. No shortness of breath noted with normal physical activity.	Regular exercise. Smoking cessation. Treatment of hypertension. Treatment of hyperlipidemia. Discontinuation of alcohol or illegal drug use. Possible addition of ACE inhibitor or angiotensin II receptor blocker (ARB), or beta-blocker to medication regime.
II (mild)	Some physical limitations due to fatigue, shortness of breath, or palpitations. Client comfortable at rest.	Class I interventions. ACE inhibitor or ARB, and beta-blocker as indicated. Surgical options include coronary artery repair and valve repair or replacement.
III (moderate)	Increased physical limitations. Less than normal physical activity results in fatigue, shortness of breath, or palpitations. Client comfortable at rest.	Class I interventions. Addition of diuretic, ACE inhibitor, ARB, and/or beta-blocker to medication regime. Additional drugs may include aldosterone inhibitor, digitalis, hydralazine, nitrates. Restrict dietary sodium. Monitor weight. Restrict fluids, as needed. Discontinue drugs that worsen condition. Surgical options may include biventricular pacing or implantable defibrillator.
IV (severe)	Any degree of physical activity results in increased discomfort. Client exhibits symptoms of cardiac insufficiency at rest.	Interventions for Classes I, II, and III. Evaluation for available options. Interventions include heart transplant, ventricular assist devices, surgery, research therapies, continuous infusion of intravenous heart pump medication, and palliative or hospice care.

Multisystem Effects of Heart Failure

Neurologic
- Confusion
- Impaired memory
- Anxiety, restlessness
- Insomnia

Respiratory
- Dyspnea on exertion
- Shortness of breath
- Tachypnea
- Orthopnea
- Dry cough
- Crackles (rales) in lung bases

Potential Complications
- Pulmonary edema
- Pneumonia
- Cardiac asthma
- Pleural effusion
- Cheyne-Stokes respirations
- Respiratory acidosis

Cardiovascular
- Activity intolerance
- Tachycardia
- Palpitations
- S_3, S_4 heart sounds
- Elevated central venous pressure
- Neck vein distention
- Hepatojugular reflux
- Splenomegaly

Potential Complications
- Angina
- Dysrhythmias
- Sudden cardiac death
- Cardiogenic shock

Gastrointestinal
- Anorexia, nausea
- Abdominal distention
- Liver enlargement
- Right upper quadrant pain

Potential Complications
- Malnutrition
- Ascites
- Liver dysfunction

Genitourinary
- Decreased urine output
- Nocturia

Integumentary
- Pallor or cyanosis
- Cool, clammy skin
- Diaphoresis

Potential Complications
- Increased risk for tissue breakdown

Musculoskeletal
- Fatigue
- Weakness

Metabolic Processes
- Peripheral edema
- Weight gain

Potential Complication
- Metabolic acidosis

Diagnostic Tests

Diagnosis of heart failure is based on the history, physical examination, and diagnostic findings. Relevant diagnostic tests include the following:

- *Atrial natriuretic peptide (ANP), also called atrial natriuretic hormone, and brain natriuretic peptide (BNP)* are hormones released by the heart muscle in response to changes in blood volume. Blood levels of these hormones increase in heart failure. BNP levels, in particular, have been shown to positively correlate with pressures in the left ventricle and the pulmonary vascular system. The level of BNP in the blood increases as the symptoms of heart failure worsen and decreases when the heart failure stabilizes. BNP levels may be elevated in women and clients over age 60 who do not have a diagnosis of heart failure. Therefore, they should not be considered as the primary diagnostic tool.

- *Serum electrolytes* are measured to evaluate fluid and electrolyte status. Serum osmolarity may be low because of fluid retention. Sodium, potassium, and chloride levels provide a baseline for evaluating the effects of treatment; serum calcium and magnesium are measured as well.

- *Urinalysis, blood urea nitrogen, and serum creatinine* are obtained to evaluate renal function.

- *Liver function tests,* including alanine aminotransferase, aspartate aminotransferase, lactate dehydrogenase, serum bilirubin, and total protein and albumin levels, are obtained to evaluate possible effects of heart failure on liver function.

- *Thyroid function tests* can indicate hyperthyroidism and hypothyroidism, which can produce symptoms resembling those of heart failure.

- *Arterial blood gas* levels are determined to evaluate gas exchange in the lungs and tissues in the client with acute heart failure.

- *Chest x-ray* may show pulmonary vascular congestion and cardiomegaly in heart failure.

- *Electrocardiography* is used to identify ECG changes associated with ventricular enlargement and to detect dysrhythmias, myocardial ischemia, or infarction.

- *Echocardiography with Doppler flow studies* are performed to evaluate left ventricular function. Either transthoracic echocardiography or transesophageal echocardiography may be used.

Hemodynamic Monitoring

Hemodynamics is the study of forces involved in blood circulation. Hemodynamic monitoring is used to assess cardiovascular function in the client who is critically ill or unstable. The main goals of invasive hemodynamic monitoring are to evaluate cardiac and circulatory function and the response to interventions.

Hemodynamic parameters include heart rate, arterial blood pressure, central venous or right atrial pressure, pulmonary pressures, and cardiac output. Direct hemodynamic parameters are obtained straight from the monitoring device (e.g., heart rate and arterial and venous pressures). Indirect or derived measurements are calculated using the direct data (e.g., the cardiac index, mean arterial blood pressure, and stroke volume). Invasive hemodynamic monitoring is routinely used in critical care units.

Hemodynamic monitoring systems measure the pressure within a vessel and convert this signal into an electrical waveform that is amplified and displayed. The electrical signal may be recorded on graph paper and displayed digitally on the monitor. System components include an invasive catheter threaded into an artery or vein connected to a transducer by stiff, high-pressure tubing. The pressure transducer translates pressures into an electrical signal that is relayed to the monitor. Additional components of the system include stopcocks and a continuous flush system with normal saline or heparinized saline and an infusion pressure bag to prevent clots from forming in the catheter. **Figure 16–43** ● illustrates a pressure transducer and typical hemodynamic monitoring system.

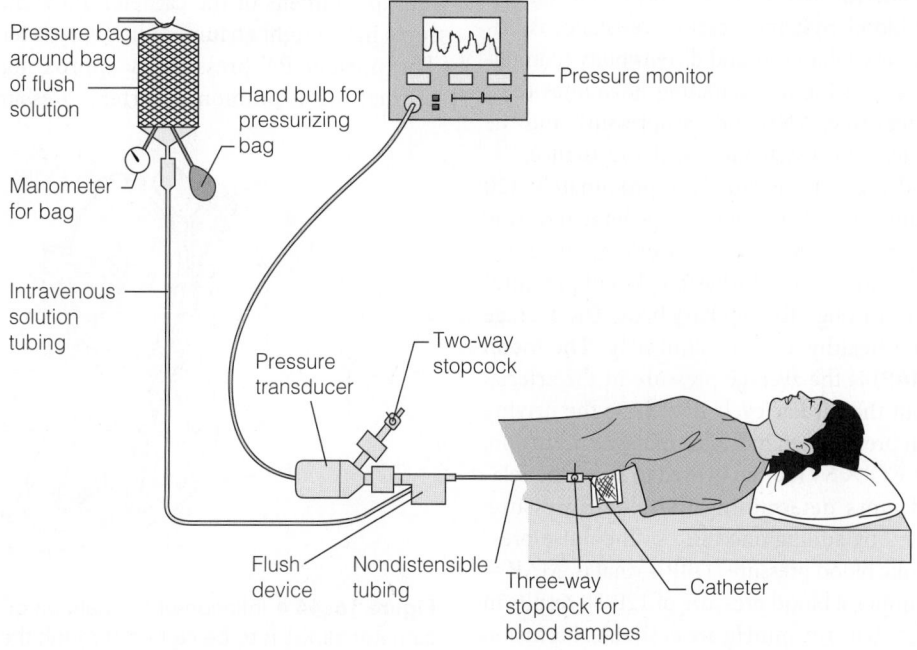

Pressure bag around bag of flush solution
Hand bulb for pressurizing bag
Pressure monitor
Manometer for bag
Intravenous solution tubing
Pressure transducer
Two-way stopcock
Flush device
Nondistensible tubing
Three-way stopcock for blood samples
Catheter

Figure 16–43 ● A hemodynamic monitoring setup.

Box 16–15   Potential Complications of Central Catheters

- Bleeding
- Hematoma
- Pneumothorax
- Hemothorax
- Arterial puncture
- Dysrhythmias
- Venospasm
- Infection
- Air embolism
- Thromboembolism
- Brachial nerve injury
- Thoracic nerve injury

Hemodynamic pressure monitoring may be used to measure peripheral artery pressures or central pressures, such as central venous pressure or right atrial pressure and pulmonary artery pressure. Although the information obtained from invasive monitoring is valuable, the procedure is not without risk. Box 16–15 ● lists potential complications of central pressure monitoring.

INTRA-ARTERIAL PRESSURE MONITORING   Intra-arterial pressure monitoring is commonly used in intensive and coronary care units. An indwelling arterial line, commonly called an art line or an A line, allows direct and continuous monitoring of systolic, diastolic, and mean arterial blood pressures and provides easy access for arterial blood sampling. Arterial lines are used to assess blood volume, to monitor the effects of vasoactive drugs, and to obtain frequent ABG determinations. Because the invasive catheter is inserted directly into the artery, it offers immediate access for blood gas measurements and blood testing.

The arterial blood pressure reflects the cardiac output and the resistance to blood flow created by the elastic arterial walls (systemic vascular resistance [SVR]). Cardiac output is determined by the blood volume and the ability of the ventricles to fill and effectively pump that blood. Systemic vascular resistance is primarily determined by vessel diameter and distensibility (compliance). Factors such as SNS input, circulating hormones (e.g., epinephrine, norepinephrine, ANP, and vasopressin), and the renin–angiotensin system affect systemic vascular resistance.

The systolic blood pressure, normally approximately 120 mmHg in healthy adults, reflects the pressure generated during ventricular systole. During diastole, elastic arterial walls keep a minimum pressure within the vessel (diastolic blood pressure) to maintain blood flow through the capillary beds. The average diastolic pressure in a healthy adult is 80 mmHg. The **mean arterial pressure (MAP)** is the average pressure in the arterial circulation throughout the cardiac cycle. It reflects the driving pressure, or perfusion pressure, an indicator of tissue perfusion. The formula MAP = CO × SVR often is used to show the relationships between factors determining the blood pressure. MAP can be calculated by adding one third of the pulse pressure (PP) to the diastolic blood pressure (DBP)—that is, MAP = DBP + PP/3. For example, a blood pressure of 120/80 results in a MAP of 93. MAPs of 70 to 105 mmHg are desirable. Perfusion to vital organs is severely jeopardized at MAPs of 50 or less;

MAPs of greater than 105 mmHg may indicate hypertension or vasoconstriction.

VENOUS PRESSURE MONITORING   Central venous pressure (CVP) and right atrial pressure are measures of blood volume and venous return. They also reflect right-heart filling pressures. Pressures are elevated in right-sided heart failure. CVP and right atrial pressure are primarily used to monitor fluid volume status. To measure venous and atrial pressures, a catheter is inserted in the internal jugular or subclavian vein. The distal tip of the catheter is positioned in the superior vena cava just above or just inside the right atrium. CVP may be measured in either centimeters of water (cm H_2O) or millimeters of mercury (mmHg). A water manometer is a clear tube with calibrated markings that is attached between a central catheter and the intravenous fluid bag. Pressure in the venous system causes fluid in the manometer to rise or fall. The CVP is recorded by noting the fluid level in the manometer. If the central line is connected to a pressure transducer, venous pressure is displayed digitally in millimeters of mercury.

The normal range for CVP is 2–8 cm H_2O or 2–6 mmHg, but CVP varies in individual clients. Hypovolemia and shock decrease the CVP; fluid overload, vasoconstriction, and cardiac tamponade increase CVP.

PULMONARY ARTERY PRESSURE MONITORING   The pulmonary artery (PA) catheter is a flow-directed, balloon-tipped catheter first used in the early 1970s. The PA catheter is often called a Swan–Ganz catheter, after the physicians who developed it. The PA catheter is used to evaluate left ventricular and overall cardiac function. The PA catheter is inserted into a central vein, usually the internal jugular or subclavian vein, and threaded into the right atrium. A small balloon at the tip of the catheter allows the catheter to be drawn into the right ventricle and, from there, into the pulmonary artery (**Figure 16–44 ●**). The inflated balloon carries the catheter forward until the balloon wedges in a small branch of pulmonary vasculature. Once in place, the balloon is deflated, and multiple lumens of the catheter allow measurement of pressures in the right atrium, pulmonary artery, and left ventricle. The normal PA pressure is approximately 25/10 mmHg; normal mean pulmonary artery pressure is approximately

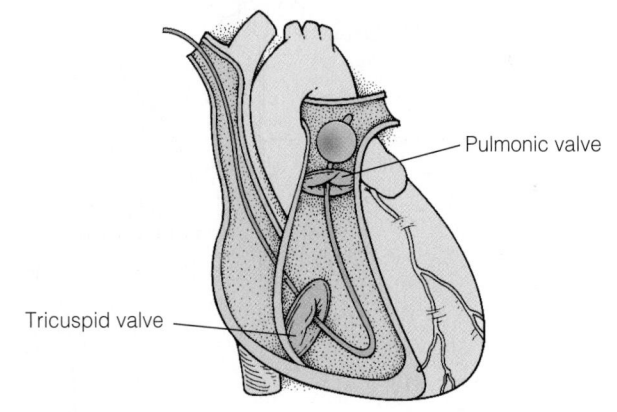

Figure 16–44 ● Inflation of the balloon on the flow-directed catheter allows it to be carried through the pulmonic valve into the pulmonary artery.

Right Ventricular (RV) Pressure

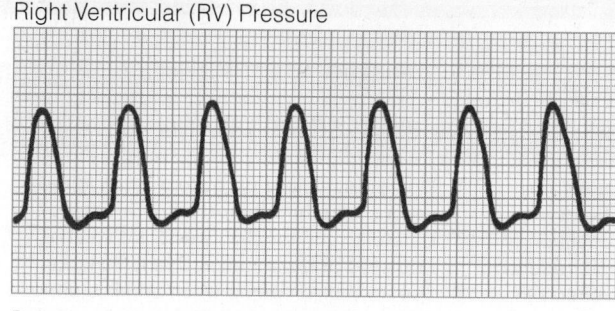

Pulmonary Artery Pressure (PAP)

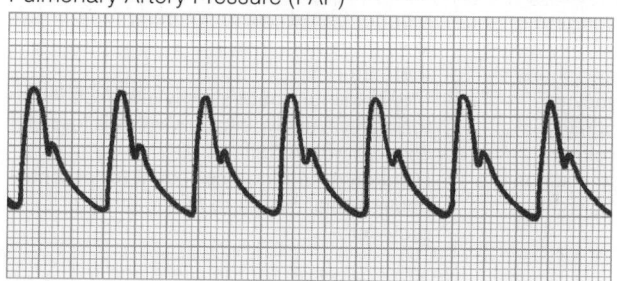

....

Figure 16–45 ● Typical waveforms seen when measuring, *A*, pulmonary artery pressure and, *B*, pulmonary wedge pressure.

15 mmHg (**Figure 16–45A** ●). Pulmonary artery pressure is increased in left-sided heart failure.

Inflation of the balloon effectively blocks pressure from behind the balloon and allows measurement of pressures generated by the left ventricle. This is known as the pulmonary artery wedge pressure (PAWP) and is used to assess left ventricular function. The normal PAWP is 8–12 mmHg (Figure 16–45*B*). PAWP is increased in left ventricular failure and pericardial tamponade, and decreased in hypovolemia.

Cardiac output also can be measured with the PA catheter using a technique called thermodilution. Cardiac output and the cardiac index are used to assess the heart's ability to meet the body's oxygen demands. Because body size affects overall cardiac output, the cardiac index is a more precise measure of heart function. The cardiac index is a calculation of cardiac output per square meter of body surface area. The normal cardiac index is 2.8–4.2 L/min/m^2.

Pharmacologic Therapy

Clients with heart failure often receive multiple medications to reduce cardiac work and improve cardiac function. The main drug classes used to treat heart failure are the ACE inhibitors, ARBs, beta-blockers, diuretics, positive inotropic medications (including digitalis, sympathomimetic agents, and phosphodiesterase inhibitors), direct vasodilators, and antidysrhythmic drugs. Medication administration for heart failure is summarized in the Medications feature.

ANGIOTENSIN-CONVERTING ENZYME INHIBITORS

Angiotensin-converting enzyme inhibitors interrupt the conversion of angiotensin I to angiotensin II by inhibiting the enzyme that mediates the conversion (i.e., ACE). Angiotensin II causes intense vasoconstriction, increasing afterload and ventricular wall stress and increasing preload and ventricular dila-

tion. It also stimulates aldosterone and ADH production, causing fluid retention. ACE inhibitors block this renin–angiotensin system activity, decreasing cardiac work and increasing cardiac output. They dilate the blood vessels, which results in increased blood flow and decreased cardiac workload.

ANGIOTENSIN II–RECEPTOR BLOCKERS

In contrast to ACE inhibitors, ARBs do not block the production of angiotensin II; instead, they block its action. The pharmacologic effect is similar, and they also are used in heart failure to slow its progression, reduce manifestations, and prevent cardiac complications.

BETA-BLOCKERS

Beta-blockers improve cardiac function in heart failure by inhibiting SNS activity. This prevents the long-term deleterious effects of sympathetic stimulation. Because beta-blockers reduce the force of myocardial contraction and may actually worsen symptoms, they are used in low doses. The combination of ACE inhibitors and beta-blockers improves client outcomes.

DIURETICS

Clients with symptomatic heart failure often are treated with diuretics, which relieve symptoms related to fluid retention. Diuretics may, however, cause significant electrolyte imbalances and rapid fluid loss. Clients with severe heart failure are often treated with a loop, or high-ceiling, diuretic, such as furosemide (Lasix), bumetanide (Bumex), torsemide (Demadex), or ethacrynic acid (Edecrin). These drugs have a rapid onset of action, inhibiting chloride reabsorption in the ascending loop of Henle and thus prompting sodium and water excretion. Their major drawback is their efficacy in promoting diuresis; loss of vascular volume can stimulate the SNS. Thiazide diuretics may be used for clients with less severe manifestations of heart failure. These agents promote fluid excretion by blocking sodium reabsorption in the terminal loop of Henle and the distal tubule.

VASODILATORS

Vasodilators relax smooth muscle in blood vessels, causing dilation. Arterial dilation reduces peripheral vascular resistance and afterload, reducing myocardial work. Venous dilation reduces venous return and preload. Pulmonary vascular relaxation reduces pulmonary capillary pressure, allowing reabsorption of fluid from interstitial tissues and the alveoli. Vasodilators include nitrates, hydralazine, and prazosin, an alpha-adrenergic blocker.

Nitrates produce both arterial and venous vasodilation. They may be given by nasal spray or the sublingual, oral, or intravenous route. Sodium nitroprusside is a potent vasodilator that may be used to treat acute heart failure. It can cause excessive hypotension, however, so it is often given along with dopamine or dobutamine to maintain the blood pressure. Isosorbide or nitroglycerin ointment may be used in long-term management of heart failure.

In 2005, the U.S. Food and Drug Administration (FDA) approved a new drug for treatment of heart failure in African Americans. This drug, known as BiDil, is a combination of two vasodilators, hydralazine and isosorbide, in fixed doses. BiDil has proven beneficial in extending life, improving heart failure symptoms, and decreasing hospital readmissions related to heart failure.

DIGITALIS

Digitalis glycosides are used judiciously in symptomatic heart failure. Digitalis has a positive inotropic effect on the heart, increasing the strength of myocardial contraction by increasing the intracellular calcium concentrations. Digitalis

Medications **Heart Failure**

CLASSIFICATION AND DRUG EXAMPLES	MECHANISMS OF ACTION	NURSING CONSIDERATIONS
Angiotensin-Converting Enzyme (ACE) Inhibitors *Drug examples:* ▪ enalapril (Vasotec) ▪ lisinopril (Prinivil, Zestril) ▪ captopril (Capoten) ▪ fosinopril (Monopril) ▪ moexipril (Univasc) ▪ quinapril (Accupril) ▪ ramipril (Altace) ▪ trandolapril (Mavik) **Angiotensin II Receptor Blockers (ARBS)** *Drug examples:* ▪ candesartan (Atacand) ▪ irbesartan (Avapro) ▪ losartan (Cozaar) ▪ telmisartan (Micardis) ▪ valsartan (Diovan)	ACE inhibitors and ARBs prevent acute coronary events and reduce mortality in heart failure. ACE inhibitors interfere with production of angiotensin II, resulting in vasodilation, reduced blood volume, and prevention of its effects in the heart and blood vessels. In heart failure, ACE inhibitors reduce afterload and improve cardiac output and renal blood flow. They also reduce pulmonary congestion and peripheral edema. ACE inhibitors suppress myocyte growth and reduce ventricular remodeling in heart failure. Although the pharmacologic effect of ARBs is similar, they block the action of angiotensin II at the receptor rather than interfering with its production.	▪ Do not give these drugs to women in the second and third trimesters of pregnancy. ▪ Carefully monitor clients who are volume depleted or have impaired renal function. ▪ Use an infusion pump when administering ACE inhibitors intravenously. ▪ Monitor blood pressure closely for 2 hr following the first dose and as indicated thereafter. ▪ Monitor serum potassium levels; ACE inhibitors can cause hyperkalemia (this is less of a concern with ARBs). ▪ Monitor white blood cell count for potential neutropenia. Report to the healthcare provider. *Health education for the client and family:* ▪ Take the drug at the same time every day to ensure a stable blood level. ▪ Monitor your blood pressure and weight weekly. Report significant changes to your healthcare provider. ▪ Avoid making sudden position changes (e.g., rise from bed slowly). Lie down if you become dizzy or light-headed, particularly after the first dose. ▪ Report any signs of easy bruising and bleeding, sore throat or fever, edema, or skin rash. Immediately report swelling of the face, lips, or eyelids and any itching or breathing problems. ▪ A persistent, dry cough may develop if you are taking an ACE inhibitor. Contact your healthcare provider if this becomes a problem. ▪ Take captopril or moexipril 1 hr before meals.
Diuretics *Drug examples:* ▪ chlorothiazide (Diuril) ▪ spironolactone (Aldactone) ▪ furosemide (Lasix) ▪ triamterene (Dyrenium) ▪ ethacrynic acid (Edecrin) ▪ amiloride (Midamor) ▪ bumetanide (Bumex) ▪ acetazolamide (Diamox) ▪ hydrochlorothiazide (HydroDIURIL)	Diuretics act on different portions of the kidney tubule to inhibit the reabsorption of sodium and water and promote their excretion. With the exception of the potassium-sparing diuretics (spironolactone, triamterene, and amiloride) diuretics also promote potassium excretion, increasing the risk of hypokalemia. Spironolactone, an aldosterone receptor blocker, reduces symptoms and slows progression of heart failure. Aldosterone receptors in the heart and blood vessels promote myocardial remodeling and fibrosis, activate the sympathetic nervous system, and promote vascular fibrosis (which decreases compliance) and baroreceptor dysfunction.	▪ Obtain baseline weight and vital signs. ▪ Monitor blood pressure, intake and output, weight, skin turgor, and edema as indicators of fluid volume status. ▪ Assess for volume depletion, particularly with loop diuretics (furosemide, ethacrynic acid, and bumetanide): dizziness, orthostatic hypotension, tachycardia, and muscle cramping. ▪ Report abnormal serum electrolyte levels to the healthcare provider. Replace electrolytes as indicated. ▪ Do not administer potassium replacements to clients receiving a potassium-sparing diuretic. ▪ Evaluate renal function by assessing urine output, blood urea nitrogen, and serum creatinine. ▪ Administer intravenous furosemide slowly, no faster than 20 mg/min. Evaluate for signs of ototoxicity. Do not administer this drug or ethacrynic acid concurrently with aminoglycoside antibiotics (e.g., gentamicin), which are also ototoxic.

Medications **Heart Failure** (continued)

CLASSIFICATION AND DRUG EXAMPLES	MECHANISMS OF ACTION	NURSING CONSIDERATIONS
		Health education for the client and family: - Drink at least six to eight glasses of water per day. - Take your diuretic at times that will be least disruptive to your lifestyle, usually in the morning and early afternoon if a second dose is ordered. Take with meals to decrease gastric upset. - Monitor your blood pressure, pulse, and weight weekly. Report significant weight changes to your healthcare provider. - Report any of the following to your healthcare provider: severe abdominal pain; jaundice; dark urine; abnormal bleeding or bruising; flulike symptoms; and signs of hypokalemia, hyponatremia, or dehydration (e.g., thirst, salt craving, dizziness, weakness, and rapid pulse). - Avoid sudden position changes because they may cause dizziness, light-headedness, or feelings of faintness. - Unless you are taking a potassium-sparing diuretic, integrate potassium-rich foods into your diet. Limit sodium use.
Positive Inotropic Agents *Drug examples:* - digitalis glycosides - digoxin (Lanoxin)	Digitalis improves myocardial contractility by interfering with adenosine triphosphatase in the myocardial cell membrane and increasing the amount of calcium available for contraction. The increased force of contraction causes the heart to empty more completely, increasing stroke volume and cardiac output. Improved cardiac output improves renal perfusion, decreasing renin secretion. This decreases preload and afterload, reducing cardiac work. Digitalis also has electrophysiological effects, slowing conduction through the atrioventricular node. This decreases the heart rate and reduces oxygen consumption.	- Assess apical pulse before administering. Withhold digitalis and notify the healthcare provider if heart rate is below 60 bpm and/or manifestations of decreased cardiac output are noted. Record apical rate on medication record. - Evaluate the electrocardiogram for scooped (spoon-shaped) ST segment, AV block, bradycardia, and other dysrhythmias (especially premature ventricular contractions and atrial tachycardias). - Report manifestations of digitalis toxicity: anorexia, nausea and vomiting, abdominal pain, weakness, vision changes (e.g., diplopia, blurred vision, or yellow-green or white halos seen around objects), and new-onset dysrhythmias. - Assess potassium, magnesium, calcium, and serum digoxin levels before giving digitalis. Hypokalemia can precipitate toxicity even when the serum digitalis level is in the "normal" range (*adult:* 0.5–2 ng/mL, 0.5–2 nmol/L [SI units]; *infants:* 1–3 ng/mL). - Monitor clients with renal insufficiency or renal failure and older adults carefully for digitalis toxicity. - Prepare to administer digoxin immune Fab (Digibind) for digoxin toxicity. *Health education for the client and family:* - Take your pulse daily before taking your digoxin. Do not take the digoxin if your pulse is below 60 bpm or if you are weak, fatigued, light-headed, dizzy, short of breath, or having chest pain. Instead, notify your healthcare provider immediately.

(continued on next page)

Medications **Heart Failure** (continued)

CLASSIFICATION AND DRUG EXAMPLES	MECHANISMS OF ACTION	NURSING CONSIDERATIONS
		■ Contact your healthcare provider if you develop manifestations of digitalis toxicity: palpitations, weakness, loss of appetite, nausea and vomiting, abdominal pain, blurred or colored vision, or double vision. ■ Avoid using antacids and laxatives; they decrease digoxin absorption. ■ Notify your healthcare provider immediately if you develop manifestations of potassium deficiency: weakness, lethargy, thirst, depression, muscle cramps, or vomiting. ■ Incorporate potassium-rich foods into your diet: fresh orange or tomato juice, bananas, raisins, dates, figs, prunes, apricots, spinach, cauliflower, and potatoes.
Sympathomimetic Agents *Drug examples:* ■ dopamine (Intropin) ■ dobutamine (Dobutrex)	Sympathomimetic agents stimulate the heart, improving the force of contraction. Dobutamine is preferred in managing heart failure because it does not increase the heart rate as much as dopamine and it has a mild vasodilatory effect. These drugs are given by intravenous infusion and may be titrated to obtain their optimal effects.	■ Monitor blood pressure, pulse, peripheral pulses, and urinary output. ■ Immediately report reduced urine flow rate in absence of hypotension, dysrhythmias, marked changes in blood pressure, signs of peripheral ischemia, and ascending tachycardia. ■ Monitor for therapeutic effectiveness (e.g., loss of pallor, capillary refill time, reversal of confusion or coma).
Phosphodiesterase Inhibitors *Drug examples:* ■ amrinone (Inocor) ■ milrinone (Primacor)	Phosphodiesterase inhibitors are used in treating acute heart failure to increase myocardial contractility and cause vasodilation. The net effects are an increase in cardiac output and a decrease in afterload.	■ Use an infusion pump to administer these agents. Monitor hemodynamic parameters carefully. ■ Avoid discontinuing these drugs abruptly. ■ Change solutions and tubing every 24 hr. ■ Amrinone is given as an intravenous bolus over 2–3 min, followed by an infusion of 5–10 mg · kg^{-1} · min^{-1}. ■ Amrinone may be infused full strength or diluted in either normal or half-strength saline. Do not mix this drug with dextrose solutions. After dilution, amrinone can be piggybacked into a line containing a dextrose solution. ■ Monitor liver function and platelet counts; amrinone may cause hepatotoxicity and thrombocytopenia. *Health education for the client and family:* ■ Notify the healthcare provider if you experience abdominal pain or notice a skin rash or bruising.

also decreases SA node automaticity and slows conduction through the AV node, increasing ventricular filling time.

Digitalis has a narrow therapeutic index; in other words, therapeutic levels are very close to toxic levels. Early manifestations of digitalis toxicity include anorexia, nausea and vomiting, headache, altered vision, and confusion. A number of cardiac dysrhythmias are also associated with digitalis toxicity, including sinus arrest, supraventricular and ventricular tachycardias, and high levels of AV block. Low serum potassium levels increase the risk of digitalis toxicity, as do low magnesium and high calcium levels. Older adults are at particular risk for digitalis toxicity.

Digitalis levels may be affected by a number of other drugs. The nurse should check for potential interactions.

ANTIDYSRHYTHMICS   Dysrhythmias are common in clients with heart failure. Although premature ventricular contractions may be frequent, they are often not associated with an increased risk of ventricular tachycardia and fibrillation. Because many antidysrhythmic medications depress left ventricular function, premature ventricular contractions are frequently left untreated in heart failure. Amiodarone is the drug of choice to treat nonsustained ventricular tachycardia, which is associated with a poor prognosis.

Nutrition and Activity

A sodium-restricted diet is recommended to minimize sodium and water retention. Intake is generally limited to 1.5–2 g of

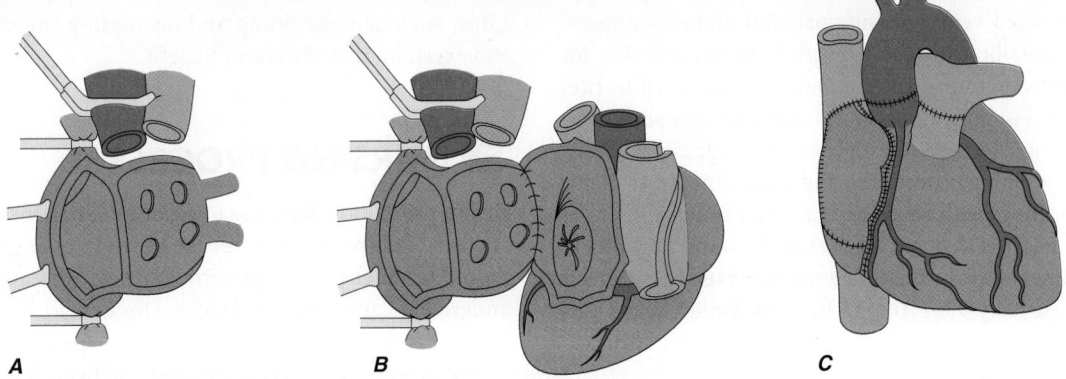

Figure 16–46 ● Cardiac transplantation. *A,* The heart is removed, leaving the posterior walls of the atria intact. *B,* The donor heart is anastomosed to the atria and, *C,* the great vessels.

sodium per day, a moderate restriction. See the exemplar on Fluid and Electrolyte Imbalance in the module on Fluids and Electrolytes for a list of high-sodium foods to avoid and for client teaching regarding a sodium-restricted diet.

Exercise intolerance (decreased ability to participate in activities using large skeletal muscles because of fatigue or dyspnea) is a common early manifestation of heart failure. Activity may be restricted to bed rest during acute episodes of heart failure to reduce cardiac workload and allow the heart to recompensate. Prolonged bed rest and continued activity limitations, however, are not recommended. A moderate, progressive activity program is prescribed to improve myocardial function. Aerobic exercise should be performed 3–7 days per week, and each session should include a 10- to 15-minute warm-up period, 20–30 minutes of exercise at the recommended intensity, and a cool-down period. It is important for clients to listen to their bodies by working with the cardiac rehab team in order to develop an awareness of the target heart rate. Flexibility exercises and weight training should be incorporated into the exercise routine.

Surgery

In end-stage heart failure, devices to provide circulatory assistance or surgery may be required. Surgery may be used to treat the underlying cause of failure (e.g., replacement of diseased valves) or improve quality of life. Heart transplant is currently the only clearly effective surgical treatment for end-stage heart failure; however, its use is limited by the availability of donor hearts.

CIRCULATORY ASSISTANCE Devices such as the intra-aortic balloon pump or a left-ventricular assist device may be used when the client is expected to recover or as a bridge to transplant. Newer devices that will allow longer-term support outside the hospital are in the developmental stages. These devices will either serve as a bridge to transplant or allow the myocardium to heal over an extended period of time.

CARDIAC TRANSPLANTATION Heart transplant is the treatment of choice for end-stage heart disease. Approximately 85%–90% of cardiac transplantation clients are living 1-year posttransplant. The estimated 3-year survival rate is 75%.

The most frequently used transplant procedure leaves the posterior walls of the atria, the superior and inferior venae cavae, and

the pulmonary veins of the recipient intact (**Figure 16–46A** ●). The atrial walls of the donor heart are then anastomosed to the recipient's atria (Figure 16–46B), and the donor pulmonary artery and aorta are anastomosed to the recipient vessels (Figure 16–46C). Care is taken to avoid damaging the sinus node of the donor heart and to ensure integrity of the suture line to prevent postoperative bleeding. Donor organs typically are obtained from young accident victims with no evidence of cardiac trauma.

Nursing care of the client with a heart transplant is similar to care of the client with any cardiac surgery. Bleeding is a major concern during the early postoperative period. Chest tube drainage is frequently monitored (initially every 15 minutes), as are the cardiac output, pulmonary artery pressures, and CVP. **Cardiac tamponade** (compression of the heart) can develop, presenting as either a sudden event or a gradual process. Chest tubes are gently milked (not stripped) as needed to maintain patency. Atrial dysrhythmias are relatively common following cardiac transplant. Temporary pacing wires are placed during surgery because the conduction system may be disrupted by surgical manipulation or postoperative swelling. Hypothermia is induced during surgery; postoperatively, the client is gradually rewarmed over a 1- to 2-hour period. Prevention of rapid rewarming and shivering are important to maintain hemodynamic stability and reduce oxygen consumption. Cardiac function is impaired in up to 50% of transplanted hearts during the early postoperative period. After the transplant procedure, recipients may be placed on a combination of inotropic agents while the donor heart regains energy stores and is able to maintain adequate cardiac output.

Infection and rejection are major postoperative concerns; these are the chief causes of mortality in clients with a transplant. Rejection may develop immediately after transplant (a rare occurrence), within weeks to months, or years after the transplant. Acute rejection usually presents within weeks of the transplant, developing when the transplanted organ is recognized by the immune system as foreign. Lymphocytes infiltrate the organ, and myocardial cell necrosis can be detected on biopsy. Clients are started on immunosuppression therapy soon after surgery and are maintained on a regimen that typically includes one to three drugs. Although immunosuppressive medications help prevent organ rejection, they impair the client's defenses against infection. Early postoperative infections commonly are bacterial or fungal (*Candida* sp.). Multiple invasive lines, prolonged ventilator support, and immunosuppressive therapy contribute to the transplant recipient's risk for infection. Infection control interventions are required to prevent healthcare-associated infections. Nursing care should be aimed at reducing exposure to exogenous pathogens, maintaining strict hand washing procedures, and instituting neutropenic precautions for those with weakened immune systems.

The donor heart is denervated during the transplant procedure. Lack of innervation by the autonomic nervous system affects the heart rate (usually 90–110 bpm in transplanted hearts), its response to position changes, stress, exercise, and certain drugs.

OTHER PROCEDURES   Other surgical procedures, such as cardiomyoplasty and ventricular reduction surgery, do not improve the prognosis or quality of life in clients with end-stage heart failure. Cardiomyoplasty involves wrapping the latissimus dorsi muscle around the heart to support the failing myocardium. The muscle is stimulated in synchrony with the heart, providing a more forceful contraction and increasing cardiac output. In ventricular reduction surgery (or partial ventriculectomy), the size of the damaged heart is reduced by excising a portion of the left ventricular wall. This procedure increases the ventricular diameter to a more optimal size. The efficiency of the remaining left ventricle improves and the failing heart pumps more effectively.

Complementary and Alternative Therapy

Strong evidence supports the use of several complementary therapies for heart failure. Hawthorn, a shrubby tree, contains natural cardiotonic ingredients in its blossoms, leaves, and fruit. It increases the force of myocardial contraction, dilates blood vessels, and has a natural ACE inhibitor. Studies have shown that adding extract of hawthorn to standard heart failure medications might worsen early disease progression. Hawthorn should not be used without consultation with the primary care provider and experienced herb practitioner. Nutritional supplements of coenzyme Q10, magnesium, and thiamine may be used in conjunction with other treatments. Coenzyme Q10 improves mitochondria function and energy production.

End-of-Life Care

Unless the client receives a cardiac transplant, chronic heart failure is ultimately a terminal disease. The client and family need honest discussions about the anticipated course of the disease and treatment options. It is important to discuss advance directives, such as the living will and medical power of attorney, and differentiating potential acute events from which recovery would be anticipated (e.g., a reversible exacerbation of heart failure or a sudden cardiac arrest) from prolonged life support without reasonable expectation of functional recovery. Hospice services are available for clients with heart failure and should be offered when appropriate. Severe dyspnea is common in the final stages of the disease and may be one of the most distressing symptoms for healthcare providers and family members. Treatment is symptomatic and may involve the administration of narcotic analgesic and/or diuretics. Nonpharmacologic measures, such as positioning and decreasing the client's anxiety and exertion, may also be of benefit.

NURSING PROCESS

Health promotion activities to reduce the risk for and incidence of heart failure are directed at lifestyle changes. The nurse should teach clients about coronary heart disease, the primary underlying cause of heart failure. Discuss risk factors for coronary heart disease and ways to reduce those risk factors.

Hypertension also is a major cause of heart failure. The nurse should routinely screen clients for elevated blood pressure, and refer clients to a primary care provider as indicated. Discuss the importance of effectively managing hypertension to reduce the future risk for heart failure. Likewise, stress the relationship between effective diabetes management and reduced risk for heart failure.

Heart failure affects the client's quality of life, interfering with such daily activities as self-care and role performance. Reducing the oxygen demand of the heart is a major nursing care goal for the client in acute heart failure. This includes providing rest and carrying out prescribed treatment measures to reduce cardiac work, improve contractility, and manage symptoms. Provide information on and offer assistance with smoking cessation and substance abuse recovery.

Assessment

Obtain the following subjective and objective data when assessing the client with heart failure:

- *Health history.* Complaints of increasing shortness of breath, dyspnea with exertion, decreasing activity tolerance, or paroxysmal nocturnal dyspnea; number of pillows used for sleeping; recent weight gain; presence of a cough; chest or abdominal pain; anorexia or nausea; history of cardiac disease or previous episodes of heart failure; other risk factors, such as hypertension or diabetes; current medications; usual diet and activity as well as any recent changes.
- *Physical examination.* General appearance; ease of breathing, conversing, and changing positions; apparent anxiety; vital signs, including apical pulse; color of the skin and mucous membranes; neck vein distention, peripheral pulses, capillary refill, and presence and degree of edema; heart and breath sounds; abdominal contour, bowel sounds, and tenderness; right upper abdominal tenderness and liver enlargement.

Diagnosis

Nursing diagnoses appropriate for the client diagnosed with heart failure may include the following:

- *Decreased Cardiac Output*
- *Excess Fluid Volume*
- *Activity Intolerance*
- *Deficient Knowledge.*

(NANDA-I © 2015)

Planning

Goals of care for the client with heart failure often include the following:

- The client will describe the purpose of each medication prescribed and which symptoms to report.
- The client will maintain adequate oxygenation, as demonstrated by respiratory status, breath sounds, oxygen saturation, and vital signs.
- The client will maintain adequate tissue perfusion and myocardial function, as demonstrated by capillary refill, hemodynamic monitoring, assessment of pulses, and vital signs.
- The client will meet the body's energy needs through adequate and appropriate nutrition.

Implementation

Nursing care is focused on promoting perfusion, improving oxygenation, and reducing fear and anxiety. A diagnosis of a disorder related to the heart often produces great fear of death and disability in the client because the heart is vital to life. Helping the client and family to cope with this fear is an important component of nursing care. Anxiety secondary to hypoxia is also anticipated and requires nursing intervention.

Maintain Cardiac Output

As the heart fails as a pump, stroke volume and tissue perfusion decrease. The nurse should do the following:

- Monitor the client's vital signs and oxygen saturation as indicated. Decreased cardiac output stimulates the SNS to increase the heart rate in an attempt to restore output. Tachycardia at rest is common. Diastolic blood pressure may initially be elevated because of vasoconstriction; in late stages, compensatory mechanisms fail and blood pressure falls. Oxygen saturation levels provide a measure of gas exchange and tissue perfusion.
- Monitor the client's BNP levels, reporting trends. BNP levels indicate the severity of heart failure: As the cardiac index decreases and left ventricular pressures increase, BNP levels increase. Noting trends provides additional information about cardiac output and effectiveness of the cardiac pump.
- Auscultate the client's heart and breath sounds according to unit policy and clinical indications. The S_1 and S_2 heart sounds may be diminished if cardiac function is poor. A ventricular gallop (S_3) is an early sign of heart failure; an atrial gallop (S_4) may also be present. Crackles are often heard in the lung bases; increasing crackles, dyspnea, and shortness of breath indicate worsening failure.
- Administer supplemental oxygen as ordered. This improves oxygenation of the blood, decreasing the effects of hypoxia and ischemia.
- Administer prescribed medications as ordered. Drugs are used to decrease the cardiac workload and increase the effectiveness of contractions.
- Encourage rest, explaining the rationale. Elevate the head of the bed to reduce the work of breathing. Provide a bedside commode, and assist with ADLs. Instruct to avoid the Valsalva maneuver. These measures reduce cardiac workload.

Monitor Fluid Volume

As cardiac output falls, compensatory mechanisms cause salt and water retention, increasing blood volume. This increased fluid volume places additional stress on the already failing ventricles, making them work harder to move the fluid load. The nurse should do the following:

- Assess the client's respiratory status and auscultate lung sounds at least every 4 hours. Notify the healthcare provider of significant changes in condition. Declining respiratory status indicates worsening left heart failure.
- Monitor the client's intake and output. Notify the healthcare provider if urine output is less than 30 mL/hr. Weigh the client daily. Careful monitoring of fluid volume is important during treatment of heart failure. Diuretics may reduce circulating volume, producing hypovolemia despite persistent peripheral edema. A fall in urine output may indicate significantly reduced cardiac output and renal ischemia. Weight

---

Community-Based Care Home Care for a Client With Heart Failure

Heart failure may be a chronic condition requiring active participation by the client and family for effective management. In preparation for home care, include the following topics:

- The disease process and its effects on the client's life
- Warning signals of cardiac decompensation that require treatment
- Desired and adverse effects of prescribed drugs, monitoring for effects, and importance of compliance with drug regimen to prevent acute and long-term complications of heart failure
- Prescribed diet and sodium restriction, practical suggestions for reducing salt intake, and AHA materials and recipes

- Exercise recommendations to strengthen the heart muscle and improve aerobic capacity (**Box 16–16** ●)
- The importance of keeping scheduled follow-up appointments to monitor disease progression and effects of therapy.

The nurse should provide referrals for home health care and household assistance (shopping, transportation, personal needs, and housekeeping) as indicated. Referrals to community agencies, such as local cardiac rehabilitation programs, heart support groups, or the AHA, can provide the client and family with additional materials and psychosocial support.

Box 16–16 Home Activity Guidelines for the Client With Heart Failure

- Perform as many activities as independently as you can.
- Space your meals and activities.
  - a. Eat six small meals a day.
  - b. Allow time during the day for periods of rest and relaxation.
- Perform all activities at a comfortable pace.
  - a. If you get tired during any activity, stop what you are doing and rest for 15 minutes.
  - b. Resume activity only if you feel up to it.
- Stop any activity that causes chest pain, shortness of breath, dizziness, faintness, excessive weakness, or sweating. Rest. Notify your healthcare provider if your activity tolerance changes and if symptoms continue after rest.
- Avoid straining. Do not lift heavy objects. To prevent constipation, eat a high-fiber diet and drink plenty of water. Use laxatives or stool softeners, as approved by your healthcare provider, to avoid constipation and straining during bowel movements.
- Begin a graded exercise program. Walking is good exercise that does not require any special equipment (except a good

pair of walking shoes). Plan to walk twice a day at a comfortable, slow pace for the first couple of weeks at home, and then gradually increase the distance and pace. Below is a suggested schedule—but progress at your own speed. Take your time. Aim for walking at least three times per week (every other day).

Week 1	200–400 feet	Twice a day, slow and leisurely pace
Week 2	1/4 mile	15 minutes, minimum of three times per week
Weeks 2–3	1/2 mile	30 minutes, minimum of three times per week
Weeks 3–4	1 mile	30 minutes, minimum of three times per week
Weeks 4–5	1 1/2 mile	30 minutes, minimum of three times per week
Weeks 5–6	2 miles	40 minutes, minimum of three times per week

is an objective measure of fluid status: 1 L of fluid is equal to 2.2 lb of weight.

- Record the client's abdominal girth every shift. Note complaints of a loss of appetite, abdominal discomfort, or nausea. Venous congestion can lead to ascites and may affect gastrointestinal function and nutritional status.
- Monitor and record the client's hemodynamic measurements. Report significant changes and negative trends. Hemodynamic measurements provide a means of monitoring condition and response to treatment.
- Restrict fluids as ordered. Allow choices of fluid type and timing of intake, scheduling most fluid intake during morning and afternoon hours. Offer ice chips and frequent mouth care; provide hard candies if allowed. Providing choices increases the client's sense of control. Ice chips, hard candies, and mouth care relieve dry mouth and thirst and promote comfort.

Monitor Activity

Clients with heart failure have little or no cardiac reserve to meet increased oxygen demands. As the disease progresses and cardiac function is further compromised, activity intolerance increases. The low cardiac output and inability to participate in activities may hinder self-care. The nurse should do the following:

- Organize nursing care to allow rest periods. Grouping activities together allows adequate time to "recharge."
- Assist the client with ADLs as needed. Encourage independence within prescribed limits. Assisting with ADLs helps ensure that care needs are met while reducing cardiac workload. Involving the client promotes a sense of control and reduces helplessness.
- Plan and implement progressive activities. Use passive and active ROM exercises as appropriate. Consult with the physical therapist on an activity plan. Progressive activity slowly increases exercise capacity by strengthening and improving

cardiac function without strain. Activity also helps prevent skeletal muscle atrophy. ROM exercises prevent complications of immobility in severely compromised clients.

- Provide written and verbal information about activity after discharge. Written information provides a reference for important information. Verbal information allows clarification and validation of the material.

Provide Low-Sodium Diet

Diet is an important part of long-term management of heart failure to manage fluid retention. The nurse should do the following:

- Discuss with the client the rationale for sodium restrictions. Understanding fosters compliance with the prescribed diet.
- Consult with a dietitian to plan and teach a low-sodium and, if necessary for weight control, low-kilocalorie diet. Provide a list of high-sodium, high-fat, high-cholesterol foods to avoid. Provide AHA materials. Dietary planning and teaching increase the client's sense of control and participation in disease management. Food lists are useful memory aids.

Evaluation

Client progress toward goals is evaluated on the basis of the following suggested expected outcomes:

- The client describes each medication prescribed along with the symptoms that should be reported to provider immediately.
- The client explains the importance of daily weights and keeping a log along with the importance of reporting significant weight gain.
- The client chooses appropriate foods from a menu reflecting a low sodium diet.
- The client modifies the daily routine to allow adequate periods of rest and activity.

NURSING CARE PLAN A Client With Heart Failure

ASSESSMENT

One year ago, Arthur Jackson, 67 years old, had a large anterior wall MI and underwent subsequent coronary artery bypass surgery. On discharge, he was started on a regimen of enalapril (Vasotec), digoxin, furosemide (Lasix), and a potassium chloride supplement. He is now in the cardiac unit complaining of severe shortness of breath, hemoptysis, and poor appetite for 1 week. He is diagnosed with acute heart failure.

Mr. Jackson refuses to settle in bed, preferring to sit in the bedside recliner in the high-Fowler position. He states, "Lately, this is the only way I can breathe." Mr. Jackson states that he has not been able to work in his garden without getting short of breath. He complains of his shoes and belt being too tight.

When Sonya Takashi, RN, Mr. Jackson's nurse, obtains his nursing history, Mr. Jackson insists that he takes his medications regularly. He states that he normally works in his garden for light exercise. In his diet history, he reports eating bacon daily and takeout Chinese food twice this week. He states that he has stopped salting his food but endorses not knowing how to track sodium intake.

Mr. Jackson's vital signs are as follows: temperature 97.5°F (36.5°C); pulse 124 bpm and irregular; respirations 28/min and labored; and blood pressure 95/72 mmHg. The cardiac monitor shows atrial fibrillation. An S_3 is noted on auscultation; the cardiac impulse is left of the midclavicular line. Mr. Jackson has crackles and diminished breath sounds in the bases of both lungs. Significant jugular venous distention, 3+ pitting edema of feet and ankles, and abdominal distention are noted. Liver size is within normal limits by percussion. Skin is cool and diaphoretic. Chest x-ray shows cardiomegaly and pulmonary infiltrates.

DIAGNOSES

- *Excess Fluid Volume* related to impaired cardiac pump and salt and water retention
- *Activity Intolerance* related to impaired cardiac output
- *Impaired Health Maintenance* related to lack of knowledge about diet restrictions

(NANDA-I © 2015)

PLANNING

Goals of care include the following:

- The client will demonstrate loss of excess fluid by weight loss and decreases in edema, jugular venous distention, and abdominal distention.
- The client will demonstrate improved activity tolerance.
- The client will verbalize understanding of diet restrictions.

IMPLEMENTATION

- Take hourly vital signs and hemodynamic pressure measurements.
- Administer and monitor the effects of prescribed diuretics and vasodilators.
- Weigh the client daily; strictly monitor the client's intake and output.
- Monitor the client for edema
- Enforce fluid restriction of 1,500 mL/24 hr (600 mL day shift, 600 mL evening shift, and 300 mL at night).
- Auscultate heart and breath sounds every 4 hours and as indicated.
- Administer oxygen via nasal cannula at 2 L/min. Monitor oxygen saturation continuously; notify the healthcare provider if it falls below 94%.

- Place the client in a high-Fowler or other position of comfort.
- Notify the healthcare provider of significant changes in laboratory values or vital signs.
- Teach the client about all medications and how to take and record pulse.
- Design an activity plan that incorporates preferred activities and scheduled rest periods.
- Instruct the client about sodium-restricted diet. Let client select meal choices within allowed limits.
- Consult a dietitian for planning and teaching the client about a low-sodium diet.

EVALUATION

Mr. Jackson is discharged after 3 days in the cardiac unit. He has lost 8 lb during his stay, and he states that it is much easier to breathe and his shoes fit better. He is able to sleep in the semi-Fowler position with only one pillow. His peripheral edema has resolved. While Mr. Jackson was in the cardiac unit, he and his wife met with a dietitian, who helped them develop a realistic eating plan to limit sodium, sugar, and fats. The dietitian also provided a list of high-sodium foods to avoid. Mr. Jackson is relieved to know that he can still enjoy Chinese food prepared without monosodium glutamate (MSG) or added salt. Ms. Takashi and the physical therapist designed a progressive activity plan with Mr. Jackson that he will continue at home. He remains in atrial fibrillation, a chronic condition. His knowledge of digoxin and Coumadin has been assessed and reinforced. Ms. Takashi confirms that he is able to accurately check his pulse and can list signs of digoxin toxicity.

CRITICAL THINKING

1. Mr. Jackson's medication regimen remains the same after discharge. What specific teaching does he need related to potential interactions of these drugs?
2. Mr. Jackson tells you, "Talk to my wife about my medications—she's Tarzan and I'm Jane now." How would you respond?
3. Design an exercise plan for Mr. Jackson to prevent deconditioning and conserve energy.
4. Mr. Jackson tells you, "Sometimes I forget whether I have taken my aspirin, so I'll take another just to be sure. After all, they are only baby aspirin. One or two extra a day shouldn't hurt, right?" What is your response?
5. Mr. Jackson is admitted to the neuro unit 6 months later with a cerebral vascular accident. What is the probable cause of his stroke?

◢ REVIEW Heart Failure

RELATE Link the Concepts and Exemplars

Linking the exemplar of heart failure with the concept of oxygenation:

1. What is the nursing priority of care for a client with heart failure and pulmonary edema? Explain your answer.

2. What impact does heart failure have on a client's oxygenation status if pulmonary edema is not found?

Linking the exemplar of heart failure with the concept of cognition:

3. Why might heart failure induce confusion in the older client?

4. What teaching would you provide the family of an older client diagnosed with heart failure who becomes suddenly confused and disoriented?

READY Go to Companion Skills Manual

REFER Go to Pearson Nursing Student Resources
nursing.pearsonhighered.com

- Additional review materials

REFLECT Case Study

Dr. Danilo Ocampo is a 74-year-old retired pathologist. He lives in his home with Lydia, his wife of 51 years. Their only child was killed some years ago in a motor vehicle crash. Dr. Ocampo was born and raised in the Philippines and came to the United

States when he was 23. He has a few nephews and nieces in the Philippines, but no relatives live nearby.

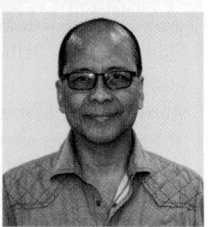

Dr. Ocampo's health has been declining for the past few years. He has a medical history that includes hypertension, myocardial infarction, angina, and class II heart failure. Because of these cardiovascular disorders, he takes multiple medications, including metoprolol, lisinopril, spironolactone, furosemide (intermittently as needed), potassium supplements (when taking furosemide), aspirin, isosorbide dinitrate, and nitroglycerin. He is concerned his current treatment plan may not be effective; he experiences a number of side effects from his medications and has been admitted multiple times to the hospital. He usually feels better after a few days in the hospital but typically checks himself out of the hospital before his physicians are ready to discharge him.

Dr. Ocampo spends most of his time and energy managing the household and caring for his wife, who has dementia.

1. What interventions can you initiate to help Dr. Ocampo minimize the side effects of the multiple medications he is taking?

2. What nutritional assessment would be appropriate for Dr. Ocampo? Why?

3. Should you intervene to help Dr. Ocampo accept help with the care of Lydia to decrease his own stress and improve his health? Explain your answer.

◣ EXEMPLAR 16.7 Hypertension

EXEMPLAR KEY TERMS

Blood flow, *1163*
Blood pressure, *1163*
Diastolic blood pressure, *1163*
Hypertension, *1162*
Hypertensive emergency, *1166*
Hypertensive encephalopathy, *1167*
Mean arterial pressure
   (MAP), *1163*
Peripheral vascular
   resistance, *1163*
Primary hypertension, *1165*
Pulse pressure, *1163*
Secondary hypertension, *1165*
Step-down therapy, *1173*
Systolic blood pressure, *1163*

EXEMPLAR LEARNING OUTCOMES

After reading about this exemplar, you will be able to:

1. Describe the pathophysiology, etiology, clinical manifestations, and direct and indirect causes of hypertension.

2. Identify risk factors and prevention methods associated with hypertension.

3. Illustrate the nursing process in providing culturally competent care across the life span for individuals with hypertension.

4. Formulate priority nursing diagnoses appropriate for an individual with hypertension.

5. Summarize therapies used by interdisciplinary teams in the collaborative care of an individual with hypertension.

6. Plan evidence-based care for an individual with hypertension and his or her family in collaboration with other members of the healthcare team.

7. Evaluate expected outcomes for an individual with hypertension.

▶ OVERVIEW

Hypertension is defined as systolic blood pressure of 140 mmHg or higher or diastolic blood pressure of 90 mmHg or higher based on the average of three or more readings taken on separate occasions (NHLBI, 2013d). Higher levels may be tolerated in clients who are being treated for hypertension. **Table 16–27** ● identifies classifications of blood pressure for adults ages 18 and older as defined by the Joint National Committee on the Prevention, Detection, Evaluation, and Treatment of High Blood Pressure.

Hypertension is an important public health issue. Although it rarely causes symptoms or noticeably limits the client's functional health, hypertension is a major risk factor for coronary heart disease, heart failure, stroke, and renal failure. Hypertension and its consequences are not unique to the United States. The World Health Organization identifies blood pressure above optimal levels (systolic >115 mmHg) as being responsible for 62% of cerebrovascular disease and 49% of ischemic heart disease worldwide (NHLBI, 2013d).

Although the identification and treatment of hypertension in the United States have improved significantly during the past

TABLE 16–27 Classification of Blood Pressure for Adults[a]

CATEGORY	SYSTOLIC (mmHG)		DIASTOLIC (mmHg)
Normal	<120	and	<80
Prehypertension	120–139	or	80–89
Hypertension[b]			
Stage 1	140–159	or	90–99
Stage 2	≥160	or	≥100

Source: Adapted from National Heart, Lung, and Blood Institute. (2013b). *The seventh report of the Joint National Committee on Prevention, Detection, Evaluation, and Treatment of High Blood Pressure (JNC 7).* Retrieved from http://www.nhlbi.nih.gov/guidelines/hypertension.

[a]When systolic and diastolic blood pressures fall into different categories, the reading that is highest or most out of acceptable range is used to classify blood pressure status.

[b]Based on the average of two or more readings taken at each of two or more visits after an initial screening.

25 years, approximately 30% of adults with hypertension remain unaware of their condition. Although 59% of adults with hypertension are being treated for the disorder, effective blood pressure control is achieved in only about 34% (NHLBI, 2013d).

▶ PATHOPHYSIOLOGY AND ETIOLOGY

The factors that affect arterial circulation are blood flow, peripheral vascular resistance, and blood pressure. **Blood pressure** is the force exerted against the walls of the arteries by the blood as it is pumped from the heart. It is most accurately referred to as **mean arterial pressure (MAP)**, which specifically denotes the average pressure in the arterial circulation throughout the cardiac cycle. The highest pressure exerted against the arterial walls at the peak of ventricular contraction (systole) is called the **systolic blood pressure**. The lowest pressure exerted during ventricular relaxation (diastole) is the **diastolic blood pressure**.

Mean arterial blood pressure is regulated mainly by cardiac output (CO) and peripheral vascular resistance (PVR), as represented in this formula: MAP = CO × PVR. For clinical use, the MAP may be estimated by calculating the diastolic blood pressure plus one third of the pulse pressure (the difference between the systolic and diastolic blood pressure) or 1/3 of the systolic pressure + 2/3 of the diastolic pressure.

Blood flow refers to the volume of blood transported in a vessel, in an organ, or throughout the entire circulation over a given period of time. It is commonly expressed as liters or milliliters per minute or as cubic centimeters per second. Blood flow through the circulatory system requires sufficient blood volume to fill the blood vessels and pressure differences within the system to allow blood to move forward.

The arterial, or supply, side of the circulation has relatively high pressures created by the thick elastic walls of the arteries and arterioles. The venous, or return, side of the system is a low-pressure system of thin-walled, distensible veins. Blood flows through the capillaries linking these two systems from the higher-pressure arterial side to the lower-pressure venous side.

The arterial blood pressure is created by the ejection of blood from the heart during systole (cardiac output) and the tension (resistance to blood flow) created by the elastic arterial walls (systemic vascular resistance). The blood pressure (the force exerted against the walls of the arteries by the blood as it is pumped from the heart) rises as the heart contracts during systole, ejecting its blood. This pressure wave, or systolic blood pressure, is felt as the peripheral pulse and is heard as Korotkoff sounds during blood pressure measurement. In healthy adults, the average systolic pressure is less than 120 mmHg. During diastole (cardiac relaxation and filling), elastic arterial walls maintain a minimum pressure, or diastolic blood pressure, to maintain blood flow through the capillary beds. The average diastolic pressure in a healthy adult is less than 80 mmHg. The difference between the systolic and diastolic pressure (normally ~40 mmHg) is known as the **pulse pressure**. The MAP is the average pressure in the arterial circulation throughout the cardiac cycle; it can be calculated by using the formula [systolic blood pressure + 2(diastolic blood pressure)]/3.

Cardiac output is determined by the blood volume and the ability of the ventricles to fill and effectively pump that blood. A number of factors contribute to systemic vascular resistance, including vessel length, blood viscosity, and vessel diameter and distensibility (compliance). While vessel length and blood viscosity remain relatively constant, vessel diameter and compliance are subject to normal regulatory activities and disease. These factors also affect **peripheral vascular resistance**, which refers to the opposing forces or impedance to blood flow as the arterial channels become more and more distant from the heart.

Peripheral vascular resistance is determined by three factors:

1. **Blood viscosity.** The greater the viscosity, or thickness, of the blood, the greater its resistance to moving and flowing.
2. **Length of the vessel.** The longer the vessel, the greater the resistance to blood flow.
3. **Diameter of the vessel.** The smaller the diameter of a vessel, the greater the friction against the walls of the vessel, leading to greater impedance of blood flow.

Factors Influencing Arterial Blood Pressure

The arterioles normally determine the systemic vascular resistance as their diameter changes in response to a variety of stimuli. These stimuli include the following:

■ **Sympathetic nervous system (SNS) stimulation.** Baroreceptors in the aortic arch and carotid sinus signal the SNS via the cardiovascular control center in the medulla when the MAP changes. A drop in MAP stimulates the SNS, increasing the heart rate and cardiac output and constricting arterioles (except in skeletal muscle). As a result, blood pressure rises. A rise in MAP has the opposite effect, decreasing the heart rate and cardiac output and causing arteriolar vasodilation.

■ **Circulating epinephrine and norepinephrine** from the adrenal medulla (e.g., the fight-or-flight response) have the same effect as SNS stimulation.

■ **Renin–angiotensin–aldosterone system** responds to renal perfusion. A drop in renal perfusion stimulates renin release. Renin converts angiotensinogen to angiotensin I, which is subsequently converted to angiotensin II in the lungs by ACE. Angiotensin II is a potent vasoconstrictor. It also promotes sodium and water retention, both directly and by stimulating the adrenal gland to release aldosterone. Both systemic vascular resistance and cardiac output increase, raising blood pressure.

- *Atrial natriuretic peptide (ANP) and brain natriuretic peptide (BNP):* ANP is released from atrial cells (sometimes the ventricles) and BNP is released from ventricular cells in response to stretching by excess blood volume. These hormones promote vasodilation and sodium and water excretion, lowering blood pressure.

- *Adrenomedullin* is a peptide synthesized and released by endothelial and smooth muscle cells in blood vessels. It is a potent vasodilator.

- *Vasopressin or antidiuretic hormone (ADH),* from the posterior pituitary gland, promotes water retention and vasoconstriction, raising blood pressure.

- *Local factors,* such as inflammatory mediators and various metabolites, can promote vasodilation, affecting blood pressure.

Other factors that can affect vessel compliance are the extent of arteriosclerosis (hardening of the arteries) and the extent of atherosclerosis (plaque accumulation). **Figure 16–47** ● summarizes the interrelationships of major factors regulating blood pressure. The cardiovascular system adapts to increased blood volume by increasing cardiac output. Autoregulatory mechanisms in the systemic arteries react to the increased volume, causing vasoconstriction. The increased systemic vascular resistance causes hypertension.

Blood flow, peripheral vascular resistance, and blood pressure, which influence arterial circulation, are in turn influenced by various factors. These factors include the following:

- The sympathetic and parasympathetic nervous systems are the primary mechanisms that regulate blood pressure. Stimulation of the SNS exerts a major effect on peripheral resistance by causing vasoconstriction of the arterioles, thereby increasing blood pressure. Parasympathetic stimulation causes vasodilation of the arterioles, lowering blood pressure.

- Baroreceptors and chemoreceptors in the aortic arch, carotid sinus, and other large vessels are sensitive to pressure and chemical changes and cause reflex sympathetic stimulation, resulting in vasoconstriction, increased heart rate, and increased blood pressure.

- The kidneys help maintain blood pressure by excreting or conserving sodium and water. When blood pressure decreases, the kidneys initiate the renin–angiotensin mechanism. This stimulates vasoconstriction, resulting in the release of the hormone aldosterone from the adrenal cortex, increasing sodium ion reabsorption and water retention. In addition, pituitary release of ADH promotes renal reabsorption of water. The net result is an increase in blood volume and a consequent increase in cardiac output and blood pressure.

- Temperatures may also affect peripheral resistance: Cold causes vasoconstriction, whereas warmth produces vasodilation. Many chemicals, hormones, and drugs influence blood pressure by affecting CO and/or peripheral vascular resistance. For example, epinephrine causes vasoconstriction and increased heart rate; prostaglandins dilate blood vessel diameter (by relaxing vascular smooth muscle); endothelin, a chemical released by the inner lining of vessels, is a potent vasoconstrictor; nicotine causes vasoconstriction; and alcohol and histamine cause vasodilation.

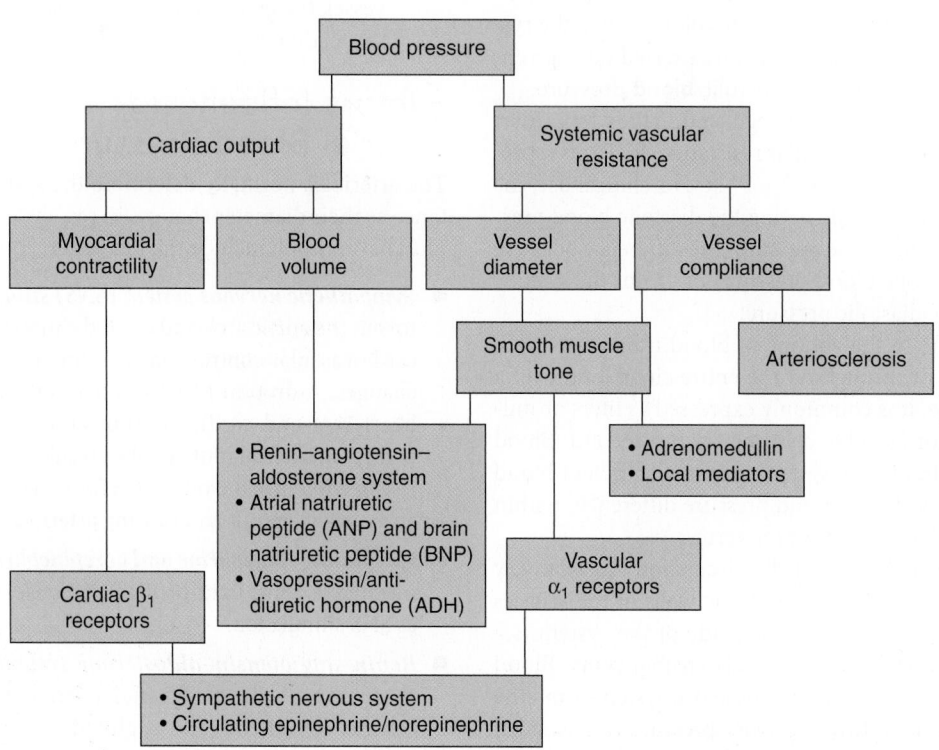

Figure 16–47 ● Factors affecting blood pressure.

- Dietary factors, such as intake of salt, saturated fats, and cholesterol, elevate blood pressure by affecting blood volume and vessel diameter.

- Race, gender, age, weight, time of day, position, exercise, and emotional state may also affect blood pressure. These factors influence the arterial pressure. Systemic venous pressure, though it is much lower, is also influenced by such factors as blood volume, venous tone, and right atrial pressure.

Primary Hypertension

Primary hypertension, formerly known as essential hypertension, is a persistently elevated systemic blood pressure. Approximately 50–65 million individuals in the United States have hypertension (NHLBI, 2013d). More than 90% of these individuals have primary hypertension, which has no identified cause.

Primary hypertension is thought to develop from complex interactions among factors that regulate cardiac output and systemic vascular resistance. These interactions may include the following:

- Excess SNS with overstimulation of alpha- and beta-adrenergic receptors, resulting in vasoconstriction and increased cardiac output.

- Altered function of the renin–angiotensin–aldosterone system and its responsiveness to factors such as sodium intake and overall fluid volume. The renin–angiotensin–aldosterone system affects vasomotor tone as well as salt and water excretion. Chronically high levels of angiotensin II lead to arteriolar remodeling, which permanently increases systemic vascular resistance. In approximately 20% of individuals with primary hypertension, renin levels are lower than normal. Increased sodium intake increases the blood pressure in these clients. Low plasma renin levels are more often seen in people of Sub-Saharan African ancestry than in those of European, North African, or Southwest Asian descent. Another 15% of clients with hypertension have higher-than-normal plasma renin levels. For these clients, salt intake has less of an effect on blood pressure (Longo et al., 2011). Most individuals with hypertension have normal levels of renin activity.

- Other chemical mediators of vasomotor tone and blood volume, such as ANP, also play a role by affecting vasomotor tone and sodium and water excretion. Vascular endothelium itself produces hormones (endothelins) that also affect vasomotor tone. Endothelin-1 is a potent vasoconstrictor (Copstead & Banasik, 2010).

- The interaction between insulin resistance, hyperinsulinemia, and endothelial function may be a primary cause of hypertension. Excess insulin has several effects that potentially contribute to hypertension: sodium retention by the kidneys, increased SNS activity, hypertrophy of vascular smooth muscle, and changes in ion transport across cell membranes (Longo et al., 2011).

The result of these interactions is sustained increases in blood volume and peripheral resistance. The cardiovascular system adapts to increased blood volume by increasing cardiac output. Autoregulatory mechanisms in the systemic arteries react to the increased volume, causing vasoconstriction. The increased systemic vascular resistance causes hypertension.

It appears unlikely that one single cause and pathological process will be found to account for essential hypertension. Increasingly, evidence points to hypertension as a diverse group of pathophysiological mechanisms resulting in the common manifestation of elevated blood pressure.

Secondary Hypertension

Secondary hypertension is elevated blood pressure resulting from an identifiable underlying process. It accounts for only 5%–10% of identified cases of hypertension.

The pathophysiology of selected causes of secondary high blood pressure can be summarized as follows:

- *Kidney disease.* Any disease that affects renal blood flow (e.g., renal artery stenosis) or renal function (e.g., glomerulonephritis, renal failure) can lead to hypertension. Disruption of the blood supply stimulates the renin–angiotensin–aldosterone system, with resulting vasoconstriction as well as sodium and water retention. Altered kidney function affects the elimination of water and electrolytes, leading to hypertension.

- *Coarctation of the aorta.* Coarctation of the aorta is narrowing of the aorta, usually just distal to the subclavian arteries. Reduced renal and peripheral blood flow stimulates the renin–angiotensin–aldosterone system and local vasoconstrictive responses, raising the blood pressure. A marked difference between pressures in the upper and lower extremities is common, with weak pulses and poor capillary refill in the lower extremities.

- *Endocrine disorders.* Adrenal gland disorders, such as Cushing syndrome and primary aldosteronism, can cause hypertension. A rare tumor of the adrenal medulla, pheochromocytoma, causes persistent or intermittent hypertension. Other endocrine disorders, such as hyperthyroidism and pituitary disorders, also can lead to hypertension.

- *Neurological disorders.* Increased intracranial pressure causes an elevated blood pressure as the body attempts to maintain cerebral blood flow. Disorders that interfere with autonomic nervous system regulation (e.g., high spinal cord injury) may allow the SNS to dominate, increasing systemic vascular resistance and blood pressure.

- *Drug use.* Estrogen and oral contraceptive use may lead to hypertension, possibly by prompting sodium and water retention and affecting the renin–angiotensin–aldosterone system. Stimulant drugs, such as cocaine and methamphetamines, increase systemic vascular resistance and cardiac output, resulting in hypertension. Decongestants, weight loss medications, glucocorticoids, cyclosporine, tricyclic antidepressants, and long term NSAID use also contribute to secondary hypertension (Basile and Bloch, 2014).

- *Pregnancy.* Approximately 10% of all pregnant women are hypertensive. Hypertension may predate pregnancy, or it may occur as a direct response to the pregnancy. The mechanism of gestational hypertension is unclear. It is a significant cause of maternal and fetal morbidity and mortality, and it requires careful perinatal management. (See Exemplar 16.10 for more details about gestational hypertension.)

- *Hypothyroidism.* Twenty to 40% of patients with hypothyroidism are hypertensive. Thyroid hormone is a smooth muscle relaxant, therefore, hypothyroidism may lead to increased vascular resistance as well as increases in serum norepinephrine and aldosterone, and decreases in endothelial relaxation factor production. Hypothyroidism is also associated with coronary artery disease.

- **Obstructive sleep apnea.** Sleep apnea has an adverse effect on the autonomic nervous system, as shown by increased levels of plasma catecholamines. The incidence and degree of hypertension is directly proportional to the frequency and severity of apneic episodes. Sleep apnea also interrupts the normal pattern of blood pressure reduction during sleep.

The pattern of secondary hypertension varies depending on its cause. Pheochromocytoma may cause attacks of hypertension that last for minutes to hours, accompanied by anxiety, palpitations, diaphoresis, pallor, and nausea and vomiting. Primary aldosteronism may cause hypertension, weakness, paresthesias, polyuria, and nocturia. Symptoms of kidney disease accompany hypertension when a renal disorder is the cause.

Hypertensive Emergency

Some clients with hypertension may, for reasons that are not clearly understood, develop rapid, significant elevations in systolic and/or diastolic pressures. In a **hypertensive emergency** (or *malignant hypertension*), the systolic pressure is greater than 180 mmHg and the diastolic pressure higher than 120 mmHg. Immediate treatment (within 1 hour) is vital to prevent cardiac, renal, and vascular damage and to reduce morbidity and mortality. Intense cerebral artery spasms help protect the brain from excess pressure; however, cerebral edema often develops. Prolonged severe hypertension damages walls of the arterioles and renal blood vessels and may lead to intravascular coagulation and acute renal failure.

Hypertension and Pregnancy

Hypertension affects roughly 10% of pregnancies and may be either chronic (pre-existing) or gestational. Gestational hypertension develops after 20 weeks gestation and may persist through the six week postpartum period. Women who experience gestational hypertension are at greater risk for developing chronic hypertension later in life.

Hypertension may progress to preeclampsia in 2-3% of pregnancies. Early signs of preeclampsia include high blood pressure and evidence of protein in the urine. Additional symptoms include swelling of the face, eyes, or hands and sudden weight gain of more than 0.9 kg (2 lb) per week. As preeclampsia progresses, more severe symptoms become evident. These include persistent headache, right-sided abdominal or shoulder pain, irritability, decreased urine output, nausea and vomiting, and vision changes. Preeclampsia is potentially fatal. Eclampsia, a serious complication of preeclampsia, is characterized by one or more seizures during pregnancy or the postpartum period. Accompanying severe epigastric pain may indicate hepatic involvement, which is commonly associated with HELLP syndrome. The characteristics of HELLP are hemolysis (H), elevated liver enzymes (EL), and low platelet count (LP). The most common reasons for critical illness and death related to eclampsia are stroke or rupture of the mother's liver.

The cure for preeclampsia is to deliver the baby by either induction or cesarean section. If the baby has not reached a safe gestational age, the mother may be monitored in the hospital and given medications to control her blood pressure. When the mother has severe preeclampsia, the baby's well-being is threatened, and the baby must be delivered.

Etiology

Hypertension primarily affects middle-aged and older adults: More than 50% of individuals ages 60–69 and approximately 75% of those age 70 and older are hypertensive (NHLBI, 2013d). An age-related increase in the systolic blood pressure is the primary factor leading to the high incidence of hypertension in older adults. Unlike the diastolic blood pressure, which tends to rise until approximately age 50 and then level off, the systolic blood pressure continues to rise with age (NHLBI, 2013d).

The prevalence of hypertension is significantly higher in Blacks than in Whites and Hispanics. Nearly 40% of Black adults are hypertensive, whereas fewer than 30% of adult White and Hispanic individuals are affected. In Whites and Hispanics, more males than females are hypertensive; in Blacks, more women than men are affected (NHLBI, 2013d). Native Americans and Alaska Natives are also at high risk for hypertension-related illnesses. This population is 1.3 times as likely as White adults to have high blood pressure (Office of Minority Health, 2010).

Risk Factors

A number of risk factors have been identified for primary hypertension (**Box 16–17** ●). Genetics plays a role, as do environmental factors.

Specific risk factors for hypertension include the following:

- **Family history.** Studies show a genetic link in approximately one third of individuals diagnosed with primary hypertension. Genes involved in the renin–angiotensin–aldosterone system and other genes that affect vascular tone, salt and water transportation in the kidney, obesity, and insulin resistance likely are involved in the development of hypertension, although no consistent genetic linkages have been found.

Box 16–17 Factors Contributing to Hypertension

MODIFIABLE FACTORS

- High sodium intake
- Low potassium, calcium, and magnesium intake
- Obesity
- Excess alcohol consumption
- Insulin resistance
- Low activity level
- Hypothyroidism
- Low vitamin D levels
- Depression
- Tobacco use

NONMODIFIABLE FACTORS

- Genetic factors
- Age
- Family history
- Race

- **Age.** The incidence of hypertension rises with increasing age. Aging affects baroreceptors involved in blood pressure regulation as well as arterial compliance. As the arteries become less compliant, pressure within the vessels increases. This is often most apparent as a gradual increase in the systolic pressure with aging.

- **Race.** Primary hypertension is more common and more severe in African Americans than in individuals of other ethnic backgrounds (see the Focus on Diversity and Culture feature). It also tends to develop at an earlier age and is associated with more cardiovascular and renal damage. More African Americans with hypertension have low renin levels and altered renal excretion of sodium at normal blood pressure levels. This genetic tendency to conserve salt may have developed as an adaptation to working in a warm environment, where salt and water conservation are beneficial (Porth, 2010).

- **Mineral intake.** High sodium intake often is associated with fluid retention. Hypertension related to sodium intake involves a number of different physiological mechanisms, including the renin–angiotensin–aldosterone system, nitric oxide, catecholamines, endothelin, and ANP (Copstead & Banasik, 2010). Low potassium, calcium, and magnesium intakes also contribute to hypertension by unknown mechanisms. The ratio of sodium to potassium intake appears to play a role, possibly through the effects of increased potassium intake on sodium excretion. Potassium also promotes vasodilation by reducing responses to catecholamines and angiotensin II. Calcium has a vasodilator effect as well. Although magnesium has been shown to reduce the blood pressure, its mechanism of action is unclear.

- **Obesity.** Central obesity (fat cell deposits in the abdomen), as determined by an increased waist-to-hip ratio, has a stronger correlation with hypertension than does body mass index or skinfold thickness. Although a clear correlation exists between obesity and hypertension, the relationship may be one of common cause. Genetic factors appear to play a role in the common triad of obesity, hypertension, and insulin resistance.

- **Insulin resistance.** Insulin resistance with resulting hyperinsulinemia is linked with hypertension through its effects of excess circulating insulin on the SNS, vascular smooth muscle, renal regulation of sodium and water, and ion transport across cell membranes. Insulin resistance may be a genetic or an acquired trait. Although it is more commonly seen in individuals who are obese, insulin resistance also has been found in individuals of normal weight.

- **Excess alcohol consumption.** Regular consumption of three or more drinks a day increases the risk of hypertension. Decreasing or discontinuing alcohol consumption reduces the blood pressure, particularly systolic readings. Lifestyle factors associated with excessive alcohol intake (obesity and lack of exercise) may contribute to hypertension as well.

- **Stress.** Physical and emotional stress cause transient elevations of blood pressure, but the role of stress in primary hypertension is less clear. Blood pressure normally fluctuates throughout the day, increasing with activity, discomfort, or emotional responses such as anger. Frequent or continued stress may cause vascular smooth muscle hypertrophy or affect the central integrative pathways of the brain (Porth, 2010).

- **Physical inactivity.** Regular exercise is proven to reduce blood pressure.

- **Vitamin D deficiency.** Current research demonstrates an association between decreased vitamin D levels and hypertension.

- **Depression.** Hypertension is more common in individuals with depression and other personality traits such as impatience and hostility.

Most hypertensive emergencies occur when clients suddenly stop taking their medications or their hypertension is poorly controlled. Younger clients (30–50 years), African American men, pregnant women with preeclampsia, and individuals with collagen or renal disease also are at higher risk for a hypertensive emergency (Porth, 2010).

► CLINICAL MANIFESTATIONS

The early stages of primary hypertension typically are asymptomatic, marked only by elevated blood pressure. Blood pressure elevations initially are transient but eventually become permanent. When symptoms do appear, they are usually vague. Headache, generally in the back of the head and neck, may be present on awakening, subsiding during the day. Other symptoms result from target organ damage and may include nocturia, confusion, nausea and vomiting, and visual disturbances. Examination of the retina of the eye may reveal narrowed arterioles, hemorrhages, exudates, and papilledema (swelling of the optic nerve). The Clinical Manifestations and Therapies feature lists the etiology and clinical manifestations of life-threatening hypertension along with recommended treatments.

Sustained hypertension affects the cardiovascular, neurological, and renal systems. The rate of atherosclerosis accelerates, increasing the risk for coronary heart disease and stroke. The workload of the left ventricle increases, leading to ventricular hypertrophy, which then increases the risk for coronary heart disease, dysrhythmias, and heart failure. The diastolic blood pressure is a significant cardiovascular risk factor until age 50; the systolic pressure then becomes the more important factor contributing to cardiovascular risk (NHLBI, 2013d). More than 348,000 American deaths in 2009 included hypertension as a primary or contributing cause (CDC, 2013d).

Clinical Manifestations and Therapies **Hypertension**

ETIOLOGY	CLINICAL MANIFESTATIONS	CLINICAL THERAPIES
Hypertensive crisis	■ Rapid onset ■ Blurred vision ■ Papilledema ■ Systolic pressure >180 mmHg; diastolic pressure >120 mmHg ■ Headache, confusion, motor or sensory deficits	■ Administer medications: vasodilators, calcium-channel blockers, angiotensin-converting enzyme inhibitors, or adrenergic blockers. ■ Blood pressure (BP) should be lowered gradually to prevent shock. ■ Monitor client's BP continuously. ■ Reduce client anxiety, which can cause BP to rise. ■ Teach importance of maintaining treatment for hypertension.
Stroke	■ Sudden onset of loss of sensation and/or movement: may be hemiplegia, hemiparesis, flaccidity, spasticity, or sensory loss of vision, hearing, taste, touch, proprioception, or smell	■ Monitor client's level of consciousness. ■ Administer medications: anticoagulants, thrombolytics, corticosteroids, or antihypertensives. ■ Prepare for surgery: carotid endarterectomy, extracranial–intracranial bypass, or carotid angioplasty. ■ Reduce client's intracranial pressure to prevent further damage.

Accelerated atherosclerosis associated with hypertension increases the risk for cerebral infarction (stroke). Increased pressure in the cerebral vessels can lead to development of microaneurysms and an increased risk for cerebral hemorrhage. **Hypertensive encephalopathy**, a syndrome characterized by extremely high blood pressure, altered level of consciousness, increased intracranial pressure, papilledema, and seizures, may develop. Its etiology is unclear.

Hypertension also can lead to nephrosclerosis and renal insufficiency. Proteinuria and microscopic hematuria develop, as do signs of chronic renal failure. African Americans experience hypertensive kidney disease more frequently than Caucasians. Hypertension is a major contributor to end-stage renal disease.

Clients presenting with a hypertensive emergency may have manifestations such as headache, confusion, swelling of the optic nerve (papilledema), blurred vision, restlessness, and motor and sensory deficits. Manifestations of hypertensive emergencies are listed in **Box 16–18** ●.

▶ COLLABORATION

Although primary hypertension cannot be cured, it can be controlled. Management of hypertension focuses on reducing the blood pressure to less than 140 mmHg systolic and 90 mmHg diastolic. The ultimate goal of hypertension management is to reduce cardiovascular and renal morbidity and mortality. The

risk of cardiovascular complications (coronary heart disease, heart failure, and stroke) decreases when the average blood pressure is less than 140/90 mmHg; when the client also has diabetes or renal disease, the treatment goal is a blood pressure of less than 130/80 mmHg. Most individuals with hypertension will require a combination of two or more drugs along with lifestyle changes to achieve recommended blood pressure levels (NHLBI, 2013d). **Figure 16–48** ● shows the recommended algorithm for hypertension management.

Diagnostic Tests

The client with hypertension is evaluated for the presence of identifiable causes of hypertension, cardiovascular risk factors, and the presence or absence of target organ damage (heart, brain, kidneys, peripheral vascular systems, and retina of the eye). Before treatment is started, the following diagnostic tests are performed:

■ ECG

■ Urinalysis

■ Blood glucose

■ Hematocrit

■ Serum potassium, creatinine, vitamin D, and calcium

■ Cholesterol and lipoprotein profile, including HDL, LDL, and triglycerides.

Additional tests that may be done include urinary albumin excretion, evaluation of the glomerular filtration rate (e.g., creatinine clearance), and tests for emerging cardiovascular risk factors, such as C-reactive protein and homocystine levels.

The following diagnostic tests may be ordered to differentiate primary from secondary hypertension:

■ *Renal function studies and urinalysis* can identify renal causes of hypertension. Elevated serum creatinine and blood urea nitrogen, reduced creatinine clearance, and hematuria, proteinuria, and casts often indicate kidney disease.

■ *The serum potassium* level is decreased in hyperaldosteronism.

Box 16–18   Manifestations of Hypertensive Emergencies

■ Rapid onset
■ Blurred vision, papilledema
■ Systolic pressure >180 mmHg
■ Diastolic pressure >120 mmHg
■ Headache
■ Confusion
■ Motor and sensory deficits

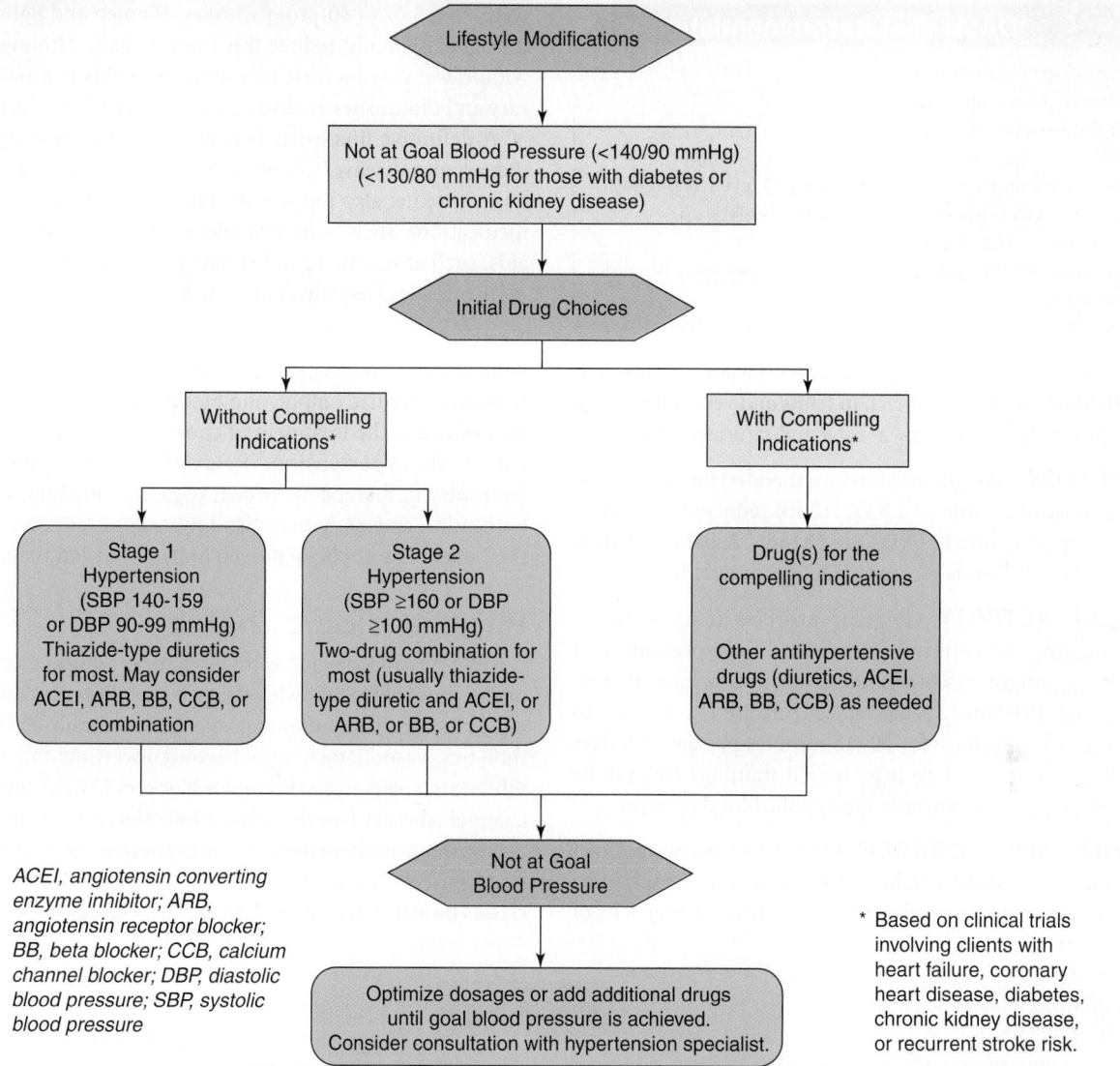

Figure 16–48 ● Algorithm for treating hypertension.

Source: Adapted from National Heart, Lung, and Blood Institute. (2004). *The seventh report of the Joint National Committee on Prevention, Detection, Education, and Treatment of High Blood Pressure* (NIH Publication No. 04-5250). Bethesda, MD: National Institutes of Health.

■ **Blood chemistries,** including serum electrolytes, glucose, and lipid studies, can detect abnormalities indicative of endocrine or cardiovascular disease.

■ **Intravenous pyelography, renal ultrasonography, renal arteriography, and computed tomography (CT) or magnetic resonance imaging (MRI)** tests are conducted when secondary hypertension is suspected.

Lifestyle Modifications

Lifestyle modifications are recommended for all clients whose blood pressure falls within the prehypertension range (120–139/80–89 mmHg) and for everyone with intermittent or sustained hypertension. These modifications include weight loss, dietary changes, restricted alcohol use and cigarette smoking, increased physical activity, and stress reduction (**Box 16–19** ●).

DIET   Dietary approaches to managing hypertension focus on reducing sodium intake, maintaining adequate potassium and calcium intakes, and reducing total and saturated fat intake. A mild to moderate sodium restriction (no added salt) lowers blood pressure and potentiates the effect of antihypertensive drugs for most clients. The DASH (Dietary Approaches to Stop Hypertension) diet has proven beneficial in lowering blood

---

Box 16–19   Lifestyle Modifications for Hypertension

■ Maintain normal body weight; lose weight if overweight.
■ Dietary modifications:
  a. Eat a diet rich in fruits, vegetables, and low-fat dairy products.
  b. Reduce sodium intake.
  c. Reduce intake of cholesterol and of total and saturated fat.
■ Limit alcohol intake to no more than 1 oz of ethanol (1/2 oz for women and lighter-weight individuals) per day.
■ Engage in aerobic exercise for 30 minutes most days of the week (5–6 days/week).
■ Stop smoking.
■ Use stress management techniques, such as relaxation therapy.

Box 16–20   DASH Diet Recommendations

- Grains: 6–8 servings per day
- Vegetables: 4–5 servings per day
- Fruits: 4–5 servings per day
- Fat-free or low-fat milk and milk products: 2–3 servings per day
- Meats, poultry, and fish: 6 or fewer servings (1 oz each) per day
- Nuts, seeds, and legumes: 4–5 servings per week
- Fats and oils: 2–3 servings per day
- Sweets and added sugars: 5 or fewer servings per week (should be low in fat)

pressure. This diet (**Box 16–20** ●) focuses on whole foods rather than individual nutrients. It is rich in fruits and vegetables (up to 10 servings per day) and is low in total and saturated fats.

WEIGHT LOSS   Weight loss is recommended for clients who are obese. Loss of as little as 4.5 kg (10 lb) reduces blood pressure in many individuals (NHLBI, 2013d). A balanced diet, such as the DASH diet, is recommended for weight loss.

PHYSICAL ACTIVITY   Regular exercise (e.g., walking, cycling, jogging, or swimming) reduces blood pressure and contributes to weight loss, stress reduction, and feelings of overall well-being. Previously sedentary clients are encouraged to engage in aerobic exercise for 30–45 minutes per day 5–6 days per week. Isometric exercise (e.g., weight training) may not be appropriate, because it can raise the systolic blood pressure.

ALCOHOL AND TOBACCO USE   The recommended alcohol intake for clients with hypertension is no more than 1 oz of ethanol or two drinks per day. A drink is 12 oz of beer, 5 oz of wine, or 1.5 oz of 80-proof whiskey. Women and lighter-weight individuals should reduce this limit by half. Although alcohol withdrawal may increase blood pressure, this is usually temporary and diminishes as abstinence or restricted intake continues.

A definitive link exists between cigarette smoking and cardiovascular disease. Clients who smoke are strongly urged to quit. Smoking also reduces the effect of some antihypertensive medications, such as propranolol (Inderal). Smoking cessation aids, such as nicotine patches and gum, contain lower amounts of nicotine and usually do not raise blood pressure.

STRESS REDUCTION   Stress stimulates the systemic nervous system, increasing vasoconstriction, systemic vascular resistance, cardiac output, and blood pressure. Regular, moderate exercise is the treatment of choice for reducing stress in clients with hypertension. Relaxation techniques, such as biofeedback, therapeutic touch, yoga, and meditation, to relax both mind and body may also lower blood pressure, although their effect has not been proven in hypertension management.

Pharmacologic Therapy

Current pharmacologic treatment of hypertension involves using one or more of the following drug classes: diuretics, alpha-adrenergic blockers, beta-adrenergic blockers, centrally acting sympatholytics, vasodilators, angiotensin-converting enzyme (ACE) inhibitors, angiotensin II receptor blockers (ARBs), and calcium-channel blockers (see the Medications feature). For most clients, two or more antihypertensive drugs selected from different drug classes are necessary to achieve effective control. These drug classes have different sites of action (see **Figure 16–49** ●).

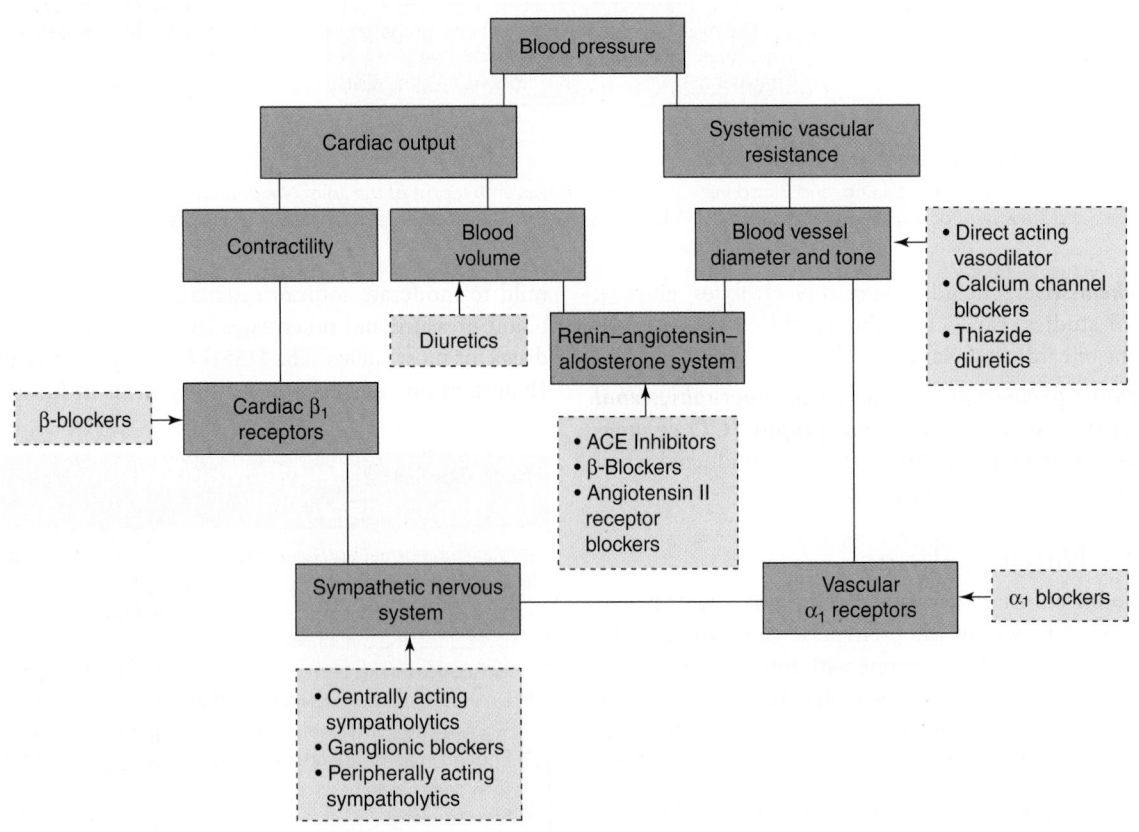

Figure 16–49 ● Sites of antihypertensive drug action.

Medications **Hypertension**

CLASSIFICATION AND DRUG EXAMPLES	MECHANISMS OF ACTION	NURSING CONSIDERATIONS
Alpha-Adrenergic Blockers *Drug examples:* ▪ doxazosin (Cardura) ▪ prazosin (Minipress) ▪ terazosin (Hytrin)	Block alpha-receptors in vascular smooth muscle. Decrease vasomotor tone and vasoconstriction. Reduce serum levels of low- and very-low-density lipoproteins.	▪ Monitor client for orthostatic hypotension, tachycardia, and palpitations. ▪ Give first dose at bedtime to minimize "first-dose" syncope. ▪ Encourage client to change positions slowly. ▪ Instruct client to notify primary care provider if nasal congestion or impotence develops. ▪ Notify primary care provider before discontinuing medication.
Angiotensin-Converting Enzyme (ACE) Inhibitors *Drug examples:* ▪ benazepril (Lotensin) ▪ captopril (Capoten) ▪ enalapril (Vasotec) ▪ fosinopril (Monopril) ▪ lisinopril (Prinivil, Zestril) ▪ ramipril (Altace) ▪ perindopril (Aceon)	Lower BP by preventing conversion of angiotensin I to angiotensin II. Prevent vasoconstriction and sodium and water retention.	▪ Monitor client for "first-dose" syncope, persistent cough, hyperkalemia. ▪ Less effective in African American clients. ▪ Report changes in WBC count, differential, serum potassium, BUN, or serum creatinine. ▪ Contraindicated in renal artery stenosis and pregnancy. ▪ Monitor client for manifestations of angioedema. ▪ Encourage client to change positions slowly. ▪ Administer orally 1 hr before meals.
Angiotensin II Receptor Blockers (ARBs) *Drug examples:* ▪ losartan (Cozaar) ▪ valsartan (Diovan)	Block vasoconstriction and promote relaxation of blood vessels, thereby lowering blood pressure.	▪ Monitor client for headache, dizziness, orthostatic hypotension, rash, and diarrhea ▪ Monitor client for manifestations of angioedema ▪ Encourage client to change positions slowly ▪ Contraindicated in pregnancy
Beta-Adrenergic Blocking Agents *Drug examples:* ▪ acebutolol (Sectral) ▪ atenolol (Tenormin) ▪ metoprolol Tartrate (Lopressor) ▪ nadolol (Corgard) ▪ propranolol (Inderal) *May be combined with alpha-adrenergic blocking agent:* ▪ carvedilol (Coreg) ▪ labetalol (Normodyne)	Reduce BP by preventing beta-receptor stimulation in the heart, resulting in decreased heart rate and cardiac output. Interfere with renin release by kidneys, decreasing the effects of angiotensin and aldosterone.	▪ Monitor client for bronchospasm, fatigue, sleep disturbances, nightmares, bradycardia, heart block, worsening heart failure, GI disturbances, impotence, and increased triglyceride levels. ▪ Use is contraindicated in asthma, chronic lung disease, bradycardia, or heart block. ▪ Assess blood pressure and apical pulse prior to administration. ▪ Report vital signs outside of parameters prior to administration. ▪ Encourage client to change positions slowly. ▪ Notify physician with development of shortness of breath, cough, or extremity swelling. ▪ Do not discontinue without discussing with physician.
Calcium-Channel Blockers *Drug examples:* ▪ amlodipine (Norvasc) ▪ diltiazem (Cardizem) ▪ felodipine (Plendil) ▪ isradipine (DynaCirc) ▪ nicardipine (Cardene) ▪ nifedipine (Procardia) ▪ nisoldipine (Sular) ▪ verapamil (Isoptin)	Inhibit flow of calcium ions across the cell membrane of vascular tissue and cardiac cells. Relax arterial smooth muscle, lowering peripheral resistance through vasodilation.	▪ Monitor client for impaired cardiac function and worsening heart failure. ▪ Prior to administration, assess blood pressure, apical pulse, and liver and renal function. ▪ Do not administer verapamil or diltiazem to clients with severe hypotension or sinus or atrioventricular blocks. ▪ Administer with caution in clients also taking digoxin or a beta-blocker. ▪ Monitor vital signs and report bradycardia, atrioventricular block, or heart failure to primary care provider. ▪ May cause constipation. Client should adjust diet as needed. ▪ Encourage client to report shortness of breath, weight gain, or extremity swelling to primary care provider.

(continued on next page)

Medications **Hypertension** (continued)

CLASSIFICATION AND DRUG EXAMPLES	MECHANISMS OF ACTION	NURSING CONSIDERATIONS
Centrally Acting Sympatholytics *Drug examples:* ■ clonidine (Catapres) ■ guanfacine (Tenex) ■ methyldopa (Aldomet) ■ reserpine	Stimulate the apha$_2$-receptors in the central nervous system to suppress sympathetic outflow to the heart and blood vessels. They decrease cardiac output and vasodilation, reducing BP.	■ Severe reflex hypertension may occur if medication is abruptly discontinued. ■ Dry mouth and sedation are common adverse effects. ■ Clonidine is contraindicated in pregnancy. ■ Methyldopa is contraindicated for clients with active liver disease. ■ Obtain baseline vital signs, CBC, a Coombs test, and liver function studies. ■ Administer oral doses at bedtime to minimize effects of sedation. ■ Promptly report lab value changes to physician. ■ Discontinue methyldopa if manifestations of liver dysfunction develop. ■ Take with meals to avoid GI upset. ■ Do not discontinue medication or skip doses. ■ Report signs of depression or decreased mental acuity. ■ Encourage the client to avoid driving if medication causes drowsiness.
Vasodilators *Drug examples:* ■ hydralazine (Apresoline) ■ minoxidil (Loniten)	Reduce blood pressure by relaxing vascular smooth muscle and decreasing peripheral vascular resistance. Often prescribed in combination with a diuretic or beta-blocker because they can cause reflex tachycardia and fluid retention.	■ Monitor vital signs prior to administration. ■ Report peripheral edema and symptoms of volume overload and heart failure. ■ Immediately report muffled heart sounds or paradoxic pulse. Pericardial effusion and possible cardiac tamponade may develop with minoxidil therapy. ■ Discontinue hydralazine if lupus-like manifestations occur. ■ Encourage client to change positions slowly. ■ Headache, palpitations, and rapid pulse may develop, but should subside within 10 days. ■ Minoxidil may cause excessive hair growth.
Thiazide Diuretics *Drug example:* ■ hydrochlorothiazide	Prevent tubular reabsorption of sodium, promoting sodium and water excretion and reducing blood volume. Reduce systemic vascular resistance.	■ Preferred treatment for systolic hypertension in older adults ■ Effective in African American clients ■ Adverse effects tend to be dose related. ■ Monitor client for hypokalemia.
Loop Diuretics *Drug example:* ■ furosemide (Lasix)	Inhibit sodium and chloride reabsorption from the loop of Henle. Act on kidneys to increase flow of urine. May be used alone or in conjunction with other antihypertensives.	■ Monitor client for hyponatremia, hypokalemia, or hypomagnesemia. ■ Encourage client to change positions slowly.
Potassium-Sparing Diuretics *Drug example:* ■ spironolactone (Aldactone)	These receptor antagonists cause water and sodium excretion by the kidneys.	■ Monitor client for skin rash, headache, dizziness, and GI upset.

DRUG CLASSES Diuretics are the preferred treatment for systolic hypertension in older adults. Diuretics are relatively safe and well-tolerated drugs; in addition, most are relatively inexpensive. Thiazide diuretics, such as hydrochlorothiazide (Hydro-DIURIL), are widely used. In major clinical studies, treatment with a single diuretic controlled blood pressure in approximately 50% of clients and reduced hypertension-linked morbidity and mortality related to coronary heart disease. Diuretics control hypertension primarily by preventing tubular reabsorption of sodium, thus promoting sodium pend water excretion and reducing blood volume. Thiazide diuretics also reduce systemic vascular resistance through an unknown mechanism. Diuretics are particularly effective in African Americans and in clients who are obese, are older, or have increased plasma volume or low renin activity. The adverse effects of diuretics generally are dose related. In addition to hypokalemia, diuretics may affect serum levels of glucose, triglycerides, uric acid, LDLs, and insulin.

Clients with heart failure, coronary heart disease, or diabetes may initially be treated with a beta-blocker. These drugs lower blood pressure, apparently by reducing peripheral vascular resistance. They may also reduce the amount of renin released by the kidneys by blocking beta$_1$-receptors in the kidney. Beta-blockers reduce the risk of complications such as heart failure and stroke. They are, however, relatively contraindicated for clients with asthma or chronic obstructive pulmonary disease because they promote bronchial constriction.

The ACE inhibitors and ARBs also are commonly used in the initial treatment of hypertension, particularly for clients with diabetes or heart failure, a history of MI, or chronic kidney disease. ACE inhibitors block formation of angiotensin II by inhibiting the action of ACE. Angiotensin II is a potent vasoconstrictor that also stimulates aldosterone release from the adrenal gland; blocking its action prevents vasoconstriction and sodium and water retention resulting from aldosterone release. ARBs have a very similar effect, although their action is to block angiotensin II receptors, thus preventing its vasoconstrictive and volume expansion effects.

Several drug classes work through their ability to promote vasodilation and reduce peripheral vascular resistance. Alpha-blockers, such as prazosin and terazosin, block stimulation of alpha₁-receptors on arterioles and veins, preventing vasoconstriction. Because of their ability to dilate both arterioles and veins, alpha-blockers can cause significant orthostatic hypotension, particularly following the initial dose. Calcium-channel blockers promote dilation of arterioles, the primary regulators of peripheral vascular resistance. These drugs can cause reflex tachycardia. Some calcium-channel blockers (verapamil and diltiazem in particular) also suppress heart function, reducing stroke volume and cardiac output. Reflex tachycardia is minimal with these calcium-channel blockers. Direct-acting vasodilators, such as hydralazine and minoxidil, also directly affect the arterioles, reducing peripheral vascular resistance. These drugs have little effect on veins, so the risk of orthostatic hypotension is minimal. They are, however, associated with reflex tachycardia and fluid retention, so they are rarely administered as in single-drug treatment regimens.

Other factors that are considered in selecting drugs for treating hypertension include demographic characteristics of the client, concurrent conditions, quality of life, cost, and possible interactions among prescribed drugs. In general, diuretics and calcium-channel blockers are more effective for treating hypertension in African Americans than beta-blockers or ACE inhibitors. Beta-blockers are preferred to treat hypertension with concurrent coronary heart disease and angina but are contraindicated for clients who have asthma or depression. Beta-blockers also reduce exercise tolerance and may adversely affect lifestyle for some clients.

DRUG REGIMENS Treatment usually is initiated by using a single antihypertensive drug at a low dose. Unless otherwise indicated, a diuretic is recommended as the initial drug of choice. The dose is slowly increased until optimal blood pressure control is achieved. If the drug does not effectively lower the blood pressure or has troubling side effects, a different drug from another class of antihypertensive medications is substituted. If, on the other hand, the drug is tolerated well but does not lower blood pressure to the desired level, a second drug from another class may be added to the treatment regimen.

Treatment of clients with stage 2 hypertension generally is more aggressive to minimize the risk of MI, heart failure, or stroke. When the client's average blood pressure is greater than 200/120 mmHg, immediate therapy (and possible hospitalization) is vital.

After a year of effective hypertension control, an effort may be made to reduce the dosage and number of drugs. This is known as **step-down therapy**. It is more successful in clients who have made lifestyle modifications. Careful blood pressure monitoring is necessary during and after step-down therapy because the blood pressure often rises again to hypertensive levels.

Complementary and Alternative Therapy

Behavioral and mind–body therapies may be helpful for some clients in lowering blood pressure. Blood pressure increases in response to physiological and psychological stress and anxiety. Mind–body therapies, such as yoga and tai chi, meditation, and guided imagery, are designed to modify both physiological and cognitive aspects of the stress response. In a study of older African American men and women with moderate hypertension, transcendental meditation was shown to reduce the blood pressure. Eastern exercises such as yoga and tai chi are gaining popularity as a means to reduce sympathetic nervous system activity. These treatments have not been fully explored but do not appear to be harmful. However, they should not replace a physician's advice regarding medication and aerobic exercise.

■ NURSING PROCESS

Health promotion teaching and activities focus on modifiable risk factors for hypertension. The nurse should advise all clients (as well as children and adolescents) to stop smoking or never start. Discuss the risks of obesity, excess alcohol intake, and a sedentary lifestyle with clients. Encourage all clients to eat a diet rich in fruits and vegetables and low in total and saturated fat. Discuss the potential benefits of following the DASH diet or a similar eating plan. Advise all clients to remain active and engage in aerobic exercise 5 days or more each week. Discuss the stress-reducing benefits of exercise. Offer blood pressure screening, and refer clients for follow-up. The Client Teaching feature lists topics for the nurse to cover in discussions about controlling a client's hypertension.

Assessment

Obtain the following information during focused assessment of the client with hypertension:

- *Health history.* Complaints of morning headache or cervical pain; cardiovascular or central nervous system manifestations; history of hypertension, renal disease, or diabetes; family history of high blood pressure, heart failure, or kidney disease; current medications.
- *Physical examination.* Vital signs, including blood pressure in both arms as well as apical and peripheral pulses; ophthalmological exam of retinal fundus as appropriate.

Diagnosis

Nursing diagnoses that may apply to the client with primary hypertension include the following:

- *Ineffective Health Maintenance*
- *Risk for Noncompliance*
- *Imbalanced Nutrition: More Than Body Requirements*
- *Excess Fluid Volume.*

(NANDA-I © 2012)

Planning

Goals of nursing care for the client with primary hypertension include the following:

- The client will describe lifestyle choices that can prevent, reduce, or resolve hypertension.
- The client's blood pressure will remain within the acceptable range for age and condition.

Client Teaching Control of Hypertension

Effective control of hypertension requires the client not only to participate in the plan of care but also to take an active role in managing the disease. Include the following topics when teaching the client and family about hypertension:

- Specific lifestyle changes recommended for the client and suggestions for implementing them, such as the following:
  a. Increase activity gradually. Develop a realistic exercise program that is enjoyable and fits into the individual's lifestyle. Identify an exercise buddy for additional motivation. Activity and exercise, through a gradual conditioning of muscles and blood vessels, lower blood pressure by reducing peripheral vascular resistance. As the heart becomes conditioned and pumps more efficiently, kidney perfusion improves and intravascular volume falls, further reducing blood pressure. Exercise also reduces stress and contributes to weight loss and maintenance. Aerobic exercise, such as walking, jogging, swimming, and cycling, are appropriate; isometric activities (e.g., such as weight lifting) should be avoided without physician approval.
  b. Adopt healthy eating patterns, following a low-fat, low-cholesterol, moderate-sodium diet that also is rich in fruits and vegetables and includes at least two servings of low-fat milk or milk products daily. Do not give up if you slip into old eating habits on occasion; use such occasions to identify ways to avoid future lapses.
  c. Stop smoking. Participating in organized smoking cessation programs or using aids such as nicotine patches can help.

  d. Use alcohol in moderation if at all, consuming no more than 1.5 oz of hard liquor, 5–10 oz of wine, or 12–20 oz of beer per day.
  e. Use stress-reducing techniques, such as meditation, relaxation, deep breathing, and exercise, to manage stress. Anger and hostility intensify vasoconstriction; channeling these emotions into more positive responses, such as using a change process to modify factors that provoke these emotions, can reduce their harmful effects on blood pressure.

- Prescribed medications, their intended effect, dose and timing, interactions, and possible adverse effects. Discuss effects that should be reported to the healthcare provider and those that can be managed by the client or that will diminish over time.
- The importance of monitoring blood pressure and regular visits to the healthcare provider or hypertension clinic to monitor treatment. During follow-up visits, assess the client's blood pressure and specific laboratory work (e.g., serum creatinine, blood urea nitrogen, and serum electrolytes) to evaluate the disease and the effects of antihypertensive medications.

Refer the client to community blood pressure clinics and to home health services as needed for regular follow-up and reinforcement of teaching. Refer the client to a dietitian or an organized weight loss program as indicated for further teaching and weight loss support.

- The client will reduce sodium consumption.
- The client will maintain fluid balance.
- The client will verbalize understanding of medication regimen and potential side effects.

Implementation

Primary nursing interventions for the client with primary hypertension are aimed at preventing hypertension through client teaching. Secondary interventions are aimed at controlling blood pressure to prevent complications.

Promote Health Maintenance

An unhealthy lifestyle and behaviors can contribute to health problems such as hypertension. When hypertension has been identified in a client, knowledge about the disease and its management is vital for the client. The client's willingness to take responsibility for hypertension management is central to effective blood pressure control. Adopting healthy lifestyle changes enhances drug therapy; in some cases, the need for medications may be eliminated or reduced. Because hypertension is often an asymptomatic disease and many antihypertensive drugs have unpleasant side effects, it is vital that the client understand the chronic progressive nature of the disease and its long-term consequences. The nurse's role in this process includes the following:

- Assist the client in identifying current behaviors that contribute to hypertension. The client must first identify contributory behaviors before being able to change them. Using knowledge of hypertension risk factors, the nurse can help identify behaviors and factors contributing to hypertension that can

be changed. Including the family in this process is important to reduce potential sabotage of the client's efforts to adopt healthier behaviors.

- Assist the client in developing a realistic health maintenance plan. Preparing a health maintenance plan for the client does little to encourage personal responsibility for health. However, the nurse can guide the client in developing realistic goals and expectations for the treatment plan and for modifying risk factors such as smoking, exercise, diet, and stress.
- Help the client and family identify strengths and weaknesses in maintaining health. Discussing areas of the health maintenance plan that are working well and those that present difficulties can help identify necessary changes in the plan and additional strategies for implementing it.

Promote Compliance

Noncompliance, or failure to follow the identified treatment plan, is a continuing risk for any client with a chronic disease. Recommended lifestyle changes, such as diet, exercise, restricted alcohol intake, stress reduction, and smoking cessation, often are difficult to maintain on a continuing basis. In addition, prescribed medications may have undesirable effects, whereas hypertension itself often has no symptoms or noticeable effects. If a client is not complying with the treatment plan, the nurse can take the following steps:

- Inquire about reasons for noncompliance with the recommended treatment plan. Listen openly and without judging. Nonthreatening discussion of factors contributing to noncompliance validates the client's self-esteem and partnership in the treatment plan.

- Evaluate knowledge regarding hypertension, its long-term effects, and treatment. Provide additional information and reinforce teaching as needed. Knowledge increases the sense of control, which also increases the likelihood of compliance with treatment.
- Assist the client to develop realistic short-term goals for lifestyle changes. Attempting to lose weight, exercising daily, stopping smoking, and dramatically changing the diet all at the same time may be overwhelming, leading to a sense of failure. Smaller, gradual changes are more easily incorporated into lifestyle and daily activities, improving compliance.
- Help the client identify cues and develop reminders (e.g., written notes or a medication box filled weekly) to assist with maintaining a schedule for exercise and medications. Cues and other devices provide helpful reminders of activities and schedules until they are incorporated into habits.
- Reassure the client that relapse into old habits and behaviors is common. Encourage the client to avoid feelings of guilt associated with relapse and use the circumstance to renew efforts to comply with treatment. Guilt and feelings of failure can lead to further noncompliance unless the event is used to identify reasons for noncompliance and ways to prevent it from recurring in the future.

Promote Balanced Nutrition

The relationship between obesity, excess alcohol intake, and hypertension is well documented. Hypertension is particularly associated with central obesity, identified by waist circumference greater than hip circumference. Although weight loss is difficult and takes commitment to changing both eating and exercise habits, most clients can achieve it. The nurse can assist in this effort by doing the following:

- Assess the client's usual daily food intake, and discuss with the client possible contributing factors to excess weight, such as a sedentary lifestyle or using food as a reward or stress reliever. Inquire about diversional activities, exercise patterns, and previous weight reduction efforts (e.g., participation in weight reduction programs or using fad or crash diets). Assessment data provide clues about factors contributing to obesity and about the client's knowledge base about the relationship between eating and exercise habits and weight as well as safe weight loss strategies. This provides direction for further teaching and for developing a realistic weight reduction plan.
- Mutually determine with the client a realistic target weight (e.g., loss of 10% of current body weight over a 6-month period). Regularly monitor the client's weight. Encourage a system of nonfood rewards for achieving small, incremental goals. Setting weight loss goals helps formalize the process and provides motivation for continued progress. Developing realistic goals may be difficult; unrealistic goals, however, set the client up for failure. Continuous incremental weight loss provides reassurance that the goal can be achieved and promotes permanent weight reduction.
- Refer the client to a dietitian for information about low-fat, low-calorie foods and eating plans. Focus on changing eating habits rather than "following a diet." Focusing on changing eating habits promotes the sense that low-fat, low-calorie

eating patterns should become a part of the client's lifestyle rather than a short-term measure to be endured until the weight loss goal is achieved.

- Recommend that the client participate in an approved weight loss program such as Weight Watchers, Overeaters Anonymous, or Take Off Pounds Sensibly (TOPS). Organized weight loss programs provide structure for a balanced weight reduction program as well as mutual support from others trying to lose weight.

Maintain Fluid Volume

Excess fluid volume often contributes to hypertension by increasing cardiac output. A number of factors associated with hypertension can cause excess fluid volume, including sodium retention and disruption of the renin–angiotensin–aldosterone system. In addition, some antihypertensive drugs, such as calcium-channel blockers and vasodilators, can contribute to excess fluid in the interstitial spaces and peripheral edema.

- Monitor the client's intake and output, and weigh the client daily (if in an acute or long-term care facility) or weekly (in the community). Rapid weight changes (over days) more accurately reflect fluid balance than intake and output records do. One liter of fluid weighs 1 kg (2.2 lb). Weight changes and intake and output records help in monitoring the effects of therapy.
- Monitor the client for peripheral edema (sacral edema in the client who is bedridden). Drugs such as vasodilators can cause fluid accumulation in interstitial tissues, leading to peripheral or dependent edema. Adding a diuretic to the treatment plan may be necessary.
- Discuss the relationship between sodium intake and fluid retention. Provide opportunities to choose low-sodium foods from simulated menus. Refer the client to a dietitian for teaching about a restricted sodium diet. Support the client's efforts, and reassure the client that lifestyle changes such as consuming less sodium take time. Knowledge provides the power to take control of sodium intake. Patience and perseverance are needed to succeed; positive reinforcement of efforts to change long-standing dietary patterns is important.
- Discuss the importance of adhering to treatment plans, such as dietary restrictions and medication schedules. Understanding the rationale for treatment measures promotes the client's sense of control and encourages compliance with the treatment regimen.

Evaluation

Evaluation of the effectiveness of client care may be based on the following expected outcomes:

- The client describes strategies for maintaining normal blood pressure, including exercising, quitting smoking, losing weight, and managing stress.
- The client describes expected actions of medications, side effects to report to the healthcare provider, and the importance of taking medication every day.
- The client demonstrates accurate performance of blood pressure monitoring and maintains a log of readings to share with the healthcare provider.
- The client demonstrates the ability to choose foods that are low in sodium.

NURSING CARE PLAN A Client With Hypertension

ASSESSMENT

Margaret Spezia is a married, 49-year-old Italian American with eight children whose ages range from 3 to 18 years. For the past 2 months, Mrs. Spezia has had frequent morning headaches as well as occasional dizziness and blurred vision. At her annual physical examination 1 month ago, her blood pressure was 168/104 and 156/94 mmHg. She was instructed to reduce her fat and cholesterol intake, to avoid using salt at the table, and to start walking for 30–45 minutes daily. Mrs. Spezia returns to the clinic for follow up.

While escorting Mrs. Spezia to the exam room and obtaining her weight, blood pressure, and history, Lisa Christos, RN, notices that Mrs. Spezia seems restless and upset. Ms. Christos says, "You look upset about something. Is everything OK?" Mrs. Spezia responds, "Well, my head is throbbing, and I'm sort of dizzy. I think I'm just overdoing it and not getting enough rest. You know, raising eight children is a lot of work and expense. I just started working part-time so we wouldn't get behind in our bills. I thought the extra money might relieve some of my stress, but I'm not so sure that's really happening. I'm not getting any better, and I'm worried that I'll lose my job or become disabled and that my husband won't be able to manage the children by himself. I really need to go home, but first, I want to get rid of this awful headache. Would you please get me a couple of aspirin or something?"

Mrs. Spezia's history shows a steady weight gain during the past 18 years. She has no known family history of hypertension. Physical findings include the following: height 63 in. (160 cm); weight 225 lb (102 kg); temperature 99°F (37.2°C); pulse 100 bpm and regular; respirations 16/min; and blood pressure 180/115 mmHg (lying), 170/110 mmHg (sitting), and 165/105 mmHg (standing). Her skin is cool and dry, with capillary refill of 4 seconds in the right hand and 3 seconds in the left hand. Mrs. Spezia's total serum cholesterol is 245 mg/dL (normal: <200 mg/dL). All other blood and urine studies are within normal limits. Based on analysis of the data, Mrs. Spezia is started on amlodipine, 20 mg, and benazepril, 5 mg and is placed on a low-fat, low-cholesterol, no-added-salt diet.

DIAGNOSES

- *Fatigue* related to effects of hypertension and stresses of daily life
- *Imbalanced Nutrition: More Than Body Requirements* related to excessive food intake
- *Ineffective Health Maintenance* related to inability to modify lifestyle
- *Deficient Knowledge* related to effects of prescribed treatment

(NANDA-I © 2012)

PLANNING

Goals of care include the following:

- The client will reduce her blood pressure readings to less than 140 mmHg systolic and 90 mmHg diastolic by the return visit next week.
- The client will incorporate into her diet low-sodium and low-fat foods from a list provided.
- The client will develop a plan for regular exercise.
- The client will verbalize understanding of the effects of the prescribed drug, dietary restrictions, exercise, and follow-up visits to help control hypertension.

IMPLEMENTATION

- Teach to take own blood pressure daily and record it, bringing the record to scheduled clinic visits.
- Teach name, dose, action, and side effects of her antihypertensive medication.
- Instruct to walk for 15 minutes each day this week and to investigate swimming classes at the local pool.

- Discuss strategies for achieving a realistic weight loss goal.
- Refer to a dietary consultation for further teaching about fat and sodium restrictions.
- Discuss stress-reducing techniques, helping identify possible choices.

EVALUATION

Mrs. Spezia returns to the clinic 1 week later. Her average blood pressure is now 148/88 mmHg. She has lost 0.7 kg (1.5 lb) and states that her oldest daughter has suggested they join a weight reduction program together. Mrs. Spezia is walking for an average of 20 minutes at a local mall each day. She verbalizes an understanding of her medication and is taking it before dinner each day. She met with the dietitian and discussed ways to reduce the sodium and fat in her diet. The dietitian provided a list of low-fat, low-sodium foods and recommended cookbooks to help Mrs. Spezia modify her cooking. Mrs. Spezia tells Ms. Christos, "I just can't believe how much better I feel already. My headaches are gone, and I've actually lost some weight—and I feel motivated to keep going. If I had only known how much better I could feel! I don't expect I'll ever go back to my old habits again; it's just not worth it!"

CRITICAL THINKING

1. *Identify the factors that contributed to Mrs. Spezia's hypertension. Which were modifiable, and which were not?*
2. *What is the rationale for reducing sodium and fat in Mrs. Spezia's diet?*
3. *Suppose your client with hypertension is homeless and has no source of income. How could you help ensure your client would follow the treatment plan? What would you do if the client did not follow it?*
4. *Discuss the role of stress in hypertension. What factors in Mrs. Spezia's life contribute to her stress level?*
5. *Develop a plan of care for the nursing diagnosis Low-Self Esteem related to obesity.*

REVIEW Hypertension

RELATE Link the Concepts and Exemplars

Linking the exemplar of hypertension with the concept of metabolism:

1. Create a plan of care, including nutrition, for the client diagnosed with both hypertension and type 2 diabetes mellitus.

2. You receive a call from a client who has been diagnosed with hypertension and diabetes mellitus. He is asking what over-the-counter medications would be safe to take to treat a mild upper respiratory infection (a cold). How will you respond to this question?

Linking the exemplar of hypertension with the concept of fluid and electrolytes:

3. Explain the impact hypertension has on urinary elimination.

4. What teaching will you provide the client diagnosed with hypertension to reduce this impact on the renal system?

READY Go to Companion Skills Manual

REFER Go to Pearson Nursing Student Resources
nursing.pearsonhighered.com

- Additional review materials

REFLECT Case Study

Yvonne Genmar is a 42-year-old female with primary hypertension. She is married to Tom, who has a 17-year-old son, Paul, from a previous marriage. The Genmars have two children together, Sabrina, 14, and Charlie, 3. Mr. Genmar runs his own business installing sprinkler systems, and Mrs. Genmar is a real estate agent and home inspector. She spends a great deal of time in her car showing houses and taking the kids to their various after-school activities.

Mrs. Genmar's mother has type 2 diabetes; her father is fairly healthy. Mrs. Genmar has been prescribed several different antihypertensives, but her blood pressure remains elevated. Most recently, she was placed on captopril 50 mg twice a day, which seems to be maintaining her blood pressure within acceptable limits.

1. What precautions would you teach Mrs. Genmar regarding captopril in conjunction with her lifestyle?

2. If you admitted Mrs. Genmar to the provider's office before captopril was prescribed, what interview questions would you want to explore in order to determine lifestyle factors that may be contributing to her continued hypertension?

3. What nutritional recommendations will you make to Mrs. Genmar to help her control her hypertension?

EXEMPLAR 16.8   Life-Threatening Dysrhythmias

EXEMPLAR KEY TERMS

Atrial kick, *1178*
Cardiac arrest, *1192*
Cardiopulmonary resuscitation (CPR), *1193*
Couplet, *1185*
Defibrillation, *1188*
Dysrhythmia, *1177*
Ectopic beats, *1178*
Heart block, *1178*
Multifocal, *1185*
Normal sinus rhythm (NSR), *1182*
Pacemaker, *1190*
Paroxysmal, *1183*
Premature junctional contractions, *1184*
Retrograde conduction, *1184*
Sudden cardiac death (SCD), *1192*
Synchronized cardioversion, *1188*
Torsades de pointes, 1185
Triplet, *1185*
Unifocal, *1185*
Valsalva maneuver, *1192*
Ventricular bigeminy, *1185*
Ventricular trigeminy, *1185*

EXEMPLAR LEARNING OUTCOMES

After reading about this exemplar, you will be able to:

1. Describe the pathophysiology, etiology, clinical manifestations, and direct and indirect causes of life-threatening dysrhythmias.

2. Identify risk factors and prevention methods associated with life-threatening dysrhythmias.

3. Illustrate the nursing process in providing culturally competent care across the life span for individuals with life-threatening dysrhythmias.

4. Formulate priority nursing diagnoses appropriate for an individual with a life-threatening dysrhythmia.

5. Summarize therapies used by interdisciplinary teams in the collaborative care of an individual with a life-threatening dysrhythmia.

6. Plan evidence-based care for an individual with a life-threatening dysrhythmias and his or her family in collaboration with other members of the healthcare team.

7. Evaluate expected outcomes for an individual with a life-threatening dysrhythmia.

DYSRHYTHMIAS

▶ OVERVIEW

Heart muscle contracts in response to electrical stimulation. In the normal heart, electrical stimulation produces a synchronized, rhythmic heart muscle contraction that propels blood into the vascular system. Changes in cardiac rhythm affect this synchronized activity and the heart's ability to effectively pump blood to body tissues.

A cardiac **dysrhythmia** is an abnormal heart rate or rhythm; more specifically, it is a disturbance or irregularity in the electrical system of the heart. Cardiac dysrhythmias may be benign or have lethal consequences. Prompt recognition of a lethal dysrhythmia and quick action can truly be lifesaving.

Dysrhythmias develop for many reasons. Not all are pathological; some alterations in cardiac rhythm occur in response to events such as exercise or fear. For example, a rapid heart rate as a result of exercise, fever, or excitement is a normal response to the body's demand for oxygen or to stimulation of the sympathetic nervous system (SNS). Slow heart rates also may be normal. Athletic heart syndrome, which results from long-term training of the heart muscle, allows the heart to beat more slowly and forcefully while maintaining adequate cardiac output and tissue perfusion at a slower rate. Many athletes have a heart rate of less than 60 beats per minute (bpm), and the heart rate in a very-well-conditioned athlete may be as low as 44–48 bpm.

Aging affects cardiac rhythm as well. The natural pacemaker of the heart loses some of its cells, resulting in a slightly slower heart rate. In older adults, the left ventricle tends to increase in size. This leads to an increase in overall heart size but a decrease in the heart's filling capacity. The ECG of a normal, healthy older adult may appear slightly different from that of a younger individual. Arrhythmias are seen more often and may be caused by heart disease. Heart murmurs may result from valve stiffness caused by the degeneration of muscle cells.

Regardless of cause, a dysrhythmia can significantly affect cardiac performance, depending on the health of the heart muscle. The client's response to the dysrhythmia is key in determining the urgency and type of treatment needed.

▶ PATHOPHYSIOLOGY AND ETIOLOGY

Five unique properties of cardiac cells allow effective heart function. Four of these properties are electrical; the fifth is cardiac muscle's mechanical response to electrical stimulation. These five properties are as follows:

1. *Automaticity* is the ability of pacemaker cells to spontaneously initiate an electrical impulse (action potential). The sinoatrial (SA) node is the dominant pacemaker, generating impulses at 60–100 times a minute. Myocardial muscle cells do not possess this ability.
2. *Excitability* is the ability of myocardial cells to respond to stimuli generated by pacemaker cells.
3. *Conductivity* is the ability to transmit an impulse from cell to cell. When one cell is stimulated, the impulse spreads rapidly throughout the heart muscle.
4. *Refractoriness* is the inability of cardiac cells to respond to additional stimuli immediately following depolarization. In the absolute refractory period, depolarization will not occur in response to any stimulus. A stronger-than-normal stimulus is required to initiate depolarization during the relative refractory period. This is followed by the supernormal period, during which a mild stimulus will cause depolarization.
5. *Contractility* is the ability of myocardial fibers to shorten in response to a stimulus. Heart muscle responds in an all-or-nothing manner: Stimulation of one muscle fiber causes the entire muscle mass to contract to its fullest extent as one unit.

Electrical activity of the heart is normally controlled by the cardiac conduction system (see Figure 16–10 earlier in this module). The impulse spreads through the atria, is briefly delayed at the atrioventricular (AV) node, then spreads through conduction pathways of the ventricles and to ventricular muscle. The AV nodal delay allows the atria to contract, delivering an extra bolus of blood to the ventricles before they contract (the **atrial kick**). The AV node also controls the number of impulses that reach the ventricles, preventing extremely rapid heart rates.

Dysrhythmias arise through disruption of the very properties that stimulate and control the heartbeat: automaticity, excitability, conductivity, and refractoriness. Dysrhythmias that result from altered impulse formation include changes in rate and rhythm and the development of ectopic beats. This category includes tachydysrhythmia (rapid heart rates), bradydysrhythmia (slow heart rates), and ectopic rhythms. These dysrhythmias result from a change in the automaticity of cardiac cells. The rate of impulse formation may abnormally increase or decrease. Aberrant (abnormal) impulses may originate outside normal conduction pathways, causing ectopic beats. **Ectopic beats** interrupt the normal conduction sequence and may not initiate a normal muscle contraction. Depending on the site and timing of abnormal impulses, they may have little effect on the client or pose a significant threat.

Ischemia, injury, and infarction of myocardial tissue affect its excitability and ability to conduct and respond to an electrical stimulus. Conduction abnormalities cause varying degrees of **heart block** (a block in the normal conduction pathways). Myocardial injury or infarction (MI) can obstruct or delay impulse conduction. Bundle branch blocks are common in acute MI.

The reentry phenomenon, a phenomenon of normal and slow conduction, is a major cause of tachydysrhythmia. A stimulus such as an ectopic beat triggers the reentry phenomenon. The impulse is delayed in one area of the heart (e.g., an area of ischemia or injury), but is conducted normally through the rest. Muscle that has been depolarized by the normally conducted impulse is repolarized by the time the impulse traveling through the area of slow conduction reaches it, thus initiating another cycle of depolarization (Huether & McCance, 2011). The result is a dysrhythmia that propagates itself.

Several forms of reentry may occur. The impulse may travel through a set pathway to reenter repolarized tissue. Many atrial dysrhythmias follow this pattern, including atrial flutter. In functional reentry, local differences in the conduction of an impulse interrupt the normal wave of depolarization, sending it back upon itself in a spiral pattern and setting up a permanent rotation. This type of pattern suppresses normal pacemaker activity and can lead to atrial fibrillation (Huether & McCance, 2011).

Cardiac rhythms are classified according to the site of impulse formation or the site and degree of conduction block. Supraventricular rhythms arise above the ventricles. These rhythms usually produce a QRS complex within the normal range. Sinus rhythms, atrial rhythms, and junctional (arising from the AV junction) rhythms are all supraventricular rhythms. Ventricular rhythms originate in the ventricles and may prove fatal if left untreated. AV conduction blocks result from a defect in impulse transmission from the atria to the ventricles. The major normal and abnormal cardiac rhythms are summarized in **Table 16–28** ●.

Lifespan Considerations Cardiac Dysrhythmias

Children

Cardiac arrhythmias (abnormal heart rhythms or dysrhythmias) occur frequently in children but less commonly than in adults. Arrhythmias can cause decreased cardiac output and congestive heart failure or can progress further to an even more serious arrhythmia that could result in sudden death.

Tachyarrhythmias (e.g., sinus tachycardia) often occur with acute conditions, such as hypoxia, anemia, hypovolemia, shock, hyperkalemia or hypokalemia, hyperthyroidism, catecholamine medications, and stimulant or illicit drug use. Causes of bradycardia include specific medications, vagal stimulation, metabolic imbalances, hypoxia, hypothyroidism, hypothermia, and acute myocardial infarction (AMI). These types of arrhythmias generally resolve once the underlying condition is treated. Some arrhythmias result from genetic conditions, such as forms of supraventricular tachycardia (SVT) and long-QT syndrome. Less common arrhythmias are often associated with congenital heart disease, especially as many more children are now surviving surgeries for complex defects.

Neonates and young children may be predisposed to SVT because of a congenital heart defect or Wolff–Parkinson–White (WPW) syndrome. Short periods of arrhythmia (several seconds), which may be caused by paroxysmal atrial tachycardia, are rarely dangerous; however, prolonged episodes (>24 hours) of continuous SVT may be life threatening and can progress to congestive heart failure or cardiogenic shock. Cardiac output is affected because blood returning during diastole cannot keep pace with such a rapid heart rate.

Nursing Assessment

- The child suspected of having an arrhythmia should be monitored for level of consciousness, heart rate, and other vital signs. A cardiorespiratory monitor and pulse oximetry should be used to identify deterioration of the child's condition.
- An early indicator of cardiopulmonary compromise is a change in the child's mental status or level of consciousness. Changes in color, weakness, irritability, and feeding patterns may indicate the development of hypoxia.
- Any child in the community found to have an abnormal ECG finding, unusual heart rhythm, syncope (especially with exercise), or dizziness with palpitations should be referred to a pediatric cardiologist for evaluation.

Home Care Teaching

Episodes of arrhythmia are frightening for both child and parents, as are the unpredictability of recurrent episodes and the risk for sudden cardiac death with some arrhythmias. The nurse should provide support, encourage the parents to promote the child's normal development between episodes, and emphasize that medications help prevent or reduce episode frequency. Other nursing interventions include the following:

- Carefully explain the treatment plan and home care.
- Teach parents to take the child's apical pulse. Make sure parents are trained in CPR and use of the Valsalva maneuver.
- Provide telephone numbers of emergency medical facilities, and help parents plan how to seek emergency care.
- Make sure the parents and child with SVT understand the need to avoid using cardiac stimulant drugs, such as decongestants, because these drugs might trigger an episode.

- Describe and provide written instructions about the danger signs indicating a recurrence of the acute condition and how to seek emergency care.
- Prepare the child and family for procedures such as radiofrequency ablation or implantation of a pacemaker or cardioverter–defibrillator.

Older Adults

Aging affects the heart and the cardiac conduction system, increasing the incidence of dysrhythmias and conduction defects. Older adults may experience dysrhythmias even when no evidence of heart disease is found.

Older adults have a higher incidence of both ventricular and supraventricular dysrhythmias without detrimental effects compared with younger individuals. Ectopic beats, including short runs of ventricular tachycardia, occur more commonly during exercise in older adults. These dysrhythmias do not affect cardiac morbidity or mortality. Fibrosis of the bundle branches can lead to atrioventricular blocks; a prolonged PR interval is common in clients over the age of 65. Older adults also have a higher incidence of diseases that may affect heart rhythm. An older client with hyperthyroidism, for example, may present with atrial fibrillation, syncope, and confusion instead of the usual manifestations of goiter, tremor, and exophthalmos.

Nursing Assessment

Assessment of the older adult for problems related to cardiac dysrhythmias focuses on the effect of the dysrhythmia on functional health status. In assessing the older adult, the nurse should do the following:

- Ask about a history of cardiovascular disease and current medications.
- Inquire about symptoms such as episodes of dizziness, light-headedness, fainting, palpitations, chest pain, or shortness of breath.
- Ask about the relationship between symptoms such as palpitations and intake of certain foods and caffeine-containing beverages.
- Evaluate for other contributing factors, such as smoking or alcohol intake.
- Inquire about a history of falls, particularly any that occurred without apparent reason.

Home Care Teaching

Teach measures to reduce the risk of cardiac dysrhythmias and potential adverse consequences of dysrhythmias:

- Emphasize the importance of taking medications as prescribed. Discuss possible effects of over-the-counter (OTC) medications on the heart.
- Encourage the client to reduce or eliminate caffeine intake. Caffeine increases the risk of ectopic beats and rapid heart rates.
- Encourage the client to participate in a smoking cessation program and reduction or elimination of alcohol intake if appropriate.
- Encourage the client to engage in regular exercise. Discuss the beneficial effects of exercise to maintain muscle mass, including cardiac muscle, and cardiovascular health.
- Instruct the client to contact the primary care provider for evaluation of symptoms such as dizziness, fainting, frequent palpitations, shortness of breath, unexplained falls, or chest pain.

TABLE 16–28 Characteristics of Selected Cardiac Rhythms and Dysrhythmias

RHYTHM/ECG APPEARANCE	ECG CHARACTERISTICS	MANAGEMENT
Supraventricular Rhythms		
Normal sinus rhythm (NSR)	Rate: 60–100 bpm Rhythm: regular P:QRS: 1:1 PR interval: 0.12–0.20 sec QRS complex: 0.06–0.10 sec	None; normal heart rhythm.
Sinus arrhythmia	Rate: 60–100 bpm Rhythm: irregular, varying with respirations P:QRS: 1:1 PR interval: 0.12–0.20 sec QRS complex: 0.06–0.10 sec	Generally none; considered a normal rhythm in the very young and very old.
Sinus tachycardia	Rate: 101–150 bpm Rhythm: regular P:QRS: 1:1 (with very fast rates, P wave may be hidden in preceding T wave) PR interval: 0.12–0.20 sec QRS complex: 0.06–0.10 sec	Treated only if symptomatic or client is at risk for myocardial damage. Treat underlying cause (e.g., hypovolemia, fever, pain). Beta-blockers or verapamil may be used.
Sinus bradycardia	Rate: <60 bpm Rhythm: regular P:QRS: 1:1 PR interval: 0.12–0.20 sec QRS complex: 0.06–0.10 sec	Treated only if symptomatic. Intravenous atropine or isoproterenol, and/or pacemaker therapy may be used.
Premature atrial contractions (PACs)	Rate: variable Rhythm: irregular, with normal rhythm interrupted by early beats arising in the atria P:QRS: 1:1 PR interval: 0.12–0.20 sec, but may be prolonged QRS complex: 0.06–0.10 sec	Usually require no treatment. Advise to reduce alcohol and caffeine intake, to reduce stress, and to stop smoking. Beta-blocker may be prescribed.
Paroxysmal supraventricular tachycardia (PSVT)	Rate: 100–280 bpm (usually 150–200 bpm) Rhythm: regular P:QRS: P waves often not identifiable PR interval: not measured QRS complex: 0.06–0.10 sec	Treat if symptomatic. Treatment may include vagal maneuvers (Valsalva, carotid sinus massage), oxygen therapy, adenosine or a beta-blocker, temporary pacing, or synchronized cardioversion.

TABLE 16–28 Characteristics of Selected Cardiac Rhythms and Dysrhythmias (*continued*)

RHYTHM/ECG APPEARANCE	ECG CHARACTERISTICS	MANAGEMENT
Atrial flutter 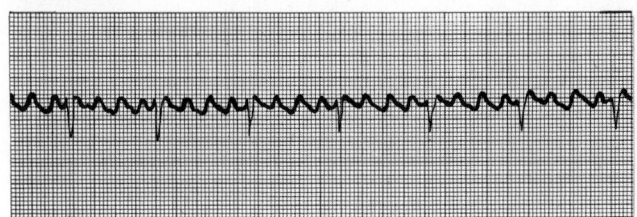	Rate: atrial, 240–360 bpm; ventricular rate depends on degree of atrioventricular block and usually is <150 bpm Rhythm: atrial, regular; ventricular, usually regular P:QRS: 2:1, 4:1, 6:1; may vary PR interval: not measured QRS complex: 0.6–0.10 sec	Medications to slow ventricular response, such as a beta-blocker or calcium-channel blocker, followed by a class I antidysrhythmic agent or amiodarone; synchronized cardioversion.
Atrial fibrillation 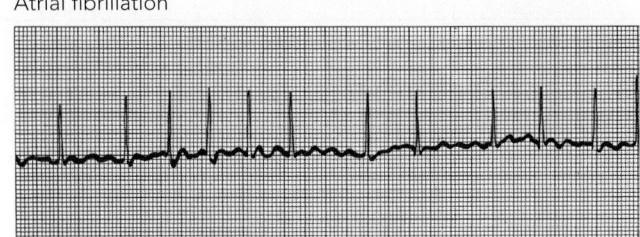	Rate: atrial, 300–600 bpm (too rapid to count); ventricular, 100–180 bpm in untreated clients Rhythm: irregularly irregular P:QRS: variable PR interval: not measured QRS complex: 0.06–0.10 sec	Synchronized cardioversion; medications to reduce ventricular response rate: metoprolol, diltiazem, or digoxin; anticoagulant therapy to reduce risk of clot formation and stroke.
Junctional escape rhythm 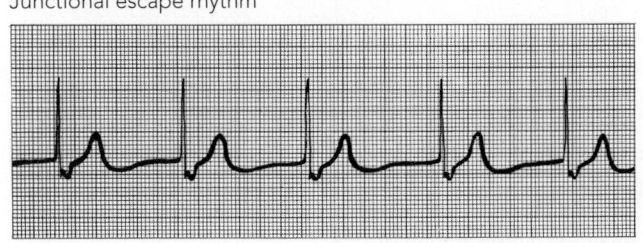	Rate: 40–60 bpm; junctional tachycardia, 60–140 bpm Rhythm: regular P:QRS: P waves may be absent, inverted and immediately preceding or succeeding QRS complex, or hidden in QRS complex PR interval: <0.10 sec QRS complex: 0.06–0.10 sec	Treat cause if symptomatic.
Ventricular Rhythms		
Premature ventricular contractions (PVCs) 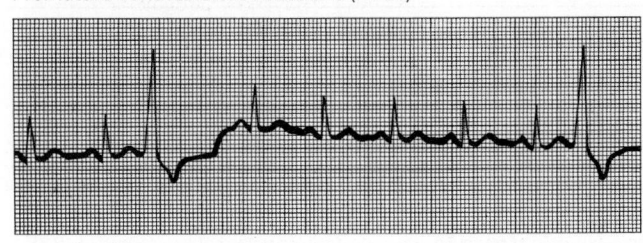	Rate: variable Rhythm: irregular, with PVC interrupting underlying rhythm and followed by a compensatory pause P:QRS: no P wave noted before PVC PR interval: absent with PVC QRS complex: wide (>0.12 sec) and bizarre in appearance; differs from normal QRS complex	Treat if symptomatic or in presence of severe heart disease. Advise against stimulant use (caffeine, nicotine). Beta-blockers or class I or III antidysrhythmic agents may be used in clients with severe heart disease who are symptomatic.
Ventricular tachycardia (VT, V tach) 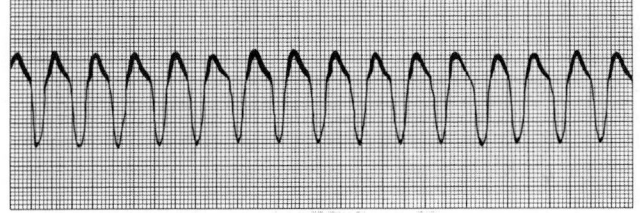	Rate: 100–250 bpm Rhythm: regular P:QRS: P waves usually not identifiable PR interval: not measured QRS complex: ≥0.12 sec; bizarre shape	Treat if VT is sustained, symptomatic, or associated with organic heart disease. Treatment includes DC cardioversion or intravenous procainamide, lidocaine, or a class III antidysrhythmic agent if hemodynamic instability accompanies; surgical ablation or antitachycardia pacing with an implanted cardioverter–defibrillator for repeated episodes. If no pulse, treat as ventricular fibrillation. Begin CPR, if needed and follow advanced cardiac life support algorithm.

(*continued on next page*)

TABLE 16–28   Characteristics of Selected Cardiac Rhythms and Dysrhythmias (*continued*)

RHYTHM/ECG APPEARANCE	ECG CHARACTERISTICS	MANAGEMENT
fibrillation (VF, V fib)	Rate: too rapid to count Rhythm: grossly irregular P:QRS: no identifiable P waves PR interval: none QRS: bizarre, varying in shape and direction	Immediate cardioversion/defibrillation.
Atrioventricular (AV) Conduction Blocks		
First-degree AV block	Rate: usually 60–100 bpm Rhythm: regular P:QRS: 1:1 PR interval: >0.21 sec QRS complex: 0.06–0.10 sec	None required.
Second-degree AV block, type I (Mobitz I, Wenckebach)	Rate: 60–100 bpm Rhythm: atrial, regular; ventricular, irregular P:QRS: 1:1 until P wave blocked with no subsequent QRS complex PR interval: progressively lengthens in a regular pattern QRS complex: 0.06–0.10 sec; sudden absence of QRS complex	Monitoring and observation; rarely progresses to a higher degree of block or requires treatment.
Second-degree AV block, type II (Mobitz II)	Rate: atrial, 60–100 bpm; ventricular, <60 bpm Rhythm: atrial, regular; ventricular, irregular P:QRS: typically 2:1, may vary PR interval: constant PR interval for each conducted QRS complex QRS complex: 0.06–0.10 sec	Atropine or isoproterenol; atropine should be used with caution if MI suspected; pacemaker therapy.
Third-degree AV block (complete heart block)	Rate: atrial, 60–100 bpm; ventricular, 15–60 bpm Rhythm: atrial, regular; ventricular, regular P:QRS: no relationship between P waves and QRS complexes; independent rhythms PR interval: not measured QRS complex: 0.06–0.10 sec if junctional escape rhythm; >0.12 sec if ventricular escape rhythm	Immediate pacemaker therapy.

▶ CLINICAL MANIFESTATIONS

Cardiac dysrhythmias occur when the normal sinus rhythm of the heart is disturbed. **Normal sinus rhythm (NSR)** is the normal heart rhythm, in which impulses originate in the SA (sinus) node and travel through all normal conduction pathways without delay. All waveforms are of normal configuration, look alike, and have consistent (fixed) durations. The rate is between 60 and 100 bpm.

The signs and symptoms associated with cardiac dysrhythmias often range from none to sudden cardiac death. More severe symptoms tend to occur in clients having evidence of structural disease. Common symptoms include light-headedness, dizziness, fluttering, pounding, quivering, shortness of breath, dizziness, chest discomfort, and painful extra beats (Jaeger, n.d.).

To improve understanding, rhythms are categorized according to the site of origination. Sinus node dysrhythmias originate in the sinus node. Supraventricular rhythms are those that originate above the ventricle. Junctional rhythms originate at the AV node. Ventricular rhythms originate below the AV node and are the most life–threatening because of their impact on cardiac output.

Sinus Node Dysrhythmias

Sinus node, also called sinoatrial node, dysrhythmias may occur as a normal compensatory response (e.g., to exercise) or because of altered automaticity. In these rhythms, as in normal sinus rhythm, the initiating impulse is from the SA node. They differ from normal sinus rhythms in rate or regularity of the rhythm. Sinus dysrhythmias include sinus arrhythmia, sinus tachycardia, and sinus bradycardia.

SINUS ARRHYTHMIA   *Sinus arrhythmia* is a sinus rhythm in which the rate varies with respirations, causing an irregular rhythm. The rate increases during inspiration and decreases with expiration. Sinus arrhythmia is common in the very young and the very old. It can be caused by an increase in vagal tone, by digitalis toxicity, or by morphine administration.

SINUS TACHYCARDIA   *Sinus tachycardia* has all of the characteristics of NSR, except that the rate is greater than 100 bpm. Tachycardia arises from enhanced automaticity in response to changes in the internal environment. Sympathetic nervous system stimulation or blocked vagal (parasympathetic) activity increases the heart rate. Tachycardia is a normal response to any condition or event that increases the body's demand for oxygen and nutrients, such as exercise or hypoxia. In the client on bed rest, tachycardia is an ominous sign. Sinus tachycardia may be an early sign of cardiac dysfunction, such as heart failure. Tachycardia is detrimental in clients with cardiac disease because it increases cardiac work and oxygen use.

Common causes of sinus tachycardia include exercise, excitement, anxiety, pain, fever, hypoxia, hypovolemia, anemia, hyperthyroidism, myocardial infarction (MI), heart failure, cardiogenic shock, pulmonary embolism, caffeine intake, and certain drugs, such as atropine, epinephrine (Adrenalin), or isoproterenol (Isuprel).

Manifestations of sinus tachycardia include a rapid pulse rate. The client may complain of feeling that the heart is "racing," shortness of breath, and dizziness. In the presence of heart disease, sinus tachycardia may precipitate chest pain.

SINUS BRADYCARDIA   *Sinus bradycardia* has all of the characteristics of NSR, but the rate is less than 60 bpm. Sinus bradycardia may result from increased vagal (parasympathetic) activity or from depressed automaticity due to injury or ischemia to the sinus node. Sinus bradycardia may be normal (e.g., in clients with athletic heart syndrome). The heart rate also normally slows during sleep because the parasympathetic nervous system is dominant at this time. Other causes of sinus bradycardia include pain, increased intracranial pressure, sinus node disease, AMI (especially with inferior wall damage), hypothermia, acidosis, and certain drugs.

Sinus bradycardia may be asymptomatic; it is important to assess the client before treating the rhythm. Manifestations of decreased cardiac output, such as decreased level of consciousness, syncope (faintness), or hypotension, indicate a need for intervention.

SICK SINUS SYNDROME   *Sick sinus syndrome (SSS)* results from sinus node disease or dysfunction that causes problems with impulse formation, transmission, and conduction. Sick sinus syndrome is often found in older adults. It may be caused by direct injury to sinus tissue, fibrosis of conduction fibers associated with aging, and such drugs as digitalis, beta-blockers, and calcium-channel blockers.

ECG characteristics of SSS include sinus bradycardia, sinus arrhythmia, sinus pauses or arrest, and atrial tachydysrhythmias such as atrial fibrillation, atrial flutter, or atrial tachycardia. Bradycardia-tachycardia syndrome, characterized either by **paroxysmal** (occurring in bursts with an abrupt onset and termination) atrial tachycardia followed by prolonged sinus pauses or alternating periods of bradycardia and tachycardia, also may indicate sinus node dysfunction.

Manifestations of sinus node dysfunction often are intermittent, related to a drop in cardiac output caused by the irregular rhythm. Fatigue, dizziness, light-headedness, and syncope are common. The heart rate may not increase in response to stressors such as exercise or fever.

Supraventricular Dysrhythmias

When an action potential originates in atrial tissue outside the SA node, the resulting rhythm is classified as a supraventricular rhythm. In these dysrhythmias, an ectopic pacemaker takes over, or overrides, the SA node. They may also occur when the SA node fails; an escape rhythm develops as a fail-safe mechanism to maintain the heart rate. The most common supraventricular dysrhythmias are premature atrial contractions, paroxysmal supraventricular tachycardia, atrial flutter, and atrial fibrillation. These rhythms may be paroxysmal.

PREMATURE ATRIAL CONTRACTIONS   A *premature atrial contraction (PAC)* is an ectopic atrial beat that occurs earlier than the next expected sinus beat. PACs can arise anywhere in the atria. They are usually asymptomatic and benign, but they may initiate paroxysmal supraventricular tachycardia in susceptible individuals. PACs are common in older adults, often occurring without an obvious cause. Strong emotions, excessive alcohol intake, tobacco, and stimulants such as caffeine can precipitate PACs. They also may be associated with MI, heart failure and other cardiac disorders, hypoxemia, pulmonary embolism, digitalis toxicity, and electrolyte or acid–base imbalances. In clients with underlying heart disease, PACs may precede a more serious dysrhythmia.

The ECG tracing shows interruption of the underlying rhythm by a premature complex that looks similar to the underlying beats. The ectopic impulse of the PAC is usually conducted normally, leading to depolarization of cardiac muscle and a normal QRS complex. Because the impulse arises above the ventricles, it follows normal conduction pathways through the ventricles. The QRS complex is narrow or matches those of the underlying rhythm. The shape of the P wave of a PAC differs from normal P waves because its impulse arises outside the sinus node. A *noncompensatory pause* usually follows, as the

PAC resets the SA node rhythm. Occasionally, the ectopic impulse may not be conducted through the heart, resulting in a lone P wave without a QRS, or a nonconducted PAC.

PACs cause few manifestations. If frequent, they may cause palpitations or a fluttering sensation in the chest. Early beats may be noted on auscultating or palpating the pulse.

PAROXYSMAL SUPRAVENTRICULAR TACHYCARDIA

Paroxysmal supraventricular tachycardia (PSVT) is tachycardia of sudden onset and termination. PSVT is usually initiated by a reentry loop in or around the AV node; that is, an impulse reenters the same section of tissue over and over, causing repeated depolarizations.

PSVT occurs more frequently in women than men. Sympathetic nervous system stimulation and stressors such as fever, sepsis, and hyperthyroidism may precipitate PSVT. It also may be associated with heart diseases such as coronary heart disease (CHD), MI, rheumatic heart disease, myocarditis, or acute pericarditis. Abnormal conduction pathways associated with WPW syndrome may account for PSVT.

PSVT affects ventricular filling and cardiac output, and decreases coronary artery perfusion. Its manifestations include complaints of palpitations and a "racing" heart, anxiety, dizziness, dyspnea, anginal pain, diaphoresis, extreme fatigue, and polyuria (urine output may reach up to 3 L in the first few hours after PSVT onset).

ATRIAL FLUTTER

Atrial flutter is a rapid and regular atrial rhythm thought to result from an intra-atrial reentry mechanism. Causes include sympathetic nervous system stimulation due to anxiety or caffeine and alcohol intake; thyrotoxicosis; CHD or MI; pulmonary embolism; and abnormal conduction syndromes, such as WPW syndrome. Older adults with rheumatic heart disease or valvular disease are especially vulnerable.

Two types of atrial flutter have been identified. Type I atrial flutter has an atrial rate of 240–340 bpm. It develops due to a reentry mechanism in the right atrium. The mechanism leading to type II atrial flutter has not been identified. In this type of flutter, the atrial rate is faster, up to 350 bpm.

Clients with atrial flutter may complain of palpitations or a fluttering sensation in the chest or throat. If the ventricular rate is rapid, manifestations of decreased cardiac output, such as decreased level of consciousness, hypotension, decreased urinary output, and cool clammy skin, may be noted. The atrial kick (additional ventricular filling with atrial contraction) is lost because of inadequate atrial filling.

ECG characteristics include a "sawtooth" or "picket fence" appearance of P waves, which are labeled flutter (F) waves. The atrial rate is rapid, often around 300 bpm. As a protective mechanism, many impulses are blocked at the AV node, and the ventricular rate is rarely greater than 150–170 bpm. Usually, atrial impulses are evenly conducted through the AV node, for example, two impulses to one QRS complex (2:1), four impulses to one QRS complex (4:1), or six impulses to one QRS complex (6:1). A constant conduction ratio results in a regular ventricular rhythm; the ventricular rhythm is irregular if the conduction ratio varies. The ventricular rate usually ranges from 150 to 170 bpm in 2:1 conduction and 60 to 75 bpm for lower conduction ratios. The T wave is usually hidden by overriding F waves; some F waves may be hidden in the QRS complex.

ATRIAL FIBRILLATION

Atrial fibrillation is a common dysrhythmia characterized by disorganized atrial activity without discrete atrial contractions. Multiple small reentry circuits develop in the atria. Atrial cells cannot repolarize in time to respond to the next stimulus (Huether & McCance, 2011). Extremely rapid atrial impulses bombard the AV node, resulting in an irregularly irregular ventricular response. Atrial fibrillation may occur suddenly and recur, or it may persist as a chronic dysrhythmia. Atrial fibrillation is commonly associated with heart failure, rheumatic heart disease, CHD, hypertension, and hyperthyroidism.

Manifestations of atrial fibrillation relate to the rate of the ventricular response. With rapid response rates, manifestations of decreased cardiac output such as hypotension, shortness of breath, fatigue, and angina may develop. Clients with extensive heart disease may develop syncope or heart failure. Peripheral pulses are irregular and of variable amplitude (strength).

The specific ECG characteristics of atrial fibrillation include an irregularly irregular rhythm and the absence of identifiable P waves. The atrial rate is so rapid that it is not measurable. The ventricular rate varies.

Atrial fibrillation increases the risk for formation of thromboemboli. Organ infarction may occur as a result; the incidence of stroke is high.

Junctional Dysrhythmias

Rhythms that originate in AV nodal tissue are termed *junctional*. The AV junction includes the AV node and the bundle of His, which branches into the right and left bundle branches. An impulse arising from the AV junction may occur in response to failure of higher pacemakers, as in a *junctional escape rhythm*, or it may result from an abnormal mechanism, such as altered automaticity. An impulse arising from the AV junction may or may not be conducted back up to the atria. This conduction against the normal flow or pattern is called **retrograde conduction**. The resulting atrial wave, called a P′ wave, may be found before, during, or after the QRS complex, depending on the speed of conduction. The P′ wave is inverted in some ECG leads because the impulse moves from the AV node up to the atria instead of from the SA node down toward the AV node. In addition, the P′R interval is shorter than normal (<0.12 second). The QRS complex is typically narrow.

A junctional rhythm may be due to drug toxicity (e.g., digitalis, beta-blockers, or calcium-channel blockers) or other causes such as hypoxemia, hyperkalemia, increased vagal tone or damage to the AV node, MI, and heart failure. Loss of synchronized atrial contraction and the atrial kick may affect cardiac output, leading to manifestations of decreased cardiac output and impaired myocardial tissue perfusion. Heart failure may develop.

Premature junctional contractions occur before the next expected beat of the underlying rhythm. Isolated premature junctional contractions may occur in healthy individuals and are insignificant. Junctional tachycardia is a junctional rhythm with a rate greater than 60 bpm. It is caused by increased automaticity of AV nodal tissue. The ventricular rate is usually less than 140 bpm. Both rhythms are most commonly associated with digitalis toxicity, hypoxia, ischemia, or electrolyte imbalances.

Ventricular Dysrhythmias

Ventricular dysrhythmias originate in the ventricles. Because the ventricles pump blood into the pulmonary and systemic vasculature, any disruption of their rhythm can affect cardiac output and tissue perfusion. A wide and bizarre QRS complex (>0.12 second) is a characteristic feature of ventricular dysrhythmias. This occurs because ventricular ectopic impulses begin and travel outside normal conduction pathways. Other characteristics include no relationship between the QRS complex and a P wave, increased amplitude of the QRS complex, an abnormal ST segment, and a T wave deflected in the opposite direction from the QRS complex.

PREMATURE VENTRICULAR CONTRACTIONS Premature ventricular contractions (PVCs) are ectopic ventricular beats that occur before the next expected beat of the underlying rhythm. They usually do not reset the atrial rhythm and are followed by a full compensatory pause. PVCs often have no significance in individuals without heart disease. Frequent, recurrent, or multifocal PVCs may be associated with an increased risk for lethal dysrhythmias. PVCs result from either enhanced automaticity or a reentry phenomenon. They may be triggered by anxiety or stress; tobacco, alcohol, or caffeine use; hypoxia, acidosis, and electrolyte imbalances; sympathomimetic drugs; CHD; heart failure; mechanical stimulation of the heart (e.g., the insertion of a cardiac catheter); or reperfusion after fibrinolytic therapy. The incidence and significance of PVCs is greatest after MI.

Premature ventricular contractions may be isolated or may occur in a specific pattern. Two PVCs in a row are called a **couplet**, or paired PVCs. Three consecutive PVCs (a **triplet**, or salvo) are a short run of ventricular tachycardia. **Ventricular bigeminy** is characterized by a PVC following each normal beat; a PVC noted every third beat is called **ventricular trigeminy**. When the ventricular impulse arises from one ectopic site, all PVCs look the same (monomorphic) and are called **unifocal** PVCs. **Multifocal** PVCs arise from different ectopic sites and appear different from one another on the ECG (polymorphic).

The frequency and patterns of PVCs can be indicative of myocardial irritability and the risk for a lethal dysrhythmia. The following are considered warning signs in the client with acute heart disease (e.g., an acute MI):

- PVCs that develop within the first 4 hours of an MI
- Frequent PVCs (six or more per minute)
- Couplets or triplets
- Multifocal PVCs
- R-on-T phenomenon (PVCs falling on the T wave).

In individuals without heart disease, isolated PVCs usually are insignificant and do not require treatment. In clients with preexisting heart disease, PVCs may indicate drug toxicity or an increased risk for lethal dysrhythmias and cardiac arrest. The risk is greatest following acute MI.

VENTRICULAR TACHYCARDIA Ventricular tachycardia is a rapid ventricular rhythm defined as three or more consecutive PVCs. Ventricular tachycardia may occur in short bursts, or "runs," or it may persist for more than 30 seconds (sustained

ventricular tachycardia). The rate is greater than 100 bpm, and the rhythm is usually regular. Reentry is the usual electrophysiological mechanism responsible for ventricular tachycardia. Myocardial ischemia and infarction are the most common predisposing factors for ventricular tachycardia. VT also is associated with cardiac structural disorders such as valvular disease, rheumatic heart disease, or cardiomyopathy. It may occur in the absence of heart disease and with anorexia nervosa, metabolic disorders, and drug toxicity.

Nonsustained ventricular tachycardia may occur paroxysmally and convert back to an effective rhythm spontaneously. The client may experience a fluttering sensation in the chest or complain of palpitations and brief shortness of breath. Clients in sustained VT generally develop signs and symptoms of decreased cardiac output and hemodynamic instability, including severe hypotension, a weak or nonpalpable pulse, and loss of consciousness. Allowed to continue, VT can deteriorate into ventricular fibrillation. Sustained ventricular tachycardia is a medical emergency that requires immediate intervention, particularly in clients with cardiac disease.

Torsades de pointes is a type of ventricular tachycardia associated with long-QT syndrome (a prolongation of the QT interval). Long-QT syndrome may be genetic or acquired, occurring secondarily to electrolyte disruptions, MI, cocaine use, liquid protein diets, medications, or other conditions. In *torsades de pointes*, the QRS complexes vary in size, shape, and amplitude (**Figure 16–50 ●**). Clients with *torsades de pointes* typically present with recurrent episodes of palpitations, dizziness, and syncope. It is important to note that sudden cardiac death can occur with the first episode.

VENTRICULAR FIBRILLATION Ventricular fibrillation is extremely rapid, chaotic ventricular depolarization that causes the ventricles to quiver and cease contracting; the heart does not pump. This is known as cardiac arrest; it is a medical emergency requiring immediate intervention with CPR. Death will follow the onset of ventricular fibrillation within 4 minutes if the rhythm is not recognized and terminated and an effective perfusing rhythm reestablished.

Ventricular fibrillation is usually triggered by severe myocardial ischemia or infarction. It occurs without warning 50% of the time. It is the terminal event in many disease processes or

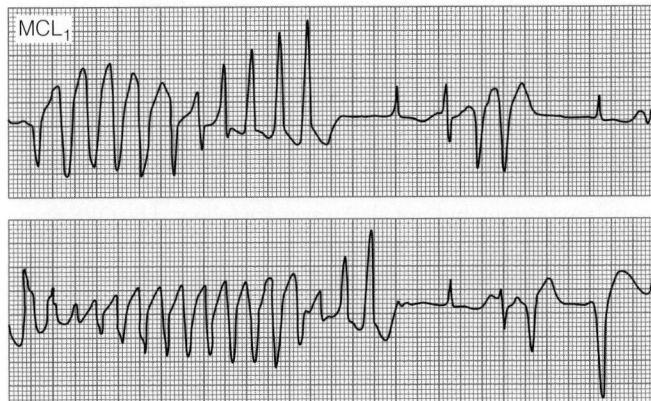

Figure 16–50 ● *Torsades de pointes.* Note the wide and bizarre QRS complexes of varying size, shape (morphology), and amplitude.

traumatic conditions. Ventricular fibrillation may be precipitated by a single PVC or may follow ventricular tachycardia. Other causes of ventricular fibrillation include digitalis toxicity, reperfusion therapy, use of antidysrhythmic drugs, hypokalemia and hyperkalemia, hypothermia, metabolic acidosis, mechanical stimulation (as with the insertion of cardiac catheters or pacing wires), and electric shock.

Clinically, loss of ventricular contractions results in the absence of a palpable or audible pulse. The client loses consciousness and stops breathing as perfusion ceases. The ECG shows grossly irregular, bizarre complexes with no discernible rate or rhythm.

Atrioventricular Conduction Blocks

Conduction defects that delay or block transmission of the sinus impulse through the AV node are called AV conduction blocks. Impaired conduction may result from tissue injury or disease, increased vagal (parasympathetic) tone, drug effects, or a congenital defect. AV conduction blocks vary in severity from benign to severe.

FIRST-DEGREE ATRIOVENTRICULAR BLOCK First-degree AV block is a benign conduction delay that generally poses no threat, has no symptoms, and requires no treatment. Impulse conduction through the AV node is slowed, but all atrial impulses are conducted to the ventricles. It may result from injury or infarct of the AV node, other cardiac diseases, or drug effects. The ECG shows all characteristics of normal sinus rhythm, except that the PR interval is greater than 0.20 second.

SECOND-DEGREE ATRIOVENTRICULAR BLOCK Second-degree AV block is characterized by failure to conduct one or more impulses from the atria to the ventricles. Two patterns of second-degree AV block are seen, identified as type I and type II.

Second-Degree Atrioventricular Block—Type I Type I second-degree AV block (Mobitz type I or Wenckebach phenomenon) is characterized by a repeating pattern of increasing AV conduction delays until an impulse fails to conduct to the ventricles. On the ECG, PR intervals progressively lengthen until one QRS complex is not conducted (or dropped). The ventricular rate remains adequate to maintain cardiac output, and the client usually is asymptomatic. Mobitz type I AV block usually is transient, associated with acute MI or drug intoxication (e.g., digitalis, beta-blockers, or calcium-channel blockers). It rarely progresses to complete heart block.

Second-Degree Atrioventricular Block—Type II Type II second-degree AV block (Mobitz type II) involves intermittent failure of the AV node to conduct an impulse to the ventricles without preceding delays in conduction. The PR interval remains constant, but not all P waves are followed by QRS complexes (e.g., there may be two P waves for every QRS). With second-degree AV block, the bundle of His and/or lower regions of the conduction system are blocked. Mobitz type II block is frequently associated with acute anterior wall MI and a high rate of mortality (Huether & McCance, 2011). Manifestations of Mobitz type II block depend on the ventricular rate. Pacemaker therapy may be required to maintain the cardiac output.

THIRD-DEGREE ATRIOVENTRICULAR BLOCK Third-degree AV block (complete heart block) occurs when atrial impulses are completely blocked at the AV node and fail to reach the ventricles. As a result, the atria and ventricles are controlled by different and independent pacemakers, with separate rates and rhythms. The ventricular impulse arises from either junctional fibers (with a rate of 40–60 bpm) or a ventricular pacemaker at a rate of less than 40 bpm. The width of the QRS complex depends on the location of the escape pacemaker. The QRS is wide and the rate is slow when the rhythm arises distal to the bundle of His.

Third-degree AV block is frequently associated with an inferior or anteroseptal MI. Other causes include congenital conditions, acute or degenerative cardiac disease or damage, drug effects, and electrolyte imbalances. The slow escape rhythm significantly affects cardiac output, causing manifestations such as syncope (known as a *Stokes-Adams attack*), dizziness, fatigue, exercise intolerance, and heart failure. Third-degree AV block is life threatening and requires immediate intervention to maintain adequate cardiac output.

ATRIOVENTRICULAR DISSOCIATION Complete dissociation of atrial and ventricular rhythms can occur in conditions other than third-degree AV block. The two primary factors leading to AV dissociation are severe sinus bradycardia and a lower pacemaker (junctional or ventricular) that competes with or exceeds the normal sinus rhythm. AV dissociation may result from acute myocardial ischemia or infarction, cardiac surgery, or drug effects. The ECG shows separate and competing atrial (P waves) and ventricular (QRS complexes) rhythms.

Intraventricular Conduction Blocks

Once the impulse enters the ventricles, its conduction through the right and left bundle branches may be impaired (bundle branch block). As a result, the impulse is conducted more slowly than normal through the ventricles. On the ECG, the QRS complex is prolonged. Its appearance varies, depending on the affected bundle (right or left). Typically, no clinical manifestations are associated with bundle branch block unless it occurs in conjunction with an AV block.

The Clinical Manifestations and Therapies feature lists the etiology and clinical manifestations of life-threatening dysrhythmias along with recommended treatments.

▶ COLLABORATION

Cardiac dysrhythmias may be either benign or critical. Recognizing lethal dysrhythmias is a matter of life and death. Major goals of care include identifying the dysrhythmia, evaluating its effect on physical and psychosocial well-being, and treating the underlying causes. This may involve correcting fluid and electrolyte or acid–base imbalances; treating hypoxia, pain, or anxiety; administering antidysrhythmic medications; or performing mechanical and surgical interventions.

Diagnostic Tests

Diagnostic tests for dysrhythmias include ECG, cardiac monitoring, and electrophysiology studies. Laboratory tests, such as serum electrolytes, drug levels, and arterial blood gases (ABGs), may be done to help identify the cause of the dysrhythmia.

Clinical Manifestations and Therapies **Life-Threatening Dysrhythmias**

ETIOLOGY	CLINICAL MANIFESTATIONS	CLINICAL THERAPIES
Decreased cardiac output	■ Changes in level of consciousness (LOC) ranging from dizziness to complete loss of consciousness ■ Ischemia ■ Reduced tissue perfusion ■ Hypotension	■ Administer antiarrhythmic medications. ■ Perform defibrillation or cardioversion (external or implanted). ■ Install pacemaker (external or implanted). ■ Reduce cardiac workload.
Alterations in oxygenation	■ Cyanosis ■ Shortness of breath ■ Hypoxemia ■ Hypercapnia ■ Altered LOC ■ Death	■ Administer oxygen. ■ Provide mechanical ventilation. ■ Reduce activity to decrease oxygen demands on the body.
Stasis of blood in the heart	■ Increased risk of emboli formation that manifests differently depending on where the thrombus occurs ■ May result in myocardial infarction, stroke, or deep venous thrombosis	■ Administer anticoagulants. ■ Treat the underlying dysrhythmia to promote movement of blood through the chambers of the heart.
Sudden cardiac death	■ Pulselessness ■ Absence of respirations ■ Death	■ Perform cardiopulmonary resuscitation. ■ Administer antiarrhythmic medications. ■ Administer oxygen. ■ Conduct cardiorespiratory monitoring after successful resuscitation.

ELECTROCARDIOGRAM   The 12-lead ECG may be required to accurately diagnose a dysrhythmia. It also provides information about underlying disease processes, such as MI or other cardiac disease. The ECG may also be used to monitor the effects of treatment.

CARDIAC MONITORING   Cardiac monitoring allows continuous observation of the cardiac rhythm. It is used in many different circumstances (**Box 16–21** ●). Different types of ECG monitoring are employed for different situations.

Continuous Cardiac Monitoring   Continuous monitoring of the cardiac rhythm is provided by bedside and central monitoring stations. Electrodes placed on the client's chest attach to cables connected to a monitor. The heart rate and rhythm are visually displayed on a bedside monitor connected to a central monitoring station. The central station allows simultaneous monitoring of multiple clients within a nursing unit. Alarms on both bedside and central monitors warn of potential problems, such as very rapid or very slow heart rates. Alarm limits are preset by the nurse for the individual client.

Telemetry may be used in acute care settings when the client is ambulatory. Chest electrodes are connected to a portable transmitter worn around the neck or waist, and the ECG is transmitted electronically to a central monitoring station for continuous monitoring.

Home Monitoring   Clients often complain of palpitations or other heart symptoms but are asymptomatic during evalua-

tion in a hospital or community-based setting. Ambulatory or Holter monitoring may be used to identify intermittent dysrhythmias, to detect silent ischemia, to monitor the effects of treatment, and to assess pacemaker or automatic cardioverter–defibrillator function. Electrodes are applied and the leads attached to the portable telemetry monitor that records and stores all electrical activity. Clients are instructed to leave the

---

Box 16–21   Indications for Cardiac Monitoring

■ Perioperative monitoring of heart rate and rhythm
■ Detecting and identifying dysrhythmias
■ Monitoring the effects of cardiac and noncardiac diseases on the heart
■ Monitoring clients with potentially life-threatening conditions:
  a. Major trauma (especially cardiac trauma)
  b. Dissecting aneurysm
  c. Acute myocardial infarction
  d. Heart failure
  e. Shock
  f. Other emergency conditions
■ Evaluating responses to procedures and interventions:
  a. Drug therapies
  b. Diagnostic procedures
  c. Ablative techniques
  d. Angioplasty or cardiac catheterization
  e. Cardiac surgery
  f. Pacemaker function
  g. Automatic implantable cardioverter–defibrillator function

electrode pads in place during monitoring and record any cardiac symptoms or events (e.g., chest pain, palpitations, or syncope) in a journal. After the prescribed period, usually 48–72 hours, the client returns to the clinic, and the monitor is removed. Diary entries are compared to the recorded heart rhythms to identify the effects of dysrhythmias.

ELECTROPHYSIOLOGY STUDIES Diagnostic cardiac electrophysiology procedures are performed to identify dysrhythmias and their causes. Electrophysiology studies are used to analyze components of the conduction system, identify sites of ectopic stimulation, and evaluate the effectiveness of treatment. Electrophysiology procedures can be employed for both diagnosis and as a therapeutic intervention.

In the electrophysiology laboratory, electrode catheters are guided by fluoroscopy into the heart through the femoral or brachial vein. The timing and sequence of electrical activation during normal and abnormal (aberrant) rhythms are observed and measured. Providers may use electrical stimulation to induce dysrhythmia similar to what the client is experiencing. Following diagnosis, an electrophysiology procedure may be used to treat the dysrhythmia—for example, by overdrive pacing (stimulating the client's heart to a rate faster than that of the tachydysrhythmia) to break the dysrhythmia cycle or ablative therapy to destroy the ectopic site. (See further information in the Cardiac Mapping and Catheter Ablation section later in this exemplar.)

Nursing care for the client undergoing an electrophysiology procedure is similar to that for the client undergoing percutaneous coronary revascularization. (See the discussion in the Revascularization Procedures section in Exemplar 16.3 for more details.) The procedure and expected sensations are explained. The client remains awake during the procedure; antianxiety medications or sedatives are given to reduce apprehension. Intravenous heparin may be given during the procedure to reduce the risk of thromboembolism.

Pharmacologic Therapy

The goal of drug therapy is to suppress dysrhythmia formation. No drug has been found to be completely safe and effective. Antidysrhythmic drugs are primarily used for acute treatment of dysrhythmias, although they may also be used to manage chronic conditions. The overall goal of therapy is to maintain an effective cardiac output by stabilizing cardiac rhythm. See the Medications feature.

It is important to remember that many antidysrhythmic drugs also have prodysrhythmic effects; that is, they can worsen existing dysrhythmias and precipitate new ones. Prior to administering antidysrhythmic medications, the nurse will want to obtain a thorough drug and medical history and measure baseline vital signs and cardiac rhythm. Labs should also be reviewed prior to initiating antidysrhythmic therapy.

Most antidysrhythmic drugs are classified by their effects on the cardiac action potential. Most are class I drugs, or fast sodium-channel blockers. By blocking sodium channels, these drugs slow impulse conduction in the atria and ventricles. This class is further divided into subclasses A, B, and C. Class II drugs are beta-blockers, which decrease SA node automaticity,

AV conduction velocity, and myocardial contractility. Class III agents block potassium channels, delaying repolarization and prolonging the relative refractory period. Class IV drugs are calcium-channel blockers. Their effect is similar to that of beta-blockers. Adenosine and digoxin do not fit within the major classes. Both drugs reduce SA node automaticity and slow AV conduction. Ibutilide and magnesium also fall outside the major classes but are used to treat dysrhythmias. The Medications feature identifies common antidysrhythmic drugs within each class and the nursing implications in caring for clients receiving these drugs.

Drugs that affect the autonomic nervous system may also be used to treat dysrhythmias. Sympathomimetics, such as epinephrine, stimulate the heart, increasing both heart rate and contractility. Anticholinergic agents, such as atropine, are used to decrease vagal tone and increase heart rate. Magnesium sulfate is an unclassified drug that has been shown to be safe and effective in treating ventricular tachycardias.

Countershock

Countershock is used to interrupt cardiac rhythms that compromise cardiac output and the client's welfare. Delivery of a direct current charge depolarizes all cardiac cells at the same time. This simultaneous depolarization may stop a tachydysrhythmia and allow the SA node to recover control of impulse formation. The two types of countershock are synchronized cardioversion and defibrillation.

SYNCHRONIZED CARDIOVERSION **Synchronized cardioversion** delivers direct electrical current synchronized with the client's heart rhythm. Synchronization of the shock with the QRS complex prevents ventricular fibrillation by avoiding current delivery during the vulnerable period of repolarization. Cardioversion is usually done as an elective procedure to treat supraventricular tachycardia, atrial fibrillation, atrial flutter, or hemodynamically stable ventricular tachycardia.

The nurse assists with cardioversion by preparing the client before the procedure; obtaining any laboratory tests ordered; obtaining and documenting ECG strips before, during, and after treatment; setting up the equipment; and monitoring the client's response.

Clients in atrial fibrillation are at high risk for thromboembolism following cardioversion. Loss of atrial contractions with atrial fibrillation leads to blood pooling in the atria, increasing the risk of clot formation. When the atria begin to contract following successful cardioversion, clots may be dislodged, embolizing to the pulmonary or systemic circulation. If possible, anticoagulants are given for several weeks before cardioversion is attempted.

DEFIBRILLATION Unlike carefully synchronized cardioversion, **defibrillation** is an emergency procedure that delivers direct current without regard to the cardiac cycle. Ventricular fibrillation is immediately treated as soon as the dysrhythmia is recognized. Early defibrillation has been shown to improve survival in clients experiencing ventricular fibrillation.

Defibrillation can be delivered by external paddles or pads or internal paddles. Conductive gel pads or paste is applied,

Medications **Antidysrhythmic Drugs**

CLASSIFICATION AND DRUG EXAMPLES	MECHANISMS OF ACTION	NURSING CONSIDERATIONS

Class I Drugs: Sodium-Channel Blockers
 	
Class IA
 	
Drug examples:
■ quinidine (Cardioquin, Quinidex, Quinaglute)
■ procainamide (Pronestyl, Procan SR)
■ disopyramide (Norpace, Norpace CR)
	Decrease the flow of sodium into the cell and prolong the action potential.
	
	Decrease automaticity, slow the rate of impulse conduction. and prolong refractoriness.
	
	Used to treat both supraventricular and ventricular tachycardias.
		■ Obtain baseline data, including vital signs, cardiac rhythm (including rate, PR and QT intervals, and QRS duration), and physical assessment (especially cardiac, neurological, and respiratory status).
		■ Assess medication regimen to identify drugs that may interfere with antidysrhythmic therapy.
		■ Monitor electrocardiogram to evaluate the effectiveness of therapy and assess for possible dysrhythmias precipitated by treatment.
		■ Immediately report to the physician any manifestations of drug toxicity:
		  • Procainamide: signs of heart failure; conduction delays or ventricular dysrhythmias; skin rash, myalgias or arthralgias, flu-like symptoms
		  • Disopyramide: urinary retention, heart failure, eye pain
		  • Lidocaine: changes in neurological status, such as agitation, confusion, dizziness, nervousness
		  • Amiodarone: pulmonary fibrosis (increasing dyspnea, cough, hepatic dysfunction—changes in liver function tests, jaundice); vision changes, photosensitivity
		  • Digoxin: anorexia, nausea, vomiting; blurred or double vision; yellow-green halos; new-onset dysrhythmias.
		■ Use an infusion pump to administer intravenous infusions. Monitor the dose, and assess its appropriateness (in mg/min or mcg/kg/min).
		
		Heath education for the client and family:
		■ Take the drug exactly as prescribed. Do not skip or double doses. Check with your physician if a dose is missed.
		■ Take your pulse and record the rate daily before rising. Count the pulse for a full minute. Bring the record with you to each office or clinic visit.
		■ Report the following to the physician: irregular pulse rate or rhythm, dizziness, eye pain, changes in vision, skin rashes or color changes, wheezing or other respiratory problems, and changes in behavior.

Class IB *Drug examples:* ■ lidocaine (Xylocaine) ■ mexiletine (Mexitil) ■ phenytoin (Dilantin) ■ moricizine (Ethmozine)	Decrease the refractory period but have little effect on automaticity. Used primarily to treat ventricular dysrhythmias, including premature ventricular contractions and ventricular tachycardia.	
Class IC *Drug examples:* ■ flecainide (Tambocor) ■ propafenone (Rythmol)	Slow impulse conduction velocity. Have little effect on refractoriness. Used to reduce or eliminate tachydysrhythmias associated with reentry. May be used to treat supraventricular tachycardia.	
Class II Drugs: Beta Blockers *Drug examples:* Esmolol (Brevibloc), Propranolol (Inderal), Metoprolol (Toprol)	Decrease automaticity through the AV node. Reduce the heart rate and myocardial contractility. Used to treat supraventricular tachycardia and to slow the ventricular response rate to atrial fibrillation. May cause bronchospasm and are contraindicated for clients with asthma, COPD, or other restrictive or obstructive.	
Class III Drugs: Potassium-Channel Blockers *Drug examples:* ■ sotalol (Betapace) ■ amiodarone (Cordarone) ■ ibutilide (Corvert) ■ dofetilide (Tikosyn)	Block potassium channels, prolonging repolarization and the refractory period. Primarily used to treat ventricular tachycardia and ventricular fibrillation. Amiodarone may be used to treat supraventricular tachycardias.	
Class IV Drugs: Calcium-Channel Blockers *Drug examples:* ■ verapamil (Calan, Isoptin, Verelan) ■ diltiazem (Cardizem, Dilacor XR)	Decrease automaticity and AV nodal conduction. Used to manage supraventricular tachycardias. Reduce myocardial contractility.	
Other Drugs *Drug examples:* ■ adenosine (Adenocard) ■ digoxin	Decrease conduction through the AV node. Used to treat supraventricular tachycardias.	

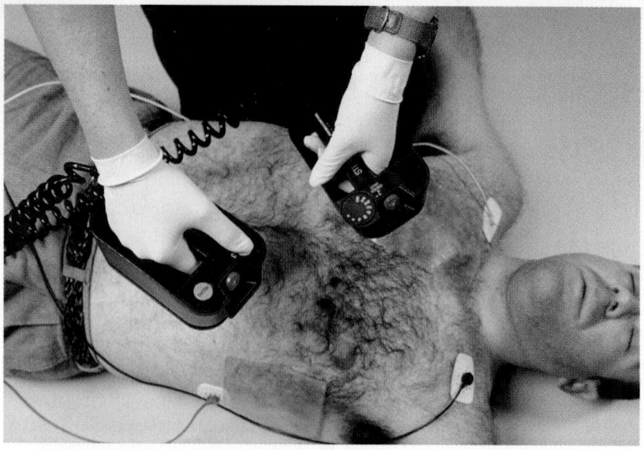

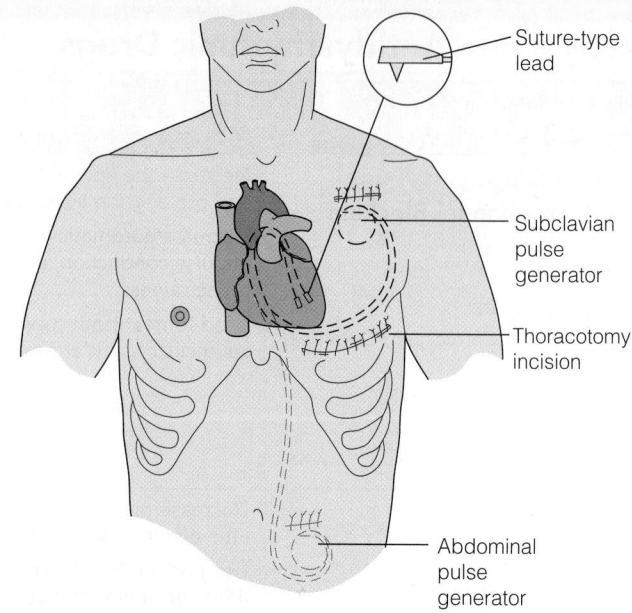

Figure 16–51 ● Placement of paddles for defibrillation.
Source: © Blend Images/Alamy.

and external paddles or pads are placed on the chest wall at the apex and base of the heart (**Figure 16–51** ●). Internal paddles are applied directly on the heart and may be used in surgery, the emergency department, or critical care. Internal defibrillation is done only by a physician; external defibrillation may be performed by any healthcare provider who has been trained in the procedure. Automatic external defibrillators are available on most hospital units to allow early defibrillation for cardiac arrest.

Pacemaker Therapy

A **pacemaker** is a pulse generator used to provide an electrical stimulus to the heart when the heart fails to generate or conduct its own stimulus at a rate that maintains the cardiac output. The pulse generator is connected to leads (insulated wires) passed intravenously into the heart or sutured directly to the epicardium. The leads sense intrinsic electrical activity of the heart and provide an electrical stimulus to the heart when necessary (pacing).

Pacemakers are used to treat both acute and chronic conduction defects, such as third-degree AV block. They also may be used to treat bradydysrhythmias and tachydysrhythmias.

Temporary pacemakers use an external pulse generator attached to a lead threaded intravenously into the right ventricle, to temporary pacing wires implanted during cardiac surgery, or to external conductive pads placed on the chest wall for emergency pacing. Permanent pacemakers use an internal pulse generator placed in a subcutaneous pocket in the subclavian space or abdominal wall. The generator connects to leads sewn directly onto the heart (epicardial) or passed transvenously into the heart (endocardial). Epicardial pacemakers (**Figure 16–52** ●) require surgical exposure of the heart. Leads may be placed during cardiac surgery or by using a small subxiphoid incision to expose the heart. Transvenous pacemaker leads are positioned in the right heart via the cephalic, subclavian, or jugular vein (**Figure 16–53** ●). Local anesthesia can be used for permanent pacemaker insertion.

Pacemakers are programmed to stimulate the atria or the ventricles (single-chamber pacing) or both (dual-chamber pacing). **Table 16–29** ● defines terms used to describe pacemaker modes and functions. The most commonly used pacemakers

Figure 16–52 ● A permanent epicardial pacemaker. The pulse generator may be placed in subcutaneous pockets in the subclavian or abdominal regions.

either sense activity in and pace the ventricles only or sense activity in and pace both the atria and the ventricles. Dual-chamber or atrioventricular sequential pacing stimulates both chambers of the heart in sequence. AV pacing imitates the normal sequence of atrial contraction followed by ventricular contraction, improving cardiac output.

✳ Go to *nursing.pearsonhighered.com* to see Chart 3: Nursing Care of the Client Having a Permanent Pacemaker Implant.

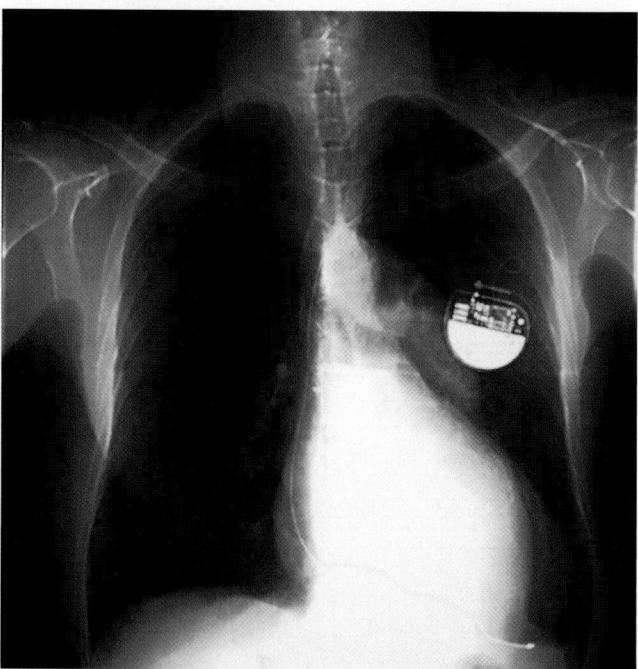

Figure 16–53 ● A permanent transvenous (endocardial) pacemaker with the lead placed in the right ventricle via the subclavian vein.
Source: Living Art Enterprises/Science Source.

TABLE 16–29 Terms Used to Describe Pacemaker Functions

TERM	DEFINITION
Asynchronous pacing	Pacemaker delivers a pacing stimulus at a set rate regardless of intrinsic cardiac activity.
Base rate	Rate at which the pacemaker paces when no cardiac activity is sensed.
Capture	The ability of the pacing stimulus to generate a cardiac depolarization.
Demand pacing	Pacemaker delivers a pacing stimulus only when the intrinsic rate falls below the pacemaker's base rate.
Dual-chamber pacing	Allows both the atria and the ventricles to be paced; most frequently used permanent pacing mode.
Output	The electrical stimulus delivered by the pulse generator.
Pacing spike	A small vertical spike noted on the electrocardiogram with every pacemaker stimulus.
Rate-responsive pacing	Pacemaker has sensors that detect changes in the client's physical activity and adjust the pacing rate accordingly.
Sensing	The pacemaker's ability to identify and respond to intrinsic cardiac activity.
Single-chamber pacing	Pacing of only the atria or the ventricles, not both; most commonly used temporary pacing mode.

Pacing is detected on the ECG strip by the presence of a pacing artifact (**Figure 16–54** ●). A sharp spike is noted before the P wave with atrial pacing and before the QRS complex with ventricular pacing. Pacing spikes are seen before both the P wave and QRS complex in AV sequential pacing. Capture is noted if a contraction of the chamber occurs immediately following the pacer spike. Problems in sensing, pacing, and capture are noted in **Table 16–30** ●.

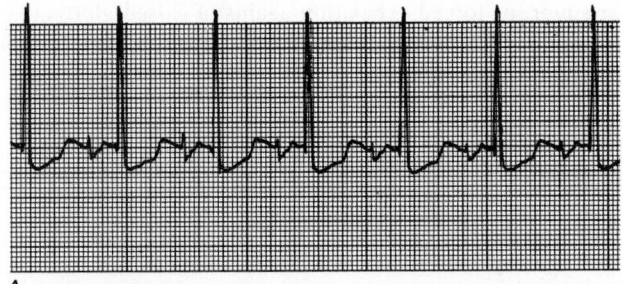

A

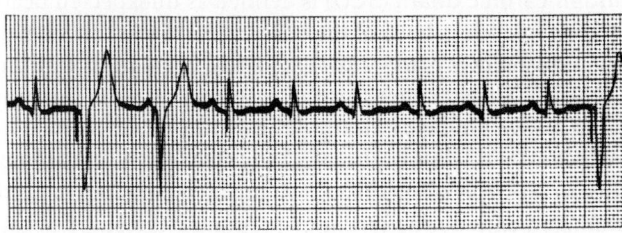

B

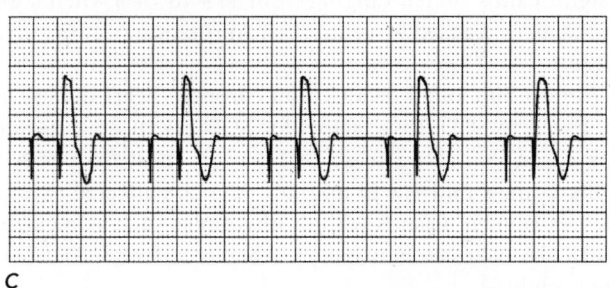

C

Figure 16–54 ● Pacing artifacts. *A,* Atrial pacing and ventricular sensing. Note the pacer spike preceding the P wave. *B,* Ventricular demand pacing. Note the absence of pacer spikes when the client's natural rhythm dominates. *C,* Atrioventricular pacing. Note the pacer spikes preceding both P waves and QRS complexes.

Care of the client with a temporary or permanent pacemaker focuses on monitoring for pacemaker malfunctioning, maintaining safety (**Box 16–22** ●), and preventing infection and postoperative complications.

Implantable Cardioverter–Defibrillator

The implantable cardioverter–defibrillator (ICD) detects life-threatening changes in the cardiac rhythm and automatically delivers an electric shock to convert the dysrhythmia back into a normal rhythm. ICDs are used for survivors of sudden cardiac death (SCD), clients with recurrent ventricular tachycardia, and clients with demonstrated risk factors for SCD. ICDs can deliver a shock as needed, provide pacing on demand, and store ECG records of tachycardic episodes.

A pulse generator connected to lead electrodes for rhythm detection and current delivery is implanted in the left pectoral region. The lead is threaded transvenously to the apex of the right ventricle. The ICD is programmed to sense a change in heart rate or rhythm. When it detects a potentially lethal

---

Box 16–22 Safety for Clients With a Temporary Pacemaker

- Ensure that all electrical equipment in use has a grounded plug; do not use adapters or extension cords.
- Encourage use of battery-powered equipment (e.g., electric razor).
- Remove any damaged electrical equipment from the unit, including equipment that
  a. has been abused (e.g., has been dropped or in which liquid has been spilled).
  b. has given anyone a shock.
  c. has frayed, worn, or otherwise damaged electrical cords or plugs.
  d. has other evidence of impaired function, such as a hot smell during use or control knobs that are loose or do not consistently produce the expected response.
- Wear gloves when handling the pacemaker electrodes or wires.
- Insulate pacemaker terminals and pacing wires with nonconductive, moisture-proof material (e.g., a rubber glove).
- Test the pacemaker battery before use.
- Keep a spare pacemaker, cable, batteries, and battery tester available at all times.
- Immediately report any apparent deviation from expected pacemaker function.

TABLE 16–30 Potential Pacemaker Problems and Considerations for Preventing Complications

DEVICE COMPLICATION	CONSIDERATIONS FOR PREVENTING COMPLICATIONS
Lead dislodgement	Active and passive fixation mechanisms.
Pneumothorax, hemothorax, or air embolism	Fluoroscopic guidance of the subclavian puncture used with careful technique. Use of introducers with hemostatic valves.
Myocardial perforation during lead placement	Consideration of lead design prior to implantation. Physician experience. Client condition.
Extracardiac stimulation	Decrease voltage output or pulse width. Pacemaker may need to be reprogrammed or leads repositioned.
Venous thrombosis and superior vena cava syndrome	Asymptomatic clients are usually not treated. Specific treatment for thrombosis or fibrosis is causative. Varies from heparin therapy to percutaneous angioplasty or open surgical procedure. Surgery is last resort.
Twiddler syndrome (leads become displaced due to the pacemaker box)	Size of the pacemaker pocket should be limited, with the device sutured to the fascia. Clients should be instructed not to manipulate device pockets.
Postpacemaker implant pericarditis	Anti-inflammatory medications. Possible repositioning of pacemaker leads and/or removal.

rhythm, it shocks the heart to convert the rhythm. The device can be programmed or reprogrammed at the bedside as necessary. The ICD may be tested before discharge.

Local or general anesthesia is used, and the client may be discharged within 24 hours. The lithium-powered battery must be surgically replaced every 5 years. Complications and nursing care are similar to those for a client having a permanent pacemaker implant.

The client may briefly lose consciousness before the device discharges but typically regains consciousness quickly after the episode. Some clients report significant discomfort with ICD discharge (like a "blow to the chest"). Anyone in direct contact with the client when the device discharges may experience a tingling sensation.

Cardiac Mapping and Catheter Ablation

Cardiac mapping and catheter ablation are used to locate and destroy an ectopic focus. These diagnostic and therapeutic measures use electrophysiology techniques and can be performed in a cardiac catheterization laboratory. Cardiac mapping is used to identify the site of earliest impulse formation in the atria or ventricles. Intracardiac and extracardiac catheter electrodes and computer technology are used to pinpoint the ectopic site on a map of the heart. These same catheters can be used to deliver the ablative intervention.

Ablation destroys, removes, or isolates an ectopic focus. In most instances, radio-frequency energy produced by high-frequency alternating current is used to create heat as it passes through tissue. Catheter ablation is used to treat supraventricular tachycardias, atrial fibrillation and flutter, and in some cases, paroxysmal ventricular tachycardia. Anticoagulant therapy may be started after catheter ablation to reduce the risk of clot formation at the ablation site.

Other Therapies

In addition to medications and interventional techniques, other measures may be used to treat selected dysrhythmias. Vagal

maneuvers that stimulate the parasympathetic nervous system may be used to slow the heart rate in supraventricular tachycardias. These maneuvers include carotid sinus massage and the Valsalva maneuver. Excessive slowing of the heart rate may result from carotid sinus massage, and it is performed only by a physician during continuous cardiac monitoring. The **Valsalva maneuver**, or forced exhalation against a closed glottis (e.g., bearing down), increases intrathoracic pressure and vagal tone, slowing the pulse rate.

SUDDEN CARDIAC DEATH

▶ OVERVIEW

Sudden cardiac death (SCD) is defined as unexpected death occurring within 1 hour of the onset of cardiovascular symptoms. It usually is caused by ventricular fibrillation and cardiac arrest. **Cardiac arrest** is the cessation of heart function that precedes biological death. Worldwide, fewer than 6% of out-of-hospital victims of cardiac arrest survive. In communities of North America that have organized lay rescuer and automated external defibrillator programs, the survival rate is significantly better, ranging from 49% to 74% when a witnessed arrest caused by ventricular fibrillation occurs (AHA, 2013e).

Almost 50% of all deaths from coronary heart disease are attributed to SCD. Risk factors for SCD are those associated with coronary heart disease. SCD occurs most frequently in adults in their mid-30s to mid-40s. Men are affected twice as often as women. Clients with dysrhythmias such as recurrent ventricular tachycardia may have a higher risk of SCD. SCD is rare in children.

Evidence of coronary heart disease with significant atherosclerosis and narrowing of two or more major coronary arteries is found in 75% of SCD victims. Although most have had a previous MI, only 20%–30% have had a recent acute MI. An acute change in cardiovascular status precedes cardiac arrest by up to 1 hour; however, the onset often is instantaneous or abrupt. Tachycardia develops, and the number of PVCs increases. Ventricular tachycardia occurs, progressing to ventricular fibrillation (Perrin & MacLeod, 2012). This causes blood flow to the brain to be reduced. Death follows unless emergency treatment occurs immediately.

Abnormalities of myocardial structure or function also contribute. Structural abnormalities include infarction, hypertrophy, myopathy, and electrical anomalies. Functional deviations are caused by such factors as ischemia followed by reperfusion, altered homeostasis, autonomic nervous system and hormone interactions, and toxic effects. The interactions of the two cause myocardial instability and may precipitate fatal dysrhythmias.

▶ PATHOPHYSIOLOGY AND ETIOLOGY

Etiology

Almost 50% of all deaths due to coronary heart disease are attributed to SCD. Coronary heart disease causes up to 80% of all sudden cardiac deaths in the United States. Other cardiac pathologies, such as cardiomyopathy and valvular disorders, also may lead to SCD. Noncardiac causes of sudden death include electrocution, pulmonary embolism, and rapid blood loss from a ruptured aortic aneurysm.

Ventricular fibrillation is the most common dysrhythmia associated with SCD, accounting for 65%–80% of cardiac arrests. Survival in these cases is largely dependent on potentially controllable or reversible electrophysiological disturbances, in contrast to SCD due to advanced heart disease. Selected cardiac and noncardiac causes of SCD are listed in **Box 16–23** ●.

Risk Factors

Risk factors for sudden death are similar to those that cause coronary artery disease or any cardiac dysfunction. Smoking,

---

Box 16–23 Selected Causes of Sudden Cardiac Death

CARDIAC CAUSES
- Coronary heart disease
- Reperfusion following ischemia
- Myocardial hypertrophy
- Cardiomyopathy
- Inflammatory myocardial disorders
- Valve disorders
- Primary electrical disorders
- Dissecting or ruptured aortic or ventricular aneurysm
- Cardiac drug toxicity

NONCARDIAC CAUSES
- Pulmonary embolism
- Cerebral hemorrhage
- Autonomic dysfunction
- Choking
- Electrical shock
- Electrolyte and acid–base imbalances

---

obesity, hypertension, diabetes mellitus, sedentary lifestyle, and high-fat diets can result in cardiac disease. Alterations in cardiac function can affect the electrical activity, resulting in dysrhythmias.

▶ CLINICAL MANIFESTATIONS

Sudden cardiac death may be preceded by typical manifestations of acute coronary syndrome or MI, including severe chest pain, dyspnea or orthopnea, and palpitations or lightheadedness. The event itself is abrupt, with complete loss of consciousness and death within minutes. If ventricular tachycardia precedes cardiac arrest, consciousness and mentation may be impaired prior to collapse and loss of consciousness.

▶ COLLABORATION

The goal of care for the client with SCD is to restore cardiac output and tissue perfusion. Treatment measures are initiated as soon as clinical cardiac arrest is verified by the absence of respirations and carotid or femoral pulses. Basic and advanced cardiac life support measures must be instituted within 2–4 minutes of cardiac arrest to prevent permanent neurological damage and ischemic injury to other organs.

Basic Life Support

Basic life support begins with identification of the cardiac arrest and initiation of an emergency response. Providers trained in use of an automated external defibrillator (AED) should immediately defibrillate the client who is in ventricular fibrillation. Self-adhesive conductive pads attached to connecting cables are positioned on the chest (**Figure 16–55** ●). The AED analyzes the rhythm and advises the provider to charge the device if ventricular fibrillation is detected. After all personnel have been warned to stand clear, the shock button is depressed to deliver a shock. Following the shock, CPR is immediately initiated. After approximately 2 minutes, or five cycles of CPR, the rhythm is evaluated and circulation checked. The sequence of analysis, shock, CPR is continued, and advanced cardiac life support protocols are initiated (AHA, 2013e).

Cardiopulmonary resuscitation (CPR) is a mechanical attempt to maintain tissue perfusion and oxygenation using oral resuscitation and external cardiac compressions. All healthcare providers need to be proficient in CPR. The technique should be performed according to AHA guidelines and hospital protocol. Research demonstrates a clear benefit from sustained, effective chest compressions, yet compressions often are interrupted for ventilation, assessment of pulses, and other measures. The 2010 AHA CPR guidelines reflect changes that align with current research findings.

Cardiopulmonary resuscitation carries a high risk for both cardiac and noncardiac trauma. CPR-related complications include injuries to the skin, thorax, upper airway, abdomen, lungs, heart, and great vessels. These complications can be minimized by adhering to accepted CPR techniques.

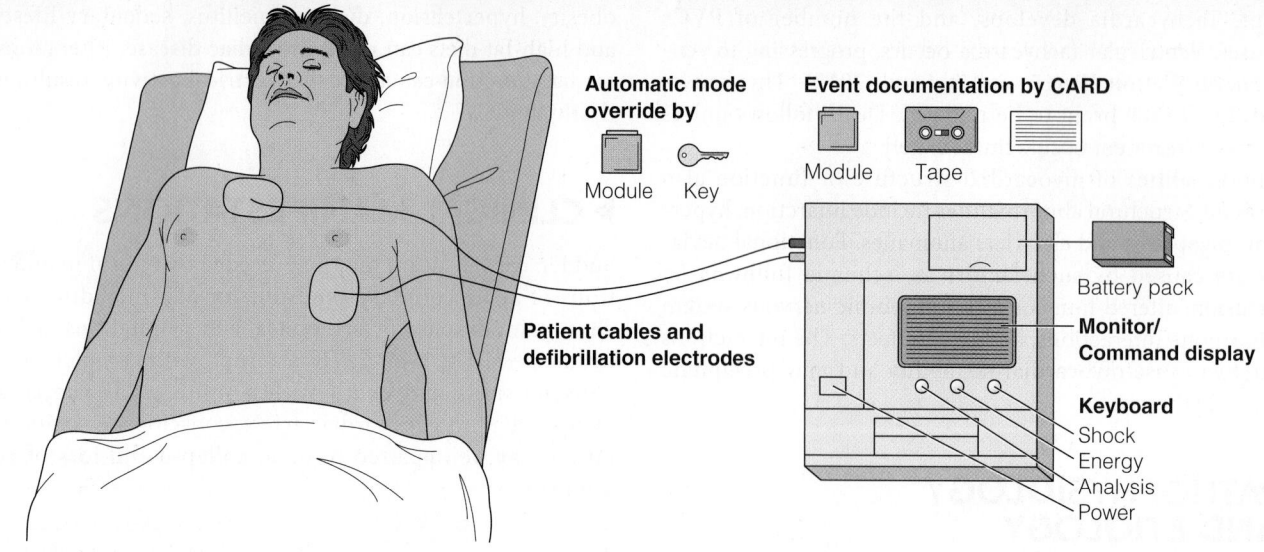

Figure 16–55 ● Schematic of an automated external defibrillator attached to a client.

Stay Current: Visit the Web site of the American Heart Association at **www.heart.org** to stay abreast of their latest recommendations. Note the new hands-only CPR that is recommended for use outside of hospital settings: **www.heart. org/HEARTORG/CPRAndECC/HandsOnlyCPR/LearnMore/ Learn-More_UCM_440810_FAQ.jsp**.

Advanced Life Support

Advanced life support, provided by specially trained healthcare personnel, includes advanced airway support (insertion of a laryngeal mask airway, esophageal–tracheal Combitube, or endotracheal intubation) to maintain the airway and oxygenation, use of intravenous drugs following specific protocols, and additional interventions, such as repeated defibrillation procedures and cardiac pacing. Epinephrine, vasopressin, sodium bicarbonate, and antidysrhythmic drugs, such as amiodarone, lidocaine, procainamide, magnesium sulfate, and atropine are used to attempt to restore and maintain an effective cardiac rhythm.

Postresuscitation Care

Clients experiencing sudden cardiac arrest continue to have a poor prognosis, even with advances in the treatment of heart disease. Treatment depends on the underlying diagnosis. Specific considerations for client care are found in **Box 16–24** ●.

After successful resuscitation, the nurse provides care specific to the client's underlying disease processes and needs. Intravenous infusions, such as lidocaine, or dopamine, may be ordered to prevent further dysrhythmias and maintain hemodynamic stability.

Care for the Family

Nursing care of the client experiencing sudden cardiac arrest includes providing care to the family. The nurse provides honest information about the client's condition to the family in a supportive manner and assesses the family's coping abilities and resources.

If family members are present, they are usually offered a private consultation room in which to await the outcome. If the

Box 16–24   Nursing Care of Clients Experiencing Sudden Cardiac Arrest

Nursing care of the client experiencing sudden cardiac arrest requires prompt recognition of the event and immediate initiation of basic and advanced life support protocols. Fast and effective cardiac compressions and early defibrillation of unstable ventricular tachycardia and fibrillation are the most important keys to the survival of a cardiac arrest event. Important concepts of emergency cardiac care include the following:

■ Treat the client, not the monitor. Recognize signs and symptoms of cardiac compromise early.
■ Activate the emergency medical services system (call a code or 911).
■ Begin and continue basic cardiac life support principles throughout the resuscitation effort.
■ Continually assess the effectiveness of emergency interventions.
■ Defibrillate pulseless ventricular tachycardia or fibrillation as soon as possible.
■ Initiate advanced life support protocols early.

family members are not present, they are notified that their family member is not doing well and are asked to come to the hospital as soon as possible. The situation is presented in a careful manner to prevent the family from racing to the hospital, possibly precipitating an automobile crash. The nurse offers pastoral care or the family's choice of spiritual support during this difficult time. Attendance of family members during resuscitation efforts is controversial and depends on institutional protocols and family desires.

If the client does not survive the arrest, the nurse provides postmortem care to the client and emotional and spiritual support to the family.

■ NURSING PROCESS

Caring for the client with cardiac dysrhythmias requires the ability to recognize, identify, and in some cases, promptly treat the dysrhythmia. The urgency of intervention is determined by the effects of the dysrhythmia on the client. Nursing care focuses on maintaining cardiac output, monitoring the response to therapy, and teaching. Nurses working in critical care areas are likely to care for clients with dysrhythmias on a regular basis and should be certified in advanced cardiac life support.

Health promotion measures to prevent coronary heart disease also reduce the risk for dysrhythmias. In most cases, dysrhythmias develop as a result of ischemic or structural changes in the heart rather than develop in isolation. The nurse should advise clients who are at risk or who complain of occasional palpitations or "flutters" in their chest to reduce their intake of caffeine and other SNS stimulants, such as excess chocolate.

Assessment

Assessment is vital before treating any suspected dysrhythmia. What appears to be ventricular tachycardia on the monitor may be the result of the client scratching or even brushing teeth. Apparent asystole on the monitor may be the result of a loose electrode patch. Similarly, a heart rate of 52 bpm may not affect the overall cardiac output in some clients.

The nurse obtains the following data when assessing the client with a dysrhythmia:

- *Health history.* Complaints of palpitations (the nurse should ask for further definition of palpitations), "fluttering" sensations, or a sensation of the heart racing; episodes of dizziness, light-headedness, or syncope (fainting); timing (duration, time of day); correlation with food or beverage intake or activity; presence of chest pain, shortness of breath, or other associated symptoms; history of heart or endocrine disease (e.g., hyperthyroidism); current medications.
- *Physical examination.* Level of consciousness; vital signs, including apical pulse for a full minute; regularity and amplitude of peripheral pulses; color; presence of dyspnea or adventitious lung sounds; ECG rhythm analysis; oxygen saturation levels.

Diagnosis

Potential diagnoses for the client experiencing a cardiac dysrhythmia include the following:

- *Ineffective Tissue Perfusion: Cerebral*
- *Decreased Cardiac Output*
- *Activity Intolerance*
- *Impaired Spontaneous Ventilation*
- *Spiritual Distress*
- *Disturbed Thought Processes*
- *Fear.*

(NANDA-I © 2012)

Planning

Goals for client care of the client with cardiac dysrhythmia may include the following:

- The client will receive supplemental oxygen to maintain or improve oxygenation; the client may be intubated and mechanically ventilated.
- The client's oxygen demands will be minimized with bed rest and limited activity.

- The client will be monitored for dysrhythmias related to anemia, hypovolemia, electrolyte imbalances, and acidosis.
- The client will comply with medications.
- The client will demonstrate knowledge of the disease process by verbalizing treatment goals.

Implementation

Addressing the effect of the dysrhythmia on cardiac output is the priority of nursing care.

Assess and Monitor Cardiac Output

Dysrhythmias can affect cardiac output. Bradycardias decrease cardiac output if the stroke volume does not increase to compensate for the slow heart rate. Tachycardia reduces diastolic filling time, affecting stroke volume and coronary artery perfusion. Loss of the atrial kick in junctional rhythms, atrial fibrillation, and AV blocks also decreases ventricular filling and cardiac output. In ventricular fibrillation, loss of ventricular contractions causes cardiac arrest and no cardiac output. Nursing interventions related to decreased cardiac output include the following:

SAFETY ALERT Before treating any dysrhythmia, assess the client, not just the monitor. Loose electrode pads, disconnected leads or cables, and muscle movement can simulate critical dysrhythmias. The client's condition is the best indicator of the need for treatment.

- Assess the client for decreased cardiac output: decreased level of consciousness; tachycardia; tachypnea; hypotension; low oxygen saturation; diaphoresis; low urine output; cool, clammy, mottled skin; pallor or cyanosis; and diminished peripheral pulses. Initial signs of decreased cardiac output may be subtle, such as decreased level of consciousness. Early recognition of the dysrhythmia's effect on cardiac output facilitates appropriate treatment and may prevent further adverse effects.
- Monitor the client's ECG; post the ECG strip every shift and when rhythm changes occur. Documenting cardiac rhythm provides a record of disease progression and treatment effectiveness.

SAFETY ALERT Assess the client's vital signs, ECG, and oxygen saturation every 5–15 minutes during acute dysrhythmic episodes and during antidysrhythmic drug infusions. These data provide a record of cardiac output during the dysrhythmia. Antidysrhythmic drugs can adversely affect heart rate, rhythm, and blood pressure, further decreasing cardiac output.

- Assess the client for underlying causes of dysrhythmias, such as hypovolemia, hypoxia, anemia, vagal stimulation, or medications. Sinus tachycardia often develops in response to tissue hypoxia. Vagal stimulation (e.g., the Valsalva maneuver) can precipitate bradycardia.
- Assess the client's serum electrolytes (especially potassium, calcium, and magnesium) and digitalis and antidysrhythmic drug levels as indicated. Report abnormal values. Electrolyte imbalances affect cardiac depolarization and repolarization

and may cause dysrhythmias. Toxic levels of digitalis and antidysrhythmic drugs can precipitate further dysrhythmias. Impaired renal or hepatic function increases the risk for toxicity, as does aging.

■ Be prepared to administer antidysrhythmic medications as indicated. Implement advanced cardiac life support protocols as needed. Emergency drugs should be readily available, especially on units with high-risk clients. See the Medications feature on page 1189 for drugs used to treat common dysrhythmias that may affect cardiac output.

■ If appropriate, instruct the client to perform the Valsalva maneuver (bear down as if straining or coughing) for supraventricular tachycardia or ventricular tachycardia without angina. Vagal maneuvers stimulate the parasympathetic system and may terminate some dysrhythmias. The Valsalva maneuver is contraindicated if chest pain occurs with the dysrhythmia.

■ Prepare to assist the client with cardioversion. Prepare the client per orders or hospital protocol. Explain the procedure to reduce anxiety. Have emergency equipment readily available. Elective or emergency cardioversion is a treatment of choice for certain dysrhythmias.

SAFETY ALERT
On recognizing ventricular fibrillation and cardiac arrest, begin emergency procedures. Call for help. Obtain a defibrillator and immediately defibrillate the client. If the defibrillator will be brought by another healthcare provider, begin CPR. Initiate ACLS protocols and assist with resuscitation measures as directed. Cardiac output ceases with ventricular fibrillation. Immediate or early defibrillation has been shown to have the greatest positive impact on survival following cardiac arrest.

■ After cardiac arrest, transfer the client to critical care. Perform and document head-to-toe assessment; obtain laboratory tests, 12-lead ECG, and chest x-ray as ordered. Monitor and maintain oxygenation and intravenous infusions, and monitor vital signs and cardiac rhythm. The period following resuscitation is critical, necessitating careful monitoring. Postarrest assessment allows comparison of the client's condition with prearrest status and may identify CPR-related injuries. Correcting electrolyte disturbances, hypoxia, and acid–base imbalances is important to prevent further dysrhythmias and potential adverse effects on cardiac output. Intravenous access is crucial to maintain drug infusions. Hemodynamic monitoring may be instituted. The 12-lead ECG documents myocardial status, and the chest x-ray provides information about pulmonary status and possible thoracic injury resulting from CPR.

■ Notify the client's family of significant changes in the client's condition or cardiac arrest, providing up-to-date information. Prepare family members before visits by explaining interventions (e.g., invasive tubes, a ventilator, or additional equipment) implemented since the last visit. Concern for the family and significant others is part of holistic nursing. Clients and families need and appreciate honest communication, information about their loved one's condition, and compassionate care. Preparing the family for critical changes in the client's condition and plan of care helps them to cope with a situational crisis.

Plan for Discharge

Discharge planning for the client diagnosed with a dysrhythmia includes client education directed toward following the prescribed treatment plan and managing risk factors. The nurse should instruct the client to take all medications as prescribed and to report any side effects to the healthcare provider when they first appear. The client should also be taught how to monitor pulse daily and keep a diary of the recordings. Substances containing caffeine, tobacco, and alcohol should be avoided because they can contribute to an irregular heartbeat. Specific risk factors to control include reducing high blood pressure, monitoring cholesterol levels, losing weight, following a heart healthy diet, stopping smoking, and engaging in regular physical activity as tolerated. The Client Teaching features list topics that are particularly relevant for the client with dysrhythmia and the client at risk for sudden cardiac arrest.

Evaluation

Expected outcomes of nursing care include the following:

■ The client experiences reduced frequency of dysrhythmic episodes through adherence to medication regimen.
■ The client and family respond appropriately to an episode of dysrhythmia.

Client Teaching Home Care for Clients With Dysrhythmias

Dysrhythmias have a significant physical and psychological impact on the client and all family members. Many of these clients and their families are under a great deal of stress from frequent hospitalizations, various treatment modalities, frustration, and the fear of sudden cardiac death. It is important for the nurse to introduce coping strategies addressing these fears. The nurse should review the following topics when educating the client and family for home care:

■ Function, maintenance, precautions, and signs of malfunction or complications of any implanted device, such as a pacemaker or implantable cardioverter–defibrillator
■ Monitoring of pulse rate and rhythm
■ Activity or dietary restrictions, and any potential effects of the dysrhythmia or its treatment on lifestyle

■ Medication management to reduce the risk of dysrhythmias, including the desired and potential adverse effects of antidysrhythmic drugs
■ Specific instructions related to planned diagnostic tests or procedures
■ The importance of follow-up visits with the cardiologist
■ The importance of and where to obtain training in cardiopulmonary resuscitation for the client and family members.
■ If the client has a cardioverter–defibrillator implanted, discharge instructions should address fears, interference from magnets, carrying proper identification, and when to notify the healthcare provider.

Client Teaching   Home Care for Clients at Risk for Sudden Cardiac Arrest

The risk for a future episode of sudden cardiac arrest requires careful and effective teaching for home care before discharge. The nurse should discuss the following topics with the client and family:

- Risk factor reduction for coronary heart disease
- Planned diagnostic studies to identify the cause of sudden cardiac arrest and possible interventions
- The risks and benefits of an implantable cardioverter–defibrillator if appropriate

- The importance of carrying a card at all times listing all current medications and the healthcare provider
- Early manifestations or warning signs of cardiac arrest
- The importance of training and maintaining proficiency in performing CPR (provide referral to local training providers or scheduled classes through the American Heart Association or American Red Cross).

NURSING CARE PLAN   A Client With Supraventricular Tachycardia

ASSESSMENT

Elisa Vasquez, 53 years old, is admitted to the cardiac unit with complaints of palpitations, light-headedness, and shortness of breath. Her history reveals rheumatic fever at age 12, with subsequent rheumatic heart disease and mitral stenosis. An intravenous line is in place, and she is receiving oxygen. Marcia Lewin, RN, is assigned to Ms. Vasquez.

Ms. Lewin's assessment reveals that Ms. Vasquez is moderately anxious. Her ECG shows supraventricular tachycardia with a rate of 154 bpm. Vital signs are as follows: temperature 37.1°C (98.8°F); respirations 26/min; and blood pressure 95/60 mmHg. Peripheral pulses are weak but equal. Mucous membranes are pale pink, and skin is cool and dry. Fine crackles are noted in both lung bases. A loud S_3 gallop and a diastolic murmur are noted. Ms. Vasquez is still complaining of palpitations and tells Ms. Lewin, "I feel so nervous and weak and dizzy." Ms. Vasquez's cardiologist orders 2.5 mg of verapamil to be given slowly via intravenous push and tells Ms. Lewin to prepare to assist with synchronized cardioversion if drug therapy does not control the ventricular rate.

DIAGNOSES

- *Decreased Cardiac Output* related to inadequate ventricular filling associated with rapid tachycardia
- *Ineffective Tissue Perfusion* related to decreased cardiac output
- *Anxiety* related to unknown outcome of altered health state

(NANDA-I © 2012)

PLANNING

Goals of care include the following:

- The client will maintain adequate cardiac output and tissue perfusion.
- The client will demonstrate a ventricular rate within normal limits and stable vital signs.
- The client will verbalize reduced anxiety.
- The client will verbalize an understanding of the rationale for the treatment measures to control the heart rate.

IMPLEMENTATION

- Provide oxygen per nasal cannula at 4 L/min.
- Continuously monitor the client's ECG for rate, rhythm, and conduction. Assess vital signs and associated symptoms with changes in ECG. Report findings to the physician.
- Explain the importance of rapidly reducing the heart rate. Explain the cardioversion procedure, and encourage questions.
- Encourage the client to verbalize fears and concerns. Answer questions honestly, correcting misconceptions about the disease process, treatment, or prognosis.
- Administer intravenous diazepam as ordered before cardioversion.

- Document pretreatment vital signs, level of consciousness, and peripheral pulses.
- Place an emergency cart with drugs and airway management supplies in the client's unit.
- Assist with cardioversion as indicated.
- Assess the client's level of consciousness, level of sedation, cardiovascular and respiratory status, and skin condition following cardioversion.
- Document the procedure and postcardioversion rhythm and the client's response to intervention.

EVALUATION

Intravenous verapamil lowers Ms. Vasquez's heart rate to 138 bpm for a short time, after which it increases to 164 bpm, with a blood pressure of 82/64 mmHg. Her cardiologist, Dr. Mullins, performs carotid sinus massage. The ventricular rate slows to 126 bpm for 2 minutes, revealing atrial flutter waves, and then returns to a rate of 150 bpm. Dr. Mullins explains the treatment options, including synchronized cardioversion. Ms. Vasquez agrees to the procedure.

Ms. Vasquez is lightly sedated, and synchronized cardioversion is performed. One countershock converts Ms. Vasquez to regular sinus rhythm at 96 bpm, with a blood pressure of 112/60 mmHg.

Ms. Vasquez is sleepy from the sedation but recovers without incident. She states that she feels "much better," and her vital signs return to her normal levels. She remains in normal sinus rhythm, with a rate of 86–92 bpm for the remainder of her hospital stay. Dr. Mullins places Ms. Vasquez on furosemide to treat manifestations of mild heart failure.

(continued on next page)

NURSING CARE PLAN   *(continued)*

CRITICAL THINKING

1. What is the scientific basis for using carotid massage to treat supraventricular tachycardias? Was this an appropriate maneuver in the case of Ms. Vasquez?

2. What other treatment options might the physician have used to treat Ms. Vasquez's supraventricular tachycardia if she had been asymptomatic with stable vital signs?

3. Develop a teaching plan for Ms. Vasquez related to her prescription for furosemide.

◤ REVIEW Life-Threatening Dysrhythmias

RELATE Link the Concepts and Exemplars

Linking the exemplar of life-threatening dysrhythmias with the concept of safety:

1. What safety teaching will you provide the client with atrial fibrillation?

2. Your client has an internal pacemaker in place secondary to third-degree heart block. When you are providing safety instructions, the client asks why battery-powered equipment is used rather than electrically powered equipment. How will you respond?

Linking the exemplar of life-threatening dysrhythmias with the concept of addiction:

3. What information will you provide the client with supraventricular tachycardia who plans to continue smoking cigarettes?

4. What alterations will you make to your plan of care for the client with a dysrhythmia who also abuses cocaine?

READY Go to Companion Skills Manual

REFER Go to Pearson Nursing Student Resources
nursing.pearsonhighered.com

- Additional review materials

- Chart 3: Nursing Care of the Client Having a Permanent Pacemaker Implant

REFLECT Case Study

Regina Moss, a 24-year-old female, is 6 weeks postpartum after delivering her first baby, Mickey. The delivery was uncomplicated; Mickey weighed 8 pounds at birth. Mickey has adapted well to the home environment, eating and sleeping well. Ms. Moss lives with Greg Mackinnon, a foreman for a construction crew. Ms. Moss has taken 3 months leave from her job as a legal secretary. She is enjoying her time at home with Mickey and is not sure she wants to return to work full time when her leave is up. Both her parents and Mr. Mackinnon's live in town, and they have all offered to care for Mickey when Ms. Moss goes back to work.

This morning Mickey is pale and seems to be lethargic and is having trouble eating. Ms. Moss calls Mr. Mackinnon, and they go to the hospital, where they are told that Mickey has supraventricular tachycardia. The emergency department physicians have given Mickey propranolol (Inderal) and are planning to admit him to the pediatric ICU.

1. What is your priority nursing diagnosis for Mickey?

2. What teaching will you provide Ms. Moss and Mr. Mackinnon?

3. How will you respond to Ms. Moss when she states that she must have done something wrong because Mickey had been so healthy?

EXEMPLAR 16.9 Peripheral Vascular Disease

EXEMPLAR KEY TERMS
Arteriosclerosis, *1198*
Atherosclerosis, *1198*
Chronic venous insufficiency (CVI), *1199*
Intermittent claudication, *1199*
Peripheral vascular disease (PVD), *1198*
Rest pain, *1199*
Venous stasis, *1199*

EXEMPLAR LEARNING OUTCOMES
After reading about this exemplar, you will be able to:

1. Describe the pathophysiology, etiology, clinical manifestations, and direct and indirect causes of peripheral vascular disease.

2. Identify risk factors and prevention methods associated with peripheral vascular disease.

3. Illustrate the nursing process in providing culturally competent care across the life span for individuals with peripheral vascular disease.

4. Formulate priority nursing diagnoses appropriate for an individual with peripheral vascular disease.

5. Summarize therapies used by interdisciplinary teams in the collaborative care of an individual with peripheral vascular disease.

6. Plan evidence-based care for an individual with peripheral vascular disease and his or her family in collaboration with other members of the healthcare team.

7. Evaluate expected outcomes for an individual with peripheral vascular disease.

▶ OVERVIEW

Peripheral vascular diseases are conditions affecting the peripheral arteries and veins. **Arteriosclerosis**, which is characterized by thickening, loss of elasticity, and calcification of arterial walls, is the most common chronic arterial disorder.

Atherosclerosis is a form of arteriosclerosis in which deposits of fat and fibrin obstruct and harden the arteries. In the peripheral circulation, these pathological changes impair the blood supply to peripheral tissues, particularly the lower extremities. This is known as **peripheral vascular disease (PVD)** or peripheral artery disease.

Chronic venous insufficiency (CVI) is a disorder of inadequate venous return over a prolonged period. It is a long-term condition that occurs because of a vein blockage or valve leakage in the leg veins making it difficult for blood to return to the heart from the legs. Blood pools in the veins causing stasis. Deep venous thrombosis (DVT) is the most common cause of CVI.

▶ PATHOPHYSIOLOGY AND ETIOLOGY

Atherosclerotic lesions involve both the intima and the media of the involved arteries. Thromboses occur in the lower extremities more often than in the upper extremities. Arteriosclerosis in the abdominal aorta leads to the development of aneurysms as plaque erodes the vessel wall.

Plaque tends to form at arterial bifurcations. The vessel lumen is progressively obstructed, decreasing blood flow to the lower extremities. Tissue hypoxia or anoxia results. With gradual obstruction of the vessel, collateral circulation often develops. However, the collateral circulation is usually not adequate to supply tissue needs, especially when metabolic demand increases (e.g., during exercise). Manifestations typically develop only when the vessel is occluded by 60% or more.

Chronic venous insufficiency results when venous blood collects and stagnates in the lower leg (**venous stasis**). Venous pressures in the calf and lower leg increase, particularly during ambulation. This increased pressure impairs arterial circulation to the lower extremities as well. The body's ability to provide sufficient oxygen and nutrients to the cells and remove metabolic waste products diminishes. Eventually, there is so little oxygen and nutrients that cells begin to die. The skin atrophies, and subcutaneous fat deposits necrose. Breakdown of red blood cells in the congested tissues causes brown skin pigmentation (Porth, 2010). Venous stasis ulcers develop. Congested tissues impair the body's ability to increase the supply of oxygen, nutrients, and metabolic energy to heal the ulcer. As a result, the condition worsens and, over time, the ulcers enlarge. The congested venous circulation also prevents the blood from mounting effective inflammatory and immune responses, significantly increasing the risk for infection in the ulcerated tissue (McCance & Huether, 2010).

Etiology

Peripheral vascular disease affects individuals in their 60s and 70s. Men are more often affected than women. African American clients are associated with an increased risk, whereas those of Hispanic origin seem to have similar to slightly higher rates of peripheral artery disease when compared to non-Hispanic Whites. Overall, approximately 8 million people in the United States are estimated to have PVD. Of those, 12%–20% are over the age of 60 (CDC, 2013e).

Risk Factors

Risk factors for PVD are similar to those for atherosclerosis and coronary heart disease; they include smoking, hypertension, high cholesterol, diabetes, family history of vascular disease, being overweight, and physical inactivity. Clients over the age of 50 also have an increased risk.

Box 16–25   Manifestations of Peripheral Atherosclerosis

- Intermittent claudication
- Rest pain
- Paresthesias (numbness, decreased sensation)
- Diminished or absent peripheral pulses
- Pallor with extremity elevation; redness of skin or rubor when dependent
- Thin, shiny, hairless skin; thickened toenails
- Areas of discoloration or skin breakdown

Several risk factors predispose a client to the development of venous insufficiency. Thrombophlebitis sometimes results in damage to the valves of the deep veins. Obesity and occupations that require prolonged standing or sitting can also lead to venous insufficiency.

▶ CLINICAL MANIFESTATIONS

Pain is the primary symptom of peripheral atherosclerosis. **Intermittent claudication** (a cramping or aching pain in the calves of the legs, the thighs, and the buttocks that occurs with a predictable level of activity) is characteristic of PVD. The pain is often accompanied by weakness and is relieved by rest.

Rest pain, in contrast, occurs during periods of inactivity. It is often described as a burning sensation in the lower legs. Rest pain increases when the legs are elevated and decreases when the legs are dependent (e.g., hanging over the side of the bed). The legs also may feel cold or numb along with the pain. Sensation is diminished, and the muscles may atrophy.

Peripheral pulses may be decreased or absent. A bruit (unusual sound made by blood rushing past an obstruction) may be heard over large affected arteries, such as the femoral artery and the abdominal aorta. The legs are pale when elevated but often are dark red (dependent rubor) when dependent. The skin often is thin, shiny, and hairless, with discolored areas. Toenails may be thickened. Areas of skin breakdown and ulceration may be evident. Edema may develop with severe PVD.

Box 16–25 ● lists the manifestations of peripheral atherosclerosis. Complications of peripheral atherosclerosis include gangrene and extremity amputation, rupture of abdominal aortic aneurysms, and possible infection and sepsis.

Manifestations of chronic venous insufficiency include lower leg edema, itching, and discomfort of the affected extremity that increases with prolonged standing (**Box 16–26** ●). The

---

Box 16–26   Manifestations of Chronic Venous Insufficiency

- Lower extremity edema that worsens with standing
- Itching, dull leg discomfort or pain that increases with standing
- Thin, shiny, atrophic skin
- Cyanosis and brown skin pigmentation of lower leg and foot
- Possible weeping dermatitis
- Thick, fibrous (hard) subcutaneous tissue
- Recurrent ulcerations of medial or anterior ankle

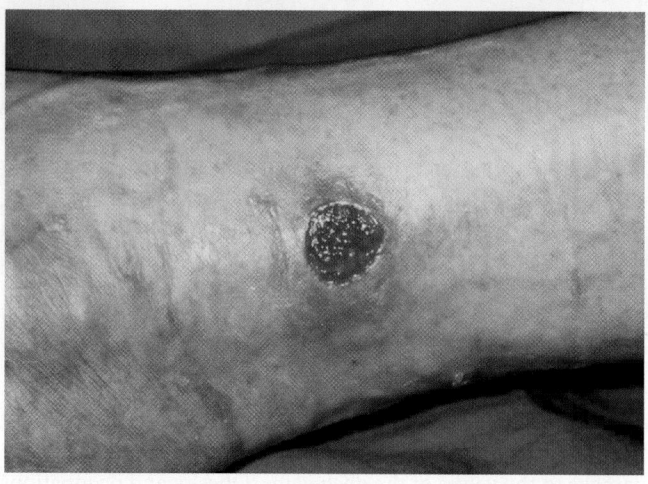

Figure 16–56 ● Chronic venous insufficiency. Note the discoloration of the ankle and the stasis ulcer.
Source: Dr. P. Marazzi/Science Source.

extremity is cyanotic. Recurrent stasis ulcers develop (**Figure 16–56** ●), usually forming just above the ankle, on the medial or anterior aspect of the leg. They heal poorly, forming scar tissue that breaks down easily. Tissue surrounding the ulcer is shiny, atrophic, and cyanotic, and there is a brownish pigmentation to the skin. Other skin changes, such as eczema or stasis dermatitis, also may develop. Necrosis and fibrosis of subcutaneous tissue cause the affected area of the leg to feel hard and somewhat leathery to the touch, but even the slightest trauma to the area can produce serious tissue breakdown. **Table 16–31** ● compares venous and arterial ulcers.

▶ COLLABORATION

Management of PVD focuses on slowing the atherosclerotic process and maintaining tissue perfusion. Collaborative care for the client with venous insufficiency focuses on relieving symptoms, promoting adequate circulation, and healing and preventing tissue damage.

The history and physical examination often establish the diagnosis of chronic venous insufficiency. Because a history of DVT is a major risk factor, careful evaluation of the medical history and questioning of the client is important. There are no specific diagnostic tests to confirm the diagnosis of CVI.

Conservative management of venous insufficiency focuses on reducing edema and treating ulcerations. Prolonged standing or sitting is discouraged. Graduated compression hosiery is ordered for daytime use, and frequent elevation of the legs and feet during the day is recommended. At night, the legs and feet should be elevated above the level of the heart by raising the foot of the mattress.

Treatment of associated stasis dermatitis varies, based on the duration of the condition. Wet compresses of boric acid, buffered aluminum acetate (Burow solution), or isotonic saline solution are applied to acute weeping dermatitis four times a day for 1-hour periods. Following the compress, a topical corticosteroid (e.g., 0.5% hydrocortisone cream) is applied. Bed rest is prescribed during the acute period.

Stasis pigmentation is very difficult to treat even when the underlying stasis dermatitis is well controlled with topical therapy. Some researchers have reported benefits from treatment with a noncoherent intense pulsed light (IPL) source.

The ulcer may be treated by using a semirigid boot applied to the foot and lower leg. This device may be made of Unna paste or Gauzetex bandage. Bony prominences must be well padded. The boot must be changed every 1–2 weeks, depending on the amount of drainage from the ulcer. This device often allows ambulatory treatment. A very large, chronic ulcer may require surgery. In this case, the incompetent veins are ligated, the ulcer is excised, and the area is covered with a skin graft.

Diagnostic Tests

Although PVD often can be diagnosed on the basis of the history and physical examination, diagnostic tests may be ordered to evaluate its extent. Noninvasive studies often are sufficient. Diagnostic tests for PVD include the following:

■ **Segmental pressure measurements** use sphygmomanometer cuffs and a Doppler device to compare blood pressures between the upper and lower extremities (normally similar) and within different segments of the affected extremity. In PVD, the blood pressure may be lower in the legs than in the arms.

TABLE 16–31   Comparison of Arterial and Venous Leg Ulcers

FACTOR	ARTERIAL ULCERS	VENOUS ULCERS
Location	Toes, feet, shin	Over medial or anterior ankle
Ulcer appearance	Deep, pale	Superficial, pink
Skin appearance	Normal to atrophic	Brown discoloration
	Pallor on elevation	Stasis dermatitis
	Rubor on dependency	Cyanosis on dependency
Skin temperature	Cool	Normal
Edema	Absent or mild	May be significant
Pain	Usually severe	Usually mild
	Intermittent claudication	Aching pain
	Rest pain	
Gangrene	May occur	Does not occur
Pulses	Decreased or absent	Normal

- *Stress testing* using a treadmill provides functional assessment of limitations. In PVD, pressure at the ankle may decline even further with exercise, confirming the diagnosis. This may be done simultaneously for testing related to cardiovascular illness.

- *Doppler ultrasound* uses sound waves reflected off moving red blood cells within a vessel to evaluate blood flow. The impulses may be translated into an audible signal or a graphic waveform. With significant PVD, the waveform becomes progressively flatter as the transducer is moved distally along the affected vessel. Segmental pressures may be used to locate the site of obstruction.

- *Duplex Doppler ultrasound* combines the audible or graphic Doppler ultrasound with ultrasound imaging to identify arterial or venous abnormalities. Ultrasonic imaging provides views of the affected vessel while Doppler ultrasound evaluates blood flow. *Color-flow Doppler ultrasound* provides color images of the vessel and blood flow.

- *Transcutaneous oximetry* evaluates oxygenation of tissues.

- *Angiography or magnetic resonance angiography* is done before revascularization procedures to locate and evaluate the extent of arterial obstruction. For angiography, a contrast medium is injected and vessels are visualized using fluoroscopy and x-rays. Magnetic resonance angiography does not require injection of a contrast medium and may replace angiography.

Pharmacologic Therapy

Drug treatment of peripheral atherosclerosis is less effective than that for coronary heart disease. Medications to inhibit platelet aggregation, such as aspirin or clopidogrel (Plavix), are ordered to reduce the risk of arterial thrombosis. Cilostazol (Pletal), a platelet inhibitor with vasodilator properties, increases blood flow to the extremities, thereby improving claudication. Pentoxifylline (Trental) decreases blood viscosity and increases red blood cell flexibility, increasing blood flow to the microcirculation and tissues of the extremities.

Nonpharmacologic Therapy

Smoking cessation is vital for the treatment of PVD. Nicotine not only promotes atherosclerosis, it also causes vasospasm, further reducing blood flow to the extremities.

Meticulous foot care is vital to prevent ulceration and infection. Elastic support hose, which reduce circulation to the skin, are avoided. Elevating the head of the bed on blocks may help relieve rest pain. Regular, progressively strenuous exercise, such as 30–45 minutes of walking daily, is important. The client is taught to rest at the onset of claudication, resuming activity when the pain resolves.

Other measures to slow the process of atherosclerosis, such as controlling diabetes and hypertension, lowering cholesterol levels, and weight loss, also are recommended.

Surgery

Revascularization may be performed if symptoms are progressive, severe, or disabling. Other indications for surgery include symptoms that significantly interfere with ADLs, rest pain, and pregangrenous or gangrenous lesions. Either nonsurgical revascularization procedures or surgery may be performed.

Nonsurgical procedures include percutaneous transluminal angioplasty, stent placement, or atherectomy. Techniques may include balloon angioplasty to dilate the narrowed lumen, mechanical atherectomy to remove plaque, or laser or thermal angioplasty to vaporize the occluding material. In either case, a stent typically is placed at the time of angioplasty to maintain vessel patency. Iliac and femoral–popliteal percutaneous transluminal angioplasty initially reestablish good blood flow and relieve symptoms in more than 80% of clients. Practitioners may also insert a mesh framework, or stent, to help keep the artery open.

Surgical options include endarterectomy (to remove occlusive plaque from the artery) and bypass grafts. Knitted Dacron bypass grafts are commonly used. Both immediate graft patency and long-term graft patency are better with bypass grafting than with nonsurgical revascularization procedures. However, the risks for operative complications must be considered.

Complementary Therapy

Complementary therapies for PVD include interventions to improve circulation and reduce stress. A number of complementary therapies may improve peripheral circulation: aromatherapy with rosemary or vetiver; biofeedback; healing or therapeutic touch and massage; herbals, such as ginkgo, garlic, cayenne, hawthorn, and bilberry; and exercise including yoga. Aromatherapy and yoga also may reduce stress, as can breathing exercises, meditation, and counseling. In addition, complementary therapies to reduce atherosclerosis and lower cholesterol levels may slow the progress of PVD. Measures such as a very low fat or vegetarian diet, including antioxidant nutrients or using vitamin C, vitamin E, or garlic supplements, and traditional Chinese medicine may be useful.

◼ NURSING PROCESS

The nurse can help to reduce the incidence and slow the progression of atherosclerosis by discussing healthy lifestyle habits with community and religious groups, with schoolchildren (grades K–12), and through the print media. The nurse should strongly encourage all clients to avoid smoking in the first place and to stop all forms of tobacco use. Discuss the adverse effects of smoking and the benefits of quitting. Provide information about dietary recommendations to maintain a healthy weight and optimal cholesterol levels. Discuss the benefits and importance of regular exercise. Finally, encourage clients with cardiovascular risk factors to undergo regular screening for hypertension, diabetes, and hyperlipidemia.

Nursing care for the client with chronic venous insufficiency is primarily educative and supportive. Client teaching includes the following recommendations:

- Elevate the legs while resting and during sleep.
- Walk as much as possible, but avoid sitting or standing for long periods of time.
- When sitting, do not cross your legs or allow pressure on the back of the knees (e.g., sitting on the side of the bed).
- Do not wear anything that pinches your legs (e.g., knee-high hose, garters, or girdles).

Client Teaching   Foot and Leg Care for the Client With Peripheral Atherosclerosis

1. Keep legs and feet clean, dry, and comfortable.
   - Wash legs and feet daily in warm water, using mild soap.
   - Pat dry using a soft towel; be sure to dry between the toes.
   - Apply moisturizing cream to prevent drying.
   - Use powder on the feet and between the toes.
   - Buy shoes in the afternoon (when feet are largest); never buy shoes that are uncomfortable. Toes should not touch the tip of the shoe.
   - Wear a clean pair of cotton socks each day.
2. Prevent accidents and injuries to the feet.
   - Always wear shoes or slippers when getting out of bed.
   - Walk on level ground and avoid crowds, if possible.
   - Do not go barefoot.

- Inspect legs and feet daily; use a mirror to examine backs of legs and bottoms of feet.
- Have a professional foot care provider trim toenails and care for corns, calluses, ingrown toenails, or athlete's foot.
- Always check the temperature of the water before stepping into a tub.
- Do not let the legs or tops of the feet get sunburned.
- Report leg or foot problems (increased pain, cuts, bruises, blistering, redness, or open areas) to your healthcare provider.

3. Improve blood supply to the legs and feet.
   - Do not cross legs.
   - Do not wear garters or knee stockings.
   - Do not swim or wade in cold water.

- Wear elastic hose as prescribed. The elastic hose should be tighter over the feet than at the top of the leg. Be sure the tops of the elastic hose do not cut into your legs. Put on the hose after you have had your legs elevated.
- Keep the skin on your feet and legs clean, soft, and dry.
- Follow guidelines in the Client Teaching feature for care of the legs and feet.

Assessment

Focused assessment related to peripheral atherosclerosis includes the following:

- **Health history.** Complaints of pain, its relationship to exercise or rest, timing, associated symptoms, and relief measures; history of coronary heart disease, PVD, hyperlipidemia, hypertension, or diabetes; current medications; smoking history; usual diet and activity patterns
- **Physical examination.** Vital signs; strength and equality of peripheral pulses of all extremities; capillary refill; skin color, temperature, hair distribution, and presence of any discolorations or lesions; movement and sensation of lower extremities.

Diagnosis

Nursing diagnoses that may be useful for the client with PVD include the following:

- *Tissue Perfusion: Peripheral, Ineffective*
- *Pain*
- *Skin Integrity, Impaired*
- *Activity Intolerance.*

(NANDA-I © 2015)

Nursing diagnoses that may apply to the client with chronic venous insufficiency include the following:

- *Body Image, Disturbed*
- *Health Maintenance, Ineffective*
- *Infection, Risk for*
- *Mobility: Physical, Impaired*
- *Skin Integrity, Impaired*
- *Tissue Perfusion: Peripheral, Ineffective.*

(NANDA-I © 2015)

Planning

Goals of nursing care for the client with chronic venous insufficiency may include the following:

- The client will stop smoking.
- The client will learn appropriate foot and wound care.
- The client will maintain adherence with medications and wound care.
- The client will maintain activity and exercise as tolerated.

Implementation

Nursing care for the client with chronic venous insufficiency is focused on improving tissue perfusion and preventing tissue damage. Any time tissues receive inadequate blood supply, the client will experience very severe pain. As a result, pain management until perfusion can be improved is also a primary nursing focus.

Promote Tissue Perfusion

Impaired blood flow to the lower extremities affects gas, nutrient, and waste product exchange between the capillaries and cells. Oxygen and nutrient deprivation impairs cell function and tissue integrity, causing pain and impaired healing. Pain develops with exercise and when extremities are elevated. To promote tissue perfusion, the nurse should do the following:

- Assess peripheral pulses, pain, color, temperature, and capillary refill every 4 hours and as needed. Use a Doppler device if pulses are not palpable. Mark pulse locations with an indelible marker. Assessment data provide a baseline for evaluating the effectiveness of interventions and identifying changes in arterial blood flow.
- Position the client with extremities dependent. Gravity promotes arterial flow to the dependent extremity, increasing tissue perfusion and relieving pain.
- Discuss the benefits of regular exercise. Exercise promotes the development of collateral circulation to ischemic tissues and slows the process of atherosclerosis.
- Use a foot cradle and lightweight blankets, socks, and slippers to keep extremities warm. Avoid electric heating pads

Client Teaching   Home Care for Clients With Peripheral Vascular Disease

The nurse should discuss the following topics when preparing the client and family for home and community-based care:

- Smoking cessation strategies and ways to avoid second-hand smoke
- Prescribed medications and anticoagulants, their purpose, doses, and desired and adverse effects
- Signs of excess bleeding to report to the practitioner
- Skin surveillance and foot care (see the Client Teaching feature on page 1202)
- Recommended diet and exercise
- Weight loss strategies if appropriate.

If revascularization or surgery has been performed, include the following topics as appropriate:

- Incision care
- Manifestations of complications (e.g., infection, graft leakage, or thrombosis) to be reported to the practitioner
- Activity limitations.

Provide referrals to home health services, physical or occupational therapy, and home maintenance assistance services as indicated. Consider resources such as Meals-on-Wheels for clients who are severely limited by their disease.

---

or hot water bottles. Keeping extremities warm conserves heat, prevents vasospasm, and promotes arterial flow. External heating devices are avoided to reduce the risk of burns in the client with impaired sensation. The foot cradle protects tissues from compression by linens.

- Encourage frequent position changes. Instruct the client to avoid crossing the legs or using a pillow under the knees. Position changes promote blood flow and reduce damage caused by pressure. Leg crossing and excessive flexion of the hip or knee joints can compress partially obstructed arteries and impair blood flow to distal tissues.

Manage Pain

Impaired blood flow results in tissue ischemia. Metabolism shifts from an efficient aerobic process to an anaerobic process. Lactic acid and metabolic waste products accumulate in tissues, causing pain. Severe and cramping pain generally occurs with exercise early in the disease. Rest initially produces relief, similar to the process of angina. As the disease progresses, pain develops with less exercise and often occurs even at rest. Rest pain disrupts sleep and the client's sense of well-being and has significant disruptive effects on life roles. The following nursing interventions may help to control the client's pain:

- Assess pain at least every 4 hours using a standard pain scale. Pain is a subjective experience. Using a standard pain scale allows evaluation of treatment measures in relieving pain and restoring blood flow. Examples of pain scales can be found in the exemplar on Acute and Chronic Pain in the module on Comfort and in the Companion Skills Manual.
- Keep the extremities warm. Cooling leads to vasoconstriction, increasing pain. Warming the extremities promotes vasodilation and improves arterial flow, reducing pain.
- Teach pain relief and stress reduction techniques, such as relaxation, meditation, and guided imagery. Pain increases stress. The stress response leads to vasoconstriction, increasing pain. Stress reduction techniques, when combined with other measures to promote blood flow, can help reduce pain.

Promote Skin Integrity

Clients with PVD are at risk for impaired skin integrity as a result of oxygen and nutrient deprivation. Chronic tissue ischemia leads to dry, scaly, and atrophied skin. Pruritus can lead to scratching; minor injuries may go unnoticed because of impaired sensation. Impaired tissue healing can lead to ulceration, infection, and potential gangrene. The following are appropriate nursing interventions to promote skin integrity in these clients:

- Provide meticulous daily skin care, keeping the skin clean and dry. Apply a moisturizing cream to dry or scaly areas. Intact skin is the body's first defense against bacterial invasion. Ischemic tissues of the injured extremity provide an excellent medium for microorganism growth. Clean, dry, supple skin decreases the risk of breakdown.
- Apply a bed cradle. The bed cradle suspends bed linens over the legs, preventing them from placing pressure on extremities and injured tissues. Minimizing pressure on the tissues promotes capillary blood flow.
- Provide an egg-crate mattress, flotation pad, sheepskin, or heel protectors. Ischemic tissues may be damaged by minor trauma, such as that created by the shearing forces of skin against bed linens.

Encourage Activity

Pain and impaired perfusion of peripheral tissues may limit the client's ability to engage in desired activities, even impairing self-care. The nurse can take the following actions to encourage the client to be active:

- Assist with care activities as needed. Severe claudication or rest pain may limit activities. Muscle atrophy of affected extremities is common, leading to fatigue and weakness.
- Unless contraindicated, encourage gradual increases in duration and intensity of exercise. Teach the client to rest with the extremities dependent when claudication develops, resuming activity after pain has abated. Gradual increases in the duration and intensity of exercise promote development of collateral circulation, improve exercise tolerance, provide a sense of well-being, and support self-esteem.

■ Provide diversional activities during periods of prescribed bed rest. Encourage relaxation techniques to reduce muscle tension. Diversional activities help prevent the boredom and stress associated with enforced rest. Relaxation techniques reduce vasoconstriction induced by stress, improving peripheral circulation.

■ Encourage frequent position changes and active range-of-motion (ROM) exercises. Encourage self-care to the extent possible. Position changes relieve pressure on tissues, improving capillary circulation and reducing tissue ischemia. ROM exercises help prevent muscle atrophy and joint contractures. Self-care supports self-esteem.

Evaluation

The client's progress toward goals may be evaluated based on the following expected outcomes:

■ The client provides a return demonstration of proper positioning of the affected extremity.

■ The client begins a smoking cessation program.

■ The client verbalizes proper wound care techniques to the nurse.

■ The client verbalizes signs and symptoms of infection prior to discharge.

REVIEW Peripheral Vascular Disease

RELATE Link the Concepts and Exemplars

Linking the exemplar of peripheral vascular disease with the concept of infection:

1. What factors related to PVD would increase the risk for infection in wounds to the lower extremities?

2. What client teaching will you provide the client with PVD to reduce the risk of infection?

Linking the exemplar of peripheral vascular disease with the concept of comfort:

3. Explain the relationship between physical exercise and pain in the client with PVD.

4. Compare the pain experienced during exercise by a client with PVD to that of a client with angina.

READY Go to Companion Skills Manual

REFER Go to Pearson Nursing Student Resources
nursing.pearsonhighered.com

• Additional review materials

REFLECT Case Study

Vincent D'Angelo is a 69-year-old male who retired recently from Ford Motor Company where he worked on the assembly line in a truck factory. He and his wife Pat are enjoying retirement and spending time together. Mr. and Mrs. D'Angelo own their own home. Their children, Laurie and Peter, live nearby. Mr. D'Angelo has not had any major health issues until recently, when he started experiencing pain during evening walks with his wife.

Mr. D'Angelo drinks an occasional glass of wine at special functions. Ten years ago, he quit a two-pack-a-day smoking habit. The D'Angelos eat relatively healthy meals, mostly cooked by Mrs. D'Angelo. She has finally convinced Mr. D'Angelo to see his primary care provider to find out why he is having leg pain.

1. Describe the noninvasive diagnostic tests that the physician might order to confirm Mr. D'Angelo's diagnosis of PVD.

2. What nursing assessments will you perform to support the diagnosis of PVD?

3. Create a teaching plan to reduce the risk of complications associated with PVD for Mr. D'Angelo.

EXEMPLAR 16.10   Hypertensive Disorders in Pregnancy

EXEMPLAR KEY TERMS
Chronic hypertension, *1205*
Eclampsia, *1206*
Gestational hypertension, *1205*
HELLP syndrome, *1205*
Preeclampsia, *1205*
Superimposed preeclampsia, *1205*

EXEMPLAR LEARNING OUTCOMES
After reading about this exemplar, you will be able to:

1. Describe the pathophysiology, etiology, clinical manifestations, and direct and indirect causes of pregnancy-induced hypertension.

2. Identify risk factors and prevention methods associated with pregnancy-induced hypertension.

3. Illustrate the nursing process in providing culturally competent care for individuals with pregnancy-induced hypertension.

4. Formulate priority nursing diagnoses appropriate for an individual with pregnancy-induced hypertension.

5. Summarize therapies used by interdisciplinary teams in the collaborative care of an individual with pregnancy-induced hypertension.

6. Plan evidence-based care for an individual with pregnancy-induced hypertension and his or her family in collaboration with other members of the healthcare team.

7. Evaluate expected outcomes for an individual with pregnancy-induced hypertension.

▶ OVERVIEW

Hypertension is the most common medical disorder among pregnant women and one of the major causes of pregnancy-related maternal deaths in the United States (Mustafa et al., 2012). Hypertension is said to complicate up to 1 in 10 pregnancies and affects an estimated 240,000 women in the United States each year (Mustafa et al., 2012). Elevated blood pressures and the results of the disease process in pregnancy can cause harm to both the mother and fetus and range in severity from minor complications to death.

The National High Blood Pressure Education Program classifies pregnancy-related hypertensive disorders as follows: chronic hypertension, gestational hypertension, preeclampsia, and preeclampsia superimposed on chronic hypertension (NHLBI, 2013d). The diagnosis of **chronic hypertension** is based on a known history of hypertension prior to pregnancy, hypertension that is discovered during the pregnancy prior to 20 weeks gestation, or hypertension that persists for more than 12 weeks postpartum (King et al. 2015). **Gestational hypertension** occurs in the second half of pregnancy in a previously normotensive mother. The diagnosis is made when the client has a blood pressure greater than or equal to 140/90 on at least two occasions that are at least six hours apart, after 20 weeks gestation (King et al. 2015). **Preeclampsia** is defined according to the same criteria as gestational hypertension, accompanied by signs of end organ damage (see Clinical Manifestations). Preeclampsia superimposed onto chronic hypertension (**superimposed preeclampsia**) occurs when a women previously diagnosed with chronic hypertension develops worsening hypertension that is resistant to treatment or hypertension related end organ dysfunction in pregnancy (August and Sibai, 2015).

Preeclampsia occurs in 3%–7% of nulliparous women and in 1%–3% of multiparous women (Uzan et al., 2011). Preeclampsia continues to be a major cause of maternal mortality, preterm births, perinatal death, and intrauterine growth restriction (Uzan et al., 2011).

▶ PATHOPHYSIOLOGY AND ETIOLOGY

The exact cause of preeclampsia is unknown. However, it has been identified as a disorder of placental dysfunction leading to a syndrome of endothelial dysfunction with associated vasospasm (Carson, 2013). Research has demonstrated abnormal placental development or placental damage from diffuse microthrombosis as playing a role in the development of maternal hypertension. An altered maternal immune response to fetal/placental tissue may also contribute to preeclampsia (Carson, 2013).

The vasculature of normal pregnant women typically demonstrates a decreased response to vasoactive peptides, such as angiotensin II and epinephrine, whereas women with preeclampsia demonstrate hyperresponsiveness to the same hormones. Blood pressures may be labile in preeclampsia.

Research suggests that inadequate trophoblast invasion during formation of the placenta leads to incomplete remodeling of the uterine spiral arteries and placental hypoxia. The poorly perfused placenta then releases increased amounts of vasoactive factors leading to a widespread activation of the maternal endothelium that, ultimately, results in elevated maternal blood pressure, increased vascular permeability, vasospasm, and coagulopathies. The clinical manifestations and sequelae of preeclampsia are a result of vasospasm and increased permeability of the blood vessels (August and Sibai, 2015).

HELLP Syndrome

HELLP syndrome (hemolysis, elevated liver enzymes, and low platelet count) is most often related to severe preeclampsia and usually occurs as a complication of preeclampsia. However, in some documented cases HELLP syndrome has occurred without a diagnosis of preeclampsia. Differential diagnoses include hepatitis, gallbladder disease, or idiopathic/thrombocytopenic purpura (ITP). HELLP syndrome is a multisystem disorder that is resolved only with delivery of the baby and placenta.

The hemolysis that occurs in HELLP syndrome is a microangiopathic hemolytic anemia. As red blood cells pass through small, damaged blood vessels, they become distorted, resulting in vascular damage. Vasospasm occurs, and platelets begin to aggregate at the sites of injury, resulting in low platelet counts. Hepatic blood flow is impeded, causing an elevation in liver enzymes. The hepatic obstruction may then lead to periportal necrosis or intrahepatic hemorrhage. The client may present with hyperbilirubinemia and jaundice. Signs of impending hepatic rupture include severe epigastric pain, liver distention, nausea, and vomiting. It is suspected that disseminated intravascular coagulopathy (DIC) is the primary process in HELLP syndrome. The risk factors for HELLP syndrome vary from those associated with preeclampsia. HELLP usually presents in the third trimester but has also been seen in both the second trimester and postpartum clients. Symptoms of HELLP in the postpartum period typically present within the first 48 hours but may be seen as long as 7 days after delivery.

Prompt diagnosis and initiation of therapy will ensure the best outcomes for the mother and fetus. Laboratory values typically worsen after delivery and peak within 24–48 hours after delivery. The peak lactate dehydrogenase level signals the beginning of recovery. The platelet count and coagulation studies may be used as predictive indicators for hemorrhagic complications. Complaints of severe right upper quadrant pain, neck pain, or shoulder pain should be considered for prompt evaluation.

Preeclampsia and HELLP syndrome are progressive and never resolve until after delivery of the placenta. In spite of this, about 5% of cases are atypical and are first recognized in the postpartum period (August and Sibai, 2015).

Risk Factors

The risk of preeclampsia is greater in pregnant women with a personal or family history of the illness. Other risk factors include a medical history of chronic hypertension or kidney disease, nulliparity, diabetes, coagulation disorders, obesity, African ethnicity, age 35 years or older, and pregnancy characteristics such as twin or molar pregnancy, or fetal congenital abnormality (Uzan et al., 2011). Women without any identifiable risk factors may develop hypertensive disorders in pregnancy, thus routine screening for all pregnant women is imperative.

▶ CLINICAL MANIFESTATIONS

Preeclampsia is distinguished from chronic or gestational hypertension by the presence of abnormal proteinuria defined as 2+ or greater on urine dipstick, random urine protein/ creatinine ratio of 0.3 or greater, and/ or 0.3 grams of protein or greater in a 24-hour urine collection.

Severe features of preeclampsia include any or all of the following:

- Blood pressure greater than or equal to 160/110
- Persistent or debilitating headache
- Persistent right upper quadrant or epigastric pain
- Serum creatinine greater than 1.1 mg/dL or double the client's baseline
- Platelet count less than 100,000/ microliter
- Liver enzymes elevated to at least twice the upper limit of normal
- Pulmonary edema
- Visual disturbances (scotomata, blurry vision, and rarely, blindness)

■ Altered mental status or seizure

Eclampsia, or eclamptic seizure is a serious complication of preeclampsia, which manifests with convulsions as in a grand mal seizure (August and Sibai, 2015).

Although they are not a diagnostic criteria, edema and rapid weight gain may increase suspicion for preeclamsia because they are found in the presence of increased capillary permeability that causes leakage of intravascular fluid into interstisial space, where it is retained instead of being excreted by the kidneys. The Clinical Manifestations and Therapies feature provides more information about the signs and symptoms of preeclampsia and their treatment.

Fetal complications related to preeclampsia and eclampsia have a direct correlation with gestational age and the severity of maternal disease. Onset of preeclampsia prior to 34 weeks gestation and preeclampsia with severe features place the fetus at a higher risk for perinatal morbidity and death (August and Sibai, 2015). Infant prematurity is a major complication (Suppo de Souza Rugolo, Bentlin, & Trindade, 2011).

▶ COLLABORATION

The goal of medical management of the client diagnosed with hypertension in pregnancy depends on gestational age and severity of disease. The primary objective of treatment is to maintain the safety of the mother with delivery of a healthy baby. Prior to 34 weeks, corticosteroids may be administered to the mother accelerate fetal lung maturity and reduce morbidity in the preterm infant. The severity of maternal disease should be weighed against the risks of infant prematurity.

Antepartum Management

Women with chronic hypertension who become pregnant are at a higher risk for the maternal and fetal complications associated with hypertension in pregnancy in addition to stroke and left ventricular hypertrophy. Many antihypertensive medications are contraindicated in pregnancy, so clients who require medication may be switched to methyldopa or labetalol. Women with chronic

Clinical Manifestations and Therapies **Hypertensive Disorders in Pregnancy**

ETIOLOGY	CLINICAL MANIFESTATIONS	CLINICAL THERAPIES
Cerebral edema and cerebral vasospasm	■ Hyperreflexia ■ Headache ■ Seizures ■ Visual disturbances ■ Presence of clonus ■ Stroke ■ Hypertensive encephalopathy	■ Reduce external stimuli. ■ Administer anticonvulsant: magnesium sulfate. ■ Consider prompt delivery.
Increased vascular permeability	■ Pulmonary edema ■ Edema of the face, hands, and lower extremities ■ Hemoconcentration	■ Monitor breath sounds and oxygen saturation. ■ Elevate extremities to reduce edema. ■ Administer IV fluid to maintain intra-vascular volume and circulation. ■ Monitor intake and output.
Loss of normal vasodilation of uterine arterioles	■ Decreased placental perfusion ■ Fetal growth restriction ■ Decreased fetal movement ■ Fetal hypoxia	■ Provide regular antenatal fetal surveil-lance and continuous intrapartum fetal monitoring. ■ Teach the client to report decreased fetal movement. ■ Nonreassuring fetal status may re-quire prompt delivery.
Vasospasm	■ Elevated serum creatinine, blood urea nitro-gen, uric acid. Decreased serum albumin. ■ Oliguria ■ Proteinuria ■ Elevated serum transaminases (liver enzymes) ■ HELLP syndrome or coagulopathies ■ Right upper quadrant or epigastric pain ■ Palpable liver enlargement ■ Hypertension ■ Abruptio placentae	■ Frequently monitor blood pressure. ■ Elevate extremities to reduce edema. ■ Monitor laboratory values. ■ Monitor intake and output.

hypertension or a history of preeclampsia in prior pregnancies should be placed on a low dose aspirin regimen (August, 2015). The normal, physiologic changes in the cardiovascular system related to pregnancy may cause a reduction in maternal blood pressure and decreased medication requirements in the first 20 weeks. If the client was on a sodium-restricted diet prior to pregnancy, she should continue this. Baseline laboratory studies should be done early in pregnancy and at regular intervals determined by the healthcare provider. Bi-weekly nonstress tests or biophysical profiles and ultrasound to evaluate fetal growth should be done in the third trimester (Norwitz and Repke, 2015).

Antepartum management for preeclampsia may include hospitalization to evaluate new-onset maternal and fetal conditions. Preeclampsia with severe features requires continued hospitalization for medical management of hypertension, seizure prophylaxis with intravenous magnesium sulfate, steroid administration, fetal surveillance, and ongoing assessment of the need for prompt delivery. There is no evidence in favor of antihypertensive medication unless maternal blood pressure is in the severe range. Management at home may be considered for stable clients. If she remains at home, the client will need to assess her blood pressure daily. She will also need to log daily fetal movement. Activity restriction and dietary modifications do not alter the course or outcome of preeclampsia. When at rest, the client may be encouraged to lie on her left side in order to maximize uterine and renal perfusion. She should avoid lying supine. Nonstress tests (NSTs) and biophysical profiles are ordered bi-weekly by the attending provider. The client will be weighed, her blood pressure taken, and home blood pressure log reviewed at these visits. Weekly laboratory studies and monthly ultrasounds for growth may also be ordered (Norwitz and Repke, 2015). The client and family members should be educated to report worsening signs and symptoms of preeclampsia.

Intrapartum Management

Induction of labor is initiated at term (at least 37 weeks) or if the risks to the mother and fetus outweigh the benefits of avoiding preterm delivery. Induction of labor is always preferable to cesarean delivery unless there's a category III fetal heart tracing.

Assessment for signs and symptoms of worsening preeclampsia should be ongoing. If the client is on magnesium sulfate, the nurse is responsible for monitoring for symptoms of magnesium toxicity. Laboratory values do not correlate well with adverse client responses, so the diagnosis of magnesium toxicity is based on clinical observations. The first sign is usually loss of deep tendon reflexes. Other signs are shortness of breath, adventitious lung sounds, and decreased oxygen saturation. Magnesium is excreted by the kidneys, so oliguria should be promptly reported to the attending provider (Norwitz and Repke, 2015). The client may also feel flushed, weak, or nauseated but these are not signs of toxicity. Severe range blood pressures may be treated with intravenous labetalol or hydralazine.

Epidural and spinal anesthesia may be contraindicated in the presence of a low platelet count. Pain management options include intravenous medication, pudendal block, labor support, and maternal position changes.

Fetal status should be assessed continuously via electronic fetal monitoring. Magnesium easily crosses the placenta and the fetal heart tracing may show a slightly decreased baseline rate and minimal variability. Toxicity can be reversed in the mother and infant with the administration of calcium gluconate (Norwitz and Repke, 2015). A pediatric team should be present at the delivery and the nurse should anticipate that the baby may have difficulty breathing immediately after birth.

Postpartum Management

The client with preeclampsia usually improves rapidly after giving birth, although seizures can still occur up to 48 hours postpartum. The nurse will need to monitor the client for the same signs of toxicity discussed previously.

Magnesium is a mild tocolytic and smooth muscle relaxer, so the risk for uterine atony and postpartum hemorrhage is higher. The mother still requires vigilant monitoring of maternal vital signs, deep tendon reflexes (DTRs), respiratory and neurological status as there is still a risk for seizure up to 48 hours postpartum. Magnesium infusion will continue for 24 hours after delivery in severe cases (ACOG, 2011).

Strict monitoring of input and output (I & O) is important because diuresis should occur with the return of normal kidney function, as the disease process starts to reverse itself. Monitoring of lab values will also confirm the progression of improvement.

Many factors influence whether preeclampsia will recur. Illness severity, underlying illness, and the client's genetic tendencies are all contributing risk factors. Additionally, the client with preeclampsia during pregnancy may be hypertensive or at risk for kidney disease later in life.

Clients who have undergone long hospitalization, induction of labor, and continuous magnesium infusion may have difficulty breastfeeding. Delayed initiation of breastfeeding and separation of mother and baby are known to have a negative effect on breastfeeding success (King et al., 2015). The infant may be unable to leave the special care nursery due to the effects of prematurity and magnesium toxicity and the mother's condition may not be stable for transport to the nursery for several days.

■ NURSING PROCESS

When caring for the pregnant woman with preeclampsia, it is important to remember that the nurse is caring for two clients, mother and baby. The needs of both individuals must be identified and met for a successful outcome.

Assessment

Blood pressure is taken and recorded during each antepartum visit. Abnormal readings should be reported to the physician or midwife. Monitor respiratory status for respiratory rate, rhythm, signs of respiratory distress, and abnormal or absent lung sounds at every visit. Urine is also monitored for protein at each visit and serum labs my be repeated weekly.

If the client is admitted to the hospital, the nurse should monitor the following:

- ■ **Respiratory status.** Lung sounds and pulse oximetry should be assessed frequently.
- ■ **Blood pressure.** Blood pressure should be assessed at least every 1–4 hours. More frequent monitoring is needed with changes in client status.
- ■ **Temperature.** Temperature should be monitored at least every 4 hours.

- *Pulse and respirations.* Pulse rate and respirations should be monitored every 4 hours or hourly if the client is on magnesium.
- *Fetal heart rate.* The fetal heart rate should be checked with maternal vital signs or continuously intrapartum or if the client is on magnesium. Increase frequency of monitoring if changes are noted.
- *Urinary output.* Intake and output should be monitored and recorded every shift or more frequently per physician's order. Output should be at least 30 mL/hr.
- *Urine protein.* The urine is monitored for protein after each void. High level of protein in the urine is indicated by 300 mg/24-hour urine, greater than 1+ on urine dip, or urine protein/creatinine ratio of greater than or equal to 0.3.
- *Urine specific gravity.* Specific gravity of the urine with each voiding. Findings over 1.040 correlate with oliguria and proteinuria.
- *Edema.* Periorbital swelling and swelling of the face should be reported but are not considered diagnostic criteria.
- *Weight.* The client is weighed daily at the same time.
- *Pulmonary edema.* Monitor the client for signs and symptoms of pulmonary edema.
- *Deep tendon reflexes.* Assess for evidence of hyperreflexia. The patellar reflex is the easiest to assess. Clonus should also be assessed by dorsiflexing the foot while the knee is held in a fixed position. Normally no clonus is present.
- *Placental separation.* The client should be monitored for vaginal bleeding or educated to report the signs and symptoms of placental abruption if at home.
- *Headache.* Headaches should be reported, including their location, duration, and intensity.
- *Visual disturbance.* Visual changes should be reported.
- *Epigastric pain.* Complaints of epigastric pain should be reported and further examined. It is important to differentiate epigastric pain from simple heartburn, which tends to be less intense.
- *Laboratory blood tests.* Laboratory tests include hematocrit, blood urea nitrogen, creatinine, and uric acid levels to assess kidney function; clotting studies for any indication of thrombocytopenia or disseminated intravascular coagulation; liver enzymes; and electrolyte levels.
- *Level of consciousness.* Any changes in level of consciousness mental status should be reported.
- *Emotional well-being and level of understanding.* The nurse should consider the emotional needs of the client who is experiencing the illness and facing possible premature delivery of her infant.

Diagnosis

Possible nursing diagnoses for the client with preeclampsia include the following:

- *Fluid Volume Excess* related to fluid retention
- *Risk for Injury* related to the possibility of seizure secondary to cerebral vasospasm or edema
- *Interrupted Breastfeeding* related to maternal fatigue and infant condition, secondary to labor induction process, prematurity, and the effects of magnesium therapy.

(NANDA-I © 2015)

Planning

Goals of nursing care for the client with preeclampsia may include the following:

- The client will participate in monitoring fetal perfusion, including observing tracking fetal movement.
- The client will be encouraged to maintain position on her left side when lying in bed and avoid lying supine.
- The client will maintain safety of herself and fetus.
- The client will have adequate fluid intake.
- The client will have adequate urine output.

Implementation

In caring for a client with preeclampsia, the focus of nursing care is to reduce the effects of the disease process while supporting the pregnancy. However, if blood pressure continues to rise or remains elevated, delivery of the premature fetus may be unavoidable. In that case, nursing care is focused on optimizing outcomes for both the client and the newborn.

Community-Based Nursing Care

The client with preeclampsia must cope with several concerns. She may fear losing her unborn child, and she may be preoccupied with her spouse and other children. If placed on limited activity, she may experience concerns regarding finances and other aspects of family life. The nurse should help the client identify and discuss these concerns. The nurse can offer information regarding community resources and support groups.

The client needs to know how to monitor her symptoms and immediately report signs of a worsening condition. She should be prepared to make frequent visits to the provider if requested.

Hospital-Based Nursing Care

Severe preeclampsia is a cause for increased concern for the client and her family. Immediate concerns are usually aimed at providing positive outcomes for both the mother and infant. The nurse should keep the client and significant other informed of fetal status and be available to discuss other concerns that may arise. Spiritual support can also be provided to the family if requested.

The occurrence of a convulsion is frightening to observers. It is important for the nurse to inform significant others of the possibility that a seizure may occur. A grand mal seizure has both a tonic phase, marked by pronounced muscular contraction and rigidity, and a clonic phase, marked by alternate contraction and relaxation of the muscles. During the tonic phase of the seizure, the client should be turned on her side to aid circulation to the placenta. The nurse should monitor the client's airway clearance in case the client experiences vomiting. In an attempt to prevent injury, the side rails should be padded.

The nurse should monitor fetal heart tones continuously. Monitoring of maternal vital signs should be increased to every 5 minutes until they are stable.

Nursing Management During Labor and Birth

During labor, the nurse should continuously monitor deep tendon reflexes, breath sounds, level of consciousness, and intake and output. Continual assessment of the central nervous system is also crucial, because changes could progress to eclamptic seizures. The mother should be observed for signs of placental abruptions. Laboratory values should be monitored for changes or abnormal values. The nurse should also assess for fetal heart rate variability and accelerations. Late decelerations or a decrease or absence of variability indicate fetal distress.

A nonstimulating, quiet environment is recommended. The client and significant other should be educated on the disease process and how care of a client with preeclampsia may differ from that of a client experiencing a normal pregnancy. The client should be positioned on her left side as much as possible. Lying on the left side promotes improved circulation to the heart, fetus, uterus, and kidneys.

If the client is unable to push while lying on her left side, she should be encouraged to move into a semisitting position. If able, she can rest in the left lateral position during contractions.

A family member or other significant person is encouraged to remain with the client during hospitalization to offer support. For continuity of care, the client should be cared for by the same nurses throughout her stay.

Nursing Management During the Postpartum Period

The nurse must assess vaginal bleeding and observe the client for signs of hypovolemic shock. Vital signs are monitored every 4 hours for 48 hours or hourly for 24 hours if the client is on magnesium. Pertinent labs are checked daily. Intake and output are measured.

Normal postpartum diuresis helps eliminate edema and is a favorable sign. However, the nurse continues to monitor the client for signs of worsening preeclampsia in the postpartum period.

The client should be monitored for signs and symptoms of postpartum depression. The nurse will provide opportunities for frequent maternal–infant contact, breastfeeding support, and encourage family members to visit. The client and significant other may have many questions, and the nurse should be available for discussion. They should be given family planning information. Oral contraceptives may be used if the woman's blood pressure has returned to normal by the time they are prescribed (usually 4–6 weeks after birth).

Evaluation

Expected outcomes of nursing care include the following:

- The client is able to verbalize the signs and symptoms of preeclampsia, the treatment plan, and the implications as they specifically relate to her pregnancy.
- The client remains seizure free through the pregnancy and into the postpartum period.
- The client and significant other can verbalize and report the signs and symptoms of worsening preeclampsia.
- The delivery has a positive outcome for both mother and newborn.

NURSING CARE PLAN — A Client With Preeclampsia

ASSESSMENT

Dianne Hardison, a 35-year-old primigravida, is 34 weeks pregnant. Three days ago, during a routine prenatal visit, her blood pressure was 138/90 mmHg. Mrs. Hardison's last in-office blood pressure reading was 118/74 mmHg. She has also gained 2.3 kg (5 lb) since her visit last month. A trace level of protein was found in her urine. Mrs. Hardison also reported experiencing some headaches during the past week. They were not relieved by acetaminophen. The certified nurse midwife explained the signs and symptoms of preeclampsia and encouraged the client to call the clinic if her condition worsened during the next few days. Mrs. Hardison was sent home and scheduled to return to the office in 3 days.

Mrs. Hardison returned to the clinic today with a blood pressure of 144/92 and has been admitted to the hospital with worsening preeclampsia. She is placed on her left side when lying in bed. The nurse monitors her closely for worsening hypertension, proteinuria, oliguria, cerebral or visual disturbances, pulmonary edema, epigastric pain, and sudden onset of severe edema. She is also placed on seizure precautions. The fetus is assessed by biophysical profile and monitoring. The nurse reassures Mrs. Hardison that everything will be done to make her comfortable and ensure the well-being of her baby.

Mrs. Hardison later reports headache, scotomata, and irritability. Other findings are as follows: blood pressure of 146/92 mmHg; deep tendon reflexes are 3+; 600 mL of urine collected during the past 24 hr with a protein level of 5 g/L; weight gain of 1.8 kg (4 lb) during past 4 days; and 2+ pitting edema on lower extremities.

DIAGNOSES

- *Deficient Fluid Volume* related to fluid shift from intravascular to extravascular space secondary to vasospasm
- *Risk for Injury* to fetus related to uteroplacental insufficiency secondary to vasospasm

(NANDA-I © 2015)

PLANNING

Goals of care include the following:

- The client's blood pressure will remain below the severe range. Signs and symptoms of preeclampsia will remain stable or decrease.
- Adequate oxygenation and perfusion to the fetus will be maintained. Supplemental oxygen will be provided, if necessary.
- The client will maintain adequate urine output.

(continued on next page)

NURSING CARE PLAN (continued)

IMPLEMENTATION

- Avoid placing the client in a supine position.
- Increase frequency of vital signs monitoring, as ordered.
- Monitor strict intake and output, and monitor each urine specimen for protein.
- Assess deep tendon reflexes and clonus.
- Assess for worsening edema.
- Administer magnesium sulfate per infusion pump as ordered.

- Monitor signs of magnesium sulfate toxicity.
- Consult with a dietitian to provide a nutritionally sound meal plan.
- Educate the client on how to monitor and record fetal movement throughout the day.
- Inform the client of various tests that may be performed for fetal monitoring. Assure her that a nurse will be there to offer support during testing.

EVALUATION

Mrs. Hardison's blood pressure remains below the severe range. Her urine protein levels remain stable. Her deep tendon reflexes remain at 2+. Tests measuring fetal status are within normal limits, indicating that uteroplacental sufficiency is maintained.

CRITICAL THINKING

1. A woman gives birth at 36 weeks of gestation after induction of labor for preeclampsia with severe features. The birth weight is graphed in the 5th percentile. What is the most likely reason for the low birth weight? How does preeclampsia affect the fetus as it grows and develops?
2. You are interviewing a client diagnosed with preeclampsia without severe features at a follow up outpatient visit. Upon questioning, the client admits to having a headache most of the time for the past 5 days. What counseling would you provide for this client on reporting new symptoms? Why?
3. Three women are being admitted to the antepartum unit. Two rooms are available: one private room and one double occupancy room. One woman being admitted is in preterm labor, the second has preeclampsia with severe features, and the third has third-trimester bleeding. Which room assignment would be most appropriate for the woman with preeclampsia? Why?
4. After performing your initial assessment on a client with preeclampsia on a magnesium drip, you report the following findings: nausea and vomiting, blurred vision, absent deep tendon reflexes (previously deep tendon reflexes were 3+), and 70 mL of total urine output over 4 hours. Are these findings normal? What actions would you take, if any?

REVIEW   Hypertensive Disorders in Pregnancy

RELATE Link the Concepts and Exemplars

Linking the exemplar of hypertensive disorders in pregnancy with the concept of intracranial regulation:

1. What independent nursing interventions might you initiate to reduce the risk of seizures in the client with preeclampsia who is 28 weeks pregnant?
2. When caring for a woman with preeclampsia that does not have severe features, what teaching would you provide to reduce disease advancement?

Linking the exemplar of hypertensive disorders in pregnancy with the concept of oxygenation:

3. What impact might preeclampsia have on fetal oxygenation?
4. List short- and long-term goals for the client with preeclampsia aimed at optimizing client and fetal oxygenation.

READY Go to Companion Skills Manual

REFER Go to Pearson Nursing Student Resources
nursing.pearsonhighered.com

- Additional review materials

REFLECT Case Study

Ginny Sims is a 36-year-old primigravida at 34 weeks' gestation. She is married to Paul, whose job as a buyer for a major department store chain requires a great deal of travel. The Simses had plans to have children when they first married, but they had trouble conceiving. Ms. Sims is the manager of a coffee shop. When she began feeling very tired and nauseated in the mornings, she decided that she was in early menopause because her period was late. As fatigue continued to impede her ability to concentrate at work, Ms. Sims finally made an appointment with her OB/GYN and found out she was pregnant. She and her husband are thrilled and can't wait to greet their newborn. Mr. Sims is investigating the possibility of taking a job that doesn't involve so much travel so he can spend more time with his family.

Ms. Sims is seeing the nurse practitioner today for her routine prenatal examination. The nurse takes Ms. Sims's blood pressure and it is 140/92, increased from her baseline of 110/70. Ms. Sims's ankles are slightly swollen, and she admits to an occasional recurrent nagging headache. Her urine dip shows 2+ protein.

1. What further physical assessments would you perform to support the diagnosis of pregnancy-induced hypertension?
2. What teaching will you provide before sending Ms. Sims home from the office?
3. What assessment findings would indicate worsening preeclampsia in this client?

EXEMPLAR 16.11   Pulmonary Embolism

EXEMPLAR KEY TERMS

Dead space, *1212*
Embolus, *1211*

Lyse, *1214*
Pulmonary embolism (PE), *1211*
Thromboemboli, *1211*

EXEMPLAR LEARNING OUTCOMES

After reading about this exemplar, you will be able to:

1. Describe the pathophysiology, etiology, clinical manifestations, and direct and indirect causes of pulmonary embolism.

2. Identify risk factors and prevention methods associated with pulmonary embolism.

3. Illustrate the nursing process in providing culturally competent care across the life span for individuals with pulmonary embolism.

4. Formulate priority nursing diagnoses appropriate for an individual with pulmonary embolism.

5. Summarize therapies used by interdisciplinary teams in the collaborative care of an individual with pulmonary embolism.

6. Plan evidence-based care for an individual with pulmonary embolism and his or her family in collaboration with other members of the healthcare team.

7. Evaluate expected outcomes for an individual with pulmonary embolism.

▶ OVERVIEW

Pulmonary embolism (PE), or pulmonary thromboembolism, is the obstruction of blood flow in part of the pulmonary vascular system by an **embolus** (a particle or aggregate of blood, fat, or pathogens or a bubble of air) traveling from one area of the body to another. **Thromboemboli** (emboli created by a blood clot) that develop in the venous system or right side of the heart are the most frequent cause of pulmonary embolism. Other sources of emboli include tumors that have invaded the venous circulation, fat or bone marrow entering the circulation as a result of fracture or other trauma, amniotic fluid released into the circulation during childbirth, and intravenous injection of air or other foreign substances.

Pulmonary embolism is a medical emergency. Fifty percent of deaths from pulmonary embolism occur within the first 2 hours following embolization. In many cases, deep venous thrombosis (DVT) has not been recognized or treated; often, embolization also goes undetected. Prompt diagnosis and treatment can help save lives and prevent complications associated with PE.

▶ PATHOPHYSIOLOGY AND ETIOLOGY

The right side of the heart receives deoxygenated blood from the systemic venous circulation. The entire output of the right ventricle enters the pulmonary circulation via the pulmonary artery. This artery branches into successively smaller arteries, arterioles, and capillaries of the pulmonary vascular system. Each alveolus of the lungs is surrounded by a meshwork of capillaries. Oxygen and carbon dioxide readily diffuse across the alveolar–capillary membrane, driven by a concentration gradient. The partial pressure of oxygen in the alveolus is greater than that in the capillary; therefore, oxygen diffuses into the blood. Carbon dioxide diffuses from the capillaries into the alveoli, driven by the higher pressure of dissolved carbon dioxide in venous blood.

A match between blood flow through the pulmonary vascular system (perfusion) and lung ventilation is necessary for effective respiration (gas exchange) (**Figure 16–57** ●). Local factors regulate ventilation and perfusion to maintain this match. A low alveolar PO_2 constricts alveolar capillaries, directing blood flow to better-ventilated areas of the lung. A high alveolar PCO_2 causes local bronchodilation, increasing airflow and eliminating excess carbon dioxide.

Thrombi that affect only the deep veins of the calf rarely embolize to the pulmonary circulation. However, thrombi often propagate proximally to the popliteal and ileofemoral veins, and there, they may break loose to become an embolus. As vessels of the venous system become progressively larger, the

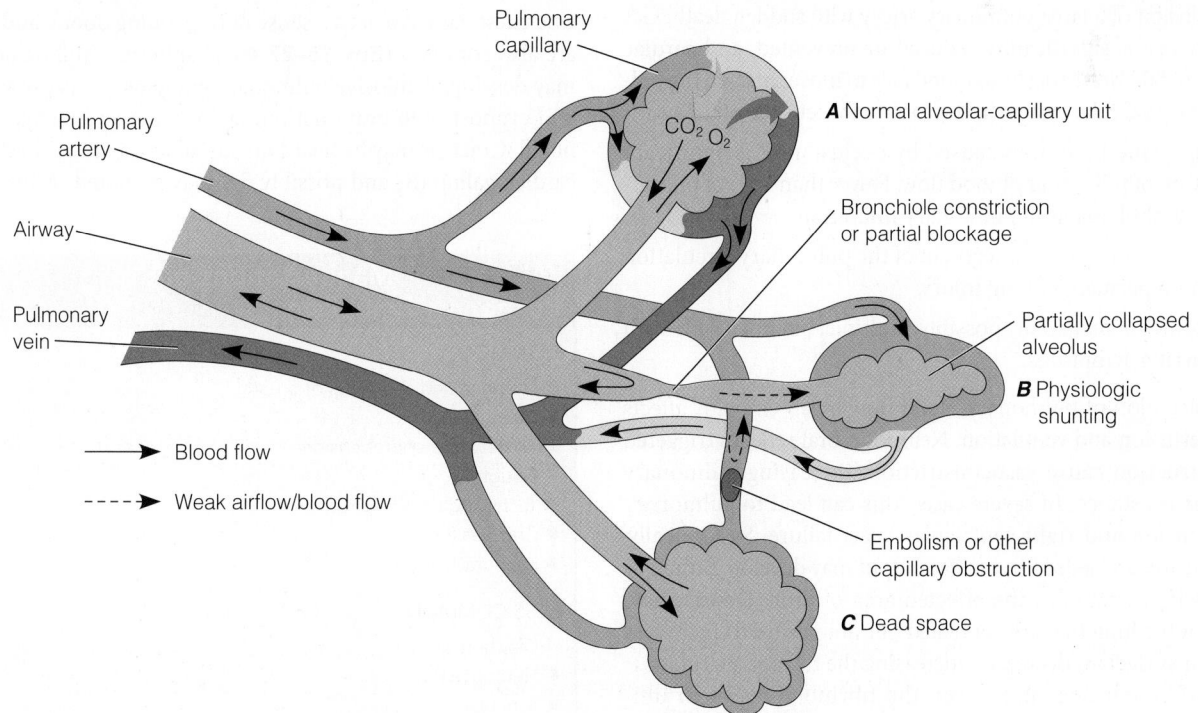

Figure 16–57 ● Ventilation-perfusion relationships. *A,* Normal alveolar–capillary unit with an ideal match of ventilation and blood flow. Maximum gas exchange occurs between alveolus and blood. *B,* Physiological shunting: a unit with adequate perfusion but inadequate ventilation. *C,* Dead space: a unit with adequate ventilation but inadequate perfusion. In the latter two cases, gas exchange is impaired.

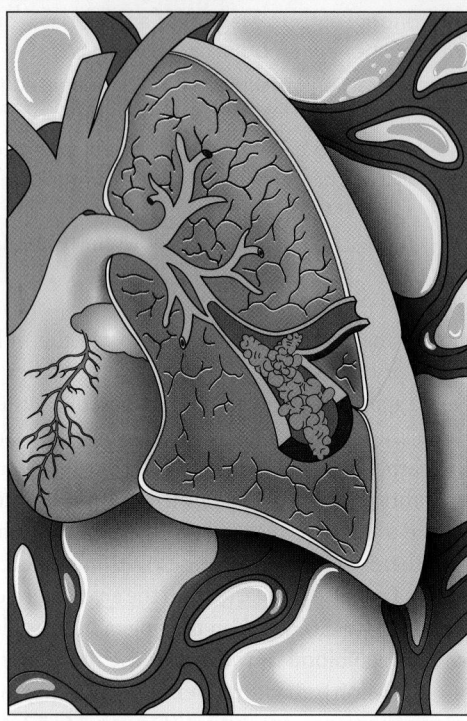

Figure 16–58 ● A thromboembolism lodged in a pulmonary vessel.

embolus moves freely until it enters the pulmonary arterial system, with its progressively smaller vessels leading to the pulmonary capillary beds (**Figure 16–58** ●).

The impact of a pulmonary embolus depends on the extent to which pulmonary blood flow is obstructed, the size of the embolus, its nature, and any secondary effects of the obstruction. The effects can range widely:

- Occlusion of a large pulmonary artery with sudden death. Gas exchange is significantly reduced or prevented, and cardiac output falls dramatically as blood fails to move through the pulmonary vascular system and return to the left side of the heart.

- Lung tissue infarction caused by occlusion of a significant portion of pulmonary blood flow. Fewer than 10% of pulmonary emboli result in pulmonary infarction.

- Obstruction of a small segment of the pulmonary circulation with no permanent lung injury.

- Chronic or recurrent, possibly multiple, small emboli with recurring symptoms.

Obstruction of pulmonary blood flow by an embolus affects both perfusion and ventilation. Neurohumoral reflexes triggered by obstruction cause vasoconstriction, increasing pulmonary vascular resistance. In severe cases, this can lead to pulmonary hypertension and right ventricular heart failure. Systemically, hypotension and a drop in cardiac output may develop. Bronchoconstriction occurs in the affected area of lung. **Dead space** (areas of the lung that are ventilated but not perfused) increases. Alveolar surfactant decreases, increasing the risk for atelectasis.

If infarction does not occur, the fibrinolytic system ultimately dissolves the clot, and pulmonary function returns to normal. If infarction does occur, the infarcted tissue becomes scarred and fibrotic.

Fat emboli are the most common nonthrombotic pulmonary emboli. A fat embolism usually occurs after fracture of long bone (typically the femur) releases bone marrow fat into the circulation. Adipose tissue or liver trauma may also lead to fat emboli.

Etiology

Thrombus arising from the deep veins of the legs is the leading cause of pulmonary embolism. A less common source of emboli is fatty tissue that enters the circulatory systems as the result of surgery or trauma. This is most commonly seen when fatty marrow enters the circulation after a fracture to a large bone, most often the femur or pelvis.

Risk Factors

The risk factors for pulmonary embolus are similar to those for DVT, including stasis of venous blood flow, vessel wall damage, and altered blood coagulation. Inherited thrombophilias and certain cancers which produce coagulation factors make clot formation more likely (Porth, 2015). Risk factors for DVT include prolonged immobility; trauma, including hip and femur fractures; surgery (orthopedic, pelvic, and gynecological surgery in particular); MI and heart failure; obesity; and advanced age. Women who use oral contraceptives or estrogen therapy are at risk, as are women during pregnancy and childbirth. Smoking cigarettes also increases the risk of pulmonary emboli.

▶ CLINICAL MANIFESTATIONS

The clinical manifestations of pulmonary embolism depend on the size and location of the emboli. Small emboli may be asymptomatic. Manifestations usually develop abruptly, over a period of minutes. The most common symptoms are dyspnea and pleuritic chest pain. Anxiety, a sense of impending doom, and cough are also common (**Box 16–27** ●). Diaphoresis and hemoptysis may develop. A massive pulmonary embolus can cause syncope and cyanosis. On examination, tachycardia and tachypnea are noted. Crackles may be heard on auscultation of the chest, and a cardiac gallop (S_3 and possibly S_4) may be noted. A low-grade

---

Box 16–27 Manifestations of Pulmonary Embolism

COMMON
- Dyspnea and shortness of breath
- Chest pain
- Anxiety and apprehension
- Cough
- Tachycardia and tachypnea
- Crackles (rales)
- Low-grade fever

LESS COMMON
- Diaphoresis
- Hemoptysis
- Syncope
- Cyanosis
- An S_3 and/or S_4 gallop

Clinical Manifestations and Therapies **Pulmonary Embolism**

ETIOLOGY	CLINICAL MANIFESTATIONS	CLINICAL THERAPIES
Hypoxia due to blockage of alveoli by thrombus	■ Restlessness ■ Chest pain ■ Dyspnea ■ Cyanosis ■ Use of accessory muscles when breathing ■ Respiratory acidosis ■ Tachycardia ■ Tachypnea ■ Feeling of impending doom	■ Administer oxygen. ■ Reposition client to decrease work of breathing. ■ Prepare client for the possibility of intubation and mechanical ventilation. ■ Begin anticoagulant therapy as ordered. ■ Monitor lab values. ■ Maintain a low-stimulus environment to decrease oxygen demands.
Rupture of small arterioles due to arterial congestion	■ Auscultation of coarse crackles in the affected lobe ■ Cough with or without the presence of blood ■ Dyspnea	■ Explain hemoptysis to help alleviate client and family member concerns. ■ Administer oxygen as ordered. ■ Maintain patent airway. Suction PRN.
Alveolar collapse related to tissue necrosis and inflammatory process	■ Hypoxia ■ Dyspnea ■ Productive cough ■ Chest pain	■ Administer oxygen. ■ Reposition client to facilitate adequate air exchange. ■ Promote use of an incentive spirometer to facilitate postural drainage.
Inflammatory process	■ Elevated temperature ■ Tachycardia ■ Tachypnea ■ Dehydration ■ Cough	■ Administer antipyretics. ■ Conduct laboratory testing to aid in diagnosis of causative agent. ■ Administer antibiotics and IV fluids as ordered.

fever may develop. It is difficult to differentiate pulmonary embolism from MI or pneumonia by manifestations.

Characteristic manifestations of fat emboli include sudden onset of cardiopulmonary and neurological symptoms: dyspnea, tachypnea, tachycardia, confusion, delirium, and decreased level of consciousness. Petechiae often develop on the chest and arms. See the Clinical Manifestations and Therapies feature for more information.

▶ COLLABORATION

Because DVT may not be identified until pulmonary embolism occurs, prevention is the primary goal in treating PE. Early ambulation of medical and surgical clients is an effective means of preventing venous stasis and reducing the incidence of PE. External pneumatic compression of the legs is also effective for clients undergoing neurosurgery, urological surgery, or major surgery of the hip or knee, or when anticoagulant therapy is contraindicated. Other preventive measures include elevating the legs and active and passive leg exercises.

When pulmonary embolism occurs, treatment is supportive. Oxygen therapy is initiated, and analgesics may be ordered to relieve severe pleuritic pain and anxiety. Pulmonary artery and wedge pressures are monitored with a balloon (Swan-Ganz) catheter. Cardiac outputs also may be assessed. Cardiac rhythm is monitored to detect dysrhythmias.

Diagnostic Tests

The studies performed to diagnose pulmonary emboli differ from those used to diagnose DVT and include the following:

■ *Plasma D-dimer levels* are highly specific to the presence of a thrombus. *D-dimer* is a fragment of fibrin formed during lysis of a blood clot; elevated blood levels indicate thrombus formation and lysis (e.g., DVT and pulmonary embolism).

■ *Chest CT with contrast* is the principal test used to diagnose pulmonary embolism. Chest CT effectively shows large, central pulmonary emboli; newer-generation scanners also can detect peripheral emboli.

■ *Lung scans,* including perfusion and ventilation scans, may be used. In a perfusion lung scan, radiotagged albumin is injected intravenously and distributed in the lungs by the pulmonary blood flow. The lungs are then scanned for distribution of the isotope. An area of lung in which the isotope cannot be detected is suggestive of occluded blood flow and pulmonary embolism. For a ventilation scan, a radiotagged gas is inhaled and the lungs are scanned for gas distribution. Combined perfusion and ventilation scans allow identification of areas of the lungs that are ventilated but not perfused, a characteristic of pulmonary embolism.

■ *Pulmonary angiography* is the definitive test for pulmonary embolism when other, less invasive tests are inconclusive. It is possible to detect very small emboli with angiography. A contrast medium injected into the pulmonary arteries illustrates the pulmonary vascular system on x-ray.

■ *Chest x-ray* often shows pulmonary infiltration and occasionally pleural effusion.

■ *Electrocardiography* is ordered to rule out acute MI as the cause of symptoms. Electrocardiographic findings commonly associated with pulmonary embolism include tachycardia and nonspecific T-wave changes.

■ *Arterial blood gas* measurements usually show hypoxemia ($PaO_2 < 80$ mmHg) and often respiratory alkalosis (pH > 7.45, $PaCO_2 < 35$ mmHg) caused by tachypnea and hyperventilation.

■ *$ETCO_2$* (end-tidal carbon dioxide, a measurement of carbon dioxide exhaled) may be measured to evaluate alveolar perfusion. The normal $ETCO_2$ reading is 35–45 mmHg; it is decreased when pulmonary perfusion is impaired.

■ *Coagulation studies* are ordered to monitor the response to therapy. The activated partial thromboplastin time (aPTT; also called PTT) is used to assess the intrinsic clotting pathway and the response to heparin therapy. Desired levels with anticoagulant therapy are 1.5–2 times the control value. The risk of recurrent thromboembolism is high at lower levels; the risk of bleeding increases at higher levels. The International Normalized Ratio (INR) is used to assess the extrinsic clotting system and oral anticoagulation with warfarin (Coumadin). The goal of anticoagulant therapy is to achieve a therapeutic INR range of 2.0–3.0.

Pharmacologic Therapy

Anticoagulant therapy is the standard treatment for preventing pulmonary emboli. It is often instituted in high-risk clients who have no evidence of pulmonary embolism in order to prevent possible devastating effects. In the client with DVT or a pulmonary embolus, anticoagulants are administered to prevent further clotting and embolization.

For the client with a pulmonary embolus, heparin therapy is initiated with an intravenous bolus of 5,000–10,000 U, followed by continuous infusion at the rate of 1,000–1,500 U/hr. The aPTT or PTT is monitored frequently until stabilized. Heparin therapy is typically continued for approximately 5 days, or until oral anticoagulant therapy has become fully effective.

Oral anticoagulant therapy with warfarin sodium (Coumadin) is initiated at the same time as heparin. Warfarin sodium alters the synthesis of vitamin K–dependent clotting factors and requires 5–7 days to be fully effective. Anticoagulant therapy is continued for 2–3 months when few risk factors for thromboemboli exist; long-term therapy is used when chronic disorders that increase the risk of thromboemboli are present.

Bleeding is a risk associated with anticoagulant therapy. Although major hemorrhage is uncommon, it occurs in approximately 5% of clients receiving intravenous heparin. Cardiac, hepatic, and renal disease all increase the risk of significant bleeding, as does age over 60 years. The use of fractionated and low molecular weight heparin is associated with fewer adverse effects and may be considered. Current research suggests that Factor X inhibitors are also effective and result in fewer side

effects and drug interactions (Porth, 2015). Protamine, a protein that combines with heparin to inactivate it, is used to stop its anticoagulant effect if major bleeding occurs. Vitamin K is given to treat bleeding associated with Coumadin therapy.

Fibrinolytic therapy may be used to treat a massive pulmonary embolus and hypotension. Streptokinase, urokinase, or tissue plasminogen activators are used to **lyse** (disintegrate) the embolus, restore pulmonary blood flow, and reduce pulmonary artery and right heart pressures. Although fibrinolytic therapy may not reduce the mortality associated with pulmonary embolus, it may reduce the incidence of pulmonary hypertension, which can develop 3–5 years after an embolism. Fibrinolysis significantly increases the risk of bleeding, particularly cerebral bleeding. Contraindications to fibrinolysis include intracranial disease, recent stroke, active bleeding or a bleeding disorder, pregnancy, severe hypertension, and recent surgery or trauma. Because of the increased risk of hemorrhage, invasive procedures are avoided after fibrinolysis.

Surgery

When anticoagulant therapy fails to prevent recurrent emboli or is contraindicated, an umbrella-like filter may be inserted into the inferior vena cava to trap large emboli while allowing continued blood flow (see Figure 16–39 on page 1134). The filter usually is inserted percutaneously, via either the femoral or jugular vein.

■ NURSING PROCESS

The nurse plays a primary role in preventing pulmonary embolism. Encouraging clients to ambulate after surgery or illness, applying compression stockings or pneumatic compression devices, teaching and encouraging leg exercises, and discouraging the use of pillows under the knees all help prevent DVT and subsequent pulmonary emboli.

The nurse can teach clients to reduce the risks associated with long periods of immobility. For example, to prevent venous stasis and pooling, the client may stop every 1–2 hours during long automobile trips for a brief stretch and walk, get up every hour or so and do leg exercises while seated during long flights, avoid sitting for long periods of time during work or leisure time, and avoid crossing the legs. Regular exercise, such as walking, also reduces the risk for DVT. Instruct clients who stand for long periods to use well-fitted elastic stockings, being careful to avoid hose that bind around the knee or thigh. Nurses can also assist clients with smoking cessation and identifying alternatives to oral contraceptives and hormone replacement therapies.

Assessment

Because pulmonary embolism can be a medical emergency, assessment may be very focused. In other instances, when emboli are small and not life threatening, a more extensive nursing assessment may be done. The nurse should obtain the following data when assessing the client with, or at risk for, a pulmonary embolus:

■ *Health history.* Chest pain, shortness of breath, and other symptoms, including onset, severity, and precipitating factors; history of recent surgery, venous thrombosis, or other risk factor, such as childbirth or malignancy; current medications

- *Physical examination.* Level of consciousness, presence of respirations and pulse; skin color, temperature, and moisture; vital signs, including apical pulse and temperature; breath sounds and heart sounds; oxygen saturation level; neck vein distention and peripheral edema.

Diagnosis

Nursing diagnoses appropriate for a client with pulmonary embolism may include the following:

- *Impaired Gas Exchange*
- *Decreased Cardiac Output*
- *Ineffective Protection*
- *Anxiety.*

(NANDA-I © 2015)

Planning

Goals of nursing care for the client with pulmonary embolism are individualized on the basis of the client's specific needs and may include the following:

- The client will demonstrate an oxygen saturation that remains greater than 94%.
- The client will verbalize fears resulting from respiratory distress.
- The client will obtain relief from pain to allow for adequate rest and comfort.
- The client will demonstrate adequate tissue perfusion.
- The client's vital signs will remain within normal limits.

Implementation

The primary and most emergent focus of nursing care for the client with pulmonary embolism is to promote oxygenation and gas exchange. Other considerations include pain management and reduction of the anxiety that often results from hypoxia.

Compensate for Impaired Gas Exchange

Pulmonary embolism results in areas of the lung that are ventilated but not perfused; these areas receive no capillary blood flow. If the embolus is large and a major segment of the lung is not perfused, gas exchange is significantly affected. Nursing interventions are directed toward compensating for impaired gas exchange and include the following:

- Frequently assess the client's respiratory status, including rate, depth, effort, lung sounds, and oxygen saturation. Impaired ventilation will further compromise gas exchange and worsen hypoxemia. Oxygen saturation can be monitored continuously and noninvasively to evaluate gas exchange.
- Place the client in the Fowler or high-Fowler position with the lower extremities dependent (e.g., hanging over the side of the bed). This position facilitates maximal lung expansion and reduces venous return to the right side of the heart, lowering pressures in the pulmonary vascular system.
- Monitor the client's arterial blood gas results, reporting abnormal findings as indicated. Arterial blood gas results are used to assess gas exchange and tissue oxygenation. An arterial line may be inserted for monitoring arterial pressure and arterial blood sampling.
- Maintain the client on bed rest. Bed rest reduces metabolic demands and tissue needs for oxygen.

Client Teaching Pulmonary Embolism

Discuss the following topics when preparing the client with pulmonary embolism and family members for home care:

- Use of prescribed anticoagulant, including drug interactions, scheduled laboratory testing, and manifestations of bleeding to report to the primary care provider
- Using a soft toothbrush and electric razor to reduce the risk of bleeding
- Avoiding aspirin (unless prescribed) and other over-the-counter medications unless approved by the physician
- Importance of wearing a medic alert tag for anticoagulant use
- Health promotion measures to reduce the risk of recurrent pulmonary embolism
- Symptoms of recurrent pulmonary embolism, such as sudden chest pain, shortness of breath, and possibly bloody sputum.
- Strategies for smoking cessation.

Preserve Cardiac Output

The impact of a large pulmonary embolus on hemodynamic status can be significant. Pressures in the pulmonary vascular system and right side of the heart increase; blood return to the left side of the heart and cardiac output may significantly decrease. A central line for hemodynamic monitoring may be instituted. Nursing interventions focus on preserving adequate blood pressure and organ function until cardiopulmonary status stabilizes and may include the following:

- Auscultate the client's heart sounds every 2–4 hours, and report any abnormalities. Sounds such as an S_3 or S_4 gallop may indicate cardiac compromise.
- Assess the client's skin color and temperature. These assessments monitor tissue perfusion.
- Monitor the client's cardiac rhythm. A drop in cardiac output and other hemodynamic alterations resulting from pulmonary embolism can precipitate dysrhythmias, which in turn can further impair cardiac output.
- Administer vasopressors and other medications as ordered. Carefully monitor the response to prescribed medications. Drugs may be prescribed to maintain adequate arterial pressure and tissue perfusion. Potent drugs, such as vasopressors, require careful monitoring for desired and adverse effects.
- Monitor the client's pulmonary arterial pressures, neck vein distention, and peripheral edema. Report findings as indicated. Right-sided heart failure is a potential complication of pulmonary embolism because of increased pulmonary arterial pressures.
- Maintain intravenous and arterial access sites as well as central lines. The client may be in unstable and critical condition, potentially needing immediate interventions to maintain life.
- Instruct the client to report chest pain or other symptoms. Decreased cardiac output and an increased workload resulting from pulmonary hypertension may cause anginal pain.

Promote Safety

Fibrinolytics and anticoagulant therapy impair normal clotting mechanisms, increasing the risk for bleeding and hemorrhage.

This risk is particularly acute during the first 24–48 hours following fibrinolytic drug administration. Nursing interventions that promote safety include the following:

- Assess the client frequently for overt and covert signs of bleeding: bleeding gums; hematuria; obvious or occult blood in stool or vomitus; incisional bleeding, bleeding or bruising of injection sites or with minor trauma; joint pain or immobility; and abdominal or flank pain. Careful monitoring is necessary to identify early signs of abnormal bleeding and prevent potential hemorrhage.
- Report coagulation study results outside the desired range for anticoagulant therapy. Levels less than the target range may indicate an increased risk for further clot development and pulmonary emboli; levels above the target range indicate an increased risk for bleeding.
- Keep protamine sulfate available for heparin therapy and vitamin K available for warfarin (Coumadin) therapy. Bleeding or hemorrhage resulting from excess anticoagulant may require antidote administration to rapidly reverse the anticoagulant effects.
- Assess the client's medication regimen for possible drug interactions that could potentiate or inhibit anticoagulant effects. Drug interactions can increase the risk for hemorrhage or further embolus formation.
- Avoid invasive procedures, injections, and venous punctures when possible, particularly during and following fibrinolytic therapy. Invasive procedures increase the risk of tissue trauma and bleeding.
- Maintain firm pressure on injection and venipuncture sites. Maintain pressure for 30 minutes following arterial puncture. Firm pressure reduces the risk for bleeding into the tissues.
- Maintain adequate fluid intake. Administer stool softeners as ordered. These measures help prevent constipation and straining, which may precipitate bleeding of hemorrhoids.

Relieve Anxiety

Pulmonary embolism is a physiological and psychological threat to safety and integrity. It is a major physiological stressor, eliciting a strong neuroendocrine stress response. The feeling of suffocation and inability to catch one's breath that accompanies a pulmonary embolus is also a strong psychological stressor. Fear, anxiety, and apprehension are common responses. The following nursing interventions will help in relieving the client's anxiety:

- Assess the client's anxiety level. Appropriate interventions are determined by the level of anxiety.
- Remain with the client as much as possible. The presence of a caring nurse helps reduce fear.
- Explain procedures and treatments, using short, simple sentences. Providing clearly understood, simple instructions reduces fear of the unknown.
- Reduce environmental stimuli, and use a calm, reassuring manner. These measures help reduce anxiety for both the nurse and the client.
- Allow supportive family members to remain with the client as much as possible. Calm, supportive family members provide further reassurance.
- Administer morphine sulfate as ordered. Morphine is given to reduce pain and anxiety.

Evaluation

The client's progress toward meeting the goals set during the planning stage of care is evaluated on the basis of the following expected outcomes:

- The client maintains adequate tissue perfusion to promote oxygenation and healing.
- The client's pain is controlled to facilitate rest and recovery.
- The client maintains effective airway clearance.

NURSING CARE PLAN   A Client With Pulmonary Embolism

Frank Marlin, 52 years old, is traveling home with his wife from their 3-week vacation in Australia. The flight is 14 1/2 hours long. As they approach their destination, Mr. Marlin experiences a sharp, stabbing pain in his right chest, which he assumes is a pulled muscle that resulted from a sudden cough he developed a few hours ago. When the plane lands, Mr. and Mrs. Marlin gather their carry-on luggage and walk through the concourse toward the baggage area. As they walk, Mr. Marlin notices that he feels short of breath. He tells his wife he needs to sit down for a minute, secretly worried that he might be having a heart attack, but the pain remains on the right side of his chest. He begins to feel increasingly anxious, and Mrs. Marlin notices that her husband is breathing rapidly and perspiring. She asks for help from a customer service clerk, who calls the paramedics. They transport Mr. Marlin to the local emergency department.

ASSESSMENT	DIAGNOSES	PLANNING
On admission to the emergency department, the nurse collects the following data: temperature 99.2°F tympanic; pulse 98 bpm; respirations 26/min; and BP 142/84 mmHg. Mr. Marlin's oxygen saturation is 87%. His breath sounds clear and equal, with fine rales in the upper right base. His lips and fingernails are mildly cyanotic. Mr. Marlin is alert, oriented, and anxious, asking the nurses, "Am I going to die?" His chest x-ray is normal; however, computed tomography (CT) with contrast shows obstructed pulmonary circulation in the right upper lobe. His D-dimer level is elevated. Mr. Marlin is diagnosed with right upper lobe pulmonary emboli.	■ *Impaired Gas Exchange* ■ *Pain* ■ *Anxiety* (NANDA-I © 2012)	Goals of care include the following: ■ The client's gas exchange will improve, as evidenced by an oxygen saturation of greater than 90%. ■ The client will have his pain controlled to improve his comfort, as evidenced by a reported pain level of 3 or less. ■ The client will experience reduced anxiety, as evidenced by his ability to sleep and to express less fear.

NURSING CARE PLAN   *(continued)*

IMPLEMENTATION

- Apply oxygen via face mask.
- Place cardiorespiratory monitor and oxygen saturation monitor on the client to allow for continuous monitoring of vital signs and oxygen saturation.
- Administer analgesics, per orders, and evaluate client's response to medication.
- Teach the client and family about risk factors contributing to development of pulmonary emboli.
- Answer client and family questions about the diagnosis of pulmonary emboli.

- Promote deep breathing.
- Position the client in the semi-Fowler position, lying on the right side to maximize expansion of healthy lungs.
- Remain with the client until vital signs normalize and oxygen saturation improves.
- Administer anticoagulants, and teach the client how to reduce bleeding risk.

EVALUATION

Mr. Marlin remains hospitalized for 5 days and is discharged on oral warfarin. Follow-up CT with contrast shows resolution of the emboli without permanent scarring or damage to lung tissue.

CRITICAL THINKING

1. On the basis of Mr. Marlin's symptoms, rate the severity of his pulmonary emboli.
2. What measures might you implement to reduce the client's anxiety?
3. Could Mr. Marlin's vital signs have been monitored manually instead of with placement of a cardiorespiratory monitor? Why is the monitor placed?

REVIEW   Pulmonary Embolism

RELATE Link the Concepts and Exemplars

Linking the exemplar of pulmonary embolism with the concept of acid–base balance:

1. What impact on acid–base balance would you anticipate finding when reviewing the results of an arterial blood gas drawn from a client with a significant pulmonary embolism?
2. What assessment findings would you anticipate when examining the client described in Question 1?

Linking the exemplar of pulmonary embolism with the concept of comfort:

3. Contrast the effectiveness of pharmacologic and nonpharmacologic therapies to control the pain associated with pulmonary embolism.
4. What risk is associated with administration of narcotics to a client with pulmonary emboli? How would you reduce these risks?

READY Go to Companion Skills Manual

REFER Go to Pearson Nursing Student Resources
nursing.pearsonhighered.com

- Additional review materials

REFLECT Case Study

Jennifer Walker is a 20-year-old female who is attending college in the Midwest. She is majoring in business and lives with her boyfriend, Sam Yoshida, age 21, in an off-campus apartment. Ms. Walker had an annual physical with a physician on campus at the beginning of the school year and obtained a prescription for oral contraceptives. Ms. Walker and Mr. Yoshida enjoy walking around the campus with their dog, Shelby, and are very active playing tennis and golf. Mr. Yoshida's parents are both physicians, and Ms. Walker's mother is a nurse.

Ms. Walker begins to notice that she has pain in her left leg when she walks Shelby and when she is playing tennis. Mr. Yoshida suggests that she return to the physician for a checkup.

Ms. Walker's physician admits her to the hospital with a diagnosis of thrombophlebitis and places her on heparin and bed rest. Ms. Walker is on her third day in the hospital, and she and Mr. Yoshida are studying together in her room when she develops dyspnea and chest pain and becomes very apprehensive. Mr. Yoshida goes to the nurse's station to inform the staff of Ms. Walker's new symptoms.

1. What is the priority intervention for Ms. Walker at this time?
2. What is the physiological rationale for pain control for Ms. Walker?
3. Create a plan of care for Ms. Walker and Mr. Yoshida regarding teaching interventions needed for discharge.

EXEMPLAR 16.12   Shock

EXEMPLAR KEY TERMS
Anaphylactic shock, *1224*
Cardiac output (CO), *1218*
Cardiogenic shock, *1223*
Distributive shock, *1224*

Hypovolemic shock, *1222*
Mean arterial pressure (MAP), *1218*
Neurogenic shock, *1224*
Obstructive shock, *1224*
Septic shock, *1224*

EXEMPLAR LEARNING OUTCOMES
After reading about this exemplar, you will be able to:

1. Describe the pathophysiology, etiology, clinical manifestations, and direct and indirect causes of shock.
2. Identify risk factors and prevention methods associated with shock.
3. Illustrate the nursing process in providing culturally competent care across the life span for individuals with shock.
4. Formulate priority nursing diagnoses appropriate for an individual with shock.
5. Summarize therapies used by interdisciplinary teams in the collaborative care of an individual with shock.
6. Plan evidence-based care for an individual with shock and his or her family in collaboration with other members of the healthcare team.
7. Evaluate expected outcomes for an individual with shock.

▶ OVERVIEW

Shock is a clinical syndrome characterized by a decrease in blood flow resulting in inadequate oxygenation. This imbalance results in a state of inadequate blood flow to body organs and tissues, causing life-threatening cellular dysfunction.

To maintain cellular metabolism, the cells of all body organs and tissues require a regular and consistent supply of oxygen and removal of metabolic wastes. This homeostatic regulation is maintained primarily by the cardiovascular system and depends on four physiological components:

1. A cardiac output sufficient to meet bodily requirements
2. An uncompromised vascular system, in which the vessels have a diameter sufficient to allow unimpeded blood flow and have good **tone** (the ability to constrict or dilate to maintain normal pressure)
3. A volume of blood sufficient to fill the circulatory system, and a blood pressure adequate to maintain blood flow
4. Tissues that are able to extract and use the oxygen delivered through the capillaries.

In a healthy individual, these components function as a system to maintain tissue perfusion. During shock, however, one or more of the components are disrupted. An understanding of basic hemodynamics is necessary to understand the pathophysiology of shock:

- **Stroke volume (SV)** is the amount of blood pumped into the aorta with each contraction of the left ventricle.
- **Cardiac output (CO)** is the amount of blood pumped per minute into the aorta by the left ventricle. It is determined by multiplying SV by the heart rate (HR): $CO = SV \times HR$.
- **Mean arterial pressure (MAP)** is the average pressure in the arterial circulation throughout the cardiac cycle. It is the product of CO and systemic vascular resistance (SVR): $MAP = CO \times SVR$. When CO, SVR, or total blood volume rises, MAP and tissue perfusion increase. Conversely, when CO, SVR, or total blood volume falls, MAP and tissue perfusion decrease.
- The *sympathetic nervous system (SNS)* maintains the smooth muscle surrounding the arteries and arterioles in a state of partial contraction called **sympathetic tone**. Increased sympathetic stimulation increases vasoconstriction and systemic vascular resistance; decreased sympathetic stimulation allows vasodilation, which decreases systemic vascular resistance.
- *Pulse pressure* (the difference between systolic and diastolic blood pressure) is often an early indicator of shock. Narrow-

ing pulse pressure is consistent with hypovolemic and cardiogenic shock as a result of reduced cardiac output, whereas septic shock causes a widening pulse pressure.

▶ PATHOPHYSIOLOGY AND ETIOLOGY

When one or more cardiovascular components do not function properly, the body's hemodynamic properties are altered. Consequently, tissue perfusion may be inadequate to sustain normal cellular metabolism. The result is the clinical syndrome known as shock.

The manifestations of shock result from the body's attempts to maintain vital organs (heart and brain) and to preserve life following a drop in cellular perfusion. However, if the injury or condition triggering shock is severe enough or of long enough duration, then cellular hypoxia and cellular death occur.

Shock is triggered by a sustained drop in MAP. This drop can occur after a decrease in cardiac output, a decrease in the circulating blood volume, or an increase in the size of the vascular bed as a result of peripheral vasodilation. If intervention is timely and effective, the physiological events that characterize shock may be stopped; if not, shock may lead to death. See **Table 16–32** ● for classifications of shock.

Stage I: Early, Reversible, and Compensatory Shock

The initial stage of shock begins when baroreceptors in the aortic arch and the carotid sinus detect a sustained drop in MAP of less than 10 mmHg from normal levels. The circulating blood volume may decrease (usually to <500 mL), but not enough to cause serious effects in an adult client. See the Lifespan Considerations feature for blood volume in children.

> **Lifespan Considerations**
> **Blood Volume in Children**
>
> The child's total blood volume varies by weight. The child has approximately 80 mL of blood for every kilogram of body weight.
>
> - *Newborn:* 3 kg × 80 mL = 240 mL (1 cup)
> - *5-year-old:* 25 kg × 80 mL = 2,000 mL (2 quarts)
> - *13-year-old:* 50 kg × 80 mL = 4,000 mL (1 gallon)

TABLE 16–32 Classification of Hemorrhagic Shock and Client Presentation

	COMPENSATED/CLASS I	MILD/CLASS II	MODERATE/CLASS III	SEVERE/CLASS IV
Blood loss	<750 mL	750–1,500 mL	1,500–2,000 mL	>2,000 mL
% of blood volume loss	<15%	15%–30%	30%–40%	>40%
Heart rate	<100	>100	>120	>140
Blood pressure	Normal or increased	Normal	Decreased	Markedly decreased
Pulse pressure	Normal or increased	Decreased	Decreased	Decreased
Capillary refill	Normal	Mild increase	Usually delayed	Delayed
Respiratory rate	Normal	Mild increase	Moderate tachypnea	Marked tachypnea
Urine output (mL/hr)	>30 mL	20–30 mL	5–15 mL	Anuria
Mental status	Normal–slightly anxious	Mildly anxious–agitated	Anxious–confused	Lethargic–obtunded

The body reacts to the decrease in arterial pressure as it would to any physical stressor. The cerebral integration center initiates the body's response systems, causing the SNS to increase the heart rate and the force of cardiac contraction, thus increasing cardiac output. Sympathetic stimulation also causes peripheral vasoconstriction, resulting in increased systemic vascular resistance and a rise in arterial pressure. The net result is that the perfusion of cells, tissues, and organs is maintained.

Symptoms are almost imperceptible during the early stage of shock. The pulse rate may be slightly elevated. If the injury is minor or of short duration, arterial pressure is usually maintained, and no further symptoms occur.

Compensatory shock in adults begins after the MAP falls 10–15 mmHg below normal levels. The circulating blood volume is reduced by 25%–35% (1,000 mL or more), but compensatory mechanisms are able to maintain blood pressure and tissue perfusion to vital organs, thereby preventing cell damage. Pediatric clients can often maintain their blood pressure until they are in profound shock. Hypotension in children is a late finding of shock. These compensatory mechanisms of shock include the following:

- Stimulation of the SNS results in the release of epinephrine from the adrenal medulla and the release of norepinephrine from the adrenal medulla and the sympathetic fibers. Both hormones rapidly stimulate the alpha- and beta-adrenergic fibers. Stimulated alpha-adrenergic fibers cause vasoconstriction in the blood vessels supplying the skin and most of the abdominal viscera. Perfusion of these areas decreases. Stimulated beta-adrenergic fibers cause vasodilation in vessels supplying the heart and skeletal muscles (beta$_1$ response) and increase the heart rate and force of cardiac contraction (beta$_2$ response). Furthermore, blood vessels in the respiratory system dilate, and the respiratory rate increases (beta$_2$ response). Thus, stimulation of the SNS results in increased cardiac output and oxygenation of these tissues.

- The renin–angiotensin response occurs as the blood flow to the kidneys decreases. Renin released from the kidneys converts a plasma protein to angiotensin II, which causes vasoconstriction and stimulates the adrenal cortex to release aldosterone. Aldosterone causes the kidneys to reabsorb water and sodium and to lose potassium. The

absorption of water maintains circulating blood volume while increased vasoconstriction increases systemic vascular resistance, maintaining central vascular volume and raising blood pressure.

- The hypothalamus releases adrenocorticotropic hormone, causing the adrenal glands to secrete aldosterone. Aldosterone promotes the reabsorption of water and sodium by the kidneys, preserving blood volume and pressure.

- The posterior pituitary gland releases antidiuretic hormone, which increases renal reabsorption of water to increase intravascular volume. The combined effects of hormones released by the hypothalamus and posterior pituitary glands work to conserve central vascular volume.

- As MAP falls in the compensatory stage of shock, decreased capillary hydrostatic pressure causes a fluid shift from the interstitial space into the capillaries. The net gain of fluid raises the blood volume.

- In children, vasoconstriction causes the blood flow to be shunted away from the nonvital organs. Extremities are cold and mottled, capillary refill is prolonged, and tachycardia occurs. If shock is left untreated, uncompensated shock develops. If the compensatory mechanisms fail, death will occur.

Working together, these compensatory mechanisms can maintain MAP for only a short period of time. During this period, the perfusion and oxygenation of the heart and brain are adequate. If effective treatment is provided, the process is arrested, and no permanent damage occurs. However, unless the underlying cause of shock is reversed, these compensatory mechanisms soon become harmful, and shock perpetuates shock.

Stage II: Intermediate or Progressive Shock

The progressive stage of shock occurs after a sustained decrease in MAP of 20 mmHg or more below normal levels and a fluid loss of 35%–50%. Although the compensatory mechanisms in the previous state remain activated, they are no longer able to maintain MAP at a level sufficient to ensure perfusion of vital organs.

The vasoconstriction response that first helped sustain MAP eventually limits blood flow to the point at which cells become oxygen deficient. To remain alive, the affected cells switch from aerobic to anaerobic metabolism. The lactic acid formed as a by-product of anaerobic metabolism contributes to an acidotic state at the cellular level. As a result, adenosine triphosphate, the source of cellular energy, is produced inefficiently. Lacking energy, the sodium–potassium pump fails. Potassium moves out of the cell, while sodium and water move inward. As this process continues, the cell swells, cell membrane integrity is lost, and cell organelles are damaged. Lysosomes within the cell spill out their digestive enzymes, which disintegrate any remaining organelles. Some enzymes spread to adjacent cells, where they erode and rupture cell membranes.

The acid by-products of anaerobic metabolism dilate the precapillary arterioles and constrict the postcapillary venules. This causes increased hydrostatic pressure within the capillary, and fluid shifts back into the interstitial space. The capillaries also become increasingly permeable, allowing serum proteins to shift from the vascular space into the interstitium. The buildup of plasma proteins increases the osmotic pressure in the interstitium, further accelerating the fluid shift out of the capillaries.

Throughout this period, the heart rate and vasoconstriction increase; however, perfusion of the skin, skeletal muscles, kidneys, and gastrointestinal organs is greatly diminished. Cells in the heart and brain become hypoxic, while other body cells and tissues become ischemic and anoxic. A generalized state of acidosis and hyperkalemia ensues. Unless this stage of shock is treated rapidly, the client's chances of survival are poor.

Stage III: Refractory or Irreversible Shock

If shock progresses to the irreversible stage, tissue anoxia becomes so generalized and cellular death so widespread that no treatment can reverse the damage. Even if MAP is temporarily restored, too much cellular damage has occurred to maintain life. Death of cells is followed by death of tissues, which results in death of organs. Death of vital organs contributes to subsequent death of the body.

Effects of Shock on Body Systems

Whatever its causes, shock produces predictable effects on the body's organ systems. See the Multisystem Effects of Shock feature on page 1221.

CARDIOVASCULAR SYSTEM The perfusion and oxygenation of the heart are adequate in the early stages of shock. As shock progresses, myocardial cells become hypoxic, and myocardial muscle function diminishes. Initially, the blood pressure may be normal or even slightly elevated (as a result of compensatory mechanisms), and the heart rate may be only slightly increased. Sympathetic stimulation increases the heart rate (a sinus tachycardia of 120 bpm is common) in an effort to increase cardiac output. As a result of vasoconstriction and decreased blood volume, the palpated pulse is rapid, weak, and thready; as shock progresses, peripheral pulses are usually nonpalpable.

Tachycardia reduces the time available for left ventricular filling and coronary artery perfusion, further reducing cardiac output. With progressive shock, altered acid–base balance, hypoxia, and hyperkalemia damage the heart's electrical systems and contractility. Consequently, cardiac dysrhythmias may develop. Decreased blood volume with decreased venous return also decreases cardiac output, and blood pressure falls.

The blood pressure changes produced by shock are characterized by a progressive decrease in both systolic and diastolic pressures and a narrowing pulse pressure. Auscultation of blood pressure is often difficult or impossible and is an inaccurate reflection of blood pressure status. For this reason, hemodynamic monitoring is usually instituted to follow the client's cardiovascular status accurately.

RESPIRATORY SYSTEM During shock, oxygen delivery to cells may be impaired by a drop in circulating blood volume or, in the case of blood loss, by an insufficient number of red blood cells that carry oxygen. Although the respiratory rate increases because of compensatory mechanisms that promote oxygenation, the number of alveoli that are perfused decreases, and gas exchange is impaired. As a result, oxygen levels in the blood decrease, and carbon dioxide levels increase. As perfusion of the lungs diminishes, carbon dioxide is retained, and respiratory acidosis occurs.

A complication of decreased perfusion of the lungs is acute respiratory distress syndrome (ARDS), or "shock lung." The exact mechanism that produces ARDS is unknown, but some contributing factors have been identified. The pulmonary capillaries become increasingly permeable to proteins and water, resulting in noncardiogenic pulmonary edema. Production of surfactant, which controls surface tension within alveoli, is impaired, and the alveoli collapse or fill with fluid. This potentially lethal form of respiratory failure may result from any condition that causes hypoperfusion of the lungs, but it is most common in shock caused by hemorrhage, severe allergic responses, trauma, and infection.

GASTROINTESTINAL SYSTEM The gastrointestinal organs normally receive 25% of the cardiac output through the splanchnic circulation. Shock constricts the splanchnic arterioles and redirects arterial blood flow to the heart and brain. Consequently, gastrointestinal organs become ischemic and may be irreversibly damaged.

Gastric mucosa tends to ulcerate when it becomes ischemic. Lesions of the gastric and duodenal mucosa (stress ulcers) can develop within hours of severe trauma, sepsis, or burns (Huether & McCance, 2013). Gastrointestinal ulcers may hemorrhage within 2–10 days following the original cause of shock. In addition, the permeability of damaged mucosa increases, allowing enteric bacteria or their toxins to enter the abdominal cavity and then progress to the circulation, resulting in sepsis.

Gastric and intestinal motility is impaired during shock, and paralytic ileus may result. If the episode of shock is prolonged, necrosis of the bowel may occur. In many cases, alterations in the structure and function of the gastrointestinal tract impair absorption of nutrients, such as protein and glucose.

Multisystem Effects of Shock

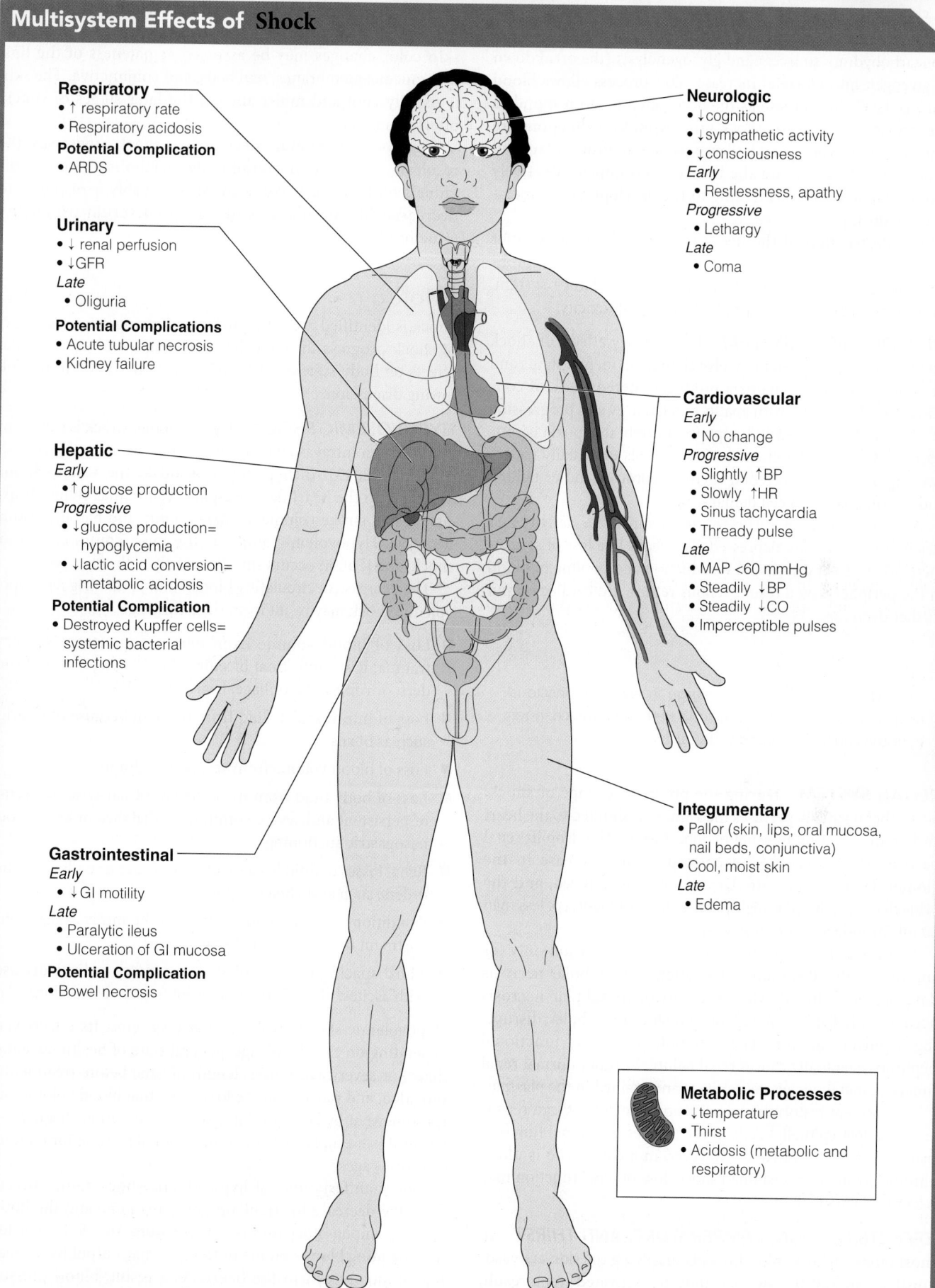

Respiratory
- ↑ respiratory rate
- Respiratory acidosis

Potential Complication
- ARDS

Urinary
- ↓ renal perfusion
- ↓GFR

Late
- Oliguria

Potential Complications
- Acute tubular necrosis
- Kidney failure

Hepatic

Early
- ↑ glucose production

Progressive
- ↓glucose production= hypoglycemia
- ↓lactic acid conversion= metabolic acidosis

Potential Complication
- Destroyed Kupffer cells= systemic bacterial infections

Gastrointestinal

Early
- ↓ GI motility

Late
- Paralytic ileus
- Ulceration of GI mucosa

Potential Complication
- Bowel necrosis

Neurologic
- ↓cognition
- ↓sympathetic activity
- ↓consciousness

Early
- Restlessness, apathy

Progressive
- Lethargy

Late
- Coma

Cardiovascular

Early
- No change

Progressive
- Slightly ↑BP
- Slowly ↑HR
- Sinus tachycardia
- Thready pulse

Late
- MAP <60 mmHg
- Steadily ↓BP
- Steadily ↓CO
- Imperceptible pulses

Integumentary
- Pallor (skin, lips, oral mucosa, nail beds, conjunctiva)
- Cool, moist skin

Late
- Edema

Metabolic Processes
- ↓temperature
- Thirst
- Acidosis (metabolic and respiratory)

Shock also alters the metabolic functions of the liver. Initially, gluconeogenesis (the process of forming glucose from noncarbohydrate sources) and glycogenolysis (the breakdown of glycogen into glucose) increase. This process allows blood glucose levels to increase as the body attempts to respond to the stressor; however, as shock progresses, liver functions are impaired and hypoglycemia develops. Metabolism of fats and protein is impaired, and the liver can no longer effectively remove lactic acid, contributing to the development of metabolic acidosis.

The destruction of the liver's reticuloendothelial Kupffer cells (phagocytes that destroy bacteria) causes a further problem. Bacteria may proliferate within the circulatory system, causing overwhelming bacterial infection and toxicity.

NEUROLOGICAL SYSTEM   The primary effects of shock on the neurological system involve changes in mental status and orientation. Cerebral hypoxia produces altered levels of consciousness, beginning with apathy and lethargy and progressing to coma. A common early symptom of cerebral hypoxia is restlessness. Continued ischemia of brain cells eventually causes swelling, resulting in cerebral edema, neurotransmitter failure, and irreversible brain cell damage.

As cerebral ischemia worsens, the sympathetic activity and vasomotor centers are depressed. This leads to a loss of sympathetic tone, causing systemic vasodilation and pooling of blood in the periphery. As a result, venous return and cardiac output further decrease.

> **SAFETY ALERT**
> An early sign of shock is a change in level of consciousness. Late signs of shock include mental status changes, hypotension, and marked tachycardia.

RENAL SYSTEM   During the progressive stage of shock, blood that normally perfuses the kidneys is shunted to the heart and brain, resulting in renal hypoperfusion. The drop in renal perfusion is reflected in a corresponding decrease in the glomerular filtration rate. Urine output is reduced, and the urine that is produced is highly concentrated. Oliguria of less than 20 mL/hr indicates progressive shock.

Healthy kidneys can tolerate a drop in perfusion only for approximately 20 minutes; thereafter, acute tubular necrosis develops (Huether & McCance, 2013). As tubular necrosis occurs, epithelial cells slough off and block the tubules, disrupting nephron function. The accumulating loss of functional nephrons eventually causes renal failure. Without normal renal function, metabolic waste products are retained in the plasma.

If treatment restores renal perfusion, the kidneys can regenerate the lost epithelial cells in the tubules, and renal function usually returns to normal. However, in a client who is older, chronically ill, or in sustained shock, loss of renal function may become permanent.

EFFECTS ON SKIN, TEMPERATURE, AND THIRST   In most types of shock, blood vessels supplying the skin are vasoconstricted, and the sweat glands are activated. As a result, changes in skin color occur. The skin of Caucasian clients

becomes pale. In individuals with darker skin (e.g., those of African, Hispanic, or Mediterranean descent), shock-related skin color changes may be assessed as paleness of the lips, oral mucous membranes, nail beds, and conjunctiva. The skin is usually cool and moist and, in the later stages of shock, often edematous.

The body temperature decreases as shock progresses, the result of a decrease in overall body metabolism. Some individuals with shock become thirsty, probably a response to decreased blood volume and increased serum osmolality (Huether & McCance, 2013).

Etiology

Shock is identified according to its underlying cause. All types of shock progress through the same stages and exert similar effects on body systems. Any differences are noted in the following discussion.

HYPOVOLEMIC SHOCK   **Hypovolemic shock** is caused by a decrease in intravascular volume of 15% or more (Huether & McCance, 2013). In hypovolemic shock, the venous blood returning to the heart decreases, and ventricular filling drops. As a result, stroke volume, cardiac output, and blood pressure decrease. Hypovolemic shock is the most common type of shock, and it often occurs simultaneously with other types.

The decrease in circulating blood volume that triggers hypovolemic shock may result from the following:

- Loss of blood volume from hemorrhage (from surgery, trauma, gastrointestinal bleeding, blood coagulation disorders, or ruptured esophageal varices)
- Loss of intravascular fluid from the skin because of injuries such as burns
- Loss of blood volume from severe dehydration
- Loss of body fluid from the gastrointestinal system because of persistent and severe vomiting or diarrhea or continuous nasogastric suctioning
- Renal losses of fluid because of diuretic use or endocrine disorders, such as diabetes insipidus
- Conditions causing fluid shifts from the intravascular compartment to the interstitial space
- Third spacing because of such disorders as liver diseases with ascites, pleural effusion, or intestinal obstruction

Hypovolemic shock affects all body systems. Its effects vary depending on the client's age, general state of health, extent of injury or severity of illness, length of time before treatment is provided, and rate of volume loss. Note that blood volume varies somewhat by age. The Lifespan Considerations feature earlier in this exemplar lists the typical blood volume for children of various ages.

The manifestations of hypovolemic shock result directly from the decrease in circulating blood volume and the initiation of compensatory mechanisms (**Figure 16–59 ●**). The loss of circulating blood volume reduces cardiac output by decreasing venous return to the heart. As a result, blood pressure drops. The carotid and cardiac baroreceptors sense the decrease

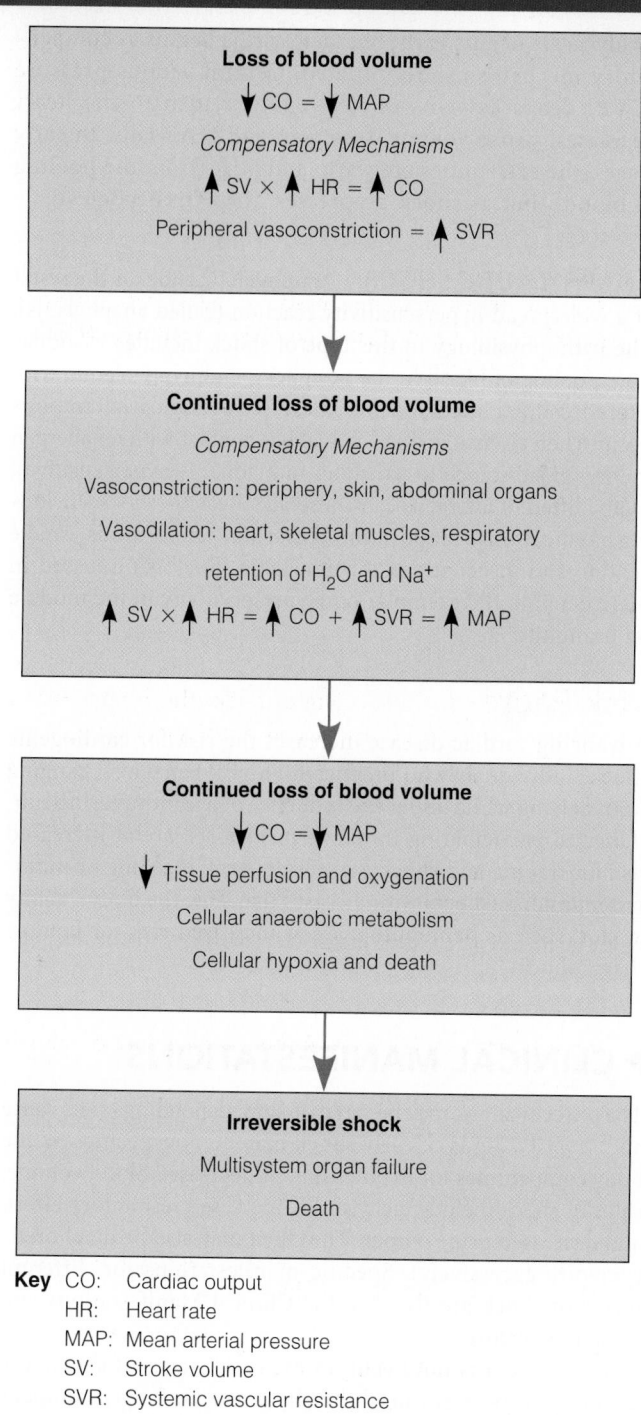

Loss of blood volume

$\downarrow$ CO = $\downarrow$ MAP

Compensatory Mechanisms

$\uparrow$ SV × $\uparrow$ HR = $\uparrow$ CO

Peripheral vasoconstriction = $\uparrow$ SVR

Continued loss of blood volume

Compensatory Mechanisms

Vasoconstriction: periphery, skin, abdominal organs

Vasodilation: heart, skeletal muscles, respiratory

retention of H_2O and Na^+

$\uparrow$ SV × $\uparrow$ HR = $\uparrow$ CO + $\uparrow$ SVR = $\uparrow$ MAP

Continued loss of blood volume

$\downarrow$ CO = $\downarrow$ MAP

$\downarrow$ Tissue perfusion and oxygenation

Cellular anaerobic metabolism

Cellular hypoxia and death

Irreversible shock

Multisystem organ failure

Death

Key CO: Cardiac output
HR: Heart rate
MAP: Mean arterial pressure
SV: Stroke volume
SVR: Systemic vascular resistance

Figure 16–59 ● Stages of hypovolemic shock.

in blood pressure and communicate it to the vasomotor centers in the brainstem. The vasomotor centers then induce the sympathetic compensatory responses. If the fluid loss is less than 500 mL in adults, activation of the sympathetic response is generally adequate to restore cardiac output and blood pressure to near normal, although the heart rate may remain elevated.

With a sustained loss of blood volume (1,000 mL or more in adults), the shock stage progresses. Heart rate and vasoconstriction increase, and blood flow to the skin, skeletal muscles, kidneys, and abdominal organs decreases. Several renal mech-

anisms and a decline in capillary pressure help conserve blood volume. Eventually, the amount of blood flowing to cells is too low to oxygenate them and sustain production of cellular energy. Anaerobic metabolism begins, producing an acidotic environment for cells. As a result, cells lose their physical integrity. If untreated, shock causes multiple organ failure, and death results.

With aging comes a relative decrease in sympathetic activity in relation to the cardiovascular system. Cardiac compliance also decreases with age. Atherosclerosis affects many vital organs' sensitivity to even the slightest reduction in blood flow. Many older adults experience secondary volume depletion because of chronic diuretic use or malnutrition. Also, clients taking beta-blockers may not present with tachycardia as an early indicator of shock. This important sign can be masked because of beta-adrenergic blockade. These clients will require early invasive monitoring in order to avoid excessive or inadequate volume restoration. This should be considered early in the treatment phase.

CARDIOGENIC SHOCK   **Cardiogenic shock** occurs when the heart's pumping ability is compromised to the point at which it cannot maintain cardiac output and adequate tissue perfusion. The loss of the pumping action of the heart may be caused by the following conditions:

- MI
- Cardiac tamponade
- Restrictive pericarditis
- Cardiac arrest
- Dysrhythmias, such as fibrillation or ventricular tachycardia
- Pathological changes in the valves
- Cardiomyopathies from hypertension, alcohol, bacterial or viral infections, or ischemia
- Complications of cardiac surgery
- Electrolyte imbalances, especially changes in normal potassium and calcium levels
- Drugs affecting cardiac muscle contractility
- Head injuries causing damage to the cardioregulatory center.

Myocardial infarction is the most common cause of cardiogenic shock. Clients admitted to the hospital for treatment of MI or cardiac surgery are at risk for cardiogenic shock. The severity and progression of shock are related to the amount of myocardial damage.

Whatever the cardiogenic cause, the decrease in cardiac output causes a decrease in MAP. Heart rate may increase in response to compensatory mechanisms. However, tachycardia increases myocardial oxygen consumption and decreases coronary perfusion. The myocardium becomes progressively depleted of oxygen, causing further myocardial ischemia and necrosis. The typical sequence of shock is essentially unchanged in cardiogenic shock.

Cyanosis, however, is more common in cardiogenic shock, because stagnating blood increases extraction of oxygen from the hemoglobin at the capillary beds. As a result, the skin, lips, and nail beds may appear cyanotic. As cardiac failure and cardiogenic shock progress, left ventricular end-diastolic pressure increases. The increase is transmitted to the pulmonary capillary bed, and pulmonary edema may occur. Retention of blood in the right side of the heart increases right atrial pressure, which leads to jugular venous distention as a result of backflow through the vena cava.

OBSTRUCTIVE SHOCK **Obstructive shock** is caused by an obstruction in the heart or great vessels that either impedes venous return or prevents effective cardiac pumping action. The causes of obstructive shock are impaired diastolic filling (e.g., pericardial tamponade or pneumothorax), increased right ventricular afterload (e.g., pulmonary emboli), and increased left ventricular afterload (e.g., aortic stenosis or abdominal distention). The manifestations are the result of decreased cardiac output and blood pressure, with reduced tissue perfusion and cellular metabolism.

DISTRIBUTIVE SHOCK **Distributive shock**, also called **vasogenic shock**, includes several types of shock that result from widespread vasodilation and decreased peripheral resistance. Because the blood volume does not change, relative hypovolemia results.

SEPTIC SHOCK **Septic shock**, also known as septicemia, is the leading cause of death for clients in intensive care units (ICUs). It is one part of a progressive syndrome called systemic inflammatory response syndrome. This condition is most often the result of gram-negative bacterial infections (e.g., *Pseudomonas*, *Escherichia coli*, or *Klebsiella*) but may also follow gram-positive infections from *Staphylococcus* and *Streptococcus* bacteria. Septic shock is discussed in more detail in the exemplar on Sepsis in the module on Infection.

NEUROGENIC SHOCK **Neurogenic shock** is the result of an imbalance between parasympathetic and sympathetic stimulation of vascular smooth muscle. If parasympathetic overstimulation or sympathetic understimulation persists, sustained vasodilation occurs, and blood pools in the venous and capillary beds.

Neurogenic shock causes a dramatic reduction in systemic vascular resistance as the size of the vascular compartment increases. As systemic vascular resistance decreases, pressure in the blood vessels becomes too low to drive nutrients across capillary membranes, and cellular metabolism is impaired.

The following conditions can cause neurogenic shock by increasing parasympathetic stimulation or inhibiting sympathetic stimulation of the smooth muscle of blood vessels:

- Head injury
- Trauma to the spinal cord
- Insulin reactions (which cause hypoglycemia, decreasing glucose to the medulla)
- Central nervous system depressant drugs (e.g., sedatives, barbiturates, or narcotics)
- Anesthesia (spinal and general)
- Severe pain
- Prolonged exposure to heat.

Bradycardia occurs early, but tachycardia begins as compensatory mechanisms are initiated. Central venous pressure (CVP) drops as veins dilate, venous return to the heart decreases, stroke volume decreases, and MAP falls. In early stages, the extremities are warm and pink (from the pooling of blood), but as shock progresses, the skin becomes pale and cool.

ANAPHYLACTIC SHOCK **Anaphylactic shock** is the result of a widespread hypersensitivity reaction (called anaphylaxis). The pathophysiology in this type of shock includes vasodilation, pooling of blood in the periphery, and hypovolemia with altered cellular metabolism. These physiological alterations occur when a sensitized individual has contact with an allergen (a foreign substance to which an individual is hypersensitive). Many different allergens can cause anaphylactic shock, including medications, blood administration, latex, foods, snake venom, and insect stings. Anaphylactic shock is discussed in more detail in the exemplar on Hypersensitivity in the module on Immunity.

Risk Factors

Advancing cardiac disease increases the risk for cardiogenic shock. Individuals who practice high-risk behaviors, ranging from driving while under the influence of a mind-altering substance to participating in dangerous sports, are at increased risk for trauma and shock that results from bleeding or multisystem injury. Clients with diseases that slow the body's ability to clot, such as hemophilia, are at increased risk for hemorrhagic shock.

▶ CLINICAL MANIFESTATIONS

The onset of shock may be rapid or slow, depending on its cause and severity. Signs of early shock may be nonspecific. As the body compensates for hypotension or decreased blood volume, signs of shock include tachycardia, increased respiratory effort, and decreased urine output. The client may also be diaphoretic (perspire excessively). Specific manifestations for different forms of shock are listed in the Clinical Manifestations and Therapies feature.

If treatment is not begun in the early stages of shock, the condition progresses until the client can no longer compensate. At that time, the systolic blood pressure drops, and the pulse pressure narrows. Reduced cerebral blood flow ultimately results in a decreased level of consciousness. If shock is not reversed, the condition progresses to cardiopulmonary failure.

▶ COLLABORATION

Medical care for the client with shock focuses on treating the underlying cause, increasing arterial oxygenation, and improving tissue perfusion. Depending on the cause and type of shock, interventions include emergency care measures, oxygen therapy, fluid replacement, and medications. Emergency care is often the first course of collaborative action taken to arrest shock.

Clinical Manifestations and Therapies **Shock**

ETIOLOGY	CLINICAL MANIFESTATIONS	CLINICAL THERAPIES
Hypovolemic shock	**Initial Stage** ■ Blood pressure: normal to slightly decreased ■ Pulse: slightly increased from baseline ■ Respirations: normal (baseline) ■ Skin: cool, pale (in periphery), moist ■ Mental status: alert and oriented ■ Urine output: slight decrease ■ Other: thirst, decreased capillary refill time **Compensatory and Progressive Stages** ■ Blood pressure: hypotension ■ Pulse: rapid, thready ■ Respirations: increased ■ Skin: cool, pale (includes trunk); poor turgor with fluid loss, edematous with fluid shift ■ Mental status: restless, anxious, confused, or agitated ■ Urine output: oliguria (<30 mL/hr) ■ Other: marked thirst, acidosis, hyperkalemia, decreased capillary refill time, decreased or absent peripheral pulses **Irreversible Stage** ■ Blood pressure: severe hypotension (systolic pressure often is <80 mmHg) ■ Pulse: very rapid, weak ■ Respirations: rapid, shallow; crackles and wheezes ■ Skin: cool, pale, mottled with cyanosis ■ Mental status: disoriented, lethargic, comatose ■ Urine output: anuria ■ Other: loss of reflexes, decreased or absent peripheral pulses	■ Administer blood. ■ Administer intravenous (IV) fluid and volume expanders. ■ Keep client NPO until gastrointestinal (GI) function returns to normal. ■ Administer oxygen. ■ Support vital functions until perfusion is restored. ■ Assess level of consciousness (LOC). ■ Monitor effectiveness of respiratory effort—may require mechanical ventilation to meet the body's oxygen demands. ■ Monitor lab data, including hemoglobin and hematocrit, arterial blood gases (ABGs), and serum electrolytes, and blood urea nitrogen (BUN). ■ Administer medications as ordered (e.g., diuretics, sodium bicarbonate, antidysrhythmic agents, cardiotonic glycoside).
Cardiogenic shock	■ Blood pressure: hypotension ■ Pulse: rapid, thready; distention of veins of hands and neck ■ Respirations: increased, labored; crackles and wheezes; pulmonary edema ■ Skin: pale, cyanotic, cold, moist ■ Mental status: restless, anxious, lethargic progressing to comatose ■ Urine output: oliguria to anuria ■ Other: dependent edema; elevated CVP; elevated pulmonary capillary wedge pressure; dysrhythmias	■ Administer IV fluid cautiously to avoid fluid overload placing more stress on the heart. ■ Keep client NPO until GI function returns to normal. ■ Treat underlying cause. ■ Medications may include diuretics, sodium bicarbonate, antidysrhythmic agents, cardiotonic glycoside. ■ Administer oxygen. ■ Support vital functions until perfusion is restored. ■ Assess LOC. ■ Monitor effectiveness of respiratory effort—may require mechanical ventilation to meet the body's oxygen demands.

(continued on next page)

Clinical Manifestations and Therapies **Shock** (continued)

ETIOLOGY	CLINICAL MANIFESTATIONS	CLINICAL THERAPIES
		■ Monitor lab data including ABGs, serum electrolytes, BUN, creatinine, cardiac enzymes, CVP, pulmonary wedge pressure, and cardiac output.
Obstructive shock	■ Tachycardia ■ Tachypnea ■ Hypotension ■ Delayed capillary refill in extremities ■ Decreased urine output ■ Peripheral edema	■ Treat underlying cause. ■ Reduce cardiac workload. ■ Administer oxygen. ■ Support vital functions until perfusion is restored. ■ Assess LOC. ■ Monitor effectiveness of respiratory effort—may require mechanical ventilation to meet the body's oxygen demands.
Distributive (vaso-genic) shock	■ Tachycardia ■ Tachypnea ■ Hypotension ■ Delayed capillary refill in extremities ■ Decreased urine output ■ Peripheral edema ■ Absent or weak peripheral pulses	■ Treat underlying cause. ■ Administer vasoconstricting medications to increase peripheral vascular resistance and restore perfusion.
Septic shock	**Early (Warm) Septic Shock** ■ Blood pressure: normal to hypotension ■ Pulse: increased, thready ■ Respirations: rapid and deep ■ Skin: warm, flushed ■ Mental status: alert, oriented, anxious ■ Urine output: normal ■ Other: increased body temperature; chills; weakness; nausea, vomiting, diarrhea; decreased CVP **Late (Cold) Septic Shock** ■ Blood pressure: hypotension ■ Pulse: tachycardia, arrhythmias ■ Respirations: rapid, shallow, dyspneic ■ Skin: cool, pale, edematous ■ Mental status: lethargic to comatose ■ Urine output: oliguria to anuria ■ Other: normal to decreased body temperature; decreased CVP	■ Treat underlying cause. ■ Administer antibiotics and IV fluids. ■ Assess for potential disseminated intra-vascular coagulation. ■ Support vital functions until perfusion is restored. ■ Assess LOC. ■ Monitor effectiveness of respiratory effort—may require mechanical ventilation to meet the body's oxygen demands. ■ Obtain cultures prior to administration of antibiotics to determine source of infection and pathogen involved.
Neurogenic shock	■ Blood pressure: hypotension ■ Pulse: slow and bounding ■ Respirations: vary ■ Skin: warm, dry ■ Mental status: anxious, restless, lethargic progressing to comatose ■ Urine output: oliguria to anuria ■ Other: lowered body temperature	■ Treat underlying injury. ■ Reduce parasympathetic stimulation or sympathetic understimulation. ■ Medications may include corticosteroids and vasoactive agents.

Clinical Manifestations and Therapies **Shock** (continued)

ETIOLOGY	CLINICAL MANIFESTATIONS	CLINICAL THERAPIES
Anaphylactic shock	■ Blood pressure: hypotension ■ Pulse: increased, dysrhythmias ■ Respirations: dyspnea, stridor, wheezes, laryngospasm, bronchospasm, pulmonary edema ■ Skin: warm, edematous (lips, eyelids, tongue, hands, feet, genitals) ■ Mental status: restless, anxious, lethargic to comatose ■ Urine output: oliguria to anuria ■ Other: paresthesias; pruritus; abdominal cramps, vomiting, diarrhea	■ Treat underlying cause. ■ Medications may include corticosteroids and albuterol to treat histamine-induced bronchospasm. ■ Remove allergen. ■ Monitor blood pressure and respirations. ■ Insertion of an artificial airway may be required to maintain a functional airway if tracheal edema occurs. ■ Administer oxygen.

Diagnostic Tests

The following diagnostic tests can help identify the type of shock and assess the client's physical status:

■ **Blood hemoglobin and hematocrit.** Changes in hemoglobin and hematocrit concentrations usually occur in hypovolemic shock. These changes reflect the underlying etiology. In hypovolemic shock resulting from hemorrhage, the hemoglobin and hematocrit concentrations are lower than normal. In hypovolemic shock resulting from intravascular fluid loss, the hemoglobin and hematocrit concentrations are higher than normal.

■ **Arterial blood gases** to determine oxygen and carbon dioxide levels and pH. The effects of shock and of the body's compensatory mechanisms cause a decrease in pH (indicating acidosis), a decrease in the PaO_2 and in total oxygen saturation, and an increase in $PaCO_2$.

■ **Serum electrolytes** to monitor the severity and progression of shock. As shock progresses, glucose levels decrease, sodium levels decrease, and potassium levels increase.

■ **Blood urea nitrogen, serum creatinine levels, urine specific gravity, and osmolality** to check renal function. As perfusion of the kidneys is decreased and renal function is reduced, the blood urea nitrogen and creatinine levels increase, as does urine specific gravity and osmolality.

■ **Blood cultures** to identify the causative organism in septic shock.

■ **White blood cell count and differential** in the client with septic or anaphylactic shock. The total white blood cell count is increased in septic shock. Elevated neutrophils indicate acute infection, increased monocytes indicate a bacterial infection, and increased eosinophils indicate an allergic response.

■ **Serum cardiac enzymes,** which are elevated in cardiogenic shock: lactate dehydrogenase, creatine phosphokinase, and serum glutamic-oxaloacetic transaminase.

■ **Central venous catheterization** to aid in the differential diagnosis of shock and provide information about the preload of

the heart. A pulmonary artery catheter may be inserted to monitor cardiac dynamics, fluid balance, and the effects of vasoactive medications.

Other diagnostic tests may be ordered to determine the extent of injury or damage or to locate the site of internal hemorrhage. These tests might include x-ray studies, CT scans, MRI, endoscopic examinations, and echocardiograms. Newer diagnostic methods for hypoperfusion include gastric tonometry and sublingual $PaCO_2$. Gastric tonometry measures $PaCO_2$ in the gastric lumen. The measurement of sublingual carbon dioxide correlates well with decreased mean arterial pressure.

Pharmacologic Therapy

When fluid replacement alone is not sufficient to reverse shock, vasoactive drugs (drugs causing vasoconstriction or vasodilation) and inotropic drugs (drugs improving cardiac contractility) may be administered. When used to treat shock, these drugs increase venous return through vasoconstriction of peripheral vessels; they also improve the pumping ability of the heart by facilitating myocardial contractility and by dilating coronary arteries to increase perfusion of the myocardium.

Drugs used to treat shock are listed in the Medications feature. Other drugs that may be administered to the client with shock include the following:

■ Diuretics to increase urine output after fluid replacement has been initiated

■ Sodium bicarbonate to treat acidosis

■ Calcium to replace calcium lost as a result of blood transfusions

■ Antidysrhythmic agents to stabilize heart rhythm

■ Broad-spectrum antibiotics to suppress organisms responsible for septic shock

■ Epinephrine, antihistamines, and inhaled beta2-agonists to treat anaphylactic shock

■ Morphine to dilate veins and decrease anxiety.

Medications **Shock**

CLASSIFICATION AND DRUG EXAMPLES	MECHANISMS OF ACTION	NURSING CONSIDERATIONS
Adrenergics (Sympathomimetics) *Vasoconstrictors* *Drug examples:* ■ norepinephrine (Levophed) ■ metaraminol (Aramine) *Inotropes* *Drug examples:* ■ dopamine (Intropin) (receptors are dose dependent) ■ dobutamine (Dobutrex) ■ isoproterenol (Isuprel)	Adrenergic drugs (also called sympathomimetics) mimic the fight-or-flight response of the SNS, selectively stimulating alpha-adrenergic and beta-adrenergic receptors. Many of these drugs have both vasopressor (vasoconstricting) effects and positive inotropic effects (**Table 16–33 ●**). Stimulation of alpha-adrenergic receptors results in vasoconstriction and increased systemic blood pressure. Stimulation of beta-adrenergic receptors increases the force and rate of myocardial contraction. The physiological effect of these drugs includes improved perfusion and oxygenation of the heart, with increased stroke volume and heart rate, and increased cardiac output. In turn, increased cardiac output increases tissue perfusion and oxygenation. The major disadvantage is that increases in stroke volume and heart rate also increase the oxygen requirements of the myocardium. These drugs may be used during the early stages of shock, especially in types of shock characterized by vasodilation.	■ Carefully monitor responses in the older adult, who may be especially sensitive to sympathomimetics and require lower doses. ■ When administering these drugs by the subcutaneous route, carefully aspirate the injection site to avoid injecting the drug directly into a blood vessel. ■ Use the intravenous route only with continuous-infusion pumps. Carefully adjust the dose to accommodate the client's cardiovascular status (as ordered by the physician or by written protocol). ■ Document lung sounds, vital signs, and hemodynamic parameters before starting the medication and then according to institutional policy (usually every 5–15 min). ■ Record and monitor urine output. Report output of less than 30 mL/hr. ■ Be aware that the sympathomimetics are incompatible with sodium bicarbonate or alkaline solutions. ■ When administering drugs that cause vasoconstriction, such as norepinephrine (Levophed) and metaraminol (Aramine), monitor the intravenous insertion site for infiltration. If infiltration does occur, stop the infusion and notify the physician immediately. (Infiltration may cause ischemia and necrosis of tissue.) *Health education for the client and family:* ■ Because these drugs mimic a physiological reaction to stress, they may cause feelings of anxiety. ■ Close monitoring to adjust the dose will be carried out by qualified nurses using written protocols. ■ Report heart palpitations or chest pain immediately.
Vasodilators *Drug example:* ■ nitroglycerin (Tridil) ■ nitroprusside (Nipride)	Drugs that cause vasodilation act directly on smooth muscle, affecting both arterioles and veins. Peripheral resistance, cardiac output, and pulmonary wedge pressure are all reduced as a result of the vasodilation. These effects decrease the oxygen need of the heart and decrease pulmonary congestion. Vasodilators are used primarily in the treatment of cardiogenic shock and may be combined with a sympathomimetic (e.g., dopamine).	■ Protect these drugs from light by wrapping the intravenous bag in the package that is provided. ■ Mix only with 5% dextrose in water. ■ Infuse with an infusion pump, and use within 4 hr of reconstitution. ■ Do not add other medications to the solution. ■ Assess mental status, blood pressure, and pulse before initiating medication. Thereafter, assess blood pressure and pulse according to institutional policy (usually every 5 min initially, then every 15 min until stable, and then every hour). ■ Monitor client for confusion, dizziness, tachycardia, dysrhythmias, hypotension, and adventitious breath sounds. If they occur, report immediately, and slow the infusion to a keep-open rate. ■ Monitor client receiving nitroprusside for signs of thiocyanate poisoning (nausea, disorientation, muscle spasms, and decreased or absent reflexes) if infusion lasts longer than 72 hr. ■ Keep client in bed with side rails up. *Health education for the client and family:* ■ It is important to stay in bed and change positions slowly to avoid dizziness. ■ The blood pressure and pulse are taken frequently to assist in adjusting the dose of medication. ■ Headache is a common side effect.

Medications Shock (continued)

CLASSIFICATION AND DRUG EXAMPLES	MECHANISMS OF ACTION	NURSING CONSIDERATIONS
Colloid Solutions (Plasma Expanders) *Drug examples:* ■ albumin 5% (Albuminar-5, Buminate 5%) ■ albumin 25% (Albuminar-25, Buminate 25%) ■ dextran 40 (Gentran 40) ■ dextran 70 (Gentran 70, Macrodex) ■ dextran 75 (Gentran 75) ■ hetastarch (Hespan [HES]) ■ plasma protein fraction (Plasmanate, Plasma-Plex, Plasmatein, Protenate)	These solutions are blood volume expanders and are used to treat hypovolemic shock caused by surgery, hemorrhage, burns, or other trauma. Albumin and plasma protein fraction are prepared from healthy blood donors. Dextran and hetastarch are synthetically prepared large molecules. The solutions promote circulatory volume and tissue perfusion by rapidly expanding plasma volume. Dextran solutions are infrequently used.	■ Before infusion begins, establish a baseline of vital signs, lung sounds, heart sounds, and (if possible) CVP and pulmonary artery wedge pressure. ■ Start administration of ordered intravenous fluids, using a large-gauge (18- or 19-gauge) infusion needle. ■ Take and record vital signs as required by institutional policy (usually every 15–60 min) and client status. ■ Take and record intake and output every 1–2 hr. ■ Monitor client for manifestations of congestive heart failure or pulmonary edema (dyspnea, cyanosis, cough, crackles, or wheezes). If these manifestations appear, stop the fluids, and notify the physician immediately. ■ Monitor client for bleeding from new sites; an increase in blood pressure may cause bleeding in severed vessels that did not bleed with decreased blood pressure. ■ Monitor client for manifestations of dehydration (dry lips; scant, dark-colored urine; loss of skin turgor). Increased intravenous fluids are usually ordered if the client becomes dehydrated. ■ Monitor client for manifestations of circulatory overload (jugular vein distention, increase in CVP, or increase in pulmonary artery wedge pressure). If these manifestations occur, slow the rate of infusion and notify the physician. ■ Monitor prothrombin time, partial thromboplastin time, and platelet counts. ■ If administering dextran or plasma protein fraction, have epinephrine and antihistamines readily available for any manifestations of a hypersensitivity reaction (fever, chills, rash, headache, wheezing, or flushing). ■ Maintain client on bed rest with side rails elevated. *Health education for the client and family:* ■ The solutions are given to replace lost serum protein, which helps maintain the volume of blood. ■ The vital signs are taken frequently to ensure the safety of the client.

Oxygen Therapy

Establishing and maintaining a patent airway and ensuring adequate oxygenation are critical nursing interventions in reversing shock. All clients with shock (even those with adequate respirations) should receive oxygen therapy (usually by mask or nasal cannula) to maintain the PaO$_2$ at greater than 80 mmHg during the first 4–6 hours of care. If a client cannot maintain the PaO$_2$ at this level with unassisted respiration, ventilatory assistance may be necessary.

Fluid Replacement Therapy

The most effective treatment for the client with hypovolemic shock is to administer intravenous fluids or blood. Fluids are also used to treat septic and neurogenic shock. However, the client with cardiogenic shock may require either fluid replacement or restriction, depending on pulmonary artery pressure.

Various fluids may be administered alone or in combination as part of fluid replacement therapy in treating shock. Whole blood or blood products increase the oxygen-carrying capacity of the blood and thus increase oxygenation of cells. Fluid replacements, such as crystalloid and colloid solutions, increase circulating blood volume and tissue perfusion. Fluid replace-

TABLE 16–33 Adrenergic Drugs Used to Treat Shock

ACTION	DRUG	RECEPTOR
Vasoconstrictors	Norepinephrine (Levophed)	A
	Metaraminol (Aramine)	A
Inotropes	Dopamine (Intropin)*	A, B1
	Dobutamine (Dobutrex)	B1
	Isoproterenol (Isuprel)	B1, B2

*Receptors are dose dependent.

ments are administered in massive amounts through two large-bore peripheral lines or through a central line.

CRYSTALLOID SOLUTIONS Crystalloid solutions contain dextrose or electrolytes dissolved in water; they are hypertonic, isotonic or hypotonic. Hypertonic solutions include 3% saline. Isotonic solutions include normal saline (0.9%), lactated Ringer's solution, and Ringer's solution. Hypotonic solutions include one-half normal saline (0.45%) and 5% dextrose in water.

Hypertonic crystalloid solutions pull fluid into the vascular space to promote excretion. Isotonic and hypotonic crystalloid solutions increase fluid volume in both the intravascular and the interstitial space. Of the total amount infused, only approximately 25% remains in the intravascular system; the remaining 75% moves into the interstitial space. Consequently, fluid volume is only minimally expanded by infusion of crystalloid solutions, and the potential for peripheral edema is increased when they are used. However, lactated Ringer's solution (an electrolyte solution) and 0.9% saline are the fluids of choice in treating hypovolemic shock, especially during the emergency phase of care while blood is being typed and crossmatched. Large amounts of these solutions may be infused rapidly, increasing blood volume and tissue perfusion.

COLLOID SOLUTIONS Colloid solutions contain substances (colloids) that should not diffuse through capillary walls. Hence, colloids tend to remain in the vascular system and increase the osmotic pressure of the serum, causing fluid to move into the vascular compartment from the interstitial space. As a result, plasma volume expands. Colloid solutions used to treat shock include 5% albumin, 25% albumin, hetastarch, plasma protein fraction, and dextran (see the Medications feature).

Colloid products reduce platelet adhesiveness and have been associated with reductions in blood coagulation. Consequently, the client's prothrombin time (PT), INR, platelet count, and aPTT should be monitored when these solutions are administered. Normal values are as follows:

PT	10–15 sec
INR	1–1.2 sec
Platelets	150,000–400,000/mm^3
aPTT	<35 sec

BLOOD AND BLOOD PRODUCTS If hypovolemic shock is caused by hemorrhage, the infusion of blood and blood products may be indicated. The goal of blood administration is to keep the hematocrit at 30%–35% and the hemoglobin level between 12.5 and 14.5 g/100 mL for adults. Available blood and blood products include fresh whole blood, stored whole blood, packed red blood cells, platelet concentrate, fresh-frozen plasma, and cryoprecipitate. Often, packed red blood cells are given to provide hemoglobin concentration and are supplemented with crystalloids to maintain an adequate circulatory volume.

▌ NURSING PROCESS

The priority of nursing care for the client with shock often requires rapid assessment and reaction to subtle symptoms in order to prevent a downward cascade of events. Anticipating the potential for shock to occur can promote rapid intervention when symptoms are caught early.

Assessment

Nursing assessments are critical in preventing shock. Identifying clients at risk and making focused assessments are essential. Although shock can occur at any age, physiological changes with aging make older adults a high-risk population. Assessments depend on the type of shock the client is experiencing:

- *Hypovolemic shock.* Clients who have undergone surgery, have sustained multiple traumatic injuries, or have been seriously burned are most likely to develop hypovolemic shock. Monitoring fluid status is essential to prevent shock and includes daily assessments of weight, fluid intake by all routes, measurable fluid loss (e.g., urine, vomitus, wound drainage, gastric drainage, and chest tube drainage), and fluid loss that must be estimated, such as fluid lost via profuse perspiration and wound drainage. Assessments for the critically ill client are ongoing and include fluid balance, hemodynamic values, and vital signs.
- *Cardiogenic shock.* Clients with left anterior wall MIs are at risk for developing cardiogenic shock. Nursing care to prevent the development of cardiogenic shock focuses on maintaining or improving myocardial oxygen supply by providing immediate pain relief, maintaining rest, and administering supplemental oxygen.
- *Neurogenic shock.* The risk of neurogenic shock is increased in clients who have spinal cord injuries and those who have received spinal anesthesia. Preventive nursing care includes maintaining immobility of the client with spinal cord trauma and elevating the head of the bed 15–20 degrees following spinal anesthesia. Elevations of more than 20 degrees, however, can potentiate headaches following spinal anesthesia and should be avoided.
- *Anaphylactic shock.* The nurse can prevent anaphylactic shock by collecting information about allergies and drug reactions during the health history, noting these allergies clearly on all documents, and placing a special armband on the client. Careful and frequent assessments during blood administration may prevent serious reactions to blood or blood products.
- *Septic shock.* Clients who are hospitalized, are debilitated, are chronically ill, or have undergone invasive procedures or tube insertions are at high risk for septic shock. Nursing care to prevent septic shock includes careful and consistent hand washing, the use of aseptic techniques for procedures (e.g., catheterizations, suctioning, changing dressings, starting and maintaining intravenous fluids or medications), and monitoring for local and systemic manifestations (e.g., white blood cell and differential counts) of infection.

Diagnosis

Different types and causes of shock will determine which nursing diagnoses are most appropriate. Priority nursing diagnoses that may be appropriate for the client with any type of shock include the following:

- *Decreased Cardiac Output*
- *Ineffective Tissue Perfusion*
- *Anxiety.*

(NANDA-I © 2012)

Planning

Goals for nursing care for the client with shock may include the following:

- The client's airway, breathing, and circulation will be maintained.
- The client's perfusion will be maintained adequately to meet the body's needs.
- The client will understand all procedures.
- The client will verbalize feelings to reduce anxiety.
- The client's cardiac workload will be reduced.

Implementation

Nurses in the emergency department and ICU participate in the resuscitation of clients in hypovolemic shock and often have guidelines or protocols for nursing actions. Assist with the client's assessment and the establishment of intravenous access. Calculate and prepare the amount of intravenous fluid needed for administration. Ensure rapid fluid administration by intravenous push or pressure bag. Monitor the client's physiological response to the fluid bolus within 5 minutes. Prepare a second and third fluid bolus. Warmed intravenous fluids are used for resuscitation, because hypothermia may interfere with the client's response to treatment.

When packed red blood cells are administered, verify that the correct blood has been obtained for the client. Change the intravenous fluid to normal saline solution to prevent clotting during blood administration. Assess the client carefully for a transfusion reaction. Monitor the client's physiological circulatory responses for improvement or deterioration in status. Notify the physician of any deterioration.

Preserve Cardiac Output

Decreased cardiac output is the primary problem for the client with shock. Although much of the care related to this diagnosis is collaborative, many independent nursing interventions are critical to the care of the client with shock. These include the following:

- Assess and monitor cardiovascular function via the following:
  a. Blood pressure
  b. Heart rate and rhythm
  c. Pulse oximetry
  d. Peripheral pulses
  e. Hemodynamic monitoring of arterial pressures, pulmonary artery pressures, and CVPs.

A baseline assessment is necessary to establish the stage of shock. If palpable peripheral pulses and audible (to ausculta-

tion) blood pressure are lost, inserting central arterial, venous, and pulmonary artery catheters is essential to establish progression of shock accurately and to evaluate the client's response to therapy.

- Measure and record the client's intake and output (total output and urinary output) hourly. A decrease in circulating blood volume with hypotension and the effect of the compensatory mechanisms associated with shock can cause renal failure. Urinary output of less than 30 mL/hr in an acutely ill adult indicates reduced renal blood flow.
- Monitor the client's bowel sounds, abdominal distention, and abdominal pain. Decreased splanchnic blood flow reduces bowel motility and peristalsis; paralytic ileus may result.
- Monitor the client for sudden, sharp chest pain and for dyspnea, cyanosis, anxiety, and restlessness. Hemoconcentration and increased platelet aggregation may result in pulmonary emboli.
- Maintain bed rest, and provide (to the extent possible) a calm, quiet environment. Place the client in a supine position with the legs elevated to approximately 20 degrees, trunk flat, and head and shoulders elevated higher than the chest (≈10 degrees) (**Figure 16–60** ●). Limiting activity and ensuring rest decrease the workload of the heart. The supine position with legs elevated increases venous return; however, this position should not be used for clients with cardiogenic shock. The Trendelenburg position is no longer recommended, because it causes the abdominal organs to press against the diaphragm (limiting respirations), decreases filling of the coronary arteries, and initiates aortic and carotid sinus reflexes.

Promote Tissue Perfusion

As shock progresses, diminished tissue perfusion causes ischemia and hypoxia of major organ systems. As shock worsens, blood flow and oxygenation of the lungs, heart, and brain are also impaired. Hypoxia and ischemia result from decreased tissue perfusion in the kidneys, brain, heart, lungs, and gastrointestinal tract and the periphery. The following nursing interventions address tissue perfusion:

- Monitor the client's skin color, temperature, turgor, and moisture. Decreased tissue perfusion is evidenced by the skin becoming pale, cool, and moist; as hemoglobin concentrations decrease, cyanosis occurs.

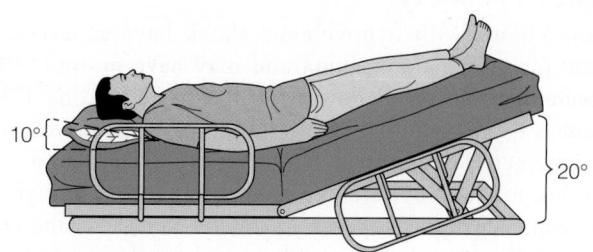

Figure 16–60 ● The client in shock should be positioned with the lower extremities elevated approximately 20 degrees (knees straight), and the head elevated about 10 degrees.

- Monitor the client's cardiopulmonary function by assessing/monitoring the following:
  a. Blood pressure (by auscultation or by hemodynamic monitoring)
  b. Rate and depth of respirations
  c. Lung sounds
  d. Pulse oximetry
  e. Peripheral pulses (brachial, radial, dorsalis pedis, and posterior tibial); include presence, equality, rate, rhythm, and quality (if unable to palpate pulses, use a device such as a Doppler ultrasound flowmeter to assess peripheral arterial blood flow)
  f. Jugular vein distention
  g. CVP measurements.

Baseline vital signs are necessary to determine trends in subsequent findings. As shock progresses, the blood pressure decreases, and the pulse becomes rapid, weak, and thready. As perfusion of the lungs decreases, crackles, wheezes, and dyspnea are commonly assessed. Capillary refill is prolonged, and peripheral pulses are weak or nonpalpable. Neck veins that cannot be seen when the client is in the supine position indicate decreased intravascular volume. CVP is an accurate means of determining fluid status in the client with shock; the findings will be low (5–15 cm H_2O or 2 to 6 mm Hg is normal) in hypovolemic shock because of the decreased blood volume.

- Monitor the client's body temperature. An elevated body temperature increases metabolic demands, depleting energy reserves. It also increases myocardial oxygen demand and may place the client with previous cardiac problems at even greater risk for hypoperfusion.
- Monitor the client's urinary output per indwelling urinary catheter hourly, using a urometer. Urine output is a reliable indicator of renal perfusion.
- Assess the client's mental status and level of consciousness. The appropriateness of the client's behavior and responses reflects the adequacy of cerebral circulation. Restlessness and anxiety are common early in shock; during later stages, the client may become lethargic and progress to a comatose state. Altered levels of consciousness are the result of both cerebral hypoxia and the effects of acidosis on brain cells.

Relieve Anxiety

Many clients with hypovolemic shock have experienced some form of major trauma and may have multiple life-threatening injuries. Following on-the-scene treatment, the client is usually admitted to the healthcare setting through the emergency department. Surgery may be required to treat injuries, followed by care in a critical care unit. Throughout this sequence of crisis events, treatment is invasive, and contact with family is minimal. Client and family responses to these situations of uncertainty, instability, and change include anxiety, fear, and powerlessness. These responses are affected by age, developmental level, cultural and ethnic group, experience with illness and the healthcare system, and support

systems. The nurse can help to relieve the client's anxiety by doing the following:

- Assess the cause(s) of the anxiety, and manipulate the environment to provide periods of rest. Reducing stimuli that cause anxiety is calming and facilitates rest, which is necessary for the client at risk for bleeding.
- Administer prescribed pain medications on a regular basis. Pain precipitates and/or aggravates anxiety.
- Provide interventions to increase the client's comfort and reduce restlessness:
  a. Maintain a clean environment.
  b. Provide skin and oral care.
  c. Monitor the effectiveness of ventilation or oxygen therapy.
  d. Eliminate all nonessential activities.
  e. Remain with the client during procedures.
  f. Speak slowly and calmly, using short sentences.
  g. Use touch to provide support.

Unfamiliar sounds, sights, and odors can increase anxiety. Damp skin or a dry mouth increases discomfort. Inadequate gas exchange with a decrease in oxygen or an increase in carbon dioxide in the blood may cause the client to experience a "feeling of doom." Activity increases the body's need for oxygen. Listening and touch provide support in an environment in which the client often feels alone and abandoned. Severe anxiety interferes with the ability to understand others and to respond appropriately.

- Provide support for the client and family:
  a. Provide time, space, and privacy for family members.
  b. Allow family members access to the client when feasible.
  c. Encourage the client to express feelings and concerns. Provide anticipatory guidance to prepare for recovery or death and to support realistic hope.
  d. Acknowledge the beliefs, values, and expectations of the client and family.

Allowing the family access to the client reduces anxiety and gives both the client and the family some feeling of control. If the client's prognosis is poor, access and involvement allow the family to begin the grieving process. If recovery is expected, contact provides the client and family with a feeling of hope. Supporting the client and family facilitates concrete problem solving, promotes acceptance of the illness and its implications, and helps them begin to establish ways of managing the illness experience.

- Provide information about the current setting to both the client and family; give the family information about available resources (e.g., pastoral care, social services, temporary housing, and meals). Knowing what to expect and how to control the environment to meet basic needs reduces anxiety.

Evaluation

Examples of expected nursing care outcomes include the following:

- The client does not progress to uncompensated shock
- The family copes with the stress of the client's injury.

NURSING CARE PLAN A Client With Septic Shock

ASSESSMENT

Huang Mei Lan is a 43-year-old, unmarried female who lives alone in a major West Coast city. Ms. Huang came to America 15 years ago from China; she speaks English well. Her family still lives in China. She worked in a neighborhood sewing shop until 3 years ago, when she was diagnosed with breast cancer. Her treatment included mastectomy of the affected breast and follow-up chemotherapy.

Last month, Ms. Huang experienced a recurrence of cancer in the liver. Surgery to remove the tumor and a lobe of the liver was performed and chemotherapy is planned. Ms. Huang has a central line, a urinary catheter, and a midline abdominal surgical incision. She is underweight, weak, and depressed.

Ms. Huang's primary nurse enters her room early in the morning to make an initial assessment and finds Ms. Huang huddled in the middle of the bed. Ms. Huang reports that she feels cold. The nurse finds Ms. Huang's dressing saturated with bright red blood. She rolls Ms. Huang onto her side and finds the bed filled with blood. The nurse measures the size of the blood stain and records it (18 × 38 inches). Her vital signs are T_O 99.2°F; P 110 bpm; R 30/min; BP 106/66 mmHg. Her pulse is weak and regular. Her skin is cool, dry, and pale with poor turgor. She is alert and oriented but restless and appears anxious. Ms. Huang states she is nauseated and suddenly begins vomiting and is incontinent of liquid stool. Laboratory data indicate leukocytosis, respiratory alkalosis, and reduced red blood cell, hemoglobin, and hematocrit.

Plasma expanders in the form of albumin are administered while a type and crossmatch for four units of blood can be performed. The IV fluid rate is increased and the client's vital signs are monitored. Ms. Huang is taken back to surgery to repair the source of the bleeding and loses an additional 2 pints of blood. She receives three units of blood in the operative suite and returns to the unit with the fourth unit running. The physician's orders indicate dopamine is to be started if her blood pressure falls below 90/60 mmHg following administration of the fourth unit of blood. Despite treatment, Ms. Huang's condition worsens. Her blood pressure continues to drop, her skin becomes cool and cyanotic, and she begins to have periods of disorientation. She is transferred to the critical care unit. As she is being prepared for the transfer, she begins to cry and asks, "Am I going to die?"

DIAGNOSES

- *Deficient Fluid Volume* related to bleeding, vomiting, diarrhea, and shift of intravascular volume to interstitial spaces
- *Ineffective Breathing Pattern* related to rapid respirations and progression of hypovolemic shock
- *Ineffective Tissue Perfusion* related to progression of hypovolemic shock with decreased cardiac output, hypotension, and massive vasodilation
- *Anxiety* related to hypoxia, serious health status, and transfer to critical care unit

(NANDA-I © 2012)

PLANNING

Goals of care include the following:

- Maintain adequate oxygenation.
- Maintain adequate circulating blood volume.
- Promote breathing to maintain acid–base within acceptable parameters.
- Promote stable hemodynamic status.
- Assist client to verbalize increased ability to cope with stressors.

IMPLEMENTATION

- Continuously monitor oxygenation status to include pulse oximetry, skin color, and breathing pattern.
- Monitor neurological status, including mental status and level of consciousness.
- Continuously monitor cardiovascular status, including arterial blood pressure; rate, rhythm, and quality of pulses; central venous pressure; pulmonary artery pressure; and cardiac output.
- Monitor color and character of skin, wound dressing for further bleeding.

- Monitor results of arterial blood gases, blood counts, clotting times, and platelet counts.
- Monitor respiratory status, including respiratory rate, rhythm, and breath sounds.
- Monitor urinary output hourly, reporting any output of less than 30 mL/hr.
- Administer blood and IV fluids as ordered.
- Explain procedures, and provide comfort measures (e.g., oral care, skin care, turning, and positioning).

EVALUATION

After administration of the fourth unit of blood, Ms. Huang's blood pressure has stabilized above the defined parameters. Her urine output is less than 30 mL/hr for 3 hours, and fluid administration is increased until her urine output improves and hemodynamic status stabilizes. She remains in the critical care area for 2 days and is then transferred back to the oncology unit.

CRITICAL THINKING

1. Vasopressors may be used in the treatment of shock. Explain the rationale for their use.
2. While monitoring Ms. Huang's arterial blood gases, the nurse notes that her PaO_2 is less than 60 mmHg and her $PaCO_2$ is greater than 50 mmHg. What do these findings indicate, and why have they occurred?
3. Ms. Huang has been given large amounts of colloids intravenously. Hemodynamic monitoring indicates higher-than-normal central venous pressure and pulmonary artery pressure. What do these findings indicate? What physical assessments would you make to confirm the changes?

▌ REVIEW **Shock**

RELATE Link the Concepts and Exemplars

Linking the exemplar of shock with the concept of spirituality:

1. You are caring for a pediatric client in hypovolemic shock following a bicycle crash. The family members refuse blood, explaining that it is against their religious beliefs. How will you respond?

2. What options for treatment might be considered for this child that do not conflict with the family's religious beliefs?

Linking the exemplar of shock with the concept of fluids and electrolytes:

3. Contrast the administration of IV fluids for the client in hypovolemic shock versus the client in cardiogenic shock.

4. Contrast the administration of colloids versus crystalloids in treating the client with hypovolemic shock.

READY Go to Companion Skills Manual

REFER Go to Pearson Nursing Student Resources
nursing.pearsonhighered.com

- Additional review materials

REFLECT Case Study

Stacie Horton is a 15-year-old client who required a heart transplant 5 years ago to repair damage done by a viral illness. She is compliant with her medication regimen and adheres to the prescribed diet. She lives with her parents and her older brother. While she appreciates the watchfulness of her parents, Stacie sometimes wishes that her family wouldn't hover over her as much as they do. Stacie is captain of the cheerleading squad at her school where she is also an honor student.

Stacie is in class and begins to feel faint and nauseated. Her skin is cold and clammy, and her color is slightly cyanotic. Her respirations are 30 breaths per minute and her pulse is weak and thready at a rate of 124 bpm. Knowing her history, the teacher alerts the school nurse who immediately calls 911 and Stacie's family.

1. What interventions will you initiate for Stacie until the paramedics arrive?

2. If you were the nurse admitting Stacie in the emergency department what would your priority assessment include?

3. When Stacie's parents arrive, what family teaching will you initiate?

▌ EXEMPLAR 16.13 **Stroke**

EXEMPLAR KEY TERMS

Agnosia, *1237*
Aneurysm, *1236*
Aphasia, *1238*
Apraxia, *1237*
Contralateral deficit, *1235*
Dysphagia, *1245*
Flaccidity, *1239*
Hemianopia, *1237*
Hemiparesis, *1239*
Hemiplegia, *1239*
Neglect syndrome, *1237*
Penumbra, *1235*
Proprioception, *1237*
Spasticity, *1239*
Stroke, *1234*
Transient ischemic attack (TIA), *1235*

EXEMPLAR LEARNING OUTCOMES

After reading about this exemplar, you will be able to:

1. Describe the pathophysiology, etiology, clinical manifestations, and direct and indirect causes of stroke.

2. Identify risk factors and prevention methods associated with stroke.

3. Illustrate the nursing process in providing culturally competent care across the life span for individuals with stroke.

4. Formulate priority nursing diagnoses appropriate for an individual with stroke.

5. Summarize therapies used by interdisciplinary teams in the collaborative care of an individual with stroke.

6. Plan evidence-based care for an individual with stroke and his or her family in collaboration with other members of the healthcare team.

7. Evaluate expected outcomes for an individual with stroke.

▶ OVERVIEW

A **stroke** (also known as a cerebrovascular accident or brain attack) is a condition in which neurological deficits result from a sudden decrease in blood flow to a localized area of the brain. Strokes may be ischemic, occurring when the blood supply to a part of the brain is suddenly interrupted by a thrombus (blood clot), embolus (foreign matter traveling through the circulation), or stenosis (narrowing); or may be hemorrhagic, occurring when a blood vessel breaks open, spilling blood into spaces surrounding neurons. The neurological deficits caused by ischemia and the resultant necrosis of cells in the brain vary according to the area of the brain involved, the size of the affected area, and the length of time blood flow is decreased or stopped. A major loss of blood supply to the brain can cause severe disabil-

ity or death. When the duration of decreased blood flow is short and the anatomical area involved is small, the individual may not be aware that damage has been done.

On average, someone in the United States has a stroke every 40 seconds and someone dies of a stroke every 4 minutes. Stroke is the fourth leading cause of death and disability in North America, where approximately 795,000 individuals suffer a new or recurrent stroke each year. Of those, 160,000 die, and many who survive are left with some type of functional impairment. Although strokes occur in every age group, the highest incidence occurs in individuals over 65 years of age; 28% of strokes occur in individuals under the age of 65. Strokes occur more frequently in men than women, although the risk of stroke may be greater in women during pregnancy and for the 6 weeks following birth (American Stroke Association, 2012).

▶ PATHOPHYSIOLOGY AND ETIOLOGY

The brain, which makes up only 2% of total body weight, receives approximately 20% of the cardiac output each minute ($\approx$750 mL) and accounts for 20% of the body's oxygen consumption. Cerebral blood flow, especially in the deep cerebral vessels, is largely self-regulated by the brain to meet metabolic needs. This self-regulation (also called autoregulation) allows the brain to maintain a constant blood flow despite changes in systemic blood pressure. However, autoregulation is not effective when systemic blood pressure falls below 50 mmHg or rises above 160 mmHg. In the latter case, the increased systemic pressure (as in hypertension) causes an increase in cerebral blood flow with resultant overdistention of cerebral vessels. Cerebral blood flow also increases in response to increased carbon dioxide concentrations, increased hydrogen ion concentrations, and decreased oxygen concentrations.

When blood flow to cerebral neurons and their oxygenation are decreased or interrupted, pathophysiological changes at the cellular level take place in 4–5 minutes. Cellular metabolism ceases as glucose, glycogen, and adenosine triphosphate are depleted and the sodium–potassium pump fails. Cells swell as sodium draws water into the cell. Cerebral blood vessel walls also swell, further decreasing blood flow. Even if circulation is restored, vasospasm and increased blood viscosity can continue to impede blood flow. Severe or prolonged ischemia leads to cellular death. A central core of dead or dying cells is surrounded by a band of minimally perfused cells, called the **penumbra**. Although cells in the penumbra have impaired metabolic activities, their structural integrity is maintained. The survival of these cells depends on a timely return of adequate circulation, the volume of toxic products released by adjacent dying cells, the degree of cerebral edema, and alterations in local blood flow. The potential survival of cells in the penumbra has led to the use of fibrinolytic agents in the early treatment of ischemic stroke (Porth, 2010).

The neurological deficits that occur as a result of a stroke can often be used to identify its location. Because the motor pathways cross at the junction of the medulla and spinal cord (decussation), strokes lead to loss or impairment of sensorimotor functions on the side of the body opposite the side of the brain that is damaged. Because of this effect, known as a **contralateral deficit**, a stroke in the right hemisphere of the brain is manifested by deficits in the left side of the body, and a stroke in the left hemisphere is manifested by deficits in the right side.

A stroke is characterized by a gradual or rapid onset of neurological deficits caused by compromised cerebral blood flow. Strokes may result from a variety of problems, including cerebral thrombosis, cerebral embolism, and cerebral hemorrhage.

Ischemic Strokes

Ischemic strokes result from blockage and/or stenosis of a cerebral artery, decreasing or stopping blood flow and ultimately causing a brain infarction. The blockage may result from a blood clot (either as a thrombus or an emboli) or from stenosis of a vessel caused by a buildup of plaque. Plaque may cause stenosis in large blood vessels (called large vessel disease) or small blood vessels (called small vessel disease). Large vessel disease usually is the result of thrombi. Small vessel strokes, called lacunar infarcts, are small to very small infarcts in the deep, noncortical areas of the brain or the brainstem. Ischemic strokes are classified as transient, thrombotic, or embolic.

TRANSIENT ISCHEMIC ATTACK   A **transient ischemic attack (TIA)**, sometimes called a mini-stroke, is a brief period of localized cerebral ischemia that causes neurological deficits lasting for less than 24 hours (Hickey, 2013). The deficits may be present for only minutes or may last for hours. TIAs are often warning signals of an ischemic thrombotic stroke. One or many TIAs may precede a stroke, with the time between the TIA and a stroke ranging from hours to months. Of the 50,000 Americans who have a TIA each year, approximately one third will have an acute stroke some time in the future (National Institute of Neurological Disorders and Stroke, 2013).

The etiology of TIA includes inflammatory artery disorders, sickle cell disease, atherosclerotic changes in cerebral blood vessels, thrombosis, and emboli. Neurological manifestations of a TIA vary according to the location and size of the cerebral vessel involved. Manifestations have a sudden onset and often disappear within minutes or hours. Commonly occurring deficits include contralateral numbness or weakness of the leg, hand, forearm, and corner of the mouth (because of middle cerebral artery involvement); aphasia (because of ischemia of the left hemisphere); and visual disturbances, such as blurring (because of involvement of the posterior cerebral artery) (Porth, 2010). The client may also experience a visual disturbance called amaurosis fugax (a fleeting blindness of one eye, described as a shade coming down over vision with the affected eye).

THROMBOTIC STROKE   A thrombotic stroke is caused by occlusion of a large cerebral vessel by a thrombus (blood clot). Thrombotic strokes most often occur in older individuals who are resting or sleeping. The blood pressure is lower during sleep, so there is less pressure to push the blood through an already narrowed arterial lumen, and ischemia may result.

Thrombi tend to form in large arteries that bifurcate and have narrowed lumens as a result of deposits of atherosclerotic plaque. The plaque involves the intima of the arteries, causing the internal elastic lamina to become thin and frayed with exposure of underlying connective tissue. This structural change causes platelets to adhere to the rough surface and release the enzyme adenosine diphosphate. This enzyme initiates the clotting sequence, and the thrombus forms. A thrombus may remain in place and continue to enlarge, completely occluding the lumen of the vessel, or a part of it may break off and become an embolus.

The most common locations of thrombi are the internal carotid artery, the vertebral arteries, and the junction of the vertebral and basilar arteries. Thrombotic strokes affecting the smaller cerebral vessels are called lacunar strokes, because the infarcted areas slough off, leaving a small cavity or "lake" in the brain tissue. A thrombotic stroke usually affects only one region of the brain, supplied by a single cerebral artery.

A thrombotic stroke occurs rapidly but progresses slowly. It often begins with a TIA and continues to worsen over 1–2 days; the condition is called a stroke-in-evolution. When maximum neurological deficit has been reached, usually in 3 days, the condition is called a completed stroke. At that time, the damaged area of brain tissue is edematous and necrotic.

EMBOLIC STROKE An embolic stroke occurs when a blood clot or clump of matter traveling through the cerebral blood vessels becomes lodged in a vessel that is too narrow to permit further movement. The area of the brain supplied by the blocked vessel becomes ischemic. The most frequent sites of cerebral emboli are at bifurcations of vessels, particularly those of the carotid and middle cerebral arteries. This type of stroke is typically seen in clients who are younger than those experiencing thrombotic strokes, and it occurs when the client is awake and active.

Many embolic strokes originate from a thrombus in the left chambers of the heart, formed during atrial fibrillation. These are referred to as cardiogenic embolic strokes. Emboli result when parts of the thrombus break off and are carried through the arterial system to the brain. Cerebral emboli may also be the result of carotid artery atherosclerotic plaque, bacterial endocarditis, recent MI, rheumatic heart disease, and ventricular aneurysm.

An embolic stroke has a sudden onset and causes immediate deficits. If the embolus breaks up into smaller fragments and is absorbed by the body, manifestations will disappear in a few hours to a few days. If the embolus is not absorbed, manifestations will persist. Even if the embolus is absorbed, the vessel wall where the embolus lodges may be weakened, increasing the potential for cerebral hemorrhage.

Hemorrhagic Stroke

A hemorrhagic stroke, or intracranial hemorrhage, occurs when a cerebral blood vessel ruptures. It occurs most often in individuals with a sustained increase in systolic–diastolic blood pressure. It can also occur due to an **aneurysm** (a bulging weak area in the wall of an artery that supplies blood to the brain) that ruptures, releasing blood into the brain. There are two types of hemorrhagic strokes: intracerebral hemorrhage and subarachnoid hemorrhage. Intracerebral hemorrhage results from bleeding within the brain and subarachnoid hemorrhage results from bleeding into the spaces around the brain. As a result of the blood vessel rupture, blood enters the brain tissue, the cerebral ventricles, or the subarachnoid space, compressing adjacent tissues and causing blood vessel spasm and cerebral edema. Blood in the ventricles or subarachnoid space irritates the meninges and brain tissue, causing an inflammatory reaction and impairing absorption and circulation of cerebrospinal fluid (CSF).

A hemorrhagic stroke usually occurs suddenly, often when the affected individual is engaged in some activity. Although hypertension is the most common cause, a variety of factors may contribute to a hemorrhagic stroke, including rupture of a brittle, plaque-encrusted artery wall; a ruptured intracranial aneurysm; trauma; erosion of blood vessels by tumors; arteriovenous malformations; anticoagulant therapy; and blood disorders. Hemorrhagic stroke is most commonly linked with poor outcomes.

The onset of manifestations from a hemorrhagic stroke is rapid. Manifestations depend on the location of the hemorrhage but may include vomiting, headache, seizures, hemiplegia, and loss of consciousness. Pressure on the brain tissue from increased intracranial pressure may cause coma and death.

Risk Factors

Specific stroke risk factors include the following:

- *Hypertension.* Hypertension is the leading cause of stroke (AHA, 2013f). Increased systolic and diastolic blood pressure is associated with damage to all blood vessels, including the cerebral vessels. Individuals with hypertension have a four to six times greater risk for stroke than do those without hypertension.
- *Heart disease.* Atrial fibrillation increases the risk for stroke. The heart's upper chambers do not beat effectively, which can lead to pooling or clotting of the blood. If a clot dislodges into the bloodstream and travels to the brain, a stroke can occur. Heart failure, dilated cardiomyopathy, heart valve disease, and some types of congenital heart defects increase the risk of stroke.
- *Diabetes mellitus.* Diabetes leads to vascular changes in both the systemic and cerebral circulation. Clients with diabetes often have high blood pressure and high blood cholesterol and are overweight, all of which raise the risk for stroke.
- *Sleep apnea.* Considered a major risk for stroke, sleep apnea increases blood pressure and causes decreased oxygen and increased carbon dioxide in the blood.
- *Blood cholesterol levels.* Increased blood cholesterol levels contribute to the risk of atherosclerosis, including in arteries in the cerebral circulation.
- *Smoking.* Cigarette smoking doubles an individual's risk for ischemic stroke and increases the risk for cerebral hemorrhage. The use of oral contraceptives combined with smoking greatly increases the risk for stroke.
- *Sickle cell disease.* Changes in the shape of the red blood cells increase blood viscosity and produce erythrocyte clumps that may occlude small cerebral vessels.
- *Substance abuse.* The injection of unpurified substances increases the risk for a stroke, and abuse of certain drugs can decrease cerebral blood flow and increase the risk for intracranial hemorrhage. Substances associated with strokes include marijuana, anabolic steroids, heroin, amphetamines, and cocaine.

Focus on Diversity and Culture
Risk Factors for Stroke Among African Americans and Hispanics

African Americans
- African Americans have almost twice the number of first-ever strokes compared to Whites.
- The prevalence of hypertension in African Americans is the highest in the world.
- African Americans are more likely to die following a stroke than Whites (CDC, 2013f).

Hispanics
- Hispanic Americans have an increased incidence of intracerebral hemorrhage, subarachnoid hemorrhage, ischemic stroke, transient ischemic attack, and transient ischemic attack at a younger age when compared to non-Hispanic Whites.
- As a result of language barriers and lack of transportation, Hispanics are more likely to delay or drop out of care.

Source: Centers for Disease Control and Prevention. (2013d). *Stroke facts.* Retrieved from http://www.cdc.gov/stroke/facts.htm.

■ *Living in the stroke belt.* Individuals living in the southeastern United States have the highest stroke mortality rate in the country. The reason for this has not been identified.

Other risk factors include a family history of stroke, obesity, a sedentary lifestyle, recent viral and bacterial infections, and previous TIAs. Risk factors specific to women are oral contraceptive use, pregnancy, childbirth, menopause, migraine headaches with aura, autoimmune disorders (e.g., diabetes and lupus), and clotting disorders. Some risk factors specific to ethnic groups are listed in the Focus on Diversity and Culture feature.

Within 5 years of the first stroke, the risk for a recurrent stroke can increase more than 40% (National Stroke Association, 2013a). The risk is highest immediately after a stroke, then decreases with time.

▶ CLINICAL MANIFESTATIONS

Manifestations of a stroke vary according to the cerebral artery involved and the area of the brain affected. Women with stroke are more likely to report nontraditional manifestations (disorientation, confusion, or loss of consciousness) than men. Manifestations are always sudden in onset and focal and are usually one sided. The most common manifestation is weakness involving the face and arm and sometimes the leg. Other common manifestations are numbness on one side, loss of vision, speech difficulties, a sudden severe headache, and difficulties with balance. The various deficits associated with involvement of a specific cerebral artery are collectively referred to as stroke syndromes, although the deficits often overlap, as shown in **Box 16–28 ●**. Specific manifestations of stroke are discussed in the subsections under Pathophysiology and Etiology.

Complications

Typical complications of a stroke include sensory–perceptual deficits, cognitive and behavioral changes, communication disorders, motor deficits, and elimination disorders. These may be transient or permanent, depending on the degree of ischemia and necrosis as well as time of treatment. As a result of the neurological deficits, the client with a stroke may have complications that involve many different body systems. The disabilities resulting from a stroke often cause serious alterations in the client's functional health status (**Box 16–29 ●**).

SENSORY–PERCEPTUAL DEFICITS   A stroke may involve pathological changes in neurological pathways that alter the ability to integrate, interpret, and attend to sensory data. The client may experience deficits in vision, hearing, equilibrium, taste, and sense of smell. The ability to perceive vibration, pain, warmth, cold, and pressure may be impaired, as may **proprioception** (the body's sense of its position). The loss of these sensory abilities increases the risk for injury.

Sensory–perceptual deficits may include the following:

■ **Hemianopia** is the loss of half of the visual field of one or both eyes. When the same half is missing in each eye, the condition is called homonymous hemianopia (**Figure 16–61 ●**).

■ **Agnosia** is the inability to recognize one or more subjects that were previously familiar; agnosia may be visual, tactile, or auditory.

Box 16–28   Manifestations of a Stroke by Involved Cerebral Vessel

INTERNAL CAROTID ARTERY
■ Contralateral paralysis of the arm, leg, and face
■ Contralateral sensory deficits of the arm, leg, and face
■ If the dominant hemisphere is involved: aphasia
■ If the nondominant hemisphere is involved: apraxia, agnosia, unilateral neglect
■ Homonymous hemianopia

MIDDLE CEREBRAL ARTERY
■ Drowsiness, stupor, coma
■ Contralateral hemiplegia of the arm and face
■ Contralateral sensory deficits of the arm and face
■ Global aphasia (if the dominant hemisphere is involved)
■ Homonymous hemianopia

ANTERIOR CEREBRAL ARTERY
■ Contralateral weakness or paralysis of the foot and leg
■ Contralateral sensory loss of the toes, foot, and leg
■ Loss of ability to make decisions or act voluntarily
■ Urinary incontinence

VERTEBRAL ARTERY
■ Pain in the face, nose, or eye
■ Numbness and weakness of the face on the involved side
■ Problems with gait
■ Dysphagia

■ **Apraxia** is the inability to carry out some motor pattern (e.g., drawing a figure or getting dressed) even when strength and coordination are adequate.

Another form of sensory–perceptual deficit is the **neglect syndrome** (or unilateral neglect), in which the client has a disorder of attention. In this syndrome, the individual cannot integrate and use perceptions from the affected side of the body or from the environment on the affected side and therefore ignores that part. In severe cases, the client may even deny the paralysis. This deficit is more common following a stroke of the right hemisphere, where damage to the parietal lobe (a center for mediation of directed attention) results in perceptual deficits.

Pain and discomfort may accompany a stroke, with the client experiencing acute pain, numbness, or strange sensations. Although not common, damage to the thalamus may cause central stroke pain or central pain syndrome. The pain in this syndrome includes hot and cold, burning, tingling, and sharp, stabbing pain, most often in the extremities. It is worsened by movement and temperature changes. The painful sensations are not relieved by pain medications, nor are there any specific treatments.

COGNITIVE AND BEHAVIORAL CHANGES   A change in consciousness, ranging from mild confusion to coma, is a common manifestation of a stroke. This change may result from tissue damage following ischemia or hemorrhage involving either the carotid or vertebral arteries. Altered consciousness may also be the result of cerebral edema or increased intracranial pressure.

Behavioral changes include emotional lability (in which the client may laugh or cry inappropriately), loss of self-control (manifested by behavior such as swearing or refusing to wear clothing), and decreased tolerance for stress (resulting in anger or depression). Intellectual changes may include memory loss,

Box 16–29   Complications of Stroke

INTEGUMENT
- Decubitus (pressure) ulcers

NEUROLOGICAL
- Hyperthermia
- Neglect syndrome
- Seizures
- Agnosias
- Communication deficits:
  - a. Expressive aphasia
  - b. Receptive aphasia
  - c. Global aphasia
  - d. Agraphia
- Visual deficits:
  - a. Homonymous hemianopia
  - b. Diplopia
  - c. Decreased acuity
- Cognitive changes:
  - a. Memory loss
  - b. Short attention span
  - c. Distractibility
  - d. Poor judgment
  - e. Poor problem-solving ability
  - f. Disorientation
- Behavioral changes:
  - a. Emotional lability
  - b. Loss of social inhibitions
  - c. Fear
  - d. Hostility
  - e. Anger
  - f. Depression
- Increased intracranial pressure
- Alterations in consciousness
- Sensory loss (touch, pain, heat, cold, pressure)

RESPIRATORY
- Respiratory center damage
- Airway obstruction
- Decreased ability to cough

GASTROINTESTINAL
- Dysphagia
- Constipation
- Stool impaction

GENITOURINARY
- Incontinence
- Frequency
- Urgency
- Urinary retention
- Renal calculi

MUSCULOSKELETAL
- Hemiplegia
- Contractures
- Bony ankylosis
- Disuse atrophy
- Dysarthria

decreased attention span, poor judgment, and an inability to think abstractly.

COMMUNICATION DISORDERS   Communication is a complex process involving motor functions, speech, language, memory, reasoning, and emotions. Communication disorders are usually the result of a stroke affecting the dominant hemi-

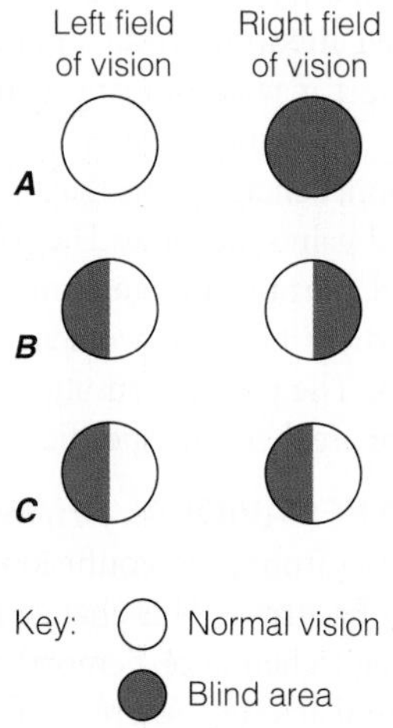

Figure 16–61 ● Abnormal visual fields. *A,* Normal left field of vision with loss of vision in right field. *B,* Loss of vision in temporal half of both fields (bitemporal hemianopia). *C,* Loss of vision in nasal field of right eye and temporal field of left eye (homonymous hemianopia).

sphere. The left hemisphere is dominant in approximately 95% of individuals who are right-handed and 70% of individuals who are left-handed (Huether & McCance, 2011).

Many different impairments may occur, and most are partial. Disorders of communication affect both speech (the mechanical act of articulating language through the spoken word) and language (the vocal or written formulation of ideas to communicate thoughts and feelings). Language involves oral and written expression as well as auditory and reading comprehension. Among these disorders are the following:

- **Aphasia.** The inability to use or understand language; aphasia may be expressive, receptive, or mixed (global):
  - *Expressive aphasia.* A motor speech problem in which one can understand what is being said but can respond verbally only in short phrases; also called Broca aphasia.
  - *Receptive aphasia.* A sensory speech problem in which one cannot understand the spoken (and often written) word. Speech may be fluent but with inappropriate content; also called Wernicke aphasia.
  - *Mixed or global aphasia.* Language dysfunction in both understanding and expression.
- *Dysarthria.* Any disturbance in muscular control of speech.

MOTOR DEFICITS   Body movement results from a complex interaction between the brain, spinal cord, and peripheral nerves. The motor areas of the cerebral cortex, the basal ganglia, and the cerebellum initiate voluntary movement by sending messages to the spinal cord, which then transmits the

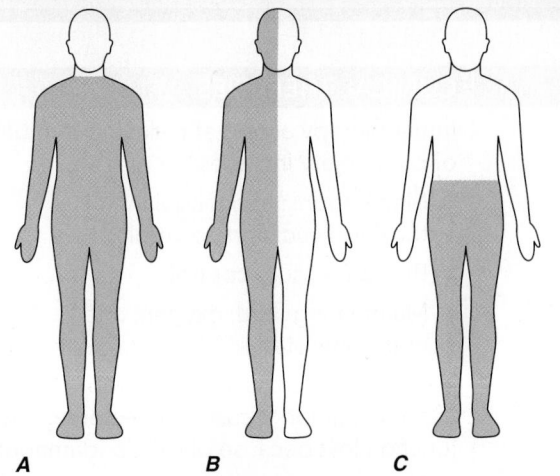

Figure 16–62 ● Types of paralysis. *A,* Quadriplegia is complete or partial paralysis of the upper extremities and complete paralysis of the lower part of the body. *B,* Hemiplegia is paralysis of one-half of the body when it is divided along the median sagittal plane. *C,* Paraplegia is paralysis of the lower part of the body.

messages to the peripheral nerves. A stroke may interrupt the central nervous system component of this relay system and produce effects in the contralateral side ranging from mild weakness to severe limitation of any kind of movement.

Depending on the area of the brain involved, a stroke may cause weakness, paralysis, and/or spasticity. Specific motor deficits include the following:

■ **Hemiplegia:** paralysis of the left or right half of the body (Figure 16–62 ●)
■ **Hemiparesis:** weakness of the left or right half of the body
■ **Flaccidity:** absence of muscle tone (hypotonia)
■ **Spasticity:** increased muscle tone (hypertonia), usually with some degree of weakness. The flexor muscles are usually more strongly affected in the upper extremities, and the extensor muscles are more strongly affected in the lower extremities.

When the corticospinal tract is involved, the affected arm and leg almost always are initially flaccid and then become spastic within 6–8 weeks. Spasticity often causes characteristic body positioning: adduction of the shoulder, pronation of the forearm, flexion of the fingers, and extension of the hip and knee. There is often foot drop, outward rotation of the leg, and dependent edema in the involved extremities.

The motor deficits may result in altered mobility, further impairing body function. The complications of immobility involve multiple body systems and include orthostatic hypotension, increased thrombus formation, decreased cardiac output, impaired respiratory function, osteoporosis, formation of renal calculi, contractures, and decubitus ulcer formation.

ELIMINATION DISORDERS Disorders of bladder and bowel elimination are common. A stroke may cause partial loss of the sensations that trigger bladder elimination, resulting in urinary frequency, urgency, or incontinence. Control of urination and changes in bowel habits may be altered as a result of cognitive deficits, immobility, and dehydration.

▶ COLLABORATION

The type of treatment a client with a stroke receives depends on the stage of the disease. In general, there are three treatment stages:

1. Stroke prevention
2. Acute care immediately after a stroke
3. Rehabilitation after a stroke.

The client with an acute stroke may receive medical and/or surgical treatment. The focus in the acute care phase is on diagnosing the type and cause of the stroke, supporting cerebral circulation, and controlling or preventing further deficits. The goals of stroke care, defined by the AHA (2013g), are to minimize brain injury and maximize client recovery by the following:

■ Rapid recognition and reaction to stroke warning signs
■ Rapid emergency medical services (EMS) dispatch
■ Rapid EMS system transport and hospital prenotification
■ Rapid diagnosis and treatment in the hospital. (The focus of care has shifted from the nearest hospital to certified stroke centers if available where clients with a stroke can be provided appropriate care from entrance to the emergency department to discharge following rehabilitation.)

Diagnostic Tests

Diagnosis begins with a complete history and careful physical assessment, including a thorough neurological examination. The time of the onset of stroke manifestations is a critical part of assessment. The National Institutes of Health Stroke Scale is a clinical evaluation tool widely used to assess neurological outcome and degree of recovery. Part of the scale is illustrated in **Table 16–34 ●**. The tool measures level of consciousness, vision, facial paralysis, motor abilities, ataxia, sensation, language, and attention.

Imaging tests are used to identify an increased risk for a stroke or to identify pathophysiological changes after a stroke has occurred. CT is the first imaging technique used to demonstrate the presence of hemorrhage, tumors, aneurysm, ischemia, edema, and tissue necrosis. A CT scan can also demonstrate a shift in intracranial contents and is useful in distinguishing the type of stroke (e.g., a hemorrhagic stroke results in an increase in density). Cerebral infarctions usually are visible with a CT scan 6–8 hours poststroke; hemorrhage is visible immediately. Other imaging tests that may be used for diagnosis include cerebral arteriography, transcranial Doppler ultrasound, MRI, magnetic resonance angiography, positron emission tomography, and single photon emission CT. A perfusion- and diffusion-weighted imaging (DWI) test can be used to identify cerebral ischemia immediately after onset of the stroke and also identify areas of possible reversible damage (the penubra).

In addition to imaging tests, a blood test has recently been approved to screen for recurrent stroke risk. The PLAC test scans the blood for high levels of lipoprotein-associated phospholipase A_2, which is more common in individuals who have had strokes. A lumbar puncture may be performed to obtain CSF for examination if there is no danger of increased intracranial pressure. (Removal of CSF when intracranial pressure is increased can result in herniation of the brainstem.) A thrombotic stroke may elevate CSF pressure; after a hemorrhagic stroke, frank blood may be seen in the CSF.

Clinical Manifestations and Therapies Stroke

ETIOLOGY	CLINICAL MANIFESTATIONS	CLINICAL THERAPIES
Damage to neurons, depending on number and location, often results in loss of sensory and/or motor function.	■ Hemiplegia, hemiparesis ■ Flaccidity ■ Paresthesias ■ Spasticity, weakness, paralysis	Initial therapy aimed at reducing amount of brain injury includes: ■ Medications: anticoagulant, thrombolytic, corticosteroids ■ Blood pressure control ■ Maintaining fluid, oxygen, and nutritional status. Following the initial insult, therapy is aimed at rehabilitation focused on restoring any function lost because of cellular damage: ■ Physical therapy ■ Occupational therapy ■ Home health assessment.
Alterations in ability to communicate often results if the cellular damage occurs on the dominant side of the brain.	■ Aphasia (expressive aphasia, receptive aphasia, mixed or global aphasia) ■ Dysarthria	Develop alternate means of communicating: ■ Use of hand signals ■ Speech therapy ■ Allow client time to express thoughts.
Sensory–perceptual deficits may occur if the neurological pathways are involved.	■ Vision, hearing, equilibrium, taste, or sense of smell deficits ■ Ability to perceive vibration, pain, warmth, cold, and pressure ■ Altered proprioception ■ Hemianopia, agnosia, apraxia, neglect syndrome	■ Provide reassurance and support. ■ Provide physical and occupational therapy when condition stabilizes. ■ Maintain client safety.
Pain or strange sensations may result with damage to the thalamus.	■ Pain that may be hot, cold, burning, tingling, or sharp and stabbing in the extremities, worsened by movement or temperature changes, and not relieved by analgesics	No treatment has been found.
Cognitive and behavioral changes can result from ischemia or hemorrhage involving either the carotid or vertebral arteries, cerebral edema, or increased intracranial pressure.	■ Emotional lability ■ Loss of self-control ■ Decreased tolerance for stress ■ Memory loss, decreased attention span ■ Poor judgment, lack of ability for abstract thought	■ Behavioral and cognitive therapy

Pharmacologic Therapy

Medications are administered to prevent a stroke in clients with TIAs or a previous stroke and to treat the client during the acute phase of a stroke.

PREVENTION   Antiplatelet agents are often used to treat clients with TIAs or those who have had a previous stroke. Platelets are concentrated in high-blood-flow arteries, where they adhere to endothelial tissue damaged by atherosclerosis and occlude the vessel. The drugs used to prevent clot formation and blood vessel occlusion include aspirin, clopidogrel (Plavix), dipyridamole (Persantine), and ticlopidine (Ticlid).

Daily low-dose aspirin reduces TIA occurrence and stroke risk by interfering with platelet aggregation. Ticlopidine (Ticlid)

is a platelet-aggregation inhibitor that reduces thrombotic stroke risk.

ACUTE STROKE   Medications are used to treat the client during the acute phase of an ischemic stroke to prevent further thrombosis formation, increase cerebral blood flow, and protect cerebral neurons. The type of medication used varies according to the type of stroke.

Anticoagulant drug therapy is often ordered for an ischemic stroke. The most commonly used anticoagulants are warfarin sodium (Coumadin), heparin, and enoxaparin (Lovenox). Anticoagulants are never administered to a client with a hemorrhagic stroke. Anticoagulants do not dissolve an existing clot; they prevent further extension of the clot and formation of new clots.

TABLE 16–34 National Institutes of Health Stroke Scale: Assessment of Level of Consciousness

INSTRUCTIONS	SCALE DEFINITION	SCORE
1a. Level of Consciousness (LOC): The investigator must choose a response, even if a full evaluation is prevented by such obstacles as an endotracheal tube, language barrier, orotracheal trauma/bandages. A 3 is scored only if the client makes no movement (other than reflexive posturing) in response to noxious stimulation.	0 = Alert, keenly responsive 1 = Not alert, but arousable by minor stimulation to obey, answer, or respond 2 = Not alert, requires repeated stimulation to attend, or is obtunded and requires strong or painful stimulation to make movements (not stereotyped) 3 = Responds only with reflex motor or autonomic effects or totally unresponsive, flaccid, areflexic	_____
1b. LOC Questions: The client is asked the month and his or her age. The answer must be correct. There is no partial credit for being close. Aphasic and stuporous clients who do not comprehend the questions will score a 2. Clients unable to speak because of endotracheal intubation, orotracheal trauma, severe dysarthria from any cause, language barrier, or any other problem not secondary to aphasia are given a 1. It is important that only the initial answer be graded and that the examiner not "help" the client with verbal or nonverbal cues.	0 = Answers both questions correctly. 1 = Answers one question correctly. 2 = Answers neither question correctly.	_____
1c. LOC Commands: The client is asked to open and close the eyes and then to grip and release the nonparetic hand. Substitute another one-step command if the hands cannot be used. Credit is given if an unequivocal attempt is made but not completed because of weakness. If the client does not respond to the command, the task should be demonstrated (pantomime) and the results scored (i.e., follows none, one, or two commands). Clients with trauma, amputation, or other physical impediments should be given suitable one-step commands. Only the first attempt is scored.	0 = Performs both tasks correctly. 1 = Performs one task correctly. 2 = Performs neither task correctly.	_____

Note: This is a sample of only one part of the National Institutes of Health Stroke Scale. The entire scale may be viewed as a PDF file at www.ninds.nih.gov/doctors/NIH_Stroke_Scale.pdf.

Sodium heparin may be given subcutaneously or by continuous intravenous drip, or warfarin sodium may be given orally.

Fibrinolytic therapy, using a tissue plasminogen activator such as the recombinant tissue plasminogen activator alteplase (rt-PA, tPA), sometimes given concurrently with an anticoagulant, is used to treat thrombotic stroke. The drug converts plasminogen to plasmin, resulting in fibrinolysis of the clot. To be effective, it should be given intravenously within 3 hours of the onset of manifestations, after CT scan to confirm the occurrence of an ischemic stroke. A European study found that tPA administered between 3 and 4.5 hours after the onset of manifestations significantly improved clinical outcomes although it also increased the risk of intracranial hemorrhage. The Evidence-Based Practice feature discusses the use of tPA in treating stroke.

Antithrombotic drugs, which inhibit the platelet phase of clot formation, have been used as a preventive measure for clients at risk for embolic and thrombotic stroke. Both aspirin and dipyridamole have been used for this purpose. These drugs are sometimes also used in combination with other drugs during acute treatment. Antiplatelet agents are contraindicated in clients with a hemorrhagic stroke.

Management of hypertension during the acute phase of stroke is controversial, but if the client is eligible for fibrinolytic therapy, blood pressure control is necessary to decrease the risk for bleeding. If the blood pressure is sustained at systolic levels greater than 185 mmHg or diastolic levels greater than 110 mmHg the client cannot be treated with IV tPA. Many clients do not recognize the early warning signs of stroke. Because of a delay in treatment, typically greater than 3 hours, clients may be deemed medically inappropriate for treatment with tPA. Corticosteroids, such as prednisone or dexamethasone, have been used to treat cerebral edema, but the results are not always positive. If the client has increased intracranial pressure, hyperosmolar solutions (e.g., mannitol) or diuretics (e.g., furosemide) may be administered. Anticonvulsants, such as phenytoin (Dilantin), and barbiturates may be prescribed if increased intracranial pressure causes seizures.

Surgery

Surgery may be performed to prevent the occurrence of a stroke, to restore blood flow when a stroke has already occurred, or to repair vascular damage or malformations. In individuals who have had TIAs or are in danger of having another stroke, a carotid endarterectomy at the carotid artery bifurcation may be performed to remove atherosclerotic plaque (**Figure 16–63 ●**).

When an occluded or stenotic vessel is not directly accessible, an extracranial–intracranial bypass may be performed. Bypass of the internal carotid, middle cerebral, or vertebral arteries may be required. The indications for the bypass are manifestations of ischemia caused by TIAs or a mild completed stroke. The procedure reestablishes blood flow to the affected area of the brain.

A carotid angioplasty with stenting is an option for treating cerebral stenosis. During the procedure, a balloon catheter is inserted through an artery in the client's arm or leg. Under fluoroscopy, the catheter is advanced to the area of carotid artery stenosis, and a small filter is inserted to catch any clots or pieces of debris that might break loose. The balloon is inflated to widen the artery, and a permanent stent is inserted.

Evidence-Based Practice Treating Stroke With tPA

Problem

Stroke is a leading cause of severe, long-term disability in the United States (American Stroke Association, 2012). The risk of disability and death can be reduced in individuals who experience a sudden ischemic stroke by the administration of thrombolytics given to dissolve blood clots.

Evidence

Tissue plasminogen activator (tPA) is the most commonly administered drug used in thrombolytic therapy (National Library of Medicine, 2013). In ideal situations, clients should receive tPA within 90 minutes after arriving in the emergency department, but positive outcomes have been seen when administered as long as 12 hours from initial symptoms. To be effective, tPA must be administered within 3 hours of the warning signs of a stroke to increase the chances of recovery (National Stroke Association, 2013b). tPA restores the brain's blood flow by dissolving the blood clot causing the stroke.

tPA was the first therapy for the treatment of acute ischemic stroke to be approved by the Federal Food and Drug Administration (National Stroke Association, 2013b). An enzyme found naturally in the body, tPA converts plasminogen, another enzyme that dissolves blood clots. Physicians administer additional tPA intravenously to speed up this process. The most commonly occurring complication of tPA therapy is brain hemorrhage (National Stroke Association, 2013b). Early identification of stroke warning signs and early thrombolytic therapy are instrumental in assisting clients to achieve a full recovery.

Implications

Vital signs should be monitored frequently by the nurse following the administration of tPA. Clients are at an increased risk for bleeding and should not be given anticoagulants or antiplatelet agents for 24 hours after administration. It is also important for the client to avoid foods that influence the body's clotting mechanism. These include spinach, lettuce, broccoli, cabbage, cauliflower, and vegetable oil. Acute care may be delivered via a specialized team of nurses and other interdisciplinary members. Level of consciousness and neurological status are important indicators of further brain hemorrhage and should be monitored continuously during the hospitalization.

Critical Thinking Application

1. A client arrives in the emergency department with an ischemic stroke and receives tPA. What is the priority nursing assessment?

2. Prior to administering tPA to a client admitted with a diagnosis of CVA, what serum lab value should the nurse check? Why?

3. Think of a slogan for the public that increases awareness of the 3-hour time limit recommended for treatment with tPA.

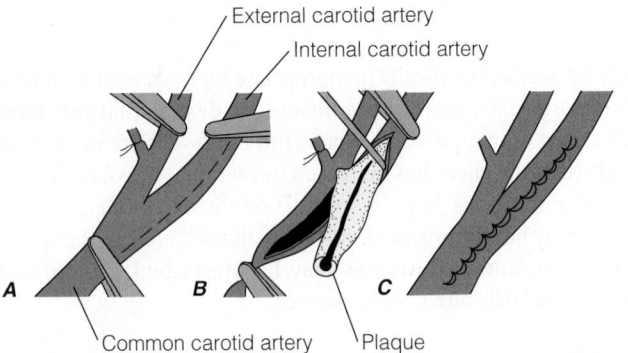

Figure 16–63 ● Carotid endarterectomy. *A,* The occluded area is clamped off and an incision is made in the artery. *B,* Plaque is removed from the inner layer of the artery. *C,* To restore blood flow through the artery, the artery is sutured, or a graft is completed.

Rehabilitation

Various types of therapy are necessary for poststroke rehabilitation. The types and goals of the therapies used are as follows:

- *Physical therapy* may help prevent contractures and improve muscle strength and coordination. Physical therapists teach exercises to enable the client to relearn how to walk, sit, lie down, and change from one type of movement to another.

- *Occupational therapy* provides assistive devices and a plan for regaining lost motor skills that greatly improve quality of life after a stroke. These skills include eating, drinking, bathing, cooking, reading, writing, and toileting.

- *Speech and language therapy* is provided to help the client relearn language and communication skills as well as improve swallowing.

◼ NURSING PROCESS

Even though many individuals who have a stroke experience full recovery, a substantial number are left with disabilities that affect their physical, emotional, interpersonal, and family status. The required nursing care is often complex and multidimensional, requiring consideration of continuity of care for clients in acute care settings, long-term care settings, rehabilitation centers, and the home.

The nurse caring for a client who has had a stroke requires knowledge and skill to meet client needs during both the acute and rehabilitative phases of care. The client may have losses in multiple areas: mobility, ability to provide self-care, communications, concept of self, and interpersonal or intimate relationships with others. Holistic, individualized nursing care is essential in all settings and focuses on promoting the achievement of maximum potential and quality of life.

The client's family often faces many changes. The young to middle-aged adult with a family member who has had a stroke may face economic difficulties and social isolation. The middle-aged adult family member may become the caretaker for an older parent, in essence switching roles with the parent. An older adult may not be able to care for a spouse and may have to accept nursing home placement. In addition, the older adult who has no family may have to struggle alone to regain the ability to function independently. Although not all of these problems are amenable to nursing solutions, the nurse is most often the healthcare provider who assesses and identifies the needs of each individual and who provides information and referrals to clients and families to help meet those needs.

Because a stroke has the potential to cause many different health problems, a wide variety of nursing diagnoses may be appropriate. It is important to remember that each individual will be affected differently, depending on the degree of ischemia and the area of the brain involved. Nursing diagnoses discussed in this section focus on problems with cerebral tissue perfusion (specific to nursing care during the acute phase), physical mobility, self-care, communication, sensory–perceptual deficits, bowel and urine elimination, and swallowing (specific to prevention of complications and rehabilitation).

Health promotion activities focus on stroke prevention, especially for individuals with known risk factors. It is important to discuss with clients of all ages the importance of stopping smoking and drug use, as appropriate. Maintaining a normal weight through diet and exercise can help reduce obesity, thus decreasing the risk of hypertension and type 2 diabetes mellitus (both of which increase the risk for stroke). Cholesterol levels should be screened regularly to monitor for hyperlipidemia. Regular health care to monitor for and treat cardiovascular disorders and to detect and treat infections such as infective endocarditis is important. It is also important to increase public awareness of the signs of a TIA or stroke and of the need to call 911 or seek care immediately if any of the following warning signs or symptoms occur:

- Sudden weakness or numbness of the face, arm, or leg, especially on one side of the body
- Sudden confusion, difficulty speaking, or difficulty understanding speech
- Sudden trouble walking, dizziness, or loss of coordination
- Sudden difficulty with vision in one or both eyes
- Sudden severe headache without a cause.

A public awareness campaign by the National Stroke Association provides symptoms that should be reported. The campaign, How to Detect Stroke Symptoms and Act F.A.S.T. include the following:

F = Face: is there facial drooping?
A = Arm: is there arm weakness?
S = Speech: is speech slurred?
T = Time: call 911 if these are present

Assessment

The nurse collects the following data through the health history and physical examination:

- **Health history.** Risk factors, previous stroke, drug use (prescribed, over-the-counter, and street drugs), smoking history, when manifestations began, severity of manifestations, presence of incontinence, level of consciousness, family support system
- **Physical assessment.** Level of consciousness, motor strength, coordination, communication, cranial nerves, sensory function, stroke scale, vital signs, cranial nerves, skin integrity, mobility status.

If the client is a woman, her risks for stroke are different than those of a man, and she should be asked questions specific to her gender. Questions relating to the uniqueness of women's symptoms include inquiries regarding sudden face and limb pain, sudden nausea, sudden hiccups, sudden shortness of breath, palpitations, and generalized weakness.

Diagnosis

Nursing diagnoses that may apply to the client with stroke include the following:

- *Ineffective Tissue Perfusion: Cerebral*
- *Impaired Physical Mobility*
- *Self-Care Deficit*
- *Impaired Verbal Communication*
- *Impaired Urinary Elimination and Risk for Constipation*
- *Impaired Swallowing.*

(NANDA-I © 2012)

Planning

Goals of care for the client who has had a stroke include the following:

- The client's blood pressure will be maintained within prescribed limits.
- The client will understand the importance of cardiac rehabilitation.
- The client will ambulate and increase activity as tolerated.
- The client will participate in therapies that maximize communication techniques.

Implementation

The focus of care for the client who has had a stroke is determined by the severity of the stroke, the neurological deficits that result, and whether the client is in the acute or rehabilitative stage of the event. In the acute phase, ensuring airway, breathing, and circulation are the priority focus. Once the ABCs of care are met, the nurse's priority shifts to reducing loss of neurological function. Psychosocial support for the client and family also is an important role of the nurse.

Maintain Cerebral Perfusion

The initial assessment and care of a client admitted for intensive care focus on identifying changes that may indicate altered cerebral perfusion. The nurse monitors the client's airway, breathing, circulation, and neurological status and provides interventions to maintain cerebral perfusion. Nursing interventions related to maintaining cerebral perfusion are as follows:

- Monitor the client's respiratory status and airway patency. Auscultate pulmonary sounds, and monitor respiratory rate and results of studies of arterial blood gases. The client is often unconscious, and breathing may be impaired. Respiratory complications develop rapidly, as manifested by crackles and wheezes, rapid respirations, and respiratory acidosis.
- Suction as necessary, using care to avoid prolonged suctioning, which can increase intracranial pressure.
- Place the client in a side-lying position.
- Administer oxygen as prescribed. Administration of oxygen decreases the risk for hypoxia and hypercapnia, which can increase cerebral ischemia and intracranial pressure.

- Monitor the client's mental status and level of consciousness: restlessness, drowsiness, lethargy, inability to follow commands, unresponsiveness. Frequent monitoring of neurological status is necessary to detect changes. Alterations in mental status, level of consciousness, and movement indicate increased intracranial pressure (IICP), the major cause of death in the acute phase of a stroke.
- Monitor the client's strength and reflexes, and assess for pain, headache, decreased muscle strength, sluggish pupillary reflexes, absent gag or swallowing reflexes, hemiplegia, a Babinski sign, and decerebrate or decorticate posturing. Alterations in strength and reflexes indicate IICP.
- Continuously monitor the client's cardiac status, observing for dysrhythmias. A stroke may cause cardiac dysrhythmias, including bradycardia, PVCs, tachycardia, and AV block. Characteristic ECG changes include a shortened PR interval, peaked T waves, and a depressed ST segment.
- Monitor the client's body temperature. Hyperthermia may develop if the hypothalamus is affected.
- Maintain accurate intake and output records; measure urinary output via an indwelling catheter. A stroke may damage the pituitary gland, resulting in diabetes insipidus and the possibility of dehydration from greatly increased urinary output.
- Monitor the client for seizures. Pad the side rails, and administer prescribed anticonvulsants. Seizures may be the result of cerebral tissue damage or IICP. Padded side rails prevent injury if a seizure occurs. Anticonvulsants prevent or treat seizures.

Promote Physical Mobility

The goals of care for clients with impaired mobility are to maintain and improve functional abilities (by maintaining normal function and alignment, preventing edema of extremities, and reducing spasticity) and to prevent complications. Nursing interventions related to physical mobility include the following:

- Encourage active range-of-motion (ROM) exercises for unaffected extremities, and perform passive ROM exercises for affected extremities every 4 hours during day and evening shifts and once during the night shift. Support the joint during passive ROM exercises. Active ROM exercises maintain or improve muscle strength and endurance and help maintain cardiopulmonary function. Passive ROM exercises do not strengthen muscles but do help maintain joint flexibility.
- Turn the client every 2 hours around the clock, following a posted schedule for side-to-side and supine-to-prone position changes (verify prone positioning with the physician). Maintain body alignment, and support the extremities in the proper position with pillows. Elevate the head of the bed 30 degrees. Turning on a regular basis, accompanied by proper positioning, maintains joint function, alleviates pressure on bony prominences that can lead to skin breakdown, decreases dependent edema in hands and feet, reduces intracranial pressure, and reduces the risk of complications resulting from immobility (**Figure 16–64** ●).
- Monitor the client's lower extremities each shift for symptoms of thrombophlebitis. Assess for increased warmth and redness in calves; measure the circumference of the calves and thighs. Clients on bed rest (especially those with loss of

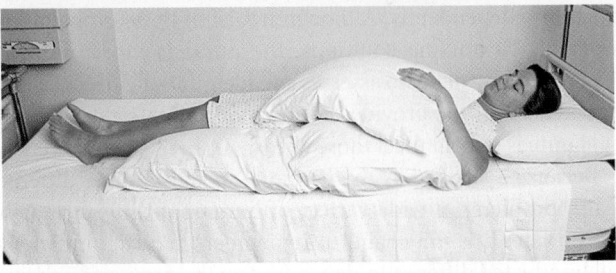

A

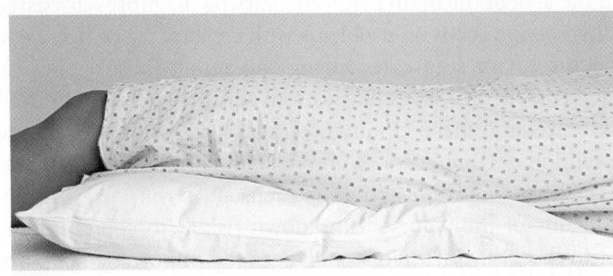

B

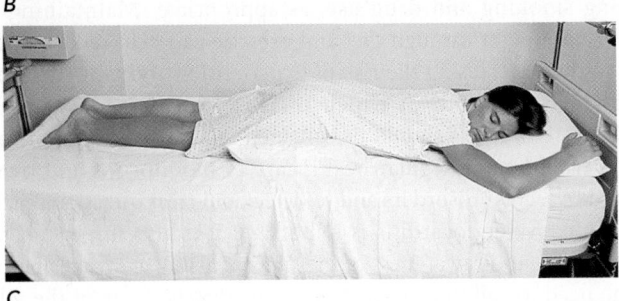

C

Figure 16–64 ● Positioning the client with hemiplegia is important in preventing deformity of the affected extremities. *A*, With the client in a supine position, place a pillow in the axilla (to prevent adduction) and under the hand and arm, with the hand higher than the elbow (to prevent flexion and edema). *B*, When the client is lying supine, use a pillow from the iliac crest to the middle of the thigh to prevent external rotation of the hip. *C*, When the client is in the prone position, place a pillow under the pelvis to promote hip hyperextension.

muscle strength and tone) are particularly prone to the development of deep venous thrombosis. Promptly report manifestations of thrombophlebitis.
- Collaborate with the physical therapist as the client gains mobility, using consistent techniques to move the client from the bed to the wheelchair and to help the client ambulate. The use of consistent techniques facilitates rehabilitation.

Promote Self-Care

The client who has had a stroke may have a self-care deficit as a result of impaired mobility or mental confusion. It is important for clients to perform as much of their own physical care and grooming as possible to promote functional ability, increase independence, decrease feelings of powerlessness, and improve self-esteem. Nursing interventions to promote self-care include the following:

- Encourage the client to use the unaffected arm to bathe, brush teeth, comb hair, dress, and eat. Use of the unaffected arm promotes functional ability and independence.

- Teach the client to put on clothing by first dressing the affected extremities and then dressing the unaffected extremities. This technique facilitates self-dressing with minimal assistance.
- Collaborate with the occupational therapist in scheduling times for training to promote the upper extremity functioning necessary for ADLs. Encourage the use of assistive devices (if required) for eating, physical hygiene, and dressing. Following a regular schedule in daily routines promotes learning. Use of assistive devices promotes independence and decreases feelings of powerlessness. Optimal grooming facilitates positive self-concept.

Before establishing a plan to increase self-care, determine which hand was dominant before the stroke. If the client's dominant side is affected, self-care will be more difficult.

Promote Verbal Communication

The client who loses communication abilities requires intensive speech therapy and emotional support. It is important for the nurse to determine the specific nature of the impairment when planning interventions and helping family members understand specific problems. Although the speech therapist is usually most involved with speech rehabilitation, nurses must plan interventions to meet communication needs during all phases of care. These interventions may include the following:

- Communicate with the client using the following guidelines:
  a. Approach and treat the client as an adult.
  b. Do not assume that the client who does not respond verbally cannot hear. Do not use a raised voice when addressing the client.
  c. Allow adequate time for the client to respond.
  d. Face the client, and speak slowly.
  e. When you do not understand the client's speech, be honest and say so.
  f. Use short, simple statements and questions.

Accepting the client and providing dignity and respect enhances the nurse–client relationship. Allowing adequate response time and using short verbal statements or questions while facing the client motivates the client to communicate and decreases frustration.

- Accept the client's frustration and anger as a normal reaction to the loss of function. Anger represents the client's frustration at the inability to control the loss of function.
- Try alternative methods of communication, including writing tablets, flash cards, and computerized talking boards. Clients who are unable to communicate verbally may be able to use other methods effectively.

Promote Urinary and Bowel Elimination

Both urinary and bowel elimination may be altered because of neurological deficits, impaired mobility, cognitive impairment, communication deficits, or preexisting problems (especially if the client is an older adult). Other causes can include changes in food and fluid intake and side effects of medications. Urinary incontinence or retention, constipation, and fecal impaction are the usual manifestations. Nursing interventions to promote normal elimination include the following:

- Assess for urinary frequency, urgency, incontinence, nocturia, and voiding in small amounts. In addition, assess the client's ability to respond to the need to void, the ability to use the call light, and the ability to use toileting equipment.
- Encourage bladder training by having client void on schedule, such as every 2 hours, rather than in response to the urge to void. Voiding every 2 hours or on schedule promotes bladder tone and urine storage.
- Teach Kegel exercises. To perform Kegel exercises, the client contracts the perineal muscles as though stopping urination, holds the contraction for 5 seconds, and then releases. Kegel exercises increase pubococcygeal muscle tone and bladder control, decreasing incontinence.
- Use positive reinforcement (verbal praise) for successful management of urinary elimination. Positive reinforcement can be a useful part of the teaching program.
- Discuss prestroke bowel habits as well as the pattern of bowel elimination since the stroke.
- If the client is able to swallow without difficulty, encourage fluids (up to 2,000 mL/day) and a high-fiber diet. Increased fluids and fiber stimulate intestinal motility.
- Increase physical activity as tolerated. Increased activity stimulates intestinal motility.
- Assist in using the toilet facilities at the same time each day (based on usual patterns of bowel elimination), ensuring privacy and having the client sit in an upright position if at all possible. Establishing a regular daily time for bowel movements in the upright position and in privacy promotes normal bowel elimination.
- Administer prescribed stool softeners if the client is following a bowel elimination routine or is not drinking sufficient fluids. Stool softeners help prevent the formation of hard stool that is more difficult to expel.

Maintain Safety

A stroke may impair the ability to swallow. Weakness or lack of coordination of the tongue, attention deficits, and deficits involving the swallowing reflex all play a role. **Dysphagia** (difficulty swallowing) may result in choking, drooling, aspiration, or regurgitation. Nursing care focuses on maintaining safety by preventing aspiration and ensuring adequate nutrition, using the following interventions:

- Monitor results of swallowing studies before providing oral food and fluids.
- Ensure safety when the client is eating.
  a. Position the client in an upright sitting position with the neck slightly flexed.
  b. Order puréed or soft food. Liquids should be of the same consistency as honey.
  c. Feed or teach the client to eat by putting food behind the front teeth on the unaffected side of the mouth and tilting the head slightly backward. Teach the client to swallow one bite at a time.
  d. Assess the client for coughing with eating or drinking.
  e. Have suction equipment available at the bedside in case of choking or aspiration.

Sitting upright with the head and neck first slightly flexed and then tilted back helps the client swallow. The client can usually swallow puréed or soft foods more easily than liquid or solid foods. Using the unaffected side of the mouth helps prevent food from collecting in the mouth and makes swallowing safer;

in addition, food is less likely to fall out of the mouth. Coughing may be indicative of dysphagia.

- Monitor the client's lung sounds. Coarse lung sounds heard in the right upper and/or lower lobes may indicate aspiration because the right bronchus is the first division of the bronchi and where the majority of aspirations occur.
- Minimize distractions and, if necessary, give the client step-by-step instructions for eating. Distractions increase the risk of aspiration. Complex activities are easier to perform when broken down into small steps.

Evaluation

Client outcomes may be evaluated based on the following expected outcomes:

- The client participates in assigned therapies.
- The client can communicate effectively.
- The client's significant other and family members participate in the client's care.
- The client experiences minimal complications resulting from immobility, dysphagia, and reduced motor or sensory function.

NURSING CARE PLAN   A Client With a Stroke

ASSESSMENT

Orville Boren is a 63-year-old African American male who had a stroke caused by right cerebral thrombosis 1 week ago. He is a history instructor at the local community college. His hobbies are wood carving and gardening. Mr. Boren is also an active member of his church. For the past 2 years, Mr. Boren has been taking medication for hypertension, but his wife Emily reports that he often forgets to take it and that his blood pressure was high at his last physical examination. Mrs. Boren tells the staff that she has never had to worry about her husband's health before and that she wants to learn everything she can to care for him at home. However, she says that her husband was always the one to make the decisions and pay the bills. Mrs. Boren adds that all the children, grandchildren, neighbors, and family pastor want to see Mr. Boren back at home as soon as possible.

Carol Merck, RN, the nurse assigned to Mr. Boren, completes a health history and physical assessment, with Mrs. Boren providing information for the history. Mrs. Boren reports that her husband did have several spells of dizziness and blurred vision the week before his stroke, but they lasted only a few minutes and he believed them to be caused by "old age and working out in the sun." On the morning of admission, Mr. Boren woke up and could not move his left arm or leg; he also could not speak sensibly. Mrs. Boren called 911, and an ambulance took her husband to the hospital.

Physical assessment findings include the following: Mr. Boren is drowsy but responds to verbal stimuli. Although he does not respond verbally, he can nod his head to indicate "yes" when asked questions. Flaccid paralysis is present in his left arm and left leg, with no response noted to touch in those extremities (he is left-handed). Visual fields are decreased in a pattern consistent with homonymous hemianopia. A computed tomographic scan, negative on admission, is repeated on the day after admission and confirms the medical diagnosis of a right-brain stroke caused by a thrombus of the middle cerebral artery.

Mr. Boren's medical treatment includes heparin sodium administered by continuous intravenous drip, with clotting studies to be performed every 4 hours and the dose adjusted accordingly.

DIAGNOSES

- *Feeding Self-Care Deficit* related to loss of the ability to use the left hand and arm
- *Impaired Physical Mobility* related to neurological deficits causing left hemiplegia
- *Risk for Impaired Skin Integrity* related to inability to change position
- *Impaired Verbal Communication* related to cerebral injury

(NANDA-I © 2012)

PLANNING

Goals of care include the following:

- The client will learn to use his right hand to feed himself.
- The client will participate in exercises necessary to maintain muscle strength and tone.
- The client will maintain skin integrity.
- The client will practice and implement speech therapy activities while at the same time using alternative methods of communication.

IMPLEMENTATION

- Arrange mealtimes so that Mr. Boren is sitting up by the window in a clean and private environment.
- Provide adaptive devices (silverware with thick handles and nonslip plates).
- Encourage Mrs. Boren to visit at mealtimes, to assist with meals, and periodically to bring a favorite food from home.
- Conduct passive ROM exercises on the left arm and leg; schedule active ROM exercises for the right extremities as well as quadriceps and gluteal sets every 4 hours during waking hours.

- Keep the skin clean and dry at all times.
- Establish and maintain a regular schedule for turning when Mr. Boren is in bed.
- Place objects (e.g., call bell and tissues) on the unaffected side, and approach Mr. Boren from that side.
- Support attempts to communicate verbally; when Mr. Boren is not understood, he prefers to use a large marker and tablet.

NURSING CARE PLAN   (continued)

EVALUATION

Mr. Boren is discharged to his home after being in the hospital for 10 days. During the first 2 months after discharge, Martha Grimes, RN, the home health nurse, visits Mr. and Mrs. Boren at home. At the end of 2 months, Mr. Boren is using his right hand to feed himself. He has regained partial use of his left arm and leg and is using a walker to move around the house and yard; he is even able to work in his flower garden. His skin has remained intact, and his vision is back to normal. He is slowly relearning speech; this has been the most difficult change for him to accept. Once he writes on his tablet, "I think God has forgotten me."

CRITICAL THINKING

1. Hypertension is sometimes referred to as the "silent killer." Provide justifications for this statement.
2. The functional changes Mr. Boren has experienced may make a return to teaching difficult. What other uses of his knowledge and abilities might you suggest?
3. What would be your reply if, after you had completed passive ROM on Mr. Boren's left arm, he wrote: "I just ignore that part of my body—it doesn't work anyway"?

REVIEW   Stroke

RELATE Link the Concepts and Exemplars

Linking the exemplar of stroke with the concept of thermoregulation:

1. What impact related to thermoregulation might be seen in the client who has had a massive stroke?
2. You are caring for a client who had a stroke. The client requires mechanical ventilation due to inadequate breathing patterns. The client's temperature is 106.2°F axillary. What are your priorities of care? Will over-the-counter antipyretics be effective? Explain your answer.

Linking the exemplar of stroke with the concept of safety:

3. You are caring for a 56-year-old male client in the rehabilitation facility who experienced a stroke 6 months ago resulting in hemiplegia of the left side. What risks to safety do you anticipate for this client?
4. What interventions, including client teaching, will you provide to reduce this client's risk of injury?

READY Go to Companion Skills Manual

REFER Go to Pearson Nursing Student Resources
nursing.pearsonhighered.com

- Additional review materials

REFLECT Case Study

Ted Marist is a 68-year-old man who lives with his wife Maggie in a condominium on the sixth floor of a high-rise building. Ted is recently retired from the police force. Mr. Marist smoked two packs a day until 1 year ago when his physician discovered a bruit in his right carotid artery. The physician placed Mr. Marist on Coumadin (1.5 mg/day), and his wife insisted that he quit smoking. He still smokes an occasional cigarette when he's out with friends, but he no longer smokes regularly. The Marists have three grown children and five grandchildren.

Mrs. Marist attempts to regulate her husband's diet and encourages him to take a walk with her every night after dinner. The Marists have come to the physician's office today to have Mr. Marist's clotting times checked. Mrs. Marist says she is very concerned because her husband has had two episodes of staring off into space and not responding to her questions. She says his eyes were open but he looked like "there was nobody home behind his eyes" and even when she screamed he did not respond. When the episode stopped, he complained of a headache and insisted on taking a nap, saying he felt much better when he awoke.

1. What do you suspect is causing Mr. Marist's symptoms?
2. How will you respond to Mrs. Marist's concerns when she tells you about these events?
3. What orders do you anticipate receiving from the provider related to these symptoms?
4. Considering Mr. Marist's history, for what type of stroke is he most at risk?

■ REFERENCES

American Congress of Obstetricians and Gynecologists (ACOG). 2011. *Committee opinion. Emergent therapy for acute-onset, severe hypertension with preeclampsia or eclampsia.* Retrieved from http://www.acog.org/Resources_And_Publications/Committee_Opinions/Committee_on_Obstetric_Practice/Emergent_Therapy_for_Acute-Onset_Severe_Hypertension_with_Preeclampsia_or_Eclampsia.

American Congress of Obstetricians and Gynecologists (ACOG). 2013. *Ob-gyns issue task force report on hypertension in pregnancy.* Retrieved from http://www.acog.org/About_ACOG/News_Room/News_Releases/2013/Ob-Gyns_Issue_Task_Force_Report_on_Hypertension_in_Pregnancy.

American Heart Association (AHA). (2013a). *Cardiomyopathy in adults.* Retrieved from http://www.heart.org/HEARTORG/Conditions/More/Cardiomyopathy/Cardiomyopathy_UCM_444459_SubHomePage.jsp.

American Heart Association (AHA). (2013b). *Congenital heart defects.* Retrieved from http://www.heart.org/HEARTORG/Conditions/CongenitalHeartDefects/

Congenital-Heart-Defects_UQCM_001090_SubHomePage.jsp.

American Heart Association (AHA). (2013c). *African-Americans and heart disease, stroke.* Retrieved from http://www.heart.org/HEARTORG/Conditions/More/MyHeartandStrokeNews/African-Americans-and-Heart-Disease-Stroke_UCM_444863_Article.jsp.

American Heart Association. (2013d). *African Americans and cardiovascular disease: Statistical fact sheet, 2013 update.* Retrieved from http://www.heart.org/idc/groups/heart-public/@wcm/@sop/@smd/documents/downloadable/ucm_319568.pdf.

American Heart Association (AHA). (2013e). *2010 American Heart Association guidelines for cardiopulmonary resuscitation and emergency cardiovascular care science.* Retrieved from http://circ.ahajournals.org/content/122/18_suppl_3/S787.full.

American Heart Association (AHA). (2013f). *Stroke and high blood pressure.* Retrieved from http://www.heart.org/HEARTORG/Conditions/HighBloodPressure/

WhyBloodPressureMatters/Stroke-and-High-Blood-Pressure_UCM_301824_Article.jsp.

American Heart Association (AHA). (2013g). *Stroke treatments.* Retrieved from http://strokeassociation.org/STROKEORG/AboutStroke/Treatment/Stroke-Treatments_UCM_310892_Article.jsp.

American Stroke Association. (2012). *What is stroke?* Retrieved from http://www.strokeassociation.org/STROKEORG/AboutStroke/About-Stroke_UCM_308529_SubHomePage.jsp.

August, P. (2015). Management of hypertension in pregnant and postpartum women. *Up To Date.* http://www.uptodate.com/contents/management-of-hypertension-in-pregnant-and-postpartum-women?source=machineLearning&search=hypertension+in+pregnancy&selectedTitle=1%7E150&sectionRank=1&anchor=H53704432#H53704432

August, P., Sibai, B.M. (2015). Preeclampsia: Clinical features and diagnosis. *Up To Date.* http://www.uptodate.com/contents/preeclampsia-clinicalfeaturesanddiagnosis?

source=machineLearning&search=preeclampsia&selectedTitle=1%7E150&sectionRank=1&anchor=H6#H6

Braunwald, E., Antman, E. M., Beasley, J. W., Califf, R. M., Cheitlin, M. D., & Hochman, J. S. (2002). *ACC/AHA 2002 guideline update for the management of patients with unstable angina and non-ST-segment elevation myocardial infarction: A report of the American College of Cardiology/American Heart Association Task Force on Practice Guidelines (Committee on the Management of Patients with Unstable Angina)*. Retrieved from http://circ.ahajournals.org/content/106/14/1893.full.

Carson, M. (2013). *Peripartum cardiomyopathy*. Retrieved from http://emedicine.medscape.com/article/153153-overview.

Centers for Disease Control and Prevention (CDC). (2011). *Physical activity for a healthy weight: Why is physical activity important?* Retrieved from http://www.cdc.gov/healthyweight/physical_activity/index.html.

Centers for Disease Control and Prevention (CDC). (2015). *Heart disease facts*. Retrieved from http://www.cdc.gov/heartdisease/facts.htm.

Centers for Disease Control and Prevention (CDC). (2013b). *Heart failure fact sheet*. Retrieved from http://www.cdc.gov/dhdsp/data_statistics/fact_sheets/fs_heart_failure.htm.

Centers for Disease Control and Prevention (CDC). (2013c). *Facts about hypoplastic left heart syndrome*. Retrieved from http://www.cdc.gov/ncbddd/heartdefects/hlhs.html.

Centers for Disease Control and Prevention (CDC). (2013d). *High blood pressure facts*. Retrieved from http://www.cdc.gov/bloodpressure/facts.htm.

Centers for Disease Control and Prevention (CDC). (2013e). *Peripheral arterial disease (PAD) fact sheet*. Retrieved from http://www.cdc.gov/dhdsp/data_statistics/fact_sheets/fs_pad.htm.

Centers for Disease Control and Prevention (CDC). (2013f). *Stroke facts*. Retrieved from http://www.cdc.gov/stroke/facts.htm.

Chumaeva, N., Hintsanen, M., Hintsa, T., Ravaja, N., Juonala, M., Raitakari, O., & Keltikangas-Jarvinen, L. (2010). Early atherosclerosis and cardiac autonomic responses to mental stress: A population-based study of the moderating influence of impaired endothelial function. *BMC Cardiovascular Disorders, 10*(16). Retrieved from http://www.biomedcentral.com/1471-2261/10/16.

Cleveland Clinic. (2013). *Dilated and restrictive cardiomyopathies*. Retrieved from http://www.clevelandclinicmeded.com/medicalpubs/diseasemanagement/cardiology/dilated-restrictive-cardiomyopathy/#cesec1.

Clinical Guidelines Committee of the American College of Physicians. (2011). Venous thromboembolism prophylaxis in hospitalized patients: A clinical practice guideline from the American College of Physicians. *Annals of Internal Medicine, 155*(9). Retrieved from http://annals.org/article.aspx?articleid=1033137.

Connolly, D., McClowry, S., Hayman, L., Mahony, L., & Artman, M. (2004). Posttraumatic stress disorder in children after cardiac surgery. *Journal of Pediatrics, 144*(4), 480–484.

Copstead, L. C., & Banasik, J. L. (2010). *Pathophysiology* (4th ed.). St. Louis, MO: Saunders.

Corbett, J. V. (2013). *Laboratory tests and diagnostic procedures with nursing diagnoses* (8th ed.). Upper Saddle River, NJ: Prentice Hall.

Cunningham, F. G., Leveno, K. J., Bloom, S. L., Spong, C. Y., Dashe, J., Hoffman, B. L., Casey, B. M., & Sheffield, J. S. (2014). *Williams obstetrics* (23rd ed.). New York, NY: McGraw-Hill.

Ebomoyi, E. W. (2010). Framingham Heart Study: The legacy and health education implications in the age of genomic medicine. *Researcher, 2*(6), 33–54.

Framingham Heart Study (FHS). (2013). *Welcome to the Framingham Heart Study*. Retrieved from http://www.framinghamheartstudy.org.

Gordon, M. C. (2012). Maternal physiology. In S. G. Gabbe, J. R. Niebyl, & J. L. Simpson (Eds.), *Obstetrics: Normal and problem pregnancies* (6th ed.). Philadelphia, PA: Saunders.

Gorler, H., Ono, M., Thies, A., Lunkewitz, E., Westhoff-Bleck, M., Haverich, A., . . . & Boethig, D. (2011). Long-term morbidity and quality of life after surgical repair of the great arteries: Atrial versus arterial switch operation. *Interactive Cardiovascular Thoracic Surgery, 12*(4), 569–574. doi:10.1510/icvts.2010.253898.

Guy, A. M. (2012). *Pulmonic valvular stenosis*. Retrieved from http://emedicine.medscape.com/article/759890-overview.

Heart Failure Society of America. (2013). *Quick facts and questions about heart failure*. Retrieved from http://www.hfsa.org/heart_failure_facts.asp.

Helfricht, S., Latal, B., Fischer, J. E., Tomaske, M., & Landolt, M. (2008). Surgery-related posttraumatic stress disorder in parents of children undergoing cardiopulmonary bypass surgery: A prospective cohort study. *Pediatric Critical Care Medicine, 9*(2), 217–223.

Hickey, J. V. (2013). The clinical practice of neurological and neurosurgical nursing (7th ed.). Philadelphia, PA: Lippincott Williams & Wilkins.

Huether, S. E. & McCance, K. L. (2011). Understanding pathophysiology (5th ed.). St. Louis, MO: Mosby Elsevier.

Jaeger, F. J. (n.d.). *Cardiac arrhythmias*. Retrieved from http://www.clevelandclinicmeded.com/medicalpubs/diseasemanagement/cardiology/cardiac-arrhythmias.

Kasper, D. L., Braunwald, E., Fauci, A. S., Hauser, S. L., Longo, D. L., & Jameson, J. L. (Eds.). (2005). *Harrison's principles of internal medicine* (16th ed.). New York, NY: McGraw-Hill.

King, T., Brucker, M.C., Kriebs, J.M., Ofahey, J.O., Gegor, C.L., Varney, H. (2015) *Varney's Midwifery, 5th ed.* Jones & Bartlett: Burlington, MA.

Levi, M. M., & Schmaier, A. H. (2012). *Disseminated intravascular coagulation*. Retrieved from http://emedicine.medscape.com/article/199627-overview.

Longo, D., Fauci, A., Kasper, D., Hauser, S., Jameson, J., & Loscalzo, J. (2011). *Harrison's principles of internal medicine* (18th ed.). New York, NY: McGraw-Hill.

Majnemer, A., Limperopoulos, C., Shevell, M. I., Rohlicek, C., Rosenblatt, B., & Tchervenkov, C. (2008). Developmental and functional outcomes at school entry in children with congenital heart disease. *Journal of Pediatrics, 153*, 55–60.

Majnemer, A., Limperopoulos, C., Shevell, M. I., Rohlicek, C., Rosenblatt, B., & Tchervenkov, C. (2008). A new look at outcomes of infants with congenital heart disease. *Pediatric Neurology, 40*(3), 197–204.

Markham, L. W., Cribbs, M. G., & Willis, P. W. (2011). *Atrial septal defect*. Retrieved from http://emedicine.medscape.com/article/162914-overview.

Mayo Clinic. (2014). *Orthostatic hypotension*. Retrieved from http://www.mayoclinic.com/health/orthostatic-hypotension/DS00997.

McCance, K., & Huether, S. (2010). *Pathophysiology: The biologic basis for disease in adults and children*. St. Louis, MO: Mosby.

McDonald-McGinn, D. M., Emanuel, B. S., & Zacai, E. H. (2013). *22q11.2 Deletion syndrome*. Retrieved from http://www.ncbi.nlm.nih.gov/books/NBK1523.

McElhinney, D. B., & Wernovsky, G. (2012). *Truncus arteriosus*. Retrieved from http://emedicine.medscape.com/article/892489-overview.

Medline Plus. (2012). *Peripartum cardiomyopathy*. Retrieved from http://www.nlm.nih.gov/medlineplus/ency/article/000188.htm.

Morton, P. G., & Fontaine, D. K. (2013). *Critical care nursing: A holistic approach*. New York, NY: Wolters Kluwer/Lippincott Williams & Wilkins.

Mustafa, R., Ahmed, S., Gupta, A., & Venuto, R. (2012). A comprehensive review of hypertension in pregnancy. *Journal of Pregnancy, 2012*. doi:10.1155/2012/105918.

National Cholesterol Education Program (NCEP). (2013). *Third report of the National Cholesterol Education Program (NCEP) Expert Panel on detection, evaluation, and treatment of high blood cholesterol in adults (Adult Treatment Panel III): Final report*. Bethesda, MD: National Institutes of Health.

National Cholesterol Education Program (NCEP). (2013). *Program description*. Retrieved from www.nhlbi.nih.gov/about/ncep/ncep_pd.htm.

National Heart, Lung, and Blood Institute (NHLBI). (2013a). *What is coronary artery disease?* Retrieved from http://www.nhlbi.nih.gov/health/health-topics/topics/cad.

National Heart, Lung, and Blood Institute (NHLBI). (2013b). *What is disseminated intravascular coagulation?* Retrieved from http://www.nhlbi.nih.gov/health/health-topics/topics/dic.

National Heart, Lung, and Blood Institute (NHLBI). (2013c). *What is heart failure?* Retrieved from http://www.nhlbi.nih.gov/health/health-topics/topics/hf.

National Heart, Lung, and Blood Institute (NHLBI). (2013d). *The seventh report of the Joint National Committee on Prevention, Detection, Evaluation, and Treatment of High Blood Pressure (JNC 7)*. Retrieved from http://www.nhlbi.nih.gov/guidelines/hypertension.

National Institute of Neurological Disorders and Stroke. (2013). *Transient ischemic attack information page*. Retrieved from http://www.ninds.nih.gov/disorders/tia/tia.htm.

National Library of Medicine. (2013). *Stroke*. Retrieved from http://www.nlm.nih.gov/medlineplus/stroke.html.

National Stroke Association. (2013a). *Am I at risk for a stroke?* Retrieved from http://www.stroke.org/site/PageServer?pagename=RISK.

National Stroke Association. (2013b). *Stroke treatment*. Retrieved from http://www.stroke.org/site/PageServer?pagename=treatment.

Norwitz, E,, Funai, E. (2015). Expectant management of preeclamsia with severe features. *UpToDate*. http://www.uptodate.com/contents/expectant-management-of-preeclampsia-with-severe-features?source=see_link.

Norwitz, E., Repke, J.T., (2015). Preeclampsia: Management and prognosis. *UpToDate*. http://www.uptodate.com/contents/preeclampsia-management-and-prognosis?source=search_result&search=magnesium+sulfate&selectedTitle=3%7E118.

O'Connor, R. E., Brady, W., Brooks, S. C., Diercks, D., Egan, J., Ghaemmaghani, C., . . . Yannopoulis, D. (2010). 2010 American Heart Association guidelines for cardiopulmonary resuscitation and emergency cardiovascular care science. Part 10: Acute coronary syndromes. *Circulation, 122*, 5787–5817. doi:10.1161/CIRCULATIONAHA.110.971028.

Office of Minority Health. (2010). *Heart disease and American Indians/Alaskan natives*. Retrieved from http://minorityhealth.hhs.gov/templates/content.aspx?ID=3025.

Perrin, K. O. & Macleod, C. E. (2012). Understanding the essentials of critical care nursing (2nd ed.). Upper Saddle River, NJ: Pearson Prentice Hall.

Porth, C. M. (2010). *Pathophysiology: Concepts of altered health states* (3rd ed.). Philadelphia, PA: Lippincott.

Porth, C. M., & Matfin, G. (2009). *Essentials of pathophysiology: Concepts of altered health states* (8th ed.). Philadelphia, PA: Lippincott Williams & Wilkins.

Ramaswamy, P., & Srinivasan, K. (2011). *Ventral septal defects*. Retrieved from http://emedicine.medscape.com/article/892980-overview.

Sliwa, K., Hilfiker-Keiner, D., Tetrie, M. C., Mebazza, A., Peiske, B., Buchman, E., . . . McMurray, J. J. (2010). Current state of knowledge on aetiology, diagnosis, management, and therapy of peripartum cardiomyopathy: A position statement from the Heart Failure Association of the European Society of Cardiology Working Group on peripartum cardiomyopathy. *European Journal of Heart Failure, 12*, 767–778. Retrieved from http://cdn.intechopen.com/pdfs/27268/InTech-Peripartum_cardiomyopathy_a_systematic_review.pdf.

Suppo de Souza Rugolo, L. M., Bentlin, M. R., & Trindade, C. E. (2011). Preeclampsia: Effect on the fetus and newborn. *NeoReviews, 12*, e198–e206. doi:10.1542/neo.12-4-e198.

Tierney, L. M., McPhee, S. J., & Papadakis, M. A. (2005). *Current medical diagnosis & treatment* (44th ed.). New York, NY: Lange Medical Books/McGraw-Hill.

Trelogan, S. (2011). *What is cardiomyopathy?* Retrieved from http://www.genetichealth.com/HD_What_is_Cardiomyopathy.shtml.

Uzan, J., Carbonnel, M., Piconne, O., Asmar, R., & Ayoubi, J. (2011). Pre-eclampsia: Pathophysiology, diagnosis, and management. *Vascular Health Risk Management, 7*, 467–474. doi:10.2147/VHRM.S20181.

Van der Rijken, R., Hulstijn-Dirkmaat, G., Kraaimaat, F., Nabuurs-Kohrman, L., Daniëls, O., & Maassen, B. (2009). Evidence of impaired neurocognitive functioning in school-age children awaiting cardiac surgery. *Developmental Medicine and Child Neurology, 52*(6), 552–558.

Woods, S. L., Froelicher, E. S., Motzer, S. A., & Bridges, E. (2010). *Cardiac nursing* (6th ed.). Philadelphia, PA: Lippincott.

Zafari, A. M., Reddy, S. V., Jeroudi, A. M., & Garas, S. M. (2013). *Myocardial infarction*. Retrieved from http://emedicine.medscape.com/article/article/155919.

17 Perioperative Care

◰ THE CONCEPT OF PERIOPERATIVE CARE

Perioperative is the term used to describe the three phases of surgical procedures: the preoperative phase, intraoperative phase, and postoperative phase. The **preoperative** phase is the phase preceding surgery in which the client is identified as a candidate for surgical or procedural intervention. During the preoperative phase, the client is assessed and prepared for surgery. Preoperative interventions include, but are not limited to, lab tests, medication administration, and physical assessment. The **intraoperative** phase is the actual surgical intervention phase. During the intraoperative phase, clients are often anesthetized, prepped, draped, and the surgical procedure takes place. If necessary, a tracheal tube is inserted (**intubation**). On completion of the surgery or procedure, after the client is stable and breathing effectively the client is prepared for the postoperative phase. The **postoperative** phase is the recovery phase. It begins when the client leaves the surgical suite and continues until the client meets all discharge criteria. Postoperative nursing care is tailored to meet the patient's specific needs. Considerations that shape postoperative care include the specific procedure performed and the patient's response to the procedure; the type of anesthetic administered and the patient's response to anesthesia; the patient's medical history; and any complications that develop during the postoperative period.

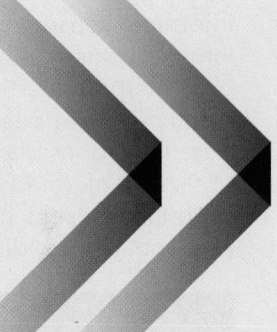

(continued on next page)

Concept Learning Outcomes

After reading about this concept, you will be able to:

1. Describe each perioperative phase.
2. Identify the various roles within each of the three perioperative phases.
3. Identify the nursing diagnoses within each perioperative phase.
4. Conduct a comprehensive client assessment within each perioperative phase.
5. Demonstrate an understanding of perioperative documentation.
6. Explain differences between surgical procedures.
7. Summarize the surgical impact of a client's related physiology and pathophysiology.
8. Demonstrate the nursing process in providing culturally competent and caring interventions across the life span for individuals undergoing a surgical procedure.

Concept Key Terms

Adhesions, *1258*

Allogeneic blood transfusion, *1270*

ASA Physical Status Classification System, *1266*

Autologous blood transfusion, *1270*

Extubation, *1256*

Hyperthermic, *1256*

Hypothermic, *1256*

Intraoperative, *1249*

Intubation, *1249*

Massive transfusion, *1252*

Malignant hyperthermia, *1271*

Normothermia, *1256*

Perioperative, *1249*

Postoperative, *1249*

Preoperative, *1249*

Time-out, *1251*

Universal protocol, *1251*

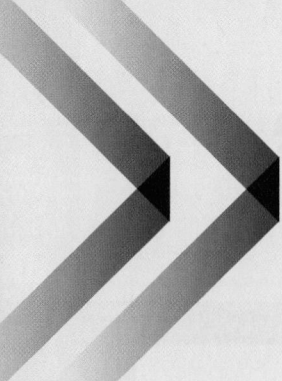

With the growth of outpatient surgical settings and other changes in the healthcare industry, nurses working in a variety of settings must be knowledgeable about perioperative care. For example, nurses working in dermatology offices are likely to assist with the removal of basal cell carcinomas, surgical procedures that generally involve local anesthesia. In pediatric offices, nurses may be required to provide nursing care for clients with minor wounds that require sutures. In medical-surgical units, nurses provide postoperative care to clients following a number of procedures. Labor and delivery nurses provide postoperative care for women who deliver via cesarean section. Because of its applicability across settings and across the life span and because of the risks involved, surgical nursing care carries a number of implications across concepts and exemplars. See the Concepts Related to Perioperative Care feature for examples. **<<**

Concepts Related to **Perioperative Care**

All surgical procedures require clients to provide informed consent. Children and adolescents require informed parental consent for most procedures and in all but emergent life-threatening situations. Although the healthcare provider who will be conducting the procedure is responsible for providing the information and obtaining informed consents, nurses are responsible for ensuring consent has been obtained, witnessing the appropriate individual signing the consent, and making sure all questions have been answered by appropriate personnel. Nurses also act to ensure that clients who do not speak English have been provided an interpreter and that these clients fully understand all aspects of the procedure, including their right to decline. Surgical procedures carry a risk for infection, and nurses work to lower this risk threshold by following infection control protocols and providing client teaching related to wound care and following discharge instructions.

CONCEPT	RELATIONSHIP TO PERIOPERATIVE CARE	NURSING IMPLICATIONS
Legal Issues		
■ Selected laws that affect nursing practice	Informed consent is required prior to surgical procedures.	■ Nurses must know the policies for informed consent in their place of employment as well as applicable federal and state laws.
Infection		
■ Healthcare-associated infections ■ Healthcare worker precautions ■ Sterile technique	Failure to follow proper safety protocols, including appropriate infection control measures, increases the client's risk for infection. Postoperative infections may occur as a result of improper wound care or healthcare-associated infections as a result of infection control protocols not being followed.	■ Nurses must follow infection control protocols. ■ Nurses providing postoperative care must provide excellent wound care. For clients who will care for their own wounds following discharge, discharge teaching must include wound care and return demonstrations confirming the client's ability to care for the wound.
Perfusion		
■ Perfusion assessment	Adequate perfusion enhances wound healing and perioperative recovery.	■ Perioperative nurses must be aware of blood transfusion policies at their place of employment. ■ Nurses must be aware of the client's hemodynamic status and understand the guidelines for transfusion.
Stress and Coping		
■ Assessment of stress and coping responses	Inadequate control of stress and coping mechanisms can prolong the perioperative healing process and a client's prognosis.	■ Perioperative care includes assessing client stress and coping mechanisms during the preoperative phase and reassessing following the procedure.

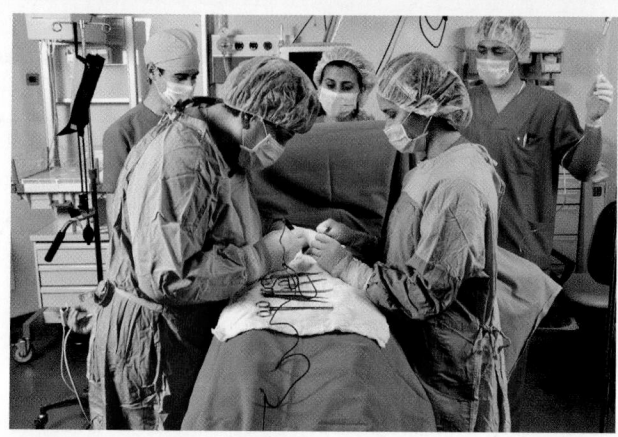

Figure 17–1 ● Surgical team in the OR.
Source: Levent Konuk/Shutterstock.

▶ INTRODUCTION TO PERIOPERATIVE NURSING

This module covers each surgical phase in the order in which the phases occur for the client, and includes a discussion of the documentation inclusive of the three phases of perioperative care. According to the Association of periOperative Registered Nurses (AORN) (2013), the perioperative documentation should include all steps of the nursing process, including assessment, diagnosis, identified outcome, planning, implementation, and evaluation.

The Interdisciplinary Team

The surgical client is cared for by an interdisciplinary team (**Figure 17–1** ●). For clients receiving anesthesia, this typically includes all of the disciplines below. It is the role of the team to assist the client back to health and to maintain client safety.

■ *Anesthesia personnel.* Delivers anesthesia during the procedure and continually monitors the client's physiological status. May be an anesthesiologist (medical doctor), certified registered nurse anesthetist (CRNA), or anesthesia assistant (AA).

■ *Circulating nurse.* Perioperative registered nurse who manages nursing care during the surgical procedure.

■ *Interpreter.* When the client's primary language is not English, an interpreter needs to be contacted. The interpreter gathers pertinent information in the preoperative phase and interprets information between the client and the nurse in the postoperative care phase.

■ *Scrub nurse.* Chooses and passes surgical instruments and supplies to the surgeon during the procedure.

■ *Preoperative nurse.* Cares for the client prior to the surgical event.

■ *Postoperative nurse.* Cares for the client after the surgical procedures.

■ *Radiology personnel.* Takes or evaluates radiological films or tests during operative or invasive procedures.

■ *Referral or specialty physician.* Specialists already caring for the client will play a role in the client's surgical care as appropriate by, for example, monitoring the client during the postoperative period in order to assist in attaining improved client outcomes.

■ *Respiratory therapist.* Assists in maintaining the client's airway and oxygen status as needed during the postoperative period.

■ *Social worker.* Assists in accessing resources for additional care of the client as an inpatient and/or outpatient. For example, if the client requires a walker to assist with mobility upon postoperative discharge, the social worker will work with the client's insurance company and the walker manufacturer to obtain the walker for the client.

■ *Surgeon.* Performs the surgical procedure.

■ *Surgical technician/first assistant.* Assists the surgeon with sterile handling of instruments and supplies during the procedure.

■ *Wound, ostomy, and continence nurse (WOCN).* Assists the client with effective wound healing.

■ *Additional disciplines.* Can include any healthcare staff from another area of the healthcare facility, such as cardiology, to complete additional testing throughout the perioperative phase. For example, an echocardiogram or an ultrasound of the cardiac system may be needed. Can also include clergy to provide spiritual/religious support to the family.

Perioperative Diagnostic Tests

Lab work is completed in the preoperative, intraoperative, and postoperative phases as needed. In all phases, the results of the blood work are analyzed by the nurse as well as the anesthesiologist and surgeon. Once analyzed, the interdisciplinary team communicates any concerns regarding abnormalities within the client's lab results. The ranges for each serum test differ depending on whether the client is female or male or an adult or pediatric client.

✳ *Go to* **nursing.pearsonhighered.com** *to see Appendix B for additional information about diagnostic tests including lab values.*

Additional diagnostic tests are ordered depending on the surgical procedure and client history, such as a pregnancy test, chest x-ray, or electrocardiogram (ECG) (**Table 17–1** ●).

Perioperative Safety Protocols and Precautions

Nurses and the interdisciplinary team engage in a variety of interventions to ensure the safety of the client throughout the perioperative phases, such as time-outs and medication preparation and administration. The Association of periOperative Registered Nurses (AORN), American Society of PeriAnesthesia Nurses (ASPAN), and the World Health Organization (WHO) have created guidelines and safe practice recommendations for the perioperative staff to utilize during the care of the perioperative client. In addition, the Joint Commission has established a **universal protocol**, guidelines for healthcare professionals that are designed to prevent errors during surgical procedures including wrong site surgery. Each of these organizations emphasizes the need for preprocedure verification (often termed a **time-out**) to ensure the correct procedure is being performed on the right site for the right client. Healthcare facilities take these guidelines and recommendations into account while creating protocols and policies for the perioperative staff to follow.

VERIFICATION/HAND-OFF REPORT A preprocedure verification process or hand-off report is performed in all three perioperative phases (**Table 17–2** ●). The length of the verification

TABLE 17–1 Perioperative Diagnostic Tests

DIAGNOSTIC TEST	IMPLICATION
Prothrombin time (PT)—time required for the client's plasma to clot	■ Due to bleeding risk, this can be the determining factor on whether the surgical procedure occurs.
Partial thromboplastin time (PTT)—time required for the client's blood to clot	
Bleeding time—time required for platelets to effectively stop bleeding; requires creation of a superficial skin wound	
Hematocrit (Hct)—measurement of the percentage of red blood cells in whole blood	■ Indications for transfusion of blood or blood products include substantial blood loss that causes a significant decrease in hemoglobin, hematocrit, and/or platelet count. In severe cases, a massive transfusion may be needed. A **massive transfusion** involves administration of a large volume of blood or blood products over a relatively short period of time.
Hemoglobin (Hgb)—measurement of hemoglobin, which is a protein found in red blood cells that binds and carries oxygen	
Red blood cells (RBC)—measurement of the red blood cells in the blood; red blood cells contain hemoglobin, which transports oxygen throughout the body	
Platelets—Assist in the formation of blood clots	

Sodium (Na⁺)—Regulates blood and body fluids, nerve impulses, muscle activity and metabolic functions in the body	■ Hyponatremia:
	    Nausea
	    Vomiting
	    Cramping
	    Edema
	    Muscle twitching
	    Signs of hypovolemia
	    Headache
	■ Hypernatremia:
	    Thirst
	    Orthostatic hypotension
	    Dry mouth and mucous membranes
	    Concentrated urine
	    Lethargy
	    Irritability
	    Fatigue
	See Table 17–10 for potential intraoperative complications.

Potassium (K⁺)—Plays an important role in muscle and nerve activity. Potassium also assists in the transfer of nutrients and waste in the cells.	■ Hypokalemia:
	    Abdominal distention
	    Loss of bowel sounds
	    Weakness
	    Severe arrhythmias
	■ Hyperkalemia:
	    Weakness
	    Nausea
	    Intestinal cramps
	    Diarrhea
	    Arrhythmias
	See Table 17–10 for potential intraoperative complications.

pH—test of the acidity or alkalinity of cells	■ The normal range of blood pH is 7.35 to 7.45.
pCO₂—measure of arterial CO_2 level ■ Decreased CO_2 = respiratory alkalosis. *Note:* Releasing too much CO_2 (hyperventilation), client is releasing too much CO_2; breathing too fast. ■ Increased CO_2 = respiratory acidosis. *Note:* Retaining too much CO_2 (hypoventilation), client is not expelling sufficient CO_2.	■ When the body attempts to compensate for a primary acid-base alteration, a secondary imbalance may occur. For example, respiratory acidosis (which is caused by an excess of CO_2) may lead to increased retention of bicarbonate (HCO_3^-) by the kidneys as the body attempts to bring the pH to a more alkaline state and restore homeostasis.
HCO₃— ■ Decreased HCO_3 = metabolic acidosis ■ Increased HCO_3 = metabolic alkalosis	

TABLE 17–1 Perioperative Diagnostic Tests (*continued*)

DIAGNOSTIC TEST	IMPLICATION
Human chorionic gonadotropin (HCG) or pregnancy test	■ A pregnancy test is usually performed in the preoperative setting on all women of childbearing age. Medications administered during the perioperative phases can be harmful to an unborn fetus because the effects on the mother are also transmitted to the fetus. Certain anesthetic medications may negatively affect fetal development. If a client is scheduled for an elective procedure, and the client is pregnant, the procedure may be cancelled. If the client is scheduled for an emergent procedure, the procedure typically will proceed, however, special precautions will be taken to decrease any side effects on the fetus. Special precautions may include the client undergoing the procedure with an anesthetic block instead of general anesthesia.
Chest x-ray	■ A chest x-ray is performed to assess for any respiratory problems, such as pneumonia. If a client has a respiratory infection, the infection could cause complications during anesthesia as well as the postoperative recovery period. The client ultimately may experience a longer hospital stay and unnecessary complications, such as a surgical site infection.
(Electrocardiogram) ECG—diagnostic test that evaluates the client's cardiac rhythm	■ A baseline ECG is conducted in the preoperative phase. If an abnormal rhythm is detected, consultation with a cardiology specialist, as well as medical treatment, may be required before the client can proceed with surgery.
Total protein—tests for albumin and globulin levels	■ Albumin levels are reflective of liver and kidney function. This is important because medications are excreted by the liver and kidneys. ■ Globulin determines whether the client is at a higher risk of acquiring an infection. Globulin transports nutrients in the blood which fight infection.
Blood glucose—a measurement of the blood glucose (sugar) level in the client's blood	■ Increased blood glucose may be indicative of diabetes. Clients with diabetes are at greater risk for poor wound healing.

TABLE 17–2 Preprocedure Verification Process/Hand-Off Report

PHASE	PARTICIPATING SURGICAL TEAM MEMBERS	PROCEDURE (CONTENT COVERED DURING PREPROCEDURE VERIFICATION PROCESS/HAND-OFF REPORT)
Preoperative	Preoperative nurse Circulating nurse Anesthesia team Interpreter if applicable	■ Correct client ■ Correct surgical procedure ■ Correct surgical site ■ Surgical site is marked by surgeon ■ Review of pertinent client history, including medications, allergies, health history, and abnormal labs.
Intraoperative	Entire surgical team	Prior to initial surgical incision, change in surgeon and/or change in position: ■ Name of client ■ Consented procedure ■ Allergies ■ Antibiotic administered ■ Any applicable implants, radiology records are present and in the room ■ Surgical prep is dry On conclusion of surgical procedure: ■ Name of client ■ Consented procedure and actual procedure completed match ■ All specimens acknowledged and approved by surgeon ■ Surgical instrument count correct
Postoperative	Postoperative (PACU) nurse Circulating nurse Anesthesia Interpretation services if applicable	■ Name of client ■ Surgical procedure completed ■ Surgical side (if applicable) ■ Review of pertinent client history, including medications, allergies, health history, and abnormal labs. ■ Drains ■ Implants placed ■ Inform of any complications during intraoperative phase

process or hand-off report is based on the history of the client and the content that needs to be covered. Preprocedure verification and hand-off reports are designed to prevent errors, including wrong client or wrong site surgery.

MEDICATIONS   On average, the hospitalized client can be subject to one or more medication errors daily (Institute of Medicine, 2006). Medication errors are costly: Approximately 1.5 million Americans are injured annually as a result of medication errors, at an estimated cost of $3.5 billion (Anderson & Townsend, 2010). Medication errors occur worldwide; however, only the reported or observed errors are noted within the data findings. Miscommunication or errors in labeling medication can result in incorrect dosages, which can result in adverse reactions and in medication being administered to the wrong client (Hicks, Wanzer, & Denholm, 2012). All staff should follow the **six rights** of safe medication practices:

1. Right client
2. Right medication
3. Right dose
4. Right time
5. Right route
6. Right documentation.

Note that Hicks and colleagues (Hicks et al., 2012) recommend a seventh right: right indication.

AORN (2013) and ASPAN (2012) created recommended practices and position statements to assist with client safety practices during medication preparation and administration for perioperative nurses to follow. AORN focuses on six phases of medication use: procuring, prescribing, dispensing, transcribing, administering, and monitoring. AORN recommendations include, but are not limited to, the perioperative nurse following the seven rights of medication administration, following clear and concise medication orders, and continually assessing the therapeutic and adverse effects of the medication being administered. According to ASPAN, additional guidelines the perioperative nurse should follow to ensure safe medication practices include adopting the two client identifier method during the preparation of the medication and prior to the administration of the medication, utilizing standard abbreviations if used by the healthcare facility, and restricting unnecessary noise or distractions during client care. These recommendations and guidelines should be followed by the perioperative nurse in all three perioperative phases.

> **SAFETY ALERT**
> The two client identifier method requires nurses and clinicians to identify the client and match the treatment to the client using two methods of identification. For example, a client wearing a wristband typically will have her or his name and a bar code or ID number on the wrist band. These two identifiers are compared to the medical order, which should match *both* identifiers.

Medications are ordered for clients based on health history including medication history, physical assessment, the systems involved in the surgical procedure, and the ongoing assessment of the client's needs throughout perioperative care. Common medications administered to clients receiving surgical procedures include antiemetics, analgesics, anxiolytics, antibiotics, and anesthetics (see the Medications feature).

Lifespan and Development Considerations

Perioperative care requires that nurses assess client needs related to lifespan and developmental considerations. For example, nurses assess the client's ability to understand the surgery and provide education according to developmental level that takes into consideration differences in learning style and abilities (see the Lifespan Considerations feature). Priorities for care include maintaining airway patency and tissue perfusion, monitoring the client's temperature and vital signs, and ensuring safe administration of medications.

PREOPERATIVE NURSING

Nursing care of the client undergoing a surgical procedure begins with communication, which is critical throughout the perioperative phases. Preoperative nursing care begins immediately when a client is notified of the need for surgery. Nurses employ therapeutic communication to educate the client about the upcoming procedure and to assess the client's health history and current physical status.

▶ PREPARING THE CLIENT

Preparing the client begins when the client is identified as needing surgery and includes any number of nursing interventions from client teaching to discharge planning. Nurses provide early client teaching and reinforce preoperative instructions related to:

- Nature and anticipated length of the procedure, including expectations related to recovery time. For example, a single mother who will need to be hospitalized overnight will need to make arrangements for her children to be cared for until she returns home.

- Whether or not to stop taking current medications in advance of the procedure.

- Communication with the surgical team prior to the procedure.

In the preoperative phase, when the client is alert and oriented, nurses provide client teaching regarding:

- Deep breathing and coughing exercises
- Surgical incision care
- Prevention of postoperative constipation
- Pain control
- Prevention of clot formation, with the application of thromboembolism-deterrent (TED) hose if appropriate.

Education continues through discharge. Some healthcare facilities offer clients classes on preparing for surgery (see Lifespan Considerations).

🔵 **Stay Current:** *The Mayo Clinic offers a 45-minute class called Preparing for Surgery for their clients:* **www.mayoclinic. org/patienteducation-rst/surgeryadults.html**.

Medications **Perioperative**

CLASSIFICATION AND DRUG EXAMPLES	MECHANISMS OF ACTION	NURSING CONSIDERATIONS
Antiemetic *Drug examples:* ■ metoclopramide hydrochloride (Reglan)	Antiemetic administered in the preoperative phase. Resting tone of esophageal sphincter and tone of the upper GI (Wilson, Shannon, & Shields, 2013). *May also be used for:* ■ Preventing nausea and vomiting associated with anesthesia postoperatively.	■ Monitor fluid and electrolytes. ■ Diarrhea is an adverse effect. ■ Monitor client cardiovascular status (for tachycardia and angina). *Administered in:* 1. Preoperative phase 2. Postoperative phase
Nonnarcotic Analgesics *Drug example:* ■ IV acetaminophen	Provides temporary analgesia for mild to moderate pain (Wilson et al., 2013). Decreases the client's pain level in the postoperative phase.	■ Monitor for signs and symptoms of hepatotoxicity. *Administered in:* 1. Preoperative phase 2. Postoperative phase
Antianxiety *Drug examples:* ■ midazolam (Versed) ■ diazepam (Valium)	Benzodiazepines: Produce CNS depression resulting in sedation, musculoskeletal relaxation, and anticonvulsant activity. Sedatives relax the client, but they do not relieve pain.	■ Monitor for adverse CNS effects (e.g., sedation). ■ Flumazenil (Romazicon) is used to reverse adverse effects of sedatives. ■ Complete baseline and periodic liver function tests. *Administered in:* 1. Preoperative phase 2. Intraoperative phase
Narcotic Analgesics *Drug examples:* ■ morphine sulfate ■ fentanyl ■ hydromorphone (Dilaudid)	Control of moderate to severe pain, but does not alter pain threshold. May be used for sedation and/or pain relief.	■ Can cause respiratory depression. ■ Naloxone hydrochloride (Narcan) reverses the effects of opiates, including respiratory depression, sedation, and hypotension (Wilson et al., 2013). *Administered in:* 1. Intraoperative phase 2. Postoperative phase
Sedative-Hypnotic Agents *Drug example:* ■ propofol (Diprivan)	Short acting; commonly used during induction and maintenance of anesthesia.	■ Propofol should be inspected prior to use for particulate matter, discoloration, or evidence of separation of the emulsion. ■ Unused propofol should be discarded within 6 hours of filling the syringe or 12 hours after spiking a large volume for infusion. ■ No reversal agent. *Administered in:* 1. Intraoperative phase
Antibiotics ■ aminoglycosides ■ macrolides ■ tetracyclines ■ cephalosporins ■ penicillins ■ sulfonamides ■ fluoroquinolones *Drug examples:* ■ penicillin ■ vancomycin ■ levofloxacin (Levaquin)	Decreases the risk for surgical site infections (SSIs).	■ Monitor for signs of allergic reaction. ■ Assess renal and hepatic function and vital signs. *Administered in:* 1. Preoperative phase 2. Intraoperative phase 3. Postoperative phase

Lifespan Considerations Perioperative

Pediatric

For all clients under the age of 18:

- Maintaining **normothermia** (normal temperature) can be difficult. Monitor and maintain the client's temperature to determine which actions need to be taken if the client is **hyperthermic** (temperature above 37.8°C [100°F]) or **hypothermic** (temperature below 36.1°C [97°F]).
- Assess the client's developmental level and understanding of surgery.
- Educate the client according to developmental level and most beneficial learning style for the individual.
- Depending on developmental level and age of client, include the family as much as possible in perioperative care plan.
- Identify proper electrocautery pad size for the client prior to transporting the client to surgery.
- Continuously monitor airway patency, and be alert to signs and symptoms of respiratory distress, including after **extubation** (withdrawal of the breathing tube on completion of anesthesia and the surgical case).
- Teenagers may emerge from anesthesia very anxious, hyperactive, combative, and vocal. The perioperative team must be prepared to implement additional safety measures as needed to protect the client from injury, including falls or dislodged intravenous devices, and to promote safe emergence from anesthesia.
- To promote safety, pediatric clients may be assigned a one-to-one perioperative nurse ratio. Younger clients may bring a comfort item, such as a stuffed animal or blanket. If the client is unable to get comfortable in any of the perioperative phases, including prior to induction in the intraoperative phase, the client's parent or caregiver may be allowed to sit with the client, especially if the client becomes agitated and disruptive.

Older Adults

For all adults ages 65 and older:

- Dementia, confusion, risk for falls, and depression need to be considered with older surgical clients (Hilsgen, 2013).
- The older adult is at a higher risk for acquiring a surgical site infection.
- Maintaining normothermia is challenging.
- A skin assessment is essential. The perioperative team must take special precautions in removing adhesives from the older adult client's skin to prevent tearing of the skin.
- Special care needs to be taken to prevent the formation of pressure sores.
- The geriatric client is at higher risk for developing a venous thromboembolism (VTE).
- Deep breathing and coughing education starts in the preoperative phase. Deep breathing and coughing assists in the prevention of pneumonia and other respiratory conditions related to surgery. (See the module on Oxygenation for a discussion of deep breathing exercises and a client teaching feature on effective coughing techniques.)
- Preexisting conditions related to the normal aging process can result in perioperative complications in the older surgical client (Bashaw & Scott, 2012).

Preparing the client for a surgical procedure often calls for the client to participate in preparations that are specific to the surgery being performed, the site of the surgery, and the postoperative recovery. For example, abdominal or pelvic surgical procedures may require bowel preps, which are completed by the client the day prior to surgery. Bowel cleansing allows the surgeon to have a better view of the client's intestines in procedures such as a colonoscopy. This allows for better visualization of the inner lining of the intestines, which assists in diagnosing abnormalities, such as a polyp.

The preoperative nurse reviews all surgical documents such as the surgical consent form with the client in preparation for surgery. If the patient has questions about the scheduled surgical procedure, the nurse should notify the surgeon that additional information is needed by the client. The preoperative phase also provides time for the preoperative nurse to establish a level of trust and confidence with the client, which will help ease anxiety and carry forward through the other perioperative phases.

Lifespan Considerations Preparing the Pediatric Client

Nurses preparing children for surgery consider the child's developmental level when communicating information. For hospitalized children, nurses understand that the child's hospital room needs to be a non-threatening place, and in many cases procedures such as drawing blood or starting an IV are performed in a treatment or procedure room rather than in the client's hospital room.

Surgical procedures create stress for both the pediatric client and family members. Preoperative assessment includes assessing stress and coping skills and being cognizant of fear. Nurses should be honest, especially regarding expectations about postoperative pain and how the care team is ready to respond and treat pain.

⊙ *Stay Current: Many pediatric hospitals have information on their Web sites, including lists of books that can help families prepare for a child's surgery. For example, see the Web site of the Children's Hospital of Philadelphia:* **www.chop.edu/healthinfo/preparing-the-preschooler-for-surgery.html**

► ASSESSMENT

Accurate and complete preoperative assessment is critical to ensuring clients achieve good outcomes during and following the surgical procedure.

Data Collection

During the preoperative phase, the nurse gathers important data regarding the client's health history and current physical status (**Table 17–3 ●**). Assessment information gathered during the preoperative phase informs the plan of care that is implemented in the preoperative area and continues to inform the care plan through the intraoperative and postoperative phases. Vital signs, including blood pressure, pulse, respiration, and oxygen saturation, are obtained throughout the perioperative period with the baseline vital signs obtained during the preoperative phase.

Physical Assessment

The surgeon is responsible for completing a full physical assessment on the client in the immediate preoperative period. Any component of a physical assessment is reassessed any time there is an apparent change from the client's baseline. Depending on the surgical procedure, a focused assessment is completed on the specific system(s) involved in the procedure. Baseline assessment data serves to provide a background for nurses to discern physiological changes during the perioperative period, but additional focused diagnostic testing may include a capillary blood glucose (CBG) test for clients who have been previously diagnosed with diabetes (see Table 17–1).

Psychosocial Assessment

Psychosocial assessment of the client includes gathering information about the client's current levels of stress and coping mechanisms. For clients needing assistance with postoperative care following discharge, the nurse will assess the presence of competent help and the degree to which the caregiver is able to provide client support. When working with older adults, ensure that cognitive function is sufficient to participate in informed consent. Nurses should follow their agency's guidelines for clients who disclose that they are in an abusive situation at home (**Box 17–1 ●**).

Questions to ask the client as part of the psychosocial assessment that directly relate to surgery include the following:

- I have some questions I will need to review with you as part of our perioperative assessment. Would you like for us to go through the questions by ourselves or would you like your family member present?
- How are you feeling about the surgical procedure?
- Do you feel safe in your home environment?
- Do you have any concerns you would like to address? For example, financial?
- Do you have any cultural beliefs that the healthcare team needs to take into account while creating your perioperative plan of care?
- Do you have anyone who can assist you with daily routine care, such as bathing and preparation of food, upon discharge?

Box 17–1 Assessing for Abuse

During the perioperative phases there are multiple opportunities to assess and determine if a client is being abused. For example, a thorough perioperative skin assessment provides an opportunity for the perioperative nurse to use critical thinking skills and determine if a bruise pattern on the client and comments made by the client require further assessment to determine any potential abuse at home. Clients often do not want to verbalize or admit to abuse, but the nurse is required to follow the healthcare organization's protocol on abuse when the nurse determines abuse is present. This is critical because abuse affects the plan of care for the client through all perioperative phases. For example, if a client is being abused, he may present with additional fears of being injured or harmed during surgery, because fears of injury and harm become "normal" for the abuse victim. The client may not trust that the healthcare team will be respectful and treat him with care throughout the perioperative phase. Also, discharge planning begins in the preoperative phase and continues until the client is discharged.

If an abuse situation is missed and the client is discharged home, there is a very good chance the client may return to the hospital through the emergency department with complications, such as a surgical site infection. An infection may occur if the client does not receive assistance with care from the abusive caregiver. See the module on Violence for detailed discussions of interpersonal violence and abuse.

Many clients preparing to undergo surgery are concerned about their appearance. Older clients are often reluctant to part with wigs or hairpieces. Clients with limited mobility may be anxious about parting with prostheses or assistive devices. Reassure these clients by giving these important items to a family member who will return the item following surgery.

Nutritional Assessment

A client's nutritional assessment will determine certain outcomes during and after surgery, including postoperative healing of the surgical wound. For example, clients with a high body mass index (BMI) are at increased risk for poor wound healing and surgical site infection. Perioperative nutritional assessment includes weight, BMI, food preferences, and total protein serum levels.

Pain Assessment

Assessment of the client's pain begins in the preoperative phase and continues throughout all perioperative phases. The pain assessment scale is based on the client's age, maturity level, and basic understanding of the question being asked. For example, a mature 12-year-old client could use the numerical pain scale (1–10, with 1 = little to no pain and 10 = the maximum pain intensity), instead of the Wong-Baker FACES Pain Rating Scale. (See the module on Comfort for a full discussion of pain rating scales.) Also, a client with a primary language other than English may find it easier to understand the facial pain scale.

Client Medication Review

Prescription medications are any medications that are prescribed by a licensed healthcare provider and dispensed

TABLE 17–3   Essential Preoperative Assessment Data Collection

ASSESSMENT DATA	NURSING IMPLICATIONS
Allergies	■ Prior to transporting the client to surgery, the preoperative nurse confirms all client allergies with the client and updates the preoperative documentation accordingly, including adding any allergies not listed or deleting incorrect allergy information.
Previous surgeries: any invasive procedure for the client	The nurse reviews all previous surgeries with the client to determine: ■ The presence of any metal implants in the client, which is important information when using electrocautery ■ The presence of **adhesions** (scar tissue) from previous surgeries ■ Helpful information, such as client history of being combative or nauseous when waking up from anesthesia.
Personal or family history with anesthesia	■ The nurse assesses personal and family history regarding anesthesia to determine client risk of presenting with malignant hyperthermia, allergies, or any adverse events.
Hearing aids, glasses, and contact lenses	■ Contact lenses are removed to prevent any potential damage to the eyes during surgery. ■ If the client is wearing a hearing aid or has an implanted hearing aid such as a cochlear implant, the circulating nurse needs to be alerted. Electrosurgical units can deactivate hearing aids.
Loose teeth, crowns, caps, dentures, etc.	■ The surgical team must be notified if the client has any loose teeth, cracks, crowns, and/or caps for liability reasons as well as client safety.
NPO status (The client has to be NPO or have nothing to eat or drink by mouth 8 hours prior to surgery. These instructions vary for infants and very young children.)	■ If the client has had anything to eat or drink within 8 hours prior to surgery, the surgical procedure may be cancelled, especially if the surgery is elective. ■ Eating or drinking anything other than clear liquids within the 8 hours prior to surgery increases the client's risk of aspiration. ■ If the procedure is an emergency case, appropriate steps are taken to prevent complications such as aspiration.
Retained hardware or metal	■ To prevent client injury, including burns, any metal on the client, including all jewelry, needs to be removed in the preoperative setting. ■ The nurse conducting the assessment also alerts the intraoperative team to the presence of any metal implants inside the client, such as a metal rod or pin placed as part of orthopedic repair of a bone. ■ Assess older adult males for implanted penile prosthesis, due to increased risk for injury during urinary catheterization.
Venous thromboembolism (VTE) assessment/prophylaxis	■ The preoperative nurse should assess the client for a history of VTEs. Certain factors may place the client at higher risk for VTEs such as a surgical procedure that lasts 30 minutes or longer. ■ Longer procedures can cause stasis or slowing of the blood, which can cause a VTE or emboli to form. For this reason, the client falls into the high-risk category. Pharmacologic and/or mechanical prophylaxis can be ordered by the physician. ■ Pharmacologic prophylaxis, such as heparin or Lovenox, interferes with coagulation and helps prevent stasis and emboli creation. ■ Mechanical prophylaxes, such as sequential hose, intermittently squeeze the leg, enhancing circulation.
Cultural assessment	■ Perioperative nurses should be aware of cultural differences among the client populations at their healthcare facility, including assessment of cultural beliefs and practices that may impact the client postoperatively. (See the module on Culture and Diversity for more information.) For example, many Jehovah's Witness clients, due to their beliefs, do not receive blood, even if it is a lifesaving measure. Some Jehovah's Witness clients consent to receiving only autologous blood. The perioperative nurse needs to understand and support this belief. Therefore, when the nurse presents the Jehovah's Witness client with the blood consent form to sign, the nurse cannot try to persuade the client. ■ Depending on the generation of the client, cultural conflicts can arise. For example, some older adults may agree with the surgical staff and do as instructed regardless of whether or not they understand the procedure or agree with the surgical staff. ■ In patriarchal cultures, the husband speaks for his wife even if she is the client. In this scenario, the surgical team needs to be aware of the client's culture in order to distinguish if the husband is speaking related to his cultural role in the family, or if there is a possibility that the relationship is abusive, with the husband exerting control over his wife's decisions.

TABLE 17–3   Essential Preoperative Assessment Data Collection (*continued*)

ASSESSMENT DATA	NURSING IMPLICATIONS
Communication assessment	■ It is imperative for the client to understand the questions being asked and to answer to the best of his or her ability. If English is not the client's primary language, the perioperative nurse is required to ask for assistance from a trained interpreter who speaks the client's primary language. If an interpreter is not available, the hospital should provide interpretation via telephone or the Internet. ■ If the client's family is present and they do not speak English, the nurse also is required to obtain assistance to communicate with the family. This is required for all age groups. ■ The perioperative nurse should not allow a family member to interpret for the client due to the risk of incorrect or incomplete translation, which could lead to the client not having all of the required information necessary for surgery. ■ Age and developmental characteristics also influence communication with the client and family (see the modules on Communication and Development).
Drug and alcohol assessment	■ Drug and alcohol use can require an increased amount of anesthetic medications to be utilized. ■ Clients who abuse drugs and alcohol may present with signs and symptoms of withdrawal in the postoperative setting. The postoperative nurse must be able to identify and assess for signs/symptoms of withdrawal.

by a pharmacy. The preoperative nurse documents the prescription medications the client is taking, including the last dose and time the medication was administered. Examples of high-alert drugs for perioperative clients include beta-blockers, which affect blood pressure, and anticoagulant medications such as Coumadin, which place the client at risk for bleeding. In addition, medication delivered by skin patches, such as nicotine, estrogen, or fentanyl, must also be documented.

Over-the-counter (OTC) medications are any medication (e.g., vitamin E, ibuprofen, and aspirin) that the client can obtain without a prescription. OTC medications are evaluated to assess if the client is at risk for any complications during surgery. Clients are instructed, if indicated, to stop taking any medication or supplement that can place the client at a bleeding risk prior to surgery.

Herbal products include teas, dietary supplements, and some cosmetics, and can cause serious complications during surgery. For example, ginseng can increase the client's level of nausea and can increase or decrease blood pressure. Nurses should inquire about ginseng and use of any other supplements that can cause complications during surgery.

▶ INFORMED CONSENT

A client is required to give informed consent prior to any surgical procedure. The nurse's role in informed consent is to verify the surgeon or healthcare provider has discussed the surgical procedure with the client and has obtained the client's signature on the informed consent form. Informed consent is required for the procedure itself, but also for administration of anesthesia and blood products. In addition, the client is required to consent to financial responsibility for the procedure, to any photos or video to be taken, and to additional activities such as additional personnel being present in the room during the

procedure. See the module on Legal Issues for more information regarding informed consent.

▶ PREOPERATIVE NURSING DIAGNOSES

Once the preoperative assessment is complete, the nurse begins creating the preoperative care plan. Some preoperative diagnoses include, but are not limited to, the following:

■ *Anticipatory Grieving* related to impending surgery
■ *Anxiety* related to the unknown
■ *Knowledge Deficit* related to surgical experiences.

(NANDA-I © 2012)

The nursing plan of care is based on the nursing assessment and diagnoses and will incorporate orders from the surgeon as well as care considerations for the client's family.

▶ PREPARING THE SURGICAL SITE

The preoperative nurse either oversees or assists with preparation of the surgical site. According to AORN (2013) and the Centers for Disease Control and Prevention (CDC) (2013), site preparation is time sensitive. For example, clipping a client's hair around the surgical site the morning of surgery (as opposed to the day before) has been shown to result in fewer surgical site infections (SSIs). See **Table 17–4** ● for an overview of surgical site preparation.

▶ PREOPERATIVE INTERVENTIONS

Preoperative nursing interventions assist in preparing the client for surgery and can save valuable time and improve client outcomes following surgery. While the client is waiting for surgery,

TABLE 17–4   Preoperative Surgical Site Preparation

TYPE OF PREPARATION	EXPLANATION
Clipping of client's hair	■ Recommended practices for preoperative client skin antisepsis: Hair at the surgical site should not be removed whenever possible. However, if necessary, the client's hair should be clipped in the preoperative setting in order to decrease the amount of hair contaminating the field. In some circumstances (e.g., gynecological procedures) the client's surgical site area is clipped during the intraoperative phase. ■ Hair is clipped with electric clippers (not shaved) immediately before the procedure.
Cast removal	■ The client's cast should be removed in the preoperative setting in order to decrease the amount of dust contaminating the surgical arena.
Showers the day prior to surgery	■ Clients undergoing open class I surgical procedures below the chin should complete two preoperative showers with chlorhexidine gluconate (CHG) before surgery. When appropriate, the surgeon will instruct the client accordingly in the physician's office. ■ Preoperative showers help remove microorganisms from the skin. ■ Cleaning with a special soap before surgery can assist in the prevention of SSIs.

Sources: Based on Association of periOperative Registered Nurses (2013). *Perioperative standards and recommended practices.* Denver, CO: Author; Centers for Disease Control and Prevention. (2011). *Having surgery? What should you know before you go?* Retrieved from http://www.cdc.gov/features/safesurgery; Kamel, C., McGahan, L., Polisena, J., Mierzwinski, M., & Embil, J. M. (2012). Preoperative skin antiseptic preparations for preventing surgical site infections. *Infection Control and Hospital Epidemiology, 33*(6), 608–617.

the nurse can provide essential client teaching related to postoperative care and expectations (see the Lifespan Considerations feature). Depending on the surgical procedure, the preoperative nurse may:

■ Implement medical orders, such as starting an IV, administering insulin, inserting a nasogastric tube, or applying TED hose (see the *Companion Skills Manual*).

■ Provide distraction techniques (e.g., music, television, or games) and other psychosocial interventions.

■ Provide skills training (e.g., deep breathing, coughing, splinting incisions with a pillow).

■ Inform family members of where they can wait during the surgery and when they will be informed of the client's status.

Information gathered during the preoperative assessment is documented according to agency protocol and is used as the baseline for care of the client (see **Box 17–2 ●**).

CASE STUDY \\ A

William Marstellar is a 2-year-old, African American male who is scheduled to undergo left tympanoplasty and adenoidectomy. He has had chronic otitis media with perforation of tympanic membrane. His mother and father are very anxious and tearful about him undergoing anesthesia. While taking the family history, you learn that William's father had an uncle die while having his appendix removed approximately 20 years ago. There is also a family history of sickle cell disease. William's vital signs are within normal limits; his lab work indicates his WBC count is 14,000. His mother tells you that he just drank some apple juice 6 hours ago.

Critical Thinking Questions Level I

1. What are your next steps?
2. What additional assessment data would it be helpful to have at this time? Why?

Lifespan Considerations Preoperative Assessment and Teaching for Older Adults

■ Assess hearing. Make sure the client can hear the information to be presented or provide information through alternative means.

■ Reinforce teaching related to moving, deep breathing, and coughing exercises. Older adults are at greater risk for pneumonia and other postoperative complications.

■ Assess and initiate plans for care following discharge. This includes arranging for necessary medical equipment (e.g., walkers, raised toilet seats), help with transportation, or extended care.

■ Assess for risks for pressure ulcers, for example, poor nutritional status, diabetes or cardiovascular illness, history of steroid use (which increases bruising, skin breakdown).

Box 17–2   Preoperative Documentation

Preoperative documentation includes, but is not limited to, the following:

1. History and physical
2. Social assessment
3. Nutritional assessment
4. Systems assessment
   a. Integumentary
   b. Neurological
   c. Cardiovascular
   d. Respiratory
   e. Gastrointestinal/abdominal
   f. Musculoskeletal
5. Pain assessment
6. Medication review
7. Medications administered in the preoperative setting
8. Perioperative care plan.

Critical Thinking Questions Level II

3. Would your "next steps" change if William's temperature were 38.3°C (101°F)? If so, how?

4. *Referring to the module on Development,* how would you explain the surgery to William? How would your strategies differ for a 7- or 8-year-old?

INTRAOPERATIVE NURSING

Intraoperative nursing includes all aspects of a surgical or invasive procedure, within the operating or procedure room. Constant monitoring of both the surgical environment and the client is necessary to ensure client safety. The intraoperative environment is a high-risk area, carrying high risk for infection, surgical errors, wrong site surgery, retained instruments, burns, and incorrect specimen labeling.

▶ INTRAOPERATIVE NURSING DIAGNOSES

The intraoperative nursing diagnoses are created after the intraoperative assessment but before the intraoperative planning. The intraoperative diagnoses may include, but are not limited to, the following:

- *Risk for Infection* related to hypothermia, break in skin integrity or decreased nutritional status

- *Anxiety* related to loss of control during induction of anesthesia

- *Risk for Deficient Fluid Volume* related to blood loss during surgery and NPO status

- *Risk for Injury* related to intubation and extubation during anesthesia, surgical burns, foreign body retention, or incorrect client positioning

- *Risk for Electrolyte Imbalance* related to anesthetic agents

- *Ineffective Breathing Pattern* related to anesthetic agents.

(NANDA-I © 2012)

▶ TYPES OF SURGICAL PROCEDURES

Surgical procedures may be *open*, such as an abdominal hysterectomy, or *laparoscopic*, such as a laparoscopic hysterectomy. Closed procedures, such as closed reduction of a bone fracture, require no incision. Surgical procedures may be performed for a variety of reasons (see **Box 17–3** ●).

Laparoscopic procedures usually include three small incisions approximately 1 cm in size to allow for insertion of thin surgical instruments into the client's body. A laparoscope allows for visualization of internal body structures through use of a tiny video camera that transmits images to a monitor. Other instruments may be inserted for various purposes, including manipulating organs for exploration of the site, removing tissue, or cauterizing blood vessels. Laparoscopic surgeries are less invasive than open surgeries and usually require a shorter hospital stay and recovery. Also, due to the

---

Box 17–3   Types of Surgical Procedures

The various surgical procedures may be open or laparoscopic, depending on the purpose of the procedure:

-ectomy—This suffix indicates removal of an organ. For example, in a hysterectomy, the client's uterus is removed.

-oscopy—This suffix indicates an organ or body part is being viewed. In a hysteroscopy, the client's uterus is being viewed. This type of procedure typically is used for diagnostic purposes.

Reconstructive surgery may be performed to restore lost or reduced appearance or function. Facial reconstruction following a motor vehicle crash is an example of constructive surgery.

Diagnostic procedures are conducted to determine or confirm a diagnosis. A biopsy of a mass is an example of a diagnostic procedure.

Elective surgery is a procedure that is the recommended treatment for a condition that is not life threatening. Hip replacement surgery is an example of an elective surgery.

Emergency surgery is performed when a condition creates the risk of loss of life or limb. Surgery to control internal hemorrhage is an example of emergency surgery.

Palliative surgery may be performed to alleviate pain or symptoms associated with a disease. Palliative surgery does not cure or stop the course of the disease.

Transplant surgery replaces malfunctioning organs or other structures.

---

small incision sites the client is at a lower risk for acquiring a surgical site infection (SSI) and experiences less blood loss. Surgeons have the option to convert to an open procedure from a laparoscopic procedure depending on the initial findings under laparoscope. For example, an extensive amount of scar tissue and adhesions can impair laparascopic visualization of the surgical site, making it necessary to convert to an open procedure.

Open surgical cases are procedures for which a surgical incision is required. Open procedures usually require a longer hospital stay and longer recovery period. Open procedures also place the client at a higher risk for blood loss. Larger incisions place the client at a higher risk for complications, such as hypothermia and SSIs.

▶ LENGTH OF SURGICAL PROCEDURE

Longer procedure times are associated with an increased risk for complications. Shorter procedures benefit clients of all ages: Less exposure time decreases the risk for physiological complications and reduces the time required for healing. Generally speaking, the longer the procedure:

- The longer the client is exposed to anesthesia, which may lengthen recovery time and increase the risk for complications.

- The greater the client's risk of hypothermia, which can increase the time required for healing and increases the risk for venous thromboembolism (VTE). It is imperative for the client to maintain normothermia.

- Procedures lasting 30 minutes or longer may call for clients to wear SCDs (mechanical method used to prevent VTE).

Review the VTE prophylaxis guidelines or parameters, including pharmacologic and mechanical prophylaxis, at your healthcare facility.

- The greater the risk for blood loss that may necessitate a blood transfusion, either intraoperatively or on admission to the medical unit.

▶ STERILE FIELD AND HAND WASHING

The sterile field consists of the area utilized for the procedure and is handled only by intraoperative personnel who have completed the required hand scrub according to their healthcare facility's surgical hand scrub guidelines or policy. Many facilities follow the "Recommended Practices for Sterile Technique" which is outlined in the AORN guidelines (2013). AORN recommends a 3- to 5-minute surgical hand scrub take place prior to donning sterile gloves to reduce the microorganisms on the skin of personnel involved in the procedure. In addition, hand washing should be completed at various times, such as on completion of the case and when surgical gloves are removed; before and after eating and using the restroom; when hands are visibly soiled; and before and after caring for clients (AORN, 2013). See the module on Infection for more information on hand washing and preventing infection in the clinical setting.

▶ DURING SURGERY

The nurse's responsibilities during surgery will vary according to the nature of the procedure and the composition of the surgical team. At all times, nurses act to promote the physiological health of the client by guarding against infection and preventing potential complications, including but not limited to complications during positioning of the client, SSIs, and hypothermia.

Continuous Surveillance

Within the intraoperative setting the perioperative nurse is required to maintain continuous surveillance. A perioperative nurse becomes responsible for the senses temporarily lost by the client during surgery, such as sight and hearing. Nurses are taught that they are client advocates. In the operating room, the client is unconscious and the circulating nurse becomes the protector of that client. The perioperative nurse needs to have self-confidence, which comes with experience, in order to be comfortable being the spokesperson for the client. Also with experience, the nurse will learn the sounds of the operating room, for example, the anesthesia monitors and the conversations between the anesthesia team and the surgeon. Nurses learn by experience to recognize changes in the client's heart rhythm, a change in blood pressure, or even a drop in oxygen saturation. The circulating nurse vigilantly monitors intraoperative events, including the client's volume of blood loss, as well as other safety-related concerns. The learning of these skills begins in nursing school and is built on as the nurse gains experience.

Intraoperative Safety Precautions

The intraoperative phase includes many dangerous combinations for both the client and the healthcare team. For example, if a combustible skin cleansing solution comes in contact with a spark from an electrosurgical unit and high-flowing oxygen, there is a very good chance a surgical fire may be ignited; this could result in burns, possibly severe ones, to the client or to the surgical team. See **Table 17–5** ● for specific safety precautions that must be followed during the intraoperative phase.

SAFETY ALERT
During surgical procedures, an electrosurgery machine that uses electrical current for cutting or cauterization is often used. During the preoperative nursing assessment, the nurse inquires if the client has any metal in her or his body. If so, the surgical nurse needs to be alerted, due to the risk for injury to the client if the electrical current comes in contact with implanted metal.

Positioning

Intraoperatively, clients are positioned for access to the surgical site (see **Table 17–6** ●). Joints, nerves and skin must be protected during movement and final positioning. Typically, padding is used under pressure points to prevent nerve injuries and protect the skin. Positioning the client correctly is extremely important for the safety of the client. For example, the brachial plexus can be damaged if the arm is not positioned correctly:

- When positioning the client in the prone position, the intraoperative nurse has to rotate the arm with the natural flow of the arm or the client's shoulder can be dislocated.

- When placing a client in the lithotomy position, both legs need to be lifted and positioned in the stirrups at the same time or the client's hips can potentially be dislocated.

- Depending on the procedure the surgical bed may have to be placed in a specific position. For example, for a gynecology procedure, the client is placed in the lithotomy position, but the bed is placed in the gynecological position. This allows the client's buttocks to be specifically placed at an opening in the bed and the bottom section of the surgical bed to be lowered or removed once the client's legs are placed in the stirrups, for easier access to the operative site.

William Marstellar (Case Study A on page 1260), will be placed in the supine position with his arms tucked (see Table 17–6) for his left tympanoplasty and adenoidectomy procedure. A tympanoplasty and adenoidectomy are considered ear, nose, and throat (ENT) procedures; therefore, the bed will be placed in an ENT position. An ENT position is when the client remains supine, but the entire bed is turned so that the client's head is directly accessible to the surgeon and the client's feet are positioned by the anesthesia provider. The bed is placed in this position to allow the ENT surgeon easier access to the client, easy placement for a portable x-ray to be taken, and placement of the microscope.

TABLE 17–5 Intraoperative Safety Precautions

PROCEDURE	NURSING IMPLICATIONS	NOTES

Electrosurgery—an electrical method used to cut and cauterize tissue	■ Always follow manufacturer guidelines.
	■ The combination of alcohol-based preps, oxygen, and electrosurgery creates an ideal environment for surgical fires, increasing the risk for client burns. The surgical team must ensure that the surgical prep is dry prior to draping.
	■ The appropriate electrosurgery pad size (e.g., pediatric or adult) must be obtained for the client.
	■ The preferred site for the electrosurgery pad is an area of large muscle or fat tissue.
	■ The pad should be placed as close to the surgical site as possible.
	■ The pad should never be placed in the following locations:
	  a. Over metal implants
	  b. Over tattoos or scars
	  c. Over skin that is not intact, (e.g., abrasions, burns).
	■ Any metal on the client, including all jewelry, hearing aids, and eyeglasses, needs to be removed in the preoperative setting.
	■ If the client is either wearing a hearing aid or has an implanted hearing aid such as a cochlear implant, the circulating nurse needs to be alerted. Electrosurgical units can deactivate hearing aids.
		■ There are two types of electrosurgery handpieces:
		Bipolar: The electrical current flows between the two points on the handpiece.
		Monopolar: The current is able to flow through the client.
		■ If the client has a pacemaker, the surgical team should use a bipolar handpiece if possible and refer to the facility's pacemaker guidelines during surgical procedures if applicable.
		■ When the pad is removed, the circulating nurse must assess the site for any changes from the client's baseline skin assessment (e.g., burns, abrasions).

Light amplification by stimulated emission of electromagnetic radiation (LASER)—a method used to cut body structures (e.g., tissue, kidney stones) Healthcare lasers are defined according to their relative hazard and the appropriate controls. Class 3 and 4 lasers are primarily used in healthcare organizations. Class 4 lasers are hazardous to the eyes and skin and can also cause fires; Class 3 lasers are hazardous under direct contact or exposure through reflection of a beam off of a reflective source, such as a mirror (AORN, 2013).	■ Always follow manufacturer guidelines. ■ Wear laser-approved protective goggles. ■ Place laser-approved protective goggles on the client. ■ Cover all windows and reflective surfaces with towel.	■ Lasers can damage the lens of the eye and cause sight damage. ■ Laser beams can go through windows and injure staff outside the operative room. Laser beams can also bounce off of reflective surfaces, causing fires and/or damage to staff's eyesight. ■ A laser safety officer (LSO) should be appointed as part of a laser safety program implemented by the healthcare organization administrators to monitor and oversee the control of laser hazards (AORN, 2013).
Pneumatic tourniquet—a method used to obliterate circulation to an extremity (e.g., circulation to the knee during a total knee replacement)	■ Always follow manufacturer guidelines. ■ Complete a baseline skin assessment on the site prior to placing the tourniquet. ■ Always pad under the tourniquet prior to securing. ■ Use an appropriately sized tourniquet on the client. ■ Follow the guidelines for the length of time the tourniquet is to be inflated. ■ Document the times when the tourniquet is inflated and deflated.	
Radiology—a method used to take intraoperative photos or accomplish surgical placement of radiation for oncology clients	■ Always follow manufacturer guidelines.	■ Perioperative staff must make sure they place lead shields to cover their bodies, including ovaries for women and testicles for men, because radiation can cause sterility. The staff should also wear a neck shield to protect the thyroid gland. ■ Staff should request a radiometer from their facility to measure their dose of radiation exposure.

(continued on next page)

TABLE 17–5   Intraoperative Safety Precautions (*continued*)

PROCEDURE	NURSING IMPLICATIONS	NOTES
Chemicals *Preps*—specific chemicals that are applied to a surgical site prior to incision to decrease the amount of pathogens on the skin surface and to decrease the chance of an SSI *Chemotherapy agents*—chemicals used in intraoperative oncology cases (e.g., hyperthermic intraperitoneal chemotherapy)	■ Always follow manufacturer guidelines because procedures may vary.	
Immobilizing units—equipment used to immobilize a part of the client's body (e.g., halo device used to immobilize the client's skull during a head procedure).	■ Always follow manufacturer guidelines. ■ When the immobilizing unit punctures the client's skin during placement, make sure the surgeon always maintains aseptic technique.	

Source: Based on Association of Perioperative Registered Nurses (2013). *Perioperative standards and recommended practices.* Denver, CO: Author; Board of Laser Safety. (2013). *Certified medical laser safety officer: Policies & procedures manual.* Retrieved from https://www.lasersafety.org/uploads/pdf/cmlso_pp_manual.pdf; Meeks, S. (2011). *Immobilization from rigid to non-rigid. MD Anderson Center.* Retrieved from www.aapm.org/meetings/2011SS/documents/Meeksrigidtononrigid.pdf.

TABLE 17–6   Surgical Positions

CLIENT POSITION	STEPS TO BE TAKEN TO SAFELY POSITION CLIENT
Supine. The circulating nurse places the client on his back and ensures that the accompanying steps are completed. 	1. Arms are gently secured on padded arm boards at less than a 90-degree angle with palms up. 2. Alternatively, tucked arms may be secured at the client's side (only if necessary) with palms of hands facing in toward the thighs, elbows and hands protected and padded, and hands and wrists anatomically aligned. 3. Pillows are placed under the client's knees. 4. Bony prominences (e.g., heels) are elevated from surface of bed using pillows and a padded foot board for leg positioning. 5. A wedge is placed under a pregnant client's right hip/flanks to displace the uterus to the left.
Semi-Fowler (sitting). The circulating nurse places the client in the sitting position and ensures that the accompanying steps are completed. 	1. Arms are gently secured on padded arm boards at less than a 90-degree angle with palms up. 2. Pressure points are protected by properly positioning and padding the buttocks/sacrum and other bony prominences. 3. Bony prominences (e.g., heels) are elevated from surface of bed using pillows and a padded foot board for leg positioning. 4. The foot of the bed is lowered slightly to allow the knees to flex. 5. The client's feet are supported on a padded foot board to prevent plantar flexion and stretching of the tibial nerve. 6. The back of the OR bed is raised to become the back rest, supporting the shoulders and torso with safety restraints.
Prone and jackknife. The circulating nurse places the client on his stomach and ensures that the accompanying steps are completed. 	1. Cervical neck is maintained in alignment. 2. Toes are elevated from the surface of bed. 3. Eyes are protected to prevent ocular injury (e.g., pressure, corneal abrasion). 4. Female breasts and male genitalia are not compressed.

TABLE 17–6 Surgical Positions (*continued*)

CLIENT POSITION	STEPS TO BE TAKEN TO SAFELY POSITION CLIENT
Lateral. The circulating nurse places the client on her side (left or right) and ensures that the accompanying steps are completed. 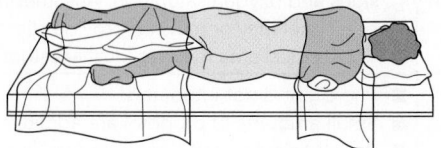	1. The correct surgical side is initialed before the client is transferred to the OR and the initials are visible after positioning, prepping, and draping. 2. The client is positioned on the nonoperative side. 3. Pressure points are padded on the dependent side (e.g., ear, acromion process, iliac crest, greater trochanter, lateral knee, malleolus). 4. Correct spinal alignment is maintained when turning and stabilizing client in position. 5. Axillary roll or other devices are needed to safely position arms and prevent brachial plexus injury.
Trendelenburg or reverse Trendelenburg. The circulating nurse places the client on his back with padded shoulder braces in place and ensures that the accompanying steps are completed. This position displaces the intestines into the upper abdomen. 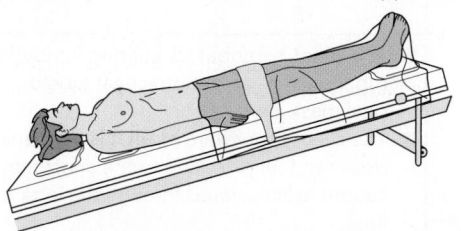	1. Time in the head-down position is monitored to identify physiological shifts. 2. The client is prevented from sliding and sheering injuries. 3. Injuries are prevented to the client's shoulders. 4. The feet are supported on a padded foot board to prevent plantar flexion and stretching of the tibial nerve. 5. Injury to the client's brachial plexus is prevented. 6. Injury to the client's feet is prevented.
Lithotomy. This is a gynecological position. The circulating nurse places the client on her back with both legs elevated in stirrups and ensures that the accompanying steps are completed. 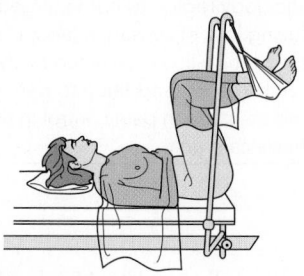	1. Ankles and heels are padded. 2. Stretching of the perineal nerve is prevented by ensuring that the hip and knee joints are not overextended. 3. Arms are padded on arm boards at less than a 90-degree angle with palms up. 4. The client's legs are removed from stirrups slowly and brought together simultaneously to prevent lumbosacral strain. 5. The client's legs are raised and lowered slowly and simultaneously to maintain hemodynamic status.
For all procedures: Prior to draping the client, the circulating nurse must complete the accompanying steps for all surgical positions.	1. Pressure is evenly distributed over bony prominences. 2. The client's body alignment is always assessed to prevent musculoskeletal compromise. 3. Placement of safety straps is assessed. 4. Tissue perfusion is assessed. 5. The client's skin integrity is assessed and the nurse ensures that there is no pooling of solutions or wet surfaces. 6. The client's circulatory, neurological, and respiratory systems are not compromised.
For each surgical procedure, the circulating nurse must evaluate the client postoperatively covering all of the accompanying steps.	1. Skin injuries (e.g., reddened, bruised, tears). 2. Musculoskeletal and nerve injuries (e.g., aberrations in circulation, movement, and sensation). 3. Pressure ulcer development (e.g., identifies the stages of pressure ulcer development). 4. Eye injuries.

Source: Based on Association of periOperative Registered Nurses (2012). *Perioperative job descriptions and competency evaluation tools.* Denver, CO: Author; Meeks, S. (2011). *Immobilization from rigid to non-rigid. MD Anderson Center.* Retrieved from http://www.aapm.org/meetings/2011SS/documents/Meeksrigidtononrigid.pdf; Osborn, K. S., Wraa, C. E., Watson, A. B., & Holleran, R. (2014). Intraoperative nursing. In *Medical-surgical nursing: Preparation for practice* (2nd ed., Chap. 18). Upper Saddle River, NJ: Pearson Education.

TABLE 17–7 Types of Anesthesia

TYPE OF ANESTHESIA	USED FOR	DEFINITION
Local anesthesia—localized specifically to surgical site	■ Invasive procedures that can be completed in the surgeon's office, but are completed instead in a procedural setting for various reasons, such as the client's anxiety level.	■ The client is awake during entire procedure. ■ A circulating nurse monitors the client's vital signs and oxygen saturation. Anesthesia personnel may or may not provide client care. ■ The surgical area receives local anesthetics.
Conscious sedation/monitored anesthesia care (MAC)	■ Older adults who are more prone to decreased renal function are good candidates for this type of anesthesia. ■ Carpal tunnel syndrome ■ Stapedectomy ■ May also be utilized for clients who will need to communicate with the surgeon at any point of the procedure. For example, when a client has a stapedectomy, the surgeon will ask the client a question after the stapes is implanted to see if the client's hearing level has improved.	■ The client is not intubated. ■ Small amounts of propofol are administered. ■ Anesthesia personnel monitor the client. ■ Anesthesia personnel must be prepared to provide advanced airway management (e.g., tracheal intubation) and to convert to using general anesthesia if needed.
General anesthesia—a medically induced coma A paralytic agent is commonly administered in conjunction with the anesthetic agent.	■ Total abdominal hysterectomy ■ Craniotomy ■ Nephrectomy	■ The client is intubated, utilizing intubation tubes such as an endotracheal tube or laryngeal mask airway. ■ The client is unaware of what is happening and does not feel pain, due to the anesthetic medications administered through the intravenous line. ■ The client is monitored by anesthesia personnel.
Regional anesthesia (e.g., spinal anesthesia, epidural anesthesia, femoral nerve block)—a specific region of the client is anesthetized	■ Cesarean birth ■ Toe/partial foot amputation ■ Hip replacements	■ The client may be awake or sedated. ■ An anesthetic medication is injected into a specific body region to bathe targeted nerves, producing loss of sensation (and, in some cases, loss of mobility) in selected body regions. ■ Can be used in addition to general anesthesia. This assists with pain control in the postanesthesia care unit.

SAFETY ALERT
Older adults are at greater risk for development of pressure ulcers. The nurse positioning the client must take care to check the appropriate pressure points of the position and providing padding as appropriate.

Anesthesia

Generally speaking, clients undergoing surgical procedures require anesthesia. The type of anesthesia varies, from local anesthesia to general anesthesia. The type of anesthesia used depends on many variables and the combinations of variables, such as the type of surgical procedure and the level of systemic illness. For example, high blood pressure and obesity increase the risk level of anesthesia and therefore conscious sedation (also known as monitored anesthesia care [MAC]) may be preferred over general anesthesia. See **Table 17–7** ● for an overview of types of anesthesia.

ASA PHYSICAL CLASSIFICATION CATEGORY The American Society of Anesthesiologists (ASA) (n.d.) created the **ASA Physical Status Classification System**, a physical risk classification category that helps describe the patient's

present state of physical illness. The ASA level is not used to estimate the possibility of anesthetic complications, nor does it dictate the type of anesthetic that will be administered. The ASA system is described as follows:

ASA I: The client is healthy, i.e., the client is free of health conditions or systemic disease.
ASA II: The client demonstrates mild systemic disease; e.g., obesity, uncomplicated diabetes, or controlled hypertension.
ASA III: The client has one severe systemic illness; e.g., coronary artery disease, angina, or poorly-controlled hypertension.
ASA IV: The client has a life-threatening severe illness, i.e., the client has a severe illness such as pulmonary dysfunction.
ASA V: The client is not expected to survive for more than 24 hours unless surgery occurs.
ASA VI: The client is brain dead; may be an organ donor.

LARYNGEAL MASK AIRWAYS AND ENDOTRACHEAL TUBES If general anesthesia is to be used, then the type of airway management device to be used is determined. In certain instances, the anesthesia provider may opt to insert a laryngeal mask airway (LMA). (**Figure 17–2** ●). An LMA is inserted

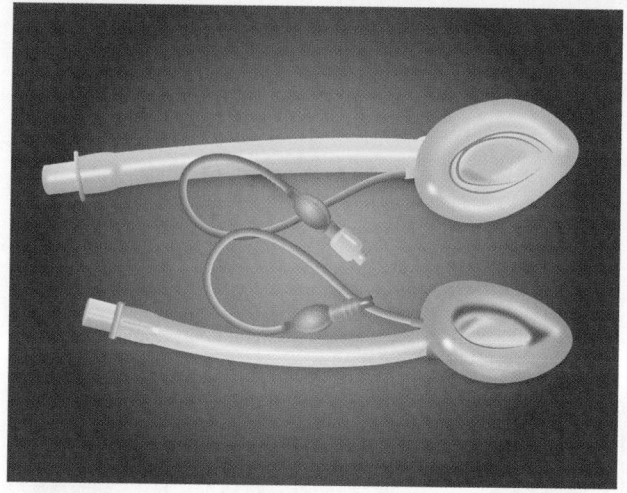

Figure 17–2 ● Laryngeal mask airway.

TABLE 17–8   Commonly Used Surgical Prep Solutions

SURGICAL PREP SOLUTIONS	USES AND PRECAUTIONS
Betadine scrub	■ Used for the initial wash or prep of surgical area. Cannot be used on mucous membranes.
Betadine paint	■ Used for the final Betadine prep of the surgical area. Can be used on mucous membranes.
ChloraPrep, DuraPrep	■ Alcohol based; needs to be completely dry before draping the client. Not to be used on mucous membranes. Avoid contact with ears and eyes.
Ultradex scrub	■ Used when the client has iodine and latex allergies.

blindly into the pharynx, forming a seal around the laryngeal inlet and creating positive-pressure ventilation. As an alternative to an LMA, an endotracheal tube (ET) may be used to manage the client's airway. An ET is inserted through the vocal cords into the trachea with the use of a laryngoscope (**Figure 17–3 ●**).

Surgical Site Preparation

Preparation of the surgical site occurs in the intraoperative setting, just prior to sterile draping of the client. The purpose of a surgical prep is to help prevent surgical site infections. When prepping, the circulating nurse always starts the prep at the surgical incision site and moves outward. Surgical preparation solutions are given an opportunity to completely dry before draping in order to prevent serious consequences from occurring, such as a surgical fire, which can burn the client. Completing the surgical preparation just prior to draping decreases the chance of the surgical site being contaminated, which decreases the risk of acquiring a surgical site infection. See **Table 17–8 ●** for a list of commonly used surgical prep solutions and **Figure 17–4 ●** for skin preparation for common surgical sites.

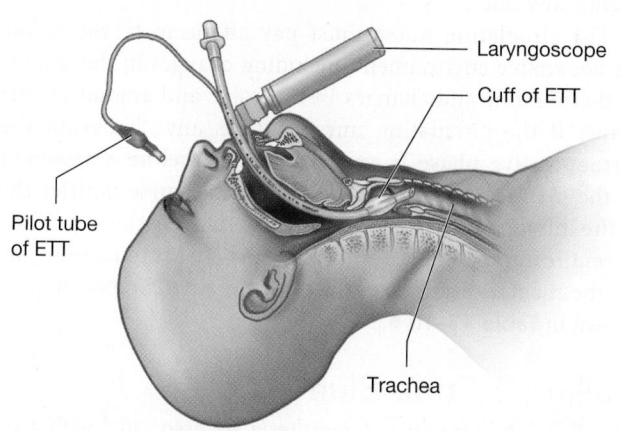

Laryngoscope

Cuff of ETT

Pilot tube of ETT

Trachea

Figure 17–3 ● Using a laryngoscope to insert an endotracheal tube.

Surgical Safety Checklist

Safety checklists are used by many hospitals to ensure client safety. These models require the entire surgical team to periodically cease all other activities (a surgical time-out) and verbally verify such information as the client name; the surgery to be performed; the side or site of surgery; whether prophylactic medications have been administered; whether all instruments, sponge, and needle counts are correct; and that any lab specimens have been correctly labeled. Often, the circulating nurse is charged with conducting the checklist time-outs. The World Health Organization (2009) created a Surgical Safety Checklist in order to assist perioperative staff in achieving best practice and maintaining the safety of the client (**Figure 17–5 ●**). The checklist ensures that the nurse documents confirmation of essential perioperative tasks.

Intraoperative Documentation

One of the responsibilities of the circulating nurses is to provide thorough documentation about the intraoperative period. The intraoperative documentation records all aspects of occurrences during the surgical procedure (see **Box 17–4 ●**).

Infection

Many factors influence a client's healing process, especially age, nutrition, and physical health of the client. Pediatric clients and older adult clients are at higher risk of surgical complications for various reasons, including decreased immune status. Clients with poor health or poor nutrition status also are at greater risk for infection. Clients who have diabetes, take immunosuppressants, or have an increased BMI have an increased risk of acquiring an infection. Nurses and other members of the surgical team act to reduce the risk of infection by maintaining aseptic technique at all times. Any break in aseptic technique increases the client's chance for infection and prolonged healing period.

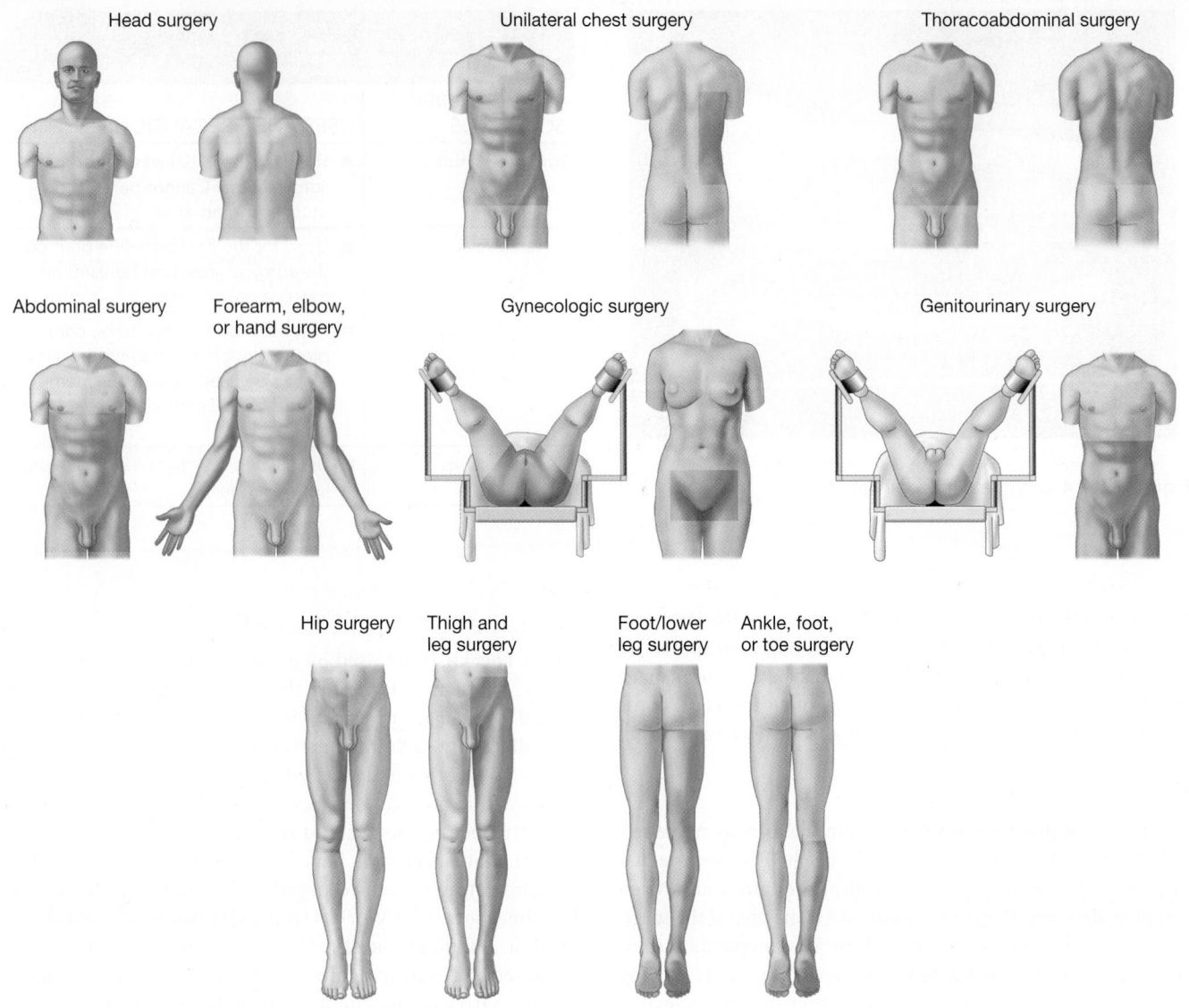

Figure 17–4 ● Skin preparation for common surgical sites.

Surgical Wound Classification

Surgical wound classification is determined for all surgical procedures (**Table 17–9** ●). Classification of surgical wounds (including incisions) is used in predicting the risk of surgical site infection (Zinn, 2012). The wound classification needs to be determined at the end of the surgical procedure to capture any events that may have occurred that would affect the wound classification (Zinn, 2012). As shown in Table 17–9, if there is a minor break in sterile technique, the wound class increases one level. The more breaks in sterile technique, the higher the wound class, which correlates with the client's risk of an SSI.

Potential Intraoperative Complications

For all clients undergoing a surgical procedure, the nurse has to pay close attention to possible physiological changes occurring within the client. The nurse cannot assume another team mem-

ber is monitoring the client. In the intraoperative setting, the nurse truly becomes the spokesperson for the client and is the client's advocate.

The circulating nurse must pay attention to the whole intraoperative environment, including changes in the sounds of the monitor and changes in the color and amount of the urine. If the circulating nurse notices any change in the intraoperative phase from the client's baseline assessment in the preoperative phase, the circulating nurse notifies the entire intraoperative team. Communicating any client issues to the entire intraoperative team ensures a better surgical outcome for the client. A list of potential intraoperative complications is shown in **Table 17–10** ●.

Calling a Code Blue

For all clients, surgery and anesthesia are associated with serious risks. Should the client's condition deteriorate during the intraoperative period, the surgical team members will work together as needed to implement appropriate interventions. In

World Health Organization

SURGICAL SAFETY CHECKLIST (FIRST EDITION)

Before induction of anaesthesia ▸▸▸▸▸▸▸▸▸ Before skin incision ▸▸▸▸▸▸▸▸▸▸▸▸▸▸ Before patient leaves operating room

SIGN IN

- ☐ PATIENT HAS CONFIRMED
  - • IDENTITY
  - • SITE
  - • PROCEDURE
  - • CONSENT
- ☐ SITE MARKED/NOT APPLICABLE
- ☐ ANAESTHESIA SAFETY CHECK COMPLETED
- ☐ PULSE OXIMETER ON PATIENT AND FUNCTIONING

DOES PATIENT HAVE A:

KNOWN ALLERGY?
- ☐ NO
- ☐ YES

DIFFICULT AIRWAY/ASPIRATION RISK?
- ☐ NO
- ☐ YES, AND EQUIPMENT/ASSISTANCE AVAILABLE

RISK OF >500ML BLOOD LOSS (7ML/KG IN CHILDREN)?
- ☐ NO
- ☐ YES, AND ADEQUATE INTRAVENOUS ACCESS AND FLUIDS PLANNED

TIME OUT

- ☐ CONFIRM ALL TEAM MEMBERS HAVE INTRODUCED THEMSELVES BY NAME AND ROLE
- ☐ SURGEON, ANAESTHESIA PROFESSIONAL AND NURSE VERBALLY CONFIRM
  - • PATIENT
  - • SITE
  - • PROCEDURE

ANTICIPATED CRITICAL EVENTS
- ☐ SURGEON REVIEWS: WHAT ARE THE CRITICAL OR UNEXPECTED STEPS, OPERATIVE DURATION, ANTICIPATED BLOOD LOSS?
- ☐ ANAESTHESIA TEAM REVIEWS: ARE THERE ANY PATIENT-SPECIFIC CONCERNS?
- ☐ NURSING TEAM REVIEWS: HAS STERILITY (INCLUDING INDICATOR RESULTS) BEEN CONFIRMED? ARE THERE EQUIPMENT ISSUES OR ANY CONCERNS?

HAS ANTIBIOTIC PROPHYLAXIS BEEN GIVEN WITHIN THE LAST 60 MINUTES?
- ☐ YES
- ☐ NOT APPLICABLE

IS ESSENTIAL IMAGING DISPLAYED?
- ☐ YES
- ☐ NOT APPLICABLE

SIGN OUT

NURSE VERBALLY CONFIRMS WITH THE TEAM:
- ☐ THE NAME OF THE PROCEDURE RECORDED
- ☐ THAT INSTRUMENT, SPONGE AND NEEDLE COUNTS ARE CORRECT (OR NOT APPLICABLE)
- ☐ HOW THE SPECIMEN IS LABELLED (INCLUDING PATIENT NAME)
- ☐ WHETHER THERE ARE ANY EQUIPMENT PROBLEMS TO BE ADDRESSED
- ☐ SURGEON, ANAESTHESIA PROFESSIONAL AND NURSE REVIEW THE KEY CONCERNS FOR RECOVERY AND MANAGEMENT OF THIS PATIENT

THIS CHECKLIST IS NOT INTENDED TO BE COMPREHENSIVE. ADDITIONS AND MODIFICATIONS TO FIT LOCAL PRACTICE ARE ENCOURAGED.

Figure 17–5 ● WHO Surgical Safety Checklist.

Source: World Alliance for Patient Safety (2008). WHO surgical safety checklist and implementation. Retrieved from http://www.who.int/patientsafety/safesurgery/ss_checklist/en/index/html.

Box 17–4 Intraoperative Documentation

Intraoperative documentation includes, but is not limited to, the following:

1. Recognition that the hand-off from the preoperative nurse to the intraoperative nurse is complete
2. Preoperative medical diagnosis
3. Postoperative medical diagnosis
4. Completion of consented surgical procedure
5. Type of anesthesia administered (e.g., general anesthesia)
6. ASA level
7. Intraoperative team members (Names of all individuals present for the surgical procedure. This should also include medical sales representatives. All individuals are to be listed on the intraoperative nurse's notes in case an unexpected event occurs. The individuals on the nurse's notes can be questioned as references for each individual's recognition of the specific outline of event.) Observing students will also be entered in the OR records and can be called as witnesses.
8. Times
   a. Start and stop times of anesthesia
   b. Start and stop times of procedure
   c. Antibiotic infusion times
9. Surgical preparation site
   a. Prep used
10. Skin assessment
    a. Initial
    b. Postoperative
11. Position or positions of client
12. Positioning aids utilized
13. Foley insertion
14. Surgical instrument count: Documenting correct or incorrect count. If an incorrect count occurs, documentation is to be completed on the steps taken to ensure the missing instrument or sponge does not remain in the client's body, for example, an x-ray can be taken to locate within the client).
    a. Initial
    b. Ongoing
    c. Closing
    d. Shift change
15. Time-out(s)
    a. Name of individual completing the time-out
    b. Time the time-out is completed
16. Equipment used during procedure
17. Specimens collected
    a. Pathology (e.g., appendix)
    b. Laboratory (e.g., diagnostic testing)
18. Tubes or drains placed
    a. Location
    b. Type
    c. Number
19. Dressing placed
    a. Location
    b. Type
20. Total fluid intake and output that occurred intraoperatively.
    a. Intake
    b. Output
21. Medications used on the surgical field or given by the circulating nurse
22. Additional notes if necessary.

TABLE 17–9   Surgical Wound Classifications

WOUND CLASSIFICATION LEVEL	DEFINITION
Class I—clean	A surgical wound that is not infected and no inflammation is present. The alimentary, respiratory, genital and urinary tract are not entered.
Class II—clean contaminated	There is no sign of infection, but the alimentary, respiratory, genital, or urinary tracts are entered under controlled conditions. There is no break in sterile technique.
Class III—contaminated	Gross spillage from the GI tract occurs. A major break in sterile technique will also cause a wound to be placed in this category.
Class IV—dirty, infected	Pus or evidence of bacterial inflammation is found. Tissue necrosis may be present.

1. If there is a minor break in sterility, the wound class level increases to the next level.
2. A major break in sterility automatically increases the wound class level to a Class III.
3. An open drain left in place also increases the wound class one level.

Sources: Based on Centers for Disease Control and Prevention. (2011). Guideline for prevention of surgical site infection, 1999. Retrieved from http://www.cdc.gov/hicpac/SSI/table7-8-9-10-SSI.html; Chard, R. (2012). Wound classifications. Retrieved from http://bcpsqc.ca/documents/2012/11/2008-AORN-wound-classifications.pdf; Medscape Multispecialty. (2013). Classification and risk of SSI. Retrieved from http://www.medscape.org/viewarticle/448981_4.

the event of cardiopulmonary arrest, the circulating nurse should follow hospital protocols to announce a code blue. Within the intraoperative phase the anesthesia team runs the code and the remaining interdisciplinary team members assist in the code blue, including drawing up medications and code blue documentation.

Blood Transfusions

Blood transfusions are primarily administered in the intraoperative and postoperative phases. Blood transfusions can be obtained from two sources: The client can donate his own blood, which is known as an **autologous blood transfusion**, or the client can receive blood that has been donated by the community, known as **allogeneic blood transfusion**.

The three methods of autologous blood transfusion include preoperative donation, normovolemic hemodilution, and perioperative salvage of autologous blood: for example, blood recovery during the intraoperative phase (Chimutengwende-Gordon, Khan, & Maruthainar, 2010). Preoperative blood donation is when the surgical client donates his or her own blood before the surgical procedure for use during upcoming surgery. Preoperative blood donation was once promoted to decrease the need for allogeneic blood transfusions (Shander et al., 2012). However, blood donated prior to surgery is labor intensive, more costly than allogeneic blood, and has an increased risk for bacterial contamination and ABO incompatibility error. In addition, a high percentage of preoperative blood goes to waste because the client is hemodynamically stable (Joyce, 2008).

Normovolemic hemodilution consists of drawing two to four units of red blood cells from the client just before surgery and replacing it with acellular fluid (Waters & Yazer, 2008). Normovolemic hemodilution results in a lower concentration of red blood cells being lost during surgery (Waters & Yazer, 2008). At the end of the procedure, the red blood cells withdrawn before the procedure are replaced along with platelets and plasma, which assist in coagulation.

The final type of autologous blood is perioperative blood recovery. Perioperative blood recovery is completed through the use of blood recovery equipment in the intraoperative suite during surgery. The blood recovery equipment captures red cells shed through low suction pressures and washing of surgical sponges (Waters & Yazer, 2008).

CASE STUDY // B

Rachel Poole is a 20-year-old female in her junior year of nursing school. Rachel was recently diagnosed with stage II breast cancer and is scheduled to have a bilateral total mastectomy with a free transverse rectus abdominis myocutaneous (TRAM) breast reconstruction. She is healthy except for her recent diagnosis and has been given an ASA 2 classification. Her vital signs in the preoperative area are T_O 98.6°F, P 72 bpm, R 14/min, and BP 110/70 mmHg. Rachel is 5 feet 4 inches and weighs 125 pounds. A type and screen is ordered. Rachel has signed all of her consents and is now slightly anxious as she will be going to the operating room shortly. The preoperative nurse administers midazolam (Versed) 2 mg IV. Rachel is monitored until she is transported to the intraoperative suite.

Rachel is transferred to the operating room where she is assisted onto the operating room bed and placed in the supine position with her arms laterally abducted less than 90 degrees and pressure points padded. A safety strap is placed over her upper thighs. Rachel is medicated and intubated by anesthesia. A Foley catheter is placed. A pillow is placed under her knees and soft gel pads are placed under her ankles. The circulating nurse completes the intraoperative skin prep for the breast and reconstructive surgery because the breast surgeon and plastic surgeon will be performing surgery concurrently. The surgeons and surgical technologists drape the client, and the circulating nurse completes the preprocedure verification process for both procedures. During the procedure Rachel loses 2,500 mL of blood, which is replenished with three units of blood from the blood bank.

When the procedure is completed, the anesthesia provider extubates Rachel. Rachel's blood pressure drops to 70/30, pulse drops to 45, respiratory rate to 8, and her oxygen saturation drops to 70% on 2 liters oxygen through nasal cannula. A code blue is

TABLE 17–10 Potential Intraoperative Complications

POTENTIAL COMPLICATIONS	NURSING IMPLICATIONS
Hypovolemia	
<ul><li>Decreased fluid volume (e.g., blood volume)</li><li>Decreased blood pressure</li><li>Decreased urine output</li><li>Increased heart rate</li><li>Increased respiratory rate</li></ul>	<ul><li>Assess the client to determine any underlying cause.</li><li>Replenish fluid volume (e.g., crystalloids, colloids, blood transfusion). See the module on Fluids and Electrolytes for discussion of intravenous fluid therapy.</li></ul>
Hypervolemia	
<ul><li>Increased fluid volume (e.g., excessive amounts of intravenous fluids)</li><li>Increased blood pressure</li><li>Increased heart rate</li><li>Increased respiratory rate</li><li>Decreased urine output</li></ul>	<ul><li>Assess the client to determine any underlying cause.</li><li>Administer medications as ordered to decrease volume (e.g., antidiuretics).</li></ul>
Hyponatremia	
<ul><li>Decreased sodium</li><li>Edema (swelling)</li><li>Muscle twitching</li><li>Signs of hypovolemia</li></ul>	<ul><li>Assess the client to determine any underlying cause.</li><li>If the cause of hyponatremia is fluid volume overload, intravenous fluids may be restricted to allow for concentration effect. Severe hyponatremia may require administration of hypertonic saline. See the module on Fluids and Electrolytes for discussion of intravenous fluid therapy.</li></ul>
Hypernatremia	
<ul><li>Increased sodium</li><li>Concentrated urine</li><li>Dry mucous membranes</li></ul>	<ul><li>Assess the client to determine any underlying cause.</li><li>If the cause of hypernatremia is dehydration, intravenous fluids may be administered to create a dilutional effect.</li></ul>
Hypokalemia	
<ul><li>Decreased potassium</li><li>Abdominal distention</li><li>Severe arrhythmias</li></ul>	<ul><li>Assess the client to determine any underlying causes.</li><li>Administer medications as ordered to increase potassium level (e.g., potassium intravenously).</li></ul>
Hyperkalemia	
<ul><li>Increased potassium</li><li>Arrhythmias</li></ul>	<ul><li>Assess the client to determine any underlying cause.</li><li>Administer medications as ordered to decrease potassium level (e.g., kayexalate or intravenous glucose and insulin).</li></ul>
Increased intracranial pressure	
<ul><li>Increased blood pressure</li><li>Decreased heart rate</li><li>Hyperthermia may increase ICP</li></ul>	<ul><li>Administer medications as ordered to decrease ICP (e.g., antidiuretics).</li><li>Use methods to decrease temperature if client has an increased temperature.</li></ul>
Hypothermia	
<ul><li>Decreased body temperature</li><li>Decreased heart rate</li><li>Decreased circulation</li></ul>	<ul><li>Assess the client to determine any underlying cause.</li><li>Utilize warming methods (e.g., body warmer).</li><li>Administer warmed intravenous fluid.</li></ul>
Hyperthermia	
<ul><li>Increased body temperature</li><li>Increased heart rate</li><li>Increased blood flow</li></ul>	<ul><li>Monitor client's temperature in all perioperative phases.</li><li>Identify cause of hyperthermia and implement appropriate interventions.</li></ul>
Malignant hyperthermia	
<ul><li>Genetic disorder that produces a life-threatening hypermetabolic state; manifestations include hypercarbia (increased CO_2), tachycardia, muscle rigidity, rhabdomyolysis (breakdown of skeletal muscle fibers), and hyperthermia.</li><li>The primary cause of malignant hyperthermia is the client's exposure to certain anesthetic agents, including succinylcholine and anesthetic gases.</li><li>Triggered by inhalation anesthetic gases and depolarizing muscle relaxants.</li></ul>	<ul><li>Perioperative nurses must review the client's history as well as the client's familial history regarding any complications with anesthesia during previous procedures.</li><li>Treatment includes administration of dantrolene.</li><li>Nurses must know the early signs of malignant hyperthermia (e.g., hypercarbia and tachycardia).</li><li>Perioperative nurses must be familiar with their institution's protocols for treatment of clients with suspected malignant hyperthermia.</li></ul>

initiated. Rachel is re-intubated. A stat arterial blood gas (ABG) is collected. The circulating nurse brings the crash cart into the operating room and is responsible for drawing up the medications ordered during the code until the pharmacist arrives. At that time, the circulating nurse documents all interventions, as well as Rachel's responses.

After 3 minutes of medications and chest compressions, Rachel continues to be hypotensive and bradycardic. ABG results include PCO_2 50 mmHg and pH 7.25. Rachel remains intubated and is transferred to the intensive care unit (ICU).

Critical Thinking Questions Level I

1. Determine alternative steps that could have been taken to prevent Rachel's complex extubation.

2. Explain the reason for Rachel being re-intubated and a code blue initiated.

POSTOPERATIVE NURSING

The postoperative phase begins with admission to designated post-surgical recovery area and concludes upon the client's transfer to a hospital unit or discharge to home. Clients receiving general anesthesia typically are transferred to a postanesthesia care unit (PACU). Clients who emerge from surgery in a more critical state may be transferred to the ICU. While the client recuperates from anesthesia, ensuring airway patency is a priority of care. The nurse places the client on an electrocardiogram monitor and pulse oximeter, checks vital signs on a regular basis, and administers medications to control pain and to assist the client through the recovery period. Following recovery, the client may be transferred to a medical-surgical floor or, depending on the nature of the procedure, the client may be discharged home.

▶ NURSING CARE

Surgery and anesthesia produce numerous physiologic effects. A detailed, thorough hand-off in the postoperative phase is imperative and occurs between the postoperative nurse, the intraoperative circulating nurse, and the anesthesia provider. Once the postoperative care nurse receives report, the nurse assesses the client, adds additional goals to the client's care plan, and then continues with the implementation of the care plan.

Immediate postoperative assessment of the client postanesthesia includes:

- Airway patency, oxygen saturation, and ventilation
- Cardiovascular status: blood pressure, heart rate and rhythm
- Protective reflexes (e.g., gag reflex, cough reflex)
- Skin assessment
- Fluid status
- Operative site: dressing, drainage (amount, type, color)
- Pain, nausea, vomiting
- Safety.

Significant findings must be reported to the surgeon or anesthesiologist. These may include, but are not limited to:

- Prolonged unresponsiveness
- Change in level of consciousness
- Oxygen saturation <93%
- Respiratory rate <10 breaths per minute
- Tachycardia
- Hypertension or hypotension
- Weak or absent peripheral pulses
- Urine output <30 mL/hr
- More than the expected amount of bleeding at the incision site.

The postoperative diagnoses include, but are not limited to the following:

- *Pain* related to surgical procedure
- *Risk for Impaired Gas Exchange* related to decreased respiratory rate secondary to effects of opiate medications and anesthetic agents
- *Anxiety* related to the unknown of surgical procedure and unfamiliar environment
- *Risk for Decreased Cardiac Output* related to intraoperative fluid volume loss
- *Risk for Deficient Fluid Volume* (e.g., hypovolemia due to massive blood loss and NPO status).

(NANDA-I © 2012)

Nursing interventions in the postoperative phase will vary according to the client, the procedure, and the client's evolving postoperative status. At all times, the nurse acts to ensure airway management, reduce the potential for postoperative complications (e.g., infection), and address client pain and anxiety.

Risk Monitoring

Clients who undergo certain surgical procedures, such as colorectal surgery, are at a high risk for acquiring a urinary tract infection and or urinary retention (Kang et al., 2012). Urinary tract infection is the leading cause of healthcare-associated infections in the United States and increase the client's mortality rate and healthcare costs (Kang et al., 2012). When applicable, it is imperative that the postoperative nurse complete a thorough assessment of the indwelling urinary (e.g., Foley) catheter, including maintaining strict intake and output calculations and documentation. For example, if the client has received 1000 mL of fluid, but has only excreted 30 mL into the Foley bag and the client's abdomen is starting to distend, the postoperative nurse uses critical thinking skills to assess the source of the problem. The problem could be as simple as a bend in the Foley tubing that needs to be straightened, or it may be that the client is truly retaining fluid and the surgeon and anesthesia personnel need to be notified. Also, the postoperative nurse should be alert to changes in the appearance of the client's urine, such as cloudiness or the presence of blood. All abnormalities should be reported to the client's attending physician. Prior to the client being discharged home, the postoperative nurse ensures that the client is able to excrete an acceptable amount of urine without straining. The client's urine flow must be normal for the client. For example, if the client states, "I really did not pass as much urine as I usually do at home," the postoperative nurse continues to assess the client.

> **SAFETY ALERT**
> Maintain IVs as ordered to replace body fluids lost as a result of the surgical procedure. Once oral intake is permitted, offer only small sips of water. Anesthetics and narcotic analgesics impair mobility of the stomach, and large amounts of water may induce vomiting. For clients who cannot yet drink water, the surgeon may permit sucking on ice chips.

Cultural Considerations

Cultural considerations must be incorporated into the client's plan of care. Cultural influences may affect every aspect of the client's response to care. It is essential for the postanesthesia care unit nurse to incorporate the client's cultural needs and preferences into the plan of care whenever possible. For example, a client arrives in the postoperative phase after a dilation and curettage for her unborn child whom she unexpectedly lost at 13 weeks' gestational age. The client requests to take the products of conception home with her due to religious beliefs, as she does not want to send the unborn child's remains to a funeral home. With regard to miscarriage, most healthcare facilities have protocols in place to guide the process of care during instances in which a client chooses to take home the remains for the purpose of burial. The nurse should follow organizational policy while seeking to safely incorporate the client's cultural preferences into the plan of care.

Postoperative Medications

Within the postoperative phase, the client recovers from anesthesia. Two types of medications typically are administered within the postanesthesia phase: pain medications and antiemetic medications for complaints of nausea or vomiting. Pain medications administered include, but are not limited to, hydromorphone (Dilaudid), morphine, and sometimes fentanyl (Sublimaze). (See the Medications feature). Pain medications assist in lowering the client's pain level and, in turn, decrease elevated blood pressure and pulse rate. Antiemetic medications assist in decreasing nausea and vomiting.

Airway

On completion of the intraoperative phase, most clients are extubated prior to transport to the postoperative phase. Many times if the client is not stable enough to be extubated and the plan is to place the client on a ventilator, the client remains intubated and is transferred to the unit, usually the ICU, to be placed on a ventilator. If the client is extubated in the intraoperative phase and is stable, the client is transferred to the postoperative phase on completion of the surgery or invasive procedure. On arrival to the postoperative care unit, the client is drowsy and is placed in a sitting position—if the surgeon's orders allow—to decrease the work of breathing. At times the

client may need to be stimulated in order to independently maintain the airway. Stimulation may include various interventions to assist the client to wake up post operatively; for example, the nurse may rigorously rub the client's sternum. Also, the postoperative nurse may have to perform a chin lift maneuver to open the airway or administer Narcan to reverse respiratory depression caused by narcotics previously administered to the client.

Cardiac Rhythm

Clients receiving general anesthesia are hooked up to an electrocardiogram (ECG) monitor upon arrival to the postoperative care unit. Postoperative nurses all have Advanced Cardiovascular Life Support (ACLS) certification. ACLS prepares the postoperative nurse to recognize the various heart rhythms, causes for the specific heart rhythms, and a course of action the nurse must take to return the client to a normal rhythm or the client's baseline rhythm prior to surgery. Depending on the client's heart rhythm, postanesthesia care nurses are trained to complete algorithms, including the administration of medications. For example, the client arrives in the postoperative phase and is placed on the ECG monitor. The ECG monitor shows the client presents with a pulse of 45 beats per minute and demonstrates labored breathing. Based on the assessment data, the nurse follows the bradycardia algorithm, including identifying and treating any underlying causes. The primary care provider who is in directing the PACU should be immediately notified of any changes in the client's condition.

In the event that the client goes into cardiac or respiratory arrest, a code blue is called and followed per the healthcare facility's set guidelines. Within the perioperative arena, the anesthesia team runs the code blue.

Wound Management

The surgeon may write orders for a dressing change prior to the client being discharged. Depending on the surgeon's preferences, the order may specifically state that the surgeon or the surgeon's assistant (e.g., physician assistant or the nurse practitioner) will complete the first dressing change and the client's nurse will only reinforce the dressing if necessary prior to discharge. An example of this is when the initial dressing placed at the completion of surgery creates a pressure pack to the wound. This assists in decreasing bleeding from the incision.

If the postoperative nurse is provided the order to change the dressing, the nurse will use clean technique to change the client's surgical dressing to decrease the chance of the client having a surgical site infection. See the module on Tissue Integrity for a discussion of wound care and healing.

Line and Drain Management

Postoperative clients typically have infusion lines and may have surgical drains that need to be managed by postoperative nurses (**Figure 17–6 ●**). All tubing is labeled with the name of the line or drain, the date and time the line or drain was placed, and the initials of the individual who initiated the line and/or drain. Lines and drains are labeled to prevent serious errors, such as attaching suction to an intravenous line. Lines and

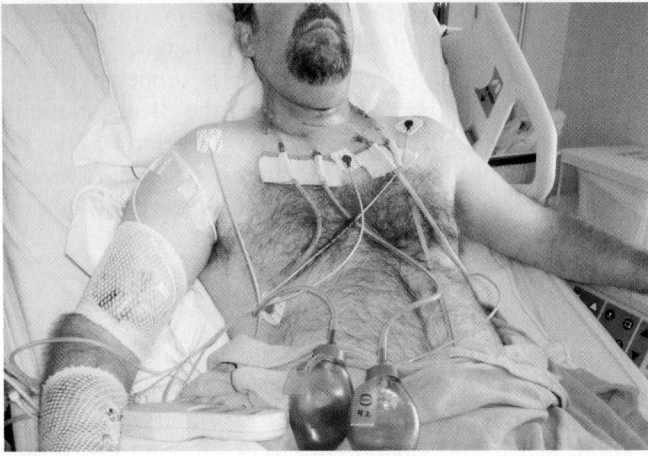

Figure 17–6 ● Jackson-Pratt drains.
Source: Ann E. F. Sievers, RN.

drains can include, but are not limited to, an intravenous line, chest tubes, urinary catheters, and closed wound drainage systems. Drains are inserted to allow excessive fluid and purulent material to drain and to promote healing of underlying tissues. Without a drain, a wound may heal on the outside, but trap discharge and purulent material internally, increasing the risk for abscess formation.

Maintenance of all lines and drains is imperative and is the responsibility of the nurse. For example, consider the intravenous line used to administer medications, fluids, and blood products. The nurse must make sure the intravenous line does not infiltrate, causing fluids to enter surrounding tissue. This can cause excessive pain for the client and tissue damage around the intravenous site, depending on the medication being administered. When drains are used, nurses are responsible for maintaining wound suction, which helps drain excess discharge. This, in turn, assists in the formation of granulation tissue. In closed wound drainage systems, the drain is connected to electric suction or a portable suction device (e.g., a Jackson-Pratt drain). Directions for use are printed on the container and must be followed carefully to ensure the container is emptied and the drainage plug replaced correctly in order to restore the vacuum function that is required for the closed drainage system to work.

> **SAFETY ALERT**
> Note that the presence of blood in drainage tubes or more than the expected amount of drainage in chest tubes or drainage sites requires a report to the surgeon or anesthesia provider.

Sutures and Staples

Sutures can be absorbable or nonabsorbable. The human body considers both types of sutures a foreign body. Sutures are chosen depending on the type of body tissue being sutured; for example, silk and nylon sutures are used in cardiovascular or neurological procedures, whereas surgical gut sutures are used for soft tissues that heal quickly (Weis, 2009). Sutures are used to close internal incisions and external skin closures.

> **Box 17–5   Postoperative Documentation**
>
> Postoperative assessment and management include, but are not limited to, the review and documentation of the following (ASPAN, 2012):
>
> 1. Review of history and physical
> 2. Systems assessment
>   a. Respiratory
>   b. Cardiovascular
>   c. Neurological
>   d. Gastrointestinal/abdominal
>   e. Urinary
>   f. Musculoskeletal
>   g. Integumentary
> 3. Pain assessment
> 4. Sedation assessment
> 5. Psychosocial assessment
> 6. Medication review and administration
> 7. Care of postoperative lines and drains (e.g., a Foley catheter)
> 8. Intake and output of fluids
> 9. Laboratory testing
> 10. Blood administration
> 11. Dressing changes
> 12. Discharge education.

Staples are mainly utilized to close the skin. Staples decrease the length of time in the operating room due to faster closure of the surgical incision (Weis, 2009). Injury to the skin is decreased when staples are used because there is uniform tension and less distortion along the closure line (Weis, 2009). Another benefit to using staples to close the skin compared to sutures is that the skin heals better and is cosmetically more appealing.

Documentation

A thorough postoperative assessment is imperative to minimize disruption to the client's physiological processes (see **Box 17–5** ●).

▶ CLIENT RECOVERY AND DISCHARGE

According to ASPAN (2012), each healthcare organization should create discharge criteria using the discharge assessment parameters created by ASPAN, while consulting with the anesthesia department and medical staff. Many healthcare facilities follow a discharge scoring record, which assists in the measurement of whether the client is physically able to be discharged. For example, the Aldrete scoring system, which measures the client's circulation, respiration, activity level, and oxygen saturation, is commonly used (**Box 17–6** ●). The Aldrete scoring system identifies two recovery phases: Phase 1 occurs with the discontinuation of anesthesia. Phase 2 begins when the client's protective reflexes and motor functioning return, indicating the client is effectively recovering from anesthesia.

If discharge criteria are not met, the client is transferred to a specified unit, such as an extended recovery or medical-surgical unit, for further monitoring until the discharge criteria are met. The postoperative nurse and anesthesia personnel determine

Box 17–6   The Aldrete Score

This system is designed to assess a client's transition from Phase 1 recovery to Phase 2 recovery, from discontinuation of anesthesia until return of protective reflexes and motor function.

Respiration

2 = Able to take deep breath and cough
1 = Dyspnea/shallow breathing
0 = Apnea

O$_2$ Saturation

2 = Maintains >92% on room air
1 = Needs O$_2$ inhalation to maintain O$_2$ saturation >90%
0 = Saturation <90% even with supplemental oxygen

Consciousness

2 = Fully awake
1 = Arousable on calling
0 = Not responding

Circulation

2 = BP ±20 % preop
1 = BP ±20–49 % preop
0 = BP ±50 % preop

Activity

2 = Able to move 4 extremities
1 = Able to move 2 extremities
0 = Able to move 0 extremities

The total score is 10. Clients scoring ≥8 (and/or are returned to similar preop status) are considered fit for transition to Phase 2 recovery.

Client Teaching
Postoperative Discharge Instructions

- Use pain medications as ordered; do not allow pain to become severe before taking the prescribed dose. Pain inhibits healing.
- Avoid using alcohol while taking opioids or other narcotic analgesics.
- Contact your primary care provider if you experience an increase in pain following increasing discomfort.
- Change dressings and perform wound care as instructed to promote healing and reduce the risk of infection.
- Promptly report any increase in redness, swelling, pain, or discharge from the incision or drain site.
- Gradually increase activities as ordered by the surgeon or primary care provider.
- Adequate rest, nutrition, and hydration are important to promote healing and immune function.

the team and equipment necessary for transport of the client according to the client's postoperative stability (ASPAN, 2012). For example, if the client is having difficulty breathing and maintaining his oxygen saturation level and needs to be transported on oxygen, a licensed professional would transport the client. Once the discharge criteria are met, the surgeon writes discharge orders, which include specific information on medications, wound care, nutrition, and physical activity. Prior to discharge, the postoperative nurse educates the client and the individual driving the client home (see the Client Teaching feature).

Wound Care

Clients are usually allowed to have a shower within 24 hours, but they cannot soak in a bath until the Steri-Strips (thin adhesive strips used to close wounds) have fallen off, due to the possible occurrence of a surgical site infection. Steri-Strips are placed on most wounds. The client is instructed by the postoperative nurse to allow surgical dressings to fall off naturally, which may take up to about 1 week.

Clients will also be instructed on suture or staple care to prevent a surgical site infection. Clients are taught to report the signs and symptoms of infection to their surgeon. The client will be given specific instructions on when to return to the surgeon's office for a postoperative appointment. During the postoperative appointment, the sutures or staples will be removed and a dressing change completed by the surgeon.

Nutrition

To help prevent nausea and vomiting, clients are encouraged to start with bland foods and gradually advance to a normal diet. Depending on the surgery, a specific diet may be prescribed for a period of time. For example, a client receiving bariatric surgery will be prescribed a specific serving size and type of food. Typically clients are encouraged to increase their fluid intake on discharge. Increasing the fluid intake assists the physiological systems to return to normal, maintaining hydration and electrolytes necessary for homeostasis.

Physical Activity

The surgical client is not allowed to drive or handle heavy machinery within 24 hours of procedures that require anesthesia administration. The surgeon also instructs the client on the appropriate time to resume physical activities, such as running, cycling, or sexual activity.

REVIEW   The Concept of Perioperative Care

RELATE Link the Concepts

Linking the concept of perioperative care with the concept of development:

1. What strategies could you use to explain a diagnostic surgical procedure to a 5-year-old child?

2. Prepare a client teaching plan for a 10-year-old client who must refrain from sports-related activities for 2 weeks following surgery.

Linking the concept of perioperative care with the concept of nutrition:

3. Why is it necessary to provide client teaching related to withholding food prior to surgery?

4. Why does altered nutrition status or malnutrition increase the risks associated with surgery?

Linking the concept of perioperative care with the concept of informatics:

5. What are the advantages of a surgical team using uniform language?

6. How might telehealth be used to assist clients to prepare for surgery prior to the day of the procedure?

READY Go to Companion Skills Manual

REFER Go to Pearson Nursing Student Resources

nursing.pearsonhighered.com

- Additional review materials
- **Chart:** Nursing Care of the Client Having an Ileostomy

REFLECT Case Study

Mary, a 25-year-old female, arrives in the postoperative phase. Mary's mother died of colon cancer, and Mary had a colonoscopy that revealed three precancerous polyps and one malignant polyp. Mary had a partial colectomy to remove the malignant section of her colon. The physician placed a closed drain system in Mary's abdominal incision. The abdominal drain has 20 mL of blood-tinged drainage. Mary has a urinary catheter in place that is draining 30 mL of clear urine every hour. During intubation, Mary sustained a 3 mm laceration to her upper lip. Bleeding is controlled. Mary's heart rate is 48 bpm, indicating bradycardia. Mary remains drowsy from the anesthesia, but she appears to be comfortable with a limited amount of pain. The postanesthesia nurse raises Mary's head and places her in the sitting position. The nurse supports Mary with pillows and provides a pillow for her to place on her stomach when she takes deep breaths.

Mary sits up for 1 hour. Her vital signs include: T 98.6°F, P 65 bpm, R 14/min, and BP 117/72 mmHg and her respirations are regular and non-labored. Mary is transferred to the medical-surgical unit for further observation for 24 hours prior to being discharged home.

1. What procedure could have been performed to assist in Mary's prognosis? Explain why.

2. Name some topics for discharge instructions that the postoperative nurse should anticipate.

◼ REFERENCES

American Society of Anesthesiologists. (n.d.). *ASA Physical Status Classification System.* Retrieved from http://www.asahq.org/Home/For-Members/Clinical-Information/ASA-Physical-Status-Classification-System.

American Society of PeriAnesthesia Nurses (ASPAN). (2012). *2012–2014 Perianesthesia nursing standards, practice recommendations and interpretive statements.* Cherry Hill, NJ: Author.

Anderson, P., & Townsend, T. (2010). Medication errors: Don't let this happen to you. *American Nurse Today.* Retrieved from http://www.americannursetoday.com/assets/0/434/436/440/6276/6334/6350/6356/8b8dac76-6061-4521-8b43-d0928ef8de07.pdf.

Association of periOperative Registered Nurses (AORN). (2012). *Perioperative job descriptions and competency evaluation tools.* Denver, CO: Author.

Association of periOperative Registered Nurses (AORN). (2013). *Perioperative standards and recommended practices.* Denver, CO: Author.

Bashaw, M., & Scott, D. (2012). Surgical risk factors in geriatric perioperative patients. *AORN Journal, 96*(1), 58–74. doi:10.1016/j.aorn.2011.05.025.

Board of Laser Safety. (2013). *Certified medical laser safety officer: Policies & procedures manual.* Retrieved from https://www.lasersafety.org/uploads/pdf/cmlso_pp_manual.pdf.

Centers for Disease Control and Prevention (CDC). (2011). *Having surgery? What should you know before you go?* Retrieved from http://www.cdc.gov/features/safesurgery.

Centers for Disease Control and Prevention (CDC). (2013). *Frequently asked questions about surgical site infections.* Retrieved from http://www.cdc.gov/HAI/pdfs/ssi/SSI_tagged.pdf.

Chimutengwende-Gordon, M., Khan, W. S., & Maruthainar, N. (2010). Perioperative blood transfusion: The role of allogenous and autologous transfusions, and pharmacological agents. *Journal of Perioperative Practice, 20*(8), 283–287. Retrieved from http://search.proquest.com/docview/741865537?accountid=12774.

Hicks, R., Wanzer, L., & Denholm, B. (2012). Implementing AORN recommended practices for medication safety. *AORN Journal, 96*(6), 605–622. doi:org/10.1016/j.aorn.2012.09.012.

Hilsgen, J. (2013). Geriooperative nursing care: Principles and practices of surgical care for the older adult. *AORN Journal, 97*(1), 154–155. doi: http://dx.doi.org/10.1016/j.aorn.2012.10.002.

Institute of Medicine. (2006). *Preventing medication errors.* Retrieved from http://iom.edu/~/media/Files/Report%20Files/2006/Preventing-Medication-Errors-Quality-Chasm-Series/medicationerrorsnew.pdf.

Joyce, J. (2008). Toward reducing perioperative transfusions. *AANA Journal, 76*(2), 131–137. Retrieved from http://search.proquest.com.libproxy.northgeorgia.edu/docview/222233897?accountid=12 774.

Kamel, C., McGahan, L., Polisena, J., Mierzwinski, M., & Embil, J. M. (2012). Preoperative skin antiseptic preparations for preventing surgical site infections. *Infection Control and Hospital Epidemiology, 33*(6), 608–617.

Kang, C., Chaudhry, O., Halabi, W., Nguyen, V., Carmichael, J., Mills, S., & Stamos, M. (2012). Risk factors for postoperative urinary tract infection and urinary retention in patients undergoing surgery for colorectal cancer. *American Surgeon, 78*(10), 1100–1104.

Meeks, S. (2011). Immobilization from rigid to non-rigid. *MD Anderson Center.* Retrieved from http://www.aapm.org/meetings/2011SS/documents/Meeksrigidtononrigid.pdf.

Osborn, K. S., Wraa, C. E., Watson, A. B., & Holleran, R. (2014). Intraoperative nursing. In *Medical-surgical nursing: Preparation for practice* (2nd ed., Chap. 18). Upper Saddle River, NJ: Pearson Education.

Shander, A., Van Aken, H., Colomina, M. J., Gombotz, H., Hofmann, A., Krauspe, R., & Spahn, D. R. (2012). Patient blood management in Europe. *British Journal of Anesthesia, 109*(1), 55–68. Retrieved from http://search.ebscohost.com/login.aspx?direct=true&db=rzh&AN=2011585895&site=ehost-live.

Waters, J. H., & Yazer, M. H. (2008). Why blood management? In Waters, J. H (Ed.), *Blood management: Options for better patient care* (pp. 1–17). Bethesda, MD: AABB Press.

Weis, M. (2009). Handle tissue with instruments. In M. L. Phippen, B. C. Ulmer, & M.P. Wells (Eds.), *Competency for safe patient care during operative and invasive procedures* (pp. 465–498). Denver, CO: Competency and Credentialing Institute.

Wilson, B., Shannon, M., & Shields, K. (2013). *Pearson: Nurse's drug guide, 2013.* Upper Saddle River, NJ: Pearson Education.

World Health Organization. (2009). *Surgical safety checklist.* Retrieved from http://www.who.int/patientsafety/safesurgery/en/.

Zinn, J. (2012). Surgical wound classification: Communication is needed for accuracy. *AORN Journal, 95*(2), 274–278. doi:10.1016/j.aorn.2011.10.013.

18 Sensory Perception

◤ THE CONCEPT OF SENSORY PERCEPTION

Our sensory organs provide pathways for stimuli to reach the brain, allowing us to experience the world in which we live. Sensory stimuli give meaning to events in the environment. The five senses—vision, hearing, touch, smell, and taste—are essential for growth, development, and survival. Normal sensory function enables or affects nearly every human activity, from reading a book to alerting to smoke from a fire. **Sensory perception** is protective—think of a mother sensing the bath water is too hot as she sees the steam rise from the water. It is also complex, allowing individuals to master activities that require the use of multiple senses at once, such as driving a car.

(continued on next page)

Concept Learning Outcomes

After reading about this concept, you will be able to:

1. Summarize the physiology of the body systems and structures involved in sensory perception.

2. Examine the relationship between sensory perception and other concepts/systems.

3. Identify commonly occurring alterations in sensory perception and their related therapies.

4. Differentiate common assessment procedures used to examine sensory perception across the life span.

5. Describe diagnostic and laboratory tests to determine the individual's sensory perception status.

6. Explain management of sensory perception health and prevention of altered sensory perception.

7. Demonstrate the nursing process in providing culturally competent and caring interventions across the life span for individuals with common alterations in sensory perception.

8. Compare and contrast common independent and collaborative interventions for clients with alterations in sensory perception.

Concept Key Terms

Accommodation, *1287*
Auditory, *1278*
Awareness, *1278*
Cerumen, *1285*
Color blindness, *1279*
Convergence, *1287*
Corneal reflex, *1289*
Gustatory, *1278*
Hyperopia, *1286*
Impulse conduction, *1278*
Kinesthetic, *1278*
Myopia, *1286*
Nystagmus, *1286*
Olfactory, *1278*

Perception, *1278*
Presbyopia, *1286*
Ptosis, *1288*
Receptor, *1278*
Refraction, *1281*
Sensory perception, *1277*
Sensory reception, *1278*
Stereognosis, *1278*
Stimulus, *1278*
Tactile, *1278*
Vertigo, *1279*
Visceral, *1278*
Visual, *1278*

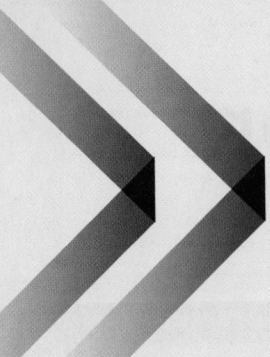

Alterations in sensory functions can affect an individual's ability to experience the world; they may limit self-care, mobility, safety, independence, communication, and relationships with others. Some deficits, such as mild vision impairment, may only require simple compensatory behaviors or assistive devices to overcome (e.g., eyeglasses). Other deficits, such as full hearing loss, present greater challenges. Some clients may experience impairments that put them at risk in institutional settings such as schools or assisted living facilities. The role of the nurse working with a client with an alteration in sensory perception is to help the client find ways to function safely in what are often confusing environments. **<<**

▶ NORMAL SENSORY PERCEPTION

The sensory process involves two components: reception and perception. **Sensory reception** is the process of receiving stimuli or data. These stimuli are either external or internal to the body. External stimuli are **visual** (sight), **auditory** (hearing), **olfactory** (smell), **tactile** (touch), and **gustatory** (taste). Gustatory stimuli can be internal as well. Other types of internal stimuli are kinesthetic and visceral. **Kinesthetic** refers to awareness of the position and movement of body parts. For example, an individual walking is aware of which leg is forward. A related sense is **stereognosis**, the ability to perceive and understand an object through touch by its size, shape, and texture. An individual holding a tennis ball is aware of its size, round shape, and soft surface without seeing it. **Visceral** means of or relating to any large organ within the body. Visceral organs may produce stimuli that make an individual aware of them (e.g., a full stomach). Sensory perception involves the conscious organization and translation of the data or stimuli into meaningful information.

For an individual to be aware of his surroundings, four aspects of the sensory process must be present:

- **Stimulus.** This is an agent or act that stimulates a nerve receptor.
- **Receptor.** A nerve cell acts as a receptor by converting the stimulus to a nerve impulse. Most receptors are specific; that is, sensitive to only one type of stimulus, such as visual, auditory, or touch.
- **Impulse conduction.** The impulse travels along nerve pathways to the spinal cord or directly to the brain. The cranial nerves (listed in **Table 18–1 ●** along with their functions) are important nerves that control many actions required for sensory perception (**Figure 18–1 ●**). For example, auditory impulses travel to the organ of Corti in the inner ear. From there, the impulses travel along the eighth cranial nerve to the temporal lobe of the brain.
- **Perception.** Perception, or awareness and interpretation of stimuli, takes place in the brain. Specialized brain cells interpret the nature and the quality of the sensory stimuli. The level of consciousness affects the perception of the stimuli.

The brain has the capacity to adapt to sensory stimuli. For example, an individual living in a city may not notice traffic noise that someone from a rural area finds loud and disturbing. The brain does not act on all stimuli immediately; some stimuli are stored in the memory to be used at a later date. Sensory processing is not the same as cognition or awareness. Cognition is the process by which an individual learns, stores, retrieves, and uses information. **Awareness** is the ability to perceive environmental stimuli and body reactions and to respond appropriately through thought and action. The normal, alert individual can assimilate many kinds of information at one time.

Understanding of sensory function and alterations in sensory perception requires familiarity with the normal anatomic structure and physiological function of each system involved in sensory perception. Knowledge of related

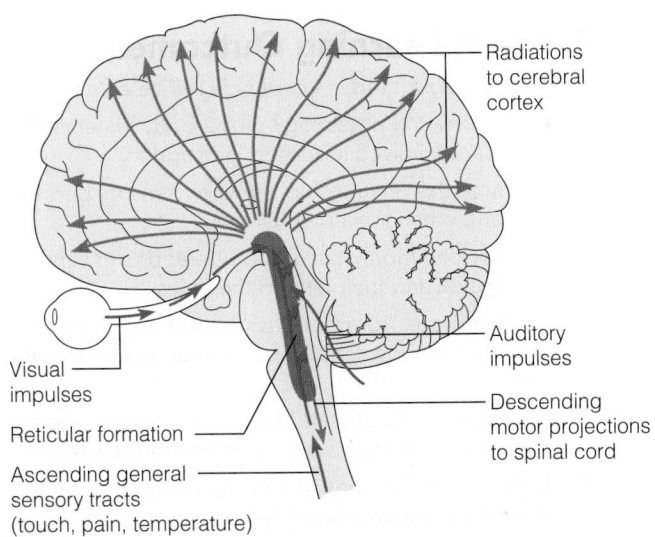

Figure 18–1 ● The nerve impulses run along the ascending sensory tracts to reach the reticular activating system (RAS); then certain impulses reach the cerebral cortex where they are perceived.

Source: From Marieb, E. N., & Hoehn, K. (2007). *Human anatomy & physiology* (7th ed., p. 455). Benjamin Cummings Publishing Company. Reprinted by permission of Pearson Education, Inc.

TABLE 18–1 Cranial Nerves and Their Functions

NAME	FUNCTION
I Olfactory	Sense of smell
II Optic	Vision
III Oculomotor	Eyeball movement: *moves eye medially,* elevates eye or rolls it superiorly, depresses eye or rolls it inferiorly, elevates eye and turns it laterally
	Raising of upper eyelid
	Constriction of pupil
	Proprioception
IV Trochlear	Eyeball movement: depresses eye and turns it laterally
V Trigeminal	Sensation of the upper scalp, upper eyelid, nose, nasal cavity, cornea, and lacrimal gland
	Sensation of the palate, upper teeth, cheek, top lip, lower eyelid, and scalp; sensation of the tongue, lower teeth, chin, and temporal scalp
	Chewing
VI Abducens	Eyeball movement: Moves eye laterally
VII Facial	Movement of facial muscles
	Secretions of lacrimal, nasal, submandibular, and sublingual glands
	Sensation of taste
VIII Acoustic/ Vestibulocochlear	Sense of balance
	Sense of hearing
IX Glossopharyngeal	Swallowing
	Gag reflex
	Secretions of parotid salivary gland
	Sense of taste
	Touch, pressure, and pain from pharynx and posterior tongue
	Pressure from carotid arteries
	Receptors to regulate blood pressure
X Vagus	Swallowing
	Regulation of cardiac rate
	Regulation of respirations
	Digestion
	Sensation from thoracic and abdominal organs
	Proprioception
	Sense of taste
XI Accessory	Movement of head and neck
	Proprioception
XII Hypoglossal	Movement of tongue for speech and swallowing

structures and functions, and how they may differ along the life span, helps nurses provide timely and accurate assessment to reduce the individual's risk for injury or complications when alterations occur.

✱ Go to **nursing.pearsonhighered.com** *for a minimodule on the review of the physiology of sensory perception, including lifespan considerations.*

▶ ALTERATIONS OF SENSORY PERCEPTION

Alterations in sensory perception are common. Nurses work with clients with a variety of alterations from color blindness to eye injury to altered sense of taste. Alterations in sensory perception can affect clients and client care in a number of ways (see the Concepts Related to Sensory Perception feature). Specific alterations are offered as exemplars to this concept: hearing impairment, cataracts, eye injury, glaucoma, and macular degeneration. An overview of some nonspecific alterations, such as vertigo, is provided here.

Alterations and Manifestations

A number of nonspecific alterations may occur due to aging, genetic factors, or underlying illness. Lifestyle factors, such as tobacco use, can also affect sensory perception. In all cases, identification of the cause begins with a thorough client assessment. Some common nonspecific alterations in sensory perception include vertigo, color blindness, impaired olfactory (sense of smell) function, and taste disturbances.

Vertigo is a feeling of rotation or imbalance. It can be acute or chronic and can range from being merely distracting to completely debilitating. It may or may not be accompanied by nausea. A client with vertigo may have difficulty with balance and/or nystagmus. Vertigo is difficult to diagnose: It can be caused by strokes, brain tumors, head trauma, viruses, or it can be idiopathic with no identifiable cause. A common cause of vertigo is vestibular neuritis. In about 50% of cases of vestibular neuritis, the client will report a prior bout of the common cold. One common type of vertigo is benign paroxysmal positional vertigo (BPPV), which is caused by a disruption of the orientation of ear otoliths. Up to 42% of cases of vertigo will be diagnosed as BPPV. Treatment and prognosis for the resolution of vertigo depend on the etiology; some clients will experience resolution within a few days, but others will experience recurring symptoms throughout their lifetime.

Color blindness affects approximately 1 in 10 men but very few women. It occurs when one or more pigments are missing within the cones in the retina. The most common variant is the inability to distinguish between red and green. Less common is the inability to distinguish between blue and yellow. Many people with the blue-yellow variant also have problems distinguishing between green and red. *Achromatopsia* is a rare form a color blindness in which the individual cannot distinguish any color at all and sees only shades of gray.

Impaired sense of smell can occur for a number of reasons. It is commonly associated with respiratory illnesses such as the common cold. As mentioned previously, a decreased sense of smell is part of the normal aging process. Some medications, such as cholesterol-lowering medications and antibiotics, may alter smell temporarily. Clients who smoke tobacco or have undergone radiation treatment for head and neck cancers will have a decreased sense of smell. Because serious conditions such as brain tumors, Parkinson disease, or multiple sclerosis also may result in loss of smell, clients reporting a prolonged alteration in their sense of smell require further assessment.

Taste disturbances are an often overlooked abnormality. Although a decrease in sense of taste is a normal part of aging,

Concepts Related to **Sensory Perception**

The loss or dysfunction of a sense can sometimes be difficult to diagnose and treat, especially in older adults who may accept loss of function as a normal part of the aging process even in cases when pathology is present. In any stage of development, the loss of one or more senses can impact daily functioning and increase the client's risk for injury. Even minor impairments can cause overload of other senses, creating stress for the client. Long-term impairment may lead to loss of independence and a sense of dignity or to depression, especially in clients who are not able to return to a normal level of functioning or who experience a change in their ability to perform familiar tasks or roles. Alterations in sensory perception can increase risk for confusion, especially when clients find themselves in unfamiliar settings. Disorientation may result from either sensory deprivation or sensory overload. Infection may also play a role: Untreated or chronic ear infections may lead to structural changes in the ear and permanent hearing impairment. Infection also is one of many potential causes of peripheral neuropathy. The role of the nurse is to provide thorough assessment, aid in an accurate diagnosis, support a safe environment, and assist the client in achieving optimal functioning.

CONCEPT	RELATIONSHIP TO SENSORY PERCEPTION	NURSING IMPLICATIONS
Cognition		
■ Mental Assessment ■ Assessment interview: Cognition ■ Confusion	Alterations in sensory perception can cause confusion. Disorientation can be caused by sensory deprivation or overload.	■ Assess for sensory function by obtaining complete client history and performing physical exam. ■ Pay close attention to mental status; loss or decrease in one or more senses can mimic senility in older adults. ■ Provide reorientation as needed. ■ Involve other members of healthcare team if deficits are noted.
Stress and Coping		
■ Types of stressors ■ Manifestations of stress	Loss of one or more senses can cause sensory overload as the other senses adapt to fill in the deficit. A client may become overwhelmed by loss of function and/or sensory overload. Unresolved anger over the loss may impact relationships with others, especially immediate family members.	■ Note if client looks bored or confused because the client may not communicate feeling over- or underwhelmed. ■ Eliminate extra noise and stimulus as needed. ■ Provide meaningful interaction and stimulation to reduce emotional or physical isolation. ■ Encourage verbalization of positive and negative feelings related to loss.
Self		
■ Self-concept ■ Self-esteem ■ Self-awareness	Alterations in one or more senses can cause loss of independence or dignity.	■ Encourage verbalization of positive and negative feelings related to loss. ■ Teach client how to adapt to sensory deficit. ■ Provide for client safety. ■ Encourage involvement with social and community groups to increase feelings of self-worth and contribution. ■ Provide referrals to organizations that may assist with involvement and interaction; assess for the need for referral related to lack of transportation.
Safety		
■ Safety considerations across the lifespan	Sensory deficits may increase a client's risk for injury, especially falls and burns.	■ Assess extent to which deficit impacts function, particularly safe movement. ■ Assist client to determine what coping mechanisms or assistive devices may promote safety. ■ Educate client, caregivers about increased risk for injury and provide client teaching related to safety; schedule an in-home safety assessment as necessary.

Concepts Related to **Sensory Perception** (*continued*)

CONCEPT	RELATIONSHIP TO SENSORY PERCEPTION	NURSING IMPLICATIONS
Infection		
■ Complications of infectious diseases	May lead to vision loss, hearing damage, peripheral neuropathy.	■ Provide client education regarding the need to take antibiotics as prescribed. ■ Provide client teaching related to preventing infection, for example, hand washing. ■ Treatment of illnesses that increase risk for sensory deprivation is one of the best methods of prevention.

Alterations and Therapies **Sensory Perception**

ALTERATION	DESCRIPTION	MANIFESTATIONS	INTERVENTIONS AND THERAPIES
Eye injuries	Damage to the structure of the eye; a common cause of vision loss in children. Common causes include sports injuries and chemical exposure.	Manifestations vary based on type of injury, but can range from redness and edema due to corneal abrasion to complete loss of vision (and/or eye) due to penetrating injury.	■ All eye injuries should be considered medical emergencies requiring immediate evaluation and intervention. ■ Treatment varies due to type and severity of injury; treatments may include irrigation, foreign body removal, and surgery.
Cataracts	A breakdown of proteins within the lens results in the lens no longer being able to change shape to focus.	Opacification of the eye prevents **refraction** of light rays onto the retina; may be congenital or acquired.	■ If vision is not affected, client will be monitored. If vision becomes impaired, the lens may be surgically removed and a new lens implanted.
Glaucoma	Optic neuropathy with gradual loss of peripheral vision; the two main types are open-angle and angle-closure glaucoma. Both types are associated with an increase in intraocular pressure.	Open-angle may cause gradual loss of peripheral vision or "tunnel" vision in both eyes. Closed-angle may cause severe eye pain, sudden onset of visual disturbances, and blurred vision.	■ Medications to control intraocular pressure and preserve vision in open-angle glaucoma ■ Surgical procedures include: Laser trabeculoplasty Photocoagulation Gonioplasty Laser iridotomy.
Age-related macular degeneration (AMD)	Progressive disorder involving loss of central vision due to damage to the retina; the two types are nonexudative and exudative.	Symptoms usually develop gradually and include needing more light to read, blurriness of print, or a blurred or blind spot in central vision.	■ High-dose antioxidants and zinc (early-to-intermediate dry AMD) ■ Laser surgery or photodynamic therapy (wet AMD)
Peripheral neuropathy	Occurs when trauma or disease processes interfere with innervation of peripheral nerves. Peripheral blood vessels constrict, peripheral nerve endings in the affected area suffer effects of decreased blood flow, and neuropathy develops.	Manifestations depend on the affected nerve(s) and the amount of damage. Manifestations may include aching, shooting, or burning pain; weakness, imbalance.	■ Interventions and therapies focus on treating the underlying cause and promoting safety and comfort.

it is also associated with medication use, smoking, and infection. Gum disease can also affect taste. Because taste and smell are closely related, they may share an etiology when impaired. Clients reporting prolonged taste impairment require further assessment. In older adults, decreased taste sensation can lead to weight loss requiring intervention. Impairment of vision and hearing and peripheral neuropathies are discussed in more detail in the exemplars in this module.

Genetic Considerations and Nonmodifiable Risk Factors

Although lifestyle choices, such as wearing vision protection while woodworking or refraining from smoking, can reduce the risk for sensory impairment, genetic predisposition to illness and the pathology of certain coexisting disorders also can lead to alterations in sensory perception.

CONGENITAL AND HEREDITARY CONDITIONS Many conditions lead to temporary or permanent impairment of sensory perception. Infants who are premature; whose mothers were infected prenatally with rubella, toxoplasmosis, or other viruses; or who have certain congenital and hereditary conditions are at a high risk for visual and/or hearing problems. More than 50% of all cases of hearing loss at birth can be linked to genetic abnormalities. Some occur in the absence of other problems. Others occur in conjunction with other genetic syndromes such as Treacher Collins syndrome and Down syndrome. Retinopathy of prematurity, low birth weight, and congenital cataracts are common causes of blindness or visual impairment in children. Fetal alcohol syndrome (FAS) is a major cause of prenatal visual and hearing disturbances.

Auditory processing disorder, a condition in which the individual has difficulty differentiating individual sounds in words, is one of several hearing disorders with which a child may be born. It creates difficulty for individuals in some environments, especially school. Its cause is unknown.

In older adults, prevalence of some visual disorders may have a cultural or genetic component. African Americans and Hispanic/Latinos have the highest prevalence of open-angle glaucoma.

Visual impairment due to refractive error occurs twice as often in American Indian/Alaskan Natives compared to Caucasians or African Americans (Lighthouse International, 2013).

ILLNESS Diseases such as atherosclerosis restrict blood flow to the receptor organs and the brain, thereby decreasing awareness and slowing responses. Hypertension, especially uncontrolled, can contribute to vision loss. Cerebrovascular accidents (strokes) can cause blindness, hearing loss, changes in taste or smell, or other sensory disturbances based on the location of damaged brain tissue. Uncontrolled diabetes mellitus can impair vision and is a leading cause of blindness in the United States. Maternal diabetes can also cause hearing loss in infants. Some central nervous system diseases cause varying degrees of paralysis and sensory loss. Repeated bouts of otitis media can cause permanent hearing loss in children.

CASE STUDY \\ PART 1

Simon Thompson is a 10-year-old Caucasian male who is currently in the fifth grade. He has always been a good student, but this year his grades haven't been very good. During a parent–teacher conference, Simon's teacher reported that he seemed to be squinting a lot. His parents scheduled an appointment with their primary care provider's office.

The nurse practitioner performs an ophthalmoscope exam and tests Simon's vision using a Snellen chart. Based on her findings, she advises Simon's parents to take him to see an ophthalmologist. The ophthalmologist determines that Simon's visual acuity is 20/100 and that he needs glasses to correct his vision. When he starts wearing his glasses, his 13-year-old sister and her friends tease Simon every chance they can, and he becomes embarrassed at having to wear his glasses.

Clinical Reasoning Questions Level I

1. This scenario features a nurse practitioner. What is the role of the registered nurse in assessing sensory perception?
2. What are some possible nursing diagnoses for Simon at this time?

Clinical Reasoning Questions Level II

3. Given Simon's visual acuity of 20/100, what condition does he most likely demonstrate?
4. What nursing interventions could help Simon cope with his embarrassment over wearing glasses?

▶ PREVENTION

Some loss of functioning is inevitable as part of the normal aging process. Individuals can lower their risk for loss of function related to sensory perception through awareness of risk factors and engaging in appropriate prevention activities.

Modifiable Risk Factors

Modifiable risk factors are those that can be changed or controlled, such as health-related behaviors and choice of environment. For certain alterations in sensory perception, individual choices can significantly influence the development of a disorder or impairment.

SMOKING Tobacco use can cause problems with taste and smell. It can also cause problems with vision because it constricts the blood vessels that supply the eyes and optic nerve. Encourage smoking cessation in all clients.

ULTRAVIOLET LIGHT EXPOSURE Although often overlooked, unprotected UV exposure can cause serious eye problems. In the short term, minor symptoms such as irritation or photokeratitis (corneal burn) may occur. Long-term effects of UV exposure can include serious visual disturbances (some of which will be discussed further in the exemplars in this module). Several types of cancers, such as melanoma, basal cell, and squamous cell, can occur on the skin near the eye or the eye itself. Long-term UV exposure also increases rates of cataracts and age-related macular degeneration (AMD). Advise clients to wear UVA/UVB blocking sunglasses and hats and to minimize sun exposure and avoid tanning beds.

MEDICATION   Certain medications can alter an individual's awareness of environmental stimuli. Narcotics and sedatives, for example, can decrease awareness of stimuli. Some antidepressants can alter perceptions of stimuli. Anyone taking several medications concurrently may show alterations in sensory function. Older adults are especially at risk and need to be monitored carefully, particularly if they are simultaneously taking multiple medications for a variety of conditions.

STRESS   During times of increased stress, individuals may find their senses overloaded and seek to decrease sensory stimulation. For example, a client dealing with physical illness, pain, hospitalization, and diagnostic tests may wish to have only close support people visit. The client may also need the nurse's help in reducing unnecessary stimuli (e.g., noise) as much as possible. Some clients, however, may seek sensory stimulation during times of low stress.

ISOLATION   Much research has been done to document the importance of touch in early life. Infants in incubators who are not touched will stop eating and fail to thrive. The same may be true for older adults, especially those with cognitive or sensory impairments. Institutionalized older adults deprived of caring touch and nurturing physical contact experience a diminishing quality of life, a lessening of their desire to relate to others, and a weakening of what may already be a fragile relationship with physical reality (Prieto-Flores et al., 2011).

INJURIES   Injuries that may damage sensory organs can occur anywhere—at home, in the workplace, or at school. Each year more than 38 million children participate in an organized sport. More than 1 in 10 will end up with an injury that requires a visit to the emergency department (Safe Kids USA, 2012).

Many eye injuries are minor, but without timely and appropriate intervention, even a minor injury can threaten vision. For this reason, all eye injuries should be considered medical emergencies requiring immediate evaluation and intervention. Eye injuries will be explored in more detail in the Eye Injuries exemplar later in this module.

Ear injuries of many types are common in children. Lacerations, infections, and hematomas may occur in the external ear structures, especially the pinna. Children may place foreign objects in the ear, and insects may enter the ear canal. Rupture of the tympanic membrane may result from head injuries, blows to the ear, or insertion of objects into the ear canal. Serous drainage from the ear can indicate a basilar skull fracture. Ruptured tympanic membranes in combination with conjunctival and retinal hemorrhage are indicative of shaken baby syndrome. Retinal hemorrhage rarely occurs with any other type of injury. A nurse who suspects child abuse should follow agency protocol for reporting to Child Protective Services.

Regardless of age, any injury resulting in earache, decreased hearing, persistent bleeding, or other discharge should be evaluated by a physician.

Screenings

Often, changes that occur within the domain of sensory perception happen very slowly or without the client noticing any symptoms. Careful routine screening is imperative; early detection can result in improved outcomes for clients.

HEARING   Most newborns are routinely screened for hearing loss prior to leaving the hospital. Guidelines vary by state, but preschoolers and school-age children undergo periodic screening at their schools or healthcare provider's office. Early detection of hearing problems is critical for children's everyday functioning and school performance. Adults should be screened at least every 10 years until the age of 50 and then every 3 years. Any client who experiences an abnormal hearing screening or feels that there has been a change in hearing should be referred to a certified audiologist for a comprehensive evaluation (American Speech-Language-Hearing Association [ASLHA], 2013d).

VISION   Current guidelines recommend all children between the ages of 3 and 5 receive a vision screening at least once. Like hearing screening, many states establish their own guidelines and periodically offer vision screening at school or as part of routine well-child visits. Any child suspected of having visual difficulties should be referred for a comprehensive ophthalmological evaluation (U.S. Preventive Services Task Force, 2011). Beyond the age of 40, 1 in 28 adults in the United States is visually impaired. Annual or biannual screenings are recommended for individuals without comorbidities. Annual screenings are recommended for adults with diabetes or hypertension (Pelletier, Thomas, & Shaw, 2009).

TASTE, SMELL, AND TOUCH   There are currently no recommended screening guidelines for taste, smell, or touch. Most abnormalities with these senses are found when clients present to their healthcare providers with complaints of alterations.

▶ ASSESSMENT

Nursing assessment of sensory-perceptual functioning includes six components: (a) nursing history, (b) mental status examination, (c) identification of clients at risk, (d) the client's environment, (e) social support network, and (f) physical assessment.

Nursing Assessment

The nursing assessment begins with obtaining a thorough history from the client. Inquire about the client's current sensory functioning, sensory deficits, and any recent changes. Include questions designed to obtain information related to noise exposure—loud, constant sounds from any type of equipment, for example—as well as hobbies or work that can cause burns or injuries. Assess for chronic diseases or illness as well as medications taken by the client, regardless of the type of impairment suspected. The following Assessment Interview provides examples of interview questions to elicit data about the client's sensory-perceptual functioning.

In some instances, significant others or family members can provide data the client cannot. For example, family members may discuss recent changes in the client's hearing ability, such as inattention to others, recent mood swings, difficulty following clear instructions, frequent requests to have something repeated, and unusually loud radio or television volumes.

Because sensory alterations can cause changes in mental status and cognitive functioning, assessment of these areas is essential (Snyderman & Rovner, 2009). Assessment of mental status

Assessment Interview   Sensory-Perceptual Functioning

Visual

- How would you rate your vision (excellent, good, fair, or poor)?
- Do you wear eyeglasses or contact lenses?
- Describe any recent changes in your vision.
- Do you have any difficulty seeing near or far objects?
- Do you have any difficulty seeing at night? Have you ever experienced blurred vision, double vision, spots moving in front of your eyes, blind spots, light sensitivity, flashing lights, or halos around objects?
- When did you last visit an eye doctor?

Auditory

- How would you rate your hearing (excellent, good, fair, or poor)?
- Do you wear a hearing aid?
- Describe any recent changes in your hearing.
- Can you locate the direction of sounds and distinguish various voices?
- Are you having any trouble with balance?
- Do you experience any dizziness or vertigo? Do you experience any ringing, buzzing, humming, crackling noises, or fullness in the ears?
- Do you listen to loud music on a regular basis?
- Are you exposed to any loud noises at work? If so, what are they? How much or how often?

Gustatory

- Have you experienced any changes in taste (e.g., difficulty in differentiating sweet, sour, salty, and bitter tastes)?
- Do you enjoy the taste of foods as you did previously?

Olfactory

- Have you experienced any changes in smell?
- Do things (foods, flowers, perfumes, and so on) smell the same as previously?
- Can you distinguish foods by their odors and tell when something is burning?
- Have you experienced any changes in appetite? (Changes in appetite may be related to an impaired sense of smell.)

Tactile

- Are you experiencing any pain or discomfort?
- Have you experienced any decrease in your ability to perceive heat, cold, or pain in your limbs?
- Do you have any numbness or tingling in your extremities?

Kinesthetic

- Have you noticed any difficulty in perceiving the position of parts of your body?
- Do you need any assistance standing or sitting down?

---

includes inquiring about any recent history of mood alterations or delirium. Assess for problems with cognitive function, including level of consciousness, orientation, memory, and attention span.

CLIENT ENVIRONMENT   The nurse assesses the client's environment for quantity, quality, and type of stimuli. Inadequate environmental stimulation may place the client at risk for sensory deprivation, whereas excessive stimulation may increase the risk for sensory overload. Nonstimulating environments include those that severely restrict physical activity and limit social contact with family and friends. Because appropriate or meaningful stimuli decrease the incidence of sensory deprivation, the nurse must consider the client's healthcare environment for the presence of stimuli such as reading materials, auditory devices (e.g., television, MP3 player, iPod, iPad), number and compatibility of roommates (which may affect level of overall noise), and number of visitors.

To assess a healthcare environment that produces excessive stimuli, the nurse also considers factors such as bright lights, noise, therapeutic measures, and frequency of assessments and procedures.

SOCIAL SUPPORT NETWORK   The degree of isolation an individual feels is significantly influenced by the quality and quantity of support from family members and friends. The nurse assesses (a) whether the client lives alone, (b) who visits and when, and (c) any signs indicating social deprivation. Signs of social deprivation may include withdrawal from

contact with others to avoid embarrassment or dependence on others, negative self-image, reports of lack of meaningful communication with others, and absence of opportunities to discuss fears or concerns that facilitate coping mechanisms.

Physical Assessment

Physical assessment determines whether the senses are impaired. During the physical examination, the nurse assesses vision (including color vision) and hearing, and the olfactory, gustatory, tactile, and kinesthetic senses. The examination should include assessment of the client's visual and hearing abilities; perception of heat, cold, light touch, and pain; and awareness of the position of the body parts (proprioception). Specific sensory tests include the following:

- Visual acuity, using a Snellen chart or other reading material such as a newspaper, and visual fields, using picture charts for those with limited reading or language proficiency
- Hearing acuity, by observing the client's conversation with others and by performing the whisper test and the Weber and Rinne tuning fork tests
- Olfactory sense, by identifying specific aromas
- Gustatory sense, by identifying three tastes such as lemon, salt, and sugar
- Tactile sense, by testing light touch, sharp and dull sensation, two-point discrimination, hot and cold sensation, vibration sense, position sense, and stereognosis.

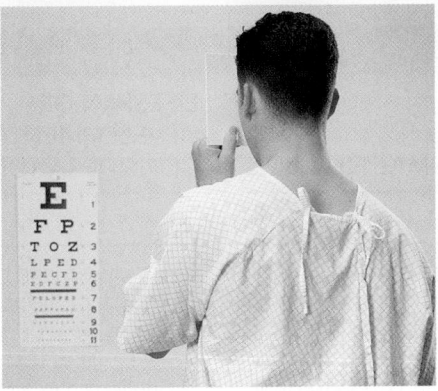

Figure 18–2 ● Testing distant vision using the Snellen eye chart.

If the client uses sensory adaptive devices such as eyeglasses or a hearing aid, the nurse should determine whether or not these function properly and if the client is compliant in using them.

EYE AND VISION ASSESSMENT   Visual acuity is assessed with an eye chart, such as the Snellen chart or the E chart for testing distance vision, and the Rosenbaum chart for testing near vision. The Snellen chart contains rows of letters in various sizes, with standardized numbers at the end of each row. The number at the end of the row indicates the visual acuity of a client who can read the row at a distance of 20 feet. (If the client is unable to read or does not read English, an E chart can be used to test visual acuity.) The top number at the end of the row is always 20, representing the distance between the client and the chart. The bottom number is the distance (in feet) at which an individual with normal vision can read the line. An individual with normal vision can read the row marked 20/20. To conduct the assessment, ask the client to stand 20 feet from the chart in a well-lit area. Ask the client to cover one eye with an opaque cover (**Figure 18–2 ●**). Then ask the client to read each row of letters, moving from largest letters to the smallest ones that the client can see. Measure visual acuity in the other eye in the same way, and then assess visual acuity while the client has both eyes uncovered. Test the client who wears corrective lenses with and without the lenses.

The Rosenbaum chart is held at a distance of from 12 to 14 inches from the eyes, with visual acuity measured in the same manner as with the Snellen chart (**Figure 18–3 ●**). A gross estimate of near vision may also be assessed by asking the individual to read from a magazine or newspaper.

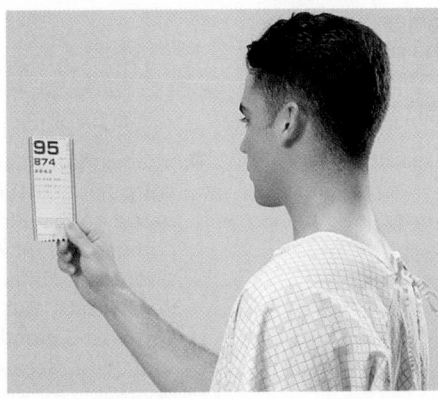

Figure 18–3 ● Testing near vision using Rosenbaum eye chart.

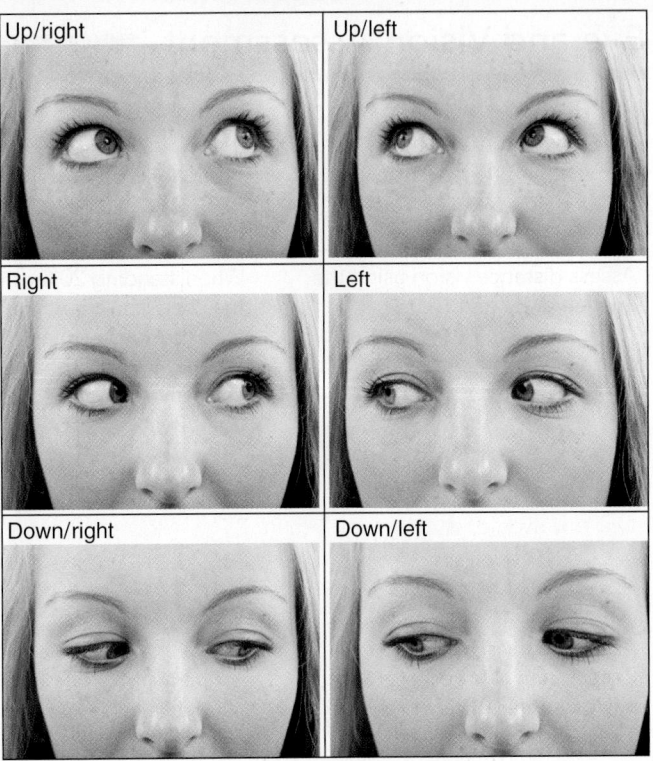

Figure 18–4 ● The six cardinal fields of vision.

The cardinal fields of vision are assessed to gain information about extraocular eye movements. Ask the client to follow a pen or your finger while keeping the head stationary. Move the pen or your finger through the six fields one at a time, returning to the central starting point before proceeding to the next field (**Figure 18–4 ●**).

The internal structures of the eye are assessed by using the ophthalmoscope, an instrument that allows visualization of the lens, the vitreous humor, and the retina.

See the Eye and Vision Assessment feature for assessment methods, normal and abnormal findings, and lifespan and development considerations.

EAR AND HEARING ASSESSMENT   Assessment of the ear and hearing usually starts with inspection of the external ear. The ears are usually equal in size and of the same skin color as the face and without palpable lesions. The otoscope is used to inspect both the external auditory canal and the tympanic membrane. The external ear canal should be pink and smooth and without lesions. The presence of **cerumen** is expected, but the amount present should not interfere with the exam or have a foul smell. The tympanic membrane should be shiny and translucent and pearly gray in color. A well-defined cone of light (light reflex) should be visible on the surface of the tympanic membrane. Any distortion or dullness of the cone of light may signal an infection or the presence of fluid behind the tympanic membrane.

The whisper test can be used to evaluate the client's level of hearing. While the client occludes one ear with a finger, the nurse stands 1–2 feet away from the client on the unoccluded side, whispers words, and then asks the client to repeat them. The test is then repeated on the other side. If hearing loss is noted, either unilaterally or bilaterally, a further evaluation can be performed with a tuning fork.

Eye and Vision Assessment

ASSESSMENT/METHOD	NORMAL FINDINGS	ABNORMAL FINDINGS	LIFESPAN OR DEVELOPMENTAL CONSIDERATIONS
Vision Assessment			
Assess distance vision using the Snellen or E chart.	When standing 20 feet from the chart, the client can read the smallest line of letters with or without corrective lenses (recorded as 20/20).	■ Changes in distance vision are most commonly the result of **myopia** (near-sightedness). For example, a reading of 20/100 indicates impaired distance vision. An individual has to stand 20 feet from the chart to read a line that an individual with normal vision could read 100 feet from the chart.	■ For clients with limited English proficiency or whose developmental level makes using the Snellen chart a challenge, the E chart may be a more appropriate tool.
Assess near vision, using a Rosenbaum chart or a card with newsprint held 12–14 inches from the client's eyes.	Normal near visual acuity is 14/14 with or without corrective lenses.	■ The client can only read lines larger than the 14/14 line with one or both eyes. ■ Tilting the head, squinting, or moving the card around may indicate the client has difficulty reading print.	■ Changes in near vision, especially in clients over age 45, can indicate **presbyopia**, an impairment in near vision resulting from a loss of elasticity of the lens related to aging. In younger clients, this condition is referred to as **hyperopia** (farsightedness). ■ Clients with low literacy levels may be embarrassed to admit they do not know the letters on the card.
Eye Movement Assessment			
Assess the cardinal fields of vision (see Figure 18–4).	The eyes should move through each field without involuntary movements.	■ Failure of one or both eyes to follow the object in any given direction may indicate extraocular muscle weakness or cranial nerve dysfunction. ■ An involuntary rhythmic movement of the eyes, **nystagmus**, is associated with neurological disorders and the use of some medications.	■ In infants or toddlers, use a brightly colored object or toy to capture the child's attention.
Assess for strabismus using the cover–uncover test: Hold a pen or your finger about 1 foot from the eyes and ask the individual to focus on that object. Cover one of the client's eyes and note any movement in the uncovered eye; as you remove the cover, assess for movement in the eye that was just uncovered. Repeat the procedure with the other eye.	The uncovered eye should remain fixed straight ahead. The covered eye should remain fixed straight ahead after being uncovered.	■ One eye will deviate from the other when the individual is focusing on an object.	■ Strabismus can occur at any point in the life span, based on the underlying pathology. It may be considered a normal finding in newborns, but if it persists past 3 months it should be assessed by an ophthalmologist.

Eye and Vision Assessment (continued)

ASSESSMENT/METHOD	NORMAL FINDINGS	ABNORMAL FINDINGS	LIFESPAN OR DEVELOPMENTAL CONSIDERATIONS
Assess **convergence**. Ask the client to follow an object as you move it toward the client's eyes.	Normally both eyes converge toward the center.	■ Failure of the eyes to converge equally on an approaching object may indicate a neuromuscular disorder or improper eye alignment.	■ Problems with convergence are usually diagnosed in school-age children when they have difficulty reading and may be interpreted as a learning disability rather than a visual problem.
Assess the corneal light reflex. Direct a light source onto the bridge of the nose from 12 to 15 inches away.	Observe for equal reflection of the light from each eye.	■ Reflections of the light from different sites on the eyes reveal improper alignment.	■ May be difficult to assess in children because looking straight ahead requires cooperation.

Pupillary Assessment

ASSESSMENT/METHOD	NORMAL FINDINGS	ABNORMAL FINDINGS	LIFESPAN OR DEVELOPMENTAL CONSIDERATIONS
Observe pupil size and equality.	Pupils should be of equal size, 3–5 mm.	■ Pupils that are unequal in size (anisocoria) may indicate a severe neurological problem, such as increased intracranial pressure. ■ Pupils that are unequal in size may also be a normal finding, especially in newborns. If there are no other symptoms, then there may be no underlying pathology.	■ One in five healthy clients will have a difference in pupil size up to 1 mm at any point in the life span. In older adults, the use of eyedrops to treat various eye disorders may also cause pupil size to be unequal.
Assess direct and consensual pupil response. Ask the client to look straight ahead. Shine a light obliquely into one eye at a time. Observe for constriction of the pupil in the illuminated eye. Test both eyes. To test consensual pupil response, again shine a light obliquely into one eye at a time as the client looks straight ahead. Observe constriction of the pupil in the opposite eye.	The normal direct and consensual pupillary response is constriction.	■ Failure of the pupils to respond to light may indicate degeneration of the retina or destruction of the optic nerve. ■ A client who has one dilated and unresponsive pupil may have paralysis of the oculomotor nerve. ■ Some eye medications may cause unequal dilation, constriction, or inequality of pupil size. Morphine and narcotic drugs may cause small, unresponsive pupils, and anticholinergic drugs such as atropine may cause dilated, unresponsive pupils.	■ This test requires cooperation, which may be difficult to obtain in newborns.
Test for **accommodation**. Hold an object at a distance of a few feet from the client. The pupils should dilate. Ask the client to follow the object as you bring it to within a few inches of the client's nose.	The pupils should constrict and converge as they change focus to follow the object.	■ Failure of accommodation along with lack of pupil response to light may signal a neurological problem. ■ Lack of response to light with appropriate response to accommodation is often seen in clients with diabetes.	■ Consider using a brightly colored object or toy to get the attention and cooperation of a young child.

(continued on next page)

Eye and Vision Assessment (continued)

ASSESSMENT/METHOD	NORMAL FINDINGS	ABNORMAL FINDINGS	LIFESPAN OR DEVELOPMENTAL CONSIDERATIONS
External Eye Assessment			
Inspect the eyelids. **Figure 18–5** ● Ptosis. *Source:* © Medical-on-Line/Alamy	Eyelids should be the color of the client's facial skin, without redness, discharge, or drooping. The sclera should not be visible.	■ Unusual redness or discharge may indicate an inflammatory state due to trauma, allergies, or infection. ■ Drooping of one eyelid, called **ptosis**, may be the result of a stroke, indicate a neuromuscular disorder, or be congenital (**Figure 18–5** ●). ■ Unusual widening of the lids may be due to exophthalmos, protrusion of the eyeball. Exophthalmos is often associated with hyperthyroid conditions. ■ An acute localized inflammation of a hair follicle is known as a hordeolum (sty) and is generally caused by staphylococcal organisms. ■ A chalazion is an infection or retention cyst of the meibomian glands.	■ Yellow plaques noted on or near the lid margins are referred to as xanthelasma and may indicate high lipid levels. ■ This can occur between the ages of 15 and 73 but most commonly occurs during the 40s and 50s.
Inspect the puncta.	The puncta should be free of redness or discharge.	■ Unusual redness or discharge from the puncta may indicate an inflammation due to trauma, infection, or allergies.	
Inspect the bulbar and palpebral conjunctiva.	The conjunctiva should be clear, moist, and smooth. The upper and lower palpebral conjunctiva should be clear, without redness or swelling.	■ Increased erythema or the presence of exudate may indicate acute conjunctivitis. ■ A cobblestone appearance is often associated with allergies.	■ A fold in the conjunctiva, called a pterygium, may be seen as a clouded area that extends over the cornea. This is an abnormal growth of the bulbar conjunctiva, usually seen on the nasal side of the cornea. It may interfere with vision if it covers the pupil. ■ This occurs most often in clients between the ages of 20 and 40.
Inspect the sclera.	The sclera is white in Caucasians; people with darker skin normally have yellow sclera.	■ Unusual redness may indicate an inflammatory state as a result of trauma, allergies, or infection. ■ Yellow discoloration of the sclera in clients with fair skin may be seen in conditions involving the liver, such as hepatitis.	

Eye and Vision Assessment (*continued*)

ASSESSMENT/METHOD	NORMAL FINDINGS	ABNORMAL FINDINGS	LIFESPAN OR DEVELOPMENTAL CONSIDERATIONS
		■ Bright red areas in the sclera are often subconjunctival hemorrhages and may indicate trauma or bleeding disorders. They may also occur spontaneously.	
Inspect the cornea.	The cornea is normally transparent.	■ Dullness, opacities, or irregularities of the cornea may be abnormal.	■ Corneal arcus is a thin, grayish-white arc seen toward the edge of the cornea. It is normal in older clients.
Assess corneal sensitivity. Lightly touch a wisp of cotton to the client's cornea.	This action should cause a **corneal reflex** (blinking of the eye).	■ Failure of the corneal reflex may indicate a neurological disorder.	
Inspect the iris.	The iris is normally round, flat, and evenly colored.	■ Lack of clarity of the iris may indicate cloudiness of the cornea. ■ Constriction of the pupil accompanied by pain and circumcorneal redness indicates acute iritis.	

Internal Eye Assessment

ASSESSMENT/METHOD	NORMAL FINDINGS	ABNORMAL FINDINGS	LIFESPAN OR DEVELOPMENTAL CONSIDERATIONS
Using the ophthalmoscope, inspect for the red reflex.	The red reflex should be clearly visible.	■ Absence of a red reflex often indicates improper positioning of the ophthalmoscope, but also may indicate total opacity of the pupil by a cataract or a hemorrhage into the vitreous humor.	■ Ophthalmoscopic examination may be difficult in children under the age of 3 because it requires some degree of cooperation.
Using the ophthalmoscope, inspect the lens and vitreous body.	The lens should be clear.	■ A cataract is an opacity of the lens, often seen as a dark shadow on ophthalmoscope examination. It may be due to aging, trauma, diabetes, or a congenital defect.	■ Although cataracts may occur at any point on the life span, they are more common in older adults.
Using the ophthalmoscope, inspect the retina.	There should be no visible hemorrhages, exudate, or white patches.	■ Findings of hemorrhage, exudate, or white patches are abnormal and require further workup.	■ Areas of hemorrhage, exudate, and white patches may be a result of diabetes or long-standing hypertension.
Using the ophthalmoscope, inspect the optic disc.	The optic disc should be round to oval in shape with clear, well-defined borders.	■ Loss of definition of the optic disc, as well as an increase in the size of the physiological cup, is seen in papilledema from increased intracranial pressure.	

(*continued on next page*)

Eye and Vision Assessment (continued)

ASSESSMENT/METHOD	NORMAL FINDINGS	ABNORMAL FINDINGS	LIFESPAN OR DEVELOPMENTAL CONSIDERATIONS
Using the ophthalmoscope, inspect the blood vessels of the retina.	The retinal blood vessels should be distinct.	■ Glaucoma often results in displacement of blood vessels from the center of the optic disc due to increased intraocular pressure.	■ Hypertension may cause a narrowing of the vein where an arteriole crosses over. ■ Engorged veins may occur with diabetes, atherosclerosis, and blood disorders. ■ Underlying pathologies are more common in older clients.
Using the ophthalmoscope, inspect the retinal background.	The retina should be a consistent red-orange color, becoming lighter around the optic disc.	■ Variations in color or a pale color overall may indicate disease.	
Using the ophthalmoscope, inspect the macula.	The macula should be visible on the temporal side of the optic disc.	■ Deposits called drusen may be visible.	■ Absence of the fovea centralis is common in older clients. It may indicate macular degeneration, a cause of loss of central vision. ■ Appearance of drusen occurs as the older client develops age-related macular degeneration.
Palpate over the lacrimal glands, puncta, and nasolacrimal duct.	There should be no tenderness, drainage, or excessive tearing.	■ Tenderness over any of these areas or drainage from the puncta may indicate an infectious process. (Wear gloves if you see any drainage.) ■ Excessive tearing may indicate a blockage of the nasolacrimal duct.	

Tuning forks are used to determine whether a hearing loss is conductive or perceptive (sensorineural) (**Figures 18–6** ● and **18–7** ●). Hold the tuning fork at the base and make it ring softly by stroking the prongs or by lightly tapping them on the heel of the opposite hand. The vibrating tuning fork emits sound waves of a particular frequency, measured in hertz (Hz). Tuning forks with a frequency of 512–1024 Hz are preferred for auditory evaluation, because that range corresponds to the range of normal speech. The Rinne test and the Weber test are performed to determine if the cause of hearing loss is either conductive or sensorineural.

Many of the hearing tests performed in a general practitioner's office are difficult to do with newborns and young children because they require a degree of cooperation. Some tests of basic hearing can be performed by clapping or using another means to create a noise and see if the child looks for the source. For older children, letting them examine the otoscope or other diagnostic tools before use may help to alleviate fear and gain more cooperation. Further evaluation typically is performed by an audiologist and/or an otolaryngologist (ENT physician).

The Ear and Hearing Assessment feature lists the techniques and methods used for assessing hearing, gives the normal and abnormal findings, and presents lifespan and developmental considerations.

TASTE, SMELL, AND TACTILE ASSESSMENT One reason decreased sense of smell fails to be detected is that it is not adequately tested. Most physical examination records state "cranial nerves II–XII intact," completely omitting cranial nerve I. The nurse can examine the mucous membranes of the nares using a penlight or an otoscope and speculum, taking care not to touch the septum. The mucous membranes of the nares should be free from polyps, slightly red in color, and without ulceration or copious exudates. The nurse can then ask the client to occlude one side of the nose, close the eyes, and identify a familiar smell such as vanilla, coffee, or an alcohol swab. This maneuver is repeated on the opposite side using a different odor. Using familiar odors enhances the validity of the test. Commercially prepared scratch-and-sniff tests are available in some smell assessment clinics. These tests contain over 40 odorants and

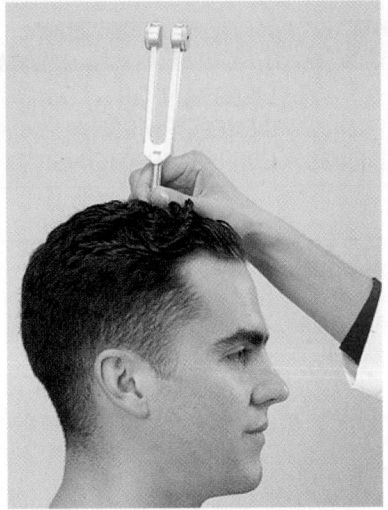

Figure 18–6 ● Performing the Weber test with a tuning fork.

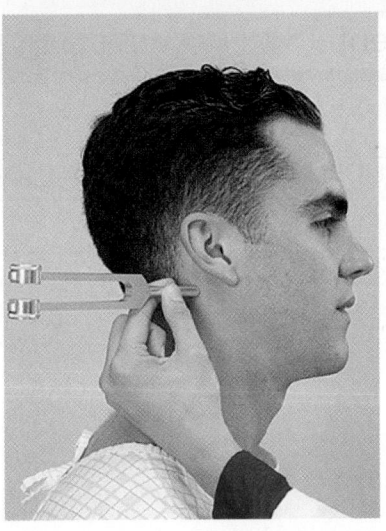
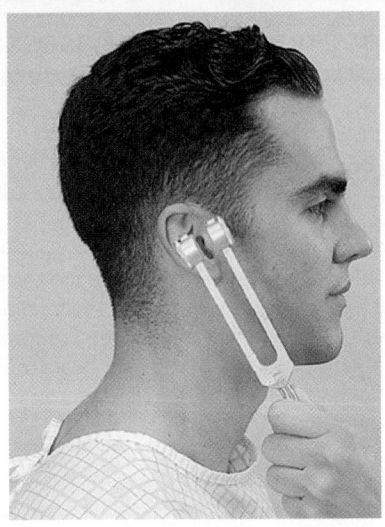

Figure 18–7 ● Performing the Rinne test with a tuning fork.

provide more complete information regarding deficits in smell. Clients with obvious deficits in smell should be referred to their primary care provider, an otolaryngologist, and a neurologist.

There are many different ways to test for tactile function. Regardless of the chosen assessment method, the key component of the exam is establishing the presence or absence of symmetry. A sharp object (such as a broken tongue blade) or a dull object (the bottom of a pen) can be touched to the skin along various points on a client's arms, legs, or face. This can also be repeated with warm objects (warm washcloth) or cold objects (ice cube). Stereognosis is the ability to recognize a common object through just the use of touch. It is tested by placing keys or a closed safety pin or coins in the client's hand and having him identify the object with his eyes closed. Graphesthesia is the ability to recognized a letter that is "written" on the skin through touch. Two-point discrimination is performed by asking a client to close her eyes and report if she feels one or two points of contact on her skin. The examiner can use special calipers or a bent paper clip and randomly make contact with only one or two points on the skin.

An inability to identify superficial touch and pain sensation may indicate sensory loss. Identify the extent of sensory loss, such as all areas below the knee. Other sensory function tests (temperature, vibratory, deep pressure pain, and position sense) are performed when sensory loss is found.

Assessment of taste is not usually done as part of a normal sensory examination. A client can be asked as a history question to comment on ability to distinguish between salty, sour, sweet, and bitter, but any deviations from normal would require referral to a specialist. Most alterations of taste are found when the client presents to the healthcare provider with a complaint of decrease in taste.

For specific considerations related to assessment of tactile function in infants and children, see the Lifespan Considerations feature.

The Cranial Nerve Assessment feature lists the testing methods and techniques, the normal and abnormal findings, and lifespan and development considerations for testing smell, taste, and tactile impairments.

Lifespan Considerations Assessing Sensory Function in Children

Infant Sensory Function

An infant's sensory function is not routinely assessed. Withdrawal responses to painful stimuli indicate normal sensory function.

Superficial Tactile Sensation

Stroke the skin on the lower leg or arm with a cotton ball or a finger while the child's eyes are closed. Cooperative children over 2 years of age can normally point to the location touched.

Superficial Pain Sensation

Break a tongue blade to get a sharp point. After asking the child to close the eyes, touch the child in various places on each arm and leg, alternating the sharp and dull ends of the tongue blade. A paper clip may also be used. Children over 4 years of age can normally distinguish between a sharp and dull sensation each time. To improve the child's accuracy with the test, let the child practice telling you the difference between the sharp and dull stimulation.

Taste

As with adults, a child's sense of taste is not part of a normal physical assessment. Any alteration reported by the client or client's parent/guardian is cause for referral to a specialist.

Other Diagnostic Tests

Additional diagnostic tests may be necessary to diagnose a specific injury or disease process, to provide information to inform selection of medications or assistive devices, and to help nurses monitor the client's responses to treatment and nursing interventions. Examples include the use of retinoscopy and or refractometry to diagnose refractive errors of the eye that require corrective lenses or audiometry to evaluate the extent of hearing impairment.

Ear and Hearing Assessment

ASSESSMENT/METHOD	NORMAL FINDINGS	ABNORMAL FINDINGS	LIFESPAN OR DEVELOPMENTAL CONSIDERATIONS
Hearing Assessment			
Perform the Weber test. Place the base of a vibrating tuning fork on the midline vertex of the client's head (see Figure 18–6). Ask whether the client hears the sound equally in both ears or better in one than the other.	Sound is normally heard equally in both ears.	■ Sound heard in, or lateralized to, one ear indicates either a conductive loss in that ear or a sensorineural loss in the other ear. The sound will be louder on the impaired side with a conductive hearing loss. The sound will be softer on the impaired side with a sensorineural hearing loss. ■ Conductive losses may be due to a buildup of cerumen, an infection such as otitis media, or perforation of the eardrum.	■ Will probably not be able to perform until school aged as it requires cooperation. ■ Consider clapping or using an item that makes a noise to see if the child will look to find the source. In some clients with autism, sudden loud noises are perceived as painful and may elicit a strong response.
Perform the Rinne test. Place the base of a vibrating tuning fork on the client's mastoid bone. Ask the client to indicate when the sound is no longer heard. When the client does so, quickly reposition the tuning fork in front of the client's ear close to the ear canal. Ask whether the client can hear the sound. If the client says yes, ask the client to indicate when the sound is no longer heard. Repeat over the opposite mastoid bone (see Figure 18–7).	The client with no conductive hearing loss will hear the sound twice as long by air conduction as by bone conduction.	■ Bone conduction is greater than air conduction in the ear with a conductive loss. The normal pattern is AC > BC (air conduction greater than bone conduction).	■ Will probably not be able to perform until school aged because it requires cooperation. ■ Consider clapping or using an item that makes a noise to see if the child will look to find the source. In some clients with autism, sudden loud noises are perceived as painful and may elicit a strong response.
Perform the whisper test. Ask the client to occlude one ear with a finger. Stand 1–2 feet away from the client, on the side of the unoccluded ear. Softly whisper numbers and ask the client to repeat them. Repeat the procedure, having the client occlude the other ear. Note whether you need to raise your voice or to stand closer to make the client hear you.	The client should be able to repeat the numbers or words whispered by the nurse without difficulty. Note whether the nurse has to raise her voice or if there is difficulty with one or both ears.	■ This test provides a rough estimate of hearing loss.	■ This test may be difficult to perform in young children, because it requires cooperation and understanding of the words being spoken.
Use a tympanogram to measure the pressure of the middle ear and observe the tympanic membrane's response to waves of pressure. Insert the device into the ear canal. Ask the client not to speak, move, swallow, or jump when hearing a sound. Tell the client he or she will hear a loud tone as the measurements are taken. Repeat for the other ear.	The normal pressure inside the middle ear is a 100 daPa (a very small amount).	■ Abnormal findings may include fluid in the middle ear, a perforated eardrum, impacted earwax, or a tumor of the middle ear.	■ Young children may be more cooperative with this test if given the chance to examine the equipment first.

Ear and Hearing Assessment *(continued)*

ASSESSMENT/METHOD	NORMAL FINDINGS	ABNORMAL FINDINGS	LIFESPAN OR DEVELOPMENTAL CONSIDERATIONS
External Ear Assessment			
Inspect the auricle.	External ears are normally bilateral, equal in size, of equal color with the client's face, without redness or lesions.	■ Unusual redness or drainage may indicate an inflammatory response to infection or trauma. ■ Scales or skin lesions around the rim of the auricle may indicate skin cancer.	■ Small, raised lesions on the rim of the ear are known as tophi and indicate gout.
Inspect the external auditory canal with an otoscope.	Canal walls should be pink and smooth without lesions. Cerumen is normally present in small, odorless amounts.	■ Unusual redness, lesions, or purulent drainage may indicate an infection. ■ Cerumen varies in color and texture, but hardened, dry, or foul-smelling cerumen may indicate an infection or an impaction of cerumen that requires removal. People with darker skin tend to have darker cerumen.	
Inspect the tympanic membrane. **Figure 18–8** ● Scarring of the tympanic membrane. *Source:* Professor Tony Wright, Institute of Laryngology and Otology/SPL/Science Source.	The tympanic membrane should be pearly gray, shiny, and translucent without bulging or retraction.	■ White, opaque areas on the tympanic membrane are often scars from previous perforations **(Figure 18–8 ●)**. ■ Inconsistent texture and color may be due to scarring from previous perforations caused by infection, allergies, or trauma. ■ Bulging membranes are indicated by a loss of bony landmarks and a distorted light reflex. Such bulges may be the result of otitis media or malfunctioning auditory tubes. ■ Retracted tympanic membranes are indicated by accentuated bony landmarks and a distorted light reflex. Such retraction is often due to an obstructed auditory tube.	
Palpate the auricles and over each mastoid process.	There should be no pain or swelling on palpation.	Tenderness, swelling, or nodules may indicate inflammation of the external auditory canal or mastoiditis.	

CASE STUDY \\ PART 2

Simon has been trying to ignore the teasing from his sister and her friends. His grades are improving, and he's happy that he can see better. All of Simon's friends have started to skateboard. For his 11th birthday, he asks his parents for a skateboard and is excited when he gets one.

He has been hanging out with his friends and skateboarding on the playground after school. Simon is afraid of breaking his glasses, so he takes them off and sets them by the slide. He has learned a new trick and is eager to show his friends. While he is showing them, he falls off of his skateboard and lands in a pile of sand. He feels like he has sand in his left eye, so he rubs it really hard. This makes his eye hurt, and his friends point out that his eye is now all red and watery. Simon gathers his glasses and his skateboard and heads home. By that evening, Simon is crying because his eye hurts so badly and the lights are bothering it. His parents note that his left eyelid is swollen

and crusty. His mother takes him to the urgent care clinic, where he is diagnosed with a left corneal abrasion. Simon is given antibiotic drops, and his mother is instructed on how to apply an eye patch to protect the eye because Simon won't stop rubbing it.

Clinical Reasoning Questions Level I

1. What nursing diagnoses would be appropriate for Simon at this time?
2. What independent nursing interventions can the nurse do with Simon and his mother?

Clinical Reasoning Questions Level II

3. *Refer to the exemplar on Eye Injury within this module.* What data indicate that Simon has a corneal abrasion?
4. What is the proper method for instilling eyedrops?
5. What additional client education would you provide to Simon and his mother prior to discharge?

Cranial Nerve Assessment

ASSESSMENT/METHOD	NORMAL FINDINGS	ABNORMAL FINDINGS	LIFESPAN OR DEVELOPMENTAL CONSIDERATIONS
Assess Smell			
Test cranial nerve (CN) I. Note client's ability to smell scents (e.g., soap, coffee) with each nostril. This test is usually done only if a problem with the ability to smell is reported.	Sense of smell should be equal in both nostrils.	■ Anosmia (an inability to smell) may be seen with lesions of the frontal lobe and may also occur with impaired blood flow to the middle cerebral artery.	■ Smell decreases as part of the normal aging process. ■ Tobacco use can alter this sense.
Assess Tactile Sensation			
Assess the ability to perceive sensations. Touch both sides of the body (the chest, abdomen, arms, and legs) with one or more of the following: ■ Cotton wisp ■ Sharp object ■ Dull object ■ Vibrating tuning fork placed on bony prominences.	Client should be able to differentiate between soft and sharp, and feel vibrations appropriately.	■ Decreased sensation of pain occurs with injury to the spinothalamic tract. ■ Decreased vibratory sensations are seen with injuries to the posterior column tract. ■ Transient numbness of face, arm, or hand is seen with transient ischemic attacks. ■ Sensory loss on one side of the body is seen with lesions of higher pathways to the spinal cord. ■ Bilateral sensory loss is seen in polyneuropathy (a disease in which multiple peripheral nerves are affected, such as Guillain-Barré syndrome or diabetes mellitus). Sensations are impaired with strokes, brain tumors, and spinal cord trauma or compression.	■ Withdrawal to noxious stimulation is assessed in newborns. ■ Identification of specific stimuli requires understanding and cooperation and may not be able to be assessed in young children or those with developmental delays. ■ Clients diagnosed with autism spectrum disorder may have unexpected responses ranging from little or no response to exaggerated reactions that are disproportionate to the amount of stimulation.

Cranial Nerve Assessment (continued)

ASSESSMENT/METHOD	NORMAL FINDINGS	ABNORMAL FINDINGS	LIFESPAN OR DEVELOPMENTAL CONSIDERATIONS
Assess Kinesthesia			
Assess sense of position (kinesthesia). Move the client's finger or big toe up or down. Ask the client to describe the movement.	Client should be able to accurately describe position of finger or toe when moved up or down.	■ Lesions of the posterior column of the spinal cord may affect sense of position.	■ Requires understanding and cooperation and may be difficult to assess on younger clients or those with developmental delays.
Assess Ability to Discriminate Fine Touch			
Ask the client to identify the following: ■ Object in hand, such as a coin or key (tests stereognosis) ■ Number written on hand (tests graphesthesia) ■ Two points of simultaneous pinpricks on the hand (tests two-point discrimination) ■ Where he or she is being touched (tests localization) ■ How many sensations are felt when touched simultaneously on both sides of the body (tests extinction).	Client should be able to identify and discriminate fine touch.	■ Inability to discriminate fine touch (stereognosis, graphesthesia, two points, point localization, and extinction) may occur with injury to the posterior columns or sensory cortex.	■ Requires understanding and cooperation and may be difficult to assess on younger clients or those with developmental delays.
Assess Taste			
Usually not performed as part of a routine physical assessment, but can be assessed through a questionnaire.	Client should be able to distinguish between sweet, salty, bitter, sour, and umami.	■ Client is not able to distinguish among one or more tastes. Related closely to sense of smell.	■ A decrease in taste is a common part of the aging process. ■ Tobacco use and certain medications can alter this sense.

▶ INTERVENTIONS AND THERAPIES

Care of the client with impaired sensory perception includes both independent and collaborative interventions. Independent interventions focus on education, injury prevention, and wellness promotion. Collaborative interventions include facilitating medical management of the client's condition, as well as interacting with other members of the healthcare team to optimize the client's outcomes.

Independent

Many of the independent therapies relevant to care for the client with alterations in sensory perception involve assessing the individual's understanding of both the alteration and the appropriate treatment. Client teaching is essential, especially with regard to promoting safety.

Client education includes teaching the client about appropriate use of any prescribed medications. If the plan of care calls for use of assistive devices, the nurse may be involved with providing instruction and verifying the client's effective use of the device. Common goals of care for clients with an alteration in sensory perception include preventing injury, restoring or maintaining function, promoting comfort, and preventing sensory overload or deprivation.

PROMOTING HEALTHY SENSORY FUNCTION   Healthy sensory function can be promoted with environmental stimuli that provide appropriate sensory input that varies and is neither too excessive nor too limited. Various colors, sounds, textures, smells, and body positions can provide multisensory stimulation. Nurses can teach parents to stimulate infants and children, and teach family members to stimulate an older adult and others in the home with sensory deficits. Nurses should explain that initially some trial and error may be necessary because it takes time to learn what materials and activities stimulate the client and which activities the client enjoys. Exercise and social activities often help stimulate the mind and the senses.

Nurses should also teach clients at risk of sensory loss how to prevent or minimize the loss. Teaching topics include general health measures, such as getting regular eye examinations and controlling chronic diseases such as diabetes. Avoiding known risk factors, such as hot temperatures for the individual with impaired tactile senses, is also critical.

PREVENTING SENSORY OVERLOAD For clients who are at risk of overstimulation, nurses should assist with reducing the number and type of environmental stimuli. The nurse can counteract sensory overload by blocking stimuli and by helping the client organize the stimuli and alter responses to the stimuli.

Dark glasses with ultraviolet (UVA and UVB) light protection can partially block light rays, and a window shade or drape can reduce visual stimulation. Earplugs reduce auditory stimuli, as do soft background music and earphones. To further reduce sensory overload, the nurse may need to schedule a quiet period following implementation of several nursing measures together. By explaining the significance of environmental sounds, such as an IV pump alarm, the nurse can help the client organize them mentally. Encourage clients to employ relaxation techniques to reduce anxiety and stress despite continual sensory stimulation.

PREVENTING SENSORY DEPRIVATION For clients at risk for sensory deprivation, newspapers, books, music, and television can be provided to stimulate the visual and auditory senses. Objects that are pleasant to touch, including soft fabrics, can provide tactile stimulation. Clocks that use color to differentiate night from day can help orient a client to time. Fresh flowers or a fragrant plant can also stimulate the olfactory sense.

Arrangements should also be made for people to visit and talk with the client regularly. Many church and community groups provide people who will visit individuals who are confined to their homes or who reside in nursing homes.

MANAGING ACUTE SENSORY DEFICITS Nursing care of clients who have a sensory deficit includes (a) encouraging the use of sensory aids to support residual sensory function, (b) promoting the use of other senses, (c) communicating effectively, and (d) ensuring client safety. Nurses also teach clients and families how to find freedom within the limitations imposed by the client's sensory loss. For example, clients with visual impairments, for example, may find comfort and joy in attending live music performances, listening to podcasts, and in downloading reading material that has been converted into spoken word via the Internet. Clients with hearing impairments may experience frustration when talking on the phone, even if they have a hearing aid that works well. These clients may increase use of communication via e-mail and text messages in order to minimize frustration with audio communications.

Sensory Aids Sensory aids can be used in the healthcare setting as well as in the home. Many sensory aids are available for clients who have visual and hearing deficits. Examples are listed in **Box 18–1** ●. Service dogs are a popular, but expensive, example. Service dogs protect individuals with sensory impairments from risk and also assist them with activities of daily living, such as opening doors and fetching objects. Raising and training service dogs can cost upwards of $40,000 before the dog is ready to go into active service. The cost along with the shortage of trainers sometimes results in long waiting lists for service dogs. Some training programs provide dogs to individuals with sensory impairments free of charge.

Promoting the Use of Other Senses For some individuals, when one sense is lost, one or more intact senses may be heightened to compensate for the impairment. To promote com-

---

Box 18–1 Sensory Aids for Visual and Hearing Deficits

VISUAL

- Eyeglasses of the correct prescription, clean and in good repair
- Adequate room lighting, including night-lights
- Sunglasses or shades on windows to reduce glare
- Bright contrasting colors in the environment
- Magnifying glass
- Phone dialer with large numbers
- Clock with large numbers or auditory device
- Color code or texture code on stoves, washer, medicine containers, and so on
- Colored or raised rims on dishes
- Reading material with large print
- Braille or recorded books; podcasts
- Seeing-eye dog

HEARING

- Hearing aid in good order
- Lip reading
- Sign language
- Amplified telephones
- Telecommunication device for the deaf (TDD)
- Amplified telephone ringers and doorbells
- Flashing alarm clock
- Flashing smoke detectors

---

pensation, sensory stimulation techniques are used that are similar to those used to prevent sensory deprivation, as discussed earlier. However, the type of stimulation needs to be adapted in accordance with the client's specific deficit. For example, for a client with a visual impairment, stimulation of hearing, taste, smell, and touch can be encouraged. A radio, audiotapes of music or books, clocks that chime, music boxes, and wind chimes can be used for auditory stimulation. Diets that include a variety of flavors, temperatures, and textures stimulate the taste buds. Taking sips of water between foods and eating foods separately can enhance the taste sensation. Fresh flowers, scented candles (safely used), room fragrances, brewing coffee, and baking can stimulate the sense of smell. Massage, hair brushing, grooming, different textures in clothing and upholstery fabrics, and pets can stimulate touch receptors.

Communicating Effectively Communication with clients who have sensory deficits should convey respect, enhance the individual's self-esteem, and ensure the exchange of correct information. For the client with a hearing impairment, communication often requires concentrated effort. Fatigue compounded by an illness can further reduce the individual's ability to hear. An individual with impaired vision is unable to observe most nonverbal cues during communication and relies largely on the spoken word and tone of voice. Guidelines for communicating with people who have visual or hearing impairments are shown in **Box 18–2** ●.

PROMOTING EFFECTIVE COPING Moderate to acute sensory deficits impact the client's quality of life. Mobility, ability to perform activities of daily living (ADLs), and independence may all be affected by sensory deficits. Clients who develop successful coping mechanisms are less likely to experience injury and more likely to experience greater quality of life. Depending on the extent of the individual's limitations, eliciting

Box 18–2 Communicating With Clients Who Have a Visual or Hearing Deficit

VISUAL DEFICIT

- Always announce your presence when entering the client's room and identify yourself by name.
- Stay in the client's field of vision if the client has a partial vision loss.
- Speak in a warm and pleasant tone of voice. Some people tend to speak louder than necessary when talking to someone who is blind.
- Always explain what you are about to do before touching the individual.
- Explain the sounds in the environment.
- Indicate when the conversation has ended and when you are leaving the room.

HEARING DEFICIT

- Before initiating conversation, convey your presence by moving to a position where you can be seen or by gently touching the individual.
- Decrease background noises (e.g., television) before speaking.
- Talk at a moderate rate and in a normal tone of voice. Shouting does not make your voice more distinct and in some instances makes understanding more difficult.

- Address the individual directly. Do not turn away in the middle of a remark or story. Make sure the individual can see your face easily and that it is well lighted.
- Avoid talking when you have something in your mouth, such as chewing gum. Avoid covering your mouth with your hand.
- Keep your voice at about the same volume throughout each sentence without dropping the voice at the end of each sentence.
- Always speak as clearly and accurately as possible. Articulate consonants with particular care.
- Do not "overarticulate"; mouthing or overdoing articulation is just as troublesome as mumbling. Pantomime or write ideas, or use sign language or finger-spelling as appropriate.
- Use longer phrases, which tend to be easier to understand than short ones. For example, "Would you like a drink of water?" presents much less difficulty than "Would you like a drink?" Word choice is important: "Fifteen cents" and "fifty cents" may be confused, but "half a dollar" is clear.
- Pronounce every name with care. Make a reference to the name for easier understanding, for example, "Joan, the girl from the office" or "Sears, the big downtown store."
- Change to a new subject at a slower rate, making sure that the individual follows the change to the new subject. A key word or two at the beginning of a new topic is a good indicator.

---

the help of the client's family or an outside source such as social workers and physical therapists may be helpful.

Impaired Vision Research has established an association between vision impairment and greater disability in ADLs (e.g., bathing, dressing, eating) and instrumental tasks (e.g., shopping, housekeeping). Studies have also shown that visual impairment increases the risk of depression among older adults living in the community, with some studies citing the rate of depression in older adults with visual disturbances as high as 30% in North America (Margrain et al., 2012). Explanations for this relationship vary. One explanation is that vision loss leads to increased disability, which leads to depression. Another explanation is that loss of vision causes fear—a fear of losing one's autonomy and becoming dependent on another or others. Visual loss also affects how an individual obtains information (e.g., reading the newspaper). In addition, reading is often a leisure activity and its loss can affect an individual's quality of life. It is important for the nurse to be aware of and assess for signs of depression and intervene as appropriate if an older adult is experiencing depression as a result of a visual impairment.

In the healthcare setting, nursing interventions for clients with visual impairments should include optimizing safety through environmental organization. For individuals outside the healthcare setting, the nurse should teach clients and their families the importance of organizing the client's living environment. Organizing the environment reduces the risk for injury and increases opportunities for independence. Features of a safe environment for the client with a visual impairment include the following:

- An uncluttered environment with plenty of lighting
- Clear pathways (chairs pushed under tables, things put away); furniture should not be rearranged without orienting the client
- Organizing self-care articles within the client's reach
- Orienting the client to a new location when traveling or running errands

- Keeping call lights and assistive devices within easy reach
- Assisting with ambulation (as necessary) by standing at the client's side, walking about 1 foot ahead, and allowing the individual to grasp your arm. Confirm whether the client prefers grasping your arm with the dominant or nondominant hand.

IMPAIRED HEARING For home safety, clients with impaired hearing need to obtain devices that either amplify sounds or respond to sounds with flashing lights. These devices can be obtained from hearing aid dealers, telephone companies, and appliance stores. In most areas, television providers offer closed caption TV, which can allow individuals with a hearing impairment to continue to enjoy their favorite television programs and access important news and weather updates.

Impaired Olfactory Sense Clients with an impaired sense of smell should be taught about the dangers of cleaning with chemicals such as ammonia. Strong chemicals such as ammonia used in confined spaces such as a bathroom may affect the client before they are smelled. Because a gas leak can go undetected, clients should keep gas stoves and heaters in good working order. Food poisoning is a concern with clients who have difficulty detecting spoiled meat or dairy products. Clients need to carefully inspect food for freshness (check its color and texture) and check expiration dates on food packages.

Impaired Tactile Sense Clients with an impaired sense of touch may not be aware of hot temperatures, which can cause burns, or pressure on bony prominences, which can produce pressure ulcers. Clients with impaired temperature perception should have the temperature adjusted on their hot water heater and test water temperature with a thermometer before bathing. Clients with decreased sensation to pressure must change their position frequently.

Collaborative

Treatment of altered sensory perception is based on the cause and severity of the problem. Clients are referred to specialists (neurologists, ophthalmologists, otolaryngologists) and ancillary services (physical therapy, occupational therapy) as appropriate.

PHARMACOLOGIC THERAPY The eye is vulnerable to a variety of conditions, many of which can be prevented, controlled, or reversed with proper treatment. Pharmacotherapy is of particular importance in the treatment of glaucoma and macular degeneration. Medications used to treat these alterations are discussed in their respective exemplars.

Treatment of olfactory impairment generally may be resolved by treating the underlying cause of the impairment. However, olfactory impairment sometimes presents with the onset of serious illnesses, such as diabetes, hypertension, and Parkinson disease. Treatment of the underlying disease does not always restore olfactory function.

Unfortunately, no medications are available to help clients experiencing permanent hearing loss or alterations of taste or smell.

◢ REVIEW **The Concept of Sensory Perception**

RELATE Link the Concepts

Linking the concept of sensory perception with the concept of development:

1. How might an alteration in sensory perception interfere with an infant/toddler's ability to meet developmental milestones?

2. How would your assessment of hearing for a 40-year-old male be different form your assessment of hearing for a 6-year-old girl?

Linking the concept of sensory perception with the concept of safety:

3. Discuss how different alterations in sensory perception might affect the safety of a 76-year-old woman.

4. Discuss how different alterations in sensory perception might affect the safety of a 4-year-old boy.

READY Go to Companion Skills Manual

REFER Go to Pearson Student Nursing Resources
nursing.pearsonhighered.com

- Additional review materials
- Minimodule: Physiology of Sensory Perception

REFLECT Case Study \\ Part 3

Simon has been instructed to keep his eye patch on for 3 days for comfort and to prevent him from rubbing his eye. His friends have been doing a new jump trick on the skateboard that Simon really wants to try. He borrows his friend's skateboard at the playground after school. He is having a hard time focusing with just one eye but doesn't want to look foolish in front of his friends. Simon is able to do the jump trick, but loses control and crashes into a metal bike rack on the playground. His friends rush over and notice that his right eye is puffy and swollen. Simon's nose begins bleeding.

His friends help him to get home, and his mother takes him to the emergency department where Simon is diagnosed with a right maxillary fracture. He is still continuing to experience epistaxis. He is scheduled for a surgical repair tomorrow.

Clinical Reasoning Questions Level I

1. What are some appropriate nursing diagnoses for Simon at this time?

2. What are some appropriate nursing diagnoses for Simon's mother at this time?

Clinical Reasoning Questions Level II

3. What diagnostic studies could have been ordered to diagnose Simon's maxillary fracture?

4. How could the nurse check to make sure that Simon doesn't have a basilar skull fracture?

5. What independent nursing interventions can be done to decrease swelling and maintain Simon's safety until surgery?

6. What additional client education do you anticipate Simon will need at his post operative follow-up appointment?

◢ EXEMPLAR 18.1 **Hearing Impairment**

EXEMPLAR KEY TERMS
Decibels (dB), *1298*
Noise-induced hearing loss (NIHL), *1300*
Presbycusis, *1299*
Tinnitus, *1301*

EXEMPLAR LEARNING OUTCOMES
After reading about this exemplar, you will be able to:

1. Describe the pathophysiology, etiology, clinical manifestations, and direct and indirect causes of hearing impairment.

2. Identify risk factors associated with hearing impairment.

3. Illustrate the nursing process in providing culturally competent care across the life span for individuals with hearing impairment.

4. Formulate priority nursing diagnoses appropriate for an individual with hearing impairment.

5. Summarize therapies used by interdisciplinary teams in the collaborative care of an individual with hearing impairment.

6. Plan evidence-based care for an individual with hearing impairment and his or her family in collaboration with other members of the healthcare team.

7. Evaluate expected outcomes for an individual with hearing impairment.

▶ OVERVIEW

Approximately 1 million children in the United States have some form of hearing impairment. Hearing loss is present in 2 to 3 out of every 1,000 births (National Institute on Deafness and Other Communication Disorders [NIDOCD], 2010). Hearing impair-

ments are expressed in terms of **decibels (dB)**, which are units of loudness, and rated according to severity (**Table 18–2 ●**). Children who have only a mild hearing loss (35–40 dB) may miss as much as 50% of everyday conversation and are considered at high risk for difficulty in school. Anyone with a hearing loss of more than 90 dB is considered legally deaf.

TABLE 18–2 Severity of Hearing Loss

TYPE OF LOSS	DECIBEL LEVEL (DB)	HEARING ABILITY
Slight/mild	26–40	Some speech sounds are difficult to perceive, particularly unvoiced consonant sounds.
Moderate	41–60	Most normal conversational speech sounds are missed.
Severe	61–80	Speech sounds cannot be heard at a normal conversational level.
Profound	81–90	No speech sounds can be heard.
Deaf	>90	No sound at all can be heard.

Hearing loss is a significant problem for adults as well, affecting an estimated 36 million adults (17%) in the United States. The problem of hearing loss is particularly significant in older adults, affecting about 30% of adults between the ages of 65 and 74, and 47% of those over age 75 (NIDOCD, 2010). As many as 70% of nursing home residents have impaired hearing.

Hearing loss impairs the ability to communicate in a world filled with sound and hearing individuals. A hearing deficit can be partial or total, congenital or acquired. It may affect one or both ears. In some types of hearing loss, the ability to perceive sound at specific frequencies is lost. In others, hearing is diminished across all frequencies.

▶ PATHOPHYSIOLOGY AND ETIOLOGY

Alterations in hearing may be due to one or more factors. For example, lesions in the outer ear, middle ear, inner ear, or central auditory pathways can result in hearing loss. The process of aging also can affect the structures of the ear and hearing.

Etiology

Hearing loss is classified as conductive, sensorineural, or mixed, depending on what portion of the auditory system is affected. Profound deafness is often a congenital condition.

CONDUCTIVE HEARING LOSS Anything that disrupts the transmission of sound from the external auditory meatus to the inner ear results in a conductive hearing loss. The most common cause of conductive hearing loss is obstruction of the external ear canal. Impacted cerumen, edema of the canal lining, stenosis, and neoplasms all may lead to canal obstruction. Other causes of conductive loss include a perforated tympanic membrane, disruption or fixation of the ossicles of the middle ear, fluid, scarring, and tumors of the middle ear. Conductive loss also occurs if the tympanic membrane does not fully vibrate, as in otitis media. In these cases, loss may be restored after the infection clears. Chronic and untreated ear infections may lead to ear structural changes and permanent hearing impairment. The loss of acuity may be gradual or rapid and results in diminished hearing in all ranges.

SENSORINEURAL HEARING LOSS Disorders that affect the inner ear, the auditory nerve, or the auditory pathways of the brain may lead to a sensorineural hearing loss. In this type of hearing loss, sound waves are effectively transmitted to the inner ear. In the inner ear, however, lost or damaged receptor cells, changes in the cochlear apparatus, or auditory nerve abnormalities decrease or distort the ability to receive and interpret stimuli. Conditions leading to sensorineural hearing loss may be congenital, genetic, or acquired. In sensorineural hearing loss, high-frequency sounds are most affected.

A significant cause of sensorineural hearing deficit is damage to the hair cells of the organ of Corti. In the United States, noise exposure is the major cause. Damage may result from either loud impulse noise (e.g., an explosion) or loud continuous noise (e.g., machinery). Exposure to a high level of noise (e.g., standing close to the stage or speakers at a rock concert) on an intermittent or continuing basis damages the hair and supporting cells of the organ of Corti. Other sources of potential damage to hearing include certain types of work (first responders, construction workers) and play (fireworks, concerts, firearms, and loud toys). Ototoxic drugs also damage the hair cells of the organ of Corti; when combined with high noise levels, the damage is greater and resultant hearing loss more profound.

Other potential causes of sensory hearing loss include prenatal exposure to rubella, viral infections, meningitis, trauma, Ménière disease, and aging. Tumors such as acoustic neuromas (vestibular schwannomas), vascular disorders, demyelinating or degenerative diseases, infections (bacterial meningitis in particular), or trauma may affect the central auditory pathways and produce a neural hearing loss.

PRESBYCUSIS With aging, the hair cells of the cochlea degenerate, producing a progressive sensorineural hearing loss. In **presbycusis**, hearing acuity begins to decrease in early adulthood and progresses as long as the individual lives. Higher-pitched tones and conversational speech are lost initially.

Risk Factors

About 50% of hearing loss in children is genetically caused, usually with a recessive inheritance pattern with *GJB2* gene abnormalities. Another 25% is due to environmental causes around the time of birth; the remainder is due to unknown causes. Although many infants with hearing loss have no known risk factors, identified risks include the following (ASLHA, 2013a):

- Family history of congenital hearing loss
- Positive titer for TORCH infections (toxoplasmosis, rubella, cytomegalovirus, syphilis, herpes)
- Craniofacial abnormalities
- Very low birth weight (<1500 g)
- Bilirubin greater than 16 mg/dL
- Aminoglycoside medication administration for more than 5 days
- Low Apgar score at 1 or 5 minutes
- Bacterial meningitis
- Mechanical ventilation for over 5 days
- Presence of syndromes associated with hearing loss (Down syndrome, Pierre Robin syndrome, Arnold-Chiari malformation).

TABLE 18-3 Decibel Levels of Everyday Sounds ●

CATEGORY	DECIBEL LEVEL (DB)	EXAMPLES
Faint	20	Leaves rustling in a breeze
	30	Quiet library
		Whisper
Moderate	50	Moderate rainfall
	60	Dishwasher
		Clothes dryer
		Normal conversation
Very loud	70	Alarm clock
		Vacuum cleaner
	80–90	Hair dryer
		Food processor
		Snowblower
Extremely loud	90	Passing motorcycle
	106	Snow blower
		Gas-powered lawn mower
		Sporting event
Painful	120	Siren
	124	Maximum volume of MP3 ear buds
		MRI scanner
	140	Jet engine
		Firearms

Sources: Based on American Speech-Language-Hearing Association. (2013b). *Noise.* Retrieved from http://www.asha.org/public/hearing/Noise; American Speech-Language-Hearing Association. (2013c). *Noise and hearing loss prevention.* Retrieved from http://www.asha.org/public/hearing/Noise-and-Hearing-Loss-Prevention; Center for Hearing, Speech and Language. (2012). *How loud is it?* Retrieved from http://www.chsl.org/soundchart.php; University of Iowa. (2012). *Sound levels.* Retrieved from http://www.uiowa.edu/~ui-safe/sound-levels.html.

Prevention

Both the loudness of the noise and the length of exposure contribute to hearing damage. The level of noise is measured in decibels (dB). The louder the noise, the higher the decibel level. The use of ear buds and head phones in young children puts them at a higher risk of hearing loss. Permanent damage can occur at volumes louder than 85 dB.

Although young children may be at higher risk, hearing impairment associated with the use of ear buds and head phones can affect individuals of any age group. Due in part to the popular practice of listening to portable media devices (e.g., MP3 players and cellular phones), **noise-induced hearing loss (NIHL)** continues to be a serious public health concern. This condition is associated with prolonged exposure to sounds of greater than or equal to 85 dB over an extended time period, including listening to loud music. NIHL may also be caused by a single exposure to an intense impulse sound at a volume of 120 dB or more, such as an explosive blast (Centers for Disease Control and Prevention [CDC], 2013). Prevention of NIHL includes avoiding situations that pose known risks and wearing ear protection when in environments that may involve exposure to known risks.

Warning signs that may suggest auditory damage include the inability to hear another individual's voice from a distance of 3 feet away and muffled sound perception. Ringing in the ears (tinnitus) and ear pain are warning signs, as well. Some examples of decibel levels of everyday sounds are shown in **Table 18–3 ●**.

TABLE 18-4 Ototoxic Medications

MEDICATION CATEGORY AND DRUG EXAMPLES	USES
AMINOGLYCOSIDES *Drug examples:* –tobramycin –gentamicin –amikacin	These drugs are used in the treatment of advanced bacterial infections and tuberculosis. Hearing loss is more likely to occur in clients with renal disease or previous hearing difficulty.
LOOP DIURETICS *Drug examples:* –Bumex –Lasix	These drugs are diuretics that affect the ascending limb of the loop of Henle in the kidney.
NONSTEROIDAL ANTI-INFLAMMATORY DRUGS (NSAIDs) *Drug examples:* –ibuprofen –naproxen –salicylates	These are some of the most commonly used drugs in our society today. They can be used as antipyretics, analgesics, and anti-inflammatory agents and for their antiplatelet effects. Ototoxic effects are likely to occur with higher doses.

Sources: American Academy of Audiology. (2009). *Position statement and clinical practice guidelines: Ototoxicity monitoring.* Retrieved from http://www.audiology.org/resources/documentlibrary/documents/otomonpositionguideline.pdf; Bisht, M., & Bist, S. (2011). Ototoxicity: The hidden menace. *Indian Journal of Otolaryngology and Head and Neck Surgery, 63*(3), 255–259; WebMD. (2011). *Ear-damaging (ototoxic) medications.* Retrieved from http://www.webmd.com/a-to-z-guides/ear-damaging-ototoxic-medicines.

Medications can also cause hearing disorders (**Table 18–4 ●**). The decision to discontinue a medication based on potential for ototoxicity should be made in collaboration with the prescribing physician. Some drugs cannot be discontinued despite their potential to damage hearing. The nurse should be aware of medication groups that can cause hearing damage and teach clients to monitor their hearing while they are taking these medications. One group requires special mention: platinum coordination complexes (cisplatin). These drugs are used in the treatment of many solid cancerous tumors, and are the most ototoxic and widely prescribed drugs in clinical practice.

▶ CLINICAL MANIFESTATIONS

Conductive hearing loss involves an equal loss of hearing at all sound frequencies. If the level of sound is greater than the threshold for hearing, speech discrimination is good. Because of this, the client with a conductive hearing loss benefits from amplification by a hearing aid.

Sensorineural hearing losses typically affect the ability to hear high-frequency tones more than low-frequency tones. This loss makes speech discrimination difficult, especially in a noisy environment. Hearing aids are often not useful, because they amplify both speech and background noise. The increased sound intensity may actually cause discomfort for the client.

Because the hearing loss of presbycusis is gradual, the client and family may not realize the extent of the deficit. The individual with a hearing impairment may be described as

Focus on Diversity and Culture
Hearing Loss

Caucasians are twice as likely as African Americans to have hearing loss. Hispanics are less likely than non-Hispanics to experience difficulty with hearing. Very little research, however, has examined ethnic diversity and hearing impairment. An interesting phenomenon that has emerged is the existence of a "deaf culture." Some people who are deaf identify with this "deaf culture" because they share historical traditions and a unique language. All people with hearing loss must interact with the hearing world, and this interaction may be beneficial to some and stressful to others. This will continue to be an evolving model (Sign Media, 2011).

Tinnitus

Tinnitus is the perception of sound or noise in the ears without stimulus from the environment. The sound may be steady, intermittent, or pulsatile and is often described as a buzzing, roaring, or ringing.

Tinnitus is usually associated with hearing loss (conductive or sensorineural); however, the mechanism producing the sound is poorly understood. It is often an early symptom of noise-induced hearing damage and drug-related ototoxicity. Tinnitus is especially associated with salicylate, quinine, or quinidine toxicity. Other etiologies include obstruction of the auditory meatus, presbycusis, middle or inner ear inflammations and infections, otosclerosis, and Ménière disease. Most tinnitus, however, is chronic and has no pathological importance. Tinnitus can be very stressful and cause anxiety and/or depression for the individual experiencing it. Individuals with chronic tinnitus should not have their distress minimized (American Tinnitus Association, 2013).

Stay Current: *You can hear some of the sounds that someone with tinnitus might experience by visiting the American Tinnitus Association at* **www.ata.org/sounds-of-tinnitus**.

Early identification of hearing loss is a key element in successful treatment. Detection of hearing loss in infants is important to ensure optimal development. Clients need to know the risk for hearing damage and how to prevent it. Awareness of the effects of noise exposure, especially when combined with the ototoxic effects of aspirin or other drugs, is important in preventing sensorineural hearing loss.

unsociable or paranoid. The family may worry that the individual is becoming increasingly forgetful, absentminded, or perhaps "senile." Depression, confusion, inattentiveness, tension, and negativism have been noted in older adults with hearing impairments. Functional problems such as poor general health, reduced mobility, and impaired interpersonal communication are also associated with hearing loss. Caregivers need to be alert for signs of impaired hearing such as cupping an ear, difficulty understanding verbal communication when the individual cannot see the speaker's face, difficulty following conversation in a large group, and withdrawal from social activities. Hearing aids and other amplification devices are useful for most clients with presbycusis.

Clinical Manifestations and Therapies **Hearing Impairment**

ETIOLOGY	CLINICAL MANIFESTATIONS	CLINICAL THERAPIES
Conductive hearing loss	■ Equal loss of hearing at all sound frequencies	■ Hearing aid ■ Treat underlying conditions such as otitis media. ■ Steroids and/or decongestants to reduce inflammation ■ Surgery
Sensorineural hearing loss	■ Decreased ability to hear high-frequency tones more than low-frequency tones ■ Difficulty discriminating speech	■ Cochlear implant
Presbycusis	■ Cognitive and affective manifestations such as confusion, forgetfulness, and depression; poor health, reduced mobility; withdrawal; signs of impaired hearing, such as cupping a hand around the ear	■ Hearing aid ■ Steroids or decongestants to reduce inflammation
Tinnitus (mechanism not fully understood; etiology varies to include noise, ototoxicity, infection or inflammation, underlying conditions such as Ménière disease).	■ Buzzing, roaring, or ringing in the ears	Treat underlying cause. ■ Tinnitus maskers such as ambient noise

▶ COLLABORATION

To properly treat an alteration in hearing, the client needs to be diagnosed with the correct type of hearing loss. Nurses can help clients with explanations about the types of tests that will be performed and providing any education if an alteration is found.

Diagnostic Tests

Assessment protocols that can be performed for initial screening were presented in the Concept of Sensory Perception section earlier in this chapter. These include the whisper test, otoscope examination, tympanogram, and use of a tuning fork to perform the Rinne and Weber tests.

Surgery

Reconstructive surgeries of the middle ear, such as a stapedectomy or tympanoplasty, may help restore hearing with a conductive hearing loss. Stapedectomy is the removal and replacement of the stapes. This procedure is used to treat hearing loss related to otosclerosis.

In a tympanoplasty, the structures of the middle ear are reconstructed to improve conductive hearing deficits. Chronic otitis media with necrosis and scarring of the middle ear is a common indication for this type of surgery.

In myringotomy, a small hole is made in the tympanic membrane and then tympanostomy tubes are placed. This procedure is common among young children with repeated episodes of otitis media but can also be performed on older adults for chronic presence of middle ear fluid (effusion). The tubes allow equalization of air within the middle ear or prevent fluid accumulation.

For the client with a sensorineural hearing loss, a cochlear implant may be the only hope for restoring sound perception. The cochlear implant consists of a microphone, speech processor, transmitter, receiver/stimulator, and electrodes (**Figure 18–9 ●**). Its function is more similar to the way the ear normally receives and processes sounds than it is to that of a hearing aid. The microphone picks up sounds, sending them to the speech processor, which selects and processes those that are useful. The receiver/stimulator and transmitter receive signals from the speech processor, convert them to electrical impulses, and send these impulses to the electrodes for transmission to the brain.

Cochlear implants provide sound perception but not normal hearing. The client is able to recognize warning sounds such as automobiles, sirens, telephones, and doors opening or closing. Clients also receive stimuli to alert them to incoming communication so they can focus on the individual speaking. Many clients learn to interpret perceived sounds as words, especially when the hearing loss is acquired as an adult.

Pharmacologic Therapy

For hearing loss that is caused by upper respiratory infections or seasonal allergies, decongestants may be helpful. Sudden sensorineural hearing loss may initially be treated with steroids. For cases of otitis media, antibiotics may be prescribed. There are currently no medications available to treat permanent hearing loss.

Medications used for temporary hearing loss are presented in the Medications feature.

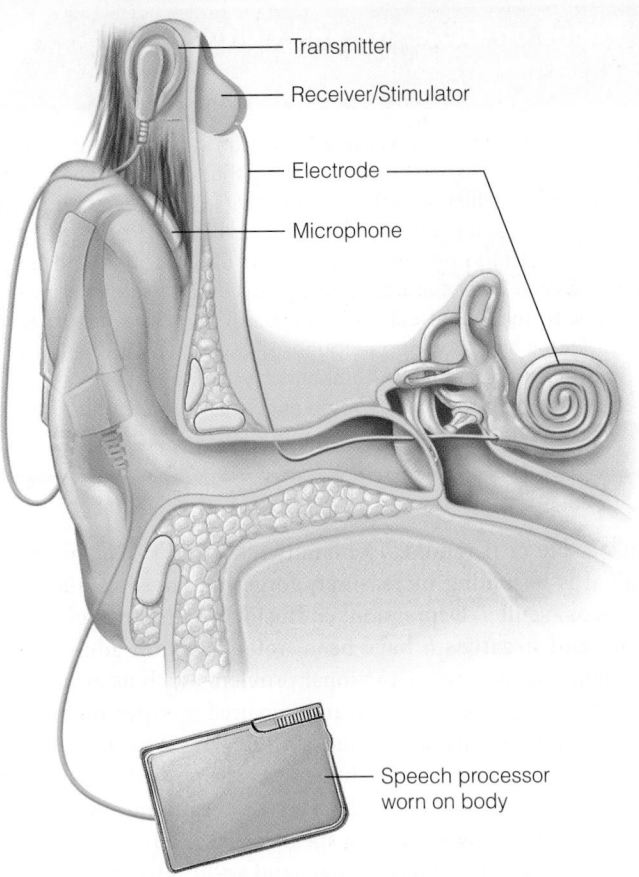

Figure 18–9 ● A cochlear implant for sensorineural hearing loss.
Source: Courtesy of National Eye Institute, National Institutes of Health.

Nonpharmacologic Therapy

If hearing loss in a client is permanent, a multidisciplinary team is formed to assist the client and family with adaptation to the disability. Team members may include any of the following: physician, nurse, a speech/language, occupational, or physical therapist, audiologist, teacher, social worker, and family members and caregivers. The team may provide strategies and accommodations for a client whose loss is correctable until surgery is completed or other treatments take effect. Therapists and social workers can often assist clients in accessing assistive technology devices at relatively low cost, especially if they are not covered by insurance, as well as help the client learn how to use these tools.

AMPLIFICATION A hearing aid or other amplification device can help many clients with hearing deficits. These assistive devices do nothing to prevent, minimize, or treat the hearing loss itself. They amplify the sound presented to the hearing apparatus of the ear, which may bring the level of sound above the hearing threshold, allowing more accurate perception and interpretation of its meaning. When sound perception is distorted, a hearing aid may be less helpful, because it simply amplifies the distorted sound. Hearing aids must be individually prescribed by an audiologist. Proper design, proper fit, and regular maintenance are necessary to maintain their effectiveness.

Unfortunately, less than one fifth of older clients with a hearing deficit have or use a hearing aid. Denial of the deficit, other health problems, poor visual acuity, and decreased manual

Medications **Temporary Hearing Loss**

CLASSIFICATION AND DRUG EXAMPLES	MECHANISMS OF ACTION	NURSING CONSIDERATIONS
Decongestants *Drug example:* ■ pseudoephedrine	Enhance norepinephrine and epinephrine activity by stimulating alpha-adrenergic receptors. This causes vasoconstriction and reduces inflammation.	■ Use with caution in clients with hyperthyroidism, hypertension, or heart disease. ■ Instruct client to limit caffeine use because it can lead to hypertension and tachycardia.
Corticosteroids *Drug examples:* ■ prednisone ■ methylprednisolone	Mimic hormones produced by the adrenal gland. Reduces inflammation and the immune response system.	■ Warn client that grapefruit or grapefruit juice may alter the drug's uptake. ■ Barbiturates may decrease effectiveness. ■ Live vaccines should be avoided while taking corticosteroids.
Antibiotics *Drug examples:* ■ cephalosporins ■ penicillins ■ macrolides ■ aminoglycosides ■ tetracyclines ■ fluoroquinolones ■ sulfonamides	Used to treat bacterial infection. Choice of antibiotic is based on bacteria causing infection.	■ Teach importance of finishing full course of antibiotics. ■ Observe for signs of allergic reactions. ■ Encourage adequate fluid intake. ■ Monitor renal and/or hepatic function if long-term use. ■ Monitor for ototoxicity. ■ Warn clients taking macrolides that grapefruit or grapefruit juice may alter the drug's uptake.

dexterity all contribute to this low usage. Cost is another factor. Health insurance plans typically cover only one pair of hearing aids within a certain time frame, and in most states Medicare does not pay for hearing aids at all. Some clients choose not to pay for hearing aids.

All hearing aids include a microphone, amplifier, speaker, earpiece, and volume control. Many include an option to turn off the microphone when using the telephone; others can be adjusted for the client's pattern of hearing loss. Hearing aids are available in a variety of styles, each with advantages and disadvantages:

■ Canal hearing aids (in-canal and completely-in-canal) are the least noticeable style, fitting in the ear canal. They are appropriate for mild to moderately severe hearing loss. These small and unobtrusive devices allow use of the telephone and can be worn during exercise. Because of their small size, the client must have good manual dexterity to insert, clean, and change the batteries in canal hearing aids. For this reason, older clients or clients with impaired dexterity may be unable to use them.

■ The in-ear style of hearing aid fits into the external ear and is used for mild to severe hearing loss (**Figure 18–10** ●). Its larger size makes manipulation somewhat easier, although it still may be difficult for less dexterous individuals. A greater degree of amplification is possible with the in-ear aid. Many have a toggle switch for telephone usage.

■ The behind-ear hearing aid allows finer adjustment of the level of amplification and is easier for the client to manipulate (**Figure 18–11** ●). This device can be used by clients with mild to profound hearing loss. For the client who wears glasses, this style can be modified, with all components fitting into the temple of the eyeglasses.

With both the in-canal and in-ear style, cleaning is important. Small portals may become plugged with cerumen, interfering with sound transmission.

For the client who does not have a hearing aid, an assistive listening device, or "pocket talker," with a microphone and earpieces is useful. Pocket talkers are available over-the-counter or

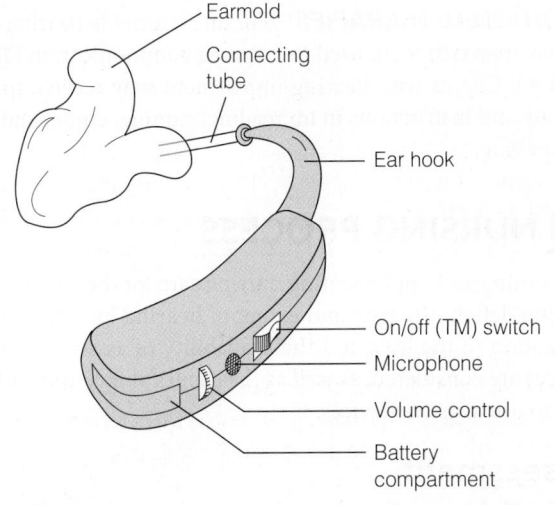

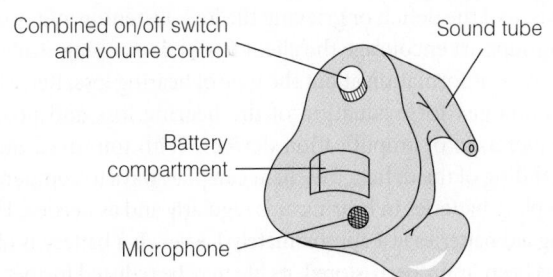

Figure 18–10 ● An in-ear hearing aid.

Figure 18–11 ● A behind-ear hearing aid.

TABLE 18–5 Communication Techniques for Clients Who Have a Hearing Impairment

TECHNIQUE	DESCRIPTION
Cued speech	Supplement to lip reading; eight hand shapes represent groups of consonant sounds and four positions about the face represent groups of vowel sounds; based on the sounds the letters make, not the letters themselves; client can "see-hear" every spoken syllable a hearing person hears.
Oral approach	Uses only spoken language for face-to-face communication; avoids use of formal signs; uses hearing aids and residual hearing.
Total communication	Uses speech and sign, finger-spelling, lip reading, and residual hearing simultaneously; client selects communication technique depending on the situation.
Sign language	A separate language that allows the user to communicate quickly and accurately with others who understand signs. The signs or hand movements represent words or concepts. When a sign is not available, the word can be spelled out using signs. American Sign Language (ASL) is most often used; however, British Sign Language (BSL) is common in Europe.

through an audiologist and are relatively inexpensive. The earpiece requires no special fitting, and the external microphone allows the client to focus on the desired sound rather than simply amplifying all sounds. Assistive listening devices may also be used in conjunction with a hearing aid.

Clients with tinnitus may find a white or pink noise–masking device helpful to promote concentration and rest. These devices conduct a pleasant sound to the affected ear, allowing the client to block out the abnormal sound.

TTD/TTY telephones and phones with amplifiers are available to assist clients who are deaf or hearing impaired in communicating with the outside world. Accessibility to the Internet can make an extraordinary difference in the quality of life to an individual with a hearing impairment, who can now make restaurant and airplane reservations by computer, as well as communicate by e-mail.

ADDITIONAL THERAPIES For uncorrectable hearing loss, several approaches are used to enhance communication (**Table 18–5** ●). Clients with hearing impairment may receive speech therapy and instructions in lip reading, signing, cuing, and finger-spelling.

■ NURSING PROCESS

In planning and implementing nursing care for the client with a hearing deficit, the type and extent of hearing loss, the client's adaptation to the loss, and the availability of assistive hearing devices are considered, as well as the client's ability and willingness to use assistive devices.

Assessment

- *Health history.* Perceived ability to hear; effect of hearing loss on function and lifestyle; risk factors such as use of oto-

toxic medications; upper respiratory tract or frequent ear infection; noise exposure; presence of vertigo, tinnitus, unsteadiness, or imbalance.
- *Physical examination.* Apparent perception of normal speech; inspection of external ear, tympanic membrane; whisper, Rinne, and Weber tests; tests of balance and cranial nerve function.

Diagnoses

Possible nursing diagnoses for the client with hearing impairment may include the following:

- *Risk for Injury*
- *Impaired Verbal Communication*
- *Social Isolation.*

(NANDA-I © 2012)

Planning

Appropriate outcomes for the client with hearing impairment are based on the extent of the deficit and may include the following:

- The client will remain free from injury.
- The client will wear hearing protection and have no further loss of hearing.
- The client will find the best method of communication with others including sign language, hearing aids, writing, and lip reading.
- The client will remain involved in his community and not experience social isolation or decreased feelings of self-worth.

Implementation

All hearing loss can cause safety concerns for the client and contribute to feelings of isolation and lowered self-esteem. Therefore, the goals of nursing care are to promote client safety, encourage social interaction, and promote feelings of self-worth.

Promote Optimal Wellness

Whether the client's hearing deficit is partial or total, impaired sound perception is the primary problem. The client needs to understand what causes the deficit and what to expect for the future. Nursing interventions focus on maximizing available hearing and preventing further deterioration to the extent possible:

- Encourage the client to talk about the hearing loss and its effect on activities of daily living. Hearing loss affects each individual in a different way. The client may be denying the extent of the deficit or grieving the loss. Listening and providing support encourage the client to develop coping strategies.
- Provide information about the type of hearing loss. Refer to an audiologist for evaluation of the hearing loss and possible exploration of amplification devices. With improved understanding of the deficit, the client can plan ways to compensate.
- Replace batteries in hearing aids regularly and as needed. Hearing aid batteries last approximately 1 week. If a battery is old or has been improperly stored, its life may be reduced further.
- Talk with the family members about techniques they can use to make communication with the client easier. The same

techniques the nurse employs, as listed in Box 18–2, can be used by family members.

■ Check hearing aids for patency, cleaning out cerumen as necessary.

Facilitate Communication

A hearing deficit impairs the client's ability to receive and interpret verbal communication. A hearing loss affects the client's ability to follow conversations, use the telephone, and enjoy television or other forms of entertainment. Use the following techniques to improve communication:

■ Wave your hand or tap the client on the shoulder before beginning to speak.
■ If the client wears corrective lenses, ensure that they are clean, and encourage the client to wear them.
■ When speaking, face the client and keep your hands away from your face.
■ Keep your face in full light.
■ Reduce the noise in the environment before speaking.
■ Use a low voice pitch with normal loudness.
■ Use short sentences and pause at the end of each sentence.
■ Speak at a normal rate, and do not overarticulate.
■ Use facial expressions or gestures.
■ Provide a magic slate for written communication.

Individuals with hearing impairments often lip read, making good visibility of the speaker's face necessary. Excessive environmental noise interferes with the ability to perceive the message. Higher tones are typically lost with presbycusis and other types of hearing loss. Using short sentences and pausing give the client time to interpret the message. Overarticulating makes it more difficult to follow the flow and to lip read. Non-verbal cues and written messages enhance the client's understanding.

Additional techniques include the following:

■ Do not place intravenous catheters in the dominant hand. The client may need to use that hand to write.
■ Rephrase sentences when the client has difficulty understanding. Hearing losses may affect different sound tones, making some words more difficult to comprehend. Using alternative words and phrases may increase the client's ability to perceive the message.
■ Repeat important information. The nurse must make sure that the client understands the information.
■ Inform other staff about the client's hearing deficit and effective strategies for communication. Consistent use of effective strategies for communication decreases the client's frustration.

Encourage Socialization

The client with impaired hearing often becomes socially isolated. This isolation may be self-imposed because of difficulty communicating, especially in a group. Often, however, the isolation comes about gradually and without intention. The client finds social settings such as family dinners or community gatherings increasingly difficult. Friends and family become frustrated trying to communicate with someone who has a hearing impairment, and invitations to participate in social activities dwindle.

Community-Based Care
Clients With Hearing Loss

Teaching for home and community-based care for the client with hearing loss focuses on managing the deficit and developing coping strategies. Many adults with hearing loss are not employed and those who are typically work in low-skilled jobs. The loss of the ability to communicate with other people can have a profound impact on everyday life and create feelings of frustration and loneliness. This is especially prevalent in clients with congenital hearing loss if they have not been given the ability to learn sign language.

Early detection and intervention is critical for children with hearing loss or deafness to minimize the impact of this deficit. Screening by their healthcare provider as well as school screenings can help with early detection. Speech/language therapists can work closely with children, their parents and their schools to maximize their educational success. Families of children with hearing loss should be given the opportunity to learn sign language with their child. Hearing aids (if appropriate), development of lip-reading skills, sign language, and use of printed text can help a child be successful at school (World Health Organization, 2013).

■ Identify the extent and cause of the social isolation. Help to differentiate the reality of the isolation and its cause from the client's perception of isolation. Clients with impaired hearing may be unaware that they are isolated. Identifying factors that contribute to isolation may provide the needed impetus to remedy the hearing loss.
■ Encourage client to interact with friends and family on a one-to-one basis in quiet settings. Clients with impaired hearing are more successful in understanding conversations that take place in small groups and quiet settings.
■ Treat the client with dignity and remind friends and family that a hearing deficit does not indicate loss of mental faculties. Inappropriate responses due to a hearing deficit can cause others to perceive the client as "stupid" or demented.
■ Involve client in activities that do not require acute hearing, such as checkers and chess. The client has an opportunity to interact socially without the stress of straining to hear.
■ Refer the client to an audiologist for evaluation and possible hearing aid fitting.
■ Refer to resources such as support groups and senior citizen centers. These groups provide new social outlets.

Evaluation

Expected outcomes of nursing care for a client with hearing impairment may include the following:

■ The client demonstrates successful establishment of a communication method.
■ The client manifests growth and developmental milestones to maximum potential.
■ The client and family demonstrate positive methods of coping.

REVIEW Hearing Impairment

REVIEW Hearing Impairment

RELATE Link the Concepts and Exemplars

Linking the exemplar of hearing impairment with the concept of development:

1. When caring for a young child who receives a cochlear implant after being deaf from birth to age 5, how will the child's speech patterns differ from those of a normal 5-year-old?

2. What strategies can the nurse employ to help this 5-year-old client improve speech patterns?

Linking the exemplar of hearing impairment with the concept of cognition:

3. How might hearing loss impact an older client's cognition?

4. What can the nurse implement to promote cognition in an older adult who has a hearing impairment?

READY Go to Companion Skills Manual

REFER Go to Pearson Nursing Student Resources
nursing.pearsonhighered.com

- Additional review materials

REFLECT Case Study

Mrs. Smith is an 87-year-old woman who recently moved into an assisted living home after hospitalization for uncontrolled diabetes. She enjoyed reading, but for a long time she has not been able to read due to poor vision acuity. During the admission assessment, the nurse also documents a hearing loss.

1. Discuss the importance of a thorough sensory assessment in this client.

2. Describe the benefits of improving Mrs. Smith's sensory deficits.

3. What recommendations will the nurse make to Mrs. Smith to improve her hearing?

4. How does diabetes mellitus impact her sense of hearing?

EXEMPLAR 18.2 Cataracts

EXEMPLAR KEY TERMS
Cataract, *1306*
Congenital cataracts, *1307*
Extracapsular extraction, *1308*
Radiation cataracts, *1307*
Secondary cataracts, *1307*
Traumatic cataracts, *1307*

EXEMPLAR LEARNING OUTCOMES
After reading about this exemplar, you will be able to:

1. Describe the pathophysiology, etiology, clinical manifestations, and direct and indirect causes of cataracts.

2. Identify risk factors associated with cataracts.

3. Illustrate the nursing process in providing culturally competent care across the life span for individuals with cataracts.

4. Formulate priority nursing diagnoses appropriate for an individual with cataracts.

5. Summarize therapies used by interdisciplinary teams in the collaborative care of an individual with cataracts.

6. Plan evidence-based care for an individual with cataracts and his or her family in collaboration with other members of the healthcare team.

7. Evaluate expected outcomes for an individual with cataracts.

▶ OVERVIEW

A **cataract** is an opacification (clouding) of the lens of the eye; it can significantly interfere with light transmission to the retina and the ability to perceive images clearly. Cataracts are a common cause of visual deficits, and by age 80, nearly half of the population is affected. In many cases, however, cataracts do not significantly impair vision.

▶ PATHOPHYSIOLOGY AND ETIOLOGY

The incidence of cataracts within the population is so common that even if it is not the primary diagnosis, most nurses will take care of clients who have either had cataracts or had them surgically removed at some point in their life. Nurses should recognize that not all cataracts need to be removed in the early stages, but many clients will eventually have them surgically corrected.

The majority of cataracts form as a result of the aging process. As the lens ages, its fibers and proteins change and degenerate. The proteins clump, clouding the lens and reducing light transmission to the retina. This process generally begins at the periphery of the lens, gradually spreading to involve the central portion. As the cataract continues to develop, the entire lens may become opaque. When only a portion of the lens is affected,

the cataract is called immature. A mature cataract is opacity of the entire lens. In addition to clouding, the lens may discolor over time, affecting the ability to accurately discriminate colors.

Etiology

The prevalence of cataracts in the United States increases rapidly with aging. Approximately 50% of individuals between the ages of 65 and 74 will develop a cataract; that increases to 70% of individuals over the age of 70. Men are affected less frequently than women. African Americans with cataracts lose

Lifespan Considerations
Cataracts in Children

- Some cataracts are present at birth, whereas others are acquired during childhood.

- Some of the causes of acquired cataracts include retinopathy of prematurity, metabolic diseases such as galactosemia, and long-term use of corticosteroids.

- A major cause of congenital cataracts in the past was congenital rubella syndrome, the mother's infection with rubella during gestation. Now that children and women receive the rubella vaccine, very few cases of cataracts result from congenital rubella syndrome.

their vision at a rate twice that of Caucasians, due to lack of or delay in treatment (Health Communities, 2011).

Additionally, four types of cataracts occur independent of the aging process. **Secondary cataracts** can form after surgery to treat another eye disorder, such as glaucoma, or as an effect of medication or another primary disorder. Clients who require regular or recurring doses of corticosteroids, for example, are at risk for secondary cataracts. **Traumatic cataracts** may result from an injury to the eye. **Radiation cataracts** may result from long-term exposure to radiation. **Congenital cataracts** may appear in a child at birth or in childhood, usually in both eyes (National Eye Institute [NEI], 2009b).

Risk Factors

Age is the greatest single risk factor for cataracts. Genetics may contribute to the risk, although the link is unclear. Environmental and lifestyle factors play a role. Long-term exposure to sunlight (UVB rays) increases the risk for cataracts; cigarette smoking and heavy alcohol consumption are associated with earlier cataract development. Eye trauma, including injury to the lens capsule by a foreign body, blunt trauma, or exposure to heat or radiation, can precipitate cataract formation. Diabetes mellitus is associated with earlier development of cataracts, especially when the blood glucose level is not carefully controlled at or near normal levels. Certain drugs, such as systemic or inhaled corticosteroids, lovastatin (Mevacor), phenytoin (Dilantin), chlorpromazine (Thorazine), and busulfan (Myleran) also prompt the formation of cataracts.

▶ CLINICAL MANIFESTATIONS

Cataracts tend to occur bilaterally unless related to eye trauma. Fortunately, they tend to develop at different rates, and one cataract generally matures more rapidly than the other. As a cataract interferes with light transmission through the lens, visual acuity decreases, affecting both close and distance vision. Light rays are scattered as they pass through the lens, causing complaints of glare. Glare affects the ability to adjust between light and dark environments. Color discrimination is impaired, particularly in the blue to purple range. When the cataract is mature, the pupil may appear cloudy gray or white rather than black.

The diagnosis of a cataract is made based on the history and eye examination. Ophthalmoscope examination confirms the diagnosis by identifying the location and extent of a cataract. As the cataract matures, ophthalmoscopy reveals a dark area instead of the red reflex.

Clinical Manifestations and Therapies **Cataracts**

ETIOLOGY	CLINICAL MANIFESTATIONS	CLINICAL THERAPIES
Congenital cataracts ■ Rare ■ Usually unknown cause ■ May occur with other birth defects such as: ■ Congenital rubella ■ Trisomy 21 (Down syndrome) ■ Pierre Robin Syndrome ■ Trisomy 13 (Patau syndrome)	■ May be different from age-onset cataracts ■ Gray or white cloudy pupils ■ May have nystagmus ■ May not have "red eye" glow in photos	■ Diagnosis confirmed by ophthalmologist. ■ Treatment depends on severity. ■ If mild and doesn't seem to affect vision, it may just be monitored, especially if bilateral. ■ If moderate to severe and seems to affect vision or if unilateral, surgical removal is usually recommended. ■ In most cases an intraocular lens is also implanted at the time of surgery.
Age-related cataracts ■ Aging causes proteins in the lens to deteriorate and become cloudy. ■ By age 75, most people will have cataracts that affect vision. ■ Factors that speed formation: ■ Diabetes ■ UVA/UVB exposure ■ Smoking ■ Family history.	■ Cloudy/opaque lens ■ May cause cloudy vision, halos, diplopia, or photophobia	■ Early cataracts or those with minimal effect on vision may require no surgical intervention. ■ Encourage UVA/UVB protection. ■ Utilize safety measures for decreased visual acuity. ■ Surgery is recommended if cataract interferes with ADLs.

▶ COLLABORATION

Providing a safe environment is a priority nursing intervention for any client with cataracts, whether or not it is the client's primary diagnosis. With the increasing age of the overall population, the prevalence of cataracts will continue to increase.

Diagnostic Tests

The simplest test to aid in the diagnosis of cataracts is the visual acuity test. The Snellen and Rosenbaum charts are used. A dilated eye exam with either an ophthalmoscope or slit-lamp examination provides a magnified view of the structures of the eye.

Surgery

Surgical removal is the only treatment used at this time for cataracts; no medical treatment is available to prevent or treat them. If the client presents with bilateral cataracts, surgery is performed on only one eye at a time. If an intraocular lens (an artificial lens to replace the diseased lens of the eye) is to be implanted during surgery, the corneal curvature will be measured via keratometry and the anteroposterior diameter of the eye will be measured via A-scan prior to surgery. This allows the healthcare team to determine the proper lens needed for the intraocular lens implant. Various lens choices are available, based on the client's vision pathology and needs. These include monofocal lenses, multifocal (accommodative) lenses, and toric lenses. The surgeon must make more careful measurements for a patient who has previously undergone LASIK surgery (American Academy of Ophthalmology [AAO], 2013a).

Surgical removal of the cataract and lens is indicated when the cataract has developed to the point that vision and activities of daily living are affected. A mature cataract also may be removed when it causes a secondary condition such as glaucoma or uveitis.

Cataract surgery typically is done on an outpatient basis using local anesthesia. If general anesthesia is required, the client may be hospitalized overnight. **Extracapsular extraction**, in which the anterior capsule, nucleus, and cortex of the lens are removed leaving the posterior capsule intact, is the procedure of choice (**Figure 18–12 ●**). Using an operating microscope, the surgeon makes a small incision at the edge of the cornea and extracts the lens intact or via emulsification and aspiration. In the latter technique, ultrasound vibrations are used to break the lens material into fragments (phacoemulsification), which are then suctioned out of the eye (AAO, 2013a). Phacoemulsification lens removal requires a smaller incision and usually is preferred over extracting the lens intact (AAO, 2011b). The remaining capsule supports the lens implant and protects the retina.

After removal of the lens, the eye can no longer focus light on the retina and vision is seriously affected. Usually a plastic, acrylic, or silicone intraocular lens is implanted at the time of surgery. This implant rapidly restores binocular vision and depth perception. In most cases, following extracapsular lens removal, the intraocular lens is positioned in the posterior capsule behind the iris (see Figure 18–12). This is called a posterior chamber lens. In some cases, the intraocular lens is positioned in front of the iris with an anterior chamber lens.

A secondary procedure called a limbal relaxing incision can be performed at the same time as the cataract surgery or at another time. This helps clients reduce or even eliminate the need for eyeglasses. Small incisions are made at opposite ends of the cornea, which allows its shape to be rounder or more symmetrical.

If an intraocular lens cannot be implanted, convex corrective glasses or contact lenses may be used to correct vision after cataract removal. Although contact lenses can provide excellent vision correction following cataract surgery, they may be difficult for some clients to adapt to or manipulate. The client with a preexisting refractive error may continue to

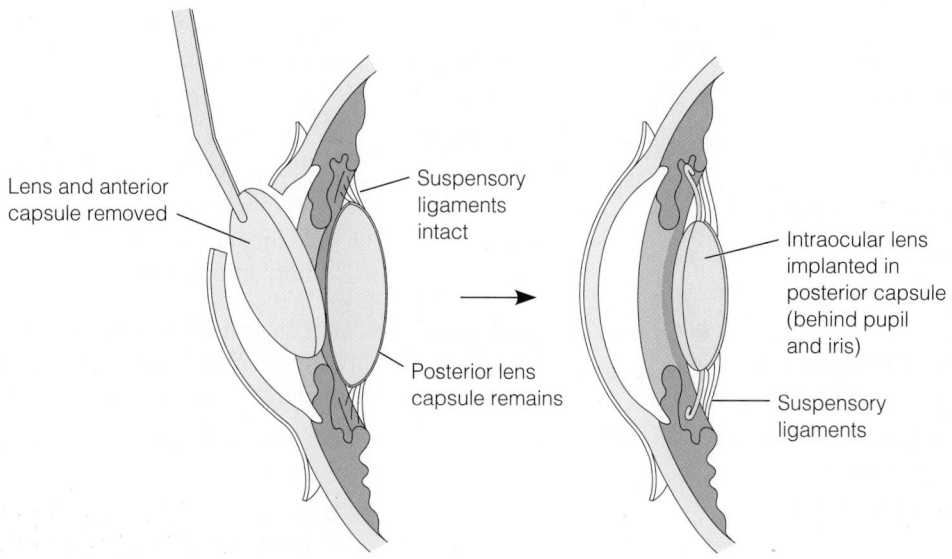

Figure 18–12 ● Extracapsular cataract extraction with removal of the lens and anterior capsule, leaving the posterior capsule intact. The intraocular lens is implanted within the posterior capsule.
Source: Courtesy of National Eye Institute, National Institutes of Health.

require corrective lenses and often needs a prescriptive change after surgery.

Complications of cataract surgery are unusual and occur in less than 1% of the surgeries. Potential complications include loss of vitreous humor, corneal edema, increased intraocular pressure, hemorrhage, inflammation or infection, retinal detachment, and displacement of the implanted lens. Between 10% and 50% of clients who undergo extracapsular extraction may develop opacification of the remaining posterior capsule 3–5 years after surgery (secondary cataract). Vision can be restored with a posterior capsulotomy (creation of an opening with a laser for light to pass through the opacified capsule) or surgical incision into the posterior capsule to allow light to reach the retina (AAO, 2013a; Eballe et al., 2011).

Nonpharmacologic Therapy

Currently, no medications are available for treating cataracts. If a cataract does not interfere with the ability to perform activities of daily living or is not associated with other eye pathology, then surgical removal is not necessary. Early cataracts can be managed with magnifying glasses, stronger prescription lenses, brighter lighting, or antiglare sunglasses (NEI, 2009b).

Complementary and Alternative Therapies

Insufficient data exists to support the treatment of cataracts with alternative therapies, although some clients may find that acupuncture relieves perceived symptoms of discomfort. Some complementary and alternative medicine (CAM) practitioners believe that antioxidants improve cataracts because they reduce the amount of free radicals that can cause damage to the eyes. There may be a link between lactose and cataract formation, but more studies in this area are needed (National Library of Medicine, 2011b).

■ NURSING PROCESS

Because aging is the single greatest risk factor for the development of cataracts, older adults are especially vulnerable to this impairment. However, as previously discussed, other factors may increase the risk for cataract development. From the standpoint of promoting wellness, all clients may benefit from client teaching regarding risk factors and preventive measures. For the client who has developed cataracts, the nursing process is geared toward both treatment and prevention of injury.

Assessment

- *Health history.* Effect of vision changes on lifestyle and activities (e.g., ability to read, watch television, participate in work and recreational activities); history of smoking, diabetes, use of prescription drugs associated with increased risk of cataracts.
- *Physical examination.* General health; visual acuity (using corrective lenses and Snellen chart) in each eye; presence of red reflex, cloudy gray or white pupil.

Diagnosis

The client with cataracts has few physical care nursing needs. Client advocacy, psychological and emotional support, and teaching/learning needs are typically of high priority for these clients.

Nursing diagnoses for the client with cataracts may include the following:

- *Risk for Injury related to visual impairment*
- *Decisional Conflict: Cataract removal*
- *Risk for Ineffective Health Maintenance.*

(NANDA-I © 2012)

Planning

Appropriate outcomes for the client diagnosed with cataracts include the following:

- The client will remain free from injury.
- The client will be able to articulate an understanding of the reasons for and risks involved with surgery.
- The client will participate in self-care activities to protect eyes from further damage and to maximize safety.
- The client will follow self-care instructions following surgery to ensure healing and to maximize benefits of surgery.

Implementation

With the initial diagnosis, teaching focuses on the disorder, indications for surgery, and vision restoration following cataract removal. Teaching adaptive strategies to deal with effects of the cataract on vision and depth perception also are useful.

Prevent Injury

Prior to surgery, the client can use a number of self-care activities to minimize further damage and to maximize safety. The nurse should teach the client to:

- Wear sunglasses with UVA/UVB protection when outdoors.
- Use reading or prescription glasses or contact lenses as necessary.
- Maximize lighting for reading, cooking, and other indoor activities.
- Limit or discontinue nighttime driving.

After surgery, the client may experience mild to moderate discomfort and some fluid discharge. The nurse should explain that these symptoms normally subside in 1 or 2 days but that the client should call the office if the symptoms persist or become intolerable. Instruct the client to continue to wear eye protection as ordered and to avoid rubbing the eye. In most cases, healing will be complete in 7–8 weeks.

Facilitate Informed Decision Making

- Explain the nonemergent nature of the condition and help the client determine the extent to which the cataract is affecting daily life. This helps the client decide when to proceed with surgery. Providing information about cataracts and their surgical removal also assists with decision making.

- Attend to verbalized concerns about surgery and its outcome. Address questions factually and completely. Fear of blindness is second only to fear of cancer for many clients. Careful listening and teaching and a caring, understanding attitude can help the client deal with this fear prior to surgery.

Teach Principles of Self-Care

- Assess for factors that may interfere with the client's ability to provide self-care postoperatively. A chronic condition that may affect the ability to administer eyedrops, such as arthritis, may indicate the need to include a family member in teaching.
- Assess for other care needs that may be impacted by vision changes in the early postoperative period. Other care needs, such as insulin injections, may suggest the need for home health or nursing care postoperatively.

When surgery is scheduled, provide pre- and postoperative teaching. Include a significant other in teaching sessions. Reinforce the following information with written instructions:

- Limitations such as avoiding reading, lifting, bending to pick up objects, strenuous activity, and sleeping on operative side
- Importance of not disturbing the eye dressing
- Prescribed medications and side effects
- Importance of follow-up appointments
- Manifestations of postoperative complications such as eye pain, decreased visual acuity or other change in vision, headache, nausea, or itching and redness of the affected eye
- Administration of eyedrops and application of eye patch or shield
- Care, insertion, and removal of contact lenses as appropriate
- Visual changes associated with thick-lensed eyeglasses as appropriate.

Promote Wellness

Care of the client in the community revolves around prevention. Advise all clients about the importance of wearing eye protection during potentially hazardous activities, such as welding, and about wearing sunglasses with UVA/UVB protection when outdoors. Discuss the link between heavy smoking and cataract development. Provide education to encourage clients to refrain from starting to smoke or to help them stop smoking.

- Encourage clients with diabetes, previous history of visual problems, or disorders that require frequent use of corticosteroids to see an ophthalmologist at least every 2 years.
- Encourage clients who smoke to enroll in a smoking cessation program.
- Encourage all clients to use appropriate eye protection when using tools and when spending time outside.
- Conduct an eye and vision assessment at each healthcare interaction with clients ages 65 years and older; inquire about any problems with vision and date of last appointment with an ophthalmologist or optometrist.

Evaluation

Criteria that may reflect attainment of identified outcomes and successful resolution of nursing diagnoses include the following:

- The client remains free from injury.
- The client makes an informed decision regarding cataract surgery.
- The client verbalizes concerns about home care.
- The client verbalizes appropriate home care activities.
- The client demonstrates correct medication administration.

REVIEW Cataracts

RELATE Link the Concepts and Exemplars

The nurse is caring for a client undergoing surgery for cataracts. The client is 78 years old and lives alone on a third-floor walk-up with no elevator.

Linking the exemplar of cataracts with the concept of safety:

1. What safety issues will the nurse address when teaching this client?
2. What issues place this client at increased risk for injury?

Linking the exemplar of cataracts with the concept of development:

3. How might the development of cataracts interfere with the older adult's ability to meet developmental milestones?
4. Prior to cataract repair, what interventions might the nurse initiate to help the older adult meet his or her developmental needs?

READY Go to Companion Skills Manual

REFER Go to Pearson Nursing Student Resources
nursing.pearsonhighered.com

- Additional review materials

REFLECT Case Study

Mary Martin, a 75-year-old widow with osteoporosis, has an appointment with her ophthalmologist this week. The ophthalmologist notes that Mrs. Martin's cataracts continue to worsen and recommends that she consider surgery. Mrs. Martin does not admit the fact that she is afraid to have surgery on her eyes. She tells the physician that she might have the surgery at some point but that she is too busy to do it right now. The physician gives Mrs. Martin a new prescription for her eyeglasses, knowing that this will help her vision at least for a little while. Mrs. Martin is told to increase the amount of light and to use reading glasses or a magnifying glass for reading.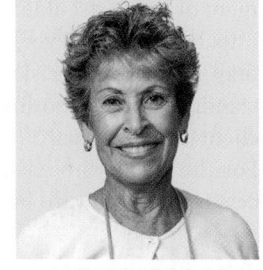

1. What nursing diagnosis would be appropriate for this client?
2. How will the nurse address the client's concerns regarding surgery?
3. What factors may impact Mrs. Martin's home care?

EXEMPLAR 18.3   **Eye Injuries**

EXEMPLAR KEY TERMS

EXEMPLAR LEARNING OUTCOMES
After reading about this exemplar, you will be able to:

1. Describe the pathophysiology, etiology, clinical manifestations, and direct and indirect causes of eye injuries.

2. Identify risk factors associated with eye injuries.

3. Illustrate the nursing process in providing culturally competent care across the life span for individuals with eye injuries.

4. Formulate priority nursing diagnoses appropriate for an individual with an eye injury.

5. Summarize therapies used by interdisciplinary teams in the collaborative care of an individual with an eye injury.

6. Plan evidence-based care for an individual with an eye injury and his or her family in collaboration with other members of the healthcare team.

7. Evaluate expected outcomes for an individual with an eye injury.

▶ OVERVIEW

Any part of the eye may be affected by trauma, with the exposed parts being particularly vulnerable. Abrasions, lacerations, and foreign bodies are the most common types of eye injury. Traumatic injury also may be caused by penetrating object, blunt force, or burns.

▶ PATHOPHYSIOLOGY AND ETIOLOGY

The majority of eye injuries are preventable. Nurses can take the opportunity to teach eye safety to clients throughout their entire life span during well visits as well as when discussing alterations in vision with clients. The pathophysiology of a given eye injury depends on the nature of the injury. Later in this exemplar, the pathophysiology of selected injuries is discussed in conjunction with their clinical manifestations.

Etiology

Eye injuries affect more than 2.5 million Americans every year, with around 73% occurring in males; almost half of all eye injuries will happen to individuals ages 18–45. Each year 50,000 people will permanently lose all or part of their vision due to injury. Recreational sports, workplace injuries, fireworks, automobile accidents, and home accidents are all settings where eye injuries can occur (AAO, 2009).

In the United States, approximately 2,000 workers each day sustain a work-related eye injury that requires medical treatment (National Institute for Occupational Safety and Health, 2010). Adults at greatest risk of eye injuries include contractors, woodworkers, welders, and electricians. Sources of eye trauma in the workplace include chemicals, flying objects, particles, and tools (American Optometric Association, n.d.).

Certain sports are associated with eye injuries. The most common sports where eye injuries occur are boxing and other full-contact martial arts, paintball, baseball, lacrosse, basketball, hockey, football, soccer, and racquet sports (AAO, 2013c).

External eye injuries are very common in children and, by themselves, rarely indicate some form of abuse or nonacciden-tal trauma. Two black eyes, however, rarely occur by accident, and raccoon eyes accompanied by swelling and skin injury are likely to accompany nonaccidental fracture at the base of the skull (Becker & Dutelle, 2013).

Prevention

Protective eyewear is estimated to prevent more than 90% of all injuries (AAO, 2011a). Yet, more than 78% of individuals with eye injuries reported not wearing eyewear at the time of injury. The type of eye protection that is required is dependent on the type of activity an individual is doing. Each home should have at least one pair of eyewear (glasses or goggles, depending on the activity) that is certified by the American National Standards Institute (ANSI). For home use, look for eyewear labeled "ANSI Z87." Standards for eye protection for sports and recreation are set by the American Society for Testing and Materials. Various types of protection are available based on the sport being played. Proper UV protection is recommended to shield eyes from glare while water or snow skiing. The Occupational Safety and Health Administration determines what type of eye protection is required in the workplace. This information should be readily available through an individual's employer (AAO, 2013f).

▶ CLINICAL MANIFESTATIONS

The nurse should remember that eye injuries can range from minor, with no loss of vision, to catastrophic, with complete loss of vision in one or both eyes. People are very dependent on their sense of sight, so the nurse should be cognizant of how impairments can affect functioning, safety, and client self-image.

Corneal Abrasion

Corneal abrasion is disruption of the superficial epithelium of the cornea. Objects commonly causing corneal abrasion include contact lenses, eyelashes, small foreign bodies such as dust and dirt, and fingernails. Drying of the eye surface and chemical irritants also may result in a corneal abrasion.

Superficial abrasions of the cornea are extremely painful but generally heal rapidly without complication or scarring. Photophobia and tearing are commonly present. When the stroma is damaged by a deep abrasion or laceration, there is an increased risk of infection, slowed healing, and scar formation.

Burns

The outer surface of the eye may be subjected to burns caused by heat, radiation, or explosion, but chemical burns are most common. Both acid and alkaline substances can burn the eye. Ammonia, products that contain lye (such as oven and drain cleaners), acids from car batteries, and other sources are often implicated in eye injuries. Burns caused by alkaline substances are particularly serious because tiny particles of the chemical may remain in the conjunctival sac, causing progressive damage. Acid causes rapid damage to the eye, but generally causes less serious burns than alkaline substances.

Explosions and flash burn injuries pose the greatest risk for thermal burns of the eye. Ultraviolet rays also can cause corneal damage ranging in severity from mild to extensive. Depending on the source of the ultraviolet light, these burns may be referred to as snowblindness, welder's arc burn, or flash burn.

The client who experiences a burn to the eye will give a history of face and eye contact with a caustic substance or another burning agent and will complain of eye pain and decreased vision. The client's eyelids may be swollen; his or her face and lips may be affected. The appearance of the client's eye may vary depending on the type of burn. Typically, the conjunctiva is reddened and edematous. Sloughing may be seen, particularly with chemical burns. The cornea often appears cloudy or hazy, and ulcerations may be evident.

Penetrating Trauma

Perforation of the eye has a variety of causes. Metal flakes or other particles produced by high-speed drilling or grinding, glass shards, or other substances may penetrate the eye. Bullets (including BBs), arrows, and knives can penetrate the eye. In a **penetrating injury**, the layers of the eye spontaneously reapproximate after entry of a sharp-pointed object or small missile (e.g., a BB) into the globe. Penetrating eye injuries are those that have a single entrance wound from the injury. There can be multiple wounds but they would have been caused by multiple sources. These injuries may not be readily apparent when the eye is inspected. In a **perforating injury**, the layers of the eye do not spontaneously reapproximate, resulting in rupture of the globe and potential loss of ocular contents. A perforating eye injury involves an entrance and exit wound, both of which are caused by the same source (Scott, 2011).

Penetrating injuries may be hidden because of tissue swelling. They may be missed when the client has other significant injuries that command attention. When the eyelid is lacerated or has a puncture wound, it is vital to inspect the underlying eye tissue for possible damage. Eye perforations cause pain, partial or complete loss of vision, and possibly bleeding or extrusion of eye contents.

Blunt Trauma

Sports injuries are a common cause of blunt trauma to the eye, which may be struck with a ball (baseballs, tennis balls, racquet balls, and handballs are frequently implicated) or injured during contact sports such as basketball, football, boxing, and wrestling. Motor vehicle crashes, falls, and physical assault are examples of other causes of blunt eye trauma.

Blunt trauma may lead to a minor eye injury such as lid ecchymosis (black eye) or subconjunctival hemorrhage, which is caused by rupture of a blood vessel in the conjunctiva. With subconjunctival hemorrhage, a well-defined bright area of erythema appears under the conjunctiva. No pain or discomfort is associated with the hemorrhage, and no treatment is necessary. The blood typically reabsorbs within 2–3 weeks.

Hyphema, bleeding into the anterior chamber of the eye, is a potential result of blunt eye trauma. When the highly vascular uveal tract of the eye is disrupted by blunt force, hemorrhage may result, filling the anterior chamber. The client complains of feeling eye pain, experiencing decreased visual acuity, and seeing a reddish tint. Blood is visible in the anterior chamber.

An orbital blowout fracture is another potential result of blunt eye trauma. Although any part of the eye orbit may be fractured, the ethmoid bone on the orbital floor is the most likely site. Orbital contents, including fat, muscles, and the eye itself, may herniate through the fracture into the underlying maxillary sinus. The client complains of diplopia (double vision), pain with upward movement of the affected eye, and decreased sensation on the affected cheek. The eye appears sunken (**enophthalmos**) and has limited movement on examination.

Detached Retina

Separation of the retina, or sensory portion of the eye, from the choroid, the pigmented vascular layer, is known as a **retinal detachment**. Although retinal detachment may be precipitated by trauma, it usually occurs spontaneously. The vitreous humor normally adheres to the retina at the optic disc, the macula, and the periphery of the eye. With aging, the vitreous humor shrinks and may pull the retina away from the choroid. Therefore, aging is a common risk factor, as are myopia, glaucoma, trauma, previous retinal detachment, and **aphakia**, absence of the lens (e.g., following lens removal for cataracts) (University of Michigan Kellogg Eye Center, 2012).

Focus on Diversity and Culture
Eye Injuries in Migrant Workers

Eye injuries among migrant farm workers are underreported. These individuals are exposed to a variety of risks: chemicals, machinery, tools, and airborne soil and particulates. Most migrant workers do not have jobs that provide workers' compensation coverage. They are also faced with tremendous pressure to support their families in either the United States or their country of origin. Because a limited number of clinics serve this population, many injuries go both unreported and untreated (Quandt et al., 2012).

Clinical Manifestations and Therapies Eye Injuries

ETIOLOGY	CLINICAL MANIFESTATIONS	CLINICAL THERAPIES
Corneal abrasion	■ Intense pain and redness ■ Photophobia ■ Tearing	■ Superficial corneal abrasions are diagnosed by touching a sterile fluorescein strip to lower conjunctiva; dye remains where corneal epithelial cells are disrupted. ■ Most corneal abrasions heal spontaneously. Antibiotic ointment may be prescribed and eyes patched in some clients.
Burns (Alkaline burns readily penetrate the cornea and are more serious than acid burns.)	■ Pain and/or complaints of "blindness" or vision loss ■ Swollen eyelids ■ Red, edematous conjunctiva ■ Cloudy or hazy conjunctiva ■ Possible presence of ulcerations	■ For chemical burns, eyes are irrigated, preferably with normal saline. ■ Pupils are dilated to reduce pain and prevent adhesions; after irrigation is complete, eyes are patched and antibiotics are prescribed. ■ Topical anesthetic is applied.
Penetrating and perforating injuries	■ Pain ■ Partial or complete vision loss ■ Possible bleeding or extrusion of eye contents	■ *Note:* If foreign object is embedded in or sticking out of eye, do not remove. Immobilize object and protect eye until ophthalmologist arrives. Manage pain. ■ Irrigate. ■ Remove object using a sterile cotton-tipped applicator or a sterile needle or other equipment. ■ Apply antibiotic ointment after removal. ■ Apply eye patch. ■ Surgery
Blunt trauma	■ Pain and redness ■ Ecchymosis ■ Subconjunctival hemorrhage ■ Hyphema ■ Possible diplopia, enophthalmos ■ Personnel should be aware that retinal hemorrhage is a common presentation of the type of child abuse called shaken-baby syndrome.	■ Client is placed in semi-Fowler's position. ■ Eye is protected with eye shield; also, unaffected eye is patched to minimize eye movement. ■ A carbonic anhydrase inhibitor may be prescribed.
Subconjunctival hemorrhage (caused by coughing, mild trauma, or increased physical activity)	■ Reddened area in conjunctiva	■ Usually heals spontaneously; client should see ophthalmologist if most of sclera is covered or if condition does not clear up in 1–2 weeks.
Periorbital ecchymosis	■ Black eye or bruising of the skin around the eye	■ Ice is applied to eye area (both eyes) for 5–15 minutes every hour for the first 1–2 days after injury (even if only one eye is affected, both eyes may discolor); then warm compresses are applied beginning the second day after injury.
Foreign body on conjunctiva	■ Intense pain or feeling of something in the eye	■ Client must not rub eye; material on surface of eye is removed by closing upper lid over lower lid, irrigating or everting upper lid, visualizing material, and removing it with a slightly damp handkerchief. Eye is patched and client transported to emergency department if foreign body cannot be removed.

(continued on next page)

Clinical Manifestations and Therapies Eye Injuries (continued)

ETIOLOGY	CLINICAL MANIFESTATIONS	CLINICAL THERAPIES
Detached retina	■ Floaters: irregular dark lines or spots in the field of vision ■ Flashes of light ■ Blurred vision ■ Progressive deterioration of vision ■ Sensation of a curtain or veil being drawn across the field of vision ■ If macula is involved, loss of central vision	■ Prompt treatment to preserve vision ■ Proper positioning ■ Cryotherapy ■ Laser photocoagulation ■ Scleral buckling ■ Laser therapy

The retina may actually tear and fold back on itself, or the retina may remain intact but no longer adhere to the choroid. A break or tear in the retina allows fluid from the vitreous cavity to enter the defect. This, along with fluid that escapes from choroid vessels, the pull of gravity, and traction exerted by the vitreous humor, separates the retina from the choroid. The detached area may rapidly increase in size, increasing loss of vision. Unless contact between the retina and choroid is reestablished, the neurons of the retina become ischemic and die, causing permanent vision loss. For that reason, retinal detachment is a true medical emergency, requiring prompt ophthalmological referral and treatment.

When the retina detaches, the client experiences floaters, or spots, and lines or flashes of light in the visual field. Often the client describes the sensation of having a curtain drawn across the vision, much like a curtain being drawn over a window. The area of the visual field affected is directly related to the area of detachment. For example, because light rays cross as they pass through the lens, a retinal tear in the superior portion of the eye results in a deficit in the lower part of the visual field. The client feels no pain, and the eye appears normal to visual inspection.

▶ COLLABORATION

Diagnostic tests and nursing and medical interventions vary widely based on the extent of an eye injury. The nurse can reinforce the importance of protective eyewear, especially in the occurrence of minor injuries.

Diagnostic Tests

Diagnostic testing for eye injuries should begin with tests of visual acuity. Extraocular movements should be evaluated. The pupil should be tested for reactivity and size with a flashlight or ophthalmoscope. The ophthalmoscope should also be used to exam the fundus to check for presence of the red reflex (Family Practice Notebook, 2013). A slit-lamp is a high-intensity light source combined with a low-power microscope. It can be focused to shine a blue light in a thin beam. It is often used in conjunction with fluorescein stain. Fluorescein is orange/yellow in color. When applied to the eye, it fills in any defect on the cornea. The defect will fluoresce under the cobalt blue light of the slit-lamp. For eye injuries it can be useful in identifying corneal injuries and retinal detachment (National Library of Medicine, 2011c). Facial

x-rays and CT scans are used to identify orbital fractures or foreign bodies in the globe. Ultrasonography may be employed to detect a detached retina or vitreous hemorrhage.

Surgery

Usually, surgery is not necessary in the treatment of corneal abrasion, subconjunctival hemorrhage, or periorbital ecchymosis. For eye injuries due to severe chemical burns, surgery may include debridement, tissue grafting, or even corneal transplant (Allina Health System, 2012). Penetrating wounds of the eye generally require surgical intervention by an ophthalmic surgeon. Surgical management of blunt trauma depends on the extent and type of injury, which may include corneal abrasions, globe rupture, retinal detachment, and lens dislocation (Sponsel et al., 2011). Conjunctival foreign bodies do not usually lead to injuries that require surgical treatment. However, nonsurgical removal of the foreign body, which is often performed in the emergency department, may be required.

Retinal detachment is a medical emergency; early diagnosis and treatment are essential in order to preserve vision. The manifestations and examination of the ocular fundus by ophthalmoscopy establish the diagnosis of retinal detachment. If the condition is left untreated, the detached portion will become necrotic because of separation from the vascular supply of the choroid. Permanent blindness in that portion of the eye results. Interventions are directed toward bringing the retina and choroid back into contact and reestablishing the blood and nutrient supply to the retina. Either cryotherapy, using a supercooled probe, or laser photocoagulation may be used to create an area of inflammation and adhesion to "weld" the layers together. **Scleral buckling**, during which an indentation or fold is surgically created in the sclera, may be performed to restore contact between the choroid and retina. Contact is maintained with a local implant on the sclera or an encircling strap or "buckle." In a procedure called **pneumatic retinopexy**, air is injected into the vitreous cavity. The client is positioned so that the air bubble pushes the detached portion of the retina into contact with the choroid.

Pharmacologic Therapy

For treatment of corneal abrasion and following removal of a conjunctival foreign body, antibiotic ointment, such as erythromycin or sulfacetamide sodium, may be applied. Pharmacologic

Client Teaching Administering Eyedrops and Eye Ointments

To ensure safe, effective delivery of eye medication, client teaching should include the following:

- Wash hands with soap and water. Rinse and dry hands.
- Read directions if drops need to be gently shaken.
- Check applicator/dropper tip for cracks or chips.
- Avoid touching the applicator tip to your eye or hands. It must be kept clean.
- Tilt your head back slightly, and pull down the lower eyelid with your index finger to form a pocket.
- Hold the applicator with the other hand, tip facing down, as close to the eye as possible without touching it.
- Use the other fingers on that hand as a brace against your face to stabilize your hand.
- Look up and gently squeeze medication into the lower eyelid pocket. Instill the prescribed amount of medication.
- Tip your head slightly down and close your eyes for 2–3 minutes. Try not to squint or blink.
- Apply gentle pressure to the lacrimal duct.
- Wipe any excess medication from your face with a tissue.
- Replace and tighten the applicator lid.
- To remove any medication, wash your hands

treatment of burns may include pain medications (oral or eyedrops), steroids (to decrease inflammation), and cycloplegic drops, such as atropine, tropicamide, or cyclopentolate, to cause pupillary dilation to decrease pain (Allina Health System, 2012).

Following irrigation, a topical antibiotic ointment, such as gentamicin ophthalmic, is applied.

For penetrating and perforating injuries, pain is managed using narcotic analgesics (e.g., morphine). The client also may require sedation (e.g., diazepam) and antiemetic medications to prevent vomiting. Antibiotics such as intravenous cefazolin (Ancef) and gentamicin (Garamycin) are prescribed to prevent infection. Blunt trauma to the eye may require reduction of intraocular pressure with a carbonic anhydrase inhibitor, such as acetazolamide (Diamox) or dichlorphenamide (Daranide). Following surgical repair of retinal detachment, steroid medications may be used to reduce inflammation (Koerner, Koerner-Stiefbold, & Garwig, 2012). Treatment of subconjunctival hemorrhage and periorbital ecchymosis does not usually include medication.

Additional Therapies

CORNEAL ABRASION Foreign bodies are removed using irrigation, a sterile cotton-tipped applicator, or a sterile needle or other instrument. In clients with corneal abrasions and large foreign bodies in the eye, an eye patch is applied firmly after application of the antibiotic to keep the eye closed for approximately 24 hours.

BURNS Remove any clothing that may still contain the chemical. If further risk of injury can be avoided, bring the container with the chemical information to the healthcare setting (Allina Health System, 2012). The immediate priority of care for clients with chemical burns is flushing the affected eye with copious amounts of fluid. Normal saline is preferred; however, water may be used if saline is not available. Rinse eye immediately for at least 30 minutes. A special contact lens irrigating

Medications Eye Injuries

CLASSIFICATION AND DRUG EXAMPLES	MECHANISMS OF ACTION	NURSING CONSIDERATIONS
Antibiotic Drops or Ointments *Drug examples:* - gentamicin - neomycin - tobramycin - erythromycin	Used to treat or prevent bacterial infection. Choice of antibiotic depends on bacteria suspected.	- Instruct client on the proper use of eyedrops or ointments.
Cycloplegics *Drug examples:* - atropine - tropicamide - cyclopentolate	Block responses of the sphincter muscles of the iris and muscles of ciliary body to cholinergic stimulation. Causes pupillary dilation.	- Instruct client on the proper use of eyedrops. - Should not be used in clients with narrow-angle glaucoma.
Carbonic Anhydrase Inhibitors *Drug examples:* - acetazolamide (Diamox): oral medication - methazolamide (Neptazane): oral medication - brinzolamide (Azopt) - dorzolamide (Trusopt)	Decrease the production of aqueous humor into the eye. Related to sulfa drugs.	- Oral medications may cause periorbital numbness and tingling in the fingers and toes. - May cause loss of potassium; assess daily weight, electrolytes. - Allergy to sulfa is a contraindication. - Use with caution in clients with renal or hepatic disease.

unit (Morgan lens) or a bottle of irrigant with intravenous tubing held to flush all eye surfaces may be useful. The eyelid is everted to identify and remove material from the conjunctival sac. A topical anesthetic, such as tetracaine drops, helps relieve pain, making inspection and irrigation easier. During irrigation, fluid is directed from the inner to the outer canthus of the eye. Move eyeball in all directions to properly irrigate. Slightly tipping the client's head to the affected side prevents contamination of the unaffected eye. Irrigation is continued until the pH of the eye is normal (in the range of 7.2–7.4). Following irrigation, a topical antibiotic ointment, such as gentamicin ophthalmic, is applied.

PENETRATING AND PERFORATING INJURIES Immediate care focuses on relieving pain and protecting the eye from further injury. To prevent loss of intraocular contents, do not place pressure on the eye itself, but gently cover it with sterile gauze or an eye pad. If a foreign body is embedded in or sticking out of the eye, no attempt should be made to remove it. The object should be immobilized and the eye protected with a metal eye shield until an ophthalmologist can see the client. A paper cup or another protective device may be used if the object is too large for an eye shield. Patching the unaffected eye will help decrease ocular movement.

BLUNT TRAUMA Interventions for the client with blunt trauma to the eye include placing the client on bed rest in semi-Fowler's position and protecting the eye from further injury with an eye shield. The unaffected eye should be patched to minimize eye movement. With subconjunctival hemorrhage, healing usually occurs without intervention. Instruct the client to seek follow-up if healing has not occurred within 1–2 weeks.

FOREIGN BODY ON CONJUNCTIVA Foreign bodies are removed using irrigation, a sterile cotton-tipped applicator, or a sterile needle or other instrument.

DETACHED RETINA If an ophthalmologist is not readily available, position client's head so that gravity pulls the detached portion of the retina into closer contact with the choroid. The client should lay flat in bed with the head midline. This position may not be tolerated by clients with certain cardiorespiratory diseases.

▮ NURSING PROCESS

The nursing role involves educating people about the prevention of eye injuries and providing direct care to clients with eye injuries.

Assessment

Ocular injuries require immediate interventions simultaneously with assessment and collection of an accurate history. Determine the time, type, and extent of injury and the circumstances under which it occurred. In addition, ask about preexisting visual problems.

If the client normally wears corrective lenses, perform a vision assessment while the client is wearing lenses. Evaluate eye movement unless a penetrating object is present, and inspect the lid and eye for lacerations. Perform inspection using strong light and magnification with a headband loupe

or slit-lamp. Topical anesthesia may be used prior to inspection if eye pain and photophobia make opening the eye difficult. Fluorescein staining can help identify foreign bodies and abrasions. Note any conjunctival or anterior chamber hemorrhage as well as the presence or absence of the red reflex.

For the client with a detached retina, the nursing focus is on early identification and treatment. Because early intervention is vital to preserve the client's sight, nurses must recognize early manifestations of retinal detachment and intervene appropriately to obtain definitive treatment for the client. Retinal detachment can be successfully treated on an outpatient basis, often in an ophthalmologist's office.

Diagnosis

Nursing diagnoses for the client with an eye injury may include the following:

- *Impaired Tissue Integrity: Ocular*
- *Acute Pain*
- *Anxiety*
- *Ineffective Tissue Perfusion: Retinal.*

(NANDA-I © 2012)

Planning

Planning with the client is based on the nature and extent of the injury. Typical outcomes may include the following:

- The client will be free of pain associated with the injury.
- The client will articulate and follow instructions regarding eye protection and the healing process.
- The client will describe when to call the primary care provider in the event of worsening symptoms or condition.
- The client will experience healing and restoration of vision to the maximum extent possible.

Implementation

All types of eye trauma pose the risk of violating the integrity of the eye, threatening vision. Therefore, the goals of nursing care are preserving vision and the integrity of the eye and preventing further damage.

Reduce Risk for Impaired Vision

- Assess vision in each eye and both eyes, with and without corrective lenses, upon client's entry to the emergency department or primary care setting. An initial assessment provides valuable information about the effect of the injury on the client's vision and a baseline for future comparisons.
- Inspect eye(s) carefully for evidence of foreign bodies, burns, penetrating injury, or blunt trauma. Note whether lacerations, burns, or other trauma are evident in tissues surrounding the eye. Eye trauma may be hidden by other injuries and thus remain untreated.
- If a burn or foreign body is present, consider administering anesthetic drops and irrigating the eye before or after the physician evaluates the client. **Blepharism** (spasms that cause the eye to blink continuously) and eye pain may prevent assessment of the injured eye. Irrigation to

Client Teaching Eye Injuries: Prevention and First Aid

Teaching individuals and groups how to prevent eye injuries is an important nursing role, especially for clients involved in hazardous occupations and activities. Children in particular are at risk for eye injuries.

Although sports injuries readily come to mind, many eye injuries in children happen at home. All chemicals should be in a childproof area. Toys that can cause eye injury such as bows and arrows, darts, and BB guns should be used under careful adult supervision or avoided. Common items around the house such as scissors, paper clips, pencils, and rubber bands can also cause serious eye injury.

Whenever the extent of injury is not clear, recommend that the child be evaluated in an emergency care facility. Protective eyewear should be used by participants in all sports with a risk of eye injury. Stress the importance of using seat belts and air bags to prevent eye injury in automobile crashes. Small children should not be left alone with dogs. When a dog bites a child age 4 or younger, eye injuries occur in about 15% of cases. Most often it is a dog that the child is familiar with.

Instruct clients and their families about steps to take for a variety of eye injuries. If a chemical splash occurs, they should immediately flush the eye with copious amounts of water. They can remove loose, visible foreign bodies using a clean, moistened cotton-tipped swab. If an abrasion, penetrating, or blunt injury is suspected, they should cover the eye loosely with sterile gauze and seek immediate medical attention. Instruct clients and their families not to remove objects that penetrate the eye (AAO, 2013b).

---

remove the chemical is of higher priority than assessment of the eye.

■ Remove any loose foreign bodies using a moist, sterile cotton-tipped applicator. Prompt removal of foreign bodies may prevent corneal abrasion.

■ For a severe or penetrating injury, promote rest and stabilize the injured eye by applying an eye pad or gauze dressing loosely over both the affected and unaffected eye. Stabilize any penetrating object if possible. These measures reduce eye movement and can help preserve the client's vision.

■ Following treatment, apply eyedrops or ointment as prescribed and apply an eye pad or shield if ordered. Apply an eye pad to the affected eye to reduce pain and photophobia and to promote healing.

■ Following an injury, discuss the following topics with the client and family:
   a. Prescribed medications and possible adverse effects
   b. Strategies to prevent further trauma
   c. Application of the eye pad or shield
   d. Avoidance of activities that increase intraocular pressure
   e. Importance of activity restrictions.

Interventions for Retinal Detachment

Restoring contact between the retina and choroid is a priority of nursing and medical care for the client with retinal detachment. Vitreous humor may leak through a retinal tear, and fluid exudate may collect behind the tear, causing further detachment. If the macula is detached, central vision is lost, and the likelihood of restoring full vision decreases.

■ Notify physician and ophthalmologist immediately. To preserve vision, immediate medical intervention is required in clients with retinal detachment.

■ Position the client so the area of detachment is inferior. For instance, for a superior temporal retinal detachment of the right eye (with corresponding vision loss in the inferior medial visual field of that eye), place the client supine with head turned to the right. Correct positioning allows the contents of the posterior portion of the eye to place pressure on the detached area, bringing the retina in closer contact with the choroid.

■ Maintain a calm, confident attitude while carrying out priority interventions. Administering care in a calm, although urgent, manner helps reassure the client that the problem is treatable and that appropriate measures are being taken.

■ Reassure the client that most retinal detachments are successfully treated, usually on an outpatient basis. Reassurance can help allay the client's fear of permanent vision loss.

■ Explain all procedures fully, including the reason for positioning. Explanations facilitate understanding and help relieve anxiety in unfamiliar settings.

■ Allow supportive family members or friends to remain with the client as much as possible. Additional support helps lower the client's anxiety level.

Teaching for the client undergoing surgical repair of retinal detachment is similar to that for clients experiencing other types of eye surgery. If the retina remains detached, provide instructions about the change in peripheral vision or other visual fields and changes in depth perception.

✳ Go to **nursing.pearsonhighered.com** to see a chart on nursing care of the client having eye surgery.

Discuss the following topics with the client and family to prepare for home care:

■ Limitations on positioning the head before or following repair
■ Activity restrictions such as no bending or straining at stool
■ Use of eye shield
■ Early manifestations and importance of seeking immediate treatment
■ Follow-up treatment with the ophthalmologist.

Evaluation

Criteria that reflect the client's achievement of identified outcomes and successful resolution of nursing diagnoses may include the following:

■ The client maintains optimal vision following injury.
■ The client experiences no loss of vision as the result of preventable complications.
■ The client reports pain management to acceptable levels.

REVIEW Eye Injuries

RELATE Link the Concepts and Exemplars

Mr. Callahan was admitted to the medical surgical unit with a retinal detachment and is scheduled for a scleral buckling procedure in the morning.

Linking the exemplar of eye injuries with the concept of safety:

1. What is Mr. Callahan's priority nursing diagnosis?

2. What post-op teaching does the nurse include for Mr. Callahan and his wife prior to discharge to reduce his risk of injury?

Linking the exemplar of eye injuries with the concept of cognition:

3. When caring for an older adult client with an eye injury, how might his or her cognition be impacted?

4. What nursing interventions might the nurse initiate to reduce the impact of reduced vision on an adult client's cognition?

READY Go to Companion Skills Manual

REFER Go to Pearson Nursing Student Resources
nursing.pearsonhighered.com

- Additional review materials
- **Chart:** Nursing Care of the Client Having Eye Surgery

REFLECT Case Study

Seth Moore, age 17, presents to the emergency department with his parents after he was hit in the eye with a paintball. Seth was running through an outdoor course with his friends when his right eye was struck. At the time of his injury, Seth was not wearing the eye protection provided to him at the course.

Seth reports eye pain and decreased visual acuity. Examination reveals visible blood in the right eye.

1. What are the potential nursing diagnoses?

2. What are the immediate nursing interventions?

3. What teaching might help Seth avoid injury in the future?

EXEMPLAR 18.4 Glaucoma

EXEMPLAR KEY TERMS

Angle-closure glaucoma, *1319*
Glaucoma, *1318*
Intraocular pressure, *1318*
Mydriasis, *1319*
Open-angle glaucoma, *1319*
Photophobia, *1319*

EXEMPLAR LEARNING OUTCOMES

After reading about this exemplar, you will be able to:

1. Describe the pathophysiology, etiology, clinical manifestations, and direct and indirect causes of glaucoma.

2. Identify risk factors associated with glaucoma.

3. Illustrate the nursing process in providing culturally competent care across the life span for individuals with glaucoma.

4. Formulate priority nursing diagnoses appropriate for an individual with glaucoma.

5. Summarize therapies used by interdisciplinary teams in the collaborative care of an individual with glaucoma.

6. Plan evidence-based care for an individual with glaucoma and his or her family in collaboration with other members of the healthcare team.

7. Evaluate expected outcomes for an individual with glaucoma.

▶ OVERVIEW

Glaucoma is a condition characterized by optic neuropathy with gradual loss of peripheral vision and (usually) increased intraocular pressure of the eye (force within the eye causing tissue damage). Glaucoma is a silent thief of vision. The client typically experiences no manifestations other than narrowing of the visual field, which occurs so gradually that it often goes unnoticed until late in the disease process. In the United States, glaucoma affects about 3 million people over the age of 40; it remains undetected in approximately 50% of these cases.

▶ PATHOPHYSIOLOGY AND ETIOLOGY

Aqueous humor, a thick fluid, occupies the anterior and posterior chambers of the eye. The normal **intraocular pressure** of approximately 12–22 mmHg is maintained by a balance between the production of aqueous humor in the ciliary body, its flow through the pupil from the posterior to the anterior chamber of the eye, and its outflow or absorption through the trabecular meshwork and canal of Schlemm. When this balance is disrupted, usually because of a decrease in the outflow or

absorption of aqueous humor, intraocular pressure increases. Although the exact relationship is unclear, it appears that increased intraocular pressure injures the optic nerve. Axons in the periphery of the optic disc are damaged first. As optic fibers are destroyed, the rim of the optic disc shrinks and the normal depression in its center (the optic cup) becomes larger and deeper (called optic "cupping"). These changes to the optic disc are visible before changes in the visual field can be detected (AAO, 2013g; Glaucoma Foundation, 2013b). As the disease progresses, the individual experiences a painless, progressive narrowing of the visual field and eventual blindness. Vision loss is often significant before the client seeks treatment and glaucoma is diagnosed.

Primary glaucoma in adults has two major forms: open-angle glaucoma and angle-closure glaucoma. Both terms refer to the angle formed at the point where the iris meets the cornea in the eye's anterior chamber (**Figure 18–13 ●**).

Pediatric glaucoma can fall into one of two categories: primary or secondary. Primary congenital glaucoma occurs in about 1 in every 10,000 births in the United States. It is caused by an abnormal development in the ocular drainage system. Approximately 10% of cases are diagnosed at birth, with the majority (80%) diagnosed by age 1. Secondary congenital glaucoma may

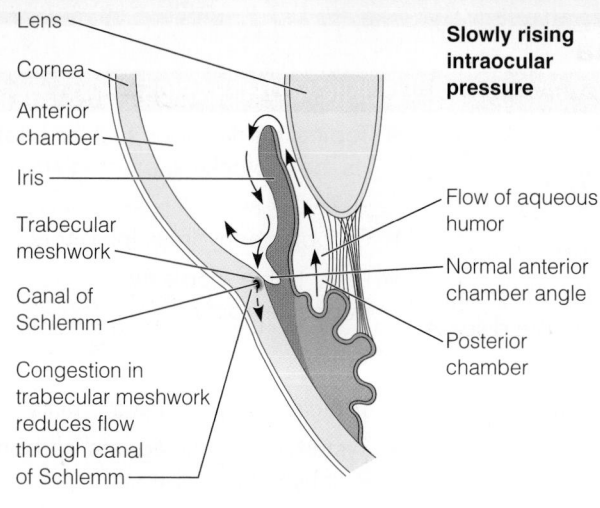

Slowly rising intraocular pressure

Lens
Cornea
Anterior chamber
Iris
Trabecular meshwork
Canal of Schlemm
Congestion in trabecular meshwork reduces flow through canal of Schlemm

Flow of aqueous humor
Normal anterior chamber angle
Posterior chamber

A

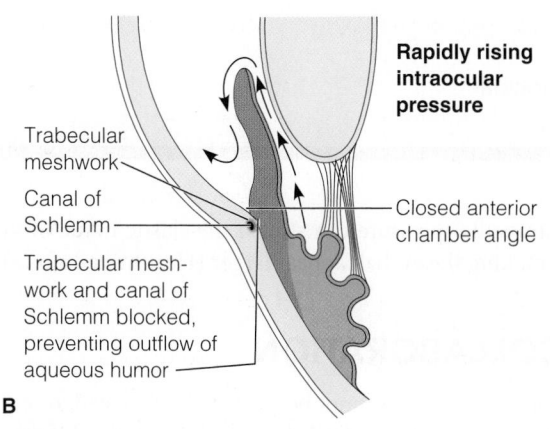

Rapidly rising intraocular pressure

Trabecular meshwork
Canal of Schlemm
Trabecular meshwork and canal of Schlemm blocked, preventing outflow of aqueous humor

Closed anterior chamber angle

B

Figure 18–13 ● Forms of primary adult glaucoma. *A,* In chronic open-angle glaucoma, the anterior chamber angle remains open, but drainage of aqueous humor through the canal of Schlemm is impaired. *B,* In acute angle-closure glaucoma, the angle of the iris and anterior chamber narrows, obstructing the outflow of aqueous humor.
Source: Courtesy of National Eye Institute, National Institutes of Health.

or may not have genetic origins. It results from disorders of the eye or the body (Glaucoma Foundation, 2013a). Secondary glaucoma can occur in adults as well. It can develop in individuals who have been on long-term steroid therapy or as the result of an eye injury (AAO, 2013g).

Open-Angle Glaucoma

Glaucoma is usually a primary condition without an identified cause. **Open-angle glaucoma**, often called chronic simple glaucoma, is the most common form in adults, accounting for approximately 90% of all glaucomas. Its cause is unknown; it is thought to have a hereditary component, but no clear inheritance pattern can be identified. Open-angle glaucoma occurs more frequently in Latinos and African Americans; cardiovascular disease or diabetes may contribute to its formation (Glaucoma Research Foundation, 2012b).

Open-angle glaucoma tends to be a chronic, gradually progressive disease. It typically affects both eyes, although the pressures and progression may not be symmetric. In open-

angle glaucoma, the anterior chamber angle between the iris and cornea is normal (thus the term *open angle*). However, the flow of aqueous humor through the trabecular meshwork and into the canal of Schlemm is relatively obstructed; the cause of this obstruction is unknown. The trabecular meshwork increasingly inhibits the outflow of aqueous humor, and the intraocular pressure gradually increases. The result is neuronal ischemia and optic nerve degeneration, leading to gradual loss of vision.

Angle-Closure Glaucoma

Acute **angle-closure glaucoma** (also called narrow-angle or closed-angle glaucoma) is the other, less common form of primary glaucoma in adults. It occurs between 1 and 40 times for every 1,000 Americans with a higher incidence among certain ethnic groups (Freedman et al., 2012).

Narrowing of the anterior chamber angle (see Figure 18–13A for an illustration of the normal anterior chamber angle) occurs because of corneal flattening or bulging of the iris into the anterior chamber. When the lens thickens during accommodation or the iris thickens during pupil dilation, this angle can close completely. Closure of the angle blocks the outflow of aqueous humor through the trabecular meshwork and canal of Schlemm, and the intraocular pressure rises abruptly (Figure 18–13B). This increase in intraocular pressure damages the neurons of the retina and the optic nerve, leading to a rapid and permanent loss of vision if not treated promptly.

Episodes of angle-closure glaucoma are typically unilateral. However, a history of angle-closure glaucoma of one eye increases the risk that it will occur in the other eye.

Because of the effect of pupil dilation on aqueous outflow in angle-closure glaucoma, episodes often occur in association with darkness, emotional upset, or other factors that cause the pupil to dilate. Clients may have intermittent episodes lasting several hours before they have a more typical prolonged attack of angle-closure glaucoma. Clients with a history of the condition must avoid medications, such as atropine and other anticholinergics, that can cause **mydriasis**, or dilation of the pupil.

Risk Factors

Glaucoma is a leading cause of blindness worldwide. Age and race are the primary identified risk factors. Glaucoma is 6 to 8

Clinical Manifestations and Therapies **Glaucoma**

GLAUCOMA TYPE	CLINICAL MANIFESTATIONS	CLINICAL THERAPIES
Open-angle glaucoma	■ No initial manifestations ■ Frequent lens changes in glasses ■ Impaired dark adaptation ■ Halos around lights ■ Gradual reduction of visual fields with preservation of central vision until late in the disease ■ Mild to severe increased intraocular pressure	■ Topical medications such as miotics, beta-blockers, prostaglandin analogs ■ Carbonic anhydrase inhibitors ■ Laser trabeculoplasty, trabeculectomy
Angle-closure glaucoma	■ Abrupt onset of eye pain, headache ■ Decreased visual acuity ■ Nausea and vomiting ■ Reddened conjunctiva ■ Cloudy cornea ■ Fixed pupil ■ Rapid, significant increase in intraocular pressure	■ Topical miotics or beta-blockers ■ Systemic osmotic agents, carbonic anhydrase inhibitors ■ Laser iridotomy or peripheral iridectomy

times more likely to occur in African Americans than in Caucasians, and it is about 15 times more likely to cause blindness in African American than in Caucasians (Glaucoma Research Foundation, 2011; Office on Women's Health, 2010). The prevalence of glaucoma rises rapidly in Mexican Americans over age 60 (NEI, 2009b). People of Asian descent are at higher risk (see the Focus on Diversity and Culture feature). Clients with an immediate family member with glaucoma have a 9 times higher chance of developing the disease. Long-term steroid use may be a contributing factor. Prior eye injuries, especially blunt trauma or penetrating injuries, may cause secondary glaucoma years later (Glaucoma Research Foundation, 2011).

▶ CLINICAL MANIFESTATIONS

In many cases of open-angle glaucoma, there are no symptoms. Vision will even remain normal for a while. Then, as the nerve becomes more damaged, blank spots will start to appear in the visual field. Almost 50% of clients with glaucoma will not have high intraocular pressure on examination, so a single pressure reading may miss the diagnosis. An optic nerve examination is an essential part of a comprehensive eye examination (AAO, 2013g).

Symptoms such as experiencing severe eye and face pain, general malaise, nausea and vomiting, seeing colored halos around lights, and experiencing an abrupt decrease in visual acuity are associated with acute episodes of angle-closure glaucoma. The conjunctiva of the affected eye may be reddened and the cornea clouded with corneal edema. The pupil may be fixed (nonreactive to light) at midpoint.

Congenital glaucoma can be more difficult to diagnose. Parents and healthcare professionals should be alert for photophobia, excessive tearing, and larger than normal eyes. The increase

in intraocular pressure can stretch the elastic tissue of the cornea, making the eyeball appear larger (Healthline Info, 2012).

▶ COLLABORATION

Although glaucoma cannot be predicted, prevented, or cured, in most cases it can be controlled and vision preserved if diagnosed early. Because the most prevalent type of glaucoma, open-angle glaucoma, has few symptoms, routine eye examinations are recommended for early detection. Measurement of intraocular pressure, funduscopy to assess the optic disc, and visual field testing are used to diagnose glaucoma and monitor the effectiveness of treatment.

Diagnostic Tests

The following diagnostic studies are used to detect and evaluate the presence, severity, type, and effects of glaucoma:

■ *Tonometry* indirectly measures intraocular pressure. Contact or noncontact tonometry may be used. Routine tonometry screening is recommended for everyone over the age of 60. A single elevated pressure reading does not warrant a diagnosis of glaucoma; variations in intraocular pressure occur throughout the day.

■ *Funduscopy* (visual inspection of the optic fundus using an ophthalmoscope) identifies pallor and an increase in the size and depth of the optic cup on the optic disc. These changes are significant for a diagnosis of glaucoma.

■ *Gonioscopy* uses a gonioscope to measure the depth of the anterior chamber. This test differentiates open-angle from angle-closure glaucoma.

■ *Visual field testing* identifies the degree of central visual field narrowing and peripheral vision loss. The client with glaucoma may retain 20/20 central vision even when there is severe peripheral vision loss.

Surgery

Surgical management of chronic open-angle glaucoma involves improving the drainage of aqueous humor from the anterior chamber of the eye or decreasing aqueous humor production. Surgical options include goniotomy, trabeculectomy, combined trabeculotomy with trabeculectomy, and trabeculotomy ab externo. Trabeculoplasty and trabeculectomy filtration surgery are the most commonly used procedures.

In a laser trabeculoplasty, an argon laser is aimed through a gonioscope to create multiple laser burns spaced evenly around the trabecular meshwork. As the burns heal, the scars they create cause tension, stretching and opening the meshwork. This noninvasive technique requires no incision and can be performed as an outpatient procedure, making it the treatment of choice.

Trabeculectomy is a type of filtration surgery in which a permanent fistula is created to drain aqueous humor from the anterior chamber of the eye. A portion of trabecular meshwork is removed, and a flap of sclera is left unsutured to create a channel, or fistula, between the anterior chamber and the subconjunctival space. Aqueous humor drains into the space under the conjunctiva, where it can be absorbed into the systemic circulation. A trabeculectomy is usually performed under general anesthesia and requires hospitalization.

If these procedures are not effective, photocoagulation using an argon laser (heat) or cyclocryotherapy using a probe to freeze tissue may be employed to destroy portions of the ciliary body. This destruction of tissue reduces the production of aqueous humor, subsequently reducing intraocular pressure. Another surgical procedure involves inserting a glaucoma drainage device that regulates the outflow of aqueous humor.

Surgical procedures used in the treatment of acute angle-closure glaucoma include gonioplasty, laser iridotomy, and peripheral iridectomy. Because of the high risk for a future attack of angle-closure glaucoma in the unaffected eye, these procedures are often performed prophylactically.

In gonioplasty (also known as iridoplasty), the healing and scarring of microscopic lesions created at the periphery of the iris draw the iris away from the cornea, widening the anterior chamber. This widening of the chamber increases the angle and opens drainage channels for aqueous humor.

Laser iridotomy is a noninvasive procedure in which a laser is used to create multiple small perforations in the iris of the eye. These perforations allow aqueous humor to drain from the posterior chamber to the anterior chamber and out through the trabecular meshwork and the canal of Schlemm. During an iridectomy, a small segment of the iris is removed to facilitate the flow of aqueous humor between the posterior and anterior chambers and to open the anterior chamber angle.

Pharmacologic Therapy

Topical medications are effective for many clients. Which therapy is prescribed depends on a number of factors, including client health history. For example, beta-blockers are contraindicated for clients with heart failure, asthma, or COPD. To help doctors, pharmacists, and clients identify their glaucoma eye-

TABLE 18–6 FDA-Approved Color Coding for Glaucoma Eyedrop Bottle Tops

MEDICATION	BOTTLE TOP COLOR
Beta-blockers	Yellow or light blue
Prostaglandin analogs	Light green or teal
Alpha-adrenergic agents	Purple
Carbonic anhydrase inhibitors	Orange
Miotics	Dark green
Combination drops	Dark blue

Source: American Academy of Ophthalmology (AAO). (2010a). *Policy statement: Color codes for topical ocular medications.* Retrieved from http://www.aao.org/about/policy/upload/color-codes-for-topical-ocular-medications-2010.pdf; American Glaucoma Society. (2011). *Position statement of color coded caps for glaucoma drops.* Retrieved from http://www.americanglaucomasociety.net/patients/position_statements/color_coded_caps_for_glaucoma_drops; Food and Drug Administration. (1999). *Guidance for industry: Container closure systems for packaging human drugs and biologics,* p. 27. Retrieved from http://www.fda.gov/downloads/Drugs/Guidances/ucm070551.pdf.

drops easier, the U.S. Food and Drug Administration has mandated that the tops of the eyedrops be color coded. Some generics and all brand name drops adhere to the guidelines shown in **Table 18–6**.

Topical beta-adrenergic blocking agents reduce intraocular pressure by decreasing the production of aqueous humor in the ciliary body. Beta-adrenergic blockers may be prescribed for use once or twice a day depending on the specific drug and dosage form. Selected beta-adrenergic blockers reduce intraocular pressure by decreasing the production of aqueous humor. Because beta-blockers do not affect pupil size and lens accommodation, they do not have the adverse effects on visual acuity that adrenergic agonists do. Their systemic effects, however, may limit their usefulness for certain clients.

When administering beta-blockers or teaching about their use, remember that they can produce systemic effects, including bronchospasm, bradycardia, and heart failure.

The prostaglandin analog drugs relax the ciliary muscle, improving the outflow of aqueous humor and reducing intraocular pressure. These drugs have the advantage of requiring only a single daily dose. However, they do have some adverse effects, such as blurred vision and stinging, and when used long term, they cause permanent darkening of the iris of the eye and eyebrows, increased growth of eyelashes, and conjunctival hyperemia (redness).

Prostaglandin analogs such as latanoprost (Xalatan) are a newer class of ophthalmics used to increase aqueous outflow. They are similar to beta-blockers in that their longer duration of action means they require only a daily dose.

Adrenergic agonists dilate the pupil, reduce the production of aqueous humor, and increase its absorption, effectively reducing intraocular pressure in open-angle glaucoma.

The adrenergic agonist brimonidine may be prescribed along with a beta-blocker or in cases when beta-blockers are contraindicated. Another adrenergic agonist, apraclonidine, may be prescribed when other drugs do not sufficiently reduce intraocular pressure, but adverse effects make it inappropriate for long-term use. The side effects have led to a reported 15% discontinuation rate (Drugs.com, 2012).

Medications **Glaucoma**

CLASSIFICATION AND DRUG EXAMPLES	MECHANISMS OF ACTION	NURSING CONSIDERATIONS
Beta-Adrenergic Blockers *Drug examples:* ■ timolol (Timoptic) ■ levobunolol (Betagan) ■ carteolol (Ocupress) ■ metipranolol (OptiPranolol)	Decrease the production of aqueous humor in the eye, thus decreasing intraocular pressure.	■ Systemic absorption may occur; assess for hypotension, bradycardia, shortness of breath. ■ Assess client for contraindications to beta-blocker medications (asthma, COPD, heart block, or heart failure). ■ Teach client to close eye and occlude lacrimal duct after administration to help reduce systemic absorption.
Prostaglandin Analogs *Drug examples:* ■ latanoprost (Xalatan) ■ bimatoprost (Lumigan) ■ travoprost (Travatan)	Increase drainage of aqueous humor through the uveoscleral pathway. Reduce intraocular pressure by about 30%.	■ Client may experience change in iris color. ■ Blurred vision, eye pain, eye redness may be noted by the client.
Alpha$_2$-Adrenergic Agonists *Drug examples:* ■ brimonidine tartrate (Alphagan) ■ apraclonidine (Iopidine)	Decrease production of aqueous humor in the eye and increase drainage of aqueous humor through the uveoscleral pathway.	■ Assess client for contraindications such as acute angle-closure glaucoma, hypertension, CAD, and dysrhythmias. ■ Assess for CNS side effects such as anxiety, nervousness, and muscle tremors. ■ Allergic reactions are common with this class of drug; assess for eye and eyelid erythema.
Carbonic Anhydrase Inhibitors *Drug examples:* ■ acetazolamide (Diamox): oral medication ■ methazolamide (Neptazane): oral medication ■ brinzolamide (Azopt) ■ dorzolamide (Trusopt)	Decrease the production of aqueous humor into the eye. Related to sulfa drugs.	■ Oral medications may cause periorbital numbness and tingling in the fingers and toes. ■ May cause loss of potassium; assess daily weight, electrolytes. ■ Allergy to sulfa is a contraindication. ■ Use with caution in clients with renal or hepatic disease.
Combination Medications *Drug examples:* ■ Cosopt (beta-blocker plus carbonic anhydrase inhibitor) ■ Combigan (beta-blocker with alpha$_2$-adrenergic agonist)	Mechanism of action depends on medication combination.	■ Same nursing implications as for individual medications. ■ May be beneficial to clients to only have one eye medication instead of two and may be at a reduced cost.
Miotics (Parasympathomimetics) *Drug examples:* ■ pilocarpine (Isopto Carpine, Pilopine, Pilostat) ■ carbachol (Isopto Carbachol)	Increase drainage of aqueous humor through the trabecular meshwork via pupillary constriction.	■ Rarely used routinely due to side effects. ■ May be beneficial in narrow-angle glaucoma. ■ Myopic clients have increased risk of retinal detachment. ■ Assess for headaches, eye pain, and dim vision, especially in low light.

The carbonic anhydrate inhibitors lower intraocular pressure and are used primarily as adjunctive therapy. Dorzolamide and brinzolamide are administered as eyedrops, whereas acetazolamide may be given orally, intramuscularly, or intravenously.

Dorzolamide (Trusopt), a carbonic anhydrase inhibitor, decreases the production of aqueous humor and reduces intraocular pressure. It is used with other drugs to control pressures and in clients for whom beta-blockers are contraindicated because of heart failure or reactive airway disease. Acetazolamide (Diamox), a systemic carbonic anhydrase inhibitor, also may be used for some clients.

Nursing implications for medications used to control chronic glaucoma are outlined in the Medications feature.

In acute angle-closure glaucoma, diuretics may be administered intravenously to achieve a rapid decrease in intraocular pressure prior to surgical intervention. Both the carbonic anhydrase inhibitor acetazolamide and osmotic diuretics, such as mannitol, are used. Fast-acting miotic drops, such as acetylcholine, also are administered to constrict the pupil and draw the iris away from the angle and from the canal of Schlemm.

The role of the nurse in teaching clients to recognize side effects of these medications is critical. The nurse should ensure that the client has been instructed on and understands how to properly instill eyedrops (refer to the Client Teaching feature in the Eye Injuries exemplar).

■ Surgery to reduce intraocular pressure is the treatment of choice because medications used to combat glaucoma in adults are not as effective in children.

■ Treatment is not always successful, especially if the child has congenital glaucoma. So parents' feelings regarding care of a child with a visual disability should be explored.

■ If treatment is not successful, the nurse should refer the family to resources for families with children with visual impairments and, when appropriate, for counseling. School-age children are eligible for services from the public school system. Young children may receive early intervention services through agencies such as pre-school developmental day centers.

■ Approximately 80%–90% of infants who receive prompt diagnosis and treatment will do well and have normal or near-normal vision throughout their lifetime.

■ Primary congenital glaucoma will result in blindness for 12%–15% of clients. Those that do not receive prompt diagnosis and treatment will have more visual damage.

psychosocial well-being. In the hospitalized client, glaucoma is typically a concurrent diagnosis rather than the primary reason for seeking care, unless the diagnosis is acute angle-closure glaucoma.

Although glaucoma cannot be prevented, its severity and potentially deleterious permanent effects can be limited with early visual screening. The nurse assumes an important role in educating the public about the risk factors for glaucoma and encouraging clients over the age of 40 to receive an eye examination every 2–4 years that includes tonometry screening. Those with a predominant family history or another risk factor, such as frequent use of corticosteroids, should be evaluated more frequently, every 1–2 years. After the age of 65, yearly ophthalmological examinations are recommended.

Assessment

Collect the following data through a health history and physical examination:

■ *Health history.* Family history; presence of altered vision, halos, and excessive tearing; sudden, severe eye pain; use of corrective lenses; most recent eye examination; history of chronic illness; medication history.

■ *Physical examination.* Distant and near vision, peripheral fields, retina for optic nerve cupping.

Diagnosis

Nursing care planning focuses on problems associated with the temporary or permanent visual impairment, the resul-

NURSING PROCESS

When planning and providing nursing care for the client with glaucoma, nurses must consider the specific form of the disease and its actual or potential effects on the client's vision, lifestyle, safety, and

Problem

The number of Americans with glaucoma is estimated to be more than 2.2 million (Glaucoma Research Foundation, 2012a). Eyedrops that help to lower intraocular pressure are a primary treatment for glaucoma, but evidence suggests that around only 30% of clients can properly instill eyedrops (AAO, 2010b). More Americans are also turning to alternative and complementary medicine. An estimated 38% of adults have used some form of alternative treatment (National Institutes of Health, 2009). It has been suggested that exercise can help with glaucoma.

Evidence

A recent study measured intraocular pressure of 25 participants without glaucoma using tonography prior to exercise, after the participants walked 1,046 meters (3,431 feet) at a brisk pace, and again after a 20-minute rest period. The exercise reduced the intraocular pressure by a significant amount immediately after exercise and the 20-minute rest period (Hamilton-Maxwell & Feeney, 2012). Another study had a combination of 145 participants, some with glaucoma (45) and some without (100). It also introduced the use of various antiglaucoma eyedrops in both study groups. Intraocular pressure was measured using tonography prior to exercise and 5 minutes after 10 minutes of exercise on a cycle ergometer. A statistically significant decrease in intraocular pressure was found in all groups (Natsis et al., 2009). Aerobic and resistance exercise was studied in a group of 21 healthy partici-

pants. Aerobic exercise was performed on a cycle ergometer for 30 minutes and resistance exercise included leg curl and butterfly machines. Tonography measurements were taken prior to exercise, during exercise, and 10 minutes after exercise. There was a statistically significant decrease in intraocular pressure during aerobic exercise, but not during resistance exercise (Rufer et al., 2013).

Implications

Studies have shown that aerobic exercise can reduce intraocular pressure and may benefit clients with glaucoma. Clients should be counseled that certain exercises that involve inversion (scuba diving, bungee jumping, and certain yoga poses) or Valsalva maneuver (weight lifting or yoga or Pilates without proper breathing techniques) may be harmful because they increase intraocular pressure (Glaucoma Foundation, 2010). Additionally, the effects of decreased intraocular pressure are only gained if the client continues to exercise regularly. The benefits may be lost after 2 weeks of not exercising (University of Maryland Medical Center, 2009).

Critical Thinking Application

Consider the needs of a client who is morbidly obese and newly diagnosed with glaucoma. Identify two forms of activity that this client can perform to help reduce intraocular pressure. Suggest two nursing interventions that can be applied to the care of this client.

tant increased risk for injury, and the psychosocial problems of anxiety and coping. Potential diagnoses include the following:

- *Risk for Injury*
- *Risk for Ineffective Self Health Management*
- *Anxiety.*

(NANDA-I © 2012)

Planning

Appropriate outcomes for the client with glaucoma include the following:

- The client will follow glaucoma care guidelines and have no further vision loss.
- The client will remain free from injury.
- The client will report control over environment and reduced anxiety.

Implementation

Whether glaucoma and resulting impaired vision is the client's primary problem or a preexisting condition in a client with another disorder, it must be a primary consideration in nursing care planning.

Prevent Injury

The following measures help ensure the client's safety while providing mobility and helping prevent complications associated with immobility:

- If the client's vision loss is unilateral and recent, provide instructions related to unilateral vision loss and change in depth perception as follows:
  a. Caution the client about the loss of depth perception and teach safety precautions such as reaching slowly for objects and using visual cues as to distance, especially when driving.
  b. Teach the client to scan, turning the head fully toward the affected side to identify potential hazards and looking up and down to compensate for the loss of depth perception.

The client with a unilateral vision loss is often unaware of its effect on peripheral vision and depth perception.

Clients who are experiencing a sudden loss of vision due to acute angle-closure glaucoma or are experiencing significant visual impairment due to inadequately managed chronic glaucoma face increased risk for injury. Clients who have had surgical interventions for glaucoma are at even greater risk.

- Assess the client's ability to perform activities of daily living. Clients may be reluctant to request assistance, believing that they should be able to perform these familiar tasks. Carefully assessing and providing needed assistance helps prevent injury and maintain the client's self-esteem.
- Discuss possible adaptations in the home to help the client remain as independent as possible and to prevent falls or other injuries. Often minor changes in the home environment, such as removing scatter rugs and small items of furniture, allow the client to navigate safely in this already familiar environment.

For the hospitalized client:
- Notify housekeeping and place a sign on the client's door to alert all personnel not to change the arrangement of the client's room. The client with impaired vision is at high risk for falling in an unfamiliar environment. It is important to maintain a safe, familiar room.
- Raise two or three side rails on the client's bed. Raised rails remind clients to ask for assistance before ambulating in an unfamiliar environment.

Facilitate Orientation and Environmental Modifications

- Address the client by name and identify yourself with each interaction. Orient the client to time, place, person, and situation as indicated. State the purpose of your visit. The client with impaired vision must rely on input from the other senses. A lack of visual cues increases the importance of verbal ones. For example, the client with impaired vision cannot see the nurse checking an intravenous infusion and needs a verbal explanation of who is in the room and why. When the client's normal daily routine is disrupted by illness or hospitalization, additional sensory input such as a radio, a television, and explanations of the routine and activities is useful to maintain the client's orientation.
- Provide any visual aids that are routinely used. Keep them close to the client, making sure the client knows where they are and can reach them easily. Easy access encourages the client to use these items and enhances the ability to provide self-care.
- Orient the client to the environment. In the hospital setting, explain the location of the call bell, personal items, and furniture in the room. If the client is able, provide a tour of the client's room, including the bathroom and sink. Clients with visual impairments are usually capable of providing self-care in a known environment.
- Provide other tools or items that can help compensate for diminished vision, as follows:
  a. Bright, nonglare lighting
  b. Books, magazines, and instructions in large print
  c. Books on tape
  d. Telephones with oversize push buttons
  e. A clock with numbers and hands that can be felt.
- Assist with meals by:
  a. Reading menu selections and marking choices.
  b. Describing the position of foods on a meal tray according to the clock system. For example, "On the plate, the peas are at 9 o'clock, the mashed potatoes are at 1 o'clock, and the chicken breast is at 6 o'clock. The milk glass is at 2 o'clock on the tray above the plate, and coffee is at 11 o'clock."
  c. Placing the utensils in a readily accessible position.
  d. Removing lids from containers, buttering the bread, and cutting meat as needed.

Client Teaching Managing Glaucoma at Home

Clients with glaucoma must be provided with strategies for managing the disease at home. They need to understand the importance of lifetime therapy to control the disease and prevent blindness. If a permanent visual impairment has resulted, the client needs information on achieving maximum independence while maintaining safety. The following topics should be discussed with the client and family:

- Importance of not taking certain prescription and over-the-counter medications without consulting a physician
- Prescribed medications, including proper way to administer eyedrops

- Periodic eye examinations with measurement of intraocular pressure
- Risks, warning signs, and management of acute angle-closure glaucoma
- Possible surgical options
- Community resources such as the National Association for Local Societies of Visually Impaired People, local libraries, and transportation services
- Helpful resources such as the Glaucoma Foundation, Young and Under Pressure, the Glaucoma Research Foundation, and Prevent Blindness America.

---

e. Feeding the client or providing continued assistance as needed during the meal if the client's visual impairment is new or temporary.

Providing assistance during eating is important to maintain the client's nutritional status. The client may be ashamed of needing help or embarrassed to request it and may respond by not eating or by claiming not to be hungry.

- As needed, assist with mobility and ambulation as follows:
  a. Have the client hold your arm or elbow and walk slightly ahead as a guide. Do not hold the client's arm or elbow.
  b. Describe the surroundings and progress as you proceed. Warn in advance of potential hazards, turns, and steps.
  c. Teach the client to feel the chair, bed, or commode with the hands and the back of the legs before sitting.

Promote Psychosocial Wellness

The actual or potential loss of sight threatens the client's self-concept, role functioning, patterns of interaction, and, potentially, environment. The client with impaired vision who functions well in a familiar environment will feel anxious in the unfamiliar setting of a hospital or care facility.

- Assess for verbal and nonverbal indications of anxiety level and for normal coping mechanisms. Repeated expressions of concern or denial that the vision change will affect the client's life indicate anxiety. Nonverbal indicators

include tension, difficulty concentrating or thinking, restlessness, and changes in vocalization (rapid speech, quivering voice). Physical indicators include tachycardia, dilated pupils, cool and clammy skin, and tremors. The client may not recognize this feeling as anxiety. Identifying and acknowledging the anxiety can help the client recognize and deal with it.

- Encourage the client to verbalize fears, anger, and feelings of anxiety. Verbalizing helps externalize the anxiety and allows fears to be addressed.
- Discuss the client's perception of the eye condition and its effects on lifestyle and roles. Discussion provides an opportunity to correct misperceptions and introduce alternative activities and assistive devices for clients with visual impairments.
- Identify coping strategies that have been useful in the past and adapt these strategies to the present situation. Previously successful coping strategies may be employed to increase the client's sense of control.

Evaluation

Expected outcomes for the client with glaucoma may include:

- The client demonstrates proper self-administration of eyedrops.
- The client describes need for compliance with plan of care and follow-up care to avoid complications or vision loss.
- The client lists resources available within the community.

NURSING CARE PLAN A Client With Glaucoma and Cataracts

Lila Rainey is an 80-year-old widow who lives alone in the house she and her late husband built 50 years ago. She has worn glasses for nearsightedness since she was a young girl; she now wears bifocals to correct her near vision as well. She was diagnosed 4 years ago with chronic open-angle glaucoma, for which she takes timolol maleate (Timoptic) 0.5%. Recently she has noticed difficulty reading and watching television despite a new lens prescription. Because she is unable to see clearly, she has stopped reading or watching television; instead, she listens to the radio. She also has stopped driving at night because the glare of oncoming headlights makes it difficult for her to see. Mrs. Rainey's ophthalmologist has told her that she has cataracts but that they do not need to come out until they bother her. Although her glaucoma is still controlled with timolol maleate 0.5%, one drop in each eye twice a day, her intraocular pressure measurements have been gradually increasing. Mrs. Rainey has taken 325 mg of aspirin daily since a transient ischemic attack 8 years ago. She is being admitted to the outpatient surgery unit for cataract removal and intraocular lens implant in her right eye.

(continued on next page)

NURSING CARE PLAN   (continued)

ASSESSMENT

Mrs. Rainey is admitted to the eye surgery unit by Susan Schafer, RN. In her assessment, Ms. Schafer finds Mrs. Rainey to be alert and oriented, although apprehensive about her upcoming surgery. Assessment findings include temperature 97.8°F oral; pulse 86 bpm; respirations 18/min; and BP 134/72 mmHg. Mrs. Rainey's neurological, respiratory, cardiovascular, and abdominal assessments are essentially normal. However, she reports that she experiences occasional constipation. Her pupils are round and equal and react briskly to light and accommodation. Her conjunctivae are pink; sclera and corneas, clear. Using the ophthalmoscope, Ms. Schafer notes that the red reflex in Mrs. Rainey's right eye is diminished. Ophthalmic examination shows visual acuity of 20/150 OD (right eye) and 20/50 OS (left eye) with corrective lenses. Her intraocular pressures are 21 mmHg OD and 17 mmHg OS. On fundoscopic exam, no disease of the blood vessels, retina, macula, or disc is found. Ms. Schafer reviews the operative procedure with Mrs. Rainey, answering her questions and telling her what to expect after surgery. Following preoperative protocols, Mrs. Rainey is prepared and transported to surgery.

DIAGNOSES

- *Risk for Injury* related to myopia and lens extraction
- *Anxiety* related to anticipated surgery
- *Deficient Knowledge* related to lack of information regarding postoperative care
- *Impaired Home Maintenance* related to activity restrictions and impaired vision

(NANDA © 2012)

PLANNING

Goals of nursing care may include:
- The client will avoid injury.
- The client will regain sufficient visual acuity to maintain activities of daily living, including reading and watching television for enjoyment.
- The client will demonstrate a reduced level of anxiety.
- The client will demonstrate the procedure for instilling eyedrops postoperatively.
- The client will demonstrate knowledge of the home care she will require after surgery, signs of complications, and actions to take if complications occur.
- The client will use appropriate resources to assist with home maintenance until vision stabilizes and activity restrictions are lifted.

IMPLEMENTATION

- Provide a safe environment, placing the call light and personal care items within easy reach.
- Encourage Mrs. Rainey to express her fears about surgery and its potential effect on vision.
- Explain all procedures related to surgery and recovery.
- Instruct Mrs. Rainey to avoid shutting the eyelids tightly, sneezing, coughing, laughing, bending over, lifting, or straining to have a bowel movement. Teach her to wear glasses during the day and an eye shield at night to prevent injury to the surgical site until the site is healed.

- Explain and demonstrate the procedure for administering eyedrops.
- Provide verbal and written instructions about postoperative care, including a schedule of follow-up examinations, potential complications, and actions to take in response.
- Refer Mrs. Rainey to a discharge planner or social worker to help establish a plan for home maintenance.

EVALUATION

Mrs. Rainey is preparing for discharge 2 hours after her surgery. She is able to relate the recommended activity restrictions. Mrs. Rainey administers her own eyedrops before discharge and relates an understanding of the prescribed postoperative care and safety precautions. She verbalizes understanding of the need to wear a protective eye shield on the operative eye for 24 hours. Mrs. Rainey's daughter, Janice, is transporting Mrs. Rainey home. Janice states she plans to visit her mother two or three times a week to help with laundry and vacuuming until Mrs. Rainey can resume all of her household activities. Mrs. Rainey says that she won't "be so scared when I need my other eye done." She understands the chronic nature of her glaucoma and says that her vision is too important for her to neglect her timolol drops and routine eye exams.

CRITICAL THINKING

1. *How has Mrs. Rainey's impaired vision affected her activities of daily living? Should she expect a full return to normal activities once her eye is healed? Why or why not?*
2. *Aside from books, television, and radio, what other form of media entertainment might Mrs. Rainey enjoy?*
3. *Explain why constipation could be a source of complications following Mrs. Rainey's surgery.*
   Describe dietary modifications that could be implemented to ensure that Mrs. Rainey avoids complications related to bowel elimination.
4. *Describe the purpose of a plan for home maintenance. What safety-related concerns should the discharge planner or social worker prioritize when creating a home maintenance plan for Mrs. Rainey?*

▌REVIEW **Glaucoma**

RELATE Link the Concepts and Exemplars

Linking the exemplar of glaucoma with the concept of safety:

1. What interventions are appropriate for the nurse to initiate to ensure safety for the client with glaucoma?

2. Why would it be important for the nurse to give anticipatory guidance to the client with glaucoma?

Susan Parkerson is a 40-year-old woman with severe, persistent asthma. In addition to receiving bimonthly immunotherapy, she takes an inhaled corticosteroid with a long-acting beta-agonist and an antihistamine daily. Each year she has four or five acute exacerbations of asthma that usually require a taper of oral prednisone.

Linking the exemplar of glaucoma with the concept of oxygenation:

3. What are Ms. Parkerson's risk factors for glaucoma?

4. What client teaching should the nurse provide Ms. Parkerson to reduce her risk of developing glaucoma?

READY Go to Companion Skills Manual

REFER Go to Pearson Nursing Student Resources
nursing.pearsonhighered.com

- Additional review materials

REFLECT Case Study

Jane Baker is a 75-year-old female who was recently widowed. She and her husband were married 40 years when he died from cancer. She has limited income because her husband's pension terminated when he died. She receives $652 a month in Social Security benefits.

Mrs. Baker does not see particularly well. She is in excellent health; the only health-related problems she is aware of are osteoporosis and glaucoma, for which she sees an ophthalmologist on a regular basis. The only prescription drugs and over-the-counter supplements she uses are Fosamax, calcium, and latanoprost ophthalmic solution (Xalatan) eyedrops to manage her glaucoma (her dose is 1 drop in each eye once a day). Her only complaint about the eyedrops is the cost. Although Mrs. Baker has a car and a driver's license, she does not drive very often due to problems with vision. She prefers that friends and family members take her places she needs to go.

At her latest visit to the ophthalmologist, the doctor notes increased intraocular pressure.

1. Based on the information provided, what might be the cause of Mrs. Baker's increased intraocular pressure?

2. What is the priority nursing diagnosis?

3. What resources might be available to help Mrs. Baker meet her needs?

▌EXEMPLAR 18.5 **Macular Degeneration**

EXEMPLAR KEY TERMS
Age-related macular degeneration (AMD), *1327*
Exudative macular degeneration, *1327*
Nonexudative macular degeneration, *1327*

EXEMPLAR LEARNING OUTCOMES
After reading about this exemplar, you will be able to:

1. Describe the pathophysiology, etiology, clinical manifestations, and direct and indirect causes of macular degeneration.

2. Identify risk factors associated with macular degeneration.

3. Illustrate the nursing process in providing culturally competent care across the life span for individuals with macular degeneration.

4. Formulate priority nursing diagnoses appropriate for an individual with macular degeneration.

5. Summarize therapies used by interdisciplinary teams in the collaborative care of an individual with macular degeneration.

6. Plan evidence-based care for an individual with macular degeneration and his or her family in collaboration with other members of the healthcare team.

7. Evaluate expected outcomes for an individual with macular degeneration.

▶ OVERVIEW

The leading cause of legal blindness and impaired vision in people over the age of 60 is **age-related macular degeneration (AMD)**, a gradual process of degeneration in the macular area of the retina. Among individuals ages 75 years or older, approximately one third are affected by AMD (BrightFocus Foundation, 2012a).

▶ PATHOPHYSIOLOGY AND ETIOLOGY

The macula is the area of the retina that provides sharp central vision, which it does by receiving light from the center of the visual field. Two forms of AMD are identified, a nonexudative (dry) form and an exudative (wet) form. Although both are progressive disorders, their manifestations and management differ.

Nonexudative, or dry, macular degeneration is the more common form of AMD. It is the early or intermediate stage of AMD and accounts for 90% of all cases. **Nonexudative macular degeneration** begins with the accumulation of deposits called drusen beneath the pigment epithelium of the retina. Over time, these deposits enlarge and increase in number. The pigment epithelium detaches in small areas and becomes atrophic, interfering with sensory function of the macula. Typically, vision loss is not significant, and the disorder progresses slowly. However, there is a risk that the disorder will progress to an exudative stage of the disease.

Exudative macular degeneration (wet) is characterized by the formation of new, weak blood vessels in the potential space between the choroid (vascular layer of the eye) and the retina

Clinical Manifestations and Therapies **Macular Degeneration**

TYPE OF MACULAR DEGENERATION	CLINICAL MANIFESTATIONS	CLINICAL THERAPIES
Nonexudative macular degeneration (dry)	■ Slow progression ■ Need for increasingly brighter light when reading ■ Possible blurriness of printed words ■ Difficulty recognizing faces ■ Overall haziness in vision ■ Blurred or blind spot in the center of visual field; activities, such as reading and sewing, are affected.	■ High-dose antioxidants and zinc
Exudative macular degeneration (wet)	■ Possible abrupt onset ■ Visual distortions ■ Visual hallucinations ■ Impaired color vision ■ Blurred spot in the center of visual field	■ Laser surgery ■ Photodynamic therapy

(neurosensory layer). These new vessels are prone to leak, elevating the retina from the choroid and distorting vision. Although exudative macular degeneration typically is a gradual process, bleeding can lead to acute vision loss in some cases. All clients with exudative macular degeneration had the intermediate stage of the dry form first. With significant or repeated bleeding episodes, scar tissue forms and central vision is permanently lost. Luckily, this form only accounts for about 10% of all cases of AMD (NEI, 2009a).

Etiology

Approximately 15 million Americans have AMD, with approximately 200,000 new diagnoses occurring each year. AMD is the number one cause of severe vision loss and legal blindness in Americans over the age of 60 (Macular Degeneration Partnership, n.d.). There are indications that the risk for AMD is much lower for Asians, leading credence to the theory that diet and sun exposure may play a role, because Asians typically have an aversion to sun exposure and have diets high in dark leafy greens (Chang, 2009). Darker pigmentation also may play a part, because those with darker skin are less likely to develop AMD.

Risk Factors

Although the exact cause of AMD is unknown, factors associated with it include aging, smoking, race, cardiovascular health, and possibly genetic factors. Caucasians have a significantly higher risk of developing AMD than do African Americans, Hispanics, and people of Asian ancestry. However, the destructive changes in the macula occur most often as a response to the aging process. AMD affects males and females equally. Evidence suggests that the risk for developing AMD may be reduced by consumption of certain antioxidant nutrients, including vitamin C, vitamin E, beta-carotene, and zinc (NEI, 2009a).

▶ CLINICAL MANIFESTATIONS

Clients with AMD will often report blurred vision, blind or blurry spots within their central visual field, and colors appearing less bright. They will also need brighter light for activities that require close central vision (e.g., reading or sewing) and have difficulty adjusting when going from bright light to lower light situations. Clients with AMD will also report difficulty in recognizing people's faces. Because central visual fields are affected, the individual must learn to rely on peripheral fields in order to function.

The Amsler grid was developed as a diagnostic tool for AMD (**Figure 18–14 ●**). Clients with wet AMD will report the same symptoms as those with dry AMD with the addition of visual distortions. Lines that are straight will appear crooked, bent, or irregular. Also, there may be a difference in the appearance of the size of objects between eyes (AAO, 2013e).

▶ COLLABORATION

The client's quality of life is affected proportionately as AMD progresses. An interdisciplinary approach will assist the client in learning to manage the disease and adapt to the resulting change in circumstances. In addition to the ophthalmologist, the healthcare team may include an occupational therapist and a social

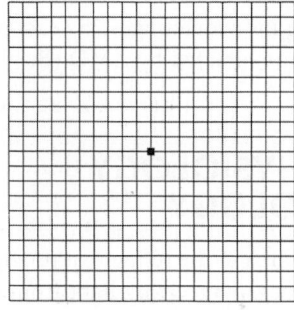

Figure 18–14 ● The Amsler grid.

Medications **Macular Degeneration**

CLASSIFICATION AND DRUG EXAMPLES	MECHANISMS OF ACTION	NURSING CONSIDERATIONS
Antiangiogenic Drugs *Drug examples:* ■ aflibercept (Eylea) ■ pegaptanib (Macugen) ■ ranibizumab (Lucentis)	Block vascular endothelial growth factor (VEGF). VEGF stimulates angiogenesis and vasculogenesis and causes blood vessels to grow in the retina, which causes damage. Useful in treating wet form of AMD.	■ Must be given by injection into the eye. ■ Teach clients to be aware of and seek treatment for serious side effects: eye pain, erythema, edema, photophobia, headache, confusion, weakness or numbness.

worker. Adaptive technology specialists can help find assistive and adaptive devices that may benefit the client (NEI, 2009a).

Diagnostic Tests

AMD is diagnosed through vision and retinal examination. Diagnostic tests for AMD usually involve pupillary dilation, which can be an unsettling experience the first time the examination is performed. The nurse can instruct the client on how the exam is performed, what to expect, and that the dilation is temporary. The nurse should encourage the client to wear dark sunglasses until the pupils have returned to normal size (the client will experience photophobia with pupil dilation).

The Amsler grid may be used to identify distortion of central vision caused by AMD. If treatment for wet AMD is planned, a fluorescein angiogram may be done. Pictures are taken as the dye passes through the blood vessels of the retina, allowing detection of leaks.

Optical coherence tomography (OCT) is relatively new. It is noninvasive and involves taking cross-sectional images of the retina to measure its thickness. Areas with thinning are noted in clients with advanced AMD (BrightFocus Foundation, 2012b).

Surgery

Wet AMD is treated with laser surgery or photodynamic therapy. Although these treatments do not cure the disease, they may slow the rate of vision loss. In laser surgery, fragile blood vessels are destroyed, preventing bleeding. In photodynamic therapy, verteporfin, a drug that tends to adhere to the surface of new blood vessels, is injected systemically. Shining a light into the affected eye activates the drug and destroys new blood vessels. Risks include damage to surrounding healthy tissue, some vision loss, and continued growth of new vessels. Since the introduction of antiangiogenic drug therapy, surgical therapy is less common.

Pharmacologic Therapy

Antiangiogenic drugs are the primary therapy used in the treatment of wet AMD. These drugs must be injected into the eye by a physician. Vascular endothelial growth factor (VEGF) causes growth of abnormal blood vessels in the macula, causing the visual changes associated with AMD. Antiangiogenic drugs block the production of VEGF, thus slowing the progression of the disease. Some examples of antiangiogenic drugs used in AMD are ranibizumab (Lucentis), bevacizumab (Avastin) and pegaptanib (Macugen) (Casey Eye Institute, 2013). See the Medications feature for nursing considerations.

Nonpharmacologic Therapy

In its early or intermediate stages, the progress of dry AMD can be slowed through the use of high-dose antioxidants and zinc. Research demonstrated a benefit when vitamin C, vitamin E, beta-carotene (vitamin A), zinc, and copper were administered daily.

Assistive devices that may be helpful to clients include magnifiers, large-print books and magazines, and high-intensity lighting to help the client cope with the reduced vision of macular degeneration. Computers and handheld electronic devices, such as iPads and Kindles, allow users to increase text size for easier reading and come equipped with audio functionality, which enables use of audiobooks and podcasts. Talking clocks or watches may also be helpful.

■ NURSING PROCESS

Nurses should be alert for clients demonstrating new and rapid onset of macular degeneration and promptly refer these clients for ophthalmological evaluation. Early intervention may preserve a greater degree of vision and slow the progress of the disease.

Assessment

■ *Health history.* Effect of vision changes on lifestyle and activities (e.g., ability to read, watch television, participate in work and recreational activities); family history of macular degeneration, nutrient intake, history of cigarette smoking
■ *Physical examination.* General health; visual acuity, including Amsler grid.

Diagnosis

For clients with slowly progressive manifestations, the nursing focus is on helping the client and family members adapt to the gradual decline in vision by recommending visual aids and other coping strategies. Client education materials should be in a large-print format. Client advocacy, psychological and emotional support, and teaching/learning needs are typically of higher priority for these clients.

Nursing diagnoses for the client with macular degeneration may include the following:

■ *Risk for Injury*
■ *Risk for Ineffective Self Health Management*
■ *Fear.*

(NANDA-I © 2012)

Planning

Identified outcomes of relevant to caring for the client with AMD may include:

- The client will remain free from injury.
- The client will express feelings related to diagnosis and reduced vision.
- The client will identify strategies to promote client's self-care and daily routine.

Implementation

Screening and education are central to nursing care for the client with AMD. Routine ophthalmic examinations should be encouraged to detect many forms of age-related eye pathologies. A diet that is high in antioxidant vitamins and zinc may help slow the vision loss in AMD. Healthy unsaturated fats such as olive oil may help prevent vision loss. Nurses should also emphasize the importance of UVA/UVB blocking eyewear, smoking cessation, and exercise to support vision health and also to reduce the risk of cardiovascular disease.

When working with the client who is experiencing severe vision loss due to AMD, nurses should assess the client for grief or fear related to the client's loss of vision and anxiety related to the disease and treatment options.

- Explain the nature of the condition and help the client determine the extent to which it is affecting daily life.
- Attend to verbalized concerns. Address questions factually and completely. For many clients, fear of blindness is second only to fear of cancer. Careful listening and teaching and a caring, understanding attitude can help the client deal with this fear.
- Assess for factors that may interfere with the client's ability to provide self-care, including environmental barriers that compromise safety.

- Recommend visual aids when appropriate (e.g., magnifying glass and large-type books).
- Teach client and caregiver about the benefits of a diet high in antioxidants, such as leafy green vegetables and fish; also offer information about supplements.
- Offer resources on smoking cessation.
- Explain the need for regular eye exams.
- Assess for other care needs that may be impacted by vision changes. Some healthcare needs, such as insulin injections, may suggest the need for home health or nursing care postoperatively.
- Encourage use of other senses, such as touch. Touch allows the client to become familiar with objects.
- Encourage use of electronic audio equipment. Radio and television can help the client remain aware of day and time and ensure the client access to emergency news services.
- As necessary, consult with occupational therapy for assistive devices.
- Make referrals to appropriate home health agency.
- Educate family and caregivers and provide resources.

Evaluation

Evaluation criteria that reflect successful achievement of identified outcomes for the client with macular degeneration may include the following:

- The client verbalizes concerns and identify appropriate resources.
- The client demonstrates the ability to safely compensate for visual deficits.
- The client describes strategies to promote self-care.

◢ REVIEW Macular Degeneration

RELATE Link the Concepts and Exemplars

Linking the exemplar of macular degeneration with the concept of health, wellness, and illness:

1. What challenges might the client with late-stage AMD experience related to physical activity?

2. What effect might AMD have on the client's ability to maintain good dental hygiene?

Linking the exemplar of macular degeneration with the concept of cognition:

3. What effect might advancing macular degeneration have on a client's cognition?

4. What strategies can the nurse implement to promote cognitive functioning?

READY Go to Companion Skills Manual

REFER Go to Pearson Nursing Student Resources
nursing.pearsonhighered.com

- Additional review materials

REFLECT Case Study

Margaret Marlborough, 58 years old, is a librarian in good health. She has never smoked and has no history of heart disease. She has made an appointment with her ophthalmologist because she has noticed pages getting blurry and she sometimes can't see her coworkers' faces clearly.

1. Based on the information above, what visual examinations will be performed?

2. What type of AMD is Ms. Marlborough likely to have?

3. What is the priority nursing diagnosis?

4. What interventions will be of most benefit to Ms. Marlborough?

EXEMPLAR 18.6 **Peripheral Neuropathy**

EXEMPLAR KEY TERMS

Guillain-Barré syndrome (GBS), *1331*
Mononeuropathies, *1331*
Paresthesias, *1331*
Peripheral neuropathy, *1331*
Polyneuropathies, *1331*

EXEMPLAR LEARNING OUTCOMES

After reading about this exemplar, you will be able to:

1. Describe the pathophysiology, etiology, clinical manifestations, and direct and indirect causes of peripheral neuropathy.

2. Identify risk factors associated with peripheral neuropathy.

3. Illustrate the nursing process in providing culturally competent care across the life span for individuals with peripheral neuropathy.

4. Formulate priority nursing diagnoses appropriate for an individual with peripheral neuropathy.

5. Summarize therapies used by interdisciplinary teams in the collaborative care of an individual with peripheral neuropathy.

6. Plan evidence-based care for an individual with peripheral neuropathy and his or her family in collaboration with other members of the healthcare team.

7. Evaluate expected outcomes for an individual with peripheral neuropathy.

▶ OVERVIEW

Peripheral neuropathy results when trauma or a disease process interferes with innervation of peripheral nerves. The overall effectiveness of blood vessels decreases, and superficial blood vessels constrict to divert blood to larger vessels. With the constriction of peripheral blood vessels, peripheral nerve endings in the constricted area suffer effects of decreased blood flow, and neuropathy develops. Although most peripheral neuropathies progress slowly over time, the symptoms, including pain and muscle weakness, can significantly affect quality of life. It is estimated that more than 20 million Americans suffer from some form of peripheral neuropathy (Neuropathy Association, 2013).

▶ PATHOPHYSIOLOGY AND ETIOLOGY

The peripheral nervous system (PNS) links the central nervous system (CNS) with the rest of the body. The PNS is responsible for receiving and transmitting information from and about the external environment. It consists of nerves, ganglia (groups of nerve cells), and sensory receptors located outside—or peripheral to—the brain and spinal cord. The PNS is divided into a sensory (afferent) division and a motor (efferent) division. Most nerves of the PNS contain fibers for both divisions, and all nerves are classified regionally as either spinal nerves or cranial nerves. Damage to these nerves can interrupt communication between the brain and the body, affecting normal muscle movement and sensory perception and causing pain.

The main components of peripheral nerves are the axon and myelin. Peripheral neuropathy can be classified according to the predominant pathology: axonal degeneration or segmental demyelination.

The peripheral neuropathies (also called somatic neuropathies) include polyneuropathies and mononeuropathies. **Polyneuropathies**, the most common types of neuropathy associated with diabetes, are bilateral sensory disorders. The manifestations appear first in the toes and feet and progress upward. The fingers and hands also may be involved, but usually only in later stages of diabetes. The manifestations of polyneuropathies depend on the nerve fibers involved.

Mononeuropathies are isolated peripheral neuropathies that affect a single nerve. Injury or trauma is the most common cause, although repetitive motions, such as those resulting in carpal tunnel syndrome, also can cause mononeuropathies.

Etiology

Neuropathies are classified by one of three causes: acquired, hereditary, or idiopathic. Acquired neuropathies include those caused by disease or illness, nutritional deficits, infection, trauma, and toxins. Hereditary, or inherited, neuropathies include Charcot-Marie-Tooth disease. Idiopathic neuropathies are from an unknown cause and account for up to 30% of neuropathies.

The etiology of polyneuropathy is varied; it often is caused by complications of diseases such as diabetes, exposure to toxins, and poor nutrition (in particular, vitamin B deficiency). One of the most serious polyneuropathies is **Guillain-Barré syndrome (GBS)**, an acute inflammatory demyelinating disorder of the peripheral nervous system characterized by an acute onset of motor paralysis (usually ascending). The classification of Guillain-Barré subtypes includes acute inflammatory demyelinating polyradiculoneuropathy, acute axonal motor neuropathy, and acute motor and sensory axonal neuropathy.

Guillain-Barré syndrome is one of the most common peripheral nervous system disorders, affecting approximately 3,000–6,000 people annually in the United States (CDC, 2012). The cause is unknown, but precipitating events include a respiratory or gastrointestinal viral or bacterial infection 1–3 weeks prior to the onset of manifestations, surgery, viral immunizations, and other viral illnesses. In 60% of cases, *Campylobacter jejuni* is identified as the cause of the preceding infection. Approximately 80%–90% of clients with GBS have a spontaneous recovery with little or no residual disabilities.

The disease is characterized by progressive ascending flaccid paralysis, accompanied by **paresthesias** (a subjective feeling of a change in sensation, such as numbness or tingling) and numbness. About 20% of clients have respiratory involvement to the point that ventilatory assistance is required. GBS is often a medical emergency.

The primary pathophysiological process in GBS is the destruction of myelin sheaths covering the axons of peripheral nerves. The demyelination is thought to be the result of both a

Clinical Manifestations and Therapies **Peripheral Neuropathy**

ETIOLOGY	CLINICAL MANIFESTATIONS	CLINICAL THERAPIES
Motor nerve damage	■ Muscle weakness ■ Cramps ■ Fasciculations ■ Muscle loss	■ Treatment of underlying cause ■ Physical therapy ■ Necessity for surgery (e.g., to remove tumor causing compression)
Sensory nerve damage	■ Numbness ■ Pain ■ Burning or shooting pain ■ Impaired touch, temperature, and pain sensation	■ Treatment of underlying cause ■ Medication ■ Physical therapy

humoral- and cell-mediated immunological response. The loss of myelin results in poor conduction of nerve impulses, causing sudden muscle weakness and loss of reflex response. Other manifestations occur when nerve conduction to various muscles is interrupted.

Systemic diseases often are the cause of peripheral neuropathy. Damage from disease processes such as metabolic and endocrine disorders affects the body's ability to process waste products and utilize nutrients. Conditions that decrease oxygen supply may cause a thickening of the walls of blood vessels that supply nerves, resulting in a reduced blood flow. Between 60% and 70% percent of individuals with diabetes develop some type of neuropathy (National Diabetes Information Clearinghouse, 2012). Autoimmune disorders and infections also can cause peripheral neuropathy. Viruses and bacteria can attack nerve tissues (or cause the body to attack nerve tissues), resulting in the destruction of nerve axons or the myelin sheath.

Sensory neuropathies with manifestations of numbness, tingling, and pain in the lower extremities affect about 30% of clients with AIDS. A Guillain-Barré type of inflammatory demyelinating polyneuropathy also can occur, resulting in progressive weakness and paralysis. In addition, untreated Lyme disease can cause extensive peripheral nerve damage.

Other disease processes that can result in peripheral neuropathy include the following:

■ Alcoholic neuropathy is damage to the nerves that results from long-term excessive use of alcohol. Malnutrition is a serious complication of chronic alcoholism; thiamine (B_1) deficiency that may be associated with chronic alcoholism is characterized by progressive cognitive deterioration, confabulation, myopathy, and peripheral neuropathy.

■ Inflammation, cancer, and toxins, including some types of chemotherapy, other medications, and environmental chemicals, such as lead, can damage nerve tissue and fibers, resulting in peripheral neuropathy.

■ Inflammation and swelling in tendon sheaths can lead to peripheral neuropathy. The carpal tunnel is a canal through which flexor tendons and the median nerve pass from the wrist to the hand. Carpal tunnel syndrome develops from narrowing of the tunnel and compression of the median nerve as a result of inflammation and swelling of the synovial lining of the tendon sheaths.

The prognosis for clients with peripheral neuropathy ranges from the neuropathy resolving (e.g., the underlying cause is successfully treated) to cases in which the client does not respond to treatment or the cause is not identified and the condition persists indefinitely.

Risk Factors

Risk factors for acquired peripheral neuropathies include the following:

■ Diabetes

■ Alcohol abuse

■ Vitamin deficiencies, particularly B vitamins

■ Immune system suppression

■ Autoimmune diseases

■ Kidney, liver, or thyroid disorders

■ Exposure to toxins, including some medications.

Age also appears to have a role in risk for peripheral neuropathy. Studies show that the incidence of peripheral neuropathy increases significantly in older adults. A survey conducted in 1999 discovered that 8%–9% of Medicare recipients have a primary or secondary diagnosis of peripheral neuropathy (Neuropathy Association, 2013). Although some changes in the peripheral system are due to the normal aging process, they are not usually associated with changes in functional status.

Prevention

Controlling medical conditions that increase risk for peripheral neuropathy is one of the best prevention methods. A healthy diet of vegetables, fruits, and whole grains can help improve nerve health. Intake of vitamin B_{12} can be helpful as well. Avoiding triggers that contribute to nerve damage, such as repetitive motions, smoking, toxic chemicals, and cramped positions, will also help in prevention of neuropathies (Mayo Clinic, 2011).

Infants

- Infants have an onset of rapidly progressive severe hypotonia, possible respiratory distress, irritability, and feeding difficulties.

Children

- Older children exhibit rapidly progressive symmetric weakness and muscle pain with varying degrees of distal paresthesia and numbness in the legs. This ascending weakness spreads to the upper extremities, trunk, chest, neck, face, and head. Deep tendon reflexes may be diminished or absent. The child may develop acute ataxia or an inability to walk.
- Difficulty swallowing and facial weakness are signs of impending respiratory failure. Respiratory effort may be inadequate for proper ventilation.
- Cranial nerves may be affected, causing Bell's palsy, for example. A dysfunctional autonomic nervous system may cause such symptoms as a labile blood pressure and cardiac rate, postural hypotension, or profound bradycardia (DiFazio et al., 2012).

▶ CLINICAL MANIFESTATIONS

Clinical manifestations of peripheral neuropathy depend on the affected nerve or nerves and the amount of damage. The primary goal of treatment is to correct or manage the underlying cause so that symptoms are controlled and further nerve damage is minimized.

The client with polyneuropathy commonly has distal paresthesias; pain described as aching, burning, or shooting; and feelings of cold feet. Other manifestations may include impaired sensations of pain, temperature, light touch, two-point discrimination, and vibration. With GBS, there is frequently a "stocking–glove" pattern—feeling as though stockings and gloves are being worn when they are not—with pain in the hands, feet, and legs.

Weakness in the arms or legs is often caused by damage to motor nerves; clients may report difficulty walking or running, stumbling, dropping things, and tiring easily. A general feeling of lack of coordination or clumsiness may be reported, and the client may compensate by changing the walking pattern to maintain balance.

Charcot-Marie-Tooth syndrome, the most common inherited peripheral neuropathy in the world, is characterized by a slowly progressive degeneration of the muscles of the foot, lower leg, hand, and forearm. Symptoms usually present between adolescence and young adulthood.

▶ COLLABORATION

Because peripheral neuropathy can involve multiple systems, collaboration is likely to include specialists (e.g., a neurologist or an endocrinologist, physical or occupational therapists, and pain specialists).

Diagnostic Tests

In addition to a medical history and neurological exam, diagnostics for peripheral neuropathy may include the following:

- Electromyography
- Complete blood count (CBC)
- Thyroid function tests
- Serum levels for B_{12} and thiamin
- Metabolic panel
- Urine screening
- Nerve biopsy.

Lyme disease and HIV tests also may be indicated.

Surgery

Surgical intervention may be appropriate when peripheral neuropathies are caused by compression, as in the case of nerve tumors, carpal tunnel syndrome, and peripheral nerve injuries. Neuropathies caused by medical pathologies cannot be treated with surgery.

Pharmacologic Therapy

There is no single drug to treat pain resulting from peripheral neuropathy, because drug therapy is individualized and based on comorbidities, extent of nerve damage, and nerve affected. Medications used include pain relievers, anticonvulsants, and antidepressants.

- ***Pain relievers.*** For mild symptoms, over-the-counter medications such as acetaminophen or ibuprofen may be helpful. More severe symptoms may require the use of an opiate.

- ***Anticonvulsants.*** In recent years the use of anticonvulsants to treat nerve pain has increased. The mechanism of action related to nerve pain is poorly understood, but it is thought that anticonvulsants may block pain receptors in the CNS. Some examples of anticonvulsants used in treating nerve pain include carbamazepine (Carbatrol, Tegretol), gabapentin (Neurontin), pregabalin (Lyrica), and topiramate (Topamax). *Antidepressants:* Tricyclic antidepressants are thought to activate a descending serotonergic (5-HT1) antinociceptive pathway that creates an endogenous pain modulation system. This action is different from how tricyclic antidepressants work in the treatment of depression. Some examples of tricyclic antidepressants are amitriptyline (Elavil) and nortriptyline (Pamelor). The serotonin-norepinephrine reuptake inhibitor (SNRI) duloxetine (Cymbalta) blocks the depletion of serotonin and norepinephrine in the CNS, which may help modulate pain receptors. Both tricyclic antidepressants and SNRIs take 4–6 weeks to reach therapeutic plasma levels. They also have side effects that include dizziness, drowsiness, nausea, and decreased appetite.

- ***Lidocaine patch.*** A local anesthetic that is absorbed through the skin. Serious side effects can occur including hives, confusion, weakness, fainting, and swelling of the lips, face, tongue, or throat (Mayo Clinic, 2011).

Medications **Peripheral Neuropathy**

CLASSIFICATION AND DRUG EXAMPLES	MECHANISMS OF ACTION	NURSING CONSIDERATIONS
Anticonvulsants *Drug examples:* ■ carbamazepine (Carbatrol, Tegretol) ■ gabapentin (Neurontin) ■ pregabalin (Lyrica) ■ topiramate (Topamax)	Mechanism of action in controlling nerve pain is poorly understood. May block pain receptors in the CNS. *May also be used for:* —Treatment of epilepsy.	■ Teach client about side effects of dizziness and drowsiness. ■ Teach client to avoid grapefruit and grapefruit juice. ■ Teach client to avoid antacids. ■ Women who are breastfeeding or may become pregnant should avoid using these drugs.
Tricyclic Antidepressants *Drug examples:* ■ amitriptyline (Elavil) ■ nortriptyline (Pamelor)	Thought to activate a descending serotonergic (5-HT1) antinociceptive pathway, which creates an endogenous pain modulation system. *May also be used for:* —Treatment of depression.	■ Teach clients about side effects of dizziness and drowsiness, nausea, and decreased appetite. ■ May take 4–6 weeks for therapeutic plasma levels to be achieved. ■ Take at bedtime to avoid drowsiness.
Serotonin-Norepinephrine Reuptake Inhibitors *Drug examples:* ■ duloxetine (Cymbalta)	Block the depletion of serotonin and norepinephrine in the CNS, which may help to modulate pain. *May also be used for:* —Treatment of depression.	■ Teach clients about side effects of dizziness and drowsiness, nausea, and decreased appetite. ■ May take 4–6 weeks for therapeutic plasma levels to be achieved. ■ Administer with food.

Nonpharmacologic Therapy

There is no specific treatment for polyneuropathy, because it is a symptom with many potential causes. The primary goals of treatment are to care for and manage the underlying cause. However, a combination of medication, lifestyle modifications, and physical therapy can be effective in treating symptoms and increasing quality of life. Physical or occupational therapy may help the client maintain mobility and avoid further changes in functional status.

Changes in daily life may be required to maintain or restore health. These include:

■ Compliance with therapeutic regimen for primary condition (e.g., maintain blood glucose control)

■ A healthy, well-balanced diet (vitamin supplements may be necessary)

■ Maintenance of optimal weight

■ Regular exercise to increase/maintain muscle strength

■ Smoking cessation

■ Limits on alcohol intake

■ Daily foot care.

Complementary and alternative therapies include acupuncture, biofeedback, transcutaneous electrical nerve stimulation (TENS), and massage.

■ NURSING PROCESS

Application of the nursing process to care of the client with known or suspected peripheral neuropathy requires significant collaboration with the client. Because the assessment interview may reveal aspects of the client's condition that are not made evident through physical assessment, it is essential for the nurse to establish effective communication with the client.

Assessment

A health assessment to determine problems with the peripheral nervous system may be conducted during a health screening, may focus on a chief complaint (such as tingling), or may be part of a total health assessment. Analyze onset, characteristics, course, severity, precipitating and relieving factors, and any associated symptoms, noting the time and circumstances. For example, ask the client the following questions:

■ Describe the location and intensity of the pain you have been experiencing in your left leg. Is it made worse by coughing, sneezing, or walking?

■ When did you first notice that you were having numbness in your fingers?

Questions about present health status include information about numbness, tingling sensations, tremors, problems with coordination or balance, and loss of movement in any part of the body. Carefully assess older adults for impaired balance and fall risk. Ask the client about difficulty with other senses, including detecting odors. In addition, assess for mood and anxiety, changes in sleep patterns, and ability to perform self-care and activities of daily living, sexual activity, and weight. Inquire about use of medications, including over-the-counter products and herbal supplements.

Ask about past history of seizures; fainting; dizziness; headaches; infection and any trauma; tumors; and surgery of the brain, spinal cord, or nerves. Discuss illnesses that may cause neurological manifestations, including cardiac disease, strokes, pernicious anemia, sinus infections, liver disease, and/or renal failure. Also ask the client about family history of neurological health problems, diabetes mellitus, hypertension, seizures, or mental health problems.

Question the client about occupational hazards, such as exposure to toxic chemicals or materials, and the amount of time spent performing repetitive motions (e.g., data entry and assembly). Information about the client's diet, use of tobacco, alcohol, or drugs, and use of safety and protective equipment also may be helpful.

A physical exam should include cranial nerve and sensory/motor assessments.

Diagnosis

Nursing diagnoses for the client with peripheral neuropathy will differ based on the type of neuropathy and comorbidities. They may include the following:

- *Risk for Injury*
- *Ineffective Peripheral Tissue Perfusion*
- *Pain*
- *Anxiety.*

(NANDA-I © 2012)

Planning

Identified outcomes relevant to the plan of care for the client with peripheral neuropathy may include the following:

- The client will remain free from injury.
- The client will report effective pain management through use of a predetermined pain rating scale.
- The client will verbalize feelings and concerns related to sensory loss.

Implementation

Nursing care is focused on promoting client safety and comfort. While the nursing plan of care is tailored to meet the needs of each individual client, general interventions relevant to the plan of care for the client with peripheral neuropathy target injury prevention and comfort promotion in both the physiological and psychosocial realms.

Prevent Injury

Ensure client safety. Those with compromised feeling in the extremities may be unaware that they have sustained injury.

- Teach clients and their families preventive and comfort measures. Clients with GBS may require frequent teaching if anxiety interferes with ability to understand. When possible, include the client and family in decision making; for example, seek their input when planning a daily schedule of care that incorporates various therapies.

Teaching topics, depending on the type of peripheral neuropathy and the extent of nerve damage, may include:

- Foot care, as the client may not feel injuries to the feet—especially important for clients with diabetes

- Exercise
- Smoking cessation
- Avoidance of toxic chemicals
- Nutrition, stressing its importance and identifying sources of B_{12}
- Avoidance of repetitive motion and/or prolonged pressure
- Massage to improve circulation, stimulate nerves, and reduce pain
- Referrals as appropriate.

Promote Comfort

Pain experienced with peripheral neuropathy varies. Pain and tenderness in muscles can be severe; interventions must be individualized to client needs. The intense pain combined with altered sensations leads to anxiety. Nursing interventions can make a difference in breaking the cycle of increasing pain that leads to increased anxiety, which can cause more pain.

- Listen to the description of pain; determine presence of triggers or a pattern. Acknowledging the client's perception of pain is a basis for treatment; listening establishes trust.
- Use a pain scale for determining extent of pain. Consistent measurement is essential to evaluate degree of pain and effectiveness of intervention.
- Use the following complementary therapies to help manage pain:

  a. Application of heat/cold
  b. Guided imagery
  c. Relaxation techniques
  d. Massage.

Presenting options for managing pain gives the client control over the situation and helps reduce anxiety. Noninvasive interventions may augment the therapeutic benefit of medications.

- Provide analgesics as indicated; administer on a regular schedule rather than waiting until pain becomes severe. Anticipating and managing pain before it becomes severe decreases anxiety and averts the cycle of increased anxiety leading to increased pain.
- For clients with GBS, monitor for side effects of analgesics, particularly respiratory depression; assess respirations and lung sounds. Perform routine pulmonary care measures and monitor for aspiration. Frequent respiratory monitoring is indicated.

Evaluation

Nursing care is evaluated based on client progress in meeting expected outcomes, which may include:

- The client experiences pain control to allow for rest and comfort.
- The client lists strategies to reduce the risk of injury and promote safety.
- The client describes a treatment plan to reduce further deterioration of sensation.

◢ **REVIEW** **Peripheral Neuropathy**

RELATE Link the Concepts and Exemplars

Linking the exemplar of peripheral neuropathy with the concept of comfort:

1. How would nursing interventions for pain differ for a client with GBS and a client with carpal tunnel syndrome?

2. What client teaching would you provide each client to prevent and/or manage pain?

Linking the exemplar of peripheral neuropathy with the concept of metabolism:

3. What client teaching would you provide the client newly diagnosed with diabetes to reduce the risk of later development of peripheral neuropathy?

4. Describe the pathophysiology of diabetes that contributes to the development of peripheral neuropathy.

READY Go to Companion Skills Manual

REFER Go to Pearson Student Resources
nursing.pearsonhighered.com

- Additional review materials

REFLECT Case Study

Bob Bender is an assembly line worker who started to feel numbness in his feet at work, where he stands 8–10 hours a day. Lately, he has noticed that he tires more easily, but he has been ignoring it "for a while" because he fears losing his job if he complains. He called in sick today because "I feel like my feet are freezing and on fire at the same time." Bob is 55 years old and lives alone on the second floor of an apartment complex. He is 6 feet tall and weighs 195 pounds. He eats "mostly junk," drinks four or five beers a night, and has smoked a pack of cigarettes a day for 30 years. Despite this, he reports "good health." Mr. Bender was adopted and has no knowledge of his family's health history. His vital signs are temperature 98.9°F oral; pulse 80 bpm; respirations 20/min; and BP 130/80 mmHg.

1. What laboratory and diagnostic tests would you expect to be performed?

2. What nursing diagnosis would be appropriate for this client?

3. What interventions would you initiate for this client?

4. What teaching will this client need prior to discharge?

■ REFERENCES

Allina Health System. (2012). *Chemical eye burns.* Retrieved from http://www.allinahealth.org/mdex/ND1420G.HTM..

American Academy of Audiology. (2009). *Position statement and clinical practice guidelines: Ototoxicity monitoring.* Retrieved from http://www.audiology.org/resources/documentlibrary/documents/otomonpositionguideline.pdf.

American Academy of Ophthalmology (AAO). (2009). *Eye injuries: Recent data and trends in the United States.* Retrieved from http://www.aaoo.org/newsroom/guide/upload/Eye-Injuries-BkgrnderLongVersFinal-l.pdf.

American Academy of Ophthalmology (AAO). (2010a). *Policy statement: Color codes for topical ocular medications.* Retrieved from http://www.aao.org/about/policy/upload/color-codes-for-topical-ocular-medications-2010.pdf.

American Academy of Ophthalmology (AAO). (2010b). *Surprising new treatment for glaucoma: Get the drops in the eye.* Retrieved from http://www.aao.org/publications/eyenet/201004/glaucoma.cfm- Surprising new treatment for glaucoma: get the drops in the eye.

American Academy of Ophthalmology (AAO). (2011a). *Eye health statistics at a glance.* Retrieved from http://www.aao.org/newsroom/upload/Eye-Health-Statistics-April-2011.pdf.

American Academy of Ophthalmology (AAO). (2011b, October). *Preferred practice pattern guidelines: Cataract in the adult eye PPP.* Retrieved from http://one.aao.org/CE/PracticeGuidelines/PPP_Content.aspx?cid=a80a87ce-9042-4677-85d7-4b876deed276.

American Academy of Ophthalmology (AAO). (2013a). *Cataract surgery.* Retrieved from http://www.geteyesmart.org/eyesmart/diseases/cataract-surgery.cfm.

American Academy of Ophthalmology (AAO). (2013b). *Children's eye injuries: Prevention and care.* Retrieved from http://www.geteyesmart.org/eyesmart/living/children-preventing-eye-injuries.cfm.

American Academy of Ophthalmology (AAO). (2013c). *Eye health in sports and recreation.* Retrieved from http://www.geteyesmart.org/eyesmart/living/sports.cfm.

American Academy of Ophthalmology (AAO). (2013d). *IOL implants: Lens replacement and cataract surgery.* Retrieved from http://www.geteyesmart.org/eyesmart/diseases/iol-implants.cfm.

American Academy of Ophthalmology (AAO). (2013e). *Macular degeneration symptoms.* Retrieved from http://www.geteyesmart.org/eyesmart/diseases/amd-symptoms.cfm.

American Academy of Ophthalmology (AAO). (2013f). *Protective eyewear.* Retrieved from http://www.geteyesmart.org/eyesmart/living/protective-eyewear.cfm.

American Academy of Ophthalmology (AAO). (2013g). *What is glaucoma?* Retrieved from http://www.geteyesmart.org/eyesmart/diseases/glaucoma.cfm#congenital.

American Glaucoma Society. (2011). *Position statement of color coded caps for glaucoma drops.* Retrieved from http://www.americanglaucomasociety.net/patients/position_statements/color_coded_caps_for_glaucoma_drops.

American Optometric Association. (n.d.). *Caring for your vision: Protecting your eyes at work.* Retrieved from http://www.aoa.org/patients-and-public/caring-for-your-vision/protecting-your-vision.

American Speech-Language-Hearing Association (ASLHA). (2013a). *Causes of hearing loss in children.* Retrieved from http://www.asha.org/public/hearing/disorders/causes.htm.

American Speech-Language-Hearing Association (ASLHA). (2013b). *Noise.* Retrieved from http://www.asha.org/public/hearing/Noise.

American Speech-Language-Hearing Association (ASLHA). (2013c). *Noise and hearing loss prevention.* Retrieved from http://www.asha.org/public/hearing/Noise-and-Hearing-Loss-Prevention.

American Speech-Language-Hearing Association (ASLHA). (2013d). *Who should be screened for hearing loss?* Retrieved from http://www.asha.org/public/hearing/Who-Should-be-Screened.

American Tinnitus Association (2013). *Sounds of tinnitus.* Retrieved from http://www.ata.org/sounds-of-tinnitus.

Becker, R. F., & Dutelle, A. W. (2013). *Criminal investigation.* Burlington, MA: Jones & Bartlett.

Bisht, M., & Bist, S. (2011). Ototoxicity: The hidden menace. *Indian Journal of Otolaryngology and Head and Neck Surgery, 63*(3), 255–259.

BrightFocus Foundation. (2012a). *Macular degeneration prevention and risk factors.* Retrieved from http://www.brightfocus.org/macular/about/risk.html.

BrightFocus Foundation. (2012b). *Macular degeneration screening & diagnosis.* Retrieved from http://www.brightfocus.org/macular/about/screeningdiagnosis.html.

Casey Eye Institute. (2013). *Macular degeneration center: Treatment.* Retrieved from http://www.ohsu.edu/xd/health/services/casey-eye/clinical-services/macular-degeneration/amd-treatment.cfm.

Center for Hearing, Speech and Language. (2012). *How loud is it?* Retrieved from http://www.chsl.org/soundchart.php.

Centers for Disease Control and Prevention (CDC). (2012). *Guillain-Barré syndrome (GBS).* Retrieved from http://www.cdc.gov/flu/protect/vaccine/guillainbarre.htm.

Centers for Disease Control and Prevention (CDC). (2013). *Adolescent and school health: About hearing loss.* Retrieved from http://www.cdc.gov/healthyyouth/noise/signs.htm.

Chang, T. (2009). Eye diseases in Asians. Paper presented at the Federation of Chinese American and Chinese Canadian Medical Studies 9th Annual Conference on Health Care of the Chinese in North America. Retrieved from http://www.fcmsdocs.org/HealthResources/FCMSConferences/1998/Document/TChang.php.

DiFazio, M., Patel, N., Patel, M., & Chibber, S. (2012). *Pediatric Guillain-Barré syndrome.* Retrieved from http://www.emedicine.medscape.com/article/1180594-overview#aw2aab6b2b5.

Drugs.com. (2012). *Apraclonidine ophthalmic side effects.* Retrieved from http://www.drugs.com/sfx/apraclonidine-opthalmic-side-effects.html.

Eballe, A., Ellong, A., Ella, G., Dohvoma, V., Bella, A., & Mvogo, C. (2011). Secondary cataract: An epidemiological and clinical survey at the Yaounde Gynaeco-obstetric and Paediatric Hospital. *Clinical Ophthalmology, 5,* 847–851.

Family Practice Notebook. (2013). *Eye injury*. Retrieved from http://www.fpnotebook.com/eye/exam/Eyinjry.htm.

Food and Drug Administration. (1999). *Guidance for industry: Container closure systems for packaging human drugs and biologics*, p. 27. Retrieved from http://www.fda.gov/downloads/Drugs/Guidances/ucm070551.pdf.

Freedman, J., Aherne, A., Sinert, R., & Ervin, M. (2012). *Acute-angle closure glaucoma: Epidemiology*. Retrieved from http://www.emedicine.medscape.com/article/798811-overview#a0199.

Glaucoma Foundation. (2010). *Exercise and glaucoma: Staying fit is good for your eyes*. Retrieved from http://www.glaucomafoundation.org/news_detail.php?id=154_Glaucoma Foundation News Story.

Glaucoma Foundation. (2013a). *Childhood glaucoma*. Retrieved from http://www.glaucomafoundation.org/childhood_glaucoma.htm.

Glaucoma Foundation. (2013b). *Frequently asked questions*. Retrieved from http://www.glaucomafoundation.org/info_new.php?id=156&cat=16.

Glaucoma Research Foundation. (2011). *Are you at risk for glaucoma?* Retrieved from http://www.glaucoma.org/glaucoma/are-you-at-risk-for-glaucoma.php.

Glaucoma Research Foundation. (2012a). *Glaucoma facts and stats*. Retrieved from http://www.glaucoma.org/glaucoma/glacoma-facts-and-stats.php.

Glaucoma Research Foundation. (2012b). *Symptoms of open-angle glaucoma*. Retrieved from http://www.glaucoma.org/glaucoma/symptoms-of-primary-open-angle-glaucoma.php.

Hamilton-Maxwell, K., & Feeney, L. (2012). Walking for a short distance at a brisk pace reduces intraocular pressure by a clinically significant amount. *Journal of Glaucoma, 21*(6), 421–425.

Health Communities. (2011). *Cataracts: Basics of cataracts*. Retrieved from http://www.healthcommunities.com/cataracts/overview-of-cataracts.shtml.

Healthline Info. (2012). *Glaucoma: Symptoms, causes, diagnosis and treatment*. Retrieved from http//:www.healthlineinfo.com/glaucoma-symptoms-causes- diagnosis-and-treatment.html.

Heiting, G., Haddrill, M., & Slonim, C. (2010). *Narrow-angle glaucoma*. Retrieved from http://www.allaboutvision.com/conditions/narrow-angle-glaucoma.htm.

Holt, J., Hotto, S., & Cole, K. (2012). *Demographic aspects of hearing impairment*. Center for Assessment and Demographic Studies, Gallaudet University. Retrieved from http://www.research.gallaudet.edu/Demographics/factsheet.php.

Koerner, F., Koerner-Stiefbold, U., & Garwig, J. (2012). Systemic corticosteroids reduce the risk of cellophane membranes after retinal detachment surgery: A prospective randomized placebo-controlled double-blind clinical trial. *Graefe's Archive for Clinical and Experimental Ophthalmology, 250*(7), 981–987.

Lighthouse International. (2013). *Vision impairment: Racial & ethnic differences*. Retrieved from http://www.lighthouse.org/research/statistics-on-vision-impairment/racial-ethnic-differences.

Macular Degeneration Partnership. (n.d.). *Macular degeneration*. Retrieved from http://www.amd.org.

Margrain, T., Nollett, C., Shearn, J., Stanford, M., Edwards, R., Ryan, B., et al. (2012). The Depression in Visual Impairment Trial (DEPVIT): Trial design and protocol. *BMC Psychiatry, 12*(57). doi:10.1186/1471-22X-12-57.

Mayo Clinic. (2011). *Peripheral neuropathy: Treatments and drugs*. Retrieved from http://www.mayoclinic.com/health/peripheral-neuropathy/DS00131/DSECTION=treatments%2Dand%2Ddrugs.

National Diabetes Information Clearinghouse. (2012). *Diabetic neuropathies: The nerve damage of diabetes*. Retrieved from http://www.diabetes.niddk.nih.gov/dm/pubs/neuropathies.

National Eye Institute (NEI). (2009a). *Facts about cataracts*. Retrieved from http://www.nei.nih.gov/health/cataract/cataract_facts.asp.

National Eye Institute (NEI). (2009a). *Facts about age-related macular degeneration*. Retrieved from http://www.nei.nhi.gov/health/maculardegen/armd_facts.asp#a.

National Eye Institute (NEI). (2009b). *Facts about cataract*. Retrieved from http://www.nei.nih.gov/health/cataract/cataract_facts.asp.

National Eye Institute (NEI). (2009c). *Facts about glaucoma*. Retrieved from http://www.nei.nih.gov/health/glaucoma/glaucoma_facts.asp.

National Institute on Deafness and Other Communication Disorders (NIDOCD). (2010). *Quick statistics*. Retrieved from http://www.nidcd.nih.gov/health/statistics/Pages/quick.aspx.

National Institute for Occupational Safety and Health. (2010). *Workplace safety & health topics: Eye safety*. Retrieved from http://www.cdc.gov/niosh/topics/eye/.

National Institutes of Health. (2009). *Americans continue to use complementary, alternative medicine*. Retrieved from http://www.nihrecord.od.nih.gov/newsletters/2009/02_20_2009/story8.htm-Americans Continue to Use Complementary, Alternative Medicine-The NIH Record-February 20, 2009.

National Library of Medicine. (2011a). *Cataract*. Retrieved from http://www.nlm.nih.gov/medlineplus/ency/article/001001.htm.

National Library of Medicine. (2011b). *Congenital cataract*. Retrieved from http://www.nlm.nih.gov/medlineplus/ency/article/001615.htm.

National Library of Medicine. (2011c). *Slit-lamp exam*. Retrieved from http://www.nlm.nih.gov/medlineplus/ency/article/003880.htm.

Natsis, K., Asouhidou, A., Nousios, G., Chatzibalis, T., Vlasis, K., & Karabatakis, V. (2009). Aerobic exercise and intraocular pressure in normotensive and glaucoma patients. *BMC Ophthalmology, 9*, 6.

Neuropathy Association. (2013). *About peripheral neuropathy: Facts*. Retrieved from http://www.neuropathy.org/site/PageServer?pagename=About_Facts.

Office on Women's Health, U.S. Department of Health and Human Services. (2010). *Minority women's health: Glaucoma and cataracts*. Retrieved from http://www.womenshealth.gov/minority-health/african-americans/glaucoma-cataracts.cfm.

Pelletier, A., Thomas, J., & Shaw, F. (2009). Vision loss in older persons. *American Family Physician, 79*(11), 963–970.

Prieto-Flores, M., Forjaz, M., Fernandez-Mayoralas, G., Rojo-Perez, F., & Martinez-Martin, P. (2011). Factors associated with loneliness of noninstitutionalized and institutionalized older adults. *Journal of Aging and Health, 23*(1), 177–194.

Quandt, S., Schulz, M., Talton, J., Verma, A., & Arcury, T. (2012). Occupational eye injuries experienced by migrant farmworkers. *Journal of Agromedicine, 17*(1), 63–69.

Rufer, F., Schiller, J., Klettner, A., Lanzl, I., Roider, J., & Weisser, B. (2013). Comparison of the influence of aerobic and resistance exercise of the upper and lower limb on intraocular pressure. *Acta Opthalmologica*. doi:10.1111/aos.12051.

Safe Kids USA. (2012). *Sports and recreation safety*. Retrieved from http://www.safekids.org/fact-sheet/sports-and-recreation-safety-fact-sheet-pdf.

Scott, R. (2011). The injured eye. *Philosophical Transactions of the Royal Society of Biological Sciences, 366*(1562), 251–260.

Sign Media. (2011). *American Deaf culture*. Retrieved from http://www.signmedia.com/info/adc.htm.

Snyderman, D., & Rovner, B. (2009). Mental status examination in primary care: A review. *American Family Physician, 80*(8), 809–814.

Sponsel, W., Gray, W., Scribbick, F., Stern, A., Weiss, C., Groth, S., & Walker, J. (2011). Blunt eye trauma: Empirical histopathological paintball impact thresholds in fresh mounted porcine eyes. *Investigative Ophthalmology & Visual Science, 52*(8), 5157–5166.

University of Iowa. (2012). *Sound levels*. Retrieved from http://www.uiowa.edu/~ui-safe/sound-levels.html.

University of Maryland Medical Center. (2009). *Glaucoma—Lifestyle changes*. Retrieved from http://www.umm.edu/patiented/articles/what_life_style_changes_help_manage_glaucoma_000025_10.htm-Glaucoma-Lifestyle Changes.

University of Michigan Kellogg Eye Center. (2012). *Detached retina*. Retrieved from http://www.kellogg.umich.edu/patientcare/conditions/detached.retina.html.

U.S. Preventive Services Task Force (2011). Vision screening for children one to five years of age: Recommendation statement. *American Family Physician, 84*(2), 221–222.

WebMD. (2011). *Ear-damaging (ototoxic) medications*. Retrieved from http://www.webmd.com/a-to-z-guides/ear-damaging-ototoxic-medicines.

World Health Organization. (2013). *Deafness and hearing loss*. Retrieved from http://www.who.int/mediacentre/factsheets/fs300/en/index.html

19 Sexuality

MODULE AT-A-GLANCE

◼ THE CONCEPT OF SEXUALITY

Sexuality is an important part of being human. It contributes to healthy relationships and a sense of well-being. Sexuality is an individually expressed and highly personal phenomenon whose meaning evolves from life experiences. Physiological, psychosocial, religious, and cultural factors influence an individual's sexuality and lead to the wide range of attitudes and behaviors seen in humans. There are no normal, universal sexual behaviors. Satisfying or "normal" sexual expression can generally be described as whatever behaviors give mutual pleasure and satisfaction to the adults involved, without threat of coercion or injury to self or others.

✳ Visit **nursing.pearsonhighered.com** *for a review of the anatomy and physiology of reproduction.* <<

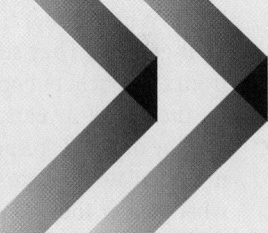

Concept Learning Outcomes

After reading about this concept, you will be able to:

1. Summarize the physiology of the reproductive system related to sexuality.

2. Examine the relationship between sexuality and other concepts/systems.

3. Identify commonly occurring alterations in sexuality and their related therapies.

4. Differentiate common assessment procedures used to examine sexual health across the life span.

5. Describe diagnostic and laboratory tests to determine the individual's reproductive system status.

6. Explain management of sexual health and prevention of alterations in sexuality.

7. Demonstrate the nursing process in providing culturally competent and caring interventions across the life span for individuals with common alterations in sexuality.

8. Compare and contrast common independent and collaborative interventions for clients with alterations in sexuality.

Concept Key Terms

Anal stimulation, *1346*
Anorgasmia, *1354*
Body image, *1345*
Climacteric, *1343*
Cryptorchidism, *1357*
Cystocele, *1360*
Desire phase, *1346*
Dissatisfaction problem, *1351*
Dysmenorrhea, *1342*
Dyspareunia, *1344*
Excitement phase, *1346*
Female orgasmic disorder, *1349*
Female sexual arousal disorder, *1349*
Galactorrhea, *1359*
Gender identity, *1345*
Gender-role behavior, *1345*

Genital intercourse, *1346*
Gynecomastia, *1356*
Hirsutism, *1360*
Hydrocele, *1357*
Hypoactive sexual desire disorder, *1349*
Impotence, *1353*
Intimacy, *1343*
Male erectile disorder, *1349*
Male orgasmic disorder, *1350*
Masturbation, *1346*
Menarche, *1340*
Menopause, *1343*
Menstrual cycle, *1354*
Menstruation, *1342*
Nabothian cysts, *1361*
Nocturnal emissions, *1340*
Oral–genital sex, *1346*
Orgasmic phase, *1346*

(continued on next page)

▶ DEVELOPMENT AND SEXUALITY

The development of sexuality begins at conception and continues throughout the life span. Although this concept section discusses development in terms of sexuality, nurses need to consider sexuality in the larger context of the development of the individual. The module on Development discusses the various stages of individual development. Sexual development throughout the life span is discussed in the Lifespan Considerations feature.

Birth to 12 Years

The ability of the human body to experience a sexual response is present before birth. As evidenced by ultrasound, males have erections several months before birth. They continue to experience erections after birth. Because females have vaginal lubrication at birth, it is assumed that lubrication also occurs prior to birth. When babies find their fingers and toes, they also find their genitals. They seem to experience a pleasurable sensation from the touch, but one would not call this a sexual experience. By the age of 3 years, more purposeful masturbation begins, and the orgasmic response is quite common, although males do not ejaculate until after puberty. By age $2^1/_2$ or 3, children know what gender they are and have beginning awareness of genital differences between males and females.

Around age 9 or 10, the first physical changes of puberty begin: the development of breast buds (**thelarche**) in girls and the growth of pubic hair in both girls and boys. As the adrenal glands mature, they produce more **testosterone** and estradiol, which contribute to the first experiences of sexual attraction to another individual. Sexual maturity rating based on Tanner stages may be assigned depending on the growth of the breasts and pubic hair in girls and the genitalia and pubic hair in boys. **Figure 19–1** ● depicts Tanner stages for breasts. **Figure 19–2** ● depicts Tanner stages for pubic hair changes in girls, and Figure **19–3** ● demonstrates the Tanner stages in genital growth and pubic hair changes in boys.

Adolescence

During early adolescence (ages 12–13), primary and secondary sex characteristics continue to develop, necessitating more information about body changes. For boys, the testes and scrotum increase in size, the skin over the scrotum becomes darker, pubic hair grows, and axillary sweating begins. Development of the genitals to adult size takes about 5–6 years. At about ages 13–15, boys experience **nocturnal emissions** (spontaneous orgasm), or "wet dreams," which are the beginning of puberty in boys (Mannheim, 2013). The boy's voice changes as the genitals grow, and he experiences a dramatic growth in height when nocturnal emissions and puberty begin.

Boys mature later than girls by about 2 years. Boys are often awkward, self-conscious, and concerned about body changes. Since the onset of puberty for boys is not marked by an event as

apparent as menses in girls, parents are less likely to talk with boys about sex and sexual changes occurring in the body (Ball, Bindler, & Cowen, 2012).

For girls, the pelvis and hips broaden, breast tissue develops, pubic hair grows, axillary sweating begins, and vaginal secretions become milky and change from an alkaline to an acid pH. **Menarche** (first menses) usually occurs within about 2 years after breast and pubic hair changes. In the United States, the average age of menarche is 12.5 years (Mannheim, 2013).

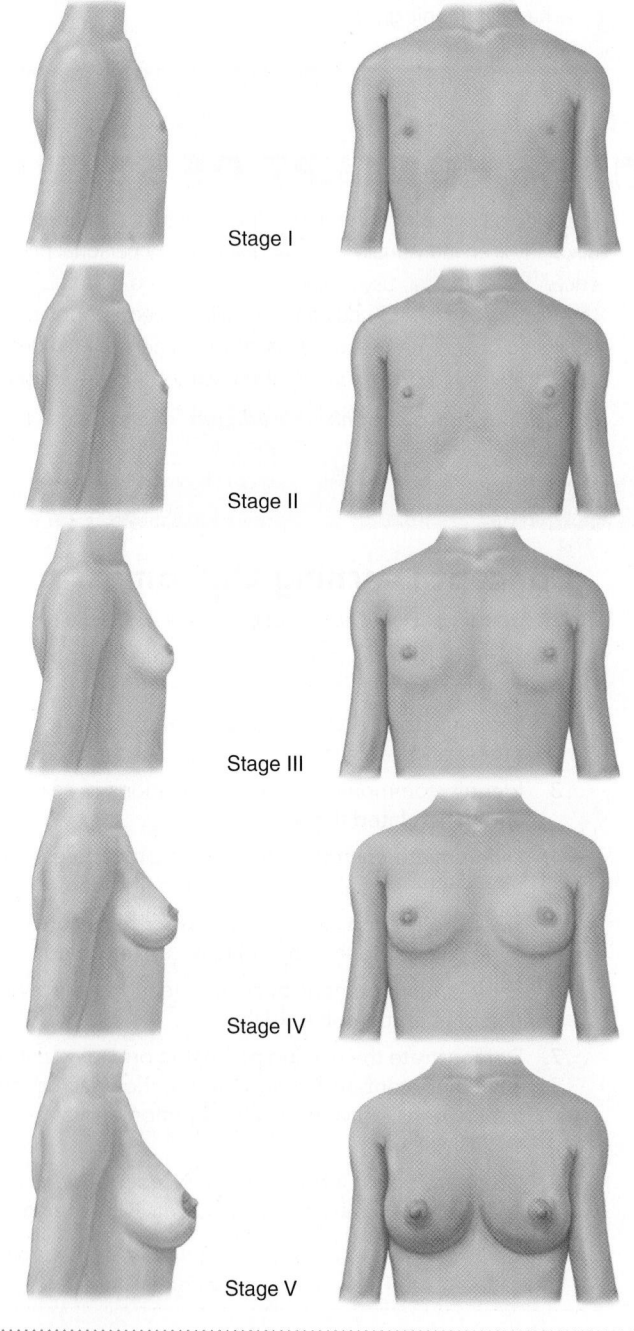

Stage I

Stage II

Stage III

Stage IV

Stage V

Figure 19–1 ● Tanner stages for the breasts.

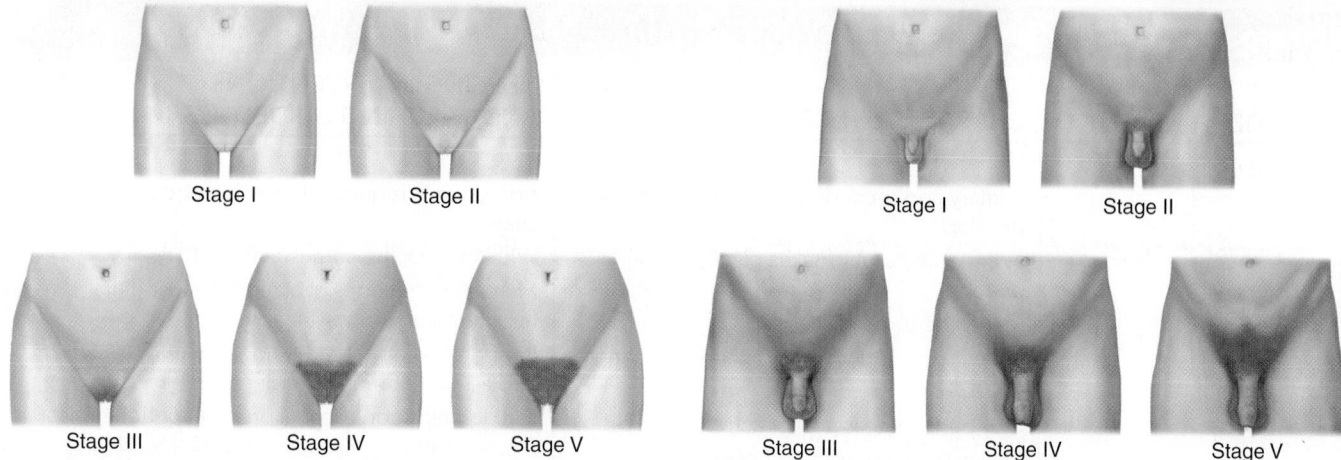

Figure 19–2 ● Tanner stages for pubic and axillary hair changes in girls.

Figure 19–3 ● Tanner stages for genital and pubic hair changes in boys.

Lifespan Considerations Sexual Development Throughout the Life Span

STAGE	CHARACTERISTICS	NURSING INTERVENTIONS AND TEACHING GUIDELINES
INFANCY Birth to 18 months	Given gender assignment of male or female. Differentiates self from others gradually. External genitals are sensitive to touch. Male infants have penile erections; females, vaginal lubrication.	Self-manipulation of the genitals is normal. Caregivers need to recognize these behaviors as common in children.
TODDLER 1–3 years	Continues to develop gender identity. Able to identify own gender.	Body exploration and genital fondling are normal. Use names for body parts. Children from single-parent homes should have contact with adults of both sexes.
PRESCHOOLER 4–5 years	Becomes increasingly aware of self. Explores own and playmates' body parts. Learns correct names for body parts. Learns to control feelings and behavior. Focuses love on parent of the other sex.	Answer questions about "where babies come from" honestly and simply. Parental overreaction to exploration of genitals and masturbation can lead to feelings that sex is "bad."
SCHOOL AGE 6–12 years	Has strong identification with parent of same gender. Tends to have friends of the same gender. Has increasing awareness of self. Increased modesty, desire for privacy. Continues self-stimulating behavior. Learns the role and concepts of own gender as part of the total self-concept. At about 8 or 9 years of age, becomes concerned about specific sex behaviors and often approaches parents with explicit concerns about sexuality and reproduction.	Provide parents and children with opportunities to express their concerns and ask questions regarding sex. Answer all questions with factual data and perhaps follow up with appropriate books and other material. Advise parents to discuss basic information about sexual intercourse, menstruation, and reproduction with children at about 10 years of age. Give children reading material and then discuss it with them.

(continued on next page)

Lifespan Considerations Sexual Development Throughout the Life Span (continued)

STAGE	CHARACTERISTICS	NURSING INTERVENTIONS AND TEACHING GUIDELINES
ADOLESCENCE 12–18 years	Primary and secondary sex characteristics develop. Spermarche usually takes place early in puberty. Menarche usually takes place. Develop relationships with interested partners. Masturbation is common. May participate in sexual activity. May experiment with homosexual relationships. Are at risk for pregnancy and sexually transmitted infections.	Adolescents require information about body changes. With spermarche comes male fertility. Menarche precedes ovulation in most girls; fertility occurs with ovulation. Peer groups have great importance at this time and assist in forming gender roles. Dating helps adolescents prepare for adult roles. Parents influence values and beliefs regarding behavior. Teenagers require information about contraceptive measures and precautions to take with regard to sexually transmitted infections.
YOUNG ADULTHOOD 18–40 years	Sexual activity is common. Establishes own lifestyle and values. Homosexual identity usually established by mid-20s. Many couples share financial obligations and household tasks.	Young adults often require information about measures to prevent unwanted pregnancies (i.e., abstinence or contraceptive devices). Information is required to prevent sexually transmitted infections. Regular communication is required to understand partner's sexual needs and to work through problems and stresses.
MIDDLE ADULTHOOD 40–65 years	Men and women experience decreased hormone production. Climacteric occurs in men and women. Menopause occurs in women, usually anywhere between 40 and 55 years. The climacteric occurs gradually in men. Quality rather than number of sexual experiences becomes important. Individuals establish independent moral and ethical standards.	Women and men may need help adjusting to new roles. Individuals may require counseling to help them reevaluate and direct their energies. Encourage couples to look at the positive aspects of this time of life.
LATE ADULTHOOD 65 years and over	Interest in sexual activity often continues. Sexual activity may be less frequent. Women's vaginal secretions diminish, and breasts atrophy. Men produce fewer sperm and need more time to achieve an erection and to ejaculate.	Older adults often continue to be sexually active. Couples may require counseling about adapting their affection and sexual needs to physical limitations.

Teenage girls may have irregular **menstruation** initially, which can lead to embarrassment because of stained clothing. They can be taught to be aware of subtle signs of impending menstruation, such as tender breasts, water retention or bloating, or the appearance of skin eruptions or pimples. Girls should also be counseled regarding the variety of feminine hygiene products available (e.g., sanitary pads and tampons) so that they can make intelligent choices about their use. Parents and nurses should advise teenage girls to wash their hands thoroughly before inserting a tampon, to change tampons frequently, to alternate tampons with sanitary pads, and to use

pads at night. These measures will help to decrease the risk of infection, including the risk of toxic shock syndrome, a particular type of *Staphylococcus aureus* infection. Thorough cleaning of the genital area and wiping from front to back will also decrease infection and prevent odors.

Dysmenorrhea (painful menstruation) is prevalent among adolescent females. Cramping, lower abdominal pain radiating to the back and upper thighs, nausea, vomiting, diarrhea, and headaches may occur for a few hours or up to 3 days. Dysmenorrhea results from powerful uterine contractions, which cause ischemia and, in turn, cramping pain. The symptoms of dysmenorrhea are treated with bed rest, application of heat to the abdomen, certain exercises such as abdominal muscle strengthening, biofeedback, and administration of nonsteroidal anti-inflammatory medications, such as ibuprofen. Masturbation to orgasm also eases cramping through the associated uterine contractions and increased blood flow.

Although it is difficult to apply statistical data about large populations to local populations, it is generally accepted that sexual experimentation is currently occurring at younger ages than in previous decades. The 2011 Youth Risk Behavior Survey conducted by the Centers for Disease Control and Prevention (CDC) revealed that of the 15,000 high school students surveyed, 6.2% had experienced sexual intercourse before age 13. Within this group, African American boys were the most likely to have experienced sexual intercourse (CDC, 2013a). In addition, of the 15,000 students surveyed, 47.4% had had sexual intercourse at least one time. The high incidence of sexual intercourse puts teenagers at risk for sexually transmitted infections (STIs) and unintended pregnancies. In 2009, about 10 million individuals ages 15–24 experienced an STI and about 400,000 adolescent girls gave birth (CDC, 2013a).

All adolescents want to know about sexual behaviors, but are often uneasy about discussing these concerns with their parents. Nurses, the schools, and the family need to provide accurate information. During the nursing assessment, teenagers should be asked directly what they know about sex, contraception, and reproduction. Sometimes a lot of a teenager's information is based on popular myths and little, if any, fact. The nurse should discuss factual information about sex, sexual actions and their consequences, the individual's right to make a decision regarding ways to express oneself sexually, and the responsibilities of each individual with respect to sexual activity.

Young and Middle Adulthood

In young adulthood, many individuals begin to form intimate relationships with long-term implications. These relationships may take the form of dating, cohabitation, or marriage. Note, however, that some individuals do not form intimate relationships until late adulthood and that some never form these types of relationships.

Young adult men and women are often concerned about normal sexual response for both themselves and their partners. In heterosexual relationships, problems may arise because of basic differences in male and female expectations and responses. Gay and lesbian couples often fare better in this respect. Couples need to communicate their needs to one another early in their courtship so that a successful intimate relationship can develop and grow. Young adults should also be aware that because sexual needs and responses may change, each partner should listen and respond to the needs of the other.

During middle adulthood, both men and women experience decreased hormone production, causing the **climacteric** (transitional period in reproductive life). In men, the transition involves a reduction in Leydig cells and androgen with continued spermatogenesis. In women, the climacteric includes perimenopause and ends in **menopause** (cessation of menses) and end of fertility (Blackburn, 2013). These events often affect the individual's sexual self-concept, body image, and sexual identity.

Older Adulthood

Research during the past decade has demonstrated that many older adults are enjoying sex well into their eighth decade. Reasons for this increase include the following:

- The population of the United State is aging as "baby boomers" reach retirement age.
- Individuals are living longer, heather lives.
- An aging population means that more widowed and divorced singles are looking for mates.
- Older women do not have to worry about pregnancy.
- The availability of male and female treatment for sexual dysfunction has increased.
- The media are more inclined to acknowledge that older adults have sex.
- Society is increasingly accepting of sexual activity among older adults (Foster et al., 2012; Poynten, Grulich, & Templeton, 2013; Stewart & Graham, 2013).

Even with these changes, however, it is important to recognize that older adults may experience some significant changes in sexual response. For men, more time may be needed to achieve an erection and to ejaculate (the erection may last longer than at a younger age), more direct genital stimulation is required to achieve an erection, the volume of ejaculated fluid decreases, and the intensity of contractions with orgasm may decrease. The time to the next erection will be longer.

Older women remain capable of multiple orgasms and may, in fact, experience an increase in sexual desire after menopause. However, vaginal lubrication and elasticity decrease with menopause and decreased estrogen, and phases of the sexual response cycle may take longer to occur.

Many products are available to assist older adults with enhancing their sexual experiences. These range from simple lubricants to surgically implanted devices that enable penile erections. Although older adults' technique may require modification, the nurse should never assume that older adults are less interested in sex or less motivated to have an active sex life.

Older adults may define sexuality far more broadly and may include in their definition such things as touching, hugging, romantic gestures (e.g., giving or receiving roses), comfort, warmth, dressing up, joy, spirituality, and beauty.

Older adults continue to need **intimacy**, that is, chosen emotional interconnectedness between two individuals that includes mutual caring and responsibility, although there may be fewer opportunities and strong social sanctions against this. Intimacy may entail close body contact, hand holding, kissing, eye contact, closeness, companionship, social support, and meaningful activity (Ryan et al., 2011). Close friendships, sexual relationships, strong ties to family members, and beloved pets can all contribute to meeting the older adult's need for intimacy but are not always available.

The age-related changes in sexual response in both men and women do not preclude a satisfying sex life. Because arousal takes longer in both sexes, foreplay is even more important in older adults than in younger adults. Hugging, kissing, and caressing are sexual activities that both men and women enjoy. They can be preludes to sexual intercourse or satisfying activities in themselves (DeLemater, 2012). The older adults described in the review presented by DeLemater were generally open minded and knowledgeable about sexual matters, but loss of a partner or problems with health status were barriers to sexual expression.

Chronic pain and osteoarthritis are two common problems that have deleterious effects on sexual activity in older adults. Arthritis in the hip joint presents the greatest challenge to satisfying sexual activity (DeLemater, 2012), but it can be ameliorated by changes in coital position, use of heat applications, and timing sexual activity during the day when joints are less painful. Warm baths can also help relieve pain and can be incorporated as foreplay (Eustice, 2013).

Many older adults who suffer from cardiovascular disease are concerned about the safety of sex. In general, if an older adult can climb two flights of stairs or walk at a rate of 2 miles per hour without chest pain or shortness of breath, the individual should have no cardiac problems during sexual intercourse (Levine et al., 2012). Consideration should be given to the partner with the less stable vital signs, particularly blood pressure, and that partner should not be positioned on top. Older adults with heart failure who develop fatigue or shortness of breath will be more comfortable in a semi-reclining position or lying under their partner during sex (Levine et al., 2012).

Dyspareunia (painful intercourse) for the older woman may be related to decreased vaginal lubrication (Stiles et al., 2012). Penetration may be difficult because the vaginal opening may be partially obscured by the labia, tightened by atrophy, and lacking in the lubrication needed for smooth entrance of the penis. The older couple might be advised to use a vaginal lubricant as part of their sexual activity and to have the woman use her hand to guide her partner's penis into the vagina.

Diabetes mellitus can have negative effects on the sexual expression of both men and women. It is correlated with low libido in both men and women, erectile dysfunction in the man, and even greater reduction of lubrication in the woman (Neithercott, 2012). Both vascular and nerve damage may affect sexual arousal and orgasm. Alternative expressions of sexuality, such as body caressing, manipulation of the partner's genitals with the hand, or mutual masturbation, may be suggested.

DISCUSSING SEXUALITY WITH OLDER ADULTS The **PLISSIT** model of intervention for sexual concerns, developed over 30 years ago, is still a valid method for the nurse to use with older adults (Annon, 1976; Kazer, 2012):

P stands for permission, in which the nurse validates the older adult's desire for sexual activity. The nurse may start the conversation with a neutral phrase such as "Many people think older adults aren't interested in sex any more, but that's not true. I wonder if you have questions that I might answer for you." The permission phase is concerned with normalizing the older adult's feelings and concerns.

LI is limited information, and the nurse offers specific, factual information pertinent to the older client. For example, an older man may appreciate knowing that although his erection is not as firm as it once was, he can still satisfy himself and his partner.

SS stands for specific suggestions, such as coital positions or timing of pain medication.

IT is intensive therapy, which requires a referral to an advanced practice nurse or other expert.

▶ SEXUAL HEALTH

Sexual health is an individual and constantly changing phenomenon falling within the wide range of human sexual thoughts, feelings, needs, and desires. For most individuals, sexual health is not considered until its absence or an impairment is noticed. An individual's degree of sexual health is best determined by that individual, sometimes with the assistance of a qualified professional. The World Health Organization (WHO) defined **sexual health** in 2006 as:

[A] state of physical, emotional, mental and social well-being in relation to sexuality; it is not merely the absence of disease, dysfunction or infirmity. Sexual health requires a positive and respectful approach to sexuality and sexual relationships, as well as the possibility of having pleasurable and safe sexual experiences, free of coercion, discrimination and violence. For sexual health to be attained and maintained, the sexual rights of all individuals must be respected, protected and fulfilled (WHO, 2013a).

This definition recognizes the biological, psychological, and sociocultural dimensions of sexuality. Sexual rights recognized by such organizations as the World Health Organization (2013c) and the World Association for Sexual Health (2013) are listed in **Box 19–1** ●.

Components of Sexual Health

Five critical components of sexual health are sexual self-concept, body image, gender identity, gender-role behavior, and freedoms and responsibilities.

An individual's **sexual self-concept** (how an individual values him- or herself as a sexual being) determines with whom the individual will have sex; the gender and kinds of individuals the person is attracted to; and the values about when, where, with whom, and how the individual expresses his or her sexuality. A positive sexual self-concept enables individuals to form intimate relationships throughout life. A negative sexual self-concept may impede the formation of relationships.

Box 19–1 **Sexual Rights**

- The right to sexual freedom, including the right to decide to be sexually active or not, and the right to choose sexual partners
- The right to sexual autonomy, integrity, privacy, and equity
- The right to sexual and reproductive healthcare services for the prevention and treatment of all sexual concerns, problems, and disorders
- The right to sexual education to seek, receive, and impart information in relation to sexuality
- The right to make free and responsible reproductive choices, including the decision of whether or not, and when, to have children

Body image, a central part of the sense of self, is constantly changing. Pregnancy, aging, trauma, disease, and therapies can alter an individual's appearance and function, which can affect body image. How an individual feels about his or her body is related to his or her sexuality. Individuals who feel good about their bodies are likely to be comfortable with and enjoy sexual activity. Individuals who have a poor body image may respond negatively to sexual arousal. A major influence on body image for women is the media focus on physical attractiveness and large breasts. Similarly, many men worry about penis size. The myth that "larger is better," particularly if it is erect and has staying power, is pervasive in North America. An individual's body image can suffer when the individual is unable to achieve these expectations.

Gender identity refers to an individual's self-image as a female or male. More than just the biological component, it also includes social and cultural norms. Gender identity is the result of a long series of developmental events that may or may not conform to an individual's apparent biological sex. Once gender identity has been established, it cannot be easily changed.

Gender-role behavior is the outward expression of an individual's sense of maleness or femaleness as well as the expression of what is perceived as gender-appropriate behavior. Each society defines its roles for males and females; boys are given reinforcement for behaving in a "masculine" way, and girls receive reinforcement for exhibiting "feminine" behaviors.

Physical structure, variations in the internal sense of what is male or female, family values, and cultural values all influence gender-role behavior. In North America, expected adult male roles include breadwinner, heterosexual lover, father, and athlete. Expected male behaviors include wearing trousers, demonstrating physical strength, and expressing feelings in a controlled fashion. Women are expected to express their emotions more freely and to be gentler in their physical responses; they also have a broader choice of clothing than men do.

Sexual health includes both *freedoms* and *responsibilities*. Sexually healthy individuals engage in activities that are freely chosen, including both self-pleasuring and shared-pleasuring activities. Individuals also have freedom of their sexual thoughts, feelings, and fantasies. Sexually healthy individuals are ethically motivated to exercise behavioral, emotional, economic, and social responsibility for themselves (Dixon-Mueller et al., 2009).

Varieties of Sexuality

There are many varieties of sexuality and a tremendous range of variation in how individuals experience and express their sexuality. There are also many differences in the priority individuals place on sexuality in their lives. Sexual varieties include sexual orientation, gender identity, erotic preferences, and sexual lifestyles.

SEXUAL ORIENTATION
An individual's attraction to people of the same sex, the other sex, or both sexes is referred to as **sexual orientation**. Sexual orientation lies along a continuum with a wide range between the two extremes of exclusively heterosexual attraction and exclusively homosexual attraction. Individuals who are attracted to individuals of both genders are referred to as *bisexuals*.

The origins of sexual orientation are still not well understood. Some biological theories describe sexual orientation in terms of the genetic composition of the individual. Psychological theories stress the role of early learning experiences and cognitive processes. Other theories acknowledge the confluence of genetics and the environment in the development of sexual orientation.

According to the Williams Institute of the University of California at Los Angeles School of Law, about 9 million individuals in the United States are gay, lesbian, bisexual, or transgender in orientation (Johnson, 2013). Because these individuals grow up acutely aware of the discrimination they face in North America, many do not disclose their sexual orientation; therefore, actual figures are not available.

GENDER IDENTITY
Western culture is deeply committed to the idea that there are only two sexes. Biologically speaking, however, there are many gradations running from female to male; this is known as **transgenderism**. In some cases, gender is clear; in other cases, there is a blending of both genders within the same individual; and in some cases, gender is unclear.

Intersex   About 1 in every 2,000 babies is born with an intersex condition, in which contradictions are seen among chromosomal gender, gonadal gender, internal organs, and external genital appearance. The gender of such an infant is ambiguous. What this means is that an intersexed individual has some parts usually associated with males and some parts usually associated with females. Intersex anatomy may not be apparent at birth. Sometimes it is undetected until puberty, until the individual is identified as an infertile adult, or until the individual dies and is autopsied.

Stay Current: *For more information, see the Intersex Society of North America at* **www.isna.org**.

Transsexuals   For the **transsexual** individual, sexual anatomy is not consistent with gender identity. Those who are born physically male but are emotionally and psychologically female are called male-to-female (MTF) transsexuals. Those who are born female but are emotionally and psychologically male are called female-to-male (FTM) transsexuals. The medical profession considers transsexuals to have a condition called gender dysphoria (strong and persistent feelings of discomfort with one's assigned gender) or gender identity disorder.

Most transsexuals report that they have felt gender dysphoria since early childhood. They often suffer for many years and try to hide the situation from family and friends for fear of being considered "crazy." Being transgendered puts women and men at extreme risk of the following:

- Ridicule and humiliation
- Discrimination in hiring and employment practices
- Eviction without cause from restaurants and stores
- Discrimination in housing
- Being refused medical treatment (Bradford et al., 2012).

As self-understanding and acceptance increase, many transsexuals live part or full time as members of the other sex. Cross-dressing (dressing in the clothing of the other sex) not only makes their outward appearance consistent with their inner identity and gender role, but also increases their comfort with themselves. Their sexual orientation may be heterosexual, homosexual, or bisexual.

EROTIC PREFERENCES Over a lifetime, sexual fantasies and single-partner sex are the most common sexual outlets for women and men, single and coupled individuals, and heterosexual, gay, lesbian, and bisexual individuals.

Masturbation is the self-stimulation of one's genitals for sexual pleasure. It may be an expression of the ongoing love affair that each of us has with ourselves throughout our lifetime. It is the way we discover our erotic feelings and learn about our sexual response. Mutual masturbation can provide sexual pleasuring and intimacy without hurrying to genital interaction before both partners are ready. Masturbation shared with a partner is a safe alternative to unprotected genital sex.

Male-to-female or female-to-female **oral–genital sex** is known as *cunnilingus.* This involves kissing, licking, or sucking of the female genitals, including the mons pubis, vulva, clitoris, labia, and vagina. *Fellatio* is female-to-male or male-to-male oral stimulation of the penis by licking and sucking. *Sixty-nine* is simultaneous oral–genital stimulation by two individuals. Preconceptions and myths are a major deterrent for individuals who have not tried oral sex. However, like most sexual activity, oral–genital sex is not completely free of the potential for transmission of infection, and safe sex practices must be used.

Anal stimulation can be a source of sexual pleasure because the anus has a rich nerve supply. Stimulation may be applied by fingers, mouth, or sex toys such as vibrators. The anus is surrounded by strong muscles, and the rectum contains no natural lubrication. Therefore, inserting a finger or penis into the rectum requires relaxation of the muscles and water-soluble lubricant.

A common form of sexual activity for heterosexual couples is **genital intercourse**. Various positions are used for penile–vaginal intercourse (coitus); the most common is lying face to face (with the female or male on top). Side-lying, standing, sitting, and rear-entry positions are also used. Side-lying, female-on-top, and rear-entry positions facilitate clitoral stimulation, by either penile or manual contact. The choice of intercourse positions and activities depends on physical comfort and beliefs, values, and attitudes about different practices.

During intercourse, the man moves the penis back and forth along the vaginal walls by rhythmic thrusting movements of his hips. At the same time, the woman may move her own body to match the partner's hip movements. Movements usually continue until orgasm is achieved by one or both partners. Simultaneous orgasm can be difficult to achieve. After coitus, caressing, hugging, and kissing can increase the shared intimacy.

The other form of genital intercourse is *anal intercourse,* during which the penis is inserted into the anus and rectum of the partner. Anal intercourse is commonly practiced by gay men, but a number of heterosexual couples engage in it as well. Positions for anal intercourse are similar to those for penile–vaginal intercourse, with minor differences due to the position of the anus.

Current practice dictates the use of a condom in both forms of intercourse to prevent the transmission of disease. Because anorectal tissue is not self-lubricating, a lubricant must be used on the condom. Also, because normal bacterial flora from the bowel can produce infection in other parts of the body, the used condom should be removed and another applied before inserting the penis into other body orifices.

There are many other varieties of sexuality that are beyond the scope of this module. These include several or many part-ners, nudism, swinging, group sex, fetishism, sexual sadism, and sexual masochism.

Sexual Response Cycle

Commonly occurring phases of the human sexual response follow a similar sequence in females and males regardless of sexual orientation. It does not matter whether the motive for being sexually active is true love or passionate lust. **Table 19–1** ● provides a summary of the physiological changes associated with each phase of the cycle.

The response cycle starts in the brain, with conscious sexual desires called the **desire phase**. Sexually arousing stimuli, often called *erotic stimuli,* may be real or symbolic. Sight, hearing, smell, touch, and imagination (sexual fantasy) can all invoke sexual arousal. Sexual desire fluctuates within each individual and varies from individual to individual. Someone who suppresses or blocks out conscious sexual desires may not experience any physiological response. Although psychological issues are the more common causes of lack of sexual desire, medications, drugs, and hormone imbalances can also interfere.

The **excitement phase** involves two primary physiological changes. *Vasocongestion* is an increase in the blood flow to various body parts resulting in erection of the penis and clitoris and swelling of the labia, testes, and breasts. Vasocongestion stimulates sensory receptors within these body parts, which in turn transmit messages to the conscious brain, where they are usually interpreted as pleasurable sensations. When stimulation is continued, vasocongestion increases until it either is released by orgasm or fades away. Likewise, *myotonia,* an increase of tension in muscles, may increase until released by orgasm, or it may also simply fade away.

The **orgasmic phase** is the involuntary climax of sexual tension, accompanied by physiological and psychological release. This phase is considered the measurable peak of the sexual experience (see **Figure 19–4** ●). Although the entire body is involved, the major focus of the orgasm is felt in the pelvic region. Male orgasms usually last 10–30 seconds, whereas female orgasms last

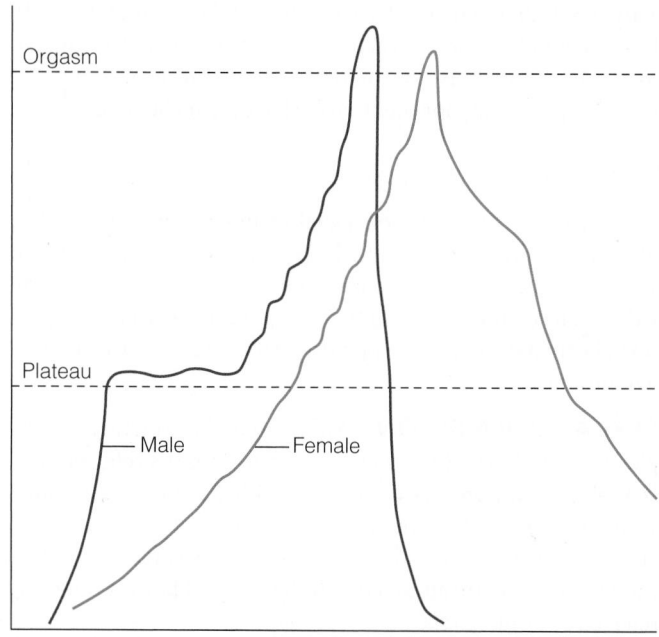

Figure 19–4 ● Phases of the sexual response cycle.

TABLE 19–1 Physiological Changes Associated With the Sexual Response Cycle

PHASE OF THE SEXUAL RESPONSE CYCLE	SIGNS PRESENT IN BOTH SEXES	SIGNS PRESENT IN MALES ONLY	SIGNS PRESENT IN FEMALES ONLY
Excitement/plateau	Muscle tension increases as excitement increases.	Penis becomes erect, testicles swell, scrotum tightens, glans size increases as excitement increases.	Erection of the clitoris.
	Sex flush, usually on chest.	Appearance of a few drops of lubricant, which may contain sperm.	Vaginal lubrication.
	Nipple erection.		Labia may increase two to three times in size.
			Breasts enlarge.
			Inner two thirds of vagina widens and lengthens; outer third swells and narrows.
			Uterus elevates.
Orgasmic	Respirations may increase to 40 breaths per minute.	Rhythmic, expulsive contractions of the penis at 0.8-second intervals.	Approximately 5–12 contractions in the orgasmic platform at 0.8-second intervals.
	Involuntary spasms of muscle groups throughout the body.	Emission of seminal fluid into the prostatic urethra from contraction of the vas deferens and accessory organs (stage 1 of the expulsive process).	Contraction of the muscles of the pelvic floor and the uterine muscles.
	Diminished sensory awareness.	Closing of the internal bladder sphincter just before ejaculation to prevent retrograde ejaculation into bladder.	Varied pattern of orgasms, including minor surges and contractions, multiple orgasms, or a simple intense orgasm similar to that of the male.
	Involuntary contractions of the anal sphincter.	Orgasm may occur without ejaculation.	
	Increased heart rate, respiratory rate, and blood pressure.	Ejaculation of semen through the penile urethra and expulsion from the urethral meatus.	
		The force of ejaculation varies from man to man and at different times, but diminishes after the first two to three contractions (stage 2 of the expulsive process).	
Resolution	Reversal of vasocongestion in 10–30 minutes; disappearance of all signs of myotonia within 5 minutes.	A refractory period during which the body will not respond to sexual stimulation; varies, depending on age and other factors, from a few moments to hours or days.	
	Genitals and breasts return to their preexcitement states.		
	Sex flush disappears in reverse order of appearance.		
	Heart rate, respiratory rate, and blood pressure return to normal.		
	Other reactions include sleepiness, relaxation, and emotional outbursts such as crying or laughing.		
	General sense of well-being; enhanced intimacy.		

Source: Based on Bridges, D. (Reviewer). (2012). Your guide to the sexual response cycle. *WebMD: Sex & Relationships.* Retrieved from http://www.webmd.com/sex-relationships/guide/sexual-health-your-guide-to-sexual-response-cycle.

10–50 seconds. Men usually have an *ejaculation* and expel **semen** as part of their orgasm. Before puberty and in later years, males experience orgasms without ejaculation.

The **resolution phase**, the period of return to the unaroused state, may last 10–15 minutes after orgasm or longer if there is no orgasm. This phase in females is quite varied; some women experience multiple successive orgasms followed by a longer period of resolution.

▶ ALTERATIONS IN SEXUAL FUNCTION

The ability to engage in sexual behavior is of great importance to most individuals, but many individuals experience transient problems with their ability to respond to sexual stimulation or to maintain the response. A small percentage of individuals will experience lifelong problems. The problems may be generalized to all sexual interactions and settings, or they may be situational, occurring in a specific setting or with specific types of sexual activity.

Alterations in other concepts/systems affect sexuality. Four of the most common are elimination, infection, mobility, and perfusion. See the Concepts Related to Sexuality feature.

It is often difficult to sort out the multiple factors contributing to an individual's or a couple's sexual problems. Generally a number of past and current factors are involved.

Past and Current Factors

Sociocultural factors interfering in sexual function include a very restrictive upbringing accompanied by inadequate sex

---

Concepts Related to **Sexuality**

Sexuality may be a source of pleasure and a sense of well-being or a source of psychological or physical problems. In addition, poor health or psychological problems can cause sexual difficulties. Sexuality, like most human experiences, is intricately related to psychological and physical elements. Psychological factors that may impact sexuality include anxiety, depression, anger, a history of sexual abuse, religious taboos, conflicts with a partner, poor communication with a partner, poor self-esteem, an inability to express needs, or a lack of knowledge about sexual arousal and stimulation

(Berge & Ward, 2012; Burri, Cherkas, & Spector, 2009; Zamboni, 2011).

Physical factors that may impact sexuality include aging, chronic disease, poor perfusion, sexually transmitted infection, and inflammation. Individuals with mobility issues related to musculoskeletal or neurological disabilities may have difficulty with sexual relations and responses. The proximity and interrelatedness of the sexual organs and organs of elimination may lead to difficulties such as urinary tract infections, urinary retention, ejaculatory issues, or anal/rectal problems and constipation.

CONCEPT	RELATIONSHIP TO SEXUALITY	NURSING IMPLICATIONS
Elimination		
■ Urinary assessment ■ Bowel assessment	*Males:* Shared outlet for urine and semen *Females:* Proximity of urethra to vagina	■ In men with prostate issues, observe for urine retention and ejaculatory issues. ■ Postcoital urinary infection is common in women.
Infection		
■ Urinary tract infection ■ Sexually transmitted infection (STI)	Infection acquired via sexual relations may affect the genitals and anus in males and females. HIV/AIDS may be acquired via sexual relations and cause immunodeficiency.	■ Be alert to signs and symptoms of STI such as penile or vaginal discharge, fever, or genital lesions. ■ Provide education in safe sex practices.
Mobility		
■ Mobility assessment ■ Assessment interview: mobility	Alterations in mobility can affect sexual relations.	■ Educate clients with mobility alterations about changes in positions that may facilitate coitus. Discuss other ways to share intimacy.
Perfusion		
■ Perfusion assessment ■ Assessment interview: perfusion ■ Coronary artery disease	Alterations in perfusion can cause erectile dysfunction due to arterial and/or venous flow.	■ Arteriosclerosis will affect the vascular supply of the penis and may lead to erectile dysfunction.

education. Rigid gender-role socialization may inhibit exploration of sexual activities, positions, toys, and other lovemaking behaviors. If the religion with which an individual is affiliated believes that sex is only for procreation, the individual may have great difficulty in celebrating the pleasure and fun of a loving sexual relationship. Another factor may be parental punishment for normally exploring one's genitals or for normal childhood sex play. In our current culture, the pressures of family and work often leave couples with too little time and not enough energy to enjoy sex.

Psychological factors may include negative feelings, such as guilt, anxiety, or fear, that interfere with the ability to experience pleasure and joy. Some individuals experience guilt when they simply enjoy sex or when they participate in what they label "unusual" sexual activities or guilt regarding the choice of the partner. Adults who have been sexually abused at any time of their lives may experience overwhelming anxiety when faced with the decision to engage in sex. Fears may include pregnancy, STIs, or pain. Because vulnerability and intimacy are inherent in most sexual relationships, fear of these may lead to an avoidance of sex. Fear of failure in sexual performance often becomes a vicious cycle; that is, fear of failure creates actual failure, which in turn produces more fear. Spectatoring is the detached appraisal of sexual performance or the body during a sexual act: "Am I going to lose my erection?" "Am I going to have an orgasm this time?" "My stomach is too flabby." "When did his thighs get that fat?" Depressed individuals lose interest in sexual activity and often experience a complete loss of sexual desire and fulfillment.

Cognitive factors include the internalization of negative expectations and beliefs. Those with low self-esteem may not understand how another individual could value and love them and also find them sexually attractive. For those who have not yet accepted their sexual orientation or gender identity, this cognitive conflict may interfere with sexual relationships.

Sexual problems may also be symptomatic of *relationship* problems. Being in conflict with or angry with one's partner is not conducive to positive sexual interaction. Some individuals lose the physical attraction to their partner or feel more attracted to someone else.

Lack of intimacy and feeling like a sex object inhibit the feeling of communion and connection that is an important part of making love. Another factor is expecting one's partner to read one's mind about sexual needs. Failure to communicate may result in one or both partners not knowing how to please the other. Unless the partners experiment, sex may, in time, become boring. Disagreements in sexual frequency and/or sexual activities may lead to further relationship conflict.

Alterations and Manifestations

Health factors can interfere with individuals' expression of sexuality. Physical changes brought on by illness, injury, or surgery may inhibit full sexual expression. Throughout your program of nursing education, you will learn about the sexual side effects of a number of diseases such as heart disease, diabetes mellitus, joint disease, cancer, and mental disorders. You will also study the impact of surgeries such as hysterectomy, prostate surgery, and radical surgeries that alter an individual's body image. Spinal cord

injuries, traumatic amputations, or disfiguring accidents negatively affect sexual functioning. The presence of an STI in one partner induces fear of transmission in the other, often resulting in abstinence from sexual contact. In some situations, the presence of an STI is unknown and transmission occurs.

Many prescription medications beyond those intended to affect sexual functioning have side effects that affect such functioning. Most frequently, the impact is negative, but sometimes there is a positive impact. **Table 19–2** provides an overview of the effects of medications on sexual function. For example, antidepressants may slow ejaculation. This may be a problem for the man who finds himself suddenly feeling unable to ejaculate. If the man is suffering from rapid ejaculation, however, the antidepressant may "cure" this problem. Some street drugs, such as marijuana, amphetamines, and cocaine, enhance sexual functioning. Others, such as opioids and anabolic steroids, interfere with sexual functioning.

SEXUAL DESIRE DISORDERS   For most individuals, sexual desire varies from day to day as well as over the years. Some individuals, however, report a deficiency in or absence of sexual fantasies and persistently low interest or a total lack of interest in sexual activity; these clients suffer from **hypoactive sexual desire disorder**. If the two individuals in a relationship are similarly uninterested in sex, there really is no problem. More typically, there is a disparity of sexual needs, and the partner with the greater desire becomes dissatisfied with the sexual relationship. The key issue in the relationship is not frequency but rather the negotiating of both partners' needs.

Sexual aversion disorder is a severe distaste for sexual activity or the thought of sexual activity, which then leads to a phobic avoidance of sex. It occurs in both women and men. Intense emotional dread of an impending sexual interaction also can trigger the physiological symptoms of anxiety: sweating, increased heart rate, and extreme muscle tension. The individual then stops the sexual interaction or prevents it from even beginning. The cause of sexual aversion disorder is usually sexual stimuli accompanied by pain. Both childhood sexual abuse or adult rape have the potential to lead to sexual aversion. More severe trauma can lead to a phobic response to sexual activity (Brotto, 2010).

SEXUAL AROUSAL DISORDERS   Sexual arousal refers to the physiological responses and subjective sense of excitement experienced during sexual activity. Lack of lubrication and failure to attain or maintain an erection are the major disorders of the arousal phase. In **female sexual arousal disorder**, the lack of vaginal lubrication causes discomfort or pain during sexual intercourse. The diagnosis of **male erectile disorder** is usually made when the man has erection problems during 25% or more of his sexual interactions. Arousal disorder may also be diagnosed even when lubrication and erection are adequate if individuals report a persistent or recurring lack of subjective sexual excitement or pleasure.

ORGASMIC DISORDERS   The term commonly applied in the past to women who did not experience orgasm, *frigid*, implied that the woman was totally incapable of responding sexually. The more accurate and objective term is **female orgasmic disorder**, which simply means that the sexual response

TABLE 19–2   Effects of Medications on Sexual Function

MEDICATION	POSSIBLE EFFECTS*
ACE inhibitors	Erectile dysfunction
Alcohol	Moderate amounts: increased sexual functioning. Large amount or chronic use: loss of inhibitions, at risk for unsafe sex, decreased sexual desire, orgasmic dysfunction, and erectile dysfunction
Alpha-blockers like prazosin (Minipress)	Inability to ejaculate due to inhibition of smooth muscle contraction in vas deferens and ejaculatory duct
Amphetamines	Increased sex drive, delayed orgasm; at risk for unsafe sex
Anabolic steroids	Decreased sex drive; shrinking of testicles and infertility in men
Antianxiety agents	Decreased sexual desire; orgasmic dysfunction in women; delayed ejaculation
Anticonvulsants like carbamazepine (Tegretol)	Decreased sexual desire; erectile dysfunction
Antidepressants	Women: decreased sexual desire, orgasmic delay or dysfunction Men: erectile dysfunction, delayed or failed ejaculation, painful erection; Desyrel may cause priapism
Antihistamines	Decreased vaginal lubrication; decreased desire
Antipsychotics	Women: decreased sexual desire, orgasmic dysfunction Men: Delayed ejaculation; ejaculatory failure; Thorazine may cause priapism
Antiulcers (e.g., cimetidine [Tagamet] and omeprazole [Prilosec])	Decreased libido; erectile dysfunction in men
Barbiturates	In low doses, increased sexual pleasure; in large doses, decreased sexual desire, orgasmic dysfunction, and erectile dysfunction
Beta-blockers like metoprolol (Toprol)	Decreased sexual desire; erectile dysfunction
Cardiotonics (Beta agonists)	Decreased sexual desire; erectile dysfunction, ejaculatory failure
Cocaine	Increased intensity of sexual experience; with chronic use, decreased sexual desire and sexual dysfunction
Diuretics	Decreased sexual desire; erectile dysfunction
Fibrates	Erectile dysfunction
Marijuana	As above for cocaine, but prolonged use reduces testosterone levels and reduces sperm production
Narcotics	Inhibited sexual desire and response; erectile dysfunction

Sources: Based on Dean, J. (Reviewer). (2012). Are your medicines disrupting your sex life? *Netdoctor.* Retrieved from http://www.netdoctor.co.uk/sexandrelationships/medicinessex.htm; Adams, M., & Koch, R. (2010). *Pharmacology: Connections to nursing practice.* Upper Saddle River, NJ: Pearson; Delvin, D. (2012). Sex and alcohol. *Netdoctor.* Retrieved from http://www.netdoctor.co.uk/sex_relationships/facts/sexalcohol.htm; and WebMD Editorial Team. (2013). Erectile dysfunction and priapism. *Erectile Dysfunction Health Center.* Retrieved from http://www.webmd.com/erectile-dysfunction/guide/erectile-dysfunction-priapism.

The nurse and client must familiarize themselves with the specific medication prescribed or used, because effects vary in each category of drug.

stops before orgasm occurs. *Preorgasmic* women have never experienced an orgasm. Studies indicate that 10%–15% of women are preorgasmic, and another 20%–22% report irregular orgasms. Compounding the orgasmic difficulty is the associated anxiety. In the preoccupation with orgasm, the real goal of being sexual—mutual pleasuring and intimacy—is lost, and the interchange can become one of anxiety, frustration, and anger (Dahir, 2013; McKay, 2011).

Some men suffer from **male orgasmic disorder**. Men with this disorder can maintain an erection for long periods (an hour or more) but have extreme difficulty ejaculating, referred to as *retarded ejaculation*. In heterosexual intercourse, the difficulty may be limited to ejaculation in the vagina. Some men ejaculate after self-stimulation or manual or oral stimulation by the partner; others have great difficulty ejaculating with any type of stimulation. This disorder is much less common than rapid ejaculation.

Rapid ejaculation is one of the most common sexual dysfunctions among men. There are many definitions, with descriptions including ejaculating before being touched, ejaculating before penetration, ejaculating with one internal thrust,

and ejaculating within a minute or two of penetration. A more helpful description is the absence of voluntary control of ejaculation. The problem is best self-defined, as when a man is concerned about his ejaculatory control or the couple agrees that ejaculation is too rapid for mutual satisfaction.

SEXUAL PAIN DISORDERS   Both women and men can experience dyspareunia, which is associated with many physiological causes, especially those that inhibit lubrication. Thus, skin irritations, vaginal infections, estrogen deficiencies, and use of medications that dry vaginal secretions can cause women to experience discomfort with intercourse.

Pelvic disorders, such as infections, lesions, endometriosis, scar tissue, or tumors, can result in painful intercourse. In males, infection or inflammation of the glans penis or other genitourinary organs can cause pain with intercourse. Also, some contraceptive foams, creams, sponges, or latex products can irritate either the vagina or the penis.

Vaginismus is the involuntary spasm of the outer one third of the vaginal muscles, making penetration of the vagina painful and sometimes impossible. The woman often experiences desire, excitement, and orgasm with stimulation of the external sexual structures. Attempts at intercourse, however, elicit the involuntary spasm. The woman may have similar difficulty undergoing pelvic exams and inserting tampons or a diaphragm.

Vulvodynia is constant, unremitting burning that is localized to the vulva with an acute onset. The girl or woman has problems in sitting, standing, and sleeping related to the intensity of pain. **Vestibulitis** causes severe pain only on touch or attempted vaginal entry. Half of the women with vestibulitis report lifelong dyspareunia. Women with either of these disorders report a negative impact on their sexual functioning and partner relationships, as well as their self-esteem and mental health (Dahir, 2013).

PROBLEMS WITH SATISFACTION   Some individuals experience sexual desire, arousal, and orgasm yet feel dissatisfied with their sexual relationships. These sexual problems are more commonly related to the emotional tone of the relationship than to the physiological response. Because giving and receiving pleasure in a mutually intimate relationship are the primary goals of sex for most individuals, **dissatisfaction problems** may be more disturbing than other types of sexual dysfunctions.

At times, satisfaction problems may be situational. For example, one partner may choose an inconvenient time, or a partner may feel anxious and therefore cannot experience much pleasure or joy. Some individuals describe their problems as being related to lack of extragenital satisfaction. These individuals describe how much they miss and continue to need all the touching and caressing of their earlier lovemaking experiences. Unfortunately, couples who have been relating sexually for a long time often become genitally focused and neglect the rest of the body. One or both partners may feel touch starved, long for more extragenital loving, and become dissatisfied with sex.

Satisfaction problems are often related to relationship difficulties. The inability to communicate effectively in other relationship areas frequently results in sexual frustration. Partners who are angry with each other and make love without resolving the conflict may feel unhappy about the relationship despite having experienced arousal and orgasm. Couples who define their relationship in terms of rigid, unequal power and gender roles may have difficulty negotiating and compromising about sexual issues. Not infrequently, the individual with the least amount of power feels helpless and dissatisfied with the sexual interchanges.

Lack of intimacy or a feeling of connectedness is understandably related to satisfaction problems. If an individual has sex with a stranger, the body may function well, but there is often a sense of something missing after the sexual experience. Making love to one individual while feeling more attracted to or in love with another individual can result in feelings of emptiness or disconnection. Even couples in a committed relationship may complain of lack of intimacy. Dissatisfaction issues include lack of romance, love, tenderness, and nurturance. Fulfillment of sexuality, then, depends on the ability to relate to a partner in an intimate and mutually pleasing manner that is compatible with one's values and chosen lifestyle.

Clients at risk for altered sexual patterns include those experiencing the following:

- Altered body structure or function due to trauma, pregnancy, recent childbirth, anatomical abnormalities of the genitals, or any of a variety of diseases
- Physical, psychosocial, emotional, or sexual abuse; sexual assault
- Disfiguring conditions, such as burns, skin conditions, birthmarks, scars (e.g., mastectomy), and ostomies
- Specific medication therapy that causes sexual problems (see Table 19–2)
- Temporary or long-term impaired physical ability to perform grooming and maintain sexual attractiveness
- Value conflicts between personal beliefs and religious doctrine
- Loss of a partner
- Lack of knowledge about or misinformation about sexual functioning and expression.

Prevalence

Numerous studies have attempted to determine the prevalence of sexual dysfunction in specific populations. The general agreement in these studies is that sexual dysfunction is more prevalent in women than in men (Dahir, 2013). Some of these studies indicate that hypoactive sexual desire disorder occurs in 1%–38% of the men studied and 31%–49% of women studied (Zamboni, 2011). The most prevalent male sexual dysfunction is erectile dysfunction (ED). About 30 million men are reported to have been affected by ED. The incidence is age related with an estimated 52% of men between the ages of 40 and 70 reporting ED (Meng, Stoller, & Walsh, 2011).

The prevalence of female sexual dysfunction (FSD) has been more widely studied, but is very difficult to measure because of the variation in definitions and the varying degrees of perceived severity of dysfunction that women may experience (Burri et al., 2009). Shifren and colleagues (2008) conducted a landmark national survey of 31,581 adult female respondents and determined that the prevalence rate for any sexual problem, including desire, arousal, and orgasm problems, was 43.1%. This finding is similar to the findings of several smaller population studies (Berge & Ward, 2012).

Genetic Considerations

Recently reported gene studies indicate that there is a genetic influence on female sexual functioning (Burri et al., 2009, 2012). A genome-wide association study on polymorphisms in more than 1,000 adult female twin pairs corresponded with data on the twins' lifelong sexual functioning revealed an association on the phenotypic dimension of arousal with a serotonin receptor gene previously shown to be involved in female sexuality (Burri et al., 2012). Although not conclusive, this research does implicate serotonin and GABA pathways as potential sources of FSD symptoms. Successful identification of genes underlying FSD will help medical scientists identify, diagnose, and treat FSD. It will also help to destigmatize societal opinions about FSD (Burri et al., 2009).

Alterations and Therapies **Sexuality**

ALTERATION	DESCRIPTION	MANIFESTATIONS	INTERVENTIONS AND THERAPIES
Priapism	Persistent penile erection unrelated to sexual stimulation	▪ Erection of the penis lasting 4 hours or longer; can lead to scarring and permanent erectile dysfunction.	▪ Ice packs to reduce swelling ▪ Surgical ligation of artery ▪ Intracavernous injection ▪ Aspiration ▪ Surgical shunt of blood flow
Orgasmic disorder	Inability to reach a satisfactory conclusion or orgasm from sexual activity	▪ Unable to attain orgasm.	▪ Assess for possible physical cause. ▪ Cognitive behavioral therapy, psychotherapy
Sexual arousal disorder	Lack of a normal sexual response to stimuli	▪ No vaginal lubrication in response to stimulation; unable to attain or maintain an erection; no sexual excitement	▪ Lubricants for the vagina ▪ Medications for erection (e.g., Viagra)
Sexual pain disorders	Pain during or immediately after intercourse	▪ Pain at entry of penis to vagina; pain with deep thrusting ▪ Painful vulva all the time ▪ Vaginismus (tight introitus)	▪ Screens for vaginal infection or STI ▪ Topical lidocaine; topical estrogen ▪ Pelvic floor physical therapy ▪ Use of dilators to gradually increase vaginal size ▪ Psychological counseling
Menstrual dysfunction	Abnormal vaginal bleeding or pain during or immediately after menstruation	▪ Vaginal bleeding at times other than menses or heavy bleeding at menses ▪ Painful menses	▪ Hormonal therapy including oral contraceptives ▪ Dilation and curettage ▪ Hysterectomy
Sexually transmitted infections	Infections obtained through sexual contact	▪ May be no manifestations ▪ Abnormal drainage from vagina or penis ▪ Chancre sores, herpes blisters, warts	▪ Bacterial infection treated with antibiotics ▪ Viral infection treated with antivirals ▪ Fungal infection treated with antifungals ▪ Surgery for removal of genital warts

Sources: Based on WebMD Editorial Team. (2013). Erectile dysfunction and priapism. *Erectile Dysfunction Health Center.* Retrieved from http://www.webmd.com/erectile-dysfunction/guide/erectile-dysfunction-priapism; Dahir, M. (2013). Women and sexuality. In E. Youngkin, M. Davis, D. Schadewald, & C. Juve (Eds.), *Women's health: A primary care clinical guide* (4th ed., pp. 119–149). Boston, MA: Pearson; and Workowski, K. & Berman, S. (2010). Sexually transmitted diseases treatment guidelines, 2010. *Morbidity and Mortality Weekly Report, 59*(RR12), 1–110.

CASE STUDY \\ PART 1

The Jarvis family lives in a comfortable home in the suburb of a large city. Ralph Jarvis, 45, has his own construction business and has prospered, particularly in the past 5 years. His wife Betty, 42, is a homemaker and hospital volunteer. They have two children. Matthew, 15, is into sports at school and is very popular. Jolene, 12½, is doing well in school and is friendly and outgoing. Eileen, Ralph's mother, came to live with the Jarvises when her husband Tom was killed in a car crash 2 years ago.

Today, Betty Jarvis has brought Jolene to the pediatrician's office for a check-up and her immunizations. In the interview with

the nurse before seeing the nurse practitioner, Mrs. Jarvis explains that she is concerned because Jolene has not started her periods. She tells the nurse, "My sister and I started when we were eleven."

Clinical Reasoning Questions Level I

1. What is the first physical sign that Jolene is beginning puberty?
2. What Tanner stage evidence would be seen if Jolene is nearing menarche?
3. What is the average age for menarche in the United States?

Clinical Reasoning Questions Level II

4. What is the priority nursing diagnosis for Jolene and her mother? Why?

5. *Refer to the exemplar on Menstrual Dysfunction within this module*: At what age would a girl with secondary sexual characteristics who has not started her periods be diagnosed as having primary amenorrhea?

6. *Refer to the exemplar on Sexually Transmitted Infections within this module*: The immunization to prevent a sexually transmitted virus and cervical cancer could be administered to Jolene today. What is that immunization?

▶ PREVENTION

Sexual relationships depend on one's health. Choosing a healthy lifestyle similar to life choices that enhance heart health will help prevent sexual dysfunction. These choices should include good nutrition, regular exercise, and avoidance of tobacco products, illicit drugs, and excessive alcohol.

Screening tests related to sexuality include regular physical checkups and screening for hypercholesterolemia and hypertension. Screenings specific to the reproductive system for women include Pap tests, clinical breast exams, mammography, screenings for STIs, and offering of HIV testing at each visit. These screenings should occur at regular intervals depending on the age of the woman. Screening tests specific for men include screening for prostate cancer with digital rectal examination after age 50 and prostate specific antigen (PSA) testing for men at high risk.

Two vaccines (Gardasil and Cervarix) to protect against infection from the human papilloma virus are now available. Both protect women from cervical cancer, and Gardasil also protects against genital warts and cancer of the anus, vagina, and vulva, and it is available for females and males. Human papillomavirus (HPV) vaccines offer the best protection when three vaccine doses are delivered on the approved schedule before clients become sexually active. Therefore, vaccination with Gardasil is recommended for preteen girls and boys. It is also recommended for teen boys and girls who were not vaccinated when they were younger, and for young women up to age 26 and young men up to age 21 (CDC, 2013d).

▶ ASSESSMENT

Nursing Assessment

ASSESSING MEN   The history or health assessment interview involves what the client shares about his sexual concern or problems with the reproductive system. The interview may be conducted during a health screening, it may focus on a chief complaint (such as a discharge from the penis), or it may be part of a total health assessment. Ideally, the health assessment interview precedes the physical examination. The interview is a time when the nurse can establish a relationship with the client that is professional and nonthreatening. A man may perceive the interview as less threatening if the discussion begins with more general questions and then progresses to specific questions and if questions are asked in a way that gives him permission to describe behaviors and manifestations. For example, rather than asking a man whether he has difficulty achieving or

---

Assessment Interview **Male Sexuality**

Current Sexuality Problem

■ When did you first notice difficulty having an erection?

■ Describe the changes in your ability to have an erection after you started taking medicine for high blood pressure.

■ Have you tried any medications or remedies to help achieve an erection?

Past Medical History

■ Do you have any chronic diseases such as diabetes, cardiovascular disease, or thyroid disease?

■ Have you ever had surgery of the penis or prostate?

Psychosocial History

■ Do you use tobacco products? If so, how much and how often?

■ Do you use alcohol? If so, how much and how often?

■ Do you use illegal drugs? If so, how much and how often?

---

maintaining an erection, the nurse could ask him to describe any changes he has noticed in his erections.

Men may be embarrassed to discuss health problems or concerns involving their reproductive organs. The nurse can help men feel more comfortable by asking questions in a nonthreatening, matter-of-fact manner. It is best to consider the psychological, social, and cultural factors that affect sexuality and sexual activity during the interview. Use words that the man can understand, and do not be embarrassed or offended by the words he uses.

If the man has a health problem, analyze its onset, characteristics and course, severity, precipitating and relieving factors, and any associated symptoms, noting the timing and circumstances. Examples of questions to ask appear in the Assessment Interview feature.

The nurse should ask about any medications, over-the-counter drugs, herbal supplements, or vitamins the man may be taking in order to determine if any of these substances may be affecting the reproductive system. This is also a good time to assess what the man may be using in an effort to relieve the symptoms. Men may be reluctant to discuss the use of Viagra, but it is important to ask because of the potential drug interactions that may occur.

It is a very good practice to ask clients about their allergies during the interview in anticipation of any medications that may be ordered. If a procedure is planned, the nurse should also determine if the client has a latex allergy.

In questioning a man about his medical history, ask about chronic illnesses such as diabetes, cardiovascular disease, and thyroid disease. The effects of these illnesses and the treatments prescribed may cause **impotence** (the inability to achieve or maintain an erection). Drugs that affect sexuality are listed in Table 19–2 earlier in this module.

If a man was born to a woman who was treated during pregnancy with diethylstilbestrol (DES), a drug used from 1938 to 1971 to prevent miscarriage, he may be prone to benign epididymal cysts (American Cancer Society [ACS], 2012).

Past surgical procedures affecting the genitoreproductive system may affect sexuality. For instance, prostatectomy may lead to impotence. If a man had mumps as a child, sterility is possible. The risk for testicular cancer is greatest in White men between the ages of 20 and 34, born in the United States or Europe. Other risk factors include history of an undescended testicle and a brother with testicular cancer (slight risk) (ACS, 2013b).

Explore the man's lifestyle, stressors, and social history. Ask about the use of alcohol, tobacco products, or street drugs that may affect sexual function. Frequent sexual intercourse, especially if unprotected, increases the potential for STIs, including HIV infection. Ask about sexual preference. Sexual intercourse with same-sex partners further increases the risk for HIV infection. Other questions about sexuality may include number of sexual partners; history of premature ejaculation, impotence, or other sexual problems; any history of sexual trauma; use of condoms or other contraceptives; and current level of sexual satisfaction.

ASSESSING WOMEN The history or health assessment interview involves what the client shares about her sexual concern or problems with the reproductive system. The interview may be conducted during a health screening, it may focus on a chief complaint (such as a discharge from the vagina), or it may be part of a total health assessment. Ideally, the health assessment interview precedes the physical examination. The interview is a time when the nurse can establish a relationship with the client that is professional and nonthreatening. The woman may perceive the interview as less threatening if the discussion begins with more general questions and then progresses to specific questions. Questions should be asked in a way that gives the client permission to describe behaviors and manifestations. For example, ask about menstrual and childbirth history before asking questions about STIs.

Women may be embarrassed to discuss health problems or concerns involving their reproductive organs. To help women feel more comfortable the nurse should ask questions in a nonthreatening, matter-of-fact manner. Consider the psychological, social, and cultural factors that affect sexuality and sexual activity. Use words that the woman can understand, and do not be embarrassed or offended by the words she uses.

The focused interview for the female reproductive system should be tailored to the woman's specific health problem. As with the assessment of other body systems, analyze and document the onset of the problem, its duration, frequency, precipitating and relieving factors, any associated symptoms, treatment, self-care, and outcomes. The Assessment Interview feature lists some specific examples of questions to ask.

The nurse should ask about any medications, over-the-counter drugs, herbal supplements, or vitamins the woman may be taking in order to determine whether any of these substances may be affecting the reproductive system. This is also a good time to assess what the woman may be using in an effort to relieve the symptoms. The nurse should ask specifically about birth control pills or other hormonal methods because many women forget to mention taking birth control pills or using a progestin intrauterine device. It is a very good practice to ask clients about their allergies during the interview in anticipation of any medications that may be ordered. If a procedure is planned, the nurse should also determine if the client has a latex allergy.

Assessment Interview **Female Sexuality**

Current Sexuality Problem
- When did you first experience painful intercourse?
- Is the pain occurring just as the penis enters the vagina or is it with deep thrusting?
- Have you tried any medications or remedies for the pain? Have these things helped?
- When was your last menstrual period?

Past Medical History
- Do you have or have you had endometriosis?
- Have you ever had gynecological surgery?

Psychosocial History
- Do you use tobacco, alcohol, or drugs?
- Is there anyone at home who is hurting you?

Taking a client's past medical history includes asking questions about chronic illnesses, gynecological surgery, menstrual history, and obstetrical history. Chronic illnesses may affect the function of the female reproductive system. For instance, diabetes mellitus increases the risk of vaginal infections and vaginal dryness, both of which interfere with sexual pleasure. Chronic heavy menstrual flow may result in anemia. Thyroid and adrenal disorders may affect secondary sex characteristics, the **menstrual cycle**, and the ability to become pregnant.

Obtaining any family history of cancer is important. The risk for endometrial cancer is higher in women with a family history of endometrial, breast, or colon cancer; the risk for ovarian cancer is higher in women with a family history of ovarian or breast cancer; and the risk for breast cancer is higher in women with a family history of breast cancer. Other aspects of family history may also be important. Exposure to diethylstilbestrol (DES) in utero increases the risk of cancer of the cervix and vagina (ACS, 2012).

Psychosocial information should be assessed also. This would include asking about the use of condoms during intercourse; unprotected sexual intercourse increases the risk of STIs, including HIV infection. Also ask about smoking; a history of smoking increases the risk of circulatory problems in the woman taking oral contraceptives. Smoking also increases the risk for cancer of the cervix. Exposure to asbestos poses a risk of cancer of the ovary.

Questions about sexuality may include sexual preference, number of sexual partners; history of **anorgasmia** (absence of orgasm), dyspareunia (painful intercourse), or other problems with intercourse; history of sexual trauma; use of contraceptives or condoms; and current level of sexual satisfaction.

ASSESSING ADOLESCENTS The approach to the adolescent client should be guided by a consideration of the teen's cognitive and social development, especially when making decisions about issues such as parental involvement during the history interview and physical examination. As with adults, a nonjudgmental attitude is very important. It is also important to show a genuine interest in the teen and to sustain that interest throughout the encounter. Try to focus on the adolescent, not the problem. When discussing sexual organs, use specific language and choose words that the adolescent understands.

Often the teen it too shy, embarrassed, or scared to ask questions about sex or sexual organs. The nurse may have to start the discussion (Satterwhite, 2013). It is important to end the history interview with asking the teen what other questions he or she may have about sex.

It is a good practice to ask parents to leave the room during part of the history beginning around ages 10–11. Time alone with the nurse will allow the teen to discuss issues that he or she does not want to discuss in front of the parent (Szilagyi, 2013). Teens should understand that everything discussed is confidential unless it affects the safety of the teen.

The examination of the adolescent is much the same as for the adult with the exception of the addition of assigning a sex maturity rating based on Tanner staging. For girls, changes in the breasts are the first sign of puberty. When the breasts develop to stage 3 or 4, menarche is expected and the growth spurt is over (Szilagyi, 2013). Pelvic examination of teen girls is done only when necessary due to a problem. The technique of speculum examination is the same as for an adult, however, the nurse should show the teen the speculum, let her handle it, and explain the procedure carefully before proceeding. A gentle, unhurried approach is needed and a chaperone should be present.

For adolescent males, the examination is much the same as for the adult with the addition of assigning sex maturity ratings based on secondary sexual characteristics. Increased size of the testes is the first sign of puberty and is seen between the ages of 9 and 13 (Szilagyi, 2013). Increasing amounts of pubic hair and progressive growth of the penis are expected sexual characteristics and will reach adult proportions by about ages 16–17. The nurse should have a chaperone present during the examination of adolescent boys.

Physical Assessment

In performing a physical assessment involving the breasts, genitalia, and rectum, the nurse should be very professional in approach in order to reduce the client's anxiety. These parts of the body are considered by most as very personal and private, making it very important that the nurse be nonjudgmental, gentle, and empathetic. The nurse must also use caution to avoid misperception by the client of sexual harassment or sexual abuse. This can be accomplished by touching in a nonintimate fashion, obtaining consent from the client before performing any assessment or procedure, and explaining what will happen before proceeding. It is always best to have another healthcare provider in the room during physical examination of the genitalia.

See the features on Male Reproductive System Assessment and Female Reproductive System Assessment.

Lifespan and Cultural Considerations

Many factors influence an individual's sexuality. Discussed here are family, culture, religion, and personal expectations and ethics.

FAMILY   For the majority of us, the family is the earliest and most enduring social relationship. Families are the fabric of our day-to-day lives and shape the quality of our lives by influencing our outlooks on life, our motivations, our strategies for

achievement, and our styles for coping with adversity. It is within our families that we develop our gender identity, body image, sexual self-concept, and capacity for intimacy. Through family interactions, we learn about relationships and gender roles and our expectations of others and ourselves.

From earliest beginnings, children observe their parents and model themselves after these adults. If parents are able to share affection with one another and other family members, children will most likely become adults who are able to give and receive affection. If parents seldom hug, hold hands, or kiss each other, their children may become adults who are very uncomfortable with romantic touch. If family gender-role behavior is very rigid, arguments and hurt feelings will abound if an individual from this system is partnered with an individual who grew up in an androgynous family system. Family messages about sex range from "sex is so shameful it shouldn't be talked about" to "sex is a joyful part of adult relationships." The following are some common sexual messages children get from their families:

- Sex is dirty.
- Premarital sex is sinful.
- Good girls don't do it.
- Masturbation is disgusting.
- Men should be the sexual experts.
- Sex is mainly for procreating.
- Bodies, including genitals, are beautiful.
- Sex should be fun for both women and men.
- Sexual thoughts and feelings are natural.
- Masturbation is a common, pleasurable activity.
- There is great variety in sexual behaviors.

CULTURE   Sexuality is regulated by the individual's culture. For example, culture influences the sexual nature of dress, rules about marriage, expectations of role behavior and social responsibilities, and specific sex practices. Societal attitudes vary widely. Attitudes about childhood sexual play with self or with children of the same gender or other gender may be restrictive or permissive. Premarital and extramarital sex and homosexuality may be unacceptable or tolerated. Polygamy (several marriage partners) or monogamy (one marriage partner) may be the norm. Gender-role behavior also varies from culture to culture. Culture is so much a part of everyday life that it is taken for granted. We tend to assume that others share our own perspective, including those for whom we provide care. It is impossible to provide sensitive nursing care if we believe that our own culture is more important than, and preferable to, any other culture.

Cultures differ with regard to which body parts they find to be erotic. In some cultures, legs are erotic and breasts are not. Body weight may also be a determinant of sexual attractiveness. There is a great deal of pressure in American culture to be very thin. Women who would be considered obese in America are considered highly attractive in other cultures. The degree of public nudity ranges from women's entire bodies and faces being covered in Islamic societies to complete nudity in some cultures in New Guinea and Australia.

Male Reproductive System Assessment

ASSESSMENT/ METHOD	NORMAL FINDINGS	ABNORMAL FINDINGS	LIFESPAN OR DEVELOPMENTAL CONSIDERATIONS
Breast and Lymph Node Assessment			
Inspect and palpate the breasts and lymph nodes.	Breasts in men are flat with an erect nipple and an areola that is darker than the surrounding skin. The axillary area should be free of lesions and masses. Axillary and infraclavicular lymph nodes are usually nonpalpable.	■ An enlarged, smooth, firm, mobile, tender disk of breast tissue behind the areola indicates **gynecomastia** (abnormal enlargement of the breasts in men). ■ A hard, irregular nodule in or near the nipple area suggests carcinoma. ■ Enlarged axillary nodes are common with infections of the hands or arms but may be caused by cancer of the breast. Enlarged supraclavicular nodes may indicate breast cancer metastasis.	■ Adolescent boys may have gynecomastia related to changes in hormones. Most cases will resolve without treatment.
External Genitalia Assessment			
Inspect inguinal and femoral area for hernias. Ask the man to bear down or cough as you palpate (**Figure 19–5 ●**). Inspect and palpate the inguinal lymph nodes.	There should be no bulging in these areas. Inguinal lymph nodes are normally nonpalpable.	■ A bulge that increases with cough or straining suggests a hernia. ■ Palpable or tender inguinal lymph nodes suggest infection of the lower abdomen, external genitalia, perianal area, leg, and foot.	■ Indirect hernia is the most common hernia in all ages and both genders. ■ Direct hernias are more common in men older than age 40.
Inspect the glans. If uncircumcised, ask him to retract the foreskin.	When nonerect, the penis is soft, flaccid, nontender, without lesions.	■ **Phimosis** (tightness of the foreskin that prevents retraction) may be congenital or due to recurrent inflammation. Narrow or inflamed foreskin may cause paraphimosis if the retraction of the foreskin becomes trapped over the glans and tightens on the penis, causing painful swelling. ■ Balanitis (inflammation of the glans) is associated with infection, irritation, or trauma. ■ Ulcers, vesicles, or warts suggest the presence of an STI. ■ Nodules or sores on the glans seen in uncircumcised men may be cancer.	■ Although phimosis and paraphimosis can occur at any age, both are more common in children.
Inspect the external urinary meatus. Press the glans between the thumb and forefinger to inspect inside (**Figure 19–6 ●**). Replace foreskin if appropriate.	The external urinary meatus is in the center of the glans, without lesions, redness, or discharge.	■ Erythema or discharge indicates inflammatory disease. Further assessment is required.	

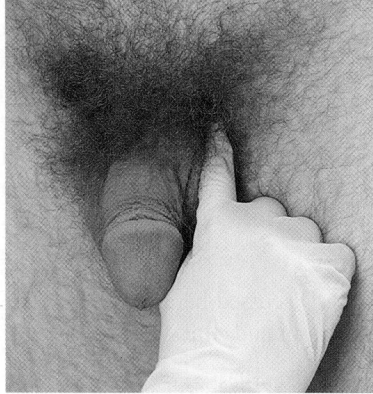

Figure 19–5 ● Palpating the male inguinal area for bulges.

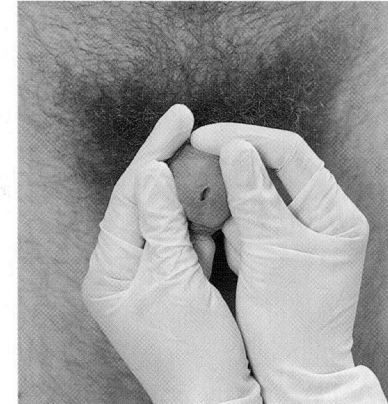

Figure 19–6 ● Inspecting the external urinary meatus of the male.

Male Reproductive System Assessment (continued)

ASSESSMENT/ METHOD	NORMAL FINDINGS	ABNORMAL FINDINGS	LIFESPAN OR DEVELOPMENTAL CONSIDERATIONS
Inspect and palpate the shaft of the penis.	Skin on shaft should be without lesions or redness. The shaft should be free of masses and nontender.	■ Excoriation or inflammation suggests lice, scabies, or fungal infection. ■ Vesicles or chancre suggests herpes or syphilis. ■ Fibrous plaques may be palpable in Peyronie disease.	■ The penis decreases in size with age.
Inspect the scrotum. If swollen, use transillumination: Darken room and place lighted flashlight behind and against the scrotum.	The scrotum hangs freely from the perineum. It is usually covered with hair. Testes and epididymis do not transilluminate.	■ A unilateral or bilateral poorly developed scrotum suggests **cryptorchidism** (failure of one or both testes to descend into the scrotum). ■ Swelling of the scrotum may indicate hernia, **hydrocele** (accumulation of fluid), or scrotal edema. Serous swelling will transilluminate; blood or tissue will not. ■ A scrotal mass may be hernia where bowel loops have descended into the scrotum. ■ A unilateral scrotal mass that feels like a "bag of worms" is a **varicocele** (varicosities of the spermatic cord).	■ Cryptorchidism is usually detected in infant boys. ■ Hydrocele is more common in newborn males. ■ The scrotum of older men sags and the testicles are smaller and lower in the scrotum. ■ Adult men with varicocele may have difficulty with fertility because of increased heat in the scrotum.
Palpate each testis and epididymis.	Testes are smooth, firm, slightly tender. The epididymis is a comma-shaped organ on the posterior of each testis.	■ Tender, painful scrotal swelling occurs in acute epididymitis, orchitis, testicular torsion, and strangulated hernia. ■ A painless nodule in the testis is associated with testicular cancer and needs to be further investigated.	■ Testicular torsion is more common in adolescents and is a surgical emergency. ■ Testicular cancer occurs infrequently and is more likely to affect teens and young adults.

Prostate Assessment

Assess the prostate via digital rectal examination (DRE). Inspect the anal area before DRE. Have the client lean over the exam table or lie on left side with right knee drawn up to expose anal area. With gloved, well-lubricated index finger, palpate the anterior rectal wall for the rounded, two-lobed posterior prostate. The single anterior lobe is nonpalpable.	The anal area should be free of lesions or excoriation. The prostate is nontender, smooth, about 2.5 cm long with a palpable median sulcus between the lobes.	■ Inflammation or excoriation of the anal area indicates infection, excoriation, or trauma. ■ Prostate enlargement with obliteration of the median sulcus suggests benign prostatic hyperplasia. ■ Painful enlargement with asymmetry and tenderness suggests prostatitis. A hard, irregular nodule is suspicious of carcinoma.	■ Disorders of the prostate affect adult men. Benign prostatic hyperplasia affects nearly all men ages 85 and older.

Sources: Adapted from Bickley, L., & Szilagyi, P. (2013). *Bates' guide to physical examination and history taking* (11th ed.). Philadelphia, PA: Wolters Kluwer/Lippincott Williams & Wilkins; and Caudle, P., & Osborn, K. (2014). Caring for the patient with male reproductive disorders. In K. Osborn, C. Wraa, A. Watson, & R. Holleran (Eds.), *Medical–surgical nursing: Preparation for practice* (2nd ed., pp. 1286–1311). Boston, MA: Pearson.

Female Reproductive System Assessment

ASSESSMENT/METHOD	NORMAL FINDINGS	ABNORMAL FINDINGS	LIFESPAN OR DEVELOPMENTAL CONSIDERATIONS
Breast Assessment			
Inspect both breasts with woman sitting with arms at sides, arms overhead, hands pressed on hips, leaning forward. Lift breasts and inspect underneath.	Breasts vary in size and shape and one breast may be normally larger than the other. Color is same as other skin; tone is firm, texture smooth.	■ Retractions, dimpling (*peau d'orange*), erythema, and prominent venous patterns suggest underlying lesions and should be further investigated.	■ Thelarche (beginning of breast development) occurs around ages 9–11. ■ Breasts enlarge during pregnancy. ■ Breasts lose fat and begin to sag in older women.
Inspect the areolae and nipples.	Color is slightly darker than surrounding skin (dark pink to dark brown). Montgomery tubercles (sebaceous glands) may be present. Nipples are usually equal in size and position bilaterally. Nipples are usually everted, but may be normally inverted or flat.	■ Lesions, excoriation, or discharge may denote skin infection, mechanical injury, or lactation. *Peau d'orange* may appear first on the areola. Recent unilateral inversion of the nipple or asymmetry in pointing direction suggests underlying malignancy.	
Palpate both breasts. **Figure 19–7** ● illustrates a pattern for breast palpation. It is important that every part of the breast, including the axillary tail (tail of Spence) be palpated. The breasts are palpated with the woman in a supine position, one at a time, with a small pillow under the shoulder and the arm extended over the head.	Breasts should feel smooth, firm, and elastic. Many women have nodularity or lumpiness that is uniform in both breasts (fibrocystic changes related to cyclic hormones).	■ Tenderness may be related to premenstrual fullness, fibrocystic changes, inflammation. Tenderness has also been associated with cancer. ■ Nodules in the tail of the breast may be enlarged lymph nodes (pectoral nodes of the axilla). Hard, irregular, fixed unilateral masses that are poorly delineated suggests carcinoma. Bilateral, single or multiple, round, mobile, well-delineated masses are consistent with fibrocystic breast changes or fibroadenoma. Swelling, tenderness, erythema, and heat may be seen with mastitis or inflammatory breast cancer.	■ Breast cancer occurs more often among older women.

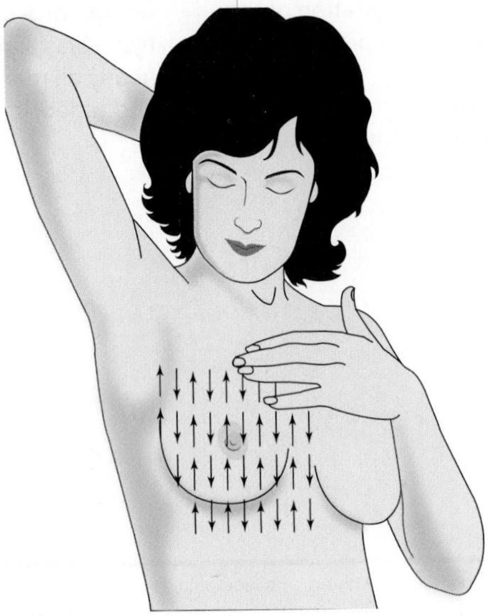

Figure 19–7 ● Pattern for palpation of the breast.

Female Reproductive System Assessment (continued)

ASSESSMENT/METHOD	NORMAL FINDINGS	ABNORMAL FINDINGS	LIFESPAN OR DEVELOPMENTAL CONSIDERATIONS
Palpate the nipple and areola.	Nipples should be firm and elastic; without discharge.	■ Loss of nipple elasticity is seen in cancer. Bloody or serous discharge is associated with intraductal papilloma. ■ Bilateral milky discharge not due to pregnancy or lactation is known as **galactorrhea**, which may be associated with pituitary tumor or certain drugs. Unilateral discharge from one or two ducts may be seen in fibrocystic breast changes, intraductal papilloma, or carcinoma.	■ The nipple ducts of middle-aged and older women are more palpable.

Axillary and Clavicular Lymph Node Assessment

With the client sitting, inspect the axilla and clavicular areas. Palpate the axillary nodes in the central, lateral, pectoral, and subscapular areas (**Figure 19–8 ●**). Palpate the supraclavicular (above the clavicle) lymph nodes.	The axillary areas are covered in hair unless shaved. The skin is the color of surrounding skin and free of lesions. Axillary and supraclavicular nodes are usually nonpalpable.	■ Redness, rash, irritation, or lesions may be due to allergy, shaving, or infection of the sweat glands or hair follicles. ■ Enlarged axillary nodes may be due to infection in the hand or arm or may be caused by breast malignancy. Enlarged supraclavicular nodes are associated with metastasis from abdominal or thoracic carcinoma or generalized lymph swelling from systemic disease.	

Hernia and Lymph Node Assessment

Inspect inguinal and femoral area with the woman standing. Palpate for inguinal lymph nodes.	The inguinal and femoral areas should be free of bulging masses. Inguinal lymph nodes are normally nonpalpable.	■ Bulge above the inguinal ligament denotes indirect inguinal hernia. Femoral hernia occurs medially to the femoral artery and may feel like an enlarged lymph node. ■ Palpable or tender inguinal lymph nodes suggest infection in the lower vagina, external genitalia, lower abdomen, anal area, and perineum.	■ Indirect hernia is the most common hernia in all ages and both genders.

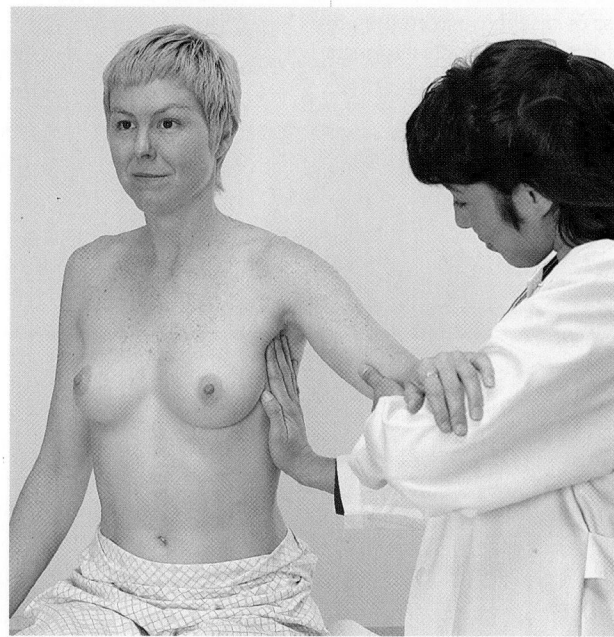

Figure 19–8 ● Palpating the axillary lymph nodes.

(continued on next page)

Female Reproductive System Assessment (continued)

ASSESSMENT/METHOD	NORMAL FINDINGS	ABNORMAL FINDINGS	LIFESPAN OR DEVELOPMENTAL CONSIDERATIONS
External Genitalia Assessment			
Help the woman into lithotomy position with knees flexed and separated. Vaginal examinations can also be done with the woman in a side-lying position with one leg drawn up. Inspect and palpate labia majora and labia minora.	Labia majora are equal in size and covered with public hair. Labia minora are smooth, symmetric, and hairless.	■ Excoriation, rashes, vesicles, nodules, or other lesions suggest inflammatory or infective processes. ■ Hair distribution toward the umbilicus or down the thighs suggests **hirsutism** (male pattern hair growth). ■ Varicosities may be present on the labia majora, especially during pregnancy. ■ Caking of discharge or smegma in tissue folds suggests vaginal infection or poor hygiene. ■ Chancres, ulcers, and vesicles may be signs of an STI such as syphilis or herpes. ■ Small, firm, cystic nodules suggest sebaceous cysts. Wartlike lesions suggest condylomata acuminate (genital warts). Ulcerated or red raised lesions suggest vulvar carcinoma.	■ Older women or women with mobility issues may have difficulty assuming the lithotomy position. ■ Pubic hair growth begins to change in puberty from fine, vellus hair to coarse curly hair. As a woman ages, pubic hair becomes more sparse and gray. ■ The labia majora loses fat as the woman ages. ■ Vulvar carcinoma is a disease of older women. ■ The labia and clitoris of older women become thin, pale, and dry.
Inspect the clitoris and vaginal opening (introitus).	The clitoris is small, very sensitive, and made up of erectile tissue. The vaginal opening varies in size depending on age and parity.	■ Clitoral enlargement may be a sign of masculinizing condition. Swelling and discoloration of lacerations for the introitus may be due to trauma. ■ Bulging of the anterior vaginal wall with or without urine incontinence at the introitus suggests **cystocele**. Bulging of the posterior wall of the vagina at the introitus suggests **rectocele**. ■ Yellowish discharge or lesions at the vaginal opening are signs of infection.	
Palpate urethra, Skene glands and Bartholin glands. Place gloved index finger under the urinary meatus and press up and toward the examiner to examine the urethral opening and the Skene ducts. (**Figure 19–9 ●** demonstrates exam of Skene ducts and urinary meatus.) Palpate the Bartholin glands by pressing with the thumb and index finger at 5 o'clock and 7 o'clock to the introitus (**Figure 19–10 ●**).	The urinary meatus opens just over the vagina. The Skene ducts open at the posterior portion of meatus and are usually not visible. The Bartholin glands are on either side of the posterior introitus and are usually not palpable or visible.	■ Tenderness or discharge from the urethral meatus or Skene ducts suggests infection. A nontender mass at 5 or 7 o'clock to the posterior introitus suggests a Bartholin cyst.	

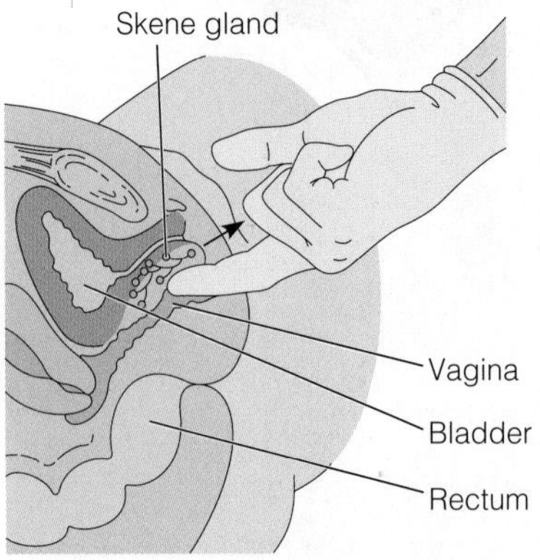

Figure 19–9 ● Palpating the Skene glands.

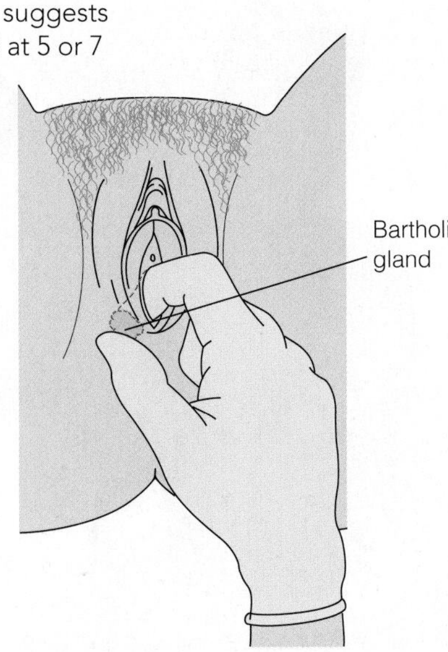

Figure 19–10 ● Palpating the Bartholin glands.

Female Reproductive System Assessment (*continued*)

ASSESSMENT/METHOD	NORMAL FINDINGS	ABNORMAL FINDINGS	LIFESPAN OR DEVELOPMENTAL CONSIDERATIONS
		■ Unilateral swelling, redness, and severe tenderness at 5 or 7 o'clock to the introitus indicates an abscess of a Bartholin gland.	
Inspect and palpate the perineum.	Area between vaginal opening and anus is same color as surrounding skin. Episiotomy or laceration from birth scars is a normal finding.	■ Inflammation, excoriations, lesions, or growths may be seen in infection or cancer. ■ Fistula or fissures may be the result of injury, trauma, infection, or spreading cancer.	
Vaginal and Cervical Assessment			
Use vaginal speculum to inspect vagina and cervix. Select size of speculum most appropriate for size of introitus.	Vaginal wall and fornices are pink and moist with rugae (accordion-like folds). The cervix is smooth and pink with a central os that may normally be scarred from childbirth. The cervix is firm like the tip of the nose.	■ Bluish color of the cervix and vaginal fornices may be a sign of pregnancy. A pale cervix may be seen if the woman is anemic. A cervix to the right or left of the midline may indicate a pelvic mass, uterine adhesions, or uterine mass. ■ Transverse or star-shaped cervical scars may reflect trauma, causing tearing of the cervix. ■ An enlarged cervix is associated with parity or infection. ■ **Nabothian cysts** (small, white or yellowish raised, round cystic areas on the cervical surface) are benign but may become infected. ■ Cervical polyps seen at the cervical os may be cervical or endometrial in origin.	■ In older women, the vagina narrows and the mucosa loses the rugae and becomes pale and dry due to decreased estrogen. ■ Pelvic organ prolapse is more common in older women. ■ The uterus and ovaries are much smaller in older women. ■ Reproductive system cancers are much more prevalent in older women.
Insert the fingers of the gloved dominant hand into the vagina. Palpate and move the cervix. Palpate the uterus and adnexa bimanually with fingers of one hand at the cervix and the other hand on the lower abdomen.	The cervix is firm like the nose in nonpregnant females and softer like the lips in pregnancy. There is normally drainage from the os that changes in consistency depending on the menstrual cycle. The uterus is mobile may be anteverted (tilted to the front), anteflexed (flexed to the front), retroverted (tilted to the back), retroflexed (flexed to the back), or midline. Uterine size varies with age and parity. The adnexa is the space on either side of the uterus where the fallopian tubes and ovaries are located. If palpable, the ovary is the size of an almond, firm, mobile, smooth, slightly tender.	■ Pain on movement of the cervix suggest cervicitis or pelvic inflammatory disease. ■ Firm, irregular nodules on the uterine surface are likely to be myomas (fibroids). ■ Unilateral or bilateral smooth, compressible adnexal masses are usually cysts. Tumors of the ovary are firm or nodular. ■ Palpable ovaries in an older, postmenopausal woman are abnormal and warrant further investigation.	■ Cancer of the ovary occurs most often in women over age 50.

Sources: Adapted from Bickley, L., & Szilagyi, P. (2013). *Bates' guide to physical examination and history taking* (11th ed.). Philadelphia, PA: Wolters Kluwer/Lippincott Williams & Wilkins; and Hain, D. (2013). Assessing older women's health. In E. Youngkin, M. Davis, D. Schadewald, & C. Juve (Eds.), *Women's health: A primary care clinical guide* (4th ed., pp. 119–149). Boston, MA: Pearson.

Female circumcision, also known as female genital mutilation (FGM) or female ritual cutting, is a dangerous practice that is common in parts of Africa. Some of the cultural beliefs behind the practice include the following: Female genitals are offensive to men, if not removed the clitoris will become the size of a penis, the labia get in the way of intercourse, the cutting enhances fertility, and the procedure prepares the woman for childbirth. Removal of the clitoris may or may not be accompanied by removal of the labia and closure of the vaginal entrance except for a small opening. Long-term medical complications include urinary incontinence, chronic urinary tract infections, vaginal scarring, pain syndromes, infertility, and sexual dysfunctions. FGM is illegal in several African and European countries and in Canada and the United States; however, female emigrants from countries where FGM is practiced often need medical care. In 1980, the World Health Organization and the United Nations Children's Fund (UNICEF) unanimously recommended that all forms of female circumcision be abolished. This effort did raise awareness in countries where FGM is practiced. In 2010, the WHO and several UN agencies and professional organizations issued a global request to stop healthcare providers from performing FGM. There has been an overall global decline in FGM (WHO, 2011a).

Male circumcision is controversial. The American Academy of Pediatrics (AAP) Committee on the Fetus and Newborn stated in 1971 that there were no valid medical indications for circumcision for newborns. The academy's current policy is that "Existing scientific evidence demonstrates potential medical benefits of newborn male circumcision; however, these data are not sufficient to recommend routine neonatal circumcision" (AAP Task Force on Circumcision, 2012). It supports informed decision making on the part of parents. The change in the rate of circumcisions is variably reported. The National Hospital Discharge Summary found that 65% of newborn males were circumcised in 1999. This number dropped to 55% in 2007. Similar studies reported by the CDC show the highest rates in the Midwest segment of the country (81%) and the lowest rates in the West (37%) in 1999 (CDC, 2012b).

RELIGION Religion influences sexual expression. It provides guidelines for sexual behavior and acceptable circumstances for the behavior, as well as prohibited sexual behavior and the consequences of breaking the sexual rules. The guidelines or rules may be detailed and rigid or broad and flexible. For example, some religions view forms of sexual expression other than male–female intercourse as unnatural and hold virginity before marriage to be the rule.

Many religious values conflict with the more flexible values of society that have developed during the past few decades (often labeled the "sexual revolution"), including the acceptance of premarital sex, unwed parenthood, homosexuality, and abortion. These conflicts create marked anxiety and potential sexual dysfunctions in some individuals.

PERSONAL EXPECTATIONS AND ETHICS Although ethics is integral to religion, ethical thought and ethical approaches to sexuality can be viewed separately from religion. Cultures have developed written or unwritten codes of conduct based on ethical principles. Personal expectations concerning sexual behavior come from these cultural norms. What one individual or culture views as bizarre, perverted, or wrong may be completely natural and right to another. Examples include values regarding masturbation, oral or anal intercourse, and cross-dressing. Many individuals accept a variety of sexual expressions if they are performed by consenting adults, are practiced in private, and are not harmful. Couples need to explore and communicate clearly about various types of acceptable sexual expression to prevent domination of sexual decision making by one member of the couple.

Diagnostic Tests

Diagnostic tests related to sexuality and the genitoreproductive system disorders include laboratory tests and imaging studies. For the male client, laboratory tests that may be used include CBC with differential, urinalysis, sperm analysis, culture and sensitivity to identify causative organisms in infection, blood tests for syphilis, HIV, or herpes; serum hormone studies; and a PSA test to screen for prostate cancer. None of these tests requires that the client be fasting. Teaching the client about these tests involves describing the venous puncture, the collection process for sperm or urine, and the reason for the various tests. Laboratory tests for women related to sexuality and genitoreproductive system disorders would also include CBC with differential, urinalysis, culture and sensitivity, blood tests for STIs, and serum hormone studies. Other laboratory tests for women include pregnancy tests (urine or blood) and the Papanicolaou test (Pap test). Because the Pap test involves a pelvic examination, teaching about the procedure and the test is required. The pregnancy tests and Pap test do not require that the woman be fasting.

Focus on Diversity and Culture
Selected Facts on Sexual Health

- Female circumcision or female genital mutilation (FGM) is a traditional or cultural practice in Africa, Asia, and Middle Eastern countries.
- FGM is increasingly found in the United States and Canada among immigrants from Africa, Asia, and the Middle East.
- The death rate from cervical cancer is higher than average in African Americans, Hispanics, and Native Americans.
- Leiomyosarcoma, one form of uterine cancer, occurs with greater frequency in African Americans than in other groups.
- In many cultures and religions, physical examination by a healthcare provider of the opposite sex is prohibited.
- Discussion of sexual activity and reproductive function is unacceptable in many cultures.
- Language barriers often prevent females from seeking or obtaining information or actual care associated with female reproductive issues.

Both men and women may require biopsies of the breasts or genitals that would require special procedures and education based on how extensive the procedure is. Both men and women may require imaging studies such as ultrasound, CT scan, or laparoscope. These may be done on an outpatient basis in most cases nurses are involved with teaching clients and with assisting other healthcare providers with the procedure. Women may also need hysteroscopic examinations or mammograms. In a hysteroscopic examination, an endoscope is used to visually inspect the uterine lining. Mammograms are x-rays of the breast.

CASE STUDY \\ PART 2

Ralph Jarvis, age 45, has "not been himself" for about a month, and his wife is worried about him. He smokes about 10 cigarettes per day and has smoked since he was 19. He has gained a little weight and doesn't seem to have much energy. The only exercise he gets is walking around the construction site. His wife convinces him to go to Ms. Walker, the family's nurse practitioner, for a checkup. He is reluctant but agrees to go if she will go with him. During the interview, Ms. Walker determines that Mr. Jarvis is a healthy man, but there is something he is not willing to discuss. Ms. Walker asks, "Mr. Jarvis, some of my male clients who are your age and smoke tell me that they are having sexual difficulties. Is this a concern for you?" Mr. Jarvis looks at his wife, who reaches for his hand and says, "Tell her, Ralph." This helps him to admit that he was unable to attain an erection a couple of times and this has him worried.

Clinical Reasoning Questions Level I

1. What model of intervention is Ms. Walker using?
2. What further assessment questions might she ask Mr. and Mrs. Jarvis?
3. In thinking about male gender and culture, is Mr. Jarvis's reluctance to talk about sex expected? Explain.

Clinical Reasoning Questions Level II

4. What is the priority nursing diagnosis for Mr. Jarvis at this time?
5. *Refer to the exemplar on Erectile Dysfunction within this module:* How will Ms. Walker determine whether Mr. Jarvis's sexual problem is a matter of sexual desire or the physical ability to attain and maintain an erection? Give two examples of history questions the nurse would ask.
6. *Refer to the exemplar on Erectile Dysfunction within this module:* What are some lifestyle changes that Mr. Jarvis can make that will improve his health and enhance his sexual performance?

▶ INTERVENTIONS AND THERAPIES

Before providing care related to sexuality, nurses should examine their own feelings about sexuality to ensure they can establish a therapeutic relationship and maintain a nonjudgmental attitude while providing care. Caring for the client with an alteration related to sexuality may include the following independent and collaborative interventions and therapies.

Independent

Independent therapies are focused on client teaching:

- Teaching related to prevention of STIs or prevention of transmission of STIs
- Teaching the client to perform breast or testicular self-examination
- Providing sexual health teaching
- Counseling for altered sexual function.

Collaborative

Nurses assist healthcare providers with various tests and examinations such as pelvic examinations and Pap tests.

SURGERY   Surgery for sexual dysfunction is limited to surgical treatment of erectile dysfunction (ED). These surgeries include implantation of prosthetic devices such as rods or inflatable balloons within the penis, reconstructing arteries within the penis to help blood flow, and blocking veins that drain the blood from the penis so that an erection is sustained (National Kidney and Urologic Diseases Information Clearinghouse [NKUDIC], 2009).

PHARMACOLOGIC THERAPY   Several different types of medications may be used to help clients maintain sexual health and ability. Oral contraceptives and female infertility medications affect the woman's reproductive system in decidedly different ways. Hormone replacement and hormone replacement therapy may help maintain hormone levels and are sometimes used in the treatment of certain cancers. Refer to the Medications feature for examples and nursing considerations.

Dealing With Inappropriate Sexual Behavior

Nurses, both male and female, may encounter a variety of sexually inappropriate behaviors for a number of reasons. The behavior may be either aggressive or nonaggressive. Clients may act out sexually by doing the following:

- Exposing themselves
- Asking the nurse to provide intimate physical care, such as bathing genital areas, when they are capable of doing this themselves
- Touching or grabbing the nurse's breasts, genitals, or buttocks
- Making blatant sexual statements to the nurse
- Offering the nurse sex
- Whistling and/or making comments about the nurse's attractiveness or desirability
- Making sexual comments to another client in the same room or to visitors about the "sexy" nurse or what they would like to do sexually with the nurse.

Following are some possible reasons for this inappropriate behavior:

- Fear or anxiety over future ability to function sexually
- Unmet needs for intimacy and sexual closeness because of hospitalization, injury, illness, treatment, lack of a partner, or lack of privacy

Medications Sexuality and Reproduction

CLASSIFICATION AND DRUG EXAMPLES	MECHANISMS OF ACTION	NURSING CONSIDERATIONS
Hormonal Contraceptives *Drug examples:* ■ estrogen/progestin combination (oral, patch, vaginal ring): • Ortho-Novum • Ortho-Tri-Cyclen • Triphasil • Alesse • Nuva Ring • Ortho Evra patch	Inhibits ovulation by inhibiting release of follicle-stimulating hormone (FSH) and luteinizing hormone (LH). Causes thickening of cervical mucus and thinning of the endometrium.	■ Teach how the medication works and importance of daily dosage for pills and what to do if dose is missed. ■ Teach how to use pills, patches, or vaginal ring. ■ Effectiveness declines with anticonvulsants and some antibiotics. Client may need backup method if using these drugs. ■ Avoid use in women over age 35 or those who smoke due to increased risk of deep venous thrombosis. ■ Screen for pregnancy prior to use. ■ Monitor blood pressure because hypertension is a potential side effect. ■ Consider increased risk for gallbladder disease, depression, and rare liver problems. ■ Benefits include decrease in acne, decreased bleeding, and decreased menstrual pain.
■ progestin only (oral, IM, subcutaneous, intrauterine device): • Micronor • Ovrette • Depo-Provera • Mirena intrauterine system • Implanon subcutaneous rod	Inhibits ovulation in variable cycles. Causes thickening of cervical mucus to prevent sperm penetration.	■ Teach drug action, how to use, and potential side effects. ■ Stress to client the importance of taking every day at same time. ■ May be used in clients with history of hypertension and deep venous thrombosis. ■ Irregular bleeding or amenorrhea is common.
Female Hormone Replacement *Drug examples:* ■ conjugated equine estrogen (Premarin [oral, IM, IV, intravaginal]) ■ chemical estrogen (Ogen [oral, patches])	Replaces estrogen that declines in perimenopause and menopause. May be used to treat hormone-dependent cancers.	■ Contraindicated if client has had breast cancer or any estrogen-dependent cancer or thromboembolic episodes. ■ Contraindicated in pregnancy. ■ Short-term use for hot flashes may be of benefit. Long-term use is contraindicated. ■ Teach importance of regular screening due to increased risk for cancer. ■ If used in male client, teach about potential feminizing changes. ■ Teach client to immediately report calf tenderness, chest pain, dyspnea. ■ Take with food if gastrointestinal upset occurs.
■ progestin (Provera, Prometrium)	Decreases action of estrogen on endometrial lining, thereby decreasing risk for endometrial cancer in women who still have a uterus.	■ Teach that combination estrogen/progestin is needed if client has not had hysterectomy. ■ Teach that combination with estrogen increases risks for myocardial infarction, stroke, breast cancer, dementia, and deep venous thrombosis. ■ Side effects include depression, weight gain, fluid retention.
Male Hormone Replacement *Drug examples:* ■ androgens (Danazol, Fluoxymesterone, Nandrolone)	Used to treat hypogonadism resulting in insufficient testosterone. Used to increase sperm count when low testosterone is the cause. Used as androgen replacement in aging men. Used in women with endometriosis to suppress LH and FSH, thereby causing anovulation and amenorrhea. Used to treat estrogen-dependent breast cancer.	■ Monitor liver enzymes and serum electrolytes. ■ Has virilizing effects—deepening voice, hirsutism, etc.—that may persist in women after therapy is stopped. ■ Teach that side effects may include weight gain, hyperglycemia, increased sperm count, priapism, renal stones, jaundice.
■ leuprolide acetate	Inhibits gonadotropin release, thereby suppressing ovulation or spermatogenesis. Is a gonadotropin-releasing hormone analog with antitumor effect and contraceptive effect. Used for endometriosis and severe uterine bleeding.	■ Warn client of pain at injection site. ■ Teach client to report hematuria or decreased urine output immediately. ■ Teach client to expect hot flashes.

Medications **Sexuality and Reproduction** (continued)

CLASSIFICATION AND DRUG EXAMPLES	MECHANISMS OF ACTION	NURSING CONSIDERATIONS
Female Infertility Medications *Drug example:* ▪ clomiphene	Stimulates ovulation and acts as an antiestrogen, nonsteroidal selective estrogen receptor modulator. Blocks normal negative feedback of circulating estradiol on hypothalamus, preventing the release of gonadotropin-releasing hormone and thereby stimulating release of FSH and LH and ovarian stimulation.	▪ Encourage client to take medication at same time every day. ▪ Warn client of increased risk for a multiple birth. ▪ Teach client to report pelvic pain, visual changes, unusual vaginal bleeding, uterine contractions, jaundice, or calf tenderness.
▪ bromocriptine	Is an ergot alkaloid and dopamine receptor agonist. Reduces increased prolactin in men and women by activating postsynaptic dopaminergic receptors in hypothalamus. Restores ovulation in amenorrheic women, correcting infertility due to increased prolactin.	▪ Monitor CBC, liver, and renal function in long-term treatment. ▪ Teach client to avoid hazardous activities or driving until effect of drug is known.
▪ antidiabetic agent metformin (Glucophage)	Lowers testosterone production in women with polycystic ovary syndrome.	▪ Monitor for hypoglycemia and GI distress. ▪ Is a Pregnancy Category B drug.

Sources: Based on Wilson, B., Shannon, M., & Shields, K. (2013). *Pearson nurse's drug guide 2013.* Upper Saddle River, NJ: Pearson; and Adams, M., & Koch, R. (2010). *Pharmacology: Connections to nursing practice.* Upper Saddle River, NJ: Pearson.

▪ Misinterpretation of the nurse's behavior as sexual or provocative

▪ Need for reassurance that they are still sexual beings and still sexually attractive

▪ Need for attention

▪ Confusion; neurological impairment or trauma can lead clients to use profane sexual language, engage in masturbation, expose themselves, or inappropriately touch or grab at the nurse

▪ Need to control; clients may be experiencing loss of control over their lives because of hospitalization, injury, or illness

▪ Need for power

▪ Belief that flirtatious behavior is expected because of media portrayals of nurses as sexy, available, and experienced.

Before implementing any nursing interventions, the nurse should first determine whether the behavior is inappropriate or an attempt to communicate a physical need. For example, clients may expose themselves if they are febrile, pull at the penis if a catheter is uncomfortable or irritating, or reach for the nurse if unable to communicate verbally. Nursing strategies to deal with inappropriate sexual behavior are listed in **Box 19–2 ●**.

Maintaining sexual health is important for both sexual pleasure and physical health. A number of issues in sexual health can cause anxiety, embarrassment, and physical discomfort. Some issues, such as sexually transmitted infections, can present a physical danger to the client. The exemplars that follow offer guidelines for the provision of culturally competent nursing care in a range of issues affecting individual sexuality.

Box 19–2   Nursing Strategies for Inappropriate Sexual Behavior

▪ Communicate that the behavior is not acceptable by saying, for example, "I really do not like the things you are saying" or "I see you are not dressed. I will be back in 10 minutes and will help you with breakfast when you get your clothes on."

▪ Tell the client how the behavior makes you feel: "When you act like that toward me, I am very uncomfortable. It embarrasses me and makes it hard for me to give you the kind of nursing care you need."

▪ Identify the behavior you expect: "Please call me by my name, not 'honey'" or "I expect you to keep yourself covered when I am in the room."

▪ Set firm limits: Take the client's hand and move it away, use direct eye contact, and say, "Don't do that!"

▪ Try to refocus clients from the inappropriate behavior to their real concerns and fears; offer to discuss sexuality concerns: "All morn-

ing you have been making very personal sexual comments about yourself. Sometimes individuals talk like that when they are concerned about the sexual part of their life and how their illness will affect them. Are there things that you have questions about or would like to talk about?"

▪ Report the incident to your nursing instructor, charge nurse, or clinical nurse specialist. Discuss the incident, your feelings, and possible interventions.

▪ Assign a nurse who will confront the behavior and relate to the client in a consistent manner.

▪ Clarify the consequences of continued inappropriate behavior (avoidance, withdrawal of services, no chance to help resolve the client's underlying concerns).

REVIEW The Concept of Sexuality

RELATE Link the Concepts

Linking the concept of sexuality with the concept of mood and affect:

1. Explain how psychological factors may impact sexuality and how problems with sexuality may impact psychological well-being.

2. What are appropriate referral resources for individuals with mood disorders who are experiencing sexual dysfunction?

Linking the concept of sexuality with the concept of elimination:

3. Explain how the proximity of sexual organs and organs of elimination may put clients at risk for problems with elimination.

4. What are the nursing interventions for clients with elimination problems related to sexuality?

Linking the concept of sexuality with the concept of perfusion:

5. Explain how poor perfusion may affect sexuality for both men and women.

6. What nursing interventions are indicated for men and women experiencing sexual difficulty related to poor perfusion?

READY Go to Companion Skills Manual

REFER Go to Pearson Nursing Student Resources
nursing.pearsonhighered.com

- Additional review materials
- MiniModule: Reproductive Anatomy and Physiology

REFLECT Case Study \\ Part 3

Eileen Jarvis, 65, has lived with her son Ralph and his wife Betty for the past 2 years. She has become much more active in the past 6 months as she has recovered from the shock and grief of losing her husband of 44 years. She volunteers at the hospital with Betty and goes to the Senior Center to walk and to socialize with old friends. Eileen has met a man, Tom Lane, at the Senior Center and they have been going out together. A couple of days ago, Tom asked Mrs. Jarvis to marry him. She has decided to say yes. She has come to Ms. Walker for her annual checkup. After her examination, Mrs. Jarvis tells Ms. Walker of her marriage plans and asks about sex. Ms. Walker congratulates Mrs. Jarvis and asks her about Tom and her relationship with Tom. Ms. Walker asks, "Have you and Tom talked about sex?" and "Do you both know each other's sexual history?"

Clinical Reasoning Questions Level I

1. Communication about sexual needs and expectations promotes a successful intimate relationships. Do you think Ms. Walker has helped Mrs. Jarvis to plan better communication with her fiance?

2. Why do you think it is important for a couple planning a sexual relationship to know about each other's sexual history before having sexual intercourse?

3. Menopause and decreased estrogen can cause two physical changes that may make sexual intercourse uncomfortable. What are these two changes?

Clinical Reasoning Questions Level II

4. What health screening for gynecological cancer may be appropriate for Mrs. Jarvis during this clinic visit?

5. *Refer to the exemplar on Menopause within this module:* If Mrs. Jarvis has dyspareunia related to sexual intercourse, one cause may be atrophic vaginitis. What are some interventions that may relieve this problem?

6. *Refer to the exemplar on Sexually Transmitted Infections within this module:* Ms. Walker knows that the incidence of STIs is increasing among older adults, but at the same time she does not want to cause undue anxiety or problems in the relationship between Mrs. Jarvis and Tom. Now that Mrs. Jarvis has initiated the conversation about sex, what would you suggest Ms. Walker teach Mrs. Jarvis about discussing this very private issue with her fiance?

EXEMPLAR 19.1 Erectile Dysfunction

EXEMPLAR KEY TERMS
Erectile dysfunction (ED), *1366*
Libido, *1366*

EXEMPLAR LEARNING OUTCOMES
After reading about this exemplar, you will be able to:

1. Describe the pathophysiology, etiology, clinical manifestations, and direct and indirect causes of erectile dysfunction.
2. Identify risk factors associated with erectile dysfunction.
3. Illustrate the nursing process in providing culturally competent care across the life span for individuals with erectile dysfunction.

4. Formulate priority nursing diagnoses appropriate for an individual with erectile dysfunction.
5. Summarize therapies used by interdisciplinary teams in the collaborative care of an individual with erectile dysfunction.
6. Plan evidence-based care for an individual with erectile dysfunction and his family in collaboration with other members of the healthcare team.
7. Evaluate expected outcomes for an individual with erectile dysfunction.

▶ OVERVIEW

Erectile dysfunction (ED) is the inability of a male to attain and maintain an erection sufficient to permit mutually satisfactory sexual intercourse with his partner. ED may involve a total inability to achieve erection, an inconsistent ability to achieve erection, or the ability to sustain only brief erections. ED may or may not be associated with a loss of **libido** (sexual desire).

The incidence of ED is difficult to estimate because many affected men may not report the disorder. It has been estimated that about 30 million men in the United States have ED. The incidence increases with age with about 4% of men ages 50–59 years affected, 17% of men ages 60–69, and about 47% of men over age 75 (NKUDIC, 2009). However, ED is not inevitable in all men, and it is treatable at any age.

▶ PATHOPHYSIOLOGY AND ETIOLOGY

Normal, physiological erection that enables the penis to enter the vagina is a neurovascular event that requires functional autonomic and somatic nerves, smooth and striated muscles in the penile shaft and pelvic floor, and adequate arterial blood flow (Meng et al., 2011). The erectile reflex to sexual stimulation occurs when the chambers within the erectile tissue of the penis become filled with blood via arterioles that relax and dilate in response to nitrous oxide. At the same time, contractions of pelvic muscles help increase the rigidity of the penis and veins of the penis constrict, blocking blood outflow until orgasm or removal of the sexual stimuli occurs (Deneris & Huether, 2010).

Etiology

The causes of ED are multiple and can be divided into psychological and physical causes. Physical causes can be further divided into vascular, neurogenic, hormonal, and iatrogenic. Table 19–3 ● lists the most common causes of ED.

Although age alone may not cause ED, age-related cellular and tissue changes in the penis, decreased sensory activity, hypogonadism, and the effects of chronic illness that tend to occur with aging do increase the risks for developing ED. In the penis, a change from elastic collagen to a more rigid collagen results in decreased distensibility (a less rigid erection). This, in turn, interferes with the veno-occlusive mechanism, which prevents blood from "leaking" out of the penis into the general vasculature prematurely. Problems with this mechanism result in incomplete erections. Vibrotactile sensation over the skin of the penis declines with age. This decline may explain why some older men require longer stimulation to achieve an erection. Hypogonadism, common in aging men, results in decreased testosterone levels. There may be a relationship between lower androgen levels and erectile function.

Damage to arteries, smooth muscles, and fibrous tissues are the most common causes of ED. Diseases such as diabetes, kidney disease, chronic alcoholism, atherosclerosis, and vascular disease are often responsible for organic ED. Iatrogenic causes, that is, problems that result from treatment and therapy, must always be considered. For example, innervation and blood flow to the penis may be damaged during surgery, prostate surgery in particular. Given the effects of vasculature damage on the penis, the increased incidence of chronic illness, and the multiple medications and treatments required to manage those illnesses, it is not surprising that many older men have problems with ED.

Risk Factors

The risk factors mirror the causes for ED and are numerous. They include advancing age, diseases such as heart disease and diabetes, trauma, the use of prescription or illicit drugs, and excessive use of alcohol. Essentially, all the causes listed in Table 19–3 are risk factors.

▶ CLINICAL MANIFESTATIONS

Erectile dysfunction can manifest as either the complete inability to attain an erection or the inability to sustain an erection. A man may achieve erection but be unable to sustain it, or the penis may become semierect but lack rigidity sufficient for intercourse. Erectile dysfunction can occur in men of any age and can be chronic, intermittent, or episodic. A medical diagnosis of ED requires that the problem be present at least 3 months (Meng et al., 2011).

▶ COLLABORATION

The management of men with ED is growing in importance and scale, because the U.S. population as a whole is aging, so the incidence is increasing proportionately. Another factor is the gradual change in the willingness of men and their partners to discuss sexual concerns. Although sexuality is still a very sensitive and private area for most individuals, the knowledge that help is available is causing men to seek answers. Many older men are coming to believe that loss of erectile function is not an inevitable part of aging.

The interdisciplinary team necessary for the management of the care for men with ED may include physicians, nurse practitioners, and nurses who educate, counsel, offer emotional support,

TABLE 19–3 Causes of Erectile Dysfunction

VASCULAR	NEUROGENIC	HORMONAL	LIFESTYLE CHOICES	PSYCHOLOGICAL	IATROGENIC
Atherosclerosis	Spinal cord injury	Low levels of testosterone, prolactin	Smoking	Stress	*Side effects of:*
Hypertension	Stroke	Alterations in thyroid function	Alcohol use	Anxiety	Antihypertensives
Heart disease	Nerve disease		Overweight	Guilt	Antihistamines
Hyperlipidemia	Multiple sclerosis		Not exercising	Depression	Antidepressants
Chronic obstructive lung disease	Parkinson disease			Low self-esteem	Tranquilizers
Diabetes mellitus	Alzheimer disease			Fear of sexual failure	Appetite suppressants
Direct injury to penis that affects vascular supply or nerves					Cimetidine
					Surgery:
					Radical prostate and bladder surgery

Sources: Based on National Kidney and Urologic Diseases Information Clearinghouse (NKUDIC). (2009). *Erectile dysfunction* (NIH Publication No. 09-3923). Retrieved from http://kidney.niddk.nih.gov/KUDiseases/pubs/ED/index.aspx; and Leslie, S. (2013). Causes of erectile dysfunction. *eMedicinehealth.* Retrieved from http://www.emedicinehealth.com/causes_of_erectile_dysfunction/article_em.htm.

prescribe drugs, perform procedures, and provide physical care. Psychologists and mental health counselors may be called on to help men with mental and emotional consequences or causes of ED. Cognitive behavioral therapy and sex therapy may help relieve psychogenic ED. Pharmacists help men with ED to understand their medications and use them properly. Medication education should include how quickly the man will feel results from the medication and the potential side effects. Community support groups may be available in the area where the man resides. These groups help the man and his partner feel less isolated and help them to cope with any long-term problems. The most important team member, however, is the man's partner. It is essential for the man to have a loving relationship with his partner and for the couple to maintain open communication with each other.

Treatment for men with ED usually starts with the least invasive methods; these may be lifestyle changes such as quitting smoking, reducing alcohol intake, losing weight, and more exercise. The next step is to assess the medications the man is taking and determine whether a drug can safely be decreased or replaced. If these interventions are not working, then oral medications are recommended (NKUDIC, 2009).

Diagnostic Tests

Medical management of ED begins with a medical and sexual history to determine the degree of the problem and to reveal disease, lifestyle habits, or medication use that may be contributing to ED. It has been estimated that about 25% of all cases of ED are medication related (Meng et al., 2011). The physical examination will provide clues about any systemic problems, signs of low androgen, and any structural problems within the penis (NKUKIC, 2009).

The diagnostic tests that may be ordered include blood studies, penile monitoring, and penile blood flow. Blood chemistry, CBC, urinalysis, lipid profile, kidney and liver function testing, testosterone, prolactin, thyroxin, and PSA levels are measured to identify metabolic and endocrine problems that may be causing the dysfunction. Nocturnal penile tumescence and rigidity monitoring helps differentiate between psychogenic and organic causes. Physically healthy men have involuntary erections during sleep. These tests can be performed in a sleep laboratory, although home testing with portable devices is an alternative. Tests for nocturnal erections are not completely reliable but do give more information about the problem (NKUDIC, 2009). The number and quality of erections occurring during REM sleep can be determined. At this point, a trial of oral medications may be prescribed to determine response. If an inadequate response to oral medication is determined, injections into the penis may be used. If injections do not produce the effect desired, then vascular studies with duplex ultrasound, penile cavernosometry, and cavernosography of the corpora or pudendal arteriography can be done to determine whether the problem is arterial or venous. These studies also determine whether or not the client is a candidate for vascular surgery (Meng et al., 2011).

Pharmacologic Therapy

Erectile dysfunction can be treated with medications taken orally, injected directly into the penis, or inserted into the urethra at the tip of the penis.

ORAL MEDICATIONS The oral medications used to treat erectile dysfunction include sildenafil citrate (Viagra), vardenafil hydrochloride (Levitra), tadalafil (Cialis), and avanafil (Stendra) (Drugs.com Editorial Team, 2012; Wilson, Shannon, & Shields, 2013). All of these drugs are selective phosphodiesterase type 5 inhibitors that enhance erections only when sexual stimulation is present. These drugs act within 30–60 minutes, so they should be taken about an hour before sexual activity. The action will persist for up to 36 hours. All four drugs enhance the effects of nitrous oxide to facilitate relaxation of the smooth muscle in the penis during sexual stimulation to increase blood flow. These drugs should be taken no more than once a day and should not be taken by men who are also taking nitrate-based drugs (for heart problems) or alpha-blockers (used to treat hypertension and prostate enlargement).

INJECTABLE MEDICATIONS Hormone replacement therapy with testosterone injections (200 mg IM every 3 weeks) or topical patches may be used for men who have documented androgen deficiency and do not have prostate cancer. Injectable medications, including papaverine and prostaglandin E injections, may be used. When injected directly into the penis using a tuberculin syringe or metered-dose injection device, prostaglandin E and papaverine relax the arterioles and smooth muscles of the cavernosum, thus inducing tumescence (swelling). An erection usually develops that lasts from 30 minutes to 4 hours. Side effects can include bruising, local pain, infection, and priapism. Priapism would require medical attention (Meng et al., 2011).

One problem with this type of treatment is its mode of delivery. There is a high attrition rate, and clients report dissatisfaction with lack of spontaneity, loss of interest in sex, physical limitations, cost, and occasionally pain. These injectables are rarely used today except in clients who cannot take oral drugs like Viagra (Adams & Koch, 2010). Alprostadil (Caverject) may be given as a minisuppository into the urethra or as an injection into the cavernosa. It works like papaverine but does not work as well. The strength of the erection produced with this drug can be enhanced with the use of a constriction ring (O-ring) at the base of the penis (Adams & Koch, 2010).

Mechanical Devices

A frequently prescribed mechanical device for ED is the vacuum constriction device (VCD). The VCD draws blood into the penis with a vacuum, trapping it there with a constricting band at the base of the penis. After the device is removed for intercourse, the band, often called an O-ring, is left at the base of the penis to maintain the erection. If the man can typically attain an erection but cannot maintain it, then an O-ring alone can be used.

Surgery

Surgical treatment for ED involves either revascularization procedures or implantation of prosthetic devices. Venous or arterial procedures are generally not successful. The result is often temporary, because the underlying cause of the vascular insufficiency is usually not corrected. Implantation of penile prostheses is now common (**Figure 19–11 ●**). The prosthesis may consist of malleable rods placed inside the two corpora cavernosa or inflatable implants that can be filled with water from a

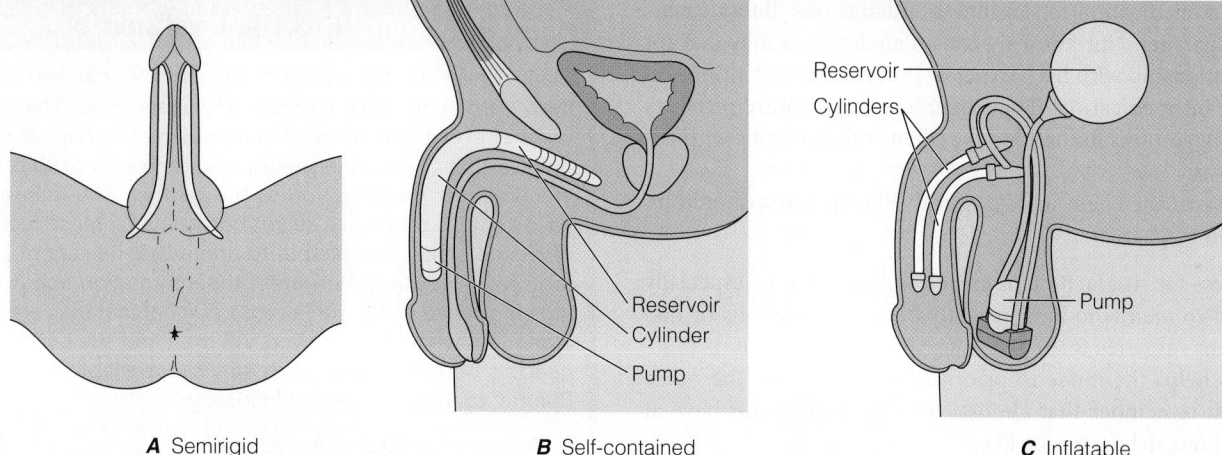

A Semirigid   **B** Self-contained   **C** Inflatable

Figure 19–11 ● Types of penile implants: *A,* With semirigid rods implanted in the corpora cavernosa, the penis is always in a state of semierection, which may not be acceptable to the man. *B,* With a self-contained penile implant, the penis remains flaccid until the man compresses a pump at the head of the penis, which transfers fluid from a reservoir to a cylinder within the penis to achieve an erection. The man presses a release valve to return the fluid to the reservoir. *C,* With an inflatable penile implant, the penis remains flaccid until the man compresses a pump in the scrotum, which transfers fluid from an abdominal reservoir to cylinders in the corpora cavernosa to achieve an erection. Pressing a release valve returns the fluid to the reservoir.

reservoir in the pelvis via a pump placed in the skin of the scrotum. Men are generally satisfied with their prostheses; they rank the inflatable type highest because, when not in use, they leave the penis in a more natural flaccid state. Problems that occur with these implants include mechanical malfunction and infection, but these do not occur frequently (NKUDIC, 2009). Partners are also more likely to report satisfaction with the penile implant, although not to the same degree as clients. Some partners report that the implanted penis is harder than a normal erect penis and therefore causes pain. Also, the man can have intercourse for a prolonged period of time, and some partners do not find prolonged penetration enjoyable. Client and partner teaching is mandatory. Counseling by a sex therapist may be needed to facilitate adaptation to the implant.

■ NURSING PROCESS

The nurse in any healthcare setting may encounter men with erectile dysfunction, either through routine examinations or through careful assessment of clients' conditions and treatments that may incidentally cause ED. Nurses employed in clinics, operating rooms, and surgical units with urological services commonly encounter men being treated for ED. Nurses in a variety of settings, including long-term care, encounter men who have had surgical interventions, such as penile implants.

Because nurses often complete a client's health history, they are most likely to discover problems of erectile dysfunction. Once a problem is known, nurses are involved in giving information, providing emotional support, and referring clients to physicians or counselors.

Assessment

Whether the client presents with reports of erectile dysfunction or it is discovered during the nursing interview, it is important to perform a complete physical examination to reveal data that may contribute to the problem. The client should be asked

questions to determine all medications, social habits, surgical history, and procedures that may be contributing factors.

Diagnosis

Appropriate nursing diagnoses for clients with erectile dysfunction often include the following:

■ *Sexual Dysfunction*
■ *Deficient Knowledge* related to ED and treatments
■ *Situational Low Self-Esteem.*

(NANDA-I © 2012)

Planning

Goals of nursing care include the following:

■ The client will discuss concerns about erectile difficulties without embarrassment or anxiety.
■ The client will understand the diagnosis and medication teaching to prevent discontinuing necessary medications.
■ The client will understand treatment options and make an informed decision.

Implementation

Although interventions will vary based on the individual client's needs, the nurse typically will provide ongoing assessment and client teaching regarding the nature of erectile dysfunction and its treatments. It is important for the nurse to maintain a very professional affect when discussing sensitive sexual dysfunction issues with clients, recognizing that clients may find it difficult to discuss sexual performance with a young nurse of either sex.

Discuss Sexual Dysfunction

Many men who lose erectile function are not aware of the cause. Often the man blames the loss on unrelated factors, such as age, a medication for an illness, a dangerous illness, or his sexual partner. Not knowing causes anxiety and may disrupt the relationship with his partner or lead him to discontinue an important medication. The Client Teaching feature provides some suggestions for helping the client come to terms with the diagnosis.

To assist the client in coping with ED, the nurse should do the following:

- Assess for risk factors for erectile dysfunction. Be especially alert to men who have recently begun medications or had recent surgeries that could cause ED. Awareness of risk factors helps the nurse to prioritize care, although the nurse must remember that almost all aging male clients have at least one risk factor for ED.

- Assess for sexual dysfunction. Men have shown increasing willingness to discuss sexual concerns and expect the nurse to be aware of the physiological effects of their disease and side effects of treatment on all aspects of their health. If a problem exists, information obtained in a sexual assessment guides the nurse in deciding whether the next step should be client teaching, referral, or both.

- Perform a detailed assessment of the client's current sexual practices. It is essential for healthcare providers to understand the client and partner's sexual pattern in order to provide appropriate, individualized care.

- Discuss the client's previous methods of coping with erectile dysfunction. Awareness of coping strategies can provide insight for the nurse and guide teaching.

- Provide information about treatment options. The client needs to know the details of the intervention, the chances for success, and the possible complications.

Promote Self-Esteem

The man with erectile dysfunction often believes himself to be "less than a man." In addition, the insertion of a penile implant with a semirigid prosthesis may result in disturbances in body image related to changes in sexual activity as well as the appearance and embarrassment of a permanent semierection. Nursing interventions that may help the client in this regard are as follows:

- Collect data during the health history, in a nonjudgmental manner, about physiological function, other chronic illnesses, and feelings about sexual inadequacy. This informa-

Client Teaching Erectile Dysfunction

Many nurses find that men with ED and their partners have lived in isolation with the problem for many years. The partner may even be unaware of the problem. The partner may believe that the man is seeing someone else or that the man has lost his attraction to the partner. The man may have kept his problem a secret because an intense feeling of shame makes him unable to admit that he cannot perform sexually. Many men greet the information about the high incidence of ED with a sense of relief that they are not alone in having this problem. All men and their partners need to be aware of support services available to them. Referral sources include the following:

- American Urological Association
- American Association of Sex Educators, Counselors, and Therapists.

tion is necessary to establish the database for individualized interventions.

- If the man has had a penile implant, teach him and his partner how to use the pump, including how to inflate and deflate the device. Suggest that he practice inflation and deflation during the postoperative period. Suggest wearing snug-fitting underwear with the penis placed in an upright position on the abdomen and loose trousers. Provide information about length of healing time, and inform the client that sexual activity may resume within 6–8 weeks following surgery. Practice using the pump will maintain the pump position and promote tissue growth around the implant. The type of clothing worn can improve the ability to conceal a semirigid prosthesis and decrease embarrassment. Recovery from surgery is necessary before resuming sexual activity.

Evaluation

Client outcomes may be evaluated based on the following expected outcomes:

- The client makes informed decision regarding treatment options.
- The client understands that the problem is not related to his masculinity.

REVIEW Erectile Dysfunction

RELATE Link the Concepts and Exemplars

Linking the exemplar of erectile dysfunction with the concept of self:

1. Why might a client's self-concept be negatively affected by ED?
2. What can the nurse do to help reduce this negative impact?

Linking the exemplar of erectile dysfunction with the concept of perfusion:

3. What effect does arteriosclerosis have on a man's ability to attain an erection?

4. What preventive teaching can the nurse provide to younger men to prevent ED as the result of altered perfusion?

READY Go to Companion Skills Manual

REFER Go to Pearson Nursing Student Resources
nursing.pearsonhighered.com

- Additional review materials

REFLECT Case Study

Steve Young is a 41-year-old African American male in excellent health. He has been married to his wife Angie for 8 years.

They have two children, Kelsey and Marcus. The Youngs met in college and were married shortly after Steve graduated with a degree in accounting. Following graduation, he took the CPA exam, and he has worked for a large corporate accounting firm ever since. He has been extremely successful in his firm and has an income that easily supports his family. He is pleased that his wife is able to be a stay-at-home mother, but his success requires long working hours. Mr. Young has few outside interests and rarely exercises. His world revolves around work and home. He recognizes that his inactivity has led to weight gain during the past few years, but is not concerned about it.

Mr. Young began smoking at age 17 and now has a 10 pack/year smoking history. He knows he should quit, but he likes it and figures he can probably get away with it for a little while longer without complications. Because he knows that it is a source of irritation for his wife, he plans to quit smoking eventually.

1. What risk factors does Mr. Young have for developing erectile dysfunction?
2. What client teaching can you provide to reduce Mr. Young's risk for erectile dysfunction?
3. How might you approach Mr. Young to discuss any sexual function issues he may have experienced?

EXEMPLAR 19.2 **Family Planning**

EXEMPLAR KEY TERMS

Autosomes, *1374*
Carrier, *1376*
Cervical cap, *1382*
Coitus interruptus, *1379*
Combined oral contraceptives
   (COCs), *1383*
Condom, *1379*
Depo-Provera, *1384*
Diaphragm, *1381*
Emergency contraception (EC), *1385*
Estrogen, *1379*
Fertility awareness–based methods, *1378*
Genotype, *1376*
In vitro fertilization (IVF), *1389*
Infertility, *1372*
Intrauterine contraception (IUC), *1382*
Karyotype, *1374*
Mendelian (single-gene) inheritance, *1376*
Monosomic, *1374*
Monosomies, *1375*
Mosaicism, *1374*
Non-Mendelian (multifactorial) inheritance, *1376*
Operative sterilization, *1386*
Pedigree, *1376*
Phenotype, *1376*
Progesterone, *1379*
Secondary infertility, *1372*

Spermicide, *1379*
Subfertility, *1372*
Therapeutic insemination, *1388*
Trisomic, *1374*
Trisomies, *1374*
Tubal ligation, *1386*
Vasectomy, *1386*

EXEMPLAR LEARNING OUTCOMES

After reading about this exemplar, you will be able to:

1. Describe decisions to be made by couples prior to beginning preconception counseling.
2. Identify factors associated with family planning, infertility, and preconception counseling.
3. Describe the pathophysiology, etiology, clinical manifestations, and direct and indirect causes of infertility.
4. Identify risk factors and prevention methods associated with infertility.
5. Summarize therapies used by interdisciplinary teams in the collaborative care of an individual or couple seeking help with family planning, preconception counseling, or infertility.
6. Plan evidence-based care for an individual or couple who seek family planning, preconception counseling, or infertility assistance.
7. Evaluate expected outcomes for the individual or couple seeking family planning, preconception counseling, or infertility assistance.

▶ OVERVIEW

Some of the most serious decisions couples must make relate to family planning and reproduction: whether and when to have children as well as how many children they want. Information provided by nurses and other health professionals can help clients make informed decisions about contraception and childbearing. Some couples are unable to fulfill their dream of having the desired baby because of infertility or genetic problems. Developments in medicine can help growing numbers of couples overcome infertility issues. Preconception planning can help couples to plan for and accomplish the perfect pregnancy and newborn for them.

Contraception

The decision to use a method of contraception may be made individually by a woman or man or jointly by a couple. The decision may be motivated by a desire to avoid pregnancy, to gain control over the number of children conceived, or to determine the spacing of future children. In choosing a specific method, consistency of use outweighs the absolute reliability of the given method.

Decisions about contraception should be made voluntarily, with full knowledge of advantages, disadvantages, effectiveness, side effects, contraindications, and long-term effects. Many outside factors influence this choice, including cultural practices, religious beliefs, attitudes and personal preferences, cost, effectiveness, misinformation, practicality of method, and self-esteem. Different methods of contraception may be appropriate at different times for individuals and couples.

Preconception Counseling

Making the decision to have children is the first step a couple makes in the process of conception. For some couples, this decision is part of discussions during the dating process. Others do not make the decision to have children until later in their relationship. This decision involves consideration of each individual's goals, expectations of the relationship, and desire to be a parent. Sometimes one individual wishes to have a child, but the other does not. In such situations, an open discussion is essential to reach a mutually acceptable decision.

Couples who wish to have children face a decision about the timing of pregnancy. At what point in their lives do they believe it would be best to become parents? Pregnancy is a life-changing event and never proceeds just as the couple anticipates, even when the pregnancy is planned and the timing is convenient.

For couples who have religious beliefs that do not support contraception or who feel that fertility planning is unnatural, planning the timing of the pregnancy is unacceptable and irrelevant. These couples can still take steps to ensure that they are in the best possible physical and mental health if and when pregnancy occurs.

PRECONCEPTION HEALTH MEASURES   Most preconception recommendations focus on helping the couple attain their best possible health state so that they do not enter pregnancy with unnecessary risks. The nurse begins by teaching the couple about known or suspected health risks.

The nurse advises the woman to stop smoking or at least to limit her cigarette intake as much as possible. Because of the hazards of secondhand smoke, it is helpful for the woman to avoid environments where secondhand smoke is common and to ask her partner to refrain from smoking around her. Although the effects of caffeine are less clearly understood, the woman is advised to avoid or limit her intake of caffeine. Alcohol, social drugs, and street drugs pose a real threat to the fetus. A woman who uses any prescription or over-the-counter medications needs to discuss the implications of their use with her healthcare provider.

Women with chronic health problems, such as thyroid disorders, seizures, hypertension, and diabetes, should have a preconception visit with the appropriate specialist to determine whether pregnancy is advised and medication changes or treatment plan changes warranted. Because of the possible teratogenic effects of environmental hazards, the nurse should urge the couple contemplating pregnancy to determine possible exposure to any environmental hazards, such as radiation or chemical exposure, at work or in their community.

PHYSICAL EXAMINATION   It is advisable for both partners to have a physical examination to identify any health problems so that these can be corrected if possible. These problems might include medical conditions, such as high blood pressure, diabetes, or obesity; problems that pose a threat to fertility, such as certain sexually transmitted infections (STIs); or conditions that keep the individual from achieving optimal health, such as anemia or colitis. If the family history indicates previous genetic disorders or if the couple is planning pregnancy when the woman is over age 35, the nurse may suggest that the couple consider genetic counseling. In addition to the history and physical exam, the woman may have a variety of laboratory tests. Before conception, the woman is also advised to have a dental examination and any necessary dental work to avoid

exposure to x-rays, local anesthetics, and the risk of infection while pregnant.

NUTRITION   Before conception, it is advisable for the woman to be at an average weight for her body build and height. Women who are underweight should be advised to gain weight, whereas women who are overweight should try to get their weight down because maternal obesity is a risk factor for numerous pregnancy complications. The woman is advised to follow a nutritious diet that contains ample quantities of all the essential nutrients. Some nutritionists advocate emphasizing calcium, protein, iron, B complex vitamins, vitamin C, and magnesium. Folic acid supplementation before conception is recommended, as these supplements decrease the risk of neural tube defects. Intake of vitamins in greater than the recommended dietary allowance (RDA) can cause severe fetal problems and should be avoided. Unique dietary practices that can affect nutrition should be explored during the assessment. Cultural norms that affect nutritional intake should also be assessed.

EXERCISE   A woman is advised to continue her present pattern of exercise or to establish a regular exercise plan beginning at least 3 months before she attempts to become pregnant. An exercise routine that she enjoys and maintains will provide the best results. Exercise that includes some aerobic conditioning and some general muscle toning will improve the woman's circulation and general health. Once an exercise program is well established, the woman is generally encouraged to continue it during pregnancy. During pregnancy, at least 30 minutes of moderate exercise daily or at least most days is recommended (Cunningham et al., 2010).

IMMUNIZATIONS   All women of reproductive age need to be up to date with immunizations prior to pregnancy. When a pregnancy is planned, immunizations for diphtheria, tetanus, pertussis, measles, mumps, rubella, and varicella should be reviewed. If any immunizations need to be initiated or boosters given, they should be finished 3 months prior to conception (Blackburn, 2013). It is important for the pregnant woman to be immunized against flu, especially if she will be pregnant during flu season (CDC, 2012c). The flu vaccine can be given during pregnancy if needed.

Infertility Counseling

Infertility, a lack of conception despite unprotected sexual intercourse for at least 12 months (Latendresse, McCance, & Morgan, 2010), has a profound emotional, psychological, and economic impact on affected couples and society. The term *sterility* is applied when there is an absolute factor preventing reproduction. **Subfertility** is used to describe a couple who has difficulty conceiving because both partners have reduced fertility. The term **secondary infertility** is applied to couples who have been unable to conceive after one or more successful pregnancies or who cannot sustain a pregnancy.

Fertility may be at risk in men who abuse alcohol, use tobacco or drugs, are exposed to environmental toxins, take certain prescription drugs for health problems, or have had treatment for cancer. Age is also a risk factor for men, but age is a much higher risk for women. Other risk factors for female infertility include excess alcohol consumption, tobacco use, stress, poor diet, being overweight or underweight, athletic training, health problems that affect hormones, or being infected with a sexually transmitted infection (Eisenberg & Brumbaugh, 2012).

Approximately 15% of couples in their reproductive years in the United States are infertile (Latendresse et al., 2010). Public perception is that the incidence of infertility is increasing, but in fact there has been no significant change in the proportion of infertile couples in the United States to the increasing population. Understanding the elements that are essential for normal fertility can help the nurse identify the many factors that may cause infertility. The components that must be present for normal fertility are discussed in **Box 19–3** ●.

The normal findings listed in Box 19–3 are correlated with possible causes of deviation in **Table 19–4** ●. With timing and environment playing such crucial roles in conception, it is an impressive natural phenomenon that the majority of couples in the United States are able to conceive. The remaining couples suffer infertility because of a male factor (30%), a female factor (30%), or either an unknown cause (unexplained infertility) or a problem with both partners (30%) (CDC, 2012a). Professional intervention can help infertile couples achieve pregnancy. In fact, the CDC reports that about 1% of infants born in the United States are conceived via assisted reproductive technology (CDC, 2013b).

Young couples with no history that is suggestive of reproductive disorders should be referred for infertility evaluation if they have been unable to conceive after at least 1 year of attempting to achieve pregnancy. An earlier workup is indicated in couples with positive history for fertility-lowering disease or advancing maternal age (Eisenberg & Brumbaugh, 2012). If the woman is over age 35, she is less likely to become pregnant because her ovaries contain a smaller number of eggs, the eggs that are left may not be as healthy, and she is more prone to miscarriage.

Box 19–3 Components Necessary for Normal Fertility

FEMALE PARTNER

- The cervical mucus must be favorable to ensure survival and passage of spermatozoa to the upper genital tract.
- The fallopian tubes must be patent and have normal fimbriae with peristaltic movements toward the uterus to facilitate transport and interaction of ovum and sperm.
- The ovaries must produce and release normal ova in a regular, cyclic fashion.
- There must be no obstruction between the ovaries and the uterus.
- The endometrium must be in a physiological state to allow implantation of the blastocyst and to sustain normal growth.
- Adequate reproductive hormones must be present.

MALE PARTNER

- The testes must produce spermatozoa of normal quality, quantity, and motility.
- The male genital tract must not be obstructed.
- The male genital tract secretions must be normal.
- Ejaculated spermatozoa must be deposited in the female vaginal tract in such a manner that they reach the cervix.

▶ GENETICS

Even when conception has been achieved, families can have special reproductive concerns. The desired and expected outcome of any pregnancy is the birth of a healthy, "perfect" baby. Parents experience grief, fear, and anger when they discover that their baby has been born with a defect or a genetic disease. Such an abnormality may be evident at birth or may not appear for some time. The baby may have inherited a disorder from one parent or both, creating guilt and strife within the family.

TABLE 19–4 Possible Causes of Infertility

NECESSARY NORMS	DEVIATIONS FROM NORMAL
Female	
Favorable cervical mucus	Cervicitis, cervical stenosis, use of coital lubricants, antisperm antibodies (immunological response)
Clear passage between cervix and tubes	Myomas, adhesions, adenomyosis, polyps, endometritis, cervical stenosis, endometriosis, congenital anomalies (e.g., septate uterus, diethylstilbestrol [DES] exposure)
Patent tubes with normal motility	Pelvic inflammatory disease, peritubal adhesions, endometriosis, intrauterine contraception (IUC), salpingitis (e.g., chlamydia, recurrent STIs), neoplasm, ectopic pregnancy, tubal ligation
Ovulation and release of ova	Primary ovarian failure, polycystic ovarian disease, hypothyroidism, pituitary tumor, lactation, peri-ovarian adhesions, endometriosis, premature ovarian failure, hyperprolactinemia, Turner syndrome
No obstruction between ovary and tubes	Adhesions, endometriosis, pelvic inflammatory disease
Endometrial preparation	Anovulation, luteal phase defect, malformation, uterine infection, Asherman syndrome
Male	
Normal semen analysis	Abnormalities of sperm or semen, polyspermia, congenital defect in testicular development, mumps after adolescence, cryptorchidism, infections, gonadal exposure to x-rays, chemotherapy, smoking, alcohol abuse, malnutrition, chronic or acute metabolic disease, medications (e.g., morphine, aspirin, ibuprofen), cocaine use, marijuana use, constrictive underclothing, heat
Unobstructed genital tract	Infections, tumors, congenital anomalies, vasectomy, strictures, trauma, varicocele
Normal genital tract secretions	Infections, autoimmunity to semen, tumors
Ejaculate deposited at the cervix	Premature ejaculation, impotence, hypospadias, retrograde ejaculation (e.g., as can happen with diabetes), neurological cord lesions, obesity (inhibiting adequate penetration)

Source: Based on Valentine, M., & Gardella, J. (2013). Infertility. In E. Youngkin, M. Davis, D. Schadewald, & C. Juve (Eds.), *Women's health: A primary care clinical guide* (4th ed., pp. 273–305). Boston, MA: Pearson.

Regardless of the type or scope of the problem, parents will have many questions: "What did I do?" "What caused it?" "How do I cope with it?" "Will it happen again?" The nurse must anticipate the couple's questions and concerns and guide, direct, and support the family. To do so, the nurse must have a basic knowledge of genetics and genetic counseling. Professional nurses can help expedite this process if they understand the principles involved and can direct the family to the appropriate resources.

Genetic Disorders

All hereditary material is carried on tightly coiled strands of deoxyribonucleic acid (DNA) found in genes that are housed in chromosomes within a cell's nucleus. Genes are the smallest units of inheritance (Jorde, 2010a). The Human Genome Project has made remarkable advances toward determining the exact DNA sequence of human genes and the precise genes that are associated with certain abnormalities such as fragile X syndrome and cystic fibrosis (Jorde, 2010a).

All *somatic (body) cells* contain 46 chromosomes, which is the *diploid* number; the sperm and egg contain half as many (23) chromosomes, or the *haploid* number. There are 23 pairs of homologous chromosomes (a matched pair of chromosomes, one inherited from each parent). Twenty-two of the pairs are **autosomes** (nonsex chromosomes), and one pair is made up of the sex chromosomes, X and Y. A normal female has a 46, XX chromosome constitution; a normal male has a 46, XY chromosome constitution.

The **karyotype**, or pictorial analysis of these chromosomes, is usually obtained from specially treated and stained peripheral blood lymphocytes. Placental tissue taken from a site near the insertion of the cord and deep enough to include chorion can also be sent for karyotyping of the fetus.

Chromosome abnormalities can occur in either the autosomes or the sex chromosomes and can be divided into two categories: abnormalities of number and abnormalities of structure. Even small alterations in chromosomes can cause problems, especially those associated with delayed growth and development. Some of these abnormalities can be also passed on to other offspring. Thus, in some cases, chromosomal analysis is appropriate even if clinical manifestations are mild.

ABNORMALITIES OF CHROMOSOMAL NUMBER

Abnormalities of chromosomal number are most often caused by nondisjunction, a failure of paired chromosomes to separate properly during cell division. If nondisjunction occurs in either the sperm or the egg before fertilization, the resulting zygote (fertilized egg) will have an abnormal chromosome makeup in all of the cells. In other words, each cell that develops from the zygote will be **monosomic** (having only one copy of a particular chromosome) or **trisomic** (having three copies of a particular chromosome). If nondisjunction occurs after fertilization, the developing zygote will have cells with two or more different chromosomal makeups, evolving into two or more different cell lines (**mosaicism**). Chromosome mosaics have trisomy occurring in some but not all of the cells of the body, in which case the manifestations are not as severe (Jorde, 2010a).

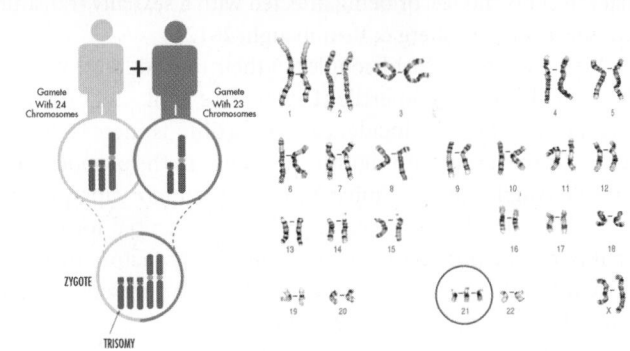

Figure 19–12 ● Karyotype of a female who has trisomy 21, Down syndrome. Note the extra chromosome 21.
Source: Courtesy of Greenwood Genetics Center. (2007). *Genetic counseling aids* (5th ed.). Greenwood, SC: Author.

Trisomies are the product of the union of a normal gamete (egg or sperm) with a gamete that contains an extra chromosome. When this happens the individual will have 47 chromosomes and be trisomic for whichever chromosome is extra (**Table 19–5** ●). Down syndrome is the most common trisomy abnormality seen in children (see **Figure 19–12** ●). The presence of the extra chromosome 21 produces distinctive clinical features (**Figure 19–13** ●). Although children born with Down syndrome have a variety of physical ailments, advances in medical science have extended their life expectancy.

Risks for having a child with Down syndrome increase when the mother is 35 years or older because the ovum has been in a suspended state for a long time. This time span increases the likelihood of errors that lead to nondisjunction (Jorde, 2010a).

Two other trisomies are trisomy 18 (Edwards syndrome) and trisomy 13 (Patau syndrome) (refer to Table 19–5). The prognosis for both trisomies 13 and 18 is extremely poor. Most children with these trisomies die within the first 3 months of life secondary to complications related to respiratory and cardiac abnormalities. However, 5%–10% survive the first year of life; therefore, the family needs to plan for the possibility of

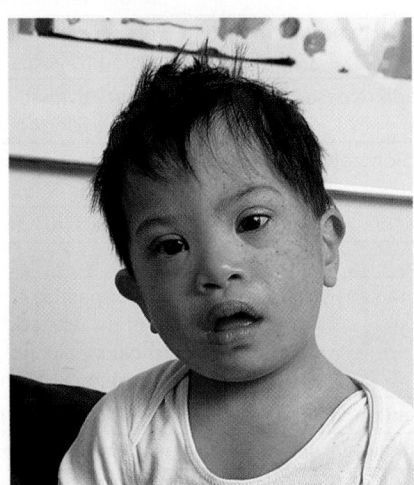

Figure 19–13 ● A boy with Down syndrome.
Source: Joni Hofmann/Fotolia.

TABLE 19–5 Chromosomal Syndromes

ALTERED CHROMOSOME	GENETIC DEFECT AND INCIDENCE	CHARACTERISTICS
5P	*Genetic defect:* deletion of short arm of chromosome 5 (cri du chat, or cat-cry syndrome) *Incidence:* 1 in 20,000 live births	*CNS:* severe mental retardation; a catlike cry in infancy *Head:* microcephaly; hypertelorism (widely spaced eyes); epicanthal folds; low-set ears *Other:* failure to thrive; various organ malformations
13	*Genetic defect:* trisomy 13 *Incidence:* 1 in 5,000 live births	*CNS:* mental retardation; severe hypotonia; seizures *Head:* microcephaly; microphthalmia, and/or coloboma (keyhole-shaped pupil); malformed ears; aplasia of external auditory canal; micrognathia (abnormally small lower jaw); cleft lip and palate *Hands:* polydactyly (extra digits); abnormal posturing of fingers; abnormal dermatoglyphics *Other:* congenital heart defects; hemangiomas; gastrointestinal tract defects; various malformations of other organs
18	*Genetic defect:* trisomy 18 *Incidence:* 1 in 3,000 live births	*CNS:* mental retardation; severe hypotonia *Head:* prominent occiput; low-set ears; corneal opacities; ptosis (drooping eyelids) *Hands:* third and fourth fingers overlapped by second and fifth fingers; abnormal dermatoglyphics; syndactyly (webbing of fingers) *Other:* congenital heart defects; renal abnormalities; single umbilical artery; gastrointestinal tract abnormalities; rocker-bottom feet; cryptorchidism; various malformations of other organs
21	*Genetic defect:* trisomy 21 (Down syndrome) (secondary nondisjunction or 14/21 unbalanced translocation) *Incidence:* average 1 in 700 live births, incidence variable with age of woman	*CNS:* mental retardation; hypotonia at birth *Head:* flattened occiput; depressed nasal bridge; mongoloid slant of eyes; epicanthal folds; white specking of the iris (Brushfield spots); protrusion of the tongue; high, arched palate; low-set ears *Hands:* broad, short fingers; abnormalities of finger and foot; dermal ridge patterns (dermatoglyphics); transverse palmar crease *Other:* congenital heart disease
XO (sex chromosome)	*Genetic defect:* only one X chromosome or partially missing second X chromosome in female (Turner syndrome) *Incidence:* 1 in 300 to 7,000 live female births	*CNS:* no intellectual impairment; some perceptual difficulties *Head:* low hairline; webbed neck *Trunk:* short stature; cubitus valgus (increased carrying angle of arm); excessive nevi (congenital discoloration of skin because of pigmentation); broad, shieldlike chest with widely spaced nipples; puffy feet; no toenails *Other:* fibrous streaks in ovaries; underdeveloped secondary sex characteristics; primary amenorrhea; usually infertile; renal anomalies; coarctation of the aorta
XXY (sex chromosome)	*Genetic defect:* extra X chromosome in male (Klinefelter syndrome) *Incidence:* 1 in 1,000 live male births, approximately 1%–2% of institutionalized males	*CNS:* mild mental retardation *Trunk:* occasional gynecomastia (abnormally large male breasts); eunuchoid body proportions (lack of male muscular and sexual development) *Other:* small, soft testes; underdeveloped secondary sex characteristics; usually sterile

Source: Based on Genetic Science Learning Center. (2012, August 6). Learn.Genetics™. *Learn.Genetics.* Retrieved from http://learn.genetics.utah.edu.

long-term care of a severely affected child and for family support (U.S. Library of Medicine, 2012a, 2012b).

Monosomies occur when a normal gamete unites with a gamete that is missing a chromosome. The most common monosomy is Turner syndrome, 45X, caused by the loss of the paternal X chromosome (Jorde, 2010a). If the fetus with monosomy survives, it is due to mosaicism. These individuals are sterile females (see Table 19–5).

ABNORMALITIES OF CHROMOSOME STRUCTURE

Abnormalities of chromosome structure involve only parts of the chromosome and occur in two forms: translocation and deletions or additions. Some children born with Down syndrome have an abnormal rearrangement of chromosomal material known as a *translocation*. Clinically, the two types of Down syndrome are indistinguishable; the only way to distinguish them is to do a chromosome analysis.

Structure abnormality is also caused by additions or deletions of chromosomal material. Any portion of a chromosome may be lost or added, generally leading to some adverse effect. Depending on how much chromosomal material is involved, the clinical effects may be mild or severe. Many types of additions and deletions have been described, such as the deletion of the short arm of chromosome 5 (*cri du chat*, or cat-cry syndrome) or the deletion of the long arm of chromosome 18 (Edwards syndrome). Table 19–5 lists other chromosomal syndromes.

SEX CHROMOSOME ABNORMALITIES To better understand abnormalities of the sex chromosomes, the nurse should know that in a female, at an early embryonic stage, one of the two normal X chromosomes becomes inactive. The inactive X chromosome forms a dark staining area known as the *Barr body*. The normal female has one Barr body, because one of her two X chromosomes has been inactivated. The normal male has no Barr bodies because he has only one X chromosome.

The most common sex chromosome abnormalities are Turner syndrome in females (45, XO with no Barr bodies present) and Klinefelter syndrome in males (47, XXY with one Barr body present). See Table 19–5 for clinical descriptions of these abnormalities. Klinefelter syndrome is usually the result of nondisjunction of the X chromosome in the ovum. Maternal age over 35 years increases the risks for this abnormality (Jorde, 2010a).

The mosaic form of the XO chromosome is associated with daughters of women who took the drug DES during pregnancy. The fertility of women with the mosaic form of the XO chromosome may not be impaired; however, there is a higher percentage of uterine malformation and hormonal difficulty associated with it and therefore a high degree of miscarriage.

Modes of Inheritance

Many inherited diseases are produced by an abnormality in a single gene or pair of genes. In such instances, the chromosomes are normal on the gross level. The defect is at the gene level. Some of these gene defects can be detected by technologies such as DNA and other biochemical assays.

The two major categories of inheritance are **Mendelian (single-gene) inheritance** and **non-Mendelian (multifactorial) inheritance**. Each single-gene trait is determined by a pair of genes working together. These genes are responsible for the observable expression of the traits (e.g., brown eyes, dark skin), referred to as the **phenotype**. The total genetic makeup of an individual is referred to as the **genotype** (pattern of the genes on the chromosomes).

One of the genes for a trait is inherited from the mother, the other from the father. An individual who has two identical genes at a given locus is considered to be *homozygous* for that trait. Individuals are considered to be *heterozygous* for a particular trait when they have two different alleles (alternative forms of the same gene) at a given locus on a pair of homologous chromosomes. A parent may be a **carrier** for a single-gene disorder without having any of the manifestations; that is, he or she is phenotypically normal (Jorde, 2010a).

The best known modes of single-gene inheritance are autosomal dominant, autosomal recessive, and X-linked (sex-linked) recessive. There is also an X-linked dominant mode of inheritance and fragile X syndrome, both of which are uncommon.

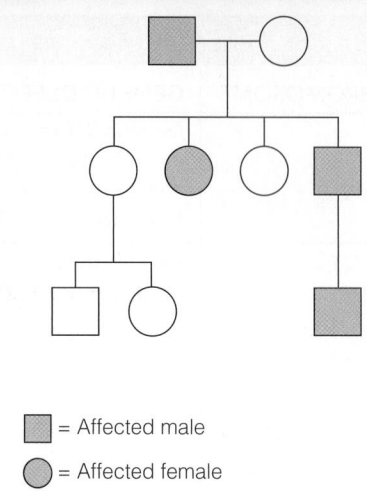

■ = Affected male

● = Affected female

Figure 19–14 ● Autosomal dominant pedigree. One parent is affected. Statistically, 50% of offspring will be affected regardless of gender.

AUTOSOMAL DOMINANT INHERITANCE An individual is said to have an autosomal dominant inherited disorder if the disease trait is heterozygous; that is, if the abnormal gene overshadows the normal gene of the pair to produce the trait. It is essential to remember that in autosomal dominant inheritance the following occurs:

■ An affected individual generally has an affected parent. Thus the family **pedigree** (graphic representation of a family tree) usually shows multiple generations with the disorder.

■ Affected individuals have a 50% chance of passing on the abnormal gene to each of their children (**Figure 19–14 ●**).

■ Males and females are equally affected, and a father can pass the abnormal gene on to his son. This is an important principle when distinguishing autosomal dominant disorders from X-linked disorders.

■ Autosomal dominant inherited disorders have varying degrees of presentation. This is an important factor in counseling families concerning autosomal dominant disorders. Although a parent may have a mild form of the disease, the child may have a more severe form.

Autosomal dominant conditions such as phocomelia (a developmental anomaly characterized by the absence of the upper portion of the limbs; a hand may be attached to a shoulder) can have minimal expression in a parent but severe effects in a child. Other common autosomal dominant inherited disorders are Huntington disease, polycystic kidney disease, neurofibromatosis (von Recklinghausen disease), and achondroplastic dwarfism.

AUTOSOMAL RECESSIVE INHERITANCE In an autosomal recessive inherited disorder, the individual must have two abnormal genes (one from the mother and one from the father) to be affected. It is essential to remember that in autosomal recessive inheritance, the following occur:

■ An affected individual may have clinically normal parents, but both parents are carriers of the abnormal gene (**Figure 19–15 ●**).

■ When both parents are carriers, there is a 25% chance that the abnormal gene will be passed on to any of their offspring.

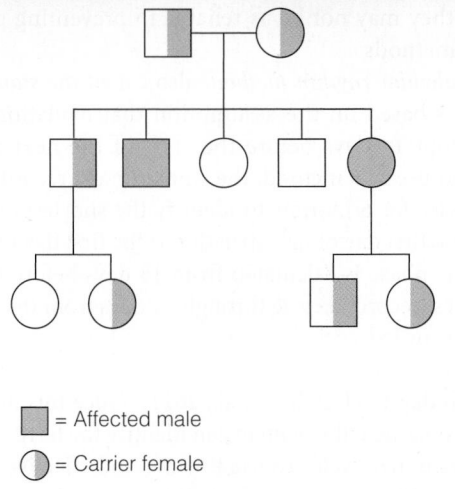

= Affected male

= Carrier female

Figure 19–15 ● Autosomal recessive pedigree. Both parents are carriers. Statistically, 25% of offspring are affected regardless of gender.

Each pregnancy has a 25% chance of resulting in an affected child.

■ If a child of two carrier parents is clinically normal, there is a 50% chance that the child is a carrier of the gene.

■ Both males and females are equally affected.

■ There is an increased history of consanguineous matings (mating of close relatives).

Some common autosomal recessive inherited disorders are cystic fibrosis, phenylketonuria, galactosemia, sickle cell disease, Tay–Sachs disease, and most metabolic disorders.

X-LINKED RECESSIVE INHERITANCE X-linked, or sex-linked, disorders are those in which the abnormal gene is carried on the X chromosome. Thus an X-linked disorder is manifested in a male who carries the abnormal gene on his X chromosome. His mother is considered to be a carrier when the normal gene on one X chromosome overshadows the abnormal gene on the other X chromosome. It is essential to remember that in X-linked recessive inheritance the following occur:

■ There is no male-to-male transmission. Affected males obtain the abnormal gene through the female line (see **Figure 19–16** ●).

■ There is a 50% chance that a carrier mother will pass the normal gene to each of her sons, who will thus be unaffected.

■ There is a 50% chance that a carrier mother will pass the abnormal gene to each of her daughters, who become carriers.

■ Fathers affected with an X-linked disorder cannot pass the disorder to their sons, but all their daughters become carriers of the disorder.

Common X-linked recessive disorders are hemophilia, Duchenne muscular dystrophy, and color blindness.

X-LINKED DOMINANT INHERITANCE The X-linked dominant disorders are rare, the most common being vitamin D–resistant rickets and fragile X syndrome. When X-linked dominance does occur, the pattern is similar to that of X-linked recessive inheritance except that heterozygous females are

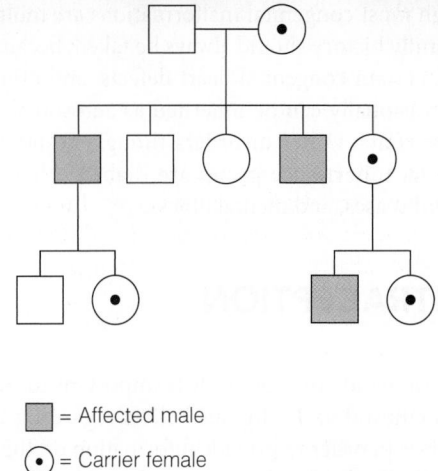

= Affected male

= Carrier female

Figure 19–16 ● X-linked recessive pedigree. The mother is the carrier. Statistically, 50% of male offspring are affected, and 50% of female offspring are carriers.

affected. It is essential to remember that in X-linked dominant inheritance there is no male-to-male transmission. Affected fathers will have affected daughters; however, because they pass only the Y chromosome to male offspring, any sons will not be affected.

Fragile X Syndrome Fragile X syndrome is an inherited form of mental retardation; it is second only to Down syndrome among all causes of moderate mental retardation in males. Fragile X syndrome is a central nervous system disorder linked to a "fragile" site on the X chromosome. It is characterized by moderate mental retardation, large protuberant ears, and large testes after puberty. The carrier females do not have the abnormal features, but about one third are mildly retarded.

MULTIFACTORIAL INHERITANCE Many common congenital malformations such as cleft palate, heart defects, spina bifida, dislocated hips, clubfoot, and pyloric stenosis are caused by an interaction of many genes and environmental factors. They are, therefore, multifactorial in origin. It is essential to remember that in multifactorial inheritance the following occurs:

■ The malformations may vary from mild to severe. For example, spina bifida may range in severity from mild (spina bifida occulta) to more severe (myelomeningocele). It is believed that the more severe the defect, the greater the number of genes present for that defect.

■ There is often a sex bias. For example, pyloric stenosis is more common in males, whereas cleft palate is more common in females. When a member of the less commonly affected sex shows the condition, a greater number of genes must usually be present to cause the defect.

■ In the presence of environmental influences (such as seasonal changes, altitude, radiation exposure, chemicals in the environment, or exposure to toxic substances), fewer genes are needed to manifest the disease in the offspring.

■ In contrast to single-gene disorders, multifactorial inheritance has an additive effect. The more family members who have the defect, the greater the risk that the next pregnancy will also be affected (Jorde, 2010b).

Although most congenital malformations are multifactorial, a careful family history should always be taken, because cleft lip and palate, certain congenital heart defects, and other malformations occasionally can be inherited as autosomal dominant or recessive traits. Other disorders thought to be within the multifactorial inheritance group are diabetes, hypertension, some heart diseases, and mental illness.

▶ CONTRACEPTION

Many couples use contraception to allow them to plan pregnancy and/or avoid conception. It is important to understand the client's cultural and religious beliefs regarding the use of contraceptives in order to provide information on the best contraceptive choices for the client or couple.

Fertility Awareness Methods

Fertility awareness–based methods, also known as *natural family planning*, are based on an understanding of the changes that occur throughout a woman's ovulatory cycle. Fertility awareness methods take into account the life span of sperm (3–6 days) and the ovum (1–3 days) in the female reproductive tract. Maximum fertility for the woman occurs approximately 6 days before ovulation and decreases rapidly the day after (Hatcher et al., 2011). All these methods require periods of abstinence and recording of certain events throughout the cycle; therefore, cooperation of the partner is important.

Fertility awareness methods are free, safe, and acceptable to many individuals whose religious beliefs prohibit other methods. They provide increased awareness of the body, involve no artificial substances or devices, encourage a couple to communicate about sexual activity and family planning, and are useful in helping a couple plan a pregnancy.

However, these methods require extensive initial counseling to be used effectively. They may interfere with sexual spontaneity; they require careful maintenance of records for several cycles before beginning to use them; they may be difficult or impossible for women with irregular cycles to use; and although theoretically they should be very reliable, in practice they may not be as reliable in preventing pregnancy as other methods.

The *calendar rhythm method*, also called the *standard days method*, is based on the assumption that ovulation tends to occur about 14 days before the start of the next menstrual period. To use this method, the woman must record her menstrual cycles for 6 months to identify the shortest and longest cycles. The first day of menstruation is the first day of the cycle. The fertile phase is calculated from 18 days before the end of the shortest recorded cycle through 11 days from the end of the longest recorded cycle. For example, if a woman's cycle lasts from 24 to 28 days, the fertile phase would be calculated as day 6 through day 17 (Hatcher et al., 2011). Once this information has been obtained, the woman can identify the fertile and infertile phases of her cycle. To use this method effectively for contraception, she must abstain from intercourse during the fertile phase. The calendar method is the least reliable of the fertility awareness methods and has largely been replaced by other, more scientific approaches.

The *basal body temperature (BBT) method* to detect ovulation requires that a woman take her BBT every morning upon awakening (before any activity) and record the readings on a temperature graph. To do this, she uses a basal body temperature thermometer, which shows tenths of a degree rather than the two tenths shown on standard thermometers. She may also use tympanic thermometry (an "ear thermometer"). After 3–4 months of recording temperatures, a woman with regular cycles should be able to predict when ovulation will occur. The method is based on the fact that the temperature sometimes drops just before ovulation and almost always rises and remains elevated for several days afterward. The temperature rise occurs in response to the increased progesterone levels that occur in the second half of the cycle. **Figure 19–17 ●** shows a sample BBT chart. To avoid conception, the couple abstains from intercourse on the day of the temperature rise and for 3 days afterward. Because the temperature rise does not occur until after ovulation, a woman who had intercourse just before the rise is at risk of pregnancy. To decrease this risk, some couples abstain from intercourse for several days before the anticipated time of ovulation and then for 3 days afterward.

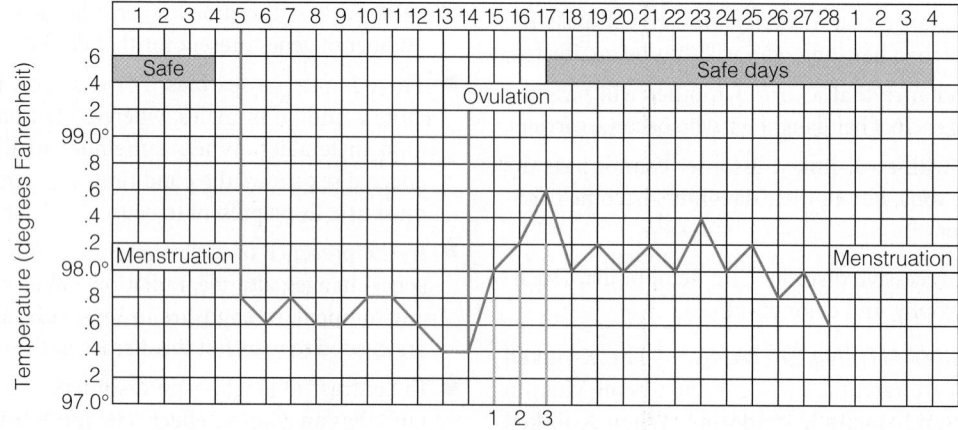

Figure 19–17 ● Sample basal body temperature chart.

The *ovulation method*, sometimes called the *cervical mucus method* or the *Billings method*, involves the assessment of cervical mucus changes that occur during the menstrual cycle. The amount and character of cervical mucus change because of the influence of **estrogen** and **progesterone**. At the time of ovulation, the mucus (estrogen-dominant mucus) is clearer, more stretchable (a quality called *spinnbarkeit*), more permeable to sperm and can prolong sperm life (Walcker & Pederson, 2013). It also shows a characteristic fern pattern when placed on a glass slide and allowed to dry. During the luteal phase, the cervical mucus is thick and sticky (progesterone-dominant mucus) and forms a network that traps sperm, making their passage more difficult.

To use the cervical mucus method, the woman abstains from intercourse for the first menstrual cycle. Each day she assesses her cervical mucus for amount, feeling of slipperiness or wetness, color, clearness, and spinnbarkeit, with the goal of becoming familiar with varying characteristics. The peak day of wetness and clear, stretchable mucus is assumed to be the time of ovulation. To use this method correctly, the woman should abstain from intercourse from the time she *first* notices that the mucus is becoming clear, more elastic, and slippery until 4 days *after* the last wet mucus (ovulation) day. Because this method evaluates the effects of hormonal changes, it can be used by women with irregular cycles.

The *symptothermal method* consists of various assessments made and recorded by the couple. These include information regarding cycle days, coitus, cervical mucus changes, and secondary signs such as increased libido, abdominal bloating, *mittelschmerz* (midcycle abdominal pain), and basal body temperature. Through the various assessments, the couple learns to recognize signs that indicate ovulation. This combined approach tends to improve the effectiveness of fertility awareness as a method of birth control.

Situational Contraceptives

Abstinence can be considered a method of contraception, and, partly because of changing values and the increased risk of infection with intercourse, it is gaining increased acceptance.

Coitus interruptus, or withdrawal, is one of the oldest and least reliable methods of contraception. This method requires that the male withdraw from the female's vagina when he feels that ejaculation is impending. He then ejaculates away from the woman's external genitalia. Failure tends to occur for two reasons: (1) This method demands great self-control on the part of the man, who must withdraw just as he feels the urge for deeper penetration with impending orgasm, and (2) some preejaculatory fluid, which can contain sperm, may be released from the penis during the excitement phase before ejaculation. The fact that the quantity of sperm in this preejaculatory fluid is increased after a recent ejaculation is especially significant for couples who engage in repeated episodes of intercourse within a short period of time. Couples who use this method should be aware of postcoital contraceptive options in case the man fails to withdraw in time.

Douching after intercourse is an ineffective method of contraception and is not recommended. It may actually facilitate conception by pushing sperm farther up the birth canal.

Spermicides

The **spermicide** nonoxynol-9 (N-9), which is approved for use in the United States, is available as a cream, jelly, foam, vaginal film, and suppository. A spermicide is inserted into the vagina before intercourse. It destroys sperm by disrupting the cell membrane. A spermicide that effervesces in a moist environment offers rapid protection, and coitus may take place immediately after it is inserted. A suppository may require up to 30 minutes to dissolve and will not offer protection until it has done so. The nurse instructs the woman to insert any of these spermicide preparations high in the vagina and to maintain a supine position.

N-9 is minimally effective when used alone. Its effectiveness increases in conjunction with a diaphragm, sponge, or condom. The major advantages of spermicides are their wide availability and low toxicity. Skin irritation and allergic reactions to spermicides are the primary disadvantages. In 2007 the Food and Drug Administration (FDA) issued a ruling requiring that a warning and label information be added for all over-the-counter vaginal contraceptives containing N-9. The ruling states that N-9 does not offer protection against infection from the human immunodeficiency virus, which causes HIV/AIDS, or against any other STI. Moreover, N-9 may actually increase a woman's risk of HIV infection because it irritates vaginal tissue, making it more susceptible to invasion by organisms such as HIV (FDA, 2009).

Barrier Methods of Contraception

Barrier methods of contraception prevent the transport of sperm to the ovum, immobilize sperm, or are lethal against sperm.

MALE AND FEMALE CONDOMS The male **condom** offers a viable means of contraception when used consistently and properly (**Figure 19–18 ●**). Acceptance of condom use has been increasing as a growing number of men are assuming responsibility for regulation of fertility. The condom is applied to the erect penis, rolled from the tip to the end of the shaft, before vulvar or vaginal contact. A small space must be left at the end of the condom to allow for collection of the ejaculate, so that the condom will not break at the time of ejaculation. If the condom or vagina is dry, water-soluble lubricants such as K-Y jelly should be used to prevent irritation and possible condom breakage.

Care must be taken when removing the condom after intercourse. For optimal effectiveness, the man should withdraw his penis from the vagina while it is still erect and hold the condom rim to prevent spillage. If after ejaculation the penis becomes flaccid while still in the vagina, the male should hold onto the edge of the condom while withdrawing to avoid spilling the semen and to prevent the condom from slipping off.

The effectiveness of male condoms is largely determined by their use. The condom is small, disposable, and inexpensive; it has no side effects (if neither partner is allergic to latex), requires no medical examination or supervision, and offers visual evidence of effectiveness. Most condoms are made of latex, although polyurethane and silicone rubber condoms are available for individuals who are allergic to latex. All condoms except natural "skin" condoms, made from lamb's intestines, offer protection

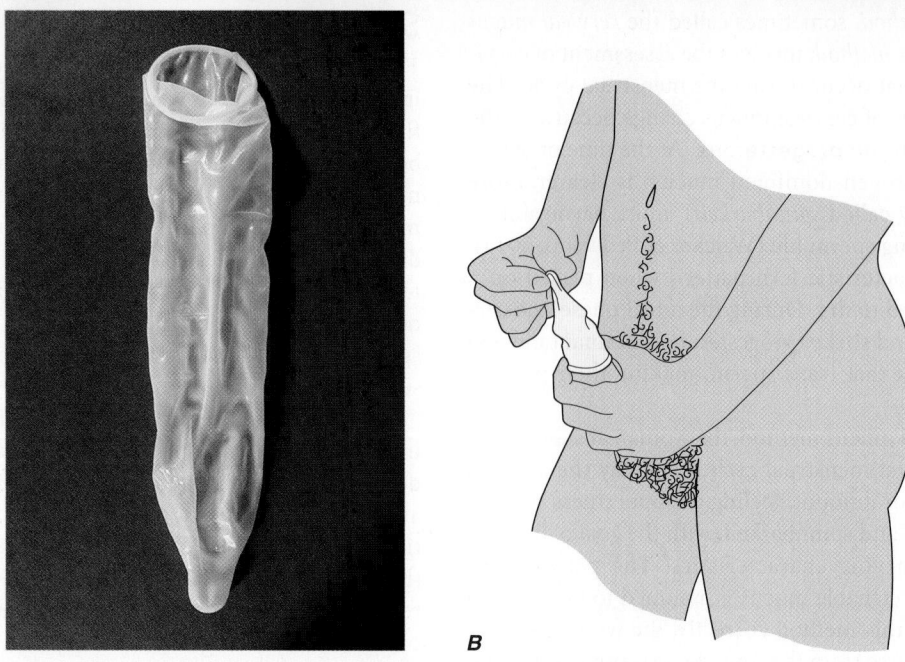

A   *B*

Figure 19–18 ● *A,* An unrolled condom with reservoir tip. *B,* Correct use.

against both pregnancy and STIs. Breakage, displacement, perineal or vaginal irritation, and dulled sensation are possible disadvantages. Condoms should not be stored in hot conditions because heat accelerates their deterioration, making them more susceptible to breaking. Thus, men should avoid placing them in a car glove box or in a wallet in a rear pants pocket.

The male condom is becoming increasingly popular because of the protection it offers from infections. For women, an STI increases the risk of pelvic inflammatory disease and resultant infertility. Many women are beginning to insist that their sexual partners use condoms, and many women carry condoms with them.

The *Reality female condom* (**Figure 19–19** ●) is a thin polyurethane sheath with a flexible ring at each end. The inner ring,

at the closed end of the condom, serves as the means of insertion and fits over the cervix like a diaphragm. The second ring remains outside the vagina and covers a portion of the woman's perineum. It also covers the base of the man's penis during intercourse. Available over the counter and designed for one-time use, the condom may be inserted up to 8 hours before intercourse. The inner sheath is prelubricated but does not contain spermicide and is not designed to be used with a male condom. Because it also covers a portion of the vulva, it probably provides better protection than other contraceptive methods against some pathogens. High cost, noisiness during intercourse, and the cumbersome feel of the device make acceptability a problem for some couples.

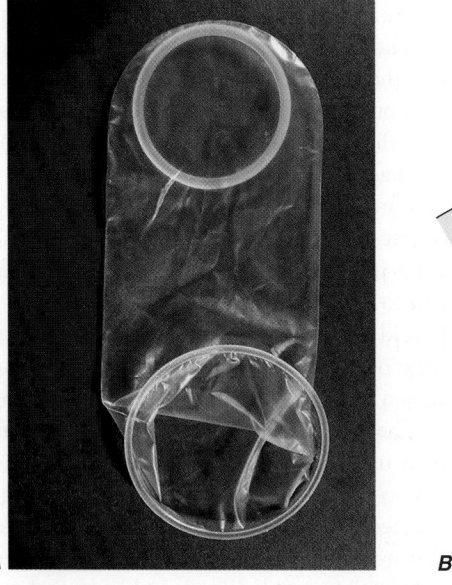

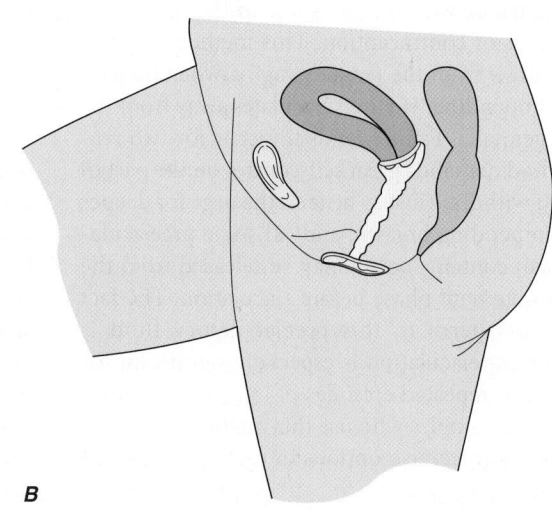

A   *B*

Figure 19–19 ● *A,* The female condom. *B,* When properly inserted, the outer ring should rest on the folds of the skin around the vaginal opening, and the inner ring (closed end) should fit loosely against the cervix.

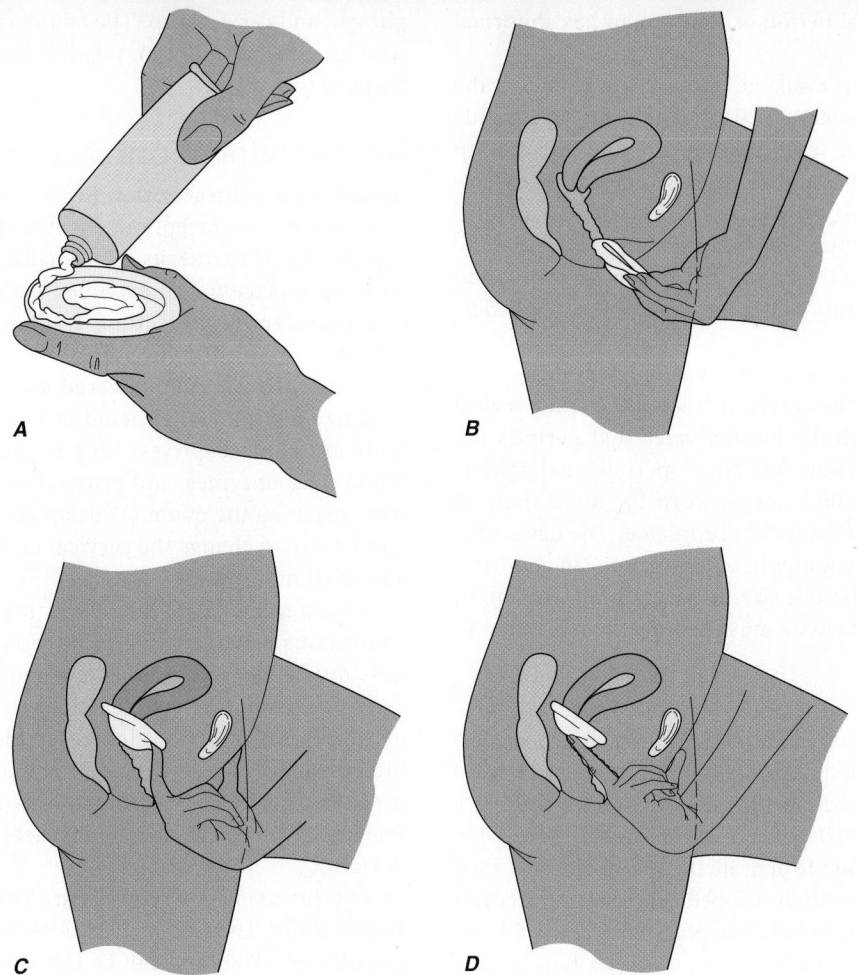

Figure 19–20 ● Inserting the diaphragm: *A*, Apply jelly to the rim and center of the diaphragm. *B*, Insert the diaphragm. *C*, Push the rim of the diaphragm under the pubic symphysis. *D*, Check placement of the diaphragm. The cervix should be felt through the diaphragm.

DIAPHRAGM AND CERVICAL CAP   A **diaphragm** (Figure 19–20 ●) is used with spermicidal cream or jelly and offers a good level of protection from conception. The woman must be fitted with a diaphragm and instructed in its use by trained personnel. The diaphragm should be rechecked for correct size after each childbirth and whenever a woman has gained or lost 10–15 pounds or more.

The diaphragm must be inserted before intercourse, with approximately 1 teaspoonful (or 1.5 inches as squeezed from the tube) of spermicidal jelly placed around its rim and in the cup. This chemical barrier supplements the mechanical barrier of the diaphragm. The diaphragm is inserted through the vagina and covers the cervix. The last step in insertion is to push the edge of the diaphragm under the symphysis pubis. When fitted properly and correctly in place, the diaphragm should not cause discomfort to the woman or her partner. Correct placement of the diaphragm can be checked by touching the cervix with a fingertip through the cup. The center of the diaphragm should be over the cervix. If more than 6 hours elapse between insertion of the diaphragm and intercourse, additional spermicidal cream should be used. It is necessary to leave the diaphragm in place for at least 6 hours after coitus. If intercourse is desired again within the 6 hours, another type of contraception must be used or additional spermicidal jelly placed in the vagina with an applicator,

taking care not to disturb the placement of the diaphragm. The diaphragm should not remain in the vagina for more than 24 hours. Periodically, the diaphragm should be held up to the light and inspected for tears or holes.

Some couples feel that the use of a diaphragm interferes with the spontaneity of intercourse. The nurse can suggest that the partner insert the diaphragm as part of foreplay. The woman can then easily verify the placement herself.

Diaphragms are an excellent contraceptive method for women who are lactating, who cannot or do not wish to use the pill (oral contraceptives), who are smokers over age 35, or who have infrequent sexual intercourse. A silicone diaphragm is available for women with latex allergy.

Women who object to touching their genitals to insert the diaphragm, check its placement, and remove it may find this method unsatisfactory. Women who are very obese or who have short fingers may find the diaphragm difficult to insert. The diaphragm is not recommended for women with a history of urinary tract infection (UTI), because pressure from the diaphragm on the urethra may interfere with complete bladder emptying and lead to recurrent UTIs. Women with a history of toxic shock syndrome should not use diaphragms or any of the barrier methods because they are left in place for prolonged periods. For the same reason, the diaphragm should not be used during a menstrual period or if a woman has abnormal vaginal discharge.

The only **cervical cap** available in the United States is the FemCap (Walcker & Pederson, 2013). The FemCap is made of silicone, looks like a small sailor's cap, and has a strap placed over the dome that allows for easy removal. The Fem-Cap does not have to fit on the cervix because it is held in place by vaginal wall muscles. Spermicide is placed in the dome and in the brim of the cap so that sperm are exposed to spermicide without getting under the cap (Walcker & Pederson, 2013).

Lea's shield is a reusable silicone vaginal barrier method that completely covers the cervix. It is similar to the cervical cap but contains a centrally located valve that permits the passage of cervical secretions and air. A spermicide should be used with it, and it should not be worn for more than 48 hours with a single application of spermicide. The device has been available over the counter in several European countries for over a decade because one size fits virtually all women. In the United States, a woman must see her practitioner to obtain one.

VAGINAL SPONGE   The *Today vaginal sponge,* available without a prescription, is a pillow-shaped, soft, absorbent synthetic sponge containing spermicide. It is made with a concave or cupped area on one side that fits over the cervix and has a loop for easy removal. The sponge is moistened thoroughly with water before insertion to activate the spermicide and then inserted into the vagina with the cupped side against the cervix (**Figure 19–21 ●**). It should be left in place for 6 hours following intercourse and may be worn for up to 24 hours, then removed and discarded.

The sponge has the following advantages: Professional fitting is not required, it may be used for multiple acts of coitus for up to 24 hours, one size fits all, and it acts as both a barrier and a spermicide. Problems associated with the sponge include difficulty removing it and irritation or allergic reactions. Some women report a problem because the sponge absorbs vaginal secretions, contributing to vaginal dryness. For women without children the failure rate is comparable to that of the dia-phragm and cervical cap. The failure rate is higher for women who have borne children, possibly because of changes in the shape of the cervix.

Intrauterine Contraception

Intrauterine contraception (IUC) is a safe, effective method of reversible contraception. An IUC device is designed to be inserted into the uterus by a qualified healthcare provider and left in place for an extended period, providing continuous contraceptive protection. Traditionally IUC was believed to act by preventing the implantation of a fertilized ovum. Therefore, IUC was considered an abortifacient (abortion-causing) method. This belief is not accurate. IUC devices truly are contraceptives; they trigger the release of white blood cells, enzymes, and prostaglandins that prevent sperm from reaching the ovum (Walcker & Pederson, 2013). IUC is also known to change the cervical mucus, endometrial lining, and tubal motility.

Advantages of IUC include its high rate of effectiveness, continuous contraceptive protection, relative inexpensiveness over time, and it does not require any coitus-related activity. Possible adverse reactions to an IUC device include discomfort at insertion, increased bleeding during menses, increased risk of pelvic infection for about 3 weeks following insertion, perforation of the uterus during insertion, intermenstrual bleeding, dysmenorrhea, and expulsion of the device.

Two forms of IUC devices are currently available in the United States. The Copper T380A (ParaGard) is nonhormonal, is highly effective, and can be left in place for up to 10 years. Mirena and Skyla are levonorgestrel-releasing intrauterine systems (LNG-IUS), small, T-shaped frames with reservoirs that release levonorgestrel gradually (**Figure 19–22 ●**). They are

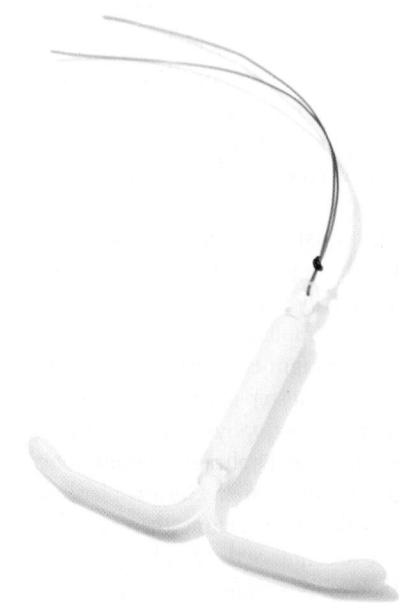

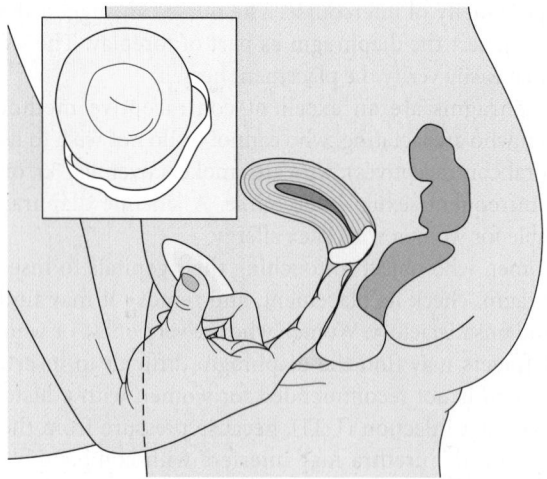

Figure 19–21 ● The contraceptive sponge is moistened well with water and then inserted into the vagina with the concave portion positioned over the cervix.

Figure 19–22 ● Levonorgestrel intrauterine system (LNG-IUS). The section near the string is a reservoir for the progestin that is slowly released into the uterine cavity.
Source: © Timothy Hogan/Corbis.

comparable in effectiveness to the Copper T380A and may be left in place for up to 5 years (Mirena) and 3 years (Skyla). After 3 months of use of the LNG-IUS, the amount of bleeding and the length of menstrual cycles are reduced, and some women experience amenorrhea. Most women welcome this once they know that the absence of menses is safe and not an indication of pregnancy.

Formerly, IUC was recommended only for women who had at least one child and were in a stable, mutually monogamous relationship, because these women have the lowest risk of developing a pelvic infection. Research indicates that, contrary to common belief, IUC is reliable and effective for women who have never been pregnant; it is effective against ectopic pregnancy because of its overall effectiveness in preventing any pregnancy. Moreover, the copper device is a good choice for women who cannot use hormonal forms of contraception (Walcker & Pederson, 2013). Note that women should be encouraged to use a barrier method of contraception as well to protect against STIs.

The IUC device is inserted into the uterus with its string or tail protruding through the cervix into the vagina. It may be inserted at any time during a woman's cycle, provided that she is not pregnant, or during the 4- to 6-week postpartum check. The copper device may be inserted up to 5 days after unprotected intercourse as a method of emergency contraception. After insertion, the clinician instructs the woman to check for the presence of the string once a week for the first month and then after each menses. She is told that she may have some cramping or bleeding intermittently for 2–6 weeks and that her first few menses may be irregular. Follow-up examination is suggested 4–8 weeks after insertion.

Women using IUC should contact their healthcare providers if they are exposed to an STI or if they develop the following warning signs: late period, abnormal spotting or bleeding, pain with intercourse, abdominal pain, abnormal discharge, signs of infection (fever, chills, and malaise), or missing string. If the woman becomes pregnant with an IUC device in place, the device should be removed as soon as possible to prevent spontaneous miscarriage (Walcker & Pederson, 2013).

Hormonal Contraceptives

Hormonal contraceptives are available in a variety of forms. The hormones used are progestin, a synthetic progesterone, and estrogen, usually estradiol. Progestins may be used alone or in combination with estrogen.

COMBINED ESTROGEN–PROGESTIN APPROACHES

Combined hormonal approaches work by inhibiting the release of an ovum, by creating an atrophic endometrium, and by maintaining a thick cervical mucus that slows sperm transport and inhibits the process that allows sperm to penetrate the ovum.

Combined Oral Contraceptives Combined oral contraceptives (COCs), also called *birth control pills*, are a combination of estrogen and progestin. COCs are safe, highly effective, and rapidly reversible. COCs are generally taken daily for 21 days, typically beginning on the Sunday after the first day of the menstrual cycle. The woman can also start on day 1 of her menstrual cycle or use

---

Box 19–4 Quick Start

Healthcare providers should consider suggesting the Quick Start method to clients, which allows them to start the hormonal contraceptive method on any day during the menstrual cycle. This provides clients with protection faster and more reliably, rather than waiting for days or weeks from receiving the prescription to starting contraceptive use.

To use Quick Start:

■ If the last menstrual period (LMP) was within the past 5 days, start the pills immediately.

■ If LMP was more than 5 days ago and a pregnancy test is negative, assess the last episode of unprotected sex to determine whether emergency contraception is needed before starting the pills.

■ If the woman had unprotected sex within the past 2 weeks, start the pills and advise the client to return for a pregnancy test in 3 weeks.

■ Instruct the client whose LMP was more than 5 days ago to use backup contraception for 7 days.

Sources: Based on Association of Reproductive Health Professionals. (2011). *Choosing a birth control method.* Retrieved from http://www.arhp.org/Publications-and-Resources/Quick-Reference-Guide-for-Clinicians/choosing/Initiation-Hormonal-Contraceptives; New York City Department of Health and Hygiene. (2012). *Quick guide to contraception.* Retrieved from http://www.nyc.gov/html/doh/downloads/pdf/ms/contra-guide.pdf; and Options for Sexual Health. (2013). *Using the pill.* Retrieved from https://www.options-forsexualhealth.org/birth-control-pregnancy/birth-control-options/hormonal-methods/combined-hormonal-contraceptives/using-pill.

---

the Quick Start method (see **Box 19–4** ●). In most cases, menses occurs 1–4 days after the last pill is taken. Seven days after taking her last pill, the woman restarts the pill. Thus, the woman always begins the pill on the same day. Some companies offer a 28-day pack with seven "blank" pills so that the woman never stops taking a pill. The pill should be taken at approximately the same time each day—usually upon arising or before retiring in the evening.

Research has demonstrated that with today's low-dose COCs, the 7 hormone-free days may result in failure to completely suppress ovarian function, resulting in the development of an ovarian follicle and possible ovulation (Hatcher et al., 2011). Consequently, some brands of low-dose COCs now have shortened or modified intervals. For instance, Loestrin 24 Fe has 24 active pills and only 4 placebo pills that contain iron. Extended-cycle COCs are available for women who would rather not have a monthly period. Seasonale and Seasonique are the first FDA-approved extended-cycle COCs. They both are 91-day regimens in which a woman takes an active pill daily for 84 consecutive days followed by 7 days of inactive tablets, during which the woman has a period. Thus, a woman has only four periods a year. Extended use reduces the side effects of COCs, such as bloating, headache, breast tenderness, and cramping (Hatcher et al., 2011). Another COC, Lybrel, has been approved by the FDA for continuous 365-day use with no scheduled hormone-free periods.

Although they are highly effective when taken correctly, COCs may produce a variety of side effects, which can be either progesterone or estrogen related (**Table 19–6** ●). The use of low-dose (35 mcg or less estrogen) preparations has reduced many of the side effects. The newer 20- or 25-mcg pills have even fewer side effects, but they may result in less contraceptive effectiveness and in weaker cycle control. The Evidence-Based Practice feature addresses the issue of weight gain that some women associate with use of hormonal contraceptives.

TABLE 19–6 Side Effects Associated With Oral Contraceptives

ESTROGEN EFFECTS	PROGESTIN EFFECTS
Alterations in lipid metabolism	Acne, oily skin
Breast tenderness; engorgement; increased breast size	Breast tenderness; increased breast size
Cerebrovascular accident	Decreased high-density lipoprotein (HDL) cholesterol levels
Changes in carbohydrate metabolism	Decreased libido
Chloasma	Depression
Fluid retention; cyclic weight gain	Fatigue
Headache	Hirsutism
Hepatic adenomas	Increased appetite; weight gain
Hypertension	Increased low-density lipoprotein (LDL) cholesterol levels
Leukorrhea, cervical erosion, ectopia	Oligomenorrhea, amenorrhea
Nausea	Pruritus
Nervousness, irritability	Sebaceous cysts
Telangiectasia	
Thromboembolic complications: thrombophlebitis, pulmonary embolism	

Source: Hatcher, R., Trussell, J., Nelson, A., Cates, W., Kowal, D., & Policar, M. (2011). *Contraceptive technology* (20th rev. ed.). New York, NY: Ardent Media.

The following side effects, remembered by the mnemonic **ACHES**, are less common but more serious:

Abdominal pain
Chest pain
Headache (severe)
Eye problems (blurred vision)
Swelling or aching in the legs and thighs.

Absolute contraindications to the use of oral contraceptives include pregnancy, previous history of thrombophlebitis or thromboembolic disease, acute or chronic liver disease of cholestatic type with abnormal function, presence of estrogen-dependent carcinomas, undiagnosed uterine bleeding, heavy smoking, gallbladder disease, hypertension, diabetes, and hyperlipidemia. In addition, women with the following relative contraindications need to be monitored frequently: migraine headaches, epilepsy, depression, oligomenorrhea, and amenorrhea. Women who choose this method of contraception should be fully advised of its potential side effects.

COCs also have some important noncontraceptive benefits. Many women experience relief of uncomfortable menstrual symptoms. Cramps are lessened, flow is decreased, and cycle regularity is increased. Mittelschmerz is eliminated, and the incidence of functional ovarian cysts is decreased. There is also a substantial reduction in the incidence of ectopic pregnancy, ovarian cancer, endometrial cancer, iron deficiency anemia, and benign breast disease. COCs are considered a good solution to the physiological problems some women experience during perimenopause. However, because of the increased risk of myocardial infarction (heart attack), women over age 35 who smoke should not take COCs. The woman using oral contraceptives should contact her healthcare provider if she becomes depressed, becomes jaundiced, develops a breast lump, or experiences any of the following warning signs: severe abdominal pain, severe chest pain or shortness of breath, severe headaches, dizziness, changes in vision (vision loss or blurring), speech problems, or severe leg pain.

Another oral contraceptive is the progestin-only pill, also called the *mini-pill*. It is used primarily by nursing mothers because it does not interfere with breast milk production. It is also used by women who have a contraindication to the estrogen component of the combination preparation, such as a history of thrombophlebitis, but are strongly motivated to use this form of contraception. The major problems with this preparation are amenorrhea or irregular spotting and bleeding patterns.

Other Combined Hormonal Methods Hormones for contraception may be administered transdermally via a polyester *contraceptive skin patch*. The woman applies the patch weekly for 3 weeks to one of four sites: her abdomen, buttocks, upper outer arm, or trunk (excluding the breasts). During the fourth week, no patch is worn and menses occurs. The patch causes a more sustained serum level of hormone and contraceptive serum levels persist at least 9 days after the patch has been used for 2 weeks (Hatcher et al., 2011). The patch is highly effective in women who weigh less than 198 pounds. The patch has a better rate of compliance than COCs and is generally considered as safe and reliable as COCs with similar concerns about the possibility of thrombophlebitis and pulmonary embolism (see Table 19–6).

The *vaginal contraceptive ring* is another form of low-dose, sustained-release hormonal contraceptive. It is a flexible, soft ring that the woman inserts into her vagina. The ring is left in place for 3 weeks and then removed for 1 week to allow for withdrawal bleeding. If the woman forgets to change the ring, blood levels remain therapeutic for over 2 weeks (Hatcher et al., 2011). One size fits virtually all women. The ring is highly effective and has minimal side effects. The ring can be worn during intercourse and is comfortable for both the woman and her partner. Replacement rings that need to be stored for more than 4 months should be kept in the refrigerator to maintain hormone levels.

LONG-ACTING PROGESTIN CONTRACEPTIVES
Subdermal implants prevent ovulation in most women. They also stimulate the production of thick cervical mucus, which inhibits sperm penetration. *Implanon*, a single 2-inch-long permeable rod implant, is inserted under the skin of the inner upper arm. It is effective for up to 3 years. It is impregnated with etonogestrel, a progestin. Implanon provides effective continuous contraception removed from the act of coitus. Possible side effects include spotting, irregular bleeding or amenorrhea, an increased incidence of ovarian cysts, weight gain, headaches, mood changes, and vaginal dryness (Hatcher et al., 2011).

Depot medroxyprogesterone acetate (DMPA) (**Depo-Provera**), another long-acting progesterone, provides highly

Evidence-Based Practice Issues of Weight Gain Associated With Contraception

Problem

In the United States about half of all pregnancies are unintended and many end in therapeutic abortion. Many women who could use hormonal contraception do not initiate contraception or stop contraception prematurely because of their perception that hormonal birth control methods cause weight gain. Healthcare providers can provide better information and contraceptive care with a good understanding of the research evidence available about weight gain associated with hormonal contraceptive use.

Evidence

Lopez et al. (2011), conducted a review of research trials available concerning progestin-only contraceptives and their effect on weight. They found 15 studies that examined progestin-only pills, implants, and injectables. Overall, when compared with groups with no hormonal birth control methods, progestin-only groups did have weight changes. In one study, users of injectable Depo-Provera had an increase in body fat and a decrease in lean body mass as compared to the participants not using a hormonal method. The mean weight gain for all the progestin-only groups was 2 kg (4 pounds 6 ounces). This compared very closely with the average weight gain in groups using other hormonal methods.

In a prospective study of 76 women new to intrauterine contraception (IUC) use, the women were divided into two groups, one using a levonorgestrel (LNG) intrauterine system (Mirena) and one using the Copper T380A. The women were paired by age and body mass index and were evaluated at the time of IUC insertion and again at 1 year of use. The women in the LNG group gained an average of 6 pounds 6 ounces with an increase in fat mass in 1 year. In that same year, women in the Copper T380A group gained an average of 3 pounds 1 ounce

with an increase in lean body mass. This study was limited, owing to the small number of participants and no monitoring of daily caloric intake or physical activity (Dal'Ava et al., 2012).

In a review of 49 research reports, Gallo et al. (2011) found few studies that compared combination oral contraception (COC) methods with placebo or no hormonal method use. In the four studies reviewed that did compare COC with placebo or no intervention, no appreciable weight gain differences in the two groups were seen. The reviewers explained that it was difficult to measure a causal relationship between COC use and weight gain because women tend to gain weight over time regardless of the method of birth control they use. Also, withholding a method or using placebo would be unethical.

Implications

All the researchers agree that it is important for healthcare providers to give appropriate counseling about typical weight gain over time so that women are less likely to stop using hormonal contraceptive methods because of perceptions of weight gain. In addition, early counseling may help women to choose lifestyles that prevent weight gain. If a woman taking Depo-Provera experiences excessive weight gain that cannot be controlled with diet and exercise, then another birth control method should be chosen.

Critical Thinking Application

Consider the learning needs of women choosing hormonal birth control methods. Formulate a teaching plan for a woman who is going to use Depo-Provera for birth control. If a woman who is about to use a low-dose COC asks about weight gain associated with its use, how will the nurse reply using the evidence presented by these studies?

---

effective birth control for 3 months when given as a single injection of 150 mg. DMPA, which acts primarily by suppressing ovulation, is safe, convenient, private, and relatively inexpensive. It also separates birth control from the act of coitus. It can safely be given to nursing mothers because it contains no estrogen. DMPA works in the same way progestin-only pills do in preventing conception. Side effects include menstrual irregularities, headache, weight gain, breast tenderness, and depression.

In a review of 15 different research studies, Lopez et al. (2011) found that average weight gain in 12 months of progestin-only use was about 4 pounds. Consequently, each woman choosing Depo-Provera for long-acting birth control needs counseling on typical weight gain, nutrition, and exercise. Return of fertility may be delayed for an average of 9–12 months (Hatcher et al., 2011).

Depo-Provera is not recommended for use for longer than 2 years without specific informed consent by the woman. It has been associated with calcium loss from the bones that may not resolve after discontinuing use. Women who remain on DMPA longer than 2 years must be educated about this serious side effect and need to exercise and take 1,200 mg of calcium daily.

Depo-Provera 104 mg subcutaneously is an alternative to Depo-Provera 150 mg. Originally approved by the FDA for the treatment of endometriosis, it subsequently was approved as a contraceptive. Because there is 30% less drug available compared with the 150-mg preparation, it may result in less bone density loss for long-term users. It is administered subcutaneously every 10–13 weeks.

EMERGENCY CONTRACEPTION **Emergency contraception (EC)** (contraception that is used after sexual activity) is indicated when a woman is worried about pregnancy because of unprotected intercourse, rape, or possible contraceptive failure (e.g., broken condom, slipped diaphragm, missed COCs, or too long a time between DMPA injections). Currently, three emergency contraception methods are used in the United States: Plan B, an oral progestin-only (levonorgestrel) method; ulipristal acetate (Ella), a progesterone receptor modulator; and insertion of the Copper T380A IUC device.

The phrase "morning-after pill" is misleading. The woman actually takes a dose of Plan B or Ella as soon after intercourse as possible (but not longer than 120 hours postcoitus). Emergency contraception taken within 72 hours can reduce the risk of pregnancy after a single act of intercourse by 59%–94% (Hatcher et al., 2011). Plan B works by stopping or delaying ovulation, causing changes in the endometrium to make it less receptive to implantation, thickening the cervical mucus, and slowing the transport of the sperm and ovum, a direct prevention of fertilization (Walcker & Peterson, 2013). In 2005, the FDA approved Plan B for use as emergency contraception.

Ulipristal acetate (Ella) is given as a single oral dose of 30 mg. It prevents or delays ovulation and decreases the thickness of the endometrium by binding to the progesterone receptors and producing an antiprogesterone effect. Progesterone is necessary for pregnancy to occur (Kim & Bridgeman, 2011). This drug is available via prescription only.

Placement of the Copper T380A IUC device within 5 days of unprotected intercourse may reduce pregnancy risk. The IUC device produces an inflammatory response that interferes with fertilization and makes the endometrium change so that implantation does not occur (Walcker & Pederson, 2013). The Mirena IUS is not recommended for postcoital use.

Use of emergency contraceptives is controversial and may be declined by some women with strong beliefs about right to life. If ovulation occurs and the sperm reaches the ovum, there is a remote chance when ECs have been used that a fertilized ovum will reach the endometrium and attempt to implant. Some individuals view this as similar to abortion and prefer not to take the medication.

Operative Sterilization

Operative sterilization is an inclusive term that refers to surgical procedures that permanently prevent pregnancy. Before sterilization is performed on either partner, the physician provides a thorough explanation of the procedure to both. Each needs to understand that sterilization is not a decision to be taken lightly or entered into when psychological stresses, such as separation or divorce, exist. Even though both male and female procedures are theoretically reversible, the permanence of the procedure should be stressed and understood.

The decision to have a sterilization procedure is the client's. The nurse's responsibility is to provide client teaching about the procedure, its permanence, and side effects (if any). The nurse should not impose his or her beliefs about sterilization on the client and should accept the client's decision. In addition, the nurse should not provide information in a way that makes the procedure sound intimidating or conveys any implication about the morality of the procedure. The nurse must support the client in his or her decision, regardless of the nurse's personal beliefs about the procedure.

Male sterilization is achieved through a relatively minor procedure called a **vasectomy**. This procedure involves surgically severing the vas deferens in both sides of the scrotum. It takes about 20 ejaculations to clear the remaining sperm from the vas deferens. This can take 8 weeks or longer (Hatcher et al., 2011). During that period, the couple is advised to use another method of birth control and to bring in two or three semen samples for a sperm count. Possible side effects of a vasectomy include pain, injury to other organs, and swelling. Infection and hematoma may occur but are rare (Hatcher et al., 2011).

Vasectomies can sometimes be reversed by using expensive, highly specialized microsurgery techniques. Restored fertility, as measured by subsequent pregnancy, ranges from 38% to 89% (Hatcher et al., 2011).

Female sterilization is most frequently accomplished by **tubal ligation**, in which the tubes are located through a small subumbilical incision or by minilaparotomy techniques and are clipped, ligated, electrocoagulated, banded, or plugged. Tubal ligation may be done at any time; however, the postpartum period is an ideal time to perform the procedure because the tubes are somewhat enlarged and easily located.

Complications of female sterilization procedures are uncommon but may include coagulation burns on the bowel, perforation of the bowel, pain, infection, hemorrhage, and adverse anesthesia effects. Reversal of a tubal ligation depends on the type of procedure performed. All reversals are expensive and require major surgery and a skilled surgeon.

The *Essure* method of permanent sterilization requires no surgical incision. Insertion requires about 35 minutes in an outpatient setting. Under hysteroscopy, stainless steel microinserts are placed in the tubes, stimulating the growth of local tissue, which results in tubal blockage by 1 year for 99.95% of women and 2 years postprocedure for 99.84% (Lessard & Hopkins, 2011). Essure eliminates the need for transabdominal surgery, but it does require some specialized training and a hysterosalpingogram (HSG) 3 months following the procedure to confirm that the tubes are occluded. The woman should use a backup contraceptive method until the HSG confirms that the tubes are occluded.

Male Contraception

The vasectomy and the condom, discussed previously, are currently the only forms of male contraception available in the United States. Hormonal contraception for men has yet to be developed, although studies are under way. Developing safe, effective, and reversible male contraceptives is challenging: It is easier to interrupt a woman's cyclic process than to interrupt a man's continuous fertility.

Discontinuing Contraception

A woman who uses hormonal contraception—such as COCs, mini-pills, the vaginal ring, the patch, or Depo-Provera—is advised to complete the current cycle before discontinuing contraception and attempting to get pregnant. Some healthcare providers advise women to have anywhere from one to three normal menstrual periods before attempting to conceive. A woman using an intrauterine device is advised to have it removed and wait 1 month before attempting to conceive. During the waiting period she can use barrier methods of contraception (condoms, diaphragm, or cervical cap with spermicides). Women who have used Depo-Provera should be advised that it could take up to 18 months to conceive after discontinuation.

▶ COLLABORATION

Care of the client or couple seeking family planning or infertility, genetic, or contraceptive care often involves several members of the healthcare team. Geneticists, psychologists, gynecologists, urologists, and infertility experts may be included in the client's healthcare team. The care given by these specialists is supplemented by nurses, counselors, and community resources such as support groups and family planning clinics. Open communication among all members of the healthcare team ensures that the client or couple will receive the best, most sensitive care.

Diagnostic Tests

Diagnostic testing that may be used in the care of a client with infertility includes the following:

- Basal body temperature recording
- Cervical mucus
- Hormonal assessments of ovulatory function (FSH, LH, estrogen, progesterone levels)
- Pregnancy tests—urine and blood human chorionic gonadotropin (hCG)

- Sperm analysis
- Antisperm antibody test
- Postcoital test to determine sperm motility in cervical mucus
- Commercial urine test for ovulation (measures LH level)
- Endometrial biopsy
- Transvaginal and pelvic ultrasound
- Hysterosalpingography
- Hysteroscopy
- Laparoscopy.

Diagnostic tests that may be used for potential genetic issues include the following:

- Genetic screening
- Genetic ultrasound including nuchal translucency

- Genetic amniocentesis
- Percutaneous umbilical cord sampling and chorionic villus sampling
- Alpha-fetoprotein, hCG, inhibin, estradiol (Quad testing)
- Preimplantation genetic testing.

Fertility Medications

Pharmacologic agents are commonly used for ovarian stimulation in the follicular phase, control of midcycle release, and support of the luteal phase. The pharmacologic treatment chosen depends on the specific cause of infertility. **Table 19–7** ● lists some of the drugs commonly used and indications for use.

Clinical Interruption of Pregnancy

Although abortion was legalized in the United States in 1973, the associated controversy over moral and legal issues continues.

TABLE 19–7 Drugs Commonly Used to Treat Infertility and Indications for Use

DRUGS	WOMEN	MEN
Clomiphene citrate (Clomid, Serophene)	■ Polycystic ovarian syndrome (PCOS) ■ Hyperandrogenemia ■ Premature follicle rupture	■ Low levels of gonadotropins ■ Hypothalamic hypogonadism
Human menopausal gonadotropin (hMG), (Repronex, Bravelle)	■ Hypothalamic ovulatory dysfunction (after failure of clomiphene) ■ Hypopituitarism ■ PCOS (rarely) ■ Luteinized unruptured follicle syndrome (after failure of hCG alone) ■ Inadequate cervical mucus ■ In vitro fertilization, GIFT, ZIFT ■ Controlled superovulation ■ Hypothalamic pituitary failure due to Kallmann syndrome or delayed puberty ■ Hypogonadotrophic hypogonadism (deficiency of FSH and LH)	
Recombinant follicle-stimulating hormone (rFSH) (Follistim, Gonal-F)	■ PCOS ■ Too-long cycles ■ In vitro fertilization, GIFT, ZIFT	
Human chorionic gonadotropin (hCG) (Pregnyl, Novarel, A.P.L.)	■ Induces dominant follicle to release egg ■ Luteinized unruptured follicle syndrome	
Bromocriptine (Parlodel)	■ Pituitary adenoma	■ Hyperprolactinemia (functional or pituitary adenoma)
Cabergoline (Dostinex)	■ Hyperpituitarism	
Gonadotropin-releasing hormone (GnRh) (Factral, Lutre-pulse)	■ Hypothalamic ovulatory dysfunction—to ensure a pulsatile release of GnRH by a small pump	■ Hypothalamic pituitary failure due to Kallmann syndrome or delayed puberty (pulsed infusion)
GnRh analogs ■ Leuprolide acetate (Lupron) ■ Nafarelin acetate (Synarel) ■ Goserelin acetate (Zoladex)	■ Premature follicular rupture ■ In vitro fertilization, GIFT, ZIFT ■ Endometriosis	■ Hypogonadotrophic hypogonadism
GnRH antagonists ■ Ganirelix acetate (Antagon) ■ Progesterone (Crinone, Prometrium, progesterone in oil)	■ Same as GnRH analogs ■ Luteal phase dysfunction ■ Luteal phase support	
Antidiabetic (metformin [Glucophage])	■ PCOS	

Sources: Based on Valentine, M., & Gardella, J. (2013). Infertility. In E. Youngkin, M. Davis, D. Schadewald, & C. Juve (Eds.), *Women's health: A primary care clinical guide* (4th ed., pp. 273–305). Boston, MA: Pearson; Adams, M., & Koch, R. (2010). *Pharmacology: Connections to nursing practice.* Upper Saddle River, NJ: Pearson; and Wilson, B., Shannon, M., & Shields, K. (2013). *Pearson nurse's drug guide 2013.* Upper Saddle River, NJ: Pearson.

This controversy is as readily apparent in the medical and nursing professions as in other groups.

Some individuals are strongly opposed to abortion for religious, ethical, or personal reasons. Some individuals believe that access to a safe, legal abortion is every woman's right. A number of physical and psychosocial factors influence a woman's decision to seek an abortion. The presence of a disease or health state that jeopardizes the mother's life and serious, life-threatening fetal problems are frequently suggested as indications for abortion. In other instances, the timing or circumstance of the pregnancy creates an inordinate stress on the woman and she chooses an abortion. Some of these situations may involve contraceptive failure, sexual assault, or incest.

Medical abortion, now available in the United States, provides an effective alternative to surgical abortion for many women with unintended pregnancy. *Mifepristone* (Mifeprex), originally called RU-486, may be used to induce abortion medically during the first 7 weeks of pregnancy (up to 49 days following conception). The American College of Obstetricians and Gynecologists has endorsed an evidence-based protocol for the administration of mifepristone that can be used up to 63 days' gestation (Pazol et al., 2012).

Mifepristone blocks the action of progesterone, thereby altering the endometrium. After the length of the woman's gestation is confirmed, she takes a dose of mifepristone. Between 1 and 3 days later (depending on length of gestation), she returns to her healthcare provider and takes a dose of the prostaglandin misoprostol, which induces contractions that expel the embryo/fetus. About 14 days after taking the misoprostol, the woman is seen a third time to confirm that the abortion was successful.

Shortly after being approved for use by the FDA, several deaths were associated with the use of mifepristone. Four of these were related to an infection caused by a rare organism, *Clostridium sordelli* (FDA, 2011). The FDA has determined since that this is a rare occurrence (1 in 100,000 women who use mifepristone). However, *any* woman who has taken the oral mifepristone/vaginal misoprostol regimen within the last 24 hours who develops stomach pain, weakness, nausea, vomiting or diarrhea, with or without fever, should contact her healthcare provider *immediately*. Currently, mifepristone is considered safe, and use of routine prophylactic antibiotics is not recommended.

In the first trimester, surgical abortion may be performed by dilation and curettage (D&C), minisuction, or vacuum curettage. The major risks include perforation of the uterus, laceration of the cervix, systemic reaction to the anesthetic agent, hemorrhage, and infection. Second-trimester abortion may be done using dilation and extraction (D&E), hypertonic saline, systemic prostaglandins, and intrauterine prostaglandins. Surgical abortion in the first trimester is technically easier and safer than abortion in the second trimester.

Important aspects of nursing care for a woman who chooses to have an abortion include providing information about the methods of abortion and associated risks; counseling regarding available alternatives to abortion and their implications; encouraging verbalization by the woman; providing support before, during, and after the procedure; monitoring vital signs, intake, and output; providing for physical comfort and privacy throughout the procedure; and health teaching about self-care, the importance of the postabortion checkup, and contraception review. It is also important to note that the American Nurses Association (ANA) Code of Ethics allows nurses to refuse to participate in a procedure, such as abortion, on moral grounds. However, the nurse is obliged to provide for the client's safety, to avoid client abandonment, and to withdraw only when assured that alternative sources of nursing care are available to the client (ANA, 2010).

Therapeutic Insemination

Therapeutic insemination (previously known as *artificial insemination*) involves the depositing of semen at the cervical os or in the uterus by mechanical means. *Therapeutic donor insemination (TDI)* is the current term for use of donor semen, and *therapeutic husband insemination (THI)* is the current term for use of the husband's semen.

THI is generally indicated for such seminal deficiencies as oligospermia (low sperm count), asthenospermia (decreased motility), and teratospermia (low percentage, abnormal morphology); for anatomical defects accompanied by inadequate deposition of semen such as hypospadia (a congenital abnormal male urethral opening on the underside of the penis); and for ejaculatory dysfunction (such as retrograde ejaculation). THI is also indicated in cases of unexplained infertility and some cases of female factor infertility, such as scant or inhospitable mucus, persistent cervicitis, or cervical stenosis. In some cases, intrauterine insemination (IUI) would be indicated to bypass the cervical factor. Seminal fluid contains high levels of prostaglandins, which can cause nausea, severe cramps, abdominal pain, and diarrhea when absorbed by the uterine lining. Therefore, sperm preparation for IUI involves washing sperm from the seminal plasma. IUI, with or without ovulation induction therapy, is an option for many couples before more aggressive treatments such as in vitro fertilization are employed.

TDI is considered in cases of azoospermia (absence of sperm), severe oligospermia or asthenospermia, inherited male sex-linked disorders, and autosomal dominant disorders. In the past several years, indications for donor insemination have expanded to include single women or lesbians desirous of pregnancy. Some states have specified the parental rights of single women and donors, but most states are silent on this issue.

TDI has become more complicated and expensive in the past decade because of the need for strict screening and processing procedures to prevent transmission of a genetic defect or STI to the offspring or recipient. Guidelines have been established that include mandatory medical (genetic) and infectious disease screening of both donor and recipient, the need for informed consent from all parties, the need to limit the number of pregnancies per donor, and the need for accurate means of record keeping. Finally, because of the risk of transmitting infectious diseases, donated sperm must be frozen and quarantined for 6 months from the time of acquisition, and the donor must be retested before sperm can be released for use.

Numerous factors need to be evaluated before TDI is performed. Has every possible effort been made to diagnose and treat the cause of the male infertility? Do tests indicate normal fertility and sperm–ovum transport in the woman? Has the couple had an opportunity to discuss this option with an infertility counselor to explore the issues of secrecy, disclosure, and potential feelings of loss the couple (particularly the male partner) may feel about not having a genetic child? Are there any religious constraints? After making the decision, the couple should allow themselves time to further assess their concerns and explore their feelings individually and together to ensure that this option is acceptable to both.

In Vitro Fertilization

In vitro fertilization (IVF) is selectively used in cases when infertility has resulted from tubal factors, mucus abnormalities, male infertility, unexplained infertility, male and female immunological infertility, and cervical factors. In IVF, a woman's eggs are collected from her ovaries and fertilized in the laboratory, and one or more embryos are placed into her uterus after normal development has begun. If the procedure is successful, the embryo continues to develop in the uterus, and pregnancy proceeds naturally (**Figure 19-23 ●**).

The potential for a successful pregnancy with IVF is maximized when three to four embryos (rather than one) are placed into the uterus. For this reason, fertility drugs are used to induce ovulation before the process. Follicular development and oocyte maturity are monitored frequently with ultrasound and hormonal assays. Monitoring usually begins around cycle day 5, and medications are titrated according to individual response. When follicles appear mature, hCG is given to stimulate final egg maturation and control the induction of ovulation. Egg retrieval is performed approximately 35 hours later, before ovulation occurs.

In the majority of cases, egg retrieval is performed by a transvaginal approach under ultrasound guidance (**Figure 19-24 ●**). This outpatient procedure is performed with intravenous sedation and a cervical block for anesthesia. Many follicles can be aspirated with only one puncture, and the procedure generally lasts no more than 30 minutes. Once the eggs have been fertilized and progressed to the embryo stage, the embryos are placed in

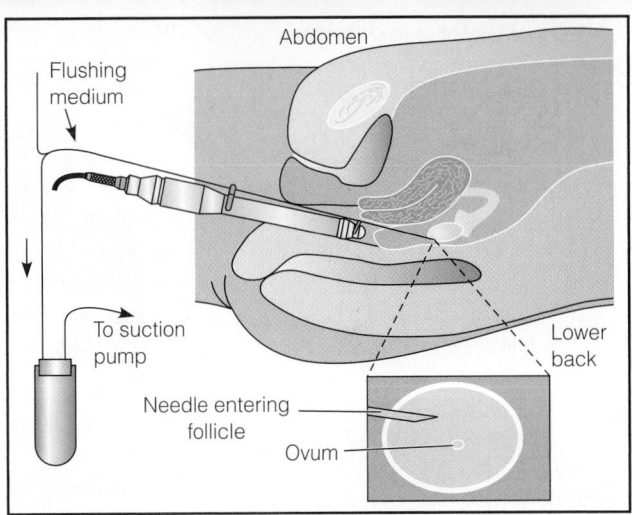

Figure 19-24 ● Transvaginal ultrasound-guided oocyte retrieval.
Source: Courtesy of Serono, Inc., Rockland, MA.

the uterus. This occurs 1–2 days after conception. After the procedure, the woman is advised to engage in only minimal activity for 12–24 hours, and progesterone supplementation is prescribed. The progesterone supplementation is given to promote implantation and support the early pregnancy; therefore, the woman will not have a period even if she is not pregnant. The pregnancy is usually determined by transvaginal ultrasound.

Sperm used to fertilize the eggs in vitro can be obtained naturally or via microsurgical epididymal sperm aspiration (MESA) or testicular sperm aspiration (TESA). These are procedures that address severe male factor infertility. MESA and TESA involve the retrieval of sperm from the gonadal tissue of men who have azoospermia or an ejaculatory disorder (**Figure 19-25 ●**). Percutaneous epididymal sperm aspiration (PESA) and TESA are replacing MESA as the preferred techniques for retrieval of sperm because they are not surgical procedures. Intracytoplasmic sperm injection (ICSI) is a microscopic procedure to inject a single sperm into the outer layer of an ovum so that fertilization will occur (Eisenberg & Brumbaugh, 2012).

Success with IVF depends on many factors, especially the woman's age and the specific indication. Women have a good chance of achieving pregnancy with an average of three cycles of IVF. Many couples find the emotional, physical, and financial costs of going beyond three cycles too great. Costs vary by treatment and by region of the country; one cycle of assisted reproductive technology (ART) averages $8,300 for the procedure and $3,000 plus $65 monthly for sperm storage (American Society of Reproductive Medicine [ASRM], 2012). Births attributed to ART and reported by the Society of Assisted Reproductive Technology from data from 379 clinics who performed 154,412 ART cycles was 59,446 (ASRM, 2013). This means that only about 38% of ART cycles result in a live birth. Increased use of single-embryo transfer has led to lower rates of multiple fetuses, particularly in younger couples.

Other Assisted Reproduction Techniques

Other assisted reproductive techniques include procedures for transfer of gametes, zygotes, or embryos; cryopreservation of

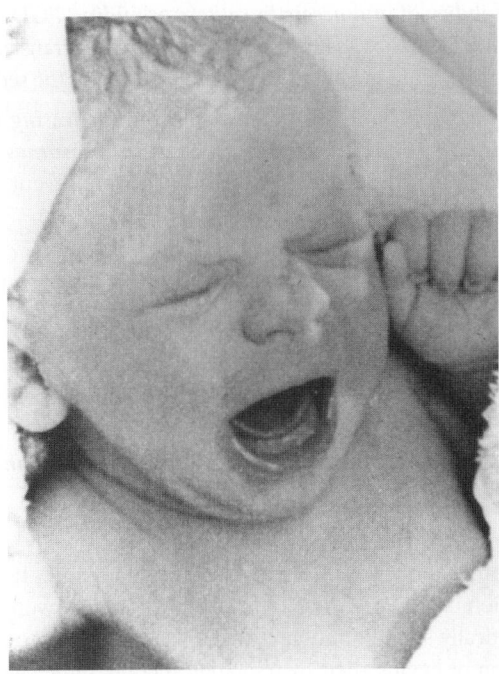

Figure 19-23 ● Louise Joy Brown, the world's first "test tube baby," shown shortly after her birth by cesarean section on July 25, 1978. IVF was pioneered by Drs. Bob Edwards and Patrick Steptoe.
Source: Keystone/Getty Images.

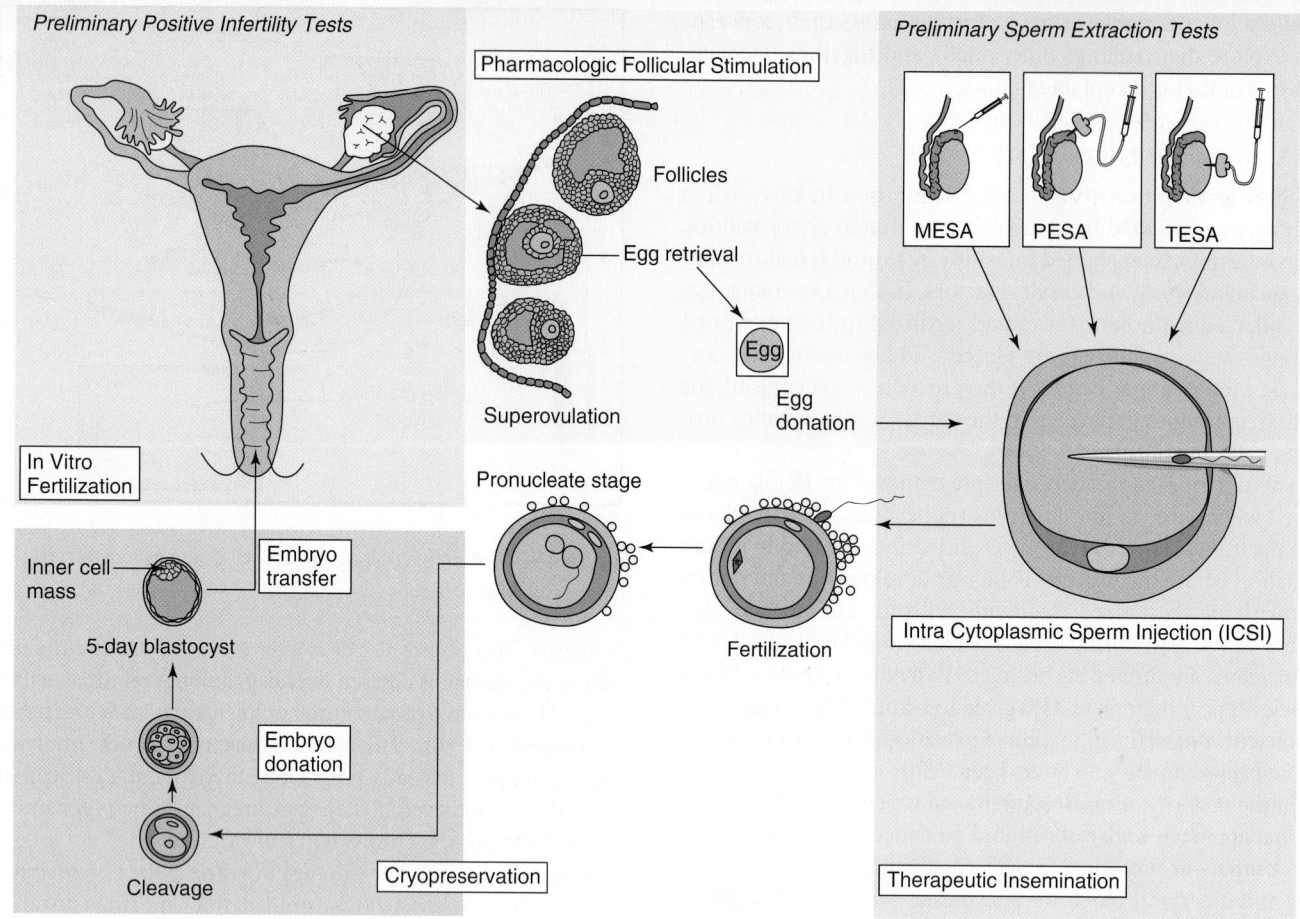

Preliminary Positive Infertility Tests

Pharmacologic Follicular Stimulation

Follicles

Egg retrieval

Superovulation

Egg

Egg donation

In Vitro Fertilization

Pronucleate stage

Inner cell mass

Embryo transfer

5-day blastocyst

Embryo donation

Cleavage

Cryopreservation

Fertilization

Preliminary Sperm Extraction Tests

MESA   PESA   TESA

Intra Cytoplasmic Sperm Injection (ICSI)

Therapeutic Insemination

Figure 19–25 ● Assisted reproductive techniques.

embryos; IVF using donor oocytes; micromanipulation techniques; and surrogacy and use of a gestational carrier.

Preimplantation Genetic Diagnosis

Other recent advances in micromanipulation allow a single cell to be removed from the embryo for genetic study. Couples at risk for having a detectable single gene or chromosomal anomaly may wish to undergo such preimplantation genetic testing, called *blastomere analysis* or, more recently, *preimplantation genetic diagnosis (PGD)*. The single cell is obtained from a six- to eight-cell embryo by a process known as *blastomere biopsy*. The genetic content of the cell is examined using the polymerase chain reaction (PCR) technique or fluorescence in situ (FISH). Results of genetic testing on the preimplantation embryos are available in 4–24 hours, so unaffected embryos may still be transferred via IVF during the required biological window of time without the need for cryopreservation.

The diagnosis of genetic disorders before implantation provides couples with the option of forgoing the attempt to establish a pregnancy and thereby avoiding a difficult decision about terminating an affected pregnancy (Scriven & Ogilvie, 2010). This technology also raises several ethical issues, including the following:

■ *Identification of couples at risk.* Criteria are needed to identify couples at risk for diseases that constitute significant hardship and suffering so that "wrongful birth" cases can be avoided.

■ *Availability of and access to centers providing PGD.* Should society provide access for those at risk for genetic transfer of disease but without the financial resources to pay for the services?

■ *Analysis of blastomeres for sex chromosome testing when a genetic disorder carried on the sex chromosomes is suspected.* In X-linked diseases, the only way to prevent the disorder is to select only females.

■ *Identification of late-onset diseases.* The Human Genome Project has aided in the identification of genetic markers for late-onset disease. Couples may wish to choose to implant blastomeres that do not carry these markers.

■ *Effect on the offspring as a result of removing cells from the embryo.*

■ *Selection for nonmedical reasons and potential concern of eugenics ("designer babies").*

A micromanipulation procedure called *assisted embryo hatching* has proved to be an effective adjunct therapy in IVF. In vitro fertilization using a *gestational carrier* allows infertile women who are genetically sound but unable to carry a pregnancy to exercise the option of having their own biological child. Other technologies involve oocyte donation and cryopreservation of the embryo.

Genetic Counseling Referral

Genetic counseling is a communication process in which a genetic counselor, physician, or specially trained and certified nurse provides a family with the most complete and accurate current information about the occurrence or the risk of recurrence of a genetic disease in that family. Genetic counseling is an appropriate course of action for any family wondering "Will it happen again?"

A genetic counseling referral is advised for any of the following categories:

- *Congenital abnormalities, including intellectual disability.* Any couple who has a child or a relative with a congenital malformation may be at increased risk and should be so informed. If intellectual disability of unidentified cause has occurred in a family, there may be an increased risk of recurrence.

- *Familial disorders.* Families should be told that certain diseases may have a genetic component and that the risk of their occurrence in a particular family may be higher than that in the general population. Such disorders as diabetes, heart disease, cancer, and mental illness fall into this category.

- *Known inherited diseases.* Families may know that a disease is inherited but not know the mechanism or the specific risk for them. An important point to remember is that family members who are not at risk for passing on a disorder should be as well informed as family members who are at risk.

- *Metabolic disorders.* Any families at risk for having a child with a metabolic disorder or biochemical defect should be referred for genetic counseling. Because most inborn errors of metabolism are autosomal recessively inherited, a family may not be identified as being at risk until the birth of an affected child; for example, a child with cystic fibrosis or sickle cell disease. Carriers of the sickle cell trait and cystic fibrosis can be identified before conception or a pregnancy has occurred, and the risk of having an affected child can be determined. Prenatal diagnosis of an affected embryo is available via chorionic villus sampling.

- *Chromosomal abnormalities.* As discussed previously, any couple who has had a child with a chromosomal abnormality may be at increased risk of having another child similarly affected.

After a couple has been referred to the genetics clinic, they are sent a form requesting information on the health status of various family members. This information assists the genetic counselor in creating the family's pedigree.

Together, the pedigree and history facilitate identification of other family members who might also be at risk for the same disorder (**Figure 19–26 ●**). The family being counseled may wish to notify relatives at risk so that they, too, can begin genetic counseling. When done correctly, the family history and pedigree can be powerful tools for determining a family's risk. It is important to keep in mind that attitudes toward infertility and its treatment are culturally determined. The Focus on Diversity and Culture feature discusses some religious beliefs related to fertility and acceptable fertility treatments.

NURSING PROCESS

The priority of nursing care for the client with family planning considerations is to identify specific needs, provide emotional support, and teach the client about options so he or she can make the best informed decision.

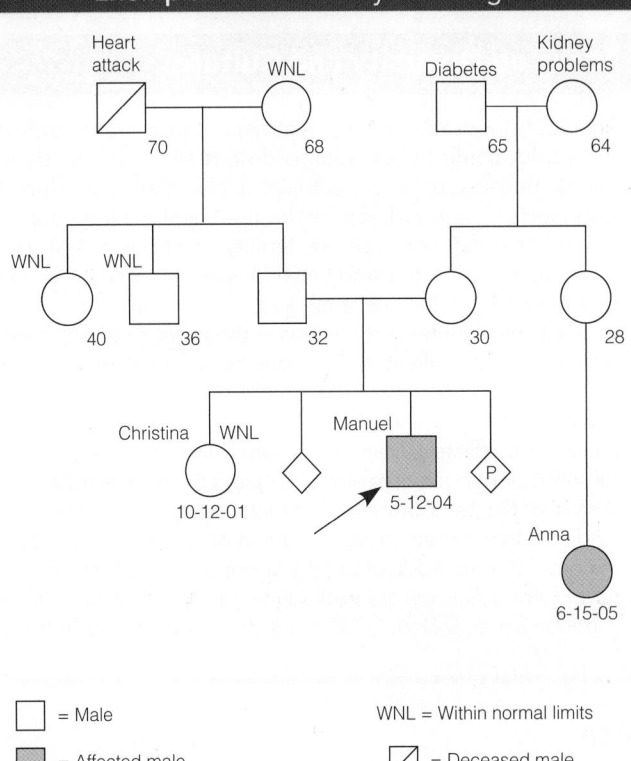

Figure 19–26 ● Screening pedigree. Arrow indicates the nearest family member affected with the disorder being investigated. Basic data have been recorded. Numbers refer to the ages of the family members.

Assessment

When assessing men and women for reproductive issues, the nurse must use a nonjudgmental attitude and open communication. Many clients are uncomfortable discussing their sexuality and sexual activity. The nurse must approach the topic in a matter-of-fact manner, with reassurance of confidentiality within the law. Some questions are the same for both genders:

- Ask about history of sexual activity, including the age at first sexual intercourse.
- Ask about the number of sexual partners, currently and in the past.
- Ask about the use of contraceptives.
- Ask about the use of barriers to prevent STIs.
- Ask about a history of sexual trauma, including abuse, rape, or incest.

Women

- Ask about risk factors for breast cancer, including family history.
- Ask about menstrual history, including onset of menstruation, the date of the last menses, and any irregularities.
- Perform breast and genital examination, including external and internal structures.

Focus on Diversity and Culture Belief Systems and Infertility Treatments

The acceptance of infertility treatments varies widely around the world. Some belief systems do not allow various treatments, because using a treatment is considered interfering with God's design or because the treatment itself is seen as tainted or sinful. For example, fertility practices in Arab cultures are influenced by traditional Muslim values that support beliefs that God decides family sizes.

In Islamic cultures, procreation is the purpose of marriage. If a couple is infertile, it is often considered the woman's problem regardless of the cause. Motherhood is considered the primary role of women, and women who do not conceive are considered afflicted. Maintaining family lineage is very important, and donor gametes and surrogacy confuse the lineage of the child. Contemporary Islamic religious opinion forbids any kind of egg, embryo, or semen donation as well as surrogacy (Inhorn, 2002). In addition, using donor gametes from unmarried individuals is considered adultery in some sects of Islam (Connor, Sauer, & Doll, 2012). For individuals in these cultures,

the approved methods for treating infertility are limited to use of therapeutic insemination using the husband's sperm and in vitro fertilization involving the fertilization of the wife's ovum by the husband's sperm (Greil et al., 2010). Sterility in a woman can lead to rejection and divorce. Also with the use of ICSI, male-initiated divorce is becoming more common for aging wives of infertile husbands (Inhorn, 2002).

In Jewish cultures, infertile couples are to try all possible means to have children, including egg and sperm donation. Jews believe that the ideal production of human life comes from the sex act between a husband and wife but accept both artificial insemination (AI) and IVF (Zivotofsky & Jotkowitz, 2009).

Roman Catholics oppose the use of AI and IVF. According to Vatican directives published in 2009 (*Dignitas Personae*), any method that substitutes for the conjugal act between a husband and wife is not permissible (Greil et al., 2010; Zivotofsky & Jotkowitz, 2009).

Men

- Ask about difficulty voiding, including difficulty starting or stopping and the size of the stream. Include symptoms of burning, frequency, urgency, or nocturia.
- Ask about sexual functioning, including premature ejaculation, impotence, or other sexual problems.
- Perform a genital examination, palpating for masses and inspecting for lesions and drainage, if warranted.

Diagnosis

Possible nursing diagnoses that may be appropriate for clients with family planning needs include the following:

- *Risk for Disturbed Body Image*
- *Sexual Dysfunction*
- *Deficient Knowledge* related to family planning, infertility, contraception, or genetics.

(NANDA-I © 2012)

Planning

Goals of nursing care for the client with family planning considerations include the following:

- The client will describe options available for treatment and choose the option that best fits his or her needs, beliefs, and values.
- The client will acknowledge the impact of the situation on existing personal relationships and lifestyle.
- The client will describe actual changes in body function.
- The client will maintain close social interactions and personal relationships.

Implementation

Family planning considerations can cause a great deal of stress for the couple or client. By providing a nonjudgmental, accepting atmosphere and thorough client teaching, the nurse can help clients resolve difficult decisions in a way that suits the

client best. This facilitates both the nurse–client relationship and the client's ability to learn and act on information.

Promote Healthy Body Image

- Encourage verbalization of feelings.
- Provide resources (pamphlets, books, tapes, referrals to support groups and counselors) as appropriate.
- Teach the client (and significant other if appropriate) about reproductive physiology as it applies to use of contraceptives, infertility issues, or genetics issues.

Promote Healthy Sexual Function

- Encourage discussion of sexual function among client, partner, and healthcare provider.
- Provide information given by the healthcare provider regarding treatment options.
- Encourage the client to discuss concerns about sexuality with a therapist or counselor.

Discuss Knowledge of Sexual and Reproductive Health

- Teach the client about risk factors for reproductive dysfunction. For example, STIs increase the risk of infertility.
- Teach the client about disease prevention. For example, teach about the application of condoms. Clients who understand disease prevention can take measures to protect themselves.
- Teach the client (and significant others if appropriate) about their specific disease and prescribed treatment.

Evaluation

Clients may be evaluated according to the following expected outcomes:

- The client makes informed decisions about treatment based on the disorder and individual choice.
- The client verbalizes understanding of information presented.
- The client expresses feelings openly.

NURSING CARE PLAN   A Client Requesting Preconception Counseling

Donner Everson and her significant other, Mola Langerson, had a child born with Tay–Sachs disease who died at 3 years of age 2 years ago. They would love to have another child but fear having another child with this genetic disorder. They've considered adoption but would like to know whether there is any chance of having a normal child. They report that they have attempted to conceive a few times throughout the past year, but when it didn't happen immediately, they decided to return to use of contraceptives. Mr. Langerson says he is willing to "throw the dice," but Ms. Everson says she would rather be childless than deliver another child with Tay–Sachs disease. Neither of them would want to risk having to make a decision about aborting a child conceived with Tay–Sachs. They want to make sure that if a pregnancy occurs, the child is healthy. They have come to talk with their healthcare provider to learn about their options.

ASSESSMENT

Both Ms. Everson and Mr. Langerson are healthy with no significant current, chronic, or past medical or surgical history. Vital signs are within normal limits, their weights are appropriate for their heights, and they are both physically active. Neither client has a substance abuse issue or history, and they report an occasional glass of wine, perhaps twice a week. They are both orthodox Jews whose grandparents lived in Germany prior to World War II.

Ms. Everson's family history includes two children born with Tay–Sachs disease, one born to her maternal aunt and one to her paternal aunt. She has no siblings. Mr. Langerson had a brother who was born with Tay–Sachs disease, but there is no other family history of congenital or genetic anomalies.

Their family provider collects blood for genetic testing and refers them to a genetic counselor.

DIAGNOSES

- *Anxiety*
- *Readiness for Enhanced Childbearing Process*
- *Decisional Conflict*
- *Deficient Knowledge* related to options for having a child without a genetic disorder

(NANDA-I © 2012)

PLANNING

- Clients will determine their chance of having a child born without Tay–Sachs disease.
- Clients will develop coping strategies for reducing anxiety.
- Clients will make an informed decision related to pregnancy, considering their risks related to genetic disorders.
- Clients will understand their options as related to conception and delivery of a healthy child.

IMPLEMENTATION

The nurse's role in caring for these clients is largely supportive. The nurse may provide the necessary teaching to help them understand what they are told and about any options that they are provided.

- Encourage the clients to verbalize their feelings.
- Suggest coping strategies to reduce anxiety.

- Recommend that the clients delay making a decision regarding pregnancy until they have time to gather facts and determine the options available to them.
- Describe the role of the genetic counselor and the type of information the geneticist can provide based on the blood tests collected.

EVALUATION

Ms. Everson and Mr. Langerson spoke with the genetic counselor and learned that there was a 50% chance that a baby conceived naturally would be born with Tay–Sachs disease. The genetic counselor told them about in vitro fertilization that could be performed, allowing the physician to choose only the sperm and ova that were free of the genetic mutation. Once conception takes place, the blastocyst could be implanted into Ms. Everson's uterus, allowing the couple a 100% likelihood of conceiving a child without Tay–Sachs disease. However, the genetic counselor cautioned that this method would not eliminate risks related to other congenital or pregnancy-induced disorders. They opted to try this procedure, and Ms. Everson became pregnant and delivered a healthy baby girl.

CRITICAL THINKING

1. One of the implementations for this couple is to encourage them to delay conception until they receive information related to their options. Is this an appropriate nursing implementation? Explain your answer.
2. Define the role of the genetic counselor and explain what information genetic counseling can provide this couple.
3. Describe the in vitro process and explain how this process can reduce the risk of having a child born with Tay–Sachs disease.

REVIEW   Family Planning

RELATE Link the Concepts and Exemplars

Linking the exemplar of family planning with the concept of addiction:

1. You are working with a young couple who are planning to have a baby. The potential father smokes cigarettes. What teaching regarding the effects of paternal smoking on planned children will you provide?

2. What information about risks associated with alcohol consumption would you provide the woman who plans to become pregnant and drinks an average of four alcoholic drinks a week?

Linking the exemplar of family planning with the concept of immunity:

3. What client teaching will you provide a client diagnosed with systemic lupus erythematosus who plans to become pregnant?

4. What is your priority of care for the woman diagnosed with rheumatoid arthritis who is anticipating pregnancy?

READY Go to Companion Skills Manual

REFER Go to Pearson Nursing Student Resources
nursing.pearsonhighered.com

- Additional review materials

REFLECT Case Study

Lisa Daniels is an 18-year-old woman recently married to her high school sweetheart, Willis. Ms. Daniels is planning to begin college in the fall to study interior decorating. Mr. Daniels is 24 and is working as the manager of a local fast-food restaurant. Ms. Daniels's family lives a few towns away and is thrilled with her marriage to Willis. Her younger brother, Tom, enjoys playing basketball with him. Mr. Daniels's family lives across the country but are very fond of Lisa and excited about the marriage.

Mr. and Ms. Daniels have come to the OB/GYN clinic to talk about planning for a family. Neither of the two has any health issues that would put them or a child at risk. Ms. Daniels feels that she can handle going to school part time and also care for a baby. Both Mr. and Ms. Daniels are very excited about the prospect of starting their family. They have just bought a house and have furnished it with hand-me-downs from family and friends. They both laugh when they talk about living paycheck to paycheck.

1. What topics will you raise with Mr. and Ms. Daniels as they consider starting a family?

2. What preconceptual counseling will you provide Ms. Daniels to help her optimize her status before becoming pregnant?

3. If Mr. and Ms. Daniels decide to begin attempting to conceive, what teaching will you provide this couple?

EXEMPLAR 19.3 Menopause

EXEMPLAR KEY TERMS
Hormone replacement therapy (HRT), *1395*
Menopause, *1394*

EXEMPLAR LEARNING OUTCOMES
After reading about this exemplar, you will be able to:

1. Describe the physiology, etiology, and clinical manifestations of menopause.

2. Identify risk factors associated with menopause.

3. Illustrate the nursing process in providing culturally competent care for individuals experiencing menopause.

4. Formulate priority nursing diagnoses appropriate for a woman transitioning into menopause.

5. Plan evidence-based care for the individual entering menopause and her family in collaboration with other members of the healthcare team.

6. Evaluate expected outcomes for the individual experiencing menopause.

▶ OVERVIEW

Menopause is the permanent cessation of menses. The *climacteric*, or *perimenopausal*, period denotes the time during which reproductive function gradually ceases. For most women, the perimenopausal period lasts several years. It begins with a decline in the production of the hormone estrogen, includes the permanent cessation of menstruation due to loss of ovarian function, and extends for 1 year after the final menstrual period, at which time a woman is said to be *postmenopausal*. The average woman will live one third of her life after menopause.

Menopause is neither a disease nor a disorder, but a normal physiological process. It is included here because it does increase the risk of physical disorders and does affect various aspects of women's health. Many women welcome the freedom from monthly menstrual periods and have relatively minor physical effects from the estrogen depletion. However, the hormonal changes that occur can be accompanied by side effects. Wide variation is seen in how individual women experience these side effects. In the United States, most women stop menstruating between 48 and 55 years of age. Earlier menopause is associated with genetics, smoking, higher altitude, and obesity (Deneris & Huether, 2010). Certain health risks increase after menopause, including heart disease, osteoporosis, macular degeneration, cognitive changes, and breast cancer.

▶ PHYSIOLOGY AND ETIOLOGY

The menopausal period marks the natural biological end of reproductive ability. *Surgical menopause* occurs when the ovaries are removed in premenopausal women, dramatically reduc-

ing the production of estrogen and progestins. *Chemical menopause* often occurs during cancer chemotherapy, when cytotoxic drugs arrest ovarian function.

As ovarian function decreases, the production of estradiol (E_2), the most biologically active estrogen, decreases and is ultimately replaced by estrone as the major ovarian estrogen. Estrone is produced in small amounts and has only about one tenth the biological activity of estradiol. With decreased ovarian function, the second ovarian hormone, progesterone, which is produced during the luteal phase of the menstrual cycle, also is markedly reduced.

▶ CLINICAL MANIFESTATIONS

Although menopause is an age-related process, not a pathological one, some women have troublesome health experiences after the cessation of menses. As estrogen decreases, various tissues are affected. Breast tissue, body hair, skin elasticity, and subcutaneous fat decrease. The ovaries and uterus become smaller, and the cervix and vagina decrease in size and become pale in color. These changes may result in problems with vaginal dryness, dyspareunia, urinary stress incontinence, urinary tract infections (UTIs), and vaginitis. Atrophic vaginitis may lead to urogenital infection, ulceration, and uncomfortable sexual intercourse. Vasomotor instability often results in hot flashes, palpitations, dizziness, and headaches. Other problems resulting from vasomotor instability include insomnia, frequent awakening, perspiration (night sweats), osteoporosis, and increased cardiovascular disease (Deneris & Huether, 2010). The woman may experience irritability, anxiety, and depression as a result of these events. Long-term estrogen deprivation

Clinical Manifestations and Therapies **Menopause**

ETIOLOGY	CLINICAL MANIFESTATIONS	CLINICAL THERAPIES
Increase in vaginal pH	■ Risk of urinary tract infection (burning, frequency, hesitancy, and urgency to urinate) ■ Vaginal infection (vaginitis, vaginal drainage)	■ Medications (antibiotics or antifungals) may be prescribed. ■ Encourage adequate fluid intake. ■ Teach importance of wiping from front to back. ■ Teach symptoms to report.
Reduced vaginal lubrication	■ Dyspareunia, injury, and fungal infections	■ Teach use of artificial water-based lubricant to reduce symptoms. ■ Treat fungal infection.
Vasomotor instability	■ Hot flashes ■ Diaphoresis ■ Increased risk of heart disease	■ Teach women to dress in layers, wear cotton underwear, drink cool liquids. ■ If severe, hormone supplements may be prescribed.
Osteoporosis	■ Fractures, increased bone fragility ■ Kyphosis	■ Teach importance of calcium, vitamin D, and phosphorus intake. ■ Suggest weight-bearing exercises.

Source: Based on Juve, C. (2013). The menopausal transition. In E. Youngkin, M. Davis, D. Schadewald, & C. Juve (Eds.), *Women's health: A primary care clinical guide* (4th ed., pp. 425–459). Boston, MA: Pearson.

results in an imbalance in bone remodeling and osteoporosis, leading to fractures and kyphosis. The risk for cardiovascular diseases increases in response to an increase in atherosclerosis (from an increase in the LDL-to-HDL cholesterol ratio).

Menopause, however, is a very individual experience that involves biocultural variation. Each woman experiencing menopause has had decades of physiological responses to her environment. Nutrition, smoking, body mass index, immune, reproductive, social, and cultural history all affect how each woman will respond to this physiological transition (Melby & Lampl, 2011). Emotionally, some women may celebrate menopause; others may experience negative feelings about themselves and their body image; others may attach no significance to it.

Manifestations of the perimenopausal period are listed in **Box 19–5** ●. These manifestations vary widely. Some women experience severe symptoms, others experience moderate symptoms, and some women experience few or no symptoms.

▶ COLLABORATION

Care of the woman experiencing menopausal symptoms focuses on relieving symptoms and minimizing postmenopausal health risks. Healthcare team members who may be involved include physicians, gynecologists, nurse practitioners, nurses, and community support groups. Most women entering this transitional period need reassurance, education, and support from the healthcare team.

Diagnostic Tests

As estrogen secretion diminishes, levels of follicle-stimulating hormone (FSH) and luteinizing hormone (LH) rise and remain elevated. A woman who has not menstruated for 1 full year or who has an increased FSH blood level is considered menopausal (Deneris & Huether, 2010). FSH and LH levels are not routinely measured but are used if the diagnosis is in question.

Pharmacologic Therapy

Before 2002, **hormone replacement therapy (HRT)** was a common medical choice for relieving the symptoms of menopause. The choices of HRT included estrogen/progestin combinations

---

Box 19–5   Manifestations of the Perimenopausal Period

■ Menstrual cycles become erratic. Menstrual flow varies widely in amount and duration and eventually ceases.

■ Vaginal, vulval, and urethral tissues begin to atrophy.

■ Vaginal pH rises, predisposing the woman to bacterial infections.

■ Vaginal lubrication decreases, and vaginal rugae decrease in number. This may result in dyspareunia, injury, and fungal infections.

■ Vasomotor instability due to a decrease in estrogen may result in hot flashes and night sweats. A hot flash starts in the chest and moves upward toward the face and may last from seconds to several minutes.

■ Psychological symptoms may include moodiness, nervousness, insomnia, headaches, irritability, anxiety, inability to concentrate, and depression.

Sources: Juve, C. (2013). The menopausal transition. In E. Youngkin, M. Davis, D. Schadewald, & C. Juve (Eds.), *Women's health: A primary care clinical guide* (4th ed., pp. 425–459). Boston, MA: Pearson; and Deneris, A., & Huether, S. (2010). Structure and function of the reproductive system. In K. McCance & S. Huether (Eds.), *Pathophysiology: The biologic basis for disease in adults and children* (6th ed., pp. 781–812). St. Louis, MO: Mosby/Elsevier.

(EPT) for women who still had a uterus and estrogen only (ET) for women who had a history of hysterectomy. Research evidence had proven that the addition of progestin protects the endometrium from estrogen-induced hyperplasia and cancer. This routine medication for women experiencing menopausal symptoms changed when a landmark study, the Women's Health Initiative (WHI), came to an early halt based on data concerning women who were using the EPT. The early data (3 years before the planned ending of the study) revealed that women using EPT were at greater risk for congestive heart failure, breast cancer, pulmonary embolism, and stroke than the women who were taking placebos. The ET arm of the study continued but was halted 1 year prior to the planned ending because the women in this part of the study were having more strokes than women on placebos and the incidence of breast cancer had increased (Juve, 2013).

This abrupt stop to this large government-sponsored study led many women to choose to stop HRT. It also led to a marked decrease in the numbers of prescriptions for HRT that physicians were willing to write.

In the years that have passed since the WHI, experts have debated and studied the safety and efficacy of HRT for menopausal symptoms. Most recently, the Kronos Early Estrogen Prevention Study (KEEPS) results have been made available. This is a 4-year study that included 727 participants. It demonstrated that lower dose estrogen/progestin started soon after menopause appears to be safe, relieves hot flashes and vaginal dryness, improves mood and bone density, and decreases risks for cardiovascular disease (North American Menopause Society [NAMS], 2012b).

As a result of research findings such as this and the expert opinions available, the North American Menopause Society has issued a position statement on HRT. The U.S. Preventive Services Task Force has also issued a recommendation statement (Moyer, 2012; NAMS, 2012a, 2013). The two documents are consistent in the recommendations made, which include the following:

- Most healthy, recently menopausal women (up to age 59 or within 10 years of menopause) can use HRT for relief of hot flashes and vaginal dryness, if they choose. Treatment choices should be individualized.

- HRT is the most effective treatment of menopausal hot flashes and vaginal dryness.

- If vaginal dryness or dyspareunia are the only symptoms, then low-dose vaginal estrogen is preferred.

- Risks for blood clots in the legs and lungs are increased with HRT, but occurrence is rare in women ages 50–59. The risk is further lowered by using low-dose estrogen pills or transdermal patches, gels, or sprays.

- Increased risk in breast cancer does occur when continuous EPT is used for 5 or more years or ET is used for 7 years or more, but the risk stops when the hormone is stopped.

Complementary and Alternative Therapies

As a result of the controversy surrounding the use of HRT, nontraditional or alternative therapies have been more popular. The following complementary therapies, some of which are more effective than others, are examples of those used by menopausal women to reduce associated discomforts:

- *Acupuncture.* Randomized, placebo-controlled trials are scarce, and the evidence about the efficacy of acupuncture is unconvincing (Borrelli & Ernst, 2010).

- *Massage.* Both massage and aromatherapy massage are effective in decreasing menopause symptoms (Darsareth et al., 2012).

- *Bioidentical hormones.* There is insufficient evidence that bioidentical hormone therapy is safe or effective. There are concerns about the content, purity, and labeling of these products (Stuenkel et al., 2012).

- *Meditation.* Randomized clinical trial evidence suggests that mindful meditation relieves vasomotor symptoms of menopause (Carmody et al., 2011).

- *Yoga.* A review of seven studies from 14 databases determined that the evidence is insufficient to suggest that yoga relieves vasomotor symptoms (Lee et al., 2009).

- *Botanicals.* See the Complementary and Alternative Therapy feature.

NURSING PROCESS

Nursing care during and after the menopausal period focuses on minimizing the symptoms associated with hormonal changes; reducing the risk of cardiovascular disease, cancer, and osteoporosis; and educating the client about lifestyle changes important to health and well-being.

The American Cancer Society (2013a) recommends periodic cancer-related checkups after the age of 20. This checkup includes examination for cancers of the thyroid, ovaries, lymph nodes, oral cavity, and skin. Other important checkups include screening for cervical, breast, and colorectal cancer. The current recommendation for screening for breast cancer includes yearly clinical breast exam and mammograms after age 40. Breast self-exam is an option for women (ACS, 2013a). To screen for colorectal cancer, a yearly fecal occult blood test or fecal immunochemical test is recommended unless there is family history or other risk factors for colorectal cancer. Women over age 65 who have had normal Pap test results on a regular basis should *not* be tested for cervical cancer. If there is history of cervical precancer, the Pap test should be done annually for 20 years after the diagnosis is made, even if it extends past age 65 (ACS, 2013a).

Health counseling should also include information about alcohol and tobacco use, sun exposure, diet and nutrition, exercise, risk factors, sexual practices, and environmental and occupational exposures. It is important to discuss the benefits of rest and exercise, as well as a diet that includes fruits, vegetables, and fiber. In addition, the nurse should suggest the following resources for further information:

- National Institute on Aging
- Centers for Disease Control and Prevention
- North American Menopause Society
- Association of Reproductive Health Professionals

Complementary and Alternative Therapy   Use of Botanicals for Menopausal Symptoms

Several botanicals have been touted as being effective in the management of menopausal symptoms. Following are some of the most popular botanicals for this use and the most recent research evidence related to the efficacy of their use to relieve hot flashes associated with menopause.

- *Black cohosh.* This botanical has been a popular alternative to HRT for hot flashes and other menopausal symptoms for many years. Some early studies showed that it did improve symptoms for up to 6 months. A new study from the Cochrane Database (Leach & Moore, 2012) reviewed 16 studies for a total of 2,027 participants who were perimenopausal. The studies compared black cohosh supplementation to placebo, hormone replacement therapy, red clover, and fluoxetine. Compared to placebo, black cohosh did not decrease hot flashes and other symptoms. The authors concluded that evidence for use of black cohosh is lacking and further research is needed.
- *Red clover.* In a study conducted to assess the safety and efficacy of black cohosh and red clover for the management of vasomotor symptoms of menopause, Geller et al. (2009) randomized 89 women with hot flashes into four groups. In the group where red clover was compared to placebo, there was a slight decrease in vasomotor symptoms, but the difference between red clover and placebo was insignificant. Red clover does appear to decrease anxiety over time and it is safe.

- *Soy.* Researchers in China evaluated the efficacy of soy in relieving menopausal hot flashes (Ye et al., 2012). The participants were 90 women, ages 45–60, randomly assigned to three groups. One group was given low-dose soy germ, one group was given high-dose soy germ, and the third group was given placebos. The researchers found that all the women studied had a reduction in vasomotor symptoms after 12 and 24 weeks. The women in both the soy groups, however, experienced much fewer hot flashes than the women in the placebo group. The researchers concluded that soy germ is beneficial in reducing hot flashes during menopause but more evidence is needed before soy may be recommended as an alternative to hormonal replacement.
- *Dong quai.* In a *Natural Standard Professional Monograph,* this botanical has been given an evidence grade of D for use for menopausal symptoms (Conquer et al., 2013). This means that there is statistically significant evidence to suggest that dong quai is of no benefit in controlling menopausal symptoms.
- *Ginseng.* This botanical has a lot of good qualities; however, it has been given an evidence grade of C for menopausal symptom control (Basch et al., 2013). This means that there is unclear or conflicting scientific evidence from multiple randomized trials that ginseng alleviates hot flashes in menopausal women.

- Women's Health Initiative
- National Women's Health Information Center.

Assessment

The nurse collects the following data through the health history and physical examination. When assessing the older woman, be aware of normal changes with aging.

- *Health history.* Problems with urinary frequency, urgency, or incontinence; menstrual history; sexual history; dyspareunia; use of alcohol, nicotine, and drugs; medications, sleep patterns, hot flashes, night sweats, changes in emotional responses
- *Physical assessment.* Height and weight, posture, vital signs, breast examination, pelvic examination, abdominal assessment.

Diagnosis

The nursing diagnoses that may apply to the client with menopause include the following:

- *Deficient Knowledge*
- *Ineffective Sexuality Pattern*
- *Situational Low Self-Esteem*
- *Disturbed Body Image.*

(NANDA-I © 2012)

Planning

Goals of client care may include the following:

- The client will understand the process of menopause.
- The client will learn strategies to reduce and cope with symptoms.

- The client will undertake a program of weight-bearing exercises.

Implementation

Menopause is viewed differently by different women, and it is important for the nurse to determine what it means to each client before beginning implementation. While some women may view menopause as a relief, others may see it as the end of their youth and the beginning of old age. Implementations should be aimed at helping the woman understand the process of menopause, cope with symptoms as they arise, and make healthy lifestyle choices.

Discuss Knowledge of Menopause

Because manifestations of menopause vary widely, it is difficult to predict their effect on an individual woman. However, the well-informed woman is better prepared to deal with whatever symptoms she experiences. To prepare the client, the nurse should do the following:

- Discuss physiological manifestations, such as hot flashes and night sweats. The underlying cause of hot flashes is the rapid change in estrogen levels (Deneris & Huether, 2010; Melby & Lampl, 2011). Many physiological effects of menopause are amenable to either HRT or nonpharmacologic methods of relief, such as lifestyle changes.

SAFETY ALERT
When hot flashes occur at night and are accompanied by perspiration, they are called night sweats. Night sweats often interfere with normal sleep patterns, leading to increased fatigue and irritability.

- Provide information about dietary recommendations. The recommended daily intake of calcium for women over age 50 is 1,200 mg. This dosage helps to prevent osteoporosis. Some women need to use calcium supplements or calcium-containing antacid tablets to meet this requirement.
- Emphasize the importance of weight-bearing exercise. Weight-bearing exercise reduces the rate of bone loss, helps maintain optimum weight, and reduces cardiovascular risk.
- Provide information about the benefits and risks of HRT. Not every woman will need or want it. Every woman needs to understand both the risks and the benefits before deciding whether to use HRT.
- Encourage the woman to obtain yearly mammograms, clinical breast examinations, and Pap tests until 65 years old. The increased risk for cancer of the breast and pelvic reproductive organs makes healthcare provider screening during and after menopause even more important.

Promote Effective Sexuality Pattern

Vaginal dryness and atrophy, together with the emotional effect of menopause, can interfere with sexual expression and satisfaction. Suggesting measures to help the woman and her partner cope with these changes can enable them to continue or resume a mutually satisfying sexual relationship.

- Encourage expression of feelings and concerns about how menopause is changing her sex life. Midlife and older women may not be comfortable discussing their intimate sexual behavior.
- Suggest ways to increase vaginal lubrication, such as spending more time in foreplay and/or using water-soluble gels (e.g., Replens) for vaginal lubrication. A more leisurely approach to sexual activity can be mutually gratifying for the woman and her partner. Use of water-soluble gels can prevent vaginal pain and irritation and improve the quality of the sexual experience. Plant estrogens, found in food such as brown rice, sweet potatoes, carrots, apples, corn, green beans, lemon and orange peels, and tofu, are mildly estrogenic and may improve vaginal dryness.
- Explain that as women age, it may take longer for vaginal lubrication and orgasm to occur. This information is important to prevent the woman from believing something is wrong with her or to prevent her partner from believing he or she is no longer interesting or sexually exciting.

Promote Self-Esteem

Each woman responds to the aging process in her own way, and most women have coping skills that adequately equip them to deal with the gradual changes associated with aging. Among the factors that may provoke a self-esteem disturbance are the loss of youth, a sense of emptiness as children leave home, and the need to redefine one's self-concept and roles as parenting becomes less important. Women who place a high value on their physical attractiveness may experience a painful psychological response to the physical changes of menopause. The nurse can help the client to negotiate the changes to her self-image by doing the following:

- Encourage expression of fears and concerns related to changes in interpersonal and family functions. Many women associate aging with "uselessness" and unattractiveness.
- Suggest volunteer activities or employment for the woman who has extra time. This enables the woman to feel that she is still a contributing member of society. Volunteering for activities involving young people can help reduce anxiety about the loss of reproductive ability or any late regrets about not having had children.
- Discuss the importance of a healthy lifestyle in maintaining physical attractiveness. Identify risk factors and high-risk behaviors. Lifestyle habits and behaviors affect many body systems and physical appearance. For example, cigarette smoking and overexposure to the sun make the skin age faster, contributing to wrinkles. Active women who exercise and eat a well-balanced diet look and feel better.

Promote Healthy Body Image

As a woman progresses through the perimenopausal period, changes in appearance and the loss of childbearing ability may combine to make her feel "old," "ugly," and "useless." Although this is far from the truth, with women living at least one third of their lives after menopause in productive careers and activities, it nevertheless is the perception of women as well as society. The physical changes the woman often experiences include growth of facial hair, excessive perspiration and flushing of the face, and weight gain. The nurse can help the woman deal with physical changes of menopause by doing the following:

- Encourage the woman to describe her perceptions of her own body. This information is necessary to obtain data to establish an individualized plan of care.
- Encourage verbalization of feelings of concern, anger, anxiety, loss, and fear over body changes. Expressing these emotions can facilitate the grieving process and acceptance of change.
- Stress that certain physical characteristics of an individual cannot be changed; emphasize the importance of learning to recognize and appreciate one's own special strengths. These help the woman gain acceptance and a realistic appraisal of self.
- Refer, as appropriate, for dietary management, exercise, stress management, and cosmetic assistance (e.g., for aggravating facial hair). These actions increase wellness and a positive sense of self.

Evaluation

Expected outcomes to evaluate the client's progress toward goals may include the following:

- The client demonstrates a positive sense of self as evidenced by stable weight, participation in a regular exercise program, and ability to manage stress.
- The client verbalizes feelings related to changes that have occurred.
- The client describes strategies for maintaining health.

REVIEW Menopause

RELATE Link the Concepts and Exemplars

Linking the exemplar of menopause with the concept of self:

1. What interventions will you initiate for the woman entering menopause who feels that she is no longer attractive and has lost her femininity?

2. What is your priority of care for the woman experiencing menopause who has low self-esteem?

Linking the exemplar of menopause with the concept of health, wellness, and illness:

3. What health promotion interventions will be a priority for the client entering menopause?

4. What nutritional and exercise behaviors would you promote for the woman in menopause? Explain your answer.

READY Go to Companion Skills Manual

REFER Go to Pearson Nursing Student Resources
nursing.pearsonhighered.com

- Additional review materials

REFLECT Case Study

Marly Cutler is a 51-year-old woman who is married to Fred. They live in a small rural community and own their farm. Mr. and Mrs. Cutler have two adult children who live in the city. Mr. Cutler has hypertension that is being treated with lisinopril, 10 mg/day, and high cholesterol for which he takes simvastatin 20 mg/day. Mrs. Cutler has no real health issues and has yearly screening examinations. Last year her physician told her to take calcium 1,200 mg/day to reduce the risk of osteoporosis.

Mrs. Cutler has come to the OB/GYN clinic today because she has missed some periods, is having night sweats, and is experiencing mood swings that are affecting her relationship with her husband. She wonders whether she has caught the flu.

1. What client teaching will you provide for Mrs. Cutler?

2. What strategies might you suggest to reduce the severity of the symptoms she reports?

3. How will you assess Mrs. Cutler's mental status?

EXEMPLAR 19.4 Menstrual Dysfunction

EXEMPLAR KEY TERMS

Amenorrhea, *1400*
Dysfunctional uterine bleeding (DUB), *1400*
Dysmenorrhea, *1399*
Endometriosis, *1400*
Menorrhagia, *1400*
Metrorrhagia, *1400*

EXEMPLAR LEARNING OUTCOMES

After reading about this exemplar, you will be able to:

1. Describe the pathophysiology, etiology, clinical manifestations, and direct and indirect causes of menstrual dysfunction.

2. Identify risk factors associated with menstrual dysfunction.

3. Illustrate the nursing process in providing culturally competent care across the life span for individuals with menstrual dysfunction.

4. Formulate priority nursing diagnoses appropriate for an individual with menstrual dysfunction.

5. Summarize therapies used by interdisciplinary teams in the collaborative care of an individual with menstrual dysfunction.

6. Plan evidence-based care for an individual with menstrual dysfunction and her family in collaboration with other members of the healthcare team.

7. Evaluate expected outcomes for an individual with menstrual dysfunction.

▶ OVERVIEW

Every woman, except in rare instances, will have monthly menstrual periods. Many women experience minor discomforts associated with the menstrual cycle such as breast tenderness, uterine cramping, low back pain, and mood swings. Other women will experience more serious changes in the menstrual cycle that will lead to visits with healthcare providers. In general, menstrual dysfunction may manifest as pain, bleeding, or both. In this exemplar, various common menstrual dysfunctions and their treatment will be described.

▶ PATHOPHYSIOLOGY, ETIOLOGY, AND CLINICAL MANIFESTATIONS

Pain associated with menses, called **dysmenorrhea**, is one of the most common menstrual dysfunctions. Primary dysmenorrhea is very common among women with normal menstrual function. It is caused by the release of prostaglandins that cause the contractions of the uterus needed to expel menstrual fluid and tissue.

Primary dysmenorrhea begins within the first three or four menstrual periods after menarche and will occur with each ovulatory cycle during the teens and twenties of a woman's life. The pain decreases over time and is often much less after childbirth. It is estimated that 50%–90% of women ages 15–25 have experienced primary dysmenorrhea, and many have missed school or work because of it (Latendresse et al., 2010). The main symptom of primary dysmenorrhea is pelvic pain that radiates to the groin just before and during the first day of menses. Women also complain of low backache, diarrhea, headache, and anorexia. **Box 19–6** ● lists the manifestations of primary dysmenorrhea.

Secondary dysmenorrhea is related to pathology or diseases that affect the uterus and pelvic area. These disorders are more likely to occur among women ages 30–50 and the pain may occur at any time with the menstrual cycle. Disorders that may cause secondary dysmenorrhea include endometriosis, tumors, cysts, pelvic adhesions, pelvic inflammatory disease, infections, cervical stenosis, uterine leiomyomas, or adenomyosis (Alswanger & Durler, 2013). The pain and discomfort associated with these disorders can be very severe. Often it is described as

Box 19–6 Manifestations of Primary Dysmenorrhea

- Abdominal pain beginning with onset of menses and lasting 12–48 hours
- Pain radiating to lower back and thighs
- Headache
- Nausea
- Vomiting
- Diarrhea
- Fatigue
- Breast tenderness

dull lower abdominal pain that radiates to the back and down the thighs. The pain gets progressively worse with each menstrual cycle (McKay, 2011).

A prime example of a disorder that causes secondary dysmenorrhea is endometriosis, potentially one of the most painful of gynecological disorders. **Endometriosis** is a condition in which cells from endometrial tissue implant and grow outside the uterus. These tissue implants respond to estrogen and progesterone just as the endometrial lining does. Each month the implants mature, open, and bleed into the pelvic cavity causing pain, fibrosis, and adhesions (Laubach, Lorntson, & Forrest, 2013).

Endometriosis may occur anywhere in the body, but the endometrial tissue is most likely to be seen attached to organs in the lower parts of the pelvis such as the uterus, ovaries, fallopian tubes, uterine ligaments, pelvic peritoneum, bladder, rectum, and rectovaginal septum (Latendresse et al., 2010; McKay, 2011). It is estimated that between 2% and 20% of women of childbearing age have endometriosis. Approximately half of all women who are examined because of pelvic pain are diagnosed with endometriosis (Latendresse et al., 2010). The incidence is higher among infertile women (McKay, 2011).

The cause of endometriosis is unknown, but it is thought to be due to impaired cellular and humoral immunity or it may be an autoimmune disorder. Evidence suggests a genetic predisposition, and the disease seems to be more severe among women with relatives who have the disease (Latendresse et al., 2010).

Clinical manifestations of endometriosis include dysmenorrhea that worsens each month, and, depending on where the implants are, dyspareunia, menorrhagia, postcoital bleeding, urinary complaints, and rectal pain. The pain is usually described as beginning a few days before onset of menses and becoming much worse as the period begins to decrease and stop. If the problem is long standing or there are complications such as adhesions, the pain may be constant (McKay, 2011). Risk factors for endometriosis are listed in **Box 19–7** ●. The Clinical Manifestations and Therapies feature lists common types of menstrual dysfunction, their etiologies, and treatments.

Box 19–7 Risk Factors for Endometriosis

- Menarche before age 11
- Cycle length less than 27 days
- Heavy, prolonged menses
- Sedentary lifestyle
- Increased dietary fat
- First-degree relative with the disorder

Abnormal uterine bleeding has several forms and may be called **dysfunctional uterine bleeding (DUB)** in some settings. However, abnormal uterine bleeding refers to bleeding from all causes, including but not limited to uterine tumors, endometrial or cervical cancer, polyps, ovarian cysts, bleeding disorders, and complications of pregnancy. DUB is heavy, prolonged or irregular bleeding most often associated with anovulatory cycles. The healthcare provider must eliminate tumors, polyps, and other causes before a diagnosis of DUB can be made (Latendresse et al., 2010).

Pathophysiologically, DUB is irregular episodes of profuse, painless bleeding preceded by long stretches of amenorrhea (Alswager & Durler, 2013). The cause is a hormonal disruption that results in failure of the ovarian follicle to mature. Without ovulation, there is no corpus luteum and, therefore, a lack of progesterone. This causes changes in the endometrial lining and a loss of control of regular, complete shedding. Over time this produces a thickened endometrial lining that will eventually begin irregular sloughing and prolonged heavy bleeding.

There are several patterns of abnormal uterine bleeding including amenorrhea, oligomenorrhea, menorrhagia, metrorrhagia, menometrorrhagia, and postmenopausal vaginal bleeding.

- **Amenorrhea** (absence of menses), like dysmenorrhea, may be primary or secondary. Primary amenorrhea is the absence of menstruation by age 14 without secondary sexual characteristics or age 16 with sexual characteristics such as breast growth and pubic hair changes (Latendresse et al., 2010). This disorder may arise from central nervous system disorders, a dysfunctional hypothalamic–pituitary–ovarian axis, tumors of the pituitary, genetic disorders such as Turner syndrome, and congenital abnormalities such as the absence of the vagina or uterus. Secondary amenorrhea has occurred when a previously menstruating woman does not spot or bleed for a period of time that is three times that of her normal cycle length. Secondary amenorrhea may be pathological or physiological. It may be due to severe weight loss related to excessive exercise or poor diet; thyroid disorders; hyperprolactinemia; polycystic ovary syndrome (PCOS); or as the result of hormonal changes during early adolescence, pregnancy, or the perimenopausal period. The most common causes of secondary amenorrhea are pregnancy, breastfeeding, menopause, and contraceptive use (Hatcher et al., 2011).
- Oligomenorrhea (scant menses) occurs when cycles are longer than 6–7 weeks and usually is related to hormonal imbalances such as those seen in polycystic ovary syndrome.
- **Menorrhagia** (excessive or prolonged menstruation that occurs at regular intervals) is one form of bleeding seen in DUB.
- **Metrorrhagia** (bleeding of variable amount between menstrual periods) may be mild spotting at ovulation or breakthrough bleeding due to combination oral contraception. Or, it may be very severe, causing anemia or hypovolemic shock. This is another form of bleeding seen in DUB.
- Menometrorrhagia (irregular, excessive, prolonged menstruation) is another form of DUB.
- Postmenopausal bleeding may be caused by endometrial polyps, endometrial hyperplasia, or uterine cancer. The possibility of cancer makes early evaluation and treatment essential.

Clinical Manifestations and Therapies **Menstrual Dysfunction**

ETIOLOGY	CLINICAL MANIFESTATIONS	CLINICAL THERAPIES
Shock due to uterine bleeding	■ Hypotension ■ Delayed capillary refill ■ Cyanosis, hypoxia, dizziness, change in LOC ■ Low urine output ■ Diminished bowel motility ■ Pale skin ■ Activity intolerance ■ Tachycardia, tachypnea	■ Provide blood transfusions. ■ Administer IV fluids. ■ Administer IV estrogen. ■ Monitor ABCs. ■ Administer oxygen. ■ Measure intake and output. ■ Increase fluid intake as tolerated.
Anemia	■ Pale skin ■ Activity intolerance, fatigue	■ Blood transfusions may be needed. ■ Administer iron supplements. ■ Promote diet high in iron. ■ Encourage fluid intake.
Dysmenorrhea	■ Grimacing ■ Lying still with legs drawn up ■ On pain scale of 0–10, may range from 4 to 10	■ Administer analgesics as appropriate. ■ Place heating pad on lower abdomen. ■ Increase fluids.

Risk Factors

A number of factors may predispose a woman to DUB. These factors include stress, extreme weight changes, and use of oral contraceptive agents or an IUC device. Dysfunctional uterine bleeding is usually related to hormonal imbalances.

▶ COLLABORATION

Care of the woman with menstrual pain focuses on identifying the underlying cause of the pain, reestablishing the woman's functional capacity, and managing pain.

A careful history and physical assessment are performed to rule out any underlying organic cause of dysmenorrhea. If no organic cause can be found, the diagnosis is primary dysmenorrhea. In addition, attitudes and expectations about menstruation and lifestyle disruption are identified and explored.

The care of the woman with abnormal uterine bleeding focuses on identifying and treating the underlying disease or hormonal disorder. A careful history and physical examination are performed. Abdominal and pelvic examinations are performed to rule out abdominal masses. All women with abnormal bleeding should keep a diary of menstrual patterns to help in diagnosing the cause of the abnormal bleeding.

Diagnostic Tests

Various diagnostic tests are performed to identify structural abnormalities, hormonal imbalances, and pathological conditions that could cause menstrual pain and abnormal uterine bleeding.

Diagnosis is made on the basis of findings from a pelvic examination and diagnostic procedures, including a Pap test for cervical dysplasia or cancer; cervical and vaginal cultures to screen for STIs or other infections; and abdominal and transvaginal ultrasound for depth of the endometrium, intrauterine or ectopic pregnancy, ovarian cysts, adnexal masses, leiomyomas, or cancer. Hysteroscopy may be used, in which a scope is placed into the uterine cavity for inspection of the endometrial lining. Another procedure is saline infusion sonohysterography, in which saline is injected into the endometrial cavity via a catheter and transvaginal ultrasound is used to assess for polyps or myomas. Colposcopy is a procedure in which a large electric microscope is used to inspect the cervix under magnification and identify areas for biopsy. Endometrial biopsy may be done to obtain tissue from the endometrium for pathological examination. Endocervical curettage and biopsy may be done to remove tissue from inside the cervical canal to look for evidence of dysplasia or cancer. CT scan or MRI may also be used to detect structural abnormalities, benign myomas, adenomyomas, malignancy, or infections.

Laboratory tests used to assess possible causes of dysmenorrhea and abnormal uterine bleeding are as follows:

■ A pregnancy test determines whether bleeding or pain is a complication of pregnancy.

■ FSH and LH levels are measured to assess the function of the pituitary gland. The results are correlated with the follicular phase or the luteal phase of the menstrual cycle.

■ Progesterone and estradiol levels are measured to assess ovarian function.

■ The thyroid-stimulating hormone test screens for thyroid dysfunction. If positive, then further testing of the thyroid is needed.

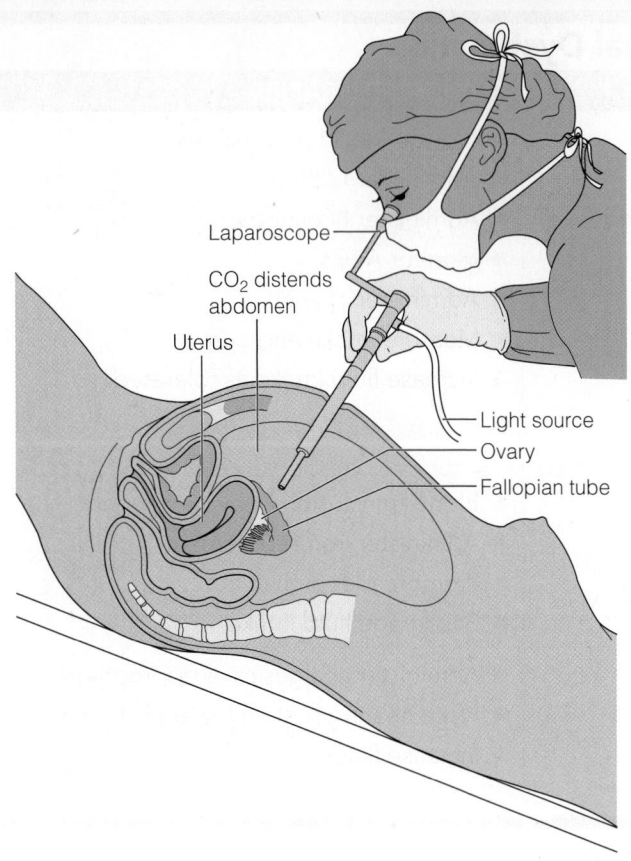

Laparoscope

CO_2 distends abdomen

Uterus

Light source

Ovary

Fallopian tube

Figure 19–27 ● Laparoscopy. In this surgical procedure, a flexible, lighted instrument (laparoscope) is inserted through a periumbilical incision. Laparoscopy allows visualization of the pelvic cavity.

■ A complete blood count (CBC) with differential can provide evidence of anemia or infection.

■ Coagulation studies reveal possible von Willebrand disease or other coagulation abnormalities (McKay, 2011).

Laparoscopy is used to diagnose structural defects and blockages caused by scarring, endometriosis, tumors, and cysts (**Figure 19–27** ●). A dilation and curettage (D&C) of the uterus may be performed to obtain tissue for evaluation or to relieve dysmenorrhea and heavy menstrual bleeding.

Pharmacologic Therapy

If the manifestations of secondary dysmenorrhea or abnormal uterine bleeding are severe or incapacitating, ovulation may be suppressed by the use of combined oral contraceptives (COCs), Depo-Provera, danazol, or GnRH agonists. Use of COCs, progesterone injections, and nonsteroidal anti-inflammatory drugs (NSAIDs) may help relieve cramping and the amount of bleeding that occurs. Diuretics may be prescribed to relieve bloating. Selective serotonin reuptake inhibitors (SSRIs) such as fluoxetine (Prozac), sertraline (Zoloft), and paroxetine (Paxil) may be used to manage mood or to help the client cope with chronic pelvic pain.

For many women with DUB, hormonal agents can correct menstrual irregularities. For anovulatory DUB, COCs may be prescribed for 3–6 months. An alternative to COCs is oral medroxyprogesterone acetate (Provera), which may be prescribed for 12 days each month to regulate uterine bleeding. The Mirena intrauterine system is another option used to control abnormal uterine bleeding. In cases of very heavy bleeding, conjugated estrogens may be given intravenously (McKay, 2011).

Oral iron supplements are often prescribed to replace iron lost through menstrual bleeding.

Surgery

Surgical intervention emphasizes the least invasive method that provides effective relief, beginning with a therapeutic D&C, then endometrial ablation, and, finally, hysterectomy.

THERAPEUTIC DILATION AND CURETTAGE   In a therapeutic D&C, the cervical canal is dilated and the uterine wall is scraped. D&C is used to diagnose and treat DUB and other disorders of the female reproductive system. D&C is contraindicated in any woman who has been taking anticoagulant drugs or whose condition precludes the use of regional or general anesthesia.

ENDOMETRIAL ABLATION   Endometrial ablation to destroy the uterine lining may be done in the office setting or in surgery under general anesthesia. This procedure stops bleeding completely in most cases. Ablation may be done with extreme cold, heated fluids, microwave energy, or high-energy radio-frequency waves that vaporize the endometrial lining within 80–90 seconds (Mayo Clinic, 2012). Ablation is not recommended for women who want to become pregnant, who were recently pregnant, or who are postmenopausal.

HYSTERECTOMY   Hysterectomy, or removal of the uterus, may be performed when medical management of bleeding disorders is unsuccessful or malignancy is present, particularly if the woman no longer wishes to bear children. In premenopausal women, the ovaries are usually left in place; in postmenopausal women, a total hysterectomy, or panhysterectomy, may be performed; this procedure involves removal of the uterus, fallopian tubes, and ovaries.

Hysterectomy may involve either an abdominal or a vaginal approach. The choice depends on the underlying disorder, the need to explore the abdominal cavity, and the preference of the surgeon and the client. Nursing care of the woman undergoing a hysterectomy is described in **Box 19–8** ●.

Abdominal hysterectomy is performed when a preexisting abdominal scar is present, when adhesions are thought to be present, or when a large operating field is necessary. For example, the woman with endometriosis is more likely to have an abdominal hysterectomy because endometrial tissue implants that may be present on other abdominal organs need to be removed. The surgical incision may be either longitudinal, made in the midline from umbilicus to pubis, or a Pfannenstiel incision, also known as the bikini cut.

Vaginal hysterectomy, removal of the uterus through the vagina, is desirable when the uterus has descended into the vagina or if the urinary bladder or rectum has prolapsed into the vagina. Laparoscopy-assisted vaginal hysterectomy (LAVH) is most often performed.

Box 19–8   Nursing Care of the Client Having a Hysterectomy

PREOPERATIVE CARE

■ Assess the woman's understanding of the procedure. Provide explanation, clarification, and emotional support as needed. Reassure that the anesthesia will eliminate any pain during surgery and that medication will be administered postoperatively to minimize discomfort. *The woman who understands the procedure to be performed and what to expect after surgery will be less anxious.*

■ Cleanse the abdominal and perineal area, and, if ordered, shave the perineal area.

■ If ordered, administer a small cleansing enema and ask the woman to empty her bladder. *This precaution helps prevent contamination from the bowel or bladder during surgery.*

■ Administer preoperative medications as ordered. Start IV fluids.

■ Check the chart to ensure that the consent form has been signed.

POSTOPERATIVE CARE

■ Assess for signs of hemorrhage. *Hemorrhage is more common after vaginal hysterectomy than after abdominal hysterectomy.*

■ Monitor vital signs every 4 hours, auscultate lungs every shift, maintain IV fluids and measure intake and output. *These data are important indicators of hemodynamic status and complications.*

■ Once the catheter has been removed, measure the amount of urine voided.

■ Assess for complications, including infection, ileus, shock or hemorrhage, thrombophlebitis, and pulmonary embolus.

■ Assess vaginal discharge; instruct the woman in perineal care.

■ Assess incision and bowel sounds every shift.

■ Encourage turning, coughing, deep breathing, and early ambulation.

■ Encourage fluid intake.

■ Teach the woman to splint the abdomen and cough deeply. Teach the use of the incentive spirometer.

■ Instruct the woman to restrict physical activity for 4–6 weeks. Heavy lifting, stair climbing, douching, tampons, and sexual intercourse should be avoided. The woman should shower, avoiding tub baths, until bleeding has ceased. *Infection and hemorrhage are the greatest postoperative risks; restricting activities and preventing the introduction of any foreign material into the vagina help reduce these risks.*

■ Explain to the woman that she may feel tired for several days after surgery and will need to rest periodically.

■ Explain that appetite may be depressed and bowel elimination may be sluggish. *These are aftereffects of general anesthesia, handling of the bowel during surgery, and loss of muscle tone in the bowel while empty.*

■ Teach the woman to recognize signs of complications that should be reported to the physician or nurse:

  a. Temperature greater than 37.7°C (100°F)

  b. Vaginal bleeding that is greater than a typical menstrual period or is bright red

  c. Urinary incontinence, urgency, burning, or frequency

  d. Severe pain.

■ Encourage the woman to express feelings that may signal a negative self-concept. Correct any misconceptions. *Some women believe that hysterectomy means weight gain, the end of sexual activity, and the growth of facial hair.*

■ Provide information on risks and benefits of estrogen replacement therapy, if indicated. *If the ovaries have also been removed, the woman is immediately thrust into menopause and may want or need estrogen replacement therapy.*

■ Reinforce the need to obtain gynecological examinations regularly even after hysterectomy.

Whatever the etiology and treatment of any dysmenorrhea, the nurse's teaching role is important. The Client Teaching feature lists some of the ways in which the nurse can help the client cope with abnormal uterine bleeding.

Client Teaching
Abnormal Uterine Bleeding

The nurse should provide support, appropriate reassurance, and information to help the woman and her family better understand her disorder and the therapeutic interventions indicated. Teaching also includes self-care measures that help minimize the effects of abnormal uterine bleeding on the daily functioning of the woman. The following topics should be included:

■ Administration and side effects of prescribed medications, including iron

■ The need to maintain a balanced diet, increasing iron-rich foods such as eggs, beans, liver, beef, and shrimp (Inform the woman that, although orange juice may improve the absorption of iron, foods high in calcium and oxalic acid, such as spinach, may reduce its absorption.)

■ Importance of maintaining a fluid intake of 2,000–3,000 mL/day

■ The need to immediately report recurring episodes of abnormal uterine bleeding, particularly in postmenopausal women, to the healthcare provider.

Complementary and Alternative Therapies for Dysmenorrhea

Alternative and complementary therapies the woman with dysmenorrhea may find helpful focus on diet, exercise, relaxation, and stress management. Some of these therapies are as follows:

■ The use of rose hips for dysmenorrhea has been given an evidence grade of B (good scientific evidence) (Bryan et al., 2013).

■ Fish oil plus B_{12} relieves dysmenorrhea by affecting the metabolism of prostaglandins (NYU Langone Medical Center [NYULMC], 2012).

■ Vitamin E and magnesium in separate studies have been shown to be more effective than placebo in treating dysmenorrhea (NYULMC, 2012).

■ Exercise, adequate rest, stress management, and good nutrition are also beneficial.

◼ NURSING PROCESS

Nursing care for the woman with primary dysmenorrhea focuses on controlling manifestations and providing education about the normal physiology of the menstrual cycle and self-care measures. Care of the woman with secondary dysmenorrhea varies according to the underlying cause.

Abnormal uterine bleeding usually causes the woman anxiety. Her self-image, sexuality, or reproductive capacity may be threatened, and she may fear the possibility of cancer. She may be embarrassed to discuss her menstrual history and hygiene practices.

Assessment

Menstrual habits of the client should be assessed whenever the woman seeks health care. Determination of last menstrual period, normal length of menstruation and time between periods, and any symptoms associated with menstruation should be assessed. Cultural influences often play a role in how the women views and responds to menstruation and should also be assessed.

It is essential to create an atmosphere that facilitates open communication and comfort for the client. Clients commonly experience anxiety, fear, and embarrassment when questioned about a topic that, in most clients' minds, is very personal. These emotions may be expressed either verbally or nonverbally. The nurse should approach the client in as nonthreatening a manner as possible and assure the client that the information provided and the results of the physical examination will remain confidential.

Throughout the assessment process, the nurse gathers subjective and objective data reflecting the client's state of health:

- *Objective data.* Results of Papanicolaou test, examination of genitalia, hemoglobin and hematocrit levels
- *Subjective data.* Date of last menstrual period and length of cycle; age at which menses began; date of last OB-GYN exam; date of last sexual encounter and typical sexual practices, including types of birth control used; medications; preexisting conditions; obstetric history.

Diagnosis

The nursing diagnoses for a client with dysmenorrhea include the following:

- *Acute Pain*
- *Ineffective Coping.*

(NANDA-I © 2012)

Nursing diagnoses that may be appropriate for the client with abnormal uterine bleeding include the following:

- *Anxiety*
- *Risk for Ineffective Perfusion* related to blood loss
- *Fatigue* related to blood loss
- *Sexual Dysfunction.*

(NANDA-I © 2012)

Planning

Goals of nursing care include the following:

- The client's pain and discomfort will be reduced to an acceptable level.
- The client will experience physical comfort and energy-saving rest.
- The client will increase intake of fluids and iron-rich foods.

- The client will become more comfortable discussing sexual dysfunction.
- The client will identify coping strategies to reduce anxiety.
- The client will maintain a journal of symptoms.

Implementation

Nursing interventions for the woman with dysmenorrhea focus on relieving symptoms and providing client teaching to decrease anxiety and increase coping skills. Assisting the client to identify lifestyle choices that may be contributing to menstrual disorders such as heavy lifting, nutrition, and substance abuse can help the nurse implement the most effective plan of care.

Relieve Acute Pain

The woman with dysmenorrhea may have pain from headache (including migraine), lower abdominal cramps, excessive fluid retention, and backache. The nurse should do the following to help the woman cope with her pain:

- Teach effective pharmacologic and nonpharmacologic self-care measures to relieve pain: application of heat, relaxation techniques (such as breathing exercises, imagery techniques, or meditation), and exercise. Heat relieves muscle spasms and dilates blood vessels, increasing blood supply to the pelvis and uterine muscles. Relaxation and exercise aid the release of naturally produced pain relievers called endorphins.

Relieve Anxiety

The anxiety associated with abnormal uterine bleeding can be intense. Until the cause of the bleeding is identified and has been addressed, the woman may fear cancer or other life-threatening conditions. The following nursing interventions can help the woman to cope with such anxiety:

- Discuss the results of tests and examinations with the woman. This allows for open exchange of information.
- Provide information about the causes, treatments, risks, long-term effects of treatments, and prognosis. This allows the woman to assume responsibility for her own health and become involved in her own treatment plan.
- Evaluate coping strategies and psychosocial support systems. Teach coping strategies if indicated. The possibility of surgery or cancer represents a crisis for the woman and her support system. Support groups can provide assistance for the woman through crisis intervention.
- Review how fatigue may be affecting the woman's activities of daily living and suggest ways to balance rest and activity. Encourage her to ask for help with daily chores from her family.

Promote Sexual Function

The woman with DUB may be unwilling to express herself sexually, particularly if bleeding is frequent or heavy. Additionally, fatigue may prevent her from participating in sexual activity. Following are some nursing interventions that address sexual dysfunction related to DUB:

- Offer information about engaging in sexual activity during menstruation. Explain that conception is possible during this time if she has a 21-day menstrual cycle. Explain that orgasm may help relieve symptoms. Some women mistakenly believe that birth control measures are unnecessary during menstruation. Orgasm causes a release of tension and vascular congestion and frequently provides at least temporary relief of symptoms.

■ Provide an opportunity for the expression of concerns related to alterations in lifestyle and sexual functioning. Some women have had a prolonged period of sexual abstinence related to DUB. Allowing women to verbalize concerns can assist them in working collaboratively with the healthcare provider to minimize the impact of illness and optimize function.

■ Encourage frequent rest periods. This conserves energy and may allow sexual activities to resume.

■ Provide information about alternative methods of sexual expression. Methods of sexual expression other than vaginal intercourse may satisfy the needs of both partners.

Evaluation

Client progress toward goals is evaluated on the basis of appropriate learning outcomes, which may include the following:

■ The client experiences less pain, allowing her to perform activities of daily living.
■ The client experiences less fatigue.
■ The client reports reduced anxiety.
■ The client reports return to baseline menstruation.
■ The client is able to participate in sexual activity without symptoms.

NURSING CARE PLAN | A Client With Menstrual Dysfunction

Angela Hall is a 31-year-old married accountant, who relates a history of severe dysmenorrhea and menorrhagia, a feeling of pelvic heaviness, and pain that radiates down her thighs. Because of her discomfort, her husband has complained about the quality of their sex life and has expressed concerns about their plans for having children. Mrs. Hall reports being so tired she doesn't care whether she has sex or not and, in fact, would really prefer not to: "Sex hurts so much, I just can't stand it." Her healthcare provider suspects endometriosis, and a diagnostic laparoscopy has been scheduled.

ASSESSMENT

Christine Brigham, RN, NP, interviews Mrs. Hall and makes the following assessments: T_O 36.7°C (98.2°F); P 68 bpm; R 18/min; BP 110/70 mmHg. Mrs. Hall's weight is 59 kg (130 lb) and within normal limits for her height. Review of laboratory findings indicates a hemoglobin level of 9.8 g/dL (normal range: 12–15 g/dL) and a hematocrit of 33.1% (normal range: 36%–46%). Physical examination reveals pelvic tenderness on manipulation of the cervix and small masses that are palpable on abdominal/pelvic examination.

DIAGNOSES

■ *Chronic Pain* related to endometrial pelvic implants
■ *Anxiety* related to effect of endometriosis on fertility
■ *Deficient Knowledge* related to diagnosis and treatment options
■ *Ineffective Sexuality Pattern* related to the manifestations of endometriosis
(NANDA-I © 2012)

PLANNING

■ The client will use effective self-care measures to deal with the pain and discomfort.
■ The client will verbalize decreased anxiety.
■ The client will demonstrate understanding of the disease and treatment options.
■ The client will articulate an improvement in sexual functioning and a decrease in interpersonal stress between herself and her husband.

IMPLEMENTATION

■ Identify the location, type, duration, and history of the pain.
■ Recommend analgesics and heat therapy.
■ Provide information on biofeedback, relaxation, and imagery to lessen pain.
■ Discuss with Mr. and Mrs. Hall the causes of endometriosis and its manifestations.

■ Encourage the Halls to discuss their feelings about the effect of the disease on their sex life, lifestyle, and fertility.
■ Refer the couple to the local mental health center if appropriate.

EVALUATION

Two years after the initiation of treatment, Mr. and Mrs. Hall have become parents of a baby girl. Mrs. Hall states that the discomfort and other manifestations of endometriosis have eased. Relaxation and imagery have effectively minimized her pain and brought about improvement in her function as wife, mother, and sexual partner. Counseling has improved the interpersonal and sexual relations between the Halls. Dietary management has improved Mrs. Hall's anemia, although the menorrhagia persists. The Halls are trying to have a second child, understanding the advantages of rapid succession of pregnancies. They will be followed in the nursing clinic and referred to an infertility clinic if conception does not occur within 1 year.

CRITICAL THINKING

1. *Explain the pathophysiological basis for Mrs. Hall's anemia.*
2. *How would you handle the situation if Mr. and Mrs. Hall were extremely uncomfortable and embarrassed about discussing their sexual problems?*
3. *Develop a plan of care for Mrs. Hall for the nursing diagnosis Situational Low Self-Esteem related to the manifestations of endometriosis.*

REVIEW **Menstrual Dysfunction**

RELATE Link the Concepts and Exemplars

Linking the exemplar of menstrual dysfunction with the concept of elimination:

1. What teaching will you initiate for the client with premenstrual syndrome regarding urinary health?

2. What nutritional counseling will you offer the client with premenstrual syndrome to prevent constipation?

Linking the exemplar of menstrual dysfunction with the concept of stress and coping:

3. What assessment data would alert you that the client with dysfunctional uterine bleeding is experiencing anxiety?

4. What priority interventions will you implement to help the woman with dysfunctional uterine bleeding to cope with fears?

READY Go to Companion Skills Manual

REFER Go to Pearson Nursing Student Resources

REFLECT Case Study

Angie Able is a 35-year-old woman married to Joe. The Ables have four children: Ted, age 12; Adam, age 10; Susie, age 8; and Linda, age 4. Mr. Able is a chef who owns a very successful restaurant in town. Ms. Able is an administrative assistant to the CEO of the largest bank in the area. She is a well-organized, detail-oriented individual with high energy. She manages the children, her home, her husband, and her job with aplomb. She has enjoyed good health with only mild seasonal colds.

Ms. Able has been having heavier than usual menstrual periods during the past 6 months, and this is beginning to interfere with her work. She has needed to leave work to change clothes several times and has begun carrying extra clothing with her during her menstrual period. Besides being very embarrassed, Ms. Able is afraid that there is something seriously wrong with her. She feels tired all the time and is always thirsty. Ms. Able decides to visit her gynecologist before her next menstrual period begins.

1. What could explain Ms. Able's symptoms of fatigue and thirst?

2. What diagnostic tests do you anticipate will be ordered?

3. What teaching will you provide Ms. Able to reduce her current symptoms?

EXEMPLAR 19.5 Responsible Sexual Behavior

EXEMPLAR KEY TERMS

Date rape, *1407*
Dating violence, *1406*

EXEMPLAR LEARNING OUTCOMES

1. Describe responsible sexual behavior.

2. Demonstrate client teaching to reduce the risk of sexually transmitted infections.

▶ OVERVIEW

The increase in the incidence of sexually transmitted infections, especially HIV/AIDS and genital herpes, has caused many individuals to modify their sexual practices and activities. Women frequently ask questions or voice concerns about these issues to the nurse in a clinic or ambulatory setting. The nurse working in these settings may need to assume the role of counselor on sexual and reproductive matters.

All sexually active individuals need to know how to reduce the spread of HIV and other STIs. The only totally safe sex practices are abstinence, long-term mutually monogamous sexual relations between two uninfected individuals, and mutual masturbation without direct contact.

Responsible sexual behavior involves more than just the physical act of sex itself. It also involves knowing how to identify the warnings signs of, and how to protect oneself from, both dating violence and date rape. Refer to the module on Violence for more information.

▶ SAFER SEX

Clients who do engage in sexual activity need to know and practice safer sex (**Box 19–9 ●**). Reducing the number of sexual partners—for example, by entering into and remaining in a long-term mutually monogamous relationship with an uninfected partner—reduces the risk. Clients should not engage in unprotected sex, especially if the HIV status of the partner is unknown. Latex condoms have been shown to reduce the risk of transmitting HIV and other infections. Their effectiveness is improved when nonoxynol-9 (a spermicide) is used for lubrication; however, nonoxynol-9 may cause genital ulcers, which can facilitate transmission of bloodborne diseases, such as HIV and hepatitis. To be effective, condoms must be used with every sexual encounter involving vaginal, oral, or anal intercourse. They also need to be applied and removed properly. A female condom is also available for use.

▶ DATING VIOLENCE

Dating violence is another type of intimate partner abuse, which occurs in relationships among youth. Most dating violence is directed at females, and studies have focused largely on girls. Over 9% of high school boys and girls report being victims of dating violence. African American girls report dating violence more commonly than Hispanic or Caucasian girls (CDC, 2012f; Howard, Wang, & Yan, 2007; MMWR, 2006). Girls who report dating violence were also more likely to report other at-risk behaviors, such as feeling sad, having attempted suicide, or having used substances such as tobacco and drugs. Early sexual activity, having a higher number of

Box 19–9 Guidelines for Safer Sex

- Practice mutual monogamy. If you are not in a mutually monogamous relationship, limit the number of sexual partners.
- Do not engage in unprotected sex, especially if the HIV status of your partner is unknown. Remember that an individual may be infected, and infective, for up to 6 months before converting to seropositive status.
- When entering into a new monogamous relationship, both partners should undergo HIV testing initially. If both are negative, practice abstinence or safer sex for 6 months, followed by retesting. If results still indicate that both partners are negative, sexual activity can probably be considered safe.
- Use latex condoms for oral, vaginal, or anal intercourse; avoid natural or animal skin condoms, which allow passage of HIV.
- For vaginal or anal sex, lubricate the condom with the spermicidal agent nonoxynol-9 for additional protection.
- Do not use an oil-based lubricant such as petroleum jelly, which can result in condom damage; water-based lubricants are acceptable.

- Women should carry and use a female condom.
- Remember that other means of birth control, such as oral contraceptives, provide no protection against HIV; barrier protection with a condom is necessary.
- Engage in safer sexual practices that are less damaging to sensitive tissues (e.g., mutual masturbation, avoiding anal or oral sex).
- Do not use drugs or alcohol.
- Do not share needles, razors, toothbrushes, sexual toys, or other items that may be contaminated with blood or body fluids.
- If HIV positive:
  a. Do not engage in unprotected sexual activity.
  b. Inform all current and former sexual partners of HIV status.
  c. Inform all healthcare personnel—primary care providers, physicians, and dentists in particular—of HIV status.
  d. Do not donate blood, plasma, blood products, sperm, organs, or tissue.
  e. If female, do not become pregnant.

Box 19–10 Early Warning Signs of Teenage Dating Violence

The teenage perpetrator:

- Believes that men should be in control and women should be submissive.
- Is jealous and possessive of his girlfriend, won't let her have friends, and checks up on her.
- Tries to control his girlfriend by giving orders and making all the decisions.

- Threatens his girlfriend with violence.
- Uses or owns weapons.
- Has a history of losing his temper quickly and fighting.
- Brags about mistreating others.
- Blames his girlfriend when he is violent; says she provoked him and made him do it.
- Has a history of abusive relationships.

sex partners, and being less likely to use birth control are also associated with higher incidences of dating violence. A cluster risk profile may therefore put adolescents more at risk for dating violence. **Box 19–10** ● lists early warning signs of teenage dating violence.

When dating violence takes the form of rape, the term **date rape** is used. This can be particularly harmful to females who often do not want to discuss the event or press charges against the attacker. See the exemplar on Rape and Rape-Trauma Syndrome in the module on Violence.

REVIEW Responsible Sexual Behavior

RELATE Link the Concepts and Exemplars

Linking the exemplar of responsible sexual behavior with the concept of infection:

1. How can responsible sexual behaviors reduce the risk of infection?
2. How can the nurse teach responsible sexual behaviors to the geriatric client?

Linking the exemplar of responsible sexual behavior with the concept of ethics:

3. The nurse is caring for a client who is HIV/AIDS positive. The client says that it is not his responsibility to protect his sexual partners and that everyone needs to look out for themselves. How would you respond to this comment?
4. The nurse is caring for a male client who says he wants to be sexually responsible. What information would you provide this client based on his ethical concerns?

READY Go to Companion Skills Manual

REFER Go to Pearson Nursing Student Resources
nursing.pearsonhighered.com

- Additional review materials

REFLECT Case Study

Qualyndria Gunderson, 14 years old, comes to the physician's office with her mother and requests to be seen alone while her mother sits in the waiting area. The nurse escorts Qualyndria back to the examination room. Qualyndria says she has become sexually active and would like a prescription for birth control pills but doesn't want her mother to know about it. She says her mother thinks she's here to discuss menstrual pain.

When the nurse goes out to the waiting room to escort another client into the examination area, Mrs. Gunderson asks to speak to the nurse. After escorting Mrs. Gunderson to an area where they can talk privately, the nurse learns that Mrs. Gunderson has been dodging questions from her daughter about sexuality. Mrs. Gunderson says she doesn't want her daughter to know about such matters until she is older, at least not until she is 18 years old.

Mrs. Gunderson says she is warning the nurse because she thinks her daughter may ask these questions of the healthcare team, and she asks the nurse to avoid answering the questions or supplying her daughter with information about sex, explaining that she believes this information should come from her and that she'll provide it when she feels her daughter is old enough to understand.

1. How would you respond to this mother?

2. How would this mother's request affect what you teach Qualyndria about responsible sexual behavior?

3. What would you tell this mother about her daughter's sexual activity?

EXEMPLAR 19.6 Sexually Transmitted Infections

EXEMPLAR KEY TERMS

Chancre, *1413*
Chlamydia, *1412*
Genital herpes (HSV), *1410*
Genital warts, *1411*
Gonorrhea, *1412*
Sexually transmitted diseases (STDs), *1408*
Sexually transmitted infections (STIs), *1408*
Syphilis, *1413*

EXEMPLAR LEARNING OUTCOMES

After reading about this exemplar, you will be able to:

1. Describe the pathophysiology, etiology, clinical manifestations, and direct and indirect causes of sexually transmitted infections (STIs).

2. Identify risk factors and prevention methods associated with STIs.

3. Illustrate the nursing process in providing culturally competent care across the life span for individuals with STIs.

4. Formulate priority nursing diagnoses appropriate for an individual with an STI.

5. Summarize therapies used by interdisciplinary teams in the collaborative care of an individual with an STI.

6. Plan evidence-based care for an individual with an STI and his or her family in collaboration with other members of the healthcare team.

7. Evaluate expected outcomes for an individual with an STI.

▶ OVERVIEW

Sexually transmitted infections (STIs) are disorders that are transmitted by vaginal, oral, and anal intimate contact and intercourse. They can be treated and cured. **Sexually transmitted diseases (STDs)** are typically viruses that cannot be cured, such as human papillomavirus (HPV), herpes simplex virus (HSV), and HIV. These terms are often used interchangeably; in this exemplar we will use the term STI to include infections and systemic diseases such as hepatitis and HIV/AIDS that can be transmitted sexually. The STIs discussed in this exemplar are genital herpes, human papillomavirus infections, chlamydia, gonorrhea, and syphilis.

Sexually transmitted infections may be caused by bacteria, viruses, fungi, protozoa, and parasites. Portals of entry for these infectious agents include the mouth, genitalia, urinary meatus, anus, rectum, and skin. STIs have many consequences, and the nurse has the responsibility of teaching sexually active clients how to prevent STIs, regardless of the client's gender, age, or sexual orientation. The nurse also has a critical role in the treatment of STIs and the complications of these common infections.

Incidence and Prevalence

The incidence of STIs has reached epidemic proportions worldwide (**Box 19–11** ●). In the United States it is estimated that 20 million new cases of STI occurs each year. STIs affect men and women of all ages, backgrounds, and socioeconomic levels. Of the 20 million new STI cases each year, half occur among individuals ages 15–24 (CDC, 2013e). Females have higher rates of gonorrhea and Chlamydia, whereas men, especially men who have sex with men, have higher rates of syphilis (CDC, 2012e).

Women and infants are disproportionately affected by STIs. Many STIs are more easily transmitted from a man to a woman than from a woman to a man because the woman is the receptor of sexual fluids. Women often experience few early manifesta-

tions of the infection, delaying diagnosis and treatment. Furthermore, women are at greater risk for complications of STIs such as pelvic inflammatory disease (PID), genital cancers, and reproductive complications. Infants are at risk because their mothers can transmit infections to them. The recognized routes of transmission include transplacental, intrapartum, and postpartum exposure (Treadwell, 1994; WHO, 2013b).

Adolescents are considered an at-risk population in terms of their physiology, inexperience, and lack of knowledge about STIs. Adolescents are more likely to engage in sexual risk behaviors to conform to their peer group or they may seek to imitate what they see in the media. Adolescent females have a more vulnerable cervix because of the exposure of the columnar cells at the cervical os (ectopy). In addition, adolescents as a group are less likely to have health insurance or the ability to pay for healthcare services. They may be very concerned about their sexual problems being confidential and some may not trust local clinics to provide confidential care (CDC, 2012e). The incidence of STIs is highest among young people of color. Sexual health is more vulnerable in those who are subject to higher rates of poverty, unemployment, low education, and income inequality. Many minorities do not have health insurance or access to health care. Areas where minorities live have higher rates of STIs, thereby increasing the risks with each sexual encounter that a young individual has (CDC, 2012e).

In this decade, older adults are living longer, healthier lives and are engaging in sex more than previous generations. Along with this increase in sexual activity is an increase in STIs (Poynten et al., 2013). Although the numbers of older adults affected is not nearly as high as those among young people, older adults are faced with barriers to prompt recognition and treatment. Many healthcare providers do not think of their older clients as sexually active and do not assess for STIs or provide education about safe sex (Stewart & Graham, 2013). This delays diagnosis of disease such as HIV that mimics other diseases more

Box 19–11 Selected Facts About Sexually Transmitted Infections

- The CDC estimates that approximately 20 million new STI cases occur each year in the United States. Half of these are among young people 15–24 years of age.
- The WHO (2011b) estimates that worldwide 448 million new infections of curable STI occur yearly.
- Biological factors place women at greater risk than men for the severe health consequences of STIs.
- Worldwide STIs are the main preventable cause of infertility, particularly in women.
- STIs increase the risk for acquisition and transmission of HIV.

Sources: Based on Centers for Disease Control and Prevention. (2012e). *Sexually transmitted disease surveillance 2011.* Retrieved from http://www.cdc.gov/std/stats11/Surv2011.pdf; and World Health Organization. (2011b). *Sexually transmitted infections: Fact sheet No. 110.* Retrieved from http://www.who.int/mediacentre/factsheets/fs110/en/index.html.

frequently seen among older clients. In 2010, 14% of new HIV diagnoses were among individuals 50 years and older (Poynten et al., 2013). According to the CDC (2012d), the number of individuals ages 65 and older newly diagnosed with HIV was estimated to increase from 926 to 948 between 2008 and 2011. It is more important than ever that older adults learn about negotiating safe sex with new partners, including condom use.

Risk factors for contracting an STI are listed in **Box 19–12** ●.

SAFETY ALERT

When a child younger than 10 years is found to have gonorrhea or other sexually transmitted infection, it is important to consider the possibility of sexual abuse. When anorectal symptoms or disease or trauma are found, suspect molestation (see the module on Violence for a discussion of child abuse).

The emergence of HIV/AIDS has created a kind of "epidemiological synergy" among all STIs. STIs such as syphilis and HSV facilitate the transmission of HIV/AIDS, and the immune suppression caused by HIV potentiates the infectious process of other STIs. In fact, individuals who are infected with STIs are at greater risk of being infected with HIV if they are exposed to the virus. This is the result of several factors: Genital ulcers create a portal of entry for HIV, nonulcerative STIs increase the concentration of cells in genital secretions that can be targets for HIV, and infection with both an STI and HIV results in an increased likelihood of having HIV in genital secretions and semen.

Box 19–12 Risk Factors for Contracting an STI

- Multiple sexual partners or a new sexual partner
- Sex with someone who has sex with one or more others
- Exchange of sex for money or drugs
- Poverty, unemployment, low education
- Young female under 25 years of age
- Drug or alcohol use that lowers inhibitions

Source: Based on Centers for Disease Control and Prevention (CDC). (2012d). *Sexually transmitted disease: Fact sheets.* Retrieved from http://www.cdc.gov/std/healthcomm/fact_sheets.htm.

Characteristics

Although STIs are caused by various organisms, they have several characteristics in common:

- Most can be prevented by the use of latex condoms.
- They can be transmitted during both heterosexual and homosexual activities, including nonpenetrating intimate exposure.
- For treatment to be effective, sexual partners of the infected individual must also be treated.
- Two or more STIs frequently coexist in the same client.

Bacterial STIs can be cured through appropriate early treatment with antibiotics. Viruses, such as genital herpes, are chronic conditions that can be managed but not cured. The most serious STI is AIDS, which is incurable. Treatment guidelines for STIs are updated regularly and are available from the CDC (Workowski & Berman, 2010).

Prevention and Control

The prevention and control of STIs are based on the principles of education, detection, effective diagnosis, and treatment of infected individuals and the evaluation, treatment, and counseling of sex partners of individuals who are infected. The ability of the healthcare provider to obtain an accurate sexual history is essential to prevention and control efforts. One approach to collecting accurate sexual histories is available from the CDC (n.d.). This approach includes the **Five Ps**:

1. **P**artners
2. **P**revention of pregnancy
3. **P**rotection from STIs
4. **P**ractice
5. **P**ast history of STIs.

Stay Current: *Suggested questions to use when obtaining a sexual history can be found on the CDC Web site:* **www.cdc.gov/std/treatment/SexualHistory.pdf**.

The most effective way to prevent sexual transmission of STIs is to avoid sexual intercourse with an infected partner. It is recommended that both partners be tested for STIs, including HIV, before beginning to have sexual intercourse. If an individual chooses to have intercourse with an infected partner or one whose infection status is unknown, a new condom should be used for each act of intercourse.

SAFETY ALERT

Eliminating further transmission and reinfection of STIs is critical to control. For treatable STIs, this means that referral of sex partners for diagnosis, treatment, and counseling is essential. STIs are reportable diseases in every state. When a healthcare professional refers infected clients to a local or state department of health, every effort is made to identify and contact sex partners. Reports of STI and HIV infections are maintained in strictest confidence, and are protected by law from subpoena.

Suggested resources for individuals with STIs are listed in **Box 19–13** ●.

▶ COMMON SEXUALLY TRANSMITTED INFECTIONS

Sexually transmitted infection is a general term used to describe many different infections. Each infection has a distinct pathophysiology, etiology, risk factors, and clinical manifestations, so each will be addressed separately.

Genital Herpes

Genital herpes (HSV) are caused by the herpes simplex viruses HSV-1 and HSV-2. Like most STIs, genital herpes are most commonly found in young, sexually active adults and are associated with early onset of sexual activity and multiple sexual partners. According to the CDC, about 776,000 individuals in the United States will contract a new infection with HSV this year. This accounts for 1 in 6 individuals 14–49 years of age; 1 in 5 women and 1 in 9 men (CDC, 2012d). There is no cure; the antivirals used to treat HSV simply lessen the severity of an outbreak and shorten its duration by a day or two.

PATHOPHYSIOLOGY There are two types of HSV that cause genital herpes. HSV-1 is associated with cold sores but may be transmitted to the genital area by oral intercourse or by self-inoculation through poor hand washing practices. HSV-2 is transmitted by sexual activity or during childbirth from an infected woman. HSV-2 causes most genital herpes cases.

HSV gains entry via mucocutaneous surfaces or small abrasions and begins to multiply causing cell destruction and vesicle formation. It continues to spread cell to cell and eventually enters the sensory nerves to be transported to the dorsal root ganglia. Here the virus enters into a latent period. During the latent period the viral DNA is maintained in the neural cell nucleus until it is reactivated. Reactivation is thought to occur due to stress or to hormonal or immunological changes. Once reactivated, the virus moves back to the skin surface via peripheral sensory nerves. The virus is shed during activation beginning before the client has symptoms or lesions. It is spread by intimate contact. The incubation period for the initial infections is 2–14 days. Women are at a greater risk because they have more mucous membrane exposure (Kaloczi, Latendresse, & Morgan, 2010).

MANIFESTATIONS Within 2–14 days after exposure to the herpes virus, painful small vesicles appear in the genital area. In men, the lesions generally occur on the glans or shaft of the penis. In women, the lesions commonly occur on the labia, perineum, vagina, and cervix (**Figure 19–28** ●). Anal intercourse or oral–anal sexual contact may result in lesions in and around the anus.

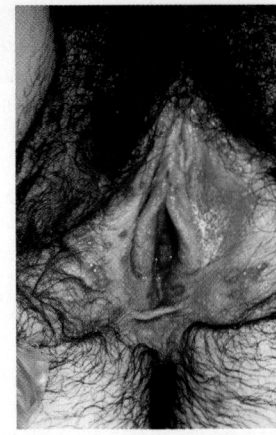

Figure 19–28 ● Genital herpes blisters as they appear on the labia.
Source: © Wellcome Image Library/Custom Medical Stock Photo.

The blisters break, shedding the highly infectious virus and creating patches of painful ulcers that last 10–20 days. Touching these blisters and then rubbing or scratching in another place can spread the infection to other areas of the body (*autoinoculation*).

Subsequent occurrences, usually less severe, produce vesicles, then shallow ulcers that crust in 4–5 days and heal without scarring. During the period between episodes, viral shedding can occur (Kaloczi et al., 2010).

The manifestations of genital herpes are listed in **Box 19–14** ●. Prodromal symptoms of recurrent outbreaks of genital herpes can include burning, itching, tingling, or throbbing at the sites where lesions commonly appear. These sensations may be accompanied by pain in the legs, groin, or buttocks. Some authorities believe that prodromal symptoms signal increased levels of infectiousness, during which sexual contact should be avoided.

DIAGNOSIS AND TREATMENT Presumptive diagnosis of genital herpes is based on history and physical examination of the client, including lesions and patterns of recurrence. Because there is no cure for genital herpes, treatment focuses on relieving symptoms and preventing spread of the infection. Client education is essential to prevent further transmission of the disease and to help clients integrate management of a chronic disease into their lifestyles.

Box 19–14 **Manifestations of Genital Herpes**

■ May have no symptoms
■ One or more vesicles on or around the genitals, rectum, or mouth
■ Blisters break and leave shallow ulcers that take 10–20 days to heal without scars
■ First outbreak is accompanied by flu-like symptoms—fever, body aches
■ Regional lymphadenopathy
■ Dysuria
■ Urinary retention
■ Vaginal discharge
■ Urethral discharge (men)

Source: Based on Centers for Disease Control and Prevention (CDC). (2012d). *Sexually transmitted disease: Fact sheets.* Retrieved from http://www.cdc.gov/std/healthcomm/fact_sheets.htm.

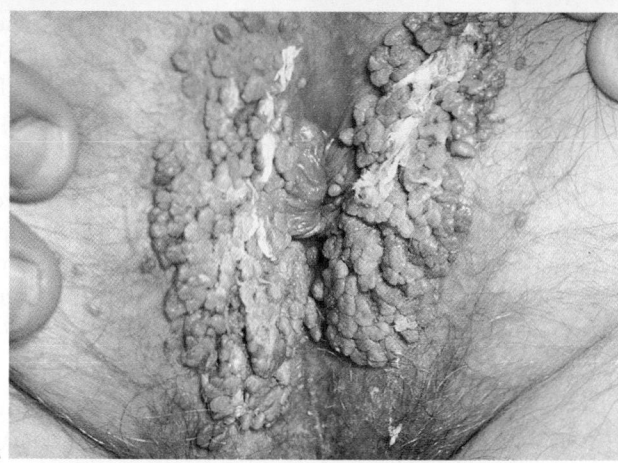
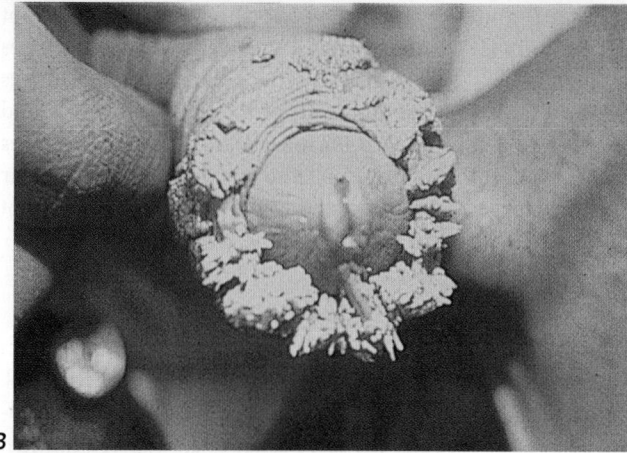

A   *B*

Figure 19–29 ● Genital warts (condyloma acuminatum) on the *A*, vulva and *B*, penis.
Source: A, © English/Custom Medical Stock Photo. *B,* Library of Congress.

DIAGNOSTIC TESTS   A virological test for the virus, virus antigen, or viral nucleic acid are available. Viral culture is the most definitive. Nucleic acid amplification techniques (NAAT), such as a PCR test for viral DNA or RNA, give more rapid results than culture. Serological tests for antibodies are available, but older tests do not differentiate HSV-1 from HSV-2. The newer HSV-1 enzyme-linked immunosorbent assay (ELISA) antibody test is reliable for HSV-1 but the HSV-2 ELISA produces false positives (CDC, 2012d).

PHARMACOLOGIC THERAPY   There is no cure for herpes. Antiviral medications such as acyclovir (Zovirax) help reduce the length and severity of each outbreak and are the treatment of choice for genital herpes. Antivirals are also used to suppress the virus, thereby decreasing the number of outbreaks. The oral form is considered most effective for the first episode and recurrences and is given for 7–10 days or until lesions heal. It may also be administered intravenously. Evidence shows that some strains of HSV are becoming resistant to acyclovir, particularly in HIV-positive individuals. In those clients, foscarnet (Foscavir) is used. Other antivirals used for treatment and suppression are valacyclovir (Valtrex) and famciclovir (Famvir).

Human Papillomavirus

Human papillomavirus (HPV) is the most common STI in the United States. There are about 40 types that can infect the genitals of men and women (CDC, 2012d). One form of HPV infection is **genital warts**, which are painless, soft, raised or flat, large or small, flesh-colored bumps in the vulvovaginal area, perineum, penis, urethra, anus, groin, or thigh (**Figure 19–29** ●). More important, HPV has been identified as the causative agent in many genital cancers (**Box 19–15** ●).

Most HPV infections are asymptomatic or unrecognized. An estimated 79 million Americans are infected with the virus, and up to 14 million new cases are diagnosed annually (CDC, 2012d) (see Box 19–14). Women are at greater risk for HPV genital infections because they have a larger mucosal surface area exposed in the genital area.

In 90% of cases, HPV will clear with no intervention within 2 years (CDC, 2012d). However, when HPV persists genital

warts, cervical cancer, and, less often, vulvar, penile, anal, and oropharyngeal cancers may occur.

PATHOPHYSIOLOGY   HPV is transmitted by vaginal, anal, or oral–genital contact. This virus can be transmitted even when the infected individual has no symptoms. The incubation period is 2–3 months (Kaloczi et al., 2010).

MANIFESTATIONS   Although some individuals with HPV may not have manifestations, others exhibit genital warts. In women, the growths may be in the vagina or on the cervix and may be apparent only during a speculum examination.

DIAGNOSIS AND TREATMENT   Diagnosis of genital warts can be made on the basis of the clinical appearance on physical examination. Regular screening using Pap tests will identify precancerous lesions on the cervix early, and treatment in this early stage will prevent cancer.

PHARMACOLOGIC THERAPY   No drug is available that can cure the virus itself, but the warts can be removed with treatments applied by a healthcare provider or by the client. Healthcare providers may use cryoprobes to freeze the warts or a chemical burn with trichloroacetic acid or podophyllum resin in the office setting that will remove the warts. Clients may use imiquimod, an immune response modifier, at home to remove the warts. Extensive warts will require CO_2 laser removal (McKay, 2011).

Box 19–15   Selected Facts About Genital HPV Infection

- HPV is so common that nearly all sexually active individuals will get at least one type of HPV at some time in their lives.
- About 12,000 women develop cervical cancer each year.
- Most individuals with a genital HPV infection do not know they are infected; most infections in women are diagnosed by abnormal Pap tests.
- Other HPV-caused cancers include vulvar, vaginal, penile, anal, and oropharyngeal cancer.

Source: Based on Centers for Disease Control and Prevention. (2012d). *Sexually transmitted disease: Fact sheets.* Retrieved from http://www.cdc.gov/std/healthcomm/fact_sheets.htm.

Gardasil and Cervarix are vaccines developed to prevent infection with HPV and cervical cancer. Gardasil prevents types 6, 11, 16 and 18. Types 6 and 11 cause genital warts, and types 16 and 18 cause cervical cancer. Cervarix prevents types 16 and 18. Both are recommended for males ages 11–21 and females ages 11–26. Both are administered by three intramuscular injections given over a 6-month period. The vaccine does not protect against the effects of an existing HPV infection.

Chlamydia

Chlamydia is caused by *Chlamydia trachomatis*, a bacterium that behaves like a virus, reproducing only within the host cell. The bacterium is spread by any sexual contact and to the neonate by passage through the birth canal of an infected mother. The infections caused by *C. trachomatis* include acute urethral syndrome, nongonococcal urethritis, mucopurulent cervicitis, and PID.

Chlamydia is the most commonly reported bacterial STI in the United States, affecting an estimated 2.86 million individuals each year (CDC, 2012d). Chlamydia occurs three times more often in 14- to 24-year-olds than in 25- to 39-year-olds. Approximately 1 in 15 sexually active teenage girls has chlamydia (CDC, 2012d). Risk factors for this STI are listed in **Box 19–16** ●.

Because chlamydia is asymptomatic in most women until the uterus and fallopian tubes have been invaded, treatment may be delayed, resulting in devastating long-term complications. Chlamydia is the leading cause of preventable infertility and ectopic pregnancy (Kaloczi et al., 2010). Infants born to mothers with untreated chlamydia are at risk for chlamydial conjunctivitis, which may cause blindness and chlamydial pneumonia.

Nearly a third of men with urethral chlamydia are also asymptomatic. However, reactive arthritis (formally Reiter syndrome) is a complication that is most likely to occur in men (Hellmann & Imboden, 2011).

PATHOPHYSIOLOGY   *C. trachomatis* is an intracellular bacterium that resembles viruses in that it can reproduce only within a host cell. It requires squamous-columnar or columnar epithelial cells of the urogenital tract, eye, nasopharynx, and rectum. The organism enters the body as an elementary body, a form in which it is capable of entering uninfected cells. The infection begins when the organism enters a cell, becomes a parasite, and reproduces until the cell ruptures and about 1,000 new elemental bodies are disseminated to adjoining cells. This process causes an inflammatory reaction that will lead to permanent scarring (Kaloczi et al., 2010).

MANIFESTATIONS   The incubation period is 1–3 weeks; however, chlamydia may be present for months without producing noticeable symptoms in men or women. Chlamydia typically invades the same target organs as gonorrhea (cervix and male urethra) and results in similar manifestations (dysuria, urinary frequency, and discharge). Even if asymptomatic, an infected individual can spread the disease.

COMPLICATIONS   If a chlamydial infection in a woman is not treated, it ascends into the upper reproductive tract, causing such complications as PID, which includes endometritis and salpingitis. Chronic pelvic pain, scarring of the fallopian tubes, and systemic dissemination and septicemia may result. Scarring of the fallopian tubes may lead to ectopic pregnancy, another potentially life-threatening disorder in women. Complications of chlamydial infections in men include epididymitis, prostatitis, sterility, and reactive arthritis. The CDC has suggested routine screening for sexually active adolescent females to minimize these serious complications (Kaloczi et al., 2010).

DIAGNOSIS AND TREATMENT   The diagnostic tests available can identify *C. trachomatis* in urine or fluids from the female endocervix and urethra or from the male urethra. The PCR test is considered the most sensitive test for chlamydia. Another test is the nucleic acid hybridization test (DNA probe), which can test for both chlamydia and gonorrhea at the same time (Kaloczi et al., 2010).

C. trachomatis is treated with antibiotics. Screening and diagnostic testing usually precede treatment; however, symptomatic individuals are often treated on a presumptive basis.

PHARMACOLOGIC THERAPY   The antibiotic recommended by the CDC for chlamydial infections in men and nonpregnant women is azithromycin (Zithromax), orally in a single dose, or doxycycline (Adoxa, Apo-Doxy), orally for 7 days, or levofloxacin orally daily for 7 days. Both sexual partners must be treated at the same time or prior to resuming sexual intercourse (Workowski & Berman, 2010).

Gonorrhea

Gonorrhea, also known as "GC" or "the clap," is caused by *Neisseria gonorrhoeae*, a gram-negative diplococcus. Gonorrhea is the most common reportable communicable disease in the United States. The CDC (2012e) estimates that approximately 820,000 new cases occur annually, but only 321,849 were reported in 2011. This is a 4% increase from 2010.

Gonorrhea rates for African Americans are higher than rates for non-Hispanic Whites. Other risk factors include residence in large urban areas, being transient, early onset of sexual activity, multiple serial or consecutive sex partners, drug use, prostitution, and previous gonorrheal or concurrent STI.

PATHOPHYSIOLOGY   The causative organism of gonorrhea is a pyogenic (pus-forming) bacteria that causes inflammation characterized by purulent exudate. Humans are the only

---

Box 19–16   Risk Factors for Chlamydial Infection

- Any sexually active individual, especially females ages 14–19
- Personal or partner history of STI
- Cervical ectopy
- Adolescent sexual activity; serial monogamy or multiple partners
- Oral contraceptive use increases risk for cervicitis but decreases risk for PID
- Unprotected sexual activity, especially inconsistent condom use
- Drug or alcohol use that increases risky sexual behavior

Sources: Based on Centers for Disease Control and Prevention. (2012d). *Sexually transmitted disease: Fact sheets.* Retrieved from http://www.cdc.gov/std/healthcomm/fact_sheets.htm; and Hatcher, R., Trussell, J., Nelson, A., Cates, W., Kowal, & Policar, M. (2011). *Contraceptive technology* (20th rev. ed.). New York, NY: Ardent Media.

host for the organism. Gonorrhea is transmitted by direct heterosexual and homosexual intercourse and during delivery as the neonate passes through an infected birth canal. The portal of entry can be the genitourinary tract, eyes, oropharynx, anorectum, or skin. The incubation period is 3–10 days after exposure in men and within 10 days in women (Kaloczi et al., 2010). The organism initially targets the female cervix and the male urethra. Without treatment, the disease ultimately disseminates (spreads widely) to other organs. In men, gonorrhea can cause acute, painful inflammation of the prostate, epididymis, and periurethral glands and can lead to sterility. In women, it can cause PID, endometritis, salpingitis, and pelvic peritonitis.

MANIFESTATIONS   Manifestations of gonorrhea in men include dysuria and serous, milky, or purulent discharge from the penis. Some men also experience regional lymphadenopathy. About 20% of men and 80% of women remain asymptomatic until the disease is advanced. Women with symptoms experience dysuria, urinary frequency, abnormal menses (increased flow or dysmenorrhea), increased vaginal discharge, and dyspareunia.

Anorectal gonorrhea is seen most often in homosexual men. The manifestations include pruritus, mucopurulent rectal discharge, rectal bleeding and pain, and constipation. Gonococcal pharyngitis occurs primarily in homosexual or bisexual men or heterosexual women after oral sexual contact (fellatio) with an infected partner. The manifestations mimic those of strep throat and include fever, sore throat, and enlarged lymph glands.

COMPLICATIONS   The complications of untreated gonorrhea in both men and women may be permanent and serious. They include the following:

- PID in women, which may lead to internal abscesses, chronic pain, ectopic pregnancy, and infertility
- Blindness, infection of joints, and potentially lethal infections of the blood in the newborn, contracted during delivery
- Epididymitis and prostatitis in men, resulting in infertility and dysuria
- Spread of the infection to the blood and joints
- Increased susceptibility to and transmission of HIV.

DIAGNOSIS AND TREATMENT   Diagnosis of gonorrhea may be obtained via cultures from the infected mucous membranes (cervix, urethra, rectum, or throat), examination of urine from an infected individual, and a Gram stain to visualize the bacteria under the microscope. The DNA probe may be used to test for both gonorrhea and chlamydia at the same time. Testing for other STIs (especially chlamydia and syphilis) at the same time is recommended. Pregnant women are routinely screened during their first prenatal visit and again at 36 weeks' gestation.

The goals of treatment for the client with gonorrhea include eradication of the organism and any coexisting disease and prevention of reinfection or transmission. The nurse must emphasize the importance of taking all medications as prescribed and abstaining from sexual contact until the infection is cured in both client and partners. Condom use to prevent future infections is essential, particularly for pregnant women whose partners may be infected.

Syphilis

Syphilis is a complex systemic STI caused by the spirochete *Treponema pallidum*, an anaerobic bacteria. It can infect almost any body tissue or organ. It is transmitted from open lesions during any sexual contact (genital, oral–genital, or anal–genital). The incubation period ranges from 12 to 90 days, averaging 21 days (Kaloczi et al., 2010). If not treated appropriately, syphilis will progress into four stages and ultimately can lead to blindness, paralysis, mental illness, cardiovascular damage, and death. Syphilis may occur with one or more other STIs, such as HIV/AIDS or chlamydial infection.

In 2011, about 46,000 new cases of syphilis were reported. This is fewer cases than HIV/AIDS in the United States. Men who have sex with men accounted for about 72% of primary and secondary syphilis cases reported (CDC, 2012d). In addition, 360 cases of congenital syphilis were reported in 2011, mostly among Black and Hispanic families (CDC, 2012d).

PATHOPHYSIOLOGY   Any break in the skin or mucous membrane is vulnerable to invasion by *T. pallidum*. Once it has entered the system, the spirochete is spread through the blood and lymphatic system. Congenital syphilis is transferred to the fetus through the placental circulation.

MANIFESTATIONS   Syphilis is generally characterized by four clinical stages: primary, secondary, latent, and tertiary. Each stage has characteristic manifestations.

Primary Syphilis   The primary stage of syphilis is characterized by the appearance of a **chancre** (**Figure 19–30** ●) and by regional enlargement of lymph nodes; little or no pain accompanies these warning signs. The chancre appears at the site of inoculation (such as the genitals, anus, mouth, breast, fingers) 3–4 weeks after the infectious contact. In women, a genital chancre may go unnoticed, disappearing within 4–6 weeks. In both primary and secondary stages, syphilis remains highly infectious, even if no symptoms are evident.

Secondary Syphilis   Secondary syphilis is systemic, with the spirochete spreading to all major organ systems. Manifestations of secondary syphilis usually appear around 6 weeks after the initial chancre (Kaloczi et al., 2010). These symptoms can include a skin rash, especially on the palms of the hands or soles of the feet; mucous patches in the oral cavity; sore throat;

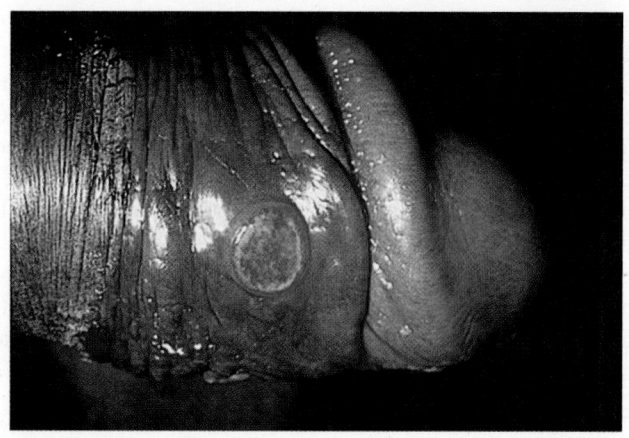

Figure 19–30 ● Chancre of primary syphilis on the penis.
Source: Biophoto Associates/Getty Images.

generalized lymphadenopathy; condyloma lata (flat, broad-based papules, unlike the pedunculated structure of genital warts) on the labia, anus, or corner of the mouth; flulike symptoms; and alopecia. These manifestations generally disappear within 2–6 weeks, and an asymptomatic latency period begins.

> **SAFETY ALERT**
> Always wear gloves when examining a client with a rash.

Latent Syphilis   Without treatment, the secondary lesions resolve and a latent period occurs during which the infected individual has no symptoms. During the early part of this stage, sexual transmission is possible. The latent period may last 1 year to a lifetime (Kaloczi et al., 2010).

Tertiary Syphilis   Unless treated, the remaining one third of infected individuals progress to late-stage or tertiary syphilis.

Two types of late-stage syphilis occur. Benign late syphilis, of rapid onset, is characterized by localized development of infiltrating tumors (*gummas*) in skin, bones, and liver, generally responding promptly to treatment. Of more insidious onset is a diffuse inflammatory response that involves the central nervous system and the cardiovascular system. Though the disease can still be treated at this stage, much of the cardiovascular and central nervous system damage is irreversible. These tertiary manifestations are rare since antibiotics cure syphilis discovered in the other stages.

DIAGNOSIS AND TREATMENT   Diagnosis of syphilis is complex because it mimics many other diseases. A careful history and physical examination are obtained, as well as laboratory evaluations of lesions and blood.

The VDRL (Venereal Disease Research Laboratory) and RPR (rapid plasma reagin) blood tests measure antibody production. Individuals with syphilis become positive about 4–6 weeks after infection. However, these tests are not specific for syphilis, and other diseases may also cause positive results. Additional tests are required for definitive diagnosis.

The FTA-ABS (fluorescent treponemal antibody absorption) test is specific for *T. pallidum* and can be used to confirm VDRL and RPR findings. It may be used for clients whose clinical picture indicates syphilis but who have negative VDRL results. In immunofluorescent staining, a specimen is obtained from early lesions or aspiration of lymph nodes and is specially treated and examined microscopically for the presence of *T. pallidum*. Darkfield microscopy involves examining a specimen from the chancre for the presence of *T. pallidum* using a darkfield microscope.

The goals of treatment are to inactivate the spirochete and educate the client about how to prevent reinfection or further transmission. Treatment includes antibiotic therapy and identification and referral of partners for testing and treatment if necessary, follow-up testing, and education about condom use to prevent reinfection of self and transmission of disease to partners. In addition, the client should be screened for chlamydial infection and advised to have an HIV test.

PHARMACOLOGIC THERAPY   The treatment of choice for all stages of syphilis in adults is penicillin G, given intramuscularly (IM). The dosage and the length of treatment depend on the stage and clinical manifestations of the disease. Clients

allergic to penicillin are given oral doxycycline or tetracycline for 14 days. Doxycycline is preferred because it has fewer GI side effects (Workowski & Berman, 2010).

Treatment of syphilis may result in a severe reaction called the *Jarisch-Herxheimer reaction*, which involves fever, musculoskeletal pain, tachycardia, and sometimes hypotension. This is a reaction not to the penicillin itself, but to the sudden and massive destruction of spirochetes by the penicillin and the resulting release of toxins into the bloodstream. The Jarisch-Herxheimer reaction generally begins within 24 hours of treatment and subsides in another 24 hours. Treatment should not be discontinued unless symptoms become life threatening.

■ NURSING PROCESS

In providing nursing care for the client with a sexually transmitted infection, the nurse needs to consider both short-term and long-term implications. Although the immediate priority is symptom relief, treatment, and prevention of further transmission, the client may need assistance in dealing with the diagnosis if the STI is a chronic disease, or the client may require repeated screening for potential complications. Note that treatment of STIs is most often done in community-based clinics (see the Community-Based Care feature).

Although this nursing process focuses on the client with genital herpes, the principles addressed may be applied to clients with any STI.

Assessment

The focused interview of the female client concerns data related to her sexual practices and health history, including menstrual cycle, forms of birth control used, number of partners, frequency of sexual encounters, medication use, and preexisting conditions. Open-ended or closed questions are used to obtain information. Often a number of follow-up questions

> **Community-Based Care**
> **Sexually Transmitted Infections**
>
> Family planning, preconceptual counseling and care, infertility care, and treatment of STIs are most often done in community-based clinics including physicians' offices, health department clinics, or Planned Parenthood settings. These community-based clinics are manned by physicians and nurses who specialize in this type of care.
>
> A client who has been diagnosed with syphilis while in the hospital would be referred to the Health Department for care. This communicable disease requires review by the Health Department physician. The nurse in this setting would administer the medication, counsel the client about the disease, its potential complications, and the side effects of the injection. The nurse would arrange the follow-up visits needed to test for cure and to give any further treatments. The nurse would also assign a community worker to act as case finder. The community worker would search for individuals who have had sexual relations with the infected client and all their sexual partners, and have all contacts come to the clinic for evaluation and treatment as needed.

or requests for descriptions are required to clarify data or gather missing information. Follow-up questions are aimed at identifying the source of problems, duration of difficulties, measures to alleviate problems, and clues about the client's knowledge of her own health.

Information about the genital areas, reproduction, and sexual activity is generally considered very private. The nurse must be sensitive to the client's need for privacy and carefully explain that all information is confidential. A conversational approach with the use of open-ended statements is often helpful in a situation that promotes anxiety and embarrassment. The client's terminology about body parts and functions should guide the nurse's questions.

The focused interview guides the physical assessment. The information is always considered in relation to normal parameters and expectations about the health of the system. Therefore, the nurse must consider age, gender, race, culture, environment, health practices, past and concurrent problems, and therapies when framing questions and using techniques to elicit information.

The nurse must consider the client's ability to participate in the focused interview and physical assessment of the reproductive system. If a client is experiencing pain or anxiety, attention must focus on relief of these symptoms. Because of the proximity of some of the female reproductive structures to the urethra and bladder, data gathered during the focused interview will relate to the status of the urinary system as well.

Abnormal vaginal discharge, pelvic pain, inflammation, infection, and suspicion of contracting an STI are some of the more frequent problems that the female reports. Examination of the perianal area is included in assessment of the female reproductive system. Related problems include hemorrhoids, fissures, and infectious processes.

Diagnosis

Nursing diagnoses that may be appropriate for clients diagnosed with a sexually transmitted infection may include the following:

- *Acute Pain*
- *Sexual Dysfunction*
- *Knowledge Deficit.*

(NANDA-I © 2012)

Planning

In planning care of the client with a diagnosed or suspected STI, the following goals may be appropriate:

- The client will describe strategies for reducing the risk of contracting an STI.
- The client will develop a plan to contact anyone who may have been exposed to the diagnosed STI through sexual contact.
- The client will abstain from sexual activity until the STI is resolved or take appropriate actions to avoid infecting others.
- The client's pain will be reduced to a tolerable level.

Implementation

Nursing diagnoses discussed in this section focus on pain and sexual dysfunction.

Relieve Acute Pain

For the client with genital herpes, herpetic lesions are very painful and can become infected. If the lesions are near the urinary meatus, dysuria and urinary retention may occur. Because the virus resides in the nerve ganglia, pain may also occur in the legs, thighs, groin, or buttocks. Although acyclovir diminishes the pain of herpes and accelerates the healing process, additional measures can relieve the discomfort further:

- Oral analgesics such as acetaminophen or ibuprofen.
- Teach the client how to keep herpes blisters clean and dry. Wash the area with mild soap and water daily. Lesions should be dried using a hair dryer turned to a cool setting. It is important to wear loose cotton clothing that will not trap moisture and to avoid wearing panty hose and tight jeans. Keeping the lesions clean and dry reduces the possibility of secondary infection and speeds the healing process.
- For dysuria and urinary retention, suggest pouring water over the genitals to start urination and to dilute the urine. Drinking additional fluids also helps dilute the urine. Diluting the urine reduces the burning sensation.
- Suggest the use of sitz baths (with tepid water) for 15–30 minutes several times a day. The warm water is soothing and decreases pain from ulcers and an irritated urethral meatus. It facilitates wound healing and facilitates urination.

Discuss Sexual Function

Clients who learn that they are infected with an incurable STI may believe they can no longer have a normal sex life. Fortunately, many individuals have learned to live with and manage genital herpes without infecting their partners or their children. The nurse should do the following:

- Provide a supportive, nonjudgmental environment for the client to discuss feelings and ask questions about what this diagnosis means to future sexual relationships. Feelings of guilt, shame, and anger are natural responses to such a diagnosis and can lead to a total avoidance of sexual intimacy.
- Offer information about support groups and other resources for individuals with herpes such as the National Herpes Information Hotline (www.herpesonline.org/herpes-hotline). Information about how others cope with this disease can offset feelings of shame and hopelessness.

Discuss Disease Management

Health teaching for clients with genital herpes involves helping them manage this chronic disease with the least possible disruption in lifestyle and relationships. Understanding the disease process and factors that affect it helps the client regain a sense of control and see the potential for future sexual intimacy without transmission of infection. The following topics should be addressed:

- How to recognize prodromal symptoms of recurrence and factors that seem to trigger recurrences (such as emotional stress)
- The need for abstinence from sexual contact from the time prodromal symptoms begin until 10 days after all lesions have healed

- If lesions become infected, a culture and sensitivity is performed and treated with the appropriate antibiotic
- Use of latex condoms due to viral shedding at any time and careful hygiene practices (such as not sharing towels or other personal items) even during latency periods
- The need to discuss the herpes infection with the significant other
- The importance of thorough hand washing to avoid autoinoculation of other areas.

Evaluation

Client care may be evaluated on the basis of the following expected outcomes:

- The client is free of the STI (for those STIs that can be treated and cured by antibiotics).
- The client explains strategies to prevent infection of others.
- The client abstains from sexual activity until the STI is treated.
- The client describes barrier methods to reduce the risk of contracting an STI.

NURSING CARE PLAN   A Client With Gonorrhea

Janet Cirit, a 33-year-old legal secretary, lives in a suburban midwestern community. She is unmarried but dating a man named Jim Adkins, who lives in an adjacent suburb. Ms. Cirit visits her gynecologist because her periods have become irregular and she is experiencing pelvic pain and an abnormal amount of vaginal discharge. Recently she has developed a sore throat. The pelvic pain has begun to disrupt her sleeping pattern, and she is concerned that she might have cancer because her mother recently died of ovarian cancer.

ASSESSMENT

When Ms. Cirit arrives for her appointment at the gynecologist's office, Marsha Davidson, the nurse practitioner, interviews her. Ms. Davidson completes a thorough medical and sexual history, including questions about her menstrual periods, pain associated with urination or sexual intercourse, urinary frequency, most recent Pap test, birth control method, history of STI and drug use, and types of sexual activity. Ms. Cirit reports her symptoms and her concern about ovarian cancer. She also indicates that she is taking oral contraceptives and therefore sees no need for her boyfriend to use a condom because she believes their relationship is monogamous.

Physical examination reveals both pharyngeal and cervical inflammation and lower abdominal tenderness. Her temperature is 37.0°C (98.5°F). There are no signs or symptoms of pregnancy.

The nurse practitioner completes a Pap test and cultures of the cervix and pharynx to evaluate for gonorrhea and chlamydial infection. Blood is drawn for a white blood cell (WBC) count. Test results are positive for gonorrhea and negative for chlamydia. The WBC count is slightly elevated, indicating possible salpingitis. Because Mr. Adkins has been Ms. Cirit's only sexual partner, it is clear that he is the source of infection and needs to be treated as well.

DIAGNOSES

- *Acute Pain* related to the infectious process
- *Anxiety* related to fear about possible cancer
- *Situational Low Self-Esteem* related to shame and guilt about having an STI
- *Ineffective Sexuality Patterns* related to the impaired relationship and fear of reinfection

(NANDA-I © 2012)

PLANNING

- The client will experience relief of pain, indicating that the infection has been eradicated.
- The client will articulate that she has nothing to be ashamed of and that she has been wise to seek treatment as soon as symptoms occurred.
- The client will verbalize that she will insist her partner use condoms during future sexual activity.

IMPLEMENTATION

- Administer ceftriaxone IM as ordered.
- Emphasize the need for regular pelvic examinations because of the family history of ovarian cancer.
- Discuss feelings and concerns about the diagnosis of gonorrhea. Stress that such a diagnosis does not reflect on one's worth as an individual.

- Teach the client how to talk with a future sexual partner about condom use.

EVALUATION

A week later during her follow-up visit, Ms. Cirit states that she is feeling much better and sleeping well at night since the pain has ended. She has terminated her relationship with Mr. Adkins and is considering joining a health club in the hope of increasing her level of fitness and perhaps meeting someone new.

CRITICAL THINKING

1. How are Ms. Cirit's manifestations related to the infectious process of gonorrhea?
2. Should the nurse have suggested that Ms. Cirit also be tested for syphilis and HIV? Why or why not?
3. Develop a care plan for Ms. Cirit for the nursing diagnosis of Impaired Social Interaction.

NURSING CARE PLAN | A Client With Syphilis

Eddie Kratz, age 22, works as a bellman at a large hotel. For the past year, he has shared a small apartment with Maria Jones, who is 5 months pregnant with his child. Although he intends to marry Ms. Jones before the baby is born, he has continued a previous relationship with a woman named Justine Simpson. His sexual activities with Ms. Simpson have increased in frequency as Ms. Jones's pregnancy has advanced. Recently Mr. Kratz has noticed a swelling in his groin and a sore on his penis.

ASSESSMENT

When Mr. Kratz comes to the community clinic, he is interviewed by the nurse practitioner, Sally Morovitz. She takes a thorough medical and sexual history, including questions about drug use, allergies, difficulty with urination, urinary frequency, itching or discharge from the penis, recent sexual activities, precautions taken against infection, history of STIs, and sexual function. She determines that Mr. Kratz has been having unprotected sex with both Ms. Jones and Ms. Simpson. He believes that Ms. Jones is not having sex with anyone except him, but he is not sure.

Physical assessment reveals a classic syphilitic chancre on the shaft of the penis and regional lymphadenopathy. A specimen of exudates from the chancre is sent for darkfield examination. Ms. Morovitz discusses with Mr. Kratz the likelihood that he has syphilis and the need to tell both Ms. Jones and Ms. Simpson so that they can be tested and, if necessary, treated. Ms. Morovitz also suggests that Mr. Kratz be tested for HIV, since he has been having unprotected sex with two women, at least one of whom may be sexually active with other partners. He agrees, and blood is drawn for an ELISA test. Darkfield analysis of the chancre exudate confirms the diagnosis of syphilis; the ELISA results are negative for HIV.

DIAGNOSES

- *Risk for Injury* to the client, his partners, and the infant, related to the disease process
- *Ineffective Health Maintenance* related to a lack of knowledge about the disease process, its transmission, and the need for treatment
- *Interrupted Family Processes* related to the effects of the diagnosis of syphilis on the couple's relationship
- *Anxiety* related to the effects of the infection on the unborn child

(NANDA-I © 2012)

PLANNING

- The client will receive prompt treatment to cure the syphilis.
- The client will articulate understanding of the need to abstain from sexual contact during treatment, complete all medications, return for follow-up visits, and use condoms to prevent reinfection.
- The client will verbalize an ability to cope with the effect of diagnosis and treatment on the relationship.
- The client will verbalize decreased anxiety following education and treatment.

IMPLEMENTATION

- Administer IM injection of penicillin G as ordered.
- Discuss the importance of abstaining from sexual activity until he and his partners are cured and of using condoms to prevent reinfection.
- Explain the need to return for follow-up testing in 3 months and again at 6 months. Provide a copy of the STI prevention checklist, and document that reminders need to be sent at 3- and 6-month intervals.

- Notify sexual partners that they need to come to the clinic for testing.
- Refer the client to a social worker for counseling about the effect of the disease on the couple's relationship.
- Teach the couple about the importance of treatment to the health of their infant.

EVALUATION

At the 3-month follow-up visit, the chancre on Mr. Kratz's penis has healed, and he reports that he is using a condom any time he has sex. Ms. Jones has also tested positive for syphilis and negative for HIV, so she, too, is given penicillin G, and verbal and written follow-up instructions, including follow-up until the infant is born. The couple meets every other week with the social worker and say that their relationship is improving. Ms. Simpson has received similar test results and is given a prescription for doxycycline because she is allergic to penicillin.

CRITICAL THINKING

1. What manifestations might a client with early syphilis experience?
2. List some appropriate questions for taking a sexual history when you suspect the presence of one or more STIs.
3. How might you counsel Mr. Kratz to help him break the news of the diagnosis to Ms. Jones?

REVIEW Sexually Transmitted Infections

RELATE Link the Concepts and Exemplars

Linking the exemplar of sexually transmitted infections with the concept of reproduction:

1. How will care of the pregnant client with genital herpes differ from the care provided to a pregnant client who does not have this infection?

2. What is your priority nursing diagnosis for the young couple contemplating pregnancy who are both diagnosed with genital warts?

Linking the exemplar of sexually transmitted infections with the concept of elimination:

3. Create a plan of care addressing pain management and prevention of urinary retention for the client diagnosed with herpes.

4. What teaching will you provide a client about using sitz baths for facilitated urination when the pain of herpes causes urinary retention?

READY Go to Companion Skills Manual

REFER Go to Pearson Nursing Student Resources

REFLECT Case Study

Maggie Lynch is a 14-year-old who has a 6-month-old daughter, Amy. Maggie lives with her single mother, Marcia Lynch, who has become very controlling of Maggie since she became pregnant. Mrs. Lynch has forced Maggie to go back to school, which Maggie was very much against. Maggie participates very little in Amy's care. Mrs. Lynch treats Amy as if she were her own child. There is a great deal of friction between Maggie and her mother.

Maggie has been skipping class occasionally to be with her 16-year-old boyfriend, Brett, who is Amy's father. Brett has no interest in Amy, but his parents make the effort to see Amy often. Maggie and Brett have resumed their physical relationship despite objections from both families.

Mrs. Lynch accidentally interrupts Maggie in the bathroom and notices a foul odor in the room. She questions Maggie and learns that Maggie has noticed a frothy yellow vaginal discharge in addition to the foul odor. Mrs. Lynch arranges for Maggie to be seen by her gynecologist.

1. The nurse calls Maggie from the waiting room. Should she allow Maggie's mother to accompany them to the exam room? Explain your answer.

2. What teaching will you initiate for Maggie once diagnosis has been made and treatment ordered?

3. How will you respond to Mrs. Lynch when she demands that you tell her what is wrong with Maggie?

■ REFERENCES

Adams, M., & Koch, R. (2010). *Pharmacology: Connections to nursing practice.* Upper Saddle River, NJ: Pearson.

Alswager, K., & Durler, C. (2013). Menstruation and related problems and concerns. In E. Youngkin, M. Davis, D. Schadewald, & C. Juve (Eds.), *Women's health: A primary care clinical guide* (4th ed., pp. 203–226). Boston, MA: Pearson.

American Academy of Pediatrics (AAP) Task Force on Circumcision. (2012). Circumcision policy statement. *Pediatrics, 130*(3), 585–586. doi:10.1542/peds.2012-1989 http://pediatrics.aappublications.org/content/early/2012/08/22/peds.2012-1989.

American Cancer Society (ACS). (2012). *DES exposure: Questions and answers.* Retrieved from http://www.cancer.org/cancer/cancercauses/othercarcinogens/medicaltreatments/des-exposure.

American Cancer Society (ACS). (2013a). *American Cancer Society guidelines for the early detection of cancer.* Retrieved from http://www.cancer.org/healthy/findcancerearly/cancerscreeningguidelines/american-cancer-society-guidelines-for-the-early-detection-of-cancer.

American Cancer Society (ACS). (2013b). *Testicular cancer.* Retrieved from http://www.cancer.org/cancer/testicularcancer/detailedguide/testicular-cancer-risk-factors.

American Nurses Association (ANA). (2010). *Code of ethics.* Silver Spring, MD: Author.

American Society of Reproductive Medicine (ASRM). (2012). *IVF is efficient and cost-effective. Highlights from the 68th annual meeting of the ASRM.* Retrieved from http://www.asrm.org/IVF_Is_Efficient_and_Cost_Effective.

American Society of Reproductive Medicine (ASRM). (2013). *Newest assisted reproductive technologies outcomes data released: SART reports 59,466 ART babies born; ART multiple birth rates continue to decline.* Retrieved from http://www.asrm.org/Newest_Assisted_Reproductive_Technologies_Outcomes_Data_Released.

Annon, J. (1976). The PLISSIT model: A proposed conceptual scheme for the behavioral treatment of sexual problems. *Journal of Sex Education and Therapy, 2*(2), 1–15.

Association of Reproductive Health Professionals. (2011). *Choosing a birth control method.* Retrieved from http://www.arhp.org/Publications-and-Resources/Quick-Reference-Guide-for-Clinicians/choosing/Initiation-Hormonal-Contraceptives.

Ball, J., Bindler, R., & Cowen, K. (2012). *Principles of pediatric nursing* (5th ed.). Boston, MA: Pearson.

Basch, E., Brigham, A., Bryan, J., Conquer, J., Costa, D., Culwell, S., . . . & Windsor, R. (2013). Ginseng. *Natural Standard Professional Monograph.* Retrieved from http://naturalstandard.com.ezproxy.midwives.org/databases/herbssupplements/ginseng.asp?

Berge, J., & Ward, R. (2012). Sexual dysfunction (female). In *Essential Evidence.* Retrieved from http://www.essentialevidenceplus.com.ezproxy.midwives.org/content/eee/632.

Bickley, L., & Szilagyi, P. (2013). *Bates' guide to physical examination and history taking* (11th ed.). Philadelphia, PA: Wolters Kluwer/Lippincott Williams & Wilkins.

Blackburn, S. (2013). *Maternal, fetal, and neonatal physiology: A clinical perspective* (4th ed.). St. Louis, MO: Elsevier.

Borrelli, F., & Ernst, E. (2010). Alternative and complementary therapies for menopause. *Maturitas, 66*(4), 333–343. doi:10.1016/j.maturitas.2010.05.010.

Bradford, J., Reisner, S., Honnold, J., & Xavier, J. (2012, November 15). Experiences of transgender-related discrimination and implications for health: Results from the Virginia Transgender Health Initiative study. *American Journal of Public Health,* pp. e1–e10. doi:10.2105/AJPH.2012.300796.

Bridges, D. (Reviewer). (2012). Your guide to the sexual response cycle. *WebMD: Sex & Relationships.* Retrieved from http://www.webmd.com/sex-relationships/guide/sexual-health-your-guide-to-sexual-response-cycle.

Brotto, L. (2010). The DSM diagnostic criteria for sexual aversion disorder. *Archive of Sexual Behavior, 39*(2), 271–277. doi:10.1007/s10508-009-9534-2.

Bryan, J., Costa, D., Jancar, P., Rapp, C., Seamon, E., Tanguay-Colucci, S., ... & Woods, J. (2013). Rose hip. *Natural Standard Professional Monograph.* Retrieved from http://naturalstandard.com.ezproxy.midwives.org/databases/herbssupplements/rosehip.asp?

Burri, A., Hysi, P., Clop, A., Rahman, Q., & Spector, T. (2012). A genome-wide association study of female sexual dysfunction, *PLoS ONE, 7*(4), e35041. doi:10.1371/journal.pone.0035041.

Burri, A., Cherkas, L., & Spector, T. (2009). The genetics and epidemiology of female sexual dysfunction: A review. *Journal of Sexual Medicine, 6*(3), 646–657. doi:10.1111/j.1743-6109.2008.01144.x.

Carmody, J. F., Crawford, S., Salmoirago-Blotcher, E., Leung, K., Churchill, L., & Olendzki, N. (2011). Mindfulness training for coping with hot flashes: Results of a randomized trial. *Menopause, 18*(6), 611–620.

Caudle, P., & Osborn, K. (2014). Caring for the patient with male reproductive disorders. In K. Osborn, C. Wraa, A. Watson, & R. Holleran (Eds.), *Medical–surgical nursing: Preparation for practice* (2nd ed., pp. 1286–1311). Boston, MA: Pearson.

Centers for Disease Control and Prevention (CDC). (2012a). *FastStats: Infertility.* Retrieved from http://www.cdc.gov/nchs/fastats/fertile.htm.

Centers for Disease Control and Prevention (CDC). (2012b). *HIV/AIDS: Male circumcision.* Retrieved from http://www.cdc.gov/hiv/malecircumcision.

Centers for Disease Control and Prevention (CDC). (2012c). *Preconception care and health care: Clinical care of women—Immunization.* Retrieved from http://www.cdc.gov/preconception/careforwomen/immunization.html.

Centers for Disease Control and Prevention (CDC). (2012d). *Sexually transmitted disease: Fact sheets.* Retrieved from http://www.cdc.gov/std/healthcomm/fact_sheets.htm.

Centers for Disease Control and Prevention (CDC). (2012e). *Sexually transmitted disease surveillance 2011.* Retrieved from http://www.cdc.gov/std/stats11/Surv2011.pdf.

Centers for Disease Control and Prevention (CDC). (2013a). *2011 Youth risk behavior survey results.* Retrieved from http://www.cdc.gov/features/yrbs and http://www.cdc.gov/healthyyouth/yrbs/slides/sexual_slides_yrbs.ppt.

Centers for Disease Control and Prevention (CDC). (2013b). *Assisted reproductive technology: What is assisted reproductive technology?* Retrieved form http://www.cdc.gov/ART.

Centers for Disease Control and Prevention (CDC). (2013c, April 15). *HIV/AIDS: Diagnosis of HIV infections in the United States and dependent areas, 2011* (HIV Surveillance Report, Vol. 23). Retrieved from http://www.cdc.gov/hiv/pdf/statistics_2011_HIV_Surveillance_Report_vol_23.pdf#Page=17.

Centers for Disease Control and Prevention (CDC). (2013d). *HPV vaccines.* Retrieved from http://www.cdc.gov/hpv/vaccine.html.

Centers for Disease Control and Prevention (CDC). (2013e). *Sexually transmitted disease: STD awareness month.* Retrieved from http://www.cdc.gov/std/sam/default.htm?s_CID=govd-std-012.

Centers for Disease Control and Prevention (CDC). (2012f). *Teen dating violence.* Retrieved from http://www.cdc.gov/violenceprevention/intimatepartnerviolence/teen_dating_violence.html.

Centers for Disease Control and Prevention (CDC). (n.d.). *A guide to taking a sexual history* (CDC Publication No. 99-8446). Retrieved from http://www.cdc.gov/std/treatment/SexualHistory.pdf.

Connor, J., Sauer, C., & Doll, K. (2012). Assisted reproductive technologies and world religions: Implications for couples therapy. *Journal of Family Psychotherapy, 23,* 83–98. doi:10.1080/08975353.2012.679899.

Conquer, J., Guilford, J., Isaac, R., Nummy, K., Varghese, M., & Zhou, S. (2013). Dong quai (*Angelica sinensis*). *Natural Standard Professional Monograph.* Retrieved from http://naturalstandard.com.ezproxy.midwives.org/databases/sports/all/dongquai.asp?#evidence-grades.

Cunningham, F., Leveno, K., Bloom, S., Hauth, J., Rouse, D., & Spong, C. (2010). *Williams obstetrics* (23rd ed.). New York, NY: McGraw-Hill Medical.

Dahir, M. (2013). Women and sexuality. In E. Youngkin, M. Davis, D. Schadewald, & C. Juve (Eds.), *Women's health: A primary care clinical guide* (4th ed., pp. 119–149). Boston, MA: Pearson.

Dal'Ava, N., Bahamondes, L., Bahamondes, M., Santos, A., & Monteiro, I. (2012). Body weight and composition in users of levonorgestrel-releasing intrauterine system. *Contraception, 86*(2012), 350–353. doi:10.1016/j.contraception.2012.01.017.

Darsareh, F., Taavoni, S., Joolaee, S., & Haghani, H. (2012). Effect of aromatherapy massage on menopausal symptoms: A randomized placebo-controlled clinical trial. *Menopause, 19*(9), 995–999. doi:10.1097/gme.0b013e318248ea16.

Dean, J. (Reviewer). (2012). Are your medicines disrupting your sex life? *Netdoctor.* Retrieved from http://www.netdoctor.co.uk/sexandrelationships/medicinessex.htm.

DeLemater, J. (2012). Sexual expression in later life: A review and synthesis. *Journal of Sex Research, 49*(2–3), 125–141. doi:10.1080/00224499.2011.603168.

Delvin, D. (2012). Sex and alcohol. *Netdoctor.* Retrieved from http://www.netdoctor.co.uk/sex_relationships/facts/sexalcohol.htm.

Deneris, A., & Huether, S. (2010). Structure and function of the reproductive system. In K. McCance & S. Huether (Eds.), *Pathophysiology: The biologic basis for disease in adults and children* (6th ed., pp. 781–812). St. Louis, MO: Mosby/Elsevier.

Dixon-Mueller, R., Germain, A., Fredrick, B., & Bourne, K. (2009). Towards a sexual ethics of rights and responsibilities. *Reproductive Health Matters, 17*(33), 111–119.

Drugs.com Editorial Team. (2012). *Stendra: Prescribing information.* Retrieved from http://www.drugs.com/pro/stendra.html.

Eisenberg, E., & Brumbaugh, K. (Reviewers). (2012). *Infertility fact sheet.* Retrieved from http://www.womenshealth.gov/publications/our-publications/fact-sheet/infertility.html.

Eustice, C. (2013). Arthritis & joint conditions: Guide to sexuality and arthritis. *About.com.* Retrieved from http://arthritis.about.com/cs/sex/a/sexualityarth.htm.

Food and Drug Administration (FDA). (2009). *New warning for nonoxynol 9 OTC contraceptive products re: STDs and HIV/AIDS.* Retrieved from http://www.fda.gov/ForConsumers/ByAudience/ForPatientAdvocates/HIVandAIDSActivities/ucm124023.htm.

Food and Drug Administration (FDA). (2011). *Drugs: Mifeprex (mifepristone) information.* Retrieved from http://www.fda.gov/drugs/drugsafety/postmarketdrugsafetyinformationforpatientsandproviders/ucm111323.htm.

Foster, V., Clark, P., Holstad, M., & Burgess, E. (2012). Factors associated with risky behaviors in older adults. *Journal of the Association of Nurses in AIDS Care, 23*(6), 487–499.

Gallo, M., Lopez, L., Grimes, D., Schulz, K., & Helmerhorst, F. (2011). Combination contraceptives: Effects on weight. *Cochrane Database of Systematic Reviews,* Issue 9. Art. No.: CD003987. doi:10.1002/14651858.CD003987.pub4.

Geller, S., Shulman, L., van Breemen, R., Banuvar, S., Zhou, Y., Epstein, G., . . . & Farnsworth, N. (2009). Safety and efficacy of black cohosh and red clover for the management of vasomotor symptoms: A randomized controlled trial. *Menopause, 16*(6), 1156–1166. doi:10.1097/gme.0b013e3181ace49b.

Genetic Science Learning Center. (2012, August 6). Learn. Genetics™. *Learn.Genetics.* Retrieved from http://learn.genetics.utah.edu.

Greil, A., McQuillan, J., Benjamins, M., Johnson, D., Johnson, K., & Heinz, C. (2010). Specifying the effects of religion on medical helpseeking: The case of infertility. *Social Science & Medicine, 71*(2010), 734–742. doi:10.1016/j.socscimed.2010.04.033.

Hain, D. (2013). Assessing older women's health. In E. Youngkin, M. Davis, D. Schadewald, & C. Juve (Eds.), *Women's health: A primary care clinical guide* (4th ed., pp. 119–149). Boston, MA: Pearson.

Hatcher, R., Trussell, J., Nelson, A., Cates, W., Kowal, D., & Policar, M. (2011). *Contraceptive technology* (20th rev. ed.). New York, NY: Ardent Media.

Hellmann, D., & Imboden, J. (2011). Musculoskeletal and immunologic disorders. In S. McPhee & M. Papadakis (Eds.), *2011 Current medical diagnosis & treatment* (50th ed., pp. 779–840). New York, NY: McGraw-Hill/Lange.

Howard, D. E., Wang, M. Q., & Yan, F. (2007). Psychosocial factors associated with reports of dating violence among U.S. adolescent females. *Adolescence, 42*(166), 311–324. Retrieved from http://www.ncbi.nlm.nih.gov/pubmed/17849938.

Inhorn, M. C. (2002). "Local" confronts the "global": Infertile bodies and the new reproductive technology in Egypt. In M. C. Inhorn & F. Van Balen (Eds.), *Infertility around the globe: New thinking on childlessness, gender, and reproductive technologies.* Los Angeles, CA: University of California Press.

Johnson, R. (2013). Gay life: Gay population statistics. *About.com.* Retrieved from http://gaylife.about.com/od/comingout/a/population.htm.

Jorde, L. (2010a). Genes and genetic diseases. In K. McCance & S. Huether (Eds.), *Pathophysiology: The biologic basis for disease in adults and children* (6th ed., pp. 781–812). St. Louis, MO: Mosby/Elsevier.

Jorde, L. (2010b). Genes, environment, and common diseases. In K. McCance & S. Huether (Eds.), *Pathophysiology: The biologic basis for disease in adults and children* (6th ed., pp. 164–182). St. Louis, MO: Mosby/Elsevier.

Juve, C. (2013). The menopausal transition. In E. Youngkin, M. Davis, D. Schadewald, & C. Juve (Eds.), *Women's health: A primary care clinical guide* (4th ed., pp. 425–459). Boston, MA: Pearson.

Kaloczi, L., Latendresse, G., & Morgan, K. (2010). Sexually transmitted infection. In K. McCance & S. Huether (Eds.), *Pathophysiology: The biologic basis for disease in adults and children* (6th ed., pp. 923–951). St. Louis, MO: Mosby/Elsevier.

Kazer, M. (2012). Sexuality assessment for older adults. *Try this: Best practices in nursing care of older adults* (General Assessment Series). Retrieved from http://consultgerirn.org/uploads/File/trythis/try_this_10.pdf.

Kim, A., & Bridgeman, M. (2011). Ulipristal acetate (Ella): A selective progesterone receptor modulator for emergency contraception. *Pharmacy and Therapeutics, 36*(6), 329–331.

Latendresse, G., McCance, K., & Morgan, K. (2010). Alterations of the reproductive system. In K. McCance & S. Huether (Eds.), *Pathophysiology: The biologic basis for disease in adults and children* (6th ed., pp. 781–812). St. Louis, MO: Mosby/Elsevier.

Laubach, J. M., Lorntson, R. P., & Forrest, D. E. (2013). Common gynecological pelvic disorders. In E. Youngkin, M. Davis, D. Schadewald, & C. Juve (Eds.), *Women's health: A primary care clinical guide* (4th ed., pp. 273–305). Boston, MA: Pearson.

Leach, M., & Moore, V. (2012). Black cohosh (Cimicifuga spp.) for menopausal symptoms. *Cochrane Database of Systematic Reviews,* Issue 9. Art. No.: CD007244. doi:10.1002/14651858.CD007244.pub2.

Lee, M., Kim, J., Ha, J., Boddy, K., & Ernst, E. (2009). Yoga for menopausal symptoms: A systematic review. *Menopause, 16*(3), 602–608. doi:10.1097/gme.0b013e31818ffe39.

Leslie, S. (2013). Causes of erectile dysfunction. *eMedicinehealth.* Retrieved from http://www.emedicinehealth.com/causes_of_erectile_dysfunction/article_em.htm.

Lessard, C., & Hopkins, M. (2011). Efficacy, safety, and patient acceptability of Essure™ procedure. *Patient Preference and Adherence, 5,* 207–212. doi:10.2147/PPA.S12400.

Levine, G., Steinke, E., Bakaeen, F., Bozkurt, B., Cheitlin, M., Conti, J., . . . & Stewart, W. (2012). Sexual activity and cardiovascular disease: A scientific statement from the American Heart Association. *Circulation, 125,* 1058–1072. doi:10.1161/CIR.0b013e3182447787.

Lopez, L., Edelman, A., Chen-Mok, M., Trussell, J., & Helmerhorst, F. (2011). Progestin-only contraceptives: Effects on weight. *Cochrane Database of Systematic Reviews,* Issue 4. Art. No.: CD008815. doi:10.1002/14651858.CD008815.pub2.

Mannheim, J. (Reviewer). (2013). Adolescent development. *Medline Plus.* Retrieved from http://www.nlm.nih.gov/medlineplus/ency/article/002003.htm.

Mayo Clinic. (2012, October 11). *Endometrial ablation.* Retrieved from http://www.mayoclinic.com/health/endometrial-ablation/MY01113.

McKay, H. (2011). Gynecologic disorders. In S. McPhee & M. Papadakis (Eds.), *2011 Current medical diagnosis & treatment* (50th ed., pp. 721–753). New York, NY: McGraw-Hill/Lange.

Melby, M., & Lampl, M. (2011). Menopause: A biocultural perspective. *Annual Review of Anthropology, 40,* 53–70.

Meng, M., Stoller, M., & Walsh, T. (2011). Urologic disorders. In S. McPhee & M. Papadakis (Eds.), *2011 Current medical diagnosis and treatment* (50th ed., pp. 904–926). New York, NY: McGraw-Hill/Lange.

MMWR. (2006). Youth risk behavior surveillance—United States. (2005). *Morbidity and Mortality Weekly Report, 55*(SS05), 1–108.

Moyer, V. (2012). Menopausal hormone therapy for the primary prevention of chronic conditions: U.S. Preventive Services Task Force recommendation statement. *Annals of Internal Medicine, 158*(1), 47–54.

National Kidney and Urologic Diseases Information Clearinghouse (NKUDIC). (2009). *Erectile dysfunction* (NIH Publication No. 09-3923). Retrieved from http://kidney.niddk.nih.gov/KUDiseases/pubs/ED/index.aspx.

Neithercott, T. (2012). Sex and diabetes. *Diabetes Forecast, 65,* 48–51.

New York City Department of Health and Hygiene. (2012). *Quick guide to contraception.* Retrieved from http://www.nyc.gov/html/doh/downloads/pdf/ms/contra-guide.pdf.

North American Menopause Society (NAMS). (2012a). The 2012 hormone therapy position statement of the North American Menopause Society. *Menopause, 19*(3), 257–271. doi:10.1097/gme.0b013e31824b970a.

North American Menopause Society (NAMS). (2012b). *KEEPS report.* Retrieved from http://www.menopause.org/annual-meetings/2012-meeting/keeps-report.

North American Menopause Society (NAMS). (2013). *NAMS & USPSTF statements consistent.* Retrieved from http://www.menopause.org/publications/other-resources/nams-and-uspstf-statements-consistent.

NYU Langone Medical Center (NYULMC). (2012). *Dysmenorrhea: Principal proposed natural treatments.* Retrieved from http://www.med.nyu.edu/content?ChunkIID=21602.

Options for Sexual Health. (2013). *Using the pill.* Retrieved from https://www.optionsforsexualhealth.org/birth-control-pregnancy/birth-control-options/

hormonal-methods/combined-hormonal-contraceptives/using-pill.

Pazol, K., Creanga, A., Zane, S., Burley, K., & Jamieson, D. (2012). Abortion surveillance—United States, 2009. *Morbidity and Mortality Weekly Report, 61*(SS08), 1–44.

Poynten, I., Grulich, A., & Templeton, D. (2013). Sexual transmitted infections in older populations. *Current Opinion in Infectious Disease, 26*(1), 80–85. doi:10.1097/QCO.0b013e32835c2173.

Ryan, P., Dudley, J., MacMahon, C., Feeney, L., & Bonham, A. (2011). Aging, relationships and sexuality. In P. Ryan & B. Coughlan (Eds.), *Aging and older adult mental health: Issues and implications for practice* (pp. 192–213). New York, NY: Routledge/Taylor & Francis Group.

Satterwhite, C. (2013). *CDC expert commentary: Talking to adolescents and young adults about sexuality.* Podcast retrieved from http://www.medscape.com/viewarticle/782515.

Scriven, P., & Ogilvie, C. (2010). FISH for pre-implantation genetic diagnosis. *Methods in Molecular Biology, 659,* 269–282. doi:10.1007/978-1-60761-789-1_20.

Shifren, J. L., Monz, B. U., Russo, P. A., Segreti, A., & Johannes, C. B. (2008). Sexual problems in United States women: Prevalence and correlates. *Obstetrics & Gynecology, 112*(5), 970–978. doi:10.1097/AOG.0b013e3181898cdb.

Stewart, A., & Graham, S. (2013, April). Sexual risk behavior among older adults. *Clinical Advisor,* pp. 28, 32, 34, 38.

Stiles, M., Redmer, J., Paddock, E., & Schrager, S. (2012). Gynecologic issues in geriatric women. *Journal of Women's Health, 21*(1), 4–9. doi:10.1089/jwh.2011.2803.

Stuenkel, C., Gass, M., Manson, J., Lobo, R., Pal, L., Rebar, R., & Hall, J. (2012). A decade after the Women's Health Initiative—The experts do agree. *Menopause, 19*(8), 1–2. doi:10.1097/gme.0b013e31826226f2.

Szilagyi, P. (2013). Assessing children: Infancy through adolescence. In L. Bickley and P. Szilagyi, *Bates' Guide to physical examination and history taking* (11th ed., pp. 765–875). Philadelphia, PA: Wolters Kluwer/Lippincott Williams & Wilkins.

Treadwell, P. (1994). Sexually transmitted diseases in neonates and infants. *Seminars in Dermatology, 13*(4): 256–261.

U.S. Library of Medicine. (2012). Trisomy 13. *Genetics Home Reference.* Retrieved from http://ghr.nlm.nih.gov/condition/trisomy-13.

U.S. Library of Medicine. (2012). Trisomy 18. *Genetics Home Reference.* Retrieved from http://ghr.nlm.nih.gov/condition/trisomy-18.

Valentine, M., & Gardella, J. (2013). Infertility. In E. Youngkin, M. Davis, D. Schadewald, & C. Juve (Eds.), *Women's health: A primary care clinical guide* (4th ed., pp. 273–305). Boston, MA: Pearson.

Walcker, B., & Pederson, C. (2013). Managing contraception and family planning. In E Q. Youngkin, M. S. Davis, D. M. Schadewald, & C. Juve (Eds.), *Women's health: A primary clinical guide* (4th ed., Chap. 12). Boston, MA: Pearson.

WebMD Editorial Team. (2013). Erectile dysfunction and priapism. *Erectile Dysfunction Health Center.* Retrieved from http://www.webmd.com/erectile-dysfunction/guide/erectile-dysfunction-priapism.

Wilson, B., Shannon, M., & Shields, K. (2013). *Pearson nurse's drug guide 2013.* Upper Saddle River, NJ: Pearson.

Workowski, K., & Berman, S. (2010). Sexually transmitted diseases treatment guidelines, 2010. *Morbidity and Mortality Weekly Report, 59*(RR12), 1–110.

World Association of Sexual Health. (2013). *Declaration of sexual rights.* Retrieved from http://www.worldsexology.org/resources/declaration-of-sexual-rights/

World Health Organization (WHO). (2002). WHO declaration of sexual rights. *Magnus Hirschfeld Archive for Sexology.* Retrieved from http://www2.hu-berlin.de/sexology/ECE5/who_declaration_of_sexual_righ.html.

World Health Organization (WHO). (2011a). *An update on WHO's work on female genital mutilation (FGM): Progress report.* Retrieved from http://whqlibdoc.who.int/hq/2011/WHO_RHR_11.18_eng.pdf.

World Health Organization (WHO). (2011b). *Sexually transmitted infections: Fact sheet No. 110.* Retrieved from http://www.who.int/mediacentre/factsheets/fs110/en/index.html.

World Health Organization (WHO). (2013a). *Defining sexual health.* Retrieved from http://www.who.int/reproductivehealth/topics/sexual_health/sh_definitions/en/index.html.

World Health Organization (WHO). (2013b). *Sexually transmitted infections (STIs).* Retrieved from http://www.who.int/mediacentre/factsheets/fs110/en.

World Health Organization. (2013c). *Gender and human rights: Sexual health.* Retrieved from http://www.who.int/reproductivehealth/topics/gender_rights/sexual_health/en/

Ye, Y., Wang, Z., Zhuo, S., Lu, W., Liao, H., Verbruggen, M., . . . & Su, Y. (2012). Soy germ isoflavones improve menopausal symptoms but have no effect on blood lipids in early menopausal Chinese women: A randomized placebo-controlled trial. *Menopause, 19*(7), 791–798. doi:10.1097/gam.0b013e31823dbeda.

Zamboni, B. (2011). Sexual dysfunction (male). In *Essential Evidence.* Retrieved from http://www.essentialevidenceplus.com.ezproxy.midwives.org/content/eee/633.

Zivotofsky, A., & Jotkowitz, A. (2009). A Jewish response to the Vatican's new bioethical guidelines. *American Journal of Bioethics, 9*(11), 26–30. doi:10.1080/15265160903197515ch.

20 Thermoregulation

◢ THE CONCEPT OF THERMOREGULATION

Body temperature reflects the balance between the heat produced and the heat lost from the body, and is measured in heat units called degrees. The body's surface temperature—the temperature of the skin, subcutaneous tissues, and fat—fluctuates in response to environmental factors and is therefore unreliable for monitoring a client's health status. The nurse should monitor core body temperatures (or the deep tissues of the body) for a more reliable assessment. This temperature remains relatively constant at about 37°C, or 98.6°F. ◀◀

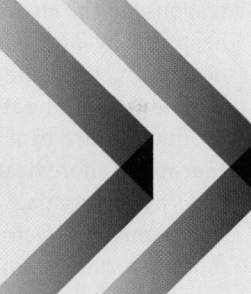

Concept Learning Outcomes

After reading about this concept, you will be able to:

1. Summarize the physiology of thermoregulation.
2. Examine the relationship between thermoregulation and other concepts/systems.
3. Identify commonly occurring alterations in thermoregulation and their related therapies.
4. Differentiate common assessment procedures used to examine thermoregulation across the life span.
5. Describe diagnostic and laboratory tests to determine the individual's thermoregulation status.
6. Explain management of thermoregulation and prevention of alterations to thermoregulation.
7. Demonstrate the nursing process in providing culturally competent and caring interventions across the life span for individuals with common alterations in thermoregulation.
8. Compare and contrast common independent and collaborative interventions for clients with alterations in thermoregulation.

Concept Key Terms

Afebrile, *1423*
Basal metabolic rate (BMR), *1422*
Chemical thermogenesis, *1422*
Conduction, *1422*
Convection, *1422*
Evaporation, *1422*
Febrile, *1423*
Fever, *1422*
Heat balance, *1422*

Heat transfer, *1422*
Hyperthermia, *1422*
Hypothermia, *1422*
Malignant hyperthermia, *1426*
Neutral thermal environment (NTE), *1423*
Normothermia, *1423*
Radiation, *1422*
Thermoregulation, *1422*

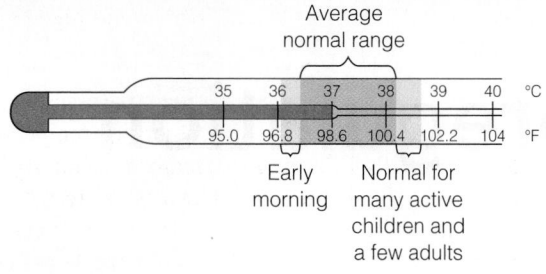

Figure 20–1 ● Average body temperature (taken orally) in normal individuals.

▶ NORMAL THERMOREGULATION

Thermoregulation is the body process that balances heat production and heat loss to maintain the body's temperature. The two kinds of body temperature are core temperature and surface temperature. Core temperature remains relatively constant. The normal core body temperature is a range (**Figure 20–1** ●). The surface temperature rises and falls in response to the environment. The body continually produces heat as a by-product of metabolism. When the amount of heat produced by the body equals the amount of heat lost, the individual is in **heat balance** (**Figure 20–2** ●). If the body produces more heat than is lost, the client displays **hyperthermia**. If more heat is lost than is produced, the client displays **hypothermia**.

A number of factors affect the body's heat production. The most important are these five:

1. ***Basal metabolic rate (BMR).*** The **basal metabolic rate (BMR)** is the rate of energy utilization the body requires to maintain essential activities such as breathing. Metabolic

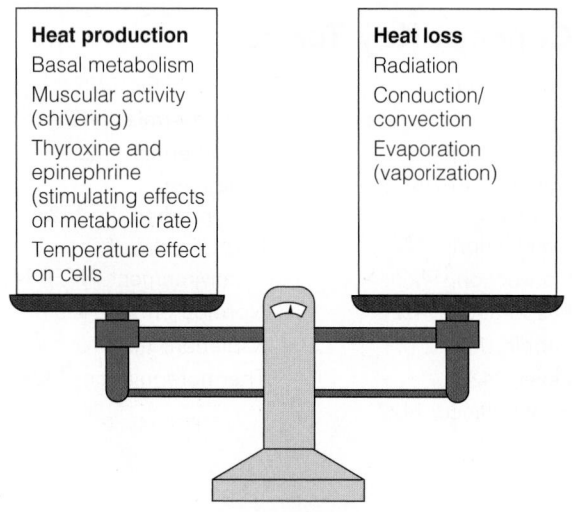

Figure 20–2 ● As long as heat production and heat loss are properly balanced, body temperature remains constant. Factors contributing to heat production (and temperature rise) are shown on the left side of the scale; those contributing to heat loss (and temperature fall) are shown on the right side of the scale.

Source: From *Human Anatomy and Physiology*, 9th ed., by E. N. Marieb and K. Hoehn, 2012, San Francisco, CA: Benjamin Cummings. Adapted with permission.

rates decrease with age. In general, the younger the individual, the higher the BMR.

2. ***Muscle activity.*** Muscle activity, including shivering, increases the metabolic rate. All muscle activity produces heat.
3. ***Thyroxine output.*** Increased thyroxine output increases the rate of cellular metabolism throughout the body. This effect is called **chemical thermogenesis**, the stimulation of heat production in the body through increased cellular metabolism.
4. ***Epinephrine, norepinephrine, and sympathetic stimulation/stress response.*** These hormones are neurotransmitters that mount a sympathetic nervous system response that can immediately increase the rate of cellular metabolism in many body tissues. Epinephrine and norepinephrine directly affect liver and muscle cells, thereby increasing cellular metabolism.
5. ***Fever.*** **Fever** is a protective immune response to foreign antigens within the body that increases the cellular metabolic rate, thus increasing the body's temperature.

To be able to predict how clients of all ages and clinical status will react to their thermal environment, the nurse should know the four ways in which **heat transfer** takes place, that is, the ways in which heat moves from one place or object to another thing:

1. **Conduction** is the process of heat transfer through physical contact of one surface with another surface. For example, if a newborn is placed on a metal changing table, the heat from the baby would transfer to that surface, making the baby's body colder.
2. **Convection** is the process of heat transfer through the fluid motion of air or water across the skin. For example, in aquatic exercises, water flows against the moving body, and because the water is colder than the body, heat from the body is transferred to the water. The exerciser must keep moving to avoid becoming chilled.
3. **Radiation** is the process of heat transfer with no physical contact. Sunshine transfers heat to individuals enjoying the warm outdoors.
4. **Evaporation** is the process of converting water to a vapor. The evaporation of sweat, in which the heat in the sweat is transferred to the air, is a natural process to cool a heated body (Vella & Kravitz, n.d.).

Physiology Review

The system that regulates body temperature has three main parts: sensors, the hypothalamus, and an effector system that adjusts the production and loss of heat. Most sensors or sensory receptors are in the skin. The skin has more receptors for cold than warmth; therefore, skin sensors detect cold more efficiently than warmth.

When the skin becomes chilled over the entire body, three physiological processes occur as the body attempts to regulate its temperature:

1. Shivering increases heat production.
2. Sweating is inhibited to decrease heat loss.
3. Vasoconstriction decreases heat loss.

The hypothalamus is the center that controls the core temperature, specifically the preoptic area of the hypothalamus. When the sensors in the hypothalamus detect heat, they send out signals intended to reduce the temperature, that is, to decrease heat production and increase heat loss. In contrast, when the cold sensors are stimulated, they send out signals to increase heat production and decrease heat loss.

Genetic and Lifespan Considerations

As with many of the processes in the human body, temperature is age related. The nurse should understand the differences that can be present when dealing with clients.

INFANTS Infants are greatly influenced by the temperature of the environment and must be protected from extreme changes. Infants also have what is known as brown fat when they are first born that helps to protect all of the organs from extreme temperature changes.

Newborns are *homeothermic*; that is, they attempt to stabilize their internal (core) body temperatures within a narrow range in spite of significant temperature variations in their environment. Thermoregulation in the newborn is closely related to the rate of metabolism and oxygen consumption.

- The newborn has less subcutaneous fat than an adult and a thin epidermis.

- Blood vessels in the newborn are closer to the skin than those of an adult. Therefore, the newborn's circulating blood is more influenced by changes in environmental temperature, and this in turn influences the hypothalamic temperature-regulating center.

- The flexed posture of the term newborn decreases the surface area exposed to the environment, reducing heat loss. Size and age may also affect the establishment of a **neutral thermal environment (NTE)**, which is produced by "any method or apparatus to maintain the normal body temperature to minimize oxygen consumption and caloric expenditure, such as an incubator" (*Mosby's Medical Dictionary*, 2012). For example, the preterm or small-for-gestational-age (SGA) newborn has less adipose tissue and is hypo-flexed, therefore requiring higher environmental temperatures to achieve an NTE. Larger, well-insulated newborns may be able to cope with lower environmental temperatures. If the environmental temperature falls below the lower limits of the NTE, the newborn responds with increased oxygen consumption and metabolism, which results in greater heat production. Prolonged exposure to the cold may result in depleted glycogen stores and acidosis. Oxygen consumption also increases if the environmental temperature is above the NTE.

Neonates are adversely affected by heat loss through conduction, so the nurse should be sure to place padding on any surface used for diapering or examination of the newborn.

CHILDREN Until they reach puberty, children's temperatures continue to be more variable than those of adults. Children often have extreme high temperatures and tolerate them

well. A healthy child can handle a temperature as high as 41°C (106°F) without difficulty.

OLDER ADULTS Many older individuals, particularly those over 75 years of age, are at risk for hypothermia (temperatures below 36°C, or 96.8°F) for a variety of reasons, including inadequate diet, loss of subcutaneous fat, lack of activity, and reduced thermoregulatory efficiency. Older adults are particularly sensitive to extremes in the environmental temperature owing to decreased thermoregulatory controls.

▶ ALTERATIONS TO THERMOREGULATION

The usual range of body temperature is called **normothermia**. The normal range for adults is between 36° and 37.5°C (96.8° and 99.5°F). The two primary alterations in body temperature are called hyperthermia and hypothermia. A body temperature above the usual range is called *hyperthermia* or, in lay terms, fever. This starts at 38°C (100.4°F) up to 41°C (106°F). The client who has a fever is referred to as **febrile**; one who does not is **afebrile**. *Hypothermia* is a core body temperature below the lower limit of normal. Hypothermic temperatures are below 35°C (95°F). At about 34°C (93.2°F), the body cannot function; death occurs. (See **Figure 20–3** ●.) The three physiological mechanisms of hypothermia are (1) excessive heat loss, (2) inadequate heat production to counteract heat loss, and (3) impaired hypothalamic thermoregulation.

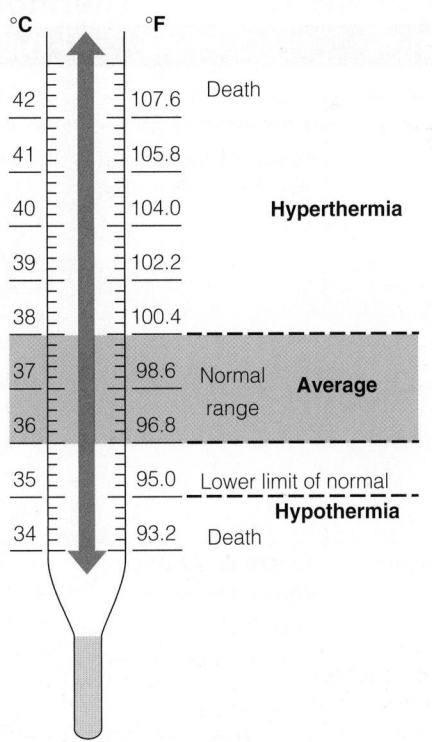

Figure 20–3 ● Terms used to describe alterations in body temperature (oral measurements) and ranges in Celsius (centigrade) and Fahrenheit scales.

The concept of thermoregulation affects many other concepts/body systems. See selected examples in the Concepts Related to Thermoregulation feature.

Prevalence

On average, there are 658 deaths in the United States every year from exposure to excessive natural heat. The very young and the very old are most susceptible (Centers for Disease Control and Prevention [CDC], 2013a). Participation in sports during the hot and humid summer months can be dangerous if signs and symptoms of hyperthermia are not heeded. High school athletes lose an estimated 9,000 days of play time each year due to heat-related illness; football participation causes the most frequent problems (CDC, 2010).

On average, 37 children die each year in the United States from heatstroke after being left in a closed vehicle. Data analysis has shown that even mild temperatures (in the 70s) can cause death because the vehicle's interior temperature rises rapidly when all windows are closed (Null, 2013).

On average, there are 1,300 deaths in the United States every year from exposure to excessive natural cold (CDC, 2013b).

Studies found that, compared to other emergency department (ED) clients, those with hypothermia were more likely to be older and uninsured (CDC, 2012). Clients with hypothermia were also more likely to be transferred to a critical care unit than other ED clients. The CDC concluded that "all hypothermia deaths are preventable" (CDC, 2005).

Fever is the most common complaint among pediatric clients of the ED, bringing over 28 million children under age 18 to the ED every year. A 2013 retrospective study from Singhal et al. identified a critically ill subgroup of these clients. The investigators analyzed data from over 95,000 pediatric clients diagnosed with severe sepsis during an ED visit, looking at triage vital signs of fever and hypotension as well as ICD-9 codes to accurately support the diagnosis. They found the following correlations in children under age 18:

- *Age.* One third of fevers were in children ages 31 days to 1 year.
- *Season of the year.* Most (37%) fevers occurred during winter months.
- *Not having health insurance.* Over half of these clients were self-pay or insured by Medicaid.
- *Geographical location.* Many (44%) of these clients were located in the Southern region of the United States.

The most common cause of fever in children is infection. The most common infections in children that produce a rise in the body temperature are colds, gastroenteritis, ear infections, croup, bronchiolitis, and urinary tract infections (Ward, 2013).

Alterations and Therapies **Thermoregulation**

ALTERATION	DESCRIPTION	THERAPIES
Hyperthermia	Increase in temperature as a result of more heat produced than lost	<ul><li>Monitor vital signs.</li><li>Assess skin color and temperature.</li><li>Monitor white blood cell count, hematocrit value, and other pertinent laboratory reports for indication of infection or dehydration.</li><li>Reduce covering (clothing, blankets, etc.) to allow heat loss.</li><li>Lower room temperature.</li><li>Administer antipyretic medications.</li><li>Increase fluid intake and provide adequate nutrition.</li><li>Measure intake and output.</li><li>Reduce physical activity to limit heat production.</li><li>Provide oral hygiene to keep mucous membranes moist.</li><li>Administer tepid sponge bath to increase heat loss through convection.</li><li>Provide dry clothing and bed linens if client is perspiring.</li><li>Use hypothermia blanket.</li></ul>
Hypothermia	Decrease in body temperature as a result of more heat lost than produced	<ul><li>Monitor vital signs.</li><li>Assess skin color and temperature.</li><li>Apply warm blankets or warm clothing.</li><li>Provide warm environment.</li><li>Provide dry clothing if heat loss is due to evaporation.</li><li>Keep limbs close to body.</li><li>Cover scalp with cap or turban.</li><li>Use hyperthermia blanket.</li><li>Administer warmed oral or IV fluids.</li><li>Use heat lamps, hot water bottles, or heating pad.</li></ul>

Concepts Related to **Thermoregulation**

The relationship of thermoregulation to other concepts is quite straightforward. Hyperthermia is related to fluid and electrolyte balance, infection, and inflammation. Both hyperthermia and hypothermia are related to comfort. The risk of clinical problems with temperature alterations varies with age; the risk is increased at both ends of the age spectrum, the very young and the very old.

CONCEPT	RELATIONSHIP TO THERMOREGULATION	NURSING IMPLICATIONS
Fluids and Electrolytes		
■ Fluid and electrolyte imbalance	Increased temperature leads to increased sweating, which leads to fluid and electrolyte loss.	■ Assess intake and output; act immediately to provide fluid replacement. ■ Treat the underlying cause. ■ Be alert for signs of dehydration or electrolyte imbalance.
Comfort		
■ Acute and chronic pain	As temperature increases or decreases significantly, comfort level and tolerance of pain decrease.	■ Assess temperature and treat symptoms to help keep the client comfortable.
Infection		
■ Prevention of infection	Most bacteria and viruses that produce infections thrive at normal temperatures. An increase in body temperature helps the body fight the infection. Also, a fever alerts the immune system to increase production of white blood cells and antibodies.	■ Focus on prevention and health maintenance and promotion. ■ Assess the client's risk for infection based on concurrent conditions, immune system functioning, and healthcare provision, such as immunizations. ■ Be sure to do and teach proper hand hygiene, use standard precautions with all clients, and follow isolation techniques, when indicated.
Inflammation		
■ Stages of inflammation	In the first stage of inflammation, blood vessels constrict, then dilate. The increased blood flow (hyperemia) causes redness and heat at the injury site (localized thermic response).	■ Do ongoing observation at the site of injury, such as monitoring to prevent IV phlebitis or to ensure wound healing. ■ The goal is to prevent the second stage of inflammation, exudate production.
Development		
■ Growth and development through the life span	Infants are more susceptible to problems caused by temperature changes both within bodies (infections) and the outer environment (e.g., a car with the windows closed). Children tolerate a wider range of temperature than infants. From puberty until old age, clients have fewer problems with temperature changes. After age 75, clients have an increased risk of hypothermia.	■ Know the important role that age plays in temperature regulation; monitor clients at greater risk more often. ■ Teach home care monitoring and basic treatment of symptoms to caregivers of infants, children, and older adults.

Genetic Considerations

Considerable progress has recently been made in identifying causative genes for hereditary periodic fever syndromes. These are rare clinical conditions characterized by short but repeated fevers and severe localized inflammation. Diagnosis depends on ruling out the usual childhood infections. The good news for clients is that, with time, even without treatment, the fevers do not return. Also, between episodes, clients can continue normal daily activities (Shinawi, 2013).

Malignant hyperthermia is a potentially fatal inherited disorder that produces a serious reaction to volatile inhalational anesthetic gases and succinylcholine, a depolarizing neuromuscular blocker. The temperature rises rapidly to as high as 43°C (109.4°F) as a result of sustained hypermetabolism. Cardiac dysrhythmias develop, and oxygen and ATP are rapidly consumed. Lactate and carbon dioxide, by-products of metabolism, are produced in excess (Porth & Matfin, 2009). If unchecked, the condition will progress to a change in consciousness level (coma), cardiac dysfunction, pulmonary edema, renal dysfunction, disseminated intravascular coagulation, and hepatic dysfunction. Researchers have documented a 35% morbidity rate (Larach et al., 2010).

CASE STUDY \\ PART 1

Caleb Kleinlein is a 30-year-old businessman who returned from a trip to South Africa 2 weeks ago. He has come into the physician's office today with complaints of fever and general malaise. As the intake nurse, you perform an assessment that includes taking his temperature. Mr. Kleinlein has a temperature of 38.6°C (101.5°F). He has not taken any medication for the fever today. You find out from Mr. Kleinlein that he has no allergies to any medication, and he prefers to take ibuprofen (Motrin) for his fevers. History reveals that Mr. Kleinlein has had this fever for 3 days and has been unable to eat or drink as he normally would. The physician prescribes ibuprofen 800 mg every 6 hours, increased fluid intake and rest.

Clinical Reasoning Questions Level I

1. What precautions should Mr. Kleinlein use to prevent side effects when taking his Motrin?
2. If Mr. Kleinlein's fever gets higher, what should you as the nurse tell him to do?

Clinical Reasoning Questions Level II

3. What education should the nurse give to Mr. Kleinlein about management of his fever?
4. What symptoms of dehydration should the nurse educate Mr. Kleinlein about? What advice should the nurse give to prevent a fluid volume deficit?

▶ PREVENTION

Modifiable Risk Factors

HYPERTHERMIA Being aware of the harmful combination of hot weather and dehydration, especially when the humidity is also high, will reduce the risk of heat exhaustion.

Factors that can increase the risk are age, obesity, medication, and unfamiliarity with a climate. Signs experienced by individuals with this condition include paleness, dizziness, nausea and vomiting, and fainting. Although they have uncomfortable symptoms, the rise in their temperatures is usually moderate (38.3°–38.9°C [101°–102°F]). The Mayo Clinic (2011) believes that interventions should begin when the outside temperature reaches 33°C (91°F). They offer these suggestions for prevention:

- Wear loose-fitting, lightweight, light-colored clothing.
- Avoid getting sunburned by using sunscreen.
- Make sure your fluid intake is sufficient to make up for sweating and other water loss.
- Know if your medications predispose you to sensitivity to heat.
- Take time to let your body acclimate to the heat.

If those suggestions are not followed, an even more dangerous condition, heat stroke, can occur.

HYPOTHERMIA Both healthcare providers and community members need to learn about individuals who could suffer frostbite without recognizing that they are in danger. One example is otherwise healthy young individuals who drink a large amount of alcohol, which decreases their alertness to outside weather changes. Another example is people with diabetes who experience hypoglycemia, which makes them less aware of their surroundings (KARE, 2013). So the modifiable risk factors can include ingestion of alcohol and other drugs and the untoward effects of acute illness and chronic diseases. Older adults with a decreased metabolic rate who use sedative medications face additional risk.

Screenings

HYPERTHERMIA The Malignant Hyperthermia Association of the United States (2013) is committed to educating both professionals and laypeople about the two methods of screening for malignant hyperthermia. The first method is genetic testing, which can be done by sending a sample through the mail to the two American healthcare facilities that have been approved to perform the tests. Health insurance coverage of the testing might prove an issue for clients. Reasons to have the genetic test done include the following:

- Having a positive muscle biopsy test from the client or a relative
- Having relatives with the known genetic mutation
- Having a clinical episode.

The second method of screening is by muscle biopsy. Only five facilities in the United States and Canada are approved to do the testing, which needs to be performed on freshly biopsied tissue. The caffeine halothane contracture test (CHCT) is the gold standard for determination of having the inherited disorder.

Stay Current: *Visit the Web site of the Malignant Hyperthermia Association of the United States at* **www.mhaus.org** *to learn more about the condition, testing for it, and how to manage a malignant hyperthermia crisis.*

TABLE 20–1 Advantages and Disadvantages of Sites for Body Temperature Measurement

SITE	ADVANTAGES	DISADVANTAGES
Mouth (oral)	Accessible and convenient	Thermometer can break if bitten. Inaccurate if client has just ingested hot or cold food or fluid or has just smoked. Could injure the mouth following oral surgery.
Rectum	Reliable measurement	Inconvenient and more unpleasant for clients; difficult for client who cannot turn to the side. Could injure the rectum following rectal surgery. Presence of stool may interfere with thermometer placement. If the stool is soft, the thermometer may be embedded in stool rather than against the wall of the rectum. May be contraindicated in clients with cardiac problems.
Axillary	Safe and noninvasive	The thermometer must be left in place a long time to obtain an accurate measurement.
Tympanic membrane	Readily accessible; reflects the core temperature; very fast; may be less scary for small children	Can be uncomfortable and involves risk of injuring the membrane if the probe is inserted too far. Repeated measurements may vary. Right and left measurements can differ. Presence of cerumen can affect the reading.
Temporal artery	Safe and noninvasive; very fast; less scary for small children	Requires electronic equipment that may be expensive or unavailable; variation in technique is needed if the client has perspiration on the forehead.

HYPOTHERMIA The American College of Physicians (2013) created a list of risk factors for hypothermia. They pointed out that neonates and older adults are more susceptible to developing hypothermia than other people. Seven of the eight factors they focused on were outdoor exposure, drugs, trauma, alcohol or drug abuse, endocrine disorders, previous neurological impairment or autonomic dysfunction, and dermatological disorders or pathology. The eighth factor of importance was multisystem disorders, including malnutrition, sepsis, shock, and hepatic or renal failure. Nurses should be mindful of the age of their clients and whether they are at risk for hypothermia due to age or the listed risk factors.

▶ ASSESSMENT

Thermoregulation is assessed primarily by measuring body temperature. Body temperature is measured on two scales: degrees Celsius (centigrade), abbreviated °C, and degrees Fahrenheit, abbreviated °F.

Nursing Assessment

The most common sites for measuring body temperature are the mouth, rectum, armpit, tympanic membrane, and temporal artery, which is accessed through the skin of the forehead. Each of the sites has advantages and disadvantages (see **Table 20–1** ●). Oral and tympanic thermometers are shown in **Figure 20–4** ●. See also the Lifespan Considerations feature on temperature.

Diagnostic Tests

Diagnostic tests may be indicated if the cause of fever is not obvious on physical examination. For example, a client suspected of having an infection might require a complete blood count with differential to diagnose the type of infection, or a client whose fever is believed to be related to head trauma may require imaging studies to determine degree and location of trauma.

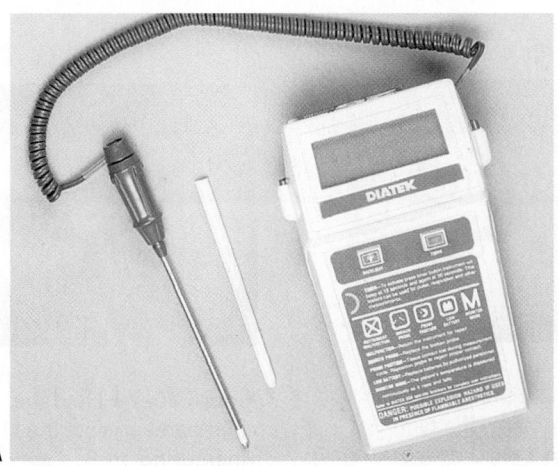

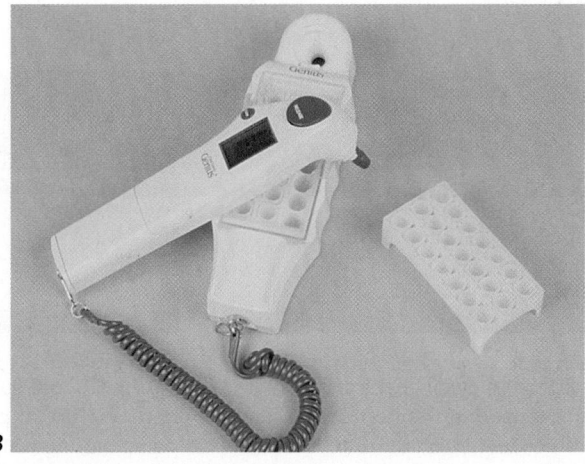

Figure 20–4 ● *A,* Oral thermometer. Note the probe and probe cover. *B,* An infrared (tympanic) thermometer used to measure the tympanic membrane temperature

Lifespan Considerations Temperature

Infants

- The body temperature of newborns is extremely labile; newborns must be kept warm and dry to prevent hypothermia.
- Many parents rely on palpation of the infant's skin as a usual method of fever determination in young infants, including nearly half of parents who own a thermometer. Palpation overestimates the incidence of elevated temperatures; however, it has been shown to be accurate in nonfebrile infants (Katz-Sidlow, Rowberry, & Ho, 2009).
- In using the axillary site, the infant's arm must be held against the chest. The axillary route may not be as accurate as other routes for detecting fevers in children (Bindler, Ball, & Cowen, 2011).
- The tympanic route is fast and convenient. The infant is placed supine, and the head is stabilized. The pinna is pulled straight back and slightly downward. The probe tip is directed anteriorly and inserted far enough to seal the canal. The tip will not touch the tympanic membrane. The tympanic route should be avoided in a child with active ear infection or tympanic membrane drainage tubes.
- In using a temporal artery thermometer, it is necessary only to touch the forehead or behind the ear.
- The rectal route is least desirable in infants.
- A pacifier thermometer (**Figure 20–5 ●**) may be used in the home. The manufacturer's instructions must be followed closely.

Children

- Currently, no consistent data or consensus reports support an evidence-based practice about the most accurate way to monitor a child's temperature. Batra and Goyal (2013) found that the temporal artery route is as accurate as the rectal route in children ages 2–12 years. However, Penning et al. (2011) found the exact opposite results in their study of children ages 0–18 years.
- For the tympanic route, the child should be held on an adult's lap with the child's head held gently against the adult for support. The pinna is pulled straight back and

upward for children over age 3 (**Figure 20–6 ●**). The tympanic route should be avoided in a child with active ear infection or tympanic membrane drainage tubes.

- For the axillary route, the child's arm is held against the chest (**Figure 20–7 ●**).
- The oral route may be used for children over age 3, but a nonbreakable, electronic thermometer is recommended.
- For a rectal temperature, the child is placed prone across the adult's lap or in a side-lying position with the child's knees flexed. The thermometer is inserted 1 inch into the rectum.

Adults

In critically ill adult clients with core temperature over 37.5°C (99.5°F), tympanic and oral thermometers are recommended to provide accurate measures of core temperatures within the febrile range. Rectal thermometers were not found to be as accurate (Jeffries et al., 2011).

Older Adults

- Older adults' temperatures tend to be lower than those of middle-aged adults.
- Older adults' temperatures are strongly influenced by both environmental and internal temperature changes. Their thermoregulation control processes are not as efficient as those of younger adults, and they are at higher risk for both hypothermia and hyperthermia.
- Older adults can develop significant buildup of ear cerumen that may interfere with tympanic thermometer readings.
- Older adults are more likely to have hemorrhoids. The anus should be inspected before a rectal temperature is taken.
- Older adults' temperatures may not be a valid indication of the seriousness of the pathology of a disease. The older adult may have pneumonia or a urinary tract infection and exhibit only a slight temperature elevation. Other symptoms, such as confusion and restlessness, may be presented and need follow-up to determine whether an underlying disease process is present.

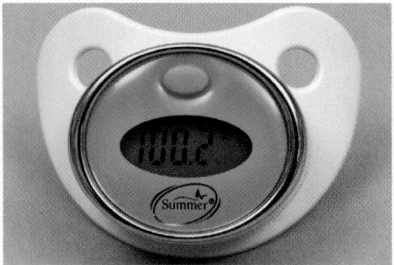

Figure 20–5 ● A pacifier thermometer can be used in the home. Parents should be cautioned to follow the manufacturer's instructions carefully for reading the temperature.

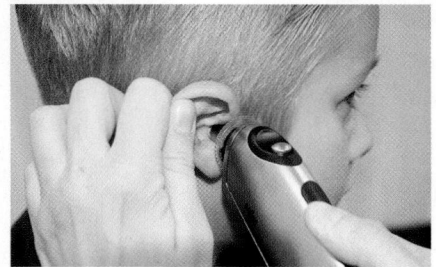

Figure 20–6 ● Pull the pinna of the ear back and up for placement of a tympanic thermometer in a child over 3 years of age; back and down for children under age 3.
Source: © Christina Kennedy/Alamy.

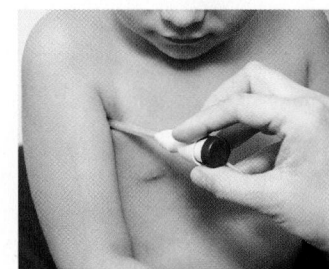

Figure 20–7 ● Hold the child's arm against the chest when using an axillary thermometer.
Source: Oscar Burriel/ Science Source.

CASE STUDY \\ PART 2

Mr. Kleinlein has been home for 24 hours since his visit to the physician's office. You are the triage nurse today and call to check on him. Mr. Kleinlein mentions that the ibuprofen has not been completely working and that his temperature fluctuates between 37.3° and 38.9°C (99.1° and 102°F). Mr. Kleinlein mentions that he still has no appetite and is struggling to remember to drink fluids. He says that he has been lying in bed since he got home yesterday and does not remember getting up at all. As the triage nurse, you speak with the physician and determine that Mr. Kleinlein needs to be hospitalized for treatment. You tell Mr. Kleinlein to have someone bring him to the emergency department and that the physician will have orders waiting for him.

Clinical Reasoning Questions Level I

1. Why did you as the triage nurse want to speak with the physician?
2. What factors led to the decision to admit Mr. Kleinlein to the hospital?

Clinical Reasoning Questions Level II

3. What nursing diagnosis would be priority for Mr. Kleinlein?
4. What further questions could you have asked Mr. Kleinlein to determine his fluid volume status?

▶ INTERVENTIONS AND THERAPIES

Independent

It is important for the nurse to support the client's environment to maintain thermoregulatory mechanisms. Older adult clients and young infants may require a warmer environmental temperature than other clients. Infants and children can gain and lose more heat than adults through their disproportionately larger heads, so they should wear a hat when exposed to temperature extremes. Adequate hydration should be maintained, especially when ambient temperatures are very hot. Dehydration can present with a low-grade fever that will resolve when hydration status is corrected. The nurse should teach the client the importance of maintaining adequate hydration during times of strenuous exercise and monitor the temperature of the highly stressed or anxious client for potential temperature elevation. In addition, when the opportunity for client education presents itself, the nurse should teach all clients how to take and record their temperature (see the Client Teaching feature).

Collaborative

Collaborative care can be divided into five types:

■ *Prehospital care.* Singhal et al. (2013) found that 11% of pediatric clients with severe sepsis were transported to an emergency department by ambulance. Emergency medical service personnel pay immediate attention to the ABCs (airway, breathing, and circulation). For toxic-appearing children (children who are pale or cyanotic, and lethargic or irritable), initiating IV access is important. Seizure precautions should be followed in children with a history of febrile seizures (Graneto, 2013).

At the other end of the age range, in older adults, the same considerations hold similar importance.

■ *Emergency department care.* Again, the ABCs are the first priorities. In addition to temperature, pulse, and respiration, blood

Client Teaching Taking Temperature

■ Teach the client accurate use and reading of the type of thermometer to be used. Examine the thermometer the client uses in the home for safety and proper functioning. Encourage and facilitate the replacement of mercury-in-glass thermometers with other types.

■ Observe the client or caregiver taking and reading a temperature. Reinforce the importance of reporting the site and type of thermometer used and the value of using these consistently.

■ Discuss means of keeping the thermometer clean, such as warm water and soap, and avoiding cross-contamination.

■ Ensure that the client has water-soluble lubricant when using a rectal thermometer.

■ Instruct the client or family member to notify the healthcare provider if the client's temperature is 37.7°C (100°F) or higher.

■ When making a home visit, take a thermometer with you in case the client does not have a functional thermometer.

■ Check that the client knows how to record the temperature. Provide a recording chart/table if indicated.

■ Discuss environmental control modifications that should be taken during illness or extreme climate conditions (e.g., heating, air conditioning, appropriate clothing and bedding).

pressure and pulse oximetry readings are recorded. In children, weight is measured to calculate appropriate antipyretic medication dosages. For all ages, antipyretics should be given as soon as possible after the client enters the ED. If the medication brings down the fever, the lower temperature still does not signal the absence of bacterial disease (Graneto, 2013).

■ *Inpatient care to pediatric, geriatric or other designated care settings.* The client's age does make a significant difference. Newborns up to 28 days old with fevers should be admitted to the hospital (Graneto, 2013). After that age, hospitalization depends on factors in the individual assessment, and the decision is often guided by protocols. Home care is often the treatment of choice because it avoids exposing the client to healthcare-associated infections. Cagatay et al. (2010) studied 185 clients hospitalized for acute fever in an infectious disease unit. The causes could not be established in 10% of the clients. Of the rest, 80% of clients had infectious diseases, mainly respiratory illnesses; the other 20% had fevers precipitated by noninfectious agents, such as cancer, autoimmune diseases, and other noncontagious diseases.

■ *Admission to an intensive care unit (ICU).* Launey et al. (2011) found a large range (23%–70%) of reported incidence of fevers in ICUs. Only half of those fevers were caused by infectious diseases.

■ *Outpatient and follow-up care.* If the client or caregiver has access to further communication with the primary care healthcare provider, continued monitoring can take place at home. Protocols should be in place that guide notification of positive laboratory results after discharge from the ED or leaving the outpatient clinic or physician's office.

Medications for lowering temperature are outlined in **Table 20–2** ●.

TABLE 20–2 Over-the-Counter (OTC) Antipyretics

CHEMICAL NAME	ACETAMINOPHEN	IBUPROFEN OR NAPROXEN	ACETYLSALICYLIC ACID (ASA)
Brand Names			
	Tylenol Tempra Panadol	Advil Motrin Midol Aleve Naprosyn	House brands
Category			
	Acetaminophen	Nonsteroidal anti-inflammatory drugs (NSAIDs)	Salicylates
Uses			
	Pain or fever, not inflammation	Pain, inflammation, or fever	Pain, inflammation, fever, or prevention of stroke and heart disease
Mechanism of Action			
	Direct action at the level of the hypothalamus and dilation of peripheral blood vessels. Resultant sweating dissipates heat. Also, inhibition of production of brain prostaglandins to reduce pain	Inhibition of COX-1, necessary for production and release of brain prostaglandins and COX-2, responsible for inflammation	Inhibition of COX-1, necessary for production and release of brain prostaglandins and COX-2, responsible for inflammation
Common Side Effects			
	Generally safe and adverse effects uncommon. Causes less gastric irritation than NSAIDs and does not affect blood coagulation.	Stomach upset, ulcer formation, bleeding	Stomach upset, ulcer formation, bleeding
Precautions			
	Potential liver damage with high doses or chronic use, especially with consumption of large amounts of alcohol	Bleeding	Bleeding Chronic use: Ringing in the ears or hearing loss needs immediate attention.
Pregnancy/Lactation			
	Relatively safe in all trimesters Detected in breast milk, but no adverse effects known, so American Academy of Pediatrics says compatible with breastfeeding	Avoid during pregnancy, since Category C prior to 30 weeks' gestation, and Category D after that No known effect on lactation	Relatively safe in intermittent dose in first and second trimesters. Avoid use in third semester. Detected in breast milk, so American Academy of Pediatrics urges caution on breastfeeding.
Nursing Implications			
	Not recommended for malnourished clients where it can cause acute toxicity and renal failure. High doses put client at risk for liver failure.	With client use of hypoglycemic agent or insulin, may increase hypoglycemic effect. Administer with food or a full glass of water to decrease gastric irritation. Assess clients taking anticoagulants to monitor increased risk of bleeding.	Avoid use in children under age 18 due to increased risk of Reye syndrome, particularly with flu virus and varicella infections.

◣ REVIEW **The Concept of Thermoregulation**

RELATE Link the Concepts

Linking the concept of thermoregulation with the concept of fluids and electrolytes:

1. What can the nurse do to provide adequate hydration to the client?

2. Why is the nurse concerned about the client's urine output?

Linking the concept of thermoregulation with the concept of safety:

3. What teaching should the nurse perform when talking with clients about hypothermia?

4. Does the teaching change when the nurse is working with adults rather than children?

Linking the concept of thermoregulation with the concept of nutrition:

5. Why is it important to maintain the client's nutritional status while the client has increased temperatures?

6. If the client is unable to eat or drink, how would the nurse anticipate the client receiving adequate nutrition?

READY Go to Companion Skills Manual

REFER Go to Pearson Nursing Student Resources
nursing.pearsonhighered.com

• Additional review materials

REFLECT Case Study \\ Part 3

Reread Parts 1 and 2 of the Case Study. Mr. Kleinlein has been in the hospital now for 48 hours. He has been receiving antibi-otics and Motrin every 6 hours since admission. He is also receiving NS IV at 125 mL/hr. His output is 80 mL/hr. His appetite has increased, and he is able to eat about half of every meal.

Clinical Reasoning Questions Level I

1. Looking at the IV intake and the urine output, what would you document for intake and output?

2. What other assessments might you need to perform?

Clinical Reasoning Questions Level II

3. What is the priority nursing diagnosis for Mr. Kleinlein?

4. How would you determine whether the fluid volume deficit is resolving?

EXEMPLAR 20.1 Hyperthermia

EXEMPLAR KEY TERMS
Constant fever, *1431*
Endogenous pyrogens, *1432*
Febrile seizure, *1434*
Fever phobia, *1436*
Fever spike, *1431*
Heat exhaustion, *1431*
Heat stroke, *1431*
Intermittent fever, *1431*
Relapsing fever, *1431*
Remittent fever, *1431*

EXEMPLAR LEARNING OUTCOMES
After reading about this exemplar, you will be able to:

1. Describe the pathophysiology, etiology, clinical manifestations, and direct and indirect causes of hyperthermia.

2. Identify risk factors associated with hyperthermia.

3. Illustrate the nursing process in providing culturally competent care across the life span for individuals with hyperthermia.

4. Formulate priority nursing diagnoses appropriate for an individual with hyperthermia.

5. Summarize therapies used by interdisciplinary teams in the collaborative care of an individual with hyperthermia.

6. Plan evidence-based care for an individual with hyperthermia and his or her family in collaboration with other members of the healthcare team.

7. Evaluate expected outcomes for an individual with hyperthermia.

▶ OVERVIEW

A body temperature above the usual range is called *hyperthermia* or, in lay terms, fever. The client who has a fever is referred to as *febrile*; the one who does not is *afebrile*.

Four common types of fevers are intermittent, remittent, relapsing, and constant. During an **intermittent fever**, the body temperature alternates at regular intervals between periods of fever and periods of normal or subnormal temperatures. Intermittent fever is common with some illnesses, such as malaria. During a **remittent fever**, such as with a cold or influenza, a wide range of fluctuating temperatures (more than 2°C [3.6°F]), all of which are above normal, occurs over a 24-hour period. In a **relapsing fever**, short febrile periods of a few days are interspersed with periods of 1–2 days of normal temperature. During a **constant fever**, the body temperature fluctuates minimally but always remains above normal. This can occur with typhoid fever. A temperature that rises to fever level rapidly, following a normal temperature, and then returns to normal within a few hours is called a **fever spike**. Bacterial blood infections often cause fever spikes.

In some conditions, an elevated temperature is not a true fever. Two such conditions are heat exhaustion and heat stroke. **Heat exhaustion** is a result of excessive heat exposure and dehydration. Signs of heat exhaustion include paleness, dizzi-ness, nausea, vomiting, fainting, and a moderately increased temperature (101°–102°F). Individuals experiencing **heat stroke**, a more serious form of heat exhaustion that can be life threatening, generally have been exercising in hot weather, have warm, flushed skin, and often do not sweat. They usually have a temperature of 106°F or higher and may be delirious, unconscious, or having seizures.

▶ PATHOPHYSIOLOGY AND ETIOLOGY

The clinical signs of fever vary with the onset, course, and abatement stages. These signs occur as a result of changes in the set point of the temperature control mechanism regulated by the hypothalamus. Under normal conditions, whenever the core temperature rises, the rate of heat loss increases, resulting in a decrease in temperature toward the set-point level. Conversely, when the core temperature falls, the rate of heat production increases, resulting in a rise in temperature toward the set point.

In a fever, however, the set point of the hypothalamic thermo-stat changes suddenly from the normal level to a higher than normal value (e.g., 39.5°C [103.1°F]). This results from the effects on the hypothalamus of tissue destruction, pyrogenic substances, or dehydration. Although the set point changes rapidly, the core body temperature (i.e., the blood temperature) reaches this new set point only after several hours. During this interval, the usual heat production responses that elevate the body temperature occur: chills, feeling of coldness, cold skin due to vasoconstriction, and shivering. This is referred to as the chill phase.

When the core temperature reaches the new set point, the client feels neither cold nor hot and no longer experiences chills (the plateau phase). Depending on the degree of temperature elevation, other signs may occur during the course of the fever. Very high temperatures, such as 41°–42°C (106°–108°F), damage the parenchyma of cells throughout the body, particularly in the brain, where destruction of neuronal cells is irreversible. Damage to the liver, kidneys, and other body organs can also be great enough to disrupt functioning and eventually cause death.

When the cause of the high temperature is suddenly removed, the set point of the hypothalamic thermostat is suddenly reduced to a lower value, perhaps even back to the original normal level. In this instance, the hypothalamus now attempts to lower the temperature, and the usual heat loss responses causing a reduction of the body temperature occur: excessive sweating and a hot, flushed skin due to sudden vasodilation. This is referred to as the flush phase.

In response to an infection, macrophages release **endogenous pyrogens** (interleukins, interferons, and tumor necrosis factor). These pyrogens travel through the circulatory system to the hypothalamus, the control center for body temperature regulation. In the hypothalamus, the pyrogens trigger the production of prostaglandins, which are believed to raise the body's thermoregulatory set point, thus causing the fever to occur. See **Figure 20–8 ●**.

Heat loss from the body is reduced, and the body temperature rises to the new temperature set point. When the temperature is elevated, the heart rate increases. One degree of temperature elevation causes an increase in respiratory rate by four breaths per minute and increases the metabolic need for oxygen by 7%. Vasodilation occurs and the skin flushes, becoming warm to the touch.

As mentioned earlier, malignant hyperthermia (MH) is a potentially fatal inherited disorder that produces a serious reaction to volatile inhalational anesthetic gases and succinylcholine, a depolarizing neuromuscular blocker (Larach et al., 2010). MH can develop during an operation or when the client returns to the postanesthetic care unit. If the early symptoms of MH (e.g., escalating temperature, increased carbon dioxide production) are identified, suspected triggering agents are immediately discontinued. The nurse should immediately administer 100% oxygen with a nonrebreather mask, stay with the client, ensure good intravenous (IV) access, and summon the anesthesia provider. The anesthesia provider will order dantrolene, a muscle relaxant, which can be given via IV push. The dantrolene can be repeated every 4–6 hours until the signs and symptoms of MH diminish. Measures to decrease core body temperature should be started at once and continued until core temperature is 36.0°C. A urinary catheter should be placed to monitor urine output, and blood should be drawn for testing. Blood gases should be drawn to measure pH, and sodium bicarbonate is given to correct metabolic acidosis. Insulin may be ordered to decrease serum potassium. The client is typically transferred to the ICU for continued monitoring (LeMone, Burke, & Bauldoff, 2011).

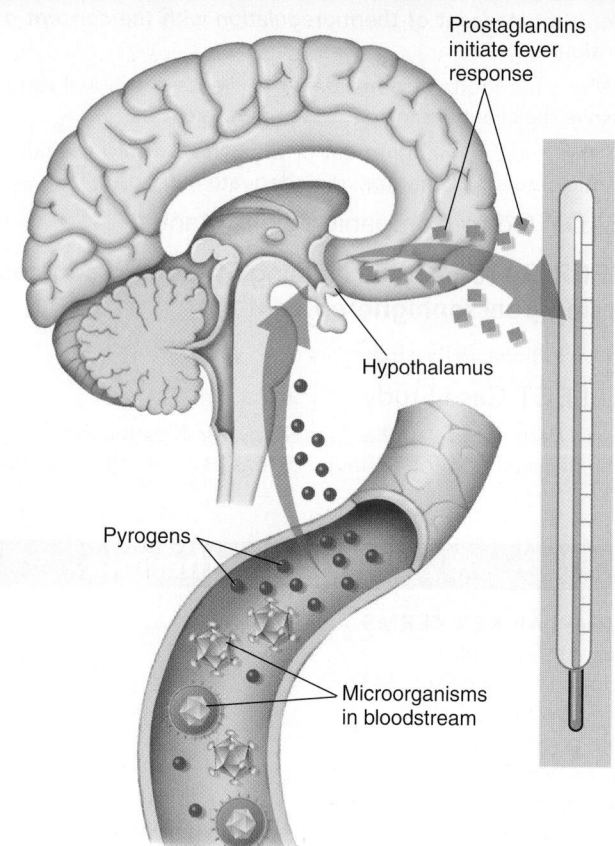

Figure 20–8 ● The hypothalamus functions as the body's thermostat, directing the body to conserve or dissipate heat. When microorganisms invade the body, endogenous pyrogens are released into the bloodstream. These substances travel to the hypothalamus, where they trigger the production and release of prostaglandins, which initiate the fever response. Blood is diverted from the extremities to more central vessels. This helps increase the core body temperature by decreasing heat loss. Shivering increases the metabolic action and heat production. The hypothalamus then maintains the temperature at the new set point.

Etiology

Hyperthermia may occur in response to viral or bacterial infections, or from tissue breakdown following myocardial infarction, malignancy, surgery, or trauma.

Risk Factors

Clients at risk for fever are those at risk for conditions resulting in fever. Diminished immune response increases the risk of infection, which increases the risk for fever. The very young and very old have diminished immunity, placing them at risk for fever. Adolescents who practice risky behavior resulting in infections or neurological trauma are also at risk for resulting fevers.

Fevers are most frequently seen in children, especially those in day care or otherwise exposed to many other children, because children have not developed immunity to common contagious diseases of childhood. Infections such as otitis media, upper respiratory infections, chickenpox, and other common diseases of childhood frequently result in fevers. The nurse should assure parents that bundling a child in many clothes and blankets might cause a slight increase in temperature but will not cause a fever.

Prevention

Vital signs such as body temperature should be looked on as only one piece of the needed data. They have to be used with awareness of the client's present and past health status as well as the client's usual vital sign results (if known by the family or previous medical records) and compared to accepted normal standards.

In situations in which monitoring for infections and inflammation is called for, measuring vital signs at regular intervals is important. This is to avoid having to take dramatic interventions in a crisis situation. Often the most effective prevention activities start with graphing the vital sign data to become aware of a pattern or trend in the temperature rising or falling over time.

▶ CLINICAL MANIFESTATIONS

The clinical manifestations of fever are frequently due, at least in part, to the cause of the fever. Signs and symptoms common to all fevers include flushing, skin that is warm or hot to the touch, increased metabolic rate resulting in an increased need for fluids, tachycardia, and tachypnea (see the Clinical Manifestations and Therapies feature). Fatigue, malaise, weakness, decreased responsiveness, difficulty concentrating, skin rash, poor appetite, malaise, vomiting and/or diarrhea, and body aches are some common signs and symptoms that may accompany a fever.

Clinical Manifestations and Therapies **Hyperthermia**

CLINICAL MANIFESTATIONS	CLINICAL THERAPIES	RATIONALES
Flushing	Correction of temperature elevation	As body temperature rises, the blood vessels vasodilate to bring more blood flow to the surface of the body. This allows the air's cooler temperature to reduce the temperature of the blood flow as heat dissipates through convection.
Warm skin	Correction of temperature elevation	As body temperature rises, the blood vessels vasodilate to bring more blood flow to the surface of the body. This causes the skin to feel warm secondary to the warmth of the blood flow.
Tachycardia	Correction of temperature elevation	With the increase in temperature, there is an increased metabolic rate resulting in increased pulse rate and respiratory rate.
Tachypnea	Correction of temperature elevation	With the increase in temperature, the metabolic rate increases, resulting in and increased pulse rate and respiratory rate.
Increased fluid requirement	Increasing oral fluid intake or provide intravenous fluids; monitoring hydration status	Insensible water loss increases as the result of perspiration, tachypnea, and increased metabolic rate. Dehydration can occur quickly, especially in young children and older adults, if extra fluid intake is not provided.
Elevated body temperature	Ranges from no treatment for a low-grade fever (<38.9°C [102°F] in children; <38.3°C [101°F] in adults) to the following for higher temperatures: ■ Antipyretic ■ Tepid bath ■ Reducing clothing and skin covering ■ Increasing fluid intake (at least 2,000 mL/day with additional fluids in hot weather or during strenuous exercise) ■ Applying cool washcloths or ice bags to axilla, groin, forehead, and nape of neck ■ Cooling blanket ■ For malignant hyperthermia, keeping emergency equipment nearby ■ Using a circulating fan in client's room	

Evidence-Based Practice Treating Fevers in Children With Alternating Ibuprofen and Acetaminophen

Problem

Should children with fever be treated with alternating doses of ibuprofen and acetaminophen?

Evidence

Recent clinical studies about the efficacy of alternating doses of ibuprofen and acetaminophen have shown mixed results. A small study by Paul et al. (2010) in children 6 months to 7 years old supported that method of lowering elevated temperatures. Sullivan et al. (2011) advocate antipyretic alternation for most children, believing that it provides enhanced fever relief, with longer-lasting fever reduction than solo medications. Another systematic review of four studies by Pereira, Dagostini, and Dal Pizzol (2012) in children 6 months to 8 years old found a tendency to affirm that approach, but the results were not conclusive. Other work by Sherman and Sood (2012) concluded that the practice of alternating antipyretics was "of limited value." Purssell (2011) performed a systematic review of six studies. The results showed a small, marginally clinically significant benefit after 4 hours. However, the researcher's conclusion was that alternating medication was unnecessary, given the effectiveness of solo drugs.

Implications

Regardless of the medication(s) chosen or pattern of administration, the nurse has a critical role in caregiver education. Because the amount of each drug contained in different preparations of the same medication may vary, the nurse must ensure that parents understand the importance of reading labels carefully, measuring doses correctly, and spacing administration with adequate intervals between doses. Liquid preparations call for particular attention to detail. Inadvertent double dosing needs to be avoided. This would happen if OTC cough and cold remedies, which often include acetaminophen, are given concurrently.

Critical Thinking Application

1. If a parent comes to you, questioning the child's healthcare provider's approach to fever reduction, what would be your best response?
2. What factors about the participation of children in clinical studies might have an influence on their results?
3. What is the effect of media (newspapers, TV advertisements, magazine articles) on the perception of the need to take action to reduce fevers?

Treatment for fever is not always indicated. A fever can be a beneficial physiological response, helping to slow the growth of organisms that thrive at lower body temperatures. A fever helps mobilize the immune response by increasing neutrophil production and T-cell proliferation.

Fever is not inherently harmful until it reaches 41°C (105.9°F). For this reason, medical management may include postponing treatment of low-grade fevers—those under 38.9°C (102°F) in otherwise healthy children and 38.3°C (101°F) in adults—to promote the body's natural defenses against infection. Fevers are more likely to be treated if they are associated with discomfort.

Acetaminophen and ibuprofen are the preferred antipyretics for children. Aspirin is no longer recommended for children because of its association with Reye syndrome. Antipyretics reduce fever by inhibiting prostaglandin synthesis, which results in lowering of the body's temperature set point. See the Evidence-Based Practice feature for a discussion of alternating acetaminophen and ibuprofen when treating children with fever.

SAFETY ALERT

In August 2013, the Food and Drug Administration (FDA) ordered a new warning label on all prescription products containing acetaminophen. The label says: "In rare cases, acetaminophen causes serious skin reactions." In looking at the previous history of reported reactions to acetaminophen, the FDA found evidence of a dozen fatalities and five times that many hospitalizations (FDA, 2013; Lowes, 2013). Manufacturers of over-the-counter products that contain acetaminophen will also be asked to use the label.

Antibiotics may also be administered for infectious diseases. Antibiotics have been responsible for decreases in morbidity and mortality from infections among children. However, some strains of bacteria have developed resistance to many antibiotics. Children with chronic illnesses such as cystic fibrosis, sickle cell disease, and AIDS are particularly susceptible to infection by drug-resistant pathogens.

Lifespan and Cultural Considerations

Febrile seizures are generalized seizures that usually occur in children as the result of rapid temperature rise above a rectal reading of 39°C (102°F) in association with an acute illness. No evidence of intracranial infection or other defined cause is found. These seizures are usually seen in children between the ages of 6 months and 5 years, with a peak incidence in toddlers. One in every 25 children will have at least one febrile seizure. Risk factors include an immediate family history of febrile seizures, first febrile seizure at a young age (less than 15 months), and frequent fevers. More than one third of children who have one febrile seizure will have a future seizure. The older the child is when an initial seizure occurs, the less likely that child is to have additional seizures (National Institute of Neurological Disorders and Stroke, 2013).

Fever is viewed differently by various cultures. See the Complementary and Alternative Therapy feature for information about the hot and cold theory of disease that many cultures use to guide home treatment of fever. The Focus on Diversity and Culture feature discusses how Latino and African American parents respond to their children's fevers.

Many cultures subscribe to the hot and cold theory of disease causation. "Hot" and "cold" do not refer to temperature, but to categories. Fever, a hot condition, is treated by giving the client cold substances (foods or medicines). Cold foods include vegetables, fruits, and fish. Cold medicines include orange flower water, linden, and sage.

▶ COLLABORATION

Collaboration related to hyperthermia or fever will generally revolve around the underlying cause of the fever. Since the causes are often closely related to the age of the client, looking at the history of a child with febrile seizures is relevant. The nurse from the child's pediatrician's office or public health clinic should collaborate with the child's parents as well as with the child's preschool or classroom teacher. They need to work together to ensure that all staff working with the child know what to do in the event the child has a seizure and how to prevent the onset of a febrile seizure. Adequate hydration, access to refrigerated fluids, shortened recess periods outside during hot weather, and shade are reasonable measures school staff can use to help prevent febrile seizures in children.

■ NURSING PROCESS

Assessment

In caring for a client with hyperthermia, the nurse assesses the client's hydration status and fluid intake, vital signs, comfort level, and appetite, and observes for seizures and a toxic appearance (lethargy, poor perfusion, hypoventilation or hyperventilation, and cyanosis), especially in the pediatric client. The client with a fever may be irritable and restless, sleep fitfully, and have nonspecific muscular pain. The nurse should identify clients who may be at higher risk for a serious illness in association with a fever, in particular the following:

- Infants and children with a toxic appearance
- Neonates under 28 days of age with a temperature greater than 38°C (100.4°F)
- Children under 4 years of age with a temperature greater than 41°C (105.8°F)
- Children with conditions such as a ventriculoperitoneal shunt, congenital heart disease, asplenia, and sickle cell disease
- Clients with immunosuppression, such as those receiving chemotherapy, undergoing organ transplantation, or diagnosed with HIV/AIDS
- Clients with chronic conditions such as diabetes mellitus, congestive heart failure, or pulmonary diseases.

The client should be observed for other signs of infection, such as a rash, nausea and vomiting, or diarrhea, as well as generalized symptoms of a poor appetite and malaise.

Cohee et al. (2010) studied the responses of Latino and African American parents to their children's fevers. They found that Latino parents were least likely to distinguish between a nonfebrile and a febrile condition. One the other hand, African American parents were least likely to believe that a child's fever could cause death or brain damage. However, African Americans parents were more likely to give their children more frequent doses of ibuprofen than are recommended. Individuals of both ethnicities were equally likely to unnecessarily treat normal temperatures and to dose acetaminophen too frequently. The study affirms the need for continued education of caregivers about hyperthermia and its treatment.

Diagnosis

Nursing diagnoses that may be appropriate for clients with febrile illnesses include the following:

- *Hyperthermia* related to infectious disease process
- *Risk for Deficient Fluid Volume* related to hypermetabolic state
- *Impaired Skin Integrity* related to hyperthermia and self-mutilation of skin lesions
- *Impaired Oral Mucous Membrane* related to infectious disease process
- *Deficient Fluid Volume* related to repeated episodes of vomiting and diarrhea.

(NANDA-I © 2012)

Planning

Care is planned for the client with hyperthermia based on the specific needs of the client and the cause of the temperature elevation. Goals specific to fever may include the following:

- The client's temperature will approach normal limits within 60 minutes of administration of an antipyretic.
- The client's temperature will remain within normal limits within 48–72 hours of beginning antibiotic therapy.
- The client's temperature will be maintained within acceptable limits within 4 hours of application of a hypothermia blanket.
- The client or caregiver will describe temperature elevations to be reported to the healthcare provider immediately.
- The client or caregiver will recognize symptoms requiring consultation with the healthcare provider.

Implementation

Nursing interventions for a client who has a fever are designed to support the body's normal physiological processes, provide comfort, and prevent complications. During the course of fever, the nurse needs to monitor the client's vital signs closely.

Nursing measures during the chill phase are designed to help the client decrease heat loss. At this time, the body's physiological processes are attempting to raise the core temperature to the new set-point temperature. During the flush or crisis phase, the body processes are attempting to lower the core temperature to the reduced or normal set-point temperature. At this time, the nurse takes measures to increase heat loss and decrease heat production.

Nursing interventions for the client with a fever can include the following:

- Monitor temperature every 2 hours, as appropriate.
- Promote adequate fluid and nutritional intake.
- Monitor intake and output.
- Apply ice bag covered with a towel to groin.
- Cover the client with only a sheet.

Nursing care for treatment of fever includes administering antipyretics, removing unnecessary clothing, and careful continued monitoring of temperature progression. Identify clear fluids the client prefers to drink, and encourage the intake of extra fluids.

Care in the Community

The nurse teaches parents to care for their child at home, including how and when to give antipyretics. Parents often fear a fever, believing it is a disease rather than a symptom of an illness. Their greatest fears about the harmful effects of fever typically include seizure, brain damage, and death. The situation of caregivers being scared about these negative results has been labeled **fever phobia**. Research in a pediatric emergency department has shown a correlation between lower educational level and more heightened concern about children's febrile condition (Poirier, Collins, & McGuire, 2010). Research by Rupe and Ahlers-Schmidt (2010) confirmed that correlation and found that more than half (57%) of surveyed parents reported being "very worried" when their child had a fever. Evidence of fever phobia was significantly higher in cases of younger children. In the study population, Hispanic ethnicity of parents was the single most predictive factor for fever phobia. Given the effect that this fever phobia has on the whole family, the nurse should provide information and reassurance, helping parents to recognize signs of the child's condition becoming better as a result of treatment efforts (see the Client Teaching feature for more information that is helpful to parents of children with fever).

Evaluation

Expected outcomes for the client with hyperthermia include the following:

- The client's fever is effectively managed with antipyretics. Alternatively, without medication, the client's own defenses maintain both the skin and body temperature in the expected range. For example, the client sweats when hot.
- The client maintains adequate hydration as evidenced by skin turgor, moist mucous membranes, sufficient urine output, and hematocrit within normal range.

Client Teaching   Evaluating and Treating Fever in Children

About Fevers

- A fever is not a disease; it is the body's response to an infection. It means the child's body is using natural defenses to fight an infection.
- If the child has a fever and does not look sick, it may be better to let the body's natural defenses fight off the virus or bacteria causing the fever. Follow guidelines about when to contact the child's healthcare provider.

Treating the Fever

- Use a thermometer to check the child's temperature every 2 hours.
- Administer either acetaminophen or ibuprofen to lower a fever. Check the label to make sure the correct dosage is given—drops and syrups do not have the same concentration. Do not alternate medications.
- Remove all but a light layer of the child's clothing.
- Monitor the child's behavior and response to fever medication. The fever medication will reduce the child's temperature, but the temperature may not return to normal until the child is recovering from the illness.
- If sponging the child, give fever medication first, and then use tepid water to sponge the child. Cool water may increase shivering and discomfort. Alcohol should not be used.
- The child's temperature may rise again 4 hours after acetaminophen or 6 hours after ibuprofen is given. Check the temperature and give another dose of acetaminophen or ibuprofen medicine. Follow the recommendations on the bottle for the maximum number of doses allowed per day.

Call Your Healthcare Provider *Immediately* If Any of the Following Occur

- The infant is under 2 months old and has a fever greater than 38.0°C (100.4°F).
- The child has a fever greater than 40.1°C (104.2°F) and any of the symptoms below are present:
  - The child is crying inconsolably or whimpering. The child cries when moved or otherwise touched by the parent or other family members.
  - The child is difficult to awaken.
  - The child's neck is stiff.
  - Purple spots are present on the child's skin.
  - The child's breathing is difficult and no better after the nose is cleared.
  - The child is drooling saliva and is unable to swallow anything.
  - The child has a convulsion or seizure.
  - The child acts or looks very sick.

Call Your Healthcare Provider Within 24 Hours If Any of the Following Occur

- The child is 2–4 months old (unless fever occurs within 48 hours of a DTaP shot and the infant has no other serious symptoms).
- The fever is higher than 40.1°C (104.2°F) (especially if the child is under 3 years old).
- The child complains of burning or pain with urination.
- The fever has been present for more than 24 hours without an obvious cause or location of infection.
- The fever went away for more than 24 hours and then returned.

REVIEW **Hyperthermia**

RELATE Link the Concepts and Exemplars

Linking the exemplar of hyperthermia with the concept of infection:

1. Do all infections result in fevers? Explain your answer.

2. When treating a 4-year-old client with a viral infection and a temperature of 39.9°C (103.8°F), measured via axillary site, what independent nursing actions would you initiate? What collaborative interventions would you anticipate?

Linking the exemplar of hyperthermia with the concept of fluids and electrolytes:

3. Explain the physiology that would cause a client to run a fever when dehydrated.

4. How does a client's fluid requirement change when the client has a fever? Explain the physiology behind your answer.

READY Go to Companion Skills Manual

REFER Go to Pearson Nursing Student Resources
nursing.pearsonhighered.com

- Additional review materials

REFLECT Case Study

Carrie Holmes is 6 weeks old, born at 38 weeks' gestation by vaginal delivery secondary to a small placental abruption

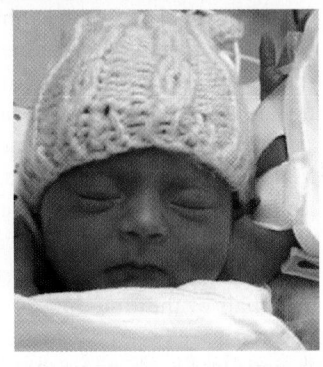

attributed to her father, Casey Holmes, hitting her mother, Jessica Riley, in the abdomen. When Carrie and her mother come home from the hospital, they move into her grandmother's house with her 3-year-old brother Ryan. By 6 weeks of age, Carrie is starting to become accustomed to the daily routine. Her grandmother Evelyn Riley cares for her when her mother goes to work at a restaurant. Mrs. Riley feeds Carrie a bottle and lets her sit in her infant seat to watch her big brother play with his toys.

1. What factors would increase Carrie's risk of developing a fever?

2. If Ms. Riley called the pediatrician's office to report that Carrie had a fever of 38.6°C (101.4°F), taken rectally, what directions would you provide for her care? Explain the rationale for your answer.

3. If Ryan developed a fever of 38.6°C (101.4°F) taken via the axillary site, what instructions would you provide his mother and grandmother for his care?

EXEMPLAR 20.2 **Hypothermia**

EXEMPLAR KEY TERMS
Brown adipose tissue (BAT), *1438*
Chemical thermogenesis, *1438*
Frostbite, *1439*
Hyperthermia blanket, *1441*
Nonshivering thermogenesis, *1438*
Piloerection, *1440*

EXEMPLAR LEARNING OUTCOMES
After reading about this exemplar, you will be able to:

1. Describe the pathophysiology, etiology, clinical manifestations, and direct and indirect causes of hypothermia.

2. Identify risk factors associated with hypothermia.

3. Illustrate the nursing process in providing culturally competent care across the life span for individuals with hypothermia.

4. Formulate priority nursing diagnoses appropriate for an individual with hypothermia.

5. Summarize therapies used by interdisciplinary teams in the collaborative care of an individual with hypothermia.

6. Plan evidence-based care for an individual with hypothermia and his or her family in collaboration with other members of the healthcare team.

7. Evaluate expected outcomes for an individual with hypothermia.

▶ OVERVIEW

Hypothermia is a condition in which the core body temperature falls below 35°C (95°F). This occurs when the heat the body produces is less than the heat lost. Hypothermia can be a life-threatening emergency and can occur in any season and any geographic location.

▶ PATHOPHYSIOLOGY AND ETIOLOGY

Hypothermia may be induced or accidental. Induced hypothermia is the deliberate lowering of the body temperature to decrease the metabolic rate, reducing the body's need for oxygen. Accidental hypothermia may occur as the result of immersion in cold water, exposure to cold environments, or damage to the body's thermoregulatory processes.

As the body's core temperature falls, the body tries to conserve the core temperature at the expense of the extremities. Two major routes of heat loss are from the internal core of the body to the body surface and from the external surface to the environment. The core temperature is usually higher than the skin temperature, resulting in continuous transfer or conduction of heat to the surface. The greater the difference in temperature between core and skin, the more rapidly heat transfers. The transfer is accomplished through an increase in oxygen consumption, depletion of glycogen stores, and, in the newborn, metabolization of brown fat.

Induced Hypothermia

Hypothermia may be induced for a variety of reasons. The most frequent reason for this treatment is to reduce metabolic rates and lower the cellular demand for oxygen in the tissues, particularly in the brain. Historically, induced hypothermia has been used to reduce neurological damage following head trauma or strokes or during cardiac surgery. Hypothermia has been shown to improve the neurological recovery of clients resuscitated in out-of-hospital ventricular fibrillation. As a result, research is being conducted to determine whether emergency responders should initiate hypothermia in clients while they are still in the field (Gavrielatos et al., 2010).

Other research about induced hypothermia has focused on its use with in-hospital cardiac arrests. Nichol et al. (2013) studied over 8,000 clients who experienced a heart attack while hospitalized. The survival rate was 30%. Even with considerable efforts to achieve hypothermia in about 3% of the clients, not even half of the time (40%) were those clients' temperatures lowered to between 32° and 34°C (889.6° and 93.2°F). Hypothermia had neither a positive nor a negative effect on survival or prevention of neurological damage.

Accidental Hypothermia

Accidental hypothermia can result from (a) exposure to a cold environment, (b) immersion in cold water, or (c) lack of adequate clothing, shelter, or heat. Hypothermia is associated with near-drowning episodes because body heat is lost more quickly in water than in air. Other causes of hypothermia include ingestion of alcohol or barbiturates, trauma or a brain disorder that interferes with temperature regulation, and overwhelming sepsis. If skin and underlying tissues are damaged by freezing cold, frostbite results.

HYPOTHERMIA IN INFANTS   A newborn is at a distinct disadvantage in maintaining a normal temperature. With a large body surface in relation to mass and a limited amount of insulating subcutaneous fat, the full-term newborn loses about four times more heat than an adult. The newborn's poor thermal stability is primarily due to excessive heat loss rather than impaired heat production. Because of the risk of hypothermia and possible cold stress, minimizing heat loss in the newborn after birth is essential. Once the infant has been dried after birth, the highest losses of heat generally result from convection because of the newborn's large body surface compared with weight. Thermal conduction is also a risk because of the marked difference between the newborn's core temperature and skin temperature. The newborn can respond to the air's cooler temperature with adequate peripheral vasoconstriction, but this mechanism is not entirely effective because of the minimal amount of fat insulation present, the large body surface, and ongoing thermal conduction. Minimizing the baby's heat loss and preventing hypothermia are imperative.

The newborn has several physiological mechanisms that increase heat production, or thermogenesis. These mechanisms include increased basal metabolic rate, muscular activity, and **chemical thermogenesis** (also called **nonshivering thermogenesis** or NST) (Rozance & Rosenberg, 2012). NST is an important mechanism of heat production unique to the newborn. It occurs when skin receptors perceive a drop in the environmental temperature and, in response, transmit sensations to stimulate the sympathetic nervous system. NST uses the newborn's stores of **brown adipose tissue (BAT)** (also called brown fat) to provide heat. Brown fat receives its name from its dark color, which is caused by its enriched blood supply, dense cellular content, and abundant nerve endings. These characteristics of brown fat cells promote rapid metabolism, heat generation, and heat transfer to the peripheral circulation. The

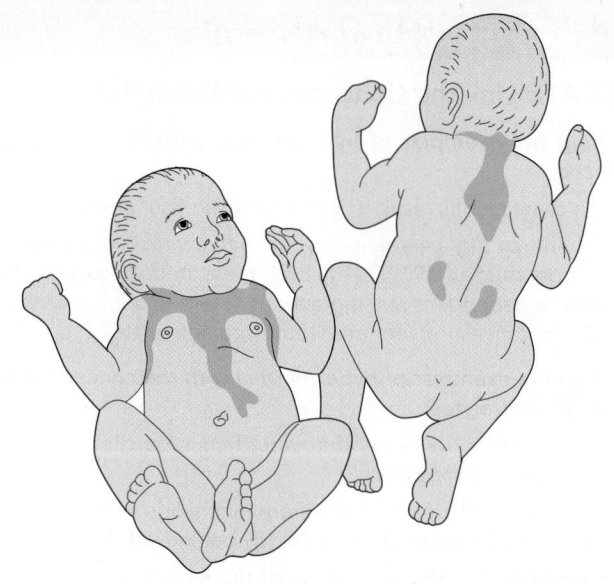

Figure 20–9 ● The distribution of brown adipose tissue (brown fat) in the newborn.
Source: Adapted from Davis, V. (1980, November–December). Structure and function of brown adipose tissue in the neonate. *Journal of Obstetric, Gynecologic, and Neonatal Nursing, 9,* p. 364.

large numbers of brown fat cells increase the speed with which triglycerides are metabolized to produce heat.

NST from BAT is the primary source of heat in the hypothermic newborn. It first appears in the fetus at about 26–30 weeks' gestation and continues to increase until 2–5 weeks after the birth of a term infant, unless the fat is depleted by cold stress. Brown fat is deposited in the midscapular area, around the neck, and in the axillae, with deeper placement around the trachea, esophagus, abdominal aorta, kidneys, and adrenal glands (**Figure 20–9** ●). BAT constitutes 2%–6% of a newborn's total body weight.

Shivering, a form of muscular activity common in the cold adult, is rarely seen in the newborn, although it has been observed at ambient temperatures of 15°C (59°F) or less (Polin, Fox, & Abman, 2010). If the newborn shivers, it means the newborn's metabolic rate has already doubled. The extra muscular activity does little to produce needed heat. Thermographic studies of newborns exposed to cold show an increase in the skin heat produced over the newborn's brown fat deposits between 1 and 14 days of age (Polin et al., 2010). However, if the brown fat supply has been depleted, the metabolic response to cold is limited or lacking. An increase in basal metabolism as a result of hypothermia results in an increase in oxygen consumption. A decrease in the environmental temperature of 2°C, from 33° to 31°C (91.4° to 87.8°F), is sufficient to double the oxygen consumption of a term newborn. Keeping the normal newborn warm promotes normal oxygen requirements, whereas chilling can cause signs of respiratory distress in the newborn.

When exposed to cold, the normal term newborn is usually able to cope with the increase in oxygen requirements. The preterm newborn, however, may be unable to increase ventilation to the necessary level of oxygen consumption. Because oxidation of fatty acids depends on the availability of oxygen, glucose, and adenosine triphosphate (ATP), the newborn's ability to generate heat can be altered by pathological events, such as hypoxia, acidosis, and hypoglycemia, or by medications that block the release of norepinephrine.

Meperidine (Demerol) given to a laboring woman or as an analgesic for a newborn can slow or prevent metabolism of newborn brown fat and lead to a greater decrease in the newborn's body temperature during the neonatal period. This effect of meperidine on brown fat is lessened if the mother and the newborn are well hydrated and in a neutral thermal environment. The newborn's body temperature has an effect on medication activity. Newborn hypothermia prolongs and potentiates the effects of many analgesic and anesthetic drugs in the newborn.

The core temperature of infants is highly responsive to changes in the external environment; therefore, infants need extra protection from even mild variations in temperature. The core body temperature of children is more stable than that of infants but less so than that of adolescents or adults. However, older adults are more sensitive than young and middle-aged adults to variations in environmental temperature. This increased sensitivity may be due to the decreased thermoregulatory control and loss of subcutaneous fat common in older adults, or it may be due to environmental factors such as lack of activity, inadequate diet, or lack of central heating. Illness or a central nervous system disorder may impair the thermostatic function of the hypothalamus.

FROSTBITE   **Frostbite** is an injury of the skin resulting from freezing. If the exposure to freezing temperatures is limited, only the skin and subcutaneous tissues become involved. However, as exposure increases, deeper structures freeze. The skin freezes when the temperature falls below 0°C (32°F), with the freezing point of skin being slightly below the freezing point of water (Castellani et al., 2010). Frostbite is most common on exposed or peripheral areas of the body, such as the nose, ears, feet, and hands.

As human tissues freeze, ice crystals form, increasing the intracellular sodium content. Small blood vessels initially vasoconstrict but then vasodilate and become more permeable, causing cells and tissues to swell. With continued exposure, vasoconstriction and increased viscosity of the blood cause infarction and necrosis of the affected tissue.

Superficial frostbite causes numbness, itching, and prickling. The skin appears cyanotic, reddened, or white. Deeper frostbite causes stiffness and paresthesias. As the skin and tissues thaw, the skin becomes white or yellow and loses its elasticity. The client experiences burning pain. Edema, blisters, necrosis, and gangrene may appear.

Rapid thawing may significantly decrease tissue necrosis. The following are general guidelines for rewarming areas of frostbite:

- Outdoors, treat superficial frostbite by applying firm pressure with a warm hand or by placing frostbitten hands in the axillae. If the feet are frostbitten, remove wet footwear, dry the feet, and put on dry footwear. Do not rub the areas with snow.

- In the hospital, rapidly rewarm affected areas in circulating warm water, 40°–40.5°C (104°–105°F), for 20–30 minutes. Do not rub or massage the areas.

Following rewarming, the client should kept on bed rest, with the affected parts elevated. The nurse should administer pain medications and anti-inflammatory agents and debride any blisters. Whirlpool therapy may be used to clean the skin and debride necrotic tissue. Recovery from frostbite is usually complete if the involved area has not become necrotic. Necrotic tissue may require amputation.

SAFETY ALERT
Frostbite can occur if a chemical ice pack (found in many first aid kits) is left in contact with the skin for too long. Avoid using these chemical packs in children if possible. When using a chemical ice pack, cover it with a few layers of clothing or towels and monitor the skin under the pack frequently. Remove the chemical ice pack if the skin starts to looks white or has decreased sensation. Remove the ice pack periodically to allow the skin to rewarm.

RISK FACTORS   Certain clients are at greater risk for accidental hypothermia. As individuals age, the metabolic rate slows, placing the older adult at risk of hypothermia. This can be complicated further by reduced sensory perception, use of medications such as sedatives, and financial issues resulting in the inability to adequately heat their homes. Many older adults suffer and die each year from hypothermia. A lowered metabolism and loss of normal insulation from thinning subcutaneous tissue decrease the older client's ability to retain heat. Older clients frequently prefer a warmer environment than younger adults do. The older adult who spends time outdoors in cold weather or does not turn on the heat in the home is at significant risk for hypothermia.

Infants and young children are at risk because of immature temperature regulatory mechanisms, thinner skin, limited subcutaneous fat, and high ratios of skin surface area to body mass. Adolescents are at risk because they are prone to risk-taking behaviors including drug and alcohol use and engaging in remote outdoor activities without proper equipment or clothing. Alcohol causes peripheral vasodilation, which exposes the circulating bloodstream to more rapid cooling, resulting in a faster decrease in temperature. Drug and alcohol use may reduce the ability to sense cold, further exacerbating risk.

Other risk factors include damage to the hypothalamus, decreased ability to shiver, decreased metabolic rate, evaporation from skin in cool environments, exposure to a cool environment, illness, inactivity, inadequate clothing, malnutrition, medications, and trauma. Hypothyroidism, immaturity of a newborn's temperature regulatory system, and ineffective thermoregulation can all contribute to hypothermia.

▶ CLINICAL MANIFESTATIONS

Symptoms of mild hypothermia (32°–35°C [90°–95°F]) include fatigue, slurred speech, poor coordination and clumsiness, confusion and poor judgment, inappropriate behavior, shivering, tachycardia, and tachypnea. Symptoms of moderate hypothermia (28°–32°C [82°–90°F]) include depressed mental status, no shivering, depressed respirations, slow pulse or irregular heartbeat, low blood pressure, pale or cyanotic color, hallucinations, and coma. Profound hypothermia (body temperature below 28°C [82°F]) results in absence of respirations and pulse, ventricular fibrillation, dilated and unresponsive pupils, and coma.

Clinical Manifestations and Therapies **Hypothermia**

ETIOLOGY	CLINICAL MANIFESTATIONS	CLINICAL THERAPIES
Reduction in temperature results in decreased metabolic rate and reduced oxygen demands, slowing respirations and pulse rate. The body's compensatory mechanism initiates shivering to produce heat from muscle activity.	■ Decreased body temperature, pulse, and respirations ■ Severe shivering (initially) ■ Feelings of cold and chills	■ Provide a warm environment. ■ Provide dry clothing. ■ Apply warm blankets. ■ Keep limbs close to body. ■ Cover the client's scalp with a cap or turban. ■ Supply warm oral or intravenous fluids. ■ Apply warming pads.
Hypothermia causes vasoconstriction to reduce exposure of the circulating bloodstream to the cold environment.	■ Pale, cool, waxy skin	
Vasoconstriction caused by hypothermia reduces peripheral circulation. Reduced heart rate reduces cardiac output. Blood flow to the kidneys is reduced. Blood flow to the brain is reduced secondary to slowed metabolic rate and reduced cardiac output.	■ Frostbite (nose, fingers, toes) ■ Hypotension ■ Decreased urinary output ■ Lack of muscle coordination ■ Disorientation ■ Drowsiness progressing to coma	■ Rapidly rewarm affected areas in circulating warm water, 40°–40.5°C (104°–105°F), for 20–30 minutes. ■ Do not rub or massage the areas. ■ Following rewarming, keep the client on bed rest with the affected parts elevated. ■ Administer analgesics and anti-inflammatory agents. ■ Debride blisters. ■ Administer whirlpool therapy to clean skin and debride necrotic tissue. ■ Necrotic tissue may require amputation. ■ Support respiratory and cardiac function. ■ Place the client on a cardiorespiratory monitor. ■ Reduce handling, because handling increases the risk of cardiac fibrillation.

SAFETY ALERT
It is important to note that a client who is hypothermic should not be declared dead. Hypothermia reduces oxygen demands, and clients with hypothermia can survive cardiac arrest for far longer than those at normal temperature. As a result, clients in cardiac arrest who are hypothermic should be warmed and resuscitated. Only if resuscitation fails after warming should the client be declared dead.

▶ **COLLABORATION**

Clients with severe hypothermia may require hemodialysis, peritoneal dialysis, or colonic irrigation in order to increase core body temperature. These interventions are typically used when hypothermia is the result of damage to the hypothalamus, usually due to trauma or cerebrovascular accidents. Such damage to the hypothalamus may make return of thermoregulation physiologically impossible.

Social service referrals may be indicated to assess the parents' ability to meet newborn or infant home care needs as well as for the client who experiences hypothermia because he or she is unable to provide a comfortable environmental temperature due to financial constraints or homelessness.

■ **NURSING PROCESS**

Assessment

The nurse assesses the client for defining characteristics of hypothermia, including the following:

■ Lowered body temperature below normal range
■ Cool skin
■ Cyanotic nail beds due to vasoconstriction, resulting from the body's attempt to raise temperature and prevent further heat loss
■ Hypertension
■ Pallor
■ **Piloerection** (goosebumps)
■ Shivering
■ Slowed capillary refill
■ Tachycardia.

Diagnosis

Nursing diagnoses for the client with hypothermia may include the following:

- *Imbalanced Body Temperature*
- *Hypothermia.*

(NANDA-I © 2012)

Planning

Prevention is a primary nursing goal.

- Thermoregulation: balance among heat production, heat gain, and heat loss
- Thermoregulation in the neonate: balance among heat production, heat gain, and heat loss during the first 28 days of life
- Vital signs: extent to which temperature is within normal range.

Implementation

Managing hypothermia involves removing the client from the cold and rewarming the client's body. For mild hypothermia, warm the client by applying blankets; for severe hypothermia, apply a **hyperthermia blanket** (an electronically controlled blanket that provides a specified temperature) and give warm intravenous fluids. Wet clothing, which increases heat loss because of the high conductivity of water, should be replaced with dry clothing. See the Clinical Manifestations and Therapies feature for nursing interventions used to treat clients with hypothermia. Monitor vital signs and urine output during active rewarming, and assess the client for cold-related injuries.

Newborns

The amount of heat an infant loses depends to a large extent on the actions of the nurse or caregiver. During the transfer of a newborn in the neonatal intensive care unit from one bed to another, a transient (although not significant) decrease in temperature may be noted for up to 1 hour. Prevention of heat loss is especially critical in very-low-birth-weight (VLBW) infants. Place the VLBW newborn in a polyethylene wrapping immediately following birth to decrease the postnatal drop in temperature that normally occurs. The use of head coverings made of insulated fabrics, wool, or polyolefin or lined with Gamgee can significantly decrease heat loss after childbirth (Blackburn, 2012). Convective, radiant, and evaporative heat losses can all be reduced (Blackburn, 2012). Swaddling and nesting maintain flexion, which reduces exposed surface area and thus convective and radiant losses. The nurse observes all newborns for signs of cold stress, including increased movement and respirations, decreased skin temperature and peripheral perfusion, development of hypoglycemia, and possible development of metabolic acidosis. Vasoconstriction is the initial response to cold stress; because it initially decreases skin temperature, the nurse should monitor and assess skin temperature instead of rectal temperature. A decrease in rectal temperature means that the infant has long-standing cold stress. By monitoring skin temperature, the nurse will be able to detect a possible decrease before the infant's core temperature is affected. If a decrease in skin temperature is noted, the nurse determines whether hypoglycemia is present. Hypoglycemia is a result of the metabolic effects of cold stress

and is suggested by glucometer values below 40 mg/dL, tremors, irritability or lethargy, apnea, or seizure activity.

If hypothermia occurs with a newborn, the following nursing interventions should be initiated (Blackburn, 2012; Cloherty et al., 2011):

- Maintain a neutral thermal environment (NTE); adjust based on the gestational age and postnatal age.
- Warm the newborn slowly because rapid temperature elevation may cause hypotension and apnea.
- Increase the air temperature in hourly increments of 1°C until the infant's temperature is stable.
- Monitor skin temperature every 15–30 minutes to determine whether the newborn's temperature is increasing.
- Remove plastic wrap, caps, and heat shields while rewarming the infant so that cool air as well as warm air is not trapped.
- Warm intravenous fluids before infusion.
- Initiate efforts to block heat loss by evaporation, convection, and conduction; maintain the newborn in NTE such as a heated incubator for transport and radiant heater for procedures.

The nurse assesses for the presence of anaerobic metabolism and initiates interventions for the resulting metabolic acidosis. Attempts to burn brown fat increase oxygen consumption, lactic acid levels, and metabolic acidosis. Hypoglycemia may be reversed by adequate glucose intake.

Children

The nurse should educate parents to layer their children's clothing and use hats in cold climates, recognize signs of hypothermia, decrease time of exposure to cold, and know how to treat mild hypothermia. The nurse teaches school-age children and adolescents who go on camping, fishing, and hunting trips how to recognize and manage hypothermia in themselves and others. The nurse should teach preventive techniques, such as avoiding riding snowmobiles or walking on ice that may not be deep enough to support the child's weight. First aid for hypothermia includes moving the child to a dry area, removing any wet clothing, and protecting the child from further environmental exposure. The nurse should wrap the child in dry blankets or dress the child in warm, dry clothing and encourage the child to drink a warm, high-calorie liquid, if the child is able.

Older Adults

Older adults are at increased risk for hypothermia because their bodies are less able to maintain a constant internal temperature. Chronic conditions (e.g., problems with the circulatory or neurological systems, hypothyroidism), medication use, reduced sensory perception, and cognitive disorders can all increase risk still further. Initial treatment is similar to treatment for hypothermia at any age, including removing wet clothing, increasing environmental temperatures, applying more clothing or blankets, and providing warm liquids. However, once the initial hypothermia is resolved, the nurse should assess for other issues that may place the older adult client at increased risk for recurrent hypothermia. These may include nutritional status, financial concerns limiting their ability to heat their homes, and self-care deficits.

NURSING CARE PLAN A Client With Hypothermia

ASSESSMENT	DIAGNOSIS	PLANNING
Jerry Karpinski, an 87-year-old Caucasian male, is brought to the emergency department after his son found him unresponsive. The son reports that the client has lived alone in a single-family home in Minnesota since his wife died 3 years ago. Mr. Karpinski depends on his Social Security income as his sole means of financial support and has been trying to keep his utility bills low by setting his thermostat to 60°F (about 15°C). His son checks on him every day and today he found Mr. Karpinski lying on the kitchen floor near the stove. Mr. Karpinski has a history of hypothyroidism and hypertension. He recently began taking sedatives to help him sleep at night. Vital signs: temperature 29°C (84.2°F) rectal; BP 82/36 mmHg. Height: 183 cm (6'). Weight: 72.7 kg (160 lb). Skin pale, cool to touch; nail beds cyanotic; breath sounds diminished throughout; pulse weak and thready. Nonresponsive to voice or stimulation. (Deep pain response not evaluated secondary to hypothermia.)	■ *Hypothermia* as evidenced by rectal temperature of 29°C (NANDA-I © 2012)	Mr. Karpinski will demonstrate thermoregulation as evidenced by the following indicators: ■ Body temperature within normal limits ■ Skin color becoming pink and less pale ■ No signs of piloerection or shivering ■ Reported thermal comfort.

IMPLEMENTATION

- Gradually rewarm Mr. Karpinski using a heating blanket until his temperature reaches 36°C (96.8°F).
- Administer warm IV solutions to maintain hydration.
- Utilize continuous core temperature monitoring device.
- Monitor continuously and record vital signs and cardiac rhythm on cardiorespiratory monitor.

- Make a referral to social services.
- Teach the client and family how to prevent hypothermia.
- Teach the client and family indications of hypothermia and appropriate emergency treatment.
- Reduce manual stimulation.

EVALUATION

Mr. Karpinski's core temperature is approaching the normal range, he is increasingly more alert, and his vital signs have returned to normal ranges. Mr. Karpinski was at increased risk for hypothermia due to his age and poorly controlled hypothyroidism. Prior to discharge, Mr. Karpinski and his son were able to explain signs of early hypothermia, strategies for preventing hypothermia, and the importance of taking his thyroid hormone supplement every day. Social services contacted a local agency that can help Mr. Karpinski pay for his prescription medications, freeing him to pay his utility bills to maintain an acceptable environmental temperature.

CRITICAL THINKING

1. *What factors contributed to Mr. Karpinski's development of hypothermia?*
2. *The care plan focuses on the acute care of Mr. Karpinski's hypothermia. Once the client's temperature returns to normal range, what nursing care will this client require? Why will that care be required?*
3. *What client teaching (other than that mentioned in the plan of care) would the nurse initiate? Why?*
4. *Does this event indicate that Mr. Karpinski is no longer able to care for himself? Explain the assessments you would perform to reach a decision about his competence for self-care.*

Evaluation

Expected outcomes for the client with hypothermia include the following:

- The client does not exhibit piloerection or shivering.
- The client maintains core temperature within normal ranges.

- The client reports thermal comfort.
- The client describes adaptive measures to minimize fluctuations in body temperature.
- The client reports early signs and symptoms of hypothermia (Wilkinson & Ahern, 2013).

REVIEW Hypothermia

RELATE Link the Concepts and Exemplars

Linking the exemplar of hypothermia with the concept of safety:

1. When teaching a class on safety at a long-term care facility, what teaching points would the nurse discuss regarding prevention of hypothermia in the older adult client?
2. What safety measures should the nurse teach the new mother of a baby born prematurely to avoid hypothermia?

Linking the exemplar of hypothermia with the concept of addiction:

3. Why is the client who abuses alcohol at increased risk for hypothermia?
4. A client is brought to the emergency department with no pulse, an elevated blood alcohol level, and a core temperature of 31.3°C (88.4°F). What is the priority nursing action? Explain the rationale for your answer.

READY Go to Companion Skills Manual
REFER Go to Pearson Nursing Student Resources
nursing.pearsonhighered.com

- Additional review materials

REFLECT Case Study

Baby girl Cho is born at 34 weeks' gestation to Jenny and Brian Cho. This is their first child. The parents attended Lamaze classes because they wanted to deliver the baby using natural childbirth methods, and they avoided all medications during labor. The baby has made a successful transition to extrauterine life and is

breathing independently and maintaining oxygenation without assistance. After spending 30 minutes bonding with her parents, the baby is taken to the newborn nursery. The baby's axillary temperature is 34.2°C (93.6°F), and she begins to demonstrate mild substernal and intercostal retractions and nasal flaring. Her respiratory rate is 52, and her apical pulse is 148.

1. What factors may contribute to the baby's development of respiratory distress?
2. What are the priority nursing interventions for this newborn?
3. What nursing interventions would be appropriate to warm the newborn?

◼ REFERENCES

American College of Physicians. (2013). *Risk factors for hypothermia.* Retrieved from http://pier.acponline.org/physicians/public/d598/tables/d598-t1.html#.

Batra, P., & Goyal, S. (2013, January). Comparison of rectal, axillary, tympanic, and temporal artery thermometry in the pediatric emergency room. *Pediatric Emergency Care, 29*(1), 63–66. doi:10.1097/PEC.0b013e31827b5427.

Bindler, R. C., Ball, J. W., & Cowen, K. J. (2011). *Clinical skills manual for pediatric nursing: Caring for children* (5th ed.). Upper Saddle River, NJ: Prentice Hall.

Blackburn, S. T. (2012). *Maternal, fetal, & neonatal physiology: A clinical perspective* (4th ed.). St. Louis, MO: Saunders.

Cagatay, A. A., Tufan, F., Hindilerden, F., Aydin, S., Elcioglu, O. C., Karadeniz, A., . . . & Taranoglu, O. (2010). The causes of acute fever requiring hospitalization in geriatric patients: Comparison of infectious and noninfectious etiology. *Journal of Aging Research.* Retrieved from http://www.hindawi.com/journals/jar/2010/380892.

Castellani, J. W., Young, A. J., Duchame, M. B., Giesbrecht, G. G., Glickman, E., & Sallis, R. E. (2010). *Prevention of cold injuries during exercise.* Retrieved from http://www.medscape.com/viewarticle/717044_5.

Centers for Disease Control and Prevention (CDC). (2005). *Hypothermia-related deaths—United States, 2003–2004.* Retrieved from http://www.cdc.gov/mmwr/preview/mmwrhtml/mm5407a4.htm.

Centers for Disease Control and Prevention (CDC). (2010). *Study examines heat related illness in high school athletes.* Retrieved from http://www.cdc.gov/media/pressrel/2010/r100819a.htm.

Centers for Disease Control and Prevention (CDC). (2012). *Winter weather frequently asked questions.* Retrieved from http://emergency.cdc.gov/disasters/winter/faq.asp.

Centers for Disease Control and Prevention (CDC). (2013a). *CDC urges everyone: Get ready to stay cool before temperatures soar.* Retrieved from http://www.cdc.gov/media/releases/2013/p0606-extreme-heat.html.

Centers for Disease Control and Prevention (CDC). (2013b). *Quickstats: Number of hypothermia-related deaths, by sex—National Vital Statistics System, United States, 1999–2011.* Retrieved from http://www.cdc.gov/mmwr/preview/mmwrhtml/mm6151a6.htm.

Cloherty, J. P., Eichenwald, E. C., Hansen, A. R., & Stark, A. R. (2011). *Manual of neonatal care* (7th ed.). Philadelphia, PA: Lippincott Williams & Wilkins.

Cohee, L. M., Crocetti, M. T., Serwint, J. R., Sabath, B., & Kapoor, S. (2010). Ethnic differences in parental perceptions and management of childhood fever. *Clinical Pediatrics, 49*(3), 221–227. doi:10.1177/0009922809336209.

Food and Drug Administration (FDA). (2013, August). *FDA warns of rare acetaminophen risk.* Retrieved from http://www.fda.gov/downloads/ForConsumers/ConsumerUpdates/UCM363067.pdf.

Gavrielatos, G., Werner, K. D., Voridis, E., & Kremastinos, D. T. (2010, October). Contemporary practices in post-cardiac arrest syndrome: The role of mild therapeutic

hypothermia. *Therapeutic Advances in Cardiovascular Disease, 4*(5), 325–333. doi:10.1177/1753944710373786.

Graneto, J. W. (2013). Emergent management of pediatric patients with fever. *Medscape Reference.* Retrieved from http://emedicine.medscape.com/article/801598-overview.

Jefferies, S., Weatherall, M., Young, P., & Beasley, R. (2011). A systematic review of the accuracy of peripheral thermometry in estimating core temperatures among febrile critically ill patients. *Critical Care and Resuscitation, 13*(3), 194–199.

KARE. (2013). *Frostbite and hypothermia risk high as temperatures dip.* Retrieved from http://www.kare11.com/news/news_article.aspx?storyid=1007005.

Katz-Sidlow, R. J., Rowberry, J. P., & Ho, M. (2009). Fever determination in young infants: Prevalence and accuracy of parental palpation. *Pediatric Emergency Care, 25*(1), 12–14. doi:10.1097/PEC.0b013e31819dac6.

Larach, M. G., Gronert, G. A., Allen, G. C., Brandom, B. W., & Lehman, E. B. (2010). Clinical presentation, treatment, and complications of malignant hyperthermia in North America from 1987 to 2006. *Anesthesia and Analgesia, 110*(2), 498–507. doi:10.1213/ANE.0b013e3181c6b9b2.

Launey, Y., Nesseler, N., Malledant, Y., & Seguin, P. (2011). Clinical review: Fever in septic ICU patients—Friend or foe? *Critical Care, 15,* 222. doi:10.1186/cc10097.

LeMone, P., Burke, K., & Bauldoff, G. (2011). *Medical-surgical nursing: Critical thinking in client care* (5th ed.). Upper Saddle River, NJ: Pearson.

Lowes, R. (2013). Acetaminophen poses risk for rare but fatal skin reactions. *Medscape Multispecialty.* Retrieved from http://www.medscape.com/viewarticle/808807.

Malignant Hyperthermia Association of the United States. (2013). *Testing for MH.* Retrieved from http://www.mhaus.org/testing.

Mayo Clinic. (2011, November). *Heat exhaustion.* Retrieved from http://www.mayoclinic.com/health/heat-exhaustion/DS01046.

Mosby's medical dictionary. (2012). (9th ed.). St. Louis, MO: Mosby Elsevier.

National Institute of Neurological Disorders and Stroke. (2013, April). *Febrile seizures fact sheet.* Retrieved from http://www.ninds.nih.gov/disorders/febrile_seizures/detail_febrile_seizures.htm.

Nichol, G., Huszti, E., Kim, F., Fly, D., Parnia, S., Donnino, M., … & Callaway, C. W. (2013, May). Does induction of hypothermia improve outcomes after in-hospital cardiac arrest? *Resuscitation, 84*(5), 620–625. doi:10.1016/j.resuscitation.2012.12.009.

Null, J. (2013). *Heatstroke deaths of children in vehicles.* Retrieved from http://www.ggweather.com/heat.

Paul, I. M., Sturgis, S. A., Yang, C., Engle, L., Watts, H., & Berlin, C. M., Jr. (2010). Efficacy of standard doses of ibuprofen alone, alternating, and combined with acetaminophen for the treatment of febrile children. *Clinical Therapeutics, 32*(14), 2433–2440. doi:10.1016/j.clinthera.2011.01.006.

Penning, C., van der Linden, J. H., Tibboel, D., & Evenhuis, H. M. (2011, June). Is the temporal artery thermometer a reliable instrument for detecting fever in children? *Journal of Clinical Nursing, 20*(11–12), 1632–1639. doi:10.1111/j.1365-2702.2010.03568.x.

Pereira, G. L., Dagostini, J. M., & Dal Pizzol ,T. S. (2012, July). Alternating antipyretics in the treatment of fever in children: A systematic review of randomized clinical trials. *Journal of Pediatrics, 88*(4), 289–296. doi:10.2223/JPED.2204.

Poirier, M. P., Collins, E. P., & McGuire, E. (2010). Fever phobia: A survey of caregivers of children seen in a pediatric emergency department. *Clinical Pediatrics, 49*(6), 530–534. doi:10.1177/0009922809355312.

Polin, R. A., Fox, W. W., & Abman, S. H. (2010). *Fetal and neonatal physiology* (4th ed.). Philadelphia, PA: Saunders.

Porth, C. M., & Matfin, G. (2009). *Essentials of pathophysiology: Concepts of altered health states* (8th ed.). Philadelphia, PA: Lippincott Williams & Wilkins.

Purssell, E. (2011). Systematic review of studies comparing combined treatment with paracetamol and ibuprofen, with either drug alone. *Archives of Disease in Childhood, 96*(12), 1175–1179. Retrieved from http://www.ncbi.nlm.nih.gov/pubmed/21868405.

Rozance, P. J., & Rosenberg, A. A. (2012). The neonate. In S. G. Gabbe, J. R. Niebyl, H. L. Galan, E. R. M. Jauniaux, M. B. Landon, J. L. Simpson, & D. A. Driscoll (Eds.), *Obstetrics: Normal and problem pregnancies* (6th ed., p. 528). Philadelphia, PA: Saunders.

Rupe, A., & Ahlers-Schmidt, C. R. (2010). A comparison of perceptions of fever and fever phobia by ethnicity. *Clinical Pediatrics, 49*(2), 172–176. doi:10.1177/0009922809336208.

Sherman, J. M., & Sood, S. K. (2012, June). Current challenges in the diagnosis and management of fever. *Current Opinion in Pediatrics, 24*(3), 400–406. doi:10.1097/MOP.0b013e32835333e3.

Shinawi, M. (2013). Hereditary periodic fever syndromes. *Medscape Reference.* Retrieved from http://emedicine.medscape.com/article/952254-overview.

Singhal, S., Allen, M. W., McAnnally, J. R., Smith, K. S., Donnelly, J. P., & Wang, H. E. (2013). National estimates of emergency department visits for pediatric severe sepsis in the United States. *Peer Journal, 1,* e79. doi:10.7717/peerj.79.

Sullivan, J. E., Farrar, H. C., & Section on Clinical Pharmacology and Therapeutics, Committee on Drugs. (2011). Clinical report: Fever and antipyretic use in children. *Pediatrics, 127*(3), 580–587. doi:10.1542/peds.2010.3852.

Vella, C. A., & Kravitz, L. (n.d.). *Staying cool when your body is hot.* Retrieved from http://www.unm.edu/~lkravitz/Article%20folder/thermoregulation.html.

Ward, M. A. (2013). Patient information: Fever in children. *UpToDate.* Retrieved from http://www.uptodate.com/contents/fever-in-children-beyond-the-basics.

Wilkinson, J. M., & Ahern, N. R. (2013). *Nursing diagnosis handbook* (10th ed.). Upper Saddle River, NJ: Prentice Hall.

21 Tissue Integrity

◢ THE CONCEPT OF TISSUE INTEGRITY

The largest organ in the body, the skin serves a variety of important functions in maintaining health and protecting the individual from injury. The skin is part of the body's **integumentary system**, which includes the skin, hair, and nails and the sebaceous, sweat, and mammary glands. Important nursing functions are maintaining skin integrity and promoting wound healing. Impaired skin integrity—that is, alterations to the dermis and epidermis—is not a serious problem for most healthy individuals but is a threat to older adults; to clients with restricted mobility, chronic illnesses, or trauma; and to those undergoing invasive healthcare procedures. To protect the skin and manage wounds effectively, the nurse must understand the factors that affect skin integrity, the physiology of wound healing, and specific measures that promote optimal conditions for the skin.

Tissue integrity includes integumentary, mucous membrane, corneal, or subcutaneous tissues uninterrupted by wounds. Tissue integrity is influenced by internal factors such as genetics, age, and the underlying health of the individual, as well as by external factors such as activity and injury. ◀◀

Concept Learning Outcomes

After reading about this concept, you will be able to:

1. Summarize the physiology of the integumentary system related to tissue integrity.
2. Examine the relationship between tissue integrity and other concepts/systems.
3. Identify commonly occurring alterations in tissue integrity and their related therapies.
4. Differentiate common assessment procedures used to examine tissue integrity across the life span.
5. Describe diagnostic and laboratory tests to determine the individual's tissue integrity status.
6. Explain management of tissue integrity and prevention of impaired tissue integrity.
7. Demonstrate the nursing process in providing culturally competent and caring interventions across the life span for individuals with common alterations in tissue integrity.
8. Compare and contrast common independent and collaborative interventions for clients with alterations in tissue integrity.

Concept Key Terms

Alopecia, *1458*
Dermis, *1447*
Edema, *1455*
Epidermis, *1446*
Erythema, *1457*
Hirsutism, *1458*
Hypodermis, *1447*
Integumentary system, *1445*

Keratin, *1446*
Lesion, *1448*
Lichenification, *1448*
Melanin, *1446*
Pruritus, *1453*
Subcutaneous tissue, *1447*
Urticaria, *1457*

▶ NORMAL PRESENTATION OF THE SKIN

The skin performs several essential functions. It protects underlying tissues from invasion by microorganisms and from trauma. The nerves in the skin enable the perception of touch, pain, pressure, heat, and cold. The skin also assists the body in regulating its temperature. Dilation of blood vessels and the secretion of sweat by the eccrine sweat glands, functioning under the control of the central nervous system, enable the body to release excess heat. The sweat glands, secreting a solution of water, electrolytes, and urea, also help rid the body of toxins. The skin supplements the body's intake of vitamin D by synthesizing this vitamin from ultraviolet light.

Physiology Review

The skin has three distinct layers: the epidermis, the dermis, and the subcutaneous fatty layer that separates the skin from the underlying tissue (**Figure 21–1 ●**).

EPIDERMIS   The **epidermis**, which is the surface or outermost part of the skin, consists of epithelial cells. The epidermis has either four or five layers, depending on its location: five layers over the palms of the hands and the soles of the feet and four layers over the rest of the body.

The outermost layer of the epidermis, the stratum corneum, is also the thickest, making up about 75% of the total thickness of the epidermis. It consists of about 20–30 sheets of dead cells filled with keratin fragments arranged in "shingles" that flake off as dry skin. **Keratin** is a fibrous, water-repellent protein that gives the epidermis its tough, protective quality.

In areas of thick skin, such as the palms of the hands and the soles of the feet, the stratum lucidum lies below the stratum corneum. The stratum lucidum is made up of dead, flattened cells called *keratinocytes*, which produced keratin prior to their death.

The stratum granulosum is the next innermost layer and is only two to three cells thick. The cells of the stratum granulosum contain a glycolipid that slows water loss across the epidermis. Keratinization, a thickening of the cells' plasma membranes, begins in the stratum granulosum.

The next layer of the epidermis is the stratum spinosum. Several cells thick, this layer contains abundant cells that arise from the bone marrow and migrate to the epidermis. Mitosis occurs at this layer, although not as abundantly as in the deepest epidermal layer, the stratum basale.

The stratum basale contains keratinocytes and melanocytes, which are the cells that produce the pigment melanin. **Melanin** forms a shield that protects the keratinocytes and the nerve endings in the dermis from the damaging effects of ultraviolet light. Melanocyte activity probably accounts for the difference

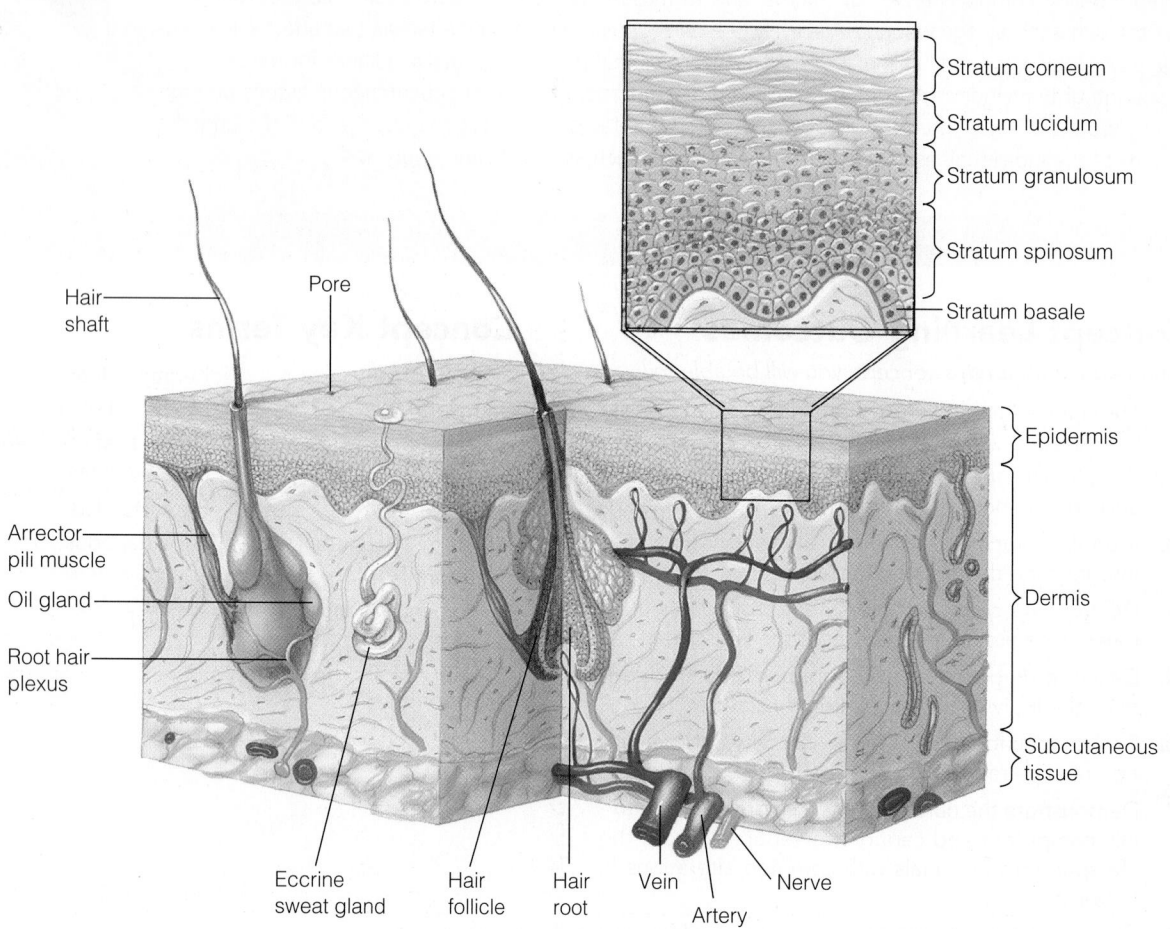

Stratum corneum
Stratum lucidum
Stratum granulosum
Stratum spinosum
Stratum basale
Epidermis
Dermis
Subcutaneous tissue

Hair shaft
Pore
Arrector pili muscle
Oil gland
Root hair plexus
Eccrine sweat gland
Hair follicle
Hair root
Vein
Artery
Nerve

Figure 21–1 ● Three-dimensional view of the skin, subcutaneous tissue, glands, and hairs.

in skin color in humans. As keratinocytes mature, they move upward through the epidermal layers, eventually becoming dead cells at the surface of the skin. Millions of these cells are worn off by abrasion each day, but millions more are simultaneously produced in the stratum basale.

DERMIS   The **dermis** is the second, deeper layer of skin. Made of a flexible connective tissue, this layer is richly supplied with blood cells, nerve fibers, and lymphatic vessels. Most of the hair follicles, sebaceous glands, and sweat glands are located in the dermis.

The dermis consists of a papillary and a reticular layer. The papillary layer contains ridges that indent the overlying epidermis. It also contains capillaries and receptors for pain and touch. The deeper, reticular layer contains blood vessels, sweat and sebaceous glands, deep pressure receptors, and dense bundles of collagen fibers. The regions between these bundles form lines of cleavage in the skin. Surgical incisions parallel to these lines of cleavage heal more easily and with less scarring than do incisions or traumatic wounds across cleavage lines.

SUBCUTANEOUS TISSUE   The **hypodermis**—more commonly known as the **subcutaneous tissue**—lies below the dermis. This layer consists of loose connective tissue and stores roughly half the fat cells in the body. Subcutaneous tissue serves as both an insulator and a cushion for the body. It also stores energy in the form of fat.

Genetic and Lifespan Considerations

The newborn's skin is covered by vernix caseosa in utero, a greasy substance containing sebum and shed cells that covers and protects the fetal skin from amniotic fluid and loss of fluids and electrolytes. It has many important properties, including anti-infective, antioxidant, moisturizing, and wound-healing agents (Singh & Archana, 2008).

The newborn's skin is between 40% and 60% thinner than an adult's skin at birth and has little underlying subcutaneous fat. As a result, the infant loses heat more rapidly, has greater difficulty regulating body temperature, and becomes chilled more quickly than an older child or an adult. The infant's thinner skin also allows increased absorption of harmful chemical substances and topical medications. It also contains more water than an adult's and has loosely attached cells. As the infant grows, the skin toughens and becomes less hydrated, so it is less susceptible to bacteria (Ball, Bindler, & Cowen, 2012).

Skin changes are a normal part of the aging process (see Table 21–1 ●); most changes occur slowly. Skin's thickness and collagen content decrease with age, causing skin to become thinner and less elastic over time. Epidermal cell turnover

TABLE 21–1   Age-Related Skin Changes

AGE-RELATED CHANGE	SIGNIFICANCE
Epidermis: ↓ thickness and miotic activity	■ Skin more fragile and at greater risk for tears or injury ■ Delayed wound healing ■ Hyperkeratoses and skin cancers in sun-exposed areas more evident
Epidermis: ↑ permeability, ↓ Langerhans cells	■ Increased risk of reactions to irritants ■ Decreased inflammatory response
Epidermis: ↓ number of active melanocytes	■ Increased susceptibility to skin damage from sun exposure
Epidermis: hyperplasia of melanocytes, especially in sun-exposed areas	■ Small areas of hyperpigmentation (liver spots) and hypopigmentation (age spots), especially on the hands
Epidermis: ↓ vitamin D production	■ Increased risk of osteomalacia and osteoporosis
Epidermis: flattened dermal-epidermal junction	■ Increased risk of skin tears, purpura, and pressure ulcers
Dermis: ↓ perfusion	■ Greater susceptibility to dry skin ■ Decreased sensation (pain, touch, temperature, and peripheral vibration) ■ Increased risk of injury
Dermis: ↓ vasomotor response	■ Greater risk of hyperthermia and hypothermia
Dermis: elastic fiber degeneration	■ Decreased tone and elasticity, with wrinkle formation
Dermis: proliferation of capillaries	■ Cherry hemangiomas common
Subcutaneous skin layer: thinning	■ Greater risk of hypothermia ■ Increased risk of pressure ulcers
Subcutaneous skin layer: redistribution of adipose tissue	■ Cellulite formation ■ Bags over and under the eyes ■ Double chin formation ■ Increase in abdominal fat ■ Sagging of breasts ■ Skin slower to return to normal when pinched (tenting)
Glands: ↓ eccrine and apocrine activity	■ Dry skin common ■ Absent perspiration

slows, and subcutaneous fat decreases and is redistributed. These variations result in a number of functional changes, including decreased sensation, increased healing time, and decreased thermoregulation (Nigam & Knight, 2008). They also give rise to wrinkled and sagging skin on the face, neck, and upper arms; these cosmetic changes often receive more attention than the functional changes, carry a social stigma, and can negatively affect self-esteem. Environmental factors such as sun exposure, chemical exposure, and nutrition can also affect skin's function and appearance.

The epidermis of the older individual is atrophic; atrophy is the result of decreased epidermal cell turnover. As a result, stratum corneum replacement slows and skin takes on a rough, dry appearance. Reduced cell turnover also has negative effects on the skin's barrier function and healing processes. In addition, surface contact between the dermal and epidermal layers decreases, causing decreased exchange of nutrients between the layers (Nigam & Knight, 2008). This decrease also leads to increased likelihood of skin tearing. Melanocyte activity, function, and distribution decrease as well. This process may cause light-skinned individuals to take on a pale complexion and may lead to uneven pigmentation and dark spots on the hands, arms, and face (Murray, Zentner, & Yakimo, 2009).

The dermis becomes thinner with aging, and fibroblasts, which produce both collagen and elastin, decrease in number. Collagen decreases and the remaining collagen becomes less organized and shows signs of degradation (Helfrich, Sachs, & Voorhees, 2010). Elastin loses quality but increases in volume. The combination of these changes causes skin to sag, wrinkle, and lose turgor. In addition, the number of dermal blood cells decreases and capillary loops shorten. These changes contribute to pale coloration, alterations in body temperature, and increased susceptibility to bruising. The loss of sensory nerve endings, in addition, changes sensations of pressure and touch and increases the likelihood of injury (Nigam & Knight, 2008).

The subcutaneous tissue loses fat during the aging process. In addition, the distribution of the remaining fat changes. This process is especially noticeable in the face and hands, which lose fat, and in the thighs and abdomen, which gain it. These changes make older individuals more prone to fractures and pressure sores over bony areas (Nigam & Knight, 2008). Changes in fat cells also contribute to problems with thermoregulation (Murray et al., 2009).

▶ ALTERATIONS TO SKIN INTEGRITY

In its role as the body's primary protective barrier, the skin is subject to a vast number of environmental agents and insults. Alterations in tissue integrity can influence the client's level of wellness in numerous areas, including immunity, infection, and mobility (see Concepts Related to Tissue Integrity).

Alterations and Manifestations

The term *intact skin* refers to the presence of normal skin and skin layers uninterrupted by wounds. The appearance of the

skin and skin integrity are influenced by internal factors such as genetics, age, and the underlying health of the individual, as well as by external factors such as activity.

SKIN DISORDERS   Skin disorders are diverse, and symptoms are often vague, such as itching, inflammation, and redness. As a result, skin disorders can be difficult to classify. One common, simple classification method groups disorders into three categories:

- ■ *Infectious.* Caused by bacterial, fungal, viral, or parasitic agents. Examples include impetigo (bacterial), athlete's foot (fungal), chickenpox (viral), and lice (parasitic).
- ■ *Inflammatory.* Caused by pathologies such as acne, burns, eczema, dermatitis, and psoriasis. Examples include atopic, seborrheic, and stasis dermatitis.
- ■ *Neoplastic.* Caused by skin cancers. Examples include squamous cell carcinoma, basal cell carcinoma, and malignant melanoma. Melanoma is the most serious type of neoplasm. (For further discussion of skin cancer, see the exemplar on Skin Cancer in the module on Cellular Regulation.)

The infectious classification covers the most diverse collection of disorders. Bacterial and viral agents are the most common causes of infectious skin disease; however, fungal infections can be especially damaging to immunocompromised clients. In addition, certain viral skin infections increase clients' likelihood of developing cancerous tumors in the genital and intestinal tracts (Marini & Hengge, 2009).

Overactive glands and increased hormone production are common in inflammatory disorders, as are itching and cracking of the skin. Interestingly, the inflammatory classification includes conditions caused by exposure to environmental stresses and injury to skin, such as sunburn; prolonged exposure to sunlight can also give rise to the cancerous cells found in neoplastic skin disorders.

Not all skin abnormalities indicate skin disorders; in fact, the skin often reflects disease processes elsewhere in the body. For example, dry skin accompanied by loss of body hair on the arms and legs can indicate hypothyroidism. Skin **lesions**, or observable changes from normal skin structure, may also indicate disorders in other systems and organs. Skin lesions vary in size, shape, color, and texture characteristics. Primary lesions arise from previously healthy skin and include macules, patches, papules, nodules, tumors, vesicles, pustules, bullae, and wheals. Secondary lesions result from changes in primary lesions. They include crusts, scales, **lichenification** (thickening of the skin), scars, keloids, excoriation, fissures, erosion, and ulcers. It is important for the nurse to be able to identify and describe the primary and secondary skin lesions and understand their underlying cause and treatment.

Primary and secondary skin lesions are described and illustrated in **Tables 21–2** ● and **21–3** ●. The terms from these tables are used throughout this module.

WOUNDS   Body wounds are either intentional or unintentional. *Intentional* trauma occurs during therapy; examples are

Concepts Related to **Tissue Integrity**

The immune system and the skin are intricately linked through their roles as protectors of the body. Impaired tissue integrity can lead to immune response. Conversely, immune responses—such as allergic reactions and inflammation—can lead to issues with tissue integrity. For example, when allergic reactions occur, they may result in contact dermatitis; the resulting discomfort may lead to scratching that leads to impaired skin integrity. When inflammation occurs, scars or abscesses may form; if healing is slow or impaired, these breaks in the skin can lead to infection.

Infection is the invasion of body tissue by microorganisms that have the potential to cause illness. Microorganisms grow on intact skin and can enter the body through a number of portals. The majority of microorganisms on the skin are harmless; however, if their growth is unchecked or if they enter the body through breaks in the skin, even normally harmless microorganisms can cause disease. These problems are further compounded if the immune system is compromised.

Clients with alterations in mobility may be at an increased risk for impaired skin integrity—and subsequently infection—as a result of pressure ulcers. Pressure ulcers are areas of skin that break down as a result of pressure on that particular area. Essentially, this pressure reduces blood flow to that area of skin, causing the skin to die. The weight of the body pressing down on areas such as the buttocks, shoulders, and elbows of bedridden clients can lead to ulcerations. Bony protuberances are particularly susceptible. Repeated irritation of the skin—as from constant friction of bed linens or moisture from urinary incontinence—can lead to ulcerations as well.

CONCEPT	RELATIONSHIP TO TISSUE INTEGRITY	NURSING IMPLICATIONS
Immunity		
■ Immune system assessment	Impaired tissue integrity triggers immune responses; immune responses can also lead to impaired tissue integrity.	■ Assess for rash and inflammation. ■ Be alert to topical and latex allergies that could worsen symptoms. ■ Be alert to abscess formation. ■ *Anticipate:* Aspirin, antipyretics, cold packs
Infection		
■ Chain of infection ■ Standard precautions ■ Infection assessment	Microorganisms grow on the skin, and breaks in the skin serve as portals for these microorganisms to enter the body.	■ Assess for complications of infectious disease. ■ Exercise infection control measures and use personal protective equipment. ■ *Anticipate:* Blood cultures, antibiotics, and isolation practices
Mobility		
■ Mobility assessment ■ Independent interventions and therapies	Impaired mobility may lead to skin breakdown and the development of pressure ulcers.	■ Assess for skin breakdown at least once per shift; pay special attention to bony prominences. ■ *Anticipate:* Repositioning, wound care, comfort measures, hygiene care, and infection control measures ■ Educate client about how to care for impaired skin.

operations or venipunctures. Although removing a tumor, for example, is therapeutic, the surgeon must cut into body tissues, thus traumatizing them. *Unintentional* wounds are accidental. For example, an individual's arm may be fractured in an automobile collision or a bicycle accident. When the tissues are traumatized without a break in the skin, the wound is closed. When the skin or mucous membrane surface is broken, the wound is open.

Wounds may be described according to how they are acquired (Table 21–4 ●). They also can be described according to the likelihood and degree of wound contamination.

■ **Clean wounds** are uninfected wounds in which minimal inflammation is encountered and the respiratory, alimentary, genital, and urinary tracts are not entered. Clean wounds are primarily closed wounds.

TABLE 21–2 Primary Skin Lesions

LESION	DESCRIPTION AND EXAMPLES	LESION	DESCRIPTION AND EXAMPLES
Macule, patch	Flat, nonpalpable change in skin color. Macules are smaller than 1 cm, with a circumscribed border, and patches are larger than 1 cm and may have an irregular border. *Examples:* Macules: freckles, measles, and petechiae. Patches: Mongolian spots, port-wine stains, vitiligo, and chloasma.	Vesicle, bulla	Elevated, fluid-filled, round or oval-shaped, palpable mass with thin, translucent walls and circumscribed borders. Vesicles are smaller than 0.5 cm; bullae are larger than 0.5 cm. *Examples:* Vesicles: herpes simplex/zoster, early chickenpox, poison ivy, and small burn blisters. Bullae: contact dermatitis, friction blisters, and large burn blisters.
Papule, plaque	Elevated, solid, palpable mass with circumscribed border. Papules are smaller than 0.5 cm; plaques are groups of papules that form lesions larger than 0.5 cm. *Examples:* Papules: elevated moles, warts, and lichen planus. Plaques: psoriasis, actinic keratosis, and lichen planus.	Wheal	Elevated, often reddish area with irregular border caused by diffuse fluid in tissues rather than free fluid in a cavity, as in vesicles. Size varies. *Examples:* Insect bites and hives (extensive wheals).
Nodule, tumor	Elevated, solid, hard or soft palpable mass extending deeper into the dermis than a papule. Nodules have circumscribed borders and are 0.5–2 cm; tumors may have irregular borders and are larger than 2 cm. *Examples:* Nodules: small lipoma, squamous cell carcinoma, fibroma, and intradermal nevi; tumors: large lipoma, carcinoma, and hemangioma.	Pustule	Elevated, pus-filled vesicle or bulla with circumscribed border. Size varies. *Examples:* Acne, impetigo, and carbuncles (large boils).
		Cyst	Elevated, encapsulated, fluid-filled or semisolid mass originating in the subcutaneous tissue or dermis, usually 1 cm or larger. *Examples:* Varieties include sebaceous cysts and epidermoid cysts.

- *Clean contaminated wounds* are surgical wounds in which the respiratory, alimentary, genital, or urinary tract has been entered. Such wounds show no evidence of infection.

- *Contaminated wounds* include open, fresh, accidental wounds and surgical wounds that involve a major break in sterile technique or a large amount of spillage from the gastrointestinal tract. Contaminated wounds show evidence of inflammation.

- *Dirty* or *infected wounds* include wounds containing dead tissue and wounds with evidence of a clinical infection, such as purulent drainage.

Wounds, excluding pressure ulcers and burns, are classified by depth, that is, the tissue layers involved in the wound (**Box 21–1 ●**).

Untreated Wounds Untreated wounds usually are seen shortly after an injury (e.g., at the scene of an accident or in an emergency center). The following are guidelines for treatment:

- Control severe bleeding by (a) applying direct pressure over the wound and (b) elevating the involved extremity.

- Prevent infection by (a) cleaning or flushing abrasions or lacerations with normal saline and (b) covering the wound with a clean dressing if possible (a sterile dressing is preferred). When applying a dressing, wrap the wound tightly enough to apply pressure, and approximate the wound edges if possible. If the first layer of dressing becomes saturated with blood, apply a second layer. Do so without removing the first layer of dressing, because removing it might disturb blood, resulting in more bleeding.

- Control swelling and pain by applying ice over the wound and surrounding tissues.

- If bleeding is severe or internal bleeding is suspected and if emergency equipment is available, assess the client for signs of shock (rapid, thready pulse; cold, clammy skin; pallor; lowered blood pressure).

TABLE 21–3   Secondary Skin Lesions

LESION	DESCRIPTION AND EXAMPLES	LESION	DESCRIPTION AND EXAMPLES
Atrophy	A translucent, dry, paperlike, sometimes wrinkled skin surface resulting from thinning or wasting of the skin due to loss of collagen and elastin. *Examples:* Striae, aged skin	Ulcer	Deep, irregularly shaped area of skin loss extending into the dermis or sub cutaneous tissue. May bleed. May leave scar. *Examples:* Decubitus ulcers (pressure sores), stasis ulcers, chancres
Erosion	Wearing away of the superficial epidermis causing a moist, shallow depression. Because erosions do not extend into the dermis, they heal without scarring. *Examples:* Scratch marks, ruptured vesicles	Fissure	Linear crack with sharp edges, extending into the dermis. *Examples:* Cracks at the corners of the mouth or in the hands, athlete's foot
Lichenification	Rough, thickened, hardened area of epidermis resulting from chronic irritation such as scratching or rubbing. *Examples:* Chronic dermatitis	Scar	Flat, irregular area of connective tissue left after a lesion or wound has healed. New scars may be red or purple; older scars may be silvery or white. *Examples:* Healed surgical wound or injury, healed acne
Scales	Shedding flakes of greasy, keratinized skin tissue. Color may be white, gray, or silver. Texture may vary from fine to thick. *Examples:* Dry skin, dandruff, psoriasis, and eczema	Keloid	Elevated, irregular, darkened area of excess scar tissue caused by excessive collagen formation during healing. Extends beyond the site of the original injury. Higher incidence in individuals of African descent. *Examples:* Keloid from ear piercing or surgery
Crust	Dry blood, serum, or pus left on the skin surface when vesicles or pustules burst. Can be red-brown, orange, or yellow. Large crusts that adhere to the skin surface are called scabs. *Examples:* Eczema, impetigo, herpes, or scabs following abrasion		

TABLE 21–4   Types of Wounds

TYPE	CAUSE	DESCRIPTION AND CHARACTERISTICS
Incision	Sharp instrument (e.g., knife or scalpel)	Open wound; deep or shallow
Contusion	Blow from a blunt instrument	Closed wound; skin appearing ecchymotic (bruised) because of damaged blood vessels
Abrasion	Surface scrape, either unintentional (e.g., scraped knee from a fall) or intentional (e.g., dermal abrasion to remove pockmarks)	Open wound involving the skin
Puncture	Penetration of the skin and often the underlying tissues by a sharp instrument, either intentional or unintentional	Open wound
Laceration	Tissues torn apart, often from accidents (e.g., with machinery)	Open wound; edges often jagged
Penetrating wound	Penetration of the skin and the underlying tissues, usually unintentional (e.g., from a bullet or metal fragments)	Open wound

- *Partial thickness.* Confined to the skin, that is, the dermis and epidermis; heal by regeneration.
- *Full thickness.* Involving the dermis, epidermis, subcutaneous tissue, and possibly muscle and bone; require connective tissue repair.

Treated Wounds   Treated or sutured wounds usually need to be observed for determination of the progress of healing. These wounds may be inspected when a dressing is changed. If the wound itself cannot be directly inspected, the dressing is inspected and other data regarding the wound (e.g., the presence of pain) are assessed. See the exemplar on Wound Healing in this module for more information.

Prevalence

Skin disorders are common among the U.S. population; in fact, an estimated one in three individuals in the United States has a skin disorder at any given time (Davila, Christenson, & Sontheimer, 2010). Some of the most common disorders in the general population are dermatitis, inflammatory reactions to topical drugs, and infectious diseases of the skin. Acne is one of the most common skin disorders, affecting approximately 45–50 million Americans; close to 100% of adolescents have at least mild acne. Other common skin diseases include contact dermatitis (72.3 million), hair and nail disorders (70.5 million), herpes simplex/herpes zoster (165 million), warts (58.5 million), seborrheic keratosis (83.8 million), and damage from solar radiation (123.1 million). Skin disorders also include fungal infections (29.4 million), rosacea (14.7 million), psoriasis (3.1 million), and skin ulcers and wounds (4.8 million; SID & AADA, 2006). Skin cancer is the most common form of cancer in the United States; an estimated 61,646 individuals were diagnosed with and 9,199 individuals died from melanoma in 2009, the most recent year for which the Centers for Disease Control and Prevention (CDC) has statistics (CDC, 2012).

Genetic Considerations and Nonmodifiable Risk Factors

Genetics affects an individual's likelihood of developing skin disorders; having one or both parents, siblings, or other closely related family members with a particular disorder increases an individual's likelihood of also developing that disorder. Skin conditions often occur as part of a genetically related metabolic disorder or a disease that affects multiple body systems (Uitto, 2012). Heritable skin disorders include epidermolysis bullosa (a blistering disorder), ichthyosis (a disorder in which the skin becomes thick and scaly), and albinism (a disorder in which too little melanin is produced). Ethnicity and age are also nonmodifiable risk factors for a number of skin diseases.

Gender and age also play a role in the development of some skin disorders. Men are generally more affected by infectious skin disorders, while women more commonly experience pigmentary and autoimmune disorders (Chen et al., 2010). The underlying causes of these differences are hard to pinpoint, but research suggests a correlation with sex hormones. In addition, as the amount of sex hormones decreases with age, the changes in skin thickness, surface pH, and quality of wound healing make older adults more susceptible to a number of skin disorders (Dao & Kazin, 2007).

Skin color also determines an individual's risk for certain skin disorders. Keloids, pseudofolliculitis, and dermatosis papulosa nigra are more common among clients with dark skin tones, and conditions such as vitiligo and depigmentation are more difficult to treat among this population. In addition, psoriasis, atopic dermatitis, and eczema present differently in clients with dark skin tones than in clients with light skin tones (Ogunyemi, 2011). While darker toned skin is less susceptible to sun damage, all types and tones of skin can be damaged by exposure to ultraviolet light. It is important, therefore, to encourage all clients to use sunscreen, cover their heads, and wear protective clothing whenever possible outdoors to prevent sunburn and the future development of skin cancer.

CASE STUDY \\ PART 1

Arthur Sullivan is a 52-year-old Caucasian male who was scheduled for neurosurgery to remove a pituitary tumor. Mr. Sullivan is a large man, standing 6'3" tall and weighing 342 pounds. After surgery, an external ventricular drainage device was inserted to prevent cerebrospinal fluid accumulation at the surgical site to promote healing. Upon the surgeon's orders, Mr. Sullivan must remain on restricted mobility in a supine position at a 20-degree angle or less for 3 days after surgery. Because of his restricted mobility, intermittent pneumatic compression pumps are placed on his legs to stimulate blood flow. However, because of Mr. Sullivan's large size, the pumps do not fit well even though they are the largest size available in the ICU.

Two days after surgery, Mr. Sullivan develops deep vein thrombosis in his left leg. Because it is too soon after surgery to administer anticoagulant or thrombolytic drugs, the physician decides that the best course of treatment is insertion of an inferior vena cava filter to prevent thromboses from traveling to the lungs, heart, and brain. As the filter clogs with additional blood clots, Mr. Sullivan experiences severe edema in both legs. In spite of continued use of the compression pumps, Mr. Sullivan does not obtain relief from the edema. One week after surgery, he is placed on IV heparin (titrated to a PTT of 60) to prevent further DVT. Three days after the heparin regimen has been initiated, Mr. Sullivan calls the nurse because his lower left leg has suddenly started "squirting blood." Upon inspection, the nurse finds that a varicose vein has ruptured over Mr. Sullivan's mid tibia.

Clinical Reasoning Questions Level I

1. What assessment techniques are required to determine the source of the bleeding?
2. What are the immediate nursing priorities for Mr. Sullivan?
3. What risk factors does Mr. Sullivan have for developing edema after insertion of the IVC filter?

Clinical Reasoning Questions Level II

4. What factors may have contributed to the rupture of a vein?
5. Once the bleeding is controlled, what responsibilities does the nurse have in caring for Mr. Sullivan's wound?
6. What additional nursing interventions should have been implemented after surgery to prevent blood clots and edema?

Alterations and Therapies **Tissue Integrity**

ALTERATION	DESCRIPTION/ DEFINITION	MANIFESTATIONS	INTERVENTIONS AND TREATMENTS
Impaired skin integrity	Disruption or damage to the epidermal and/or dermal layers of skin as a result of a cut, scrape, burn, or other injury	▪ Open wound of varying severity, depth, and size (e.g., incision, severe burn, ulcer) ▪ Closed wound affecting the superficial (e.g., sunburn) or deeper (e.g., bruise) layers of skin ▪ Changes in skin color, especially after burn	▪ Cleanse wound. ▪ Close open wounds with sutures or staples if edges can be approximated. ▪ Use moist wound management. ▪ Apply sterile bandage. ▪ Apply ointment, cream, or gel as prescribed. ▪ Promote good nutrition and fluid intake; administer enteral or parenteral nutrition or IV fluids as ordered. ▪ Refer to a nutritionist or dietician if needed. ▪ Monitor for infection and other complications.
Pain	Discomfort related to impaired skin integrity	▪ Acute pain at the site of injury ▪ Pain rating of higher than 1 on a 0–10 scale ▪ Elevated blood pressure ▪ Increased heart rate ▪ Anxiety ▪ Decreased ability to perform ADL	▪ Opioid or nonopioid analgesics ▪ Nonpharmacologic pain management techniques (e.g., relaxation, distraction)
Inflammation	Innate immune response to tissue damage or foreign organisms or particles	▪ Pain ▪ Redness ▪ Swelling ▪ Heat ▪ Impaired function	▪ Heat/ice ▪ Compression ▪ Analgesics ▪ Movement/exercise
Infection	Invasion of the wound with microorganisms such as bacteria, viruses, fungi, or parasites	▪ Inflammation ▪ Purulent drainage ▪ Foul smell ▪ Elevated body temperature ▪ Impaired oxygenation (if infection is in the lungs) ▪ Restlessness ▪ Fatigue ▪ Sweating/chills	▪ Obtain culture of wound exudate for sensitivity testing. ▪ Treat with topical or oral antibiotics as prescribed. ▪ If not bacterial infection, administer other anti-infective agents as needed. ▪ Debride wound. ▪ Use good wound hygiene. ▪ Administer antipyretics as ordered. ▪ Provide cool compress or blankets as needed.
Pruritus	Itching of the skin	▪ Rash ▪ Redness ▪ Rough, dry skin ▪ Scaly skin	▪ Administer medications as ordered: ▪ Topical or oral corticosteroids ▪ Antihistamines ▪ Topical anesthetics

(continued on next page)

Alterations and Therapies **Tissue Integrity** (*continued*)

ALTERATION	DESCRIPTION/ DEFINITION	MANIFESTATIONS	INTERVENTIONS AND TREATMENTS
			▪ Apply soothing lotions or creams to affected site. ▪ Teach client to avoid scratching. ▪ Monitor for open wounds caused by scratching. ▪ Monitor for infection. ▪ Apply cool compresses or give a cool bath. ▪ Avoid substances that stimulate pruritus (e.g., perfumes, soaps, jewelry).
Eschar	Hard crust covering an open wound consisting of dried plasma proteins and dead cells	▪ Leathery and rigid crust over wound ▪ Circumferential constriction of the torso or extremity ▪ Gangrene (severe cases)	▪ Removal by debridement ▪ Escharotomy ▪ Hydrotherapy
Edema	Fluid accumulation under the skin	▪ Swelling ▪ Spongy or boggy skin upon palpation ▪ Increased compartment pressure ▪ Pitting upon pressure ▪ In lungs: ▪ Atelectasis ▪ Labored breathing ▪ Stridor	▪ Elevate edematous area. ▪ Apply compression to stimulate blood flow (contraindicated if pressure will cut off blood flow). ▪ Administer diuretics (contraindicated in clients at risk for deficient fluid volume). ▪ Maintain patent airway ▪ Ensure adequate fluid intake. ▪ Monitor fluid intake and output ▪ Use vacuum-assisted closure.
Exudate	Fluid drainage from a wound	▪ Clear or straw-colored exudate (serous) ▪ Milky exudate full of cells and necrotic debris (purulent); color may be blue, green, or yellow ▪ Bright or dark red exudate containing red blood cells (sanguineous)	▪ Cleanse exudate from wound. ▪ Cover with sterile, absorptive bandage. ▪ Collect purulent exudate for culture. ▪ Apply antibacterial ointments as prescribed. ▪ Apply pressure to bleeding wound, or cover with pro-coagulant bandage.
Bruising	Bleeding underneath the epidermal layer of skin caused by broken blood vessels or capillaries	▪ Discoloration of skin at the site of injury ("black-and-blue," red, or purple for fresh bruises, yellow or green for older bruises) ▪ Discomfort upon movement or pressure	▪ Apply ice to bruised area. ▪ Administer analgesics if ordered. ▪ Most bruises heal on their own with no treatment.

▶ PREVENTION

Skin disorders can cause intense pain and discomfort for clients and can affect their overall health and self-concept. Many of these disorders are preventable; even individuals with genetic predispositions for certain disorders can benefit from taking simple preventive measures.

Modifiable Risk Factors

Proper skin care and maintenance are important for preventing many infectious disorders, especially for clients with compromised immune systems, diabetes, HIV/AIDS, or obesity. Skin should be kept clean, dry, and moisturized; when wounds occur, they should be kept clean and covered to decrease the risk of infection. Children and others who are in close contact in a community setting should be coached to avoid sharing personal items—such as combs, brushes, and hats—with others to decrease the likelihood of parasitic transfer.

Risk for inflammatory disorders can be decreased through avoidance of irritants or allergens known to inflame clients' skin, such as harsh chemical cleaners and certain metals. Skin should be kept clean, but excessive cleansing should be avoided as it can cause the skin to become overly dry. Use of moisturizers may also be helpful. Parents of children in diapers should be taught proper diaper-area care and coached to change wet or soiled diapers as soon as the parent becomes aware of them.

Many chronic illnesses and their treatments increase the risk for impaired skin integrity. Impaired peripheral arterial circulation in the lower extremities may produce skin that appears shiny, has lost its hair distribution, and damages easily. Some medications, such as corticosteroids, cause thinning of the skin, making it much more easily harmed. Many medications increase sensitivity to sunlight and can predispose the individual to severe sunburns. Some of the most common medications that cause this kind of damage are certain antibiotics, chemotherapy drugs for cancer, and some psychotherapeutic drugs. Poor nutrition alone can also interfere with the appearance and function of normal skin.

Screenings

All clients benefit from regular self-examination of the skin. The benefits of these examinations are twofold: Clients are able identify and recognize problems as they occur, and clients develop a familiarity with their skin. This familiarity makes it easier for clients to identify changes (such as the appearance of new wounds in clients with diabetic neuropathy). Examinations should focus on areas that receive the most exposure to sunlight and toxins: the face, neck, ears, scalp, arms, and legs. The trunk, chest, and feet should also be examined.

Next to self-examinations of the skin, professional examinations are perhaps the most common screening method for identifying skin disorders. During a professional examination, a physician—often a dermatologist—conducts a head-to-toe inspection of the skin and identifies any problem areas. Diagnostic tests—such as biopsy, cultures, and patch tests—are ordered on the basis of these findings. These and other common diagnostic tests are discussed in detail later in the module.

▶ ASSESSMENT

General physical assessment always includes the integumentary system. Even when providing routine care, such as assisting with personal hygiene, the nurse should be alert to skin abnormalities. Antiembolic stockings, braces, or other medical or assistive devices must be removed for assessment of the skin condition underneath. Detection of variations in skin color and identification of lesions require good lighting.

Nursing Assessment

During the review of systems as part of the history, the nurse obtains information about skin diseases, previous bruising, general skin condition, skin lesions, and usual healing of sores. Inspection and palpation of the skin focus on determining skin color distribution, skin turgor, presence of **edema** (swelling caused by excess fluid trapped in bodily tissue; see **Figure 21–2 ●**), and characteristics of any lesions that are

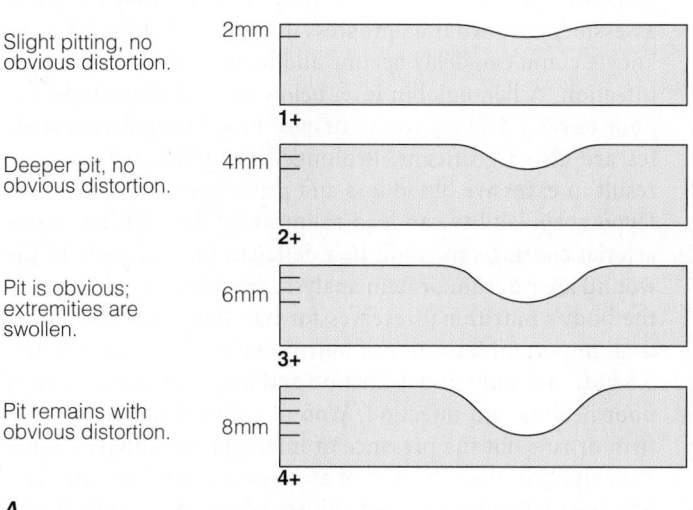

Slight pitting, no obvious distortion. 2mm 1+

Deeper pit, no obvious distortion. 4mm 2+

Pit is obvious; extremities are swollen. 6mm 3+

Pit remains with obvious distortion. 8mm 4+

A

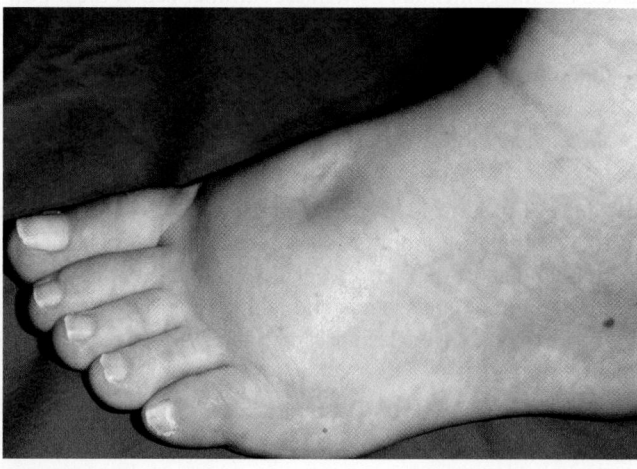

B

Figure 21–2 ● *A,* Degrees of pitting in edema. *B,* 4+ pitting.
Source: B, Dr. P. Marazzi/Science Photo Library/Photo Researchers, Inc.

Assessment Interview Skin and Tissue Integrity

Following are questions the nurse asks in assessing the client's skin and tissue integrity:

- Do you have a history of skin problems? If so, what were the problems and when did they occur?
- If the problems were acute, have they ever recurred? If the problems were chronic, how are you currently managing them?
- What treatments have been effective for previous skin problems?
- Are lesions, sores, ulcers, or rashes on your skin slow to heal?
- When did you first notice your current skin problem? Where did it originate? Where and when did it spread?
- Is your skin problem accompanied by other symptoms, such as fever or chills?
- Do you notice the problems occurring after exposure to certain chemicals, toxins, items of clothing, or items of jewelry?
- Have you recently switched soap, shampoo, detergent, or moisturizer, or started taking new medications? Has your diet changed recently?

- Have you traveled or been exposed to extreme temperatures recently?
- Have you noticed any drainage from affected areas? If so, what did it look and smell like?
- How frequently is your skin exposed to direct sunlight? Do you take proper protective measures—such as sunscreens, protective clothing, and hats—during exposure?
- How does your skin react to sun exposure? Does it burn or become red easily? Have you ever developed blisters as a result of exposure?
- Do you have any tattoos, piercings, or brands? How long have you had your tattoos, piercings, or brands, and have you ever noticed any skin problems in those areas?
- Have you noticed any long-term changes in your skin over the past few years?
- Are you under a high level of stress, or have you ever experienced intermittent or prolonged anxiety?
- Do your skin problems negatively affect your personal or social relationships in any way?

present. Particular attention is paid to skin condition in areas that are most likely to break down: in skin folds such as under the breasts; in areas that are frequently moist, such as the perineum; and in areas that receive extensive pressure, such as the bony prominences.

Diagnostic Tests

The results of diagnostic tests of the structure and function of the integumentary system are used to support the diagnosis of a specific injury or disease. Diagnostic tests also provide information used to identify or modify the appropriate medications or treatments for the disease and help the nurse monitor the client's responses to nursing care interventions. Diagnostic tests to assess the integumentary system are summarized in the following list:

- One of the most common diagnostic tests is a skin biopsy, which is used to differentiate a benign skin lesion from a skin cancer. Skin biopsies can be obtained by a punch technique, incision, excision, or shaving.
- Cultures used to identify infections may be conducted on tissue samples, on drainage and exudate (material, such as fluid and cells, that has escaped from blood vessels during the inflammatory process and is deposited in tissue or on tissue surfaces) from lesions, and (if an illness is generalized) on serum.
- Tests that are used to identify infections include immunofluorescent studies, Wood lamp, potassium hydroxide, and the Tzanck test.
- Patch tests or scratch tests may be used to determine allergies.

Some studies are conducted to identify bacterial carriers. For example, if clients have repeated bacterial skin infections or if a healthcare unit or agency experiences numerous bacterial infections of clients, nasal cultures may be performed to determine whether the clients or healthcare workers are carriers of the bacteria. Regardless of the type of diagnostic test, the nurse is responsible for explaining the procedure to the client; explaining any special preparation needed, including fasting or avoiding allergy medications prior to testing; assessing for medication use that may affect the outcome of the tests; supporting the client during the examination as necessary; documenting the procedures as appropriate; and monitoring the results of the tests.

Laboratory data can also support the nurse's clinical assessment of a wound's progress in healing. A decreased leukocyte count can delay healing and increase the possibility of infection. A hemoglobin level below normal range indicates poor oxygen delivery to the tissues. Blood coagulation studies are also significant. Prolonged coagulation times can result in excessive blood loss and prolonged clot absorption. Hypercoagulability can lead to intravascular clotting. Intraarterial clotting can result in a deficient blood supply to the wound area. Serum protein analysis provides an indication of the body's nutritional reserves for rebuilding cells. Albumin is an important indicator of nutritional status. A value below 3.5 g/dL indicates poor nutrition and may increase the risk of poor healing and infection. Wound cultures can either confirm or rule out the presence of infection. Sensitivity studies are helpful in the selection of appropriate antibiotic therapy. The nurse obtains a wound culture whenever an infection is suspected.

Integumentary Assessment

ASSESSMENT/METHOD	NORMAL FINDINGS	ABNORMAL FINDINGS	LIFESPAN OR DEVELOPMENTAL CONSIDERATIONS
General Assessment			
Inspect the skin color and note any odors coming from the skin.	Skin color should be even, appropriate to the age and race of the client, and without foul odors.	■ A strong odor of perspiration may indicate poor hygiene. ■ A foul odor may indicate a disorder of the sweat glands. ■ Pallor or cyanosis is seen with exposure to cold and with decreased perfusion and oxygenation. ■ Redness, swelling, and pain are seen with various rashes, inflammations, infections, and burns. ■ First-degree burns cause areas of **erythema** (redness of the skin) and swelling; second-degree burns cause red, painful blisters; third-degree burns cause white or blackened areas. ■ Abnormal loss of melanin in patches of the face, hands, or groin may indicate the autoimmune disorder vitiligo.	■ Hormone fluctuations during pregnancy may cause skin discoloration, which is more pronounced in women with darker skin tones. In most cases, the discoloration resolves itself postpartum without treatment. Oral contraceptives causes similar discoloration in some women.
Assessment of Skin With Impaired Integrity			
Inspect skin for lesions and alterations, including calluses, scars, tattoos, and piercings. Include inspection of skin creases and folds.	Skin should be intact without abnormal lesions.	■ Primary, secondary, and vascular lesions. ■ Pearly edged nodules with a central ulcer may indicate basal cell carcinoma. ■ Scaly, red, fast-growing papules may indicate squamous cell carcinoma. ■ Dark, asymmetrical, multicolored patches with irregular edges may indicate malignant melanoma. ■ Circular lesions may indicate ringworm or tinea versicolor. ■ Grouped vesicles may be seen in contact dermatitis. ■ Linear lesions may indicate poison ivy or herpes zoster. ■ In herpes zoster, vesicles appear along sensory nerve paths, turn into pustules, and crust over. ■ **Urticaria** (also known as hives) appears as patches of pale, itchy wheals in an erythematous area. ■ In psoriasis, scaly red patches appear on the scalp, knees, back, and genitals. ■ Bruises in various stages of healing may be indicators of trauma or abuse.	■ Some skin conditions, such as psoriasis, eczema, and atopic dermatitis, are more difficult to diagnose in darker skin. If undiagnosed or treated improperly, lesions can darken. These dark spots often remain for years. ■ Pseudofolliculitis barbae (razor bumps) is common in individuals who have darker skin or curly hair. In some cases, this condition results in scarring, infection, and keloid formation.
Skin Temperature Assessment			
Palpate skin temperature.	Skin should be warm.	■ Warm, red skin indicates inflammation and elevated body temperature. ■ Decreased skin temperature indicates decreased blood flow to the skin; may be generalized (as in shock) or localized (as in arteriosclerosis).	■ Temperature regulation in infants is inefficient, and skin may feel warm or cool in the absence of inflammation or decreased blood flow.

(continued on next page)

Integumentary Assessment (continued)

ASSESSMENT/METHOD	NORMAL FINDINGS	ABNORMAL FINDINGS	LIFESPAN OR DEVELOPMENTAL CONSIDERATIONS
Skin Texture Assessment			
Palpate skin moisture.	Skin should be dry.	■ Excessively dry skin may be present in older adults and clients with hypothyroidism. ■ Oily skin may be present in adolescents and young adults; finding may be normal or may indicate a skin disorder like acne vulgaris. ■ Excessive perspiration may be associated with shock, fever, increased activity, or anxiety.	■ In darker skin tones, an ashy appearance indicates excessive dryness.
Skin Turgor Assessment			
Palpate skin turgor. Pinch skin gently over the sternum or collarbone.	Skin fold should return rapidly to the normal positions.	■ Skin turgor is decreased in dehydration. It is increased in edema and scleroderma.	■ Tenting, in which the skin remains pinched for a few moments before resuming its normal position, is common among thin older adults.
Edema Assessment			
Assess edema by depressing the client's skin (see Figure 21–2) Record findings on a four point scale: ■ 1+: Slight pitting, no obvious distortion ■ 2+: Deeper pit, no obvious distortion ■ 3+: Pit is obvious; extremities are swollen ■ 4+: Pit remains with obvious distortion	No edema should be present.	■ Edema commonly occurs in cardiovascular disorders, renal failure, and cirrhosis of the liver.	■ Edema is a side effect of some medications, including calcium channel blockers, NSAIDS, and estrogens. Pregnant women may also exhibit mild edema.
Assessment of Hair Distribution and Quality			
	Hair should be evenly distributed for client's gender.	■ **Alopecia** (hair loss) may be related to changes in hormones, chemical or drug treatment, or radiation. ■ **Hirsutism** (increased growth of coarse hair on the face and trunk) is seen in Cushing syndrome, acromegaly, and ovarian dysfunction. ■ A deviation in normal hair distribution in the genital area may indicate an endocrine disorder.	■ In adult males whose hair loss follows the normal male pattern, the cause is usually genetic. ■ Excess hair is a common problem for individuals with darker skin; laser hair removal should be used cautiously, because certain types of lasers cause changes in skin pigment.

Integumentary Assessment (continued)

ASSESSMENT/METHOD	NORMAL FINDINGS	ABNORMAL FINDINGS	LIFESPAN OR DEVELOPMENTAL CONSIDERATIONS
Hair Texture Assessment			
Palpate hair texture.	Hair should be of even texture.	■ Systemic diseases cause changes to the texture of the hair. ■ Hypothyroidism causes the hair to coarsen. ■ Hyperthyroidism causes the hair to become fine.	■ Gradual changes in hair texture normally occur across the life span. Infants have fine soft hair that thickens in diameter through childhood and adolescence. During middle and old age, the diameter gradually decreases, and hair becomes finer again.
Scalp Assessment			
Inspect the scalp for lesions.	There should be no lesions on the scalp.	■ Mild dandruff is normal, but excessive or greasy flakes indicate seborrhea. ■ Hair loss, pustules, and scales appear on the scalp in tinea capitis. ■ Red, swollen pustules that appear around infected hair follicles indicate folliculitis. ■ Head lice may be seen as oval nits adhering to the base of the hair shaft. Head lice are usually accompanied by itching.	■ Head lice are common among children but may be particularly embarrassing for those in late elementary school or middle school. Children in this age group may be subject to ridicule by their peers.
Nail Assessment			
Inspect nail curvature.	Nail surfaces should be smooth and nail folds firm, without redness.	■ Inflammation and transverse rippling of the nail are associated with chronic paronychia and/or eczema. ■ The nail plate may separate from the nail bed in trauma, psoriasis, and *Pseudomonas* and *Candida* infections. This separation is called *oncolysis*. ■ Nail grooves may be caused by inflammation, planus, or nail biting. ■ Nail pitting may be seen with psoriasis. ■ A transverse groove (Beau line) may be seen in trachoma or acute disease. ■ Thin, spoon-shaped nails are common in anemia.	■ Spoon-shaped concave nails occur normally in young children and usually resolve themselves with age.
Inspection of Nail Color			
	Nail color should be even.	■ The sudden appearance of a pigmented band may indicate melanoma in Caucasians. ■ Yellowish nails are seen in psoriasis and fungal infections. ■ Dark nails occur with trauma, *Candida* infections, and hyperbilirubinemia. ■ Blackish-green nails are apparent in injury and in *Pseudomonas* infection. ■ Red splinter longitudinal hemorrhages may be seen in injury and/or psoriasis.	■ Pigmented bands are normally found in more than 90% of African Americans. ■ Certain foods, chemicals, and nail polishes can stain the nails yellow; this condition may be particularly noticeable in individuals who wear nail polish the majority of the time.

(continued on next page)

Integumentary Assessment (continued)

ASSESSMENT/METHOD	NORMAL FINDINGS	ABNORMAL FINDINGS	LIFESPAN OR DEVELOPMENTAL CONSIDERATIONS
Inspection of Nail Thickness			
	Nails should not be excessively thick.	■ Trauma to the nails usually causes thickening. Other causes of thick nails include psoriasis, fungal infections, and decreased peripheral vascular blood supply.	■ Thickening of the nails is common in older clients and not necessarily indicative of disease in this population.

Focus on Diversity and Culture

Skin Color

- Skin color and skin care are emotionally charged subjects for many clients, as is exposure of skin through either removal of clothing or removal of makeup. It is imperative that the nurse be sensitive to these emotions when discussing clients' skin conditions and care regimens and when examining the skin itself.

- Variations in skin color are tied to the amount of melanin in the skin. In general, individuals with light skin tones produce less melanin than individuals with dark skin tones. Melanin helps protect skin from UV damage, and the darkest skin tones are found in individuals from the hottest climates or whose ancestors lived in the hottest climates.

- Because increased melanin levels make darker toned skin less susceptible to problems associated with overexposure, some clients may mistakenly believe they are not at risk of developing skin cancer. All clients, regardless of skin tone, should understand the risks and be coached on preventive measures.

- Dark skin tones differ from light skin tones in terms of certain biological characteristics, such as sebum production. These differences tend to make dark skin more prone to inflammation than light skin. Therefore topical medications that are effective in treating certain disorders in lighter toned skin may be too harsh to treat the same conditions in darker toned skin (Davis & Callendar, 2010).

- Many mainstream skin and hair care products do not adequately address the health needs of culturally diverse clients. As a result, clients may rely on home remedies and alternative products that contain ingredients like olive oil, honey, or lemon juice; some of these remedies and products are culturally significant. It is important to understand individual clients' skin care regimens and the potential impact of these regimens on medical treatments.

- The increased amount of pigment in darker toned skin makes it prone to discoloration in areas where lesions have healed. In addition, clients with darker skin tones are prone to a condition called *melasma*, in which too much melanin is produced, causing discolored patches on the face. Clients may be sensitive or embarrassed about these areas and seek to cover them with make up or treat them with bleaching creams. These treatments may irritate the skin or negatively interact with topical medications (Davis & Callendar, 2010).

CASE STUDY \\ PART 2

Because of Mr. Sullivan's complications, his hospital stay extends to 8 weeks. His surgical site is healing well, and he is no longer on restricted mobility. Mr. Sullivan is undergoing physical therapy to regain his ability to walk after the extended bed rest and edema. Treatment to reduce edema in his legs includes elevation of his legs; compression stockings (custom-fit stockings have been ordered and fit well); furosemide 80 mg, 4 times daily; and sustained ambulation of 15 minutes or more at least three times daily. Edema has steadily decreased over the weeks but is still significant. He is now on oral warfarin 4 mg daily (adjusted to maintain PT of 1.5) to prevent additional DVT.

Over the 6 weeks since his varicose vein ruptured, Mr. Sullivan has been diagnosed with chronic venous disease. He has experienced four episodes of hemorrhage from the site, and bleeding is difficult to stop because of the anticoagulant he is taking for DVT. The site of rupture has developed into a grade C6 (open venous ulcer) on the CEAP venous disease scale. The ulcer is 2.8 cm long, 2.3 cm wide, and 0.6 cm deep. When the ulcer is not bleeding profusely, it is exuding a dark reddish-brown serosanguineous fluid. No signs of infection are present. The surrounding skin has turned purple in an area approximately 19 cm long and 11 cm wide. However, there is no sign of additional ulceration in the area. Daily care of the wound includes cleansing the area with sterile saline and applying an alginate dressing and topical sucralfate. The wound site is then wrapped in an elastic bandage, and the compression stocking is placed over the top.

Clinical Reasoning Questions Level I

1. What nursing assessments are necessary to monitor the status of the venous ulcer?
2. Why has the skin around the venous ulcer turned purple?
3. Based on the location and dimensions of Mr. Sullivan's ulcer, which layers of skin may be affected? What implications does this have for any symptoms he may experience and how the ulcer should be treated?

Clinical Reasoning Questions Level II

4. How would Mr. Sullivan's nursing plan change if the ulcer develops an infection?
5. What other treatments are available to help heal the venous ulcer?

6. Mr. Sullivan's case is complicated because he needs both anticoagulation to prevent DVT and procoagulation to prevent hemorrhage of the ulcer. Which treatment is a higher priority for Mr. Sullivan at this point in his healing process? Why?

▶ INTERVENTIONS AND THERAPIES

Medical and nursing management of alterations in tissue integrity is based on the cause and severity of the condition. The goals of treatment are to control the severity of the disease, prevent infection, and promote healing. Palliative care may also be necessary, depending on the severity of the problem and the level of discomfort it presents for the client.

Independent

The nurse should ask questions to determine whether the client is doing anything at home to relieve discomfort that could unintentionally inhibit healing. The nurse should also provide information about home remedies that may provide comfort while promoting healing.

Where appropriate, the nurse should teach the client about good hygiene, that is, daily bathing for the purpose of keeping skin clean and free of odors. Children and older adults may need to bathe only every other day. Because soap can cause the skin to become dry, the client should be encouraged to rinse thoroughly; liquid cleansers may be appropriate rather than bar soap for individuals with very dry skin. Use of moisturizing lotions after bathing should also be encouraged.

The client with impaired skin integrity or chronic skin conditions should be taught infection prevention measures. These include proper cleaning and dressing of wounds; use of antibiotic ointments on wounds may also be appropriate. The client should be taught proper hand washing technique and instructed to wash the hands before and after touching the wound; the client should also be taught how to properly dispose of soiled dressings. In addition, the nurse should teach the client how to recognize a wound that has become infected or necrotic and emphasize the importance of contacting a healthcare provider if infection occurs.

Exercise and nutrition should also be emphasized. Exercise improves blood flow and is important for maintaining overall well-being. Clients who are bedridden and susceptible to pressure ulcers should do simple exercises appropriate to their condition that can be performed while seated or lying down. Proper nutrition is also important for wound healing. During the healing process, the body requires increased amounts of calories, proteins, and vitamins A and C (Cleveland Clinic, 2013). Eating a variety of foods—including whole grains, leafy vegetables, citrus fruits, fortified dairy products, and lean proteins—enables the client to get these vitamins and minerals. If the client has difficulty consuming the necessary calories and nutrients in three large meals per day, the nurse should encourage the client to eat smaller, more frequent meals or healthy snacks between meals. Nutritional supplements and multivitamins may also be appropriate for some clients.

Collaborative

In some cases, treatment of skin disorders requires pharmacologic therapy. Over-the-counter medications are suitable for less serious conditions, such as lice infestation, minor sunburns, and mild to moderate acne. The majority of over-the-counter medications are topical; the efficacy of these medications depends upon the severity of the disorder, the client's skin type, and the client's skin care practices. For example, there are a variety of over-the-counter acne medications on the market with active ingredients ranging from benzoyl peroxide to salicylic acid to sulfur; these ingredients may effectively treat acne in some clients but cause excessive dryness, redness, or burning sensations in others.

More serious disorders, such as eczema, dermatitis, and psoriasis, often require extensive or prolonged prescription therapy. These regimens are used under a doctor's supervision and may include a combination of oral and topical preparations. In some cases, alternative therapies are used to complement prescriptions regimens The Medications feature provides information about the different classes and actions of drugs used to treat skin disorders.

Medications **Tissue Integrity**

CLASSIFICATION AND DRUG EXAMPLES	MECHANISM OF ACTION	NURSING CONSIDERATIONS
Topical Corticosteroids ▪ alcometasone ▪ amcinonide ▪ betamethasone ▪ clobetasol ▪ clocortolone ▪ difluorasone ▪ desonide ▪ desoximetasone ▪ fluocinolone ▪ fluocinonide ▪ halcinonide ▪ hydrocortisone ▪ mometasone ▪ triamcinolone	Relieve inflammatory and pruritic manifestations of corticosteroid-responsive dermatoses. *May also be used for:* —Immunosuppression	▪ Encourage the client to apply a thin layer of medication after bathing. ▪ Advise the client against self-diagnosis and treatment with OTC preparations for more than 7 days. ▪ Monitor for skin thinning and atrophy, acne, hypo- and hyperpigmentation, and allergic reaction; these effects are more severe on areas of thin skin, such as the face. ▪ Assess for systemic toxicity in small children; do not use in children younger than 2.

(continued on next page)

Medications **Tissue Integrity** (continued)

CLASSIFICATION AND DRUG EXAMPLES	MECHANISM OF ACTION	NURSING CONSIDERATIONS
Drug examples: Alclovate, Cyclocort, Diproline, Clobex, Cloderm, Florone, Tridesilon, Topicort, Fluoderm, Vanos, Halog, Cetacort, Elocon, Triderm		
Antiacne ■ adapalene ■ tazarotene ■ tretinoin **Drug examples:** Differin, Tazorac, Avita	Promote cell turnover and prevent blocking of follicles. May be used in combination with antibiotics. *May also be used for:* —Treatment of plaque psoriasis —Treatment of hypo- and hyperpigmentation	■ Advise the client that acne may worsen during the initial weeks of treatment. ■ Encourage the client not to use in combination with OTC preparations containing salicylic acid, benzoyl peroxide, or sulfur. ■ Advise the client to minimize sun exposure during treatment. ■ Monitor for pruritus, erythema, inflammation, and contact dermatitis.
Antibacterials ■ erythromycin ■ methotrexate ■ tetracycline **Drug examples:** EryDerm, MTX, Novo-Tetra	Interfere with bacterial DNA and protein synthesis, causing cell death. *May also be used for:* —Prophylaxis for neonatal eye infection (erythromycin) —Treatment of rheumatoid arthritis (methotrexate) —Treatment of chlamydia and rickettsial infections (tetracycline)	■ Encourage the client using oral medications to take with a full glass of water on an empty stomach; if stomach upset occurs, medications can be taken with foods that are not high in calcium. ■ Advise the client to avoid exposure to sunlight and ultraviolet light. ■ Encourage the client to check expiration dates on antibacterial medications and dispose of those that have expired. ■ Monitor for urticaria, pruritus, and skin eruptions.
Antibiotics ■ bacitracin ■ gentamicin ■ polysporin ■ silver sulfadiazine **Drug examples:** Silvadene	Interfere with bacterial replication and synthesis; used to treat infection. *May also be used for:* —Superficial infection of external eye —Prevention and treatment of sepsis in burns	■ Encourage the client to clean affected area prior to application and cover with a sterile bandage or gauze after application. ■ Advise the client against applying to large areas because of risk of systemic absorption and toxicity. ■ Monitor for hypersensitivity, local allergic reaction, and photosensitivity.
Antifungals ■ clotrimazole ■ ketoconazole ■ miconazole ■ nystatin **Drug examples:** Lotrimin, Nizoral, Monistat, Mycostatin	Alter fungal membrane structure, causing cell death; each preparation is specific to a particular organism.	■ Emphasize the importance of keeping affected areas clean and dry. ■ Advise the client against covering areas with occlusive dressings unless instructed by the physician. ■ Monitor for erythema, irritation, pruritus, contact dermatitis, and allergic reaction.
Antivirals ■ acyclovir ■ famciclovir **Drug examples:** Zovirax, Famvir	Inhibit viral DNA replication. *May also be used for:* —Prophylaxis for cytomegalovirus —Prophylaxis for varicella	■ Advise the client that full therapeutic effect may take several weeks. ■ Encourage adequate fluid intake. ■ Explain that antivirals do not cure the herpes virus. ■ Teach the client about standard precautions to prevent the spread of infection. ■ Monitor for effectiveness and viral resistance. ■ Monitor for urticaria, pruritus, burning, and irritation.
Anesthetics ■ lidocaine hydrochloride **Drug examples:** ■ Xylocaine	Decrease pain through reversible nerve conduction blockade. *May also be used for:* —Treatment of postherpetic neuralgia	■ Advise the client against applying to large areas or broken skin. ■ Advise the client to avoid contact with eyes.

Medications **Tissue Integrity** (continued)

CLASSIFICATION AND DRUG EXAMPLES	MECHANISM OF ACTION	NURSING CONSIDERATIONS
Creams *Drug examples:* ■ Aquacare ■ Curel ■ Nutraderm	Moisturize the skin.	■ Encourage the client to apply after bathing while skin is slightly damp. ■ Advise the client to rub cream in completely. ■ Monitor for redness and itching.
Ointments *Drug examples:* ■ Aquaphor ■ Vaseline	Lubricate the skin; retard water loss.	■ Advise the client to cleanse the affected area with warm water and soap prior to application. ■ Encourage the client to apply in a thin layer so air can reach the wound. ■ Advise the client to avoid the nose and mouth area. ■ Monitor for redness and itching.
Lotions *Drug examples:* ■ Alpha-Keri ■ Dermassage ■ Lubriderm	Moisturize the skin; lubricate the skin.	■ Encourage the client to apply after bathing while the skin is slightly damp. ■ Advise the client to rub lotion in completely. ■ Monitor for redness and itching.
Alternative therapies ■ aloe vera gel (topical) ■ chamomile (topical) ■ evening primrose oil (oral)	Soothe irritation and discomfort associated with skin inflammation and eczema; promote healing of superficial burns, wounds, and abrasions (NCCAM, 2012). *May also be used for:* ■ Treatment of sleeplessness ■ Treatment of gastrointestinal conditions	■ Ask the client about any alternative or complementary therapies used; be mindful of interactions with prescription medications or other alternative therapies. ■ Monitor for allergic reaction.

REVIEW **The Concept of Tissue Integrity**

RELATE Link the Concepts

Linking the concept of tissue integrity with the concept of comfort:

1. You are caring for a 2-year-old client with nonbullous impetigo. What actions can you take to improve the child's comfort?

2. What client teaching would you provide the child's caretaker to improve the child's comfort?

Linking the concept of tissue integrity with the concept of development:

3. You are caring for a 12-year-old who was just diagnosed with vitiligo. How can you explain the child's condition to him in a developmentally appropriate way? What psychosocial considerations are especially important for a client in this age group?

4. What psychological and cognitive aspects should you consider when explaining impaired tissue integrity related to pressure ulcers to a bedridden client in his 80s?

READY Go to Companion Skills Manual

REFER Go to Pearson Student Nursing Resources
nursing.pearsonhighered.com

• Additional review materials

REFLECT Case Study \\ Part 3

Three years after his release from the hospital following his neurosurgery, Mr. Sullivan's venous ulcer has improved but is still not healed completely. The ulcer is now 2.5 cm long, 1.8 cm wide, and 0.4 cm deep. The purple area around the ulcer has measured at 22 cm long and 13 cm wide for the past 2 years. Mr. Sullivan has experienced no further episodes of hemorrhage since he was taken off all anticoagulants. However, because of the open wound and skin discoloration, Mr. Sullivan has developed a disturbed body image.

Mr. Sullivan has been seeing a dermatologist for treatment of his ulcer, and several treatments have been tried and failed over the years. Therefore his dermatologist has scheduled sclerotherapy to collapse the damaged veins. After the procedure, Mr. Sullivan continues treatment with daily topical sucralfate covered by simple gauze. Compression with an elastic bandage and compression stockings also continues. Six months after sclerotherapy, the ulcer measures 1.3 cm long, 0.8 cm wide, and 0.2 cm deep. However, the purple area surrounding the wound has not decreased. Mr. Sullivan and his dermatologist hope that the ulcer will be completely healed within a year of the procedure.

Clinical Reasoning Questions Level I

1. As the dermatologist's nurse, what client teaching will you perform prior to sclerotherapy?

2. How does ablation of damaged veins contribute to ulcer healing?

3. Once Mr. Sullivan's ulcer has healed completely, what maintenance therapy may be beneficial for continued healing of the damaged area?

Clinical Reasoning Questions Level II

4. What may be the long-term consequences of Mr. Sullivan's venous ulcer?

5. What client teaching is necessary to help Mr. Sullivan prevent future development of venous ulcers?

6. What nursing interventions are appropriate for the nursing diagnosis *Disturbed Body Image*?

EXEMPLAR 21.1 Burns

EXEMPLAR KEY TERMS

Allograft, *1479*
Autografting, *1478*
Burn, *1464*
Burn shock, *1471*
Compartment syndrome, *1471*
Contractures, *1468*
Curling ulcers, *1472*
Debridement, *1473*
Eschar, *1472*
Escharotomy, *1477*
Fascial excision, *1478*
Fasciectomy, *1478*
Fluid resuscitation, *1476*
Full-thickness burn, *1468*
Heterograft, *1479*
Homograft, *1479*
Hypertrophic scar, *1470*
Keloid, *1470*
Partial-thickness burn, *1467*
Superficial burn, *1467*

Surgical debridement, *1478*
Tangential excision, *1478*
Xenograft, *1479*

EXEMPLAR LEARNING OUTCOMES

After reading about this exemplar, you will be able to:

1. Describe the pathophysiology, etiology, clinical manifestations, and direct and indirect causes of burns.
2. Identify risk factors and prevention methods associated with burns.
3. Illustrate the nursing process in providing culturally competent care across the life span for individuals with burns.
4. Formulate priority nursing diagnoses appropriate for an individual with burns.
5. Summarize therapies used by interdisciplinary teams in the collaborative care of an individual with burns.
6. Plan evidence-based care for an individual with burns and his or her family in collaboration with other members of the healthcare team.
7. Evaluate expected outcomes for an individual with burns.

▶ OVERVIEW

A **burn** is a type of injury caused by exposure to heat, certain chemicals, radiation, or electricity. When energy from one of these sources is transferred to an individual's body, it initiates a sequence of physiological events that, in the most severe cases, lead to irreversible tissue destruction. Burns range in severity from minor losses of small segments of the epidermis to complex multisystem injuries. Accordingly, treatment may involve anything from simple first aid to delivery of complex, interdisciplinary team care in the aseptic environment of a hospital burn center.

▶ PATHOPHYSIOLOGY AND ETIOLOGY

Burns are among the most common types of injuries, in part because they arise from many different causes. Although burns affect individuals from all walks of life, some individuals are at elevated risk because of factors such as age, occupation, and preexisting conditions.

Types of Burns

Burns may be caused by heat, chemicals, electricity, or radiation. Although all four types of burns can result in generalized tissue damage and multisystem involvement, each type exhibits unique characteristics and requires unique priority treatment measures.

THERMAL BURNS As their name suggests, thermal burns result from exposure to heat, either dry (such as flames) or moist (such as steam and hot liquids). Thermal burns are the most common type of burn injury and most often affect children and older adults (**Figure 21–3** ●). With thermal burns,

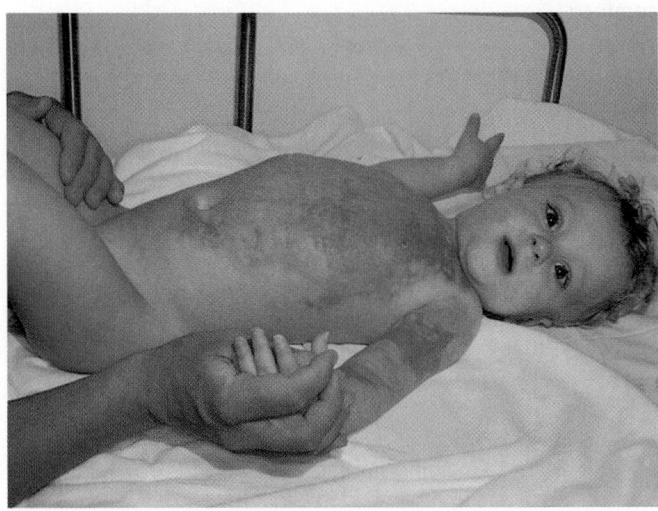

Figure 21–3 ● Thermal (scald) burns are the most common burn injury in infants. Notice the distribution of the burned skin, a wide area on the upper chest and arm where the hottest liquid fell, with a narrower area near the umbilicus, indicating that the liquid cooled as it traveled down the chest.

direct exposure to the heat source causes cellular destruction and may result in charring of vascular, bony, muscle, and nervous tissue.

CHEMICAL BURNS Chemical burns result from direct contact between skin and certain acids, alkaline agents, or organic compounds. The destruction that these chemicals cause in the proteins in the individual's tissues leads to necrosis.

More than 25,000 products found in the home or workplace can cause chemical burns, including those listed in **Box 21–2** ●. Of these products, acids (such as hydrochloric acid) produce burns via tissue coagulation, alkalis (such as lye) produce burns via liquefaction necrosis, and organic compounds (such as petroleum distillates) produce burns by dissolving cells' lipid membranes. Burns from alkalis are more difficult to neutralize than burns caused by acids and tend to be deeper and more severe. Organic compound burns also pose a special threat because their causative agents may trigger renal and liver failure if absorbed. For all chemical burns, the severity of an individual's injury is related to the type and concentration of chemical agent, the mechanism of action, the duration of contact, and the amount of body surface area exposed (Palao et al., 2010; Veenema, 2007).

ELECTRICAL BURNS Electrical burns vary in severity depending on the type and duration of current and the amount of voltage. Assessment of electrical burn injuries is difficult because electricity follows the path of least resistance. This path tends to lie along muscles, bone, blood vessels, and nerves, so that the extent and depth of an individual's injury may not be evident until weeks after the initial burn event. Furthermore, the small entry and exit wounds from electricity mask widespread tissue damage underneath the outer layer of the skin. Frequently, tissue necrosis results from impaired blood flow secondary to blood coagulation at the site of an electrical injury. If this necrosis is severe, an individual may develop gangrene that necessitates amputation (Yale School of Medicine, 2013).

The nurse should be aware that different types of electric current tend to produce characteristic patterns of injury. Generally, alternating current (AC), like that found in most U.S. households, produces repeated electrical surges that lead to tetanic muscle contractions. These sustained contractions inhibit an individual's respiratory efforts for the duration of contact and may result in respiratory arrest. The contractions may also cause the individual to clamp down on the power source (such as an electrical cord) and thereby increase the duration of contact with the source. In comparison, direct current, as in injury from a lightning bolt, exposes the body to very high voltage for an instant. High-voltage injury usually results in entry and exit wounds. In some high-voltage lightning

strikes, however, a phenomenon known as the *flashover effect* occurs. Here, the lightning bolt flashes over the individual, the current traveling over the moist surface of the skin rather than through deeper structures, often saving the individual from death. Individuals who are struck by lightning may experience instantaneous cardiopulmonary arrest. Other possible outcomes include brain injury resulting in loss of consciousness or coma; injuries to the eyes and ears; temporary paralysis; nerve damage; and burns from metal jewelry or coins that are heated by the lightning. Many who survive have no memory of the event but may experience ongoing symptoms, including seizures (Cooper, 2009a).

RADIATION BURNS Radiation burns are usually associated with sunburn or radiation treatment for cancer. These kinds of burns tend to be superficial, involving only the outermost layers of the epidermis. All functions of the skin remain intact. Symptoms are limited to mild systemic reactions, including headache, chills, local discomfort, nausea, and vomiting.

More extensive exposure to radiation or radioactive substances, as in nuclear power accidents, leads to the same degree of tissue damage and multisystem involvement associated with other types of burns.

Etiology

Researchers estimate that U.S. hospitals and emergency departments treat 450,000 individuals with burn injuries each year. Of these, approximately 40,000 require hospital admission, 30,000 receiving care in specialized burn centers (American Burn Association, 2012). Annually, nearly 3,500 Americans die from burns, 3,000 of these fatalities being caused by fires and the remainder by other sources (Burn Survivor Resource Center, 2011). Burn injuries are the second leading cause of accidental death in the United States, after motor vehicle crashes (Centers for Disease Control and Prevention, 2011).

Burns are especially common among children. Around 88,000 children receive hospital-based emergency treatment for burns each year, and most of these burns involve thermal causes. For example, scalds (65%) and contact burns (20%) together account for 85% of burn injuries in children age 4 and under. Hot tap water is the leading cause of scald burns in children, and residential fires are the leading cause of contact burns (Boston Children's Hospital, 2011). Sadly, fires kill approximately 600 children under age 14 each year, and 85% of these blazes occur in residences. Another 47,000 children are injured by fires but do not die from their wounds (Burn Survivor Resource Center, 2011).

For children and adults alike, residential fires are the most common cause of fire-related burns. Although cooking equipment accounts for more house fires than any other source, fires in bedrooms and living areas are responsible for more deaths. Typical causes of these fires include cigarettes, portable heating equipment, and unsupervised child's play with matches and lighters. Up to two thirds of fatal residential fires occur in homes without working smoke detectors—a sobering statistic that highlights the importance of properly installing and maintaining such equipment (Boston Children's Hospital, 2011).

Risk Factors

Several factors increase an individual's likelihood of burns. Chief among these is age, with children age 4 and younger and adults age 65 and older at greatest risk (Centers for Disease Control and Prevention, 2011). One reason young children are so vulnerable to burns is that they simply don't understand the dangers presented by everyday objects such as hot tap water and electrical outlets. Children are also innately curious and therefore apt to play with items such as matches, lighters, fireworks, microwaves, and stoves if left unattended. In addition, children's lower height places them at increased risk of burns from spills. Very young children also lack the ability to react appropriately and/or escape from dangerous situations, such as residential fires. For this reason alone, children ages 5 and under are twice as likely to perish in a house fire than are individuals in any other age group (Burn Survivor Resource Center, 2011). Finally, abuse is a factor in many childhood burn injuries; experts estimate that between 1% and 35% of children who are admitted to burn units are suffering from intentional burns (Hornor, 2012).

Older adults are also at increased risk for burns. Slower reaction times, impaired mobility, and sensory impairment account for much of this risk. Dementia is another age-related factor that can increase an individual's likelihood of injury. Furthermore, age-related thinning of the skin means that older adults are more susceptible to deep burns, even from sources that would cause minor to moderate burns in a younger individual.

Other factors associated with heighted burn risk include the following:

- *Gender.* Males are more likely to suffer serious burns than females. In fact, between 2002 and 2011, roughly 69% of all burn center admissions were male clients (American Burn Association, 2012).

- *Socioeconomic status.* Poor individuals are at increased risk for burns, often because they live in unsafe homes, lack smoke detectors, and/or rely on portable heating devices.

- *Race/ethnicity.* African Americans and Native Americans have a higher incidence of burn injury, in part because they are more likely to be socioeconomically disadvantaged.

- *Rural location.* Rural dwellers are often located far from fire departments and other emergency responders.

- *Drug, alcohol, and/or tobacco use.* Smoking increases an individual's burn risk for obvious reasons. Drug and alcohol abuse, on the other hand, increases individuals' risk by impairing their judgment and reaction time.

- *Physical and/or mental disability.* Individuals with physical and/or mental disabilities may not understand the risk posed by various hazards, may have decreased reaction times, and/or may be physically unable to escape fires and other dangers.

- *Occupation.* Individuals who work with chemicals, gasoline, electricity, or extreme heat sources are more likely to be burned than individuals in other occupations.

The nurse should also be aware that certain conditions can increase a client's risk of burn-related complications and morbidity. Examples include preexisting cardiac, pulmonary, or renal disorders; diabetes mellitus; and alcoholism.

Lifespan Considerations
Children and Burns

Children at different developmental stages are at risk for different types of burns.

- Infants are most often injured by thermal burns, such as burns from scalding liquids, excessively hot bathwater, and house fires.

- Toddlers are at risk for thermal burns (e.g., from pulling hot liquids or grease onto themselves), electrical burns (e.g., from biting electrical cords), contact burns, and chemical burns (e.g., from ingesting cleaning agents and other substances) associated with exploring the environment.

- Pre-school-age children are most often injured by scalding or contact with hot appliances such as curling irons and ovens.

- School-age children are at risk for thermal burns (e.g., from playing with matches and fireworks), electrical burns (e.g., from climbing high-voltage towers or climbing trees and making contact with electrical wires), and chemical burns (e.g., from conducting combustion experiments) associated with their curiosity and interest in experimentation.

- Adolescents also experience thermal, chemical, and electrical burns, as well as radiation burns associated with sunbathing.

Prevention

Methods for preventing burns vary by setting and causative agent. Many of these measures involve taking proper precautions in the home, especially when children are present. See **Box 21–3** ● for examples. Other methods are specific to the workplace. For instance, individuals who work with hazardous chemicals should be aware of proper handling protocols and

Box 21–3   Burn Prevention in the Home

The following measures can greatly reduce burn risk in the home:

- Be sure working smoke detectors are installed in each level of the home. Test the devices monthly, and change the batteries at least once per year.
- Create an emergency escape plan and practice it with all members of the household.
- When cooking, do not wear clothes with loose-fitting sleeves, and keep pot handles turned away from the front of the stove.
- Never leave cooking food or open flames (even in a grill or fireplace) unattended.
- Keep fire extinguishers near possible sources of ignition.
- Use caution when carrying hot foods and liquids around children.
- Install childproofing devices on electrical outlets, oven knobs, and cabinets that contain hazardous chemicals. Keep matches, lighters, and fireworks stored out of children's reach.
- Set the home's water heater temperature at 120°–130°F.
- Keep electrical appliances away from water, and unplug them when they are not in use.
- Check all electrical cords for wear and replace them as needed.
- Avoid overloading outlets and extension cords.
- Always test the temperature of a child's bathwater before placing the child in the tub.
- Never leave young children in the bathroom or kitchen unsupervised.

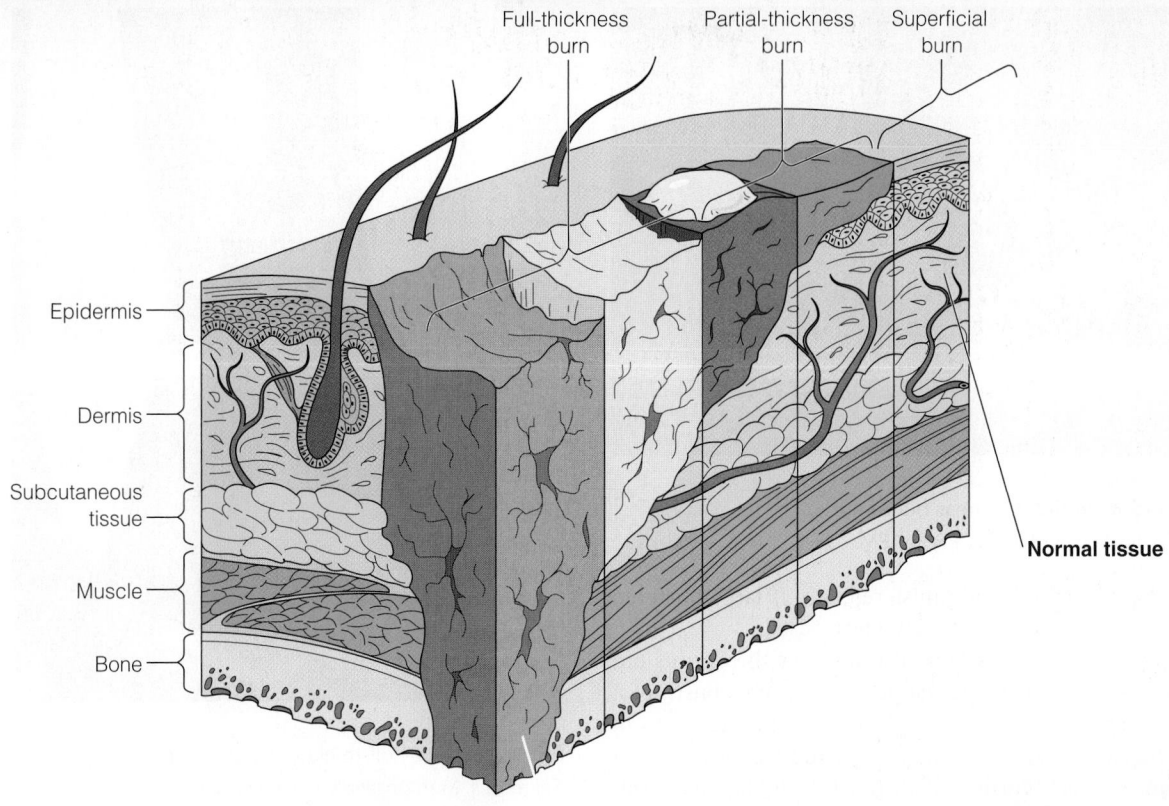

Figure 21–4 ● Characteristics of burns by depth of thermal injury.

what to do if a spill, fire, or other accident occurs, and individuals who work with electricity should be sure to use proper safety equipment at all times. Of course, all employees in all workplaces should know and be familiar with a planned escape route in case of fires or other emergencies.

Other burn prevention tips apply specifically to individuals who smoke. Smokers should always use safe, heat-resistant ash trays, and they should be sure all ashes, butts, used matches, and related materials are completely cool before placing them in the trash. Individuals should also avoid smoking in bed, as well as during periods when they are sleepy or under the influence of alcohol or medications that can induce drowsiness. Finally, matches and lighters should be kept out of children's reach, and working smoke detectors should be installed in rooms where smoking most often occurs.

▶ CLINICAL MANIFESTATIONS

Regardless of their cause, all burns are classified according to the same basic system and heal by way of a similar process. Still, different burns can affect an individual's body systems in a number of different ways depending on their source, type, and severity.

Classification of Burns

Tissue damage following a burn is determined primarily by two factors: the depth of the burn (i.e., how many layers of underlying tissue are affected) and the extent of the burn (i.e., the percentage of body surface area involved).

DEPTH OF THE BURN The depth of a burn injury is determined by which elements of the skin have been damaged or destroyed. Burn depth depends on the temperature of the burning agent and the length of contact. Based on depth, burns are classified as superficial, partial thickness, or full thickness (**Figure 21–4** ●).

Superficial burns involve only the epidermal layer of the skin. They most often result from sunburn, ultraviolet light, minor flash injury (from a sudden ignition or explosion), or mild radiation associated with cancer treatment. Because the skin remains intact, superficial burns are not calculated into estimates of burn extent.

Skin affected by superficial burns ranges in color from pink to bright red and may be accompanied by slight edema over the burned area. If a significant portion of the body is burned, additional symptoms may include chills, headache, nausea, and vomiting. Superficial burns usually heal in 3–6 days, with dryness and peeling of the outer layer of skin and no scar formation. Treatment typically involves administration of mild analgesics and application of water-soluble lotions. However, extensive superficial burns may require intravenous (IV) fluid treatment, especially in older adults.

Partial-thickness burns are deeper than superficial burns, involving both the epidermis and the dermis. Depending on their depth, partial-thickness burns may be further categorized as either superficial or deep.

A *superficial partial-thickness burn* (**Figure 21–5** ●) extends from the skin's surface into the papillary layer of the dermis. This type of burn may result from brief exposure to a flash flame or dilute chemical agents or contact with a hot surface. Superficial partial-thickness burns are often bright red and have a moist, glistening appearance with blister formation. The burned area blanches on pressure, and touch and pain sensation remains intact. Pain in response to temperature and air exposure is usually severe. These burns typically heal within 21 days with minimal or no scarring, but pigment changes are com-

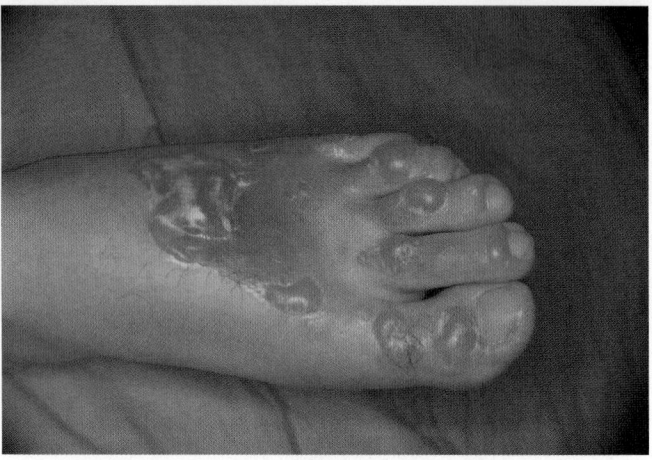

Figure 21–5 ● Partial-thickness burn injury.
Source: Charles Stewart MD FACEP, FAAEM.

mon. Analgesics may be administered, and if large blistered areas are disrupted, skin substitutes may be used.

A *deep partial-thickness burn* also involves the dermis but extends deeper than a superficial partial-thickness burn, past the papillae and into the reticular layer. Despite the depth of damage, hair follicles, sebaceous glands, and epidermal sweat glands remain intact (Porth & Matfin, 2010). Hot liquids or solids, flash flame, direct flame, intense radiant energy, or chemical agents may cause this level of burn wound. The surface of a deep partial-thickness burn appears pale and waxy and may be moist or dry. Large, easily ruptured blisters may be present, or the blisters may look like flat, dry tissue paper. Capillary refill is decreased. The wound is less painful than a superficial partial-thickness burn because sensation is decreased at the site. However, areas of pain may be present, and sensation to deep pressure will remain intact. Deep partial-thickness burn wounds often require more than 21 days for healing and may convert to full-thickness injuries if necrosis extends the depth of the wound. **Contracture**, or permanent shortening of connective tissue, is possible, as are hypertrophic scarring and functional impairment (**Figure 21–6** ●). Excision of the wound and skin grafting may be necessary to decrease scarring and loss of function.

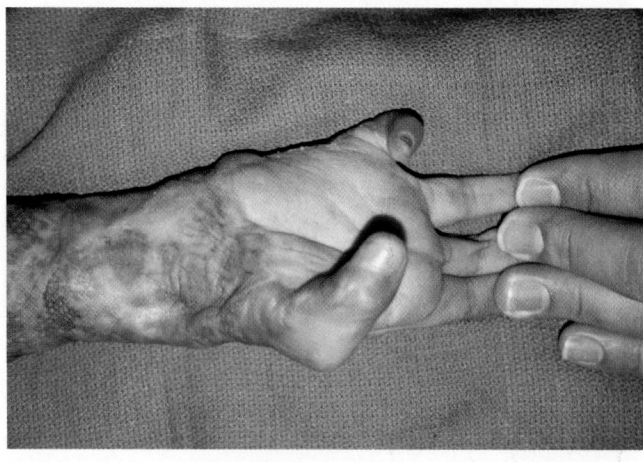

Figure 21–6 ● Burn contracture.
Source: JPD/Custom Medical Stock Photo, Inc.

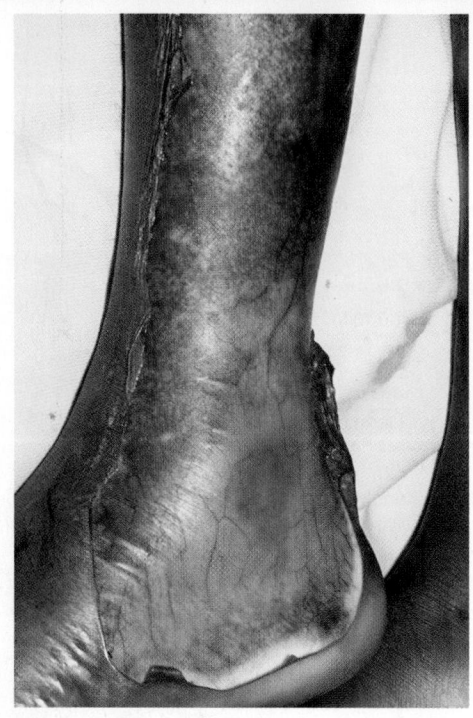

Figure 21–7 ● Full-thickness burn injury.
Source: Dr. M.A. Ansary/Science Source.

Full-thickness burns involve all layers of the skin, including the epidermis, the dermis, and the epidermal appendages (**Figure 21–7** ●). The wound may extend below the skin into subcutaneous fat, connective tissue, muscle, and bone. Full-thickness burns are caused by prolonged contact with flames, steam, chemicals, or high-voltage electric current.

Depending on the cause of injury, a full-thickness burn wound may appear pale, waxy, yellow, brown, mottled, charred, or non-blanching red. The wound's surface is dry, leathery, and firm to the touch. Thrombosed blood vessels may be visible under the surface of the wound. There is no sensation of pain or light touch at the site because pain and touch receptors have been destroyed. Full-thickness burns require skin grafting to heal.

EXTENT OF THE BURN　The extent of a burn injury is expressed as a percentage of the affected individual's total body surface area (TBSA). Several methods are used to determine this percentage. The *rule of nines* is a quick method of estimation used during the prehospital and emergency care phases. In the rule of nines method, the adult body is divided into five surface areas—head, trunk, arms, legs, and perineum—and percentages that equal or total a sum of nine are assigned to each body area; different percentages are assigned for children (**Figure 21–8** ●). For example, an adult client with burns of the face, anterior right arm, and anterior trunk would have burn injury involving 27% of the TBSA. (In this example, face = 4.5%, arm = 4.5%, and trunk = 18%, for an overall total of 27%.) Again, only partial- and full-thickness burns are included in the estimation.

Later, upon the client's admission to the hospital, critical care unit, or burn center, more accurate methods for estimating the extent of injury can be employed. For example, the Lund and Browder method (**Figure 21–9** ●) determines surface area measurements for each body part according to the age of the client.

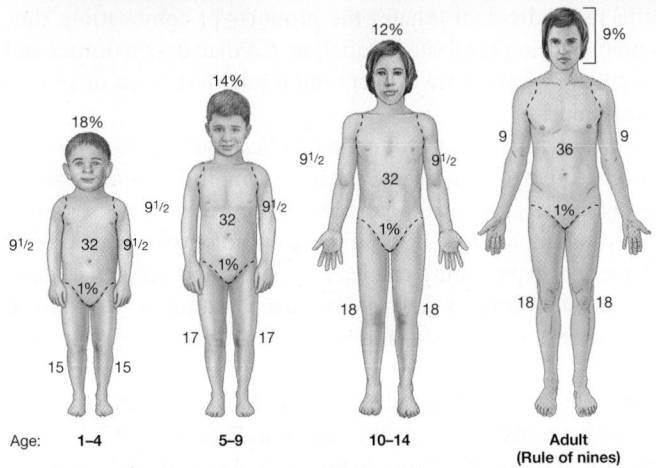

Area	Age (years) 0–1	1–4	5–9	10–15	Adult	% 1°	% 2°	% 3°	% Total
Head	19	17	13	10	7				
Neck	2	2	2	2	2				
Ant. trunk	13	13	13	13	13				
Post. trunk	13	13	13	13	13				
R. buttock	2½	2½	2½	2½	2½				
L. buttock	2½	2½	2½	2½	2½				
Genitalia	1	1	1	1	1				
R.U. arm	4	4	4	4	4				
L.U. arm	4	4	4	4	4				
R.L. arm	3	3	3	3	3				
L.L. arm	3	3	3	3	3				
R. hand	2½	2½	2½	2½	2½				
L. hand	2½	2½	2½	2½	2½				
R. thigh	5½	6½	8½	8½	9½				
L. thigh	5½	6½	8½	8½	9½				
R. leg	5	5	5½	6	7				
L. leg	5	5	5½	6	7				
R. foot	3½	3½	3½	3½	3½				
L. foot	3½	3½	3½	3½	3½				
					Total				

Figure 21–8 ● The rule of nines is one method for quickly estimating the percentage of TBSA affected by a burn injury. Although useful in emergency care situations, the rule of nines is not accurate for estimating TBSA for adults who are short, obese, or very thin.

Another widely recognized system for describing burn injuries, developed by the American Burn Association, uses both the extent and the depth of injury to classify burns as minor, moderate, or major (see **Table 21–5** ●). See also the Clinical Manifestations and Therapies feature later in this exemplar for information on therapeutic measures appropriate for each class of burn.

Burn Wound Healing

Burns heal through the same processes as do other wounds, but the healing phases occur more slowly and last longer. There are three phases in the burn healing process: inflammation, proliferation, and remodeling (Porth & Matfin, 2010).

INFLAMMATION The inflammation phase begins immediately following a burn injury, as platelets come into contact with the damaged tissue and start to aggregate. Fibrin is deposited, trapping additional platelets, and a thrombus forms. The thrombus, combined with local vasoconstriction, causes hemostasis, which walls off the wound from the systemic circulation.

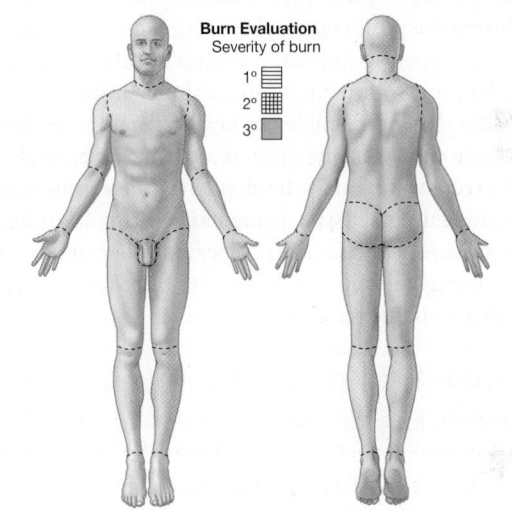

Figure 21–9 ● The Lund and Browder burn assessment chart. This method of estimating TBSA affected by a burn injury is more accurate than the rule of nines because it accounts for changes in body surface area across the life span.

TABLE 21–5 American Burn Association Classification of Burn Injury

MINOR BURN INJURY	MODERATE BURN INJURY	MAJOR BURN INJURY
Excludes electrical injury, inhalation injury, complicated injuries (such as multiple trauma), and all clients who are considered at high risk (such as older adults and those with chronic illnesses).	Excludes electrical injury, inhalation injury, complicated injuries (such as multiple trauma), and all clients who are considered at high risk (such as older adults and those with chronic illnesses).	Includes all burns of the hands, face, eyes, ears, feet, and perineum; all electrical injuries, inhalation injuries, and multiple-trauma injuries; and all clients who are considered at high risk.
Includes partial-thickness burns of less than 15% of TBSA in adults.	Includes partial-thickness burns of 15%–25% of TBSA in adults.	Includes partial-thickness burns of greater than 25% of TBSA in adults.
Includes full-thickness burns of less than 2% of TBSA not involving special care areas (i.e., eyes, ears, face, hands, feet, joints, perineum).	Includes full-thickness burns of less than 10% of TBSA not involving special care areas (i.e., eyes, ears, face, hands, feet, joints, perineum).	Includes all full-thickness burns of 10% or greater of TBSA.

Note: The injuries described in this table (except minor burns) should be treated in a specialized burn center. These criteria have been established by the American Burn Association.

Local vasodilation and an increase in capillary permeability follow hemostasis. Neutrophils infiltrate the wound and peak in about 24 hours, at which point monocytes predominate. The monocytes are converted into macrophages, which consume pathogens and dead tissue and secrete various growth factors. These growth factors stimulate the proliferation of fibroblasts and the deposit of a provisional wound matrix.

PROLIFERATION   The proliferation phase begins about 2–3 days postburn. At this point, the wound primarily contains fibroblasts. Their number peaks about 14 days after the injury. Granulation tissue begins to form, with complete reepithelialization occurring during this stage. Epithelial cells gradually cover the wound as each cell stretches across the wound's surface to join with other epithelial cells on the opposite side of the wound. The proliferation phase lasts until complete reepithelialization occurs by epithelial cell migration, surgical intervention, or a combination of the two.

REMODELING   With burn wounds, the remodeling phase may last for years. Over time, collagen fibers that were laid down during the proliferative phase reorganize into more compact areas. Scars also gradually contract and fade in color. In normal healing following a minor burn injury, the newly formed skin closely resembles its neighboring tissue. However, when a burn injury extends into the dermal layer of skin, two types of excessive scar may develop. A **hypertrophic scar** is an overgrowth of dermal tissue that remains within the boundaries of the wound. A **keloid** is a scar that extends beyond the boundaries of the original wound. Clients with dark skin are at greater risk for hypertrophic scars and keloids.

Systemic Effects of Burn Injuries

The pathophysiological changes that result from major burn injuries involve all body systems. Extensive loss of skin (the body's protective barrier) can result in massive infection, fluid and electrolyte imbalances, and hypothermia. Often, the affected individual inhales the products of combustion, thus compromising respiratory function. Cardiac dysrhythmias and circulatory failure are also common manifestations of serious burn injuries.

Meanwhile, the profound catabolic state associated with a severe burn dramatically increases an individual's caloric expenditure and nutritional deficiencies. Alterations in gastrointestinal motility predispose the client to developing paralytic ileus, and hyperacidity can lead to gastric and duodenal ulcerations. Dehydration slows glomerular filtration rates and renal clearance of toxic wastes and may lead to acute tubular necrosis and renal failure. Thanks to all these effects, a significant burn injury may profoundly alter an individual's metabolism. Systemic responses to burns are shown in **Figure 21–10 ●**. More specific systemic responses to burns are discussed in the following sections.

RESPIRATORY SYSTEM   Pulmonary damage sometimes results from the systemic response to a burn injury. More commonly, however, breathing in hot gases and smoke causes direct damage to an individual's pulmonary tissues. In fact, inhalation injury is a frequent and often lethal complication of burns. The injury may range from mild respiratory inflammation to massive pulmonary failure, such as acute respiratory distress syndrome (ARDS).

Exposure to heat, asphyxiants, and smoke initiates the pathophysiological process associated with inhalation injury. Inflammation occurs at localized sites in the airway and is manifested as hyperemia (increased blood supply). As a result, cells are destroyed and the bronchial cilia are rendered inactive. Because the mucociliary transport mechanism no longer functions, the client may develop bronchial congestion and infection. Interstitial pulmonary edema develops secondary to the escape of fluid from the pulmonary vasculature into the interstitial compartment of the lung tissue. Surfactant is inactivated, and the result is atelectasis (collapse of lung tissue) and alveolar collapse. Sloughing of the damaged and dead lung tissue occasionally produces debris that may lead to complete airway obstruction.

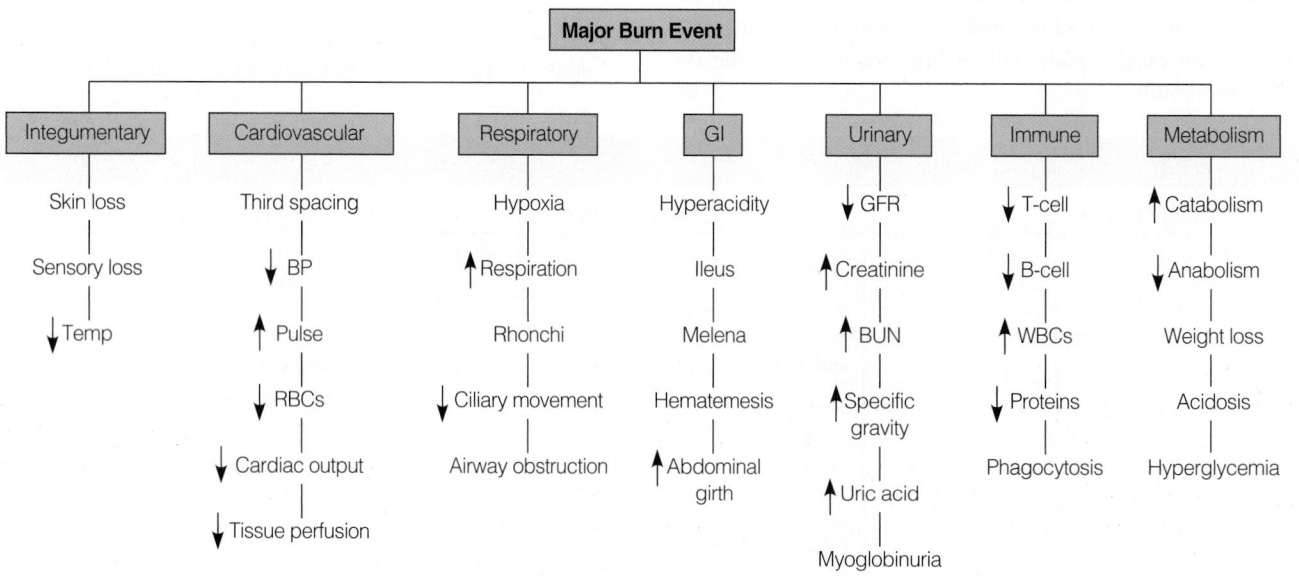

Figure 21–10 ● Effects of a severe burn on major body systems and metabolism.

Upper airway thermal injury (above the level of the glottis) can also result from the inhalation of heated air or chemicals dissolved in water. This type of injury should be suspected when a client has singed facial, scalp, or nasal hair. Physical findings include the presence of soot, charring, edema, blisters, and ulcerations along the mucosal lining of the oropharynx and larynx. The resulting edema in the airway peaks within the first 24–48 hours of injury. Ominous signs of hoarseness, labored breathing, or stridor indicate possible airway obstruction due to edema.

Lower airway thermal injury is a more rare occurrence. Because the lower airway is protected by laryngeal reflexes, thermal injury below the vocal cords is uncommon. When it does occur, it is typically associated with the inhalation of steam or explosive gases or the aspiration of hot liquids. Sputum containing soot or carbon particles is a classic manifestation of lower airway thermal injury (Bishop & Maguire, 2012).

Smoke poisoning results when toxic gases and particulate matter, the products of incomplete combustion, deposit directly on the pulmonary mucosa. The composition of the products of combustion depends on the combustible material, the rate at which the temperature increases, and the amount of ambient oxygen present. Irritant gases and particulate matter have a direct cytotoxic effect. The degree of injury is determined by the solubility in water of the irritant, the duration of exposure, and the size of the particulate or aerosol droplet.

One product of combustion that deserves special mention is carbon monoxide, which is an extremely common asphyxiant. Carbon monoxide is a colorless, tasteless, odorless gas that has a 200 times greater affinity for hemoglobin than does oxygen. Thus carbon monoxide easily displaces oxygen to bind with hemoglobin, forming a complex called *carboxyhemoglobin*. When this occurs, the resulting decrease in an individual's arterial oxyhemoglobin produces tissue hypoxia. Carbon monoxide impairs both oxygen delivery and cellular oxygen use. Clinical manifestations of carbon monoxide poisoning range from headache, nausea, and dizziness to coma and death.

Another notable product of combustion is cyanide gas, which is released when plastic, polyurethane, nylon, or silk is burned. Cyanide gas impedes cellular respiration. Of the various organs, the brain and heart are most vulnerable to cyanide poisoning. Manifestations of this condition include headache, dizziness, seizures, tachycardia, and lethal dysrhythmias.

CARDIOVASCULAR SYSTEM The effects of a major burn are also manifested in all components of the vascular system. These effects include hypovolemic shock (burn shock), cardiac dysrhythmias (such as ventricular fibrillation), cardiac arrest, and vascular compromise.

Hypovolemic Shock (Burn Shock) Within minutes of a major burn injury, a cascade of cellular events is initiated, and a massive amount of fluid shifts from the intracellular and intravascular compartments into the interstitium. This shift is a type of hypovolemic shock called **burn shock**, which continues until capillary integrity is restored, usually within 24–36 hours of the injury.

Although the pathophysiological mechanisms of postburn vascular changes and fluid volume shifts are not clearly under-stood, three processes occur early in the postburn phase in clients who have burns involving 40% or more of their TBSA:

1. An increase in microvascular permeability at the burn wound site
2. Generalized impairment of cell wall function, resulting in intracellular edema
3. An increase in osmotic pressure of the burned tissue, leading to extensive fluid accumulation

During burn shock, the shifting of fluid directly results from a loss of cell wall integrity at the site of injury and in the capillary bed. Fluid leaking from the capillaries into interstitial compartments located at the wound site and throughout the body result in a decrease in fluid volume within the intravascular space. The escape of plasma proteins and sodium into the interstitium enhances edema formation. Blood pressure falls as cardiac output diminishes.

Vasoconstriction results as the vascular system attempts to compensate for fluid loss. Abnormal platelet aggregation and white blood cell (WBC) accumulation result in ischemia (insufficient blood supply) in the deeper tissue below the burn, leading to eventual thrombosis. Red blood cells (RBCs) and WBCs remain in the circulation, producing an elevation in erythrocyte and leukocyte counts secondary to hemoconcentration.

The leakage of fluid into the interstitium compromises the lymphatic system, resulting in intravascular hypovolemia and edema at the burn wound site. Edematous body surfaces impair peripheral circulation and result in necrosis of the underlying tissue. During burn shock, potassium ions leave the intracellular compartment, a process that puts the client at risk for cardiac dysrhythmia due to hypokalemia. The process of burn shock continues until capillary integrity is restored, usually within 24 hours of the injury.

Burn shock reverses when fluid is reabsorbed from the interstitium into the intravascular compartment. As this happens, the client's blood pressure rises, cardiac output increases, and urinary output improves. Diuresis continues from several days to 2 weeks postburn. During this phase, the extra cardiac workload may predispose older clients or clients with cardiovascular disease to fluid volume overload.

Cardiac Rhythm Alterations Burns on more than 40% of an individual's TBSA cause significant myocardial dysfunction, with a decrease in myocardial contractibility and cardiac output. These changes, which occur prior to a decrease in plasma volume, are believed to be due to the release of substances and oxygen-free radicals from the burn wound and from ischemic myocardial cells. In addition, electrical burns often result in cardiac dysrhythmias or cardiopulmonary arrest caused by heat damage to the myocardium or by electrical interference with cardiac electrical activity.

Peripheral Vascular Compromise Circumferential burns are those that result from injury that encircles an extremity. As scar tissue develops, the circumferential burn tightens, much like a rubber band, reducing or eliminating blood supply below the burn. Circulation to extremities may be further impaired by edema and by peripheral vasoconstriction that occurs during burn shock. In addition, **compartment syndrome** may result. With this condition, tissue pressure in a muscle compartment exceeds microvascular pressure, interrupting cellular perfusion.

INTEGUMENTARY SYSTEM   The loss of skin in burn injuries interrupts normal integumentary functions and protective mechanisms. Thus common results of burn injuries include the following:

■ Loss of water secondary to evaporation

■ Infection secondary to loss of skin integrity, which allows pathogens to enter the body

■ Difficulty maintaining body temperature due to heat loss from open wounds

Heat transfer to skin is a complex phenomenon. If the skin's microcirculation remains intact during burning, it both cools and protects the deeper portions of the skin and cools the skin's outer surface once the heat source is removed. With extensive burn injury, however, the integrity of the microcirculation is lost, and the burning process continues even after the heat source is removed. For this reason, stopping the burning process is critical in extensive burn injuries.

Burns have a characteristic surface appearance that resembles a bull's-eye, with the most severe part of the burn located centrally and the less severe portions of the burn located along the peripheral wound edges. Depending on their intensity, burns consist of one, two, or three concentric three-dimensional zones closely corresponding on the skin surface to the depth of the burn (**Figure 21–11 ●**):

■ The outer zone of hyperemia consists of unburned tissue, blanches on pressure, and heals in 2–7 days postburn.

■ The medial zone of stasis is initially moist, red, and blistered, and it blanches on pressure. It may recover or become pale

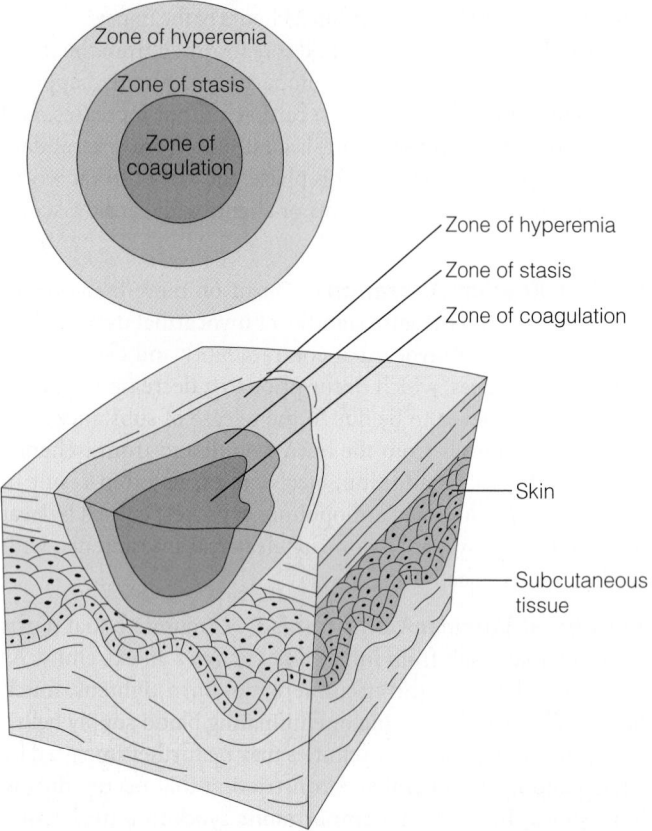

Figure 21–11 ● The zones of injury.

and necrotic between 3–7 days postburn due to decreased perfusion or infection.

■ The inner zone of coagulation immediately appears leathery and coagulated. It may merge with the zone of stasis from 3–7 days postburn.

The overall thickness of the dermis and epidermis varies considerably from one area of the body to another. For example, in adults, the skin covering the medial aspect of the forearm is thinner and more easily damaged than the skin covering the back of the body. As a result, similar temperatures produce different depths of injury in different body parts. Skin dissipates heat maximally in the areas of greatest vascularization. When heat absorption exceeds the rate of dissipation, cellular temperatures rise and skin tissue is destroyed.

Burn injuries result in the formation of necrotic skin and subcutaneous tissue. During the acute stage of a burn injury, a hard crust called an **eschar** forms, covering the wound and harboring necrotic tissue. The eschar is characteristically leathery and rigid. Removal of the eschar facilitates healing.

GASTROINTESTINAL SYSTEM   Dysfunction of the gastrointestinal system is directly related to the size of a burn wound. Clients with burns involving 20% or more of their TBSA experience decreased peristalsis, with resultant gastric distention and increased risk of aspiration. A decrease in or absence of bowel sounds is a manifestation of paralytic ileus (adynamic bowel) secondary to burn trauma. The resulting cessation of intestinal motility leads to gastric distention, nausea, vomiting, and hematemesis.

Stress ulcers (**Curling ulcers**) are acute ulcerations of the stomach or duodenum that may form after a burn injury. Abdominal pain, acidic gastric pH levels, hematemesis, and blood in the stool may all indicate a gastric ulcer.

URINARY SYSTEM   During the early stages of a burn injury, renal blood flow and glomerular filtration rates are greatly reduced due to decreased intravascular blood volume and the release of antidiuretic hormone by the posterior pituitary. Thus urine output decreases, and serum creatinine and blood urea nitrogen increase.

Dark brown concentrated urine may indicate myoglobinuria or hemoglobinuria, the result of underlying muscle damage or the release of large amounts of dead or damaged erythrocytes after a major burn injury. When large amounts of these pigments are released, the liver cannot keep pace with conjugation, and the pigments pass through the glomeruli. These pigments can occlude the renal tubules and cause renal failure, especially when dehydration, acidosis, or shock also is present.

IMMUNE SYSTEM   The function of the immune system is to protect the body from invasion by foreign microorganisms. Unfortunately, this system may be impaired as a result of burn injury. Specifically, the capillary leak that occurs in the early stages of a burn continues throughout the burn shock phase and impairs the active components of both the cell-mediated and the humoral immune systems.

The humoral immune system relies on B cells to produce antibodies or immunoglobulins. However, in the client with burns, the serum levels of all immunoglobulins are significantly diminished. Serum protein levels remain persistently low throughout the clinical course until wound closure occurs. At the same time, a marked decrease in T-cell counts results in reduction of cytotoxic activity and suppression of the cell-mediated immune system.

Burn-related compromises in the humoral and cell-mediated immune systems cause a state of acquired immunodeficiency, which places the client at risk for infection. The period of vulnerability is transient and may last from 1–4 weeks after the onset of the burn injury. During this time, opportunistic infections may be fatal despite aggressive antimicrobial therapy.

METABOLISM Two distinct phases characterize the body's metabolic response to a burn injury. The *ebb phase*, which occurs during the first 3 days of the injury, is manifested by decreased oxygen consumption, fluid imbalance, shock, and inadequate circulating volume. These responses protect the body from the initial impact of the injury.

The second phase, called *the flow phase*, occurs when adequate burn resuscitation has been accomplished. This phase is characterized by increases in cellular activity and protein catabolism, lipolysis, and gluconeogenesis. The client's basal metabolic rate (BMR) significantly increases, reaching twice the normal rate. Meanwhile, body weight and heat drop dramatically. Total energy expenditure may exceed 100% of the client's normal BMR. Hypermetabolism persists until after wound closure has been accomplished, and it may reappear if complications occur.

Lifespan and Cultural Considerations

Age has a significant impact on an individual's response to burn injury, with older adults at greatest risk for death as a result of their wounds. In fact, studies reveal a mortality rate of 13%–30% among older adult burn clients, as compared to roughly 2% of pediatric clients (Brusselaers, Monstrey, Vogelaers, Hoste, & Blot, 2010).

Several factors account for the higher rate of mortality in the older adult population. For one, older adults are more likely to suffer burns to a greater percentage of their TBSA, largely because their skin is so much thinner and therefore more delicate than that of younger individuals. The greater the amount of TBSA affected, the more likely an individual is to die from a burn. Older adults also tend to experience inhalation injury at greater rates than members of other age groups, and inhalation injury is a leading cause of burn-related mortality (Davidge & Fish, 2008). Finally, older clients are far more likely to have preexisting conditions that increase their risk of complications and impair their ability to heal from burn wounds. Common examples of such conditions are diabetes, cardiovascular disease, respiratory disease, malnutrition, and alcoholism (Brusselaers et al., 2010).

▶ COLLABORATION

A burn team is an interdisciplinary group of healthcare professionals who plan the care and treatment of the burn-injured client during the acute and rehabilitative stages. This team typically consists of the nurse, physician, physical therapist, dietitian, and social worker. The team members meet regularly to discuss client progress and collaboratively determine the most effective regimen of care and psychosocial support.

Treatment for burns depends on the amount of body surface area involved, the depth of skin damage, and the location of the burn. Burns that involve the airway require more careful monitoring than those involving extremities. Treatment often begins on scene, where it may be provided by family members, emergency services personnel, or specially trained personnel in occupational settings. Later, the client may receive more advanced treatment in an outpatient facility, hospital, or burn center.

Minor Burns

Minor burn injuries are usually treated on an outpatient basis. The goals of therapy are to promote wound healing, eliminate discomfort, maintain mobility, and prevent infection.

Sunburn is one of the most common types of minor burns. Independent nursing interventions relevant to care of the client with a sunburn generally consist of applying mild lotions, increasing liquid intake, and maintaining warmth. Older adults and young children should be monitored for evidence of dehydration. The client should be taught that using sunscreen properly and limiting sun exposure to the less hazardous hours of the day (before 10 a.m. and after 3 p.m.) can prevent sunburn. For all types of minor burns, client education should also include teaching regarding the application of skin dressings and antibiotic solutions as ordered by the primary care provider. Additionally, the nurse should reinforce the need to maintain adequate nutritional intake for promotion of wound healing.

Collaborative nursing interventions may include administration of mild analgesics as ordered by the primary care provider. In addition, if blistering is present, the lesions may be either left intact or debrided. **Debridement** is the process of removing necrotic material (including all loose tissue, wound debris, and eschar) from the wound. Follow up care for the minor burn injury includes twice daily wound cleansing with application of a topical ointment, range-of-motion (ROM) exercises for affected joints, and weekly clinic appointments until the wound heals completely.

Severe Burns

The clinical course of treatment for a client with a severe burn injury is divided into three stages: emergent/resuscitative, acute,

Focus on Diversity and Culture
Litargirio Use

When taking a history about methods used to treat minor burns in children, the nurse should inquire about the use of *litargirio*, a powder that is sold in small packets at specialty stores that serve Spanish-speaking populations. This traditional remedy is used as a treatment for burns and wounds and as a deodorant and foot fungicide in the Dominican Republic. However, its high lead content places the client at risk for lead poisoning (Chandran & Cataldo, 2010). The nurse who determines a client has been using *litargirio* should provide client teaching regarding the use of this medication, and the client's lead levels should be checked. If the blood test indicates that treatment is necessary, the physician may prescribe DMSA (dimercaptosuccinic acid), an oral medicine that binds to lead and mercury (Chandran & Cataldo, 2010).

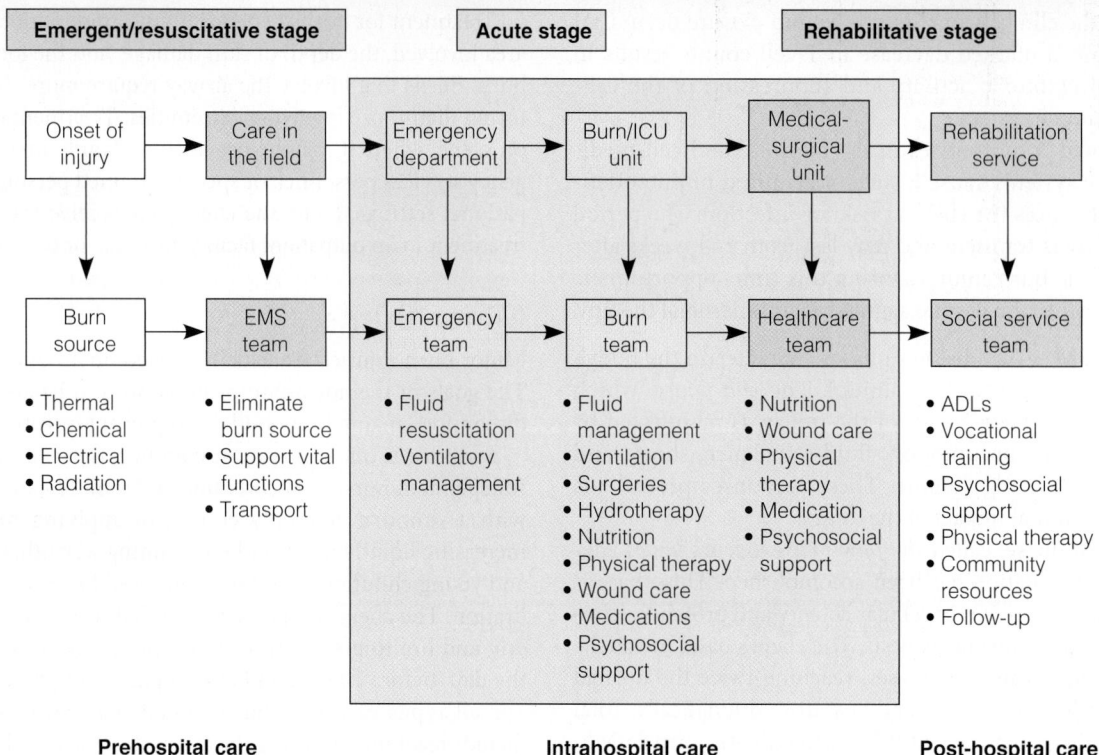

| Emergent/resuscitative stage | Acute stage | Rehabilitative stage |

Figure 21–12 ● The client's progression through the healthcare system during the emergent, acute, and rehabilitative stages of burn injury.

and rehabilitative. Although these stages are useful in helping plan the client's care, it is important to recognize that the process of burn injury is dynamic and that, in many cases, the clinical stage may not be clearly delineated. This is one of the many reasons ongoing assessment is necessary throughout the course of treatment. **Figure 21–12** ● shows the burn client's typical progression through the healthcare system. During each stage of care, different groups of nurses, physicians, and other healthcare specialists collaborate to manage the client's recovery as described in the following sections.

EMERGENT/RESUSCITATIVE STAGE The emergent/resuscitative stage lasts from the onset of a burn injury through successful fluid resuscitation. During this stage, healthcare workers estimate the extent of the burn injury, institute first aid measures, and implement fluid resuscitation therapies. The client is assessed for shock and evidence of respiratory distress. If indicated, IV lines are inserted, and the client may be prophylactically intubated. Frequently, these actions are performed at the scene of the injury rather than in a hospital setting. See **Box 21–4** ● for more information on prehospital client management.

Toward the end of the emergent/resuscitative stage, healthcare workers must often determine whether the client is to be transported to a burn center for the complex intervention strategies of the professional interdisciplinary burn team. According to American Burn Association guidelines, adult clients who should be treated at burn centers include the following:

■ Individuals older than age 50 who have second- or third-degree burns on more than 10% of their TBSA

■ Individuals younger than age 50 who have second- or third-degree burns on more than 20% of their TBSA

■ Adults of any age who have third-degree burns on more than 5% of their TBSA

■ Individuals with electrical (including lightning), chemical, and inhalation injuries

■ Individuals with circumferential burns of the extremities and/or chest

■ Any burned individuals with extenuating problems, preexisting illness, fractures, or other trauma

ACUTE STAGE The acute stage begins with the start of diuresis and ends with closure of the burn wound (either by natural healing or by use of skin grafts). During this stage, the following therapies are implemented:

■ *Wound care.* Hydrotherapy and excision and grafting of full-thickness wounds are performed as soon as possible after injury.

■ *Nutrition therapy.* Enteral and parenteral nutritional interventions are started early in the treatment plan to address caloric needs resulting from extensive energy expenditure.

■ *Infection prevention.* Measures to combat infection are also implemented during this stage, including administration of topical and systemic antimicrobial agents.

■ *Pain management.* Pain management constitutes a significant segment of the nursing care plan throughout the entire course of burn treatment. Administration of opioid analgesics must precede all invasive procedures to maximize client comfort and reduce anxiety associated with wound debridement and intensive physical therapy.

REHABILITATIVE STAGE The rehabilitative stage begins with wound closure and ends when the client returns to the

Box 21–4   Prehospital Client Management

Treatment at the scene of a burn injury includes measures to limit the severity of the burn and to support vital functions. Before attempting to remove the client from the source of injury, rescuers must ensure their own safety. Depending on the causative agent, the rescuers may need to consult with experts to determine the best way to eliminate the source of the injury.

Once the safety of the rescuers has been established, all prehospital interventions are aimed at eliminating the burn source, stabilizing the client's condition, identifying the type of burn, preventing heat loss, reducing wound contamination, and preparing for emergency transport. Any restrictive jewelry and clothing should be removed from the client at the scene to prevent circumferential constriction of the torso and extremities.

Ideally, emergency personnel will be called to provide prehospital treatment for a client with burns. In the case of a workplace injury, onsite treatment may be provided by a specially trained employee, and the injured client may or may not be treated and transported by emergency services.

STOPPING THE BURNING PROCESS

Regardless of who is providing care, one of the most important elements of prehospital client management is stopping continuation of the burning process. Appropriate emergency measures vary by type of injury and include the following:

- *Thermal burns.* If a thermal injury has been caused by dry heat, smother inflamed clothing or lavage with water. Help the client to "stop, drop, and roll" to extinguish the flame and limit the extent of burn. Once the flame has been extinguished, cover the client's body to prevent hypothermia. If the thermal injury has been caused by moist heat, lavage the area with cool water. Ice should not be used for cooling because it causes vasoconstriction and may result in further injury. Tar and asphalt can be removed from the skin with mineral oil, petroleum ointments, Medisol (a citrus and petroleum distillate with hydrocarbon structure), or Crisco.
- *Chemical burns.* For chemical burns, immediately remove the client's clothing and use a hose or shower to lavage the involved area thoroughly for a minimum of 20 minutes. Many chemicals come in powder form, and as much dry chemical as possible needs to be removed from the skin before its surface is flushed with water. Unusual chemicals may require consultation with a Poison Control Center about appropriate treatment. The rescuer should wear protective clothing during this portion of the care process for personal protection from chemical exposure. Chemical splashes in or near the eye require immediate eye irrigation with clean, cool water or saline solution.
- *Electrical burns.* Electrical injuries pose the potential of serious harm to both rescuer and burn victim. Thus, before assisting the victim, ensure that the source of electrical current has been disconnected. If this isn't possible, move the client to safety away from the energy source using a nonconductive device such as an unpainted nonmetal broomstick. Assess an unresponsive client for the presence of cardiac and respiratory function. If indicated, begin cardiopulmonary resuscitation (CPR). Keep in mind a pos-

sible spinal cord injury secondary to the forceful contraction of the muscles of the neck and back during exposure to the current. If possible, place the client in a cervical collar and transport him on a spinal board.

- *Radiation burns.* Radiation injuries are usually minor and involve only the epidermal layer of skin. Treatment therefore focuses on helping normal body mechanisms promote wound healing. However, for severe radiation burns, such as those caused by industrial radiation accidents, trained personnel may need to render the area safe for entry prior to beginning rescue efforts. In such cases, appropriate interventions are aimed at shielding, establishing distance, and limiting the time of exposure to the radioactive source.

SUPPORTING VITAL FUNCTION

Once the burning process has been stopped, rescue personnel should take steps to support the client's respiratory and circulatory function. Initial assessment of the client's respiratory and hemodynamic status begins with an evaluation of the client's airway, breathing, and circulation, as well as her disability status and exposure to the source of the burn. Collectively, these five elements (airway, breathing, circulation, disability, and exposure) are known as the **ABCDE** bundle of trauma care:

Airway
Breathing
Circulation
Disability
Exposure

Depending on the results of the ABCDE evaluation, one or more of the following actions may be appropriate:

- If the client has no pulse and is not breathing, begin CPR. Establish an airway and start mouth-to-mouth breathing and chest compressions. Continue CPR until spontaneous cardiopulmonary function returns or the emergency management team takes over.
- Position the client with his head elevated more than 30 degrees, and administer 100% humidified oxygen by face mask. Use nasotracheal suction as necessary to maintain a patent airway. Endotracheal intubation may be necessary if the client has facial edema and inhalation injury. Auscultate the lungs often on-site to monitor respiratory status. If available, continuous pulse oximetry can be used to provide ongoing assessment of the client's oxygen saturation levels.
- Monitor for cardiac dysrhythmias or arrest. When one is available, connect the client to a cardiac monitor and observe for dysrhythmias. Elevate any burned extremities above the level of the heart to facilitate circulation.
- Initiate fluid replacement therapy for burn wounds that involve more than 20% of the client's TBSA. Continuously assess heart and lung sounds and observe level of consciousness, cardiac rate and rhythm, blood pressure, and urine output.
- Cover the client to maintain body temperature and to prevent further wound contamination and tissue damage.

---

highest level of health restoration, which may take years. During this stage, the primary focus is the biopsychosocial adjustment of the client, which may include the following measures:

- Prevention of contractures and scars
- The client's successful resumption of work, family, and social roles through physical, vocational, occupational, and psychosocial rehabilitation
- ROM exercises to enhance mobility and to support injured joints

Emergency and Acute Care

Immediately upon the client's arrival at the hospital, the nurse should assess the client's airway and efficacy of breathing, including thorough auscultation of breath sounds and continuous pulse oximetry monitoring. Clients who sustain severe burns or who may be at risk for inhalation injury often are tracheally intubated by emergency medical personnel prior to hospital arrival. Assessment of circulatory status includes obtaining and continuing to monitor the client's blood pressure, heart rate, and ECG. The nurse should obtain a history of the injury (including any medical interventions already implemented), estimate the depth and extent of the burn, begin fluid resuscitation as per medical orders, and continue to support ventilation according to protocol. These measures generally precede diagnostic testing and any surgical or pharmacologic therapies, with the exception of administration of analgesics.

After stabilization in the emergency department, the client is transferred to the critical care unit or a facility that specializes in the treatment of clients with burns. In both settings, continuous support and monitoring of the client's physiological status, administration of medications, pain control, wound management, and nutrition support therapies constitute the initial plan of care.

AIRWAY AND VENTILATORY MANAGEMENT Intubation is indicated for all clients with burns of the chest, face, or neck. The primary treatment plan is oriented toward preventing atelectasis and maintaining alveolar oxygen exchange. The following interventions should be initiated:

■ Maintain the head of the bed at 30 degrees or greater to maximize the client's ventilatory efforts. Turn the client from side to side every 2 hours to prevent hypostatic pneumonia.

■ To keep airway passages clear, suction the client frequently, encourage the client to use incentive spirometry hourly, and help the client perform coughing and deep-breathing exercises every 2 hours.

■ In the face of impending airway obstruction, the client will require immediate intubation. Nasotracheal tube placement is the preferred route because it seems to be better tolerated and can be more effectively secured. If the client has suffered nasolabial burns, however, the orotracheal route is preferred. Nasotracheal and orotracheal intubation are reserved for short-term ventilatory management. For long-term ventilatory management (i.e., greater than 3 weeks), a tracheostomy should be performed.

■ Humidification of either room air or oxygen helps prevent drying of tracheal secretions. The choice of ambient air or oxygen flow is based on ABG results. The client may be placed on a face mask, steam collar, T-piece, mechanical ventilation with positive end-expiratory pressure, pressure support ventilation, or high-frequency jet ventilation. The goal of all therapies is to maintain adequate tissue oxygenation with the least amount of inspired oxygen flow necessary.

■ Medications to dilate constricted bronchial passages may be administered intravenously and/or as inhalants to control bronchospasms and wheezing. Mucolytic agents can be used to liquefy tenacious sputum and aid in expectoration.

■ An arterial line is placed in the client with a major burn injury for continuous assessment of ABGs. Pulmonary artery pressure (PAP) catheters may be inserted to measure pulmonary vascular resistance (PVR), PAP, pulmonary artery wedge pressure (PAWP), and mixed venous oxygen saturation (SvO_2). The client's PVR and PAP rises in the presence of hypoxia. The SvO_2 is the average percentage of hemoglobin bound with oxygen in the venous blood, and it reflects overall tissue utilization of oxygen. Pulse oximetry may also be used to monitor arterial oxygen saturation levels.

■ In the presence of carbon monoxide (CO) poisoning, the client's carboxyhemoglobin (COHgb) levels must be monitored. Pulse oximetry cannot distinguish between oxyhemoglobin and COHgb; thus a false normal or high pulse oximetry reading is seen. High-flow 100% oxygen should be given immediately by nonrebreather mask. Clients with COHgb greater than 15% may also require hyperbaric oxygen therapy to replace the CO.

SAFETY ALERT
High levels of carbon monoxide in the bloodstream can skew pulse oximetry readings, giving the appearance of adequate oxygen saturation even in hypoxic clients. Make client assessment your primary data source, and do not rely on monitors as a replacement for assessment.

CIRCULATORY SUPPORT AND FLUID RESUSCITATION
Fluid resuscitation is the administration of IV fluids to restore the circulating blood volume during the acute period of increasing capillary permeability, thus counteracting the effects of burn shock. Fluid replacement is necessary for all burn wounds that involve 20% or more of the TBSA.

During fluid resuscitation, crystalloid fluids are administered through two large-bore (14- to 16-gauge) catheters, preferably inserted through unburned skin. Because it most closely approximates the body's extracellular fluid composition, warmed lactated Ringer solution is the IV fluid most widely used during the first 24 hours after burn injury. Several formulas may be used to replace fluid loss, including Parkland formula and ABLS Consensus formula. These formulas specify the volume of fluid to be infused over the first 24 hours from the time of the burn injury, with 50% of the fluid to be infused during the first 8 hours, followed by the remaining 50% during the next 16 hours (25% per 8 hours; Stander & Wallis, 2011; University of Washington Harborview Medical Center, 2011).

Hourly urine output is considered the most effective indicator of fluid resuscitation. In adult clients with burn injuries, urine production of 0.5–1 mL/kg/hr is considered adequate. In pediatric clients with burns, the targeted hourly urine output is 1–1.5 mL/kg/hr (Emergency Nurses Association, 2010). Clients who sustain electrical burns often have injuries that are not visible. For these clients, conventional fluid resuscitation formulas, which rely upon calculation of the percentage of the client's body that is burned, may underestimate their fluid requirements and generally are not used. Instead, administration of intravenous fluids is titrated to maintain urine output of approximately 100 mL/h in adult clients and 1.5 mL/kg/h in pediatric clients (Cooper, 2009b).

Another indicator is heart rate; if fluid resuscitation is adequate, the rate should be less than 110 beats per minute or in the upper limits of normal for age. However, underlying conditions and the fear, anxiety, and pain that accompany burn injuries often increase heart rate. Blood pressure changes are less reliable because significant hypotension does not develop until volume losses exceed 30% due to the body's compensatory mechanisms. Rather, assessment for narrowed pulse pressure (which indicates shock earlier) should be considered along with urine output to monitor adequate fluid resuscitation (Latenser, 2009).

During the fluid resuscitation stage, the client may require invasive hemodynamic monitoring. A pulmonary artery catheter may be used to monitor cardiac output, cardiac index, and PAWPs. All measurements must be maintained within normal limits to effect adequate fluid resuscitation.

Diagnostic Tests

Upon the client's admission to the emergency department, following assessment and management of all acute life-threatening issues, several diagnostic tests should be completed. The following tests are particularly useful in establishing a baseline and evaluating the burn client's response to therapeutic interventions throughout the entire hospitalization period:

- *Pulse oximetry* generally allows for continuous assessment of oxygen saturation levels, except in clients with carbon monoxide poisoning. For these clients, pulse oximetry readings may be falsely elevated due to carbon monoxide that is bound to hemoglobin.

- *Carboxyhemoglobin measurement*, which may be performed using venous or arterial blood, measures the percentage of hemoglobin that is bound to carbon monoxide.

- *Serial ABGs* indicate the presence of hypoxia and acid–base disturbances and help measure client response to changes in oxygen therapies. The burn-injured client may demonstrate elevated or lowered pH, decreased PCO_2, decreased PO_2, and low-normal bicarbonate levels.

- *Serial 12-lead electrocardiograms (ECGs)* are necessary to monitor the development of dysrhythmias, especially those associated with hypokalemic and hyperkalemic states.

- *Serial chest x-ray studies* document changes within the first 24–48 hours after injury that may reflect the presence of atelectasis, pulmonary edema, or ARDS.

- *Urinalysis* indicates the adequacy of renal perfusion and the client's nutritional status. In catabolic states, nitrogen is excreted in large amounts into the urine. Nitrogen loss is measured through 24-hour urine collection and testing for total nitrogen, urea nitrogen, and amino acid nitrogen. Myoglobinuria, which manifests as dark brown or wine-colored urine, signals the development of acute tubular necrosis. Loss of plasma protein and dehydration often lead to proteinuria and elevated urine specific gravity. Glycosuria is also a transient development following major burn injury, and it indicates a need to adjust the nutritional program.

- *Complete blood count (CBC)* must be monitored regularly. Hematocrit may be elevated secondary to hemoconcentration and fluid shifts from the intravascular compartment, and hemoglobin may be decreased secondary to hemolysis. WBCs are also elevated if infection is present.

- *Serum electrolytes* should also be regularly monitored. Sodium levels are generally decreased secondary to massive fluid shifts into the interstitium. Potassium levels are initially elevated during burn shock as a result of cell lysis and fluid shifts into the extracellular space. However, potassium levels decrease after burn shock resolves as fluid shifts back to the intracellular and intravascular compartments.

- *Renal function* test results are critical. In burn clients, blood urea nitrogen (BUN) is elevated secondary to dehydration. Creatinine is also elevated in the presence of renal insufficiency.

- *Total protein, albumin, transferrin, prealbumin, retinol binding protein, alpha one-acid glycoprotein, and C-reactive protein levels* indicate protein synthesis and nutritional status. However, because of the fluid shifts that occur during the early stages of a burn injury, these measurements are more useful during the rehabilitative phase of care.

- *Creatine phosphokinase (CPK)* is elevated following an electrical burn, secondary to extensive muscle damage.

- Finally, *blood glucose* is transiently elevated after any major burn injury.

Surgery

Three surgical interventions are commonly employed to manage burn wounds: escharotomy, surgical debridement, and autografting.

ESCHAROTOMY   When burn eschar forms circumferentially around the torso or extremities, it acts as a tourniquet, impairing circulation. If this eschar is left unchecked, the affected body part will become gangrenous. To prevent circumferential constriction of the torso or extremity, the physician may perform an **escharotomy**, removing the eschar with a scalpel or by electrocautery (**Figure 21–13 ●**). During this procedure, a sterile surgical incision is made longitudinally along the extremity or trunk to release taut skin and allow for expansion caused by edema formation. In the first 24 hours following the

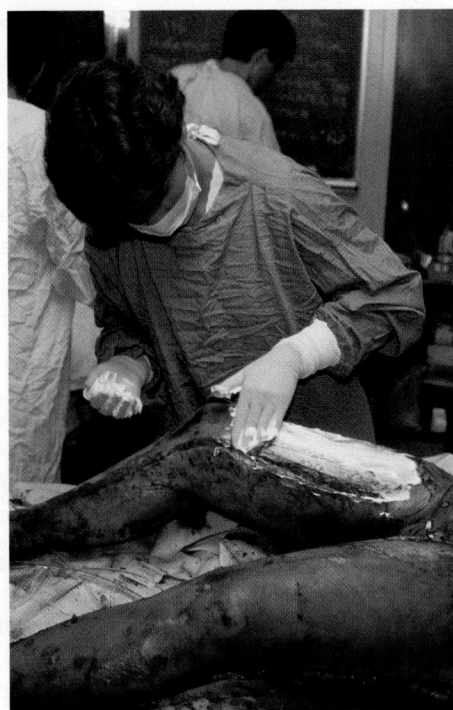

Figure 21–13 ● Escharotomy, the surgical procedure that removes the eschar formed on the skin and underlying tissue following severe burns. The procedure is particularly helpful in restoring circulation to the client's extremities when scar tissue forms a tight, constrictive band around the circumference of a limb.
Source: © English/Custom Medical Stock Photo.

procedure, the incision should be gently packed with fine-mesh gauze. After 24 hours, the site may be treated with direct application of a topical antimicrobial agent.

SURGICAL DEBRIDEMENT

Surgical debridement is the process of excising a wound to the level of fascia (**fascial excision**) or sequentially removing thin slices of the wound to the level of viable tissue (**tangential excision**). Because fascial excision, or **fasciectomy**, sacrifices potentially viable fat and lymphatic tissue, its use is reserved for clients with extensive or full-thickness burns. The most common technique is electrocautery with cutting and coagulating current capabilities. Tangential excision, by contrast, is performed with the use of a dermatome. Shallow burns and some burns of moderate depth bleed briskly after one slice. If bleeding does not occur, the procedure is repeated until a viable bed of dermis or subcutaneous fat is reached. Following surgical debridement, the client is returned to the burn unit.

AUTOGRAFTING

Autografting is a procedure performed in the surgical suite in which part of the client's healthy skin is removed and used to effect permanent skin coverage over the wound area. Early burn wound excision and skin grafting decrease the client's hospital stay and enhance rehabilitation.

During an autografting procedure, skin is removed from healthy tissue (the donor site) of the burn-injured client and applied to the burn wound. After the autograft is applied, the grafted area is immobilized. The site is assessed daily for evidence of adherence. The client resumes ROM exercises 5 days postgraft. As the wound heals, the client may complain of itching, which can be treated with mild lotions.

Cultured epithelial autografting is a technique in which skin cells are removed from unburned sites on the client's body, then minced and placed in a culture medium for growth. Over a 5- to 7-day period, the cells grow to 50–70 times the size of the initial biopsies. The cells are again separated out and placed in a new culture medium for continued growth. With this technique, enough skin can be grown over a period of 3–4 weeks to cover an entire human body. The cells are prepared in sheets and attached to petroleum jelly gauze backing, which is applied to the burn wound site. Although this procedure is often successful, problems with infection and lack of attachment may occur.

Pharmacologic Therapy

Clients with burns typically receive medications to control pain, prevent infection (including tetanus), and reduce the risk of peptic ulcer disease. IV fluids and other medications to support vital functions may also be indicated in individuals with severe burns.

ANALGESIA

Burns often cause excruciating pain. In the emergent stages of care, opioid analgesics such as morphine, oxycodone, or fentanyl are the best means of managing pain. Morphine is generally the drug of choice, and it may be given orally or intravenously. Oxycodone is an effective alternative to morphine, and it, too, may be administered either orally or intravenously. While also a fast-acting opiate, fentanyl differs from morphine and oxycodone in that it may be given intravenously, orally, or transmucosally (often via intranasal sprays or lozenges that permit absorption through the buccal mucosa). For all three drugs, it's best to avoid oral administration until the client has resumed hemodynamic stability and normal gastric emptying. IV and/or transmucosal preparations also offer

the benefit of faster pain relief and are thus preferred during the early stages of care.

Later, during the acute stage of burn care, various opioids may be administered around the clock to decrease pain that occurs at rest. Prior to undergoing any procedures, the client typically receives a larger dose of these medications. Ongoing pain management may also be provided by simple analgesics such as acetaminophen (which has an enhanced effect when combined with opiates) and nonsteroidal anti-inflammatory drugs (NSAIDs). In many cases, patient-controlled analgesia (PCA) enhances the client's ability to cope with pain. Because burn treatments and the trauma associated with experiencing a major burn can produce high levels of anxiety, antianxiety agents such as midazolam and lorazepam may also be helpful, especially when administered 1 hour before wound care (Richardson & Mustard, 2009).

ANTIMICROBIALS

Systemic infection is a leading cause of death in clients with major burns. Gram-positive organisms such as *Staphylococcus* and *Streptococcus* colonize the burn surface during the first week postburn; gram-negative enteric organisms become more common with longer periods of hospitalization, as do yeast and other fungal infections. To determine whether infectious organisms are present—and if so, what they are—routine wound cultures should be obtained at least once a week while a client is in the hospital or burn center (Weber & McManus, 2004).

Depending on protocol, topical antimicrobial therapy may be used to eliminate infection on the surface of a burn wound. Generally, topical antimicrobials are not applied until the client is admitted to a burn unit. Of the many antimicrobial agents available, the most widely used are mafenide acetate (Sulfamylon) cream, silver nitrate 0.5% soaks, and silver sulfadiazine (Silvadene) cream. All three are broad-spectrum antibiotics. The choice of topical antibiotic is based on the extent of the burn wound; the presence of identified bacterial organisms; the method of treatment (that is, whether open to the air or closed using bulky dressings); and client response.

Despite antimicrobial therapy, clients with major burn assault have a greater risk for sepsis and septic shock. Thus clients with major burns are usually given prophylactic antibiotics. Systemic antimicrobial therapy is indicated in the immediate preoperative and postoperative periods associated with excision and autografting. Postoperatively, antibiotic therapy is discontinued as soon as the client's hemodynamic status returns to normal, usually within the first 24 hours. In the long-term treatment of identified infectious processes, drug administration is limited to the least amount of time required to eradicate the infection.

TETANUS PROPHYLAXIS

If the client's immunization status is in doubt, tetanus toxoid should be administered intramuscularly early in the acute phase of care to prevent *Clostridium tetani* infection. If the client's tetanus immunization is older than 5 years, a booster should be administered.

ANTACIDS

With burn clients, hyperacidity must be controlled to prevent Curling ulcer. A nasogastric tube is placed during the emergent phase of care, and gastric aspirant is obtained hourly. The gastric pH should be assessed and maintained at levels above 5. To control gastric acid secretion during the acute phase of care, histamine H_2 blockers (e.g., famotidine [Pepcid]) or proton pump inhibitors (e.g., pantoprazole [Protonix]) can be administered intravenously, either intermittently or as continuous infusions. As soon as bowel sounds become audible, the client is placed on an antacid regimen.

Nonpharmacologic Therapy

Clients with burn wounds can benefit from a range of nonpharmacologic interventions delivered by a multidisciplinary team of professionals. In general, these interventions revolve around proper wound management and nutritional therapies.

WOUND MANAGEMENT The main goal of burn wound management is to close the wound as soon as possible (Latenser, 2009). To help clients with major burns achieve this goal, the healthcare team must prevent and treat infection through daily topical wound care, wound monitoring, and wound excision and closure. This treatment includes proper debridement and use of dressings, as described in the following sections.

Debridement Burned tissue releases chemical mediators that stimulate phagocytosis in an attempt to digest debris left by decaying necrotic tissue. Necrotic tissue that remains despite phagocytic action retards healing and prolongs inflammation. To prevent this from happening, the necrotic tissue must be removed by one of three methods: mechanical, enzymatic, or surgical debridement.

As was previously described, surgical debridement is the cutting away of necrotic tissue. Mechanical debridement also involves the removal of dead tissue, but in this case, the nurse does so by applying and removing gauze dressings (wet-to-dry or wet-to-moist) or by using hydrotherapy, irrigation, or scissors and tweezers (sharp debridement). Although removal of gauze dressings is perhaps the simplest method, it can cause pain and possibly damage granulation tissue. To prevent these problems, hydrotherapy is sometimes preferable. During hydrotherapy (in an immersion tank, in a shower, or on a spray table), the burn injury is gently washed with a mild, non-perfumed antimicrobial soap or wound cleanser solution to remove dead skin and to separate eschar. The solution is then rinsed off with warm saline or tap water. Within the burn, body hair (except for eyebrows) is shaved to within 2.5 cm of the wound edges. Blistered skin is then grasped with dry gauze and gently removed. Next, the edges of blisters or eschar are trimmed with blunt scissors, and the wound is covered with a topical antimicrobial agent.

Enzymatic debridement is similar but involves the use of a topical agent to dissolve and remove necrotic tissue and lift eschar. An enzyme preparation such as collagenase (Santyl), papain, papain-urea, or fibrinolysis-deoxyribonuclease (Elase) is applied in a thin layer only within the wound area and covered with one layer of fine-mesh gauze. A topical antimicrobial agent is then applied and covered with a bulky wet dressing, and the wound is immobilized with expandable mesh gauze. Enzymatic agents are discontinued once the eschar is removed and granulation tissue appears.

Dressing the Wound Once the burn wound has been cleaned and debrided, it may be dressed by one of two methods. In the open method, the wound remains open to air, covered only by a topical antimicrobial agent. This method allows easy access to the wound. Topical agents must be reapplied frequently because they tend to rub off onto the bedding. The open method also increases the risk for hypothermia.

In the closed method, a topical antimicrobial agent is applied to the wound site, and the site is then covered with gauze or a nonadherent dressing and gently wrapped with a gauze roll bandage. With the closed method, burn wounds are usually dressed twice daily and as needed. Dressings are applied circumferentially in a distal-to-proximal manner. All fingers and toes are wrapped separately. Dressings are held in place with stockinettes rather than tape to prevent further skin injury. The closed method decreases heat loss but may impair ROM.

Applying uniform pressure can prevent or reduce hypertrophic scarring. Accordingly, tubular support bandages may be applied 5–7 days postgraft to maintain tension ranging from 10 to 20 mmHg. The client may also wear custom-made elastic pressure garments (e.g., Jobst garments) for 6 months to a year postgraft.

Using Biological and Biosynthetic Dressings The terms *biological dressing* and *biosynthetic dressing* refer to any temporary material that rapidly adheres to the wound bed, promotes healing, and/or prepares the burn wound for permanent autograft coverage. Ideally, these kinds of dressings are inexpensive, nonantigenic, elastic, and easy to apply and remove. They should also reduce pain, serve as a bacterial barrier, and enhance the natural healing process. Such dressings are applied to the burn wound as soon as possible. Covering the wound eliminates the loss of water through evaporation, reduces infection, and promotes wound healing. Types of biological and biosynthetic dressings currently in use include homograft (allograft), heterograft (xenograft), amnionic membranes, and synthetic materials.

Homograft, also called **allograft**, is human skin that has been harvested from cadavers. It is stored in skin banks located throughout the nation. The development of methods to achieve prolonged storage of viable frozen skin has increased use of this dressing; however, its short supply and high expense still pose problems. Homograft is cut to match the pattern of a client's burn and applied by the use of sterile technique. As with any transplanted tissue, rejection is always a concern. Under normal circumstances, a homograft demonstrates rejection within 14–21 days following application if it is not accepted. Still, even with rejection, the homograft acts as a covering to reduce infection and promote healing for as long as it remains in place.

Heterograft, or **xenograft**, is skin obtained from an animal, usually a pig. Although fresh porcine heterograft is available at some centers, frozen heterograft is more commonly used. Once applied, heterograft appears to undergo early softening and lysis from enzymatic action in the wound. As a result, frequent changes of the heterograft dressing are necessary. Because of high infection rates associated with this type of dressing, researchers have developed silver-nitrate–treated porcine heterograft to help retard microbial growth.

The multiple problems associated with the use of biological dressings have driven the development of synthetic substitutes. One such material is Biobrane, a composite material consisting of nylon mesh bonded to silicone that has been used successfully in the temporary coverage of second- and third-degree burns. Whereas Biobrane adheres well to moderately clean wounds, it unfortunately cannot adhere to, or lower bacterial counts in, grossly contaminated wounds. Biobrane dressing is supplied in various sizes, cut to fit the wound site, and secured with tape or Steri-Strips. It spontaneously separates from the wound when the underlying tissue heals. Hydrocolloid dressings are another type of biosynthetic dressing that consists of occlusive wafers of gumlike materials that provide a water-resistant outer layer for coverage of the donor site. Hydrocolloid dressings protect healing tissue from excessive drying, liquefy necrotic tissue, and absorb wound drainage.

If dermal thickness is lost in deep partial-thickness or full-thickness burns, several products can serve as a dermal replacement. Integra is a synthetic dermal substitute, and AlloDerm is human cadaver allograft dermis that is nonimmunogenic. These products are placed in the wound, and split-thickness autografts are then placed over the dermal replacement. They provide temporary wound coverage, reduce pain, and facilitate healing.

Two more recently developed temporary skin substitutes are TransCyte and Apligraf. TransCyte is a bioengineered substance derived from human fibroblast cells grown within mesh. As the cells grow, they secrete human dermal collagen, matrix proteins, and growth factors. The product is produced, extensively tested for infectious agents, and then frozen. It is used as a temporary covering for surgically debrided full-thickness and deep partial-thickness burn wounds and is an alternative to silver sulfadiazine and cadaver skin. TransCyte forms a transparent protective barrier over the wound surface and is typically applied only once. The best results have been obtained when TransCyte was applied within 24 hours of injury. Apligraf is a bilayered skin substitute cultured from neonatal foreskin, and it is used similarly.

An even newer treatment method for burn wounds involves use of a vacuum-assisted closure (VAC) device. With this method, sponge that has tubing connecting it to a pump is placed over the wound. An occlusive adhesive dressing covers the wound and tubing, sealing the wound to create negative pressure. VAC has shown positive results in reducing wound edema, removing exudate, and improving healing in partial-thickness burns. It also helps shorten the time required to prepare burn wounds prior to skin grafting (Bollero et al., 2010).

NUTRITIONAL SUPPORT The client with a major burn is in a hypermetabolic and catabolic state. In fact, an individual's resting energy expenditure after severe burn injury can increase by as much as 100% over normal levels depending on the extent of catabolism and the client's physical activity, size, age, and gender. This increase is believed to be due to heat loss from the burn wound, an increase in beta-adrenergic activity, pain, and infection. As a result, the client's total caloric needs may be as great as 4,000–6,000 kcal/day.

Traditional dietary management based on oral intake seldom meets the kilocalorie requirements necessary to reverse negative nitrogen balance and begin the healing process. Therefore enteral feedings with a nasointestinal feeding tube are instituted within 24–48 hours of the burn injury to offset hypermetabolism, improve nitrogen balance, decrease sepsis, and decrease length of hospital stay. A nasointestinal feeding tube is placed under fluoroscopy, with the tip extending past the pylorus to prevent reflux and aspiration.

Although enteral feeding is the preferred nutritional therapy, it is contraindicated in Curling ulcer, bowel obstruction, feeding intolerance, pancreatitis, and septic ileus. When the enteral route cannot be used, a central venous catheter is inserted via the subclavian or jugular vein for administration of total parenteral nutrition.

NURSING PROCESS

The client with a major burn has complex multisystem needs. During the acute phase, life support and monitoring take priority. While beginning to heal, the client must cope with scarring, hair loss, and powerlessness. Thus the nurse must consider altered body image and loss of independence for a significant period of time, sometimes lifelong, when planning care.

Assessment

Nursing assessment is continuous from the initial contact with the client with a burn injury. Once the client arrives at the emergency department, the staff must act quickly to obtain the history of the burn injury, including the time of occurrence, causative agents, and any early treatment that has been provided. The nurse should also inquire about the client's medical history (including medication use), age, and body weight. In most cases, the client is awake and oriented and can relate the information during the emergent phase of care. Because changes in sensory abilities become evident within the first few hours following a major burn injury, the nurse must obtain as much information as possible immediately upon the client's arrival. Some guidelines for information gathering are as follows:

- *Time of injury.* In many cases, the client is admitted to the emergency department an hour or more after the injury occurred. The time of the burn injury must be documented as precisely as possible at the scene because all fluid resuscitation calculations are based on the time of the injury, *not* on the client's time of arrival at the emergency department.

- *Cause of the injury.* Because the type of burn injury determines which nursing measures take priority, it is important to identify the specific causative agent. This information allows the nurse to establish the appropriate plan of care.

- *First-aid treatment.* Prior to the arrival of medical personnel, the client or family may have applied home remedies to treat the burn wound. It is important for the nurse to ascertain and document the nature of all home treatment interventions, including the application of neutralizing agents, liquids, and immobilizing devices used to splint associated injuries.

- *Past medical history.* Obtaining a medical history is important because more intense observation is required for the client with a history of respiratory, cardiac, renal, metabolic, neurological, gastrointestinal, or skin diseases; alcohol abuse; or altered immune states. The nurse must also obtain information about known allergies.

- *Medications.* Any drugs (either prescribed or recreational) taken by the client prior to the burn injury may further complicate the treatment regimen. Drugs that affect any of the major body systems or cause mood alterations need to be factored into the treatment plan. Thus, as part of the early assessment, the nurse must obtain and document blood levels of therapeutic pharmaceutical agents and mood-altering substances.

- *Age.* Age is an important consideration in the treatment of burn clients, as children and older adults tend to require more supportive care.

- *Body weight.* During the acute and rehabilitative phases of the burn injury, the client loses as much as 20% of her preburn weight. This fact has significant implications for all clients, especially those who are underweight at the time of injury.

Clinical Manifestations and Therapies **Burns**

ETIOLOGY	CLINICAL MANIFESTATIONS	CLINICAL THERAPIES
Superficial burns	■ Only the epidermis is affected. ■ Skin is dry and pink to bright red. ■ Slight edema may be present over the burned area. ■ May be accompanied by chills, headache, nausea, and vomiting. ■ Usually heals in 3–6 days with no scarring.	■ Administration of mild analgesics ■ Regular cleaning ■ Application of water-soluble lotions and topical agents ■ If burns are extensive, IV fluid may be required
Partial-thickness burns *Superficial partial-thickness burn*	■ Both epidermis and dermis (papillary layer) are affected. ■ Skin is bright red and has a moist appearance. ■ Blister formation is common. ■ Burned area blanches upon pressure. ■ Client may experience severe pain in response to temperature and air exposure. ■ Usually heals within 21 days with minimal to no scarring.	■ Administration of analgesics ■ Regular cleaning ■ Use of skin substitutes if large area is burned ■ Administration of antipyretics in case of fever associated with thermal burns
Deep partial-thickness burn	■ Both epidermis and dermis (papillary and reticular layers) are affected. ■ Burn area is pale and waxy and may be moist or dry. ■ Blisters are present and may be large and easily ruptured or flat and dry like tissue paper. ■ Capillary refill is decreased. ■ Sensation to deep pressure remains intact, although other forms of sensation (including pain) are decreased. ■ May require more than 21 days to heal. ■ May convert to full-thickness injury if necrosis extends to depth of wound. ■ Contractures are possible. ■ Hypertrophic scarring and functional impairment may occur.	■ Therapeutic measures generally the same as those used for superficial partial-thickness burns ■ Excision and grafting possibly necessary to decrease scarring and lack of function
Full-thickness burns	■ Epidermis, dermis, and underlying tissues are all affected. ■ Burn area may appear pale, waxy, yellow, brown, mottled, charred, or nonblanching red. ■ Wound surface is dry and leathery, with thrombosed vessels visible. ■ Sensation to pain and light touch is absent at the burn site. ■ Skin grafting is required for the wound to heal.	■ Regular cleaning ■ Application of topical agents ■ Use of skin substitutes ■ Excision of eschar ■ Skin grafting

Diagnosis

Each client's condition warrants individualized nursing diagnoses based on assessment data. Nursing diagnoses that may be appropriate for inclusion in the plan of care for the client with burns include the following:

- *Ineffective Airway Clearance*
- *Impaired Gas Exchange*
- *Risk for Aspiration*
- *Risk for Decreased Cardiac Tissue Perfusion*
- *Deficient Fluid Volume*
- *Risk for Ineffective Renal Perfusion*

- *Risk for Infection*
- *Imbalanced Nutrition: Less Than Body Requirements*
- *Acute Pain*
- *Impaired Physical Mobility*
- *Powerlessness*

(NANDA-I © 2012)

Planning

A major burn affects virtually every body system, as well as the client's social, cultural, economic, psychological, and spiritual well-being. As was discussed earlier in this exemplar, for the

Lifespan Considerations Assessing a Child With a Burn Injury

Interviewing a parent about a child's burn injury can be difficult. If the injury was preventable, the parent may be emotionally stressed by feelings of guilt. The nurse must therefore use caution to avoid sounding accusatory when questioning the parent about the injury.

The nurse should also be alert to signs of child abuse when the history does not match the burn injury (e.g., glove and stocking burns; burns that spare flexor surfaces; contact burns from objects such as curling irons, cigarettes, and irons; and zebra burn lines from contact with a hot grate; **Figure 21–14 ●**). Photographs may be taken to document these burn injuries. Child neglect may be a factor in the burn of a child who was not adequately supervised.

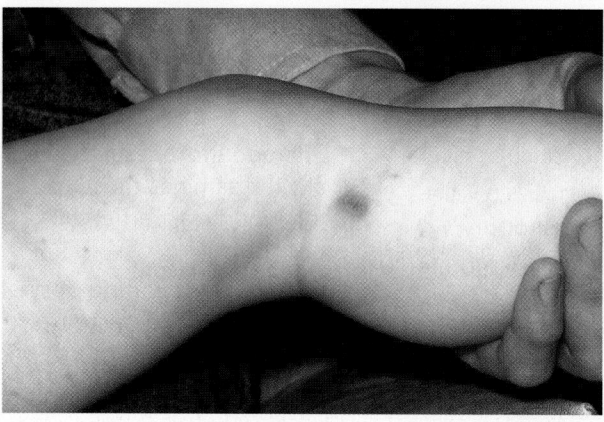

Figure 21–14 ● Burn injuries associated with child abuse.
Source: © Medical-on-Line/Alamy.

client who has sustained life-threatening injuries, the three priorities of care are ensuring proper airway management, maintaining effective breathing, and promoting adequate cardiovascular circulation. The plan of care changes as the client moves from stage to stage, and it requires frequent updating in response to the client's changing condition. For the stable client who has sustained a burn, goals of client care often include the following:

- The client will maintain a clear, unobstructed airway.
- The client will maintain ABG values and pulse oximetry readings that are within normal limits.
- The client will demonstrate no cardiac dysrhythmias.
- The client will receive adequate nutrition to meet body needs.
- The client will maintain adequate fluid volume, as evidenced by hourly urine output that meets minimum acceptable guidelines.
- The client's blood pressure and heart rate will range within acceptable limits.
- The client will demonstrate adequate wound healing.
- The client will maintain adequate pain control, reporting pain as a 3 or less on a scale of 0–10.
- The client will not develop a healthcare-associated infection.
- The client will maintain full ROM following recovery.

Implementation

Nursing interventions related to ensuring airway patency, effective ventilation, and adequate circulation, were described earlier in this exemplar. Additional elements included in the care of the client who sustains a burn injury include fluid and nutritional considerations, pain management, wound care, and infection prevention. Continuous assessment is necessary until well into the healing process and should include assessment of client and family feelings regarding the injury and its long-term effects.

Promote Fluid Volume Balance

Fluid resuscitation rates are adjusted periodically throughout the emergent stage of care. The nurse should be particularly aware of several situations that may warrant administration of fluids at rates in excess of the calculations needed to maintain adequate urine output. These situations include initial underestimation of burn size, sequestration of fluid into lung tissue in an inhalation injury, electrical injury full-thickness burns, and inordinately delayed starts of fluid resuscitation. To most effectively promote fluid volume balance, the nurse should also do the following:

- Monitor intake and output hourly. Report decreased or inadequate urine output.
- Regularly assess narrowed pulse pressure, which is an earlier and more accurate indicator of shock than blood pressure or heart rate.
- Monitor hemodynamic status; inadequate fluid resuscitation is manifested by a drop in central venous pressure (CVP) and PAWP.
- Follow prescribed protocols for IV fluid resuscitation. Therapy for burn shock is aimed at supporting the client through the period of hypovolemic instability.
- Weigh the client daily. Body weight is used to calculate fluid requirements.
- Test all stools and emesis for the presence of blood. Occult blood in emesis or stool indicates gastrointestinal bleeding.
- Maintain a warm environment. Hypothermia leads to shivering and further loss of body fluid through increased energy expenditure and catabolism.
- Monitor for fluid volume overload. Older clients and clients with underlying cardiac disease may demonstrate symptoms of heart failure during the fluid resuscitation stage.

SAFETY ALERT

Major burn clients receive 10 or more liters of fluid and gain weight due to fluid shifts. When their capillary membrane integrity resumes, these clients have a high CVP and urine output that necessitates monitoring of urine electrolytes.

Provide Effective Pain Management

All partial-thickness burns, along with extensive superficial burns, can cause excruciating pain, as can wound care and physical therapy. Increased levels of anxiety about treatments and outcomes may increase a client's perception of pain. To help manage this pain, the nurse should take the following actions:

- Measure the client's level of pain using a consistent measurement tool. The term *pain tolerance* refers to the duration and

Lifespan Considerations Burns in the Older Adult

Older adults are at greater risk for burns of all degrees of severity, burns and fires being a major cause of death. Most burns are accidental, resulting from slower reaction times, decreased mobility, visual deficits, decreased sense of smell, forgetfulness, and impaired sensation. Many older adults are burned by stoves, hot water, hot food, irons, cookware, and heating pads. Older adults with cognitive impairment or dementia may start fires by leaving foods cooking unattended. The most common burns in this age group result from clothing catching fire and from tap water that is too hot.

Care of the older adult with burns often presents unique challenges. Older adults may delay seeking treatment, thus increasing the risk of infection. Care is also often complicated by the presence of other chronic illnesses. In addition, older adults may live alone and have no one to care for them dur-

ing rehabilitation. Thus even small burns have the potential to become lethal in older adults.

To help prevent burn injuries, the nurse should be sure to emphasize the following topics when working with older adults:

- Have a relative or neighbor routinely check for the odor of gas.
- Check the smoke detector battery once a month.
- Wear close-fitting clothing when cooking.
- Use a cooking timer with a loud alarm.
- Do not lay anything over a heating device.
- Set the temperature of the hot water heater no higher than 120°F.
- Install antiscald devices in bathroom plumbing.
- Encourage no smoking in the house.

intensity of pain that the client is able to endure. Pain tolerance differs from one client to the next and may vary in the same client in different situations. A description of pain management tools can be found in the exemplar on Acute and Chronic Pain in the module on Comfort.

- Administer pain medication before painful procedures and determine when PCA is appropriate. Remember that inability to manage pain often results in feelings of despair and frustration for the client.
- Administer IV opioid analgesics as prescribed. Nurses' fears of precipitating addiction often make them reluctant to administer narcotics. During the acute stage of burn injury, however, invasive procedures and exposed neurosensory nerve endings dictate the need for narcotic pharmaceutical agents.
- Explain all procedures and expected levels of discomfort. Clients experience less stress when they are prepared for painful procedures and know beforehand the actual sensations they will feel.
- Use methods of nonopioid pain control in combination with medications for pain. Noninvasive pain relief measures (e.g., relaxation, massage, distraction) can enhance the therapeutic effects of pain relief medications.
- Allow the client to verbalize the pain experience. Be aware that every individual experiences and expresses pain differently, using various sociocultural adaptation techniques.

SAFETY ALERT
Narcotics should be administered intravenously (rather than orally, subcutaneously, or intramuscularly) in the emergent or acute stage of a burn due to decreased circulation and absorption of medications.

Protect Skin Integrity

A burn injury significantly impairs the client's skin integrity, although the severity of impairment varies according to the depth and extent of the burn. General treatment measures are designed to restore normal skin function as quickly as possible. Nursing care focuses on assessing and cleaning the wound and

controlling infection. In this capacity, the nurse generally does the following:

- Estimate the extent and depth of the burn wound and recalculate the extent of unhealed burns weekly. The severity of the burn injury is the basis for determining which types of interventions are appropriate. Regular reassessment is necessary to monitor the healing process.
- Provide daily wound care (including debridement, dressing, and medication administration) as prescribed to remove dead tissue, control infection, and promote reepithelialization as soon as possible. During all wound care, steps must be taken to avoid cross-contamination of wounds.
- Elevate burned or newly skin-grafted extremities at or above heart level to increase venous return and prevent edema formation.
- Immobilize skin graft sites for 3–5 days or as ordered to promote graft adherence and prevent loss of newly grafted skin.

SAFETY ALERT
Move the client slowly and carefully across bed sheets to prevent shearing or dislodging new skin grafts.

- Provide special skin care to sensitive body areas as follows:
  a. Clean burns involving the eyes using normal saline or sterile water to prevent corneal and conjunctival drying and adherence. If contracture of the eyelid develops, apply drops or ointment to the eye to prevent corneal abrasion.
  b. Gently wipe burns of the lips with saline-soaked pads. Apply an antibiotic ointment as prescribed. Assess the mouth frequently, and perform mouth care routinely. If an oral endotracheal tube is in place, reposition it often to prevent pressure ulcer formation.
  c. Gently debride burns of the nose and apply mafenide acetate (Sulfamylon) cream. Position nasogastric and nasotracheal tubes to prevent excessive pressure.
  d. Apply mafenide acetate (Sulfamylon) cream to burns of the ear. Gently debride and thoroughly clean the wound with a water spray. Do not cover ears with dressings. Do not use pillows; to reduce pressure to the area, use a foam

doughnut instead. Burns of the ears are prone to infection, and special positioning devices are necessary to decrease pressure ulcer formation.

Prevent Infection

From the onset of a burn injury, loss of the body's natural barrier to the external environment increases the risk of infection. Appropriate nursing interventions therefore focus on controlling infectious processes and include the following:

- Monitor daily for manifestations of wound infection. Be sure to remove topical medications and wound exudate and examine the entire wound. Early manifestations of infection include swelling and inflammation of intact skin surrounding the wound; a change in the color, odor, or amount of exudate; increased pain; and loss of previously healed skin grafts.

> **SAFETY ALERT**
> An increase in body temperature without other manifestations of infection does not indicate infection in clients with large burn wounds, because the hypermetabolic response resets their core temperature to a higher level.

- Monitor for positive blood cultures, which indicate bacteremia.
- Monitor for hyperemia, cough, chest pain, wheezing, rhonchi, decreased oxygen saturation, and purulent sputum, all of which are manifestations of pneumonia.
- Monitor for the presence of bacteriuria, fever, urgency, frequency, dysuria, and superpubic pain, which are all manifestations of urinary tract infection.

> **SAFETY ALERT**
> If the client has an indwelling catheter, assess the urine for cloudiness and a foul odor, and obtain a urine culture and sensitivity at least weekly.

- Obtain daily WBC counts. Leukocyte counts are indicators of immune system function and increase in the presence of infection.
- Determine tetanus immunization status. Burn clients are at risk for anaerobic infection caused by *Clostridium tetani*.
- Maintain a high-kilocalorie intake. Nutritional support provides the nutrients needed to maintain the body's defense mechanisms.
- Maintain an aseptic environment using standard precautions (including gloving, gowning, and sterile procedures). Strict isolation technique deters the development of healthcare-associated infections.
- Culture all wounds and body secretions per protocol. Culture and sensitivity reports identify the presence of infectious microbes and indicate appropriate antimicrobial therapies.
- Administer prescribed antimicrobial medications to decrease invasive wound infections.

Maintain Physical Mobility

As a client's burn wound heals and new skin tissue forms, the involved area tends to shrink. Contractures often form at the site and significantly limit mobility, especially when a joint is involved. Physical therapy is therefore important beginning in the early stages of treatment. The nurse plays an important role in physical therapy and preservation of client mobility by way of the following interventions:

- Perform active or passive ROM exercises to all joints every 2 hours and assist the client in ambulating once she is stable. Regular exercise prevents further loss of motion, restores movement, and improves functional status.
- Apply splints as prescribed. Maintain antideformity positions and reposition the client hourly. Splinting and positioning retard the formation of contractures.
- Maintain limbs in functional alignment to preserve joint mobility.
- Anticipate the need for analgesia. Administering analgesics promotes the client's comfort during exercise sessions.

> **SAFETY ALERT**
> Assess all clients, especially older adults, for indications of pressure ulcer formation under splints.

Promote Balanced Nutrition

A burn injury initiates a complex series of events that have a profound effect on the body's use of nutrients and expenditure of energy. The dietitian determines a client's daily kilocalorie requirements, and as soon as possible, enteral or parenteral feedings are initiated. Associated nursing measures focus on assessing feeding tolerance and use of nutrients and include the following:

- Maintain nasogastric/nasointestinal tube placement. Correct tube placement ensures appropriate absorption of nutrients and prevents aspiration.
- Maintain enteral/parenteral nutritional support as prescribed. Observe and report any evidence of feeding intolerance, such as diarrhea, vomiting, excessive gastric residual, abdominal distention, absent bowel sounds, and constipation. The dietitian, in collaboration with the physician, selects and individualizes the feeding formula according to the client's daily energy expenditure requirements and feeding tolerance. Failure to maintain rates of infusion predisposes the client to continued catabolism and negative nitrogen balance.
- Weigh the client daily. Weight indicates the adequacy of nutritional support therapies.
- Obtain daily laboratory values for protein, iron, CBC, glucose, and albumin. Decreased serum values indicate inadequate nutritional intake.

Facilitate Empowerment

Usually, the client with a major burn injury endures a lengthy hospital stay involving many treatments and care protocols that are beyond the client's control. During the early stages, much of the care regimen involves excruciating pain. Further, the foreign environment of the burn unit makes it difficult for the client to relate to the immediate surroundings. For example, the need to control infection in the burn unit requires hospital personnel and family members to don sterile clothing before coming to the client's bedside. Family members and nursing personnel appear radically different when they are masked and gowned, and their odd appearance can add to the burn-injured client's sense of alienation. Furthermore, the client's body image is often altered depending on the extent and location of the

TABLE 21–6   Interventions in Various Stages of Burn Injury

STAGE OF BURN INJURY	ONSET	END POINT	INTERVENTIONS
Emergent/resuscitative	Occurrence of burn injury	Successful fluid resuscitation	Remove client from heat source. Initiate first aid. Assess extent of burn injury. Prevent hypothermia. Assess for shock. Determine need for intubation. Determine need for IV therapy. Follow protocol for fluid resuscitation. Obtain history. Transport to tertiary care facility.
Acute	Diuresis	Wound closure	Begin hydrotherapy. Determine need for excision of burn wound. Control spread of infection. Institute wound care. Start nutrition support. Graft burn wound. Initiate physical therapy. Manage pain.
Rehabilitative	Wound closure	Return to highest level of health restoration	Prevent scar formation. Continue physical therapy. Address psychosocial, cultural, and spiritual needs. Consider occupational therapy. Consider vocational training. Assess home maintenance management.

burn injury. To help address feelings of powerlessness, the nurse should take the following actions:

- Allow the client as much control over surroundings and daily routine as possible. For example, allow the client to choose times of dressing changes. Powerlessness derives from the belief that one is unable to influence the outcome of a situation.
- Keep needed items (e.g., call bell, urinal, water pitcher, and tissues) within the client's reach to reinforce the client's feelings of control.
- Encourage the client to express feelings. The nurse can help the client cope by therapeutically listening, displaying a caring presence, clarifying misconceptions, and providing positive feedback.
- Set short-term, realistic goals for the client (e.g., to ambulate from bedside to chair twice daily). Small incremental gains are easiest to achieve and allow for frequent positive reinforcement.

Table 21–6 ● lists overall interventions for the emergent, acute, and rehabilitative stages of burn injury.

Evaluation

The client with a severe burn must be constantly evaluated, and the plan of care changes to meet emerging or diminishing needs. It is not unusual for a client with a severe burn to be hospitalized for extended periods of time, requiring new care plan modifications as the client moves through the recovery process. Expected outcomes used to evaluate client progress may include the following:

- The client maintains stable vital signs, as evidenced by values within normal limits.
- The client receives adequate pain management to allow for comfort, as evidenced by being able to rest and reporting a pain level of 3 or less.

- The client's nutritional needs are being met, as evidenced by stable weight, balanced intake and output, and laboratory values within normal range.
- The client is infection-free, as evidenced by CBC within normal range and wound healing.

Lifespan Considerations
Recovery From Burns

Children

Play therapy is encouraged for children even if they can only observe initially. Play therapy serves the following purposes for the child with a major burn:

- It provides an outlet for frustration, independence, and creativity.
- It promotes activities that challenge ROM.
- It normalizes the child's daily routine.
- It encourages the child, who sees the progress that other children make day by day.

Family

Families of children with major burns are at risk for emotional stress. They should be forewarned to expect edema and changes in the child's body with the injury response. Fear usually results from lack of knowledge about the severity of the burn and the child's status, especially in the early stages of burn care and admission to the hospital's ICU.

Include the family in the child's care when possible. The family must be given information and frequent updates to promote the development of trust between the family and the healthcare team. Parents often feel guilty and responsible for the child's injury. It is important to help parents focus on recovery rather than past actions.

Client Teaching Burn Care

Client and family teaching is an important component of all phases of burn care. As treatment progresses, the nurse encourages family members to assume more responsibility in providing care. However, many burn centers perform dressing changes in a burn clinic because parents find it difficult to perform procedures they know will inflict pain on their child. If parents perform dressing changes, the nurse should provide client teaching regarding how to change the dressing(s) and how soon before the dressing change to give pain medication. Specific guidelines for dressing changes should be outlined so that parents and healthcare team members have the same focus.

From admission to discharge, the nurse teaches the client and family to assess all findings, implement therapies, and evaluate progress. The nurse should address the following topics when preparing the client and family for home care:

- Long-term goals of rehabilitation care (including preventing soft tissue deformity, protecting skin grafts, maintaining physiological function, managing scars, and returning the client to an optimal level of independence)

- Necessity of avoiding exposure to individuals with colds or infections and meticulously following aseptic technique when caring for the wound
- Need for progressive physical activity
- Procedures for applying splints, pressure support garments, and other assistive devices
- Dietary requirements with increased kilocalorie amounts
- Alternative pain control therapies such as guided imagery, relaxation techniques, and diversional activities
- Care of the graft and donor sites
- Referral for occupational therapy, social services, clergy, and/or psychiatric services as appropriate
- Referral to any of the following organizations dedicated to helping burn survivors:
  - American Burn Association (www.ameriburn.org)
  - International Society for Burn Injuries (www.worldburn.org)
  - American Academy of Facial Plastic and Reconstructive Surgery (www.aafprs.org)
  - The Phoenix Society for Burn Survivors (www.phoenix-society.org)

NURSING CARE PLAN   A Client With a Severe Burn

Craig Howard, a 39-year-old truck driver, is admitted to the hospital following an accident in which the cab of his truck caught fire. Mr. Howard was freed from the truck by a passing motorist, who stayed with him until the rescue team arrived to transport him to a local emergency department. Mr. Howard's wife, Mary, and twin daughters, Jessica and Jane, age 10, have been notified of the accident.

ASSESSMENT

On his admission to the emergency department, Mr. Howard is diagnosed with deep partial-thickness and full-thickness burns of the anterior chest, arms, and hands. A quick assessment based on the rule of nines estimates the extent of his burn injury at 36% of TBSA. His vital signs are as follows: T 35.6°C rectal (96.2°F), P 140 bpm, R 40/min, BP 98/60 mmHg. In the field, the paramedics inserted a large-bore central line into Mr. Howard's right subclavian vein and started the rapid infusion of lactated Ringer solution. Mr. Howard is also receiving 40% humidified oxygen via face mask. Initial ABGs are pH 7.49, pO$_2$ 60 mmHg, pCO$_2$ 32 mmHg, and bicarbonate 22 mEq/L. Lung sounds indicate inspiratory and expiratory wheezing, and a persistent cough reveals sooty sputum production. A Foley catheter is inserted and initially drains a moderate amount of dark concentrated urine. A nasogastric tube is connected to low intermittent suction. Mr. Howard is alert and oriented and complains of severe pain associated with the burn injuries. The burn unit is notified, and Mr. Howard is transferred there.

DIAGNOSES

- *Risk for Ineffective Airway Clearance* related to increasing lung congestion secondary to smoke inhalation
- *Deficient Fluid Volume* related to abnormal fluid loss secondary to burn injury
- *Risk for Ineffective Tissue Perfusion* (peripheral) related to peripheral constriction secondary to circumferential burn wounds of the arms

(NANDA-I © 2012)

PLANNING

Goals of nursing care include the following: Mr. Howard will

- Demonstrate a patent airway as evidenced by clear breath sounds; absence of cyanosis; and vital signs, chest x-ray findings, and ABGs within normal limits.
- Demonstrate adequate fluid volume and electrolyte balance as evidenced by urine output, vital signs, mental status, and laboratory findings within normal limits.
- Demonstrate adequate tissue perfusion as evidenced by palpable pulses, warm extremities, normal capillary refill, and absence of paresthesia.

IMPLEMENTATION

- Prepare for prophylactic nasotracheal intubation to maintain airway patency.
- Initiate fluid resuscitation therapy using the Parkland formula to calculate IV fluid rate for the first 24 hours postburn.
- Assist the physician in performing escharotomies of both upper extremities.

NURSING CARE PLAN (continued)

EVALUATION

The nurse anesthetist inserted a nasotracheal tube and connected Mr. Howard to a T-piece delivering 40% oxygen. Vigorous respiratory toileting has significantly improved his ABGs. Bronchodilators have been parenterally administered and mucolytic agents added to his respiratory treatments. Mr. Howard's tracheal secretions have begun to show evidence of clearing. Hourly urine outputs indicate adequate fluid resuscitation. Urine output has been maintained at 50 mL/h, and color and concentration have improved. CVP readings have been maintained at 6 cm H_2O, and blood pressure has increased to 100/64 mmHg. Pulse rate has decreased to 100 bpm.

To improve tissue perfusion of both arms, the physician has performed bilateral escharotomies, and the wounds have been dressed by sterile procedure. Consequently, the extremities have demonstrated improved circulation.

CRITICAL THINKING

1. Explain the rationale for the immediate insertion of a Foley catheter and nasogastric tube.
2. An escharotomy was performed on both arms. Why was this procedure necessary in Mr. Howard's case?
3. What is the rationale supporting the IV administration of narcotics to control Mr. Howard's pain?
4. Explain the sequence of events that led to a fluid and electrolyte shift during the first 24–48 hours after Mr. Howard sustained his injury.

REVIEW Burns

RELATE Link the Concepts and Exemplars

Linking the exemplar of burns with the concept of comfort:

1. When providing care to the client with deep full thickness burns involving the entire right arm, will the nurse need to administer analgesics? Explain your answer.

2. A client is brought to the emergency department with partial-thickness burns of the chest and neck. The client is crying in pain. What nursing considerations will affect the plan for pain management for this client?

Linking the exemplar of burns with the concept of development:

3. In the care of a 12-year-old client admitted following a major burn, what pain scale is most appropriate for assessing pain? Explain your choice.

4. Once this client's physical condition stabilizes, how can the nurse address the client's developmental issues?

READY Go to Companion Skills Manual

REFER Go to Pearson Student Nursing Resources
nursing.pearsonhighered.com

- Additional review material

REFLECT Case Study

David Newton, age 54, was smoking a cigarette and fell asleep, dropping the cigarette and igniting his bed linens. A neighbor saw the fire and called 911, and Mr. Newton was rescued by the fire department. He sustained full-thickness burns over the upper half of his chest and back and the posterior aspects of both upper arms. He also sustained superficial partial-thickness burns to his anterior and posterior head and neck.

Mr. Newton was initially treated in the local emergency department and then transported via life flight to a specialized burn unit located 150 miles from his home. Upon his arrival in the burn unit, 5 hours after injury, the nurse notes the presence of a Foley catheter that is draining burgundy-colored urine. Mr. Newton also has a nasogastric tube that is draining dark yellow-green liquid. He was intubated in the emergency department and is now placed on a ventilator in the burn unit. Upon admission to the burn unit, Mr. Newton's vital signs are as follows: temperature 99.9°F oral; pulse 102 bpm; respirations 24/min; and BP 98/52 mmHg. His pain level is reported as a 9 on a 1–10 scale, and he is medicated with morphine sulfate 10 mg IV by the physician's order.

1. The initial assessment in the emergency department is that Mr. Newton has sustained burns over 36% of his body. Using the rule of nines, how does the nurse analyze this total percentage?

2. Mr. Newton is in the phase of burn shock. His urinary output for the past 5 hours has been 150 mL. On the basis of his urinary output and vital signs, what is the nurse's explanation for the physiology of shock related to a major burn injury?

3. Mr. Newton's diagnosis is *Impaired Gas Exchange* related to swelling secondary to inhalation injury manifested by need for intubation and mechanical ventilation. Why was intubation necessary for Mr. Newton? What important nursing interventions are related to this choice?

4. Why was Mr. Newton's Foley catheter draining burgundy-colored urine at the time of admission to the burn unit?

5. Mr. Newton is put on enteral feeding during the recovery phase of the burn injury, and the related nursing diagnosis is *Imbalanced Nutrition: Less Than Body Requirements* related to hypermetabolic and catabolic stage secondary to a major burn. What is the rationale for this diagnosis?

EXEMPLAR 21.2 Contact Dermatitis

EXEMPLAR KEY TERMS
Allergic contact dermatitis, *1488*
Contact dermatitis, *1488*
Irritant contact dermatitis, *1488*
Patch testing, *1490*

EXEMPLAR LEARNING OUTCOMES
After reading about this exemplar, you will be able to:

1. Describe the pathophysiology, etiology, clinical manifestations, and direct and indirect causes of contact dermatitis.

2. Identify risk factors and prevention methods associated with contact dermatitis.

3. Illustrate the nursing process in providing culturally competent care across the life span for individuals with contact dermatitis.

4. Formulate priority nursing diagnoses appropriate for an individual with contact dermatitis.

5. Summarize therapies used by interdisciplinary teams in the collaborative care of an individual with contact dermatitis.

6. Plan evidence-based care for an individual with contact dermatitis and his or her family in collaboration with other members of the healthcare team.

7. Evaluate expected outcomes for an individual with contact dermatitis.

▶ OVERVIEW

Contact dermatitis is an inflammation of the skin caused by direct contact with an allergen or irritant. It typically manifests as a localized rash or irritation in the superficial layers of the skin. Contact dermatitis may not appear until several days after exposure and may take several weeks to heal. Healing is slowed if the skin is continually exposed to the allergen or irritant.

> ### SAFETY ALERT
> - The increased use of latex gloves among healthcare providers has resulted in increased reporting of latex allergies. It is estimated that 8–12% of healthcare providers are allergic to latex (Occupational Safety and Health Administration, 2008).
> - The most common type of allergic response to latex gloves is type IV, T-cell–mediated contact dermatitis.
> - Type I, IgE-mediated hypersensitivity, manifested by urticaria, rhinoconjunctivitis, asthma, or anaphylaxis, is far more serious than the T-cell–mediated type.
> - All clients with a latex allergy should be treated in a latex-free environment.
> - Healthcare providers with severe allergic responses to latex may have to seek a different type of employment.

▶ PATHOPHYSIOLOGY AND ETIOLOGY

Contact dermatitis is characterized by damage to the dermis and epidermis. This damage typically takes the form of a red, itchy rash. The rash is usually confined to the area of skin that came into contact with the allergen or irritant. Bullae, vesicles, and wheals may also form and often take on the pattern or shape of the object that caused the irritation. For example, a client who has an allergic reaction to the nickel used in the case and band of a metal watch may develop lesions around the wrist where the watch touched it. Edema may also occur in some cases.

Etiology

There are two types of contact dermatitis: allergic contact dermatitis and irritant contact dermatitis. **Allergic contact dermatitis** is a cell-mediated or delayed hypersensitivity to a wide variety of allergens. Sensitizing antigens include microorganisms, plants, chemicals, drugs, metals, and foreign proteins. On initial contact with the skin, the allergen binds to a carrier protein, forming a sensitizing antigen. The antigen is processed and carried to the T cells, which in turn become sensitized to the antigen. The first exposure is the sensitizing contact; the individual does not experience manifestations until subsequent exposures. Manifestations include erythema, swelling, and pruritic vesicles.

Irritant contact dermatitis is an inflammation of the skin from irritants; it is not a hypersensitivity response. Common sources of irritant contact dermatitis are chemicals (such as acids), soaps, and detergents. The skin lesions are similar to those seen in allergic contact dermatitis.

The major sources known to cause contact dermatitis are dyes, perfumes, poison plants (ivy, oak, sumac), chemicals, and metals (**Box 21–5** ●). Latex (glove) dermatitis is a contact dermatitis that is common in the healthcare field.

Risk Factors

Risk factors for contact dermatitis include allergies; family history of eczema; regular exposure to a moist environment; burns; and exposure to plants, chemicals, and metals. Occupations that require frequent hand washing also increase the risk of developing contact dermatitis. Older clients are at greater risk for contact dermatitis.

▶ CLINICAL MANIFESTATIONS

Allergic contact dermatitis is characterized by erythema, edema, pruritus, vesicles, or bullae that rupture, ooze, and crust (**Figure 21–15** ●). Symptoms of allergic contact dermatitis can develop several hours to 3 days after exposure, when the immunological response has been activated. The rash may take 2–3 weeks to resolve (Usatine & Riojas, 2010).

In contrast, irritant contact dermatitis is a discrete area of redness that corresponds to the exposure location. The rash usually develops within a few hours of contact, peaks within 24 hours, and quickly resolves with removal of the irritant. Reactions to

---

> ## Box 21–5 Common Causes of Contact Dermatitis
>
> - Acids
> - Alkalis: soaps, detergents, household ammonia, lye, cleaners
> - Bromide
> - Chlorine
> - Cosmetics: perfumes, dyes, oils
> - Dusts of lime, arsenic, wood
> - Hydrocarbons: crude petroleum, lubricating oil, mineral oil, paraffin, asphalt, tar
> - Iodine
> - Insecticides
> - Fabrics: wool, polyester, dyes, sizing
> - Metal salts: calcium chloride, zinc chloride, copper, mercury, nickel, silver
> - Plants: ragweed, poison oak, poison sumac, poison ivy, pine
> - Coloring agents
> - Rubber products
> - Soot

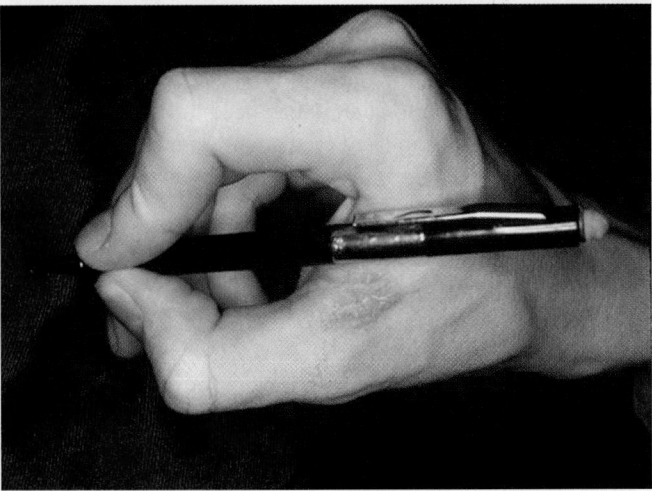

Figure 21–15 ● Contact dermatitis.

TABLE 21–7   Distribution of Lesions by Type of Allergen

DISTRIBUTION OF LESION	ALLERGEN
Face, eyelids, and neck	Cosmetics, skin and hair care products, nail polish, metal jewelry containing nickel, perfumes, cell phones
Lips, mouth	Oral hygiene products, dental materials, foods, medications
Extremities	Rubber, leather chemical in shoes or gloves, moisturizers, plants, metal keys or coins
Trunk	Snaps on pants, belt buckles, elastic band on undergarments, moisturizers, cleansers, sunscreens

Sources: Based on Taylor, J. S., & Amado, A. (2010). Contact dermatitis and related conditions. *Cleveland Clinic Center for Continuing Education Disease Management Project.* Retrieved from http://www.clevelandclinicmeded.com/medicalpubs/diseasemanagement/dermatology/contact-dermatitis-and-related-conditions/; Mayo Clinic. (2011). Contact dermatitis. Retrieved from http://www.mayoclinic.com/health/contact-dermatitis/DS00985/DSECTION=causes; American Academy of Dermatology. (2013). Saving face: Dermatologists helping patients identify source of facial allergic contact dermatitis. Retrieved from http://www.aad.org/stories-and-news/news-releases/saving-face-dermatologists-helping-patients-identify-source-of-facial-allergic-contact-dermatitis-

irritants include painful erythema, edema, vesiculation, dryness of the skin, scaling, fissuring, and necrosis.

The distribution of the lesions provides clues about the source and identity of the allergen or irritant (**Table 21–7** ●). The diagnosis is often based on the manifestations of the disorder and a history of exposure to a known allergen. Scratch tests and intradermal tests are used to identify a specific allergen.

Lifespan and Cultural Considerations

The nature of an allergen or irritant, its toxicity, and the degree and frequency of exposure are the primary factors in the development of contact dermatitis (Taylor & Amado, 2010). Individuals with impaired skin barrier function and slower healing processes are at an increased risk of developing contact dermatitis; for this reason, normal aging of the skin can put older clients at increased risk of developing contact dermatitis.

Interestingly, research suggests that older clients are more likely to develop allergic contact dermatitis than younger clients but less likely to develop irritant contact dermatitis. One possible explanation for the higher likelihood of the allergic type is greater exposure and sensitization to allergens over time; another is older clients' frequent use of topical medications for longer periods (Zhai et al., 2012a). Irritant response, on the other hand, is enhanced in young skin while older skin has a slower, less intense reaction; the decreased efficiency of the circulatory system and slower turnover of the stratum corneum with age may account for this slowed response (Zhai et al., 2012b).

▶ COLLABORATION

Treatment begins with identifying the causative agent (e.g., clothes, plant, soap) and ending the client's exposure to it. The client should be educated about potential sources of exposure; education should include information about products that contain the agent as well as reasonable substitutes for those products. In some cases, it may not be possible to completely end exposure to the causative agent. In these situations, education should focus on methods for limiting exposure, such as through use of protective clothing and cleansing of exposed areas (Taylor & Amado, 2010).

Clinical Manifestations and Therapies **Contact Dermatitis**

ETIOLOGY	CLINICAL MANIFESTATIONS	CLINICAL THERAPIES
Allergic contact dermatitis	Urticaria with intense pruritus and erythema; lesions may rupture, ooze, and crust. Symptoms are usually limited to the area of contact and may occur up to 3 days after exposure to the allergen.	■ Topical corticosteroids ■ Antihistamines ■ Cool, wet compresses or dressings ■ Soothing lotions that promote drying
Irritant contact dermatitis	Painful erythema, edema, and dryness of the skin; lesions may form scales or fissures or become necrotic. Symptoms typically appear in the exposure location and peak within 24 hours of exposure.	■ Topical calcineurin inhibitors ■ Occlusive dressings ■ Petroleum-based emollients

Diagnostic Tests

Patch testing, in which an adhesive patch with common allergens is placed on the back between the scapulae, may be used to identify the allergen. The patch is generally removed after several days; if there is no reaction to a particular allergen, that allergen is eliminated as a possible cause of dermatitis.

Skin prick testing—sometimes called *scratch testing*—involves applying small amounts of allergens to the skin (usually on the back). A control substance, such as saline, may also be applied. Needles are then used to penetrate the skin under the allergens. The skin is observed for allergic reactions after 15 minutes. Reactions are indicated by the formation of wheals.

Skin injection testing uses needles to inject small amounts of allergen into the skin on the arm; it is sometimes referred to as *intradermal testing*. As in a skin prick test, the test site is examined for a reaction after 15 minutes. Injection testing is especially common for suspected allergies to penicillin or insect venom. Skin prick and skin injection tests are used to check for immediate reactions to allergens; patch tests are used to test for delayed reactions.

Skin testing is not appropriate for all individuals, especially those who have had life-threatening allergic reactions in the past, are taking medication that could trigger false positive results, have very large areas of contact dermatitis, or have certain skin conditions. For these clients, blood tests for IgE antibodies are preferable.

> ### SAFETY ALERT
> The patch for allergy testing stays on for 48–72 hours, and the client is not permitted to shower or exercise to the point of perspiring while the patch is in place. Most clients can tolerate the patch; however, if intense burning, itching, or discomfort occurs, the client should contact the healthcare provider for early removal (Massachusetts General Hospital, 2013).

Pharmacologic Therapy

Calamine lotion can be applied to the affected skin. Cool compresses with aluminum acetate (Burow solution) promote drying. Wet dressings or colloidal oatmeal soaks relieve itching. Antihistamines may be given to reduce itching or for a sedative effect when the itching makes the client too uncomfortable to sleep.

Acute allergic contact dermatitis is managed with medium-potency topical corticosteroids when less than 10% of the body surface area is affected; however, this topical medication should not be applied to open lesions. The topical corticosteroids limit the production of cytokines, stop lymphocyte proliferation, and limit the inflammatory response to the allergens. The topical corticosteroid is applied to the affected area twice a day for 2–3 weeks. Stopping the treatment too soon can cause rebound dermatitis. Reactions to poison ivy or other allergens covering more than 10% of the body surface area require treatment with oral corticosteroids for 7–10 days and a tapered dose over another 7–10 days. An antibiotic may be required if the area becomes infected (see the Medications feature in The Concept of Tissue Integrity).

Nonpharmacologic Therapy

Collaborative care may be required for the client who experiences repeated episodes of contact dermatitis. For example, if a client is exposed to irritants at work, the nurse may need to encourage the client to speak with the employer or to contact an organization that provides training in the regulations of the Occupational Safety and Health Administration (OSHA). A client who has repeated episodes due to allergy may need to be referred to an allergist for further testing and evaluation. A nurse working with a school-age child might want to speak with the school nurse or the child's classroom teacher to ensure that follow up care is maintained at school and that the child is adequately hydrated.

Complementary and Alternative Therapy

Clients with chronic contact dermatitis often rely on alternative therapies for relief from symptoms. In general, alternative therapies are used to complement pharmacologic therapies, not to replace them. Topical treatments are common, and traditional examples include aloe vera and chamomile; rice bran broth (similar to oatmeal baths or treatments) and vitamin B12 are more recent examples. Use of many topical treatments is not well researched, though some studies suggest that certain treatments, such as vitamin B12, can aggravate contact dermatitis in some cases (Mayo Clinic, 2012).

Dietary therapies may also be used and are typically intended to control symptoms associated with allergic contact dermatitis. One therapy of particular interest among pediatric clients involves the use of probiotics as a dietary supplement. Proponents of probiotic supplementation posit that children with allergic disorders harbor different microflora than children without these disorders; supplementation promotes colonization of organisms common in allergy-free children. These organisms, in turn, influence immune response. Research on probiotic supplementation suggests that this therapy helped control symptoms in some clients but was limited to the period when the probiotics were ingested; in other words, the positive effect diminished shortly after therapy was discontinued (Michail, 2009).

◼ NURSING PROCESS

Nursing care related to contact dermatitis is primarily directed toward identifying causative agents and developing strategies to avoid them. The nurse is also responsible for teaching the client what to do in the event that exposure does occur; this includes postexposure prophylaxis and treatment and comfort measures in the event that dermatitis does occur.

Assessment

A health assessment interview for a condition such as contact dermatitis focuses on a chief complaint (e.g., itching or a rash). If the client has a skin problem, the nurse analyzes its onset, characteristics and course, severity, and precipitating and relieving factors; the nurse also notes the timing and circumstances of any associated symptoms. The following are specific questions to ask the client:

- What type of itching have you experienced? When did it begin?
- Have you changed any household products lately? Have you changed any personal products lately, such as soap?

- Have you been anywhere unusual, for example, hiking in a new place?
- Do you have any allergies? Have you been in contact with anything to which you are allergic?

The nurse should ask about any change in health, rashes, itching, color changes, and the presence of lesions. Possible precipitating causes, such as medications, the use of new soaps and detergents, skin care agents, cosmetics, pets, travel, stress, or dietary changes, should be explored.

The examination should be conducted in a warm, private room. The client removes all clothing and puts on a gown or drape. Fully expose the area to be examined, but protect the client's modesty by keeping other areas covered. The client may be standing, sitting, or lying down at various times in the examination. Wear disposable gloves when palpating open lesions, skin surfaces that are suggestive of infections or infestations, or discharge from lesions of the skin and mucous membranes. Adhere to standard precautions when conducting a skin assessment. Use a ruler to measure the size of the lesions and a flashlight to help examine them.

Diagnosis

Possible nursing diagnoses for the client with contact dermatitis include the following:

- *Impaired Skin Integrity related to contact dermatitis as evidenced by pruritus and rash*
- *Deficient Knowledge*

(NANDA-I © 2012)

Planning

Appropriate goals for the client with contact dermatitis may include the following:

- The client's skin integrity will be restored and protected.
- The client's triggers will be identified and eliminated.
- The client will remain free of infection.

Implementation

Nursing care of the client with contact dermatitis focuses primarily on providing information for self-care at home. The cli-

ent is responsible for managing skin problems and requires education and support. The nurse should ensure that the client is familiar with the symptoms of infection in the affected area (e.g., increased redness, oozing, fever) and knows when to return for follow up care. The nurse should also address the following topics:

- Medications and treatments do not cure the disease; they only relieve the symptoms.
- Dry skin increases pruritus, which stimulates scratching. Scratching may in turn cause excoriation, which increases the risk of infection.
- It may be necessary to change the diet or environment to prevent contact with allergens. If a nickel allergy exists, the client should make sure not to use nickel jewelry and belt buckles.
- The client should remove clothing worn after outside activities where suspected allergens may be present and shower immediately after those activities.
- The client should wash all clothes before the first wearing and rinse the clothes an extra time to remove all soap. Mild soap should be used to clean the skin.
- The client should place a barrier between the allergen and the skin. For example, cover all metal snaps on clothing with cloth, and wear socks to avoid exposure to tanning chemicals left on shoe leather. If barriers do not reduce the dermatitis, it may be necessary to try to find clothing without nickel or shoes with specific tanning chemicals.
- The client should apply topical corticosteroids and keep using the ointment for 2–3 weeks, even when the skin shows signs of healing. When using steroid preparations, only a thin layer should be applied to slightly damp skin (e.g., after taking a bath). Caution the client using oral corticosteroids never to stop taking the medication abruptly and to follow instructions to taper the dosage gradually.
- Wet dressings may be soothing and can help to loosen crusts. Applying Burow or Domeboro solution to blistered or oozing lesions for 15–30 minutes, three to four times per day, helps dry lesions (Sasseville, 2011). Caution the client that using oatmeal soaks will make the tub slippery. Advise the client to pat the body dry to leave the oatmeal film in place.

Client Teaching   How to Reduce Dry Skin and Relieve Pruritus

- Wash clothing in a mild detergent and rinse twice; do not use fabric softeners.
- Avoid using perfumes and lotions containing alcohol.
- Apply skin lubricants after a bath to help retain moisture.
- Because soaps and hot water are drying, clean the skin with tepid water and either a mild soap or cleansing creams. If soap is used, rinse it off carefully.
- It is not necessary to take a bath every day.
- If bath oils are used, add them to the bath water at the end of the bath (the moist skin is more likely to retain the oil). Bath oils make the tub surface slippery, so they may be contraindicated for use by clients with poor balance and clients who are already at risk for falls.

- Use a humidifier to humidify the air.
- Apply creams and lotions when the skin is slightly damp after bathing.
- Increase fluid intake.
- Keep nails trimmed short, wear loose clothing, and keep the environment cool.
- A brief application of pressure or cold may relieve pruritus.
- Cotton gloves may be worn at night if scratching during sleep causes skin excoriation.
- Distraction or relaxation techniques may prove helpful.

- If occlusive dressings are necessary, a plastic suit may be used.
- Antihistamines cause drowsiness. Caution the client using these medications to avoid alcohol and use great care when driving or working around machinery.

See the Client Teaching feature for suggestions on how to avoid drying of skin and how to relieve pruritus.

Evaluation

Expected outcomes of nursing care include the following:

- Control of the dermatitis is maintained, and no infection occurs.
- Triggers have been identified and eliminated.
- The client's sleep is minimally disturbed by itching.

REVIEW Contact Dermatitis

RELATE Link the Concepts and Exemplars

Linking the exemplar of dermatitis with the concept of immunity:

1. What is your priority nursing diagnosis for a client with contact dermatitis related to hypersensitivity?

2. How would your priority of care differ for this client if the contact dermatitis is located on or around the head and neck? Why?

Linking the exemplar of dermatitis with the concept of infection:

3. How would you respond to a client who insists on antibiotics for contact dermatitis?

4. When would a client with contact dermatitis need to be placed on an antibiotic? What physical assessment findings would support the need for antibiotic therapy?

READY Go to Companion Skills Manual

REFER Go to Pearson Student Nursing Resources
nursing.pearsonhighered.com

- Additional review material

REFLECT Case Study

Nichole Worley, a 21-year-old female college student, reported "an itchy rash" on the right side of her face. Examination revealed erythema, vesicles, and pruritus below her ear. Testing revealed a reaction to nickel. However, Ms. Worley wore no nickel items. During the course of the assessment, she took three calls on a cell phone; her placement of the phone covered the rash.

1. Is it possible that the cell phone cause the reaction? Explain.

2. What kind of testing would determine a nickel allergy?

3. What can Ms. Worley do to reduce the risk of future reactions?

EXEMPLAR 21.3 Pressure Ulcers

EXEMPLAR KEY TERMS
Debridement, *1497*
Eschar, *1497*
Excoriation, *1493*
Immobility, *1493*
Maceration, *1493*
Necrosis, *1492*
Pressure ulcers, *1492*
Shearing forces, *1493*

EXEMPLAR LEARNING OUTCOMES
After reading about this exemplar, you will be able to:

1. Describe the pathophysiology, etiology, clinical manifestations, and direct and indirect causes of pressure ulcers.

2. Identify risk factors and prevention measures associated with pressure ulcers.

3. Illustrate the nursing process in providing culturally competent care across the life span for individuals with pressure ulcers.

4. Formulate priority nursing diagnoses appropriate for an individual with pressure ulcers.

5. Summarize therapies used by interdisciplinary teams in the collaborative care of an individual with pressure ulcers.

6. Plan evidence-based care for an individual with pressure ulcers and his or her family in collaboration with other members of the healthcare team.

7. Evaluate expected outcomes for an individual with pressure ulcers.

▶ OVERVIEW

Pressure ulcers are ischemic lesions of the skin and underlying tissue caused by external pressure that impairs the flow of blood and lymph (Porth & Matfin, 2010). The ischemia causes tissue **necrosis** (dead tissue) and eventual ulceration. These ulcers, also called *bedsores* or *decubitus ulcers*, tend to develop over a bony prominence (such as the heels, greater trochanter, sacrum, and ischia), but they may appear on the skin of any part of the body that is subjected to external pressure, friction, or shearing forces.

The incidence of pressure ulcers in hospitals, long-term care facilities, and home settings is high enough to warrant concern among healthcare providers. The incidence in hospitals has been reported to be as high as 8%; the incidence in long-term care facilities is reported to range from 2.4% to 23% (Porth & Matfin, 2010). Little research has been done to determine the extent of the problem in the home setting. However, with increasing numbers of clients (especially older adult clients) being cared for in the home, it is probable that the incidence is great enough to warrant plans of care to prevent their occurrence.

▶ PATHOPHYSIOLOGY AND ETIOLOGY

When an individual lies or sits in one position for an extended length of time without moving, pressure on the tissue between a bony prominence and the external surface of the body distorts capillaries and interferes with normal blood flow. If the pressure is relieved, blood flow to the area increases, and a brief period of reactive hyperemia occurs without permanent damage. If the pressure continues, platelets aggregate in the endothelial cells surrounding the capillaries and form microthrombi. These microthrombi impede blood flow; the result is ischemia and hypoxia of tissues. Eventually, the cells and tissues of the immediate area of pressure and of the surrounding area die and become necrotic.

Alterations in the involved tissue depend on the depth of the injury. Injury to superficial layers of skin results in blister formation; injury to deeper structures causes the pressure ulcer area to appear dark reddish-blue. As the tissues die, the ulcer becomes an open wound that may be deep enough to expose the bone. The necrotic tissue elicits an inflammatory response, and the client experiences increases in temperature, pain, and white blood cell count. Secondary bacterial invasion is common. Enzymes from bacteria and macrophages dissolve necrotic tissue; the result is a foul-smelling drainage.

Etiology

Pressure ulcers develop from external pressure that compresses blood vessels or from friction and shearing forces that tear and injure vessels. Both types of pressure cause traumatic injury and initiate the process of pressure ulcer development.

External pressure that is greater than capillary pressure and arteriolar pressure interrupts blood flow in capillary beds. When pressure is applied to skin over a bony prominence for 2 hours, tissue ischemia and hypoxia from external pressure cause irreversible tissue damage. For example, when the body is in the supine position, the body's weight applies pressure to the sacrum. A given amount of pressure causes more damage when it is applied to a small area than when it is distributed over a large surface.

Shearing forces result when one tissue layer slides over another. The stretching and bending of blood vessels cause injury and thrombosis. The client in a hospital bed is subject to shearing forces when the head of the bed is elevated and the torso slides down toward the foot of the bed. Pulling the client up in bed also subjects the client to shearing forces. (For this reason, always lift the client up in bed instead of pulling.) In both cases, friction and moisture cause the skin and superficial fascia to remain fixed to the bedsheet, while the deep fascia and bony skeleton slide in the direction of body movement.

Risk Factors

Although a pressure ulcer may develop in any adult who has impaired mobility, those who are most at risk are older adults with limited mobility, individuals with quadriplegia, and clients in the critical care setting (Porth & Matfin, 2010).

Several factors contribute to the formation of pressure ulcers: immobility and inactivity, inadequate nutrition, fecal and urinary incontinence, decreased mental status, diminished sensation, excessive body heat, advanced age, and the presence of certain chronic conditions.

IMMOBILITY   Immobility is a reduction in the amount and control of one's movement. Normally, individuals move when they experience discomfort from pressure on an area of the body. Healthy individuals rarely exceed their tolerance to pressure. However, paralysis, extreme weakness, pain, or any cause of decreased activity can hinder an individual's ability to change positions independently and relieve the pressure, even if the individual can perceive the pressure.

INADEQUATE NUTRITION   Prolonged inadequate nutrition causes weight loss, muscle atrophy, and the loss of subcutaneous tissue. These processes reduce the amount of padding between the skin and the bones, thus increasing the risk of pressure ulcer development. More specifically, inadequate intake of protein, carbohydrates, fluids, zinc, and vitamin C contributes to pressure ulcer formation.

Hypoproteinemia (abnormally low protein content in the blood), due to either inadequate intake or abnormal loss, predisposes the client to dependent edema. Edema (swelling caused by excess fluid trapped in bodily tissue) makes skin more prone to injury by decreasing its elasticity, resilience, and vitality. Edema increases the distance between the capillaries and the cells, thereby slowing the diffusion of oxygen to the tissue cells and of metabolites away from the cells.

FECAL AND URINARY INCONTINENCE   Moisture from incontinence promotes skin **maceration** (tissues softened by prolonged wetting or soaking) and makes the epidermis more easily eroded and susceptible to injury. Digestive enzymes in feces, gastric tube drainage, and urea in urine also contribute to skin **excoriation** (the area of loss of the superficial layers of the skin, also known as a *denuded area*). Any accumulation of secretions or excretions is irritating to the skin, harbors microorganisms, and makes the skin prone to breakdown and infection.

DECREASED MENTAL STATUS   Individuals with a reduced level of awareness, including those who are unconscious, are heavily sedated, or have dementia, are at risk for pressure ulcers because they are less able to recognize and respond to pain associated with prolonged pressure.

DIMINISHED SENSATION   Paralysis, stroke, or other neurological disease may cause loss of sensation in a body area. Loss of sensation reduces an individual's ability to respond to trauma, to injurious heat and cold, and to the tingling ("pins and needles") that signals loss of circulation. Sensory loss also impairs the body's ability to recognize and provide healing mechanisms for a wound.

EXCESSIVE BODY HEAT   Body heat is another factor in the development of pressure ulcers. An elevated body temperature increases the metabolic rate, thus increasing the cells' need for oxygen. This increased need is particularly severe in the cells of an area under pressure, which are already oxygen deficient. Severe infections with accompanying elevated body temperatures may affect the body's ability to deal with the effects of tissue compression.

ADVANCED AGE The aging process brings about several changes in the skin and its supporting structures, making the older individual more prone to impaired skin integrity. These changes include the following:

- Loss of lean body mass
- Generalized thinning of the epidermis
- Decreased strength and elasticity of the skin due to changes in the collagen fibers of the dermis
- Increased dryness due to a decrease in the amount of oil produced by the sebaceous glands
- Diminished pain perception due to a reduction in the number of cutaneous end organs responsible for the sensation of pressure and light touch
- Diminished venous and arterial flow due to aging vascular walls

CHRONIC MEDICAL CONDITIONS Certain chronic conditions, such as diabetes and cardiovascular disease, are risk factors for skin breakdown and delayed healing. These conditions compromise oxygen delivery to tissues; the result is poor and delayed healing and increased risk of pressure sores.

OTHER FACTORS Other factors contributing to the formation of pressure ulcers are poor lifting and transferring techniques, incorrect positioning, hard support surfaces, and incorrect application of pressure-relieving devices.

Prevention

Preventing pressure ulcer development requires a multifaceted approach. Nursing interventions combine actively promoting optimal skin integrity with educating the client, support people, and caregivers about how to prevent pressure ulcers. Key preventive measures incorporate topics including nutrition, skin hygiene and protection, and use of supportive devices.

PROVIDING NUTRITION Because an inadequate intake of calories, protein, vitamins, and iron is believed to be a risk factor for pressure ulcer development, nutritional supplements should be considered for nutritionally compromised clients. The diet should be similar to one that supports wound healing, as was discussed earlier. The nurse should monitor weight regularly to help assess nutritional status. Pertinent lab work should also be monitored, including lymphocyte count, protein (especially albumin), and hemoglobin.

MAINTAINING SKIN HYGIENE The nurse should obtain baseline data using the established tool and then reassess the skin at least daily in the hospital and weekly at home. When bathing the client, the nurse should minimize the force and friction applied to the skin, using mild cleansing agents that minimize irritation and dryness and do not disrupt the skin's "natural barriers." Also, the nurse should avoid using hot water, which increases skin dryness and irritation. The nurse can minimize dryness by avoiding exposure of the client's skin to cold and low humidity. Dry skin is best treated with moisturizing lotions applied while the skin is moist after bathing. The client's skin should be kept clean and dry and free of irritation and maceration by urine, feces, sweat, or incomplete drying after a bath. The nurse applies skin protection if indicated. Dimethi-

cone-based creams or alcohol-free barrier films, which are available in liquid, spray, and moist wipe preparations, are very effective in preventing moisture or drainage from collecting on the skin. In most cases, the nurse can apply these without a primary care provider's order. Use of petroleum-based creams and ointments is no longer advised because of their poor overall skin protection and interference with diaper/incontinence product absorption.

AVOIDING SKIN TRAUMA Providing the client with a smooth, firm, and wrinkle-free foundation on which to sit or lie helps to prevent skin trauma. To prevent injury due to friction and shearing forces, the client must be positioned, transferred, and turned correctly. For a bedridden client, shearing force can be reduced by elevation of the head of the bed to no more than 30 degrees if this position is not contraindicated by the client's condition (for example, a client with respiratory disorders may find it easier to breathe in Fowler position). When the head of the bed is raised, the skin and superficial fascia may stick to the bed linen, while the deep fascia and skeleton slide down toward the bottom of the bed. As a result, blood vessels in the sacral area become twisted, and the tissues in the area can become ischemic and necrotic. Baby powder and cornstarch are never used for friction or moisture prevention. These powders create harmful abrasive grit that is damaging to tissues, and they are considered a respiratory hazard when airborne. Instead, moisturizing creams and protective films, such as transparent dressings and alcohol-free barrier films, are used.

Frequent shifts in position, even if only slight, effectively change pressure points. The client who is able should shift weight 10–15 degrees every 15–30 minutes and, whenever possible, exercise or ambulate to stimulate blood circulation.

When lifting a client to change position, the nurse should use a lifting device such as a trapeze rather than dragging the client across or up in bed. The friction that results from dragging the skin against a sheet can cause blisters and abrasions, which may contribute to more extensive tissue damage. Therefore using a device that lifts the client's weight off the bed surface is the method of choice. To deter shearing forces, the nurse should place a draw sheet that covers the bed from an individual's chest to buttocks and is folded to be wide enough to tuck under the mattress on either side when not in use.

Any at-risk client who is confined to bed—even when a special support mattress is used—should be repositioned at least every 2 hours, depending on the client's need, to allow another body surface to bear the weight. Six body positions can usually be used: prone, supine, right and left lateral (side-lying), and right and left Sims positions. When a lateral position is used, the nurse should avoid positioning the client directly on the trochanter and should instead position the client at a 30-degree angle. A written schedule should be established for turning and repositioning.

PROVIDING SUPPORTIVE DEVICES For circulation to remain uncompromised, pressure on the bony prominences should remain below capillary pressure for as much time as possible through a combination of turning, positioning, and use of pressure-relieving surfaces. Mean capillary pressure can be estimated at 20 mmHg, although it varies. Some

TABLE 21–8   Mechanical Devices for Reducing Pressure on Body Parts

DEVICE	DESCRIPTION/COMMENTS
Gel flotation pads	Polyvinyl, silicone, or Silastic™ pads are filled with a gelatinous substance similar to fat.
Pillows and wedges (foam, gel, air, fluid)	Support positioning and offloads bone-on-bone contact.
Heel protectors (sheepskin boots, padded splints, off-loading inflatable boots, foam blocks)	Can raise or "float" a body part (e.g., heels) off of the surface; prevent shearing and limit pressure on heel area.
Memory foam mattress/chair pad	Distributes weight over bony areas evenly; molds to the body.
Alternating pressure mattress	Are composed of a number of cells in which the pressure alternately increases and decreases; uses a pump.
Water bed	Support surface is filled with water; water temperature is controllable.
Static low-air-loss (LAL) bed	Consists of many air-filled cushions divided into four or five sections. (Separate controls permit each section to be inflated to a different level of firmness; thus pressure can be reduced on bony prominences but increased under other body areas for support.)
Active or second-generation LAL bed	Is like the static LAL but in addition gently pulsates or rotates from side to side, thus stimulating capillary blood flow and facilitating movement of pulmonary secretions.
Air-fluidized (AF) bed (static high-air-loss bed)	Consists of millions of tiny silicone-coated beads, around which forced temperature-controlled air circulates, producing a fluidlike movement; provides uniform support to body contours; decreases skin maceration by its drying effect. (Moisture from the client penetrates the linens and soaks the beads. Air flow forces the beads away from the client and rapidly dries the sheet. A major disadvantage is that the head of the bed cannot be elevated. Some beds are a unique combination of air-fluidized therapy and low-air-loss therapy on an articulating frame. These are used with clients who require head elevation.)

research has evaluated the effectiveness of pressure-reducing support surfaces in preventing pressure ulcers in clients at low, intermediate, or high risk; however, the results have been inconclusive (McInnes et al., 2011). The nurse should review the manufacturer's product descriptions that report the amount of time that the pressure between the surface and the bony prominence is above or below specified levels and determine whether this amount of time is adequate to protect a particular client.

For clients who are confined to bed, three types of support surfaces can be used to relieve pressure:

1. The overlay mattress is applied on top of the standard bed mattress. Use a replacement mattress instead of the standard mattress; most overlay mattresses are made of foam and gel combinations.
2. Specialty beds replace hospital beds. They provide pressure relief, eliminate shearing and friction, and reduce moisture. Examples are high-air-loss beds, low-air-loss beds, and beds that provide kinetic therapy.
3. Kinetic beds provide continuous passive motion or oscillation therapy, both of which are intended to counteract the effects of a client's immobility.

When a client is confined to bed or to a chair, pressure-reducing devices, such as pillows made of foam, gel, air, or a combination of these, can be used. When the client is sitting, weight should be distributed over the entire seating surface so that pressure does not center on just one area. To protect a client's heels in bed, supports such as wedges or pillows can be used to raise the heels completely off the bed. Doughnut-type devices should not be used, since they limit blood flow and can

cause tissue damage to the areas in direct contact with the device. Table 21–8 ● lists mechanical devices for reducing pressure on body parts.

▶ CLINICAL MANIFESTATIONS

Pressure ulcers take on many different forms depending upon their severity. They range from discoloration to blisters or areas of denuded superficial skin to deep tissue damage with necrosis. As a result, pressure ulcers are graded or staged to classify the degree of tissue damage. The stages are listed in Table 21–9 ●.

▶ COLLABORATION

The primary objective for the client at risk for developing pressure ulcers is prevention. Members of the healthcare team should assess clients for ulcer development regularly and reposition them following an established schedule. In repositioning, proper technique is essential to prevent injuries related to shear. When ulcers develop, they should be regularly assessed to ensure that they do not advance to a more severe stage. The client and family members should be taught how to protect and treat ulcers and assess for stage changes.

Diagnostic Tests

Diagnostic tests are conducted to determine the presence of a secondary infection and to differentiate the cause of the ulcer. If the ulcer is deep or appears infected, drainage or biopsied tissue is cultured to determine the causative organism.

TABLE 21–9 Pressure Ulcer Staging

STAGE		DESCRIPTION
STAGE I	 *Source:* © Medical-on-Line/Alamy.	Nonblanchable erythema of intact skin; the heralding lesion of skin ulceration. Usually occurs in a localized area over a bony prominence. Identification of stage I pressure ulcers may be difficult in clients with darkly pigmented skin. *Note:* Affected areas may be painful and a different temperature and consistency than surrounding skin.
STAGE II	 *Source:* © Medical-on-Line/Alamy.	Partial-thickness skin loss involving the dermis. Presents as a shallow open ulcer without slough; may also present an intact or open pus- or blood-filled blister or a shiny, dry ulcer without slough. *Note:* Skin tears, tape burns, incontinence-associated dermatitis, maceration, and excoriation are not included in this classification.
STAGE III	 *Source:* © Medical-on-Line/Alamy.	Full-thickness skin loss involving damage or necrosis of subcutaneous tissue; bone, tendon, and muscle are not exposed. The ulcer presents clinically as a deep crater with or without undermining and tunneling of adjacent tissue; slough may be present. *Note:* Depth of a stage III ulcer varies by anatomical location; in areas without adipose tissue, the ulcer may be very shallow.
STAGE IV	 *Source:* © SPL/Custom Medical Stock Photo.	Full-thickness skin loss with extensive tissue damage and necrosis. Muscle, tendon, and bone are exposed and directly palpable; slough or eschar may be present. Undermining and tunneling are usually present. *Note:* Ulcers can extend into muscle and supporting structures (including fascia, tendons, or joint capsules) increasing the likelihood of osteomyelitis.

TABLE 21–9 Pressure Ulcer Staging *(continued)*

STAGE		DESCRIPTION
UNSTAGEABLE	*Source:* BSIP/UIG Via Getty Images.	Full-thickness tissue loss with depth completely obscured by slough or eschar in the wound bed. Depth of the wound cannot be determined until slough or eschar is removed; once it is removed, ulcer will be classified as stage III or IV. *Note:* Stable eschar on the heels serves as a natural biological cover and should not be removed.
SUSPECTED DEEP TISSUE INJURY	*Source:* © SPL/Custom Medical Stock Photo.	Intact skin with purple discoloration or blood-filled blister. Indicates damage of underlying soft tissue from pressure or shear. May rapidly evolve into a thin blister over a dark wound bed or develop thin eschar. May be difficult to detect in clients with darkly pigmented skin. *Note:* Discoloration or blister may be preceded by painful tissue that is a different temperature and consistency than surrounding skin.

Source: Adapted from National Pressure Ulcer Advisory Panel (NPUAP). (2007). *NPUAP pressure ulcer stages/categories.* Retrieved from http://www.npuap.org/resources/educational-and-clinical-resources/npuap-pressure-ulcer-stagescategories/.

Surgery

Nonviable tissue must be removed from a wound before the wound can be staged or heal. Surgical **debridement** (removal of necrotic material) may be necessary if the pressure ulcer is deep, if subcutaneous tissues are involved, or if **eschar** (a scab or dry crust consisting of dried plasma proteins and dead cells that forms over skin damaged by burns, infections, or excoriations) has formed over the ulcer, preventing healing by granulation.

In addition to the surgical, mechanical, and enzymatic methods of debridement discussed in the exemplar on Burns in this module, autolytic debridement may be used to treat pressure ulcers. In *autolytic debridement,* dressings that contain wound moisture, such as hydrocolloid and clear absorbent acrylic dressings, trap the wound drainage against the eschar. The body's own enzymes in the drainage break down the necrotic tissue. Although this method takes longer than the other three, it is the most selective and therefore causes the least damage to healthy surrounding and healing tissues.

Recently, the use of fly larvae (maggots, *Phaenicia sericata*) has received increased attention. Larval therapy can be extremely effective in cleansing chronic wounds because the maggots secrete enzymes that break down necrotic tissue (while leaving healthy tissue untouched), eat bacteria, and reduce bacterial growth by the increasing surface pH that results from

their presence (Wang et al., 2010). Large wounds may require skin grafting for complete closure.

Pharmacologic Therapy

Topical and systemic antibiotics specific to the infectious organism eradicate any infection present. Additionally, a variety of topical products promote healing. Many of these products come in the form of dressings. For ulcers that are clean and granulating, dressings that maintain moisture are typically used, such as hydrocolloid and transparent film dressings. In addition to maintaining moisture, these dressings protect the wound from friction and bacterial colonization. Dressings may be impregnated with substances that offer microbial benefits, such as silver sulfadiazine and medical-grade honey. For deep, exudative wounds, alginate, foam, and iodine dressings may be preferable. The type of dressing used change over time as the wound either heals or worsens (EPUAP & NPUAP, 2009). Some examples of common dressings and the stages at which they are used are listed in **Table 21–10** ●.

Nonpharmacologic Therapy

Pressure ulcers are a challenge for nurses because of the number of variables involved (e.g., risk factors, types of ulcers, and degrees of impairment) and the numerous treat-

Clinical Manifestations and Therapies **Pressure Ulcers**

ETIOLOGY	CLINICAL MANIFESTATIONS	CLINICAL THERAPIES
Pressure ulcers with nonblanchable erythema (stage I)	Intact skin with localized redness that does not blanch (lose redness) when pressed	■ Cleansing of ulcer and surrounding area ■ Application of barrier cream ■ Application of protective dressing ■ Introduction of appropriate support surfaces and other measures to redistribute pressure ■ Frequent repositioning
Pressure ulcers with partial-thickness loss of dermis (stage II)	Shallow open wound, blister, or dry ulcer without slough	■ Cleansing of ulcer and surrounding area ■ Application of moisture-retaining protective dressing ■ Assessment for necrosis and infection ■ Frequent repositioning ■ Comfort measures
Pressure ulcers with full-thickness tissue loss (stages III and IV; unstageable)	Deep, open wound bed; necrosis of subcutaneous tissue and possible exposure of underlying bone, muscle, and support structures; slough or eschar present	■ Cleansing of ulcer and surrounding area ■ Debridement of wound bed and edges ■ Surgical removal of necrotic tissue ■ Application of medicated moisture-retaining dressing that maintains contact with skin ■ Assessment for and treatment of infection ■ Pain management
Suspected deep tissue injury	Intact skin with localized purple discoloration; possibly quick development of a thin blister or eschar	■ Cleansing of injury and surrounding area ■ Application of moisturizers or barrier creams ■ Application of nonadhesive protective dressing ■ Introduction of appropriate support surfaces and other measures to remove all pressure ■ Elevation of affected area (if possible) ■ Monitoring for pressure ulcer development

TABLE 21–10   Products Used to Treat Pressure Ulcers

STAGE	PRODUCT	PURPOSE
I	Skin prep Granulex	Toughens intact skin and preserves skin integrity. Prevents skin breakdown, increases blood supply, adds moisture, contains trypsin to aid in removal of necrotic tissue.
	Hydrocolloid dressing (e.g., DuoDerm) Transparent dressing (e.g., Tegaderm)	Prevents skin breakdown and promotes healing without the formation of a crust over the ulcer; is permeable to air and water vapor; prevents the growth of anaerobic organisms. Prevents skin breakdown; prevents entrance of moisture and bacteria but allows oxygen and moisture vapor permeability.
II	Transparent dressing Hydrocolloid dressing	Enhances healing (see transparent dressing for stage I). Enhances healing (see hydrocolloid dressing for stage I). Note: If infection is present, these types of dressings are contraindicated. A sterile dressing should be applied instead.
III	Wet-to-dry gauze dressing with sterile normal saline	Allows necrotic material to soften and adhere to the gauze, so that the wound is debrided.
	Hydrocolloid dressing Proteolytic enzymes (such as Elase)	Enhances healing (see above). Serve as debriding agents in inflamed and infected lesions.
IV	Wet-to-dry gauze dressing with sterile normal saline Vacuum-assisted closure (VAC)	Enhances healing (see above). Note: Transparent or hydrocolloid dressings or skin barriers are contraindicated. Creates a negative pressure to help reduce edema, increase blood supply and oxygenation, and decrease bacterial colonization; it also helps promote moist wound healing andthe formation of granulation tissue.

Box 21–6 Treating Pressure Ulcers

Following are the nursing care activities in treating pressure ulcers:

- Minimize direct pressure on the ulcer. Reposition the client at least every 2 hours. Make a schedule and record position changes on the client's chart. Provide devices to minimize or float pressure areas.
- Clean the pressure ulcer with every dressing change. The method of cleaning depends on the stage of the ulcer, the products available, and agency protocol.
- Clean and dress the ulcer using surgical asepsis. Never use alcohol or hydrogen peroxide, as they are cytotoxic to tissue beds.
- If the pressure ulcer is infected, obtain a sample of the drainage to culture and test for sensitivity to antibiotic agents.
- Teach the client how to move to alleviate pressure. Even slight movements can be beneficial; provide assistive devices such as trapeze bars to facilitate movement.
- Provide range-of-motion (ROM) exercises and mobility out of bed as the client's condition permits.

ment measures advocated. Infection is the most serious complication of pressure ulcers. When treating pressure ulcers, the nurse should follow the agency protocols and the primary care provider's orders. Prompt treatment can prevent further tissue damage and pain and can facilitate wound healing. See **Box 21–6** for more information about treating pressure ulcers.

Nurses may find themselves collaborating with a number of individuals when providing care for a client who has or is at risk for pressure ulcers. Nurses frequently collaborate with physical therapists, especially in hospitals, rehabilitation centers, and nursing homes. When caring for a client who is living at home, the nurse often collaborate with the individual's primary caregiver, be that a family member or a hired professional. Because many clients with pressure ulcers are older or have other serious illnesses, a caregiver may require teaching in the following areas:

- Definition and description of pressure ulcers
- Common locations of pressure ulcers
- Risk factors for the development of pressure ulcers
- Skin care
- Ways to avoid injury
- Diet

Depending on the stage of the pressure ulcer, the nurse teaches the client or caregiver how to care for ulcers that are already present: how to change dressings, apply skin barriers, and avoid injury and infection. Referrals to a home health agency or community health department can help the family through the lengthy healing process.

■ NURSING PROCESS

Prevention is the goal for the client at risk for pressure ulcers. The client with one or more pressure ulcers not only has impaired skin integrity but also is at increased risk for infection, pain, and decreased mobility. Pressure ulcers prolong treatment for other health problems, increase healthcare costs, and diminish the client's quality of life.

Assessment

It is important to ensure that the lighting is good; natural or fluorescent lighting is preferable, because incandescent lights can create a transilluminating effect. The room should be neither too hot nor too cold. Heat can cause the skin to flush; cold can cause the skin to blanch or become cyanotic.

The nurse should inspect pressure areas for discoloration (**Figure 21–16** ●), which can result from impaired blood circulation to the area. The pressure areas should have brisk capillary refill or blanch response when gently palpated with the end of a finger or thumb.

Inspect pressure areas for abrasions and excoriations. An abrasion can occur when skin rubs against a sheet (e.g., when the client is pulled). Excoriations can occur when the skin has

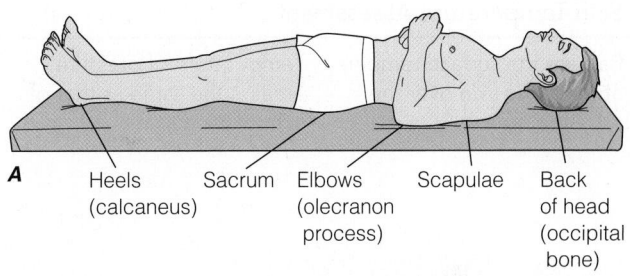

A Heels (calcaneus) | Sacrum | Elbows (olecranon process) | Scapulae | Back of head (occipital bone)

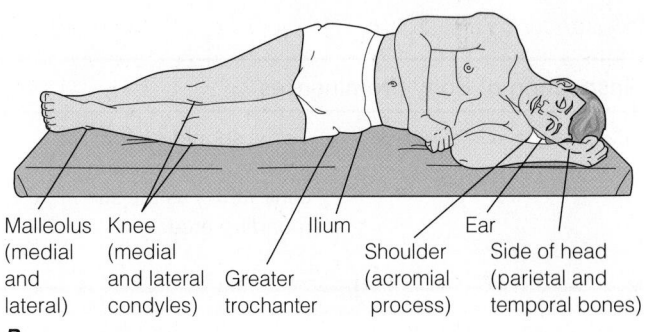

B Malleolus (medial and lateral) | Knee (medial and lateral condyles) | Greater trochanter | Ilium | Shoulder (acromial process) | Ear | Side of head (parietal and temporal bones)

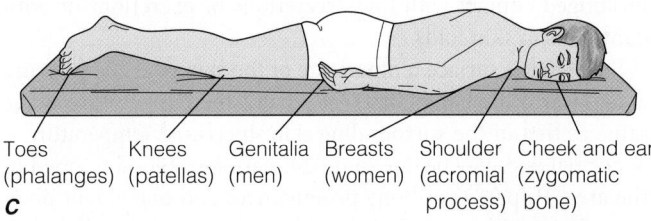

C Toes (phalanges) | Knees (patellas) | Genitalia (men) | Breasts (women) | Shoulder (acromial process) | Cheek and ear (zygomatic bone)

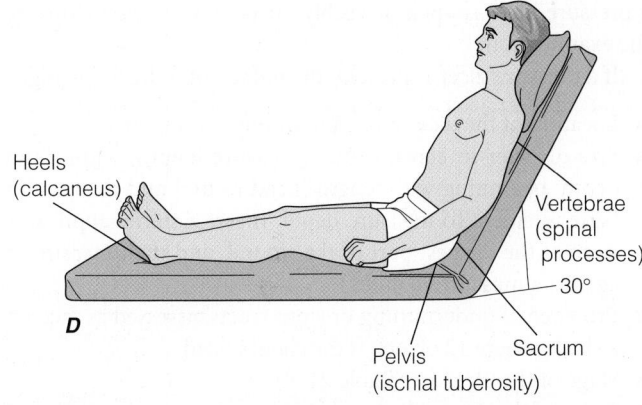

D Heels (calcaneus) | Pelvis (ischial tuberosity) | Sacrum | Vertebrae (spinal processes) | 30°

Figure 21–16 ● Body pressure areas in *A*, supine position; *B*, lateral position; *C*, prone position; *D*, Fowler position.

Pressure Ulcer Assessment

ASSESSMENT/METHOD	NORMAL FINDINGS	ABNORMAL FINDINGS	LIFESPAN OR DEVELOPMENTAL CONSIDERATIONS
Pressure Area Assessment			
Inspect pressure areas for discoloration, abrasion, and excoriation.	Pressure areas should have brisk capillary refill or blanch response when gently palpated with the end of a finger or thumb. Skin over pressure areas should be intact.	■ Nonblanching redness ■ Abrasions in areas where skin rubs on linens or bedding ■ Excoriations in areas exposed to bodily secretions or excretions and in skin folds	■ Older clients—even those in generally good health—may have mobility limitations. Do not discount early signs of pressure ulcers in clients who are not bedridden.
Skin Temperature Assessment			
Palpate the surface temperature of the skin over the pressure area.	Temperature of pressure areas is the same as that of surrounding skin.	■ Increased temperature indicates inflammation or trapping of blood in the pressure area. ■ Decreased temperature indicates lack of blood flow.	■ Because of decreased subcutaneous tissue in the extremities, older clients may have trouble regulating body temperature and have skin that is cool to the touch. Cool skin on its own does not necessarily indicate a problem; always compare the temperature of the pressure area to that of the surrounding skin.
Inspection of Bony Prominences			
Palpate the skin over bony prominences.	Tissue should be firm but not hard and have the same consistency as the surrounding area.	■ Spongy or boggy tissue or skin is indicative of edema.	■ Regardless of age, clients with spinal cord injuries who rely on wheelchairs are prone to pressure ulcers over the bony prominences of the pelvic bones.

prolonged contact with body secretions or excretions or with dampness in skin folds.

Palpate the surface temperature of the skin over the pressure areas (warm the hands first). Normally, the temperature is the same as that of the surrounding skin. Increased temperature is abnormal and may be due to inflammation or blood trapped in the area. Palpate over bony prominences and dependent body areas for the presence of edema, which feels spongy or boggy. If a pressure ulcer is open or visibly infected, wear gloves during the examination.

If a pressure ulcer is present, the nurse notes the following:

■ Location of the ulcer related to a bony prominence
■ Size of ulcer in centimeters. (Measure length, width, and depth, beginning with length [head to toe] and then width [side to side]. To measure depth, insert a sterile applicator swab at the deepest part of the wound, and then measure it against a measuring guide.)
■ Presence of undermining or sinus tracts, assessed as face on a clock, where 12 o'clock is the client's head
■ Stage of the ulcer (see Table 21–9)
■ Color of the wound bed and location of necrosis or eschar
■ Condition of the wound margins

■ Integrity of surrounding skin
■ Clinical signs of infection, such as redness, warmth, swelling, pain, odor, and exudate (note color of exudate)
■ Client complaints of pain or discomfort at the wound site
■ Signs of infection, such as fever, chills, or elevated white blood cell (WBC) count.

The nurse should document the status of the client's skin and wounds on the standard agency form. It is important to be able to determine how these change over time.

Several available risk assessment tools provide the nurse with systematic means of identifying clients at high risk for pressure ulcer development. The National Pressure Ulcer Advisory Panel (NPUAP, 2007) recommends that these tools consider mental status; exposure to moisture; incontinence; device-related pressure, friction, and shear; immobility; inactivity; and nutritional deficits.

The most commonly used assessment tool in the United States is the Braden Scale for Predicting Pressure Sore Risk. The scale was developed in 1987 by Bergstrom, Braden, Laguzza, and Holman and consists of six subscales: sensory perception, moisture, activity, mobility, nutrition, and friction and shear (**Figure 21–17** ●). A total of 23 points is possible. An

BRADEN SCALE FOR PREDICTING PRESSURE SORE RISK

Patient's Name _____   Evaluator's Name _____   Date of Assessment _____

SENSORY PERCEPTION

Ability to respond meaningfully to pressure-related discomfort

1. Completely Limited:
Unresponsive (does not moan, flinch, or grasp) to painful stimuli, due to diminished level of consciousness or sedation,
OR
limited ability to feel pain over most of body surface.

2. Very Limited:
Responds only to painful stimuli. Cannot communicate discomfort except by moaning or restlessness,
OR
has a sensory impairment which limits the ability to feel pain or discomfort over 1/2 of body.

3. Slightly Limited:
Responds to verbal commands but cannot always communicate discomfort or need to be turned,
OR
has some sensory impairment which limits ability to feel pain or discomfort in 1 or 2 extremities.

4. No Impairment:
Responds to verbal commands. Has no sensory deficit which would limit ability to feel or voice pain or discomfort.

MOISTURE

Degree to which skin is exposed to moisture

1. Constantly Moist:
Skin is kept moist almost constantly by perspiration, urine, etc. Dampness is detected every time patient is moved or turned.

2. Moist:
Skin is often but not always moist. Linen must be changed at least once a shift.

3. Occasionally Moist:
Skin is occasionally moist, requiring an extra linen change approximately once a day.

4. Rarely Moist:
Skin is usually dry; linen requires changing only at routine intervals.

ACTIVITY

Degree of physical activity

1. Bedfast:
Confined to bed.

2. Chairfast:
Ability to walk severely limited or nonexistent. Cannot bear own weight and/or must be assisted into chair or wheelchair.

3. Walks Occasionally:
Walks occasionally during day but for very short distances, with or without assistance. Spends majority of each shift in bed or chair.

4. Walks Frequently:
Walks outside the room at least twice a day and inside room at least once every 2 hours during waking hours.

MOBILITY

Ability to change and control body position

1. Completely Immobile:
Does not make even slight changes in body or extremity position without assistance.

2. Very Limited:
Makes occasional slight changes in body or extremity position but unable to make frequent or significant changes independently.

3. Slightly Limited:
Makes frequent though slight changes in body or extremity position independently.

4. No Limitations:
Makes major and frequent changes in position without assistance.

NUTRITION

Usual food intake pattern

1. Very Poor:
Never eats a complete meal. Rarely eats more than 1/3 of any food offered. Eats 2 servings or less of protein (meat or dairy products) per day. Takes fluids poorly. Does not take a liquid dietary supplement,
OR
is NPO and/or maintained on clear liquids or IV's for more than 5 days.

2. Probably Inadequate:
Rarely eats a complete meal and generally eats only about 1/2 of any food offered. Protein intake includes only 3 servings of meat or dairy products per day. Occasionally will take a dietary supplement,
OR
receives less than optimum amount of liquid diet or tube feeding.

3. Adequate:
Eats over half of most meals. Eats a total of 4 servings of protein (meat, dairy products) each day. Occasionally will refuse a meal, but will usually take a supplement if offered,
OR
is on a tube feeding or TPN regimen, which probably meets most of nutritional needs.

4. Excellent:
Eats most of every meal. Never refuses a meal. Usually eats a total of 4 or more servings of meat and dairy products. Occasionally eats between meals. Does not require supplementation.

FRICTION AND SHEAR

1. Problem:
Requires moderate to maximum assistance in moving. Complete lifting without sliding against sheets is impossible. Frequently slides down in bed or chair, requiring frequent repositioning with maximum assistance. Spasticity, contractures, or agitation leads to almost constant friction.

2. Potential Problem:
Moves feebly or requires minimum assistance. During a move skin probably slides to some extent against sheets, chair, restraints, or other devices. Maintains relatively good position in chair or bed most of the time but occasionally slides down.

3. No Apparent Problem:
Moves in bed and in chair independently and has sufficient muscle strength to lift up completely during move. Maintains good position in bed or chair at all times.

Total Score _____

Figure 21–17 ● Braden Scale for Predicting Pressure Sore Risk.

Source: Clinical Practice Guideline, Pressure Ulcers in Adults: Prediction and Prevention, by U.S. Department of Health and Human Services, PPPPUA Pub No. 92-0047, pp. 16–17, 1992, Rockville, MD: Public Health Service. Copyright © Barbara Braden and Nancy Bergstrom, 1988. Reprinted with permission.

adult who scores below 18 points is considered at risk (AHCRQ, 2012). For best results, the nurse should be trained in proper use of the scale.

The Norton Scale for pressure area risk assessment was developed in the United Kingdom in 1962 and includes the categories of general physical condition, mental state, activity, mobility, and incontinence. With the addition of a medications category in 1987, the possible score is 24. Scores of 15 or 16 should be viewed as indicators—not predictors—of risk.

A third assessment tool, the Waterlow Score, was developed by clinical nurse teacher Judy Waterlow in 1985. The Waterlow explores nine areas; six general categories are scored for all clients and three special risk categories are scored only in the highest risk clients. The general categories include build/weight for height, skin type and assessment, sex and age, malnutrition screening, continence, and mobility. The three special risk categories include tissue malnutrition, neurological deficit, and major surgery or trauma (AHCRQ, 2012). Scores can range from 1 to 64, with scores of 10 or above indicating different levels of risk for developing pressure ulcers. The Waterlow Score was developed—and continues to be used primarily—in the United Kingdom.

Assessment tools should be used when the client first enters the healthcare agency and whenever the client's condition changes. In some long-term care facilities, a risk assessment scale such as the Braden or Norton scale is used on admission and then on a regular basis, usually weekly. This schedule increases awareness of specific risk factors and provides assessment data to use in planning goals and interventions to either maintain or improve skin integrity.

Professional organizations advocate the use of assessment tools, but the effectiveness of these scales in clinical practice is unclear. Research assessing the outcomes of at-risk clients scored with these tools is limited; the research that is available does not show a strong correlation between tool use and positive outcomes (AHCRQ, 2012). The research does suggest, however, that the Braden scale is the best indicator of pressure ulcer risk (Pancorbo-Hidalgo et al., 2006).

Diagnosis

The following NANDA diagnoses may be appropriate for the client with a pressure ulcer:

- *Risk for Impaired Skin Integrity*
- *Impaired Skin Integrity*
- *Risk for Infection*
- *Imbalanced Nutrition: Less Than Body Requirements*
- *Risk for Compromised Human Dignity*
- *Situational Low Self-Esteem*

(NANDA-I © 2012)

Planning

Outcomes to be developed in collaboration with the client and caregivers include the following:

- The client who is immobile or on bed rest will be repositioned every 2 hours. Appropriate positioning devices may be used.
- The client who is mobile will maintain or improve activity levels.

- The client will report any alterations such as changes in pain level, redness, numbness, tingling, or increased drainage.
- The client will articulate the importance of maintaining adequate nutrition and hydration.
- The client will describe measures to protect and heal tissue.

Implementation

Nursing implementations depend on the client's mobility, risk factors for developing pressure ulcers, and staging of existing ulcers. Nursing care focuses on ulcer and infection prevention.

Maintain Skin Integrity

To assist the client at risk for or with *Impaired Skin Integrity*, the nurse should consider the following:

- Conduct a systematic skin inspection at least once a day, paying particular attention to the bony prominences. Systematic, comprehensive, and routine skin care may decrease pressure ulcer incidence (although the exact role is unknown). Skin inspection provides data the nurse uses in designing interventions to reduce risk and in evaluating outcomes of those interventions.
- Clean the skin at the time of soiling and at routine intervals, as frequently as the client's need or preference dictates. Avoid hot water, use a mild cleansing agent, and clean the skin gently, applying as little force and friction as possible. Metabolic wastes and environmental contaminants accumulate on the skin; these potentially irritating substances should be removed frequently. Feces and urine cause chemical irritation and should be removed as soon as possible. Hot water may cause skin injury. Mild cleansing agents are less likely to remove the skin's natural barrier.
- Minimize environmental factors leading to skin drying, such as low humidity and exposure to cold. Treat dry skin with moisturizers. Well-hydrated skin resists mechanical trauma. Hydration decreases as the ambient air temperature decreases, especially when the air humidity is low. Poorly hydrated skin is less pliable, and severe dryness is associated with fissuring and cracking of the stratum corneum. Moisturizers reduce dry skin.
- Avoid massage over bony prominences. Although massage has been practiced for years, evidence now suggests that massage over bony prominences may lead to deep tissue trauma in clients at risk for, or with beginning, skin manifestations of a pressure ulcer.
- Minimize skin exposure to moisture due to incontinence, perspiration, or wound drainage. When these sources of moisture cannot be controlled, use underpads or briefs made of materials that absorb moisture and present a quick-drying surface to the skin. Change underpads and briefs frequently. Do not place plastic directly against the skin. Moisture from incontinence, perspiration, or wound drainage may contain factors that irritate the skin; moisture alone can increase the susceptibility of the skin to injury.
- To minimize skin injury due to friction and shearing forces, use proper positioning, transferring, and turning techniques. Lubricants (such as creams), protective films (such as trans-

parent dressings and skin sealants), protective dressings (such as hydrocolloids), and protective padding may also reduce friction injuries. Shear injury occurs when skin remains stationary and the underlying tissue shifts. This shift diminishes the blood supply to the skin; the result is ischemia and tissue damage. Proper positioning, however, can eliminate most shear injuries. Friction injuries occur when the skin moves across a coarse surface, such as bed linens. Most friction injuries can be prevented by the use of appropriate techniques to move the client so that the skin is never dragged across the linens. Any agent that eliminates contact or decreases the friction between the skin and the linens reduces the potential for injury.

■ For the client who is immobile or on bed rest, provide interventions against the adverse effects of external mechanical forces of pressure, friction, and shear:

a. Reposition the at-risk client at least every 2 hours, using a written schedule for systematic turning and repositioning.

b. For the client on bed rest, use positioning devices, such as pillows or foam wedges, to protect bony prominences.

■ For the completely immobile client, use devices to totally relieve pressure on the heels (the most common method is to raise the heels off the bed). Do not use doughnut-type devices.

■ Avoid placing the client in the side-lying position directly on the trochanter.

■ Maintain the head of the bed at the lowest degree of elevation consistent with the client's medical condition and other restrictions. Limit the amount of time the head of the bed is elevated.

Evidence-Based Practice Treating Pressure Ulcers

Problem

Despite advances in health care to extend life and improve functional status, individuals with chronic illnesses and impaired mobility are at increased risk of developing pressure ulcers. The older adult, with age-related compromised cellular activity, is especially vulnerable to impaired healing of injured tissue, including pressure ulcers. An estimated 2.5 million clients in the United States are treated for pressure ulcers each year (Lynch & Vickery, 2010). Preventing pressure ulcers during hospitalizations and maintaining skin integrity after discharge require the cooperation and collaboration of the entire healthcare team.

Evidence

A study conducted at a 166-bed acute rehabilitation center with a 2.8% rate of hospital-acquired pressure ulcers in 2007 focused on identifying common causative factors. The most significant factor was misidentification of pressure ulcers at admission, which progressed to more severe staging. It was discovered that admitting clinicians did not perform thorough skin assessments, in part because they were not educated about what constitutes a through visual assessment. This omission, in turn, led to inaccurate application of pressure ulcer prevention and care protocols. Priorities identified for improving outcomes included staff education, wound care workshops, documentation, case studies, benchmarks, evaluations, surveys, staff newsletters, and client education (Lynch & Vickery, 2010).

A similar study was conducted in 2009 at a 560-bed teaching hospital with a pressure ulcer acquisition rate above the national average. Protocols for care were discovered to be problematic for staff, particularly as they addressed support surfaces. Specifically, staff were not fully educated in the protocols, and the protocols themselves were not appropriately streamlined. This situation created a lag between identification of pressure ulcers or at-risk tissues and treatment. This problem was compounded by difficulty in procuring proper support surfaces for clients with pressure ulcers. Priorities for improving client outcomes focused on developing staff education and awareness campaigns, streamlining existing protocols, and providing support surfaces to all clients (Middaugh, 2011).

A study conducted at a large California medical center in 2009 yielded similar results. The center, in turn, launched an initiative to improve staff education and continuing training on ulcer identification and care; as part of this initiative, each unit was assigned a designated wound care specialist. Screening processes were also revamped and support surfaces were replaced (California Hospital Association, 2011).

In all three of these cases, the facilities experienced a dramatic decrease in hospital-acquired pressure ulcer incidence after addressing the priorities identified.

Implications

Education is paramount for preventing pressure ulcers. Staff must be taught how to properly screen and examine clients at the time of admission and to stage ulcers after they are identified. Continuing education should be offered to keep skin integrity issues at the forefront of care and to keep staff abreast of protocol changes. Protocols should be clear and easy to implement; they should also address issues related to reassessment to ensure that ulcers are being regularly assessed for changes. Finally, support surfaces should be readily available and easily accessible. Staff should be trained on the proper use of these devices and how to identify the types of devices appropriate to specific clients' condition.

In addition, because pressure ulcers can occur both in and out of the hospital setting, education should extend beyond hospital staff. Clients and their family or at-home healthcare providers should also understand how to screen for ulcers and how to identify changes in stage or condition. They should also be educated on care protocols and the use of support surfaces.

Critical Thinking Application

Consider the at-home care of a wheelchair-reliant older client with a spinal cord injury who has a stage II pressure ulcer at the time he is released from the hospital into the care of his wife, who is in her 80s and mobile but frail. Identify potential issues that may result in the worsening of the ulcer, and develop interventions appropriate to the age and condition of the client and his wife. Suggest two resources that the client and his wife could utilize to aid in his care and potentially improve the staging of his ulcer.

- Use assistive devices, such as a trapeze or bed linen, to move the client in bed who cannot assist during transfers and position changes.
- Place the at-risk client on a pressure-reducing device, such as a foam, static air, alternating air, gel, or water mattress. Data indicates that the more spontaneous movements bedridden older adult clients make, the lower the incidence of pressure ulcers. Studies reveal that fewer pressure ulcers develop in at-risk clients who are turned every 2–3 hours. Proper positioning can reduce pressure on bony prominences. It is difficult to redistribute pressure under heels; suspending the heels is the best method. Do not use doughnut cushions, which are more likely to cause than to prevent pressure ulcers. Shearing forces are exerted on the body when the head of the bed is elevated. Lifting (rather than dragging) is less likely to cause injury from friction. Pressure-reducing devices and beds can reduce the incidence of pressure ulcers.
- For the chair-bound client, use pressure-reducing devices. Consider postural alignment, distribution of weight, balance and stability, and pressure relief when positioning the chair-bound client. Avoid uninterrupted sitting in a chair or wheelchair. Reposition the client every hour. Teach clients who can do so to shift their weight every 15 minutes. Use a written plan for positioning, movement, and the use of positioning devices. Do not use doughnut devices. Prolonged, uninterrupted mechanical pressure results in tissue breakdown.

Prevent Infection of Pressure Ulcers

Untreated pressure ulcers can become infected quickly. The nurse working with a client who is at risk for pressure ulcers should teach the client to guard against infection by doing the following:

- Maintaining skin hygiene
- Maintaining appropriate nutrition and hydration
- Recognizing the early stages of a pressure ulcer
- Contacting the healthcare provider at the earliest appearance of a pressure ulcer or change in skin integrity
- Maintaining or improving current activity levels

Prevent Nutritional Imbalance

Although the role nutrition plays in the development of (and to a lesser degree, the healing of) pressure ulcers is not well understood, poor dietary intake of kilocalories, protein, and iron has been associated with the development of pressure ulcers. The nurse should do the following:

- Assess factors involved in inadequate dietary intake of protein or kilocalories.
- Offer nutritional supplements, and support the client during mealtimes as necessary to ensure adequate dietary intake.
- If dietary intake remains inadequate, consult with a dietitian about other dietary interventions.

Prevent Compromised Human Dignity and Situational Low Self-Esteem

The immobile or nearly immobile client is at the mercy of the individuals who are responsible for caregiving. If family members or caregivers do not implement interventions necessary to inhibit the growth of pressure ulcers and maintain client hygiene, the client is at risk for compromised human dignity, which can affect a client's moods and perception of self, in turn putting the client at risk for situational low self-esteem. Depression can follow quickly. The nurse can assist the client in these areas by doing the following:

- Conduct a physical examination at each healthcare interaction that includes examining the client for indicators of abuse or neglect.
- Develop a caring, trusting relationship with the client in order to get the client to discuss issues related to human dignity and self-esteem. Refer for counseling as appropriate.
- Teach family members and caregivers the importance of repositioning the client every 2 hours, and teach them about skin hygiene and how to position the client properly.
- Assist family members and caregivers with obtaining supportive devices to help maintain appropriate positioning of the client.

Evaluation

For the client who is immobile or on bed rest, the treatment plan may need to be evaluated and modified as often as daily, depending on the assessment of the client's skin integrity, client comfort and pain level, and whether or not the written repositioning plan has been followed. Clients who are in bed for long periods of time can experience a diminished appetite. For a client who is not maintaining adequate dietary intake even with changes to the nutrition plan, the nurse may need to consult with a nutritionist or dietician. The nurse should inform clients who are mobile when to call the office if they discover another potential pressure ulcer or change in skin integrity.

NURSING CARE PLAN A Client With a Pressure Ulcer

Agnes Pimm, age 74, recently underwent knee replacement surgery. She was hospitalized for a week following her surgery, after which she spent 4 weeks at a rehabilitation facility. She returned to her home earlier this week and has arranged for a home health agency nurse to visit her daily. Her surgical incision and the bone are healing nicely; during her time at the rehabilitation facility, however, she developed a stage III pressure ulcer on the leg where her supportive knee brace rubs against her skin. She does not want to take the brace off because she doesn't want to leave her knee unsupported; however, the ulcer is causing her a great deal of pain, especially since she has been weaned off the prescription pain medication she was taking postoperatively.

NURSING CARE PLAN (continued)

ASSESSMENT

Jessi Fletcher, RN, is the agency nurse assigned to Ms. Pimm. During her visit to Ms. Pimm's home, she obtains a history and does a physical examination. Ms. Fletcher notes that Ms. Pimm's husband died 6 months ago after a lengthy battle with prostate cancer; since her husband's death, Ms. Pimm hasn't "felt much like eating" and states that what she does eat is canned or frozen. As a result, Ms. Pimm's diet is high in sodium and low in protein. The sodium is of particular concern in light of Ms. Pimm's history of hypertension. Ms. Pimm also indicates that she is a smoker; she has smoked on and off for 50 years, having quit for several years at a time during that span. She indicates that she always returned to smoking during particularly stressful times; her most recent return to cigarettes came during her husband's illness. Ms. Pimm is very proud that her husband remained at home for the duration of his illness, and she wants to be as independent as possible during her own recovery; therefore she has turned down an offer from her son to stay with him until she recovers. She also does not want to return to the rehabilitation facility because it made her feel "very cramped and claustrophobic."

Ms. Pimm is clean and well-groomed, and her home is tidy. She is thin but is very strong and shows no signs of frailty. She is capable of performing most ADLs but mentions that the surgery and the pain from the ulcer have slowed her down and that she "sometimes takes all day" to get washed and dressed and the house picked up. Ms. Pimm's vital signs include temperature 98.3°F oral; pulse 75 bpm; respirations 20/min; and BP 141/84 mmHg.

Upon inspection of the pressure ulcer, Ms. Fletcher notes that it is a roughly 4-cm by 4-cm stage III ulcer that involves full-thickness skin loss with damage to the subcutaneous tissue. No necrotic tissue is present, and the underlying bone, tendon, and muscle are not exposed. Undermining and tunneling are not present, and there are no signs of inflammation or infection. She cleanses the wound and applies a hydrocolloid dressing, which should be changed every third day. Ms. Fletcher then contacts Ms. Pimm's surgeon, who indicates that she no longer needs to wear the immobilizer brace she has been wearing. He states that if Ms. Pimm feels more comfortable with some kind of support on the area, she can wear a soft elastic sleeve-type brace and should wear it only when sleeping or walking. He also indicates that over-the-counter ibuprofen is appropriate for both postoperative and ulcer pain if needed, and that it should be taken according to the directions on the package.

DIAGNOSES

- *Risk for Infection* related to pressure ulcer
- *Impaired Tissue Integrity* related to prolonged pressure, inadequate nutrition, and decreased vascular perfusion associated with smoking
- *Acute Pain* related to stage III ulcer and postoperative recovery
- *Imbalanced Nutrition: Less than Body Requirements* related to loss of appetite and grieving
- *Grieving* related to loss of spouse

(NANDA-I © 2012)

PLANNING

Goals for Ms. Pimm's care include the following:

- The client will describe measures to protect and heal the tissue.
- The client will demonstrate no signs or symptoms of infection.
- The client will report any additional symptoms or changes immediately.
- The client will demonstrate an understanding of nutritional that supports wound healing.
- The client will decrease her per day consumption of cigarettes.
- The client will remain in her home and maintain independence.

IMPLEMENTATION

- Administer antibiotics as ordered.
- Teach about wound care and infection prevention, and demonstrate the proper method for cleaning and dressing the pressure ulcer.
- Describe changes to the wound that indicate the development of infection or a deterioration of the wound site.

- Demonstrate how to use a soft elastic brace, and review when and how it should be used.
- Teach about nutrition that promotes wound healing.
- Provide information about smoking cessation and support groups.

EVALUATION

Initially, Ms. Fletcher changes Ms. Pimm's dressing and cleanses her wound every third day. Over time, Ms. Pimm takes over this responsibility and is very serious about wound care and infection prevention. Ms. Fletcher is able to decrease the frequency of her visits to Ms. Pimm's home from every day to three times per week. The wound remains infection free and, after a month with the hydrocolloid dressings, is restaged as a stage II ulcer. At this point, treatment continues with hydrocolloid dressings that require changing every fifth day, rather than every third day.

Ms. Fletcher also refers Ms. Pimm to a dietician, who outlines a meal plan that promotes wound healing, appeals to Ms. Pimm's tastes, is appropriate for someone with hypertension, and is easy to prepare. Ms. Pimm struggles with her diet a bit because it is difficult for her to visit the store and purchase fresh foods and because she continues to struggle with a lack of appetite. However, she verbalizes an understanding of the need to eat a healthier diet and makes an effort to follow the dietician's meal plan as best she can.

(continued on next page)

NURSING CARE PLAN   *(continued)*

Finally, Ms. Pimm continues to struggle with smoking cessation. She has tried several different methods to decrease her cigarette consumption but states that continued stress about her husband's death and her current condition prevents her from making much progress. Ms. Fletcher refers Ms. Pimm to several community resources for smoking cessation.

CRITICAL THINKING

1. *How would you adapt Ms. Pimm's care plan if the surgeon indicated that she was required to wear the brace that caused the ulcer?*
2. *Suppose that Ms. Pimm's ulcer had progressed to stage IV after a month of treatment rather than improving to stage II. How would her treatment regimen change? Would the goals and implementation for her care change as well?*
3. *Develop a care plan for the nursing diagnosis Impaired Tissue Integrity related to physical immobilization.*

REVIEW   Pressure Ulcers

RELATE Link the Concepts and Exemplars

Linking the exemplar of pressure ulcers with the concept of infection:

1. What assessment findings would cause you to believe a pressure ulcer is infected?
2. What nursing interventions can be implemented to reduce the risk of infection of a pressure ulcer?

Linking the exemplar of pressure ulcers with the concept of mobility:

3. Contrast appropriate nursing interventions to prevent pressure ulcers in clients age 6, 30, and 80 with limited mobility.
4. You are caring for a child who was involved in a bicycle accident resulting in below-the-waist paraplegia. How will you teach the parents to reduce the risk of pressure ulcers?

READY Go to Companion Skills Manual

REFER Go to Pearson Student Nursing Resources
nursing.pearsonhighered.com

- Additional review material

REFLECT Case Study

Lydia Ocampo is a 69-year-old widow who has recently been moved from a rehabilitation center to the skilled nursing wing of a nursing facility. She is still receiving care related to surgery on a

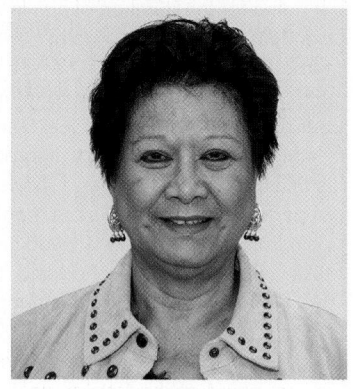

broken hip a couple of months before. Before that, she had lived in the home that she shared with her husband of 50 years. Her husband died a few weeks ago. Ms. Ocampo has Alzheimer disease. At the nursing home, she exhibits intermittent confusion and is alternately passive and uncooperative with the staff. Over the course of the next month, her condition deteriorates. She eats very little and is fairly unresponsive to caregivers. She sleeps often.

1. What data suggest that Ms. Ocampo is particularly vulnerable to pressure ulcer development?
2. What additional information do you need in order to use the Braden scale to determine Ms. Ocampo's potential for pressure ulcer development?
3. What independent measures can you take to protect Ms. Ocampo's skin from further breakdown?
4. Considering that Ms. Ocampo does not have any areas of skin breakdown, why is it important to institute treatment for pressure ulcers at this time?

EXEMPLAR 21.4   Wound Healing

EXEMPLAR KEY TERMS

Approximated, *1507*
Collagen, *1508*
Dehiscence, *1509*
Evisceration, *1509*
Exudate, *1509*
Fibrin, *1508*
Granulation tissue, *1508*
Hematoma, *1508*
Hemorrhage, *1508*
Hemostasis, *1508*
Keloid, *1508*
Macrophages, *1508*
Phagocytosis, *1508*
Primary intention healing, *1507*
Purulent exudate, *1509*

Pus, *1509*
Pyogenic bacteria, *1509*
Regeneration, *1507*
Sanguineous (hemorrhagic) exudate, *1509*
Secondary intention healing, *1507*
Serosanguineous exudate, *1509*
Serous exudate, *1509*
Suppuration, *1509*
Tertiary intention healing, *1507*

EXEMPLAR LEARNING OUTCOMES
After reading about this exemplar, you will be able to:

1. Describe the pathophysiology and clinical manifestations of wound healing and the etiology and direct and indirect causes of impaired wound healing.

2. Identify risk factors and prevention methods associated with open wounds.

3. Illustrate the nursing process in providing culturally competent care across the life span for individuals with a wound.

4. Formulate priority nursing diagnoses appropriate for an individual with a wound.

5. Summarize therapies used by interdisciplinary teams in the collaborative care of an individual with a wound.

6. Plan evidence-based care for an individual with a wound and his or her family in collaboration with other members of the healthcare team.

7. Evaluate expected outcomes for an individual with a wound.

▶ OVERVIEW

Healing is a quality of living tissue; it is also referred to as **regeneration** (renewal) of tissues. Healing can be considered in terms of *types of healing*, having to do with the caregiver's decision about whether to allow the wound to seal itself or to purposefully close the wound, and *phases of healing*, which refer to the steps in the body's natural processes of tissue repair. The phases are the same for all wounds, but the rate of healing depends on factors such as the type of healing, the location and size of the wound, and the client's health.

▶ PHYSIOLOGY

There are two types of healing, each influenced by the amount of tissue loss. **Primary intention healing** occurs where the tissue surfaces have been **approximated** (closed) and there is minimal or no tissue loss; it is characterized by the formation of minimal granulation tissue and scarring. It is also called *primary union* or *first intention healing*. An example of wound healing by primary

intention is a closed surgical incision. Another example would be the use of tissue adhesive, a liquid "glue," to seal clean lacerations or incisions (Coulthard et al., 2010).

A wound that is extensive and involves considerable tissue loss and in which the edges cannot or should not be approximated heals by **secondary intention healing**. An example of wound healing by secondary intention is a pressure ulcer. Secondary intention healing differs from primary intention healing in three ways: The repair time is longer, the scarring is greater, and the susceptibility to infection is greater.

Those wounds that are left open for 3–5 days to allow edema or infection to resolve or to permit exudate to drain and then are closed with sutures, staples, or adhesive skin closures, undergo **tertiary intention healing**. This is also called *delayed primary intention healing*.

Phases of Wound Healing

Wound healing can be broken down into three phases: inflammatory, proliferative, and maturation or remodeling (**Figure 21–18 ●**).

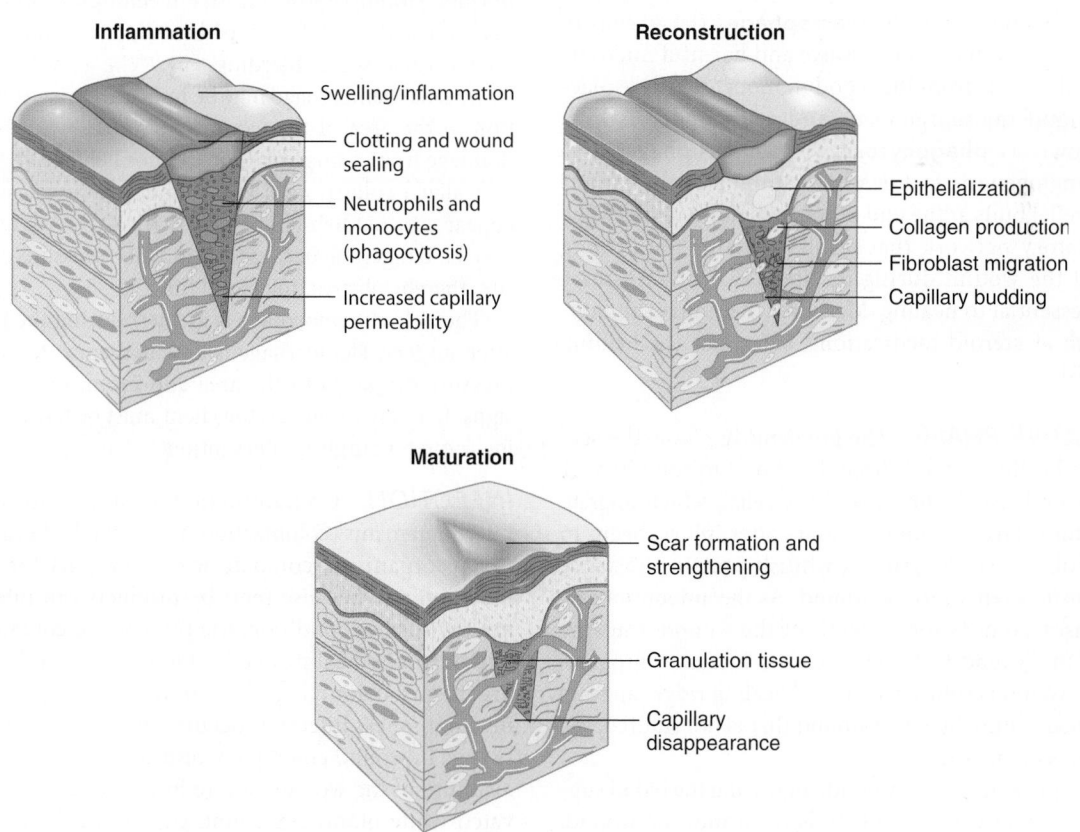

Figure 21–18 ● Wound healing occurs in three overlapping phases.

Source: Based on Nicol, N. H., Heuther, S. E., & Weber, R. (2006). Structure, function, and disorders of the integument. In K. L. McCance & S. E. Huether (Eds.), *Pathophysiology: The biologic basis for disease in adults and children* (5th ed., pp. 1573–1607). St. Louis, MO: Elsevier Mosby.

INFLAMMATORY PHASE The *inflammatory phase* is initiated immediately after injury and lasts 3–6 days. Two major processes occur during this phase: hemostasis and phagocytosis.

Hemostasis (the cessation of bleeding) results from vasoconstriction of the larger blood vessels in the affected area, the retraction (drawing back) of injured blood vessels, the deposition of **fibrin** (connective tissue), and the formation of blood clots in the area. The blood clots, formed from blood platelets, provide a matrix of fibrin that becomes the framework for cell repair. A scab also forms on the surface of the wound. Consisting of clots and dead and dying tissue, the scab aids hemostasis and inhibits contamination of the wound by microorganisms. Below the scab, epithelial cells migrate into the wound from the edges. The epithelial cells serve as a barrier between the body and the environment, preventing the entry of microorganisms.

The inflammatory phase also involves vascular and cellular responses intended to remove any foreign substances as well as dead and dying tissues. The blood supply to the wound increases, bringing with it oxygen and nutrients needed in the healing process. As a result, the area appears reddened and edematous. Exudate of fluid and cell debris is a normal accumulation and helps cleanse the wound. Overproduction of this exudate and other factors can impair wound healing, especially of chronic wounds (Bianchi, 2012).

During cell migration, leukocytes (specifically, neutrophils) move into the interstitial space. These are replaced about 24 hours after injury by **macrophages** (large cells of the immune system that remove waste and harmful microorganisms), which arise from the blood monocytes. These macrophages engulf microorganisms and cellular debris by a process known as **phagocytosis**. The macrophages also secrete an angiogenesis factor, which stimulates the formation of epithelial buds at the end of injured blood vessels. The microcirculatory network that results sustains the healing process and the wound during its life. This inflammatory response is essential to healing. Measures that impair inflammation, such as steroid medications, can place the healing process at risk.

PROLIFERATIVE PHASE The *proliferative phase,* the second phase in healing, extends from day 3 or 4 to about day 21 postinjury. Fibroblasts (connective tissue cells), which migrate into the wound starting about 24 hours after injury, begin to synthesize collagen. **Collagen** is a whitish protein substance that adds tensile strength to the wound. As the amount of collagen increases, so does the strength of the wound; thus the chance that the wound will remain closed increases progressively. If the wound is sutured, a raised "healing ridge" appears under the intact suture line. In a wound that is not sutured, the new collagen is often visible.

Capillaries grow across the wound, increasing the blood supply. Fibroblasts move from the bloodstream into the wound, depositing fibrin. As the capillary network develops, the tissue becomes a translucent red. This tissue, called **granulation tissue**, is fragile and bleeds easily.

When the skin edges of a wound are not sutured, the area must be filled in with granulation tissue. When the granulation tissue matures, marginal epithelial cells migrate to it, proliferating over this connective tissue base to fill the wound. If the wound does not close by epithelialization, the area becomes covered by a scab or dry crust, called *eschar*, formed by dried plasma proteins and dead cells. Initially, wounds healing by secondary intention seep blood-tinged (serosanguineous) drainage. Later, if they are not covered by epithelial cells, they become covered with thick, gray, fibrinous tissue that is eventually converted into dense scar tissue.

MATURATION PHASE The *maturation phase* begins about day 21 and can extend 1 or 2 years after the injury. Fibroblasts continue to synthesize collagen. The collagen fibers themselves, which were initially laid haphazardly, reorganize into a more orderly structure. During maturation, the wound site is remodeled and contracted. The scar becomes stronger, but the repaired area is never as strong as the original tissue. In some individuals, particularly those with dark skin, an abnormal amount of collagen appears. The result can be a hypertrophic scar or **keloid**.

Risk Factors for Complications

Several untoward events can interfere with the healing of a wound: hemorrhage, infection, dehiscence, and evisceration.

HEMORRHAGE Some escape of blood from a wound is normal. **Hemorrhage** (massive bleeding), however, is abnormal. A dislodged clot, a slipped stitch, or erosion of a blood vessel may cause severe bleeding.

Internal hemorrhage may be indicated by swelling or distention in the area of the wound and, possibly, by sanguineous drainage from a surgical drain. Some clients have a **hematoma**, a localized collection of blood underneath the skin that may appear as a reddish blue swelling (bruise). A large hematoma may be dangerous because it can place pressure on blood vessels, thereby obstructing blood flow.

The risk of hemorrhage is greatest during the first 48 hours after surgery. Hemorrhage is an emergency; the nurse applies pressure dressings to the area and monitors the client's vital signs. In many instances, the client must be taken to the operating room for surgical intervention.

INFECTION Contamination of a wound surface with microorganisms (colonization) is inevitable. Because the colonizing organisms compete with new cells for oxygen and nutrition and because their by-products can interfere with a healthy surface condition, the presence of contamination can impair wound healing and lead to infection. When the microorganisms colonizing the wound multiply excessively or invade tissues, infection occurs. Infection is suggested by a change in wound color, pain, or drainage and is confirmed by a culture of the wound. Severe infection causes fever and elevated white blood cell count. Clients who are immunosuppressed, such as those with HIV or those receiving myelosuppressive treatment for cancer, are especially susceptible to wound infections.

A wound can be infected with microorganisms at the time of injury, during surgery, or postoperatively. Wounds that occur as a result of injury (e.g., bullet and knife wounds) are most likely to be contaminated at the time of injury. Surgery involving the intestines can also result in infection from microorganisms inside the intestine. Surgical infection becomes apparent 2–11 days postoperatively.

DEHISCENCE WITH POSSIBLE EVISCERATION

Dehiscence is the partial or total rupture of a sutured wound. Dehiscence usually involves an abdominal wound in which the layers below the skin also separate. **Evisceration** is the protrusion of the internal viscera through an incision. A number of factors, including obesity, poor nutrition, multiple trauma, failure of suturing, excessive coughing, vomiting, and dehydration heighten a client's risk of wound dehiscence. Wound dehiscence is most likely to occur 4–5 days postoperatively, before extensive collagen has been deposited in the wound.

Sudden straining, such as coughing or sneezing, may precede dehiscence. It is not unusual for a client to feel that "something has given way." When dehiscence or evisceration occurs, the wound should be supported quickly by large sterile dressings soaked in sterile normal saline. The nurse should place the client in bed with knees bent to decrease pull on the incision. The surgeon must be notified because immediate surgical repair of the area may be necessary.

Prevention

Characteristics of the individual such as age, nutritional status, lifestyle, and medications influence the speed of wound healing. The modifiable factors among this group affect the overall health of an individual. In general, habits that promote overall good health—like eating a balanced diet and exercising—promote wound healing; conversely, habits that do not promote good health can lead to impaired healing.

NUTRITION
Wound healing places additional demands on the body. The client requires a diet rich in protein, carbohydrates, lipids, vitamins A and C, and minerals such as iron, zinc, and copper. Malnourished clients may require time to improve their nutritional status—before surgery, if possible. Obese clients are at increased risk of wound infection and slower healing because adipose tissue usually has a minimal blood supply.

LIFESTYLE
Clients who exercise regularly tend to have good circulation and are more likely to heal quickly because blood brings oxygen and nourishment to the wound. Smoking constricts arterioles and reduces the amount of functional hemoglobin in the blood, thus limiting the oxygen-carrying capacity of the blood. As a result, smokers are at risk for delayed healing.

MEDICATIONS
Anti-inflammatory drugs (e.g., steroids and aspirin) and antineoplastic agents interfere with healing. Prolonged use of antibiotics may make an individual susceptible to wound infection by resistant organisms.

▶ CLINICAL MANIFESTATIONS

Exudate is material, such as fluid and dead phagocytic cells, that has escaped from blood vessels during the inflammatory process and is deposited in tissue or on tissue surfaces. The nature and amount of exudate vary according to the tissue involved, the intensity and duration of the inflammation, and the presence of microorganisms.

There are three major types of exudate: serous, purulent, and sanguineous (hemorrhagic). A **serous exudate** typically accompanies mild inflammation and presents as clear or straw colored. It is thin and watery and has few cells. An example is the fluid in a blister from a burn.

A **purulent exudate** is thicker than serous exudate and consists of a large quantity of cells and necrotic debris; it is usually opaque or milky in appearance. The formation of purulent exudate, commonly known as **pus**, is referred to as **suppuration**, and the bacteria that produce pus are called **pyogenic bacteria**. Not all microorganisms are pyogenic. Purulent exudates can vary in color, some acquiring tinges of blue, green, or yellow. The color may depend on the causative organism.

A **sanguineous (hemorrhagic) exudate** consists of large amounts of red blood cells, indicating damage to capillaries that is severe enough to allow the escape of red blood cells from plasma. Bright sanguineous exudate indicates fresh bleeding, while dark sanguineous exudate denotes older bleeding. This type of exudate is frequently seen in open wounds.

Mixed types of exudates are often observed. A **serosanguineous exudate** (consisting of clear and blood-tinged drainage) is commonly seen in surgical incisions. A *purosanguineous* discharge (consisting of pus and blood) is often seen in a new wound that is infected.

Lifespan and Cultural Considerations

Healthy children and adults often heal more quickly than do older adults, who are more likely to have chronic diseases that hinder healing. For example, reduced liver function can impair the synthesis of blood clotting factors. Older adults are also at an increased risk of developing nutritional deficiencies. These deficiencies may reduce the numbers of red blood cells and leukocytes, thus impeding the delivery of oxygen and the inflammatory response essential for wound healing. Diabetes, chronic lung disease, and cardiovascular disease also impair oxygen delivery to body tissues. In addition, vascular changes—such as atherosclerosis and atrophy of capillaries in the skin—impair blood flow to wounds.

Older adults who do not have chronic diseases may still experience slowed healing as a result of normal cellular and molecular changes. Chief among these changes is a delayed inflammatory response with fewer macrophages and decreased phagocytic activity. Cell renewal and collagen synthesis also slow with age, and collagen tissue is less flexible and more susceptible to damage from pressure, friction, and shearing. Scar tissue is also less elastic. Interestingly, research suggests that even though the healing process is slowed, the quality of healing in healthy older adults is the same as that in younger individuals (Guo & DiPietro, 2010).

Clinical Manifestations and Therapies Impaired Wound Healing

ETIOLOGY	CLINICAL MANIFESTATIONS	CLINICAL THERAPIES
Massive bleeding (hemorrhage)	Swelling, wound distention, sanguineous drainage, and hematoma indicate internal hemorrhage. Rapid loss of blood and the onset of shock indicate external hemorrhage.	■ Pressure dressings ■ Emergency surgery
Infection by colonized microorganisms	Wound color changes, and pain or drainage increases. Edema may develop, and skin may become red and warm to the touch.	■ Antibiotics ■ Debridement ■ Protective dressings ■ Infection prevention measures
Rupture of a sutured wound (dehiscence)	Spontaneous Wound opens spontaneously with possible bleeding, pain, or inflammation. Protrusion of underlying tissue or organs indicates evisceration.	■ Supportive dressings ■ Positioning to decrease pressure ■ Antibiotics ■ Debridement ■ Emergency surgery

▶ COLLABORATION

Under normal circumstances, collaborative efforts related to wound healing are wellness oriented. Efforts should focus on promoting healing and preventing infection. The client should be taught how to recognize signs of infection and other complications of impaired healing and be coached to contact the healthcare provider immediately if symptoms develop. When healing is impaired, the first priority is addressing any life-threatening complications, such as hemorrhage or evisceration. The focus then shifts back to promotion of healing and prevention of infection. Impaired healing may also result in significant discomfort for the client, so pain management strategies may also be appropriate.

Diagnostic Tests

If infection is suspected, a culture and sensitivity test may be performed. The culture identifies the causative organism and the sensitivity test determines which medication is most appropriate for treating the infection. For a culture, drainage or tissue is collected from the wound and placed it in a medium that promotes bacterial growth. In most cases, the sensitivity test indicates an antibiotic.

Surgery

In the event of life-threatening complications, surgery may be performed to repair damaged tissues or vessels and to reclose the wound. In nonemergency situations, surgery may also be indicated if healing is ineffective. The presence of slough, eschar, or necrotic tissue indicate ineffective healing.

Surgical debridement is appropriate for wounds with large amounts of infected and necrotic tissue. It may also be used to treat wounds that abscess. During this procedure, the wound is flushed with saline solution and topical anesthetic is applied. Forceps are used to grip the necrotic tissue, which is then cut away with a scalpel. Depending upon the extent of the necrosis and the amount of living tissue affected, debridement may take place in multiple sessions. In

some cases, a laser rather than a scalpel is used to cut away the dead tissue.

Escharotomy is performed to treat full-thickness wounds that encircle or nearly encircle a body part and have formed eschar; these wounds are often caused by burns. The inelasticity of the eschar restricts the flow of blood and extracellular fluids and can lead to fluid accumulation and increased pressure inferior to the wound. If left untreated, this pressure can cause compartmental tissue damage. Escharotomy is the surgical removal of the eschar. During the procedure, incisions are made along the damaged area to release pressure; the swelling of the tissue causes the incisions to spread and exposes the underlying tissue and structures. The client is usually sedated during the procedure, and the wound is covered with a moist dressing after the procedure.

Pharmacologic Therapy

Pharmacologic therapy of wounds depends upon whether wound healing is normal or impaired. For normal wound healing, therapies may include antibacterial ointments, prophylactic antibiotics, and analgesics for pain.

Treatment for wounds with impaired healing depends upon the particular complication. Infected wounds are treated with antibiotics specific to the causative organism. In some cases, growth factors may be prescribed to promote healing; these factors simulate the body's own growth factors and stimulate collagen and keratinocyte production and migration to wound sites. Growth factors often come in the form of topical gels that are applied directly to the wound, though some may be administered via injection (Barrientos et al., 2008). Opioids and NSAIDs may also be appropriate for management of pain associated with the wound.

Nonpharmacologic Therapy

Nonpharmacologic therapies for wound healing are diverse and include a number of techniques and procedures. For wounds with normal healing, these may include infection

Evidence-Based Practice Aloe Vera and Wound Healing

Problem

Many alternative therapies are available for promotion of wound healing, including honey, iodine, aloe vera, phenytoin, and electrical stimulation. However, the research that supports the use of these alternative practices is variable, and solid scientific evidence for their use is often lacking. It is the nurse's responsibility to understand the benefits and risks of using alternative therapies for wound healing.

Evidence

One of the most widely accepted alternative therapies for wound healing is application of aloe vera. It is used for burns, sunburns, frostbite, psoriasis, cold sores, surgical wounds, pressure ulcers, inflammatory skin disorders, and other minor wounds (NIH, 2011; WHO, 2013). Indeed, many FDA-approved wound dressings and over-the-counter topical gels contain aloe vera. Aloe vera (*Aloe barbadensis miller*) is a cactuslike plant that produces a clear gel and yellow latex. Active components of aloe vera include vitamins A, B, C, and E, enzymes, minerals, sugars, anthraquinones, fatty acids, hormones, amino acids, lignin, saponins, and others. These components give aloe vera its healing properties, including reducing inflammation, neutralizing free radicals, preventing infection, reducing pain, stimulating fibroblast proliferation and activity, promoting wound closure, and binding moisture into the skin (Surjushe, Vasani, & Saple, 2008). Multiple studies have investigated the usefulness of aloe vera for treating a variety of acute and chronic wounds. One study of 30 clients showed a beneficial effect of aloe gel compared to silver sulfadiazine for clients with second-degree burns (Khorasani et al., 2009), whereas another study showed no difference between the two treatments (Dat et al., 2012). A benefit of aloe vera application was also seen when it was applied to hemor-

rhoidectomy incisions (Eshghi et al., 2010) but not to skin biopsy wounds or pressure ulcers (Dat et al., 2012). When it was applied to other surgical wounds, one study found that aloe vera actually delayed wound healing (Schmidt & Greenspoon, 1991).

Implications

Although generally safe when applied topically to minor wounds and burns, aloe vera is not clinically supported for all wounds. Before applying aloe, the nurse should fully research its known effects for the client's specific type of wound. Because many products that contain aloe are available over-the-counter and do not require a prescription, the nurse must use best judgment based on clinical research and personal experience before providing this treatment to clients. In addition, adverse reactions to aloe vera have been reported, including contact dermatitis, burning sensations, and allergic reaction. These reactions appear to be associated with anthraquinones found in the aloe latex. Aloe should not be used in clients with a known allergy to plants in the Liliaceae family (WHO, 2013). Before applying a lotion, cream, gel, or wound dressing containing aloe, the nurse should ask the client about any known allergies or previous adverse reactions to aloe.

Critical Thinking Application

1. What are the advantages and disadvantages of using aloe vera to treat open wounds (e.g., cuts, surgical wounds) versus closed wounds (e.g., sunburns, psoriasis)?

2. What nursing interventions would you implement for a client who develops contact dermatitis after being treated with a wound dressing containing aloe vera?

3. Develop a strategy for teaching clients about three alternative wound-healing treatments using clinical evidence that supports or opposes each treatment.

prevention measures; compression bandages or hosiery; and diets high in protein, carbohydrates, and vitamins to promote healing.

For wounds with impaired healing, vacuum-assisted closure may be used. This noninvasive procedure uses negative pressure to remove excess fluid from the wound, thus improving oxygenation and blood flow to the area and promoting formation of granulation tissue. Similarly, hyperbaric oxygen therapy improves oxygenation in nonhealing wounds (Samalonis, 2011).

Other regenerative therapies include cellular therapies that introduce rapidly regenerating new cells—such as stem cells—into wounds to promote healing (Samalonis, 2011). Skin or tissue grafts—either of the client's own skin or of donor skin—may also be appropriate in some cases.

Biosurgery may be used in nonhealing wounds with necrotic tissue or slough; in this procedure, sterile maggots are placed on the wound and digest the damaged tissue. The damage to surrounding healthy tissue is minimal. In some cases, biosurgery is preferable to surgical debridement of necrotic wounds.

For many clients, a combination of therapies is used. As a result, clients with wounds may receive care from a number of healthcare providers. Surgeons, nurses, scrub persons, anesthetists, phlebotomists, x-ray technicians, registration clerks, and emergency transporters are often involved in securing the safety and health of clients. Case managers and social workers are available based on client needs postdischarge. This interdisciplinary approach focuses on placing the client in the best possible health status to achieve successful wound healing.

◼ NURSING PROCESS

Nursing care related to wounds is primarily directed toward promotion of healing and prevention of infection and other complications. This goal involves not only care and aseptic procedures when the client is in the healthcare setting, but client teaching focused on ongoing care of the wound at home. The client should understand not only how to clean, dress, and promote healing of wounds, but also how to identify signs of complications in the healing process.

Assessment

Nurses commonly assess both untreated and treated wounds. Untreated wounds usually are seen shortly after an injury (e.g., at the scene of an accident or in an emergency center). Assessment for these wounds is as follows:

- Assess the location and extent of tissue damage (e.g., partial thickness or full thickness). Measure the length, width, and depth of the wound.
- Inspect the wound for bleeding. The amount of bleeding varies with the type of wound and its location. Penetrating wounds may cause internal bleeding.
- Inspect the wound for foreign bodies (soil, broken glass, shreds of cloth, or other foreign substances).
- Assess associated injuries such as fractures, internal bleeding, spinal cord injuries, or head trauma.
- If the wound is contaminated with foreign material, determine when the client last had a tetanus toxoid injection. A tetanus immunization or booster may be necessary.

Assessment of a treated (sutured) wound involves observation of its appearance, size, and drainage and the presence of swelling, pain, and status of drains or tubes. In some long-term facilities, home care situations, and outpatient clinics, photographs are taken weekly for a visual record of the progress of pressure ulcers and wounds. Other assessments are documented and dated along with the photograph.

Estimating the amount of wound drainage can be difficult. One recommendation is to describe the degree to which the dressing is saturated. Minimal drainage only stains the dressing; moderate drainage saturates the dressing without leakage prior to scheduled dressing changes; and heavy drainage overflows the dressing prior to scheduled changes (WUHS, 2007). These terms, plus the description of the drainage and the amount and type of dressing material used, should be well understood by all care providers.

Sometimes the wound reaches under the skin surface (called *undermining*). The edges of the wound around an open center may be raw or appear healed, but the undermining can result in a sinus tract or tunnel that extends the wound many centimeters beyond the main wound surface. To assess the size of the wound, gently explore the undermined area with a thin, flexible probe. Do not use a cotton-tipped swab, since it can leave fibers in the wound. Once the end of the tract is reached, gently raise the probe so that the bulge created by the end can be seen and its length can be measured on the skin surface. Sinus tracts are often caused by infection and have significant drainage. They may be treated with antibiotics, irrigation, surgical incision to open and drain the tract, or vacuum therapy for large tracts.

Diagnosis

The following nursing diagnoses relate to clients who have skin wounds or who are at risk for skin breakdown:

- *Risk for Infection*
- *Risk for Impaired Skin Integrity*
- *Impaired Skin Integrity*
- *Impaired Tissue Integrity*
- *Acute Pain*

(NANDA-I © 2012)

If the skin impairment is severe, the client is immunosuppressed, or the wound is caused by trauma, the potential for infection is even greater.

Impaired Skin Integrity commonly applies to pressure ulcers and wounds that extend through the epidermis but not through the dermis. *Impaired Tissue Integrity* applies to pressure ulcers and wounds that extend into subcutaneous tissue, muscle, or bone. Pain is also a concern, particularly related to nerve involvement within the tissue impairment or as a consequence of procedures used to treat the wound.

Planning

The major goals for the client at *Risk for Impaired Skin Integrity* are to maintain skin integrity and avoid potential associated risks. The outcomes associated with these goals may be as follows:

- The client will demonstrate progressive wound healing and regain intact skin within a specified time.

Client education for home care management focuses on maintaining skin integrity.

Implementation

The four major areas in which the nurse can help the client develop optimal conditions for wound healing are maintaining moist wound healing, providing sufficient nutrition and hydration, preventing wound infections, and proper positioning. Interventions addressing these four areas differ depending upon the age and condition of the client. For more information, see the Lifespan Considerations feature.

Facilitate Wound Healing

The dressing and frequency of change should support moist wound bed conditions. Wound beds that are too dry or disturbed too often fail to heal. See the Evidence-Based Practice feature in the exemplar on Cellulitis in the module on Infection for more information about moist wound management.

Promote Optimal Nutrition and Hydration

The client should be assisted to take in at least 2,500 mL of fluids a day unless other health conditions contraindicate this amount. Although there is no evidence that excessive doses of vitamins or minerals enhance wound healing, adequate amounts are extremely important. The nurse should ensure that the client receives sufficient protein, vitamins C, A, B, and B5, and zinc. A consultation with a registered dietitian helps to ensure that correct supplementation needs are met. The nurse and those planning the client's meals should take into account the client's personal and religious food preferences.

Prevent Infection

There are two main aspects to controlling wound infection: preventing microorganisms from entering the wound and preventing the transmission of bloodborne pathogens between the client and others.

Lifespan Considerations   Wound Care

Infants

- The skin of infants is more fragile than that of older children and adults and is more susceptible to infection, shearing from friction, and burns.

Children

- *Staphylococcus* and fungus are two major infectious agents affecting the skin of children. Abrasions or small lacerations, commonly experienced by children, provide an entry in the skin for these organisms. Clean minor wounds with warm, soapy water, and cover them with a sterile bandage. Instruct children not to touch the wound.
- With more serious skin lesions, remind the child not to touch the wound, drains, or dressing. Cover with an appropriate bandage that will remain intact during the child's usual activities. Cover a transparent dressing with opaque material if viewing the site is distressing to the child. Restrain the child only when all alternatives have been tried and when absolutely necessary.

- For younger children, demonstrate wound care on a doll. Reassure the child that the wound will not be permanent and that nothing will fall out of the child's body.

Older Adults

- Hold wrinkled skin taut during application of a transparent dressing. Obtain assistance if needed.
- The older adult's skin is more fragile and can easily tear with removal of tape (especially adhesive tape). Use paper tape and tape remover as indicated, keeping tape use to the minimum required. Use extreme caution during tape removal.
- Older adults in long-term care facilities often have the following factors: immobility, malnutrition, and incontinence. All of these increase the risk for development of skin breakdown.
- Skin breakdown can occur as quickly as within 2 hours, so assessments should be done with each repositioning of the client.
- A thorough assessment of a client's heels should be done every shift. The skin can break down quickly from friction of movement in bed.

Position to Minimize Pressure on the Wound

To promote wound healing, position the client to keep pressure off the wound (sometimes referred to as *off-loading*). Changes of position and transfers can be accomplished without shear or friction damage. In addition to proper positioning, assist the client to be as mobile as possible because activity enhances circulation. If the client cannot move independently, range-of-motion exercises and a turning schedule are implemented. See the Nursing Care Plan and Community-Based Care features.

Evaluation

Regular evaluation during the wound healing process is important for a client at *Risk for Impaired Skin Integrity*. Expected outcomes of nursing care include the following:

- Skin and tissue integrity is maintained.
- The wound has decreased in size.
- The client demonstrates an understanding of preventive care measures.

Community-Based Care   Home Care for Clients With Wounds

In planning home care for the client with a wound, the nurse needs to assess the following factors.

Client and Environment

- Client's current level of knowledge: understanding of the cause of the wound or risk for developing a pressure ulcer; prevention or treatment strategies
- Client's self-care abilities for mobility: physical ability to change position, ambulate, and transfer, including the use of assistive devices
- Client's self-care abilities for wound care: manual dexterity and visual acuity necessary to perform skin assessments and wound treatments
- Facilities: bathroom with running water and garbage container needed to perform wound care and contain potentially infectious materials
- Client's current level of nutrition: eating habits and preferences, laboratory values indicating need for teaching or other intervention

Family

- Caregiver availability, skills, and responses: understanding of the cause of the wound or risk for developing a pressure ulcer, prevention or treatment strategies, willingness to assist with wound care, and actions to prevent pressure ulcers
- Family role changes and coping: effect on financial status, parenting and spousal roles, sexuality, and social roles
- Alternative potential primary or respite caregivers: for example, other family members, volunteers, church members, paid caregivers, or housekeeping services; available community respite care (adult day care, senior centers, etc.)

Community

- Resources: availability and familiarity with possible sources of assistance such as equipment and supply companies, organizations that offer medical supplies or financial assistance, home health agencies, and transportation to and from medical appointments, if needed

NURSING CARE PLAN   A Client With a Postoperative Wound

ASSESSMENT

Tara Overbeck, 44 years old, underwent bariatric surgery 4 days ago. She says she knew it was time to do something dramatic when her doctor diagnosed both hypertension and type 2 diabetes mellitus on the same day. She has an 8-inch midline abdominal incision that appeared slightly red and began to ooze purulent drainage yesterday. The incision is stapled and has dissolvable sutures internally. Ms. Overbeck is NPO due to absent bowel sounds with an intravenous solution of dextrose and water infusing at 100 mL/h per infusion pump. The antibiotic ciprofloxacin hydrochloride (Cipro) is to be administered every 6 hours IV. Other medications include Regular Humulin insulin administered on a sliding scale based on finger-stick glucose levels, clevidipine butyrate (Cleviprex) administered PRN for hypertension, acetaminophen suppository PRN for fever greater than 100°F, and morphine sulfate PRN for pain.

Assessment findings include:
- Ms. Overbeck is drowsy but arousable and oriented.
- Skin is pale and slightly cool.
- Ms. Overbeck states that she is cold and requests additional covers.
- Ms. Overbeck states that she is in no pain and would like to sleep.
- Her respirations are unlabored.
- Vital signs: temperature 101.2°F oral; pulse 96 bpm; respirations 18/min; and BP 122/86 mmHg.
- She has a large abdominal dressing over a midline abdominal incision with purulent drainage the size of a silver dollar and a Jackson Pratt suction device connected to a drain with 10 mL dark red serosanguineous drainage coming from the distal part of the wound.
- An indwelling catheter is in place with 210 mL clear amber urine.
- This morning's lab results include: fasting blood sugar 110 mg/dL, hemoglobin within normal limits, WBC 12,400 mm^3 serum albumin 2.6 g/dL.

DIAGNOSES

- *Ineffective Thermoregulation* related to surgical procedure
- *Risk for Fluid Volume Deficit* related to altered postoperative intake
- *Impaired Skin Integrity* related to surgical incision
- *Delayed Surgical Recovery* related to postoperative surgical site infection

(NANDA-I © 2012)

PLANNING

Goals for Ms. Overbeck's plan of care include:
- The client will engage in activities that promote wound healing.
- The client will maintain adequate hydration.
- The client's temperature will be controlled within acceptable limits until fever subsides.
- The client's risk for complications secondary to wound infection will be reduced.

IMPLEMENTATION

- Use aseptic technique while changing the client's dressing.
- Monitor the client's temperature every 4 hours, with repeat measurement in 1 hour following administration of antipyretic if elevated higher than 100°F.
- Assess the wound every 4 hours for purulent drainage and odor; assess edges of wound for approximation, edema, redness, inflammation.
- Teach the client how to use aseptic technique when caring for her wound.
- Promote comfort through appropriate pain management, both pharmacologic and nonpharmacologic.

- Monitor intake and output, daily weight, and hydration status.
- Assess blood glucose four times per day and administer insulin on a sliding scale as ordered.
- Empty the Jackson Pratt wound drain every 4 hours, and notify the primary care provider if drainage increases beyond acceptable limits based on baseline drainage to date.
- Assist the client to change positions at least every 2 hours.
- Teach the client proper nutrition to promote wound healing in keeping with postop bariatric surgical requirements.

EVALUATION

Expected outcomes for Ms. Overbeck include the following:
- The client attains skin integrity of the abdominal incision.
- The client demonstrates proper aseptic technique while performing dressing changes.
- The client reports control of pain at incision site.
- The client's temperature returns to acceptable limits within 1 hour of receiving antipyretic.

CRITICAL THINKING

1. In addition to the nursing diagnoses identified in this plan of care, what other nursing diagnoses would be appropriate for Ms. Overbeck's care?
2. Assess Ms. Overbeck's nutritional status based on the data provided. Is it adequate to promote wound healing? Explain your answer and devise interventions as needed based on your response.
3. What impact will Ms. Overbeck's preexisting conditions of hypertension and type 2 diabetes mellitus have on her wound healing?
4. Other than the implementations listed in the plan of care, what else could you do to promote wound healing?
5. What discharge teaching will you provide Ms. Overbeck to promote wound healing?

REVIEW Wound Healing

RELATE Link the Concepts and Exemplars

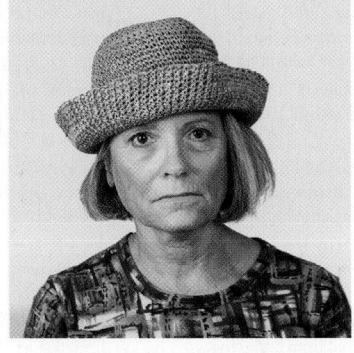

Norma James, a 65-year-old widow who lives alone, presents at the geriatric nursing clinic at the local senior center with a wound on her ankle about the size of a quarter. The wound is sore, with yellowish drainage. The skin around the wound is red and inflamed. Ms. James says that she has had the sore about 3 weeks and that she treated it with butter for a while but that that seemed to make it worse. Ms. James says that her foot hurts when she walks on it. The nurse at the clinic smells cigarette smoke on Ms. James clothing. When asked, Ms. James reports that she smokes about a pack a day. In response to a question from the nurse, Ms. James says that she has diabetes and high blood pressure. Ms. James is not able to say what medicines she takes but estimates that she takes "about four different ones."

Linking the exemplar of wound healing with the concept of metabolism:

1. What metabolic factors will increase the risk of delayed wound healing?
2. What teaching can the nurse provide Ms. James to promote wound healing in relation to metabolic concerns?

Linking the exemplar of wound healing with the concept of perfusion:

3. What factors related to perfusion will increase the risk of delayed wound healing for Ms. James?
4. What teaching will you provide Ms. James to reduce these risks related to perfusion?

READY Go to Companion Skills Manual

REFER Go to Pearson Student Nursing Resources
nursing.pearsonhighered.com

- Additional review material

REFLECT Case Study

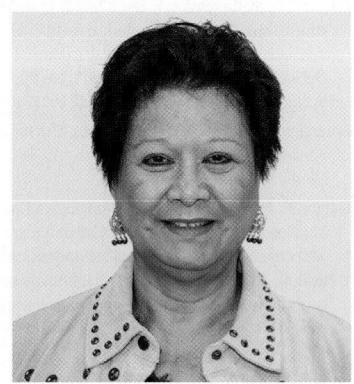

Lydia Ocampo, 69, wakes during the night to urinate but falls on the way to the bathroom. An ambulance takes her to the emergency department, where she is diagnosed with a left hip fracture. She is sent to the operating room for an open reduction internal fixation of the left hip. She is admitted to the medical-surgical floor following surgery.

Ms. Ocampo remains at the hospital because she has developed an infection in her incision and needs intravenous antibiotics and dressing changes. Her oral intake has been inadequate, but she has been well hydrated by intravenous fluids. She has been incontinent ever since the Foley catheter was removed. Attempts at physical therapy have been unproductive. The physical therapists are successful at transferring her from the bed to a chair, but this maneuver requires nearly full assistance.

1. Identify priority nursing diagnoses for Ms. Ocampo.
2. List factors that put Ms. Ocampo at risk for *Impaired Tissue Integrity*.

REFERENCES

Agency for Healthcare Research and Quality. (2012). Pressure ulcer risk assessment and prevention: A comparative effectiveness review. *Evidence-Based Practice Center Systematic Review Protocol.* Retrieved from http://effectivehealthcare.ahrq.gov/index.cfm/search-for-guides-reviews-and-reports/?pageaction=displayproduct&productid=926.

American Burn Association. (2012). Burn incidence and treatment in the United States: 2012 fact sheet. Retrieved from http://www.ameriburn.org/resources_factsheet.phpBall, J. W., Bindler, R. C., & Cowen, K. J. (2012). *Principles of Pediatric Nursing: Caring for Children* (5th ed.). Upper Saddle River, NJ: Prentice Hall.

Ball, J. W., Bindler, R. C., & Cowen, K. (2012). *Principles of pediatric nursing: Caring for children* (5th ed.). Upper Saddle River, NJ: Pearson Prentice Hall.

Barrientos, S., Stojadinovic, O., Golinko, M. S., Brem, H., & Tomic-Canic, M. (2008). Growth factors and cytokines in wound healing. *Wound Repair and Regenerations, 16*(5), 585–601. doi: 10.1111/j.1524-475X.2008.00410.x.

Bianchi, J. (2012). The effective management of exudate in chronic wounds. *Wounds International, 3*(4). Retrieved May 7, 2013 from http://www.woundsinternational.com/practice-development/the-effective-management-of-exudate-in-chronic-wounds.

Bishop, S., & Maguire, S. (2012). Anaesthesia and intensive care for major burns. *Continuing Education in Anaesthesia, Critical Care, and Pain, 12*(3), 118–122.

Bollero, D., Driver, V., Glat, P., Gupta, S., Lazaro-Martinez, J. L., Lyder, C., Ottonello, M., . . . Woo, K. (2010). The role of negative pressure wound therapy in the spectrum of wound healing. *Ostomy Wound Management, 56*(Suppl 5), 1–118.

Boston Children's Hospital. (2011). Fire safety and burn injury statistics. Retrieved from http://www.childrens-hospital.org/az/Site903/mainpageS903P0.html. The Braden Scale for Predicting Pressure Sore Risk. (1987). *Nursing Research, 36*(4), 205–210.

Brusselaers, N., Monstrey, S., Vogelaers, D., Hoste, E., & Blot, S. (2010). Severe burn injury in Europe: A systematic review of the incidence, etiology, morbidity, and mortality. *Critical Care, 14*(R188). doi:10.1186/cc9300.

Burn Survivor Resource Center. (2011). *Medical care guide: Burn statistics.* Retrieved from http://www.burnsurvivor.com/burn_statistics.html.

California Hospital Association. (2011). Evidence-based practices are resulting in fewer pressure ulcers for patients in California hospitals. *PR Newswire.* Retrieved from http://www.prnewswire.com/news-releases-test/evidence-based-practices-are-resulting-in-fewer-pressure-ulcers-for-patients-in-california-hospitals-132494828.html.

Centers for Disease Control and Prevention. (2011). *Fire deaths and injuries: Fact sheet.* Retrieved from http://www.cdc.gov/homeandrecreationalsafety/fire-prevention/fires-factsheet.html.

Centers for Disease Control and Prevention. (2012). *Skin cancer.* Retrieved from http://www.cdc.gov/cancer/skin/.

Chandran, L., & Cataldo, R. (2010). Lead poisoning: Basics and new developments. *Pediatrics in Review, 31*(10), 399–405.

Chen, W., Mempel, M., Traidl-Hofmann, C., Al Khusaei, S., & Ring, J. (2010). Gender aspects in skin disease. *Journal of the European Academy of Dermatology and Venerology, 24*(12), 1378–1385. doi: 10.1111/j.1468-3083.2010. 03668.x.

Cleveland Clinic. (2013). *Nutrition guidelines to improve wound healing.* Retrieved from http://my.cleveland-clinic.org/healthy_living/nutrition/hic_nutrition_guidelines_to_improve_wound_healing.aspx.

Cooper, M. A. (2009a). *Lightning injuries.* Retrieved from http://www.merckmanuals.com/home/injuries_and_poisoning/electrical_and_lightning_injuries/lightning_injuries.html?qt=&sc=&alt=.

Cooper, M. A. (2009b). *Electrical injuries.* Retrieved from http://www.merckmanuals.com/professional/injuries_poisoning/electrical_and_lightning_injuries/electrical_injuries.html.

Coulthard, P., Esposito, M., Worthington, H. V., van der Elst, M., van Waes, O. J., & Darcey, J. (2010). Tissue adhesives for closure of surgical incisions. *Cochrane Database Systematic Reviews, May 12*(5). doi: 10.1002/14651858.CD004287.pub3.

Dat, A. D., Poon, F., Pham, K. B., & Doust, J. (2012). Aloe vera for treating acute and chronic wounds. *Cochrane Database of Systematic Reviews, 2*, CD008762. doi:10.1002/14651858.CD008762.pub2.

Davidge, K., & Fish, J. (2008). Older adults and burns. *Geriatrics and Aging, 11*(5), 270–275.

Davila, M., Christenson, L. J., & Sonteimer, R. D. (2010). Epidemiology and outcomes of dermatology in-patient consultations in a midwestern U.S. university hospital. *Dermatology Online Journal, 16*(2), 12. Retrieved from http://dermatology.cdlib.org/1602/commentary/outcomes/sontheimer.html.

Davis, E. C., & Callendar, V. D. (2010). A review of acne in ethnic skin: Pathogenesis, clinical manifestations, and management strategies. *Journal of Clinical Aesthetic Dermatology, 34*, 24–38. Retrieved from http://www.ncbi.nlm.nih.gov/pmc/articles/PMC2921746/.

Emergency Nurses Association. (2010). *Sheehy's emergency nursing: Principles and practice* (6th ed.). St. Louis, MO: Mosby Elsevier.

Eshghi, F., Hosseinimehr, S. J., Rahmani, N., Khademloo, M., Norozi, M. S., & Hojati, O. (2010). Effects of aloe vera cream on posthemorrhoidectomy pain and wound healing: Results of a randomized, blind, placebo-control study. *Journal of Alternative and Complementary Medicine, 16*(6), 647–650. doi:10.1089/acm.2009.0428.

European Pressure Ulcer Advisory Panel and National Pressure Ulcer Advisory Panel. (2009). *Treatment of pressure ulcers: Quick reference guide.* Washington, DC: National Pressure Ulcer Advisory Panel.

Guo, S., & DiPietro, L. A. (2010). Factors affecting wound healing. *Journal of Dental Research, 89*(3), 219–229. doi: 10.1177/0022034509359125.

Helfrich, Y. R., Sachs, D. L., & Voorhees, J. J. (2010). The biology of skin aging. *U.S. Dermatology, 4*(1), 48–51. Retrieved from http://www.touchdermatology.com/articles/biology-skin-aging?page=0,2.

Hornor, G. (2012). Medical evaluation for child physical abuse: What the PNP needs to know. *Journal of Pediatric Health Care, 26*(3), 163–170.

Khorasani , G., Hosseinimehr, S. J., Azadbakht, M., Zamani, A., & Mahdavi, M. R. (2009). Aloe versus silver sulfadiazine creams for second-degree burns: A randomized controlled study. *Surgery Today, 39*(7), 587–591. doi:10.1007/s00595-008-3944-y.

Latenser, B. A. (2009). Critical care of the burn patient: The first 48 hours. *Critical Care Medicine, 37*(10), 2819–2826.

Lynch, S., & Vickery, P. (2010). Steps to reducing hospital-acquired pressure ulcers. *Nursing, 40*(11), 61–62. doi: 10.1097/01.NURSE.0000387754.83476.77.

Marini, A., & Hengge, U. R. (2009). Important viral and bacterial infections of the skin and mucous membrane. *Internist, 50*(2), 160–170. doi:10.1007/s00108-008-2209-6.

Mayo Clinic. (2012). *Dermatitis: Alternative medicine.* Retrieved from http://www.mayoclinic.com/health/dermatitis-eczema/DS00339/DSECTION=alternative-medicine.

McInnes, E., Jammali-Blasi, A., Bell-Syer, S. E. M., Dumville, J. C., & Cullum, N. (2011). Can pressure ulcers be prevented by using different support surfaces? *Cochrane Database of Systematic Reviews, 4*. doi: 10.1002/14651858.CD001735.pub4.

Michail, S. (2009). The role of probiotics in allergic diseases. *Allergy, Asthma, and Clinical Immunology, 5*(5). doi:10.1186/1710-1492-5-5.

Middaugh, S. (2011). ABC'Skin holds it all together: Nurses use evidence-based practice to reduce pressure ulcers. *Johns Hopkins Nursing Magazine,* (Fall/Winter). Retrieved from http://magazine.nursing.jhu.edu/2011/12/abc%E2%80%99skin-holds-it-all-together/.

Murray, R. B., Zentner, J. P., & Yakimo, R. (2009). *Health promotion through the life span* (8th ed.). Upper Saddle River, NJ: Prentice Hall.

National Center for Complementary and Alternative Medicine. (2012). *Herbs at a glance.* Retrieved from http://nccam.nih.gov/health/herbsataglance.htm?nav=gsa.

National Institutes of Health. (2011). Aloe. *MedlinePlus.* Retrieved from http://www.nlm.nih.gov/medlineplus/druginfo/natural/607.html.

National Pressure Ulcer Advisory Panel. (2007). *Pressure ulcer prevention points.* Retrieved from http://www.npuap.org/resources/educational-and-clinical-resources/pressure-ulcer-prevention-points/.

Nigam, Y., & Knight, J. (2008). Exploring the anatomy and physiology of aging: 11, The skin. *Nursing Times, 104*(49), 24–25. Retrieved from http://www.nursingtimes.net/nursing-practice/clinical-zones/older-people/exploring-the-anatomy-and-physiology-of-ageing-part-11-the-skin/1944136.article.

Occupational Safety and Health Administration. (2008). *Latex Allergy.* Retrieved April 30, 2013, from http://www.osha.gov/SLTC/latexallergy/index.html.

Ogunyemi, B. (2011). Ethnic dermatology: Social and medical challenges. *Dermanities, 7*(1). Retrieved from http://www.dermanities.com/detail.asp?article=316.

Palao, R., Monge, I., Ruiz, M., & Barret, J. P. (2010). Chemical burns: Pathophysiology and treatment. *Burns, 36*(3), 295–304.

Pancorbo-Hidalgo, P. L., Garcia-Fernandez, F. P., Lopez-Medina, I. M., & Alvarez-Nieto, C. (2006). Risk assessment scales for pressure ulcer prevention: A systematic review. *Journal of Advanced Nursing, 54*(1), 94–110. Retrieved from http://www.ncbi.nlm.nih.gov/pubmed/16553695.

Porth, C., & Matfin, G. (2010). *Pathophysiology: Concepts of altered health states* (8th ed.). Philadelphia, PA: Lippincott Williams & Wilkins.

Richardson, P., & Mustard, L. (2009). The management of pain in the burn unit. *Burns, 35*(7), 921–936.

Samalonis, L. B. (2011). New integrated therapies for wound healing on the horizon. *Dermatology Times.* Retrieved from http://dermatologytimes.modernmedicine.com/dermatology-times/news/modernmedicine/modern-medicine-feature-articles/new-integrated-therapies-woun?id=&sk=&date=&&pageID=1.

Sasseville, D. (2011). Occupational contact dermatitis (in Chapter 12, Skin Diseases). In J. M. Stellman (Ed.), *Encyclopedia of occupational health and safety.* Geneva, Switzerland: International Labour Organization. Retrieved from http://www.ilo.org/oshenc/part-i/skin-diseases/item/470-occupational-contact-dermatitis.

Schmidt, J. M., & Greenspoon, J. S. (1991). Aloe vera dermal wound gel is associated with a delay in wound healing. *Obstetrics and Gynecology, 78*(1), 115–117.

Singh, G., & Archana, G. (2008). Unravelling the mystery of vernix caseosa. *Indian Journal of Dermatology, 53*(2), 54–60. doi:10.4103/0019-5154.41645.

Society of Investigative Dermatology and American Academy of Dermatology Association. (2006). *The burden of skin diseases: 2004.* Retrieved from http://www.sidnet.org/pdfs/burden%20of%20skin%20diseases%202004.pdf.

Stander, M., & Wallis, L. A. (2011). The emergency management and treatment of severe burns. *Emergency Medicine International, 2011,* 15. doi:10.1155/2011/161375.

Surjushe, A., Vasani, R., & Saple, D. G. (2008). Aloe vera: A short review. *Indian Journal of Dermatology, 53*(4), 163–166. doi:10.4103/0019-5154.44785.

Taylor, J. S., & Amado, A. (2010). Contact dermatitis and related conditions. *Cleveland Clinic Center for Continuing Education Disease Management Project.* Retrieved from http://www.clevelandclinicmeded.com/medicalpubs/diseasemanagement/derma.

Uitto, J. (2012). Milestones in genetics of structural skin disorders. *Journal of Investigative Dermatology, 132,* E1. doi:10.1038/skinbio.2012.

University of Washington Harborview Medical Center. (2011). *Burn stabilization protocol.* Retrieved from http://www.uwmedicine.org/patient-care/locations/hmc/clinical-services/specialty-areas/burn/documents/burn-stabilization-protocol.pdfUsatine, R. P., & Riojas, M. (2010). Diagnosis and management of contact dermatitis. *American Family Physician, 82*(3), 249–255. Retrieved from http://www.aafp.org/afp/2010/0801/p249.html.

Veenema, T. G. (Ed.). (2007). *Disaster nursing and emergency preparedness for chemical, biological, and radiological terrorism and other hazards.* New York, NY: Springer.

Wang, S., Wang, J., Lu, D., Diao, Y., & Zhang, Z. (2010). Clinical research on the bio-debridement effect of maggot therapy for treatment of chronically infected lesions. *Orthopaedic Surgery, 2*(3), 201–206. Retrieved from http://onlinelibrary.wiley.com/doi/10.1111/j.1757-7861.2010.00087.x/pdf.

Weber, J., & McManus, A. (2004). Infection control in burn patients. *Burns, 30*(8), A16–A24.

World Health Organization. (2013). *Aloe vera gel.* Retrieved from http://apps.who.int/medicinedocs/en/d/Js2200e/6.html#Js2200e.6.

World Union of Healing Societies. (2007). *Principles of best practice: Wound exudate and the role of the dressing, a consensus document.* London: MEP Ltd. Retrieved from http://www.kendallhq.com/imageServer.aspx?contentID=18608&contenttype=application/pdf.

Yale School of Medicine. (2013). *Gangrene.* Retrieved from http://www.yalemedicalgroup.org/stw/Page.asp?PageID=STW048448. Zhai, H., Meier-Davis, S. R., Cayme, B., Shudo, J., & Maibach, H. (2012a). Allergic contact dermatitis: Effect of age. *Cutaneous and Ocular Toxicology, 31*(1), 20–25. doi: 10.3109/15569527.2011.595749.

Zhai, H., Meier-Davis, S. R., Cayme, B., Shudo, J., & Maibach, H. (2012b). Irritant contact dermatitis: Effect of age. *Cutaneous and Ocular Toxicology, 31*(2), 138–143. doi:10.3109/15569527.2011.618472.

NANDA-Approved Nursing Diagnoses 2012–2014

Activity, Deficient Diversional
Activity Intolerance
Activity Intolerance, Risk for
Activity Planning, Ineffective
Activity Planning, Risk for Ineffective
Adaptive Capacity: Intracranial, Decreased
Adverse Reaction to Iodinated Contrast Media, Risk for
Airway Clearance, Ineffective
Allergy Response, Latex
Allergy Response, Latex, Risk for
Allergy Response, Risk for
Anxiety
Anxiety, Death
Aspiration, Risk for
Attachment, Risk for Impaired
Bleeding, Risk for
Blood Glucose Level, Risk for Unstable
Body Image, Disturbed
Body Temperature: Imbalanced, Risk for
Bowel Incontinence
Breast Milk, Insufficient
Breastfeeding, Ineffective
Breastfeeding, Interrupted
Breastfeeding, Readiness for Enhanced
Breathing Pattern, Ineffective
Cardiac Output, Decreased
Caregiver Role Strain
Caregiver Role Strain, Risk for
Childbearing Process, Ineffective
Childbearing Process, Readiness for Enhanced
Childbearing Process, Risk for Ineffective
Comfort, Impaired
Comfort, Readiness for Enhanced
Communication, Readiness for Enhanced
Communication: Verbal, Impaired
Confusion, Acute
Confusion, Chronic

Confusion, Risk for Acute
Constipation
Constipation, Perceived
Constipation, Risk for
Contamination
Contamination, Risk for
Coping: Community, Ineffective
Coping: Community, Readiness for Enhanced
Coping, Defensive
Coping: Family, Compromised
Coping: Family, Disabled
Coping: Family, Readiness for Enhanced
Coping, Ineffective
Coping: Readiness for Enhanced
Decision Making, Readiness for Enhanced
Decisional Conflict (Specify)
Denial, Ineffective
Dentition, Impaired
Development: Delayed, Risk for
Diarrhea
Disuse Syndrome, Risk for
Dry Eye, Risk for
Dysreflexia, Autonomic
Dysreflexia, Autonomic, Risk for
Electrolyte Imbalance, Risk for
Energy Field, Disturbed
Environmental Interpretation Syndrome, Impaired
Failure to Thrive, Adult
Falls, Risk for
Family Processes, Dysfunctional
Family Processes, Interrupted
Family Processes, Readiness for Enhanced
Fatigue
Fear
Fluid Balance, Readiness for Enhanced
Fluid Volume: Deficient
Fluid Volume: Deficient, Risk for

Fluid Volume: Excess

Fluid Volume: Imbalanced, Risk for

Gas Exchange, Impaired

Gastrointestinal Motility, Dysfunctional

Gastrointestinal Motility, Risk for Dysfunctional

Grieving

Grieving, Complicated

Grieving, Risk for Complicated

Growth: Disproportionate, Risk for

Growth and Development, Delayed

Health: Community, Deficient

Health Behavior, Risk-Prone

Health Maintenance, Ineffective

Home Maintenance, Impaired

Hope, Readiness for Enhanced

Hopelessness

Human Dignity, Risk for Compromised

Hyperthermia

Hypothermia

Immunization Status, Readiness for Enhanced

Impulse Control, Ineffective

Infant Behavior: Disorganized

Infant Behavior: Disorganized, Risk for

Infant Behavior: Organized, Readiness for Enhanced

Infant Feeding Pattern, Ineffective

Infection, Risk for

Injury, Risk for

Insomnia

Jaundice, Neonatal

Jaundice, Neonatal, Risk for

Knowledge, Deficient

Knowledge, Readiness for Enhanced

Lifestyle, Sedentary

Liver Function, Risk for Impaired

Loneliness, Risk for

Maternal/Fetal Dyad, Risk for Disturbed

Memory, Impaired

Mobility: Bed, Impaired

Mobility: Physical, Impaired

Mobility: Wheelchair, Impaired

Moral Distress

Mucous Membrane: Oral, Impaired

Nausea

Neglect, Unilateral

Neurovascular Dysfunction: Peripheral, Risk for

Noncompliance

Nutrition, Imbalanced: Less Than Body Requirements

Nutrition, Imbalanced: More Than Body Requirements

Nutrition, Imbalanced: More Than Body Requirements, Risk for

Nutrition, Readiness for Enhanced

Pain, Acute

Pain, Chronic

Parenting, Impaired

Parenting, Readiness for Enhanced

Parenting, Risk for Impaired

Perfusion: Gastrointestinal, Risk for Ineffective

Perfusion: Renal, Risk for Ineffective

Perioperative Positioning Injury, Risk for

Personal Identity: Disturbed

Personal Identity: Disturbed, Risk for

Poisoning, Risk for

Post-Trauma Syndrome

Post-Trauma Syndrome, Risk for

Power, Readiness for Enhanced

Powerlessness

Powerlessness, Risk for

Protection, Ineffective

Rape-Trauma Syndrome

Relationship, Ineffective

Relationship, Readiness for Enhanced

Relationship, Risk for Ineffective

Religiosity, Impaired

Religiosity, Readiness for Enhanced

Religiosity, Risk for Impaired

Relocation Stress Syndrome

Relocation Stress Syndrome, Risk for

Resilience: Individual, Impaired

Resilience, Readiness for Enhanced

Resilience, Risk for Compromised

Role Conflict, Parental

Role Performance, Ineffective

Self-Care, Readiness for Enhanced

Self-Care Deficit: Bathing

Self-Care Deficit: Dressing

Self-Care Deficit: Feeding

Self-Care Deficit: Toileting

Self-Concept, Readiness for Enhanced

Self-Esteem, Chronic Low

Self-Esteem, Chronic Low, Risk for

Self-Esteem, Situational Low

Self-Esteem, Situational Low, Risk for

Self-Health Management, Ineffective

Self-Health Management, Readiness for Enhanced

Self-Mutilation

Self-Mutilation, Risk for

Self-Neglect

Sexual Dysfunction

Sexuality Pattern, Ineffective

Shock, Risk for

Skin Integrity, Impaired

Skin Integrity, Risk for Impaired

Sleep, Readiness for Enhanced

Sleep Deprivation

Sleep Pattern, Disturbed

Social Interaction, Impaired

Social Isolation

Sorrow, Chronic

Spiritual Distress

Spiritual Distress, Risk for

Spiritual Well-Being, Readiness for Enhanced

Stress Overload

Sudden Infant Death Syndrome, Risk for

Suffocation, Risk for

Suicide, Risk for

Surgical Recovery, Delayed

Swallowing, Impaired

Therapeutic Regimen Management:
    Family, Ineffective

Thermal Injury, Risk for

Thermoregulation, Ineffective

Tissue Integrity, Impaired

Tissue Perfusion: Cardiac, Risk for Decreased

Tissue Perfusion: Cerebral, Risk for Ineffective

Tissue Perfusion: Peripheral, Ineffective

Tissue Perfusion: Peripheral, Risk for Ineffective

Transfer Ability, Impaired

Trauma, Risk for

Trauma: Vascular, Risk for

Urinary Elimination, Impaired

Urinary Elimination, Readiness for Enhanced

Urinary Incontinence, Functional

Urinary Incontinence, Overflow

Urinary Incontinence, Reflex

Urinary Incontinence, Stress

Urinary Incontinence, Urge

Urinary Incontinence, Urge, Risk for

Urinary Retention

Ventilation: Spontaneous, Impaired

Ventilatory Weaning Response, Dysfunctional

Violence: Other-Directed, Risk for

Violence: Self-Directed, Risk for

Walking, Impaired

Wandering

GLOSSARY

Abortion Loss of pregnancy before the fetus is viable outside the uterus. Also called *miscarriage*.

Absorption The process of moving nutrients and fluid from the external environment of the gastrointestinal tract to the internal environment. May also refer to the intake of any specific nutrient.

Abstinence Voluntarily going without alcohol, drugs, or other pleasurable substances or activities.

Abuse of power An attempt by an individual to use his or her position or authority in a manner that shames, controls, demeans, humiliates, or denigrates another individual to gain emotional, psychological, or physical advantage over that individual.

Accelerations A transient increase in the fetal heart rate normally caused by fetal movement.

Accommodation 1. The ability of the eye to adjust to variations in distance. **2.** The process of a change whereby cognitive processes mature sufficiently to allow an individual to solve problems that were unsolvable before.

Accountability The ability and willingness of an individual to assume responsibility for his or her actions and to accept the consequences of his or her behavior.

Accreditation A peer review process that evaluates and certifies the quality of an organization.

Acculturation The process of adapting to the majority culture and accepting it as one's own.

Acid indigestion A condition in which an individual can taste the stomach acid when it flows back into the esophagus.

Acidosis The condition that results when hydrogen ion concentration increases above normal, causing the pH to drop below 7.35.

Acids Substances that release hydrogen ions in solution.

Acquaintance phase The first few days after a child's birth, when the new mother applies herself to the task of getting to know her baby.

Acquaintance rape A broad term used to describe a rape committed by an acquaintance or other familiar individual.

Acquired immunity Immunity developed after exposure to a pathogen.

Acquired immunodeficiency syndrome (AIDS) An immune system deficit induced by infection with the human immunodeficiency virus (HIV). AIDS is characterized by opportunistic infections.

Acrocyanosis A bluish discoloration of the hands and feet.

Acromegaly Excessive growth of bone from growth hormone hypersecretion.

Actinic keratosis An epidermal skin lesion directly related to chronic sun exposure and photodamage. Also called *senile keratosis* or *solar keratosis*.

Action potential The electrical activity produced by movement of ions across cell membranes that stimulates muscle contraction.

Active acquired immunity Antibodies formed in response to an illness or an immunization while a female is pregnant.

Active euthanasia Actions to bring about a client's death directly, with or without client consent.

Active immunity Production of antibodies or development of immune lymphocytes against specific antigens.

Active transport A method that requires additional energy (in the form of adenosine triphosphate) to move substances against the concentration gradient (from low concentration to high concentration).

Activities of daily living (ADLs) Activities used routinely in daily life, such as grooming, eating, bathing, and dressing.

Activity-exercise pattern An individual's routine of exercise, activity, leisure, and recreation, including activities of daily living that require energy expenditure.

Activity tolerance The type and amount of exercise or daily living activities that an individual is able to perform without experiencing adverse effects.

Actual loss A change in or unavailability of something or someone of value that can be recognized by others.

Acute coronary syndrome (ACS) Any condition that develops due to sudden, reduced blood flow to the heart.

Acute fatigue A sudden onset of physical and mental exhaustion or weariness, particularly after a period of mental or physical stress.

Acute illness An alteration in health or functioning characterized by severe symptoms of relatively short duration.

Acute infection An infection that appears suddenly and lasts for a short time.

Acute kidney injury (AKI) Proposed as a more accurate term for *acute renal failure*, AKI is defined as a sudden decline in kidney function that causes disturbances in fluid, electrolyte, and acid–base balances.

Acute lymphocytic leukemia (ALL) The most common type of leukemia in children and adolescents, marked by the proliferation of malignant cells that resemble immature lymphocytes.

Acute myeloid leukemia (AML) A disorder characterized by uncontrolled proliferation of myeloblasts and hyperplasia of the bone marrow and spleen.

Acute myocardial infarction (AMI) A life-threatening condition that occurs when blood flow to a portion of the cardiac muscle is blocked. If circulation to the affected myocardium is not promptly restored, loss of functional myocardium affects the heart's ability to maintain an effective cardiac output, ultimately leading to cardiogenic shock and death.

Acute pain Temporary, localized, and sudden pain that lasts for less than 6 months and has an identifiable cause, such as trauma, surgery, or inflammation.

Acute pancreatitis An inflammatory disorder that involves self-destruction of the pancreas by its own enzymes through autodigestion.

Acute postinfectious glomerulonephritis (APIGN) Inflammation of the glomerular capillary membrane that is most often seen in children as a response to a group A beta-hemolytic streptococcal infection of the skin or pharynx or as a result of infection by the *Staphylococcus, Pneumococcus,* or *Coxsackie* viruses.

Acute renal failure (ARF) A rapid decline in renal function with azotemia, fluid, and electrolyte imbalances. ARF may be reversed with prompt intervention.

Acute respiratory distress syndrome (ARDS) A disorder with rapid onset characterized by noncardiac pulmonary edema and progressive refractory hypoxemia. ARDS is a life-threatening emergency.

Acute retroviral syndrome (ARS) Primary human immunodeficiency virus infection.

Acute stress disorder A condition that may occur following an individual experiencing, learning of, or witnessing an extremely stressful event that involves the threat of death, actual or threatened serious injury, or actual or physical or sexual violation.

Acute tubular necrosis (ATN) The destruction of tubular epithelial cells, which causes an abrupt and progressive decline of renal function.

Adaptation 1. The ability to handle the demands made by the environment. Also called *coping behavior.* **2.** The return to normal functioning, even when homeostasis cannot be regained.

Adaptation phase The phase during a crisis in which the individual meets the challenges presented and uses his or her resources to successfully resolve the crisis.

Adaptive behavior Everyday skills including conceptual skills, social skills, and practical skills.

Adaptive functioning The ability of an individual to meet the standards expected for his or her cultural group.

Adaptive mechanisms Methods the ego uses to fulfill the needs of the id in a socially acceptable manner. Also called *defense mechanisms.*

Addiction A psychological or physical need for a substance (such as alcohol) or process (such as gambling) to the extent that the individual will risk negative consequences in an attempt to meet the need.

Addictive behaviors Compulsive, problematic patterns of action resulting in psychological and/or physiological dependence.

Adherence Commitment or attachment to a regimen. Also called *compliance.*

Adhesions Fibrous bands of scar tissue.

Adjustment disorder with depressed mood A maladaptive reaction to an identifiable psychosocial stressor or stressors that occurs within 3 months after the onset of the stressor and has persisted for no longer than 6 months. Also called *adjustment disorder* or *situational depression.*

Adjustment phase Initial phase experienced in response to crisis, characterized by disorganization and unsuccessful attempts to meet the crisis.

Adjustment reaction to depressed mood See Postpartum blues.

Administrative information system A system designed to provide support and management to the business side of health care. This includes human resources, financial data, materials management, risk management, and quality performance.

Administrative laws Responsibilities that may be interpreted and enforced by an agency that has been delegated the power of oversight by the governing legislation.

Adolescent family A family in which one or more parents are adolescents.

Advance healthcare directives Legal documents that allow an individual to plan for healthcare and/or financial affairs in the event of incapacity. Also called *advance directives* or *healthcare advance directives.*

Advocacy Protecting an individual by expressing and defending the individual's cause on his or her behalf.

Advocate An individual who expresses and defends the cause of another.

Aerobic exercise An activity during which the amount of oxygen taken into the body is greater than that used to perform the activity.

Aesthetic knowing The subjective elements and personal style a nurse uses when delivering care, including empathy, holistic thinking, compassion and sensitivity.

Afebrile Without fever.

Affect The immediate and observable emotional expression of mood, which people communicate verbally and nonverbally; the outward manifestation of what the individual is feeling.

Affective commitment An attachment to a profession that includes identification with and involvement in the profession.

Affective domain The learning domain encompassing an individual's emotional response to tasks, including feelings, emotions, interests, attitudes, and appreciation. Also called the *feeling domain.*

Afterload The force that ventricles must overcome to eject their blood volume.

Afterpains Cramp-like pains caused by intermittent contractions of the uterus that occur after childbirth.

Age-related macular degeneration (AMD) A gradual degeneration in the macular area of the retina that is the leading cause of blindness in people over age 65.

Ageism A deep and profound prejudice in American society against older adults.

Aggravated assault An unlawful attack by one individual on another for the purpose of inflicting severe or aggravated bodily injury. This type of assault usually is accompanied by the use of a weapon or by means likely to produce death or great bodily harm.

Aggression Any form of behavior directed toward the goal of harming or injuring another living being.

Aggressive behavior Behavior directed toward getting what one wants without considering the feelings of others.

Aggressive communicators Individuals who tend to focus on their own needs and become impatient when these needs are not met.

Agnosia The inability to recognize one or more objects that previously were familiar.

Agnostic An individual who doubts the existence of God or a supreme being or believes the existence of God has not been proved.

Agoraphobia A condition that is characterized by anxiety associated with two or more of the following situations: being in enclosed spaces, being in open spaces, utilizing public transportation, being in a crowd or standing in a line of people, or being alone outside the home environment.

Agraphia The inability to write properly.

AIDS dementia complex The most common cause of mental status changes for clients with HIV infection. This dementia results from a direct effect of the virus on the brain and affects cognitive, motor, and behavioral functioning. Fluctuating memory loss, confusion, difficulty concentrating, lethargy, and diminished motor speed are typical manifestations.

Air trapping Decreased airflow with exhalation caused by edema of the air passages.

Airborne precautions Used for clients who are known to have or suspected of having serious illnesses transmitted by airborne droplet nuclei smaller than 5 microns, such as tuberculosis.

Airway remodeling Structural changes of the airway caused by a disease, such as asthma, resulting in progressive or permanent loss of lung function.

Airway resistance The effort or force needed to move oxygen through the trachea to the lungs.

Akathisia Restlessness.

Alcohol dependence A primary, chronic disease characterized by use or abuse of alcohol; genetic, psychosocial, and environmental factors influence its development and manifestations. Also called *alcoholism*.

Alcohol poisoning A toxic condition that results from excessive consumption of large amounts of alcohol in a very short period of time.

Alcohol withdrawal delirium A medical emergency usually occurring 3–5 days following alcohol withdrawal and lasting 2–3 days. Characterized by paranoia, disorientation, delusions, visual hallucinations, elevated vital signs, vomiting, diarrhea, and diaphoresis. Also known as *delirium tremens (DTs)*.

Alcohol withdrawal syndrome Condition that typically begins about 6–8 hours after an individual with alcoholism takes his or her last drink. Early symptoms include irritability, anxiety, insomnia, tremors, sweating, and a mild tachycardia.

Alcoholic cirrhosis A progressive, irreversible liver disorder resulting from excessive consumption of alcohol. Also called *Laënnec cirrhosis*.

Alcoholism A primary, chronic disease characterized by use or abuse of alcohol; genetic, psychosocial, and environmental factors influence its development and manifestations. Also called *alcohol dependence*.

Alkalosis The condition that results when hydrogen ion concentration falls below normal and the pH level rises above 7.45.

Allen test A measurement of radial or ulnar patency; either the radial or ulnar artery is digitally compressed by the examiner after blood has been forced out of the hand by clenching it into a fist.

Allergen An environmental or exogenous antigen that provokes a hypersensitivity response.

Allergic contact dermatitis A cell-mediated or delayed hypersensitivity to a wide variety of allergens.

Allergy A hypersensitivity response to environmental or exogenous antigens.

Allogeneic blood transfusion A transfusion using blood that has been donated by the community.

Allogeneic bone marrow transplant A transplant using bone marrow from a matched donor.

Allografts Grafts between members of the same species who have different genotypes and HLA antigens. Human skin that has been harvested from cadavers is usually used. Also called *homograft*.

Alloimmunization The reaction of the immune system to donated tissue.

Allostasis Necessary changes that must occur to achieve the characteristic stability of homeostasis.

Allostatic load The physical cost of adaptation to physiological or psychosocial stressors.

Alogia Limited speech, associated with catatonic inhibition.

Alopecia Hair loss.

Alternative therapies A term used to describe use of these diverse therapies *instead of* conventional therapies including acupuncture; cultural practices related to food preparation or practices at specific times of the day or during the week.

Altruism A concern for the welfare and well-being of others.

Alzheimer disease (AD) The most common kind of dementia, Alzheimer disease involves progressive dementia, memory loss, and the inability to care for one's self.

Ambulation The ability to walk from place to place independently with or without an assistive device.

Amenorrhea The absence of menstruation.

Amniocentesis A procedure used to obtain amniotic fluid for genetic testing to determine fetal abnormalities or fetal lung maturity in the third trimester of pregnancy.

Amnion A thin protective membrane that contains amniotic fluid.

Amniotic fluid The liquid surrounding the fetus in utero. It absorbs shocks, permits fetal movement, and prevents heat loss.

Amphetamine A powerful stimulant that, when used improperly or abused, poses a severe health risk due to its devastating physical and neurological consequences, including amphetamine-induced mental disorders.

Ampulla The outer third of the fallopian tube, where fertilization usually occurs.

Amyloid plaques Seen in Alzheimer disease and formed when groups of nerve cells degenerate and clump around the amyloid core in the spaces between the neurons in the brain. Amyloid plaques consist primarily of insoluble deposits of beta-amyloid, a protein fragment from a larger protein called amyloid precursor protein, mixed with other neurons and non-nerve cells.

Anaerobic exercise Activity in which the muscles cannot draw out enough oxygen from the bloodstream, and anaerobic pathways are used to provide additional energy for storing for a short time.

Anal stimulation The stimulation of the anus with the fingers, mouth, or sex toys for sexual pleasure.

Anaphylactic shock Shock resulting from a widespread hypersensitivity reaction. Also called *anaphylaxis*.

Anaphylaxis An acute systemic type I hypersensitivity (allergic) response that may result in shock and death. It occurs in highly sensitive persons following exposure to a specific antigen, usually through injection or ingestion.

Anaplasia The regression of a cell to an immature or undifferentiated cell type.

Anasarca Severe, generalized edema.

Andragogy The art and science of teaching adults.

Androgen A hormone that stimulates the development and maintenance of male sex characteristics.

Androgyny Flexibility in gender roles.

Anemia An abnormally low number of circulating red blood cells, low hemoglobin concentration, or both.

Anergic Unable to react to common antigens.

Anergy Fatigue and decreased energy associated with a depressive disorder. Also called *anergia*.

Anger A subjective sense of intense displeasure, irritation, or animosity.

Angina pectoris Chest pain resulting from reduced coronary blood flow caused by a temporary imbalance between myocardial blood supply and demand. Also called *angina*.

Angle-closure glaucoma A type of glaucoma that results from a narrowing of the anterior chamber angle due to corneal flattening or bulging of the iris into the anterior chamber. Also called *narrow-angle* or *closed-angle glaucoma*.

Anhedonia The inability to feel pleasure.

Animism Giving lifelike qualities to nonliving things.

Anion Ion that carries a negative charge.

Anomia Difficulty naming people and things.

Anorexia Loss of appetite.

Anorexia nervosa (AN) A potentially life-threatening disorder characterized by extreme perfectionism, weight fear, significant weight loss, body image disturbances, strenuous exercising, peculiar food-handling patterns, and reductions in heart rate, blood pressure, metabolic rate, and the production of estrogen or testosterone.

Anorgasmia Absence of orgasm.

Antagonism One of the six trait domains associated with personality disorders that is comprised of manipulativeness, deceitfulness, callousness, hostility, grandiosity, and attention seeking.

Antepartum Time between conception and the onset of labor; usually used to describe the period during which a woman is pregnant.

Anthropometric measurements Measurements that can help identify individuals who are at risk for undernutrition or overnutrition. Specific measurements include height, length (in babies), weight, body mass index, waist-to-hip circumference, and skinfold thickness.

Antibodies Proteins that work against antigens.

Antibody-mediated (humoral) immune response Activation of B cells to produce antibodies to respond to antigens such as bacteria, bacterial toxins, and free viruses.

Anticipatory grief Grief experienced in advance of a loss, such as the wife who grieves before her ailing husband dies.

Anticipatory guidance Information about developmental changes that can be expected in the future. Including the recognition of the potential for a crisis and assistance with identifying potential methods for averting the crisis.

Anticipatory learning Learning necessary to effectively reach a desired outcome or in anticipation of a need for information that has not yet occurred.

Anticipatory loss A loss that is experienced before the loss actually occurs. For example, the gradual decline and eventual death of a family member who has Alzheimer disease.

Anticipatory problem solving Initial information is presented to a learner, who is then asked a question or presented with a situation related to the information. The learner applies the new information to the situation and decides what to do.

Antigen Foreign substance that triggers the immune response.

Antigen-antibody complex The complex formed by the binding of an antibody to an antigen.

Antigenic drift Describes small changes that occur continuously as a virus makes copies of itself.

Antigenic shift When two different strains of a virus infect the same cell and exchange genetic material to create a new subtype of the virus.

Antiretroviral therapies Pharmacologic therapies that stop or suppress the activity of a retrovirus, preventing further weakening of the immune system and thereby minimizing opportunistic infections.

Antiseptics Agents that inhibit the growth of some microorganisms.

Antisocial personality disorder (ASPD) One of several types of personality disorders defined by the DSM-5, it is characterized by a pattern of disregard for and violation of the rights of others.

Anuria The failure of the kidneys to produce urine, resulting in a total lack of urination or output of less than 100 mL/day in an adult.

Anxiety A stress response characterized by feelings of apprehension, dread, mental uneasiness, and a sense of helplessness in response to an actual or perceived threat to the well-being of oneself or others.

Anxious distress A combination of symptoms often associated with anxiety, including restlessness, impaired concentration due to worry, fear of something awful happening, and fear of losing control. Anxious distress often manifests in clients with depression and bipolar disorders and is associated with an increased risk for suicide.

Aortic stenosis Narrowing of the aortic valve that obstructs blood flow to systemic circulation.

Apathy A lack of interest or enthusiasm.

Apgar score A physical assessment of a newborn at 1 minute and 5 minutes after birth on a scale from 1 to 10 that includes heart rate, respiratory effort, muscle tone, reflex irritability, and skin color.

Aphakia Absence of the lens of the eye (e.g., after surgical removal of a cataract).

Aphasia Defective or absent language function.

Apical-radial pulse A comparison of the apical and radial pulses, which are normally identical. A pulse deficit can indicate certain cardiovascular disorders.

Aplastic anemia A disorder that results when the bone marrow fails to produce all three types of blood cells.

Apnea Absence of breathing.

Apnea of prematurity Absence of breathing for 20 seconds or longer, or for less than 20 seconds when associated with cyanosis, pallor, and bradycardia. A common problem in a preterm infant of less than 36 weeks' gestation, usually presenting between day 2 and day 7 of life.

Appendectomy Surgical removal of the appendix.

Appendicitis Inflammation of the vermiform appendix.

Appendicular skeleton Pectoral girdles, upper limbs, pelvic girdle, and lower limbs.

Approach-coping The use of confrontation to change the stressor by taking direct action.

Approximated Closed.

Apraxia The inability to perform purposeful movements and use objects correctly.

Areflexia The loss of reflex function.

Areola Pigmented ring surrounding the nipple of the breast.

Arrhythmogenic tissue Tissue that affects the generation and conduction of electrical impulses in the heart.

Arrogance Excessive pride and a feeling of superiority.

Arterial blood gas (ABG) A laboratory test used to evaluate oxygen and carbon dioxide exchange and the acid–base balance within the blood.

Arterial blood pressure A measure of the pressure exerted by the blood as it flows through the arteries.

Arteriosclerosis An arterial disorder characterized by thickening, loss of elasticity, and calcification of arterial walls.

Arteriovenous (AV) fistula An artificial connection between a vein and an artery created for long-term vascular access.

Arthrodesis A procedure that permanently fuses two or more bones together at a joint using pins, plates, screws, and rods. Also called *joint fusion*.

Arthroplasty Total joint replacement.

Arthroscopy A surgical procedure in which a thin, lighted tube with a camera in one end is inserted into a joint in order to allow a surgeon to visualize joint structure more easily.

Artificial disc surgery Surgery to replace a herniated disc with an artificial disc in order to maintain flexibility of the spinal joint.

Artificial rupture of membranes A process of rupturing of the membranes by the certified nurse-midwife or physician using an instrument called an amniohook. Completed if spontaneous rupture of membranes does not occur.

ASA Physical Classification Scale A physical risk classification category that determines the type and dosage of sedation a client can receive.

Ascites Excess fluid in the peritoneal cavity.

Asepsis The absence of disease-causing organisms.

Assault The action of creating an apprehension of offensive, insulting, or physically injurious touching.

Assertive behavior Behavior that consists of expressing one's wishes and opinions, or taking care of oneself, but not at the expense of others.

Assertive communicators Individuals who tend to declare and affirm their opinions. In doing this, however, they respect the rights of other to communicate in the same fashion.

Assertive community treatment (ACT) A therapeutic regimen for individuals with moderate to severe mental illness that provides clients with individually tailored services within their communities.

Assessment The systematic and continuous collection of data about a client for the purpose of determining the client's current and ongoing health status, predicting the client's health risks, and identifying appropriate health-promoting activities.

Assignment The transfer of responsibility to accomplish a task, without the transfer of authority.

Assimilation **1.** The process of adapting to and integrating characteristics of the dominant culture as one's own. **2.** The process by which humans encounter and react to new situations by using the mechanisms they already possess.

Assisted suicide Self-administration of a lethal dose of medication provided by a physician or healthcare provider in order to intentionally end a client's life with the goal of relieving pain and suffering.

Associative play A stage of play in which children play together or share tasks during play.

Astereognosis The inability to identify objects by touch.

Asthma A chronic inflammatory disease of the lungs characterized by recurrent episodes of wheezing, breathlessness, chest tightness, and coughing.

Asynclitism A condition that occurs when the sagittal suture is directed toward either the symphysis pubis or the sacral promontory and is felt to be misaligned.

Asystole Cardiac standstill.

Ataxia Lack of muscle coordination.

Atelectasis Collapse of lung tissue following obstruction of the bronchus or bronchioles.

Atheist An individual who does not believe in God.

Atherosclerosis A form of arteriosclerosis in which deposits of fat and fibrin obstruct and harden the arteries.

Atrial gallop (S_4) A heart sound produced by atrial contraction and ejection of blood into the ventricle during late diastole. Also called the *fourth heart sound*.

Atrial kick An extra bolus of blood delivered to the ventricles before they contract.

Atrial natriuretic factor (ANF) A peptide hormone released from cells in the atrium of the heart in response to excess blood volume and stretching of the atrial walls.

Atrial septal defect (ASD) An opening in the atrial septum that permits left-to-right shunting of blood.

Atrioventricular (AV) canal defect A combination of defects in the atrial and ventricular septa and portions of tricuspid and mitral valves. A complete AV canal defect allows blood to travel freely among all four chambers of the heart. Also called *endocardial cushion defect*.

Atrophy The wasting away or decrease in size of an organ, muscle, or tissue.

Attention deficit disorder (ADD) A variation in central nervous system processing characterized by developmentally inappropriate behaviors involving inattention.

Attention-deficit/hyperactivity disorder (ADHD) A variation in central nervous system processing characterized by developmentally inappropriate behaviors involving inattention, hyperactivity, and impulsivity.

Attention impairment A condition marked by an inability to process information and respond to such information appropriately; a client with attention impairment will have poor concentration and be easily distracted.

Attentive listening The process of listening actively, using all the senses. Also called *mindful listening*.

Audiologist A healthcare professional specializing in identifying, diagnosing, treating, and monitoring disorders of the auditory and vestibular portions of the ear.

Audit An examination of records to verify accuracy and proper use.

Auditory Of or relating to hearing.

Aura An olfactory or visual sensory sensation that may provide an early warning sign of a seizure.

Auscultation Listening to the sounds produced within the body. Auscultation can be direct using the unaided ear or indirect using a stethoscope or other listening device.

Authority **1.** The power to command other individuals and direct their activities. **2.** The right to act or to accomplish the task.

Autism spectrum disorders (ASDs) A developmental disorder in which individuals have persistent deficits in social communication and social interaction, and restricted, repetitive patterns of behavior, interest, or activities.

Autoantibodies Antibodies that react to the individual's own tissues.

Autocratic (authoritarian) leader A leader who makes decisions for the group based on the belief that individuals are externally motivated and are incapable of independent decision making.

Autografting A procedure performed in the surgical suite in which part of a client's healthy skin is removed and used to effect permanent skin coverage over a wound area.

Autoimmune disorder/disease Failure of immune system to recognize itself, resulting in normal host tissue being targeted by immune defenses.

Autologous blood transfusion A blood transfusion using a client's own blood.

Autologous bone marrow transplant Bone marrow transplant using a client's own bone marrow.

Automatism A repetitive reaction that occurs automatically, without conscious thought. Examples include lip smacking, eyelid fluttering, aimless walking, picking at clothing, and swallowing.

Autonomic dysreflexia An abrupt onset of excessively high blood pressure as the result of an overactive autonomic nervous system. An exaggerated sympathetic response that occurs in clients with spinal cord injuries at or above the T6 level. Also called *autonomic hyperreflexia*.

Autonomy **1.** The state of being independent and self-directed without outside control. **2.** The right to make one's own decisions.

Autosomal chromosomes Genetic material found in a cell nucleus that determines physical characteristics (excluding gender) of the individual.

Autosome A single chromosome from any one of the 22 pairs of chromosomes not involved in sex determination (X or Y); humans have 22 pairs of autosomes.

Avascular necrosis The death of bone tissue due to lack of blood supply. Also called *osteonecrosis*.

Avian influenza Also known as "bird flu," it is a form of influenza that commonly infects birds. This virus has not yet demonstrated the ability to spread among humans; however, concerns are that it will mutate to allow person-to-person spread. This viral strain has a mortality rate of greater than 50% in people who have been infected due to close association with infected birds.

Avoidance-coping The use of both behaviors and cognitive processes to avoid a stressor.

Avoidant personality disorder (APD) One of several types of personality disorders recognized by the DSM-5, APD is characterized by a pattern of social withdrawal along with a sense of inadequacy, fear, and hypersensitivity to potential rejection or shame.

Avolition The inability to persist in goal-directed activities.

Awareness The ability to perceive environmental stimuli and body reactions and to respond appropriately through thought and action.

Axial loading The application of vertical force to the spinal column.

Axial skeleton Ribs, sternum, vertebral column, and skull.

Axon A nerve fiber.

Azotemia Increased levels of nitrogenous wastes in the blood.

B lymphocytes (B cells) Integral to specific immune response, they are activated and mature into either plasma cells, which secrete antibodies, or memory cells.

Babinski reflex The fanning and extension of the toes or flexion of the toes due to gentle stroking on the sole of the foot. Also called the *Babinski response*.

Bacilli Rod-shaped bacteria.

Background questions General questions asked of a client that seek more information about a topic, such as diseases and medications.

Bacteremia The presence of bacteria in the blood.

Bacteria The most common category of infection-causing microorganisms.

Bactericidal agent Destroys bacteria.

Bacteriostatic agent Prevents the growth and reproduction of some bacteria.

Balloon tamponade The inflation of the balloon tip of a multiple-lumen nasogastric tube to control bleeding.

Barlow maneuver A procedure used to evaluate an infant for hip dislocation or instability in which the healthcare provider grasps and adducts the infant's thigh and then applies gentle downward pressure.

Barotrauma Lung injury caused by alveolar overdistention. Also called *volutrauma*.

Barrel chest An increase in the anteroposterior chest diameter resulting from air trapping and hyperinflation.

Basal cell carcinoma An epithelial tumor believed to originate either from the basal layer of the epidermis or from cells in the surrounding dermal structures. Also called *basal cell cancer*.

Basal metabolic rate (BMR) The amount of energy expended by the body at rest.

Base excess (BE) A calculated value also known as *buffer base capacity*. The BE measures substances that can accept or combine with hydrogen ions. It reflects the degree of acid–base imbalance by indicating the status of the body's total buffering capacity.

Baseline rate The average fetal heart rate rounded to increments of 5 bpm observed during a 10-minute period of monitoring. This excludes periodic or episodic changes, periods of marked variability, and segments of the baseline that differ by more than 25 bpm.

Bases Substances that accept hydrogen ions in solution. Also called *alkalis*.

Basic needs The physical needs of an individual, such as eating, sleeping, resting, self-care, and physical stability.

Battery The willful touching of another individual, an individual's clothes, or even something the individual is carrying that is unwanted, embarrassing, or unwarranted.

Behavioral therapy A form of therapy in which clients learn techniques to modify or change maladaptive behaviors.

Behaviorist theory A theory that suggests that learning takes place when an individual's reaction to a stimulus is either positively or negatively reinforced.

Belief An interpretation or conclusion that one accepts as true.

Belief system The way in which a culture explains the mysteries of the universe and life.

Belt restraint Restraint used to ensure the safety of clients who are transported by wheelchair or gurney, or to protect clients confined to a bed or a chair. Also called *safety strap body restraint*.

Benchmarking A method used to compare the performance of an individual or organization to industry standards.

Beneficence The act of doing good or beneficial actions.

Benign Referring to a growth or tumor that does not endanger life or health and tends to not recur after treatment.

Benign prostatic hyperplasia (BPH) Nonmalignant enlargement of the prostate gland commonly seen in the aging male.

Bereavement The subjective response experienced by the surviving loved ones after the death of an individual with whom they have shared a significant relationship.

Bias The favoring of a group or individual over another.

Bidirectional influence Influences exerted between an individual and his or her family that may negatively affect the emotional health of the individual, the family, or both.

Bilevel ventilator (BiPAP) Mechanical ventilation that provides inspiratory positive airway pressure as well as airway support during expiration.

Biliary colic A severe, steady pain in the epigastric region or right upper quadrant of the abdomen.

Binge drinking The consumption of five or more drinks containing alcohol in a single session.

Binge eating The ingestion of huge amounts of food (about 3,500 kcal) within a short time (about 1 hour).

Binge eating disorder (BED) An eating disorder characterized by recurring episodes of binge eating, a sense of lack of control, and negative feelings about oneself, but without intervening periods of behavior such as self-induced vomiting, purging by laxatives, fasting, or prolonged exercise.

Binuclear family A postdivorce family in which the biological children are members of two nuclear households—that of the father and that of the mother—and the children alternate between the two homes.

Bioethics The application of ethics to issues of human life or health (e.g., to decisions about abortion or euthanasia).

Biological rhythm A cyclical event or function that consists of repeated occurrences and repeated, regular intervals between occurrences. Biological rhythms can refer to both physical and psychological patterns.

Biomedical informatics The interdisciplinary science that deals with biomedical information's structure, acquisition, and use.

Bioterrorism The deliberate release of viruses, bacteria, or other microbes as weapons.

Bipolar disorder A mood disorder characterized by alternating depression and elation, with periods of normal mood in between. Formerly called *manic–depressive disorder*.

Birthing room A single room in a hospital where a pregnant woman and her partner or other family members will stay for the labor, birth, recovery, and possibly the postpartum period.

Bisexual An individual who is attracted to members of both sexes.

Bisphosphonates Drugs used to treat osteoporosis that inhibit bone reabsorption by suppressing osteoclast activity.

Blackouts A form of amnesia about events that occurred during a drinking period. This is often seen in the early stages of alcoholism.

Bladder training Gradually increases the bladder capacity by increasing the intervals between voidings and resisting the urge to void.

Blame-free environment An environment in which healthcare providers can report errors or near misses without the fear of punishment.

Blended family A family formed after the death or divorce of a parent, may include stepparents on both sides, stepchildren, half-siblings.

Blepharism Spasms that cause the eye to blink continuously.

Blighted ovum One of the most common causes of miscarriage, it occurs when the egg has been fertilized and both the membrane and placenta have formed, but the embryo has not formed.

Blood flow The volume of blood transported in a vessel, in an organ, or throughout the entire circulation over a given period of time.

Blood pressure The force that blood exerts against the walls of the arteries as it is pumped from the heart.

Blood urea nitrogen (BUN) A measure of blood level of urea, the end product of protein metabolism.

Bloodborne pathogens Microorganisms carried in blood and body fluids that are capable of infecting other individuals with serious and difficult to treat viral infections.

Bloody show The pink-tinged secretions resulting from a small amount of blood loss from the exposed cervical capillaries during pregnancy.

Blunt trauma Trauma that occurs without any communication between the damaged tissues and the outside environment.

Body fluid Any fluid that is essential to homeostasis; water is the primary body fluid.

Body image The mental image of the physical self.

Body mass index (BMI) A method of comparing weight to height as an indirect measure of body fat.

Body substance isolation (BSI) System that employs generic infection control precautions for all clients, except those with the few airborne diseases.

Body surface area (BSA) The relationship between height and weight measured in square meters.

Body temperature The core or surface measurement of a client's internal heat production and loss.

Bone marrow transplant The treatment of disease by infusing a client with his or her own bone marrow or that of a healthy donor.

Borborygmus Hyperactive, high-pitched, tinkling, rushing, or growling bowel sounds heard in diarrhea or at the onset of bowel obstruction.

Borderline personality disorder (BPD) One of several personality disorders defined in the DSM-5, BPD is marked by unstable interpersonal relationships, self-image, affect, and impulsiveness.

Bouchard nodes Bony lumps in the middle joint of the digit.

Boundaries The invisible lines that define the amount and kind of contact allowable among members of a family and between the family and outside systems.

Boutonnière deformity A flexion deformity of the PIP joints with extension of the DIP joint.

Bowel incontinence The inability to voluntarily control the passage of fecal contents and intestinal gas through the anal sphincter. Also called *fecal incontinence*.

Brachytherapy Radiation treatment given by placing radioactive material directly in or near the target, which is often a tumor.

Bradycardia A heart rate in an adult of less than 60 bpm.

Bradydysrhythmia Abnormally slow rhythms.

Bradykinesia Slowed movements due to muscle rigidity.

Bradyphrenia Slowed thinking and a decreased ability to form thoughts, to plan, or to make decisions.

Bradypnea A respiratory rate of less than 10 breaths per minute in adults.

Brain death The cessation and irreversibility of all brain functions, including those of the brainstem.

Brainstem Contains the midbrain, pons, and medulla oblongata. Located between the cerebrum and spinal cord, the brainstem connects pathways between the higher and lower structures. Ten of the 12 pairs of cranial nerves originate in the brainstem.

Brainstorming A decision-making method in which group members meet and generate diverse ideas about the nature, cause, definition, or solution to a problem.

Braxton Hicks contractions Intermittent painless uterine contractions that may occur every 10–20 minutes and occur more frequently near the end of pregnancy.

Brazelton neonatal behavioral assessment scale A scale developed to assess a newborn's state changes, temperament, and individual behavioral patterns.

Breach of care See Breach of duty.

Breach of duty A deviation from the standard of care owed a client. Also called *breach of care*.

Breakthrough pain A sudden flare or increase in pain despite comfort with or without baseline analgesia.

Breast Mammary gland.

Breast cancer The unregulated growth of abnormal cells in breast tissue.

Breathing exercises Techniques used to slow the breathing rate by focusing on taking regular and deep breaths from the diaphragm.

Brief psychotic disorder Rapid onset of at least one of the following psychotic symptoms: delusions, hallucinations, disorganized speech, or disorganized behavior. The episode lasts at least 1 day but less than 1 month, after which the person returns to the premorbid level of functioning.

Bronchiectasis Chronic dilation of the bronchi and bronchioles.

Bronchiolitis A lower respiratory tract illness that occurs when an infecting agent (virus or bacterium) causes inflammation and obstruction of the small airways.

Bronchitis Inflammation of the mucous membranes of the bronchial tubes.

Bronchogenic carcinomas Tumors of the airway epithelium.

Bronchoscopy A procedure that allows direct visualization of the lungs by inserting a bronchoscope orally into the trachea and advancing it to the bronchi bifurcation.

Bronchovesicular sound The sound created as air moves within the bronchial tree.

Brown adipose tissue (BAT) A specific store of fat in newborn infants that appears dark brown due to enriched blood supply, dense cellular content, and abundant nerve endings.

Bruits Blowing sound sometimes heard due to restriction of blood flow through the vessels.

Buffers Substances that prevent major changes in pH by releasing hydrogen ions.

Bulimia nervosa (BN) A type of eating disorder characterized by an obsessive focus on weight and body size and cycles of binge eating followed by purging.

Bureaucratic leader A leader who relies on the organization's rules, policies, and procedures to direct the group's work efforts.

Burn An injury resulting from exposure to heat, chemicals, radiation, or electric current.

Burn shock Hypovolemic shock resulting from the shift of a massive amount of fluid from the intracellular and intravascular compartments into the interstitium following burn injury. Also called *hypovolemic shock*.

Burnout A complex syndrome resulting from unmanaged stress that manifests as physical and emotional depletion, a negative attitude and self-concept, and feelings of helplessness and hopelessness.

Cachexia Physical wasting from weight loss and loss of muscle mass due to the rapid growth and reproduction of cancer cells and their need for increased nutrients.

Caffeine A stimulant that increases the heart rate and acts as a diuretic.

Calcium oxalate A chemical compound from which kidney stones may form.

Calcium phosphate A chemical compound from which kidney stones may form.

Calculi Renal stones.

Cancellous bone The spongy tissue of bone.

Cancer A family of complex diseases with manifestations that vary according to body system and type of tumor cells.

Cancer pain Pain that may result from the direct effects of the cancerous disease and its treatment, or it may be unrelated to the disease and its treatment in individuals with cancer.

Candidiasis A common, opportunistic fungal infection in clients with AIDS.

Cannabis sativa The plant source of marijuana.

Caput succedaneum A localized, easily identifiable, soft area of the scalp, generally resulting from a long and difficult labor or vacuum extraction.

Carbohydrate One of the three major macronutrients primarily derived from plant foods. These foods contain simple and complex sugars, and starches.

Carcinogen A substance that causes cancer.

Carcinogenesis The production or origin of cancer.

Cardiac arrest The cessation of heart function that precedes biological death.

Cardiac cycle One contraction and relaxation of the heart; a single heartbeat.

Cardiac index The cardiac output adjusted for the client's body size or body surface area (BSA).

Cardiac markers Proteins released from necrotic heart muscle.

Cardiac output (CO) The amount of blood pumped by the ventricles into the pulmonary and systemic circulations in 1 minute.

Cardiac rehabilitation A medically supervised program designed to aid people with their recovery from heart attacks, heart surgeries, and percutaneous coronary interventions.

Cardiac reserve The heart's ability to respond to the body's changing need for cardiac output.

Cardiac tamponade Compression of the heart caused by collected blood or fluid in the pericardium.

Cardinal ligament Major ligament of the uterus containing the uterine artery and vein.

Cardinal movements A series of changes in position that allow the fetus to move through the birth canal. Also called *mechanisms of labor*.

Cardiogenic shock Shock that occurs when the heart's pumping ability is compromised to the point that it cannot maintain cardiac output and adequate tissue perfusion.

Cardiomyopathy Disease that affects the heart muscle's ability to pump effectively. Primary abnormality of the heart muscle that affects its structural or functional characteristics.

Cardiopulmonary resuscitation (CPR) A mechanical attempt to maintain tissue perfusion and oxygenation using oral resuscitation and external cardiac compressions.

Care coordination The means by which a multidisciplinary team works with a client to ensure that the care received across the healthcare continuum meets the client's needs.

Care management model Planning, assessment, and coordination of health services to provide an integrated continuum of clinical services including medical care, health promotion, disease prevention, costs, and use of resources.

Care map Expected outcomes and care strategies developed through collaboration by the healthcare team. Also called a *critical pathway*.

Caring To feel interest, concern, and respect for a client while demonstrating sensitivity, sincerity, honesty, and patience.

Caring for the dying The act of helping clients live as comfortable as possible until death and helping the client's support individuals cope with death.

Carpal spasm Involuntary contraction of the hand and fingers due to decreased calcium levels.

Carphologia Involuntary, repeated lint picking.

Carrier Human or animal reservoir of a specific infectious agent that usually does not manifest any clinical signs of the disease.

Cartilage A type of flexible connective tissue found throughout the body.

Case management (CM) The process of coordinating, facilitating, and following a client's use of an array of health and social services over time.

Case managers Individuals who help manage the care of certain client populations including clients with chronic medical conditions, such as diabetes; clients recovering from acute conditions, such as those receiving joint replacement; and clients managing psychiatric disorders.

Caseation necrosis A process in which tissue infected with *Mycobacterium tuberculosis* dies and forms a cheeselike center in the infectious bacilli.

Cast A rigid device applied to immobilize injured bones and promote healing.

Catabolism The breakdown of body proteins.

Cataract An opacification (clouding) of lens of the eye due to a breakdown of proteins within the lens.

Catatonia Unresponsiveness to the environment or others.

Catatonic excitement Includes hyperactivity and bizarre behavior and is a positive symptom of schizophrenia.

Catatonic inhibition involves decreased activity level; limited speech; minimal self-care; and, at times, a trancelike state. Catatonic inhibition is a negative symptom of schizophrenia.

Cation Ion that carries a positive charge.

Cauda equina syndrome (CES) A condition that occurs when the nerve roots of the cauda equine are compressed. It may result in permanent neurological impairment, including urinary incontinence and paralysis.

Causation To make a successful claim for malpractice, an injury must have occurred as a direct consequence of a nurse's or professional's breach of duty.

Cavitation Formation of a cavity or bubble.

Celiac disease A chronic immune-mediated disorder of the small intestine in which the absorption of nutrients, particularly fats, is impaired. Also known as celiac sprue or nontropical sprue.

Cell cycle The four phases of cell growth and development.

Cell-mediated (cellular) immune response Direct or indirect inactivation of antigen by lymphocytes.

Cellulitis An acute bacterial infection of the dermis and underlying connective tissue. Cellulitis is characterized by red or lilac, tender, warm, edematous skin that may have an ill-defined, nonelevated border.

Central nervous system (CNS) One of two principal parts of the neurological system, the central nervous system consists of the brain and the spinal cord.

Central nervous system (CNS) depressants A type of drug that acts to slow brain function, decreasing levels of alertness and awareness. CNS depressants include barbiturates, benzodiazepines, paraldehyde, meprobamate, and chloral hydrate.

Central pain 1. A type of pain related to a lesion in the brain that may spontaneously produce high-frequency bursts of impulses that are perceived as pain. 2. A type of pain caused by damage to the central nervous system that may manifest in constant pain, pain paroxysms, evoked pain, or allodynia. Clients may describe their pain as "pins and needles," aching, or lacerating.

Centration Focusing only on one particular aspect of a situation or the ability to concentrate.

Cephalocaudal development Growth that proceeds in the direction from head to toe.

Cephalohematoma A collection of blood resulting from ruptured blood vessels between the surface of a cranial bone and the periosteal membrane. Also called an *entrapped hemorrhage*.

Cerebellum Located below the cerebrum and behind the brainstem, it coordinates stimuli from the cerebral cortex to provide precise timing for skeletal muscle coordination and smooth movements.

Cerebral palsy (CP) A group of chronic conditions affecting body movement, coordination, and posture that results from a nonprogressive abnormality of the immature brain.

Cerebral perfusion pressure (CPP) The pressure it takes for the heart to provide the brain with blood. It is calculated by finding the difference between arterial pressure and intracranial pressure. Normal CPP is 0–95 mmHg.

Cerebrum The largest portion of the brain, it is composed of gray matter and has two hemispheres divided into four regions or lobes.

Certification The credentialing process by which a nongovernmental agency or association recognizes the professional competence of an individual who has met the predetermined qualifications specified by the agency or association.

Cerumen Earwax.

Cervical cap A latex cup-shaped contraceptive device, used with spermicidal cream or jelly, that fits snugly over the cervix and is held in place by suction.

Cervical collar A device that stabilizes and maintains neutral alignment of the cervical spine; it is used with clients with potential or suspected cervical spine injury. Also called *C-collar.*

Cervical ripening The softening and effacing of the cervix.

Cervix The narrow neck of the uterus.

Cesarean birth The birth of an infant through an abdominal and uterine incision.

Chain of command The hierarchy of authority and responsibility within an organization.

Chancre A painless ulceration formed during the first stage of syphilis.

Change-of-shift report A type of handoff communication given to all nurses on the next shift.

Channel A medium used to convey messages.

Charismatic leader A rare type of leader who is characterized by a strong, emotional relationship between the leader and the group members.

Chart A formal, legal document that provides evidence of a client's care. Also called a *client record* or a *clinical record.*

Charting The process of making an entry on a client record. Also called *recording* or *documenting.*

Charting by exception (CBE) A documentation system in which only abnormal or significant findings or exceptions to norms are recorded.

CHCT A biopsy of thigh skeletal muscle tissue to determine sensitivity to caffeine and halothane.

Cheilosis Cracking of lips.

Chemical conjunctivitis An irritation of the conjunctiva by chemicals used to treat the eyes.

Chemical restraints Pharmacologic agents administered for the purpose of controlling hyperactive behavior in agitated clients.

Chemical thermogenesis The stimulation of heat production in the body through increased cellular metabolism. Also called *nonshivering thermogenesis* or *NST.*

Chemotaxis The movement of cells in response to a chemical stimulus.

Chemotherapy Cancer treatment involving the use of cytotoxic medications to decrease tumor size, adjunctive to surgery or radiation therapy; or to prevent or treat suspected metastases.

Chest x-ray Allows for two-dimensional visualization of the contents of the thoracic cavity.

Child abuse Any act or failure to act on the part of a parent or caretaker which results in the death, serious physical or emotional harm, sexual abuse, or exploitation of a child.

Child Health Insurance Program (CHIP) State and federal funded healthcare coverage for children under the age of 19 whose families earn more than the Medicaid limits but cannot afford to purchase private healthcare coverage.

Childhood traumatic grief A grief reaction that occurs when an important person in a child's life dies as the result of a traumatic event or circumstances the child views as traumatic.

Childless family A family without children. Also called a *child-free family.*

Chlamydia A group of sexually transmitted infections caused by *Chlamydia trachomatis.*

Chloasma Brownish pigmentation over the bridge of the nose and the cheeks during pregnancy and in some women who are taking oral contraceptives. Also called *melasma gravidarum* or *mask of pregnancy.*

Cholangitis Duct inflammation.

Cholecystitis Inflammation of the gallbladder.

Cholelithiasis The formation of stones (*calculi* or *gallstones*) in the gallbladder or biliary duct system.

Chromosomes Tightly coiled strands of DNA within the nucleus that contain genetic information.

Chronic bronchitis A disorder of excessive bronchial mucous secretion.

Chronic fatigue Profound fatigue of long duration that is not improved by rest.

Chronic fatigue syndrome A complex disorder in which the client experiences unrelenting fatigue and associated symptoms that are not alleviated by substantial rest and that cannot be otherwise explained for a period of 6 months or longer. Also called *myalgic encephalomyelitis.*

Chronic illness An alteration in health or function that lasts for an extended period of time, usually 6 months or longer, and often for the duration of the individual's life.

Chronic infection An infection that develops slowly and persists for months or sometimes years.

Chronic intermittent colitis A recurrent form of ulcerative colitis characterized by insidious onset, few systemic manifestations, and attacks lasting 1–3 months that occur at intervals of months to years.

Chronic kidney disease A type of renal failure that progresses slowly with few symptoms until the kidneys are severely damaged and unable to meet the excretory needs of the body. Also called *chronic renal failure.*

Chronic lymphocytic leukemia (CLL) A disorder characterized by the proliferation and accumulation of small, abnormal, mature lymphocytes in the bone marrow, peripheral blood, and body tissues.

Chronic myeloid leukemia (CML) A disorder characterized by abnormal proliferation of all bone marrow elements.

Chronic obstructive pulmonary disease (COPD) A specific progressive disorder that slowly alters the structures of the respiratory system over time, irreversibly affecting lung function.

Chronic pain Prolonged pain, usually lasting longer than 6 months. It is not always associated with an identifiable cause and is often unresponsive to conventional medical treatment.

Chronic pancreatitis An irreversible process characterized by chronic inflammation, fibrosis, and gradual destruction of functional pancreatic tissue.

Chronic renal failure See Chronic kidney disease.

Chronic venous insufficiency (CVI) A disorder of inadequate venous return over a prolonged period of time.

Chvostek sign Facial grimacing caused by repeated contractions of the facial muscle. A test used to check for hypocalcemia.

Circumcision A surgical procedure in which the prepuce, an epithelial layer covering the penis, is separated from the glans penis and excised. This procedure permits exposure of the glans for easier cleaning.

Cirrhosis The end stage of chronic liver disease. It is a progressive, irreversible disorder, eventually leading to liver failure.

Civil law The area of law that deals with the rights and duties of private persons or citizens and is most often enforced through the awarding of damages or compensation.

CK-MB A subset of CK enzyme specific to cardiac muscle. Elevated CK-MB is an indicator of myocardial infarction. Also called *MB-bands*.

Clang Repetition of rhyming words without apparent meaning.

Classism The oppression of groups of people based on their socioeconomic status.

Clean A state of medical asepsis in which almost all microorganisms are absent.

Client An individual who engages the advice or services of another person who is qualified to provide this service.

Client advocate An individual who acts to protect the client and defend the client from harm.

Client-focused care A delivery model that organizes health care around the expressed physical and emotional needs of the client.

Client record A formal, legal document that provides evidence of a client's care. Also called a *chart* or a *clinical record*.

Clinical decision support system A system that analyzes data and provides information about evidenced-based practices. These systems can help improve client safety and quality of care when used with sound nursing and medical judgment.

Clinical information system A software-based system that allows multiple disciplines to simultaneously access the client's chart and record data that can be viewed and analyzed by a number of healthcare providers in real time. These systems are designed to provide the most accurate and current information about the client so that the best decisions concerning the care of that client can be made.

Clinical pathway A standardized, evidence-based, multidisciplinary plan that outlines the expected care required for clients with common, predictable—usually medical—conditions.

Clonic phase Typically the second phase in a generalized or tonic-clonic seizure, characterized by alternating muscular contraction and relaxation.

Closed fracture A bone fracture in which the skin remains intact. Also called a *simple fracture*.

Closed questions Restrictive questions in an interview that require only a "yes" or "no" or short, specific answer.

Club drugs Substances popular among adolescents and young adults who frequent dance clubs and "raves." The most common is MDMA (methylenedioxymethamphetamine), better known as ecstasy.

Coaching The process that encourages the development of individuals through personal interaction within an organization.

Coanalgesics Drugs that have analgesic properties, potentiate the effects of pain medications, relieve other discomforts, or reduce the side effects of analgesic drugs. Coanalgesics are especially effective at reducing neuropathic pain.

Coarctation of the aorta Narrowing or constriction in the descending aorta, often near the ductus arteriosus or left subclavian artery, which obstructs the systemic blood outflow.

Cobb angle A technique to estimate the degree of curvature of the spine using lines drawn from the vertebrae at the upper and lower limits of the curve that tilt most dramatically toward the apex of the curve.

Cocaine A powerful stimulant of natural origin that acts at the nerve terminals to prevent the reuptake of dopamine and norepinephrine, which in turn results in vasoconstriction, tachycardia, and hypertension.

Code of ethics A general guide for a profession's membership and a social contract with the public that it serves.

Codependence A cluster of maladaptive behaviors exhibited by significant others of a substance-abusing individual that serves to enable and protect the abuse at the expense of living a full and satisfying life.

Cognition The complex set of mental activities through which individuals acquire, process, store, retrieve, and apply information.

Cognitive appraisal The process of appraising, sorting, assessing, categorizing, evaluating, and framing the significance of an event or stressor with respect to an individual's own well-being.

Cognitive behavioral therapy (CBT) The use of cognitive techniques and behavior modification to change detrimental beliefs and thought patterns.

Cognitive development The manner in which people learn to think, reason, and use language.

Cognitive domain The learning domain that includes the six intellectual abilities and thinking processes: knowing, comprehending, applying, analysis, synthesis, and evaluation. Also called the *thinking domain*.

Cognitive skills Intellectual skills or thought processes that include problem solving, decision making, critical thinking, and creativity.

Cognitive theory A learning theory that recognizes the developmental level of learners and acknowledges the learner's motivation and environment. Also called *cognitivism*.

Coitus interruptus A method of contraception in which the male withdraws from the female's vagina when he feels that ejaculation is impending.

Cold zone When a disaster occurs, this zone, located outside the warm zone, is where decontaminated victims are triaged and treated. Also called the *green zone* or the *support zone*.

Colectomy Surgical resection and removal of the colon.

Collaboration Two or more people working toward a common goal.

Collaborative intervention The actions a nurse carries out in collaboration with other healthcare team members, such as physical therapists, social workers, dietitians, and physicians.

Collagen A whitish protein substance that adds tensile strength to a wound.

Collateral channels Small blood vessels that develop to connect small arteries. Also called *collateral circulation.*

Colloid osmotic pressure A pulling force exerted by colloids that helps maintain the water content of blood by pulling water from the interstitial space into the vascular compartment. Also called *oncotic pressure.*

Colloids Substances such as large protein molecules that do not readily dissolve into true solutions.

Colon cancer Cancer of the third segment of the large bowel that may or may not include the anus.

Colonization The process by which strains of microorganisms become resident flora, capable of growing and multiplying.

Colorectal cancer Cancer of both the colon and rectum.

Colostomy A surgical opening into the colon.

Colostrum The initial milk that begins to be secreted during mid-pregnancy and that is immediately available to the baby at birth.

Column plan A nursing care plan that uses columns to categorize data for each phase of the nursing process. This type of care plan may include four columns: (1) nursing diagnoses, (2) goals/desired outcomes, (3) nursing interventions, and (4) evaluation. Some include only three columns.

Combined oral contraceptives (COCs) A safe, highly effective contraceptive pill combining estrogen and progestin. Also called *birth control pills.*

Comfort To ease the grief or trouble of others; to give hope.

Commitment The state or an instance of being obligated or emotionally impelled.

Communicable disease An illness that is transmitted directly from one person or animal to another by contact with body fluids, or that is indirectly transmitted by contact with contaminated objects or vectors.

Communication The exchange of information, feelings, thoughts, and ideals through verbal or other techniques.

Communication deviance Communication patterns that are distracting and confusing to listeners who are trying to share a common focus or meaning with a speaker. Communication deviance has been identified as a social-environmental trigger for schizophrenia symptoms.

Communicator style The manner in which an individual communicates; includes the way the individual interacts with others.

Community-based care Care that focuses on the political, social, institutional, and physical environments of the client.

Community Emergency Response Team (CERT) program A Federal Emergency Management Agency–organized program that prepares participants to safely assist themselves, their families, and their neighbors in case of a diaster.

Comorbidity The presence of two or more disease processes.

Compartment syndrome A condition in which the tissue pressure in a muscle compartment exceeds the microvascular pressure, interrupting cellular perfusion.

Compassion An awareness of and concern for other individuals' suffering.

Competence Possessing the knowledge and skills necessary to perform one's job appropriately and safely.

Complementary therapies Any of the diverse array of practices, therapies, and supplements that are not considered part of conventional or traditional medicine that are used in addition to conventional treatments.

Complete spinal cord injury An injury that involves a total loss of all sensory and motor function below the level of the injury; usually the damage is irreversible.

Compliance 1. The relationship between the volume of the intracranial components and intracranial pressure. 2. The amount of distention or expansion the ventricles can achieve to increase stroke volume. 3. The extent to which an individual's behavior coincides with medical or health advice.

Complicated grief A form of grief in which the individual's strategies to cope with a loss are maladaptive. Also called *prolonged grief disorder (PGD).*

Compression A condition that occurs when a vertical force is applied to the spinal column, such as occurs by falling and landing on the feet or buttocks or diving into shallow water.

Compromised host An individual who is at increased risk of infection.

Compulsion A repetitive behavior or mental activity used in response to obsessive thoughts that helps the individual lower his or her anxiety level.

Compulsivity One of the six trait domains associated with personality disorders that is distinguished by extreme inflexibility in a quest for perfection, both in relation to the individual's own actions and others' behaviors.

Computer vision syndrome The most common sequela of computer use. Symptoms include eye fatigue, headaches, blurred vision, dry eyes, and changes in color perception. Also called *eye strain.*

Concept map A visual representation of a nursing plan of care in a patterned diagram with data and ideas. Various shapes and colors are used to show relationships and connections in combination with lines or arrows.

Concrete thinking A type of thinking characterized by a focus on facts and details coupled with an inability to generalize or think abstractly.

Concurrent audit An evaluation of the adequacy of the nursing care a client is receiving and a determination of whether desired outcomes are being met while the individual is still undergoing care at the healthcare facility.

Condom A sheath of synthetic material that covers the penis to prevent conception or disease.

Conduction The process of heat transfer through physical contact of one surface with another surface.

Confabulation Making up information to fill memory gaps; used as a defensive mechanism to protect the person's attempt to protect self-esteem when confronted with memory loss.

Confidentiality The assurance the client has that private information will not be disclosed without the client's consent.

Conflict A situation that occurs when an agreement cannot be reached with regard to significant issues and concerns or when emotional opposition creates discord within an individual or among individuals, groups, or organizations.

Confusion An alteration in cognition that makes it difficult to think clearly, focus attention, or make decisions.

Confusion assessment method (CAM) A two-part test that differentiates between delirium and dementia. It is specifically designed to account for and control ageism.

Congenital cataracts A type of cataract that may appear in a child at birth or in childhood, usually in both eyes.

Congenital heart defect A defect of the heart or great vessels that is present at birth.

Congruent communication Communication in which the verbal and nonverbal aspects of the message match.

Conjugate vera The true conjugate, which extends from the middle of the sacral promontory to the middle of the pubic crest.

Conjunctiva The thin, transparent membrane that covers the anterior surface of the eye and lines the inner surfaces of the eyelids.

Conjunctivitis Inflammation of the conjunctiva. The most common eye disease, conjunctivitis is usually caused by a bacterial or viral infection.

Connective tissue Tissue made of fiber that forms the framework for support of the body's tissue and organs.

Consciousness A condition in which the individual is aware of self and environment and is able to respond appropriately to stimuli. Full consciousness requires both normal arousal and full cognition.

Consequence-based (teleological) theories Theories that look to the outcomes (consequences) of an action in judging whether that action is right or wrong.

Conservation The concept that matter is not changed when its form is altered.

Consolidation Solidification of damaged cells and tissue during immune response to inflammation, specifically in the lungs.

Constant fever A condition that occurs when the body temperature fluctuates minimally but always remains above normal.

Constipation Fewer than three bowel movements per week or the difficult passage of stools.

Constructivism A collection of theories with the common thread of individuals actively constructing knowledge in order to solve realistic problems, often in collaboration with others.

Consumer An individual, a group of people, or a community that uses a service or commodity.

Consumer-driven healthcare plan (CDHP) A type of employer-sponsored coverage that combines a private insurance plan with a Health Savings Account (HSA) or Health Reimbursement Account (HRA).

Contact dermatitis An inflammation of the skin that occurs in response to direct contact with an allergen or irritant.

Contact precautions Used for clients who are known to have or suspected of having serious illnesses that are easily transmitted by direct contact with the client or by contact with items in the environment, such as *shigella*.

Contingency contracts A reinforcement process. Contingency contracts operate by "if–then" rules. If the client performs a targeted response, such as abstinence from the addictive behavior (gambling, drug use, cutting, etc.), then the client receives desired reinforcers.

Contingency planning The process of identifying and managing unplanned and unexpected events that interfere with getting work done efficiently, effectively, and timely.

Continuance commitment The awareness of costs associated with leaving a profession that inhibit an individual from leaving that profession. Considered the weakest type of commitment to a profession.

Continuous bladder irrigation (CBI) A method used to prevent the formation of blood clots.

Continuous positive airway pressure (CPAP) Mechanical ventilation that applies positive pressure to the airways of a client who is breathing spontaneously. Breathing is client triggered and pressure controlled. CPAP is used to help maintain open airways and alveoli, decreasing the work of breathing.

Continuous quality improvement (CQI) A structured organizational process for involving personnel in planning and executing a continuous flow of improvements to provide quality health care that meets or exceeds expectations.

Continuous renal replacement therapy (CRRT) A form of dialysis in which blood is continuously circulated through a highly porous hemofilter from artery to vein or vein to vein.

Contractility The inherent capability of the cardiac muscle fibers to shorten.

Contraction stress test (CST) A method of evaluating the respiratory function (oxygen and carbon dioxide exchange) of a placenta.

Contracture Permanent shortening of connective tissue.

Contralateral deficit Loss or impairment of sensorimotor functions on the side of the body opposite the side of the brain that is damaged by stroke.

Controlled Substance Act (CSA) A federal law that requires drugs to be classified based on the substance's medical use, potential for abuse, and safety risks.

Controlling The managerial process of comparing actual results with projected results, similar to the evaluation step in the nursing process. Controlling includes establishing performance standards, determining how to measure performance and creating the tools that will permit consistent measurement, evaluating performance, and providing feedback.

Convection The process of heat transfer through the fluid motion of air or water across the skin.

Convergence The medial rotation of the eyeballs so that each is directed toward the viewed object.

Co-occurring disorders Concurrent diagnosis of a substance use disorder and a psychiatric disorder. One disorder can precede and cause the other, such as the theorized relationship between alcoholism and depression.

Cooperative play The stage of play in which children work together to contribute to a unified whole, such as forming a sports team or dancing in an ensemble.

Copayment The set payment owed by an insured individual at the time a covered service is rendered.

Coping A dynamic process through which an individual applies cognitive and behavioral measures to handle internal and external demands that are perceived by the individual as exceeding available resources.

Cor pulmonale Right-sided heart failure.

Corneal abrasion Disruption of the superficial epithelium of the cornea.

Corneal reflex Closure of eyelids (blinking) due to corneal irritation.

Cornu The elongated portion of the uterus where the fallopian tubes enter.

Coronary artery disease (CAD) The most common type of heart disease, CAD is caused by impaired blood flow to the myocardium.

Coronary circulation A network of vessels that supply the heart muscle.

Corpus The upper triangular portion of the uterus. Also called the *uterine body*.

Corpus luteum A small yellow body that develops within a ruptured ovarian follicle.

Corrective action The steps taken to overcome a job performance problem.

Coryza Inflammation of the mucous membranes lining the nose usually associated with nasal discharge.

Countershock phase The second part of an alarm reaction during which the sympathetic nervous system stimulation triggers the body's defenses.

Couplet Two premature ventricular contractions in a row.

Couvade In some cultures, the male's observance of certain rituals and taboos to signify the transition to fatherhood.

Covert conflict Conflict that is avoided, ignored, or not discussed openly.

Crack A form of freebase cocaine that is made of baking soda, water, and cocaine mixed into a paste and microwaved to form a rock.

Crackles High-pitched popping sounds heard on inspiration due to fluid associated with or resulting from inflammation, or exudates, within the lung fields, or localized atelectasis.

Creatinine clearance A test that uses 24-hour urine and serum creatinine levels to determine the glomerular filtration rate; a sensitive indicator of renal function.

Creativity The ability to find or create a unique solution to a unique problem when traditional interventions are not effective.

Credentialing The formal identification of professionals who meet predetermined standards of professional skill or competence.

Credibility The quality of being truthful, trustworthy, and reliable.

Crepitation A grating or cracking sound.

Crime An act prohibited by statute or by common law principles.

Criminal law The area of law that deals with conduct that is harmful to another individual or to society as a whole and that may be punishable by fines or imprisonment.

Crisis An event or circumstance that overwhelms an individual's inherent ability to resolve, manage, or process the event or circumstance.

Crisis counseling A meeting that focuses on brief solutions, focused interventions, and supportive care during or after a crisis. It also considers the individual's physical vulnerability and degree of emotional stability.

Crisis intervention An emergent approach to care that is intended to assist clients with recognizing a crisis situation, and identifying and implementing an immediate, short-term solution.

Crisis intervention centers Organizations that provide telephone counseling for clients in crisis. Some organizations also provide consultation through e-mail and online chatting.

Critical pathway Expected outcomes and care strategies developed through collaboration by the healthcare team. Also called a *case map*.

Critical thinking All or part of the process of questioning, analysis, synthesis, interpretation, inference, inductive and deductive reasoning, intuition, application, and creativity.

Crohn disease A chronic, relapsing inflammatory bowel disorder affecting the gastrointestinal tract. Also known as *regional enteritis*.

Cross-dressing Occurs when an individual of one gender (typically male) dresses in clothing specific to the opposite gender.

Crowning During birth, the appearance of the newborn's head or presenting fetal part at the vaginal orifice.

Crystalloids Salts that dissolve readily into true solutions.

Cultural deprivation A lack of culturally assistive, supportive, or facilitative acts.

Cultural groups Racial, ethnic, religious, or social groups with specific group behaviors and characteristics that are learned and shared, including language, customs, beliefs, and values.

Cultural humility The recognition that a healthcare provider's personal cultural values are not superior over the cultural values of others, thus preventing an abuse of power.

Cultural values Preferred ways of behaving or thinking that are sustained over time and used to govern a cultural group's actions and decisions.

Culture The patterns of behavior and thinking that people living in social groups learn, develop, and share.

Cultures Laboratory cultivations used to identify probable microorganisms by their characteristics, such as shape, growth patterns, and Gram-staining qualities.

Curling ulcers Acute ulcerations of the stomach or duodenum that form following a burn injury.

Cyanosis Gray to blue or purple skin color caused by deoxygenated hemoglobin.

Cycle of violence Violence that occurs with a patterned frequency, usually in three phases: initial tension due to communication failures, an abusive incident, and a honeymoon stage in which the aggressor may show love and affection. Cycle of violence may also refer to violence that spans multiple generations in a family.

Cyclothymic disorder A type of bipolar disorder characterized by chronic, fluctuating mood disturbances involving numerous periods of hypomanic symptoms and numerous periods of depressive symptoms.

Cystitis Inflammation of the urinary bladder.

Cystoscopy Endoscopy of the urinary tract. Also called *catheterization*.

Cytokines Proteins that carry messages for immune system function.

Damages Compensation sufficient to restore the plaintiff to his or her original position, so far as is financially possible.

Dashboard An interface that gathers, organizes, and displays a healthcare facility's key performance indicators in an easy-to-read format, often with charts or graphs.

Dashboard knee Tearing of the posterior cruciate ligament or any knee injury resulting from an individual's knee slamming into the dashboard or back of a seat during a motor vehicle crash.

Database A compilation of all information about a client including the nursing health history, physical assessment, primary care provider's history, physical examination, and test results.

Date rape A term used when dating violence takes the form of rape.

Dating violence A type of intimate partner abuse; this type occurs most often in relationships among youth.

Dawn phenomenon A rise in blood glucose between 4 a.m. and 8 a.m. that is not a response to hypoglycemia.

Dead space Areas of the lung that are ventilated but not perfused.

Death anxiety Worry or fear related to death or dying.

Debridement The process of removing painful or necrotic material, including all loose tissue, wound debris, and dead tissue from a wound.

Decelerations The periodic decreases in fetal heart rate from the normal baseline.

Decerebrate posturing An abnormal posture adopted by an unconscious individual that indicates deteriorating brain function. It is characterized by an extended neck; clenched jaw; arms pronated, extended, and close to the sides; legs extended and feet plantar flexed.

Decibels (dB) Units of loudness.

Declarative memory Memory that is related to people and facts, is consciously accessible, and can be verbally expressed.

Decode The process of relating the message perceived to the receiver's storehouse of knowledge and experience and sorting out the meaning of the message.

Decompensation Loss of effective compensation.

Decorticate posturing An abnormal posture adopted by an unconscious individual that indicates deteriorating brain function. It is characterized by the upper arms kept close to the sides; the elbows, wrists, and fingers flexed; the legs extended and internally rotated; and the feet plantar flexed.

Deductible A set annual cost for healthcare paid by an individual or family participating in a health insurance plan.

Deductive reasoning A "top-down" method of logical thinking that starts with a conclusion and analyzes the situation for valid, significant cues. One of two methods of logical thinking that are used to determine if decisions are reasonable.

Deep brain stimulation (DBS) A procedure in which a neurostimulator is implanted into the individual to send electrical signals to one of three brain regions—the subthalamic nucleus, the globus pallidus, or the thalamus—in order to reduce symptoms of Parkinson disease.

Deep venous thrombosis (DVT) A blood clot that forms along the intimal lining of a large vein, usually in a leg.

Defecation The expulsion of feces from the anus and rectum.

Defense mechanism See Adaptive mechanisms.

Defibrillation An emergency procedure that delivers an electrical shock to stop ventricular fibrillation and return to a rhythm that promotes cardiac output sufficient to sustain life.

Deficiency A term used to describe when intake of a nutrient is less than recommended.

Defining characteristics The cluster of signs and symptoms that indicate the presence of a particular diagnostic label.

Deformation The alteration of the spinal cord and soft tissues caused by abnormal movement.

Dehiscence An unintended separation of wound margins due to incomplete healing.

Dehydration A condition that occurs when a body does not take in as much water as it loses or lacks sufficient reserves to maintain proper function.

Delayed union The delayed healing of bones beyond the expected time period.

Delegate An individual who assumes responsibility for the actual performance of an assigned task or procedure.

Delegation The transfer of responsibility and authority for completing an activity to a qualified individual.

Delegator An individual who assigns a task to another individual to perform, but retains accountability for the outcome.

Delirium An acute cognitive disorder that affects functional independence.

Delirium tremens (DTs) A medical emergency usually occurring 3–5 days following alcohol withdrawal and lasting 2–3 days. Characterized by paranoia, disorientation, delusions, visual hallucinations, elevated vital signs, vomiting, diarrhea, and diaphoresis. Also known as *alcohol withdrawal delirium*.

Delphi technique Data gathering technique that averages comments or ratings off of anonymous interviews and questionnaires.

Delusions False ideas or beliefs not based in reality.

Dementia The progressive, irreversible loss of cognitive function.

Democratic leader A leader who assumes that individuals are internally motivated, are capable of making decisions, and value independence. Democratic leaders typically provide constructive feedback, offer information, make suggestions, and ask questions to gain information or to help group members grow in their ability to make decisions.

Demography The study of population, including statistics about distribution by age and place of residence, mortality, and morbidity.

Demyelination A condition in which cells of the immune system, such as lymphocytes and macrophages, cross the blood–brain barrier and attack and destroy the myelin sheath.

Denominations Groups of members that adhere to the same practices and beliefs.

Dental caries Cavities.

Deoxyribonucleic acid (DNA) One of two types of nucleic acid made by cells, DNA contains the genetic instructions for the development and functioning of human beings.

Dependence A physiological need for a substance that the client cannot control, and which results in withdrawal symptoms if the substance is withheld.

Dependent intervention Activities carried out under a physician's orders or supervision, or according to specified routines or protocols.

Dependent personality disorder (DPD) One of several personality disorders defined in the DSM-5, it is marked by a pervasive, excessive, and unrealistic need to be cared for; fear of separation; lack of self-confidence; an inability to make decisions; and an inability to function independently.

Depersonalization A feeling of strangeness or unreality about the physical self.

Depolarization 1. The rapid inflow of sodium ions, causing an electrical change in which the inside of a cell becomes positive in relation to the outside. **2.** The phase in which the heart contracts as a result of ion channel functions.

Depo-Provera A long-acting progesterone that provides highly effective birth control for 3 months when given as a single injection.

Depression A disorder characterized by a sad or despondent mood or loss of interest in usual activities.

Depressive disorder with peripartum onset See Postpartum depression.

Derealization A feeling of disconnection from an individual's own body or the environment.

Dermatome An area of skin innervated by the cutaneous branch of one spinal nerve.

Dermis The second layer of skin, which is made of a flexible connective tissue. It is richly supplied with blood cells, nerve fibers, and lymphatic vessels, as well as most of the hair follicles, sebaceous glands, and sweat glands.

Desaturated blood Blood that is low in oxygen as a result of oxygenated and deoxygenated blood mixing due to a congenital heart defect.

Desire phase The first phase of the sexual response cycle is the arousal of sexual interest by means of real or symbolic stimuli.

Detachment One of the six trait domains associated with personality disorders that is broken down into withdrawal, intimacy avoidance, anhedonia, and restricted affectivity.

Detrusor muscle The smooth muscle layers of the bladder wall, the detrusor muscle allows the bladder to expand as it fills with urine and contract as it releases urine during voiding.

Development An increase in the complexity and function of skill progression, the individual's capacity and skill to adapt to the environment. Related to growth.

Developmental disability Any of a variety of chronic conditions characterized by mental and/or physical impairment.

Developmental stage A level of achievement for a particular segment of an individual's life.

Developmental task A skill or behavior pattern learned during stages of development.

Device integration Real-time, accurate data is recorded in the client's chart directly from a device (e.g., blood pressure monitor). Device integration allows the nurse to more quickly analyze and interpret that data and make adjustments to the plan of care based on the most current information.

Diabetes mellitus Group of chronic disorders of the endocrine pancreas, all categorized under a broad diagnostic label. The condition is characterized by inappropriate hyperglycemia caused by a relative or absolute deficiency of insulin or by a cellular resistance to the action of insulin. Also called *diabetes*.

Diabetic ketoacidosis (DKA) A form of metabolic acidosis that develops when there is an absolute deficiency of insulin and an increase in the insulin counterregulatory hormones. It may also induced by stress in an individual with type 1 diabetes.

Diabetic nephropathy Disease of the kidneys in clients with diabetes that is characterized by the presence of albumin in the urine, hypertension, edema, and progressive renal insufficiency.

Diabetic neuropathy A disorder of the peripheral nerves and the autonomic nervous system in clients with diabetes, which manifests in one or more of the following: sensory and motor impairment, muscle weakness and pain, cranial nerve disorders, impaired vasomotor function, impaired gastrointestinal function, and impaired genitourinary function.

Diabetic retinopathy The collective name for the changes in the retina that occur in the person with diabetes. The retinal capillary structure undergoes alterations in blood flow, leading to retinal ischemia and a breakdown in the blood retinal barrier.

Diagnosis-related groups (DRGs) A system of price control regulation that classifies client illnesses based on diagnoses and pays hospitals a predetermined sum for each specific diagnosis regardless of the actual cost of services, the length of stay, or the acuity or complexity of the client's illness.

Diagnostic label Standardized NANDA names for nursing diagnoses.

Diagonal conjugate Distance from the lower posterior border of the symphysis pubis to the sacral promontory.

Dialysate Dialysis solution.

Dialysis A process by which fluids and molecules pass through a semipermeable membrane from an area of higher solute concentration to one of lower solute concentration according to the rules of osmosis. Dialysis is used to remove excess fluid and metabolic waste products in renal failure.

Diaphragm A flexible disc that covers the cervix to prevent conception.

Diaphysis The shaft of a bone.

Diarrhea The passage of liquid feces and an increased frequency of defecation.

Diastasis recti abdominis A separation of the abdominal muscle.

Diastole The phase of ventricular relaxation between heartbeats.

Diastolic blood pressure The minimum pressure within the arteries during diastole.

Diathermy Treatment with heat generated by high-frequency electrical currents.

Diet recall Client history of intake over a specified period of time.

Dietary Reference Intakes (DRIs) A standardized, recommended nutrient intake to support a healthy diet often provided by health organizations.

Differentiated practice A system in which each nurse's educational preparation and skill sets are evaluated and used to determine how he or she will be best utilized.

Differentiation A process occurring over many cell cycles that allows cells to specialize in certain tasks.

Diffusion The continual intermingling of molecules in liquids, gases, or solids brought about by the random movement of the molecules.

Digestion The conversion of food by means of its mechanical and chemical breakdown into absorbable substances in the gastrointestinal tract.

Digital rectal examination (DRE) An examination to detect for abnormalities in the rectum that can be detected through palpation.

Dihydrotestosterone (DHT) The androgen that mediates prostatic growth at all ages; formed in the prostate from testosterone.

Dilated cardiomyopathy The most common form of cardiomyopathy, it is characterized by the dilation of the heart chambers and impaired ventricular contraction.

Directing The managerial process of effectively motivating, communicating, and delegating tasks in order to complete an organization's work.

Directive interview A highly structured interview that elicits specific information about health information.

Dirty In medical asepsis, a term used to indicate that microorganisms are likely to be present.

Disaster An event that occurs with little or no warning in which available personnel and emergency services are initially overwhelmed and a serious threat to life, public health, and the environment is posed.

Discharge planning A plan of care that prepares the client for discharge, including training in any necessary health skills.

Discipline A method of teaching children the rules for how to behave in society and what is expected in different circumstances.

Discoid lesions Raised, scaly, circular lesions with an erythematous rim.

Discovery The legal process of obtaining information before a trial.

Discrimination The differential treatment of individuals or groups, based on categories such as race, age, weight, gender, or social class, that occurs when an individual acts on prejudice and denies other people one or more of their fundamental rights.

Discussion An informal oral consideration of a subject by two or more healthcare personnel to identify a problem or establish strategies to resolve a problem.

Disease A detectable alteration in body function resulting from infection by microorganisms that causes a reduction of capacities or a shortening of the normal life span. Also called *pathogenesis*.

Disease surveillance Monitoring patterns of disease occurrence from cases of infections and communicable diseases reported by healthcare workers to state officials.

Diseases of adaptation Stress-related illnesses, such as peptic ulcers and hypertension.

Disenfranchised grief Grief that occurs when an individual is unable to acknowledge a loss to other persons. Also called *ambiguous loss*.

Disinfectants Agents that destroy pathogens other than spores.

Disinhibition One of the six trait domains associated with personality disorders that is noted for the presence of irresponsibility, impulsivity, and risk taking.

Disc Fluid-filled "shock absorber" that holds together and insulates the vertebrae. Also called *spinal disc*.

Discectomy The removal of all or part of the nucleus pulposus of an intervertebral disc.

Dismissal Termination of employment.

Disorganized behavior The inability to start or finish goal-oriented activities to a degree that it interferes with an individual's ability to lead a normal life.

Disorganized thinking Difficulty logically connecting thoughts, leading to garbled speech.

Dissatisfaction problems Issues that arise from unmet sexual needs and expectations.

Disseminated intravascular coagulation (DIC) A disruption of hemostasis characterized by widespread intravascular clotting and bleeding. It may be acute and life threatening, or it may be relatively mild.

Distracted driving The act of driving a motor vehicle while doing any activity that takes attention away from the road. Activities include texting, talking on the phone, eating, drinking, reading a map, talking to passengers, looking at a GPS, and adjusting the radio.

Distress A stress that is associated with inadequacy, insecurity, and loss.

Distributive shock Shock that results from widespread vasodilation and decreased peripheral resistance. Also called *vasogenic shock*.

Diuresis The production and excretion of abnormally large amounts of urine. Also called *polyuria*.

Diuretics Pharmacologic agents that increase urine formation and secretion.

Diversity The unique variations among and between individuals, variations that are informed by genetics and cultural background, but that are refined by experience and personal choice.

Diverticula Saclike projections of mucosa through the muscular layer of the colon.

Documenting The process of making an entry on a client record. Also called *recording* or *charting*.

Domestic partner An unmarried partner of the same or opposite sex.

Do-not-intubate (DNI) order Usually written by the physician for the client who has a terminal illness or is near death, this order is usually based on the wishes of the client and family that no life-saving measures be provided once the client stops breathing.

Do-not-resuscitate (DNR) order Usually written by the physician for the client who has a terminal illness or is near death, this order is usually based on the wishes of the client and family that no cardiopulmonary resuscitation be performed for respiratory or cardiac arrest. Also called a *no-code order*.

Dopamine A brain neurotransmitter that regulates voluntary movement, reward-seeking behavior, memory and learning, attention, sleep, affect, and many other functions.

Dormant Temporarily inactive but not dead.

Double-bind theory The theory that schizophrenia symptoms are partially an expression of contradictory family interactions.

Double depression A term used to describe a situation in which an individual experiences dysthymic disorder in combination with major depressive disorder.

Doula A paid caregiver who has typically received special training and may even be certified in caring for laboring women.

Down syndrome A developmental disorder that occurs when an individual is born with an extra full or partial chromosome. Down syndrome is associated with intellectual disability and a wide variety of physical impairments that can range from mild to severe.

Dramatic play The stage of play in which individuals use props to act out the drama of human life.

Droplet nuclei Residue of evaporated droplets emitted by an infected host; can remain in the air for long periods of time.

Droplet precautions Used for clients who are known to have or suspected of having serious illnesses transmitted by particle droplets larger than 5 microns, such as pertussis or pneumonia.

Dubowitz tool A tool for assessing newborns that includes neuromuscular tone assessments, such as head lag, ventral suspension, and leg recoil.

Dullness A thudlike sound produced by dense tissue such as the liver, spleen, or heart.

Duodenal ulcer A peptic ulcer occurring in the duodenum.

Durable power of attorney A legal document that can delegate the authority to make health, financial, and/or legal decisions on an individual's behalf.

Durable power of attorney for health care A legal designation of another individual, usually a family member, significant other, or close personal friend, to make healthcare decisions on an individual's behalf.

Duration 1. The length of a sound. 2. The length of time from the beginning of a contraction to the completion of that same contraction.

Duty A legally enforceable obligation to conform to a particular standard of conduct that is owed to the client.

Dwarfism Excessively short stature caused by insufficient growth hormone, typically resulting from a genetic abnormality.

Dysfunctional uterine bleeding (DUB) Vaginal bleeding that is usually painless but abnormal in amount, duration, or time of occurrence. Also called *abnormal uterine bleeding.*

Dysmenorrhea Painful menstruation.

Dyspareunia Painful intercourse.

Dysphagia Difficulty swallowing.

Dysplasia A loss of DNA control over differentiation occurring in response to adverse conditions.

Dyspnea Shortness of breath or difficulty breathing that is uncomfortable or painful; or when breathing is insufficient to meet oxygen demand.

Dysrhythmia Abnormal heart rate or rhythm. Also called *arrhythmia.*

Dysthymic disorder A chronic disorder in which periods of depressed mood are interspersed with normal mood. Also called *persistent depressive disorder* or *dysthymia.*

Dystonia Severe muscle spasms, particularly of the back, neck, tongue, and face.

Dysuria Difficult or painful urination.

Early deceleration During birth, a condition that occurs when the fetal head is compressed and cerebral blood flow decreases, causing central vagal stimulation. Usually associated with the onset of uterine contractions.

Eating disorder A set of maladaptive responses to stress or anxiety characterized by obsessions with food and weight, often to the extent that daily functioning is impaired and physical and psychological health are threatened.

Echolalia The compulsive parroting of a word or phrase just spoken by another.

Echopraxia The compulsive imitation of the movements of another.

Eclampsia A major complication of pregnancy characterized by hypertension, albuminuria, oliguria, tonic and clonic convulsions, and coma.

Ecological theory A theory of development that emphasizes the presence of mutual interactions between the individual and all of life's settings.

Ecomap Visual representation of how the family unit interacts with the external community environment, including schools, religious institutions, occupational duties, and recreational pursuits.

Ectopic beats Impulses originating outside normal conduction pathways of the heart that interrupt the normal conduction sequence and may not initiate a normal muscle contraction.

Edema Swelling caused by excess fluid trapped in body tissue.

Effacement The drawing up of the internal os and the cervical canal into the uterine side walls.

Effectiveness In health care, effectiveness is providing services based on scientific knowledge to all who could benefit and refraining from providing services to those not likely to benefit.

Efficiency In health care, efficiency is avoiding waste of equipment, supplies, ideas, and energy.

Ego The realistic part of the individual, the ego balances the gratification demands of the id with the limitations of social and physical circumstances.

Ego defense mechanisms Unconscious psychological processes developed for the purpose of defending the personality. Also called *defense mechanisms.*

Egocentrism Ability to see things only from one's own point of view.

Ego-syntonic The perception that one's behaviors and beliefs are normal and any difficulties with other people are external to themselves.

E-health Electronic information that can be retrieved and transferred online or through a mobile device to improve a person's health or health care.

Ejection fraction The fraction or percentage of the diastolic volume that is ejected from the heart during systole.

Elasticity of the arterial wall An indicator of the health of an artery. A healthy, normal artery feels straight, smooth, soft, and pliable. Older adults often have inelastic arteries that feel twisted (tortuous) and irregular upon palpation.

Elder abuse The intentional physical, emotional, or sexual mistreatment or neglect of an individual 65 years of age or older.

Elderspeak A speech style similar to baby talk, which communicates a message of dependence and incompetence to older adults.

Elective surgery Performed when surgical intervention is the preferred treatment for a condition that is not imminently life threatening (but may ultimately threaten life or well-being) or to improve the client's life.

Electrocardiogram (ECG) A graphic record of the heart's activity.

Electrocardiography A diagnostic test of cardiac function.

Electroconvulsive therapy (ECT) A treatment procedure during which an electric current is passed through the brain. It is useful to clients with severe depression, acute mania, some psychotic conditions, and those who are acutely suicidal.

Electroencephalogram (EEG) Measures and records the brain's electrical activity.

Electrolyte A charged ion capable of conducting electricity.

Electromyogram A diagnostic technique that measures the electrical activity of the muscles at rest and during contraction.

Electronic communication Transmitting information though e-mail, social networking, text messaging, and other electronic means.

Electronic fetal monitoring (EFM) The measurement and tracing of the fetal heart rate (FHR), which allows many characteristics of the FHR to be visually assessed.

Electronic health record (EHR) A health record system that is designed so that multiple clinicians from multiple disciplines (e.g., family practice, nursing, pharmacy, specialists) can all have simultaneous access to the client's health information.

Electronic medical record (EMR) A system focused on diagnosis and treatment. EMRs track information over time (weight, blood pressure, cholesterol readings) and identify when clients are due for routine preventive health maintenance such as vaccines and mammograms.

Elimination The secretion and excretion of body wastes from the kidneys and intestines.

Embolus A particle or aggregate of blood, fat, or pathogens or a bubble of air that obstructs a blood vessel.

Embryo The early stage of development of the young of any organism. In humans the embryonic period is from about 2–8 weeks' gestation and is characterized by cellular differentiation and predominantly hyperplastic growth.

Embryonic membranes The amnion and chorion.

Emergency A sudden, often unforeseen event that threatens health or safety.

Emergency preparedness The act of making plans to prevent, respond to, and recover from emergencies.

Emergency response The implementation of emergency preparedness plans.

Emergency surgery Surgery that is performed immediately to preserve function or the life of the client.

Emigration The movement of leukocytes through the blood vessel wall into affected tissue spaces in response to illness or injury.

Emotion-focused coping The regulation of emotional responses to distress when the stressor is perceived to be beyond the individual's control.

Emotional availability The quality of parent–child interactions, including parental sensitivity, structuring, and degree of intrusiveness and hostility.

Emotions Feeling responses to a wide variety of emotional stimuli.

Emphysema A progressive pulmonary disease characterized by destruction of the walls of the alveoli, with resulting enlargement of abnormal air spaces.

Empirical knowing The twofold understanding of facts and observations relevant to nursing, and of the analyses and theories that attempt to explain them. Also called the *science of nursing*.

Empyema Accumulation of purulent (infected) exudate in a space, for example, the pleural cavity or the gallbladder.

Enabling behavior Any action by an individual that consciously or unconsciously facilitates substance dependence.

Encapsulated Enclosed.

Encoding The selection of specific signs or symbols to transmit a message, such as which language and words to use, how to arrange the words, and what tone of voice and gestures to use.

Encopresis Abnormal elimination pattern characterized by recurrent soiling or passage of stool at inappropriate times.

Enculturation The process by which children learn culture from adults. Also called *cultural transmission*.

End-of-dose medication failure Pain experienced at the end of one dose of medication before the next dose is scheduled.

End of life The final weeks of life when death is imminent.

End-of-life care The nursing care provided to a client who is dying or who is near death.

End-stage renal disease (ESRD) The final stage of chronic kidney disease, when the kidneys are unable to excrete metabolic wastes and regulate fluid and electrolyte balance adequately.

Endocardial cushion defect A combination of defects in the atrial and ventricular septa and portions of the tricuspid and mitral valves. A complete AV canal defect allows blood to travel freely among all four chambers of the heart. Also called *atrioventricular (AV) canal defect*.

Endocardial cushions Fetal growth centers for mitral and tricuspid valves and AV septum.

Endogenous Developing from within.

Endogenous insulin Insulin that is produced by an individual's own body.

Endogenous pyrogens Interleukins, interferons, and tumor necrosis factor released by macrophages in response to an infection.

Endometriosis A condition that occurs when endometrial tissue implants on organs outside the uterus, causing pain, fibrosis, and adhesions.

Endometrium The innermost mucosal layer of the uterus.

Endotoxins Found in the cell wall of gram-negative bacteria, endotoxins are released only when the cell is disrupted. They act as activators of many human regulatory systems, producing fever, inflammation, and potentially clotting, bleeding, or hypotension when released in large quantities.

Engagement The passing of the fetus into the pelvic inlet in preparation for birth.

Engrossment The characteristic sense of absorption, preoccupation, and interest in an infant demonstrated by fathers during early contact.

Enophthalmos Sunken appearance of the eyes.

Enteral nutrition Tube feeding used to meet calorie and protein requirements in clients who are unable to consume enough food on their own.

Entropion Inversion of the eyelid.

Enuresis Involuntary passing of urine in children after bladder control is achieved.

Enzymes Chemicals that induce a chemical reaction in order to assist in the breakdown of nutrients.

Eosinophil A type of leukocyte found in large numbers in the respiratory and gastrointestinal tracts. Eosinophils are thought to be responsible for protecting the body from parasitic worms. They also play a role in the hypersensitivity response by inactivating some of the inflammatory chemicals released during the inflammatory response.

Epidemic Widespread outbreak of infectious disease with many infected people.

Epidermis The surface or outermost part of the skin consisting of four to five layers of epithelial cells.

Epigenetic External factor's effects on internal genetic results.

Epilepsy A chronic disorder characterized by recurrent, unprovoked seizures secondary to a central nervous system disorder.

Epiphyseal plate Cartilage between the epiphysis and diaphysis found in the long bones of children.

Episiotomy A surgical incision of the perineal body to enlarge the outlet.

Epstein's pearls Small, glistening, white specks that feel hard to the touch on the hard palate and gum margins

Erb-Duchenne paralysis Damage affecting the upper arm between the fifth and sixth cervical nerves, causing paralysis. Also called *Erb's palsy*.

Erectile dysfunction (ED) The inability of a male to attain and maintain an erection sufficient to permit satisfactory sexual intercourse.

Ergonomics The science of fitting workplace conditions and job demands to the capabilities of the working population.

Erik Erikson A German-born psychologist and psychoanalyst who created a theory of development comprised of eight stages or age-related tasks faced by an individual throughout the life span.

Erythema A reddening of the skin.

Erythema toxicum An eruption of lesions in the area surrounding a hair follicle that are firm, vary in size from 1 to 3 mm, and consist of a white or pale yellow papule or pustule with an erythematous base. Also called *newborn rash* or *flea bite dermatitis*.

Eschar Hard, leathery crust that covers a burn wound and harbors necrotic tissue.

Escharotomy Surgical removal of eschar from the torso or extremity to prevent circumferential constriction.

Essential nutrients The macro- and micronutrients needed for the body's survival.

Estimated date of birth (EDB) The approximated date of childbirth. Also called *due date*.

Estrogen The primary hormone responsible for female sex characteristics.

Ethical knowing Understanding and applying the ethical codes by which nurses are expected to abide, as well as upholding the various philosophical, cultural, and moral frameworks of the institution and of the client. Also called the *moral component*.

Ethics The rules or principles that govern right or moral conduct.

Ethnic group Group of individuals who have common racial characteristics and share a cultural heritage.

Etiology A causal relationship between a problem and its related or risk factors.

Eupnea Breathing within the expected respiratory rates.

Eustachian tube Connects the middle ear with the nasopharynx to help equalize the pressure in the middle ear with the atmospheric pressure.

Eustress Good stress that is associated with accomplishment and victory.

Euthanasia From the Greek for *painless, easy, gentle,* or *good death*, now commonly used to signify a killing prompted by a humanitarian motive.

Euthyroid A normal thyroid state.

Evaluation statement A written comment on the care plan or in the nurse's notes about progress following an evaluation. An evaluation statement must contain the date and time evaluation was done; a conclusion statement determining goal met, partially met, or not met; and a supporting statement giving the results of how the client did or did not achieve the goal.

Evaporation The process of converting water to a vapor.

Evidence Clinical knowledge, expert opinion, or information resulting from research.

Evidence-based nursing An integration of the best evidence available, nursing expertise, and the values and preferences of the individuals, families, and communities who are served.

Evidence-based practice The application of research in areas that are of interest to nursing and in the actual practice of nursing.

Evisceration Protrusion of internal viscera through a surgical wound.

Exacerbation A reappearance of symptoms of a chronic illness. Also called a *flare*.

Excess More than is needed in order for the body to survive and remain productive.

Excitement phase This second phase of the sexual response cycle is marked by an increase in blood flow to various body parts, resulting in erection of the penis and clitoris and swelling of the labia, testes, and breasts.

Excoriation Area of loss of the superficial layers of the skin. Also called *denuded area*.

Exercise Physical activity that is planned, structured, and involves repetitive body movements; the goal is to improve or maintain one or more components of physical fitness.

Exercise intolerance Decreased ability to participate in activities using large skeletal muscles because of fatigue or dyspnea.

Exogenous Developing from outside sources.

Exogenous insulin Insulin from a source outside the body.

Exophthalmos Protruding eyes.

Exotoxins Soluble proteins that microorganisms secrete into surrounding tissue. Exotoxins are highly poisonous, causing cell death or dysfunction.

Expectorate To expel or spit out.

Expiration The act of exhaling air in respiration.

Expressed consent An oral or written agreement.

Expressive jargon Using unintelligible words with normal speech intonations as if truly communicating in words.

Expressive speech The ability to speak and be understood by others.

Extended family The relatives of nuclear families, such as grandparents, aunts, and uncles.

Extended kin network family A form of extended family in which two nuclear families of primary or unmarried kin live in proximity to each other and share a social support network, goods, and services.

External environmental stressors Triggers outside of an individual that demand change or disrupt homeostasis.

External locus of control The belief that an individual's health is controlled by forces outside of his or her control such as chance or fate.

Extracapsular extraction A surgical treatment for cataracts in which the anterior capsule, nucleus, and cortex of the lens are removed, leaving the posterior capsule intact.

Extracapsular hip fracture A hip fracture involving the trochanteric region between the neck and diaphysis of the femur.

Extracellular fluid (ECF) Fluid found outside the cells. It accounts for about one third of total body fluid and is subdivided into compartments. The two main compartments of ECF are intravascular and interstitial.

Extracorporeal shock wave lithotripsy (ESWL) A noninvasive technique for fragmenting kidney stones using shock waves generated outside the body.

Extrapulmonary tuberculosis Results when tuberculosis spreads through the blood and lymph system to other organs.

Extrapyramidal side effects (EPS) A particularly serious set of adverse reactions to antipsychotic drugs. EPS includes acute dystonia, akathisia, parkinsonism, and tardive dyskinesia.

Extubation The process of withdrawing a breathing tube on completion of anesthesia and the surgical case.

Exudate Material, such as fluid and cells, that has escaped from blood vessels during the inflammatory process and is deposited in tissue or on tissue surfaces.

Exudative macular degeneration A form of macular degeneration characterized by the formation of new, weak blood vessels in the potential space between the choroid and the retina. Also referred to as the wet form of macular degeneration.

Eye movement desensitization and reprocessing (EMDR) A form of psychotherapy that contains elements of a number of types of therapy, including cognitive-behavioral therapy and body-centered therapy.

Failure to thrive (FTT) 1. Inability to meet or maintain developmental milestones related to physical growth due to undernutrition. **2.** A syndrome in which an infant falls below the fifth percentile for weight and height on a standard growth chart or is falling in percentiles on a growth chart.

Faith To believe in or be committed to something or someone.

Fallopian tubes Tubes that extend from the lateral angle of the uterus and terminate near the ovary. Also called *oviducts* and *uterine tubes.*

False imprisonment The unjustifiable detention of an individual without legal warrant to confine the person.

False pelvis The portion of the pelvis above the linea terminalis that supports the enlarged pregnant uterus.

Familial AD (FAD) One of the two basic types of Alzheimer disease, it has a strong inherited component and usually manifests before the age of 65. Also called *early-onset Alzheimer disease.*

Family Individuals who are joined together by marriage, blood, adoption, or residence in the same household.

Family burden The overall level of distress experienced by a family as a result of a family member's illness.

Family-centered care A model of healthcare service that is provided in partnership with the client and family.

Family-centered nursing Nursing that considers the health of the family as a unit in addition to the health of individual family members.

Family cohesion The emotional bonding between family members.

Family communication Includes listening, speaking, self-disclosure, and tracking abilities of the family as a group.

Family coping mechanisms The behaviors families use to deal with stress or changes imposed from either within or without the family.

Family development The dynamics or changes a family experiences over time, including changes in relationships, communication patterns, roles, and interactions.

Family flexibility The amount of change in a family's leadership, role relationships, relationship rules, and ability to respond to stress.

Family recovery Family response to a member's mental illness.

Family support Support from family members as they care for other family members; for example, one sister relieves another to care for their aging mother over the weekend.

Family therapy A form of therapy in which the family system is treated as a unit and the focus is on family dynamics.

Fascial excision Excising a wound to the level of fascia. Also called *fasciectomy.*

Fasciculation An irregular movement or a twitch.

Fasciectomy Excising a wound to the level of fascia. Also called *fascial excision.*

Fat embolism syndrome (FES) Occurs when fat globules lodge in the pulmonary vascular bed or peripheral circulation.

Fatigue A condition characterized by a lack of energy and motivation that may or may not be accompanied by drowsiness.

Fear A sense of apprehension triggered by a perceived threat to safety or well-being, including a painful stimuli or dangerous event.

Febrile Having a fever.

Febrile seizures Generalized seizures that usually occur in children as the result of rapid temperature rise above 39°C (102°F), usually in association with an acute illness. No evidence of intracranial infection or other defined cause is found in relation.

Fecal impaction A mass or collection of hardened feces in the folds of the rectum.

Fecal incontinence The loss of voluntary ability to control fecal and gaseous discharges through the anal sphincter. Also called *bowel incontinence.*

Fecalith A hard mass of feces.

Feces Body wastes and undigested food eliminated from the bowel. Also called *stool.*

Feedback 1. The mechanisms by which some of the output of a system is returned to the system as input. **2.** The response a receiver of a message gives to the message's sender.

Female orgasmic disorder A sexual arousal cycle that stops before orgasm.

Female reproductive cycle (FRC) The monthly rhythmic changes in sexually mature women; composed of the ovarian cycle, during which ovulation occurs, and the uterine cycle, during which menstruation occurs.

Female sexual arousal disorder Discomfort or pain during sexual intercourse caused by a lack of vaginal lubrication.

Fertility awareness-based methods Contraception based on an understanding of the changes that occur throughout a woman's ovulatory cycle. Also called *natural family planning.*

Fertilization The process by which a sperm fuses with an ovum to form a new diploid cell, or zygote.

Festination Rapid, small steps, as if an individual is trying to run.

Fetal alcohol spectrum disorder See Fetal alcohol syndrome (FAS).

Fetal alcohol syndrome (FAS) A developmental disorder that occurs when a developing fetus is exposed to ethyl alcohol. Fetal alcohol syndrome is associated with physical, intellectual, behavioral, and/or learning disabilities. Also called *fetal alcohol spectrum disorder.*

Fetal attitude The flexion or extension of the fetal body and extremities.

Fetal bradycardia A fetal heart rate of less than 110 bpm during a 10-minute period or longer.

Fetal demise Death of a fetus that occurs after 20 weeks' gestation. Also called a *stillbirth* or *intrauterine fetal death (IUFD).*

Fetal heart rate (FHR) The number of times the fetal heart beats per minute; normal range is 120–160.

Fetal lie The relationship of the cephalocaudal axis, or spinal column, of the fetus to the cephalocaudal axis, or spinal column, of the woman. The fetus may be in a longitudinal or transverse lie.

Fetal movement record A noninvasive technique that enables the pregnant woman to monitor and record movements easily and without expense.

Fetal position The relationship of the landmark on the presenting fetal part to the front, sides, or back of the maternal pelvis.

Fetal presentation The body part of the fetus entering the pelvis in a single or multiple pregnancy.

Fetal tachycardia A fetal heart rate of 161 bpm or more during a 10-minute period of continuous monitoring.

Fetoscope An adaptation of a stethoscope that facilitates auscultation of the fetal heart rate.

Fetoscopy A technique for directly observing the fetus and obtaining a sample of fetal blood or skin.

Fetus The child in utero from about the seventh to ninth week of gestation until birth.

Fever A protective immune response to foreign antigens within the body that increases the cellular metabolic rate, thus increasing the body's temperature.

Fever phobia Fear felt by caregivers about the harmful effects of a fever on a child, such as seizure, brain damage, and death.

Fever spike A temperature that rises to fever level rapidly, following a normal temperature, and then returns to normal within a few hours.

Fiber A polysaccharide that contributes to disease prevention, especially in the gastrointestinal tract and the cardiovascular system.

Fibrin Connective tissue.

Fibrin degradation products Potent anticoagulants.

Fibromyalgia A chronic disorder characterized by widespread musculoskeletal pain, fatigue, and multiple tender points.

Fidelity A moral principle that obligates an individual to be faithful to agreements and responsibilities one has undertaken.

Filtration A process whereby fluid and solutes move together across a membrane from a compartment with higher pressure to a compartment with lower pressure.

Filtration pressure The pressure in the compartment that results in the movement of the fluid and substances dissolved in fluid out of the compartment.

Fimbria A funnel-like enlargement of the fallopian tube with many fingerlike projections (fimbriae) reaching out to the ovary.

First heart sound (S_1) The heart sound produced by the closure of the AV valve; characterized by the syllable "lub."

Five P's neurovascular assessment An assessment checklist for pain, pulse, pallor, paralysis/paresis, and paresthesia.

Fixation The immobilization or inability of an individual to proceed to the next developmental stage because of anxiety.

Flaccidity Absence of muscle tone. Also called *hypotonia.*

Flashbacks The recurrence of images, sounds, smells, or feelings from a traumatic event; often triggered by daily events, such as a car backfiring on the street or the smell of a perpetrator's cologne.

Flat affect Minimal facial expression and movement, sometimes monotone speech patterns.

Flatness An extremely dull sound produced by very dense tissue, such as muscle or bone.

Flatulence The presence of excessive amounts of gas in the stomach or intestines.

Flatus Gas or air normally present in the stomach or intestines.

Flight of ideas Rapidly changing, fragmentary thoughts.

Flow sheet A specific assessment criteria in a particular format, such as human needs or functional health patterns.

Fluid resuscitation The administration of intravenous (IV) fluids to restore circulating blood volume during an acute period of increasing capillary permeability.

Fluid volume deficit (FVD) Substantial loss of both water and electrolytes in similar proportions from the extracellular fluid. Also called *hypovolemia.*

Fluid volume excess (FVE) Excessive fluid retained by the body. The retention of both water and sodium in similar proportions to normal extracellular fluid (ECF). Also called *hypervolemia.*

Fluoroscope A scope used to project visual examination images on a fluorescent screen.

Focal seizures Seizures that are caused by abnormal electrical activity in one hemisphere or in a specific area of the cerebral cortex, most often the temporal, frontal, or parietal lobes. The seizure may spread regionally, and the symptoms are related to the region of the cortex that is affected. Also known as *partial seizures.*

Focus charting Date and time, focus, and progress notes are recorded for a specific condition, nursing diagnosis, and behavior to make the client and the client's concerns and strengths the focus of care.

Folic acid A vitamin that is required for normal growth, reproduction, and lactation and that prevents the macrocytic, megaloblastic anemia of pregnancy.

Follicle-stimulating hormone (FSH) Hormone produced by the anterior pituitary during the first half of the menstrual cycle, stimulating development of the graafian follicle.

Fontanelles The intersections of membranous spaces between the cranial bones of a fetus.

Food choice An individual's decision of what and how much to eat of a specific food. This decision can be influenced by a number of conscious and unconscious factors such as taste, preparation, smell, habits, convenience, availability, and cost.

Food insecurity Results when one or more members of a household must reduce their eating patterns due to a lack of money or lack of resources to access appropriate amounts and varieties of food.

Food security Results when all members of a household have sufficient resources to access appropriate amounts and varieties of food.

Foramen ovale An opening between the atria of the fetal heart.

Foraminotomy An enlargement of the opening between the disc and the facet joint to remove bony overgrowth.

Forced expiratory volume in 1 second (FEV1) The amount of air that can be exhaled in 1 second as measured by a spirometer.

Forceps-assisted birth The use of forceps to assist the birth of a fetus by providing traction or by providing the means to rotate the fetal head to an occiput-anterior position. Also called an *instrumental delivery*, *operative delivery*, or *operative vaginal delivery*.

Forceps marks Reddened areas over the cheeks and jaws on an infant caused by a difficult forceps birth.

Foreground question Questions that are narrow in focus about a specific clinical issue.

Foreseeability The ability to foresee events that reasonably may be expected to cause specific results.

Formal group A group with formalized goals, designated management, and only partly voluntary membership.

Formal leader A leader who is selected by an organization and given official authority to make decisions and act.

Formation The process that facilitates the transformation of an individual from a layperson to a professional nurse.

Foster family A family consisting of one or more adults caring for one or more children from other families when the children can no longer live with their birth parents.

Fourth heart sound (S4) A heart sound produced by atrial contraction and ejection of blood into the ventricle during late diastole. Also called *atrial gallop*.

Fracture A break in the continuity of a bone.

Fragile X syndrome A developmental disorder caused by a single recessive gene abnormality on the X chromosome. Fragile X syndrome is associated most notably with intellectual disability, often accompanied by ADHD and other behavioral problems.

Frank–Starling mechanism An increase in venous return increases ventricular filling and myocardial stretch, which increases the force of contraction.

Free-floating anxiety Excessive worry about everyday events; worry that is hard to control and the focus of which may shift from moment to moment.

Freezing A condition in which an individual feels like his or her feet are stuck to the floor.

Frequency The time between the beginning of one contraction and the beginning of the next contraction.

Friend support Support or assistance from nonfamily members, such as friends or coworkers, for a family during a time of illness or stress.

Frostbite An injury of the skin resulting from freezing.

Frustration An emotion that occurs when an individual is prevented from reaching a desired goal. Intense frustration may trigger violent aggressive tendencies resulting in assault or homicide.

Fulguration A procedure that destroys tissue with electrical current.

Full-thickness burn A burn that involves all layers of the skin, including the epidermis, the dermis, and the epidermal appendages.

Fulminant colitis An acute form of ulcerative colitis that involves the entire colon; manifestations include severe bloody diarrhea, acute abdominal pain, and fever.

Functional assessments Typically a combination of assessments that includes observations of child behavior, responses, and abilities. It is used to assess how a child functions on a daily basis in his or her environment and to determine if the child has any developmental delays or special needs.

Functional nursing A task-oriented approach to care delivery used in situations of inadequate staffing or nursing shortages.

Functional strength The body's ability to perform work.

Fundus The rounded, uppermost portion of the uterus.

Fungi A type of microorganism capable of producing infection. Yeasts and molds are common types of fungi.

Galanin A neuropeptide that is released by neurons as they are injured or die. Often associated with Alzheimer disease, although the exact role galanin plays in the disease is unknown.

Gallstone ileus A large gallstone.

Gamete Female or male germ cell; contains a haploid number of chromosomes.

Gametogenesis The process by which germ cells are produced.

Gastric lavage Irrigation of the stomach with large quantities of normal saline.

Gastric outlet obstruction Obstruction of the pyloric region of the stomach and duodenum that impairs gastric outflow; a potential complication of peptic ulcer disease.

Gastric ulcer A peptic ulcer that occurs in the stomach.

Gastrocolic reflex The increased peristalsis of the colon after food has entered the stomach.

Gastroesophageal reflux disease (GERD) A disease in which stomach contents flow back up into the esophagus.

Gate control theory Melzack and Wall's 1965 theory that states the perception of pain is controlled by the overall activity of small-diameter (pain) fibers vs. large-diameter (heat, cold, mechanical) fibers.

Gender identity One's self-image as a female or male.

Gender-role behavior The outward expression of an individual's sense of maleness or femaleness as well as the expression of what is perceived as gender-appropriate behavior.

General adaptation syndrome (GAS) A three-stage chain of events in an individual's stress response.

Generalized anxiety disorder (GAD) A condition that occurs when an individual experiences intense tension and worry, even if no external stressors are present.

Generalized seizures The result of diffuse electrical activity that often begins in both hemispheres of the brain simultaneously, then spreads throughout the cortex into the brainstem. As a result, movements and spasms displayed by the client are bilateral and symmetric.

Generational cohort Individuals born in the same general time span who share key life experiences, including historical events, public heroes, pastimes, and early work experiences.

Genital herpes A sexually transmitted infection caused by the herpes simplex virus.

Genital intercourse Penetration of the vagina by the penis. Also called *coitus*.

Genital warts A sexually transmitted infection caused by the human papillomavirus (HPV).

Genogram Visual representation of gender showing lines of birth descent through the generations.

Genotype The pattern of genes on chromosomes.

Geographic information system (GIS) A system that relies on satellite imaging and global positioning systems to capture, manage, and analyze geographical data.

Geragogy The process of stimulating and helping older adults to learn.

Geriatric failure to thrive (GFTT) A condition in which older clients experience a multidimensional decline in physical functioning that is characterized by weight loss of more than 5% of baseline body weight, decreased appetite, undernutrition, dehydration, depression, and cognitive and immune impairment.

Gestation Period of intrauterine development from conception through birth; pregnancy.

Gestational age assessment tools Methods to determine an infant's age at birth assessing external physical characteristics and neurological or neuromuscular development.

Gingiva The gum.

Gingivitis Red, swollen gingiva.

Glaucoma A condition characterized by optic neuropathy with gradual loss of peripheral vision and, usually, increased intraocular pressure of the eye.

Global evaluative dimension of the self The degree to which an individual likes him- or herself overall, as a whole being. Also called *global self-esteem*.

Global self The collective beliefs and images an individual holds about him- or herself.

Global self-esteem See Global evaluative dimension of the self.

Glomerular filtration rate (GFR) The rate at which fluid is filtered through the kidneys.

Glomerulonephritis Inflammation of the glomerular capillary membrane.

Glomerulus Found in the nephrons of the kidneys, a tuft of capillaries surrounded by the Bowman capsule.

Glucagon A hormone that stimulates the breakdown of glycogen in the liver, the formation of carbohydrates in the liver, and the breakdown of lipids in both the liver and adipose tissue.

Gluconeogenesis The formation of glucose from fats and proteins.

Glucosuria The excretion of glucose in the urine.

Glycogenolysis The breakdown of liver glycogen.

Glycosuria The excretion of carbohydrates into the urine.

Goiter An enlarged thyroid gland

Gonadotropin-releasing hormone (GnRH) A hormone secreted by the hypothalamus that stimulates the anterior pituitary to secrete follicle-stimulating hormone and luteinizing hormone.

Gonorrhea A sexually transmitted infection caused by *Neisseria gonorrhoeae*.

Good Samaritan laws Specific laws designed to protect healthcare workers from potential liability when volunteering their skills outside of an employment contract.

Goodpasture syndrome A rare autoimmune disorder of unknown etiology that is characterized by formation of antibodies to the glomerular basement membrane.

Governance The establishment and maintenance of social, political, and economic arrangements by which professionals control their practice, their self-discipline, their working conditions, and their professional affairs.

Graafian follicle The ovarian cyst containing the ripe ovum, which secretes estrogens.

Grading A standardized method of judging a tumor's aggressiveness based on the level of differentiation and mitotic rate; where the least malignant cells are classified grade 1 and the most aggressive malignant cells are classified grade 4.

Graft-versus-host disease (GVHD) A series of immunological reactions in response to transplanted cells.

Gram stain A diagnostic test conducted to identify infecting organisms in urine by shape and characteristic.

Granulation tissue Young connective tissue with new capillaries formed in the healing process.

Grasping reflex The closing and grasping of an infant's fingers in response to a finger placed in the palm of the infant's hand.

Graves disease An autoimmune disorder marked by an enlarged thyroid and signs of hyperthyroidism.

Grief The total psychological, biological, and behavioral response to the emotional experience related to loss.

Group Three or more individuals who have a common purpose, interact with each other, influence each other, and are interdependent.

Group therapy A form of therapy that allows group members to help each other with psychological, cognitive, behavioral, and spiritual dysfunctions through a process of change, aided by a professional group therapist.

Groupthink A type of decision making characterized by a group's failure to critically examine their own processes and practices or to recognize and respond to change.

Growth Physical change and increase in size.

Guillain-Barré syndrome (GBS) An acute inflammatory demyelinating disorder of the peripheral nervous system characterized by an acute onset of motor paralysis (usually ascending).

Gustatory Of or relating to taste.

Gynecomastia Abnormal enlargement of the breast(s) in men.

H_1 receptors Cellular histamine receptors that are present in the smooth muscle of the vascular system, the bronchial tree, and the digestive tract. Stimulation of these receptors results in itching, pain, edema, bronchoconstriction, and other characteristic symptoms of inflammation and allergy.

H1N1 influenza A form of the influenza virus that consists of avian genes, human genes, and genes from flu viruses typically found in pigs from Asia and Europe. Once mistakenly called *swine flu*, it can be spread through human-to-human transmission.

H_2 receptors Cellular histamine receptors present primarily in the stomach; their stimulation results in the secretion of large amounts of hydrochloric acid.

Habit training Attempts to keep clients dry by having them void at regular intervals.

Habituation The newborn's ability to process and respond to complex stimulations.

Hallucination The perception of seeing, hearing, or feeling something that is not present in reality.

Hallucinogen A type of drug that induces the same types of thoughts, perceptions, and feelings that occur in dreams. Hallucinogens include PCP, 3,4-MDMA, D-lysergic acid diethylamide (LSD), mescaline, dimethyltryptamine (DMT), and psilocin.

Hand restraints A device used to protect confused clients from scratching or injuring their skin, or dislodging intravenous access devices. Also called *mitt restraints.*

Handoff The transfer of information along with authority and responsibility during transitions in care across the continuum.

Handoff communication A verbal or written exchange of information. It encompasses the nursing team and all other members of the healthcare team who care for a client at any given time.

Hardware The physical component of technology, including computers, keyboards, and display screens.

Harlequin sign A reddening of the skin on one side of an infant's body while the other side remains pale. Also called *clown color change.*

Hashimoto thyroiditis An autoimmune disorder in which antibodies destroy thyroid tissue.

Hassles Day-to-day tension/stressors.

Health A state of complete physical, mental, and social well-being.

Health beliefs Concepts about health that an individual believes are true, regardless of whether or not they are founded in fact.

Health Insurance Portability and Accountability Act (HIPAA) Legislation enacted by Congress to minimize the exclusion of preexisting conditions as a barrier to healthcare insurance, designate special rights for those who lose other health coverage, and eliminate medical underwriting in group plans. The act includes the Privacy Rule, which creates a national standard for of the disclosure of private health information.

Health Level Seven (HL7) A framework designed for the exchange, integration, sharing, and retrieval of electronic health information that supports clinical practice and the management, delivery, and evaluation of health services.

Health literacy The ability to read, understand, and act on health information, including such tasks as comprehending prescription labels, interpreting appointment slips, completing health insurance forms, and following instructions for diagnostic tests.

Health maintenance organization (HMO) The most restrictive type of private health insurance plan. HMO participants must select a primary care provider who provides basic medical services and, as the gatekeeper to care, refers the client to in-network hospitals and specialists when additional care is needed.

Health policy The actions and decisions by government bodies and professional organizations that affect whether or not healthcare organizations and individuals working within the healthcare system can achieve their healthcare goals.

Health promotion A way of thinking and acting in order to increase individuals' overall health and well-being regardless of their health and illness status or age.

Health restoration Care focusing on the ill client that extends from early detection of disease through helping the client during the recovery period.

Healthcare advance directive Legal document that allows an individual to plan for healthcare and/or financial affairs in the event of incapacity. Also called *advance directive* or *advance healthcare directive.*

Healthcare-associated infection (HAI) Infections associated with the delivery of healthcare services in a facility such as a hospital or nursing home. Also called a *nosocomial infection.*

Healthcare disparity A difference in a measurement of access to or quality of healthcare services between an individual or group possessing a defined characteristic when other variables have been controlled, such as individual health choices, disease courses, and other variations from the normative measure.

Healthcare proxy An individual selected to speak to physicians and other healthcare providers on behalf of a client to determine the best course of treatment.

Healthcare surrogate An individual selected to make medical decisions when someone is no longer able to make them for him- or herself.

Heart block A block in the normal electrical conduction of the heart.

Heart failure The inability of the heart to pump adequate blood to meet the metabolic demands of the body.

Heart murmur Harsh, blowing sounds caused by disruption of blood flow into the heart, between the chambers of the heart, or from the heart into the pulmonary or aortic systems.

Heartburn A burning sensation in the chest or throat. Also called *pyrosis.*

Heat balance When the amount of heat produced by the body equals the amount of heat lost.

Heat exhaustion Excessive heat exposure and dehydration that causes paleness, dizziness, nausea, vomiting, fainting, and a moderately increased temperature (38.3°–38.9°C [101°–102°F]).

Heat stroke A serious form of heat exhaustion that can be life threatening, generally caused by exercising in hot weather. Clients will have warm, flushed skin, often do not sweat, and have a temperature of 41°C (106°F) or higher. A client may be also delirious, unconscious, or having seizures.

Heat transfer The four ways heat moves from one place or object to another place or object.

Heaving Lifting of the chest wall during contraction.

Heberden nodes Bony lumps on the end joint of a digit.

Helper T cells Play a vital role in normal immune system function, recognizing foreign antigens and infected cells and activating antibody-producing B cells. They are the primary cells infected by the human immunodeficiency virus.

HELPP syndrome A cluster of changes including hemolysis, elevated liver enzymes, and low platelet count, sometimes associated with preeclampsia.

Hematochezia Bright blood in the stool.

Hematocrit The proportion of cells and plasma in blood. Also refers to the laboratory test that measures the hematocrit. This test can also be used to detect severe dehydration or overhydration.

Hematogenous spread Describes the spread of infection or disease through the blood.

Hematoma A localized collection of blood underneath the skin that may appear as a bruise.

Hematopoiesis Blood cell formation.

Hematuria The presence of blood in the urine.

Hemianopia The loss of half of the visual field of one or both eyes.

Hemiarthroplasty Hip replacement that involves replacement of the ball, the head, or the femur.

Hemiarthroscopy The surgical replacement of the femoral head with a smooth metal sphere.

Hemiparesis Weakness of the left or right half of the body.

Hemiplegia Paralysis of the left or right half of the body.

Hemispheres The two halves created by the division of the cerebrum by the deep fold.

Hemodialysis A process by which a client's blood flows through vascular catheters, passes by the dialysate in an external machine, and then returns to the client.

Hemodynamics The study of forces involved in blood circulation.

Hemoglobin The oxygen-carrying molecule within red blood cells; a laboratory test to measure the amount of hemoglobin.

Hemoglobinopathy A disorder of hemoglobin.

Hemolysis The destruction of red blood cells; releases hemoglobin into the circulation.

Hemolytic anemia A disorder that results from the premature destruction of red blood cells.

Hemoptysis Bloody sputum.

Hemorrhage Rapid or excessive bleeding.

Hemosiderosis The storage of excessive iron in tissues and organs.

Hemostasis The cessation of bleeding.

Hemotympanum Bleeding into or behind the tympanic membrane.

Hepatitis The inflammation of the liver triggered by a virus, alcohol, medications, toxins, autoimmune disorder, or other pathogens.

Here-and-now concept A concept used in group therapy that recognizes that only in the present moment of a group's experience can change be made.

Hernia A protrusion in the intestine through the inguinal wall or canal.

Herniated intervertebral disc A rupture of the cartilage surrounding the intervertebral disc with protrusion of the nucleus pulposus. Also called a *ruptured disc, slipped disc,* or *herniated nucleus pulposus.*

Heroin An illicit, central nervous system depressant narcotic that alters perception and produces euphoria.

Heterograft Skin used for transplantation that was obtained from an animal, usually a pig. Also called a *xenograft.*

Heterosexism The view that heterosexuality is the only correct sexual orientation.

Heterosexual An individual who is attracted to members of the opposite sex.

Highly active antiretroviral therapy (HAART) Effective treatment of AIDS that combines at least three medications to inhibit HIV replication.

Hip fracture A fracture of the femur at the head, neck, or trochanteric regions.

Hippocampus A small, curved body in the brain. Part of the limbic system, it plays a major role in memory formation.

Hirsutism An increased growth of coarse hair on the face and trunk.

Histamine A key chemical mediator of inflammation.

Histrionic personality disorder (HPD) One of several personality disorders defined in the DSM-5, it is characterized by a lifelong tendency for dramatic, egocentric, attention-seeking response patterns.

Hoarding compulsion An excessive collection and accumulation of objects, extreme cluttering of the living environment, accompanied by a lack of regard for the embarrassment of family member or others whose living is impacted.

Holism An approach to health care that considers more than the physiological health status of an individual.

Holosystolic Term used to describe the sounds heard during the entire phase of systole.

Holy day A day set aside for special religious observance.

Homan sign Pain in the calf when the foot is dorsiflexed.

Homeostasis The body's ability to maintain a state of physiological balance in the presence of constantly changing conditions.

Homicide The killing of one individual by another; for legal purposes, this act is further specified by whether the act was intentional or due to negligence.

Homocysteine An amino acid that is a homologue of cysteine.

Homograft Grafts between members of the same species who have different genotypes and HLA antigens. Usually human skin that has been harvested from cadavers. Also called an *allograft.*

Homologous chromosomes The two paired chromosomes that are inherited, one from each parent.

Homophobia The fear, hatred, or mistrust of gays and lesbians often expressed in overt displays of discrimination.

Homosexual An individual who is attracted to members of the same sex.

Hope To expect or desire with confidence.

Horizontal violence (HV) Aggressive acts committed against a nurse by one or more nursing colleagues.

Hormone replacement therapy (HRT) Administration of hormones, usually estrogen and a progestin, to alleviate the symptoms of menopause.

Hormones Chemical messengers secreted by various glands that exert controlling effects on the cells of the body.

Hospice An organization that provides end-of-life care for clients either in their homes or in a hospital setting.

Hospice care The support and care for persons in the last phase of an incurable disease so that they may live as fully and comfortably as possible until their death.

Hot zone When a disaster occurs, the hot zone is the most dangerous zone because it is located immediately adjacent to the site of the disaster. All responders who enter the area must be protected by personal protective equipment.

Human chorionic gonadotropin (HCG) A hormone produced by the chorionic villi that is found in the urine of pregnant women. Also called *prolan.*

Human dignity The inherent worth and uniqueness of individuals and populations.

Human immunodeficiency virus (HIV) A primary immunodeficiency disorder that is spread primarily through sexual contact with an infected person. HIV is the virus that causes acquired immunodeficiency syndrome (AIDS).

Human leukocyte antigen (HLA) The major histocompatibility complex gene.

Humanistic learning theory A learning theory that focuses on the unique cognitive and affective qualities of a learner.

Humoral immune response Hyperreactive response of B cells characteristic of systemic lupus erythematosus (SLE).

Hunger The feeling that makes individuals think of food and encourages them to satisfy this feeling by eating.

Hyaluronic acid (HA) A lubricating substance in cartilage and joint synovial fluid.

Hydrocephalus A condition characterized by enlargement of the head caused by inadequate drainage of cerebrospinal fluid.

Hydronephrosis An accumulation of urine in the renal pelvis as a result of obstructed outflow.

Hydrostatic pressure The pressure a fluid exerts within a closed system on the walls of its container. The hydrostatic pressure of blood is the force blood exerts against the vascular walls (e.g., the artery walls). The principle involved in hydrostatic pressure is that fluids move from an area of greater pressure to an area of lesser pressure.

Hydroureter Distention of the ureter with urine.

Hyperalgesia Increased response to a pain stimulus because of peripheral sensitization.

Hypercalcemia Elevated blood levels of calcium.

Hypercapnia A condition marked by a $PaCO_2$ level above 45 mmHg.

Hypercarbia An increased level of carbon dioxide in the blood that drives the impulse to breathe.

Hyperchloremia Elevated chloride levels in the blood.

Hypercyanotic episode A potentially life-threatening episode of hypoxia. Also called a *tet episode*.

Hyperemia Increased blood flow to an area.

Hyperextension Forcible backward bending.

Hyperflexion Forcible forward bending.

Hyperglycemia Elevated glucose levels.

Hyperkalemia Elevated potassium levels in the blood.

Hypermagnesemia Elevated magnesium levels in the blood.

Hypernatremia Elevated sodium levels in the blood.

Hyperopia Farsightedness.

Hyperosmolar hyperglycemic state (HHS) A disorder characterized by a plasma osmolarity of 340 mOsm/L or greater, greatly elevated blood glucose levels, and altered levels of consciousness. It occurs in individuals who have type 2 diabetes mellitus.

Hyperphosphatemia Increased blood levels of phosphate.

Hyperplasia An increase in the number or density of normal cells.

Hyperresonance An abnormal, booming sound that can be heard over an emphysematous lung.

Hyperresponsiveness An exaggerated response, as with bronchoconstriction in asthma.

Hypersensitivity An overreaction of the immune system to an antigen or antigens.

Hypersomnia The inability to stay awake during the day, despite obtaining sufficient sleep at night.

Hypertension Excess pressure in the arterial portion of the circulatory system, specifically a systolic blood pressure of 140 mmHg or higher or a diastolic blood pressure of 90 mmHg or higher.

Hypertensive emergency A systolic blood pressure greater than 180 mmHg and diastolic blood pressure higher than 120 mmHg. Also called *malignant hypertension*.

Hypertensive encephalopathy A syndrome characterized by extremely high blood pressure, altered level of consciousness, increased intracranial pressure, papilledema, and seizures.

Hyperthermia A condition that occurs when a body produces more heat than is lost.

Hyperthermia blanket An electronically controlled blanket that provides a specified temperature

Hyperthermic A body temperature above 37.8°C (100°F).

Hyperthyroidism A disorder caused by excessive delivery of thyroid hormone to the peripheral tissues. Also called *thyrotoxicosis*.

Hypertonic Refers to solutions that have a higher osmolality than body fluids; 3% sodium chloride is a hypertonic solution.

Hypertonic dehydration Occurs when sodium loss is proportionately less than water loss. Also called *hypernatremic dehydration*.

Hypertrophic cardiomyopathy A disorder characterized by decreased compliance of the left ventricle and hypertrophy of the ventricular muscle mass.

Hypertrophic scar An overgrowth of dermal tissue that remains within the boundaries of the wound.

Hypertrophy An enlargement of glandular cells or muscles.

Hyperventilation Unusually fast respirations, or overbreathing causing an imbalance of oxygen and carbon dioxide.

Hypervolemia The excessive retention of both water and sodium in similar proportions to normal extracellular fluid (ECF). Also called *fluid volume excess*.

Hyphema Bleeding into the anterior chamber of the eye.

Hypoactive sexual desire disorder A deficiency in or absence of sexual fantasies and persistently low interest or a total lack of interest in sexual activity.

Hypocalcemia Decreased blood levels of calcium.

Hypocapnia A condition that results when $PaCO_2$ falls below 35 mmHg.

Hypochloremia Decreased blood levels of chloride.

Hypodermis The layer of loose connective tissue and fat cells that lies below the dermis. Also called *subcutaneous tissue*.

Hypodermoclysis Fluid administered subcutaneously.

Hypoglycemia Diminished glucose levels.

Hypokalemia Decreased blood levels of potassium.

Hypomagnesemia Decreased blood levels of magnesium.

Hypomania A less extreme form of mania that is not severe enough to markedly impair functioning or require hospitalization.

Hyponatremia Decreased blood levels of sodium.

Hypoperfusion Decreased blood flow.

Hypophonia A lowered voice volume.

Hypophosphatemia Decreased blood levels of phosphate.

Hypoplastic left heart syndrome (HLHS) One of the most severe congenital heart defects, characterized by absence or stenosis of mitral and aortic valves, an abnormally small left ventricle, a small aorta, and aortic or mitral stenosis or atresia.

Hypotension A below-normal blood pressure reading between 85 and 110 mmHg.

Hypothermia A condition that occurs when a body loses more heat than it produces.

Hypothermic A body temperature below 36°C (97°F).

Hypothyroidism A disorder resulting when the thyroid gland produces an insufficient amount of thyroid hormone.

Hypotonic Refers to solutions that have a lower osmolality than body fluids, such as one half normal saline.

Hypotonic dehydration Occurs when fluid loss is characterized by a proportionately greater loss of sodium than water. Also called *hyponatremic dehydration*.

Hypovolemia Loss of both water and electrolytes in similar proportions from extracellular fluid. Also called *fluid volume deficit*.

Hypovolemic shock Shock caused by a decrease in intravascular volume of 15% or more.

Hypoxemia Decreased oxygen levels in the blood that result when PaO_2 falls below 80 mmHg.

Iatrogenic Refers to a condition induced by the effects of treatment.

Iatrogenic infection A type of infection that results directly from diagnostic or therapeutic procedures.

Id In Freudian terms, the source of instinctive and unconscious psychological urges.

Ideal body image A mental representation of what an individual believes his or her body should look like.

Ideal self How the individual thinks he or she should be or would prefer to be.

Idiopathic pain A type of pain that occurs unpredictably and is not associated with any known cause, making it difficult to treat.

Ileostomy A surgical opening made in the ileum of the small intestine.

Ileus A condition that causes a temporary cessation of the passage of material through the intestines, usually lasting 24–48 hours.

Illness A state in which an individual's physical, emotional, intellectual, social, developmental, or spiritual functioning is diminished.

Illness behavior A coping mechanism that includes the ways in which an individual describes, monitors, and interprets symptoms, and the individual's ability to take remedial action and use the healthcare system.

Illness prevention Health care focusing on maintaining optimal health by preventing disease through programs on immunizations, prenatal and infant care, and prevention of sexually transmitted infections.

Illusion A distorted perception of actual sensory stimuli.

Imagery A relaxation technique in which the client focuses on pleasant images such as a beach or a garden to replace negative images such as pain and darkness. Also called *guided imagery*.

Imitation The process by which individuals copy or reproduce what they have observed.

Immobility A reduction in the amount and control of one's movement.

Immunity The body's natural or induced response to infection and the conditions associated with its response.

Immunization Introduces an antigen into the body, allowing immunity against a disease to develop naturally.

Immunocompetent Term used to describe clients who have an immune system that identifies antigens and effectively destroys or removes them.

Immunodeficiency A condition that develops when the immune system is incompetent or unable to respond effectively.

Immunoglobulin (Ig) A protein that functions as an antibody.

Immunosuppression Inability of the immune system to respond to an antigen. Occurs in response to disease or medications; may be intentional to prevent rejection of transplants or a side effect of some medications.

Implied consent Nonverbal consent indicated by a client's cooperative actions.

Impotence Inability to achieve or maintain an erection.

Impulse conduction The transmission of an impulse along the nerve pathways to the spinal cord and directly to the brain.

Impulsiveness Acting without considering the consequences of one's behavior. Also called *impulsivity*.

In vitro fertilization A process in which a woman's eggs are collected from her ovaries, fertilized in the laboratory, and then placed into her uterus after normal embryo development has begun.

Incentive spirometry Measures the forced emptying of alveolar gas.

Incident pain A type of breakthrough pain that is predictable because it is precipitated by an event or activity such as coughing or changing position.

Incident report An agency record of an accident or incident occurring within the agency. This record is designed to collect adequate information to assist personnel in preventing future incidents or occurrences. Also called *variance reports* or *unusual occurrence reports*.

Incomplete spinal cord injury An injury that involves only a partial loss of sensory and motor function below the level of the injury.

Increased intracranial pressure (IICP) Sustained, elevated pressure (15 mmHg or higher in adults) in the cranial cavity.

Indemnity plan A type of health insurance program that allows the insured to self-select healthcare providers and has no predefined network.

Independent intervention The activities that nurses are licensed to do within their scope of practice; in other words, areas of health care that are unique to nursing and separate and distinct from medical management.

Indicator A statistic that reflects the organization's performance in a specific area.

Inductive reasoning A "bottom-up" method of logical thinking that starts with putting significant cues together in order to reach a conclusion. It is a method of logical thinking that is used to determine if decisions are reasonable.

Infection An invasion of the body tissue by microorganisms with the potential to cause illness or disease.

Infectious disease Any communicable disease that is caused by microorganisms that are commonly transmitted from one person to another or from an animal to an individual.

Infertility A lack of conception despite unprotected sexual intercourse for at least 12 months.

Inflammation An adaptive response to what the body sees as harmful, such as an allergen, illness, or injury. Inflammation typically is characterized by pain, heat, redness, and swelling. Also called *inflammatory response.*

Inflammatory bowel disease (IBD) Chronic inflammation of the bowel common to a group of conditions that includes Crohn disease and ulcerative colitis.

Influenza A highly contagious viral respiratory disease characterized by coryza (inflammation of the mucous membranes lining the nose usually associated with nasal discharge), fever, cough, and systemic symptoms such as headache and malaise (vague feeling of physical discomfort).

Informal groups A type of group that functions with much less structure than a formal or semiformal group. Characteristics of informal groups include easily recognized, basic objectives; rotational leadership; and no set of written rules or regulations.

Informal leader A leader who is not officially appointed to direct the activities of others but, because of seniority, age, or special abilities, is recognized by the group as a leader and plays an important role in influencing colleagues, coworkers, or other group members to achieve the group's goals.

Informed consent **1.** A client's legal and ethical rights to be informed of and give permission for any healthcare procedure or treatment. **2.** A study volunteer's legal right to be informed with full disclosure of the study's purpose, required procedures, length of the study, expectations, risks, and possible benefits before consenting to participate. Informed consent also includes the right to withdraw from the study at any time.

Infundibulopelvic ligament A ligament that suspends and supports the ovaries.

Inhalant A substance inhaled to produce euphoria. Categorized into three types: anesthetics, volatile nitrites, and organic solvents.

Input Information, material, or energy that enters a system.

Inquiry A search for knowledge or facts in order to gain clarification and find solutions to problems.

Insensible fluid loss Fluid loss that is not perceptible to the individual and cannot be measured.

Insomnia The inability to fall asleep or remain asleep.

Inspection A visual, auditory, and olfactory examination or assessment of a client to note health condition.

Inspiration The act of inhaling air in respiration.

Insubordination Defiance of authority, such as the refusal to complete a task as assigned.

Insulin A hormone that facilitates the uptake and use of glucose by cells and prevents an excessive breakdown of glycogen in the liver and muscle.

Insulin reaction Low blood glucose levels, or hypoglycemia. Also called *insulin shock.*

Integrity Adherence to a strict moral or ethical code.

Integumentary system The body's system that includes skin, hair, and nails and the sebaceous, sweat, and mammary glands.

Intellect The ability to learn and understand knowledge; the capacity for thinking and reasoning intelligently.

Intellectual disability Significant limitations in intellectual functioning and adaptive behavior prior to the age of 18. Previously called *mental retardation.*

Intellectual functioning General intelligence or mental capacity, including an individual's abilities to learn, use logic, and solve problems.

Intensity **1.** The amplitude of a sound produced. **2.** The strength of the contraction during acme, the peak of a uterine contraction during the birth process.

Interdisciplinary team A team that seeks to achieve a common goal, though the team members are professionals with varied backgrounds. Also called *interprofessional team.*

Intergroup conflict Conflict that occurs between teams that are in competition or opposition to one another.

Intermittent claudication A cramping or aching pain in the calves of the legs, the thighs, and the buttocks that occurs with a predictable level of activity

Intermittent fever Occurs when body temperature alternates at regular intervals between periods of fever and periods of normal or subnormal temperatures.

Internal environment The physical, spiritual, cognitive, emotional, and psychological well-being of an individual that depends on the satisfaction of these basic human needs.

Internal locus of control A belief that an individual can impact her or his own health and well-being.

Interorganizational conflict Usually conflict that occurs between two organizations that exist within one market.

Interpersonal conflict Conflict that occurs between two or more individuals due to differences, competition, or concern about territory, control, or loss.

Interpersonal violence Violence that occurs within relationships, between family members, intimate partners, acquaintances, or strangers that does not aim to further the goals of a formal group or cause.

Interprofessional team A team that seeks to achieve a common goal, though the team members are professionals with varied backgrounds. Also called *interdisciplinary team.*

Intersex A general term used to describe a variety of conditions in which reproductive or sexual anatomy does not fit the typical definitions of male or female.

Interstitial fluid Accounts for approximately 75% of extracellular fluid; interstitial fluid surrounds the cells.

Intervention A personalized confrontation that prevents an addict from denying the addiction problem and forces them to face the negative aspects of their behavior and enroll in treatment.

Intimacy A relationship that entails commitment, companionship, affective intimacy, social support, physical closeness, and mutuality.

Intimate distance Communication that is characterized by body contact, heightened sensations of body heat and smell, and vocalizations that are low.

Intimate partner violence (IPV) The act of inflicting sexual, emotional, or physical harm on a current or previous partner or spouse.

Intracapsular hip fracture A hip fracture involving the head or neck of the femur.

Intracellular fluid (ICF) Fluid found within the body cells that contains solute vital to the metabolic processes of the cells. Also called *cellular fluid*.

Intracranial hypertension A sustained state of increased intracranial pressure that is potentially life threatening.

Intracranial regulation The processes that affect intracranial compensation and adaptive neurological function.

Intractable seizures Seizures that continue to occur even with optimal medical management.

Intradiscal electrothermal therapy (IDET) The use of thermal energy to treat pain from a bulging spinal disc.

Intradisciplinary assessment An evaluation that occurs within a group of individuals with a similar position in the healthcare system, such as a group of nurses or a group of surgeons, to identify areas of improvement at each level of care.

Intradisciplinary team A team that seeks to achieve a common goal with team members from the same background.

Intragenerational family A family in which more than two generations live together.

Intranet A smaller version of the Internet that is meant to be used by a smaller group of people, such as employees within a company or members of an organization.

Intraocular pressure A force within the eye that causes tissue damage.

Intraoperative The phase of an operative process in which the surgical procedure actually takes place.

Intrapartum The time from the onset of true labor until the birth of the infant and expulsion of the placenta.

Intrapersonal conflict Conflict that occurs within an individual, arising from stress or tension that results from real or perceived pressure generated by incompatible expectations or goals.

Intrauterine contraception (IUC) A safe, effective method of reversible contraception that is designed to be inserted into the uterus by a qualified healthcare provider and left in place for an extended period, providing continuous contraceptive protection.

Intrauterine device (IUD) A small plastic or metal form that is placed in the uterus to prevent implantation of a fertilized ovum.

Intrauterine fetal death (IUFD) Death of a fetus that occurs after 20 weeks' gestation. Often referred to as *stillbirth* or *fetal demise*.

Intrauterine pressure catheter (IUPC) A device that measures the pressure in the uterine cavity.

Intravascular fluid Accounts for approximately 20% of the extracellular fluid and is found within the vascular system. Also called *plasma*.

Intravenous pyelography (IVP) A diagnostic test used to evaluate the structure and excretory function of the kidneys, ureters, and bladder.

Introspection The personal exploration and evaluation of one's own thoughts, emotions, behaviors, and values incorporating both verbal and nonverbal feedback from others.

Intubation The process of inserting a breathing tube.

Intuition The use of nursing knowledge, experience, and expertise for understanding without the conscious use of reasoning.

Invasion Occurs when cancerous cells overtake adjacent tissues.

Involuntary admission The detention of a client in a psychiatric or medical facility against the client's will, normally reserved for cases in which the client is a danger to himself or others.

Involution The rapid reduction in size of the uterus and the return of the uterus to a nonpregnant state.

Ions Electrically charged particles.

Iron deficiency anemia A disorder that results when the supply of iron in the body is insufficient for the formation of red blood cells.

Irritant contact dermatitis An inflammation of the skin from irritants; it is not a hypersensitivity response.

Ischemia Insufficient blood supply.

Ischemic Deprived of oxygen.

Ischial spines Prominences that arise near the junction of the ilium and ischium and jut into the pelvic cavity.

Isoelectric line A straight line on an electrocardiograph that indicates the absence of electrical activity.

Isokinetic exercises Resistive exercises that involve muscle contraction or tension against resistance; can be either isotonic or isometric.

Isolation Measures designed to prevent the spread of infection to health personnel, clients, and visitors.

Isometric exercises Static or sitting exercises in which muscles contract without moving the joint.

Isotonic A solution that has the same osmolality as body fluids. Normal saline, 0.9% sodium chloride, is an isotonic solution.

Isotonic dehydration A type of fluid imbalance that occurs when fluid loss is not balanced by intake and the losses of water and sodium are in proportion. Also called *isonatremic dehydration*.

Isotonic exercises Dynamic exercises in which the muscle shortens to produce muscle contractions and active movement.

Isotonic fluid volume deficit A type of fluid imbalance that occurs when electrolytes are lost along with fluid.

Isotonic imbalance A fluid imbalance that occurs when water and electrolytes are lost or gained in equal proportions, so that the osmolality of body fluids remains constant.

Isthmus That portion of the uterus between the internal cervical os and the endometrial cavity.

Jaundice A yellow pigmentation of body tissues caused by the presence of bile pigments.

Joint arthroplasty The reconstruction or replacement of a joint.

Joint custody Occurs when two parents who are not married have equal responsibility and legal rights for their shared children.

Joint fusion A procedure that permanently fuses two or more bones together at a joint using pins, plates, screws, and rods. Also called *arthrodesis*.

Joint irrigation A fluid injected into the joint to allow the surgeon to visualize joint structures more easily and to help remove debris and infection in the joint.

Joint resurfacing A procedure in which a little bone is removed at the articulating surface of the joint and a metal replacement is fitted over the end of the bone.

Just culture An attempt to balance the blame-free environment with appropriate accountability by focusing on correcting problems that lead individuals to engage in unsafe behavior while maintaining individual accountability by establishing zero tolerance for reckless behavior.

Justice Fairness.

Juvenile idiopathic arthritis (JIA) See juvenile rheumatoid arthritis (JRA).

Juvenile rheumatoid arthritis (JRA) A chronic inflammatory autoimmune disease diagnosed in children that is characterized by joint inflammation resulting in decreased mobility, swelling, and pain.

Kaposi sarcoma (KS) Often the presenting symptom of AIDS, it remains the most common cancer associated with the disease. Kaposi sarcoma is caused by a virus called the Kaposi sarcoma–associated herpes virus, also known as human herpes virus 8.

Kardex A widely used, concise method of organizing and recording data about a client, making information quickly accessible to all healthcare professionals.

Karyotype A pictorial analysis of chromosomes.

Kcalorie See Kilocalories.

Kegel exercises The act of tightening the perineal muscle in order to strengthen the pubococcygeus muscle and increase its elasticity.

Keloid A scar that extends beyond the boundaries of the original wound.

Keratin A fibrous, water-repellent protein that gives the epidermis its tough, protective quality.

Keratotic basal cell carcinoma A type of skin cancer.

Ketonuria The presence of ketones in the urine.

Ketosis An accumulation of ketone bodies produced during oxidation of fatty acids.

Kilocalories A term used to identify the energy-producing ability of nutrients. Also called Kcalories or kcal.

Kindling Long-term changes in brain neurotransmission that occur after repeated detoxifications.

Kinesthesia The ability to perceive movement and sense of position.

Kinesthetic A term referring to awareness of the position and movement of body parts.

Korotkoff sounds The series of sounds identified while taking a blood pressure using a stethoscope.

Korsakoff psychosis A condition typically seen in alcoholics that is characterized by intact intellectual functioning but an inability to retrieve long-term memory events or retain new information.

Kosher Acceptable to or prepared according to Jewish law.

Kussmaul respirations Deep, rapid respirations associated with compensatory mechanisms.

Kyphosis A convex curvature of the spine that may decrease mobility.

Labor induction The stimulation of uterine contractions before the spontaneous onset of labor, with or without ruptured fetal membranes, for the purpose of accomplishing birth.

Labyrinthitis Inflammation of the inner ear. Also called otitis interna.

Lactase deficiency An individual's inability to digest lactose because of a deficiency of lactase, the enzyme that breaks down lactose into monosaccharides. Also called lactose intolerance.

Lacto-ovovegetarians Vegetarians who include milk, dairy products, and eggs in their diets.

Lactose intolerance An individual's inability to digest lactose because of a deficiency of lactase, the enzyme that breaks down lactose into monosaccharides. Also called lactose deficiency.

Lactovegetarians Vegetarians who include dairy products but no eggs in their diets.

Laënnec cirrhosis A progressive, irreversible liver disorder resulting from excessive alcohol consumption. Also called alcoholic cirrhosis.

Laissez-faire leader A leader who recognizes a group's need for autonomy and self-regulation. The leader assumes a "hands-off" approach, being less directive and more permissive than other types of leaders.

Lamellar A type of bone that is stronger and more compact with better blood circulation compared to woven bone.

Laminectomy The surgical removal of the vertebral lamina.

Laminotomy The surgical removal of part of the vertebral lamina.

Lanugo A large quantity of fine hair found on some newborns.

Laparoscopic cholecystectomy Removal of the gallbladder using an endoscope.

Late deceleration A condition caused by uteroplacental insufficiency resulting from decreased blood flow and oxygen transfer to the fetus through the intervillous spaces during uterine contractions.

Law The sum total of the rules and regulations by which a society is governed.

Laxatives Medications that stimulate bowel activity and assist in fecal elimination.

Lead An insulated wire that connects an electrocardiograph to the electrodes attached to a client.

Leader An individual with the ability to rule, guide, or inspire others to think or act as that individual recommends.

Leading question A closed question that gives the client an opportunity to decide whether the answer is true or not.

Lean Six Sigma A methodology used to reduce waste and provide consistency in the quality of care.

Learning A change in human disposition or capability that persists and that cannot be solely accounted for by growth.

Learning disabilities Disorders that impair an individual's ability to receive and process information, causing reduced functioning in verbal, linguistic, reasoning, and academic skills; neurological conditions in which the brain cannot receive or process information normally.

Learning need A desire or a requirement to know something that is presently unknown to the learner.

Lecithin/sphingomyelin (L/S) ratio The measurement of lecithin and sphingomyelin in order to determine the lung maturity of a fetus.

Leopold maneuvers A systematic way to evaluate the maternal abdomen.

Lesbian A woman who prefers relationships with other women.

Lesion An observable change in skin structure that may indicate disorders in other systems and organs.

Leukemia A group of chronic malignant disorders of white blood cells (WBCs) and WBC precursors.

Leukocytes The primary cells involved in both nonspecific and specific immune system responses. Also known as white blood cells (WBCs).

Leukocytosis An increase in the number of leukocytes in the blood (above 10,000/mm^3), in response to infection or inflammation.

Leukopenia A decrease in the number of circulating leukocytes.

Level of injury The vertical location of an injury along the spinal column.

Lewy bodies Abnormal aggregates of proteins, including alpha-synuclein.

Liability The state of being legally obliged and responsible.

Libido 1. Sexual desire. 2. The psychic energy that, according to Freud, provides the underlying motivation to human development.

Licensed practical nurses (LPNs) Members of a nursing team who provide direct client care under the direction of an RN, physician, or other licensed practitioner.

Lichenification The thickening of the skin.

Lifestyle An individual's general way of living, including living conditions and individual patterns of behavior that are influenced by sociocultural factors and personal characteristics.

Ligaments Connective tissue between bones to create joints.

Lightening The effects that occur when the fetus begins to settle into the pelvic inlet.

Limb restraints A device typically made of cloth that may be used when limb immobilization is needed for therapeutic purposes, for example, to prevent dislodgement of an intravenous infusion device.

Limbic system A set of structures located deep inside the brain; includes the hippocampus.

Limit setting Establishing clear and consistent rules or guidelines for child or client behavior.

Line authority The power to direct the activities of subordinates within an organization.

Lipids The macronutrient that provides most of the body's energy at 9 kcal/g. There are three categories of lipids: triglycerides, phospholipids and sterols. Also called *fats*.

Lipoatrophy Atrophy of subcutaneous tissues.

Lipodystrophy Excessive growth of subcutaneous tissue.

Lithiasis Stone formation.

Lithotripsy The preferred treatment for urinary calculi; uses sound or shock waves to crush a stone.

Living will A document that provides written directions about life-prolonging procedures to provide instructions when an individual can no longer communicate in a life-threatening situation.

Lobes Specialized cognitive regions in the hemispheres of the brain.

Local adaptation syndrome (LAS) A stress response that affects only one organ or body system.

Local emergency management agency (LEMA) A governmental agency with expertise in public safety, emergency medical services, and management.

Local infection Invasion by a microorganism that is limited to the specific part of the body where the microorganism remains.

Localized responses Common manifestations of type I hypersensitivity, they are typically atopic responses; that is, they have a strong genetic predisposition. Atopic reactions are the result of localized, rather than systemic, IgE-mediated responses to an allergen. They are prompted by contact of the allergen with IgE in the bronchial tree, nasal mucosa, and conjunctival tissues.

Lochia The discharge through which the uterus rids itself of the debris remaining after birth. The discharge should change appearance and contents as healing commences.

Lochia alba The final discharge as the uterus completes healing; composed primarily of leukocytes, decidual cells, epithelial cells, fat, cervical mucus, cholesterol crystals, and bacteria.

Lochia rubra The dark red initial discharge as the uterus eliminates epithelial cells, erythrocytes, leukocytes, shreds of decidua, and occasionally fetal meconium, lanugo, and vernix in the first 1–2 days following birth.

Lochia serosa A light pink discharge of serous exudate, shreds of degenerating decidua, erythrocytes, leukocytes, cervical mucus, and numerous microorganisms from the uterus 3–10 days following birth.

Locked-in syndrome A state of consciousness in which the client is alert and fully aware of the environment and has intact cognitive abilities but is unable to communicate through speech or movement because of blocked efferent pathways from the brain. Motor paralysis affects all voluntary muscles, although the upper cranial nerves (I through IV) may remain intact, allowing the client to communicate through eye movements and blinking.

Locus of control (LOC) The extent to which clients believes their health status is under their own or others' control.

Long-term memory The repository for information stored for periods longer than 72 hours and usually weeks and years.

Longboard spinal immobilization A device that provides support and immobilization of the entire spine below the level of the neck, instituted for clients with a potential or suspected spinal cord injury from a motor vehicle crash.

Loose association An indication of disordered thinking characterized by the shifting of verbal ideas from one topic to another, with no apparent relationship between thoughts, and the person speaking being unaware that the topics are unconnected. Commonly seen in schizophrenia.

Lordosis A concave curvature of the spine that may decrease mobility.

Loss A situation in which someone or something that is valued becomes altered or no longer available.

Lower body obesity Identified by a waist-to-hip ratio of less than 0.8; more commonly seen in women. Also called *peripheral obesity*.

Lumpectomy Removal of a tumor and the surrounding margin of breast tissue followed by radiation therapy. Also called *segmental mastectomy* or *breast conservation surgery*.

Lung abscess A local area of necrosis and pus formation within the lung.

Lupus nephritis Inflammation of the kidneys resulting from systemic lupus erythematosus (SLE).

Luteinizing hormone (LH) Anterior pituitary hormone responsible for stimulating ovulation and for development of the corpus luteum.

Lymphadenopathy The enlargement of lymph nodes with or without tenderness. It may be caused by inflammation, infection, or malignancy of the nodes or the regions drained by the nodes.

Lymphangitis Inflammation of a lymph vessel.

Lymphedema Accumulation of fluid in the soft tissues of the arm caused by removal of lymph channels.

Lymphocytes The principal effector and regulator cells of specific immune responses to protect the body from microorganisms, foreign tissue, and cell mutations or alterations.

Lyse Disintegrate.

Maceration Tissues softened by prolonged wetting or soaking.

Macronutrients Essential nutrients needed by the body in large amounts to survive: carbohydrates, proteins, and fats.

Macrophages Large phagocytes that are important in the body's defense against chronic infections.

Macular degeneration A progressive disorder involving loss of central vision due to damage to the retina.

Magical thinking Believing that events occur because of one's thoughts or actions.

Major depressive disorder (MDD) A mood disorder characterized by loss of interest in life and unresponsiveness, moving from mild to severe, with severe symptoms lasting at least 2 weeks. Also called *unipolar depression*.

Major depressive episode Characterized by a change in several aspects of an individual's emotional state and functioning consistently over a period of 14 days or longer.

Malabsorption A condition in which the intestinal mucosa is unable to absorb nutrients, resulting in nutrients being excreted in the stool.

Malaise Vague feeling of physical discomfort.

Maldigestion A condition in which there is inadequate preparation of chyme for absorption of nutrients; also can result in malabsorption.

Male erectile disorder A condition that occurs when a male has erection problems during 25% or more of his sexual interactions.

Male orgasmic disorder A condition that occurs when a male can maintain an erection for long periods, but has difficulty ejaculating.

Malignant Term used to refer to a cell or growth that, if not treated, will recur, continue to grow, and spread to other sites in the body, ending in death.

Malignant hyperthermia A musculoskeletal disorder resulting from an inherited cellular deficit that places the client in a hypermetabolic state.

Malnutrition Health effects due to insufficient nutrient intake or stores. Also called *undernutrition*.

Malpractice Conduct deviating from the standard of practice dictated by a profession.

Malpresentation A condition that occurs when a fetus passes into the pelvic inlet with a breech or shoulder presentation. These presentations are associated with difficulties during labor.

Malunion The healing of bones in an anatomically incorrect position. Surgical correction may be needed.

Managed care A healthcare delivery system designed to provide cost-effective, high-quality care for groups of clients from the time of their initial contact with the health system through the conclusion of their health problem.

Manager An individual employed by an organization and granted the required authority, responsibility, accountability, and power to accomplish the organization's goals.

Mandatory health insurance Health insurance is provided by large, nonprofit health organizations centered around large employers or work-based associations or else is provided by government-sponsored programs. Everyone belongs to one of these two types of insurance plans, thus ensuring universal coverage.

Mandatory reporting A legal requirement to report an act, event, or situation that is designated by state or local law as a reportable event.

Mania An abnormal and persistently elevated, expansive, or irritable mood lasting at least 1 week, significantly impairing social or occupational functioning and generally requiring hospitalization.

Manipulation Controlling behavior used to exploit others for personal gain.

Margination The accumulation of leukocytes along the inner surface of blood vessels. Occurs as part of the inflammatory process.

Marital rape Rape that occurs when one spouse forces the other to have sex against his or her will.

Maslow's hierarchy of needs A concept proposed by Abraham Maslow in which he proposed the existence of levels of human needs that could be organized into five categories: physiological, safety, love and belonging, esteem, and self-actualization.

Massage therapy The scientific manipulation of the soft tissues of the body for the purposes of promoting healing and wellness.

Massive transfusion A series of blood parcels, including packed red blood cells, fresh frozen plasma, cryo units, and platelet pheresis administered to a client who has lost a substantial amount of blood.

Mast cells Leukocytes that detect foreign agents or injury and respond by releasing histamine, thereby activating the inflammatory process.

Masturbation The self-stimulation of one's genitals for sexual pleasure.

Maternal role attainment (MRA) The process by which a woman learns mothering behaviors and becomes comfortable with her identity as a mother.

Maturational crisis A crisis that occurs normally as an individual progresses through the life cycle.

Mature milk A white or slightly blue-tinged color milk that presents by 2 weeks postpartum and continues thereafter until lactation ceases.

McDonald sign A probable sign of pregnancy characterized by an ease in flexing the body of the uterus against the cervix.

Mean arterial pressure (MAP) The average pressure in the arterial circulation throughout the cardiac cycle.

Meaning-focused coping The use of revaluation to reduce the appraisal of a threat.

Meatus A body passage or opening.

Meconium The first fecal material passed by a newborn, normally within 8–24 hours after birth.

Medicaid A state-administered health insurance program available to certain lower-income individuals and families, older adults, and people with disabilities.

Medical asepsis All practices intended to confine a specific microorganism to a specific area, thus limiting the number, growth, and transmission of the microorganism.

Medicare A federally funded health insurance program available to people ages 65 or older, younger people with disabilities, and people with end-stage renal disease.

Medigap policy A private health insurance plan designed to supplement Medicare coverage. It may pay copayments, coinsurance, deductibles and "gaps" in Medicare coverage (i.e., noncovered healthcare costs). Also called *Medicare supplemental insurance*.

Meditation The act of focusing one's thoughts or engaging in self-reflection or contemplation.

Meiosis A reductive division of sex cells, producing ova or sperm with a half set (haploid) of chromosomes.

Melanin A shield that protects the keratinocytes and the nerve endings in the dermis from the damaging effects of ultraviolet light.

Melanoma A type of malignant skin cancer.

Melasma gravidarum See **Chloasma**.

Mendelian inheritance Traits that are passed on by a single gene. Also called *single-gene inheritance*.

Meninges Three connective tissue membranes that cover, protect, and nourish the central nervous system.

Menopause The permanent cessation of menses.

Menorrhagia Excessive or prolonged menstruation that occurs at regular intervals.

Menstrual cycle The cyclic phases of menstruation that normally occur about every 28 days.

Menstruation The periodic shedding of the uterine lining in a woman of childbearing age who is not pregnant.

Mental retardation See **Intellectual disability**.

Mentor A competent, experienced professional who develops a relationship with a novice for the purpose of providing advice, support, information, and feedback in order to encourage development of the individual.

Message Content that is actually said or written, the body language that accompanies the words, and how the words are transmitted.

Metabolic acidosis This bicarbonate deficit is characterized by a low pH (<7.35), low bicarbonate (<24 mEq/L), and $PaCO_2$ less than 38 mmHg. It may be caused by excess acid in the body or loss of bicarbonate from the body.

Metabolic alkalosis This bicarbonate excess is characterized by a high pH (>7.45), a high bicarbonate (>28 mEq/L), and $PaCO_2$ higher than 45 mmHg. It may be caused by loss of acid or excess bicarbonate in the body.

Metabolic syndrome A disorder characterized by the presence of three or more of the following: increased waist circumference, hypertension, elevated blood triglycerides and fasting blood glucose, and low HDL cholesterol.

Metabolism The complex process of biochemical reactions occurring in the body's cells necessary to produce energy, repair cells, and sustain life.

Metaphysis The portion of the bone between the diaphysis and the epiphysis.

Metaplasia A change in the normal pattern of differentiation such that dividing cells differentiate into cell types not normally found at that location in the body.

Metastasis The process by which spreading of malignant neoplasms occurs; the transfer of disease from one organ or part to another.

Metrorrhagia Bleeding between menstrual periods.

Microalbuminuria An abnormally low level of albumin in the urine.

Micronutrients Essential nutrients needed by the body in small quantities, such as vitamins and minerals.

Microstaging The assessment of the level of invasion of a malignant melanoma and the maximum tumor thickness.

Micturition Releasing urine from the urinary bladder. Also called *voiding* or *urination*.

Middle ear effusion Results when negative pressure in the middle ear causes sterile serous fluid to move from the capillaries into the space.

Milia Exposed sebaceous glands that appear as raised white spots on the face, especially across the nose on infants within the first month after birth.

Miliary tuberculosis Results from hematogenous spread (through the blood) of the tuberculosis bacilli throughout the body.

Milieu therapy A therapeutic recovery environment that supports behavior changes, teaches new coping skills, and helps the client move from addiction to sobriety.

Milliequivalent The chemical combining power of the ion, or the capacity of cations to combine with anions to form molecules.

Minerals Salts dissolved in water that carry electrical charge and work with other nutrients to maintain fluid balance throughout the body. Also called *electrolytes*.

Minimal enteral nutrition Small-volume feedings of formula or human milk (usually $<24 \text{ mL} \cdot \text{kg}^{-1} \cdot \text{day}^{-1}$) designed to "prime" the premature infant's intestinal tract and stimulate many of its hormonal and enzymatic functions.

Minor trauma Trauma that affects a single part or system of the body and is usually treated in a physician's office or in a hospital's emergency department.

Miscarriage The loss of a fetus prior to 20 weeks' gestation. Also called a *spontaneous abortion*.

Mitigation A phase that takes place before and after an emergency that consists of identifying potential hazards, minimizing effects, and reducing the likelihood of their occurrence.

Mitosis The process of cell division.

Mitt restraints A device used to protect confused clients from scratching or injuring their skin or dislodging intravenous access devices. Also called *hand restraints*.

Modeling Observing the behavior of people who have successfully achieved a goal that they have set for themselves and, through observing, acquiring ideas for behavior and coping strategies.

Modified radical mastectomy The removal of the breast tissue and lymph nodes under the arm, leaving the chest wall muscles intact.

Molding The asymmetrical appearance of an infant's head caused by overlapping of the cranial bones during labor and birth.

Mongolian spots Macular areas of bluish-black or gray-blue pigmentation on the dorsal area and the buttocks; common in newborns of Asian, Hispanic, and African descent and in newborns of other dark-skinned races.

Monoamine oxidase inhibitor (MAOI) A drug that inhibits monoamine oxidase, an enzyme that terminates the actions of neurotransmitters such as dopamine, norepinephrine, epinephrine, and serotonin. These drugs are used to treat individuals who have not responded to typical treatments for depression.

Mononeuropathies Isolated peripheral neuropathies that affect a single nerve.

Monophasic A term used to describe rheumatoid arthritis when it occurs for a limited time and then improves.

Monopolizing The domination of a discussion by one member of a group.

Monosomy Absence of a chromosome.

Monotheism The belief in the existence of one God.

Monro-Kellie hypothesis A hypothesis that states if the volume of any of the three intracranial components (the brain, cerebrospinal fluid, and blood) increases, the volume of the others must decrease to maintain normal pressures in the cranial cavity.

Mood An individual's internal, subjective, sustained emotional state.

Mood stabilizers Drugs used for treatment of bipolar disorder because they moderate extreme shifts in emotions between mania and depression.

Moral behavior The way in which an individual perceives and responds to society's requirements.

Moral development **1.** The process of learning to tell the difference between right and wrong and of learning what ought and ought not to be done. **2.** The pattern of change in moral behavior that occurs with age.

Moral rules Specific prescriptions for actions.

Morality Private, personal standards of what is right and wrong in conduct, character, and attitude; the requirements necessary for people to live together in society.

Morbid obesity A condition in which an individual weighs more than 200% of his or her ideal body weight or has a BMI >40 kg/m^2.

Morning sickness A term that refers to the nausea and vomiting that a woman may experience in early pregnancy. This lay term is sometimes used because these symptoms frequently occur in the early part of the day and disappear within a few hours.

Moro reflex In response to being lifted, then suddenly lowered or surprised by a loud noise, a newborn will straighten the arms and hands outward while the knees flex. Slowly, the arms return to the chest, as in an embrace. The fingers spread, forming a "C," and the newborn may cry.

Morpheaform basal cell carcinoma A type of skin cancer.

Morula Developmental stage of the fertilized ovum in which there is a solid mass of cells.

Mosaicism The expression of two cell lines, each with a different chromosomal number, in an individual.

Motility The process of moving food and fluid through the gastrointestinal tract from the mouth to the anus.

Motivation to learn The individual's personal desire and need to learn that affects how much and how fast the individual will learn.

Motor vehicle crash (MVC) The unintentional collision of one or more motor vehicles with another vehicle or object.

Mottling A lacy pattern of dilated blood vessels under the skin.

Mourning The behavioral process through which grief is eventually resolved or altered; it is often influenced by culture, spiritual beliefs, and custom.

Movement disorder A disorder associated with schizophrenia. There are two general forms: The first involves increased body movements that may appear agitated, repetitious, or purposeless. The second form involves catatonia, or unresponsiveness to the environment or others.

Movement technique A relaxation technique, such as yoga or tai chi, designed to improve strength, balance, and mental calmness.

Multiculturalism Characterized by many subcultures coexisting within a given society in which no one culture dominates.

Multidisciplinary team approach An approach to health care in which team members work together to deliver client care, but a single team member—usually a physician—makes the treatment decisions.

Multifocal A term used to describe premature ventricular contractions (PVCs) that arise from different ectopic sites and appear distinct on the ECG.

Multigravida Term used to describe a woman who has been pregnant more than once.

Multipara Term used to describe a woman who has had more than one pregnancy in which the fetus was viable.

Multiple pregnancy More than one fetus in the uterus at the same time.

Multiple sclerosis (MS) A chronic demyelinating neurological disease of the central nervous system associated with an abnormal immune response to an environmental factor.

Multiple trauma Trauma that involves serious single-system injury or multiple-system injuries. Also called *major trauma.*

Mural thrombi Blood clots in the heart wall.

Muscle relaxation A relaxation technique that involves consciously tightening and then relaxing each muscle progressively from either head to toe or toe to head.

Mutual recognition model A licensing system that allows a nurse to have a single license that confers the privilege to practice in other states that are part of the Nurse Licensure Compact.

Mutual respect A state in which two or more individuals show or feel honor or esteem toward one another.

Mycobacterium tuberculosis The bacteria that causes tuberculosis.

Mydriasis Abnormal or excessive dilation of the pupil of the eye, usually caused by a disease or drug.

Myelin The fatty, segmented wrappings that normally protect and insulate nerves. Also called *myelin sheath.*

Myelogram A diagnostic technique in which dye is injected into the spinal fluid and visualized by x-ray in order to identify areas of pressure on the spinal cord or nerves due to herniated discs.

Myocardial hypertrophy An increase in the size of muscle cells of the myocardium.

Myometrium The middle muscular layer of the uterus.

Myopia Nearsightedness.

MyPlate A nutrient intake guide from the U.S. Department of Agriculture that outlines suggested food intake by food groups.

Myringotomy A surgical incision of the tympanic membrane.

Myxedema The hypothyroid state with characteristic accumulation of nonpitting edema in the connective tissues throughout the body.

Myxedema coma A life-threatening complication of long-standing, untreated hypothyroidism, usually triggered by an acute illness or trauma.

Nägele rule The most common method of determining the estimated date of birth using the first day of the last menstrual period, subtracting 3 months, and adding 7 days.

NANDA The acronym for North American Nursing Diagnosis Association.

Narcissism Self-centered behavior in which the individual feels entitled to special favors due to a mistaken perception that they are superior to others.

Narcissistic personality disorder (NPD) One of several personality disorders defined in the DSM-5, it is marked by in a pattern of grandiosity, difficulty regulating self-esteem, and the need for admiration and attention from others.

Narcolepsy A disorder characterized by daytime sleep attacks or excessive daytime sleepiness.

Narcotics See **Opioids**.

Narrative charting A traditional part of the source-oriented record. It consists of written notes that include routine care, normal findings, and client problems.

National Institute for Occupational Safety and Health (NIOSH) An organization that focuses on generating new knowledge in the field of occupational safety and health and transferring that knowledge into practice for the betterment of workers.

National Patient Safety Goals (NPSGs) Formulated goals to assist accredited organizations with specific topics about client safety.

Natural killer (NK) cells Large, granular cells found in the spleen, lymph nodes, bone marrow, and blood. NK cells provide immune surveillance and resistance to infection, and they play an important role in the destruction of early malignant cells.

Nature The genetic or hereditary capability of the individual.

Nausea A vague, but unpleasant, subjective sensation of sickness or queasiness.

Necrosis Dead tissue.

Negative affectivity One of the six trait domains associated with personality disorders that is distinguished by anxiousness, emotional lability, separation insecurity, depressive tendencies, perseveration, and suspicion.

Negative airflow room A room where airflow is controlled to prevent the air from circulating into the hallway or other rooms. Multiple fresh-air exchanges dilute the concentration of droplet nuclei in a negative airflow room. Also called *negative flow room*.

Negative feedback Output of a system that returns to the system as input and which inhibits system change.

Negative pressure ventilators A device that creates negative pressure externally to draw the chest outward and air into the lungs, mimicking spontaneous breathing.

Negative punishment The removal of a positive reward if an undesirable behavior occurs.

Negative symptom Loss or absence of a normal function seen in mentally healthy adults, such as the ability to care for one's self; commonly seen in schizophrenia.

Neglect syndrome A disorder of attention that can result from stroke, which is characterized by the inability to integrate and use perceptions from the affected side. Also called *unilateral neglect*.

Negligence Any conduct that deviates from what a reasonable person would do in a particular circumstance.

Neologisms Use of meaningless words that only have meaning to the individual using them.

Neonatal abstinence syndrome (NAS) A combination of neonatal signs and symptoms caused by withdrawal of gestational opioid exposure.

Neonatal anemia A disorder caused by blood loss, hemolysis, and impaired red blood cell production related to birth.

Neonatal mortality risk An infant's chance of death within the first 28 days of life.

Neonatal transition The first few hours after birth, in which a newborn's body systems adapt to extrauterine life.

Neonatology The field of medicine providing care for sick and premature infants.

Neoplasm A mass of new tissue that grows independently of its surrounding structures and has no physiological purpose.

Nephrectomy Removal of a kidney.

Nephritis Inflammation of the kidneys.

Nephrolithiasis The formation of stones in the kidney.

Nephrolithotomy A procedure for removal of a staghorn calculus that invades the calyces and renal parenchyma.

Nephrotoxins Substances that damage nerves or nerve tissue.

Nerve block A chemical interruption of a nerve pathway, effected by injecting a local anesthetic into the nerve.

Networking The act of developing and maintaining relationships with others within and outside of the nursing profession and affiliated organizations to improve nursing practice, advance career goals, offer support, share information, and provide advice.

Neurofibrillary tangles Seen in clients with Alzheimer disease, they are thick, insoluble clots of protein inside the damaged brain cells or neurons.

Neurogenic bladder Interference with the normal mechanisms of urine elimination in which the client does not perceive bladder fullness and is unable to control the urinary sphincters; usually the result of impaired neurological function.

Neurogenic shock The result of an imbalance between parasympathetic and sympathetic stimulation of vascular smooth muscle.

Neuroleptic malignant syndrome (NMS) A potentially fatal condition caused by antipsychotic medications that block dopamine receptors. It is characterized by fever, rigidity, and increased prolactin levels.

Neuron The basic or specialized cell of the nervous system that carries electrical impulses throughout the body.

Neuropathic pain A type of pain experienced by people who have damaged or malfunctioning nerves.

Neurotransmitters Chemical messengers that carry information between neurons.

Neutral question An open-ended question the client can answer without direction or pressure.

Neutral thermal environment (NTE) A specific environmental temperature range in which the rates of oxygen consumption and metabolism are minimal and the internal body temperature is maintained because of thermal balance.

Nevi Moles.

Nevus flammeus A capillary angioma directly below the epidermis. It is a nonelevated, sharply demarcated, red-to-purple area of dense capillaries. In infants of African descent, it may appear as a purple-black stain. Also called *port-wine stain*.

Nevus vasculosus A capillary hemangioma consisting of newly formed and enlarged capillaries in the dermal and subdermal layers. It is a raised, clearly delineated, dark red, rough-surfaced birthmark commonly found in the head region. Also called a *strawberry mark*.

New Ballard score Specific criteria designed for accurate assessment of the gestational age of newborns between 20 and 28 weeks of gestation and weighing less than 1,500 g.

Newborn Infant from birth through the first 28 days of life.

Nicotine A highly addictive chemical that is found in tobacco and enters the body via the lungs (cigarettes, pipes, and cigars) and oral mucous membranes (chewing tobacco as well as smoking).

Nicotine replacement therapy (NRT) A pharmacologic therapy designed to relieve some of the physiological effects of withdrawal, including cravings, for clients trying to quit smoking or using tobacco. NRT transdermal patches and gums are available over the counter; nicotine inhalers and nasal sprays are available by prescription only.

Nicotinic receptors Found in the hippocampus and involved with new sensory information and memory formation, they are thought to be impaired in clients with schizophrenia.

Nidation The cyclical preparation of the uterine lining by steroid hormones for implantation of the embryo.

Nociceptive pain A type of pain resulting from external stimuli on an uninjured, fully functional nervous system.

Nociceptors The nerve receptors for pain.

Nocturia Voiding two or more times at night.

Nocturnal emissions Orgasm and emission of semen during sleep. Also called *wet dreams*.

Nocturnal enuresis Involuntary urination at night after bladder control has been achieved. Also called *bed wetting*.

Nocturnal frequency The need for older adults to arise during the night to urinate.

Nodular basal cell carcinoma A type of skin cancer.

Noise-induced hearing loss (NIHL) A condition associated with prolonged exposure to sound of greater than or equal to 85 dB.

Nolo contendere A term used when an individual neither admits to nor denies committing a crime but agrees to a punishment as if guilty.

Nominal group technique (NGT) A process that alternates between individual work and group work. Individuals meet as a group, but they write their responses without any discussion.

Nondirective interview An unstructured interview in which the nurse allows the client to control the purpose, subject matter, and pacing.

Nonexudative macular degeneration The most common form of macular degeneration, it is characterized by the accumulation of deposits beneath the pigment epithelium of the retina, causing the pigment epithelium to detach and interfere with the sensory function of the macula. Also referred to as the dry form of macular degeneration.

Noninvasive ventilation (NIV) Ventilator support using a tight-fitting face mask, thus avoiding intubation.

Nonmaleficence The duty to do no harm.

Non-Mendelian inheritance Traits that are passed on by the influence of multiple genes. Also called *multifactorial inheritance*.

Nonshivering thermogenesis (NST) The stimulation of heat production in the body through increased cellular metabolism. Also called *chemical thermogenesis*.

Non-small-cell carcinoma Lung cancers other than small-cell carcinoma.

Nonstress test (NST) A widely used method of evaluating fetal status; may be used alone or as part of a more comprehensive diagnostic assessment called a biophysical profile.

Nonunion Failure of the ends of a fracture to heal together after at least 3 months.

Nonverbal communication Transmitting information through gestures, facial expressions, or touch.

Normal sinus rhythm (NSR) The normal heart rhythm, in which impulses originate in the sinus node and travel through all normal conduction pathways without delay.

Normative commitment A feeling of obligation to continue in the profession due to benefits or positive experiences derived from the profession.

Normothermia Normal body temperature.

Nosocomial infections Infections that are associated with the delivery of healthcare services in a facility such as a hospital or nursing home. Also called *healthcare-associated infections (HAIs)*.

NREM Sleep Non-rapid-eye-movement sleep occurs when activity in the *reticular activating system* is inhibited.

Nuclear family A family structure consisting of a husband and wife and their biological children.

Nucleation The formation of a crystal from a liquid.

Nucleotomy The surgical removal of the nucleus pulposus.

Nulligravida Term used to describe a woman who has never been pregnant.

Nullipara Term used to describe a woman who has not given birth to a viable fetus.

Nurse practice act (NPA) State-level statutes that define and regulate nursing practices.

Nursing clinical research Research that seeks to answer questions that ultimately will improve client care.

Nursing diagnosis A clinical judgment about individual, family, or community responses to actual and potential health problems/life processes.

Nursing ethics Ethical issues that occur in nursing practice.

Nursing informatics (NI) A specialty that integrates nursing science, computer science, and information science to manage and communicate data, information, knowledge, and wisdom in nursing practice.

Nursing plan of care A written or electronic guideline that organizes information about an individual client's or family's care.

Nursing process The process used to identify a client's health status and actual or potential healthcare problems or needs, to establish plans to meet the identified needs, to deliver specific nursing interventions to meet those needs, and to evaluate the success of those interventions.

Nursing research A systematic and strict scientific process that tests hypotheses about health-related illness and conditions and processes of nursing care practices.

Nursing transactional model The relationship among the nurse, the client, and the environment in which they interact.

Nurture The effects of the environment on an individual's performance.

Nutrient density The ratio of good nutrients to calories a food contains.

Nutrients Substances found in food used by the body to promote growth, maintenance, and repair.

Nutrition The process by which the body ingests, absorbs, transports, uses, and eliminates nutrients in food.

Nutritional health The physical result of the balance between nutrient intake and nutritional requirements.

Nystagmus Involuntary rapid eye movement.

Obesity An excess of adipose tissue.

Object permanence The ability to understand that when something is out of sight it still exists.

Objective data Information that is detectable by an observer or can be measured or tested against an accepted standard. Also called *overt data* or *signs.*

Objective family burden Actual, identifiable family problems associated with the mental illness of a family member.

Obligatory losses Essential fluid losses required to maintain body functioning.

Observational learning The acquisition of new skills or the alteration of old behaviors simply by watching other children and adults.

Obsession A recurrent, unwanted, and often distressing thought or image that leads to feelings of fear and anxiety.

Obsessive-compulsive disorder (OCD) A disabling disorder characterized by obsessive thoughts and compulsive, repetitive behaviors that dominate an individual's life.

Obsessive–compulsive personality disorder (OCPD) One of several personality disorders defined in the DSM-5, it is marked by fear and anxiety concerning loss of control over situations, objects, or people.

Obstetric conjugate The distance from the middle of the sacral promontory to an area approximately 1 cm below the pubic crest.

Obstructive shock Shock caused by an obstruction in the heart or great vessels that either impedes venous return or prevents effective cardiac pumping action.

Occult blood Blood in stool that cannot be seen with the naked eye.

Occupational exposure Skin, eye, mucous membrane, or parenteral contact with blood or other potentially infectious materials that may result from the performance of an employee's duties.

Occupational Safety and Health Administration (OSHA) An organization that enforces the guidelines presented in the OSHA Act of 1970, requiring its covered employees to report specific incidents and illnesses in a timely manner.

Olfactory Of or relating to smell.

Oligodendrocytes Cells that produce myelin.

Oliguria The production of abnormally small amounts of urine by the kidney.

On–off effect A sudden lack of symptom control and unexpected dyskinesias appearing as drug effectiveness diminishes.

Oncogenes Genes that promote cell proliferation and are capable of triggering cancerous characteristics.

Oncology The study of cancer.

Oncotic pressure A pulling force exerted by colloids that helps maintain the water content of blood by pulling water from the interstitial space into the vascular compartment. Also called *colloid osmotic pressure.*

Oogenesis The process that produces the female gamete, called an ovum (egg).

Open-angle glaucoma The most common form of glaucoma, it is a chronic, gradually progressive disease that typically affects both eyes.

Open-ended question A question that allows clients to discover, explore, elaborate, clarify, or illustrate their thoughts or feelings.

Open fracture A fracture in which the skin integrity is disrupted. Also called a *compound fracture.*

Open reduction and internal fixation (ORIF) The surgical insertion of nails, screws, plates, or pins to hold fractured bones in place.

Opiates A type of drug derived from natural or synthetic opiates that is used as a pain reliever. Opiates include morphine, meperidine, codeine, hydrocodone, and oxycodone.

Opioids Drugs that act on one or more of three opioid receptors: mu, delta, and kappa. They are controlled substances due to their potential for abuse. Also called *narcotics.*

Opportunistic infection An invasion of the body tissue by microorganisms appearing in an individual with immunodeficiency that would normally not affect an individual with an intact immune system.

Opportunistic pathogen A microorganism that causes disease only in susceptible individuals.

Optimism A feeling that things will turn out for the best.

Oral–genital sex Kissing, licking, or sucking of the genitals for sexual pleasure.

Orchiectomy Surgical removal of the testes.

Organizational chart A chart that depicts the formal hierarchical structure and related responsibilities within a traditional organization.

Organizational commitment The relative strength of an individual's relationship and sense of belonging to an organization

Organizing The process of coordinating the work to be done. Formally, it involves identifying the work of the organization, dividing the labor, developing the chain of command, and assigning authority.

Orgasmic phase The third phase of the sexual response cycle that is marked by the involuntary release of sexual tension accompanied by physiological and psychological release.

Orientation 1. A structured program of activities to help new employees adapt to their new workplace; it is geared toward helping newly employed nurses to be successful. **2.** A newborn's ability to be alert to, follow, and fixate on appealing and attractive, complex visual stimuli.

Orthopnea Difficulty breathing when supine.

Orthopneic position A body position with the head and arms supported on the overbed table to facilitate breathing.

Orthotic devices Orthopedic devices that may include splints or braces applied to reduce strain on a joint.

Ortolani maneuver A procedure used to evaluate an infant for developmental dysplastic hip.

Osmolality A measure of the concentration of solutes in body fluids. Osmolality is determined by the total solute concentration within a fluid compartment and is measured as parts of solute per kilogram of water.

Osmolar imbalance A fluid imbalance that involves the loss or gain of only water, so that the osmolality of the serum is altered.

Osmosis The movement of water across cell membranes, from a less concentrated solution to a more concentrated solution.

Osmotic pressure The power of a solution to draw water across a semipermeable membrane.

Ossification The development of bone.

Osteoarthritis (OA) The most common form of arthritis in older adults. It is caused by chronic degenerative changes in the cartilage and synovial membranes of the joints.

Osteoblasts Cells that form bone.

Osteoclasts Cells that resorb bone.

Osteocytes Cells that maintain bone matrix.

Osteodystrophy A complex bone disease process of chronic kidney disease in which chronic hyperparathyroidism causes increased resorption of bone.

Osteomyelitis Infection of the bone in a compound fracture.

Osteophytes Bony spurs that form as cartilage deteriorates.

Osteoporosis A metabolic bone disorder characterized by loss of bone mass, increased bone fragility, and increased risk of fractures.

Osteotomy 1. Surgical removal of a wedge of bones above or below a joint to realign the joint and shift weight away from the damaged potion of a joint. 2. An incision into or transection of the bone.

Otitis externa Inflammation of the ear canal. It is often called *swimmer's ear* because it is most frequently found in people who spend significant time in the water.

Otitis interna An inflammation of the inner ear. Also called *labyrinthitis*.

Otitis media Inflammation of the middle ear.

Otoscope A handheld instrument with a light and a cone-shaped attachment; known as an *ear speculum*.

Outcome The specific, observable criteria used to evaluate whether goals have been met and the effectiveness of nursing actions.

Outcome standards Standards that focus on the performance of a process, such as the number of bedridden clients who develop a pressure ulcer.

Outcomes management Management process that uses client experiences to guide improvement in all areas of health care by providing a link between medical interventions and health outcomes and between health outcomes and the cost of care.

Output Energy, material, or information that a system gives out as a result of its processes.

Ovarian cycle The three cyclical phases of oogenesis that occur about every 28 days.

Ovarian ligaments Ligaments that anchor the lower pole of the ovary to the uterus.

Ovaries Female sex glands in which the ova are formed and in which estrogen and progesterone are produced. Normally, a woman has two ovaries.

Overdelegation A situation that occurs when a delegator loses control over a situation by providing a delegate with too much authority or too much responsibility. This places the delegator in a risky position, increasing the potential for liability.

Overnutrition Health effects caused by excesses in nutrient intake or stores, such as obesity, hypertension, hypercholesterolemia, or toxic levels of stored vitamins or minerals.

Overt conflict Conflict that is addressed openly and is generally obvious to the individuals involved.

Ovulation Normal process of discharging a mature ovum from an ovary approximately 14 days before the onset of menses.

Oxygenation The mechanism that facilitates or impairs the body's ability to supply oxygen to all cells of the body.

Pacemaker An external or implanted pulse generator used to provide an electrical stimulus to the heart when the heart fails to generate or conduct its own stimulus at a rate that maintains the cardiac output.

$PaCO_2$ A measure of the pressure exerted by dissolved carbon dioxide in the blood; it reflects the respiratory component of acid–base regulation and balance because it is regulated by the lungs.

Pain An unpleasant sensory and emotional experience associated with actual or potential tissue damage.

Pain threshold The point at which pain is initially perceived.

Pain tolerance The duration of time or intensity of pain an individual will endure before demonstrating pain responses.

Palliation Measures taken not to cure a disease, but to relieve disease-related symptoms and enhance the client's quality of life. See also **Palliative care**.

Palliative care Nursing care that improves the quality of life of clients and their families facing life-threatening illness by preventing, assessing, and treating pain and other physical, psychosocial, and spiritual problems.

Palliative procedure A surgical or interventional cardiac catheterization procedure that does not create normal anatomical or hemodynamic results but allows adequate blood flow to oxygenate the tissues.

Pallidotomy A surgical technique for Parkinson disease in which the neurosurgeon locates the affected areas of the globus pallidus and destroys the involved tissue in order to improve tremors and mobility.

Palpation A method of assessment that involves touching the areas related to the body system to determine symmetry, equality of the size, shape, or condition of opposite sides of the body.

Pancreatitis Inflammation of the pancreas that occurs when pancreatic enzymes are released into the pancreas itself, causing autodigestion of pancreatitic tissues.

Pandemic Widespread global outbreak of an infectious disease.

Panic disorder A sudden attack of terror, sometimes accompanied by a pounding heart, sweating, fainting, or dizziness.

Pannus An abnormal tissue layer that includes newly formed blood vessels. Pannus leads to scar tissue formation that immobilizes joints.

PaO_2 A measure of the pressure exerted by oxygen that is dissolved in the plasma.

Para Term used to describe a woman who has borne offspring who reached the age of viability.

Paracentesis Aspiration of fluid from the peritoneal cavity.

Parallel play A stage of play in which toddlers play side by side with similar objects, but do not play together.

Paranoia An extreme suspicion that others are "out to get you" and delusions that one is being followed and that others are trying to harm oneself; experienced by some individuals with psychosis.

Paranoid personality disorder (PPD) One of several personality disorders defined in the DSM-5, it is characterized by the inability to trust others, hypervigilance, pathological jealousy, and prejudicial and judgmental tendencies.

Paraplegia Paralysis of all or part of the lower portion of the body.

Parasite One of the four categories of microorganisms, parasites live on other organisms.

Parasomnias Abnormal behaviors that may interfere with sleep and may occur during sleep

Parenteral nutrition (PN) The intravenous administration of amino acids, often with added carbohydrates, fats, electrolytes, vitamins, and minerals.

Parenting The ongoing act of guiding children to learn acceptable behaviors, morals, and rituals of the family and of teaching them to become socially responsible, contributing members of society.

Paresis Weakness.

Paresthesia Sensation of prickling, tingling, or numbing.

Parkinson disease (PD) A degenerative disorder of the central nervous system resulting from the death of neurons that produce the brain neurotransmitter dopamine.

Parkinsonian gait Altered gait characterized by small, shuffling steps, as well as bradykinesia or festination.

Parkinsonism The motor symptoms of Parkinson disease: tremors, muscle rigidity, postural instability, and bradykinesia.

Paroxysmal Occurring in bursts with an abrupt onset and termination.

Paroxysmal nocturnal dyspnea A sudden episode of shortness of breath occurring at night during sleep.

Partial-thickness burns Burns that involve the entire dermis and the papillae of the dermis (superficial partial-thickness burns) or extend into the hair follicles (deep partial-thickness burns).

Passive acquired immunity A condition that occurs when a pregnant woman passes IgG antibodies to a fetus in utero.

Passive behavior Behavior that seeks to avoid conflict at any cost, even at the expense of one's own happiness.

Passive communicators Individuals who focus on the needs of others. They often deny themselves any sort of power, which causes them to become frustrated.

Passive immunity Temporary protection—provided by antibodies produced by other people or animals—against disease-producing antigens. Protection is gradually lost when these acquired antibodies are used up either by natural degradation or by combining with the antigen.

Patch testing A test used to identify allergens causing dermatitis. An adhesive patch with common allergens is placed on the back between the scapulae. The patch is generally removed after several days; if there is no reaction to a particular allergen, that allergen is eliminated as a possible cause of dermatitis.

Patent airway An airway that is open and free of obstruction.

Patent ductus arteriosus (PAD) A congenital connection between the great vessels that normally closes after birth, allowing blood from the right and left side of the heart to mix.

Pathogen A microorganism that causes disease.

Pathogenicity The ability to produce disease.

Pathological fracture A fracture that results from disease that has weakened the bone.

Patient An individual who is waiting for or undergoing medical treatment and care.

Patient-controlled analgesia (PCA) A pump with a control mechanism that allows the client to self-manage pain.

Patient Protection and Affordable Care Act (PPACA or ACA) A law that regulates health care and attempts to make health care affordable for all Americans. Also called *Obamacare* after President Barak Obama, the U.S. president when the ACA was enacted.

Patient Self-Determination Act (PSDA) A federal law that requires every competent adult to be informed in writing on admission to a healthcare institution about his or her rights to accept or refuse medical care and to use advance directives.

Pauciarticular arthritis A form of juvenile rheumatoid arthritis that primarily affects the knees, ankles, and elbows; it occurs more frequently in females.

Peak expiratory flow rate (PEFR) A measurement used to monitor the ability of an individual to exhale a specific volume of air related to the individual's age, gender, height, and weight.

Pedagogy The study or science of teaching, specifically referring to children and adolescents.

Pedigree The graphic representation of a family tree, usually to trace genetic abnormalities.

Peer review A method to professionally critique a colleague's work based on predetermined standards.

Pelvic cavity Bony portion of the birth passage; a curved canal with a longer posterior than anterior wall.

Pelvic diaphragm Part of the pelvic floor, composed of deep fascia and the levator ani and the coccygeal muscles.

Pelvic inlet Upper border of the true pelvis.

Pelvic outlet Lower border of the true pelvis.

Pelvic tilt An exercise that helps prevent or reduce back strain as it strengthens abdominal muscles. Also called *pelvic rocking*.

Penetrating injury A type of eye injury in which the layers of the eye spontaneously reapproximate after entry of a sharp-pointed object or small missile (e.g., a BB) into the globe.

Penetrating trauma Trauma that occurs when a foreign object enters the body, causing damage to body structures.

Penta screen Maternal screening that measures five indicators whose presence may suggest fetal complications: AFP, beta hCG, unconjugated estriol, inhibin A, and invasive trophoblast antigen.

Penumbra A band of minimally perfused cells that surrounds a central core of dead or dying cells.

Peplau, Hildegard A nursing theorist who is widely considered the mother of psychiatric nursing; she presented nursing as a therapeutic interpersonal process, rather than as a task-oriented process.

Peptic ulcer A break in the mucosal lining of the GI tract exposed to acid-pepsin secretions, including the esophagus, stomach, and duodenum.

Peptic ulcer disease (PUD) A break in the mucous lining of the GI tract where it comes in contact with gastric juice.

Perceived loss A loss that is experienced by one person but cannot be verified by others.

Perception Awareness and interpretation of stimuli; the ability of the individual to interpret the environment.

Percussion A method of tapping the chest or back to assess underlying structures. Forceful striking of the skin with cupped hands, sometimes called *clapping*.

Perforating injury A type of eye injury in which the layers of the eye do not spontaneously reapproximate after the entry of a sharp-pointed object or small missile (e.g., a BB) into the globe, which results in rupture of the globe and potential loss of ocular contents.

Perforation Rupture, as in the penetration of ulcer through mucosal wall.

Performance improvement Quality of care improvement is directly linked to the performance of an individual, team, unit, or organization.

Pericarditis Inflammation of the pericardial tissue surrounding the heart.

Pericardium A double layer of fibroserous membrane that encases and anchors the heart.

Perimetrium The outermost layer of the uterus.

Perinatal loss Death of a fetus or infant that occurs between the time of conception and the end of the newborn period 28 days after birth.

Perineal body The wedge-shaped mass of fibromuscular tissue between the lower part of the vagina and the anus.

Periodic breathing A breathing pattern characterized by pauses lasting 5–15 seconds.

Periodontal disease Gum disease.

Perioperative The three phases of a surgical procedure: the pre-operative phase, intraoperative phase, and postoperative phase.

Perioperative nursing care Nursing care provided during any or all of the three phases of surgery: preoperative, intraoperative, and postoperative.

Peripartum cardiomyopathy A rare but serious dysfunction of the left ventricle that occurs in the last month of pregnancy or the first 5 months postpartum in a woman with no previous history of heart disease.

Peripheral nervous system (PNS) One of two principal parts of the neurological system, the peripheral nervous system consists of the cranial nerves and the spinal nerves.

Peripheral neuropathy A condition that results when trauma or a disease process interferes with innervation of peripheral nerves.

Peripheral pulse A pulse located away from the heart, in the foot or the wrist.

Peripheral vascular disease (PVD) A disorder in which arteriosclerosis and atherosclerosis affect circulation to peripheral tissues, particularly the lower extremities.

Peripheral vascular resistance The opposing forces or impedance to blood flow as the arterial channels become more and more distant from the heart.

Peristalsis The process of wavelike muscular contractions that propels food and digestive products through the digestive tract.

Peritoneal dialysis The process by which dialysate is instilled into the abdominal cavity through a catheter, allowed to rest there while fluids and molecules exchange, and then removed through the catheter.

Peritonitis Inflammation and bacterial infection of the abdominal area.

Pernicious anemia A disorder that results from a failure to absorb dietary vitamin B_{12}.

Perseveration Use of the same words or phrases repetitively.

Persistent A term used to describe a disease or disorder (such as rheumatoid arthritis) that lasts for a period of 3–6 months or longer.

Persistent bacteriuria The reappearance of bacteria in urine due to a persistent source of infection causing repeated infection after the initial cure.

Persistent depressive disorder Chronic depression that affects an individual for the majority of most days for at least 2 years (1 year for children and adolescents). May be interrupted by periods of normal mood that do not exceed 2 months over the course of the 2 years. Also called *dysthymic disorder*.

Persistent vegetative state A permanent condition of complete unawareness of self and the environment and loss of all cognitive functions. Also called *irreversible coma*.

Personal distance Communication characterized by moderate voice tones, less noticeable body heat and smell. Physical contact such as a handshake or touching a shoulder is possible.

Personal identity The conscious sense of individuality and uniqueness that is continually evolving throughout life.

Personal knowing A nurse's commitment to ongoing, individual self-exploration and self-actualization.

Personal space The distance people prefer in interactions with others.

Personality The individual qualities, including habitual behavior patterns, that make an individual unique; the outward expression of the inner self.

Personality disorder (PD) Rigid, stereotyped behavioral patterns that deviate markedly from the norm of an individual's culture and persist throughout the person's life. Personality disorders are characterized by a lifelong maladaptive pattern of perceiving, thinking, and relating that impairs social or occupational functioning.

Personality traits The elements and patterns that comprise an individual's personality.

Pessimism A feeling that a situation is always bad and may become worse.

pH A measurement of the hydrogen ion concentration of a solution.

Phagocytosis A process by which a foreign agent or target cell is engulfed, destroyed, and digested. Neutrophils and macrophages, known as phagocytes, are the primary cells involved in phagocytosis.

Phantom pain A confusing pain syndrome that occurs following surgical or traumatic amputation of a limb. The client experiences pain in the missing body part even though there is complete mental awareness that the limb is gone. Also called *phantom limb syndrome*.

Phase of mutual regulation Time period during which a mother and her infant seek to determine the degree of control each partner in their relationship will exert. In this phase of adjustment, a balance is sought between the needs of the mother and the needs of the infant.

Phenotype The observable expression of genetic traits.

Philadelphia chromosome The balanced translocation of chromosome 22 to chromosome 9; associated with chronic myeloid leukemia.

Phimosis Tightness of the prepuce that prevents retraction of the foreskin.

Phobia An intense, persistent, irrational fear of a simple thing or social situation that compels the individual to avoid the stressor that elicits the fear.

Photophobia Sensitivity to light.

Physical activity Body movement produced by skeletal muscle contraction that increases energy expenditure.

Physical attending The conveyed act of being with another individual through physical posturing.

Physical restraint Any manual method, material, device, or equipment that is attached to the client's body with the intention of limiting or restricting free movement of the client's head, arms, legs, or body.

Physiological anemia of infancy A type of anemia that occurs as a result of the normal, gradual drop in hemoglobin for the first 6–12 weeks of life.

Physiological anemia of pregnancy Apparent anemia that results because during pregnancy the plasma volume increases more than the erythrocytes increase. Also called *pseudoanemia.*

Physiological jaundice A yellow discoloration of the skin caused by accelerated destruction of fetal red blood cells, impaired conjugation of bilirubin, and increased bilirubin reabsorption from the intestinal tract.

Physiological pain Experienced when an intact, properly functioning nervous system sends signals that tissues are damaged, requiring attention and proper care.

Pica The craving for and persistent eating of nonnutritive substances not ordinarily considered to be edible or nutritionally valuable, such as soil, clay, and soap.

PICOT A mnemonic method used by clinicians to define and formulate a clinical question driving the search for evidence-based practice. PICOT stands for Population of a group, Intervention or activity focus, Comparison group, Outcome(s) or desired effects, and Time frame.

Pigmented basal cell carcinoma A type of skin cancer.

Pill-rolling Rubbing of the thumb and fingers together accompanying other tremors.

Piloerection Goosebumps.

Pitch The frequency of vibrations in a sound.

Pitfalls A hidden trap that catches people unaware and undermines their plans.

Pitting edema Edema that retains indentation caused by pressure.

Placenta A flat, disc-shaped organ that is highly vascular and normally forms in the upper segment of the endometrium of the uterus; exchanges nutrients and gases between the fetus and the mother.

Placenta previa Occurs when the placenta partially or totally covers the mother's cervix; can result in severe bleeding before or during delivery.

Placental abruption A condition that occurs when the placenta detaches from the uterine wall before delivery. May or may not result in fetal demise, but a fetus's survival depends on the stage of development and prompt medical treatment.

Plan–do–study–act (PDSA) A system of quality improvement most often associated with total quality management.

Planning The four-stage, managerial process that establishes objectives, evaluates the present situation in order to predict future trends and events, formulates a planning statement, and converts the plan into an action statement.

Plaque 1. An invisible soft film that adheres to the enamel surface of teeth. Consists of bacteria, saliva molecules, and remnants of epithelial cells and leukocytes. 2. Scar tissue on myelin sheath due to repeated attacks by the immune system.

Plasmapheresis Removal of a harmful component from plasma. Also called *plasma exchange therapy.*

Play therapist A therapist who designs and provides recreational activities to promote emotional and/or physical healing and wellness.

Pleural effusion Accumulation of excess fluid in the pleural cavity.

Pleuritic pain Sharp localized chest pain that increases with breathing and coughing.

Pleuritis Local extension of an infection to involve the pleura.

Pleximeter The middle finger of the nondominant hand. Often used in indirect percussion techniques.

Plexor The middle finger of the dominant hand. Often used in indirect percussion techniques.

Pneumatic retinopexy A surgical procedure to correct retinal detachment in which air is injected into the vitreous cavity and the client is positioned so that the air bubble pushes the detached portion of the retina into contact with the choroid.

Pneumocystis carinii pneumonia (PCP) An opportunistic infection that is not pathogenic in those with intact immune systems.

Pneumomediastinum The presence of air in the mediastinum.

Pneumonia Inflammation of the lung parenchyma (the respiratory bronchioles and alveoli).

Pneumopericardium Air in the pericardial sac.

Pneumothorax A partial lung collapse due to air or gas collecting in the lung or in the pleural space that surrounds the lungs.

Point of care Interventions or testing that provides on-the-spot information about the client rather than having to send blood or urine samples down to the laboratory and wait for results to be returned.

Point of maximal impulse (PMI) A pulse located at the apex of the heart. Also called the *apical pulse.*

Point-of-service (POS) plan An insurance plan that allows the insured to choose between a health maintenance organization or a preferred provider organization each time they seek health care.

Polyarticular arthritis A form of juvenile rheumatoid arthritis that involves many joints (five or more), particularly the small joints of the hands and fingers. It may also affect the hips, knees, feet, ankles, and neck.

Polycyclic Describes a periodically recurring course of rheumatoid arthritis.

Polycythemia An increase in the production of red blood cells.

Polydipsia Excessive thirst.

Polyneuropathies Bilateral sensory disorders; they are the most common types of neuropathy associated with diabetes.

Polyp A small vascular growth on the surface of any mucous membrane.

Polyphagia Excessive hunger.

Polysomnography (PSG) A recording of the biophysical changes that a client experiences during sleep.

Polysubstance abuse The simultaneous use of many substances.

Polytheism The belief in more than one god.

Polyuria The production of abnormally large amounts of urine. Also called *diuresis*.

Pop-ups Unexpected things or events occurring during the day that require time and attention in addition to the regular plan for the day.

Positive end-expiratory pressure (PEEP) Mechanical ventilation in which a positive pressure is maintained in the airways during exhalation and between breaths to help keep alveoli open.

Positive feedback Output of a system that returns to the system as input and which promotes system change.

Positive pressure ventilator A mechanical device that pushes air into the lungs through an invasive device such as an endotracheal tube or tracheostomy tube, rather than drawing air in by negative pressure.

Positive punishment The addition of a negative consequence if undesirable behavior occurs.

Positive reinforcement Giving rewards such as praise or encouragement for a learner's achievements.

Positive symptoms Excessive or added behaviors that are not normally seen in healthy adults, such as delusions; commonly seen in schizophrenia.

Postcoital contraception A drug taken after intercourse to avoid pregnancy. Also called *Plan B* or the *morning after pill*.

Postconception age periods Period of time in embryonic/fetal development calculated from the time of fertilization of the ovum.

Postictal period A period immediately following seizure activity in which level of consciousness is decreased. The length of the postictal period varies.

Postoperative The third phase of an operative process in which recovery occurs.

Postpartal hemorrhage A loss of blood of greater than 500 mL following birth. The hemorrhage is classified as *early* if it occurs within the first 24 hours and *late* if it occurs after the first 24 hours.

Postpartum After childbirth.

Postpartum blues A maternal adjustment reaction occurring in the first few postpartum days, characterized by mild depression, tearfulness, anxiety, headache, and irritability. Also called *adjustment reaction to depressed mood*.

Postpartum depression A severe form of depression that affects new mothers, often beginning within 3 months of delivery but which may strike at any time during the first year after having a child. Also called *depressive disorder with peripartum onset*.

Postpartum psychosis Severe psychosis occurring within the first 3 months after birth that usually requires hospitalization.

Postterm labor Labor that occurs after 42 weeks' gestation.

Postterm newborn Any infant born after 42 weeks' gestation.

Postterm pregnancy Pregnancy that lasts beyond 42 weeks' gestation.

Posttraumatic stress disorder (PTSD) A trauma- and stressor-related disorder that can evolve after exposure to a traumatic or overwhelming event in which an individual's physical health was endangered.

Postural drainage The drainage by gravity of secretions from various lung segments.

PPD Tuberculin skin test. See **Purified protein derivative**.

Prader–Willi syndrome (PWS) A congenital disorder of the 15th chromosome that causes an unrelenting feeling of hunger, but also low muscle tone, short stature, incomplete sexual development, mild to severe mental retardation, and behavioral problems.

Prayer Human communication with divine and spiritual entities.

Preceptor An experienced nurse who provides knowledge and emotional support, as well as a clarification of role expectations, on a one-to-one basis.

Precipitating factor A practice, behavior, or environmental factor that gives rise to a specific incident of violence.

Predisposing factor A practice, behavior, or environmental factor that increases the potential of an individual's risk of violent victimization or perpetration of violence.

Preeclampsia An increase in blood pressure after 20 weeks of gestation accompanied by proteinuria. May also be accompanied by albuminuria and edema. Also called *toxemia of pregnancy*.

Preferred provider organization (PPO) A type of health insurance program that does not require its insureds to select a primary care provider. PPOs usually have larger networks of providers than health maintenance organizations (HMOs) and provide financial incentives that encourage insureds to seek care from in-network providers. They are less restrictive than HMOs but typically have higher copayments.

Prejudice A negative belief or preference that is generalized about a group that leads to prejudgment.

Preload The amount of cardiac muscle fiber tension, or stretch, that exists at the end of diastole.

Premature junctional contractions Heartbeats that occur before the next expected beat of the underlying rhythm.

Premature rupture of membranes (PROM) Spontaneous rupture of membranes and leakage of amniotic fluid before the onset of labor at any gestational age.

Premenstrual syndrome (PMS) A complex of manifestations (e.g., mood swings, breast tenderness, fatigue, irritability, food cravings, and depression) that occurs to 3–14 days before menstruation and is relieved by the onset of menses.

Prenatal education Programs offered to expectant families, adolescents, women, or partners to provide education regarding the pregnancy, labor, and birth experience.

Preoperative The first phase of an operative process in which the client is identified as a candidate for surgical intervention, assessed, and prepared for surgery.

Preparedness The phase that takes place before an emergency occurs during which risks are assessed and plans are developed to address them.

Presbycusis Age-related loss of the ability to hear high-frequency sounds; may occur because of cochlear hair cell degeneration or loss of auditory neurons in the organ of Corti.

Presbyopia Impaired near vision resulting from a loss of elasticity of the lens related to aging.

Presencing Being present with a client and being open, receptive, and available at all levels without judging or labeling.

Presenting part The first part of the fetus to enter and settle in the pelvic inlet during fetal presentation.

Pressure ulcer Ischemic lesions of the skin and underlying tissue caused by external pressure that impairs the flow of blood and lymph.

Preterm infant An infant born at less than 37 completed weeks of gestation.

Preterm premature rupture of the membranes (PPROM) A condition that occurs when membranes rupture and amniotic fluid leaks from the vagina before 37 weeks of gestation.

Pretibial myxedema The bilateral formation of edematous, erythematous, and sometimes hyperpigmented plaques and nodules over the shins and dorsal surface of the feet. A characteristic sign of Graves disease.

Priapism Persistent, painful erection of the penis.

Primary appraisal The evaluation of an event or circumstance in terms of its potential to harm, benefit, threaten, or challenge the individual.

Primary care provider (PCP) A healthcare provider who provides basic medical service and acts as a gatekeeper to more specialized care, referring clients to in-network hospitals and specialists.

Primary group A small, intimate group in which the relationships among members are personal, spontaneous, sentimental, cooperative, and inclusive.

Primary hypertension A persistently elevated systemic blood pressure. Also called *essential hypertension.*

Primary immune response When an individual is exposed to antigen, the B-lymphocyte system produces antibodies that react specifically with that antigen over the first 3 days.

Primary intention healing Healing that occurs where the tissue surfaces have been closed and there is minimal or no tissue loss. It is characterized by the formation of minimal granulation tissue and scarring. Also called *primary union* or *first intention healing.*

Primary nursing A model in which one nurse has 24/7 authority and responsibility for the care of an assigned group of clients.

Primary prevention Methods designed to focus on health promotion and illness prevention.

Primigravida A woman who is pregnant for the first time.

Primipara Term used to describe a woman who has given birth to her first child (past the point of viability), whether or not that child is living or was alive at birth.

Principles-based (deontological) theories Theories that involve logical and formal processes and emphasize individual rights, duties, and obligations.

Prioritizing care A process that helps nurses manage time and establish an order for completing responsibilities and care interventions for a single client or for a group of clients.

Priority Something given or meriting attention before competing alternatives.

Privacy The right of individuals to keep their personal information from being disclosed.

Private insurance Health insurance provided by private or publicly owned companies such as Blue Cross Blue Shield, Kaiser, or Aetna.

Problem-focused coping Managing or altering a stressor, event, or circumstance in response to distress.

Problem, intervention, evaluation (PIE) An assessment system consisting of client care flow sheets and progress notes.

Problem-oriented medical record (POMR) A recording system in which data are arranged according to the problems the client has rather than the source of the information. Also called *problem-oriented record (POR).*

Problem-oriented record (POR) See Problem-oriented medical record (POMR).

Procedural memory Recall of information that does not require conscious awareness and involves the memory of motor skills and procedures.

Process addictions Compulsive behaviors that serve to reduce anxiety such as workaholism, gambling, shopping, cutting, pornography, spending and indebtedness, Internet surfing or gaming, eating disorders, and sexual addictions.

Process standards Standards that focus on the steps used to lead to a particular outcome. It is used to determine if a set of steps exists and if those steps are being followed.

Productivity The performance measure of both the effectiveness and efficiency of nursing care.

Profession An occupation that requires extensive education or a calling that requires special knowledge, skill, and preparation.

Professional behaviors Effective nursing actions based on ethical principles, clinical reasoning, and technical knowledge and expertise that form helping relationships.

Professional development Continued staff education, planned activities to enhance role performance, and defined goals to improve client outcomes. Also called *staff development.*

Professional support Assistance provided by professionals in the community who exhibit a nonblaming and respectful attitude toward families and clients and who provide information and help locating community resources.

Professionalism Acting with the knowledge, skill, and preparation of a professional.

Professionalization The process of establishing qualifications, ethical guidelines, and a standardized knowledge base by which an occupation transforms itself into a profession.

Progesterone Hormone produced by the corpus luteum, adrenal cortex, and placenta whose function is to stimulate proliferation of the endometrium to facilitate growth of the embryo.

Projectile vomiting Vomiting in which emesis may be spewed up to 2–3 feet out of a baby's mouth. A major symptom of pyloric stenosis.

Prone Face-down.

Proprioception The body's sense of its position.

Proptosis Forward displacement of the eye.

Prospective payment system (PPS) A system in which hospitals determine the amount to be billed to the insurance company before the client is ever admitted to the hospital.

Prostaglandins (PGs) Complex lipid compounds synthesized by many cells of the body.

Prostate specific antigen (PSA) A protein produced in the cells of the prostate gland.

Prostatectomy Surgical removal of part or all of the prostate gland.

Prostatitis An inflammation of the prostate gland.

Prostatodynia A condition in which the client experiences the symptoms of prostatitis, but shows no evidence of inflammation or infection.

Protected health information Personal information or healthcare data that could identify an individual. This information is protected and defined by HIPAA's Privacy Rule.

Protective factor 1. A practice, behavior, or environmental factor that provides strength and assistance to children and families in dealing with crises and risk factors. 2. A practice, behavior, or environmental factor that decreases the potential of individual to perpetuate violence or victimization.

Protein A macronutrient that contains nitrogen and is a critical component of all tissues in the human body, including muscle, bone, and blood.

Protein-calorie malnutrition Problem of clients with long-term deficiencies in caloric intake; characteristics include depressed visceral proteins (e.g., albumin), weight loss, and visible muscle and fat wasting.

Proteinuria Excess protein in urine.

Proxemics The study of distance between people in their interactions.

Proximodistal Growth that proceeds from the center of the body outward.

Proximodistal development Development that proceeds from the center of the body outward.

Pruritus Itching of the skin.

Pseudoaddiction A term applied to clients who display drug-seeking behaviors but differ from addicts in that they have true underlying pain for which they are seeking relief. These behaviors will generally stop when adequate pain control is achieved.

Pseudoexacerbation A temporary aggravation of symptoms that is directly related to a trigger and subsides as soon as the trigger is removed.

Pseudomenstruation Blood or whitish discharge may occasionally be observed on the diapers of female newborns caused by the withdrawal of maternal hormones.

Purified protein derivative (PPD) Used to screen for tuberculosis in a tuberculin test. A small amount of the PPD is injected and the body's response interpreted.

Purulent exudate A large quantity of cells and necrotic debris that form an opaque or milky discharge that is thicker than serous exudate. Also called *pus* or *suppuration*.

Pus The common name for *purulent exudate*.

Psychoanalytic theory A framework for personality development that emphasizes the presence of unconscious impulses and their influence on behaviors and the formation of self; developed by Sigmund Freud (1856-1939).

Psychogenic pain Pain that is experienced in the absence of any diagnosed physiological cause or event.

Psychomotor domain The learning domain that includes fine motor skills. Also called the *skill domain*.

Psychomotor retardation A state in which thinking and body movements are noticeably slower than normal and speech is slowed or absent.

Psychosis A mental health condition characterized by delusions, hallucinations, illusions, disorganized behavior, and a difficulty relating to others. Also called *psychotic disorder*.

Psychosocial skills Skills that enable an individual in crisis to maintain relationships with family and friends throughout and after the crisis period.

Psychostimulants Stimulants that have a high potential for abuse. Psychostimulants include cocaine and amphetamines.

Psychoticism One of the six trait domains associated with personality disorders that is composed of eccentricity, cognitive and perceptual dysregulation, and unusual beliefs and experiences.

Ptosis Drooping of the eyelid.

Ptyalism Excessive, often bitter salivation.

Puberty The stage during which an individual reaches sexual maturity.

Pubis Pertaining to the pubes or pubic area.

Public distance Communication that requires loud, clear vocalizations with careful enunciation.

Public insurance Health insurance financed by the government.

Public self How the individual wishes to be perceived by others.

Puerperium That time immediately following childbirth during which physiological changes that occurred during pregnancy begin to return to normal. Also called *postpartum period*.

Pulmonary atresia The absence of communication between the right ventricle and the pulmonary artery.

Pulmonary circulation Circulation through the right side of the heart, the pulmonary artery, the pulmonary capillaries, and the pulmonary vein.

Pulmonary edema An abnormal accumulation of fluid in the interstitial tissue and alveoli of the lung.

Pulmonary embolism (PE) The obstruction of blood flow in part of the pulmonary vascular system by an embolus. Also called *pulmonary thromboembolism*.

Pulmonary function test (PFT) A test designed to provide information about ventilation airflow, lung volume, and the capacity and diffusion of gas.

Pulmonary vascular resistance The force or resistance of the blood in the pulmonary circulation.

Pulse A wave of blood created by the contraction of the left ventricle of the heart.

Pulse oximetry A noninvasive method of assessing arterial blood oxygenation.

Pulse pressure The difference between the systolic and diastolic pressure.

Pulse rhythm The pattern of the beats and the intervals between the beats.

Punctual On time.

Punishment 1. Action taken to enforce rules when a child misbehaves. 2. Consequences that lead to a decrease in undesirable behavior.

Pupillary light reflex Reflex in which the pupil contracts in response to a bright light.

Purging Self-induced vomiting or misuse of laxatives, diuretics, or enemas.

Pursed-lipped breathing Exhaling through a narrow opening between the lips to prolong the expiratory phase in an effort to promote more alveolar emptying while maintaining open alveoli.

Pyelolithotomy An incision into and removal of a stone from the kidney pelvis.

Pyelonephritis Inflammation of the renal pelvis and parenchyma, the functional kidney tissue.

Pyloric stenosis A thickening of the pyloric muscle resulting in a narrowing of the pyloric sphincter between the stomach and small intestine.

Pyogenic bacteria Bacteria that produces purulent exudate or pus.

Pyorrhea Advanced periodontal disease.

Pyuria Cloudy or pus-filled urine.

Quadriplegia Complete loss of function of the upper and lower body, including the arms, trunk, legs, and pelvic organs. Also called *tetraplegia*.

Quadruple screen The most widely used test to screen for Down syndrome (trisomy 21), trisomy 18, and neural tube defects.

Qualifiers Words that have been added to some NANDA nursing diagnosis labels to give additional meaning to the diagnostic statement.

Qualitative research Investigates a question through narrative data from interviews, storytelling, and description of observation to provide a better understanding of the client's perspective.

Quality 1. A subjective description of a sound, for example: whistling, gurgling, or snapping. 2. The degree to which health services for individuals and populations increase the likelihood of desired health outcomes and are consistent with current professional knowledge.

Quality and Safety Education for Nurses (QSEN) A program designed to identify and standardize the six core competencies or nursing: patient-centered care, teamwork and collaboration, evidence-based practice, quality improvement, safety, and informatics.

Quality assurance The process of collecting data related to a problem and then analyzing the data based on benchmark standards to determine if standards are being met.

Quality improvement The process of using systematic and continuous actions that lead to measurable improvement in healthcare services and the health status of targeted client groups.

Quality management The evaluation of medical and nursing processes for quality and effectiveness compared to accepted standards in order to correct problems before they harm clients and to prevent errors in treatment.

Quantitative research Uses precise measurements for data collection and employs statistical analysis to provide specific and objective data about a topic.

Quickening The mother's perception of fetal movement.

Race A term used to describe socially defined populations that share genetically transmitted physical characteristics, such as skin color and bone structure.

Racism The oppression of a group of people based on their perceived race.

Radiation The process of heat transfer with no physical contact.

Radiation cataracts A type of cataract that may result from long-term exposure to radiation.

Radical mastectomy The removal of an entire affected breast, its underlying chest muscles, and the lymph nodes under the arms. Compare with **Simple mastectomy**.

Range of motion (ROM) The degree to which a joint can be moved; a measurement of flexion and extension.

Range-of-motion (ROM) exercises Exercises designed to take each joint through all possible movements to maintain flexibility and movement in the joint.

Rape Any penetration, no matter how slight, of the vagina or anus with any body part or object, or oral penetration by a sex organ of another person, without the consent of the victim.

Rape-trauma syndrome (RTS) A series of psychological sequelae that many victims experience following rape in addition to physiological sequelae.

Rapport An understanding between two or more people.

Readiness to learn The demonstration of behaviors or cues that reflect a learner's motivation to learn at a specific time.

Real self The perceived true self.

Reappraisal An individual's ongoing evaluation and reinterpretation of an event or circumstance, as well as continued evaluation of the efficacy of the coping strategies.

Receiver This is the third component of the communication process. The receiver is the listener, who listens, observes, and attends.

Receptive speech The ability to understand the spoken word.

Receptor A nerve cell that converts a stimulus to a nerve impulse. Most receptors are specific, that is, sensitive to only one type of stimulus.

Record A formal, legal document that provides evidence of a client's care. Also called a *client record* or a *clinical chart*.

Recording The process of making an entry on a client record. Also called *charting* or *documenting*.

Recovery 1. Return to (or exceed) preillness levels of functioning. 2. A continued state of voluntary sobriety in which an individual maintains personal health and functions normally.

Recurrence A later recurrence of a disorder after recovery.

Red blood cells (RBCs) Blood cells shaped like biconcave discs that contain the hemoglobin required for oxygen transport to body tissues; the most common type of blood cell. Also called *erythrocytes*.

Reduction Surgical placement of a broken bone in the correct alignment.

Referred pain Pain that is perceived in an area distant from the site of the stimuli.

Reflection The action of making sense of occurrences, situations, or decisions by carefully considering the totality of the experience: what worked or did not work, what could have been done differently to achieve better outcomes, what was done well, what necessary resources were available, and so on.

Reflexes The rapid, involuntary, predictable motor responses to a stimulus.

Reflux A backward flow of acidic secretions into the lower esophagus.

Refraction The bending of light rays as they pass from one medium to another medium of different optical density.

Refractory hypoxemia The decrease of particle arterial oxygen despite administration of oxygen at high flow rates.

Refractory period A phase during which myocardial cells resist stimulation.

Refractory septic shock A persistently low mean arterial blood pressure despite vasopressor therapy and adequate fluid resuscitation.

Regeneration The replacement or renewal of destroyed tissue cells by cells that are identical or similar in structure and function.

Registered nurses (RNs) The members of a nursing team who are specially licensed and trained to deliver direct client care, including client assessment, identification of health problems, and development and coordination of care.

Regurgitation The backflow of blood into the atria during systole.

Reinfection The development of a new infection with a different pathogen following successful treatment.

Reinforcement Consequences that lead to an increase in a particular behavior.

Relapse Return of a disorder soon after recovery.

Relapsing fever Short febrile periods of a few days are interspersed with periods of 1–2 days of normal temperature.

Relationship-based (caring) theories Theories that stress courage, generosity, commitment, and the need to nurture and maintain relationships.

Relaxation response A healthful physiological state that can be elicited through deep relaxation breathing with emphasis on a prolonged exhalation phase.

Religion A set of doctrines accepted by a group of people who gather together regularly to worship that offers a means to relate to God or a higher power; an organized system of beliefs and practices.

REM sleep Rapid-eye-movement sleep that occurs during sleep about every 90 minutes and lasts 5–30 minutes. The brain is highly active in this phase, and most dreams will take place during REM sleep.

Remission 1. A period during a chronic illness in which the symptoms of the illness disappear. 2. A sustained recovery lasting 8 weeks or more.

Remittent fever A wide range of fluctuating temperatures (more than 2°C [3.6°F]), all of which are above normal and occur over a 24-hour period.

Remyelination Repair of the damaged myelin sheath by oligodendrocytes.

Renal colic Acute, severe flank pain on an affected side that develops when a stone obstructs the ureter, causing ureteral spasm.

Renal failure A condition in which the kidneys are unable to remove accumulated metabolites from the blood or produce urine, resulting in altered fluid, electrolyte, and acid–base balance.

Renal insufficiency Decrease in the kidneys' ability to conserve sodium and concentrate the urine.

Renin–angiotensin–aldosterone system System initiated by specialized receptors in the juxtaglomerular cells of the kidney nephrons that respond to changes in renal perfusion.

Repetitive strain injury A nerve, tendon, or muscle condition that occurs when the limbs are subjected to repetitive use, awkward positions, or forced positions. Also called *repetitive motion disorder.*

Repolarization The process that returns the cell to its resting, polarized state.

Report An oral, written, or electronic communication intended to convey information to others.

Research participants Volunteers for a specific study project that meet all the inclusion criteria, have been informed of all aspects of the study, and have signed informed consent.

Reservoir A source of microorganisms.

Residual urine Urine that remains in the bladder after voiding.

Resilience/resiliency The ability to function with healthy responses, even when experiencing significant stress or adversity; the personal patterns, behaviors, or processes that promote an individual's recovery from or adaptation to adversity.

Resolution phase The fourth and final phase of the sexual response cycle is marked by a return to an unaroused state.

Resonance A hollow sound, such as the sound produced by lungs filled with air.

Resource An asset that helps nurses meet client needs.

Resource allocation The distribution of resources among competing groups of people or programs.

Respiration The act of inhaling (inspiration) and exhaling (expiration) air to transport oxygen to the alveoli so that oxygen may be exchanged for carbon dioxide, and the carbon dioxide expelled from the body.

Respiratory acidosis A condition that is caused by an excess of dissolved carbon dioxide, or carbonic acid. It is characterized by a pH of less than 7.35 and a $PaCO_2$ greater than 45 mmHg. It may be caused by hypoventilation.

Respiratory alkalosis A condition that results when pH rises above 7.45 and $PaCO_2$ falls below 35 mmHg. It is caused by hyperventilation (unusually fast respiration, or overbreathing), leading to a carbon dioxide deficit.

Respiratory syncytial virus (RSV) A highly contagious respiratory infection that affects almost all children before 2 years of age.

Response This is the fourth component of the communication process; it is the message that the receiver returns to the sender. Also called *feedback.*

Responsibility The specific accountability or liability associated with the performance of duties of a particular role.

Rest pain Cramping or aching pain in the calves of the legs, the thighs, and the buttocks that occurs while at rest.

Restless leg syndrome A neurological sensorimotor disorder that is characterized by an overwhelming urge to move the legs when at rest.

Restraints Any devices or medications intended to protect the client from injuring self or others through partially or fully limiting the client's mobility.

Restrictive cardiomyopathy A disorder characterized by rigid ventricular walls that impair diastolic filling.

Retinal detachment Separation of the retina or sensory portion of the eye from the choroid.

Retractions Visible sinking of the chest wall, or sunken areas seen between the ribs during inspiration.

Retrograde conduction Cardiac conduction against the normal flow or pattern.

Retropulsion The tendency to topple backward when bumped or when rising, standing, or turning.

Retrospective audit An evaluation performed after a client's discharge comparing the care provided to the client with care provided to clients with similar conditions.

Reverse delegation A situation that occurs when someone with a lower rank delegates to someone with more authority.

Reverse triage A method in which the most severely injured or ill victims who require the greatest resources are treated last to allow the greatest number of victims to receive medical attention.

Revision surgery The replacement of an artificial joint after 10 years or more.

Reward deficiency syndrome The decreased ability to experience pleasure. Reward deficiency syndrome drives the person to seek external forms of gratification through the use of substances, pathological gambling, or other high-risk behaviors.

Rh disease A rare condition where the mother is Rh negative while the child is Rh positive. If this condition arises, the mother's body will see the Rh-positive cells in the fetus as foreign, and will then produce antibodies to fight off the Rh-positive cells. May result in fetal demise in extreme cases.

Rheumatoid arthritis (RA) A chronic systemic autoimmune disease that causes inflammation of connective tissue, primarily in the joints.

Rhinorrhea Drainage of mucus from the nose. Commonly known as a runny nose.

Rhonchi A long, low-pitched sound that continues throughout inspiration suggesting a blockage of large airway passages.

Ribonucleic acid (RNA) One of two types of nucleic acid made by cells. Ribonucleic acid is made up of ribose rather than deoxyribose and contains information that has been copied from DNA (the other type of nucleic acid).

Rigidity Resistance to movement because of the involuntary contraction of all skeletal muscles.

Risk diagnosis A clinical judgment that a problem does not exist, but the presence of risk factors indicates a problem is likely to develop unless the nurse intervenes.

Risk factor A practice, behavior, or environmental factor that increases the potential of negative effects on an individual's health.

Risk management Preventive policies and processes that focus on limiting a healthcare agency's financial and legal risk associated with the delivery of care, particularly in terms of lawsuits.

Role A set of expectations about how an individual occupying one position behaves.

Role ambiguity Occurs when expectations are unclear and when people do not know how to perform their roles and/or are unable to predict the reactions of others to their behavior.

Role conflict Emotional conflict arising when competing demands are made on an individual in the fulfillment of his or her multiple social roles.

Role development Teaching and modeling the behaviors needed to successfully assume a particular role.

Role mastery Occurs when an individual's behaviors meet or exceed social expectations.

Role performance The demonstration of behaviors or actions associated with a given role.

Role strain The stress or strain experienced by an individual when incompatible behavior, expectations, or obligations are associated with a single social role.

Root cause analysis An evaluation required by the Joint Commission that is focused on identifying areas of improvement that would decrease the likelihood of future adverse events and to develop an action plan for improvement.

Rooting reflex In response to a light touch of a finger on an infant's cheek close to the mouth, the infant's head will rotate toward the stimulation and attempt to suck the finger.

Rotational injury An injury caused by lateral flexion or twisting of the head and neck.

Round ligaments The ligaments that hold the ovaries in place.

Rupture of membranes The rupturing of amniotic membranes before the onset of labor.

Sacral promontory A projection into the pelvic cavity on the anterior upper portion of the sacrum, which serves as a landmark for pelvic measurements.

Sarcopenia The process of atrophy due to age.

Safety strap body restraint Restraints used to ensure the safety of clients who are transported by wheelchair or gurney, or to protect clients confined to a bed or a chair. Also called *belt restraint.*

Salient cue The leading, most noticeable, or most important information about a client's health status.

Saline An isotonic solution of 0.9% sodium chloride.

Sanguineous exudate A large amount of red blood cells that form a bright or dark red discharge indicating new or old damage to capillaries. Also called *hemorrhagic exudate.*

Satiety The sensation of fullness and satisfaction that should inhibit eating until the next meal.

Saturated fat A triglyceride fat that contains all of the hydrogen ions it is capable of holding.

Scaling The rating of the severity of symptoms or problems.

Scapegoat An individual who has been selected to take the blame for another individual or for a group.

Scheduled toileting Toileting at regular intervals.

Schemes Adaptive cognitive structures formed in response to environmental stimuli according to Jean Piaget's theory of cognitive development.

Schistocytes Fragmented red blood cells.

Schizoaffective disorder A psychotic disorder with features of both schizophrenia and mood disorders.

Schizoid personality disorder (SPD) One of several personality disorders defined in the DSM-5, it is characterized by a lifelong pattern of indifference to others, absence of humor, and social isolation.

Schizophrenia The most common psychotic disorder, schizophrenia is a combination of disordered thinking, perceptual disturbances, behavioral abnormalities, affective disruptions, and impaired social competency.

Schizophreniform disorder A disorder with rapid onset of psychotic symptoms, very similar to schizophrenia, lasting less than 6 months.

Schizotypal personality disorder One of several personality disorders defined in the DSM-5, it is characterized by a pattern of disturbed interpersonal relationships, thought patterns, appearance, and behavior.

Sciatica Lumbar back pain that radiates down the posterior leg to the ankle due to irritation or compression of all or part of the sciatic nerve.

Scleral buckling A surgical procedure to correct retinal detachment.

Scoliometer A diagnostic test used to measure a client's rib hump when in the Adam position.

Scoliosis A lateral, or sideways, curvature of the spine.

Seasonal affective disorder (SAD) A mood disorder typically characterized by depression during fall and winter and normal mood or hypomania during spring and summer.

Second heart sound (S_2) The heart sound produced by closure of the semilunar valves; characterized by the syllable "dub."

Secondary appraisal Evaluation of an individual's available coping resources and potential options for responding to an event or circumstance.

Secondary cataracts A type of cataract that may form after surgery to treat another eye disorder, such as glaucoma, or as an effect of medication or another primary disorder.

Secondary group A group that is larger, more impersonal, and less sentimental than a primary group.

Secondary hypertension Elevated blood pressure resulting from an identifiable underlying process.

Secondary immune response Subsequent encounters with an antigen following the primary immune response that result in triggering memory cells.

Secondary infertility The inability to conceive after one or more successful pregnancies, or the inability to sustain a pregnancy.

Secondary intention healing Healing that occurs when a wound's edges cannot or should not close. Repair time is typically longer, scarring is greater, and susceptibility to infection is greater.

Secondary prevention Methods that focus on the diagnosis and treatment of disease.

Segmental mastectomy See *Lumpectomy*.

Seizures Periods of abnormal electrical discharges in the brain that cause involuntary movement, as well as behavior and sensory alterations.

Selective perception The process of filtering out unnecessary and distracting information in order to focus on what is important at any given moment.

Selective serotonin reuptake inhibitor (SSRI) A drug that selectively inhibits the reuptake of serotonin into nerve terminals; used mostly for depression.

Selectively permeable Refers to membranes separating body fluid compartments across which solutes can move with relative ease.

Self-awareness The relationship between an individual's perception of himself or herself and others' perceptions of him or her.

Self-concept The personal perception of the self formed in response to interactions with others and the environment throughout the course of an individual's lifetime.

Self-efficacy The expectation that someone can produce a desired outcome.

Self-esteem One's judgment of one's own worth.

Self-help group A group of individuals who come together to face a common problem or difficulty.

Self-quieting ability The ability of newborns to use their own resources to quiet and comfort themselves.

Semen Sperm mixed with seminal fluid, ejaculated during sexual activity.

Semiformal group A group with formalized structure, delineated hierarchy, and voluntary, but selective, membership.

Sender An individual or group who wishes to convey a message to another; can be considered the *source-encoder*.

Sensitization An increased reaction to pain over time, or a reduced threshold for reaction to painful stimuli.

Sensory memory The momentary perception of stimuli from the environment.

Sensory overload An overabundance of sensory stimulation that cannot be correctly processed.

Sensory perception The conscious organization and translation of external data or stimuli into meaningful information.

Sensory reception The process of receiving external stimuli or data. External stimuli are visual (sight), auditory (hearing), olfactory (smell), tactile (touch), and gustatory (taste).

Sentinel event An unexpected occurrence involving death or serious physical or psychological injury, or the risk thereof.

Sepsis 1. A whole-body inflammatory process resulting in acute illness. 2. A state of infection.

Septal defect A congenital heart defect that connects the right and left side of the heart.

Septic shock Altered perfusion resulting from a systemic infection that manifests with hypotension, delayed capillary refill, and inadequate perfusion and oxygenation of vital body tissues. Also called *septicemia*.

Septicemia See **Septic shock**.

Seroconversion Antibody response to a disease or vaccine.

Serosanguineous exudate A clear or blood-tinged discharge commonly seen in surgical incisions.

Serotonin syndrome A condition that may occur in individuals taking two or more medications that increase serotonin levels. Symptoms include hypertension or hypotension, agitation, shivering, changes in mental status, symptoms of gastrointestinal distress, restlessness, tremor, muscle rigidity, unreactive pupils, and tachypnea.

Serous exudate A watery, clear or straw-colored discharge that accompanies mild inflammation.

Serum bicarbonate (HCO_3) A value that reflects the renal regulation of acid–base balance. The normal HCO_3 value is 24–28 mEq/L.

Serum sickness A systemic type III hypersensitivity response, usually in response to a drug such as penicillin or a sulfonamide.

Severe sepsis Sepsis associated with acute organ failure.

Sex chromosomes The 23rd pair of chromosomes found in a cell's nucleus; it determines an individual's gender.

Sexism When male values, beliefs, or activities are preferred over female ones.

Sexual abuse Any sexual act that is perpetrated against someone's will including rape, attempted sexual acts, unwanted sexual contact, voyeurism, and sexual harassment. Also called *sexual violence*.

Sexual aversion disorder A disorder characterized by severe distaste for sexual activity or the thought of sexual activity.

Sexual health A state of physical, emotional, mental, and social well-being in relation to sexuality, not merely the absence of disease, dysfunction, or infirmity. Sexual health requires a positive and respectful approach to sexuality and sexual relationships.

Sexual orientation The sexual attraction of an individual to the same sex, the opposite sex, or both sexes.

Sexual self-concept How one values oneself as a sexual being.

Sexually transmitted infections (STIs) Infections transmitted by vaginal, oral, and anal intimate contact and intercourse.

Shared governance A method that aims to distribute decision making among a group of people.

Shared leadership The concept that a professional workplace is made up of many leaders.

Shared psychotic disorder A condition that results when an individual who is in a close relationship with another person who is delusional comes to share the delusional beliefs.

Shearing force A condition that results when one tissue layer slides over another.

Shock A clinical syndrome characterized by a systemic imbalance between oxygen supply and demand.

Shock phase The initial part of an alarm reaction during which the sympathetic nervous system is suppressed and an individual may experience manifestations such as hypotension, decreased body temperature, and decreased muscle tone.

Short bowel syndrome A condition in which the transit time of ingested foods and fluids is reduced and digestive processes are impaired because of a resection of significant portions of the small intestine.

Short-term memory Information held in the brain for immediate use; what an individual has in mind at a given moment.

Shunt A natural or artificially created tunnel or passage that allows blood to flow through an area.

Sickle cell anemia An inherited chronic hemolytic anemia, sickle cell anemia is the most common form of sickle cell disease.

Sickle cell crisis Severe episodes of fever and intense pain that are the hallmark of sickle cell disease. Also called *vaso-occlusive crisis*.

Sickle cell disease A hereditary hemoglobinopathy characterized by replacement of normal hemoglobin with abnormal hemoglobin S (Hgb S) in RBCs.

Sickle cell trait Carrying one copy of the defective sickle cell gene, which can be passed on to children but does not usually cause the illness.

Sickling A process in which red blood cells take on the characteristic sickle shape following deoxygenation in clients who have sickle cell disease.

Signs See Objective data.

Simple assault An unlawful physical attack by one person upon another in which neither the offender displays a weapon, nor the victim suffers any obvious severe or aggravated bodily injury involving apparent broken bones, loss of teeth, possible internal injury, severe laceration, or loss of consciousness.

Simple mastectomy The removal of a complete breast only. Compare with **Radical mastectomy**.

Single-parent family A family in which only one parent resides in the home and is the primary caretaker and provider for the family.

Situational crisis A crisis that involves an unexpected stressor or circumstance that occurs in the course of daily living.

Situational depression A maladaptive reaction to an identifiable psychosocial stressor or stressors that occurs within 3 months after the onset of the stressor and has persisted for no longer than 6 months. Also called *adjustment disorder with depressed mood*.

Situational leader A leader who is flexible in task and relationship behaviors, considers the staff members' abilities, knows the nature of the task to be done, and is sensitive to the context or environment in which the task takes place.

Six Sigma A quality improvement program originally implemented by Motorola and General Electric that focuses on reducing variation within a process to produce a near-perfect product.

Skin turgor The elasticity of skin.

Sleep An altered state of consciousness in which an individual's perception and reaction to the environment are decreased.

Sleep apnea A disorder characterized by frequent short breathing pauses during sleep.

Sleep architecture The basic organization of normal sleep.

Sleep hygiene Interventions used to promote quality sleep at night.

Sleep loss A duration of sleep shorter than the recommended 7–8 hours a night for an adult.

Small cell carcinoma A highly malignant cancer usually associated with the lung.

SMART An acronym to provide assistance in writing a client-centered goal statement. SMART is Single action (choose a specific, singe action to focus on), Measurable result (observable or measurable result), Attainable (level appropriate), Relevant (customized specifically for client's needs), and Time-limited (specific time frame for goal to be completed).

SOAP An acronym for collective data in a progress note; it stands for subjective data, objective data, assessment, and planning.

Sobriety A state of habitual refrain from using alcohol or drugs.

Social distance Communication characterized by a clear visual perception of the whole person. Body heat and odor are imperceptible, eye contact is increased, and vocalizations are loud enough to be overheard by others.

Social justice A framework in which to explore the complexities surrounding the variety of factors that impact diverse and vulnerable populations.

Social microcosm The concept that group members eventually behave in a therapy group the same way they behave with family and friends.

Social phobia A condition that is characterized by a pervasive, extreme fear of one or more social situations that may lead to scrutiny by others. Also called *social anxiety disorder*.

Socialization The process by which individuals learn to become members of groups and society and learn the social rules defining relationships into which they will enter.

Socialized insurance A system in which all medically necessary services are covered, including physician care, hospital services, and to some extent, prescription drugs.

Socialized medicine State government-owned and -controlled healthcare services.

Software The operating systems and application components of technology.

Solitary play A stage of play in which an infant still plays primarily alone, but enjoys the presence of others.

Solute Substance that dissolves in liquid.

Solvent The component of a solution that can dissolve a solute.

Somatic cells Cells that make up the tissue of the body, with a full complement (diploid) of chromosomes, as opposed to sex cells.

Somatic pain Pain arising from nerve receptors originating in the skin or close to the surface of the body.

Somatization The process by which psychological distress is experienced and communicated in the form of somatic symptoms.

Somatostatin A substance, believed to be a neurotransmitter, that inhibits the production of both glucagon and insulin.

Somnology The study of sleep.

Somogyi phenomenon A combination of hypoglycemia during the night with a rebound, morning rise in blood glucose to hyperglycemic levels.

Source-oriented record Client record in which each health-care provider or department member makes notations in a separate section or sections of the client's chart.

Spasticity Increased muscle tone, usually with some degree of weakness.

Specific defenses Immune system responses directed against identifiable bacteria, viruses, fungi, or other infectious agents.

Specific gravity An indicator of urine concentration that can be performed quickly and easily by nursing personnel.

Specific phobia An intense or extreme fear with regard to a particular object or situation.

Specific self-esteem How much one approves of a certain parts of oneself.

Spermatogenesis The process by which mature spermatozoa are formed.

Spermicide A cream, jelly, foam, vaginal film, or suppository that is inserted into the vagina before intercourse to destroy sperm and prevent conception.

Spinal cord A continuation of the medulla oblongata, it has the ability to transmit impulses to and from the brain via the ascending and descending pathways.

Spinal cord injury (SCI) Trauma to the spinal cord that results from excessive force to the spinal column.

Spinal cord stimulation (SCS) A form of therapy used with persistent pain that has not been controlled with less invasive therapies. SCS involves the insertion of an electrode (a single channel or multichannel device) adjacent to the spinal cord in the epidural space. The electrode(s) is attached to an impulse-generator (external or implanted) that sends electric impulses to the spinal cord to control pain.

Spinal fusion The insertion of a wedge-shaped piece of bone or bone chips between the vertebrae to stabilize them and reduce pain.

Spinal shock A condition that is characterized by spinal cord swelling, decreased blood flow and blood pressure, and complete loss of motor function, spinal reflexes, and autonomic function below the level of injury.

Spiritual distress A challenge to the spiritual well-being or to the belief system that provides strength, hope, and meaning to life; a feeling of being separated from interconnectedness with others or with a higher power.

Spiritual health The overall feeling of strength, hope, and fulfillment that encourages people to find life-sustaining and enriching opportunities.

Spiritual skills Skills that help an individual find meaning in and understand the personal significance of an unexpected event.

Spiritual support Assistance to clients and families in providing meaning and sustaining courage during difficult times.

Spiritual well-being A feeling of inner peace and of being generally alive, purposeful, and fulfilled; the feeling is rooted in spiritual values and/or specific religious beliefs.

Spirituality The part of being human that seeks meaningfulness through personal connection, which may include belief in or relationship with some higher power, creative force, driving being, or infinite source of energy.

Splint An easily adjustable device that stabilizes injuries, usually before swelling has subsided or after the reparative phase of healing.

Splitting 1. The inability to integrate contradictory experiences. **2.** The inclination to perceive people or situations as one extreme or the other.

Spontaneous abortion The loss of a fetus prior to 20 weeks of gestation. Also called *miscarriage.*

Spontaneous rupture of membranes (SROM) The rupturing of membranes during the height of an intense contraction with a gush of fluid out of the vagina.

Sporadic AD One of the two basic types of Alzheimer disease, it shows no clear pattern of inheritance, although genetic factors may contribute to the disorder. Sporadic AD typically does not develop until after the age of 65. Also called *late-onset Alzheimer disease.*

Sprain A stretching or tearing of ligaments.

Sputum Mucus or mucopurulent matter expectorated from the lungs.

Squamous cell carcinoma A malignant tumor of the squamous epithelium of the skin or mucous membranes.

Staff authority The power to provide advice and support to employees or departments but not to assign tasks.

Staff development Continued staff education, planned activities to enhance role performance, and defined goals to improve client outcomes. Also called *professional development.*

Stage of exhaustion Stage in which the body ceases to maintain its adaptation to a stressor; the stressor overwhelms the individual's ability to cope or mount a continued defense, resulting in the depletion of energy and resources.

Stage of resistance Stage in which the body attempts to move toward restoration of homeostasis while continuing to respond to the stressor.

Staghorn stones A type of calculi associated with a urinary tract infection caused by urease-producing bacteria such as *Proteus.* These stones can grow to become very large, filling the renal pelvis and calyces. Also called *struvite stones.*

Staging A system of classifying cancer according to the size of the tumor, involvement of lymph nodes, and metastasis to distant sites.

Standard precautions Safety guidelines, such as proper hand hygiene, use of proper protective equipment, safe injection practices, and effective management of potentially contaminated surfaces or equipment, that are designed to decrease the risk of transmitting unidentified pathogens. Also called *universal precautions* and *body substance isolation (BSI)*.

Standardized plan A nursing care plan that specifies the nursing care for groups of clients with common needs (e.g., all clients with myocardial infarction).

Standards Models of high-quality performance that may reflect the performance of industry leaders, scientific or clinical research, or recommendations of professional organizations such as the ANA.

Standards of care Guidelines used to determine what a nurse should or should not do, and may be defined as a benchmark of achievement based on a desired level of excellence.

Standards of practice A standardized description of the responsibilities for which nurses are responsible.

Standards of professional performance The behaviors expected in the professional nursing role by the American Nurses Association.

Station The location of the fetal presenting part in the maternal pelvis in relation to the ischial spine.

Status asthmaticus A severe, prolonged form of asthma that is difficult to treat.

Status epilepticus A continuous seizure that lasts for more than 30 minutes or a series of seizures during which time consciousness is not regained.

Statutory laws Laws made by any legislative branch of the government, including the U.S. Congress, state legislatures, and city and county governments.

Steatorrhea Fatty, frothy, foul-smelling stools caused by a decrease in pancreatic enzyme secretion.

Stem cell transplant The infusion of immature stem cells to replenish a client's blood cell lines; used as an alternative to bone marrow transplantation.

Stenosis Narrowing of the valve, valve area, or great artery above the valve.

Step-down therapy A gradual reduction in the dosage and number of drugs used in a therapeutic regimen.

Stepfamily Consists of a biological parent with children and a new spouse who may or may not have children.

Stereognosis The ability to perceive and understand an object through touch.

Stereotaxic thalamotomy An x-ray taken during neurosurgery to guide the insertion of a needle into a specific area of the brain.

Stereotyping The act of generalizing that all people in a group are the same.

Stereotypy Rigid and obsessive behavior.

Sterile field An area free of microorganisms.

Sterile technique Practices that keep an area or object free of all microorganisms. Also known as *surgical asepsis*.

Sterilization 1. A process that destroys all microorganisms, including spores and viruses. 2. An inclusive term that refers to surgical procedures that permanently prevent pregnancy.

Stigma A collection of negative attitudes and beliefs that lead people to fear, reject, avoid, and discriminate against people with mental illness.

Stillbirth Death of a fetus that occurs after 20 weeks of gestation. Also called *fetal demise* or *intrauterine fetal death (IUFD)*.

Stimulus The agent or act that stimulates a nerve receptor.

Stimulus-based stress model A model that defines stress as being a life event that requires change or adaptation on the part of the individual who is experiencing the life event.

Stoma An artificial opening in the abdominal wall; it may be permanent or temporary.

Stool Body wastes and undigested food eliminated from the bowel. Also called *feces*.

Strain A stretching or tearing of a muscle or tendon.

Strategic planning The process of continual assessment, planning, and evaluation to guide future decisions and developments.

Stress The body's general, nonspecific response to the demands placed upon it by a stressor.

Stress fracture A fracture that results from disease that has weakened the bone.

Stress mediators Hormonal triggers that are intended to promote adaptation through mechanisms such as triggering a necessary increase in heart rate and blood pressure when faced with physical danger.

Stress response Physiological changes triggered by stress; includes activation of the neural, neuroendocrine, and endocrine systems, as well as activation of target organs.

Stressor An external influence that threatens to disrupt the equilibrium that is needed to maintain homeostasis.

Striae Whitish-silver stretch marks seen in obesity and during or after pregnancy.

Stridor A high-pitched sound within the trachea and larynx that suggests narrowing of the tracheal passage.

Stroke A condition in which neurological deficits result from a sudden decrease in blood flow to a localized area of the brain. Also called *cerebrovascular accident* or *brain attack*.

Stroke volume (SV) The amount of blood pumped into the aorta with each contraction of the left ventricle that is measured by the difference between the end-diastolic volume and the end-systolic volume.

Structural-functional theory Focuses on family structure and function, examining family relationships and how they affect the functions of the family and relationships with other systems.

Structure standards Standards related to material resources, human resources, and general organizational structure.

Struvite stones A type of calculi associated with a urinary tract infection caused by urease-producing bacteria such as *Proteus*. These stones can grow to become very large, filling the renal pelvis and calyces. Also called *staghorn stones*.

Subconjunctival hemorrhage Temporary, nonpathogenic hemorrhages that are caused by the changes in vascular tension or ocular pressure during birth.

Subculture groups Minority groups characterized by specific norms, beliefs, and values that coexist with a dominant culture.

Subcutaneous tissue The layer of loose connective tissue and fat cells that lies below the dermis. Also called *hypodermis*.

Subdermal implant Capsules implanted within the skin that slowly release medication, such as for contraception.

Subfertility Occurs when both partners of a couple have reduced fertility.

Subinvolution A slowing of the descent of the uterus during the postpregnancy healing process.

Subjective data Information that is apparent to only the client affected and can be described or verified by only that client. Also called *symptoms* or *covert data*.

Subjective family burden The psychological distress of family members in relation to the objective family burden of having a family member with a mental illness.

Substance abuse The use of any chemical in a fashion inconsistent with medical or culturally defined social norms despite physical, psychological, or social adverse effects.

Substance dependence A condition in which the client can no longer control use of the substance, continues to use it despite adverse effects, and experiences withdrawal symptoms without continued use of the substance.

Subsystem A component of a larger system.

Sucking reflex Occurs in response to a finger or nipple inserted into an infant's mouth; the infant responds by beginning to rhythmically suck on the finger.

Suctioning Aspirating secretions through a catheter connected to a suction machine or wall suction outlet.

Sudden cardiac death (SCD) Unexpected death occurring within 1 hour of the onset of cardiovascular symptoms.

Sudden infant death syndrome (SIDS) The sudden death of an apparently healthy infant that remains unexplained after other possible causes have been ruled out through autopsy, death scene investigation, and review of the medical history.

Suicidal ideation A case of an individual constantly considering, planning, or thinking about suicide.

Suicide An act of an individual inflicting self-harm resulting in death.

Suicide attempt An act of an individual inflicting self-harm with the intent to cause death that is not successful.

Sundowning A behavioral change commonly seen in clients with dementia, characterized by increased agitation, time disorientation, and wandering behaviors during afternoon and evening hours; it is accelerated on overcast days.

Superego The third aspect of the personality that contains the conscience and the ego ideal. The superego is the source of feelings such as guilt, shame, and inhibition.

Superficial basal cell carcinoma A type of skin cancer.

Superficial burn A burn that involves only the epidermal layer of the skin.

Supersaturated urine A condition that results when the concentration of an insoluble salt in the urine is very high.

Supine On the back.

Suppuration A large quantity of cells and necrotic debris that form an opaque or milky discharge that is thicker than serous exudate. Also called *pus* or *purulent exudate*.

Suprasystem An overarching system to which smaller systems or subsystems belong. For example, the family is the suprasystem of the individual.

Surface temperature Body temperature taken at the skin's surface that may rise or fall in response to the environment.

Surfactant Specialized cells that control surface tension and keep alveoli from collapsing and sticking to themselves.

Surge capacity A community's ability to rapidly meet the increased demand for qualified personnel and resources, including healthcare resources, in the event of a disaster.

Surgical asepsis Practices that keep an area or object free of all microorganisms. Also called *sterile technique*.

Surgical debridement The process of excising a wound to the level of fascia or sequentially removing thin slices of a burn wound to the level of viable tissue.

Sutures The membranous spaces between the cranial bones of a fetus.

Swan-neck deformity Caused by rheumatoid arthritis, it is characterized by hyperextension of the proximal interphalangeal joints with compensatory flexion of the distal interphalangeal joints.

Switching A term used in disorders of mood and affect to describe a new illness phase (manic or depressed) without recovery.

Symmetry Equality of the size, shape, or condition of opposite sides of the body.

Sympathetic tone A state of partial smooth muscle contraction around arteries and veins.

Symphysis pubic Fibrocartilaginous joint between the pelvic bones in the midline.

Symptom See **Subjective data**.

Synchronized cardioversion Delivery of direct electrical current synchronized with the client's heart rhythm.

Synclitism A condition that occurs when the sagittal suture is midway between the symphysis pubis and the sacral promontory and is felt to be aligned.

Syncope Transient loss of consciousness and muscle tone after exercise or activity.

Syndrome diagnosis A cluster of nursing diagnoses that occur together and may result in best client outcomes if addressed at the same time.

Synovectomy Excision of synovial membrane, this procedure is used as a treatment for rheumatoid arthritis.

Synovitis Inflammation of the synovial membrane lining the articular capsule of a joint.

Syphilis A complex systemic sexually transmitted infection caused by the spirochete *Treponema pallidum*.

System A set of interacting identifiable parts or components.

Systematized delusions A manifestation of schizophrenia characterized by an extensively developed central delusional theme from which conclusions are deduced.

Systemic arthritis A form of juvenile rheumatoid arthritis that characteristically is manifested by high fever, polyarthritis, and rheumatoid rash. Systemic arthritis also affects internal organs and joints.

Systemic circulation Circulation through the left side of the heart, the aorta and its branches, the capillaries that supply the brain and peripheral tissues, the systemic venous system, and the vena cava.

Systemic infection Occurs when an invading microorganism spreads and damages different parts of the body.

Systemic inflammatory response syndrome (SIRS) Describes the body's response to a critical illness that can result from an infectious or noninfectious cause precipitating a whole-body inflammatory process.

Systemic lupus erythematosus (SLE) A chronic, inflammatory connective tissue disease.

Systemic response Results because of a widespread antibody-antigen reaction. Systemic responses include anaphylaxis, urticaria, or angioedema.

Systemic vascular resistance The force or resistance of the blood in the body's blood vessels that helps return blood to the heart.

Systems theory The study of how a system operates, including how it interacts with other systems and how its components interact with each other within the system itself.

Systole The phase of ventricular contraction.

Systolic blood pressure The maximum pressure exerted within the arteries when the heart compresses.

T lymphocyte (T cells) A type of leukocyte that matures in the thymus gland and is integral to the specific immune response.

Tachycardia An excessively fast heart rate greater than 100 bpm in an adult.

Tachypnea A respiratory rate greater than 20 bpm in adults.

Tactile Of or relating to touch.

Tangential excision The sequential removal of thin slices of a burn wound to the level of viable tissue.

Tardive dyskinesia A condition characterized by repetitive, involuntary body movement of varying severity that may not cease after medication cessation; includes unusual tongue and face movements such as lip smacking and wormlike motions of the tongue.

Tartar A visible, hard deposit of plaque and dead bacteria that forms at the gumlines. Also called *dental calculus*.

Tau A protein found in the neurons.

Teaching A system of activities intended to produce learning.

Team Two or more individuals who agree to work in tandem to accomplish a common goal.

Team nursing The delivery of individualized nursing care to a group of clients by a team led by a professional nurse.

Telangiectatic nevi Pale pink or red spots frequently found on the eyelids, nose, lower occipital bone, and nape of the neck of young children. These areas have no clinical significance and usually fade by the second birthday. Also called *stork bites*.

Telecommunication The transmission of information from one site to another, using equipment to send information in the form of signs, signals, words, or pictures by cable, radio, or other systems.

Telehealth A system that employs the use of telecommunications technologies (e.g., videoconferencing, streaming media, real-time forwarding imaging, and land-based and wireless communications) to allow clients access to care that they might not otherwise be able to obtain. Also called *telemedicine* or *remote client monitoring*.

Temperament The combination of biological and physical characteristics that influence personality and behavior specific to each individual.

Tender points Tenderness that occurs in precise, localized areas, particularly in the neck, spine, shoulders, and hips.

Tendon Tissue that connects bones to muscles and carries the contractile forces from the muscle to the bone to cause movement.

Tendonitis Inflammation of a tendon.

Teratogen Any chemical that has the potential to harm the fetus, including pesticides, viruses, and medications.

Terminal weaning The gradual withdrawal of mechanical ventilation when survival without assisted ventilation is not expected.

Territoriality A concept of the space and things that an individual considers as belonging to the self.

Tertiary intention healing Healing that occurs after closing a wound that has been left open for 3–5 days to allow edema or infection to resolve. Also called *delayed primary intention*.

Tertiary prevention Methods that focus on the restoration of health following an illness or accident and include rehabilitation and palliative services.

Testosterone The primary male sex hormone produces by the testes.

Tetany Tonic muscle spasms.

Tetralogy of Fallot A rare disease that consists of four defects: pulmonic stenosis, right ventricular hypertrophy, ventricular-septal defect, and an overriding aorta.

Tetraplegia Complete loss of function of the upper and lower body, including the arms, trunk, legs, and pelvic organs. Also called *quadriplegia*.

Thalassemia Inherited disorder of hemoglobin synthesis in which either the alpha or beta chains of the hemoglobin molecule are missing or defective.

Therapeutic communication An interactive process between the nurse and the client that helps the client to overcome temporary stress, to get along with other people, to adjust to situations that cannot be altered, and to overcome any psychological blocks that may stand in the way of self-realizations.

Therapeutic insemination The process of depositing semen at the cervical os or in the uterus by mechanical means.

Therapeutic relationship Nurse–client relationship that is focused on helping clients manage problems and become better at helping themselves.

Thermoregulation The body process that balances heat production and heat loss to maintain the body's temperature.

Third heart sound (S$_3$) Heart sound that is sometimes heard after the second heart sound in children, young adults, and pregnant females during the third trimester. Also called a *ventricular gallop*.

Third spacing A shift of fluid from the vascular space into an area where it is not available to support normal physiological processes.

Thoracentesis Needle insertion into the pleural space to remove fluid accumulation.

Thoracolumbar sacral orthosis (TLSO) A brace contoured to conform to the body and support the spine. Also called an *underarm brace* or *Boston brace*.

Thought blocking Speech stopped in midsentence as if the thought disappeared from the individual's head.

Thought disorders Disorders associated with schizophrenia that involve an abnormal way of thinking, such as disorganized thinking, sensory overload, thought blocking, neologisms, loose association, clang, and perseveration.

Threshold potential The point at which an action potential is capable of being generated.

Thrill A palpable vibration over the precordium or an artery.

Thromboemboli Emboli created by a blood clot.

Thrombophlebitis See Venous thrombosis.

Throughput The process by which information, energy, or material that enters a system (input) is used by the system.

Thrush White patches that look like milk curds that adhere to the mucous membranes usually caused by an infected vaginal tract during birth, antibiotic use, or poor hand hygiene. Bleeding may occur if patches are removed.

Thyroid crisis See **Thyroid storm.**

Thyroid storm An extreme state of hyperthyroidism. Now extremely rare due to improved diagnosis and treatment methods. Also called *thyroid crisis.*

Thyroidectomy Surgical removal of all or part of the thyroid gland.

Thyroiditis Inflammation of the thyroid gland.

Thyrotoxicosis A disorder caused by excessive delivery of thyroid hormone to the peripheral tissues. Also called *hyperthyroidism.*

Time constraints Deadlines for completion.

Time-out A preprocedure verification to ensure the correct procedure is being performed at the right site on the right client.

Time priority A time constraint to complete an action.

Tine test Test in which a multiple-puncture device is used to introduce tuberculin into the skin.

Tinea pedis Fungal infection of the feet. Also called *athlete's foot.*

Tinnitus The perception of sound or noise in the ears without stimulus from the environment.

Token economies Formalized programs of contingency contracts.

Tolerance State in which a particular dose elicits a smaller response than it formerly did. With increased tolerance, the individual needs higher and higher doses to obtain the desired response.

Tone 1. The amount of tension or resistance to movement in a muscle. 2. The ability of vessels to constrict or dilate to maintain normal pressure.

Tonic-clonic seizures Alternating contraction (tonic phase) and relaxation (clonic phase) of muscles during seizure activity.

Tonic neck reflex In response to an infant's head being turned to one side while the infant lies on the back, the infant will extend the arm and leg on the side the infant faces while the opposite arm and leg will be flexed.

Tonic phase Initial phase of a generalized seizure, manifested by unconsciousness and continuous muscular contraction.

Tonicity The osmolality of a solution. Solutions may be termed *isotonic, hypertonic,* or *hypotonic.*

Torsades de pointes A type of ventricular tachycardia associated with a prolongation of the QT interval.

Tort A civil wrong committed against an individual or an individual's property.

Total anomalous pulmonary venous return The pulmonary veins empty into the right atrium or into veins leading to the right atrium, rather than into the left atrium.

Total lymphoid irradiation A procedure sometimes used in the treatment of rheumatoid arthritis; it decreases total lymphocyte levels.

Total quality management (TQM) A comprehensive management philosophy that improves quality and productivity by utilizing data and statistics to improve system processes.

Toxic multinodular goiter A tumor characterized by small, discrete, independently functioning nodules in the thyroid gland tissue that secrete excessive amounts of thyroid hormone.

Toxoplasmosis Space-occupying lesions common in clients with AIDS that may cause headache, altered mental status, and neurological deficits.

Trachoma A chronic conjunctivitis caused by *Chlamydia trachomatis.* It is a significant preventable cause of blindness worldwide.

Traction The application of a straightening or pulling force to return or maintain fractured bones in their normal anatomical position.

Traditional family An autonomous unit in which both parents reside in the home with their children, the mother assuming the nurturing role and the father providing the necessary economic resources.

Transactional leader A leader who has a relationship with followers based on an exchange of some resource valued by the follower.

Transcellular fluid One of the compartments where extracellular fluid is found. Examples of transcellular fluid are cerebrospinal, pericardial, pancreatic, pleural, intraocular, biliary, peritoneal, and synovial fluids.

Transcendence A person's recognition that there is something other or greater than the self and a seeking and valuing of that greater other, whether it is an ultimate being, force, or value.

Transcranial magnetic stimulation (TMS) A promising alternative therapy for individuals with schizophrenia that uses electromagnetic stimulus to affect brain activity in the cerebral cortex.

Transductive reasoning Connecting two events in a cause-and-effect relationship simply because they occur together in time.

Transection An injury that occurs when an individual is injured by a gunshot, stabbing, or similar force, which may partially or completely sever the spinal cord.

Transference The transfer of feelings that were originally evoked by one's parents or significant others to people in the present setting.

Transformational leader A leader who fosters creativity, risk taking, commitment, and collaboration by empowering a group to share in an organization's vision. The leader inspires others with a clear, attractive, and attainable goal and enlists them to participate in attaining the goal.

Transfusion reaction A type II or cytotoxic hypersensitivity reaction to blood of an incompatible type.

Transgender Gradations of human characteristics running from female to male; more commonly, an individual who expresses a gender identity different from that with which he or she was born.

Transient ischemic attack (TIA) A brief period of localized cerebral ischemia that causes neurological deficits lasting for less than 24 hours. Also called a *mini-stroke.*

Transitional milk A light yellow milk that is more copious than colostrum and contains more fat, lactose, water-soluble vitamins, and calories; it usually presents between the second and fifth day following birth.

Transjugular intrahepatic portosystemic shunt (TIPS) An expandable metal stent inserted through a transcutaneous needle to channel blood from the portal vein into the hepatic vein, bypassing the cirrhotic liver.

Transplacental immunity Passive immunity transferred from mother to infant.

Transposition of the great arteries (TGA) A congenital heart defect in which the pulmonary artery, the outflow tract for the left ventricle, and the aorta, the outflow tract for the right ventricle, are transposed.

Transsexual An individual who feels his or her sexual anatomy is not consistent with his or her gender identity.

Transurethral incision of the prostate (TUIP) Small incisions are made in the smooth muscle where the prostate is attached to the bladder in order to reduce pressure on the urethra.

Transurethral needle ablation (TUNA) A procedure that uses low-level radio-frequency through twin needles to burn away a region of the enlarged prostate in order to improve the flow of urine.

Transurethral resection of the prostate (TURP) A procedure that removes obstructing prostate tissue using the wire loop of a resectoscope and electrocautery inserted through the urethra.

Transverse diameter The largest diameter of the pelvic inlet; helps determine the shape of the inlet.

Trauma An injury to human tissues and organs resulting from the transfer of energy from an external environmental source, such as a motor vehicle, a fire, or a sharp object.

Traumatic cataracts A type of cataract that may result from an injury to the eye.

Tremors Rhythmic, involuntary movements or twitching of the extremities.

Triage The process of identifying priorities for implementing care.

Tricuspid atresia The absence of the tricuspid valve.

Tricyclic antidepressant (TCA) A class of drugs that inhibit the reuptake of both norepinephrine and serotonin into presynaptic nerve terminals. TCAs are primarily used in the pharmacotherapy of depression.

Triglycerides Substances converted from dietary fats and carbohydrates to store energy in fat cells.

Triplet Three premature ventricular contractions in a row.

Tripod position A position of sitting and leaning forward; often used by clients who are having difficulty breathing.

Trisomy An extra chromosome.

Trisomy 21 A condition that occurs when an individual born with Down syndrome has an additional full chromosome present.

Troponins Proteins released during a myocardial infarction that are sensitive indicators of myocardial damage.

Trousseau sign Spasmodic contraction of the hand and fingers in response to occlusion of the blood supply by a blood pressure cuff; caused by decreased blood calcium levels. A test used to check for hypocalcemia.

True pelvis The portion that lies below the linea terminalis; made up of the inlet, cavity, and outlet.

Truncus arteriosus A heart defect in which a single large vessel empties both ventricles and provides circulation for the pulmonary, systemic, and coronary circulations.

Trunk incurvation In response to stroking an infant's spine, the infant's pelvis will turn toward the stimulated side. Also called *Galant reflex.*

Tubal ligation A surgical procedure to clip, tie off, band, or plug the fallopian tubes to sterilize a female client.

Tubercle A granulomatous lesion (a sealed-off colony of bacilli) formed from *Mycobacterium tuberculosis.*

Tuberculosis (TB) A chronic, recurrent infectious disease caused by *Mycobacterium tuberculosis.* TB usually affects the lungs, but any organ can be affected.

Tubular sound The sound air makes moving through a clear and functioning trachea.

Tumor lysis syndrome (TLS) A condition that occurs when tumor cells dissolve and release intracellular contents into circulation, causing hyperkalemia, hyperuricemia, and hyperphosphatemia.

Tumor marker A protein molecule detectable in serum or other body fluids that is used to highlight suspicious regions for follow-up.

TURP syndrome A condition that is characterized by hyponatremia, decreased hematocrit, hypertension, bradycardia, nausea, and confusion.

Two-career family A family in which both partners are employed by choice or necessity. A two-career family may or may not have children.

Tympanic membrane A thin, tense membrane that separates the middle ear from the external auditory canal, protecting the middle ear from the external environment.

Tympanocentesis A surgical incision of the tympanic membrane. Also called *myringotomy.*

Tympanogram A test that provides a graph of the middle ear's ability to transmit sound.

Tympanostomy tubes Pressuring-equalizing tubes inserted to provide the middle ear with ventilation and drainage during healing.

Tympany A musical or drumlike sound produced from an air-filled stomach.

Ulcer A break in the GI mucosa that develops when the mucosal barrier is unable to protect the mucosa from damage by hydrochloric acid and pepsin, the gastric digestive juices.

Ulcerative colitis A chronic inflammatory bowel disorder that affects the mucosa and submucosa of the colon and rectum.

Ultrafiltration Removal of excess body water using a hydrostatic pressure gradient.

Ultrasound A test using intermittent ultrasonic waves transmitted by an alternating current to a transducer and applied to the abdomen.

Unconscious mind The part of an individual's mental life of which he or she is unaware.

Underinsured Individuals whose healthcare coverage is insufficient to meet their needs.

Undernutrition Health effects due to insufficient nutrient intake or stores. Also known as *malnutrition.*

Unifocal When a ventricular impulse arises from one ectopic site.

Unilateral lobar pneumonia A pattern of pneumonia in which bacteria tend to be distributed evenly throughout one or more lobes of a single lung.

Uninsured Individuals who are without any type of healthcare coverage.

Unipolar depression A mood disorder characterized by loss of interest in life and unresponsiveness, moving from mild to severe, with severe symptoms lasting at least 2 weeks. Also called *major depressive disorder (MDD)*.

Universal precautions (UP) Safety guidelines, such as proper hand hygiene, use of proper protective equipment, safe injection practices, and effective management of potentially contaminated surfaces or equipment, that are designed to decrease the risk of transmitting unidentified pathogens. Also called *standard precautions* and *body substance isolation (BSI)*.

Universal protocol Established guidelines for healthcare professionals to prevent errors during surgical procedures including wrong-site surgery.

Unlicensed assistive personnel (UAP) Members of a nursing team who assume delegated aspects of basic client care such as bathing, assisting with feeding, and collecting specimens. UAPs include certified nurse assistants, hospital attendants, nurse technicians, and orderlies.

Unresolved bacteriuria The presence of bacteria in urine that fails to resolve with treatment.

Unsaturated fat A triglyceride fat that does not contain all of the hydrogen ions it is capable of holding.

Upper body obesity Identified by a waist-to-hip ratio of greater than 1 in men or 0.8 in women. Also called *central obesity*.

Uremia Excessive amounts of urea in the blood.

Uremic fetor A urine-like breath odor often associated with a metallic taste in the mouth.

Uremic frost Crystallized deposits of urea on the skin.

Ureteral stent A thin catheter inserted into the ureter to provide for urine flow and ureteral support.

Ureterolithotomy An incision in the affected ureter to remove a calculus.

Ureteroplasty The surgical repair of a ureter.

Urgency The sudden, strong desire to void.

Urgency factor A way to illustrate how much time can safely lapse before doing interventions without compromising client outcomes.

Uric acid stones Develop when the urine concentration of uric acid is high.

Urinary calculi Stones in the urinary tract.

Urinary drainage system Those organs required to drain urine from the kidneys, including the ureters, urinary bladder, and urethra.

Urinary frequency The need to urinate often, specifically more than four to six times a day.

Urinary hesitancy A delay and difficulty in initiating voiding; often associated with dysuria.

Urinary incontinence Involuntary urination due to the temporary or permanent inability of the external sphincter muscles to control the flow of urine from the bladder. Also called *involuntary urination*.

Urinary reflux Backward flow of urine.

Urinary retention The accumulation of urine in the bladder and inability of the bladder to empty itself, resulting in overdistention of the bladder.

Urinary stasis Stagnation of urinary flow.

Urination Releasing urine from the urinary bladder. Also called *voiding* or *micturition*.

Uroflowmetry A method of measuring urine flow rate.

Urolithiasis The formation of stones in the urinary tract.

Urticaria Patches of pale, itchy wheals in an erythematous area. Also known as *hives*.

Uterine atony The relaxation of uterine muscle tone.

Uterosacral ligaments Ligaments that provide support for the uterus and cervix at the level of the ischial spines.

Uterus The hollow muscular organ in which the fertilized ovum is implanted and in which the developing fetus is nourished until birth.

Utilitarianism A form of consequentialist theory that views a good act as one that brings the most good and the least harm for the greatest number of people. This is called the principle of utility.

Utility See Utilitarianism.

Utilization review An evaluation of the use of resources to identify areas of overuse, misuse, and underuse.

Uveitis Inflammation of the middle layer of the eye called the uvea.

Vaccine Suspensions of whole or fractionated bacteria or viruses that have been treated to make them nonpathogenic; introduced by immunization to provoke active immunity.

Vacuum extraction An obstetric procedure used by physicians and CNMs to assist the birth of a fetus by applying suction to the fetal head.

Vagina The muscular and membranous tube that connects the external genitals with the uterus.

Vaginal birth after cesarean (VBAC) A trend in which a mother could choose a trial of labor and vaginal birth after having a cesarean for a previous child, provided the previous cesarean was required due to a nonrecurring indication and the mother met the guidelines established by the American College of Obstetricians and Gynecologists.

Vaginismus The involuntary spasm of the outer one third of the vaginal muscles, making penetration of the vagina painful and sometimes impossible.

Validation The act of verifying the accuracy and factuality of data.

Valsalva maneuver Forced exhalation against a closed glottis.

Values Personal beliefs about truth and the worth of behaviors or objects; standards that influence behavior.

Variability Change or wavering; more specifically, a change in fetal heart rate over a few seconds to a few minutes.

Variable decelerations A condition that occurs if the umbilical cord becomes compressed, reducing blood flow between the placenta and fetus. Fetal hypertension stimulates the baroreceptors in the aortic arch and carotid sinuses, slowing the fetal heart rate.

Variance 1. An unmet goal. 2. An incident or accident that affects a client or a visitor in a healthcare facility.

Vasectomy A procedure to surgically sever the vas deferens on both sides of the scrotum to sterilize a male client.

Vasogenic shock Shock that results from widespread vasodilation and decreased peripheral resistance. Also called *distributive shock*.

Vaso-occlusive crisis See Sickle cell crisis.

Vegan A type of vegetarian diet that excludes all animal and fish products, including dairy, meat, eggs, and honey.

Venous stasis The collection and stagnation of blood in the lower extremities.

Venous thrombectomy Surgical removal of a blood clot from the femoral vein to prevent pulmonary embolism or gangrene.

Venous thrombosis A condition in which a blood clot (thrombus) forms on the wall of a vein, accompanied by inflammation of the vein wall and some degree of obstructed venous blood flow. Also called *thrombophlebitis*.

Ventilation The exchange of oxygen and carbon dioxide.

Ventilation-perfusion (V-Q) The movement of oxygen across the alveolar–capillary membrane into a well-perfusing capillary.

Ventricular aneurysm An outpouching of the ventricular wall that does not contract during systole, causing stroke volume to decrease.

Ventricular bigeminy A premature ventricular contraction following each normal beat.

Ventricular gallop (S₃) Heart sound sometimes heard after the second heart sound in children, young adults, and pregnant females during the third trimester. Also called the *third heart sound*.

Ventricular septal defect (VSD) An opening in the ventricular septum that causes increased pulmonary blood flow.

Ventricular trigeminy A premature ventricular contraction every third beat.

Veracity A moral principle that holds that an individual should tell the truth and not lie.

Verbal abuse The use of berating, humiliating, ridiculing, blaming, or threatening language toward an individual.

Verbal communication Transmitting information through the spoken or written word.

Vernix caseosa A whitish, cheeselike substance that covers a fetus while in utero.

Vertical rotation The degree of rotation of the vertebrae.

Vertical transmission Perinatal transmission of an infection, such as the human immunodeficiency virus, from mother to infant.

Vertigo A sensation of whirling or rotation

Very-low-calorie diets A program providing a protein-sparing modified fast (400–800 kcal/day or less) under close medical supervision.

Vesicoureteral reflux A condition in which urine moves from the bladder back toward the kidney. A common risk factor in children who develop pyelonephritis that may also be seen in adults whose bladder outflow is obstructed.

Vesicular sounds The soft and breezy sounds of air moving in and out of the lobes at the alveolar level.

Vestibulitis Pain of the outer portion of the vagina upon touch or attempted penetration.

Vibration A series of vigorous quiverings produced by hands that are placed flat against the client's chest wall.

Violence The use of excessive force against other individuals or oneself, often resulting in physical or psychological injuries or death.

Virchow triad Three factors associated with thrombophlebitis: stasis of blood, vessel damage, and increased blood coagulability.

Virions Virus particles unable to grow and reproduce outside a host.

Virulence The ability of a microorganism to produce disease.

Virus A type of microorganism that must enter living cells in order to reproduce.

Visceral Of or relating to any large organ in the body.

Visceral pain Pain arising from body organs. It is dull and poorly localized because of the low number of nociceptors.

Viscosupplementation A treatment for osteoarthritis of the knee that involves injecting lubricating substances directly into the knee.

Visual Of or relating to sight.

Vitamin Micronutrient compounds that are involved in regulating body functioning. Most vitamins, with the exceptions of vitamins D and K, cannot be manufactured within the body and must be consumed through dietary intake.

Vitiligo An autoimmune disorder that results in loss of melanin in patches of the face, hands, or groin.

Voiding Releasing urine from the urinary bladder. Also called *urination* or *micturition*.

Voiding cystourethrography Use of a contrast medium and x-rays to assess the bladder and urethra when filled and during voiding.

Volatile acid Acids eliminated from the body as a gas.

Volkmann contracture The impaired mobility of the arm and inability to extend the arm completely, which is a common complication of elbow fractures.

Voluntary admission The detention of a client in a psychiatric or medical facility at the client's request.

Voluntary insurance Health care that provides no guarantee of universality because coverage may be expensive and difficult to purchase.

Vomiting The forceful expulsion of the contents of the upper gastrointestinal tract resulting from contraction of muscles in the gut and abdominal wall.

Vulnerability An individual's susceptibility to react to a specific stressor.

Vulnerability factors A practice, behavior, or environmental factor that increases the potential of an individual becoming a victim of violence.

Vulnerable populations Social groups with inadequate access to health care because they lack resources and are exposed to more risk factors.

Vulva The external female genitals.

Vulvodynia Constant, unremitting burning that is localized to the vulva with an acute onset.

Wandering baseline A smooth, meandering, unsteady baseline in the normal range without variability.

Warm zone When a disaster occurs, this zone, located at least 300 feet from the outer edge of a hot zone, is where decontamination occurs and rapid triage and emergency treatment are given to stabilize victims. Also called the *yellow zone, contamination zone,* or *contamination reduction zone.*

Water An essential nutrient for the body's survival, it contributes to fluid balance and plays an important role in nerve and muscle functioning and in the transport of nutrients to all body systems.

Weaning 1. The process of removing ventilator support and reestablishing spontaneous, independent respirations. **2.** The process of discontinuing breastfeeding and accustoming an infant to another feeding method.

Well-being A subjective perception of feeling well that can be described objectively and measured.

Wellness A state of well-being that encompasses self-responsibility, dynamic growth, nutrition, physical fitness, emotional health, preventive health care, and the whole being of the individual.

Wellness diagnosis A term that describes human responses to levels of wellness in an individual, family, or community that have a readiness for enhancement. For example, *Readiness for Enhanced Coping*.

Wernicke encephalopathy A condition typically seen in people with alcoholism that is characterized by ataxia (lack of coordination), abnormal eye movements, and confusion.

Wheezing A high-pitched whistling sound most often heard on expiration and caused by the narrowing of bronchi; wheezes can also be heard on inspiration.

Whiplash An injury that results from sudden impact to a motor vehicle that causes an individual's head and neck to be forcibly contorted, resulting in injury to the spine.

Whistleblower A nurse or other individual who goes outside of an organization for the public's best interest when the organization fails to follow procedures regarding safety and client care.

Whistleblowing The act of going outside of an organization for the public's best interest when an organization fails to follow procedures regarding safety and client care.

White blood cells (WBCs) See Leukocytes.

Withdrawing or withholding life-sustaining therapy (WWLST) The withdrawal of extraordinary means of life support, such as removing a ventilator or withholding special attempts to revive a client, and allowing the client to die of the underlying medical condition.

Work ethic A belief in the importance and moral worth of work.

Workplace bullying Malicious, repeated, harmful mistreatment of an individual with whom one works, regardless of whether that individual is an equal, a superior, or a subordinate.

Workplace violence Any physical assault, threatening behavior, or verbal abuse occurring in the workplace.

Worldview The way in which people in a culture perceive ideas and attitudes about the world, other people, and life in general.

Wrong-site surgery (WSS) A surgical operation that is performed at the wrong location on a client's body due to error.

Xenograft Skin used for transplantation that was obtained from an animal, usually a pig. Also called *heterograft*.

Xenophobia The fear or dislike of people different from one's self.

Xerostomia Dry mouth that occurs when an individual's supply of saliva is reduced.

Zollinger-Ellison syndrome A form of peptic ulcer disease caused by a gastrinoma, or gastrin-secreting tumor of the pancreas, stomach, or intestines.

Zygote A fertilized egg.

COMBINED INDEX

interventions, 1435–1436
lifespan and cultural considerations, 1434
malignant, 1426, 1432
manifestations, 1433–1434, 1433t
modifiable risk factors, 1426
nursing process, 1435–1436
outcome evaluation, 1436
overview of, 1431
pathophysiology and etiology, 1431–1433
prevalence of, 1424
prevention of, 1426–1427, 1433
risk factors, 1432–1433
screenings, 1426
therapies, 1424t
Hyperthermia blanket, 1441
Hyperthermic, 1256t
Hyperthyroidism. See also Thyroid disease
antepartum care and, 2078t
assessment, 810
body image and, 811
cardiac input monitoring and, 810
care planning, 810
collaborative care, 808–810
defined, 806
diagnosis, 810
diagnostic tests, 808–809
excess TSH stimulation and, 808
Graves disease and, 806–808, 806f
interventions, 810–811
laboratory findings in, 809t
manifestations, 806–808, 809t
multisystem effects of, 807t
Nursing Care Plan, 811–812t
nursing process, 810–811
nutrition and, 811
outcome evaluation, 811
pathophysiology and etiology, 806
pharmacologic therapy, 809
radioactive iodine therapy, 809
risk factors, 806
surgery, 809–810
thyroid storm and, 808
thyroiditis and, 808
toxic multinodular goiter and, 808, 808f
visual health and, 810–811
Hypertonic dehydration, 355
Hypertonic labor, 2138t
Hypertonic solutions, 337
Hypertrophic cardiomyopathy, 1077t, 1078
Hypertrophic scar, 1470
Hypertrophy, 285, 421
Hyperventilation
asthma and, 991
causes of, 25, 26
defined, 25, 991, 2163
labor and, 2163–2164
Hypervolemia, 363
Hyphema, 1312
Hypnotics/sedatives, 151t
Hypoactive sexual desire disorder, 1349
Hypocalcemia
defined, 372, 378
serum calcium, 372
uremia and, 395
Hypocalcemic tetany, 737t
Hypocapnia, 6
Hypochloremia, 372
Hypodermis, 1447

Hypodermoclysis, 352
Hypoglycemia
alcohol and, 772, 772t
in children with type 1 DM, 772
hospitalization criteria, 748
immediate treatment of, 748
manifestations of, 747
in newborns, 2210t
Hypoglycemic agents, 756
Hypokalemia
defined, 352
metabolic alkalosis and, 17–18
serum potassium, 372
Hypomania, 1776, 1809
Hyponatremia
acute renal failure (ARF) and, 387
defined, 263, 352
serum sodium, 370–371
Hypoperfusion, 374
Hypophonia, 897
Hypoplastic left heart syndrome (HLHS), 1093–1094t
Hypotension, 1067–1068, 1759
Hypothalamus, 1423, 1432, 1432f
Hypothermia
accidental, 1438–1439
assessment, 1440
care planning, 1441
in children, 1441
collaborative care, 1440
defined, 1422, 1423, 1437
diagnosis, 1441
frostbite, 1439
induced, 1437–1438
in infants, 1438–1439, 1438f
interventions, 1441
manifestations, 1439, 1440t
modifiable risk factors, 1426
in newborns, 1441
Nursing Care Plan, 1442t
nursing process, 1440–1441
in older adults, 1441
pathophysiology and etiology, 1437–1438
physiological mechanisms, 1423
prevalence of, 1424
prevention of, 1426–1427, 1441
risk factors, 1439
screenings, 1427
therapies, 1424t
Hypothermic, 1256t
Hypothyroidism. See also Thyroid disease
antepartum care and, 2078t
assessment, 815
cardiac output monitoring and, 815
care planning, 815
collaborative care, 813
constipation prevention and, 815
defined, 728–729, 812
diagnosis, 815
diagnostic tests, 813
fatigue and, 188t
Hashimoto thyroiditis and, 812–813
interventions, 815–816
iodine deficiency and, 812
laboratory findings in, 813
lifespan considerations, 815t
manifestations, 813, 813t
multisystem effects of, 814t

myxedema coma and, 813
Nursing Care Plan, 816–817t
nursing process, 815–816
outcome evaluation, 816
pathophysiology and etiology, 812–813
pharmacologic therapy, 813
risk factors, 812–813
skin integrity and, 815–816
surgery, 813
Hypotonic dehydration, 355
Hypotonic labor, 2138t
Hypotonic solutions, 337
Hypovolemia, 376, 1044
Hypovolemic shock
assessment, 1230
as burn shock, 1471
defined, 1222–1223
manifestations, 1225t
Hypoxemia
asthma and, 991
cyanosis and, 1046
defined, 6, 596, 957
infection and, 596
interventions and therapies, 960t
manifestations, 960t
refractory, 975
Hysterectomy
abdominal, 1402
defined, 1402
nursing care, 1403t
vaginal, 1402

I

IABP (intra-aortic balloon pump), 1123, 1123f
Iatrogenic, 365
Iatrogenic infections, 531
IBD. See Inflammatory bowel disease
Ibuprofen, fever and, 1434, 1434t
ICD (implantable cardioverter-defibrillator) and, 1191–1192
ICF (intracellular fluid), 336
ICH (intracranial hemorrhage), 2002
ICN code of ethics, 2568t
ICP (intracranial pressure), 2002
Id, 1649
Ideal body image, 1833
Ideal self, 1832–1833
Identification, 1905t
Idiopathic pain, 156
IEPs (individualized education plans), 768
IgE-mediated (type I) hypersensitivity, 482–483, 482f, 483t
IICP. See Increased intracranial pressure
Ileal pouch-anal anastomosis (IPAA), 662, 662f
Ileostomy, 662–663
Ileus, 274
Illegal, immoral, or unethical activities of professionals, 2561
Illicit drug use, 1522f
Illness
acute, 408
behaviors, 408
chronic, 408, 1731
defined, 408
effects on client and family, 408–409
sensory perception and, 1282

Lymph nodes
assessment
female, 1359t
male, 1356t
defined, 443
palpating, 452, 452f
Lymphadenopathy, 560
Lymphatic drainage, 365
Lymphedema, 79
Lymphocytes
B (B cells), 441
defined, 440
development and differentiation of, 441f
NK (natural killer cells), 441
T (T cells), 441
Lymphoid system, 443–444, 443f
Lymphoid tissues, 444
Lymphomas, 464
Lysine, 2184t
Lysosomes, 31

M

Maceration, 1493
Macronutrients, 927
Macrophages, 440, 1508
Macrosomia, 2046
Macrosystem, 1657
Macular degeneration
Amsler grid and, 1328, 1328f
assessment, 1329
care planning, 1330
collaborative care, 1328–1329
defined, 1327
diagnosis, 1329
diagnostic tests, 1329
exudative, 1327–1328, 1328t
interventions, 1281t, 1330
manifestations, 1281t, 1328, 1328t
nonexudative, 1327, 1328t
nonpharmacologic therapy, 1329
nursing process, 1329–1330
outcome evaluation, 1330
overview of, 1327
pathophysiology and etiology, 1327–1328
pharmacologic therapy, 1329, 1329t
risk factors, 1328
surgery, 1329
Magical thinking, 1665t
Magnesium (Mg²⁺)
function in the body, 342t, 931
locations in the body, 341–342
regulation of, 342t
Magnetic resonance cholangiopancreatography
(MRCP), 247
Magnetic resonance imaging (MRI)
cancer and, 55
congenital heart defects and, 1098t
deep venous thrombosis (DVT) and, 1132
HIV/AIDS testing and, 468
multiple sclerosis testing and, 880
peripheral vascular disease (PVD) and, 1201
in violence assessment, 1961
Mahoney, Mary, 2547
Maintenance phase, acute renal failure (ARF), 378
Major depressive disorder (MDD)
bipolar disorder comparison, 1811f
characteristics of, 1800f
defined, 1778, 1798
diabetes and, 750

DSM-5 diagnostic criteria for, 1799t
key facts about, 1799t
manifestations, 1800t
prevalence of, 1782–1783
therapies, 1800t
Major depressive disorder with peripartum onset,
1817
Major depressive episodes, 1798
Major histocompatible complex (MHC), 447
Malabsorption
causes of, 211t
defined, 211, 240
Malabsorption disorders
celiac disease, 240–243
lactase deficiency, 243–244
lifespan considerations, 240t
manifestations and therapies, 213t
overview of, 240
short bowel syndrome, 244–245
Malaise, 570
Maldigestion, 211, 211t
Male circumcision, 1362
Male condoms, 1379–1380, 1380f
Male contraception, 1386
Male erectile disorder, 1349
Male genitals, in gestational age,
2218, 2218f
Male hormone replacement, 1364t
Male orgasmic disorder, 1350
Male reproductive assessment
breast and lymph node, 1356t
external genitalia, 1356–1357t
prostate, 1357t
Malignant cells, 43, 43t
Malignant hyperthermia, 1426, 1432
Malignant neoplasms, 42–44, 43t, 53t
Malnutrition
alcohol abuse and, 1536
assessment, 218t
Malpractice
client safety and, 2657
communication and, 2658
defined, 2653, 2655
elements of, 2656
examples of negligence that result in,
2656t
failure to observe and take appropriate
action, 2657
medication errors and, 2658
professional liability insurance and, 2658
related doctrines, 2656
statute of limitations, 2656–2657
strategies to prevent incidents of,
2657–2658
Malpresentations, 2115
Malunion fractures, 857
Managed care, 2457, 2599
Management principles
accountability, 2476
authority, 2476
conflict management, 2477
controlling, 2475–2476
directing, 2475
effectiveness, 2477
efficiency, 2477
employee performance enhancement
and, 2476
functions, 2475–2476
leaders and mangers, 2474–2475
organizing, 2475

overview of, 2474
planning, 2475
productivity, 2477
resource management, 2476
responsibility, 2476
team building and management,
2476–2477
time management, 2477
Managers, 2474–2475
Managing care
case management, 2457
case method, 2458
client-focused care, 2457
concept of, 2455
concepts related to, 2456t
differentiated practice, 2457
functional method, 2458
healthcare systems and, 2601t
managed care, 2457
nursing practice, 2459
primary nursing, 2459
shared governance, 2457–2458
team nursing, 2458–2459
Mandatory health insurance, 2463
Mandatory reporting
abuse and neglect, 2674, 2674t
defined, 2674
good faith immunity, 2674, 2674t
injuries and illnesses, 2675
nurses in violation of NPA, 2674–2675
other examples of, 2675–2676
overview of, 2674
Mania
defined, 1776, 1809
nurse reactions and, 1814t
Manic episodes, 1809, 1811f
Manipulation, 1852
MAO (monoamine oxidase), 1784
MAO-B inhibitors, 899t, 900
MAOIs. See Monoamine oxidase inhibitors
MAP (mean arterial pressure), 1163, 1218
Maple syrup urine disease, 2208t
Marasmus, 930, 930t
Marfan syndrome, 2049
Margination, 634
Marijuana, pregnancy and, 1554
Marital rape, 1984
MARs (medication administration records),
2648, 2649f
Maslow's hierarchy of needs
in assessment, 2282
defined, 142
illustrated, 142f, 1899f
in prioritizing care, 2365–2366
in self-care in nursing, 2308–2310
sequencing of, 1899
Mass in Motion (MiM), 2702–2703
Massage
antenatal perineal, 2132t
infant, 2259
Massage therapy
for anxiety disorders, 1925
for end-of-life care, 182t
for herniated discs, 843
for menopause, 1396
Massive transfusion, 1252t
MAST (Michigan Alcohol Screening Test), 1540
Mast cell stabilizers
for asthma, 999t
for hypersensitivity, 490

outcome evaluation, 429
overview of, 424
periodontal disease and, 424
plaque and, 425–426
in preschoolers, 427–428
pyorrhea and, 426
in school-age children, 427–428
special needs, 428
tartar and, 426
in toddlers, 427, 427t
tooth decay prevention and, 427t
Oral rehydration, 360–361
Oral thermometers, 1427f
Oral-genital sex, 1346
Orchiectomy, 115
Organ Procurement and Transplantation Network
 (OPTN), 2608
Organ transplantation, 2573
Organizational charts, 2550, 2550f
Organizational commitment, 2486
Organizing, 2475
Organizing data, 2282
Orgasmic disorders, 1349–1350, 1352t
Orgasmic phase, sexual response cycle,
 1346–1348, 1347t
Orientation
 in newborn assessment, 2235
 newborns, 2204
 in professional development, 2528–2529
ORIF (open reduction and internal fixation),
 860, 860f
Orlistat (Xenical), 793
Oropharyngeal airways, 983, 983f
Orthopnea, 365, 959, 960t, 1148
Orthopneic position, 1002
Orthostatic hypotension, 901, 1067–1068
Orthotic devices, 504
Ortolani maneuver, 2232
OSA (obstructive sleep apnea), 195, 429
OSHA. *See* Occupational Safety and Health
 Administration
Osmolality, 337, 351, 1227
Osmolar imbalances, 354
Osmosis, 337–338, 337f
Osmotic diuretics, 712t
Osmotic pressure
 colloid, 338, 364
 defined, 337–338
 interstitial, 364–365
Osteoarthritis
 arthroplasty and, 888
 arthroscopy and, 888
 assessment, 891
 Bouchard nodes, 886
 care planning, 891
 characterization, 825
 children and, 887t
 collaborative care, 887–891
 comfort promotion, 891–893
 complementary and alternative therapy, 891t
 complications of, 887
 culture and, 887t
 defined, 496, 824t, 886
 diagnosis, 891
 diagnostic tests, 887t
 evaluation areas, 893
 exercise and, 890, 891t
 Heberden nodes, 886
 home care, 890t
 hyaluronic acid injections and, 890t

interventions, 824t, 891–893
joint fusion and, 888
joint resurfacing and, 888
juvenile, 887t
manifestation comparison, 496t
manifestations, 824t, 887, 892–893t
nonpharmacologic therapy, 889–891
Nursing Care Plan, 893t
nursing process, 891–893
nutrition and, 893
obesity and, 890
osteophytes, 886
osteotomy and, 888
overview of, 886
pathophysiology and etiology, 886–887
pharmacologic therapy, 888–889
physical mobility optimization and, 893
prevention of, 887
risk factors, 887
sleep/rest and, 890
surgery, 888
Osteoblasts, 820
Osteoclast, 821
Osteodystrophy, 380
Osteomyelitis, 854
Osteophytes, 886
Osteoporosis
 assessment, 802
 bisphosphonates for, 802t
 care planning, 802–803
 collaborative care, 800–802
 defined, 729, 799
 diagnosis, 802
 diagnostic tests, 800–801
 dietary management for, 801
 drugs for, 802t
 exercise and, 803–804
 genetic considerations and nonmodifiable risk
  factors, 731
 healthy behaviors and, 804
 hormonal agents for, 802t
 injury prevention, 803
 interventions, 733, 803–804
 manifestations, 800
 modifiable risk factors, 799–800
 Nursing Care Plan, 804–805t
 nursing process, 802–804
 nutrition and, 803
 outcome evaluation, 804
 overview of, 799
 pain management, 803
 pathophysiology and etiology, 799–800
 pharmacologic therapy, 801–802
 physical therapy for, 801
 prevalence of, 729
 risk factors, 799–800
 spinal changes caused by, 801f
 unmodifiable risk factors, 799
Osteotomy, 888
Otitis externa, 576
Otitis interna, 576
Otitis media
 acute, 576
 assessment, 581
 care planning, 581
 caregiver support, 582
 in children, 581, 581f
 chronic, 576
 collaborative care, 578–580
 communication facilitation, 582

complementary and alternative therapy, 580t
defined, 576
diagnosis, 581
diagnostic tests, 579
diversity and culture, 577
education, 582
with effusion, 578f
interventions, 581–582
manifestations, 577–578, 580t
Nursing Care Plan, 583t
nursing process, 581–582
outcome evaluation, 582
overview of, 576
pain management, 582
pathophysiology and etiology, 576–577
pharmacologic therapy, 579–580
prevention, 577
risk factors, 577
serous, 576
surgery, 579
tympanic membrane, 576, 578f
types of, 576
vertigo and, 577
Otoscope, 577, 581
Ototoxic medications, 1300, 1300t
Outcome standards, 2686
Outcomes
 defined, 2341t
 evaluation example of, 2352t
 goals versus, 2341t
 management, 2685
Ovarian cycle, 2018, 2018f
Ovaries, 2030
Overdelegation, 2472
Overdose
 alcohol, 1539
 drug abuse, 1565–1567
Overflow incontinence, 299t
Overnutrition, 936, 2290
Overt conflicts, 2387
Ovulation
 defined, 2018
 postpartum changes, 2173
Ovulation method, 1379
Oxygen administration
 defined, 972
 delivery system summary, 973t
 with nasal cannula, 972, 972f
 with nonrebreather mask, 972, 973f
 with simple face mask, 972, 972f
 with Venturi mask, 972, 973f
Oxygen therapy
 in COPD, 1011
 in sepsis, 602
 in shock, 1229
Oxygen transport, 2193–2194
Oxygenation
 alterations, 957–961
 alterations and therapies, 960t
 assessment, 962–968, 963–964t
 assessment interview, 962
 breathing muscles inspection, 964t
 in cardiac functioning, 1046
 in children, 1046
 collaborative interventions and therapies,
  970–973
 concepts related to, 958–959
 defined, 953
 diagnostic tests, 965–966, 967t
 disorders

PEARSON SOURCES

The following authors from Pearson generously allowed us to repurpose their work for this project:

- Priscilla LeMone and Karen Burke, *Medical-Surgical Nursing: Critical Thinking in Client Care,* Fifth Edition
- Audrey Berman, Shirlee J. Snyder, Barbara Kozier, and Glenora Erb, *Kozier & Erb's Fundamentals of Nursing: Concepts, Process, and Practice,* Ninth Edition
- Jane W. Ball and Ruth C. Bindler, *Pediatric Nursing: Caring for Children,* Fifth Edition; and *Child Health Nursing,* Third Edition, along with Kay J. Cowen
- Patricia A. Tabloski, *Gerontological Nursing,* Second Edition
- Patricia A. Wieland Ladewig, Marcia L. London, and Michele R. Davidson, *Contemporary Maternal-Newborn Nursing Care,* Eighth Edition
- Donita D'Amico and Colleen Barbarito, *Health & Physical Assessment in Nursing,* Second Edition
- Karen Lee Fontaine, *Complementary and Alternative Therapies for Nursing Practice,* Third Edition
- Karen Lee Fontaine, *Mental Health Nursing,* Sixth Edition
- Michael Patrick Adams, Leland Norman Holland, Jr., and Carol Urban, *Pharmacology for Nurses: A Pathophysiologic Approach,* Fourth Edition
- Kathleen Koerning Blais, Janice S. Hayes, Barbara Kozier, and Glenora Erb, *Professional Nursing Practice: Concepts and Perspectives,* Sixth Edition
- Carol Ren Kneisl and Eileen Trigoboff, *Contemporary Psychiatric-Mental Health Nursing,* Third Edition
- Eleanor J. Sullivan, *Effective Leadership and Management in Nursing,* Eighth Edition
- Anita W. Finkelman, *Leadership and Management in Nursing,* Second Edition
- Sherry Makely, *Professionalism in Health Care: A Primer for Career Success,* Fourth Edition
- Michele Davidson, Marcia London, and Patricia Ladewig, *Olds' Maternal-Newborn Nursing & Women's Health Across the Lifespan,* Ninth Edition

SPECIAL FEATURES

CLINICAL MANIFESTATIONS AND THERAPIES

COMMUNITY-BASED CARE

COMPLEMENTARY AND ALTERNATIVE THERAPY

CONCEPTS RELATED TO …

EVIDENCE-BASED PRACTICE

FOCUS ON DIVERSITY AND CULTURE

LIFESPAN CONSIDERATIONS